618.9212 AND

Accession no.
36088929
MCHT

JET LIBRARY

Paediatric Cardiology

Paediatric Cardiology

3rd Edition

EDITORS

Robert H. Anderson, MD
Emeritus Professor of Pediatric Cardiac Morphology
Institute of Child Health
London, UK

Edward J. Baker, MA, MD, FRCP, FRCPCH
Senior Lecturer and Consultant Paediatric Cardiologist
Guy's Hospital
London, UK

Daniel J. Penny, MD
Director of Cardiology
The Royal Children's Hospital Melbourne
Murdoch Children's Research Institute
Department of Paediatrics
University of Melbourne
Melbourne, Australia

Andrew N. Redington, MD
Division Head, Department of Cardiology
Hospital for Sick Children
Senior Associate Scientist
University of Toronto
Toronto, Ontario, Canada

Michael L. Rigby, MD
Consultant Paediatric Cardiologist
Royal Brompton Hospital
London, UK

Gil Wernovsky, MD
Staff Cardiologist, Cardiac Intensive Care Unit
Director, Program Development, The Cardiac Center
The Children's Hospital of Philadelphia
Professor of Pediatrics
University of Pennsylvania School of Medicine
Philadelphia, Pennsylvania, USA

ILLUSTRATOR

Gemma Price

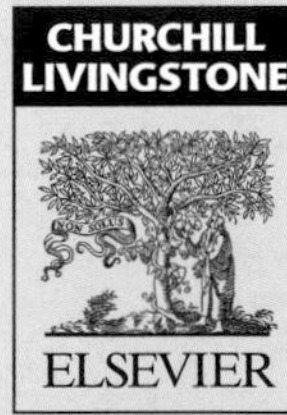

Churchill Livingstone/Elsevier Philadelphia, PA

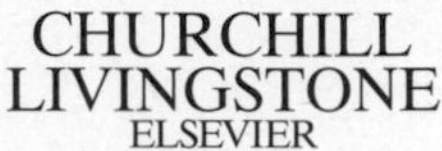

1600 John F. Kennedy Boulevard
Suite 1800
Philadelphia, PA 19103-2899

PAEDIATRIC CARDIOLOGY, 3rd EDITION

ISBN: 978-0-7020-3064-2

Copyright © 2010 by Churchill Livingstone, an imprint of Elsevier Ltd.

All rights reserved. No part of this publication may be reproduced or transmitted in any form or by any means, electronic or mechanical, including photocopying, recording, or any information storage and retrieval system, without permission in writing from the publisher. Permissions may be sought directly from Elsevier's Rights Department: phone: (+1)215 239 3804 (U.S.) or (+44)1865 843830(UK): fax: (+44)1865 853333: e-mail:healthpermission@elsevier.com. You may also complete your request online via the Elsevier (U.S.) website at http://www.elsevier.com/permissions.

Notice

Knowledge and best practice in this field are constantly changing. As new research and experience broaden our knowledge, changes in practice, treatment and drug therapy may become necessary or appropriate. Readers are advised to check the most current information provided (i) on procedures featured or (ii) by the manufacturer of each product to be administered, to verify the recommended dose or formula, the method and duration of administration, and contraindications. It is the responsibility of the practitioner, relying on their own experience and knowledge of the patient, to make diagnoses, to determine dosages and the best treatment for each individual patient, and to take all appropriate safety precautions. To the fullest extent of the law, neither the Publisher nor the Editors assume any liability for any injury and/or damage to persons or property arising out or related to any use of the material contained in this book.

The Publisher

Previous editions copyrighted 1987, 2002.

Library of Congress Cataloging-in-Publication Data
Paediatric cardiology / Robert H. Anderson ... [et al.]. -- 3rd ed.
p. ; cm.
Includes bibliographical references and index.
ISBN 978-0-7020-3064-2
1. Pediatric cardiology. I. Anderson, Robert Henry. II. Title.
[DNLM: 1. Heart Defects, Congenital. 2. Adolescent. 3. Child. 4. Heart Diseases. 5. Infant. WS 290 P126 2009]

RJ421.P333 2009
618.92'12--dc22 2009012419

Executive Publisher: Natasha Andjelkovic
Developmental Editor: Pamela Hetherington
Project Manager: David Saltzberg
Design Direction: Steven Stave

Printed in China

Last digit is the print number: 9 8 7 6 5 4 3 2 1

Working together to grow
libraries in developing countries

www.elsevier.com | www.bookaid.org | www.sabre.org

ELSEVIER BOOK AID International Sabre Foundation

Contents

Preface to the Third Edition

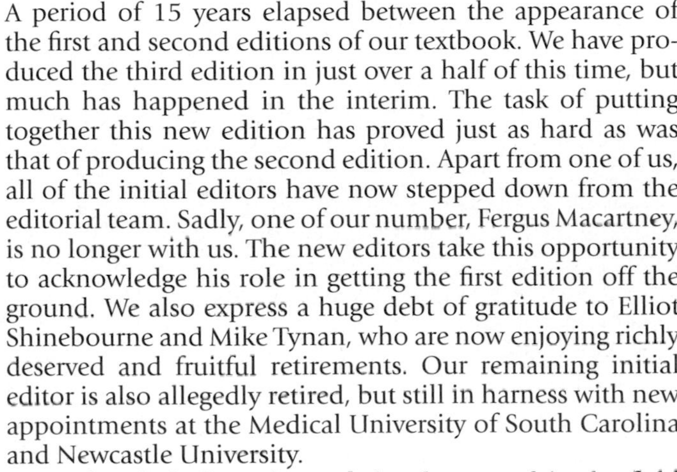

A period of 15 years elapsed between the appearance of the first and second editions of our textbook. We have produced the third edition in just over a half of this time, but much has happened in the interim. The task of putting together this new edition has proved just as hard as was that of producing the second edition. Apart from one of us, all of the initial editors have now stepped down from the editorial team. Sadly, one of our number, Fergus Macartney, is no longer with us. The new editors take this opportunity to acknowledge his role in getting the first edition off the ground. We also express a huge debt of gratitude to Elliot Shinebourne and Mike Tynan, who are now enjoying richly deserved and fruitful retirements. Our remaining initial editor is also allegedly retired, but still in harness with new appointments at the Medical University of South Carolina and Newcastle University.

As already indicated, much has happened in the field of cardiac disease in the young since the turn of the millennium. All of these changes are reflected in this third edition, which is markedly changed from our second offering. One of the major changes is the geographic representation of the editorial team, with editorial input now provided from Europe, North America and Australasia. To further offer a worldwide perspective, we have invited authors from five continents to contribute their cutting-edge expertise to the new edition.

Readers will note multiple changes in the format of the book, thanks to the suggestions of our publisher. Thankfully, we are now able to include color illustrations throughout the book. The influence of this change on the figures is truly spectacular. Also, the third edition now includes access to the full content of the book via a dedicated Expert Consult website. We have chosen to include the full lists of references exclusively in this web version, closing each of the chapters in the print version with a list of annotated references. In this way, we have been able to condense the contents into a single volume, which we consider a significant advance. Although we have made these multiple changes, we hope that the overall philosophy and approach of the book is unchanged. As with the previous edition, we have sought to maintain a standard style throughout the text. We hope that the uniformity achieved, along with an avoidance of abbreviations, will make the text appreciably easier to read and assimilate. Some of the revised chapters took some time to be written, but the quality of the chapters made the wait worthwhile. It is our belief that we have produced a truly first-class third edition.

We thank all our contributing authors for their efforts in making this possible. We also thank the editorial and production teams at Elsevier for smoothing the path towards publication, in particular Pamela Hetherington, who laboured beyond the call of duty in her efforts to obtain all the chapters on time. We are also indebted to Linnea Hermanson, production editor, who made correction of the proofs a pleasurable task rather than a chore. We particularly wish to thank Gemma Price, who drew and coloured the majority of the beautiful cartoons that grace our pages. We also express our thanks to our various friends and colleagues who permitted us to use illustrations from various previous collaborative ventures. We have cited their contributions in the legends to the specific figures, hoping that we have not made any omissions. We close this preface to the third edition with the same hopes as expressed for the second edition. It is our belief that this version marks a significant step upwards in the quality of our textbook. We hope that you, the reader, share our own enthusiasm as you make your way through its pages.

Robert H. Anderson
Edward J. Baker
Daniel J. Penny
Andrew N. Redington
Michael L. Rigby
Gil Wernovsky

Contributors

Vera Demarchi Aiello, MD, PhD
Associate Professor
Cardiopneumology Department
University of São Paulo Medical School
Pathologist-in-Chief, Surgical Pathology Section
Heart Institute (InCor), University of São Paulo Medical School
São Paulo, Brazil

Fahad Al Habshan, MD
Consultant in Pediatric Cardiology
King Abdulaziz Medical City
Assistant Professor, Cardiac Sciences
King Saud Bin Abdulaziz University for Health Sciences
Riyadh, Saudi Arabia

Page A.W. Anderson, MD
Duke University School of Medicine
Durham, North Carolina, USA
[deceased]

Robert H. Anderson, MD
Emeritus Professor of Pediatric Cardiac Morphology
Institute of Child Health
London, UK

Christian Apitz, MD
Clinical Research Fellow
Division of Cardiology
The Hospital for Sick Children
Toronto, Ontario, Canada

Edward J. Baker, MA, MD, FRCP, FRCPCH
Senior Lecturer
King's College
Consultant Paediatric Cardiologist
Guy's and St Thomas' Hospital NHS Foundation Trust
London, UK

David J. Barron, MBBS, MD, FRCP, FRCS(CT)
Honorary Senior Lecturer
Department of Child Health
University of Birmingham
Consultant Cardiac Surgeon
Birmingham Children's Hospital
Birmingham, UK

Anton E. Becker, MD
Department of Pathology
University of Amsterdam
Wilhelmina Gasthuis
Amsterdam, The Netherlands

Elisabeth Bédard, MD
Adult Congenital Heart Center and Center for Pulmonary Arterial Hypertension
Royal Brompton Hospital
London, UK

Lee N. Benson, MD
Professor of Pediatrics
University of Toronto School of Medicine
Director, Cardiac Diagnostic and Interventional Unit
The Hospital for Sick Children
Toronto, Ontario, Canada

Elizabeth D. Blume, MD
Department of Cardiology
Children's Hospital of Boston
Boston, Massachusetts, USA

Philipp Bonhoeffer, MD
Professor of Cardiology
Institute of Child Health
Chief of Cardiology and Director of the Cardiac Catheterisation Laboratory
Great Ormond Street Hospital for Children
London, UK

Timothy J. Bradley, MBChB, DCH, FRACP
Staff Cardiologist
Department of Cardiovascular Surgery
The Hospital for Sick Children
Assistant Professor
Department of Paediatrics
University of Toronto
Toronto, Ontario, Canada

Nancy J. Braudis, RN, MS, CPND
Clinical Nurse Specialist
Cardiovascular ICU
Children's Hospital of Boston
Boston, Massachussetts, USA

William J. Brawn, MBBS, FRCS, FRACS
Consultant Cardiac Surgeon
Birmingham Children's Hospital
Birmingham,UK

Christian Brizard, MD
Cardiac Surgery Department
Royal Children's Hospital
Parkville, Australia

Nigel Brown, BSc, PhD
Dean, Faculty of Medicine and Biomedical Sciences
Head, Division of Basic Medical Sciences
St. George's University of London
London, UK

Benoit G. Bruneau, PhD
Associate Professor
Department of Pediatrics
University of California, San Francisco
Associate Investigator
Gladstone Institute of Cardiovascular Disease
San Francisco, California, USA

Tyra Bryant-Stephens, MD
Clinical Associate Professor
University of Pennsylvania School of Medicine
Medical Director
The Community Asthma Prevention Program
The Children's Hospital of Philadelphia
Philadelphia, Pennsylvania, USA

John Burn, PhD
Honorary Consultant Clinical Geneticist
Newcastle Hospitals NHS Trust
Medical Director and Head of Institute of Human Genetics
Newcastle University
Newcastle-upon-Tyne, UK

Marietta Charakida, MD
Clinical Research Fellow
Great Ormond Street Hospital
London, UK

Yiu-fai Cheung, MD
Professor of Paediatric Cardiology
Department of Paediatrics and Adolescent Medicine
Queen Mary Hospital
The University of Hong Kong
Hong Kong

Jack M. Colman, MD, FRCPC
Associate Professor of Medicine (Cardiology)
University of Toronto
Cardiologist
Mount Sinai Hospital and Toronto Congenital Cardiac Centre for Adults, Toronto General Hospital
Toronto, Ontario, Canada

Piers E.F. Daubeney, MA, DM, MRCP, MRCPCH
Honorary Senior Lecturer
National Heart and Lung Institute
Imperial College London
Consultant Paediatric and Fetal Cardiologist
Royal Brompton Hospital
London, UK

Andrew M. Davis, MBBS, MD
Associate Professor of Paediatrics
Faculty of Medicine, Dentistry and Health Sciences
Melbourne University
Electrophysiologist
Clinical Leader, Arrhythmia Service
Royal Children's Hospital
Melbourne, Victoria, Australia

John E. Deanfield, BA Hons, BChir, MB, FRCP
Professor
Cardiothoracic Unit
Institution of Child Health
University College London
London, UK

Joseph A. Dearani, MD
Professor of Surgery
Mayo Clinic College of Medicine
Rochester, Minnesota, USA

Graham Derrick, BM, BS, MRCP(UK)
Consultant Paediatric Cardiologist
Great Ormond Street Hospital for Children NHS Trust
London, UK

Anne I. Dipchand, MD
Associate Professor
Faculty of Medicine
University of Toronto
Head, Heart Transplant Program
Associate Director, SickKids Transplant Centre
Staff Cardiologist
Labatt Family Heart Centre
Hospital for Sick Children
Toronto, Ontario, Canada

Troy E. Dominguez, MD, FCCP
Department of Anesthesiology and Critical Care Medicine
The Children's Hospital of Philadelphia
Philadelphia, Pennsylvania, USA

Lucas J. Eastaugh
Registrar
Royal Children's Hospital
Melbourne, Australia

Tjark Ebels, MD, PhD
Professor of Cardiothoracic Surgery
University Medical Centre Groningen
Groningen, The Netherlands

Martin J. Elliott, MD, FRCS
Professor of Cardiothoracic Surgery
University College London
Chairman of Cardiothoracic Services
The Great Ormond Street Hospital for Children
London, UK

Perry Elliott, MBBS
Reader in Inherited Cardiovascular Disease
University College London
Honorary Consultant Cardiologist
The Heart Hospital UCLH
London, UK
Cardiomyopathies

Toni Ellis
Great Ormond Street Hospital for Children
London, UK

Nynke Elzenga, MD, PhD
Teaching Staff Member in Pediatric Cardiology
Consultant Pediatric Cardiologist
Division of Cardiology
Beatrix Children's Hospital
University Medical Center
Groningen, The Netherlands

Robert F. English, MD
Assistant Professor
University of Florida–Jacksonville
Jacksonville, Florida, USA

José A. Ettedgui, MD
Glenn Chuck Professor of Pediatric Cardiology
University of Florida
Director, Pediatric Cardiovascular Center
Wolfson Children's Hospital
Jacksonville, Florida, USA

Alan H. Friedman, MD, FAAP
Professor of Pediatrics
Associate Chair for Education
Director, Pediatric Residency Program
Director, Pediatric Echocardiography Laboratory
Yale University School of Medicine
New Haven, Connecticut, USA

Kimberly L. Gandy, MD, PhD
Associate Professor of Surgery
Associate Professor of Cell Biology, Neurobiology, and Anatomy
Associate Director of Children's Research Institute
Medical College of Wisconsin
Milwaukee, Wisconsin, USA

Helena M. Gardiner, PhD, MD, FRCP, FRCPCH, DCH
Senior Lecturer in Perinatal Cardiology
Institute of Reproductive and Developmental Biology
Faculty of Medicine
Imperial College London
Honorary Consultant
Royal Brompton and Queen Charlotte's and Chelsea Hospitals
London, UK

Michael A. Gatzoulis, MD, PhD, FACC, FESC
Professor of Cardiology and Congenital Heart Disease
Consultant Cardiologist and Head, Adult Congenital Heart Centre and Centre for Pulmonary Hypertension
Royal Brompton Hospital and the National Heart and Lung Institute
Imperial College, London, UK

Lars Grosse-Wortmann, MD
Hospital for Sick Children
Toronto, Ontario, Canada

Peter J. Gruber, MD, PhD
Attending Surgeon
Assistant Professor of Surgery
University of Pennsylvania School of Medicine
Philadelphia, Pennsylvania, USA

Julian P. Halcox, MD, MRCP
Al Maktoum BHF Senior Lecturer in Cardiology
Institute of Child Health UCL
Consultant Cardiologist
University College and Great Ormond Street Hospitals
London, UK

Sheila G. Haworth, MD, FRCP, FRCPATH, FRCPCH, FMedSci
Professor of Developmental Cardiology
Institute of Child Health
University College London
Honorary Consultant in Paediatric Cardiology
Great Ormond Street Hospital for Children
London, UK

Anthony M. Hlavacek, MD, MSCR
Assistant Professor of Pediatrics and Cardiology
Attending Physician
Medical University of South Carolina
Charleston, South Carolina, USA

George M. Hoffman, MD
Professor of Anesthesiology and Pediatrics
Medical College of Wisconsin
Medical Director and Chief of Pediatric Anesthesiology
Associate Director of Pediatric Critical Care
Children's Hospital of Wisconsin
Milwaukee, Wisconsin, USA

Estela S. Horowitz, MD
Associate Paediatric Cardiologist
Instituto de Cardiologia do Rio Grande do Sul
Porto Alegre, Brazil

J. Andreas Hoschtitzky, Estela S. Heroniz MSc, FRCSEd (CTh)
Consultant Cardiac Surgeon
Manchester Royal Infirmary
Manchester and Alder Hey Children's Hospital
Liverpool, UK

Tilman Humpl, MD, PhD
Assistant Professor of Paediatrics
University of Toronto
Staff Physician
Cardiac Critical Care Unit and Cardiology
Hospital for Sick Children
Toronto, Ontario, Canada

Damian Hutter, MD
Stress Signaling Unit
Laboratory of Cellular and Molecular Biology
National Institute on Aging
National Institutes of Health
Baltimore, Maryland, USA

Edgar T. Jaeggi, MD, FRCPC
Associate Professor of Paediatrics
Faculty of Medicine
University of Toronto
Head, Fetal Cardiac Program
The Hospital for Sick Children
Toronto, Ontario, Canada

Timothy J.J. Jones, MD, FRCS(CTh)
Consultant Cardiac Surgeon
Birmingham Children's Hospital
Birmingham, UK

Juan Pablo Kaski, MBBS, MRCPCH, MRCPS(Glasg)
Clinical Research Fellow
Department of Medicine
Institute of Child Health
University College London
Specialist Registrar
Royal Brompton Hospital
London, UK

Sachin Khambadkone, MBBS, DCH, MD, DNB, MRCP(UK), CCT
Honorary Senior Lecturer
Cardiac Unit
Institute of Child Health
Consultant Paediatric Cardiologist
Great Ormond Street Hospital
London, UK

Lisa M. Kohr, RN, MSN, CPNP-AC/PC, MPH
Adjunct Faculty
University of Pennsylvania Graduate School of Nursing
Pediatric Nurse Practitioner
Cardiac Intensive Care Unit
Children's Hospital of Philadelphia
Philadelphia, Pennsylvania, USA

Whal Lee, MD
Department of Radiology
Seoul National University College of Medicine
Seoul, Republic of Korea

Stavros P. Loukogeorgakis, MBBS, PhD
Vascular Physiology Unit
Institute of Child Health
University College London
London, UK

Michael G. McBride, PhD
Director of Exercise Physiology
The Children's Hospital of Philadelphia
Philadelphia, Pennsylvania, USA

Brian W. McCrindle, MD, MPH
Professor of Pediatrics
Department of Pediatrics
University of Toronto
Staff Cardiologist
The Hospital for Sick Children
Toronto, Ontario, Canada

Patrick J. McNamara, MB, BCH, BAO, DCH, MSc (Paeds), MRCP, MRCPCH
Assistant Professor
University of Toronto
Staff Neonatologist
The Hospital for Sick Children
Toronto, Ontario, Canada

Luc L. Mertens, MD, PhD
Section Head of Echocardiography
The Hospital for Sick Children
Associate Professor of Paediatrics
University of Toronto
Toronto, Ontario, Canada

Antoon F.M. Moorman, MSc, PhD
Professor of Anatomy and Embryology
Academic Medical Center
Amsterdam, The Netherlands

Cleonice C. Coelho Mota, MD, MsD, PhD
Professor of Paediatrics
Head, Department of Paediatrics
Faculty of Medicine
Consultant
Chief of Division of Paediatrics and Fetal Cardiology
Hospital das Clínicas
Federal University of Minas Gerais
Belo Horizonte, Brazil

Kathleen Mussatto, PhD, RN
Research Manager
Herma Heart Center
Children's Hospital of Wisconsin
Milwaukee, Wisconsin, USA

Jane Newburger, MD, MPH
Professor of Pediatrics
Department of Medicine
Harvard Medical School
Boston, Massachusetts, USA

Patrick W. O'Leary, MD
Associate Professor of Pediatrics
Mayo Clinic College of Medicine
Consultant, Division of Pediatric Cardiology
Mayo Clinic
Rochester, Minnesota, USA

Stephen M. Paridon, MD
Associate Professor of Pediatrics
University of Pennsylvania School of Medicine
Staff Pediatric Cardiologist
The Children's Hospital of Philadelphia
Philadelphia, Pennsylvania, USA

Daniel J. Penny, MD
Director of Cardiology
The Royal Children's Hospital Melbourne
Murdoch Children's Research Institute
Department of Paediatrics
University of Melbourne
Melbourne, Australia

Shakeel A. Qureshi, MBChB, FRCP
Honorary Senior Lecturer
Paediatric Cardiology
King's College London
Consultant Paediatric Cardiologist
Evelina Children's Hospital
Guy's and St Thomas Foundation Trust
London, UK

Marlene Rabinovitch, MD
Pediatric Cardiology Department
Stanford University School of Medicine
Stanford, California, USA

Andrew N. Redington, MD
Division Head, Department of Cardiology
Hospital for Sick Children
Senior Associate Scientist
University of Toronto
Toronto, Ontario, Canada

Christopher J.D. Reid, MBChB, MRCP (UK), FRCPCH
Honorary Senior Lecturer, Kings' College London School of Medicine
Consultant Paediatric Nephrologist
Evelina Children's Hospital
Guy's and St Thomas's NHS Foundation Trust
London, UK

John F. Reidy, MBBS, FRCR, FRCP
Consultant Radiologist
Guy's and St Thomas' Hospital
London, UK

Michael L. Rigby, MD
Consultant Paediatric Cardiologist
Royal Brompton Hospital
London, UK

Jack Rychik, MD
Professor of Pediatrics
The Children's Hospital of Philadelphia
University of Pennsylvania School of Medicine
Director, Fetal Heart Program
Cardiac Center at The Children's Hospital of Philadelphia
Philadelphia, Pennsylvania, USA

Caner Salih, MBChB, FRCS
Locum Paediatric Cardiac Surgeon
Royal Melbourne Hospital
Melbourne, Australia

Ingram Schulze-Neick, MD
Privatdozent and Senior Lecturer
Humboldt University
Berlin, Germany
Cardiac Unit
Cardiothoracic Division
Great Ormond Street Hospital for Children
Institute of Child Health
National Lead, Consultant Cardiologist
UK Service for Pulmonary Hypertension in Children
London, UK

Mathew Sermer, MD, FRCSC
Professor of Medicine and Obstetrics and Gynaecology
University of Toronto
Associate Chief, Obstetrics and Gynaecology
Head, Maternal-Fetal Medicine
Mount Sinai Hospital
Toronto, Ontario, Canada

Robert E. Shaddy, MD
Professor and Chief
Department of Pediatric Cardiology
Vice Chair
Department of Pediatrics
The Children's Hospital of Philadelphia
University of Pennsylvania School of Medicine
Philadelphia, Pennsylvania

Lara Shekerdemian, MBChB, MRCP, FRCPCH, FRACP, FJFICM, MD
Director of Intensive Care
The Royal Children's Hospital
Melbourne, Victoria, Australia

Amanda J. Shillingford, MD
Division of Cardiology
Children's Hospital of Philadelphia
Philadelphia, Pennsylvania, USA

Girish S. Shirali, MBBS, FACC, FAAP
Professor, Departments of Pediatrics and Obstetrics and Gynecology
Director, Pediatric Cardiology Fellowship Training
Vice-Chairman, Fellowship Education
Director, Pediatric Echocardiography
Medical University of South Carolina
Charleston, South Carolina, USA

Norman H. Silverman, MD, DSc Med
Professor of Pediatrics
Department of Pediatric Cardiology
Stanford University
Stanford, California
Professor of Pediatrics
Lucile Packard Children's Hospital and Stanford Hospital and Clinics
Palo Alto, California, USA

Candice K. Silversides, MD, MS, FRCPC
Assistant Professor
University of Toronto
Staff Cardiologist
University Health Network, Toronto General Hospital
Toronto Congenital Cardiac Centre for Adults
Toronto, Ontario, Canada

Manish D. Sinha, MRCP, MRCPCh
Consultant Paediatric Nephrologist
Evelina Children's Hospital
Guy's and St Thomas' NHS Foundation Trust
London, UK

Samuel C. Siu, MD, SM
Gunton Professor and Chair of Cardiology
Professor of Medicine
Schulich School of Medicine and Dentistry
University of Western Ontario
Chief of Cardiology
London Health Sciences Centre and St. Joseph's Health Care
London, Ontario, Canada

Jeffrey F. Smallhorn, MBBS, FRACP, FRCP
Professor of Pediatrics, Program Director Pediatric Cardiology
Pediatrics
University of Alberta
Head, Section of Echocardiography
Stollery Children's Hospital
Edmonton, Alberta, Canada

Deepak Srivastava, MD
Director, Gladstone Institute of Cardiovascular Disease
Professor, Departments of Pediatrics and Biochemistry & Biophysics
Wilma and Adeline Pirag Distinguished Professor in Pediatric Developmental Cardiology
University of California, San Francisco
San Francisco, California, USA

Paul Stephens, Jr., MD
Clinical Associate Professor of Pediatrics
University of Pennsylvania School of Medicine
Staff Pediatric Cardiologist
The Children's Hospital of Philadelphia
Philadelphia, Pennsylvania, USA

Elizabeth A. Stephenson, MD, MSc
Assistant Professor of Paediatrics
University of Toronto
Staff Cardiologist
The Hospital for Sick Children
Toronto, Ontario, Canada

Anita L. Szwast, MD
Department of Cardiology
Children's Hospital of Philadelphia
Philadelphia, Pennsylvania, USA

Rohayati Taib, MBChB, MRCP (UK)
Paediatric Cardiologist
RIPAS Hospital
Bandar Seri Begawan, Brunei, Darussalam

Gerald Tulzer, MD
Dozent
Medical University of Vienna
Vienna, Austria
Chief, Department of Pediatric Cardiology
Children's Heart Centre Linz
Linz, Austria

James Tweddell, MD
Professor of Surgery (Cardiothoracic) and Pediatrics
The S. Bert Litwin Chair of Cardiothoracic Surgery
Children's Hospital of Wisconsin
Chair, Division of Cardiothoracic Surgery
Medical College of Wisconsin
Milwaukee, Wisconsin, USA

Hideki Uemura, MD, FRCS
Consultant Cardiac Surgeon
Royal Brompton Hospital
London, UK

Patrick VanderWal, MSP
Department of Cardiovascular Surgery
Children's Hospital of Wisconsin and Medical College of Wisconsin
Milwaukee, Wisconsin, USA

Michael C. Vogel, MD
Pediatric Cardiologist
Munich, Germany

Gary D. Webb, MD, FRCPC, FACC
Professor of Medicine
Director of the Philadelphia Adult Congenital Heart Center
University of Pennsylvania School of Medicine
The Hospital of the University of Pennsylvania
Philadelphia, Pennsylvania, USA

Steven A. Webber, MBChB
Professor of Pediatrics
University of Pittsburgh School of Medicine
Chief, Division of Pediatric Cardiology and Co-Director, Heart Center
Children's Hospital of Pittsburgh
Pittsburgh, Pennsylvania, USA

Gil Wernovsky, MD
Staff Cardiologist, Cardiac Intensive Care Unit
Director, Program Development, The Cardiac Center
The Children's Hospital of Philadelphia
Professor of Pediatrics
University of Pennsylvania School of Medicine
Philadelphia, Pennsylvania, USA

James L. Wilkinson, MBChB, FRCP, FRACP, FACC
Professor
Department of Paediatrics
University of Melbourne
Melbourne, Victoria, Australia
Senior Cardiologist
Royal Children's Hospital
Parkville, Victoria, Australia

Shi-Joon Yoo, MD
Professor of Medical Imaging and Paediatrics
University of Toronto
Section Head of Cardiac Imaging
Department of Diagnostic Imaging
Hospital for Sick Children
Toronto, Ontario, Canada

SECTION

1

Structural and Functional Development

CHAPTER 1

Terminology

ROBERT H. ANDERSON

It might reasonably be thought that those who diagnose and treat patients with congenitally malformed hearts would, by now, have reached consensus concerning the most appropriate way of describing the malformations with which they are confronted. It is certainly the case that nomenclature is far less contentious now than when we produced the first two editions of this book, in 1987 and 1999. It would be a brave person, nonetheless, who stated that the field of description and categorisation was now fully resolved. There are still major differences of opinion as how best to cope with certain topics, such as those patients who have visceral heterotaxy (or so-called splenic syndromes). It is not our intention, in this chapter, to initiate detailed debates on the differences in the approaches to these, and other, contentious issues. Rather, we will describe our own system for description, leaving the readers to decide whether or not this is satisfactory for their needs. By and large, there is no right or wrong way of describing the hearts, simply different ways.[1,2] Even these different ways have been mitigated to considerable extent by the cross-mapping of existing systems,[3] but this should not detract from the need to resolve ongoing differences according to the nature of the abnormal anatomy as it is observed.

It may be asked, however, whether we need a system for nomenclature, since the hearts themselves have not changed since their initial descriptions. The reason that a standardised approach is preferable is that the number of individual lesions that can co-exist within malformed hearts is considerable. Add to this the possibilities for combinations of lesions, and the problem of providing pigeonholes for each entity becomes immense. We all recognise the nature of straightforward lesions, such as septal deficiencies or valvar stenoses. Almost always these entities are encountered in otherwise normally structured hearts. It is when the hearts containing the lesions are themselves built in grossly abnormal fashion that difficulties are produced. We can no longer be satisfied with a wastebasket category for so-called complex lesions. The recognition of apparent complexity does nothing to determine diagnosis or optimal treatment. If these alleged complex lesions are approached in a simple and straightforward fashion, none need be difficult to understand and describe.

The simplicity comes when we recognise that, basically, the heart has three building blocks, namely the atriums, the ventricular mass and the arterial trunks (Fig. 1-1). A system for description and categorisation based on recognition of the limited potential for variation in each of these cardiac segments was developed independently in the 1960s by two groups: one based in the United States of America, and led by Richard Van Praagh,[1] and the other, from Mexico City, headed by Maria Victoria de la Cruz.[4] Both of these systems concentrated on the different topological arrangements of the components within each cardiac segment. When Van Praagh and his colleagues[5,6] introduced the concept of concordance and discordance between atriums and ventricles, they were concerned primarily with the harmony or disharmony to be found between atrial and ventricular situs. At this time, they placed less emphasis for description on the fashion in which the atrial and ventricular chambers were joined together across the atrioventricular junctions. A similar approach, concentrating on arterial relationships, was taken by de la Cruz and colleagues[7] when they formulated their concept of arterio-ventricular concordance and discordance. These approaches were understandable, since it was often difficult, at that time, precisely to determine how the adjacent structures were linked together.

The advent of cross sectional echocardiography changed all that. Since the mid-1970s, it has been possible with precision to determine how atriums are, or are not, joined to ventricles, and similarly to establish the precise morphology found at the ventriculo-arterial junctions. Since we evolved our system concomitantly with the development of echocardiography, our approach has been to concentrate on the variations possible across the atrioventricular and ventriculo-arterial junctions. We call this system sequential segmental analysis (see Fig. 1-1). In making such analysis, we do not ignore the segments themselves. Indeed, junctional

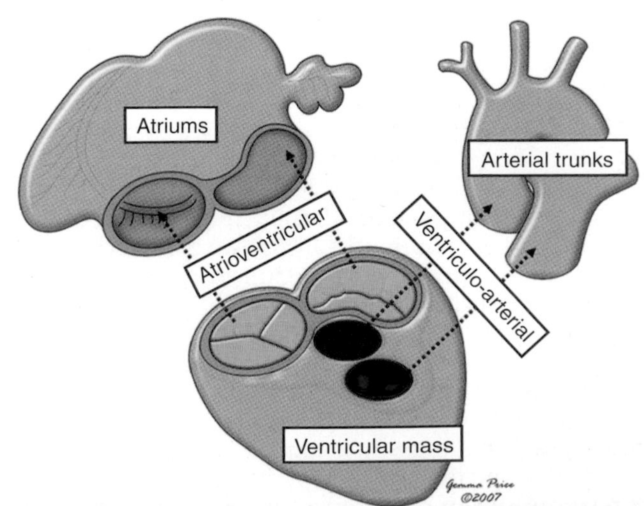

Figure 1-1 The cartoon shows the essence of sequential segmental analysis. It depends on recognition of the topological arrangement of the three cardiac segments, and combines this with analysis of the fashions in which the segments are joined or are not joined to each other.

connections cannot be established without knowledge of segmental topology. In this respect, we have acknowledged our debts to the other schools as our system has evolved.[8–12]

Our system, throughout its evolution, has followed the same basic and simple rules. From the outset, we have formulated our categories on the basis of recognisable anatomical facts, avoiding any speculative embryological assumptions. Again, from the start, we have emphasised the features of the morphology of the cardiac components, the way they are joined or not joined together, and the relations between them, as three different facets of the cardiac make-up. It still remains an undisputed fact that any system which separates out these features, does not use one to determine another, and describes them with mutually exclusive terms, must perforce be unambiguous. The clarity of the system then depends upon its design. Some argue that brevity is an important feature and have constructed formidable codifications to achieve this aim.[13] In the final analysis, however, clarity is more important than brevity. We do not shy, therefore, from using words to replace symbols, even if this requires several words. Whenever possible, we strive to use words that are as meaningful in their systematic role as in their everyday usage. In our desire to achieve optimal clarity, we have made changes in our descriptions over the years, most notably in our use of the term univentricular heart. We make no apologies for these changes, since their formulation, in response to valid criticisms, has eradicated initially illogical points from our system to its advantage. It is our belief that the system now advocated is entirely logical, and we hope it is simple. But, should further illogicalities become apparent, we would extirpate them as completely as we removed[14] univentricular heart from our lexicon as an appropriate descriptor for hearts that possess one big and one small ventricle, showing that this can produce a functionally, but not anatomically, univentricular arrangement.[15]

BASIC CONCEPTS OF SEQUENTIAL SEGMENTAL ANALYSIS

The system we advocate depends first upon the establishment of the arrangement of the atrial chambers. Thereafter, attention is concentrated on the anatomical nature of the junctions between the atrial myocardium and the ventricular myocardial mass. This feature, which we describe as a type of connection, is separate from the additional feature of the morphology of the valve or valves that guards the junctions. There are two junctions in the normally constructed heart, and usually they are guarded by two separate valves. The two atrioventricular junctions can be guarded, on occasion, by a common valve. If we are to achieve this analysis of the atrioventricular junctions, we must also determine the structure, topology, and relationships of the chambers within the ventricular mass. As with the atrioventricular junctions, the ventriculo-arterial junctions are also analysed in terms of the way the arterial trunks are joined to the ventricular mass, and the morphology of the arterial valves guarding their junctions. Separate attention is directed to the morphology of the outflow tracts, and to the relationships of the arterial trunks. A catalogue is then made of all associated cardiac and, where pertinent, noncardiac malformations. Included in this final category are such features as the location of the heart, the orientation of its apex, and the arrangement of the other thoracic and abdominal organs.

Implicit in the system is the ability to distinguish the morphology of the individual atriums and ventricles, and to recognise the types of arterial trunk taking origin from the ventricles. This is not as straightforward as it may seem, since often, in congenitally malformed hearts, these chambers or arterial trunks may lack some of the morphological features that most obviously characterise them in the normal heart. The most obvious feature of the morphologically left atrium in the normal heart, for example, is the connection to it of the pulmonary veins. In hearts with totally anomalous pulmonary venous connection, these veins connect in extracardiac fashion. In spite of this, it is still possible to identify the left atrium. It is considerations of this type that prompted the concept we use for recognition of the cardiac chambers and great arteries. Dubbed by Van Praagh and his colleagues the morphological method,[16] and based on the initial work of Lev,[17] the principle states that structures should be recognised in terms of their own intrinsic morphology, and that one part of the heart which is itself variable should not be defined on the basis of another variable structure. When this eminently sensible concept is applied to the atrial chambers, then the connections of the great veins are obviously disqualified as markers of morphological rightness or leftness since, as discussed above, the veins do not always connect to their anticipated atriums. Although Lev[17] placed great stress on septal morphology as a distinguishing feature, this morphology is of little help when the septum itself is absent, as occurs in hearts with a common atrium. Similarly, the atrial vestibule is ruled out as a marker, since it is usually lacking in hearts with atrioventricular valvar atresia. Fortunately, there is another component of the atrial chambers that, in our experience, has been almost universally present and which, on the basis of the morphology of its junction with the remainder of the chambers, has enabled us always to distinguish between morphologically right and left atriums. This is the appendage. The morphologically right appendage has the shape of a blunt triangle, and its cavity has a broad junction with the remainder of the atrium. The junction is marked externally by the terminal groove, and internally by the terminal crest. Its most significant feature is that the pectinate muscles lining the appendage extend all round the parietal atrioventricular junction (Fig. 1-2).

The morphologically left appendage, in contrast, is much narrower and tubular. It has a narrow junction with the remainder of the atrium, and one that is marked by neither terminal groove nor muscular crest. The pectinate muscles are confined within the morphologically left appendage, with the posterior aspect of the morphologically left vestibule, also containing the coronary sinus, being smooth walled as it merges with the pulmonary venous component (Fig. 1-3).

The morphological method also shows its value when applied to the ventricular mass, which extends from the atrioventricular to the ventriculo-arterial junctions. Within the ventricular mass as thus defined, there are almost always two ventricles. Description of ventricles, no matter how malformed they may be, is facilitated if they are analysed as possessing three components. These are, first, the inlet, extending from the atrioventricular junction to the distal attachment of the atrioventricular valvar tension

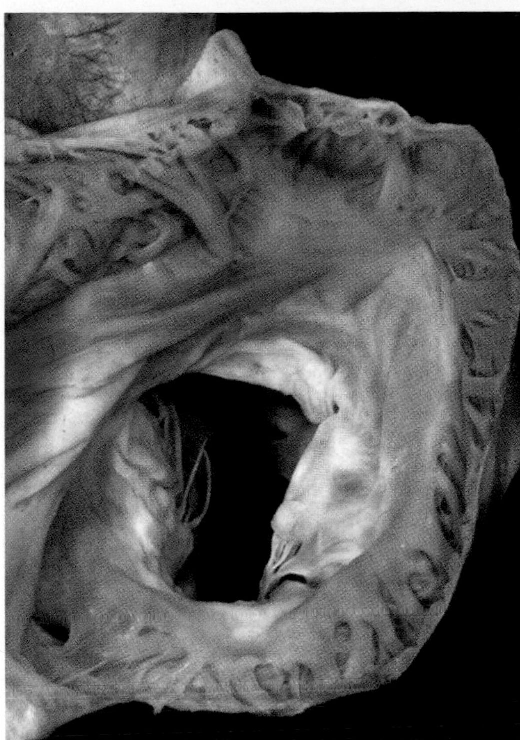

Figure 1-2 The short-axis view of the right atrioventricular junction from above, the atrium having been opened, with a cut parallel to the atrioventricular junction, and the wall of the appendage having been reflected, shows how the pectinate muscles within the appendage extend all round the vestibule of the tricuspid valve.

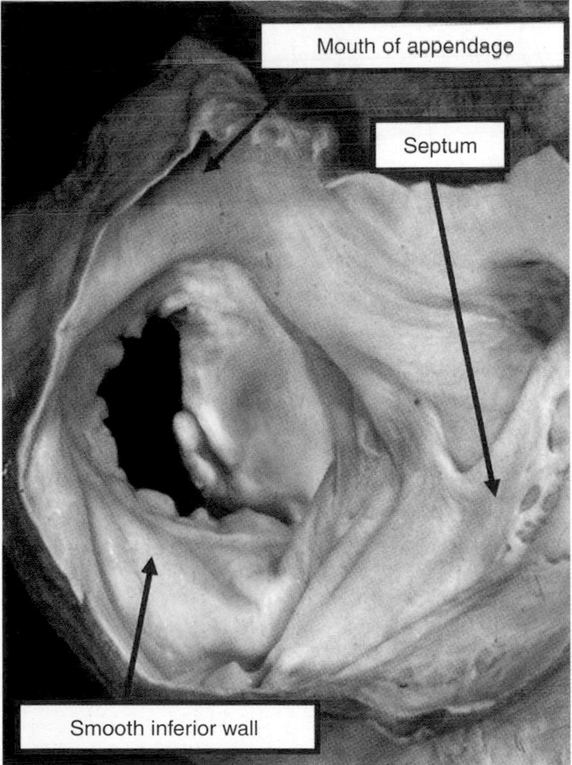

Figure 1-3 The short-axis view of the left atrioventricular junction from above, from the same heart as in Figure 1-2, shows the narrow entrance to the tubular appendage of the morphologically left atrium. The pectinate muscles are confined within the appendage, so that the inferior wall of the atrium is smooth. This contains the coronary sinus within the morphologically left atrioventricular junction. Note also the typical appearance of the morphologically left side of the septum.

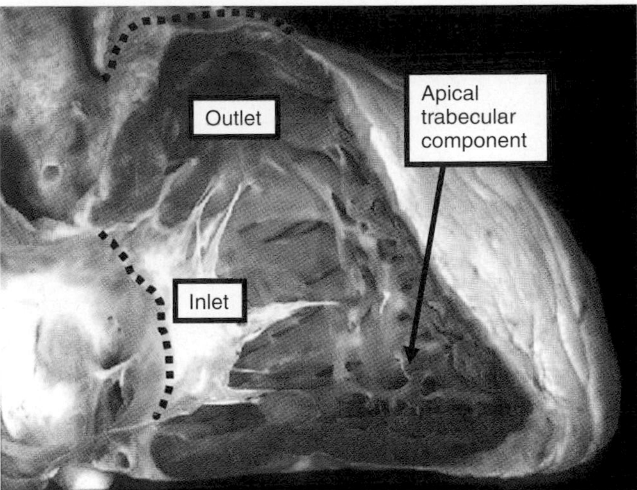

Figure 1-4 The anterior wall has been removed to show the three component parts of the morphologically right ventricle, which extends from the atrioventricular to the ventriculo-arterial junctions (*dotted red lines*). The coarse apical trabeculations are the most constant of these features.

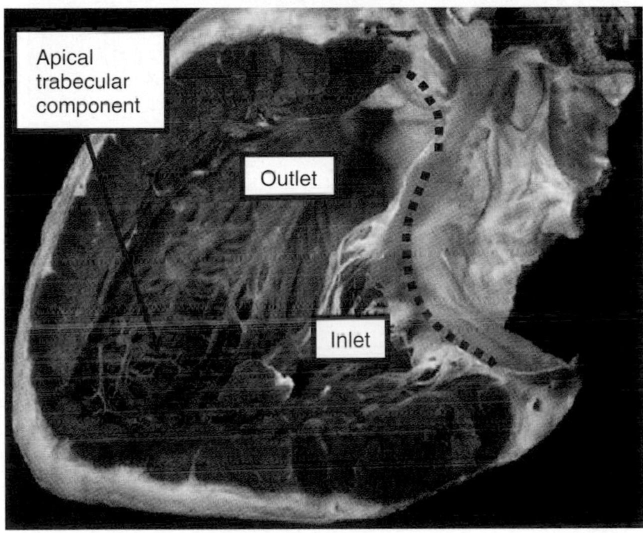

Figure 1-5 The posterior wall has been removed to show the three component parts of the morphologically left ventricle of the same heart as shown in Figure 1-4. This ventricle also extends from the atrioventricular to the ventriculo-arterial junctions (*dotted red line*), and the fine apical trabeculations are its most constant feature.

apparatus. The second part is the apical trabecular component. The third is the outlet component, supporting the leaflets of the arterial valve (Figs. 1-4 and 1-5).

Of these three components, it is the apical trabecular component that is most universally present in normal as well as in malformed and incomplete ventricles. Furthermore, it is the pattern of the apical trabeculations that differentiates morphologically right from left ventricles (see Figs. 1-4 and 1-5). This is the case even when the apical components exist as incomplete ventricles, lacking either inlet or outlet components, or sometimes both of these components (Fig. 1-6).

When the morphology of individual ventricles is identified in this fashion, all hearts with two ventricles can then be analysed according to the way in which the inlet and outlet components are shared between the apical trabecular components. In order fully to describe any ventricle,

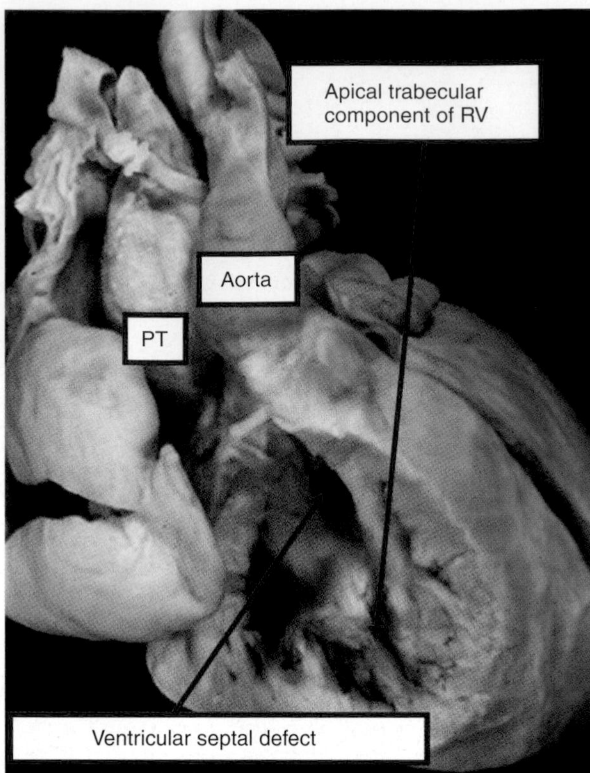

Figure 1-6 In the heart illustrated, there is double inlet to and double outlet from a dominant left ventricle. The aorta and pulmonary trunk (PT) are seen arising in parallel fashion from the left ventricle, with the aorta anterior and to the left. On the anterior and right-sided shoulder of the dominant left ventricle, however, there is still a second chamber to be seen, fed through a ventricular septal defect. This chamber is the apical trabecular component of the right ventricle (RV), identified by its coarse trabeculations.

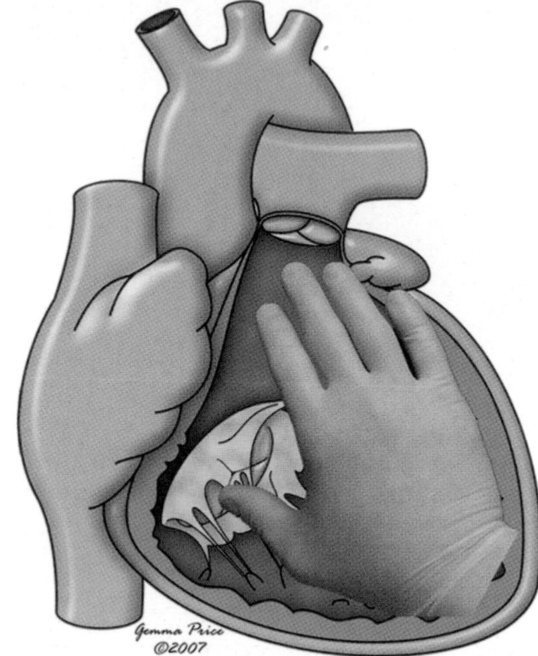

Figure 1-7 The cartoon shows how the palmar surface of the right hand can be placed on the septal surface of the normal morphologically right ventricle with the thumb in the inlet component and the fingers extending into the ventricular outlet. This is the essence of right hand ventricular topology, also known as a d-ventricular loop.

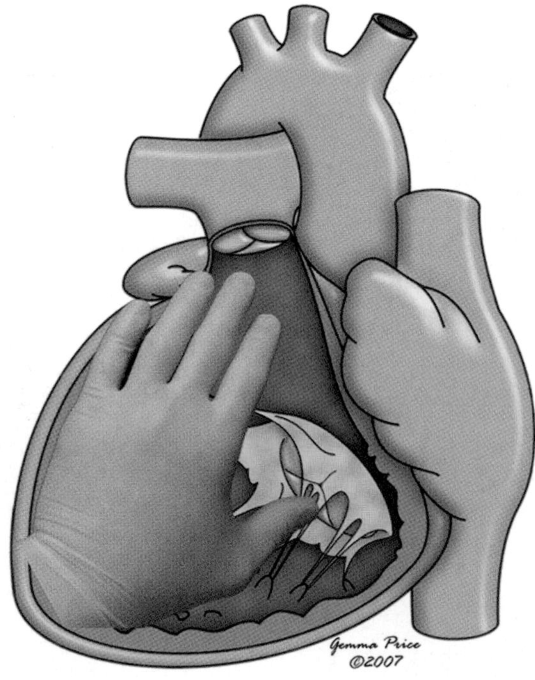

Figure 1-8 This cartoon shows the mirror-imaged normal heart. In this setting, it is the palmar surface of the left hand that can be placed on the septal surface of the morphologically right ventricle with the thumb in the inlet and the fingers in the outlet. This is the essence of left hand topology, or the l-ventricular loop. Compare with Figure 1-7.

account must also be taken of its size. It is then necessary further to describe the way in which the two ventricles themselves are related within the ventricular mass. This feature is described in terms of ventricular topology, since two basic patterns are found that cannot be changed without physically taking apart the ventricular components and reassembling them. The two patterns are mirror images of each other. They can be conceptualised in terms of the way in which, figuratively speaking, the palmar surface of the hands can be placed upon the septal surface of the morphologically right ventricle. In the morphologically right ventricle of the normal heart, irrespective of its position in space, only the palmar surface of the right hand can be placed on the septal surface such that the thumb occupies the inlet and the fingers fit into the outlet (Fig. 1-7).

The palmar surface of the left hand then fits in comparable fashion within the morphologically left ventricle, but it is the right hand that is taken as the arbiter for the purposes of categorisation. The usual pattern, therefore, can be described as right hand ventricular topology.[18] The other pattern, the mirror image of the right hand prototype, is then described as left hand ventricular topology. In this left hand pattern, seen typically in the mirror-imaged normal heart, or in the variant of congenitally corrected transposition found with usual atrial arrangement, it is the palmar surface of the left hand that fits on the septal surface of the morphologically right ventricle with the thumb in the inlet and the fingers in the outlet (Fig. 1-8).

These two topological patterns can always be distinguished irrespective of the location occupied in space by the ventricular mass itself. A left hand pattern of topology, therefore, is readily distinguished from a ventricular mass with right hand topology in which the right ventricle has

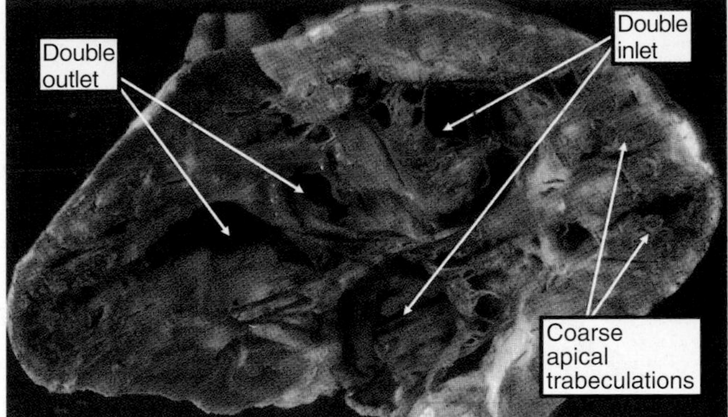

Figure 1-9 The heart is opened in clamshell fashion to show that both atrioventricular valves enter the same ventricular chamber, which also gives rise to both outflow tracts. We were unable to find a second ventricular chamber. The exceedingly coarse apical trabeculations, and the absence of the second chamber, identify this heart as having a solitary ventricle of indeterminate morphology. This is the only true single ventricle.

been rotated to occupy a left-sided position. Component make-up, trabecular pattern, topology and size are independent features of the ventricles. On occasion, all may need separate description in order to remove any potential for confusion.

Only rarely will hearts be encountered with a solitary ventricle. Sometimes this may be because a right or left ventricle is so small that it cannot be recognised with usual clinical investigatory techniques. There is, nonetheless, a third pattern of apical ventricular morphology that is found in hearts possessing a truly single ventricle. This is when the apical component is of neither right nor left type, but is very coarsely trabeculated, and crossed by multiple large muscle bundles. Such a solitary ventricle has an indeterminate morphology (Fig. 1-9).

Analysis of ventricles on the basis of their apical trabeculations precludes the need to use illogically the term single ventricle or univentricular heart for description of those hearts with one big and one small ventricle. These hearts may have a functionally univentricular arrangement, but all chambers that possess apical trabecular components can be described as ventricles, be they big or small, and be they incomplete or complete. Any attempt to disqualify such chambers from ventricular state must lead to a system that is artificial. Only hearts with a truly solitary ventricle need be described as univentricular, albeit that the connections of the atrioventricular junctions can be univentricular in many more hearts.

In determining the morphology of the great arteries, there are no intrinsic features which enable an aorta to be distinguished from a pulmonary trunk, or from a common or solitary arterial trunk. The branching pattern of the trunks themselves, nonetheless, is sufficiently characteristic to permit these distinctions (Fig. 1-10).

The aorta gives rise to at least one coronary artery and the bulk of the systemic arteries. The pulmonary trunk gives rise directly to both, or one or the other, of the pulmonary arteries. A common trunk supplies directly the coronary, systemic and pulmonary arteries. A solitary arterial trunk exists in the absence of the proximal portion of the pulmonary trunk. In such circumstances, it is impossible to state with certainty whether the persisting trunk is common or aortic. Even in the rare cases that have transgressed one of these rules, examination of the overall branching pattern has always permitted us to distinguish the nature of the arterial trunk.

ATRIAL ARRANGEMENT

The cornerstone of any system of sequential analysis must be accurate establishment of atrial arrangement, since this is the starting point for subsequent analysis. When arrangement of the atriums is assessed according to the morphology of the junction of the appendages with the rest of the atriums,[19] then since all hearts have two atrial appendages, each of which can only be of morphologically right or left type, there are only four possible patterns of arrangement (Fig. 1-11).

The most common is the usual arrangement, also called situs solitus, in which the morphologically right appendage is right-sided, and the morphologically left appendage is left-sided. The second arrangement, very rare, is the mirror image of the usual. It is often called situs inversus, even though the atrial chambers are not upside down. In these two arrangements, the appendages are lateralised, with the morphologically right appendage being to one side, and the morphologically left appendage to the other. The two other arrangements do not show such lateralisation. Instead, there is isomerism of the atrial appendages. In these patterns, the two appendages are mirror images of each other, with morphological characteristics at their

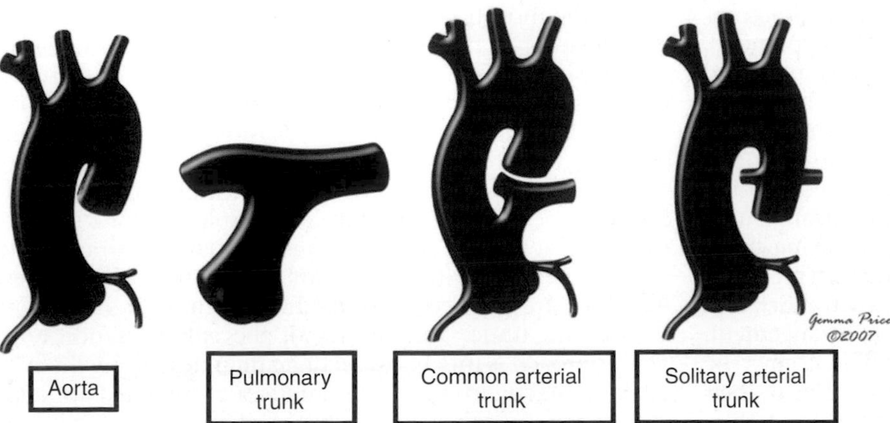

Figure 1-10 The cartoon shows how the branching pattern of arterial trunks permits their distinction. The solitary arterial trunk is described when the intrapericardial pulmonary arteries are absent, since in this setting it is impossible to determine, had they been present, whether they would have taken origin from the heart, making the trunk an aorta, or from the trunk itself, in which case there would have been a common arterial trunk with pulmonary atresia.

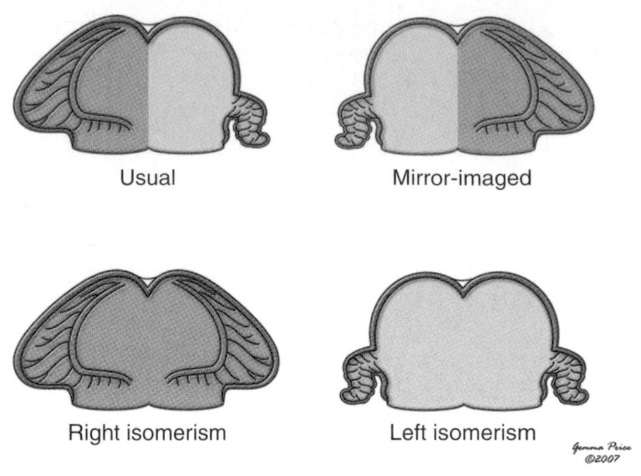

Figure 1-11 The cartoon shows how, when analysed on the basis of the extent of the pectinate muscles relative to the atrioventricular vestibules (see Figures 1-2 and 1-3), there are only four possible ways in which the two atrial appendages can be arranged. Note, however, that the venoatrial connections can show marked variation, particularly in the isomeric settings, also known collectively as visceral heterotaxy.

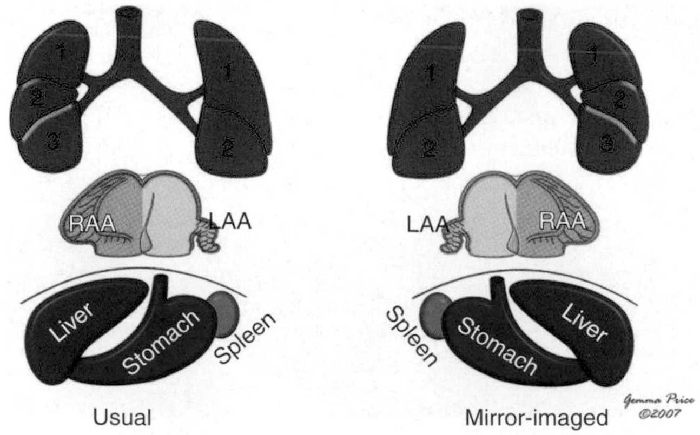

Figure 1-12 The cartoon shows the usual and mirror-imaged arrangements of the organs, which are lateralised. Almost always there is harmony between the arrangement of the right and left atrial appendages (RAA, LAA) and the remaining thoraco-abdominal organs. The numbers show the three lobes of the morphologically right lung, and the two lobes of the morphologically left lung.

junctions with the rest of the atriums on both sides of either right type or left type.

RECOGNITION OF ATRIAL ARRANGEMENT

The arrangement of the appendages, ideally, is recognised by direct examination of the extent of the pectinate muscles round the vestibules (see Figs. 1-2 and 1-3). This feature should now be recognisable using cross sectional echocardiography, particularly from the transoesophageal window. In most clinical situations, however, it is rarely necessary to rely only on direct identification. This is because, almost always, the morphology of the appendages is in harmony with the arrangements of the thoracic and abdominal organs. In patients with lateralised arrangements, that is the usual and mirror imaged patterns, it is exceedingly rare for there to be disharmony between the location of the organs (Fig. 1-12).

When the appendages are isomeric, in contrast, then the abdominal organs are typically jumbled-up (Fig. 1-13).

Even when there is such abdominal heterotaxy, the lungs and bronchial tree are almost always symmetrical, and it is rare for the bronchial arrangement to show disharmony with the morphology of the appendages. The presence of isomerism, therefore, can almost always be inferred from the bronchial anatomy. The morphologically left bronchus is long, and it branches only after it has been crossed by its accompanying pulmonary artery, making the bronchus hyparterial. In contrast, the morphologically right bronchus is short, and is crossed by its pulmonary artery only after it has branched, giving an eparterial pattern of branching. The four patterns of bronchial branching are then almost always in harmony with the arrangement of the atrial appendages. Similar inferences to those provided from bronchial arrangement can also usually be obtained non-invasively by using cross-sectional ultrasonography to image the abdominal great vessels. These vessels bear a distinct relation to each other, and to the spine, which generally reflects bodily arrangement, although not as accurately as does bronchial anatomy. The vessels can be distinguished ultrasonically according to their pattern of pulsation. When the atriums are lateralised, then almost without exception the inferior caval vein and aorta lie to opposite sides of the spine, with the caval vein on the side of the morphologically right appendage. When there is isomerism, then the great vessels usually lie to the same side of the spine, with the caval vein in anterior position in those with isomerism of the right atrial appendages, and posterior, or with the azygos vein posterior, in those having isomerism of the right atrial appendages.

Generally speaking, isomerism of the right atrial appendages is associated with absence of the spleen, while isomerism of the left atrial appendages is associated with multiple spleens. Patients with isomerism of the atrial appendages, therefore, are frequently grouped together, from the cardiac standpoint, under the banner of the splenic syndromes. This approach is much less accurate than describing the syndromes directly in terms of isomerism of the atrial appendages, since the correlation between isomerism of the right

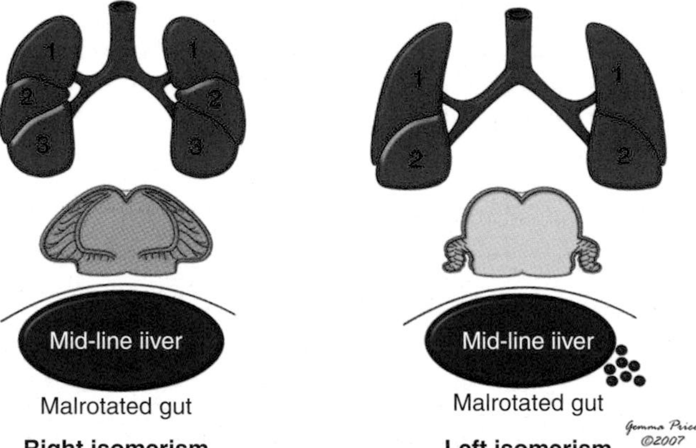

Figure 1-13 This cartoon shows the typical features of the thoraco-abdominal organs in so-called visceral heterotaxy. The abdominal organs are jumbled up, but the lungs and atrial appendages are usually isomeric, having the same morphological features on the right and left sides. It is usual for right isomerism to be associated with absence of the spleen, and left isomerism with multiple spleens, but these associations are far from constant. Thus, different pictures emerge when visceral heterotaxy is subdivided on the basis of isomersim as opposed to splenic morphology. Cardiac assessment, however, should start with analysis of atrial morphology based on the structure of the atrial appendages.

atrial appendages and absence of the spleen, and between isomerism of the left atrial appendages and multiple spleens, is far from perfect.[20] Isomerism of the right and left appendages, in contrast, describes what is there, and additionally serves to concentrate attention upon the heart.

THE ATRIOVENTRICULAR JUNCTIONS

In the normal heart, the atrial myocardium is contiguous with the ventricular mass around the orifices of the mitral and tricuspid valves. Electrical insulation is provided at these junctions by the fibrofatty atrioventricular grooves, other than at the site of the penetration of the bundle of His. In order to analyse accurately the morphology of the atrioventricular junctions in abnormal hearts, it is first necessary to know the atrial arrangement. Equally, it is necessary to know the morphology of the ventricular mass so as to establish which atrium is connected to which ventricle. With this information to hand, it is then possible to define the specific patterns of union or non-union across the junctions, and to determine the morphology of the valves guarding the atrioventricular junctions. In hearts with complex malformations, it is also necessary on occasion to describe the precise topology of the ventricular mass, and to specify the relationships of the ventricles themselves.

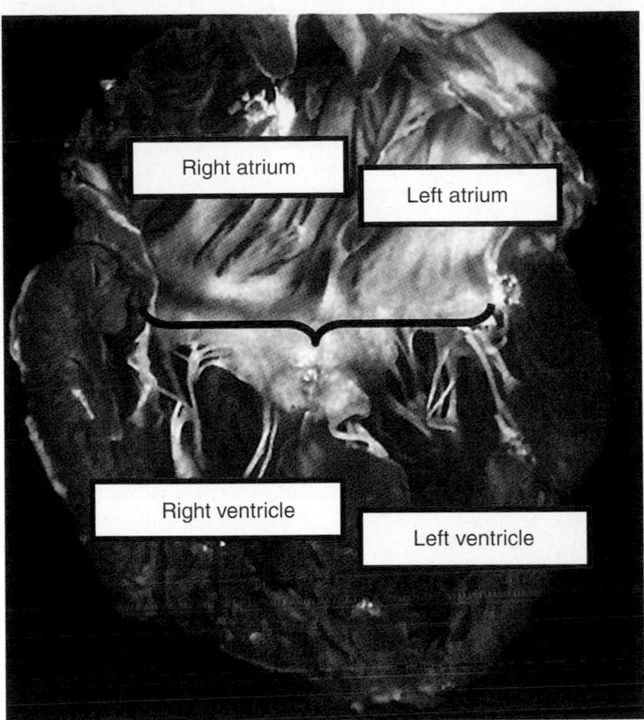

Figure 1-15 This heart has an atrioventricular septal defect with common atrioventricular junction (*red brace*). The presence of the common junction, however, does not disguise the fact that each atrium is joined to its own ventricle across paired junctions, albeit now guarded by a common valve.

PATTERNS OF UNION OR NON-UNION OF THE ATRIAL AND VENTRICULAR CHAMBERS

As already described, the patterns depend on the way that the myocardium of both atriums is joined to the ventricular myocardium around the entirety of the atrioventricular junctions, the atrial and ventricular muscle masses being separated from the electrical standpoint by the insulating fibrofatty tissues of the junctions other than at the site of the atrioventricular bundle. The cavities of the atrial chambers, therefore, are potentially connected to the underlying ventricular cavities via the atrioventricular orifices. In every heart, perforce, since there are two atrial chambers, there is the possibility for two atrioventricular connections, which will be right sided and left sided (Fig. 1-14).

This is the case irrespective of whether the junctions themselves are guarded by two valves (see Fig. 1-14) or a common valve (Fig. 1-15).

One of the junctions may be blocked by an imperforate valvar membrane, but this does not alter the fact that, in such a setting, there are still two potential atrioventricular connections (Fig. 1-16).

In some hearts, in contrast, this possibility is not fulfilled. This is because one of the connections is completely absent. Then, the atrial myocardium on that side has no connection with the underlying ventricular myocardium, being separated from the ventricular mass by much more extensive

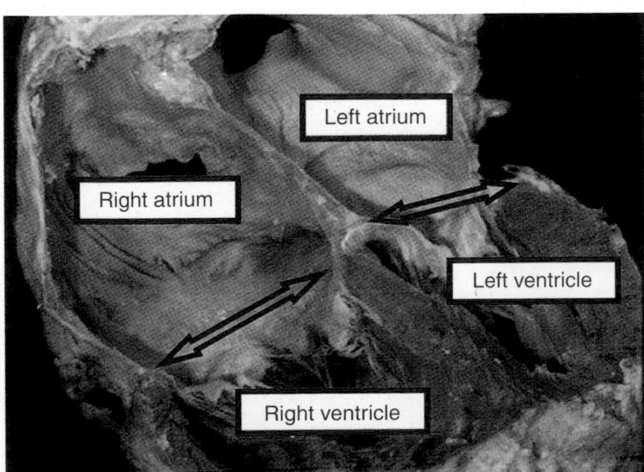

Figure 1-14 This four-chamber section of the normal heart shows the paired atrioventricular junctions (*red double-headed arrows*) across which the cavities of the atrial chambers are connected to their appropriate ventricles.

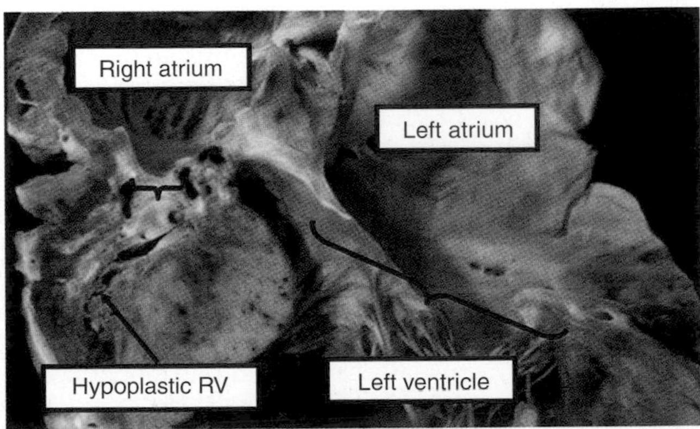

Figure 1-16 The atrioventricular junctions have ben sectioned in four-chamber fashion in this heart with combined tricuspid and pulmonary atresia. In this instance, unusually, the tricuspid atresia is the consequence of an imperforate right atrioventricular valve, shown by the *short red brace*. The *longer brace* shows the patent left atrioventricular connection, through which the left atrium drains to the left ventricle. The atrioventricular connections, therefore, are potentially concordant (compare with Fig. 1-17). RV, right ventricle.

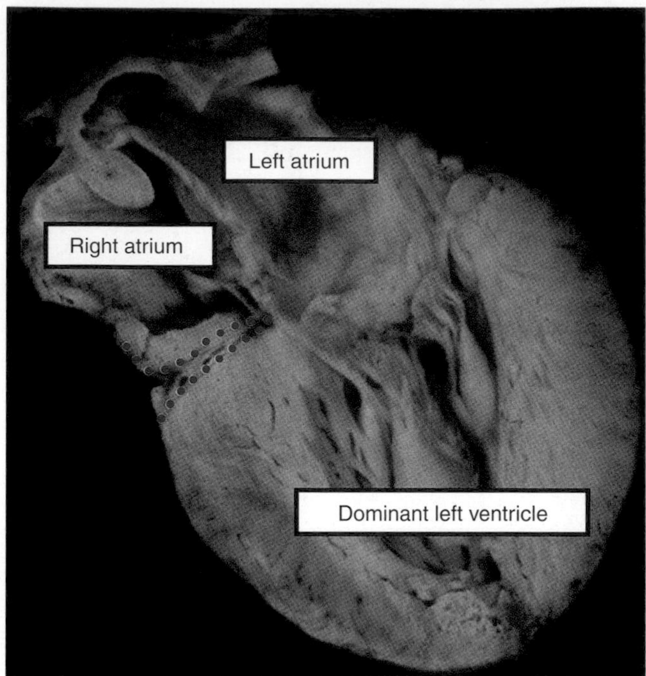

Figure 1-17 This heart, with the usual form of tricuspid atresia, has also been sectioned in four-chamber fashion. Only three chambers, however, are seen. This is because the essence of typical tricuspid atresia, and many patients with mitral atresia, is absence of an atrioventricular connection, in this instance the right atrioventricular connection (*blue dotted line*).

formation than normal of the fibrofatty tissues of the atrioventricular groove. This arrangement is the most common pattern producing atrioventricular valvar atresia (Fig. 1-17).

When atrioventricular connections are defined in this fashion, all hearts fit into one of three groups. In the first group, by far the most common, the cavity of each atrial chamber is joined actually or potentially, but separately, to that of an underlying ventricle. The feature of the second group is that only one of the ventricles, if indeed two are present, is in communication with the atrial cavities. There is then an even rarer third group. This is seen when one atrioventricular connection is absent, and the solitary atrioventricular junction, via a straddling valve, is connected to two ventricles. This arrangement is uniatrial but biventricular.

There are three possible arrangements in hearts with each atrium joined to its own ventricle. Put in another way, there are three types of biventricular atrioventricular connection. These depend on the morphology of the chambers connected together. The first pattern is seen when the atriums are joined to morphologically appropriate ventricles, irrespective of the topology or relationship of the ventricles, or of the morphology of the valves guarding the junctions. This arrangement produces concordant atrioventricular connections. Such concordant connections can be found with either usually arranged atrial appendages, or in the mirror-imaged arrangement (Fig. 1-18).

The second arrangement is the reverse of the first. It is again independent of relationships or valvar morphology. It produces discordant atrioventricular connections, and can again be found in the usual or mirror-imaged situations, albeit that, when the atrial appendages are mirror-imaged in patients with discordant atrioventricular connections,

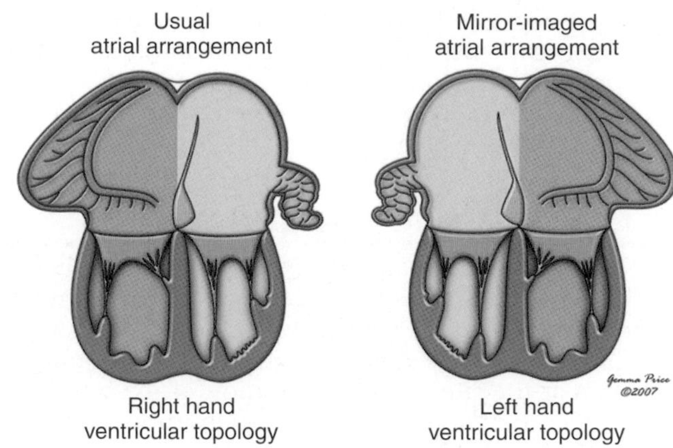

Figure 1-18 The cartoon shows how concordant atrioventricular connections can exist in usual and mirror-imaged patterns. Almost without exception, atriums with usually arranged appendages are joined to a ventricular mass with right hand topology, whilst atriums with mirror-imaged appendages are joined to a ventricular mass with left hand topology. It is only when these features are not present that it is necessary always to state the topology of the ventricles.

the ventricles are typically in their expected pattern—in other words show right hand topology (Fig. 1-19).

These first two arrangements (see Figs. 1-18 and 1-19) are found when the atrial appendages are lateralised. The other biventricular atrioventricular arrangement, in which each atrium is joined to a separate ventricle, is found in hearts with isomeric appendages, be they of right or left morphology. Because of the isomeric nature of the appendages, this third arrangement cannot accurately be described in terms of concordant or discordant connections. It is a discrete biventricular pattern in its own right, which is mixed (Fig. 1-20). It, too, is independent of ventricular relationships and atrioventricular valvar morphologies, and requires specification of ventricular topology to make the description complete.

There are also three possible junctional arrangements that produce univentricular atrioventricular connections (Fig. 1-21). The first is when the cavities of right- and left-sided atrial chambers are connected directly to the same ventricle. This is called double inlet atrioventricular connection, irrespective of whether the right- and left-sided atrioventricular junctions are guarded by two atrioventricular

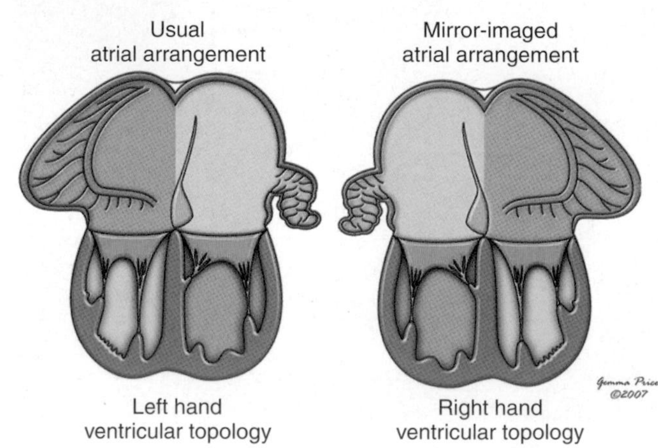

Figure 1-19 The cartoon shows the arrangements that, almost without exception, produce discordant atrioventricular connections.

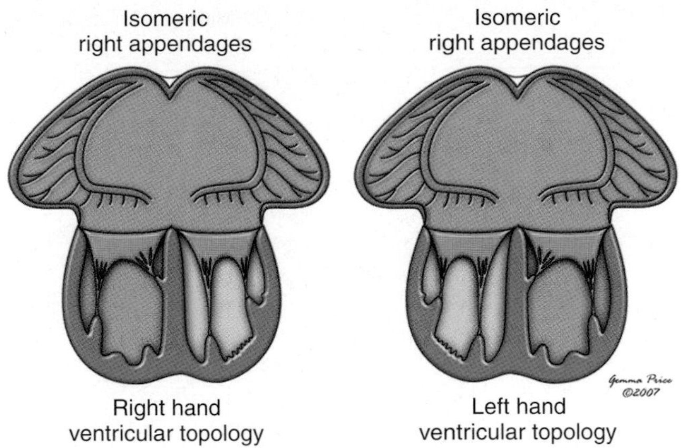

Figure 1-20 In the setting of isomeric atrial appendages, with right isomerism as shown in the cartoon, biventricular connections of necessity are mixed irrespective of ventricular topology. Fully to describe these patterns, therefore, it is necessary to specify both the morphology of the atrial appendages and the ventricular topology.

valves or a common valve. The other two arrangements exist when one atrioventricular connection is absent, giving absent right-sided and absent left-sided atrioventricular connection, respectively. The patterns across the junctions that produce univentricular atrioventricular connections are different from those found with biventricular connections. Not only are they independent of ventricular relationships and valvar morphology, but they are also independent of atrial and ventricular morphologies. Hearts with concordant or discordant atrioventricular connections can only exist when usually arranged or mirror-imaged atrial chambers are each joined to separate ventricles. A heart with biventricular mixed connection can only be found when each of two atrial chambers having isomeric appendages is joined to a separate ventricle. In contrast, double inlet, absent right-sided, or absent left-sided atrioventricular connections can be found with usually arranged, mirror-imaged or isomeric atrial appendages. Each type of univentricular atrioventricular connection can also be found with the atriums connected to a dominant right ventricle, a dominant left ventricle, or a morphologically indeterminate ventricle (see Fig. 1-21).

Ventricular morphology must always, therefore, be described separately in those hearts in which the atrial chambers are joined to only one ventricle. Although, in these hearts, only one ventricle is joined to the atriums, in most of them there is a second ventricle present. This second ventricle, of necessity incomplete, will be of complementary trabecular pattern to that of the dominant ventricle. Most frequently, the dominant ventricle is a left ventricle, and the incomplete ventricle possesses right ventricular apical trabeculations. More rarely, the dominant ventricle is morphologically right, with the incomplete ventricle being morphologically left. Even more rarely, hearts will be found with a solitary ventricular chamber of indeterminate morphology (see Fig. 1-9). In clinical practice, seemingly solitary left or right ventricles may be encountered when the complementary incomplete ventricle is too small to be demonstrated.

ARRANGEMENTS OF THE ATRIOVENTRICULAR VALVES

Describing the fashion in which the atriums are joined to the ventricles across the atrioventricular junctions accounts only for the way in which the atrial musculature inserts into the base of the ventricular mass. The morphology of the valves guarding the overall atrioventricular junctional area is independent of this feature, within the constraints

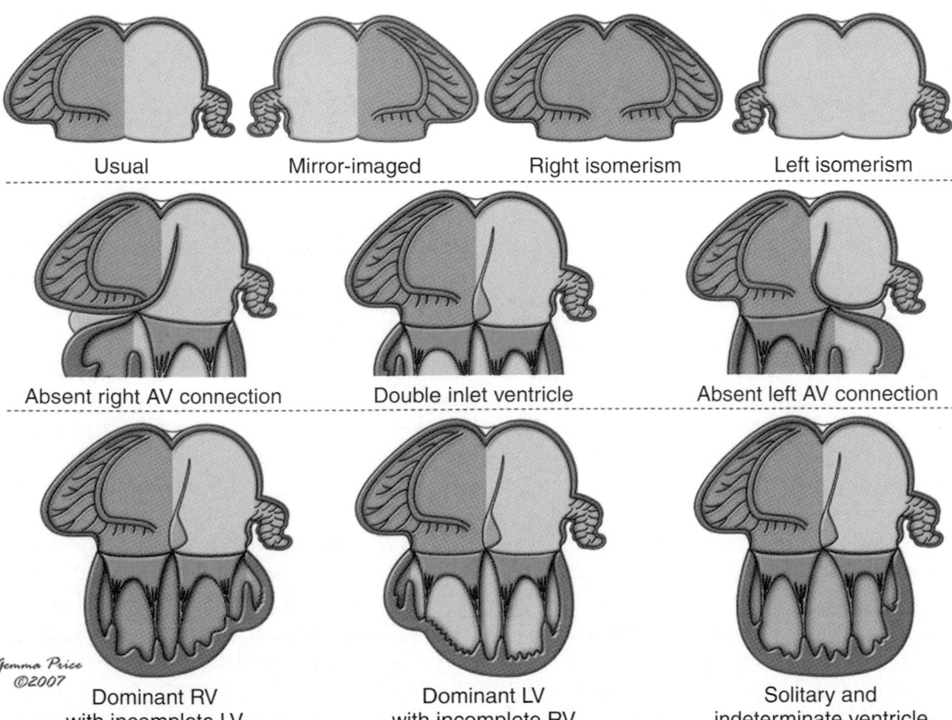

Figure 1-21 The cartoon shows some of the potential univentricular atrioventricular connections. In reality, these can exist with any arrangement of the atrial appendages (*upper row*), with double inlet, absent right or absent left atrioventricular (AV) connections (*middle row*) and with dominant left or right ventricles (LV, RV), or solitary and indeterminate ventricle (*bottom row*). The middle and bottom rows are illustrated with usual appendages simply for convenience. There is further variability with regard to the position of the incomplete ventricle, and with ventriculo-arterial connections, and so on. These hearts, therefore, exemplify the need for full sequential segmental analysis and description.

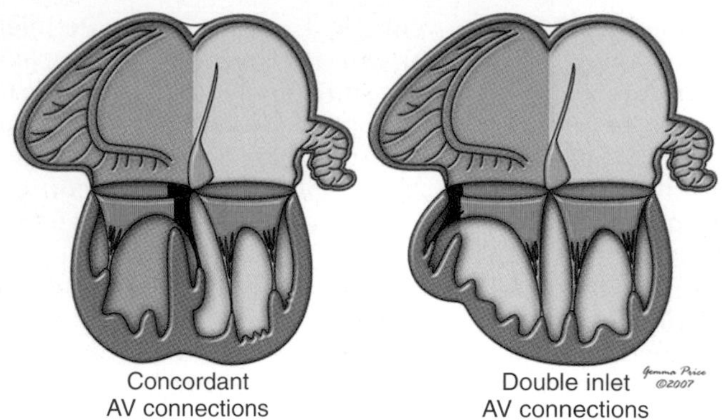

Figure 1-22 The cartoon shows the influence of an overriding atrioventricular (AV) junction on the precise arrangement of the connections. When the lesser part of the overriding junction is attached to the dominant ventricle, then the connections are effectively biventricular, and concordant in the example shown in the *left panel*. When the lesser part is committed to the incomplete ventricle, in contrast, then the connection is effectively double inlet, and to the left ventricle in the illustration (*right panel*). Any combination of atrial chambers and ventricles can be found with such straddling and overriding valves.

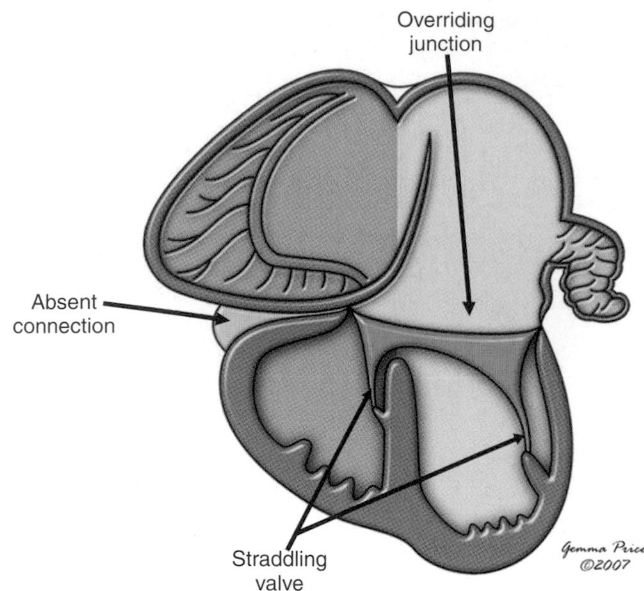

Figure 1-23 The cartoon illustrates tricuspid atresia due to absence of the right atrioventricular connection associated with straddling and overriding of the left atrioventricular valve. This produces an atrioventricular connection that is uniatrial but biventricular. The connection can be found with any combination of atrial arrangement and ventricular topology.

imposed by the pattern of the junctions itself. When the cavities of both atriums are joined directly to the ventricular mass, the right- and left-sided atrioventricular junctions may be guarded by two patent valves (see Fig. 1-14), by one patent valve and one imperforate valve (see Fig. 1-16), by a common valve (see Fig. 1-15), or by straddling and overriding valves (Fig. 1-22).

These arrangements of the valves can be found with concordant, discordant, biventricular and mixed or double inlet types of connection. Either the right- or the left-sided valve may be imperforate, producing atresia but in the setting of a potential as opposed to an absent atrioventricular connection. A common valve guards both right- and left-sided atrioventricular junctions, irrespective of its morphology. A valve straddles when its tension apparatus is attached to both sides of a septum within the ventricular mass. It overrides when the atrioventricular junction is connected to ventricles on both sides of a septal structure. A right-sided valve, a left-sided valve, or a common valve can straddle, can override, or can straddle and override. Very rarely, both right- and left-sided valves may straddle and/or override in the same heart.

When one atrioventricular connection is absent, then the possible modes of connection are greatly reduced. This is because there is a solitary right- or left-sided atrioventricular connection and, hence, a solitary atrioventricular valve. The single valve is usually committed in its entirety to one ventricle. More rarely, it may straddle, override, or straddle and override. These latter patterns produce the extremely rare group of uniatrial but biventricular connections (Fig. 1-23).

A valve that overrides has an additional influence on description. This is because the degree of commitment of the overriding atrioventricular junction to the ventricles on either side of the septum determines the precise fashion in which the atriums and ventricles are joined together. Hearts with two valves, in which one valve is overriding, are anatomically intermediate between those with, on the one hand, biventricular and, on the other hand, univentricular atrioventricular connections. There are two ways of describing such hearts. One is to consider the hearts as representing a special type of atrioventricular connection. The alternative is to recognise the intermediate nature of such hearts in a series of anomalies, and to split the series depending on the precise connection of the overriding junction. For the purposes of categorisation, only the two ends of the series are labelled, with hearts in the middle being assigned to one or other of the end-points. We prefer this second option (see Fig. 1-22). When most of an overriding junction is connected to a ventricle that is also joined to the other atrium, we designate the pattern as being double inlet. If the overriding junction is connected mostly to a ventricle not itself joined to the other atrium, then each atrium is categorised as though joined to its own ventricle, giving the possibility of concordant, discordant, or mixed connections.

In describing atrioventricular valves, it should also be noted that the adjectives mitral and tricuspid are strictly accurate only in hearts with biventricular atrioventricular connections having separate junctions, each guarded by its own valve. In this context, the tricuspid valve is always found in the morphologically right ventricle, and the mitral valve in the morphologically left ventricle. In hearts with biventricular atrioventricular connections but with a common junction, in contrast, it is incorrect to consider the common valve as having mitral and tricuspid components, even when it is divided into right and left components. These right- and left-sided components, particularly on the left side, bear scant resemblance to the normal atrioventricular valves (see Chapter 27). In hearts with double inlet, the two valves are again better considered as right- and left-sided valves rather than as mitral or tricuspid. Similarly, although it is usually possible, when one connection is absent, to deduce the presumed nature of the remaining solitary valve from concepts of morphogenesis, this is not always practical or helpful. The valve can always accurately be described as being right or left sided. Potentially contentious arguments are thus defused when the right- or left-sided valve straddles in the absence of the other atrioventricular connection, giving the uniatrial but biventricular connections.

VENTRICULAR TOPOLOGY AND RELATIONSHIPS

Even in the normal heart, the ventricular spatial relationships are complex. The inlet portions are more or less to the right and left, with the inferior part of the muscular ventricular septum lying in an approximately sagittal plane. The outlet portions are more or less anteroposteriorly related, with the septum between them in an approximately frontal plane. The trabecular portions extend between these two components, with the trabecular muscular septum spiralling between the inlet and outlet components. It is understandable that there is a desire to have a shorthand term to describe such complex spatial arrangements. We use the concept of ventricular topology for this purpose (see Figs. 1-7 and 1-8). In persons with usually arranged atriums and discordant atrioventricular connections, the ventricular mass almost always shows a left-handed topological pattern, whereas right-handed ventricular topology is usually found with the combination of mirror-imaged atriums and discordant atrioventricular connections. Although these combinations are almost always present, exceptions can occur. When noting such unexpected ventricular relationships as a feature independent of the topology, we account for right–left, anterior–posterior and superior–inferior coordinates. And, should it be necessary, we describe the position of the three ventricular components separately, and relative to each other.

In hearts with disharmonious arrangements in the setting of usual atrial arrangement and discordant atrioventricular connections, the distal parts of the ventricles are usually rotated so that the morphologically right ventricular trabecular and outlet components are to the right of their morphologically left ventricular counterparts, giving the impression of normal relationships. In such criss-cross hearts seen with usual atrial arrangement and concordant atrioventricular connections, the ventricular rotation gives a spurious impression of left-handed topology. In cases with extreme rotation, the inlet of the morphologically right ventricle may also be right sided in association with discordant atrioventricular connections. Provided that relationships are described accurately, and separately, from the connections and the ventricular topology, then none of these unusual and apparently complex hearts will be difficult either to diagnose or to categorise. In addition to these problematic criss-cross hearts, we have already discussed how description of ventricular topology is essential when accounting for the combination of isomeric appendages with biventricular mixed atrioventricular connections. This is because, in this situation, the same terms would appropriately be used to describe the heart in which the left-sided atrium was connected to a morphologically right ventricle as well as the heart in which the left-sided atrium was connected to a morphologically left ventricle. The arrangements are differentiated simply by describing also the ventricular topology.

Both the position and the relationships of incomplete ventricles need to be described in hearts with univentricular atrioventricular connections. Here, the relationships are independent of both the connections and the ventricular morphology. While, usually, the incomplete right ventricle is anterior and right sided in classical tricuspid atresia, it can be anterior and left sided without in any way altering the clinical presentation and haemodynamic findings. Similarly, in hearts with double inlet ventricle, the position of the incomplete ventricle plays only a minor role in determining the clinical presentation. While a case can be made for interpreting such hearts with univentricular atrioventricular connections on the basis of presumed morphogenesis in the setting of right- or left-handed topologies, there are sufficient exceptions to make this approach unsuitable in the clinical setting. When we describe the position of incomplete ventricles, therefore, we simply account for their location relative to the dominant ventricle, taking note again when necessary of right–left, anterior–posterior and superior–inferior coordinates. On occasion, it may also be advantageous to describe separately the position of trabecular and outlet components of an incomplete ventricle.

THE VENTRICULO-ARTERIAL JUNCTIONS

Most polemics concerning the ventriculo-arterial junctions devolved upon the failure to distinguish between the way the arterial trunks arose from the ventricular mass as opposed to their relations to each other, along with undue emphasis on the nature of the infundibulums supporting their arterial valves. When these features are described independently, following the precepts of the morphological method, then all potential for disagreement is removed.

Origin of the Arterial Trunks from the Ventricular Mass

As with analysis of the atrioventricular junctions, it is necessary to account separately for the way the arteries take origin, and the nature of the valves guarding the ventriculo-arterial junctions. There are four possible types of origin. Concordant ventriculo-arterial connections exist when the aorta arises from a morphologically left ventricle, and the pulmonary trunk from a morphologically right ventricle, be the ventricles complete or incomplete. The arrangement where the aorta arises from a morphologically right ventricle or its rudiment, and the pulmonary trunk from a morphologically left ventricle or its rudiment, produces discordant ventriculo-arterial connections. Double outlet connection is found when both arteries are connected to the same ventricle, which may be of right ventricular, left ventricular or indeterminate ventricular pattern. As with atrioventricular valves, overriding arterial valves (see below) are assigned to the ventricle supporting the greater parts of their circumference. The fourth ventriculo-arterial connection is single outlet from the heart. This may take one of four forms. A common trunk exists when both ventricles are connected via a common arterial valve to one trunk that gives rise directly to the coronary arteries, at least one pulmonary artery, and the majority of the systemic circulation. A solitary arterial trunk exists when it is not possible to identify any remnant of an atretic pulmonary trunk within the pericardial cavity. The other forms of single outlet are single pulmonary trunk with aortic atresia, and single aortic trunk with pulmonary atresia. These latter two categories describe only those arrangements in which, using clinical techniques, it is not possible to establish the precise connection of the atretic arterial trunk to a ventricular cavity. If its ventricular origin can be established, but is found to be imperforate, then the connection is described, along with the presence of an imperforate valve (see below). It is also necessary in hearts with single outlet to describe the ventricular origin of the arterial trunk. This may be exclusively from a right or a left ventricle, but more usually the trunk overrides the septum, taking its origin from both ventricles.

There are fewer morphologies for the valves at the ventriculo-arterial than at the atrioventricular junctions. A common arterial valve can only exist with a specific type of single outlet, namely common arterial trunk. Straddling of an arterial valve is impossible because it has no tension apparatus. Thus, the possible patterns are two perforate valves, one or both of which may override, or one perforate and one imperforate valve. As with overriding atrioventricular valves, the degree of override of an arterial valve determines the precise origin of the arterial trunk from the ventricular mass, the overriding valve, or valves, being assigned to the ventricle supporting the greater part of its circumference. For example, if more than half of an overriding pulmonary valve was connected to a right ventricle, the aorta being connected to a left ventricle, we would code concordant connections. If more than half the overriding aortic valve was connected to the right ventricle in this situation, we would code double outlet connections. In this way, we avoid the necessity for intermediate categories. The precise degree of override, nonetheless, is best stated whenever an overriding valve is found. This is done to the best of one's ability, using whichever techniques are available, and recognising the subjective nature of the task. In this setting, as with atrioventricular connections, we err on the side of the more usually encountered pattern.

Arterial Relationships

Relationships are usually described at valvar level, and many systems for nomenclature have been constructed on this basis. Indeed, the concept that the position of the arterial valves reflected ventricular topology[5,6] became so entrenched that it became frequent to see d-transposition used as though synonymous with all combinations of concordant atrioventricular and discordant ventriculo-arterial connections. In the same way, l-transposition was used as a synonym for congenitally corrected transposition. In reality, we now know that the relationships of the arterial valves are a poor guide to ventricular topology. Describing arterial valvar position in terms of leftness and rightness also takes no cognisance of anteroposterior relationships, an omission particularly since, for many years, an anterior position of the aorta was used as the cornerstone for definitions of transposition.[21] It is, therefore, our practice to describe arterial valvar relationships in terms of both right–left and anterior–posterior coordinates. Such description can be accomplished with as great a degree of precision as is required. A good system is the one that describes aortic position in degrees of the arc of a circle constructed around the pulmonary valve.[18] Aortic valvar position is described relative to the pulmonary trunk in terms of eight positions of a compass, using the simple terms left, right, anterior, posterior, and side-by-side in their various combinations. So long as we then remember that these describe only arterial–valvar relations, and convey no information about either the origin of the arterial trunks from the ventricular mass, or the morphology of the ventricular outflow tracts, we have no fear of producing confusion.

From the stance of positions of the arterial trunks, the possibilities are either for the pulmonary trunk to spiral round the aorta as it ascends from the base of the ventricles, or for the two trunks to ascend in parallel fashion. It is rarely necessary to describe these relationships. Spiralling trunks are associated most frequently with concordant ventriculo-arterial connections, and parallel trunks with discordant or double outlet connections, but again there is no predictive value in these relationships. In almost all hearts, the aortic arch crosses superiorly to the bifurcation of the pulmonary arteries.

An unexpected position of the aortic arch is a well-recognised associated anomaly of conditions such as tetralogy of Fallot (Chapter 36) or common arterial trunk (Chapter 41). In this respect, distinction should be made between the position of the arch and the side of the descending aorta, particularly in describing vascular rings (Chapter 47). The side of the aortic arch depends on whether it passes to the right or the left of the trachea. The position of the descending aorta is defined relative to the vertebral column.

Infundibular Morphology

The infundibular regions are no more and no less than the outlet components of the ventricular mass, but they have been the dwelling place of two of the sacred cows of paediatric cardiology. One is the so-called bilateral conus. In the past, this was often considered an arbiter of the ventriculo-arterial connection when associated with double outlet right ventricle, but ignored when each great artery with its complete muscular infundibulum was supported by its own ventricle. The other was the enigmatic crista, sought here and there as was the Scarlet Pimpernel, and just as elusive.[22] If the infundibular structures are recognised for what they are, and their morphology described as such, then they, too, provide no problems in recognition and description. The morphology of the ventricular outlet portions is variable for any heart. Potentially, each ventricle can possess a complete muscular funnel as its outlet portion, and then each arterial valve can be said to have a complete infundibulum. When considered as a whole, the outlet portions of the ventricular mass in the setting of bilateral infundibulums have three discrete parts (Fig. 1-24).

Two of the parts form the anterior and posterior halves of the funnels of muscle supporting the arterial valves. The anterior, parietal, part is the free anterior ventricular wall. The posterior part is the inner heart curvature, a structure that separates the leaflets of the arterial from those of the atrioventricular valves. We term this component the ventriculo-infundibular fold. The third part is the septum that separates the two subarterial outlets, which we designated the outlet, or infundibular, septum. The dimensions of the outlet septum are independent of the remainder of the infundibular musculature. Indeed, it is possible, albeit rarely, for both arterial valves to be separated from both atrioventricular valves by the ventriculo-infundibular fold, but for the

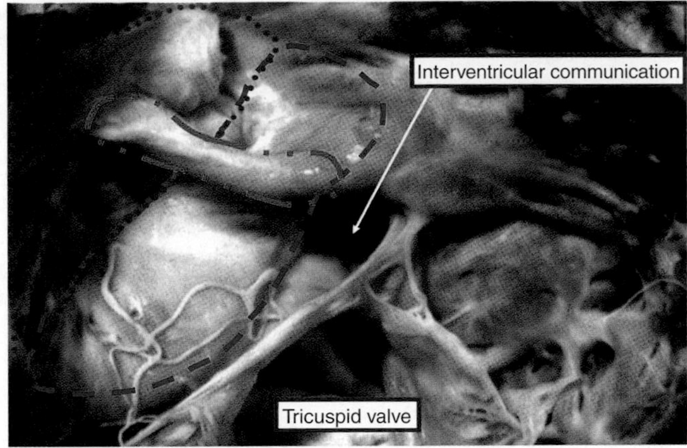

Figure 1-24 The illustration shows the complete cone of musculature supporting both arterial valves in the setting of double outlet right ventricle with bilateral infundibulums and subaortic interventricular communication. The cones have parietal parts, outlined in *red*, posterior parts adjacent to the atrioventricular junctions, outlined in *blue*, and a part that divides them, outlined in *yellow*. The posterior part is the ventriculo-infundibular fold, separating the leaflets of the atrioventricular and arterial valves, whilst the dividing part is the outlet septum, interposed between the leaflets of the arterial valves.

arterial valves to be in fibrous continuity with one another because of the absence of the outlet septum. In most hearts, however, some part of the infundibular musculature is effaced, so that fibrous continuity occurs between the leaflets of one of the arterial and the atrioventricular valves. Most frequently, it is the morphologically left ventricular part of the ventriculo-infundibular fold that is attenuated. As a result, there is fibrous continuity between the leaflets of the mitral valve and the arterial valve supported by the left ventricle. Whether the arterial valve is aortic or pulmonary will depend on the ventriculo-arterial connections present. In the usual arrangement, the morphologically right ventricular part of the ventriculo-infundibular fold persists, so that there is tricuspid-arterial valvar discontinuity. Depending on the integrity of the outlet septum, there is usually a completely muscular outflow tract, or infundibulum, in the morphologically right ventricle. When both outlet portions are connected to the morphologically right ventricle, then most frequently the ventriculo-infundibular fold persists in its entirety, and there is discontinuity bilaterally between the leaflets of the atrioventricular and arterial valves. But many hearts in which both arterial valves are connected unequivocally to the right ventricle have fibrous continuity between at least one arterial valve and an atrioventricular valve. It makes little sense to deny the origin of both arterial trunks from the right ventricle in this setting. This situation is yet another example of the controversy generated when one feature of cardiac morphology is determined on the basis of a second, unrelated, feature. When both arterial trunks take their origin from the morphologically left ventricle, the tendency is for there to be continuity between the leaflets of both arterial valves and both atrioventricular valves. Even then, in some instances the ventriculo-infundibular fold may persist in part or in its whole.

It is usually the state of the ventriculo-infundibular fold, therefore, that is the determining feature of infundibular morphology. Ignoring the rare situation of complete absence of the outlet septum, and considering morphology from the standpoint of the arterial valves, there are four possible arrangements. First, there may be a complete subpulmonary infundibulum, with continuity between the leaflets of the aortic and the atrioventricular valves. Second, there may be a complete subaortic infundibulum, with continuity between the pulmonary and the atrioventricular valves. Third, there may be bilateral infundibulums, with absence of continuity between the leaflets of the arterial and the atrioventricular valves. Fourth, there may be bilaterally deficient infundibulums, with continuity bilaterally between the arterial and the atrioventricular valves. In themselves, these terms are not specific. For specificity, it is also necessary to know which arterial valve takes origin from which ventricle. This emphasises the fact that infundibular morphology is independent of the ventriculo-arterial connections.

The above discussion has been concluded without any mention of the enigmatic crista. This is because, when used in reference to malformed hearts, the term has had so many definitions as to render it virtually meaningless. We reserve the term supraventricular crest for the normal heart, or for hearts with a normally structured right ventricular outflow tract. The crest is then the muscular ventricular roof that separates the attachments of the leaflets of the tricuspid and pulmonary valves. The greater part of this fold is made up of the right ventricular component of the ventriculo-infundibular fold, including the free-standing sleeve of subpulmonary infundibulum. Only a small part of its most medial edge is the muscular outlet septum. This cannot be distinguished in its own right when the outflow tract is normally structured. The supraventricular crest of the normal heart as thus defined is discrete and separate from the extensive muscular trabeculation that reinforces the septal surface of the morphologically right ventricle. This structure divides into two limbs, which clasp the body of the supraventricular crest. We call this extensive muscular strap the septomarginal trabeculation, but others recognise it as the septal band. These three structures, the ventriculo-infundibular fold, outlet septum, and the septomarginal trabeculation, can be so well aligned that it is not possible to say where one starts and the other finishes. In hearts with ventricular septal defects, or abnormal ventriculo-arterial connections, the three parts are frequently widely separated. Each can then be clearly recogniszed in its own right. The problem with the term crista is that, at some time or in some place, it has been used to describe each of these three different structures. It is for this reason that we restrict its use to the normal heart. In abnormal hearts, we describe each muscle bundle in its own right. Any muscular structure that interposes between the ventricular outflow portions is called the outlet septum. Any muscular structure separating the attachments of the leaflet of an arterial valve from that of an atrioventricular valve is called the ventriculo-infundibular fold. The extensive muscular strap in the morphologically right ventricle is described as the septomarginal trabeculation. We also take note of the series of muscle bundles that radiate from the anterior margin of the septomarginal trabeculation, and term these septoparietal trabeculations.

ASSOCIATED MALFORMATIONS

A majority of patients seen with congenitally malformed hearts will have their cardiac segments joined together in usual fashion, together with normal morphology and relations. In such a setting, the associated malformation will be the anomaly. The body of this book is concerned with describing the specific morphological and clinical features of these anomalies. It is also necessary, nonetheless, to pay attention to the position of the heart within the chest, and the orientation of the cardiac apex. It is also necessary to recognise that the heart may be positioned ectopically outside the thoracic cavity. An abnormal position of the heart within the chest is another associated malformation, and should not be elevated to a prime diagnosis. This is not to decry the importance of an abnormal cardiac position, if only to aid in interpretation of the electrocardiogram. Knowing that the heart is malpositioned, however, gives no information concerning its internal architecture. Full sequential segmental analysis is needed to establish the cardiac structure, and not the other way round. The heart can be located mostly in the left hemithorax, mostly in the right hemithorax, or centrally positioned in the mediastinum. The cardiac apex can then point to the left, to the right, or to the middle. The orientation of the apex is independent of cardiac position. And both of these are independent of the arrangement of the atrial appendages, and of the thoracic and abdominal organs. Describing a right-sided heart, with leftward apex, should be understandable by all, even including the patient!

The complete reference list can be found on the companion Expert Consult web site at www.expertconsult.com.

ANNOTATED REFERENCES

- Van Praagh R: The segmental approach to diagnosis in congenital heart disease. In Bergsma D (ed): Birth Defects Original Article Series, vol VIII, no 5. The National Foundation–March of Dimes. Baltimore: Williams & Wilkins, 1972, pp 4–23.

  This chapter in a volume from a series devoted to congenital malformations in general summarised the state of play with segmental analysis following the two articles discussed above. The segmental approach, with its shorthand notations, has changed little since this work was published.

- de la Cruz MV, Nadal-Ginard B: Rules for the diagnosis of visceral situs, truncoconal morphologies and ventricular inversions. Am Heart J 1972;84:19–32.

  This review summarised the thoughts of the Latin-American school headed by Maria Victoria de la Cruz, a splendid lady who based her concepts very much on her understanding of cardiac embryology. The system had much in common with the approach taken by Van Praagh and his colleagues, and was equally important in guiding further innovations.

- Van Praagh R, Ongley PA, Swan HJC: Anatomic types of single or common ventricle in man: Morphologic and geometric aspects of sixty necropsied cases. Am J Cardiol 1964;13:367–386.
- Van Praagh R, Van Praagh S, Vlad P, Keith JD: Anatomic types of congenital dextrocardia. Diagnostic and embryologic implications. Am J Cardiol 1964;13:510–531.

  These two seminal works were the first to suggest that a logical approach be adopted to so-called complex congenital cardiac malformations. Prior to these innovative publications, the complicated malformations had usually been grouped together in a miscellaneous category. These important investigations showed that the lesions were amenable to logical analysis.

- Shinebourne EA, Macartney FJ, Anderson RH: Sequential chamber localization: The logical approach to diagnosis in congenital heart disease. Br Heart J 1976;38:327–340.
- Tynan MJ, Becker AE, Macartney FJ, et al: Nomenclature and classification of congenital heart disease. Br Heart J 1979;41:544–553.

  These reviews represented the initial steps taken by the European school of nomenclaturists to refine the segmental approach to diagnosis. The Europeans shifted emphasis from the segments themselves, whilst still recognising the importance of segmental morphology, but pointing out at the same time the need to assess the way the components of the segments were joined together, or in some instances not joined together.

- Anderson RH, Becker AE, Freedom RM, et al: Sequential segmental analysis of congenital heart disease. Pediatr Cardiol 1984;5:281–288.
- Anderson RH, Becker AE, Tynan M, et al: The univentricular atrioventricular connection: Getting to the root of a thorny problem. Am J Cardiol 1984;54:822–882.

  In these two reviews, the European school, supported now also by the late Robert Freedom, recognised the wisdom of the morphological method. They pointed out that, in so-called hearts with single ventricles, or univentricular hearts, it was very rare for the ventricular mass to contain but one chamber. In fact, it was the atrioventricular connections that were univentricular in these settings. Since then, the European school has based its definitions exclusively on the morphological method, as explained at length in this chapter.

- Jacobs ML, Anderson RH: Nomenclature of the functionally univentricular heart. Cardiol Young 2006;16(Suppl 1):3–8.

  This review showed how, by the addition of a simple adverb, namely functionally, *it was possible to defuse all the multiple arguments that continued to surround so-called hearts with single ventricles. Most such hearts have one big and one small ventricle. The key point is that only the big ventricle is capable of supporting one or the other of the circulations, or in most instances both circulations. Hence, the arrangement, whilst not anatomically univentricular, is certainly functionally univentricular.*

- Van Praagh R, David I, Wright GB, Van Praagh S: Large RV plus small LV is not single LV. Circulation 1980;61:1057–1058.

  This crucial concept, stated in a letter to the Editor, identified a crucial flaw in the approach taken by the European school when analysing patients with alleged single ventricles, or univentricular hearts. The authors pointed out that it was philosophically unsound to base definitions of a given structure on one of its parts that was variable. Instead, they established the crucial principle of the morphological method, recommending that the structures be identified on the basis of their most constant components.

CHAPTER 2

Anatomy

ROBERT H. ANDERSON

It is axiomatic that, to understand abnormal anatomy and to describe it adequately, it is necessary to understand normal cardiac anatomy, including the relationships of the conduction tissues and coronary arteries to the various components of the heart. I review these features in this chapter. An appreciation of normal anatomy is the key to the understanding of the terms and concepts outlined in the previous chapter. The changes in these features of normality in congenitally malformed hearts will then be emphasised in the various chapters within the book concerned with specific lesions. At this stage, I place emphasis on the diagnostic features of the chambers that permit their recognition when the heart itself is congenitally malformed.

THE HEART WITHIN THE CHEST

My account begins with a description of the normal interrelationships of the chambers within the heart, and the location of the heart itself within the chest. The heart normally occupies the middle compartment of the mediastinum, with two-thirds of its bulk to the left of the midline (Fig. 2-1). The long axis shows a considerable obliquity relative to the long axis of the body, extending roughly along a line drawn through the right shoulder to the left hemidiaphragm. Despite this discrepancy between the planes of the body and those of the heart, the cardiac structures should still be described relative to the bodily coordinates, that is, in attitudinally appropriate orientation, although this basic rule of anatomy has not always been followed.[1] Usually described in terms of a triangle, the true shape of the heart as projecting to the frontal surface is more trapezoidal, with horizontal upper and lower borders, a more or less vertical right border just outside the edge of the sternum and a sloping left border extending out to the apex in the fifth intercostal space (Fig. 2-2). The most instructive single plane to be found within the heart is the so-called base.

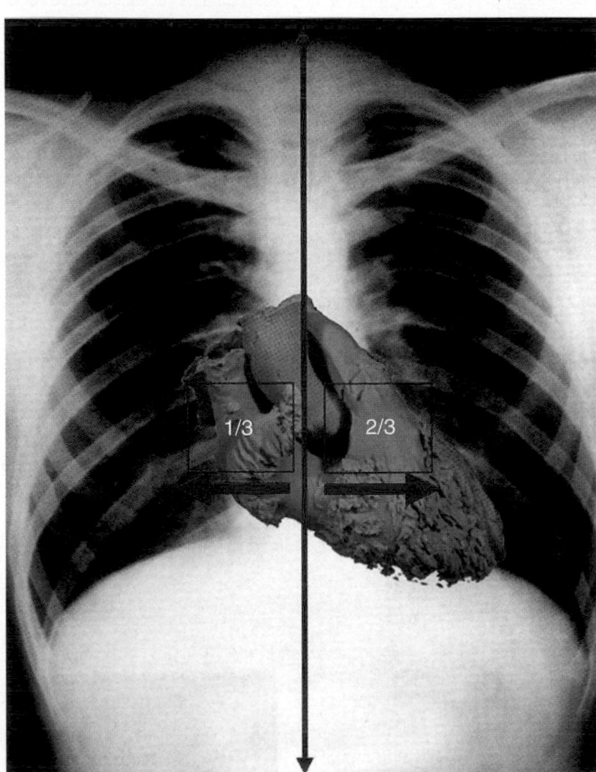

Figure 2-1 As shown by this cast of a normal heart superimposed on the frontal chest radiograph, the heart is a mediastinal structure with two-thirds of its bulk positioned to the left of the midline.

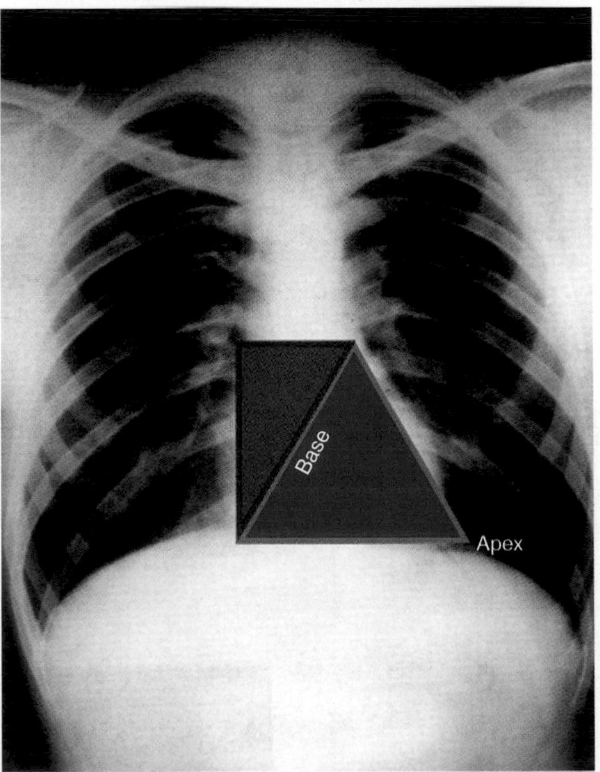

Figure 2-2 In considering the arrangement of the cardiac silhouette as seen in frontal projection as shown in Figure 2-1, it can best be likened to a trapezium, with a longer inferior border adjacent to the diaphragm. The trapezium itself can then be broken down into atrial (*red*) and ventricular (*blue*) triangles, with the ventricular triangle having its own base and apex, the latter corresponding with the cardiac apex.

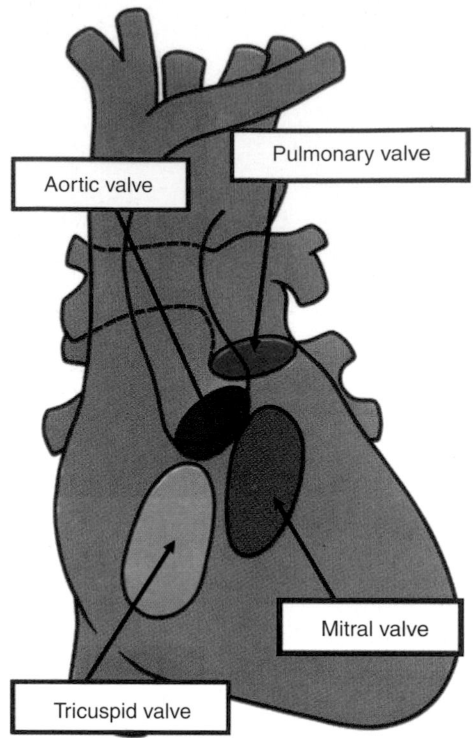

Figure 2-3 The positions of the valves are shown within the cardiac silhouette, as seen in the frontal projection.

In this respect, the term base is itself used in various ways. The true base of the heart is the posterior aspect of the atrial chambers relative to the mediastinum. More usually, the term is applied to the base of the ventricular mass. A section along the short axis across this ventricular base contains all four cardiac valves. When viewed in attitudinally appropriate fashion from the front, the pulmonary valve is seen to be located superiorly and to the left, with the aortic, mitral and tricuspid valves overlapping when traced in rightward and inferior direction (Fig. 2-3). Interrogation of the short-axis section from the atrial aspect emphasises the central location of the aortic valve, with its leaflets, and their supporting aortic sinuses, being related to all of the cardiac chambers (Fig. 2-4).

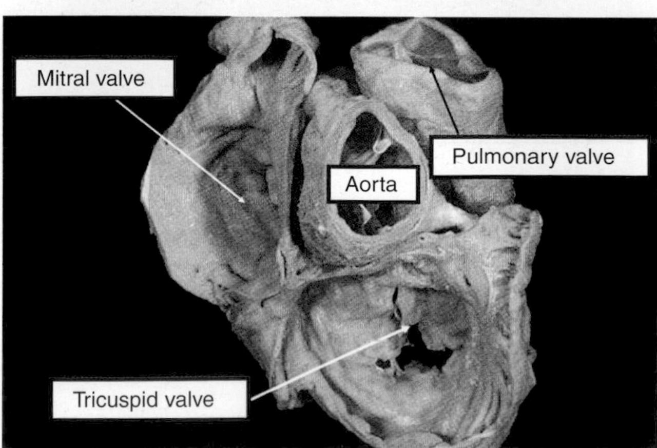

Figure 2-4 The dissection shows the short axis of the heart viewed from its atrial aspect, and illustrates the keystone location of the aortic valve relative to the other cardiac valves.

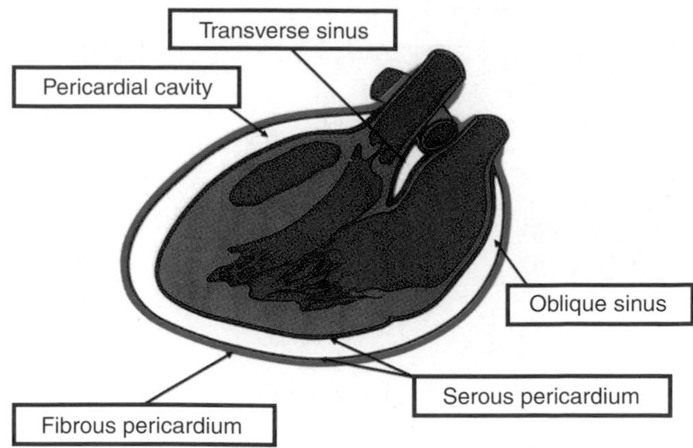

Figure 2-5 The cartoon shows the arrangement of the pericardium relative to the heart as seen in the parasternal long-axis echocardiographic cut. The transverse sinus within the pericardial cavity lines the inner curvature, while the oblique sinus is behind the left atrium.

In considering the location of the heart, note should be taken of the pericardium, and the major nerves that cross it. The fibrous pericardium can be likened to a cardiac seat belt, with its attachments to the diaphragm, along with the entrances and exits of the great veins and arterial trunks, anchoring the heart within the mediastinum. The tough fibrous pericardial sac is lined with a serous layer, the parietal pericardium, which is itself reflected onto the surface of the heart as the epicardium. Two important recesses are found within the cavity, namely the transverse and oblique sinuses (Fig. 2-5).

Coursing through the mediastinum, and embedded within the fibrous pericardium, are the vagus and phrenic nerves (Fig. 2-6). Both sets of nerves traverse the length of the heart on each side, with the phrenic nerves anterior and the vagus nerves posterior to the hilums of the lungs. Note should also be taken of the recurrent laryngeal nerves, which pass round the brachiocephalic trunk on the right side and the arterial duct, or its ligamentous remnant, on the left. The thymus gland is also a prominent structure related to the anterior and lateral aspects of the pericardial sac in the region of exit of the great arterial trunks,

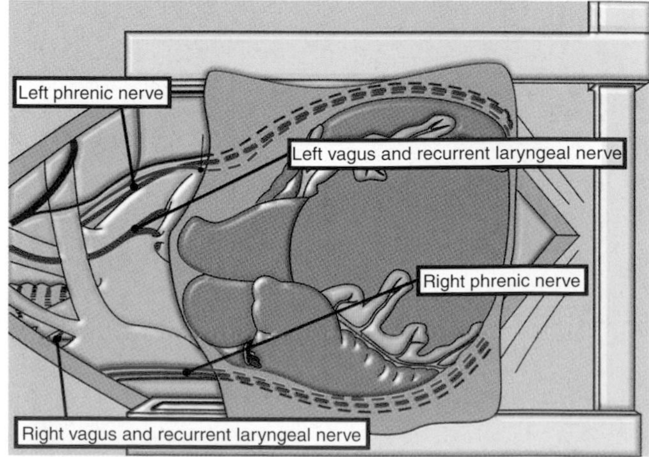

Figure 2-6 The heart is shown as seen by the surgeon through a median sternotomy. The locations of the vagus and phrenic nerves are shown relative to the opened pericardial sac.

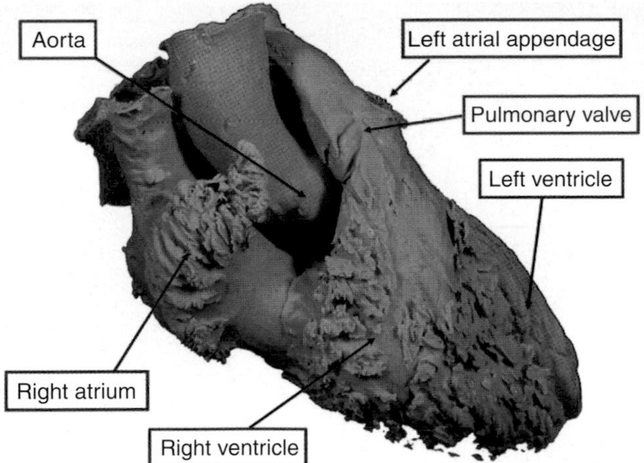

Figure 2-7 The cavities of the heart have been cast in red for the so-called right chambers, and blue for the left chambers. The casts are positioned in attitudinally correct orientation, and show that, in reality, the right chambers are positioned anterior to their supposedly left counterparts. The tip of the left atrial appendage is the only part of the left atrium that projects to the frontal silhouette, and only a small strip of left ventricle is seen when the cardiac contour is viewed in frontal projection.

particularly in neonates and infants, while the oesophagus is, perhaps, the most important mediastinal structure related directly to the heart.

The Chambers within the Heart

The key to full understanding of cardiac anatomy is the realisation that the heart is not arranged in the upright fashion of a Valentine heart.[1] Instead, the long axis of the heart extends from right to left with considerable obliquity. When seen in frontal projection, the anterior surface of the silhouette is occupied for the most part by the right atrium and ventricle. The left atrium is almost entirely a posterior structure, with only its appendage projecting to the left upper border, while only a strip of left ventricle is seen down the sloping left border. The so-called right chambers of the heart, therefore, are basically anterior, with the ventricles situated to the left and inferiorly relative to their atrial counterparts (Fig. 2-7). The aortic and mitral valves are closely related one to the other within the base of the left ventricle, while the pulmonary and tricuspid valves are separated in the roof of the right ventricle by the extensive supraventricular crest, known classically in its Latin form as the crista supraventricularis. The crest itself is intimately related on its posterior aspect to the aortic valve and root. The diaphragmatic border of the ventricular mass, made up of the right ventricle, exhibits a sharp angle between the sternocostal and inferior surfaces, known as the acute margin. In contrast, the left border of the ventricular mass, formed by the left ventricle, has a much gentler curve, and is the obtuse margin. Important grooves are found within the various surfaces, namely the atrioventricular, or coronary, grooves, which more or less mark the cardiac short axis, and the interventricular grooves, which indicate the long axis, and mark the location of the ventricular septum. A particularly important point is found on the diaphragmatic surface, positioned inferiorly rather than posteriorly when the heart is located within the body, where the interventricular groove joins the atrioventricular groove. This is the so-called cardiac crux.

The Morphologically Right Atrium

The right atrium in the normal heart is recognised most readily as the chamber receiving the systemic venous return through the superior and inferior caval veins, along with the venous return from the heart itself through the coronary sinus. These channels open into the smooth-walled venous component of the atrium. In addition, the atrial chamber possesses a smooth-walled area that we described as the vestibule. This layer of muscle inserts into the leaflets of the tricuspid valve. The atrium also has a characteristic septal surface, and the extensive and trabeculated appendage (Fig. 2-8). It is the appendage that is the most constant part. This feature, therefore, should be used to permit recognition of the chamber as the morphologically right structure in congenitally malformed hearts. Recognition of structures according to their morphology rather than their location, and using their most constant part in final arbitration, is called the morphological method.[2] As I discussed in the previous chapter, this principle is the basis of logical analysis of congenitally malformed hearts.[3]

The characteristic external feature of the right appendage is its broad triangular shape (Fig. 2-9), along with its extensive junction with the smooth-walled venous component, this being marked by the terminal groove. Internally, the groove matches with the strap-like terminal crest (Fig. 2-10). Taking origin in parallel fashion from the crest and extending laterally into the appendage are the pectinate muscles. In the morphologically right atrium, these muscles extend all round the atrioventricular junction, reaching into the diverticulum located inferior to the orifice of the coronary sinus (Fig. 2-11). Although often considered to be sub-Eustachian, this diverticulum, also described as a sinus, is sub-Thebesian when the heart is seen in attitudinally appropriate position (see Fig. 2-11). The extent of the pectinate muscles relative to the vestibule of the right atrioventricular valve is the single most characteristic feature of the right atrium in congenitally malformed hearts.[4] In many hearts, flap-like muscular or fibrous valves take origin from the extent of the terminal crest and guard the orifices of the inferior caval vein and

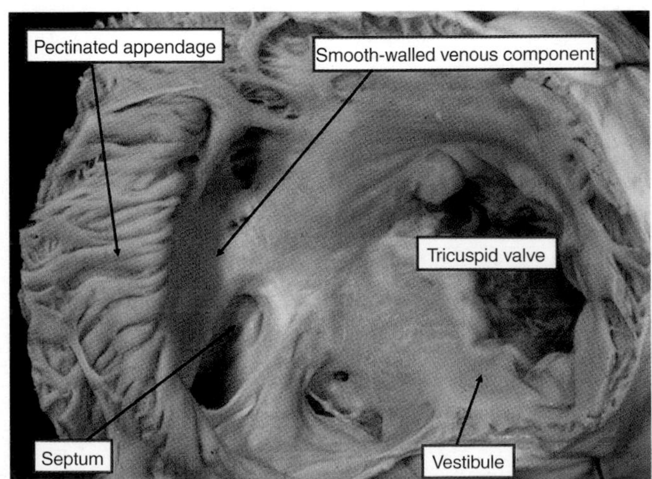

Figure 2-8 The morphologically right atrium has been opened by a cut through its appendage parallel to the right atrioventricular junction, and the wall of the appendage reflected upwards, revealing that the atrium, in addition to its appendage, possesses a vestibule along with the systemic venous sinus, and is separated by the septum from the left atrium.

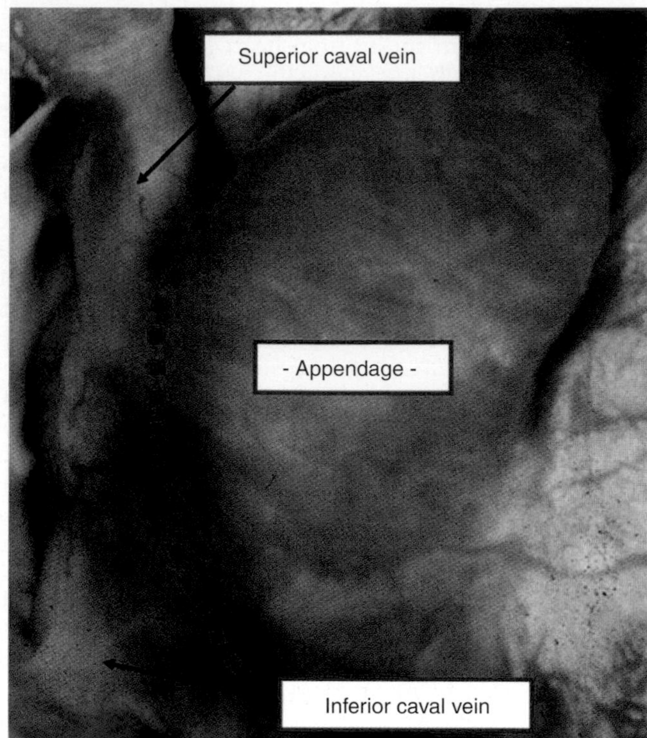

Figure 2-9 The characteristic external feature of the morphologically right atrium is the triangular shape of its appendage, with the terminal groove (*red dotted line*) separating the appendage from the termination of the systemic venous tributaries in the systemic venous sinus.

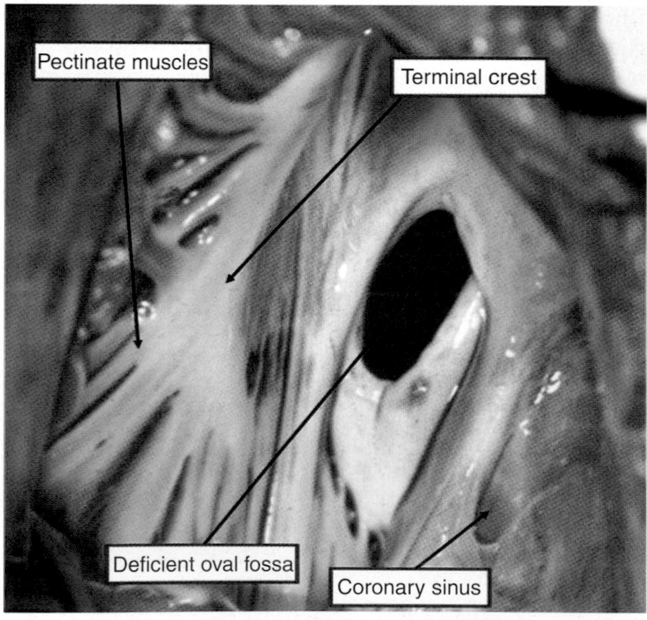

Figure 2-10 This view of the interior of the morphologically right atrium, shown in attitudinally appropriate orientation, is taken in the operating room from a patient with a septal defect in the floor of the oval fossa. It shows the extensive terminal crest giving rise to the pectinate muscles. (Courtesy of Dr. Benson R. Wilcox, University of North Carolina, Chapel Hill.)

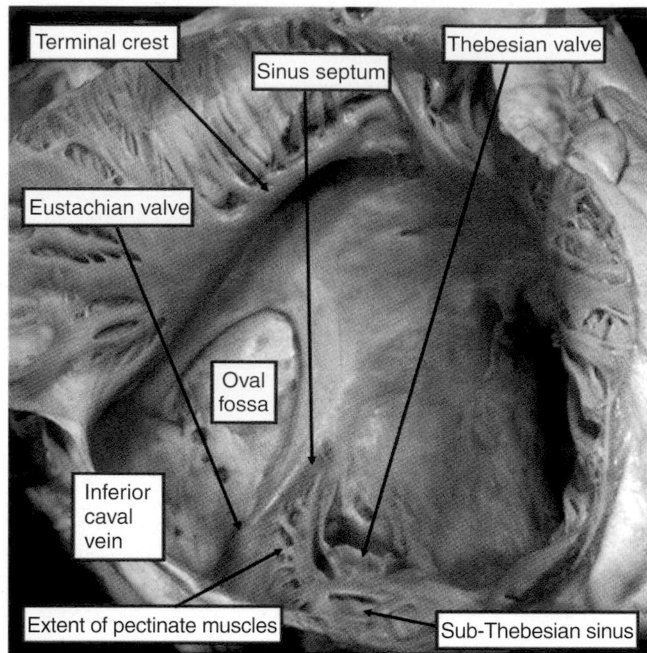

Figure 2-11 This view of the interior of the morphologically right atrium, made possible as in Figure 2-8 by making an extensive cut parallel to the atrioventricular junction, and reflecting the wall of the appendage superiorly, shows the location of the so-called venous valves, and the position of the sinus septum.

the coronary sinus. These are the Eustachian and Thebesian valves, respectively (see Fig. 2-11). The valves, however, are not uniformly present. An important structure in continuation with the Eustachian valve, nonetheless, can almost always be found. This is the tendon of Todaro,[5] which runs through the wall that separates the coronary sinus from the oval fossa, the so-called sinus septum, to insert into the fibrous root of the aorta. This tendon forms one of the borders of the triangle of Koch (see below).

At first sight, the septal surface of the right atrium is extensive, surrounding the oval fossa and incorporating the orifices of the superior caval vein and coronary sinus (see Figs. 2-8 and 2-11). This appearance is deceptive. Only the floor of the oval fossa, along with its antero-inferior rim, is made up of tissues that separate the cavities of the two atriums. The apparently extensive rims of the oval fossa, also described as the septum secundum, or the secondary septum, are largely the infolded walls of the atrial chambers.[6] This infolding is particularly prominent superiorly, where it forms the extensive fold between the superior caval and right pulmonary veins (Fig. 2-12). This superior interatrial fold is also known as Waterston's, or Sondergaard's, groove. Part of the extensive antero-inferior margin of the oval fossa is unequivocally a septal structure. This is the part formed by muscularisation of the atrial or vestibular spine, also known as the dorsal mesenchymal protrusion. The development of this part of the atrium is discussed extensively, and illustrated, in our chapter devoted to embryology (Chapter 3). Another part is an atrioventricular muscular sandwich, existing because of the more apical attachment of the leaflet of the tricuspid relative to the mitral valve (see below). In this area, an extension of the inferior atrioventricular groove separates the overlapping segments of atrial and ventricular muscle. This area is confluent with the so-called sinus septum, separating the orifices of the coronary sinus and the inferior caval vein (see Fig. 2-11). The sinus septum is no more than the adjacent walls of the two venous structures.

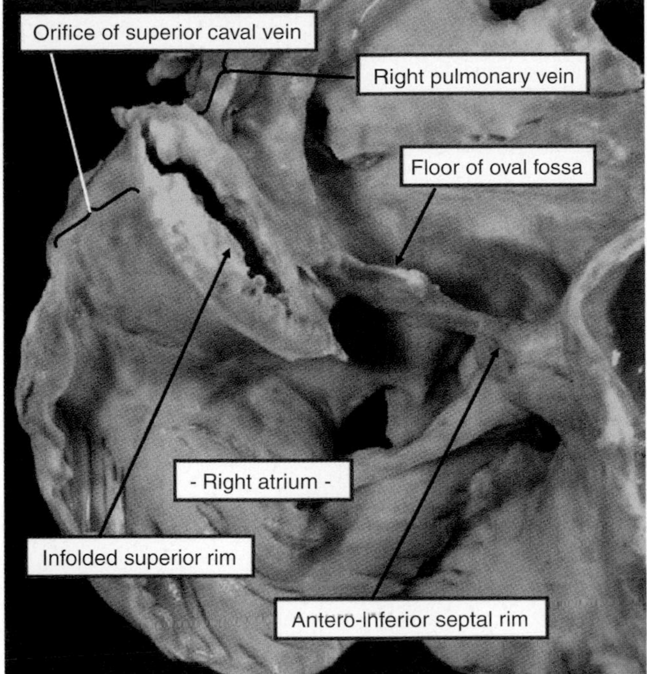

Figure 2-12 This section through the atrial chambers in four-chamber plane shows how the superior rim of the oval fossa, the so-called septum secundum, is simply the infolded walls between the origins of the superior caval vein from the right, and the right pulmonary veins from the left atriums, respectively. Note that the floor of the oval fossa, along with its antero-inferior rim, is a true septal structure interposing between the atrial cavities.

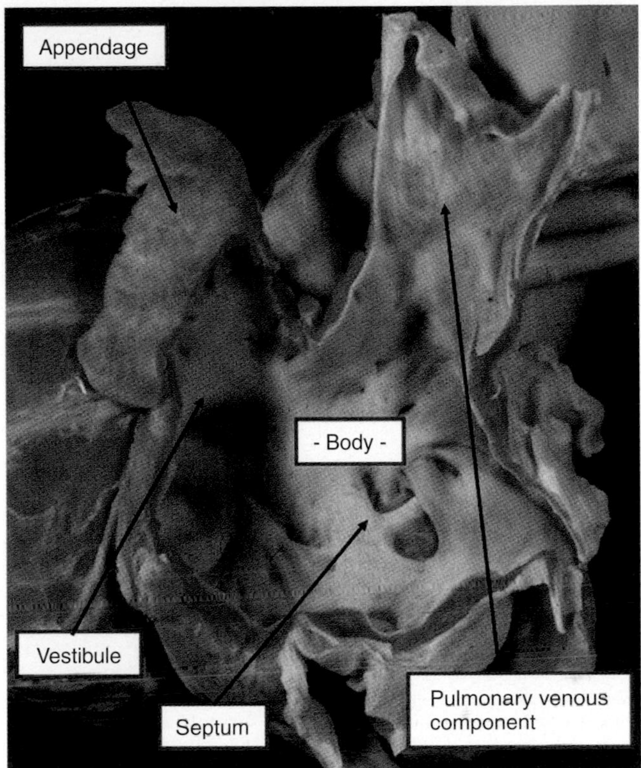

Figure 2-13 As with the right atrium, the morphologically left atrium is made up of an appendage, a venous component, a vestibule and a septal surface. In addition, the left atrium possesses an obvious body, joining together the other parts.

The Morphologically Left Atrium

The left atrium, like its right-sided counterpart, possesses a venous component, an appendage, and a vestibule (Fig. 2-13). Again, in keeping with its morphologically right partner, the morphologically left appendage is the most characteristic and constant component. It is a long tubular structure, usually with several constrictions along its length. Its opening with the venous component is restricted, but its most characteristic feature in malformed hearts is that its pectinate muscles are contained within the appendage, or else they spill only marginally onto the septal surface and the anterior part of the wall we described as the vestibule. The vestibule surrounding the posterior part of the atrioventricular groove, therefore, is smooth. The coronary sinus is located within the atrioventricular groove, and hence is an integral component of the morphologically left atrioventricular junction, even though it opens into the cavity of the morphologically right atrium (Fig. 2-14). Its walls are separate from those of the left atrium itself.[7] The pulmonary veins open into the corners of the extensive smooth-walled venous component. The septal surface is formed by the flap valve of the oval fossa, which has a characteristically roughened appearance where it overlaps the infolded superior rim (Fig. 2-15). In addition to these parts, the left atrium also possesses a significant body. The evidence for the existence of the body is seen in the setting of totally anomalous pulmonary venous connection. Even when the pulmonary venous component is lacking, there is part of the left atrial chamber that forms a site of union for the appendage, vestibule and septum. This is the body.

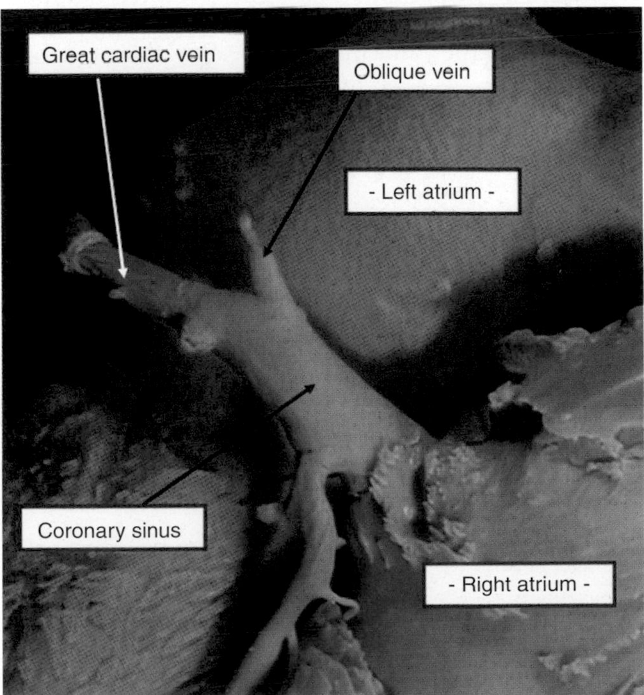

Figure 2-14 This cast of the right and left sides of the heart is photographed to show the diaphragmatic surface. The coronary sinus, formed by the union of the great cardiac and oblique veins, is an integral part of the morphologically left atrioventricular junction, but opens into the cavity of the right atrium.

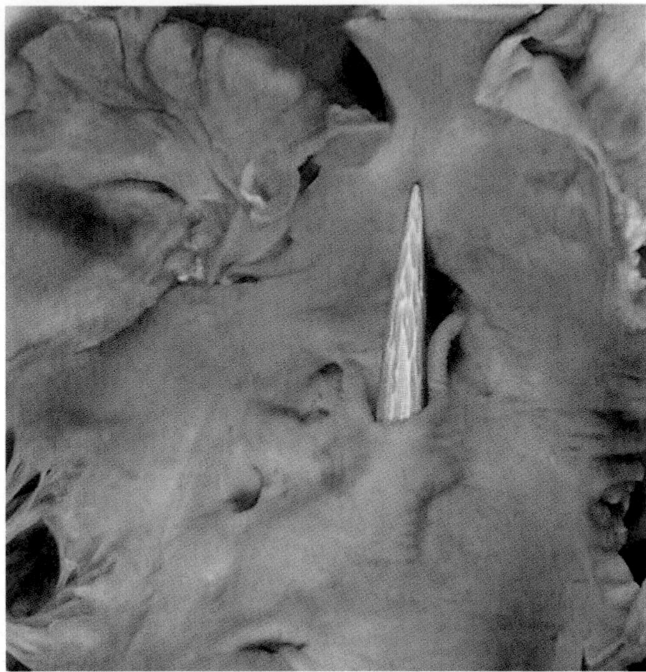

Figure 2-15 In this heart, photographed to show the septal surface of the left atrium, the oval foramen was probe-patent, as shown by the probe placed between the flap valve of the septum and the infolded superior rim.

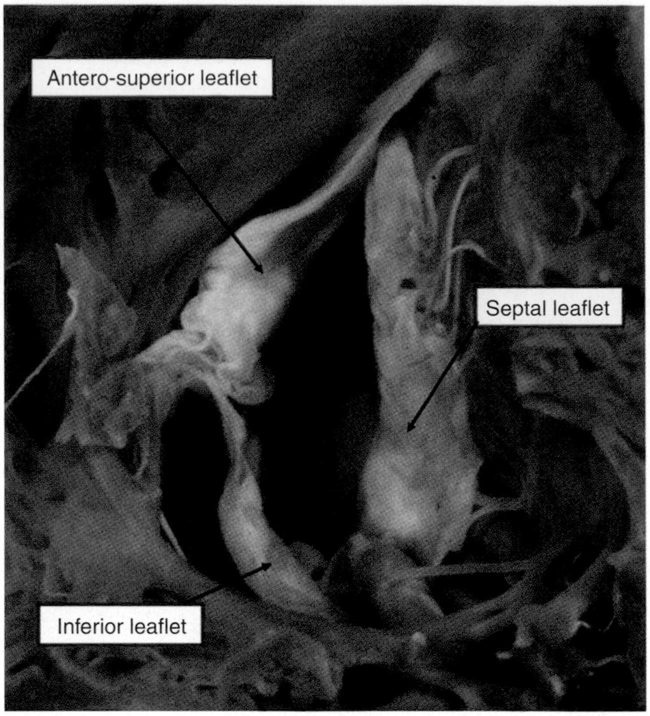

Figure 2-17 As seen from their ventricular aspect, the leaflets of the tricuspid valve occupy anterosuperior, inferior and septal positions.

The Morphologically Right Ventricle

The muscular walls of the right ventricle extend from the discrete atrioventricular junction to their union with the fibroelastic walls of the pulmonary trunk at the anatomical ventriculo-arterial junction. Within the cavity thus demarcated, there are three components, the inlet, the apical trabecular and the outlet parts (Fig. 2-16). The inlet component contains and supports the leaflets of the tricuspid valve, extending to the attachments of the valvar tension apparatus. The three leaflets of the valve take origin from the septal, inferior or mural, and anterosuperior margins of the atrioventricular junction (Fig. 2-17). The septal leaflet has multiple cordal attachments to the septum. The inferior leaflet runs along the diaphragmatic surface of the ventricle, and its margin with the anterosuperior leaflet is often indistinct. When examined in terms of its pattern of closure, however, there is no doubt about its existence as a third valvar leaflet.[8] The anterosuperior leaflet is the most extensive of the three, and extends from its zone of apposition with the septal leaflet, an area supported by the medial papillary muscle, to the acute margin of the ventricle. A characteristic anterior papillary muscle arises from the prominent apical trabeculation (see below) to support this leaflet, but not always at its site of apposition with the inferior leaflet.

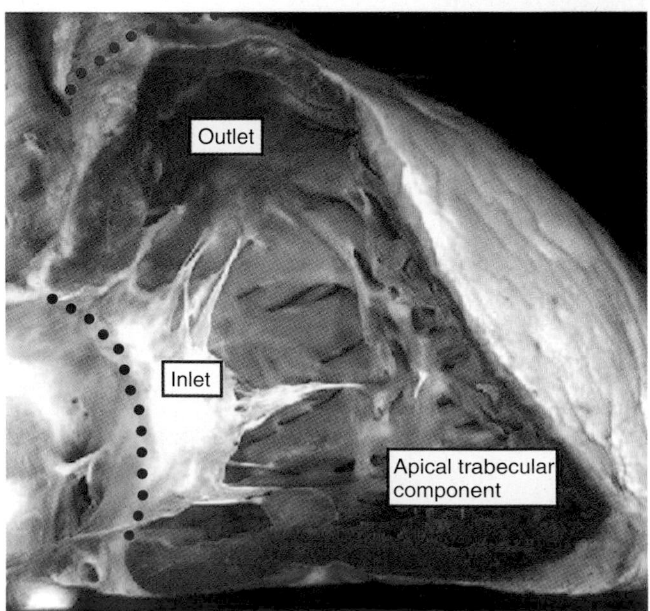

Figure 2-16 The parietal wall of the morphologically right ventricle has been cut away, showing how the ventricular myocardium extends from the atrioventricular (*blue dotted line*) to the ventriculo-arterial junction (*green dotted line*). The ventricle itself has inlet, apical trabecular, and outlet components.

The apical trabecular part of the ventricle has particularly coarse trabeculations, this being the most constant feature of the ventricle in malformed hearts. One of these trabeculations on the septal surface is particularly prominent, diverging into two limbs at the base to clasp the supraventricular crest. This is the septomarginal trabeculation, or septal band (Fig. 2-18). The medial papillary muscle arises from the posterior limb of this trabeculation, while the anterior papillary muscle springs from the body towards the ventricular apex. The moderator band continues on from the papillary muscle as a discrete muscular bundle, extending to the parietal ventricular wall. A further series of trabeculations extend from the anterior surface of the septomarginal trabeculation and run into the parietal margin of the trabecular zone. These are the septoparietal trabeculations (Fig. 2-19).

The outlet component of the ventricle is relatively smooth walled. It forms the free-standing sleeve of musculature (Fig. 2-20) that supports the leaflets of the pulmonary valve.

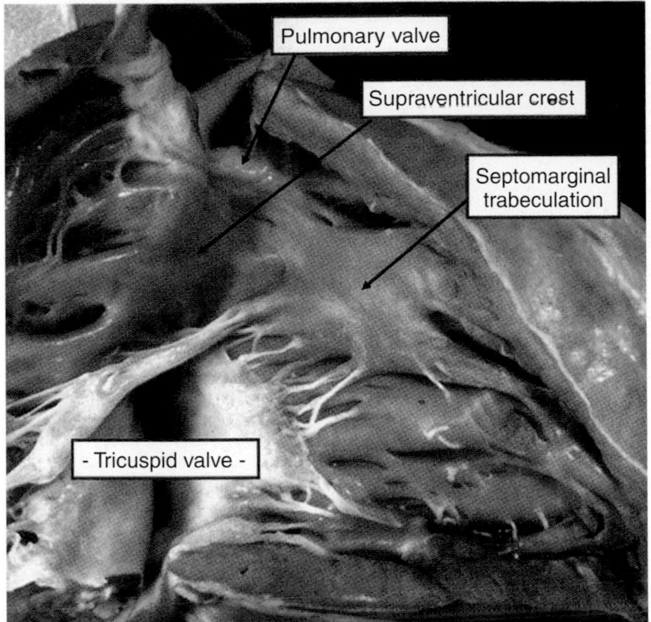

Figure 2-18 Opening the right ventricle reveals its muscular roof, the supraventricular crest, which separates the leaflets of the tricuspid and pulmonary valves. The crest inserts to the septum between the limbs of a prominent muscular landmark, the septomarginal trabeculation, or septal band.

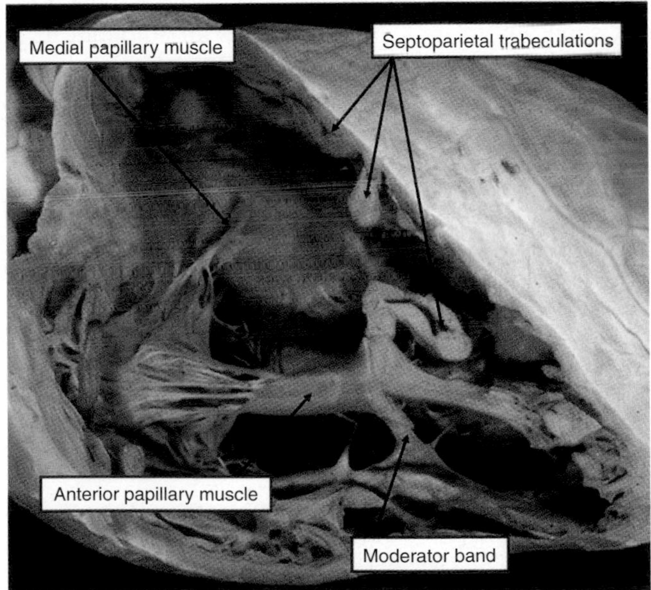

Figure 2-19 A series of further muscular structures, the septoparietal trabeculations, arise from the anterior margin of the septomarginal trabeculation, and extend to the parietal wall of the right ventricle. One of these, also extending from the anterior papillary muscle, is the moderator band.

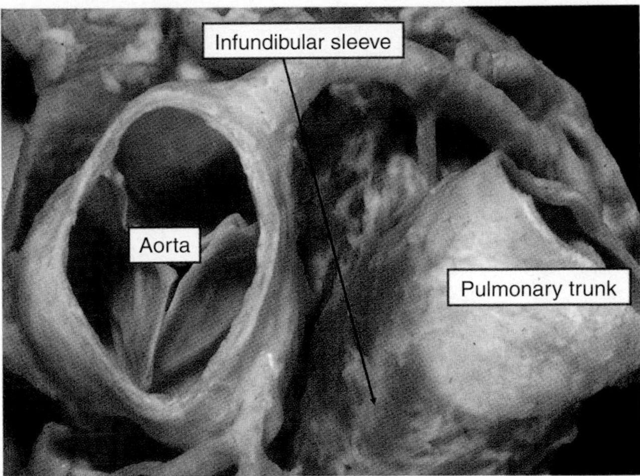

Figure 2-20 The pulmonary trunk has been reflected forward relative to the aorta, showing the extensive sleeve of infundibular musculature that lifts the trunk away from the base of the ventricular mass.

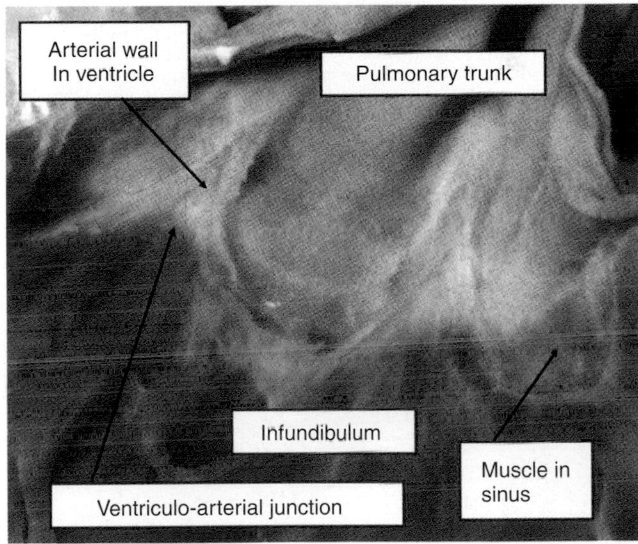

Figure 2-21 The pulmonary trunk has been opened, and the valvar leaflets removed from their attachments, revealing the semilunar nature of these attachments. The attachment of each semilunar leaflet crosses the anatomical ventriculo-arterial junction, so that crescents of infundibular musculature are incorporated into the base of each valvar sinus, and triangles of arterial wall are incorporated into the ventricular outflow tract, extending to the level of the sinutubular junction.

The leaflets of the valve themselves are attached in semilunar fashion within the sleeve, crossing the circular junction between ventricular muscle and the fibroelastic wall of the pulmonary trunk (Fig. 2-21). Because of this arrangement, three crescents of ventricular musculature are incorporated within the bases of the sinuses of the pulmonary trunk, while three triangular areas of pulmonary trunk are incorporated within the ventricular outflow tract beneath the tips of the zones of apposition between the valvar leaflets.[8] As a result, the valvar leaflets do not possess an annulus in the sense of a fibrous ring supporting their attachments in circular fashion. Indeed, the most obvious circles within the outflow tract are either the anatomical ventriculo-arterial junction, or else the junction between the valvar sinuses and the tubular pulmonary trunk, the latter best described as the sinutubular junction, and an integral part of the valvar mechanism. There is then another ring that can be constructed by joining together the most proximal parts of the three semilunar leaflets, but this is a virtual structure, with no counterpart (Fig. 2-22). Part of the free-standing subpulmonary infundibular sleeve interposes between the leaflets of the pulmonary and tricuspid valves. This is the supraventricular crest (see Fig. 2-18). It is often illustrated as representing a septal structure. In reality, as can be shown by removing the wall (Fig. 2-23), it is largely made up from the inner curvature of the right ventricular musculature. We describe this

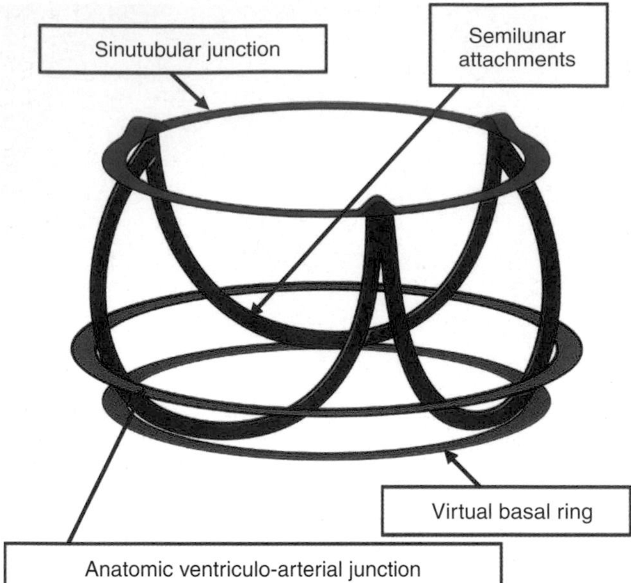

Figure 2-22 The cartoon represents the anatomy as depicted in Figure 2-21. The true rings, or annuluses, are the line over which the walls of the pulmonary trunk join the muscular infundibulum, or the anatomical ventriculo-arterial junction, depicted in *yellow*, and the sinutubular junction, shown in *blue*. A third ring can be constructed by joining together the basal attachments of the valvar leaflets, as shown in *yellow*. The *red lines* show the semilunar attachments of the valvar leaflets.

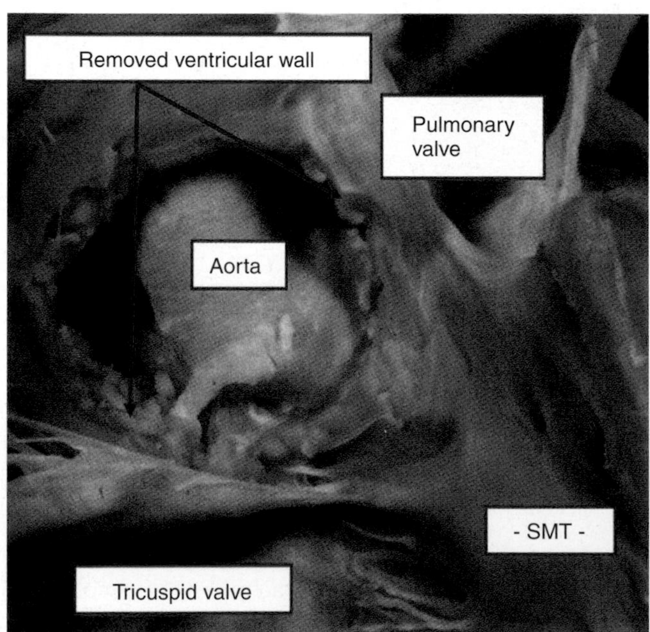

Figure 2-23 The dissection shows that the greater part of the supraventricular crest is made up of the parietal ventricular wall. As can be seen, removing this wall reveals the sinuses of the aorta.

area as the ventriculo-infundibular fold. It is also the case that a small part of the musculature between the limbs of the septomarginal trabeculation can be removed to provide access to the left ventricle, this small part truly representing a muscular outlet septum (Fig. 2-24). The outlet part, however, cannot be distinguished in normal hearts from the remainder of the muscular ventricular septum. The key feature of the infundibular area, therefore, is the sleeve of free-standing musculature that supports the leaflets of the

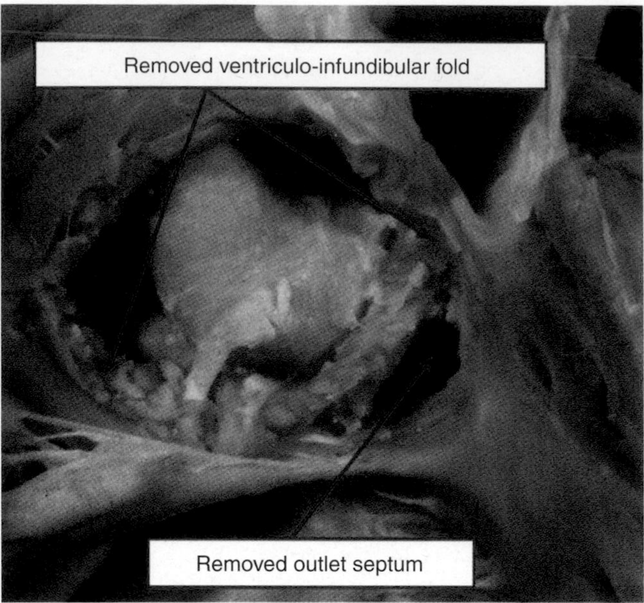

Figure 2-24 The dissection shown in Figure 2-23 has been continued, showing that it is possible to remove a very small part of the septum, immediately between the limbs of the septomarginal trabeculation, so as to gain access to the left ventricle. This small part, representing a true muscular outlet septum, cannot be distinguished from the remainder of the septum without the aid of dissection.

pulmonary valve, the presence of this sleeve making it possible surgically to remove the valve as an autograft in the Ross procedure.[8–10]

The Morphologically Left Ventricle

The inlet, apical trabecular and outlet components of the left ventricle (Fig. 2-25) are as distinct as their counterparts within the right ventricle, and each shows significant features permitting its recognition. The inlet component surrounds and supports the leaflets of the mitral valve and its paired papillary muscles. The components of the valve are best distinguished in closed rather than open position. When the valve is viewed with the leaflets adjacent to one another, the

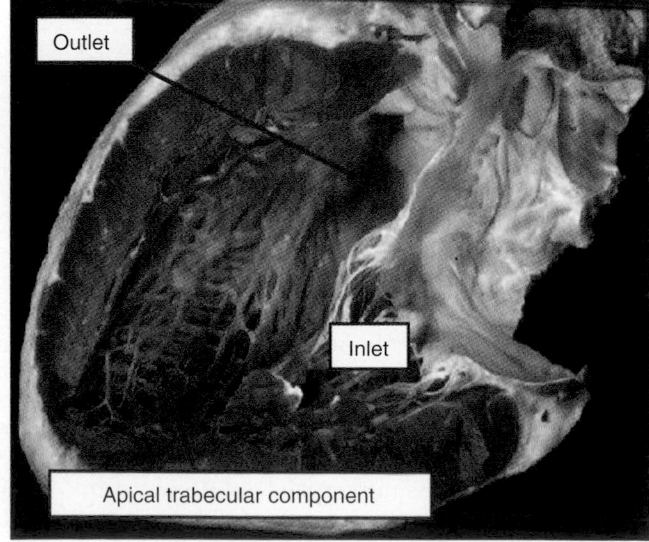

Figure 2-25 As with the morphologically right ventricle (see Fig. 2-15), the morphologically left ventricle can readily be described in terms of its inlet, apical trabecular and outlet components.

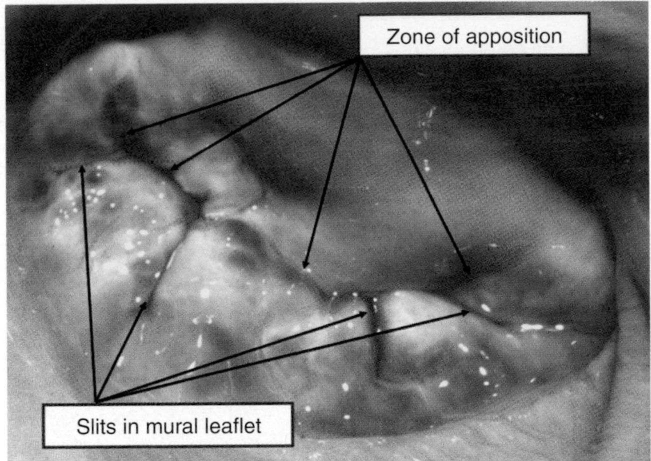

Figure 2-26 When viewed in its closed position, it can be seen that a solitary concave zone of apposition separates the leaflets of the mitral valve. The zone of apposition does not reach to the annular attachments of the leaflets. Note the slits in the mural leaflet, necessary to permit the two leaflets to close snugly.

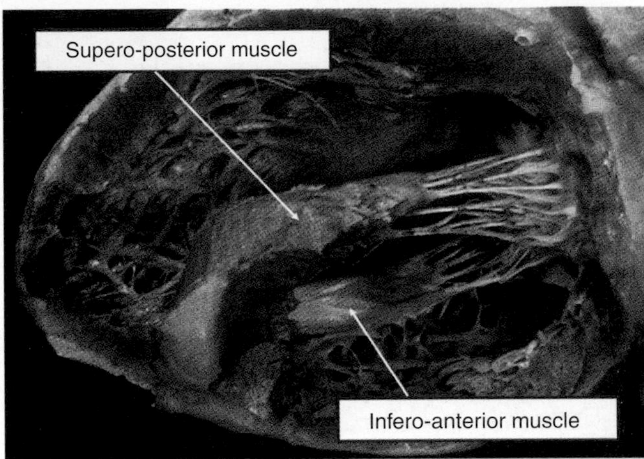

Figure 2-27 The posterior wall of the left ventricle has been removed, and the heart is photographed from behind. The dissection reveals the relations of the two papillary muscles of the mitral valve, which are positioned supero-posteriorly and infero-anteriorly.

solitary line of apposition is readily apparent (Fig. 2-26). In terms of valvar function, this zone of apposition represents the commissure between the leaflets. The mitral valve would best be described, therefore, as having one commissure. Almost always, however, the valve is illustrated in open position, and then it is the ends of the zone of apposition that are usually interpreted as the paired commissures, and typically described as being postero-medial and antero-lateral. This convention introduces major complications. Those who analyze the valve in open, rather than closed, position point to the characteristic fan-shaped pattern of branching of the tendinous cords at the ends of the zone of apposition.[11] With the passage of time, these fan-shaped structures have, by convention, become recognised as commissural cords. Similar fan-shaped ramifications, nonetheless, are found supporting the slits in the extensive mural leaflet of the valve, particularly between those well-formed components that are often identified as the scallops. Because of the resemblance of these areas to the ends of the major zone of apposition, some suggest that the valve is better viewed as possessing four leaflets.[12] The valvar architecture, however, is not sufficiently constant to support this notion, which is avoided when the leaflets of the valves are assessed in terms of their closed position. The valvar leaflets can then simply be recognised on the basis of the obvious solitary zone of apposition between them. Such inspection shows that the mural, or posterior, leaflet is a lengthy, albeit shallow, structure that guards two-thirds of the overall valvar circumference, with several slits along its length, which permit it to fit snugly against the other aortic or anterior leaflet.[13] The major feature of this other leaflet is its fibrous continuity, on its ventricular aspect, with parts of the left coronary and non-coronary leaflets of the aortic valve, hence our preferred title of the aortic leaflet. It is much deeper than the mural leaflet, but guards only one-third of the valvar circumference. The tendinous cords from the leaflets insert mostly to the paired papillary muscles, which are seated adjacent to one another on the parietal wall of the ventricle. When viewed in attitudinally appropriate position, however, they are located supero-anteriorly and infero-posteriorly (Fig. 2-27), rather than postero-medially and antero-laterally.[14] The latter descriptions hold good only when the heart is removed from the body and positioned on its apex. The oft-illustrated spread position of the leaflets is also artefactual, reflecting the way in which the ventricle has been opened.

Many anatomists have used complex systems to describe the tendinous cords that support the leaflets of the atrioventricular valves. Such categorisation is not very helpful. Suffice it to say that, in the normal heart, cords arise uniformly along the free leading edge of all the valvar leaflets, and extend to insert into the supporting papillary muscles. Each papillary muscle supports the adjacent parts of two leaflets. These cords providing uniform support to the free edges of the leaflets are then reinforced by the prominent strut cords found on the ventricular aspect of the aortic leaflet, and by basal cords that run from the undersurface of the mural leaflet to insert directly into the myocardium. Unlike the tricuspid valve, the mitral valve has no cords inserting directly into the ventricular septum. Instead, the deep subaortic outflow tract separates the aortic leaflet of the valve from the smooth septal surface of the left ventricle (Fig. 2-28).

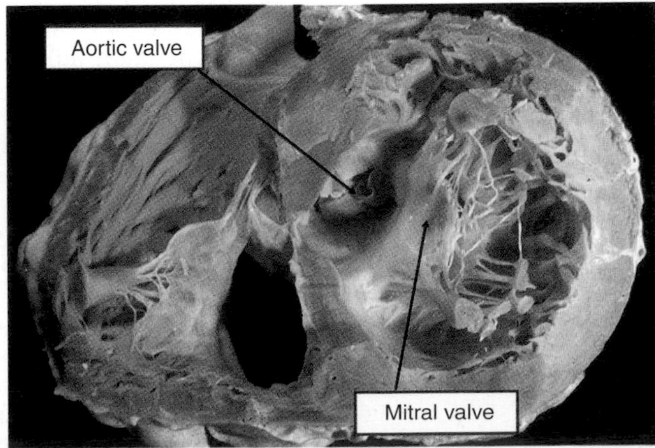

Figure 2-28 The short axis of the ventricular mass is shown as seen from the apex. Note the extensive diverticulum created by the subaortic outflow tract, which separates the mitral valve from the septum. Note also that, unlike the tricuspid valve, the leaflets of the mitral valve, best described as aortic and mural, have no direct cordal attachments to the septum.

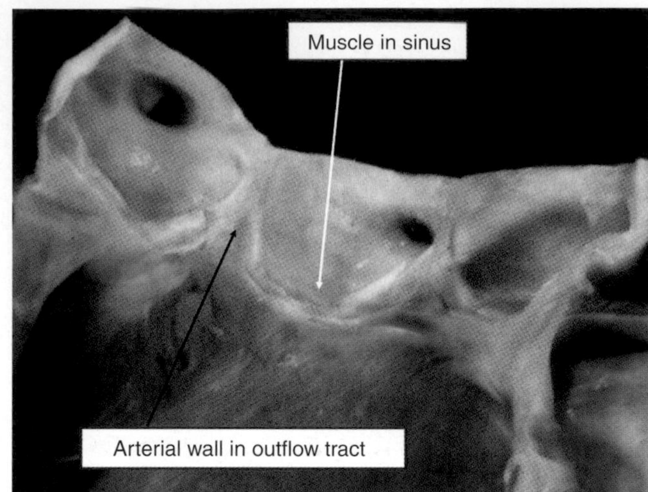

Figure 2-29 The aorta has been opened through the area of aortic-to-mitral valvar continuity, and is viewed from behind, the leaflets of the valve having been removed. Note that, as with the pulmonary valve (see Fig. 2-21), the leaflets are attached within the aortic root in semilunar fashion, so that fibrous triangles of aortic wall are incorporated within the ventricular outflow tract, and segments of ventricular musculature within the bases of the two coronary arterial sinuses.

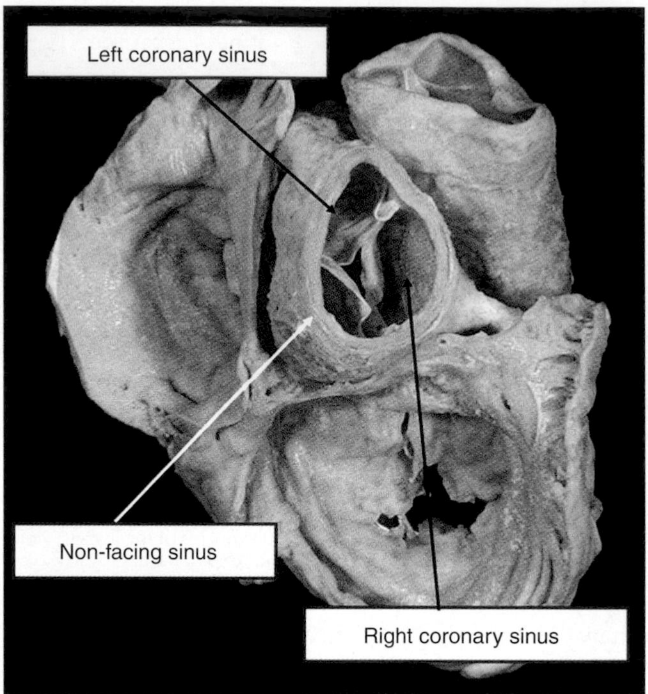

Figure 2-30 This dissection of the short axis of the heart, shown from its atrial aspect, shows how the coronary sinuses, and the leaflets of the aortic valve, can be described as right coronary, left coronary and non-facing. In almost all instances the non-facing sinus does not give rise to a coronary artery, so it can also be described as the non-coronary sinus.

The trabecular component of the left ventricle extends beyond the papillary muscles of the mitral valve, reaching to the relatively thin apical point. The trabeculations themselves are significantly finer than those of the right ventricle, and criss-cross in characteristic fashion (see Fig. 2-25). Strands often cross the cavity of the ventricle, particularly from the papillary muscles, in the fashion of telephone wires. They are of no functional significance. The surface of the septal aspect of the trabecular component is smooth, with no evidence of any structure comparable to the septomarginal trabeculation of the right ventricle. The left bundle branch descends from the crest of the muscular ventricular septum and fans out in this area.

The outlet component is significantly abbreviated in comparison to its right ventricular counterpart, with the leaflets of the aortic valve supported by musculature only around the anterior quadrants of the outflow tract (see Fig. 2-28). Posteriorly, two of the leaflets of the aortic valve are in fibrous continuity with the deep aortic leaflet of the mitral valve. Despite this difference in terms of support, the overall semilunar structure of the aortic valve is comparable to that of the pulmonary valve (Fig. 2-29). As in the right ventricle (see Fig. 2-22), the semilunar attachments incorporate crescents of ventricle within the bases of the three aortic sinuses of Valsalva, while three triangles of arterial wall are incorporated within the outflow tract beneath the apices of the zones of apposition between the valvar leaflets.

The location of these three fibrous triangles separating the zones of apposition of the leaflets helps in understanding the relationships of the aortic valve.[15] The leaflets of the valve itself are named according to the origin of the coronary arteries from the aortic sinuses. Thus, the sinuses, and the leaflets they support, can be distinguished as being left coronary, right coronary, and non-facing. Non-facing is preferable to non-coronary (Fig. 2-30) because, very rarely, the so-called non-coronary sinus can give origin to a coronary artery. In such a setting, the non-coronary title would obviously become nonsensical. Non-facing is also a good term because, without exception, and irrespective of the relationships of the arterial trunks, two of the aortic sinuses face, or are adjacent to, corresponding sinuses of the pulmonary trunk. This permits the sinuses of the pulmonary trunk similarly to be distinguished as right-facing, left-facing, and non-facing, or non-adjacent.

The fibrous triangle that separates the left coronary leaflet from the non-facing leaflet of the aortic valve separates the left ventricular outflow tract from the transverse sinus of the pericardium, forming the wall between the back of the aorta and the anterior interatrial groove (Fig. 2-31). The triangle separating the right coronary aortic leaflet from the non-coronary leaflet is directly continuous with the membranous septum. When the triangle is removed, it can be seen to separate the left ventricular outflow tract from the transverse sinus above the inner curvature of the right ventricle, specifically with the pericardial space above the supraventricular crest (Fig. 2-32). The triangle which separates the two coronary leaflets of the aortic valve separates the cavity of the left ventricle from the tissue interposing between the anterior surface of the aorta and the posterior surface of the free-standing subpulmonary infundibulum (Fig. 2-33).

The Arterial Trunks

The two great arteries leave the base of the heart at the ventriculo-arterial junctions, extending superiorly into the mediastinum, with the pulmonary trunk spiralling around the centrally located aorta as it bifurcates. Its branches then extend to the hilums of the lungs. Each arterial trunk shows a characteristic cloverleaf shape at its root, with the truncal sinuses interdigitating with the supporting ventricular structures as they support the arterial valvar leaflets in semilunar fashion (Fig. 2-34). There is then a characteristic ring-like

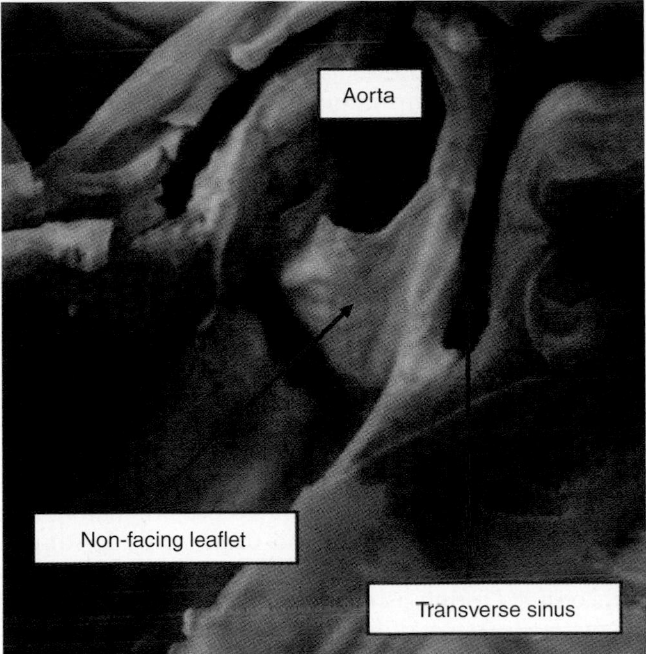

Figure 2-31 The aortic root has been opened by a cut made between the non-facing and left coronary aortic sinuses. The cut transects the fibrous interleaflet triangle, showing how this area interposes between the left ventricular outflow tract and the transverse sinus of the pericardium.

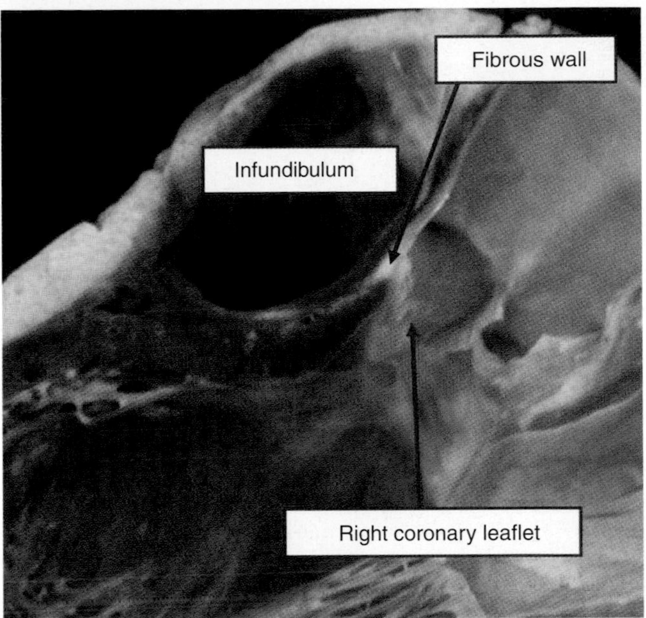

Figure 2-33 This long-axis section, paralleling the parasternal long-axis echocardiographic plane, is made between the two arterial sinuses of the aortic valve. It shows how the fibrous interleaflet triangle between these sinuses separates the left ventricular outflow tract from the fibrofatty tissue plane between the aortic wall and the free-standing subpulmonary muscular infundibulum.

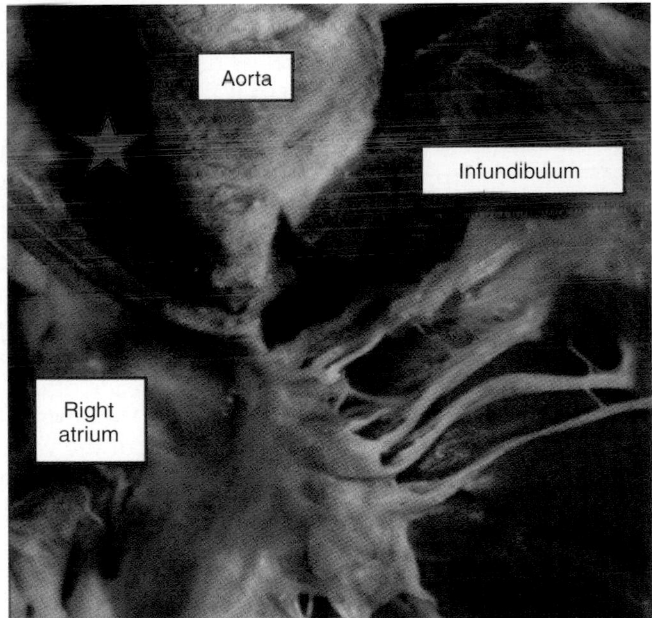

Figure 2-32 The heart is shown from the right side, the interleaflet triangle between the non-facing and right coronary aortic sinuses having been removed. Note how the top of the triangle separates the left ventricular outflow tract from the transverse sinus of the pericardium (*yellow star*), which lines the epicardial aspect of the supraventricular crest.

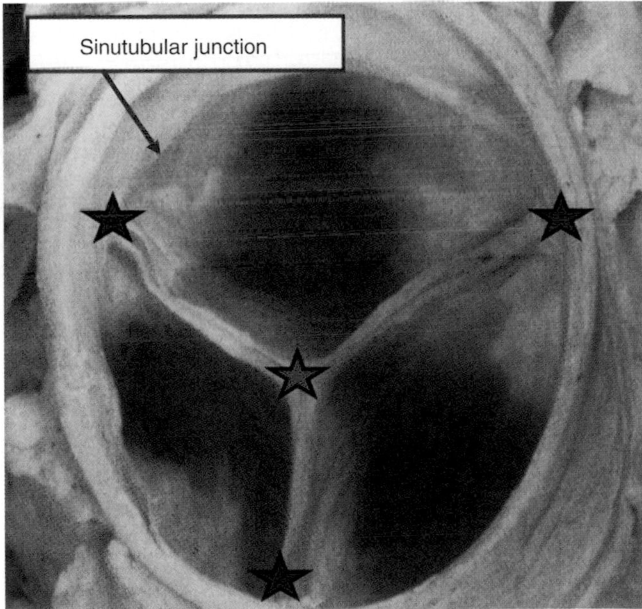

Figure 2-34 The aortic root is viewed from above, having transected the aorta. Note how the zones of apposition between the leaflets of the aortic valve close snugly along lines from the centre of the valvar orifice (*red stars*) to the attachments at the sinutubular junction (*yellow star*), making the latter attachments an integral part of the valvar complex.

junction to be found between the expanded sinuses and the tubular trunk of each great artery. The tips of the zones of apposition between the arterial valvar leaflets, usually known as the commissures, are firmly attached to this sinutubular junction, thus making it an integral part of the valvar complex. Stenosis occurring at this level, therefore, is valvar rather than supravalvar. The arrangement of the closed valve also show that the entirety of the zones of apposition between the leaflets should be considered to represent the commissures, rather than merely their peripheral attachments.

The pulmonary trunk runs only a short course before bifurcating into the right and left pulmonary arteries, which then extend to the respective lung hilums. The aorta continues through its ascending component above the sinutubular

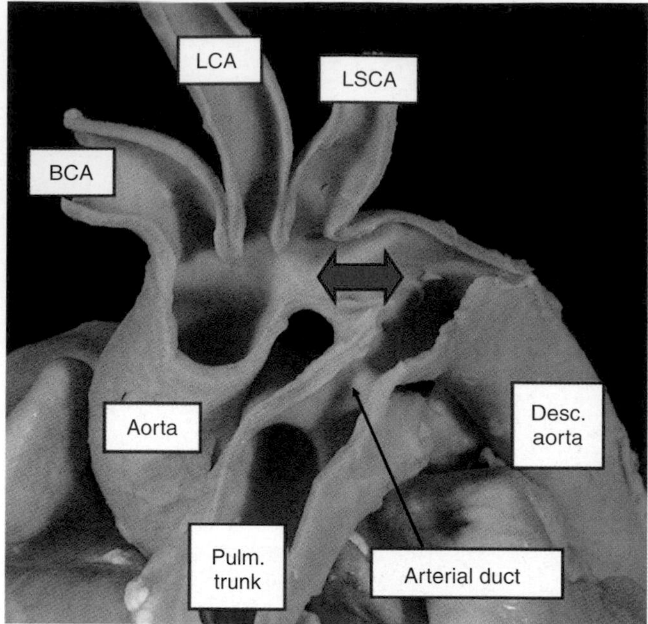

Figure 2-35 The intrapericardial arterial trunks spiral round one another as they extend from the base of the heart. The aorta, having exited the pericardial cavity, gives rise to the brachiocephalic (BCA), left common carotid (LCA) and left subclavian (LSCA) arteries. Note the arterial duct extending from the left pulmonary artery to the underside of the aortic arch, delimiting the distal end of the aortic isthmus (*double-headed arrow*). Desc., descending; Pulm., pulmonary.

junction until it runs horizontally as the transverse arch, giving rise to the brachiocephalic, left common carotid and left subclavian arteries (Fig. 2-35). The zone between the origins of the left subclavian artery and the arterial ligament, or the junction with the arterial duct prior to closure of this structure, is known as the isthmus. Beyond this point, the arch becomes the descending thoracic aorta. The arterial duct, or ligament after its closure, runs from the underside of the arch to the upper surface of the left pulmonary artery. The left recurrent laryngeal nerve turns back into the mediastinum round the duct or its ligamentous remnant.

THE VALVES OF THE HEART

Although we have already discussed the morphological features of the atrioventricular and arterial valves, these are such significant structures in normal and abnormal function of the heart that it is worthwhile reviewing the component parts of each set of valves, and the terms we use to describe them.

The Atrioventricular Valves

The atrioventricular valves guard the inlets to the ventricular mass and, as such, have to withstand the full force of ventricular contraction when in their closed position. For this reason, it is better to examine the valves in their closed position, taking care, of course, also to take note of their features when open. The overall valvar complex is made up of the annulus, the leaflets, the tension apparatus, and the papillary muscles. The annulus is a much firmer structure in the mitral than in the tricuspid valve. Even in the mitral valve, it is unusual to find a complete collagenous structure supporting the leaflets. In the tricuspid valve, it is the rule for the valvar leaflets to be suspended from the endocardial surface of the atrioventricular junction, with the fibrofatty tissue of the atrioventricular groove serving to insulate electrically the atrial from the ventricular musculature.

We distinguish the leaflets of the valves by determining the fashion in which they fit together in closed position. In this way, it can readily be seen that the mitral valve has two leaflets,[14] while the tricuspid valve has three.[8] This, of course, is no more than a restatement of well-established anatomical fact. It is the zones of apposition that are the key structures in defining the extent of the leaflets. This approach, focussing on zones of apposition, works for arterial as well as atrioventricular valves and is as useful for the valves seen in congenitally malformed as in otherwise normal hearts. We have already discussed, when describing the mitral valve, the different types of tendinous cord and the complicated categorisations that some use to describe them. In simple terms, the cords can be divided into those originating from the free edges of the leaflets and those coming from the ventricular aspects, the latter being divided into strut and basal cords.[14] Distinguishing the leaflets according to their patterns of closure avoids the need to subdivide the cords from the free edge of the leaflets into commissural or cleft variants.[8,15] This, in turn, avoids the controversies that arise in attempting to make these difficult distinctions. In the normal heart, the entire leading edges of the leaflets are uniformly supported by tendinous cords, the key feature being that the edges of adjacent leaflets at the peripheral ends of the zones of apposition are tethered to the same papillary muscle. It is also of note that, at the ends of the zones of apposition, there is a curtain of valvar tissue separating the valvar orifice from the annulus (see Fig. 2-26).

The papillary muscles of the valves are distinctive structures. The tricuspid valve is supported by a small medial muscle that arises from the posterior limb of the septomarginal trabeculation, a prominent anterior muscle, and an inferior muscle, the last named often duplicated or triplicated. The septal leaflet of the valve is characterised by its multiple direct cordal attachments to the septum. The mitral valve, in contrast, has obviously paired papillary muscles located infero-anteriorly and supero-posteriorly within the ventricular cavity, albeit that the heads of both muscles are frequently multiple. Each muscle supports the adjacent ends of the aortic and mural leaflets of the valve, being positioned beneath the two ends of the solitary zone of apposition between the leaflets.

The Arterial Valves

As with the atrioventricular valves, we view the outlet valves of the ventricular mass as complex structures with multiple components, these being the supporting ventricular walls, the leaflets, the sinuses, the interleaflet triangles, and the sinutubular junction. As such, each arterial valve extends from the basal attachment of the leaflets to the ventricular walls to the peripheral attachments of the zones of apposition between adjacent leaflets at the sinutubular junction. Within this valvar complex, most will continue to seek the annulus or ring. In reality, the entire valvar complex is a ring, or crown, and there is no cord-like collagenous circle within the valvar structure that supports the semilunar attachments of the leaflets.[16] At least three zones within the complex can justifiably be described as rings (see Fig. 2-22). The first is the sinutubular junction. The second is the anatomical ventriculo-arterial junction, this being the circular area over which the fibroelastic wall of the arterial trunk joins with the supporting ventricular walls. This anatomical junction should be distinguished from the haemodynamic boundary between ventricle and arterial trunk, this being marked self-evidently by the semilunar attachment of the valvar leaflets.[17] We have already emphasised how, in both aortic (see Fig. 2-29) and pulmonary (see Fig. 2-21) valves, this arrangement results in crescents of ventricular wall being incorporated within the truncal sinuses, and triangles of arterial wall being incorporated within the ventricular outflow tracts (see Fig. 2-22). The final ring within the valvar complex is an incomplete circle, formed by joining the basal attachments of the leaflets within the ventricles. The reason that some surgeons describe a semilunar annulus is surely because, having removed the leaflets of a diseased valve, they see the semilunar remnants, which they use as points of anchorage for the sutures that secure in place the prostheses used as valvar replacements.

The Septal Structures

Although each of the septal structures has already been described, it is worth re-emphasising their structure, the more so since only cursory mention has been made of the important membranous part of the ventricular septum. In this respect, only those parts of the cardiac walls that separate adjacent chambers should be described as septal.[18] Walls that separate the cavity of a chamber from the outside of the heart, even when folded on themselves, are not part of the septal structures.

The atrial septum, when defined in this fashion, is composed primarily of the floor of the oval fossa, this being the flap valve. In addition to the floor, only the antero-inferior rim of the fossa is a true septum in its own right, since the other margins are the infolded atrial walls, or else the atrial wall overlapping the base of the ventricular mass (see Fig. 2-12). The so-called sinus septum is no more than the branching point of the coronary sinus and the inferior caval vein.

Contiguous with both sinus septum and the inferior margin of the oval fossa is the area known as the triangle of Koch (Fig. 2-36). This important zone is the atrial aspect of an atrioventricular muscular sandwich, made up of overlapping areas of atrial and ventricular myocardium, the two separated by a fibrofatty extension from the inferior atrioventricular groove. In this area, as shown by the so-called four-chamber section, the leaflets of the tricuspid valve are attached more apically than are those of the mitral valve (Fig. 2-37). The apex of the triangle of Koch is made up of the fibrous tissue in the posterior component of the aortic root. Within this tissue is incorporated the fibrous part of the atrioventricular septum, itself a part of the membranous septum of the heart (Fig. 2-38). This is the only true atrioventricular septum. Taken overall, the membranous septum is contiguous with the fibrous triangle beneath the zone of apposition between the non-coronary and the right coronary leaflets of the aortic valve (see Fig. 2-32). It is the line of attachment of the tricuspid valve on its right aspect that divides the membranous septum into its atrioventricular and interventricular components, albeit that the proportions of the two components vary markedly from heart to heart.

The interventricular component of the membranous septum, when considered relative to the bulk of the muscular ventricular septum, is inconspicuous, but forms the keystone of the septum within the aortic root. We thought, in the past, that we were able to divide the much larger muscular ventricular septum into inlet, apical trabecular, and outlet components, thinking that these septal components matched the corresponding parts of the ventricular cavities.[19] In reality, the parts of the septum separating the inlet and

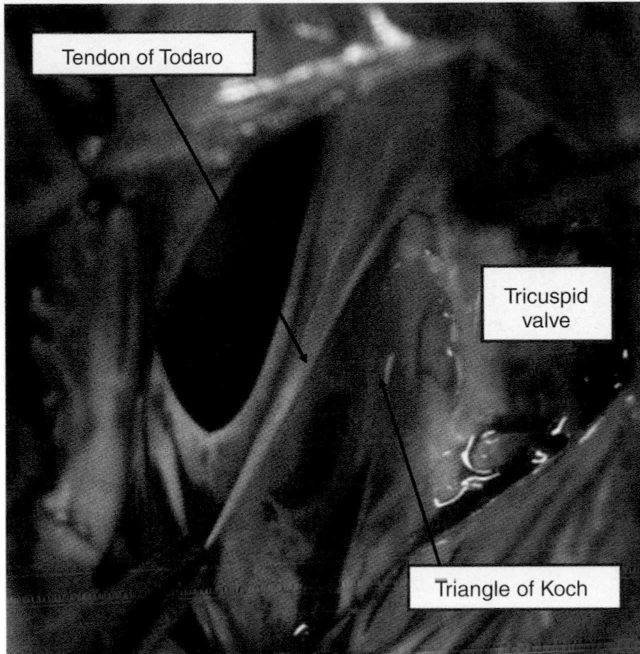

Figure 2-36 This picture shows how tension on the Eustachian valve brings into prominence the tendon of Todaro, which together with the line of attachment of the septal leaflet of the tricuspid valve forms the boundaries of the triangle of Koch. Note that the patient also has a large defect in the floor of the oval fossa. (Courtesy of Dr Benson R. Wilcox, University of North Carolina, Chapel Hill.)

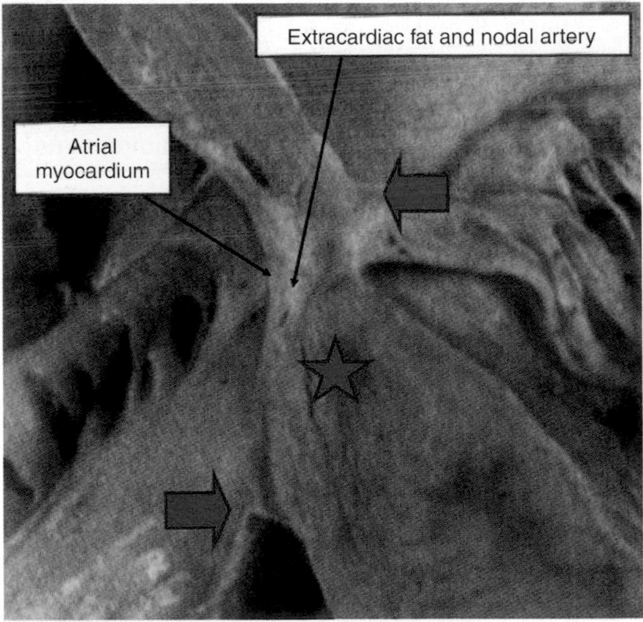

Figure 2-37 The heart has been sectioned in four-chamber plane, showing the sandwich formed by the atrial myocardium and the crest of the muscular ventricular septum (*star*) between the off-set attachments of the leaflets of the tricuspid and mitral valves (*arrows*).

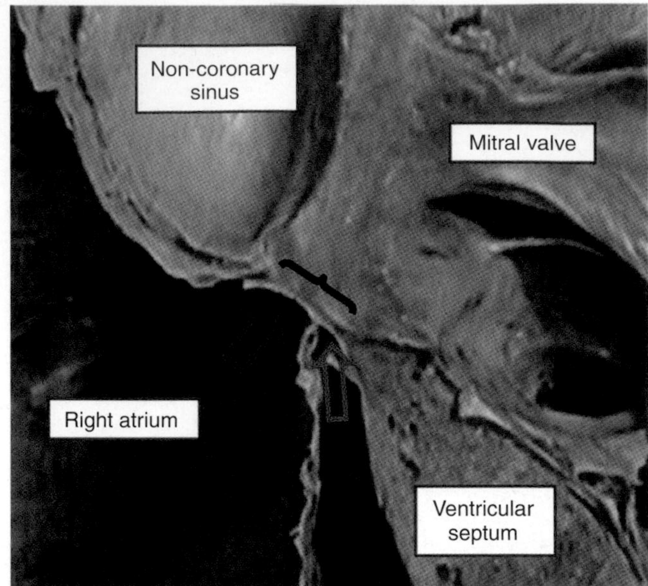

Figure 2-38 This heart has also been sectioned in four-chamber plane, but anteriorly relative to the cut shown in Figure 2-37. This cut, taken through the membranous septum, shows how the fibrous part of the septum (*bracket*) is divided into atrioventricular (*red arrow*) and interventricular (*yellow arrow*) components by the attachment of the septal leaflet of the tricuspid valve. (Courtesy of Dr Sandra Webb, St. George's Medical University, London, United Kingdom.)

outlet of the right ventricle from their comparable components in the left ventricle are not nearly so large as was initially thought. Because of the deeply wedged location of the subaortic outlet component, much of the septum supporting the septal leaflet of the tricuspid valve separates the inlet of the right ventricle from the left ventricular outlet (Fig. 2-39). In addition, because of the free-standing nature of the subpulmonary infundibulum, only a very small part of the muscular septum is a true outlet septum (see Fig. 2-24). In the normal heart, therefore, there are no obvious boundaries that divide the muscular ventricular septum into its component parts. The outlet septum seen as an anatomical entity achieves a separate existence only when the septum itself is deficient, particularly when this part is malaligned relative to the rest of the muscular septum.

THE FIBROUS SKELETON

Many textbooks illustrate the basal section of the heart as seen in the short axis containing a fibrous skeleton that embraces the origins of, and provides the attachments for, the leaflets of all four cardiac valves. There is no foundation in anatomical fact to support this notion. As already shown, the leaflets of the pulmonary valve are supported on an extensive sleeve of free-standing right ventricular musculature (see Figs. 2-20 and 2-21). Endorsing the findings of McAlpine,[20] we have been unable to identify the so-called tendon of the conus, or infundibular ligament.[21] The leaflets of the aortic valve also arise in part from the septal musculature and in part from a zone of fibrous continuity with the aortic leaflet of the mitral valve (see Fig. 2-29). It is this zone of fibrous continuity that forms the basis of the cardiac skeleton. The two ends of the zone are thickened to form the right and left fibrous trigones (Fig. 2-40). The right fibrous trigone is then continuous with the membranous septum, the conjoined structure being known as the central fibrous body. This is the strongest part of the fibrous skeleton. From the two fibrous trigones, cords of fibrous tissue extend around the orifices of the mitral valve. It is rare, however, to find these cords encircling the entirety of the valvar orifice, and providing uniform support for

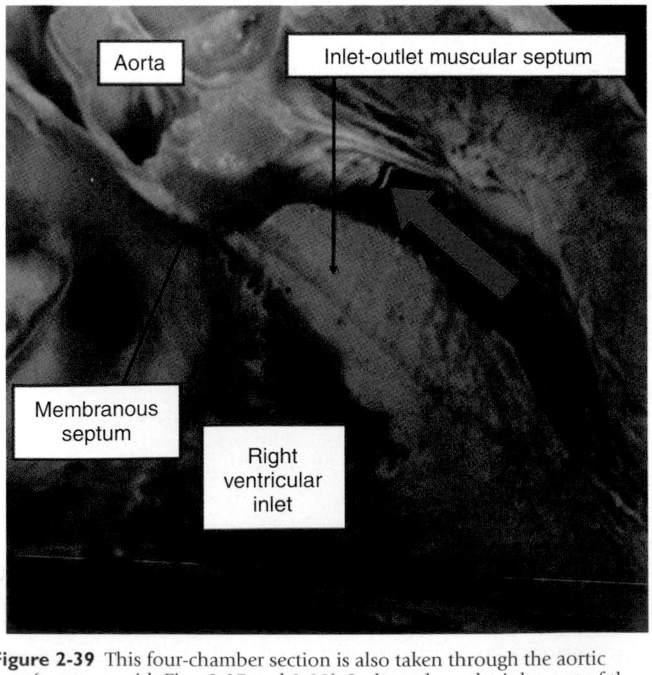

Figure 2-39 This four-chamber section is also taken through the aortic root (compare with Figs. 2-37 and 2-38). It shows how the inlet part of the muscular septum, because of the wedged location of the subaortic outflow tract (*arrow*) separates the inlet of the right ventricle from the left ventricular outlet. It is, in reality, an inlet-outlet septum.

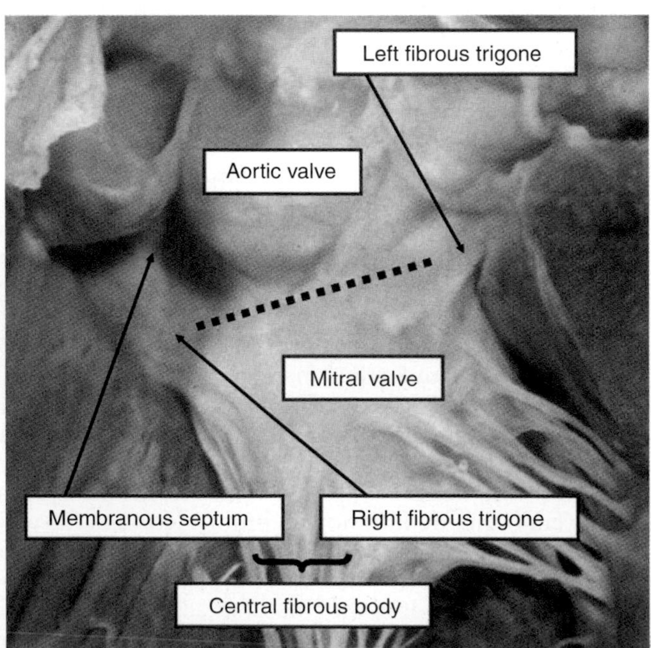

Figure 2-40 It is the right and left fibrous trigones, the thickenings at the ends of the zone of fibrous continuity between the leaflets of the aortic and mitral valves (*dotted line*), together with the membranous septum, that form the basis of the fibrous skeleton of the heart. Note that the right fibrous trigone joins with the membranous septum to form the so-called central fibrous body. The atrioventricular bundle penetrates through this part of the heart.

the attachments of mural leaflet of the mitral valve. The fibrous tissue can be well formed around the mitral valve, but frequently takes the form of a short fibrous strip, rather than a circular cord.[22] Often, the fibrous tissue fades out completely at various sites around the ring, with the atrial and ventricular muscle masses being separated one from the other by fibrofatty tissue of the atrioventricular groove in these locations. The mitral valvar leaflets then take origin from the ventricular myocardium, rather than from a fibrous skeleton. This arrangement is the rule rather than the exception in the right atrioventricular junction, where it is usually the fibrofatty tissues of the atrioventricular groove that serve to insulate the atrial from the ventricular musculature. Taken together, therefore, the fibrous skeleton of the human heart is relatively poorly formed, being a firm structure only within the aortic root.[23]

THE CONDUCTION TISSUES

The conduction tissues are small areas of specialised myocardium that originate and disseminate the cardiac impulse. Although it is only rarely possible to visualise the tissues directly, their sites are sufficiently constant for accurate anatomical landmarks to be established as a guide to their location.

The cardiac impulse is generated in the sinus node.[24] This small cigar-shaped structure is located, in a majority of individuals, subepicardially within the terminal groove, being positioned inferior to the crest of the atrial appendage (Fig. 2-41). In about one-tenth of individuals, however, the node extends across the crest of the appendage to sit like a horseshoe, with one limb in the terminal groove, and the other in the interatrial groove (see Fig. 2-41, inset). Equally important to the location of the node is the course of its arterial supply. The artery to the sinus node is the most prominent atrial artery. It arises in most individuals from the initial course of either the right or the circumflex coronary artery. It then runs through the interatrial groove, and enters the terminal groove across or behind the cavoatrial junction, with an arterial circle formed in a minority of individuals. In some individuals, the artery arises from the lateral part of the right coronary artery, or else from the distal course of the circumflex artery. The nodal artery then runs either across the lateral margin of the right atrial appendage or across the dome of the left atrium.[25] In either event, it can be at major risk when a surgeon makes a standard incision to enter the atrial chambers.

The impulse from the sinus node is conducted at the nodal margins into working atrial myocardium, and it is then carried through the working myocardium towards the atrioventricular node. Much has been written in the past concerning the presence of so-called internodal atrial tracts. Anatomical studies show that there are no narrow and insulated tracts of cells that join the cells of the sinus node to those of the atrioventricular node that are, in any way, analogous to the insulated ventricular conduction pathways (see below). There may be pathways of preferential conduction through the terminal crest and the sinus septum and around the margins of the oval fossa. The more rapid spread of conduction through these areas is simply a consequence of the more ordered packing of the myocardial fibres within these prominent muscular bundles (Fig. 2-42).

The atrioventricular node,[26] surrounded on most sides by short zones of transitional cells, is contained exclusively within the triangle of Koch. This important landmark is delineated by the tendon of Todaro, the attachment of the

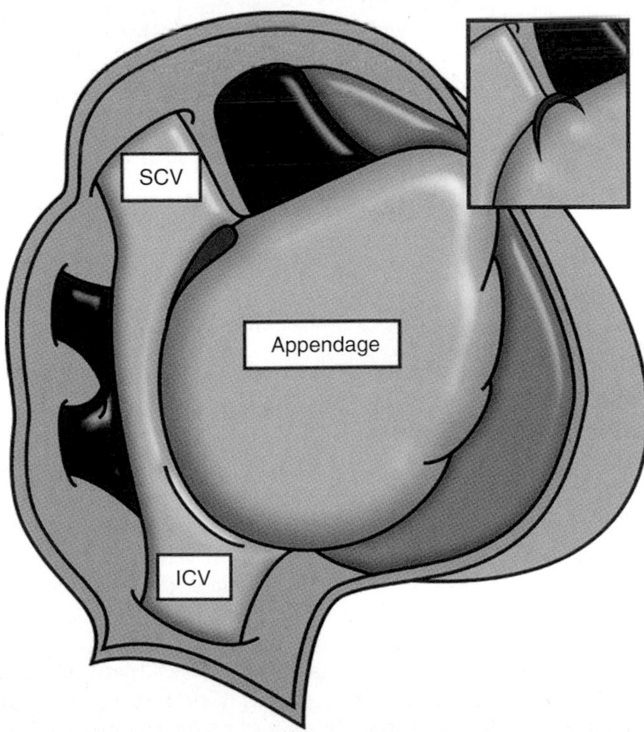

Figure 2-41 The cartoon shows the location of the sinus node, which lies immediately subepicardially within the terminal groove. In a minority of patients it occupies a horseshoe position (*inset*). IVC, inferior caval vein; SCV, superior caval vein.

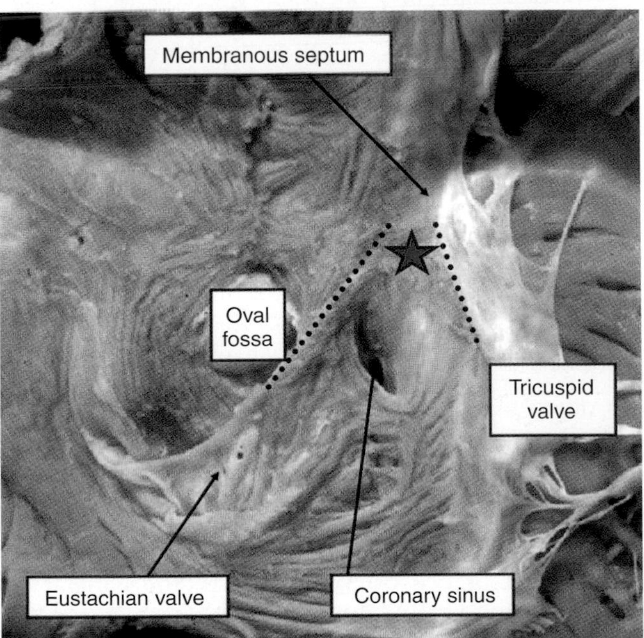

Figure 2-42 Removal of the epicardium shows well the parallel arrangement of the muscular fibres in the prominent bundles of the right atrium. It is this orderly arrangement that is responsible for the preferential nature of internodal conduction. Note also the continuation of the Eustachian valve as the tendon of Todaro. Together with the hinge of the septal leaflet of the tricuspid valve (*dotted lines*), the tendon delineates the triangle of Koch. The atrioventricular node is situated at the apex of this triangle (*star*). (Courtesy of Professor Damian Sanchez-Quintana, University of Badajoz, Spain.)

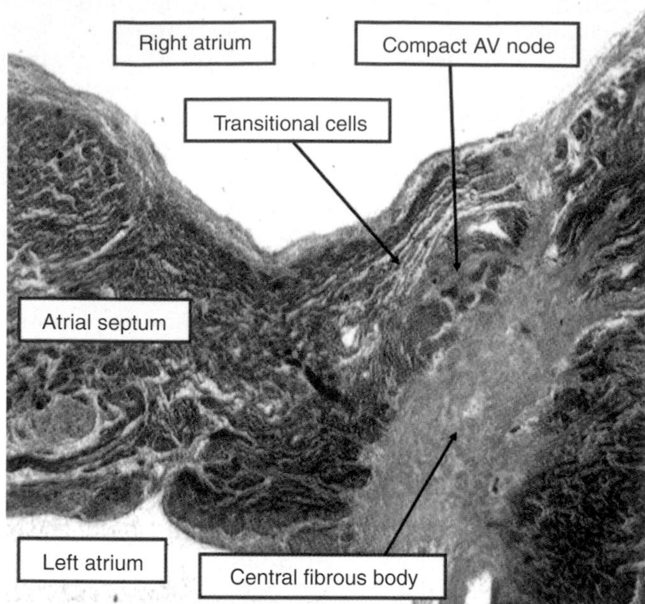

Figure 2-43 The section is taken through the junction of the atrial and ventricular septums, and is orientated attitudinally, with the right atrium uppermost. Note the cells of compact atrioventricular (AV) node set as a half-oval against the insulating fibrous tissue of the central fibrous body, with transitional cells interposing on most sides between the cells of the node and the atrial myocardium.

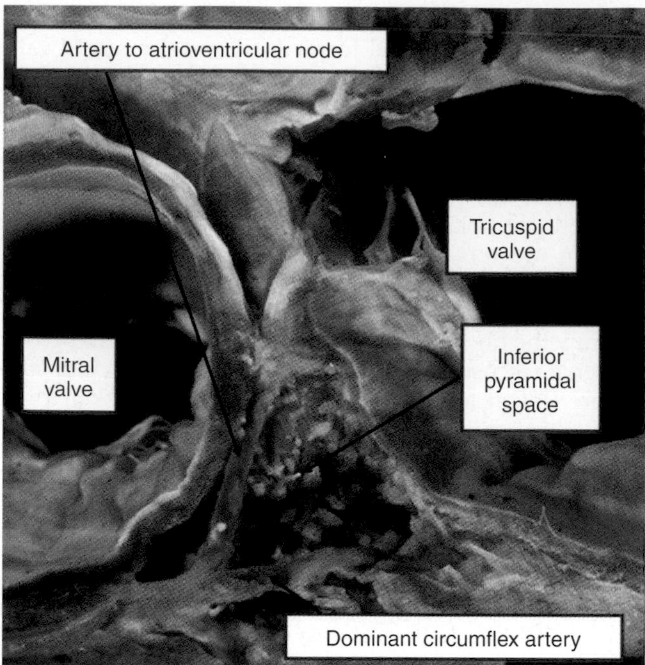

Figure 2-44 Removing the floor of the coronary sinus reveals the pyramidal space between the atrial musculature and the diverging infero-posterior margins of the ventricular walls. This space, containing the artery to the atrioventricular node, is a superior extension from the inferior atrioventricular groove.

septal leaflet of the tricuspid valve and the orifice of the coronary sinus (see Figs. 2-36 and 2-42). The specialised myocardial cells of the node, and the transitional zones, are situated within the atrial component of the atrioventricular muscular septum,[27] with the atrial myocardium approaching the node from all sides (Fig. 2-43). The floor of the coronary sinus in this area roofs the inferior pyramidal space. This space is paraseptal,[28] situated between the atrial musculature and the crest of the muscular ventricular septum (Fig. 2-44). The artery to the atrioventricular node courses anteriorly through this space into the triangle of Koch (see Fig. 2-37), having taken origin from the dominant coronary artery (see below).

From the apex of the triangle of Koch, it is but a short distance for the atrioventricular conduction axis to penetrate the central fibrous body as the bundle of His, better described as the penetrating atrioventricular bundle. Having penetrated, the bundle reaches the crest of the muscular septum beneath the non-facing leaflet of the aortic valve (Fig. 2-45), where it branches. The left bundle branch then runs down the smooth left surface of the septum, before fanning out towards the ventricular apex (see Fig. 2-45). The right bundle branch traverses the septum to emerge beneath the medial papillary muscle. It then extends as a thin insulated cord in the substance of the septomarginal trabeculation before ramifying at the ventricular apex. A prominent branch usually passes to the parietal wall through the moderator band.

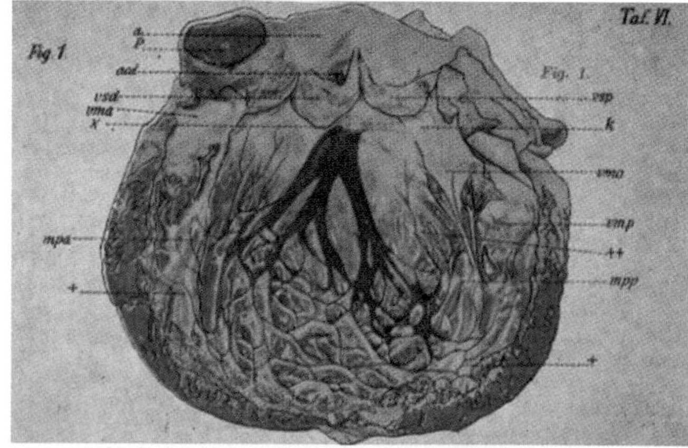

Figure 2-45 The figure shown is Figure 1 from Table 6 of the monumental monograph published by Sunao Tawara in 1906. It shows, in *dotted lines,* the location of the knoten (k), or atrioventricular node, and the penetrating atrioventricular bundle. The reconstruction shows, in *red,* the location of the trifascicular left bundle branch on the surface of the ventricular septum. Removal of the non-coronary sinus of the aorta reveals the very short distance needed to be traversed by the penetrating atrioventricular bundle (of His) as it passes from the apex of the triangle of Koch *(bullet)* to reach the crest of the muscular ventricular septum.

BLOOD SUPPLY TO THE HEART

The Coronary Arteries

The coronary arteries are the first branches of the aorta, usually taking their origin within the bulbous expansions of the aortic root proximal to the sinutubular junction known as the aortic sinuses of Valsalva. As already discussed, there are two major coronary arteries and three aortic sinuses (see Fig. 2-30). Almost without exception, the arteries arise from one or the other of the sinuses closest to the pulmonary trunk, these being the adjacent or facing sinuses. In most normal individuals, one artery arises from each of these facing sinuses, permitting them to be named the right coronary and left coronary sinuses, respectively (see Fig. 2-30). It is useful, nonetheless, to have a convention for naming the sinuses that works irrespective of the origin of the coronary arteries, and irrespective of the relationship

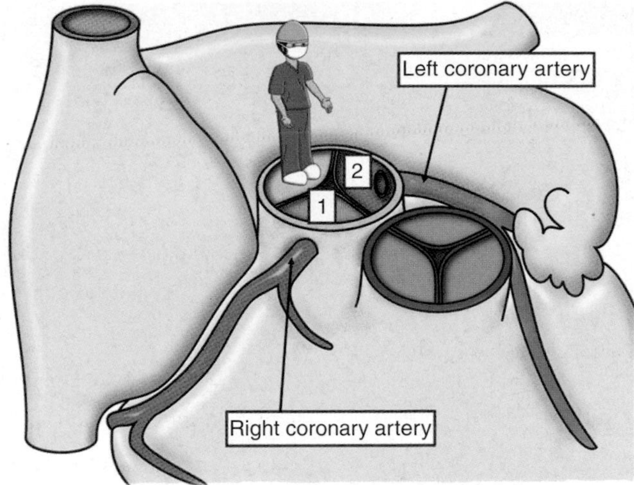

Figure 2-46 When an observer views the aortic sinuses from the non-facing sinus looking towards the pulmonary trunk, then, irrespective of the relationship of the great arteries, one aortic sinus is always to the left hand and the other to the right hand. In the normal situation, the sinus to the right hand, known as #1, gives rise to the right coronary artery, while the sinus to the left hand, known as #2, gives rise to the main stem of the left coronary artery.

of the aorta to the pulmonary trunk. This is provided by observing the aortic sinuses from the point of the non-facing sinus, and looking towards the pulmonary trunk (Fig. 2-46). One facing sinus is then to the right hand of the observer, and this is the sinus that usually gives rise to the right coronary artery. The other sinus is to the left hand of the observer, and usually gives rise to the main stem of the left coronary artery. By convention, the facing sinus to the right hand has become known as sinus 1, while the left hand facing sinus is known as sinus 2.[29] As we will see, this convention, known as the Leiden Convention, holds good for naming the aortic sinuses and the origin of the coronary arteries, even when the arterial trunks are abnormally disposed in congenitally malformed hearts.

In the normal heart, it is the right coronary artery that arises from the right hand facing sinus, usually but not always beneath the sinutubular junction, and oftentimes eccentrically positioned within the sinus. It is by no means uncommon for additional arteries to arise directly within the sinus, most frequently the infundibular artery or the artery to the sinus node. The right coronary artery itself passes directly into the right atrioventricular groove, lying in the curve of the ventriculo-infundibular fold above the supraventricular crest (Fig. 2-47). From this initial course, the artery gives rise to infundibular and atrial branches before turning round the acute margin of the ventricular mass, where it gives rise to the acute marginal origin. The main stem of the right coronary artery then continues along the diaphragmatic surface of the right atrioventricular junction, giving off additional atrial and ventricular branches until, in about nine-tenths of individuals, it gives rise to the inferior interventricular artery, described as being posterior in most current textbooks, but unequivocally positioned inferiorly when the heart is located within the chest. The right coronary artery usually continues beyond the crux to supply a variable portion of the diaphragmatic surface of the left ventricle. This arrangement is called right coronary arterial dominance.

The main stem of the left coronary artery, having taken origin from the left hand facing sinus, passes into the left atrioventricular groove beneath the orifice of the left atrial appendage. It then immediately branches into the anterior interventricular and circumflex arteries (Fig. 2-48). In some individuals a third artery, the intermediate artery, supplies directly the obtuse marginal surface of the left ventricle. It is much rarer for additional arteries to arise within the left

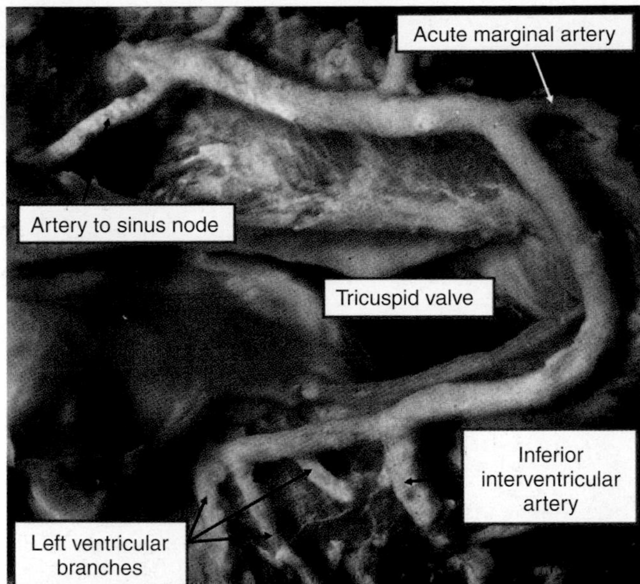

Figure 2-47 The dissection shows the course of the right coronary artery. Having arisen from its aortic sinus, the artery encircles the right atrioventricular junction, giving off atrial and ventricular branches. In nine-tenths of individuals, as in this instance, it gives rise to the inferior interventricular artery, continuing beyond the crux to supply the diaphragmatic walls of the left ventricle.

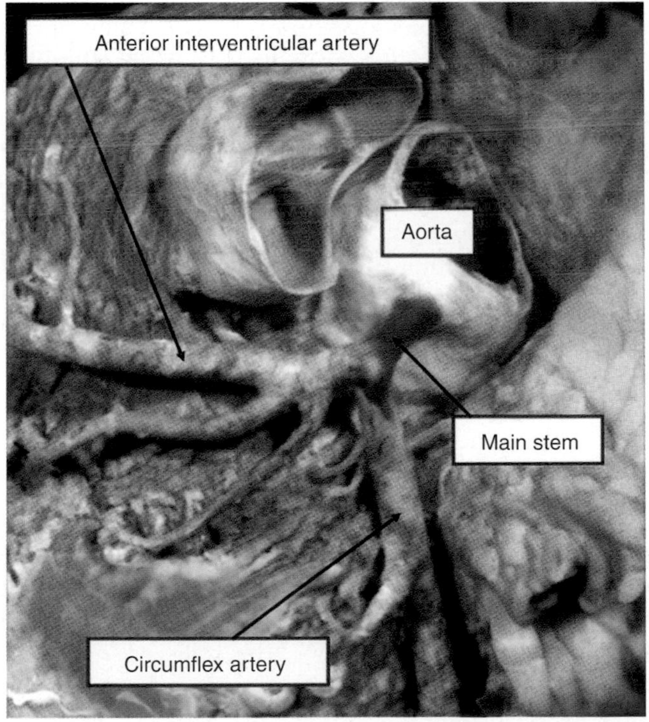

Figure 2-48 The main stem of the left coronary, having emerged from the aortic sinus, branches immediately into its anterior interventricular and circumflex branches.

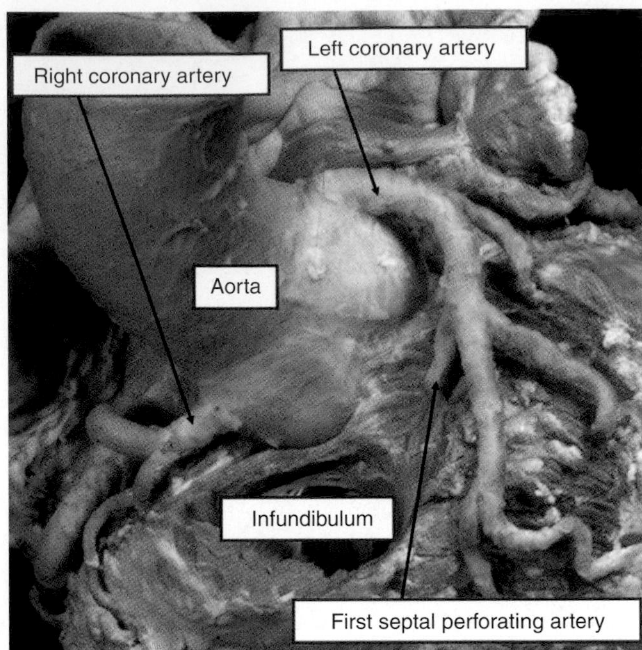

Figure 2-49 Removal of the free-standing subpulmonary infundibulum shows well the origin of the right and left coronary arteries from the aorta. Note the origin of the first septal perforating artery from the anterior interventricular artery.

hand facing sinus, but sometimes the two major arteries have independent origins. More usually, albeit still rarely, it is the sinus nodal artery that takes a separate origin from this sinus. The anterior interventricular artery, also known as the anterior descending artery, runs down the anterior interventricular groove, giving diagonal branches to the adjacent surfaces of the right and left ventricles, along with the perforating arteries, which pass perpendicularly into the ventricular septum. The first septal perforating branch is particularly significant, being located immediately posterior to the free-standing sleeve of subpulmonary infundibular musculature (Fig. 2-49). The extent of the circumflex artery depends on whether the right coronary artery is dominant. When the right artery is dominant, then the circumflex artery often terminates abruptly after it has given rise to the obtuse marginal branch or branches. Sometimes, in perhaps one-tenth of individuals, the circumflex artery is dominant. It then runs all the way round the left atrioventricular junction and continues beyond the crux to supply part of the diaphragmatic surface of the right ventricle, as well as giving rise to the inferior interventricular artery and the artery to the atrioventricular node (Fig. 2-50).

The Coronary Veins

The venous return from the heart is, for the most part, collected by the major cardiac veins, which run alongside the coronary arteries in the interventricular and atrioventricular grooves. The largest vein, termed the great cardiac vein, accompanies the anterior interventricular artery, turning beneath the left atrial appendage to join the coronary sinus. The junction between vein and sinus is the point of entrance of the oblique vein of the left atrium, or the vein of Marshall, which usually corresponds with the site of a prominent venous valve, the valve of Vieussens.

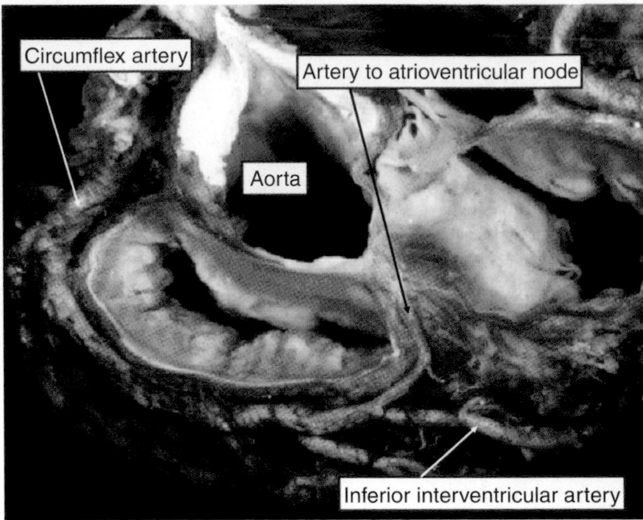

Figure 2-50 In this heart, the circumflex artery, running within the postero-inferior left atrioventricular groove, continues beyond the crux of the heart, where it gives rise to the inferior interventricular artery and the artery to the atrioventricular node.

The coronary sinus then runs within the left atrioventricular groove to the right atrium (Fig. 2-51). As it enters the right atrium, it collects the middle cardiac vein, which accompanies the inferior interventricular artery, and the small cardiac vein, which runs in the right atrioventricular groove. Further smaller veins usually drain into the sinus as it courses within the left atrioventricular groove. When there is a persistent left superior caval vein, it usually drains into the coronary sinus along the route normally occupied by the oblique vein. An additional series of veins, the minor cardiac veins, usually three to four in number, drain the blood from the anterior surface of the right ventricle

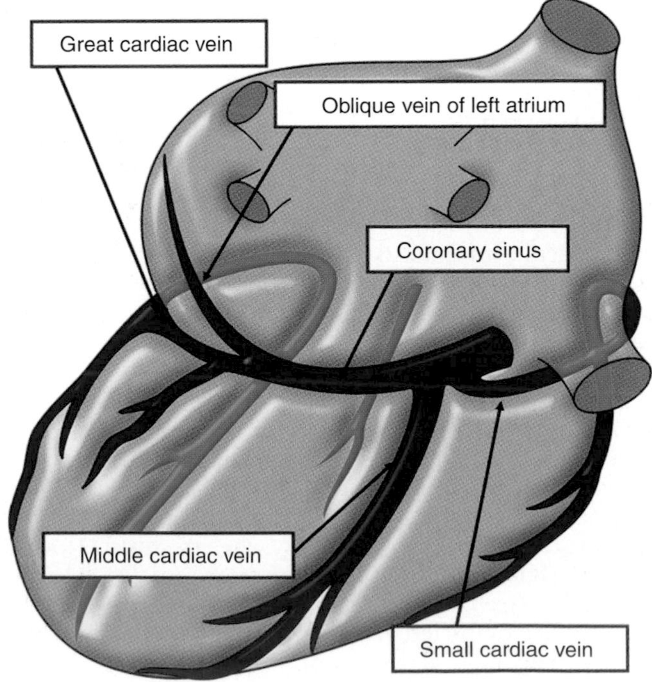

Figure 2-51 The cartoon, showing the heart viewed from behind, illustrates the arrangement of the coronary veins.

and enter directly the infundibulum. A further series of minimal cardiac veins, or Thebesian veins, then drain the blood from the walls of the right and left atriums, opening directly into the atrial cavities.

The complete reference list can be found on the companion Expert Consult web site at www.expertconsult.com.

ANNOTATED REFERENCES

- Cook AC, Anderson RH: Attitudinally correct nomenclature [editorial]. Heart 2002;87:503–506.

  Although we had indicated that, having studied the book of McAlpine, we also would use anatomically appropriate nomenclature, for a long time we failed to follow our own advice. In this editorial, we stressed again the importance of adopting the suggestions of McAlpine.

- Anderson RH, Brown NA, Webb S: Development and structure of the atrial septum. Heart 2002;88:104–110.

  In this review, we emphasised the difference between the true atrial septum, formed largely by the flap valve, which can be removed without creating a communication with the extracardiac spaces, as opposed to the so-called septum secundum, in reality the superior interatrial groove. It is possible to pass between the atrial chambers by cutting through this fold, but only by, at the same time, transgressing on the extracardiac space.

- Chauvin M, Shah DC, Haissaguerre M, et al: The anatomic basis of connections between the coronary sinus musculature and the left atrium in humans. Circulation 2000;101:647–652.

  In this study, the French group showed that the coronary sinus and the left atrium each possess their own walls. Prior to this investigation, it had been presumed that a common wall interposed between the cavities of the venous structure and the atrium.

- Merrick AF, Yacoub MH, Ho SY, Anderson RH: Anatomy of the muscular subpulmonary infundibulum with regard to the Ross procedure. Ann Thorac Surg 2000;69:556–561.

  We pointed out that, unless the pulmonary valve was truly supported by its muscular infundibular sleeve, it would be impossible to remove the valve for use as an autograft in the Ross procedure. The corollary of this finding is that there is no outlet septum interposed between the back wall of the right ventricular outflow tract and the aortic valvar sinuses.

- Victor S, Nayak VM: Definition and function of commissures, slits and scallops of the mitral valve: Analysis in 100 hearts. Asia Pacific J Thorac Cardiovasc Surg 1994;3:10–16.

  In this work, the authors pointed out that examining the mitral valve in its closed position negated the need to define commissures on the basis of the arrangement of the tendinous cords. When the value is seen in its closed position, it is obvious that there is but a solitary line of closure for the mitral valve, albeit that the mural leaflet has multiple slits along its length to permit competent closure.

- Sutton JP III, Ho SY, Anderson RH: The forgotten interleaflet triangles: A review of the surgical anatomy of the aortic valve. Ann Thorac Surg 1995;59:419–427.

  In this investigation, we showed that, because of the semilunar nature of the attachments of the arterial valvar leaflets, crescents of ventricle were incorporated into the bases of the arterial sinuses, whilst triangles of fibrous tissue extended to the sinutubular junction as parts of the ventricle. We also emphasised that, because of these anatomical arrangements, the arterial valves did not possess an annulus in terms of a circular structure supporting the leaflets in cord-like fashion. Instead, the arrangement resembled a crown.

- McAlpine WA: Heart and Coronary Arteries. An Anatomical Atlas for Clinical Diagnosis, Radiological Investigation, and Surgical Treatment. Berlin: Springer-Verlag, 1975.

  An important book, now out of print, that stressed the importance of describing the heart as it is positioned within the body. The dissections illustrated are exquisite, and it is deserving of greater recognition than it has achieved.

- Angelini A, Ho SY, Anderson RH, et al: A histological study of the atrioventricular junction in hearts with normal and prolapsed leaflets of the mitral valve. Br Heart J 1988;59:712–716.

  This investigation showed that it was the exception rather than the rule for the mural leaflet of the mitral valve to be supported by a cord-like fibrous structure that also insulated the atrial from the ventricular myocardium.

- Dobrzynski H, Boyett MR, Anderson RH: New insights into pacemaker activity: Promoting understanding of sick sinus syndrome. Circulation 2007;115:1921–1932.

  In this review, celebrating the centenary of discovery of the sinus node by Keith and Flack, we review the history of the discovery and put the antomic findings into the context of the subsequent researches into electrophysiology and developmental biology.

- Tawara S: Das Reizleitunggssystem des Saugetierherzens. Jena: Gustav Fischer, 1906.

  In this monumental monograph, Tawara clarified the arrangement of the specialised muscular axis responsible for atrioventricular conduction, demonstrating for the first time the existence of the atrioventricular node. As was emphasised by Keith in his autobiography, this research ushered in a new epoch of understanding. The book is now available in an English translation, published by Imperial College Press.

CHAPTER 3

Embryology of the Heart

ANTOON F.M. MOORMAN, NIGEL BROWN, and ROBERT H. ANDERSON

Much has been learnt since the second edition of the book was published. It remains a fact that, as was emphasised at the start of this chapter in the second edition, from the functional point of view the heart is simply a specialised part of the vascular system. The development of the heart as a specialised pump, nonetheless, is obviously of great significance, as is the formation of a coelomic cavity around the developing organ so as to aid its action. We have learnt a great deal over the past decade regarding the origin of the muscular parts of this pumping organ. In the previous edition, emphasis was placed on the so-called segments of the developing heart tube, since it was believed that the initial linear tube contained the precursors of the components as seen in the postnatal heart. We now know that this is not the case, and that tissue is continually added to the heart tube as it grows and loops. The initial straight part of the tube (Fig. 3-1) eventually forms little more than the left ventricle. This knowledge now permits us better to interpret the morphogenesis of many congenital cardiac malformations. Embryology, therefore, is no longer a hindrance in this regard, as one of us stated somewhat controversially over 2 decades ago.[1] It is the new evidence that has emerged concerning the appearance of the cardiac components that we will emphasise in the opening sections of our chapter. Thereafter, we will revert to providing an account of the various cardiac segments, as was done in the second edition.[2] In this respect, we should emphasise, again as was done in the second edition, that we do not use *segment* in its biological sense when describing the development of the cardiac components. Thus, we do not imply that each purported segment is identical to the others, as is seen in invertebrates such as annelids. As explained in Chapter 1, however, the so-called segmental approach is now the preferred means of describing the cascade of information acquired in interrogating cardiac structure during the diagnostic process. As in the previous edition, therefore, we will continue to describe the cardiac components as segments, hoping to provide the necessary background to understand the anomalous development that leads to congenitally malformed hearts with abnormal connections between them. It is also the case that there are discrepancies between the terms used by biologists to describe developing heart and the attitudinally appropriate terms used by clinicians when describing the formed organ. Biologists and embryologists use the term anterior to describe structures that are towards the head, and posterior for those towards the feet. We circumvent these problems by describing cranial and caudal structures. So as to avoid confusion, we also need to avoid use of these terms when describing those structures located towards the spine and sternum, as is the wont of clinicians. For this purpose, we will use the adjectives dorsal and ventral. Right and left, of course, retain their time-honoured usage.

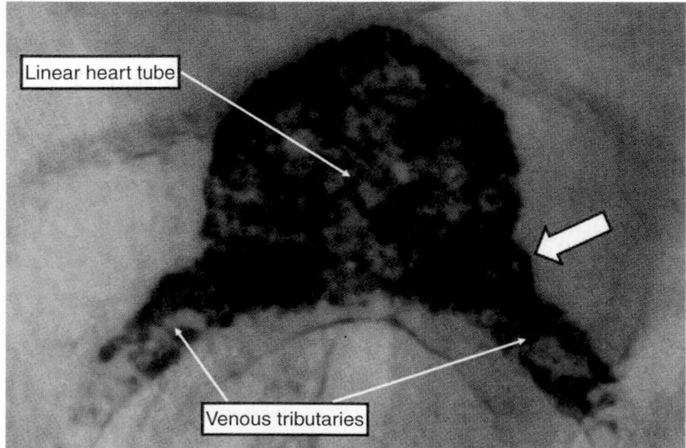

Figure 3-1 The heart tube has been visualised in the developing mouse embryo by detection of the expression of myosin heavy chain. It used to be thought that all parts of the organ were represented in the so-called linear tube. We now know that this part gives rise only to the definitive left ventricle and the ventricular septum. Note that there is already an asymmetrical arrangement of the tube, as shown by the *arrow*. The embryo is at about 8 days of development, which is comparable to about 21 days of human development.

ORIGIN OF THE HEART TUBE

Recent molecular studies[3–5] have validated the time-honoured concept[6–8] that, after formation of the linear heart tube (see Fig. 3-1), cells are continuously added at both its venous and arterial poles. The source of this new material has been called the second heart field, albeit that the difference between this purported second field and the presumptive primary field has not adequately been defined.[9] Despite this lack of adequate definition, the rediscovered information has revolutionised our understanding of the building plan of the heart. Acceptance of this concept of temporal addition of new material to the heart has also helped our understanding of cardiac morphogenesis, but new questions arise. Are there two developmental fields as opposed to just one, or three, or perhaps more? How are the alleged fields distinguished from the surrounding tissues, and from each other? Do the fields represent territories of gene expression, or of morphogenetic signaling? Most importantly, do the alleged first and second fields represent distinct cellular lineages, the descendants of which form distinct compartments within the definitive

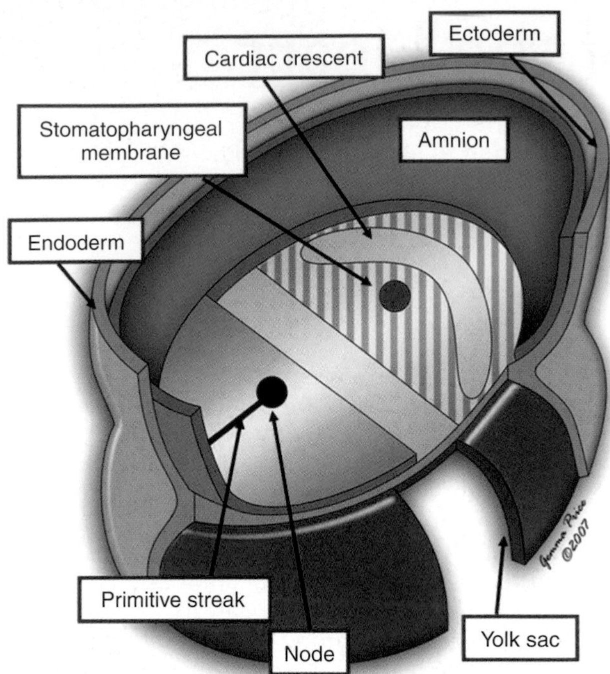

Figure 3-2 The cartoon shows how the embryonic disc is formed as a trilaminar structure, with the mesodermal structures sandwiched between the endodermal and ectodermal layers. In the cranial part of the embryonic disc, the ectoderm has been removed to visualize the cranial mesoderm. All mesoderm, including the so-called cardiac crescent, is derived from the primitive streak, as shown in Figure 3-3.

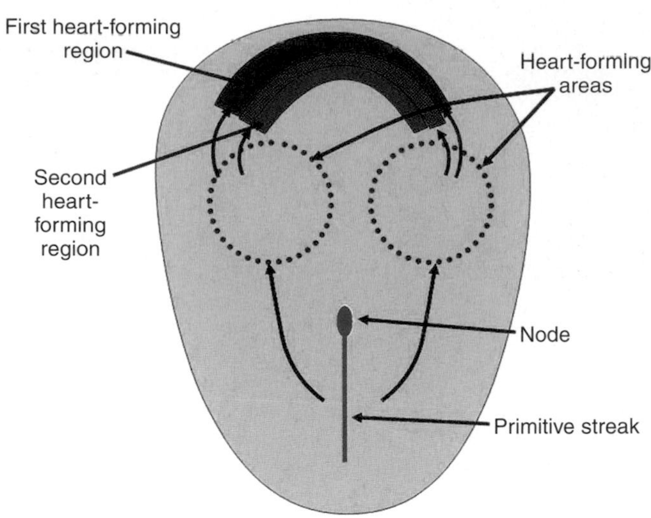

Figure 3-3 The cartoon shows how cells migrate from the primitive streak bilaterally to form first the heart-forming areas, and then the cardiac crescent. There are then temporal migrations of heart-forming cells from the cardiac crescent into the developing heart tube, with two of these migrations currently considered as the first and second heart-forming regions, or heart fields, although it is debatable whether these are discrete areas (see text for further discussion).

heart? An understanding of the mechanics of formation of the cardiac tube can provide some answers to these questions.[9]

Subsequent to gastrulation, the embryo possesses three germ layers. These are the ectoderm, which faces the amniotic cavity, the endoderm, which faces the yolk sac, and the intermediate mesodermal layer (Fig. 3-2). At this stage, we can recognise the so-called embryonic disc, marked by the junction of the developing embryo itself with the extra-embryonic tissues formed by the amnion and yolk sac. It is subsequent folding of this disc, concomitant with extensive growth, that gives the embryo its characteristic shape. Eventually, the original junction between the disc and the extraembryonic tissues becomes the navel of the embryo. As part of this process of remodelling, the parts of the disc initially positioned peripherally attain a ventral location within the embryo. At the initial stage, the region where ectoderm and mesoderm face one another without interposing mesoderm, is the stomato-pharyngeal membrane, which closes the orifice of the developing mouth. This membrane is flanked centrally by pharyngeal mesoderm that, in turn, is bordered peripherally by the cardiogenic mesoderm. The cardiac area is itself contiguous with the mesoderm of the transverse septum, in which will develop the liver. This transverse septum is the most peripheral part of the mesodermal layer of the embryonic disc and, after the completion of folding, it is located cranial to the navel.

During the process of gastrulation, the cells that will form the heart migrate from the anterior part of the primitive streak. Subsequent to their migration, they give rise to two heart-forming regions in the mesodermal germ layer. These areas are positioned on either side of the midline.[10–12] With continuing development, they join across the midline to form a crescent-shaped area of epithelium (Fig. 3-3). It is this tissue which subsequently provides the material for the heart tube, albeit in complex fashion. Initially, the crescent becomes a trough, which starts to close dorsally along the margins closest to the developing spine. Starting at the level of the part of the tube that will eventually become the left ventricle, closure proceeds by a process of zipping, the edges of the trough coming together in both cranial and caudal directions (Fig. 3-4). After the process of folding, the part of the crescent that was initially positioned centrally retains this position, becoming positioned medio-dorsally in the formed body. The peripheral part of the cresent, in contrast, becomes the ventral part of the definitive heart tube. It is the centro-medial part of the initial heart-forming area that several investigators have described as the secondary, or anterior, heart field.[3–5] Its location permits it to contribute to those parts of the heart that develop at the arterial pole, specifically the right ventricle and outflow tract, and also to those which will form at the venous pole. At the venous pole, there is formation of the so-called mediastinal myocardium,[13] this area eventually providing the site of entry for the pulmonary veins.[14,15] The peripheral part of the initial crescent flanks the transverse septum, which is the site of formation of the liver, and the location of the termination of the systemic venous tributaries.

It follows from the description given above that the tissues directly adjacent to the cardiac crescent are made of pharyngeal mesoderm. From the outset, therefore, the tissues that will form the right ventricle and outflow tract at the arterial pole are directly adjacent to the developing pharyngeal arches. This pharyngeal mesoderm, also containing cells derived from the so-called second heart field, eventually provides the tissues not only for the myocardial components of the right ventricle and outflow tract, but also for the non-myocardial intrapericardial arterial trunks and their valves and sinuses.

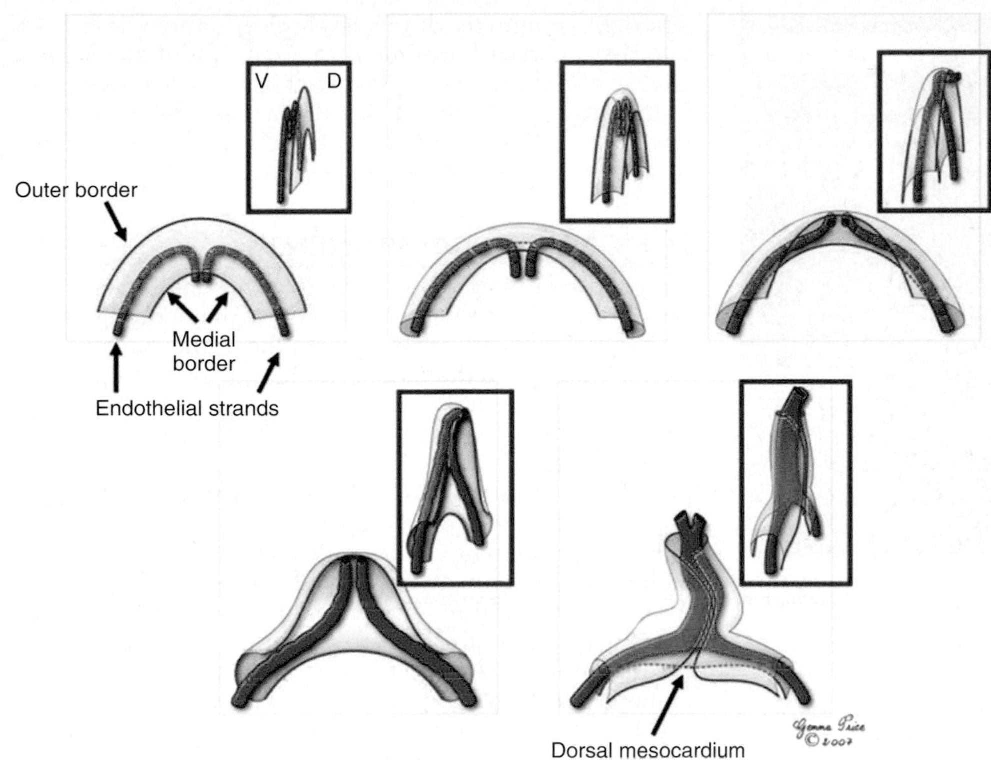

Figure 3-4 The cartoon shows the steps involved in folding of the cardiac crescent to become a tube. The heart-forming area is viewed from the dorsal aspect, with the *insets* within the *boxes* showing the arrangement as seen from the left side. Note that the initial outer part of the crescent (*red line*) becomes translocated ventrally during the process of folding, with the inner part (*blue line*) taking up a dorsal location. D, dorsal; V, ventral.

It has been analyses of molecular lineage that have demonstrated in unambiguous fashion that myocardium is added to the already functioning myocardial heart tube.[16,17] Thus, use of these techniques revealed a similar programme to that observed in the differentiation of the primary heart field, involving the transcription factors Nkx2-5, Gata4 and Mef2c, as well as fibroblast growth factors and bone morphogenetic proteins.[5] Differences in opinion remain regarding the structures formed from the so-called second field. One group has argued that this field forms only the outflow tract,[4] but another group claims that, as well as the outflow tract, the field also gives rise to the non-myocardial but intrapericardial portion of the arterial pole.[5] Such differences may be more apparent than real, since boundaries between morphological regions are not necessarily formed at subsequent stages by the same cells as were present initially. Interpretation has also been hampered by assumptions that, in avian hearts, the right ventricular precursors are derived from the initial linear heart tube, which contains the precursors of only the left ventricle in mammals.[17] It is now known that, in the developing avian heart, as in the mammalian heart, if the straight tube is labelled at the pericardial reflection of the arterial pole,[18] the entirety of the right ventricle is seen to be added to the linear heart tube later in development, consistent with the data derived in the mouse.[3]

Some authors[19] have already suggested that there is complex patterning in the primary heart field, rather than the existence of multiple fields. Based on our interpretation of the processes of folding that lead to the formation of the linear heart tube (see Fig. 3-4), we endorse this notion.[9] Acceptance of the notion, nonetheless, carries with it the implication that the cells within this solitary field initially have the capacity to form all parts of the heart, depending on their position in the field. This, in turn, is in keeping with current views on cellular diversity, since differences in the concentration of diffusing morphogens can create a number of different fates for a given cell, promoting diversity within a field that was initially homogeneous.

Even if we accept that the material from which the heart is formed is derived from the same basic field, there is an obvious temporal order in the differentiation of the alleged first and second cardiac heart-forming regions. This order does no more than reflect the evolutionary development of the cardiovascular system. When initially developed during evolution of the animal kingdom, the heart contained no more than the components of the systemic circulation, namely an atrium with left and right appendages, a ventricle, and a myocardial outflow tract. The pulmonary circulation, represented by the right ventricle, and the dorsal atrial wall, including the atrial septum, appears appreciably later in evolutionary development. Within the evolutionary tree, it is in the lungfish that the pulmonary veins are first seen to unite, and drain directly to the left atrium. This sets the scene for a separate pulmonary circulation, and also for the appearance of the atrial septum. It cannot be coincidental, therefore, that the atrial septum in mammals, along with the dorsal atrial wall, is formed from mediastinal myocardium.[13] This mediastinal myocardium, along with the right ventricle, is added to the heart relatively late in its development. The evolutionary considerations suggest strongly that novel patterning, with different temporal sequences, but within a single heart field, is sufficient to provide all the material needed to construct the four-chambered hearts of birds and mammals, albeit that not all precursors are present in the linear heart tube when it first appears (see Fig. 3-1).

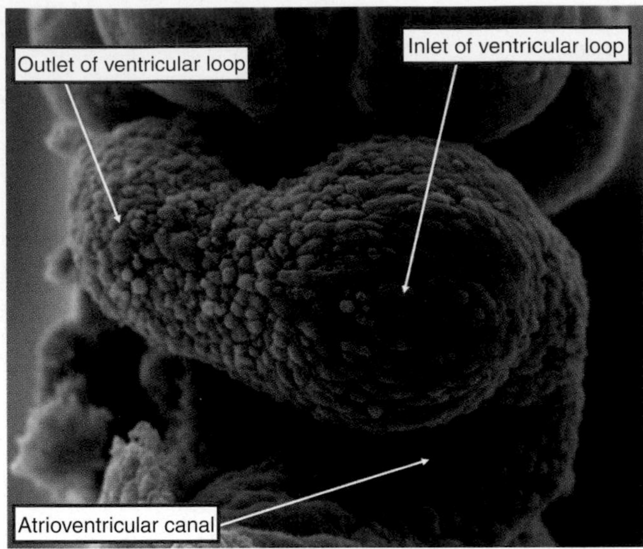

Figure 3-5 This scanning electron micrograph shows the developing mouse heart during the process of so-called looping. The ventricular part of the tube has inlet and outlet components formed in series.

FORMATION OF THE CARDIAC LOOP

When first seen, the developing heart is more or less a straight tube (see Fig. 3-1). Very soon, it becomes S-shaped (Fig. 3-5). The changes involved in producing the bends are described as looping. It had been thought that the curvatures produced were the consequence of rapid growth of the tube within a pericardial cavity that expanded much more slowly.[20] Experiments showed that the tube continues to loop even when deprived of its normal arterial and venous attachments,[21] and also loops when no longer beating, ruling out the role of haemodynamics as a morphogenetic factor.[22] Looping, therefore, is an intrinsic feature of the heart itself, albeit that the exact cause has still to be determined. Be that as it may, the tube usually curves to the right. This rightward turning is independent of the overall left–right asymmetry of the developing embryo. It is often said that rightward looping is the first sign of breaking of cardiac symmetry. This is incorrect. Asymmetry is evident in the structure of the atrioventricular canal when it is first seen (see Fig. 3-1),[23] but asymmetry can even be seen in the morphology and extent of the heart-forming fields.[13]

THE CARDIAC COMPONENTS

Only after looping of the heart tube has taken place is it possible to recognise the appearance of the building blocks of the cardiac chambers, along with the primordiums of the arterial trunks, and the venous tributaries. In the second edition of this book, it was suggested that five segments could be seen in the developing tube, on the basis of constrictions between the various parts, and that these constrictions played important roles in further development. As has been explained above, we now know that this is not the case.

The development of the cardiac chambers depends on ballooning of their cavities from the lumen of the primary heart tube. Addition of new material from the heart-forming area produces the primordiums of the right ventricle and outflow tract at the arterial pole, whilst addition of material at the venous pole produces initially the atrioventricular canal, followed by the atrial primordium, to which drain the systemic venous tributaries. The addition of this material is part and parcel of the appearance of the looped tube. Subsequent to looping, the cells making up the larger part of the tube are negative for both connexin40 and atrial natriuretic factor, permitting them to be labelled as primary myocardium (Fig. 3-6).

As the parts of the cavity begin to balloon out from both the atrial and ventricular components of the tube, so does the myocardium forming the walls of the ballooning components change its molecular nature, being positive for both connexin40 and atrial natriuretic peptide (Fig. 3-7). This myocardium is called chamber, or secondary, myocardium. The parts ballooning from the atrial component do so symmetrically with the newly formed pouches appearing to

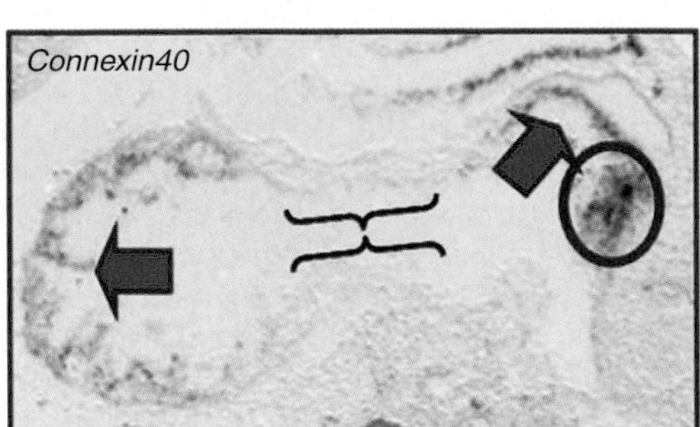
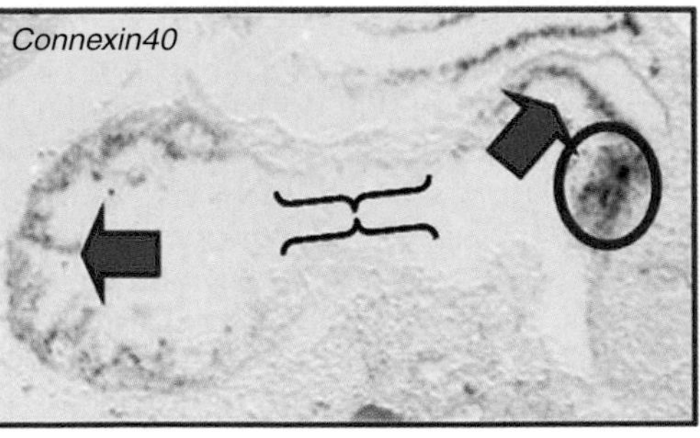

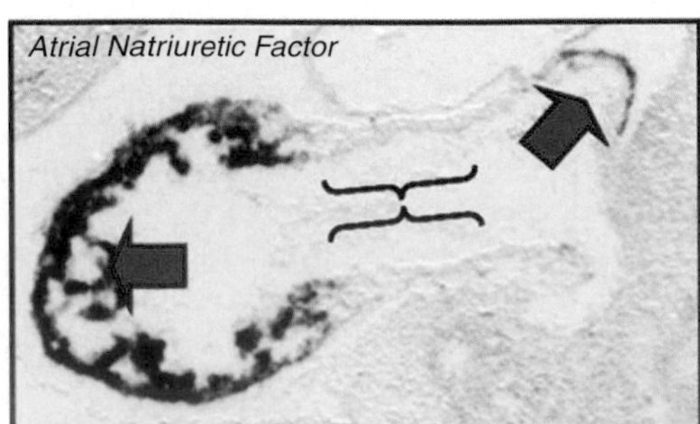

Figure 3-6 The adjacent sections processed to show expression of either connexin40 (Cx40) or atrial natriuretic factor (ANF) show how it is possible to distinguish three specific myocardial phenotypes. The mediastinal myocardium is shown in the *red oval*, the primary myocardium of the atrioventricular canal by the *braces* and the chamber myocardium by the *arrows*. The embryo is at about 9.5 days of development, which is comparable to about 4 weeks of human development.

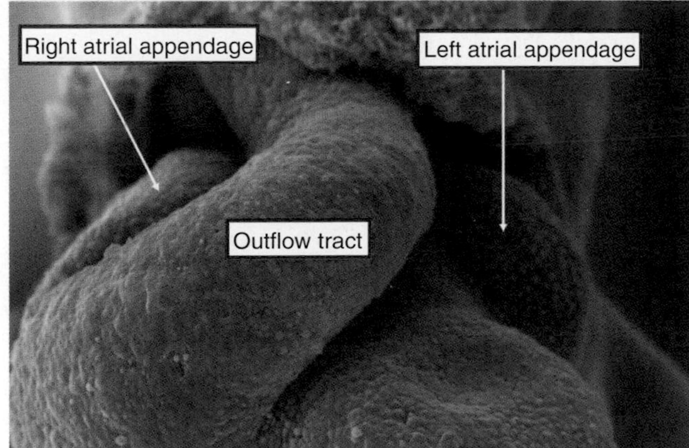

Figure 3-7 The scanning electron micrograph of a murine heart shows how the developing atrial appendages balloon forward to either side of the developing outflow tract.

either side of the outflow tract. The pouches will eventually become the atrial appendages. Examination of the atrial component of the heart at this early stage, however, reveals the presence of a third population of cells. These cells are positive for connexin40, but negative for atrial natriuretic peptide. They make up the part of the tube that retains its connection with the developing mediastinum through the dorsal mesocardium, and hence are described as being mediastinal myocardium.[13] These cells will eventually form the dorsal wall of the left atrium, or pulmonary venous component, a small part of the dorsal wall of the right atrium bordered at the right side by the left venous valve and at the left side by the primary atrial septum, which also is derived from the mediastinal component (Fig. 3-8). From the stance of lineage, the cells are derived from the mesenchyme of the mediastinum that surrounds the developing lung buds.[24] There is also ballooning of cavities from the ventricular part of the heart tube. Unlike the situation in the atrial component, where the appendages of both definitive atriums balloon in parallel, the pouches that will eventually form the apexes of the left and right ventricles balloon in sequence from the ventricular loop (Fig. 3-9). The apical part of the developing left ventricle balloons from the inlet part of the loop, whilst the apical part of the developing right ventricle takes its origin from the outlet part of the loop. Concomitant with the ballooning of these two parts, so the muscular ventricular septum is formed between the apical components (see Fig. 3-9), albeit that the cells of the septum largely belong to the left ventricle. The cells making up the walls of the ballooned segments are composed of secondary, or chamber, myocardium (see Fig. 3-6). Ballooning of the chamber myocardium sets the scene for septation of the atrial and ventricular chambers. For this to be achieved, however, appreciable remodelling is required in the initial cavity of the primary heart tube. This is because, subsequent to looping and the initial phases of ballooning, the circumference of the atrioventricular

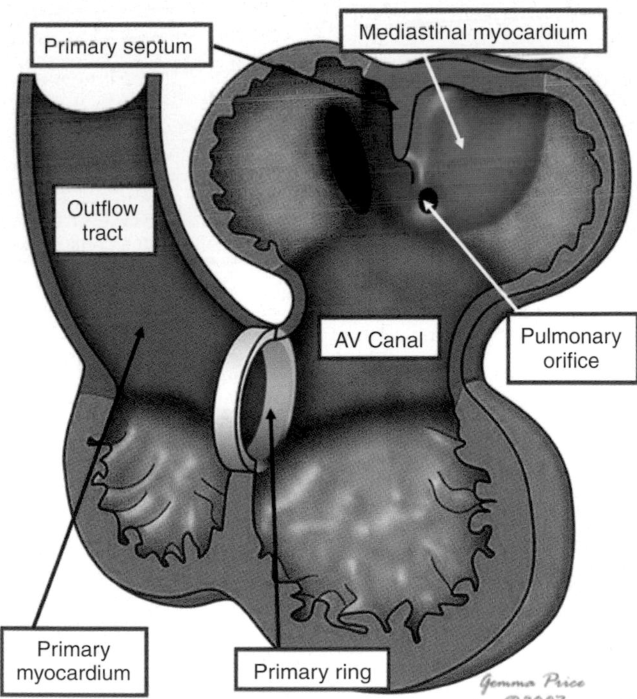

Figure 3-8 The cartoon shows how the atrial appendages, and the ventricular apical components, both coloured in *yellow*, have ballooned from the primary heart tube, shown in *grey*. The cartoon does not represent a particular stage of development but tries to bridge the transition of the primary heart tube into a four-chambered heart. The cardiac cushions are not represented in this cartoon, and the outflow tract has been bent to the *right* to visualize the inner curvature. Note the location of the mediastinal myocardium, which gives rise to the primary atrial septum, and encloses the opening of the pulmonary vein (see text for further discussion). (Modified from Moorman AFM, Christoffels VM: Cardiac chamber formation: Development, genes and evolution. Physiol Rev 2003;83:1223-1267.)

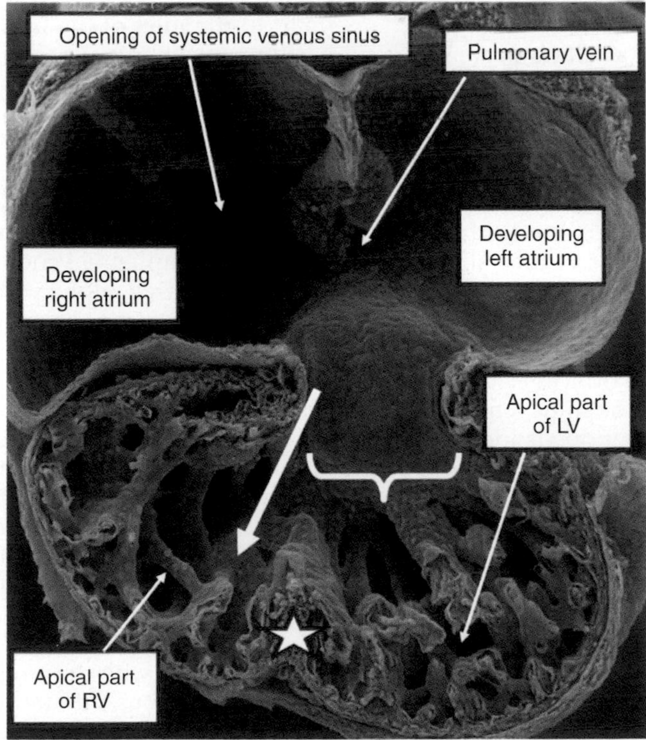

Figure 3-9 This scanning electron micrograph of a mouse heart shows how ballooning of the apical parts of the ventricles is associated with formation of the apical part of the muscular interventricular septum (*star*). Note that there is already a direct communication from the atrioventricular canal to the right ventricle (RV) (*arrow*), even though the canal is supported in its greater part by the developing left ventricle (LV) (see Fig. 3-10). The atrioventricular cushions (*brace*) occupy almost entirely the atrioventricular canal, leaving very narrow channels draining to the ventricles. The embryo is at about 10 days of development, which is comparable to 5 weeks of human development.

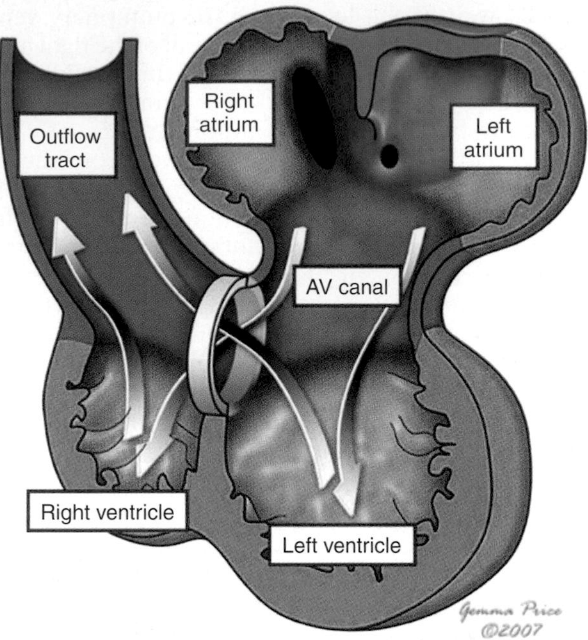

Figure 3-10 The cartoon shows how the separate streams through the heart exist from the outset of development. The outlet segment of the heart tube is supported for the most part by the outlet part of the ventricular loop, from which will form the right ventricle, but again a direct connection already exists through the lumen of the tube between the developing left ventricle and the arterial segment. It is the remodelling of the lumen of the primary tube, along with the concomitant rearrangements of the junctions with the developing atrial and arterial segments, that underscores the definitive arrangement, permitting effective closure of the plane between the bloodstreams. AV, atrioventricular.

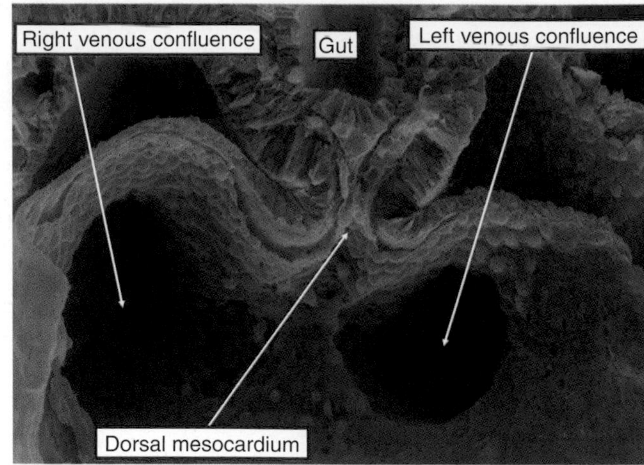

Figure 3-11 This scanning electron micrograph showing the atrial component of the developing heart reveals how the heart tube remains connected to the pharyngeal mesenchyme through the dorsal mesocardium, and how there are no boundaries at this stage between the atrial component and the systemic venous tributaries. Already, however, the confluence of the left-sided tributaries is smaller than the right-sided confluence. The embryo is at about 9 days of development, equivalent to about 4 weeks in humans.

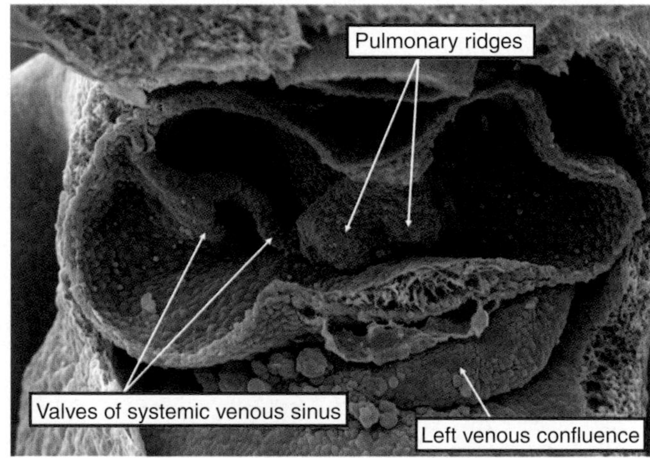

Figure 3-12 This scanning electron micrograph, at a slightly later stage than shown in Figure 3-11, shows how the systemic venous tributaries have become connected to the right side of the atrium, and how their junctions with the atrium have become distinct as the valves of the systemic venous sinus. Note the pulmonary ridges marking the site of the dorsal mesocardium (see Fig. 3-11), and the walls of the left venous confluence in the developing left atrioventricular groove. The embryo is at about 10 days of development, equivalent to 5 weeks of human development.

canal is attached in its larger part to the inlet of the heart tube, albeit that a direct connection already exists from its right side to the developing outflow tract (Fig. 3-10).

DEVELOPMENT OF THE VENOUS COMPONENTS

Subsequent to the process of looping, the venous pole of the heart tube shows a good degree of symmetry. Venous tributaries from both sides of the embryo itself, along with bilateral channels from the yolk sac, and from the placenta, drain into the atrial component of the tube through confluent orifices (Fig. 3-11). These structures are often described as the sinus venosus, with the channels draining to the atrial component identified as the horns of this venous sinus. Such a discrete component of the heart is to be found in lower animals, such as fish. No anatomically discrete structure is seen, however, in the early stages of development of the mammalian heart.[14] The venous tributaries on both sides of the embryo simply empty into the atrial component through the confluent right- and left-sided channels (see Fig. 3-11). At the initial stages, there are no landmarks indicating the junction of these venous channels with the atrial component. It is not until the systemic venous tributaries have remoulded so as to drain asymmetrically to the right side of the atrial component that structures are seen demarcating their borders, these structures then being recognised as the valves of the systemic venous sinus (Fig. 3-12). A key part of normal development, therefore, is remoulding of the systemic venous tributaries so that they open exclusively to the right side of the developing atrial component. This process involves the formation of anastomoses between right- and left-sided components of the various venous systems so that the left-sided venous return is shunted to the right side of the embryo. The major anastomosis formed in the caudal part of the embryo results in all the umbilical venous return from the placenta being diverted to the caudal part of the cardinal venous system. This anastomotic channel persists as the venous duct. The vitelline veins largely disappear, with some of these structures being incorporated into the venous system of the liver as this structure develops in the transverse septum. A second important anastomosis develops in the cranial part of the embryo, the left brachio-cephalic vein, this channel serving to divert the venous return from the left-sided to the right-sided cardinal vein. With this shift of the cranial venous return to the right-sided cardinal channel, and with the disappearance of the

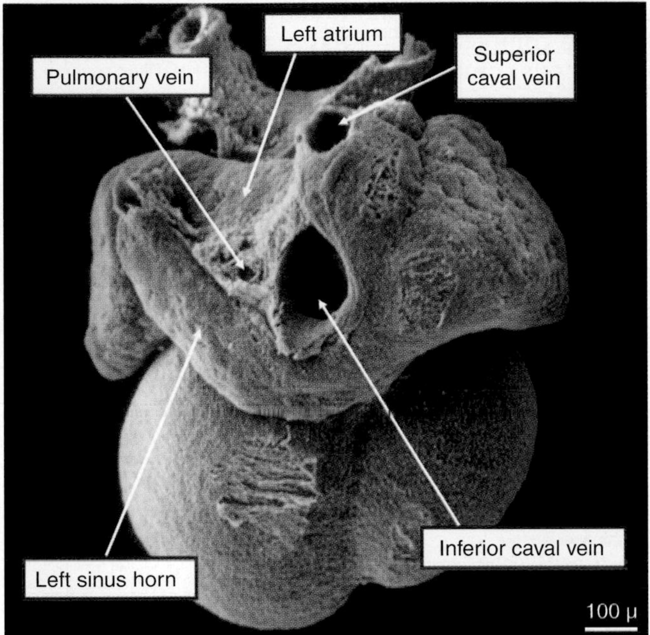

Figure 3-13 This scanning electron micrograph shows the dorsal aspect of a human heart subsequent to incorporation of the left-sided venous confluence into the left atrioventricular junction. Note that, at this stage, the pulmonary veins open through a solitary orifice immediately cranial to the left-sided venous confluence, this being the left sinus horn. The embryo is at about 6 weeks of development.

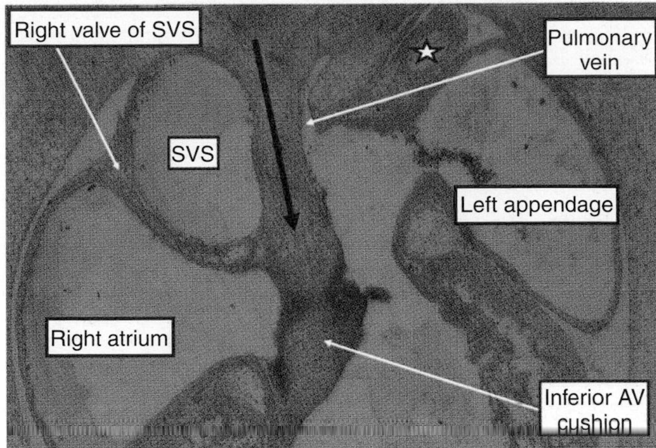

Figure 3-14 This section from a human embryo of about 5½ weeks of development, in four-chamber plane, shows the orifice of the solitary pulmonary vein sandwiched at this stage between the left-sided venous confluence (*star*), now incorporated into the left atrioventricular (AV) groove, and the remainder of the systemic venous sinus (SVS), now an integral part of the developing right atrium. Note the connection with the pharyngeal mesenchyme (*arrow*). This is the vestibular spine.

left-sided vitelline and umbilical veins, there is gradual diminution in size of the atrial orifice of the left-sided venous confluence. As this structure diminishes in size, so its walls become incorporated into the left half of the developing atrioventricular junction (Fig. 3-13). It has been suggested that a left sinuatrial wall is required to separate this channel from the left side of the developing atrium.[25] This is not the case. The left venous confluence simply retains its own walls as it is incorporated into the developing left atrioventricular groove. Subsequent to the rightward shift of the systemic venous orifices, the valvar structures appear, which then permit anatomical distinction between the systemic venous sinus and the remainder of the developing right atrium. The cranial and caudal right-sided cardinal veins, along with the orifice of the left systemic venous confluence, now open within their confines.

Remodelling of the systemic venous sinus also sets the scene for development of the pulmonary venous system. The pulmonary veins, of course, cannot appear until the lungs themselves have formed. These develop as buds on the ends of the bifurcating tracheo-bronchial tube, this structure extending from the ventral aspect of the gut, the lungs developing in the ventral part of the mediastinal mesenchyme. A further venous channel then develops from a mid-line strand formed within the mediastinal tissues.[26] This channel, when canalised, drains the developing intrapulmonary venous plexues from both lungs, and joins the heart at the site of the persisting part of the dorsal mesocardium (Fig. 3-14; see also Fig. 3-13). This part of the mesocardium persists as most of the initial structure breaks down during looping, and continues to attach the most dorsal part of the atrial component of the heart tube to the mediastinum. When the channel is viewed internally, its edges are seen as two ridges that bulge into the lumen of the atrial cavity (see Figs. 3-11 and 3-12). These are the pulmonary ridges. After the pulmonary venous channel has canalised within the mediastinum, it opens to the atrial cavity between these ridges, appearing initially as a midline structure, with its opening directly adjacent to the developing atrioventricular junction (Figs. 3-15 and 3-16).

For over a century there has been controversy as to the relationship between this newly formed pulmonary venous confluence and the tributaries of the systemic venous sinus. From the stance of the morphology,[13,27,28] and the lineage of the cells forming the pulmonary vein,[13,24,29] the evidence is now overwhelming that, during normal development, the pulmonary venous structure has never had any connection with the systemic venous tributaries. It forms as a new structure within the mediastinum, and opens within

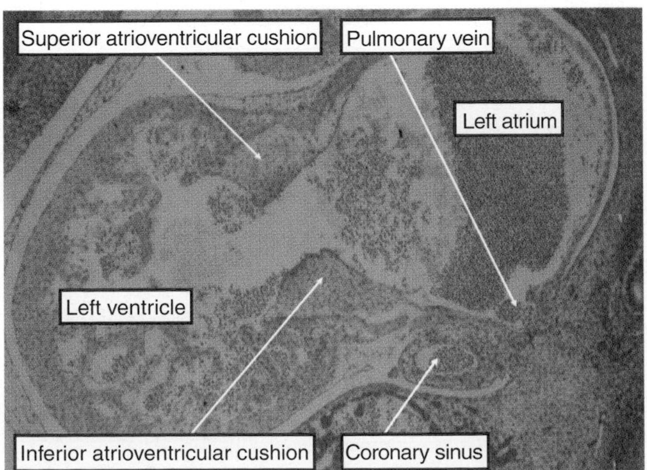

Figure 3-15 This section, also from a human embryo, and at a comparable stage to that shown in Figure 3-14, is cut in the long-axis plane. It shows the location of the solitary pulmonary venous orifice immediately cranial to the venous confluence, now incorporated into the left atrioventricular junction as the coronary sinus.

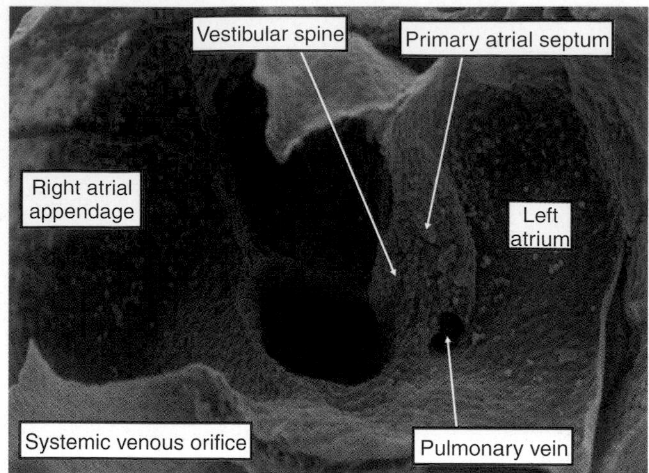

Figure 3-16 This scanning electron micrograph of a heart of a mouse embryo at 10 days of development shows the relationship of the pulmonary vein, systemic venous sinus and primary atrial septum. The atrial orifice of the pulmonary vein is directly cranial to the walls of the left venous confluence, by now incorporated into the left atrioventricular junction, and recognisable in the developing human embryo as the coronary sinus (see Fig. 3-15).

the mediastinal myocardium to the left atrium. As such, it is positioned to the left of the site of appearance of the primary atrial septum, which is also derived from mediastinal myocardium (see Fig. 3-8). The pulmonary venous structures are also recognisable from the outset as being derived from mediastinal myocardium, whereas the systemic venous tributaries initially possess a primary myocardial lineage. We have now also shown that the systemic venous tributaries can be identified in molecular terms by their expression of the transcription factor Tbx18. The pulmonary veins, in contrast, do not contain this protein.[30] When the pulmonary vein first appears, it is a mid-line structure which drains to the heart directly adjacent to the atrioventricular junction. It is only appreciably later in the development in the human heart that the venous component of the left atrium is remodelled so that, at first, separate orifices appear to drain the blood from the right and left lungs (Fig. 3-17). And it is then later still, indeed not until the completion of atrial septation, that the pulmonary venous component achieves its definitive position at the roof of the left atrium, with separate orifices on both sides for the superior and inferior veins from each of the two lungs (Fig. 3-18).

Only at this stage, when there are four pulmonary venous orifices, is it possible to see formation of the so-called secondary atrial septum. This so-called septum, in the postnatal heart, is no more than the fold between the right-sided pulmonary veins and the systemic venous tributaries (Fig. 3-19). It is not produced during development until the pulmonary channels are incorporated into the atrial roof (see Fig. 3-18). Such a superior interatrial fold is lacking in abnormal human hearts having totally anomalous pulmonary venous connection.

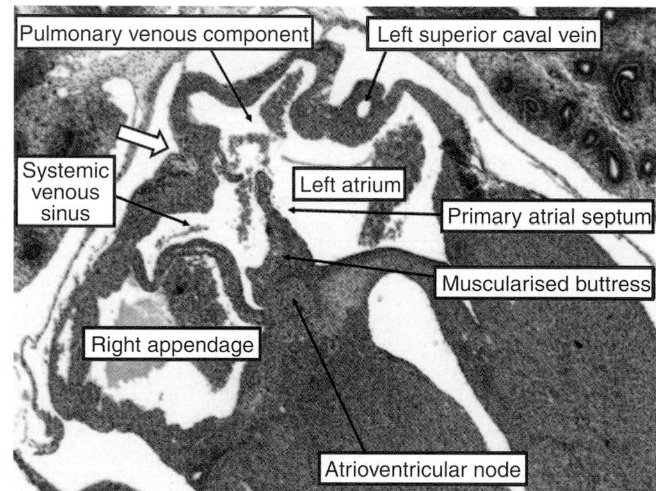

Figure 3-18 This section, again from a human embryo after the completion of septation, is at a later stage than the one shown in Figure 3-17. Note the diminution in size of the left superior caval vein, and the deepening of the superior interatrial fold, which now provides a superior buttress for the flap valve of the oval foramen. The vestibular spine and mesenchymal cushions have now muscularised to form the inferior buttress of the atrial septum.

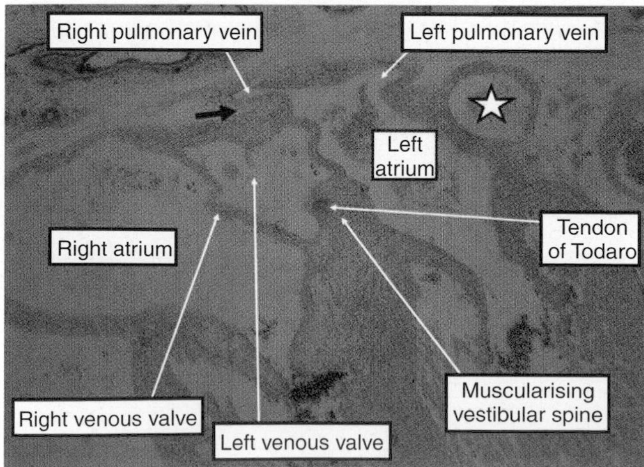

Figure 3-17 This four-chamber section is from a human heart after the completion of septation, at about 9 weeks of development, but before the pulmonary veins are completely incorporated into the atrial roof. Note the size of the coronary sinus (*star*) and that the superior interatrial infolding is as yet incomplete (*arrow*). Note also the muscularising vestibular spine and the forming tendon of Todaro.

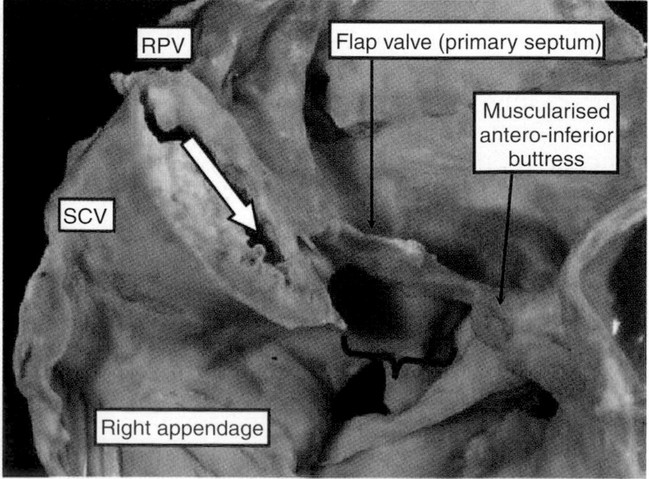

Figure 3-19 This four-chamber section is taken through the atrial chambers of an adult heart, and shows the definitive arrangement of the deep superior interatrial fold (*arrow*), the oval foramen (*brace*) and the antero-inferior muscular buttress. RPV, right pulmonary vein; SCV, superior caval vein.

SEPTATION OF THE ATRIAL CHAMBERS

With the initial rightward shift of the tributaries of the systemic venous sinus, the stage is set for septation of the atrial component of the heart. As the systemic venous sinus reorientates relative to the developing atrium, the addition of the new mediastinal myocardium forms the larger part of the body of the developing atrial component (see Fig. 3-8). The atrioventricular canal, of course, was present from the outset, and is composed of primary myocardium. The myocardium of the atrial component itself was also initially composed of primary myocardium, but as we have shown, the two appendages bud dorsocranially in symmetrical lateral fashion from this lumen, passing to either side of the developing outflow tract. With the rightward shift of the systemic venous tributaries, and the appearance of the mediastinal myocardium, so there is also a rightward shift of the dorsal corridor of primary myocardium that continues to form the floor of the systemic venous sinus. It is at this stage that we first see the appearance of the primary atrial septum, or septum primum, which grows as an interatrial shelf from the atrial roof (see Fig. 3-16). By the time that the primary atrial septum appears, endocardial cushions have also developed within the atrioventricular canal, these structure growing towards each other so as eventually to divide the canal itself into right-sided and left-sided channels (Fig. 3-20). As the cushions grow towards each other to divide the canal, so the primary septum grows towards the cushions, carrying on its leading edge a further collection of endocardial tissue, the so-called mesenchymal cap. By the time the primary septum and mesenchymal cap approach the cushions, the cranial part of the septum, at its origin from the atrial roof, has broken down, creating the secondary interatrial foramen. The primary foramen is the space between the mesenchymal cap and the fusing atrioventricular endocardial cushions (Fig. 3-21). It is then fusion of the mesenchymal cap with the endocardial cushions that obliterates the primary atrial foramen. This process occurs to the right side of the pulmonary ridges, so that the solitary opening of the newly canalised pulmonary vein is committed to the left side of the dividing atrial component, the orifices of the systemic venous tributaries, enclosed within the systemic venous valves, obviously being committed to the right side of the atrium by this selfsame process. The base of the newly formed atrial septum, formed by the mesenchymal cap, is then further reinforced by growth into the heart of mesenchymal tissue through the right pulmonary ridge (see Fig. 3-14). This process was initially illustrated by Wilhelm His the Elder, who called the protrusion seen in the caudal wall of the atrium the vestibular spine, or *spina vestibuli*.[31]

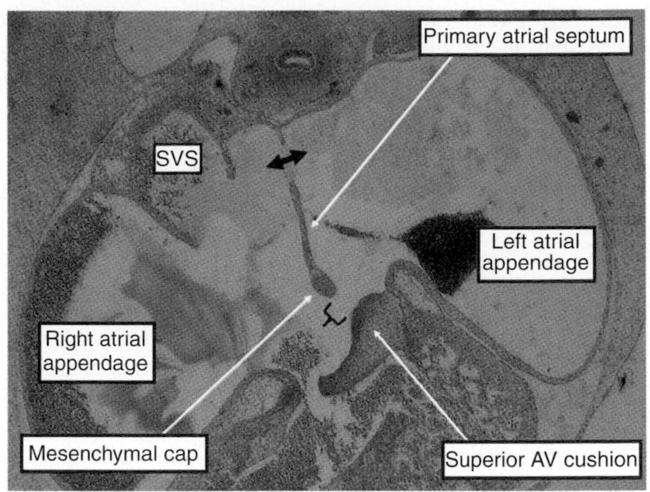

Figure 3-21 This image, in four-chamber plane, is from the same embryo as shown in Figure 3-14. This section shows the primary atrial septum, with its mesenchymal cap, growing towards the superior atrioventricular (AV) cushion. Note the primary (*brace*) and secondary (*arrow*) interatrial communications. SVS, systemic venous sinus.

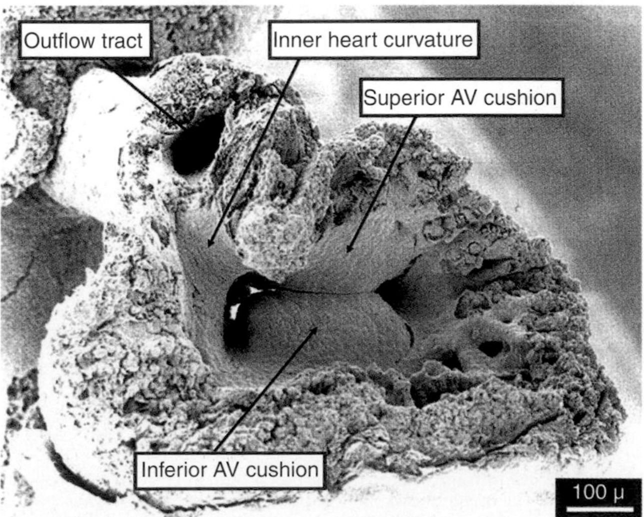

Figure 3-20 This scanning electron micrograph shows the atrioventricular junctions of the developing human heart from the ventricular aspect just prior to fusion of the atrioventricular (AV) endocardial cushions. The embryo is at about 6 weeks of development.

The mesenchymal tissue of the spine, together with the mesenchymal cap on the primary septum, then muscularises to form the buttress at the base of the atrial septum, anchoring the septum firmly against the central fibrous body, itself formed from the fused atrioventricular cushions (see Figs. 3-17 and 3-18). The so-called sinus septum is no more than the bifurcation between the orifice of the inferior caval vein and the coronary sinus within the confines of the valves of the systemic venous sinus. The right valve itself persists to varying degrees in the definitive heart, remaining as the Eustachian valve adjacent to the opening of the inferior caval vein, and the Thebesian valve in relation to the opening of the coronary sinus. These two valves join together in the musculature of the so-called sinus septum and, in the definitive heart, a fibrous structure extends through the newly muscularised buttress at the base of the atrial septum (see Fig. 3-17), extending forward to insert into the central fibrous body. This is the tendon of Todaro, an important landmark to the site of the atrioventricular conduction axis.

Subsequent to these changes, the base of the atrial septum separates the newly formed right and left atriums, but a foramen is still present at the atrial roof. This hole is an essential part of the fetal circulation, permitting the richly oxygenated placental return to reach the left side of the developing heart so as to pass to the developing brain. As explained, not until the pulmonary veins are incorporated into the atrial roof does the upper margin of this foramen become converted into the interatrial fold, often described inaccurately as the secondary atrial septum. It is the formation of the fold that provides the buttress for the flap valve

JET LIBRARY

of the definitive oval foramen, the flap itself being formed by the primary atrial septum (see Fig. 3-19). This process is not completed until well after the finish of definitive cardiac septation.[28]

After the formation of the primary atrial septum, and its reinforcement by the vestibular spine, the atrial chambers have effectively been separated one from the other. As also explained, the septum initially grows between the site of the left venous valve and the orifice of the newly formed pulmonary vein. All the tissue to the left of the venous valve is mediastinal myocardium (see Fig. 3-8), and it is this tissue which represents the body of the developing atrium. The larger part of this body is, therefore, committed to the definitive left atrium subsequent to atrial septation. If we summarise the development of the atrial components, each atrium possesses a part of the body derived from mediastinal myocardium, with the larger part committed to the morphologically left atrium. Each atrium also possesses an appendage, formed by budding from primary myocardium of the heart tube and differentiation into secondary, or chamber, myocardium, and a vestibule, derived from the initial primary myocardium of the atrioventricular canal. The venous components, in contrast, have disparate origins. The systemic venous myocardial component is formed by differentiation of Tbx18-positive mesenchyme into myocardium. The pulmonary venous myocardial component, in contrast, is derived, along with the atrial septum, from Islet1-positive mediastinal mesenchyme, itself developing from what some call the secondary heart field.

THE ATRIOVENTRICULAR CANAL

In early stages, the junction between the developing atrial component and the inlet of the ventricular loop is indeed a canal with a finite length (see Fig. 3-15). The canal itself is septated by fusion of the superior and inferior atrioventricular endocardial cushions (see Fig. 3-20). His[31] described the fused cushions as producing the intermediate septum. It is this part of the septum that is buttressed by the ingrowth of the vestibular spine, with muscularisation of the spine and mesenchymal cap forming the prominent infero-anterior rim of the oval fossa seen in the definitive heart (see Figs. 3-17 and 3-18). The cushions themselves, as we will describe subsequently, provide the foundations for formation of the aortic leaflet of the mitral valve, and the septal leaflet of the tricuspid valve. They also contribute to closure of the interventricular foramen, forming in the process the membranous part of the septum. Only subsequent to delamination of the septal leaflet of the tricuspid valve, a relatively late event, does this part become separated into atrioventricular and interventricular portions.[32]

Much has been learned in recent years concerning the endothelial to mesenchymal transformations that take place during formation of the atrioventricular cushions.[33] These events are not directly relevant to an understanding of cardiac development. It was thought, in the past, that failure of fusion of the cushions underscored the development of hearts with atrioventricular septal defect and common atrioventricular junction, for quite some time these lesions being labelled as endocardial cushion defects.[34] We now know that abnormal hearts can develop with all the features of atrioventricular septal defect subsequent to fusion of the cushions, albeit that the cushions themselves are abnormal. The problem underscoring the abnormality is one that permits the retention of the common junction, probably involving abnormal formation of the vestibular spine.[35,36] Irrespective of such niceties, there is no question but that, during normal development, the atrioventricular cushions fuse with each other to divide the atrioventricular canal into right-sided and left-sided channels (see Fig. 3-20). With ongoing development, part of the musculature of the atrioventricular canal becomes sequestrated as the atrial vestibules. We know this because of studies made using an antibody prepared against the nodose ganglion of the chicken.[37] These studies proved that this antibody, subsequent to formation of the ventricular loop, marked serendipitously a ring of cells in the developing human heart that surrounded the primary foramen (Fig. 3-22). The marked area extended from the crest of the muscular ventricular septum and included the right side of the atrioventricular canal. When human embryos were then studied subsequent to formation of the right atrioventricular junction, and commitment of the right atrium to the right ventricle, the area of the atrioventricular canal initially seen to have been marked by the antibody was located in the vestibule of the right atrium, and was separated from the ventricular myocardium by the forming insulating tissues of the right atrioventricular junction (Fig. 3-23). The insights provided by the studies using this antibody showed, therefore, that part of the atrioventricular canal musculature became sequestrated as the atrial vestibules with ongoing development. The studies also provided important insights into remodelling of the primary interventricular foramen, which we will discuss further in our next section. We now know that the parietal wall of the inlet of the left ventricle is also derived from the initial primary myocardium of the atrioventricular canal, at least in the mouse heart. This knowledge comes from the development of a mutant mouse in which the gene *Tbx2* was used to mark

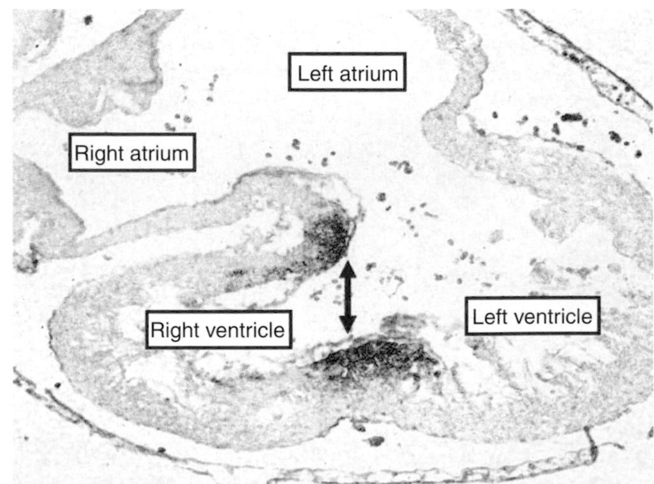

Figures 3-22 An immuno-stained section of a human embryo at 5 weeks of development. The image shows the location of the ring of cells (*double-headed arrow*) demarcated by the antibody to the nodose ganglion of the chick prior to expansion of the atrioventricular canal. This ring demarcates the myocardium surrounding the so-called primary foramen, a part of the primary heart tube that defines the outlet of the forming left ventricle and the inlet of the forming right ventricle.

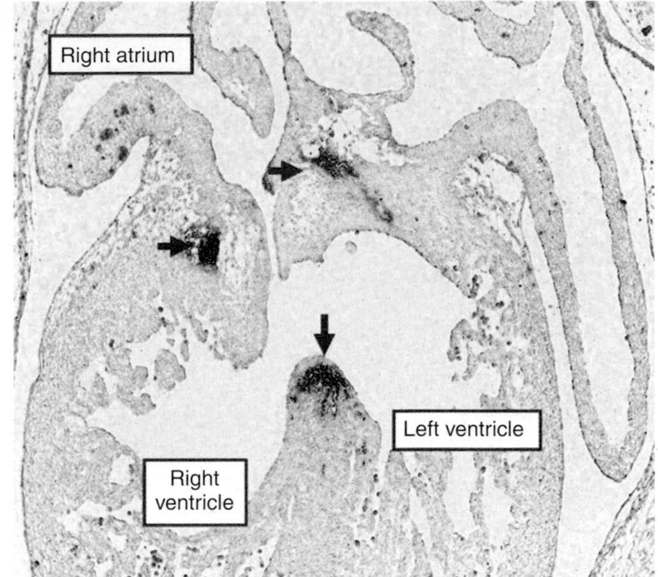

Figure 3-23 This image, also immuno-stained using the antibody to the nodose ganglion of the chick, shows how the interventricular ring (*arrows*), by 6 weeks of development has come to surround the newly formed right atrioventricular junction, along with the developing outflow tract of the aorta from the left ventricle.

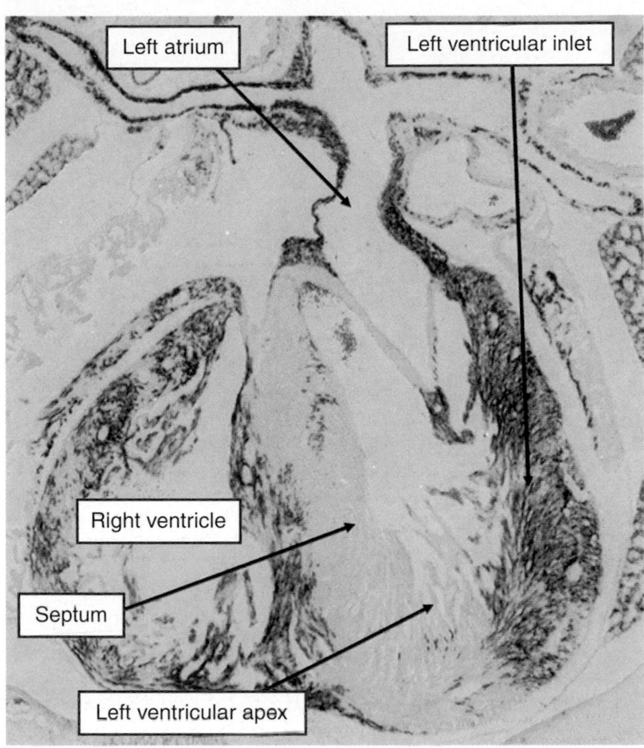

Figure 3-24 This image shows a cross section of a murine heart from an embryo at 17.5 days of development. The mouse has been created so as to show the lineage of the cells making up the atrioventricular canal and the outflow tract at 9.5 days of development, by crossing a *Tbx2 cre* mouse with an *R26R* mouse. Use of this lineage study means that all the cells derived from the atrioventricular canal, which is marked by *Tbx2* at 9.5 days of development, are subsequently coloured blue. As can be seen, the inlet part of the left ventricle is coloured blue, showing that the cells forming this part of the ventricle were derived from the atrioventriular canal. The septum, and the apical component, are largely unmarked. (Courtesy of Dr Vincent Christoffels, University of Amsterdam, Amsterdam, The Netherlands.)

the lineage of the initial myocardium in the atrioventricular canal (Fig. 3-24). The studies, as yet unpublished, showed that, whilst the parietal wall of the left ventricular inlet is marked by the gene-encoded product the greater part of the septum is free from marked cells. The septum, therefore, along with the apical component develops from the chamber myocardium of the left embryonic ventricle.

FURTHER DEVELOPMENT OF THE VENTRICULAR LOOP

The confusion that existed concerning the way in which the ventricular loop became converted into the definitive ventricles,[38] and which received considerable attention in the previous edition of this book,[2] has been resolved in part by the use of descriptive terms for the inlet and outlet parts of the loop, and in part by recognition that the apical parts of the ventricles balloon out in series from the lumen of the primary tube, the apical part of the left ventricle ballooning from the inlet, and the right ventricular apical part from the outlet (see Fig. 3-9). It had long been recognised that functional separation of the left-sided and right-sided bloodstreams had taken place long before the completion of ventricular septation, so that two parallel bloodstreams, instead of a single one, traverse the serial segments (see Fig. 3-10). Development of the ventricles simply proceeds by partitioning these bloodstreams so that the one originating from the right side of the atrioventricular canal becomes channeled to the pulmonary trunk, whilst the one commencing at the left side of the atrioventricular canal is committed to the aorta. In addition to requiring marked remodelling of the inner heart curvature, this process also requires appropriate septation of the outlet component of the primary heart tube.

Expansion of the right side of the atrioventricular junction is sufficient to place the cavity of the right atrium in more direct communication with the apical part ballooned from the outlet part of the ventricular loop. The mechanics of this expansion are well illustrated by the fate of the ring of cells marked by the antibody to the nodose ganglion of the chick, and illustrated in Figs. 3-22 and 3-23.[37] The fate of this ring of marked cells also shows that, during ongoing development, the outlet part of the heart tube is reorientated so that its dorsal half becomes the outlet from the left ventricle. Concomitant with this reorientation, the proximal parts of the cushions that have developed and fused to divide the outlet segment of the primary tube into pulmonary and aortic channels are brought into alignment with the crest of the muscular ventricular septum (Fig. 3-25), the latter structure, as we have already shown, being formed by the apical ballooning of the chamber myocardium of the right and left ventricles (see Fig. 3-9). This remodelling of the cavity of the initial heart tube, providing an effective inlet to the apical part of the right ventricle, and an outlet for the apical part of the left ventricle, then permits the middle part of the initial foramen to be closed by apposition of tissue derived from both the atrioventricular and outlet endocardial cushions[39,40] (Fig. 3-26).

Before moving on to consider the formation of the atrioventricular valves, obviously crucial features of the definitive ventricles, it is convenient first to discuss the changes that take place with the outlet segment of the heart tube, and the arteries it feeds within the developing pharyngeal mesenchyme.

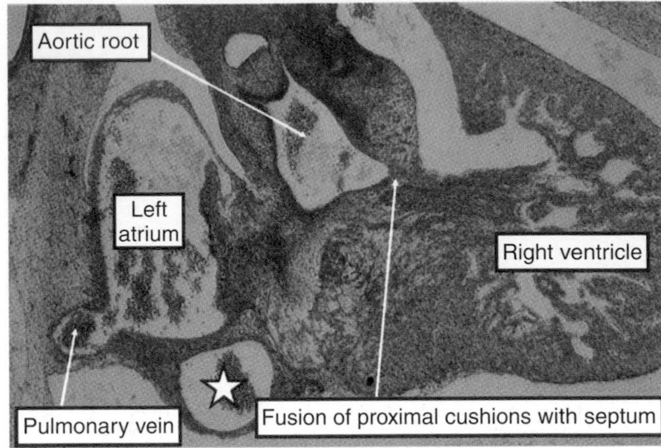

Figure 3-25 This section through a human embryo at about 7 weeks of development, cut in frontal plane, replicating the oblique subcostal echocardiographic cut, shows how fusion of the muscularising proximal cushions of the outflow tract with the ventricular septum walls the aorta into the left ventricle. The *star* shows the coronary sinus. Note the pulmonary venous orifice adjacent to the sinus at this stage of development.

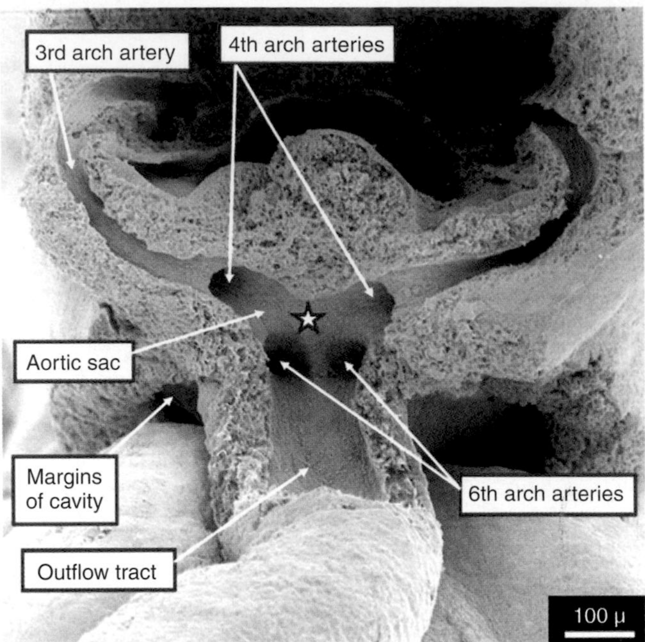

Figure 3-27 This scanning electron micrograph of a human embryo at around 6 weeks of development shows the junction of the outflow tract with the so-called aortic sac. The sac is no more than a manifold within the pharyngeal mesenchyme that gives rise to the arteries running through the pharyngeal arches, at this stage the third, fourth, and sixth arches. The *star* shows the dorsal wall of the sac, which represents the aorto-pulmonary septum.

THE OUTLET SEGMENT

It is, perhaps, the outlet segment of the heart about which we have learnt most since the appearance of the second edition of our book.[2] In the first place, as we have now emphasised several times, we now know that this part of the developing heart is derived from a secondary source, different at least in temporal terms from that producing the initial linear heart tube. In the second place, although the larger parts of the intrapericardial outflow tracts in the definitive heart have arterial walls, the entirety of the outlet segment, when initially formed, has walls made of myocardium. In the third place, we now know that the so-called aortic sac is little more than a manifold giving rise to the arteries that extend through the arches of the pharyngeal mesenchyme. In previous accounts, notions of division of this sac, and the outlet segment itself, by growth of an aortopulmonary septum have been grossly exaggerated. We also now know that migration of cells from the neural crest is crucial for normal development of this part of the heart, and for its separation into the pulmonary and aortic channels. In this section, therefore, we will seek to correlate our own findings and observations with currently existing concepts of development.

The distal extent of the developing outlet segment of the heart tube, subsequent to the completion of ventricular looping, is marked by the margins of the pericardial cavity. At this stage of development, the outlet is a tube with a solitary lumen, taking its origin from the outlet of the ventricular loop. At its distal extent, marked by the pericardial reflections, the lumen becomes confluent with the area known as the aortic sac (Fig. 3-27). At this early stage, the walls of the tube are exclusively myocardial. Endocardium is then formed in the luminal lining, again by a process of mesenchymal to endothelial transformation as occurs with the atrioventricular cushions, but the endocardial jelly

Figure 3-26 These scanning electron micrographs show the back (**A**) and the front (**B**) of a transected mouse heart at 11½ days of development, equivalent to the sixth week of development in the human. As can be seen in panel **B**, the embryonic interventricular foramen (*red dotted circle* in **B**) will be closed by adherence of the atrioventricular (AV) and outflow cushions. In this panel, the front part of the heart is viewed from behind. LV, left ventricle; RV, right ventricle.

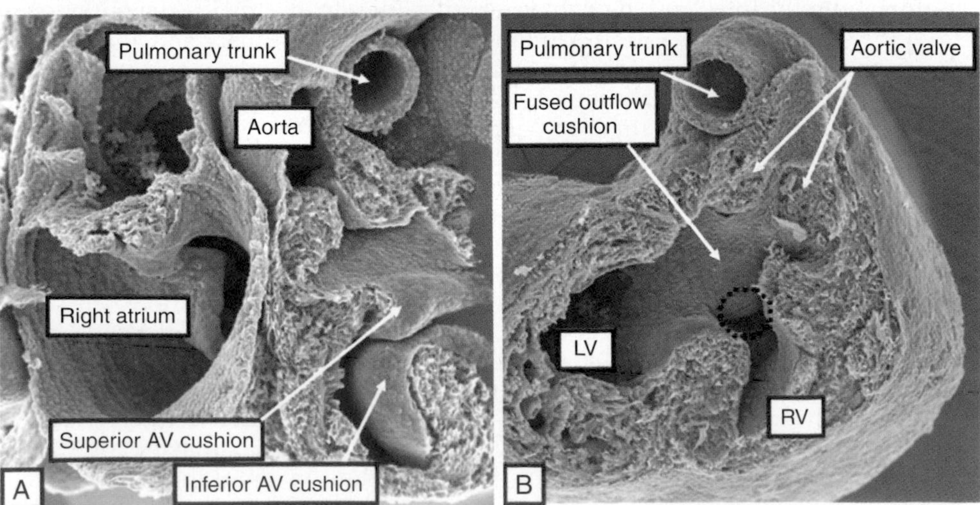

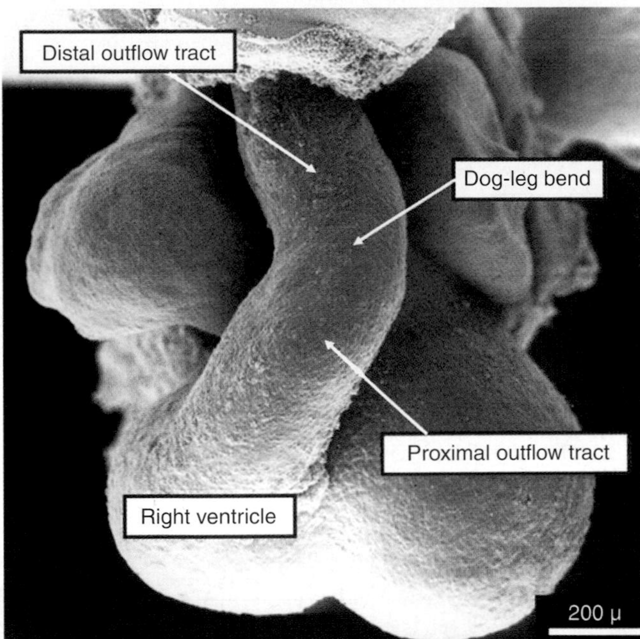

Figure 3-28 This scanning electron micrograph of a human embryo at around 6 weeks of development shows the external aspect of a human embryo when the outflow tract is a muscular tube. Note how it is divided into proximal and distal parts by the dog-leg bend.

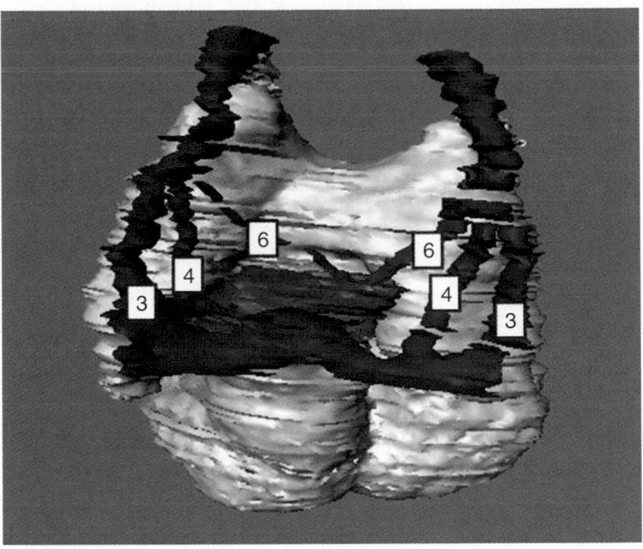

Figure 3-30 This cranial view of the developing mouse heart at 11 days of development shows the stage at which the third, fourth and sixth arteries, running through the pharyngeal arches, take their origin from the aortic sac. Note that, already, the right sixth arch artery is smaller than the left one. The *green* tissues are the arterialised component of the outflow tract, within the pericardial cavity. (Courtesy of Dr. Sandra Webb, St George's Medical University, London, United Kingdom.)

initially lines the entirety of the tube in circumferential fashion. When viewed externally at this stage, the tube has an obvious bend, permitting the distinction of proximal and distal parts (Fig. 3-28). At the margins of the pericardial cavity, the lumen is continuous with the space in the ventral pharyngeal mesenchyme from which originate the arteries that initially run symmetrically through the developing pharyngeal arches. These arteries encircle the gut and the developing tracheobronchial groove, uniting dorsally to form the descending aorta. Although it is frequent for cartoons representing this stage to show five pairs of arteries, in reality there are never more than two or three pairs of arches, along with their arteries, to be seen at any one time. At the earliest stage, at least in the mouse, the mediastinal space has right and left horns, with each horn giving rise to the arteries of the first to third arches (Fig. 3-29). These arteries rapidly become assimilated into the arterial system of the head and face. By the time it becomes possible to recognise the arteries of the fourth and sixth arches, the arteries within the fourth arch are feeding the arteries of the third arches, and it is no longer possible to recognise the arteries of the initial two arches as encircling structures (Fig. 3-30). The cavity of the so-called aortic sac by this stage is little more than the continuation of the lumen of the outlet segment beyond the pericardial boundaries. It is still possible, nonetheless, to recognise obvious proximal and distal parts of the outlet segment, with a marked dog-leg bend between them. Within the lumen, throughout the tract, the endocardial tissue has now thickened to form opposing cushions, or ridges. When traced proximally to distally, the ridges spiral. The ridge that is parietal at the proximal end of the outlet turns beneath the other ridge at the bend, and achieves a caudal location within the distal outflow tract. The ridge that is septal proximally spirals to become positioned cranially at the distal extent of the outlet. This means that, as the ridges approximate one another, fusing along their facing surfaces, the proximal outflow tract will eventually be separated into ventral and dorsal channels, whilst fusion of the ridges distally will produce right-sided and left-sided channels. Fusion of the ridges, or cushions, however, does not occur at the same time, but rather commences distally, with the act of closure moving in proximal direction. Prior to the commencement of fusion, important changes have also taken place in the aortic sac. There is marked diminution in size of the right-sided arteries running from the sac to join the descending aorta (Fig. 3-31).

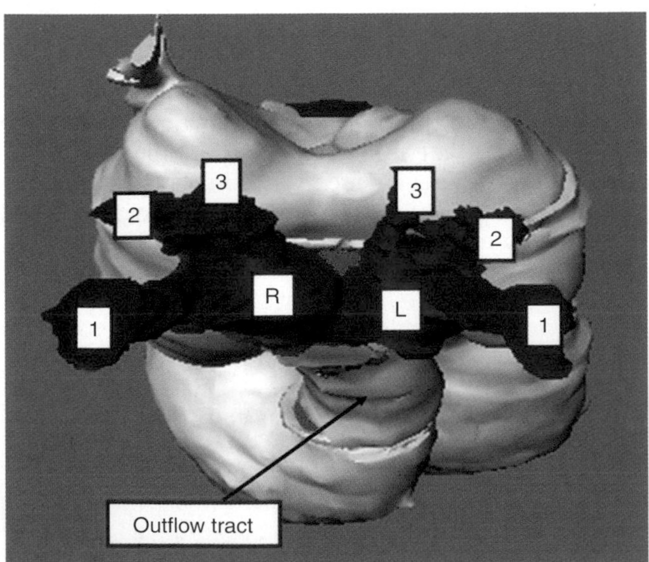

Figure 3-29 At this early stage of development of the mouse heart, at 10 days, the aortic sac gives rise to right and left horns (R, L), each of which supplies the arteries to the first three pharyngeal arches (numbered 1 to 3) in symmetrical fashion. (Courtesy of Dr. Sandra Webb, St George's Medical University, London, United Kingdom.)

As the dorsal parts of the arteries running with the right pharyngeal arches begin to involute, so it becomes possible

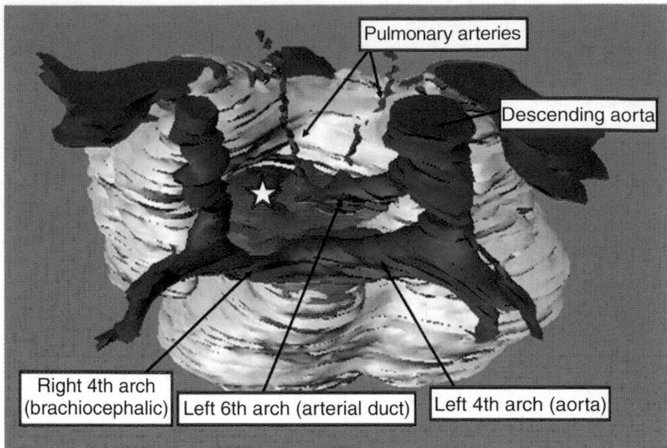

Figure 3-31 The stage in the mouse heart, at 12 days of development, after remodelling of the arteries running through the pharyngeal pouches. The heart is viewed from above. Note that the systemic arteries, namely the fourth arch, arise from the cranial and rightward part of the outflow tract, again shown in *green*, whilst the pulmonary channels, the sixth arch, arise from the leftward and caudal part. Note also the appearance of the pulmonary arteries themselves, but that the right sixth arch has involuted (*star*). Only the left fourth arch now communicates with the descending aorta, which is left sided. Compare with Figure 3-31. (Courtesy of Dr. Sandra Webb, St George's Medical University, London, United Kingdom.)

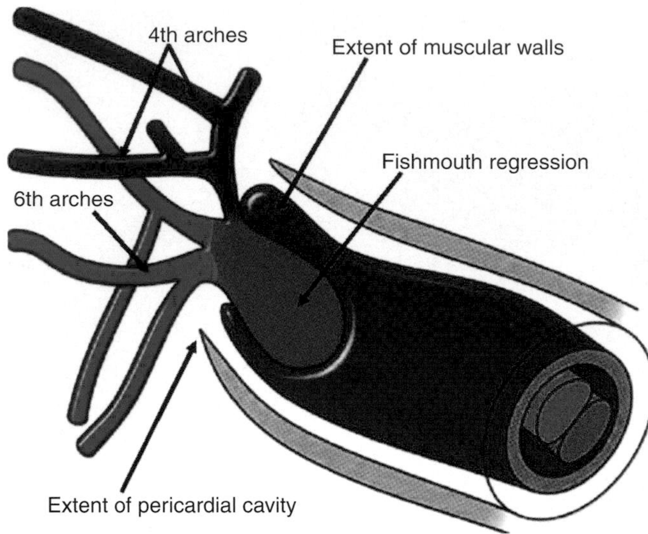

Figure 3-32 The drawing, made from the reconstruction of a human embryo reported by Bartelings and Gittenberger-de Groot,[41] shows the initial regression of the muscular walls of the outflow tract at the distal margin of the pericardial sac concomitant with invasion of the walls by non-myocardial cells from the pharyngeal mesenchyme.

to recognise the developing pulmonary arteries, which course caudally within the ventral mesenchyme of the mediastinum to feed the rapidly growing lung buds. The effect of these changes is that the aortic sac now gives rise to only two sets of arteries, located cranially and caudally, with the orifices of the left-sided arteries being appreciably larger than those seen to the right, particularly for the arteries running within the sixth arch. Throughout this process of remoulding, it has been the dorsal wall of the pharyngeal mesenchyme, separating the origins of the pairs of arteries running through the fourth and sixth arches, which represents the so-called aortopulmonary septum. It is this tissue that separates the flow from the cranial part of the outflow tract and aortic sac to the fourth arch and the developing brachiocephalic arteries from that flowing to the caudal part, which now feeds the two pulmonary arteries and the artery of the left sixth arch, representing the arterial duct, the right sixth arch having involuted (see Fig. 3-31). Concomitant with the remodelling of the arteries within the pharyngeal arches, cells have begun to grow from the pharyngeal mesenchyme into the distal ends of the outlet segment, growing parietally between the ends of the distal ridges or cushions to replace the initially myocardial walls. The tongues of tissue thus formed, which rapidly arterialise, produce at the same time a fishmouth appearance for the remaining myocardial margins of the outflow tract, as initially emphasised by Bartelings and Gittenberger-de Groot[41] (Fig. 3-32). The tongues run between the distal extents of the cranial and caudal ridge, which reach almost to the margins of the pericardial cavity.

So as finally to separate the developing channels for the pulmonary and systemic circulations, it is necessary for the right-sided channel within the distal outflow tract to be joined to the cranial part of the persisting aortic sac, and for the left-sided channel to be directed to the floor of the aortic sac, the two pulmonary arteries, and the left-sided artery running within the sixth arch. The mechanics of this process have still to be fully elucidated, but most current accounts correlate the process with growth of an aortopulmonary septum. As Los[42] emphasised, such a septum can readily be identified in reconstructions of the lumens of the arteries arising from the aortic sac, but is difficult to identify in reconstructions of the pharyngeal mesenchyme. As we have shown, supporting the findings of Los,[42] the aortopulmonary septum in reality is no more than the mesenchymal tissue separating the lumens of the arteries running through the fourth and sixth arches. And as can be seen in scanning electron micrographs,[43] this tissue is simply the most prominent of a series of interarterial structures (see Fig. 3-27).

The precise mechanics of the way in which the dorsal wall of the aortic sac, representing the aortopulmonary septum, fuses with the distal margins of the outlet ridges remains to be clarified, as does any role the ridges themselves may play in formation of the walls of the intrapericardial arterial trunks. As we have seen, nonetheless, it is the parietal portions of myocardium at the distal margins of the outflow segment that are initially replaced by ingrowths from the pharyngeal mesenchyme. Additional migrations then occur through these right and left sides of the outflow segment to populate the cushions themselves. These migrating cells are derived from the neural crest.[44] Indeed, it is the cells from the neural crest that fill the larger parts of the fusing cushions, so they could well be described as neural crest cushions, rather than endocardial cushions. The central part of the pharyngeal mesenchyme, furthermore, which forms the initial aortopulmonary septum, save for a thin luminal cap, is not populated by cells derived from the neural crest (Fig. 3-33).

It is the fusion of the distal ends of the ridges with each other, and also with the dorsal wall of the aortic sac, that serves to connect the right-sided channel within the distal outflow tract to the cranial systemic arteries, and the left-sided channel to the caudally positioned pulmonary arteries and the artery of the left sixth arch. In essence, this process obliterates a previously existing aortopulmonary foramen (Fig. 3-34). As

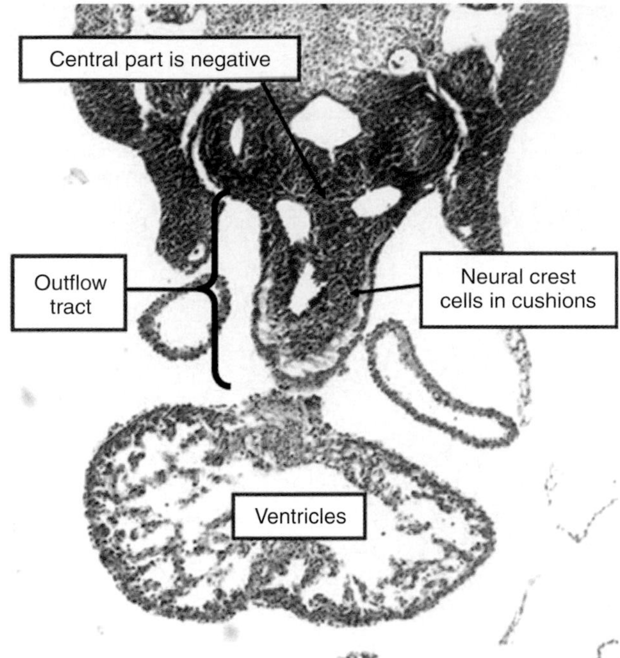

Figure 3-33 This frontal section shows the origin of the arteries feeding the fourth and sixth arches from the aortic sac in a mouse at about 11 days of development, and programmed to show cells derived from the neural crest as *blue.* The cells populate the cushions within the outflow tract, but the dorsal wall of the sac, the so-called aortopulmonary septum, does not contain cells derived from the crest. (Courtesy of Dr. Sandra Webb, St George's Medical University, London, United Kingdom.)

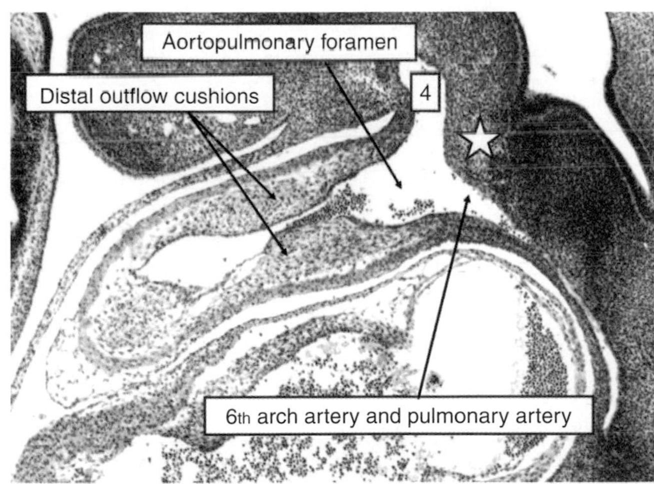

Figure 3-34 This sagittal section through a human embyo at 6 weeks of development shows how fusion of the distal cushions with each other, and with the dorsal pharyngeal mesenchyme (*star*), will close the aortopulmonary foramen, and separate the systemic (fourth arch) from the pulmonary pathways.

part of this process, there is also rapid proximal regression of the jaws of the fishmouth of outflow myocardium, so that the distal segment of the outflow tract comes to attain non-myocardial walls. There is delay in formation of the adjacent walls of the newly formed intrapericardial pulmonary trunk and aorta when compared with the parietal walls, the latter being formed, as we have described, by the initial ingrowths of non-myocardial tissue from the pharyngeal mesenchyme (Fig. 3-35). Whether the arterialising adjacent walls are derived from the distal parts of the cushions themselves, or

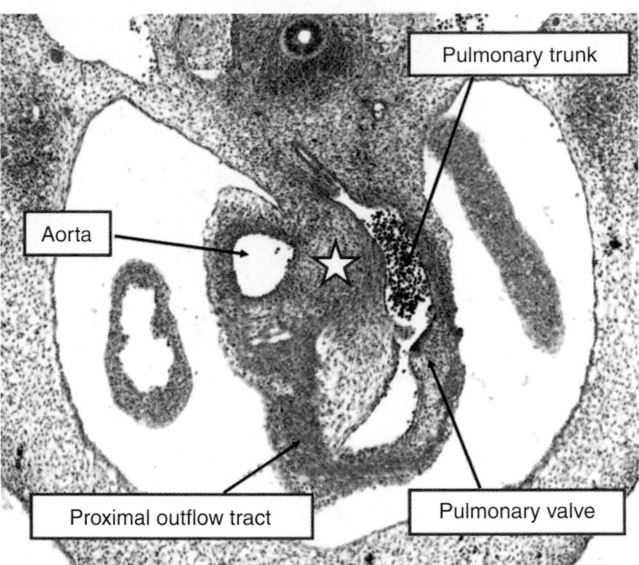

Figure 3-35 In this human embryo at about 6½ weeks of development, the aortopulmonary foramen has been closed, and the walls of the intrapericardial arterial trunks are arterialising. Note, however, that the parietal walls of both trunks are better formed than the adjacent walls, which are separated by a mass of tissue continuous with the pharyngeal mesenchyme (*star*). This tissue will eventually disappear. Note also that the cushions are still present in the proximal outflow tract, with the pulmonary valve beginning to form in the intermediate section.

are delaminated from the cranial and caudal margins of the pharyngeal mesenchyme at the margins of the pericardial cavity, has still to be determined. It is possible to recognise, nonetheless, a spur of pharyngeal mesenchyme, comparable in many ways to the vestibular spine, from which are formed at least part of the arterialising adjacent walls of the intrapericardial arterial trunks (see Fig. 3-35). This spur is the remnant of the aortopulmonary septum, which will disappear as the aorta and pulmonary trunk develop their own walls in their intrapericardial course.

At the stage at which the distal part of the outflow tract has separated into the intrapericardial parts of the aorta and pulmonary trunk, the most proximal parts of the outflow ridges remain unfused, albeit that the ridges have fused at the now separated origins of the arterial trunks. By now, additional cushions have appeared in the parietal parts of the aortic and pulmonary channels, the pulmonary cushion being placed much more cranially compared with the aortic cushion. These are the intercalated cushions. It is cavitation within the distal ends of these cushions, and also within the opposite ends of the now fused original outflow cushions, that produces the primordiums of the aortic and pulmonary valves (Fig. 3-36). This process takes place within the persisting cuff of outflow myocardium, which still encloses the outflow tract as far distally as the origins of the intrapericardial arterial trunks. The site of origin of the aorta and pulmonary trunk, in the region of the bend of the outflow tract, will become the sinutubular junctions, again with the pulmonary junction located more cranially and leftward when compared with the developing aortic sinutubular junction. As the cushions cavitate, so the outside part of the cavity, next to the myocardial cuff, arterialises to become the walls of the arterial valvar sinuses, whilst the inside part of each cavity, adjacent to the arterial lumen, remodels to become the valvar leaflets.

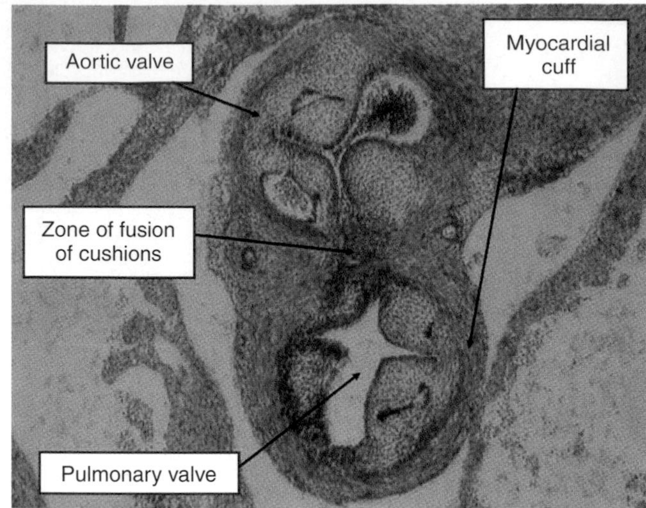

Figure 3-36 This section from a human embryo at around 7 weeks of development has cut through the short axis of the developing arterial valves. Note that both valves are still surrounded by a myocardial cuff. The sinuses and leaflets are forming by a process of cavitation of the cushions. Note also the site of the initial zone of fusion between the cushions. The arterial roots will separate at right angles to this plane.

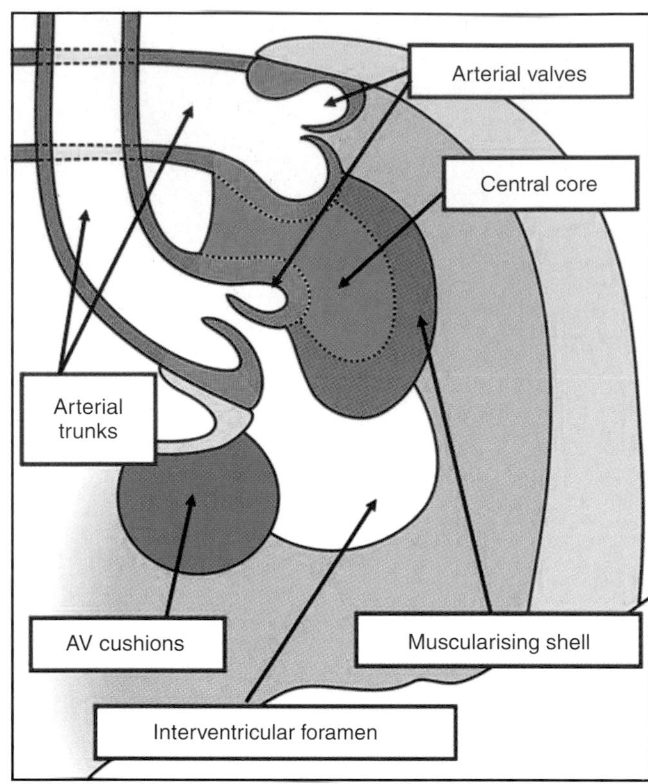

Figure 3-37 The cartoon shows how the distal part of the outflow tract has formed the intrapericardial parts of the arterial trunks (*green*), and the middle part has given rise to the valvar leaflets and their supporting sinuses (*yellow*), while the proximal parts of the cushions muscularise to form the subpulmonary infundibulum (*pink*). The core of the cushions, filled with cells from the neural crest (*purple*), disappears so as to produce the tissue plane between the infundibulum and the aorrtic root. The proximal cushions then fuse with the ventricular septum so as to wall the aorta into the left ventricle (see Fig. 3-25). AV, atrioventricular.

The opposing edges of the cushions themselves do not fuse, thus producing the trifoliate arrangement of the aortic and pulmonary valves (see Fig. 3-36). The middle part of the cushions breaks down along a line which is normal to the line of fusion so that, eventually, the newly formed aortic root is separate from the pulmonary root. This middle part of the fused cushions was initially occupied by the cells derived from the neural crest, which die during this process by apoptosis.[45]

At the initial stage of formation of the arterial valves and their supporting sinuses from the middle part of the outflow tract, the proximal parts of the cushions are themselves still unfused. As these cushions fuse with each other, so they also fuse with the crest of the ventricular septum, this having been formed concomitant with the ballooning of the apical parts of the right and left ventricles. At the same time, there is muscularisation of the most proximal part of the fused cushions, whilst the middle part, occupied by the cells migrating from the neural crest, again disappears by the process of apoptosis. In this way, the caudal part of the proximal outflow tract becomes committed to the left ventricle, taking with it the newly formed aortic valve, while the cranial part now forms the exclusive outlet from the right ventricle, feeding the newly formed pulmonary valve. The muscularised part of the fused proximal cushions becomes the subpulmonary infundibulum, while the apoptosis of the cells migrating from the neural crest creates the tissue plane which separates the subpulmonary infundibulum from the aortic root (Fig. 3-37). At the stage at which the proximal parts of the fused outflow cushions themselves fuse also with the crest of the muscular ventricular septum, so the remaining interventricular foramen is closed by apposition of the outflow cushions with the atrioventricular cushions (see Fig. 3-25).[39] At this stage, the musculature of the inner heart curvature continues to separate the developing leaflets of the aortic valve, by now committed to the left ventricle, from the forming aortic leaflet of the mitral valve. It is only at a much later stage that this muscle disappears, producing the aortic-to-mitral valvar continuity that is a feature of the postnatal heart. Similarly, it is at much later stages, once more by a process of apoptosis, that the muscular cuff surrounding the developing arterial roots disappears so that the arterial valvar sinuses form the external walls of the pulmonary and aortic roots.[46]

FORMATION OF VALVES

Valves are formed at several locations within the developing heart, in all instances preventing regurgitation to a proximal segment. This is the only common feature, since there are marked differences in both morphogenesis and final structure at the various levels.

The Sinuatrial Valves

The valve-like structures seen at the sinuatrial junction are most conspicuous during the stages of development. The left-sided valve of the systemic venous sinus reinforces the right side of the developing atrial septal structures, albeit that, when first seen, an intersepto-valvar space can be recognised, the wall of this space being formed from mediastinal myocardium. This is the body of the right atrium, but its site cannot be recognised in the mature heart. The right valve of the systemic venous sinus does remain recognisable, albeit seen to various extents postnatally in different individuals. Its ventral portion persists to guard the orifice of the coronary sinus, and is known as the Thebesian valve. The dorsal part persists as the Eustachian valve, which guards the orifice of the inferior caval vein. This valve varies considerably in postnatal life. In some individuals, it may reach sufficiently far to provide a valve also for the mouth of the superior caval vein, but this is rare unless the heart itself is malformed. More usually, the Eustachian valve is not so large, and mostly disappears, leaving only a remnant attached to the muscular terminal crest. This internal ridge corresponds with the external terminal groove, and marks the boundary between the smooth-walled systemic venous sinus, initially composed of primary myocardium, and the pectinated wall of the atrial appendage formed from secondary, or chamber, myocardium. In early stages, this right valve is a muscular structure, but it becomes a fibrous flap in the mature heart.

The Atrioventricular Valves

As we have already described, the atrioventricular canal is initially lined by a continuous mass of endocardial jelly, from which develop gradually, by the process of mesenchymal to endothelial transformation, the superior and inferior atrioventricular endocardial cushions. In the early stages, these cushions themselves have a valve-like function. They also provide the scaffold for formation of parts of the definitive valvar leaflets, with their left ventricular components fusing to form the aortic leaflet of the mitral valve, and the right ventricular parts the septal leaflet of the tricuspid valve.[47,48] Additional cushions also develop within the lateral parts of the atrioventricular canal which provide the primordiums of the other valvar leaflets. There is also initially delamination of the luminal part of the ventricular myocardium at the sites of the cushions, but analysis of lineage shows that the definitive leaflets do not have a myocardial heritage, so the delaminating myocardium must subsequently disappear. The points of attachment of the myocardium within the ventricles compact as the trabeculated part of the ventricular wall also disappears, these compacted areas persisting as the papillary muscles. Not all the leaflets mature at the same time. Formation of the septal leaflet of the tricuspid valve, in particular, is an extremely late event. As we have already described, it is the final steps of this undermining that lead to differentiation of the atrioventricular and interventricular parts of the membranous septum, a process which often remains incomplete at the time of birth.[32]

The Arterial Valves

We have already described the processes involved in formation of the arterial valves, and we will not reiterate this information, save to say that, as yet, we do not know how the cushions differentiate separately to form, on the one hand, the valvar leaflets, and, on the other hand, the supporting valvar sinuses.

THE CONDUCTION SYSTEM

It is, perhaps, knowledge regarding the development of the so-called conduction tissues of the heart that has been aided most by the recent development of genetic and molecular biological techniques. As we write this chapter, it is exactly 100 years since Keith and Flack[49] described the anatomical location of the cardiac pacemaker, and just over 100 years since Sunao Tawara, a Japanese pathologist working with Aschoff in Marburg, clarified the structure of the morphological axis responsible for atrioventricular conduction, his wonderful monograph now available in an English translation.[50] Shortly after these giants described the cardiac nodes in such splendid fashion, the first suggestion was made that histologically recognisable structures joined together the pacemaker and the node responsible for delaying the cardiac impulse.[51] This, in turn, triggered an important debate at the meeting of the German Pathological Society held in Erlangen in 1910, from which emerged the two publications that established the anatomical criteri for recognition of those structures that we now describe as the cardiac conduction tissues.[52,53] On the basis of these suggestions, which retain their currency even in the era of molecular biology as the gold standard for histological recognition of the so-called conduction tissues, we can state that specialised conduction tracts need to be histologically distinct, traced from section to section in serially prepared material, and insulated by fibrous tissue from the adjacent working myocardium. The cardiac nodes are recognised on the basis of their histological characteristics, and again the ability to follow them from section to section, since it would defeat their purpose if they, too, were insulated from the adjacent myocardial tissues.

When we examine the developing heart, areas of myocardium satisfying these criterions are not recognised until the heart is well formed. Long before these stages, however, it is possible to record an electrocardiogram from the developing embryo. This is because all myocardial cells within the heart have the ability to conduct the cardiac impulse. The electrocardiogram is seen as soon as the heart tube develops areas permitting fast as opposed to slow conduction. This is seen concomitant with the appearance of the chamber, or secondary, myocardium that balloons from the linear heart tube.[54] This chamber myocardium conducts rapidly, its cells being linked by multiple connexins that are absent from the slowly conducting primary myocardium of the linear heart tube. At this early stage, of course, the primary myocardium forms the atrioventricular canal, the outflow tract and also a corridor of myocardium extending from the atrioventricular canal to incorporate the orifices of the systemic venous tributaries. In the developing murine heart, this myocardium can be recognised by its content of the transcription factor *Tbx3* gene. This gene also marks the entirety of the atrioventricular canal at an early stage, and shows the location of the ring of cells demarcated by the Gln1 antibody in the human heart, which we know will become the atrioventricular conduction axis initially demonstrated by Tawara.[50] With ongoing development, the tissues remaining positive for the transcription factor become smaller, concomitant with the development of the mediastinal myocardium, and the commitment of the systemic venous tributaries to the right atrium. Eventually, only the atrioventricular node and the sinus node remain *Tbx3* positive, although the location of the tissues initially positive for *Tbx3* within the atrial vestibules, around the mouth of the coronary sinus and along the terminal crest offers some explanation for the origins of arrhythmic activity in patients with atrial arrhythmias.[55] Initially, the myocardium surrounding both the left and right cardinal veins displays a nodal phenotype.[30] This so-called sinus myocardium is derived from Tbx18-positive mesenchyme, and is gradually recruited to the myocardial lineage at the systemic venous tributaries. It is fundamentally different from the so-called pulmonary myocardium that, from the outset has a working myocardial phenotype, and is derived from Islet1-positive mesenchyme.[29] The tissue related to the orifice of the superior caval vein, initially the cranial cardinal vein, is known to be the site of cardiac pacemaking. We now know that it is the presence of Tbx3 that maintains the tissues added to the venous pole as the leading pacemaker,[56] and this tissue eventually forms the sinus node at the cranial cavoatrial junction, whereas the rest of the sinus myocardium differentiates into atrial working myocardium. The presence of the tracts of tissue visualised by content of Tbx3 extending between the site of pacemaking and the atrioventricular canal indicates that, early in development, all of this area was made up of primary myocardium. With ongoing growth and maturation, however, the internodal area, from the stance of histology, becomes converted into working atrial myocardium. Using the criterions established by the German pathologists, therefore, there is no evidence to support the notion that insulated tracts of histologically specialised myocardial cells join together the sinus and atrioventricular nodes. Nor does the application of these criterions lend any credence to suggestions that the cells within the pulmonary venous sleeves are histologically specialised.[57] Indeed, in this latter instance we also know that the pulmonary venous myocardium has a totally different lineage from that of the tissues forming the anatomical conduction system.[29,30] We do know, nonetheless, that the tissues of the right atrial vestibule persist as recognisable node-like structures. These are the entities recognised by Kent at the turn of the 19th century, but erroneously interpreted by him as providing multiple muscular connections across the atrioventricular junctions of the normal heart.[58] The structures can, in very rare circumstances, function as substrates for ventricular pre-excitation in otherwise normally structured hearts,[59] and can form anomalous atrioventricular nodes in the setting of congenital malformations such as congenitally corrected transposition and double inlet left ventricle (see Chapters 31 and 39). In the course of normal development, it is only the atrioventricular conduction axis described by Tawara[50] that provides muscular continuity between the atrial and ventricular muscle masses. There have also been discussions as to whether the myocardial cells making up this axis, including the so-called Purkinje cells, are derived by recruitment of working myocardial cells, or are remnants of primary myocardium. Lineage studies now show unequivocally that the so-called conduction tissues are derived from the initial primary myocardium of the heart tube.[60]

MYOCARDIAL VASCULARISATION

When the ventricular loop is first formed, there is no need for any particular system for vascularisation of the developing walls, since myocardium is broken up into a mass of individual trabeculations lined by endocardium, with little formation of a compact layer. The intertrabecular spaces, which reach almost to the epicardium, play a role subsequently in the formation of the myocardial vascular bed, albeit that it still has to be established how they are incorporated within the forming compact component of the ventricular walls. The first indication of the epicardial trunks that feed the mural vessels is the appearance of a subepicardial endothelial plexus.[61] This network subsequently establishes continuity with endothelial sprouts in the walls of the developing aortic valvar sinuses. Original theories suggested that multiple coronary arterial orifices arose from both the developing aortic and pulmonary roots.[62] The concept was disproved when it was shown that the endothelial sprouts, which together form a peritruncal ring, invade the aortic wall from the outside.[63] Only two of these multiple sprouts eventually develop a lumen, thus producing the orifices of the definitive right and left coronary arteries.

MYOCARDIAL MATURATION

The maturation of the myocardium forming the ventricular walls is intimately connected to the development of the mural coronary arterial supply. Understanding of the steps involved in establishment of the compact layer of the wall has become increasingly important since the recognition of so-called ventricular non-compaction.[64] As yet, however, our knowledge of the precise steps involved in removal of the initially extensive trabecular myocardial network, and the thickening of the compact layer, remain rudimentary. It is certainly the case that in the sixth and seventh weeks of development, immediately prior to closure of the embryonic interventricular foramen, there is an extensive trabecular meshwork filling the larger part of the ventricular lumens, and the compact layer of the myocardium is very thin in relation to the thickness of the trabeculated layer (Figs. 3-38 and 3-39). At these initial stages, there is also muscular continuity across the developing atrioventricular junctions. The inner heart curvature remains as a muscular fold between the developing leaflets of the aortic and mitral valves (see Fig. 3-39). Immediately subsequent to closure of the embryonic interventricular communication, in the eighth week of development, there is a marked reduction in the extent of the trabeculations, and a thickening of the

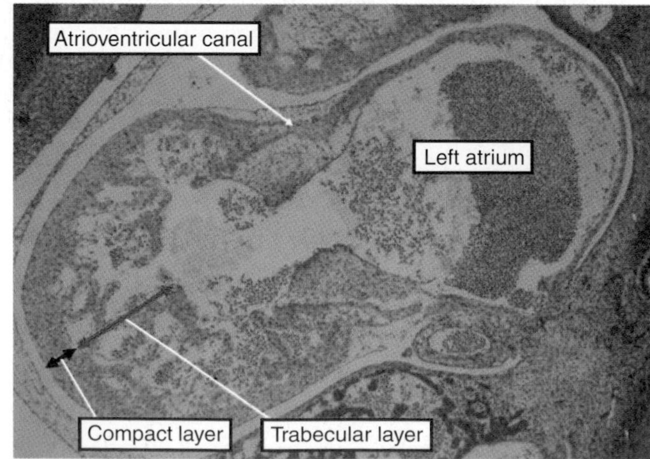

Figure 3-38 This long-axis section of the left ventricle is from a human embryo at stage 14, in the sixth week of development. Note the extensive trabecular meshwork (*yellow arrow*) filling the ventricular cavity. The compact layer (*red arrow*) is relatively thin. Note also the muscular continuity across the atrioventricular junctions through the atrioventricular canal musculature.

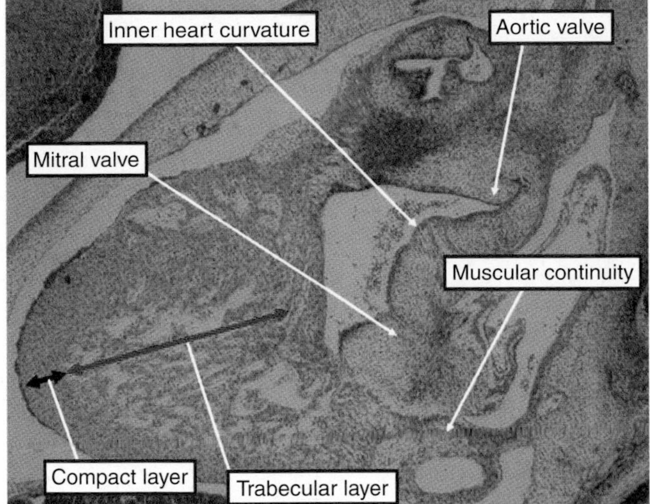

Figure 3-39 This section to be compared with Figure 3-38, and also taken through the long axis of the left ventricle, is from a human embryo in the seventh week of development. There is still an extensive trabecular meshwork (*yellow arrow*) relative to the thickness of the compact layer (*red arrow*). Note the developing leaflets of the aortic and mitral valves, which are still separated by the muscular inner heart curvature. Note also the diminishing muscular continuity across the atrioventricular junction.

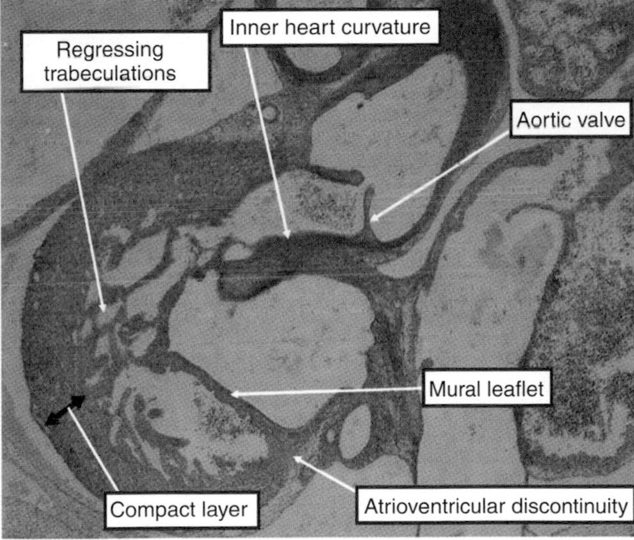

Figure 3-40 This section, again taken through the long axis of the left ventricle, is from a human embryo in the eighth week of development, subsequent to closure of the embryonic interventricular foramen. In comparison with the situation in the seventh week (see Fig. 3-39), there has been marked thickening of the compact layer (*red arrow*), and the trabeculations within the lumen are regressing. Note that the atrial myocardium is now separated from the ventricular musculature across the atrioventricular junction, but that there is still muscle between the developing leaflets of the aortic and mitral valves.

compact layer (Fig. 3-40). It seems unlikely that the trabeculations themselves coalesce to produce the compact layer, but this has still to be established with certainty. It is very likely, however, that persistence of the embryonic trabecular layer is the substrate of the morphological picture now described as ventricular non-compaction.[64,65]

ACKNOWLEDGEMENTS

We are indebted to our colleagues at the University of Amsterdam and St George's Medical University, London, United Kingdom, for granting us permission to discuss findings, and produce illustrations, from work as yet unpublished in the peer-reviewed literature, in particular Drs Vincent Christoffels and Sandra Webb.

The complete reference list can be found on the companion Expert Consult web site at www.expertconsult.com.

ANNOTATED REFERENCES

- Kelly RG, Brown NA, Buckingham ME: The arterial pole of the mouse heart forms from Fgf10-expressing cells in pharyngeal mesoderm. Dev Cell 2001;1:435–440.
- Mjaatvedt CH, Nakaoka T, Moreno-Rodriguez R, et al: The outflow tract of the heart is recruited from a novel heart-forming field. Dev Biol 2001;238: 97–109.
- Waldo KL, Kumiski DH, Wallis KT, et al: Conotruncal myocardium arises from a secondary heart field. Development 2001;128:3179–3188.

  These three investigations, appearing independently, showed that all parts of the developing heart were not represented in the initial linear heart tube. They established the importance of the so-called anterior or second heart field, although it seems unlikely that the so-called heart fields are totally discrete one from the other. It is more likely that the second field represents a later migration of cells into the heart from the cardiac crescent.
- Moorman AFM, Christoffels VM: Cardiac chamber formation: Development, genes and evolution. Physiol Rev 2003;83:1223–1267.

  This review summarised the evidence in favour of what has become known as the ballooning model for formation of the cardiac chambers. The investigations establishing the significance of the second heart field showed that the so-called segmental model for chamber formation was inappropriate. This review explained how the atrial appendages ballooned from the atrial component of the heart tube, and the ventricular apexes in sequence from the inlet and outlet components of the ventricular loop.
- Anderson RH, Brown NA, Moorman AFM: Development and structures of the venous pole of the heart. Dev Dyn 2006;235:2–9.

  A review of the controversies concerning the development of the pulmonary vein, and its relationship to the systemic venous sinus. As the review shows, the systemic venous sinus is not recognisable in mammalian embryos until the systemic venous tributaries have shifted to open within the morphologically right atrium. The pulmonary vein opens into the heart through an area of medisatinal myocardium, and has neither anatomical nor developmental connections to the systemic venous sinus.
- Lamers WH, Wessels A, Verbeek FJ, et al: New findings concerning ventricular septation in the human heart. Implications for maldevelopment. Circulation 1992;86:1194–1205.

  This important paper, describing the findings using an antibody to the nodose ganglion in the human heart, showed how the right ventricle develops entirely downstream relative to the embryonic interventricular communication.
- Odgers PNB: The development of the pars membranacea septi in the human heart. J Anat 1937–8;72:247–259.

  The classic paper describing the mechanisms of closure of the embryonic interventricular communication. Although very difficult to understand, recent studies have endorsed the accuracy of the observations.
- Bogers AJJC, Gittenberger-de Groot AC, Poelmann RE, et al: Development of the origin of the coronary arteries, a matter of ingrowth or outgrowth? Anat Embryol 1989;180:437–441.

  The investigation that showed there was no substance in the suggestion that several twigs grew out from the developing arterial roots to make contact with the developing coronary arteries. Instead, the coronary arterial primordiums grew into the developing aortic root.
- Moorman A, Webb S, Brown NA, et al: Development of the heart (1) Formation of the cardiac chambers and arterial trunks. Heart 2003;89:806–814.
- Anderson RH, Webb S, Lamers W, Moorman A: Development of the heart (2) Septation of the atriums and ventricles. Heart 2003;89:949–958.
- Anderson RH, Webb S, Brown NA, et al: Development of the heart (3) Formation of the ventricular outflow tracts, arterial valves, and intrapericardial arterial trunks. Heart 2003;89:1110–1118.

  This series of reviews discusses recent findings in cardiac development, and offers an overview for those working in clinical disciplines. The third part of the series points out the current deficiencies in concepts explaining septation of the outflow tract on the basis of growth of an aortopulmonary septum.

CHAPTER 4

Myocardium and Development

PAGE A.W. ANDERSON*

The developing heart appears to be simply a smaller version of the adult heart, based on global function. The ventricles of the adult and the developing heart fill with blood, develop pressure, eject blood, and relax (Fig. 4-1). Across development, nonetheless, ventricular myocardium differs quantitatively and qualitatively in function and structure. For example, adult myocardium develops greater active tension than does fetal myocardium, and is more compliant[1] (Fig. 4-2). When the extracellular matrix that enfolds the cells is removed, a marked developmental increase in contractility is observed in the isolated cell. The velocity and amount of sarcomeric shortening of the adult myocyte are greater than those of the immature myocyte[2] (Fig. 4-3). In this chapter, I review the structures and processes that are basic to cardiac function, and show how they are affected by development.

THE HEART

The volume and mass of the heart increase with development.[3,4] The postnatal increase in left ventricular mass in the structurally normal heart is a result of an increase in the number, or hyperplasia, and in size, or physiological hypertrophy, of the ventricular myocytes, and in the growth of the non-myocytic components of the myocardium.[5] Workload and mural stress directly affect mural thickness, as evidenced by the differences in thickness of the right and left ventricular free walls of the adult heart. With birth, the relative workloads of the ventricles change, with that of the left ventricle being increased. This postnatal change in workload is associated with an increase in left ventricular mass, relative to body weight, while that of the right ventricle remains the same or decreases.[4] The ability of the developing heart to increase ventricular mass in response to an increase in mural stress is exemplified by changes in the left ventricle of the newborn with concordant atrioventricular and discordant ventriculo-arterial connections. The normal postnatal increase in left ventricular mural mass does not occur in the presence of the normal neonatal fall in pulmonary arterial pressure. If, however, the pulmonary arterial pressure is elevated in the infant through surgical

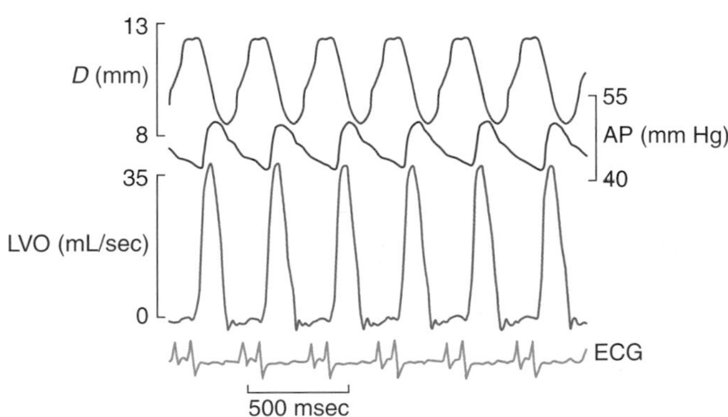

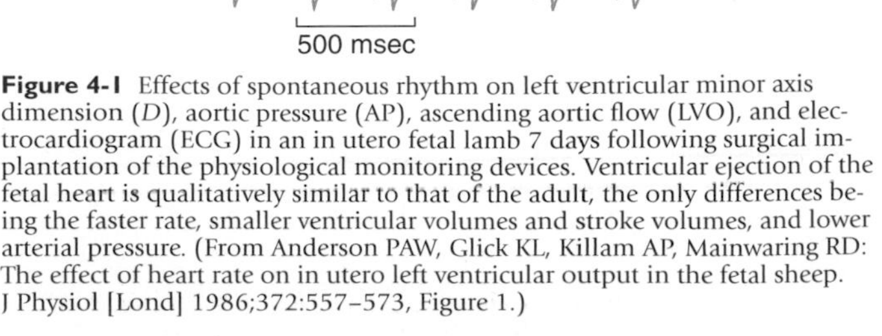

Figure 4-1 Effects of spontaneous rhythm on left ventricular minor axis dimension (*D*), aortic pressure (AP), ascending aortic flow (LVO), and electrocardiogram (ECG) in an in utero fetal lamb 7 days following surgical implantation of the physiological monitoring devices. Ventricular ejection of the fetal heart is qualitatively similar to that of the adult, the only differences being the faster rate, smaller ventricular volumes and stroke volumes, and lower arterial pressure. (From Anderson PAW, Glick KL, Killam AP, Mainwaring RD: The effect of heart rate on in utero left ventricular output in the fetal sheep. J Physiol [Lond] 1986;372:557–573, Figure 1.)

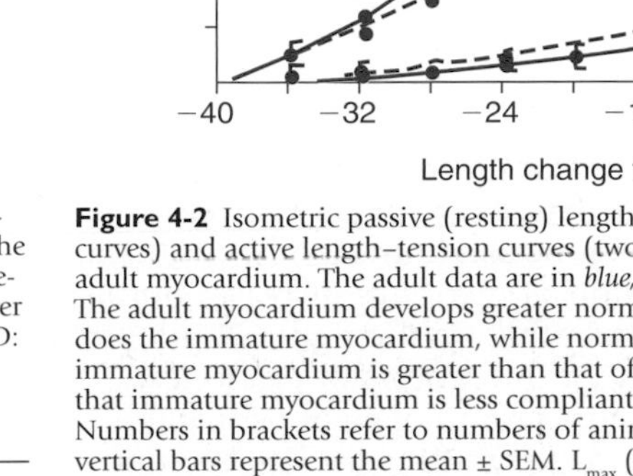

Figure 4-2 Isometric passive (resting) length–tension curves (two lower curves) and active length–tension curves (two upper curves) from fetal and adult myocardium. The adult data are in *blue*, and the fetal data are in *red*. The adult myocardium develops greater normalised active tension than does the immature myocardium, while normalised passive tension of the immature myocardium is greater than that of the adult. The latter illustrates that immature myocardium is less compliant than adult myocardium. Numbers in brackets refer to numbers of animals studied. Each point and the vertical bars represent the mean ± SEM. L_{max} (see right hand end of abscissa) is a muscle length at which the greatest active tension was developed. (From Friedman WF: The intrinsic physiologic properties of the developing heart. Prog Cardiovasc Dis 1972;15:87–111, Figure 2.)

*Sadly, Page A.W. Anderson passed on between the completion of this chapter and its production. The editors dedicate this part of the book to his eternal memory.

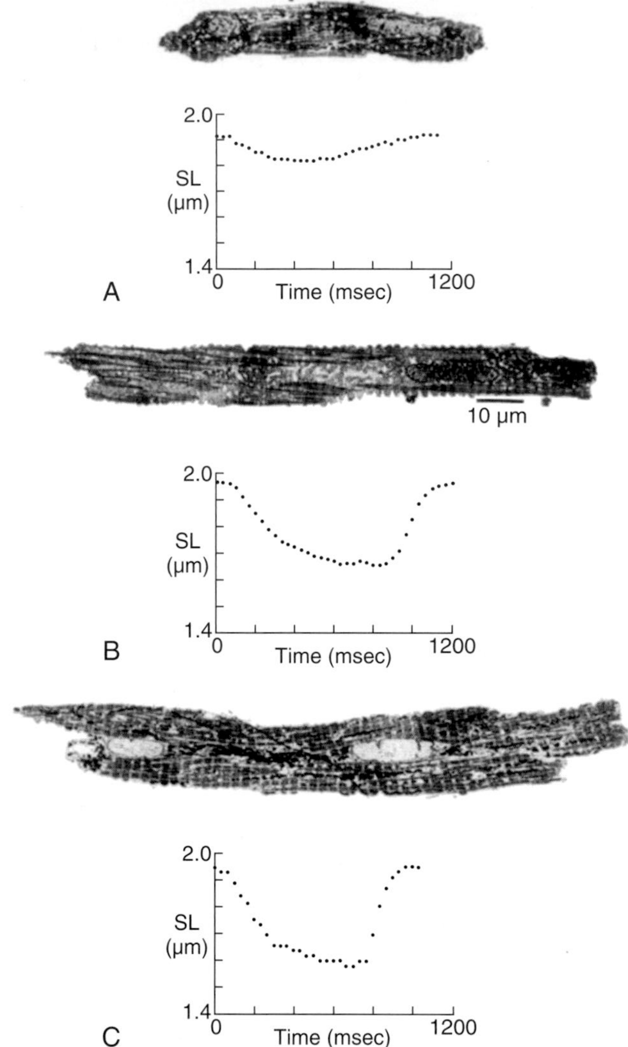

Figure 4-3 Longitudinal sections through the near central region of three myocytes from isolated rabbit hearts and their sarcomere shortening waveforms in response to field stimulation. **A,** An average-sized myocyte from the heart of a 3-week-old rabbit. **B,** A small-sized adult myocyte. **C,** An adult cell of average size. A sarcomere shortening waveform elicited from each cell is shown beneath its electron micrograph. Sarcomere length (SL) is plotted as a function of time (1 mM [Ca^{2+}]). Even the relatively small adult cell had a greater amount of sarcomere shortening and a faster rate of shortening than the average-sized immature cell. All cells are shown at identical magnification. (From Nassar R, Reedy MC, Anderson PAW: Developmental changes in the ultrastructure and sarcomere shortening of the isolated rabbit ventricular myocyte. Circ Res 1987;61:465–483, Figure 1.)

constriction of the discordantly connected pulmonary trunk, left ventricular mass increases markedly within a few days.

Hyperplasia

During fetal and early neonatal life, division of cells is the primary mechanism by which myocardial mass increases.[3,4,6] In response to the greater workload borne by the postnatal left ventricle, the population of myocytes increases during neonatal life more rapidly in than in the right. Of note, in the mammal, hyperplasia, or the process of cytokinesis, is thought to cease after the first month or so of neonatal life. Evidence for hyperplasia in the adult heart has been provided in the adult amphibian heart, nonetheless, and more recently in the mammalian heart. The extent to which these mechanisms, which may involve resident cardiac stem cells in the adult, generate additional myocytes in the adult mammalian heart remains to be established.[7–9] The potential for division of myocytes, or generation of myocytes from stem cells, and the mechanisms underlying this process are, at present, topics of great interest and debate because of the need to develop new therapies for the failing heart.[10,11]

Hypertrophy

Increasing size of the cardiac myocytes, or physiological hypertrophy, becomes the major mechanism through which ventricular mass increases after a few months of postnatal life[3,4] (Figs. 4-3 and 4-4). The stimulus is the normal developmental increase in mural stress and work.[12,13] This process is also present prenatally. Excessive pressure overload will induce hypertrophy, in addition to hyperplasia, in the fetal heart.[14]

The developmental process that results in physiological hypertrophy is associated with changes in the shape and size of the cardiac myocytes (Figs. 4-3 to 4-5). For example, the average length of the cardiac myocyte in the newborn rat is approximately 20 µm, while that of the 11-day-old rat is 45 µm.[4] Only an increase of one-fifth in cross sectional area accompanies this doubling of cell length. The immature cardiac myocyte changes from being relatively ovoid to the long tetrahedral shape of the adult myocyte (see Fig. 4-3). A further postnatal increase in cell length is seen in the adult heart, with cell lengths of 150 µm and longer being achieved in the mammal, and more than 300 µm in the bird. The cross sectional minor diameter increases from 10 to 20 µm following birth in the

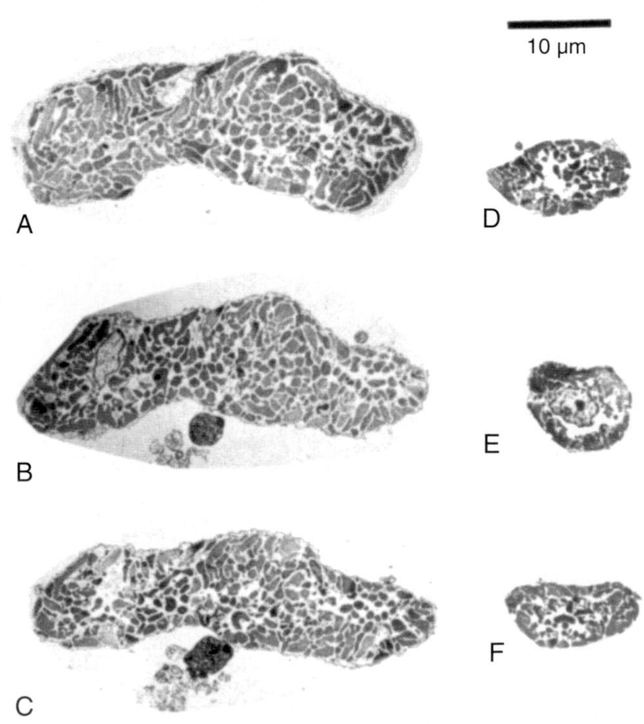

Figure 4-4 The size and complexity of shape of cardiac myocytes increases with development. Cross-sections through widely separated levels of a myocyte isolated from an adult heart (**A–C**) and a myocyte isolated from the heart of a 3-week-old rabbit (**D–F**). (From Nassar R, Reedy MC, Anderson PAW: Developmental changes in the ultrastructure and sarcomere shortening of the isolated rabbit ventricular myocyte. Circ Res 1987;61:465–483, Figure 2.)

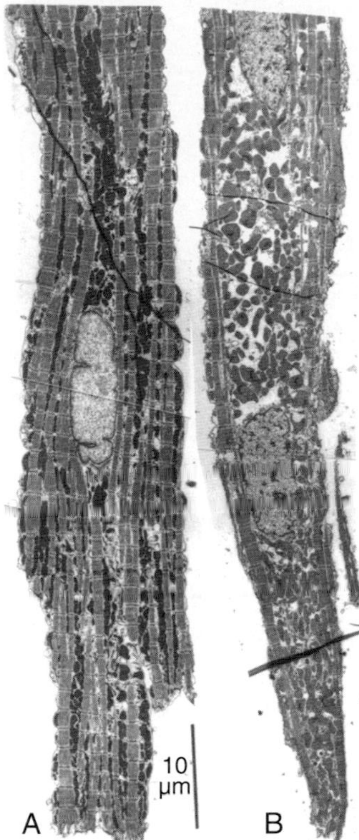

Figure 4-5 Longitudinal sections from single isolated myocytes: an adult myocyte (**A**) and a myocyte from a 3-week-old rabbit (**B**). The cell shape and myofibril organisation relative to the mitochondria and nuclei differ markedly at the two stages of development. The myofibrils of the neonatal myocyte are restricted to the subsarcolemmal region, while those of the adult are ranged in layers across the width of the cell. The second nucleus of the adult cell lies just out of view. (From Nassar R, Reedy MC, Anderson PAW: Developmental changes in the ultrastructure and sarcomere shortening of the isolated rabbit ventricular myocyte. Circ Res 1987;61:465–483, Figure 5.)

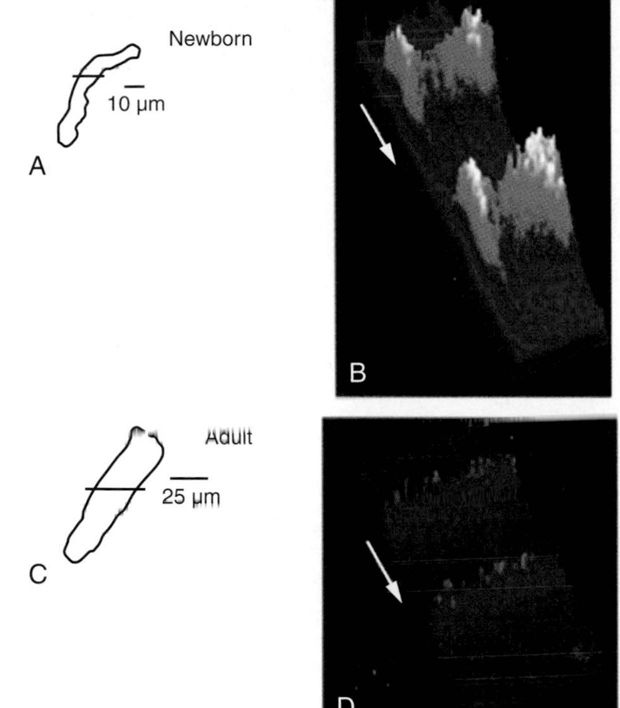

Figure 4-6 Regional changes in $[Ca^{2+}]_i$ in a newborn (**A** and **B**) and an adult (**C** and **D**) rabbit myocyte. **A,** Outline of a newborn (1-day-old) rabbit myocyte and the position of the scan line for the confocal microscope that was scanned repeatedly to monitor the rise and fall of $[Ca^{2+}]_i$ during systole and diastole, using a fluoroprobe (fluo 3). The $[Ca^{2+}]_i$ transients (*yellow*) of two contractions are illustrated in **B. B,** A three-dimensional reconstruction of the scan line. The direction of the arrow indicates time. The edges of the cell (the sarcolemma) are on the left and right sides of the image. The subsarcolemmal $[Ca^{2+}]_i$ increases before and more rapidly than $[Ca^{2+}]_i$ in the center of the cell, supporting the importance of trans-sarcolemmal influx of $[Ca^{2+}]$ during activation in the immature cell. **C,** Outline of an adult cell and position of the scan line for the confocal microscope that was repeatedly scanned to monitor the increase and fall in $[Ca^{2+}]_i$ during systole and diastole. **D,** Similar to **B,** the three-dimensional reconstruction of the time course of $[Ca^{2+}]_i$ during two sequential contractions. Unlike the newborn myocyte, $[Ca^{2+}]_i$ appears to rise uniformly across the entire width of the adult myocyte, illustrating the importance of CICR that follows from the T-tubular system and its calcium release units (see text). (From Haddock PS, Coetzee WA, Cho E, et al: Subcellular $[Ca^{2+}]_i$ gradients during excitation contraction coupling in newborn rabbit ventricular myocytes. Circ Res 1999;85:415–427).

mammal[2] (see Fig. 4-4). These developmental changes are likely to have functional consequences, for example, the greater contribution of trans-sarcolemmal movement of calcium to the systolic $[Ca^{2+}]_i$ transient in the immature myocyte versus the greater contribution of calcium release from intracellular stores to be $[Ca^{2+}]_i$ transient in the adult myocyte (Fig. 4-6). The greater contribution of trans-sarcolemmal calcium to the $[Ca^{2+}]_i$ transient in the immature myocyte may be reflected in the apparent great sensitivity of the infant heart following surgery to an increase in concentration of calcium in the plasma.

REGULATION OF CYTOSOLIC CALCIUM

The cascade underlying cardiac contraction is initiated by depolarisation of the transmembrane potential. Voltage-gated calcium channels are activated, extracellular calcium enters the myocyte, and calcium is released from intracellular stores into the cytosol.[15,16] The effects on sarcomeric function that follow from the systolic increase in cytosolic concentrations of $[Ca^{2+}]_i$ in the cytosol will be described in the section of the chapter devoted to the sarcomere. During diastole, $[Ca^{2+}]_i$ is about 100 nM, about 1/10,000 of extracellular calcium. The electrochemical gradient for entry of calcium is opposed primarily by the sarcolemmal Ca^{2+}TPase, a system with high affinity but low capacity that regulates resting or diastolic $[Ca^{2+}]_i$.

The L-type calcium channel, the dihydropyridine receptor, is the primary source for entry of calcium into the adult human cardiac myocyte.[17] With depolarisation, the L-type calcium channel is activated, and influx of calcium occurs (Fig. 4-7). Following activation, and during the contraction, the channel closes as a consequence of an increase in $[Ca^{2+}]_i$ and further depolarisation, a feedback loop that limits the calcium current (I_{Ca}). Phosphorylation of the L-type calcium channel, secondary to β-adrenoreceptor stimulation, increases the calcium current. Another calcium channel, the T-type calcium channel, which is expressed in the embryonic heart, is activated at a more negative potential.[18,19]

Exchange of calcium for sodium across the sarcolemma, through the Na^+Ca^{2+} exchanger, can occur in both directions[15,20] (see Fig. 4-7). This exchange of three sodium molecules for one calcium molecule is energy dependent. The direction of the exchange of sodium and calcium through the exchanger is based on its reversal potential. At more positive membrane potentials and higher $[Na^+]_i$, influx is favoured through the exchanger. In some species, this exchanger may provide an amount of calcium to the

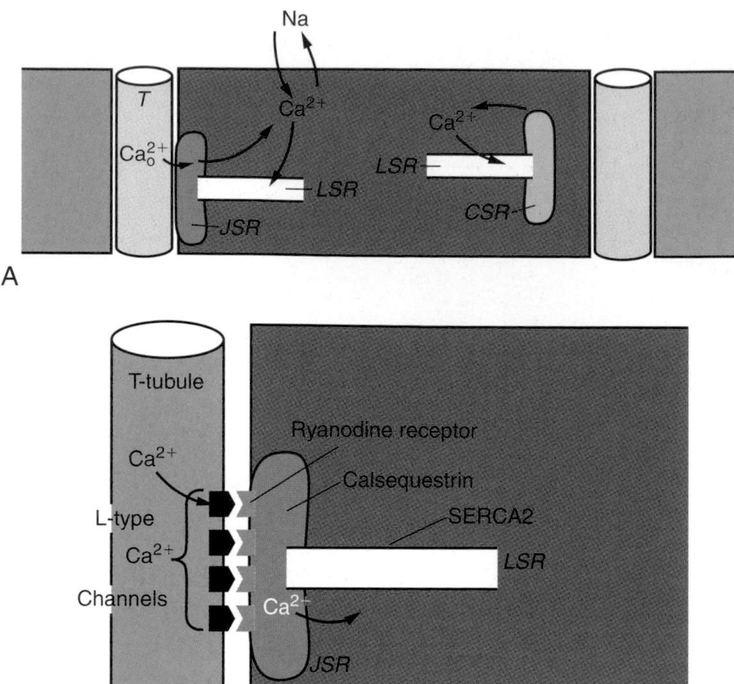

Figure 4-7 **A,** Schematic representation of the basis of the rise and fall in cytosolic calcium concentration $[Ca^{2+}]_i$ during a contraction. With activation, the voltage-dependent calcium channels located in the T-tubule open, and the inward movement of calcium results in release of calcium from the JSR (see Fig. 4-8). The calcium that is released from the CSR and JSR was obtained through LSR uptake of calcium during the previous contraction. Trans-sarcolemmal movement of calcium is also a product of the Na^+Ca^{2+} exchanger. Because of its voltage dependence, this exchanger functions primarily as an efficient mechanism for removing calcium from the cell. The Na^+Ca^{2+} exchanger also functions in reverse, providing a mechanism for entry of calcium into the cell during systole. **B,** The generally accepted model of calcium-induced calcium release (CICR) is illustrated. With activation, calcium movement through the L-type calcium channels increases the local $[Ca^{2+}]_i$ near the ryanodine receptor (RyR, the SR calcium-release channel). The local increase in calcium induces release of calcium from the JSR, markedly amplifying the increase in $[Ca^{2+}]_i$. CSR, corbular sarcoplasmic reticulum (see text); JSR, junctional sarcoplasmic reticulum; LSR, longitudinal sarcoplasmic reticulum; T, T-tubule.

systolic $[Ca^{2+}]_i$ transient similar to that provided by the L-type calcium channel. When the membrane potential is more negative, and $[Ca^{2+}]_i$ is higher, removal of calcium from the cell is favoured, helping restore $[Ca^{2+}]_i$ to diastolic levels. Operating in this mode, the exchanger demonstrates its role as a system with low affinity and high capacity, designed to deal with the intracellular loads of calcium.

The sarcoplasmic reticulum is the major intracellular site of release of calcium needed to support the $[Ca^{2+}]_i$ transient.[15] The reticulum contains specialised components, namely the junctional, corbular, and longitudinal components[2] (Figs. 4-7 to 4-9). The junctional and corbular components contain calcium-binding calsequestrin, with 40 calcium molecules bound to each calsequestrin molecule, triadin, junction, and the ryanodine receptors, known as the RyRs, and representing the calcium-permeable ion channel of the reticulum. Corbular reticulum is not associated with the sarcolemma, while the junctional part is morphologically and functionally coupled to the transverse-tubules (see Fig. 4-8), forming dyads with the T-tubule sarcolemma, and peripheral couplings with the surface sarcolemma. The junctional and corbular components are located at the level of the Z-disc, where T-tubules are located. The T-tubular system, providing sarcolemmal extensions from the surface of the myocyte to deep within its core, is acquired with development, and is present in adult mammalian ventricular myocytes (see Figs. 4-7 and 4-8).

Entry of calcium into the cell triggers calcium-induced release from the sarcoplasmic reticulum (see Fig. 4-7). The calcium release units that support the systolic $[Ca^{2+}]_i$ transient are specialised junctional domains of the reticulum containing the L-type calcium channel, dihydropyridine receptors of the surface sarcolemma, and that of the T-tubule, the RyRs, triadin and junctin, and calsequestrin, the high capacity-low affinity calcium binding protein.[21] The latter four molecules form a supramolecular quaternary complex in the junctional and corbular parts of the sarcoplasmic reticulum.[16] Junctin binds calsequestrin within the calcium release units, but is not required for its localisation to the junctional and corbular components.[22] Junctin, also, regulates contractility but is not required for contraction.[23] The predominant ryanodine receptor in the heart is RyR2. The central role of trans-sarcolemmal influx of calcium in initiating calcium-induced release of calcium is evidenced by the effect of removing extracellular calcium. Activation of membranes in the absence of extracellular calcium does not result in excitation-contraction coupling. There is no $[Ca^{2+}]_i$ transient, and the myocyte fails to contract.

The close structural relationship between the junctional component of the sarcoplasmic reticulum and the L-type calcium channel, located in the sarcolemmal T-tubules, ensures that voltage-dependent opening of the L-type channel, and the associated flow of extracellular calcium into the cytosol, produces a very high $[Ca^{2+}]_i$ ryanodine receptor (see Fig. 4-7). In response to the increase in $[Ca^{2+}]_i$ with excitation, the ryanodine receptors are activated throughout the myocyte, and calcium flows into the cytosol from the sarcoplasmic reticulum, amplifying the effect of the L-type calcium channel current on the $[Ca^{2+}]_i$ transient.[24,25] The ryanodine receptors are, also, a scaffolding protein. The associated molecules in the release units, and associated kinases, phosphatases, and calmodulin are likely to modulate their function.[16,26,27]

Cardiac relaxation follows the fall in the $[Ca^{2+}]_i$ transient to diastolic levels. Extrusion of calcium from the myocyte, and intracellular uptake of calcium, underlie this process. The major intracellular site of uptake is the longitudinal component of the sarcoplasmic reticulum (see Figs. 4-7 and 4-9). Although the mitochondria serve as a site for intracellular storage of calcium, they do not significantly contribute to the fall in the $[Ca^{2+}]_i$ transient. The longitudinal elements of the reticulum contain the sarcoplasmic version of calcium ATPase, known as SERCA, a transmembrane protein that translates calcium from the cytosol into the

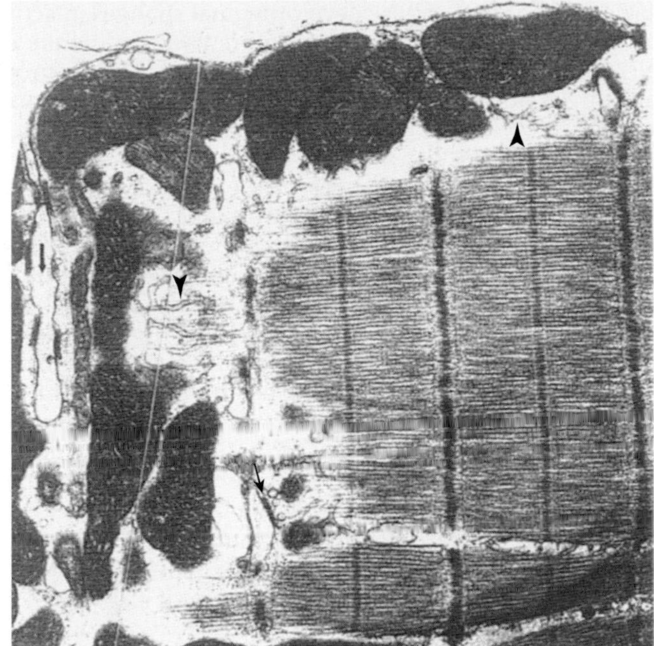

Figure 4-8 Electron micrograph of an isolated adult myocyte illustrates the membranous systems important in the beat-to-beat regulation of $[Ca^{2+}]_i$. The sarcolemma and extracellular space are at the top of the illustration. The invagination of the T-tubule in the upper part of the illustration is marked by the arrow (upper left side of image). The LSR, the membranous system that enfolds the myofilaments and removes calcium from the cytosol through its calcium ATPase, is pointed out by the arrowheads. The CSR and JSR, the sites of calcium release that support the cardiac contraction, are pointed out by the small arrow.

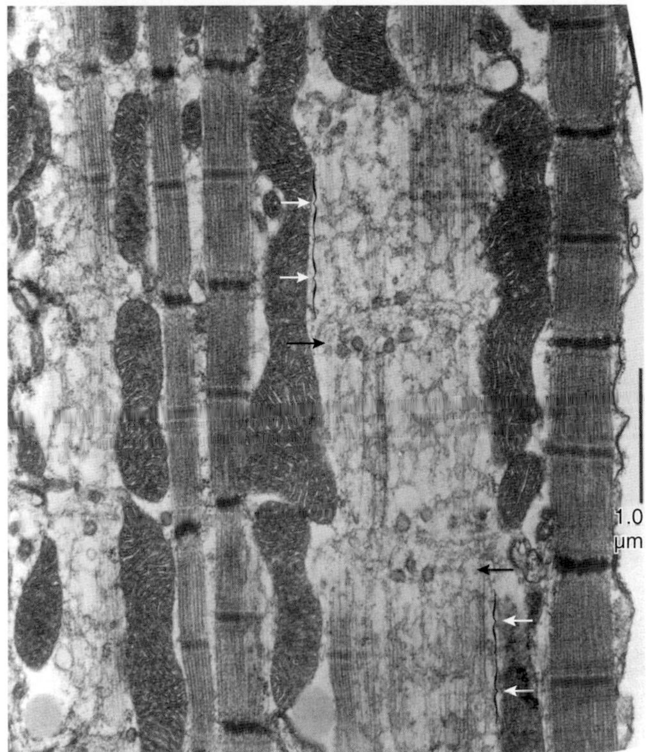

Figure 4-9 Longitudinal section of an isolated adult cell. The repetitive arrangement of CSR and LSR is typical of the mature myocyte. A myofibril passes slightly out of the section plane and reveals a ring of CSR components (*black arrows*) at each Z band and the network of LSR components (*white arrows and braces*) around each sarcomere. (From Nassar R, Reedy MC, Anderson PAW: Developmental changes in the ultrastructure and sarcomere shortening of the isolated rabbit ventricular myocyte. Circ Res 1987;61: 465–483, Figure 10.)

lumen of the sarcoplasmic reticulum.[15] Activity of SERCA is isoform dependent.[28] Of note, across development, cardiac myocytes express only SERCA2a. The longitudinal elements of the reticulum surround each sarcomere from Z-disc to Z-disc like a three-dimensional mesh, providing a system for rapid removal of the calcium bathed in the myofibrils (see Fig. 4-9). Calcium pumping is enhanced by $[Ca^{2+}]_i$ and decreased by $[Ca^{2+}]$ within the sarcoplasmic reticulum. Activity of SERCA is inhibited by phospholamban.[29] Phosphorylation of phospholamban in response to β-adrenoreceptor stimulation removes its inhibitory effect on the activity of SERCA, and leads to a greater uptake of calcium into the longitudinal sarcoplasmic reticulum, providing a larger pool of calcium for release through the ryanodine receptors in subsequent contractions.

In summary, the systolic $[Ca^{2+}]_i$ transient is driven by modulation of the L-type calcium current, SERCA activity, the volume, organisation, and content of calcium in the sarcoplasmic reticulum, the number and properties of the ryanodine receptors, the sodium calcium exchanger, and the extent to which calsequestrin is saturated with calcium. Altogether, they modulate of the systolic $[Ca^{2+}]_i$ transient, provide the basis for the heart to vary its force of contraction from beat-to-beat, in other words the ability to modulate cardiac contractility. These processes underlie the increase in contractility that occurs with increase in heart rate, and those that follow from the introduction of an extrasystole. The extrasystole leads to greater content of calcium in the sarcoplasmic reticulum, allowing greater release of calcium, and a higher $[Ca^{2+}]_i$ transient in the post-extrasystolic contraction, and so post-extrasystolic potentiation (Fig. 4-10).

DEVELOPMENT AND REGULATION OF CYTOSOLIC CALCIUM

The $[Ca^{2+}]_i$ transient increases postnatally in the mammalian ventricular myocyte[30] (Fig. 4-11). In the immature heart, the $[Ca^{2+}]_i$ transient in response to excitation-contraction coupling has a greater dependence on trans-sarcolemmal influx of calcium[31] (see Fig. 4-6). Developmental changes in the sarcoplasmic reticulum, the calcium release units, constituted in its specialised junctional domains,[2,22] and expression of the sodium calcium exchanger, are all pertinent to this observation.[32,33]

The organisation, differentiation, and relative volume of the sarcoplasmic reticulum increase with development, and the size and frequency of the specialised couplings with the surface and T-tubular sarcolemmal units that contain the elements for release of calcium increase with development.[21,22] The T-tubular system is acquired with development in the mammalian ventricular myocyte. The relative volume of the cells comprising the sarcoplasmic reticulum increases during late gestation, and following birth,[2,34] and the structure of the release units changes with development. In the immature myocyte, ryanodine receptors extend from the corbular component onto the surface of the longitudinal elements, while calsequestrin, located within the lumen of the corbular component in the adult, extends into the lumens of the longitudinal elements in the neonatal myocyte (Fig. 4-12). The expression and targeting of calsequestrin to the junctional and corbular

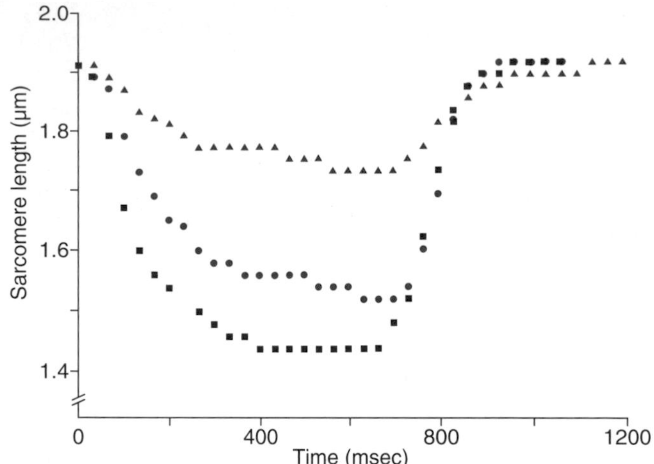

Figure 4-10 Postextrasystolic potentiation: effect of introducing an extrasystole on sarcomere shortening in a cardiac myocyte isolated from an adult rabbit heart. The previous contraction at the regular pacing rate (*blue circles*), the extrasystole (*red triangles*), and the postextrasystolic contraction (*black squares*) are superimposed. The amount and velocity of sarcomere shortening in the extrasystole are smaller than for the previous contraction at the regular pacing rate and are greater for the subsequent extrasystolic potentiated contraction.

components is an early embryonic event that is followed by the expression of junctin and triadin. The developmental localisation of calsequestrin within the junctional and corbular components may be related to a marked postnatal increase in expression of junctin, and its binding of calsequestrin within the specialised region of the sarcoplasmic reticulum.[35] The fixed structural relation between the corbular components and the Z-disc are acquired postnatally (compare Figs. 4-9 and 4-12) in mammals that are not born ready to flee the nest as neonates. The lack of differentiation of the sarcoplasmic reticulum, and its ordered relation with other membranes in the immature myocyte, prevents the close coupling of the L-type calcium channel and the ryanodine receptors. This is likely, in the presence of a lower L-type calcium current density, to contribute to the slower rates of rise and lower peak systolic $[Ca^{2+}]_i$ transient in the immature myocyte[30] (see Fig. 4-11).

Function of the sarcoplasmic reticulum also changes with development as measured by increases in activity and efficiency of SERCA. These developmental changes in activity and efficiency will result in a more effective uptake of calcium by the sarcoplasmic reticulum, providing more calcium to be released during a subsequent contraction and, so, a developmental increase in the range over which the force of contraction can be modulated.

The developmental changes in the structural and biochemical properties of the sarcoplasmic reticulum are reflected in interventions that affect release of calcium by the ryanodine receptors. Ryanodine itself, which inhibits release of calcium by the receptors, does not affect the development of force by fetal myocardium, including that of humans. Within a few days following birth, however, ryanodine markedly attenuates the force of contraction.[36,37] Caffeine, which increases release of calcium by the receptors, has little effect on neonatal myocardium, while enhancing contractility in the adult. These findings support the importance of the developmental acquisition of the components underlying calcium-induced release of calcium, and the consequent decreased dependence of the adult heart on trans-sarcolemmal influx of calcium (see Fig. 4-6).

The greater role of contribution of the sarcoplasmic reticulum to the $[Ca^{2+}]_i$ transient in the adult heart is evidenced by post-extrasystolic potentiation and the restitution of contractility (see Figs. 4-10 and 4-13). Post-extrasystolic potentiation increases with maturation.[38] In addition, the restitution of contractility following a contraction (see Fig. 4-13) is also acquired with maturation.[2,38] Altogether, these findings demonstrate that the developmental increase in the amount, organisation, and structure of the sarcoplasmic reticulum and the calcium release units have a fundamental role in the developmental increase in the peak $[Ca^{2+}]_i$ transient in response to the L-type calcium current with activation.

There are two calcium channels expressed in the myocardium during development, the T-type and the L-type, the latter being dihydropyridine-sensitive. Early in development, a T-type calcium current is present, while in the adult heart, very little, if any, T-type calcium channel is expressed.[18] The developmental changes in the L-type calcium current density are more complex. In general, it increases with development (see Fig. 4-11). This increase may be related to an increase in the number of channels, or to differential expression of the α- and β-subunit isoforms.

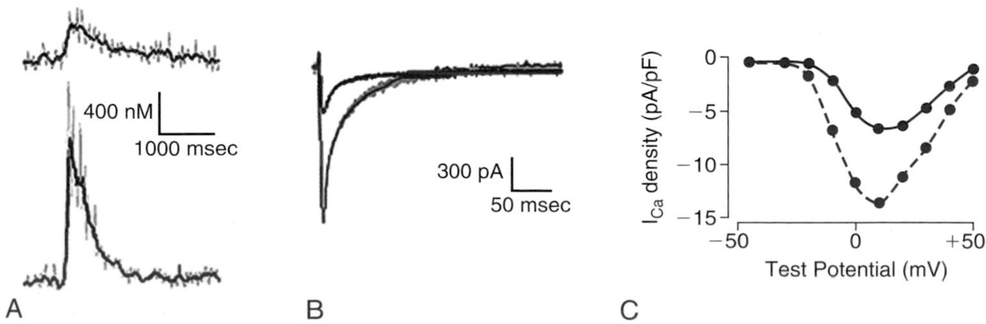

Figure 4-11 Comparison of systolic $[Ca^{2+}]_i$ transients and L-type calcium currents from 3-week-old and adult rabbit ventricular myocytes. **A,** Calcium transients from the 3-week-old (*red waveform*) show much smaller transients than the adult (*blue waveform*). Diastolic levels were 155 and 103 nmol/l respectively. **B,** L-type calcium currents (I_{Ca}) from the 3-week-old (*red waveform*) show a significantly smaller current than the adult (*blue waveform*) myocyte. **C,** I_{Ca}-voltage relations from a 3-week-old (capacitance 61 pF, *red symbols*) and an adult (capacitance 109 pF, *blue symbols*) myocyte showing a significantly lower I_{Ca} density in the immature myocyte.

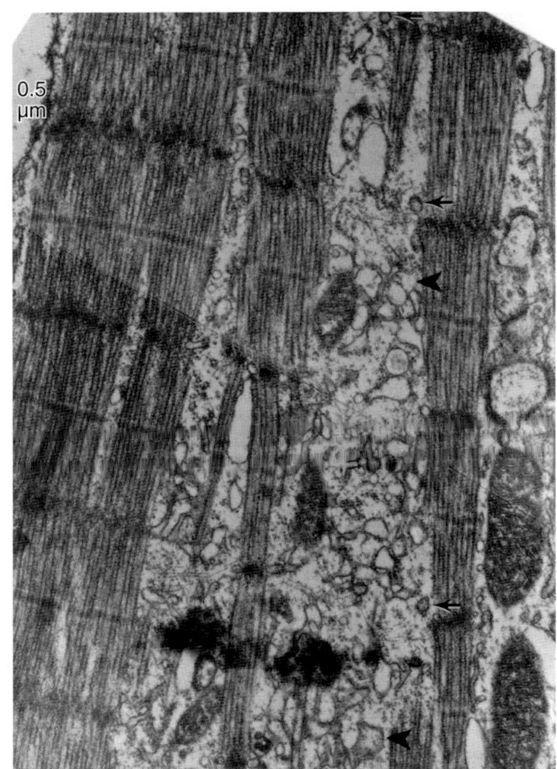

Figure 4-12 Longitudinal section of a myocyte isolated from the heart of a 3-week-old rabbit. Contrast the looser organisation of the CSR (*black arrows*) and LSR (*arrowheads*) with the tightly arranged adult arrangement (see Fig. 4-9). Also of note are the broader connections between the corbular and longitudinal components of the immature cell (*small double arrows*) and the extension of the ryanodine receptors over the LSR. Cell surface is to the left. (From Nassar R, Reedy MC, Anderson PAW: Developmental changes in the ultrastructure and sarcomere shortening of the isolated rabbit ventricular myocyte. Circ Res 1987;61:465–483, Figure 11.)

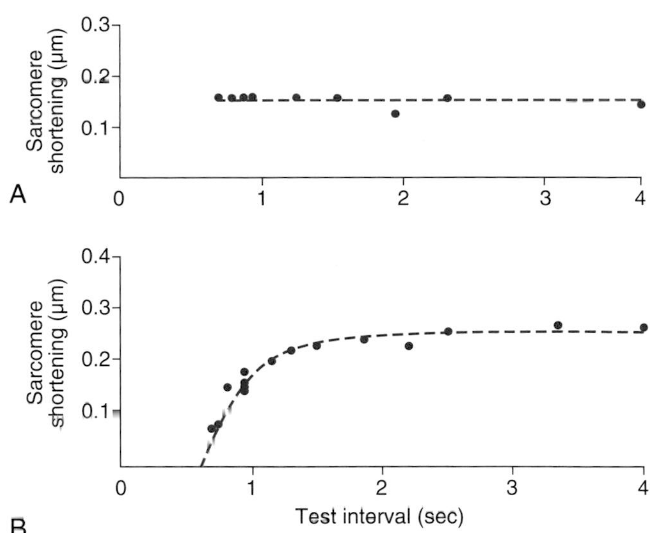

Figure 4-13 A comparison of restitution of sarcomere shortening in extrasystole between an immature (**A,** *red*) and an adult (**B,** *blue*) cell. The test interval is the time between application of the extrasystolic stimulus and the previous regular stimulus. **A,** In the immature cells, the earliest extrasystole that could be elicited exhibited the same amount of sarcomere shortening as the contraction at the regular rate. The absence of restitution in the immature myocyte is consistent with its sarcoplasmic reticulum being unable to modulate cytosolic calcium concentration, and so sarcomere shortening. **B,** In the adult cell, restitution was gradual (the *dotted line* is monoexponential curve, time constant 0.4 sec) demonstrating the ability of the adult myocyte to regulate its $[Ca^{2+}]_i$ and so sarcomere shortening over a broad range of calcium concentration and amounts of sarcomere shortening. (From Nassar R, Reedy MC, Anderson PAW: Developmental changes in the ultrastructure and sarcomere shortening of the isolated rabbit ventricular myocyte. Circ Res 1987;61:465–483, Figure 4.)

Importantly, the developmental increase in the L-type calcium current density provides a greater trigger for calcium-induced release of calcium.

The activity and expression of the sodium calcium exchanger increase during fetal life to a plateau, and subsequently fall rapidly during postnatal development.[33] The exchanger, working in a reverse mode, provides an important mechanism for influx of calcium to support the systolic $[Ca^{2+}]_i$ transient in the neonatal myocyte.[39] Working in the forward mode, the exchanger provides an effective mechanism for removal of calcium from the cytosol, bringing about relaxation.[15] Its effectiveness in removing calcium from the cell in association with a decreased uptake of calcium by the immature sarcoplasmic reticulum may result in little calcium being taken up by the immature sarcoplasmic reticulum, and so decreasing in the immature myocyte the calcium available for release from the sarcoplasmic reticulum in subsequent contractions.

Sodium potassium ATPase, a pump that regulates trans-sarcolemmal concentrations of the sodium and potassium ions, indirectly affects calcium within the cell. Cardioactive glycosides, for example digoxin, selectively bind to and inhibit the sodium potassium ATPase. Inhibition of this enzyme is thought to lead to elevation of sodium ions, with consequent increase in cellular and sarcoplasmic reticulate calcium via the exchanger.[40] Of note, other mechanisms for glycoside-induced enhancement of contractility have been suggested, including direct activation of ryanodine receptors, and increased selectivity by calcium of sodium channels.[41]

Developmental changes have been found in the relative amount of the activity of the enzyme, and expression of its isoforms. Tissue-specific developmentally regulated and differentially localised expression of the α-subunit isoforms, the catalytic subunit, and differential effects of a β-subunit isoforms on affinity for sodium suggests that these isoforms have distinct roles.[42–44] These isoforms have different sensitivities and affinities for binding to cardiac glycosides. Myocardial contractility in the immature heart is positively affected by digoxin.[45,46] The differential expression of the isoforms, and the developmental regulation of this system, suggest that, in the human, α-subunit isoforms may contribute to maturational differences in the response to digoxin.

THE SARCOMERE

The sarcomere, the force-producing unit of the heart, is present at all stages of development. It is made up of a lattice-like highly organised arrangement of thick and thin filaments (Fig. 4-14A and B). The thick filament is a bipolar structure about 1.5 μm in length containing myosin heavy chain and multiple accessory proteins (see Fig. 4-14B). Myosin is asymmetrically shaped, and is made up of two heavy chains and two pairs of associated light chains.[47] The heavy chains form two globular domains, the heads at one end of the molecule containing ATPase and a long rod-like coiled-coil domain. Molecules of the heavy chain are

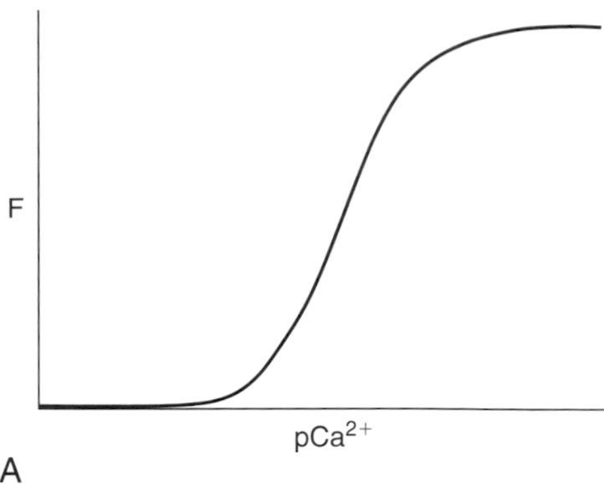

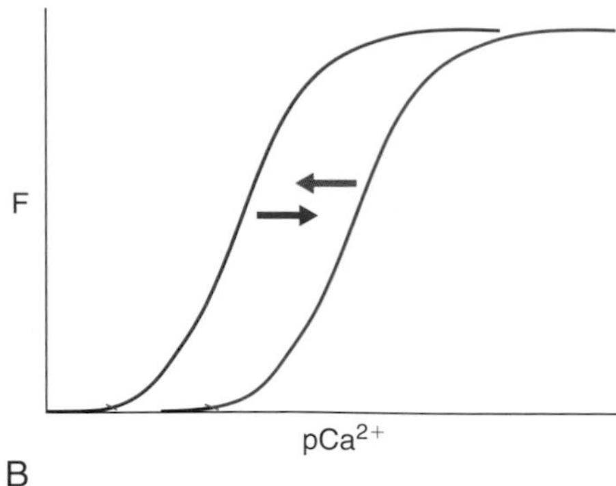

Figure 4-18 The sigmoidal relation describes the sensitivity of the myofilaments to calcium, seen here as the effect of calcium concentration on myofilament force (F) production. **A,** Calcium concentration is illustrated as pCa^{2+}, the negative log of $[Ca^{2+}]$. At low $[Ca^{2+}]$, no force is developed. Over the physiological range of $[Ca^{2+}]$ induced by activation and CICR, a steep relationship between force and $[Ca^{2+}]$ exists. At still higher $[Ca^{2+}]$, no greater force development occurs. **B,** The sensitivity of myofilaments to calcium is dependent on factors such as sarcomere length and post-translational modifications of the contractile proteins. When sarcomere length is increased, the relation is shifted to the left toward lower $[Ca^{2+}]$ (*yellow arrow*). In other words, the myofilaments become more sensitive to calcium. This effect of sarcomere length is in addition to the cross-bridge interactions described in Figure 4-15. Phosphorylation of cardiac TnI, in response to β-adrenergic stimulation, shifts the relation towards higher $[Ca^{2+}]$ (*blue arrow*) decreasing the sensitivity of the myofilaments to calcium.

Calcium-calmodulin dependent phosphorylation of the regulatory myosin light chain, and switch in expression of the myosin heavy chain isoforms, enhance myofilamentous sensitivity to calcium. Protein kinase C phosphorylation of cardiac troponin I and cardiac troponin T also modulates the sensitivity of development of force to calcium.[61] Acidic pH decreases the myofilamentous sensitivity to calcium. It also depresses the peak force of contraction. The result of this effect of acidic pH is that the same systolic $[Ca^{2+}]_i$ transient will elicit a weaker cardiac contraction.

Increasing muscular length increases the sensitivity of the myofilaments to calcium[62] (see Fig. 4-18). At longer sarcomeric lengths, cardiac troponin C has a greater affinity for calcium. Although this property is seen in both skeletal muscle and cardiac muscle, the increase in sensitivity to calcium with an increase in sarcomeric length is greater in cardiac muscle. The positive effect of sarcomeric length on myofilamentous sensitivity to calcium provides a molecular basis for the Frank–Starling relation.

DEVELOPMENT AND THE SARCOMERE

The sensitivity of myofilamentous development of force to calcium and the effect of acidic pH on this sensitivity change with development. Across phyla, the myofilamentous development of force is more sensitive to calcium in the fetal and neonatal heart as compared to the adult heart.[63,64] In contrast, acidosis has a greater negative effect on these processes in the adult compared to the fetal and neonatal situations.[65,66] Altogether, these developmental changes appear to be teleologically appropriate. The peak cytosolic transient for calcium is lower in the immature myocyte (see Fig. 4-11), requiring a greater sensitivity of the myofilaments to calcium to induce a comparable force of contraction for a given concentration The greater resistance of the immature heart to acidosis, also, seems appropriate given that episodes of acidosis are likely to occur during perinatal life.

The developmental switch in expression from slow skeletal to cardiac troponin I has an important effect on the extent to which acidic pH negatively affects myofilamentous function.[67] In the human, developmental pull in slow skeletal troponin I takes place during fetal life, and the first years of postnatal life.[68,69] The expression of the slow skeletal form in the immature heart provides a protective effect against perinatal acidosis. Development of force by myofilaments containing the slow skeletal form is more resistant to acidosis than that of myofilaments containing the cardiac version.

The complexity of the differential effects of these different forms of troponin I on the sensitivity of the myofilaments to calcium at different stages of development is reflected in several ways. First, myofilaments containing the slow skeletal form are more sensitive to calcium, as measured by active development of force, while being less sensitive to acidic pH. Second, cardiac myocytes expressing the slow skeletal form have impaired relaxation, and left ventricles expressing this form have slowed diastolic relaxation.[70] Third, expression of the cardiac form confers onto the myofilaments a more positive effect of increasing their length on myofilamentous calcium, and so enhances the Frank–Starling relation.[71] Fourth, phosphorylation of the cardiac form dependent on cyclic adenosine triphosphate, through stimulations of β-adrenoreceptors, decreases the sensitivity of the myofilaments to calcium,[72] blunting markedly the effect of increasing sarcomeric length on increasing myofilamentous sensitivity to calcium. The physiological importance of such phosphorylation of the cardiac form on sensitivity to calcium is a more rapid relaxation of myocardial contraction. This more rapid relaxation is important given the stimulation of the β-adrenoreceptors increases in the peak of the $[Ca^{2+}]_i$ transient, development of force, and heart rate. In the absence of the more rapid relaxation that follows from this phosphorylation, the increase in heart rate induced by stimulation of β-adrenoreceptors would be associated with an inappropriate decrease in diastolic filling time, and a compromise in ventricular filling, negatively affecting stroke volume. In contrast, stimulation of β-adrenoreceptors has no effect on the slow skeletal form of troponin I, making the sarcomere in the developing heart less sensitive to the effects of such stimulation, and so potentially superimposing a compounding effect on the positive effects of stimulation on heart rate and the $[Ca^{2+}]_i$ transient, while maintaining the Frank–Starling relation in a positive fashion.

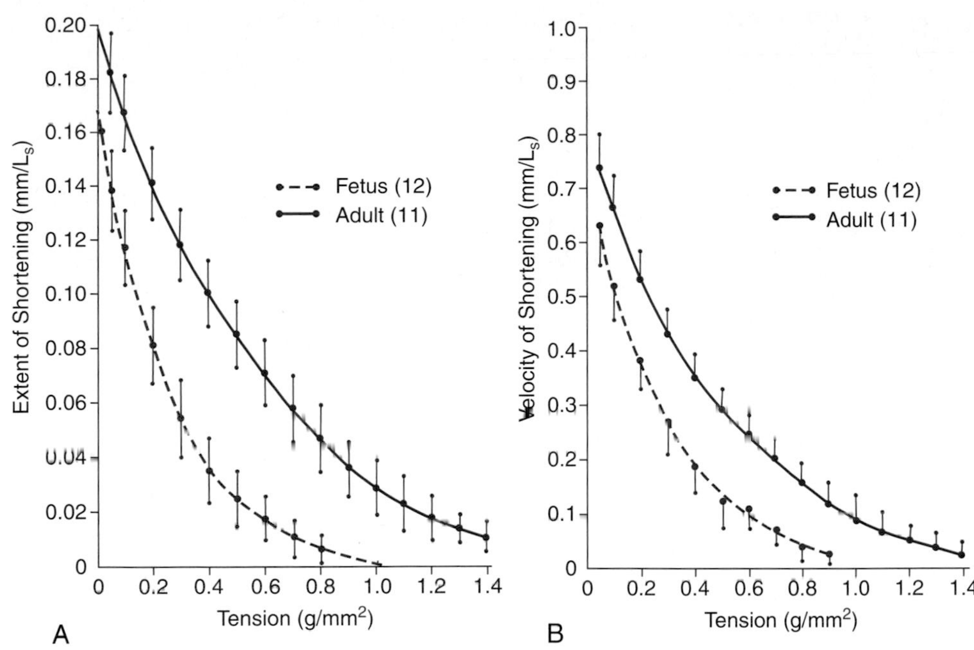

Figure 4-19 Myocardial contractility increases with development. Relationships between the extent (**A**) and velocity (**B**) of shortening and developed tension (i.e., afterload) of myocardium isolated from fetal and adult sheep (*blue,* adult data; *red,* fetal data). Both reflect the ability of the myocardium to generate tension. Fetal myocardium is not able to shorten with the same velocity and to the same extent as adult myocardium does when subjected to the same load. Each point and vertical bar represents the mean ± SEM. (From Friedman WF: The intrinsic physiologic properties of the developing heart. Prog Cardiovasc Dis 1972;15:87–111, Figure 3.)

Developmental switching in the expression of the isoforms of cardiac troponin T, also, affects the sensitivity of myofilamentous development of force to calcium.[30,63] During development, the expression of the two longest and most acidic isoforms decreases, while that of the two shorter and less acidic ones increases.[73] The calcium sensitivity of the myofilaments is greatest in the presence of the two longest isoforms.[74] I have already emphasised that the calcium transient is lower in the neonatal than in the adult myocyte[30] (see Fig. 4-11). Furthermore, the expression of the longer isoforms in the developing heart compensates for the lower calcium transient in the immature heart. The expression of the isoforms of troponin I modulates the effects of the cardiac isoforms of troponin T on the sensitivity of the myofilaments to calcium. The slow skeletal form expressed in the immature heart enhances the positive effect of the longer isoforms of cardiac troponin T, further compensating for the smaller calcium transient in the immature heart, and helping support its function.[75]

The β- and α-isoforms of tropomyosin have a differential effect on the sensitivity of the myofilaments to calcium, and also undergo changes in expression with development. In the rodent, α-tropomyosin essentially replaces β-tropomyosin in the adult heart.[76] In contrast, in the human, β-tropomyosin expression increases by half from the fetus to the adult.[77] Myofilaments containing β-tropomyosin have greater sensitivity to calcium, so that the developmental switch in the rodent to α-tropomyosin will lead to a decrease in sensitivity of development of force to calcium. Consistent with this effect, ventricles expressing β-tropomyosin have decreased rates of ventricular diastolic relaxation as compared to those expressing α-tropomyosin.[78] In contrast, in the human, the developmental increase in expression of β-tropomyosin could have a positive effect on the sensitivity of myofilamentous development of force to calcium.

The velocity of myocardial shortening increases with development. These changes are well correlated with activity of myofibrillar adenosine triphosphatase[1] (Fig. 4-19). The developmental switch in expression from the β to the α variant of myosin heavy chain in the rat heart has led to the correlation of developmental changes in shortening velocity to expression of the isozymes of myosin heavy chain. In the human, it is the β form that is expressed predominantly across maturation from fetal life through senescence, and also in the presence of hypertrophy and cardiac failure. Consequently, in the human, maturational changes in expression of isozymes are not likely to contribute to the developmental increase in myocardial contractility. There is a complex developmental pattern of expression of the α-isoform of actin.[79–81] The smooth muscle variant is expressed during cardiac embryogenesis. Subsequently, the skeletal and cardiac forms are expressed differentially with development in a species-dependent manner. In the rodent, the skeletal form is expressed in the fetus, and the cardiac form in the adult. In contrast, in human myocardium, expression of cardiac α-actin is highest during fetal development, while expression of the skeletal variant is equal to or higher to than the cardiac form in the adult heart.[82] The skeletal, and cardiac forms of α-actin differ by only a few residues. The basis for the differences in expression of the isoforms between species, and the consequences of these different patterns on function and organogenesis, remain to be determined.

THE MYOCYTIC CYTOSKELETON

The cytoskeleton is the complex meshwork of structural proteins that gives the cell its shape and organisation. In addition to the myofibrils, the microtubules, and intermediate filaments, made up of desmin, there are other major components. They connect the Z-discs to the sarcomeres, the myofibrils one to another, and the myofibrils to the T-tubules, mitochondria, and nuclei (Fig. 4-20). Myofibrils that lie just underneath the sarcolemma are

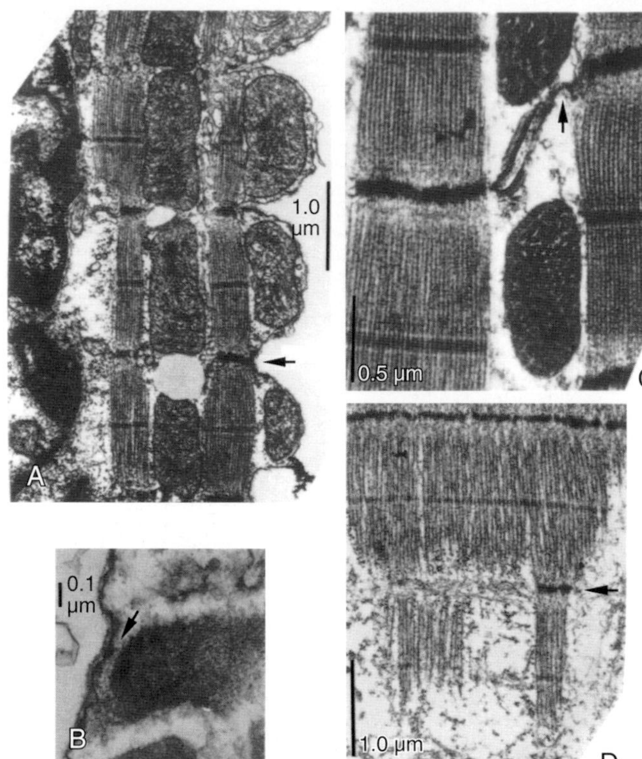

Figure 4-20 The relation of the Z-band to the sarcolemma and to the intermediate filaments in isolated adult cardiac myocytes. **A,** A longitudinal section shows two rows of myofibrils and mitochondria. The sarcolemma is on the right, and a nucleus is at the left. The sarcolemma appears fused with the Z-I area of the sarcomere at the *arrow*, the region of colocalisation of the cytoskeletal protein vinculin and the extracellular matrix protein-binding integrins. **B,** A cross-section of a comparable region of another adult cell. The density between the sarcolemma and the Z-I band area is frequently observed (*arrow*). **C,** The cytoskeletal attachment of the T-tubule to the Z-band is suggested by this image, in which the T-tubule profile maintains a close proximity to two Z-lines that are out of register (*arrow*). **D,** A slightly oblique longitudinal section of a myocyte from the heart of a 3-week-old rabbit illustrates a ring of intermediate filaments surrounding the Z-line (*arrow*). (From Nassar R, Reedy MC, Anderson PAW: Developmental changes in the ultrastructure and sarcomere shortening of the isolated rabbit ventricular myocyte. Circ Res 1987;61:465–483, Figure 9.)

attached to the sarcolemma at the Z-disc by structures called costameres, which are formed from vinculin, another cytoskeletal protein (see Fig. 4-20).[83] Desmin-containing intermediate filaments, and the vinculin-containing costameres, together with titin, provide the passive properties of length and tension of the single cardiac myocyte, and contribute to the properties of the intact myocardium[83] (Figs. 4-21 and 4-22). This scaffolding of microtubules, intermediate filaments, and costameres underlies the integrated movement of the contractile apparatus, the intracellular membranous compartments, and the sarcolemma during contraction and relaxation in the adult myocyte.

The cytoskeletal proteins spectrin and ankyrin are located in the sarcolemma near the Z-disc, and extend along the sarcolemma from Z-disc to Z-disc. The spectrins and sarcoglycan complex are thought to play a role in maintaining cellular integrity and flexibility as components of the membrane cytoskeleton.[84] α-Actinin, a major component of the Z-disc in striated muscle, and β-spectrin, have a highly conserved amino-terminal actin-binding domain.[85] Through this domain, α-actinin provides an anchor for the sarcomeric thin filaments in the Z-disc.

Integrins are transmembrane receptors for the proteins within the extracellular matrix, for example collagen, fibronectin, and laminin. They colocalise with the cytoskeletal attachments to the sarcolemma.[86] Their receptors are dimeric, containing an α- and β-subunit with the β-subunits being associated with different sets of α-subunits.[86] The multiple α-subunits appear to confer ligand specificity, in that α_1- and α_2-subunits have affinity for interstitial collagens, collagen type IV, and laminin, while the α_3-subunit interacts with fibronectin. These integrins are localised to sarcolemmal regions adjacent to the Z-discs, providing sites of attachment of collagen to the sarcolemmal Vinculin, the cytoskeletal protein that attaches the Z-discs to the sarcolemma, colocalises to the cytocollagenous attachment[87–89] (see Fig. 4-20). The integrins provide a mechanism for interaction of environmental stimuli and intracellular events.[90] In addition, the organised arrangement of the receptors on the cell surface and the proteins in the extracellular matrix provides a link for transducing production of sarcomeric force into development of ventricular pressure and ejection of blood.

DEVELOPMENT AND THE CYTOSKELETON

The organisation and numbers of myofibrils in the cardiac myocyte undergo prominent changes during embryonic and neonatal life. Early in development, the myofibrils appear to lack any particular orientation relative to other myofibrils, and do not appear to be connected. This lack of organisation is associated with a relatively low density of myofilaments. Before the content of myofibrils, expressed as a percentage of total volume of the myocyte, reaches that of the adult myocyte, the myofibrils become oriented parallel to the long axis of the myocyte.[2] Following the acquisition of this orientation, the myofibrils are linked as a thin subsarcolemmal shell surrounding a central mass of nucleus and mitochondria (see Fig. 4-5 and compare Fig. 4-22 with Fig. 4-23). In these immature cells, the large central mass of non-contractile material provided an internal load against which the myofibrils must contract. With further maturation, the myocyte achieves an ordered packing of alternating layers of myofibrils and mitochondria from one side of the myocyte to the other (see Fig. 4-5). All of these developmental changes are important in bringing about a more efficient transmission of development of force from the sarcomere.

The proteins that make up the cytoskeleton, and the sarcolemmal receptors for integrin, change with development, as does their distribution within the myocyte.[86,88,89,91] The affinity of cardiac myocytes for specific components of the extracellular matrix also changes with development. These results are consistent with developmentally regulated expression of integrin receptor α-subunit isoforms. In the human, expression of desmin increases during fetal life, with the distribution of desmin into the integrated lattice within the myocyte being acquired by the end of the first year of life.[92]

It is unclear how the developmental changes in the cytoskeleton contribute to the developmental increase in myocardial compliance (see Fig. 4-2). In isolated cardiac myocytes, the length of the sarcomeres in the neonatal myocyte is shorter than that of the adult myocyte, suggesting greater internal loads in the neonatal myocyte.[2] The perinatal

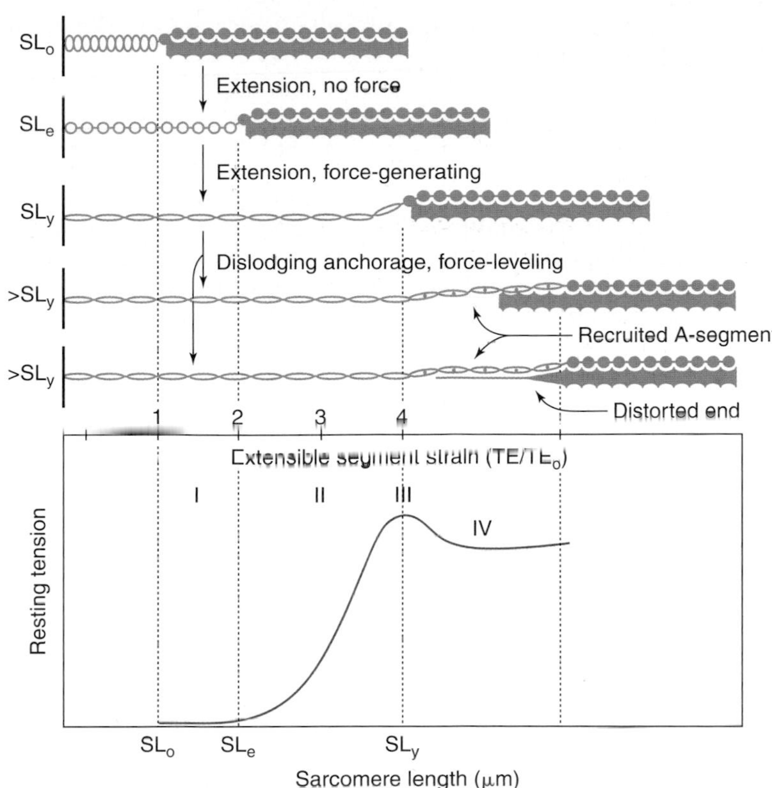

Figure 4-21 Segmental extension of titin filaments as the structural basis of passive tension-length relations of resting muscle. The titin filaments are illustrated as chains of filled circles along the top of the thick filaments and as coiled-coils extending from the end of the thick filament to the Z-disc (see also Fig. 4-16). The postulated structural events of the titin filaments that underlie the stress-strain curves are shown. The titin filament is represented as consisting of two mechanically distinct segments: an extensible segment in the I-band (*open symbols*) and an inextensible segment that is constrained by interaction with thick filaments (*solid symbols*). At slack sarcomere length (SL_o), titin maybe flaccid, and stretching to SL_e causes a small increase in force. Beyond SL_e, a linear extension of titin segment generates an exponential increase in tension. At SL_y, the extensible segment becomes longer by recruiting previously inextensible titin resulting in the leveling of tension. The net contour length of the extensible segment of titin is longer in a sarcomere expressing a larger titin isoform, for example N2BA (see Fig. 4-16). (From Wang K, McCarter R, Wright J, et al: Regulation of skeletal muscle stiffness and elasticity by titin isoforms: A test of the segmental extension model of resting tension. Proc Natl Acad Sci U S A 1991;88:7101–7105, Figure 5.)

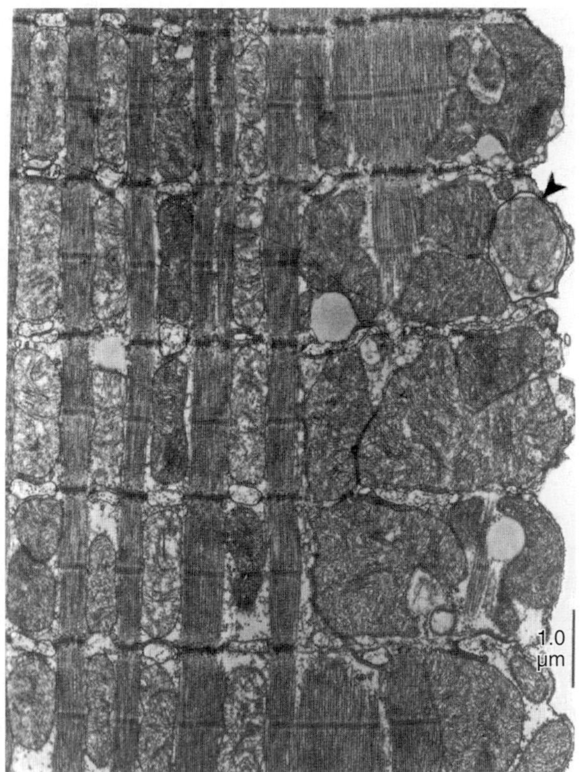

Figure 4-22 Longitudinal section of an isolated adult cardiac myocyte. T-tubule profiles are penetrating at the level of the Z-line of the cell surface, on the right, and appear as triads flanking each Z-line. Rows of mitochondria and myofibrils, which alternate across the image, typify the arrangement in the adult cell. The myofibril closest to the cell surface passes out of the section plane for a short distance, demonstrating that the mitochondria envelop each myofibril. A vesiculated gap junction is at the right (*arrowhead*). (From Nassar R, Reedy MC, Anderson PAW: Developmental changes in the ultrastructure and sarcomere shortening of the isolated rabbit ventricular myocyte. Circ Res 1987;61:465–483, Figure 7.)

switching in expression of isoforms of titin from longer highly extensible isoforms to shorter less extensible ones does not appear consistent with the developmental increase in myocardial compliance[93] (see Fig. 4-16). In that only a portion of the passive stiffness of the isolated myocyte is attributed to titin, developmental changes in the extracellular matrix, and switching of isoforms of the proteins within the extracellular matrix, may be a more important contributor to the developmental increase in passive compliance (see below).

DEVELOPMENT AND THE MITOCHONDRIA

Mitochondria undergo a developmental increase in crista thickness, number, size, and relative volume in the myocyte. These changes are most striking during early postnatal life.[4,94–96] Their highly ordered relation to the myofibrils in the adult myocyte is acquired with maturation (compare Figs. 4-5, 4-22, and 4-23). The effects of ventricular workload on this postnatal process are suggested by the more rapid increase in mitochondrial number and size in neonatal left ventricular myocytes. Fetal mitochondria contain sparse and widely spaced cristae, or crests. Soon after birth, these crests become dense and closely packed. Although acquisition of other properties during development varies among species, the postnatal timing of these changes in mitochondria is common to all mammals. The developmental changes are consistent with the mitochondria having an increased importance in postnatal life as a source of energy for sarcomeric function, the maturational increase in the ability of the myocardium to utilise long-chain fatty acids, and myocardial metabolism becoming primarily oxidative, with long chain fatty acids being the primary substrate.

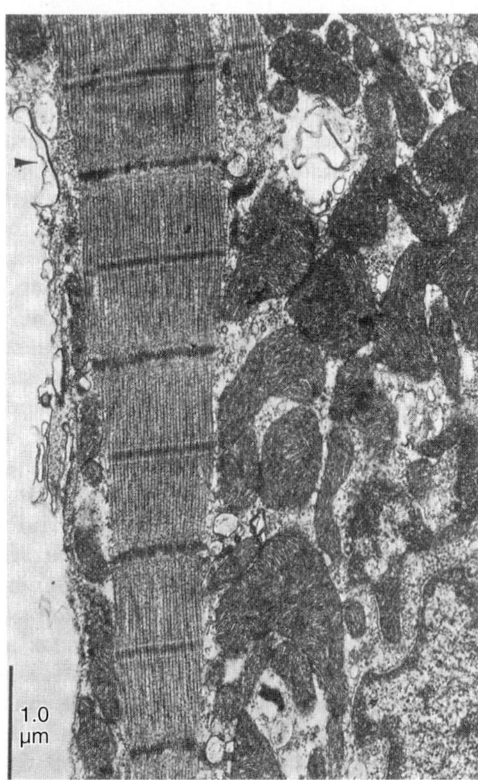

Figure 4-23 Longitudinal section of a myocyte isolated from the heart of a 3-week-old rabbit. Cell surface is to the left. A single myofibril lies just below the sarcolemma; mitochondria and a nucleus occupy the rest of the image. Note that in the immature cell, alternating rows of mitochondria and myofibrils are not present (compare Fig. 4-16). An incompletely vesiculated gap junction is seen at the *arrowhead.* (From Nassar R, Reedy MC, Anderson PAW: Developmental changes in the ultrastructure and sarcomere shortening of the isolated rabbit ventricular myocyte. Circ Res 1987;61:465–483, Figure 8.)

MYOCYTE-MYOCYTE CYTOSOLIC COMMUNICATION—GAP JUNCTIONS

Myocytes, although individual units anatomically, function as a synctium. The cytosol of adjacent myocytes is coupled directly by gap junctions in the sarcolemma that are made up of connexons containing six identical units, connexins, which surround an aqueous pore.[97,98] The channels in the sarcolemma of one cell join the channels in the adjacent cell. The intracellular communication is regulated by voltage, intracellular pH, calcium, and protein kinases.[99–101] The channels in the gap junction are of sufficient size, at 1 to 2 nm in diameter, to fulfill a signalling role, permitting the diffusion of small molecules, up to 1 kDa in size, from one cardiac myocyte to another.[11,102]

DEVELOPMENT AND MYOCYTE-MYOCYTE CYTOSOLIC COMMUNICATION

The density of gap junctions in the membranes increases during embryonic and fetal life in the mammal.[103,104] Expression of isoforms of the connexins also changes with development.[105] With development, conductances across the gap junction increase, and sensitivity to transjunctional voltage decreases. The net result of these developmental increases in the density of the gap junctions and their conductance is better coupling between the myocytes in adult myocardium, and a resultant increase in velocity of conduction.[106]

EXTRACELLULAR MATRIX

The extracellular matrix is an important contributor to the passive and active mechanical properties of the myocardium. It has multiple components, including interstitial collagen types I and III, glycoproteins, such as fibronectin and laminin, and proteoglycans, such as heparan sulphate and hyaluronic acid.[107,108] The interaction of this matrix with the cardiac myocytes requires the binding of the contained extracellular proteins to the receptors on the cell surface, the integrins.[86]

The network that makes up the extracellular matrix is considered to have four levels: the epimysium, perimysium, endomysium, and basement membrane.[108] The basement membrane is considered to be a specialised outer layer of the sarcolemma, where collagen type IV, laminin, fibronectin, and heparan sulphate are found. The epimysium is characterised as the region of the subepicardium and subendocardium. Its firm attachment to the cells makes up the epicardium and endocardium. The perimysium of the heart consists of large cable-like bundles of collagen that connect the epimysial layer with the endomysium, and give the appearance of a coiled spring. The fibroblasts, the major producers of components of the extracellular matrix, and the two interstitial collagens, collagen I and collagen III, have contacts with the endomysial collagen, adjacent fibroblasts, and myocytes, and form a three-dimensional weave that is intimately associated with myocytes and the extracellular matrix.[109] The endomysial layer itself consists of connections between fibroblasts, connections between fibroblasts and myocytes, connections between myocytes, connections between the myocytes and the capillaries, and interactions between the cells and the extracellular matrix in the overall weave. The connections include bundles of collagen that connect the adjacent myocytes, as well as attaching the myocytes to the capillaries and other components of the extracellular matrix.

DEVELOPMENT AND THE EXTRACELLULAR MATRIX

The specialised outer layer of the sarcolemma, where laminin, fibronectin, and heparan sulphate are found, undergoes prominent changes during embryonic, fetal, and perinatal development. For example, laminin is localised to distinct patches of extracellular matrix associated with the sarcolemma during fetal development, is distributed extensively over the myocyte in the neonate, and in the adult heart is localised most heavily in the area of morphological specialisation, such as the integrin-containing sarcolemmal regions that are adjacent to the Z-discs.[110] These interactions are involved in regulation of genetic expression, and myocytic differentiation.[111]

The principal elements of the network of connective tissue in the fetus are the epimysium and the perimysium. The weave is poorly developed at birth.[112] The collagenous connections between the myocytes themselves, and with the capillaries, develop rapidly in the heart during the neonatal period. In late fetal development, collagen type I and III are present in very low amounts.[112] The acquisition of the extracellular matrix during late fetal and early postnatal life with a relative increase in myocardial collagen may appear paradoxical when considered in the context of the developmental increase in myocardial compliance (see Fig. 4-2). A developmental change does occur, nonetheless, in the expression of the subtypes of collagen. Collagen type I provides rigidity, and type III provided elasticity. In the human, the ratio between these types is very high in the fetus, but falls with development.[113] This differential expression of the two types may underlie the developmental increase in compliance. Developmental changes in the expression of other proteins within the extracellular matrix, and the subunits of integrin, may also contribute to the developmental increase in myocardial compliance (see Fig. 4-2). Importantly, the developmental increase in myocardial compliance will lead to enhanced ventricular diastolic function, and potentially improved systolic function.

DEVELOPMENT, SYMPATHETIC INNERVATION, AND THE ADRENORECEPTORS

The sympathetic nervous system is important in the process of growth and differentiation of cells, control of calcium, and modulation of the response of the contractile and membrane proteins to activation of membranes and calcium. The cardiac sympathetic nerves are derived from the neural crest.[114] The response of the myocardium to β- and α-agonists precedes the acquisition of myocardial innervation.[1] The effects of exogenous catecholamines on myocardial function vary among species, and between investigations.[1,115–118] Commonly, the myocardium becomes more responsive with maturation.[1,117] The intramyocardial availability of noradrenaline, which stimulates both α- and β-adrenoreceptors, increases with the developmental acquisition of the intramyocardial adrenergic plexuses, and the associated increased storage of the neurotransmitter in their synaptic vesicles. This developmental increase in myocardial stores of noradrenaline is reflected in the human by an increased ability of the myocardium to take up noradrenaline during gestation.[119] The maturational time course of cardiac innervation varies among species. In some, innervation appears during fetal life while, in others, innervation is acquired during postnatal life.[1,120–122] In the human fetus, nerves grow into the heart along the large coronary arteries before extending into the myocardium. The developmental acquisition of sympathetic innervation provides an intrinsic system within the myocardium to enhance contractility and increase heart rate.

The functional consequences of these maturational changes are multiple. The coupling of receptors to the adenylate cyclase system is acquired with maturation, resulting in more effective phosphorylation of target proteins following adrenoreceptor stimulation. Phosphorylation of the α_1-subunit of the L-type calcium channel dependent on protein kinase, itself dependent on cyclic adenosine triphosphate, results in an increase in calcium current. Removal of phospholamban inhibition of SERCA, by way of phosphorylation of protein kinase A, results in an increase in activity of SERCA, a more rapid uptake of cytosolic calcium by the sarcoplasmic reticulum, and a greater intracellular store of calcium for release during subsequent contractions. The combination of these effects on the calcium channel and the sarcoplasmic reticulum is an increase in the peak of the calcium transient, and more rapid fall of calcium itself to diastolic levels. Phosphorylation of troponin I dependent on cyclic adenosine triphosphate results in decreased sensitivity of the myofilaments to calcium, allowing the cardiac contraction to relax more rapidly, the so-called lusotropic effect, and, in addition, a blunting of the Frank–Starling relation. These, and other examples, characterise the complex interactions that result from the developmental changes in the autonomic nervous system and the systems intrinsic to the regulation of calcium and sarcomeric function.

The complete reference list can be found on the companion Expert Consult web site at www.expertconsult.com.

ANNOTATED REFERENCES

- Nassar R, Reedy MC, Anderson PAW: Developmental changes in the ultrastructure and sarcomere shortening of the isolated rabbit ventricular myocyte. Circ Res 1987;61:465–483.

  Sarcomere shortening and the ultrastructure of intact isolated ventricular myocytes from the neonatal and adult rabbit are examined. The developmental changes in function and structure provide an understanding of the basis of increased contractility of the adult myocyte.

- Anversa P, Olivetti G, Loud AV: Morphometric study of early postnatal development in the left and right ventricular myocardium of the rat: I. Hypertrophy, hyperplasia, and binucleation of myocytes. Circ Res 1980;46:495–502.

  The absolute and differential growths of the populations of myocytes in the right and left ventricular myocardium are examined in the first days following birth. The effects of the circulatory changes occurring shortly after birth are related to the differences in hyperplasia between the right and left ventricles.

- Bers DM: Cardiac excitation-contraction coupling. Nature 2002;415:198–205.

  An excellent overview of excitation-contraction coupling is provided. The article provides a basic understanding of how calcium is moved around among the various organelles of the myocyte to bring about myocardial contraction and relaxation.

- Bodi I, Mikala G, Koch SE, et al: The L-type calcium channel in the heart: The beat goes on. J Clin Invest 2005;115:3306–3317.

  The heart does not beat in the absence of extracellular calcium. This article examines the role of extracellular calcium and the L-type voltage-dependent calcium channel in normal cardiac function and in disease.

- Flucher BE, Franzini-Armstrong C: Formation of junctions involved in excitation-contraction coupling in skeletal and cardiac muscle. Proc Natl Acad Sci U S A 1996;93:8101–8106.

  The structural organisation and composition of the intracellular junctions fundamental to release of calcium from internal stores are provided. The organisation of the L-type calcium channel and the ryanodine receptor in the sarcoplasmic reticulum is discussed in the context of the development of normal and mutant muscle.

- Gyorke I, Hester N, Jones LR, Gyorke S: The role of calsequestrin, triadin, and junctin in conferring cardiac ryanodine receptor responsiveness to luminal calcium. Biophys J 2004;86:2121–2128.

  The molecular basis of ryanodine receptor regulation by luminal sarcoplasmic reticulum calcium is investigated in the context of the luminal auxiliary proteins calsequestrin, triadin, and junctin. This biophysical study suggests that the macromolecular complex of calsequestrin, triadin, and junctin refer onto the ryanodine receptor luminal calcium sensitivity.

- McCall SJ, Nassar R, Malouf NN, et al: Development and cardiac contractility: Cardiac troponin T isoforms and cytosolic calcium in rabbit. Pediatr Res 2006;60:276–281.

  The functional consequences of the developmental changes in the expression of the cardiac troponin T isoforms are considered in the context of the cytosolic calcium transient in myocytes from the immature and the adult rabbit heart. The higher calcium sensitivity of troponin–calcium binding and force development conferred by the longest and most acidic of the cardiac troponin T isoforms suggest that the higher expression of these isoforms in the neonatal myocyte may partially compensate for the lower systolic calcium transient in the immature myocyte.

- Altamirano J, Li Y, DeSantiago J, et al: The inotropic effect of cardioactive glycosides in ventricular myocytes requires Na+-Ca2+ exchanger function. J Physiol 2006;575:845–854.

  The demonstration that sodium–calcium exchanger function is required for the inotropic effect of cardiac glycosides in ventricular myocytes is consistent with the positive effect of cardiac glycosides on myocardial contractility in the immature heart where exchanger expression may be higher.

- Gordon AM, Homsher E, Reginier M: Regulation of contraction in striated muscle. Physiol Rev 2000;80:853–924.

  The regulation by calcium of contraction in cardiac muscle is exerted primarily through effects on the thin filament. The three-state model of thin filament activation and the structural and biochemical studies that underlie this model are reviewed.

- Day SM, Westfall MV, Fomicheva E, et al: Histidine button engineered into cardiac troponin protects the ischemic and failing heart. Nat Med 2006;12:181–189.

  The molecular basis for the differential effect of acidic pH on the function of myofilaments containing cardiac troponin I and slow skeletal muscle troponin I is revealed. A single histidine residue difference between the two isoforms results in acidic pH having a greater negative effect on myofilaments containing cardiac troponin I. This difference is of fundamental importance in the developing heart, where ss is the dominantly expressed isoform during fetal and perinatal life.

- Gomes AV, Venkatraman G, Davis JP, et al: Cardiac troponin T isoforms affect the Ca^{2+} sensitivity of force development in the presence of slow skeletal troponin I: Insights into the role of troponin T isoforms in the fetal heart. J Biol Chem 2004;279:49579–49587.

  The developmental changes in the cardiac troponin T isoforms have been shown to confer onto myofilaments in the developing heart a greater sensitivity to calcium. Here, the slow skeletal muscle and cardiac forms are shown to modulate the effects of the cardiac isoforms. The contemporaneous expression of the slow skeletal muscle form in the developing heart amplifies the positive effects of the fetal cardiac isoforms.

CHAPTER 5

Physiology of the Developing Heart

HELENA M. GARDINER

The heart is the first organ to become fully functional in the developing embryo, providing the circulatory system necessary for embryogenesis and subsequent fetal development when growth can no longer be sustained by diffusion of nutrients from the surrounding tissue. The rapid advances in genetics and molecular biology have revolutionised our knowledge of the developing embryonic heart. In similar fashion, technical improvements in imaging and non-invasive physiological recording of the early human fetus have enabled us to study the human heart non-invasively from the first trimester, and build on information from studies of the chick embryo model.[1]

The drive towards a greater understanding of the molecular aspects of cardiac development during the previous decade temporarily pushed the physiologist to the sidelines in cardiovascular research.[2] The pendulum is now swinging back to a combined approach that will allow translation of information obtained from basic science into clinical practice, and provide a unique picture of human cardiovascular development along with the long-term cardiovascular responses to intra-uterine and postnatal challenges. In this chapter, I review our current understanding of the physiology and pathophysiology of the human heart in fetal life, and determinants of a successful transition in the perinatal period.

EMBRYONIC CIRCULATION

In the chick embryo, rhythmic pulsations of approximately 50 Hz begin in the ventricle, coincident with fusion of cushions in the ventriculo-arterial segment. These pulsations, although rhythmic, are insufficiently forceful to set blood in motion, or to generate recordable pressures, the onset of electrical activity preceding myofibrillogenesis.[3] The elaboration of intracellular contractile proteins is incomplete at this stage, the functional contractile units are not fully assembled, and the matrix of collagen has not yet formed.[4] Once cardiac rhythm is established, nonetheless, the myofibrils within the myocytes become aligned and, as the heart rate rises, the direction of flow of blood is established to provide a circulation for the growing embryo. Growth of the atriums and ventricles is associated with an increase in the rate of pulsation of the primitive heart tube. This establishes the direction of propagation of the peristaltic waves of contraction from atrium to ventricle.

Cardiac myocytes isolated from the venous sinus, atrium, and ventricle at this developmental stage in the chick embryo all exhibit automaticity with different intrinsic rates of contraction. The ventricle is slowest, at approximately 50 to 60 Hz, while cells from the venous sinus have the fastest rate, with the atrium being intermediate. The earliest recordings of human fetal cardiac activity have been obtained at 25 days after fertilisation by high-frequency trans-vaginal ultrasound. At this stage, only the amniotic sac is visible, and no embryonic poles are identifiable. The mean heart rate at this stage of gestation is approximately 90 beats per minute and regular. This most likely represents atrial rhythm. The mechanism responsible for the characteristic early increase in heart rate between the fifth and eighth weeks of gestation is uncertain. The initial rapid increase in the frequency of contraction is comparable to that occurring in the chick embryo. It is associated with the transition of the pacemaker, first from ventricle to atrium as fusion occurs between the two, and then to the venous sinus as this segment becomes incorporated into the right atrium. The precursor of the sinus node, which assumes the role of the cardiac pacemaker subsequently, is formed at the junction of the developing superior caval vein with the atrium.

By 8 to 10 weeks, the mean heart rate in the human fetus varies between 160 and 170 beats per minute, declining to an average of 150 beats per minute at 15 weeks. After this, the rate declines progressively towards term. This pattern of change in heart rate, seen during embryonic and fetal life in the human, parallels that occurring in the chick, in which cardiac action begins between 33 and 36 hours at a rate of 60 beats per minute, and increases to 220 beats per minute by the eighth day of gestation.

In the human, there is little variation of the mean heart rate at any particular gestational age up until 15 weeks, as the pre-innervated immature cardiovascular system does not rely on heart rate acutely to control cardiac output. The maximum cardiac output occurs at the intrinsic heart rate at each embryonic stage, suggesting that, as in the chick, cardiac function is optimised by the systolic and diastolic time intervals.[5]

Alterations in heart rate significantly affect cardiac performance,[6] and there is no compensatory change in cycle length in response to preload as is seen in the more mature heart. Human embryos die if their heart rate falls, or if they experience tachycardia.[7] This indicates that, during cardiogenesis, extremes of heart rate are not commensurate with long-term viability.[8]

AUTONOMIC CONTROL

The subsequent decline in heart rate after 10 weeks, and the increased variability in heart rate after 15 weeks of gestation, may be explained by a combination of maturational changes. These include development of the nervous control of the heart, stresses associated with cardiogenesis, and changes in the handling of calcium by the myocyte.

Innervation of the mammalian heart is similar to that in the chick heart, consisting of parasympathetic, sympathetic, and sensory components, all of which derive from the neural crest.[9] Although parasympathetic and sympathetic innervation of the heart occurs early during cardiac development, the time period between innervation, neuroeffector transmission, and functional neurotransmitter reactivity of both cholinergic and adrenergic receptors, varies greatly between species. Functional adrenergic and muscarinic cholinergic receptors have been detected in the heart of very early chick embryos.[10] These differences in the timing to achieve a balance between parasympathetic and sympathetic reflex neuroeffector transmission in varying mammalian species relates largely to the maturity and independence of the individual animal species at birth. The variability in heart rate reflects the changing status of the autonomic nervous system as the heart becomes more sensitive in response to internal and external stimuli. Spectral analysis of the variability of heart rate in the normal human fetus demonstrates gestational-related changes ascribed to the imbalance between sympathetic and parasympathetic neuroactivity consistent with cardiovascular maturity of the fetus. Maturation of autonomic control has been difficult to assess in the human fetus until relatively recently, as the cardiotocograph has been the only non-invasive tool available to measure the variability in heart rate. This system provides limited information, as it uses a mean of three fetal heartbeats, compared with beat-to-beat recordings of cardiac activity. Furthermore, it does not produce an electrical signature. New tools, such as magnetocardiography, have permitted a more detailed assessment of the developing electrophysiology in the human fetus, and will be discussed later in this chapter.

THE BIOPHYSICAL PROPERTIES OF FETAL MYOCARDIUM

The biophysical characteristics of fetal, neonatal and adult myocardium have been investigated in a number of mammalian species, but the studies in the sheep and rabbit have provided the majority of information.[11,12] (See also Chapter 4.) These studies have consistently demonstrated that active development of tension is lower in fetal than adult myocardium at all lengths, including the optimal length.[11] In addition, in the ovine fetus, resting tension was greater than that in the adult animal; consequently, operational development of peak tension was less at all lengths (Fig. 5-1). The velocity and extent of shortening in fetal myocardium were lower than in adult myocardium at every level of developed tension (Fig. 5-2). Explanations for this have been sought. Sarcomeral length is optimal, and not significantly different, in fetal and adult myocardium. The difference in developed tension, therefore, cannot be accounted for entirely by the greater proportion of non-contractile protein per unit cross sectional area of fetal myocardium. It may be explained in part by the different sensitivity of the fetal contractile proteins troponin and myosin to cytosolic calcium.[12]

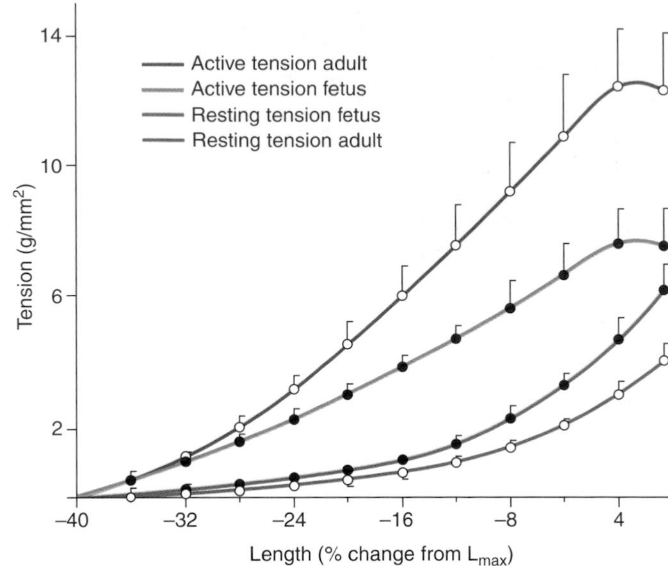

Figure 5-1 Comparison of peak isometric passive and active length–tension curves in the fetal heart and adult heart. The former had consistently higher resting tension over the range of muscle lengths. (Reproduced with permission from Friedman WF: The intrinsic physiologic properties of the developing heart. Prog Cardiovasc Dis 1972;15:87–111.)

In the early human fetus, handling of calcium depends on diffusional gradients through the sarcolemma in the absence of a developed sarcoplasmic reticulum. Sarcoplasmic calcium ATPase is expressed in a downstream gradient along the primitive heart tube, resulting in increased contraction duration in the outlet portions of the heart. By the 38th day of gestation, the early human myocardium may be divided into primary and working functional components. The primary components are characterised by slow conduction of the cardiac impulse, owing to the low density of gap junctions and the presence of slow voltage-gated calcium ion channels. The working components, found in the atriums and ventricles, permit fast conduction through the development of gap junctions and of fast voltage-gated sodium channels. The sarcoplasmic reticulum later regulates calcium release in the cell and is known to play an important role in the frequency-dependent facilitation of the L-type calcium current in the rat ventricular myocyte.[13]

The three major connexins, 40, 43, and 45, are present in cardiac myocytes and are developmentally regulated. Immunoconofocal microscopy has been used to compare the distribution of these within the developing mouse and human heart. In the human, connexin 45 is most prominent in the conduction tissues; connexin 40 is also abundant in conduction tissues, particularly in the Purkinje fibres, and in the atrial rather than in the ventricular muscle; and connexin 43 is distributed in the ventricular myocardium, and plays an important role in conduction across gap junctions.[14] Downregulation of gap junctional conduction has been demonstrated in cardiomyopathy caused by tyrosine phosphorylation of connexin 43.[15] Altered patterns of calcium ionic fluxes, and of abnormal β-adrenoreceptor stimulation in diseased adult myocardium,[16] may also occur in the developing heart exposed to chronic hypoxaemia associated

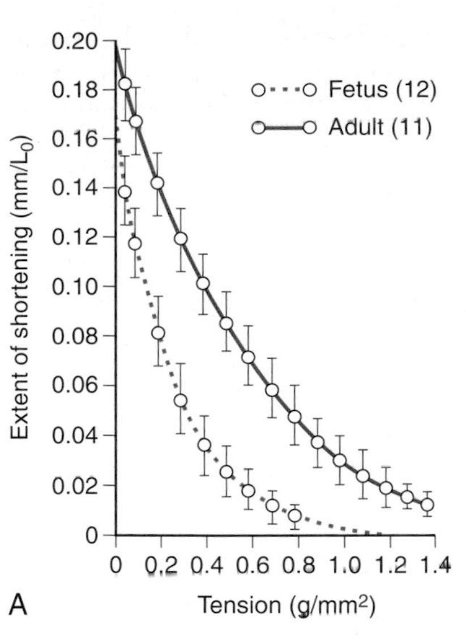

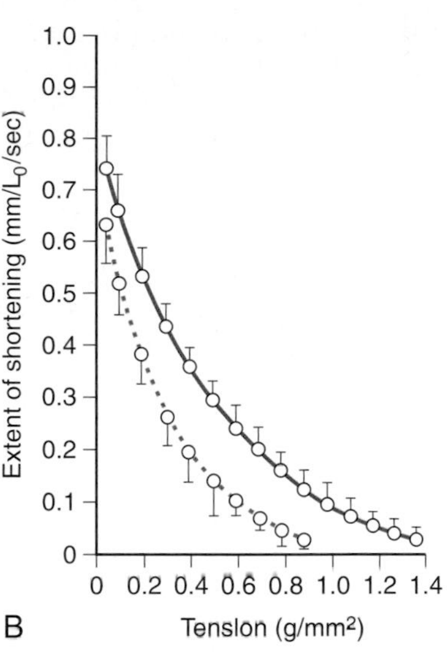

Figure 5-2 Relationships between extent (**A**) and velocity (**B**) of the shortening and developed tension in the fetal and adult sheep. These plots demonstrate a lesser degree of shortening and a lower velocity of shortening in the fetal compared with the adult sheep. (Reproduced with permission from Friedman WF: The intrinsic physiologic properties of the developing heart. Prog Cardiovasc Dis 1972;15:87–111.)

with restriction of growth, or in conditions with abnormal volume loading.

PROTEIN COMPONENTS

Troponin

The differences between fetal and adult myocardial contractile function are, in large part, related to their regulatory and structural protein components. Different isoforms of troponin and myosin heavy chain have been identified in fetal and adult myocardium from a number of mammalian species, including humans. These are genetically programmed during early embryonic development, and are modulated by specific neurohormones. Troponin T has been studied extensively and cloned. It regulates contraction in response to the concentration of ionic calcium.[17] Multiple isoforms have been recognised, the gene *TNNT2* being identified on chromosome 1q23. Slow skeletal muscle troponin T is the predominant isoform throughout fetal life, but this is lost after birth. Only troponin I is detectable by 9 months of postnatal life.[18] The genes coding for these two isoforms lie in close apposition, but show independent tissue-specific expression, although this close arrangement may complicate investigation of mutations implicated in cardiomyopathy.[19] A knock-out model of myocardial troponin I has shown that, while affected mice are born healthy, they begin to develop heart failure by 15 days. They have an isoform of troponin I that is identical to slow skeletal troponin I, and permits survival, but this isoform disappears after birth despite the lack of compensatory myocardial troponin I. Cardiac muscle is abnormal in the absence of troponin I. The ventricular myocytes have shortened sarcomeres, and elevated resting tension under relaxing conditions, and they show reduced sensitivity of their myofilaments to calcium under activating conditions.[20] Calcium is released more readily in fetal isoforms of SSTN1 than adult muscle cardiac troponin T isoforms. In its presence, troponin T shows increased calcium sensitivity of force development.[21] In contrast, a reduction in calcium sensitivity of force development is seen in individuals with dilated cardiomyopathy caused by mutation of troponin T1 in the R141W and delta K210 regions.[22]

Beta-myosin

The β-myosin heavy chain isoform predominates in all fetal mammals thus far examined, including humans. This isoform is more efficacious in the fetus, conferring biochemical and mechanical advantages on fetal myocardium, in that the β-isoform utilises less oxygen and ATP than the adult α-isoform in generating the same amount of force. Recent investigations have shown re-expression of fetal genes that downregulate adult, but not fetal, isoforms in response to increased cardiac work and subsequent mechanical unloading. This response appears to result in mechanical improvement, and may be important in future strategies for the management of cardiac failure.[23]

The myosin heavy chain carries the ATPase site. The enzymic kinetics of the ATPase are specific for each isoform. This has importance, because it is the rate at which ATPase hydrolyses ATP that primarily determines the force–velocity relationship during myocardial contraction. This explains the fundamental differences in active and passive mechanics between fetal and adult myocardium.[24] The transition from fetal to adult isoforms of myosin heavy chain around birth is similar to the controlled switch from fetal to adult haemoglobin, and represents stage-specific regulation of genetic expression of the proteins prior to birth While a number of hormones, and particularly thyroid hormone,[25,26] are known to modulate the phenotypic expression of the myosin heavy chain, the factors responsible for the precise timing of the transition from fetal to adult isoforms remain unknown.

Chronic Heart Failure

Chronic heart failure in the human adult is characterised by left ventricular remodelling and reactivation of a fetal gene programme, with alterations of expression of micro RNA closely mimicking those observed in fetal cardiac tissue.[27] Furthermore, transfection of cardiomyocytes with a set of fetal micro RNAs induced cellular hypertrophy, as well as changes in gene expression comparable to that seen in the failing heart. Re-expression of fetal genes may also be seen in mice having obstruction to the left ventricular outflow tract. The myocardium achieves stable mural stress by hypertrophic response in the presence of pressure overload. Once compensated cardiac hypertrophy had occurred in these experiments, most of the genes returned to basal levels of expression. Thus, it appears that pressure overload results in transient early changes in genetic expression, and this may reflect a beneficial response, as there is no evidence of deterioration of haemodynamic function or heart failure.[28] This response, nonetheless, may result in a decompensated hypertrophic phenotype. There is some evidence in the Wistar rat model that hearts responding in a decompensated form show activation of pro-apoptotic pathways, in contrast to those showing compensated hypertrophy, who appear to block this using p38-MAPK. In these experiments, the response occurred early after the induction of the phenotype, and thus might be one helpful early predictor of clinical outcome, potentially allowing early interventional therapy.[29]

CIRCULATORY PHYSIOLOGY IN THE NORMAL HUMAN FETUS

The Fetoplacental Circulation

Knowledge of the physiological changes in the circulatory system beyond the period of cardiogenesis and embryonic life, including growth of the cardiac chambers, haemodynamics and oxygen saturation of the fetal pathways, ventricular interaction, and distribution of the cardiac output, are largely based on studies of the ovine fetus.[30–32] These experimental investigations have provided important insights into ovine fetal circulatory dynamics, which are similar to those in the human fetus, even though there are quantitative differences in the distribution of flows of blood, especially to the brachiocephalic and uteroplacental circulations in the human fetus, that caution against unconditional extrapolation.

The fetal circulation is characterised by four shunts. These are, first, within the placenta, second, across the venous duct, which connects the intrahepatic portion of the umbilical vein to the inferior caval vein, third, through the oval foramen, which is essential for filling of the fetal left ventricle, and fourth, across the arterial duct, which directs the majority of flow through the right ventricular outflow tract into the descending aorta below the level of the isthmus in the structurally normal heart. The patterns of flow through all these structures have been studied non-invasively in health and disease states using echo Doppler.

The Placenta

The placenta plays a major role in the fetal circulation, fulfilling the functions of the lung for exchange of gases, and for the kidney and gastrointestinal tract in delivery of nutrients and excretion of metabolites. The fetal side of the placenta, which develops from the chorion, receives blood from paired umbilical arteries, which take origin from the internal iliac arteries of the fetus. The umbilical arteries within the cord spiral around the umbilical vein, and then divide into branches at the junction of the cord and the placenta. These branches have a radial disposition. The terminal branches perforate the chorionic plate, and form anastomotic plexuses within the main stem of each chorionic villus. Each main stem possesses a derivative of the umbilical artery, which penetrates the thickness of the placenta, dividing to form a huge network of capillary plexuses. These project into the inter-villus spaces that contain maternal blood.[32] As a result, there is a very extensive surface area within each chorionic villus, across which exchange of gas occurs down gradients for both oxygen and carbon dioxide. There is, essentially, no mixing of maternal and fetal blood. Following oxygenation within the chorionic villi, the blood enters the venous radicals within each main stem. These efferent venules become confluent at the junction of the placenta and umbilical cord to form the umbilical vein.

The Venous Duct

The umbilical vein carries oxygenated blood, with an oxygen saturation of between 80% and 90%, from the placenta to the umbilical cord (Fig. 5-3). The cord enters the fetal abdomen, where it divides to form the portal sinus and the venous duct. The portal sinus joins the portal vein, while the venous duct carries oxygenated blood to the inferior caval vein. The origin and proximal part of the venous duct act as a physiological sphincter, which, during hypoxaemia

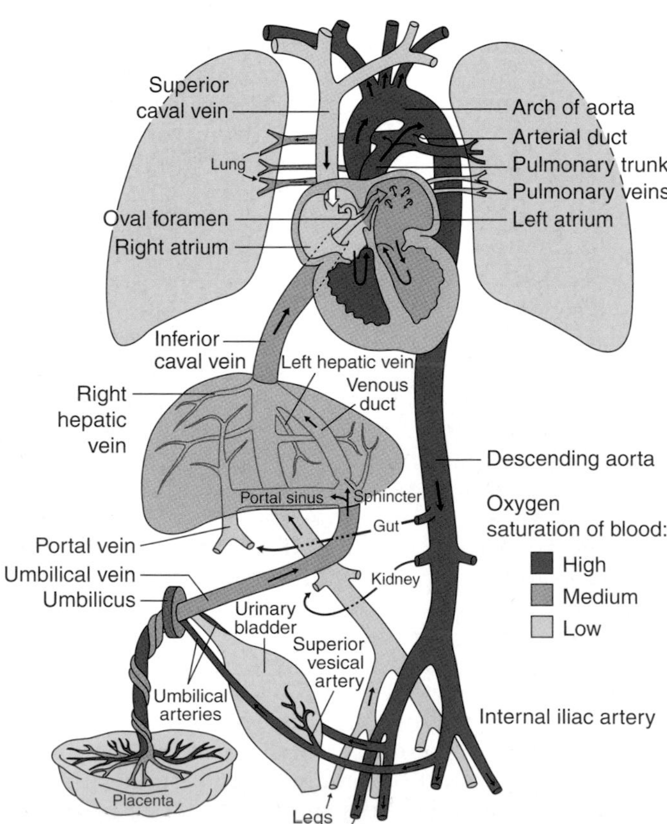

Figure 5-3 A simplified scheme of the fetal circulation. The *shading* indicates the oxygen saturation of the blood, and the *arrows* show the course of the fetal circulation. Three shunts permit most of the blood to bypass the liver and the lungs: the venous duct, the oval foramen, and the arterial duct. (Adapted with permission from Moore KL: The cardiovascular system. In The Developing Human: Clinically Oriented Embryology, 5th ed. Philadelphia: WB Saunders, 1993.)

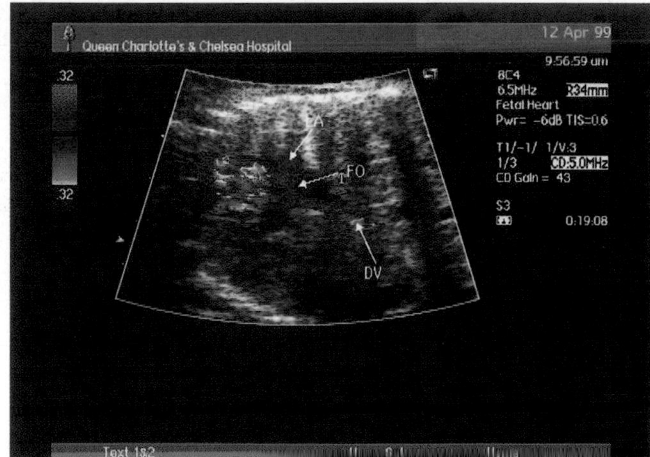

Figure 5-4 Parasagittal view of the fetal liver and heart. Colour flow mapping illustrates flow in the venous duct slipstreaming within the inferior caval vein, through the oval foramen to enter the left atrium.

or haemorrhage, results in an increased proportion of oxygenated blood passing through the duct to the inferior caval vein and to the heart, with less exiting to the portal sinus and the liver.[33] The oxygenated blood from the venous duct can be demonstrated coursing along the medial portion of the inferior caval vein after their confluence. Flow in the inferior caval vein continues towards the head into the inferior aspect of the right atrium, where a proportion of the oxygenated blood is slipstreamed by the lower border of the infolded atrial roof, also known as the dividing crest or crista dividens. This structure, therefore, acts as a baffle diverting blood into the atrium, a process which can readily be visualised during echocardiography (Fig. 5-4).

A proportion of the oxygenated blood is diverted to the heart, and this proportion varies in different mammalian species. The remainder of the mainly desaturated blood mixes with the desaturated blood from the mesenteric, renal, iliac, and right hepatic veins, and with that from the coronary sinus and the brachiocephalic veins.

The Oval Foramen

Patency of the oval foramen is essential to enable filling of the left side of the heart in the fetus, as pulmonary venous return is low. The proportion of oxygenated blood returning to the heart via the inferior caval vein that crosses the oval foramen to reach the left side of the heart also varies between species. This oxygenated blood mixes with the desaturated blood returning to the left atrium via pulmonary veins such that, after complete mixing in the left ventricle, the oxygen saturation is approximately 60%, compared with levels between 50% and 55% in the right ventricle. Blood from the left ventricle is directed to the brachiocephalic circulation, thus supplying the most oxygenated blood to the brain, which grows at a disproportionately greater rate in the human fetus compared with the rest of the body. The majority of blood ejected into the ascending aorta by the left ventricle is directed cephalad to the head and upper limbs, and only about one-third of the left ventricular stroke volume crosses the aortic isthmus to reach the descending thoracic aorta and lower body.

Although the arterial saturation of oxygen is comparatively low, extraction of oxygen by the tissues is facilitated by the leftward displacement of the dissociation curve for oxygen of fetal haemoglobin compared with that of the adult.

The Arterial Duct

The mixed venous return has an oxygen saturation of approximately 40%. This blood passes through the tricuspid valve into the right ventricle, where mixing occurs before it enters the pulmonary trunk, where the oxygen saturation is between 50% and 55%. The majority of blood in the pulmonary trunk passes through the arterial duct to the descending thoracic aorta, with only a small proportion continuing to the lungs via the right and left pulmonary arteries. The arterial duct enters the descending aorta immediately distal to the origin of the left subclavian artery, and blood is directed to the descending thoracic aorta by the geometry of its insertion, and also by a shelf-like projection at its upper insertion. The degree of patency of the arterial duct is regulated by the periductal smooth muscle cells, which produce prostaglandins. In the human fetus, ductal flow may be compromised by maternal ingestion of inhibitors of prostaglandins, such as the non-steroidal anti-inflammatory agents. Blood from the arterial duct mixes with that crossing the aortic isthmus from the aorta. This produces a saturation of oxygen between 50% and 55% in the descending aorta, from which a major proportion returns to the placenta via the umbilical arteries for reoxygenation.

FETAL DEVELOPMENTAL PHYSIOLOGY

Cardiac Growth

The first systematic study of cardiac growth in the human fetus was made using a large series of normal hearts obtained at postmortem. This established the relationship between total body weight, total heart weight, and the variability of heart weight with gestational age.[34] Detailed examination of the heart is now possible during the first trimester using trans-vaginal and transabdominal ultrasound.[35,36] These scans can provide excellent imaging of the fetal heart from 12 gestational weeks, even in multiple pregnancies. Diagnostic views at normal obstetric scanning depths can be obtained using modern ultrasound transducers with limits of resolution of about 50 μm in the axial plane at 6 MHz, and less than 100 μm in the lateral plane. As a result, morphological and physiological data have become easier to record and more reliable. *Z*-scores have been derived to take account of the effects of fetal gestation and growth on the size of vessels, valves and chambers. These are particularly useful for quantitative comparison when cardiac structures are very hypoplastic.[37,38] They are downloadable from references 37 and 38. Models derived from anatomical specimens have been superseded by three-and four-dimensional technology, which now permits assessment of volumes and morphology non-invasively in larger cohorts.[39,40] Magnetic resonance imaging, however, is still not sufficiently robust to provide cardiac imaging of comparable quality to ultrasound in the fetal heart.

Assessment of the Fetal Circulation

The fetal circulation is assessed using pulsed wave Doppler. Initial studies used blind continuous wave ultrasound of the umbilical cord. Technical improvements, including newer colour Doppler modalities such as energy and directional power, have enabled the visualisation and interrogation of smaller vessels in regional circulations and indicators of fetal wellbeing have been derived.[41,42]

In the healthy placenta, the copious villous bed allows exchange of oxygen and metabolic products. When placental function is severely reduced, as in fetuses with restricted growth, increased placental resistance leads to a reduction in total delivery of arterial oxygen to the fetus because of the reduction in mean placental return, even though the content of oxygen of the umbilical venous blood is often near normal. The fetal brain, heart and adrenal glands respond to this pathological state by drawing increased flow, thus requiring an increase in combined ventricular output to provide it. In the human fetus, the brain is the largest organ, and the healthy, responsive fetus is able to reduce cerebral resistance by arteriolar dilation.

The pulsatility index was derived in the 1970s to quantify waveforms in the umbilical cord, and assess fetal compromise. It uses the ratio of flow velocities as shown in Figure 5-5. Abnormalities of flow in the cord are characterised firstly by a reduction, and then a reversal, of diastolic velocities, thus increasing the pulsatility index. This may be accompanied by abnormalities of the umbilical vein as seen in Figure 5-6.

Initial experimental work in the fetal sheep model demonstrated a redistribution of flow in response to hypoxaemia.[43] With the availability of non-invasive Doppler techniques, the observed low diastolic flow was associated with uteroplacental insufficiency.[44] On the fetal side of the placenta, an increased resistance to flow in growth-restricted pregnancies was described.[45] Evidence of redistribution of flow in the growth-restricted human fetus during the same period was provided by a comparison of Doppler waveforms in the carotid, aortic and umbilical arteries, and also in the middle cerebral artery.[46–48] Animal work has supported the concept that, in the presence of uteroplacental insufficiency, the cerebral circulation becomes the vascular bed with the lowest impedance in the fetoplacental circulation. As systemic impedance rises, flow is directed in a retrograde manner about the arch towards the cerebral circulation.[49] Increased flow to the brain results in a decreased pulsatility index recorded usually in the middle cerebral artery. Auto-regulatory arterioles are sensitive to the local concentration of metabolic products, but will not function if the surrounding tissue is metabolically inactive. This may misleadingly manifest as a normalisation of cerebral Doppler flow waveforms in terminally sick fetuses just prior to their intra-uterine death.[50]

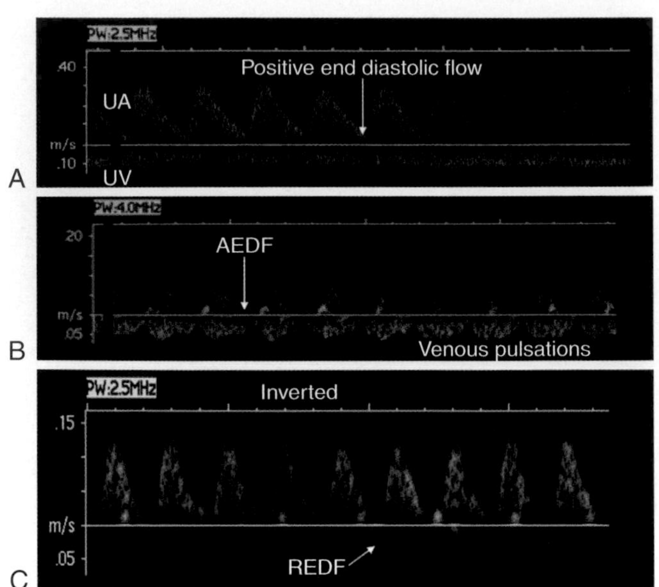

Figure 5-6 Doppler (**A**) of normal flow in the umbilical artery (UA) and vein (UV) showing prograde flow in diastole and absence of venous pulsation. **B,** Absence of end diastolic flow in the umbilical artery (AEDF) increases the pulsatility index in the umbilical artery of pregnancies suffering from placental dysfunction. The Doppler trace also shows abnormal venous pulsations associated with fetal hypoxaemia or increased systemic venous pressure. **C,** Reversed end-diastolic flow (REDF) in the umbilical artery signifying increasing placental resistance.

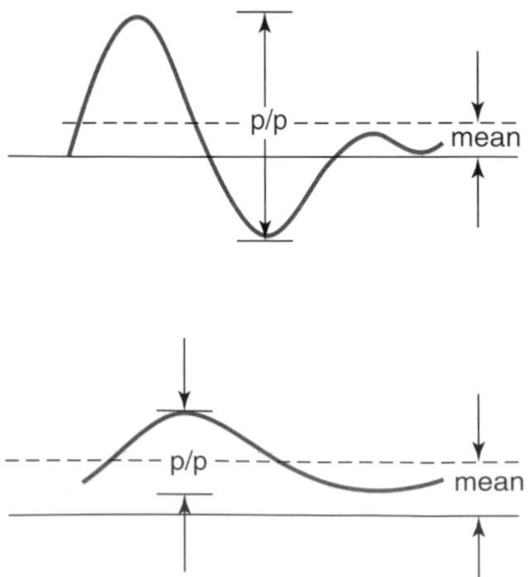

Figure 5-5 Diagram illustrating the pulsatility index calculated from the ratio of (maximum velocity – minimum velocity)/mean velocity. (With permission from Gosling RG, King DH: Ultrasonic angiology. In Harcus AW, Adamson L [eds]: Arteries and Veins. Edinburgh: Churchill Livingstone, 1975, p 71.)

Arterial and venous Doppler waveforms have become incorporated as standard measurements in surveillance of the high-risk pregnancy,[51] with the latter shown to provide a more specific predictor of fetal compromise.[52] Of the Doppler measurements used in evaluation, absence or reversal of end-diastolic flow in the descending aorta or umbilical artery of the fetus is seen first, and may be tolerated for a period of weeks in the compromised growth-restricted fetus, but once changes are seen in the systemic veins, imminent delivery is required.[53]

Flow in the Venous Duct

The venous duct has been investigated at length because it occupies a unique physiological position as a regulator of oxygen in the fetoplacental circulation. Animal studies first demonstrated streaming of oxygenated blood from the umbilical vein through the oval foramen into the left side of the heart, estimated at half of the returning flow. The degree of shunting in the human fetus is less, being estimated at between one-quarter and two-fifths.[33] The determinants of shunting include the differing resistances of the portal vasculature and venous duct, along with other influences such as blood viscosity, umbilical venous pressure, and mechanisms

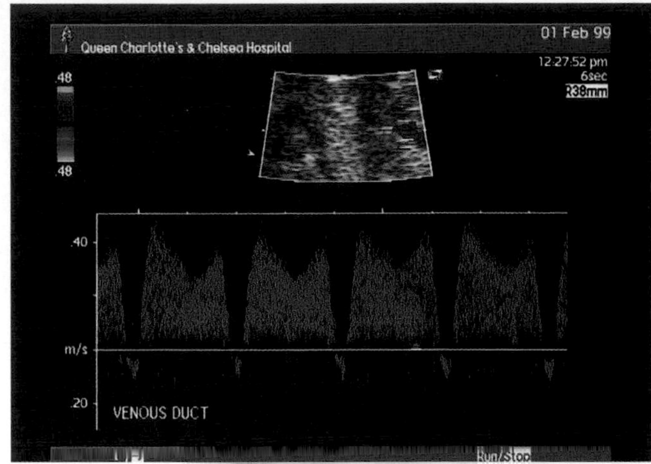

Figure 5-7 Abnormal Doppler flow in the venous duct showing reversal of flow coincident with the a wave of atrial contraction.

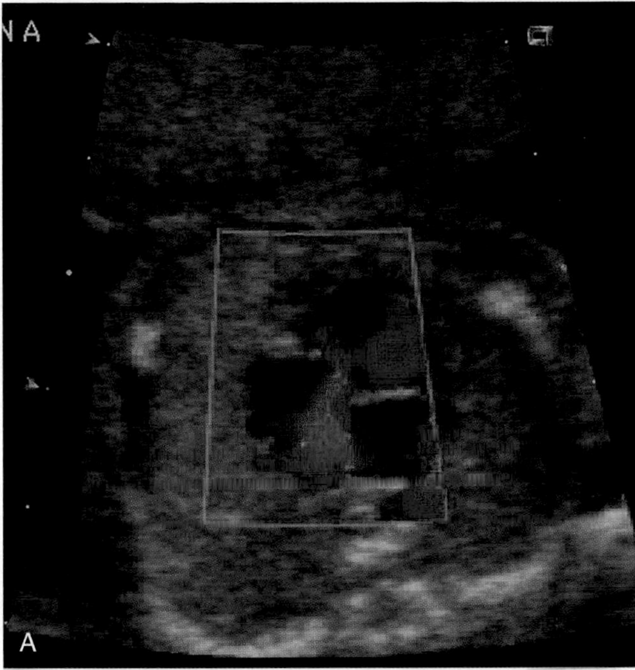

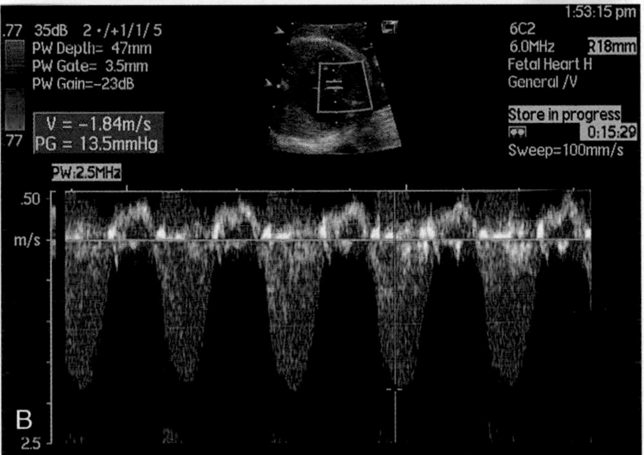

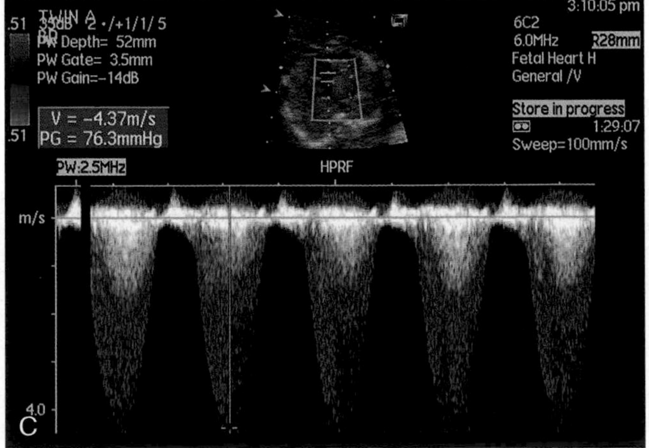

Figure 5-8 Colour flow mapping (**A**) of a fetal tricuspid regurgitant jet and Doppler velocity (**B**) measuring 1.84 m/sec and of moderate duration with sufficient time for ventricular filling. There is severe tricuspid regurgitation (**C**) at 4.37 m/sec of long duration.

of neural and endocrine control. The waveforms measured within the venous duct have been found to remain normal for long periods during placental compromise, reflecting its essential role in the fetal circulation.[54] Patterns in the umbilical vein also act as a barometer of fetal wellbeing. These are caused by the dilation of the venous duct in response to fetal hypoxaemia that reduces impedance, and allows pressure waves to travel in a retrograde fashion from the right atrium to the umbilical vein resulting in venous pulsations. Absent or reversal of flow in the venous duct is usually an ominous sign (Fig. 5-7). It reflects fetal hypoxaemia, and may result in emergency delivery by caesarean section. An alternative explanation for absent or reversed end-diastolic flow in the venous duct is increased central venous pressure, seen particularly where there is obstruction within the right heart, such as pulmonary atresia with severe tricuspid regurgitation (Fig. 5-8). This may also result in fetal hydrops and intra-uterine death.[55–57]

A combination of Doppler parameters and assessment of fetal myocardial function has been combined to create a cardiovascular profile.[58] This scoring system includes the size of the heart and venous Doppler parameters. The best predictor of adverse outcome remains abnormal venous Doppler, and may be predictive when used in isolation.[52,53]

Flow Across the Aortic Isthmus

Only approximately one-third of left ventricular output, or one-tenth of total cardiac output, flows through the aortic isthmus. One consequence of this is that the isthmal diameter is less than that of the transverse arch, and shows a characteristic Doppler pattern (Fig. 5-9). Experimental increases in systemic impedance in the lamb, mimicking placental insufficiency in the human, have been shown to reduce or stop isthmal flow.[49] In the human, where flow to the brain is 8 to 10 times that of the lamb, the hypoxic-mediated increase allows a reduction in cerebral impedance, with reversal of flow about the aortic arch that can be demonstrated on pulsed wave Doppler.[59]

In fetuses with intra-uterine restriction of growth, abnormal arterial and venous Doppler findings influence perinatal outcome. At delivery, brain sparing was associated with hypoxaemia and abnormal venous flows with acidaemia. Abnormal flow in the venous duct predicts fetal death.[51–53] Growth restricted fetuses with abnormal venous flow have worse perinatal outcome compared to those where the abnormality in flow is confined to the umbilical or middle cerebral arteries. In fetuses with low middle cerebral arterial

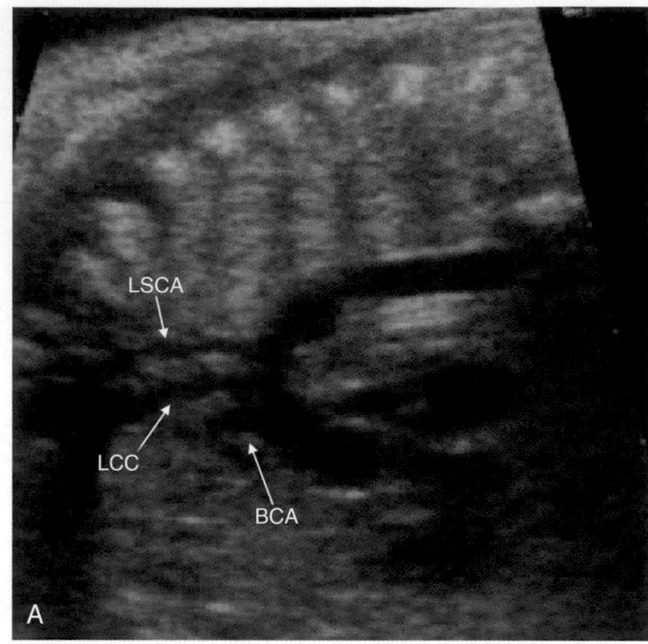

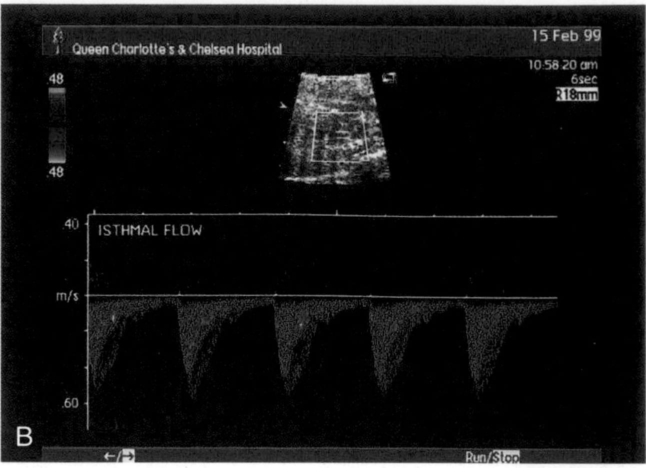

Figure 5-9 The fetal aortic arch (**A**) showing the origins of the brachiocephalic (BCA), left common carotid (LCC), and left subclavian (LSCA) arteries. Doppler of flow in the aortic isthmus (**B**) shows superimposed waveforms of earlier aortic flow and the later flow through the ductal arch.

pulsatility, an abnormal venous Doppler signal indicates further deterioration.[60]

A combination of Doppler indexes shown to be predictive of the optimal time for delivery of the sick fetus has been studied to identify whether they are predictive of early cerebral injury if combined with imaging techniques.[61] Abnormal fetoplacental flow did not appear to correlate with cerebral injury, but evidence of cerebral redistribution, as measured by the ratio of the pulsatility indexes of the umbilical artery compared to the middle cerebral artery, was associated with reduced total volume of the brain. The significance of this in neurodevelopmental outcome remains uncertain, and requires further investigation.

Flow of Blood to the Lungs

The flow of blood in the lungs of the normal human fetus has been calculated non-invasively from the difference in estimated volumes in the arterial duct and in the pulmonary trunk using Doppler ultrasound. In this way, an increase with age for pulmonary flow from 13% to 25% has been described in a cross-section of normal fetuses studied from 20 to 30 weeks of gestation, and an increase in the proportion of the cardiac output from the right side to 60% at term.[62] Pulmonary vascular resistance increases during the last trimester. This again changes the balance of the cardiac output, increasing flow into the systemic circulation.

It is clinically helpful to predict infants with important fetal pulmonary hypoplasia, both to aid counselling of parents, and to prepare the resources required for neonatal resuscitation and support. Doppler parameters such as the pulsatility index have not proven to be discriminatory for pulmonary hypoplasia, for which there is currently no good antenatal test.[63] Early echocardiographic ratios, such as the ratio of sizes of the lungs and head, were derived to predict pulmonary hypoplasia in cases with diaphragmatic hernia. A ratio below 0.6 has been associated with poor outcome, whereas one above 1.4 has been associated with survival.[64] Alternative indexes of the ratio of fetal lung volume to fetal body weight using magnetic resonance imaging in combination with ultrasonography have been devised.[65] Others have used magnetic resonance imaging alone to assess the total lung volume by comparing the signal intensity of lung to that of spinal fluid.[66] These may prove to be more promising methods for predicting fetal pulmonary hypoplasia than Doppler indexes alone.

Coronary Arterial Flow

In normal fetuses, flow in the coronary arteries is not usually seen until the third trimester. Reference ranges for velocities have been described, and do not appear to change with gestational age in the structurally normal heart.[67] Visible flow was first described in terminally sick fetuses, and proposed as an additional predictor of adverse outcome[68] (Fig. 5-10). Animal studies of myocardial flow show that coronary reserve is mediated by nitric oxide and, therefore, changes during hypoxaemia.[69] This finding has been termed fetal cardiac sparing.[70] Accordingly, visible flow in

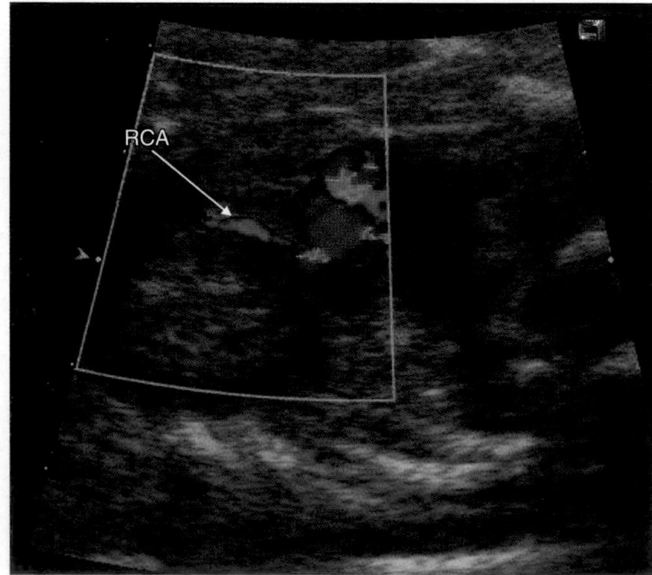

Figure 5-10 Colour flow mapping demonstrating visible coronary flow in the right coronary artery (RCA).

the coronary arteries is attributed to an increased volume of flow secondary to low fetal arterial content of oxygen.

Fetal ultrasound may demonstrate visible coronary arterial flow in conditions associated with restriction of growth, anaemia, constriction of the arterial duct, and bradycardia, thus demonstrating short-term auto-regulation and long-term alterations in myocardial flow reserve in the human fetus. It can be demonstrated in growth-restricted fetuses earlier in gestation than in appropriately grown fetuses and at higher velocity. Fetuses with anaemia show the highest velocities in the coronary arteries, perhaps reflecting increased left ventricular output due to a reduction in cerebral impedance in response to both pathological situations. Coronary arterial flow is no longer visible once the underlying cause has been treated, for example by intra-uterine fetal transfusion for anaemia, or by stopping any causative medication such as indomethacin in the case of constriction of the arterial duct. Visualisation of flow coincides with important increases in the Doppler velocity Z-scores in the umbilical artery, inferior caval veins, and venous duct. The greatest change was observed in the venous duct Z-score occurring 24 hours before visible coronary arterial flow was identified. These changes were associated with adverse perinatal outcomes.[71]

It is relatively easy to demonstrate abnormal vascular connection between the coronary arteries and ventricular cavities, particularly in association with obstructed outflow tracts. Postnatal coronary arterial steal may be predicted by reversal of flow in the aortic arch, and coronary stenoses or occlusion by the finding of retrograde flow at high velocity (Fig. 5-11). These findings are important to discuss during antenatal counselling, as outcomes for these babies may be poor, and associated with postnatal death.

Intracardiac Flows

In the early embryo, gradients across the atrioventricular orifices act as a resistance to, and regulate, the flow of blood, thus influencing ventricular development.[72] As the ventricular mass becomes trabeculated, so its mass increases while stiffness decreases, thus optimizing ventricular filling and ejection. Increasing cardiac efficiency is associated with increasing myocardial mass and competence of the atrioventricular and arterial valves.[73] Trans-vaginal Doppler ultrasound of the human fetal heart has confirmed that ventricular inflow waveforms are monophasic before 9 weeks of gestation, becoming biphasic by 10 weeks. Atrioventricular valvar regurgitation is a common finding from 9 weeks onwards.[74] Tricuspid regurgitation is commonly found in the first trimester, and is thought to be more common in fetuses suffering from aneuploidy, particularly trisomy 21. It has been incorporated into early screening programmes, and is used to adjust the age-related risk for trisomy 21.[75] It is not clear why tricuspid regurgitation is more common in these fetuses, but it may be associated with delayed development of the atrioventricular cushions, as it resolves spontaneously in most cases, and has no physiological consequences later in pregnancy or after birth. Most cases of tricuspid regurgitation reported in later gestation are also transient and trivial. They are associated with a normal outcome.[76]

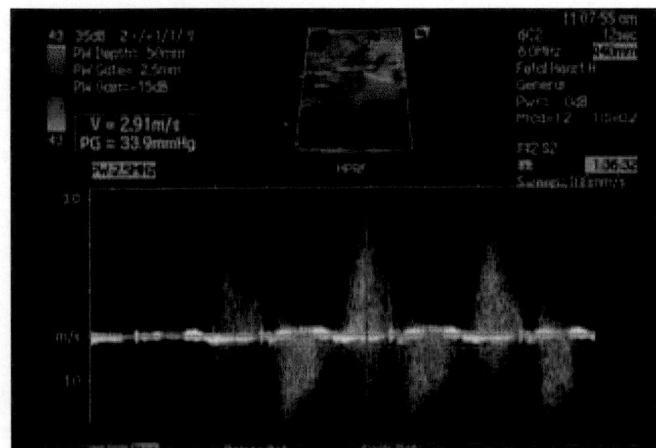

Figure 5-11 Doppler recording of abnormal coronary blood flow in a fetus with pulmonary atresia with intact ventricular septum and a right coronary artery to right ventricle fistula. The trace shows high-velocity reversal of flow along the right coronary artery at 2.9 m/sec and normal velocity forward flow.

In the absence of an obstructed right ventricular outflow tract, non-invasive estimates of the systemic fetal pressures can be estimated from the peak velocity of the jet of tricuspid regurgitation. Important tricuspid regurgitation is holosystolic, often with increased duration of the systolic Doppler envelope, with a compensatory shortening of the diastolic filling time. It may be associated with abnormal waveforms in the peripheral arterial and venous circulations, for example reversal of flow in the venous duct at end-diastole.

DEVELOPMENTAL CHANGES IN SYSTOLIC FUNCTION

In common with observations in more mature fetuses, mean velocities through the outflow tract increase with gestational age. Isovolumic relaxation and contraction times decrease, thus improving the cardiac function. The second half of pregnancy is associated with a rising ventricular stroke volume, and reduction in afterload, which affects the left side more than the right. The peak velocities in the ascending aorta are generally higher than in the pulmonary trunk, and a linear increase with increasing gestation is observed in cross sectional studies.

Cardiac output is traditionally calculated from the right and left ventricles using the velocity time integral of the maximum velocity envelopes through the valves, and a static assessment of valvar diameter measured at the hinge-points. The mean total cardiac output calculated in this way is approximately 550 mL/min/kg body weight. Various investigations in humans, supported by animal data, have shown right cardiac output to be greater than left by at least two-fifths. The major source of error in the calculation of cardiac output results from measurement error of the diameter of the vessel, particularly for clinical studies, and failure to account for pulsatility of the vessel in the equation. In one study, the upper 95% confidence limits for intraobserver variation were reduced to 0.04 mm and 0.09 mm for diameters of 0.6 mm and 6 mm, respectively, by making six repeated measurements of the vessel.[77]

DEVELOPMENTAL CHANGES IN DIASTOLIC FUNCTION

Atrial pressure exceeds ventricular pressure throughout filling, and from early gestation there is a clear distinction between passive and active filling, referred to as the E and A waves, respectively.[5] The active velocities are higher than passive velocities in the fetus and in the newborn period, resulting in a ratio between the E and A waves which is below 1 in the normal fetus. This ratio, nonetheless, is highly dependent on preload. It cannot provide a load-independent assessment of ventricular function. It is, therefore, a particularly unsuitable measure in fetal life, when direct pressures cannot easily be measured. The patterns of ventricular filling change with age, with a relative increase in early diastolic filling, represented by the E wave, compared with the late diastolic component, or A wave, reflecting increasing ventricular compliance.[78–80] Reference ranges between 8 and 20 weeks of gestation show a greater volume of flow passing through the tricuspid than mitral valve at all gestational ages. Maturational changes in ventricular properties in human fetuses accelerate after mid-gestation as diastolic filling increases mainly after 25 weeks. They are associated with a decrease in the ratio of the area of the myocardial wall to the end-diastolic diameter of the left ventricle. Thus, the decrease in left ventricular wall mass related to gestational age may be one important mechanism responsible for the alterations in diastolic properties noted in the fetal heart. These are co-incident with the reduction in placental impedance associated with normal adaptation of the spiral arteries.[81,32]

METHODS FOR NON-INVASIVE FUNCTIONAL ASSESSMENT OF THE FETAL HEART

Diastolic function of the fetal ventricles may be examined using pulsed wave Doppler, but results thus far have prompted differing conclusions. Longitudinal studies have shown that peak E and A waves both increase with gestational age, reflecting the increasing preload of the normally growing fetus, and also, more speculatively, improved maturation of ventricular function.[82–84] Some studies have reported a similar gestational increase in the waves across the mitral valve, resulting in no significant change in the ratio between them in individuals studied longitudinally.[82] A significant increase was found, however, in the ratio of the waves through the tricuspid valve in both normal and growth-restricted fetuses.[83] An alternative parameter, the velocity–time integral of flow into the ventricles during early and late diastole, has been thought to reflect more accurately changes in diastole. The ratio of the velocity time integral of the A wave to the total velocity time integral has been evaluated,[82] but no significant change was found, implying no change in diastolic function with increasing gestation. Others, however, have suggested there is an increase in right ventricular compliance.[83,85] Differences between studies may be explained, in part, by the imprecise nature and variability of these parameters, and the fact that they are poor reflectors of ventricular diastolic function. Furthermore, studies have failed to correlate changes in downstream impedance with patterns of ventricular filling.[86] Better methods may include measurement of long-axis function of the fetal heart using amplitude of displacement of the atrioventricular ring, and Doppler tissue velocities.

The Tei Index

First described in 1997 from measurements made in adult hearts,[87] the Tei index has been used in fetal echocardiography to describe changes in myocardial performance with

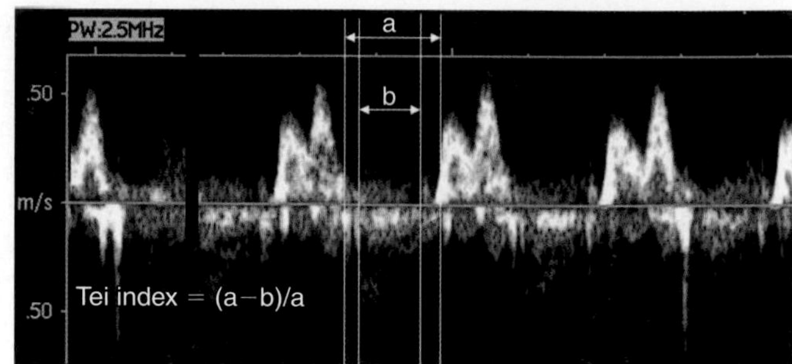

Figure 5-12 Doppler recording of simultaneous inflow into the left ventricle and flow through the aortic valve. The Tei index is calculated as shown in the figure, measurement a includes the isovolumic acceleration and relaxation times. The ratio of these to the ejection period gives the Tei or myocardial performance index. The higher this is, the worse the myocardial performance.

gestational age, and in conditions of altered loading such as twin-twin transfusion syndrome.[88–90] This index uses pulsed wave Doppler of the mitral inflow and aortic outflow waveforms. It is technically easy to record and reproducible in serial examination of the fetus (Fig. 5-12), particularly when modified by using the valvar ejection clicks,[88] and by other authors using myocardial tissue velocities to produce a Doppler tissue Tei index.[91] A reduction in the index is seen with increasing gestational age due to a reduction in isovolumic contraction and relaxation times. Although it has been shown ineffective in animal models to reflect global myocardial function, it is sensitive to afterload changes and fetal conditions complicated by differential loading can be predicted and monitored using this technique.[89,90]

Long-axis Function of the Fetal Heart

M-Mode Measures of Displacement of the Atrioventricular Ring

The pattern of arrangement of myocytes differs in the right and left ventricles, with the right ventricle lacking myocytes aggregated in circular fashion.[92] The myocytes aggregated in longitudinal fashion lie predominantly in the ventricular subendocardium, and are affected first by ischaemia.

It is difficult to assess right ventricular function in the minor axis because of poor detection of the endocardial borders, but in adults with heart failure, assessment of the amplitude in the long axis predicts exercise tolerance and survival.[93,94] Displacement of the atrioventricular ring is assessed using M-mode techniques, and reflects shortening of the myocytes aggregated in longitudinal fashion towards the apex of the ventricle in systole, and their retraction in diastole. In common with evaluation of long-axis function in the adult, M-mode measurements of amplitude of displacement of the atrioventricular ring can be made in the human fetus. The methodology is simple and reliable, and normal reference ranges have been described in the fetus and adult.[95,96] These show age-related increases in amplitude of displacement in the fetus, confirming right ventricular dominance as the right ventricular free wall shows increased displacement compared to the left or the ventricular septum.

Doppler Tissue Imaging

New Doppler imaging technologies are available to assess myocardial function, and are widely used in the assessment of the adult heart. Most of these modalities have been tested in the fetus. Some are suitable, and may increase our knowledge of maturation of the myocardium in the normal fetus and in response to pathophysiological situations.

There are, nonetheless, considerable technical limitations in applying all measurement used in adult studies to the smaller fetal heart, where there is no electronic gating and smaller tissue volumes. All Doppler modalities require high frame rates, with 200 Hz being ideal, and must be closely aligned parallel to the mural motion, ideally below 20 degrees. Accuracy of measurement requires that the sample volume is small, and velocity limits reduced to optimise the trace.

Pulsed Doppler Assessment of Long-axis Function

The simplest method in use to assess long-axis function is pulsed Doppler assessment of myocardial tissue Doppler velocities at the atrioventricular ring. These reflect shortening and lengthening velocities of the myocytes aggregated in longitudinal orientation. Ventricular long-axis shortening velocities and amplitude correlate with overall ventricular function as assessed by ejection fraction, and early and late diastolic lengthening velocities correlate with ventricular filling velocities assessed by Doppler. Reference ranges have been created in the normal fetal heart, and gestationally related values show similar increases,[95,97,98] albeit that those recorded using spectral Doppler tissue were up to one-fifth lower than those obtained in other studies (Fig. 5-13).[99]

Pulsed Doppler and M-mode measures allow quantification of long-axis cardiac function in pregnancies complicated by maternal disease, such as diabetes mellitus. Studies have reported a relationship between maternal concentrations of haemoglobin A1c in diabetic women and cardiac function in their fetuses.[100] Although free wall and septal hypertrophy was observed in the fetuses of diabetic mothers from the second trimester, this was accompanied by increased function, suggesting adaptive hypertrophy rather than the presence of a cardiomyopathy.

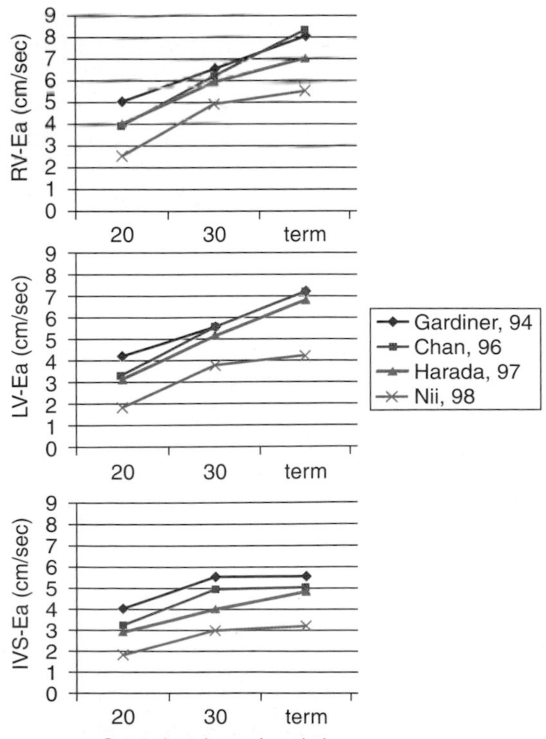

Figure 5-13 Graphs plotting gestation changes in mean or median tissue Doppler velocities of the E wave (Ea) at the base of the heart with the gate placed at the right ventricular free wall (RV), left ventricular free wall (LV), and interventricular septum (IVS): Those measured using spectral tissue Doppler were consistently 15% to 20% lower.

Colour Doppler Myocardial Imaging

Colour Doppler myocardial imaging[101] provides measurements of myocardial motion and deformation from which myocardial strain and strain rate can be calculated. This technology is based on the differences of tissue Doppler velocities in adjacent myocardial points from which strain rate and strain is estimated. This shows the extent of torsion and twist of the heart during the normal cardiac cycle. The technique is particularly useful following myocardial infarction in the adult, as it enables regional abnormalities to be detected. Strain rate has been recorded in small numbers of children with aortic valvar atresia, and in those with hypoplastic left heart syndrome.[102,103] There are particular technological difficulties using this approach in the fetus, relating to the small myocardial mass interrogated by each pixel, and also to the fact that myocytes are aligned longitudinally in the fetal right ventricle, but circumferentially in the fetal left ventricle. Doppler velocity colour coding permits the detection of motion of the aortic wall, and measurement of the velocity of the pulse wave. This technique may prove to be a useful non-invasive technique to assess fetal arterial compliance.

Speckle Tracking

Cardiac torsion and twist have been investigated using a non-Doppler method based on speckle tracking. This methodology works by tracking bright myocardial echoes, and is relatively angle independent. It has been evaluated against sonomicrometry in animal models and is currently in clinical use in the adult, where its ability to demonstrate motion of the heart during systole and diastole has been compared to magnetic resonance imaging. The method is under evaluation in the fetus, but published studies so far have insufficient power to create normal reference ranges in the fetus, and reproducibility is rather limited. Preliminary reports have shown a gestational increase in velocities, but no change in strain or strain rate. The angle independence is likely to be useful in examination of the fetal heart provided frame rates analysable by the software can be improved.

METHODS FOR ASSESSING VASCULAR PHYSIOLOGY AND VOLUME OF BLOOD

Measurement of Volumes of Flow of Blood

Accurate measurement of volumes of flow in peripheral vessels is of clinical interest because it reflects differential perfusion of organs in the fetus, both during normal growth and in response to adverse circumstances. Data on placental and cardiovascular flow and function in the human fetus are more difficult to collect and to verify than in the chick embryo and ovine models because they have to be collected non-invasively. Flow of blood can, of course, be measured with a high degree of accuracy with electromagnetic[104] or transit-time flowmeters.[105] Since these methods require an invasive approach, they cannot currently be applied in studies on human fetuses. Non-invasive methods to measure the volume of flow in the aorta are confounded by methodological difficulties, mostly in relation to accurate measurements of aortic diameter, an issue that has still not been resolved, despite improvements in the resolution of ultrasound.[77,106]

The method traditionally used to estimate volume of flow in a vessel is from the product of the velocity time integral of the Doppler signal in the vessel, the heart rate and a separate estimation of the area of the lumen from static measurements of its diameter. The inherent error in this method is estimated to be as large as one-fifth when measuring fetal arteries.[77] This error mostly results from limits of resolution of the diameter, but failure to account for changes in pulsatile flow may account for almost one-tenth of the difference in volume of flow compared with static assessment.[107] Estimations of venous flow have been reported,[108] but the potential error is further compounded by the assumption that the vessel under examination is circular.

Simultaneous measurement of the diameter of the pulsatile vessel and the mean velocity of flow allows an estimate of flow volume in the descending aorta of the healthy fetus.[106] The volume of aortic flow, measured in this way, has shown a linear increase with increasing gestation, being estimated at 225 mL/min/kg body weight in fetuses of 250 days.

Estimation of Perfusion Using Power Doppler

Methods using newer Doppler modalities have been evaluated as surrogate estimates of perfusion. Power Doppler was initially investigated as a method to estimate perfusion in the adult, but an important methodological problem was the formation of rouleaux that artificially elevated the maximal value for power Doppler amplitude. Fortunately, studies in the fetus confirm that fetal blood does not form rouleaux to any significant degree, so permitting a comparison of perfusion of different organs. Studies using quantification of power Doppler have suggested an increase in power Doppler signals from the placenta, lungs, spleen, liver and kidney up to 34 weeks of gestation, following by a decrease in all but the spleen, which remains constant. Abnormalities in the ratio of volumes in the brain and lungs were seen in high-risk pregnancies, but methodological problems using this technique may limit the conclusions drawn by such studies. Mean pixel intensity has been the traditional method of assessment of perfusion over a region of interest, but this methodology is dependent not only on the volume of flow of blood, but also depth, gain and attenuation in overlying layers of tissue.

An alternative method, the fractional moving volume, attempts to compensate for these confounding variables.[109,110] When power Doppler is applied to a region, the centre of a large fetal vessel, such as the aorta, is interrogated and assigned a value of 100% amplitude. This can be used to compare the amplitude in smaller vessels, such as those supplying the fetal kidney.[111] There are pitfalls with all imaging methods, and those limiting the reliability of the technique of the fractional moving blood volume include the depth of the imaged organ from the transducer. Phantom studies describe that the power is linearly related to velocity over a limited range, suggesting it may be useful to discriminate between normal and decreased fetal perfusion in organs such as the lung. Validation of measurements with power Doppler ultrasound has been performed in sheep using radioactive microspheres, showing good correlations in the adrenal gland.[112] Power Doppler methods may be improved by combining them with three-dimensional standardised techniques in order to identify a reproducible anatomical plane for measurement.[113]

Three- and Four-Dimensional Echocardiography

All imaging techniques depend on excellent quality of imaging, so the three-dimensional picture is only as good as the cross sectional image, and quality may be compromised by fetal movements and maternal respiration. Additionally the development of these techniques have been hampered until relatively recently by the lack of electrocardiographic gating of the fetal heart. New technology that allows live real-time three-dimensional imaging is promising, and has been reported by several groups. These techniques have been used for imaging of the fetal heart for diagnostic purposes, using technology such as spatial temporal methodology that allows the rapid acquisition of a three dimensional volume set which can be manipulated later off-line. This has potential in training and evaluation of cardiac abnormalities remotely, as the volume sets can be sent electronically for expert analysis.[114]

Three-Dimensional Quantification of Volume and Ejection Fraction

Physiological information is limited, but three-dimensional inversion mode sonography has been used to establish normal ranges for ventricular volumes and ejection fractions.[40] This may prove to be a useful methodology in the assessment of ventricular size in structural heart disease.

Fetal Vascular Physiology

Arterial Physiology

The role of the endothelium in modulating vascular responses is well recognised. A series of studies performed in children and young adults with risk factors for later disease have shown that it is possible to detect abnormalities in vascular responses to stimuli both dependent and independent of the endothelium before there are signs of overt disease.[115–117] While it is not yet possible to examine directly the responses of the fetal endothelium in this way, information is available on the pulsations of the vessel wall and the velocity of the pulse wave of the fetal aorta, which have been measured using wall-tracking devices. Pulsations of the arterial wall (Fig. 5-14) reflect impedance from distal vascular beds along the fetal arterial tree. The pulsatile change in cross sectional area of the fetal aorta during the cardiac cycle at the 20th week of gestation is approximately 22%, falling to 17% at term compared with about 9% in the adult aorta.[118] This may reflect a reduction

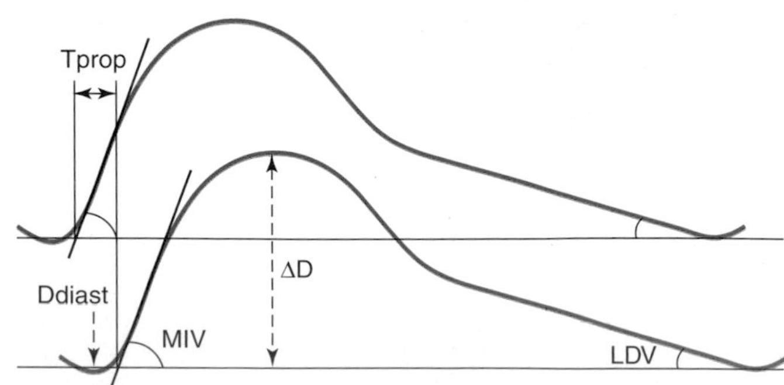

Figure 5-14 Diagram of the arterial pulse waveform, illustrating the maximum incremental velocity (MIV), the relative pulse amplitude (ΔD), and the late decremental velocity (LDV). Ddiast, diastolic diameter of the vessel; Tprop, propagation time of the pulse wave.

in arterial mural compliance with increasing blood pressure in the growing fetus, and with structural changes within the vessel wall, which alter its physical properties. Information about the fetal vascular tree may be gained from analysis of the separate parts of the wall as it moves. Studies using a feline model have correlated the diameter of the movements of the pulsating wall with invasive measures of ventricular function and afterload[119] and found the maximal incremental velocity to be the best single variable, reflecting total peripheral resistance and late decremental velocity better to reflect a lower stroke volume and reduced cardiac output. The maximum incremental velocity of the arterial pulse waveform (see Fig. 5-14) may provide additional information on ventriculo-vascular coupling in the fetal circulation. Standard arterial Doppler assessment using the ratio of acceleration to ejection periods at the level of the arterial valve is said to reflect the mean arterial pressure in that artery, and also to reflect on the ventricular function. Unfortunately, this has not proved to be reliable.[120] In contrast, the maximum incremental velocity has been shown in animal studies to correlate well with the acceleration in aortic flow, and with the rate of rise of left ventricular pressure.[119] The rate of increase in the aortic diameter in early systole is dependent on ventricular systolic function but is dependent also on distal impedance. If this can be considered to remain relatively constant for a single examination, then maximum incremental velocity may be a better non-invasive indicator of ventriculo-vascular coupling than currently available Doppler measures.

Venous Physiology

The venous system is considerably more pulsatile in the fetus than after birth. Pulsations of the wall of the inferior caval vein reflect not only the fetal central venous pressure, but also the changes in ventricular relaxation and filling. Because of the parallel arrangement of the circulation, venous pulsations also reflect the distal arterial impedance. The information derived has provided interesting physiological insights into fetal circulatory development.[118,121] In contrast to the arterial system, the relative pulse amplitude of the inferior caval vein increases with gestation.[121] The relative gestational increase in venous pulse amplitude may reflect an improvement in the filling and emptying of the right ventricle. This is supported by the findings, using Doppler, of a reduction in reversal of flow of blood away from the heart in the inferior caval vein of the healthy fetus.[51] That veno-ventricular coupling is further improved is suggested by the finding of forward diastolic flow in the pulmonary trunk in normally growing fetuses with increased venous mural pulsatility.[118] Diastolic flow in the pulmonary trunk has been reported in association with a restrictive right ventricle in children following repair of tetralogy of Fallot,[122] but these fetal Doppler indexes suggest that diastolic filling of the right ventricle improves with gestation. The Doppler findings suggest that improved filling is a consequence of reduced distal impedance drawing blood into the arterial duct at the end of diastole, before the valve opens fully.[123,124] Venous mural pulsations, therefore, may reflect the falling impedance of the arterial tree distal to the arterial duct, as well as improving cardiac compliance (Fig. 5-15).

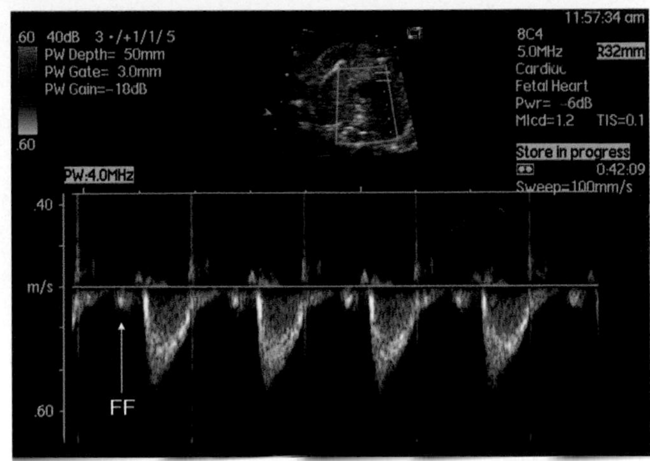

Figure 5-15 Doppler recording of flow through the pulmonary valve. Forward flow (FF) at end diastole is frequently seen in the normal fetal heart.

Pulsed Wave Velocity

Measurement of compliance or elastance of a blood vessel may be determined from the speed of propagation of a pulse travelling in its wall: The faster the velocity, the stiffer the wall. Such velocity has been shown to increase by about 1 m/sec in chick embryos from stage 18 to 29,[125] and in normal fetuses from 20 weeks to term.[118] The velocity depends on the mean distending pressure of the vessel, coupled with changes in the composition of the wall. The mean aortic blood pressure increases during gestation, as does the thickness of the aortic wall relative to the lumen and the supporting adventitial tissue. The composition of the wall changes with accelerated deposition of elastin during the last weeks of gestation. This continues during the first months of life and confers increased distensibility to the aorta.[126] The velocity of the pulse wave has been shown to increase with age, and is an important determinant of coronary arterial flow and left ventricular function.[127] It has also been shown to correlate with atherosclerosis and to be increased in coronary arterial disease.[128] Reduced arterial distensibility contributes to the pathogenesis of hypertension. A reduction in the arterial characteristic impedance results in increased pulse pressure, and the pulsatile cardiac workload is accentuated. Furthermore, the resultant increase in the velocity of the pulse wave results in early return of the reflected wave and further augments the systolic pressure.

Ventriculo-vascular Coupling

Fetal Systemic Pressures

Direct measurements of intraventricular pressure have been made in the normal heart between 18 and 29 weeks of gestation.[129] This study confirmed that ventricular systolic pressures increase with gestation. In fetuses in which it was possible to record measurements in both ventricles, the pressures were equal. End-diastolic pressures that have previously only been inferred from Doppler assessment were directly measured (Fig. 5-16).

Pressure–Volume Loops

Pressure–volume loops remain the gold standard for measuring ventricular function independently of load, but their measurement is invasive. It is possible to construct pressure–volume loops in the chick embryo (Fig. 5-17).[1] Physiological differences have been demonstrated between right and left ventricular function in the postnatal dog.[130] The shape of the pressure–volume relationship of the right ventricle differs in several ways from that of the left ventricle

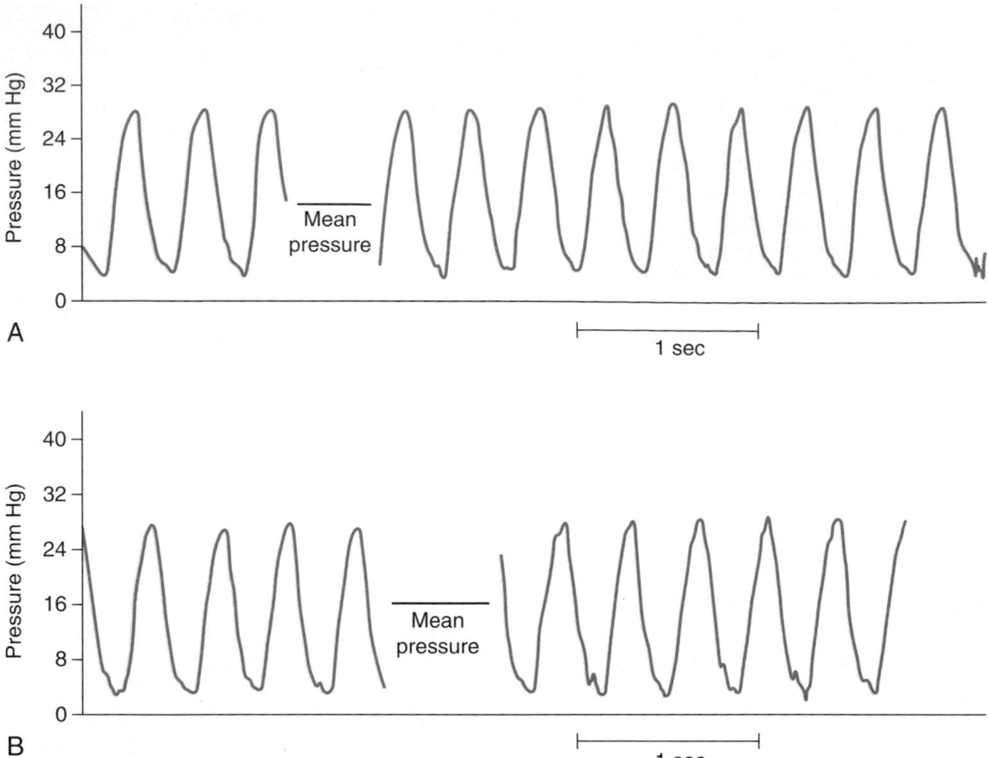

Figure 5-16 Pressure traces showing the systolic and end-diastolic measurements within the human fetal ventricle at 22 weeks of gestation for (**A**) the left ventricle and (**B**) the right ventricle. (Reproduced by permission of Heart from Johnson P, Maxwell DJ, Tynan MJ, Allan LD: Intracardiac pressures in the human fetus. Heart 2000;84:59–63.)

(Fig. 5-18). Right ventricular ejection occurs long after peak pressure has been achieved, and, for a given intraventricular volume, the pressure is less in the right ventricle.[131] The instantaneous pressure–volume relationship at end-systole is linear in both ventricles, but the correction volume, as defined by the intercept of this line with the *x* axis, is constant in the left ventricle. It does not change with contractile state, in contrast to that of the right ventricle.[130]

Similar assessment of the pressure–volume relationships, independent of load, is not yet technically possible in the healthy human fetus. Non-invasive insights into normal cardiovascular physiological development, however, have been obtained using echo-tracking equipment and Doppler ultrasound tissue imaging. Although the right ventricle deals with a greater volume load in fetal life than does the left ventricle, minor-axis ventricular systolic function and simultaneous direct pressure measurements are similar in right and left ventricles before birth.[129] More recently, studies of fetal long-axis function have reported that myocardial velocities and amplitude of motion are increased in the right ventricular free wall compared to the left or the ventricular septum.[95,97–99] This may be in response to the increased volume loading of the right ventricle compared with the left ventricle during normal maturation, and the increased number of myocytes aligned in longitudinal fashion. The relative volume loading of the right ventricle during fetal life may alter the deposition, or cause the re-expression of, essential cytoskeletal and certain heat shock proteins such as desmin, the cytokeratins, vimentin, and HSP-72. These have been described in conditions of volume and pressure loading of ventricles postnatally, and may act adversely, altering responses in the postnatal situation, thus permitting the ventricle to dilate more readily in response to volume and pressure loads, and so further prejudice its function.

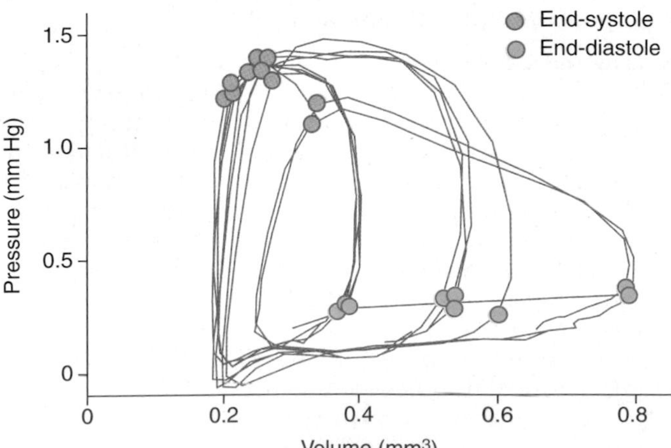

Figure 5-17 Pressure–volume loops in a stage 21 chick embryo measured during preload infusion. (With permission from Keller BB: Maturation/coupling of the embryonic cardiovascular system. In Clarke EB, Markwald RR, Takao A [eds]: Developmental Mechanisms of Heart Disease. Armonk, NY: Futura, 1995, p 375.)

Heart Rate Variability

The variability in heart rate is determined by the maturation of the autonomic system. There are major differences between species in the time at which the balance between neurotransmission of the sympathetic and parasympathetic system is accomplished. This is related to the independence of the individual species before and immediately after birth. Maladaptation, or immaturity, of neural control may manifest in acute life-threatening events in infancy. Antenatal assessment has been difficult, as measurement of beat-to-beat measurements has not been possible with existing technology such as the cardiotocograph.

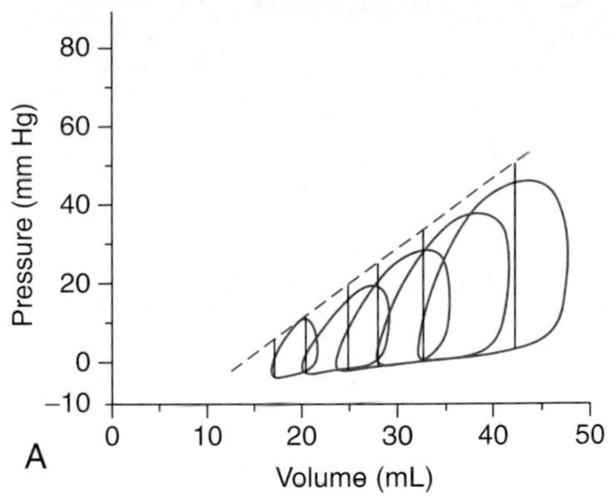

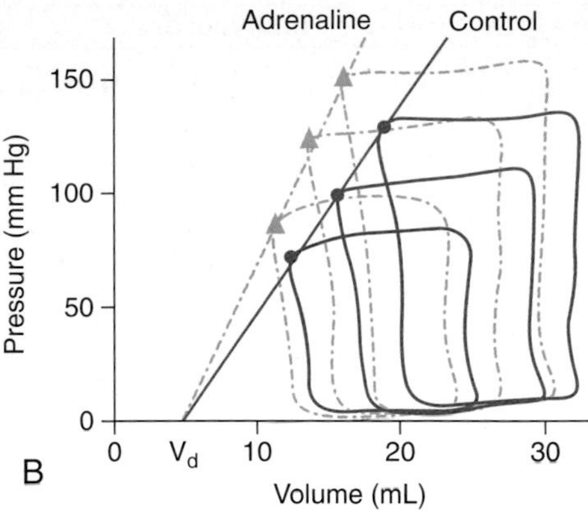

Figure 5-18 Pressure–volume loops of the right (**A**) and left (**B**) ventricles in a canine model illustrating the differences in the end-systolic pressure–volume relationship. The instantaneous pressure–volume ratio of the canine left ventricle is independent of load and is altered by adrenaline and by the heart rate. The correction volume (Vd) is constant. (**A**, With permission from Maughan WL, Shoukas AA, Sagawa K, Weisfeldt ML: Instantaneous pressure–volume relationship of the canine right ventricle. Circ Res 1979;44:309–315; **B** with permission from Suga H, Sagawa K, Shoukas AA: Load independence of the instantaneous pressure–volume ratio of the canine left ventricle and effects of epinephrine and heart rate on the ratio. Circ Res 1973;32:314–322.)

The full electrocardiogram can be recorded by use of scalp electrodes, but only once rupture of membranes has occurred. This has provided useful information during labour by analysing the ST waves.[132] Non-invasive recordings of the full fetal electrocardiogram can now be obtained from 15 weeks of gestation in the human fetus using newer techniques. These include blind signal separation from signals obtained from electrodes placed on the maternal abdomen, and magnetocardiography (Figs. 5-19 and 5-20). These studies have described reference ranges for time intervals in the fetus.[133] Use of the techniques has permitted more detailed analysis of fetal arrhythmias.[134–136] Variability may also be described using the standard deviation from the time domain, as well as other measures from the frequency domains and approximate entropy as a measure of complexity.[137] Two distinct fractal structures have been identified within this variation. They show significant gestational change in the normal fetus, and may be useful to evaluate variation in disease states.[138] Investigation into variability of the heart rate in the fetus and neonate may provide insights into developmental processes in health and disease, and refine stratification of fetuses at risk of intra-uterine death, as well as the risk of sudden infant death syndrome in those born prior to term. Neonates who have suffered apparent life-threatening events show differences in heart rate variability, suggesting altered autonomic control.[139,140]

Vascular Programming

The fetal origins hypothesis proposes that adaptation of the fetus to its intra-uterine environment and postnatal stressors may have life-long consequences, and that the fetal response to an environmental challenge may result in programming of different organs, depending on the timing of the insult. Restricted growth in the last trimester of pregnancy has been associated with later cardiovascular disease. The original concept of fetal programming has been expanded, and now encompasses both pre- and postnatal adaptation under the umbrella of the 'Developmental Origins of Health and Disease', known also by the acronym DOHaD. Environmental factors may also contribute to permanent effects resulting from altered epigenetic genetic regulation, and this has created a new field of epigenetic epidemiology.[141]

Fetal ECG Report

Name: QC50 Date: 18/7/2001

Singleton Gestation: 35 weeks
No. of sensors 12 Length of dataset: 57.9 seconds

Data used: 57.9 seconds - from 0 to 57.9 seconds
Pass band from 1 to 150 Hz

Mean heartrate: 153 bpm
Max heartrate: 157 bpm
Min heartrate: 146 bpm

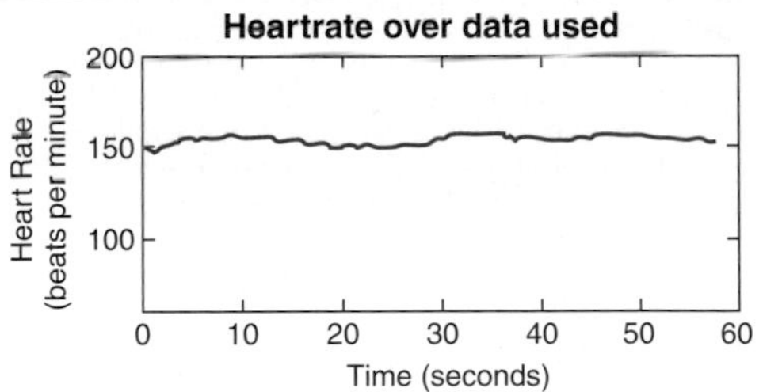

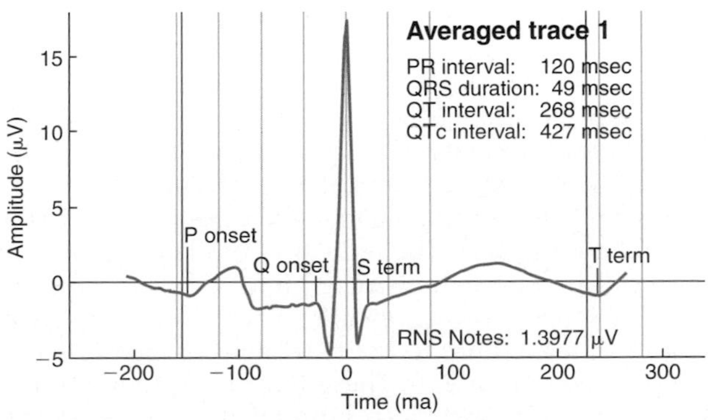

Rhythm strip trace 1: from 0 sec to 3 sec

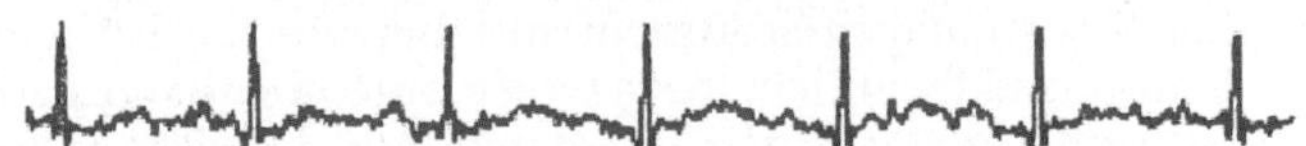

Figure 5-19 An example of a report on a fetal electrocardiogram from a singleton pregnancy at 35 weeks gestation. (Reproduced by permission of the British Journal of Obstetrics and Gynaecology, and the authors of reference #132.)

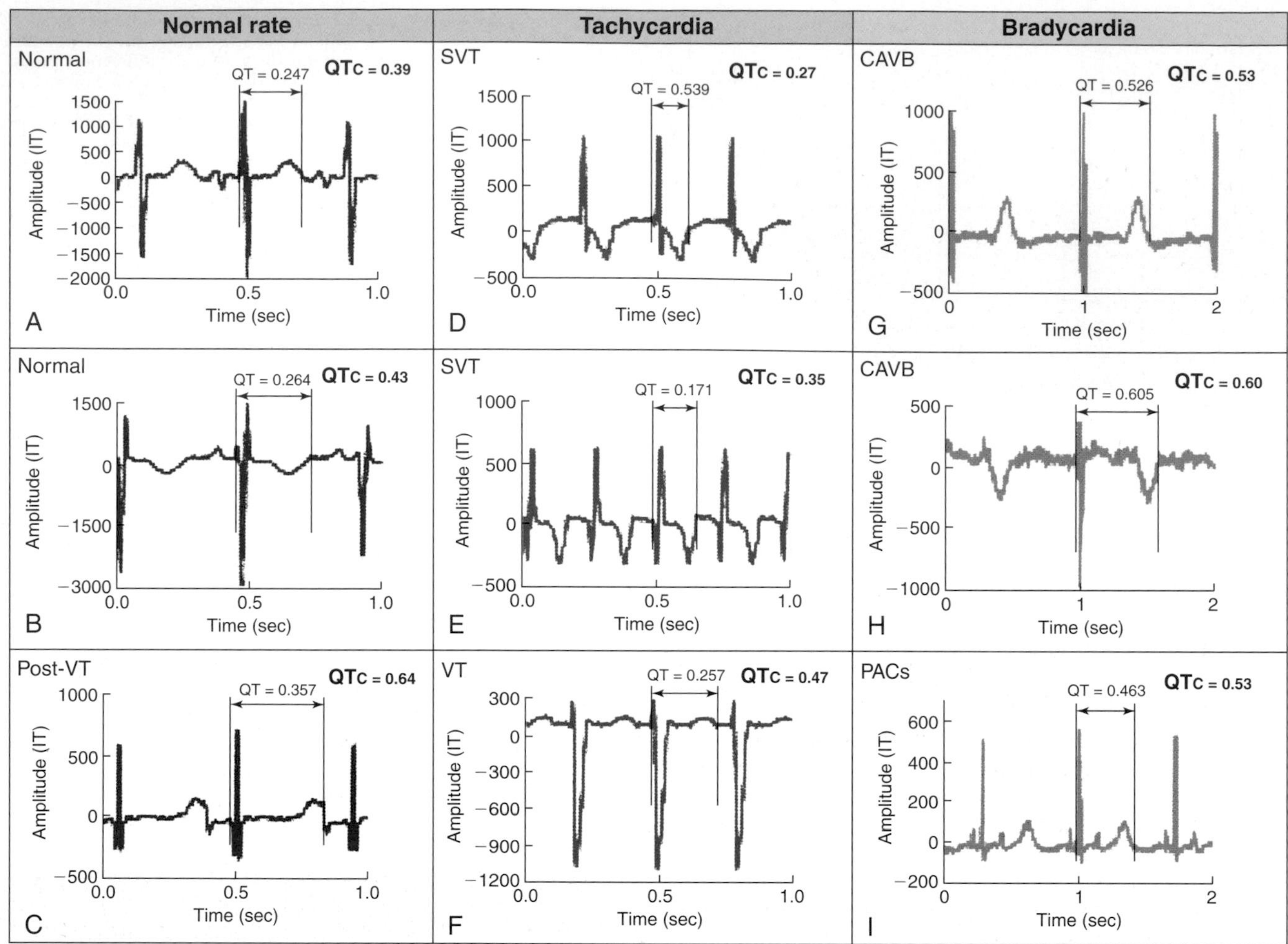

Figure 5-20 Representative averaged magnetoelectrocardiographic waveforms recorded during fetal life. **A,** A normal fetus at 39 weeks gestation. **B,** A normal fetus, but at 37 weeks gestation. **C,** Recordings from a fetus of 27 weeks gestation, but suffering ventricular tachycardia (VT) at 25 weeks gestation. **D,** A fetus of 27 weeks gestation with supraventricular tachycardia (SVT). **E,** A fetus, again with supraventricular tachycardia, at 31 weeks gestation. **F,** The fetus illustrated in panel C, but this panel reveals the tachycardia present at 25 weeks gestation. **G** and **H,** Fetuses with complete atrioventricular block (CAVB) at 30 and 25 weeks gestation, respectively. **I,** A fetus with blocked premature atrial contractions (PACs) at 20 weeks gestation. All waveforms are taken from the channel with the largest signal amplitude, the amplitude being shown in units of femtotesla, with each femtotesla equal to 10^{-5} tesla. (The image is reproduced by permission of the authors of reference #134.)

Vascular Programming in the Setting of Restricted Growth

The fetal cardiovascular system differs from that of the neonate in that the interdependence between cardiac and pulmonary physiology is less important than that of the placental vasculature. Normal placental development includes appropriate trophoblastic invasion to remodel placental spiral arteries and create a low impedance circulation. This is important in the development of normal fetal cardiovascular responses.[32] This vascular change does not occur in cases of placental dysfunction. The reduction in placental flow may then result in a growth-restricted fetus.[44,45] The fetus alters its adaptive responses to enable survival in these adverse conditions, sometimes to the detriment of later functional and adaptive responses.[46] These have been termed predictive adaptive responses.[142] This model proposes that the risk of disease depends on the degree of mismatch between the predicted postnatal environment and that which exists. The prediction usually anticipates a worse outcome than exists, which further increases the mismatch. Adverse early influences are thought to result in the so-called thrifty phenotype. This describes an individual that can match supply and demand successfully to permit survival, even though some of the adaptive mechanisms this involves may lead to later disease through disturbances of normal cardiovascular and neuro-hormonal control mechanisms. Postnatal nutrition often results in catch-up growth in growth-restricted infants, and this may further disturb the thrifty phenotype, leading to further adaptations to permit an individual to live within his or her predicted environment.

Many Doppler ultrasound studies of the growth-restricted fetus have been published. Ventricular diastolic filling is lower than normal. The increased systemic impedance, due to placental dysfunction, results in an impairment of venous flow towards the heart during diastole, with a consequent reduction of peak velocity of inward flow[51,52] and a reduction in the pulsations of the wall of the inferior caval vein. The increased central venous pressure may contribute to impairment of systemic venous return and a reduction in normal forward flow during late diastole in the pulmonary trunk. This suggests that there is abnormal veno-ventricular–vascular coupling.[83] Increased shunting through the venous duct in growth-restricted fetuses reduces umbilical blood supply to the fetal liver, which may be detrimental in those surviving with restricted growth.[143] Occlusion of the venous duct leads to a significant increase in cell proliferation in fetal skeletal muscle, heart, kidneys, and liver and possibly to an increase in expression of IgF1 and 2 and mRNA. These alterations may have a significant long-term influence on metabolism in the growth-restricted individual, lending support to the concept of altered metabolism seen in adults with reduced birth weight.[144]

Some studies have reported a reduction in systolic velocities through the arterial valves in growth-restricted fetuses. This is not a universal finding, however, and does not necessarily reflect poor ventricular function. Other authors have reported increased peak systolic velocities of flow, but found that the flow commenced later in systole than normal, thus resulting in an increased pre-ejection period and a shorter ejection time because of the increased systemic impedance, resulting in a reduced stroke volume.[145] Cardiac output corrected for weight is normal in growth-restricted fetuses, but the mean velocity of flow in the descending aorta is significantly less, and the volume of blood flowing showed a similar, but non-significant trend, suggesting more is directed cephalad.[83]

The effects of vascular programming associated with altered intra-uterine nutrition may not be obvious in individuals studied early in life. While component parts of the fetal arterial pulse waveform are significantly different in the growth-restricted fetus, no differences have been found in pulsed wave velocity.[83] The relationship between pulsed wave velocity and intra-uterine growth restriction is not yet clear, but in babies delivered at normal term, there appears to be an inverse association between the velocity of the neonatal arterial pulse wave and maternal systolic blood pressure, with a positive relationship for neonatal gestational age, birth weight, length, and neonatal blood pressure.[146] Prematurity alone does not appear to influence later the velocity of the pulse wave. Children born prior to term with a Z-score for birthweight below −2 SD had significantly higher mean blood pressure and higher pulse-wave velocity at school age than those born prior to term, but of normal weight.[147] Longitudinal studies have shown that young adults studied in fetal life because of restricted growth have smaller aortas than controls, and higher resting heart rates.[148] It may be that maturation of the aortic wall is required. Alternatively, a process of amplification[149] may need to occur during infancy before any differences can be appreciated in the properties of the aortic wall.

Vascular Programming in Twin-Twin Transfusion Syndrome

Twin-twin transfusion syndrome is an extreme model of circulatory imbalance occurring in monochorionic pregnancies where there are two genetically identical individuals. Within-pair responses in the cardiovascular response to differences in volume load and the effect of increased placental resistance can be measured. Studies have confirmed that fetal vascular programming occurs and reduced arterial distensibility is detectable in the growth-restricted donor twin during infancy.[150] Furthermore the inter-twin differences are altered by intra-uterine laser ablation of placental vascular anastomoses in the second trimester of pregnancy.[151]

Vascular Programming Following Fetal Coarctation

Coarctation of the aorta can be present in the fetus. Both a hypoplastic arch, and a coarctation shelf, can be visualised and quantified using ultrasound.[38] A continuous Doppler pattern of flow in the isthmus may be recorded, and reflects altered patterns of flow which confirm obstruction (Fig. 5-21). Studies of endothelial function in normotensive young adults undergoing repair of the coarctation as neonates and infants have demonstrated reduced endothelial-dependent and -independent function confined to the precoarctation site compared with normal controls, suggesting that early alteration of flow in fetal life may programme later function in spite of early and adequate surgical repair.[115,149,152]

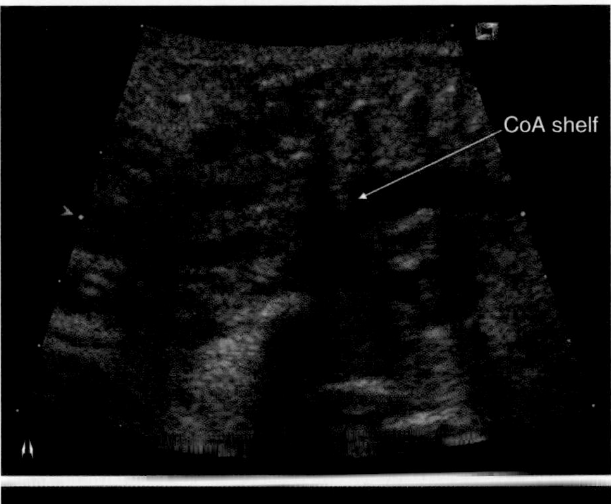

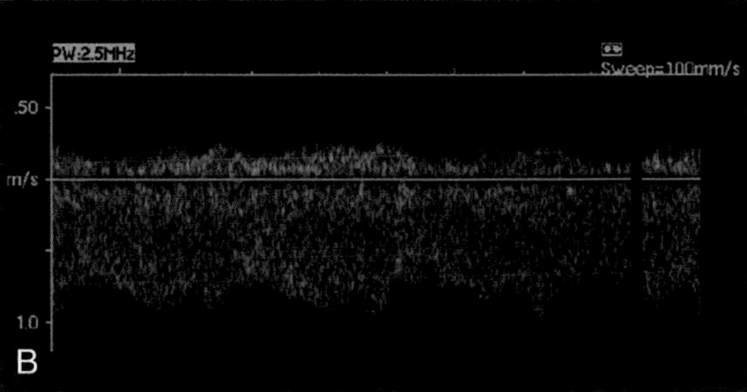

Figure 5-21 **A,** A coarctation shelf (CoA) can be visualised in the fetus using ultrasound. **B,** A continuous Doppler pattern of flow in the isthmus may be recorded, that reflects altered patterns of flow which confirms arch obstruction in fetal life.

SUMMARY

The ability to examine the physiology of the developing circulation in the human fetus non-invasively has become a reality. It provides us with the opportunity to compare developmental changes in the human with those of other species, thereby ensuring that we do not accord unquestioningly human cardiovascular development with those attributes found previously in other species using invasive methods.

Doppler ultrasound technology has enabled serial examination of the human fetus from the first trimester allowing us to observe non-invasively developmental changes in diastolic and systolic function, myocardial maturation and the responses to structural and functional disease states. More quantitative measures of perfusion, volume flow and ventricular volumes enable a better appreciation of cardiac output and organ flows in the early human fetus.

The importance of the development of the arterial tree can be examined by pulsed wave velocity and measures of endothelial function in conduit arteries. There is a convincing body of evidence that suggests early changes in volume flows and the response of the arterial wall may initiate permanent structural changes that may lead to longer term pathology such as hypertension. Early detection of vascular abnormalities may permit interventional strategies before birth and in childhood that could reverse the progression to clinically important disease in fetuses identified as being at high risk.

ACKNOWLEDGEMENT

I am grateful to Dr Constancio Medrano for permitting me to adapt his graphic of long-axis function presented at the meeting of the Association for European Paediatric Cardiology held in Warsaw in May, 2007 for Figure 5-13.

The complete reference list can be found on the companion Expert Consult web site at www.expertconsult.com.

ANNOTATED REFERENCES

- Barton PJ, Cullen ME, Townsend PJ, et al: Close physical linkage of human troponin genes: Organization, sequence, and expression of the locus encoding cardiac troponin I and slow skeletal troponin T. Genomics 1999;57: 102–109.

  The authors discovered that the genes encoding striated muscle troponin I and troponin T isoforms are closely co-located, but show independent tissue-specific expression. Their findings have important implications for characterisation of the troponin families and assessment of mutations implicated in cardiomyopathy.
- Baschat AA, Cosmi E, Bilardo CM, et al: Predictors of neonatal outcome in early-onset placental dysfunction. Obstet Gynecol 2007;109:253–261.

  This large multicentric study quantified the impact of birth weight, gestational age, and fetal cardiovascular factors on neonatal outcome.
- Kiserud T, Kessler J, Ebbing C, Rasmussen S: Ductus venosus shunting in growth-restricted fetuses and the effect of umbilical circulatory compromise. Ultrasound Obstet Gynecol 2006;28:143–114.

  This cross sectional study of growth-restricted fetuses showed that shunting across the venous duct is higher, and the flow of umbilical blood to the liver is less, in fetuses with growth restriction, particularly in those with the most severe umbilical haemodynamic compromise.
- Rasanen J, Wood DC, Weiner S, et al: Role of the pulmonary circulation in the distribution of human fetal cardiac output during the second half of pregnancy. Circulation 1996;94:1068–1073.

  This Doppler echocardiography study describe the normal distribution of human fetal combined cardiac output from the left and right ventricles and weight-indexed pulmonary and systemic vascular resistances and changes during the second half of pregnancy in 68 fetuses stressing the role of the pulmonary circulation in determining cardiac output.
- Mäkikallio K, Jouppila P, Räsänen J: Human fetal cardiac function during the first trimester of pregnancy. Heart 2005;91:334–338.

  Longitudinal first-trimester scans describe the maturation of systolic and diastolic cardiac function and report that atrioventricular valve regurgitation is commonplace and of no functional significance.
- Fouron JC, Gosselin J, Raboisson MJ, et al: Early intertwin differences in myocardial performance during the twin-to-twin transfusion syndrome. Circulation 2004;110:3043–3048.

  The Tei index was used in monochorionic twin pregnancies to distinguish between early twin-to-twin transfusion syndrome and discordant fetal growth. The recipient twin showed early alteration of the Tei index that was not seen in the larger of the twins discordant for size.
- Gardiner HM, Pasquini L, Wolfenden J, et al: Increased periconceptual maternal glycosolated haemoglobin in diabetic mothers reduces fetal long axis cardiac function. Heart 2006;92:1125–1130.

  Fetuses of mothers with type 1 and 2 diabetes showed increased Doppler tissue velocities and amplitude of motion at the base of the heart compared with normal reference ranges. These measures correlated positively with the modest hypertrophy observed, and negatively with the first HbA1c measurement in pregnancy, confirming that poor maternal diabetic control reduces fetal long-axis function, but modest hypertrophy alone does not.
- Welsh A: Quantification of power Doppler and the index 'fractional moving blood volume' (FMBV). Ultrasound Obstet Gynecol 2004;23:323–326.

  This review explores the advantages and pitfalls of assessment of multidirectional flow and hence organ perfusion using power Doppler. It discusses the important role of fractional moving blood volumes and cumulative power distribution function in standardisation of power Doppler.
- Yagel S, Cohen SM, Shapiro I, Valsky DV: 3D and 4D ultrasound in fetal cardiac scanning: A new look at the fetal heart. Ultrasound Obstet Gynecol 2007;29:81–95.

  This useful review summarises the technological advances in fetal cardiac scanning. It observes that its role in improving the accuracy of detection and fetal cardiac function has still to be evaluated.
- Gardiner HM, Celermajer DS, Sorensen KE, et al: Arterial reactivity is significantly impaired in normotensive young adults after successful repair of aortic coarctation in childhood. Circulation 1994;89:1745–1750.

  Endothelium-dependent and -independent measures of vascular function were shown to be abnormal in the precoarctation site of a cohort of young adults that had undergone early and successful repair of coarctation of the aorta.
- Johnson PJ, Maxwell DJ, Tynan MJ, Allan LD: Intracardiac pressures in the human fetus. Heart 2000;84:59–63.

  Direct ventricular pressures were recorded in the human fetal heart in a series of second-trimester fetuses. Both ventricles worked at similar pressure ranges and showed a gestational increase.
- Gardiner HM, Taylor MJO Karatza AA, et al: Twin-twin transfusion syndrome: The influence of intrauterine laser—photocoagulation on arterial distensibility in childhood. Circulation 2003;107:1906–1911.

  This study compared the vascular stiffness in 50 pairs of twins in childhood and is the first paper to show vascular programming occurs in fetal life and may be altered by intra-uterine therapy.
- de Divitiis M, Pilla C, Kattenhorn M, et al: Ambulatory blood pressure, left ventricular mass, and conduit artery function late after successful repair of coarctation of the aorta. J Am Coll Cardiol 2003;41:2259–2265.

  This study confirms the earlier findings of this group that fetal coarctation of the aorta has long-term cardiovascular consequences despite successful early surgical repair.

CHAPTER 6

Systemic Circulation

YIU-FAI CHEUNG

The systemic circulation refers to the circulation in which blood is carried from the systemic ventricle, which is the left ventricle in the setting of ventriculo-arterial concordance, through a network of arteries and arterioles to the tissue capillaries, and drained via the systemic venous system to the systemic venous atrium.

The systemic arterial system serves two important functions. First, it acts as a low-resistance conduit through which blood is distributed to different parts of the body. Second, the arterial tree buffers the pulsatile pressure to convert systemic ventricular pulsatile ejection into a steady stream of capillary flow. Additionally, the endothelium, which lines the vascular lumen, exerts important vascular homeostatic effects through production of a variety of substances. Hence, alterations of the mechanical properties of the arterial wall and function of the endothelium have significant implications on normal functioning of the systemic arterial system. Furthermore, optimal performance of the systemic ventricle depends on its favorable interaction with the systemic circulation. In the setting of congenital heart disease, the systemic ventricle may be a morphological left ventricle, morphological right ventricle, or single functional ventricular chamber of right, left or indeterminate morphology. As a result of systemic arterial dysfunction, an unfavorable ventriculo-arterial interaction may result. On the other hand, systemic ventricular dysfunction may also predispose to systemic arterial dysfunction.

In this chapter, the systemic circulation is discussed from structural, physiological, and mechanical perspectives. Measures of arterial function and paediatric conditions associated with systemic arterial dysfunction are then highlighted. Finally, the concept of ventriculo-arterial interaction and its relevance in congenital and acquired heart disease in the young are described. The systemic venous system is discussed in Chapter 23.

SYSTEMIC ARTERIAL SYSTEM

Structure

The systemic arterial tree begins with the aorta, the largest arterial trunk that arises from the left ventricle. The aorta ramifies into tributaries to perfuse all parts of the body, with the exception of hair, nails, epidermis, cartilage, and cornea. The large central arteries are protected within the thoracic and abdominal cavities, while peripheral conduit arteries run along the flexor surfaces in the upper and lower limbs where they are less exposed to injury. The fashion in which the arterial tree ramifies varies: an arterial trunk may give off several branches in succession and continue as a main trunk, give off a short trunk that subdivides into several branches, or bifurcate at its distal end. The ascending aorta arises at the base of the left ventricle and gives off the first branches, the right and left coronary arteries. It continues as the aortic arch, from which the brachiocephalic, left common carotid, and left subclavian arteries arise. The thoracic descending aorta begins as a continuation of the aortic arch and penetrates the diaphragm to continue as the abdominal descending aorta. The celiac trunk and superior and inferior mesenteric arteries arise from the abdominal descending aorta to supply the liver and gastrointestinal tract, while the renal arteries branch off at right angles to perfuse the kidneys. The descending aorta bifurcates at its distal end into the right and left common iliac arteries, the latter bifurcating into the internal iliac artery to supply the pelvic organs and the external iliac artery that continues as the femoral artery to supply the lower limbs. The systemic arterial tree is a tapering branching system. Hence, the aorta tapers from its origin to its termination at the iliac bifurcation and branched daughter vessels are always narrower than the parent vessel, which has implications on wave reflection. The arterial ramifications end in arterioles, which then usually continue as capillaries. Beyond the major arterial branches, the total cross sectional area increases progressively to the capillary bed. Apart from size, the proportion of cellular and structural components also varies along the arterial tree. Notwithstanding these variations, the arterial wall is made up of three constant layers: an internal tunica intima, a tunica media, and an external tunica adventitia.

The intima comprises the endothelium, a subendothelial layer, and an elastic membrane. The endothelium consists of a monolayer of cells that line the vascular lumen. Apart from forming a physical barrier between the circulating blood components and the vascular wall, the endothelial cells play a pivotal role in vascular homeostasis. The subendothelial layer is made up of fibroblasts and variable amount of collagen. The internal elastic membrane consists of a network of elastic fibres and forms the boundary with the media.

The media, usually the thickest layer in the arterial wall, is responsible for the mechanical properties of the vessel. Its structural components are vascular smooth muscle cells and extracellular matrix, the latter consisting of elastic lamellas, collagen fibres, structural glycoproteins, and ground substance.[1] While vascular smooth muscle cells maintain vascular tone through contraction and relaxation, the extracellular matrix of the media provides a structural framework for optimal functioning of the blood vessels.

The elastic fibres in the media, arranged in concentric lamellas that form boundaries between layers of vascular smooth muscle cells, are 90% represented by elastin. Cross-linking of elastin confers to the arteries elasticity, the ability to distend during cardiac systole and recoil during diastole. Elastin has also further been implicated in the control of proliferation and phenotype of smooth muscle cells.[2] Elastin has an estimated half-life of more than 40 years in humans, and the rate of its synthesis is thought to be negligible in adulthood.[3–5] Hence, it appears that damaged elastin, as a result of either degeneration or pathological process, is unlikely to be replaced. Other constituents of elastic fibres include microfibrillar-associated glycoproteins and fibrillin.[6–8] Fibrillin forms a microfibrillar network that serves as scaffolding for deposition of elastin and assembly of elastic fibres. A recently discovered protein, fibulin-5, also plays a critical function during elastic fibre development through its interactions with elastin and integrins.[9,10] Other structural glycoproteins in the arterial wall include fibronectin, vitronectin, lamin, entactin/nidogen, tenascin, and thrombospondin.[11,12]

Collagens are composed of three polypeptide α-chains arranged to form a triple helix, which confers tensile strength to the vessel wall. Types I and III collagen are the major fibrillar collagens in blood vessels, constituting about 90% of vascular collagens.[13] Collagen is the stiffest component of the arterial wall, with an elastic modulus of 10^8 to 10^9 dyne/cm^2.[14] By contrast, the elastic modulus of elastin is of the order of 10^6 dyne/cm.[2,15,16] Hence, the absolute and relative quantities of elastin and collagen contribute significantly to stiffness of the arterial wall. The elasticity of the arterial wall is a non-linear function of transmural pressure. To explain the non-linear elasticity, a qualitative model proposes that at low pressure, the tension is borne by elastin, and as the pressure and stretch increase, collagen fibres take on an increasing fraction of the tension with progressive stiffening of the blood vessel, hence preventing its over-distention at high pressure.[17] Indeed, increasing recruitment of collagen fibres in the human brachial artery as transmural arterial pressure increases has been shown in vivo.[18] Recent proposed models take into account the contribution of vascular smooth muscle cells, viscoelastic properties of the matrix proteins, residual stresses due to growth and remodeling, and gradual recruitment of collagen fibres with increasing pressure.[19–22]

The ground substance is filled by proteoglycans. Proteoglycans are macromolecules that possess one or more linear glycosaminoglycan chains linked to a core protein. The proteoglycans in the vessel wall are hyaluronan, versican, biglycan, decorin, lumican, syndecans, fibroglycan, and glypican.[23] The proteoglycans have diverse roles in the organisation of connective tissue structure, regulating cellular activities and metabolism, permeability, filtration, and hydration, and controlling cytokine biodisponibility and stability.[24–27] Different components of the extracellular matrix can be degraded by matrix metalloproteinases. Importantly, matrix metalloproteinases play a fundamental role in the degradation of vascular extracellular matrix[28] not only during normal physiological vascular remodeling, but also during pathological remodeling.[23,29]

The distribution of structural components within the media varies along the arterial tree, hence accounting for the difference in mechanical properties between proximal and distal arteries.[30] Of significance is the fall in elastin to collagen ratio and increase in smooth muscle cells with increasing distance from the heart.[31,32] Arteries have been categorised as elastic or muscular based on structural composition of the media. Hence, the aorta and its major branches are described as elastic arteries, while brachial and femoral arteries are regarded as muscular conduit arteries. At the arteriolar level, the media consists of essentially one to several layers of smooth muscle cells. Thus, the basic architecture of arteries justifies the division of the systemic arterial tree into a proximal compartment, in which elastin predominates, and a distal compartment, in which collagen and vascular smooth muscle cells predominate.[30] Alterations of structural components of the media as a result of degeneration, genetic mutations, or imbalanced activities of metalloproteinases and their inhibitors can have significant impact on the mechanical properties of the vessels.

The adventitia contains mainly fibroblasts and collagen fibres and some elastic fibres. Increasingly, the contribution of adventitial layer to the elastic properties of arteries is recognised.[33,34] Nutrient vessels, vasa vasorum, arise from a branch of the artery or from a neighbouring vessel to ramify and distribute to the adventitial layer.

Endothelial Function

The endothelium comprises a monolayer of endothelial cells that lines the vascular lumen. It is strategically located between circulating blood components and vascular smooth muscle cells to exert a pivotal role in vascular homeostasis. By producing a wide variety of substances, the endothelium regulates vascular tone, inhibits smooth muscle cell proliferation and migration, controls cellular adhesion, regulates inflammation, and exerts fibrinolytic and antithrombotic actions. In recent years, the concept of endothelial function has extended from the vascular lumen to the vascular wall and adventitia, which are supplied by vasa vasorum considered as an active intravascular microcirculation.[35,36]

Nitric oxide, initially identified as the endothelium-derived relaxing factor,[37] is the major vasodilating substance released by the endothelium. Nitric oxide is synthesised from L-arginine by the action of endothelial nitric oxide synthase, primarily in response to sheer stress produced by blood flow.[38] Cofactors including tetrahydrobiopterin and nicotinamide adenine dinucleotide phosphate are involved in nitric oxide production.[39] Apart from shear stress, endothelial nitric oxide synthase can also be activated by bradykinin, adenosine, vascular endothelial growth factor, and serotonin.[40] Asymmetrical dimethylarginine, on the other hand, is an endogenous inhibitor of nitric oxide synthase[41] and has been implicated in the mediation of adverse effects of traditional risk factors on endothelial vasodilator function.[42] Nitric oxide has a half-life of a few seconds in vivo. It diffuses from endothelial cells to exert its relaxation effects on vascular smooth muscle cells by activation of guanylate cyclase, which in turn increases production of cyclic guanosine monophosphate and leads to reduction of intracellular calcium concentration. Apart from regulation of vascular tone through vasodilation, nitric oxide also mediates other important vascular homeostatic functions by exerting inhibitory effects on vascular smooth muscle proliferation,[43] counteracting leucocyte adhesion to the endothelium[44,45] and inhibiting platelet aggregation.[46]

The endothelium also mediates hyperpolarisation of the vascular smooth muscle to cause relaxation.[47,48] Although the identity of the endothelium-derived hyperpolarizing factor remains elusive, its hyperpolarizing mechanism is in general considered to be mediated by calcium-activated potassium channels on vascular smooth muscle.[49–52] Candidates of endothelium-derived hyperpolarizing factor include epoxyeicosatrienoic acids,[53,54] potassium ion,[55] gap junctions,[56] and hydrogen peroxide.[57] In human forearm circulation, endothelium-derived hyperpolarizing factor appears to be a cytochrome P-450 derivative, possibly an epoxyeicosatrienoic acid,[58] and contributes to basal vascular resistance and vasodilation evoked by substance P and bradykinin.[59] There is a suggestion that endothelium-derived hyperpolarizing factor might play a compensatory role for the loss of nitric-oxide mediation vasodilation in patients with heart failure.[59,60] Other endothelium-derived vasodilators include prostacyclin and bradykinin. Prostacyclin is produced via the cyclo-oxygenase pathway and acts independently of nitric oxide to cause vasodilation.[61] It also acts synergistically with nitric oxide to inhibit platelet aggregation. Prostacyclin appears to have a limited role in humans in the control of vascular tone. Bradykinin stimulates release of nitric oxide, prostacyclin, and endothelium-derived hyperpolarizing factor.

Regulation of vascular tone by the endothelium is accomplished not only by release of vasodilators, but also by the control of vasoconstrictor tone through release of endothelin[62] and conversion of angiotensin I to angiotensin II at its surface.[63] Endothelin-1, the predominant endothelin isoform in the cardiovascular system, binds to ET_A receptors on vascular smooth muscle cells to cause vasoconstriction.[64] At lower concentration, however, endothelin-1 causes transient vasodilation in human forearm circulation,[65] probably due to stimulation of release of nitric oxide and prostacyclin via ET_B receptors located on endothelial cells.[66]

Vascular Smooth Muscle Function

The primary function of the vascular smooth muscle cells is contraction, during which the cells shorten to reduce vessel diameter, alter vascular tone, and regulate blood flow. This contractile phenotype of vascular smooth muscle cells is characterised by expression of genes that encode contractile proteins, ion channels, and other molecules involved in contraction.[67,68] Excitation-contraction coupling is the process by which cellular signaling pathways modulate activities of ion channels in the smooth muscle sarcolemma, thereby causing alterations in intracellular calcium signaling and other signaling cascades and resulting in contraction or relaxation of vascular smooth muscle cells. The regulation of smooth muscle contraction in vivo is primarily by pharmacomechanical and electromechanical activation of the contractile proteins myosin and actin.[69] Pharmacomechanical coupling refers to activation of contraction by ligands of cell surface receptors without obligatory change in plasma membrane potential. In vascular smooth muscle, the phosphoinositide signaling cascade is the common secondary messenger system utilised by the surface receptors. Electromechanical coupling, on the other hand, involves alterations in plasma membrane potential. Receptor activation may induce an activation of receptor-operated or voltage-dependent channels and lead to passive influx of calcium down its concentration gradient. Detailed discussion of the molecular mechanisms of smooth muscle contraction is beyond the scope of this chapter. Interested readers are referred to several recently published reviews.[70–74] The balance between force generation and release is responsible for the maintenance of vascular tone,[71] which can be envisaged as the sum of forces generated in the vessel wall to oppose the increase in vessel diameter. The vascular tone is influenced by local metabolic substances, humoral factors, and activity of the autonomic nervous system. In the smallest arteries and arterioles, contraction of vascular smooth muscle causes large reduction in the vascular lumen and increases peripheral vascular resistance. In large elastic and muscular conduit arteries, the change in vascular tone is accompanied by an increase in elastic modulus, and hence stiffness, of the arteries.

Apart from a contractile phenotype, vascular smooth muscle cells exhibit other phenotypes. This phenotypic diversity plays an important role in normal development, repair of vascular injury, and vascular disease process.[75,67] Hence, after vascular injury, phenotypic modulation of vascular smooth muscle cells causes upregulation of genes required for their proliferation and production of extracellular matrix and suppression of genes that characterise the contractile phenotype. On the other hand, inappropriate pathological differentiation into other mesenchymal lineages as osteoblastic, chondrocytic, and adipocytic ones may contribute to vessel calcification, altered matrix production, and abnormal lipid accumulation, respectively.[76–80] Recent studies have focused on the understanding of mechanisms that underlie the physiological control and pathologic alterations of phenotypic switching of vascular smooth muscle cells.[67,75,81]

Control of Circulation

The regulation of circulation aims to adjust precisely the blood flow in relation to tissue needs and to maintain adequate driving pressure to perfuse the various body tissues. Such control is achieved through local mechanisms, humoral factors, and neural regulation.

Local Control

Auto-regulation refers to the ability to maintain relatively constant blood flow in response to acute changes in perfusion pressure. The coronary, renal, and cerebral circulations exhibit auto-regulation. Two theories have been proposed for this auto-regulatory mechanism. The metabolic theory[82] suggests that elevated perfusion pressure increases blood flow, and hence oxygen delivery and removal of vasodilators, thereby leading to vasoconstriction and reduction of blood flow and vice versa. The myogenic theory[83] proposes that stretching of vascular smooth muscle cells by the elevated perfusion pressure increases their tension, which in turn causes vasoconstriction and reduces the blood flow back to normal. Conversely, less stretching at low pressure leads to smooth muscle relaxation and increased blood flow. The physiological relevance of myogenic constriction lies in its influence on peripheral vascular resistance, provision of vascular tone, and contribution to control of capillary pressure. However, the exact mechanisms that link intraluminal pressure generation to myogenic constriction remain uncertain.[84]

Metabolic mechanisms also contribute to the control of local blood flow. Two theories have likewise been proposed. The vasodilator theory proposes that vasodilator substances are formed and released from tissues when metabolic rate increases or oxygen and other nutrient supplies decrease. Suggested vasodilator substances include adenosine, carbon dioxide, potassium ion, hydrogen ion, lactic acid, histamine, and adenosine phosphate. The nutrient theory suggests that blood vessels dilate naturally when oxygen or other nutrients are deficient. Hence, increased metabolism causes local vasodilation by increased utilisation of oxygen and nutrients, a phenomenon known as active hyperaemia. Reactive hyperaemia is another phenomenon related to local metabolic flow control mechanism. In reactive hyperaemia, brief interruption of arterial blood flow results in transient increase in blood flow that exceeds the baseline, after which the flow returns to baseline level. Both the deprivation of tissue oxygen and accumulation of vasodilating substances probably account for this phenomenon. The duration of reactive hyperaemia depends on the duration of flow cessation and usually lasts long enough to repay the oxygen debt.

Autoregulation and metabolic mechanisms control blood flow by dilation of microvasculature. The consequent increase in blood flow dilates the larger arteries upstream via the mechanism of flow-mediated dilation. The pivotal role of endothelial cells in the transduction of shear stress secondary to increased blood flow and the release of the vasodilators has been alluded to earlier. Flow-mediated dilation has been shown to occur predominantly as a result of local endothelial release of nitric oxide.[85] The mechanisms of shear stress detection and subsequent signal transduction are unclear, but probably involve opening of calcium-activated potassium channels[86–88] that hyperpolarises endothelial cells and calcium activation of endothelial nitric oxide synthase.[85,89] Flow-mediated dilation allows flow to increase with a negligible increase in pressure gradient, thus optimizing energy losses within the circulation.[90] The phenomenon of flow-mediated dilation as induced by reactive hyperaemia has commonly been used as an assessment of endothelial function in vivo. All of the aforementioned mechanisms represent relatively acute responses to regulate local blood flow. Long-term local mechanisms involve changes in tissue vascularity, release of angiogenic factors, and development of collateral circulations.

Humoral Control

Humoral control refers to regulation by hormones or locally produced vasoactive substances that act in an autocrine or a paracrine fashion. These humoral substances act either directly via receptors on vascular smooth muscle cells or indirectly through stimulation of the endothelium to release vasoactive substances.

Circulating catecholamines, noradrenaline and adrenaline, are secreted by the adrenal medulla, which is innervated by pre-ganglionic sympathetic fibres. Sympathetic activation stimulates the release of catecholamines, about 80% being noradrenaline, from the adrenal gland. The adrenal gland and the noradrenergic sympathetic vasoconstrictor fibres provide dual control of circulation by catecholamines. Adrenergic receptors in the blood vessels are α_1, α_2, and β_2 receptors. Noradrenaline causes vasoconstriction by acting on α-receptors, while adrenaline causes vasodilation at physiological concentrations through its β-agonistic effect. At higher concentrations, adrenaline also causes vasoconstriction through activation of α-receptors.

The regulatory role of the renin-angiotensin system in the circulation is well known. The final effector of the system, angiotensin II, mediates its effects classically in an endocrine fashion. In response to decreased renal perfusion pressure or extracellular fluid volume, renin is secreted from the juxta-glomerular apparatus of the kidney and cleaves angiotensinogen, released from the liver, to form angiotensin I. By the action of angiotensin-converting enzyme, which is predominantly expressed on the surface of endothelial cells in the pulmonary circulation, angiotension I is activated to angiotensin II. Angiotensin II is a potent vasoconstrictor and acts directly by stimulating the angiotensin II type I (AT_1) receptor and indirectly by increasing sympathetic tone and release of vasopressin. Recently, it has become obvious that a local paracrine renin-angiotensin system exists in the vasculature.[91,92] Vascular production of angiotensin II has been shown to be mediated by the endothelium.[93] The tissue renin-angiotensin system has dual effects on vessel function, being mediated through opposing effects of two receptors. Stimulation of AT_1 receptor causes contraction of vascular smooth muscle by directly increasing intracellular calcium and indirectly stimulating synthesis of endothelin-1 and other vasoconstrictors.[94] Furthermore, promotion of oxidative stress via the AT_1 receptor may possibly reduce nitric oxide bioavailability.[95,96] On the other hand, stimulation of angiotensin II type 2 receptor appears to mediate vasodilation through activation of the nitric oxide pathway.[97] The local tissue angiotensin II hence also plays an important role in maintaining vascular homeostasis. Additionally, recent studies have shown that other biologically active aminopeptides of the circulating renin-angiotensin system, such as angiotensins III and IV, may act in the central nervous system to raise blood pressure through the AT_1 receptor.[98]

Three peptides of the natriuretic peptide family, atrial natriuretic peptide, brain natriuretic peptide, and C-type natriuretic peptide, participate in the control of circulation. The atrial natriuretic peptide is primarily produced by the atrial myocardium, while the brain natriuretic peptide is synthesised by the ventricular myocardium. The main stimulus for their release is stretching of the myocardium. Other stimuli include endogenous vasoactive factors, neurotransmitters, pro-inflammatory cytokines, and hormones.[99,100] The vascular effects of atrial and brain natriuretic peptides are similar. Both reduce sympathetic tone through suppression of sympathetic outflow from the central nervous system, reduction of release of catecholamines from autonomic nerve endings, and probably damping of baroreceptors.[101,102] The consequence is decreased vascular tone and increased venous capacitance. The atrial and brain natriuretic peptides also inhibit the activities of the renin-angiotension system, endothelins, cytokines, and vasopressin.[99,103,104] The renal haemodynamic effects include induction of diuresis, secondary to increased glomerular filtration rate due to vasodilation of afferent renal arterioles and vasoconstriction of the efferent arterioles,[105] and promotion of natriuresis. Despite preload reduction, reflex tachycardia is suppressed as these peptides lower the activation threshold of vagal afferents. C-type natriuretic peptide is a more potent dilator of veins than the other natriuretic peptides and acts in an autocrine or paracrine fashion.

Adrenomedullin was first isolated from human pheochromocytoma cells, identified by its ability to stimulate cyclic adenosine monophosphate in platelets.[106] It was subsequently found that adrenomedullin is produced in a wide range of cells, including vascular endothelial and smooth muscle cells.[107,108] Evidence is accumulating that adrenomedullin may function as a novel system in the control of circulation.[109,110] Infusion of adrenomedullin via the brachial artery in humans has demonstrated dose-dependent vasodilation and increase in blood flow.[111] Furthermore, the finding of variable blockade of the vasodilating effect of adrenomedullin by inhibition of nitric oxide synthase activity suggests that nitric oxide may be an important mediator for adrenomedullin.[112–114]

The endothelium-derived vasoactive substances and their role in the control of vascular tone and homeostasis were discussed earlier. While prostaglandins are produced by most tissues, prostacyclin (prostaglandin I_2) is the main prostanoid produced by the endothelium of blood vessels. Prostacyclin is a potent vasodilator and an inhibitor of platelet aggregation. Nonetheless, it appears to have a limited role in humans in the control of basal vascular tone. The balance of actions between two antagonistic prostanoids, prostacyclin and thromboxane A_2, has been the recent focus of attention in the light of reported adverse effects of selective inhibition of cyclooxgenase-2.[115,116] Prostaglandins and thromboxane are eicosanoids generated by metabolism of arachidonic acid, a major unsaturated fatty acid present in the phospholipids of cell membranes. Arachidonate is released from the membrane phospholipids by phospholipase A_2 due to a variety of mechanical and neurohumoral stimuli. Arachidonate is then converted to prostaglandin H_2 by prostaglandin H synthase, also known as cyclooxygenase. Specific synthases then produce the biologically active end products of this metabolic pathway, namely prostaglandin E_1, prostaglandin $F_2\alpha$, prostacyclin, and thromboxane A_2. The endothelial cells produce predominantly prostacyclin and lesser amounts of prostaglandin E_1, also a vasodilator, and prostaglandin $F_2\alpha$, a vasoconstrictor.[117] Thromboxane A_2, although predominately generated by platelets, is also synthesised by the endothelium[118] and induces vasoconstriction and platelet aggregation. Cyclooxygenase exists in two isoforms: cyclooxgenase-1 and cyclooxygenase-2.[119,120] Whether endothelial production of prostacyclin depends on cyclooxgenase-1 or -2 activity, however, remains debatable.[116,121,122] Under normal physiological conditions, eicosanoids, primarily prostacyclin, produced by the cyclooxygenase pathway induce vasorelaxation.[120] Furthermore, the cyclooxygenase-dependent vasodilators can compensate for the deficiency of other vasorelaxants.[123] By way of the lipoxygenase pathway, leucotrienes are produced from arachidonic acid. Leucotrienes C_4, D_4, and E_4 cause arteriolar constriction, while leucotrienes B_4 and C_4 induce pulmonary vasoconstriction by activating cyclooxygenase to produce thromboxane A_2.[117]

Several other endogenous substances affect the systemic circulation. Vasopressin, produced in the supraoptic and paraventricular nuclei of the hypothalamus, is probably the most potent known endogenous constrictor. It is released in quantities sufficient to exert a pressor effect when volume depletion is significant. It has, however, little role in normal vascular control.[124,125] Serotonin exists in large amount in the enterochromaffin cells of the gastrointestinal tract. Although serotonin exerts vasoconstrictor and vasodilator effects, depending on vasculature, its function in the regulation of circulation is unknown. Kinins are among the most potent endogenous vasodilators. Examples of kinins include bradykinins and kallidin, which are formed from the action of kallikrein on the α_2-globulin kininogen. Kinins cause vasodilation and increase capillary permeability. Bradykinin is believed to play a role in the control of blood flow in the skin, gastrointestinal glands, and salivary glands. Histamine is located in mast cells and basophils. Histamine is released from these cells upon stimulation by injury, inflammation, or allergic reaction to induce vasodilation and increase capillary permeability.

Neural Control

Neural control of the systemic circulation involves feedback mechanisms that operate in both the short and long term through the autonomic, primarily the sympathetic, nervous system.[126] Short-term changes in sympathetic activity are triggered either by reflex mechanisms involving peripheral receptors or by a centrally generated response. Long-term changes, on the other hand, are evoked through modulation of the sympathetic nervous system by other humoral factors and possibly by central mechanisms involving the hypothalamus.

Peripheral receptors that constitute the afferent limb of the reflex are arterial baroreceptors, arterial chemoreceptors, and cardiac stretch receptors. Arterial baroreceptors are located in the walls of the carotid sinus and aortic arch. Afferent fibres run in the glossopharyngeal and vagal nerves and terminate within the nucleus tractus solitarius. The nucleus tractus solitarius neurons then excite neurons within the caudal and intermediate parts of the ventrolateral medulla to cause inhibition of the sympathoexcitatory neurons in the rostral ventrolateral medulla.[127] Hence, stretching of arterial baroreceptors increases afferent input and results in reflex slowing of heart rate, decrease in cardiac contractility, and vasodilation, thereby providing a negative feedback mechanism for homeostasis of arterial pressure.[128]

Peripheral chemoreceptors are located in the carotid and aortic bodies, being stimulated primarily by decreased arterial partial pressure of oxygen. Their afferent fibres also run in the glossopharyngeal and vagus nerves. Activation of peripheral chemoreceptor results in hyperventilation and sympathetically mediated vasoconstriction of vascular beds, with the exception of those of the heart and brain.[129] Hence, oxygen conservation is attempted by increasing oxygen uptake and reducing tissue oxygen consumption. These chemoreflexes are nonetheless subjected to negative feedback interaction, with inhibition of the chemoreflex-mediated sympathetic activation through stimulation of baroceptors and thoracic afferents.[130]

Atrial receptors are located in the walls of the right and left atriums and in pulmonary venous and cavoatrial junctions.[131,132] Two types of atrial receptors are described based on their discharge pattern in relation to atrial pressure waves. Type A receptors signal atrial contraction and hence respond to increase in central venous pressure. These receptors send impulses via myelinated fibres in the vagus nerve, while the efferent portion consists of sympathetic activation. The tachycardia due to stimulation of sinoatrial node caused by atrial stretch is termed the Bainbridge reflex. Type B baroreceptors are stretch receptors stimulated by volume distention of the atriums and fire during ventricular systole. The afferents are via unmyelinated vagal fibres. Atrial distention decreases sympathetic activity. Receptors which respond to stretch and contractility are also present in the ventricles. The receptors provide afferent input to the medulla via unmyelinated C-fibres.[133] Stimulation of these fibres decreases sympathetic tone and causes bradycardia and vasodilation. Stretching of the atrial and ventricular myocardium also leads to the release of natriuretic peptides, as discussed earlier.

Apart from the reflex-triggered short-term control of circulation, the central pathways responsible for the central command responses, such as those occurring at the onset of exercise or evoked by a threatening stimulus, are increasingly understood.[126] The rostral ventrolateral medulla is traditionally regarded as the vasomotor centre that controls circulation via the autonomic, primarily sympathetic, nervous system.[134] Nonetheless, accumulating evidence suggests that the dorsomedial hypothalamic nucleus may be a critical region responsible for the integration of autonomic, non-autonomic, and cardiovascular components of the central command responses.[135] Indeed, recent data suggests that groups of neurons in the hypothalamus can project to synapse directly with sympathetic pre-ganglionic fibres in the spinal cord, implying that the medullary vasomotor centre is perhaps not the only region that directly controls sympathetic outflow.[136]

The autonomic nervous system represents the efferent component of the neural control of the circulation. Up to three types of fibres may innervate blood vessels: sympathetic vasoconstrictor fibres, sympathetic vasodilator fibres, and parasympathetic vasodilator fibres. As the size of vessel decreases, the density of autonomic innervation increases. The small arteries and arterioles are therefore the most richly innervated arteries.

Sympathetic vasoconstrictor fibres release noradrenaline upon nerve stimulation and constitute the most important components in the neural control of circulation. Postsynaptically, the α_1-adrenoceptor is the predominant receptor mediating vasoconstriction. Although noradrenaline is the principal neurotransmitter in the sympathetic nervous system, it has been observed to co-exist with adenosine triphosphate and neuropeptide Y in sympathetic neurons.[137,138] Co-transmission refers to the concept of storage and release of more than one type of neurotransmitter,[139] which is now recognised as the norm of most neurons. Hence, in most blood vessels, adenosine triphosphate and noradrenaline act synergistically to cause vasoconstriction by acting on the post-synaptic P_2 purinoreceptors and α_1-adrenoceptors, respectively. While neuropeptide Y has little direct action in most vessels, it appears to have an enhancing effect on the post-synaptic activity of adenosine triphosphate and noradrenaline and to act presynaptically to inhibit release of these transmitters.[140] Sympathetic vasoconstriction of arterioles increases vascular resistance, while constriction of capacitance vessels alters the circulating blood volume. In larger arteries, contraction of vascular smooth muscle in response to sympathetic activation causes less significant change in arterial caliber but alters vascular tone and hence arterial stiffness.

Sympathetic vasodilator fibres are scarce and are not tonically active. Evidence suggests that sympathetic vasodilator fibres regulate skeletal vascular tone in many animal species. Both cholinergic[141] and nitric oxide–dependent[142,143] mechanisms contribute to the vasodilator effect. Parasympathetic vasodilator fibres are found in blood vessels of the salivary gland, cerebral arteries, and coronary arteries. The vasodilator effect is mediated via release of acetylcholine with hyperpolarisation of the vascular smooth muscle.

Long-term neural regulation of the circulation is modulated by humoral and other factors. Angiotensin II is an important facilitator of sympathetic transmission. It may enhance neurotransmitter release at sympathetic nerve terminals, sympathetic transmission through sympathetic ganglia,[144] and perhaps central activation of sympathetic nervous activity.[145] Evidence is also accumulating that nitric oxide interacts with the autonomic nervous system at both central and peripheral levels.[146] Centrally, nitric oxide decreases sympathetic vasoconstrictor outflow. Peripherally, augmented vasoconstriction to nitric oxide synthase inhibition has been demonstrated in denervated forearm in humans.[147] Interaction between nitric oxide and cholinergic vasodilator fibres is also evidenced by significant pressor response to nitric oxide synthase inhibition with cholinergic blockade.[148] Finally, accumulating evidence suggests that the hypothalamic paraventricular nucleus in the central pathways may mediate sustained increases in sympathetic nerve secondary to a variety of stimuli.[127] It has therefore been hypothesised that stress, anxiety, or pathological conditions such as heart failure may exert long-term influence on neural control of circulation through tonic activation of sympathoexcitatory neurons located in paraventricular nuclei of the hypothalamus.[126]

MODELING OF SYSTEMIC CIRCULATION

Models

From the mechanical perspective, the systemic arterial system can be envisaged as a network of elastic tubes that receive pulsatile blood flow from left ventricular ejection and transmit it distally as a steady stream into capillaries. Hence, apart from acting as a low-resistance conduit, the systemic arterial tree functions as a cushion to smooth out pressure and flow pulsations generated by cycles of left ventricular contraction. While the success of the conduit function depends primarily on a low peripheral vascular resistance, the efficiency of cushioning function depends on the elastic properties, described in terms of stiffness, of the arterial system. Importantly, stiffness of the arterial system is related to vascular impedance, the opposition to blood flow taken to represent the afterload presented by the systemic arterial circulation to the left ventricle.

Modeling of the arterial circulation has contributed significantly to the understanding of the behaviour of the arterial system and the effects of arterial load on the systemic ventricle. The lumped model of arterial circulation, commonly termed *Windkessel* model, was first described in the eighteenth century. In his book entitled *Haemastaticks*, Hales drew an analogy between the arterial system and an air-filled dome of the fire engine compression chamber (*Windkessel*)[149] (Fig. 6-1). The dome represents the cushioning function of the arteries, which buffers intermittent spurts of water from the pump. The rigid fire hose represents the

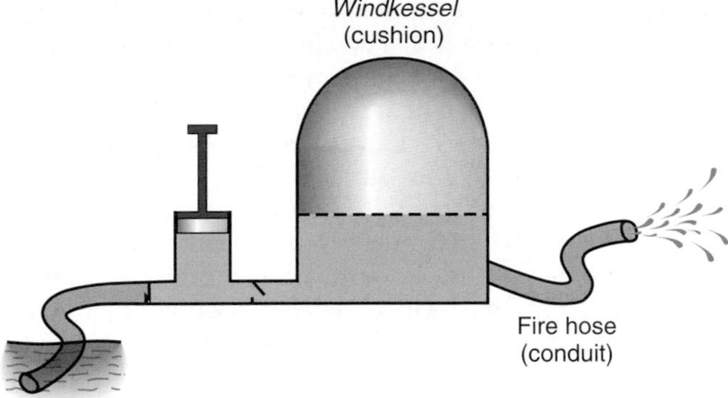

Figure 6-1 *Windkessel* model of the arterial system. The *Windkessel* buffers spurts of water from the pump, while the fire hose functions as a low resistance conduit. (Reproduced with permission from O'Rourke MF: Arterial function in health and disease. Edinburgh: Churchill Livingstone, 1982.)

conduit function, while the nozzle represents the peripheral resistance. As an analogy, blood ejected from the left ventricle distends the large elastic arteries during systole, while elastic recoil of the arteries during diastole propels blood to perfuse the peripheral resistance vessels. This cushioning function smooths out the pulsatile blood flow and protects the peripheral vascular beds from exposure to large pressure fluctuations. The electrical analogues of the systemic arterial system are shown in Figure 6-2. The two-element electrical analogue of the *Windkessel* model comprises a capacitor, which represents the arterial compliance, and a resistor, the total peripheral resistance. To better characterise the arterial system, a modified *Windkessel* model has been proposed[150] to take into account the input impedance of the proximal aorta by addition of a resistor proximal to the two-element capacitance-resistance model. A four-element *Windkessel* model, with addition of an inertial term, has further been shown to be superior to the three-element *Windkessel* as a lump model of the entire systemic tree.[151] Inertance is due to mass of the fluid and physiologically; it can be regarded as the inertial effect secondary to simultaneous acceleration of the blood mass within the vessel.

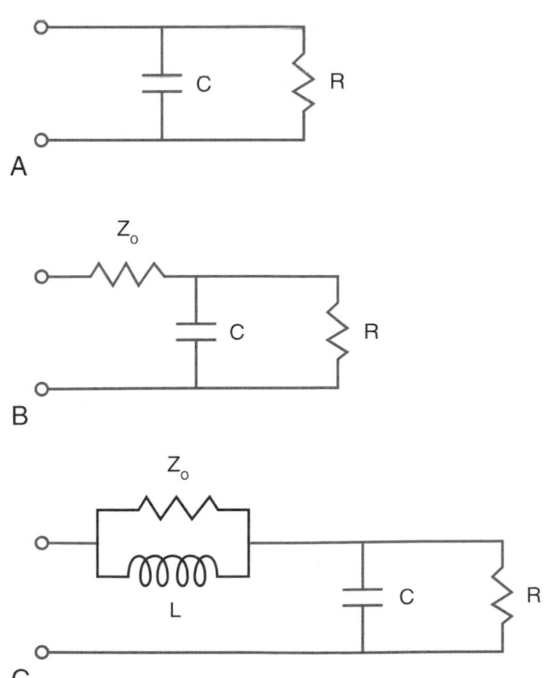

Figure 6-2 Electrical analogues of the systemic arterial system. **A**, Classic two-element *Windkessel* model with arterial compliance being represented by a capacitor (C) and the peripheral resistance by a resistor (R). **B**, A modified *Windkessel* model with addition of a proximal resistor (Z_o) to represent characteristic impedance of the proximal aorta. **C**, A four-element *Windkessel* model with incorporation of an inertance element (L).

The *Windkessel* model, albeit simple and qualitative, emphasises the elasticity of the large arteries and resistance offered by the small peripheral arteries. Nonetheless, this model has intrinsic shortcomings: limitation of vessel elasticity to one site, lack of a finite velocity of propagation of the pulse wave, and overlooking of the significance of wave reflection. In this model, the pressure generated by contraction of the systemic ventricle is assumed to be transmitted instantaneously throughout the *windkessel,* the pressure pulse is assumed to subside before the next cardiac cycle, and there is a single systolic and a single diastolic blood pressure throughout the major arteries. However, the fact that the cushioning and conduit functions of the arterial tree are combined results in two phenomena: (1) traveling of pulse wave at a finite speed along the arterial wall, and (2) wave reflection at arterial terminations and other discontinuities. A more realistic model proposed is a distensible tube with one end receiving pulsatile ejection of blood from the left ventricle and with the other end representing the peripheral resistance.[152] The pressure wave at any point along the tube is regarded as a result of the incident and reflected waves. The velocity at which the pulse travels depends on the elasticity of the tube and has implications on the timing of arrival of the reflected wave. When the tube is distensible, the wave velocity is slow and the reflected wave returns late in diastole. By contrast, when the tube is stiffened, the pulse velocity is increased and the reflected wave merges with the systolic part of the incident wave, causing a higher pressure in systole and a lower pressure in diastole. It is conceivable, therefore, that stiffness is an important mechanical property of the arterial tree and contributes to left ventricular afterload.

Arterial Impedance as Ventricular Afterload

Ventricular afterload can be conceptualised as all those external factors that oppose ventricular ejection and contribute to myocardial wall stress during systole. The hydraulic load of the systemic arterial system has therefore been taken to represent the afterload presented to the systemic ventricle.[153,154] The total arterial hydraulic load comprises three components: resistance, stiffness, and wave reflection, all of which can be obtained from impedance spectra based on analysis in the frequency domain.[155]

Vascular Resistance

Vascular resistance is commonly used in the clinical setting as an index of systemic ventricular afterload. The electrical analogue for vascular resistance is described by Ohm's law, which applies to direct electric current circuit. For a steady flow state, the vascular resistance is derived by dividing pressure gradient by volume flow. As the systemic venous pressure is very small when compared with the mean aortic pressure, the systemic arterial resistance can be approximated as mean aortic pressure divided by cardiac output. Nonetheless, as arterial blood flow is pulsatile in nature, the use of vascular resistance alone to describe afterload is deemed inadequate.

Vascular Impedance

For pulsatile flow, the corresponding pressure-flow relationship is vascular impedance. This is analogous to the voltage-current relationship of an alternating current electric circuit. To analyse the mathematical relationship between pressure and flow waves, Fourier analysis is used to decompose these complex non-sinusoidal waves into a set of sinusoidal waves with harmonic frequencies that are integral multiples of the fundamental wave frequency (Fig. 6-3). Each of the sinusoidal components is described in terms of frequency, amplitude, and phase angle.

In applying Fourier analysis to the circulatory system, two prerequisites have to be fulfilled: periodicity and linearity. Regularity of the heartbeat can generally be regarded as a type of steady-state oscillation.[156] For a linear system, when the system is driven by a pure sine wave of a certain frequency, no pressure or flow components of another frequency should be generated. By contrast, there will be interactions between harmonic components and creation of additional frequency components in a non-linear system. Hence, strictly speaking, the harmonic terms of the pressure should be related exclusively to the corresponding harmonic terms of flow if the circulatory system is linear. While non-linearities of the circulatory system do exist, their magnitude is small.[157] Importantly, the arterial system has been shown to be linear for normal physiological oscillations.[156,158]

Vascular input impedance is defined as the ratio of pulsatile pressure to pulsatile flow. The aortic input impedance is particularly relevant as it characterises the properties of the entire systemic arterial circulation and represents the hydraulic load presented by the systemic circulation to the left ventricle.[153,154] To obtain the aortic input impedance spectrum, the ascending aortic flow is usually measured by an electromagnetic flow catheter, while the pressure is measured by a micromanometer mounted onto the catheter. Noninvasive determination of aortic input impedance involves the use of Doppler echocardiography to measure flow and tonometry to obtain a carotid, subclavian, or synthesised aortic pressure waveform, the latter based on the radial arterial waveform.

An example of the human aortic input impedance spectra is shown in Figure 6-4. The vascular impedance modulus at different harmonics is the ratio of pressure amplitude to flow amplitude. For a heart rate of 60 beats/min, the fundamental frequency is 1 Hz, the second harmonic is 2 Hz, and so forth. Beyond the 10th harmonic, the magnitudes are usually small and negligible. At zero frequency, impedance is equivalent to resistance in the steady-flow state. The phase difference is the delay in phase angle between the pressure and flow harmonics, which is analogous to time delay in the time domain. When a particular pressure harmonic leads the flow harmonic, the phase angle is positive. Conversely, when the pressure harmonic lags behind the corresponding flow harmonic, the phase is negative. The aortic input impedance spectrum is characterised by a steep decrease in the magnitude of input impedance from its value at zero frequency (resistance), followed by fluctuations with maxima and minima. The fluctuations of the impedance modulus are related to peripheral wave reflection as discussed in the following section. The average of the relatively stable high-frequency components of the impedance moduli provides an approximation of characteristic impedance.

Characteristic impedance is the ratio of pulsatile pressure to pulsatile flow at a site where pressure and flow waves are not influenced by wave reflection. The concept of characteristic impedance is important as it is principally

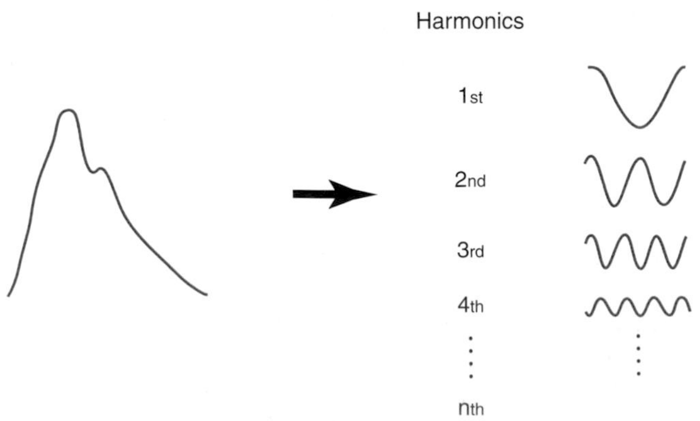

Figure 6-3 Decomposition of complex non-sinusoidal pressure and flow waves into a set of sinusoidal waves with harmonic frequencies at multiples of the frequency of heart rate (first or fundamental frequency) using Fourier analysis.

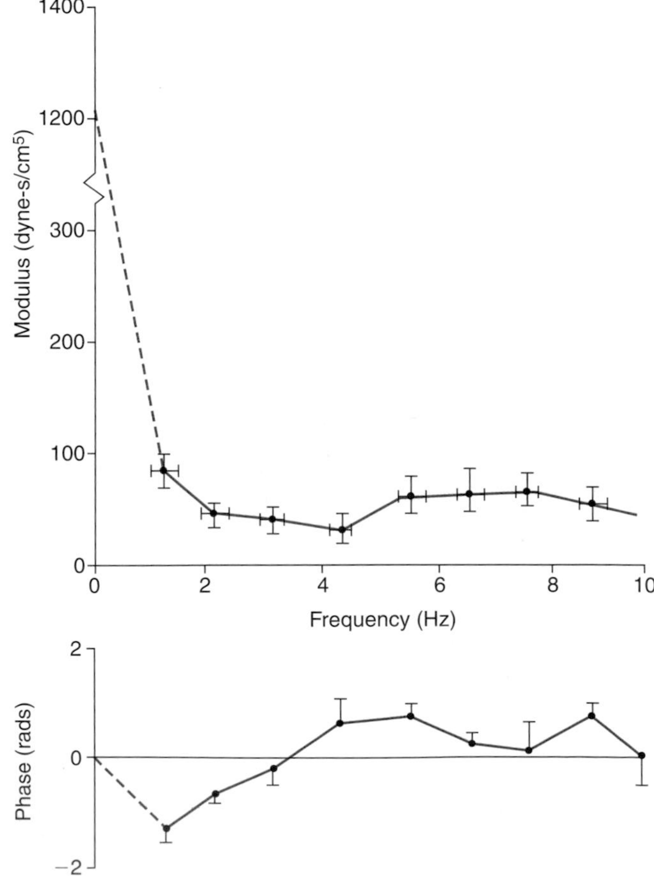

Figure 6-4 Aortic input impedance spectra obtained in normal adults. (Reproduced with permission from Nichols WW, Conti CR, Walker WE, Milnor WR: Input impedance of the systemic circulation in man. Circ Res 1977;40:451–458.)

determined by and related directly to stiffness of the major arteries distal to the site of measurement. Hence, it represents the pulsatile component of the hydraulic workload presented to the left ventricle when it is measured at the ascending aorta. As wave reflection is always present, characteristic impedance cannot be measured directly. It is usually estimated by averaging impedance moduli over a frequency range where fluctuations due to wave reflection above characteristic impedance are expected to cancel out those below.[159] Hence, characteristic impedance has been estimated as the average value of modulus between 2 and 12 Hz,[160] above 2 Hz,[161] or above the frequency of the first minimum.[152] In the time domain, the characteristic impedance can be estimated by relating the initial upstroke of the pressure wave to the upstroke of the simultaneously recorded flow wave,[162] as the effects of wave reflection are minimal with the first 20 msec of the wave.

Wave Reflection

As the velocities of pressure and flow waves transmitted in the arteries are of the order of metres per second, it is obvious that the waves have sufficient time to travel to the periphery and be reflected back before the next cardiac cycle. The existence of wave reflections is supported by several observations. A secondary pressure wave is usually obvious in arterial pressure pulse when flow is in fact decreasing. Furthermore, such secondary pressure waves show different patterns in different arteries.[163,164] Wave reflection also accounts for the observed amplification of the pulse between central and peripheral arteries.[152]

As a result of non-uniformities of geometric and elastic properties along the arterial tree and impedance mismatch at the arterial termination, wave reflection sites can exist throughout the arterial system. There is no universal agreement on the reflecting sites, with possible ones including branching points in major arteries,[165,166] areas of alterations in arterial stiffness,[167] and high-resistance arterioles.[152] Nonetheless, the terminations at which low-resistance conduit arteries terminate in high-resistance arterioles are usually regarded as the principal sites for reflection. Wave reflection in the ascending aorta hence represents the result of reflections at multiple peripheral sites of the body.

The pressure and flow waves measured at any site in the arterial system can therefore be considered as a summation of a forward or incident wave and a reflected wave. Wave reflection exerts opposite effects on pressure and flow. Reflected pressure wave increases the amplitude of the incident pressure wave, while reflected flow wave decreases the amplitude of the incident flow wave. In most experimental animals and in young human subjects who have elastic arteries, wave reflection returns to the ascending aorta from the periphery after ventricular ejection.[152] Such timing is desirable, as the reflected pressure wave augments early diastolic blood pressure, thereby boosting the perfusion pressure of the coronary arteries without increasing left ventricular afterload.

Alteration of arterial stiffness has profound effects on wave reflection. Stiffening of systemic arteries due to aging or disease processes increases pulse wave velocity and causes earlier return of the reflected wave to augment aortic blood pressure in late systole rather than in diastole, the implications of which will be discussed in the section on ventriculo-arterial interaction.

MEASURES OF ARTERIAL FUNCTION

Arterial Stiffness

Arterial stiffness describes the rigidity of the arterial wall. In the last decade, there has been increasing interest in the potential role of arterial stiffening in the development of cardiovascular disease in adults. Arterial stiffness is primarily determined by structural components of the arterial wall, elastin and collagen in particular, vascular smooth muscle tone, and transmural distending pressure.[168] Increasing evidence suggests a role for endothelium in the regulation of arterial stiffness through the influence of smooth muscle tone by release of vasoactive mediators. Indeed, the influence of basal nitric oxide production[169] and endothelin-1[170] on stiffness of the common iliac artery in an ovine model have recently been shown. Additionally, it has been shown that atrial natriuretic peptide and, to a lesser extent, brain natriuretic peptide can modify iliac artery stiffness in this animal model.[171]

The significance of arterial stiffness, as alluded to earlier, owes to its direct relationship with characteristic impedance, hence the pulsatile component of the arterial afterload, and its effect on the timing of return of the reflected waves from peripheral sites. On the one hand, atherosclerotic changes with thickening, fibrosis, and fragmentation and loss of elastin fibres can stiffen the arterial wall by causing structural alterations[172]; on the other, arterial stiffening may predispose the intima to atherosclerosis due to injury sustained from increased pulsatile pressure.[173] Indeed, aortic stiffness has been positively associated with the extent of coronary arterial plaque load in elderly subjects undergoing elective coronary angiography.[174]

The contention that arterial stiffness is a marker of vascular disease and a risk factor for cardiovascular morbidity and mortality in adults is gaining support, and the role of arterial stiffness in the development of cardiovascular disease is increasingly emphasised.[175] The association in adults of increased arterial stiffness and various pathophysiological conditions, which are themselves also associated with increased cardiovascular risk, has been extensively reviewed.[175–178] Studies have also shown that arterial stiffness is associated with end-organ alterations including left ventricular hypertrophy and arterial intima-media thickening in adults independent of systemic blood pressure.[179] Importantly, stiffness of central arteries, as assessed by aortic pulse wave velocity and carotid distensibility, has been shown to have independent predictive value for cardiovascular events in the general adult population,[180,181] in the elderly,[182] in adults with hypertension,[183–185] in end-stage renal failure,[186–189] and with impaired glucose tolerance.[190]

While central arterial stiffness has been the focus of most of the adult studies, the contribution of stiffness of the smaller peripheral arteries to total vascular impedance should not be ignored. Structural remodeling occurs also in smaller arteries and branching points. The changes in mechanical properties of conduit and resistive arteries influence wave reflections and contribute to augmentation of late systolic blood pressure in the aortic root.[191] Hence, carotid augmentation index has also been shown to have independent predictive value for cardiovascular events in adults with hypertension,[192] and end-stage renal failure[193] and in those undergoing percutaneous coronary interventions.[194] Associations between increased small artery stiffness, as assessed by pulse contour analysis, and aging, hypertension, smoking, diabetes, and cardiovascular events have also been reported.[195,196]

The increasing application of non-invasive methods to determine systemic arterial stiffness in the clinical and research arenas has significantly increased the understanding of its pathophysiological significance. With adoption of these non-invasive methodologies for use in children and adolescents,[197,198] the phenomenon and significance of arterial stiffening in the young is also beginning to unveil.

Measurement of Arterial Stiffness in Vivo

Non-invasive methods for determination of local, regional, and systemic arterial stiffness and quantification of wave reflections in vivo are available. For meaningful interpretation of these indices, their fundamental limitations have to be taken into account. First, the relationship between pressure and arterial diameter is nonlinear due to progressive recruitment of the stiffer collagen as transmural pressure increases. Arterial stiffness should therefore be quantified at a given level of pressure as the tangent to the pressure-diameter curve.[152] Importantly, comparison of arterial stiffness among different populations should take into account the potential confounding influence of the distending pressure. Second, modulation of smooth muscle tone by sympathetic nervous activity, hormones, or endothelium-derived vasoactive substances as mentioned above can alter arterial stiffness. Finally, spontaneous vasomotor changes in the muscular arteries can alter arterial diameter and stiffness.[199]

Local Arterial Stiffness

Local arterial stiffness is obtained by relating pressure changes to arterial diameter or cross sectional area changes at the site of interest. Arterial stiffness can be expressed as compliance, distensibility, Person's elastic modulus, Young's modulus, and stiffness index[175,200,201] (Table 6-1). The elastic property of the artery as a hollow, circular structure is described by distensibility, compliance, Peterson's elastic modulus, and stiffness index. The elastic property of the arterial wall, on the other hand, is estimated by Young's elastic modulus that takes into account the wall thickness, which is usually estimated by the intima-media thickness. Assumption of homogeneity of the non-homogeneous arterial wall, however, underestimates Young's elastic modulus. Among the various indices of local arterial stiffness, the stiffness index is considered relatively independent of systemic blood pressure.[202]

For superficial arteries such as the brachial, femoral, and carotid arteries, the diameter and diameter change from end-diastole to systole can be assessed by ultrasound and echo-tracking techniques. Two-dimensional ultrasound assessment is, however, limited by the precision of measurements. In contrast, echo-tracking devices process radio-frequency signals to track the displacement of the anterior and posterior arterial walls with a high precision.[203,204] The difference between displacements, which reflects changes in arterial diameter as a function of time, can then be displayed (Fig. 6-5). The precision in determining the change in diameter has been estimated to be as low as 1 μm for echo-tracking devices and about 150 μm for video-image analysis of ultrasound images.[175,203,205] Furthermore, the intima-media thickness can be estimated from the radio-frequency signals, which enable calculation of Young's elastic modulus. An additional advantage of echo-tracking

TABLE 6-1

INDICES OF LOCAL ARTERIAL STIFFNESS

		FORMULA	
Term	Definition	in Terms of Change in Vessel Diameter	in Terms of Change in Cross Sectional Area of Vessel Lumen
Compliance	Absolute change in diameter or area during systole for a given pressure change	$\Delta D/\Delta P$	$\Delta A/\Delta P$
Distensibility	Relative change in diameter or area during systole for a given pressure change	$\Delta D/(D \cdot \Delta P)$	$\Delta A/(A \cdot \Delta P)$
Peterson's elastic modulus	Inverse of distensibility, i.e., the pressure change required for a given relative change in diameter or area	$\Delta P \cdot D/\Delta D$	$\Delta P \cdot A/\Delta A$
Stiffness index (β)	Ratio of ln (systolic/diastolic pressure) to relative change to vessel diameter	$\ln(Ps/Pd)/(\Delta D/D)$	
Young's modulus or incremental elastic modulus	Elastic modulus per unit wall thickness or area; provides information on intrinsic elastic properties of the arterial wall	$\Delta P \cdot D/\Delta D \cdot h$	[3(1+A/WCSA)]/cross sectional distensibility

A, diastolic cross sectional area; ΔA, difference in systolic and diastolic cross sectional area; D, diastolic diameter; ΔD, difference in systolic and diastolic diameter; h, wall thickness; ΔP, pulse pressure; Pd, diastolic blood pressure; Ps, systolic blood pressure; WCSA, wall cross sectional area = $\pi(D/2 + \text{intima-media thickness})^2 - \pi(D/2)^2$.

devices is that a pressure-diameter curve can be plotted for determination of arterial stiffness at any given blood pressure.[168,206] For deeper arteries such as the aorta, cine magnetic resonance imaging[207] and transoesophageal echocardiography with acoustic quantification[208] have been used to determine diameter change during the cardiac cycle.

Ideally, the local pressure should be measured at the site of diameter measurements. Applanation tonometry allows noninvasive recording of the arterial pressure waveform in the carotid and peripheral conduit arteries.[209] Gentle compression of the superficial artery against the underlying bone by the pen-like tonometer allows its equalisation with the arterial circumferential pressure. The recorded pressure waveform, almost identical to that obtained intra-arterially, can then be calibrated against the cuff mean and diastolic blood pressures of the brachial artery.[210,211] Derivation of central aortic waveform from radial arterial tonometry has also been made possible by application of a transfer function, which has been validated in adults[212–214] but not in children. Although cuff brachial artery pulse pressure has

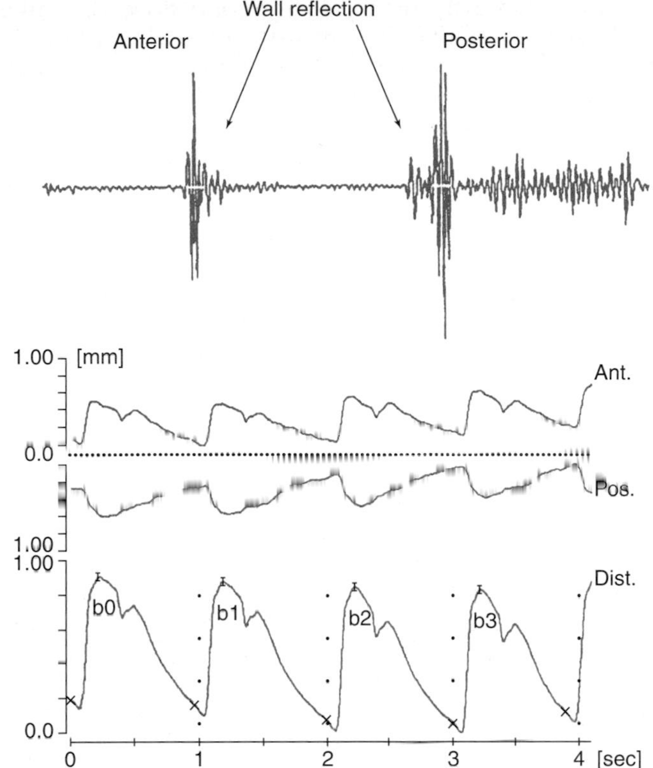

Figure 6-5 Echo-tracking technique. The upper panel shows the radiofrequency signal, while the lower panel shows displacement of the anterior (Ant.) and posterior (Pos.) walls of the artery as a function of time, and the total distention (Dist.) that reflects the change of arterial diameter. (Reproduced with permission from Reneman RS, Hoeks APG: Non-invasive assessment of artery wall properties in humans—methods and interpretation. J Vasc Invest 1996;2:53–64.)

commonly been used for the calculation of local arterial stiffness indices, amplification of pressure pulse along the arterial tree constitutes a potential source of error.

Regional Arterial Stiffness

Arterial stiffness of an arterial segment, or regional stiffness, is assessed by measuring the pulse wave velocity over the segment of interest. Pulse wave velocity is the speed at which the pressure or flow wave is transmitted along the arterial segment. It is related to Young's elastic modulus (E) by the Moens-Korteweg equation: $PWV = \sqrt{Eh/2r\rho}$, where PWV is pulse wave velocity, h is wall thickness of vessel, r is inside radius of vessel and ρ is density of blood.[152] The Bramwell and Hill[215] (1922) equation relates pulse wave velocity to arterial distensibility: $PWV = \sqrt{(\Delta P \cdot V)/\Delta V\rho} = \sqrt{1/\rho D}$, where P is pressure, V is volume, $\Delta P \cdot V/\Delta V$ represents volume elasticity, and D is volume distensibility of the arterial segment. Furthermore, pulse wave velocity is directly related to characteristic impedance (Z_c) by the formula[166] $Z_c = PWV \cdot \rho$. Pulse wave velocity is hence related directly to arterial elasticity and characteristic impedance and inversely to arterial distensibility. By providing an average stiffness of the arterial segment of interest, pulse wave velocity may provide a better reflection of the general vascular health. As aforementioned, the value of aortic pulse wave velocity as a risk for cardiovascular morbidity and mortality in adults is increasingly recognised.[175]

Pulse wave velocity is determined by dividing the distance of pulse travel by the transit time. As the pressure pulse and flow pulse propagate at the same velocity, the arterial pulse may be registered using pressure-sensitive transducers,[216] oscillometric devices,[217] applanation tonometry,[218] and Doppler ultrasound.[219,220] Furthermore, the pulse wave can be detected using magnetic resonance imaging,[221,222] which also allows accurate determination of path length and measurements to be made from relatively inaccessible arteries. Recently, determination of pulse wave velocity based on the principle of photoplethysmography[223] has also been validated.[224] By contrast to the assessment of local arterial stiffness, measurement of pulse wave velocity does not require accurate measurement of the pressure in the arterial segment of interest.

Transit time is measured as the time delay between the feet of the proximal and distal pulse waves (Fig. 6-6). The time delay can be measured by simultaneously recording the pulse waves at two sites of the arterial segment. Alternatively, the time intervals between the R-wave of the electrocardiogram and the foot of the pulse wave at the two sites may be recorded consecutively, and the transit time calculated as the difference between the two. The foot of the pulse wave is used to locate the wave front as it is relatively

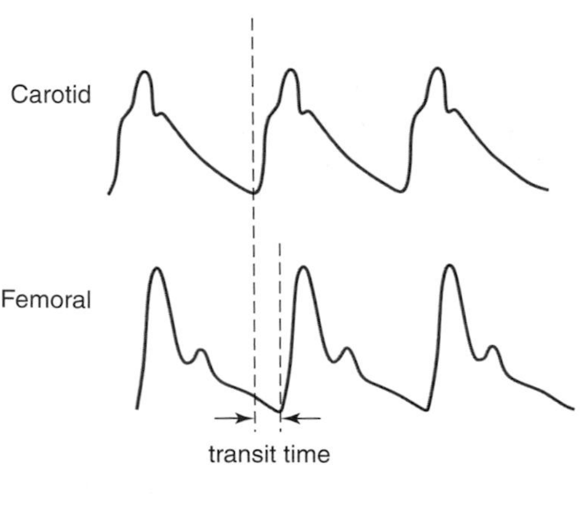

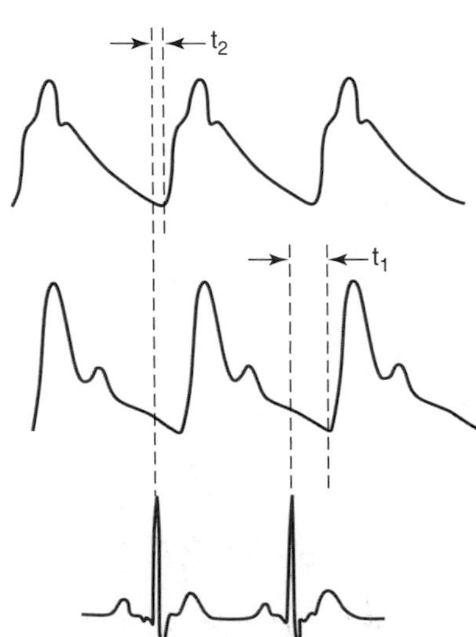

Figure 6-6 Determination of pulse transit time. The foot of the pulse wave is used to locate the wavefront as it is relatively unaffected by wave reflections. The time delay can be measured by simultaneously recording pulse waves at two sites of the arterial segment (*left*). Alternatively, the time intervals between the R-wave of the electrocardiogram and the foot of the pulse wave at two sites may be recorded consecutively, and the transit time calculated as the difference between the two (*right*).

unaffected by wave reflections. The most consistent method for determination of the foot of the pulse wave has been shown to be either the point at which its second derivative is maximal or the point formed by intersection of a line tangential to the initial systolic upstroke of the waveform and a horizontal line through the minimum point.[225]

The distance can be estimated by direct superficial measurement between the centres of the two pressure transducers or other devices in case of relatively straight segments like the brachioradial arterial segment. If arterial segments are not straight, measurement of the distance may be a source of error. Furthermore, in two sites where pulse waves propagate in opposite directions, as in the determination of carotid-femoral pulse wave velocity, the method of measuring distance varies. Some investigators recommend using the total distance between the carotid and femoral sites of measurement, while others subtract the carotid-sternal notch distance from the total distance, or subtract the carotid-sternal notch distance from the femoral-sternal notch distance.[175,226,227] Despite the limitations of the need to estimate distance by superficial measurement, pulse wave velocity is probably the most widely used technique for assessment of arterial stiffness.

Systemic Arterial Stiffness

Pulse contour analysis has been used to assess systemic or whole-body arterial stiffness non-invasively.[228–230] One of the methods, based on the electrical analogue of a modified *Windkessel* model with proximal and distal capacitance, inertance, and resistance parameters, concentrates on analysis of the diastolic pressure decay of the radial pulse contour. An algorithm is used to determine the best set of values for matching the diastolic portion of the pulse contour to a multi-exponential waveform equation. Based on these values, the capacitative compliance of the proximal major arteries and the oscillatory compliance of the distal small arteries are estimated. However, the biologic relevance of the lumped proximal and distal compliance derived from a model construct based on assumptions remains to be defined. Nonetheless, these parameters have been shown to change with aging and in diseases associated with increased cardiovascular events,[228,229] although evidence for their predictive value for the occurrence of such events is lacking.

The area method, based on a two-element *Windkessel* model, has also been used to determine systemic arterial compliance using the formula compliance = Ad/[TVR × (Pes – Pd)], where Ad is area under the diastolic portion of the arterial pressure wave from end-systole to end-diastole, TVR is total vascular resistance, Pes is end-systolic pressure, and Pd is end-diastolic pressure.[231,232] The pressure and pressure waveform can be obtained by applanation tonometry over the right common carotid artery, while total vascular resistance is calculated as mean blood pressure divided by mean aortic blood flow, the latter obtained by a velocimeter positioned at the suprasternal notch. The area method nonetheless shares similar limitations.

Wave Reflection Indices

Arterial stiffening increases pulse wave velocity and shortens the time for the pulse wave to return from the periphery. Early arrival of the reflected waves augments systolic blood pressure in stiff arteries. The effects of wave reflection can be quantified by determination of this pressure wave augmentation.[166,233] The augmentation index is defined as the ratio of difference between systolic peak and inflection point to pulse pressure (Fig. 6-7). The inflection point corresponds to the time when peak blood flow occurs in the artery. In adolescents and young adults with elastic arteries, the augmentation index is negative, as late return of reflected waves during diastole causes the peak systolic pressure to precede an inflection point. By contrast, in middle-aged and older individuals, the peak systolic pressure occurs in late systole after an inflection point and the augmentation index becomes increasingly positive with age. The aortic augmentation index is hence negative in adolescents and reaches to about 50% of pulse pressure at 80 years.[152] As height is related to reflection sites, the augmentation index is inversely related to height[234] and is paradoxically greater in infants and young children than in adolescents due to early return of reflected wave with a short body length. Rather than a direct measurement of arterial stiffness, augmentation index is a manifestation of arterial stiffness. It is also important to recognise that apart from arterial stiffness, the amplitude of reflected wave, reflectance point, heart rate, and ventricular contractility are all important determinants of augmentation index.

To determine the aortic augmentation index non-invasively, the central aortic waveform can be estimated from the common carotid artery waveform using applanation tonometry, although this is technically demanding. Alternatively, the aortic waveform can be reconstructed using a transfer function from the radial waveform, which is easier to obtain.[212–214] The radial-to-aortic transfer function has nonetheless not been validated in children, and furthermore, its accuracy for derivation of aortic augmentation index has been disputed.[235–237] The recent introduction of a carotid sensor with multiple micro-piezo-resistive transducers may facilitate the derivation of augmentation index.[217]

Contour analysis of the digital volume pulse has also been used to derive indices attributable to wave reflection.[238–240] Takazawa et al used the second derivative of the digital photoplethysmogram waveform to identify five distinct waves (Fig. 6-8) and determined their mathematical relationships. In particular, the d/a and b/a ratios have been related to age and arterial stiffness.[238,241–243] The d/a ratio is also related to aortic augmentation index.[238] However,

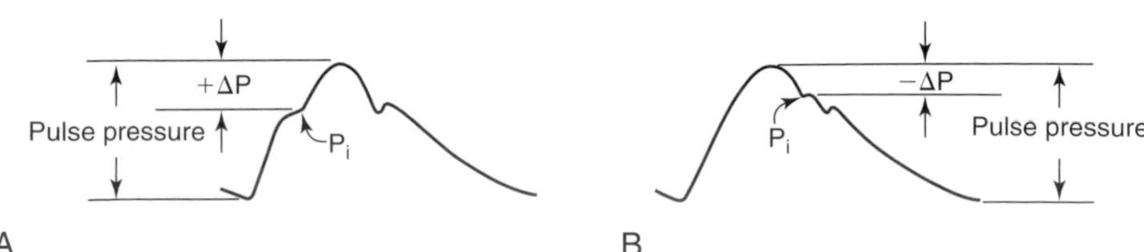

Figure 6-7 The augmentation index is calculated from pressure waveforms as the ratio of difference between systolic peak pressure and inflection point (P_i) to pulse pressure (ΔP/pulse pressure). ΔP is (**A**) positive when peak systolic pressure occurs after the inflection point and becomes (**B**) negative when peak systolic pressure precedes the inflection point.

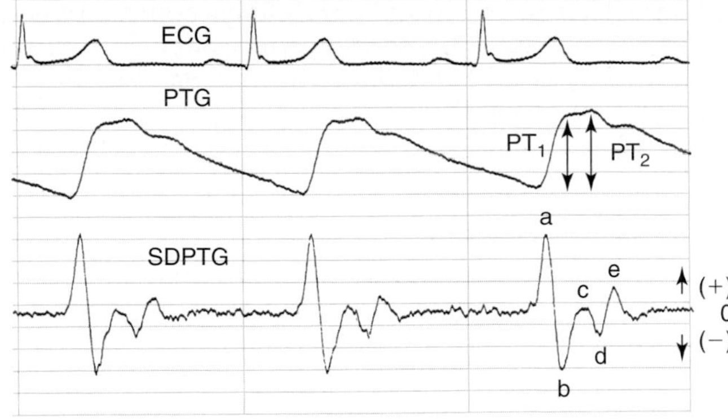

Figure 6-8 Five components of the second derivative of photoplethysmogram waveform (SDPTG). This includes four systolic waves (a–d) and one diastolic wave (e). An augmentation index based on photoplethysmogram (PTG) can also be defined as PT_2/PT_1, where PT_2 is amplitude of the late systolic component and PT_1 is amplitude of the early systolic component. (Reproduced with permission from Takazawa K, Tanaka N, Fujita M, et al: Assessment of vasoactive agents and vascular aging by the second derivative of photoplethysmogram waveform. Hypertension 1998;32:365–370.)

the physical and physiological meanings of these measurements remain unclear.

Using similarly photoplethysmographic digital volume pulse waveform, Chowienczyk et al proposed that the first peak in the waveform corresponds to a forward-traveling pressure wave from the heart to the finger, and the second peak or point of inflection to the backward-traveling reflected pressure[239,240] (Fig. 6-9). A reflection index, defined at the ratio of the magnitude of the reflected wave to the first peak, has been proposed as measure of the amount of reflection, while the peak-to-peak time has been proposed as a surrogate measure of pulse wave velocity and arterial stiffness.[239,240] An index of large arterial stiffness, defined as height divided by peak-to-peak time, has been shown to be related to pulse wave velocity.[244] The simplicity of the digital photoplethysmographic waveform analysis may facilitate large-scale epidemiological studies. These indices, nonetheless, provide at best an indirect assessment of arterial stiffness, and factors affecting their reliability and interpretation in different patient cohorts remain to be clarified.

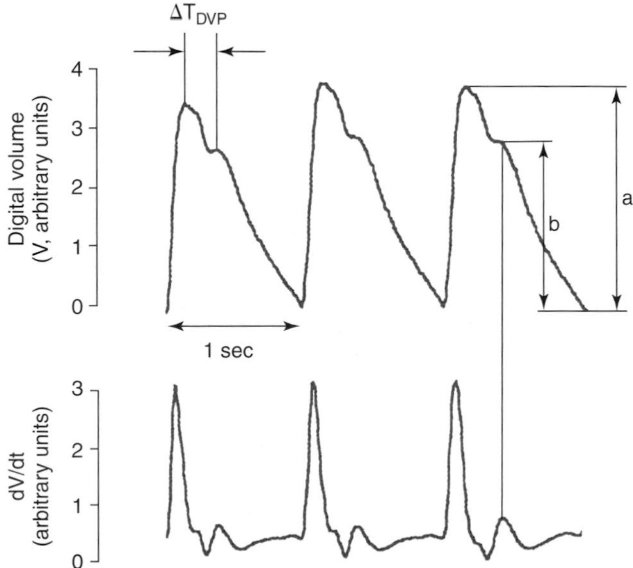

Figure 6-9 Digital volume pulse and its first derivative. The inflection point is identified by the local maximum in the first derivative. The reflection index, b/a, has been proposed as a measure of amount of reflection. The ratio of ΔT_{DVP}, the time between the first and second peaks, to body height has been used as an index of arterial stiffness. (Reproduced with permission from Chowienczyk PJ, Kelly RP, MacCallum H, et al: Photoplethysmographic assessment of pulse wave reflection. J Am Coll Cardiol 1999;34:2007–2014.)

Blood Pressure Indices

Central pulse pressure, being influenced by wave reflection amongst other factors, is often considered a surrogate of arterial stiffness.[245] It should not, however, be used interchangeably as an index of arterial stiffness as their physiological meanings differ. Similar to augmentation index, central pulse pressure is dependent on heart rate, ventricular contractility, and factors affecting the reflected wave, notably arterial stiffness and reflectance points.[175] Peripheral pulse pressure, measured usually at the brachial artery, overestimates central pulse pressure due to the amplification phenomenon, which is more prominent in more elastic arteries such as those in young subjects.[246]

Recently, an ambulatory arterial stiffness index has been proposed as a novel index of arterial stiffness.[247,248] Using ambulatory blood pressure monitoring data throughout the day, the index is calculated as 1 minus the regression slope of diastolic blood pressure on systolic blood pressure. This index is based on the concept that average distending pressure varies during the day and that the relation between diastolic and systolic blood pressure, with this changing distending pressure, largely depends on the structural and functional characteristics of the large arteries.[248] While this index has been shown to be related to pulse pressure and augmentation index and a predictor of cardiovascular mortality in adults,[247,248] its physiological meanings and its use as a marker of stiffness remain highly disputed.[175,249–251]

Endothelial Dysfunction

Endothelial dysfunction is characterised by upset of the regulation of balance between vasodilation and vasoconstriction, inhibition and promotion of vascular smooth muscle proliferation, and prevention and stimulation of platelet aggregation, thrombogenesis, and fibrolysis by the endothelium.[252] While the normal quiescent state is represented by nitric oxide–dominated endothelial phenotype and maintained primarily by laminar shear stress,[253] endothelial activation is characterised by dominance of reactive oxygen signaling.[254] The common denominator of chronic production of reactive oxygen species potentially exhausts the protective capacity of endogenous anti-inflammatory and anti-oxidative mechanisms and results in sustained endothelial dysfunction. Dysfunction of the endothelium results in loss of its protective function, increased expression of adhesion molecules, and promotion of inflammation within the vessel wall.

Given the important protective role of the endothelium against vascular injury, inflammation, and thrombosis, all of which are key events involved in the initiation and progression of atherosclerosis, it is not surprising that endothelial dysfunction has also prognostic implications. In adults with or without coronary atherosclerosis and in those with hypertension, coronary endothelial dysfunction,[255–258] impaired flow-mediated dilation of the brachial artery,[259–261] and impaired agonist-mediated increase in forearm blood flow[262,263] have been shown to predict cardiovascular events. With the introduction of a variety of non-invasive techniques as elaborated below for assessment of endothelial function, the phenomenon of endothelial dysfunction has also been documented in an increasing number of paediatric and adolescent conditions.

Assessment of Endothelial Function in Vivo

Coronary Circulation

Assessment of endothelial function in the coronary circulation was first described in 1986 by Ludmer and colleagues[264] who demonstrated that local infusion of acetylcholine dilates angiographically normal epicardial coronary arteries secondary to release of nitric oxide from an intact endothelium. By contrast, acetylcholine was found to cause paradoxical constriction of atherosclerotic coronary arteries as a result of direct muscarinic action on vascular smooth muscle. Endothelial function of the coronary resistance vessels can be assessed simultaneously using Doppler flow wires.[265] The measurement of changes in coronary arterial diameter, blood flow, and vascular resistance in response to intracoronary infusion of acetylcholine has become the gold standard against which other tests of endothelial function have been compared. Endothelial-independent changes in coronary diameter and flow reserve can be assessed by intracoronary boluses of adenosine or infusion of nitroglycerine. The response to endothelium-independent agonist is assessed to exclude insensitivity of vascular smooth muscle to nitric oxide. In children, coronary endothelial function has been mainly assessed in those with a history of Kawasaki disease. The invasive nature of this technique limits its use to patients in whom cardiac catheterisation is clinically indicated and precludes serial follow-up assessments.

Forearm Resistance Vessels

Endothelial function of forearm resistance vessels is assessed by measurement of forearm blood flow in response to intra-arterial infusion of endothelium-dependent and-independent agonists. Venous occlusion plethysmography has been widely used to measure forearm blood flow.[266] The principle of measurement is based on the premise that interruption of venous outflow from the forearm, but not arterial inflow, results in a linear increase in forearm volume with time. In this technique, blood pressure cuffs are placed around the upper arm and the wrist. The forearm is positioned above the heart level to ensure satisfactory venous emptying when cuffs in the upper arm are deflated. The contralateral arm is studied simultaneously to correct for possible changes in basal blood flow with time and to act as control. The upper arm cuff is inflated to around 40 mmHg to occlude venous outflow while allowing arterial inflow into the forearm. The hands are excluded from the circulation by inflating the wrist cuff to suprasystolic blood pressure, as they contain a high proportion of arterio-venous shunts and their blood flow is highly temperature sensitive. The change in forearm volume with continuous arterial inflow is measured using strain-gauge plethysmography. The mercury-in-rubber strain gauges, which act as resistors connected as one arm of a Wheatstone bridge,[267] are placed around the right and left forearms. With the increase in forearm volume and circumference, the strain gauges lengthen and increase in resistance, leading to a potential difference in the Wheatstone bridge circuit. The period of measurement, during which the hands are rendered ischaemic, has been up to 13 minutes in adults.[268]

A variety of agonists, which include acetylcholine, methacholine, bradykinin, 5-hydroxytryptamine, and substance P, have been used to assess the endothelial-dependent vasodilation response.[269,270] Of importance to note is that nitric oxide dependence varies among agonists, and indeed, vasodilation caused by methacholine does not appear to be nitric oxide mediated.[271,272] Apart from stimulation of nitric oxide release, these agonists also induce release of endothelium-derived hyperpolarizing factor and prostaglandins. The response to endothelium-independent agonist, like sodium nitroprusside, is assessed to exclude abnormal vascular smooth muscle function. The forearm blood flow response to endothelial-dependent agonist has been found to correlate with coronary endothelial function[272,273] and to predict independently cardiovascular events in patients with coronary artery disease.[262] The basal release of nitric oxide in the basal forearm can also be assessed using this technique by infusing NG-monomethyl-L-arginine, an L-arginine analogue that inhibits nitric oxide synthase.[274] Co-infusion of NG-monomethyl-L-arginine with specific endothelium-dependent agonist can further be used to determine upregulation of alternative vasodilator pathways in condition of endothelial dysfunction.[269] This technique is hence invaluable in elucidating mechanisms that underlie endothelial dysfunction. However, as a technique to assess endothelial function, the need for arterial cannulation limits its repeatability and its application in the paediatric population.

Conduit Artery

Non-invasive assessment of flow-mediated dilation of the brachial artery using high-resolution ultrasound was first introduced by Celermajer et al[275] in 1992, based on the principle of endothelium-dependent release of nitric oxide in response to shear stress. As alluded to earlier, flow-mediated dilation has been shown to occur predominantly as a result of local endothelial release of nitric oxide.[85]

In this technique, the brachial arterial diameter and Doppler-derived flow velocity is determined at baseline, when the patient has rested in a supine position for at least 10 minutes, and after an increase in shear stress induced by reactive hyperaemia. To induce reactive hyperaemia, a sphygmomanometer cuff, placed either above the antecubital fossa or over the forearm, is inflated to supra-systolic blood pressure and deflated after 4 to 5 minutes. Cuff occlusion of the upper arm has additional direct ischaemic effect on the brachial artery. There is no consensus, however, as to whether cuff occlusion of the upper arm or forearm provides more accurate information.[276,277] Reactive hyperemia after cuff deflation increases shear stress and leads to dilation of the brachial artery. The maximum increase in flow is assessed within the first 10 to 15 seconds after cuff release, while the brachial arterial diameter is measured at usually 60 seconds after cuff deflation, at a time when maximal dilator response occurs in normal subjects.[278] Commercially available automatic edge-detection software allows continuous monitoring of the brachial arterial diameter after cuff deflation and detection of the true peak response (Fig. 6-10). Flow-mediated dilation in the radial, femoral, and posterior tibial arteries can similarly be determined

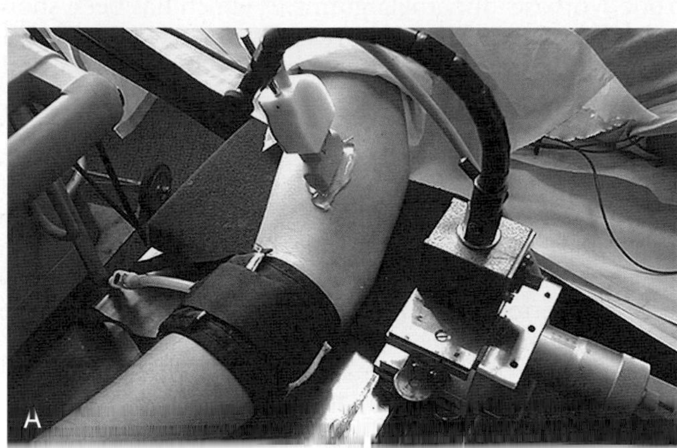

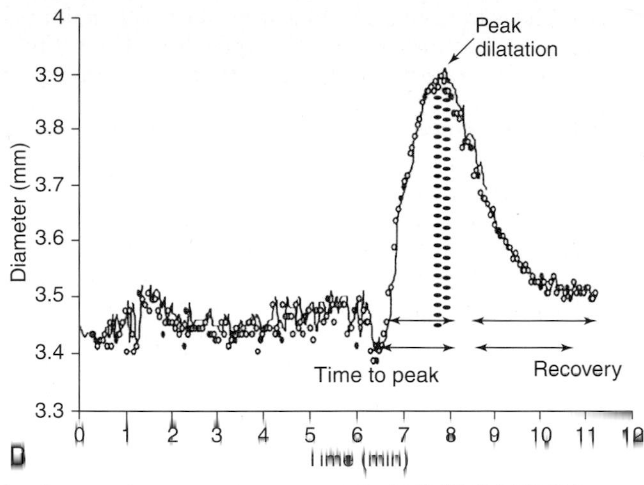

Figure 6-10 Assessment of brachial arterial flow-mediated dilation. **A**, Ultrasound probe secured in position by a stereotactic clamp for continuous imaging of brachial artery. **B**, Continuous measurement of brachial arterial diameter before and during cuff inflation and after cuff release using automatic edge-detection software. (Reproduced with permission from Deanfield JE, Halcox JP, Rabelink TJ: Endothelial function and dysfunction: Testing and clinical relevance. Circulation 2007;115:1285–1295.)

by inflating the cuff at the wrist, just beneath the popliteal fossa, and the ankle, respectively. After at least 10 minutes following cuff release, sublingual nitroglycerine is given to assess endothelium-independent vasodilation. This direct vasodilation response peaks at 3 to 5 minutes after administration of nitroglycerine.

Accurate assessment of flow-mediated dilation is nonetheless challenging. Furthermore, centres differ in the protocols used for elicitation of reactive hyperaemia. The methodological issues, strengths, and limitations of this technique have been explored in depth by the International Brachial Artery Reactivity Task Force[279] and the Working Group on Endothelin and Endothelial Factors of the European Society of Hypertension.[270] Notwithstanding the skills required and limitations of this technique, its non-invasive nature and its correlation with coronary endothelial function[280] have led to its widespread use in clinical trials and in the field of vascular epidemiology.[281–283] The technique is also widely used for the assessment of endothelial function in children and adolescents, although its application in children younger than 6 years is likely to be difficult given the cooperation needed for accurate measurement of brachial arterial diameter and flow.

Microvasculature

Laser Doppler techniques have been used for the assessment of microvascular endothelial function of the skin.[284] The principle of laser Doppler techniques is based on changes in wavelength of the reflected light after hitting moving blood cells. Rather than measuring absolute skin perfusion, these techniques determine red blood cell flux as defined by the product of velocity and concentration of the moving blood cells within the measured volume. Laser Doppler flowmetry is a single-probe technique used to assess the blood flux in a small volume of 1 mm^3 or smaller,[285] while laser Doppler imaging provides an integrated index over a larger volume by using a mirror to reflect the laser beam to scan a larger skin area.[286]

To assess microvascular endothelial function, laser Doppler flowmetry and imaging have been used to detect the increase in skin blood flow during reactive hyperaemia after brief arterial occlusion,[287,288] during local thermal hyperaemia,[289,290] and after local application of endothelial-dependent vasodilators by iontophoresis.[291,292] Nonetheless, the microvascular response to reactive hyperaemia and local heating is complex and depends on mechanisms other than those mediated by the endothelium.[293–296] Iontophoresis of acetylcholine and sodium nitroprusside has commonly been used to generate endothelium-dependent and endothelium-independent dilation respectively of the skin microvasculature. The applied current can, however, induce vasodilation directly, which is more pronounced with cathodal delivery of acetylcholine and related probably to induction of an axon reflex.[297] This effect can be reduced by the use of lower anodal current and larger iontophoresis electrodes. The usefulness of acetylcholine iontophoresis as an assessment of skin microvascular endothelial function has recently been challenged, as acetylcholine-induced vasodilation has been shown to remain unchanged or be only partially attenuated after inhibition of nitric oxide synthase.[298] While the test is non-invasive and may reflect to a certain extent the microvascular endothelial function, the poor reproducibility remains an issue of concern. Despite the limitations, acetylcholine iontophoresis coupled with laser Doppler imaging have been used to assess microvascular endothelial function in neonates.[299] The latest development of laser flowmetry is quantification of periodic oscillations of skin blood flow by spectral analysis of laser Doppler signals.[300,301] The oscillations at around 0.01 Hz have been suggested to be endothelium-dependent, although further studies are required to clarify its usefulness as a test for skin microvascular endothelial function.

Emerging Techniques

The aforementioned techniques primarily assess the endothelial-dependent nitric oxide–mediated vasodilation response to agonists. Recent techniques attempted to determine the change in arterial stiffness upon endothelial stimulation. Salbutamol, a β-2 agonist, has been demonstrated to reduce arterial stiffness in a nitric oxide–dependent manner.[302] Thus, the changes in augmentation index[303,304] and the inflection point in the photoplethysmographic digital volume pulse[239] in response to salbutamol inhalation have been used as measures of endothelial function. However, both of these techniques have been found to be much less reproducible in children when compared with brachial arterial flow-mediated dilation.[305] The upper and lower limb pulse wave velocity responses to reactive hyperaemia in the hand and foot have also been used to assess endothelial function.[306]

The change in digital pulse volume amplitude during reactive hyperaemia, so-called reactive hyperaemia peripheral arterial tonometry, has also been used to assess peripheral microvascular endothelial function[307,308] (Fig. 6-11). The pattern of the reactive hyperaemia peripheral arterial tonometry has been shown to mirror that of brachial arterial flow-mediated dilation[307] and be attenuated in adults with coronary microvascular endothelial dysfunction.[308] Recently, the central role for nitric oxide in the augmentation of pulse volume amplitude during reactive hyperaemia in humans has been demonstrated.[309]

Circulating Biomarkers

While endothelial function is commonly assessed by determining the effects of endothelium-derived nitric oxide on vessel diameter, blood flow, and arterial stiffness, assay of various circulating biomarkers of endothelial and non-endothelial origins may provide additional information on other aspects of endothelial function and magnitude of endothelial activation. These biomarkers include measures of nitric oxide availability, adhesion molecules, inflammatory cytokines, markers of inflammation and oxidative stress, pro- and anti-coagulants, and indices of endothelial cell damage and repair.

The circulating pool of nitric oxide as a measure of its bioavailability can be assessed by measuring plasma nitroso compounds and nitrite.[310–313] While the exact chemical species of this pool are unclear and their values may be confounded by diet,[314] recent studies showed that plasma nitrite reflects regional endothelial nitric oxide synthase activity.[313] Plasma nitrite reserve during reactive hyperaemia[311] and plasma nitroso compounds[310] have been found to be reduced in the presence of endothelial dysfunction. Reduced nitric oxide availability can also be inferred from elevated levels of the naturally occurring antagonist of nitric oxide synthase, dimethylarginine,[315] which has been shown to be associated with cardiovascular disease and mortality in adults.[316] Activation of endothelial cells upregulates the expression of adhesion molecules. The levels of circulation adhesion molecules, including intercellular adhesion molecule 1, vascular cell adhesion molecule 1, E-selectin, and P-selectin can be determined using commercially available assays. Interaction of the dysfunctional endothelium with circulating leucocytes, in which the adhesion molecules play a crucial role,[317,318] initiates inflammation within the vessel wall. Furthermore, oxidative stress, an important determinant of inflammation, is increasingly recognised to play an important role in compromising endothelial function.[319,320] Thus, the levels of inflammatory markers, including high-sensitivity C-reactive protein, interleukin-6, and tumor necrosis factor–α, and markers of oxidative stress, such as oxidised low-density lipoprotein and 8-iso-prostaglandin $F_2\alpha$, can be used to reflect ongoing endothelial activation and vascular inflammation.

Disturbance of the protective role of the endothelium against thrombosis in endothelial dysfunction is reflected by the imbalance between endothelium-derived tissue plasminogen activator and plasminogen activation inhibitor–1[321] and the release into circulation of von Willebrand factor.[322] Measurement of the dynamic release of tissue-plasminogen activator by agonists such as bradykinin, substance P, methacholine, and desmopressin has been used to assess endothelial function,[323–326] although data on its relationship with cardiovascular risk factors and prognostic values is limited.

There is increasing interest in the role of endothelial microparticles and endothelial progenitor cells as markers and risk factors of endothelial dysfunction and cardiovascular disease. Damage to endothelial cells can result in their detachment into the circulation in entirety or as microparticles. Endothelial microparticles have been found to be increased in vasculitis and atherosclerotic diseases.[327–330] The quantity of circulating endothelial cells and microparticles is therefore a potentially useful marker of endothelial function. Interestingly, recent evidence suggests that

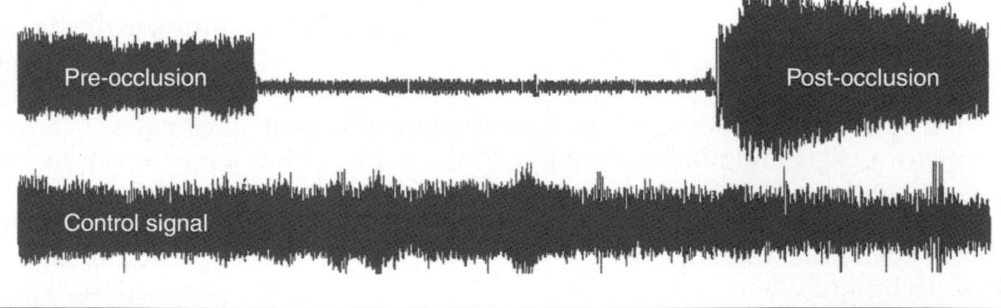

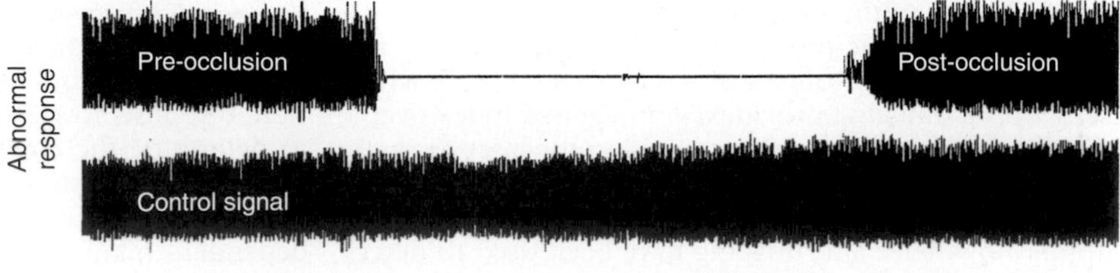

Figure 6-11 Reactive hyperaemia peripheral arterial tonometry recordings of individuals with normal and abnormal responses. (Reproduced with permission from Bonetti PO, Pumper GM, Higano ST, et al: Noninvasive identification of patients with early coronary atherosclerosis by assessment of digital reactive hyperemia. J Am Coll Cardiol 2004;44:2137–2141.)

endothelial microparticles may contribute directly to endothelial dysfunction.[328,331] With regard to the repair of damaged endothelium, apart from proliferation of local mature endothelial cells, the importance of bone-marrow derived endothelial stems cells and endothelial progenitor cells is increasingly recognised.[332–334] Mobilisation of endothelial progenitor cells is in part nitric oxide–dependent.[335] Furthermore, the number of progenitor cells has been shown to correlate negatively with the cardiovascular risk score and positively with brachial arterial flow-mediated dilation in adults.[336] The level of endothelial progenitor cells may hence be a novel marker of endothelial function, vascular dysfunction, and cardiovascular risk in adults. The usefulness of endothelial microparticles and endothelial progenitor cells as markers of endothelial function in the paediatric population awaits further clarification.

SYSTEMIC ARTERIAL DYSFUNCTION IN CHILDHOOD

Age-related Evolution

Progressive increase in aortic, upper limb, and lower limb pulse wave velocities, as measured by transcutaneous Doppler technique, with age in a cohort of subjects aged 3 to 89 years has been reported.[337] Age-dependent increase in brachio-radial arterial pulse wave velocity has similarly been demonstrated in a cohort of children and adolescents aged 6 to 18 years using the photoplethysmographic technique.[338] Using the area under the ascending aortic pressure-time curve to determine the total stiffness of the arterial tree and assuming a two-element *Windkessel* model, a non-linear increase in total arterial stiffness in children aged 6 months to 20 years has been demonstrated.[339] Although a nadir of arterial stiffness at around 10 years of age has been reported,[340] this has not been replicated in subsequent studies.

Notwithstanding the influence of the distending pressure on arterial stiffness, previous findings did not suggest that the change in pulse wave velocity with age is entirely due to differences in systemic blood pressure.[337,338] Rather, the gradual increase in arterial stiffness with age is probably related to progressive medial degeneration. With cyclical mechanical stress, fragmentation of the elastin fibres and transfer of stress to the much stiffer collagen fibres inevitably result in progressive increase in vascular stiffness.[341] Furthermore, studies of developmental changes in arterial structure during childhood have demonstrated progressive increase in intimal and medial thickness after birth.[342] Hence, the observed age-related increase in stiffness is likely related to progressive structural changes in the arterial wall during childhood.

In otherwise healthy adult subjects, endothelial function has been shown to deteriorate with aging.[343] Furthermore, progressive endothelial dysfunction appears to occur earlier in men than in women. While puberty has been speculated to be a critical period for the vascular endothelium,[344] this requires further clarification.

Cardiovascular Risk Factors

Childhood obesity has become a global epidemic. In obese children, increased stiffness of the abdominal aorta[345,346] and carotid artery[347] has been demonstrated. Endothelial dysfunction is evidenced by elevated serum biomarkers of endothelial activation[348,349] and impaired brachial arterial flow-mediated dilation.[347,350–352] Studies have further shown that in obese children, endothelial dysfunction improves with exercise training.[353–355] Concomitant cardiovascular risk factors linked with arterial dysfunction often occur in obese children and these include dyslipidaemia, diabetes mellitus, and low-grade inflammation. Indeed, endothelial dysfunction in obese prepubertal children has recently been shown to be related to insulin resistance and markers of inflammation.[356] Obese children who have concomitant metabolic syndrome were found to have stiffer common carotid artery than those without.[357] Furthermore, a strong graded inverse association between number of components of metabolic syndrome and brachial arterial distensibility has been demonstrated.[358] The effects of obesity-related peptides on vasculature are increasingly recognised.[359] Elevations in leptin have been shown to be associated with impaired arterial distensibility in healthy children[360] and in children with type 1 diabetes.[361] The effect of leptin on endothelial function in humans is, however, controversial.[362] Plasma adiponectin, on the other hand, has been shown to correlate with vasodilator response of the forearm microcirculation to reactive hyperaemia.[363,364]

In children with heterozygous familial hypercholesterolaemia increased stiffness of the common carotid artery[365,366] and modification of the aortic elastic properties[367] have been demonstrated. Impaired brachial arterial flow-mediated dilation has also been shown in these children and in those with familial combined hyperlipoproteinaemia at as young as 6 years of age.[275,368–370] Endothelial dysfunction is most pronounced in those with a positive family history of premature cardiovascular disease.[371] Early statin and antioxidant vitamins C and E therapy may potentially restore endothelial dysfunction in these children towards normal.[369,370,372] However, the relationship between flow-mediated dilation and low-density lipoprotein cholesterol levels is controversial.[365,368,369] On the other hand, in a population-based study, total and low-density lipoprotein cholesterol levels were found to relate inversely to brachial arterial distensibility,[373] suggesting the possibility that cholesterol levels in the general population during childhood may already be of relevance in the pathogenesis of arterial stiffening.

Children with type 1 diabetes have well-documented endothelial dysfunction,[374–377] which has been shown to improve by folic acid.[378] Arterial stiffening in these children is further suggested by an increase in augmentation index,[379] and has recently been found to be associated with nitric oxide synthase 3 polymorphism.[380] Offspring of parents with type 2 diabetes have a high risk of developing diabetes and atherosclerotic complications. Studies have shown increased aortic[381] and carotid-radial[382] pulse wave velocity in normoglycaemic who are offspring of parents with type 2 diabetes. Impaired brachial arterial flow-mediated dilation has similarly been shown in first-degree adult relatives of type 2 diabetic patients.[383–387] Whether such arterial dysfunction has its onset in childhood is unknown.

Structural alterations of the common carotid artery with intima-media thickening have been found in children and adolescents with a parental history of premature myocardial infarction.[388] In adults who are offspring of parents with premature cardiovascular disease, apart from intima-media thickening, impaired endothelial-dependent vasodilation of brachial artery has also been found.[389,390]

Habitual physical activity in children aged 5 to 10 years has been shown to correlate positively with flow-mediated dilation, suggesting that its cardiovascular protective effect may be mediated via the endothelium.[391] In another cohort of 10-year-old children, physical activity was found to correlate inversely with arterial stiffness as assessed by measuring the aorto-femoral and aorto-radial pulse wave velocities.[392]

Apart from the traditional cardiovascular risk factors, novel risk factors have also been shown to be associated with arterial dysfunction in children. Associations between increased baseline high-sensitivity C-reactive protein concentrations and the risks of developing cardiovascular disease in adults have been reported.[393–395] Furthermore, in vitro studies showed that C-reactive protein induces adhesion molecule expression in human endothelial cells.[396] In healthy children, serum high-sensitivity C-reactive protein concentrations have been found to have an inverse dose-dependent relationship with the magnitude of brachial arterial flow-mediated dilation.[397] Increased serum high-sensitivity C-reactive protein levels are found in obese adolescents.[351,398] Analysis of the 1999–2000 National Health and Nutrition Examination Survey indeed showed a strong independent association between body mass index and C-reactive protein level even in young children aged 3 to 17 years.[399] However, in children and adolescents who do not have much of an atherosclerotic burden, whether high-sensitivity C-reactive protein is a risk factor or a risk marker requires further clarification.

In children with homozygous homocystinuria, impaired brachial arterial flow-mediated dilation has been demonstrated in those as young as 4 years.[400] In the general paediatric population, findings of elevated homocysteine levels in children with a family history of premature cardiovascular disease are conflicting.[401–403] Although hyperhomocysteinaemia is a risk factor for endothelial dysfunction in middle-aged[404] and elderly[405] subjects, there is as yet no data to suggest a link between arterial dysfunction and serum homocysteine levels in children.

Prenatal Growth Restriction

It has almost been two decades since the report of associations between low birth weight and increased risk of cardiovascular disease.[406] These findings, having been replicated in subsequent studies,[407–409] have formed the basis of the fetal origins hypothesis that implicates the origin of cardiovascular disease from adaptations to an adverse environment in utero. These adaptations have been proposed to cause permanent alterations of cardiovascular structure and physiology through the process of programming.

There is evidence that individuals who are born small are at risk of vascular dysfunction in childhood and adulthood. Arterial endothelial dysfunction has been found in term infants,[299] children,[410] and young adults[411] with low birth weight. A recent study showed elevated uric acid in children with low birth weight and a graded inverse relationship between uric acid and flow-mediated dilation.[412] In children born at term, leanness at birth has been reported to correlate with the lowest endothelium-dependent microvascular responses and the highest carotid stiffness indices.[413] In infants with umbilical placental insufficiency before birth, the increase in afterload has been shown to result in a decrease in aortic distensibility during the neonatal period, suggesting an alteration of aortic wall structure.[414] Furthermore, reduced compliance of the aorta and conduit arteries of the legs has been shown to occur in adults born small.[415]

The risk of arterial dysfunction for individuals who are born small as a result of prematurity is controversial. An increase in systolic blood pressure has been shown in a cohort of young adults born prematurely, regardless of whether or not they had intra-uterine growth retardation.[416] On the other hand, only individuals who had been preterm babies with intra-uterine growth retardation were found to have impaired brachial arterial flow-mediated dilation.[417] Nonetheless, preterm birth has also been demonstrated to attenuate the association between low birth weight and endothelial dysfunction.[418] With regard to arterial stiffness, reduced aortic wall distensibility and whole-body compliance have been shown in very low birth weight premature infants as early as the neonatal period.[419] Other studies have demonstrated inverse relationships between systemic arterial stiffness and gestational age[420] and birth weight standardised for gestational age.[421]

In monozygotic twins with twin-twin transfusion syndrome, the growth-restricted donor twin provides a unique model for studying the effects of differing volume load and increased placental resistance on the developing cardiovascular systems in two genetically identical individuals. A previous study has shown that the peripheral conduit arterial stiffness is increased during infancy in the donor twins.[422] Such vascular programming has been shown to be ameliorated, albeit not completely abolished, by intra-uterine endoscopic laser ablation of placental anastomoses.[423] Even in monozygotic twins without twin-twin transfusion syndrome, the twin with the lower birth weight has been found to have higher systolic blood pressure and pulse pressure and impaired endothelial function in childhood.[424]

The mechanism whereby low birth weight is associated with increased arterial stiffness in childhood and adulthood remains unclear. The reported endothelial dysfunction in individuals born preterm and small-for-gestational age[299,410,411,415,417] suggests that functional alteration of arterial tone may contribute to an increase in systemic arterial stiffness. Altered haemodynamics in intra-uterine growth retardation, which result in preferential perfusion of upper part of body,[425] may affect the mechanical properties of the large arteries. Hence, selective carotid arterial atherosclerosis has been found to be more severe in elderly people with the lowest birth weight.[426] Another proposed mechanism is the impairment of synthesis of elastin in the arterial wall.[341] In the donor twin in twin-twin transfusion syndrome, the superimposed circulatory imbalance probably acts synergistically with growth restriction to cause the vascular programming, although the exact mechanism remains to be defined.[422] The exact mechanism of endothelial dysfunction in individuals with low birth weight is even more elusive.

Nutritional Issues

The associations between early growth restriction and arterial dysfunction highlight the potential importance of nutrition in antenatal and early postnatal life on long-term vascular programming. Leeson et al studied in a young adult population-based cohort the relation between duration of breast-feeding and brachial arterial distensibility.[427] They found an inverse relation between duration of breast-feeding and arterial distensibility even after adjusting for current lipid profile, body mass index, and social class. A recent study in 10-year-old children also demonstrated a positive association between breast-feeding and stiffness of the aorto-femoral arterial segment as determined by pulse wave velocity.[392] Despite these findings that evoked much comment, it is important to realise that there is to date little consistent evidence that breast-feeding influences subsequent mortality related to cardiovascular disease[428] and that the current advice on breast-feeding practise has not been altered by these findings.

In children receiving long-term parenteral nutrition, significant increase in elastic modulus of the common carotid artery and impairment of brachial arterial flow-mediated dilation have been demonstrated.[429] While the mechanisms are unclear, infusion of lipid emulsions or high-concentration dextrose has caused endothelial damage and vascular remodeling in animal models.[430,431] It remains unknown whether vascular dysfunction is reversible after reestablishment of enteral feeding.

Childhood Vasculitides

Kawasaki disease, a childhood vasculitis of unknown etiology, is the commonest cause of acquired heart disease in children in developed countries (see Chapter 52). The sequelas of inflammation involving coronary and other medium-sized muscular arteries in the acute phase of the disease are well documented.[432–434] Long-term structural alteration and functional disturbance of coronary arteries also have long been known.[432–436] Systemic arterial dysfunction is increasingly recognised in children with a history of Kawasaki long term after the acute illness. Indeed, concerns have been raised regarding the possibility of its predisposition to premature atherosclerosis in adulthood.[437–441]

Impaired brachial arterial flow-mediated dilation has been demonstrated in patients, even in those without early coronary arterial involvement, studied at a median of 11 years after the acute illness.[442] Intravenous administration of vitamin C has been shown to improve the impaired flow-mediated dilation.[443] Increased stiffness of the carotid artery[444,445] and brachioradial artery,[441] relating in a dose-dependent manner to the degree of coronary arterial involvement, has also been documented in the long-term follow-up of these patients. By measuring aortic input impedance during cardiac catheterisation, Senzaki et al[446] found that both characteristic impedance and total peripheral arterial compliance were reduced in Kawasaki patients regardless of persistence of coronary artery aneurysms, suggesting an increase in both central and peripheral arterial stiffness. Chronic low-grade inflammation, as reflected by elevated high-sensitivity C-reactive protein,[447,448] in patients with coronary aneurysm formation has been associated positively with carotid arterial stiffness.[447] Indeed, histological evidence of extensive fibro-intimal thickening and infiltration of lymphocytes and plasma cells in the coronary arterial walls has been documented in fatal cases of Kawasaki disease occurring years after apparent resolution of vascular inflammation and in the absence of early detectable coronary arterial abnormalities.[449] In vitro evidence further suggests that chronic activation of the monocyte chemoattractant protein-1/chemokine receptor CCR2 pathway and inducible nitric oxide synthase may play a role in chronic low-grade inflammation in Kawasaki patients.[450] Besides, modulating effects of mannose-binding lectin genotype on arterial stiffness are suggested by findings of patients with intermediate- or low-level expression genotypes having faster brachioradial arterial pulse wave velocity than those with high-level expression genotypes.[451]

Limited data exists for systemic arterial dysfunction in other types of childhood vasculitis. Transient impaired forearm vascular endothelium-dependent relaxation has been found in children during the acute phase of Henoch-Schoenlein purpura.[452] In children with polyarteritis nodosa, a chronic vasculitis characterised by recurrent episodes of inflammatory exacerbations, stiffening of the brachioradial artery with amplification during episodes of inflammatory exacerbation has been demonstrated.[338] Endothelial microparticles has also been found to be significantly increased in children with systemic vasculitis and to correlate with disease activity score.[453]

Vasculopathies in Syndromal Disorders

Marfan syndrome is caused by mutations of the *fibrillin-1* gene.[454] Fibrillin-1, as mentioned earlier, is a matrix glycoprotein and is the principal constituent of microfibrils. Increased aortic stiffness is well documented in patients with Marfan syndrome, as shown by the decreased distensibility and increased stiffness index,[455–463] increased pulse wave velocity,[464] and decreased tissue Doppler-derived systolic and diastolic velocities of the aortic wall.[465] Apart from structural alterations, impaired flow-mediated dilation, possibly related to a defective role of subendothelial fibrillin in endothelial cell mechanotransduction,[466] may also contribute to arterial stiffening. In an animal model of Marfan syndrome, down-regulation of signaling of nitric oxide production in the thoracic aorta has recently been shown to account for endothelial dysfunction.[467] While correlation between *fibrillin-1* genotype and aortic stiffness is poor,[468] aortic stiffness has been shown to be an independent predictor of progressive aortic dilation[469,470] and aortic dissection.[470] Beta-blocker therapy[464] and angiotensin-converting enzyme inhibition[471] appear to reduce aortic stiffness, which may in turn slow aortic dilation and delay aortic root replacement.[471]

Williams syndrome is a contiguous gene disorder with chromosomal microdeletion at 7q11.23, which encompasses the elastin gene and the genes nearby.[472,473] Haploinsufficiency of the elastin gene has been implicated in the arteriopathy of Williams syndrome.[474] Despite a biological basis for abnormal elastic fibres, results of studies exploring arterial elastic properties in patients with Williams syndrome are controversial. Studies have shown increased stiffness of the ascending aorta and aortic arch and implied that abnormal mechanical property of the arteries may contribute to systemic hypertension, which is common in patients with Williams syndrome.[475,476] By contrast, paradoxical reduction of stiffness of the common carotid artery has also been reported.[477,478] The authors speculated that abnormal elastic fibre assembly in the media may shift the load-bearing structures in the arterial wall to those with a lower elastic modulus.

Systemic arterial abnormalities are common in Turner's syndrome, which include bicuspid aortic valve, coarctation of the aorta, and aneurysmal dilation of the aortic root. Although histological evidence of cystic medial necrosis has been reported in Turner's syndrome,[479,480] these findings are not consistently present. Functionally, carotid augmentation index has been found to be increased, explainable in part by the short stature, while carotid-femoral pulse wave velocity and brachial arterial flow-mediated dilation remain normal in these patients.[481,482] It is worthwhile to note, however, that isolated bicuspid aortic valve is associated with progressive dilation of the ascending aorta in both children and adults[483] and increased aortic stiffness.[484,485]

Congenital Heart Disease

Aortic medial abnormalities with elastic fibre fragmentation have been identified in intra-operative biopsies and necropsy specimens in a variety of congenital heart disease in patients ranging from neonates to adults.[486] These congenital heart lesions include tetralogy of Fallot with or without pulmonary atresia, truncus arteriosus, complete transposition of the great arteries, coarctation of the aorta, double outlet ventricles, and univentricular hearts. Whether these abnormalities are inherent or acquired is, however, unknown.

Intrinsic histological abnormalities as characterised by medionecrosis, fibrosis, and elastic fragmentation of the aortic root and ascending aorta have been implicated in causing subsequent aortic root dilation in patients after surgical repair of tetralogy of Fallot.[487–489] The potential alterations of aortic mechanical properties have also been studied. In children and adolescents with tetralogy of Fallot, aortic stiffness has been shown to be increased and related to the aortic root dimensions.[490] A subsequent study demonstrated preferential stiffening of the central over peripheral conduit arteries as evidenced by increased heart-femoral pulse wave velocity without concomitant increase in femoral-ankle pulse wave velocity.[491] Importantly, the heart-femoral pulse wave velocity and carotid augmentation index were found to be significant determinants of the size of sinotubular junction, suggesting that central arterial stiffening may contribute to progressive aortic root dilation in these patients.

In transposition of the great arteries, abnormal aorticopulmonary septation has been hypothesised to be associated with events in elastogenesis.[492,493] As described earlier, medial abnormalities have been found in this congenital heart anomaly.[486] In patients undergoing two-stage anatomical correction, decreased distensibility of the neoaorta has been thought to be related to pulmonary arterial banding.[494] Nonetheless, even after one-stage arterial switch operation, impaired distensibility of the neoaorta has similarly been found.[495] Recent studies further documented increased stiffness index of the carotid artery in patients after both atrial and arterial switch operations,[493,496] suggesting that impaired elastogenesis may be an intrinsic component of this congenital anomaly.

Structural abnormalities of the aortic segment proximal to the site of aortic coarctation are characterised by increase in collagen and decrease in smooth muscle content.[497] Functionally, impaired flow-mediated dilation, reduced nitroglycerine-induced vasodilation, and increased pulse wave velocity were found to be confined to conduit arteries proximal to the site of coarctation despite successful surgical repair.[498–500] The distensibility of the aortic arch has likewise been shown to be significantly lower than that of the distal thoracic aorta.[501] Furthermore, analysis of the ascending pressure waveform obtained during cardiac catheterisation revealed enhanced aortic pressure wave reflection as evidenced by a short time to inflection point and increased augmentation index.[502] This has been hypothesised to be related to a major reflection point at the site of coarctation repair. The finding of an inverse relationship between the magnitude of brachial artery vasodilation response to nitroglycerine and 24-hour systolic blood pressure implicates a possible role of reduced vascular reactivity in the development of systemic hypertension and left ventricular hypertrophy in patients late after successful repair of coarctation.[500] The importance of early coarctation repair on possible prevention of late vascular dysfunction is highlighted by the inverse relationships found between age at repair and stiffness and vascular reactivity of the precoarctation arterial segments.[499,501,503] Nonetheless, the results of a recent study suggest that impaired elastic properties of the prestenotic aorta may be a primary abnormality, as evidence by increased ascending aortic stiffness index in neonates with coarctation even pre-operatively.[504]

Endothelial dysfunction has also been associated with congenital heart anomalies. In adults with cyanotic congenital heart disease, impaired forearm blood flow response to intra-arterial infusion of acetylcholine has been shown.[505] The cause is probably multi-factorial, being related to reduced nitric oxide production,[506] hypoxaemia,[507] and secondary erythrocytosis.[508] Altered levels of biomarkers of endothelial activation have been shown in a small cohort of children and adolescents with univentricular hearts who have undergone cavopulmonary connection.[509] In patients after the Fontan operation, reduced brachial arterial flow-mediated dilation,[510,511] and, in a subset, impaired nitroglycerine-induced vasodilation[511] have been demonstrated. A negative correlation, albeit weak, was found in post-Fontan patients between flow-mediated dilation and serum levels of nitric oxide pathway inhibitors, asymmetric and symmetric dimethlyarginine.[510] Furthermore, those on angiotensin-converting enzyme inhibitor tended to have better endothelial function. The usefulness of angiotensin-converting enzyme inhibitor in the post-Fontan state nonetheless remains debatable.

Systemic Diseases

Inflammation plays a pivotal role in the pathogenesis of atherosclerosis and cardiovascular disease.[512] The association between low-grade chronic inflammation and endothelial dysfunction has been discussed earlier. Rheumatoid arthritis and systemic lupus erythematosus provide clinical models for determining relationships between chronic systemic inflammation and arterial stiffness and endothelial dysfunction. In adults, rheumatoid arthritis has been associated with increased arterial stiffness[513–518] and endothelial dysfunction.[519–522] In the only available study of children with juvenile rheumatoid arthritis to date, Argyropoulou and colleagues reported increased pulse wave velocity and reduced distensibility of the aorta,[523] as determined by phase contrast magnetic resonance, although these parameters were not found to be related to disease activity parameters. Few studies have evaluated arterial function in children with systemic lupus erythematosus. In women with systemic lupus erythematosus, brachial artery flow-mediated dilation has been found to be impaired[524,525] and carotid arterial stiffness increased.[518,526] In adolescents and young adults with paediatric onset lupus, endothelial function has been found to be normal.[527] However, a recent study demonstrated increased carotid arterial stiffness, which is associated with left ventricular hypertrophy and subclinical left ventricular dysfunction.[528]

Apart from intrinsic chronic inflammatory stimuli, acute exposure to extrinsic inflammatory insult in children who had an acute infection or are convalescing from an infection in the previous 2 weeks has been shown to cause transient impairment of brachial arterial flow-mediated dilation.[529] The endothelial dysfunction was found to recover in most but not all of the children studied at follow-up 1 year later. Possible mechanisms include a direct effect of virus[530] or an indirect effect through inflammatory cytokines on endothelial function. Apart from common acute childhood infections, chronic infection with human immunodeficiency virus in children has been associated with arterial dysfunction. The functional alteration is characterised by impaired brachial arterial flow-mediated dilation[531,532] and increased elastic modulus of the carotid arterial wall.[531] Additionally, endothelial dysfunction was found to be more pronounced in children receiving protease inhibitor therapy.[532] Whether these vascular changes are related to metabolic abnormalities such as dyslipidemia and insulin resistance secondary to antiretroviral therapy[533,534] is uncertain. On the other hand, the direct virus-induced and indirect cytokine activation of endothelium[531] may account for the observed arterial dysfunction.

In adults with chronic renal failure, premature atherosclerosis is a major cause of morbidity and mortality. Recent evidence suggests that children with end-stage renal failure are similarly subjected to increased risk of cardiovascular disease.[535] Increased aortic pulse wave velocity and carotid arterial stiffness have been shown to be an independent predictor of cardiovascular mortality in adults with end-stage renal failure.[186,187,536] In children on haemodialysis, increased carotid-femoral pulse wave velocity and augmentation index have also been demonstrated,[537] although the prognostic significance of these indices in children is unknown. Even after successful renal transplantation, the carotid arterial stiffness in children and adolescents remains elevated and is found to be associated with higher daytime systolic blood pressure load and receipt of cadaveric kidney.[538] Apart from arterial stiffening, endothelial dysfunction has been shown in children with chronic renal failure, even in the absence of classic cardiovascular risk factors,[539] and in those after transplantation.[540] Limited evidence suggests that oral folic acid, but not L-arginine, may improve endothelial function in children with chronic renal failure by lowering homocysteine level and increasing resistance of low-density lipoprotein to oxidation.[541,542]

Increased iron store has been linked to the risk of atherosclerosis.[543] Iron-overloading in patients with β-thalassaemia major results in alterations of arterial structures with disruption of elastic tissue and calcification.[544,545] Functional disturbance of human vascular endothelial cells when being incubated with thalassemic serum has further been demonstrated in vitro.[546] In adolescent and adult patients with β-thalassaemia major, increased stiffness of the carotid artery, brachioradial artery, and aorta has been shown in vivo.[547,548] Importantly, systemic arterial stiffening is inversely related to brachial arterial flow-mediated dilation and positively with left ventricular mass and carotid intima-media thickness.[547,549] In a mouse model of β-thalassaemia major, the Pourcelot index, a parameter that depends on arterial compliance, downstream vascular resistance, and total peripheral vascular resistance was found to be increased.[550] This result corroborates the findings of elevated pulsatile and static afterload in patients with β-thalassaemia major.[551] Apart from oxidative damage related to iron overload, the cell-free haemoglobin in haemolytic disease has also been implicated in mediating vascular dysfunction by limiting nitric oxide availability.[552]

Sleep-related disorders are common in children and may potentially affect arterial function. While relationship between snoring and cardiovascular complications in adults has been controversial,[553–558] in children with primary snoring, higher daytime systemic blood pressure and increased brachioradial arterial stiffness has been reported.[559] In adults with obstructive sleep apnea, increased carotid-femoral pulse wave velocity and brachial-ankle pulse wave velocity have been reported.[560,561] Acute increase in radial arterial stiffness during episodes of apnea has also been shown.[562] While the exact mechanisms are unknown, hypoxia, increased vasoconstrictors, enhanced vasoconstrictor sensitivity, and increased sympathetic tone might account for the alteration of arterial elastic properties.[556–558,560,563,564] Endothelial dysfunction has been shown in adults with obstructive sleep apnea,[565–567] which is potentially reversible by nasal continuous positive airway pressure.[568,569] Whether arterial dysfunction exists in paediatric patients remains to be clarified.

In children with MELAS (mitochondrial myopathy, encephalopathy, lactic acidosis, and stroke), the level of L-arginine has been found to be significantly lower during stroke-like episodes and associated with reduced brachial arterial flow-mediated dilation.[570–572] Prolonged L-arginine supplementation has been shown to reduce the stroke-like episodes and normalise endothelial dysfunction.[571,572]

Genetic Considerations

The genetic aspect of arterial stiffness is increasingly being unveiled. The phenomenon of arterial stiffening in genetic syndromes associated with mutations or deletion of genes encoding structural proteins of the arterial wall has been alluded to earlier. Marfan and Williams syndromes are examples whereby genes exert influence on systemic arterial stiffness. Studies have demonstrated significant heritabilities of common carotid artery stiffness, augmentation index, and carotid-femoral pulse wave velocity in different ethnic populations.[573–576] Microarray analysis of the transcriptome of aortic specimens obtained from adults with coronary artery disease has revealed correlations between aortic stiffness and expression of two groups of genes, namely, those associated with cell signaling and those associated with mechanical regulation of vascular structure.[577] Indeed, the influence of *matrix metalloproteinase-3* and *-9* genotypes on aortic stiffening in healthy elderly subjects has been reported.[578,579] Studies have also related arterial stiffness to polymorphisms of candidate genes, including those involved in the renin-angiotensin-aldosterone system[580–582] and endothelin receptors.[583] In adults with coronary artery disease, *fibrillin-1* genotype is associated with aortic input and characteristic impedance and disease severity.[584] Whether *fibrillin-1* genotype is similarly associated with aortic stiffening in healthy adults is, however, controversial.[585,586] In children, gene polymorphism of the mannose-binding lectin, a body defence molecule, has been found to exert modulating influence on arterial stiffness after vasculitic damage in patients with a history of Kawasaki disease, as discussed earlier,[451] while arterial stiffening in children with type 1 diabetes is associated with *nitric oxide synthase 3* polymorphism.[380] Recently, a genome-wide scan identified linkage of carotid-femoral pulse wave velocity to several separate genetic loci in humans.[576]

Potential genetic contribution to endothelial dysfunction is evidenced by studies demonstrating that young individuals with a family history of cardiovascular disease have impaired endothelial function[389,390] and that polymorphisms of angiotensin-converting enzyme[587] and endothelial nitric oxide synthase genes[588] may influence endothelial function. In children, endothelial dysfunction has been documented in single-gene disorders including homocystinuria[400] and familial hypercholesterolemia.[275,368–370] In a large community-based sample, the estimated heritability of brachial artery flow-mediated dilation has been shown to be modest.[589] While polymorphisms of genes encoding factors involved in the regulation of nitric oxide synthesis have been implicated in endothelial dysfunction,[590] further studies are warranted before any conclusions can be drawn.

Clinical Implications

The prognostic implications of arterial dysfunction in adults have been alluded to earlier. In children and adolescents, the predictive value of these measures of arterial dysfunction for future cardiovascular events is unclear. It appears unrealistic, however, to assess prognostic value of indices of arterial function in childhood only in terms of end-points such as cardiovascular morbidity and mortality. Structural surrogate measures of atherosclerosis, such as carotid intima-media thickness, are potentially useful alternatives.[591] Indeed, increased carotid intima-media thickness has been associated with several of the aforementioned paediatric conditions including familial hypercholesterolaemia,[592–594] type 1 diabetes,[374,594] family history of premature myocardial infarction,[388] children infected with human immunodeficiency virus on antiretroviral therapy,[595] obese children with insulin resistance,[596] and thalassaemia major.[549] Nonetheless, whether arterial stiffening and endothelial dysfunction represent genuine childhood cardiovascular risk factors awaits further clarification.

Early identification of arterial dysfunction that potentially precedes and induces atherosclerotic changes provides a window for early intervention. The potential beneficial effects on endothelial function of folic acid in children with renal failure,[541,542] antioxidant vitamins and statins in those with familial hypercholesterolaemia,[369,371,372] vitamin C in those with Kawasaki disease,[443] and exercise training in obese children[353,597] were alluded to earlier. In patients with Marfan syndrome, β-blocker therapy[464] and angiotensin-converting enzyme inhibition[471] appear to reduce aortic stiffness. Longitudinal studies are required to determine whether improvement of arterial function will be translated into clinical benefits. In healthy children, whether such lifestyle and dietary modifications have any effects on the prevention of arterial dysfunction remains to be substantiated.

Given that the systemic arterial system receives and distributes output from the systemic ventricle, satisfactory performance of the systemic ventricular pump depends on not only its intrinsic properties but also its optimal interaction with the systemic circulation. Dysfunction of either of the components of the cardiovascular system would inevitably affect performance of the other. This issue of ventriculo-arterial interaction is discussed in the following section.

VENTRICULO-ARTERIAL INTERACTION

Impact of Arterial Dysfunction on Ventricular Function

From the cardiac perspective, arterial dysfunction exerts its influence on systemic ventricular afterload, energetic efficiency, structure, function, and coronary arterial perfusion. As discussed earlier, ventricular afterload is increased in the presence of systemic arterial stiffening and endothelial dysfunction, the latter through modulation of vascular tone. To generate the same stroke volume against a stiffened arterial tree, the systemic ventricle has to generate a higher end-systolic pressure. As the pressure developed during systole is a major determinant of myocardial oxygen consumption, greater energy cost to the heart is required. In a canine model in which a Dacron graft was sewn to replace the descending aorta, increased cardiac workload, increased myocardial oxygen consumption by 30% to 50%, and reduced cardiac efficiency, defined as ratio of stroke work to oxygen consumption, by an average of 16% have been found.[598,599] Structural adaptation of the left ventricle to increased afterload is also evident in the presence of arterial stiffening. In a rat model of aortic elastocalcinosis, isolated increased aortic stiffness but without changes in mean arterial blood pressure has been associated with left ventricular hypertrophy.[600] Findings in adult human studies were nonetheless often confounded by presence of concomitant systemic hypertension.[601,602] The pressure-dependent parameter such as elastic modulus, but not relatively pressure-independent stiffness index, has been shown to be associated with left ventricular hypertrophy.[602] Likewise, in an otherwise healthy population of adults, measures of arterial function including elastic modulus, distensibility, and pulse wave velocity have been shown to be significant determinants of left ventricular mass when blood pressure is removed from the statistical model.[601]

Arterial stiffening is associated with alteration of phasic coronary flow pattern.[598,603] Early return of the reflected pressure wave augments the systolic pressure and lowers the diastolic coronary perfusion pressure. In a canine model with aortic bypass by a stiff conduit, the percentage of systolic coronary flow was found to increase from a normal of 25% to almost 50%.[603] The tighter coupling of coronary perfusion to systolic pressure has important implications. As the ventricular systolic performance and pressure declines due to causes such as acute ischaemia, the fall in systolic pressure would have more pronounced effects than expected on the size of the ischaemic bed and ventricular function due to a shift to greater reliance on systolic coronary perfusion.[604]

The afterload dependence of cardiac relaxation is well recognised.[605–607] While the mechanisms remain elusive, recent evidence suggests a potential role of troponin I phosphorylation.[608] Additionally, the increased myocardial oxygen consumption, left ventricular hypertrophy, and decreased diastolic coronary perfusion pressure secondary to arterial stiffening predispose to subendocardial ischaemia and interstitial fibrosis, which in turn can impair myocardial relaxation and reduce ventricular compliance.[609,610] Indeed, the associations between arterial stiffness and left ventricular diastolic dysfunction in adults with hypertension[610–613] and diabetes mellitus[611,613,614] are well recognised. The association between arterial stiffening and left ventricular systolic function has also been reported. In adults with[615] and without[611] coronary artery disease, aortic and conduit arterial stiffness has also been inversely related to long-axis systolic left ventricular function. In adults with coronary artery disease, an inverse relationship between brachial-ankle pulse wave velocity and left ventricular ejection fraction has been reported.[615] Nonetheless, maintenance of systolic function in the presence of increased afterload may be achieved through adaptive left ventricular hypertrophy, shift of myocardial myosin heavy chain from α- to β-isoform that develops a slower, more energy efficient term of contraction,[600] facilitation of transduction of cardiomyocyte contraction into myocardial force development by the fibrillar collagen, and the Anrep effect.

Effect of Ventricular Dysfunction on Systemic Circulation

Systemic ventricular dysfunction with development of heart failure is associated with sympathoadrenal activation, activation of the renin-angiotensin system, systemic inflammation, and increased oxidative stress.[616,617] While left ventricular dysfunction occurs most commonly in acquired conditions such as ischaemic heart disease and dilated cardiomyopathy, the syndrome of heart failure in the context of systemic ventricular dysfunction complicating congenital heart lesions is increasingly recognised.[618,619]

Arterial dysfunction in adults with chronic heart failure is well documented. Despite reduced brachial arterial diameter in these patients, increased brachioradial arterial pulse wave velocity has been reported.[620] Reduced radial, carotid, and aortic distensibility, as determined by echo-tracking, has also been shown.[621] Progressive arterial stiffening is found in adults with worsening New York Heart Association functional class.[620] Furthermore, in adults with heart failure, reduced endothelial-dependent increase in forearm blood flow[622–624] and dilation of femoral arteries[625] have been demonstrated.

Several mechanisms may account for systemic arterial dysfunction in heart failure. Contraction of vascular smooth muscle secondary to activation of the sympathoadrenal and renin-angiotensin systems modulates arterial stiffness through increasing vascular tone. In a canine model of heart failure, decreased gene expressions of endothelial nitric oxide synthase and cyclooxygenase-1 have been found, suggesting reduction of release of endothelium-derived vasodilating substances.[626] Whether basal nitric oxide production is reduced or increased in heart failure is, however, controversial.[627] Nonetheless, direct evidence suggests decreased synthetic activity of the L-arginine-nitric oxide pathway.[628] Using isotope-labeled L-arginine to assess synthesis of nitric oxide, urinary excretion of isotope-labeled nitrate was found to be reduced in patients with heart failure at rest and during submaximal exercise. Increased degradation of nitric oxide can also occur in heart failure due to its inactivation by reactive oxygen species.[629] Increased angiotensin-converting enzyme activity in heart failure increases breakdown of kinins, which in turn may lead to reduction of nitric oxide release.[630]

Apart from activation of the neurohumoral system and reduced availability of endothelium-derived vasodilating substances, elevation of endothelium-derived vasoconstrictors, in particular endothelin, in congestive heart failure may also contribute to increased vascular tone and arterial stiffening.[631] Indeed, endothelin-1, the major isoform in the cardiovascular system, is elevated in adults with heart failure and related to severity of haemodynamic disturbance and symptoms.[632–634]

The elevation of circulating proinflammatory cytokine tumor necrosis factor–α in heart failure[635] may also contribute to arterial dysfunction. Administration of tumor necrosis factor–α has been shown to reduce acetylcholine-induced vascular relaxation in a rat model.[636] Possible mechanisms include increased production of reactive oxygen species, blockage of activation of endothelial nitric oxide synthase, and direct degradation of endothelial nitric oxide messenger RNA.[637–638] Importantly, tumor necrosis factor–α antagonism with etanercept in adult patients with advanced heart failure has been shown to improve the impaired systemic endothelial vasodilator capacity.[637]

Ventriculo-arterial Coupling

It is obvious from the above discussions that reciprocal interactions between the arterial system and systemic ventricle, if unfavorable, may set up a vicious cycle (Fig. 6-12). Interactions between the left ventricle and the systemic circulation have been studied under frameworks of ventriculo-arterial coupling.[639–642] Analysis of the forward- and backward-traveling wave energy has also been used to assess ventriculo-arterial interaction.[643,644] By far, the framework proposed by Sunagawa et al has been used most commonly for analysis of ventriculo-arterial coupling in humans in health and disease.[639] In this framework of ventriculo-arterial coupling, the systemic ventricle and the arterial system are considered as two elastic chambers (Fig. 6-13). The volume of blood transferred from one chamber to the other is determined by their relative elastance, expressed as the ratio of effective arterial elastance (E_a) to ventricular end-systolic elastance (E_{es}). In this model, the coupling is studied in terms of the pressure-volume relationship (Fig. 6-14).

Effective arterial elastance is defined as the ratio of end-systolic pressure to stroke volume and is used as an index of total external load opposing left ventricular ejection. Arterial elastance takes into account of both the static and pulsatile components of the arterial load, as it depends on the total peripheral resistance, total arterial compliance, and

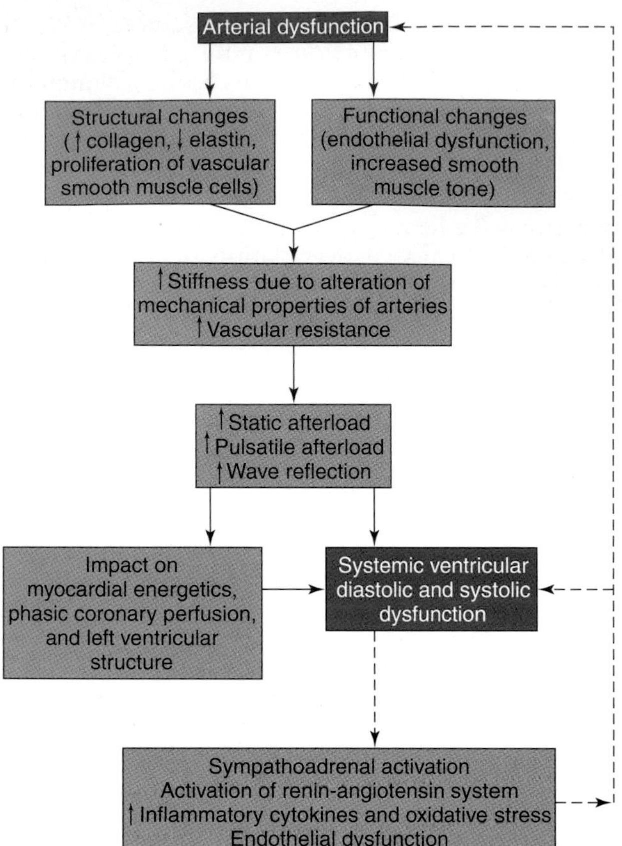

Figure 6-12 Unfavorable interactions in the presence of arterial dysfunction between the systemic circulation and left ventricle. The setting up of vicious cycles (*dashed lines*) may aggravate pre-existing arterial and ventricular dysfunction.

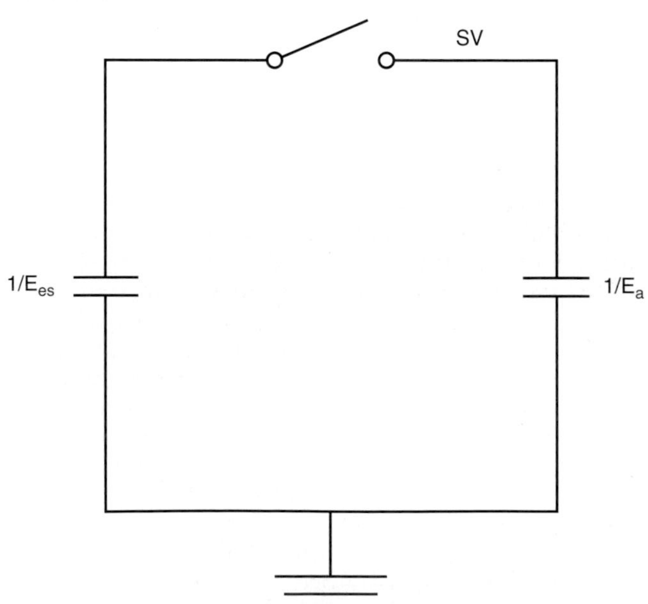

Figure 6-13 Ventriculoarterial coupling model. The systemic arterial system and systemic ventricle are considered as elastic chambers with volume elastance E_a and E_{es}, respectively. The stroke volume (SV) being transferred from the heart to the arterial system when the two are connected is determined by their relative elastance. (Adapted with modification from Sunagawa K, Maughan WL, Burkhoff D, Sagawa K: Left ventricular interaction with arterial load studied in isolated canine ventricle. Am J Physiol 1983;245: H773–H780.)

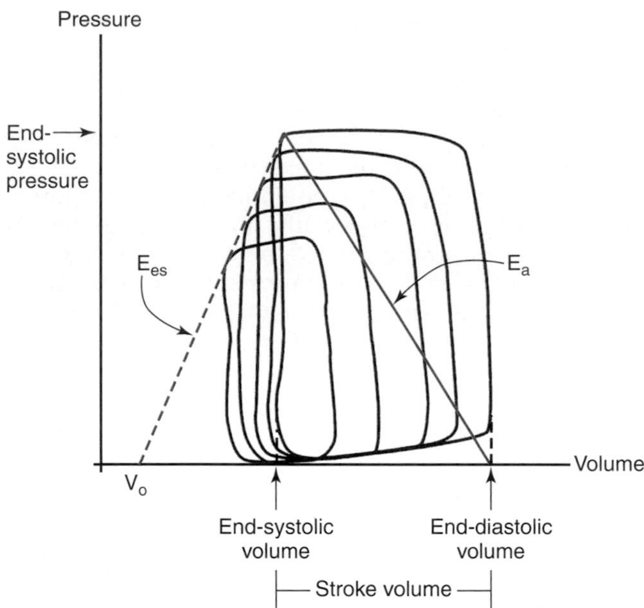

Figure 6-14 Ventriculo-arterial coupling framework based on pressure-volume relations. Left ventricular end-systolic elastance (E_{es}) is represented by the end-systolic pressure volume relationship, which can be obtained from pressure-volume loops generated at varying loads. V_o is the volume axis intercept of the end-systolic pressure volume relationship. Arterial elastance (E_a) equals the ratio of end-systolic pressure to stroke volume. The equilibrium point at which the ventricle is coupled with the arterial system lies at the intersection with a common peak end-systolic pressure.

aortic characteristic impedance. While the contribution of total peripheral vascular resistance and cardiac frequency to arterial elastance is greater than arterial stiffness,[639,645] arterial elastance has been shown to reflect pure alterations in arterial compliance, wave reflection, and characteristic impedance.[599] Importantly, the fact that arterial elastance is expressed in terms of pressure-volume relationship enables its coupling to the elastance of the left ventricle.[646]

The left ventricular elastance is represented by the slope of end-systolic pressure-volume relationship, determined from a family of pressure-volume loops and commonly regarded as a load-independent index of contractility. The intersection of the arterial end-systolic pressure-volume relationship and ventricular end-systolic pressure-volume relationship represents the equilibrium end-systolic pressure and volume where the two systems couple. The effective stroke volume being transferred can be calculated by the formula stroke volume = (end-diastolic volume − V_0)/(1 + E_a/E_{es}), where V_0 is the volume axis intercept of the end-systolic pressure-volume relationship.[639] It is worthwhile to note that both arterial elastance and ventricular elastance vary dynamically during the cardiac cycle and reach a maximum at end-systole.

The coupling ratio, E_a/E_{es}, has been used extensively in humans for characterisation of interaction between the systemic ventricle and arterial system.[599,647,648] Analytical modeling in isolated canine hearts has shown that the left ventricle delivers maximal stroke work when E_a/E_{es} approaches 1, while the mechanical efficiency of the ventricle, defined as the ratio of stroke work to myocardial oxygen consumption, is maximal when the ratio is about 0.5.[649] In normal humans, the ratio has been shown to lie between 0.7 and 1.0.[648,650] In isolated canine hearts, it has further been shown that over an E_a/E_{es} ratio spanning 0.3

and 1.3, the left ventricular stroke work and cardiac efficiency remain nearly optimal, whereas both decline at higher and lower ratios.[651] This framework of ventriculo-arterial coupling has been used commonly to analyse interactions between the arterial system and the systemic ventricle in children with congenital and acquired heart disease.

Relevance in Congenital and Acquired Heart Disease in the Young

Fontan Physiology

The Fontan physiology is characterised by connection in series of the systemic and pulmonary circulation. Theoretical modeling using the ventriculo-arterial coupling framework suggested increased arterial elastance, reduced ventricular end-systolic elastance, increased E_a/E_{es} ratio, and reduced ventricular external stroke work and mechanical efficiency.[652] In clinical studies, elevated systemic[653,654] and total vascular resistance[655] has been demonstrated consistently. The pulsatile component of the afterload, as determined from the first harmonic impedance in the impedance spectra, has also been shown to be elevated in Fontan patients.[655] Importantly, the first harmonic impedance was found to correlate negatively with cardiac index. In a canine model of Fontan circulation, the input impedance at zero harmonic and characteristic impedance were also found to be elevated.[656] The cause of increased pulsatile afterload in Fontan circulation is not entirely clear. Proposed explanations include increased wave reflections[655] and sympathetic activation as a compensatory mechanism for reduced cardiac output.[656] Documented endothelial dysfunction in these patients might also play a role through modulation of vascular tone.[657,511]

In terms of ventriculo-arterial coupling, Fontan patients have been found to have increased arterial elastance without concomitant changes in ventricular end-systolic elastance, indicating that abnormal coupling is due to increased afterload.[658] In this study, the coupling E_a/E_{es} ratio in Fontan patients was found to be around 1.5, and the reduced cardiac index at baseline was attributed to increased afterload rather than decreased ventricular contractility. Compared with biventricular circulation, Fontan circulation is found to be associated with reduced ventricular hydraulic power and higher ventricular power expenditure per unit cardiac output.[655]

Interestingly, staged total cavopulmonary connection with a preceding bidirectional Glenn procedure has been demonstrated to be associated with a smaller increment in arterial elastance after surgery and reduced E_a/E_{es} ratio, as compared to increased E_a/E_{es} ratio after primary total cavopulmonary connection.[659]

Given the findings of abnormal ventriculo-arterial coupling in Fontan physiology, the use of afterload-reducing agents should theoretically improve haemodynamics and coupling. Nonetheless, administration of enalapril for 10 weeks in a small cohort of Fontan patients was found not to alter systemic vascular resistance, resting cardiac index, and exercise capacity.[660] It is important to realise, however, that limited β-adrenergic reserve in Fontan patients induced by dobutamine[655,658] is primarily related to a limited preload, which could have been further reduced after enalapril. Further studies are required to clarify the controversial role of systemic vasodilators in optimizing the Fontan haemodynamics.

Norwood Procedure

The ventriculo-arterial coupling ratio in patients after a Norwood procedure with a right ventricular-pulmonary artery conduit has been shown to be similar to those with a systemic-pulmonary shunt.[661] This holds true even after a bidirectional Glenn procedure and total cavopulmonary connection. However, ventricular end-systolic elastance was found to be lower in the right ventricular-pulmonary artery conduit group after bidirectional Glenn procedure and total cavopulmonary connection. This has been attributed to deleterious influence of ventriculotomy on systemic right ventricular function. Afterload reduction for the lowering of arterial elastance and optimisation of coupling ratio is thought to be beneficial.

Systemic Left Ventricle in Biventricular Circulation

In a porcine model of paediatric cardiopulmonary bypass, arterial elastance was found to be increased while ventricular end-systolic elastance was found to remain unchanged.[662] The absence of compensatory increase in ventricular contractility provided an explanation for the low cardiac output syndrome in this cardiopulmonary bypass model. Importantly, this study demonstrated that milrinone or levosimendan prevented the increase in arterial elastance after bypass, probably through their systemic vasodilator properties, and protected against the reduction in cardiac output. These findings shed light on the understanding of the beneficial effects of prophylactic milrinone in the prevention of low cardiac output syndrome in infants and young children after open heart surgery.[663]

In children with coarctation of the aorta, the increased afterload is characterised by increased arterial elastance.[664] Interestingly, data suggested that clinical symptoms of heart failure are related to left ventricular contractile response to increased afterload. Increased ventricular end-systolic elastance that matches with increased arterial elastance was characteristic of asymptomatic patients, while infants with overt heart failure were found to have minimal increase in ventricular end-systolic elastance consistent with afterload mismatch. In an animal model of aortic coarctation, banding of the aortic arch has been shown to increase aortic characteristic impedance and cause concentric left ventricular hypertrophy.[665] In adolescents after successful repair of coarctation, increased stiffness of the ascending aorta has been found to correlate with the degree of impairment of left ventricular longitudinal strain rate.[666]

The response of the systemic circulation to systemic ventricular dysfunction has been alluded to earlier. Indeed, studies have shown suboptimal ventriculo-arterial coupling in adults with idiopathic non-ischaemic cardiomyopathy.[667,668] The arterial elastance was found to be elevated, which has been attributed to increased systemic vascular resistance, tachycardia, and decreased stroke volume.[668] As expected, with reduced cardiac contractility, ventricular end-systolic elastance was found to be decreased in these patients.[669] Although inotropes have been shown to improve the coupling, their effects on mechanical efficiency were found to be minimal.[667]

In adolescents and adults with β-thalassaemia major, arterial elastance has been shown to be elevated and to correlate positively with total vascular resistance and negatively with systemic vascular compliance.[551] Increased arterial elastance is probably related to arterial stiffening and endothelial dysfunction in these patients.[547] Importantly, arterial elastance was also found to be a significant negative determinant of cardiac contractility. Afterload reduction with oral enalapril has been shown to improve systolic and diastolic function in asymptomatic or minimally symptomatic thalassaemia patients with left ventricular dysfunction.[670]

Interactions between systemic arterial load and left ventricular structure and function have also been shown in adolescents and young adults with paediatric-onset systemic lupus erythematosus.[528] Carotid arterial stiffness, being increased in these patients, was found to be a significant independent determinant of mass, myocardial performance index, and relatively load independent indices of systolic and diastolic function of the left ventricle.

Systemic Right Ventricle in Biventricular Circulation

In asymptomatic adolescent and adult survivors of the Mustard operation, increased E_a/E_{es} ratio with a mean of 3.47 has been reported.[671] Increased arterial stiffness[493,496] might in part account for the suboptimal ventriculo-arterial coupling. Enhancement of systemic right ventricular contractility by dobutamine has been shown to reduce the ratio to approach unity, which suggests improved coupling.[671] Disappointingly, administration of afterload-reducing agents including enalapril[672] and lorsartan[673] did not improve exercise capacity in patients with transposition of the great arteries after atrial switch operation. Possible causes include minimal baseline activation of the renin-angiotensin system[673] and limited preload due to impairment of atrioventricular transport.[671,674]

THE FUTURE

A comprehensive understanding of the normal functioning of the systemic circulation requires its appraisal from the structural, physiological, and mechanical perspectives. Over the last decade, there has been an increasing interest in the role of systemic arterial dysfunction as a risk factor and a probable etiologic factor for cardiovascular disease in adults. Concurrent development of non-invasive methodologies for assessment of systemic arterial function, notably arterial stiffness and endothelial function, leads to its increasing utilisation in the paediatric population. The list of childhood conditions associated with arterial dysfunction has since expanded rapidly. Further studies to elucidate the underlying mechanisms of arterial dysfunction in the young are undoubtedly warranted. Additionally, longitudinal studies are required to clarify whether systemic arterial dysfunction tracks from childhood to adulthood and whether arterial dysfunction detected early in life would have an impact on cardiovascular health in the long term. Although strategies to reduce arterial stiffness and to improve endothelial dysfunction have been proposed and their potential benefits demonstrated in selected high-risk cohorts of paediatric patients, their benefits in otherwise healthy children remain unknown. Advances in molecular biology would further unveil the genetic determinants of vascular structure and function, which may provide novel targets for reversal of arterial dysfunction. It cannot be overemphasised that optimal interaction between the systemic circulation and the systemic ventricle is instrumental in ensuring the normal functioning of the cardiovascular system. Further understanding of ventriculo-arterial coupling in paediatric cardiac conditions, in particular congenital heart disease associated with systemic ventricular dysfunction, would shed light on the choice of the most appropriate management strategy.

The complete reference list can be found on the companion Expert Consult web site at www.expertconsult.com.

ANNOTATED REFERENCES

- Nichols WW, O'Rourke MF: McDonald's Blood Flow in Arteries: Theoretical, Experimental and Clinical Principles, 5th ed. London: Hodder Arnold, 2005.

  This classic text provides a theoretical basis for the understanding of arterial haemodynamics in normal and diseased conditions. The scientific basis of the complex relationship between pulsatile pressure and flow in arteries and the practical applications of such relationship are highlighted. In particular, the topics on pulse waveform analysis, pulse wave transmission and reflection, arterial impedance, and ventriculo-arterial coupling are clearly presented.

- Wamhoff BR, Bowles DK, Owens GK: Excitation-transcription coupling in arterial smooth muscle. Circ Res 2006;98:868–878.

  This review summarises the current knowledge of an important new paradigm termed excitation-transcription coupling in arterial smooth muscle. Phenotypic diversity and plasticity of vascular smooth muscle cells play an important role during normal and diseased vascular states. This article reviews recent progress in the understanding of mechanisms by which signals that regulate excitation-contraction coupling are capable of regulating selective gene expression in vascular smooth muscle cells.

- Deanfield JE, Halcox JP, Rabelink TJ: Endothelial function and dysfunction: Testing and clinical relevance. Circulation 2007;115:1285–1295.
- Deanfield J, Donald A, Ferri C, et al: Endothelial function and dysfunction. 1. Methodological issues for assessment in the different vascular beds: A statement by the working group on endothelin and endothelial factors by the European Society of Hypertension. J Hypertens 2005;23:7–17.

  These reviews summarise the current understanding of endothelial function and dysfunction in health and disease, the methodological issues for assessment of endothelial function in different vascular beds, and potential applications of different techniques in the research and clinical arenas.

- O'Rourke MF, Staessen JA, Vlachopoulos C, et al: Clinical applications of arterial stiffness: Definitions and reference values. Am J Hypertens 2002;15:426–444.

  This review summarises the definition of various terms used clinically to describe arterial stiffness, methods used for its estimation, and paediatric and adult reference values.

- Laurent S, Cockcroft J, Van Bortel L, et al: Expert consensus document on arterial stiffness: Methodological issues and clinical applications. Eur Heart J 2006;27:2588–2605.

  This review, representing the consensus document of the proceedings of meetings of the European Network for Non-invasive Investigation of Large Arteries, provides an updated overview of the methodological issues and clinical applications in the assessment of arterial stiffness.

- Aggoun Y, Szezepanski I, Bonnet D: Noninvasive assessment of arterial stiffness and risk of atherosclerotic events in children. Pediatr Res 2005;58: 173–178.
- Groner JA, Joshi M, Bauer JA: Pediatric precursors of adult cardiovascular disease: Noninvasive assessment of early vascular changes in children and adolescent. Pediatrics 2006;118:1683–1691.

  These two reviews provide summaries of the current utilisation of noninvasive methods for evaluating vascular function and discuss the potential usefulness of these techniques in the assessment of atherogenic risk in the paediatric population.

- Sunagawa K, Maughan WL, Burkhoff D, et al: Left ventricular interaction with arterial load studied in isolated canine ventricle. Am J Physiol 1983;245: H773–780.

  This paper introduces the crucial ventriculo-arterial coupling framework that has proved extremely useful in the characterisation of both vascular and ventricular properties in the prediction of functional variables such as stroke volume, and ultimately in the understanding of integrated cardiovascular performance. This framework has been used extensively in the evaluation of ventriculo-vascular interactions in congenital and acquired heart disease in the young.

- Kass DA, Kelly RP: Ventriculo-arterial coupling: Concepts, assumptions, and applications. Ann Biomed Eng 1992;20:41–62.

  This review summarises the frameworks of ventriculo-arterial coupling, examines assumptions, and provides insight in their clinical applications. It provides the basis for the application of coupling frameworks in the study of ventriculo-vascular interactions in the various congenital and acquired heart conditions as discussed at length in this chapter.

CHAPTER 7

Pulmonary Circulation

SHEILA G. HAWORTH and MARLENE RABINOVITCH

Understanding the features of the pulmonary circulation is critically important in the management of patients with congenitally malformed hearts. The past 10 years have seen remarkable advances in our understanding of its development, the genetics, pathobiology, and treatment of pulmonary vascular disease, and the physiology of this circulation. Primary intracardiac repair in infancy has become the norm, but the selection of patients suitable for intracardiac repair can still pose a problem, particularly in developing countries when many patients present late. Assessment has been facilitated by improvements in tissue Doppler imaging, computerised tomography, and magnetic resonance imaging. The patients who, in the absence of surgical correction, develop the Eisenmenger syndrome and become severely symptomatic can be helped by treatment with new medicines used to treat idiopathic pulmonary hypertension. Advances in our understanding of the pathogenesis of pulmonary vascular disease now influence our approach to the management of many patients with congenitally malformed hearts and pulmonary hypertension. In this chapter, we will focus on the normal and abnormal development of the pulmonary circulation, neonatal circulation, the hypoperfused lung, and advances made in the pathobiology and treatment of pulmonary vascular disease.

NORMAL PULMONARY CIRCULATION

Normal Anatomy of the Pulmonary Circulation

The functional unit of the lung is the acinus. An acinus is all the lung tissue supplied by a terminal bronchiolus. In the mature lung, it includes up to eight generations of respiratory bronchioluses, alveolar ducts, and the alveoluses beyond (Fig. 7-1). It is the respiratory unit of the lung. At the end of any airway, three to five acinuses are grouped to form a lobule. Each small airway is accompanied by a branch of the pulmonary artery until the arteries finally enter the capillary network of the alveolar walls. The acinuses and lobules, with their accompanying arteries, are the last part of the lung to appear before birth. It is these structures that are remodelled in the normal lung with growth, and which change most readily in disease. The bronchopulmonary segment is the basic topographical unit of the lung. It is a wedge of lung tissue supplied by a principal branch of a lobar bronchus and its accompanying pulmonary artery. The pulmonary veins and lymphatics lie in the intersegmental plane, receiving tributaries from adjacent segments.

The bronchopulmonary segment is the surgical unit of lung tissue, since a segment can be resected along its intersegmental boundaries. Familiarity with normal bronchopulmonary segmental anatomy also helps the cardiologist because, when examining pulmonary angiograms, he or she must ensure that all the bronchopulmonary segments are normally connected to the intrapericardial pulmonary arteries. Segments that are not perfused by a normal pulmonary arterial supply must be identified, and a search made for their source of systemic arterial supply. On angiography, large collateral systemic arteries arising from the aorta, often called major aortopulmonary collateral arteries, are distinguished from large bronchial arteries by their origin, distribution, and proximal connections with the hilar, lobar, or segmental arteries. The final destination of bronchial arteries is not seen angiographically, since the majority of them connect with the intra-acinar pulmonary arteries.

Bronchial Circulation

In children with congenitally malformed hearts, the bronchial circulation may provide an alternative source of arterial supply to the pulmonary capillaries when there

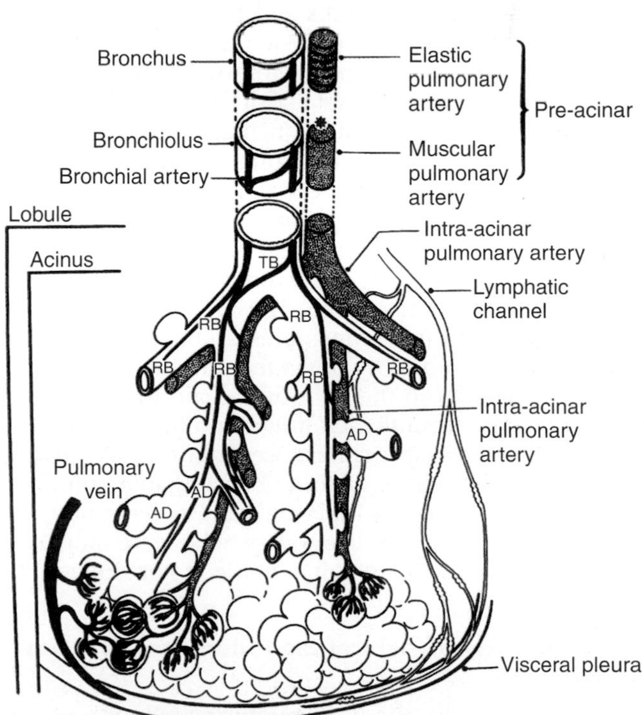

Figure 7-1 Diagram of the airway and arterial pathway, showing an elastic artery that accompanies cartilaginous lobar, segmental and subsegmental bronchi. The pulmonary artery becomes muscularised at the 7th to 9th division from the segmental hilum (*asterisk*). AD, alveolar duct; RB, respiratory bronchiolus; TB, terminal bronchiolus.

is little or no flow of blood down the lobar or segmental arteries. In the presence of obstructed or absent pulmonary veins, the bronchial veins drain oxygenated blood from the lung into the systemic veins.

The main bronchial arterial supply usually arises from the aorta directly, or from an intermediary intercosto-bronchial artery. The number of vessels arising from the aorta to supply each lung varies in the normal circulation. The most common anatomical patterns seen in one series included two posterior bronchial arteries supplying each lung in about one-third, two arteries supplying the left and one the right lung in one-fifth, with this relationship mirror-imaged in a further sixth, and a single trunk supplying each bronchus in a further tenth.[1] The successive branches of each bronchial artery are described as superior, middle, and inferior, this reference made to the relative levels of origin from the aorta, and not the ultimate level of distribution within the lung.

Additional accessory bronchial arteries may arise from the subclavian, brachiocephalic, or internal thoracic arteries. When the bronchial arterial circulation is expanded to provide an alternative source of blood supply to the lung, these and other vessels enlarge, distributing blood through the bronchial arteries via the pulmonary ligaments and retroperitoneal tissues. Blood is also distributed from the pericardiophrenic, oesophageal, and other mediastinal vessels, and occasionally from a coronary artery. Within the lung, each lobar and segmental bronchus is accompanied by two large bronchial arteries, which frequently anastomose around the bronchus.

Microscopically, the bronchial arteries are readily distinguishable from the pulmonary arteries by their position in the lung and by their mural structure. They accompany the bronchuses to supply the adventitial and mucosal layers, along with the walls of large pulmonary arteries. They lie next to the bronchial veins and the nerves that supply the large airways. As in other systemic arteries, the medial wall is thick and muscular, the internal elastic lamina is well defined, and the external elastic lamina is interrupted or absent. The structure of bronchial arteries frequently changes with age in the normal lung. Longitudinal muscle bundles develop, which may even occlude the lumen. The mechanism for this change is not understood.

There are two types of bronchial veins: the deep and the superficial, or pleurohilar, veins. Both types communicate freely with the pulmonary veins. The deep veins originate in the walls of the terminal bronchioluses, and eventually drain into the left atrium directly or via the pulmonary veins. The pleurohilar veins from the right lung drain into the azygos vein, while those from the left lung drain into the hemiazygos, superior intercostal, or brachiocephalic veins. Microscopically, a bronchial vein has a thinner wall than a pulmonary vein for a given diameter. Unlike pulmonary veins, bronchial veins contain delicate bifoliate valves, which are more commonly seen in the immature than in the mature lung.

Microscopic Assessment of the Pulmonary Arteries and Veins

In the normal child, the lung is remodelled with growth. In the abnormal lung, therefore, each structural feature must be compared with that of age-matched controls in tissues prepared and analysed in the same manner. To make such a comparison, the intrapulmonary arteries must be identified. They cannot be identified according to their size, because this changes in the normal lung with age, and may also change in disease. In a postmortem specimen, the elastic and large muscular arteries are identified by counting the number of generations that separate them from the segmental hilum, counting the segmental artery as the first generation. Their mural structure is determined by their position in the lung. Within the acinus, arteries continue to branch with the airways. On microscopic examination of both biopsy and postmortem tissue, the arteries are identified according to the type of airway they accompany, that is, terminal or respiratory bronchioluses, alveolar ducts, or ones that lie within the alveolar walls (see Fig. 7-1). Describing any part of the pathway in terms of arterioles is best avoided, because this term is open to different interpretations based on size, structure, and function, or a combination of attributes. In a large and unselected population of arteries, the mean percentage medial thickness can be calculated from measurements of medial thickness and external diameter. Other assessments include the mean ratio of arterial lumen to wall, the area of muscle present, and an index of medial muscular tissue present in the lung. Population counts reveal the relationship between mural structure, size, and the position in the arterial pathway. Arterial muscularity is usually assessed by determination of percentage medial thickness, and by finding the extent to which muscle has differentiated along the arterial pathway as judged both by the size and the position of the artery in the lung field. The number of arteries per unit area, or volume, of lung can be determined and the ratio of alveoluses to arteries calculated to overcome any difference in the degree of inflation in different lungs. In postmortem specimens, the effect of hypoperfusion on lung growth can be studied by determining the number and size of alveoluses. The veins are studied in a comparable manner.

Anastomoses Between Pulmonary and Bronchial Circulations

In the normal adult, most of the proximal connections between the pulmonary and bronchial arteries accompanying the same airway occur at the level of non-cartilaginous bronchioluses. More peripherally, the small bronchial arteries become indistinguishable as they anastomose with small pulmonary arteries around the necks of respiratory and terminal bronchioluses. In addition, branches of the bronchial arteries that accompany large and small airways anastomose with adjacent thin-walled pulmonary arteries in the surrounding lung tissue. These connections are called bronchopulmonary arteries. They are relatively common in the normal fetal and neonatal lung. Subepithelial bronchial arteries also anastomose with small precapillary pulmonary arteries.

The frequency with which the bronchial and pulmonary arterial circulations anastomose explains why accidental surgical interruption of a pulmonary artery, or ligation of a collateral artery providing the only source of blood supply to a region of lung, does not usually lead to infarction of the lung. By contrast, experimental stripping of the bronchial arteries at the hilum leads to necrosis of the bronchial wall near the hilum. In the venous circulation, there are many connections between bronchial and pulmonary veins. These enlarge in the presence of pulmonary venous hypertension. Blood may then flow from the pulmonary veins indirectly to the right atrium. Arterio-venous connections are not found in the normal lung.

Pulmonary Lymphatics

The superficial lymphatic network lies in the pleura, and the deep network lies in the interstitium. The two networks anastomose around the hilum, and drain to the hilar and tracheobronchial lymph nodes. Lymphatics are present in the pleura, in connective tissue septums, around the pulmonary arteries and veins, and in the bronchial wall, including the mucosa. Microscopically, small lymphatics consist of endothelial cells lying on a basement membrane, while in the large channels the walls are strengthened by the addition of collagen and elastic fibres, and an occasional muscle cell. The lymphatics contain delicate bicuspid valves. When pulmonary venous return is obstructed, either at the mitral valve or within the pulmonary veins themselves, the lymphatics become dilated. In the presence of long-standing obstruction, the walls of the lymphatics may be thickened by an increase in the amount of smooth muscle.

Biopsy of the Lung

A biopsy should be taken from the inflated lung. It is fixed in inflation to ensure distention of the airways, and hence their identification. The biopsy will be representative of the entire vasculature in a young child, providing that the flow of blood is evenly distributed. The lingula is best avoided, since even in the normal lung the arteries of this region tend to be more thick walled. In adults with rheumatic mitral stenosis, the lower lobe vessels are usually more severely affected than the rest of the vasculature. In any biopsy, the mural structure of the pulmonary arteries varies, as is to be expected, since the pulmonary arterial tree is a branching system. All arteries at a certain point along the pathway, in both normal and abnormal lungs, are structurally similar to, and different from, arteries proximal and distant to them.

Morphologic Assessment of Right Ventricular Hypertrophy

In the normal heart, the septum is considered as part of the left ventricle. Hypertrophy of the right ventricle, therefore, is indicated by a decrease in the ratio of the weight of the left ventricle and the septum assessed relative to the weight of the right ventricle. During fetal life, the right ventricle forms a greater proportion of the total ventricular weight than it does in the child or adult. At sea level, the ratio of between 2.3 to 1 and 3.3 to 1, as expected in the adult, is normally achieved when the infant reaches 4 months of age.[2]

DEVELOPMENT OF THE HUMAN PULMONARY VASCULATURE

Structural Development

Morphological study of the development of the pulmonary vasculature in the human describes the creative process, and provides clues about regulatory mechanisms which can be explored in other species and in experimental models. Abnormal development is informative in that it can be viewed as a vicarious experiment.

The heart tube is formed by the end of the third week of gestation, and about 5 days later the lung bud develops at the caudal end of the laryngotracheal groove. The lung bud expands laterally and divides into the two primordial lung sacs, each of which then divides first into lobes, and then into bronchopulmonary segments. In the normal lung, recent work shows that the pre-acinar arteries and post-acinar veins form by vasculogenesis from the splanchnopleural mesoderm of the lung bud.[3,4] The pre-acinar airways and post-acinar veins form in a centrifugal manner from hilum to periphery, but the vessels do not.[3,4] They form by continuous coalescence of endothelial tubes alongside the newly formed airways, which appear to provide a template for pre-acinar arterial development (Fig. 7-2). The continuous addition of endothelial tubes gradually lengthens the pulmonary arteries and veins. The heart is connected to the two lung buds from a very early stage of embryonic life. By at least 34 days of gestation, serial reconstructions demonstrate physical continuity between the aortic sac, the pulmonary arteries, the peribronchial capillary plexus, the pulmonary veins, and the atrial component of the heart. Thus, blood can circulate through the lung earlier than had been supposed, exposing the developing structures to circulating factors generated at distant sites, including angioblasts and other cells which could become incorporated into the vessel wall. The extent to which angiogenesis contributes to formation of vessels during this pseudoglandular phase is uncertain, but it may be responsible for the supernumerary vessels. Angiogenesis predominates later, and is thought to be responsible for formation of intra-acinar arteries, which starts in the canalicular phase with further development of airways and alveoluses, and continues after birth. All the pre-acinar arteries and airways have formed by the 16th week of gestation. Between a third to a half of the adult complement of alveoluses and intra-acinar arteries form before birth, with new structures then forming most rapidly within the first 6 months of life. After 3 years of age, development mainly consists of an increase in size of existing structures.

The pulmonary arterial smooth muscle cells are derived from three sites in a temporally distinct sequence[3] (Fig. 7-3). The first cells to surround the endothelial tubes migrate from the bronchial smooth muscle around the neck of each terminal bud. These cells become surrounded by the second population, which differentiates from mesenchymal cells. The third source is from endothelial cells in the most peripheral arteries, which transdifferentiate into smooth muscle cells later in gestation, from 98 to 140 days. Venous smooth muscle does not derive a contribution from bronchial smooth muscle.[4] Irrespective of their origin, all smooth muscle cells follow the same sequence of expression of smooth muscle specific cytoskeletal proteins. Maturation takes place from the subendothelium to the adventitial layers, and from hilum to periphery. In the pulmonary veins, the cytoskeletal proteins appear in the same sequence as in the pulmonary arteries, but do not express caldesmon, which might help explain why pulmonary veins are so responsive to contractile agonists.

The lymphatics originate at the hilum, and are first seen at about 56 days of gestation.[3] By the end of the pseudoglandular period, lymphatic channels have subdivided the lung periphery, positioned in the prospective connective tissue septums. The bronchial arteries develop from the dorsal aorta relatively late in gestation, at about 8 weeks

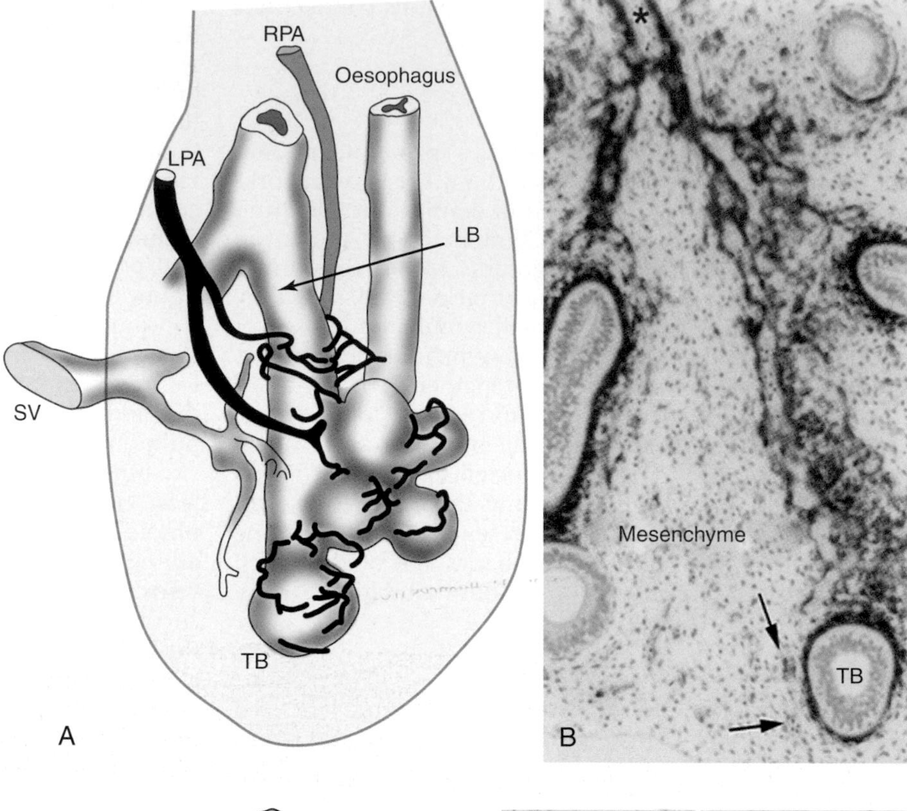

Figure 7-2 **A,** Drawing derived from a serial reconstruction of the human embryo viewed from the left side of the left lung at 38 days of gestation. Peripheral capillaries are clustered around each terminal bud. A mesenchymal sheath surrounds the lung bud and vessels, continuous with that of the trachea and oesophagus. LB, left brochus; LPA and RPA, left and right pulmonary arteries; SV, sinus venosus. **B,** Microscopic transverse section of human lung at 56 days of gestation, stained for alpha smooth muscle actin, showing terminal buds (TB) and adjacent coalescing endothelial tubes joining the newly formed pulmonary artery proximally (*asterisk*).

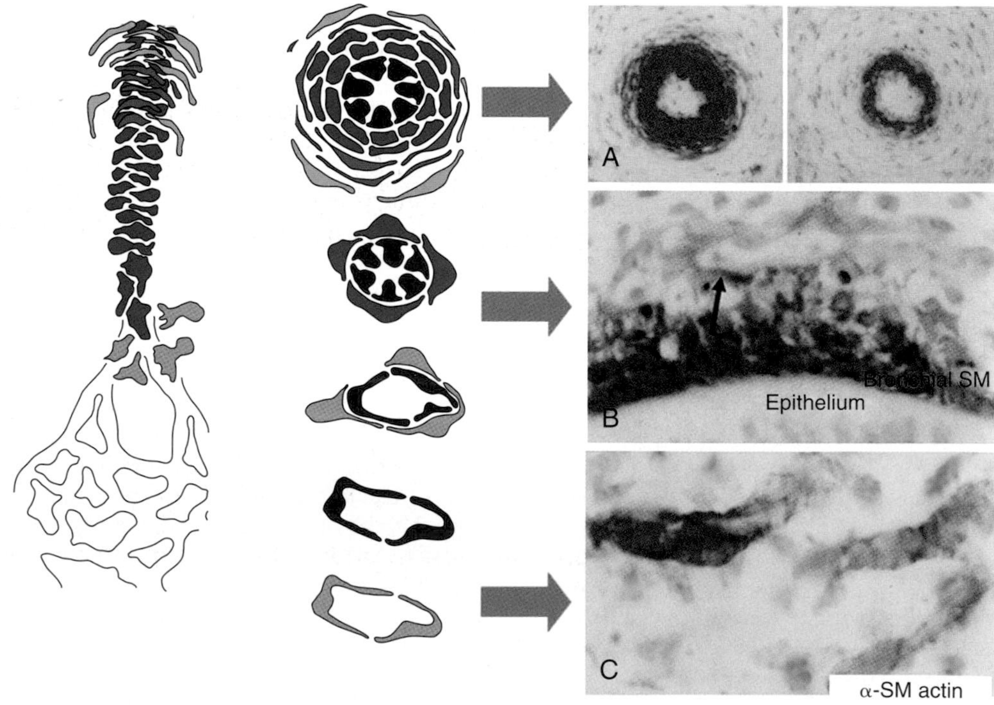

Figure 7-3 Origins of pulmonary arterial smooth muscle (SM). Tissue stained with alpha smooth muscle actin. **A,** Mesenchymal cells, as yet containing no cytoskeletal markers, aligning around first layers of muscle cells. **B,** Bronchial smooth muscle surrounding adjacent endothelial tubes. **C,** Endothelial cells undergoing transdifferentiation. Green, endothelial cells; red, pulmonary arterial smooth muscle originating from bronchial smooth muscle; purple, smooth muscle originating from mesenchymal cells; pink, endothelial cells undergoing transdifferentiation.

of gestation. When flow through the extrapulmonary arteries is abnormally diminished in late fetal life, or after birth, the bronchial arteries enlarge to supply the peripheral pulmonary arteries through connections between the pulmonary and bronchial circulations. Many such connections exist in the normal fetus and newborn, suggesting great adaptability, but they appear to decrease rapidly in size and number after birth. The structure of the pulmonary trunk reflects the high pulmonary vascular resistance of fetal life. It has a similar mural structure to that of the aorta, having concentric, compact parallel elastic fibres of uniform thickness.

Growth and Innervation after Birth

As the intrapulmonary arteries increase in size, their walls thicken to maintain a constant low relationship to the external diameter. In the arteries of the respiratory unit, smooth muscle cells differentiate from precursor intermediate cells and pericytes already in position, and as judged by light microscopy, non-muscular arteries become partially or completely muscularised. Muscle is said to have extended along the arterial pathway. The elastic laminas in the pulmonary trunk gradually become fragmented, and lose their ordered appearance. The wall of the pulmonary trunk becomes thinner relative to that of the aorta, with a ratio decreasing from unity to a mean value of 0.6 at about 8 months of age.[5] This ratio is maintained throughout life. The pulmonary vasculature is densely innervated at birth, and becomes more densely innervated with age.[6] In babies, as in adults, the nerves are predominantly of the sympathetic type. In pulmonary hypertensive infants, the abnormally thick-walled blood vessels are prematurely innervated by 3 months of age.[6]

Regulation of Pulmonary Vascular Development

The presence of a circulation through the pulmonary vasculature from early embryonic and fetal life means that the circulation is exposed to external, distal influences from an early stage in its development. Circulating cells could contribute to building the vessel walls. Angioblasts can stream to developing organ beds from a considerable distance,[7] and incorporation of marrow-derived stem cells seems likely. The extent to which such cells retain their genetic memory, and the extent to which they can be modified by environmental factors, is of fundamental importance.

The innermost medial smooth muscle cells originate by migrating from bronchial smooth muscle. They have a migratory phenotype in the setting of obstructive pulmonary vascular disease. With respect to cytoskeletal composition, regulation of the actin cytoskeleton by RhoGTPases, and contractility, the smooth muscle cells from the inner and outer medial layers retain stable phenotypic differences when cultured.[8,9]

These and other observations suggest that the cells may have been recruited into the vessel walls from afar. Because of this, they retain distinct hereditable characteristics which would enhance the heterogeneity of the vessel wall, and its potential for adaptation to environmental change.[10] The factors which determine whether an endothelial cell lying in the mesenchyme will become dedicated to either an arterial or a venous system are not understood. The tyrosine receptor EphB4, and its cognate ligand ephrin B2, discriminate between arteries and veins in the mouse, but less so in humans. Early angioblasts commit to either an arterial or a venous fate directed by a Notch gridlock signalling pathway.[11] It is possible, however, that pulmonary endothelial cells do not become committed until they have coalesced with an adjacent pulmonary artery or vein. It is at that time that the direction of flow, pressure, and circulating factors might influence commitment.

Experimental and gene targeting studies continue to emphasise the critical role of growth factors in lung development. Each appears to have a precise spatial and temporal expression pattern. In the human lung, we found eNOS, VEGF, and the VEGF receptors Flk-1and Flt-1and Tie-2, expressed in the capillary plexus at 38 days.[3] eNOS stimulates endothelial proliferation, migration, and formation of tubes, is a downstream mediator of growth factor–induced angiogenesis, and inhibits apoptosis. It is expressed on the endothelium of human arteries, capillaries, and veins throughout development. VEGF mediates vasculogenesis and angiogenesis. VEGF-A is required for vascular development throughout the embryo, and blood vessels do not form in mice deficient in the VEGF receptor Flk-1.[12,13] In cultured mouse lungs, VEGF is found at the branching points of peripheral airways. Grafting of beads coated with VEGF increases the density of the capillary bed.[14]

The tyrosine receptor kinase Tie-2, and its ligand angiopoietin, is essential in formation of the capillary networks.[15] Also, endothelial phosphorylation of the Tie-2 receptor by angiopoietin leads to proliferation of smooth muscle cells, perhaps indicating that it has a role in the neomuscularisation of newly formed pulmonary arteries.[16,17] EGFmRNA and TGFαmRNA are expressed in the mesenchymal cells surrounding airways and alveoluses in the human fetal lung from 12 to 33 weeks of gestation,[18] but the receptors for these ligands were found in the airways and were involved in differentiation. Their direct role in vascular development is uncertain. Insulin-like growth factors I and II, and IGF-IR ligands and mRNA, become apparent at 4 weeks.[19] Anti-IGF-IR neutralising antibody reduced the number of endothelial cells and increased apoptosis of endothelial and mesenchymal cells in human lung explants. IGF-1 also upregulates VEGF, further emphasising the crucial role of this growth factor. A low oxygen tension, as occurs during fetal life, stimulates vascular and airway development. This involves HIF-1α, which upregulates expression of VEGF, and plays an important role in both vasculogenesis and angiogenesis. Studies on HIF-1α emphasise the importance of cross-talk between developing arteries and airways to ensure the normal development of both structures.[20]

Functional Development in Fetal and Neonatal Life

The pulmonary endothelium plays a crucial role in adaptation to extra-uterine life. Its two most important functions are to help reduce pulmonary vascular resistance and to facilitate the clearance of alveolar fluid.[21]

During fetal life, the endothelial cells are squat, have a narrow base on the subendothelium and a low ratio of surface to volume, with considerable overlap of lateral cell borders[22] (Fig. 7-4). The small arterial lumen offers a high resistance to flow. Pulmonary vascular resistance is probably kept high during fetal life due to a significant release of vasoconstrictor substances, including endothelin-1 and leucotrienes, and low basal release of vasodilators such as nitric oxide and prostaglandin I_2 in the presence of a low oxygen tension. A mechanically induced increase in pulmonary blood flow, or exposure to vasodilators such as a raised oxygen tension, prostaglandin I_2, and acetylcholine induces only transient vasodilation.[23]

Endothelial Permeability

During fetal life, the lung is filled with fluid produced by the alveolar epithelium.[24] The liquid is absorbed by the alveolar epithelium at birth. Fetal pulmonary endothelial intercellular junctions are complex and fenestrated, while being tighter and less complex in older babies, indicative of improved barrier function. The higher endothelial permeability in fetal pulmonary vessels is probably due to the combined actions of hypoxia and a high level of circulating endothelin-1, VEGF, and angiotensin II. Endothelin-1 induces endothelial permeability, and its receptor antagonists can prevent capillary leakage.[25,26]

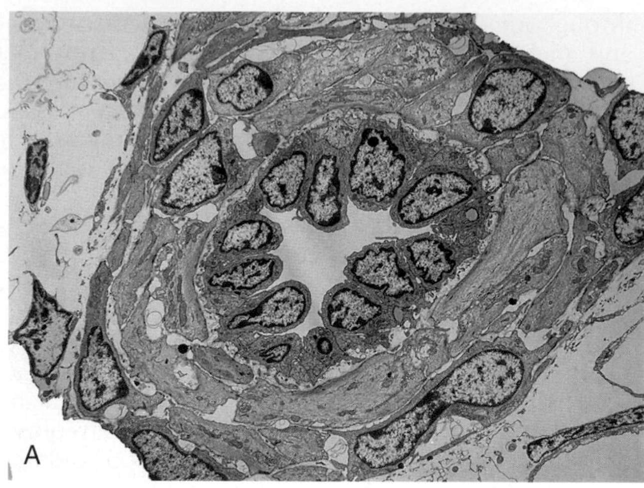

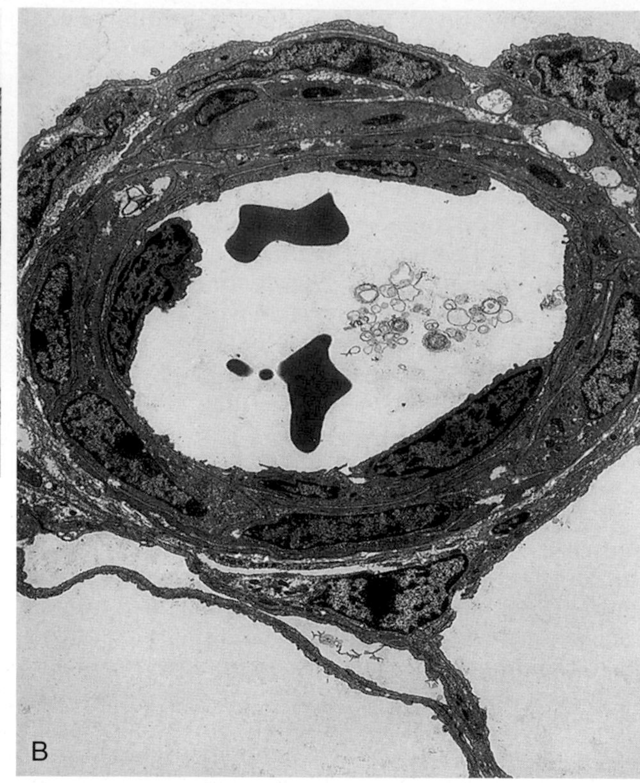

Figure 7-4 Electron micrographs of transverse sections through small muscular arteries, taken at the same magnification. **A,** Stillborn. **B,** At 5 minutes of age.

VEGF, originally identified as a vascular permeability factor, is a potent inducer of plasma extravasation. It is produced in large quantities during fetal development. Angiotensin II may affect endothelial permeability via the release of prostaglandins and VEGF.[27] By contrast, an increase in nitric oxide has been shown to prevent endothelial leakage in the lung. The postnatal increase in nitric oxide, and the simultaneous reduction in endothelin, may contribute to tightening of endothelial junctions after birth.[28] Rho GTPases play an important role in maintaining endothelial junctional integrity, emphasising the necessity of sustaining a high ratio of Rac1 to RhoA.[29]

The scaffolding proteins in the endothelial cell membrane may also change at birth, and contribute to the perinatal changes in endothelial barrier function. PECAM-1, also known as CD31, influences transendothelial migration of inflammatory cells, mechanosignal transduction, and angiogenesis.[30] Considerable amounts of this agent are expressed on fetal rat endothelial junctions, and expression decreases after birth when the barrier is formed between blood and gases. Caveolin-1 is a component of caveolas, an endothelial scaffolding protein which regulates the assembly of different signalling molecules at the plasma membrane.[31] Studies on doubly homozygous mice with caveolin-1 knocked out indicates that the protein plays a dual regulatory role in controlling lung microvascular permeability, acting as a structural protein required for formation of caveolas and caveolar transcytosis, and as a tonic inhibitor of eNOS negatively to regulate paracellular permeability.[32]

Ensuring the Postnatal Fall in Pulmonary Vascular Resistance

Immediately after birth, the pulmonary arterial smooth muscle undergoes remodelling of the cytoskeletal actin, changing shape and showing an increase in the ratio of surface to volume ratio so as to achieve an increase in luminal diameter.[33] There is a transient reduction in the content of actin, and disassembly of actin filaments, with an increase in monomeric G-actin. The smooth muscular phenotype is regulated by the transcription factor serum response, which is itself negatively regulated by YY1.[34] The brief postnatal reduction in filamentous actin causes YY1 to relocate from cytoplasm to nucleus, thereby inhibiting the expression of differentiation markers, and increasing the activity of cell cycle genes. These changes do not occur in the pulmonary hypertensive state.

The transition to breathing air stimulates several physiological actions, including drainage of fetal lung fluid, rhythmic distension of the lung, and an increase in oxygen tension, all of which contribute to the fall in pulmonary vascular resistance.[35,36] The pioneering studies of Dawes and colleagues in Oxford in the 1960s on fetal sheep showed that mechanical ventilation reduced pulmonary vascular resistance, and that the response was enhanced when the inspired gas was enriched with oxygen.[37] Forty years later, no single factor has yet been identified as being primarily responsible for the initiation of vasodilation at birth. Nor do we know whether the endothelial cell, or the smooth muscle cell, is the prime target. It is probable that the abrupt expansion of the lungs leads to a cascade of events that facilitate the activation of vasodilatory responses, and reduce vasoconstrictor stimuli from the endothelium. The onset of breathing is associated with an increase in circulating bradykinin, and the release of prostaglandin I_2 and nitric oxide.[38,39] The process is thought to be caused by the sudden increase in flow imposing a sheer stress on the endothelium to promote their release. Although the pathway involving nitric oxide appears to play a crucial role in regulating the vasoreactivity of the transitional circulation, it is not essential. Mice deficient in eNOS survive, and there is no evidence that either iNOS or nNOS compensates for the absence of eNOS.[40] Irrespective of the signalling pathway under consideration, it is generally assumed that the pulmonary arteries are solely responsible for the postnatal fall in resistance. This is unlikely, since the pulmonary veins are not passive conduits. Newborn porcine pulmonary veins respond to acetylcholine to a greater extent than do pulmonary arteries.[41]

Endothelial heterogeneity is evident even before birth. During embryonic development, the endothelial cells show high plasticity, and undergo constant changes in their expression of proteins to match the requirements of the developing vessel.[42,43] Heterogeneity is demonstrated in the newborn pulmonary circulation by the relaxant response to bradykinin, in which dependence on prostaglandin, nitric oxide, and a hyperpolarising factor differs in conduit and resistance arteries, and changes with age in each segment.[44,45] The regulation of these alternative signal transduction pathways in the immature normal and hypertensive pulmonary vasculature has still to be determined. Their tolerance to injury differs.

Role of Specific Mediators

Nitric Oxide

All three isoforms of nitric oxide synthase have been identified in the fetal lung.[46] Production of nitric oxide is regulated by transcription, post-transcriptional modification, availability of substrate, intracellular localisation, production of superoxides, and availability of co-factors.[47] Endothelial release is influenced by a variety of factors, including shear stress and tension of oxygen, which change dramatically at birth, and growth factors. The basal release of nitric oxide helps control resistance in the ovine fetal and transitional circulation.[48] Newborn isolated ovine and porcine conduit arteries and fetal and newborn porcine resistance arteries fail to relax to acetylcholine, the response maturing during the first 2 weeks of life.[23,44,49,50] By contrast, isolated fetal and newborn porcine pulmonary veins relax well in response to acetylcholine at birth, although like the arteries, the response improves with age.[41] Significant release of nitric oxide has also been demonstrated in newborn ovine pulmonary veins, possibly helping explain the experimental response of sheep to L-NAME, as noted above. A relatively poor receptor-mediated response is perhaps not surprising, given the marked changes occurring in the endothelial cell membrane as the ratio of surface to volume increases at birth. The density of muscarinic receptors increases rapidly immediately after birth, and the subtypes change.[51] But the relatively poor neonatal relaxant response is not restricted to receptor-dependant mechanisms, since the vessels do not relax in response to a calcium ionophore[49,50] Nor is the relatively poor endothelial-dependant relaxation at birth due to the pulmonary arterial smooth muscles cells being incapable of relaxation. The vessels relax in response to exogenous nitric oxide, although this response also improves significantly during the first 2 to 3 weeks of life.[49,50] There is no lack of nitric oxide synthase at birth. The expression of both the protein and the gene increases markedly towards term, and increases further to reach a maximum at 2 to 3 days of life. As in the adult, the predominant enzyme present at birth is the constitutive endothelial isoform.

There is no absolute or relative deficiency of the co-factor for nitric oxide synthase, BH4, at birth.[52] The efficacy of the enzyme, however, can be reduced by the action of endogenous inhibitors, primarily asymmetric dimethylarginine, which competes with the substrate L-arginine.[53] Levels of this inhibitor are high in amniotic fluid, increase towards term, and remain high in fetal blood. It would be expected to exert a significant tonic inhibitory effect on nitric oxide synthase at such concentrations. The inhibitor is certainly present in the urine of healthy newborn infants, and gradually declines to become undetectable by 5 days of age.[54] It is metabolised to citrulline by the dimethylarginine dimethylaminohydrolase enzymes, DDAH I and II, both of which are highly expressed in the fetal lung. Each isoform is developmentally regulated, and activity of the second increases rapidly immediately after birth.[55] Both asymmetric dimethylarginine and dimethylarginine dimethylaminohydrolase could play a significant role in the regulation of the fetal and newborn pulmonary vasculature.

The pulmonary arterial smooth muscle cell being targeted by the endothelium is itself changing rapidly. Basal accumulation of cGMP is high at birth, but falls rapidly to a lower adult level by 3 days of age.[50] This postnatal fall might be explained by the high expression of phosphodiesterase 5 (PDE5) and its hydrolytic activity found in the newborn rat lung.[56] Studies on lungs of several species also showed that PDE5 was responsible for a greater proportion of PDE activity during the first week of life than in the adult.[56,57] Despite the basal accumulation and enhanced accumulation of cyclic GMP in response to nitric oxide and its donors, the relaxation response of newborn vessels is less than might be expected. This might be accounted for by the smooth muscle cell membrane being more depolarised at birth than later.[58]

Prostacyclin

Metabolism of arachidonic acid metabolism within endothelial cells leads to the production of vasoactive eicosanoids, either prostaglandins or leucotrienes. The circulating concentration of vasoconstrictor leucotrienes C_4 and D_4 decreases at birth and that of endothelial-derived prostacyclin increases, facilitating relaxation of the smooth muscle cells. The receptor for prostacyclin belongs to the family of G-protein coupled receptors.[59] Its effects are mediated by cAMP, though there may also be a cAMP-independent coupling of the receptor to the activation of potassium channels, which are important in the relaxation of smooth muscle cells.[60] The levels of prostacyclin during early fetal life are low, and this effect may be attributed to the inhibitory action of plasma glucocorticoids on endothelial transcription of the COX-1 gene, and expression of COX via a glucocorticoid receptor.[61] Levels increase at birth, a change coinciding with increasing levels of oestrogen in the fetal plasma. Physiologic levels of estradiol 17 activate synthesis of prostacyclin.[62] We lack information, however, about the function of the different subtypes of the prostacyclin receptor during development. Whether prostacyclin is crucial to the postnatal reduction in pulmonary arterial pressure is still uncertain. Expression of prostacyclin synthase is low at birth, and increases rapidly in the first week of life. Synthesis is higher in newborn than fetal vessels in the sheep,[63] as COX-1 activity is upregulated. The sudden increase in shear stress at birth, and the fall in pulmonary vascular resistance, coincide with the increased release of nitric oxide and prostacyclin, suggesting that the two agents may act in concert to effect the vasodilatory action of shear stress. Although inhibition of nitric oxide blocks the vasodilation resulting from increased oxygen and rhythmic pulmonary distension, COX inhibitors also attenuate vasodilation caused by rhythmic distension.[64]

Endothelin

The level of circulating endothelin-1 is high in the normal fetus at term, and falls rapidly during the first week of life. Endothelial release of this potent vasoconstrictor is stimulated by hypoxia, the mechanical stimulation of shear stress and stretch, and chemical stimuli such as thrombin, norepinephrine, transforming growth factor-β, phorbol esters, and calcium ionophores. In the presence of high vascular tone, the agent has a vasodilatory effect, but similar infusions have a vasoconstrictor effect when pulmonary vascular tone is decreased during acute ventilation. It generally causes transient vasodilation followed by sustained vasoconstriction. It is abundant in the lung parenchyma and pulmonary arteries at birth, the expression decreasing initially, then increasing again, but at a lower level than in the newborn. Receptor binding sites are densely distributed over the smooth muscle cells of pulmonary vessels, with a relative increase in the B type with age. Between birth and 3 days, vasodilator receptors are transiently expressed on the pulmonary arterial endothelial cells.[65] This vasodilatory response to endothelin-1 increases after birth in both pulmonary arteries and veins.[66]

Angiotensin

The role of the vasoconstrictor angiotensin in the regulation of the perinatal circulation is not understood. It is first expressed on the endothelium of large proximal pulmonary arteries in the pseudoglandular stage of lung development, and extends distally during gestation.[67] Expression of angiotensin-converting enzyme is 10 times lower at birth than in the mature rat lung. The vasoconstricting effects of angiotensin are largely due to angiotensin-mediated increases in the production of endothelin-1,[68] suggesting that its release may decrease immediately after birth.

Failure to Adapt to Extra-uterine Life: Persistent Pulmonary Hypertension of the Newborn

This condition has a high morbidity, and the rate of mortality remains at up to one-fifth despite the advent of treatment with inhaled nitric oxide. The pulmonary arteries fail to remodel after birth, and the vessels remain thick walled. The condition can be idiopathic but is more usually associated with hypoxia. It is a feature of certain types of congenital cardiac disease. Hence, it is multi-factorial in origin, but the nature of the underlying defect causing failure to adapt is uncertain. It has been shown to involve failure of endothelial-dependent and -independent relaxation, a primary structural abnormality of the targeted smooth muscle cells, and an excess of endothelin, possibly also with an excess of other vasoconstrictor agonists such as thromboxane or an isoprostane. Hypoxia, a common cause of the condition, alters the endothelial metabolism of vasoactive agents, such as endothelial nitric oxide synthase, 5-hydroxytryptamine, and angiotensin-converting enzymes.[69–71] It also increases endothelial permeability, which facilitates leakage of growth factors and blood cells into the underlying layer of smooth muscle cells.[29]

Role of Specific Mediators

Nitric Oxide

Neonatal pulmonary hypertension affects both release of, and response to, nitric oxide in the pulmonary arteries.[41,50,72] Chronic hypoxia impairs endothelial calcium metabolism and normal coupling between the enzyme and caveolin-1, thus inactivating the enzyme.[69] Inappropriate postnatal persistence of an endogenous inhibitor of nitric oxide, such as ADMA, may also cause persistent pulmonary hypertension of the newborn, since it is known to persist at abnormally high levels after birth in such babies.[54] Arginine deficiency, absolute or relative, is a feature of the human infant with such persistent pulmonary hypertension, and an L-arginine infusion can be associated with an improvement in oxygenation.

Endothelin

The circulating levels of endothelin remain high in experimental models of hypoxia-induced persistent pulmonary hypertension. The density of binding of receptors, primarily the A type, is increased.[73] Co-constriction of pulmonary arteries and bronchuses is a well-recognised clinical feature of infants with pulmonary hypertension. Messenger RNA for preproendothelin was significantly elevated in fetal ovine lung tissue after ductal ligation during fetal life, and expression of the A type receptors was elevated.[74]

Prostacyclin

The release of this agent is reduced in many forms of pulmonary arterial hypertension in humans, and is assumed to be low in newborns with persistent pulmonary hypertension. Its administration alleviates hypoxic pulmonary vasoconstriction in both afflicted newborn infants and experimental animals. Systemic hypotension can occur when this medication is used in sick infants.

Activation of Rho GTPases

Rho GTPases are key regulators of endothelial actin dynamics, thereby influencing both vascular reactivity and endothelial permeability.[21] Activation of RhoA has been associated with the development of pulmonary hypertension,[8,75] possibly by mediating the effects of vasoconstrictors such as angiotensin II, endothelin-1, and acetylcholine, and downregulating the expression of endothelial nitric oxide synthase in endothelial cells, and hence the production of nitric oxide.[21]

Serotonin Fluoxetine

This selective inhibitor of the uptake of serotonin induced pulmonary hypertension in rats exposed to the drug during fetal life. Pulmonary arterial muscularity was increased.[76]

Endothelial Permeability in Pulmonary Hypertension

Endothelial leakage occurs in pulmonary hypertension, irrespective of aetiology. Inhalation of nitric oxide may prevent pulmonary oedema, by both improving the barrier function of the endothelium and enhancing vascular relaxation.[77] Overexpression of angiotensin-1 produces leakage-resistant vessels, and angiotensin-1 is protective when used experimentally.[78] Potential therapeutic approaches include inhibition of VEGF, RhoA, and other molecules.[79] The natural mediator sphingosine 1-phosphate activates Rac1, and has considerable therapeutic potential.[80]

Treatment

The aim is to control excessive reactivity and structural remodelling by using therapeutic agents which exploit the interactions between the signalling pathways controlling these events. Clinically, we rely on nitric oxide, inhibitors of phosphodiesterase 5, and less commonly, antagonists of the receptors to endothelin-1. Studies with guanylate cyclase activators are promising. Looking ahead, we know that in animal models the overexpression of vasodilator genes such as endothelial nitric oxide synthase, prepro-calcitonin gene-related peptide, and prostacyclin synthase, have produced promising results,[81] as has fasudil, the inhibitor of Rho kinase.[75] Statins might also be helpful, since they inhibit the prenylation and membrane translocation of Rho proteins, have anti-leakage and anti-inflammatory effects, and increase the availability of endothelial nitric oxide. Perhaps the most logical therapy would be an agent to open the potassium channels.

In summary, we are at last beginning to understand some of the mechanisms regulating pulmonary vascular development and function. Integrating clinical observations with experimental studies, taking advantage of gene targeting, and designing appropriate models of lung development present exciting challenges for the future.

PULMONARY CIRCULATION IN THE SETTING OF CONGENITALLY MALFORMED HEARTS

In children with congenitally malformed hearts, the pulmonary circulation may fail to develop normally, even before birth.

Abnormal Prenatal Development

Abnormalities of pulmonary vascular development arising during fetal life may be divided into primary developmental abnormalities that arise early in gestation and those that are probably secondary to haemodynamic changes caused by the presence of congenital heart disease and develop late in fetal life. Primary abnormalities include an absent right or left pulmonary artery, failure of some or all of the intrapulmonary arteries to connect exclusively with the central intrapericardial pulmonary arteries, a reduction in the number of generations of intrapulmonary arteries, and stenoses of the pulmonary arteries. These abnormalities may occur in children with a normal heart, when they are usually associated with disordered development of the airways. A persistent systemic arterial supply is a feature of a sequestrated segment of malformed hypoplastic lung. A reduction in the pulmonary arterial branching pattern is seen in the hypoplastic lung of renal agenesis and dysplasia, congenital diaphragmatic hernia, and rhesus isoimmunisation.[82–84] Pulmonary arterial stenoses occur in the rubella syndrome, with or without an associated intracardiac abnormality.

Absence of One Pulmonary Artery

Absence of one of the branches of the pulmonary trunk can occur in the presence of a patent pulmonary trunk when the pulmonary artery at the hilum is connected to a vessel arising from the ascending aorta or the aortic arch. This is sometimes known as a distal ductal origin of a pulmonary artery. Occasionally, the hilar pulmonary artery is connected to the right ventricle or aorta by an atretic thread in the position of a pulmonary trunk or arterial duct. In some cases, it is impossible at thoracotomy or postmortem to identify any such structure that might once have perfused the lung. In some children, serial angiographic studies show that the abnormality was acquired postnatally, usually in association with closure of the ducts. The intrapericardial pulmonary artery is then more correctly described as being interrupted rather than absent. Patients with tetralogy of Fallot are particularly vulnerable to such an acquired change. When no large systemic artery anastomoses with the hilar pulmonary artery, the pulmonary arterial supply is derived from an expanded bronchial circulation. When the intrapericardial pulmonary artery is absent or interrupted, however, the pulmonary artery is usually patent at the hilum, although it is frequently small. Consequently, all such patients should be regarded as potential candidates for correction by insertion of a prosthesis between the pulmonary trunk or right ventricle and the hilar pulmonary artery.

Failure of All Intrapulmonary Arteries to Connect Exclusively with the Intrapericardial Pulmonary Arteries

In the majority of patients with tetralogy of Fallot and pulmonary atresia, the lungs are perfused by large arteries arising from the aorta, called major systemic-to-pulmonary collateral arteries (Fig. 7-5).[85] Development of the airways is normal. The intrapericardial pulmonary arteries are usually present, although they may be extremely small, or even incompletely canalised. Systemic-to-pulmonary collateral arteries are usually easily distinguishable from the enlarged bronchial arteries seen after birth in several types of congenital disease characterised by a low flow of blood to the lungs. The distinction is, however, sometimes blurred. Occasionally, arteries as large as major collateral arteries appear to have a similar origin from the aorta as do bronchial arteries, and then connect with intrapulmonary

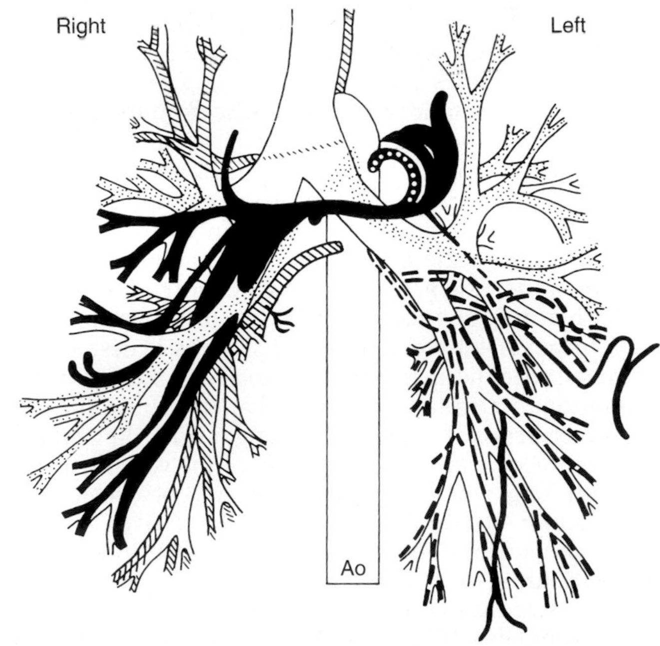

Figure 7-5 The pulmonary arterial branching pattern seen in pulmonary atresia with ventricular septal defect and major aortopulmonary collateral arteries. The solid lines indicate the central pulmonary arteries and their branches, and the cross-hatched, stippled, interrupted, and dotted lines indicate the collateral arteries and the intrapulmonary arteries with which they connect. Ao, aorta. (From Haworth SG, Macartney FJ: Growth and development of the pulmonary circulation in pulmonary atresia with ventricular septal defect and major aortopulmonary collateral arteries. Br Heart J 1980:44:14–24.)

arteries to supply the lung. If, as seems probable, pulmonary and bronchial arteries have a common origin from the embryonic pulmonary plexus, this is not surprising. In the presence of collateral arteries, the source of arterial supply to the lungs is frequently complex, and varies in different patients. The complexity of their connections with the intrapulmonary arteries, and with each other, therefore, is also not surprising. In children with tetralogy and pulmonary atresia, a collateral artery may connect with a pulmonary artery at the hilum, and so perfuse both lungs if the intrapericardial pulmonary arteries are patent (see Fig. 7-5). Alternatively, a collateral artery may anastomose end-to-end with a lobar or segmental pulmonary artery and have no connection with the intrapericardial pulmonary arteries at either the hilum or within the lung. More than one collateral artery may perfuse the same intrapulmonary artery at the hilum, which is then said to have a duplicate, or dual, blood supply. Collateral arteries that do not connect with an intrapericardial or hilar pulmonary artery run to the hilum of the lung and then accompany a lobar bronchus until they anastomose with an intrapulmonary artery. As a result, a vessel that has the basic structure of a muscular systemic artery becomes a vessel with the structure of an elastic pulmonary artery.[86] The pulmonary artery then branches with the airways in a normal manner to perfuse the capillary bed, as in the normal lung. Different bronchopulmonary segments within a lobe may be connected to several different vessels, some segments being connected to an intrapericardial pulmonary artery, and others connecting directly with collateral arteries. Several arteries may, therefore, accompany the main and lobar bronchuses. On angiography, the orderly appearance of one pulmonary artery accompanying each bronchus is lost. The only method of ensuring that the anatomy is understood in each patient is to account for the arterial supply of each bronchopulmonary segment, look for sources of a duplicate supply to each segment, and search for connections between different collateral arteries.

The collateral arteries commonly arise from the descending thoracic aorta behind the origin of the left main bronchus in the presence of a left aortic arch, and almost in the midline when the arch is on the right. They may also arise from beneath the aortic arch and, less commonly, from below the diaphragm above the coeliac axis. They frequently divide near their aortic origin. Collateral arteries are commonly stenosed where they anastomose with a hilar or intrapulmonary artery. In postnatal life, a degree of stenosis is desirable to reduce the systemic arterial pressure to a level more suited to the pulmonary circulation. Collateral arteries, however, may be severely stenosed either at their origin from the aorta or, more commonly, in the mid-portion of the vessel between aorta and lung, where the lumen may even be occluded by large mounds of proliferating intimal tissue (Figs. 7-6 and 7-7). It is not uncommon for children to become increasingly cyanosed during the first months of life, probably as a result of progressive intimal proliferation in the collateral arteries. Occasionally, children are born with minute intrapericardial and intrapulmonary arteries, and small or occluded collateral arteries. Multiple systemic-to-pulmonary collateral arteries seen in infants are best regarded as precarious fetal connections. Within the lung, the development of the pre- and intra-acinar arteries before and after birth depends on the lumen diameter of the perfusing vessels.

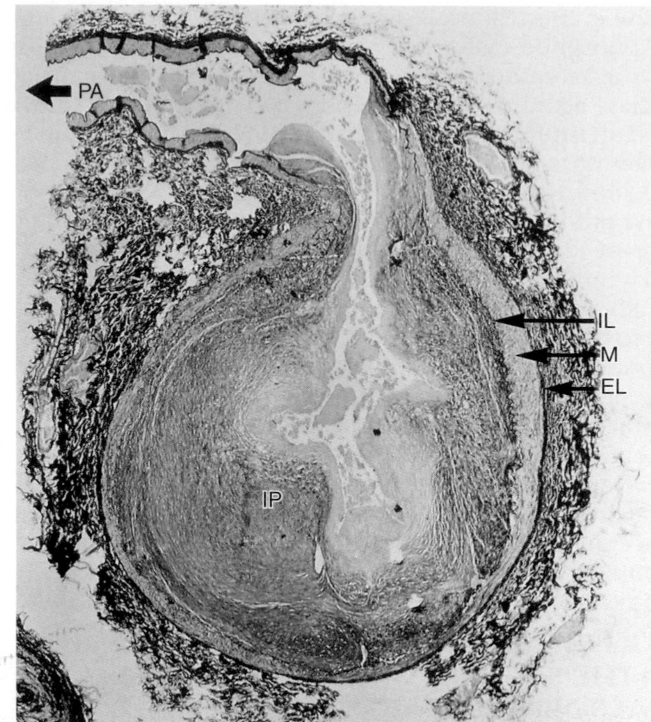

Figure 7-6 Transverse section of the mid-portion of a collateral artery at a region of segmental narrowing. The lumen of this muscular artery is almost totally obliterated by intimal proliferation (IP) and cushion formation and a layer of amorphous material containing no elastic tissue. EL, external elastic lamina; IL, internal elastic lamina; M, media; PA, pulmonary artery. (Miller's elastic stain.)

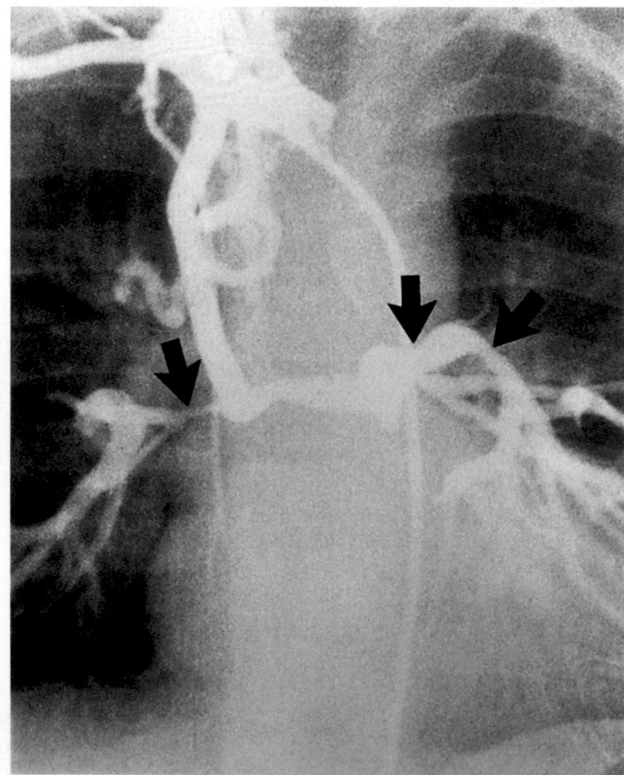

Figure 7-7 Post-operative injection into aortopulmonary anastomosis shows central pulmonary arteries, stenoses (*arrows*) and aneurysmal dilation at origin of left upper and lower lobe arteries; it also shows that central vessels perfuse only a minority of bronchopulmonary segments.

Most infants with tetralogy and pulmonary atresia suffer from the effects of hypoperfusion. Occasionally, the collateral arteries have a more elastic mural structure, being large vessels that provide a good, or even excessive, blood supply to the lung. Such patients present later. Large collateral arteries expose the distal intrapulmonary arteries to a high pressure, which can lead to the development of pulmonary vascular obstructive disease. When the lungs are perfused by an arterial duct, all the intrapulmonary arteries are usually connected to the hilum. A duct may, however, connect with a hilar pulmonary artery to perfuse some bronchopulmonary segments, while major systemic-to-pulmonary collateral arteries provide the only blood supply to other segments. Supply through bilaterally persistent arterial ducts can also be found.

Approximately two-thirds of patients present in infancy; at presentation, half are severely cyanosed and one-quarter are in heart failure.[87] In hypoperfused patients, the aim of surgery is to increase the supply to encourage growth of both intrapericardial and peripheral pulmonary arteries. All, or at least most, bronchopulmonary segments in each lung should connect, or be made to connect by unifocalisation, to an intrapericardial pulmonary artery or conduit, either as a prelude to, or at the time of, definitive repair. Collaterals should not be ligated unless an alternative source of arterial supply can be demonstrated. Since the anatomy is exceedingly variable, management must be individually tailored to each patient. The anatomy should be defined at presentation and the long-term management planned accordingly. Staged surgical procedures may be required to make a patient a candidate for complete repair. The morphological substrate is the limiting factor, and some patients will do better for longer without surgical intervention and eventually be candidates for transplantation.

Developmental Abnormalities of the Intrapulmonary Arteries

The various types of congenital cardiac disease may be regarded as vicarious experiments in which to study the relationship between changes in pulmonary arterial pressure and flow and structural development. Aortic valvar atresia, or critical stenosis, and pulmonary atresia with an intact ventricular septum, cause different and almost diametrically opposite structural abnormalities of the intra-acinar pulmonary arteries. In critical aortic stenosis or atresia, the entire cardiac output is ejected into the pulmonary trunk, and the body is perfused by the arterial duct. During fetal life, there is an increase in pulmonary arterial muscularity, and the number of intra-acinar arteries per unit area of lung may be increased.[88] At birth, the babies have severe pulmonary hypertension. It is now well established that those undergoing the Norwood sequence of operations can subsequently be converted to the Fontan circulation, indicating a marked reduction in pulmonary vascular resistance. By contrast, children with pulmonary atresia in whom the arterial duct is the only source of blood supply to the lung are born with abnormally small thin-walled pre- and intra-acinar arteries, and may have a reduction in the number of intra-acinar arteries.[89] Before birth, the pressure generated by the left ventricle is probably not transmitted to the pulmonary circulation across the rather small, abnormally angulated duct found in these patients. When the duct is relatively large, however, pulmonary arterial muscularity develops normally and intra-acinar arterial multiplication is almost normal.

Babies with totally anomalous pulmonary venous connection who present with obstructed venous return during the first week of life may show a marked increase in muscularity of both intra-pulmonary arteries and veins.[90,91] The findings are consistent with prenatal obstruction to pulmonary venous return. In those with the infradiaphragmatic type of anomaly, the descending vein can be narrowed or even occluded by fibrous tissue at birth. Also, the extrapulmonary veins may be smaller than normal and show intimal proliferation. Within the lungs, the increased muscularity is potentially reversible. In the extrapulmonary veins, however, prenatal obstruction may instigate intimal proliferation and fibrosis that can progress despite a technically successful operation. Post-operative stenosis then develops at some distance from the suture lines. Patients with the infradiaphragmatic type of anomaly are particularly vulnerable.

These findings in the pulmonary circulation of patients with aortic atresia or stenosis, pulmonary atresia, and totally anomalous pulmonary venous connection demonstrate the vulnerability of the fetal pulmonary circulation to changes in pressure and flow, and show how the structural changes in the lung can prejudice survival.

Effects of Pulmonary Hypoperfusion

The effects of hypoperfusion on the developing pulmonary circulation may be as deleterious as those of hyperperfusion. The intrapericardial pulmonary arteries may be minute. The proximal elastic arteries may contain less elastin than normal, while the intra-acinar arteries are usually smaller, and have a thinner muscle coat, than normal. Pulmonary arterial thrombosis can occur, leading to eccentric areas of intimal fibrosis, characterised by a peculiar form of recanalisation in which strands of fibrous tissue of varying thickness divide the arterial lumen into several channels. The aetiology and incidence of thrombotic lesions is uncertain, but they are thought to relate to the degree of polycythaemia. Enlargement of the bronchial arterial circulation to supplement, or even to replace, a normal pulmonary arterial blood supply occurs in many forms of cyanotic congenital heart disease, such as tetralogy of Fallot and pulmonary atresia. An enlarged bronchial arterial circulation is rarely found in newborn infants with an abnormally low pulmonary blood flow. Infants with pulmonary atresia and intact ventricular septum die when the duct closes because the bronchial arterial circulation is not sufficiently enlarged at that time. In older patients with tetralogy and pulmonary atresia, an enlarged bronchial arterial circulation is frequently seen at angiography. Serial cardiac catheterisation studies in such patients frequently show progressive enlargement of the bronchial arterial circulation. When the lung is severely hypoperfused, the development of the alveoluses can be impaired. Postmortem lung volume is reduced in children dying of tetralogy of Fallot. Performing a corrective operation before the end of the critical period of growth of the lung presumably encourages normal alveolar development. In addition, an early repair permits greater physical activity. In normal children, physical training increases total lung volume and vital capacity. Fortunately, the full impact of pulmonary hypoperfusion on the developing lung is rarely seen nowadays, since the flow can be increased as early as is necessary by medical or surgical treatment, be it palliative or corrective.

Growth of small pulmonary arteries is encouraged by surgically increasing the flow of blood through them for some time before performing the definitive repair. Whether the arteries will grow sufficiently to permit definitive repair depends upon their initial size, surgical expertise in increasing flow through them, and the extent of peripheral run-off. The potential for growth of both intrapericardial and peripheral pulmonary arteries is uncertain. Increased distensibility of a vessel consequent upon an increase in flow must be distinguished from growth. While in the reported studies the magnitude of the response and the relatively long time interval between operation and restudy suggests that growth has indeed occurred, we do not know whether or not these vessels will grow sufficiently to achieve a size appropriate to the size of the lung and that of the child. That the growth potential may not be normal is suggested by the abnormal structure of the wall of extrapulmonary vessels when pulmonary blood flow is low, abnormalities which change the mechanical properties of the wall and, hence, their physical response to an increase in flow.

PULMONARY HYPERTENSION

Pulmonary hypertension is a condition which causes immense suffering. A modest elevation in pulmonary arterial pressure is tolerable, but a high pressure is associated with obstructive pulmonary vascular disease leading to right-sided failure and death. The scene has changed so dramatically since the millennium. Improved diagnostic techniques facilitate assessment, and we now have a clinically useful classification (Table 7-1). Pulmonary arterial hypertension is subdivided into the idiopathic and familial form and the pulmonary hypertension associated with other disorders, such as congenital cardiac disease. For those with established pulmonary vascular disease, discoveries of therapeutic agents have revolutionised management. They do not, however, cure the basic problem of pulmonary vascular disease.

Pulmonary hypertension itself is defined as a mean pressure within the pulmonary arteries equal to or greater than 25 mm Hg at rest, or 30 mm Hg on exercise, a definition which applies to all but the youngest infants.

The commonest causes of pulmonary hypertension in children are congenital heart disease and persistent pulmonary hypertension of the newborn. Children can also suffer from idiopathic pulmonary arterial hypertension, previously known as primary pulmonary hypertension. The patient is said to be suffering from the idiopathic form when there is no identifiable explanation for the increase in pulmonary arterial pressure. Idiopathic pulmonary arterial hypertension has been the subject of intense research because it is the most pure form of pulmonary hypertension, and new medicines have been evaluated and studied in this condition.

Pulmonary Hypertension in Those with Congenitally Malformed Hearts

Diagnosis of unrepaired congenital cardiac malformations calls for experienced assessment of likely operative outcomes, particularly the risk of acute post-operative and of long-term sustained pulmonary hypertension with continued evolution of pulmonary vascular disease.

TABLE 7-1

CLASSIFICATION OF PULMONARY HYPERTENSION AS PROPOSED IN VENICE IN 2003

1. Pulmonary arterial hypertension (PAH)
   - 1.1 Idiopathic (IPAH)
   - 1.2 Familial (FIPAH)
   - 1.3 Associated with (APAH)
     - 1.3.1 Connective tissue disease
     - 1.3.2 Congenital systemic-to-pulmonary shunts
     - 1.3.3 Portal hypertension
     - 1.3.4 HIV
     - 1.3.5 Drugs and toxins
     - 1.3.6 Other (thyroid disorders, glycogen storage disease, Gaucher's disease, hereditary haemorrhagic telangiectasia, haemoglobinopathies, myeloproliferative disorders, splenectomy)
   - 1.4 Associated with significant venous or capillary involvement
     - 1.4.1 Pulmonary veno-occlusive disease
     - 1.4.2 Pulmonary capillary haemangiomatosis
   - 1.5 Persistent pulmonary hypertension of the newborn
2. Pulmonary hypertension associated with left heart diseases
   - 2.1 Left-sided atrial or ventricular disease
   - 2.2 Left-sided valvular heart disease
3. Pulmonary hypertension associated with respiratory disease and/or hypoxia
   - 3.1 Chronic obstructive pulmonary disease
   - 3.2 Interstitial lung disease
   - 3.3 Sleep disordered breathing
   - 3.4 Alveolar hypoventilation disorders
   - 3.5 High altitude
   - 3.6 Developmental abnormalities
4. Pulmonary hypertension due to chronic thrombotic/embolic disease
   - 4.1 Thromboembolic obstruction of proximal pulmonary arteries
   - 4.2 Thromboembolic obstruction of distal pulmonary arteries
   - 4.3 Non-thrombotic pulmonary embolism (tumour, parasites, foreign material)
5. Miscellaneous
   - Sarcoidosis, histiocytosis X, lymphangiomatosis, compression of pulmonary vessels (adenopathy, tumour, fibrosing mediastinitis)

From Simonneau G, Galie N, Rubin LJ, et al: Clinical classification of pulmonary hypertension. J Am Coll Cardiol 2004;43(12 Suppl S):5S-12S.

Pre-operative Assessment of the Hypertensive Pulmonary Circulation

The cardiologist is constantly trying to predict the structural changes present in the lungs from the clinical, radiological, and haemodynamic findings without having to resort to a biopsy of the lung. Prediction can be difficult.

The clinical history is important. Cardiac failure may appear to improve as pulmonary vascular resistance increases. High flow of blood to the lungs is frequently associated with recurrent infections of the respiratory tract. Dilated pulmonary arteries compress the main and lobar bronchuses in children with and without pulmonary hypertension, leading to the familiar problem of recurrent collapse of different lobes or segments of lung. Not infrequently, the respiratory complications of congenital cardiac disease constitute an indication for corrective surgery in infancy. After operation, the bronchial deformity may persist for some time. Indeed, in some patients, prolonged compression appears to be associated with bronchomalacia. Rarely, babies may present to the paediatrician with a history of episodic collapse, indicative of pulmonary hypertensive crises. A labile pulmonary vasculature in the presence of an intact ventricular septum can be hazardous before as well as after surgical intervention. The extent of the problem is unknown.

The chest radiograph is reassuringly plethoric when the resistance is sufficiently low to permit a high flow to the lungs, and it is depressingly evident when pulmonary vascular disease is advanced. The development of severe obstructive disease in the muscular pulmonary arteries leads to peripheral pruning and a hypertranslucent appearance in association with dilation of the hilar and proximal vessels. Wedge angiography is not widely used, but it is helpful in demonstrating advanced pulmonary vascular obstructive disease, and should always be used in concert with other examinations in assessing whether the patient may still be able to undergo corrective surgery. If performed by balloon occlusion, the abnormal pulmonary wedge angiogram is characterised by decreased arborisation, reduced background opacification, and delayed venous filling. The arteries may appear tortuous, have segments of dilation or constriction, and have marginal defects suggestive of obliterative disease. Quantitative wedge angiography represents an attempt to improve the correlation between structure and function.[92] In the normal lung, the pulmonary arteries taper towards the periphery, but the vessels narrow over a shorter distance in the presence of an elevated pulmonary vascular resistance.

Pulmonary arterial pressure can be estimated non-invasively by Doppler ultrasound, but resistance cannot. At cardiac catheterisation, the lowest determinations of pulmonary arterial pressure and vascular resistance are conventionally accepted as a guide to outcome. This is based on the premise that, if the predominant structural abnormality in the pulmonary circulation is an increase in muscularity, it will respond to vasodilator substances. To this end, the patient is usually given nitric oxide. With any vasodilator, the release of vasoconstrictor tone will lower pulmonary vascular resistance and increase the magnitude of the left-to-right shunt, and may lower the pulmonary arterial pressure. Failure to achieve this response implies fixed and organic obstruction of the pulmonary circulation. Children with Down syndrome are particularly difficult to assess because they often suffer from obstruction of the upper airways, which may contribute to the increased pulmonary vascular resistance determined at cardiac catheterisation. The pathologist will then find less pulmonary vascular damage in a lung biopsy than expected for the increase in pulmonary arterial pressure and resistance. The use of oxygen to calculate vasoreactivity is usually more problematic than the use of nitric oxide. In both cases, consumption of oxygen should be measured, and dissolved oxygen should be taken into account when oxygen is added to nitric oxide to test reactivity.

The structural abnormalities present in the lung can usually be predicted from the type of intracardiac abnormality, the age of the child, and the haemodynamic findings at cardiac catheterisation. In more complex cardiac abnormalities, and if there is ever doubt about the likely outcome of intracardiac repair, an open lung biopsy should help clarify the position. It is also helpful in predicting prognosis even if the decision is taken to go ahead with the corrective operation.

Development of Pulmonary Vascular Disease

Children are occasionally born with pulmonary vascular disease, but this is rare. Pulmonary vascular disease usually starts at birth with abnormal postnatal remodelling, abnormal muscularisation of distal pulmonary arteries, and a reduction in the number of vessels. This is followed by obstructive intimal proliferation, and ultimately to formation of plexiform lesions if the pulmonary arterial pressure is allowed to remain high (Fig. 7-8). Current thinking is that endothelial injury leads to programmed cell death and loss of small vessels. Endothelial injury is manifest as impaired endothelial dependent relaxation, defective levels of von Willebrand factor[93] and fibrinolysis. The progressive thickening of the wall of the more proximal intra-acinar and pre-acinar muscular arteries, and the obliteration associated with neointimal formation, has been related to heightened proliferation and migration of cells that have markers of smooth muscle cells because they are positive for α-smooth muscle actin. These cells may represent a specialised subpopulation, have originated as stem cells or fibrocytes, may be transformed fibroblasts or endothelial cells, or all of the above. With progressive obstruction, plexiform lesions develop. Endothelial proliferation is characteristic of this lesion, leading to the formation of aberrant channels in the obliterated lumen and in the adventitia. These lesions are thought to reflect clonal expansion of an endothelial cell resistant to death,[94] or of

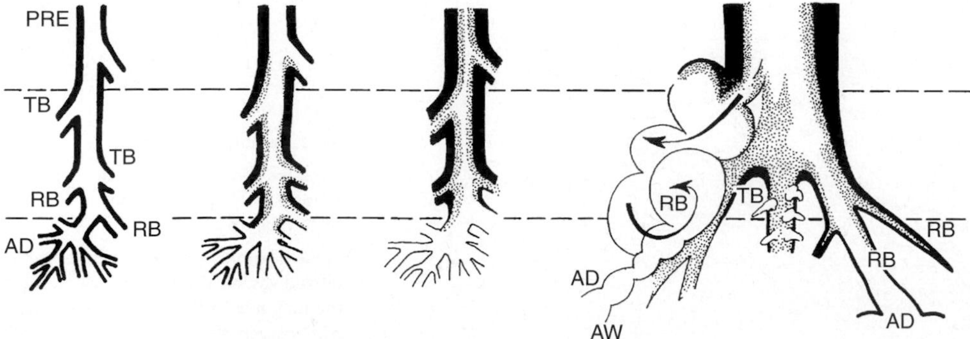

Figure 7-8 The end of four arterial pathways from the pre-acinar (PRE) and terminal bronchiolar arteries (TB) to the intra-acinar respiratory bronchiolar (RB) and alveolar duct (AD) arteries, showing the gradual development of intimal proliferation (stippling) associated with a progressive increase in wall thickness of pre-acinar arteries and decrease in alveolar wall (AW) thickness of intra-acinar arteries until dilation lesions develop. The upper interrupted line indicates the plane of section of satisfactory biopsies, and the lower line the plane of section of biopsies taken too close to the pleura to sample the distal pre-acinar and all the intra-acinar vessels.

circulating endothelial progenitor cells. Pulmonary arterial endothelial cells from patients with idiopathic pulmonary hypertension are known to produce decreased amounts of nitric oxide on the basis of high levels of arginase, show exaggerated proliferation in response to growth factors, and exhibit high rates of glycolysis.[95] Additional pathological features include thickening of the pulmonary adventitial layers and venous hypertrophy. Immunohistochemical studies have revealed increased expression of transforming growth factor beta (TGF-β), matrix proteins such as collagen, elastin, fibronectin, tenascin-C, and glycosaminoglycans, macrophages, and T cells, as well as agents associated with inflammation, such as S100A4/Mts1 and fractalkine.[96]

The intimal obstruction to flow is strategically placed at the entrance to each respiratory unit (see Fig. 7-8). As in transposition with ventricular septal defect, such obstruction can increase resistance to flow during the first months of life.[97] In babies, these changes occur before the development of marked intimal fibrosis, and other features characteristic of advanced pulmonary vascular disease in older patients, have had time to develop. Intimal proliferation in infants is cellular rather than fibrous. The cells are loosely organised rather than being arranged in a neat circumferential fashion, and the onionskin picture of laminar intimal fibrosis is uncommon. Even in older children, fibrinoid necrosis and arteritis are rare findings. As intimal proliferation increases in severity in the small muscular arteries, it narrows the lumen, and the medial thickness of the more peripheral respiratory unit arteries decreases (Fig. 7-9). The transitory near-normal appearance of the peripheral intra-acinar arteries can be misleading, because it reflects the severity of more proximal obstruction in patients with a high pressure and resistance. In order to interpret a lung biopsy with confidence, therefore, it is important that the biopsy be sufficiently deep to include some of the pre-acinar and terminal bronchiolar arteries in which intimal proliferation first develops.[98] The appearance of these arteries is crucial to the evaluation of the intra-acinar arteries beyond. If pre-acinar arteries are not present in the specimen, however, a mean medial thickness of less than one-sixth in arteries from 50 to 100 μm in diameter, particularly when associated with respiratory unit arteries slightly larger than normal for age, is suspicious of pre-dilation in patients with severe pulmonary hypertension and elevated resistance. This stage in the evolution of pulmonary vascular disease is associated with an increase in mortality and morbidity at and after intracardiac repair. The number of intra-acinar arteries is reduced in the presence of severe pulmonary hypertension. Ultrastructural examination reveals many occluded vessels.[99] This is an early change and can be seen in young infants in the presence of a low resistance. Whether there is also a primary failure of postnatal angiogenesis is unknown. When the pulmonary arterial pressure remains elevated after birth, whatever the reason, the structure of the pulmonary trunk retains its fetal appearance, and contains long, thick elastin fibres. If pulmonary hypertension develops later in life, the pulmonary trunk becomes thicker through the deposition of connective tissue, and smooth muscle cells are hypertrophic in a normally adapted vessel.

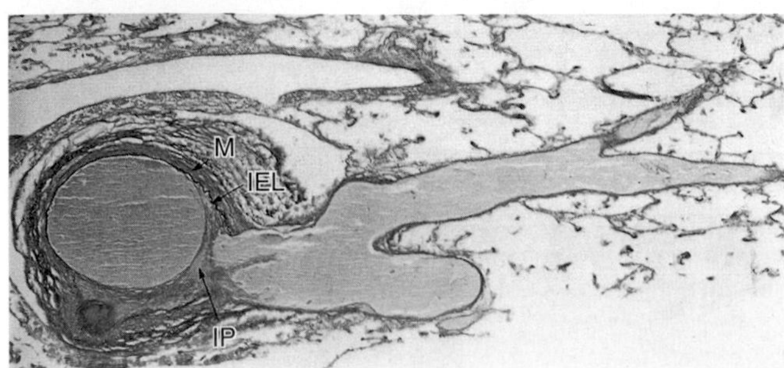

Figure 7-9 Photomicrograph of the lung of a 5-month-old infant with transposition and ventricular septal defect showing a terminal bronchiolar artery, distended by injection medium, having a thick media (M). Intimal proliferation (IP) surrounds the origin of the thin-walled branches. IEL, internal elastic lumina. (×130.)

Classification of Pulmonary Vascular Disease

In 1958, Heath and Edwards published their classical papers on the evolution of pulmonary vascular disease.[100–102] They classified pulmonary vascular disease into six grades, in order of increasing severity (Table 7-2). The structural features of each grade were related to measurements of pulmonary arterial pressure, flow, resistance and patient outcome. In Figures 7-10 and 7-11, we illustrate the first three grades, and in Figure 7-12, we show the features of the transitional fourth grade. Although the first three grades reflect a succession of structural changes, the subsequent grades probably do not. Necrotizing arteritis can precede the development of plexiform lesions. None of the advanced lesions carries a more severe prognosis than the others, save for the plexiform lesion. All the patients with congenital cardiac disease studied initially by Heath and Edwards were at least 10 months of age. Younger patients were excluded from the analysis because the lungs showed less structural change

TABLE 7-2

GRADING CLASSIFICATION FOR PULMONARY VASCULAR DISEASE

Grade	Structural Features	Characteristics
I	Medial hypertrophy	High resistance, high reserve pulmonary vascular bed still labile
II	Medial hypertrophy with cellular intimal proliferation	
III	Progressive fibrous occlusion	
IV	Progressive generalized arterial dilation with the formation of complex dilation lesions	Transitional stage
V	Chronic dilation with numerous dilated vessels throughout the lung plus pulmonary haemosiderosis	High resistance, low reserve pulmonary vascular bed no longer labile because of luminal occlusion
VI	Fibrinoid necrosis of the media Arterial dilation with the formation of complex dilation lesions	

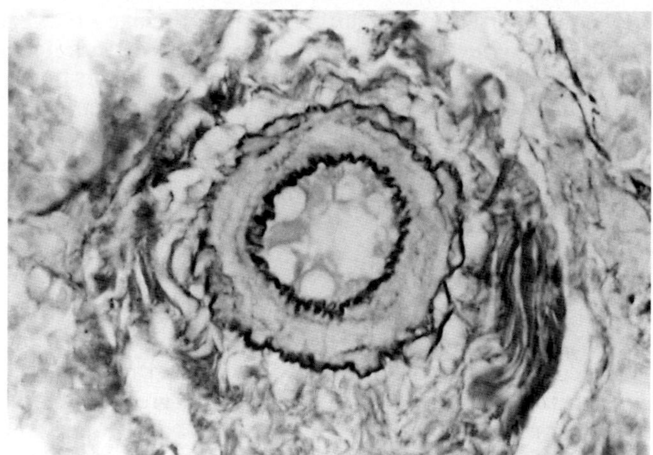

Figure 7-10 Photomicrograph of lung tissue from a 3-month-old child with a ventricular septal defect, showing severe medial hypertrophy. (×496.)

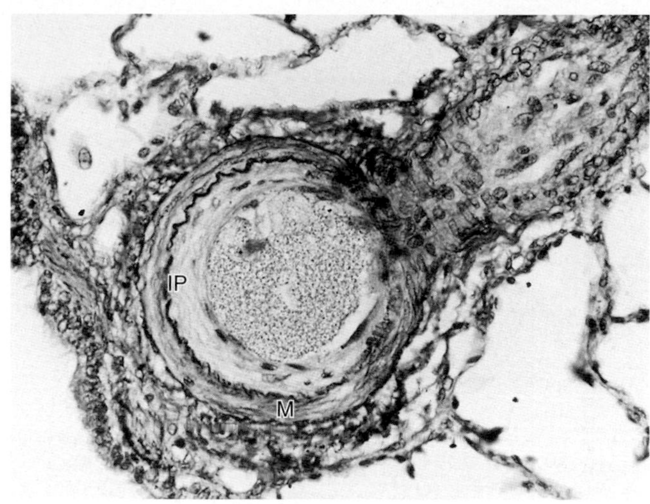

Figure 7-12 Photomicrograph of lung tissue from an 11-month-old child with a common arterial trunk. Injection medium distends an artery, showing medial hypertrophy (M) with circumferential intimal proliferation (IP). (×267.)

than was expected for the elevation in pulmonary vascular resistance. A more recent classification[103] concentrates on the early structural changes when medial hypertrophy is developing, before fibrotic intimal damage appears. All classifications have their limitations and the biopsy findings in any individual must be interpreted in the light of the clinical picture in that patient. Medial hypertrophy is usually associated with a low pulmonary vascular resistance and is potentially reversible. In young children, resistance may be high, and the children may die after a technically successful intracardiac repair because the pulmonary arterial pressure is high, either continuously or sporadically; the episode is then described as a pulmonary hypertensive crisis. Medial hypertrophy, although a potentially reversible lesion, is not necessarily a safe lesion. At the other extreme, extensive dilation plus the other features of classical pulmonary vascular disease of the sixth grade are invariably associated with a high resistance and a poor prognosis. In practice, however, most patients fall between the two extremes. The use of a semiquantitative descriptive analysis of arterial mural structure, combined with quantitative morphometry of arterial muscularity and size, has helped identify a high-risk pre-dilation phase of pulmonary vascular disease, seen most often in children younger than 2 years.[98]

Evolution of Pulmonary Vascular Disease in Common Types of Congenital Cardiac Disease

In children with severe pulmonary hypertension, the rate of development of pulmonary vascular change depends upon the type of intracardiac abnormality (Fig. 7-13). For example, both a large isolated ventricular septal defect and one associated with discordant ventriculo-arterial connections cause pulmonary hypertension, but while the former rarely causes severe pulmonary vascular disease during the first year, the latter causes irreparable damage.

Ventricular Septal Defect

In children with a hypertensive ventricular septal defect, the peripheral pulmonary vasculature fails to develop normally after birth[98] (Fig. 7-14). Pulmonary arterial muscularity increases in both pre- and intra-acinar arteries from early

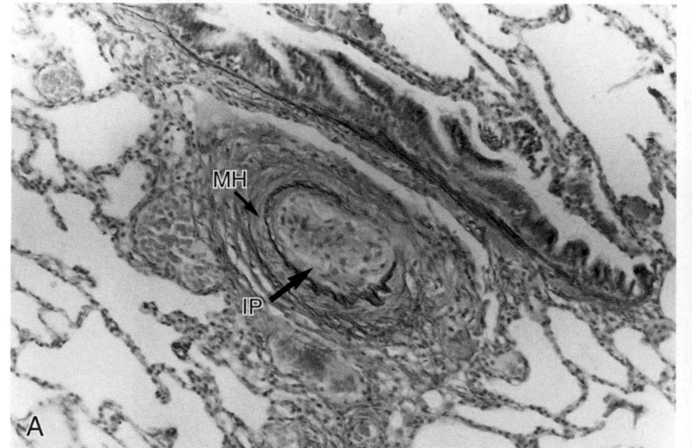

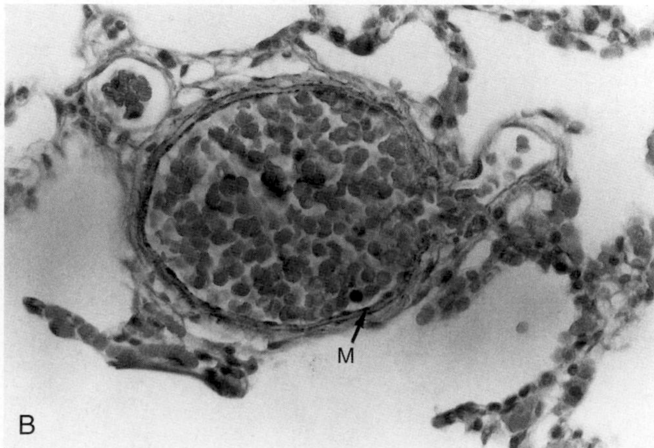

Figure 7-11 Photomicrographs of the lung biopsy of a child aged 19 months who had a ventricular septal defect and a mean pulmonary arterial pressure of 51 mm Hg, and died at operation. **A**, Cellular intimal proliferation (IP) in an artery accompanying a respiratory bronchiolus. **B**, A more peripheral vessel accompanying an alveolar duct. Note absence of medial hypertrophy. M, media; MH, medial hypertrophy.

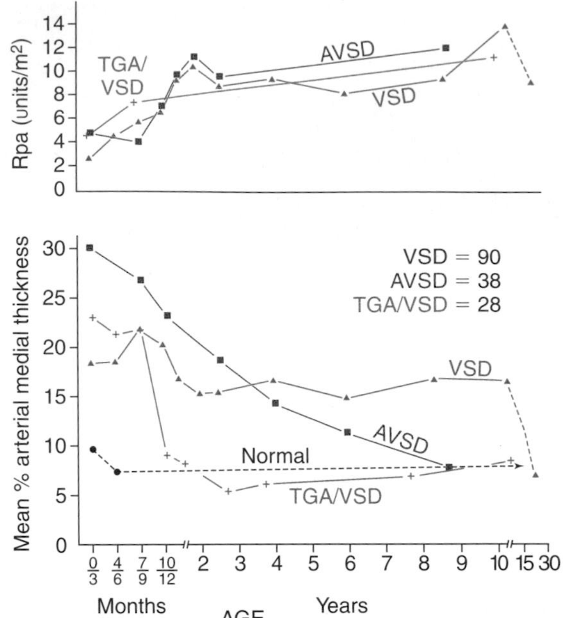

Figure 7-13 The mean percentage arterial medial thickness is given by 2(medial thickness) (external diameter) × 100. The figure shows its value in arteries 50–100 μm in diameter at various ages in 90 children with a ventricular septal defect (VSD), in 38 with an atrioventricular septal defect (AVSD), and in 28 with complete transposition and ventricular septal defect (TGA/VSD).

infancy. Occluded alveolar walls are seen on electron microscopic examination. Intimal proliferation tends to develop towards the end of the first year, and fibrosis during the third year of life. Patients with severe pulmonary hypertension should therefore undergo surgery before the age of 1 year. A few children develop severe early obstructive intimal proliferation, with the arteries beyond the obstruction having a relatively normal arterial medial thickness. This finding is associated with a pulmonary arteriolar resistance greater than 6 units/m^2 in the absence of the generalised arterial dilation or other stigmas of pulmonary vascular disease of the fourth grade.

Transposition

In the days before Rashkind septostomy, the average life expectancy was 1.3 months in cyanotic babies with transposition and an intact ventricular septum.[104] Those with a ventricular septal defect survived longer because a higher effective pulmonary blood flow ensures a greater systemic arterial saturation. The presence of a large ventricular septal defect, however, leads to the rapid development of severe pulmonary vascular disease. Persistent patency of the arterial duct also leads to the early development of pulmonary vascular disease. A duct should be closed surgically at 3 months of age if it has not closed spontaneously. In transposition as a whole, outcome correlates with the pulmonary arterial pressure.[105] With transposition and an intact ventricular septum, the pulmonary circulation usually adapts normally to extrauterine life. The bronchial circulation is enlarged, making a large but unknown contribution to total flow of blood to the lungs. Angiography suggests that the bronchial flow is high from birth. An enlarged bronchial circulation can sometimes persist after successful intracardiac repair. In the presence of a large ventricular septal defect, the pulmonary vasculature does not remodel normally after birth, and this failure to remodel marks the onset of pulmonary vascular obstructive disease[106] (see Figs. 7-9 and 7-13). Intimal proliferation is

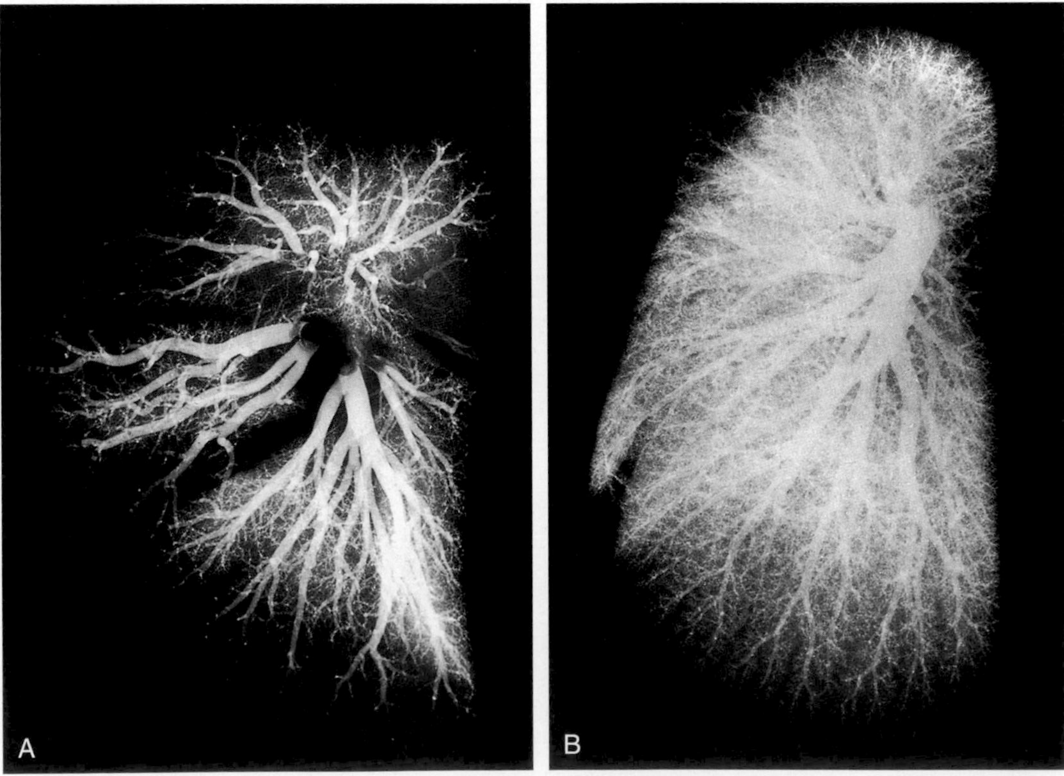

Figure 7-14 Postmortem arteriograms from a 9-month-old child with a ventricular septal defect (A) and from a normal child of the same age (B) (×0.50.). (From Haworth SG, Sauer U, Buhlmeyer K, Reid L: Development of the pulmonary circulation in ventricular septal defect: A quantitative structural study. Am J Cardiol 1977;40:781–788.

seen from 2 months of age, and is abundant by 5 months.[97] As the intimal obstruction increases in severity, the muscularity decreases in more distal vessels (see Fig. 7-13). After the age of 7 to 9 months, the medial thickness is normal, or even less than normal, in the distal vessels. These patients, without medial hypertrophy despite a high pulmonary resistance, are usually inoperable.

Atrioventricular Septal Defect

Cellular intimal proliferation develops earlier and is more severe in babies with an atrioventricular septal defect than in those with an isolated ventricular septal defect (see Fig. 7-13). Severe medial hypertrophy and intimal proliferation can be present by 6 or 7 months of age, and intracardiac repair should be carried out in early infancy.[107] Children of all ages can have a high pulmonary vascular resistance of 6 units/m^2 or more. In those under 3 months of age, however, the pulmonary arteries usually have increased muscularity, with or without intimal proliferation.

Atrial Septal Defect In the Oval Fossa

Pulmonary hypertension rarely develops in children with defects of the floor of the oval fossa. Those who develop pulmonary hypertension often have inoperable disease or do not survive surgery. Their pulmonary vasculature shows severe obstruction with intimal fibrosis. Such patients probably have idiopathic pulmonary hypertension with an associated atrial communication. The pulmonary vascular abnormalities in these children with pulmonary hypertension are unlike those seen in most middle-aged patients with defects in the oval fossa and cardiac failure, and more like those of children with a hypertensive ventricular septal defect. The pre-acinar arteries in older patients usually undergo a modest increase in pulmonary arterial muscularity and are dilated, while the dominant change at the periphery is fibrotic occlusion of small alveolar duct and the alveolar wall arteries, leading to a reduction in the capacity of the peripheral pulmonary vascular bed.

Abnormalities Causing Pulmonary Venous Obstruction

Totally anomalous pulmonary venous connection is primarily a disease of early infancy, presenting at or soon after birth. When the venous return is supradiaphragmatic, flow to the lungs is elevated for some time before obstruction develops. The intrapulmonary arteries and veins show increased mural thickness, the amount depending on the duration and severity of the obstruction. In infants with the infradiaphragmatic type of return, obstruction and vascular abnormalities are frequently present at or soon after birth, indicating intra-uterine change.[91] Pulmonary hypertension subsides after repair in almost all patients, and the pulmonary vascular changes apparently regress. Children with infradiaphragmatic return may occasionally have intrinsically small extrapulmonary veins, and pulmonary hypertension may then persist despite adequate reconstruction.[91]

In other cardiac abnormalities causing pulmonary venous obstruction, such as divided left atrium, congenital mitral stenosis, and stenosis of individual pulmonary veins at their junction with the left atrium, the vascular abnormalities are similar to those in totally anomalous pulmonary venous connection, but the arterial changes are less prominent. The lymphatic channels are dilated and abnormally thick walled, and the perivascular connective tissue is abnormally dense.

Scimitar Syndrome

Pulmonary hypertension is not usually a feature of the scimitar syndrome when the diagnosis is an incidental finding in older patients, but it can occur in babies. In four children with the syndrome presenting at between 1.5 and 4 months of age, microscopic examination showed normal development of the peripheral airways and alveolar regions.[108] The pulmonary arterial branching pattern was deficient in three, and in areas of lungs not perfused by the right pulmonary artery, the systemic arteries from the upper abdominal aorta anastomosed with the pulmonary arteries to distribute blood to a dilated capillary bed. Pulmonary arterial medial wall thickness was increased, but venous morphology was normal. Early correction is recommended.

Operability and Survival after Cardiac Repair

The outcome of a satisfactory intracardiac repair in patients with pulmonary hypertension is determined by the state of the pulmonary vascular bed at the time of repair. Operability and the reversibility of pathological lesions are not synonymous. Pulmonary arterial medial hypertrophy with or without a modest amount of cellular intimal proliferation may be potentially reversible, but it is not always a safe lesion. It is associated with pulmonary hypertensive crises. Hypoxia is probably the most common precipitating factor, but other, unrecognised and unknown, factors no doubt operate. Crises tend to cluster and can be fatal. Complete obliteration of the arterial lumen by intimal proliferation, even when highly cellular, is not usually reversible. Plexiform lesions are regarded as irreversible. It is not entirely certain whether these lesions are irreversible when present in early childhood. Given the severity of obstructive pathology with which they are associated, however, reversibility seems unlikely. The reduction in small intra-acinar arteries seen particularly in young children with severe pulmonary hypertension is probably not reversible.[99] The age at which intracardiac repair is carried out is the most crucial factor, and it is now well recognised that abnormalities are best repaired in early infancy. The emphasis in clinical management, therefore, must be on prevention of pulmonary vascular disease. When the natural history of the cardiac abnormality is that of rapidly progressive pulmonary vascular disease, as in transposition with ventricular septal defect, or hearts with univentricular atrioventricular connection in the absence of obstruction to the pulmonary outflow tract, then the child should undergo corrective or palliative surgery soon after birth. Where the natural history of pulmonary vascular disease is less aggressive, as in a ventricular septal defect, the abnormality should be corrected before 1 year of age if the pulmonary arterial pressure remains high in the presence of a large defect.

Medical Treatment of Pulmonary Hypertension

The beneficial effect of the drugs used to treat idiopathic pulmonary hypertension has encouraged extension of their use to pulmonary arterial hypertension of other aetiologies. Most children with post-operative pulmonary hypertension have a modest increase in pulmonary arterial pressure, but those symptomatic children in whom the pulmonary arterial pressure is equal to, or approaching, systemic level are treated as though they have the idiopathic form. In patients with the Eisenmenger syndrome, the clinical picture varies considerably. Many untreated patients have a good quality of life for many decades, but some are severely limited. The new specific therapies available for oral use can help. Bosentan can improve both exercise tolerance and haemodynamic parameters in these patients, without a reduction in systemic arterial saturations of oxygen.[109,110]

Effect of Palliative Surgery on the Lung

In patients with pulmonary hypoperfusion, insertion of a systemic-to-pulmonary shunt may lead to pulmonary hypertension. In patients with congenitally malformed hearts associated with pulmonary hypertension, banding the pulmonary trunk may fail adequately to reduce the pulmonary arterial pressure and flow. This may be acceptable if the repair will include a subpulmonary ventricle, but can compromise and prejudice the outcome of conversion to the Fontan circulation or cardiac transplantation.

ACQUIRED HEART DISEASE

Rheumatic Heart Disease

In developing countries, rheumatic heart disease is a common cause of pulmonary hypertension. In India, some children develop mitral stenosis very rapidly after having rheumatic fever and require intervention by 6 years of age, or less. The pulmonary vascular abnormalities in children with rheumatic mitral stenosis are generally more severe than in adults. Pulmonary arterial pressure, nonetheless, usually falls after valvotomy. Balloon mitral valvotomy has revolutionised the management of this condition.

Left Heart Disease

Long-standing disease of the left heart causes pulmonary hypertension and structural changes in the vasculature, which can prejudice cardiac transplantation. Chronic intravenous epoprostenol has reduced pulmonary vascular resistance in some of these patients, making it possible to transplant the heart rather than both heart and lungs.

IDIOPATHIC PULMONARY ARTERIAL HYPERTENSION

Interest in the condition dates back to the early 1950s, when Paul Wood identified six cases during a study of 233 patients with congenitally malformed hearts. As noted by Dresdale, a familial tendency to develop the disease was discovered by Dressler in 1954, and is now known to account for one-twentieth of cases. The therapeutic breakthrough came in 1984, when intravenous prostacyclin was first used therapeutically.[111,112] The efficacy of this treatment was subsequently proven in adults, and benefit was later demonstrated in children.[113,114] The first effective oral therapy, bosentan, was introduced in 2002,[115] followed by the inhibitor of phosphodiesterase 5, sildenafil.[116] The beneficial effect of these drugs has encouraged extension of their use to pulmonary arterial hypertension of other aetiologies. The new therapies treat arterial rather than venous disease. Left untreated, children with idiopathic pulmonary hypertension fare less well than adults. The predicted survival after diagnosis is less than a year, compared with almost 3 years in adults.[117,118]

The introduction of specific therapies has improved the prognosis in children as well as adults. Before the definitive trial of intravenous epoprostenol, the only medications available were calcium channel antagonists,[119] which we now know are efficacious in the long term in only a minority of patients. Anticoagulation was, and is, also considered helpful.[120] After the introduction of bosentan in adults, we and others showed that it was also efficacious in children.[121,122] The inhibitor of phosphodiesterase 5, known as sildenafil, was shown to be efficacious in a short 12-week trial in adults with idiopathic pulmonary hypertension.[116] Rates of survival of up to four-fifths at 5 years are now reported.[123,124] A good quality of life can be assured for many years, but ultimately lung transplantation is necessary in most patients.

Diagnostic Strategy

The patient is said to be suffering from idiopathic pulmonary arterial hypertension when there is no identifiable explanation for the increase in pulmonary arterial pressure. In any patients with pulmonary hypertension, the clinician must exclude any causation which is amenable to treatment, be it medical or surgical.

Clinical Suspicion of Pulmonary Hypertension

Pulmonary hypertension should be suspected in any child who is unduly short of breath, tires easily, or is syncopal when there is no evidence of cardiac or pulmonary disease. The disorder should also be suspected in those known to suffer from these diseases, and in whom increasing shortness of breath cannot be explained by the underlying disease process itself. The commonest misdiagnosis is asthma. The physical signs of pulmonary hypertension include a left parasternal, right ventricular lift, an accentuated pulmonary component of the second heart sound, and sometimes cool extremities. A diastolic murmur of pulmonary regurgitation may be present, but signs of overt right-sided cardiac failure are a late event in young children.

Confirming the Clinical Suspicion of Pulmonary Hypertension

An accurate and complete diagnosis is essential, remembering that dual pathology is not uncommon in pulmonary hypertensive children. A chest radiograph, an electrocardiogram, and a transthoracic echocardiogram, including Doppler interrogation, are mandatory. The classical findings include a chest radiograph showing enlarged intrapericardial pulmonary arteries, and diminished peripheral pulmonary vascular markings. The electrocardiographic findings include evidence of right ventricular dilation and hypertrophy, which can be confirmed by transthoracic echocardiography. Doppler interrogation can estimate pulmonary arterial systolic and diastolic pressures. The right ventricular systolic pressure is estimated from the velocity of the regurgitant systolic flow across the tricuspid valve, and the estimated right atrial pressure, using the Bernoulli equation in which the pressure is equal to four times the velocity squared plus the right atrial pressure.

A regurgitant jet across the tricuspid valve is found in the majority of pulmonary hypertensive patients. Echocardiographic measures of right ventricular function include the Tei index, which is the sum of the periods of isovolumetric contraction and relaxation time divided by the period of ejection. It assesses both systolic and diastolic function. The systolic excursion of the tricuspid annular plane correlates with the right ventricular ejection fraction. Blood tests may show elevation of brain natriuretic peptide, although less reliably than in adults. Functional capacity is graded according to the classification of the New York Heart Association, from the asymptomatic patient in the first class to the severely disabled in the fourth class. An objective assessment of exercise capacity is helpful. In a co-operative child of 6 years or more, the results of a 6-minute walk test can be compared with those in normal children of the same age and sex.[125] Cardiopulmonary exercise testing to determine maximum uptake of oxygen, rate of work, and anaerobic threshold can also be helpful. This test, however, should be carried out after the severity of the pulmonary hypertension has been ascertained at cardiac catheterisation, and it is known that it is safe to stress the child.

Investigations

The systemic arterial oxygen saturation is normal in the absence of interatrial shunting. Desaturation can occur in the presence of right-to-left interatrial shunting. The electrocardiographic findings are characteristic, and include right-axis deviation, evidence of right ventricular hypertrophy with or without a pattern of strain, and right atrial enlargement. In addition to an abnormal chest radiograph, contrast-enhanced spiral computed tomography of the lungs is indicated in older patients to exclude thrombus in the intrapericardial pulmonary arteries, and chronic thromboembolic disease. It is also helpful in distinguishing idiopathic pulmonary arterial hypertension from pulmonary veno-occlusive disease. Ventilation/perfusion scans can be normal in idiopathic pulmonary arterial hypertension, but may show small peripheral non-segmental defects of perfusion. Magnetic resonance imaging can help assess right ventricular function, but is not yet part of the routine work-up in children suspected of having idiopathic pulmonary arterial hypertension. The echocardiogram generally reveals dilated right heart chambers, right ventricular hypertrophy with posterior bowing of the ventricular septum and of the atrial septum when it is intact.[126]

The left ventricle may be severely compressed. In adults, right atrial size and the index of left ventricular eccentricity are predictive of outcome, and should be routinely assessed in children. Testing pulmonary function can sometimes demonstrate obstruction of the small airways. In addition to routine haematology and biochemistry, tests of thyroid function, a screen for thrombophilia, including antiphospholipid antibodies, and an auto-immune screen should all be performed. Children may seroconvert when they are older. Some children have a deficiency of immunoglobulin. They may have a low level of antithrombin III, protein S, or protein C, which may be genetic in origin, or result from a consumption coagulopathy. It is also necessary to screen siblings for the familial form of the disease.

Cardiac Catheterisation to Confirm the Diagnosis, Assess the Severity of Disease, and Guide Therapeutic Management, Including the Role of Lung Biopsy

The purpose of cardiac catheterisation in children with pulmonary hypertension is to confirm the diagnosis, and to ensure that the conclusions drawn from the non-invasive tests were complete and accurate. The catheterisation also determines the severity of the disease by determining accurately the pulmonary arterial pressure, the pulmonary vascular resistance, and the vasoreactivity of the pulmonary vasculature. The main determinant of treatment is the response to testing the potential for vasodilation with nitric oxide during cardiac catheterisation. Adequate sedation, optimal ventilation, and meticulous attention to the acid-base state and loss of blood are mandatory. The clinical history and the haemodynamic findings may indicate the need for further interventions, such as the creation of an interatrial communication by septostomy, or insertion of a Hickman line for continuous infusion of epoprostenol. Lung biopsy is rarely justified. The exceptions are to exclude pulmonary veno-occlusive disease, pulmonary capillary haemangiomatosis, and alveolar hypoplasia and dysplasia. It is also justified very rarely in children with complex congenitally malformed hearts in whom appropriate findings might indicate operability.

Treatment

All children with idiopathic pulmonary arterial hypertension need urgent treatment. Without treatment, the expected survival is less than 1 year.[114] The main determinant of treatment is the response to testing with nitric oxide at cardiac catheterisation. In those with a positive response, the pressures and resistance must fall to a near normal level, with no fall in cardiac output. Only patients with a positive response can be treated with a calcium channel antagonist. This applies to less than one-tenth of the patients. Children who improve, and are stable when receiving a calcium channel antagonist, need repeated cardiac catheterisation, since they can become resistant to the drug at any time, and need escalation of therapy before they deteriorate. The majority of negative responders present in the third or fourth classes of the categorisation made by the New York Heart Association. They may need to be treated immediately with epoprostenol delivered intravenously. In some, however, it is feasible to initiate treatment with an endothelin receptor antagonist. Most children require combination therapy. Syncopal children may need an urgent atrial septostomy. After discharge from hospital, it is essential to maintain close monitoring, principally by echocardiography, since urgent intensification of therapy is frequently necessary.

The rationale for treatment is clear. Treatment with prostacyclin is indicated, in that patients with pulmonary arterial hypertension have reduced circulating levels of this agent, which is vasodilatory and prevents proliferation of smooth muscle cells relative to levels of the vasoconstrictor and proliferative compound thromboxane.[127] Clinical studies have documented an increase in expression of endothelin in the lungs of patients with pulmonary arterial hypertension,[128] and experimental studies in rats have shown that high levels of this powerful vasoconstrictor promote proliferation of smooth muscle cells and inflammation. It is this evidence that supports the giving of antagonists of endothelin receptors. The reduced expression of nitric oxide synthase in the setting of the idiopathic pulmonary arterial hypertension also suggests that treatment with phosphodiesterase inhibitors, such as sildenafil, would be effective in dilating the pulmonary arteries.[129]

Prostacyclin and Its Analogues

In the light of the above discussion, it is not surprising that the most effective therapy to date has proved to be a continuous intravenous infusion of epoprostenol, the sodium salt of prostacyclin. It has a short half-life of 3 to 5 minutes. Hence, it is unstable, and the infusion has to be prepared every 24 hours. The principal side effects are mandibular pain and diarrhoea. The child is dosed according to response. Children need much higher doses than adults. A more stable analogue of prostacyclin, treprostinil, can also be given intravenously, but is associated with more prominent side effects, such as headaches and leg pain. Meticulous care of the Hickman line is essential to prevent local and systemic infections, the latter being extremely uncommon. Treprostinil can also be given by continuous subcutaneous infusion, but this is painful, the drug stimulating neural endings, and causing induration and sometimes ulceration of the skin. Because of these problems, it is not used in children. Iloprost is another analogue of prostacyclin, which can be given by inhalation, but small and tired children find it difficult to inhale an effective dose every 2 hours. Such frequent administration is needed, since the drug is effective for less than 2 hours.

Endothelin Receptor Antagonist

The dual endothelin receptor antagonist, bosentan (Tracleer), was the first oral drug shown to be efficacious in idiopathic pulmonary arterial hypertension. It has now been used extensively in this, and other types of pulmonary hypertension, since its introduction in 2002.[115] It is efficacious in children.[121,122] Its principal side effect is elevation of hepatic enzymes, which necessitates a monthly blood test. Interactions can occur with other drugs, and the agent decreases effective exposure to warfarin. The newer selective antagonists sitaxentan and ambrisentan have yet to be studied in children. Both drugs affect the liver less than bosentan, and interaction with other drugs is probably less likely with ambrisentan. Clinical trials are currently still under way comparing the effects of blocking both the A and B endothelin receptor subtypes and the more selective receptor A antagonists.

Inhibitors of Phosphodiesterase

Sildenafil was the first drug of this class, and is still the most commonly used, particularly in young children with associated pulmonary hypertension. In those with the idiopathic pulmonary arterial hypertension, it is given in combination with other specific therapies. Systemic hypotension can occur when high doses are used. In babies, the dose is 0.5 to 1 mg/kg given three to four times a day, rarely more.

Anticoagulation

Patients with pulmonary vascular disease are prone to develop thrombosis. Older children are given warfarin, while younger ones usually receive aspirin. For the reasons discussed above, the international normalised ratio must be monitored particularly closely in those receiving endothelin receptor antagonists.

Oxygen

The gas is a potent pulmonary vasodilator. Nocturnal supplemental oxygen is indicated if there is nocturnal desaturation, and can benefit those with high pulmonary arterial pressures.

Atrial Septostomy

This procedure is indicated in children with idiopathic pulmonary arterial hypertension and in those with post-operative pulmonary hypertension suffering from syncope or severe right-sided cardiac failure.[130] It reduces the effect of a sudden increase in the pulmonary arterial and right-sided pressures, and maintains left ventricular output.

Lung Transplantation

Patients who fail to respond to medical therapy are offered the possibility of lung transplantation. The current predicted survival for this procedure in children is just short of 4 years, with only seven-tenths surviving at 1 year.[131]

New and Emerging Therapies

The therapeutic goal is to remodel the pulmonary vasculature to its normal structure, to restore endothelial function, and induce the growth of new peripheral pulmonary arteries. New modes of administration, new formulations, new analogues of existing drugs, and new antagonists of the endothelin receptors and other inhibitors are currently in development. In addition, statins, anti-growth factor drugs, inhibitors of elastase, openers of the potassium channels, stem cell and gene therapy, and inhibitors of RhoA are all under investigation. Studies showing vasodilation and reversal of pulmonary hypertension by inhibitors of Rho kinase, such as fasudil, in rodents[75] suggest that these agents should be developed for clinical use. Fasudil has indeed shown some benefit in acute testing of patients.[132] The systemic hypotensive side effects of these agents may be reduced when the inhibitors are administered via inhalation. This issue will need to be addressed if these agents are to be useful in treating patients for a prolonged period of time. Recent attention has also focused on the vasodilator adrenomedullin and on vasoactive intestinal peptide. The latter peptide is an important vasodilator and inhibitor of proliferation of smooth muscle cells. Transgenic mice null for the peptide develop pulmonary hypertension with remodelled distal arteries. Both the haemodynamic abnormality and the pathology can be reversed with administration of the peptide.[133] At present, we can stabilise patients for many years, but new and radical medicines used in combination offer the hope of cure and greater promise of tailoring the treatment to the individual child. Novel therapies will emerge from improved understanding of the mechanisms initiating and maintaining pulmonary vascular disease.

Pathobiology of Pulmonary Vascular Disease

Our understanding of the pathobiology of pulmonary vascular disease has improved enormously in the past 10 years (Fig. 7-15). Studies in humans and animals have emphasised the role of three major signalling pathways. The idiopathic variant is characterised by a relative or absolute reduction in the release of prostacyclin and nitric oxide, and excessive release of endothelin. Present therapies target these three signalling pathways, singly or in combination.

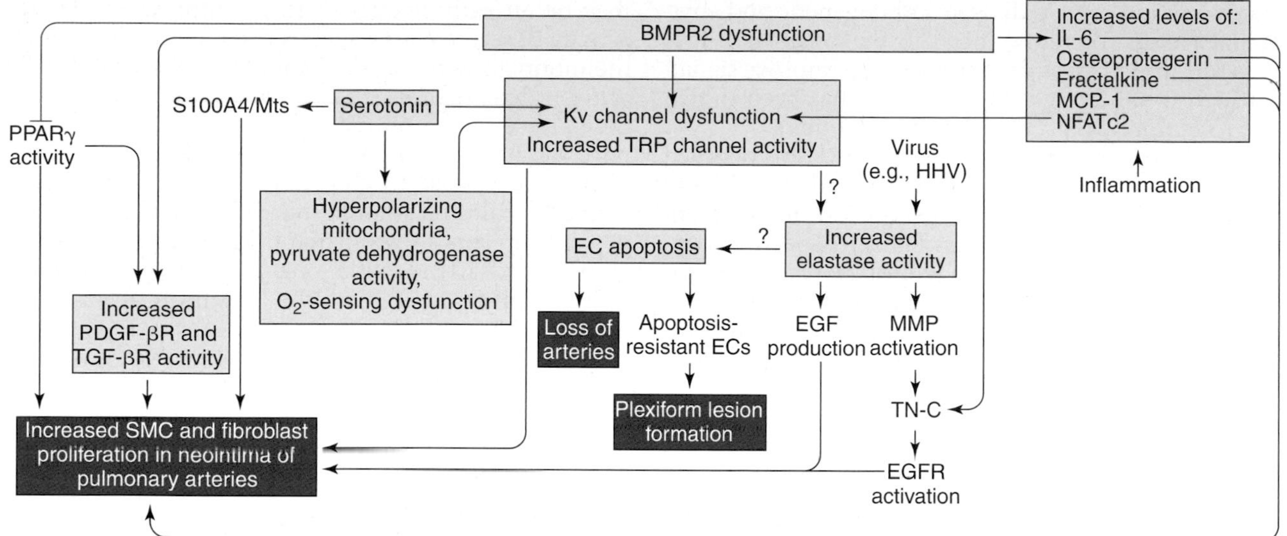

Figure 7-15 The cartoon shows factors that converge in the molecular pathogenesis of pulmonary arterial hypertension, and how these may interact with BMPR2 dysfunction, a known genetic defect associated with such hypertension. The scheme focuses on factors causing increased proliferation of smooth muscle cells (SMC) and fibroblasts, as well as apoptosis of endothelial cells (EC), causing an initial reduction in vessel number, followed by proliferation of apoptosis-resistant endothelial cells in plexiform lesions. It shows multiple levels of interaction, with numerous factors related to dysfunction of BMPR2 and the Kv channels, as described in the text. For example, serotonin, hyperpolarised mitochondria, aberrant regulation of the NFATc gene, and BMPR2 dysfunction all lead to suppression or dysfunction of Kv channels. This is related to abnormal proliferation of smooth muscle cells. BMPR2 dysfunction, serotonin, and elastase all can produce increased signals from growth factor receptors. Serotonin can induce S100A4/Mts1, which also causes proliferation of smooth muscle cells, as does fractalkine. BMPR2, bone morphogenetic protein receptor 2; EGF, epidermal growth factor; EGFR, epidermal growth factor response; HHV, human herpesvirus; IL-6, interleukin-6; Kv, voltage-gated potassium channel; MCP, mast cell proteinase; MMP, metalloproteinase; NFAT, nuclear factor of activated T cells; PDGF, platelet-derived growth factor; PPAR, peroxisome proliferator-activated receptor; TGF, transforming growth factor; TN-C, tenascin-C; TRP, transient receptor potential Ca channels.

Interestingly, clinical experience with prostacyclin preceded discovery of the scientific evidence for its use. Progress has accelerated with advances in cell and molecular biology, along with the identification of mutations in the genes for the bone morphogenetic protein receptor II, and activin-like kinase, which regulate specific signalling pathways for transforming growth factors. Exonic mutations account for half of familial and one-tenth of patients with the sporadic form of the idiopathic variant who have identifiable mutations of the bone morphogenetic protein.[134] These genetic studies have opened up new avenues for the treatment of pulmonary hypertension.

Bone Morphogenetic Protein Receptor 2

This receptor, usually described as BMPR2, is a member of the superfamily of transforming growth factor receptors. In the familial form of pulmonary arterial hypertension, the penetrance of mutations of the receptor is only about one-fifth. In other words, four-fifths of family members that carry the mutation will never develop pulmonary hypertension. The presence of a mutation is much lower, less than 10%, in patients with pulmonary hypertension acquired because of congenital left-to-right shunting.[135] Mutations have also been observed in patients with pulmonary hypertension acquired owing to ingestion of appetite suppressants, but the frequency has not been established.[136] Although the penetrance is low, the functional link between mutations and pulmonary arterial hypertension is reinforced by the fact that, independent of a mutation, all patients with the idiopathic variant have reduced expression of bone morphogenetic protein 2, as do, to some extent, patients with associated pulmonary hypertension.[137] In addition, a reduction in the expression of the coreceptor, BMPR1A, is frequently observed in patients with idiopathic pulmonary arterial hypertension.[138] The functional consequences of a reduction, or absence, of signaling for BMPR2 in endothelial and smooth muscle cells have been addressed by a number of laboratories. When loss of the receptor is induced by interference to RNA in the endothelial cells of the pulmonary arteries, they become susceptible to apoptosis.[139] Thus, it is possible that such apoptosis is responsible for the reduction in peripheral alveolar ducts and mural arteries, causing rarefaction of the precapillary vasculature.

Loss of BMPR2 also causes proliferation of the pulmonary arterial smooth muscle cells in response to agents such as TGF-β1 and the bone morphogenetic protein itself that normally inhibit their proliferation[140] and induce susceptibility to apoptosis. This observation is in keeping with the aberrant proliferative response of smooth muscle cells causing occlusive changes in the intra-acinar pulmonary arteries in patients with pulmonary hypertension. BMPR2 suppresses proliferation of smooth muscle cells in response to growth factors, such as platelet-derived growth factor, known as PDGF,[141] and possibly others implicated in the pathobiology of pulmonary arterial hypertension, such as endothelial growth factor, or EGF.[142] Signalling through BMPR2 induces differentiation of fetal lung fibroblasts into smooth muscle cells.[143] This could expand the population of fibroblasts or myofibroblasts, accounting for the adventitial and medial thickening of the hypertensive pulmonary arteries.

In view of these studies in cultured cells, it is interesting that mice with haploinsufficiency of the BMPR2[144] or with dominant negative receptor[145] develop pulmonary arterial hypertension associated with a relatively unimpressive degree of structural remodeling. This only reinforces the fact that the deficiency in the BMPR2 gene is necessary but not sufficient to induce severe disease. Other genetic and environmental factors, therefore, need to be considered. It is still possible, nonetheless, that strategies to improve signalling through BMPR2 might be helpful, as has been shown in some rodent models[146] although not in others.[147]

Also, while loss of the BMPR1A coreceptor was believed to contribute to the adverse pathology in patients with the idiopathic form of pulmonary hypertension, more recent experimental data suggest that loss of BMPR1A without concomitant reduction in BMPR2 may protect against abnormal muscularisation and loss of pulmonary arteries.[148] In addition, other members of the bone morphogenetic protein and TGF-β families, such as activin-like kinase type 1 and endoglin, that are mutated in hereditary hemorrhagic telangiectasia, are also occasionally mutated in patients with pulmonary arterial hypertension.[149] Thus, changes in the expression of BMPR2 coupled with BMPR1A, and changes in the availability of ligands that signal through these receptors, and perhaps concurrent abnormalities in downstream signalling events that influence gene expression, together with concurrent abnormalities in other members of the TGF-β superfamily of receptors, may all be required in the development of pulmonary arterial hypertension. It has been suggested that it is the loss of signals for BMPR2 that leads to an exaggeration in signals for TGF-β.[150] Downstream of BMPR2 signaling are the transcription factors that programme the genes important in vascular homeostasis. One such transcription factor is an inhibitor of DNA binding 1,[151] and another appears to be PPARγ.[141] There is evidence from the use of cultured smooth muscle cells from pulmonary arteries that BMPR2 regulates transcriptional activity of PPARγ,[141] and that apoε gene is transcribed by PPARγ. Mice with deletion of PPARγ or apoε develop pulmonary hypertension.[152] Indeed, in the smooth muscle cells from systemic arteries, apoε can repress proliferation, preventing proliferative signals through the receptor for PDGF.[153]

This is of further interest in light of work showing that repression of the PDGF receptor by imatinib can reverse monocrotaline-induced pulmonary hypertension in rats,[154] and may improve outcome in patients with end-stage pulmonary arterial hypertension.[155] In addition to apoE, other transcriptional targets of PPARγ, such as adiponectin, can sequester PDGF,[156] and repress proliferation of smooth muscle cells from the pulmonary arteries. Treatment of knock-out mice for *Apoε* with the agonist of PPARγ, rosiglitazone, increases levels of adiponectin and reverses the pulmonary arterial hypertension.[152] So, it appears that, while the antiproliferative effect of BMPR2 in smooth muscle cells could be impeded in patients with a mutation there is also the potential for rescue by activating downstream effectors such as PPARγ.

BMPR2 may also be a negative regulator of transcription factors, such as acute myelogenous leucaemia factor 1, which regulates serine elastase,[157] an enzyme that is also implicated in the pathobiology of pulmonary arterial hypertension. Other interesting targets of BMPR2 implicated in the proliferation of pulmonary arterial smooth muscles cells include osteoprotegerin and tenascin-C.

Elastase Activity and Pulmonary Arterial Hypertension

Previous studies analysing lung biopsy tissue from children with congenitally malformed hearts and associated pulmonary arterial hypertension suggest that elastolytic activity may be an early feature of this complication.[158] Elevated activity of serine elastase was subsequently documented in the monocrotaline-induced model of disease, as well as in other rodent models.[159] This led to the successful experimental use of inhibitors of elastase in preventing pulmonary vascular pathology.[160] The mechanism relating such activity of elastase to clinical practice is also based upon studies in cultured smooth muscle cells obtained from pulmonary arteries, showing that heightened activity of serine elastase leads to the release of growth factors from the extracellular matrix, along with the activation of matrix metalloproteinases, and the induction of tenascin C, this being a glycoprotein associated with activation of growth factor receptors and survival pathways. Further studies used inhibitors of elastase not only to prevent, but to also to reverse, experimental monocrotaline-induced pulmonary hypertension by inducing apoptosis of smooth muscle cells.[161] Regression was subsequently also achieved by blocking a downstream effector of elastase, the EGF receptor. In studies using either inhibitors or blockers, regeneration of the distal vasculature was demonstrated. Similarly, treatment with a dominant-negative construct of survivin[162] was also highly successful in reversing pulmonary hypertension through apoptosis of the smooth muscle cells.

Dysfunction of Potassium Channels, Mitochondrial Abnormalities, and Pulmonary Arterial Hypertension

Recent studies have related aberrant signaling through BMPR2 to other abnormalities that are relevant to the pathobiology of pulmonary arterial hypertension. For example, reduced expression and function of voltage-gated potassium channels, notably Kv1.5, is observed in smooth muscle cells obtained from the pulmonary arteries of patients with both the idiopathic and associated pulmonary arterial hypertension, and signalling through BMPR2 has been directly related to expression of the Kv channels.[163] Reduced expression of these channels favors an influx of intracellular calcium, and promotes cellular proliferation as well as vasoconstriction. Increased expression of the voltage-gated potassium channels appears necessary in mediating the apoptosis associated BMPR2 signaling in smooth muscle cells. Agents that open the channels, like dichloroacetate, as well as gene transfer of the channels, have been used as experimental strategies in animal models to prevent and reverse pulmonary arterial hypertension.[164,165] It is of interest that the fawn-hooded rat, which has a defect in serotonin metabolism, and develops pulmonary arterial hypertension in response to relative alveolar hypoxia at mile-high altitude, also has abnormal oxygen sensing in the mitochondria of smooth muscle cells, leading to reduced function of the Kv channels.[166] Reversal of the mitochondrial abnormality can be achieved through the pyruvate dehydrogenase kinase inhibitor, dichloroacetate, as described above since this reverses dysfunction of the Kv channels.[166] Consistent with this, it is reported that the serotonin can, in signaling through the 5HT2A receptor, directly inhibit voltage-gated potassium channels in the rat.[167]

Transient Receptor Potential Calcium Channels

Recent work has implicated expression of transient receptor potential types 3 and 6 in highly proliferating smooth muscle cells obtained from the pulmonary arteries of patients with the idiopathic form of pulmonary hypertension. These studies have shown that inhibition of these channels can repress the heightened proliferation.[168] Moreover, it was also shown that inhibition of protein kinase A, or activation of cAMP, might have a similar effect.[169]

Serotonin Receptor and Transporter and Pulmonary Arterial Hypertension

Elevated levels and transport of serotonin have been implicated in the pathology of pulmonary arterial hypertension, based upon studies in both animals and in humans.[170] Serotonin results in increased vasoreactivity in the fawn-hooded rat, and there is attenuated severity of pulmonary vascular disease in mice lacking the gene encoding the serotonin transporter.[171] In contrast, overexpression of the serotonin transporter in a transgenic mouse worsens hypoxia-induced pulmonary hypertension.[172] When the serotonin transporter is selectively overexpressed in the smooth muscle cells of these transgenic mice, severe pulmonary arterial hypertension ensues.[173] Moreover, haploinsufficiency of BMPR2, both in cultured smooth muscle cells from the pulmonary arteries of mice, and in transgenic mice, makes them more sensitive to the pro-proliferative effects of serotonin.[174] Loss of BMPR2 leads to impaired repression of PDGF-mediated proliferation of the smooth muscle cells. This disinhibition could be further compounded by increased activity of the serotonin transporter, since this also enhances PDGF receptor β–mediated signalling. Other studies have shown that serotonin-mediated stimulation of the serotonin transporter and the serotonin receptors induces cyclins[175] and c-fos, which are critical to the proliferative response of the smooth muscle cells. Serotonin also stimulates the production of S100A4/Mts1, a member of the S100 family of calcium-binding proteins.[176] S100A4/Mts1 stimulates proliferation and migration of smooth muscle cells,[176] and is increased in neointimal lesions from patients with both idiopathic pulmonary arterial hypertension and pulmonary hypertension associated with other conditions. Moreover, a mouse that overexpresses S100A4/Mts1 spontaneously rarely develops pulmonary arterial hypertension.[176] In one study, a gain-of-function polymorphism in the serotonin transporter characterised by two long alleles was described in two-thirds of patients with pulmonary arterial hypertension, and only one-quarter of controls.[177] This apparent modifier, however, was not observed in other studies with different populations of patients.

Proinflammatory State of the Vessel Wall and Pulmonary Arterial Hypertension

Increasing attention is being focused on the proinflammatory state of the vessel wall in the progression of pulmonary arterial hypertension, but the mechanisms involved remain poorly defined. The development of pulmonary hypertension in a subset of patients infected with the human immunodeficiency virus may be a function of the HLA class II alleles, such as HLA-DR6.[178] Also, a link was made between expression of human herpes virus–8, associated with Kaposi sarcoma, and the idiopathic variant. The mouse that overexpresses S100A4/Mts1 develops extensive and severe neointimal lesions following injection of the gamma murine herpes virus–68, this being the murine homolog of HHV-8.[179] The *nef* gene for the human immunodeficiency virus was also recently implicated in plexogenic pulmonary vascular lesions associated with pulmonary arterial hypertension in infected patients, and SIV-infected nonhuman primates.[180] Advanced occlusive lesions similar to those seen in patients with pulmonary arterial hypertension have also been produced experimentally by an immune or inflammatory mechanism dependent on T cells following injection of soluble antigens.[95] Autoantibodies against B23, a cleavage product of a nuclear protein produced by the T-cell enzyme granzyme B, can distinguish the subset of patients with scleroderma who also have pulmonary arterial hypertension from patients with scleroderma but without hypertension.[95] Although the mechanistic significance of this biomarker is not known, in the experimental setting, haploinsufficiency of BMPR2 in mice is associated with an increase in pulmonary arterial hypertension in response to an inflammatory stimulus.[95] Other experimental models of chronic inflammation, such as repeated injections of endotoxin or TNFα, result in the development of pulmonary vascular changes. A recent study has shown that, in the model of pulmonary arterial hypertension in which loss of arteries is induced by the combination of hypoxia and SUGEN, an inhibitor of VEGF, the principal growth factor for endothelial cells, depletion of subsets of T cells worsens the pathology.[181] This adverse response has been attributed to unbalanced activity of B cells. Heightened circulating levels of cytokines and their receptors have also been demonstrated in patients with idiopathic pulmonary hypertension, including fractalkine, and its cognate receptor, both of which are associated with heightened proliferation of smooth muscle cells. Other chemokines and cytokines, such as stromal derived factor 1 and monocyte chemoattractant protein 1, which are implicated in pulmonary arterial hypertension, have been found circulating in serum obtained from pulmonary hypertensive patients. Loss of function of BMPR2 is also known to lead to upregulation of the proinflammatory cytokine IL-6.[182]

Mononuclear fibrocytes have been identified as key contributors to the remodeling of the pulmonary vasculature. It is believed that these cells, which have characteristics of both fibroblasts and leucocytes, migrate into the vessel wall through the angiomata located in the expanding adventitial layers. Heightened expression of the transcription factor NFATc2, which is associated with inflammatory cells, may also underlie pulmonary hypertension. Increased nuclear content of this factor is observed in T cells from patients with the idiopathic variant of pulmonary hypertension, and in pulmonary vascular lesions, and this can lead to repression of expression of Kv1.5 channels. The factor can be inhibited by VIVT, a specific peptide which inhibits calcineurin-mediated NFAT activation. Its nuclear translocation can be suppressed by cyclosporine. These agents can also attenuate monocrotaline-induced pulmonary hypertension.

Stem Cells in the Pathobiology and Treatment of Pulmonary Arterial Hypertension

A major effort is being directed at understanding the mechanisms underlying regeneration of the pulmonary vasculature following injury. In the mouse model of pulmonary arterial hypertension induced by monocrotaline, but not hypoxia, the recruitment of circulating stem cells appears to be protective.[183] Mesenchymal stem cells can also be engineered to prevent the development of experimental pulmonary hypertension in rodents. Mesenchymal cells have also been delivered intratracheally to attenuate the monocrotaline-induced hypertension through an obscure mechanism. In addition, these cells have been engineered to improve myocardial performance following injection into the right ventricles in rodent models.[184] Endothelial progenitor cells transfected with endothelial nitric oxide synthase not only prevent, but also reverse, pulmonary arterial hypertension in rats by reestablishing connections between proximal and distal pulmonary arteries.[185] This strategy of genetically engineering endogenous cells to express endothelial nitric oxide synthase has been recently embarked upon in a clinical trial in patients with advanced pulmonary arterial hypertension. Non-engineered cells have been used to treat patients in a pilot study, which showed some short-term efficacy.[186] These results are at variance with studies indicating that these may be the very cells that induce plexiform lesions in the setting of advanced pulmonary arterial hypertension.

Right Ventricular Failure

Patients die when the subpulmonary ventricle fails. Although the focus in understanding the mechanism of pulmonary arterial hypertension has been on the small pulmonary arteries, there is evidence that changes in impedance, resulting from stiffening of the more proximal pulmonary arteries, may also be a critical determinant, not only of the pressure but also of the ability of the right ventricle to function. The right ventricle has received little attention until now, but magnetic resonance imaging gives insight into the anatomical and functional effects of a sustained increase in afterload, genetic variation may help explain patient variation in ventricular tolerance, and the molecular approaches to left ventricular dysfunction can be applied to the right ventricle. Medicinal targeting of right ventricular function demands a greater understanding of the biology of this ventricle.

PULMONARY HYPERTENSION OF VARIABLE AETIOLOGY

Pulmonary Veno-occlusive Disease and Pulmonary Capillary Haemangiomatosis

These conditions are uncommon. They can present like idiopathic pulmonary arterial hypertension, but recognition is important, because their management differs. Veno-occlusive disease usually presents with shortness of breath, sometimes accompanied by small, frequent haemoptysis. The patient may be desaturated, be clubbed, and have minimal rales on auscultation. The electrocardiogram and echocardiogram can be indistinguishable from the idiopathic variant, but the diffusing capacity is lower, and high resolution computed tomographic scans can be diagnostic to the experienced radiologist. In addition to the expected features of pulmonary hypertension, contrast computed tomography with vascular imaging shows a patchy centrilobular pattern of ground glass opacities, the lobules having the appearance of pavement because their margins are demarcated by thickened septal lines caused by oedema. Typically, mediastinal lymphadenopathy is prominent. The contrast scan also confirms the echocardiographic findings of unobstructed venous return in the large pulmonary veins. These children are usually very ill, and should be listed for transplantation without delay. Cardiac catheterisation may be indicated to confirm the diagnosis. If the child is relatively well and stable, it can be helpful to do an open lung biopsy in order to distinguish those with pulmonary capillary haemangiomatosis, who may be amenable to treatment for a short period of time, although such treatment with anti-cancer drugs must be regarded as experimental. Pulmonary veno-occlusive disease has the distinctive pathological feature of uniform fibrotic occlusion of peripheral small veins. It can be associated with an immunopathological process. There may be extensive deposits of IgG, IgA and IgM in the subendothelial basement membranes of small veins and capillaries, but not of arteries. Deposition of IgG and complement has also been observed on capillary basement membranes in veno-occlusive disease in adulthood. Diagnosis demands immediate referral for lung transplantation.

Thromboembolic Pulmonary Hypertension

Thromboembolic pulmonary hypertension in children is usually iatrogenic, caused by intravenous hyperalimentation, catheterisation of the umbilical vein in the newborn, or a ventriculo-venous shunt for hydrocephalus. Showers of embolus discharged from the tip of the catheter can gradually occlude a large proportion of the pulmonary vascular bed. Thromboembolisation also occurs in certain hypercoagulable states, such as sickle cell disease, nephrotic syndrome, and homocystinuria.

Cor Pulmonale

Lung disease in childhood damages the airways and alveoluses while they are still developing, and may have a long-standing harmful effect on the pulmonary circulation. The most common causes of cor pulmonale in childhood are chronic long-term diseases originating at birth, and cystic fibrosis. Extensive disease of the small airways and alveoluses, as occurs in bronchiolitis, fibrosing alveolitis, and the collagen vascular disorders, can lead to pulmonary vascular change and hypertension, but this is not common in childhood. Chronic obstruction of the upper airways by large tonsils and adenoids is a well-recognised cause of pulmonary hypertension and right heart failure in children, but there is rapid improvement following surgery, and no evidence of permanent pulmonary vascular damage. Deforming thoracomusculoskeletal abnormalities, such as severe scoliosis, pleural symphysis or fibrothorax, and severe weakness of the respiratory muscles, are all recognised causes of cor pulmonale.

Congenital Abnormalities of the Lung

Pulmonary hypoplasia is associated with impaired development of airways, a reduction in the number of peripheral pulmonary arteries, and excessive muscularisation of the pulmonary arterial bed. These changes are generally present at birth. Pulmonary hypoplasia occurs most commonly in congenital diaphragmatic hernia, renal dysplasia, rhesus isoimmunisation, and more rarely, in a single lung, asphyxiating thoracic dystrophy, and phrenic nerve agenesis.[82,83] In congenital diaphragmatic hernia, the degree of hypoplasia varies. In severe cases, there is a reduction in the number of pre-acinar airway and arterial generations, indicating that development was interrupted before the 16th week of intra-uterine life in both the affected and contralateral lung. This causes a marked reduction in total alveolar and peripheral arterial number. The lungs of babies who survive for some time may be emphysematous, and show evidence of barotrauma caused by long-term mechanical ventilation after repair. Pulmonary hypertension is present in many babies after surgical repair, but it usually improves considerably in early life. Persistence of pulmonary hypertension can require aggressive medical therapy with antagonists of the endothelin receptors, sildenafil, and even chronic intravenous epoprostenol.

THE FUTURE

Pulmonary vascular disease is still a major problem. Important contributions from genetics, which uncover abnormalities in modifier genes of the bone morphogenetic protein pathway, will help elucidate the process by which develops idiopathic pulmonary arterial hypertension, and shed light on the mechanisms regulating susceptibility in the associated forms. The role of chronic inflammation and autoimmunity will be important to pursue in novel models that recapitulate the features seen clinically. New clinical trials based upon rescuing altered metabolism and signaling in endothelial, smooth muscle, fibroblast, and inflammatory cells should follow from findings in experimental studies.

The complete reference list can be found on the companion Expert Consult web site at www.expertconsult.com.

ANNOTATED REFERENCES

- Wojciak-Stothard B, Tsang LY, Paleolog E, et al: Rac1 and RhoA as regulators of endothelial phenotype and barrier function in hypoxia-induced neonatal pulmonary hypertension. Am J Physiol Lung Cell Mol Physiol 2006;290: L1173–L1182.

  This paper defines the cytoskeleton and its role in the remodelling response of pulmonary arteries.
- Rabinovitch M: Molecular pathogenesis of pulmonary arterial hypertension. J Clin Invest 2008;118:2372–2379.

  This review focuses on idiopathic pulmonary arterial hypertension and the cellular and molecular mechanisms that lead to the structural changes that are observed. It indicates ways in which the pathology could be reversed in the future.
- Galie N, Beghetti M, Gatzoulis MA, et al: Bosentan therapy in patients with Eisenmenger syndrome: A multicenter, double-blind, randomized, placebo-controlled study. Circulation 2006;114:48–54.

  This study indicates that treatments for idiopathic pulmonary hypertension could be helpful in the Eisenmenger syndrome.
- Rosenzweig EB, Ivy DD, Widlitz A, et al: Effects of long-term bosentan in children with pulmonary arterial hypertension. J Am Coll Cardiol 2005;46:697–704.

  One of the few studies focusing on the response of children with idiopathic pulmonary hypertension to newer therapeutic agents.
- Humpl T, Reyes JT, Holtby H, et al: Beneficial effect of oral sildenafil therapy on childhood pulmonary arterial hypertension: Twelve-month clinical trial of a single-drug, open-label, pilot study. Circulation 2005;111:3274–3280.

  A similar study using sildenafil in children.
- Newman JH, Trembath RC, Morse JA, et al: Genetic basis of pulmonary arterial hypertension: Current understanding and future directions. J Am Coll Cardiol 2004;43(Suppl S):33S–39S.

  An important review of the genetics of pulmonary hypertension.
- Hansmann G, de Jesus Perez VA, Alastalo TP, et al: An antiproliferative BMP-2/PPARgamma/apoE axis in human and murine SMCs and its role in pulmonary hypertension. J Clin Invest 2008;118:1846–1857.

  This study helps define the pathway downstream of the mutant BMPR2 and how the genetic defect might be rescued.
- Morrell NW: Pulmonary hypertension due to BMPR2 mutation: A new paradigm for tissue remodeling? Proc Am Thorac Soc 2006;3:680–686.

  This review relates the genetics to the pathophysiology of pulmonary hypertension.
- Ghofrani HA, Seeger W, Grimminger F: Imatinib for the treatment of pulmonary arterial hypertension. N Engl J Med 2005;353:1412–1413.

  This is an interesting case report that is the basis for a current clinical trial to use growth factor receptor blockade to reverse clinical pulmonary hypertension.
- Haworth SG: The management of pulmonary hypertension in children. Arch Dis Child 2008;93:620–625.

  This review explains how to investigate and confirm the diagnosis, and how to assess the options for treatment.

Prevalence of Congenital Cardiac Disease

BRIAN W. McCRINDLE

Examination of the frequency of congenital cardiac disease, either as a rate or as a proportion, has important implications for the study of congenital cardiac malformations, as well as their clinical management. There is much confusion and misuse, however, regarding terminology and methodology, with important implications for the accuracy, validity and comparability of findings reported in the published literature. Knowledge of how critically to appraise these reports is important in defining their value when applied to issues of diagnostic likelihood, surveillance and trends, aetiologic associations, burden of disease, and requirements for resources. These issues have more recently been impacted by fetal diagnosis and termination, with individual decisions influenced by contemporary estimates of prognosis related to the natural and modified natural history. As more patients survive into adulthood, estimates of the burden of disease, and the requirements for resources, have also achieved greater importance. The question 'how much congenital cardiac disease?' therefore continues to evolve. Providing the correct answer has important relevance for both the providers of health care, and the health care system itself.

DEFINITIONS

When considering the frequency of congenital cardiac disease, strict and explicit definitions are important, but often misunderstood and misused. Critical terms to be defined include congenital cardiac disease itself, frequency, ratio, proportion, rate, incidence, and prevalence.

In looking at reports of congenitally malformed hearts, it is important to know how the lesions were defined, and what conditions were included or excluded. Congenital cardiac disease has been defined as the presence of 'a gross structural abnormality of the heart or intrathoracic great vessels that is actually or potentially of functional significance'.[1] The additional implication of this definition is that these abnormalities arose at the time of cardiovascular development, and should therefore be present at the time of delivery or, with the advent of fetal assessment, fetal diagnosis. This definition would exclude normal variants that would be of no functional consequence, such as anomalies of the systemic veins, for example, persistent patency of the left superior caval vein, or abnormal patterns of branching of the systemic arteries that have no functional consequence. Using this definition, however, does not end all controversy. There is no current consensus as to whether several groups of lesions should be considered to represent congenital cardiac malformations:

- Genetic conditions, obviously present from conception, which may not have manifest cardiovascular consequences until much later in life. Examples would include Marfan syndrome, Williams syndrome, hypertrophic cardiomyopathy, and pulmonary hypertension.
- Arrhythmic conditions with abnormalities at the physiologic or ultrastructural level, such as long QT syndrome and abnormal pathways producing ventricular pre-excitation pathways.
- Primary cardiomyopathies with a genetic or metabolic aetiology. This might also include myocardial abnormalities such as ventricular non-compaction.
- Structural defects which do not have functional significance in many, but not all, circumstances, such as the aortic valve with two leaflets, the prolapsing mitral valve, so-called silent persistent patency of the arterial duct or small septal defects, including patency of the oval foramen. This group might also include structural defects which resolve without ever becoming clinically manifest, such as small muscular ventricular septal defects. Consideration of these lesions is important because they are common, and might inflate a prevalence estimate.
- Persistent patency of the arterial duct in premature neonates.

Comparability of previous reports of congenital cardiac malformations has suffered from a lack of common and accepted nomenclature regarding their morphological and functional description, developmental aspects, and interrelationships. To some extent, there has been important work in consolidating nomenclature towards an internationally accepted standard.[2–4] This will greatly facilitate future collection of data relevant to incidence, prevalence, and prognosis. It does not resolve the current dilemma.

RATIOS, RATES, AND PROPORTIONS

Confusion and misuse regarding the terms incidence and prevalence is rooted in misunderstanding regarding what constitutes a ratio, a rate, and a proportion. A ratio has a numerator and a denominator, which are mutually exclusive. An example would be the ratio of males to females born with transposed arterial trunks. It has use when one is interested in the relative frequencies of two related categories, and is often represented as an entity called odds. A rate has both a numerator, indicating frequency of occurrence of a condition or event, and a denominator, indicating the time period over which the numerator was accumulated. Often the rate would apply to a defined population at risk for the condition, or an event specified in the numerator. An example would be the rate of the occurrence of a thrombotic episode in patients during their first year subsequent to construction of the Fontan circulation. Such a rate may give the impression that the condition or event occurs uniformly over the specified period of time, which may or may not be true. Rates are often used when assessing the risk of occurrence of a condition or event, and are often accompanied by explorations of factors that might be associated with increases or decreases in that rate. An often more appropriate method for looking at rates would be the calculation of Kaplan-Meier estimates, or parametric modeling of the time-related hazard, which would depict and reflect instantaneous changes in rates and risk over time. A proportion, likewise, has a numerator, which represents the frequency of a condition or category within the population specified in the denominator. It is frequently expressed as a fraction or percent, and is independent of any period of time. An example would be the proportion of patients with deficient ventricular septation in whom the defect itself is encased within the muscular ventricular septum. It would most frequently be used when describing the frequency of a characteristic or condition in a specified population.

INCIDENCE

This entity is a rate, and is strictly defined as the number of new occurrences of a condition or event identified over a specified period of time related to the number of the population at risk. The precondition is that the population at risk starts the period of observation with no occurrences of the condition or event. To apply this definition to individuals with congenitally malformed hearts, it would be necessary to begin the evaluation at conception, and then to follow embryos and fetuses throughout cardiac development to determine the number who develop defects. This would be an impossible task, since many conceptions may terminate spontaneously before cardiac development is complete, or even before conception has become manifest, or before a defect could be detected with current technology. This inability creates important challenges in the study of aetiology. Incidence and rates, however, are relevant in the study of prognosis and the natural and modified natural history.

PREVALENCE

This feature is a proportion, and is strictly defined as the number of pre-existing and new occurrences of a condition or event identified in a population at risk, either at a single point in time or over a specified period. What many mistakenly refer to as the incidence of congenital cardiac disease is in reality the prevalence, consisting of the number of newborns who are subsequently confirmed to have congenitally malformed hearts as observed within a defined population of live born individuals over a specified time. Such a proportion would more appropriately be called the prevalence at live birth. This prevalence at live birth reflects the incidence of congenital cardiac disease as modified by undetected conceptions, spontaneous and elective terminations, and stillbirths, all of which may occur differentially in those with specific aetiologies or defects. The recognised proportion can further be modified by the completeness and accuracy of ascertainment of disease in all those neonates born alive. Rarely, some estimates of prevalence may include stillbirths, giving the prevalence of congenital cardiac disease in completed pregnancies. Alternatively, some estimates may include fetuses assessed prenatally, some of which may be spontaneously or electively terminated. If it were possible accurately to assess disease prenatally in all fetuses from a uniform time point in gestation, then it would be possible to estimate the prevalence at fetal assessment. This is not the current reality, and the current inclusion of data relating to fetal diagnosis in estimates of prevalence creates great inaccuracy and confusion.

The prevalence at live birth is, of course, important in defining the maximal burden of congenital cardiac disease in the population. The natural and modified natural history specific to certain defects, and strategies for their management, influences the changing prevalence in the population over time, with the numerator and denominator both decreasing due to deaths, and the numerator falling due to spontaneous resolution. The absolute number and characteristics of patients at any given time is important in defining the burden posed by disease, which is a key determinant in defining the requirements for resources. With the increasing survival of patients into adulthood, and their transition into the system of health care providing for adults, this number has taken on increasing importance, but its accurate estimation is fraught with numerous methodological challenges.

RELEVANCE OF INCIDENCE AND PREVALENCE

Estimates of incidence and prevalence, and the study of factors influencing them, have relevance to many aspects of congenital cardiac disease and its management.

Aetiologic Associations

Accepting the caveats discussed above, it remains the case that knowledge of factors associated with variations in the prevalence of specific lesions, or groups of lesions, may suggest aetiologic influences. These factors might then be used to target prenatal screening and counseling, or they might be amenable to intervention, resulting in the prevention of congenital cardiac disease. In general, studies providing evidence of such associations have been difficult to perform when using an approach depending on cohorts identified at birth, since congenital cardiac disease is rare, specific lesions even rarer, and potential factors may similarly be rare. In addition, aetiologic factors may not act uniformly or consistently in respect to the lesion under investigation. Classifications of lesions on the basis of morphology may not relate to aetiology. Genetic studies have shown that specific genetic factors may be associated with a variety of lesions, which might not typically be grouped together on the basis of morphology. Studies of environmental factors have not yielded great discoveries, and have engendered few hypotheses. Focused hypotheses regarding associations between specific factors and specific lesions can more efficiently be pursued using studies based on case-control study designs.

Surveillance and Trends over Time

Related somewhat to aetiology, there is an ongoing interest in discovering trends in the prevalence of congenital cardiac disease. Ongoing surveillance is necessary to detect acute changes in prevalence that may be attributable to a specific aetiology, such as the epidemic of birth defects associated with the use of thalidomide during pregnancy. These changes in prevalence reflect a true change in the incidence of congenital cardiac disease. Many factors other than aetiologic ones, nonetheless, may contribute to a change in prevalence. Prevalence may decrease with prenatal diagnosis and elective termination. Prevalence may increase with increasing access to medical care, prenatal diagnosis, prevention of death during fetal life, improved screening and diagnostic capabilities, and their broader application. Estimates of prevalence may also change with alterations in definitions, nomenclature, and classification. Examination and comparison of prevalence across periods of time, or disparate geography and ethnic regions, requires careful attention to these details.

Likelihood of Diagnosis

Knowledge of the relative frequency of specific lesions can aid somewhat in formulating differential diagnoses and an index of suspicion. Most studies of prevalence at live birth continue to include cases that were diagnosed beyond the first few days of life, and often into the first year. In earlier studies, ascertainment relied almost exclusively on clinical manifestation and presentation. So-called critical disease is more likely to present in the neonatal period during the transition from fetal circulation with closure of the arterial duct and oval foramen, and the fall in pulmonary arterial resistance. Anomalies associated with evident syndromes are also more likely to be detected early. Some defects, such as ventricular septal defects, are not evident until further falls in pulmonary vascular resistance permit an increase in the shunting of blood, with emergence of heart murmurs and signs of cardiac failure, typically in early infancy. Still other defects, such as aortic valvar stenosis and coarctation, might initially be mild, without evident symptoms or signs, and not become manifest until the obstruction worsened weeks, months, or even years later. Some lesions, such as the aortic valve with two leaflets, or uncomplicated congenitally corrected transposition, may only present fortuitously many years later upon investigation for something else. This picture of diagnostic likelihood has changed recently. Some studies of prevalence have employed uniform early screening. Prenatal diagnosis has had an impact on age at presentation, independent of the severity or physiologic consequences of the cardiovascular defect. In addition, elective termination of more severe defects has had some impact on their relative frequency at live birth.

Burden of Disease and Requirements for Resources

Disease involving the cardiovascular system continues to be the greatest contributor to infant mortality related to congenital malformations. Trends, however, have shown significant decreases in mortality, and an increasing age at which death might occur. The greatest attributable factor to these trends has been advances in management, which have modified the natural history. To a lesser extent, decreasing prevalence of severe lesions related to prenatal diagnosis, and elective termination, may also have an impact. These factors increase the point prevalence of congenital cardiac disease at advancing ages, and have created a growing population of adults with congenitally malformed hearts, which has been predicted soon to exceed the point prevalence during childhood. There have been no studies which have specifically quantified the point prevalence beyond infancy or early childhood. These are difficult to attain, since they would require systems providing complete capture of data, and uniform ongoing contact with those providing health care. Studies in adults would be particularly problematic, in that broad-based systems for their health care do not yet exist, and many adults lose care through lack of coverage, and lack of available providers. In addition, many adults may falsely believe that their congenital cardiac malformation has been cured when it is increasingly shown to be associated with ongoing morbidity and risk of death. Current estimates of the prevalence of congenital cardiac disease in adults rely on projections and assumptions, rather than accurate and specific collection of data. Thus, beyond infancy, the true and ongoing prevalence is poorly known, and hence knowledge concerning the burden of disease on society is equally vague. In addition, while infants and children in general maintain their contact with those providing health care, and thereby influence the estimates made for requirements of resources and future planning in a well-defined system, this is not so for adults, for whom a well-defined system of care does not yet uniformly exist. Reliable estimates of prevalence in adults based on data are needed in order to plan for, and address, their needs for health care, as well as to assess their potential impact on the overall system providing care.

METHODOLOGY AND APPRAISAL

Estimates of prevalence can vary widely between different reports, depending on how the numerator was defined and ascertained, and the source of the data for the denominator. It can also be influenced by the period of time or point in time, and the absolute numbers in both the numerator and denominator. Ideally, differences in estimates of prevalence between reports should reflect true differences in prevalence related to potential aetiologic or epidemiologic factors, such as time trends or genetic or environmental differences between populations, rather than methodological discrepancies.

Denominator

When seeking to estimate prevalence, the first consideration should be the denominator, since that determines the population from which the numerator will be drawn, and also the perspective and utility of the estimate. The denominator is a key piece of information, since it defines the population to which the estimate may be applied, and suggests the population to which the estimate might be extrapolated. The most valid denominators are ones that are enumerated during the time of ascertainment of the cases, such as with a study designed on the basis of a prospective cohort. Such an approach gives the most valid and reliable value for the denominator, and also the numerator, but is intensive in terms of both time and resources. Most estimates of prevalence use, as their denominator, the total number of live births over a specified period of time derived from a geographically defined population, hence giving the prevalence at live birth. The defined population may truly be defined by geography, or may relate to a catchment area, or to a subset of the population under a specified plan or system providing health care.

A convenient, and readily available, denominator, frequently used, is the number of births reported to a governmental system for registration of births. These almost always relate to a geographically defined population, and reporting is usually mandatory. In looking at such estimates, it should be clear that the cases were ascertained from the same catchment or geographic area as the reported number of births from the birth registry. In addition, the periods over which the births occurred, and the cases were ascertained, should be identical. Information regarding the validity and reliability of the registry should also be available. Strategies by which all births were correctly identified, characterised, and reported should be explicit. Any information regarding validation, through audits of the data, should be sought. Some registries will include stillbirths and fetal deaths, and this information should be evident. Registries of births usually collect additional information, specifically demographics for the family, but may also include data regarding clinical diagnoses and characteristics at birth. Some estimates of prevalence will rely on this information for ascertainment of cases. If so, then the validity and reliability of that data needs carefully to be scrutinised.

Some studies report the prevalence of congenital cardiac disease as a contributor to overall or infant mortality. For these studies, a governmental registry of deaths may be used to define a denominator, that being the number of deaths occurring over a specified period of time within a defined geographic area. Many of the same limitations regarding validity and reliability of data for registration at birth apply to registration at death. Information regarding clinical diagnoses and cause of death are often collected. If this is used for ascertainment, then further consideration should be given to validity and reliability, particularly since the qualifications of the persons completing and submitting these data are typically unknown, as well as the definitions they might have used.

Numerator

The numerator of any estimate of prevalence will represent the number of cases of congenital cardiac disease that were identified from a population at risk over a defined period of time. To evaluate the numerator, one must know how the cases were identified and verified from the source of the data, what types of lesions were included and excluded, and what scheme was used for nomenclature and classification.

Ascertainment of Cases

The completeness of identification of the cases from the source population is a critical aspect of appraisal of the numerator of an estimate of prevalence. A comprehensive and active prospective surveillance of all sources of cases is likely to yield the most complete ascertainment, since ascertainment is a specific and planned endeavour. Most studies of this nature rely on clinical presentation, or evaluation of a living subject, as the initial point of entry. Many trivial lesions, nonetheless, such as small atrial septal defects, mild pulmonary valvar stenoses, tiny muscular ventricular septal defects, silent arterial ducts, and nonstenotic aortic valves with two leaflets, may not cause symptoms, and clinical findings may be subtle or absent. In addition, some of these lesions may resolve spontaneously without ever being detected. Still other types of severe lesions may occasionally lead to death before a clinical diagnosis is made or verified, and may not be ascertained unless autopsies are performed and the information is accessed and the case included. An important aspect of ascertainment is the interval from birth during which cases could be identified and included. This would be particularly important for cases identified initially on the basis of clinical features. The majority of patients with significant congenital cardiac disease would be expected to present early. Some lesions, however, may not become clinically manifest until the occurrence of physiologic changes, such as with a fall in pulmonary vascular resistance and increased shunting with ventricular septal defects, or with the development of pulmonary vascular disease or ventricular dysfunction with other lesions. Some lesions may become clinically manifest only with progression of the pathology over time, such as with valvar stenoses. The duration of follow-up for ascertainment must be sufficiently long that all cases are identified.

The optimal method for complete ascertainment would be a universal screening shortly after live birth with a technology with sufficient sensitivity to detect all lesions, usually echocardiography. Given the large number of newborns that would have to undergo screening to detect sufficient cases to allow such a valid and reliable estimate of prevalence, this is unlikely to be feasible. Currently, fetal ultrasound at 14 to 20 weeks of gestation seems to be universally performed for nearly all pregnancies in developed countries, particularly those with universal provisions for healthcare. This might afford the opportunity for a complete surveillance, but routine fetal ultrasound as performed has proven to have a low sensitivity, unless cardiac assessment is specifically and accurately applied. At present, fetal detection of cardiac lesions, even serious ones, is variable and imperfect. Other sources can be used to supplement cases ascertained from surveillance, including registries of deaths and autopsy records, registries of birth defects, and administrative data such as abstracts at discharge from hospital, and data from medical claims. These sources have the advantage that reporting is often mandatory, although they are limited by the validity and reliability with which diagnoses and details are reported.

Verification of Cases

Given the preceding discussion that most studies of prevalence rely on a clinical diagnosis for the majority of identification of cases, verification or confirmation is very important. Earlier studies focused on cases identified or verified by autopsy, but this would include only cases associated with a high mortality, and for whom a decision to perform an autopsy was made. Studies that have focused on cases ascertained through clinical presentation and identification have reported high estimates unless some sort of objective verification has been applied. Earlier studies have included cases verified by autopsy, surgery, or cardiac catheterisation. These estimates have been somewhat low, and skewed toward more serious lesions, but become inflated when cases with a clinical diagnosis only are included. The Baltimore–Washington Infant Study was one of the first studies to include echocardiography as a means of verification.[5] Echocardiography has since become the standard for the initial verification of cases, and has proven to have high sensitivity and specificity. In general, these early studies that used echocardiography as a means for verification have produced similar estimates to those studies which use more invasive means of verification, with larger estimates if cases with a clinical diagnosis only are also included. Broader and earlier application of echocardiography, and improved sensitivity through the application of cross sectional imaging and colour Doppler interrogation, have resulted in improved detection of haemodynamically insignificant lesions, such as tiny or small muscular ventricular septal defects, and silent arterial ducts. This improved ascertainment has largely accounted for an apparent increase in estimates of prevalence. The impact of fetal echocardiography will likely also influence ascertainment in future studies of prevalence, through both possible improved detection of cases with lesions who might succumb during fetal life, and through elective termination.

Sources of Data

Sources for the numerator vary widely in the degree to which ascertainment was passive or active, and the degree to which they accurately relate to a defined denominator. Knowledge of the details and limitations of these sources is important for critical appraisal.

Earlier studies tended to rely on registration of death and autopsy records for ascertainment. These studies were important in defining the spectrum of congenital cardiac disease and its morphologic features, particularly of complex lesions. Use of autopsy records tended to focus on cases presenting to a tertiary care centre, and were heavily weighted to more severe defects associated with a high mortality. The only valid denominator to which these cases might be applied is that of total autopsies at the given institution, and it would give the proportion of congenitally malformed hearts among deaths verified by autopsy, and may be an indicator of the contribution of congenital cardiac disease to overall mortality. Alternatively, most geopolitical regions have some sort of mandatory registration of death. There is usually an accurate enumeration of deaths, although reporting of causes of death and associated conditions may be less accurate and, therefore, less useful in determining a numerator. The accuracy of identification of cases from death certificates depends on who completes the registration, along with their knowledge of that person and their medical history, whether an autopsy was performed and the information included, and whether the congenital malformation was the primary cause of death, a contributing factor or an associated condition. One such study of death of patients with congenitally malformed hearts previously followed by paediatric cardiologists showed that only four-fifths of certificates noted cardiovascular disease, with the major defect being noted on only two-fifths of certificates.[6] This highlights the deficiencies in relying on registries of death for ascertainment.

Secondary data is that which was collected for purposes other than the research question at hand. Usually this data is collected for purposes of documenting clinical care, such as the health record, or for administrative purposes usually linked to reimbursement or statistical tracking. The findings often have the advantage that the collection itself is mandatory. Administrative data may include registries of births and deaths, and abstracts of discharge from hospital and databases of medical claims. The major limitation of using such data as the source of ascertainment is the variable completeness and accurateness by which diagnoses are recorded in a valid and reliable manner. Diagnoses recorded on registrations of births and deaths may only enumerate those present and verified at the time of registration. Ascertainment using databases of hospital discharges only identify those cases associated with hospitalisation, which might be true for only a limited number of lesions.[7] The addition of databases recording medical claims that capture outpatient assessments and diagnostic testing may be important supplements to ascertainment using administrative data. While administrative data is of limited value in specifying the numerator, as mentioned previously, it is often useful in defining the denominator, particularly of live births.

An important source of secondary data for ascertainment is the medical record. Sufficient information can often be found in the medical record to identify and verify cases. Many studies have used the medical records of tertiary care centres in such a manner in reported series, but are limited in that the denominator is difficult to define. The challenge of the denominator often precludes an accurate estimate of prevalence, but these studies are useful in defining the spectrum and distribution of congenitally malformed hearts, particularly in reference to the provision of clinical care. These types of studies are now rarely reported, except from developing countries where the only cases that may be enumerated are those presenting to a specialised centre. Some studies relate to a defined system for provision of healthcare, with the denominator being all individuals captured and registered within that system. These studies can produce an estimate of prevalence, but the degree to which it is representative of the proportion of the population not included within that system is often unknown.

The most accurate and complete source for ascertainment is from surveillance, particularly if the surveillance is an active rather than passive process. Mechanisms for passive surveillance tend to rely on voluntary reporting, which may be incomplete with variable verification of diagnoses. The most valid estimates of prevalence are derived from active surveillance, particularly if both the numerator and denominator are defined simultaneously as part of the surveillance. Such active studies tend to be designed specifically to determine an estimate of prevalence. They may also include a more focused collection of data, usually in the format of case-control design, aimed at detecting associations of a potential aetiologic nature. The completeness of ascertainment depends on the comprehensive nature of the system created for identification. This may include primary care networks, paediatric cardiologists working in both community-based and tertiary care practise, as well as all points of obstetrical delivery and care of the newborn. The reporting from these points of contact may be voluntary by the practitioners themselves, or may involve surveyors deployed to these sites. The reporting may occur as each case is identified, or after periodic assessments of logs or records. Identified cases are usually referred to experts for verification and specification, usually in centres of tertiary care. Pathology departments may also be involved. Additionally, registrations of births and deaths, and other types of administrative data, may be reviewed. The challenge to complete ascertainment is the reliance on clinical presentation and findings to initiate identification and verification of the cases, the limitations of which have been stated above.

The most complete source for ascertainment would be the active screening of a defined population. A sensitive and accurate method of identification would be universally applied to all subjects included in the denominator. Clinical assessment by paediatric cardiologists has been shown to have sufficient, though not perfect, sensitivity and specificity, while other types of providers have fared less well.[8,9] Verification and specification of clinically suspected cases with echocardiography could then be applied. Alternatively, echocardiography could be universally applied as the screening tool, ensuring complete and accurate ascertainment. These types of screenings are not feasible for application on a large scale, and the resulting estimates of prevalence would tend to be more accurate but less reliable.

Definition of Cases

Regardless of the source used for ascertainment, it must be clearly stated which specific lesions were included and excluded from the numerator. This predominately applies to lesions of minor or no functional consequence but which are common, as discussed previously. The inclusion or exclusion of these types of lesions can have an important impact on inflating the prevalence estimate. Additionally, the time period after live birth during which cases could be identified should be specified and reported. It should be clearly stated whether cases noted in stillbirths and cases diagnosed by fetal assessment, but either spontaneously or electively aborted, are included or excluded.

Nomenclature and Classification

In addition to specifying an overall prevalence, most studies provide a breakdown by specific lesions. This is challenging, in that some lesions may exist in isolation, such as partially anomalous pulmonary venous connection, or as part of a complex of lesions, such as anomalous pulmonary venous return in the setting of isomerism of the atrial appendages and complex congenital cardiac disease. Some isolated lesions may also be complicated by additional lesions, such as transposition with an associated ventricular septal defect. Some patients may have two lesions of equal importance, such as a ventricular septal defect and coarctation of the aorta. Additional lesions may be acquired as either part of the natural history, or as a result of therapeutic interventions. These distinctions make it challenging to identify primary as opposed to secondary lesions. These challenges are magnified by the lack of a uniform nomenclature. Lesions had initially been described on the basis of their first reports, such as Ebstein's malformation or the Holmes heart, and then from systematic examination of pathologic specimens. Nomenclature was therefore driven by considerations of morphology. Increasing understanding of both physiology and cardiac development have modified some of these descriptions, and have led to some controversies. As a result, individuals have used systems for description that were developed within the institutions where they had either trained or practised. Different organisations have attempted to develop consensus regarding common nomenclature, and recently have come together as the International Nomenclature Working Group.[2,3] This organisation seeks to cross-map the different systems, and to provide a common, consensus-based system.[4]

There is often a desire to group together lesions into categories that reflect a common basis in either development, morphology, physiology, management, outcome, or aetiology. A scheme aimed at both the presumed developmental mechanism and physiology was employed in the Baltimore–Washington Infant Study (Table 3.2 in their monograph).[5] It was hypothesised that this classification might reduce aetiologic heterogeneity when related to potential familial and environmental risk factors. More recent studies of genetic mechanisms have shown that a single genetic defect may be associated with a more diverse range of morphologic abnormalities, and that these may not be concordant with the scheme based on developmental mechanisms. These genetic studies have refined our understanding of mechanisms of cardiac development that may influence future schemes for classification.

Reliability of Estimates

When reporting an estimate, it is important to be clear about the methodology behind determining the numerator and the denominator. When describing an estimate, details are needed of what the number represents. Prevalence at live birth is usually reported in terms of the number of cases of congenital cardiac disease in each 1000 live births. Additional information may include the geographic location, and the years over which the numerator and denominator were derived. Not all estimates made in this fashion have the same reliability. Reliability is influenced by the duration underlying the estimate, and the absolute magnitude of the numerator and denominator. Studies in which the estimate represents a period of many years are less reliable, in that changes are likely to have occurred in the system, and influenced the estimate. The absolute magnitude of the numerator and denominator influence the width of the confidence limit. A confidence limit is a statistical derivation of an interval in which we may be 95% confident, or sometimes 70% confident, that the estimate is true. The width of the interval is highly dependent on the absolute numbers. The greater the numbers, the narrower the width of the interval, and the more reliable the estimate. Confidence limits should be reported with any estimate, and often the absolute numbers for the numerator and denominator should be given. The absolute and relative magnitude of the numerator in relation to the denominator may also influence reliability. Estimates based on small numbers of cases are less reliable, and the confidence limits enclose wider ranges of relative magnitude. For example, a 95% confidence interval around an estimate of 100 per 1000 live births might be reported as 98 to 102, or ±2% of 100. A different study of similar size noting an estimate of 10 per 1000 live births with a similar 95% confidence interval of 8 to 12 in terms of absolute magnitude, but ±20% of 10 in terms of relative magnitude, thus would be less reliable. Thus, estimates for total prevalence of congenital cardiac disease, and for common specific lesions, tend to be more precise and reliable than those for less common specific lesions. In addition to reporting confidence intervals around estimates of prevalence, such intervals should also be reported around any measure of association, such as relative risk, odds ratios, or attributable risk.

Critical Appraisal

Most studies that report estimates of prevalence are specifically designed to do so, and have it as the primary aim of the study. Before accepting the results of these studies, it is important critically to appraise the methods and reporting, in order to determine if the findings are valid, reliable, and relevant. Critical appraisal is also required when wishing to compare estimates from different studies, such as comparisons of trends over time, or different populations. Consideration must be given to all of the aspects of the denominator, numerator, and reporting already described. In Table 8-1, I have delineated questions for which the answers should be evident when critically appraising a report regarding prevalence.

FACTORS INFLUENCING ESTIMATES OF PREVALENCE

Ideally, factors should be identified that might have a true causal relationship to the development of congenital cardiac disease, and hence influence the true incidence. Other factors may alter outcomes during fetal life, and predominately affect the prevalence at live birth. Identification of these factors may allow for the prevention of congenital cardiac disease, or provide new knowledge as to aetiology and development. The identification of these associations comes mainly from observational studies.

Environmental Factors

The most commonly held belief is that congenital cardiac disease is the product of an interaction between genes and their environment. Evidence, however, has yet to progress sufficiently far to prove this notion. Numerous environmental factors have been linked to such development, independent of any already known genetic influence or predisposition. The Baltimore–Washington Infant Study provided a thorough assessment of environmental and parental risk factors for the development of congenital cardiac disease, and development of specific lesions.[5] Other research has since contributed to this growing body of knowledge. It is important to note that association does not infer causality, and that identified risk factors can be viewed only as potential risk factors. To infer causality, it would be necessary to perform a randomised controlled trial, and impose a controlled exposure on mothers with child. The ethical dilemma in asking expectant mothers intentionally to expose themselves and their unborn child to a potentially harmful agent for the purposes of a randomised controlled trial can be imagined. We must rely, therefore, on observational studies. Initial associations are usually determined from studies of cohort, where exposures are determined by recall after the child has been born and identified as having congenital cardiac disease. These studies are often subject to recall bias. Case-control studies are an efficient method to focus on a specific exposure, comparing the prevalence of congenital cardiac disease in those having a specific exposure to those not confronted by the same exposure. This is usually reported as an odds ratio, being the odds of congenital cardiac disease in those with the exposure divided by the odds of the disease in those without the exposure.

A recent Scientific Statement from the American Heart Association reviewed studies of prevalence, and summarised studies of environmental factors.[10] In Table 8-2, positive associations for maternal illnesses and maternal exposures are highlighted.

TABLE 8-1

QUESTIONS FOR CRITICALLY APPRAISING A REPORT ABOUT PREVALENCE

What was the stated purpose or aim of the study?

How accurate and valid was the estimate reported?

- How accurate and valid was the definition and completeness of the numerator?
  - What forms of congenital heart disease were included or excluded?
  - What nomenclature and system of classification was used to describe and group cases?
  - What were the methods by which cases were ascertained and reported?
  - What was the overall design of the study and data collection?
  - How were cases detected and reported from the population studied?
  - What factors, particularly relating to the system for healthcare, may have influenced the ascertainment of cases? Specifically, did everyone in the population studied have equal access to healthcare and the referral center, and was screening and verification influenced by differences in quality and availability of expertise or technology?
  - How were diagnoses confirmed or verified?
  - How long was the follow-up, and was it sufficiently long to capture cases with later clinical manifestation?
  - If a universal screening was applied, was it applied equally to the entire population at an early enough time point, was it sufficiently sensitive and specific, and was an assessment of verification performed?
- How accurate and valid was the definition and completeness of the denominator?
  - What was the definition of the population studied?
  - What were the sources of data used to derive the denominator, and were they valid and reliable?
  - How accurately and completely does the population studied reflect the target population or population at large?
  - Are the cases completed derived from the population studied as defined in the denominator? Were the cases and population characterized as part of the same study with the same methodology, as in a cohort study?

How reliable is the estimate of prevalence estimate? Are confidence intervals provided?

How does the estimate from the study compare to those reported from other studies with comparable methodology?

Is the estimate applicable to your own clinical population? Is the population studied similar to your own clinical population in terms of setting, time, geography, and demographic characteristics? Is the estimate of prevalence relevant to your own clinical or research question?

TABLE 8-2

FETAL EXPOSURES AND INCREASED RISK OF CONGENITAL HEART DEFECTS

Exposures Associated with Definite or Possible Risk of Offspring with Any Congenital Cardiovascular Defect	Odds Ratio
Maternal Illness	
Phenylketonuria[11–14]	>6
Pregestational diabetes[15–18]	3.1–18
Febrile illness[15, 19–21]	1.8–2.9
Influenza[21, 22]	2.1
Maternal rubella[23]	†
Epilepsy[24]	†
Prepregnancy overweight/obesity[25]	1.13–1.40
Maternal Therapeutic Drug Exposure	
Anticonvulsants[26, 27]	4.2
Ibuprofen[28]	1.86
Sulfasalazine[29]	3.4
Thalidomide[30]	†
Trimethoprim-sulfonamide*[29, 31]	2.1–4.8
Vitamin A congeners/retinoids*[32, 33]	†

*Risk reduced if mother took folic acid simultaneously.
†Odds ratio not available.
Adapted from Jenkins KJ, Correa A, Feinstein JA, et al: Noninherited risk factors and congenital cardiovascular defects: Current knowledge—a scientific statement from the American Heart Association Council on Cardiovascular Disease in the Young: Endorsed by the American Academy of Pediatrics. Circulation 2007;115:2995–3014.

TABLE 8-3

MATERNAL EXPOSURE TO ORGANIC SOLVENTS AND RISK OF SPECIFIC CONGENITAL HEART DEFECTS

Defect	Risk Ratio
Defects of the ventricular outflow tracts[34, 35]	2.0–3.9
Hypoplastic left heart syndrome[15]	3.4
Coarctation of the aorta[15, 36]	3.2
Pulmonary stenosis[15]	5.0
Transposition[15]	3.4
Tetralogy of Fallot[15]	2.7
Totally anomalous pulmonary venous return[15, 37]	2.0
Atrioventricular septal defect (nonchromosomal)[15]	5.6
Ebstein's malformation[15, 38]	3.6

Adapted from Jenkins KJ, Correa A, Feinstein JA, et al: Noninherited risk factors and congenital cardiovascular defects: Current knowledge—a scientific statement from the American Heart Association Council on Cardiovascular Disease in the Young: Endorsed by the American Academy of Pediatrics. Circulation 2007;115:2995–3014.

Table 8-3 shows that maternal exposure to organic solvents has frequently and consistently been reported to be associated with relatively high odds ratios for development of specific congenital cardiac malformations. In contrast to maternal illnesses and use of medications, it is feasible to avoid exposure to organic solvents, and programmes can be directed at reducing maternal exposures to these materials.

An earlier study summarised environmental associations noted from the Baltimore–Washington Infant Study.[2] The study was a large population-based surveillance with careful verification. The investigators reported results as both relative risk, representing the prevalence of congenital cardiac disease in those with the exposure divided by the prevalence in those without the exposure, and attributable fraction, this being the proportion of cases of specific defects that might be attributable to specific exposure. In Table 8-4, the identified positive associations are highlighted. Some of the significant exposures were paternal rather than maternal.

Genetic Factors

The science of genetics, genomics, and proteomics has seen rapid advancements with the application of novel technologies and improved understanding. The prevalence of congenital cardiac disease is increased in children with specific chromosomal abnormalities and syndromes. Genetic defects are also being discovered that are associated with abnormalities of cardiac development and an increased prevalence. Furthermore, with increasing survival of women into the child-bearing years who themselves have congenitally malformed hearts, the issue of recurrence in the offspring has become of importance.

Chromosomal Abnormalities

Children with chromosomal abnormalities have a greater likelihood of having a congenital cardiac malformation. A high prevalence of congenital cardiac disease has been observed among children with trisomy 21, or Down syndrome,[39] trisomy 18 or Edwards' syndrome,[40,41] trisomy 13 or Patau's syndrome,[40,42] and monosomy XO, or Turner's syndrome. These syndromes are also associated with an increased prevalence of extracardiac anomalies. Changes in the prevalence of these conditions as a result of elective termination on the basis of prenatal testing may influence the prevalence of congenital cardiac disease at live birth. These chromosomal abnormalities are also associated with a higher rate of fetal death and stillbirth. The median survival of live born infants with trisomy 13 is reported at 2.5 to 10 days,[42–44] and the median survival of live born infants with trisomy 18 is reported at 2.5 to 14.5 days.[41,43–46] Consequently, their high rate of early mortality, some of which is due to decisions to pursue only palliative care, with non-intervention, will remove them from estimates of prevalence derived at time points later in life.

The inclusion of stillbirths in estimates of prevalence is somewhat problematic, but is of importance if seeking genetic influences. Detecting the associations with congenitally malformed hearts in stillborns would require that all stillborns be autopsied and undergo genetic testing. One autopsy study found that the prevalence of congenitally malformed hearts in stillborns was 16%,[47] which is much higher than the prevalence in live born infants. Of those stillborns with congenital cardiac disease, half had more than one cardiac anomaly. The presence of a chromosomal abnormality was noted in just over half of the stillborns who had multiple or complex cardiac defects. Given the high likelihood of both congenital cardiac disease and chromosomal abnormalities in stillborns, it is, therefore, important to include them when seeking genetic associations. Likewise, inclusion of fetuses dying spontaneously prior to birth is also important, since they are also more likely to have chromosomal abnormalities in association with congenital cardiac disease. These cases, however, are difficult to capture, since abortions are usually spontaneous, and material is unlikely to be available for autopsy examination. The increasing application of fetal screening and echocardiography will likely detect more of these fetuses, and increase the likelihood of obtaining genetic material and confirmation of diagnoses.

With the average maternal age increasing, the prevalence of infants with chromosomal abnormalities is likely to rise, in particular the number of infants with trisomy 21. This is associated with congenital cardiac disease in from two-fifths to half of pregnancies.[48–55] After the age of 30 years, a mother's risk of having a child with trisomy 21 increases exponentially, such that by the time she is 35 years, the risk is 1 in 365 pregnancies.[56] A rate of selective termination of nine-tenths is reported when the syndrome is detected prenatally.[57] When used more routinely, prenatal screening for trisomy 21 may reduce the prevalence at birth of congenital cardiac disease associated with this chromosomal abnormality.

The prevalence at live birth of trisomy 21, trisomy 18, trisomy 13, and monosomy XO may reflect the impact of selective termination. Sensitive and specific techniques for prenatal screening that can detect these syndromes are now more readily available, especially for pregnancies deemed to be at high risk. Parents are opting to abort affected fetuses. This is likely to influence current estimates of prevalence at live birth. Measurements of nuchal translucency, for example, have demonstrated a modest association with congenital cardiac disease.[58,59] While not supported as an effective screening method for congenital cardiac disease,[60,61] this method does indicate a means of identifying the possible risk for the presence of a cardiac defect, and referral for more specific screening.

Non-syndromic Genetic Abnormalities

A number of genes have been implicated in the development of congenital cardiac disease, albeit that the extent of their involvement is still relatively unknown. Studies of the influence of genetics on the development and maldevelopment of the heart are still evolving, and will be facilitated by improving technology, along with the creation of large databases and banks of tissue and deoxyribonucleic acid. Specific genetic disorders can display classic mendelian inheritance, whereby a phenotype manifests as a result of mutations in one or both copies of a gene, or they can be multi-factorial disorders, whereby a host of

TABLE 8-4

ATTRIBUTABLE FRACTION OF CONGENITAL CARDIAC LESIONS TO POTENTIAL RISK FACTORS

Malformation and Potential Risk Factors	$P < 0.01$		Relative Risk
	AF (%)	95% CI	
Transposition with Intact Ventricular Septum (*N* = 106)	12.1	8.5–15.8	
Influenza	7.0	3.6–10.3	2.2
Miscellaneous solvents	4.8	3.0–6.6	3.2
Tetralogy of Fallot (*N* = 204)	6.5	4.8–8.3	
Paternal anaesthesia	3.9	2.4–5.5	2.5
Clomiphene	2.4	1.5–3.4	3.0
Atrioventricular Septal Defect with Down Syndrome (*N* = 190)	4.6	2.7–6.5	
Ibuprofen	4.6	2.7–6.5	2.4
Hypoplastic Left Heart Syndrome (*N* = 138)	8.6	6.9–10.3	
Solvent/degreasing agent	4.6	3.2–6.0	3.4
Family history of congenital heart disease	4.0	3.1–4.9	4.8
Coarctation of the Aorta (*N* = 120)	9.4	8.1–10.8	
Family history of congenital heart disease	4.6	3.5–5.7	4.6
Macrodantin	2.3	1.8–2.8	6.7
Clomiphene	2.0	1.4–2.7	4.5
Isolated/Simple Perimembranous VSD (*N* = 459)	7.9	4.2–11.6	
Paternal use of marijuana	6.0	2.2–9.7	1.4
Maternal use of cocaine	1.7	0.9–2.5	2.4
Multiple/Multiplex Perimembranous VSD (*N* = 181)	8.3	6.0–10.5	
Paternal use of cocaine	4.8	2.6–6.9	2.3
Diabetes mellitus	2.1	1.4–2.8	3.9
Metronidazole	1.4	1.1–1.7	7.6
Atrial Septal Defect (*N* = 187)	14.1	11.3–17.0	
Gestational diabetes mellitus	4.4	2.5–6.2	2.4
Paternal use of cocaine	3.7	1.9–5.4	2.3
Family history of congenital heart disease	3.4	2.4–4.3	3.9
Corticosteroids	2.6	1.9–3.2	4.8

AF, attributable fraction; CI, confidence interval; VSD, ventricular septal defect.
Adapted from Wilson PD, Loffredo CA, Correa-Villasenor A, Ferencz C: Attributable fraction for cardiac malformations. Am J Epidemiol 1998;148:414–423.

polymorphisms interact with each other and environmental factors to produce a phenotype (see Chapter 9). This makes it difficult to identify the genes responsible, and their interaction with environmental factors is very complicated. Careful studies are needed to validate hypotheses regarding aetiology. Studies of prevalence, particularly those that get closest to incidence, can contribute largely to this effort.

The deletion of the 22q11 gene has been implicated as a major contributor to the development of congenital cardiac disease, as well as other major birth defects.[62] As the occurrence of genetic testing varies from country to country, and from institution to institution, the prevalence of the deletion cannot be characterised as accurately as desired. Studies in well-defined populations have estimated the prevalence of the deletion to be around 1.5 cases in each 10,000 live births.[62,63] It has been suggested that over 1% of all congenitally malformed hearts are associated with the deletion, accounting for half of the cases with interrupted aortic arch, one-fifth of those with common arterial trunk, and one-sixth of those with tetralogy of Fallot.[63]

A newer body of research has begun to explore the genetics of folate metabolism and the effects on the development of congenitally malformed hearts. The methylenetetrahydrofolate reductase gene has recently been identified as playing a role in such development, with certain allelic variants having a protective effect,[64] while others are risk factors in the absence of periconceptional folate supplementation.[65]

Risk of Recurrence

The risk of congenital cardiac disease recurring in the offspring of affected individuals is of increasing interest as treatment and surgical correction are allowing for survival into adulthood, and affected women are reaching their child-bearing years (Table 8-5).

In the majority of cases, no single underlying cause can be identified. Some lesions, nonetheless, have displayed monogenic inheritance with relatively high concordance. In one study,[96] analysis was made of referrals for fetal echocardiography at a tertiary centre. When the reason for referral was a positive family history of congenital cardiac disease in a first-degree relative, the recurrence in offspring was 2.7%. In recurrent cases, the overall concordance was almost half between the parent and the first affected child for lesions in the same group, with exact concordance in almost two-fifths. Such exact concordance was high for laterality defects and isolated atrioventricular septal defects, at two-thirds and four-fifths, respectively. In one-fifth of families, first-, second-, and third-degree relatives were found to have congenital cardiac disease, providing evidence for dominantly inherited susceptibility genes with incomplete penetrance as contributors to recurrence. Supporting evidence for concordant recurrence of atrioventricular septal defect has been reported elsewhere.[82] Of note, affected women experience more miscarriages,[82] and congenital cardiac defects appear to occur more in the offspring of affected women than affected men,[82,97,98] suggesting that imprinted genes play a role in normal cardiac development, relying on the maternal copy of the gene.[82] With the population of affected adult females growing, future studies will be able to provide more information about the contribution of genetics to the development of congenitally malformed hearts. Information about these genetic influences on prevalence will accompany such findings.

TABLE 8-5

NON-SYNDROMIC CONGENITAL CARDIAC DEFECTS AND IMPLICATED MODES OF INHERITANCE, RISKS OF RECURRENCE, AND GENES

Congenital Cardiac Defect	Mode of Inheritance	Recurrence Risk	Gene	Reference
Atrioventricular septal defect	Multi-factorial	3%–4%	—	66–69
	Autosomal dominant	50%	*p93*	70
			CRELDI	71, 72
			GATA4	73
			PTPN11	74
Tetralogy of Fallot	Multi-factorial	2.5%–3%	—	68, 69, 75
	Autosomal dominant	50%	*NKX2.5*	76
	Autosomal recessive	25%	*Jagged 1*	77
	Three-gene model	2.5%–3%	*FOG2*	78
			—	79
			—	75, 80, 81
				82
Transposition	Multi-factorial	1%–1.8%	—	82–84
	Autosomal dominant	50%	*CFC1*	85
Congenitally corrected transposition	Multi-factorial	5.8%	—	86
Left-sided obstructions	Multi-factorial	3%	—	87
	Autosomal dominant	50%	*NOTCH1*	88
	Autosomal recessive	25%	*NKX2.5*	89
			—	90–92
Atrial septal defect	Multi-factorial	3%	—	87
	Autosomal dominant	50%	*NKX2.5*	93, 94
			GATA4	93
			MHC6	95

Adapted from Calcagni G, Digilio MC, Sarkozy A, et al: Familial recurrence of congenital heart disease: An overview and review of the literature. Eur J Pediatr 2007;166:111–116.

Multiple Pregnancies and Reproductive Technology

It is estimated that twins of a monozygotic pair have a two-fold increase in the prevalence of congenital cardiac disease compared to singletons.[99] The prevalence of a congenital heart defect in at least one twin of a monochorionic pair is estimated at almost 1 in 10,[100] with the prevalence in the second twin increasing to over one-quarter if the first twin is affected.[101,102] There is inconclusive evidence of concordancy in the lesions affecting both twins.[100,103] Possible explanations for the increased prevalence of congenital cardiac disease in monozygotic twins include the postzygotic unequal division of the inner cell mass accounting for discordant vascular anatomy,[103] and disturbances of laterality.[104,105] In twin-to-twin transfusion syndrome, there is a 12-fold increase in the prevalence of structural cardiac defects, possibly acquired in response to altered haemodynamics. It was reported that pulmonary stenosis accounted for one-third of the lesions present in the recipient in the setting of twin-to-twin transfusion.[103] With the increasing use of technologies for assisted reproduction, the prevalence of both monochorionic twinning and congenital cardiac disease is increasing, dependently and independently of each other. In vitro fertilisation is responsible for a prevalence of monozygotic twinning of over 3%, compared to less than 0.5% in the general population.[106] Multi-fetal pregnancies carry the risk of adverse neonatal outcomes resulting from premature birth,[107] low weight at birth,[107] and babies born small for their gestational age,[108] all of which carry associations with the development of congenital cardiac disease.[109] The odds ratio for a cardiovascular malformation in premature neonates has been reported to be 2.4.[110] Studies have indicated a two- to four-fold increase in the prevalence of congenital cardiac defects in infants conceived by means of in vitro fertilisation.[111,112] With more females delaying childbirth, and consequently seeking treatment for infertility, the potential impact on the prevalence of congenital cardiac disease might be important. Consequently, detailed fetal echocardiography is merited in the setting of multiple pregnancies, and in those resulting from in vitro fertilisation.

Systemic Factors

Two important factors are emerging as influences on the changing prevalence of congenital cardiac disease that are not reflective of changes in incidence, but of changes related to the systems providing health care. As mentioned repeatedly in the preceding discussion, prenatal diagnosis will improve ascertainment, but also allow for interventions, which may alter the prevalence at live birth. Improvements in management of most congenital cardiac lesions have led to improved survival, such that for the majority of patients, survival into adulthood is assured. This has resulted in dramatic changes in the point prevalence of congenital cardiac disease, its spectrum, and its demographics.

Fetal Diagnosis and Termination

The increasing use of fetal ultrasound and echocardiography has important implications for the prevalence of congenital cardiac disease. As I have pointed out, the true incidence of congenital cardiac disease would take into account all conceptions that are affected by a cardiac defect. Since many fetuses may die prior to ascertainment, they are often excluded in estimates of prevalence. The impact of fetal echocardiography on prevalence, therefore, is two-fold. Detection of lesions during fetal life may allow their inclusion should the fetus die prior to birth, the cause of death never being ascertained. Of those detected through fetal echocardiography, up to one-sixth die in this fashion.[113–115] In addition, those cases that are detected and then selectively terminated, can also be included, thus providing a higher estimate more reflective of the true incidence of congenital cardiac disease. Alternatively, cases detected during fetal life may be amenable to specific strategies for management that will prevent fetal death and stillbirth, or possibly interventions aimed at altering the development of the congenital cardiac malformation itself. At the same time, with increased use and accuracy, fetal detection is likely to increase the number of selective terminations. While these fetuses may still be counted in estimates of prevalence, information about them will have little impact on areas of antenatal and postnatal prognosis. Those cases that will be live born are of more relative importance to the systems providing healthcare than those that are terminated. Until fetal diagnosis and management is routine and clinically effective, selective termination will be an option for many parents faced with a fetal diagnosis of congenital cardiac disease, and will influence the prevalence at live birth.

Reported rates of fetal detection vary from two- to three-fifths in studies on non-selected populations,[115–117] and may be as high as five-sixths in selected populations.[118] Variation in detection may be attributed to the expertise of the sonographer,[117] the stage of pregnancy at which the ultrasound is performed,[114] and whether or not the outflow tracts are observed.[116] During late gestation, diagnosis of lesions is easier and minor lesions are more commonly found.[114,119] This is problematic for parents who would potentially opt for selective termination, as it is often unsafe to undergo therapeutic abortion beyond the first trimester. Lesions may go undetected if screening is performed in the first trimester. A further issue is the imperfect specificity of fetal ultrasound. A specificity of 99% would leave 1% of those referred with a false-positive diagnosis, which may lead to an unjustified termination. Reports on prevalence of terminations following prenatal diagnosis vary from less than one-fifth to half,[113–116,120] with the majority of pregnancies being aborted in the first trimester.[114,115] The variation is likely due to legal, social, religious, and economic factors. Termination, nonetheless, is clearly an option that parents are choosing to exercise. Some have tried to estimate the impact of fetal echocardiography on the prevalence of congenital cardiac disease at live birth.[121] Assuming a sensitivity of 35%, and subsequent termination rate of 43% for an affected fetus, this would result in an estimated 15% reduction in the prevalence of the most severe forms of congenital heart defects. If diagnosis occurred earlier, termination rates would increase 1.4-fold and the prevalence at live birth would be further reduced. There is no certainty, however, that those terminations would have all been live born had the pregnancy continued.

Given that elective termination is not certain following detection of a cardiac defect, clinicians need to respond to the needs of affected fetuses for care. Awareness of a lesion during fetal life is of no value if the outcome is no different from that of an undetected lesion presenting at live birth. Since fetal interventions are limited, and of uncertain safety and benefit, fetal diagnosis is primarily used to inform postnatal care and prognosis. For example, prenatal diagnosis is associated with a decreased risk of postnatal cardiovascular compromise and organ dysfunction, and better preoperative condition, when compared with cases diagnosed following discharge to home after hospital delivery.[122] Delivery before 36 weeks of gestation is discouraged because of associations with high morbidity and mortality for premature neonates.[123] Studies of outcomes subsequent to fetal echocardiography have recently become more frequent and important, showing that anatomical and haemodynamic factors that might predict outcomes and prognosis following live birth can inform decisions relative to management both before and after live birth.[124–129]

Adults with Congenitally Malformed Hearts

It is predicted that five-sixths of patients born with congenitally malformed hearts will now survive to adulthood. Projections suggest that this will result in the need for follow-up for over 200 extra cases per 100,000 live births each year.[130] In a representative population in 2000, there were equal numbers of children and adults alive with severe congenital cardiac disease.[131] The Congenital Cardiac Centre for Adults in Toronto, Canada, reported a significant and steady fall in the mean age of their population over the period from 1987 to 1997, reflective of the number of young adults referred to their centre who had undergone previous repair as opposed to palliation.[132] Estimates indicate that of the patients, one-quarter would have complex lesions, over half would have significant lesions, and less than one-fifth minor lesions.[131] Morbidity is still relatively high in this population, especially for those with complex defects. Overall Kaplan-Meier estimates of mortality after 5 years for patients with a congenital cardiac defect after the age of 17 have been reported at 3.0% to as high as 12.6% for patients with cyanotic defects, and 8.2% for patients with those with the Fontan circulation.[133] The overall point prevalence of congenital cardiac disease, therefore, has and will continue to increase, with the spectrum shifting towards adults with repaired or palliated lesions. This will have an important impact on increasing the need for specialised care, with services needing to expand to meet this growing need.

With the increase in prevalence, tertiary care centres with adult congenital cardiology clinics saw increases of up to three-fold in workload between 1992 and 1997.[132] Annual rates of hospitalisation for patients with all other congenital cardiac defects was also not inconsequential.[134] Expenditures have been reported to be higher for adults with congenitally malformed hearts than for the general population.[135] With the greater potential need for reoperation, and care during follow-up, an economic and logistical burden can be expected in the future.

REPORTED PREVALENCE OF CONGENITAL HEART DISEASE

It is unlikely that any single study will give the definitive estimate of the prevalence of congenitally malformed hearts. Studies differ in methodology and quality, as well as the population and period of time studied. Studies using autopsy records, or series of cases gathered in clinical centres, for ascertainment do not usually report an estimate of prevalence, since the denominator is difficult to define. These studies are useful in defining the spectrum and relative proportion of specific defects. Estimates of prevalence usually come from studies where either a passive or active strategy of surveillance was used for ascertainment from a defined population.

One of the first reports was from a cardiac substudy of the Collaborative Study of Cerebral Palsy, Mental Retardation, and Other Neurological and Sensory Disorders of Infancy and Childhood, published in 1971.[1] This study prospectively enrolled pregnant mothers at 12 participating large institutions within the United States of America, and then repeatedly assessed the infants up to the age of 7 years. The study included stillbirths. Hospital and outpatient records, and autopsy reports, were reviewed for diagnoses of congenital cardiac disease. From 56,109 births, 549 cases of definite or suspected congenital cardiac disease were identified. The cases were subsequently examined by physicians involved in the study, private paediatricians, and paediatric cardiologists, and divided into three groups. The first group, of 272 cases, was made up of those with definite heart disease. The second group, comprising 222 cases, was formed by the patients initially thought to have cardiac disease, but proved to have normal hearts on evaluation. The remaining 55 cases, making up the third group, were those with signs suggestive of cardiac disease, but who did not return for evaluation. The evaluation yielded 457 cases, with 178 diagnosed at autopsy, 36 from surgical findings, 42 from cardiac catheterisation, and 201 from clinical evaluation only. This gave an estimate of prevalence of 8.1 per 1000 births. The prevalence among live births only was 7.7, but among stillbirths only was 27.5. For those live born, the prevalence among those that died before 28 days was 73.2 per 1000 deaths, and among those that died between 28 days and 1 year was 112.6 per 1000 deaths. Ventricular septal defect was the most frequent diagnosis, occurring in 133, or three-tenths, of the 457 cases.

The New England Regional Infant Cardiac Program began in 1969 with the aim of coordinating and improving the care of infants with congenital heart disease in six states in New England.[136] Medical records from hospitals and practitioners were reviewed, and data collected relative to cardiac diagnoses, procedures, and major events. The programme aimed to tabulate and report local and regional experience, with a view to improvement of quality, but information regarding prevalence and epidemiology were secondarily reported. From 1968 through 1974, 2,251 cases were ascertained, and when related to regional vital statistics of live births, gave an estimate of prevalence of 2.08 per 1000. All cases except 18 were verified by autopsy, surgery, or cardiac catheterisation. The prevalence increased from 1.82 in 1969 to 2.20 in 1974. When cases were included that had been identified only from death certificates, the prevalence increased to 2.34 in 1969 and 2.62 in 1974. Ventricular septal defects accounted for one-sixth of the cases.

A national study from Sweden used four different registries for ascertainment of those born alive with congenitally malformed hearts during 1981.[137] Of the registries, two were involved with collecting vital statistics with mandatory reporting, namely, the Medical Birth Registry and the Registry of Death Certificates. The Medical Birth Registry of all delivery records included up to four diagnoses for the infant coded according to modified codes of the International Codes and Definitions, and added up to the time of death or discharge from hospital. The Registry of Congenital Malformations, with mandatory reporting since 1965, included cardiac defects, but only those reported within 6 months of birth, those associated with cyanosis, or cardiac failure, or death within the first week of life, and those associated with known syndromes. In 1980, a Child Cardiology Registry was established, with coordinated voluntary reporting from all five units for paediatric cardiology active in Sweden at that time. The purpose of the Registry was to provide more active surveillance, and to provide feedback to the reporting clinicians. Cases were reported if the diagnosis was made during the first year of life, with confirmation by echocardiography, cardiac catheterisation, surgery, or autopsy. Cases with isolated arterial ducts under the age of 3 months were excluded. Lesions were coded using the coding scheme of the International Society of Cardiology. Comparisons were made between the four registries regarding common cases. The Medical Birth Registry was used to define the denominator of live births. Using these sources, 853 cases were identified from 93,678 live and stillbirths, giving a prevalence at birth of 9.1 per 1000. Of the cases, however, 564 were identified only from the Medical Birth Registry data, with 75 of these being coded as suspected cardiac malformations, 2 coded as cardiac malposition, and 68 with only an arterial duct and a birth weight less than 2500 grams. Exclusion of these 145 cases gave a prevalence at birth of 7.6 per 1000. There were 17 cases that were identified from death certificates only, with 225 cases having been captured in the Child Cardiology Registry.

Perhaps the most contemporary estimate of prevalence at live birth comes from the Baltimore–Washington Infant Study.[5] This study involved an identified cohort, and was one of the first to include echocardiography as a modality for ascertainment, verification, and classification of cases. It also prospectively defined the denominator for the cohort. From 1981 to 1989, 4390 infants with congenitally malformed hearts were identified from 906,646 regional live births, giving an estimate of prevalence of 4.84 for each 1000 live births, with 95% confidence limits from 4.70 to 4.99. The prevalence increased throughout the period of study, with the proportion of cases having diagnostic confirmation by echocardiography increasing, and those confirmed by cardiac catheterisation decreasing. The prevalence in the last 3 years of the study was 5.5 for each 1000 live births. The overwhelming contributor to the apparent increase in prevalence was an increase in the number of perimembranous and muscular ventricular septal defects, reflecting better ascertainment with increasing use of and improvements in echocardiography. Ventricular septal defects accounted for one-third of the cases (Table 8-6).

TABLE 8-6

DISTRIBUTION OF DIAGNOSTIC GROUPS IN ORDER OF FREQUENCY (N = 4390)

Diagnostic Group	Number	Percent (%)
Ventricular septal defect	1411	32.1
Pulmonary stenosis	395	9.0
Atrial septal defect within oval fossa	340	7.7
Atrioventricular septal defect	326	7.4
Tetralogy of Fallot	297	6.8
Transposition	208	4.7
Coarctation of aorta	203	4.6
Hypoplastic left heart syndrome	167	3.8
Aortic stenosis	128	2.9
Patent arterial duct	104	2.4
Isomerism of atrial appendages	99	2.3
Double outlet right ventricle	86	2.0
Bifoliate aortic valve	84	1.9
Cardiomyopathy	82	1.9
Pulmonary atresia with intact septum	73	1.7
Peripheral pulmonary arterial stenosis	65	1.5
Totally anomalous pulmonary venous return	60	1.4
Common arterial trunk	51	1.2
Congenitally corrected transposition	47	1.1
Ebstein's malformation	43	1.0
Tricuspid atresia	32	0.7
Interrupted aortic arch	31	0.7
Other left-sided lesions*	26	0.6
Double inlet ventricle	18	0.4
Other right-sided lesions†	9	0.2
Divided left atrium	5	0.1

*Includes 13 cases of coronary arterial anomalies, 7 anomalies of the aortic arch, 5 instances of mitral valvar regurgitation, and 1 case with drainage of the superior caval vein to the left atrium.
†Includes eight examples of partially anomalous pulmonary venous return and one pulmonary arterial sling.
From Ferencz C, Rubin JD, Loffredo CA, Magee CA: Epidemiology of Congenital Heart Disease: The Baltimore–Washington Infant Study: 1981–1989, Vol 4. Mount Kisco, NY: Futura, 1993.

The Baltimore–Washington Infant Study included a case-control study within its design, with control infants randomly selected each year of the study from all live born infants without congenitally malformed hearts in a manner stratified by the hospital managing the births. A comprehensive questionnaire was completed by standardised interviews of mothers at home visits. The questionnaire collected data regarding demographic, maternal health, nutritional, genetic, and environmental factors. The study defined a broad spectrum of familial and genetic factors, which were present in just over one-third of cases. Table 8-7 gives the results of a multi-variable analysis of potential risk factors without inclusion of maternal reproductive history variables. When the number of previous pregnancies is included in the model, three or more pregnancies, as opposed to none, has an adjusted odds ratio of 1.29, and maternal age, race, familial noncardiac malformations, local contraceptives, and increasing number of drugs taken are no longer significantly associated with congenital cardiac disease. When associations with environmental risk factors were examined separately for cases with and without genetic risk factors in comparison to controls without genetic risk factors, a greater number of environmental risk factors with stronger associations were noted in the analysis of cases with genetic risk factors, particularly for exposures to therapeutic drugs. This suggests that environmental factors have a greater influence in those with an underlying genetic susceptibility.

TABLE 8-7

MULTI-VARIABLE MODEL OF POTENTIAL RISK FACTORS WITHOUT MATERNAL REPRODUCTIVE HISTORY VARIABLES

Variable	Adjusted Odds Ratio*	95% CI
Genetic Factors in Nuclear Family		
Familial congenital heart disease	2.20	1.69–2.85
Familial noncardiac malformations	1.27	1.02–1.57
Maternal Factors		
Diabetes (overt)	2.97	1.82–4.86
Maternal Age Score		
0 (<20 years old)	1.00	—
1 (20–29 years old)	1.13	1.05–1.22
2 (30+ years old)	1.28	1.10–1.50
Therapeutic and Recreational Drug Use		
Diazepam	2.14	1.22–3.77
Phenothiazines	1.74	1.06–2.86
Cocaine, paternal	1.62	1.26–2.08
Gastrointestinal drugs	1.36	1.05–1.76
Local contraceptives	0.82	0.72–0.94
Number of drugs taken	1.04*	1.01–1.08
Occupational and Avocational Exposures		
Extreme cold temperature, paternal	2.64	1.14–6.12
Miscellaneous solvents, maternal	1.42	1.02–1.98
Sociodemographic and Other Factors		
Race (0 = nonwhite, 1 = white)	0.88	0.79–0.98

*Odds ratio per increment in number of drugs.
CI, confidence interval.
From Ferencz C, Rubin JD, Loffredo CA, Magee CA: Epidemiology of Congenital Heart Disease: The Baltimore–Washington Infant Study: 1981–1989, Vol 4. Mount Kisco, New York: Futura, 1993.

A large-scale study using a universal screening strategy for ascertainment has yet to be performed. Investigators from Japan performed a more focussed screening of newborns with echocardiography aimed at determining the prevalence and natural history of muscular ventricular septal defects, a lesion known to inflate estimates of prevalence.[138] They screened 1028 newborns delivered at term without evident chromosomal abnormalities, and identified 21 newborns with muscular ventricular septal defects, 3 with coarctation of the aorta, and 1 with double outlet right ventricle, giving a prevalence of 24.3 cases per 1000 live births. The 95% confidence limits were wide, ranging from 15.8 to 35.7, and thus the estimate is not very reliable given the relatively small number of subjects. Only three-fifths of the ventricular septal defects were associated with a cardiac murmur, and follow-up showed that three-quarters had closed spontaneously by the age of 12 months, with the majority closing before 6 months. This has implications for strategies of ascertainment that rely on clinical presentation for identification. If diagnostic confirmation is delayed, many defects will have closed spontaneously, and escape verification.

Two teams of reviewers have examined multiple studies of prevalence with an aim of comparing, and potentially pooling, the estimates. The investigators from the Baltimore–Washington Infant Study compared their prevalence at live birth from their initial 2 years of the study, 1981 and 1982, to that of eight previously published and widely cited reports.[139] The prevalence from the Baltimore–Washington Infant Study for that period was 3.7 cases for each 1000 live births, with all cases being confirmed by autopsy, surgery, cardiac catheterisation, or echocardiography. The studies differed widely by dates, number, and characteristics of the population of births, time period after birth during which cases were accrued, and methods of ascertainment, verification, and classification. The New England Regional Infant Cardiac Program spanned 1969 to 1977, with 2251 cases of congenitally malformed hearts ascertained from follow-up up to 1 year after birth for 1,528,686 resident live births from six New England states in the United States.[136] Cases were verified by autopsy, surgery, or cardiac catheterisation, with a prevalence of 2.03.

When cases verified only by echocardiography were excluded from the estimate of prevalence made from the Baltimore–Washington Infant Study, their estimate became more similar, at 2.38. The remaining seven studies included cases for which a clinical diagnosis without verification had been made, varying from three-tenths of half of included cases, with estimates ranging from 5.51 to 8.56.[1,137,140–144] If cases that were diagnosed by clinical means only were excluded from these estimates, the prevalence then ranged from 3.75 to 4.30, which is comparable to the estimate reported by the investigators conducting the Baltimore–Washington Infant Study. The review also compared the prevalence of specific defects, and noted wider variations between studies.

A more recent review provided an analysis of a larger number of studies, with an aim at determining the sources of variability in estimates of prevalence between studies.[145] This analysis was based on review of 62 studies reported after 1955, with larger studies representing surveillance registries or cohort studies, and smaller studies usually from less developed countries representing series of cases reported from clinical centres which were based on larger geographic population-based denominators. Wide discrepancies were found in reported estimates of prevalence, ranging from 4 to 50 per 1000 live births (Fig. 8-1). Estimates were stable, at between about 4 and 8 for each 1000 live births, until 1985. The advent of widespread use of echocardiography at this point resulted in estimates becoming more diverse, and the reported prevalences began to exceed 10 for each 1000 live births (Fig. 8-2). The increases in overall estimates of prevalence reflected an overall increase in ascertained cases, but this was more marked for trivial or mild lesions, particularly ventricular septal defects, with the estimated prevalence of lesions producing cyanotic disease remaining relatively stable (Fig. 8-3). The estimated prevalence of ventricular septal defects is reflective of the modality used for ascertainment and verification, but also on the timing, since more complete early ascertainment would be expected to capture more lesions which would subsequently undergo spontaneous closure. The median prevalence of congenital heart disease was 7.7, with an interquartile range from 6.0 to 10.6, excluding nonstenotic aortic valves with two leaflets, silent arterial ducts, and isolated partially anomalous pulmonary venous connections. The median prevalence of bifoliate aortic valves was 9.2, with an interquartile range from 5.3 to 13.8. Inclusion of cases with such bifoliate aortic valves would greatly inflate estimates of prevalence. The median prevalence of congenitally malformed hearts producing cyanosis was 1.08, with an interquartile range of 1.27 to 1.53. In Table 8-8, I have summarised the statistics regarding the prevalence of specific lesions for each one million live births.

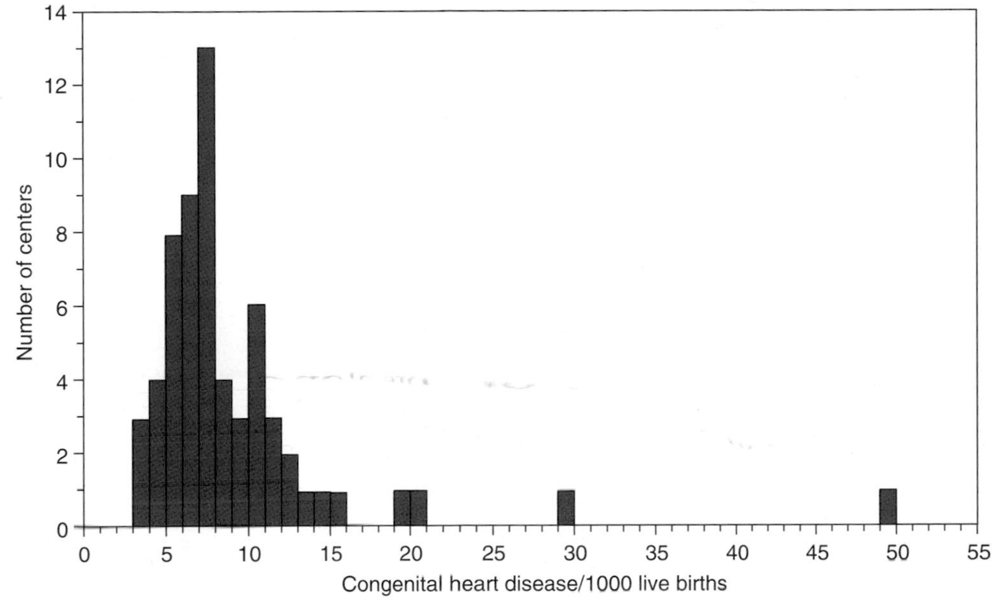

Figure 8-1 Histogram of the prevalence of congenital cardiac defects per 1000 live births, as noted in 62 reports. (From Hoffman JI, Kaplan S: The incidence of congenital heart disease. J Am Coll Cardiol 2002;39:1890–1900.)

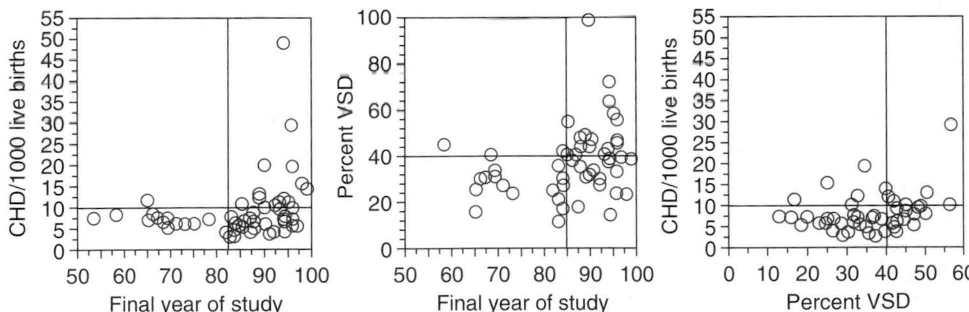

Figure 8-2 Changes in the reported prevalence of congenital heart disease (CHD) from multiple reports over time, and the influence of the proportion of ascertained cases of ventricular septal defect (VSD). Each circle represents the value derived from each report. The horizontal lines are drawn arbitrarily at a prevalence of 10/1000 live births and 40% of all congenital heart disease, and the vertical lines are drawn arbitrarily at 1985 and 40%, respectively. An increasing proportion of the high prevalence estimates are beyond 1985 and for series that have over 40% ventricular septal defects. (From Hoffman JI, Kaplan S: The incidence of congenital heart disease. J Am Coll Cardiol 2002;39:1890–1900.)

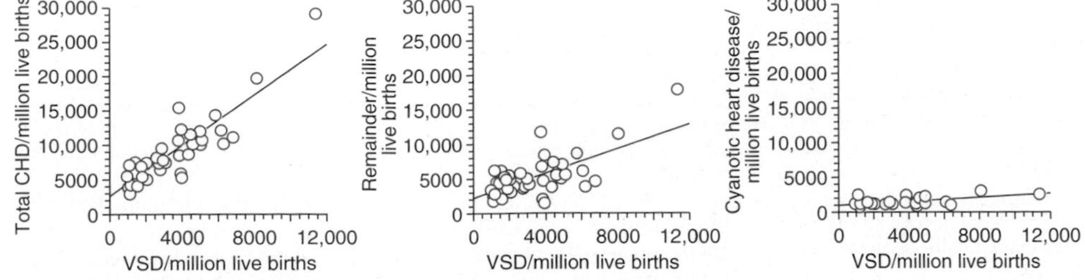

Figure 8-3 The association of the reported prevalence of ventricular septal defects to total, total exclusive of ventricular septal defects, and cyanotic cardiac disease, as assessed from reported studies. Abbreviations as in Figure 8-2. (From Hoffman JI, Kaplan S: The incidence of congenital heart disease. J Am Coll Cardiol 2002;39:1890–1900.)

TABLE 8-8

MEAN AND MEDIAN PREVALENCE OF SPECIFIC CONGENITAL CARDIAC LESIONS FOR EACH ONE MILLION LIVE BIRTHS

Lesion	Number of Studies	Mean	Lower Quartile	Median	Upper Quartile	NERICP 1975–1977	BWIS 1981–1989
Ventricular septal defect	43	3570	1757	2829	4482	345	1557
Patent arterial duct	40	799	324	567	782	135	115
Atrial septal defect	43	941	372	564	1059	65	375
Atrioventricular septal defect	40	348	242	340	396	110	360
Pulmonary stenosis	39	729	355	532	836	73	436
Aortic stenosis	37	401	161	256	388	41	141
Coarctation of the aorta	39	409	289	356	492	165	224
Tetralogy of Fallot	41	421	291	356	577	196	328
Transposition	41	315	231	303	388	218	229
Hypoplastic right heart	32	222	105	160	224	—	81
Tricuspid atresia	11	79	24	92	118	56	35
Ebstein's malformation	5	114	38	40	161	12	47
Pulmonary atresia with intact ventricular septum	11	132	76	83	147	69	81
Hypoplastic left heart	36	266	154	226	279	163	184
Common arterial trunk	30	107	61	94	136	30	56
Double outlet right ventricle	16	157	82	127	245	32	95
Double inlet ventricle	23	106	54	85	136	54	54
Totally anomalous pulmonary venous connection	25	94	60	91	120	58	66
All cyanotic	37	1391	1078	1270	1533	888	—
All congenital cardiac disease*	43	9596	6020	7669	10,567	2033	—
Bifoliate aortic valve	10	13,556	5336	9244	13,817	—	93

*Excluding bifoliate nonstenotic aortic valves, isolated partially anomalous pulmonary venous connection, and silent arterial ducts.
BWIS, Baltimore Washington Infant Study; NERICP, New England Regional Infant Cardiac Program.
Data from Hoffman JI, Kaplan S: The incidence of congenital heart disease. J Am Coll Cardiol 2002;39:1890–1900; Report of the New England Regional Infant Cardiac Program. Pediatrics 1980;65:375–461; and Ferencz C, Rubin JD, Loffredo CA, Magee CA: Epidemiology of Congenital Heart Disease: The Baltimore–Washington Infant Study: 1981–1989, Vol 4. Mount Kisco, NY: Futura, 1993.

ACKNOWLEDGEMENT

The author wishes to acknowledge the assistance of Nadia Clarizia for her contributions to this chapter.

The complete reference list can be found on the companion Expert Consult web site at www.expertconsult.com.

ANNOTATED REFERENCES

- Hoffman JI, Kaplan S: The incidence of congenital heart disease. J Am Coll Cardiol 2002;39:1890–1900.

  This comprehensive review of 62 published studies of estimated prevalence noted great variability in reported estimates, much of which was explained by methodological aspects and increasing ascertainment with echocardiography of ventricular septal defects.
- Hoffman JI, Kaplan S, Liberthson RR: Prevalence of congenital heart disease. Am Heart J 2004;147:425–439.

  The point prevalence defines the total number of cases at any given point in time, and is important for defining the requirement for resources and the burden of disease within the total population. This study applies assumptions regarding prevalence at live birth and survival to estimate this number, with particular reference to adults with congenitally malformed hearts.
- Jenkins KJ, Correa A, Feinstein JA, et al: Noninherited risk factors and congenital cardiovascular defects: Current knowledge—a scientific statement from the American Heart Association Council on Cardiovascular Disease in the Young: endorsed by the American Academy of Pediatrics. Circulation 2007;115:2995–3014.

  This is a contemporary review of studies estimating prevalence aimed at summarising non-genetic risk factors of potential aetiologic and preventive relevance.
- Wilson PD, Loffredo CA, Correa-Villaseñor A, Ferencz C: Attributable fraction for cardiac malformations. Am J Epidemiol 1998;148:414–423.

  The Baltimore–Washington Infant Study was based on active surveillance with a case-control design, and was aimed at identifying potential genetic and environmental risk factors. This report estimates the contribution to the occurrence of specific defects of familial and environmental risk factors.
- Gill HK, Splitt M, Sharland GK, Simpson JM: Patterns of recurrence of congenital heart disease: An analysis of 6,640 consecutive pregnancies evaluated by detailed fetal echocardiography. J Am Coll Cardiol 2003;42:923–929.

  The investigators examined fetal echocardiograms for pregnancies where either the mother, father, or a sibling had congenital cardiac disease. They noted a recurrence risk in the fetus of 2.7%, with variable concordance for specific lesions or groups.
- Calcagni G, Digilio MC, Sarkozy A, et al: Familial recurrence of congenital heart disease: An overview and review of the literature. Eur J Pediatr 2007;166:111–116.

  This is a contemporary review of patterns of familial recurrence and associated factors.
- Germanakis I, Sifakis S: The impact of fetal echocardiography on the prevalence of liveborn congenital heart disease. Pediatr Cardiol 2006;27:465–472.

  These investigators employed mathematical modelling of the probability of fetal screening, detection of defects, and elective termination to determine the potential impact on the prevalence at live birth.
- Marelli AJ, Mackie AS, Ionescu-Ittu R, et al: Congenital heart disease in the general population: Changing prevalence and age distribution. Circulation 2007;115:163–172.

  The investigators used administrative databases in the context of a system for health care providing universal coverage to determine the point prevalence of congenital cardiac disease in adults. In 2000, the point prevalence was 4.09 per 1000 adults for any type of defect, and 0.38 for serious lesions.
- Mitchell SC, Korones SB, Berendes HW: Congenital heart disease in 56,109 births: Incidence and natural history. Circulation 1971;43:323–332.

  This study is one of the first to use a surveillance programme involving major tertiary centres, and defined prevalence at birth of 8.14 per 1000 before verification with echocardiography was possible. Cases diagnosed at stillbirth were included, and an important proportion of cases diagnosed by clinical evaluation only were included.
- Report of the New England Regional Infant Cardiac Program. Pediatrics 1980;65(Suppl 2):375–461.

  While primarily a programme for health care, a database was maintained of cases verified by autopsy, surgery, or catheterisation from which prevalence, distribution, and clinical epidemiology were defined. The prevalence at live birth was 2.08 per 1000, with ventricular septal defects accounting for 15.7% of cases.

- Carlgren LE, Ericson A, Kallen B: Monitoring of congenital cardiac defects. Pediatr Cardiol 1987;8:247–256.

  This study used four registries to determine an estimate of prevalence and frequency of distribution of congenitally malformed hearts for Sweden, and gives limited epidemiologic features.

- Epidemiology of Congenital Heart Disease: The Baltimore-Washington Infant Study 1981–1989. In Ferencz C, Rubin JD, Loffredo CA, Magee CA (eds): Vol 4 of Perspectives in Pediatric Cardiology. Mount Kisco, NY: Futura, 1993.

  This is an important monograph providing the full results of the seminal active surveillance study incorporating echocardiography, with a case-control comparison regarding potential risk factors. The prevalence was 4.84 per 1000 live births.

- Hiraishi S, Agata Y, Nowatari M, et al: Incidence and natural course of trabecular ventricular septal defect: Two-dimensional echocardiography and color Doppler flow imaging study. J Pediatr 1992;120:409–415.

  This study universally screened 1028 newborns with echocardiography, and identified 21 with muscular ventricular septal defects, with four additional cases of congenital cardiac disease. Early screening of live births gives the highest estimates of prevalence through complete ascertainment of cases.

CHAPTER 9

Aetiology of Congenital Cardiac Disease

BENOIT G. BRUNEAU, JOHN BURN, and DEEPAK SRIVASTAVA

Perhaps one of the most vexing aspects of congenital cardiac disease is the current inability to explain its origin. Environmental causes have been invoked, and until recently only scant evidence had pointed towards a genetic component. Recent experimental data, combined with advances in human genetics, have now provided a clearer understanding of how some malformations may occur, and certainly have illuminated general concepts that are certain to apply to congenital cardiac disease in general. One of the most important developments has been the paradigm shift from grouping lesions based on clinical presentation, to understanding the anomalies based on their embryonic and genetic origins. Thus, it is now clear how an inherited mutation can result in a family where one individual has an interatrial communication, while another tetralogy of Fallot, and still be considered the same genetic defect. In this chapter, we will review the various aetiologies, environmental and genetic, with a constant eye towards the embryology of the heart, with the hope that by synthesising the current knowledge, we will provide a useful insight into the fundamental basis of congenital cardiac malformations.

EPIDEMIOLOGY OF HEART DISEASE: GENES VERSUS ENVIRONMENT

The study of the aetiology of congenital cardiac disease initially focused on epidemiological studies, which mainly incorporated the identification of factors that influence the incidence of the various lesions. This is in large part because familial inheritance is not obvious, and thus a tractable focus is environmental influence and assessment of heritability. These studies primarily led to the conclusion that there were multi-factorial influences. Several difficulties are apparent with these studies. First, intra-uterine mortality due to congenital cardiac disease is difficult to assess, and conversely, in addition to the nearly 1% of children with cardiac malformations,[1] an additional 1% to 2% of the population harbour more subtle cardiac developmental anomalies that only become apparent later in life. Second, familial associations are rarely obvious. In retrospect, this should be evident from the observations that defined mutations in a single gene can cause seemingly unrelated lesions, compounded by forme fruste or low genetic penetration.

Amongst epidemiological studies, the Baltimore–Washington Infant Study was a prospective surveillance for liveborn cases from 1981 to 1989, with a case-control study to determine aetiological associations.[2,3] More than 4000 cases were identified amongst close to 1 million live births. Some clues about inheritance were obtained,[2-4] but despite suggestive information, the focus of genetic evaluation was on chromosomal anomalies and known hereditable syndromes, and not on identification of specific mutations. Thus, although several teratogenic causes of heart defects have been documented, their underlying causes are unknown. Most recently, prenatal use of angiotensin converting enzyme has been identified as a strong risk factor for congenital defects that include cardiac lesions.[5]

Other than obvious associations with chromosomal syndromes, such as atrioventricular septal defects in the setting of Down syndrome, genetic causes have been slow in their discovery and characterisation. Some cardiac conditions have a clear familial component, and include Marfan's syndrome, Williams syndrome, and Holt-Oram syndrome.[6,7] Recognition of the syndrome produced by deletion of chromosome 22q11 has caused a paradigm shift in how clinicians now think about the genetic contribution to congenital cardiac malformations.[8,9] The deletion syndrome is associated with a host of cardiac lesions, ranging in severity, and mostly involving the ventricular outflow tracts.[7,9] The deletion has been reported in up to three-fifths of those with interrupted aortic arch, one-third of those with common arterial trunk, one-sixth of those with tetralogy of Fallot, and one-tenth of patients with ventricular septal defect. Routine testing is now standard, although its influence on cardiac outcomes is as yet unclear. It is interesting to note that the identification of the most likely causative gene came from studies in the mouse.[10-12]

In contrast to clearly defined syndromes, most congenital cardiac malformations rarely occur in families with a sufficient number of affected members to lend themselves to genetic linkage analyses. Also, when familial cases occur, they are often marked by heterogeneity of defect, and affected family members may manifest as cardiomyopathy or arrhythmia rather than congenital malformations. Decreased penetrance and variable expressivity also occur, and suggest that additional environmental and genetic factors may contribute to risk of malformation. Historically, therefore, the risk factors for reoccurrence of the lesions were based on epidemiological studies such as those described above, and were classified broadly into family inheritance and vague environmental considerations. More recently, genetic analyses have determined that even some common types of defects have a genetic component. For example, atrial septal defects, and aortic valves with two leaflets, have been shown to be inheritable.[13,14] The subsequent isolation of the causative genetic mutations substantiated this notion.[15–17]

CARDIAC DEVELOPMENT: KEY CONCEPTS

While early anatomical descriptions have provided significant insights into normal cardiac development, modern genetic experimentation with model organisms has been particularly useful in deciphering the anatomical and genetic contortions that the developing heart must undergo to become a formed and functional organ. It has become clear that the genetic pathways that operate in such diverse species as the fruitfly, zebrafish, and mouse are relevant to each other and provide important biological insights that are relevant to human disease. In particular, the fruitfly and the zebrafish have permitted the discovery of previously unknown pathways due to their use in large-scale phenotypic-based screens for discovery of genes. Similarly, genetic manipulation in the laboratory mouse, whose cardiovascular system is nearly identical to that of humans, has allowed profound insight into the mechanisms underlying human disease.

Origins of the Heart

The vertebrate heart arises from paired pools of mesodermal precursors. Cardiac differentiation begins shortly after gastrulation has begun, and the first clear markers of the differentiating heart are apparent near the end of gastrulation, this occurring during the eighth day of development in the mouse. The process demarcates a horseshoe-shaped group of cells called the cardiac crescent (see also Chapter 3). These cells will contribute to the atria and left ventricle, while another group of cells more medial within the cardiac crescent will form the so-called second heart field, or lineage, from which the right ventricle, outflow tract, and a portion of the atria will be derived.[18–24] The cells of the cardiac crescent come together at the midline of the embryos, where their fusion and anterior growth leads to the formation of the linear heart tube. This beating structure breaks the symmetry of the embryo, and loops towards the right side as distinct chambers form during the ninth day in the mouse. Looping proceeds during the tenth day, with growth of distinct chambers, giving rise to a heart composed of left and right atria and ventricles. Subsequent steps in cardiac morphogenesis refine the distinctions between each chamber, and separate the left and right sides by growth of septa.

A recent discovery is that the outflow tract, the right ventricle, and a large component of the atria arise not from cardiac crescent–derived myocardium, but from a population of cardiac cells that form more anteriorly—the so-called second heart field.[20–23,25–27] As defined by genetic lineage analysis, the second field originates very early in development from mesoderm expressing the transcription factor Isl1. This lies near the area of the heart-forming mesoderm and is displaced cranially during development of the embryo. A subset of the this area itself, initially called the anterior heart field, is marked by the presence of *Fgf10* and *Mef2c* mRNA.[21,26]

This remarkable discovery has fundamentally altered our view of cardiac morphogenesis. Instead of continued growth of a defined population of differentiated cells, uncommitted cardioblasts from the second lineage are actively recruited into the heart, where they differentiate into cardiac cells. In fact, *Isl1*-expressing precursor cells have been shown to persist postnatally as cardiac myoblasts.[28] The discovery of the second lineage is also significant from the stance of a disease. To understand lesions involving the outflow tract and right ventricle, we must understand how the factors that regulate their formation from their precursors are coordinated and integrated with the rest of the heart. In DiGeorge syndrome, the defective gene operates primarily in the second lineage, affecting its differentiation and migration.[29,30] Thus, understanding of how the switch in lineage occurs from undifferentiated myoblasts from the second field to differentiated cardiac myocytes has many implications for embryology and disease.

The lineage of the second field has also been shown to be a multi-potent precursor cell, which can give rise to all cardiovascular cell types, including myocytes, endothelial cells, and smooth muscle of the vasculature.[31–33] These multi-potent cells differentiate into the three different cell types presumably in response to local cues, such as growth factors, which instruct a particular gene programme to be activated over another. Additionally, these cardiovascular precursors restrict their potential as they further differentiate. This is a strategy similar to that employed by haematopoietic precursors, which give rise to the different cell types that form blood.

The primary heart field was initially thought to contribute to the entire heart. Although no lineage analysis has been performed, it appears that it is the left ventricle and part of the atria that derive from the primary field. Some evidence for this comes from deletion of *Tbx5*, which is largely absent from the second field and its derivatives.[34,35] Loss of *Tbx5* in the mouse results in severe hypoplasia of the caudal segment of the heart, the atria and left ventricle, leaving intact the right ventricle and outflow tract.[35] Unlike the complete absence of derivatives of the second field in *Isl1* knock-out mice, *Tbx5* mutant mice still develop primitive, albeit malformed, structures. Mutations in other genes that affect formation of the heart most severely do not affect early formation of the tube from the first heart field.[23,35–37] The determinants of the so-called primary heart field, and the importance of its differentiation for overall cardiac development, are not known.

Genes That Regulate Formation of the Heart

Beginning with the discovery of the *tinman* mutant in Drosophila in 1989, several dozen genes have been identified that are critical for various aspects of formation of the heart, from its earliest inception, through major morphogenetic steps, and into postnatal regulation of cardiac function. Most genes encode transcriptional regulators, which turn on or off other genes, or signalling molecules that activate potent intracellular signalling cascades.

Transcription Factors

The fruitfly *tinman* mutation was identified in flies that did not form any heart at all, the mutation being named after the character in *The Wizard of Oz*.[38] This mutation was in a gene belonging to a family of transcription factors called the homeodomain factors. Shortly after this discovery, vertebrate versions were identified, which were given the less colourful name of *Nkx2-5*. It turns out that *Nkx2-5* in vertebrates is not essential in itself for formation of the heart, but it does have important functions in early initiation of the cardiac genetic programme, and in formation of the cardiac chambers.[39,40] As will be discussed below, along with many other genes that were initially experimentally defined, *NKX2-5* is one of the genes that has been identified as causative in inherited human congenitally malformed hearts.[15] Considerable literature exists on the function of *Nkx2-5*, and in many of its functions it interacts with other transcription factors that are important for the normal development of the heart. For example, a factor from another gene family, *Gata4*, also plays important roles in heart differentiation, in chamber morphogenesis, and also has additional roles in bringing the two heart fields together. The last role was dramatically evident from its mutation in the mouse, which led to production of a bifid heart.[41,42] And as with *NKX2-5*, human genetics has pinpointed *GATA4* as a gene that when mutated causes inherited congenital cardiac defects. The primary role of *Nkx2-5* in the developing heart is to activate a set of target genes that will execute the correct cellular differentiation program of a variety of types of cells. For example, certain contractile protein genes rely on *Nkx2-5* for their initial activation, and the proper development of the conduction system relies on its appropriate function.

Gata4, as mentioned above, is also a key player in formation of the heart. Indeed, this gene has been shown to be important for such diverse aspects of formation as early differentiation, valvar formation, chamber maturation, and even postnatal function. In fact these same roles have also been ascribed, to varying degrees, to *Nkx2-5*. Genes that are active in the early heart usually have binding sites for *Gata4* and *Nkx2-5* in the regulatory regions, called enhancers, that confer cardiac-specific expression of genes. *Gata4* and *Nkx2-5* function together to act on these sequences of enhancers, and this interaction provides a degree of robustness and specificity to the system. Many other transcription factors have been defined as important for various aspects of cardiac formation. They often have multiple roles at various times during development, reflecting their potency and versatility.

Growth Factors

Growth factors of many different families are important for several aspects of heart development. In early development, the bone morphogenic factors and the *Wnts*, two types of developmentally important secreted factors, are key inducers of cardiac development, via their instructive cues that promote expansion of early cardiovascular precursors, and later also the induction of cardiac differentiation from these same precursors.[43–49] The picture is a bit more complicated, as some *Wnt* signals also dampen cardiogenesis, by slowing the growth of precursors, presumably so that the timing of cardiac differentiation is kept.[43–48,50]

Growth factors are also important in later stages of cardiac development, such as valvar formation and septation.[51] Bone morphogenetic proteins are critical for the initiation of the earliest steps in valvar formation, and indeed the dosage of *Bmp4*, for example, results in valvar malformations and deficient atrioventricular septation that are reminiscent of human disease.[52,53] Later regulation of valvar morphogenesis relies on a complex interplay between myocardium and endocardium which is regulated by calcineurin-dependent signalling and the repression of vascular endothelial growth factor in myocardium of the valve-forming region.[54]

MicroRNA Regulation of Cardiac Development

The transcriptional regulation of cardiac development and its modulatory and instructive signalling pathways are well studied, and their biology is becoming well understood. Less clear is the translational control of cardiac morphogenesis by small noncoding RNAs, such as microRNAs. MicroRNAs are genomically encoded 20- to 22-nucleotide RNAs that function by targeting mRNAs either for translational inhibition or for degradation, leading to an effective reduction in quantity of the protein product. Several hundred human microRNAs have been identified, and some of these have important roles in development that may be eminently relevant to congenitally malformed hearts.

The best characterised example is the microRNA-1 family, comprising *miR-1-1* and *miR-1-2*. These microRNAs are highly conserved from worms to humans, and are specifically expressed in the progenitor cells of developing cardiac and skeletal muscle as they differentiate.[55] Both are highly expressed in the cells of the outflow tract derived from the second heart field. Interestingly, expression of these microRNAs is directly controlled by well-studied transcriptional regulatory networks that promote muscular differentiation. Cardiac expression is dependent on serum response factor, and expression in skeletal muscle requires the myogenic transcription factors MyoD and Mef2. Consistent with a role in differentiation, overexpression of miR-1 in the developing mouse heart results in a decrease in expansion of ventricular myocytes, with fewer proliferating cardiomyocytes remaining in the cell cycle. Validation of *Hand2* as a target for miR-1 suggests that tight regulation of levels of protein may be involved in controlling the balance between cardiomyocyte proliferation and differentiation. MiR-1 and another microRNA, *miR-133a*, are transcribed in a polycistronic message, therefore sharing common regulation, and both are co-expressed in cardiac and skeletal muscle. As in cardiac muscle, miR-1 promotes the differentiation of skeletal myoblasts in culture, but interestingly, *miR-133a* has the opposite effect, inhibiting differentiation and promoting the proliferation of myoblasts.

Defects caused by mutations in microRNA genes range from benign to severe. Disruption of the single fly orthologue of miR-1 had catastrophic consequences, resulting in uniform lethality at embryonic or larval stages, with a frequent defect in maintaining cardiac gene expression.[56] In a subset of flies lacking miR-1, a severe defect of cardiac progenitor cell differentiation provided loss-of-function evidence that miR-1 was involved in events leading to muscular differentiation, events, similar to the gain-of-function findings in mice. miR-1 in flies regulates the Notch signalling pathway by directly targeting microRNA of the Notch ligand, Delta,[56] potentially explaining the involvement of miR-1 in deriving differentiated cardiac cells from an equivalency group of progenitor cells. Thus, miR-1 seems to be a muscle-specific microRNA that directs progenitor cells towards a cardiac cell fate by regulating central mediators of determination and differentiation. Although only three miRNAs have been deleted in mice to date, targeted deletion of miR-1-2 resulted in ventricular septal defects, although with incomplete penetrance.[57] In surviving adults, disruption of normal cardiac conduction and cell cycle control was also observed.

Haemodynamics and Formation of the Heart

As the heart forms, it soon begins to beat and pump blood. This occurs at the early stages of cardiac looping, well before chambers have formed and separations between segments of the heart are established. It would seem intuitive that the physical forces of a beating heart would affect its morphological development, but until recently this has been but a concept. In fact, haemodynamic forces are indeed important, and shape not only the normal development of the heart, but produce the secondary defects associated with major structural congenital cardiac malformations.

The initial identification of a role for haemodynamics was in zebrafish, a simple model of cardiac development in which a single atrium connects to a single ventricle. By altering the flow at the inflow or outflow of the zebrafish heart, and imaging the structure and function of the heart, it was determined that altering flow within the heart led to abnormal cardiac looping and defects in formation of the cardiac cushions, indicating that normal intracardiac flow is a key regulator of cardiac morphogenesis.[58] This was confirmed using zebrafish and mouse models in which embryonic contractility is impaired or absent.[59-61] More recent experiments, again in zebrafish, have clearly shown that intrinsic defects in contractility of cardiac myocytes, in combination with external haemodynamic forces, are essential for the normal development of the heart.[62]

The most intriguing results on haemodynamics and cardiac development have a direct connection to congenital malformations. It had been observed in a mouse model of laterality defects that include anomalies of the outflow tracts that formation of the arteries in the brachial arches is randomised between the left and right sides.[63] Normally, the arches form initially in bilateral fashion, but the left-sided brachiocephalic artery regresses, leaving only a right-sided artery. It was determined that, in this mouse model, the flow to the brachial arches was randomised to both left and right sides, unlike the usual situation where flow is preferentially directed to the right side. With a combination of surgical and morphological manipulations, it was shown that the altered flow was the likely culprit for the abnormal presence of a left-sided brachiocephalic artery. Thus a genetic defect, in this case involving *Pitx2*, not only leads to direct defects in regions of the heart where the mutated gene is expressed, but produces morphological defects secondary to altered flow. This finding has important implications for the understanding of the origin of congenital cardiac malformations.

CHROMOSOMAL DISORDERS

Each body cell contains, in its nucleus, 46 chromosomes. This is its own copy of the blueprint for the body. Of these, 44 chromosomes are common to males and females. These are the 22 pairs of autosomes. The remaining two are the sex chromosomes, X and Y. Aneuploidy is a generic term for any disturbance of the chromosomal complement other than the addition of whole extra sets, which represents polyploidy. Translated literally, aneuploidy means 'not good set' and may be defined as the loss or gain of all or part of a chromosome.

Autosomal Aneuploidy

Autosomal aneuploidy, that is, any disturbances of chromosomes other than X or Y, causes major disturbances of embryonic development, with the result that most afflicted fetuses are spontaneously aborted. Among the survivors, the most common form of aneuploidy is trisomy. This is the addition of one whole extra chromosome. Most cases are the result of non-disjunction at meiosis. When the primordial cell divides to produce an egg or sperm, the matching pairs of chromosomes separate so that the gamete contains one of each. This makes 23 in all, and this is known as a haploid set. The fusion of an egg and sperm restores the number to 46. If a pair of chromosomes fails to separate at meiosis, the gamete, and hence the embryo, will have either one too many, or one too few. The latter group abort, as do most of the former, particularly when large chromosomes are involved. Fetuses with trisomy for the smaller chromosomes may reach term, in particular those with trisomy 13, 18, or 21.

Trisomy 21

Of children born with a cardiac defect, 1 in 20 has trisomy 21.[64] It is, therefore, the largest specific aetiological category. Intelligence is rarely in the normal range, the mean quotient being about 50. Such children have an increased incidence of malformation and disease, including duodenal atresia, Hirschsprung's disease and anal atresia, leucaemia, and defects of the immune system. Those who reach adulthood tend to age prematurely. Of particular interest here is the frequency of cardiac malformations. In a large review of infants with trisomy 21 who had a cardiac defect, just over two-fifths were found to have an atrioventricular septal defect, while three-tenths had multiple anomalies, with persistence of the arterial duct being the second most common lesion, afflicting one-sixth.[65] Review of a necropsy series showed that almost half of infants with Down syndrome had a cardiac malformation, with two-thirds having an atrioventricular septal defect.[66] The strong association of atrioventricular septal defect with trisomy 21 is not seen with other chromosomal anomalies. It prompts the speculation that some important function of growth or adhesion of the endocardial cushions is determined by genes on the chromosome 21, or else abnormal genes disturb the separation of the common muscular atrioventricular junction, since it is the common junction which is the hallmark of the malformation. From a practical viewpoint, the presence of left-axis deviation in a neonate with the features of Down syndrome makes an atrioventricular septal defect very likely.

Mosaic Down Syndrome

About 3% of children with trisomy 21 have a parent who is a mosaic. This means that some of the parental cells have an extra chromosome 21, and this involved one or both gonads. If mosaicism is identified in the parent, the recurrence risk is greater than 10%.[67] It is the existence of such families that accounts for part of the 1% recurrence risk in siblings of a child with trisomy 21. In addition, some parents seem to have an increased risk of non-disjunction, since recurrences of trisomy involving chromosomes other than 21 have been described.

Trisomy 18, or Edward's Syndrome

Trisomy 18 affects 1 in 3500 newborns. Early death is almost invariable because of the multiple malformations. Survivors are severely developmentally delayed. Typical features are a prominent occiput, low-set malformed ears, and a small jaw, though the appearance is less characteristic than that seen with trisomy 21 or 13. Two additional clinical signs of great value are the unusual clenched fists, and rocker bottom feet. Cardiac defects are present in the majority, most being persistent patency of the arterial duct or ventricular septal defects. A bedside diagnosis is strengthened by examination of dermatoglyphic patterns.

Trisomy 13, or Patau's Syndrome

One in 7000 newborn infants has Patau's syndrome. The majority die as neonates. Survival beyond the first year is exceptional. The characteristic clinical features are polydactyly, cleft lip and palate, often bilateral and severe, and hypotelorism associated with malformation of the frontal lobes of the brain, also known as holoprosencephaly. There is a high incidence of cardiac defects, in particular atrial and ventricular septal defects. Abnormalities of cardiac position are relatively frequent,[68] perhaps indicating isomerism of the atrial appendages. As with atrioventricular septal defects and trisomy 21, the high incidence of disturbed cardiac position in trisomy 13 may reflect a specific role for this part of the genome in the determination of laterality.

Aneuploidy of the Sex Chromosomes

The female has two X chromosomes in each cell. The male has one X and the small Y chromosome. The latter determines maleness. The normal development of males shows that only a single copy is required for genes on the X chromosome. Females avoid having an excess by inactivating one of the two X chromosomes in each cell between the 16- and 1000-cell stages of embryonic life, a process called lyonisation. When excess of X chromosomes is present in each cell, all but one are switched off. An embryo, therefore, can tolerate chromosomal complements that contain three, four, or five X chromosomes with relatively little disturbance of development. Apart from the frequent occurrence of persistent patency of the arterial duct in the group with five X chromosomes, cardiac development is not affected. This is not the case when a single sex chromosome is present from the start, as in the 45, X karyotype.

45, X, or Turner's Syndrome

Though first described by Ullrich, the resultant syndrome is associated with the name of the American physician Turner. Despite being mild relative to most other forms of chromosomal aneuploidy, Turner's syndrome is associated with particularly heavy prenatal loss. Based on studies of aborted fetuses, it is estimated that the frequency of 1 in 10,000 births represents only 1% of conceptions with the 45, X karyotype.[69] Failure of sexual maturation, and short stature, are associated often with a webbed neck, also known as *pterygium colli*. Other features are a shark mouth, down-slanting palpebral fissures, and low-set ears. The strong association with aortic coarctation is well known. Aortic stenosis is the most common of a wide variety of other cardiac defects seen rarely in patients with Turner's syndrome. The prevalence of cardiac defects among 45, X individuals is estimated between 10% and 20%.[70]

SYNDROMES INVOLVING MICRODELETIONS: SINGLE GENES OR MORE?

22q11 Microdeletion Syndrome (DiGeorge Syndrome) and Defects of the Outflow Tracts

By far the most important example of a microdeletion is 22q11 deletion. About 3 million base pairs are normally lost in this disorder, resulting in the loss of at least 30 genes. There are segments at either end of the commonly deleted segment that have the same sequence. At meiosis, when the two copies of chromosomes 22 pair, this repeat makes them liable to misalign. If a crossover then occurs, it is possible to produce a chromosome with this segment deleted.

All individuals with this syndrome have facial features, though these may be subtle. Typically those involved will have short and narrow palpebral fissures, which may be up-slanting, a bulbous tip to the nose, which seems pinched because the supporting facial structures are flattened, a small mouth, and small rounded ears. While several acronyms have been utilised to describe this genetic disease, including Shprintzen syndrome, velo-cardio-facial syndrome, conotruncal anomaly face or Takao syndrome, Strong syndrome, and CATCH22, the most descriptive and inclusive name is 22q11 microdeletion syndrome.

A broad range of congenital cardiac malformations are seen in the setting of 22q11 microdeletion syndrome, including tetralogy of Fallot with pulmonary stenosis or atresia, common arterial trunk, and interrupted aortic arch. This range of lesions, in addition to the extracardiac defects found in the syndrome, made it difficult to pinpoint a particular causative gene or group of genes in the minimal 22q11 interval solely based on their known or perceived function. It took clever mouse chromosome engineering studies to pinpoint the likely single gene responsible for the majority of defects in 22q11 microdeletion syndrome. Taking advantage of the similar arrangement of genes between mouse and human, known as synteny, researchers utilised the power of mouse genetics to mimic the 22q11 microdeletion.[71,72] Once this rather spectacular technological feat had been achieved, the same groups refined their analysis to whittle down the interval, in effect doing in mouse what nature had not quite done in humans. These studies, combined with additional mouse models, narrowed down the likely culprit for the majority of defects in 22q11 microdeletion syndrome to a gene for a transcription factor, *Tbx1*.[10,11] *Tbx1* encodes a transcription factor that had previously not been functionally characterised, but is a member of the developmentally important T-box gene family. Significant debate surrounded this discovery, as it was considered unlikely that a single gene in the 22q11 minimal interval would result in all the defects in the syndrome, and confounding data from deletions that excluded the minimal interval, and therefore *TBX1*, further fueled the debate. The potential for *TBX1* as a major causative gene was strongly supported by the identification of *TBX1* missense mutations in patients with features of 22q11 microdeletion syndrome, but without a microdeletion.[73] Again, mouse genetics has lent support for the possibility that other genes within the 22q11 critical region probably also contribute to the disease, as deficiency of the 22q11 gene *crkl* results in similar defect in a mouse model and exacerbates loss of *Tbx1*.[74,75]

Although the congenital cardiac malformations seen in the setting of 22q11 microdeletion syndrome were attributed based on inferences to defects in migration of cells from the neural crest migration, *Tbx1* is expressed in the second heart field, and is important for its normal expansion.[29,30] The transcription factor Tbx1 appears to affect the neighbouring cells in the neural crest in a non-cell autonomous fashion by promoting secretion of fibroblast growth factor that interacts with its receptor on the cells from the neural crest to affect their proliferation or differentiation.

Williams Syndrome and Supravalvar Aortic Stenosis

The association between supravalvar aortic stenosis and the classic dysmorphic pattern known as Williams syndrome has been established in the literature for many years.[76] It led to speculation that there might be a gene responsible for the cardiac defect that was deleted as part of a microdeletion syndrome. This proved to be correct. Unlike the usual progression from deletion to discovery of the gene, the process was reversed when a patient with supravalvar aortic stenosis caused by a translocation focused attention on the elastin gene carried on chromosome 7.[77,78] Fluorescent in situ hybridisation soon revealed microdeletions in patients with Williams syndrome. Elastin is a major component of the walls of large vessels, and disruption of this gene somehow leads to excessive proliferation of cells in the vascular wall in mice.[79,80] The mechanism by which elastin regulates cellular proliferation is currently unknown. There is continuing controversy about the underlying cause of the characteristic learning disability with the outgoing personality. The chromosomal basis of the recurrent deletion appears to be a set of inversions that promotes recombination.[81]

Alagille Syndrome and Peripheral Pulmonary Arterial Stenosis

Peripheral pulmonary arterial stenosis is the hallmark of Alagille syndrome, a multi-system disorder affecting liver, cardiovascular system, spine, eyes, and face. The association of a microdeletion involving chromosome 20p12 narrowed the region of interest and led to identification of the causative gene defect, loss of *JAGGED1*.[82] Mutations in this gene, which encodes a Notch receptor, cause cardiac defects, not only in the context of Alagille syndrome, but also in isolated cases of congenital cardiac disease.[82–84] This gene encodes a ligand for the Notch family of receptors. The Notch pathway is involved in control of a variety of processes, extending from tissue patterning and morphogenesis to cancer. This discovery explains, at a superficial level, the stenotic lesions in the pulmonary vascular tree, along with the other features of the syndrome, such as hypoplasia of the biliary ductules, posterior embryotoxon of the eye, butterfly vertebrae, and the characteristic face. Much work will be needed to understand fully the relationship between the genetic error and the clinical phenotype, but the discovery of the loss of *JAGGED1* focuses attention on the correct pathway. Furthermore, the observation that loss of the whole gene produces the same phenotypic spectrum as mutations within the gene that lead to a gene product of reduced size demonstrates that this is a haplo insufficiency syndrome. In other words, the problem arises from loss of half of the gene product.

Defects of Laterality

Defects of laterality are often associated with congenital cardiac lesions, specifically those associated with isomerism of the atrial appendages, or visceral heterotaxy (see Chapter 22). The genetic cascades that regulate the situs of internal organs, including the lateralisation of the atrial appendages, have been carefully delineated using experimental models.[85] As defects of laterality in humans can be inherited, it is likely that in many cases single gene mutations are responsible. Indeed, human genetic studies have identified mutations in a few genes that lead to inherited defects of laterality.[85] A search for mutations in these genes in patients with congenital cardiac lesions but in the absence of isomerism that did not have any other feature of laterality defects identified a few rare cases, indicating that they may be a cause of isolated disease.[86,87]

SINGLE GENE DEFECTS

In the last decade, human genetic studies have identified several genes that are mutated in those with inherited cardiac disease. All of these are important regulators of cardiac morphogenesis, supporting the concept that the cardiac malformations are primarily a disease of abnormal embryonic organogenesis. These findings have also cemented the notion that most lesions have a genetic origin. In addition, these discoveries have clearly demonstrated that unrelated lesions can be caused by the same genetic defect, resulting in a need to reexamine epidemiological studies from a different perspective. In all cases, the mutations are dominant, as they affect only one of two alleles of the gene. As yet, it is not known how dominant mutations in these genes result in profound aberrations in formation of the heart. They may be related to decreased dosage, or may be due to gain of function effects. It is of paramount importance to understand the molecular consequences of disease-causing mutations, and the mechanism underlying these events, in order to be able to design in rational fashion non-surgical therapeutic interventions for those with congenitally malformed hearts. The future of our understanding of the aetiology of the lesions, therefore, lies in understanding how mutations in these important regulators leads to altered morphogenesis.

Syndromic Mutations

Mutations of *TBX5* in Holt-Oram Syndrome

Some genetic mutations have been identified in rare syndromes that include congenital cardiac malformations. For example, mutations in *TBX5* cause defects in the context of Holt-Oram syndrome.[88–90] These defects are predominantly interatrial communications, usually within the oval fossa, muscular ventricular septal defects, and abnormalities of the conduction system, but mutations can also result in more diverse abnormalities, such as hypoplastic left heart syndrome, totally anomalous pulmonary venous connection, and common atrioventricular junction (Fig. 9-1). The syndrome also includes defects in limb formation, specifically of the radial ray, the thumb, first digit, and radius. Most defects of the limbs involve the thumbs, and range in severity from mild triphalangeal thumbs, up to complete phocomelia, with defects of intermediate severity such as missing thumbs, and hypoplastic radius.

Mutations have been found throughout the *TBX5* gene,[90] although they predominantly cluster in the so-called T-box domain, which confers DNA-binding capabilities on the protein. Early studies supported the concept of genotype-phenotype correlation, whereby mutations in one part of the gene were predominantly associated with families with severe cardiac defects, while mutations in a different part of the gene were found in families that had a predominance of severe limb, but not cardiac, defects.[91] Subsequent findings, however, discounted this hypothesis. It is now believed that the difference in manifestation of disease is more likely a result of genetic background.[90,92,93]

The observation by clinical geneticists that limb anomalies often coincide with cardiac defects has led some investigators to investigate *TBX5* mutations for several related disorders. This often does not yield positive correlations. Recent work has strived to define the clinical criterion for the Holt-Oram syndrome in relation to the presence of *TBX5* mutations. Indeed, there is excellent concordance, as long as a strict definition is maintained for the components of the syndrome.[94]

Modelling of Holt-Oram syndrome in the mouse has revealed interesting and important features of the consequences of haploinsufficiency on downstream target gene regulation.[35,95,96] In particular, it is clear that some genes in the heart are exquisitely sensitive to the dosage of Tbx5, explaining the occasional severity of defects in mice or humans with reduced dosage of this gene. Some genes, such as the gap junction protein-encoding gene *Gja5*, also known as connexin 40, are targets that may explain some aspects of Holt-Oram syndrome, such as, in this case, the atrioventricular block. In other cases investigation of the mouse model has led to the intriguing observation that independent of structural lesions one can identify clear defects in diastolic function due to reduced Tbx5 activity. These functional deficits are directly due to reduced function of the calcium pump (see Chapter 4), related to reduced activity of the *Serca2a* gene, which is directly regulated by Tbx5.[96] These results, observed in the mouse, correlate to human patients with Holt-Oram syndrome, indicating that specific defects in cardiac function can accompany structural lesions while being unrelated to them except for their underlying genetic cause.[96]

Mutations of *SALL4* in Okihiro Syndrome

Mutations in the Spalt gene *SALL4* have been found to underlie Okihiro syndrome, which, as with Holt-Oram syndrome, affects the limbs as well as the heart, although it also has a broad spectrum of ocular, renal, and other defects.[93,97–101] The two syndromes are sometimes confused clinically due to very similar defects involving the heart and limbs, but molecular genetic studies have clearly outlined the distinction between the two.[93] Using mouse models, it has been shown that *Sall4* and *Tbx5* genetically and

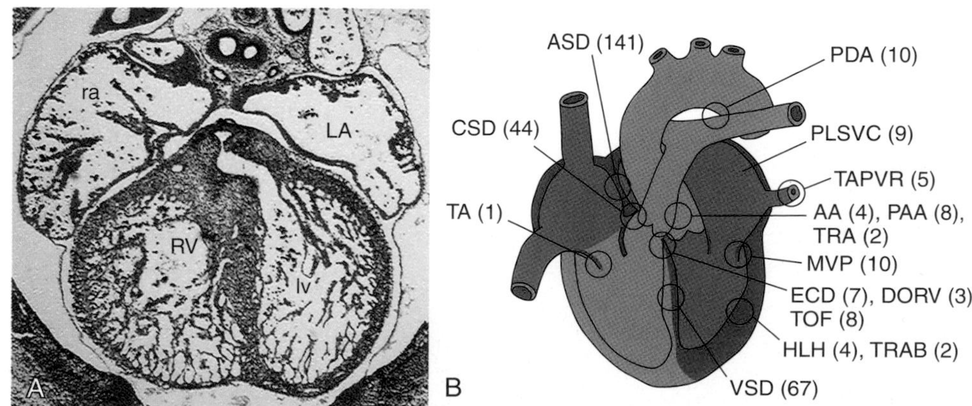

Figure 9-1 *Tbx5* expression and congenital heart defects in Holt-Oram syndrome. **A,** In situ hybridisation of *Tbx5* (red signal) in an E13.5 mouse embryo, with expression in the atria (la, ra), left ventricle (lv) and left side of the interventricular septum, and right ventricular (rv) trabeculae. **B,** A diagrammatic representation of *Tbx5* expression in a mature heart, and the location and type of congenital heart defects found in Holt-Oram syndrome patients. Numbers in parentheses represent numbers of reported cases. AA, aortic atresia; ASD, atrial septal defect; CSD, conduction system defects; DORV, double outlet right ventricle ECD, atrioventricular septal defect with common atrioventricular junction; HLH, hypoplastic left heart; LA, left atrium; MVP, mitral valve prolapse; PAA, pulmonary arterial atresia; PDA, persistent patency of arterial duct; PLSVC, persistent left superior caval vein; TA, tricuspid atresia; TAPVR, total anomalous pulmonary venous return; TF, tetralogy of Fallot; TRA, common arterial trunk; TRAB, trabecular anomalies; VSD, ventricular septal defects. (Adapted from Bruneau BG: The developing heart and congenital heart defects: A make or break situation. Clin Genet 2003;63:252–261; and Bruneau BG, Logan M, Davis N, et al: Chamber-specific cardiac expression of Tbx5 and heart defects in Holt-Oram syndrome. Dev Biol 1999;211:100–108.)

physically interact to pattern the heart and limbs,[102] thus explaining the reason for the similarities in syndromes caused by mutations in either gene.

Disruptions of the RAS Signalling Network in Noonan's Syndrome

Autosomal dominant gain of function mutations in *PTPN11*, encoding the protein tyrosine phosphatase SHP2, cause Noonan's syndrome, characterised by pulmonary stenosis, hypertrophic cardiomyopathy, and occasional atrioventricular valvar defects.[103] Most recently, hypomorphic mutations in *SOS1*, an essential RAS guanine nucleotide-exchange factor (Ras-Gef), was shown to enhance RAS-ERK activation, and this can account for as high as one-fifth of the cases of Noonan's syndrome not explained by *PTPN11* mutations.[104,105] Recent evidence implicates epidermal growth factor signalling as an important regulator of late valvar remodeling. Loss or attenuation of EGFR/ErbB1 signalling results in preferential hypercellularity of arterial but not atrioventricular valves.[106] The hyperplastic arterial valvar phenotype is augmented when crossed to mice heterozygous for a null mutation in *ptpn11*.[107] Deletion of the EGF ligand, heparin binding epidermal growth factor, results in increased size of the endocardial cushions and ridges, along with the size and proliferation of cells in both the arterial and atrioventricular valvar leaflets.[108,109]

Non-Syndromic Mutations

Mutations of *NKX2-5* Cause Septation and Other Defects

Mutations in the *NKX2-5* gene cause defects similar to those caused by mutations of *TBX5*, namely deficiencies of atrial and ventricular septation, problems with conduction, hypoplasia of the left heart, and others anomalies such as tetralogy of Fallot or Ebstein's malformation.[15,110–112] Mutations were originally identified in two families with very distinctive clinical features, namely progressive atrioventricular block in the setting of interatrial communications. Subsequent studies showed that this unusual combination was not the only type of lesion that could be caused by the mutations. Indeed, mutations in *NKX2-5* were identified in several additional families that had some members presenting with an interatrial communication and atrioventricular block, but others with ventricular septal defects in isolation, Ebsein's malformation, and tetralogy of Fallot[110] (Fig. 9-2). These results were extended to sporadic cases, which in addition to several cases of interatrial communication within the oval fossa and tetralogy of Fallot, included rare sporadic cases of common arterial trunk, double outlet right ventricle, congenitally corrected transposition, interrupted aortic arch, hypoplastic left heart syndrome, and aortic coarctation.[112] This was perhaps not surprising to developmental biologists, who would expect a broad set of defects based on the pan-cardiac expression of the *Nkx2-5* gene in the mouse, but it showed with definitive clarity that a single defined mutation could result in a wide range of clinically and anatomically unrelated defects. This finding went a long way to explain the considerable difficulties in identifying familial inheritance of congenital cardiac malformations.

As with mutations of *TBX5*, a broad range of mutations have been identified in the *NKX2-5* gene, which is made up of two rather compact exons. Functional analysis of these mutations has determined that, for the most part, mutations of *NKX2-5* result in a loss of activity for the gene, whether it be due to the production of a truncated protein, or one that cannot activate transcription by itself, or one that does not allow the gene to interact with its partner proteins such as TBX5 and GATA4.[113,114] The biochemical basis of the differential expressivity of the various *NKX2-5* mutations, therefore, has not been elucidated, and we are left once again with the potential for genetic modifiers as the modulating factors.

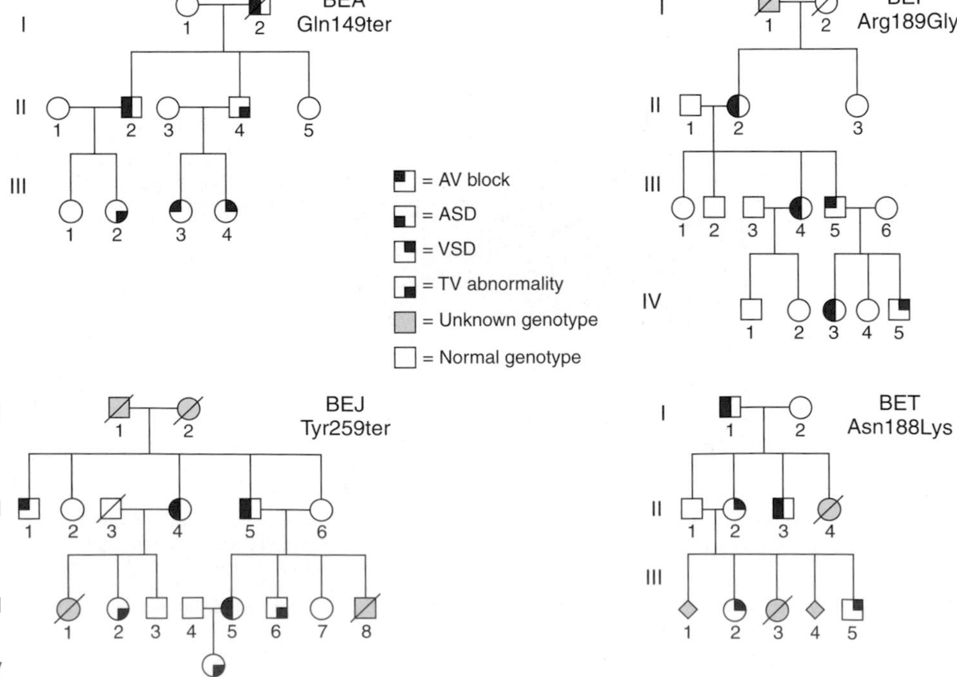

Figure 9-2 *NKX2-5* mutations cause a variety of inherited congenital cardiac malformations. Four family trees are shown, each representing a discrete mutation in *NKX2-5* that when inherited is associated with a range of defects, including atrioventricular block (AV block), atrial septal defects (ASD), ventricular septal defects (VSD), and tricuspid valvar abnormality (TV abnormality). Circles represent females, squares represent males. Roman numerals indicate generations within a family. (Adapted from Benson DW, Silberbach GM, Kavanaugh-McHugh A, et al: Mutations in the cardiac transcription factor NKX2.5 affect diverse cardiac developmental pathways. J Clin Invest 1999;104:1567–1573.)

The progressive nature of the atrioventricular block in some patients with mutations of *NKX2-5* was an important clue about one of its unexpected roles in the heart. From a clinical standpoint, this discovery suggests that patients with the familial form of atrial septal defect should be followed longitudinally to check for the appearance of problems with atrioventricular conduction even after surgical correction of the septal defect. Indeed, studies in the mouse have suggested that a primary defect in the conduction system is at the root of these problems with conduction, and that additionally the loss of *Nkx2-5* might lead to cardiomyopathy unrelated to the structural defects or the abnormalities in the conduction system.[115]

Mutations of *GATA4* Cause Problems with Septation

Families have now been identified with problems in septation as a their sole phenotype. Genetic mapping in two unrelated families with interatrial and interventricular communications have identified mutations in *GATA4*[16] (Fig. 9-3). These mutations were predicted to result in a partial loss of function of the gene, and also predicted impaired interaction with Tbx5, thus linking the function of these two transcription factors to septation of the atrial and ventricular chambers. Mutations in *GATA4* have also been identified in a few other families and individuals,[116,117] but overall they are rare in patients with congenitally malformed hearts. Mouse models previously would not have predicted that dominant mutations in *GATA4* could cause congenital cardiac disease, as mice heterozygous for *Gata4* null alleles were normal. Recent results have shown that, when bred in a particular strain, loss of one copy of *Gata4* does indeed result in significant congenital cardiac disease, which resembles to a certain degree the malformations seen in humans with mutations of *GATA4*.[117]

Mutations of *NOTCH1* Cause Bicuspid Aortic Valve

Malformations of the valves are due to improper valvogenesis, and can vary in severity. As such, they may not be recognised until adulthood, when the valves begin to malfunction. The most common cause of valvar disease is seen in patients with aortic valves having two instead of three leaflets, the so-called bicuspid aortic valve. Found with a prevalence of 1% to 2% in the population, it is the most common congenital cardiac anomaly, affecting more patients than all other defects combined. The bifoliate valve can cause disease in childhood if the valvar abnormality is severe, and can be part of the hypoplastic left heart syndrome. Indeed, one-sixth of first-degree relatives with hypoplasia of the left heart have bifoliate aortic valves not necessarily producing symptoms, suggesting a common genetic aetiology. The bifoliate aortic valve is more frequently asymptomatic until later decades of life, when premature calcification, prolapse, or bacterial endocarditis occurs. In those with calcification or regurgitation, the valve becomes stenotic, leading to dysfunction that eventually requires valvar replacement. This disease is the third most common form of cardiac disease seen in adults, and over 50,000 bifoliate aortic valves are replaced annually in the United States of America alone.

Recently, through investigation of families with autosomal dominant disease, mutations in *NOTCH1* were identified as a genetic cause of the valvar malformations and calcification.[17] Linkage studies mapped the disease

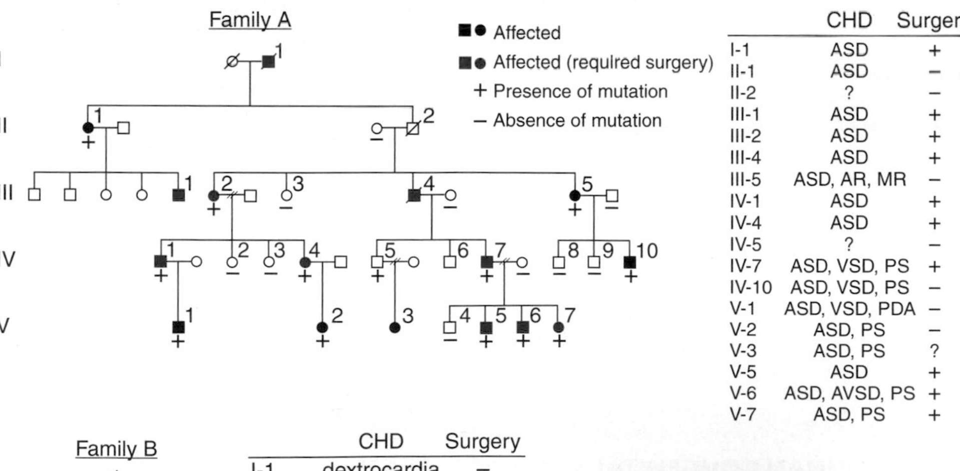

	CHD	Surgery
I-1	ASD	+
II-1	ASD	−
II-2	?	−
III-1	ASD	+
III-2	ASD	+
III-4	ASD	+
III-5	ASD, AR, MR	−
IV-1	ASD	+
IV-4	ASD	+
IV-5	?	−
IV-7	ASD, VSD, PS	+
IV-10	ASD, VSD, PS	−
V-1	ASD, VSD, PDA	−
V-2	ASD, PS	−
V-3	ASD, PS	?
V-5	ASD	+
V-6	ASD, AVSD, PS	+
V-7	ASD, PS	+

	CHD	Surgery
I-1	dextrocardia	−
II-1	ASD	+
II-2	ASD	−
II-3	ASD	+
III-1	ASD	+
III-2	ASD	+
III-3	ASD	+
IV-1	ASD	+

Figure 9-3 *GATA4* mutations cause septal defects. Family A is a five-generation kindred with several family members afflicted with congenital malformations of the heart, as listed in the table to the right of the family tree. Family B has inherited defects across four generations; defects are again listed in the table to the right of the family tree. In both families, affected members with a plus sign carry a *GATA4* mutation. An echocardiogram of one patient shows atrial and ventricular septal defects. AR, aortic regurgitation; ASD, atrial septal defect; AVSD, atrioventricular septal defect; LA, left atrium; LV, left ventricle; PS, pulmonary stenosis; PDA, patent arterial duct; RA, right atrium; RV, right ventricle; VSD, ventricular septal defect. (Adapted from Garg V, Kathiriya IS, Barnes R, et al: GATA4 mutations cause human congenital heart defects and reveal an interaction with TBX5. Nature 2003;424:443–447.)

locus to mutations in *NOTCH1* in two unrelated families with a similar valvar phenotype (Fig. 9-4), specifically severe premature calcification of a bifoliate valve. Interestingly, a subset of family members who harboured mutations in *NOTCH1* had trifoliate aortic valves, but still developed calcification that required subsequent valvar replacement. Thus, *NOTCH1* signalling may be required to suppress calcification of the mesenchymal cells of the valve under normal circumstances. Indeed, experimental studies showed that *NOTCH1* represses the osteoblast phenotype that is typical of valvar and vascular calcification. As for other familial disease, a wide spectrum of lesions was observed within family members, including tetralogy of Fallot, hypoplasia of the left heart, and ventricular septal defect, likely due to genetic background features.

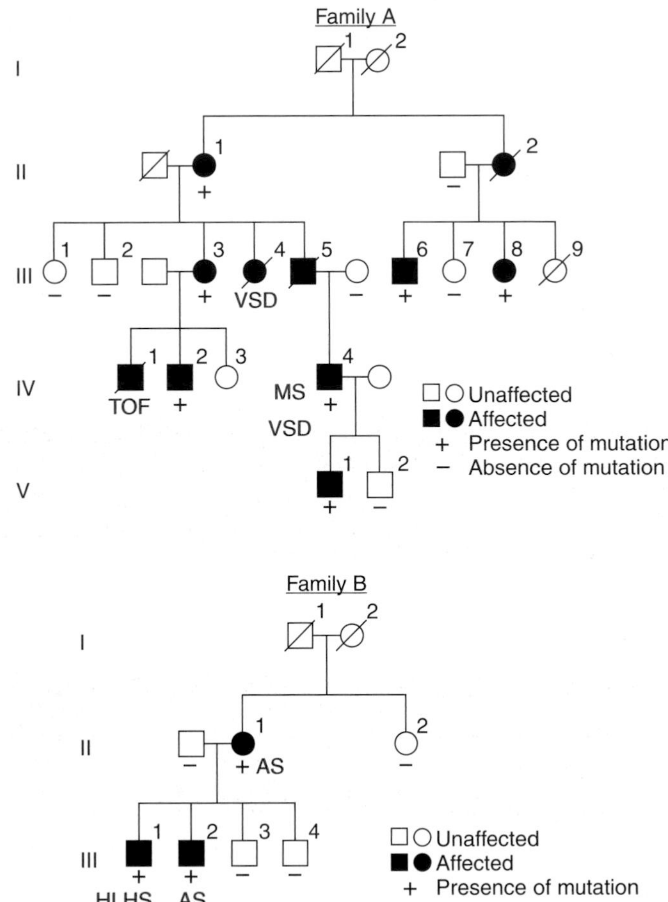

Figure 9-4 *NOTCH1* mutations cause aortic valvar disease associated with more severe congenital cardiac malformations. Family A and Family B both have inherited *NOTCH1* mutations (indicated by the plus signs). Most patients in both families have bicuspid aortic valve, but several members also have more severe defects, such as aortic stenosis (AS), hypoplastic left heart syndrome (HLHS), mitral stenosis (MS), ventricular septal defect (VSD), or tetralogy of Fallot (TOF). One patient has both mitral stenosis and a ventricular septal defect. (Adapted from Garg V, Muth AN, Ransom JF, et al: Mutations in NOTCH1 cause aortic valve disease. Nature 2005;437:270–274.)

CONCLUSIONS

So far the clinical impact of the identification of genetic mutations producing congenitally malformed hearts has not been felt, largely because of an incomplete understanding of the range of mutations and their functional significance. In some cases, pre-implantation in vitro fertilisation genetic screening has been established for those mutations that cause very severe defects.[118] Clearly, a comprehensive genomics-based examination of a much larger set of genes in a wide range of patients is required to begin to understand the genetic basis for congenital cardiac malformations.

Congenital cardiac disease, therefore, can now be conceived as not only a defect of morphogenesis, but in some cases, a failure of differentiation among subsets of lineages that contribute to the heart. We are now embarking on a phase in which knowledge of developmental pathways, and high-throughput methods of genotyping rare and common genetic variants, should allow rigorous investigation into the causes of human cardiac disease. With the increasing recognition that congenitally malformed hearts harbour a significant genetic contribution (Table 9-1), we can now imagine that genetic variation underlies both the morphogenetic defect, and the predisposition to long-term consequences that will affect clinical outcomes for the millions of survivors. Thus, vigorous efforts to identify genetic variation associated with the congenitally malformed heart, and outcomes of treatment, will be essential as therapeutic or preventive measures to alter the course of disease may be possible throughout childhood and in the adult. It may even be conceivable eventually to predict genetic risk among parents, and focus preventive strategies on those at greatest risk vertically to transmit the disease. The efficacy of folic acid in prevention of defects of the neural tube provides hope for similar prevention of congenital cardiac disease.

TABLE 9-1

FREQUENCY OF GENETIC MUTATION IN HUMAN CONGENITAL CARDIAC DISEASE

Gene Name	CHD	Numbers of Families/% CHD Population	Reference
BMPR2	PPH + CHD (ASD, VSD, AVSD)	6% (6/106 PPH + CHD cases)	119
CFC1	TGA	2% (2/86 TGA cases)	87, 120
GATA4	ASD, VSD	Five families/12% (2/16 ASD cases)	16, 121, 122
NKX2-5	ASD, AV block, TOF, Ebstein's	4% of ASDs and 4% TOF, 3/16 ASD	110–112, 121
NOTCH1	BAV, TOF, AS, VSD, HLHS, IAA	Two families	17
THRAP2	TGA	One family/3% (3/97 TGA cases)	123
ZIC3	CHD	2% (2/97 non-heterotaxy CHDs)	124

AS, aortic stenosis; ASD, atrial septal defect; AVSD, atrioventricular septal defect; AV block, atrioventricular block; BAV, bifoliate aortic valve; CHD, congenital heart disease; HLHS, hypoplastic left heart syndrome; IAA, interrupted aortic arch; PPH, pulmonary hypertension; TGA, transposition; TOF, tetralogy of Fallot; VSD, ventricular septal defect.

The complete reference list can be found on the companion Expert Consult web site at www.expertconsult.com.

ANNOTATED REFERENCES

- Hoffman JI, Kaplan S: The incidence of congenital heart disease. J Am Coll Cardiol 2002;39:1890–1900.

  This important paper synthesises the literature to provide a clear summary of the incidence of cardiac disease in children.
- Lindsay EA, Vitelli F, Su H, et al: *Tbx1* haploinsufficiency in the DiGeorge syndrome region causes aortic arch defects in mice. Nature 2001;410: 97–101.
- Merscher S, Funke B, Epstein JA, et al: *TBX1* is responsible for cardiovascular defects in velo-cardio-facial/DiGeorge syndrome. Cell 2001;104:619–629.

  These papers pinpointed, using mouse genetics, Tbx1 as the likely major gene responsible for most of the defects observed in 22q11 microdeletion syndrome.
- Schott J-J, Benson DW, Basson CT, et al: Congenital heart disease caused by mutations in the transcription factor *NKX2-5*. Science 1998;281:108–111.

  This important paper was the first demonstration of a human mutation in non-syndromic inherited congenital cardiac disease. It also placed a developmentally important gene as involved in human disease, which cemented the notion of impaired development as the cause of congenital cardiac disease.
- Garg V, Kathiriya IS, Barnes R, et al: *GATA4* mutations cause human congenital heart defects and reveal an interaction with TBX5. Nature 2003;424: 443–447.

  This important work identified mutations in the GATA4 transcription factor gene in families with abnormal atrial and ventricular septation. This finding was the first example of a human disease gene in isolated defects of septation. Molecular analyses identified defects in interaction between GATA4 and TBX5 as a potential mechanism of disease.
- Garg V, Muth AN, Ransom JF, et al: Mutations in *NOTCH1* cause aortic valve disease. Nature 2005;437:270–274.

  In this paper, mutations in the NOTCH1 gene were identified in families with inherited aortic valvar disease, which included bicuspid aortic valve, valvar calcification, and in one case, hypoplastic left heart syndrome.
- Bruneau BG, Nemer G, Schmitt JP, et al: A murine model of Holt-Oram syndrome defines roles of the T-box transcription factor Tbx5 in cardiogenesis and disease. Cell 2001;106:709–721.

  This paper describes the first mouse model of inherited congneital cardiac disease, firmly establishing the mechanism of transcription factor haploinsufficiency as a cause of disease, and established that transcription factor interactions were important for the dosage effect in the developing heart.
- Zhao Y, Ransom JF, Li A, et al: Dysregulation of cardiogenesis, cardiac conduction, and cell cycle in mice lacking miRNA-1-2. Cell 2007;129:303–317.

  This paper defines the contibution of a single microRNA gene in mouse development, which indicates that disruption of this newly discovered family of genes may underlie human disease of the heart.
- Yashiro K, Shiratori H, Hamada H: Haemodynamics determined by a genetic programme govern asymmetric development of the aortic arch. Nature 2007;450:285–288.

  A paper that clearly indicates that haemodynamics are an important epigenetic component of congenital heart disease, secondary to genetic disruptions. This work, conducted in a mouse model of outflow tract defects, elegantly distinguishes genetic from haemodynamic components, and provides the important suggestion that not all observed defects can be linked directly to an underlying genetic defect.
- Mori AD, Bruneau BG: TBX5 mutations and congenital heart disease: Holt-Oram syndrome revealed. Curr Opin Cardiol 2004;19:211–215.

  This review article summarises the range of mutations found in the TBX5 gene that cause Holt-Oram syndrome, as well as the proposed mechanisms for this disease.
- Tartaglia M, Mehler EL, Goldberg R, et al: Mutations in PTPN11, encoding the protein tyrosine phosphatase SHP-2, cause Noonan syndrome. Nat Genet 2001;29:465–468.

  In this paper, the aetiology of Noonan's syndrome was identified in the form of mutations that affect the function of an important signalling molecule.

CHAPTER 10
Fetal Echocardiography

ANITA L. SZWAST and JACK RYCHIK

Malformations of the heart and arterial trunks are the most common form of congenital anomalies found in humans. They occur in approximately 6 of every 1000 live births, and in 8 to 10 of every 1000 pregnancies. Fetal echocardiography, or the use of ultrasonic technologies to evaluate the fetal cardiovascular system, enables diagnosis of structural heart defects, and offers a way to observe complex physiological processes prior to birth. The primary benefits of fetal echocardiography include the ability to counsel parents prior to birth as to the expectations for a child born with a congenitally malformed heart, the ability to implement appropriate postnatal management strategies in an anticipatory fashion, so as to maximise outcome, and the ability to identify and treat cardiovascular diseases prior to birth.

SCREENING WITH FETAL ECHOCARDIOGRAPHY

As imaging technologies, and the skills of operators, continue to improve, a higher percentage of congenital cardiac malformations can be detected accurately before birth. Analysis of large registries has shown that rates of detection can vary from 15% to 25%.[1-5] Many studies have documented the utility of the four-chamber view of the heart in identifying the malformations during fetal life.[5-11] In these studies, rates of detection using this view alone ranged from 4.5% to 81%.[5-11] Malformations of the outflow tracts, however, and discordant ventriculo-arterial connections, may frequently be missed when this view is used in isolation. When views showing the right and left ventricular outflow tracts are included in the obstetrical screen, the reported detection rate increases to between 43.8% and 85.5%.[7,12,13] In contrast, if fetal echocardiography, defined as a detailed, focused assessment of the fetal cardiovascular system, is performed, then rates of detection are significantly higher, and diagnostic accuracy rates may exceed 85% to 90%.[12,14] Given the disparity in rates of detection between those specialising in fetal echocardiography and routine obstetrical screening, the question of who should be referred for fetal echocardiography remains an important consideration.

Currently, the American Society of Echocardiography recommends fetal echocardiography for fetal, maternal, and familial indications (Table 10-1).[15] In the past, many women were referred for fetal echocardiography due to a family history of congenital cardiac disease, an umbilical cord containing two vessels, maternal diabetes, or maternal exposure to teratogens. Patterns of referral, however, have changed on account of improved techniques becoming available for imaging. Referrals for fetal echocardiography producing a high yield now include an abnormal obstetrical ultrasound evaluation, in which up to two-thirds of referrals have congenital cardiac malformations, and a chromosomal anomaly, with half of such referrals proving to have congenital cardiac lesions.[16,17] Referrals with a low yield include presence of a single umbilical artery, or exposure to teratogens, with congenital cardiac lesions detected infrequently in mothers referred with these indications.[16,17] A family history of congenital cardiac disease accounts for between one-quarter and one-third of all referrals for fetal echocardiography, but less than one-twentieth of cases with detected malformations.[16,17] Increased nuchal translucency noted on screening during the first trimester, from 10 to 13 weeks of gestation, has now emerged as an important indication for fetal echocardiography. Indeed, increased nuchal translucency of greater than 3 mm as seen during scanning when the fetus is aged from 10 to 14 weeks is a published marker for aneuploidy.[18-23] Even in the absence of a chromosomal anomaly, fetuses found to have increased nuchal translucency on early scanning have been shown to be at increased risk for congenital cardiac disease.[24,25] Fetuses conceived via artificial fertilisation, particularly when using intracytoplasmic injection of sperm, have a twofold increased risk of major birth

TABLE 10-1

INDICATIONS FOR FETAL ECHOCARDIOGRAPHY

Maternal Indications

- Family history of congenital cardiac disease
- Metabolic disorders, such as phenylketonuria or diabetes
- Exposure to teratogens
- Exposure to inhibitors of prostaglandin synthetase, such as ibuprofen, salicylic acid, or indomethacin
- Infection with rubella
- Autoimmune disease, such as systemic lupus erythematosus, or Sjögren's syndrome
- Familial inherited disorders, such as Ellis van Creveld syndrome, Marfan's syndrome, or Noonan's syndrome
- Artificial fertilisation

Fetal Indications

- Abnormal result following obstetrical ultrasonic screening
- Extracardiac abnormality
- Chromosomal abnormality
- Arrhythmia
- Hydrops
- Increased nuchal translucency in first trimester
- Multiple gestation and twin-twin transfusion

defects, including congenital cardiac disease, compared to infants conceived naturally.[26] While somewhat controversial, it is increasingly recognised that the frequency of congenital anomalies is increased in this population, and fetal echocardiography is therefore of benefit to these families.

TIMING OF FETAL ECHOCARDIOGRAPHY

Fetal echocardiography is best performed between 18 and 22 weeks of gestation. At this gestational age, there is adequate amniotic fluid to allow good visualisation of the cardiac structures and vasculature. After 30 weeks gestation, the increase in the fetal body mass, and the shadowing effects of the fetal ribs, may make acquisition of images more difficult. Maternal transabdominal fetal imaging may be performed between 15 and 18 weeks gestation, although visualisation may be suboptimal. New interest has emerged in early maternal transabdominal or trans-vaginal scanning at 11 to 14 weeks of gestation, especially in populations known to be at high risk, such as those noted to have increased nuchal translucency during scanning at 10 to 14 weeks, those with suspected aneuploidy, or those with a family history of congenital cardiac disease. Feasibility studies have demonstrated adequate acquisition of images at these gestational ages for both maternal transabdominal and trans-vaginal imaging. Diagnostic transabdominal images have been reported in 98.7% of cases, with abnormalities detected in 13 of 226 fetuses studied.[27] In this study, only 4 of 213 minor structural abnormalities were missed on the initial scan.[27] Others have shown that the four-chamber view can be obtained using trans-vaginal imaging in all cases, with extended views of the heart obtained in almost all of these instances.[28] In this study, three cases of major congenital cardiac disease were diagnosed on the initial trans-vaginal scan, while three cases were diagnosed later in gestation.[28]

MODALITIES FOR IMAGING

Cross sectional imaging remains the gold standard for the diagnosis of structural cardiac disease during fetal life. The Pediatric Council of the American Society of Echocardiography recommends obtaining multiple cross sectional tomographic views of the heart in order to make an accurate diagnosis.[15] Fetal echocardiography should include an apical four-chamber view of the heart, an apical five-chamber view, a long-axis view of the left ventricular outflow tract, a long-axis view of the right ventricular outflow tract, a short-axis view at the level of the arterial trunks, a short-axis view at the level of the ventricles, a long-axis view of the caval veins, a view of the ductal arch, and a view of the aortic arch[15] (Table 10-2 and Figs. 10-1 and 10-2). The fetal heart rate should be documented, and any arrhythmia confirmed with M-mode imaging. The diameters of the orifices of all valves should be measured in systole at right angles to the plane of flow.[15] Reference ranges for the diameters of all valves over the course of gestation have been published.[29] Cardiac dysfunction may be assessed by cross sectional interrogation by the presence of ascites, pleural or pericardial effusions, skin oedema, and cardiomegaly, as defined by a ratio of cardiothoracic areas of greater than 0.36.[30] A ratio of cardiothoracic areas greater than 0.6 is associated with an extremely poor outcome.[31]

TABLE 10-2

ESSENTIAL COMPONENTS OF THE FETAL ECHOCARDIOGRAM

Feature	Essential Component
Anatomical overview	Fetal number and position in the uterus Establish stomach position and arrangement of abdominal organs Establish cardiac position
Biometric examination	Cardiothoracic ratio Biparietal diameter Femoral length
Cardiac imaging views/sweeps	Four-chamber view Four-chamber view angled towards great arteries (five-chamber view) Long-axis view (left ventricular outflow) Long-axis view (right ventricular outflow) Short-axis sweep, cephalad angling to include the three-vessel view Long-axis view of caval veins Ductal arch view Aortic arch view
Doppler examination	Inferior and superior caval veins Pulmonary veins Hepatic veins Venous duct Oval foramen Atrioventricular valves Arterial valves Arterial duct Transverse aortic arch Umbilical artery Umbilical vein
Measurements	Atrioventricular valvar diameter Arterial valvar diameter Pulmonary trunk Ascending aorta Right and left pulmonary arteries Transverse aortic arch Ventricular length Ventricular short-axis dimensions
Examination of rhythm and rate	M-mode of atrial and ventricular mural motion Doppler examination of patterns of atrial and ventricular flow

Colour Doppler interrogation adds to the assessment of fetal cardiovascular wellbeing by establishing the degree of valvar stenosis and regurgitation, if present. Mild tricuspid regurgitation may be seen throughout gestation, and is frequently a benign finding,[32,33] but tricuspid regurgitation detected during early scanning, from 11 to 14 weeks, may be a marker for aneuploidy, even in the absence of structural heart disease.[34] In contrast, regurgitation across the mitral, pulmonary, or aortic valves is usually not a normal finding and suggests pathology, secondary to underlying structural cardiac disease or fetal cardiac failure. Cardiovascular physiology can also be assessed by colour Doppler echocardiography by determining the direction of blood flow. In the normal fetal circulation, the direction of shunting is right to left at both the patent oval foramen and the arterial duct. Abnormal directions of flow at these sites may

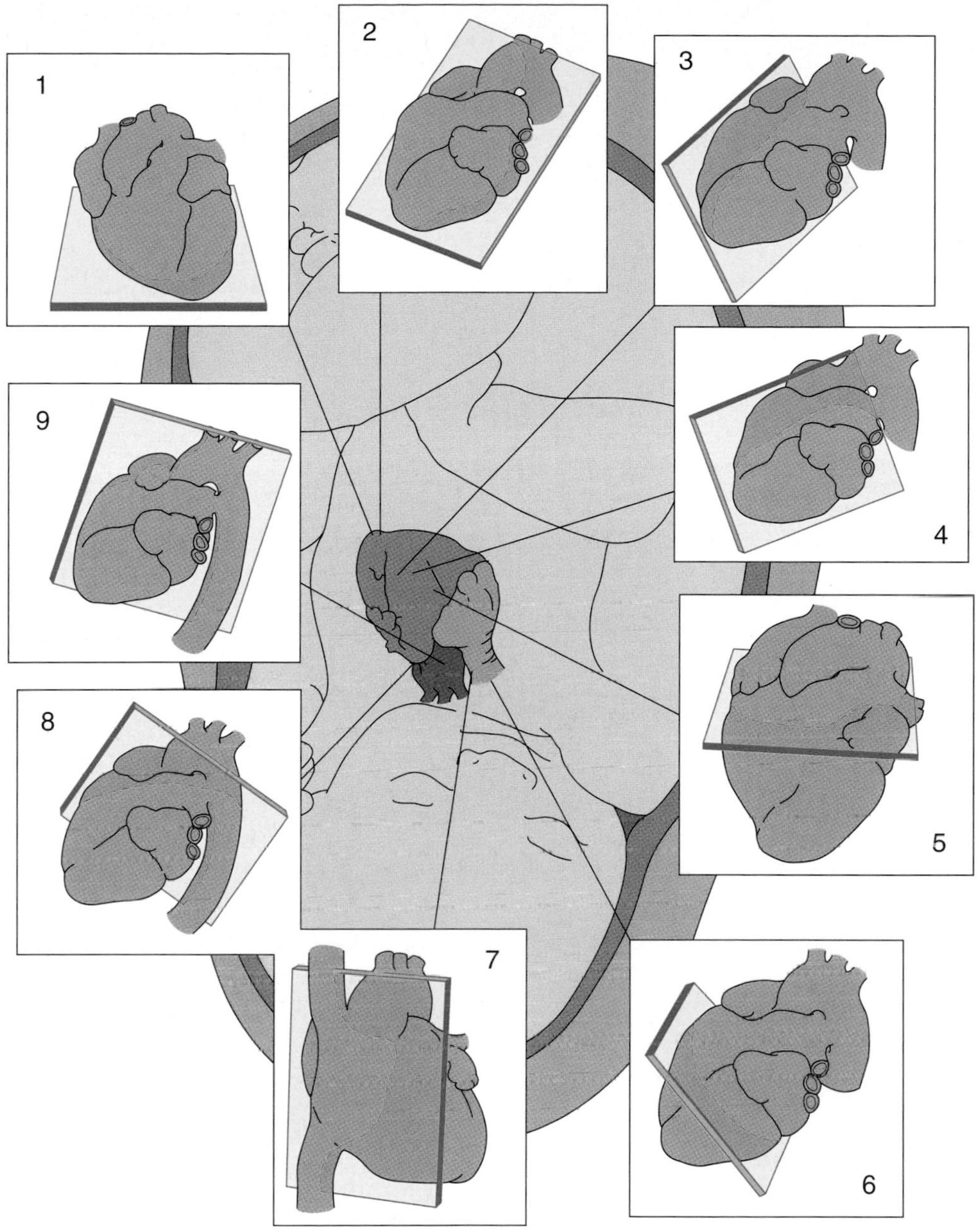

Figure 10-1 Illustration of the tomographic planes used to image the fetal cardiovascular system. Imaging planes displayed are in a normal human fetus. Starting at the top left, the following views are demonstrated in a clockwise manner: **1,** apical (four-chamber) view; **2,** apical (five-chamber) view angled towards the aorta; **3,** long-axis view of the left ventricular outflow tract; **4,** long-axis view of the right ventricular outflow tract; **5,** short-axis view at the level of the great vessels; **6,** short-axis view with caudad angling at the level of the ventricles; **7,** caval long-axis view; **8,** ductal arch view; **9,** aortic arch view. (With permission from the American Society of Echocardiography Guidelines and Standards for Performance of the Fetal Echocardiogram. J Am Soc Echocardiogr 2004;17:803–810.)

suggest cardiac disease. For example, left-to-right flow at the patent oval foramen, or bidirectional shunting through the arterial duct with reversal of flow in the transverse arch, may indicate inadequacy of the left ventricle.[35,36]

Doppler echocardiography is a powerful tool with which to assess cardiovascular physiology and function, and is an important part of the comprehensive evaluation of the fetal cardiovascular system. Pathological conditions associated with elevated central venous pressures may manifest as changes in the Doppler flow patterns in the inferior caval vein, the venous duct, and the umbilical vein. After 18 weeks gestation, flow in the venous duct should be all antegrade with atrial contraction. As central venous pressure increases, there is first decreased flow, and ultimately reversal of flow seen with atrial contraction in the venous duct (Fig. 10-3). In the umbilical vein, there is normally continuous forward flow at low velocity. As central venous pressure increases, notching is seen at the end of diastole in the umbilical venous flow. In severe cardiovascular compromise, there is absence of flow at end-diastole, with venous pulsations seen in the umbilical vein.

Doppler evaluation of the arterial system provides important information regarding fetal cardiovascular wellbeing. Doppler evaluation of the umbilical artery provides information concerning the health and state of the placental circulation (Fig. 10-4). The healthy placenta has a very low vascular resistance, and hence Doppler spectral display will demonstrate substantial antegrade flow during the diastolic phase of the cardiac cycle. Abnormally elevated placental vascular resistance, as seen in cases of intra-uterine retardation of growth, or in the donor fetus of a twin-twin transfusion syndrome, can be identified by the presence of diminished, or even reversed, flow in diastole (Fig. 10-5).

Changes in cerebrovascular resistance may be seen in conditions of altered cardiac output, and with different forms of congenital cardiac disease. These changes are a

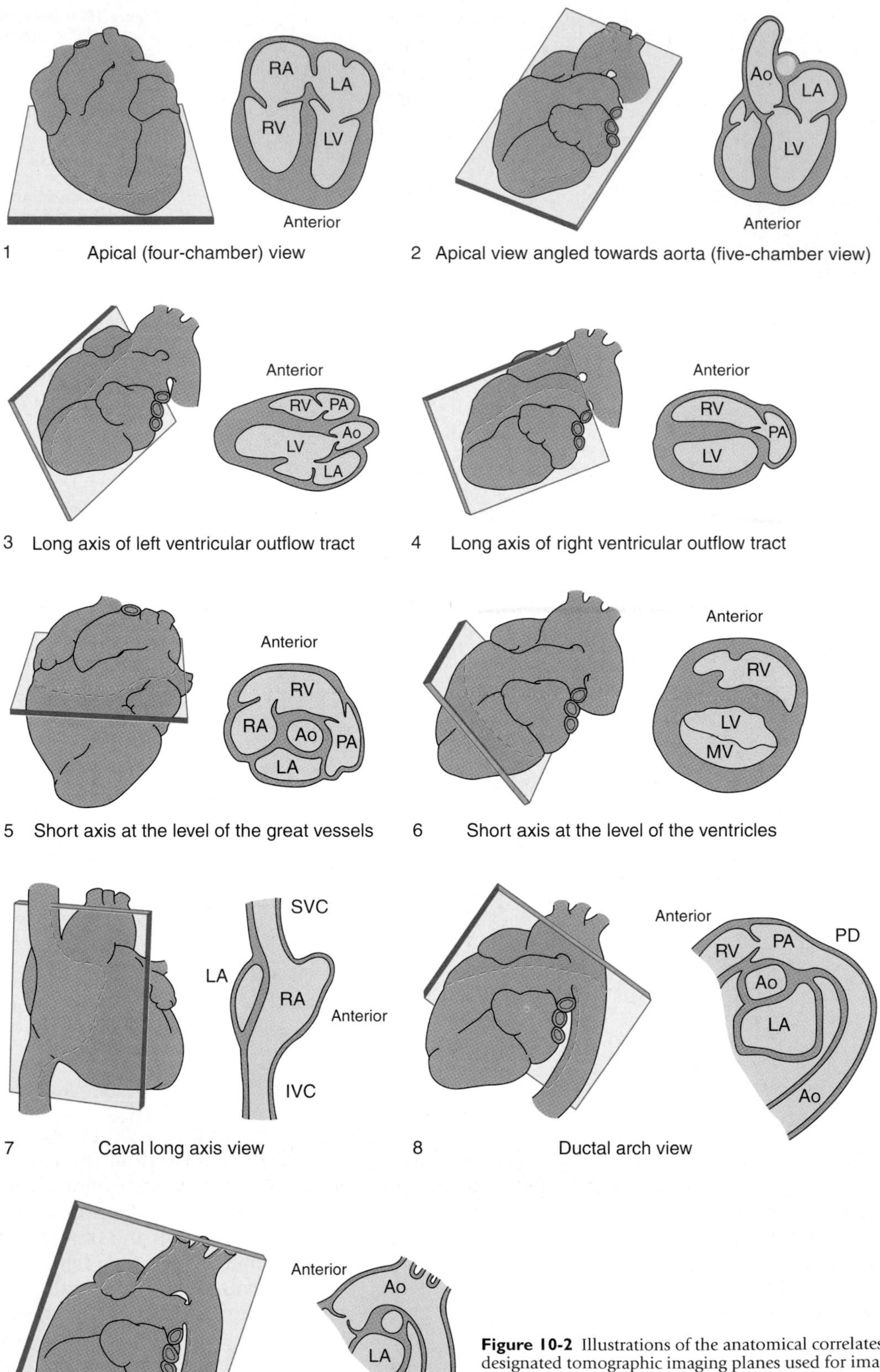

Figure 10-2 Illustrations of the anatomical correlates for each of the designated tomographic imaging planes used for imaging of the fetal cardiovascular system. Each numbered view relates to the clockwise illustration of the fetal heart in Figure 10-1. Ao, aorta; IVC, inferior caval vein; LA, left atrium; LV, left ventricle; MV, mitral valve; PA, pulmonary trunk; PD, patent arterial duct; RA, right atrium; RV, right ventricle; SVC, superior caval vein. (With permission, from the American Society of Echocardiography Guidelines and Standards for Performance of the Fetal Echocardiogram. J Am Soc Echocardiogr 2004;17:803–10.)

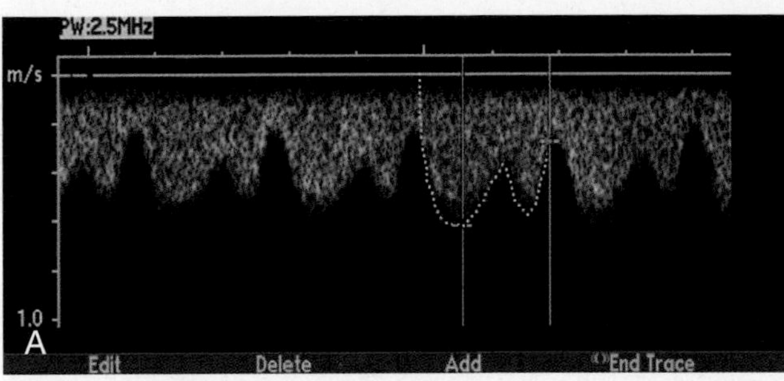

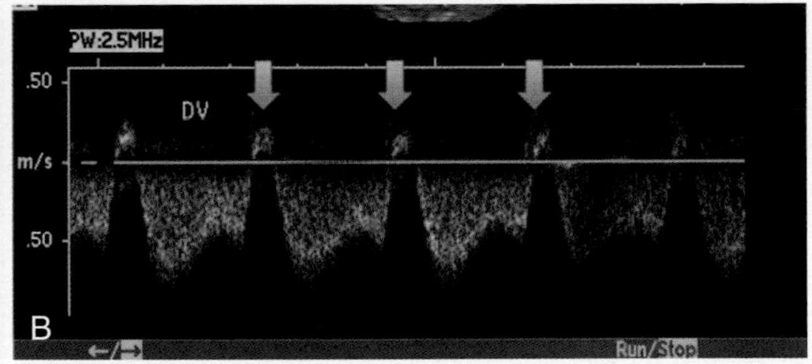

Figure 10-3 **A,** Doppler spectral display of the normal pattern of flow in the venous duct. Note that flow is phasic, but all antegrade below the baseline. **B,** An abnormal pattern of flow in the venous duct. *Arrows* point to reversal of flow (above the baseline) with atrial contraction. Such patterns are seen in the presence of an abnormal compliance of the right ventricle.

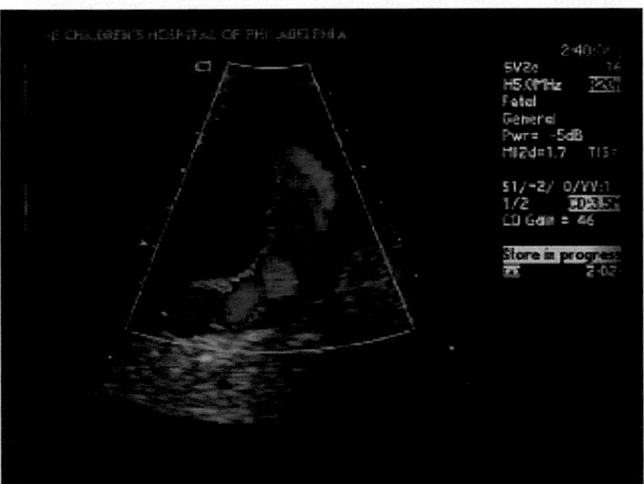

Figure 10-4 Colour Doppler image of the normal umbilical cord. Two arteries (*blue*) and one umbilical vein (*red*) are seen.

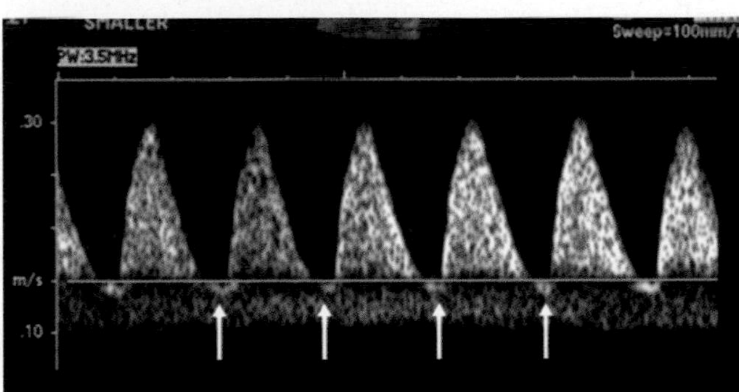

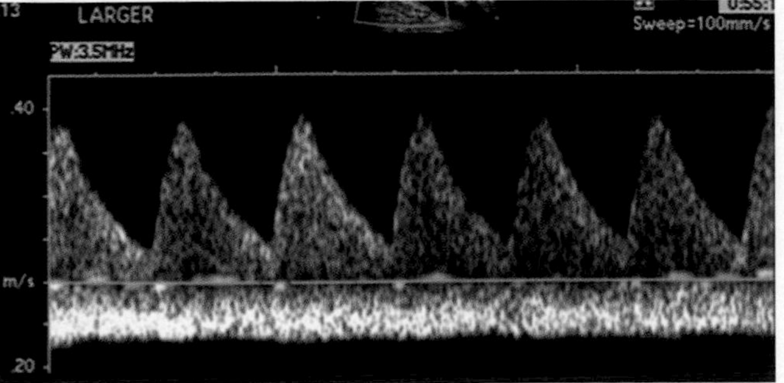

Figure 10-5 Doppler spectral display of blood flow in the umbilical cord. Umbilical artery flow is above the baseline and umbilical venous flow is below the baseline. In the top panel, the *arrows* point to reversal of flow in the umbilical artery suggesting markedly elevated placental vascular resistance. The bottom panel is obtained from a normal umbilical cord with abundant diastolic flow in the umbilical artery indicating normal placental vascular resistance.

manifestation of auto-regulatory mechanisms of the fetal cardiovascular system, in which there is a natural tendency to preserve flow of blood to vital organs such as the brain. When flow to the brain is diminished due to an overall decrease in cardiac output as a consequence of myocardial dysfunction, or due to an anatomical impediment, vascular resistance will be lower than normal in the middle cerebral artery as the brain attempts to augment volume and flow (Fig. 10-6). Hence, in the presence of left-sided obstructive lesions, the resistance measured in the middle cerebral artery decreases. In the setting of right-sided obstructive lesions, in contrast, the resistance increases.[37,38] In addition, in fetuses with cardiovascular compromise, there may be a redistribution of the cardiac output away from the placenta and toward the brain, the so called brain sparing effect.[39–41] Typically, the ratio of resistance in the middle cerebral artery compared to the umbilical artery is greater than 1. With hypoxia or inadequate cardiac output, there may be cephalisation of flow, characterised by a ratio of resistance in the middle cerebral artery compared to the umbilical artery of less than 1. Assessment of patterns of antegrade flow across the atrioventricular valves also provides important information regarding diastolic function and ventricular compliance (Fig. 10-7). Compared to mature myocardium, the fetal myocardium is comprised of greater non-contractile elements.[42] As a result, the fetal heart exhibits impaired myocardial relaxation, reflected by a lower velocity of the Doppler E wave compared to that of the A wave. Over the course of gestation, the ratio of the velocities of the E to A waves increases progressively. In severe cases of diastolic dysfunction, such as in the recipient twin with twin-twin transfusion syndrome, or in ventricles compromised by endocardial fibroelastosis, the E and A waves may merge into a single peak (Fig. 10-8).

Novel imaging techniques, such as three-dimensional echocardiographic interrogation, or use of magnetic resonance imaging, remain relatively untested in the detailed assessment of the fetal cardiovascular system, but may be of increasing importance in the future. Feasibility studies assessing the usefulness of such techniques in providing detailed information above and beyond screening are currently underway.[43–49]

CONGENITAL CARDIAC LESIONS AT RISK FOR PROGRESSION DURING FETAL LIFE

With the growing application of fetal echocardiography, it has become apparent that some malformations undergo developmental change during the second and third

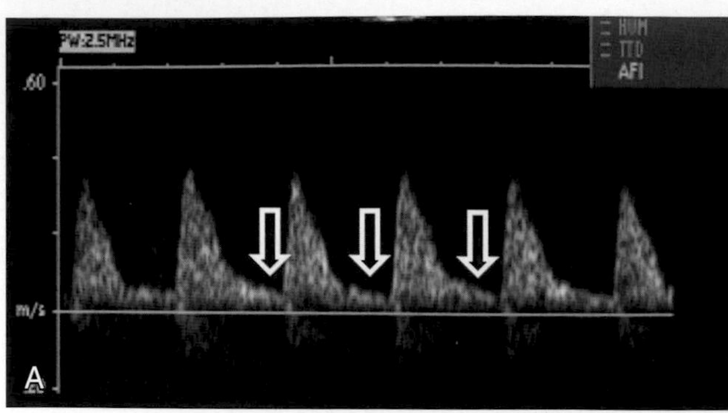

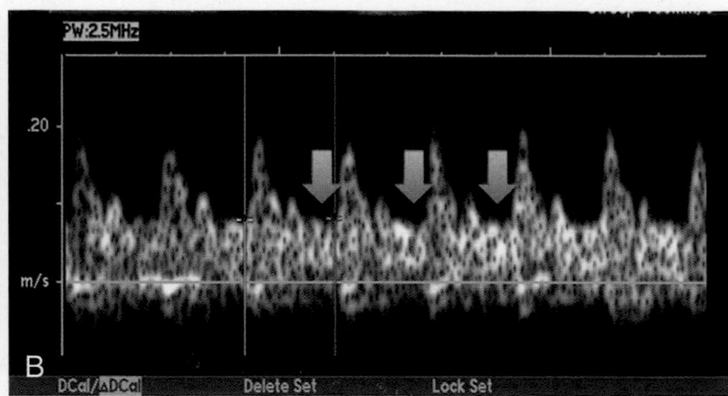

Figure 10-6 A, Doppler spectral display of normal flow in the middle cerebral artery flow. The *arrows* point to diastolic flow at low velocity suggesting elevated, normal cerebrovascular resistance. **B,** Abnormal flow. The *arrows* point to relatively elevated velocity of diastolic flow, suggesting diminished cerebrovascular resistance, an abnormal finding in a fetus with poor myocardial function and low cardiac output.

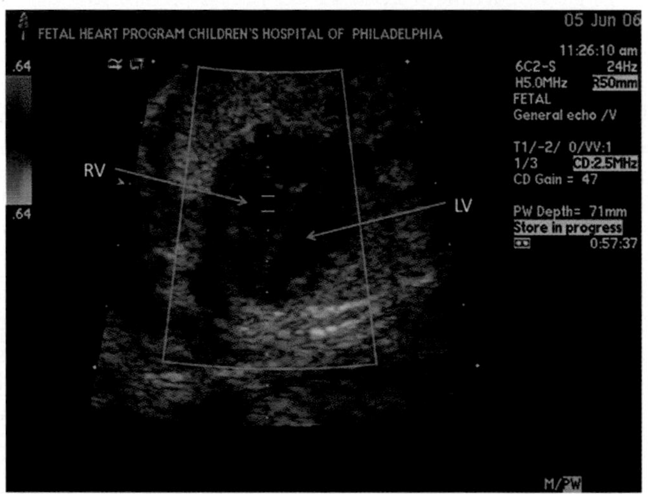

Figure 10-7 Four-chamber view with Doppler interrogation sample positioned beneath the tricuspid valve at the right ventricular inflow. LV, left ventricle; RV right ventricle.

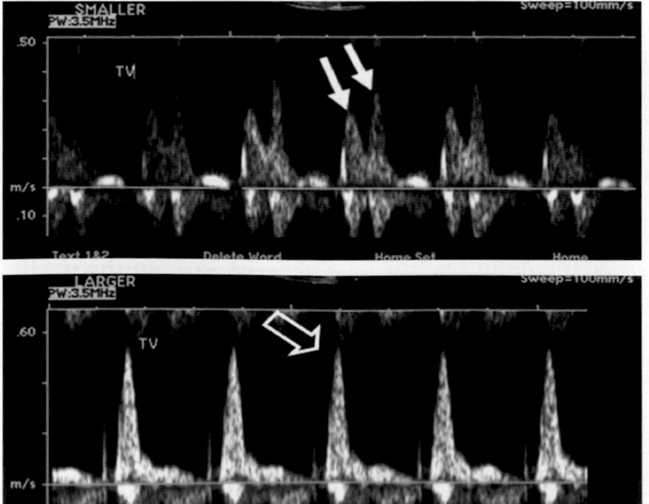

Figure 10-8 Doppler spectral display of flow across the tricuspid valve. The *arrows* in the top panel point to the normal double-peaked pattern. In the bottom panel, the *arrow* points to a fused single peak of inflow, suggesting abnormal right ventricular compliance.

trimesters of gestation. Serial evaluation from the point of initial identification is, therefore, an important part of care for these families. At present, there is a paucity of knowledge concerning the overall potential for progression of disease and the natural history of congenital cardiac disease in the fetus. In some diseases, nonetheless, progression during fetal life is known to be important.

Left-sided Obstructive Lesions

Critical aortic stenosis is readily recognisable in the early second trimester by the appearance of a dilated and dysfunctional left ventricle, lined with endocardial fibroelastosis, and a thickened and stenotic aortic valve. In fetuses recognised to have left-sided obstructive lesions, those with patency of the aortic valve who required functionally univentricular palliation at birth were shown to have either bidirectional, or left-to-right, flow across the patent oval foramen, and reversal of flow in the distal transverse arch.[50] At term, the left ventricle in many of these fetuses was found to be hypoplastic, despite findings of normal left ventricular length earlier in gestation.[50] Others have published predictors for progression of critical aortic stenosis to hypoplasia of the left heart, with left-to-right flow across the patent oval foramen, reversal of flow in the distal transverse arch, a monophasic pattern of flow across the mitral valve as shown by Doppler interrogation, and significant left ventricular dysfunction all predicting progression during fetal life from critical aortic stenosis to hypoplastic left heart syndrome.[36] In the hopes of achieving a postnatal biventricular repair for these fetuses initially having critical aortic stenosis, much interest has focused on developing techniques for fetal intervention. Different institutions have reported technical success for these fetal interventions,[51–58] although the proportion of fetuses progressing to postnatal biventricular repair remains disappointingly low.

Right-sided Obstructive Lesions

Similar to obstruction within the left-sided outflow tract, right-sided obstruction may also progress over the course of gestation. In the setting of tetralogy of Fallot or valvar pulmonary stenosis, obstruction may progress from mild to severe stenosis, or even atresia.[59–61] To prevent the development of right ventricular hypoplasia in such fetuses with critical pulmonic stenosis or atresia and impending hydrops, some have successfully dilated the pulmonary valve during fetal life, and achieved a biventricular repair postnatally.[62,63] Specific criterions for predicting the development of critical obstruction, nonetheless, remain elusive, and await a more complete understanding of the natural history of these lesions.

Regurgitant Lesions

In Ebstein's malformation, severe regurgitation across the malformed tricuspid valve may lead to decreased forward flow through the pulmonary valve, with the development of severe pulmonary stenosis, or even atresia, over the course of gestation.[64,65] These fetuses are at significant risk for the development of hydrops and death during gestation. If the fetus does survive to term, the combination of severe tricuspid regurgitation, pulmonary atresia, and pulmonary hypoplasia is associated with a particularly poor outcome, with few postnatal survivors.[64,65]

Progressive Restriction at the Patent Oval Foramen

In those with transposition, or hypoplastic left heart syndrome, the patent oval foramen may become progressively restrictive, or may even close over the course of gestation.[66–68] Closure of this interatrial communication may result in particularly poor outcomes, with the development of arrhythmias, hydrops, or fetal cardiac dysfunction.[67] Fetuses with a restrictive foramen or an intact atrial septum in the setting of transposition are at risk for profound postnatal cyanosis, and should be delivered in a centre capable of performing immediate balloon atrial septostomy after birth. Fetuses with a restrictive or intact interatrial communication in the setting of hypoplastic left heart syndrome are at risk for left atrial hypertension, with the development of lethal pulmonary vasculopathy.[69,70] Current rates of survival for neonates with hypoplasia of the left heart and an intact atrial communication remain disappointingly low, ranging from 47% to 57%.[71,72] Strategies employed to improve the neonatal rates of survival include early catheter-based interventions,[71,72] surgical atrial septotomy, or immediate cannulation for extracorporeal oxygenation after birth. At our own institution, we currently favour delivery by caesarian section in a cardiac operating room, with cardiothoracic anaesthesia available, and immediate postnatal intervention on the atrial septum either via a catheter-based or surgical approach. The initial stage of palliation is delayed for a few days to allow stabilisation. In an attempt to avoid all postnatal instability, some centres have advocated ultrasonically guided fetal atrial septoplasty[73] or laser atrial septotomy,[74] for those fetuses with hypoplasia of the left heart and a highly restrictive or intact atrial communication. Selection of candidates for fetal atrial septoplasty remains an important consideration. Direct measurement of the patent oval foramen may be unreliable during fetal life in predicting the postnatal size of the interatrial communication.[75] Multiple investigators, nonetheless, have demonstrated the value of assessing the forward and reverse patterns of flow in the pulmonary veins by Doppler interrogation to predict the need for immediate postnatal intervention.[75–78]

POSTNATAL OUTCOMES

As critical care and cardiac surgery continue to improve, rates of neonatal survival for infants born with prenatally diagnosed congenital cardiac malformations have similarly improved. Whether prenatal diagnosis of the defects alone improves neonatal survival remains controversial. A number of studies have failed to demonstrate a difference in neonatal survival after surgical repair among infants diagnosed prenatally compared to those diagnosed postnatally,[79–83] although some have reported improved survival in infants prenatally diagnosed with hypoplasia of the left heart, and transposition, respectively.[84,85] Prenatal diagnosis, nonetheless, does impact on morbidity. Numerous studies have demonstrated improved preoperative conditions in infants prenatally diagnosed with ductal-dependent lesions, with the potential for better long-term neurodevelopmental outcomes.[79,80,82,86] Multi-institutional studies are needed to assess the effect of prenatal diagnosis upon long-term neurodevelopmental outcome.

The complete reference list can be found on the companion Expert Consult web site at www.expertconsult.com.

ANNOTATED REFERENCES

- Garne E, Stoll C, Clementi M: Evaluation of prenatal diagnosis of congenital heart diseases by ultrasound: Experience from 20 European registries. Ultrasound Obstet Gynecol 2001;17:386–391.

  This article summarises data from 20 registries of congenital malformations in 12 European countries. The overall prenatal detection rate was 25%, with the rate of detection varying from 8% to 48%. The presence of associated malformations significantly increased the rate of detection.

- Rychik J, Ayres N, Cuneo B, et al: American Society of Echocardiography guidelines and standards for performance of the fetal echocardiogram. J Am Soc Echocardiogr 2004;17:803–810.

  This review article provides a standardised approach to the fetal echocardiogram. Numerous tomographic views are described in detail so that an accurate diagnosis of congenital cardiac disease may be made.

- Friedberg MK, Silverman NH: Changing indications for fetal echocardiography in a University Center population. Prenat Diagn 2004;24:781–786.

  In this article, investigators explore the changing indications for fetal echocardiography. High yield indications include a chromosomal anomaly and an abnormal obstetrical screen. Low yield indications include a family history of congenital cardiac malformation and exposure to teratogens.

- Taipale P, Hiilesmaa V, Salonen R, Ylostalo P: Increased nuchal translucency as a marker for fetal chromosomal defects. N Engl J Med 1997;337:1654–1658.

  In this study, investigators screened singleton pregnancies of 10,010 adolescents and women less than 40 years of age with trans-vaginal ultrasonography between 10 and 16 weeks gestation. A nuchal translucency greater than 3 mm in width was found to be a sensitive test for fetal aneuploidy.

- Berning RA, Silverman NH, Villegas M, et al: Reversed shunting across the ductus arteriosus or atrial septum in utero heralds severe congenital heart disease. J Am Coll Cardiol 1996;27:481–486.

  In the above study, reversed shunting across the arterial duct was found to be a sensitive echocardiographic marker for critical right-sided obstructive disease. Reversed shunting across the atrial septum was found to be a sensitive echocardiographic marker for critical left-sided obstructive disease.

- Makikallio K, McElhinney DB, Levine JC, et al: Fetal aortic valve stenosis and the evolution of hypoplastic left heart syndrome: Patient selection for fetal intervention. Circulation 2006;113:1401–1405.

  This study explores echocardiographic markers for progression to hypoplastic left heart syndrome in mid-gestational age fetuses with critical aortic stenosis. Markers predictive of progression to hypoplastic left heart syndrome included reversal of flow in the transverse aortic arch and oval foramen, monophasic inflow pattern across the mitral valve, and dysfunction of the left ventricle.

- Donofrio MT, Bremer YA, Schieken RM, et al: Autoregulation of cerebral blood flow in fetuses with congenital heart disease: The brain sparing effect. Pediatr Cardiol 2003;24:436–443.

- Kaltman JR, Di H, Tian Z, Rychik J: Impact of congenital heart disease on cerebrovascular blood flow dynamics in the fetus. Ultrasound Obstet Gynecol 2005;25:32–36.

  The above two studies demonstrate altered cerebrovascular resistance in fetuses with congenital cardiac malformations. In left-sided obstructive lesions, cerebrovascular resistance is lower than normal.

- Michelfelder E, Gomez C, Border W, et al: Predictive value of fetal pulmonary venous flow patterns in identifying the need for atrial septoplasty in the newborn with hypoplastic left ventricle. Circulation 2005;112:2974–2979.

  This study investigates the pulmonary venous Doppler flow patterns in fetuses with hypoplastic left heart syndrome and a restrictive interatrial communication. In this study, a ratio of the forward to reverse flow in the pulmonary veins less than 5 was predictive of the need for emergent atrial septectomy in the newborn period.

- Mahle WT, Clancy RR, McGaurn SP, et al: Impact of prenatal diagnosis on survival and early neurologic morbidity in neonates with the hypoplastic left heart syndrome. Pediatrics 2001;107:1277–1282.

  This study explores whether prenatal diagnosis impacts upon survival and early neurologic morbidity in neonates with hypoplastic left heart syndrome. The authors concluded that mortality was not significantly different between the group diagnosed prenatally compared to postnatally. There were fewer adverse perioperative neurologic events in those patients with a prenatal diagnosis.

- Tworetzky W, McElhinney DB, Reddy VM, et al: Improved surgical outcome after fetal diagnosis of hypoplastic left heart syndrome. Circulation 2001;103:1269–1273.

  In this study, the authors concluded that prenatal diagnosis of hypoplastic left heart syndrome was associated with improved clinical state prior to surgery, and with improved survival after the first stage of palliation in comparison with patients diagnosed after birth.

CHAPTER 11

Prematurity and Cardiac Disease

PATRICK J. McNAMARA

On average, up to one-eighth of liveborn infants in the developed world are born prior to term. These rates have increased as a consequence of assisted reproductive technology, and earlier intervention for either maternal or fetal wellbeing. The causes of birth prior to term are many (Table 11-1). The care of the premature neonate has improved dramatically over the past 100 years, during which time mortality rate has fallen from 40 deaths for each 1000 live births at the turn of the 20th century, to the current rates of 4 deaths per 1000 live births in the developed world. These improvements are a direct result of enhanced maternal health, and access to quality obstetric and neonatal intensive care. Birth weight remains the major risk factor for neonatal mortality (Fig. 11-1). The past two decades have witnessed a number of significant advancements in neonatal care, most notably maternal administration of antenatal steroids,[1] the ability to replace surfactant,[2] use of inhaled nitric oxide,[3,4] increased scientific evidence for routine practices, and superior equipment, such as ventilators and incubators. In addition, an increased number of neonatal conditions requiring intensive care are being recognised antenatally, which allows focused resuscitation, and timely intervention by specialist teams. This is particularly relevant for neonates with congenitally malformed hearts, particularly premature infants, who represent the most critical and potentially vulnerable patients. Despite regionalised perinatal health care, from one-tenth to one-third of those born with extremely low weight (Box 11-1) are delivered outside tertiary neonatal centers. Although overall survival for premature infants in general has improved, mortality remains high, particularly at the limits of viability (Table 11-2). The outcome for neonates born outside tertiary centres is less favourable when compared to those patients delivered and resuscitated at perinatal centers specialised in coping with those at high risk.[5,6] A large population-based study of mortality and disability, with the acronym EPICURE, was conducted in the United Kingdom of all infants born alive between the gestational ages of 22 and 25 weeks.[7,8] Survival at 30 months reached just over 40% in neonates born at 25 weeks of gestation, falling to 10% for those born at 23 weeks of gestation. Moderate-to-severe disability occurred in almost half of the survivors when compared to school classmates at the age of 6 years. The contribution of cardiovascular performance and systemic haemodynamics to ongoing neonatal morbidity is poorly understood. Enhanced cardiovascular monitoring, and earlier therapeutic intervention, may prove to be a necessary step towards improving survival further, and minimising adverse neurodevelopmental sequels.

THE TRANSITIONING CIRCULATION

The condition of the infant at birth is dependent, in part, on intra-uterine wellbeing and growth. Intra-uterine growth retardation is the failure of the fetus or infant to achieve his or her predetermined genetic potential. Typically, the preterm infant is below the third centile for weight, length, and head circumference. The consequences to the developing heart include cardiac hypertrophy, abnormal diastolic performance, and impaired vascular relaxation.[9–11] Doppler interrogation of fetal and neonatal mitral valvar velocities revealed lower E wave amplitude compared with normal mature mitral E peaks.[12,13] Impaired early left ventricular filling may relate to a diminished ability to relax, and higher muscular stiffness. The implications may include impaired myocardial performance, hypertension, and

TABLE 11-1

FACTORS CONTRIBUTING TO SPONTANEOUS PRETERM DELIVERY, OR THE NEED FOR EARLIER THERAPEUTIC INTERVENTION

Maternal	Placental	Fetal	Miscellaneous
Pre-eclampsia	Intra-uterine infection, or premature rupture of membranes	Chromosomal abnormality	Cervical incompetence
Systemic hypertension		Fetal distress	Idiopathic
Renal failure	Placental abruption	Hydrops fetalis	Familial
Diabetes mellitus	Antepartum haemorrhage	Congenital infection, such as toxoplasmosis, rubella, or cytomegalovirus	
Infection of the urinary tract	Uterine stretch • Multiple pregnancies • Polyhydramnios • Uterine abnormality		
Chronic disease			

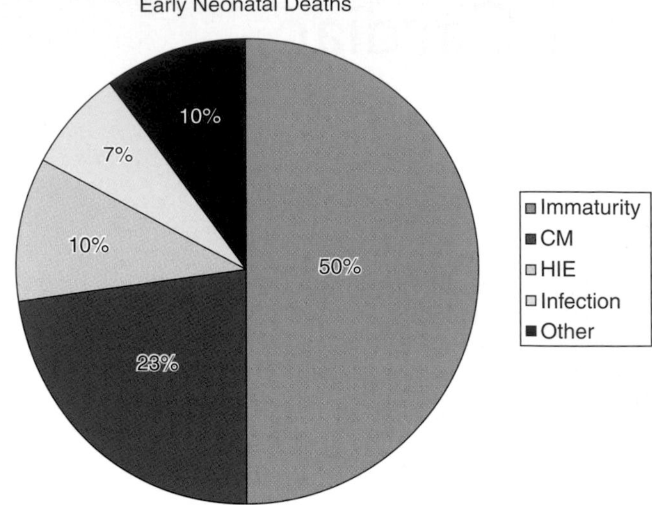

Figure 11-1 Causes of perinatal mortality (England and Wales, 1998).

BOX 11-1

Relevant Neonatal Definitions

Preterm: A neonate born prior to 37 weeks of completed gestation
Near-term: A neonate between the 34th and 37th weeks of gestation
Low birth weight: A neonate born weighing less than 2500 g
Very low birth weight: A neonate born weighing less than 1500 g
Extremely low birth weight: A neonate born weighing less than 1000 g
Perinatal mortality rate: The number of stillbirths and early neonatal deaths, those occurring within 6 days of birth, per 1000 live births and stillbirths
Neonatal mortality rate: The number of neonates dying in the first 4 weeks, specifically within 27 completed days of life, for each 1000 live births
Intra-uterine growth retardation: Growth parameters below the third centile for corrected gestational age. Asymmetric retardation is characterized by sparing of the head, the circumference of the head being greater than the third centile.

TABLE 11-2

NEONATAL MORTALITY ACCORDING TO BIRTH WEIGHT

Birth Weight (grams)	Births (%)	Neonatal Mortality per 1000 Live Births in Each Subgroup
Greater than 2500	92.4	0.9
Less than 2500	7.6	48
Less than 1000	1.4	214

hypotension. Poor glycaemic control during pregnancy, particularly in the setting of maternal diabetes, is a known risk factor for structural heart disease and hypertrophic cardiomyopathy.[14–16] In severe cases, where there is placental malfunction leading to retardation of growth, the same vascular and myocardial dysfunction may occur as described above.

PHYSIOLOGY OF THE POSTNATAL TRANSITION

The preterm infant undergoes dramatic cardiorespiratory changes at birth, which coincide with improved lung compliance and termination of the placental circulation. These critical adaptive changes:

- Include increased pulmonary blood flow, to about 20 times fetal levels
- Occur in part due to the exposure of the pulmonary vascular bed to higher alveolar concentrations of oxygen than the relatively hypoxic intra-uterine environment. Other metabolically active substances, such as metabolites of prostaglandin, bradykinins, or histamine, may play some role through inducing pulmonary vasodilation.
- Include alteration in flow through fetal channels such as the arterial duct and oval foramen, which may last for many days. The major change in flow through fetal channels is either a direct result of increased flow to the lungs, or improved systemic arterial tensions of oxygen. Increased left atrial pressure secondary to improved pulmonary venous return causes displacement of the flap of the oval foramen over the rims of the fossa, thus abolishing any right-to-left atrial flow. The pattern of flow through the arterial duct is significantly altered as lung compliance improves and pulmonary vascular resistance decreases. An increase in systemic vascular resistance also occurs once the compliant placenta is removed from the systemic circuit, and as a result of systemic vasoresponsiveness to increased tensions of oxygen. This will also contribute to increased transductal flow. The architecture of the arterial duct prior to term differs such that ductal tone is less responsive to oxygen, thus delaying closure and potentially contributing to excessive flow to the lungs and compromised systemic flow. The administration of surfactant can alter transductal flow significantly through reduced pulmonary vascular resistance. There is evidence of functional closure by 6 hours in some immature patients, although this is rare.[17]
- Include improved left and right ventricular outputs to meet the metabolic needs of immature neonate with insufficient thermoregulatory mechanisms and increased work of breathing. The transition from right to left ventricular dominance occurs over hours, and is secondary to increased left atrial preload and left ventricular afterload. In total, there is a threefold increase in left ventricular output, which is necessary to meet the increased demands of the body. The enhanced ability of the left ventricle to increase its output is related, in part, to elimination of constraint by the pressure-loaded right ventricle.

REGULATION OF MYOCARDIAL PERFORMANCE

Architecture of the Myocyte

Fetal myocardial tissue consists of 70% noncontractile tissue, compared to 40% in the mature adult heart. Histological studies have shown that the myocytes making up the left ventricular myocardium are aligned circumferentially in the mid wall, and longitudinally in the subepicardial and subendocardial layers of the walls.[18,19] Studies of isolated myocardial tissue in fetal and adult lambs suggest that fetal myocardium is less compliant. Ventricular myocytes change considerably as they transition from fetal to post-natal life. The immature sarcomere and contractile apparatus is relatively disorganised. Myofibrils are irregular and scattered along the interior of the cell. Intra-uterine and early postnatal cardiac growth is a combination of both hyperplasia and hypertrophy. Exposure of the developing rodent heart to dexamethasone led to cardiac hypertrophy, characterised by myocytes which were longer and wider, with increased volume.[20] Biventricular hypertrophy is a recognised complication of exposure of the preterm myocardium to prolonged and high doses of steroids.[21] Neonates born to mothers who had received a single antenatal course of steroids had higher systolic blood pressures, and increased myocardial thickness, suggesting modified myocardial development.[22] The nature of these changes may relate to earlier transition from a phase of hyperplasia to hypertrophy. The functional consequence of an enlarged hypertrophic myocardium, with a reduced overall number of myocytes, is unknown.

Activation of the Myocyte

In contrast to adults, immature myocytes lack transverse tubules, are smaller in size, and have a greater ratio of surface area to volume.[23] They are more reliant on trans-sarcolemmal fluxes of calcium for contraction and relaxation.[24] The high ratio of surface area to volume, and the subsarcolemmal location of myofibrils, supports direct calcium delivery to and from the contractile proteins. The sodium-calcium exchanger is the major conduit for attachment of calcium to, and release from, the contractile elements.[25]

Control of Myocytic Activation

The control mechanisms governing contraction and relaxation in the immature heart are poorly understood, but thought to be substantially different from the fully mature heart. In the mature heart, graded control of release of calcium is related to so-called L-type activity, which triggers release from the sarcoplasmic reticulum. Graded control of release in immature myocytes is thought to be related to factors influencing the activity of the sodium-calcium channel. Recently isoproterenol-induced β-adrenergic stimulation of sodium-calcium exchanger was identified in guinea-pig ventricular myocytes. An improved understanding of factors which govern myocardial contractility and relaxation may facilitate more physiologically appropriate choice of therapeutic interventions in premature infants.

Performance and Physiology of the Immature Myocardium

At physiological heart rates, the immature myocardium shows a positive relationship, albeit that contractility falls with extreme tachycardia. Both the force-rate trajectory, and the optimal heart rate, reflects myocytic function and global myocardial contractile behaviour. Developmentally, the immature myocardium has been shown to exhibit a higher basal contractile state, and a greater sensitivity to changes in afterload.[26,27] The intolerance of the immature myocardium to increased afterload may be attributable to differences in myofibrillar architecture, or immaturity of receptor development or regulation.[28] The Frank–Starling law appears less applicable to the immature myocardium.[29]

HAEMODYNAMIC ASSESSMENT AND MONITORING

The consequences of haemodynamic instability include necrotising enterocolitis, intraventricular haemorrhage, and periventricular leucomalacia, all of which may lead to mortality or adverse neurodevelopmental outcomes. Intraventricular haemorrhage occurs in up to three-tenths of infants born with very low weight, most commonly in the first 7 hours of life. The origin of the haemorrhage is the germinal matrix, an immature network of capillaries highly susceptible to hypoxaemia, hypercapnaemia, and altered cerebral blood flow. Periventricular leucomalacia is a loss of white matter in the watershed areas around the lateral cerebral ventricles secondary to hypoxic-ischaemic injury. The infant born at very low weight is highly susceptible to such morbidities, necessitating focused cardiovascular monitoring and targeted intervention in a timely fashion.

Is Blood Pressure a Reliable Measure of Circulatory Stability?

The determination of haemodynamic stability in premature infants is fraught with uncertainty, myths, and dogma without scientific validity. Suboptimal systemic blood flow is usually suspected on the basis of tachycardia, delayed capillary refill time, hypothermia, oliguria, altered blood pressure, metabolic acidosis, and increased levels of lactate in the plasma. Blood pressure readings are readily available at the bedside as a continuous stream of data from indwelling arterial lines, or periodically using a validated oscillometric cuff method.[30] The approach to monitoring and guiding therapeutic intervention has relied on using mean arterial pressure as a surrogate of the adequacy of tissue perfusion and oxygenation. This reasoning is based on an assumed proportionality between blood pressure and systemic blood flow.[31] In 1992, a report from the former British Paediatric Association stressed the importance of monitoring blood pressure in order to guide early therapeutic intervention, and thus prevent adverse neurological sequelae.[32] It was suggested that mean arterial pressure equivalent to the gestational age in weeks is adequate as a minimum value. The group also suggested the need to establish accurate normative ranges for systolic and diastolic blood pressure. Unfortunately, achieving a mean blood pressure equal to gestational age has now become dogma, and the standard on which therapy is based. Normative centiles for systolic blood pressure that take into account both gestational age at birth and postnatal age have been developed, but are rarely used.[33] Monitoring blood pressure in isolation is problematic for a number for reasons. First, blood pressure is but one surrogate of circulatory stability. Second, the concept of numerical hypotension as mean blood pressure less than gestational age in weeks has not been validated against indexes of perfusion of end-organs. Third, important changes in either systolic or diastolic blood pressure may be missed. The systolic pressure indicates the pressure generated by the left ventricle, whereas the diastolic pressure reflects local perfusion of the

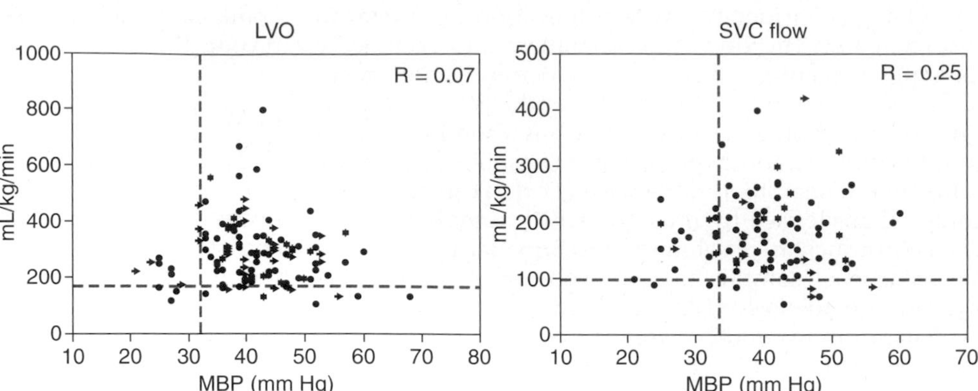

Figure 11-2 Relationship between mean arterial pressure and left ventricular output or superior vena cava flow in 46 neonates assessed at three time points following surgical ligation of the ductus arteriosus. The dashed lines represent lower acceptable limits according to gestational norms (From Teixeira LS et al: Pediatr Res 2006;59:239.).

tissues. In neonates with a haemodynamically significant arterial duct, diastolic pressure is oftentimes compromised in isolation of changes in mean arterial pressure. This may have an unappreciated adverse effect on coronary arterial perfusion, and subsequently on myocardial performance. The relationship between mean blood pressure and cardiac output is also weak (Fig. 11-2). The finding of neonates with numerical hypotension, but no clinical or biochemical signs of systemic flow, and conversely patients with normal or high blood pressure but signs of circulatory compromise, is not uncommon. It must be recognised that blood pressure is but a surrogate of perfusion, and not the end-point of interest.

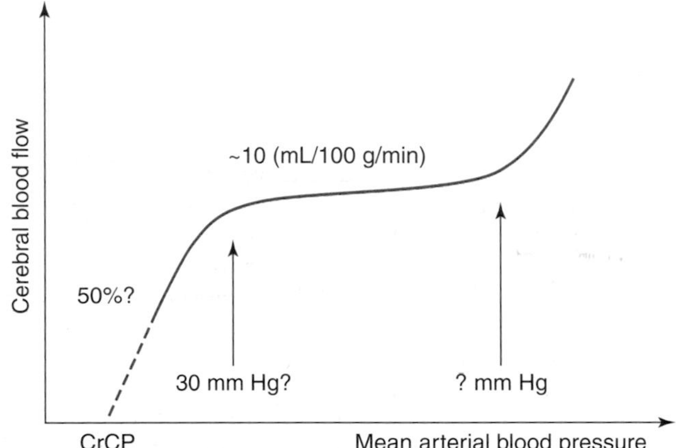

Figure 11-3 Schematic drawing of the relationship between cerebral blood flow and mean arterial pressure. The flat portion of the curve reflects the auto-regulatory plateau. Below the lower part of the plateau cerebral blood flow falls proportionate to mean arterial pressure. (From Greisen G: Autoregulation of cerebral blood flow in newborn babies. Early Hum Dev 2005;81:423–428.)

Does Hypotension Lead to Brain Injury?

The rationale for treating hypotension is based on two important considerations. First, the cerebral circulation becomes pressure-passive below a critical level for blood pressure (Fig. 11-3).[34,35] The auto-regulatory mechanism is thought to fail below a mean arterial pressure of 30 mm Hg.[36] There is also evidence suggesting that neonates with hypotension have impaired cerebral oxygenation as determined by near-infrared spectroscopy, and are at increased risk of intracranial haemorrhage or periventricular leucomalacia.[37] Other investigators have shown no relationship between blood pressure and cerebral blood flow.[38] Second, associations have been shown between adverse neurological consequences and systemic hypotension.[39–42] There is a significant body of evidence, nonetheless, which challenges these assumptions. For example, there is data suggesting that the association of hypotension to injury to the white matter and adverse neurodevelopmental outcome is not one of cause and effect, but an epiphenomenon. Studies with superior designs, and larger numbers, have failed to demonstrate any positive association between blood pressure and adverse neurological outcomes.[43–52] When corrected for associated risk factors, such as intra-uterine growth retardation, postnatal use of steroids, and chronic lung disease, the association between hypotension and abnormal neurodevelopmental outcomes was lost.[53] The discrepancy between individual studies may reflect the fact that the association is much more complex than any direct effect of blood pressure on cerebral blood flow (Fig. 11-4). There may be concurrent changes in cardiac output and regional differences

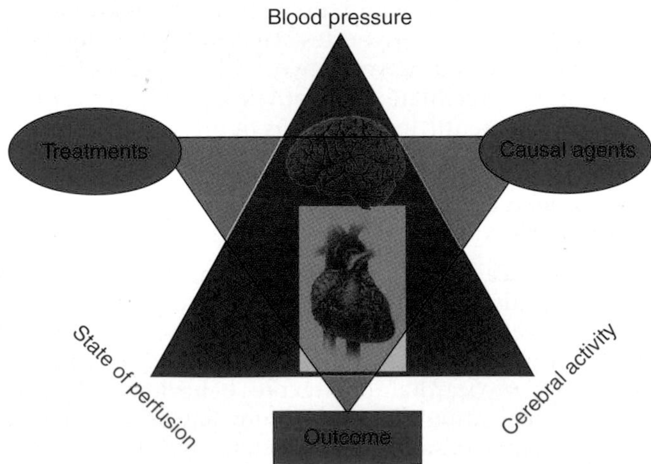

Figure 11-4 A schematic drawing of the complex relationship between disease state, blood pressure, systemic blood flow, and therapeutic intervention in neonates at risk of brain injury.

in flow of blood independent of blood pressure that are influencing cerebral perfusion, but these studies have not been performed.

How Should We Monitor the Preterm Circulation?

Failure of the neonatal transition may lead to myocardial dysfunction, low cardiac output, and hypotension, which may compromise perfusion of the end-organs with consequent damage. The vulnerability of the cerebral circulation in the first 72 hours of life increases the likelihood of injury to the brain more than any other organ. It is essential that the systemic flow be monitored adequately at all stages. Tachycardia and capillary refill time are poorly validated and non-specific measures of systemic flow. In isolation, capillary refill time is inaccurate, highly subjective, and a poor overall predictor of the adequacy of perfusion.[54] The measurement of cardiac output at the bedside is a useful adjunct to the clinical assessment and there is normative data for both right and left ventricular outputs.[55,56] The normal range for cardiac output in normal premature infants is between 170 and 320 mL/kg/min. Unfortunately these measurements are potentially inaccurate in the early neonatal period due to the effects of transductal shunting. Recently, measurement of flow in the superior caval vein has been proposed as a novel method of assessing the adequacy of systemic flow, as it is not confounded by atrial or ductal shunts.[57] As four-fifths of flow in the superior caval vein represents venous return from the head and neck, such measurements may provide novel insights into any association between regional cerebral blood flow and cerebral injury. Reduced flow in the superior caval vein is common in premature infants in the first 24 hours, reaching a nadir between 8 and 12 hours which coincides with increased systemic vascular resistance. Neonates with the lowest flow are at greatest risk of intraventricular haemorrhage (Fig. 11-5).[58] When 3-year neurodevelopmental assessment was performed, low superior caval venous flow remained significantly associated on multiple logistic regression analysis, when adjusted for gestation and birth weight, with an abnormal developmental quotient and the combined endpoint of death and abnormal developmental quotient.[59] Both blood pressure and systemic flow are important determinants of the likelihood of altered perfusion, and neither should be monitored nor treated in isolation, without consideration of the influence of the other.

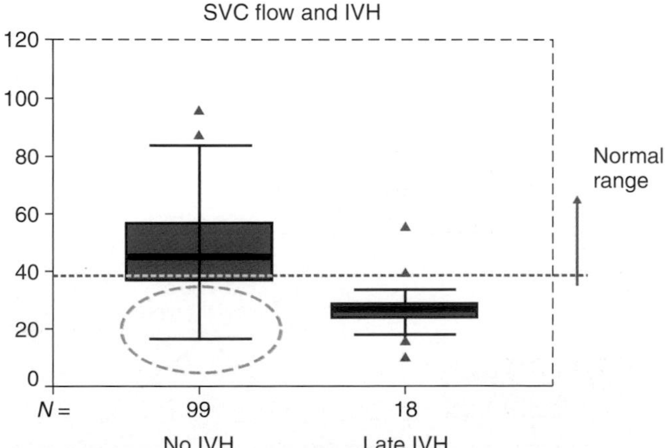

Figure 11-5 Box plot of the lowest superior caval vein (SVC) flow in the first 24 hours for neonates who developed severe intraventricular haemorrhage ($N = 18$) versus those who did not develop an intraventricular haemorrhage ($N = 99$). IVH, intraventricular haemorrhage. (From Kluckow M, Evans N: Low superior caval vein flow and intraventricular haemorrhage in preterm infants. Arch Dis Child Fetal Neonatal Ed 2000;82:188–94.)

CARDIOVASCULAR PROBLEMS UNIQUE TO THE PRETERM INFANT

The Haemodynamically Significant Arterial Duct

Patency of the arterial duct is a common problem in preterm babies, especially those born with extremely low weight. Although functionally essential for the normal fetal circulation, persistent ductal patency may have significant effects in preterm infants that include pulmonary overcirculation and systemic hypoperfusion. Persistent patency is found in about half of babies born at less than 29 weeks gestation, and/or weighing under 800 g.[60,61]

Biology of Normal Closure

Ductal closure is not immediate, particularly in infants born with extremely low weights, and occurs in two stages. Functional closure depends on the vasoconstricting action of humoral and biochemical factors on the muscular layer of the duct. This constriction results in the development of a zone of profound hypoxia in the media, which is the sentinel stimulus for irreversible closure. Anatomical closure depends on the architectural remodeling of the ductal wall.[62] It consists of extensive neointimal thickening, and loss of smooth muscle cells from the inner media.[63] The remodeling effects start at the pulmonary end, progressing toward the aortic insertion.[64] Both vasodilator prostaglandins, especially PgE_2, and nitric oxide, oppose ductal closure during fetal life.[65,66] In the second trimester, intimal cushions are formed that closely resemble the pathological intimal thickening seen in atherosclerotic disease.[67] The media is supplied with oxygen from either the lumen or its mural vessels. The thickness of the avascular zone, adjacent to the lumen, plays a critical role in determining the degree of hypoxia and subsequent remodeling of the ductal wall. Constriction of the circumferential and longitudinal muscle in the ductal wall leads to compaction, increased avascular thickness, and limits luminal supply of oxygen to both the avascular zone and the medial muscle.[63] The resultant hypoxia induces expression of vascular endothelial growth factor or cell death, depending on its severity. The geographic distribution of expression corresponds with the distribution and intensity of mural hypoxia.[68] The biologic consequences of these changes include a decline in tissue distensibility and increased contractile potential.[69] The ductal wall of fetuses during late gestation has a high level of intrinsic tone, which is further increased after delivery by unopposed oxygen-induced contractile forces.[68] After delivery, the increase in arterial content of oxygen, along with the decrease in circulating prostaglandins following placental separation,[70] and reduced intraluminal blood pressure, contribute towards ductal closure.[71,72] As transductal flow decreases, the wall becomes progressively more ischaemic, and eventually fibrotic.[73]

Ductal Closure in Infants Born with Extremely Low Weight

The duct remains patent in up to four-fifths of infants born prior to term and weighing below 1200 g. Such infants have no mural vessels in the medial layer, and are nourished entirely via transluminal diffusion or from adventitial vessels. The immature duct, when studied experimentally, has also been shown to have less intrinsic tone,[68] and lacks both intimal folds and circumferential medial musculature.[74] It is less responsive to oxygen,[68,75] and more sensitive to prostaglandin E_2 and nitric oxide.[66] It is possible for the immature infant to develop comparable hypoxia in the medial muscle, but only if transluminal flow is completely obliterated. Even when the duct constricts, profound hypoxia in the medial wall and anatomical remodeling fail to develop.[63] A progressive increase in levels of nitric oxide synthetase in the ductal mural vessels after the first 15 days of life makes the preterm duct even less sensitive to prostaglandins.[73,76] Non-steroidal anti-inflammatory agents, therefore, are less likely to be effective. In baboons, co-administration of an inhibitor of nitric oxide synthase, along with indomethacin, leads to increased contractility and luminal obliteration of the preterm duct.[77] There is data also to suggest that, in more mature preterms, those born prior to 33 weeks gestation, the arterial duct is also less sensitive to non-steroidal anti-inflammatory agents, although the mechanism has not been elucidated.[78]

The Pathophysiological Effects of a Haemodynamically Significant Arterial Duct

Failure of ductal closure, coinciding with the normal post-partum fall in pulmonary vascular resistance, results in a left-to-right transductal shunt. The consequences may include pulmonary over-circulation and/or systemic hypoperfusion, both of which may be associated with significant morbidity (Fig. 11-6). The clinical impact is dependent on the magnitude of the shunt, and the ability of the infant to initiate compensatory mechanisms. These infants are less capable of compensating, and are prone to developing left ventricular failure, which may lead to alveolar oedema and/or low cardiac output syndrome.[79] The increased pulmonary flow, and accumulation of interstitial fluid secondary to the large ductal shunt, contributes to decreased lung compliance.[80] The cumulative effects of increasing or prolonged ventilator requirements and myocardial dysfunction may increase the risk of chronic lung disease.[81,82] Systemic flow may also be compromised with ductal shunts due to retrograde diastolic flow in the aorta and the arteries supplying organs such as the kidneys and gut. The redistribution of systemic flow is significantly altered even with shunts of small volume. Oftentimes there may be significant hypoperfusion to the kidneys and gastrointestinal tract before a haemodynamically significant duct is clinically suspected. This may lead to significant morbidity, including renal insufficiency, necrotising enterocolitis, intraventricular haemorrhage, and myocardial ischemia.[83,84] Early detection and targeted intervention may potentially improve long-term neonatal outcomes.

Diagnosis of a Haemodynamically Significant Arterial Duct

Clinical Presentation

The classical clinical features include a systodiastolic murmur, hyperactive praecordium, bounding pulses, and wide pulse pressure. More commonly, a systolic murmur is audible that radiates widely across the praecordium and back. In many of those born prior to term, however, cardiac auscultation is unremarkable.[85] In the first week of life, despite the presence of a large duct, typical clinical signs are often absent. Such a situation is widely recognised as the silent duct. Surfactant, by assisting the natural post-natal fall in pulmonary arterial pressure, has been shown to alter the timing of clinical presentation, specifically, by increasing the volume of the systemic-to-pulmonary shunt, which leads to an earlier clinical presentation.[86,87] The existence of a haemodynamically significant but silent duct has been confirmed by cardiac catheterisation[88,89] and detailed echocardiographic evaluation.[90] Such a situation should be suspected in a setting of delayed hypotension during the second and third days, failure of oxygenation, increasing requirements for ventilatory support, or metabolic acidosis. The infant is more likely to present with both systolic and diastolic hypotension due to the inability of the immature myocardium to compensate for shunting at high volume throughout the cardiac cycle.[91,92]

Ancillary Tests

Although not very sensitive, chest radiography may show cardiomegaly and/or signs of pulmonary congestion, while the electrocardiogram may show signs of left atrial or ventricular enlargement.[93,94] The latter may be more useful for the identification of subendocardial ischaemia secondary to low coronary arterial perfusing pressures in neonates with a large duct, although this association has not been formally evaluated.

Echocardiographic Confirmation of the Haemodynamically Significant Arterial Duct

It is now standard of care, in many centers, to perform routine ductal and functional assessment within the first 72 hours of life due to the unreliability of clinical assessment, the increased likelihood of the ductal sensitivity to closure assisted by indomethacin, and the magnitude of the potential morbidities if left untreated. The determination of ductal significance using echocardiography involves

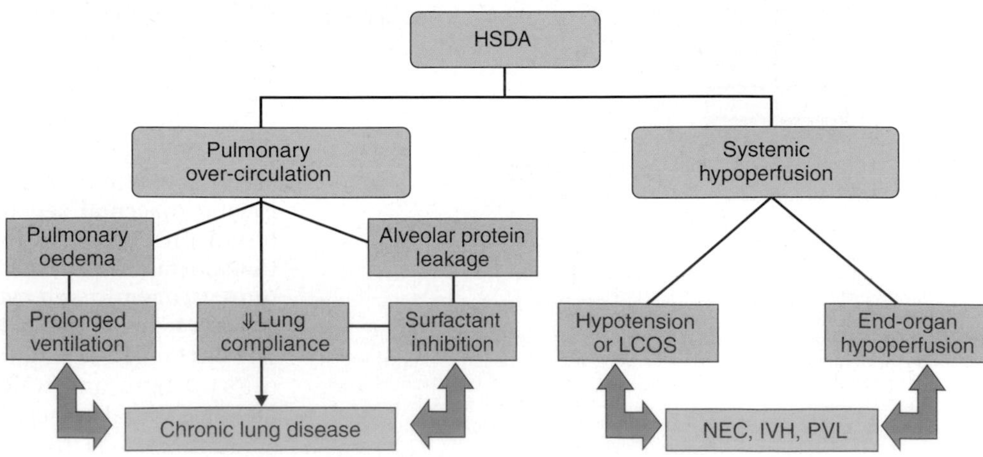

Figure 11-6 Schematic of morbidity attributed to the haemodynamically significant ductus arteriosus (HSDA) as a consequence of pulmonary over-circulation and systemic hypoperfusion. IVH, intraventricular haemorrhage; LCOS, low cardiac output syndrome; NEC, necrotising enterocolitis; PVL, periventricular leucomalacia. (Modified from Teixeira LS, McNamara PJ: Enhanced intensive care for the neonatal ductus arteriosus. Acta Paediatr 2006;95:394–403.)

assessment of size, patterns of transductal flow, systemic and/or end-organ perfusion, and characterisation of the degree of volume loading of the heart.

- The size of the duct is obtained from a suprasternal short-axis view (Fig. 11-7A) although measuring its internal diameter can be difficult, even with clear images. In addition the transductal diameter is not consistent throughout, often becoming tapered at the pulmonary end. A transductal diameter less than 1.5 mm is associated with retrograde or absent postductal aortic diastolic flow.[17] A diameter of more than 1.5 mm resulted in a positive likelihood ratio of 5.5, and a negative likelihood ratio of 0.22 for prediction of the need for therapeutic intervention. In a prospective study of 116 neonates, transductal diameter was the most accurate echocardiographic marker in predicting clinical and haemodynamic significance.[95]
- The pattern of transductal flow, estimated using pulse wave Doppler interrogation from a suprasternal short-axis view, can also be used to characterise ductal significance. High-velocity, continuous left-to-right flow is predictive of imminent functional closure, whereas a low-velocity pulsatile left-to-right flow pattern is likely to be clinically significant (Fig. 11-7B).[96]
- The effects on systemic and/or end-organ perfusion may also be examined. Large ductal shunts are associated with decreased superior caval venous flow.[58,97] This is relevant as low flow, less than 40 mL/kg/min, a surrogate of systemic perfusion, has been shown to correlate with increased risk of late intraventricular haemorrhage.[58] Evidence of end-organ hypoperfusion may be also inferred from Doppler assessment of the patterns of flow in the mesenteric, cerebral or renal arteries. Specifically, reversal or absence of diastolic perfusion is pathognomonic of a haemodynamically significant duct.[98,99]
- Cross sectional echocardiography has also been used to quantify the degree of volume overload. Specifically, estimates of left atrial or left ventricular size have been used as surrogates of pulmonary over-circulation and/or volume loading. Although the measurement is standardised, it is not very specific, and is prone to error dependent on the operator.[57] The presence of a large atrial septal defect permitting left-to-right shunting will lead to further augmentation of pulmonary flow, potentially overestimating the magnitude of the ductal shunt.

Management of the Haemodynamically Significant Duct

The aims of treatment are to reduce pulmonary over-circulation and improve systemic blood flow. The decision to treat is based on both clinical and echocardiographic findings, although the optimal time and method of ductal closure remain uncertain. Treatment should be classified as supportive intensive care strategies and therapeutic interventions aimed at closing the duct.

Focused Intensive Care

Ventilation. Strategies should be considered in attempts to minimise pulmonary over-circulation in a fashion comparable to other cardiac defects. This can be achieved by accepting P_{CO_2} between 45 and 55 mm Hg, arterial pH of 7.25 to 7.35, and oxygen saturations between 88% and 93%. Improvements in oxygenation and lung compliance may also be achieved by increasing the positive end expiratory pressure to levels that maintain optimal recruitment, minimise atelectasis-induced lung injury, and lead to improvements in myocardial performance and cardiac output by reducing left ventricular afterload.[100,101]

Cardiotropic Support. The optimal treatment for hypotension and/or systemic hypoperfusion is closure of the duct, and not cardiotropic support. Excessive α-adrenergic stimulation, by agents such as dopamine or epinephrine, should be avoided, as the increased systemic vascular resistance may lead to increased left-to-right shunting or may further compromise an already dysfunctional left ventricle. Dobutamine or newer inodilators currently under investigation, such as milrinone, may be preferred if there is associated left ventricular dysfunction.

Fluid Management and Diuretic Therapy. A recent meta-analysis suggested that restriction of water to meet the physiologic needs, whilst avoiding dehydration, may prevent the duct from becoming clinically and haemodynamically significant.[102] This strategy should not be routinely recommended, as it may lead to reduced left ventricular stroke volume and cardiac output, further compromising systemic flow. Fluid restriction may be considered in patients who become oliguric and/or volume overloaded during treatment with indomethacin. The evidence for routine diuretic therapy to promote ductal closure is also limited.[103,104] This may relate to excessive new production of prostaglandin E_2 by the kidneys in babies treated with furosemide.[105] A systematic review of the co-administration of furosemide in indomethacin-treated neonates concluded that evidence was insufficient to support its routine administration.[106] Diuretics should be restricted to the treatment of pulmonary oedema or left ventricular failure in neonates awaiting ductal ligation.

Feeding. Special consideration should be given to feeding, particularly if there is reversal or absence of perfusion in the superior mesenteric artery, or there are additional risk

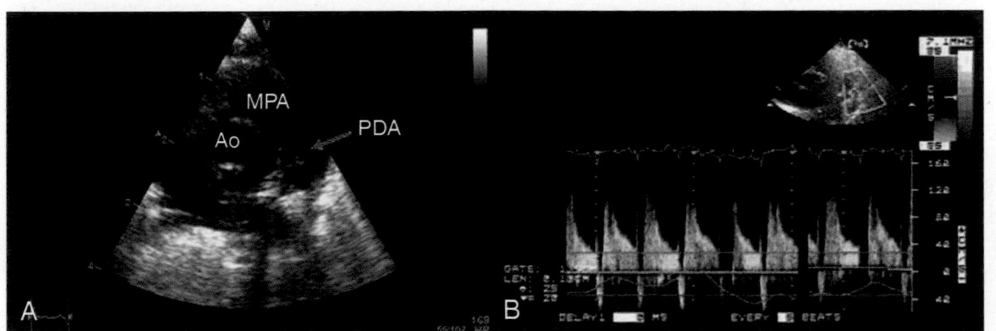

Figure 11-7 **A,** Two-dimensional echocardiographic representation of a large patent ductus arteriosus from a parasternal short-axis view. **B,** Pulsed wave Doppler interrogation at the mid-ductal level reveals unrestrictive laminar transductal flow. Ao, aorta; MPA, main pulmonary artery; PDA, patent ductus arteriosus.

factors, such as intra-uterine retardation of growth. Specifically, a more cautious feeding regime, and lower thresholds for discontinuation of feeds, or consideration to screen for necrotising enterocolitis, should be considered. It may also be advisable to withhold feeds during treatment, due to the potential effects of ductal steal and non-steroidal anti-inflammatory agents such as indomethacin on intestinal perfusion.[99]

Specific Treatment

Accepted strategies include both medical and surgical options. The decision to treat is normally made on the following basis:

- Echocardiographic confirmation of a duct with an internal diameter greater than 1.5 mm and unrestrictive left-to-right ductal shunting.
- Clinical signs of pulmonary over-circulation, myocardial dysfunction, or end-organ hypoperfusion.

Therapeutic closure is not recommended in a setting of suprasystemic pulmonary hypertension, or right heart failure where exclusive right-to-left shunting is a means to off-load a stressed right ventricle.

Non-steroidal Anti-inflammatory Drugs

As prostaglandins play a major role in preserving ductal patency, inhibitors of cyclooxygenase are conventionally used to assist its closure. Medical treatment should not be attempted, whenever possible, without prior echocardiographic evaluation and exclusion of duct-dependent cardiac lesions. Indomethacin is currently the treatment of choice for ductal closure in preterm babies, although the ideal dose, duration, and/or time to intervene remains somewhat controversial. Therapeutic options include prophylactic therapy or early targeted intervention.

Prophylactic Treatment

The merits of prophylactic treatment in the first 24 hours of life are highly questionable. Although the numbers of patent ducts are reduced, two-fifths of neonates are unnecessarily treated as the duct may have closed spontaneously.[107] In addition, ongoing ductal patency, in a transitional circulation with elevated pulmonary vascular resistance and poor right ventricular function, may be necessary for augmenting pulmonary perfusion. Severe hypoxaemia, responsive to inhaled nitric oxide, was recently reported in premature infants born prior to 28 weeks following prophylactic exposure to ibuprofen on the first day of life.[108] Prophylactic treatment in the first 24 hours of life, therefore, is not recommended, as the risks substantially outweigh the benefits as outlined previously.

Therapeutic Treatment

Early intervention, on the first to third days, is preferable to late intervention after 1 week, as the risks of necrotising enterocolitis, pulmonary morbidity and need for surgical ligation are significantly reduced.[109] The choice of dose and duration of treatment is controversial.[110] A targeted early approach to intervention appears the most effective and safest option. Treatment with indomethacin fails in up to half the infants born with extremely low weight.[61] This may reflect architectural differences and remodelling in the most immature patients, as described earlier, in addition to the severity of illness. Antenatal administration of indomethacin is also associated with postnatal hypo-responsiveness, and increased need for surgical ligation.[111] Architectural remodelling of the ductal wall, secondary to increased expression of vascular endothelial growth factor, and altered regulation of ductal tone by nitric oxide, has been demonstrated in a fetal ovine model.[69]

Complications of Medical Treatment

The decision to use indomethacin should be carefully balanced against the potential pitfalls of treatment. These include impaired renal function and compromised cerebral and/or mesenteric blood flow. Ibuprofen is a related agent that has been shown to have comparable efficacy in achieving ductal closure.[112–114] A recent meta-analysis confirmed these findings, but also demonstrated an improved safety profile with ibuprofen.[115] Specifically, those treated with ibuprofen had lower levels of creatinine, improved urinary output, and were less likely to have cerebral or mesenteric vasoconstrictive effects. There is, however, a potential greater risk of kernicterus, because ibuprofen interferes with binding of bilirubin to albumin in the serum when given in usual doses.[116]

Surgical Intervention

Surgical ligation is normally indicated after failure of medical therapy, or where medical therapy is contraindicated. The procedure is most commonly performed from a lateral subcostal approach, although video-assisted thoracoscopic ligation has been successfully performed.[117–119] Some authors have argued that ligation may be preferable over indomethacin as the initial treatment because it is associated with low morbidity and almost certain success.[120,121] A randomised controlled trial of early surgical ligation demonstrated a lowered incidence of necrotising enterocolitis.[122] An aggressive approach to ductal closure has been proposed as an effective way to reduce the incidence and severity of chronic lung disease.[123] A recent meta-analysis was inconclusive in determining whether medical or surgical intervention was preferable.[124]

Post-operative Complications

Ligation is not a benign procedure, and is oftentimes associated with significant post-operative cardiorespiratory instability. The most common complications include air-leak syndromes, pulmonary oedema,[125] hypotension requiring vasopressor support,[126] recurrent laryngeal nerve palsy,[127] and occasionally ligation of the left pulmonary artery, or even the aorta. Ligation is associated with immediate systolic and diastolic hypertension, which may contribute to reperfusion haemorrhage.[128] Although improvements in lung compliance immediately following ligation have been recorded,[80] the post-operative course is characterised by a post-ligation cardiac syndrome consisting of failure of oxygenation due to pulmonary oedema, systolic hypotension, and the need for cardiotropic support, which typically occur 8 to 12 hours after the procedure (Fig. 11-8).[129] This may relate to altered ventricular loading conditions following ligation.[130] Surgical ligation in preterm baboons is associated with a significant increase in left ventricular afterload within 12 hours of the procedure, coinciding with the development of left ventricular dysfunction and failure.[131] A number of recent publications highlight an association between ligation and an increased risk of bronchopulmonary dysplasia, severe retinopathy of prematurity, and neurosensory impairment.[132,133] It is impossible to determine whether this relationship reflects causality, or whether the need for ligation is merely a marker of the severity of illness.

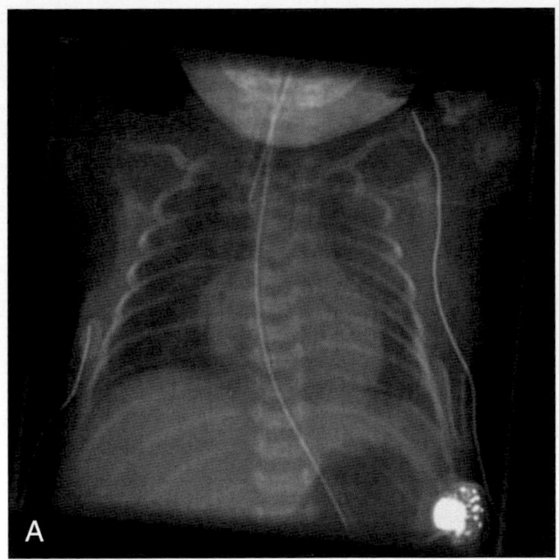

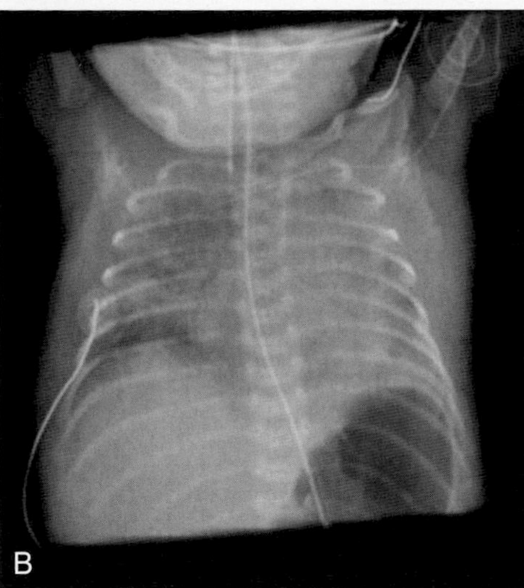

Figure 11-8 Chest radiographs before (A) and 12 hours (B) after patent ductus arteriosus ligation in a 750-g infant who required patent ductus arteriosus ligation. The post-operative chest film demonstrates a significant deterioration with evidence of cardiomegaly and lung oedema suggestive of pulmonary oedema.

Post-operative Care

On the basis of cardiovascular adaptation and other surgical complications, all neonates should be monitored closely in the post-operative period. Specifically, vital signs and urinary output should be carefully monitored, with frequent testing of arterial blood gases and/or lactate. Early commencement of diuretic therapy and increased positive end-expiratory pressure are recommended with failure of oxygenation, and radiologic evidence of pulmonary oedema or atelectasis. Inotropic agents with significant vasoconstrictive activity, such as dopamine or epinephrine, which increase systemic vascular resistance through α-adrenergic mediated mechanisms, should be avoided. Inotropes with afterload-reducing properties, such as dobutamine or milrinone, may be preferable.

Hypotension and Circulatory Collapse

Aetiology of Hypotension or Circulatory Collapse

The nature of the disease processes causing cardiovascular instability is variable, and should be considered when managing treatment. Myocardial dysfunction related to immaturity or elevated systemic vascular resistance and hypovolaemia should be considered as important aetiological factors in the immediate transitional period (Table 11-3). Beyond the first 24 hours of life the haemodynamically significant duct and sepsis are the most common causes. Hypovolaemia, adrenal suppression, and the effects of raised intrathoracic pressure may present at any stage, and should always be considered. The presence of a duct-dependent obstruction of the systemic outflow tract is just as likely for premature infants, and must be considered, particularly for those in refractory shock.

Hypovolaemia

All neonates require a normal central venous pressure to optimise pulmonary flow. The lack of a relationship between crystalloid support and blood pressure suggests that hypovolaemia is less common than previously considered as a primary aetiological agent. Nevertheless, it should be considered when there is evidence of acute maternal or neonatal blood loss, high insensible losses, or polyuria coinciding with weight loss, where there are major bodily cavity collections of fluid, such as pleural or pericardial effusions or ascites, or where there are excessive gastrointestinal fluid losses due to diseases such as necrotising enterocolitis or short bowel syndrome.

Myocardial Dysfunction

The maturational differences which make the preterm myocardium susceptible to failure have been described in a previous section. These developmental disadvantages make

TABLE 11-3

CAUSES OF HAEMODYNAMIC INSTABILITY IN PREMATURE INFANTS ACCORDING TO THEIR POSTNATAL AGE

Less Than 24 Hours	24 to 72 Hours	Older Than 72 Hours
Myocardial dysfunction, such as increased left ventricular afterload, or sepsis	Haemodynamically significant arterial duct	Haemodynamically significant arterial duct
Hypovolaemia such as birth-related blood loss, or high insensible losses	Myocardial dysfunction, due to, for example, sepsis or asphyxia	Myocardial dysfunction, due to, for example, necretising entrocolitis, or sepsis
Haemodynamically significant arterial duct	Hypovolaemia, for example due to loss of blood, or insensible losses	Relative adrenal insufficiency
Increased intrathoracic pressure, for example due to pulmonary hyperinflation, or fetal hydrops	Duct-dependent systemic disorder of flow	Post-ligation cardiac syndrome
Duct-dependent systemic disorder of flow	Increased intrathoracic pressure, such as pulmonary hyperinflation	Increased intrathoracic pressure such as lung hyperinflation, pleural or pericardial effusion
		Duct-dependent systemic disorder of flow

the neonatal myocardium vulnerable during a hypoxic-ischaemic insult or when subjected to preload or afterload compromise. The onset of left ventricular dysfunction within 8 to 12 hours of ductal ligation is one example of the intrinsic vulnerability of the immature myocardium to altered loading conditions.[130] Myocardial dysfunction is also more likely to occur during periods of metabolic acidosis, hypocalcaemia, hypokalaemia, or as a consequence of release of cytokines in the setting of sepsis or necrotising enterocolitis.

Vasomotor Regulation

The immediate postnatal period is characterised by increased systemic vascular resistance upon removal of the placenta from the systemic circuit. The placenta is a low resistance organ, and a rich source of prostaglandins and other inflammatory mediators with vasodilator properties. Beyond the transitional period, the complex regulation of vascular tone involves balancing of vasoconstrictor and vasodilator modifying factors, including nitric oxide, eicosanoids and catecholamines. Septic shock is characterised by increased production of nitric oxide due to upregulation of inducible nitric oxide synthase by endotoxins and tumor necrosis factor-α. Stores of vasopressin are also reduced in septic shock. Both of these factors may contribute to excessive systemic vasodilation and low vascular resistance leading to hypotension. Dysregulation of vasomotor tone should be considered as a possible contributory factor towards circulatory collapse particularly in the presence of isolated low diastolic pressure. The increase in left ventricular exposed vascular resistance following ductal ligation is temporally associated with impaired myocardial performance and low cardiac output. The nature of the vasomotor imbalance is an essential consideration when choosing between vasopressor and vasodilator agents.

Adrenal Gland Suppression

There is accumulating evidence from animal and human studies that the hypothalamic-pituitary-adrenal axis may be dysfunctional in some premature infants, particularly when subjected to stress.[134] Antenatal administration of multiple courses of steroids may contribute to postnatal impaired adrenal performance.[135] There is evidence that suboptimal adrenal performance is an important contributor to impaired myocardial performance and impaired cardiorespiratory adaptation in the early neonatal period.[136] The association between hypotension and levels of cortisol in the plasma is an important consideration, although assessment of the performance of the adrenal glands in clinical practice is challenging.[134]

Therapeutic Approach to Hypotension and Circulatory Collapse

The traditional approach to cardiovascular care is problematic for a number of reasons. First, it has been predominantly pressure based, and fails to consider the importance of systemic blood flow. Second, the approach to intervention is based on regimental protocols which recommend administration of volume followed by dopamine, dobutamine, and epinephrine.[137] These protocols do not take into account the nature of the underlying disease, or the acute physiologic disturbance, postnatal maturation, or inter-individual variation. Hence, they lend themselves to incorrect decisions regarding treatment. It is not logical to treat hypotension secondary to sepsis or congenitally malformed hearts in a similar fashion. It should also be recognised that there is limited clinical evidence to support any current therapeutic agent. In addition there is limited pharmacologic evidence to support the agents currently used in practice. Nevertheless, it is important to understand the mechanism of action, benefits, and limitations of commonly used agents. It is important to recognise that the goal of treatment is to ensure there is adequate oxygenation to meet the metabolic needs of the cell. Both delivery and consumption of oxygen are important considerations (Fig. 11-9). Delivery is influenced by level of circulatory haemoglobin, saturations, and factors which influence myocardial performance, such as preload, afterload, contractility, and heart rate. Consumption is subject to the influence of work of breathing, agitation, and pain.

Volume

There have been no studies of volume versus no treatment. The systematic review of trials of early expansion found no evidence of benefit.[138] There are two trials, comparing normal saline with albumin, which found no advantage of either therapy in reducing mortality or improving cardiovascular outcomes. Volume should be restricted to treating hypovolaemia where there is an identified precipitating factor, such as acute loss of blood.

Vasopressor Agents

Dopamine is a sympathetic amine and the most commonly used vasoactive agent in the neonatal intensive care unit. It has mixed β-1 and α-adrenergic effects depending on the dose. There is evidence of improved left ventricular performance at levels of less than 2.5 μg/kg/min in immature neonates.[139,140] It was previously thought that the vasoconstricting effects occur only at doses above 10 μg/kg/min. There is evidence of significant α-adrenergic effects in some premature infants at doses as low as 6 μg/kg/min, with marked elevation in systemic vascular resistance leading to decreased cardiac output and decreased flow in the superior mesenteric and middle cerebral arteries.[141] Whilst dopamine is an effective agent at increasing systemic blood pressure,[142] its effects on systemic flow and end-organ perfusion are concerning. Epinephrine is an endogenous catecholamine produced by the adrenal medulla with similar mixed β-1, at low doses, and α-, at doses greater than 0.375 μg/kg/min, adrenergic effects to epinephrine. It is an effective pressor agent in the first 24 hours of life, and may augment cerebral flow.[143] Its clinical use is normally reserved as a rescue agent, although it may be a more effective pressor agent than dopamine in septic shock or necrotising enterocolitis. High doses or prolonged treatment have been associated with ischaemia and myocardial dysfunction.[144,145] These effects may relate to direct β-1 adrenergic receptor mediated damage to the myocardium.[146,147] Vasopressin is a 9-amino acid peptide synthesised in the posterior pituitary, commonly known as anti-diuretic hormone. It displays dichotomous effects through V1 receptors. In the lung, it has pulmonary vasodilator properties via modulation of release of nitric oxide.[148] It acts as a systemic vasoconstrictor, acting through phospholipid complex mediated calcium release. In adults it is a promising systemic vasopressor in vasodilatory shock and cardiopulmonary resuscitation.[149–151] Its role in neonatal cardiovascular care is unknown, although theoretically it may be of benefit in restrictive physiologies such as the

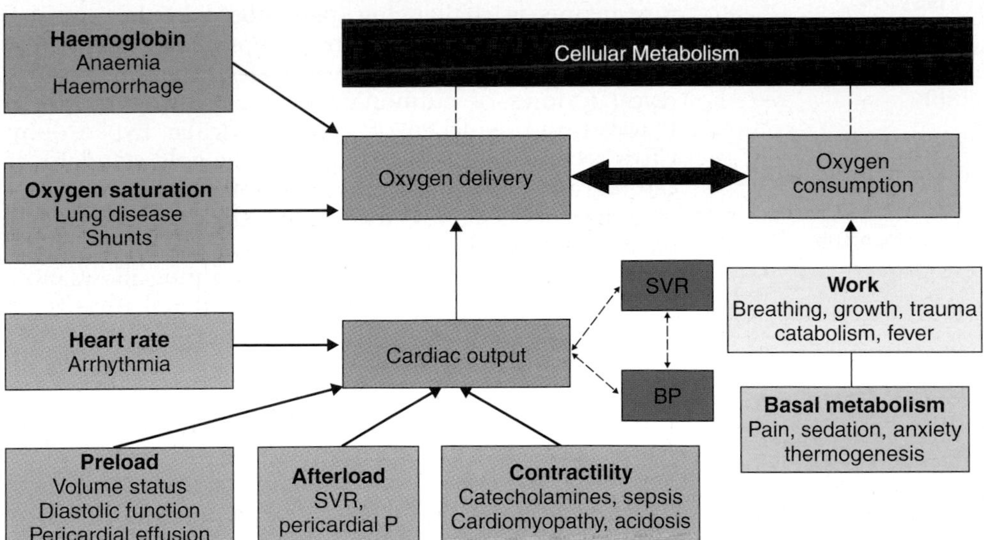

Figure 11-9 Factors governing cellular metabolism and the adequacy of tissue oxygenation subdivided according to tissue oxygen delivery and consumption. BP, blood pressure; SVR, systemic vascular resistance.

septal hypertrophy or biventricular hypertrophy that occurs in infants of diabetic mothers.

Inodilator Agents

Dobutamine is a synthetic analogue of dopamine with a predominantly β-1 adrenergic mode of action and minimal α-adrenergic properties. These translate into positive inotropic and afterload reducing effects, which are highly desirable in many neonatal settings e.g. transitional period, post-asphyxial insult, pulmonary hypertension, and following ductal ligation. A systematic review of five randomised controlled trials concluded that dopamine was superior at elevating systemic blood pressure, but there were no differences in survival or neonatal morbidity.[142] Two randomised trials have shown that dobutamine is a more effective agent at improving systemic blood flow.[152,153] In one study, dopamine was shown to lead to a decrease in left ventricular output. It can be concluded that dobutamine is a more desirable agent for neonates with hypotension and clinical signs of low cardiac output.

Milrinone is an inhibitor of phosphodiesterase III which acts through increasing the bioavailability of cyclic adenine monophosphate. It is both a systemic and pulmonary vasodilator, with positive inotropic and lusitropic properties. In infants and children undergoing cardiac surgery it has been shown to decrease the combined end-point of death and low cardiac output syndrome.[154] There is also evidence of benefit in neonates with pulmonary hypertension.[155–157] The pharmacokinetics of milrinone have been characterised in premature infants in the first 24 hours of life.[158,159] Experimental data suggests that the myocardial effects may be developmentally regulated, with negative inotropy in some species in early gestation.[160] Results of a randomised controlled trial of prophylactic treatment are awaited.

Steroids

These are normally considered as rescue therapy after failure of cardiotropic support. A number of clinical trials have demonstrated improved cardiovascular stability facilitating weaning of cardiotropic drugs after commencement of treatment.[161,162] The mechanism of action is a combination of genomic and non-genomic effects. Their merits must be considered in the context of the potential negative effects on myelination and brain maturation.[163]

In summary, the choice of a cardiovascular treatment should consider the nature of the disease, maturational factors, potential effects on both blood pressure and cardiac output (Fig. 11-10), and pharmacological properties. The complications of treatment need also be recognised, which may include tachycardia, increased myocardial consumption of oxygen, hypotension produced by vasodilator agents, regional hypoperfusion produced by vasopressors, impaired myocardial compliance, and arrhythmias.

Pulmonary Hypertension and Prematurity

Until recently, the nature and treatment of pulmonary vascular disease in premature infants have received little attention. It is not recognised that persistent pulmonary vascular disease increases morbidity and mortality associated with chronic lung disease.

	Normal/High BP	Low BP
Normal/High CO	Observe	Pressors (dopamine, epinephrine, vasopressin)
Low CO	Inodilators (milrinone, dobutamine)	Combination therapy (dobutamine, dopamine, epineprhine)

Figure 11-10 Choice of cardiovascular treatments subdivided according to whether the disturbance affects blood pressure, cardiac output, or both.

TABLE 11-4

CAUSES OF PULMONARY HYPERTENSION IN PREMATURE INFANTS

Acute	Chronic, with Variable Reversibility
Reversible	Chronic lung disease
Respiratory distress syndrome	Chronic patency of arterial duct
Pneumothorax	Congenitally malformed heart
Sepsis	Mild pulmonary hypoplasia
Irreversible	
Pulmonary hypoplasia	
Congenital diaphragmatic hernia	

Aetiology of Pulmonary Hypertension

Persistent pulmonary hypertension of the newborn is the failure of normal postnatal fall in pulmonary vascular resistance leading to problems in oxygenation, right ventricular failure, and/or pulmonary-to-systemic shunting. The regulation of pulmonary vascular resistance represents a balance between vasoconstrictor and vasodilator agents. Pulmonary hypertension is seen both acutely and chronically in premature infants (Table 11-4). This distinction is important, as the responsiveness to pulmonary vasodilator agents is dependent on the degree of pulmonary vascular remodeling. The outcome for neonates with pulmonary hypoplasia is poor. Factors contributing to pulmonary hypoplasia include prolonged rupture of membranes and renal agenesis. Neonates with significant hyaline membrane disease may develop suprasystemic pulmonary arterial pressure, which results in right ventricular loading and, as a consequence of ventricular interaction, impaired left ventricular function. Surfactant rapidly improves oxygenation by reducing pulmonary vascular resistance, which leads to further dramatic changes in pulmonary arterial pressure, right ventricular loading, and left-sided haemodynamics. The mortality rate for preterm infants with pulmonary hypertension, at 26.2%, is six times higher than matched controls.[164]

Chronic Lung Disease, Pulmonary Vascular Remodeling, and Pulmonary Hypertension

Preterm lung injury is characterised by injury to both the airspaces and vasculature.[165] The former is characterised by alveolar simplification, whereas the latter is characterised by impaired angiogenesis and pulmonary hypertension. The abnormal pulmonary vascular bed is characterised by increased muscularisation of vascular smooth muscle cells, distal extension of muscle into non-muscularised vessels, and arrested vascular growth. The vasoactivity of pulmonary vessels is characterised by increased basal vascular tone and impaired potential to relax. Factors contributing to pulmonary vascular remodeling include oxygen toxicity, hypoxaemia, and mechanical ventilation.[166] Injury to the pulmonary vascular bed may also play a role in the development of impaired alveolisation. Pulmonary angiogenesis is modulated by vascular endothelial derived growth factor. The administration of a receptor antagonist leads to impaired angiogenesis and alveologenesis in neonatal rodents.[167]

Diagnosis of Pulmonary Hypertension in Premature Infants

The diagnosis of pulmonary hypertension in premature infants is challenging, particularly in the presence of lung disease. The signs and symptoms of pulmonary hypertension are non-specific. The electrocardiogram may reveal features of pulmonary hypertension, such as tall P waves and evidence of right ventricular hypertrophy. Cross sectional echocardiography is the gold standard, as cardiac catheterisation is rarely performed. The majority of imaging studies have focused on evaluation of pulmonary haemodynamics in the early neonatal period. The presence of a patent duct and transductal shunting allows more accurate quantification of pulmonary arterial pressure.[168] Magnetic resonance imaging may provide an opportunity to study pulmonary flow and pressure more effectively.

Treatment of Pulmonary Hypertension

The primary treatment is the administration of oxygen; on the basis that hypoxaemia leads to worsening of the pulmonary hypertension. There remains uncertainty as to the most desirable saturation for premature infants. There is some justification for maintaining saturations above 93%.[169] The results of a recent randomised controlled trial of normal versus high saturations suggested a less favorable outcome at higher saturations.[170] Inhaled nitric oxide may be a more desirable therapeutic agent.[171–173] It has also been shown to protect surfactant,[174] and promote both angiogenesis and alveolarisation.[172] These properties suggest it to be an ideal agent for the treatment of pulmonary hypertension and prevention of lung alveolar or vascular injury. Acute administration leads to improved oxygenation in premature infants.[175,176] The response is developmentally regulated, with few responders less than 28 weeks gestation.[164] In total there have been 11 randomised controlled trials of inhaled nitric oxide in premature infants. Early or late rescue does not reduce the risk of chronic lung disease, improve survival, or long-term outcomes. Early routine use for mildly sick preterm infants seems to reduce the risk of severe cerebral injury, and may improve survival without chronic lung disease.[177] Routine administration in clinical practice is not yet recommended. There is some evidence in support of alternative vasodilator treatments, such as milrinone in premature infants, although there may be an increased risk of intraventricular haemorrhage.[155]

Systemic Hypertension and Prematurity

Neonatal hypertension is defined as a sustained systolic blood pressure greater than the 97th percentile for age, gender, and size according to published nomograms. The incidence of systemic hypertension is between 0.2% and 3%.[178,179] Of these, 9% had indwelling arterial catheters.

Causes of Neonatal Hypertension

In most cases the finding is coincidental on routine monitoring. Occasionally some neonates present insidiously with non-specific symptoms, such as difficulty in feeding, tachypnoea, or lethargy. In more extreme cases, seizures or congestive cardiac failure may occur. It is important to take a thorough history, make a complete cardiovascular evaluation, including testing of blood pressure in all limbs, and to screen for dysmorphisms, ambiguous genital organs, abdominal masses such as Wilms' tumour, and bruits such as produced by renal arterial stenosis. There are many causes

TABLE 11-5

CAUSES OF SYSTEMIC HYPERTENSION IN PREMATURE INFANTS GROUPED AND LISTED IN ORDER OF FREQUENCY OF PRESENTATION

Illness	Cause
Renovascular	Thromboembolism related to catheterisation, renal arterial stenosis, renal venous thrombosis, midaortic coarctation, renal arterial compression as caused by severe hydronephrosis
Congenital renal parenchymal disease	Polycystic renal disease, multi-cystic dysplastic renal disease, obstruction at uretero-pelvic junction, unilateral renal hypoplasia or agenesis, congenital nephritic syndrome
Acquired renal parenchymal disease	Acute tubular or cortical necrosis, interstitial nephritis
Drug induced	Dexamethasone, α-adrenergic agents such as dopamine, epinephrine, muscular relaxants, theophylline, ophthalmic drops with phenylephrine
Neonatal abstinence syndrome	Maternal cocaine or heroin
Cardiac	Thoracic coarctation, iatrogenic fluid overload
Endocrine	Congenital adrenal hyperplasia, hyperaldosteronism, hyperthyroidism
Neurologic	Pain, seizures, subdural hematoma
Neoplasia	Wilm's tumour, phaeochromocytoma, neuroblastoma

of hypertension, of which renovascular disease and renal parenchymal disease are the most common (Table 11-5).

Treatment of Systemic Hypertension

The urgency of therapeutic intervention with anti-hypertensive drugs is dependent on illness severity. The following general principles should be considered before embarking on specific drug therapy:

- Indwelling arterial catheters should be removed if felt to be causal.
- All current treatments should be re-evaluated as they may be contributory.
- Rapid correction of blood pressure should be avoided, particularly in the early postnatal period, as this may contribute to cerebral ischaemia or haemorrhage.
- It should be the goal of therapy to reduce blood pressure by one-third in the first 6 hours.

Intravenous agents should be used for emergent hypertension. Intravenous diuretics and vasodilators are the mainstay of treatment (Fig. 11-11). Commonly used oral maintenance treatments include diuretics, such as thiazides, inhibitors of angiotensin converting enzyme, except if the neonate exhibits renal impairment, or antagonists of the calcium channel.

CONGENITALLY MALFORMED HEARTS AND PREMATURITY

The diagnosis and pre-operative care of the preterm neonate with a congenitally malformed heart is challenging as a consequence of the additional effects of immaturity, low birth weight, and other maturational factors. The overall

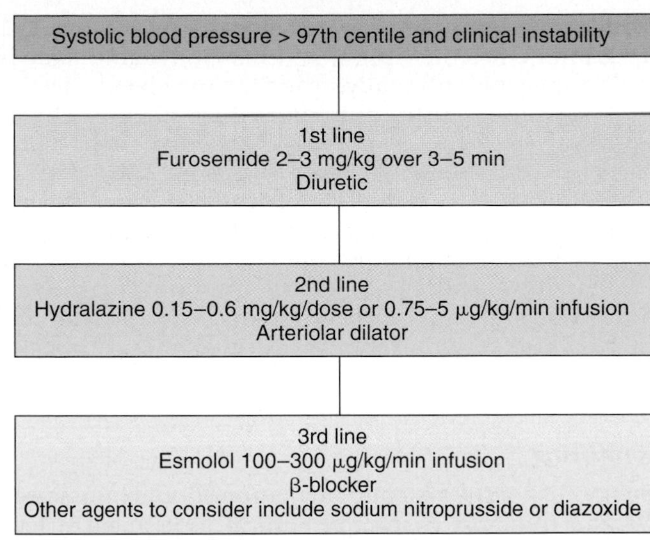

Figure 11-11 Therapeutic approach to the care of premature infants with systemic hypertension greater than 97th centile.

risk of mortality and pre-operative, peri-operative, and post-operative morbidity is significantly increased, particularly in neonates born with extremely low weight.[180–183] There is no published data or guidelines on best practice for the management of preterm neonates with congenital cardiovascular malformations. Most of the current practices incorporate best evidence for the care of preterm neonates with treatments normally used for full-term infants. More important, these neonates should be cared for in tertiary neonatal centres with a critical mass of preterm neonates with such malformations, and comprehensive cardiological services.

Echocardiography

The role of cross sectional echocardiography in the care of preterm neonates is twofold: first, to establish the anatomic diagnosis, and second, to monitor patency of the duct, myocardial performance, and pulmonary arterial pressures. Infants born with extremely low weights will often require several echocardiograms before surgical intervention to monitor cardiovascular health and the effects of the cardiac defects on pulmonary arterial pressures.

Cardiovascular Care

The care of the preterm neonate with structural heart disease should focus on those issues related to prematurity and the specific defect. These should not be considered mutually exclusive, nor should they be ranked in terms of the overall care plan, as each influences the other. Care in the early postnatal period is predominantly medical. Surgical interventions or other invasive procedures are normally delayed until the neonate reaches a maturity and weight at which the risks of an expectant approach outweigh the risks of the specific intervention.

Prostaglandin Treatment

Neonates with a duct-dependent cardiac defect require continuous intravenous prostaglandin E_2 therapy to ensure ongoing ductal patency. In the early phase of stabilisation, the dose required ranges from 0.01 to 0.2 µg/kg/min. Once the clinical and haemodynamic state is stable, the agent is normally weaned to the lowest effective dose to avoid excessive pulmonary vasodilation. This is particularly relevant for neonates with functionally univentricular physiology, where a profound or sustained fall in pulmonary vascular resistance leads to excessive pulmonary blood flow at the expense of systemic perfusion. In many cases, treatment is required for several weeks or months whilst awaiting surgical intervention. This increases the risks of complications related to chronic administration. These include apnoea, gastric outlet obstruction, and hyperostosis.

Monitoring

The stability of the systemic circulation should be assessed first and foremost by careful clinical assessment. Clinical signs of circulatory compromise include tachycardia, hypotension, and decreased urinary output. Plasma lactate, arterial pH, base deficit, and mixed venous oxygen saturations should be monitored as markers of the efficacy of tissue oxygenation. Arterial $PaCO_2$ and pH should be carefully controlled to avoid excessive pulmonary vasodilation.

Cardiovascular Support

The goal of treatment is to ensure that blood pressure is maintained within a range that sustains adequate systemic perfusion. Treatments should not be administered in any sequential, random, or ranked order but should be given based on the pathophysiology and the likelihood of the treatment to correct the abnormal physiologic state. Therapeutic options include volume expansion, inodilator drugs such as dobutamine and milrinone, or pressors such as dopamine, epinephrine, and vasopressin. Volume expansion is useful in neonates with abnormal right ventricular performance; hence it may play an important role in the care of neonates with elevated pulmonary pressures or duct-dependent pulmonary circulations such as those with pulmonary atresia or severe tetralogy of Fallot. Milrinone has been shown to reduce both mortality and low cardiac output syndrome in post-operative cardiac patients.[155]

Interventional

Cardiac catheterisation is occasionally performed. There are some reports in the literature of successful balloon dilation of the pulmonary valve in neonates as small as 690 g and implantation of stents in the left pulmonary artery which had been inadvertently ligated.[184] More commonly balloon atrial septostomy is performed at the bedside in neonates with transposition, or other conditions dependent on a transatrial shunt, such as hypoplastic left heart syndrome.

Surgical Procedures

Decisions related to the optimal timing for surgery are challenging due to the effects of immaturity, low birth weight, and co-morbidities.[180,181,185–187] Traditionally, an expectant approach has been preferred. Delaying surgery until immature neonates reach a predetermined maturity and weight increases the risks of pre-operative, peri-operative, and post-operative morbidity. This is particularly the case for neonates with established chronic lung disease. In most centres, the average weight at surgery is between 2000 and 2500 g, although with modified techniques of cardiopulmonary bypass, surgical intervention is attempted at less than 1800 g.[185] Repair of coarctation is also possible in premature neonates as cardiopulmonary bypass is not required. Valvar replacement is rarely performed in premature neonates.

FOCUSED NEONATAL CARE

Respiratory Care

Routine intubation of all neonates when prostaglandins are administered should not be considered to be mandatory, particularly when the diagnosis has been established antenatally and low doses are prescribed. The decision to intubate should be made based on the usual clinical indications. Intubation is recommended in the presence of respiratory failure, clinical signs of cardiogenic shock, the need for cardiotropic support, profound metabolic or lactic acidosis, gestational age less the 28 weeks, and an associated disorder of the airways. One of the most challenging aspects of management is supporting those neonates with evolving chronic lung disease and pulmonary hypertension secondary to pulmonary vascular remodeling. Episodic apnoea, and/or hypoxaemia, occur frequently in these patients, necessitating therapeutic intervention. Oxygen is normally administered to preterm neonates to maintain saturations above 75% due to the risks of tissue hypoxia and adverse neurodevelopmental outcomes.[188] The administration of prophylactic surfactant to those with an antenatal diagnosis of a duct-dependent systemic circulation is not without risk. An excessive fall in pulmonary vascular resistance following administration of surfactant may lead to excessive flow to the lungs at the expense of systemic perfusion. This may be particular hazardous for neonates with hypoplastic left heart syndrome, where the systemic circulation is extremely tenuous. The radiological confirmation of respiratory distress syndrome is recommended for these neonates before administering surfactant.

Neurological Care

Recent studies using magnetic resonance imaging have identified abnormalities of the cerebral white matter pre-operatively in at least half full-term neonates.[129,188] There is a strong correlation between these findings and pre-operative arterial tensions of oxygen and blood pressure. The presence of peri-operative hyperthermia or seizures, co-existing genetic abnormalities, or associated defects in other organs, also increases the risk of neurological morbidity. The preterm neonate is even more vulnerable due to the effects of chronic hypoxaemia and intermittent periods of systemic hypoperfusion on the developing brain. In full-term neonates, these events translate into poor long-term neurodevelopmental outcome. There is limited published data on the combined impact of prematurity and a congenital cardiovascular malformation.

Gastrointestinal Care

The risk of necrotising enterocolitis is significantly increased in these neonates, of whom two-fifths had functionally univentricular physiology.[183] This is most likely to be related to intestinal hypoperfusion and/or chronic hypoxaemia. Extreme immaturity, higher doses of prostaglandin, and episodic low cardiac output syndrome, are also strong predictive factors. These newborns required a focused approach to nutrition that balances the risks of prematurity within the context of a fragile circulation. Wherever possible, guidelines should be developed that focus on the unique needs of such preterm neonates with cardiac disease. Whilst growth is paramount to improve weight, they should be fed cautiously. Expressed breast milk is recommended, and feeds should be increased slowly compared to their normal gestational counterparts.

Miscellaneous

The risk of anaemia is probably increased due to more frequent sampling of blood. Although the threshold for transfusion in preterm neonates remains unclear, it is probably advisable to implement a lower than normal threshold. This is particularly relevant for neonates with functionally univentricular physiology, who are at greater risk of tissue hypoxia. The risk of infection is higher in these preterm neonates, and vigilance is required, as periods of instability are often assumed to be cardiovascular in nature. Due to the challenges of clinical assessment for dysmorphism or genetic abnormalities, routine karyotypic analysis, together with screening for 22q microdeletion, is recommended.

Outcomes

Overall mortality rates of greater than 40% for newborns weighing less than 1500 g, and a doubling of mortality for newborns less than 2.5 kg, have been reported.[182,183] These reports do not take into account the heterogeneity of the cardiovascular malformations. The literature is severely lacking with respect to long-term outcome in this high-risk population. There are reviews on heterogeneous clusters of preterm neonates with varying types of cardiovascular malformations, but none which focus on any specific defect. Physicians will use the limited information that is available on the outcome for mature infants with certain cardiovascular malformations, and combine this with data for comparable preterm neonates when discussing prognosis. Follow-up data is urgently required for preterm neonates with common cardiovascular malformations so physicians can provide parents with accurate information on the likely course and outcome for their child.

The complete reference list can be found on the companion Expert Consult web site at www.expertconsult.com.

ANNOTATED REFERENCES

- Systolic blood pressure in babies of less than 32 weeks gestation in the first year of life. Northern Neonatal Nursing Initiative. Arch Dis Child Fetal Neonatal Ed 1999;80:F38–F42.

  This study represents the largest population-based evaluation of systolic blood pressure in premature neonates. It provides normative data with both gestational and postnatal corrected population means and centiles.
- Limperopoulos C, Bassan H, Kalish LA, et al: Current definitions of hypotension do not predict abnormal cranial ultrasound findings in preterm infants. Pediatrics 2007;120:966–977.
- Martens SE, Rijken M, Stoelhorst GM, et al: Is hypotension a major risk factor for neurological morbidity at term age in very preterm infants? Early Hum Dev 2003;75:79–89.

  These two studies address the relationship between systemic blood pressure and abnormal neurological sequelae. The first study concludes that current operational definitions of blood pressure, namely that mean blood pressure approximates gestational age, are not associated with early cerebral injury. The second study demonstrates that any association between hypotension and injury to the white matter is no longer valid when corrected for confounding variables, such as retardation of growth or treatment with steroids.
- Kluckow M, Evans N: Low superior vena cava flow and intraventricular haemorrhage in preterm infants. Arch Dis Child Fetal Neonatal Ed 2000;82: F188–F194.
- Hunt RW, Evans N, Rieger I, Kluckow M: Low superior vena cava flow and neurodevelopment at 3 years in very preterm infants. J Pediatr 2004;145: 588–592.

  Conventional methods used to assess ventricular output in premature infants are confounded by shunting through the arterial duct. The measurement of flow in the superior caval vein is representative of perfusion of the head and neck, and is not confounded by ductal shunting. An association between critically low superior caval venous flow and early intraventricular haemorrhage has been demonstrated which translates into adverse neurodevelopmental outcomes at 3 years of age.
- Evans N, Moorcraft J: Effect of patency of the ductus arteriosus on blood pressure in very preterm infants. Arch Dis Child 1992;67:1169–1173.
- Kluckow M, Evans N: Early echocardiographic prediction of symptomatic patent ductus arteriosus in preterm infants undergoing mechanical ventilation. J Pediatr 1995;127:774–779

  The decision to intervene in patients with a patent arterial duct is dependent on the clinical impact. The degree of haemodynamic significance is best predicted by transductal diameter. One important early consequence of systemic-to-pulmonary transductal shunting is systemic hypotension, particularly in neonates weighing less than 1000 g.
- Van Overmeire B, Smets K, Lecoutere D, et al: A comparison of ibuprofen and indomethacin for closure of patent ductus arteriosus. N Engl J Med 2000;343:674–681.

  This randomised controlled trial demonstrates equivocal efficacy but less renal side effects with ibuprofen compared to indomethacin.
- Rowland DG, Gutgesell HP: Noninvasive assessment of myocardial contractility, preload, and afterload in healthy newborn infants. Am J Cardiol 1995;75:818–821.
- Moin F, Kennedy KA, Moya FR: Risk factors predicting vasopressor use after patent ductus arteriosus ligation. Am J Perinatol 2003;20:313–320.
- Noori S, Friedlich P, Seri I, Wong P: Changes in myocardial function and hemodynamics after ligation of the ductus arteriosus in preterm infants. J Pediatr 2007;150:597–602.

  The sensitivity of the immature myocardium to increased afterload is highlighted in these three studies. In comparison to older children, neonates function at a higher basal contractile state, and impaired myocardial contractility is more likely at higher levels of afterload. The haemodynamic instability that occurs following ligation of the arterial duct is one example of the vulnerability of the immature myocardium to increased afterload.
- Kabra NS, Schmidt B, Roberts RS, et al: Neurosensory impairment after surgical closure of patent ductus arteriosus in extremely low birth weight infants: Results from the Trial of Indomethacin Prophylaxis in Preterms. J Pediatr 2007;150:229–234.

  This study was a reanalysis of a subgroup of patients who were recruited for a trial of prophylactic indomethacin. The authors draw an important association between patients who required ligation of the arterial duct and abnormal neurodevelopmental outcomes. It is not possible to determine whether the relationship is causal, or relates to the primary problem of ductal disease.
- Osborn D, Evans N, Kluckow M: Randomized trial of dobutamine versus dopamine in preterm infants with low systemic blood flow. J Pediatr 2002;140:183–191.
- Paradisis M, Evans N, Kluckow M, et al: Pilot study of milrinone for low systemic blood flow in very preterm infants. J Pediatr 2006;148: 306–313.

  These two studies address the effect of cardiotropic agents on systemic blood flow. Dobutamine is a more effective agent than dopamine at increasing systemic blood flow. Early administration of milrinone prevents low superior caval venous flow.
- Van Meurs KP, Wright LL, Ehrenkranz RA, et al: Inhaled nitric oxide for premature infants with severe respiratory failure. N Engl J Med 2005;353: 13–22.

  Inhaled nitric oxide is a controversial treatment for hypoxaemic respiratory failure. This study shows a beneficial effect on rates of bronchopulmonary dysplasia and mortality only in neonates weighing more than 1000 g.

- McElhinney DB, Hedrick HL, Bush DM, et al: Necrotizing enterocolitis in neonates with congenital heart disease: Risk factors and outcomes. Pediatrics 2000;106:1080–1087.
- Galli KK, Zimmerman RA, Jarvik GP, et al: Periventricular leukomalacia is common after neonatal cardiac surgery. J Thorac Cardiovasc Surg 2004;127:692–704.

These studies address the impact of congenital cardiac disease on two important neonatal morbidities. The consequences of critical hypoxaemia and systemic hypoperfusion include cerebral white matter injury, and bowel necrosis. Both of these conditions compromise both survival and long-term neurodevelopmental outcomes.

SECTION

2

Special Topics

CHAPTER 12

Pharmacological and Interventional Fetal Cardiovascular Treatment

EDGAR T. JAEGGI and GERALD TULZER

With cross sectional echocardiography providing the means non-invasively to detect and monitor the evolution of anomalies occurring during pregnancy, the fetus has increasingly become the object of intended treatment. This includes the administration of pharmaceutical agents via the maternal circulation or directly into the fetus to control fetal cardiac arrhythmias, to improve congestive heart failure, to treat inflammation and infections and to prevent pulmonary immaturity. Moreover, the increasing ability to use ultrasonic and fetoscopic guidance directly to intervene on the fetus with progressive cardiovascular pathology promises to magnify the advantage offered by prenatal detection of congenital cardiac disease. We will discuss the principles, risks, and contemporary results of intra-uterine fetal treatment for specific cardiac arrhythmias, along with anomalies, which, in the absence of universally accepted guidelines for management, remains a contentious topic among experts.

FETAL ARRHYTHMIAS

Fetal arrhythmia may present as an irregularity of the cardiac rhythm, as an abnormally slow or fast heart rate, or as a combination of irregular rhythm and abnormal heart rate. In most cases, such anomalies as encountered during fetal life present as brief episodes of little clinical relevance. No treatment is usually required. This includes irregularities of the cardiac rhythm caused by blocked and conducted premature atrial contractions. Of more concern are sustained episodes of a cardiac rate that is too fast, greater than 180 beats per minute, or one that is too slow, less than 100 beats per minute. The most common causes for such problems are supraventricular tachycardia, atrial flutter, and severe bradyarrhythmias associated with complete heart block. While a persistently fast or slow rate may be well-tolerated, at the more severe end of the spectrum, it may result in low cardiac output, cerebral damage, fetal hydrops, and death. The finding of arrhythmia-related fetal hydrops is the single most important predictor of adverse fetal outcome. On the other hand, a symptomatic fetal tachyarrhythmia or bradyarrhythmia may respond to, or improve on, pharmacological treatment. Hence, if a disturbance of rhythm is suspected, it is important to determine the likely arrhythmic mechanism, to clarify the impact on the fetal circulation, and to conclude on the urgency and choice of care. Detailed fetal ultrasonic examination provides essential information on the level of fetal activity as an indicator of well-being, on the size and function of the fetal heart, and the distribution and extent of accumulation of fluid in the fetal pleural, pericardial, and abdominal spaces and the skin. Detailed fetal echocardiography is helpful to detect cardiac tumours, Ebstein's malformation of the tricuspid valve, left isomerism, and congenitally-corrected transposition, all of which may be associated with abnormally fast or slow heart rates. Key to the proper management is a clear understanding of the underlying pattern and mechanism of the arrhythmia. Stepwise analysis of the rate, rhythm, and chronology of atrial and ventricular mechanical events by means of echocardiographic techniques allows the distinction between the different anomalies (Table 12-1). The correct diagnosis will reduce the risk of unnecessary pharmacological treatment, or premature delivery of fetuses with more benign findings, and facilitate the care of those with a major disorder of rhythm. We will discuss in detail those cardiac disorders that might take advantage of transplacental treatment, specifically fetal tachyarrhythmia, fetal thyrotoxicosis, and immune-mediated isolated atrioventricular block and endocardial fibroelastosis.

FETAL TACHYARRHYTHMIA

Mechanisms

A persistent or intermittent fast fetal heart rate is usually the consequence of supraventricular tachycardia, atrial flutter, or sinus tachycardia, with atrial fibrillation, ventricular tachycardia, and junctional ectopic tachycardia as more unusual causes.[1,2] Supraventricular tachycardia itself can be produced by three different mechanisms, namely atrioventricular re-entrant tachycardia, typically involving the atrioventricular node for antegrade conduction and a fast retrograde ventriculo-atrial conducting accessory pathway, permanent junctional reciprocating tachycardia related to retrograde conduction through the slow pathway of the atrioventricular node, and atrial ectopic tachycardia due to enhanced atrial focal automaticity. These can be distinguished echocardiographically on the basis of the arrhythmic pattern and the ventriculo-atrial time relationships.[3] The most common form underscoring fetal tachycardia, atrioventricular re-entry, presents electro-mechanically as a short ventriculo-atrial arrhythmia, the atrium being activated shortly after the ventricles via the fast retrogradely conducting accessory pathway. Re-entry within the atrioventricular node, another potential mechanism of a short ventriculo-atrial tachycardia, is probably rare in the fetus. Therapeutic intervention to terminate atrioventricular or atrioventricular nodal re-entrant tachycardia is aimed at

TABLE 12-1

DIAGNOSTIC ECHOCARDIOGRAPHIC FEATURES OF MORE COMMON FETAL DISTURBANCES OF RHYTHM AND CONDUCTION

	Arrhythmia	A Rate	A-A Interval	AV Relation	V Rate	V-V Interval	V-A Interval	Relevance + Outcome
Irregular rhythm	Isolated PAC, conducted	Normal	Irregular	1:1	Normal	Irregular	Variable	Minor, transient
	Isolated PAC, blocked	Normal	Irregular	>1:1	Normal	Irregular		Minor, transient
Bradycardia	Sinus	75–90	Regular	1:1	75–90	Regular	Long VA	Depends on cause
	Atrial bigeminy, blocked	Normal	Regular irregular	2:1	65–90	Regular		Minor, transient
	2:1 AV block	Normal	Regular	2:1	60–75	Regular		Major, may progress
	Third-degree AVB	Slow–normal	Regular	Dissociated	35–80	Regular	Dissociated	Major, irreversible
Tachycardia	Sinus	160–200	Regular	1:1	160–200	Regular	Long VA	Depends on cause
	AV reentry	190–280	Regular	1:1	190–280	Regular	Short VA	Major, treatable
	Atrial flutter	300–500	Regular	Mainly 2:1	150–250	Mainly regular		Major, treatable
	AET, PJRT	180–230	Regular	1:1	180–230	Regular	Long VA	Major, treatable
	Ventricular (+VA block)	Normal	Regular	<1:1	160–260	Regular–irregular	Dissociated	Major, treatable

A, atrial; AET, atrial ectopic tachycardia; AV, atrioventricular; AVB, atrioventricular block; PAC, premature atrial contractions; PJRT, permanent junctional reciprocating tachycardia; V, ventricular; V-A, ventriculo-atrial; VA block, absence of retrograde conduction via AV node or accessory pathway.

interrupting the balance in timing between the electrical pathways required to sustain the re-entrant circuit.

In long ventriculo-atrial supraventricular tachycardia, which is considerably less common but often more difficult to control when compared to atrioventricular re-entry, the atrial contraction closely precedes the ventricular contraction. This pattern of activation is seen during atrial ectopic tachycardia and permanent junctional reciprocating tachycardia, but also characterises sinus tachycardia. Treatment of atrial ectopic tachycardia aims at the suppression of the ectopic generation of impulses. A variety of treatable conditions occurring during pregnancy may be responsible for sustained sinus tachycardia, including fetal distress, anaemia, infections, maternal β-stimulation, and fetal thyrotoxicosis. The importance of sinus tachycardia is in recognising and treating the underlying cause.

Atrial flutter is sustained by a circular macro–re-entrant pathway that is completely contained within the atrial wall. The atrioventricular node is not part of the re-entry circuit, but serves to transmit the atrial flutter waves to the ventricles. The atrial rate typically exceeds 300 beats per minute, which is sufficiently fast that only every second or third atrial re-entrant wave is conducted through the atrioventricular node, producing ventricular rates of between 150 and 250 beats per minute. Management of atrial flutter aims to terminate the atrial re-entrant circuit, or to delay atrioventricular nodal conduction to achieve a more physiologic fetal heart rate, with improved cardiac filling and output.

Reasons for Fetal Care

There is extensive experience in the management of fetal supraventricular tachycardia and atrial flutter, while data on fetal ventricular tachycardia and junctional ectopic tachycardia is limited to a handful of case reports. Irrespective of the arrhythmic mechanism, three options can be considered if a fetal tachyarrhythmia is detected. The first is not to attempt treatment. The second option is to institute intra-uterine pharmacological therapy, while the third option is to deliver the fetus and opt for neonatal care. The choice should be based on the condition of the fetus; the characteristics of the arrhythmia in terms of duration, heart rate, and mechanism; the gestational age; the condition of the mother; and the willingness of the mother to undergo treatment. The benefits and risks of the different options must be discussed with both the parents.

In the non-hydropic fetus with a new diagnosis of an intermittent, or even persistent, tachyarrhythmia after 35 weeks of gestation, observation without anti-arrhythmic pharmacologic therapy may be a safe approach, because hydrops will rarely develop, presumably due to improved intrinsic myocardial properties of the fetal heart during late gestation. On the other hand, pharmacological control of the arrhythmia will facilitate vaginal delivery by allowing the interpretation of the tracings showing the fetal heart rate during labour. If close monitoring without treatment is not feasible, delivery by caesarian section and postnatal conversion to sinus rhythm is the usual choice.

Prior to 35 weeks of gestation, the risks associated with premature delivery probably outweigh the potential hazards of pharmacological treatment to the mother and the fetus. Treatment with drugs aims prenatally to control the disturbance of rhythm in order to prevent or treat fetal cardiac failure. Irrespective of the mechanism of tachycardia and the underlying fetal heart rate, the likelihood of heart failure increases if the tachycardia is incessant and if the fetus has a lower gestational age at diagnosis.[4] It is well established, nonetheless, that an intermittent arrhythmia pattern may also result in fetal hydrops and death.[5] As a consequence, intra-uterine treatment with drugs is offered to the majority of fetuses encountered with intermittent and incessant tachyarrhythmia, even in the absence of fetal compromise. Still, for those cases presenting with only brief and occasional runs of tachycardia in the absence of haemodynamic impairment, abstention from pharmacological treatment and close monitoring for signs of progression may be a valid option, as the arrhythmia often resolves spontaneously.

While antiarrhythmic drugs are usually well-tolerated, some of the most commonly used agents, such as digoxin and flecainide, have narrow margins between levels in the serum that are therapeutic, and those that may be associated with toxicity. In addition, virtually all antiarrhythmic agents have proarrhythmic potentials to provoke new, or to exacerbate existing, arrhythmias. These risks must be factored into a common-sense analysis of risk versus benefit. To our knowledge, no serious maternal complications owing to transplacental or direct fetal anti-arrhythmic pharmacological therapy have been reported thus far in the medical literature. The rate of mortality of treated non-hydropic fetuses with supraventricular tachycardia or atrial flutter ranges between 0% and 5%, whereas up to one-fifth of hydropic fetuses will have a fatal outcome. Comprehensive data on the outcome of untreated fetal tachyarrhythmia is not available.

Treatment

There is no single medication that can safely and effectively convert all fetal tachyarrhythmias to a normal rhythm. In the absence of such a magic bullet, schemes for management are frequently based on personal preferences and experiences, and thus may significantly differ among institutions. In Table 12-2, we illustrate the pharmacokinetics and risks of agents that are commonly used to treat fetal tachyarrhythmias, while in Table 12-3 we list the published experience with first and second lines of drugs used for treatment, discussing these features later in the text.

TABLE 12-2

CARDIOVASCULAR DRUGS USED PRENATALLY, SHOWING THE INDICATIONS FOR TREATMENT, DOSAGES, AND POSSIBLE SIDE-EFFECTS

Drug	Fetal Indications	Dosage and Therapeutic Concentrations	F:M Ratio	Maternal Effects	Fetal and Neonatal Effects
Digoxin	SVT, AF	Oral loading: 0.5 mg q 12h over 2 days Oral maintenance: 0.25–0.75 mg/day TC: 1–2.5 ng/mL	0.8–1 ↓ in hydrops	Narrow therapeutic range; Nausea, anorexia, disturbed vision, fatigue, sinus bradycardia, AV block, VT	Contraindicated in WPW syndrome (not known prenatally)
Flecainide	SVT, AF	Oral 100 mg q 8h (q 6h) TC: 0.2–1 μg/mL	0.7–0.9	Proarrhythmia, blurred vision, nausea, paresthesia, headache, negative inotropy	Proarrhythmia, negative inotropy
Sotalol	SVT, AF, VT	Oral 80 mg q 12h–160 mg q 8h	0.7–2.9	Proarrhythmia, bradycardia, fatigue, hypotension, dizziness	Proarrhythmia, bradycardia
Amiodarone	SVT, VT	Oral loading: 1.6–2.4 g/day for 2–7 days Oral maintenance: 200–400 mg/day Direct: 2.5–5 mg/kg fetal weight IV over 10 min TC: Amiodarone: 1–2.5 μg/mL; DEA: 2 x ↑	0.1– 0.3 ↓ in hydrops	Proarrhythmia, bradycardia, lung fibrosis, thyroid dysfunction, hepatitis, photosensitivity; corneal micro-deposits, neuropathy, myopathy	Proarrhythmia, transient thyroid dysfunction, growth restriction
Propranolol	Thyrotoxicosis	Oral 60–120 mg q 6–8h	0.9–1.3	Bradycardia, AV block, fatigue, hypotension, worsening of diabetes, bronchospasm, cold extremities	Growth restriction, bradycardia, respiratory depression, hypoglycemia
Propylthiouracil	Thyrotoxicosis	Oral 50–200 mg/day Aim: lowest effective dose to maintain maternal FTI in high normal range	1.9	Agranulocytosis, nausea, vomiting, loss of taste, skin rash, itching, drowsiness, dizziness, headache	Risk of hypothyroidism; goiter
Dexamethasone	Immune-mediated AV block; EFE	Transplacental: 8 mg/day for 2 weeks; 4 mg/day – 30 weeks; 2 mg/day – delivery Postnatal (for carditis and EFE): prednisone for 6–8 weeks	0.3	Adrenal gland suppression, weight gain, fluid retention, hypertension, mood changes, insomnia, irritability, striae, hair growth, diabetes, impaired wound-healing, susceptibility to infections	Oligohydramnios, growth restriction, impaired wound-healing, (?) delayed brain development
β-agonists	Immune-mediated AV block	Oral salbutamol: 10 mg q 8h (–6h) (maximal dose: 40 mg/day) Oral terbutaline: 2.5–7.5 mg q 4–6 h (maximal dose: 30 mg/day)	0.5	Palpitation, tremor, diaphoresis, dyspnea, hyperglycemia, chest pain, nausea, nervousness, dizziness, arrhythmias	Neonatal hypoglycemia
Immune-globulin	Immune-mediated AV block; EFE	Maternal: 1 g/kg IVIG every 2–3 weeks (maximal dose: 70 g/dose) Neonatal: single dose of 1 g/kg IVIG + prednisone for 6–8 weeks	↑ with age	Headache, chest pain, fever, chills, nausea, malaise, anaphylaxis (rare), aseptic meningitis	Not reported

AF, atrial flutter; AV, atrioventricular; DEA, desethylamiodarone; EFE, endocardial fibroelastosis; FTI, free thyroxin index; F:M ratio, fetal to maternal fetal ratio; IVIG, intravenous immunoglobulin; SVT, supraventricular tachycardia; TC, therapeutic concentrations; VT, ventricular tachycardia.

TABLE 12-3

PUBLISHED EXPERIENCE ON TRANSPLACENTAL PHARMACOLOGICAL TREATMENT OF FETAL TACHYARRHYTHMIA

Authors	Case Numbers	Age	Hydrops	Medication	Choice	1 Drug	≥2 Drugs	Rhythm Control	Fetal Outcome	Maternal Events
Kleinman et al[9]	14 SVT	24–28	Yes: 13	Digoxin	First	6		4/6 (67)		
				+ various drugs	Second		2	5/6 (83)		
				Digoxin + verapamil	First		6	5/6 (83)		1: AV-block after verapamil
	3 AF; 1 Afib	30–38	Yes: 3	Digoxin + propranol	First		2	1/2 (50)		
				Digoxin	First	2		1/2 (50)	1 FD (H)	
				+ verapamil	Second		1	0/1 (0)		
Van Engelen et al[10]	34 SVT, 16 AF	n/m	No: 14	Digoxin	First	14		10/14 (71)		
			Yes: 10	Digoxin	First	10	7	1/10 (10)	1 FD; 1 NND (2H)	
				+ various drugs	Second			7/7 (100)		
Frohn-Mulder et al[11]	36 SVT; 14 AF	16–41	No: 22	Digoxin	First	22		16/22 (73)		
			Yes: 6	Digoxin	First	6		1/6 (17)	3 FD; 2 NND (5H)	
Simpson and Sharland[12]	105 SVT; 22 AF	21–36	No: 63	Digoxin	First	63		39/63 (62)	2 FD	
				+ various drugs	Second		17	13/17 (76)	1 FD	
			Yes: 46	Digoxin	First	5		1/5 (20)	1 FD (H)	
				Digoxin + verapamil	First		14	8/14 (57)	1 FD; 1 NND (2H)	
				Digoxin + flecainide	First		27	16/27 (59)		
Jaeggi et al[3]	19 short VA SVT	20–38	Yes: 3	Digoxin	First	14		9/14 (64)	1 FD (H)#	
				+ sotalol	Second		4	3/4 (75)		
	4 long VA SVT	24–34	Yes: 1	Digoxin	First	4		0/4 (0)		
				+ sotalol	Second		3	2/3 (66)		
Ebenroth et al[13]	34 SVT; 6 AF	n/a	Yes: 5	Digoxin	First	37		17/37 (46)		
				+ flecainide	Second		13	12/13 (92)		
Krapp et al[24]	24 SVT	26–36	Yes: 15	Digoxin	First	24		4/24 (24)		
				+ verapamil	Second		6	0/6 (0)		
				Digoxin + flecainide	First/second		20	19/20 (95)		
Fouron et al[15]	5 short VA SVT	29–35	No: 4	Digoxin		4		4/4 (100)		
		22	Yes: 1	Sotalol + digoxin			1	1/1 (100)		
	6 AF	27–36	Yes: 1	Digoxin	First	4		3/4 (75)		
			Yes: 1	Digoxin + sotalol	First		2	1/2 (50)	1 NND	
Jaeggi et al[16]	15 AF	27–38	Yes: 0	Digoxin	First	11		5/11 (45)		
				+ various drugs			2	0/2 (0)		
Allan et al[18]	12 SVT; 2 AF	23–36	Yes: 9	Flecainide	First	14		12/14 (86)	1 FD†	
Van Engelen et al[10]	34 SVT, 16 AF	n/a	No: 5	Flecainide	First	5		5/5 (100)		
			Yes: 5	Flecainide	First	5	3	2/5 (40)		2: vision anomaly + dizziness
				+ various drugs	Second			2/3 (66)		

Frohn-Mulder et al[11]	36 SVT; 14 AF	16–41	Yes: 7	Flecainide	First	7		3/7 (43)	1 ND (H)	
Simpson and Sharland[12]	105 SVT; 22 AF	21–36	Yes: 27	Flecainide	First	27		16/27 (56)	4 FD†, 1 NND (5H)	
				+ various drugs	Second		4	4/4 (100)	1 FD, 2 NND (3H)	
				+ direct treatment	Second		2	1/2 (50)		
Joannic et al[14]	22 SVT; 4 AF	19–37	Yes: 26	Flecainide	First	12		7/12 (58)	1 FD; 1 TOP; 1 NND (3H)	
Oudijk et al[17]	10 SVT	21–37	Yes: 5	Sotalol	First	10		4/10 (40)	3 FD (2H)	1: nausea
				+ digoxin	Second		3	6/10 (60)		1: dizziness
	10 AF		Yes: 3	Sotalol	First	10		5/10 (50)	1 FD (H)	
				+ digoxin	Second		4	8/10 (80)		
Oudijk et al[27]	9 SVT	n/m	Yes: 1	Sotalol	First	7		6/7 (86)	1 FD (H)	No
				Sotalol + digoxin	First		2	2/2 (100)		
	9 AF		Yes: 1	Sotalol	First	7		7/7 (100)		
				Sotalol + digoxin	First		2	0/2 (0)	1 NND (H)	
Fouron et al[15]	5 long VA SVT	31	Yes: 2	Sotalol	First	1		1/1 (100)		
		22–35		Sotalol + digoxin	First		3	3/3 (100)		No
Sonesson et al[29]	14 SVT	24–35	Yes: 8	Digoxin + sotalol	Second		14	10/14 (71)	2 FD (2H)#	No
Strasburger et al[31]	15 SVT; 9 AF		Yes: 24	Amiodarone	First	1		SVT 14/15 (93)	5 transient thyroid dysfunction	1: slow HR
	1 VT; 1 JET			Other drugs + amiodarone	Second/third		25	AF 3/9 (33)		6: AV-block
								other 2/2 (100)		1: rash
Joannic et al[14]	22 SVT; 4 AF	19–37	Yes: 26	Amiodarone	First	4		2/4 (50)	1 TOP; 1 FD (2 H)	
				Amiodarone	Second		9	5/9 (56)	2 hypothyroidism	

AET, atrial ectopic tachycardia; AF, atrial flutter; Afib, atrial fibrillation; AVB, incomplete AV block; L, loading dose; FD, fetal demise; FD (H), fetal demise associated with hydrops; JET, junctional ectopic tachycardia; M, maintenance dose; NND, neonatal death; n/m, data not mentioned; PJRT, permanent junctional reciprocating tachycardia; SVT, supraventricular tachycardia; TOP, pregnancy termination; VT, ventricular tachycardia; Yes, indicates total number of hydropic fetuses; †, #, same case of fetal demise reported in different studies.

Because of the risk of hazardous complications, each antiarrhythmic treatment other than digoxin should probably be started in an inpatient setting to allow serial monitoring of the maternal electrocardiogram and the fetal cardiac rhythm. To exclude unsafe maternal conditions, such as long-QT syndrome for class III agents, or ventricular pre-excitation for digoxin, the pregnant mother should undergo a detailed medical examination, a 12-lead electrocardiogram, and testing of the electrolytes in the maternal serum prior to administration of any medication. Thyroid function should be checked if fetal hyperthyroidism is suspected, or if treatment with amiodarone is considered. The risk of dangerous side-effects may be further reduced by restricting treatment whenever possible to a single agent, and by avoiding excessive dosages, toxic concentrations, or potentially hazardous combinations, if additional pharmacological treatment is required.

Choice of Drug

A clear understanding of the pharmacokinetics, actions, and indications of the handful of clinically relevant pharmaceuticals is essential if the tachycardia is to be treated efficiently and safely.

Digoxin

Digoxin is the preferred choice for fetal atrioventricular re-entrant tachycardia and atrial flutter in the absence of fetal hydrops. The drug has two main effects. First, it induces vagal slowing of the sinus node and atrioventricular nodal conduction, and second, it enhances myocardial contractility. The positive inotropic effect is the result of an inhibition of the sodium-potassium adenosine triphosphatase pump, which leads to an increase in the level of sodium ions in the myocytes, triggering a rise in the intracellular level of calcium ions by the exchange of sodium and calcium ions.

Dosing and Pharmacokinetics

Oral or intravenous maternal digoxin loading is recommended for more urgent fetal indications. A standard oral loading dose of digoxin is 0.5 mg given twice daily for 2 days, followed by a maintenance dose of from 0.25 to 0.75 mg daily, aiming at achieving maternal concentrations at the upper therapeutic range, namely 2 to 2.5 ng/mL. When no loading dose is given, steady-state concentrations are achieved after 5 to 7 days on maintenance therapy. Approximately four-fifths of the tablet form is absorbed from the gastrointestinal tract, and one quarter of the drug is bound to plasma proteins. Elimination occurs via the kidneys, and adjustment of dosage is required in the setting of maternal renal failure. Digoxin readily crosses the placenta, reaching similar concentrations in the fetal and maternal serums. The transplacental passage of the drug is hampered in the setting of fetal hydrops, and adequate levels are usually not obtained in the fetal serum.[6]

Interactions

There are numerous known interactions, including those with amiodarone and flecainide, both of which increase the levels of digoxin.

Adverse Effects and Precautions

Use of digoxin is contraindicated in the settings of Wolff-Parkinson-White syndrome, higher-degree atrioventricular block, and hypertrophic obstructive cardiomyopathy. The incidence of undesired symptoms correlates with the concentration of the drug achieved in the plasma. In the elderly adult treated with digoxin for cardiac conditions, adverse effects include loss of appetite, nausea, vomiting, diarrhoea, blurred vision, confusion, drowsiness, dizziness, nightmares, agitation, and depression. Uncommon symptoms are acute psychosis, delirium, amnesia, atrial or ventricular tachycardia, and atrioventricular block. No major adverse events have been reported during pregnancy.

Treatment of the Fetus

Successful transplacental treatment of fetal supraventricular tachycardia with digoxin was first reported in 1980.[7,8] The first larger case series reporting efficacy in reversing fetal supraventricular tachycardia to a normal rhythm was published 5 years later,[9] conversion to a normal rhythm being achieved in seven-tenths of cases with digoxin given either alone to the mother, or in combination with another antiarrhythmic drug. Similar results were obtained by others,[3,10–14] albeit that the rate of success declined to one-tenth if there was fetal hydrops.[10] Apart from fetal hydrops, digoxin administered transplacentally is less effective for atrial ectopic tachycardia and permanent junctional reciprocating tachycardia, while it is most efficient in atrioventricular re-entrant tachycardia.[3,15] The drug slows atrioventricular conduction and the rate of tachycardia in fetuses with atrial flutter, but is less likely to restore a normal cardiac rhythm when compared to sotalol alone, or to the combination of digoxin and sotalol.[16,17] Digoxin, therefore, is a safe and reasonably efficient first line of transplacental therapy for atrioventricular re-entrant tachycardia, the most common cause of persistent fetal tachycardia. In the presence of hydrops, atrial flutter, atrial ectopic, and permanent junctional reciprocating tachycardia, class 1c or class III agents either alone, or combined with digoxin, are more effective therapeutic choices.

Flecainide

Flecainide is the most extensively used class Ic agent for treatment of fetal supraventricular tachycardia. The drug blocks slow sodium channels, causing prolongation of the cardiac action potential. The electrophysiological effect is slowing of the electrical conduction in the His-Purkinje system and ventricular myocardium, along with reduction in ventricular contractility. The blocking effect on the cardiac sodium channels increases as the heart rate increases. This means that flecainide is potentially most useful to break an abnormal rhythm associated with a rapid heart rate.

Dosing and Pharmacokinetics

To treat a fetal arrhythmia, the standard oral dosage of flecainide is 300 mg/day, given in three doses. The drug is well-absorbed, and peak levels are obtained within 2 to 4 hours. A small amount of the drug is bio-transformed in the liver to nearly inactive metabolites. Flecainide is primarily excreted in the urine. The drug crosses the placenta readily, even in the presence of fetal hydrops.[18,19] Therapeutic levels in the mother are reached within 3 days of commencing treatment.

Interactions

There are numerous interactions with other agents. Amiodarone, for example, may increase the levels of flecainide by inhibiting cytochrome 450, which is used to metabolise flecainide. Flecainide increases the concentration of digoxin by about one-fifth.

Adverse Effects and Precautions

Flecainide depresses cardiac performance, particularly in patients with compromised myocardial function. The chance of proarrhythmia increases in the presence of major structural cardiac disease, ventricular dysfunction, ventricular arrhythmias, and hypokalemia.[20,21] Thus, flecainide should be avoided in individuals with any of these conditions. Flecainide can safely be used in predominantly healthy mothers carrying fetuses with supraventricular tachycardia.[22] Adverse events such as blurred vision, dizziness, headache, nausea, paresthesia, fatigue, tremor, and nervousness were uncommon in a placebo-controlled trial.[23] No major maternal side-effects are reported.[12–14,24]

Trans-placental Treatment

When used as the drug of choice, flecainide controlled supraventricular tachycardia and atrial flutter in two-thirds of cases.[10–12,14,18] This improved to almost four-fifths if a second antiarrhythmic drug was added.[14] No maternal adverse effects were observed, but one-quarter of fetuses died either during fetal life or as neonates. Severe fetal bradycardia causing death was observed in one fetus with only mild ascites shortly after commencing treatment with flecainide.[14] Control in excess of nine-tenths of cases was observed when flecainide and digoxin were used in combination.[13,24] When given at therapeutic doses, therefore, flecainide provides safe and effective treatment for fetal supraventricular tachycardia. When flecainide was the preferred choice to treat hydropic fetuses, however, around one-sixth of fetuses died in the perinatal period.

Sotalol

Sotalol is used to treat both fetal supraventricular tachycardia and atrial flutter. No data exist on its use in fetal ventricular tachycardia. The actions of sotalol include those of both class II agents, providing non-selective β-blockade, and class III effects, with prolongation of the duration of the cardiac action potential. The drug inhibits inward potassium channels, progressively prolonging refractoriness of the working myocardial and conduction tissues at slower heart rates.[25] Clinically, this may mean that the prolongation of the action potential is more effective at preventing the initiation of a tachycardia than in terminating one once established. Sotalol exhibits a positive inotropic effect, particularly at a slower heart rate.[26] The β-blocking potency of sotalol is up to half of that of propranolol when compared milligram per milligram. Beta-blockade decreases the heart rate, and delays atrioventricular nodal conduction.

Dosing and Pharmacokinetics

To treat the fetus, the typical starting dose given to the mother is 160 mg per day, given in two doses. If there is fetal hydrops, we would commence with 320 mg per day, either alone or in combination with digoxin. If there is no conversion to a normal rhythm within several days of administration, we would increase the dose further to a maximal daily level of 480 mg, given in three doses. The drug is completely absorbed and peak concentration in the plasma is reached within 2 to 4 hours of oral administration. The compound is secreted in the urine, and it may be necessary to regulate the dose in mothers with renal failure. Placental transfer is excellent, and the drug does not accumulate in the fetus.[27]

Adverse Effects

The most feared adverse effect is torsade de pointes, which may present with a range of clinical symptoms from palpitations to syncope to sudden death. The incidence of ventricular proarrhythmia in adults with supraventricular tachycardia is less than 2%. Probably the most effective way to prevent maternal proarrhythmia is by avoiding excessive prolongation of the QTc interval.[25] The prevalence of maternal electrocardiographic changes is unknown, but no significant prolongation of the neonatal QTc interval has been found after administration of up to 480 mg per day to the mother for treatment of fetal supraventricular tachycardia.[27] Adverse effects related to the β-blocking properties include arterial hypotension, bradycardia, worsening of asthma or obstructive lung disease, depression, fatigue, insomnia, and impaired sexual function. Its safety was assessed in a randomised, double-blind trial in adults,[28] with one-twentieth of patients discontinuing the drug because of side-effects related to β-blockade.

Treatment of the Fetus

When used as a first line agent, the drug controlled supraventricular tachycardia and atrial flutter in two-thirds of fetuses.[15,17,27] Higher rates of conversion to a normal rhythm were observed when sotalol was started jointly with digoxin when the arrhythmia was diagnosed, or eventually used as a combination to treat resistant supraventricular tachycardia.[3,17,19,29] Transient maternal side-effects, such as nausea, dizziness, and fatigue, were reported in one-tenth of mothers.[17] Conflicting data exist on the role in the fetus, even from the same investigators.[17,27] When used as a first line agent, however, the drug was shown to convert over nine-tenths of fetuses with supraventricular tachycardia or atrial flutter to a normal rhythm. Sotalol, therefore, is an efficient and safe drug with which to treat fetal supraventricular tachycardia and atrial flutter when there are no maternal contraindications to its actions. The overall rate of perinatal death in fetuses treated with transplacental sotalol was 18%.

Amiodarone

Amiodarone has mainly been used to treat drug-resistant fetal tachyarrhythmias associated with cardiovascular compromise. There is considerable data documenting its efficacy and reasonable safety in children and adults with supraventricular and ventricular tachycardias. The drug, which acts by blocking the potassium channels, lengthens the duration of the action potential and cardiac refractoriness at all heart rates. It also acts to produce β-blockade, to block the L-type calcium channels, and to slow His-Purkinje and myocardial conduction at rapid heart rates. It does not affect ventricular contractility.

Dosing and Pharmacokinetics

To achieve therapeutic fetal concentrations, oral loading doses of from 1600 to 2400 mg per day are given to the mother for from 2 to 7 days, followed by maintenance doses of 200 to 400 mg per day.[14,30,31] The drug has unusual pharmacokinetics, with absorption of the drug given orally ranging from one-third to two-thirds, and peak concentrations in the plasma being reached within 3 to 7 hours of ingestion. Amiodarone is metabolised in the liver to its major metabolite, desethylamiodarone, which also has antiarrhythmic properties. Because of their lipophilicity, the compounds accumulate in many tissues, including fat, liver, lung, skin, and myocardium. Excretion is predominantly via shedding of epithelial cells of the skin and gastrointestinal tract. The half-life for elimination is between 3 and 10 days for the first 50% of the drug, and is then slower due to slowed release from tissue stores.

As a consequence, clinically important levels may persist for several months following cessation of administration. Amiodarone and desethylamiodarone incompletely cross the placenta to the fetus, with only one-sixth reaching the fetus for amiodarone, albeit a somewhat higher ratio existing for desethylamiodarone.[32] Transplacental transfer is reduced still further in hydropic fetuses.[33]

Interactions

Amiodarone interferes with the pharmacokinetics of a large variety of drugs, such as digoxin, class Ic agents, tricyclic antidepressants, and general anaesthetics. Doses of most other drugs need to be reduced in individuals taking amiodarone.

Adverse Effects

Amiodarone has numerous side-effects. The most serious reaction is interstitial lung disease, which occurs in up to one-tenth of adults receiving doses of amiodarone greater than 400 mg per day over prolonged periods of time. Pulmonary fibrosis has also been documented during therapy at low doses and short duration. Clinical findings suggesting pulmonary toxicity include coughing, dyspnea, fever, chest pain, high sedimentation rates, and bilateral lung infiltrates. If diagnosed at an early stage, the disease may be reversible. Due to the high iodine content, and the structural similarity of amiodarone to thyroxine, thyroid dysfunction is common, being found in almost one-tenth of chronically treated individuals. Asymptomatic, reversible corneal microdeposits are almost universally present if the drug is taken for at least 6 months. Hepatitis may also occur. As a precaution, periodic ophthalmic, hepatic and thyroid function tests are recommended for patients receiving amiodarone. There is a low risk of torsade de pointes, which can be minimised by keeping the QTc interval in a near-normal range. Adverse fetal effects attributable to amiodarone include congenital hypo- and hyper-thyroidism, retardation of growth, bradycardia, and prolongation of the QTc interval.

Treatment of the Fetus

Transplacental amiodarone has been shown to restore sinus rhythm in two-thirds of hydropic fetuses with drug-refractory tachyarrhythmias.[14,31] Of the treated fetuses, one-twentieth died, and side-effects serious enough to withdraw the drug occurred in one woman, who suffered photosensitivity dermatitis and thrombocytopenia. Transient biochemical signs of thyroid dysfunction were seen in one-fifth of both fetuses and mothers. Other maternal side-effects were mild sinus bradycardia and transient incomplete atrioventricular block during loading with the drug. Because of the maternal and fetal risks, therefore, amiodarone should be reserved for drug-refractory fetal tachyarrhythmias in hydropic fetuses with ventricular dysfunction.

Direct Fetal Treatment

Direct fetal treatment is reserved for the rare, severely hydropic fetus with a drug-refractory tachyarrhythmia. As mentioned previously, the transplacental transfer of some antiarrhythmic agents is significantly hampered in the presence of fetal hydrops, and thus therapeutic levels of drugs may not be reached even with toxic maternal doses. To overcome this problem, repeated intravenous, intramuscular and intraperitoneal fetal injections of amiodarone, digoxin and adenosine, in addition to the conventional therapy, has been successfully performed to resolve multi-drug refractory fetal tachyarrhythmia complicated by fetal hydrops.[33–38] Direct intravenous adenosine may instantly terminate re-entrant supraventricular tachycardia, but because of its short duration of action, direct treatment should be combined with a longer acting antiarrhythmic agent. Amiodarone seems to be predestined for the direct use, both because of its efficiency and long-half life, limiting the number of invasive fetal procedures that are required to maintain therapeutic levels.

Other Antiarrhythmic Agents

Other antiarrhythmic agents, such as verapamil, procainamide, and quinidine are no longer used for prenatal therapy, because of substantial side-effects in both mother and fetus, and/or insufficient antiarrhythmic actions. By contrast, maternal intravenous infusion of magnesium and lidocaine, a blocker of the sodium channel that shortens the duration of the QT interval, has been used to suppress fetal torsades de pointes associated with congenital long QT syndrome diagnosed prenatally by fetal magnetocardiography.[39]

Summarising the published results, digoxin remains a drug of choice in the treatment of fetal atrioventricular re-entrant tachycardia in the absence of fetal hydrops, although some centers nowadays favour more potent and equally safe medication. In terms of converting atrial flutter to sinus rhythm, sotalol appears to be more effective than digoxin. In the setting of fetal hydrops, a class Ic or class III drug, either alone or in combination with digoxin, is the preferred treatment for supraventricular tachycardia, with the most favourable outcomes reported for amiodarone. The primary use of amiodarone, an antiarrhythmic agent with no negative inotropy, should be considered if the fetal myocardial contractility is severely hampered. Control of the rate of tachycardia, or conversion to sinus rhythm, is achieved in the majority of cases within a few days of transplacental treatment with a single drug, or with combinations of therapeutic agents. Once the arrhythmia is under control, the antiarrhythmic treatment is usually maintained to birth, with weekly monitoring of the fetal heart rate to detect arrhythmic recurrence. If supraventricular tachycardia recurs spontaneously after birth, or is easily inducible, for example by transoesophageal electrophysiological study, the antiarrhythmic treatment, usually with a β-blocker, will be continued for at least 6 to 12 months. In up to one-fifth of infants, the supraventricular tachycardia will persist beyond 1 year of age. In contrast, postnatal recurrence of atrial flutter is uncommon, and antiarrhythmic long-term prophylaxis is usually not required.[16,40]

FETAL THYROTOXICOSIS

Thyrotoxicosis, induced by maternal thyroid-stimulating antibodies, should always be considered if the fetus of a mother with active Graves' disease, or with a history of Graves' disease, presents with a persistent tachycardia of 180 to 200 beats per minute. Other findings in the fetus include hydrops, restriction of growth, and goiter.[41] Fetal ultrasonography is helpful in assessing both the fetal goiter and growth. The diagnosis of maternal Graves' disease is suggested by physical signs, such as prominent eyes, an enlarged thyroid gland, and exaggerated reflexes, and is confirmed by finding markedly elevated levels of thyroid hormone. Because fetal tachycardia and restricted growth may result from other pathological processes, some have advocated sampling of umbilical blood to measure the levels of thyroid-stimulating antibodies, thyroid-stimulating hormone, and FT_4 for definitive diagnosis.[42] The risk of fetal mortality and severe complications is high if thyrotoxicosis goes unrecognised and untreated.

Treatment

The mainstay of prenatal treatment is inhibition of the excessive fetal synthesis of thyroid hormone by propylthiouracil and slowing of the fetal heart rate by β-blockade (see Table 12-2).

Propylthiouracil

Propylthiouracil does not affect the release of thyroxin, and therefore the rapidity of response to treatment depends on the amount of colloid stored in the thyroid gland. The drug is generally well-tolerated, with side-effects occurring in about 1% of treated adults. Adverse events are mainly related to the skin, and include rash, itching, abnormal loss of hair, and dermal pigmentation. Agranulocytosis, nausea, vomiting, loss of taste, joint or muscle aches, numbness and headache are other possible reactions. The agent crosses the placenta and may produce fetal hypothyroidism even if administered in relatively low doses.[42] To limit the risk, treatment with propylthiouracil should be titrated to the lowest possible dose to maintain the maternal index for free thyroid in the high normal range. The fetal response can be monitored by serial measurement of the fetal heart rate, and by direct measurement of T_4 and thyroid-stimulating hormone in the fetal cord blood. Ultrasonography may permit assessment of changes in the size of the thyroid gland. Infants born to mothers with Graves' disease should be closely followed by a paediatrician to assess any thyroidal dysfunction. No long-term effects on intellectual or physical development from propylthiouracil or drug-induced hypothyroidism have been reported.[43]

Propranolol

Maternal propranolol, or a similar β-blocker, is used to slow the fetal sinus tachycardia, thus reducing the risk of high-output cardiac failure. Propranolol is rapidly and completely absorbed, with levels peaking in the plasma from 1 to 3 hours after oral ingestion. Despite complete absorption, propranolol has a variable bioavailability due to extensive hepatic first-pass metabolism. The agent is highly lipophilic, achieving high concentrations in the brain. The commonly observed side-effects of the drug are explained by spasm of smooth muscle, exaggerated cardiac actions, and effects on the central nervous system. Beta-blockade is contraindicated in the presence of severe bradycardia, high-degree atrioventricular block, severe asthma, or bronchospasm, Raynaud's phenomenon, and other peripheral vasculopathies. The drug readily crosses the placenta. Pharmacological β-blockade is considered relatively safe for the fetus, although a number of side-effects have been reported in neonates following the use of propranolol in pregnancy. These include restricted growth, hypoglycemia, bradycardia, and respiratory depression.[44] Thus, newborns of women consuming the drug close to delivery should be observed during the first days of life for symptoms of excessive β-blockade.

IMMUNE-MEDIATED FETAL ATRIOVENTRICULAR BLOCK

Atrioventricular block refers to a disturbance of the normal conduction of the electrical impulse through the atrioventricular node, the bundle of His, and/or the bundle branches. Depending on the severity of the blockage, the conduction is either delayed, producing first-degree atrioventricular block, intermittently conducted, giving second-degree block, conducted in alternative fashion to produce 2 to 1 atrioventricular block, or completely interrupted, producing third-degree block. Complete atrioventricular block, with independently beating atriums and ventricles, is the most common fetal presentation of conduction disorders, accounting for almost two-fifths of major fetal arrhythmias. The cardiac output is compromised by the slowed ventricular rate, by the loss of the normal atrial contribution to ventricular filling, and by co-existing structural or functional cardiovascular pathology.

In roughly half of prenatally diagnosed cases, complete atrioventricular block is associated with left isomerism of the atrial appendages or congenitally corrected transposition.[45,46] Conduction block associated with structural heart disease results from anatomical discontinuity of the electrical conduction system, either due to an initial lack of fusion of the atrial and ventricular components, or due to a secondary interruption of the atrioventricular conduction axis.[47–49] The outcome of left isomerism complicated by congenital complete heart block is particularly poor, with less than one-tenth of afflicted fetuses surviving to infancy. Transplacental treatment with a β-sympathomimetic agent to increase the fetal cardiac output has not improved the outcome of these fetuses.[45,46,50–52]

In some fetuses having heart block without congenital cardiac disease or maternal auto-antibodies, interruption of the His bundle was found on necropsy.[53] As an isolated disorder, nonetheless, congenital atrioventricular block is strongly linked to mothers with auto-antibodies to 48-kDa SSB/La, 52-kDa and/or 60-kDa SSA/Ro ribonucleoproteins. These antibodies are prevalent in nearly 2% of predominantly asymptomatic pregnant women.[54] The maternal IgG antibodies increasingly enter the fetal circulation during gestation, and may elicit an immune-mediated reaction, resulting in the progressive destruction of the fetal atrioventricular node, cardiac and extracardiac inflammation, endocardial fibroelastosis, and dilated cardiomyopathy in the susceptible offspring.[45,55,56,57] Diffuse deposition of immune-globulins, and infiltration of T-cells throughout the myocardium, leading to endocardial fibroelastosis, may occur in the absence of congenital heart block.[5] Complete atrioventricular block, the most common cardiac manifestation, affects about 1% to 2% of antibody-positive mothers, while the risk of recurrence for subsequent fetuses ranges from one-tenth to one-fifth.[55,58] Complete atrioventricular block is most commonly detected between 20 and 24 weeks of gestation, but a presentation later during the course of pregnancy, or even after birth, is not exceptional.[55] To this day, there is no reliable marker that predicts which fetus, in the absence of early anomalies, will eventually develop immune-mediated complications.

Reasons for Treatment

Untreated fetuses with isolated congenital complete atrioventricular block have a perinatal mortality of up to two-fifths.[45,53,55,59] Risk factors for death included the echocardiographic documentation of fetal hydrops, endocardial fibroelastosis, a ventricular rate below 55 beats per minute, as well as premature delivery. Hydrops, endocardial fibroelastosis, and/or a heart rate below 55 beats per minute were found in one-tenth, one-quarter, and two-fifths, respectively, of fetuses referred with isolated complete atrioventricular block to the Hospital for Sick Children, Toronto, between 1990 and 2003.[60] In one-quarter of the more severely affected cases, symptoms associated with a poor outcome became apparent, or developed, only later in pregnancy. The diagnosis of antibody-mediated myocarditis, hepatitis, and dilated cardiomyopathy was made only after delivery in cases that had been managed without prenatal anti-inflammatory treatment. These factors have led to the routine use of dexamethasone in pregnancies complicated by isolated fetal complete heart block.[60] The routine administration of transplacental glucocorticoids for fetal atrioventricular block, however, is controversial, because of concerns of toxic steroid effects on the developing fetus, and because survival is often possible without prenatal intervention. Thus, an alternative approach could be to restrict transplacental treatment to the compromised fetus.[51,61] On the other hand, the value of such an approach is unknown apart from a handful of anecdotal case reports.

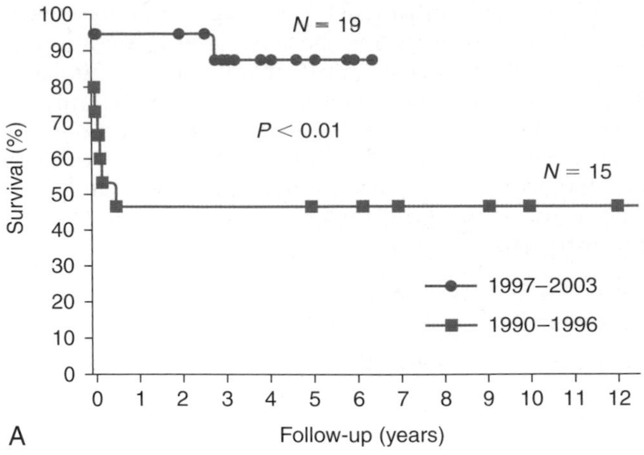

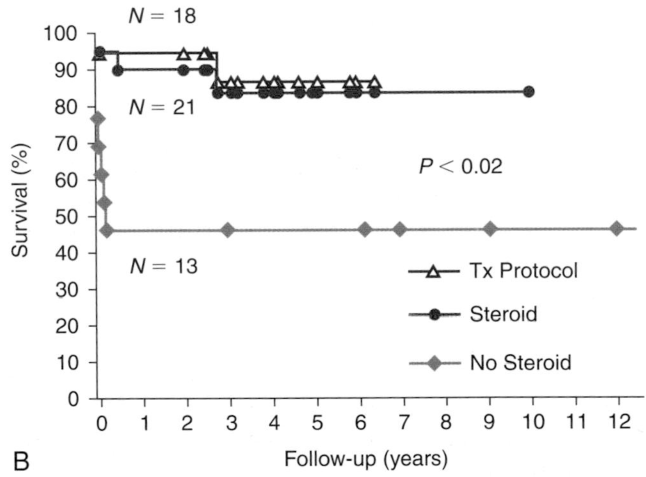

Figure 12-1 The impact of transplacental fetal treatment with (Steroid) and without (No Steroid) dexamethasone on fetal and postnatal outcome. The survival was best with the protocol-guided approach (Tx Protocol) introduced in 1997. (Reproduced with permission from Jaeggi ET, Fouron JC, Silverman ED, et al: Transplacental treatment improves the outcome of prenatally diagnosed complete atrioventricular block without structural heart disease. Circulation 2004;110:1542–1548.)

Choice of Treatment

Different prenatal strategies have been attempted with variable success, including the use of fluorinated steroids, immunoglobulin, plasmapheresis, β-inotropic agents, and pacing, either to prevent or treat immune-mediated fetal inflammation, and/or to augment fetal cardiac output. Direct ventricular pacing is technically possible, though it failed to prevent fetal death in the two cases for which it was attempted more than a decade ago. Similarly, premature delivery for immediate pacing has not been a satisfactory approach in our experience, nor in that of others, as it places the infant at the additional risks and complications of prematurity. To date, evidence of clinical usefulness has been provided only for fluorinated steroids and β-agonists (see Table 12-2). Repeated maternal injections of immunoglobulin could become a useful adjunct to lower maternal levels of antibodies, and to block their pathologic expression on the fetal heart.

Dexamethasone and Betamethasone

Dexamethasone and betamethasone are potent synthetic glucocorticoids that are only minimally metabolised by the placenta and easily pass to the fetus, making these agents useful for direct fetal treatment. Use of steroids in the treatment of isolated fetal atrioventricular block is based on the assumption that the aetiology of conduction disease is an inflammatory carditis, and that the transplacental administration of steroids may help to temper the immune-mediated tissue damage.[62] Access to the Research Registry for Neonatal Lupus then permitted study of a series of mothers with anti-Ro/La antibodies and offspring with atrioventricular block.[63] None of the fetuses with complete heart block responded to the transplacental treatment with steroids with an improvement of the conduction anomaly, and three treated fetuses with incomplete third-degree atrioventricular block progressed to complete block. Of treated fetuses with second-degree block, four reverted to first-degree block, with two remaining in first-degree block at 4 years of age. Transplacental treatment with steroids has also resulted in resolution of effusions and fetal hydrops.[53,63–68] This type of response is often observed without any improvement in heart rate, implying that accumulation of fluid in the fetus may result from immune-mediated serositis rather than cardiac failure.

There has been an improvement in outcome for fetuses with complete atrioventricular block (Fig. 12-1) simultaneous with the introduction of perinatal guidelines for treatment (Fig. 12-2).[60] At the time of diagnosis of atrioventricular block, oral dexamethasone was given in high doses and, when possible, maintained for the duration of the pregnancy. If the average fetal heart rate declined below 50 to 55 beats per minute, or if the cardiac function was reduced, a β-sympathomimetic agent was added. Pregnancies were monitored weekly by a closely collaborating team of fetal cardiologists, rheumatologists, and obstetricians. Delivery was arranged at around 37 weeks of gestation

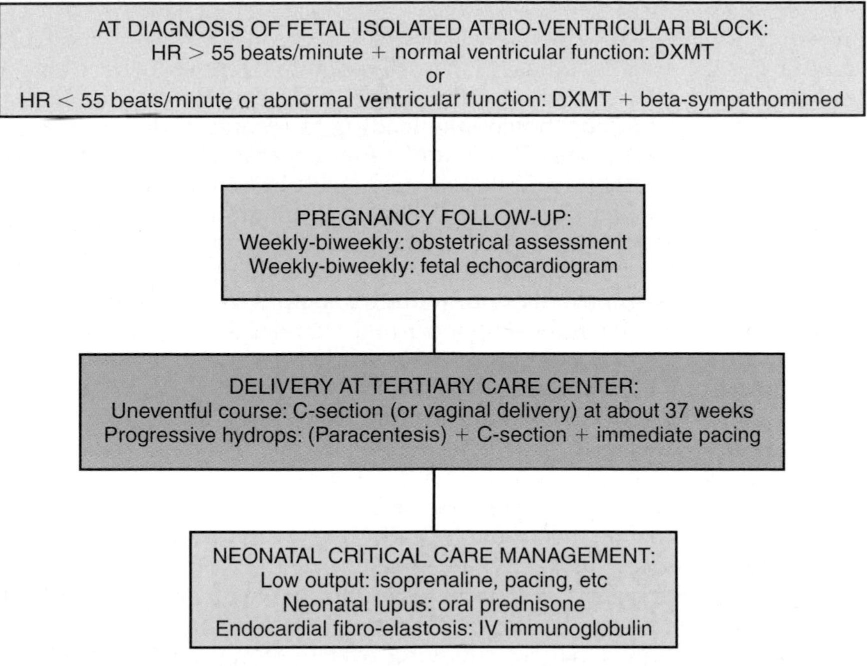

Figure 12-2 The protocol used for the management of immune-mediated fetal complete atrioventricular block at the Hospital for Sick Children. DXMT, dexamethasone; HR, heart rate. (Reproduced with permission from Jaeggi ET, Fouron JC, Silverman ED, et al: Transplacental treatment improves the outcome of prenatally diagnosed complete atrioventricular block without structural heart disease. Circulation 2004;110:1542–1548.)

in uncomplicated pregnancies, and the neonate was then transferred to the intensive care unit. Prior to 1997, pregnancies with isolated heart block had typically been followed by serial echocardiography, but without attempts to alter the perinatal outcome by transplacental fetal therapy. Survival of fetuses diagnosed prior to 1997 was 80% at birth, and 47% at 1 year, but thereafter this improved to 95% (see Fig. 12-1). Immune-mediated conditions causing postnatal death or requiring cardiac transplantation were only observed in fetuses surviving from untreated pregnancies. Prolonged administration of dexamethasone, therefore, may render a fetus with isolated complete atrioventricular block less likely to develop other disease-related manifestations such as myocarditis, cardiomyopathy, and/or hydrops, thus improving overall outcome.

We have now modified the guidelines to minimise the risk of severe oligohydramnios in the last trimester. Dexamethasone, which is now started at 8 mg per day, is reduced to 4 mg per day after two weeks, and then to 2 mg per day at around 30 gestational weeks. Moreover, maternal intravenous immunoglobulin is usually added if we detect ventricular endocardial fibroelastosis, ventricular dysfunction, and/or incomplete atrioventricular block.

Effects of Steroids on the Developing Fetus

Dexamethasone and betamethasone have been given to humans and animals in a wide range of dosages, at different gestational ages, and for various indications. While in fetuses with heart block the daily exposure does not exceed 0.05 mg per kg, the treatment is maintained over several weeks. Higher dosages were used in animal studies, for prenatal human pulmonary maturation, and for the postnatal treatment of respiratory distress syndrome. With the caveat that the published data may not be applicable to the fetus with complete atrioventricular block, steroids that cross the placenta have been shown to affect birth weight and the central nervous system with single and repeated prenatal steroid administration. Reduction in birth weight has been seen in sheep,[69] non-human primates,[70] and humans.[60,71,72] The effects on growth are more dramatic with multiple doses. Not unexpectedly, one-quarter of our newborns with isolated heart block were growth-restricted after prolonged transplacental exposure to steroids. Few, if any, other adverse effects on the fetus during the human pregnancy, however, have been documented. Neuroimaging of preterm human infants exposed to a single steroid course for lung maturation suggests a reduced incidence of intraventricular hemorrhage and white matter injury.[73,74] Multiple administration of dexamethasone before or after birth was associated with a reduction in cortical involution and in the cerebral surface area,[75,76] though the clinical significance of these findings is not known. Normal physical and mental development of children and young adults is reported, nonetheless, after prenatal exposure to steroids.[77–80] Similarly, no negative effects on neuro-psychological development and on intelligence were found in a cohort of preschool- and school-age children exposed prenatally to prolonged treatment with dexamethasone.[81]

Maternal Effects

Dexamethasone given at doses greater than 1.5 mg per day suppresses the hypothalamic-pituitary-adrenal function. Gradual reduction in dosing is required if given for more than 2 weeks. Side-effects to systemic glucocorticoids include an increased susceptibility to infections; changes in mood such as irritability, euphoria, mania, depression and anxiety; weight gain; fluid retention; arterial hypertension; glucose intolerance; insomnia; hirsutism; strias; impaired wound-healing; stomach irritation; and headache. In Toronto, we have now consecutively treated 30 pregnancies with immune-mediated fetal complete heart block. Adverse effects attributed to the use of steroids included the development of severe oligohydramnios in five pregnancies, requiring premature delivery in three cases, maternal hypertension in two cases, discontinuing the drug in one case, insulin-dependent diabetes in another case, and three women complaining about insomnia or mood changes, which resolved after reducing the dose. We now monitor carefully the volume of amniotic fluid throughout gestation, and taper the dose to 2 mg per day at around 30 weeks gestation to reduce the risk of severe oligohydramnios.

Beta-sympathomimetic Drugs

Beta$_2$-adrenergic receptor stimulation with short-acting terbutaline, ritodrine, and salbutamol has widely been used for tocolysis. Simultaneous β_1-actions may increase the fetal and maternal cardiac output by a change in heart rate and a decrease in systemic vascular resistance.[82–84] These effects have been used to treat the fetus with a slow heart rate and/or reduced myocardial function. Indeed, fetuses with complete atrioventricular block often respond to transplacental β-stimulation with a small, but persistent increase of 5 to 10 beats per minute, without necessarily improving the chance of survival of a haemodynamically compromised fetus.[52,60,67,85–89] If β-stimulation was used in combination with dexamethasone, five-sixths of fetuses with isolated complete atrioventricular block and with heart rates below 55 beats per minute survived to infancy.[60]

Dosing, Pharmacokinetics, and Adverse Events

Oral salbutamol and terbutaline, administered at or close to the maximal recommended daily doses, are the predominantly used β-agonists. The drugs are rapidly absorbed from the gastrointestinal tract, and incompletely cross the placenta, providing ratios of about 1:2 for umbilical cord and maternal samples.[90,91] While salbutamol and terbutaline are in general well-tolerated, mothers on maximal oral β-mimetic treatment regularly complain about mild tremor, palpitations and sweating.[52,60] These symptoms become better tolerated or resolve after some time of therapy. More serious maternal adverse events, or intolerable symptoms that required a change in treatment, have not been reported, nor were they observed by us. Tocolytic therapy with parenteral β-sympathomimetic agents, nonetheless, may rarely be associated with maternal pulmonary oedema, myocardial ischaemia, cardiac arrhythmias, hypotension, hyperglycemia, ketoacidosis, and hypokalemia.[92–94] Transient hypoglycemia has also been reported in newborn preterm infants after maternal treatment. Beta-agonists should be used cautiously, or not at all, in mothers with diabetes, hypertension, hyperthyroidism, and a history of seizures or tachyarrhythmias.

The outcome for fetuses with immune-mediated complete atrioventricular block, therefore, has significantly improved during the last decade, coinciding with a change in overall management of affected pregnancies that included the introduction of transplacental anti-inflammatory and β-sympathomimetic treatment. Based on the present knowledge on risks and benefits of treatment, there is no solid ground to deny the obvious improvement in survival to the fetus with newly diagnosed immune-mediated atrioventricular block. New strategies are evolving that aim at the prevention of fetal heart block. This includes echocardiographic diagnosis and pharmacological treatment closer to the onset of immune-mediated damage to the cardiac tissues.

CATHETER INTERVENTION FOR FETAL STRUCTURAL CARDIAC DISEASE

Owing to steady advances in ultrasonic imaging, congenital malformations of the heart can now accurately be diagnosed as early as the first trimester, and the progression of disease followed during the course of pregnancy. Not unexpectedly, prenatal worsening of cardiac anomalies has been well documented in both individual reports and series. For example, valves may become more incompetent, stenotic, or atretic, potentially leading to secondary damage of the heart, lungs, brain and other organs. Impaired growth of ventricles and vessels may result in a functionally univentricular circulation. Valvar regurgitation has the potential to lead to congestive cardiac failure and fetal hydrops. On the other hand, timely intra-uterine intervention may lead to improved or normalised haemodynamics, thus reducing the likelihood of abnormal fetal development, circulatory failure, and intra-uterine death.

Fetal intervention was pioneered in 1991, when Maxwell and colleagues dilated a stenotic aortic valve.[95] The previous 12 patients diagnosed with this condition at their centre had not survived postnatal treatment, so the aim of the fetal intervention was simply to ensure survival. Following this initial report, valvoplasties were undertaken at several other institutions around the world. The results of this experience were disappointing, with aortic valvoplasty technically successful in only just over half the cases, and only 1 patient surviving over the long term.[96] In light of improving surgical results in children with hypoplastic left heart syndrome, and the discouraging results of prenatal intervention, procedures were abandoned for some time. The reasons for prenatal intervention, however, have changed since 1991. The goal nowadays is no longer simply to ensure fetal survival but, more ambitiously, to reduce morbidity, for example by promoting intra-uterine ventricular, valvar and vascular growth so as to avoid development of a functionally univentricular circulation, or by restoring normal cerebral perfusion to improve the neurological outcome. The achievements of these goals depend on an evidence-based selection of suitable candidates, on the level of expertise and cooperation of the team performing the intervention, and on the availability of adequate technical equipment. Only limited cardiac lesions have the potential to benefit from prenatal interventions, specifically critical aortic valvar stenosis, critical pulmonary valvar stenosis or atresia with an intact ventricular septum, and hypoplasia of the left heart in the setting of a closed or severely restrictive oval foramen.

CRITICAL AORTIC VALVAR STENOSIS

Aortic stenosis typically leads to increased left ventricular pressure and hypertrophy. If ventricular growth and function are maintained, the patient with severe aortic stenosis is usually a good candidate for postnatal balloon dilation. In a subset of fetuses, however, the left ventricle progressively fails to overcome the increase in afterload despite generating maximal systolic pressure. As a consequence, the left ventricle progressively dilates, its contractile and filling function worsens, and signs of endocardial fibroelastosis appear. Related to the impaired diastolic function, left atrial pressure rises, and left-to-right shunting becomes visible echocardiographically across the patent oval foramen. In some fetuses, dilation of the high-pressure left ventricular cavity may severely impair right ventricular diastolic and systolic function, and cause fetal hydrops.[97] If the left ventricle is unable to eject blood into the aorta, the upper body will be supplied by the right ventricle via the patent

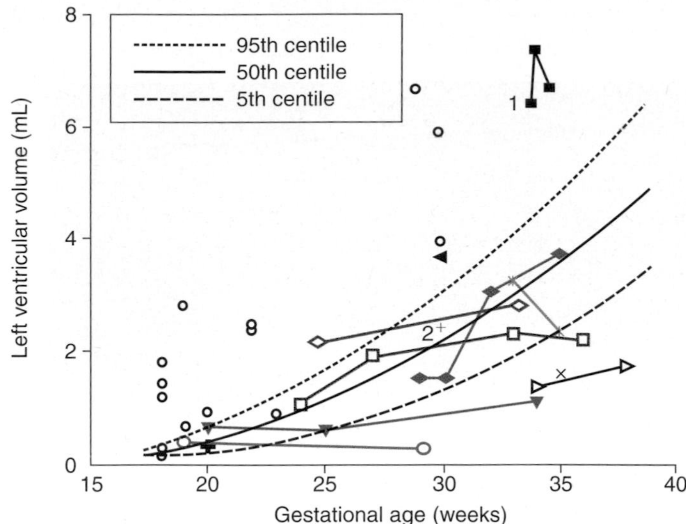

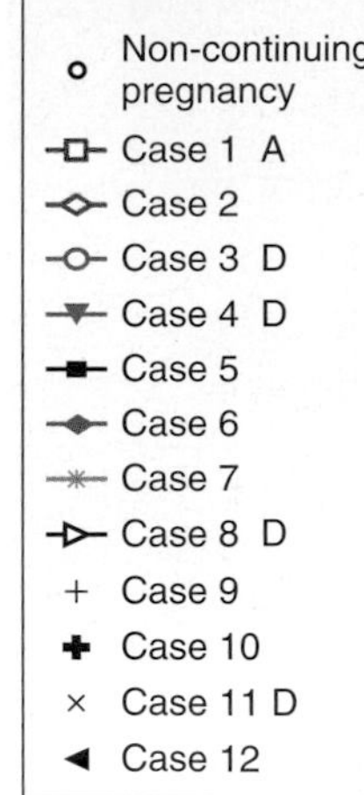

Figure 12-3 Graph of left ventricular end-diastolic volume versus gestational age in fetuses with aortic stenosis. (Reproduced with permission from Simpson JM, Sharland GK: Natural history and outcome of aortic stenosis diagnosed prenatally. Heart 1997;77:205–210.)

arterial duct. At this stage, growth of the left ventricle and aortic arch slows down or ceases (Fig. 12-3).[97–101] The typical finding at birth is a neonate with a left heart that is too small to sustain the systemic circulation, and which cannot be anatomically corrected. If the parents elect active postnatal care, this is usually done by step-wise palliative surgery involving the Norwood sequence of operations, and culminating in conversion to the Fontan circulation, or by cardiac transplantation. In a subset of fetuses, however, early relief of the obstructed aortic outflow by fetal intervention might restore left ventricular growth and function to an extent that would allow biventricular repair, rather than functionally univentricular palliation after birth. Prior to any intra-uterine intervention, nonetheless, it is important to pose three questions. First, are there evidence-based criterions to identify a suitable candidate for fetal valvoplasty? Second, can the procedure be effectively performed with minimal risks to the mother and fetus? Third, is a technically successful intervention likely to result in the desired outcome?

Reasons for Fetal Dilation of the Aortic Valve

As discussed, the primary goal of the first fetal cardiac interventions was to improve the chance of survival for a group of children with a high institutional mortality rate. As hypoplastic left heart syndrome is now surgically manageable with more acceptable results, this motivation no longer holds true. The exception is the rare circumstance of a hydropic fetus with severe right ventricular compression by a dilated left ventricle. Decompression of the left ventricle will improve right ventricular filling and output, and might prevent almost certain intra-uterine death. In the remaining cases with critical aortic stenosis, the reason for intra-uterine intervention is to preserve a biventricular circulation after birth, with a normal quality and expectancy of life. Another argument for intra-uterine aortic valvoplasty relates to cerebral perfusion and development. Flow of blood to the brain of the fetus with severe left ventricular outflow obstruction is sustained by the right ventricle via the patent arterial duct. This results in a lower than usual oxygenated cerebral blood supply, and may also alter the pattern of cerebral perfusion. Pulsed wave Doppler assessment of the mid-cerebral arterial flow may show increased end-diastolic velocities and lower pulsatility indexes, similar to the severely growth-restricted fetus with brain sparing.[102,103] The finding is explained by an auto-regulatory lowering of the cerebro-vascular resistance to enhance cerebral perfusion, and has been correlated with an impaired neurological outcome.[104] Abnormal cerebral perfusion may account for the abnormal neurodevelopment and lower circumferences of the head found in many offspring with hypoplastic left heart syndrome.[105] Other disease-related long-term risks include thrombo-embolic events, protein-losing enteropathy, plastic bronchitis, arrhythmias, and early ventricular dysfunction (see Chapter 32).

With this morbidity in mind, prevention of a functionally univentricular postnatal circulation by means of a well-timed prenatal intervention inevitably becomes an ideal goal. If significant endocardial fibroelastosis of the left ventricle is already present at the time of diagnosis, however, diastolic function may remain abnormal despite a technically successful valvoplasty. Abnormal ventricular compliance due to the diffusely thickened endocardium may lead to left atrial and pulmonary arterial hypertension, with unfavourable consequences for the child subsequent to attempted construction of a biventricular circulation. Moreover, a borderline-sized left ventricle with a narrowed left ventricular outflow tract may require a Ross or a Ross-Konno operation, with the need for further surgery later in life. The situation becomes even more complex if the mitral valve is dysplastic, stenotic, and/or hypoplastic, and will need to be repaired or replaced, in particular if the child is still at a young age. Thus, at least for some cases with more complex left ventricular pathology, the question must arise whether a well-performed functionally univentricular palliation is not superior to a malfunctioning biventricular repair.

Selection of Patients

The ideal candidate for percutaneous fetal balloon valvoplasty is the mid-trimester fetus with isolated critical aortic valvar stenosis and an adequate sized, apex-forming left ventricle that will become hypoplastic unless the obstruction is successfully relieved. In a series of patients with prenatal diagnosis of this entity at the Boston Children's Hospital, such progression to hypoplastic left heart syndrome could

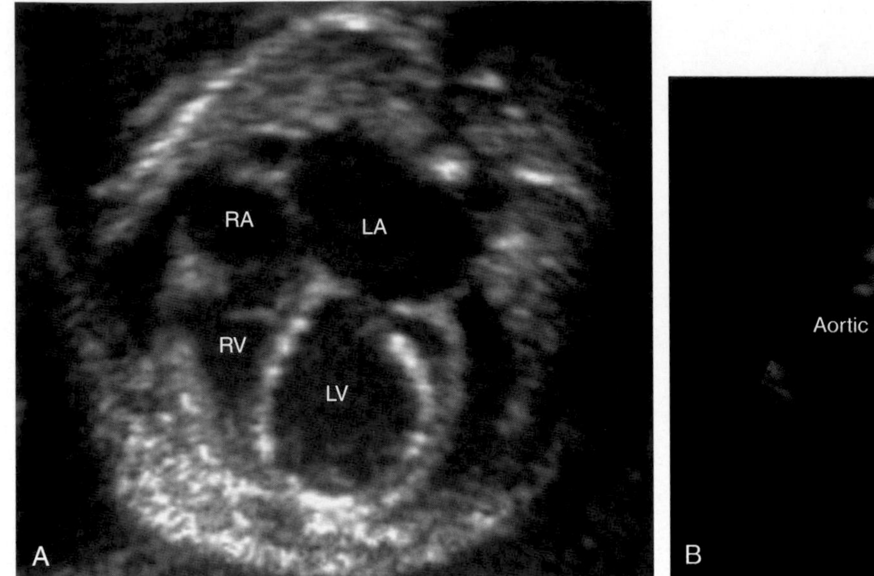

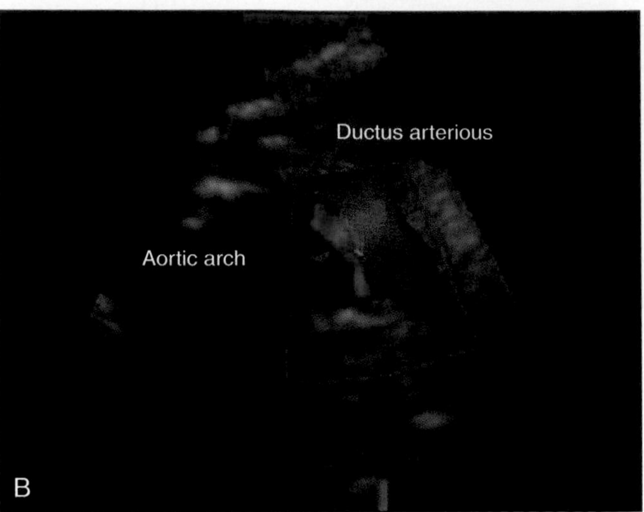

Figure 12-4 Typical appearance of a suitable candidate for fetal aortic valvoplasty. **A,** The dilated and poorly contracting left ventricle with endocardial brightness suggesting endocardial fibroelastosis. **B,** Retrograde flow in the transverse aortic arch. The fetus also had a monophasic left ventricular Doppler inflow pattern and left-to-right shunting across the patent oval foramen. LA, left atrium; LV, left ventricle; RA, right atrium; RV, right ventricle.

not be predicted by anatomical findings, but necessitated the inclusion of physiological parameters.[106] All cases with progressive left heart hypoplasia had a retrograde pattern of flow in the transverse aortic arch, while nine-tenths had left-to-right shunting across the oval foramen, monophasic mitral inflow, and significant left ventricular dysfunction on the initial fetal echocardiogram. In contrast, all fetuses with a preserved biventricular circulation after birth had normal antegrade flow in the transverse aortic arch, a biphasic mitral inflow pattern, and normal left ventricular systolic function (Fig. 12-4). Retrograde flow in the transverse aortic arch predicted neonatal hypoplastic left heart syndrome with complete sensitivity and specificity. This data supports the concept that fetal disturbances of flow contribute to the development of ventricular hypoplasia. The unsolved, yet critically important, question remains as to whether the dysfunctional left ventricle is capable of recovery after successful fetal intervention.

Technique of Fetal Aortic Valvoplasty

Fetal intracardiac interventions are the effort of a closely collaborating team that minimally includes an obstetrician with experience in ultrasonic guided fetal procedures, a fetal cardiologist, and an anaesthetist. The interventional procedure may be performed under general anaesthesia, where the fetus is anesthetised via the mother, or using local anaesthesia, where narcotics and muscle relaxants are directly injected into the fetus. The interventional techniques have been described in detail by different authors.[95,96,107] Under ultrasonic guidance a cannula and stylet needle are advanced through the maternal abdomen, the uterine wall, the amniotic cavity, the fetal chest, and into the left ventricle (Fig. 12-5). The success of valvoplasty critically depends on a suitable fetal position, and on high-quality transabdominal or transuterine fetal echocardiographic imaging. Care must be taken to insert the needle at an angle that is directly pointed towards the left ventricular outflow tract. After removal of the stylet, a floppy guide-wire is advanced across the stenotic aortic valve into the ascending aorta and aortic arch. A standard coronary balloon catheter is then advanced over the wire to perform multiple dilations of the aortic valve. Inflations to ratios of balloon to valve of between 0.8 and 1.2 have been used. Following successful dilation, stylet and balloon are removed together in one step (Fig. 12-6).

After little success with their first five cases, the team from Boston Children's Hospital added the option of a laparotomy for those cases with an unfavourable fetal position, and/or poor transabdominal fetal ultrasonic imaging.[108] Such laparotomies, performed in two-thirds of cases, improved the rate of technical success from 20% to 83%. A considerable learning curve reduced the need for a laparotomy with increasing experience. We have used exclusively a transabdominal approach, and have achieved success in five of eight cases, improved to five of our most recent six cases, highlighting the importance of a critical number of patients to attain and maintain the necessary skills and expertise for successful interventions.

Several complications have been reported during and after fetal aortic valvoplasty. Fetal bradycardia at around 50 beats per minute lasting more than 1 minute occurs in almost half of fetuses once the left ventricle is punctured. This can be prevented or abolished by fetal injection of atropine or epinephrine adjusted to the estimated fetal weight. A small pericardial effusion is observed in most cases immediately after withdrawal of the cannula, which usually resolves within a few hours. The pericardium should be drained, however, if the effusion increases in size, or haemodynamic compromise is suspected. Thrombus may form in the left ventricle, especially if the procedure takes some time. Once a thrombus has formed, the echocardiographic visibility of the fetal heart becomes poor, and the chance of successfully performing the procedure is dramatically reduced. The thrombus usually resolves within 24 hours without specific treatment. When using larger ratios of balloon to

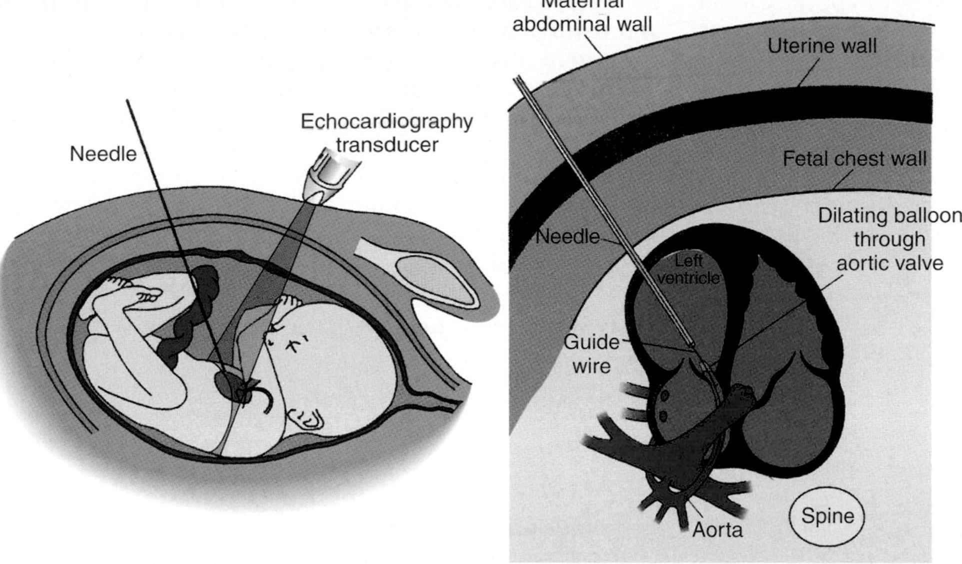

Figure 12-5 Schematic drawing showing the steps involved in fetal aortic valvoplasty. (Reproduced with permission from Tworetzky W, Wilkins-Haug L, Jennings RW, et al: Balloon dilation of severe aortic stenosis in the fetus: Potential for prevention of hypoplastic left heart syndrome. Candidate selection, technique and results of successful intervention. Circulation 2005;110:2125–2131.)

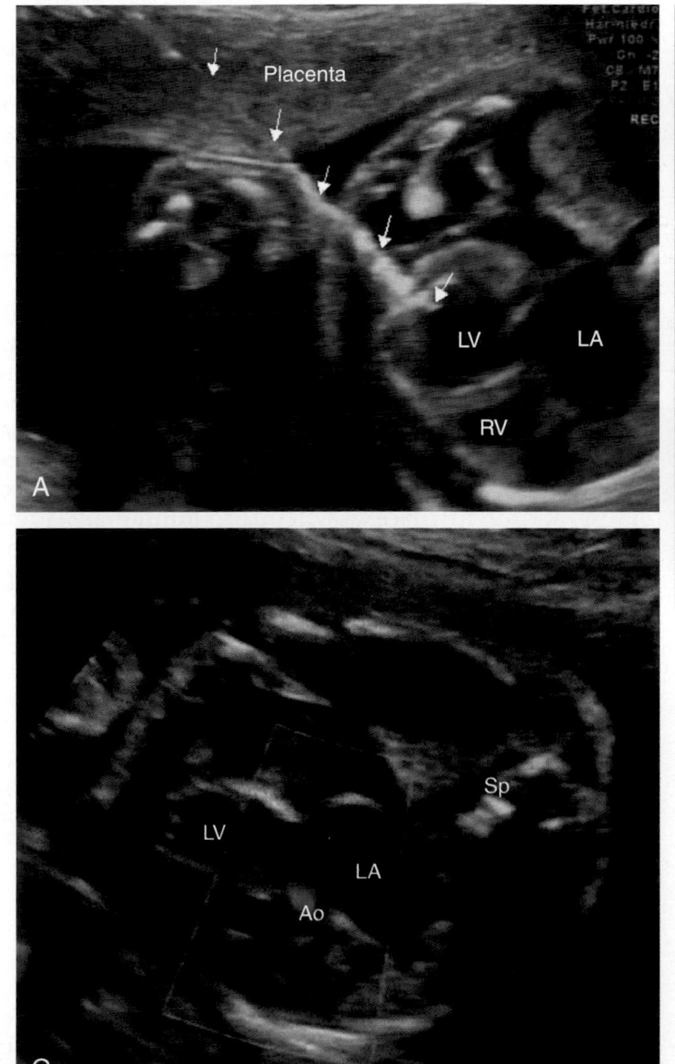

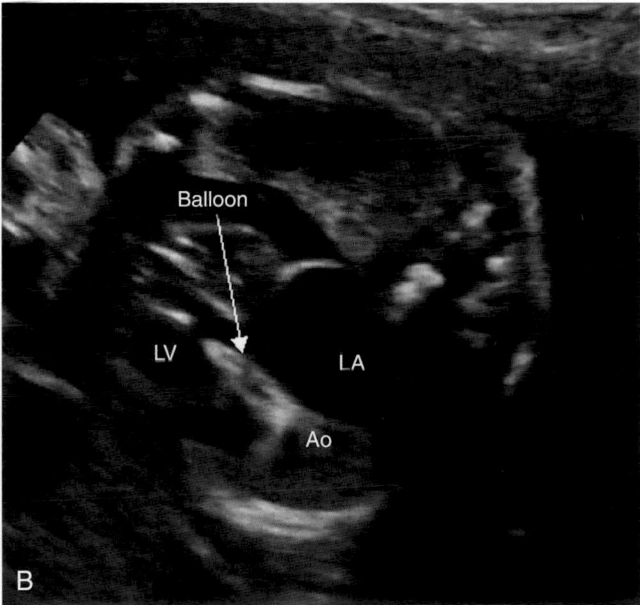

Figure 12-6 Sequential ultrasonic images of a successful fetal aortic valvoplasty. **A,** The needle (*arrows*) that is inserted through an anterior placenta into the left ventricle. **B,** The positioned balloon catheter in the aortic valve. **C,** After the successful valvoplasty, flow across the aortic valve is antegrade (*blue*). Ao, aorta; LA, left atrium; LV, left ventricle; RV, right ventricle; Sp, spine.

aortic valve, aortic regurgitation is likely to appear. Unlike the postnatal situation, even severe valvar insufficiency resolves within a few weeks. This suggests that remodelling of leaflets is possible prenatally. Whether aortic regurgitation promotes ventricular growth by increasing volume load, or further impairs left ventricular myocardial function due to a theoretical decrease in coronary arterial perfusion pressure, is unknown. Death of the fetus within 1 to 3 days after the procedure occurred in one-sixth of the procedures in the Boston experience, while this was the case with the first two of our eight patients treated in Linz. More recent unpublished data from Boston now indicates an early post-interventional rate of fetal death of approximately 10%.

Results and Outcomes

Technical success is defined by a successful positioning of the balloon catheter across the stenotic aortic valve, followed by one or several dilations resulting in a broader jet of ejection across the stenotic valve. After the initial disappointing experience, a technically successful procedure is nowadays possible in approximately four-fifths of cases if performed by experienced interventionists. The components of the left heart grow significantly better after a successful valvoplasty when compared to the fetus with an unsuccessful procedure, or with no attempt to intervene (Fig. 12-7). Unfortunately, technical success and improved left heart growth does not always produce a biventricular postnatal outcome. In the initial experience reported from Boston, biventricular repair was achieved in only 3 of 14 cases with technically successful fetal valvar dilation.[107] Their more recent report, including 26 fetuses, demonstrates several significant improvements in the fetal haemodynamics after successful valvoplasty.[109] This included re-establishment of antegrade flow in the transverse aortic arch, the change from an exclusive left-right to a bidirectional flow pattern across the oval foramen, improvement to biphasic left ventricular inflow, and an increase in the average left ventricular ejection fraction. Of five successful interventions in Linz, four patients went on to delivery, and all achieved biventricular repair, albeit including the need for Ross-Konno procedures in three, replacement of the mitral valve at 6 months in one, and redilation of the aortic valve in another.

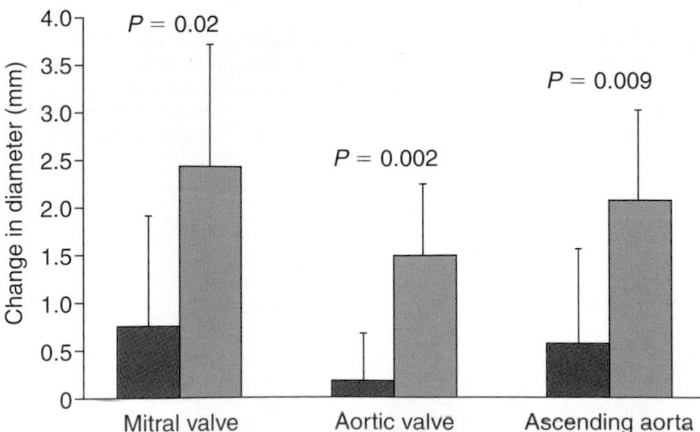

Figure 12-7 The change in dimensions of left heart structures in fetuses with a technically successful fetal aortic valvoplasty (*blue bars*) are compared to those after an unsuccessful or declined procedure (*orange bars*) (Reproduced with permission from Tworetzky W, Wilkins-Haug L, Jennings RW, et al: Balloon dilation of severe aortic stenosis in the fetus: Potential for prevention of hypoplastic left heart syndrome. Candidate selection, technique and results of successful intervention. Circulation 2005;110:2125–2131.)

Current data, therefore, suggests that an immediate biventricular repair after birth can be achieved in only about one-third of patients. In those fetuses born with components of the left heart that are too small despite a successful intra-uterine valvoplasty, larger components of the left heart, and antegrade aortic flow, may facilitate functionally univentricular palliative surgery, and reduce the risk of neuro-developmental impairment.

CRITICAL PULMONARY STENOSIS AND ATRESIA WITH AN INTACT VENTRICULAR SEPTUM

Pulmonary valvar stenosis or atresia with an intact ventricular septum presents with a variable spectrum of pathology, ranging from good-sized to variably small and dysfunctional right ventricles and tricuspid valves. Prenatal detection of this anomaly is feasible, and even anatomical details such as right ventriculo-coronary connections can be readily detected by high-resolution echocardiography.[110,111] Progression of the severity of pulmonary stenosis has been observed during the course of pregnancy.[112–114] If detected sufficiently early, up to four-fifths of those with pulmonary atresia with intact ventricular septum undergo termination, significantly reducing the incidence of this anomaly at birth in some countries.[115] Spontaneous intra-uterine death also occurs in approximately one-twentieth, but most fetuses will survive to birth without problems.

Morbidity and mortality mainly depend on whether a biventricular, functionally univentricular, or the so-called one and a half ventricular repair can be achieved after birth (see Chapter 30). Postnatal treatment includes intravenous administration of prostaglandins to prevent closure of the arterial duct. Different interventional and surgical options are then used to open the obstructed pulmonary valve, and to decompress the right ventricle in the absence of a right ventricular-dependent coronary arterial circulation, and/or to place a systemic-to-pulmonary arterial shunt. This includes radio-frequency perforation and balloon dilation of the pulmonary valve, stenting of the arterial duct, placement of a modified Blalock-Taussig shunt or a homograft from the right ventricle to the pulmonary arteries, as well as enlargement of the right ventricular outlet tract with a patch. Despite significant improvements in postnatal management, mortality remains high,[114,116–119] with only around two-thirds of cases, or less, proceeding to biventricular repair. There is evidence that, even in patients with an advantageous biventricular repair, right ventricular growth and biventricular function may be impaired, with unknown consequences for the long term.[120–122]

Reasons for Fetal Pulmonary Valvoplasty

In the fetus with critical pulmonary valvar stenosis or atresia and an intact ventricular septum, with signs of imminent cardiac failure due to restrictive right-to left shunting across the oval foramen, fetal pulmonary valvoplasty is performed to ensure survival. As most fetuses will not develop restrictive atrial flow leading to cardiac failure, the primary intention of fetal intervention in most instances is to prevent progressive hypoplasia of the right heart, thus promoting the potential for postnatal biventricular repair.

Selection of Patients

Prenatal prediction of whether or not a biventricular circulation will be achieved after birth is crucial for parental counselling, and for selection of those fetuses who may profit from fetal valvotomy to salvage the right heart. Uncertainty regarding the ultimate outcome may influence management of pregnancy, and may also lead to unnecessary fetal intervention. The question, therefore, is whether it is indeed possible accurately to predict the potential for right ventricular growth, and hence a biventricular outcome, in the fetus with pulmonary stenosis or atresia. The group from Boston studied whether measurements of tricuspid valvar size, and the respective *z*-scores, could be used in this fashion.[123] They found that biventricular repair was unlikely when the *z* score was −3 or worse, but always possible when better than −3. Almost two-thirds of those with *z* scores worse than −3 also had right ventricular dependent coronary arterial circulations, compared to none with the more favorable scores. The *z* scores noted at mid- and late-gestation also correlated with those measured after birth. Groups from Toronto and Montreal have also sought to identify ultrasonic markers for biventricular versus non-biventricular surgical outcomes.[111] Poor right ventricular function, reversal of flow in the arterial duct, the degree of tricuspid valvar regurgitation, and the Doppler pattern of flow in the inferior caval vein did not discriminate. By assessing the ratio of tricuspid to mitral valvar diameters, using 0.7 as the cut-off, the ratio of the lengths of the ventricles, with 0.6 being the break point, duration of tricuspid valvar inflow of less than three-tenths of the cardiac cycle length, and the presence of right ventricular to coronary arterial communications, it proved possible to predict a functionally univentricular outcome with sensitivity of 100% and specificity of 75% if three out of these four parameters were observed.

A subset of fetuses with pulmonary atresia and intact ventricular septum present with severe tricuspid regurgitation and a grossly enlarged right heart secondary to tricuspid valvar dysplasia or Ebstein's malformation. In this setting, pulmonary atresia may be functional as opposed to anatomic, as the right ventricle fails to generate enough force to eject the blood into the pulmonary vascular bed.[124] Dilation of the functionally closed pulmonary valve, therefore, would not improve the haemodynamic situation because the primary cause, right ventricular and tricuspid valvar dysfunction, would not be addressed. Measurement of the velocity of the jet of tricuspid regurgitation to estimate right ventricular pressure might help, nonetheless, to separate anatomic from functional pulmonary valvar occlusion.

Technique of Fetal Pulmonary Valvoplasty

The techniques used for dilation of the pulmonary valve are comparable to those used for the aortic valve. The procedure, however, is more technically challenging. The right ventricular cavity to be punctured is, in general, far smaller than the dilated left ventricle found in the setting of fetal aortic stenosis. Moreover, the optimal angle to advance the cannula from the right ventricular outflow tract across the pulmonary valve and into the pulmonary trunk is almost perpendicular to the fetal chest, and hence more difficult to achieve. The atretic pulmonary valve also needs to be perforated with a sharp needle to permit advancement of the guide-wire and balloon across the valve. This increases the risk for procedure-related complications (Fig. 12-8).[125]

Results and Outcome

The first successful intra-uterine pulmonary valvuloplasty in a fetus with an atretic pulmonary valve was achieved in our centre at Linz.[126] The fetus had been thought to develop cardiac failure secondary to a large atrial septal aneurysm that protruded into the mitral valve and obstructed the left ventricular inflow. Following successful pulmonary valvar perforation and balloon dilation, the tricuspid regurgitation disappeared, and the right ventricular inflow improved from a monophasic to biphasic pattern (Fig. 12-9). In addition, signs of cardiac failure improved, and the right ventricle

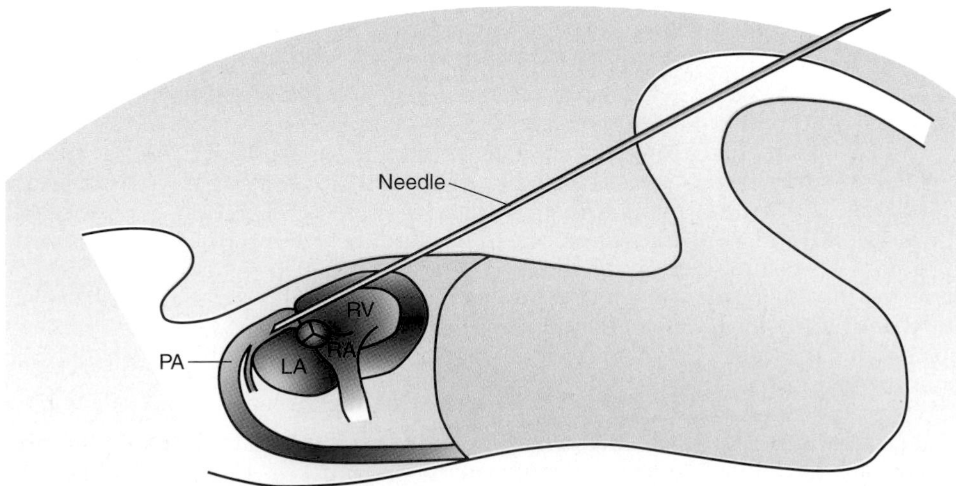

Figure 12-8 Schematic illustration of fetal pulmonary valvoplasty. LA, left atrium; PA, pulmonary artery; RA, right atrium; RV, right ventricle.

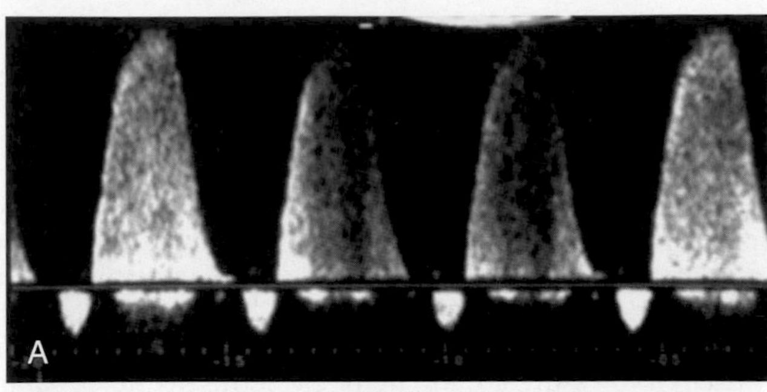

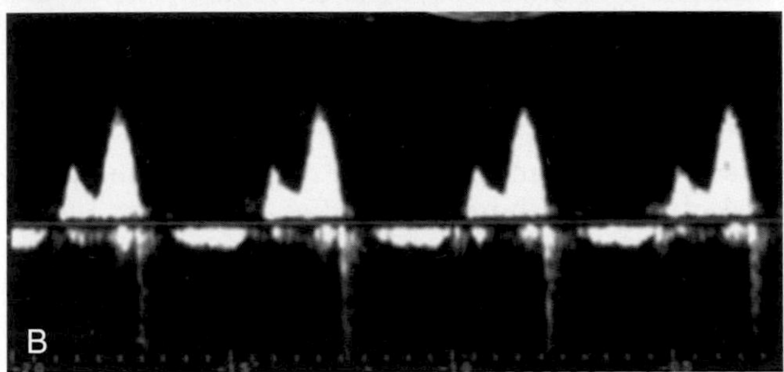

Figure 12-9 The tricuspid Doppler pattern of flow before (**A**) and after (**B**) successful pulmonary valvoplasty shows disappearance of tricuspid regurgitation and improvement of right ventricular filling from a monophasic to biphasic inflow pattern. (Reproduced with permission from Tulzer G, Arzt W, Franklin RC, et al: Fetal pulmonary valvuloplasty for critical pulmonary stenosis or atresia with intact septum. Lancet 2002;360:567–568.)

and the pulmonary valve continued to grow with advancing gestation. Several weeks after the fetal intervention, the pulmonary valve had restenosed. The newborn infant underwent successful pulmonary valvar dilation, but also required construction of a modified Blalock-Taussig shunt. At 8 months of age, it proved possible to take down the shunt and create a biventricular circulation. Subsequently, we reported the combined experience of the Children's Heart Centre in Linz and the Royal Brompton Hospital in London.[127] We attempted six interventions in five fetuses with pulmonary atresia or critical pulmonary stenosis between 23 and 30 weeks of gestation. Of the procedures, four were technically successful, but pulmonary atresia reappeared in two cases. In one fetus with a large coronary arterial fistula, the fistula remained unchanged despite successful valvotomy with right ventricular decompression. Reasons for the two technical failures included placental bleeding related to an intervention across an anterior placenta, and poor visibility in an obese mother. Biventricular repair was achieved in two of the children, one child underwent a one-and-a-half ventricle repair, while two patients died in the neonatal period. To date, eight procedures have been undertaken at Boston Children's Hospital, as yet unreported. The first four were technically unsuccessful, and the neonates required construction postnatally of a functionally univentricular circulation. The more recent attempts have been technically successful, with three fetuses proceeding to postnatal biventricular repairs, and the other requiring a modified Blalock-Taussig shunt in addition to a patch across the right ventricular outflow tract.

Echocardiographic criterions to predict univentricular versus biventricular outcomes, therefore, are available, and can be used to select suitable candidates for fetal pulmonary valvoplasty. The interventions on the pulmonary valve, however, are technically more challenging than those on the aortic valve. The benefit of the procedure in terms of improved postnatal outcomes is still to be established.

INTACT OR HIGHLY RESTRICTIVE ATRIAL SEPTUM ASSOCIATED WITH OBSTRUCTIVE ANOMALIES OF THE LEFT HEART

In the fetus with severe left ventricular inflow obstruction, unrestricted flow across the oval foramen is essential to ensure unobstructed pulmonary venous drainage from the left to the right atrium. If the left-to-right atrial shunt is restrictive, left atrial hypertension and pulmonary venous congestion develop, often with major consequences on the pulmonary vascular morphology and function.[128] Accordingly, children born with hypoplastic left heart syndrome and a restrictive or intact atrial septum have a substantial increase in morbidity and mortality, even when the obstruction is successfully relieved immediately after birth by an emergency atrial septostomy.[129]

Reasons for Intra-uterine Atrial Septostomy

The poor outcome of infants with hypoplasia of the left heart and a highly restrictive or intact oval foramen was the primary reason to intervene on the atrial septum prior to delivery. The aim of the intervention is to facilitate left-to-right shunting, thus decompressing the left atrium and pulmonary venous system. In theory, at least, this should allow for a more normal pulmonary vascular development, with an improved postnatal outcome.

Selection of Patients

Whenever a fetus with an intact or severely restrictive atrial septum in the setting of severe mitral valve stenosis or atresia is identified, the option of prenatal atrial septostomy should be considered. On cross sectional echocardiography, the atrial septum will be seen to bulge into the right atrium, and will appear thickened and muscularised, while the pulmonary veins will be dilated. Colour and pulsed wave Doppler echocardiography should be used to examine the pattern of flow and velocities across the oval foramen and in the pulmonary veins. It is well-known that the fetus with hypoplastic left heart syndrome has a Doppler pattern of pulmonary venous flow that differs from the normal fetus, even in the absence of atrial septal restriction. If the pulmonary venous flow has minimal or no early diastolic forward movement, but shows significant reversal during atrial contraction, this will indicate severe restriction of intra-atrial flow (Fig. 12-10).[130–132] Moreover, assessment of the severely restrictive atrial shunting by Doppler interrogation will show continuous left-to-right shunting at high velocity, suggesting a significant pressure gradient between the two atriums (Fig. 12-11).

Technique of Fetal Atrial Septostomy

The interventional technique is comparable to intra-uterine aortic or pulmonary valvoplasty. Using an ultrasonic guided percutaneous approach, either the right or the left atrial free wall is entered from the lateral chest wall, with

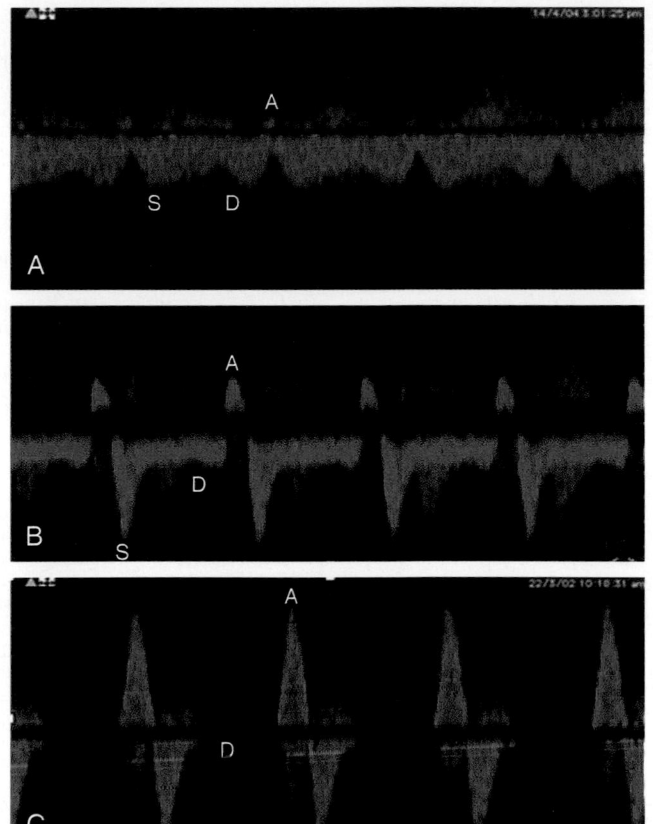

Figure 12-10 The pulmonary venous Doppler pattern of flow is seen during several cardiac cycles in a normal fetus and in a fetus (**A**) with hypoplastic left heart syndrome and un-restrictive atrial communication (**B**). Note the small amount of backward flow during atrial systole. **C**, Comparable findings in a fetus with hypoplastic left heart syndrome and an intact atrial septum: There is complete absence of early diastolic flow and increased flow reversal during atrial systole. A, late diastolic flow at the time of atrial contraction; D, early diastolic flow; S, systolic flow;.

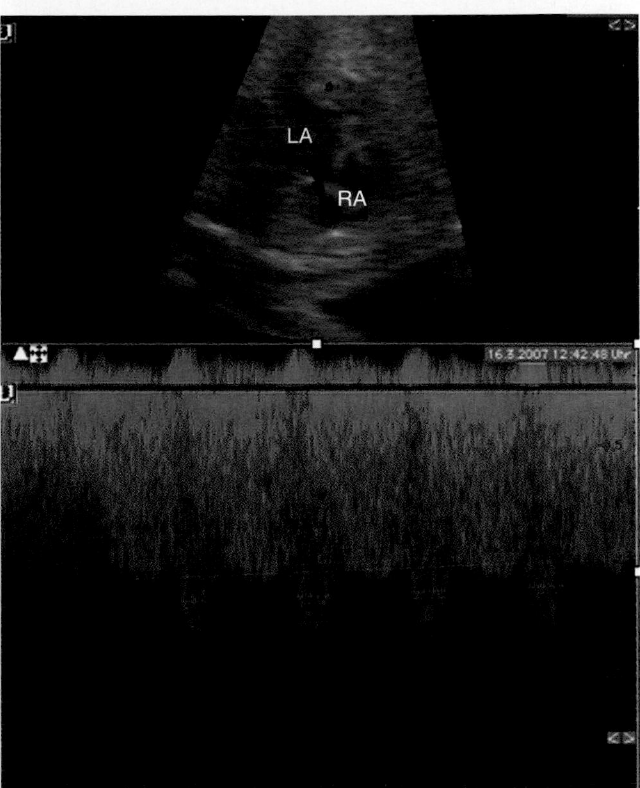

Figure 12-11 Restrictive atrial septum in a fetus with hypoplastic left heart syndrome. **Upper panel,** Color Doppler recording showing left to right shunt across a small oval foramen. **Lower panel,** Typical pulse Doppler recording of a severely restrictive atrial communication with high velocity left-right shunting that persists throughout the entire cardiac cycle. LA, left atrium; RA, right atrium.

the cannula pointing perpendicularly to the atrial septum. A sharp needle is advanced via the cannula to perforate the thickened septum. A guide-wire is then advanced across the cannula into a pulmonary vein, followed by placement of a coronary arterial balloon catheter across the atrial septum. The balloon is then inflated to its maximal diameter (Fig. 12-12). The dilation can be repeated until adequate left-to-right atrial shunting is achieved. Larger communications, nonetheless, are usually not obtained by balloon dilation. Permanent decompression of the left atrium, therefore, may not be obtained. An alternative approach that may result in larger and more persistently patent communications is to implant a coronary arterial stent within the created atrial communication. This has successfully been achieved in one fetus by the group in Boston, albeit not yet described in the literature. It is also possible to use a Neodymuim-YAG laser to fulgurate the atrial septal tissue rather than employing the needle, wire, and balloon.[133]

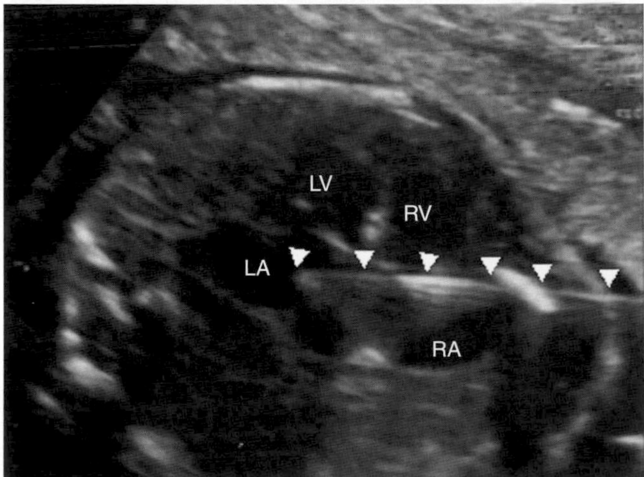

Figure 12-12 A balloon placed across the atrial septum during fetal atrial septostomy. LA, left atrium; LV, left ventricle; RA, right atrium; RV, right ventricle.

Results and Outcome

The current experience with fetal atrial septostomy is very limited, effectively representing the experience obtained in Boston.[134] Interventions were attempted on seven fetuses between 26 and 34 weeks of gestation, of which six were technically successful. There were no maternal complications. Of the fetuses, one died prior to birth, and the remaining cases were live born, albeit that all died in the neonatal period. The latest unpublished experience from Boston has extended to 18 fetal procedures, with technical success in more than nine-tenths, 17 of the fetuses being live born children, one dying prior to surgical intervention, and more than half successfully surviving postnatal surgical intervention.

Ultrasonically guided fetal atrial septostomy, therefore, is technically feasible, and can be achieved with a low risk of fetal death. Whether the procedure ensures permanent left atrial decompression, with reversal of pulmonary vascular abnormalities, and with improved postnatal outcome, remains to be established.

SUMMARY

Nowadays, a team of experienced clinicians can perform successful fetal intracardiac interventions with low risks to the mother and fetus. Identification of suitable candidates for interventions has improved in recent years. New modalities to assess myocardial function, such as tissue Doppler imaging, can provide additional information on the optimal timing of procedures, and the prediction of myocardial recovery. While technical rates of success have improved with more clinical experience, the development of more appropriate interventional tools would help further to increase the safety and efficiency of the procedures. The quality of the images obtained should not need to be improved by means of laparotomy, but rather by an improvement in ultrasonic resolution, and perhaps by adding real-time three-dimensional or transoesophageal fetal echocardiography.[135] Little is currently known about fetal resuscitation, and the application, safety, and efficacy of currently used drugs and potentially useful medication. At this stage, fetal cardiac interventions are not the standard of care, but tentative undertakings with potential pitfalls. As stated by Kleinman,[136] 'The paediatric community as a group is entering a field with complex and unique legal and ethical underpinnings that have been formulated during a period of more than 35 years. Unless it takes note of the experiences of our colleagues in maternal fetal medicine and paediatric surgery in the field of fetal intervention, it is likely that we and our patients will be doomed to revisit the errors of judgement that were made in well-intentioned efforts to treat fetal conditions such as diaphragmatic hernia, obstructive uropathy and hydrocephaly'. Only then will the future be bright for thoughtful applications of new techniques in fetuses with congenitally malformed hearts.[137]

ACKNOWLEDGEMENT

We are indebted to Dr Wayne Tworetsky, of Boston Children's Hospital, for sharing with us the extensive, but as yet unpublished, experience of himself and his colleagues with the various lesions currently amenable to fetal intervention.

The complete reference list can be found on the companion Expert Consult web site at www.expertconsult.com.

ANNOTATED REFERENCES

- Jaeggi ET, Fouron JC, Silverman ED, et al: Transplacental treatment improves the outcome of prenatally diagnosed complete atrioventricular block without structural heart disease. Circulation 2004;110:1542–1548.

  First documentation that a standardised treatment approach, including transplacental fetal administration of dexamethasone and β-stimulation at heart rates of less than 55 beats per minute, significantly improves the outcome of immune-mediated fetal complete atrioventricular block.

- Simpson JM, Sharland GK: Fetal tachycardias: Management and outcome of 127 consecutive cases. Heart 1998;79:576–581.

  To date, this is the largest review of the management and outcome of fetal tachyarrhythmias and the problems encountered with various treatment protocols.

- Fouron JC, Fournier A, Proulx F, et al: Management of fetal tachyarrhythmia based on superior vena cava/aorta Doppler flow recordings. Heart 2003;89:1211–1216.

  The authors illustrate the importance of Doppler and M-mode echocardiographic techniques in identifying electrophysiological mechanisms and in selecting the appropriate management of fetal tachyarrhythmias.

- Saleeb S, Copel J, Friedman D, Buyon JP: Comparison of treatment with fluorinated glucocorticoids to the natural history of autoantibody associated congenital heart block. Arthritis Rheum 1999;42:2335–2345.

  This publication, provided by the Research Registry for Neonatal Lupus, shows that immune-mediated incomplete fetal heart block, effusions and fetal hydrops may improve or resolve with transplacental steroid treatment. In contrast, none of the fetuses with complete atrioventricular block responded to the treatment with an improvement of the conduction anomaly, suggesting that third-degree block represents irreversible damage to the atrioventricular node.

- Mäkikallio K, McElhinney DB, Levine JC, et al: Fetal aortic valve stenosis and the evolution of hypoplastic left heart syndrome: Patient selection for fetal intervention. Circulation 2006;113:1401–1405.

  In mid-gestation, fetuses with aortic stenosis and normal left ventricular length, reversed flow in the transverse aortic arch and across the oval foramen, monophasic mitral inflow, and left ventricular dysfunction are predictive of progression to hypoplastic left heart syndrome. These features may help refine the selection of those fetuses best suited for intervention to prevent the progression of aortic stenosis to hypoplastic left heart syndrome.

- Tworetzky W, Wilkins-Haug L, Jennings RW, et al: Balloon dilation of severe aortic stenosis in the fetus: Potential for prevention of hypoplastic left heart syndrome. Candidate selection, technique and results of successful intervention. Circulation 2004;110:2125–2131.

  One of several important publications from the Children's Hospital of Boston, this one focuses on the reasons underscoring the selection of patients for, the techniques of, and the results of fetal aortic valvar dilation.

- Roman KS, Fouron JC, Nii M, et al: Determinants of outcome in fetal pulmonary valve stenosis or atresia with intact ventricular septum. Am J Cardiol 2007;99:699–703.

  Pulmonary valvar stenosis or atresia with intact ventricular septum represents a spectrum of severity. This study aimed to identify mid-gestational ultrasonic markers predicting biventricular versus non-biventricular outcome. It proved possible to identify four predictors that may be used in selecting fetuses for prenatal catheter intervention to prevent progressive right ventricular hypoplasia.

- Tulzer G, Arzt W, Franklin RC, et al: Fetal pulmonary valvuloplasty for critical pulmonary stenosis or atresia with intact septum. Lancet 2002;360:1567–1568.

  A biventricular outcome was documented in two fetal cases after successful fetal pulmonary valvoplasty for critical pulmonary stenosis.

- Marshall AC, van der Velde ME, Tworetzky W, et al: Creation of an atrial septal defect in utero for fetuses with hypoplastic left heart syndrome and intact or highly restrictive atrial septum. Circulation 2004;110:253–258.

  Infants born with hypoplastic left heart syndrome and an intact or highly restrictive atrial septum face a high postnatal mortality related to chronic pulmonary vascular disease. In this report, the group from Boston Children's Hospital demonstrated that left atrial decompression by prenatal catheter intervention is technically feasible with low risks, but were unable to find any positive clinical benefit on outcome.

Surgical Techniques

KIMBERLY L. GANDY, GEORGE M. HOFFMAN,
PATRICK VANDERWAL, and JAMES S. TWEDDELL

The conduct of an operation for palliation or repair of the congenitally malformed heart is ideally the culmination of a thorough preoperative evaluation, the careful formulation of an operative plan after interpretation of all data and the execution of this plan by a well-coordinated team. In this chapter, we review some of the issues that are common to all surgical procedures performed in patients with congenitally malformed hearts. We will describe the incisions that are used in the approach to the heart, the materials that are used to perform the necessary surgical manipulations and the strategies for intraoperative support.

SURGICAL APPROACHES TO THE HEART

There are a variety of incisions that are used in cardiac surgery. Until most recently, the majority of paediatric cardiac surgery was performed through two incisions, namely the median sternotomy and the left posterolateral thoracotomy. Over the last decade, minimally invasive strategies have resulted in the use of a variety of other incisions.

The Sternotomy

The most commonly used incision continues to be the median sternotomy (Fig. 13-1), in which the sternum is divided along its length from top to bottom. Originally described in 1897, this incision came into widespread use after the advent of coronary artery bypass grafting in the 1960s. The overlying skin and subcutaneous tissues are divided with a combination of the knife and electrocautery, and the sternum is divided with a reciprocating saw (Fig. 13-2). In neonates and young infants, scissors can be used to divide the bone. The reciprocating saw is used when opening the sternum for the first time. The blade has vertical movement through a short distance, and a protective shoe covers the tip of the blade. The shoe glides underneath the sternum, and prevents injury to the underlying cardiac structures. At the completion of the procedure, the sternum is closed with stainless steel wire, bands, or sometimes, in small children, heavy suture material. The incision provides excellent exposure, and is preferred for most intracardiac procedures. In addition to opening the sternum itself, the incision is extended for a short distance into the upper abdomen, separating the rectus muscle in the midline. Because there is minimal interruption of muscle, and because the sternum is solidly reconstructed at the end of the procedure, the incision is less painful than other commonly used incisions, such as the thoracotomy. There is minimal respiratory compromise. Early extubation, effective coughing and deep breathing are easily achieved with this incision. Long-term functional results are excellent, and lung function is minimally perturbed. This is in

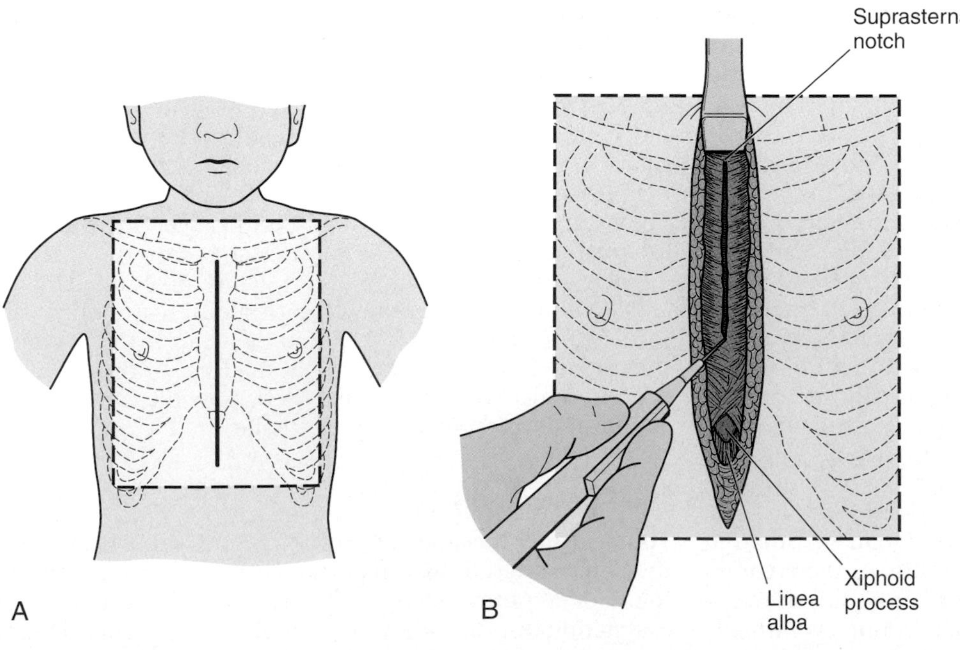

Figure 13-1 The median sternotomy. **A,** The skin, subcutaneous tissue, and presternal fascia are divided with a combination of the knife and electrocautery. The sternum is divided longitudinally with a saw. **B,** The incision is extended for a short distance into the upper abdomen, dividing the rectus abdominus muscle in the midline.

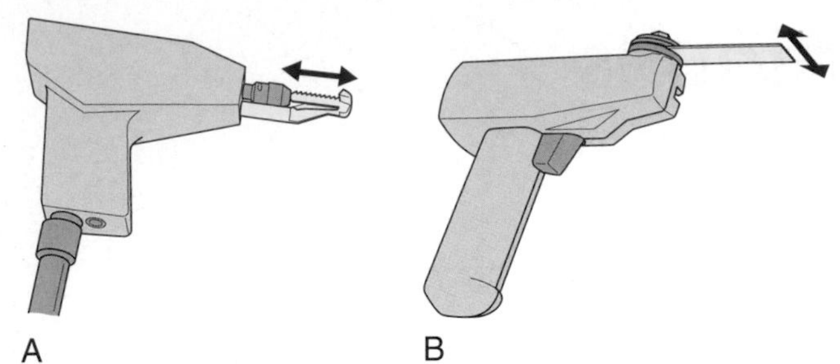

Figure 13-2 **A,** In primary sternotomies, the sternum is usually divided with a reciprocating saw. **B,** In redo sternotomies, the sternum is divided with an oscillating saw. There are a variety of sizes and shapes of blades that can be adapted for use with the oscillating saw.

contrast to the situation found after thoracotomies, where a degree of restrictive lung physiology is predictable.[1]

When it is necessary for a patient to undergo a cardiac operation through an operative field that has been previously explored, the mortality and morbidity of the operation are increased.[2] Over the last several decades, however, the morbidity and mortality of reoperative surgery in the adult have significantly decreased.[3,4] There has probably been a similar decrease in mortality of reoperative surgery in children. Resternotomy requires preparation. Careful preoperative assessment is necessary to determine if the patient is at increased risk for resternotomy haemorrhage. Axial imaging studies such as computerised tomographic scanning, and magnetic resonance imaging, can be examined to determine the relationship of structures such as the atrium, right ventricular outflow tract, and aorta to the sternum. The position of the aorta and calcified conduits can also be identified on angiography.

Preparation for emergent volume support, and identification of alternative sites of access for cardiopulmonary support, are essential. Blood should be immediately available at the time of resternotomy. In adults and older children, the femoral vessels are frequently used for access. In older patients who have had multiple previous cardiac catheterisations and cardiac surgical procedures, ultrasonic interrogation of the femoral vessels should be considered to verify patency. The brachiocephalic artery, accessed through the sternal notch, and the axillary vessels, provide alternative sites for emergency access. In infants, the common carotid and internal jugular veins may be used for emergent cardiopulmonary bypass. Preparation should also be made for external cardioversion should the patient develop an arrhythmia before direct access to the heart is obtained. Resternotomy is accomplished using an oscillating saw (see Fig. 13-2). This device has horizontal blade translating through a short distance that limits, but by no means eliminates, the risk of injury to underlying vascular structures. At the completion of a procedure, preparation for resternotomy should be made in any patient in whom resternotomy is likely. A sheet of polytetrafluoroethylene can be placed over the heart at the time of closure in a child in whom subsequent reoperation is anticipated.

Infection of the sternal wound, and mediastinitis, are rare complications in children, but do occur. For the most part these complications are more easily managed than in older patients.[5] In particular, osteomyelitis of the sternum is exceedingly rare,[6] and sternal resection, a common necessity in adults with an infected sternal wound, is virtually never required in children. In children, re-exploration, debridement, irrigation, and immediate closure over drains has been successful.[5] A variety of techniques have been used to address more significant infections including the use of vacuum dressings, omental flaps,[7] and flaps of the rectus abdominus muscle.[8] These techniques enhance drainage and neovascularisation, improving control of infection, and enhancing eventual closure. The approach to the sternum considered at high risk for dehiscence is a subject unto itself. Though this has not been an area of significant concern in paediatric cardiac surgery, as our patient population ages, it may soon become a more important consideration. The time is nearing when up to half of those undergoing surgery for congenital cardiac disease may be adults. A significant portion of these procedures will necessarily be performed through a resternotomy. When the patient is obese or diabetic or has undergone previous chest irradiation, this sternum can be considered at increased risk for dehiscence. Many of these patients will have undergone multiple previous sternotomies. As a result, blood supply to the sternum may be significantly reduced. Indeed, a large portion of these patients may have lost both internal mammary arteries during previous explorations. As such, additional measures may be taken with sternal closure. Double sternal wires, steel bands[9] and sternal plates,[10–14] which reduce movement and distribute stresses in the wound over larger areas, are strategies used to close the sternum at high risk of dehiscence.

As outcomes have improved after cardiothoracic surgery, interest in improving the cosmesis of incisions has emerged. The longitudinal skin incisions have been shortened significantly in some cases, even when the sternum is divided fully along its length. Another effort has involved abandoning the longitudinal skin incision altogether, in favor of a submammary or transverse skin incision (Fig. 13-3A).[15,16] The incision has not been widely adopted secondary to fear of wound complications and compromised exposure, but some have reported excellent results with this incision, and very low rates of complication.[17–20] It is of note that the majority of the sensory supply to the chest wall enters laterally (Fig. 13-3B). If the submammary incision is appropriately performed, sensory supply to the breast should be uninterrupted.[19] It is also important that this incision is made well below the mammary tissue. Significant compromise to development of the breasts has resulted when the incision has been made too high. In an older individual who has completed mammary development, the most inferior extent of the breast is more clearly delineated. In younger children, this line is not as clear. The future site of the mammary fold can be identified in an infant or young child by placing a hand on the anterior chest wall above the nipple and gently pushing caudad. A fold will be evident that will correspond reasonably well to the future mammary crease. In general, if the incision if made in a transverse fashion at the level of the xyphoid process, a nice cosmetic result will be possible, with preservation of developing mammary tissue.

The Thoracotomy

Thoracotomy incisions are commonly used for ligation of the patent arterial duct, repair of aortic coarctation, placement of a pulmonary artery band and construction of a systemic-to-pulmonary arterial shunt. A posterolateral

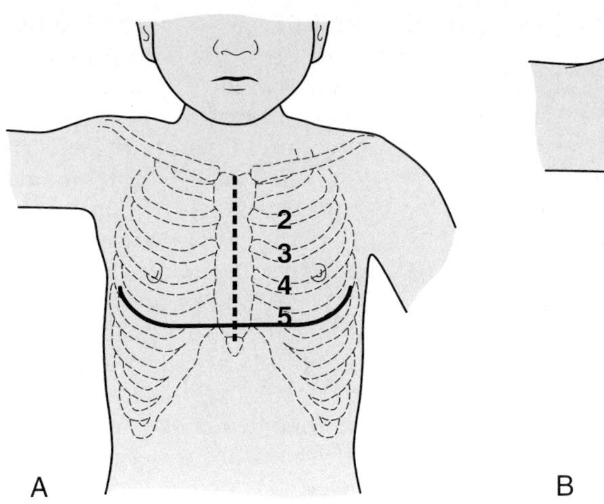

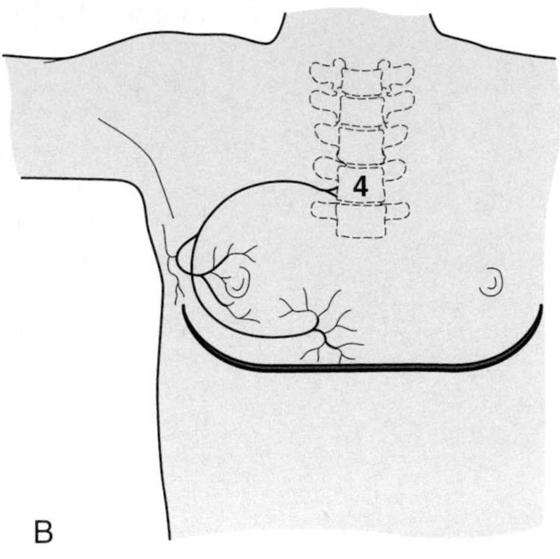

Figure 13-3 The submammary skin incision for median sternotomy. The skin and subcutaneous tissues (**A**) are divided with a combination of the knife and electrocautery (*solid black line*). The sternum is divided longitudinally, as it is in the standard median sternotomy (*dashed line*). The area is innervated (**B**) by nerves entering laterally.

thoracotomy is shown in Figure 13-4. The skin incision is made in a curvilinear fashion along the path of the ribs (Fig. 13-4A). In most instances, the latissimus dorsi muscle is divided (Fig. 13-B), but the serratus anterior is spared (Fig. 13-4C). The intercostal muscles are divided between the ribs to be spread. At times, even the latissimus can be spared, the approach to the thoracic cavity being made through a small space between these muscles, the so-called triangle of auscultation. In cases where greater exposure is necessary, especially in older patients, it may be necessary to harvest a rib to obtain ideal exposure. The skin incision can be limited compared to the length of the incision within the thoracic cavity. This incision is performed through a variety of intercostal spaces, depending on the level for which exposure is desired. The arterial duct and aortic arch are typically approached through the third or fourth intercostal space. Exposure for excision of pulmonary pathology typically involves an incision in the fourth or fifth intercostal space. Exposure for treatment of oesophageal pathology can be made through the left fifth through eighth intercostal spaces, or the right fourth or fifth intercostal spaces. Exposure to the diaphragm is usually through the seventh intercostal space.

The transverse thoracosternotomy incision is used when there is need for extensive thoracic exposure (Fig. 13-5). In this incision, both thoracic cavities are entered through bilateral anterolateral thoracotomies that are connected across the midline by a transverse sternotomy. This incision gives excellent exposure to all of the mediastinal structures anteriorly. It is most commonly used for bilateral sequential lung transplantation, but has also been used for unifocalisation of aortopulmonary collateral arteries. The skin incision can be made as indicated in the figure to preserve development of the breasts. This incision is sometimes complicated by sternal malunion, characterised by a malaligned sternal union or sternal nonunion. Some have abandoned this incision for this reason, and prefer to approach the chest through bilateral anterolateral thoracotomies without dividing the sternum.[21] The use of alternative wiring techniques or alternative materials such as cables for sternal approximation have been reported and may reduce the incidence of complications with the transverse sternotomy.[22–24]

The anterolateral thoracotomy is shown in Figure 13-6. The right anterolateral thoracotomy has been used for repair of a variety of congenital cardiac malformations, with good results.[25-30] The anterolateral thoracotomy can be placed in the mammary crease and has been used as an alternate, more cosmetically appealing approach for simple intracardiac operations such as closure of atrial septal defects.[31] There have been isolated reports, however, of compromised or asymmetric development of the breast with this incision,[32,33] and of increased pain.[34] The left anterolateral thoracotomy is often used on the haemodynamically unstable victim of thoracic trauma with suspected damage to the thoracic structures. If sufficient access is not possible

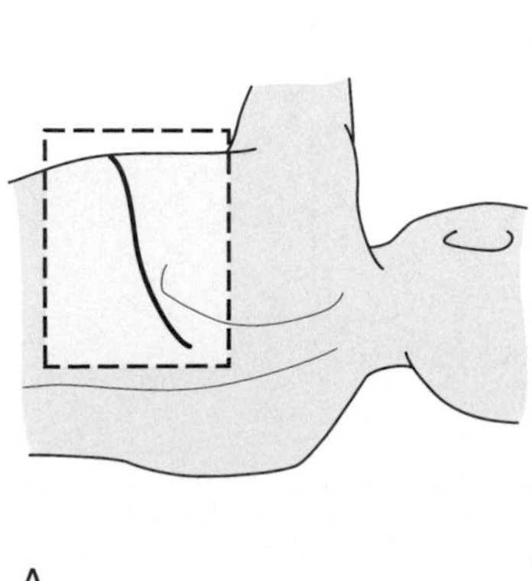

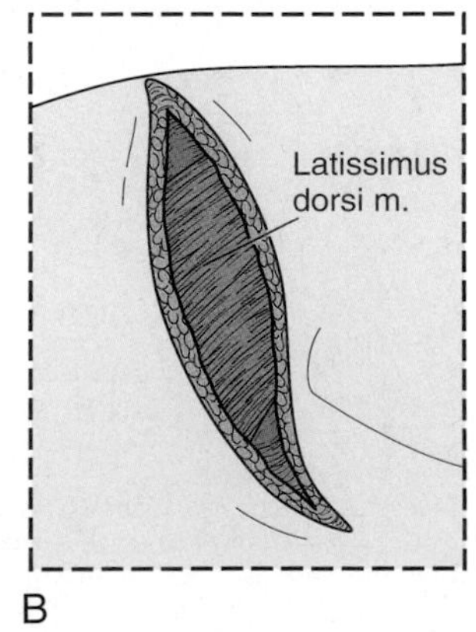

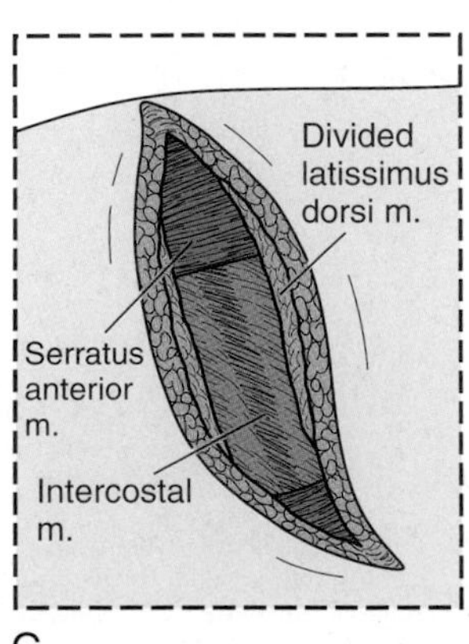

Figure 13-4 The posterolateral thoracotomy. **A,** The skin and subcutaneous tissues are divided with a combination of the knife and electrocautery along the indicated line. In the most common iteration used today, the latissimus muscle is divided and the serratus anterior is spared. The intercostal muscles in the intercostal space of entry are also divided. **B,** The undivided latissimus dorsi. **C,** The divided muscle with the spared serratus anterior.

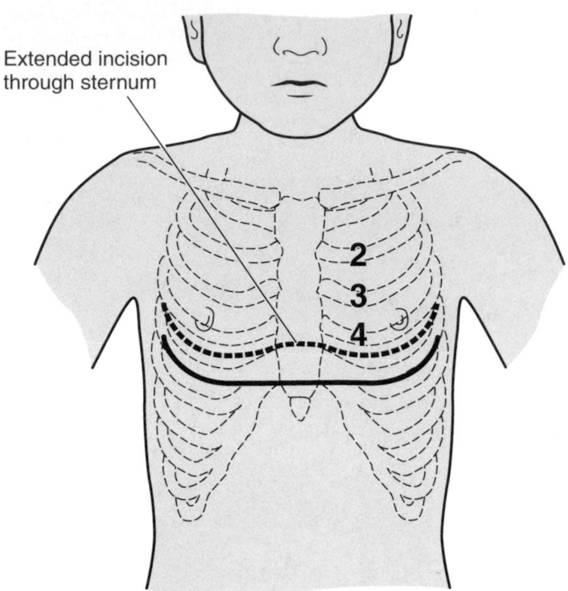

Figure 13-5 The transverse thoracosternotomy. The skin and subcutaneous tissues are divided with a combination of the knife and electrocautery along the solid line as indicated. A subcutaneous flap beneath the breast tissue is developed until the fourth or fifth intercostal space is reached. The intercostals are then divided at the desired interspace (*dashed line*). The internal mammary arteries are identified and ligated. The sternum is then divided transversely at the interspace in which the thoracic cavities were entered.

with this incision, it can be extended across the midline for further access to cardiac structures.

Minimally Invasive Approaches

In continued attempts to improve the cosmetic results after surgery, a variety of minimally invasive techniques have emerged. Originally applied to adults, they are now frequently applied to children. Among these techniques are partial upper and lower sternotomy, video assisted thoracoscopic surgery, the mini-thoracotomy, the subxiphoid approach to the heart and robotic techniques.[35-38] Use of these techniques is controversial. Opponents cite the potential for compromised exposure, and the accompanying increased risk of the procedure. Proponents cite the psychosocial benefits of smaller incisions. The potential for limited exposure must be balanced against the complexity of the case, and the likelihood of future reoperation. Partial sternotomies can consist of a partial superior sternotomy or a partial inferior sternotomy. The partial upper sternotomy has been used for such complex procedures as the arterial switch operation.[39] The inferior partial sternotomy has been commonly used for many years for procedures such as placement of epicardial pacemaker leads, where access to the anterior portion of the heart or atrium is needed. Atrial septal defects have been repaired through this incision.[40] More recently, a broader range of cardiac operations have been performed through this incision including closure of ventricular septal defects, repair of tetralogy of Fallot and atrioventricular septal defect with common junction, and procedures on the mitral valve.[39–44] In small children with more pliable sternums, a similar variety of procedures has been accomplished through a subxiphoid incision.[40]

Video assisted thoracic surgery has become a mainstay of general thoracic surgery during the last decade. In this type of procedure, one large incision is replaced by two to four smaller incisions (Fig. 13-7). A thoracoscope is placed through one incision. Others ports are used to place stapling devices, thoracoscopic scissors or instruments for dissection and retraction. The technique has been used for ligation of the arterial duct, closure of interatrial communications and division of vascular rings.[45–49] In some series, pain and postoperative stay are significantly reduced.[50–54] The relative advantages of different minimal-access procedures will vary depending on the strengths and weaknesses of individual institutions.[40,52]

There are no long-term data on the effectiveness and complications associated with many of these techniques.

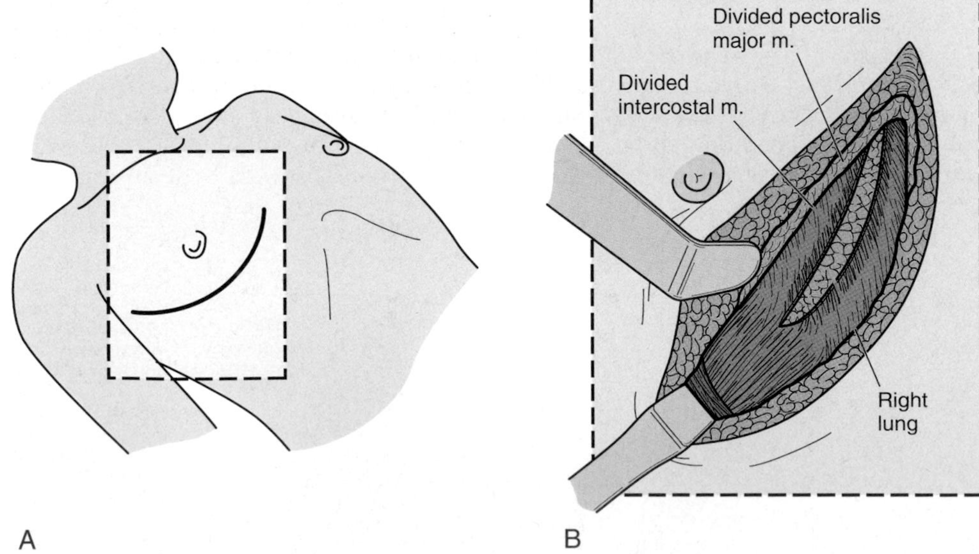

Figure 13-6 The anterolateral thoracotomy. The skin and subcutaneous tissues are divided with a combination of the knife and electrocautery along the line indicated. In some individuals, it is necessary to develop a flap beneath the subcutaneous tissue in order to reach the desired intercostal space. The pectoralis major and the intercostal muscles in the desired space of entry are then divided. In some individuals, the skin incision can be made more laterally, avoiding division of the pectoralis major.

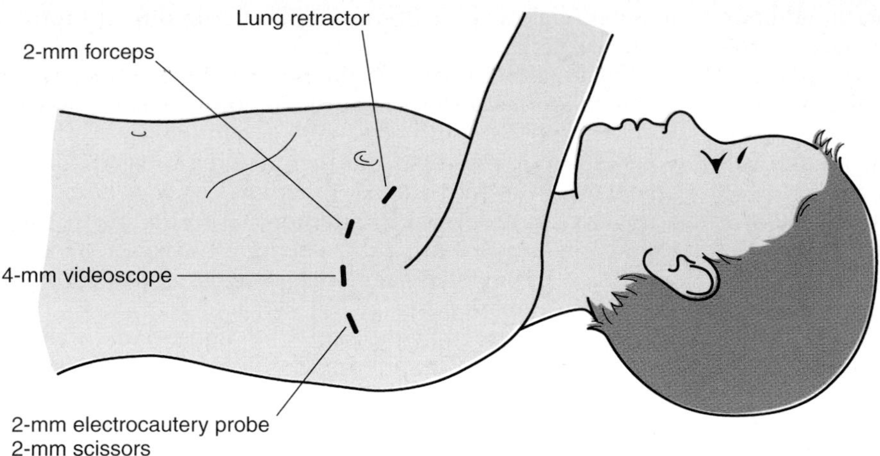

Figure 13-7 Incisions for video assisted thoracoscopic surgery. Most procedures are attempted with isolation of the lung, in which it is possible selectively to deflate the lung in the operative thoracic cavity. Two to four small incisions are made as indicated depending on the procedure to be attempted. The intercostal muscles are divided in the rib space of entry with electrocautery. (Adapted from Soukiasian HJ, Fontana GP: Surgeons should provide minimally invasive approaches for the treatment of congenital heart disease. Semin Thorac Cardiovasc Surg Pediatr Card Surg Annu 2005:185–192.)

Opponents argue that the burden of proof rests with the proponents of the newer techniques before such techniques are adopted on a widespread basis.[55] Proponents argue that the technology is quickly improving, and that there are multiple potential benefits for children, such as shortened length of stay in hospital, earlier resumption of physical activity, reduction of postoperative pain, improved respiratory function and the reduction in the long-term morbidity associated with sternotomies and thoracotomies.[56]

Open Sternum

After completion of a long, complex procedure, there may be significant accumulation of extravascular fluid in the heart, lungs, chest wall and even the peritoneal cavity. Reapproximation of the sternum can result in a significant reduction in cardiac output due to compression of the heart by adjacent structures, combined with the diastolic dysfunction that is the result of myocardial oedema. This acute restrictive physiology is similar to that seen with tamponade, and has been termed pseudotamponade physiology.[57] Because a period of decreased cardiac output is predictable following complex procedures, even the patient with initially acceptable haemodynamics may display pseudotamponade physiology within the first 12 hours following termination of cardiopulmonary bypass. Delayed sternal closure has been used commonly as a means of avoiding or managing low cardiac output syndrome in neonates and small infants undergoing complex procedures. Other indications for delayed sternal closure include ongoing bleeding that cannot be easily controlled. Occasionally, the sternal edges may be stented open to increase available space. Indications for an open sternum strategy and timing of closure vary greatly. For some, all patients undergoing the first stage of palliation for hypoplastic left heart syndrome undergo delayed sternal closure.[58,59] For others, the strategy is applied on an individual basis.[60] Closure is undertaken when haemostasis has been achieved and the patient has diuresed and been weaned from the majority of inotropic support. Some have advocated waiting until the patient has diuresed to the preoperative weight.[58] While the sternum is open, the mediastinum is covered with either Gore-Tex or a silicone sheet. This can be secured with adhesive, saving the skin edges from the injury of sutures.

MATERIALS

The job of the congenital cardiac surgeon often requires reconstruction of non-existent structures. The materials available for this task include biomaterials, synthetic materials, and combinations thereof.

Sutures

To date, sutures are necessary for any surgical task. Materials are usually classified as absorbable or nonabsorbable, and as monofilament or polyfilament. The choice of sutures depends on the specific application and stresses expected on the suture line or anastomosis. Vascular anastomoses are constructed most commonly with monofilament suture. The suture glides through the tissue easily, and this results in minimal damage to the tissue and improved haemostasis. For tasks such as fascial closure, absorbable braided sutures are commonly used, because they have a lower likelihood of tearing through tissue, and will be reabsorbed, minimising the risk of infection.

Absorbable sutures persist in the body for a limited period of time. Among the earliest absorbable sutures is gut, created from the intestines of cows or sheep. Used less commonly than in the past, the suture may be used untreated, or after treatment with chromium salts, a process which is thought to increase durability. More modern absorbable sutures include polygalactic acid (Vicryl, Johnson and Johnson, New Brunswick, NJ), and polyglycolic acid (Dexon, Tyco Healthcare, Gosport, Hampshire, UK). These polyfilament braided sutures are absorbed within 60 to 90 days. They are commonly used for closure of fascia, subcutaneous tissue and skin. Absorbable sutures are also available as monofilament. Polyglyconate (Maxon, Tyco Healthcare, Gosport, Hampshire, UK), and poliglecaprone (Monocryl, Johnson and Johnson, New Brunswick, NJ), have excellent strength when compared with other absorbable sutures, and are frequently used to close the skin. In addition to use in closing wounds, they have been used for vascular anastomoses. Polydioxanone (PDS, Johnson and Johnson, New Brunswick, NJ) is a monofilament suture that has a long duration of absorbability, and high tensile strength, with the additional advantage of maintaining its integrity in the face of infection. It appears to induce less fibrosis than polygalactic acid. As a result, it is commonly used for surgery of the airway.

Among nonabsorbable sutures, one of the oldest is silk. It is considered nonabsorbable and polyfilament, though it is ultimately degraded. Although in the past silk was used for vascular anastomoses, today it is used for retraction or to ligate small vessels. Braided polyester sutures with Teflon coating (Tevdek, Tycron) have minimal memory, hold knots well, and are used frequently to secure patches used to close ventricular septal defects, or to secure prosthetic valves. Polypropylene (Prolene) is a monofilament suture that may last from 2 to 6 years. Its long durability, easy maneuverability, and tendency to glide easily though tissue, make it the suture of choice for cardiac reconstruction and vascular anastomoses. The Gore-Tex suture, made of polytetrafluoroethylene, is a monofilament nonabsorbable suture also used for vascular anastomoses. The suture is frequently used with Gore-Tex grafts to improve haemostasis of the suture line.

Patch Material and Valveless Conduits

One of the easiest materials to use is fresh autologous pericardium. The material is easily harvested at the time of a primary operation, though it is less easily harvested during reoperation. The material is pliable, sterile, and has no likelihood of inciting an immunological reaction. Some prefer for the pericardium to have firmer texture to increase ease of handling, in which case it is fixed in glutaraldehyde. Glutaraldehyde fixation results in cross-linking of collagen, making the pericardium stiffer. Such fixation may reduce aneurysmal formation when pericardium is used for vascular reconstruction.[61] When native pericardium is not available, glutaraldehyde-treated bovine pericardium can be used. Though this tissue is readily available, and has minimal to no risk of transmission of disease, it has been known to stimulate an immune reaction, and undergo significant calcification.

Homograft aortas or pulmonary arteries, in other words cadaveric tissues, can also be used for vascular reconstruction. Such material is commonly used during reconstruction of the pulmonary arterial tree and confluence, or to relieve isolated pulmonary stenoses. They are also commonly used for reconstruction of the aortic arch in the neonate.[58,62] The material is haemostatic, and easy to handle. It is, however, expensive, and it requires time for thawing, carries a risk of calcification, and comes in varying thicknesses that are often difficult to predict. In addition, homograft material can incite an immune response resulting in a nonspecific increase in anti-human lymphocyte antibodies, potentially complicating future transplantation.[63]

Dacron, a synthetic polyester material, has been a mainstay in vascular reconstruction since its introduction in the 1950s. It is used in its tubular form to reconstruct vascular segments. It can also be used as a patch, and is commonly used for closure of ventricular septal defects. The Dacron material can incite a fibrous reaction. This is an advantage for closure of ventricular septal defects, in that such fibrous ingrowth may allow closure of the tiny residual defects at the edges of the patch. Fibrous ingrowth is even further enhanced when the Dacron is covered with velour.[64] Caution, however, should be used when Dacron is placed close to an arterial valve, as fibrous ingrowth can impair motion of the valvar leaflets.

When used as a conduit, the porosity of Dacron poses a problem for haemostasis. In order to improve haemostasis, grafts can be pre-clotted by soaking them in either autologous blood or albumin, and then heating the grafts in an autoclave. In order to make the grafts easier to use, sealants have been developed and applied to the grafts. One example is the Hemashield Dacron graft (Medox Medical, Newark, NJ), in which formaldehyde cross-linked collagen is used to decrease porosity.

Polytetrafluoroethylene, with the trade name Teflon, and produced by the DuPont Corporation, Wilmington, Delaware, can be expanded or stretched such that it carries a pore size of 20 to 30 μm, a size that has been determined to be the optimal pore size for healing.[65,66] The result is expanded polytetrafluoroethylene, commonly known as Gore-Tex (W.L. Gore and Associates, Flagstaff, AZ). It is used extensively for systemic to pulmonary artery shunts and for arterial reconstruction. Gore-Tex is thrombogenic, and a pseudointimal layer will develop over time that is the result of a combination of thrombus and cellular ingrowth.[67–71] This pseudointimal layer will decrease the caliber of small grafts, and can result in critical reduction of flow. Aspirin has been shown to improve patency of small caliber Gore-Tex grafts.[72]

Valves and Valved Conduits

Decisions concerning valvar replacement in children are complicated because of the need to accommodate growth, the desire to avoid anticoagulation and the need for durability. Options in children can be divided into four broad categories: mechanical valves, xenobioprosthetic valves, homograft valves and autograft valves.

Mechanical Valves

Significant progress has been made with mechanical valves since the introduction of the first mechanical valve in 1952. Currently manufactured mechanical valves have either a single tilting disc, such as the Medtronic Hall Valve, or a bileaflet design, such as the St. Jude (St. Jude Medical, St. Paul, MN), Carbomedics (Austin, TX), ATS (ATS Medical, Minneapolis, MN), or On-X Valves (Medical Carbon Research, Austin, TX) (Fig. 13-8A). Structural failure of prosthetic valves is currently rarely reported. To date, all mechanical valves are thrombogenic, and necessitate anticoagulation. As a result, patients with mechanical valves are at risk for thromboembolic and bleeding complications. The risk of such complications is present, even in patients with optimally managed anticoagulation, and is influenced by factors specific to the patient, along with the position of the valve.

In adults, the incidence of thromboembolic complications among patients with a mechanical valve in the aortic position varies between 1.4 to 2.7 per patient per year, and bleeding complications between 0.7 and 2.3 per patient per year.[73] The risk of these complications with mechanical valves in the aortic position in children is less well known. In one report, the freedom from thromboembolic complications after 20 years was 93%.[74] Another series reported no episodes of thromboembolic complications, and only one incident of anticoagulation-related haemorrhage at a mean follow-up of 12 ± 6 years.[75] Although these two reports suggest that replacement of the aortic valve with mechanical

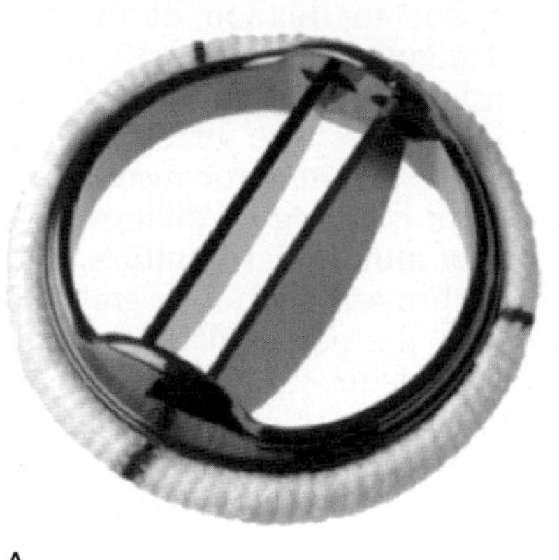
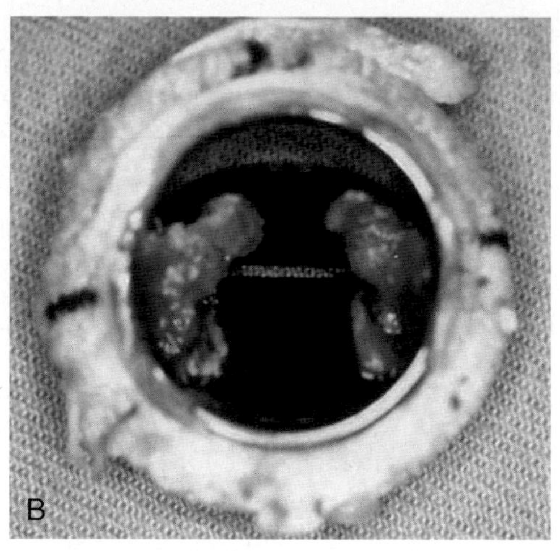

Figure 13-8 **A,** A typical bileaflet mechanical valve. Such valves are at risk for thromboembolic complications and anticoagulation is necessary. **B,** Adherent thrombus in an explanted valve. (Reproduced with permission from St. Jude Medical, Inc., St. Paul, Minnesota.)

prostheses in children has a low risk of anticoagulation-related complications, they summarise only relatively small experiences from single centres. The true risk probably falls between these reports and the larger adult experience.

The risk of complications related to anticoagulation is greatest for mechanical valves placed in atrioventricular position in the systemic circulation. Three separate reports summarising individual institutional experiences in children totaling 115 patients reported 10-year freedom from thromboembolic complications above 92%, and the risk of complications related to bleeding at between 76% and 97%.[76–78] The true incidence of thromboembolic complications in children undergoing replacement of the mitral valve with a mechanical prosthesis is probably underestimated by those reporting from single centres. A multi-centre study found that 4 of 102 survivors of such replacement required re-replacement for thrombosis at a mean follow-up of 6.0 years.[79] Prospective studies of adults, with combined enrollment of over 1000 patients, showed that bileaflet mechanical valves in the mitral position were associated with an incidence of both thromboembolic events and complications due to bleeding at a frequency between 1% and 3% per patient per year.[80,81] Freedom from thromboembolic complications after 10 years was 85.5%, and freedom from bleeding was 81.7%.[80]

The most widely used prosthetic valve of the last decade is the St. Jude valve (Fig. 13-8B). It is a low profile, bileaflet valve constructed of pyrolytic carbon. In its most recent iteration, it has a rotatable valvar mechanism. Competing bileaflet designs include the ATS, On-X, and Carbomedics valves. There has been considerable interest of late in the potential of utilising the On-X valve with aspirin as the only anti-thrombotic agent. The manufacturer claims that the lack of silicon coating on the carbon used to construct the valve makes it less thrombogenic. Controlled trials are underway to evaluate the risk of thromboembolic complications using only an antiplatelet strategy with the On-X valve.

Another major problem with mechanical valves when used in children is the limited availability of small sizes. Modifications of the sewing ring of the 19-mm Carbomedics and the 19-mm St. Jude valve have resulted in prosthetic valves that can accommodate a native annulus between 16 and 18 mm. Oftentimes, there is insufficient orifice for placement of even the smallest valve designed. Surgical techniques of annular enlargement, such as the anterior enlargement of Konno,[82] or the posterior enlargement of Nicks[83] or Manougian[84,85] are used when the diameter of the native aortic root does not permit placement of a valve sufficiently large to meet the haemodynamic needs of the patient. In the mitral position, the anatomy does not lend itself as well to annular expansion. Other techniques must be utilised. Valves can be placed in the supra-annular position, or at angles, techniques that can permit placement of modestly larger prosthesis. Significant oversizing of mitral prostheses should be avoided, as this can result in subaortic obstruction.

Xenobioprosthetic Valves

Xenobioprosthetic valves include porcine aortic valves, either stented, as in the Hancock and Mosiac Valves (Medtronic, Minneapolis, MN) (Fig. 13-9), or nonstented,

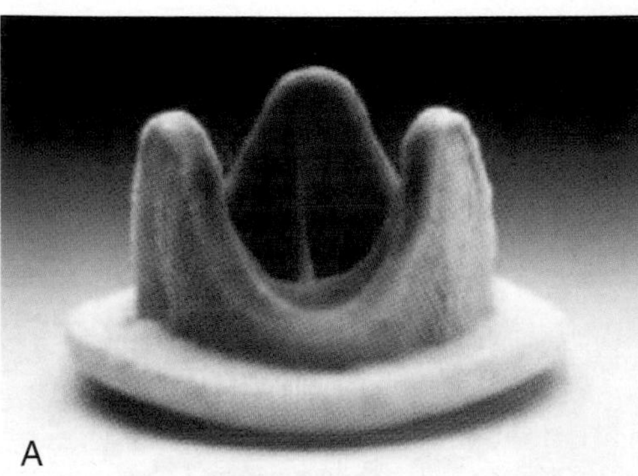
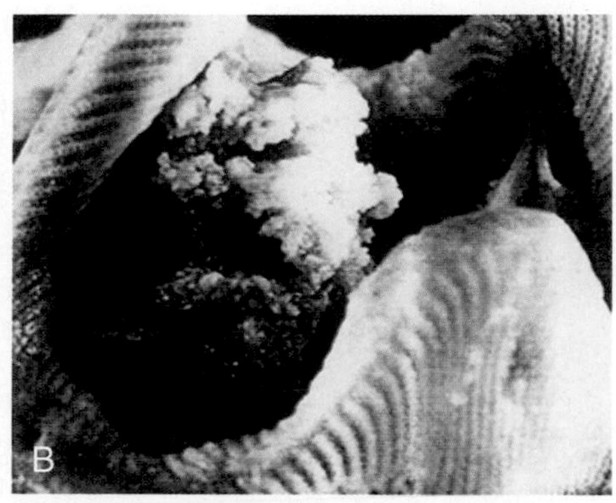

Figure 13-9 **A,** A typical xenobioprosthetic stented porcine valve. **B,** Such valves, when inserted in children, undergo rapid calcification and degeneration. (**A,** Reproduced with permission from Edwards Lifesciences, Irvine, California.)

as in the Freestyle (Medtronic, Minneapolis, MN), Toronto SPV valve (St. Jude Medical, St. Paul, MN) and valves manufactured from bovine pericardium such as the Perimount valve (Edwards Life Science, Irvine, CA).[86,87] Xenobioprosthetic material has been treated with glutaraldehyde in order to decrease immunogenicity and improve durability. In children, xenobioprosthetic valves undergo rapid calcific degeneration, limiting their use in the systemic circulation.[88] Recent efforts have been directed at newer techniques for preservation that limit this process of calcification.[89] Xenobioprosthetic valved conduits have been used for apicoaortic conduits for relief of obstruction of the left ventricular outflow tract, and in other rare circumstances where anticoagulation must be avoided, but in general xenobioprosthetic valves are rarely used in children in the systemic circulation.

Homograft Valves

Valved homograft material can also be used for valvar replacement and reconstruction (Fig. 13-10). The homograft is considered the conduit of choice for replacement of the aortic valve and aortic root in the face of endocarditis.[90–95] Small homograft valved conduits are ideal for complex reconstruction in neonates and small infants, such as repair of common arterial trunk, and tetralogy of Fallot with pulmonary atresia. In North America, however, homografts in sizes suitable for neonates and small infants are becoming less and less available. The use of homografts to join the right ventricle to the pulmonary arteries is discussed more fully when considering selection of valves.

Pulmonary Autograft Valves

The pulmonary autograft used for replacement of the aortic valve (the Ross procedure) addresses some of the limitations in other options, and involves the harvest of the native pulmonary valve for replacement of the aortic valve.[96] The native outflow tract from the right ventricle is then reconstructed with another conduit, usually a homograft. The pulmonary autograft is frequently chosen for infants and small children. Although the autograft does allow for growth, late dilatation of the neoaortic root with resultant aortic insufficiency has been identified in a subgroup of patients undergoing the Ross procedure. At least two mechanisms resulting in regurgitation appear to explain dysfunction of the autograft. Patients undergoing the Ross procedure for isolated aortic incompetence have been shown to have an increased risk for development of incompetence, primarily due to dilation of the left ventriculo-aortic junction. Patients undergoing the Ross procedure for congenital aortic stenosis have an increased incidence of ascending aortic dilation, with dilation of the sinutubular junction that also results in aortic insufficiency. Efforts to limit development of autograft dilation and insufficiency include the use of annuloplasty sutures, and placement of the autograft within a Dacron tube graft.[97,98] Both of these techniques limit the potential for growth, and are only suitable in older patients.

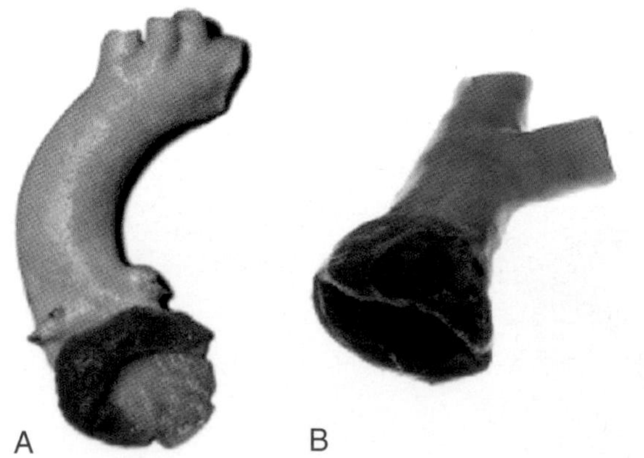

Figure 13-10 Aortic (**A**) and pulmonary (**B**) homografts. The valves are harvested along with a segment of the outflow tract and varying lengths of artery. (Reproduced with permission of Cryolite, Inc., Kennesaw, Georgia.)

The autograft compares favourably to other options for replacing the aortic valve in children, but concern persists over long-term durability. In 150 patients under the age of 21 years, freedom from autograft failure of 84% ± 4%, and freedom from all valve-related complications of 72% ± 6%, were reported at 8 years.[99] Other series from Western Europe and North America, in which it is possible to differentiate the outcome for children, report freedom from reoperation of 83% to 88% at 5 to 6 years of follow-up.[100–103] The long-term outlook of the pulmonary valve when used to replace the aortic valve remains unknown. Data from the Ross Procedure International Registry shows that the freedom from reintervention curve does not reach a plateau, and it seems likely that many of these patients will require additional procedures directed at the neoaortic valve, as well as the predictable need for reintervention on the right ventricular outflow tract. Although it is generally acknowledged that the pulmonary homograft placed during the Ross procedure has greater longevity than that used for reconstruction of the right ventricular outflow tract for other forms of congenital cardiac disease, presumably due to the orthotopic position, normal pulmonary arteries and pulmonary vascular resistance, recent data indicate that replacement still will be necessary.[104,105] Additional studies have indicated that even a mild, and apparently acceptable, gradient across the right ventricular outflow tract will increase importantly during exercise, and that exercise-induced arrhythmias are common following the Ross procedure.[106]

Selection of Valves

No consensus has been reached on selection, but some generally accepted guidelines are presented. For use in the aortic position in neonates, infants and small children, the Ross procedure is commonly chosen, because it accommodates growth and anticoagulation is not required. Furthermore, the size of the autograft matches the size of the normal left ventricular outflow tract, and lesser degrees of enlargement of the aortic root are required compared to mechanical valves. Homografts can be used in the aortic position in infants and small children, either as a first choice, or if the pulmonary valve is deemed unsuitable for use in the aortic position. For older children, some continue to advocate the Ross procedure, although mechanical valves are also frequently used. Xenobioprosthetic valves within valved conduits have been used as conduits from the left ventricular apex to the aorta for relief of severe and complex obstruction in the left ventricular outflow tract.

Mechanical valves are generally used for the mitral (or systemic atrioventricular junction) position. Despite the need for anticoagulation, these valves have the necessary durability. Mortality after such replacement continues to be high in younger children. Results, however, seem to be improving, with one study showing reduction in operative mortality from 31% to 3.6% when comparing children receiving operations at the same institution before and after 1990.[76] A recent report showed an early mortality rate of 13% in children under 2 years of age undergoing replacement of the mitral valve,[107] a figure to be compared with a mortality rate as high as 52% in a report from 1990.[108] Xenobioprosthetic valves are rarely used in the mitral position due to the high rates of calcification and failure.[109,110] Exceptions can be made, however, in extreme circumstances, such as haematological disorders or pregnancy, when the need to avoid anticoagulation is more definitive. There are advocates for the use of the pulmonary autograft in the mitral position, a procedure now known as the Ross II.[111] The autograft is placed within a Dacron tube graft. Although the viability may be good, and the need for anticoagulation diminished, there is no potential for growth. There has been some success in children,[112] but follow-up is limited.[104] More studies will be necessary to determine the long-term success of this technique.

For reconstruction of the right ventricular outflow tract, biologic valves including homograft valved conduits, and xenobioprosthetic valves, are most commonly used. Biologic valves have longer durability in the lower pressured pulmonary position compared to any position in the systemic circuit, favouring the use of biologic over mechanical valves. Furthermore, the risk of anticoagulation is avoided. Homograft conduits have excellent handling qualities, conform to the anatomy, and facilitate achievement of haemostasis. Limited durability, however, can be a problem. Homografts are commonly used for reconstruction of the right ventricular outflow tract. Early valvar insufficiency and obstruction have been reported.[113–115] In some children, homografts undergo severe calcification, with accompanying shrinkage, that can result in obstruction. Calcification appears to be more accelerated in younger children.[114,116–118] Incompatibility between donor and recipient have been proposed as contributing factors to this calcification and failure of the graft.[116,119–121]

An alternative to homografts is use of the bovine jugular venous conduit (Contegra, Medtronic, Minneapolis, MN) (Fig. 13-11). The Contegra graft has been used in reconstruction of the outflow tract in patients with common arterial trunk, tetralogy of Fallot, the Ross procedure, and pulmonary atresia.[122–127] Early and mid-term haemodynamic results are favourable,[127] with one study showing valvar regurgitation to be absent in almost half of patients at a mean follow-up of 26 months.[125] In the largest series reported to date, with a mean follow-up of 2.1 years, there was no relevant gradient detected at the level of the valves, and minimal valvar insufficiency.[127] In the large prospective multi-centre study conducted by the Congenital Cardiac Surgeon's Society, the bovine jugular vein fared well, with a lower probability of progressing to more severe forms of severe regurgitation than other types of conduit.[128,129] Aneurysmal formation,[113,130] and a particular tendency for distal stenosis,[123] however, have been reported, though it is difficult at the current time to determine if these incidences are higher than those seen with homografts.

The use of small conduits is not surprisingly a risk factor for failure,[115,131] but interestingly oversizing the valve by more than a *z* score of 2.7 has also been shown to be a risk factor for early failure.[131] This trend was confirmed in the study coordinated by the Society of Congenital Heart Surgeons, where outcomes were better when sizes with *z* scores between 1 and 3 were chosen.[129]

There is general agreement that a bioprosthetic valve is the conduit of choice in the tricuspid position when the native valve cannot be repaired.[132,133] Bioprosthetic valves appear to fair better in this position than in any other position, with freedoms of reoperation reported at 97.5% ± 1.9%, and 80.6% ± 7.6%, at 1 and 5 years, respectively.

Valvar Repair

As discussed in the preceding section, options for replacement of valves are limited during childhood. Repair, if feasible, preserves the potential for growth, avoids anticoagulation, and also the need for valvar re-replacement. The disadvantages of repair include residual lesions, such as stenosis and insufficiency, and limited durability. Decision-making regarding the suitability of a lesion for repair is complex, and must take into account the pros and cons outlined above, as well as the specific lesion and the ability of the surgeon. Repair of the mitral valve is commonly performed, and uses techniques that borrowed from the experience in adults, as well as techniques that have been developed from repair of atrioventricular septal defects. Repair of the mitral valve is frequently successful and durable.[134,135] In contrast, replacement of the mitral valve necessitates a repeated replacement in almost three-quarters of patients.[136] Mitral valvopathy amenable to surgical intervention may be the result of rheumatic heart disease, acquired and congenital cardiomyopathies, Marfan's disease, Shone's complex, and congenital mitral

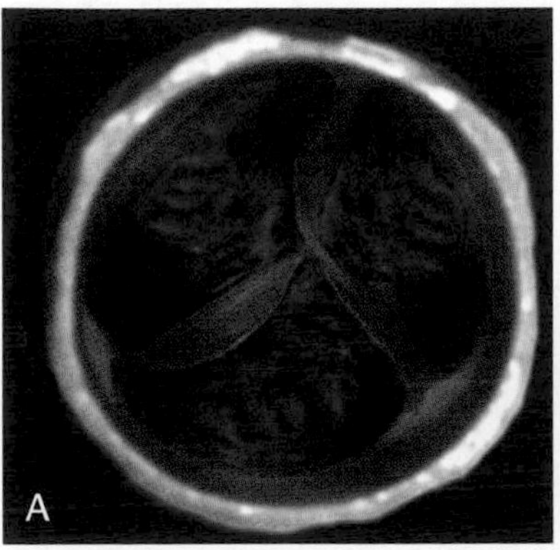

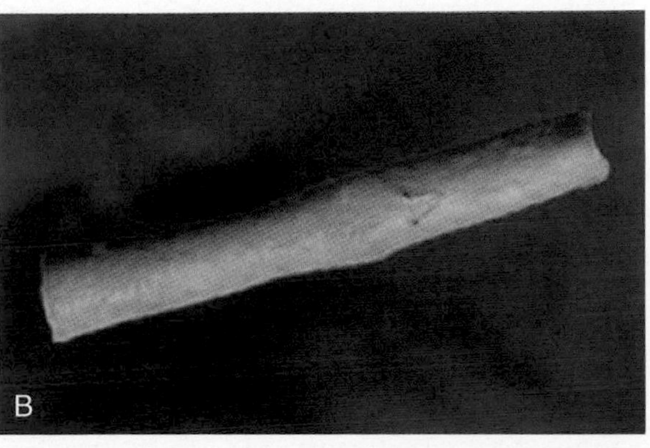

Figure 13-11 **A,** A bovine jugular vein graft. Note the tricuspid venous valve. **B,** The valve is contained within a length of jugular vein that can be tailored to the specific anatomic requirements of the patient. (Reproduced with permission from Medtronic, Inc., Minneapolis, Minnesota.)

stenosis. Techniques for repair vary depending on the aetiology of the pathology.[135] For repair of mitral stenosis, techniques include commissurotomy, valvoplasty, cordal fenestration, and splitting of papillary muscles. For mitral insufficiency, techniques include repair of clefts, resection, shortening, or augmentation of leaflets, cordal shortening, annuloplasty, and creation of a double orifice.[137] In general, mortality is low with repair in the setting of biventricular circulations.[138–141] In those with a functionally univentricular circulation, in contrast, repair carries a higher mortality.[135]

Repair of the aortic valve is less well accepted than that of the mitral valve, albeit that experience is accumulating.[142–148] Over the last decade, experience and success with repair have improved.[146–149] Techniques include repair of valvar perforations, suspension of prolapsed leaflets, annuloplasty and extension of leaflets with pericardium.[146] In particular extension of the leaflets has been used with success in patients with rheumatic aortic valve disease, with 90% of patients free from valvar related complications at 7 years. Extension has also been applied to patients with congenital pathology with improving results.[150,151]

STRATEGIES FOR CARDIOPULMONARY BYPASS AND PERFUSION

Surgical intervention inside the heart or on the great vessels normally requires significant interruption of flow of blood in regions of the surgical field to achieve adequate visualisation. To permit a more controlled surgical approach, extracorporeal circulation and oxygenation of blood has been developed. During cardiopulmonary bypass, venous blood from the great veins or right atrium is routed through an oxygenator or artificial lung, and reinfused into the aorta. A variety of specific techniques are used for cannulation and perfusion. These are intended to deliver oxygenated blood into the patient at a rate sufficient to fully support the function of the bodily organs for the duration of the surgical repair, and as such have permitted the development of extraordinary surgical reconstructive procedures. Optimal strategy permits extensive surgical intervention, with largely predictable freedom from permanent injury to the organs. Planned and unplanned modifications of techniques, however, may place organs at the risk of ischaemia.[152,153] Additionally, the nature of the interactions of blood with non-endothelialised surfaces, and the effects of associated alterations in temperature and pulse during bypass, make the technique a pathway for direct inflammatory and ischaemic injury.[154]

The Circuitry of Cardiopulmonary Bypass

One task of the perfusionist is to tailor the circuit to the specific needs of the individual child. The variability of size, anatomy, and pathophysiology in this population necessitate the use of a great number of products. Large extracorporeal surface areas and prime volumes have been identified as potential contributors to complications following bypass.[155] Multiple sizes of oxygenators, heat exchangers, reservoirs, and other components have been designed to address these issues. Much of the research and development for the child has focused on reduction in surface area and volume to reduce total prime volume, surface area, and biologic incompatibility.[156,157]

It is advisable for the circuits at a given institution to be organised in the same manner, facilitating the ability of perfusionists to provide safe and consistent service to all patients. A common configuration for bypass is to use bicaval cannulation with a single venous line for drainage into a hardshell venous reservoir with an integrated cardiotomy reservoir (Fig. 13-12). A typical strategy for a cardiac cannulation is shown in Figure 13-13. A roller pump is used to pump deoxygenated blood from the reservoir through a hollow fibre oxygenator with an integrated heat exchanger. Blood exiting the oxygenator passes through an arterial line filter, and returns to the patient via the arterial cannula placed in the ascending aorta.

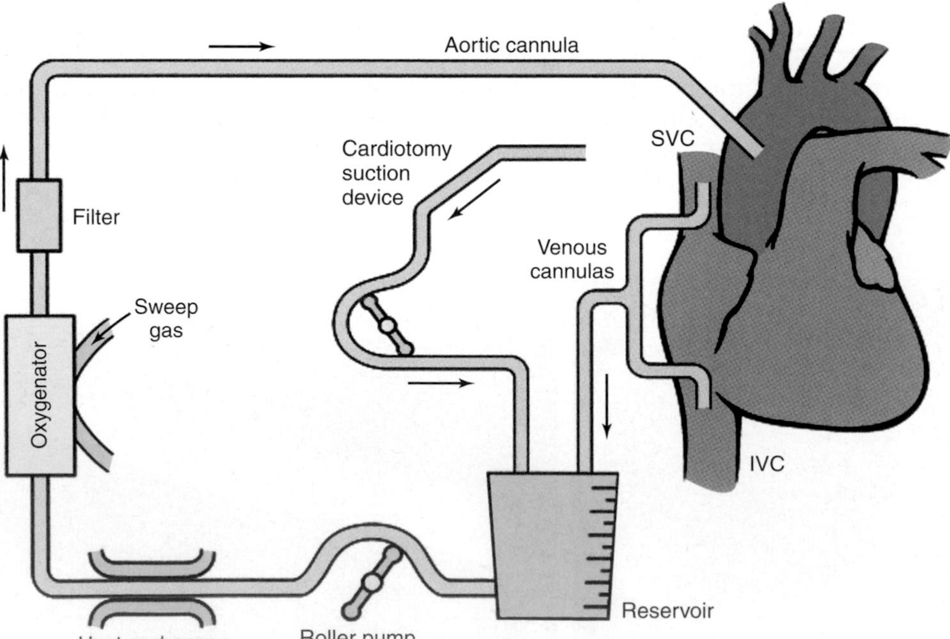

Figure 13-12 A simplified schematic of the components of a typical cardiopulmonary bypass circuit. A roller pump, an oxygenator, a heat exchanger, a venous reservoir, and a filter are included. IVC, inferior caval vein; SVC, superior caval vien.

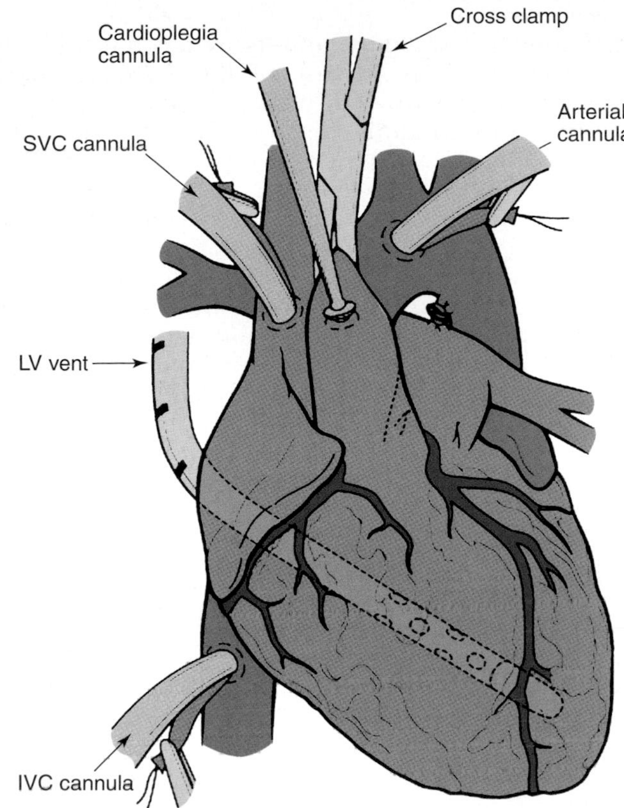

Figure 13-13 A common technique of cannulation. Cannulation for an arterial switch is shown. Venous drainage is accomplished with separate venous cannula for the superior caval vein (SVC) and inferior caval vein (IVC). Oxygenated blood is infused via the arterial cannula positioned at the junction of the ascending aorta and aortic arch. The cross clamp has been applied isolating the coronary arteries for delivery of cardioplegia via a cannula in the proximal ascending aorta. Left ventricular distension is avoided by placing a left ventricular (LV) vent through the junction of the right superior pulmonary vein and left atrium, advancing it across the mitral valve into the left ventricle. (Reproduced with permission from Tweddell JS, Litwin SB: Transposition of the great arteries. Operative Techniques in Thoracic and Cardiovascular Surgery: A Comparative Atlas 7:49–63, 2002.)

Additional roller pumps provide active suction for use as field suckers, a left ventricular vent, or a vent in the aortic root. A variety of pressure transducers, level detectors, bubble detectors, and in-line blood gas analysers are used for enhanced precision and safety.

Oxygenators

Hollow fibre membranes are manufactured to mimic the pulmonary capillary bed by packing together microporous fibres in a spiral fashion.[158] Gas delivered to the oxygenator can be manipulated by the perfusionist to optimise oxygenation and removal of carbon dioxide. Anaesthetic vapours are commonly delivered via the membrane oxygenator, although the specific function for transfer of different vapours and oxygenators is variable. Surfaces exposed to the blood can be coated with some form of a biomimetic treatment. Several types of treatments are available, all having the goal of increasing the biocompatibility of the circuit, reducing damage to blood, and minimising the impact of bypass on the inflammatory response.[157]

Reservoirs

Two types of reservoirs are utilised, venous and cardiotomy. The former is a collection chamber only for the venous blood. The latter collects all shed blood returning from the operative field via cardiotomy suction and the left ventricular vent. Both reservoirs are filtered. The cardiotomy filters are designed to remove debris such as tissue, fat, macrothrombi and suture material.[158] Many reservoirs are available that combine the venous and cardiotomy suction as a single unit. In this configuration, the separation of the chambers is made internally. After the filtration process, their volumes combine into a single outlet, which simplifies connections and permits visualisation of air and the level of fluid in the reservoir. According to the latest published survey, nine-tenths of paediatric institutions in North America use hardshell venous reservoirs.[159]

Pumps

Although many types of pumps have been described in the literature, there are primarily two types of arterial pumps in use today, namely roller and centrifugal. Roller pumps contain a length of tubing located inside a curved raceway. This raceway is placed at the travel perimeter of rollers mounted on the ends of rotating arms positioned opposite each other. These rollers are mounted in such a way that one roller is compressing the tubing at all times. By compressing a segment of the blood-filled resilient tubing, the pump pushes blood ahead of the moving roller, producing continuous flow. The output of the roller pump is determined by the revolutions per minute of the pump, and the volume displaced with each revolution. This stroke volume depends on the internal diameter of tubing and the circumferential length of the raceway.[160] The roller pump head is reusable. The flow rate is simple to determine, by multiplying stroke volume by the revolutions each minute, and multiple sizes of tubing can be used in the same pump, making it applicable to patients of all sizes. These pumps, however, do have disadvantages. The pump displaces in positive fashion, so it will pump air as well as blood, necessitating the need for a system to detect bubbles. It is an occlusive pump, so pressure transducers must be connected to the system to detect excessive pressures, reducing the risk of particulate microembolisation from tubing spallation, shear-induced blood damage or possible rupture. Establishment of the optimal setting for occlusion is imperative for accurate calculation of rates of flow, and to minimise blood trauma.

Centrifugal pumps consist of an impeller arranged with either vanes or a nest of smooth plastic cones inside a plastic housing. The sterile, disposable impeller is coupled magnetically with an electric motor spinning in the drive console. When the impeller rotates rapidly, it generates a pressure differential, causing blood to flow.[160] Centrifugal pumps are non-occlusive and pressure dependent. They generate increased flow when either the preload increases, or the afterload decreases. The non-occlusive nature of the pump eliminates the possibility of tubing wear, spallation, and excessive pressure in the lines, but since they are pressure dependent, a flow transducer is necessary to determine accurate rates of flow. If the pump slows or stops, reverse flow can occur. Centrifugal pumps require more expensive disposable parts compared to the roller pump. As a result of the described limitations of centrifugal pumps, a recent survey found that roller pumps were the predominant pump device in nine-tenths of paediatric centers.[159]

Filters and Haemoconcentrators

In addition to the cardiotomy and venous reservoir filters mentioned previously, all but 2% of paediatric institutions use arterial line filters as a last line of defense against gaseous and particulate microembolisation.[159] They come in a variety of sizes, with pre-established limits to rates of flow. They require additional volume to prime, but are excellent gross bubble traps. Because they are micropore filters, they are susceptible to obstruction. Manufacturers recommend placing a clamped bypass line around them that can be opened if the filter becomes obstructed.

Haemoconcentrators allow the perfusionist to remove water and other electrolytes, such as potassium, from the blood. They contain hollow fibres similar to those within a dialysis filter. Blood passes through the inside of hollow fibres and light vacuum is placed on the outside. Everything smaller than the size of the pores of the semipermeable membrane will be extracted, including water, electrolytes, some cytokines and drugs, and everything larger than the pores will remain in the blood stream, including red cells, platelets and most plasma proteins. Significant haemoconcentration can be achieved. Some heparin will be removed; thus adequacy of heparinisation must be monitored regularly.[160] The haemoconcentrator can be used at any time during the case, provided there is sufficient volume in the venous reservoir. This is the same type of filter used to perform modified ultrafiltration.

Conduct of Cardiopulmonary Bypass

Rates of Flow

Although the determinants of delivery of oxygen, namely concentration of haemoglobin, saturation of oxyhaemoglobin and rates of flow, are more easily measured during cardiopulmonary bypass that at any other time in the life of a neonate or infant, the adequacy of delivery of oxygen should always be continuously monitored and adjusted to avoid overt or occult injury to the organs throughout the perioperative period.[161,162] Rates of flow have typically been guided by nomograms based on body weight or surface area, and Fick's principles of delivery of oxygen and metabolism.[163] The regional distribution of blood during cardiopulmonary bypass is related to host and technical factors, and the probability of adequate flow to the whole body or organs is related to the total rate of flow.[162,164–167] Typically, full flow refers to a perfusion index of 2.8 to 3.6 L/m^2/min, which corresponds to 150 to 200 mL/kg/min in a neonate. Low flow is delivered at varying hypothermic conditions to afford metabolic protection and typically refers to rates of between one-quarter and half of full flow.[167] The rates of flow to the whole body necessary to maintain adequate cerebral perfusion range from 30 to 80 mL/kg/min.[168,169] Isolated perfusion of organs during bypass is governed by the relative distribution of vascular resistance. Reduction in temperature to 16° C to 20° C allows termination of flow for a limited amount of time to permit unobscured access to the surgical field, a condition referred to as deep hypothermic circulatory arrest. The safe duration of deep hypothermic circulatory arrest in any individual patient is unknown and highly related to the determinants of delivery of oxygen.[170] The deleterious effects of lowered flow may be more pronounced after hypothermic arrest,[171] when a higher perfusion pressure is necessary to re-establish cerebral flow.[172] Because of variability between patients and techniques it is advisable to measure indicators of cerebral oxygenation. Manipulation of the independent determinants of delivery of oxygen, such as haemoglobin, and partial pressures of carbon dioxide, can be used to restore cerebral oxygen delivery.[173]

Haemodilution

Haemodilution has almost universally accompanied cardiopulmonary bypass because of the desire to prime extracorporeal circuitry with products other than blood. Rheologic considerations for microvascular flow during hypothermia have supported this approach, and are thought to outweigh the reduction in delivery of oxygen associated with the anaemia produced by haemodilution. The weight of evidence, however, supports limiting haemodilution in neonates and children, targeting a haematocrit of at least 30% even during deep hypothermia.[174–176] While variations in prime solutions are mainly targeted at manipulation of electrolytes, oncotic pressure, and haemoglobin, the effects on prothrombotic, procoagulant and anticoagulant factors should also be recognised as important effects of haemodilution, and calculated based upon estimated blood volume and circuit volume for each patient.

Temperature Regulation

Hypothermia reduces both the cerebral metabolic rate and the availability of oxygen for transfer to the brain. The effects on cerebral metabolism are complex. The metabolism of brain and other tissue is reduced with reduction in body temperature.[177] Most data suggests an inverse exponential relationship, with as much as a 3.5-fold reduction in metabolism for a reduction of 10°C in temperature, the so-called Q10.[178] Others have found a Q10 as low at 2.3.[179] The bulk of evidence suggests a nearly-inverse exponential reduction in metabolism is reduced by an average of 2.8 fold for a 10° C change in temperature.[180] The result of metabolic suppression with hypothermia is that cerebral oxygen extraction is reduced, while flow of blood is allowed to be autoregulated, whether measured by saturations in the jugular bulb[180,181] or near-infrared spectroscopy.[182,183] Because temperature affects the solubility of oxygen and carbon dioxide in solution, and their interaction with haemoglobin, changes in temperature are coupled with changes in gas tensions and pH. In a broad range of studies, the independent effect of pH is small compared to the effect of temperature, with a small reduction in oxygen consumption in more acidotic environments.[180] Because pH responsiveness of the cerebral vasculature remains in effect at hypothermia, however, control and manipulation of pH is a critical part of temperature management.

The coupling between cerebral metabolism and blood flow seems to be reasonably maintained in the temperature range of 32° C to 37° C.[184–189] Below 30° C, however, uncoupling is commonly demonstrated, regardless of pH, such that the metabolism is reduced more than blood [181,190–192] The solubility of oxygen in plasma, and the affinity of haemoglobin for oxygen, are both increased with hypothermia, such that availability of oxygen in the tissues is reduced at any given rate of flow, the Bohr effect. The increased ratio of cerebral flow to metabolism with hypothermia is commonly viewed as cytoprotective from an energetic viewpoint,[180] but the decreased availability of oxygen may negate this apparent metabolic protection.[193,194] The result of increased solubility and leftward oxyhaemoglobin shift is that the fall in cerebral oxygenation with ischaemia is not attenuated by hypothermia, even though saturations of haemoglobin are better maintained.[195] Altogether the cytoprotective effects of mild hypothermia exceed measurable metabolic effects and likely involve other mechanisms including alterations in gene expression.[196]

In practical terms, schemes for cooling are relatively standardised in most institutions. The complexity of the defect to be corrected or palliated dictates the strategy for the temperature used during bypass, albeit that compounding anatomic features such as the presence of aortopulmonary collateral arteries may influence the strategy. Typically, mild hypothermia, at 37° C to 32° C, will be employed for simple defects such as atrial and ventricular septal defects. Moderate hypothermia, between 32° C and 28° C, is used for more complex lesions such as atrioventricular septal defect or tetralogy of Fallot. Deep hypothermia, from 28° C down to 18° C, is reserved for the most complex lesions requiring a period of circulatory arrest, such as palliation of hypoplasia of the left heart, repair of interrupted aortic arch or correction of discordant ventriculo-arterial connections.

Acid-Base Management

The management of blood gases during cardiopulmonary bypass is intertwined with that of temperature and has been widely investigated and debated. The complexity ensues because metabolic rate, the solubility of gases in blood, the ionisation of water, and therefore the pH of electroneutrality, the ionisation of intracellular buffers, and the affinity of both oxygen and carbon dioxide for haemoglobin are all dependent on temperature.[197] There are two strategies developed for management. A pH-stat strategy maintains normal levels of carbon dioxide and hydrogen ions when measured at hypothermia, or temperature corrected. An alpha-stat strategy maintains normal gas tensions and acid base balance when measured at normothermia, or temperature uncorrected. The alpha-stat approach is associated with minimal metabolic suppression, and represents the physiologic situation in homeotherms with temperature gradients across parts of the body, but with thermoregulation maintained. The pH-stat approach is associated with metabolic suppression, and more closely mimics the metabolic milieu of hibernation with induction of metabolic suppression.[198]

The pH affects the ratio of flow of blood to metabolism.[185] While levels of adenosine triphosphate in the brain are maintained during alpha-stat cooling,[183,199] with pH-stat cooling there is evidence of luxury perfusion. At temperatures below 30° C, blood flow is pressure-passive over a wider range of metabolism, with overperfusion evidenced by the appearance of oedema.[200] The increased flow with pH-stat strategy is widely utilised to increase uniformity of cerebral cooling, oxygenation[174,183,201–205] and metabolic suppression.[182,197,205] There is evidence of improved outcome in children subjected to deep hypothermic circulatory arrest[206–208] or low-flow bypass when using the pH-stat strategy.[209–211] Evidence also exists for improved myocardial function with pH-stat techniques.[212] The effects of pH on non-cerebral tissue are also important in determining the distribution of flow on cardiopulmonary bypass. A pH-stat strategy directs more blood to the brain in the presence of aortopulmonary collateral connections.[174] Approaches which combine pH-stat strategy for cooling with alpha-stat strategy for maintenance of high-flow hypothermic perfusion may represent a compromise between inadequate delivery of oxygen and metabolic suppression, and overperfusion-related formation of oedema and post-acidotic increased cerebrovascular resistance.[181,213]

Cerebral Protection and Anaesthesia

Suppression of cerebral consumption of oxygen occurs with both vapour and barbiturate-based anaesthesia, and hypoxia tolerance, based upon lactate production, is enhanced.[214] The suppression of metabolism by anesthetic vapours is accompanied by maintenance of high energy phosphates, indicating desirable energetic balance.[215] Because vapour agents are also cerebral vasodilators, the ratio of cerebral flow to metabolism is higher with these agents, and the increase in cerebral flow may be maintained for hours.[216–218] Suppression of thermoregulatory[219] responses to hypothermia may be an important role for the salutary effect of lower-stress anaesthetic strategies on survival in complex repairs.[220] Inhibition of K-ATP channels by vapours may induce preconditioning, reduce reperfusion injury and reduce apoptosis in ischaemic models.[221–223] The vasodilatory effects of vapour anesthetics can be expected to improve the uniformity of cerebral cooling and warming. Withdrawal of anaesthetic vapour is likely to induce cerebral vasoconstriction in a fashion parallel to the vasodilation seen on acute introduction. Because the neonatal brain is particularly vulnerable to apoptosis via excitotoxic injury, vapour anesthetics might be particularly indicated.[222,224–227]

Pathways of Cerebral Injury Related to Bypass

Cerebral injury is deterministically related to the delivery of oxygen, with irreversible necrotic cell death resulting from a sustained reduction in delivery below 20% of normal.[227,228] Rates of delivery above half baseline typically do not result in injury, while delivery rates of one-quarter to half of the normal range result in cellular injury, whose outcome is modifiable by other factors, such as temperature and free-radical scavenging, even when applied after the insult.[229] Apoptotic cell death ensues hours to days after subnecrotic hypoxic-ischaemic injury in susceptible populations of cells, and there exists a spectrum of ischaemic and apoptotic death in both focal and global models of ischaemia.[225,228,229] Amplification of injury through excitatory amino acid neurotransmitter-related calcium-dependent cascades of uncontrolled neuronal depolarisation may play a role in both necrotic and apoptotic cell death.[228] Modification of excitotoxicity can be demonstrated with glutamate receptor antagonists such as ketamine and dextromethorphan, receptor agonists such as anesthetic vapours and barbiturates, magnesium, and hypothermia.[228] Although therapeutic trials have generally been disappointing in profound ischaemia, an incremental effect is likely in more moderate injury.[230,231]

Although hypothermic circulatory arrest represents an obvious example of global ischaemia, it is likely that regional partial ischaemia exists during many phases of bypass and the perioperative period. In an animal model of tissue oxygenation during changing conditions of bypass, a range of levels of oxygen in the tissues was demonstrated using the phosphorescent quenching technique, even during high-flow bypass. More hypoxic regions appear during low flow and hypothermic circulatory arrest.[232] The cerebral circulation is susceptible to hypoxic injury throughout the perioperative period, and partial ischaemia is possible even during high-flow bypass, with neuronal fate modifiable by postoperative factors.[229,233,234]

Myocardial Protection and Cardioplegia

Initiation of cardiopulmonary bypass often has myocardial protective effects if the heart is properly unloaded by enhancing the availability of oxygen delivered through the coronary arteries and reducing consumption of oxygen. Hypothermia is a core component of myocardial protection. It further decreases consumption of oxygen, and preserves stores of high energy phosphates. Myocardial work can be further reduced by inducing a hyperkalaemic arrest via the administration of cardioplegia. The coronary arteries are isolated from the distal aortic circulation by placement of an aortic crossclamp distal to the cannula used to deliver cardioplegia. Cold solutions are then immediately delivered at 4° C. Aortic valvar competence is necessary to ensure the cardioplegia flows to the coronary arteries and not into the left ventricle. If the aortic valve is not competent, the aortic root can be opened and cardioplegia can be delivered directly into the orifices of the coronary arteries. Cardioplegia can also be delivered in a retrograde fashion via a catheter placed in the coronary sinus, as long as the sinus is not receiving blood from a left superior caval vein. Retrograde cardioplegia is often used as a supplementary method of cardioplegia, even when antegrade cardioplegia is possible.

Localised myocardial hypothermia can be achieved with cooling jackets and placement of ice slush in the pericardial space. This technique should be judiciously used, however, as it can result in injury to the phrenic nerves.[159] As an adjunct to hypothermia, the high concentration of potassium in the cardioplegia results in myocardial electromechanical silence and diastolic arrest. The initial arresting dose of cardioplegia at our institution is 35 mL/kg delivered at a pressure in the aortic root of 80 to 120 mm Hg. Maintenance doses of 15 mL/kg are given every 15 to 20 minutes thereafter until the repair is complete.

A crucial component of successful myocardial protection is ventricular decompression. Myocardial consumption of oxygen and impedance to subendocardial flow of blood is significantly reduced by lowering the ventricular mural tension.[235] Decompression is accomplished most commonly with the use of a catheter introduced through the right superior pulmonary vein and the left atrium. The catheter passes through the left atrium, across the mitral valve into the left ventricle. Constant suction is applied to the catheter with the use of a designated roller pump on the bypass machine. Blood returning from the venting catheter is recycled into the cardiotomy reservoir as discussed previously.

Anticoagulation

Although other anticoagulants have been used in special situations,[236–238] heparin is overwhelmingly the most commonly administered anticoagulant.[239,240] Heparin has a rapid onset of action, is easily reversed with protamine, and has important anti-inflammatory effects.[241,242] Dosing regimes include simple weight-based schemes, titration to a functional endpoint depending on activated clotting time, and measurement of concentrations with more complicated predictions. Convincing evidence for superiority of approaches is lacking. The gold standard of determining adequate anticoagulation suitable for bypass has been the activated clotting time. This test, however, does not take into account the effects of volume of blood, previous exposure to heparin, deficiency of antithrombin III, hypothermia or haemodilution. The Hepcon heparin management system (Medtronic, Inc. Minneapolis, MN) uses a pre-bypass titration of protamine to determine a patient-specific concentration of heparin to be maintained throughout the bypass run. While on bypass, samples of blood are taken every 30 minutes to determine both concentrations of heparin and activated clotting times. Additional need for heparin is based on maintaining an adequate concentration regardless of an extended activated clotting time. The Hepcon device calculates the dose of protamine needed to reverse heparin based on the circulating concentration of heparin at the end of the bypass run. The thrombotic, embolic, and inflammatory complications of cardiopulmonary bypass are increased with lower heparin effect. Adequate anticoagulation is crucial, otherwise intravascular coagulation, thrombosis, oxygenator dysfunction, and consumption of clotting factors may occur.[160] Heparin-induced thrombocytopenia, still an unusual complication in infants and children, may be more difficult to recognise.[243]

Strategies for Cooling

Surface cooling can begin with induction of anaesthesia, which promotes loss of heat and impairs thermoregulatory responses. A reduction in temperature to 35° C is generally well tolerated, and may confer protection against ischaemia in the period prior to bypass by metabolic suppression and alteration of responses to cellular injury. Further cooling on bypass is targeted based upon the anticipated level of flow required to complete the surgical repair. If deep hypothermic circulatory arrest is anticipated, a nasopharyngeal temperature of 18° C is generally the target, with evidence for increased complications at significantly higher and lower temperatures. Active cooling should be accompanied by measures of the adequacy of uniform cerebral cooling, for which measurements of surface temperature are inadequate.[244] Other indicators include jugular venous saturation, the electroencephalogram, and near infrared spectroscopy, from which evidence of metabolic suppression can be more directly ascertained.[245–249] At least 20 minutes of cooling is associated with improved outcome if hypothermic circulatory arrest is utilised.[250,251] A high flow hard-cooling pump strategy is necessary to raise the jugular venous saturation above 95%.[181] Measures which increase cerebral blood flow, such as a pH stat strategy, can improve brain cooling as previously discussed.[182]

Recent evidence-based reviews cite no advantage to hypothermia in either neurosurgery or open heart operations.[252,253] Since many operations can be completed without significant interruption in flow of blood, this finding may be unsurprising.[254] These meta-analytic reviews, nonetheless, fly in the face of overwhelming laboratory and clinical evidence of protection from ischaemic injury with hypothermia in global ischaemia.[255–259] Because the metabolic benefit of cooling and hypothermia is lost during rewarming, which may be superimposed on a period of reduced delivery of oxygen, a greater risk of ischaemia to both heart and central nervous system occurs with rewarming.[260] Given the multiple factors that may cause unexpected disruption in perfusion at full flow, some emergent in nature, most centers continue to use mild or moderate hypothermia as a protective adjunct to cardiopulmonary bypass without planned reduction of flow or circulatory arrest.[254,261] While the overall perioperative inflammatory response, although reduced during hypothermia, does not seem to be altered by strategies depending on temperature,[262] moderate hypothermia probably induces cellular adaptations at the transcriptional and translational level that result in survival programming.[263,264]

Deep Hypothermic Circulatory Arrest

Deep hypothermic circulatory arrest was first developed as a neuroprotective strategy when continuous perfusion could not be maintained. Currently, there is intense debate over the degree of protection offered by hypothermic circulatory arrest compared to hypothermic perfusion. The Boston circulatory arrest trial demonstrated that a strategy utilising hypothermic circulatory arrest compared to even low-flow bypass is associated with more immediate cerebral brain injury. Patients undergoing hypothermic circulatory arrest had more seizures, an increased tendency to have abnormal electroencephalograms,[265] and lower developmental performance at 1 year.[163] Both groups underperformed at 8 years.[165] Prolonged hypothermic circulatory arrest, greater than 40 minutes at 18° C, is associated with impaired neurodevelopmental outcome.[266,267] The relationship between a shorter duration of circulatory arrest and outcome is uncertain, but examination of the data from the Boston trial reveals a range of outcomes across the range of circulatory arrest intervals, indicating a multiplicity of determinants of outcome, including individual biologic susceptibility.[268] The safe duration of hypothermic circulatory arrest is related to the rate of use of oxygen from available stores, and can be predicted on the combination of haemoglobin, temperature, pH, and time. It is reflected uniformly by the cerebral saturation of oxygen as measured by near infrared spectroscopy.[166,170,199] The distribution of tensions of oxygen in the brain during hypothermic circulatory arrest is higher, and apoptotic regulators are lower, with a pH-stat strategy for cooling, predicting a longer safe time for hypothermic circulatory arrest.[171,269]

In an individual, the use of near-infrared spectroscopy can guide the safe duration of hypothermic circulatory arrest by limiting the time of low cerebral oxygenation.[173,174] With optimal cooling to 18° C and a circulatory arrest time of less than 30 minutes, cerebral injury is unlikely.[267] Moderate and profound hypothermia may initiate protective pro-apoptotic mechanisms that off-set the deleterious effects of sublethal ischaemic times.[270] During longer periods of circulatory arrest, intermittent reperfusion at intervals of 15 to 30 minutes has been demonstrated to maintain cytoarchitecture, cerebral distribution of oxygen, and indicators of excitotoxicity in animals.[271-273]

Selective Antegrade Cerebral Perfusion

Because of the variability in time necessary to complete repair, and the limited duration of deep hypothermic circulatory arrest, strategies have been employed to maintain continuous delivery of oxygen to the brain. Selective antegrade cerebral perfusion via the brachiocephalic artery has become widely used.[274-279] The optimal strategy for this technique remains poorly characterised, because measurements of cerebral blood flow are not readily available, and autoregulation may be altered during cold cardiopulmonary bypass and selective perfusion.[280] Most centers use pH-stat cooling to a target of 20° C to 26° C as in anticipated circulatory arrest, followed by direct perfusion of the brachiocephalic artery. Flow rates of 10 to 80 mL/kg/min have been described.[173] Flow rates of less than 30 mL/kg/min, however, are not likely to provide adequate cerebral blood flow to open all capillary beds.[281,282] Moreover, the increased affinity of haemoglobin at hypothermia may limit availability of oxygen during perfusion, partially off-setting the anticipated reduction in metabolism. The optimal temperature is not known, and is undoubtedly related to strategies of flow, although evidence supports maintenance of a deep hypothermia should a period of circulatory arrest be necessary.[283,284] Techniques to monitor adequacy of cerebral flow during this technique include trans-cranial Doppler and near infrared spectroscopy.[173]

Experimental models of continuous cerebral perfusion compared to hypothermic circulatory arrest show improved cerebral oxygenation,[169,285] better post-perfusion haemodynamics,[286] reduced apoptosis[232] with less ischaemic injury, and improved outcomes.[284,287,288] A recent comparison of cerebral perfusion versus hypothermic circulatory arrest in neonates undergoing reconstruction of the aortic arch showed no difference in neurodevelopmental outcome at 1 year. The technique for cerebral perfusion in this study, however, used a rate of flow of only 5 to 20 mL/min, and measures of cerebral oxygenation were not reported.[289] Because the rates of flow in those receiving cerebral perfusion were not likely to result in adequate delivery of oxygen, the results are not surprising, showing no difference between complete ischaemia and inadequate perfusion. Outcomes utilising an alternative approach utilising high-flow perfusion of 50 to 70 mL/kg/min show no evidence of ischaemic injury on postoperative magnetic resonance imaging.[290]

Because bypass exposes the body to a huge inflammatory stimulus, there may be a relative disadvantage of prolonged cerebral perfusion compared to circulatory arrest of shorter duration.[291-293] At present, there exists no direct comparison between cerebral perfusion at rates of flow with measured adequate cerebral oxygenation and deep hypothermic circulatory arrest. The optimal pH strategy for continuous selective perfusion is also debatable and conflicting, with some evidence favouring an alpha-stat approach,[294] and other evidence favoring a pH-stat approach.[171,269] Because of the inherent risk of prolonged ischaemia, and the unpredictable delayed effects of hypothermic cerebral perfusion and circulatory arrest on postoperative flow of blood to the brain, we favour strategies that rely both on measurement and maintenance of cerebral oxygenation throughout the operative period.[295]

Pharmacologic and Mechanical Adjuncts

Corticosteroids

Pre-treatment with corticosteroids is widely used, with broad but conflicting evidence for alteration of outcome. Pre-treatment in adults reduces postoperative levels of tumour necrosis factor-α, interleukin-6, the incidence of atrial fibrillation, and markers of myocardial ischaemia.[296-299] Evidence exists for both exacerbation and amelioration of hypoxic and ischaemic cerebral damage.[300-303] It was shown that two doses of 30 mg/kg methylprednisolone may ameliorate the inflammation-related delayed reflow and cerebral metabolism after hypothermic circulatory arrest.[304] The membrane-stabilising effect may reduce excitatory neurotoxicity,[302] and perivascular oedema may be reduced,[305] but necrotic cell death appeared to be unaffected, and apoptotic cell death may be increased.[306,307]

Aprotinin

Aprotinin is a serine protease inhibitor with a wide range of enzymatic targets. It has approval from the Food and Drug Administration to reduce the loss of blood during reoperation in adults undergoing bypass, and is widely used for conservation of blood, and for its anti-inflammatory effects.[153,308–310] As with other therapies aimed at modification of the inflammatory response, both desirable and undesirable outcomes may result, including an apparent increase in renal dysfunction related to hypotension.[311] Studies in adults have shown a reduction in both cerebral and myocardial injury in patients receiving aprotinin. This finding has been linked putatively to the anti-inflammatory effect of endothelial protection.[312,313] Administration of aprotinin to piglets undergoing hypothermic bypass and hypothermic circulatory arrest resulted in greater preservation of endothelial-dependent vasodilation, improved cerebral blood flow, and produced faster recovery of cerebral stores of high energy phosphate,[314] underscoring the impact of inflammatory microvascular injury in the pathophysiology of organ dysfunction following bypass.

Alpha-Adrenergic Blockade

The distribution of cardiac output is strongly influenced by the sympathetic nervous system, mainly through α-adrenergic mechanisms. Although deep anaesthetic strategies can alter the neurohumoral stress response to surgery,[220] evidence exists for high levels of sympathetic response during cardiac surgery, regardless of the anaesthetic regimen.[315] We have shown an improvement in whole-body economy of oxygen using phenoxybenzamine that permits and necessitates a strategy of bypass at high rates of flow.[316,317] In the presence of milrinone, α-adrenergic blockade is more effective than nitrovasodilators in improving flow both on[318] and off bypass.[281,319,320] Although outcomes seem improved with this approach,[317,321] a randomised outcome trial is lacking.[322]

Control of Glucose

Evidence for a beneficial effect of glycaemic control in paediatric cardiac surgery is distinctly lacking. The neonatal brain and heart are poorly tolerant of hypoglycaemia, which has been related to seizure activity and poor outcome in a large retrospective study of intraoperative glycaemic patterns and neurologic outcome.[323] In contrast to findings in adults, post-hypoxic supplementation of glucose may reduce neurologic injury in the developing brain.[324] Insulin has anti-oxidative, anti-apoptotic pro-survival cell programming effects, independent of its glycaemic effects.[294,325] Because deficiency of insulin is rare in infants and children, the role for exogenous insulin is not yet established.

Ultrafiltration

Modified ultrafiltration is a technique to remove excessive water from the body after restoration of the native circulation, but before removal of the cannulas used for bypass.[326,327] As an incremental strategy in adults, modified ultrafiltration reduces morbidity and post-operative use of resources.[328] In children, benefits include improved haemodynamics, pulmonary mechanics, and cerebral metabolism.[329–333] Some of these effects may be achieved by other strategies to reduce the deleterious effects of bypass-related haemodilution and activation of blood products, including conventional ultrafiltration and strategies for reduction of the prime.[334–336] A direct effect of modified ultrafiltration on inflammatory mediators, and on ultimate clinical outcome, is uncertain.[337,338] Extreme reduction in the volume of prime volume miniaturisation of the circuit may eventually replace ultrafiltration.[339] It is likely that a combination of ultrafiltration and incremental alterations in components of the circuit to improve biocompatibility can also improve outcomes.[157,329]

Preconditioning

Ischaemic preconditioning, or induction of tolerance to prolonged ischaemia by brief exposure to ischaemia, has been observed in the myocardium, brain, liver, kidney, intestine, and skeletal muscle, and probably is a feature of all mammalian cells.[340] The effect was first described by the observation of reduced size of infarcts after 40 minutes of coronary arterial occlusion if preceded by cycles of 5 minutes of occlusion.[341] The early protective window occurs within minutes, and fades within a few hours. A later second window of protection, or delayed preconditioning, opens about 24 hours after some preconditioning stimuluses.[340,342,343]

Early protective responses to sublethal ischaemia induce alteration in the flow of blood and metabolism. Within hours, signaling systems involving hypoxia-inducible factors and heat shock proteins confer resistance to apoptotic transformation.[344] Features of this characteristic response can be induced by hypoxia-ischaemia, hyperthermia, hypothermia, hypoglycaemia, a range of drugs including K-ATP channel blockers, erythromycin, volatile anaesthetics, opioids, acetylsalicylic acid, glutamate, and erythropoietin, the latter having received much attention in recent clinical trials.[345,346] The mediators of this response favouring survival can be released remotely from the target organ, and improved myocardial function has been demonstrated in humans after minimal ischaemia induced by a tourniquet placed on the leg.[347] Induction of a common signaling pathway for survival of cells, as opposed to apoptosis, has been suggested as the underlying mechanism for these findings.[348,349]

Considerations at the End of Bypass

Altered Cerebral Flow of Blood and Metabolism

The increased relative flow of blood to the brain induced by hypothermia can result in a postoperative increase in cerebrovascular resistance and cerebral oedema, although responsiveness to carbon dioxide is maintained.[350–353] Some of this impaired flow may be due to microvascular occlusion, and can be ameliorated by treatments that reduce aggregation and adhesion of platelets, such as donors of nitric oxide, antagonists of thromboxane, and antiplatelet drugs.[354–357] Modified ultrafiltration also seems to improve cerebral blood flow and metabolism, presumably by reduction of inflammatory mediators.[332]

Hypothermic circulatory arrest results in both loss of autoregulation and delayed reflow, with a prolonged suppression of flow of blood and uptake of oxygen.[358–360] This delayed recovery of cerebral metabolism may exacerbate the neurologic injury related to circulatory arrest.[164] Suppression of metabolism during hypothermic circulatory arrest using a pH-stat strategy,[201] and maintenance of a higher postoperative haematocrit,[361] can, in piglets, partially ameliorate this metabolic derangement occurring after circulatory arrest. Postoperative arterial hypoxaemia exacerbates the arrest-related injury,[362] and maintenance of delivery of oxygen to the brain with mechanical assistance may be preferable to inadequate postoperative delivery.[169,363] We have demonstrated that, following hypothermic circulatory arrest in neonates, inadequate postoperative economy for oxygen is related to poor late neurodevelopmental outcome, and that postoperative hypercapnia is protective in this setting.[234] Continuous cerebral perfusion does not eliminate the risk of post-operative cerebral desaturation,[295,364] and the interaction between intraoperative management and post-operative flows of blood remains complex.

Postconditioning

Ischaemic postconditioning describes modification of injury by interventions applied just at the time of reperfusion, and was first observed with intermittent reperfusion.[365] This may be a form of modified reperfusion, and has been observed with a variety of agents, including erythropoietin, insulin, and isoflurane, which are commonly administered in the operating room around the time of cardiopulmonary bypass and other ischaemic challenges.[340,366,367] While hypothermia and volatile anaesthetics amplify the protection afforded by preconditioning for tolerance of prolonged ischaemia, postconditioning seems to have limited effect after prolonged ischaemia.[368–370] Remote postconditioning has been described via brief occlusion of leg or kidney perfusion just at the time of reperfusion of myocardium, yielding a reduction in the size of infarcts 48 to 72 hours later.[345,371] While the application of these techniques may seem simple, and associated with minimal risk, the clinical utility remains to be elucidated. Inadvertent conditioning may result from aspects of stimulations providing pre- and postconditioning commonly present throughout the operative period. The technique of intermittent reperfusion during prolonged hypothermic circulatory arrest[273] may be a paradigm for both pre- and postconditioning. An acidotic perfusion milieu at the beginning of reperfusion may not only enhance flow, but may also be important in promoting ischaemic postconditioning and anti-apoptosis.[372]

Post-operative hyperthermia is common after cardiopulmonary bypass,[373] and has been associated with poorer neurologic outcome.[374,375] Attention to the control of temperature during rewarming, and immediately following bypass, can reduce the incidence of undesired hyperthermia. Induction of post-operative hypothermia should be strongly considered for patients experiencing uncontrolled or prolonged peri-operative ischaemia.[376] Hypothermia may afford protection independent of its effects on cerebral blood flow and metabolism. The effects of hypothermia post-injury are likely due to reduction in apoptotic cell death, and thus both intra-operative and post-operative hypothermia may provide anti-apoptotic programming. Reduction in apoptotic cell death has been demonstrated using cerebral perfusion as a supportive strategy as opposed to hypothermic circulatory arrest.[287,288] Post-operative mild hypothermia, and administration of albumin, are simple clinical interventions commonly applied which may alter outcome after incomplete ischaemia.[229,377] Evidence of focal ischaemia from gas embolism or other causes should prompt consideration of hyperbaric treatment with oxygen.[378,379]

Monitoring

Because a range of conditions can affect central haemodynamics, regional cerebral perfusion, cerebral metabolism, and flow metabolism coupling during cardiac surgery, cerebral oxygenation is likely altered in both predictable and unpredictable ways. Cerebral hypoxia, measured by jugular venous saturation or infrared spectroscopy, has been shown experimentally to be related to injury during ischaemia,[174,380] with similar findings reported in humans.[364,381] Hypoxic-ischaemic conditions cannot reliably be identified by standard haemodynamic monitoring. Because aggressive prevention of overt and occult hypoperfusion improves outcomes,[161,317,382] measurement of global and regional oxygenation is recommended as a method to prevent and treat unanticipated and unappreciated hypoxic-ischaemic conditions. This is especially crucial in the immediate perioperative period, when intervention to improve outcome is possible.[382–385]

Intra-operative Echocardiography

Transoesophageal echocardiography has become a mainstay of intra-operative management of the patient undergoing cardiac surgery. Specific guidelines have been developed as to the indications for its use in children. There is general agreement that the technique is indicated in every child over 3 kg. Some centers use the system in any infant over 2.5 kg in whom a probe is easily placed. An echo is generally performed at the beginning of every case, both to confirm the anatomy previously detected by using transthoracic windows, and to obtain real-time orientation to dynamic structures. Intra-operatively, echocardiography can be important to verify that air has been cleared from cardiac chambers prior to allowing cardiac contractions and emergence from cardiopulmonary support. It can also be very useful in delineating the source of failure when a child is not able to be weaned from bypass (i.e., residual lesions). For instance, echocardiography is very useful when differentiating hypovolaemia from functional compromise and residual structural deficits. At the termination of the procedure, echocardiography is critical in verifying the adequacy of many repairs.[386]

Post-operative Extracorporeal Support

Short-term mechanical support is occasionally necessary following complex cardiac operations. The use of extracorporeal membrane oxygenation carries a reasonable expectation of recovery for small patients in cardiopulmonary failure. In the current era, the technique is an essential component of programmes undertaking complex congenital cardiac surgery.[387,388] The circuit used by most centres is a direct descendant of the circuit initially developed for support of the neonate with pulmonary hypertension and persistent fetal circulation, and has the advantage of being standardised and well understood by the specially trained staff who manage the circuit.[389,390] Key to its success was the development of the silicone membrane oxygenator, which extended the safe duration of extracorporeal support from hours to days, providing enough time for recovery of most neonates with respiratory failure. More recently, hollow fibre membrane oxygenators have been adapted for use, and both the oxygenator and the circuit can be heparin bonded.[391] As a result the requirement for heparin is reduced, which can be helpful in controlling bleeding. The technique is still of value only in the short term, but because myocardial dysfunction is likely to recover within 96 hours, this duration of support is suitable for the post-operative patient. Survival to discharge from hospital for patients who required extracorporeal support subsequent to the operation is in the range of 40%.[392,393] Not surprisingly, among patients requiring such support, a lack of residual lesions favours survival.[393] Patients with a functionally univentricular circulation suffering acute thrombosis of a shunt are noteworthy for a high rate of survival.[393] Many centres have developed a rapid response system to permit rapid cannulation so as to salvage patients who sustained unexpected cardiac arrest.[394] The technique, however, is still suitable only for relatively short periods of treatment. The longest duration resulting in a hospital survivor without transplantation in a large series reported from the Children's Hospital of Philadelphia was 15 days. Bridging to transplantation requires long-term, low-morbidity support.

Providing mechanical support for the failing heart over longer periods has become a clinical reality in adults. Although the devices are imperfect, being subject to infection, haemolysis, and thromboembolic complications, long-term support has been possible. Patients have been bridged to transplantation with improvement in end-organ function, and reduction in pulmonary vascular resistance, ultimately resulting in a better candidate and a less complicated course following transplantation. The Heartmate and Thoratec devices, both manufactured by Thoratec (Pleasanton, CA) have been used in children. The Thoratec device in particular, an external or paracorporeal pump, has been used in patients as small as 17 kg.[395]

Devices are now available that are specifically designed for use in children. The DeBakey VAD Child (MicroMed Technology, Inc., Houston, TX) uses an axial flow pump, and is modified from a device designed for adults. The axial flow pump itself is identical to the one designed for adults, but the inflow and outflow cannulas and flow probe have been modified to accommodate smaller patients. This device was given exemption by the Food and Drug Administration for humanitarian use as a bridge to transplantation for children. It is totally implantable, and is approved for use in patients aged from 5 to 16 years, and with body surface areas greater than 0.7 m^2 and less than 1.5 m^2.[396,397] The device has now been used in six patients with an average age of 11 years, and body surface areas from 0.8 to 1.7 m^2.[398] The average duration of support was 39 days, with 84 days being the longest duration of support. Half of the patients were successfully bridged to transplantation. There are three major shortcomings with the device. The smallest size available will ideally accommodate only larger children, limiting the application in smaller children. Additionally, the intracorporeal position complicates replacement if thrombus develops in the device. Furthermore, because it is an axial flow device, reverse flow, mimicking severe acute aortic insufficiency, may occur if the device stops, a condition that can occur with formation of thrombus.

The Berlin Heart (Berlin Heart AG, Berlin, Germany) is a paracorporeal pneumatic displacement pump. The pumping ventricle is available in a variety of sizes from 10 to 80 mL. The smallest size is suitable for support of infants.[399] The experience in North America of May 2007 includes just under 100 patients. The longest duration of support is 234 days. Death occurred in one-quarter of those placed on the device, with just over half undergoing transplantation, and one-tenth being weaned from the device and a further one-tenth still being supported (personal communication). Because of the paracorporeal or external position of the pump, and the range of available cannulas, the device accommodates a range of anatomic variances. It is even possible to support patients with functionally univentricular circulations.[400] Thrombus within the device can be identified by visual inspection, and the external position permits changing of the pump without reoperation.

Placement of any assist devices puts patients at risk for bleeding and thromboembolic complications. The risk appears to be greatest in the smallest patients. Presently both the DeBakey VAD Child and the Berlin Heart permit extubation and ambulation, both necessary conditions for rehabilitation (Fig. 13-14). Although the paracorporeal

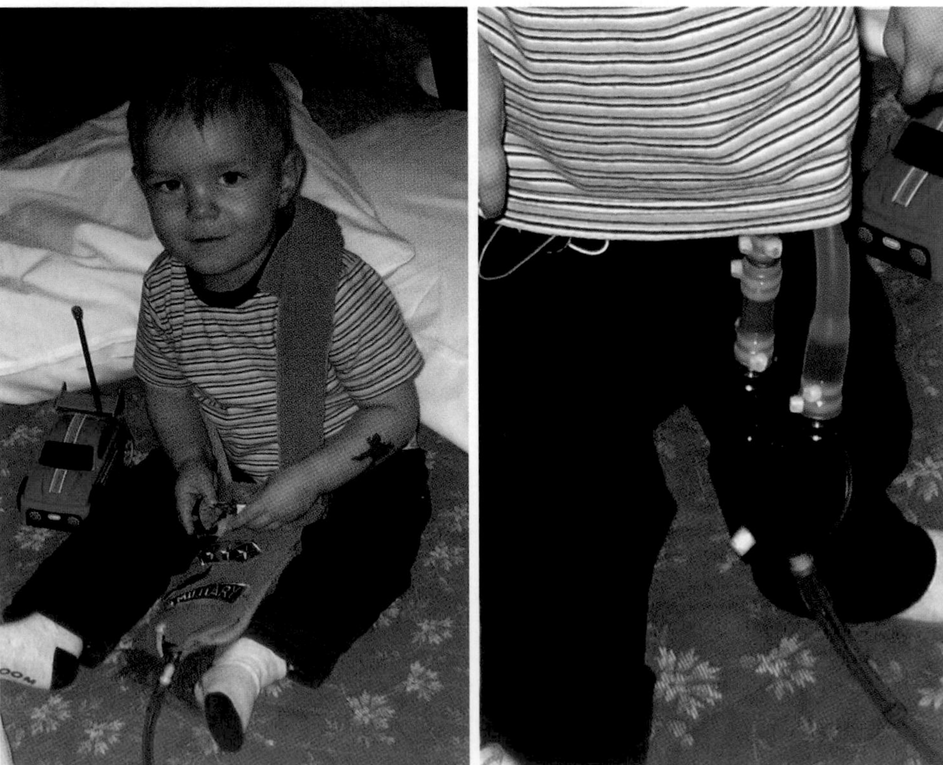

Figure 13-14 A child being assisted with a Berlin Ventricular Assist Device. The child is fully ambulatory, and is able to leave his room under supervision.

pump may be more cumbersome, at present all devices in children are placed as bridges to transplantation, and not as permanent therapy. The ease of exchange of the pump, and the ability to accommodate anatomic variances and a greater range of size, favour the paracorporeal pump for use in children.

CONCLUSIONS

The beginning of cardiac surgery can be traced to the ligation of the persistently patent arterial duct, performed by Robert Gross in 1938, and reported in 1939. Cardiac surgery began, therefore, with the treatment of congenital cardiac disease. In the last 60 years, we have seen tremendous progress. Correction or palliation of congenitally malformed hearts is now routinely performed in infants and neonates, with the expectation of survival in most instances. Our goal in this chapter has been to review issues common to all congenital cardiac operations including incisions, materials used, conduct of cardiopulmonary bypass, and the options for extracorporeal support. We have sought to provide a balanced overview of the current state of the art, and perhaps included in our discussion the mean and first standard deviation of thought. The topic of surgical techniques is vast, and obviously beyond the scope of a single chapter. We believe we have provided a background, context, and a reasonable starting point for more thorough investigation.

ACKNOWLEDGEMENT

We thank Christine Sulock for her work with the illustrations.

The complete reference list can be found on the companion Expert Consult web site at www.expertconsult.com.

ANNOTATED REFERENCES

- Jonas RA: Comprehensive Surgical Management of Congenital Heart Disease. London: Arnold, 2004.

  A recent and well-written text on the conduct of congenital cardiac surgery, with specific reference to details of the technique of congenital cardiac surgery.

- Husain SA, Brown JW: When reconstruction fails or is not feasible: Valve replacement options in the pediatric population. Semin Thorac Cardiovasc Surg Pediatr Card Surg Annu 2007:117–124.

  A nice review of the options for valvar replacement in congenital cardiac surgery.

- Gravlee GP, Davis RF, Kurusz M, Utley JR: Cardiopulmonary Bypass: Principles and Practice. Philadelphia: Lippincott Williams & Wilkins, 2000.

  A thorough text reviewing the pertinent principles for cardiopulmonary bypass in adults and infants.

- Rivers E, Nguyen B, Havstad S, et al: Early goal-directed therapy in the treatment of severe sepsis and septic shock. N Engl J Med 2001;345:1368–1377.

  A well-designed prospective comparison of standard interventions vs. SvO_2-directed interventions showing improved morbidity of the various organs and mortality in septic shock.

- Tweddell JS, Ghanayem NS, Mussato KA, et al: Mixed venous oxygen saturation monitoring after stage 1 palliation for hypoplastic left heart syndrome. Ann Thorac Surg 2007; 84:1301–1311.

  A large series evaluating the relationship between SvO_2 and morbidity and mortality in a uniform group of patients with hypoplastic left heart syndrome, with findings congruous to the study annotated above.

- Greeley WJ, Bracey VA, Ungerleider RM, et al: Recovery of cerebral metabolism and mitochondrial oxidation state is delayed after hypothermic circulatory arrest. Circulation 1991;84:III400–III406.

  Elegant investigations in neonates and infants during bypass and circulatory arrest utilising Kety-Schmidt techniques for measuring cerebral flow of blood and metabolism, showing impairment of metabolism after hypothermic arrest.

- Dexter F, Hindman BJ: Theoretical analysis of cerebral venous blood hemoglobin oxygen saturation as an index of cerebral oxygenation during hypothermic cardiopulmonary bypass: A counterproposal to the "luxury perfusion" hypothesis. Anesthesiology 1995;83:405–412.

  A mathematical analysis of the effects of temperature on the solubility and availability of oxygen in blood, revealing the dominant effects of temperature over pH on the tension of oxygen in the tissues during hypothermia.

- Amir G, Ramamoorthy C, Riemer RK, et al: Neonatal brain protection and deep hypothermic circulatory arrest: Pathophysiology of ischemic neuronal injury and protective strategies. Ann Thorac Surg 2005;80:1955–1964.

- Andropoulos DB, Stayer SA, McKenzie ED, Fraser CD Jr: Novel cerebral physiologic monitoring to guide low-flow cerebral perfusion during neonatal aortic arch reconstruction. J Thorac Cardiovasc Surg 2003;125:491–499.

  A succinct review of techniques used for monitoring neonatal bypass.

- Hoffman GM: Pro: Near-infrared spectroscopy should be used for all cardiopulmonary bypass. J Cardiothorac Vasc Anesth 2006;20:606–612.

  A comprehensive review of the application of near infrared spectroscopy to avoid cerebral hypoxia.

- Duncan BW: Pediatric mechanical circulatory support in the United States: Past, present, and future. ASAIO J 2006;52:525–529.

  A comprehensive review of the options for mechanical support in children, including extracorporeal oxygentaion and ventricular assist devices.

CHAPTER 14

Acute Circulatory Failure: Pharmacological and Mechanical Support

LARA SHEKERDEMIAN

In 1913, Sir James MacKenzie, physician in charge of the cardiac department at the London Hospital, defined cardiac failure as a condition in which 'the heart is unable to maintain an efficient circulation when called upon to meet the efforts necessary to the daily life of the individual'. The causes of such circulatory failure in children include sepsis, primary myocardial disease such as myocarditis or cardiomyopathy producing end-stage failure with acute decompensation, and congenital cardiac disease. Children with congenitally malformed hearts suffering circulatory failure can present in the unoperated state, or in the early post-operative period after surgery, when the condition is usually recoverable. Myocardial performance in children with acute circulatory failure depends upon the underlying condition, and in some cases may change with time. The unifying feature for all children with acute circulatory failure is that the heart is unable to meet the circulatory demands of the tissues. Treatment, therefore, must be directed at restoring this critical balance.

Over the past decade, there have been important advances in the approach to the treatment of acute cardiac failure. Treatment has shifted away from a focus on myocardial contractility in favour of strategies which optimise systemic perfusion, protecting the myocardium through manipulation of afterload, control of the demand for oxygen, or in the extreme by providing complete myocardial rest.

The successful management of children with acute cardiac failure depends upon providing careful and individualised treatment, which begins with establishing the underlying cause, with subsequent tailoring of available treatments. In this chapter, I begin with a broad overview of the pathophysiology of circulatory failure in children. I then discuss the spectrum of available therapies for acute circulatory failure, focusing on pharmacological agents, and non-pharmacological treatments, considering both extracorporeal support and ventilation. The principles of good, basic intensive care, and the application of understanding of the complex circulatory physiology of children with cardiac disease, will complement all of the ensuing discussions, as these are prerequisites for successful therapy.

THE PATHOPHYSIOLOGY OF ACUTE CIRCULATORY FAILURE

Acute circulatory failure in children with cardiac disease can be classified into five broad categories, according to intrinsic cardiac function, global cardiac output, and overall balance of oxygen. These categories differ significantly in their manifestations, underlying causes, and subsequent therapeutic strategies, but share a common feature, which is the phenomenon of systemic hypoperfusion.

- **Acute myocardial dysfunction with reduced cardiac output and increased afterload.** Acute myocardial dysfunction with reduced systemic delivery of oxygen characterises the low cardiac output which complicates the post-operative course of around one in four children early after cardiopulmonary bypass. A fundamental feature of this is an elevated ventricular afterload, abnormal ventriculo-vascular interactions, as well as impaired systolic and/or diastolic function. This is the most commonly encountered cause of acute circulatory failure in children with cardiac disease.
- **Preserved myocardial function with normal cardiac output but systemic hypoperfusion.** Inadequate systemic delivery of oxygen can affect infants with a functionally univentricular heart and good ventricular contractility whose total cardiac output may be normal, but is maldistributed between the pulmonary and the systemic circulations. These infants are very dependent upon the maintenance of stable pulmonary and systemic vascular resistances, and even small changes in these can precipitate rapid circulatory failure and systemic hypoperfusion.
- **Preserved systolic function with abnormalities of diastolic function.** A proportion of patients with normal systolic function after surgical repair of tetralogy of Fallot, or conversion to the Fontan circulation, can develop a low cardiac output early after surgery which is secondary to diastolic dysfunction and inadequate flow of blood to the lungs. In these patients, treatment is directed at optimising diastolic function and cardiopulmonary interactions, while avoiding interventions which increase contractility.
- **Residual anatomic lesions in post-operative patients.** In a minority of patients after cardiac surgery, a low cardiac output state may be secondary to residual anatomic problems. In the absence of targeted investigations, these are often clinically indistinguishable from other causes of a low output, but are generally resistant to, or paradoxically may be worsened by, conventional medical interventions.
- **Preserved myocardial function with normal or increased cardiac output.** Inadequate systemic delivery of oxygen in the presence of normal myocardial function, reduced afterload, and normal or increased cardiac output, is an important, though unusual cause of acute

Figure 14-1 Junctional ectopic tachycardia may be clinically indistinguishable from other causes of a low cardiac output early after cardiac surgery. Escalation of inotropes may exacerbate the arrhythmia, hence the importance of diagnostic investigations. Appropriate therapy includes measures to slow the rate, such as hypothermia or amiodarone, and pacing.

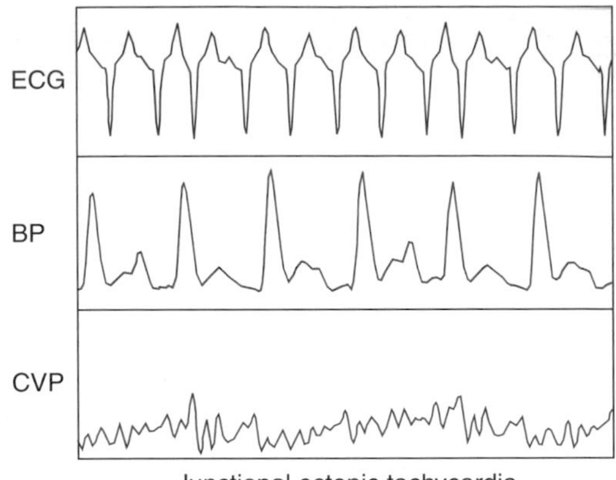

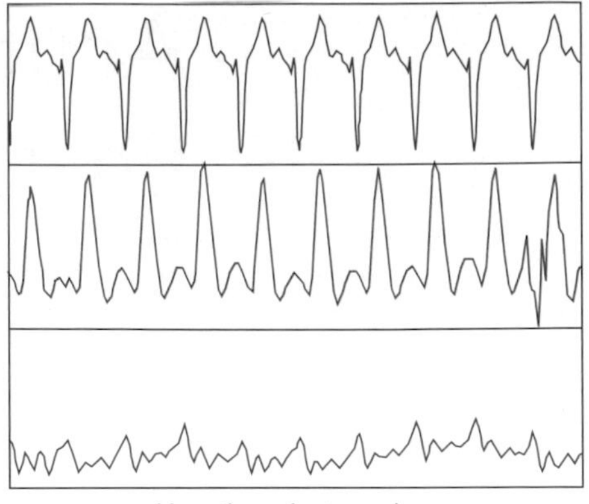

circulatory failure. In this setting, despite a seemingly normal cardiac output, the total or regional demand for oxygen is excessively high. This occurs in children with sepsis, or the systemic inflammatory response syndrome. Deceptively, the prodrome of acute myocarditis may also present in this way, but this so-called honeymoon period generally precedes a rapid circulatory collapse.

The first four categories described above generally affect infants and children with congenitally malformed hearts who are undergoing cardiac surgery. We can surmise, therefore, that circulatory failure in many infants and children with heart disease is to an extent predictable. In these patients, therefore, medical management should routinely include proactive strategies which are targeted at the prevention of this phenomenon. If circulatory failure does occur, then this should prompt early investigation and subsequent therapeutic intervention with appropriate measures.

A FRAMEWORK FOR THE MANAGEMENT OF ACUTE CIRCULATORY FAILURE IN CHILDREN

Acute cardiac failure in adults is often unexpected, whereas this condition is often predictable in many children with pre-existing cardiac disease. This unusual paradox presents a great opportunity for pre-emptive management in children who are undergoing surgery for congenitally malformed hearts, with the appropriate tailoring of post-operative management. Where anticipatory therapy is not possible, for example in acute myocarditis, or in circumstances where this does not prevent circulatory failure, then a proactive approach with early investigation, consideration of therapeutic targets, and appropriate intervention is recommended.

The Importance of Detailed Investigation

Although circulatory failure may be predictable in some settings, such as the post-operative period after cardiopulmonary bypass, it is unwise simply to accept its onset without considering early reinvestigation to guide therapy or to rule out a treatable cause. In children with circulatory instability early after cardiac surgery, echocardiography can immediately differentiate systolic and diastolic dysfunction, or may reveal an unexpected, acutely treatable cause such as a pericardial effusion. Similarly, detailed electrocardiography and atrial electrograms may demonstrate a treatable arrhythmia as the cause (Fig. 14-1). Moreover, echocardiography or additional imaging with cardiac catheterisation or computerised tomographic angiography may confirm or exclude anatomic causes for circulatory failure, such as collateral circulations, residual intracardiac shunting, or obstruction in the pulmonary or systemic circulations (Fig. 14-2).

Circulatory failure in post-operative cardiac patients can be due to different causes, which may be clinically indistinguishable, but which require very different treatments. Timely investigations, therefore, avoid the inappropriate use of therapies which may further exacerbate the underlying problem or its clinical manifestation. This is particularly relevant when circulatory failure is related to a tachyarrhythmia such as junctional ectopic tachycardia,

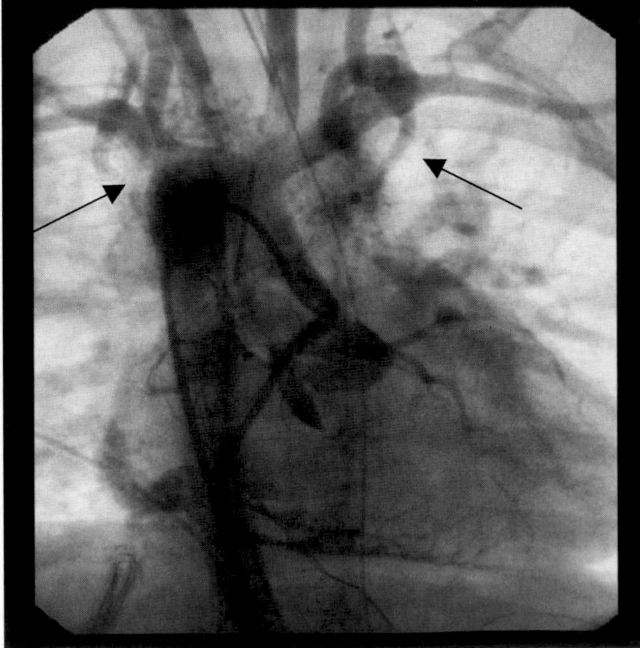

Figure 14-2 Aorto-pulmonary collateral arteries can contribute to a state of low output after surgery for congenital cardiac disease. The aortogram shows such major collateral vessels (*arrows*) in an infant with a low cardiac output, and well-preserved systolic and diastolic function after surgical repair of tetralogy of Fallot.

an undiagnosed anatomic outflow obstruction or pure diastolic dysfunction. In these situations, which may all be clinically indistinguishable from systolic myocardial dysfunction, escalating inotropic therapy generally will further potentiate the haemodynamic instability. Having highlighted the importance of diagnosing or excluding treatable causes for circulatory failure, as part of a pragmatic approach to management, we must next focus upon current therapies for primary circulatory failure.

Therapeutic Targets

The basic premise for the management of acute circulatory failure is to restore the systemic balance of oxygen, by manipulating one or more of the following:

- Systolic function
- Diastolic function
- Preload
- Afterload
- Consumption of oxygen
- Cardiopulmonary interactions

This is most often achieved using one or more of the therapeutic tools listed below.

Therapeutic Tools

A variety of tools are available for the treatment of acute circulatory failure in children. Those which will be discussed in further detail are:

- Ventilation to optimise cardiopulmonary interactions
- Pharmacological agents to improve contractility and loading conditions
- Mechanical support, such as extracorporeal membrane oxygenation, or use of devices providing temporary ventricular assistance to optimise cardiac output while allowing myocardial rest.

In the remainder of this chapter, I will discuss how these essential haemodynamic tools can be applied to infants and children with circulatory failure in the intensive care unit.

THERAPIES FOR CIRCULATORY FAILURE IN CHILDREN

Ventilation

In this section, I discuss the application of one of our most basic haemodynamic tools, namely ventilation, in relation to children with cardiac disease. In addition to its primary function, which is to maintain gas exchange, ventilation is an important haemodynamic tool in children with cardiac disease, and should routinely be used to optimise the systemic perfusion. Cardiopulmonary interactions describe the interplay between spontaneous or mechanical ventilation and the cardiovascular system. These interactions differ greatly in health and disease, and unique interactions are present in children with congenitally malformed hearts.

The application of mechanical ventilation in children with circulatory failure requires an understanding of the underlying diagnosis and physiology, and of how cardiopulmonary interactions may therefore be tailored for an individual. Similar to inotropes, an approach which may benefit one patient may be highly detrimental to another, which highlights the importance of understanding the underlying pathophysiology.

Cardiopulmonary Interactions: Ventilation and the Cardiovascular System

The modern understanding of cardiopulmonary interactions has largely followed pioneering work from Cournand and his co-workers in the mid-1900s.[1] This group carried out a number of fundamental investigations, which addressed many aspects of the complex relationship between spontaneous and mechanical respiration and the cardiovascular system. They showed that, in the healthy circulation, the fall in intrathoracic pressure during spontaneous inspiration was associated with an increase in cardiac output secondary to increased right ventricular preload. Conversely, positive pressure ventilation produced a reduction in venous return and right heart filling, resulting in a small reduction in cardiac output which was proportional to the mean airway pressure (Fig. 14-3).

The effects of ventilation are not confined to its influences on the preload of the right heart. Positive pressure ventilation can also impede the emptying of the right heart through its effects on pulmonary vascular resistance, and may also reduce left ventricular afterload through a reduction in transmural left ventricular pressure.[2] These haemodynamic effects are, in practice, of minimal importance in the healthy individual. In the presence of circulatory failure, or in patients at risk for this, cardiopulmonary interactions become much more relevant in both the genesis of the problem, and in its treatment.

Cardiopulmonary Interactions in Children with Systolic Ventricular Dysfunction

In an historic study in 1973, it was shown that some adults with systolic ventricular dysfunction following open heart surgery responded to separation from positive pressure ventilation with an unexpected fall in cardiac output which was not associated with any disturbance in gas exchange.[3] Positive pressure ventilation reduces the work of breathing, filling of the right heart, and left ventricular transmural pressure, resulting in reduced left ventricular afterload. These cardiopulmonary interactions may be very desirable in patients with impaired systolic ventricular function, and are obviously lost on extubation from positive pressure ventilation. Similar haemodynamic effects also contribute to the improved early outcomes of adults presenting with acute, decompensated cardiac failure who are treated with non-invasive positive pressure ventilation.[4]

Positive pressure ventilation should therefore routinely be considered as a form of haemodynamic support for young infants with systolic impairment early after cardiac surgical repair. Common post-operative examples where infants may benefit from the reduction in right ventricular preload, left ventricular afterload and work of breathing afforded by positive pressure ventilation include the arterial switch operation, reimplantation of an anomalous left coronary artery from the pulmonary trunk or relief of left ventricular obstruction. These infants, and others with significant cardiac dysfunction may also benefit from a period of continuous positive airways pressure as ongoing haemodynamic support following extubation. Children with acute myocardial dysfunction secondary to sepsis or

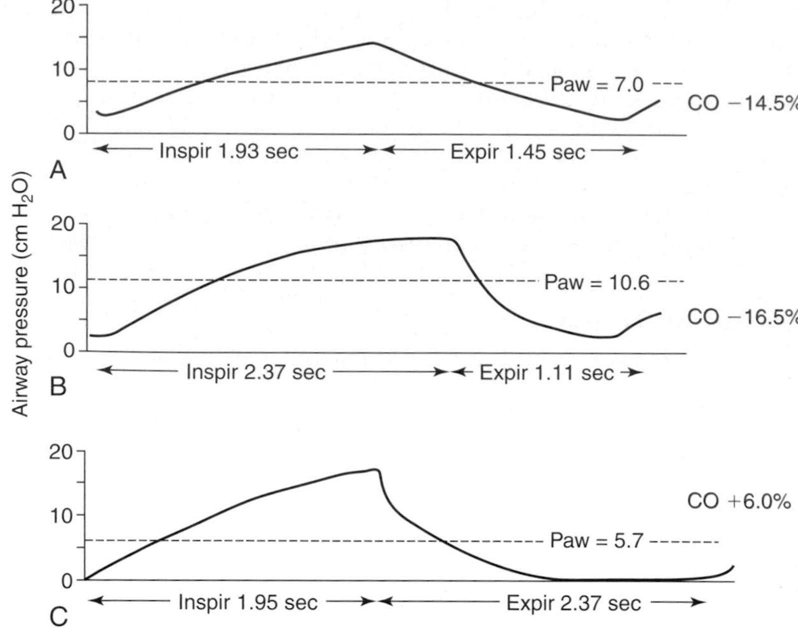

Figure 14-3 The influence of airway pressure on the cardiac output of healthy individuals. In their landmark research, Cournand and colleagues established that the reduction in cardiac output (CO) during positive pressure ventilation, was due to the effects of airway pressure on right heart filling. The graphs shown here, based on those of Cournand and colleagues,[1] show that the change in cardiac output is related to airway pressure, such that a higher mean airway pressure and longer inspiratory time (**A** and **B**) produces a significant fall in cardiac output. A low airway pressure, with a short inspiratory time (**C**), does not adversely affect cardiac output.

myocarditis may similarly benefit from positive pressure ventilation, through either an endotracheal tube or via the non-invasive route.

Cardiopulmonary Interactions in Children with Abnormalities of Diastolic Function

Infants and children with diastolic impairment associated with congenital cardiac disease respond very differently to mechanical ventilation, and this highlights, once again, the importance of anticipating or diagnosing the problem, and tailoring therapy according to the underlying physiology. A low cardiac output in the presence of normal systolic ventricular function can complicate the early post-operative period of infants and children after surgery on the right heart, specifically after repair of tetralogy of Fallot, or establishment of the Fontan circulation. Although the anatomies of these entities are very different, their cardiopulmonary physiology in the early post-operative phase is in fact very similar.

The cardiac output of patients with the Fontan circulation is critically dependent upon the pulmonary vasculature. Consequently, the low cardiac output in these patients is most often related to inadequate flow of blood to the lungs, rather than problems with systolic ventricular function. In the absence of a subpulmonary ventricle, these patients depend upon the fall in intrathoracic pressure during spontaneous respiration in order to maintain flow to the lungs. Conversely, a positive intrathoracic pressure can impede or even reverse such flow.[5] Indeed, in his original description of his operation, Fontan observed the clinical improvement that accompanied extubation, and recommended that spontaneous respiration be established early after surgery.[6]

A subgroup of patients early after repair of tetralogy of Fallot have a reduced cardiac output secondary to restrictive right ventricular physiology, and their cardiac output is very dependent upon diastolic forward flow to the pulmonary arteries. Of key importance for the intensive care of these patients, as for those with the Fontan circulation, is that their pulmonary flow is critically related to intrathoracic pressure. In children with restrictive physiology, increases in airway pressure reduce or completely obliterate the diastolic pulmonary flow, which is an important source of cardiac output. Conversely, by mimicking spontaneous respiration, negative pressure ventilation augments cardiac output.[7]

Thus, children with the Fontan circulation, and a subgroup of patients early after repair of tetralogy of Fallot, share some fundamental, and quite unique cardiopulmonary interactions in the early post-operative period. In these patients, inappropriate ventilatory management using principles applied to children with systolic dysfunction could exacerbate clinical instability. The pre-emptive or early pro-active circulatory management should include the use of low ventilatory pressures, and early extubation where possible.

Cardiopulmonary Interactions in the Functionally Univentricular Circulation

Ventilation is a very simple, and fundamental tool which can, and should, be used to manipulate the perfusion of young infants with a functionally univentricular circulation. Similar principles can be applied to infants with hypoplastic left heart syndrome and its variants before or after surgery, to infants with a common arterial trunk in the pre-operative setting, and to neonates early after a systemic-to-pulmonary shunt. The maintenance of a stable pulmonary resistance is key to the early optimisation of these infants, and this is greatly influenced by ventilation. Seemingly minor increases in pulmonary blood flow secondary to alkalosis, or excess inspired oxygen, can compromise systemic flow. A time of particularly high risk is immediately after birth, when there may be a temptation to resuscitate these infants with oxygen, or hyperventilation. Even minimal periods of supplemental oxygen can be highly detrimental to these infants, and can precipitate metabolic acidosis, shock and circulatory collapse. This is an important factor which differentiates the resuscitation of infants with a prenatal diagnosis, from those without, in whom supplemental oxygen is more likely to be administered. The outcome of these infants is in part associated with their worst acid-base state, which is critically related to ventilatory management, and is influenced by the timing of diagnosis.[8]

In infants with a functionally univentricular circulation who are haemodynamically unstable in the pre-operative period, conservative levels of positive pressure ventilation can be used to control pulmonary flow. Ventilation using high airway pressures, or slow rates, is no longer used deliberately to induce respiratory acidosis and pulmonary vasoconstriction, as acidosis is not advantageous to these infants. Instead, mechanical ventilation stabilises the pulmonary resistance, and in turn this helps to optimise the systemic perfusion.

The use of supplemental nitrogen or carbon dioxide, delivered with the ventilatory gases, to augment the systemic perfusion before or after Norwood-type operations, has also been investigated. There is limited data which suggest that, while the addition of nitrogen to achieve an inspired oxygen fraction of around 0.17 lowers the systemic arterial saturations, it also reduces the mixed venous saturation and cerebral delivery of oxygen. In contrast, the addition of 3% carbon dioxide to the ventilatory circuit improves mixed venous saturation and cerebral saturation without changing the systemic arterial saturation, suggesting that this manoeuvre does improve the systemic delivery of oxygen in high risk infants.[9,10]

Summary of Ventilation as a Haemodynamic Tool

Children with cardiac disease have complex, and varied, cardiopulmonary interactions, which depend upon the underlying diagnosis, type of surgery, and associated myocardial function. Ventilation should routinely be tailored to manipulate haemodynamic performance, and may often be of more benefit to the child than pharmacotherapy (Table 14-1).

Cardiovascular Drugs

In recent years, the approach to pharmacological therapy for acute circulatory failure has moved away from the historical premise that the default target for treatment should be myocardial contractility. A better understanding of the pathophysiology and haemodynamic manifestations of circulatory failure in children has resulted in a shift away from therapy using pure inotropes to measures which also focus on the peripheral vasculature, and the interactions between the periphery and the myocardium. Current approaches are aimed at optimising afterload and manipulating contractility with careful, not excessive, inotropic therapy, while avoiding any unwanted increases in vascular resistance or myocardial oxygen consumption.

Drug therapies for acute circulatory failure are generally categorised according to their pharmacological actions, and also by their physiological effects. The classes of drugs most commonly used to treat acute circulatory failure in children are catecholamines and phosphodiesterase inhibitors. More recently, a number of newer drugs which influence cardiovascular function through very different mechanisms including sensitisation to calcium, and neurohormonal effects, have also become available for clinical use. The physiological effects of drugs used to treat cardiac failure are inotropic, vasodilator or a combination of the two, the so-called inodilator effect.

TABLE 14-1

SUMMARY OF THE HAEMODYNAMIC EFFECTS OF SPONTANEOUS AND MECHANICAL VENTILATION IN CHILDREN WITH HEART DISEASE

		SPONTANEOUS RESPIRATION		POSITIVE PRESSURE VENTILATION/CPAP	
Nature of Cardiac Failure	Key Considerations	Cardiopulmonary Features	Haemodynamic Effect	Cardiopulmonary Features	Haemodynamic Effect
Systolic cardiac failure (post-op, myocarditis)	Increased LV afterload Systolic LV dysfunction	Increased work of breathing Exaggerated negative intrapleural pressure	Increased LV afterload Jeopardises the systemic perfusion	Reduced work of breathing Obliterates negative swings in pleural pressure	Reduced venous return Reduced LV afterload Improved LV function
Post-op tetralogy of Fallot	Good systolic function Diastolic RV dysfunction Preload dependent	Increased RV preload Improved diastolic pulmonary artery flow	Improved cardiac output	Reduced RV preload Reduced diastolic pulmonary artery flow	Reduced cardiac output
Post-op Fontan	Good systolic function Preload dependent Cardiac output depends on pulmonary blood flow	Increased preload	Improved pulmonary flow and cardiac output	Reduced preload Reduced pulmonary blood flow	Reduced cardiac output
Duct-dependent systemic flow	Excessive pulmonary flow leading to reduced systemic flow Control difficult if infant is spontaneously breathing	Respiratory alkalosis and oversaturation often associated with low pulmonary vascular resistance	May result in excessive pulmonary flow, reduced systemic perfusion	Better control of pulmonary flow, pH, and pulmonary resistance	Improved systemic cardiac output

CPAP, continuous positive airway pressure; LV, left ventricular; RV, right ventricular.

Special Considerations in Children

When approaching pharmacological treatment of cardiac failure in infants and children, it is important first to consider some unique factors affecting children, which influence the choice of therapy in specific situations.

Maturational Influences

The neonatal myocardium differs significantly from the more mature heart in its innervation, and contractile reserve. The neonatal heart is less densely supplied with sympathetic nerve terminals than older infants and adults, which results in reduced myocardial effects, and less re-uptake of catecholamines. This latter factor may also predispose to the cardiotoxicity of catecholamines which has been described in the neonatal myocardium.[11] The newborn myocardium is, conversely, more sensitive to changes in intracellular calcium such that agents which act upon this may be of greater utility.

The Pulmonary Vasculature

Pulmonary hypertension, or lability of the pulmonary vascular resistance, is commonly encountered in newborns and infants with cardiac disease, and changes in pulmonary vascular tone can play a role in the genesis of circulatory failure in some patients. Patients at increased risk of pulmonary hypertension include those with structural heart disease resulting in excessive pulmonary blood flow, pulmonary venous hypertension or a functionally univentricular circulation. Pulmonary vascular instability can be further compounded in the newborn transitional circulation, and by cardiac surgery and cardiopulmonary bypass which disturbs the balance between endogenous pulmonary vasodilators and constrictors.[12,13]

Complex Circulations

Careful control of vascular tone is a pre-requisite for the circulatory management of patients with more complex congenitally malformed hearts, in particular those with a functionally univentricular heart. In these patients, acute changes in pulmonary or systemic vascular resistance can immediately impact on the systemic delivery of oxygen, and can rapidly precipitate acute circulatory failure. In these patients, stable pulmonary vascular resistance, and an appropriately dilated systemic vasculature is highly desirable.[14,15]

The presence of severe congenital cardiac disease can also impact on the responsiveness of the heart to exogenous agents. Sympathetic dysregulation is most marked in newborns and young infants with cyanotic or critical acyanotic cardiac disease. In these infants, a reduced density of β-adrenoreceptors is associated with elevated endogenous levels of noradrenaline and a partial uncoupling of the receptor to adenylate cyclase. As a result the myocardium is less responsive to β-adrenergic stimulation.[16]

Catecholamines

Adrenaline, noradrenaline and dopamine are endogenous neurotransmitters that play a central role in the physiological response to physiological stressors including hypoxia, hypotension, hypovolaemia, acidosis, temperature, and pain. Exogenous catecholamines are commonly administered to infants and children with circulatory failure, or to those who are at risk for this.

Catecholamine Receptors

Catecholamines produce their clinical effects through their interaction with post-synaptic α- and β-adrenergic receptors, and dopaminergic receptors, which are located on the myocardium, and on the peripheral vasculature. The α_1-, α_2-, and β-adrenoreceptors were originally characterised by Ahlquist in 1948. Each is known to have at least three sub-types. The physiological effects of catecholamine receptor stimulation are produced through alterations in intracellular ionised calcium.

Physiological Effects of Individual Receptor Stimulation

Stimulation of α_1-receptors leads to increased influx of calcium to the post-synaptic effector cell, resulting in peripheral vasoconstriction; α_2- and β-adrenergic agonists bind to their respective G-protein coupled adrenoreceptors, and activate adenylate cyclase which increases intracellular cyclic-adenosine monophosphate. This produces increased contractility, heart rate, and vasodilation. Dopamine receptors are located on tissues and the peripheral vasculature. They are classified into two categories according to their structure and actions. These receptors are generally referred to as $dopamine_1$-like, specifically $dopamine_1$ and $dopamine_5$ subtypes, and $dopamine_2$-like, comprising $dopamine_{2,3}$, and $dopamine_4$ subtypes.[17–19] Stimulation of dopamine receptors results in vasorelaxation through two potential mechanisms. Stimulation of $dopamine_1$-like receptors reduces the sensitivity of the post-synaptic cell to intracellular calcium.[20] Stimulation of $dopamine_2$-like receptors, in contrast, inhibits release of noradrenaline from the nerve terminal.[21]

Pattern of Receptor Stimulation by Individual Catecholamines

Adrenaline. Adrenaline is an α- and β-agonist, which at lower doses theoretically produces predominantly β-effects, such as increased heart rate and contractility, with some reduction in peripheral resistance, and an increase in cardiac output. At higher doses, adrenaline stimulates α-receptors and increases vascular resistance, with a concomitant increase in myocardial demand for oxygen. Although the effects are in theory dose-related, in practice the degree of relative β- versus α-effects in response to adrenaline is unpredictable, and systemic vasoconstriction is common.

Noradrenaline. Noradrenaline predominantly stimulates α-receptors, resulting in systemic vasoconstriction, without directly influencing cardiac output. This may be desirable in the presence of excessive vasodilation, but can potentially worsen the cardiovascular performance in patients with elevated ventricular afterload and borderline ventricular function.

Dopamine. Dopamine was identified as an endogenous neurotransmitter in 1958,[22] and was subsequently shown to have pressor effects,[23,24] and direct cardiac effects.[25] Dopamine stimulates α, β, and dopamine receptors, and produces an array of physiological responses with vasodilation secondary to dopaminergic stimulation, and α- and β-adrenergic stimulation at higher doses. The theoretical dose-related spectrum of effects led to the labels of renal and cardiac doses being applied for lower and higher doses, respectively. This concept is now obsolete, as there is no evidence to support such specific dose-selective actions.[26] Thus, the physiological effects seen when dopamine is administered are increases in contractility, heart rate, and vascular tone, with little if any convincing evidence of systemic vasodilation.

Dobutamine. Dobutamine was originally developed as a selectively inotropic catecholamine for adults with circulatory failure.[27] The drug has primarily β-adrenergic effects, with increased contractility and peripheral vasodilation, accompanied by a modest increase in heart rate.[28] It also improves myocardial flow, which balances adverse effects on consumption of oxygen brought about by the chronotropic response.[29]

Caveats with the Administration of Catecholamines

The clinical response to catecholamines is often less clear-cut or predictable than might be hoped. This is, in part, related to the highly variable dose-response relationship which has already been described. It is also due to the intrinsic property of most agents to produce multiple physiological effects, and due to unique factors present in children.

Unpredictable Pattern of Catecholamine Receptor Stimulation. Catecholamines have multiple physiological effects, and the overall efficacy of a single agent relies on any undesirable effects being counter-balanced by beneficial effects. For example, if the chronotropic response to adrenaline or dopamine, which may result in increased myocardial consumption of oxygen, to adrenaline or dopamine is not met with an appropriate increase in myocardial flow, then myocardial ischaemia may result. Moreover, a single catecholamine may stimulate more than one receptor, which could produce exactly opposing effects. For example, exogenous dopamine may concomitantly produce α-mediated vasoconstriction and dopaminergic vasodilation. A desired effect can also prove detrimental if endogenous cardiovascular compensation is not achieved. The administration of noradrenaline can produce peripheral vasoconstriction. The resulting increase in ventricular afterload may need to be met by an increase in contractility, and if this cannot be achieved through endogenous compensation, the net result is worsening of the cardiac output.

Factors Related to the Patient. Downregulation of catecholamine receptors due to elevated endogenous levels is well-recognised in critically ill infants and children with cardiac disease. Specific circumstances include patients who have received exogenous catecholamines for prolonged periods, those with cardiac disease and overwhelming circulatory failure, and children who have recently undergone cardiopulmonary bypass.[30,31]

Clinical Application of Catecholamines in Children

Despite the factors which are listed above, catecholamines remain the first line therapy for acute circulatory failure in children. This is undoubtedly related to familiarity with these drugs and our ability to work around aspects of their inherent unpredictability, features which are somewhat off-set by their rapid onset of action and short half-life.[32,33] In addition catecholamines are widely available and relatively cheap.

Clinical Trials Comparing Effects of Catecholamines

A number of randomised studies in adults have suggested that, as a single agent, dobutamine is superior to dopamine in its haemodynamic effects in post-cardiac surgical patients,[34] after major surgery,[35] and in the setting of septic shock.[36] There are few clinical trials comparing the haemodynamic effects of catecholamines in paediatric cardiac intensive care, and none which focus on objective outcome measures. In children with cardiac disease, it is extremely important to consider not only cardiac output as a marker of the haemodynamic efficacy of a catecholamine, but equally to consider its influence on other vascular beds. While dopamine and dobutamine both improve the global cardiac output in infants and children after cardiac surgery,[37,38] dopamine, and not dobutamine, increases pulmonary vascular resistance in these patients.[39] In a model of right ventricular injury and pulmonary hypertension, dopamine, dobutamine and adrenaline all produced similar improvements in right ventricular function. Dobutamine and adrenaline, but not dopamine, reduced the pulmonary vascular impedance, and adrenaline was the only agent which improved overall pulmonary vascular and right ventricular coupling.[40]

Adrenaline

Adrenaline is generally administered as an inotropic agent in patients with poor myocardial function, for example early after cardiac surgery. Even at the lowest doses, systemic vasoconstriction may complicate the administration of adrenaline, and this can exacerbate the elevated ventricular afterload which is characteristically common in the early post-operative period. In order to overcome unwanted systemic vasoconstriction, consideration should be given to the concomitant, and careful, addition of a short-acting intravenous nitro-vasodilator.

Noradrenaline

Noradrenaline should be used carefully as a single agent in cardiac intensive care, as it generally increases the systemic vascular resistance without any compensatory enhancement of cardiovascular performance. It may, therefore, exacerbate a low cardiac output in patients with minimal myocardial reserve and borderline ventricular function. When used in low doses, nonetheless, it is useful for patients with circulatory failure secondary to a post-operative systemic inflammatory response. Noradrenaline can be used either alone, or in combination with careful inotropic support, to improve pulmonary perfusion in patients where this is critically reduced, or coronary arterial perfusion in patients with diastolic run-off. Examples are patients with a borderline cardiac output but good ventricular function after conversion to the Fontan circulation, young infants after construction of a systemic-to-pulmonary arterial shunt, or infants with a critically obstructed pulmonary circulation prior to any surgical relief.

Dopamine

The systemic and pulmonary vasoconstriction which often accompanies the administration of dopamine somewhat negates its desirable inotropic effects, and renders the agent less useful as a single agent for infants and children with circulatory failure. This can, in part, be mitigated by combining dopamine with a systemic vasodilator. Dopamine, nonetheless, is uncommonly used in paediatric cardiac intensive care.

Dobutamine

Dobutamine is arguably the most commonly used single agent for the treatment of acute circulatory failure in all age groups. The appeal of dobutamine as a single agent arises from the combination of its inotropic effects with systemic and coronary vasodilation, which unlike other catecholamines co-exist at a single dose. These properties underpin its popularity in infants and children weaning from cardiopulmonary bypass, and in the initial treatment of primary myocardial failure.

Phosphodiesterase Inhibitors

These agents are classed as inodilators, being agents with both inotropic and vasodilator properties.

The Biology of Phosphodiesterase Inhibitors

Phosphodiesterase inhibitors are derivatives of bypridine. They prevent the intracellular hydrolysis of 3′5′ cyclic adenosine monophosphate by the enzyme phosphodiesterase III, which is plentiful in the myocardium and vascular smooth muscle cells. There are three such inhibitors, namely amrinone, enoximone, and milrinone. Their pharmacological effects are mediated through an increase in intracellular cyclic adenosine monophosphate, which has been shown to result in peripheral and coronary vasodilation, increased myocardial contractility, and improved myocardial relaxation.[41–43] In theory, therefore, they are inodilators with additional lusitropic, or diastolic relaxant, effects.

Milrinone

Milrinone is the phosphodiesterase inhibitor which is most widely used at present. It improves cardiovascular performance through systemic vasodilation, and has additional pulmonary vasodilator properties, which may be particularly desirable in young infants at risk of post-operative pulmonary hypertension.[44] It is now very frequently used in paediatric cardiac intensive care as a short-term infusion, and its most common use is in the early period after cardiopulmonary bypass, where its prophylactic use has been shown to prevent the onset of a low cardiac output in patients already receiving intravenous catecholamines.[45]

Most clinicians readily refer to milrinone as an *inodilator*. There is no question that milrinone is a potent vasodilator. It is unclear whether the clinical improvement, or maintenance, of haemodynamic stability in children receiving milrinone may simply be through a reduction in afterload alone, or whether this is also attributable to its inotropic and lusitropic properties. In order to investigate this, a comparison of the haemodynamic effects of milrinone with a pure vasodilator would be necessary.

Pharmacology of Milrinone

Milrinone has a more complex pharmacokinetic profile than catecholamines. It has a slower onset of action, a much longer half-life, around 3 hours, and is excreted unchanged by the kidney. In order to achieve its maximum efficacy in a timely manner, milrinone must be administered as a loading dose followed by a continuous infusion. The dose administered should be adjusted according to both age, and renal function.[46,47] The clinical effects are generally evident for between 6 and 24 hours after discontinuing the infusion, and this important observation should influence the timing of initiating oral vasodilator therapy.

Caveats with Administration

An important consideration when administering milrinone is that the vasodilation, and the reduction in filling pressures which accompany its initial use may be substantial. This is particularly significant following cardiopulmonary bypass and ultrafiltration, when the patient is often hypovolaemic. To this end, a bolus of colloid should be available to militate against this effect during the early phase of administration. In general, its overall beneficial effects outweigh this temporary and avoidable phenomenon.

A more important consideration with all phosphodiesterase inhibitors is the confidence with which a vasodilator with a long duration of action can, or should, be administered to a given patient. For example, the use of milrinone as the first-line agent in patients with any potential for fixed cardiac outlet obstruction would not be recommended, as the fall in preload and afterload may impair subsequent systemic and/or pulmonary perfusion. In these circumstances, the initial use of a vasodilator with a short half-life, such as a nitro-vasodilator, would be advisable in order to ascertain whether vasodilation will be tolerated.

Clinical Uses of Milrinone

Milrinone is a useful agent for infants and children who have, or who are at risk of developing acute cardiac failure secondary to ventricular dysfunction, for example children immediately after cardiac surgery in whom there is no obstruction to the ventricular outlets. In this setting, milrinone can be used as a single agent, or as an adjunct to an inotropic catecholamine. Milrinone may also be useful in children who are at additional risk of developing circulatory failure secondary to post-operative pulmonary hypertension, for example after closure of a large intracardiac shunt, or after early neonatal reparative surgery. Additional clinical uses include patients with severe myocardial dysfunction which is unrelated to cardiac surgery, for example children with an acute decompensation of chronic cardiac failure.

Newer Vasoactive Agents

Sensitisers to Calcium

The role of calcium in cardiovascular regulation has been alluded to in this chapter and elsewhere. It is clear that the majority of cardiotonic drugs exert their haemodynamic effects either directly or indirectly through their influence on intracellular calcium. Most inotropes increase contractility through changing concentrations of ionised calcium within the cytoplasm or sarcoplasmic reticulum of the cardiomyocyte. An additional mechanism of action of cardiovascular agents has recently been established, which is to increase the sensitivity of the contractile apparatus to calcium without altering its total intracellular concentration.[48] Levosimendan was the first such agent to enter clinical practice, and has gained great popularity in the treatment of adults with circulatory failure.

Biology of Levosimendan

Levosimendan increases myocardial contractility through sensitisation to calcium. Levosimendan also produces coronary and peripheral vasodilation by opening the adenosine triphosphate–dependent potassium channels within the mitochondria of vascular smooth muscle.[49] Levosimendan, therefore, has very different molecular actions to those of all the drugs so far discussed, and all of these properties would make it a very appealing drug as the primary, adjunctive, or secondary therapy for children with acute circulatory failure.

Levosimendan has been widely investigated in a number of models of cardiovascular dysfunction, and is known to improve global haemodynamics and left and right ventricular systolic function, without increasing the myocardial demand for oxygen. Its effects, however, are not confined to myocardial contractility, and the agent also has been shown to optimise right and left ventriculo-vascular coupling, along with systemic and pulmonary vascular resistances, in laboratory models of myocardial injury.[50,51]

Pharmacology and Administration of Levosimendan

The concept of treating acute circulatory failure with long-acting vasoactive drugs has already been introduced. Levosimendan has much longer duration of clinical effects than milrinone, and its pharmacokinetics have dictated its unusual dosing regime. It has at least two active metabolites, which both have prolonged effects.[52] The current recommended dose regime for levosimendan in adults is for a bolus dose to be followed by an infusion for 24 hours. Thus, a single infusion of levosimendan produces haemodynamic effects which last for between 4 and 7 days. The unique pharmacokinetics of levosimendan result in the potential for its use in a cyclic manner, or potentially rotating with intermittent catecholamine administration.

Clinical Application of Levosimendan

Levosimendan has been widely investigated in adults with acute decompensated cardiac failure, and early experience suggested improved survival in these patients when compared with dobutamine.[53] This observation, however, was not borne out in the more recent SURVIVE study.[54] Levosimendan has also been shown to improve right ventricular performance in patients with acute lung injury,[55] and regional perfusion in patients with septic myocardial dysfunction.[56] In combination with dobutamine, levosimendan appears to have superior haemodynamic effects, and improves early outcome compared with milrinone in high risk adults after cardiac surgery.[57]

Levosimendan would appear to be a very appealing agent for use in infants and children requiring continued cardiovascular support, in whom prolonged treatment with catecholamines is likely to be met with tachyphylaxis. In these patients, the administration of a single dose of levosimendan should enable the discontinuation of catecholamines, with their reintroduction several days later, by which time receptor-responsiveness is likely to have been regained. This approach has been shown to improve survival when compared with a single dose of catecholamine in adults with severe cardiac failure.[58]

Levosimendan in Children

The experience with levosimendan in children is currently very limited. We have recently reported improved ejection fraction and reduced catecholamine requirements in children with severe cardiac failure who were given levosimendan (Fig. 14-4).[59] Its role in children early after cardiac surgery has not been established, though the agent shows great promise in this area. In a laboratory comparison of levosimendan and milrinone in a model of infant cardiac surgery, we have recently shown that the two agents have equivalent effects on afterload and ventricular-vascular coupling, but levosimendan has superior effects on contractility.[51] The drug, therefore, is an inodilator which shows great potential for infants and children with cardiac failure, but which warrants much more detailed investigation in this population.

Natriuretic Peptides

Atrial natriuretic peptides with potent natriuretic, diuretic, and vasodilatory properties were first identified from mammalian atrial tissue in the early 1980s.[60] In 1988, a molecule with similar properties was identified from brain tissue, and this was named brain natriuretic peptide, though its primary site of synthesis was subsequently shown to be the ventricle of the heart.[61] Brain natriuretic peptide is released from the ventricle in response to distension in patients with cardiac failure. It has been widely researched as a biomarker of severity of cardiac failure, prognostic indicator, or marker of response to therapy in a number of settings. Nesiritide, a recombinant brain natriuretic peptide, has been widely investigated as a vasodilator for the treatment of acute cardiac failure in adults.

The Biology of Nesiritide

Nesiritide is a pure vasodilator without any actual or theoretical inotropic properties. It binds to the receptors for both the atrial and brain natriuretic peptides of the endothelium and vascular smooth muscle. This leads to increased production of cyclic-guanosine monophosphate, resulting in venous and arterial, and coronary vasodilation. Nesiritide

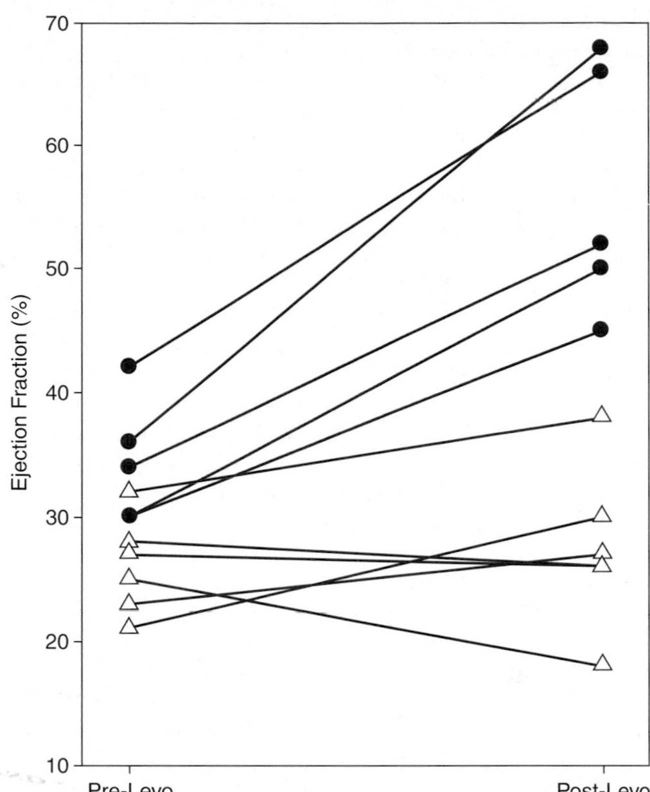

Figure 14-4 The graph illustrates our early experience with Levosimendan in children with cardiac failure. In those with acute cardiac failure (*blue circles*), a 24-hour infusion of levosimendan resulted in an improvement in ejection fraction from 30% to 41%. There was no significant change in ejection fraction in children with end-stage cardiac failure (*red triangles*). Doses of catecholamine, however, were substantially reduced in all patients.[59]

also inhibits cardiac sympathetic nervous system activity, so that its vasodilator effects are not accompanied by reflex tachycardia. It also produces important renal effects, including an increase in the rate of glomerular filtration, and inhibits reabsorption of sodium, therefore leading to diuresis and natriuresis.[62]

Clinical Effects of Nesiritide

There is mixed experience in the literature with nesiritide in adults with acute, decompensated cardiac failure. Nesiritide may be superior to dobutamine in terms of short-term survival[63]; and the Vasodilation in the Management of Acute Congestive Heart Failure trial demonstrated superior effects on cardiac preload of nesiritide compared to nitroglycerin, although there was no difference in symptomatology.[64] A more recent pooled analysis of randomised trials of nesiritide in adults not receiving additional inotropic agents suggested that its administration might be associated with a worse outcome, which may have been related to a worsening of renal function.[65]

There is growing experience of nesiritide in children, and its safety has been demonstrated in children with acute-on-chronic cardiac failure, or a low cardiac output state early after cardiac surgery. In these patients, its administration has been associated with improved urinary output, and reduction in neurohormonal markers of cardiac failure.[66,67] As with levosimendan, further research, and in particular comparative trials, will be necessary before establishing whether or not nesiritide has a role in the primary treatment of children with cardiac disease.

Summary of Pharmacological Support in Children with Acute Circulatory Failure

The emphasis on the treatment of cardiac failure has shifted from a focus on manipulating contractility to reducing afterload, controlling systemic vascular resistance, and avoiding increases in myocardial work. Unlike adults with acute circulatory failure, children with cardiac disease present a very different range of considerations, which vary greatly between individuals. These include the relative immaturity of the pulmonary vasculature and the myocardium, the lability of the pulmonary vascular resistance, the contribution of complex circulations which are most stable in the presence of systemic vasodilation and the post-bypass circulation with elevated systemic and pulmonary resistances. Accordingly, the choice of pharmacological agents must be carefully tailored and adjusted according to the underlying diagnosis and pathophysiology for the individual patient.

Extracorporeal Support

From Pharmacology to Extracorporeal Life Support: The Pragmatic Approach to Mechanical Support

In previous sections, I discussed how the pharmacological management of acute circulatory failure is shifting away from overworking the myocardium with pure inotropes towards enhancing cardiovascular performance using agents which reduce myocardial work. Thus, optimising the systemic balance of oxygen in cardiac intensive care now routinely employs approaches which are aimed at minimising myocardial work. Mechanical support, using extracorporeal membrane oxygenation or a ventricular assist device, provides assistance for children with acute circulatory failure, in whom intrinsic cardiovascular function cannot, with the assistance of carefully tailored pharmacological agents, adequately support the circulation. Moreover, the institution of mechanical support provides the opportunity for a period of almost complete myocardial rest.

Mechanical cardiac support should ideally be considered at a stage where the risk of escalating pharmacological agents outweighs the benefits of a period of myocardial rest, rather than a last resort treatment for patients who will otherwise surely die. This represents a philosophically unusual continuum for patients with circulatory failure, because escalation of therapy generally involves first a careful increase in vasoactive drugs, until a certain threshold is reached, at which point mechanical support is initiated and pharmacological agents are ceased.

Background: The Introduction of Mechanical Support into Intensive Care

In the early 1950s, C. Walther Lillehei changed the face of congenital cardiac surgery when he introduced the concept of extracorporeal circulation into clinical practice. The earliest application of this concept was the so-called cross-circulation, in which a healthy adult provided a living heart-lung machine to provide extracorporeal circulatory support for the child during open repair of congenitally malformed hearts.[68] Clearly cross-circulation was not likely to become a long-term option, due to the excessive hazards which it entailed. To this end, Gibbon developed the bubble oxygenator, which was first used in 1955 by Dewall and Lillehei during surgery for congenital cardiac disease.[69]

Cardiopulmonary bypass, cardiac surgery and intensive care practice all progressed rapidly from this point forwards, and in the 1970s mechanical cardiopulmonary support began its transition to the intensive care unit. Refinements of oxygenators ensued, such that circuits were designed which created less haemolysis, and were viable for much longer periods, and the first reports of extracorporeal membrane oxygenation in intensive care appeared in the literature thereafter.[70,71]

Temporary mechanical support in children with acute circulatory failure, using extracorporeal membrane oxygenation or ventricular assist devices, has been increasingly used since the late 1980s. In a historical context, extracorporeal membrane oxygenation has been the more commonly used modality for cardiac support in children. This bias can largely be attributed to the familiarity of clinicians with cardiopulmonary bypass, and historically, to the widespread use of extracorporeal membrane oxygenation for the treatment of neonatal hypoxaemic respiratory failure. Despite a recent increase in its use for cardiac support, the Extracorporeal Life Support Organisation registry report of 2007 states that, since 1989, only one-fifth of all paediatric extracorporeal membrane oxygenation has been for cardiac indications.

Determinants of Success of Extracorporeal Life Support: Basic Principles

Extracorporeal life support is a hazardous therapy with a high associated mortality, and is only used for critically unwell children, many of whom would otherwise not survive. Given the inherent risks of this therapy, all involved clinicians are responsible for maximising the chances of its success for each individual. This requires a streamlined approach to decision-making, optimal timing of initiating support and an ongoing commitment to investigating and optimising factors which may reduce the chances of its successful discontinuation.

A Programmatic Approach

The delivery of extracorporeal life support by a dedicated team of practitioners, with appropriate training and familiarity with the technology, and collaborative decision-making contributes to the success of this complex therapy. This is achieved in part through regular use of extracorporeal support in dedicated centres, a commitment to ongoing education and a uniform approach to the design of the circuitry, and avoiding unnecessary variables which would increase the likelihood of error. In our institution for example, all circuits for extracorporeal membrane oxygenation and short-term ventricular assist use identical tubing, driver consoles, and pump heads, regardless of the underlying condition or age of the child. This approach encourages familiarity with the circuit, and therefore minimises technical errors.

The Timely Institution of Extracorporeal Life Support

The timely institution of mechanical support, rather than its use only as a rescue therapy, contributes to improved outcomes. Thus, the survival of infants and children requiring support following surgery for congenital cardiac disease is generally better when support is instituted early in the operating room rather than later in the intensive care unit.[72] Delay in the institution of support often results in a window of opportunity for appropriate and timely intervention, and therefore the greatest chance of success, being lost. In the extreme, early intervention may prevent

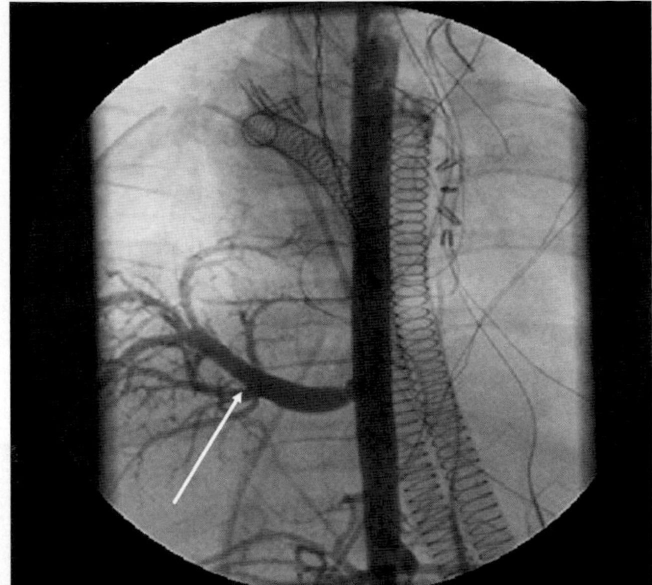

Figure 14-5 The illustrated aorto-pulmonary collateral artery *(arrow)* caused failure to wean from cardiopulmonary bypass. It was revealed by cardiac catheterisation of the patient after stabilisation with extracorporeal membrane oxygenation.

the potentially catastrophic consequence of cardiac arrest. Although extracorporeal cardiopulmonary resuscitation is now widely available, patients cannulated during cardiac arrest may have a poorer long-term prognosis than those cannulated earlier.[73]

Ongoing Reassessment of the Patient

An important contributor to the success of extracorporeal life support is a proactive approach to reassessment once support has been established. Although mechanical support can temporise an unstable patient, it is not an alternative for incomplete surgery, or a therapy for residual anatomic lesions. Indeed, it is widely accepted that children with residual anatomic or surgical problems do poorly unless the lesions are addressed and corrected (Fig. 14-5).[74]

Mode of Mechanical Support

Extracorporeal Membrane Oxygenation

Veno-arterial extracorporeal membrane oxygenation provides circulatory support and gas exchange by draining the systemic venous blood, passing it through an oxygenator which functions as a highly efficient lung, and returning oxygenated blood to the systemic arterial circulation. This can provide total cardiopulmonary rest for the heart with poor intrinsic function, or can provide partial support for a borderline, or recovering circulation.

Cannulation for extracorporeal membrane oxygenation can be through a sternotomy, or the peripheral route using neck or femoral vessels. The route for cannulation is dictated by the underlying pathophysiology, and the age or size of the patient. The risk of cerebral ischaemia related to carotid arterial cannulation increases with age, and the efficacy of support in terms of achievable flows, and avoidance of complications related to femoral cannulation decreases.[75,76] Thus, cannulation for extracorporeal membrane oxygenation without sternotomy in infants and small children is generally via the carotid artery and jugular vein, whereas for older children it is typically via the femoral route (Table 14-2).

Devices for Ventricular Assistance

Temporary mechanical ventricular assistance provides support to one or both ventricles, but does not support the lungs. The basic circuitry for this type of support requires cannulation for venous drainage, and arterial return. This can be right atrial drainage and pulmonary arterial return, for patients requiring right ventricular support, or left atrial drainage and aortic return, for patients requiring left ventricular support. Cannulation for a ventricular assist device generally requires a median sternotomy, with central cannulation of the cardiac chambers or great vessels.

The popularity of temporary support with a ventricular assist device for children with ventricular failure but preserved pulmonary function has grown over the past decade,[77,78] but still lags behind the use of extracorporeal membrane oxygenation in many institutions (Table 14-3). In contrast with extracorporeal membrane oxygenation, the circuit incorporating the ventricular assist device circuit does not include an oxygenator, which is an important source of turbulence or clot formation, and requires less systemic anticoagulation resulting in a reduced risk of bleeding.

Choice of Mechanical Support

Extracorporeal membrane oxygenation is the appropriate mode of support for patients with both cardiac and pulmonary impairment, for infants with pulmonary hypertension, or for extracorporeal cardiopulmonary resuscitation. Support with a ventricular assist device would be the preferred approach for infants or children with dysfunction of one ventricle and preserved pulmonary function, and adequate function of the contralateral ventricle. The function of the

TABLE 14-2

ROUTES OF CANNULATION FOR EXTRACORPOREAL MEMBRANE OXYGENATION

Indication	Cannulation	Comments	Reasons
Acute circulatory failure, not post-operative	Neck cannulation (carotid artery-jugular vein)	Neck cannulation for infants and younger children	Morbidity related to carotid cannulation greater in older patients.
	Femoro-femoral (femoral artery-femoral vein)	Femoro-femoral for older children (routinely consider if aged >10 yr)	Peripheral circulatory problems related to femoral cannulation greater in younger patients
	Open chest cannulation (right atrium – aorta)	Consider for overwhelming sepsis with supra-normal flow requirements	High flows achievable with larger cannulas
Post-operative circulatory failure	Open chest	If early post-operative phase	Easily accessible for rapid cannulation or conversion from cardiopulmonary bypass

TABLE 14-3

MODE OF EXTRACORPOREAL SUPPORT IN CHILDREN WITH CIRCULATORY FAILURE

Cardiac Arrest	ECMO	Default Mode of Support for Children Receiving CPR
Failure to wean from bypass		
or		
Early post-operative low cardiac output state		
Isolated ventricular dysfunction	Single VAD	
Biventricular dysfunction	BIVAD/ECMO	Institutional preference may be for ECMO, especially in smaller infants
Pulmonary hypertension	ECMO	
Functionally univentricular physiology with a systemic-to-pulmonary artery shunt	ECMO/VAD	Identical cannulation but no oxygenator for VAD Shunt restriction may be appropriate
Acute myocarditis	ECMO	With left atrial decompression
Decompensation of chronic cardiac failure	Single VAD	Unless cardiac arrest or poor lung function

BIVAD, biventricular assist device; CPR, cardiopulmonary resuscitation; ECMO, extracorporeal membrane oxygenation; VAD, ventricular assist device.

opposite ventricle does not need to be entirely normal, as inotropic therapy at low doses and/or afterload reduction, may adequately support this. Careful assessment of both ventricles, and pulmonary function is, therefore, essential prior to instituting support. The timing of the introduction of a device providing ventricular assistance is key to its success, and it is most likely to prove efficacious if commenced in the operating room, or very early after surgery in the intensive care unit. Significant delays may otherwise result in a missed window of opportunity, necessitating the more urgent institution of extracorporeal membrane oxygenation.

In patients with biventricular dysfunction and adequate pulmonary function, the decision to use extracorporeal membrane oxygenation or biventricular assist devices for temporary circulatory support is more open to debate, particularly in small children. The ultimate choice is usually dictated by institutional preference. In transplant centres where biventricular assist devices are frequently used as a bridge to transplantation in children, then this may also be the preferred modality for temporary support.[79] Others would consider that the complexity of four cannulas, significant cardiotomy and the requirement to synchronise ventricular outputs for biventricular assist devices would outweigh the potential disadvantage of an oxygenator in the circuit for extracorporeal membrane oxygenation.

Indications for Extracorporeal Life Support

The most common indication for cardiac support in infants and children is post-operative circulatory failure. Extracorporeal support has a well-established role in the acute, short-term support for infants and children with a critical low cardiac output state early after surgery for congenital heart disease,[77] the treatment of children with fulminant myocarditis,[80,81] post-operative pulmonary hypertension[82] and early graft failure after cardiac transplantation.[83] More recently, rapid-deployment extracorporeal membrane oxygenation has become established as a resuscitative tool in infants and children during cardiac arrest.[84]

At the Royal Children's Hospital, Melbourne, between 1989 and 2006, 229 infants and children received mechanical support early after cardiac surgery, which represents an overall rate of 2.9% of cardiac surgical patients. The predominant indications for support were an inability to wean from bypass or failure to respond to maximal medical therapy in the intensive care unit, which together account for more than two-thirds of patients requiring cardiac support at our centre.

Criterions for Support

The spectrum of patients for whom mechanical support is offered has broadened over the past decade, and strict criterions for support no longer exist. In principle, support should only be considered if the patient is expected to recover to a reasonable level of function with or without additional intervention.

Contra-indications to Extracorporeal Life Support

The presence of severe pre-existing cerebral injury, or a new parenchymal intracerebral haemorrhage, would be considered to be relative contra-indications to mechanical support in most centres undertaking extracorporeal life support. This is because mechanical support carries a significant risk of causing new haemorrhage, or worsening of existing bleeds, and additional ischaemic or embolic cerebral injury. Although there are well-recognised groups of patients known to be at high risk (see below), there are no diagnostic subgroups for whom mechanical support would be absolutely contra-indicated. Patients with severe residual anatomic lesions that cannot be addressed, nonetheless, would be considered poor candidates for support in most centres, for example, infants with totally anomalous pulmonary venous connection and diffuse pulmonary venous stenosis, who cannot be weaned from bypass.

Groups of Patients Known to Be at High Risk

Historically, complex palliated circulations such as the Fontan circulation were associated with poor outcomes, and therefore were considered by many to be unsuitable for extracorporeal support.[85,86] Outcomes for these patients have, however, improved somewhat since the early 1990s. Thus, while accepting that these patients still carry the highest mortality, most centres now occasionally support patients after conversion to the Fontan circulation, along with children having bidirectional cavopulmonary shunts.[87]

Young infants with a surgically palliated functionally univentricular circulation and a systemic-to-pulmonary artery shunt continue to present a challenge. This circulatory physiology was previously considered to be a relative contra-indication to mechanical support.[86] Over recent years, the overall outcomes of support for these patients has improved. This is for a combination of reasons, including earlier institution of support, the advent of programmatic rapid-deployment, the increased use of a ventricular assist device, and refined approaches to management of the shunt (see below).[88,89]

Special Considerations for Children Receiving Extracorporeal Life Support

The Systemic-to-Pulmonary Arterial Shunt

Infants with a functionally univentricular circulation, with shunt-dependent pulmonary flow, were historically considered poor candidates for mechanical support. In these infants, complete occlusion of the shunt was traditionally performed during cannulation for extracorporeal membrane oxygenation, in order to prevent the sequels of uncontrolled pulmonary flow, and compromised systemic perfusion. Although this approach was theoretically reasonable, it was proposed that an important contributory factor towards the dismal outcome for this group was their totally absent pulmonary perfusion.[90] This theory is now supported by the observations that outcomes of infants with this physiology have improved with less aggressive management of the shunt,[91] such that it is now usual practice to leave the shunt either completely patent or minimally restricted during extracorporeal membrane oxygenation.[88]

As for all patients, mechanical support with a ventricular assist device would be the modality of choice for infants with a functionally univentricular circulation and a low cardiac output who have preserved pulmonary function. However, with this mode of support, one ventricle must supply sufficient blood for both the systemic and pulmonary circulations, and hence the shunt must be completely patent. Thus, the total flows provided by a ventricular assist device must take into account this fact, and higher than standard flows should initially be used.

Decompression of the Left Heart on Extracorporeal Membrane Oxygenation

The majority of children with isolated, severe left ventricular dysfunction are placed on a left ventricular assist device. In these patients, the routine left atrial cannulation usually provides excellent decompression of the left heart, and additional intervention is not required. On some occasions, for example in the setting of fulminant myocarditis, where rapid cannulation and temporary pulmonary support may be required, patients may initially be placed on veno-arterial extracorporeal membrane oxygenation. In these patients, severe dilation of the left heart may accompany the initiation of extracorporeal membrane oxygenation. The reason for this is that continued right ventricular ejection results in pulmonary venous return to the left atrium, which in turn exacerbates left atrial and ventricular dilation. This vicious cycle of increased wall stress, left atrial hypertension, and pulmonary venous congestion defeats one of the purposes of support, which is to rest the heart and the lungs. Such dilation of the left heart may be in part be off-set by the use of higher flows, diuretics, afterload reduction, or gentle inotropic support to encourage ejection. Unfortunately these measures often prove inadequate, especially in the setting of left ventricular standstill when the aortic valve remains closed. Decompression of the left heart should therefore be routinely considered at the time of cannulation. In children with an open sternum, such decompression can be achieved by directly placing a cannula in the left atrium, which drains left atrial blood into the venous component of the extracorporeal circuit. Decompression of the left heart can also be performed via the transcatheter route, using a blade septectomy followed by either balloon septostomy or transcatheter cannulation of the left atrium.[92–94]

Anomalous Left Coronary Artery from the Pulmonary Trunk

An excellent example of a homogeneous group of patients with favourable outcomes for left ventricular assistance are infants following repair of anomalous left coronary artery from the pulmonary trunk. These patients typically have critically depressed pre-operative left ventricular function, with elevated left atrial pressures and left ventricular end-diastolic pressure, and commonly suffer from low cardiac output early after surgery. Many centres, including our own, have tended to manage borderline patients with a short period, usually 2 to 3 days, of semi-elective mechanical support with a device providing left ventricular assistance immediately after bypass, in preference to substantial doses of vasoactive drugs.

The Role of Echocardiography for Patients on Extracorporeal Life Support

Echocardiography plays an important role throughout the clinical course of infants and children receiving extracorporeal support (Table 14-4). Echocardiographic assessment of myocardial function may assist the early decision-making regarding whether or not to initiate support for a borderline patient. The careful assessment of the degree of dysfunction of one or both ventricles is critical in deciding whether single ventricular assistance will suffice, or whether biventricular assistance or extracorporeal membrane oxygenation would be better for the individual patient (Fig. 14-6). Echocardiography is also an essential tool in assessing the adequacy of surgical repair, and in identifying or excluding additional surgical or anatomic defects that may be contributing to lack of response to conventional therapy.

Once a child has been placed on support, echocardiography plays a continuing, and equally important role in the subsequent assessment of the adequacy of support, the ongoing assessment for residual anatomic defects, the response to therapy, the assessment of ventricular ejection and the presence of complications. Echocardiography is also a necessary tool to assess the clinical recovery, and response of the heart to weaning from mechanical support (see Table 14-4).

Weaning from Mechanical Support

When temporary mechanical support is initiated in children, the likely duration of support should be known, and this depends upon the indication for support. For children with acute myocarditis, or end-stage myocardial disease, there may be the expectation on initiation of support, that this will be required for up to several weeks or even as a bridge to transplantation.[80] In post-surgical patients, where support is provided for a low cardiac output state, or after cardiovascular collapse, native myocardial recovery should be achieved within 3 to 5 days of commencing mechanical support. Successful weaning and long-term survival without transplantation become much less likely when support is required beyond 7 days in post-cardiotomy patients.[73]

TABLE 14-4

THE ROLE OF ECHOCARDIOGRAPHY IN PATIENTS RECEIVING EXTRACORPOREAL LIFE SUPPORT

	Extracorporeal Membrane Oxygenation	Left Ventricular Assist Device
Pre-cannulation Echocardiography		
Ventricular function	Careful assessment essential	Right ventricular function and pressures Additional afterload reduction or inotropes may be required to assist non-supported ventricle
Atrial septal defect	Beneficial for left heart decompression	Will create right-to-left shunt
Residual defects	Early identification will lead to early attention	Early identification will lead to early attention
Aortic regurgitation	Severe regurgitation precludes good support	Severe regurgitation precludes good support
Post-cannulation Echocardiography		
Cannula position	Careful assessment essential	Careful assessment essential
Ventricular function		Right ventricular function and pressures Is single ventricular support adequate? Additional afterload reduction or inotropy may be required to assist non-supported ventricle
Adequacy of decompression	Left atrial decompression may be required	Should be excellent if cannula well-positioned
Presence of residual defects	Early identification will lead to early attention	Early identification will lead to early attention
Troubleshooting (clots, effusion)	Careful assessment essential	Careful assessment essential
Intervention	To guide atrial decompression	
Echocardiography During Weaning		
Ventricular function	Ventricular recovery during weaning and introduction of additional therapies	Ventricular recovery during weaning and introduction of additional therapies
Response to drugs, pacing	To guide timing of decannulation	To guide timing of decannulation

Successful weaning from mechanical support includes a careful assessment of the heart and circulation, with specific attention to excluding residual anatomic or surgical abnormalities. It is essential routinely to search for a remediable cause in all children who are placed on post-operative support, rather than simply assume that this is due to a long or high-risk operation. This requires detailed transthoracic or transoesophageal evaluation. If there remains suspicion that there may be an anatomic cause which is not explained by echocardiography alone, then cardiac catheterisation or further radiological evaluation, for example using computerised tomographic angiography, should be undertaken early to utilise the window of opportunity for transcatheter or surgical intervention.[95] Examples of residual lesions which may preclude successful weaning are significant aortopulmonary collateral vessels, distal pulmonary arterial obstruction, arrhythmic ablation and persisting additional intracardiac shunts.

The technical aspects of weaning from extracorporeal support vary according to the mode of support, the underlying indication, and the urgency of the need to separate from support. There are, however, some broad principles that apply for all patients, which are aimed at optimising their condition prior to separation from support. Weaning

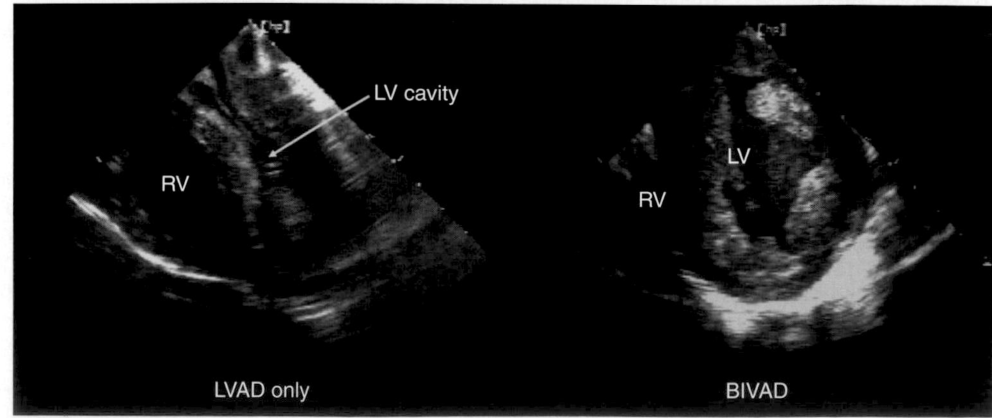

Figure 14-6 The images demonstrate the value of intra-operative transoesophageal echocardiography during institution of ventricular assistance in a child with ventricular failure. Initially, the child was placed only on left-sided support. The echo to the left shows complete obliteration of the left ventricular cavity, with the right ventricle remaining dilated and poorly functioning. Right-sided cannulation was therefore performed, and the child was placed on biventricular support (*right*).

from mechanical support is a process where the flows on the extracorporeal circuit are reduced over a period of at least several hours. During this time, the performances of the myocardium and for many patients, their lungs, are being tested. In order to maximise the chances of success, it is essential to ensure that pulmonary function is optimal prior to weaning, and that appropriate inotropic and afterload reducing agents, in some cases including inhaled nitric oxide, have been commenced and appropriately titrated. In addition, it is sensible to introduce measures aimed at reducing the consumption of oxygen, including high levels of sedation and analgesia, and muscle relaxants.

Risks of Extracorporeal Life Support

Mechanical support is a hazardous therapy, and mortality is often related to complications rather than to the underlying disease. Extracorporeal support carries a significant risk of haemorrhage, which is directly related to the level of systemic anticoagulation. In addition, the extracorporeal circuit can cause haemolysis, or can precipitate formation of thrombus, with the potential to embolise to the circulation, or to cause occlusion of the circuit. The risk of these complications is related to the complexity of the circuit and is also increased by the presence of an oxygenator, which further reinforces the use of a ventricular assist device wherever possible. Patients on mechanical support are at significant risk of sepsis. This is related to deconditioning of the patient, exposure to artificial surfaces, the presence of cannulas, multiple surgical sites, and in some the need for the chest to be kept open. All of the risks increase with the duration of mechanical support, which reinforces the need for constant reassessment of circulation, and timely weaning from support.

Survival

The worldwide survival to hospital discharge for children receiving extracorporeal life support for cardiac disease is now between 40% and 50%.[77,88,96] This figure has remained relatively stable over the past decade, though increasing proportions of patients at higher risk are now receiving support. When diagnostic subgroups are considered, survival is lowest for infants with a cavopulmonary connection, and those with functionally univentricular circulation supported with extracorporeal membrane oxygenation for a low cardiac output. Conversely, a survival of greater than 80% is reported for infants after the first stage of surgical reconstruction for hypoplastic left heart syndrome, when extracorporeal membrane oxygenation was initiated for acute shunt occlusion.[88,97] Other factors which may be associated with reduced survival include a longer duration of support, the presence of additional organ dysfunction and the development of sepsis, haemorrhage or abnormal neurology.[77,89,96,98–100] In our own institution, survival has improved over the past two decades, despite our recent use in higher-risk patients, and as a resuscitative tool (Fig. 14-7). The likely reasons for this improvement include the establishment of a dedicated team, careful selection of patients, an algorithmic approach to the choice of support for specific diagnostic groups, the earlier deployment of support in patients at high risk of acute deterioration, refinements in components of the circuit and minimising variables within the circuit. The outcome of children receiving mechanical support should not be limited to discussing survival. Extracorporeal life support carries with it substantial additional risk of long-term neurodisability,

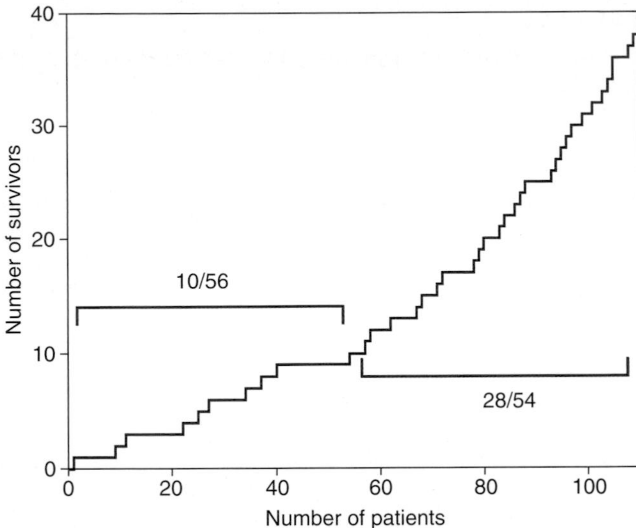

Figure 14-7 The graph shows the improved outcomes from extracorporeal membrane oxygenation in children with cardiac disease in Melbourne, illustrating survival to discharge from hospital for the first 110 infants and children who received such cardiac support at the Royal Children's Hospital, Melbourne.

and this is more common in children receiving extracorporeal membrane oxygenation than temporary support with a ventricular assist device. Long-term neuromotor and cognitive outcomes may be adversely affected in at least half of the survivors, and this reinforces the need for their continued neurodevelopmental surveillance.[101,102]

Summary of Extracorporeal Life Support for Acute Circulatory Failure

Over the past 2 decades, there have been remarkable advances in the field of extracorporeal support in children with circulatory failure, which have been associated with improved outcomes in increasingly complex groups of patients. These advances include the programmatic approach to support, refinements in circuitry, proactive decision-making and a better understanding of the circulatory physiology of patients during acute mechanical support.

When considering mechanical support for children with cardiac disease, and when talking to their families, it is essential to be fully informed that this therapy is not a panacea, but provides temporary support with the hope of enabling myocardial recovery after the insult of surgery, infection, or other causes of cardiovascular decompensation. The initiation of support should herald the start of a timer for clinicians who have a limited window of opportunity to optimise cardiovascular function, while considering additional investigation and therapeutic intervention, in order to maximise the chance of weaning from support.

When considering survival, successful decannulation should not be used as an end-point, as this step is relatively early in the protracted clinical course of most of these patients. Discharge home is a more appropriate marker of survival, but this statistic still masks a significant proportion of patients who may not be neurologically intact. The success of extracorporeal life support should ideally be defined in terms of neurologically intact survival, in a patient with adequate cardiac function.

TABLE 14-5

SUMMARY OF KEY THERAPEUTIC INTERVENTIONS FOR INFANTS AND CHILDREN WITH ACUTE CIRCULATORY FAILURE

Category	Example	Ventilation	Pharmacology	Extracorporeal Life Support
Systolic +/- diastolic dysfunction Increased afterload	Post-operative cardiac	Positive pressure ventilation is beneficial → Reduced LV afterload and RV preload)	Systemic vasodilators, careful inotrope therapy → Reduction in LV afterload, increased contractility	Early institution, usually open chest Single VAD preferable if lung function adequate and not emergency ECMO if cardiac arrest
Normal total cardiac output Maldistribution of pulmonary/systemic flow	Functionally univentricular heart	Positive pressure ventilation to stabilise the pulmonary vascular resistance (pre- and post-operative)	Systemic vasodilation Gentle inotropic support if impaired systolic function	Post-operative principles: Early institution if persisting acidosis and systemic hypoperfusion VAD if not-emergency ECMO if cardiac arrest
Normal systolic function Diastolic dysfunction	Post-operative Fontan Post-operative tetralogy of Fallot	Positive pressure ventilation is generally detrimental Aim for early extubation	Low dose noradrenaline may be beneficial Inotropes and vasodilators not generally useful	Uncommon indication Rarely necessary if appropriate use of other modalities and if residual lesions are excluded
Residual anatomic lesions	Post-operative cardiac	Routine positive pressure ventilation according to lesion	Careful use of all drugs, especially if fixed obstruction	Can be used to temporise the situation, and to enable investigations under more controlled conditions. Poor outcome if lesions are uncorrected.
Normal function Reduced afterload	Septic shock	At risk of systemic ventricular failure, and pulmonary oedema Positive pressure ventilation is beneficial.	First line: dobutamine + noradrenaline—commonly used in combination.	ECMO if systemic hypoperfusion and multi-organ dysfunction Consider sternotomy for high flow requirements.

ECMO, extracorporeal membrane oxygenation; LV, left ventricular; RV, right ventricular; VAD, ventricular assist device.

Summary of Treatment of Acute Circulatory Failure in Children

Acute circulatory failure is a multi-factorial phenomenon in children with heart disease, and its pathophysiology and haemodynamic manifestations are very variable. The successful treatment of children with circulatory failure requires a good understanding of the underlying disease and associated physiology, and a proactive approach to treatment using carefully tailored therapeutic interventions. The importance of considering the underlying physiology prior to managing circulatory failure in children cannot be over-emphasised. Indeed, the strategies for treating two patients with similar clinical manifestations of a low cardiac output may be very different, the treatment for one child being detrimental to the other.

The use of ventilation, cardiovascular drugs and mechanical support is aimed at providing short-term support for children at risk of developing circulatory failure, or for those who have developed this phenomenon. These strategies are often used in combination, and are aimed at assisting the heart and circulation to recover from an identifiable insult, but should not be expected to provide an alternative to reintervention for a significant anatomic problem (Table 14-5).

ACKNOWLEDGEMENTS

I would like to acknowledge the contributions of my friends and colleagues, Associate Professor Warwick Butt, lead in extracorporeal life support, and Mr Derek Best, coordinator for extracorporeal life support, at the Royal Children's Hospital, Melbourne, Australia.

The complete reference list can be found on the companion Expert Consult web site at www.expertconsult.com.

ANNOTATED REFERENCES

• Masip J, Roque M, Sánchez B, et al: Noninvasive ventilation in acute cardiogenic pulmonary edema: Systematic review and meta-analysis. JAMA 2005;294:3124–3130.

A systematic review of the role of non-invasive positive pressure ventilation in the treatment of acute heart failure in adults. This review considered the available evidence, from randomised controlled trials and systematic reviews, and concluded that non-invasive ventilation reduced the need for intubation and mortality.

• Shekerdemian LS, Shore DF, Lincoln C, et al: Negative-pressure ventilation improves cardiac output after right heart surgery. Circulation 1996;94(9, suppl):II49–II55.

This was the first of several clinical investigations by these authors, of negative pressure ventilation in infants and children with congenital heart disease. A brief period of negative pressure ventilation in children early after surgery, resulted in increases in cardiac output of 46% in ventilated children early after Fontan operations or tetralogy of Fallot repair. This study, and others by the same group, used a cuirass negative pressure ventilator to mimic spontaneous respiration, and conclusively demonstrated the importance of the early establishment of spontaneous respiration in these patients.

- Tworetzky W, McElhinney DB, Reddy VM, et al: Improved surgical outcome after fetal diagnosis of hypoplastic left heart syndrome. Circulation 2001;103:1269–1273.

  This retrospective cohort analysis of 88 infants with hypoplastic left heart syndrome reinforces the important role of pre-operative clinical status in determining the early outcome of these patients. Infants with a prenatal diagnosis were in better clinical condition early after birth and before surgery, and this impacted upon the subsequent clinical course after surgery. Specifically, acidosis, ventricular dysfunction and the need for inotropes, in the pre-operative period, were significant predictors of adverse outcome. These negative factors were associated with a postnatal diagnosis.

- Tweddell JS, Hoffman GM: Postoperative management in patients with complex congenital heart disease. Semin Thorac Cardiovasc Surg Pediatr Card Surg Annu 2002;5:187–205.

  Infants with complex heart disease, in particular hypoplastic left heart syndrome and its variants, present a challenge in intensive care. This review focuses upon the optimisation of the systemic delivery of oxygen in these infants early after surgery. The authors report an approach which uses vasodilator therapy to improve systemic perfusion in the context of goal-directed therapy.

- Hoffman TM, Wernovsky G, Atz AM, et al: Efficacy and safety of milrinone in preventing low cardiac output syndrome in infants and children after corrective surgery for congenital heart disease. Circulation 2003;107:996–1002.

  The low output state affects around one in four children early after cardiac surgery. An important focus of modern cardiac intensive care is the prevention of this phenomenon. Milrinone is a vasodilator with possible inotropic effects. This prospective, randomised, controlled study in 227 children undergoing complete biventricular repairs of congenital heart disease. cardiac repairs, demonstrated that prophylactic high-dose milrinone, given early after cardiopulmonary bypass, reduced the risk of a low output state from 26% to 12%.

- Stocker CF, Shekerdemian LS, Nørgaard MA, et al: Mechanisms of a reduced cardiac output and the effects of milrinone and levosimendan in a model of infant cardiopulmonary bypass. Crit Care Med 2007;35:252–259.

  In this laboratory model of infant cardiopulmonary bypass, increased afterload and impaired ventriculo-vascular coupling, without sufficient compensation, were found to be the most significant precipitants of the reduced cardiac output early after heart surgery. In this model, milrinone and levosimendan both prevented this deterioration and benefitted myocardial oxygen balance and pulmonary vascular resistance. In addition, levosimendan had additional inotropic properties which would suggest that it may be a superior agent in the peri-operative management of high-risk infants undergoing cardiopulmonary bypass.

- Chaturvedi RR, Macrae D, Brown KL, et al: Cardiac ECMO for biventricular hearts after paediatric open heart surgery. Heart 2004;90:545–551.

  The timing of institution of extracorporeal support is likely to influence outcome of this high-risk and complex therapy. This retrospective review of 81 children undergoing extracorporeal membrane oxygenation after cardiac surgery in a single centre reported a survival to hospital discharge of 49% (in keeping with worldwide experience). Survival rates were higher for patients in whom support had been initiated in the operating room (64% survival) and much lower if support was commenced in the intensive care unit (29% survival). The authors suggested that earlier institution of support was likely to prevent ongoing systemic hypoperfusion, and on occasions, the catastrophic complication of cardiac arrest.

- Duncan BW: Pediatric mechanical circulatory support. ASAIO J 2005;51: ix–xiv.

  This comprehensive review considers the extensive use of extracorporeal membrane oxygenation, and the growing (though less common) use of ventricular assist devices in children with heart disease.

- Booth KL, Roth SJ, Perry SB, et al: Cardiac catheterization of patients supported by extracorporeal membrane oxygenation. J Am Coll Cardiol 2002;40:1681–1686.

  The importance of detailed reassessment of patients requiring mechanical support cannot be overstated. This review of cardiac catheterisation of children receiving extracorporeal membrane oxygenation in a single institution demonstrates the importance of reinvestigation in this population. Sixty catheterisations resulted in an additional intervention (either transcatheter or surgical) on 50 occasions, with only minimal additional morbidity, and no directly-associated mortality.

CHAPTER 15

Chronic Cardiac Failure: Physiology and Treatment

ROBERT E. SHADDY and DANIEL J. PENNY

Chronic cardiac failure has long been recognised as a cause of considerable mortality and morbidity in the adult. The early recognition of cardiac failure in the 17th and 18th centuries was that of oedema, anasarca and dyspnoea, which was appropriately attributed to blood backing up behind an impaired pump, the heart.[1] Early descriptions of cardiac failure in children, which were rare, were usually associated with rheumatic fever. It wasn't until 1936 that Abbott mentioned cardiac insufficiency as a cause of death in children,[2] although we now recognise that chronic cardiac failure and cardiomyopathy are indeed important causes of morbidity and mortality in children. For children with cardiomyopathy entering a national population-based registry in Australia between 1987 and 1996, the freedom from either transplant or death at 5 years after diagnosis was only 83% for patients with the hypertrophic[3] and 63% for those with the dilated[4] form of the disease.

The concepts which underlie our understanding of chronic cardiac failure in both children and adults have changed considerably in recent years. In this chapter we aim to summarise some of the current concepts related to key pathophysiological processes in chronic cardiac failure and examine outcomes from its treatment. This chapter will complement comprehensive reviews related to the different types of cardiomyopathy and to the role of imaging in this condition which are presented elsewhere in this textbook.

BASIC CONCEPTS IN CHRONIC CARDIAC FAILURE

While for centuries cardiac failure was considered to be the result of a severe and irreversible injury to the heart, which led to an irremediable abnormality of the systolic function of the ventricle, it is now recognised that the syndrome of cardiac failure reflects a more complex, dynamic and progressive process which can no longer be defined in simple haemodynamic terms and which impacts, not only on the heart itself, but on a myriad of extracardiac physiological processes.

The current framework within which cardiac failure is now considered is one in which a primary insult to the heart, whether due to ischaemia, infection, altered cardiac load or tachycardia, results in a cascade of secondary responses within the heart itself and within related organs.[5,6] It appears that irrespective of the precise nature of the primary insult, for the most part, the secondary responses and the clinical evolution share common features, so that the progression of cardiac failure represents an ordered, predictable, coordinated cascade of events, which although initially reversible, in the absence of treatment may result in terminal cardiac failure and ultimately death.[6]

It appears that these secondary responses to cardiac injury may, at least in the initial phase, be adaptive and designed to preserve the flow of blood to the vital organs.[6] Thus in response to a regional injury of the myocardium, the global cardiac function is maintained by invoking a number of compensatory mechanisms. The regional function of the uninjured myocardium increases and the ventricle hypertrophies as growth factors within the myocyte accelerate the synthesis of protein and growth of the myocyte. As will be described later, within the kidneys, a reduction in renal perfusion pressure is detected by receptors in the renal arterioles which leads to the release of renin. The subsequent formation of angiotensin II results in constriction of the efferent arterioles so that the glomerular filtration pressure is maintained. Angiotensin also stimulates the synthesis of aldosterone which results in the retention of salt and water by the kidney. As a result, reductions in systemic and renal perfusion pressure are attenuated by vasoconstriction and retention of salt and water. Activation of the neuroendocrine system, manifest by the systemic release of neurohormones such as noradrenaline and adrenaline maintain cardiac output through their chronotropic and inotropic properties.

With time these mechanisms become maladaptive as the patient progresses into a phase of decompensated cardiac failure.[5] The increase in the mass of the left ventricle, combined with its dilation augment the mural stress within the myocardium and its consumption of oxygen, potentially worsening the myocardial injury. Chronic activation of the renin-angiotensin system results in oedema, elevations of pulmonary arterial pressure and increased afterload. Sympathetic activation increases the risk of arrhythmia and sudden death. While these changes may be reversed by successful treatment, it has been suggested that such treatment must be initiated before the patient reaches the so-called terminal threshold that is a point after which recovery of left ventricular function is not possible[7] (Fig. 15-1).

THE FUNCTION OF THE NORMAL AND THE FAILING HEART

The ability to accurately describe the function of the heart, its metabolic demands and its interactions with the vasculature, is of paramount importance in analysing the mechanisms of circulatory failure and the effects of interventions in patients with myocardial disease. In clinical practice our

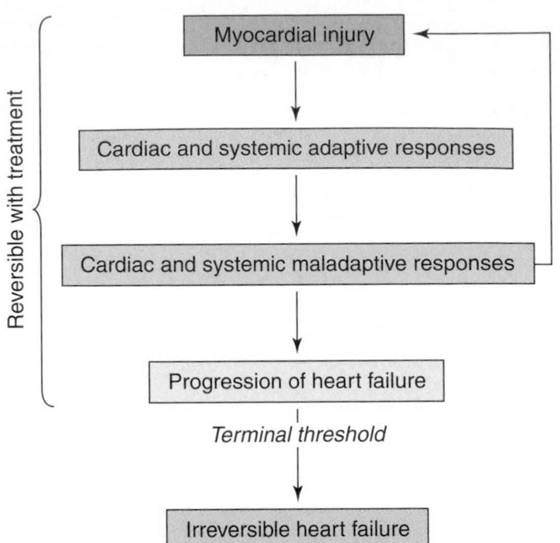

Figure 15-1 The responses to myocardial injury. Injury results in adaptive responses within the heart and within related systems. As the condition progresses, these adaptive responses become counterproductive (maladaptive) leading to progression of the disease and increasing symptoms. Treatment may reverse these maladaptive changes until a terminal threshold is reached, after which recovery of left ventricular function is not possible and irreversible cardiac failure ensues. (Modified from Delgado RM, 3rd, Willerson JT: Pathophysiology of heart failure: A look at the future. Tex Heart Inst J 1999;26:28–33.)

assessment of cardiac function is usually limited to the indirect estimation of ventricular systolic and end-diastolic pressure, ejection fraction, and in some echocardiography laboratories, the assessment of mural stress. However, a complete evaluation of cardiac function would extend further, ideally to include an indicator of ventricular systolic and diastolic performance that is relatively independent of load, an assessment of the myocardial consumption of oxygen and an examination of the relationship between ventricular performance and cardiac load.

Since Suga presented his analysis of the instantaneous pressure-volume relationship,[8] and subsequently developed the concept of time-varying elastance,[9] there has been heightened interest in the use of the pressure-volume relationship in assessing ventricular performance, especially in recent years with the introduction of the conductance catheter technique[10] which allows high-fidelity on-line measurements of ventricular pressure and volume at fast acquisition speeds.

The classic work of Wiggers[11] which described changes in left ventricular pressure and volume during the cardiac cycle has provided the foundations for our current understanding of ventricular function. In Wiggers' schema the cardiac cycle begins with the onset of depolarisation on the electrocardiogram, which is soon followed by an increase in pressure within the ventricle. When left ventricular pressure exceeds left atrial pressure the mitral valve closes. The aortic valve remains closed while aortic pressure still exceeds left ventricular pressure, and ventricular volume therefore remains constant: so-called isovolumic contraction. When left ventricular pressure exceeds aortic diastolic pressure, the aortic valve opens and the ventricle begins to eject. Consequently the volume of the left ventricle falls (Fig. 15-2).

Diastole is traditionally assumed to begin with closure of the aortic valve; however the decay in ventricular pressure (relaxation) begins before this event. After aortic valve closure, ventricular pressure continues to decay rapidly resulting from the energy-requiring mechanism, together with the passive release of myocardial elastic forces generated during contraction. As the ventricular pressure continues to decay, the mitral valve initially remains closed and the period of relaxation during which ventricular volume remains constant, is termed isovolumic relaxation.

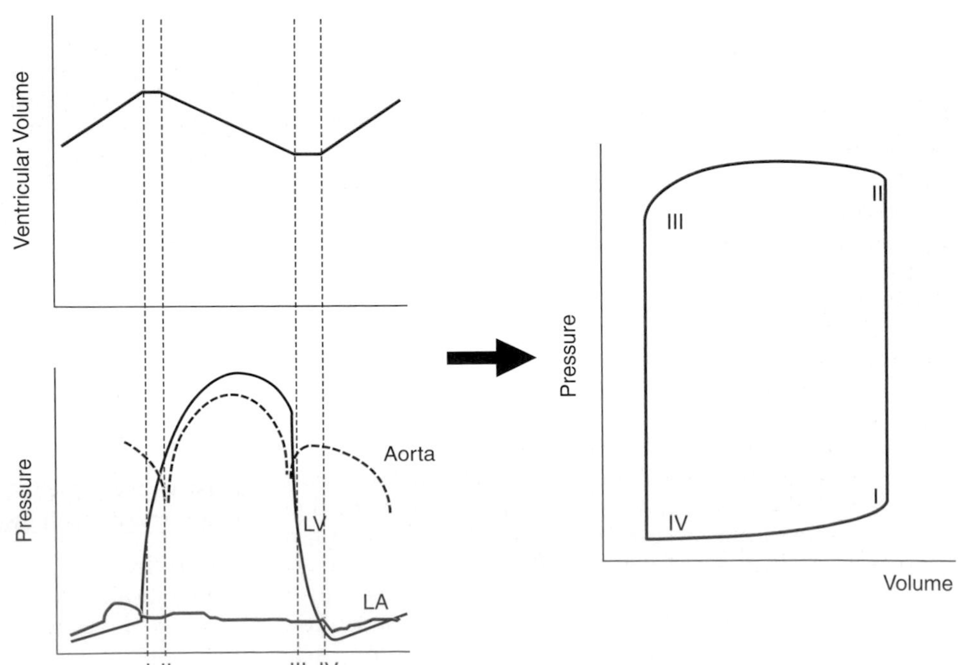

Figure 15-2 The temporal changes in the volume of the left ventricle (LV), as well as the pressures within the left atrium (LA), the left ventricle and aorta during the cardiac cycle (*left*). The onset of the isovolumic contraction time begins at I, when the pressure in the ventricle exceeds that within the atrium. This period ends at II, with the onset of ejection as the pressure within the ventricle exceeds that in the aorta. The period of isovolumic relaxation begins at III when the pressure in the left ventricle falls below that in the aorta. Filling of the ventricle begins at IV, when ventricular pressure falls below that in the atrium. The right hand panel represents the instantaneous relationship between the pressure and volume in the ventricle, with the time points represented as I to IV corresponding to the same events as those for the left hand panel.

When ventricular pressure falls below atrial pressure, the mitral valve opens and ventricular filling begins. During the early period of ventricular filling its pressure falls. This anomalous relationship between pressure and volume is thought to result from restoring forces, which attempt to restore the shape of the ventricle to that at end-diastole. After this time, both pressure and volume increase in the ventricle, which exhibits elastic behavior. Later in diastole the rate of ventricular filling is further augmented by atrial contraction.

Examination of Cardiac Function with the Pressure-Volume Loop

While until now, we have considered the temporal changes in left ventricular pressure and volume, the essence of the pressure-volume analysis is to consider the time-varying relationship between ventricular pressure and volume, represented by the pressure-volume loop. The pressure-volume loop has four characteristic phases. Beginning at its bottom right hand corner, an initial upstroke (I to II; see Fig. 15-1) represents the rapid increase in ventricular pressure, with little volume change: isovolumic contraction. There is then a rapid fall in ventricular volume, as ventricular ejection proceeds to the end-systolic point (II to III). Ventricular pressure then rapidly falls, with little volume change, as the ventricle enters the isovolumic relaxation phase (III to IV). Finally, ventricular volume increases to its end-diastolic level, reflecting ventricular filling (IV to I).

Suga noted that at constant inotropic state, alterations in ventricular load resulted in a population of pressure-volume loops in which, at any time in the cardiac cycle, the pressure-volume points follow a straight line. It was proposed therefore that cardiac contraction could be modelled as a time-varying elastance, with maximal elastance occurring at end-systole (end-systolic elastance),[9] represented by the upper left hand corner of the pressure-volume loop (Fig. 15-3).

While the end-systolic pressure-volume relationship has been considered the definitive measure of ventricular contractility, the importance of other indices should not be underestimated. It is important to emphasise that there is no single gold-standard measure, which will encompass the complex physiologic processes which determine myocardial contractility, rather, there are a number of measures, each of which provides individual pieces of a complex jigsaw.

It must be appreciated that the pressure-volume relationship provides a wealth of information about cardiovascular physiology beyond end-systolic elastance on which we will now concentrate.

The intricate coupling between the ventricle and the vasculature is an extremely important clinical determinant of cardiovascular function. While many treatments for cardiac failure are aimed at augmenting ventricular systolic performance, it is clear that without the ability of the vasculature to convert within itself the increased pressure work of the ventricle into flow work, these therapeutic strategies would be of little benefit. One measure of the efficiency of ventriculo-vascular coupling, based on an examination of the pressure-volume relationship, examines the coupling between end-systolic elastance and arterial elastance[12] to illustrate how the arterial response determines the physiological effect of an increase in contractility during inotropic stimulation.

The pressure-volume relationship can also provide important information regarding the energetic state of the ventricle. As in many critically ill patients with myocardial disease, the relationship between myocardial oxygen demand and supply is already precarious, it is imperative that any potentially desirable augmentation of ventricular performance should not be off-set by adverse effects on myocardial metabolism and energetics. Suga demonstrated that the total energy consumption of the ventricle can be quantified by the specific area in the pressure-volume diagram that is bounded by the end-systolic and end-diastolic pressure-volume relations and the systolic pressure-volume trajectory.[13] The scope of the pressure-volume diagram therefore extends beyond cardiac mechanics to include cardiac energetics and mechanoenergetic coupling under varying contractile conditions.

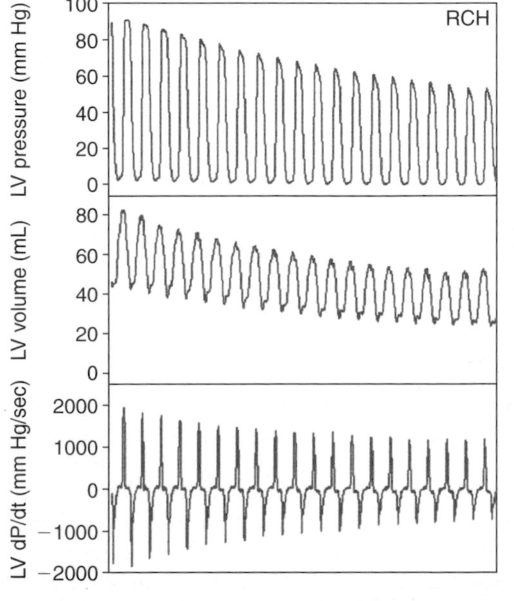

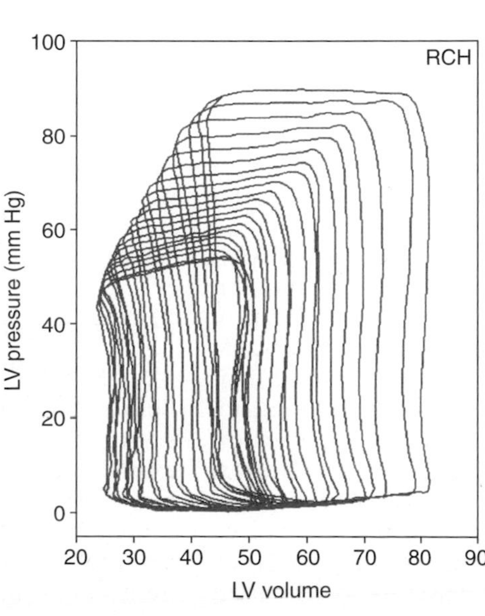

Figure 15-3 Changes in left ventricular pressure, volume, and rate of change of pressure (dP/dt) recorded with a conductance catheter during caval occlusion (*left*). A series of pressure-volume loops is generated (*right*) with a linear relationship between pressure and volume at end-systole.

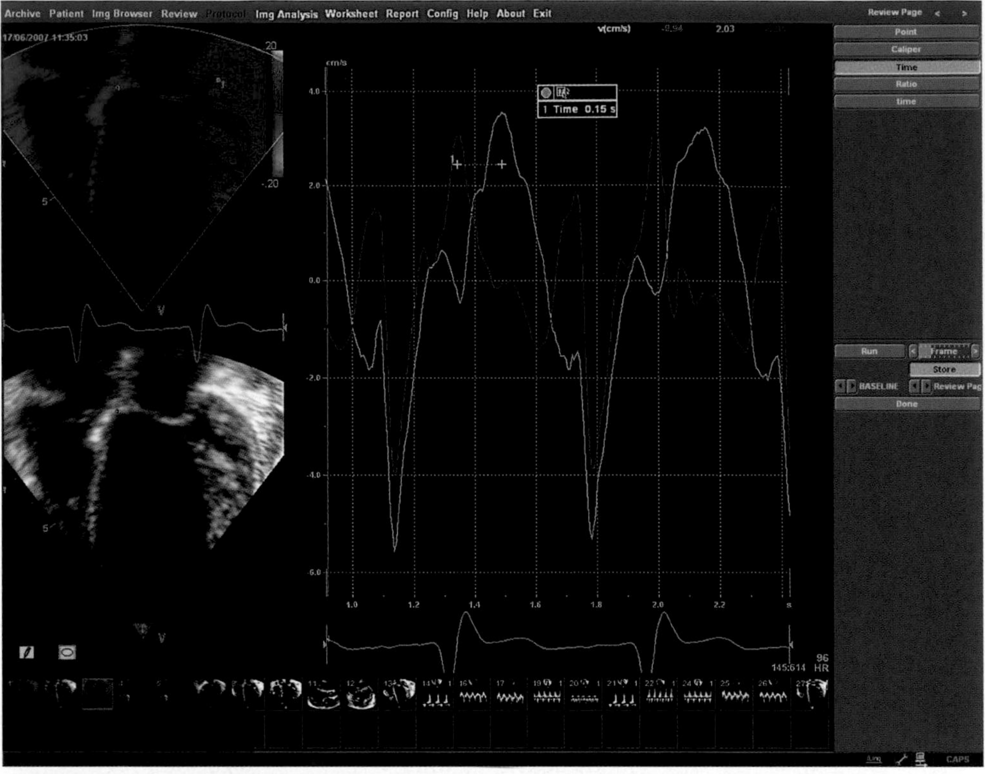

Figure 15-4 Dyssynchrony of left ventricular function, demonstrated with tissue Doppler imaging. The time to the peak of inward movement of the lateral part of the annulus occurs 150 msec after the peak inward movement of the central fibrous body.

The use of the pressure-volume relationship to assess the diastolic properties of the ventricle is based on the assumption that throughout the period during diastole when both volume and pressure are increasing, the ventricle exhibits elastic behaviour. As a result, at any point during this time, the slope of the relationship between pressure and volume represents ventricular compliance. As the normal pressure-volume relation at this time is curvilinear, chamber compliance becomes lower as filling proceeds, indicating that the cavity has become stiffer. The pressure-volume curve during this part of diastole is usually assumed to be exponential and to show behaviour characteristic of Lagrangian stress, so that, if pressure is plotted logarithmically and volume linearly, then a linear relationship will be obtained; it is then possible to calculate its slope and intercept.

There is little data which addresses the changes which occur in the ventricular pressure-volume relationship in children with myocardial failure. However, studies in adults have shown that the assessment of the pressure-volume relationship can be used to assess the effects of progressive myocardial failure on integrated cardiovascular performance.

Studies which investigated the matching of ventricular properties to arterial load, are particularly important in this respect. In normal subjects with an ejection fraction of 60% or more, ventricular elastance is nearly double arterial elastance. This condition affords an optimal coupling between ventricular work and oxygen consumption. In patients with moderate cardiac failure, with ejection fractions of 40% to 59%, ventricular elastance is almost equal to arterial elastance, a condition affording maximal stroke work from a given end-diastolic volume. However, in patients with severe cardiac failure, with ejection fraction of less than 40%, ventricular elastance is less than half of arterial elastance, which provides a suboptimal relationship between ventricular work and either oxygen consumption or stroke volume. These studies suggest that ventriculo-arterial coupling is normally set towards maximising work efficiency in terms of the relationship between left ventricular work and oxygen consumption. As cardiac function becomes impaired, in patients with moderate cardiac dysfunction, ventricular and arterial properties are initially matched, in order to maximise stroke work at the expense of work efficiency. However, as cardiac dysfunction becomes severe, the ventricle and vasculature become uncoupled, so that neither the stroke work nor work efficiency is near maximum for patients with severe cardiac dysfunction.[14,15]

While until now we have considered the function of the left ventricle as a whole, dyssynchrony of left ventricular function is frequently observed in patients with cardiac failure, in whom it results in inefficiencies in the contraction of left ventricle, a decreased cardiac output and increased risk of sudden cardiac death (Fig. 15-4). Recently, new therapies aimed at restoring mechanical synchrony in such patients have been shown to result in reductions in symptoms and improvements in outcomes.[16]

THE CELLULAR PHYSIOLOGY OF THE CARDIAC MYOCYTE

Before discussing the cellular mechanisms associated with the development of myocardial failure, it is necessary to examine the structure and function of the normal cardiomyocyte. In this section we will examine some of the principles related to this topic, although will not provide a comprehensive review of the multitude of intracellular and intercellular messengers, as these have been considered in some excellent specialist reviews.[17–19] Rather we aim to outline some of the principles.

Cardiac myofibres are composed of groups of muscle cells (cardiac myocytes) connected in series and surrounded by connective tissue. Each cardiomyocyte is bounded by a thin bilayer of lipid (the sarcolemma) and contains bundles of myofibrils, arranged along its long axis. These myofibrils, in turn, are formed of repeating sarcomeres, the basic contractile units of the cell, composed of thick and thin filaments, which provide the myocyte with its characteristic striated pattern. The thick filaments consist of interdigitating molecules of myosin and the myosin-binding proteins, while the thin filaments consist of monomers of α-actin, as well as the regulatory proteins, α-tropomyosin and troponins T, I, and C. A third filament within the myofibril is the giant protein titin.

Cardiac myocytes are joined at each end to adjacent myocytes at the intercalated disc. The intercalated disc contains gap junctions (containing connexins) which mediate electrical conduction between cells and mechanical junctions, composed of adherens junctions and desmosomes. The myocyte also contains an extensive and complex network of proteins, which links the sarcomere with the sarcolemma and in turn, with the extracellular matrix. This highly organised cytoskeleton provides support for subcellular structures and transmits mechanical and chemical signals within and between cells, by activating phosphorylation cascades.[20–22]

Myocardial activation is dependent on the phenomenon of excitation-contraction coupling. This is mediated through the release of calcium into the myocyte from the extracellular space, but more importantly from intracellular stores, particularly from an intracellular network of membranes, the sarcoplasmic reticulum. It appears that the generation of an action potential facilitates the influx of calcium from the extracellular space, through the so-called L-type calcium channels, which are particularly concentrated in specialised areas of the sarcolemma (transverse tubules) and which invaginate into the cell to reach its interior, close to receptors on the surface of the sarcoplasmic reticulum (the so-called ryanodine receptors). The increase in the intracellular concentration of calcium, which results from its influx from the extracellular space, triggers further release of calcium from the sarcoplasmic reticulum. The calcium activates myocardial contraction through its interaction with regulatory proteins on the myofibrils. Conversely, diastole is heralded by the reuptake of calcium into the sarcoplasmic reticulum through the activation of an energy-dependent mechanism which resides with the so-called sarcoplasmic reticulum calcium ATPase, which itself is regulated by a number of stimulatory and inhibitory proteins, in particular the inhibitory protein phospholamban.

The ambient level of myocardial activation is modulated by the actions of catecholamines through their interaction with specific receptors on the surface on the myocyte. Stimulation of these receptors invokes a series of complex intracellular phosphorylation cascades, which modulate not only the rate of influx of calcium from the extracellular space, but also the release and reuptake of calcium from the sarcoplasmic reticulum and the affinity of the myofibrillar proteins for calcium.

Central to the function and homeostasis of the cardiomyocyte is the mitochondrion. As the heart is the organ in the body with the highest oxygen uptake rate and an enormous demand for the continuous synthesis of adenosine triphosphate by oxidative phosphorylation, cardiac myocytes have a very high density of mitochondria. This central role for the mitochondrion as the power source for the cell and its position as the major site for the transformation of energy within the myocyte has been well-established. Energy is stored in the form of high-energy phosphate bonds in adenosine triphosphate. The free energy necessary for the formation of the adenosine triphosphate by the phosphorylation of adenosine diphosphate is derived from the oxidation of nicotinamide adenine dinucleotide by the electron transport chain.

As well as playing a central role in the metabolism of oxygen, it is also now recognised that the mitochondrion plays a crucial role in both apoptosis and necrosis, through its so-called permeability transition pores. The mitochondrion contains all the necessary machinery for apoptosis and is now acknowledged to be a key determinant in whether a myocyte will live or die after a pathological insult.[23] Central to this determination is the role of reactive oxygen species, generated by the diversion of electrons from the electron transport chain. While it has been long established that excessive levels of superoxide may result in damage to biological molecules, for example the sarcolemma and intracellular proteins, it is also established that reactive oxygen species play a central signalling role within the cell, which may not only regulate the key metabolic pathways within the cell, but also prevent apoptosis and cellular necrosis. It is clear therefore that the mitochondrion and reactive oxygen species play a central role as executioner or saviour in determining the viability of the cardiomyocyte.[24,25]

The Cardiac Myocyte in Cardiac Failure

Having considered the basic physiology of the cardiac myocyte, it is of interest to consider that any of these elements, the myofibrils, the sarcolemma, the gap junctions, the cytoskeleton, the mechanism of excitation-contraction coupling, the adrenergic receptors or the mitochondria may contribute to the pathogenesis of cardiac failure. This role may be a primary one, for example the abnormality of the mitochondrion seen in a patient with a so-called mitochondrial cardiomyopathy,[26] the abnormality of the key component of the cytoskeleton, dystrophin in the patient with muscular dystrophy[27] or the mutation in a sarcomeric protein in a patient with hypertrophic cardiomyopathy.[28] Abnormalities of these elements may also occur secondary to a primary insult originating outside the myocyte. They may thus represent the final common pathway in the development of cardiac failure[29,30] and the maladaptive myocardial response to a host of primary external insults. Thus, the development of cardiac failure secondary to ischaemia-reperfusion injury may be associated with abnormalities of the myocardial mitochondrion, in association with alterations in the expression and function of the adrenergic receptors. In patients with viral myocarditis, changes in the function of the mitochondrion may herald the onset of apoptosis, while enteroviral proteases may cleave dystrophin, leading to a secondary impairment of its function.[29]

OTHER ORGANS AND MEDIATORS IN CHRONIC CARDIAC FAILURE

It is now clear that the syndrome of cardiac failure is a multi-system disease, affecting not only the heart, but also many other organs and processes including the sympathetic nervous system, the kidney, the gastrointestinal system and nutrition,[31] haemopoiesis,[32,33] the brain,[34] and skeletal muscle.[35] Of these, we will consider only a few.

The Sympathetic Nervous System

It is now widely acknowledged that activation of the sympathetic nervous system plays a central role in the pathogenesis of congestive cardiac failure. Activation of the sympathetic nervous system occurs early in the course of the disease, even before the onset of symptoms[36] and as the syndrome evolves may play both adaptive and maladaptive roles. It appears that in the early stages of the syndrome, before the onset of symptoms, activation of the sympathetic nervous system occurs selectively within the heart[37] and kidneys. It has been suggested that this initially selective activation occurs secondary to ventricular dilation, which stimulates the release of natriuretic peptides and activation of the cardiac sympathetic nervous system. This initially adaptive response to ventricular dysfunction may preserve myocardial function. However, with worsening cardiac failure, the onset of symptoms, and as cardiac output and systemic blood pressure falls, this selective activation of the sympathetic nervous system becomes generalised as the high pressure baroreceptors within the heart and the carotid sinus become unloaded.[38,39]

Although activation of the sympathetic nervous system may play an important role in maintaining cardiac output and arterial blood pressure in the early stages of the condition (adaptive response), with time catecholamines may have detrimental effects. Elevated levels of catecholamines in the plasma[40] have been shown to correlate with decreased survival, which may be secondary to myocardial hypertrophy or activation of the renin-angiotensin system. Catecholamines are also known to be toxic to the myocyte,[41] through their effects on the intracellular levels of calcium.[42,43]

Retention of Sodium and Water

From the time that the condition was known as dropsy, retention of salt and water has been recognised to be a prominent feature of cardiac failure. Recent decades have considerably improved our understanding of the mechanisms responsible for the retention of sodium and water, and in particular have highlighted the contributions of activation of the sympathetic nervous system and the renin-angiotensin-aldosterone system, as well as the role of arginine vasopressin, aquaporins, and the natriuretic peptide systems.[44]

A pivotal trigger in the development of sodium and water retention has been attributed to arterial underfilling, secondary to a reduction in cardiac output. Unloading of the baroreceptors in the arterial tree results in activation of the sympathetic nervous activity, including to the kidneys, where it may not only impact directly on the retention of sodium and water, but may also stimulate the renin-angiotensin system.[45] Activation of the sympathetic nervous system within the supraoptic and paraventricular nuclei of the hypothalamus results in the release of vasopressin which further contributes to the retention of water by the kidney.

Activation of the renin-angiotensin system occurs early in the evolution of cardiac failure, with levels of renin within the plasma being observed before the onset of symptoms in patients with subclinical dysfunction of the left ventricle. Angiotensin plays a number of roles in the pathogenesis of cardiac failure. Although its synthesis is stimulated by sympathetic stimulation, angiotensin, in turn, enhances activity of the sympathetic nervous system, through a positive feedback loop. Angiotensin II has important vasoconstrictor properties as well as contributing directly to the development of cardiac hypertrophy and fibrosis.[46] Angiotensin II plays a central role in retaining sodium and water, through its direct effects on the tubular absorption of sodium, as well as indirectly through its effects of the secretion of aldosterone by the adrenal gland.

The natriuretic peptide system which is activated in cardiac failure is also important in the retention of sodium and water. In normal subjects, natriuretic peptides increase the rate of glomerular filtration and sodium excretion by the kidney. Although the secretion of natriuretic peptides is increased in the early stages of the evolution of cardiac failure, it is now known that cardiac failure is associated with considerable resistance to their actions.[44,47] This resistance to natriuretic peptides which may contribute substantially to the retention of sodium has been attributed to a number of factors, including a downregulation of the receptors for natriuretic peptides in the kidney, secretion of natriuretic peptide which is biologically inactive or its enhanced degradation by the enzyme neutral endopeptidase or by phosphodiesterase.[48]

While for decades, it was thought that vasopressin contributed little to the retention of water in patients with cardiac failure, it has been shown more recently that vasopressin through its actions on aquaporins within the collecting duct of the renal tubule may play a central role.[49] In animal models of congestive cardiac failure, the expression of aquaporin-2 is increased[50] and in clinical studies, antagonists of vasopressin may result in a dose-related increase in water excretion.[51]

TREATMENT OF CHRONIC CARDIAC FAILURE

The treatment of chronic cardiac failure has changed greatly over the years. Not surprisingly, once it was recognised that the cause of congestive cardiac failure was a failing pump, treatment strategies were directed toward making the pump work better. For centuries, the only treatment available for cardiac failure was digitalis. First described in his classic monograph in 1785, Withering praised the efficacy of the leaves of the common foxglove plant.[52] With the advent of the understanding of the complex neurohormonal syndrome now recognised as cardiac failure, strategies for the treatment of cardiac failure have changed from that of increasing pump function to that of decreasing the maladaptive neurohormonal stimulation associated with cardiac failure. In fact, no positive inotropic medication has ever been shown to increase survival in cardiac failure. The following discussion will focus on the current strategies for the treatment of cardiac failure, particularly as it relates to children. The development of an evidence base for the treatment of chronic cardiac failure is somewhat unique in that no drug has ever been developed solely for the treatment of cardiac failure; angiotensin converting enzyme inhibitors and β-adrenergic receptor blockers were both developed initially for the treatment of hypertension.

The use of the term cardiac failure in children can have many different implications. Patients with large left-to-right shunts with pulmonary over-circulation and tachypnea can be described as being in cardiac failure, despite that fact that ventricular performance is usually normal. Surgical outcomes for the treatment of these types of lesions, even in the smallest and youngest of infants, are now good enough to recommend early surgical correction. Thus, with few exceptions, long-term medical management of these structural lesions is unnecessary and will not be discussed in this chapter. Similarly, medical management of symptomatic valvar regurgitation is no longer routinely considered, since surgical correction is the treatment of choice in most cases. Finally, an evidence base is lacking for the treatment of patients with cardiac failure with preserved systolic function (also called diastolic cardiac failure), particularly in children. Because of this paucity of data, this type of cardiac failure will not be discussed. The remainder of this chapter will focus on the treatment of cardiac failure in children and adults as a result of decreased systemic ventricular dysfunction.

Digoxin

As stated above, digitalis has been the mainstay of chronic cardiac failure treatment for centuries. Even before physicians really knew what actually caused oedema, shortness of breath and/or anasarca, it was known that digitalis improved these maladies in addition to normalising irregular heart rates. Once it was known that this syndrome of oedema, shortness of breath, anasarca and irregular heart rate was due to poor cardiac function, then the use of digoxin as a treatment for cardiac failure needed to be studied more carefully. The mechanism of action is through inhibition of the sodium-potassium pump both within the heart and elsewhere. Within the heart such inhibition results in increased contractility; while outside, it reduces the sympathetic outflow from the central nervous system[53] and the release of renin by the kidney.[53] Several studies have helped define the role of digoxin in the treatment of cardiac failure.[54–56] These studies showed that, although digoxin does not improve survival in cardiac failure, it does indeed improve symptoms. Current recommendations in adults are that physicians can consider adding digoxin in patients with persistent symptoms of cardiac failure during therapy with diuretics, and an angiotensin converting enzyme inhibitor or angiotensin receptor blocker and a β-adrenergic blocker.[57] Toxicity from digoxin was common when serum levels exceeded 2.0 ng/mL and so early practice was to maintain levels to just below toxicity to achieve maximal benefit. More recent retrospective analyses of this and other studies suggest that lower doses may be better than higher doses.[58,59] There is now increasing evidence that lower levels of digoxin are safer and at least as efficacious as higher levels for the treatment of chronic cardiac failure. Since digoxin only appears to be helpful in the treatment of symptomatic cardiac failure, there is little if any role for it in the treatment of asymptomatic cardiac failure. In the most recent recommendations of the American Heart Association and the American College of Cardiology, digoxin is only recommended in the treatment of symptomatic cardiac failure, and actually contra-indicated in asymptomatic patients, unless atrial fibrillation is present.[57]

The indications for the use of digoxin in paediatric cardiac failure are less clear. The most recent recommendations of an expert group of paediatric cardiologists recognise that there is little data to support or refute its use in paediatric cardiac failure.[60] In patients with left-to-right shunts such as ventricular septal defects, the data is conflicting as to whether digoxin has any beneficial haemodynamic effects.[61–63] In one study, digoxin acutely worsened haemodynamics in children with cardiac failure due to left-to-right shunts.[64] There is no data to either support or refute the use of digoxin in children with cardiac failure due to ventricular dysfunction. Thus, in the absence of pediatric data, one can consider using the recommendations for digoxin in adult cardiac failure, with the caveats that these extrapolations become much less justifiable in the extremely young child or in the child with systemic ventricular dysfunction whose systemic ventricle is not of a left ventricular morphology. Major side effects include arrhythmias and gastrointestinal and neurological symptoms. Digoxin interacts with many medications (e.g., amiodarone, carvedilol, verapamil, spironolactone, flecainide, propafenone), and interactions should be explored before instituting digoxin therapy.

Diuretics

Although diuretics have never been shown (and possibly never will) to improve survival in cardiac failure, their use is considered important because of the need for anti-congestive measures in the treatment of cardiac failure. This is based largely on the significant symptomatic relief and haemodynamic improvement seen in patients with congestive cardiac failure treated with diuretics. A large number of diuretics are available, including those that act on the renal loop of Henle (loop diuretics) and those that act in the distal tubules of the kidney (thiazides). Potassium sparing diuretics will be discussed below in the section on aldosterone antagonists. Diuretics interfere with the retention of sodium in the kidney, and water follows this increased excretion of sodium passively. This causes a decrease in filling pressure of the ventricle and a reduction in right-sided (e.g., hepatic) and left-sided (e.g. pulmonary) congestion. The most common side effects are depletion of electrolytes and fluid (e.g., hyponatremia, hypokalemia), elevated urea levels in the plasma and even hypotension if excessive diuresis takes place. There is some evidence from retrospective analyses of previous trials that diuretics which do not result in sparing of potassium may actually be harmful in the treatment of cardiac failure, but further prospective studies are needed to confirm this.[65,66]

Inhibitors of the Renin-Angiotensin System

As stated above, the primary thrust of the treatment of cardiac failure over the last quarter century has been directed toward inhibition of the initially adaptive and ultimately maladaptive neurohormonal response to low cardiac output. The most studied and effectively inhibited neurohormonal system has been the renin-angiotensin system. Inhibitors of the angiotensin converting enzyme have been studied in many large, prospective randomised trials in adults with cardiac failure, in which more than 7000 adults have been enrolled.[67–70] These studies have conclusively demonstrated that these agents improve symptoms and survival in adults with cardiac failure, and delay the onset of symptoms in those asymptomatic patients with decreased systolic ventricular function. These drugs work through the inhibition of angiotensin converting enzyme which inhibits the conversion of angiotensin I to angiotensin II, a potent vasoconstrictor. Angiotensin converting enzyme is identical to kininase II, thus having an additional action of increasing bradykinin levels. This is thought to be responsible for the relatively frequent side effect of cough seen in some patients who take these agents. They also reduce afterload, preload and systolic mural stress. Angiotensin converting enzyme inhibitors are currently recommended for all adult patients with symptomatic cardiac failure and for those with a history of symptomatic cardiac failure,[57] unless the patient is intolerant of them.

The data on the efficacy of angiotensin converting enzyme inhibitors in children with cardiac failure is less robust than in adults. Many small studies from the 1980s and 1990s suggested that they may be beneficial in children with cardiac failure due to left-to-right shunts.[71–73] A few small retrospective reports also suggested a possible benefit from them in children with decreased systolic ventricular function.[74,75] One prospective, randomised trial compared the effects of enalapril with placebo in children who had undergone the Fontan operation. The primary end-point was exercise capacity, and no difference was found between the two groups after 10 weeks of therapy. In fact, the mean percent change from rest to maximal exercise was significantly decreased in the enalapril group compared to placebo.[76] Another study compared two groups of post-operative patients at two different hospitals, one receiving post-operative angiotensin converting enzyme inhibitors and one not. Those receiving inhibitors had a decreased duration and amount of pleural drainage.[77]

Angiotensin II receptor blockers have been shown to be beneficial in the treatment of cardiac failure in adults, but not superior to angiotensin converting enzyme inhibitors. Thus, angiotensin receptor blockers are currently recommended for the treatment of cardiac failure in adults, primarily those who are intolerant to angiotensin converting enzyme inhibitors. There is very little experience with angiotensin receptor blockers in children. Studies of angiotensin converting enzyme inhibitors and angiotensin receptor blockers in young adults with congenital heart disease and cardiac failure due to dysfunction of a systemic right ventricle have failed to show a clear benefit.[78,79]

Beta-Blockers

Waagstein and colleagues first reported the beneficial effects of β-blockade in a small group of adults with cardiac failure in 1975.[80] Many small studies over the next 20 years suggested some benefit from metoprolol, bisoprolol, and carvedilol in adults with stable, chronic cardiac failure.[80–82] However, it was not until 1996, that two large, prospective, randomised trials of carvedilol conclusively demonstrated that β-blockers improve symptoms, survival, and ventricular remodeling in adults with mild-to-moderate cardiac failure[81,82] (Fig. 15-5).

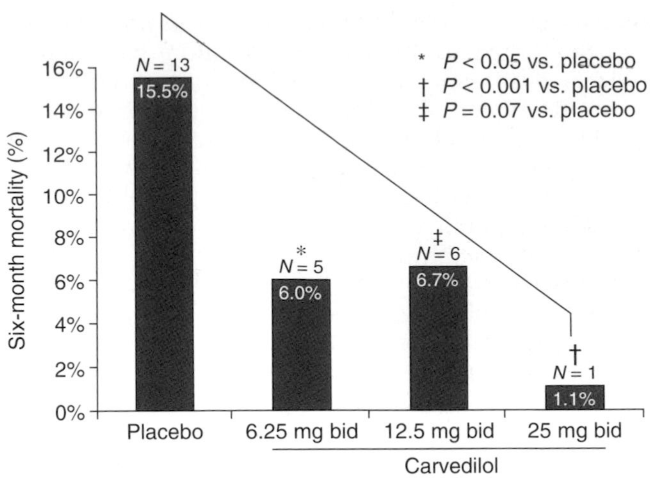

Figure 15-5 Mortality rates at 6 months (deaths per 100 patients randomised). (From Bristow MR, Gilbert EM, Abraham WT, et al: Carvedilol produces dose-related improvements in left ventricular function and survival in subjects with chronic heart failure. MOCHA Investigators. Circulation 1996;94:2807–2816.)

Subsequent studies have shown that other β-blockers, the long-acting metoprolol and bisoprolol, have similar effects to carvedilol in adults with mild-to-moderate cardiac failure.[83,84] Subsequently, carvedilol was also shown to improve survival in adults with severe cardiac failure[85] (Fig. 15-6). Based on these studies, β-blockers are now recommended for all adults with stable cardiac failure due to reduced left ventricular ejection fraction unless they have a contraindication to their use or have been shown to be intolerant to these drugs.[57]

Not all β-blockers are equally effective in the treatment of cardiac failure. In one large, randomised trial, bucindolol failed to show a survival benefit in adults with cardiac

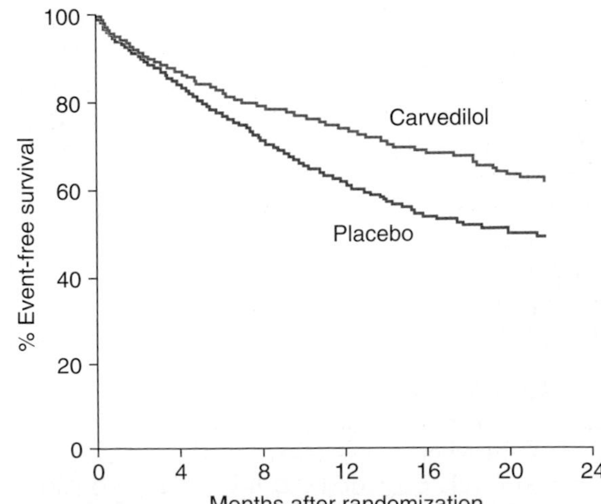

Figure 15-6 Analysis of time to death in patients receiving either placebo or carvedilol in the COPERNICUS trial. The 35% lower risk in the carvedilol group was significant: $P = 0.00013$ (unadjusted) and $P = 0.0014$ (adjusted). (Used with permission from Packer M, Fowler MB, Roecker EB, et al: Effect of carvedilol on the morbidity of patients with severe chronic heart failure: Results of the carvedilol prospective randomized cumulative survival [COPERNICUS] study. Circulation 2002;106:2194–2199.)

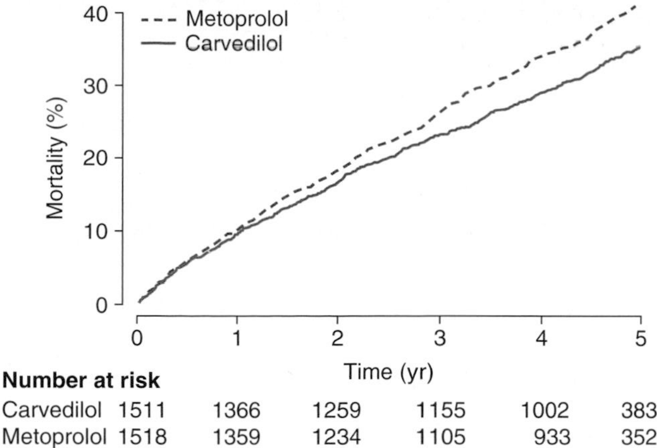

Figure 15-7 Mortality rates from all causes in patients treated with either carvedilol or metoprolol in the COMET trial. Mortality was significantly lower in the carvedilol group (34%) than the metoprolol group (40%). (Used with permission from Poole-Wilson PA, Swedberg K, Cleland JG, et al: Comparison of carvedilol and metoprolol on clinical outcomes in patients with chronic heart failure in the Carvedilol or Metoprolol European Trial [COMET]: Randomised controlled trial. Lancet 2003;362:7–13.)

failure.[86] The reason for this is unclear, but may be at least in part due to some interesting pharmacogenomic reasons that will be discussed later in this chapter. One comparison of metoprolol and carvedilol demonstrated improved survival after carvedilol compared to after metoprolol[87] (Fig. 15-7). This may be due to the broader actions of carvedilol, affecting the β-1, β-2, and α-1 receptors compared to metoprolol which is selective for the β-1 receptor.[88]

The initial reports of the use of β-blockers in children with cardiac failure suggested possible benefit of metoprolol in some children with cardiac failure due to anthracycline toxicity, dilated cardiomyopathy or congenital heart disease.[89–91] Since the FDA approved the use of carvedilol in adults, many small (mostly retrospective) studies have reported its potential benefit in children with cardiac failure due to systemic ventricular dysfunction.[92–97] However, the only multi-centre, prospective, randomised, double-blind trial of carvedilol in children with cardiac failure due to systemic ventricular dysfunction failed to detect a benefit of carvedilol over placebo in a composite end-point of clinical outcomes.[98] The half-life of carvedilol in children is shorter than in adults.[94] Thus, higher doses may be needed. Also, carvedilol increases levels of digoxin, so one needs to monitor and probably decrease doses of digoxin in children started on carvedilol.[99] Thus, it is likely that certain children with cardiac failure may benefit from β-blocker therapy, but the indications and dosing need to be defined.

Cardiac Resynchronisation Therapy

Patients with a left bundle branch block have delayed activation and contraction of the free wall of the left ventricle. It has long been recognised that this may alter regional loading conditions, myocardial blood flow, and myocardial metabolism.[100] There are regional alterations in gene expression and production of proteins involved with mechanical function and stress which lead to derangements of both contractile and non-contractile elements, resulting in ventricular remodeling, dilation, and pump failure. Early studies demonstrated that cardiac resynchronisation therapy resulted in improvements in functional class, quality of life, distances walked in 6 minutes, and ejection fraction.[101] More recently, resynchronisation therapy has been shown to improve survival in cardiac failure,[102] thus making it a class 1 recommendation for the treatment of adults with left ventricular ejection fraction lower than 35%, sinus rhythm, QRS duration of at least 120 msec, with moderate-to-severe cardiac failure on maximal cardiac failure medications.[57]

The knowledge base for cardiac resynchronisation therapy in children is small. Some series have demonstrated its feasibility in children with a resultant decrease in QRS duration and possible beneficial effects on ventricular reverse remodelling.[103,104] In the largest report to date, Dubin and colleagues reviewed their experience with this form of treatment in 103 children with cardiac failure due to dilated cardiomyopathy, congenital heart disease, or complete heart block.[105] The average change in left ventricular ejection fraction reported after treatment was about 13%, although there was no difference in this measurement between the three groups. The only discernible characteristic predictive of response versus no response was a lower ejection fraction before treatment (24% vs. 32%). However, the incidence of side effects was significant. Three percent of patients died early and 2% later. Five percent of patients had complications related to the coronary sinus electrode. Thus, as with virtually all other treatments for cardiac failure in children, the indications for resynchronisation therapy are unclear, and their potential risk-benefit ratio is still to be determined.

Treatments Primarily Aimed at Reducing Sudden Death

Mortality in patients with cardiac failure is related either to terminal end-organ failure or sudden death. While the treatment options discussed in this chapter, until now, aim to maintain stability with the patient's cardiac failure, recently there has been increasing interest in the use of therapies which aim primarily to reduce the risk of sudden death in this group of patients. As a result, implantable cardioverter-defibrillators are now widely recommended in the treatment of selected adults with chronic, stable cardiac failure.[57] Early studies with these devices suggested benefit in those patients who had suffered an aborted sudden death episode (secondary prevention)[106–108] although more recent, randomised trials have shown clear benefit in the primary prevention of sudden death in adults with a left ventricular ejection fraction less than 35%, and mild-to-moderate cardiac failure (Fig. 15-8).[109]

A meta-analysis of 13 studies in pediatric dilated cardiomyopathy demonstrated a 27% incidence of sudden death in children who died of this disease (Table 15-1).[110] Thus, appropriate application of cardioverter-defibrillator therapy to children with cardiac failure could clearly save lives, although there is a paucity of data on their use in children. Although not proven, possible indications include children with cardiac failure and the following: an aborted sudden death episode, severe, symptomatic cardiomyopathy awaiting heart transplantation, after heart transplantation with severe graft vasculopathy awaiting retransplantation.[111,112] Many of the technical challenges described above for resynchronisation therapy in children applies to implantable cardioverter-defibrillators.

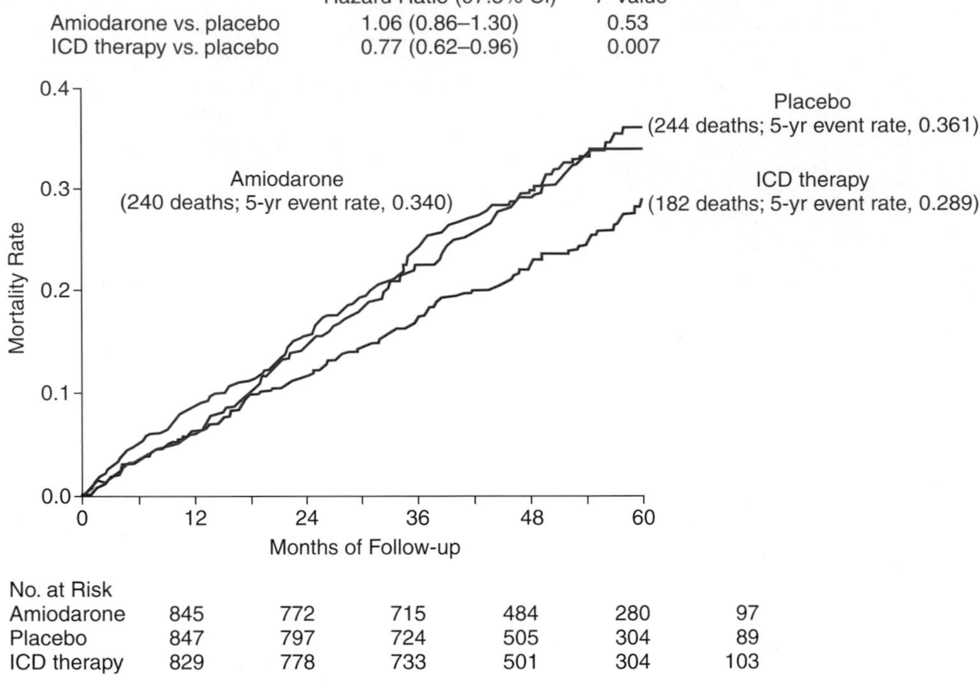

Figure 15-8 Estimates of death from any cause in the SCD-HeFT trial. (From Bardy GH, Lee KL, Mark DB, et al: Amiodarone or an implantable cardioverter-defibrillator for congestive heart failure. N Engl J Med 2005;352:225–237.)

TABLE 15-1

SUDDEN CARDIAC FAILURE AND TOTAL MORTALITY IN PAEDIATRIC SERIES OF DILATED CARDIOMYOPATHY

Year	Patients	Deaths	Mortality (%)	Mean Follow up (months)	1-Year Mortality (%)	5-Year Mortality (%)	Number of Sudden Deaths	Number of Deaths due to CHF	Risk Factors for Mortality	Risk Factors for Arrhythmia
1985	24	12	63	33	37	63	1	11	Severe MR	No
1988	32	17	53	36	15	25	7	10	Age > 2	Yes
1990	23	11	48	43	30	44	4	7	Low EF, EFE, family history	No
1991	25	18	72	12	60	80	1	17	CT ratio > 65%, EF < 30%	
1991	36	12	33	59	25	33	4	8	Undefined	Yes
1991	81	30	37	42	20	64	11	19	LVEDP > 25 mm Hg	Yes
1991	63	10	16	48	11	20	3	7	Persistent CHF	No
1994	19	7	37	39	21	36	3	4	Undefined	No
1994	63	17	27	19	21	61	7	10	Age > 2; no improvement	
1995	28	9	32	49	11	22	4	5	Undefined	No
1998	62	29	47	47	38	50	1	28	EFE, RHF	No
Total	**456**	**172**	**38**	**46**	**27**	**73**	**46** **27%**	**126** **73%**		

CHF, congestive heart failure; CT, cardiothoracic ratio on chest roentgenogram; EF, ejection fraction; EFE, endocardial fibroelastosis; LVEDP, left ventricular end diastolic pressure; MR, mitral regurgitation; RHF, right heart failure.

Adapted from Silka MJ, Szmuszkovicz JR: Arrhythmias and sudden cardiac death in pediatric heart failure. In Shaddy RE, Wernovsky G (eds): Pediatric Heart Failure. Boca Raton, FL: Taylor & Francis, 2005, p 441, with permission.

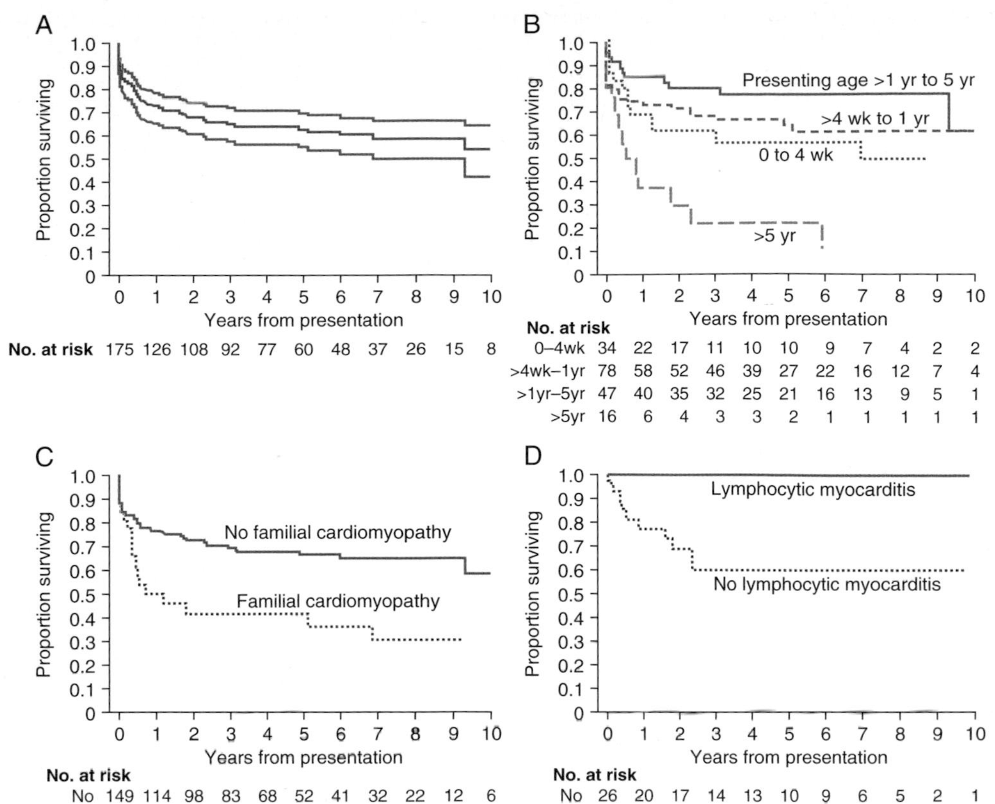

Figure 15-9 Survival to death or transplantation from time of presentation: overall, with 95% CI (**A**), with patients grouped by age at presentation (**B**), with patients grouped by presence or absence of familial cardiomyopathy (**C**), and with patients grouped by presence or absence of lymphocytic myocarditis on endomyocardial biopsy (**D**). (Used with permission from Daubeney PE, Nugent AW, Chondros P, et al: Clinical features and outcomes of childhood dilated cardiomyopathy: Results from a national population-based study. Circulation 2006;114:2671–2678.)

OUTCOME IN PAEDIATRIC CARDIAC FAILURE

There is little data which determines outcomes for all children with a diagnosis of cardiac failure. Obviously, outcome will depend upon a large number of factors, including the cause for the cardiac failure, its severity at the time of presentation and the age and possibly gender of the patient, as well as other factors. With the advent of new medications and pacing interventions, this outcome is hopefully improving over time. Preliminary data from a large prospective, multi-centre trial suggest that more than 50% of children with cardiac failure, who have been stabilised on ACE inhibitors and other oral medications for at least one month, will show improvement over an 8-month period of evaluation.[98] More long-term evaluation of outcomes is available for children with dilated cardiomyopathy, many, but not all, of which have some degree of cardiac failure.[113,114] In these studies, risk factors for death or transplantation include older age, presence of cardiac failure, worse left ventricular function (fractional shortening or ejection fraction), failure to increase left ventricular function during follow-up, familial cardiomyopathy, moderate-to-severe mitral regurgitation, and ventricular arrhythmias (Fig. 15-9).

The complete reference list can be found on the companion Expert Consult web site at www.expertconsult.com.

ANNOTATED REFERENCES

- Nugent AW, Daubeney PE, Chondros P, et al: Clinical features and outcomes of childhood hypertrophic cardiomyopathy: Results from a national population-based study. Circulation 2005;112:1332–1338.
- Daubeney PE, Nugent AW, Chondros P, et al: Clinical features and outcomes of childhood dilated cardiomyopathy: Results from a national population-based study. Circulation 2006;114:2671–2678.

  These two papers describe the clinical features and outcomes for children included within a National Registry for childhood cardiomyopathy in Australia.
- Delgado RM 3rd, Willerson JT: Pathophysiology of heart failure: A look at the future. Tex Heart Inst J 1999;26:28–33.

  This article provides an excellent overview of the concepts of adaptive and maladaptive responses during the evolution of cardiac failure.
- Towbin JA, Bowles NE: Dilated cardiomyopathy: A tale of cytoskeletal proteins and beyond. J Cardiovasc Electrophysiol 2006;17:919–926.

  This excellent review describes the important role of the cyctoskeleton in the pathogenesis of cardiomyopathy.
- Davila DF, Nunez TJ, Odreman R, de Davila CA: Mechanisms of neurohormonal activation in chronic congestive heart failure: Pathophysiology and therapeutic implications. Int J Cardiol 2005;101:343–346.

  This interesting review article summarises for clinicians the transition from the initially selective, regional and adaptive activation of the sympathetic nervous system to a generalised activation of all the neurohumoral systems.
- Re RN: Mechanisms of disease: Local renin-angiotensin-aldosterone systems and the pathogenesis and treatment of cardiovascular disease. Nat Clin Pract 2004;1:42–47.

  Accumulating evidence has made it clear that not only does the renin-angiotensin-aldosterone system exist in the circulation, but it is also active in many tissues—and likely within cells as well. These local systems affect the concentrations of angiotensin II in tissues and appear to be associated with clinically relevant physiologic and pathophysiologic actions in the cardiovascular system and elsewhere. The evidence in support of this possibility is reviewed in this article.
- Hunt SA, Baker DW, Chin MH, et al: ACC/AHA Guidelines for the Evaluation and Management of Chronic Heart Failure in the Adult: Executive Summary A Report of the American College of Cardiology/American Heart Association Task Force on Practice Guidelines (Committee to Revise the 1995 Guidelines for the Evaluation and Management of Heart Failure): Developed in collaboration with the International Society for Heart and Lung Transplantation; endorsed by the Heart Failure Society of America. Circulation 2001;104:2996–3007.

  This task force has provided essential reading related to the evaluation and management of chronic cardiac failure for all in the area.
- Bristow MR: What type of beta-blocker should be used to treat chronic heart failure? Circulation 2000;102:484–486

This editorial explores the hypothesis that clinically important differences exist among the many adrenergic blockers which might be used in the treatment of chronic cardiac failure.

- Cleland JG, Daubert JC, Erdmann E, et al: The effect of cardiac resynchronization on morbidity and mortality in heart failure. N Engl J Med 2005;352:1539–1549

  This study randomised patients with class III or IV cardiac failure to receive medical therapy alone or with cardiac resynchronisation. Cardiac resynchronisation improved symptoms and the quality of life and reduced complications and the risk of death. These benefits were in addition to those afforded by standard pharmacologic therapy.

- Bardy GH, Lee KL, Mark DB, et al: Amiodarone or an implantable cardioverter-defibrillator for congestive heart failure. N Engl J Med 2005;352: 225–237.

  In this study patients with class II or III cardiac failure and a left ventricular ejection fraction of less than 35% were treated with either conventional therapy alone, conventional therapy plus amiodarone or conventional therapy plus a conservatively programmed, shock-only, single-lead implantable defibrillator. Amiodarone was found to have no effect on survival, whereas the defibrillator reduced overall mortality by 23%.

- Towbin JA, Lowe AM, Colan SD, et al: Incidence, causes, and outcomes of dilated cardiomyopathy in children. JAMA 2006;296:1867–1876.

  This paper provides data on children who presented to 89 centres with dilated cardiomyopathy. The 1- and 5-year rates of death or transplantation were 31% and 46% respectively. Risk factors for death were older age, congestive cardiac failure, and the fractional shortening of the left ventricle. It was not possible to identify a cause for the disease in most children.

CHAPTER

16

Transplantation of the Heart, and Heart and Lungs

ANNE I. DIPCHAND and ELIZABETH D. BLUME

The first transplantation of a human heart was performed in South Africa in 1966.[1] By the end of the 1970s, transplantation was established as an effective therapy for end-stage cardiac failure. Over the next 25 years, improvements in donation and preservation of organs, selection of patients, post-operative management, and treatment of rejection have resulted in improved survival following transplantation in both adults and children. Consequently, orthotopic transplantation of the heart is now widely accepted as an important part of management for infants and children with severe forms of congenital cardiac disease and cardiomyopathy.

PATTERNS OF REFERRAL AND DEMOGRAPHICS OF TRANSPLANTATION OF THE HEART DURING CHILDHOOD

The factors affecting referral and listing of patients for cardiac transplantation are complex, but will include the availability and outcomes of alternative surgical strategies, availability of specific expertise, the patterns of referral to an individual centre, as well as societal and individual beliefs. Analysis of the natural history and outcomes must take all these factors into account. Besides reports from single centres, there are two main sources of data on outcomes for children following listing for transplantation and subsequent to transplantation. The registry of the International Society of Heart and Lung Transplantation[2] is an international registry, to which referral is voluntary except in the United States of America, where federal mandate requires all data from the United Network of Organ Sharing to be shared with the database of the International Society. The second source is the Pediatric Heart Transplant Study, a voluntary, research-based and event-driven multi-centric registry. It was established in 1993 in order to capture data relative to outcomes[3] from the Pediatric Heart Transplant Study. This source currently includes 3454 patients listed for transplantation, of whom 2452 patients underwent transplantation between January 1, 1993, and December 31, 2007. The data is supplied by 33 centres within North America and the United Kingdom.

According to the 10th annual report[2] of the International Society of Heart and Lung Transplantation registry, presented in 2007, the number of transplantations in children performed each year has remained stable, at approximately 375 to 400, since the mid-1990s, as has the distribution of ages (Figs. 16-1 and 16-2). Geographical differences exist worldwide. For example, teenagers account for half of the recipients in Europe and other areas of the world, whereas in North America more infants undergo transplantation (Fig. 16-3).

The underlying diagnoses prior to transplantation have changed over time. In infants younger than 1 year of age, congenital cardiac disease has remained the commonest underlying diagnosis, though the proportion of infant recipients with cardiomyopathy has almost doubled over time, increasing from one-sixth to one-third (Fig. 16-4). Cardiomyopathy remains the main diagnosis amongst those aged from 1 to 10 years and amongst adolescents (Figs. 16-5 and 16-6). Indications for transplantation also

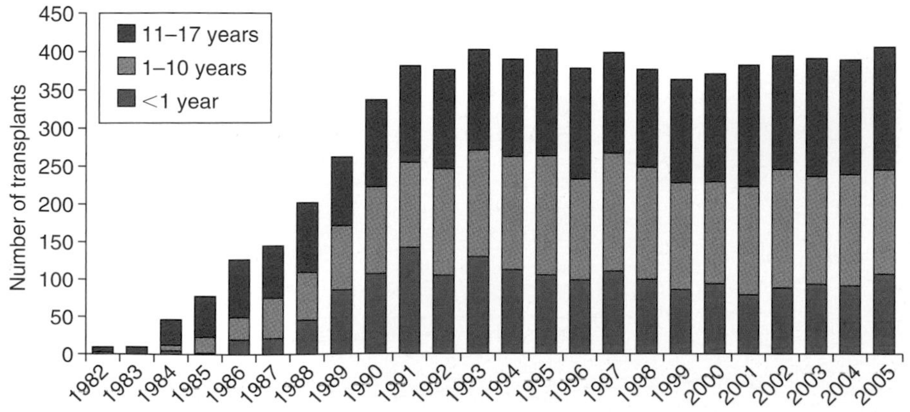

NOTE: This figure includes only the heart transplants that are reported to the ISHLT Transplant Registry. As such, this should not be construed as evidence that the number of hearts transplanted worldwide has increased or decreased in recent years.

Figure 16-1 Annual age distribution of recipients of cardiac transplantation during childhood. (From the registry of the International Society of Heart and Lung Transplantation. J Heart Lung Transplant 2007;26:796–807.)

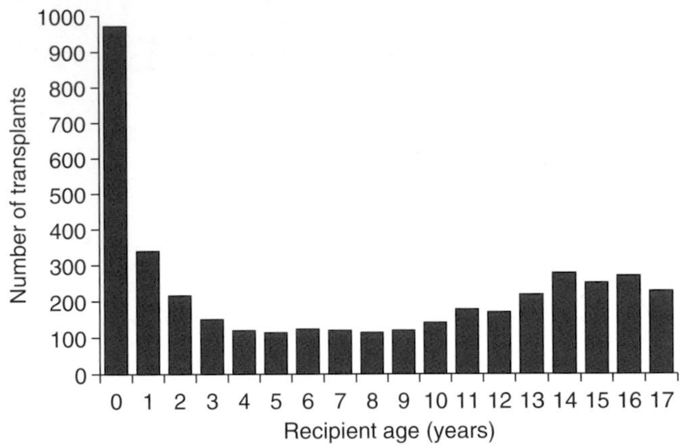

Figure 16-2 Age distribution of recipients of cardiac transplantation during childhood. (From the registry of the International Society of Heart and Lung Transplantation. J Heart Lung Transplant 2007;26:796–807.)

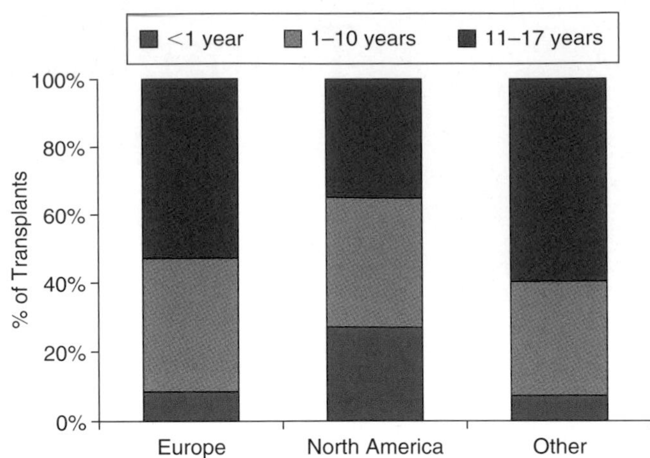

Figure 16-3 Age distribution of recipients of cardiac transplantation during childhood by geographic location. (From the registry of the International Society of Heart and Lung Transplantation. J Heart Lung Transplant 2007;26:796–807.)

Figure 16-4 Diagnosis in recipients of cardiac transplantation during childhood aged less than 1 year. CAD, coronary artery disease; ReTx, retransplantation. (From the registry of the International Society of Heart and Lung Transplantation. J Heart Lung Transplant 2007;26:796–807.)

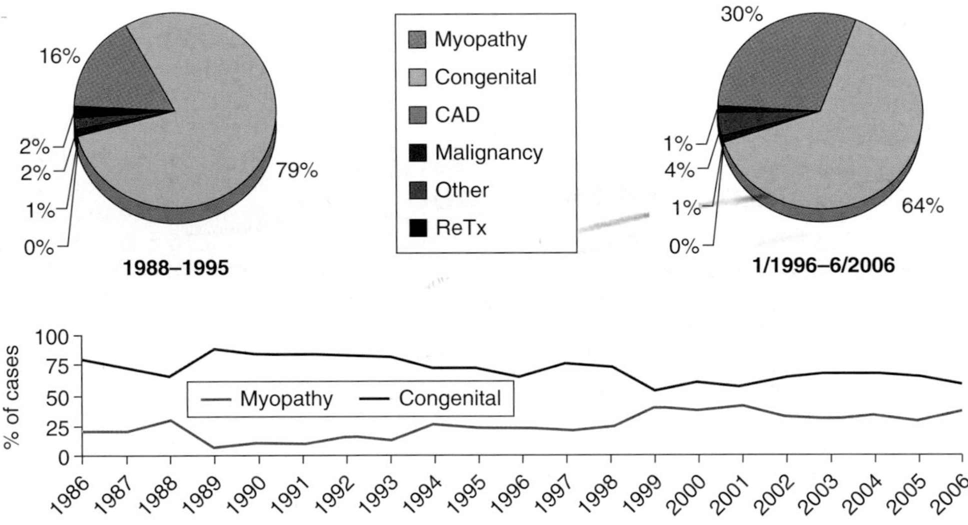

Figure 16-5 Diagnosis in recipients of cardiac transplantation aged from 1 to 10 years. CAD, coronary artery disease; ReTx, retransplantation. (From the registry of the International Society of Heart and Lung Transplantation. J Heart Lung Transplant 2007;26:796–807.)

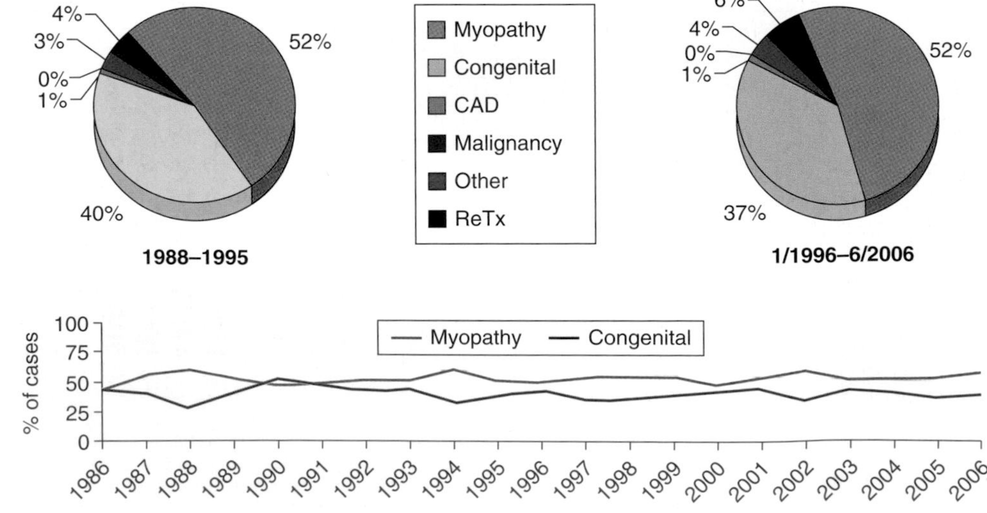

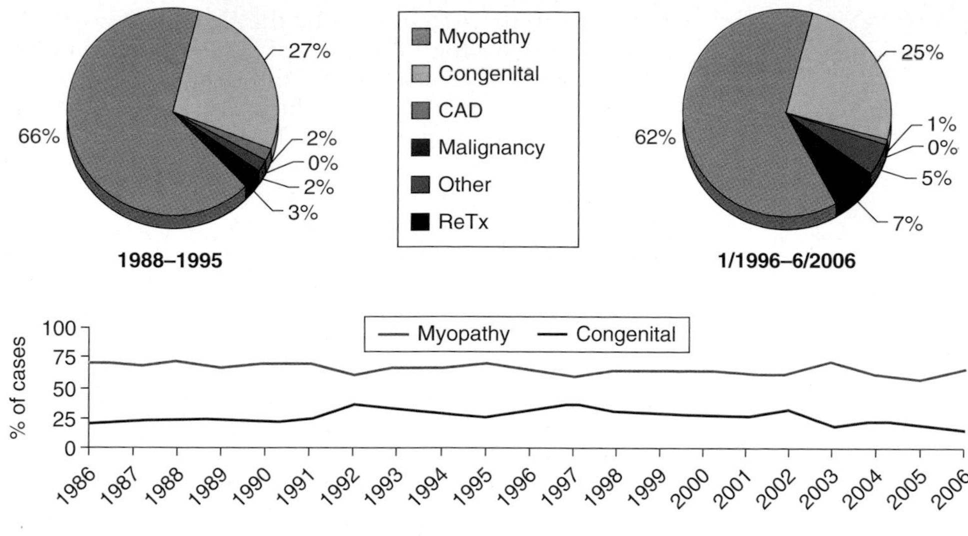

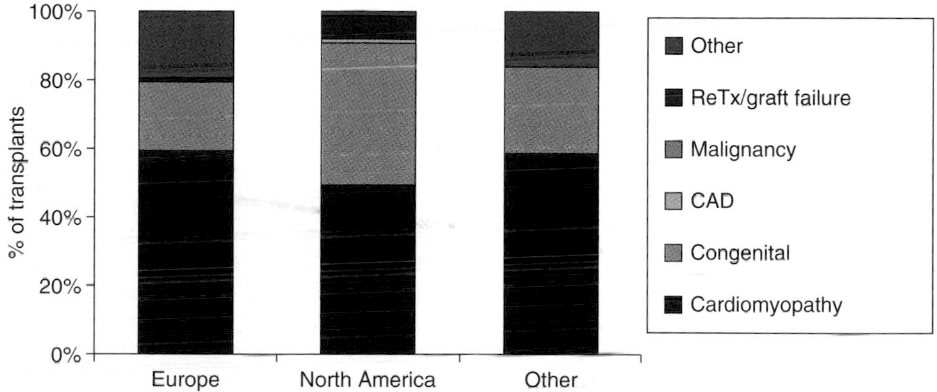

Figure 16-6 Diagnosis in recipients of cardiac transplantation aged from 11 to 17 years. CAD, coronary artery disease; ReTx, retransplantation. (From the registry of the International Society of Heart and Lung Transplantation. J Heart Lung Transplant. 2007;26:796–807.)

Figure 16-7 Diagnosis distribution of recipients of cardiac transplantation by geographic location. CAD, coronary artery disease; ReTx, retransplantation. (From the registry of the International Society of Heart and Lung Transplantation. J Heart Lung Transplant 2007;26:796–807.)

show geographic variation, with congenital cardiac disease and retransplantation both more common in North America compared with Europe (Fig. 16-7).[2]

OUTCOMES

Overall Survival

Overall survival for children listed for heart transplantation, including deaths prior to and after transplantation, as listed in the Pediatric Heart Transplant Study is 74%, 66%, and 59% at 1, 5, and 10 years respectively.[4] Overall survival from the time of listing is higher for patients with a diagnosis of cardiomyopathy compared to those with congenitally malformed hearts (Fig. 16-8).[5] There is an effect of era, with improved survival at all times after listing in the period from 2003 through 2006 (Fig. 16-9).[4]

Mortality while Awaiting Transplantation

Death whilst waiting for transplantation reflects a combination of availability of donor organs, the medical state of the recipient, the underlying diagnosis, and the blood group. While modifying availability of organs is difficult, knowledge of the other factors that influence mortality during the period of waiting plays an important role in decision-making regarding appropriate timing for listing a patient for transplantation.

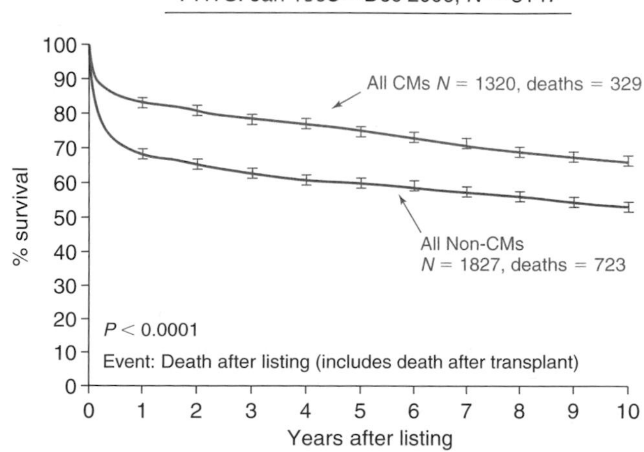

Figure 16-8 Actuarial survival curve in children aged from 0 to 18 years who underwent primary cardiac transplantation between January 1, 1993, and December 31, 2006, stratified by diagnosis, with all patients having cardiomyopathy (CM) compared with all other patients. Analysis includes death after transplantation. (Data from the registry of the Pediatric Heart Transplant Study.)

Data from the Pediatric Heart Transplant Study for the period between 1993 and 2006 demonstrates mortality for all listed patients whilst waiting of 17% at 1 year.[4] Unsurprisingly, mortality during the period of waiting varies according to the state of the patient, with those listed

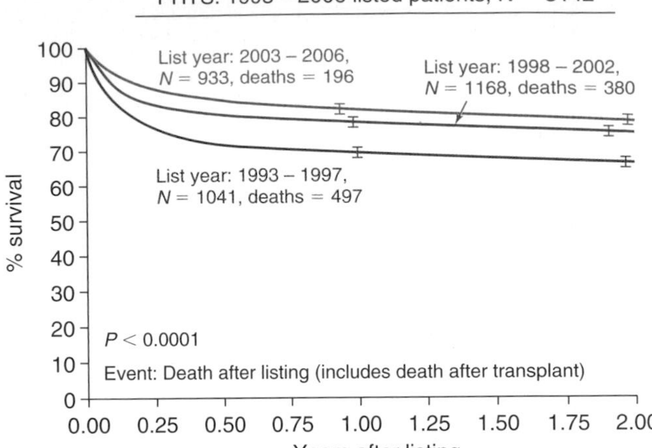

Figure 16-9 Actuarial survival curve in children aged from 0 to 18 years who underwent primary cardiac transplantation between January 1, 1993, and December 31, 2004, stratified by era. Includes death after transplantation. (Data from the registry of the Pediatric Heart Transplant Study. From Morrow RW, Kirklin JK: Survival after pediatric heart transplantation. In Canter CE, Kirklin JK: Pediatric Heart Transplantation. ISHLT Monograph Series, vol. 2. Philadelphia, Elsevier, 2007, Chap. 8, Fig. 5, p. 129.)

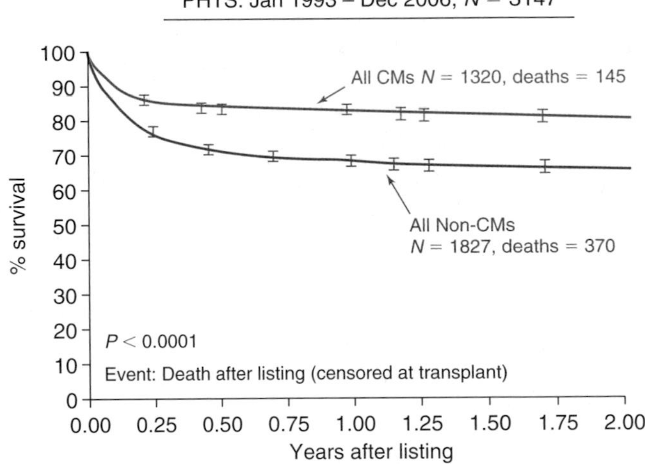

Figure 16-10 Actuarial survival curve in children aged from 0 to 18 years who underwent primary cardiac transplantation between January 1, 1993, and December 31, 2006, stratified by diagnosis, cardiomyopathic (CM) patients being compared with all others. This graph reflects overall wait-list mortality as patients are censored at the time of transplantation. (Data from the registry of the Pediatric Heart Transplant Study.)

at level 1A in the system used by the United Network for Organ Sharing having a mortality of 21%, compared to 7% for those listed as level 1B or 2.[4] A diagnosis of cardiomyopathy carries a lower mortality during this period of waiting than do other diagnoses (Fig. 16-10).[5] Blood group O, in contrast, has been associated with a higher risk of death.[6] The mortality for infants during the period of waiting, at from 25% to 30%, has consistently been higher than that reported for older patients.[7-9]

Survival after Transplantation

Data from the registry of the International Society of Heart and Lung Transplantation shows that survival after transplantation in the most recent era is 80%, 68%, and 58% for 1, 5, and 10 years respectively.[2] The survival after 20 years, while clearly reflecting transplantation during an earlier era, is 40% (Fig. 16-11).[2] Looked at a different way, the same data shows a half-life for transplantation, defined as the time to 50% survival without death or retransplantation, of 15.8 years for those aged less than 1 year at transplantation, 14.2 years for those aged from 1 to 10 years, and 11.4 years for those older than 11 years. These differences are even more marked when conditional survival is examined, excluding mortality related to the procedure itself (Figs. 16-12 and 16-13). Infants and neonates are relatively protected from later complications, while adolescents, who have lower mortality over the short term, are at increased risk of death or the need for retransplantation during long-term follow-up. Data from the Pediatric Heart Transplant Study is similar, showing that overall survival is generally good, with survival at 1 and 5 years of 85% and 75%.[4]

When survival is analysed by era, significant improvements are revealed in the results of transplantation of the heart during childhood, primarily related to a reduction in mortality immediately subsequent to transplantation (Fig. 16-14). Conditional survival for the different age groups within the period from 1999 through 2005 amplifies the difference between infants and adolescents, with infants having a conditional survival at 6 years of greater than 85%, while that of adolescents is approximately 65% (Fig. 16-15).

The diagnosis before transplantation also modifies survival. There is a significantly higher early mortality for

Figure 16-11 Kaplan-Meier survival curve out to 20 years after cardiac transplantation in childhood stratified by age at the time of transplantation. (From the registry of the International Society of Heart and Lung Transplantation. J Heart Lung Transplant 2007;26:796–807.)

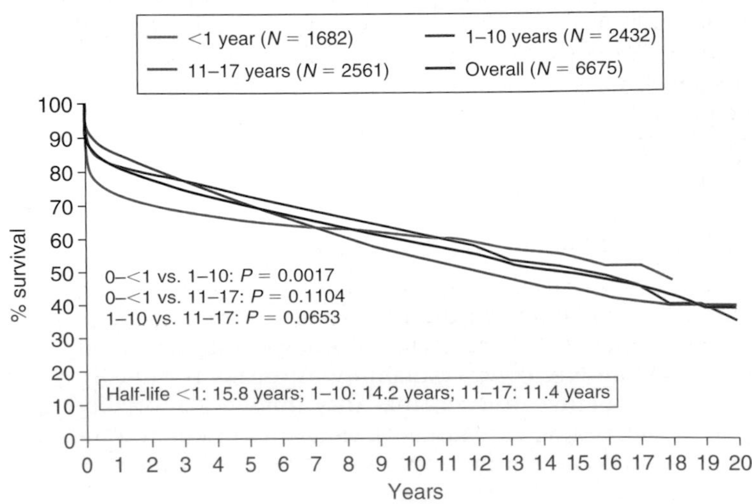

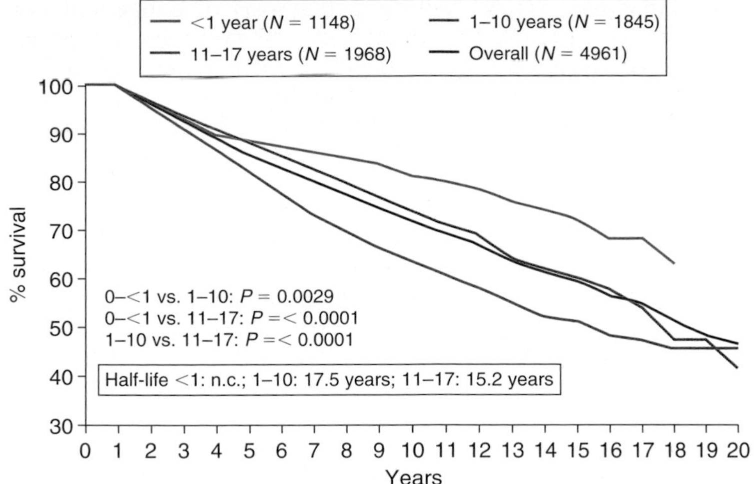

Figure 16-12 Conditional Kaplan-Meier survival, conditional on survival to 1 year subsequent to cardiac transplantation, stratified by age at transplantation. (From the registry of the International Society of Heart and Lung Transplantation. J Heart Lung Transplant 2007;26:796–807.)

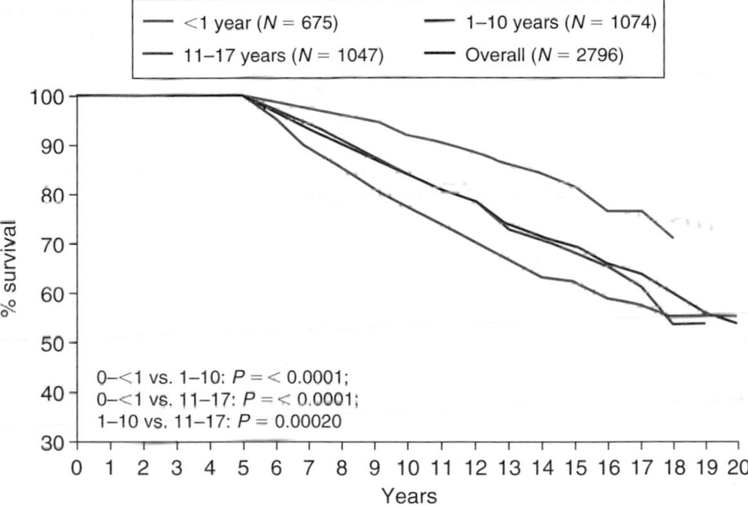

Figure 16-13 Conditional Kaplan-Meier survival conditional on survival to 5 years subsequent to cardiac transplantation stratified by age at transplantation. (From the registry of the International Society of Heart and Lung Transplantation. J Heart Lung Transplant 2007;26:796–807.)

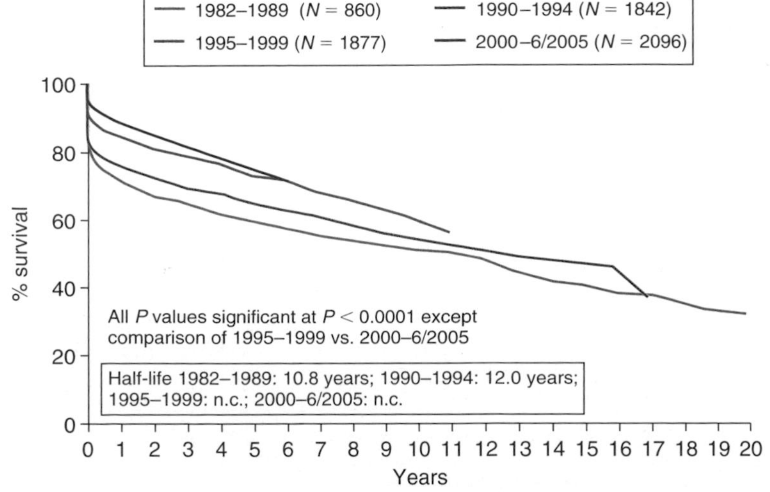

Figure 16-14 Kaplan-Meier survival curve out to 20 years after cardiac transplantation during childhood stratified by era. (From the registry of the International Society of Heart and Lung Transplantation. J Heart Lung Transplant 2007;26:796–807.)

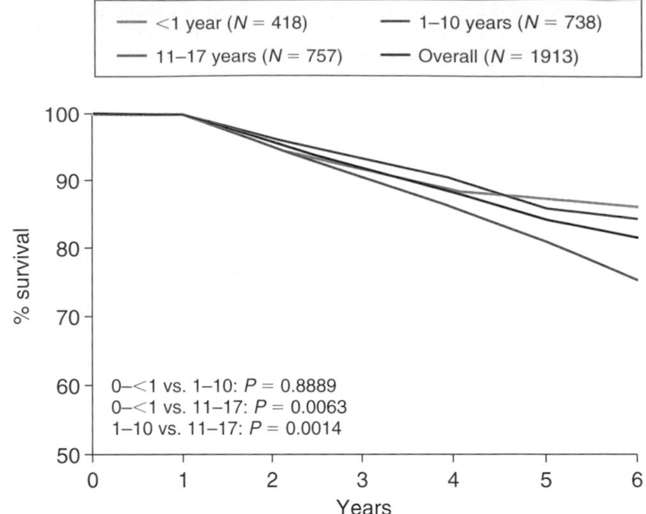

Figure 16-15 Conditional Kaplan-Meier survival conditional on survival to 1 year after cardiac transplantation for the most recent era from 1999 through 2005 stratified by age at transplantation. (From the registry of the International Society of Heart and Lung Transplantation. J Heart Lung Transplant 2007;26:796–807.)

patients with congenitally malformed hearts, compared to those transplanted for cardiomyopathy (see Fig. 16-8), with a recent analysis of patients transplanted for dilated cardiomyopathy showing an overall survival of 73% at 10 years.[5]

Risk Factors for Death

The risk factors for death in the first year following transplantation of the heart during childhood are outlined in Table 16-1. They include a diagnosis of congenital cardiac disease, need for extracorporeal mechanical support, mechanical ventilation before transplantation, and retransplantation.[2] Risk factors for mortality during the first 5 years are similar (Table 16-2), but female gender of both the recipient and the donor become additional risk factors.[2]

Causes of Death

The causes of death reported to International Society of Heart and Lung Transplantation registry, stratified by time after transplantation, are summarised in Table 16-3.[2] Similarly, the data from the Pediatric Heart Transplantation Study, outlining the causes and proportions of deaths within the first 5 years after transplantation, are summarised in Table 16-4. Rejection, infection, failure of the primary graft, and sudden cardiac death are the major causes of death in children within the first 5 years.[10-12] Graft vasculopathy remains the leading cause of death in the longer term. This, combined with failure of the graft and acute rejection, accounted for about seven-tenths of deaths between 5 and 10 years after transplantation.

INDICATIONS AND CONTRAINDICATIONS TO TRANSPLANTATION

Assessment Prior to Transplantation

Careful assessment prior to transplantation is required in order, first, to identify indications for transplantation, second, to identify potentially reversible causes of end-stage heart failure and optimise management, and third, to identify confounding factors or contraindications that may preclude candidacy for transplantation. The general components required for a comprehensive

TABLE 16-1

RISK FACTORS FOR 1-YEAR MORTALITY IN CHILDREN WITH A TRANSPLANTED HEART

Variable	N	Relative Risk	P Value	95% Confidence Interval
Congenital diagnosis, age = 0, on ECMO	51	5.66	<0.0001	3.54–9.06
Congenital diagnosis, age >0, on ECMO	48	4.30	<0.0001	2.58–7.14
Congenital diagnosis, age >0, no ECMO	710	2.23	<0.0001	1.70–2.91
Congenital diagnosis, age = 0, on PGE	201	2.12	0.0003	1.40–3.20
Retransplant	179	1.91	0.0029	1.25–2.92
Congenital diagnosis, age = 0, no PGE or ECMO	336	1.90	0.0004	1.33–2.70
On ventilator	581	1.45	0.0033	1.13–1.87
Year of transplant: 1995–1996 vs. 1999–2000	547	1.43	0.0191	1.06–1.94

ECMO, extracorporeal membrane oxygenation; PGE, prostaglandin E1.
Data from the registry of the International Society of Heart and Lung Transplantation. J Heart Lung Transplant 2007;26:796–807.

TABLE 16-2

RISK FACTORS FOR 5-YEAR MORTALITY IN CHILDREN WITH A TRANSPLANTED HEART

Variable	N	Relative Risk	P value	95% Confidence Interval
Congenital diagnosis, age = 0, ECMO	21	3.11	0.0020	1.51–6.39
Congenital diagnosis, age >0, ECMO	23	2.72	0.0127	1.24–5.96
Congenital diagnosis, age >0, no ECMO	434	2.30	<0.0001	1.66–3.18
Retransplant	104	2.17	0.0062	1.25–3.77
Ventilator	311	1.59	0.0026	1.18–2.16
Hospitalized (including ICU)	1224	1.49	0.0108	1.10–2.03
Year of transplant: 1995–1996 vs. 1999–6/2001	547	1.43	0.0139	1.08–1.91
Female recipient	808	1.27	0.0489	1.00–1.62
Female donor	800	1.27	0.0494	1.00–1.60

ECMO, extracorporeal membrane oxygenation; ICU, intensive care unit.
Data from the registry of the International Society of Heart and Lung Transplantation. J Heart Lung Transplant 2007;26:796–807.

TABLE 16-3

CAUSES OF DEATH IN CHILDREN WITH A TRANSPLANTED HEART

Cause of Death	0– 30 Days (N = 164)	31 Days– 1 Year (N = 159)	>1–3 Years (N = 144)	>3–5 Years (N = 104)	>5–10 Years (N = 184)	>10 Years (N = 96)
CAV	1 (0.6%)	11 (6.9%)	25 (17.4%)	36 (34.6%)	56 (30.4%)	30 (31.3%)
Acute rejection	19 (11.6%)	30 (18.9%)	32 (22.2%)	14 (13.5%)	27 (14.7%)	7 (7.3%)
Lymphoma		3 (1.9%)	6 (4.2%)	2 (1.9%)	19 (10.3%)	6 (6.3%)
Malignancy, other		1 (0.6%)	1 (0.7%)		2 (1.1%)	6 (6.3%)
CMV		3 (1.9%)	1 (0.7%)			
Infection, non-CMV	24 (14.6%)	22 (13.8%)	8 (5.6%)	2 (1.9%)	12 (6.5%)	8 (8.3%)
Primary failure	30 (18.3%)	5 (3.1%)	4 (2.8%)	3 (2.9%)	5 (2.7%)	2 (2.1%)
Graft failure	29 (17.7%)	15 (9.4%)	30 (20.8%)	30 (28.8%)	38 (20.7%)	23 (24.0%)
Technical	8 (4.9%)		2 (1.4%)		2 (1.1%)	
Other	14 (8.5%)	10 (6.3%)	16 (11.1%)	9 (8.7%)	14 (7.6%)	2 (2.1%)
Multiple organ failure	20 (12.2%)	31 (19.5%)	6 (4.2%)	2 (1.9%)	3 (1.6%)	6 (6.3%)
Renal failure		5 (3.1%)	1 (0.7%)			1 (1.0%)
Pulmonary	8 (4.9%)	17 (10.7%)	8 (5.6%)	6 (5.8%)	3 (1.6%)	5 (5.2%)
Cerebrovascular	11 (6.7%)	6 (3.8%)	4 (2.8%)		3 (1.6%)	

CAV, cardiac allograft vasculopathy; CMV, cytomegalovirus.
Data from the registry of the International Society of Heart and Lung Transplantation, J Heart Lung Transplant 2007;26:796–807.

assessment prior to transplantation are outlined in Box 16-1. In addition to the assessment of the heart, consultation from an interdisciplinary team, including social workers, psychiatrists, physiotherapists, occupational therapists, specialists in adolescent medicine, and key medical services including nephrology and anaesthesia, are critical to the process. For example, renal and/or hepatic dysfunction has been associated with a reduction in intermediate and long-term survival, and must therefore be integrated into the assessment of risk for child and parents. Psychosocial assessment of the entire family is paramount. This is especially important when assessing adolescents, given the increasing awareness of the impact of non-compliance and risk-taking behaviours on survival of both the graft and the patient.[13]

TABLE 16-4

PROPORTIONS OF DEATHS FROM VARIOUS CAUSES WITHIN THE FIRST 5 YEARS AFTER CARDIAC TRANSPLANTATION

	PROBABILITY (%) OF DEATH						
	0–5 yr	0–6 mo	7–12 mo	2nd yr	3rd yr	4th yr	5th yr
Early graft failure	4.7	4.7	0	0	0	0	0
Rejection	6.6	1.8	0.6	1.1	1.1	1	1
Infection	5.4	3.3	0.5	0.4	0.4	0.4	0.4
Sudden death	4.2	1.7	0.4	0.6	0.5	0.5	0.5
Nonspecific graft failure	2.4	0.3	0.3	0.5	0.5	0.5	0.4
Malignancy	1.2	0.1	0.1	0.2	0.2	0.2	0.2
Coronary artery disease	2.1	0.2	0.2	0.4	0.4	0.4	0.4
Other	2.6	1.9	0.3	0.2	0.1	0.1	0
Total	29.2	14.1	2.4	3.5	3.2	3.1	2.9

From Morrow RW, Kirklin JK: Survival after pediatric heart transplantation. In Canter CE, Kirklin JK: Pediatric Heart Transplantation. ISHLT Monograph Series, vol. 2. Philadelphia, Elsevier, 2007, Table 1, p 133.

Indications

There are no absolute indications for transplantation of the heart during childhood given the wide variability in cardiac diagnoses and pathophysiology. Indications can

BOX 16-1

General Components of the Assessment Prior to Transplantation

- Echocardiogram
- Cardiac catheterisation (haemodynamics, anatomy)
- MRI/MRA or CT angiography (anatomy)
- Exercise test
- Vascular ultrasound
- Blood group
- HLA antibody testing
- Chemistry
  - Renal function
  - Liver function
  - Lipid profile
  - Immunoglobulins
- Haematology
- Infectious serologies

be broadly divided into two groups, either life-saving (Box 16-2) or life-enhancing. Life-enhancing indications include treatment of excessive disability, unacceptably poor quality of life, usually in the setting of poor myocardial function, complex unoperated congenital cardiac disease, and failed surgical treatment.

Guidelines for listing adults for cardiac transplantation, based on a comparatively uniform population with cardiac failure and a predictable natural history, have been published by both the American Society of Transplantation[14] and the Canadian Cardiovascular Society.[1] They have limited applicability to transplantation during childhood. Specific guidelines are being developed for the populations of children and adults with congenitally malformed hearts. These strive to identify patients who are at the greatest risk of dying, and who will derive the greatest benefit from transplantation. There are two published consensus reports on the listing of children for cardiac transplantation, but these are predominantly based on the opinions of experts, and their recommendations remain the subject of debate.[15,16]

Contraindications

The contraindications to transplantation of the heart during childhood included fixed pulmonary hypertension, pulmonary venous atresia or progressive stenosis, and severe hypoplasia of the pulmonary arteries or the thoracic aorta. Other contraindications include irreversible failure of multiple organs, a progressive systemic disease with early mortality independent of cardiac function, active infection, malignancy, multi-specific and high sensitisation to HLA antigens, morbid obesity, diabetes mellitus with end-organ damage, hypercoagulable states, and severe chromosomal, neurological, or syndromic abnormalities. Complicating factors that are no longer considered contraindications to cardiac transplantation include complex congenital cardiac disease, such as abnormalities of atrial arrangement, systemic venous abnormalities, anomalous pulmonary venous drainage without stenosis, and some pulmonary arterial anomalies, previous sternotomy or thoracotomy, reversible pulmonary hypertension, more minor non-cardiac congenital abnormalities, kyphoscoliosis with restrictive pulmonary disease, non-progressive or slowly progressive systemic diseases with life expectancies into the third or fourth decade such as genetic or metabolic cardiomyopathies, and diabetes mellitus without end-organ damage.

Elevated pulmonary vascular resistance is an independent risk factor for death both early and late after transplantation.[17,18] The threshold which precludes transplantation is ill-defined, as there is a continuum of increasing risk as pulmonary vascular resistance rises. By convention, a pulmonary vascular resistance of greater than 6 Wood units per meter squared has been considered a contraindication. Intermediate outcomes have been reported nonetheless, for children with pulmonary vascular resistances greater than 6 Wood units, with mortality of 12% and a fall in resistance to less than 4 Wood units when assessed 10 days after transplantation.[18] In another experience, however, one-third of patients with resistances greater than 6 Wood units developed right ventricular failure, with mortality of 15%, with no patient having a resistance less than 6 Wood units developing right ventricular failure.[19] Despite these problems, five-sixths of patients with pulmonary vascular resistances greater than 6 and an indexed pulmonary vascular resistance greater than 9 were successfully transplanted. Both these studies concluded that it is the reactivity of the vascular bed, as opposed to the absolute measure of resistance, which is correlated with outcome. There is a role, therefore, for testing pulmonary vasoreactivity as part of the assessment prior to transplantation.

Accurate assessment of pulmonary vascular resistance and/or vasoreactivity with any diagnosis of functionally univentricular physiology, some complex malformations with variable sources of flow of blood to the lungs, or restrictive cardiomyopathy, nonetheless, may be challenging if not impossible, albeit that the risk of pulmonary hypertension and/or right-sided cardiac failure after transplantation in the population of infants with functionally univentricular hearts is low.[20] Timing of listing with a diagnosis of restrictive cardiomyopathy remains controversial. The most recent guidelines recommend listing at, or shortly after, the time of diagnosis due to the limited effect of medical therapies, and concern about the development of a non-reactive pulmonary vascular bed.[16]

BOX 16-2

Life-saving Indications for Heart Transplantation

- End-stage myocardial failure due to
  - Cardiomyopathies or myocarditis
  - Congenital heart disease
  - Post-cardiotomy heart failure
  - Malignant arrhythmias refractory to medical therapy
  - Complex congenital heart disease with no options for surgical palliation at an acceptable risk
  - Unresectable cardiac tumours causing obstruction or ventricular dysfunction (systolic or diastolic)
- Unresectable ventricular diverticula

SPECIAL CONSIDERATIONS

Neonatal Advantage and ABO-incompatible Transplantation

The published data from the registries, and specific institutional experience, increasingly show advantages to successful neonatal transplantation.[2,21,22] As outlined above, there is consistent evidence from survival curves that infants transplanted at an age of less than 6 months have improved survival when assessed up to 10 years after transplantation in comparison with older age groups (see Figs. 16-11 to 16-13). The reports from the Pediatric Heart Transplant Study show lower rates of rejection and graft vasculopathy in the population of infants.[23,24] Furthermore, data from Loma Linda University Medical Center shows that infants with hypoplastic left heart syndrome, transplanted at less than 1 month of age have a higher survival rate, 77% at 10 years, and less graft loss, than infants transplanted from 1 to 6 months of age, only 54% of this latter group surviving at 10 years.[21,22] The biggest challenge to transplantation during neonatal and infant life remains the availability of donors, which has not changed appreciably over the last decade. Consequently, strategies are being developed to expand the donor pool, or improve utilisation of available organs, one example of which is ABO-incompatible transplantation.

Such transplantation between donors and recipients incompatible for their major blood groups is usually contraindicated because of a high risk of hyperacute rejection mediated via activation of complement. Newborn infants, however, do not produce the isohemagglutinins responsible for the blood groups, and their complement system is not fully developed. It has now been shown heart transplantation across ABO blood groups is possible during infancy, reflecting the immaturity of the infant immune system or even representing the first human example of immune tolerance.[25] An advantage of such transplantation is a reduction in deaths during the period of waiting. In an analysis of risk factors relative to the strategy of listing, failure to list for an ABO-incompatible graft and high clinical status emerged as the only factors associated with mortality.[26] A strategy to accept ABO-incompatible hearts from donors for transplantation into infants significantly improved the likelihood of transplantation and reduced deaths whilst waiting, at the same time not adversely altering outcomes.

A report has now been compiled of the follow-up over 10 years of the largest cohort of recipients of ABO-incompatible transplantations.[27] Survival, the incidence of rejection, graft vasculopathy, and development of lymphoproliferative disorders subsequent to transplantation were no different from the ABO-compatible population followed in the same institution (Table 16-5). It remains to be proven whether there are immunological advantages such as tolerance or accommodation of the graft, but ABO-incompatible transplantation for infants is increasingly being adopted in centres worldwide. The optimal selection criterions for suitability for ABO-incompatible transplantation remain ill defined. In general, the younger the patient the better, but successful transplantation has been performed in recipients as old as 3 years. Antibody-mediated rejection has been reported, with titres of antibodies as low as 1 to 8, while there are reports of rejection-free survival with titres as high as 1 to 128.[28] Assessment should be made by a cardiologist experienced in ABO-incompatible transplantation on an individual basis, taking into account age, blood group, isohaemagglutinin titres, and clinical state.

TABLE 16-5

COMPARISON OF KEY OUTCOMES BETWEEN ABO-INCOMPATIBLE (ABO-I) AND ABO-COMPATIBLE (ABO-C) INFANTS AFTER CARDIAC TRANSPLANTATION

	ABO-I (*N* = 35)	ABO-C (*N* = 45)
Actuarial survival–1 yr	81%	80%
Actuarial survival–7 yr	75%	74%
EBV disease or PTLD	4 (11%)	5 (11%)
Graft vasculopathy	4 (11%)	5 (11%)
Mild	2	1
Severe	2	4
Wait-time (median)	25 days	26 days

HLA Sensitisation

Screening panel reactive antibody testing is performed on patients prior to transplantation in an effort to identify the potential presence of anti-HLA antibodies and minimise the risk of antibody-mediated rejection. High panel reactive antibody titres, greater than 10%, are associated with an increased incidence of rejection and reduced survival.[29,30] Common sensitizing events in children include repair of congenitally malformed hearts, specifically those achieved using homograft material,[31] and the use of ventricular assist devices.[32] There are many reports of transplantation in highly sensitised patients, nonetheless, and/or across a positive crossmatch, with reasonable results over the intermediate term.[28] A variety of strategies have been used to lower the titres of antibodies, and/or manage the rejection in sensitised patients. A detailed discussion is beyond the scope of this chapter, but most protocols include plasmapheresis immediately before and after transplantation with, variably, the use of intravenous immunoglobulin, rituximab, cyclophosphamide, and treatment with antimetabolites.[28,33,34]

Mechanical Support as a Bridge to Transplantation

Mechanical circulatory support is increasingly being used as a bridge to transplantation (Fig. 16-16).[35] Indications for such support continue to evolve as the availability of devices changes. In general, mechanical support should be considered when low cardiac output results in end-organ dysfunction despite maximal medical therapy. The mainstay for support in children has been extracorporeal membrane oxygenation,[36–38] which can sustain up to

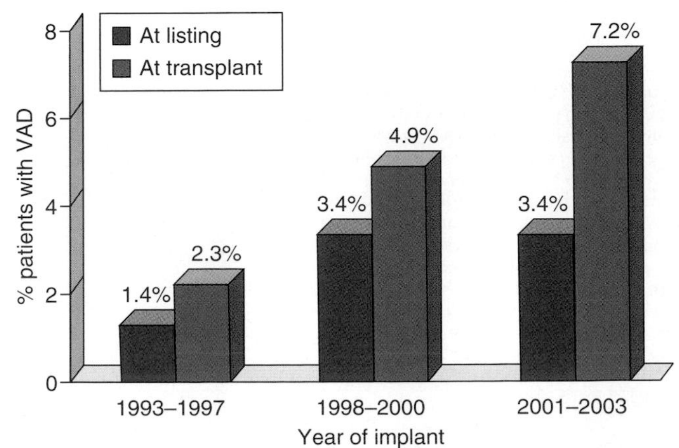

Figure 16-16 Percentage of patients with implantation of a ventricular assist device (VAD) as a bridge to cardiac transplantation. (From Blume ED, Naftel DC, Bastardi HJ, et al, for the PHTS Investigators: Outcomes of children bridged to heart transplant with ventricular assist devices: A multi-institutional study. Circulation 2006;113:2313–2319.)

three-fifths of children to transplantation.[39,40] In the experience at Toronto, the mean duration of mechanical support was 6 days, and almost four-fifths of patients survived to be discharged from hospital.[41] Higher levels of creatinine before and during extracorporeal oxygenation, fungal infection, and high exposure to blood products, were factors for poor outcome. Patients supported using extracorporeal membrane oxygenation may have successful outcomes despite circumstances that previously may have been considered relative contraindications, such as cardiac arrest, or systemic bacterial infections. The approach should still be viewed, nonetheless, as a short-term bridge to cardiac transplantation because of the time-related risks for complications, such as infection, bleeding, and impairment of end organs. Consequently, devices capable of providing assistance over a longer term are now replacing extracorporeal membrane oxygenation.

Ventricular assist devices, primarily developed for adults, have been used in adolescents and larger children,[35,42] and there is increasing experience with smaller devices[43] specifically designed for infants and children. As opposed to those receiving extracorporeal membrane oxygenation, patients supported with a ventricular assist device can usually be mobile and undergo physical and nutritional rehabilitation while awaiting transplantation. In a recent multi-centric review of outcomes, the median duration of support by ventricular assist device in children was 70 days,[35] with successful bridging in from two-thirds to four-fifths of patients.[35,42,43] As expected, results have improved with increasing experience (Fig. 16-17),[35] but serious morbidity, including stroke, bleeding, and malfunction of the devices remain common, occurring in one-third of cases. Survival is lowest in those of younger age, and in those with congenitally malformed hearts (Fig. 16-18).[35] The current devices require extracorporeal pumps and pumping consoles, making them rather cumbersome. There are several fully implantable devices in development with the aim of long-term support to bridge children to transplantation and/or recovery.[44]

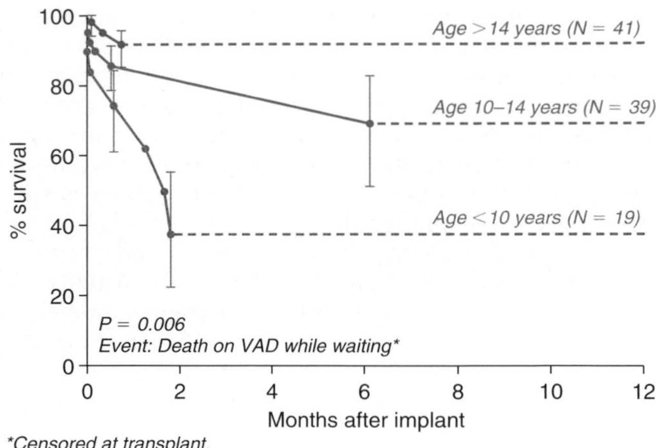

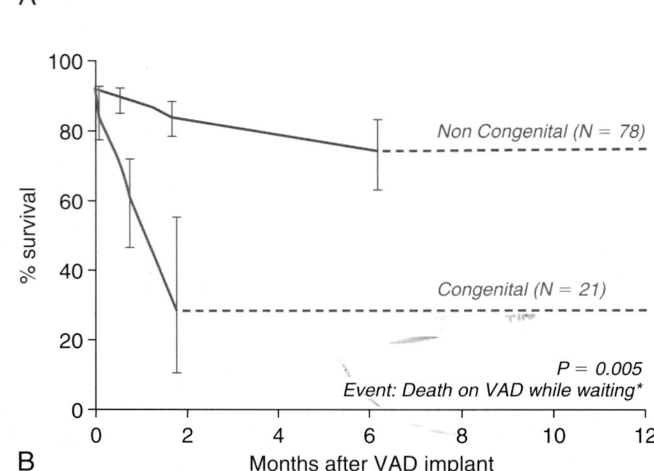

Figure 16-18 Survival to transplantation of patients after implantation of a ventricular assist device (VAD) stratified for (**A**) age at implantation and (**B**) congenital heart disease. Probability value is the unadjusted value. (From Blume ED, Naftel DC, Bastardi HJ, et al, for the PHTS Investigators: Outcomes of children bridged to heart transplant with ventricular assist devices: A multi-institutional study. Circulation 2006;113:2313–2319.)

Listing for Transplantation During Fetal Life

The improved accuracy of fetal echocardiography, and a better understanding of the natural history of cardiac disease diagnosed early in gestation, has allowed the possibility of listing for transplantation during pregnancy. Fetuses are listed, and delivered electively once a donor heart becomes available. The potential advantages of fetal listing include an

Figure 16-17 Competing outcomes analysis of cumulative proportion of patients with a ventricular assist device (VAD) who died or have received or are awaiting transplants. **A**, Early era (1993 to 1999; $N = 49$). **B**, Outcomes of the recent era (2000 to 2003; $N = 50$). The dotted line shows the percent of patients with each mutually exclusive end point at 6 months after implantation of the device. (From Blume ED, Naftel DC, Bastardi HJ, et al, for the PHTS Investigators: Outcomes of children bridged to heart transplant with ventricular assist devices: A multi-institutional study. Circulation 2006;113:2313–2319.)

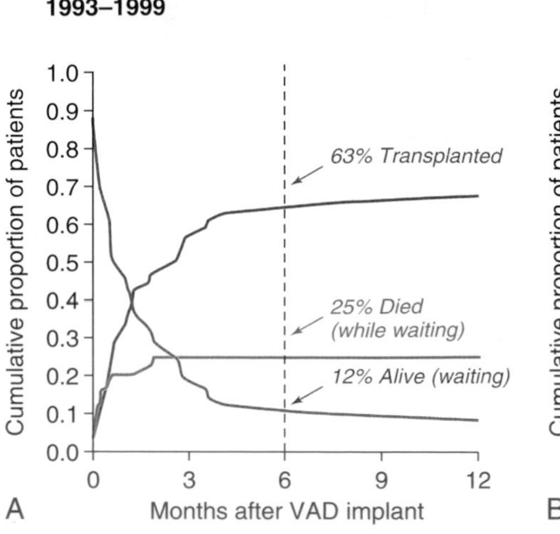

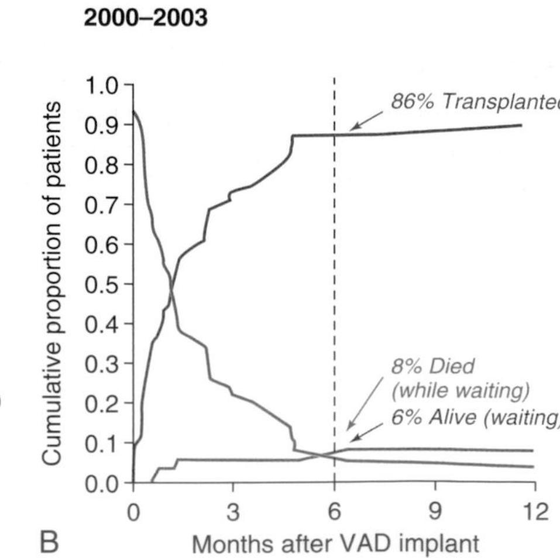

extended time to wait for a donor organ, a favourable stage of immunological maturation, and avoidance of prolonged intensive care support with all its potential complications and morbidities. Potential disadvantages include high pulmonary resistance, with potential right heart failure in the transplanted heart, uncertainty of additional extracardiac lesions and/or undiagnosed chromosomal abnormalities, and a potential risk to the mother of an expedient delivery. A cohort of 26 fetuses listed for transplantation in Toronto has been reported.[45] Diagnoses considered for antenatal listing included hypoplastic left heart syndrome, other combinations producing a functionally univentricular arrangement with risk factors for traditional surgical palliation such as severe atrioventricular valvar regurgitation or decreased ventricular function, unresectable cardiac tumours, isomerism of the right atrial appendages, and intractable arrhythmias. The prenatal assessment included a detailed fetal echocardiogram for diagnosis, a complete anatomical antenatal ultrasonic investigation for other anomalies, amniocentesis for chromosomal analysis, and testing of maternal blood for viral exposure and other infectious diseases. Listing was usually at or beyond 35 weeks of gestation, when the fetus was deemed to have reached an age of pulmonary maturity, and an estimated fetal weight of greater than 2.5 kg.

MANAGEMENT OF THE DONOR AND RECIPIENT

Considerations Relative to the Donor

The mechanism of death, resuscitation, and the type of support required have a significant bearing on the suitability of an organ for transplantation. There is accumulating knowledge on the effect of brain death on cardiac function and the best methods to support the circulation to preserve cardiac function for subsequent donation. The response to acute traumatic brain death can be a profound decrease in ventricular function, with the myocardium of the right ventricle more affected than that of the left.[46] There is potential for functional recovery and seemingly borderline organs can become acceptable for transplantation with appropriate support.[47-49] Therapy should be directed towards restoration of intravascular volume, and appropriate support of the myocardium and vascular system to ensure optimal cardiac output. Detailed discussion about the optimal management of the organ donor is published elsewhere,[50] but repeated echocardiography is essential to reassess suitability for donation.[51] Even so, studies in animals and humans provide evidence for a continued susceptibility to dysfunction in the acute post-operative period, despite apparent functional recovery.[46,52]

Much emphasis has been placed on the development of better cardioplegia and preservation solutions, and optimising temperature during transport after harvest of the donor heart. This is because an ischaemic time of more than 4 hours has been shown in multi-institutional studies to be a risk factor for poorer short- and long-term survival in adult recipients.[53] Interestingly, ischaemic times of more than 8 hours have been reported in children, without adversely affecting short- or long-term outcomes.[54,55]

Although rarely a consideration in adults, in children the donor heart must be appropriately matched in size to the recipient. Widely disparate ratios of weight between

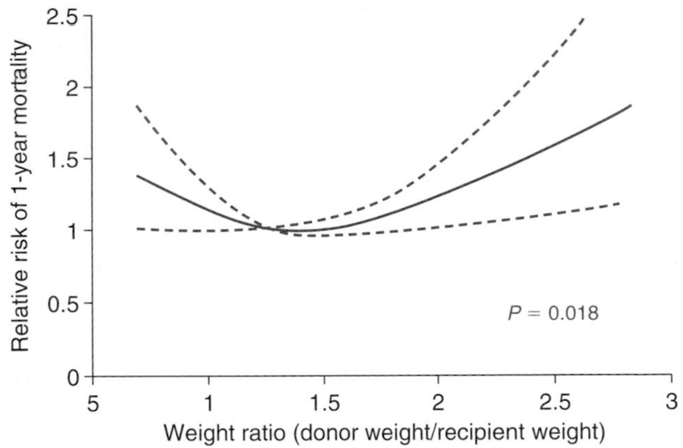

Figure 16-19 Ratio of the weight of the donor to the recipient as a risk factor for 1-year mortality. (From the registry of the International Society of Heart and Lung Transplantation. J Heart Lung Transplant 2007;26:796–807.)

donor and recipient, nonetheless, have been reported, with no adverse effect on outcome.[56,57] In another study, oversizing by greater than 2.5 times was associated with pulmonary collapse and delayed sternal closure.[58] A recent analysis of the database of the International Society for Heart Lung Transplantation database has shown a ratio of less than 0.5, or more than 2.5, to be associated with an increased risk for mortality within the first year (Fig. 16-19).[2]

Age of the donor over 40 years has also been shown to be a significant risk factor for mortality when the heart is transplanted to an adolescent,[59] with similar results produced from analysis of the registry of the International Society for Heart Lung Transplantation registry.[60] As a result, within the protocols of both the United Network of Organ Sharing and the Canadian organ allocation, hearts from adolescent donors are allocated preferentially to adolescent recipients.[13,61]

Surgical Techniques

The basic techniques for implantation of a cardiac allograft have not changed significantly since their original description.[62] In children, the size of the patient, the location of the heart, atrial arrangement, systemic venous anatomy, and pulmonary venous anatomy must all be taken into consideration when determining the surgical approach. In some complex forms of congenital cardiac disease, there may be a need to harvest portions of the right and left pulmonary arteries, aorta, inferior caval vein, or the brachiocephalic vein to facilitate the anastomoses within the recipient. These details should be planned during assessment prior to transplantation. The surgical challenges pertaining to transplantation for patients with complexly malformed hearts have recently been reviewed.[63]

Several retrospective studies have analysed outcomes related to the type of surgical approach. The bicaval approach has been reported to be associated with fewer tachyarrhythmias, slightly better haemodynamics, less tricuspid regurgitation, lower incidence of pacemaker support, and better exercise tolerance.[64,65] The biatrial technique has been associated with disturbances of conduction requiring placement of pacemakers in up to one-sixth,[66] a higher risk of thromboembolism, poor atrial synchrony, and more atrioventricular valvar regurgitation due to distortion

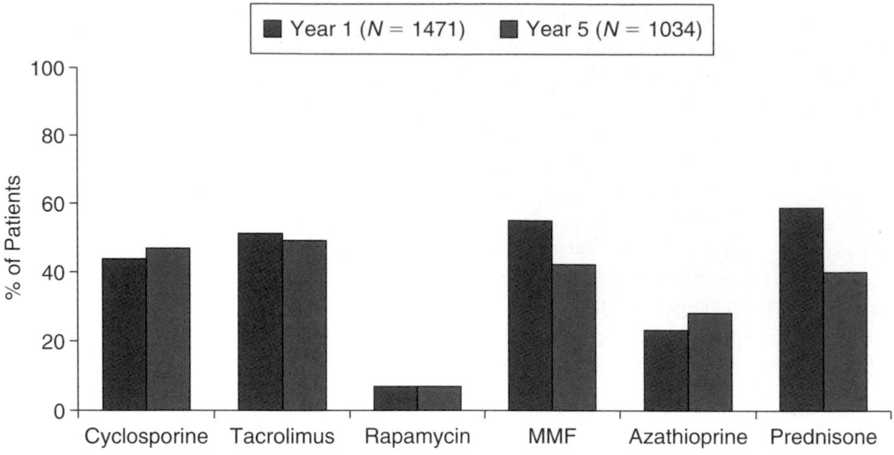

Figure 16-20 Summary of maintenance immunosuppression in children receiving transplanted hearts. MMF, mycophenolate mofetil. (From the registry of the International Society of Heart and Lung Transplantation. J Heart Lung Transplant 2007;26:796–807.)

of atrial anatomy.[67] Other studies have shown no differences,[68] or only differences in the incidence of atrial tachyarrhythmias.[69] The only randomised trial demonstrated that the bicaval technique resulted in better haemodynamics and survival.[70]

Management of the Recipient

There are several important postoperative issues that must be anticipated, and appropriately managed, in the recipient. The acutely denervated heart is frequently in slow sinus or junctional rhythm. Ventricular dysfunction as a result of ischaemia-reperfusion injury, compounded by brain death of the donor, can lead to acute decompensation of the transplanted heart, right ventricular failure being a specific concern. The latter is made more likely by elevated pulmonary vascular resistance, which commonly persists for days or weeks after transplantation. In general, strategies of post-operative management should be aimed at maintaining coronary arterial perfusion and systemic blood pressure by inotropic support, pulmonary vasodilators, chronotropy with either pacing or isoproterenol; optimising preload to the ischaemic and dilated right ventricle by limiting the circulating volume and central venous pressure, especially if there is systemic hypotension and/or low cardiac output previously unresponsive to fluid boluses; reducing the right ventricular afterload and pulmonary vascular resistance; ensuring an atrioventricular synchronous rhythm; optimizing ventilatory management to avoid hypercapnia and acidaemia by optimising peak early expiratory pressures and seeking early extubation; and providing early mechanical assistance to facilitate recovery of the transplanted hearts using extracorporeal membrane oxygenation, a ventricular assist device, or an intra-aortic balloon pump.

Specific Post-operative Complications

Stenosis can develop at the sites of the systemic venous anastomoses, the pulmonary arterial anastomoses, or the anastomosis of the reconstructed aorta. These may be amenable to interventional treatment, usually requiring implantation of stents. Less commonly, the size of the left atrial anastomosis may be a problem. If it is haemodynamically significant, and not recognised in the operating room at the time of the post-operative transoesophageal echocardiogram, it will likely cause haemodynamic instability in the immediate period subsequent to transplantation, and may require early reoperation.

IMMUNOSUPPRESSION

The goal of immunosuppressive therapy is to prevent rejection, whilst minimizing morbidities related to chronic immune suppression. There are a large number of centre specific protocols for maintenance immunosuppression, with ongoing controversy regarding the optimal regime (Figs. 16-20 and 16-21). Indeed, there are a myriad of agents, dosages, protocols, and combinations that have been used for both induction and maintenance of immunosuppression, making definitive comparisons and recommendations difficult.[2] A detailed discussion of the various protocols is beyond the scope of this chapter.

MONITORING AND SURVEILLANCE AFTER TRANSPLANTATION

The hallmark of care subsequent to transplantation is meticulous attention to detail, with a high index of suspicion for transplant-related problems. Care of children after cardiac transplantation must account for physical growth and development, the stage of immunological development, intellectual, emotional and social maturation, educational activities, and other parameters of quality of life for children. Each one of these aspects can significantly affect morbidity and mortality after transplantation.

Rejection

Rejection is the process of destruction of genetically foreign material by the immune system of the host. It varies in severity and timing between individuals, and may wax and wane within an individual patient. Although acute rejection remains an important cause of mortality and morbidity

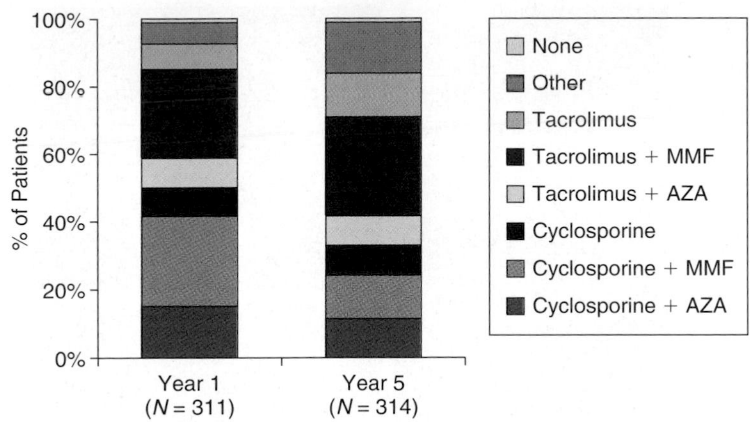

Figure 16-21 Summary of maintenance immunosuppression at 1 and 5 years after transplantation in children with transplanted hearts. AZA, azathioprine; MMF, mycophenolate mofetil. (From the registry of the International Society of Heart and Lung Transplantation. J Heart Lung Transplant 2007;26:796–807.)

after transplantation (see Table 16-3), its incidence has decreased as a result of improvements in perioperative immunosuppression. There are few identifiable risk factors for rejection prior to transplantation, other than sensitisation to HLA antigens. Pre-formed donor-specific anti-HLA antibodies can lead to humoral rejection within the first few hours after transplantation. Cellular rejection usually starts during the first few weeks, and is present to some degree in most patients. Rejection is most commonly mediated by T cells, though humoral rejection mediated by B-cell activation is increasing due to the larger number of patients sensitised to HLA antigens. There is increasing evidence for the role of both acute cellular rejection and antibody-mediated rejection on survival of the transplanted organ (Fig. 16-22)[2] and the development of vasculopathy.[71,72]

The gold standard for diagnosis of rejection remains the endomyocardial biopsy. Biopsies are graded according to the revised criterions of the International Society for Heart Lung Transplantation.[73] Grade 0 R indicates no rejection, and is unchanged from the criterions of 1990. Grade 1 R now represents mild rejection, and includes grades 1A, 1B, and 2 from 1990. Grade 2 R indicates moderate rejection, and is the same as grade 3A from the earlier system. Grade 3 R represents severe rejection, and incorporates grades 3B and 4 from the previous categorisation. There is a trend towards reducing the number of biopsies performed late after transplantation, with some centres discontinuing routine biopsies for surveillance of patients considered to be at low risk.[74,75] There have been many efforts to identify and validate non-invasive tests for diagnosing rejection, including echocardiography, intramyocardial electrography, and profiling of gene expression. As yet, no non-invasive test has been developed to consistently and accurately diagnose and/or predict rejection.[76]

The incidence of acute rejection peaks in the first month after transplantation, and then tapers off by 3 months (Fig. 16-23).[76] The early peak is delayed until the second month by the use of induction immunosuppression, but acute rejection still occurs. By 6 months after transplantation, three-fifths of patients have had at least one episode of acute cellular rejection.[2] The majority of recipients will have at least one further episode of rejection in the first year, but they are usually asymptomatic, and identified only by biopsy. These episodes are easily treated, and do not result in significant morbidity or mortality.

Of patients alive at 1 year, one-quarter will experience another episode of rejection within 3 years.[23] Mortality

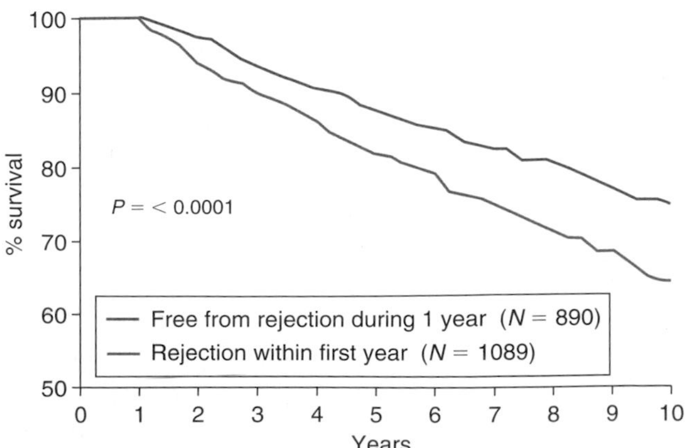

Figure 16-22 Kaplan-Meier survival in children with transplanted hearts based on the presence of rejection within the first year after transplantation. (From the registry of the International Society of Heart and Lung Transplantation. J Heart Lung Transplant 2007;26:796–807.)

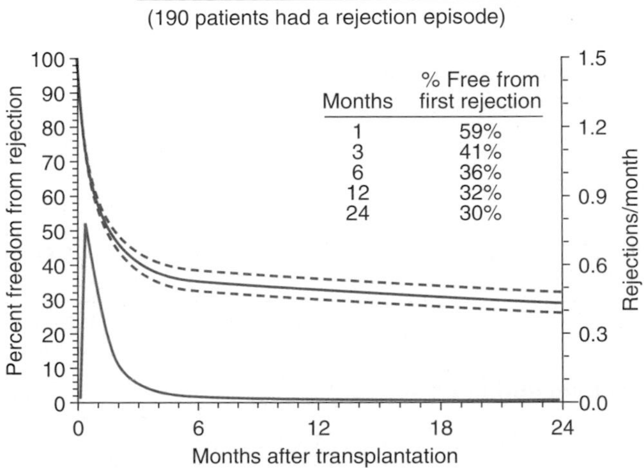

Figure 16-23 Freedom from first acute episode of rejection shown as a hazard function curve. (From Dodd DA, Cabo J, Dipchand AI: Acute rejection: Natural history, risk factors, surveillance, and treatment. In Canter CE, Kirklin JK: Pediatric Heart Transplantation. ISHLT Monograph Series, vol. 2. Elsevier, 2007, Chap. 9. Fig. 3, p. 143.)

among patients suffering late rejection is significantly higher than in those without such rejection.[77-79] Episodes of late rejection are also more often associated with haemodynamic compromise requiring inotropic support, and represent antibody-mediated rejection. Rejection with haemodynamic compromise is associated with a higher incidence of failure of the graft and mortality, with only half of patients alive at 1 year after such an episode.[23,79] Rejection often recurs, with only one-third of patients suffering one episode remaining free of subsequent episodes at 5 years following the event.[79]

Risk factors for rejection, late rejection, rejection with haemodynamic compromise, and recurrent rejection include older recipient age, black or Hispanic race, more frequent early rejection, more than one episode in the first year after transplantation, and shorter time since a previous episode.[23,77,80] More recently, interest has been focused on genetic polymorphisms affecting production of tumour necrosis factor-α and interleukin-10 and risk of rejection.[81]

Treatment of rejection depends on many factors, including the type, grade, time after transplantation, clinical and haemodynamic effect, and baseline immunosuppression. There is general agreement that mild rejection does not require specific intervention. Moderate rejection usually requires some degree of intensification of immunosuppression, which generally includes an oral or intravenous bolus of corticosteroid, and an increase in regular therapies. Any rejection with haemodynamic compromise requires haemodynamic support commensurate with the clinical presentation, and aggressive intensification of immunosuppression.

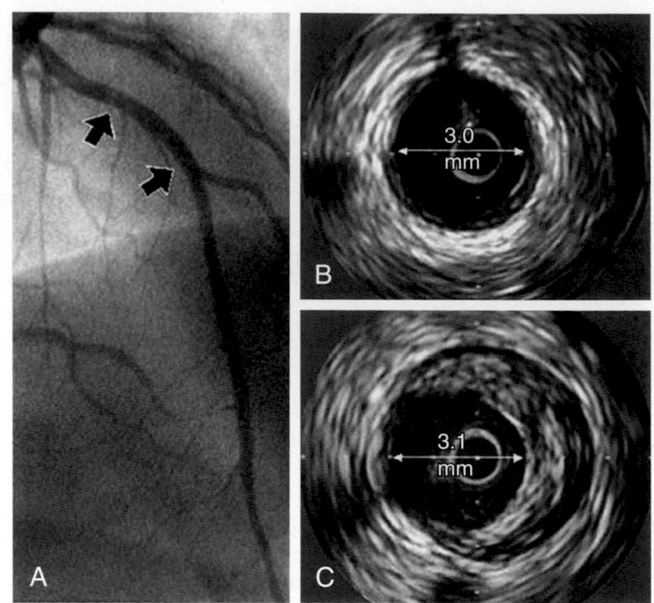

Figure 16-24 Graft vasculopathy. **A**, Coronary angiography (single plane) demonstrating a smooth calibre regular lumen (*arrows*). **B** and **C**, Intravascular ultrasound of the same vessel at the sites indicated by the black arrows. Despite the normal appearing angiogram, note the difference in intimal thickening reflecting the presence of moderate graft vasculopathy as seen by ultrasound.

Allograft Vasculopathy

Risk Factors and Diagnosis

Allograft vasculopathy is a diffuse, chronic vascular injury to the graft. Ultimately, ischaemia results from circumferential thickening of the vascular intima with stenosis or occlusion (Fig. 16-24). Classical clinical signs associated with coronary arterial disease are rare in recipients of transplanted hearts. Since the transplanted heart is denervated, they may not experience characteristic chest pain, even in the face of significant myocardial ischaemia. Consequently, the first clinical manifestations may be symptoms of advanced disease, including congestive cardiac failure, syncope, ventricular arrhythmias, and death. Transplant vasculopathy is a leading cause of death beyond 3 years after transplantation (see Table 16-4).

The pathogenesis of the vasculopathy is multi-factorial, but includes both immune and non-immune components. Commonly, there is donor-specific cell-mediated alloreactivity to vascular endothelium,[82] which appears to be promoted by a number of cytokines and growth factors.[83] There is probably some relationship between number of acute cellular rejection episodes and the risk of vasculopathy (Table 16-6).[2,84,85] Non-immune associations include infections with cytomegalovirus,[86-88] hypercholesterolemia,[89] smoking,[84,85] hypertension,[85] elevated homocysteine,[90,91] and cumulative doses of prednisone.[92]

The risk factors for vasculopathy in children are outlined in Table 16-7.[93] After the first year, allograft vasculopathy is the commonest cause of morbidity and mortality.[2] Figure 16-25 illustrates freedom from this complication for the first 9 years after transplantation, with the same data stratified by age shown in Figure 16-26. This is highly dependent on the aggressiveness of screening. Coronary angiography remains the gold standard, but it tends to underestimate the vasculopathy compared with

TABLE 16-6

RELATIONSHIP BETWEEN REJECTION AND ALLOGRAFT VASCULOPATHY (AV) IN CHILDREN WITH A TRANSPLANTED HEART

	REPORTED AV BETWEEN FIRST AND THIRD YEARS POST-TRANSPLANT			REPORTED AV BETWEEN THIRD AND FIFTH YEARS POST-TRANSPLANT		
Rejection during 1st Year	Yes	No	All	Yes	No	All
Yes	44 7.7%	529 92.3%	573 100%	23 7.7%	275 92.3%	298 100%
No	18 3.0%	588 97.0%	606 100%	15 4.8%	300 95.2%	315 100%

Data from the registry of the International Society of Heart and Lung Transplantation. J Heart Lung Transplant 2007;26:796–807.

TABLE 16-7

COMBINED DONOR/RECIPIENT RISK FACTORS FOR ALLOGRAFT VASCULOPATHY IN CHILDREN

Risk Factor	Single-centre Study	Multi-centre Study or Registry	Diagnostic Tools*
Older recipient age	Yes	Yes	Angio, IVUS
Older donor age	Yes	Yes	Angio
Acute rejection in first year after heart transplant	Yes	Yes	Angio
High acute rejection frequency rate	Yes		Angio, IVUS
Lower immunosuppression (double vs. triple)	Yes		Angio
Late (>1 yr) acute rejection with hemodynamic compromise	Yes		Angio, IVUS
Earlier year of heart transplant	Yes		Angio
Late (>1 yr) acute rejection	Yes		Angio, IVUS
Cytomegalovirus infection	Yes		IVUS
No pravastatin therapy	Yes		Angio
Viral genome by polymerase chain reaction	Yes		Angio or autopsy

Angio, angiography; IVUS, intravascular ultrasound.
From Pahl E, Caforio ALP, Kuhn MA: Allograft vasculopathy: Detection, risk factors, natural history and treatment. In Canter CE, Kirklin JK: Pediatric Heart Transplantation. ISHLT Monograph Series, vol. 2. Philadelphia, Elsevier, 2007, Table 4, p 179.

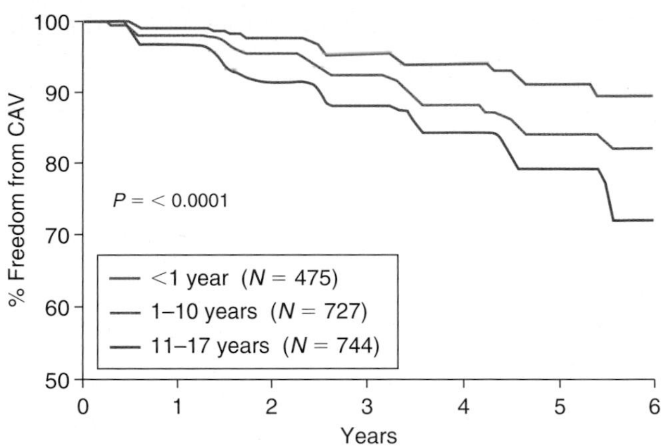

Figure 16-26 Freedom from cardiac allograft vasculopathy (CAV) in children with transplanted hearts stratified by age group. (From the registry of the International Society of Heart and Lung Transplantation. J Heart Lung Transplant 2007;26:796–807.)

pathological examination or intravascular ultrasound (see Fig. 16-24).[94,95] In addition, angiography provides minimal information on the impact of allograft vasculopathy on cardiac function. Once allograft vasculopathy is evident angiographically, short-term mortality is high (Fig. 16-27).[94,95] Supportive evidence for the presence of ischaemia may be obtained by exercise testing and nuclear medicine scintigraphy, but the application of these testing modalities is limited to older, cooperative patients and abnormalities may only be apparent at a relatively advanced stage of disease.[96]

The use of dobutamine stress echocardiography has been advocated in adult recipients for routine surveillance for allograft vasculopathy,[97] in some centres even replacing routine angiography. Several studies in adults have shown a relationship between an abnormal test and events related to allograft vasculopathy.[94,95,97] Preliminary studies in children have supported the feasibility and safety of such testing, in addition to providing preliminary evidence for a role in identifying children with allograft vasculopathy.[98–101]

Because of the limitations of angiography, intravascular ultrasound has been proposed as a better means of

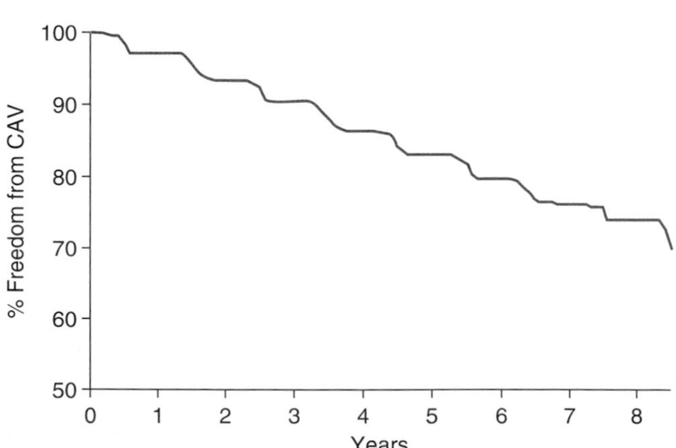

Figure 16-25 Freedom from cardiac allograft vasculopathy (CAV) in children with transplanted hearts. (From the registry of the International Society of Heart and Lung Transplantation. J Heart Lung Transplant 2007;26:796–807.)

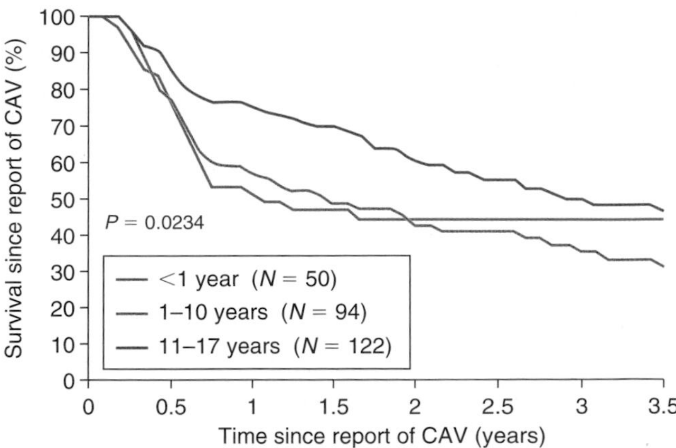

Figure 16-27 Kaplan-Meier survival following diagnosis of cardiac allograft vasculopathy (CAV) in children with transplanted hearts stratified by age group. (From the registry of the International Society of Heart and Lung Transplantation. J Heart Lung Transplant 2007;26:796–807.)

identification and study of progression of epicardial coronary arterial disease (see Fig. 16-24). The early enthusiasm has been tempered by technical issues, cost, and lack of meaningful end-points for management and/or prognosis. Its use is presently limited to older children due to the size of the available catheters.

Management

Lipid-lowering therapy, using statins, has been shown to play a role in the prevention of allograft vasculopathy. In adults, pravastatin has been shown to reduce the incidence of acute rejections associated with haemodynamic compromise, improve survival at 1 year, and reduce the development of vasculopathy.[102] This was independent of the level of cholesterol, suggesting the effect of statins extends beyond manipulation of lipids. Similar findings have been reported with simvastatin.[103] There is limited data in children, but two studies have shown a lower incidence of vasculopathy during treatment with simvastatin[104] or atorvastatin.[105] There is accumulating data in adults on the potential role of different immunosuppressant agents on the development of intimal thickening, including mycophenolate mofetil, sirolimus, and everolimus, but these are short-term studies, and do not include children.[93]

Treatment of established allograft vasculopathy is challenging, especially in children. In adults, percutaneous transluminal angioplasty and/or stenting of discrete lesions has been successfully performed.[1] The majority of patients are not amenable to these techniques due to the diffuse nature of the disease. Similarly, coronary arterial bypass grafting has also been successfully performed, but has a very limited role.[1] There are only two reports of interventions in a small number of children, making definitive recommendations impossible.[106,107] Ultimately, patients with moderate-to-severe vasculopathy and evidence of graft dysfunction may be candidates for retransplantation.

Retransplantation

The assessment of need for retransplantation is an important element of management of children undergoing their first transplantation. There has been an increasing number of retransplantations in North America over the last few years (Fig. 16-28; see also Figs. 16-4 to 16-6), with most performed more than 5 years following the initial procedure (Fig. 16-29). Review of the database of the United Network for Organ Sharing for the period between 1987 and 2004 revealed 19 children who underwent retransplantation (Table 16-8).[108]

Overall survival following retransplantation approaches that of primary transplantation, when retransplantation occurs later than 1 year after primary transplantation (Fig. 16-30). Retransplantation for early failure or acute rejection, the usual causes of death in the first year, carries a high mortality. For patients transplanted within 1 year of their first transplantation, the 1 year actuarial survival is 60%, compared to almost 90% for those retransplanted later than 3 years.

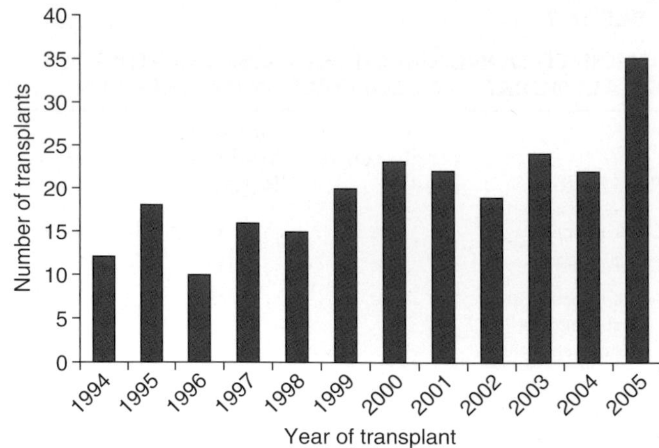

Figure 16-28 Retransplantation in children with transplanted hearts by year. (From the registry of the International Society of Heart and Lung Transplantation. J Heart Lung Transplant 2007;26:796–807.)

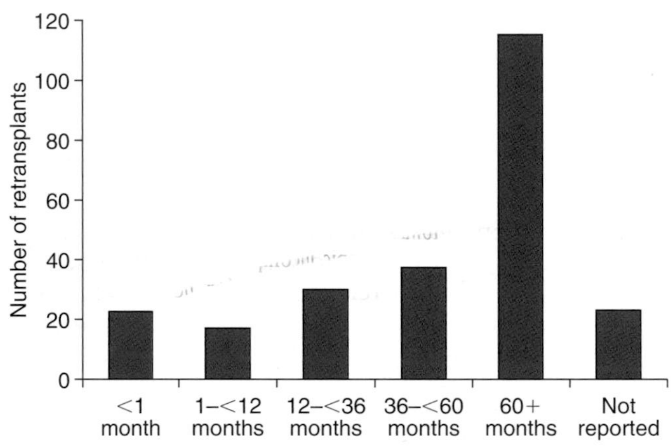

Figure 16-29 Retransplantation in children with transplanted hearts by intertransplant interval. (From the registry of the International Society of Heart and Lung Transplantation. J Heart Lung Transplant 2007;26:796–807.)

TABLE 16-8

INDICATIONS FOR RETRANSPLANTATION

	N = 219 (%)
Allograft vasculopathy	111 (51%)
Nonspecific graft failure	34 (16%)
Acute rejection	19 (9%)
Chronic rejection	16 (7%)
Primary failure	10 (5%)
Hyperacute rejection	7 (3%)
Other	22 (10%)

From Mahle WT, Vincent RN, Kanter KR: Cardiac retransplantation in childhood: Analysis of data from the United Network for Organ Sharing. J Thorac Cardiovasc Surg 2005;130:542–546.

Exercise and Aerobic Capacity

Exercise restriction is not usually necessary after transplantation. Indeed, a benefit was found when comparing a regimented monitored programme for cardiac rehabilitation and exercise in a large randomised study of adults.[97] Structured cardiac rehabilitation has also been useful for adolescents. For younger patients, and those teenagers who cannot participate in such a programme, we recommend 30 minutes of aerobic exercise three to four times a week. Children can generally return to routine exercise once their incisions have healed, this generally being after 6 to 8 weeks.

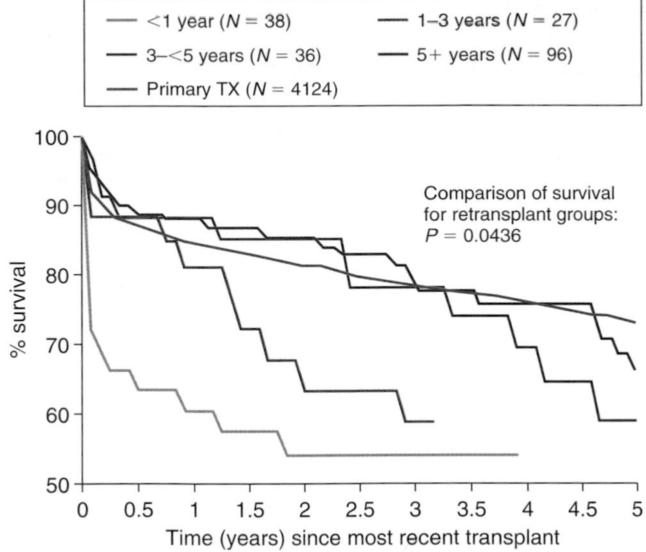

Figure 16-30 Kaplan-Meier survival for retransplantation in children with transplanted hearts by intertransplant interval. (From the registry of the International Society of Heart and Lung Transplantation. J Heart Lung Transplant 2007;26:796–807.)

Following transplantation, physiological responses to exercise may be impaired. This is related to several factors, including age at transplantation,[109] deconditioning prior to transplantation, growth of the allograft,[110,111] degree of reinnervation,[112–115] chronotropic incompetence,[116–118] comorbidities such as renal dysfunction, respiratory abnormalities, and so on, and the effects of medication such as corticosteroids and cyclosporine on skeletal muscular function. Studies examining exercise performance in children have demonstrated a blunted response of heart rate to graded exercise, and decreased maximal consumption of oxygen,[117,119,120] albeit that one group of children has been identified with heart rate responses faster and greater.[118] Despite near normalisation of rate responses in this group, maximal consumption of oxygen remained submaximal. There are a few studies demonstrating a more normal rate response and a low normal maximal consumption of oxygen.[109,121]

The largest and most recent series of serial exercise tests in children demonstrated better exercise capacity associated with younger age at transplantation, especially for infants, a positive relationship between peak heart rate and time subsequent to transplantation, good exercise capacity with a mean maximum consumption of oxygen of 30 mL/kg/min at a mean of 5.5 years after transplantation, which is but mildly reduced compared to the normal population, and a possible association with changes on serial studies and the presence of allograft vasculopathy.[96]

Infections

Analysis of the data collected by the Pediatric Heart Transplant Study showed reported infections to occur in two-fifths of patients during a period of 2 years.[122] Such infections are an important cause of morbidity and mortality after transplantation. A report from the International Society of Heart Lung Transplantation identified infection as the second commonest cause of death within the first year after transplantation (see Table 16-4).[2] Several factors determine the risk of infection (Fig. 16-31).[123] Certain infections may become reactivated following introduction of immunosuppression. Serological testing prior to transplantation helps identify the possibility, and routine surveillance can sometimes guide prophylactic or pre-emptive treatment. Not all infections are amenable to prophylactic treatment, and under those circumstances reactivation of disease may also require specific treatment. Of special mention is the impact of Epstein-Barr virus in seronegative recipients. Prophylaxis is controversial, and surveillance should include regular testing for active viral replication by polymerase chain reaction techniques. Conversion to seropositivity for Epstein-Barr virus requires consideration of anti-viral therapy, especially in the first 6 months after transplantation. Patients with a chronic viral load should be regularly investigated for the development of lymphoproliferative disorder.

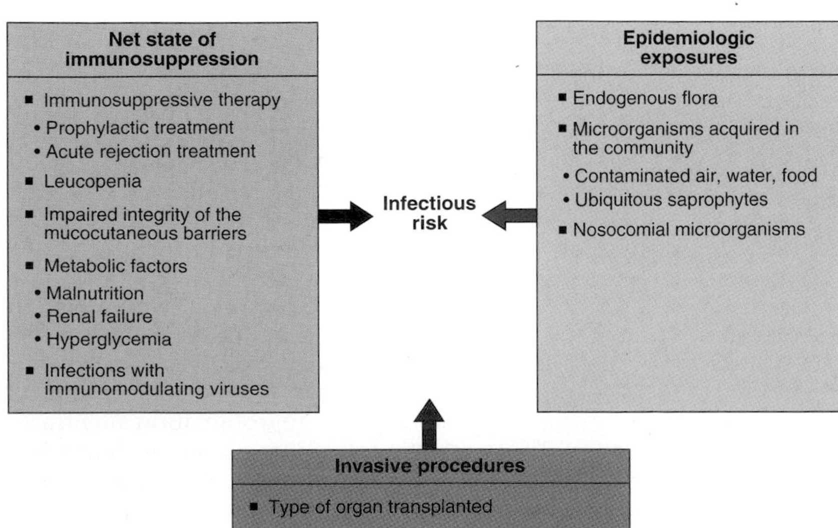

Figure 16-31 Factors that determine the risk of infection in children with transplanted hearts. (From Renoult E, Buteau C, Lamarre V, et al: Infectious risk in pediatric organ transplant recipients: Is it increased with the new immunosuppressive agents? Pediatr Transplant 2005;9:470–479.)

Most children undergoing transplantation have not finished their routine schedule of immunisations. Titres should be checked prior to transplantation. Efforts should be made to immunise with as many vaccinations as is feasible and developmentally appropriate prior to transplantation. This is particularly important with vaccines that incorporate live viruses. Vaccination schedules should be resumed approximately 6 months after transplantation. Given the suppression of the immune system and the variable responses to foreign antigen, antibody titres should be checked after vaccination in order to ensure an appropriate response. In general, live viral vaccines are avoided.

Renal Function

There is increasing awareness of the adverse effects of renal dysfunction on outcomes after transplantation. There are many causes for the gradual decline that is common in these patients. In addition to the preoperative compromise that results from low cardiac output, chronic diuretic therapy, or mechanical support, there is often an acute perioperative decline reflecting the ischaemia/reperfusion injury following cardiopulmonary bypass and the use of multiple nephrotoxic drugs. In the long term, the cumulative use of calcineurin inhibitors leads to structural changes at all levels of the kidney. This is characterised by glomerulosclerosis, tubular atrophy, interstitial fibrosis, and afferent arteriopathy.[124–127] In a comparison of inhibitors of calcineurin inhibitors, no difference was observed in the decline of calculated clearance of creatinine when tacrolimus was compared with cyclosporine.[128]

The reported incidence of renal insufficiency varies depending on the definition used and the method used for assessment.[126] In most cross sectional reviews, no more than 1% or 2% of patients have progressed to end-stage renal failure requiring dialysis and/or renal transplantation.[128] Another study showed the percentage of patients with a normal rate of glomerular filtration to be 78% at the time of transplantation, reducing to 45%, 29%, and 14% at 1, 2, and 5 years after transplantation.[127] Analysis of the database of the International Society of Heart Lung Transplantation shows the incidence of renal dysfunction to be 6.0% at 1 year, and 9.3% at 5 years (Tables 16-9 and 16-10).[2]

Close follow-up of renal function is clearly required. Clearance of creatinine may be estimated from the levels in the serum and the height of the patient, albeit that such calculated values consistently overestimate the measured rate of glomerular filtration.[126,128] Strategies to improve renal function should be directed towards reducing or eliminating exposure to nephrotoxic agents, including the inhibitors of calcineurin. Partial improvement in renal function may occur after the dose of such inhibitors is reduced, even after years of use. This reversible component of renal dysfunction is secondary to persistent afferent arteriolar constriction and decreased renal blood flow. Recently, the use of immunosuppression using sirolimus as a calcineurin sparing agent has shown some benefit in patients with moderate renal dysfunction.[129]

TABLE 16-9

PREVALENCE OF MORBIDITIES AFTER TRANSPLANTATION IN SURVIVORS AT 1 YEAR AFTER TRANSPLANTATION

Outcome	Within 1 Year	Total Number with Known Response
Hypertension	46.7%	(*N* = 2704)
Renal dysfunction	6.0%	(*N* = 2710)
Abnormal creatinine < 2.5 mg/dL	4.0%	
Creatinine > 2.5 mg/dL	1.2%	
Chronic dialysis	0.8%	
Renal transplant	0.0%	
Hyperlipidemia	11.1%	(*N* = 2838)
Diabetes	3.5%	(*N* = 2716)
Coronary artery vasculopathy	2.5%	(*N* = 2495)

Data from the registry of the International Society of Heart and Lung Transplantation. J Heart Lung Transplant 2007;26:796–807.

TABLE 16-10

PREVALENCE OF MORBIDITIES IN SURVIVORS 5 YEARS AFTER HEART TRANSPLANTATION

Outcome	Within 5 Years	Total Number with Known Response
Hypertension	63.2%	(*N* = 980)
Renal dysfunction	9.3%	(*N* = 1021)
Abnormal creatinine < 2.5 mg/dL	7.5%	
Creatinine > 2.5 mg/dL	1.0%	
Chronic dialysis	0.6%	
Renal transplant	0.2%	
Hyperlipidemia	25.6%	(*N* = 1062)
Diabetes	5.0%	(*N* = 981)
Coronary artery vasculopathy	10.9%	(*N* = 724)

Data from the registry of the International Society of Heart and Lung Transplantation. J Heart Lung Transplant 2007;26:796–807.

Lymphoproliferative Disorders

Malignancies are another important cause of morbidity and mortality after transplantation. They can occur as new events, be a reactivation of previous cancer, or result from chronic viral infections, with the latter being most important in children. The cumulative prevalence in survivors is 2% at 1 year, 5% at 5 years, and 7% at 10 years (Fig. 16-32 and Table 16-11).[2] The reported overall incidence of such disorders as analysed in the database of the Pediatric Heart Transplant Society was 5%.[130] Survival in those with the disorder was 95% at 1 month, 75% at 1 year, and 67% at 5 years.[130] There may also be a temporal relationship to incidence, Ross et al reporting a 23% incidence in survivors more than 10 years after transplantation.[131]

The lymphoproliferative disorders include all clinical syndromes associated with lymphoproliferation after transplantation. The spectrum ranges from a mononucleosis-like illness to life-threatening malignancies with clonal chromosomal abnormalities. Epstein-Barr virus plays a major role in their development, with the highest risk for development being a primary infection with the virus. As noted above, given their naivety to Epstein-Barr virus, primary infection, and consequently occurrence of the disorders, is

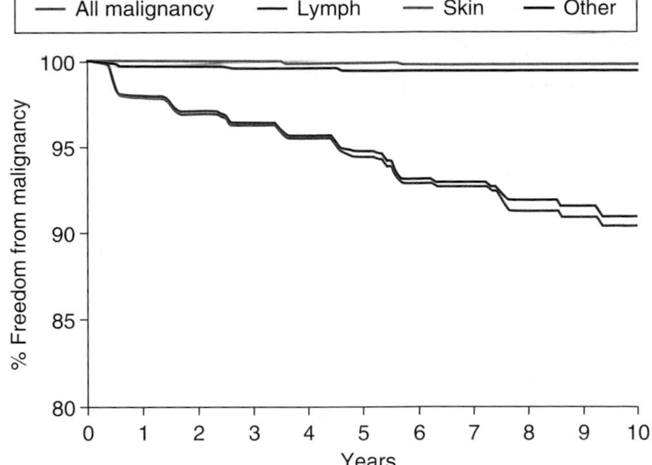

Figure 16-32 Freedom from malignancy. (From the registry of the International Society of Heart and Lung Transplantation. J Heart Lung Transplant 2007;26:796–807.)

TABLE 16-11

CUMULATIVE PREVALENCE OF MALIGNANCY IN SURVIVORS OF HEART TRANSPLANTATION

Malignancy/Type	1-Year Survivors	5-Year Survivors	10-Year Survivors
No malignancy	2771 (98.1%)	1010 (95%)	186 (93%)
Malignancy (all types combined)	55 (1.9%)	53 (5%)	14 (7%)
Malignancy type			
Lymph	51	48	13
Other	3	6	
Skin		1	
Type not reported	1		1

Data from the registry of the International Society of Heart and Lung Transplantation. J Heart Lung Transplant 2007;26:796–807.

more common in children. The risk is also clearly related to the viral load.[132]

There are no controlled clinical trials comparing interventions or therapies for these disorders. Treatments include reduction in immunosuppression, anti-viral medication, immunoglobulin therapy, monoclonal antibodies such as rituximab,[133,134] chemotherapy, tumour debulking, radiation therapy, and rarely, bone marrow transplantation.

Growth

Retarded growth is frequent in children after cardiac transplantation. In the population followed by the Pediatric Heart Transplant Society, the rate of growth fell between the time of listing and the time of transplantation. Catch-up linear growth occurred during the first year, but patients remained shorter than their age-matched peers at 6 years after transplantation. Children transplanted for reasons other than a congenital cardiac disease maintained steady linear growth after transplantation, but also failed to achieve normal height. Patients with a diagnosis of hypoplastic left heart syndrome, or those at a younger age at transplantation, showed less catch-up growth.[135]

Development

Formal assessment of infant development has been carried out in a large cohort of babies transplanted by the group in Loma Linda.[136–139] Overall, their mean developmental scores, for both mental and psychomotor indexes, fell within normal limits, though they tended to be at the lower end of normal. Reports beyond infancy demonstrate a range of variation in a spectrum of developmental parameters compared to a normal population, with overall cognitive scores at the lower limit of normal.[13,140–143] Focused studies of patients born with hypoplastic left heart syndrome all demonstrate lower scores on the scales for infant development and intelligence compared with the general population, but similar to patients undergoing the Norwood sequence of palliative procedures.[144,145]

Quality of Life, Psychosocial Issues, and Non-adherence

While most children and families report a good quality of life,[146] psychosocial and adverse functioning has been reported.[141,142,147–151] A longitudinal study of children after transplantation of either the heart or the heart and lungs showed academic cognitive functioning to be in the normal range, and not to change as a function of time from transplantation.[141] Performance at school, nonetheless, was significantly poorer than that of healthy children, and the prevalence of behavioural problems rose significantly. Similar results were reported in another longitudinal study, which followed children for more than 10 years, with psychological functioning outside the normal range in one-quarter of patients.[149] In this latter cohort, there was significant improvement in emotional functioning compared to findings prior to transplantation, and the severity of the medical disability before transplantation was not correlated to subsequent psychologic function.[148] These results concur with other studies in which the severity of illness is less important to adaptation than other factors. Illness-related stress, and symptoms of post-traumatic stress, are significant problems affecting parents of children undergoing transplantation, with nearly two-fifths of one cohort of parents declaring moderately severe to severe symptoms of post-traumatic stress.[151] Pre- and post-operative psychological assessment, and support of the patient and his or her family, is clearly an important role of any centre involved in cardiac transplantation.

Non-adherence to complicated and life-sustaining therapy is less well studied. The complex psychological issues described above, combined with normal adolescent development after cardiac transplantation, render a large population of recipients at risk of rebellious or risk-taking non-adherence.[152–153] Non-adherence has been linked to late rejection,[154] and to high rates of death in adolescents.[155] It has been suggested that high variability in trough levels of medications, with both high and low levels presumably reflecting variable adherence, was a sensitive marker for children at greater risk for recurrent rejection and hospitalisation after transplantation.[156] A coordinated effort between paediatricians, the transplant team, the

TABLE 16-12

INCIDENCE OF HYPERTENSION IN CHILDREN WITH A TRANSPLANTED HEART

Maintenance Immunosuppression at Discharge and 1 Year	HYPERTENSION (%) REPORTED BETWEEN 3 AND 8 YEARS		
	For Patients on Drug	For Patients Not on Drug	*P* Value
Azathioprine	37.0	42.3	0.6119
Cyclosporine	34.7	41.7	0.5062
MMF	38.5	37.4	0.9407
Prednisone	47.8	19.1	0.0002
Rapamycin	—	35.8	—
Tacrolimus	38.9	33.1	0.6234

MMF, mycophenolate mofetil.
Data from the registry of the International Society of Heart and Lung Transplantation. J Heart Lung Transplant 2007;26:796–807.

patient, and family must be in place to help identify those recipients at risk, particularly at the time of transition from paediatric to adult-based care.

Other Complications

Hypertension has been noted in almost half of recipients at 1 year, with this proportion increasing to two-thirds at 5 years, and almost three-quarters at 10 years after transplantation[2] (Table 16-12). Abnormalities of lipids and lipoproteins are more prevalent in children after cardiac transplantation compared to their age-matched controls.[80,157] These abnormalities are related to immunosuppressant agents such as cyclosporine, corticosteroids, and sirolimus; obesity, which is often steroid-induced; and diabetes, the latter also associated with steroids and tacrolimus. Small single-centre studies have demonstrated the safety and efficacy of treatment of children with statins after transplantation,[105,158] and some have suggested a lower incidence of allograft vasculopathy in patients treated in this fashion.[108] Other complications include hypomagnesaemia and cosmetic side effects, such as hirsutism, gingival hyperplasia, acne, and loss of hair.

TRANSPLANTATION OF THE HEART AND LUNGS

Transplantation of the heart together with the lungs has limited application in children, with this procedure peaking in the late 1980s, with 40 procedures, and reaching a nadir in 2002, with 9 procedures, according to the registry of the International Society of Heart and Lung Transplantation.[157] It is indicated for severe pulmonary vascular disease or pulmonary vascular issues when the cardiac lesions are not amenable to conventional surgery. It has also been used in end-stage lung disease with concurrent left ventricular dysfunction felt to be irreversible in nature. Most right ventricular failure in association with pulmonary vascular disease is amenable to bilateral transplantation of the lungs. Post-operative transplant-related morbidities are similar to those for isolated transplantation of the heart and the lungs, with the issues relating to transplantation of the lungs predominating, and generally guiding the clinical course and plans for treatment. Risk factors for mortality include ventilation at transplant, infection, and obliterative bronchiolitis. Long-term outcomes are well below those for transplantation of the heart, and have shown no improvement over the last decade, with a 5-year survival of less than 50%.

FUTURE DIRECTIONS

Overall, the survival for children undergoing transplantation of the heart has improved remarkably during the past 20 years, and the functional state of most patients remains good for many years following surgery. Despite this, there is a continuing risk of major late morbidity. Development of new immunosuppressant agents that decrease the morbidity for children following transplantation will be crucial to modify these late adverse outcomes. Mortality whilst waiting for transplantation remains unacceptably high. Improved management of cardiac failure, and improved technology more effectively to bridge these young patients to transplantation, will help reduce these deaths occurring during the period of waiting, but ultimately societal change will be required to widen the pool of available donors. The holy grail remains the induction of complete immune tolerance of the recipient to the implanted organ.

The complete reference list can be found on the companion Expert Consult web site at www.expertconsult.com.

ANNOTATED REFERENCES

- Boucek MM, Aurora P, Edwards L, et al: Registry of the International Society for Heart and Lung Transplantation: Tenth Official Pediatric Heart Transplantation Report—2007. J Heart Lung Transplant 2007;26:796–807.

  An excellent resource for a summary of overall statistics on a large cohort of children undergoing transplantation, including survival, deaths, immunosuppression, and morbidities.

- Blume ED, Naftel DC, Bastardi HJ, et al, for the PHTS Investigators: Outcomes of children bridged to heart transplant with ventricular assist devices: A multi-institutional study. Circulation 2006;113:2313–2319.

  This article reports the largest series of children bridged to transplantation with mechanical support.

- Canter CE, Kirklin JK: Pediatric Heart Transplantation. ISHLT Monograph Series, vol. 2. Philadelphia, Elsevier, 2007. Information available at: www.ishlt.org.

  This monograph published in 2007 is the most up-to-date and comprehensive summary of all topics relevant to cardiac transplantation in children. Each chapter is written by leaders in the field.

- Canter CE, Shaddy RE, Bernstein D, et al: Indications for heart transplantation in pediatric heart disease. Circulation 2007;115:658–676.

This scientific statement produced on behalf of the American Heart Association reviews and summarises accumulated experience with cardiac transplantation in children, and its use in unrepaired and/or repaired/palliated congenital cardiac disease, cardiomyopathies and previous transplantation, with the purpose of developing and reporting evidence-based guidelines for the indications for transplantation.

- Shemie SD, Ross H, Pagliarello J, et al, on behalf of the Pediatric Recommendations Group: Organ management in Canada: Recommendations of the Forum on Medical Management to Optimize Donor Organ Potential. Can Med Assoc J 2006:174:S13–S30.

  This report summarises the literature on the pathophysiology of brain death and effect on organ function. Best practice and evidence-based guidelines for donor resuscitation, support, and assessment are provided to maximise organ function and suitability for transplantation.

- Stewart S, Winters GL, Fishbein MC, et al: Revision of the 1990 working formulation for the standardisation of nomenclature in the diagnosis of heart rejection. J Heart Lung Transplant 2005;24:1710–1720.

  This article summarises the revised consensus for classification of cardiac allograft rejection. Recommendations are also made for the histological recognition and immunohistological investigation of acute antibody-mediated rejection.

CHAPTER 17

Interventional Techniques

SACHIN KHAMBADKONE and PHILIPP BONHOEFFER

Interventional cardiac catheterisation describes procedures where cardiac catheters are used to modify, palliate, or treat congenital or acquired cardiac disease. Evolution of interventional techniques has been a natural progression from surgical procedures used to treat such lesions. The development of newer interventional techniques has largely been possible by pushing the boundaries of established interventional procedures in order to achieve results comparable with surgical techniques. Although the aim is to do something to alter the course of disease the basics of interventional catheterisation are drawn from experience with diagnostic cardiac catheterisation. Not all interventional catheterisation techniques are therapeutic. Some do no more than modify the course of the disease, or help delay future interventional or surgical procedures. The design and organisation of the catheterisation laboratory, personnel, use of equipment, catheters and techniques are a progression of the exercise of gathering of information related to diagnostic catheterisation and angiography. In sick neonates, infants, and children, however, any catheterisation is an intervention, involving higher risks than therapeutic elective procedures performed in stable patients.

HISTORICAL BACKGROUND

The evolution of interventional techniques has followed the basic principles of cardiac catheterisation outlined by Werner Forssman in 1929. The use of interventional catheterisation was first initiated by the use of balloon dilation in pulmonary and tricuspid valvoplasty,[1] and in dilation of atherosclerotic lesions.[2] It was Rashkind and his colleagues who widened the therapeutic implications of interventional catheterisation with the first intracardiac procedure in paediatrics and congenital cardiac disease when they introduced balloon atrial septostomy.[2,3] The use of occlusive devices was first reported by Porstmann and his colleagues in 1967, when a patent arterial duct was occluded with the aid of an Ivalon plug.[4] Attempts were then made to close left-to-right shunts with other devices, such as an atrial septal occluder for atrial septal defects,[5] and the double umbrella device for the persistently patent arterial duct and atrial septal defects.[6] The application of percutaneous transluminal balloon angioplasty by Gruntzig and Hoppf in 1974[7] was a landmark that expanded the field of interventional cardiology to the situation where it became recognised as a subspecialty in its own right. The principles of percutaneous transluminal balloon angioplasty were first applied by Lock and his colleagues[8–11] in the field of congenital cardiology, when they addressed stenotic pulmonary arteries, the aorta, and systemic veins, both in animal experiments and in humans. Kan and colleagues,[12] in 1982, then reported the first use of balloons introduced percutaneously for dilation of congenital valvar pulmonary stenosis. This approach has since became an accepted first intervention for treatment of stenosed pulmonary and aortic valves. The development of balloon-expandable stents has helped overcome problems of residual stenosis and restenosis in vessel walls.[13] The development of newer materials, such as Nitinol, a nickel-titanium alloy, has revolutionised technology, and expanded its use in closure of left-to-right shunts.[14–16] The use of this shape-memory alloy has simplified the delivery and retrieval of these devices by significantly reducing the size of the catheters used for delivery, thereby increasing their application in infants and smaller children. Various designs are now available, with different characteristics, allowing the operator to choose the most appropriate device for the morphology of the defects. Transcatheter insertion of valves is the most recent development in the field of interventional catheterisation.[17] Percutaneous implantation of biological or pericardial tissue valves mounted on balloon-expandable or self-expanding stents are now clinically approved for use in treatment of stenotic and regurgitant lesions in both the left and right ventricular outflow tracts.[18–22] Transcatheter techniques for repair of the mitral valve, based on surgical principles such as the creation of dual orifices and annuloplasty, are also being actively investigated in the clinical setting.[23,24] The final frontier in interventional techniques could well be the transcatheter treatment of complex congenitally malformed hearts, replacing surgical interventions such as the Norwood procedure or completion of Fontan circulation.[25–28]

PRINCIPLES OF CATHETERISATION

The field of interventional catheterisation is rapidly expanding as newer techniques and devices appear on the market. Any description of a standard procedure is, therefore, unlikely to stand the test of time, and will soon be outdated. The basic tenets of interventional catheterisation, however, are likely to remain constant, and have already stood the test of time over the last few decades. The success of an interventional catheterisation procedure is dependent not only on the performance of the procedure, but also on good planning prior to the procedure, coupled with anticipation and preparation for unexpected events.

Pre-procedural Planning

Consent should ideally be obtained either during outpatient consultation, or in a dedicated pre-admission clinic that provides parents the opportunity to discuss relevant issues.

The consent should be obtained by a person suitably qualified, with sufficient knowledge to explain the procedural details and its risks or, ideally, by the senior cardiologist. It is unreasonable to expect to receive a blanket consent, covering all procedures, although detailed consent for specific anticipated events might be obtained. The patient and the family should have sufficient time and information to make a fully informed decision. As it is difficult to approach parents during catheterisation for consent to additional procedures, treatment of life-threatening complications, or events that may lead to significant deterioration in the health of the patient, must be performed as deemed necessary.[29]

The planning of an interventional catheterisation procedure cannot be over-emphasised. Procedural planning aids in giving sufficient time to order necessary laboratory equipment and devices not stocked on a regular basis. Admission of the patient should include a meeting with the patient and family, explaining details and risks associated with the procedure, so that any doubts and fears specifically pertaining to the procedure are reclarified. All investigations should be reviewed on the day of the procedure. A repeated clinical examination of the patient helps determine the need for any additional investigations. Imaging should be reviewed to reconfirm the diagnosis, and the decision made for the procedure. Ideally, the symptoms, findings on clinical examination, and investigations should be reviewed by a team of doctors, including the primary cardiologist, the interventional cardiologist, the imaging cardiologist, the anaesthetist and, if applicable, the cardiac surgeon, in order to maximise the information leading to the procedure. An approach based on consensus also adds to the safety and efficacy of the decision-making process, as individuals with different areas of expertise contribute in a complementary manner, maximising the benefit to every patient. Use of additional cross sectional imaging, such as three-dimensional echocardiography, magnetic resonance imaging, or computerised tomography, can add significantly to the clinical information by providing details of complex cardiac anatomy that could suggest the need for a modified approach, or even contraindicate catheterisation. Decisions regarding access, via the femoral, jugular, or bilateral jugular approach, for example, choice of sheaths, catheters, wires, dosage of contrast agents, and projections to be used, can be made with reasonable certainty before starting the procedure. It is always helpful to discuss the whole strategy in a step-wise manner with the fellow in training, scrub nurse, cardiac physiologist, anaesthetist, radiographer, and all staff involved with the procedure. Steps that can be performed quickly and safely should be identified and delegated to assistants in the interest of time, particularly for long procedures.

Vascular Access

The conventional approach, namely to have both an arterial and a venous access, works in almost all situations where interventional catheterisation is performed. Femoral, internal jugular, subclavian, axillary and hepatic vascular approaches have all been used for various interventions. The possible need for reintervention should be borne in mind, thus avoiding unnecessary access. Repeated catheterisation, prolonged periods in intensive care, and multiple operations for complex staged palliative procedures can make access difficult due to repeated use of the vessels. Ultrasonically guided access allows for visualisation of vessels, detects unusual arrangements, thrombosed veins and arteries, and also reduces the risk of inadvertent puncture. Stenosis or atresia with luminal continuity of systemic veins may have to be dealt with by crossing the site with a floppy-tipped guide-wire, and use of long sheaths, which go across the stenosis and provide access to the central circulation. On the arterial side, in small neonates or infants, vascular cut-down has been used to access the carotid or axillary arteries for interventions on the aortic valve or arch.[30,31] In neonates and small infants, the availability of small catheters and sheaths, of 3 and 4 French sizes, have facilitated procedures, and reduced the risk of vascular injury.[32]

Catheters and Guide-Wires

In infants and children, angled and curved tipped catheters are most commonly used in situations where catheters need to be manoeuvred through tight bends and small chambers and vessels. The operator needs to have sufficient knowledge of the differences in the types of catheter when performing cardiac and peripheral interventions in order to modify the approach to access difficult sites. Hydrophilic catheters, such as the Glide catheter, Medi-tech, or Boston Scientific products, track well over guide-wires into difficult sites. Balloon-tipped catheters, such as the Berman angiographic catheter, or the Arrow balloon wedge catheter, are useful for wedge injections, or to cross atrioventricular valves without entrapment in the intercordal spaces. Catheters of short length help make manipulation easy in small babies. Long catheters in older patients help to form loops in dilated proximal chambers, such as the right atrium, to provide stability, and allow tracking into distal vessels such as the pulmonary trunk.

Guide-wires are used to access vessels, stabilise catheters, and provide easy access for multiple crossings of stenotic lesions. A soft hydrophilic wire, such as the Terumo, with an angled tip, can be used to enter small tortuous vessels. A stiff exchange length wire, such as the 0.035-inch, 260-cm product from Cook (Bloomington, IN), is usually required to obtain multiple haemodynamic measurements, provide stability across a lesion, for multiple crossings after interventions, to perform angiography, and to mount balloon catheters, stents, or large sheaths.

Anti-coagulation

Heparin is used as an anti-coagulant during cardiac catheterisation to prevent thromboembolism during and after the procedure. Some operators monitor heparin effect by measuring the activated clotting time or the partial thromboplastin time, albeit that most use a standard dose based on the weight of the patient.[33]

For short procedures, a single dose of 50 units per kilogram body weight is administered after vascular access is obtained. For long procedures, between 100 and 200 units per kilogram weight is administered and may be repeated either after 2 to 3 hours or by monitoring either the activated clotting or the partial thromboplastin times. Protamine may be used to reverse the effect of heparin should there be persistent bleeding from the site of access.

INTERVENTIONAL CATHETERISATION PROCEDURES

Balloon Dilation

Balloon dilation is performed to relieve stenosis of valves, vessel walls, surgically-created pathways, or intracardiac structures such as a fenestration in the atrial septum. There have been significant advances in the size, profile, design and materials used in balloon catheters, facilitating their use in various applications. Design of co-axial balloons has reduced the time required for inflation and deflation, with only transient haemodynamic compromise. The size of the balloon used for a particular procedure not only depends on the diameter of the lesion to be dilated, but also on the diameter of the contiguous and non-contiguous normal anatomical structures. The use of an over-sized balloon increases the chance of a successful dilation of the lesion, but also increases the risk of trauma to contiguous anatomical structures. Balloons have been used to treat valvar stenosis when fusion of the leaflets along their zones of apposition is responsible for reduction in the effective valvar orificial area. The principle of creating a controlled tear or split along the zone of apposition, thus improving excursion of the leaflets, provides a better effective orificial area, and relieves the stenosis. As the valve is abnormal, competence may be affected to various degrees after balloon dilation. Pulmonary, aortic, mitral, and tricuspid valves have all been treated by balloon valvoplasty for different diseases. The technique, however, is not useful in treating valves that are hypoplastic because of narrowing at the ventriculo-arterial junction. Dilation of arterial valves is performed commonly for congenital lesions, and dilation of atrioventricular valves is performed almost exclusively for acquired lesions. The technique used in performing balloon valvoplasty also forms the basis for angioplasty and implantation of stents. High-pressure balloons have been more recently used in dilating tight lesions, such as calcified conduits or pulmonary arterial stenosis.[34,35] Cutting balloons have been used in substrates which do not respond to standard balloon angioplasty, such as severe pulmonary arterial stenosis or recurrent pulmonary venous stenosis, with encouraging results.[36] Balloon-in-balloon catheters, known as BIB, and produced by NuMed (Hopkinton, NY), have been very useful in implanting stents in the aorta and pulmonary arteries.[37] The inner balloon is an additional tool to help confirm the position before deployment of the stent. The use of two balloons inserted over a single guide-wire for valvoplasty was first introduced for dilation of the mitral valve.[38] It provides a large effective diameter of the combined balloons, and has been used in pulmonary valvoplasty in adults who have a large diameter of the pulmonary outflow tracts.[39] Stability of the balloon during inflation depends on choice of a balloon of correct length and diameter, appropriate selection of a stiff guide-wire, obtaining a good position for the guide-wire, and achieving a rapid sequence of inflation and deflation. Stability could be further aided by using techniques to reduce stroke volume, such as rapid ventricular pacing, mainly for lesions in the systemic circulation. In balloon valvoplasty, the size of the balloon is chosen based on the size of the valve measured. In pulmonary valvoplasty, the balloon size is usually one-fifth to one-quarter larger than the measured diameter of the valve at the basal hinge points of the leaflets. In aortic valvoplasty, the size is usually nine-tenths of the diameter at the hinges of the leaflets. Size for dilating the coarcted aorta equals the diameter of the proximal transverse arch, or a size is chosen not greater than three times the size of the lesion, but less than the diameter of the descending aorta at its position close to the diaphragm. The length of the balloon should not be so short as to produce instability during inflation, and not too long to cause trauma to the proximal or distal structures. The size of the patient should be taken into consideration in choosing the correct balloon. Balloons are filled with contrast medium diluted 1 in 5 with saline, and should be de-aired thoroughly to reduce the risk of air embolism, should the balloon rupture. If the margins of the balloon, at its ends, are parallel, it suggests that inflation is at nominal pressure, and any further inflation can increase the risk of rupture. After successful dilation, haemodynamics and angiography should be repeated to evaluate results and assess complications. Further evaluation by echocardiography is imperative to decide long-term management.

Stent Angioplasty

Stents are capable of maintaining patency of vessels and prevent elastic recoil after balloon dilation. There have been major advances in stent technology, and their impact can be easily observed in congenital cardiology. Typically, stents are cut from stainless steel tubes with a laser, or made from platinum alloy wires welded together. Stents can be expanded on balloons, or be self-expanding when made of shape-memory alloy and covered by a sheath. Self-expanding stents are used in patients who have already achieved their potential for growth. Balloon-expandable stents can be redilated within limits, and may be used in children. The design of the cells may be open, avoiding jailing or covering of neighbouring arterial branches, or closed. The properties of materials considered favourable for use in congenital cardiology are those with a low profile, good strength and flexibility, and ability to withstand cyclic compressive stresses of the cardiovascular system. The diameter of the stent should also have the potential to reach maximal dimensions of the vessel wall as seen in the adult. In small infants, however, a coronary arterial stent may be used in extenuating circumstances of severe haemodynamic compromise, despite its limited final maximal diameter. Stents are implanted using balloons of appropriate size through long, large-bored, sheaths to reach the lesion. Stents may be pre-mounted on the balloons, or may need to be crimped on to the balloon manually or by using a crimping device. The length of the balloon should always be longer than the length of the stent. The diameter of the balloon determines the final diameter of the stent. Stability of the stent during deployment can be improved by using the balloon-in-balloon catheters, extra-stiff wires, long sheaths, and rapid right ventricular pacing to reduce stroke volume.[40] The luminal surface of the stent endothelialises in 8 to 10 weeks, and patients may need to take anti-platelet agents or, in some situations, anti-coagulants during this period to prevent in-stent restenosis.

Risks associated with stent angioplasty include dislodgement and embolisation, trauma to the vessel walls, fracture of the stent, and restenosis. Covered stents made by suturing expanded polytetrafluoroethylene to balloon-expandable or self-expanding stents have been used in situations where the risk of vascular injury and aneurysm is considered to be high. The use of these covered stents in younger patients is limited by their size, and the calibre of the delivery systems currently available. Newer bioabsorbable stents are currently being investigated to reduce restenosis in coronary arterial lesions. If approved, these stents could prove useful in treating stenosis of small vessels in infants, albeit temporarily, thus allowing for normal growth.[41]

Closure of Septal Defects and Vascular Occlusion

The advent of shape-memory alloy has revolutionised transcatheter interventions for intra- and extracardiac shunts. Nitinol is the most common alloy used. Several devices for closing septal defects and vascular occlusion are currently available. The most commonly used occluder, produced by Amplatz at AGA Medical, has a central occluding part, with left- and right-sided discs. A Dacron polyester patch sewn into the device is responsible for thrombogenicity and complete occlusion. Sizing of a septal defect is performed by trans-oesophageal or intracardiac echocardiography, or by inflating a balloon during the procedure. Reported complications of such devices eroding through the atrial or aortic walls, and devices designed to occlude ventricular septal defects causing complete heart block, emphasise the importance of choosing a device of appropriate size. Various practices from over-sizing, to reduce the risk of embolisation, to appropriate sizing, to reduce the risk of trauma to contiguous structures, have been used.

INTRACARDIAC INTERVENTIONS

Valvar Heart Disease

Pulmonary Valve

Pulmonary Valvar Stenosis

As already discussed, the initial description of balloon dilation of pulmonary stenosis was made by Kan and her colleagues in 1982.[12] Since then, the technique has been accepted as a first-line treatment for congenital valvar pulmonary stenosis.[42–45] Balloon dilation is usually indicated when the gradient across the stenosed valve is 50 mm Hg or more, or when there is an increase in right ventricular systolic pressure by more than half of the systemic pressure. The indications for the procedure are, however, different in neonates with a duct-dependent pulmonary circulation, when gradients are unreliable. A high right ventricular systolic pressure, and the presence of a dysplastic valve, is an accepted indication for treatment.

The right ventricular pressure is measured, following which right ventricular angiography is performed in the lateral projection in order to measure the diameter of the ventriculo-arterial junction at the basal attachment of the valvar leaflets. The stenotic pulmonary valve is crossed using an end-hole catheter, such as a multi-purpose catheter, a cobra-shaped catheter, or a Judkins right coronary arterial catheter. A guide-wire, from 0.014 to 0.035 inch in diameter, is passed through the catheter across the valve, and placed in a branch of the pulmonary artery supplying the lower lobe of either lung. In neonates, the guide-wire may be placed across the patent arterial duct into the descending aorta. A balloon that is about one-fifth to one-quarter larger than the diameter of the measured valve is passed through the sheath in the femoral vein over the wire, and placed across the pulmonary valve. The balloon is rapidly inflated and deflated with dilute contrast across the stenosis. The balloon is then withdrawn, with the guide-wire still in place, and a catheter is passed into the pulmonary arteries to measure the persisting gradient. The Multitrack catheter designed by Bonhoeffer is very useful, as it allows measurement of both right ventricular pressure and the gradient across the pulmonary valve, coupled with the ability to perform angiography before and after dilation of the balloon without loss of position of the guide-wire. In patients with a very dysplastic pulmonary valve, balloons that are up to three-fifths larger than the diameter of the supporting subpulmonary infundibulum can be used, with acceptable relief of the stenosis. The technique of balloon dilation is more demanding in neonates. Although balloon dilation of pulmonary valvar stenosis carries low risks when performed in infants and children over the age of 1 year, there is a significant morbidity and mortality in the early neonatal period.[46–48] In neonates, it is the size and function of the right ventricle that determine outcome. High right ventricular pressure, an irritable myocardium with a risk of arrhythmia, and splinting of the tricuspid valve, can all lead to haemodynamic instability. This necessitates very short periods of inflation, which may be helped by using balloons with low profile.

Adequate relief of the stenosis, with a reduction in the transvalvar gradient and in right ventricular systolic pressure, is achieved in the majority of patients.[49] Occasionally, however, there may be very little immediate reduction in gradient across the pulmonary valve. This is because of associated infundibular muscular stenosis, which disappears over a period in a similar fashion to that observed after surgical pulmonary valvotomy. Repeat balloon valvoplasty, after a few months, in those patients where the initial result was suboptimal, can produce a further reduction in gradient. Serious complications of balloon dilation include a tear of the pulmonary trunk, or perforation of the heart.[50,51] In general, the complication rate, at 0.4%, is low, and reported mortality is no more than 0.2%.[52] The consequences of chronic pulmonary regurgitation, nonetheless, can be underestimated, and more conservative dilation is now recommended.

Balloon dilation of the pulmonary valve can also be carried out as a palliative procedure in patients with tetralogy of Fallot and other complex congenital cardiac malformations. It can also be performed in patients with a functionally univentricular circulation to improve the size of the pulmonary arteries prior to staged palliations or repair. The basic principles of the procedure in these situations are the same as for isolated congenital valvar pulmonary stenosis, although crossing the stenotic subpulmonary outflow tract can be challenging. Problems with atrioventricular conduction can occur if the position of the atrioventricular bundle is abnormal. A more conservative approach is followed to avoid excessive flow of blood to the lungs, and to reduce the risk of pulmonary regurgitation. Reports have also emerged for dilation for infundibular stenosis using balloons, as palliative procedures, although without consistently desired results.

Valvar Pulmonary Atresia with Intact Ventricular Septum

The transcatheter interventions available to alter the course of this lesion (see also Chapter 30) include relief of right ventricular outflow obstruction with perforation of the

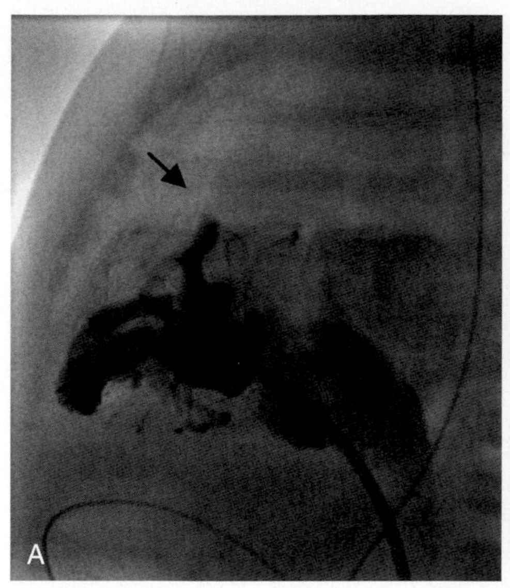

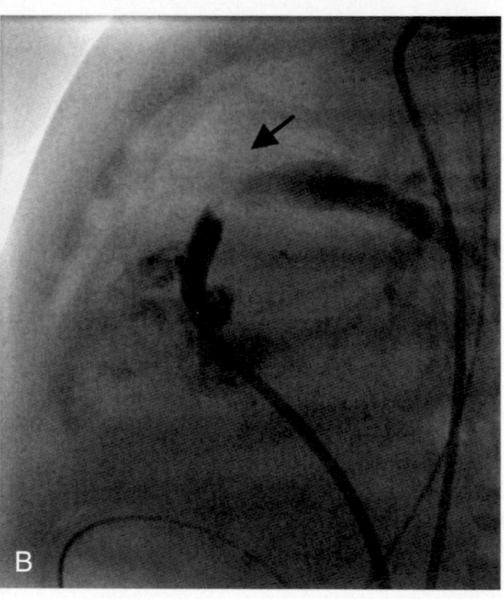

Figure 17-1 Images from a patient with pulmonary atresia with intact ventricular septum. **A,** Right ventricular contrast injection in lateral projection shows the atretic pulmonary valve (*arrow*). **B,** Simultaneous injection of contrast in the aorta delineates the pulmonary arterial surface of the atretic pulmonary valve (*arrow*) through a systemic-to-pulmonary artery shunt.

atretic valve and balloon dilation, stenting of the arterial duct to provide additional flow of blood to the lungs, enlargement of the atrial communication by balloon atrial septostomy to reduce right atrial hypertension, and occasionally, stenting of the subvalvar muscular right ventricular outflow tract in the setting of residual obstruction.

The success of interventional catheterisation, as determined by achieving a biventricular circulation, depends upon specific morphological characteristics. Patients should have a right ventricle with a tripartite cavity, a tricuspid valve with a diameter greater than 10 mm, or z score more than −1.5, a pulmonary valvar and infundibular diameter more than 7 mm, and absence of right ventricular-dependent coronary arterial circulation.[53]

The principles of catheterisation involve appropriate selection of patients, maintaining haemodynamic stability with ventilation, maintaining patency of the arterial duct with infusion of prostaglandins, careful catheterisation to avoid cardiac trauma or excessive bleeding through the catheter lumen, selection of the appropriate technique to perforate the atretic pulmonary valve, continuous monitoring of systemic arterial pressure, and anticipation and prompt management of pericardial tamponade by pericardiocentesis.

Antero-posterior and lateral projections of right and left ventricular angiography help confirm the absence of right ventricle-dependent coronary arterial circulation, delineate the right ventricular outflow and the pulmonary arterial end of the atretic valve, assess the left ventricle, and determine the morphology of the aorta and the arterial duct. Appropriate frames from the angiograms are fixed as reference images after identifying landmarks for perforation. An end-hole catheter with a curved tip, typically either cobra shaped or a Judkins right 3.5-cm curve, is used to achieve stable and precise position of the tip of the catheter in the right ventricular infundibulum, just beneath the atretic pulmonary valve. Clockwise rotation of the catheter hooks it around the ventriculo-infundibular fold, and directs the tip towards the right ventricular outflow tract. After pushing the catheter tip into the infundibulum, a counter-clockwise rotation engages it in most cases against the atretic pulmonary valve. Multiple angiograms should be performed to confirm the position of the tip of the catheter, which will determine the site of perforation (Fig. 17-1A). By attaching a Tuohy-Borst Y connector to the hub of the catheter, biplane angiography can be performed with or without simultaneous aortography, thus delineating the right ventricular and pulmonary arterial surfaces of the atretic pulmonary valve (Fig. 17-1B). Once the position of the tip of the catheter against the atretic valve is satisfactory and stable, a radio-frequency wire connected to a generator is inserted into the guiding catheter. A commercially available radio-frequency perforation generator with a perforation catheter and co-axial injectable catheter, produced by the Bayliss Medical Company, is now available, and is most commonly used. This system is designed for tissue perforation and uses high voltage at 150 to 280 volts, with low power at 5 to 10 watts, to reach very high impedance, up to 7000 ohms, for short durations of application, from 1 to 5 seconds. An earthing plate is required, and should be placed under the buttocks before draping the patient. Care should be taken to avoid pooling of the antiseptic over this plate when the groin or umbilicus is prepared for access. A wire of 0.024-inch diameter, and 260-cm length, can be connected to a customised radio-frequency generator, which cuts off if the impedance exceeds the specified range. The wire has an exposed metal tip of 2 mm that is responsible for generating the thermal energy needed for the perforation. Rest of the wire is covered with Teflon. Repeated angiography should always be performed to confirm that the position of the catheter has not changed during loading of the perforating wire. The stiff-end of a coronary arterial wire, or a fibre-optic wire such as a 0.018- or 0.021-inch trimedyne wire connected to a Nd Yag or Excimer laser generator, may be used in place of the radio-frequency wire. After confirming the final position, perforation of the atretic pulmonary valve is carried out, taking extreme caution to prevent injury to the pulmonary trunk.[53-58] The position of the radio-frequency wire beyond the perforated valve should again be confirmed before proceeding further. The position of the tip of the wire within the cardiac silhouette on both antero-posterior and lateral projections should raise suspicion of cardiac perforation suggesting that wire is in the pericardial space.

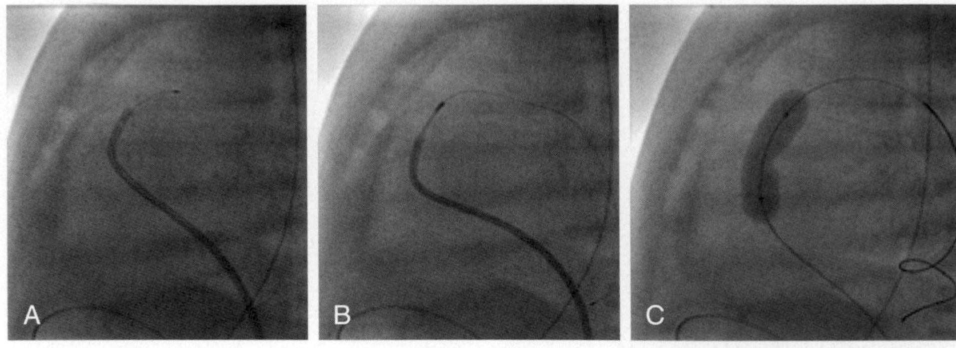

Figure 17-2 Radio-frequency perforation of atretic pulmonary valve. The lateral projection (**A**) shows perforation of the atretic pulmonary valve with a radio-frequency wire, followed by (**B**) insertion of a co-axial catheter over the radio-frequency wire, and (**C**) balloon dilation of the pulmonary valve. Note the abolition of the waist on the balloon.

In these circumstances, the wire should be promptly withdrawn and systemic arterial pressure should be monitored. If necessary, an echocardiogram should be performed to rule out cardiac tamponade. The hole made by the radio-frequency wire is usually very small, and unlikely to cause significant bleeding into the pericardial space. Once the atretic valve is successfully crossed, a fine catheter that can go over the wire is used, creating a co-axial system allowing for graded dilation of the pulmonary valve (Fig. 17-2). Various balloons are available to dilate the pulmonary valve. Pre-dilation with a small coronary arterial balloon of 2.5- to 4-mm diameter allows a larger balloon, of 7- to 10-mm diameter and 2-cm length, to be used effectively (Fig. 17-2C). An echocardiogram should be performed soon after the procedure to confirm adequate relief of right ventricular outflow obstruction. Pericardial effusion, if present, should be monitored closely after the procedure with invasive systemic arterial pressure monitoring and frequent echocardiography.

If adequate relief of obstruction has been achieved, the infusion of prostaglandin could be stopped to prevent the complications of systemic arterial steal from a large patent arterial duct. It is not, however, unusual to need prostaglandin for a few days to maintain adequate flow of blood to the lungs until right ventricular diastolic function improves, and there is effective antegrade flow across the right ventricular outflow tract. If weaning from prostaglandin fails to maintain systemic arterial saturations within an acceptable range, ductal stenting can be undertaken to provide additional pulmonary blood flow.[59] Ductal stents have a high risk of restenosis with intimal proliferation, and need close monitoring and anti-platelet therapy. Presence of infundibular muscle may contribute to dynamic obstruction after adequate relief of valvar stenosis. If severe, implantation of a stent into the outflow tract may also produce successful relief of obstruction.[60] In less severe situations, chronic treatment with oral β-blockade has been effective in providing adequate relief until regression of the muscular hypertrophy improves forward flow into the pulmonary arteries. During late follow-up, if despite an effective biventricular circulation, systemic arterial desaturation is observed due to right-to-left shunting, devices can be inserted to occlude the interatrial communication.[61]

Implantation of Pulmonary Valves

Bonhoeffer and his colleagues[62] described the first implantation of a valve in the pulmonary position, placing the device through a catheter in a dysfunctional prosthetic conduit to relieve stenosis and regurgitation. The Medtronic Melody valve was made of a bovine jugular vein sutured inside a balloon-expandable platinum-iridium stent, and was deployed using a custom-made system, now known as Ensemble, and produced by Medtronic Inc. The system contains a balloon-in-balloon catheter inside a long sheath with a dilator at the tip. Current systems have outer balloons of 18-, 20-, and 22-mm diameter. These balloons determine the final diameter of the implanted valved-stent, which should equal the diameter of the homograft conduit initially inserted surgically in the right ventricular outflow tract. The valve is suitable for insertion in right ventricular outflow tracts with diameters varying between 16 to 22 mm in patients with circumferential-valved conduits implanted surgically during their definitive repair. Magnetic resonance imaging helps to define the morphology of the outflow tract and the bifurcation of the pulmonary trunk, determine right ventricular volume and ejection fractions, and quantify the pulmonary regurgitant fraction. Echocardiography is used for surveillance and haemodynamic monitoring.

The procedure is performed under general anaesthesia. A balloon-tipped or curved-tip catheter is inserted through the femoral or jugular vein to access the distal left or right pulmonary artery with the aid of a floppy tipped Terumo wire. An Ultrastiff guide-wire, of 0.035-inch diameter and 260-cm length, with a pre-formed curve, is then positioned in one of the pulmonary arteries. A Multitrack catheter is passed over this stiff wire to measure right ventricular pressure, the gradient across the right ventricular outflow tract, and to perform angiography (Fig. 17-3A). Different projections are employed to define the morphology of the outflow tract, the bifurcation of the pulmonary arteries, and to assess the pulmonary regurgitation. Aortography performed through a pigtail catheter inserted into the femoral artery helps define the coronary arterial anatomy. If an anomalous course of a coronary artery is suspected, a selective injection into the artery, with simultaneous inflation of a balloon in the right ventricular outflow tract, is performed to rule out arterial compression. Once the outflow tract is deemed suitable for implantation, the valved-stent is washed in three different saline baths for 5 minutes each to wash off the glutaraldehyde preservative. The venepuncture is dilated in a graded fashion with 14 and 22 French dilators. The delivery system is thoroughly flushed, de-aired, and the inner and outer balloons prepared with syringes filled with diluted contrast, 10 mL for the inner balloon, and 20 ml for the outer balloon. The valved-stent is crimped on a 2.5-mL syringe by a gentle rolling action, and loaded on the balloon catheter. The outer sheath of the delivery system is brought gently over the crimped

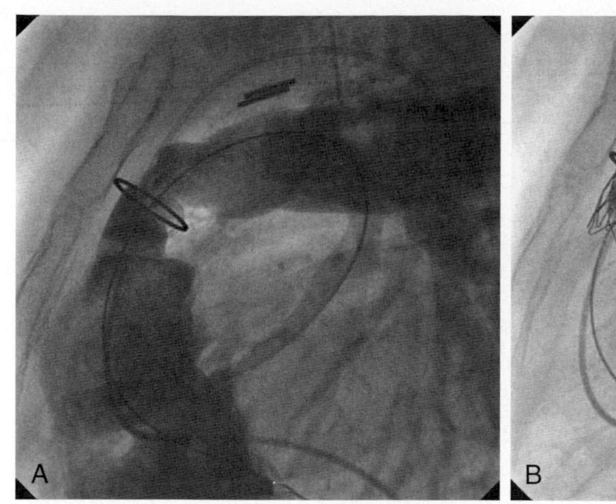

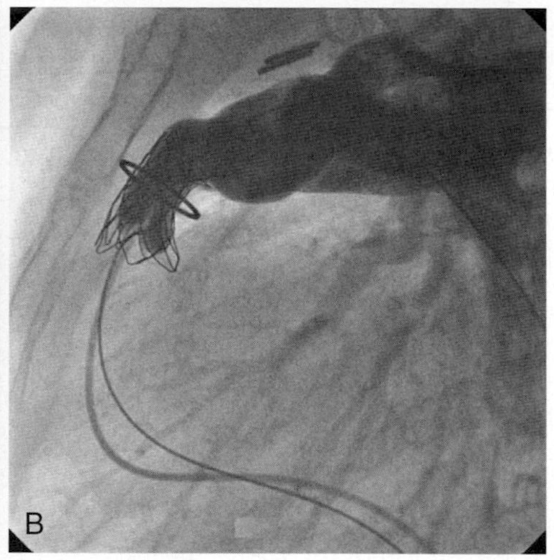

Figure 17-3 The steps involved in percutaneous implantation of the pulmonary valve. **A,** The lateral projection of the pulmonary angiogram shows free pulmonary regurgitation through a Hancock conduit. **B,** Insertion of the Melody valve has resolved the problem.

valved-stent, ensuring complete covering of the proximal struts. The sheath is then slid over the entire length of the valved-stent, which is fully covered and ready to be inserted. The tip of the delivery system has a dilator, which provides a tapered tip to facilitate entry into the vein through the skin. The flexible delivery system can be looped in the right atrium to facilitate delivery of the valved-stent into an appropriate position. Standard principles of manipulation ensure delivery of the device in the right ventricular outflow tract without losing position of the wire. In patients with severe calcification and stenosis, pre-dilation with a high-pressure balloon, or pre-stenting with a bare metal stent, such as the Max LD, Intrastent, or Cheatham-Platinum stent, may be required. Once within the conduit, the valved-stent is uncovered by pulling back on the outer sheath. Angiography confirms satisfactory position of the valved-stent (Fig. 17-3B). Calcification of the conduit, or the bare stent itself, usually provides good landmarks for optimal positioning. The valve is deployed by sequentially inflating the inner and outer balloons. Haemodynamic assessment and angiography is then performed using the Multitrack catheter after implantation. In patients with a significant residual gradient, post-dilation with a high-pressure balloon may be required, using pressures of 10 to 12 atmospheres.

Implantation has now been carried out for dysfunction of the right ventricular outflow tract in patients with repaired tetralogy of Fallot and variants, transposed arterial trunks with ventricular septal defect and pulmonary stenosis, the Ross operation for left ventricular outflow disease, and repaired common arterial trunk.[19] The majority of the patients had a homograft in the right ventricular outflow tract. There was a significant reduction in right ventricular systolic pressure, the gradient across the outflow tract, and improvement in pulmonary competence after valvar implantation, with no procedural mortality. Survival was 95.9% at 72 months.[19] The incidence of complications decreased with subsequent implantations as a result of improvements in selection of patients and design of the device. Restenosis due to a hammock effect created by the venous wall hanging within the stent was not observed after these alterations in design. Fractures remain an important cause of restenosis, being seen after one-fifth of insertions, and can be managed with a second implantation within the initial one. Early detection, and anticipatory management, of the fractured stent can be aided by chest radiography and echocardiography at regular intervals.[63]

Adults who have undergone repair of the right ventricular outflow tract without use of a conduit, but have suffered aneurysmal dilation, are not suitable for implantation of the current device. Future research to design a device that can be implanted in larger right ventricular outflow tracts, more than 22 mm in diameter, is ongoing. Self-expanding stents designed to reduce the size of the dilated aneurysmal right ventricular outflow tract can hold the valved-stent within it to provide a secure anchoring mechanism.[64] These devices are likely to be most suited to treat isolated pulmonary regurgitation in dilated outflow tracts.

Aortic Valve

Aortic Stenosis

Balloon dilation of the aortic valve was first reported by Lababidi.[65] Currently accepted indications for intervention include the presence of a peak gradient greater than 70 mm Hg on Doppler with a left ventricular strain pattern on the electrocardiogram and symptoms such as syncope, effort intolerance, or angina. Neonatal indications for intervention are based on the presence of a duct-dependent systemic circulation, a low cardiac output state with severe left ventricular dysfunction, and a dysplastic stenotic aortic valve. Asymptomatic infants with congenital valvar aortic stenosis are treated for gradients greater than 50 mm Hg in the absence of a duct-dependent systemic circulation due to the risk of progression of the stenosis and development of left ventricular dysfunction. Since the original documentation, good results of balloon dilation of the aortic valve have been reported in both the short and medium term.[66-68] There was some concern regarding femoral arterial occlusion, but this complication is less frequently seen now with the availability of low-profile balloons.

Parameters given consideration prior to the procedure, particularly in sick neonates with a low cardiac output, include achieving access, maintaining haemodynamic stability, ensuring hydration, adequate control of glycaemia and acid-base balance, ventilation, infusion of prostaglandin to maintain ductal patency, and appropriate cardiovascular drugs to maintain cardiac output. In infants and children, the procedure is performed under general anaesthesia. Heparin is used for anti-coagulation to prevent vascular thrombosis of the femoral artery or vein and systemic thromboembolism. Avoidance of cooling and loss of blood during the procedure is very important to prevent haemodynamic compromise. The procedure can be performed through femoral arterial, femoral venous, umbilical arterial, axillary or carotid arterial access.[31,67,69–71] The advent of rapid right ventricular pacing has reduced the need for an anterograde approach with trans-septal puncture with atrial septostomy. Femoral arterial puncture is used for monitoring of systemic arterial pressure when dilation is carried out anterograde through the femoral vein.

In haemodynamically stable patients, an angiogram is performed in the ascending aorta via a pigtail catheter profiled in antero-posterior and lateral projections. The aortic valvar leaflets are delineated, and the diameter of the ventriculo-arterial junction is measured and compared with those obtained on echocardiography, to avoid the risk of using an oversized balloon. Severe angulation of the left ventricular outflow tract can complicate accurate measurement of the valvar diameter. In haemodynamically unstable patients, angiography poses a risk of severe ventricular arrhythmia in the presence of left ventricular dysfunction. Hence, the diameter of the aortic valve as measured by echocardiography alone is used to determine the appropriate diameter of the balloon. Small sheaths, and catheters of 3 French diameter, are employed when using umbilical access in neonates, and 4 or 5 French catheters with angled-tip guide-wires are used in older children. A ratio of the diameter of the balloon to the outflow tract of 0.9 indicates an appropriately selected balloon, and is unlikely to cause significant regurgitation. An angiogram illustrating a jet of negative contrast through the stenotic valve serves as a reference to locate the effective orifice, which most commonly lies posteriorly and to the left in the aortic root. The valve is crossed in retrograde fashion using a curved-tip catheter, such as a Judkins right coronary catheter, a cobra-shaped catheter, or a cut-pigtail to provide a curved tip, and a floppy steerable guide-wire. Multiple rapid gentle stabs are made with the guide-wire to cross the valve. This step reduces the risk of perforating the valvar leaflets and traumatising the orifices of the coronary arteries.

When approaching in anterograde fashion, a Judkins right or a cobra-shaped balloon angiographic or wedge catheter is placed across the patent oval foramen and manoeuvered to enter the left ventricle through the mitral valve. Coronary wires are used in neonates and infants, and stiff exchange length wires are used in older patients requiring trans-septal puncture for anterograde access to the aortic valve. Similar stiff wires can be also used in the retrograde approach. The balloon-tipped catheters reduce the risk of passing through the intercordal spaces of the mitral valvar tension apparatus. A large curve is formed in the cavity of left ventricle to direct the tip of the catheter towards left ventricular outflow tract. A floppy steerable wire is then used to cross the aortic valve and achieve a good position in the descending aorta. The catheter is then threaded over the wire so that a stiff wire could be positioned for subsequent steps. Some authors believe that the anterograde approach offers a reduced risk of aortic regurgitation as a result of valvar perforation.

In patients with a low cardiac output, balloons remain stable during inflation across the stenotic aortic valve. In the absence of a state of low cardiac output, balloons can be mobile during ventricular systole, and can cause trauma

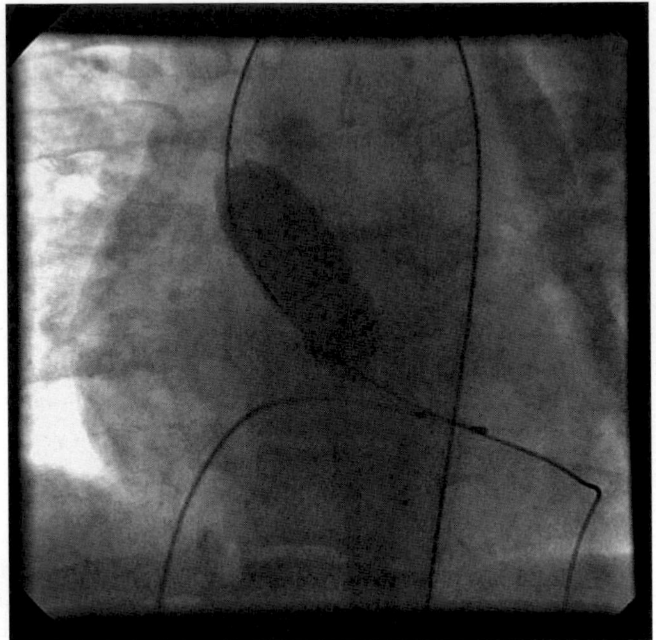

Figure 17-4 Retrograde aortic balloon valvoplasty with rapid right ventricular pacing as seen in frontal projection.

to the valvar leaflets. Stability is achieved using adenosine, and more commonly, rapid right ventricular apical pacing in older patients at fast rates of 180 to 220 beats per minute (Fig. 17-4). The anterograde approach leads to greater stability of the balloon, albeit that the risk of creating a tight loop across the atrial septum and the mitral valve increases the risk of severe haemodynamic compromise and cardiac trauma (Fig. 17-5). It is prudent to use a long balloon of 3.5 to 5 cm in older patients, as the left ventricle has a tendency to eject the balloon subsequent to inflation. Rapid inflation and deflation of the balloon are performed to minimise the duration of complete obstruction of flow through the valve.

Recent reports of long-term outcome after aortic balloon valvoplasty indicate that there is an excellent early relief of the valvar gradient, but an increase in aortic regurgitation.[72] Independent predictors of unfavourable outcome have been a small aortic root, a valve with two leaflets, poor function of the left ventricle or mitral valve, and limited experience of the operator.[73] Procedure related mortality is reported at 4.8%.[73] Although the risk of vascular injury is high, the majority of the complications are transient, and respond to thrombolysis and anti-coagulation. In critical aortic stenosis, the morphology of the aortic root, the mitral valve and presence of left ventricular endocardial fibro-elastosis have a major impact on outcome and need for reintervention. Neonatal critical aortic stenosis remains challenging despite continuing development of catheter technology for small babies. Despite effective relief of stenosis, patients may require functionally univentricular palliation if the morphology is not favourable for effective biventricular circulations (see also Chapter 44).

Implantation of the Aortic Valve

Percutaneous interventions on the aortic valve in adults with calcific aortic valvar stenosis and other co-morbidities rendering the valve inoperable are encouraging. The

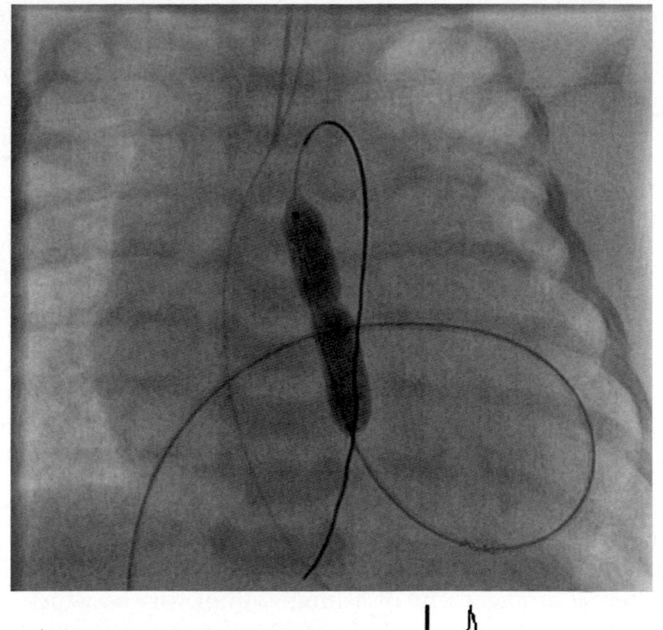

Figure 17-5 Anterograde balloon aortic valvoplasty. The balloon is introduced through the femoral vein and across the oval fossa defect, or after a trans-septal puncture, to access the left heart. The wire is placed in the descending aorta and provides stability to the balloon.

first report of insertion of bovine pericardial trifoliate valve came from Cribier and his colleagues.[74] Procedural complications in early implantations were related to the anterograde approach and the large size of the system required for delivery. The technique has been refined, with development of a retrograde approach, and implantation of the valve with rapid right ventricular pacing to reduce the risk of embolisation.[20] Self-expanding stent-mounted valves have also been used in similar clinical settings.[75] The current devices available, however, are not yet suitable for use in children and young adults.

Mitral Valve

Mitral Stenosis

Congenital mitral valvar stenosis is a complex disease, with involvement of supravalvar, valvar and subvalvar components (see Chapter 35). Balloon dilation is rarely used as first intervention, due to the high risk of restenosis or risk of injury to the valvar tension apparatus and leaflets leading to severe regurgitation. Percutaneous valvoplasty, however, has successfully replaced closed and open mitral commisurotomy for rheumatic mitral stenosis. Selection of patients based on echocardiography is fundamental in predicting outcomes, and requires a detailed assessment of the mitral valve.[76]

The approach is anterograde after trans-septal puncture. The Inoue balloon is most widely used, which consists of a coaxial balloon with a double lumen. Inflation leads to sequential dilation of the distal part, facilitating entry into the left ventricle, of the proximal part fixing the balloon across the mitral valve, and of the central part, which dilates the valvar annulus. A Multitrack technique with a monorail system with two balloons over a single guide-wire was introduced by Bonhoeffer and colleagues,[38] permitting successful dilation of the fused leaflets of the mitral valve.

Mitral Regurgitation

Percutaneous transcatheter interventions on the mitral valve to treat mitral regurgitation are being investigated in adults, permitting clipping or suture of the leaflets to produce dual orifices, or by inserting devices within the coronary sinus to improve coaptation of the leaflets.[23,24]

Tricuspid Valve

Congenital tricuspid valvar stenosis rarely occurs as an isolated lesion, and is most commonly associated with hypoplasia of the components of the right heart. Acquired stenosis in children is almost always due to rheumatic disease, and virtually never occurs as an isolated lesion.

Balloon dilation of the stenotic tricuspid valve has been reported in parts of the world with high prevalence of rheumatic fever. The basic principles of the techniques used are similar to those applied for mitral stenosis. The Inoue balloon is most commonly used, albeit that double balloons can be used. In congenital lesions, the associated hypoplasia of the right heart usually takes precedence in making management decisions.

Shunts

Atrial Septal Defects

Interventional catheterisation is the first modality of treatment to close defects in the atrial septum when increased pulmonary blood flow has caused dilation of the right heart. The morphology of the defect determines the suitability of the technique, those most suitable being the ones within the oval fossa with adequate margins at the rims. Superior and inferior sinus venosus communications, those defects in the oval fossa with deficient or floppy margins, or large defects encroaching on surrounding structures or resulting in haemodynamic compromise or trauma, are the general contraindications. Any associated lesions, such as anomalous pulmonary venous drainage, should be ruled out.

There are many devices available to close the defects, and they vary in their ease of loading and deployment, their suitability for the morphology of the defect, along with safety, efficacy and long-term behaviour. The most commonly used Amplatzer atrial septal occluder consists of two discs of Nitinol wire mesh connected by a waist of 4 mm thickness, which forms the central occluding disc (Fig. 17-6). The device is available in different sizes depending upon the diameter of the central disc. The left atrial disc is larger than the central occluding disc by 12 to 16 mm. A new Cribriform device is now available for closure of multi-fenestrated defects. This device has a much narrower waist to position it through one of the central defects, with the left and right atrial discs covering the surrounding holes. A Dacron polyester patch is sewn into the device to increase thrombogenicity. The delivery system consists of a loading sheath to help collapse the device and load it into a long delivery sheath attached to a delivery cable. The long sheath is angled at 45 degrees and has varying diameters and lengths. The device is attached to the delivery cable with a screw-on mechanism allowing release of the device after satisfactory deployment. Rates of closure are excellent when patients are selected in appropriate fashion.

The procedure is performed under general or local anaesthesia with sedation. Availability of trans-thoracic, trans-oesophageal, and intracardiac echocardiography has been crucial to the safety and success of the procedure. A catheter

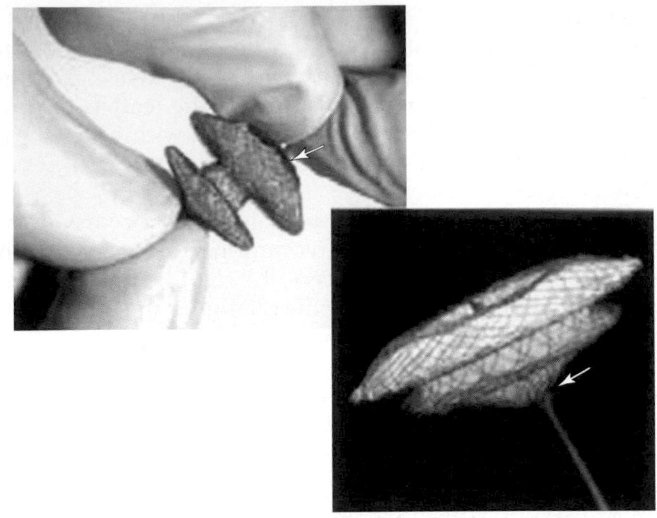

Figure 17-6 The Amplatz septal occluder, with the left and right atrial discs connected by a waist. The device is attached to a cable which is inserted through a delivery sheath. (Reproduced with permission from Seivert H, Qureshi SA, Wilson N, Hijazi ZM [eds]: Percutaneous Interventions for Congenital Heart Disease. London: Informa Healthcare, 2007, Figure 28.1.)

passed through the femoral vein is used to position the sheath across the defect. The pulmonary vein is used as the site for anchorage of a stiff guide-wire. Initially, complications of embolisation led operators to use large devices. The defect is sized using pulmonary arterial angiography, echocardiography, or with a contrast-filled balloon stretched across the defect (Fig. 17-7A). Care must be taken to avoid stretching the defect.[77] Colour flow mapping and occlusion of flow by inflating a balloon, the stop-flow technique, are also used as techniques for sizing. A device of size equal to or just larger than the size of the defect is commonly used. It is delivered through the sheath across the defect under fluoroscopic and echocardiographic guidance, ensuring appropriate deployment, absence of obstruction to contiguous structures, and lack of residual shunting (Fig. 17-7B). Successful anchorage is checked by wiggling the device whilst it is still attached to the delivery system, thus ensuring a secure position. The device can be retrieved and redeployed to the satisfaction of the operator prior to release. Various techniques used to deploy devices in larger defects include the use of specially designed sheaths with a double curve, a sheath positioned in the right upper pulmonary vein, a dilator, or balloon-assisted techniques that prevent prolapse of the left atrial disc across the defect.

Complications of the procedure include trauma leading to tamponade, embolisation, thrombosis, endocarditis, and arrhythmias. Recently, concerns have been raised about late cardiac perforations after use of the Amplatz occluders.[78,79] The risk of erosion, however, has been low, as confirmed by the registry for adverse events in clinical trials in the United States of America and in other countries.[77] Patients with a deficient aortic rim, and/or a deficient superior rim, of the oval fossa may have a higher risk of erosion. Those patients who present with a pericardial effusion within 24 hours should be monitored closely, and may require removal of the device surgically should there be an increase in the effusion.

Other devices available to close atrial septal defects include the CardioSEAL and STARflex devices, based on the double umbrella design, and with struts made from a cobalt alloy.[80] The Helex device is a new concept with a helical arrangement of a long Nitinol wire to which is attached a long curtain of expanded polytetrafluoroethylene.[81] When deployed, two circular discs form at each end of a flat helix, the curtain covering the septal defect. By pulling on the suture connecting the right atrial disc to the inner catheter of the delivery system, the whole device uncoils from its circular shape, and can be retrieved even after deployment into the delivery system (Fig. 17-8). A button device, and more recently, a frameless occlusion device, have also been described for use in defects without adequate rims.[82]

Ventricular Septal Defects

Closure of ventricular septal defects was first performed subsequent to myocardial infarction, or for congenital defects, using the Rashkind double-umbrella devices.[83] The current device of choice is the Amplatzer ventricular septal defect occluder, although various other devices have been used over the years.

The designs of the Amplatzer device can be tailored according to the morphology of the ventricular septal defect. The device used for perimembranous defects has a special asymmetrical shape with a very short waist, which forms the occluding part of the device. The left-sided disc has a deficient cephalad margin to avoid

Figure 17-7 Closure of an atrial septal defect closure with the Amplatz septal occluder. **A,** Balloon sizing of the defect. The current guidelines suggest use of stop-flow technique, rather than over-stretch the defect margins. **B,** The Amplatz device before release.

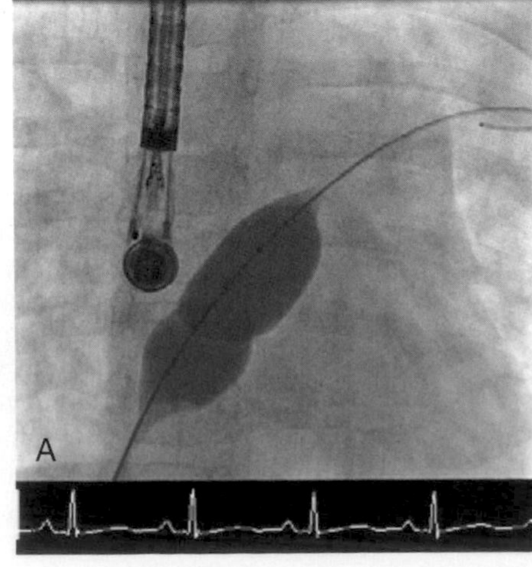

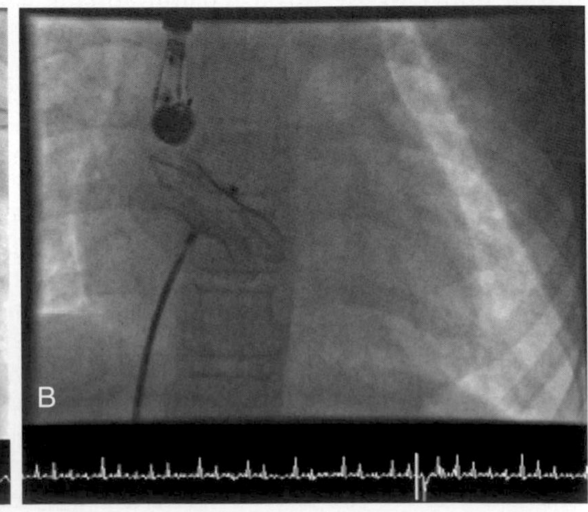

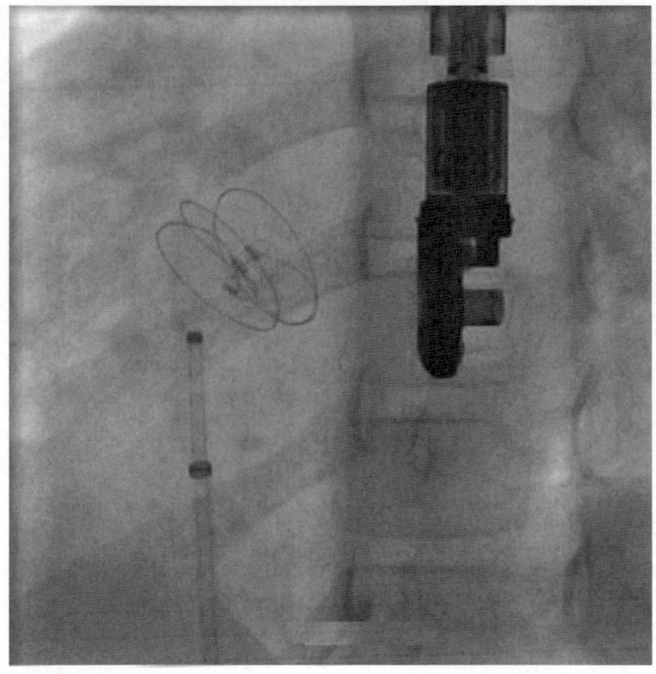

Figure 17-8 The Helex atrial septal occluder after deployment, when it is still retrievable.

contact with the aortic valve, and a platinum marker diametrically opposite, on the caudal margin, to help orientate the device correctly. Orientation is achieved using a custom-made delivery system that has a flattened segment on the circumference of the micro-screw, to which the device is attached before loading. Occluders designed for muscular defects have a longer waist depending on the size of the occluder, which varies from 6 to 24 mm in diameter (Fig. 17-9). The device is sized on the basis of the diameter of the occluding part, which is its waist.

Haemodynamic assessment is performed to quantitate the shunt and demonstrate a restrictive defect. Angiography in the long axial oblique view usually defines the location and the size of a perimembranous defect. Transoesophageal echocardiography, with views between 0 and 30 degrees and longitudinal views between 90 and 120 degrees, are best suited to define the morphology of these defects. The defect is crossed from the left ventricular side with a curved tip catheter and a glide wire, which is positioned in either the superior caval vein or the pulmonary artery. The glide wire is then exchanged with a special wire, the so-called noodle wire from AGA Medical, which is snared using a goose-neck snare from the femoral vein, and exteriorised to form an arterio-venous loop. The delivery sheath is loaded over this wire and positioned across the defect. When the defect is perimembranous, the sheath may have to be positioned in the left ventricular apex by careful manipulation in tandem with the guide-wire and the catheter. The device is deployed under fluoroscopic and echocardiographic guidance. Before release, left ventricular angiography and echocardiography help confirm a good position and secure anchorage (Fig. 17-10). Continuous monitoring of atrioventricular conduction is vital during occlusion of perimembranous defects. Persistent complete heart block is an indication either for redeployment or abandonment of the procedure.

Complications of this intervention include embolisation of the device, haemolysis, thrombo-embolism, tricuspid, and aortic regurgitation. Late complete heart block, reported particularly in perimembranous defects[84,85] due to the proximity with the conduction tissue, use of oversized devices to reduce the risk of embolisation, and continued expansion of the device, have been treated with high dose steroids and aspirin. A future review of the design of devices used to close perimembranous defects may help match the high standards of results achieved after surgical closure, and the low risks of complication of the surgical approach, such as the need for cardio-pulmonary bypass, heart block, residual defects, and mortality.

The principles for closure of muscular defects are similar to those for perimembranous defects. Single muscular defects may be crossed from the right ventricular aspect without the need for an arterio-venous loop. Apical defects may be crossed easily from a jugular approach, and outlet defects from a femoral approach. Angiography and echocardiography aid in appropriate positioning of the device (Fig. 17-11).

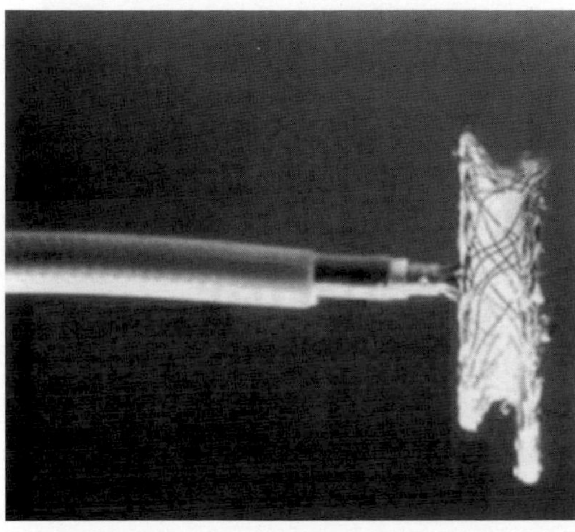

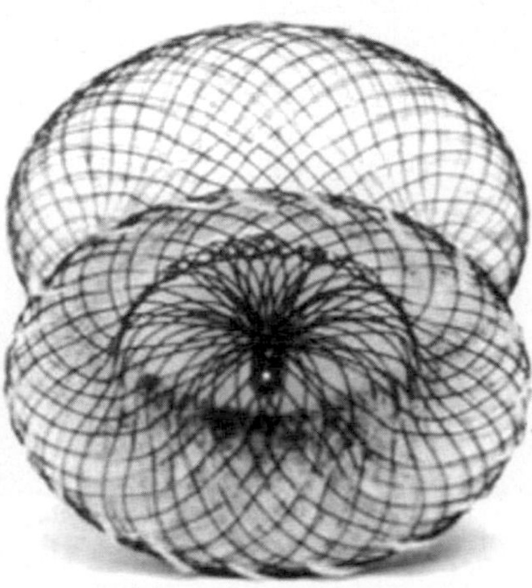

Figure 17-9 The Amplatz membranous ventricular septal defect occluder, and the muscular ventricular septal defect occluder. (Reproduced with permission from Seivert H, Qureshi SA, Wilson N, Hijazi ZM [eds]: Percutaneous Interventions for Congenital Heart Disease. London: Informa Healthcare, 2007, Figures 35.1 and 37.1.)

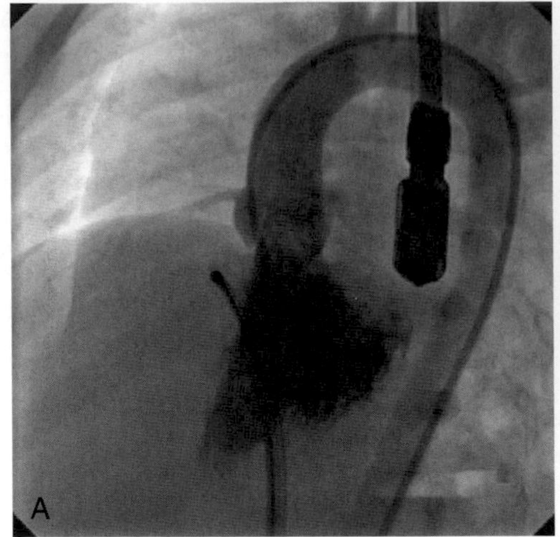

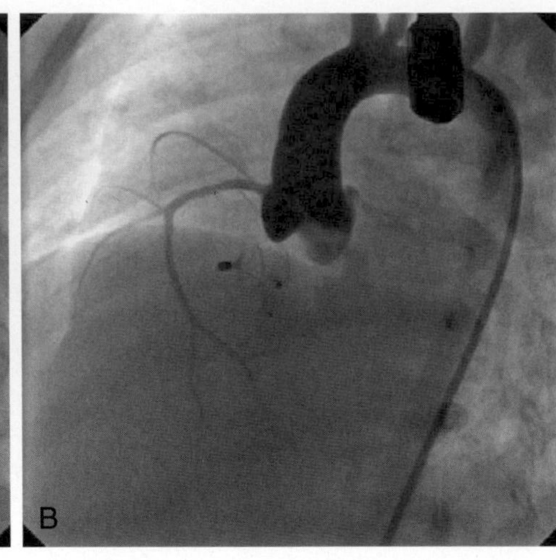

Figure 17-10 Closure of perimembranous ventricular septal defect with Amplatz membranous septal occluder. **A,** Long axial oblique projections show the left ventriculogram with the device in the defect and no residual shunt before release. **B,** The aortogram after release shows no aortic regurgitation. The orientation of the device is clearly seen, with a flattened margin to the left ventricular disc to prevent aortic valvar injury, and a platinum marker diametrically opposite to it.

Interventions on the Intact Atrial Septum

The creation of an 'atrial septal defect without thoracotomy or anaesthesia' as described by Rashkind and his colleagues was the first intervention reported on the atrial septum, and as explained in our introduction, represented the birth of interventional catheterisation.[3] Enlargement of a naturally occurring atrial communication is performed in patients with transposition to improve mixing. In other conditions, such as tricuspid atresia, double inlet ventricle with hypoplastic left or right atrioventricular valves, hypoplastic left heart syndrome, and others with the Fontan circulation, atrial septostomy is performed to relieve left or right atrial hypertension. Patients with left ventricular failure who are supported by extracorporeal membrane oxygenation may also need trans-septal puncture and atrial septostomy.

In patients with a patent oval foramen or a restrictive atrial communication, pull-back of a balloon catheter filled with saline or contrast (Fig. 17-12), or static balloon atrial septoplasty, increases the size of the interatrial communication. The flap valve of the oval fossa can be torn to enlarge the defect in a graded manner by increasing the volume of contrast or saline in the balloon. Access to the atrium may be through umbilical, femoral or hepatic veins. In neonates, this procedure can be performed even on the intensive care unit under trans-thoracic echocardiographic guidance. In patients with an intact atrial septum, a trans-septal atrial puncture is performed to gain access to left-sided structures. The use of the trans-septal needle requires experience with fluoroscopic and echocardiographic guidance. A Brockenbrough needle is used within a long sheath and dilator. The length of the needle tip protruding from the dilator should be marked by noting the distance of the proximal flange of the needle from the hub of the dilator within the sheath. The arrow on the flange, and its alignment to the needle tip, should also be checked before inserting the needle into the right heart. The long sheath with the dilator is inserted over a guide-wire to position the tip of the dilator in the superior caval vein. The wire is replaced with the trans-septal needle with its tip still sheathed in the

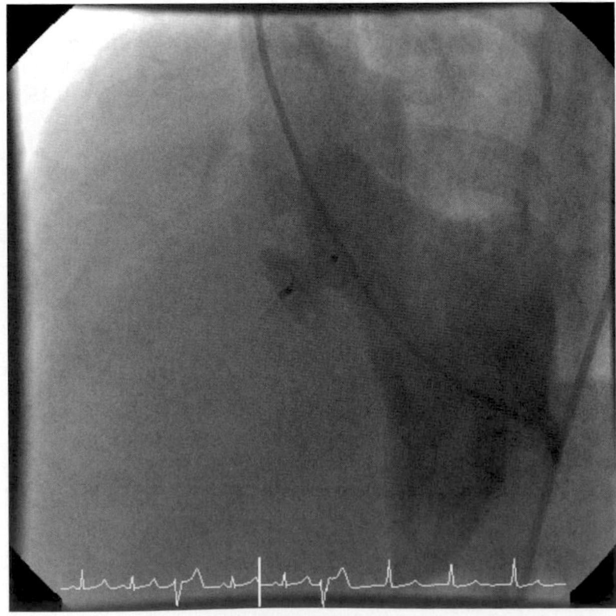

Figure 17-11 Closure of muscular ventricular septal defect with the Amplatz muscular septal occluder. Long axial oblique projection, left ventricular angiography shows no residual shunt.

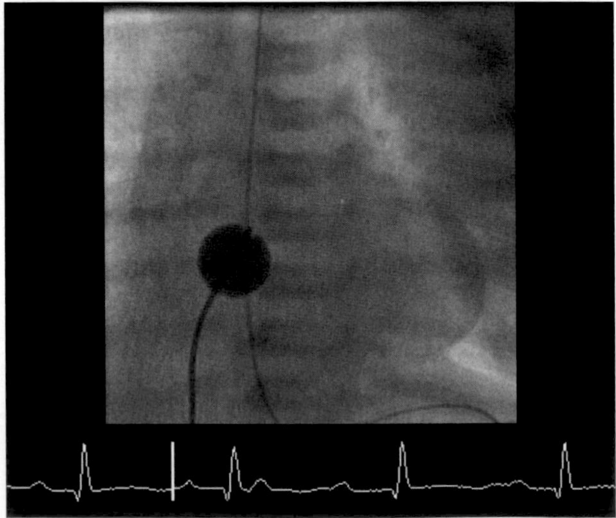

Figure 17-12 Balloon atrial septostomy by the pull-back technique. The balloon, filled with contrast, is pulled back from the left to the right atrium to enlarge the atrial communication.

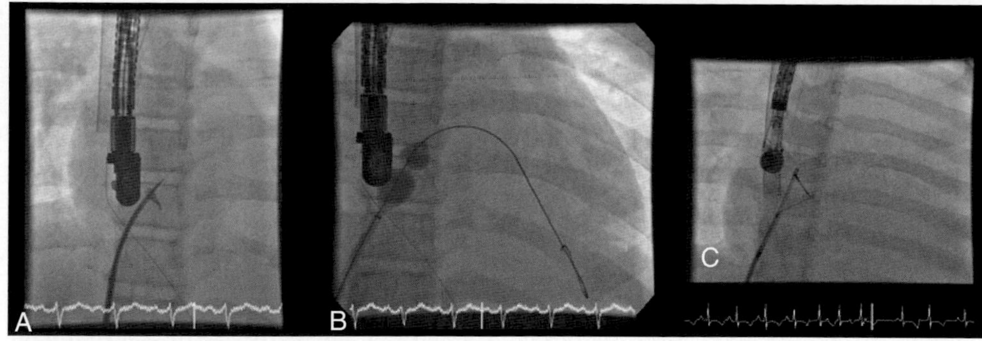

Figure 17-13 **A,** Trans-septal puncture used to decompress the left heart in a patient with dilated cardiomyopathy on extra-corporeal membrane oxygenation, illustrating fluoroscopy on frontal projection and trans-oesophageal echocardiography (probe seen). **B,** A static balloon dilation used to enlarge the atrial septal puncture. **C,** Blade atrial septostomy, with the Park blade catheter open with the blade at an angle of 45 degrees.

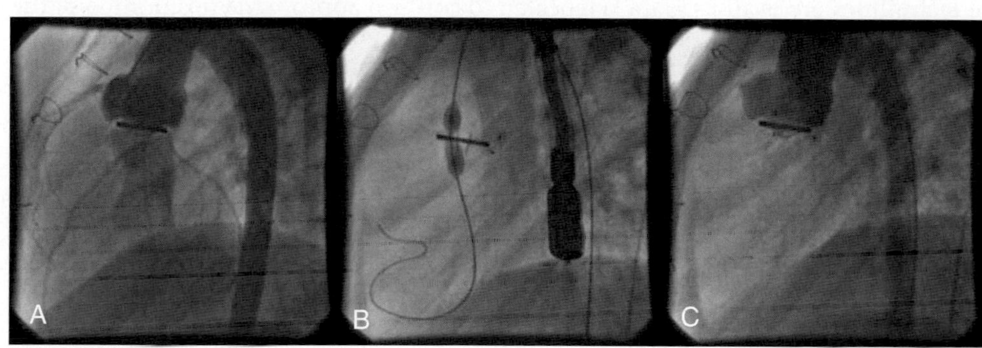

Figure 17-14 **A,** Paravalvar leak from a prosthetic aortic valve. Balloon sizing (**B**) is followed (**C**) by occlusion with the Amplatz duct occluder.

dilator. Using echocardiography and fluoroscopy in frontal and lateral projections, the whole assembly is slid down into the oval fossa, indicated by stepping over the superior limb of the margin of the oval fossa. A pigtail catheter placed in the non-coronary sinus of the aortic valve helps to identify the posterior wall of the aorta. Once the needle tip is engaged in the fossa, the septum can be stained with contrast and tented by pushing (Fig. 17-13A). A change in the waveform from right to left atrial pressure traces, injection of contrast in the left atrium, and echocardiographic and fluoroscopic guidance, all indicate entry into the left atrium. The needle should then be covered with the dilator and the sheath at all times to prevent trauma to the left atrial wall. Depending upon the indication for trans-septal puncture, the needle could be exchanged for other catheters or guide-wires. Diligent de-airing manoeuvres and anti-coagulation are required whenever operating in the left atrium and systemic circulation. Static or pull-back balloon angioplasty is then performed to create an adequate atrial communication (Fig. 17-13B). In some instances, when the atrial septum is very thick, the use of a blade catheter facilitates septostomy (Fig. 17-13C).

A newer method of creating an atrial fenestration is the use of radio-frequency wires.[86] Defects created by static balloon septoplasty, or pull-back septostomy, tend to close spontaneously within weeks or months, particularly in those with a thickened atrial septum, with a limited flap valve in the oval fossa. Various methods to keep the defect patent have been attempted, including implantation of stents and the use of fenestrated devices for atrial septal closure.[87,88]

Para-valvar Leaks

Para-valvar leaks around surgically implanted prosthetic valves in aortic or mitral position may lead to haemodynamically significant valvar regurgitation or chronic haemolysis, anaemia, and jaundice. The leaks may be single or multiple, circular or crescentic in shape, and may sometimes extend all around the circumference of the valve. Various devices have been used to close these leaks, including the Rashkind double umbrella device, the Amplatz ductal occluder, or vascular plug and coils.

For aortic para-valvar leaks, femoral arterial access is used to perform an aortogram to identify the leaks, and confirm that the origins of the coronary arteries are not in close approximation (Fig. 17-14A). The leak is crossed with an angled wire placed through a Judkins right coronary arterial catheter, and then exchanged with a stiff 0.035-inch diameter wire, which is positioned in the left ventricle. A balloon catheter is passed over the stiff wire to size the leak (Fig. 17-14B). An Amplatz ductal occluder is usually the most appropriate device for para-aortic leaks (Fig. 17-14C). The device is delivered through a long sheath. Before release, it is necessary to confirm free movement of the valvar leaflets, and unobstructed flow into the coronary arteries.

For mitral para-valvar leaks, trans-septal puncture is necessary either to cross the leak from left atrium, or to snare a guide-wire passed from the left ventricle to the left atrium through retrograde arterial access. The device is delivered through the left atrium after forming an arterio-venous loop, which is exteriorised on the venous side through the femoral or jugular vein.

EXTRACARDIAC INTERVENTIONS

Shunts

Patent Arterial Duct

Techniques for occlusion of the persistently patent arterial duct have come a long way since the first use of Ivalon plugs. The most common devices used are detachable coils for small ducts, and the Amplatz ductal occluder for larger defects. Access to the duct can be anterograde or retrograde. Use of oximetry to quantitate the shunt is not useful, and the decision for intervention relies upon echocardiography. Angiography in right anterior oblique and lateral projections profiles the length of the duct adequately. The smallest diameter along the length of the duct is used to determine suitability for interventional closure. The presence of a long restrictive duct with a good aortic ampulla is most suitable for transcatheter occlusion. Small residual leaks at the end of the procedure, particularly after occlusion with coils, close over time during follow-up.

Ducts that are less than 3 mm diameter in infants and young children, and less than 5 mm in older children, may be closed with a coil. Multiple techniques are available for use in older patients. Various coils are available depending on the diameter of the wire, the diameter of the coil when formed, and the length of the coil. Delivery of the coil can be achieved by pushing it out of the catheter with a guide-wire, as with the Gianturco system, or by using the delivery cable to which they are screwed, as with the Flipper device. The diameter of the coil should be twice the smallest diameter of the duct. Retrograde delivery is performed with the use of small catheters, with not more than three-quarters of the coil loop on the pulmonary arterial side, and the remaining loops within the aortic ampulla. No part of the loop should be hanging in the aortic lumen. Care is also taken to avoid overhanging of the origin of the left pulmonary artery, particularly in young infants (Fig. 17-15).

The most common device used for closing larger ducts, those greater than 4 mm diameter, is the Amplatz ductal occluder, made of Nitinol wire woven into a cylindrical shape with a retention disc 4 mm larger than the diameter of the device. It is available in different sizes based on the diameter of the cylindrical occluding parts at the aortic and pulmonary ends, respectively. Delivery of the device is through a long sheath with a delivery cable, which has a male end screwed on to the female thread that is welded to the pulmonary arterial end of the device. Due to this arrangement, delivery of this device is always anterograde with venous access. Arterial access is also used to perform aortography before and after closure. The device is deployed under fluoroscopy, with the aortic retention disc in the descending aorta. The assembly, including the sheath, the delivery cable and the device, are pulled back as one unit to engage the device into the aortic ampulla. The tracheal air column, and the tugging sensation experienced during delivery, provide useful landmarks for optimal delivery and positioning within the duct. The sheath is then pulled back over the device to release it across the narrowest diameter of the duct with a slight tension on the cable. An aortogram is repeated to confirm appropriate positioning of the device, and to rule out aortic or pulmonary arterial obstruction. (Fig. 17-16). It is common to have some contrast go through the device. If the position is not satisfactory, it is possible to retrieve the device into the sheath, and either redeploy or replace it with a device of more appropriate size. Angled devices, with a concave aortic rim at an angle to the occluding part, designed to prevent protrusion into the aortic lumen, may reduce the risk of aortic obstruction.[89] Multiple coils delivered with snares or bioptomes have been used in ducts of moderate size.[90]

Risks of this procedure are low in older infants and children. Residual leaks, haemolysis, or obstruction of a pulmonary artery or the aorta may occur when either coils or the ductal occluder are used. Embolisation to the pulmonary or systemic circulation can occur if the ducts are not sized appropriately. Removal of the device can be achieved by using a snare inserted through a long sheath. Late dislodgement and migration are rare. Should they occur, then surgical removal is needed. There have been no well-designed trials, to date, truly comparing the outcome of various devices.

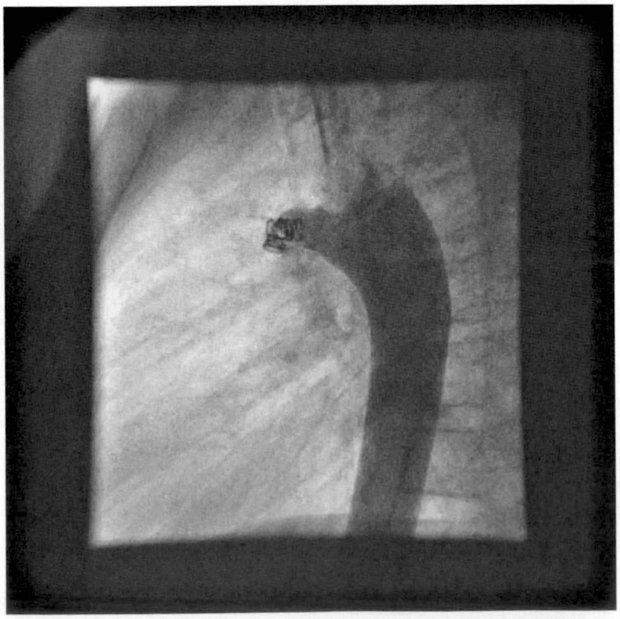

Figure 17-15 Occlusion of a patent arterial duct with multiple coils.

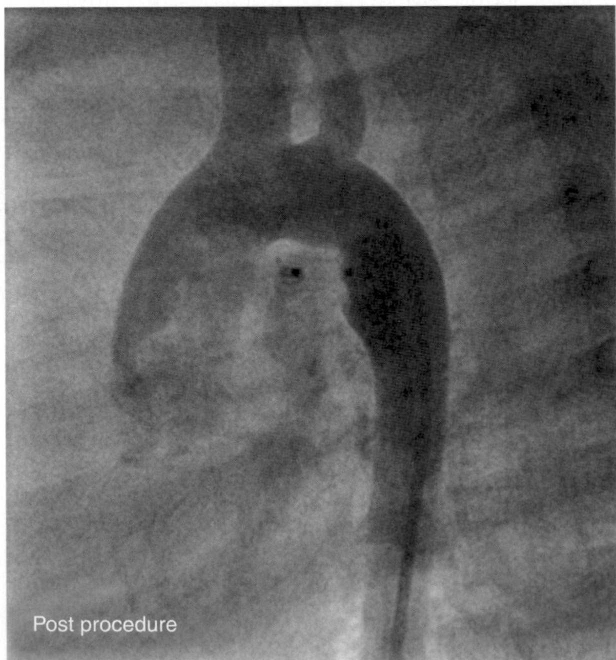

Figure 17-16 The Amplatz duct occluder has been used to close a moderate sized duct. The aortogram in lateral projection shows minimal residual flow through the device.

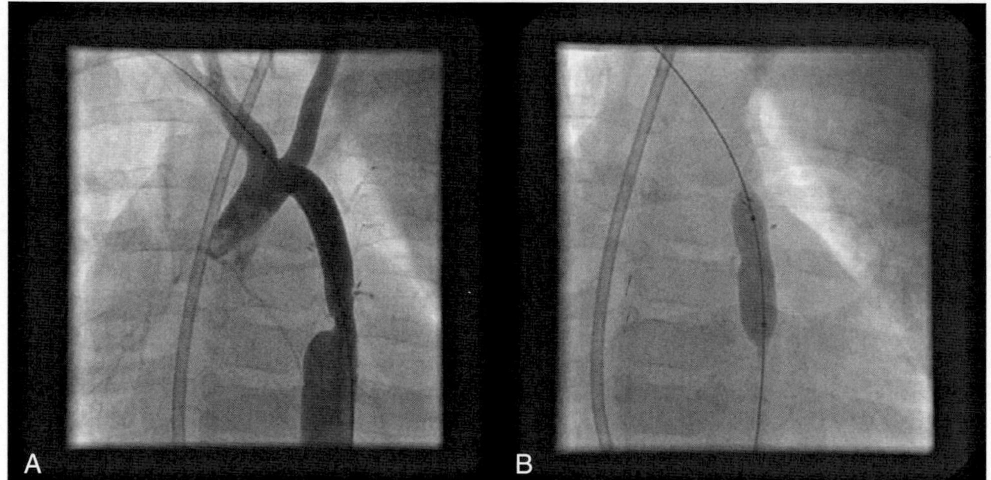

Figure 17-17 Balloon angioplasty of recoarctation. **A,** The lateral projection of the aortogram shows stenosis after a subclavian flap surgical angioplasty for coarctation. **B,** The result of balloon angioplasty, with abolition of the waist.

Aorto-pulmonary Window

The closure of small aorto-pulmonary defects was successfully attempted with the Rashkind double umbrella device.[91] The Amplatz group of occluders have also been used to close aorto-pulmonary windows, either as the primary procedure or to close residual defects after surgery.[92,93]

Arterial and Venous Obstructions

Coarctation of the Aorta

Balloon Angioplasty

Experimental angioplasty by Lock and his colleagues[10] heralded the clinical application of this technique for coarctation, while the technique first described by Singer and colleagues[94] is a widely accepted treatment for recoarctation, although a controversial treatment of native coarctation.

The procedure is performed under general anaesthesia. A haemodynamic assessment of the lesion is made through femoral access using a Multitrack catheter over a guide-wire placed in the left or right subclavian artery or within the left ventricle. Angiography is performed to measure the diameter and length of the stenosis, the proximal and distal segment of the aorta, to determine the size of the balloon, and identify presence of aneurysms from previous surgical repair. The size of the balloon is chosen to equal the proximal transverse arch, or a size is chosen not greater than three times the size of the lesion, but less than the diameter of the descending aorta at its position close to the diaphragm (Figs. 17-17 and 17-18). The Multitrack system is versatile enough to allow all procedures subsequent to dilation, avoiding recrossing of the freshly dilated site with a wire or a catheter. Risks of the procedure, particularly for those with native coarctation, include rupture of the aorta and aneurysmal formation. Presence of postoperative scar tissue makes the aorta less susceptible to disruption.

Early results of balloon angioplasty for native coarctation in infants as a temporising measure before definitive surgical intervention have been encouraging. Effective short-term palliation was reported in nine-tenths of infants less than 3 months of age, albeit that half developed recoarctation during follow-up, and required repeated intervention or surgery.[95] Balloon angioplasty has been shown to be as successful as surgery for native coarctation in selected children and adults, but for recoarctation, balloon angioplasty was more successful in children than in adults.[96]

Stent Angioplasty

The advent of stent angioplasty has challenged the usefulness of balloon angioplasty in coarctation of the aorta. Stent angioplasty is performed for both native and recoarctation of the aorta, predominantly in older patients. Its use in infants and young children is limited by the size of stents available, and their lack of growth, albeit that stent angioplasty has been used for obstruction of the arch after the Norwood operation for hypoplastic left heart syndrome[97] (Fig. 17-19). Stents provide a more effective relief of stenosis, reduce the risk of restenosis, injury to the aortic wall, and aneurysmal formation.[98] The size of the balloon is chosen using the same principles as applied for standard angioplasty, and the length of the stent is determined by the length of the stenosis. Stents should be long enough to cover the stenotic segment, extending at least

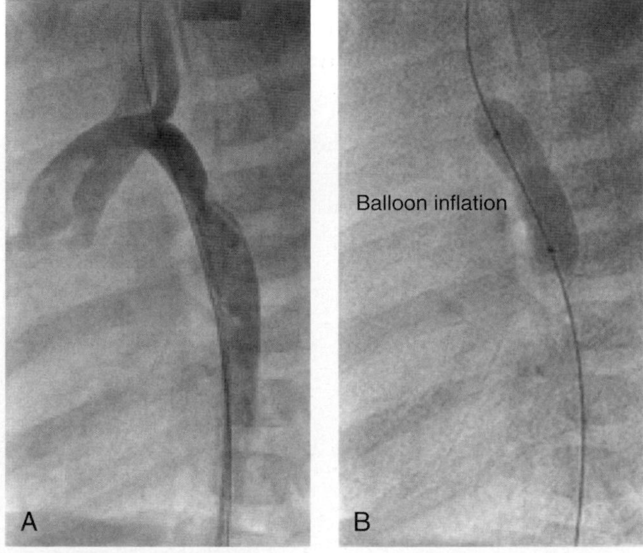

Figure 17-18 The lateral projection of an aortogram showing (**A**) recoarctation after end-to-end anastomosis for aortic coarctation, (**B**) relieved by balloon angioplasty.

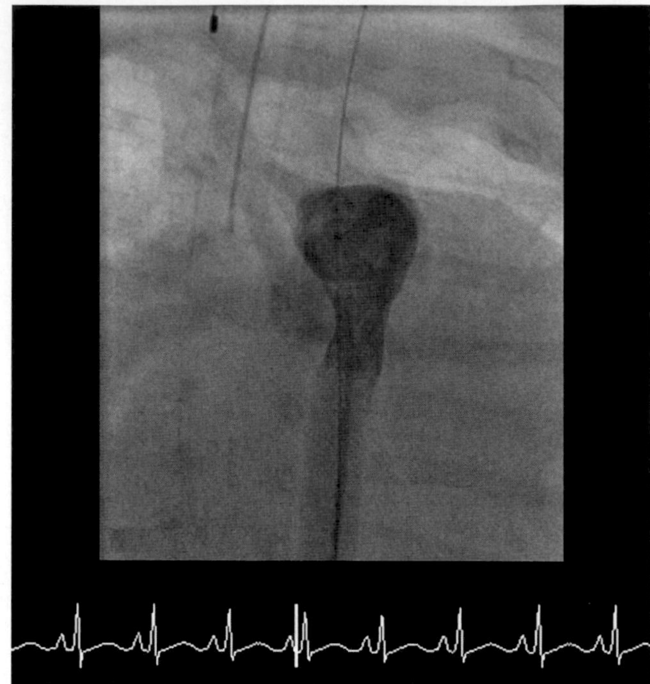

Figure 17-19 Stent angioplasty for recoarctation after Norwood operation in frontal projection aortography.

15 mm beyond the stenosis, without covering the origins of the arterial branches arising from the aortic arch. Various stents of different designs are currently available for use in the aorta, including the Palmaz, Cheatham-Platinum, and Intrastent variants.

Insertion of the stents has produced satisfactory relief of the gradient across the stenosis, with increase in the diameter of the coarcted segment, and with only minor complications.[99] Some have reported aneurysmal formation,[100] while others have noted greater reduction in gradient, lower residual gradients, and a larger diameter of the coarcted segment when comparing stent angioplasty with balloon angioplasty.[101] Use of balloon-in-balloon catheters (Fig. 17-20), graded dilation, and right ventricular pacing (Fig. 17-21) at the time of implantation, has reduced the rate of complications. Covered stents (Fig. 17-22) used for complex coarctation and near-atretic lesions have reduced the consequences of dissection or rupture. The use of polytetrafluoroethylene-coated Cheatham platinum stents has also significantly reduced the systolic gradient across the coarctation, and increased the diameter of the coarctation.[102] Despite advances in techniques, and availability of covered stents, the risk of aortic rupture, dissection, and aneurysmal formation may never be completely abolished.

Pulmonary Arterial Stenosis

Pulmonary arterial stenosis may be caused by postsurgical scarring after palliation or repair of congenitally malformed hearts, as in tetralogy of Fallot, a distally migrated pulmonary arterial band, or after the LeCompte manoeuvre as part of an arterial switch operation. Arteriopathy related to genetic factors include elastin gene mutations in Williams syndrome, Alagille syndrome, and congenital rubella syndrome, and tend to be more widespread and associated with diffuse hypoplasia of the pulmonary arterial tree. Pulmonary arterial hypoplasia due to diminished flow necessitates surgery, involving either a systemic-to-pulmonary arterial shunt or a patch across the right ventricular outflow tract extending onto the pulmonary arteries. Extension of ductal tissue to a pulmonary artery may also cause constriction in postnatal life, needing augmentation with a patch. The risk of restenosis remains high. Palliative surgery leading to a Fontan circulation often involves multiple interventions on the pulmonary arteries.

Pulmonary Arterial Balloon Angioplasty

Indications for angioplasty when the right ventricular pressures are normal or only mildly elevated are controversial. In infants and children, however, significantly diminished perfusion to one lung in spite of a normal right ventricular pressure is an accepted indication for intervention. More aggression may be needed in patients requiring staged palliation culminating in Fontan circulation in order to have good sized pulmonary arteries despite small gradients. Overall, accepted indications for balloon angioplasty include right ventricular hypertension, right ventricular dysfunction, perfusion mismatch, with less than one-quarter of flow directed to one lung, pulmonary hypertension in the unaffected lung, or presence of severe pulmonary regurgitation.[103]

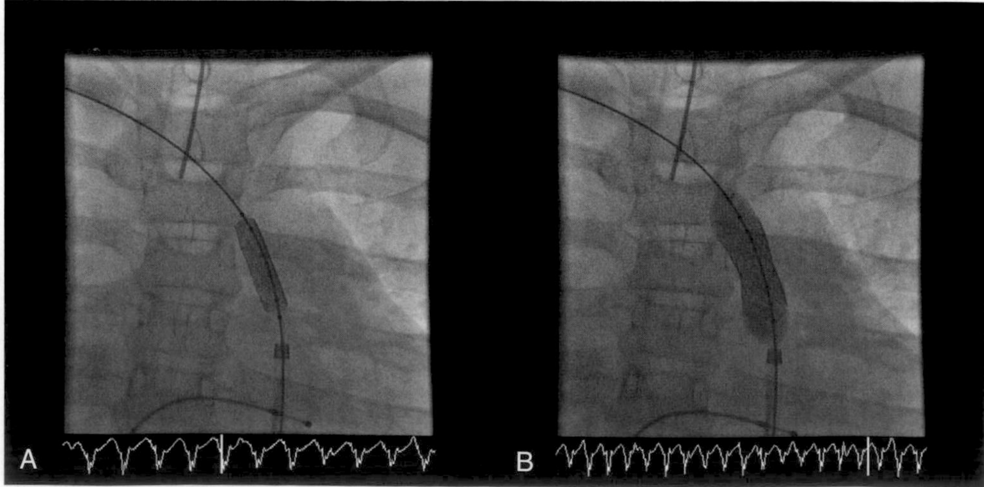

Figure 17-20 Balloon-in-balloon catheter used for stent angioplasty with (A) the inner balloon inflated first and (B) the outer balloon inflated to deploy the stent.

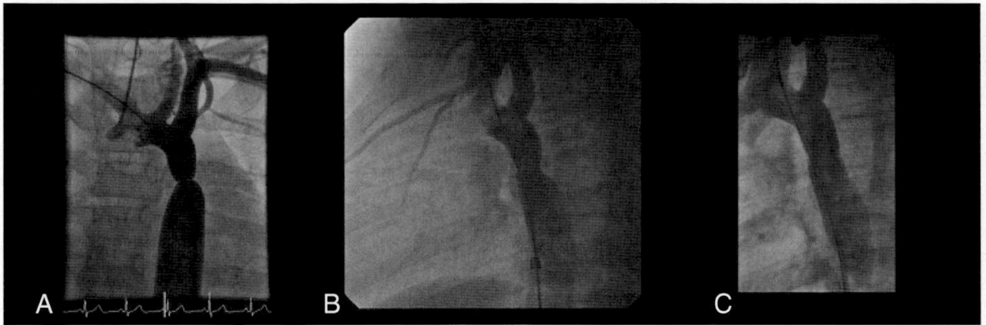

Figure 17-21 Stent angioplasty of native coarctation. **A,** Native coarctation of aorta, treated by graded dilation with stent angioplasty (**B** and **C**) to reduce the risk of aortic dissection or aneurysmal formation.

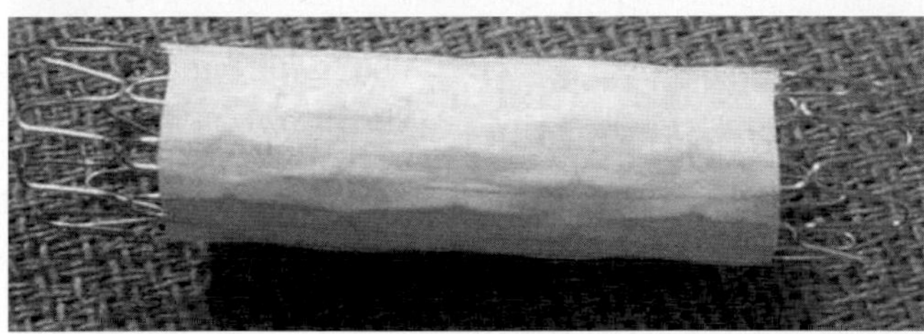

Figure 17-22 The covered Cheatham Platinum stent. (Reproduced with permission from Seivert H, Qureshi SA, Wilson N, Hijazi ZM [eds]: Percutaneous Interventions for Congenital Heart Disease. London: Informa Healthcare, 2007, Figure 53.1.)

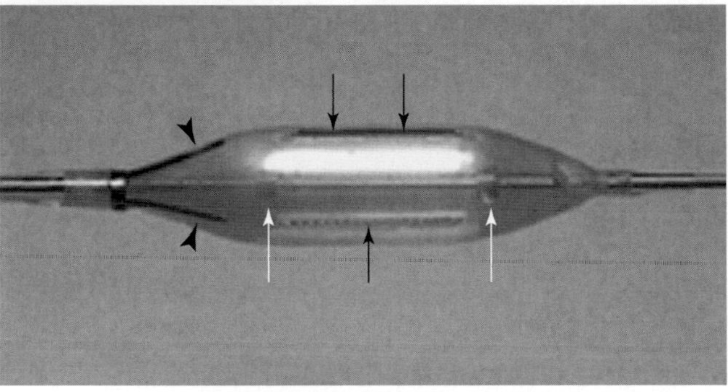

Figure 17-23 A cutting balloon with microtome blades. (Reproduced from Engelke C, Sandhu C, Morgan RA, Belli AM: Using 6-mm Cutting Balloon angioplasty in patients with resistant peripheral artery stenosis: Preliminary results. Am J Roentgenol AJR 2002;179:619–623. Copyright of American Roetgen Ray Society.)

The basic principles of balloon angioplasty are applied. After haemodynamic stabilisation, a stiff wire position is achieved in a good distal vessel of the lung. Angiography is performed and the size and length of stenosis are measured. The Multitrack catheter is useful for multiple haemodynamic measurements and performing angiography. The diameter of the balloon is determined by the diameter of a normal vessel adjacent to the stenosis. A higher ratio of balloon-to-stenosis diameter increases the chance of success, but also the risk of dissection, rupture, or aneurysmal formation. The success rate in one series was higher when the diameter of the balloon was more than 3 times the diameter of the stenosis, with a significantly greater diameter achieved after the procedure.[104] Outcome is assessed by an increase in the diameter by more than half, a reduction of the ratio of right ventricular to systemic arterial pressures, or by assessment of distribution of perfusion to the lungs.

Complications are more frequent after dilation of tight stenoses requiring oversized balloons and high pressures of inflation. Stenoses were impossible to dilate in half the patients on one series, with recurrent stenoses occurring in up to one-third.[105] The Valvuloplasty and Angioplasty registry documents an incidence of complications on one-eighth of patients, including rupture of vessels and death. Success has been achieved in two-thirds of patients unresponsive to conventional angioplasty by using high-pressure balloons.[34] Trauma can also be produced to the pulmonary arteries, usually with the tear occurring distal to the area of the stenosis.[106] Pulmonary hypertension was found to be a significant risk factor for such trauma.

Cutting balloons, as produced by Boston Scientific (Fig. 17-23), and used successfully in resistant coronary and peripheral arterial lesions, are now being used for resistant stenotic lesions in the pulmonary arteries that are undilatable even at high pressures. The balloon has three or four microtome blades, attached along the length of the balloon, that protrude on inflation to create controlled cuts on the walls of the stenosed vessels. On deflation, the balloon folds over the blades. Early results in lesions resistant to conventional balloon angioplasty have been encouraging.[107,108] Overall, cutting balloons improve the gain in luminal diameter, albeit with a slight increased risk of vascular trauma.

Pulmonary Arterial Stenting

Endovascular stenting has been increasingly used in older patients, and in haemodynamically significant stenosis in infants and young children. Stents are particularly effective in abolishing stenosis that reappears after successful balloon angioplasty due to elastic recoil and for dynamic stenosis related to folds and kinks in surgically repaired pulmonary arteries.[109]

Stenting of complex stenoses involving the pulmonary arterial bifurcation remains a challenging procedure (Fig. 17-24). Due to close proximity of the origins of the right and left pulmonary arteries, it is advisable to deploy stents simultaneously into both arteries. In patients who have undergone the LeCompte manoeuvre as part of the arterial switch operation, the pulmonary arterial bifurcation lies anterior to the ascending aorta. Coronary arteries that have been transferred during arterial switch may be in close proximity to the site of implantation of stents, and the risk of arterial occlusion should be considered.

Systemic Venous or Baffle Stenosis

Stenosis of major systemic veins, such as the superior or inferior caval vein, may be seen after injury due to cannulation in neonates or infants undergoing cardiopulmonary bypass. Systemic venous baffles constructed surgically to redirect systemic venous flow for repair of complex congenital heart disease may also develop obstruction

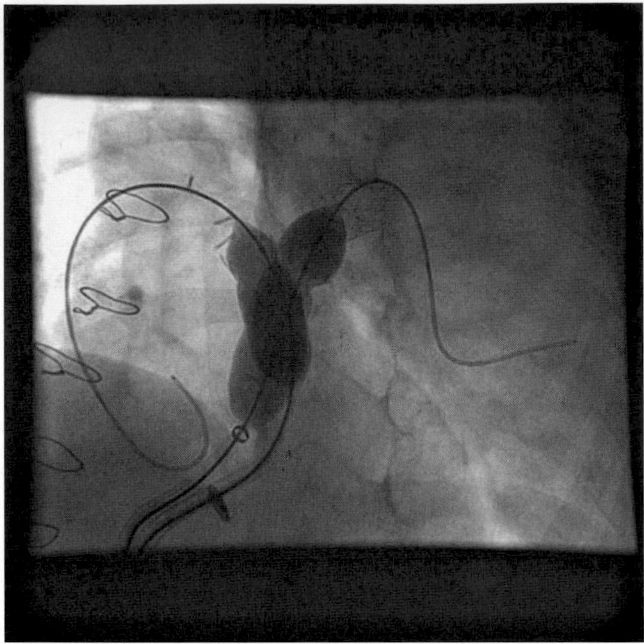

Figure 17-24 Bilateral pulmonary arterial stenting for stenosis at the bifurcation of the pulmonary trunk. Simultaneous inflation of balloons in both pulmonary arteries. The left anterior oblique projection with a cranial tilt profiles well the pulmonary arterial bifurcation.

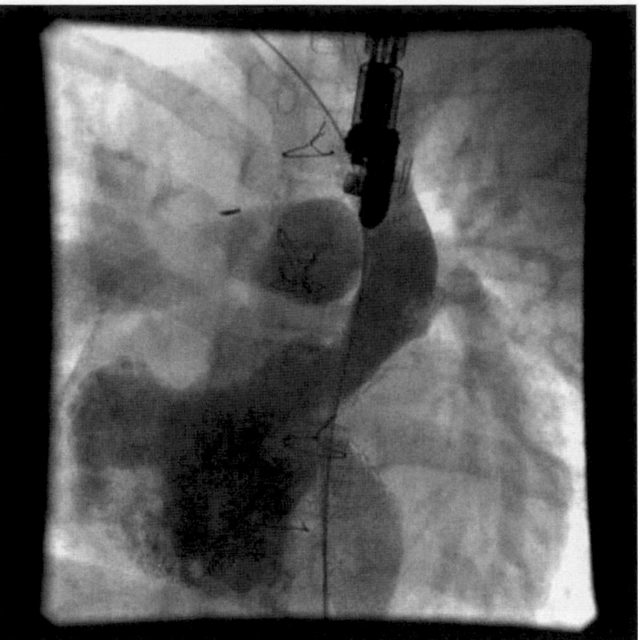

Figure 17-25 Systemic venous obstruction, with stents implanted in the obstructed superior and inferior caval pathways in a patient with a Mustard procedure.

during late follow-up. Systemic venous connections to the pulmonary circulation, which are direct, such as a superior cavopulmonary anastomosis, or through a conduit, as in the inferior cavopulmonary anastomosis, may develop stenosis with important consequences. With the advent of the arterial switch operation, the use of intra-atrial baffles for redirection of systemic veins is now used for treatment of complex lesions with abnormal systemic venous drainage in the context of isomerism, or with the double-switch operation for those with congenitally corrected transposition. The long-term survivors of Mustard and Senning operations, nonetheless, are now seen in the clinics for adults with congenital heart disease, and this intervention may be most often required in this population. Obstruction of the superior or inferior caval venous pathway may remain silent, with formation of collateral venous channels, and only be detected during routine investigations, or during placement of the permanent pacemaker because of sinus nodal dysfunction. Similarly, presence of collateral circulation may mask any pressure gradients in systemic venous baffles or conduits.

Obstruction to systemic venous drainage can be treated with balloon dilation as a palliative measure in young infants or children, or with stenting for older patients, with good long-term outcome. Angiography to delineate the stenosis is a very important step in planning the treatment. If stenosis is severe, access may be required from both ends with cannulation of femoral and jugular veins. Very thin wires may be used to cross the lesion. If there is atresia, the Brockenbrough needle may have to be used. Long sheaths are then used to cross the stenotic segment and an appropriate stent is deployed. Balloon expandable (Fig. 17-25) and self-expanding stents have also been successfully used to relieve obstruction, with good long-term results.[110–112] Transvenous pacing has also been successfully achieved through the stents.

Pulmonary Venous Stenosis

Pulmonary venous stenosis can be isolated, or can follow repair of anomalous pulmonary venous drainage, with or without other congenital cardiac disease. There has been an increasing awareness of the condition as an isolated entity, particularly, in premature infants. In infants and children, pulmonary hypertension and right-sided cardiac failure manifest over time. In adults, the aetiology may be compression by a mediastinal or pulmonary malignant neoplasm, or following interventional or surgical treatment of atrial arrhythmia. In both the congenital and acquired forms of pulmonary venous stenosis, histological findings show neo-intimal proliferation leading to occlusion of the lumen of one or more pulmonary veins.

Angioplasty and stenting of pulmonary veins are increasingly performed to treat this difficult disease. Access to the pulmonary vein is through the patent oval foramen or after trans-septal atrial puncture. A guide catheter is commonly used over a 0.014-inch coronary arterial wire if a coronary arterial or a cutting balloon is used. Angioplasty with a cutting balloon is usually followed by conventional balloon angioplasty, with or without stenting. Anti-coagulation is used during follow-up to prevent in-stent thrombosis. Failure of angioplasty, and occurrence of in-stent stenosis after stent angioplasty, are probably explained by the progressive neo-intimal proliferation.[113] Cutting balloons have been used with encouraging results, albeit that the disease substrate is progressive, and long-term benefit remains unknown.[114] Drug-eluting stents, and concomitant use of oral agents such as sirolimus, are being used to treat this fascinating and frustrating disease.[115] Intrastent sonotherapy has been used to treat restenosis.[116]

Stenting of the Arterial Duct

Stenting of arterial duct for duct-dependent systemic and pulmonary circulations has made a resurgence with improvements in technology and advances in interventional

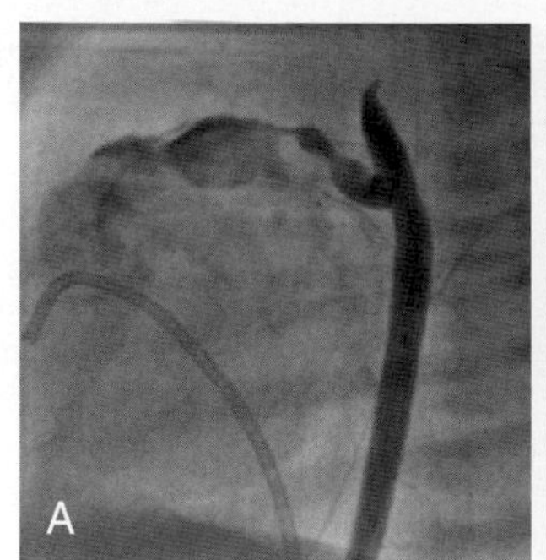

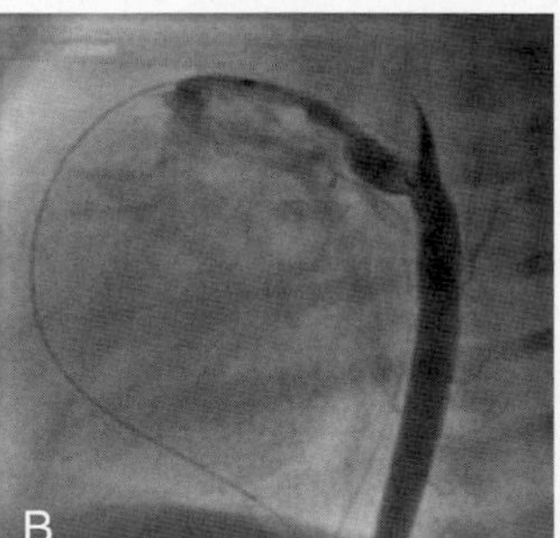

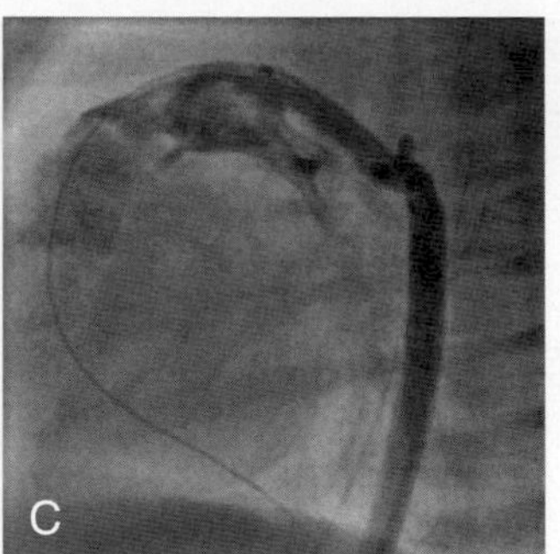

Figure 17-26 Ductal stenting in a patient with pulmonary atresia, intact ventricular septum. **A,** The lateral projection of the aortogram outlines the restrictive arterial duct. **B,** The stent is positioned in the arterial duct from the pulmonary artery with check aortography. **C,** There is good flow through the duct after implantation.

catheterisation. Patients with pulmonary atresia and intact ventricular septum amenable to transcatheter perforation of atretic pulmonary valve may need augmentation of pulmonary flow until right ventricular diastolic function, and hence filling, improves and effective forward flow can be established across the pulmonary valve. Ductal stenting as a part of hybrid procedure in hypoplastic left heart syndrome is based on similar principles. The most commonly used stents are pre-mounted coronary arterial stents 3 to 4 mm diameter, and 12 to 24 mm in length. Based on previous surgical experience, the diameter of the ductal stent is chosen to be smaller than that of a comparable modified Blalock shunt suitable for the weight of the patient. The small diameter of the stent reduces the risk of pulmonary over-perfusion.

The procedure is performed under general anaesthesia. The duct needs to constrict in order to provide a good grip on the stent, and this may require cessation of prostaglandin for at least 6 hours prior to procedure. Venous access is employed for delivery of the stent, and arterial access for angiography and monitoring of arterial pressures. Aortography is performed to identify ductal morphology, noting its diameter and length, and to identify landmarks for implantation of the stent (Fig. 17-26). A coronary arterial guide-wire is passed through the duct, and the stent is delivered through a coronary guide catheter, or directly over the wire. Angiography is performed from the aorta, or through the coronary guide catheter, to confirm a satisfactory position of the duct. The length of the stent is usually 1 to 2 mm longer than the ductal length, so as to cover the pulmonary arterial end of the duct. Compression of the origin of the pulmonary arteries, and protrusion of the stent into the descending aorta, are diligently avoided. After deployment, aortography confirms the adequate patency of the duct and the stent. Prostaglandin is then discontinued, and the patient is commenced on an anti-platelet dose of aspirin. Risks associated with stenting of the arterial duct include thrombosis and intimal proliferation, occasionally requiring redilation.[117,118]

Removal of Foreign Bodies or Devices from the Circulation

With the widespread use of in-dwelling central venous catheters for chemotherapy, hyperalimentation, and monitoring, and the use of coils and other devices for occlusion, removal of embolised foreign bodies in the central and peripheral circulation is not infrequently performed in the catheterisation laboratory. Most of the foreign bodies and devices are radio-opaque in parts, if not in their entirety, and can be easily identified on radiography. Various devices based on those used in urological practice have been used for retrieval. Depending upon the location of the foreign body to be retrieved, access is achieved in arterial or venous circulation. Usually, two routes are used for access, one with the device, and the other for multiple angiograms to assess proximity to the foreign body.

Snares are the most versatile and commonly used devices. They function like a lasso, encircling and tightening around the object to be retrieved. The snare is delivered through a large sheath to the reach the foreign body. Once snared, the foreign body is pulled into the sheath, and removed from the circulation.

Basket devices were designed for removal of biliary and renal stones. They are made of multiples wires arranged to protrude in different directions, and then converge to form a basket which can hold devices. They can be used to retrieve larger foreign bodies that can be compressed, and may need larger bore sheaths. Forceps, either specifically designed for retrieval or those used for endomyocardial biopsy, have also been used.[119] The risk of vascular trauma during retrieval should be borne in mind and surgical removal of a foreign body considered if interventional techniques fail.

INTERVENTIONS ON SURGICAL AND OTHER NATURALLY OCCURRING ABNORMAL PATHWAYS

Coils and devices made of Nitinol have been used to occlude other structures with abnormal vascular communications, including systemic or pulmonary arterio-venous fistulas, veno-venous (Fig. 17-27) or veno-arterial communications,[120] aorto-pulmonary shunts, and systemic-to-pulmonary collateral arteries (Fig. 17-28).[121,122] Closure of surgically created fenestrations in the Fontan circulation can be successfully performed with a wide variety of devices. The Amplatz atrial septal occluder (Fig. 17-29) and Helex (Fig. 17-30) are the most commonly used.[123,124] A careful haemodynamic assessment should be performed before occluding the fenestration. A test occlusion of the fenestration with a balloon catheter, with a subsequent rise in systemic arterial saturations, should be performed. Measurement of systemic venous saturations to assess the arterio-venous oxygen difference serves as a surrogate for the cardiac output. An increase of more than 16 mm Hg, a significant decrease in the cardiac output after test occlusion of the fenestration, or presence of protein losing enteropathy, are contraindications to closure of fenestration.

Conduits of different types are commonly used to repair complex congenital cardiac disease. Biological valved conduits

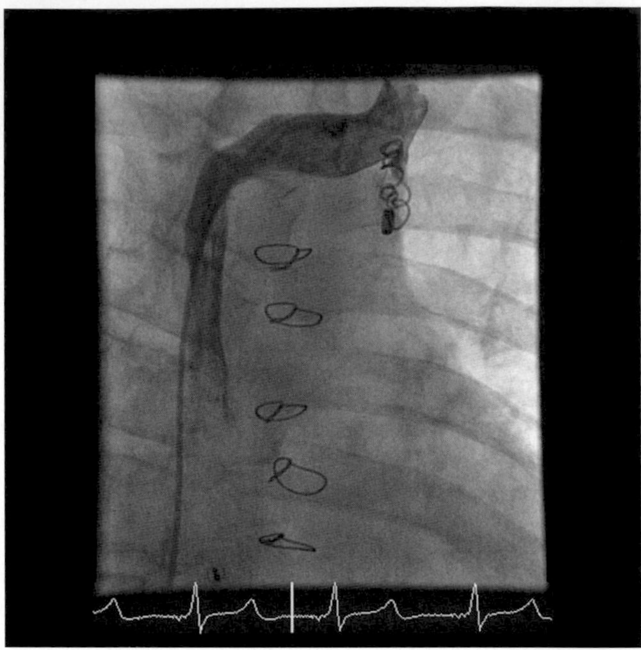

Figure 17-27 Occlusion of a systemic-to-pulmonary venous collateral vessel in the Fontan circulation to reduce systemic arterial de-saturation.

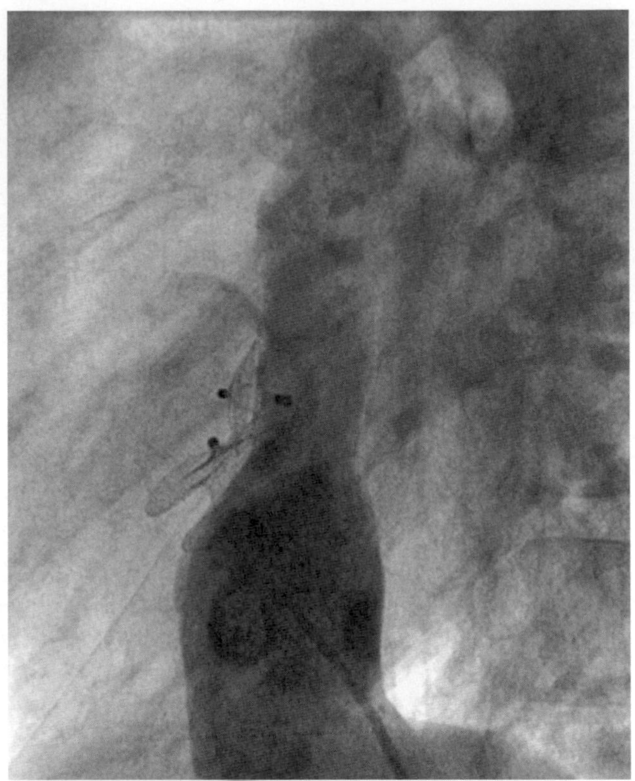

Figure 17-29 Closure of a Fontan fenestration and a baffle leak using Amplatz atrial septal occluders.

or tubes have been used to establish continuity between the right ventricle and pulmonary arteries during both definitive repairs and palliative surgery. Obstruction of the conduit may result from external anatomical constraints, twists and folds within the tubes, or degeneration with calcification. Balloon dilation usually provides only transient relief of obstruction[125] and implantation of stents is commonly used to palliate or prolong the life of the conduit,[126] especially after calcification and obstruction resulting in right ventricular hypertension. Coronary arterial stents have been used to improve flow of blood to the lungs after Norwood palliation for hypoplastic left heart syndrome. Interventional procedures on systemic-to-pulmonary conduits providing obligatory pulmonary blood flow have a high risk of morbidity and mortality. Obstructions to anastomosis of conduits involving the pulmonary bifurcation are also difficult to treat.[127]

Steps involved in stenting of conduits include assessment of the size of the conduit, selection of the balloon and stent, use of stiff exchange-length guide-wires to provide strong support to the long sheaths used to deliver the stents, and the use of high-pressure balloons for rigid conduits. The advent of balloon-in-balloon catheters has facilitated positioning of the stents. High-pressure balloons requiring 10 to 12 atmospheres, with the use of indeflators, are effective in dilating rigid calcified homografts. Pre-dilation

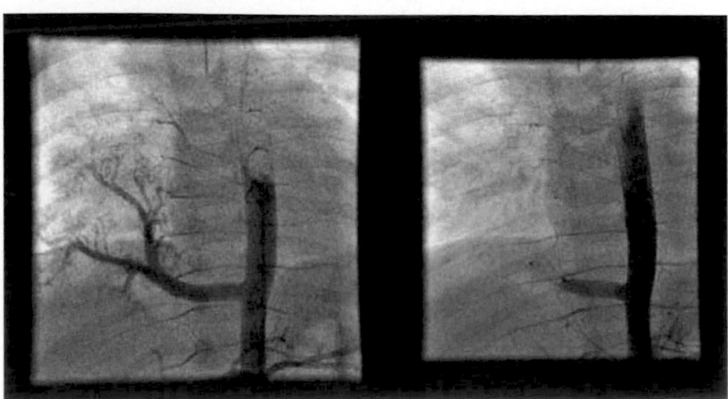

Figure 17-28 Occlusion of a systemic-to-pulmonary collateral artery from the descending aorta with an Amplatz duct occluder.

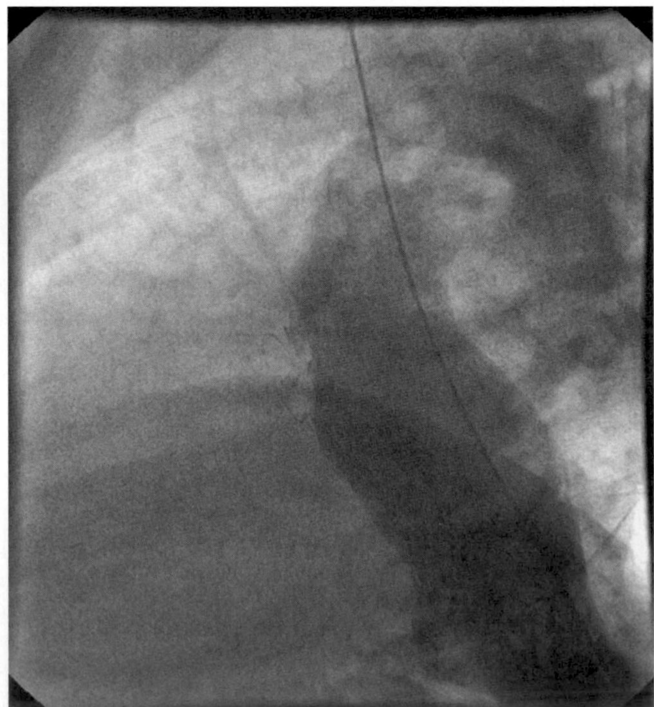

Figure 17-30 A Helex device is inserted in an intracardiac conduit providing a total cavopulmonary connection, completely occluding a fenestration.

of the conduit may be necessary in the setting of tight stenosis to facilitate delivery of the long sheath beyond the site of implantation.

Complications include embolisation, dissection, or rupture of conduits with bleeding, coronary arterial compression with myocardial ischaemia or tricuspid regurgitation.[128] Free pulmonary regurgitation is an expected consequence of dilating conduits placed from the right ventricle to the pulmonary arteries, which may prove deleterious in the long-term. Insertion of valved stents may help avoid this complication in the future.

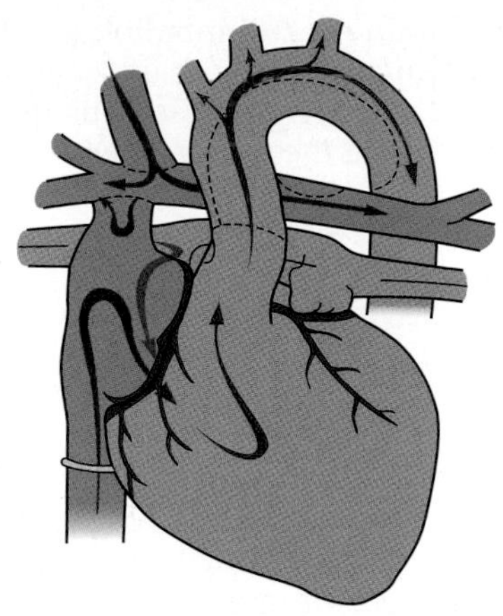

Figure 17-32 Illustration of a Comprehensive Stage 2 procedure to facilitate transcatheter completion of the Fontan circulation. (Reproduced with permission from Seivert H, Qureshi SA, Wilson N, Hijazi ZM (eds): Percutaneous Interventions for Congenital Heart Disease. London: Informa Healthcare, 2007, Figure 59.11.)

HYBRID PROCEDURES: COLLABORATION BETWEEN THE SURGEON AND THE INTERVENTIONIST

Treatment of complex congenital cardiac diseases has traditionally required close collaboration between the cardiologists and cardiac surgeons. A new relationship between the interventional cardiologist and the cardiac surgeon has led to the development of combined transcatheter and surgical therapeutic options, now called the hybrid approach. This involves complementary interventions by the interventional cardiologist and the cardiac surgeon. The principle of this approach came from treatment of hypoplastic left heart syndrome, stenting the arterial duct and performing balloon atrial septostomy or surgical septectomy, combined with bilateral banding of the pulmonary arteries to provide initial short-term palliation.[129] This hybrid approach has now been used in a systematic and reproducible manner for patients with hypoplastic left heart syndrome,[130] and the technique extended to develop truly hybrid suites in which both the interventional cardiologist and surgeons can operate together[131] (Figs. 17-31 and 17-32). A similar combined approach has been applied in closure of muscular ventricular defects.[132] The closure of single or multiple defects in the apical part of the muscular septum, which are difficult to reach through the tricuspid valve, or require a ventriculotomy, may be closed using the periventricular approach or with intra-operative interventional closure using the Amplatz muscular septal occluder. Echocardiography is extremely important to guide the operator in identifying the defects and deploying the device. The periventricular closure is performed after a median sternotomy and a right ventricular free wall needle puncture to insert a short sheath and guide-wire, into the left ventricle through the defect. Extreme caution needs to be exercised to prevent the dilator of the sheath perforating the posterior wall of the left ventricle. This part of the procedure, therefore, is performed under continuous echocardiographic guidance. An Amplatz muscular septal occluder is then deployed through the sheath in the standard fashion with echocardiographic visualisation. Meticulous de-airing and flushing of the system should be carried out throughout the procedure.

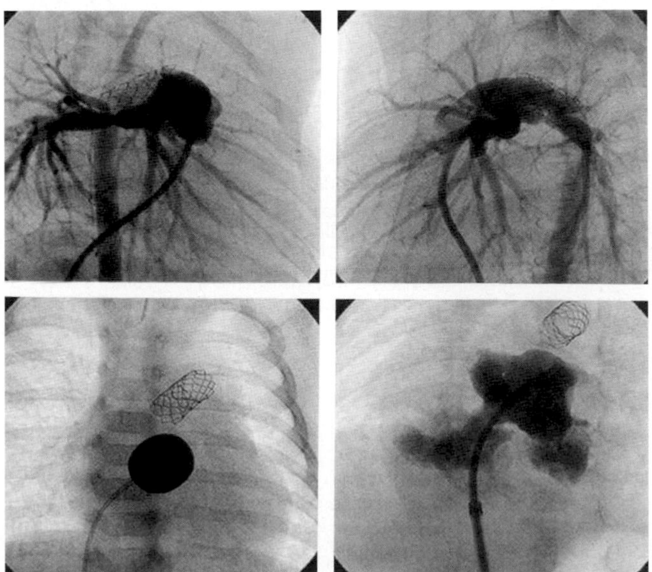

Figure 17-31 The Hybrid Norwood procedure. A ductal stent is combined with bilateral pulmonary arterial banding and balloon atrial septostomy. (Reproduced with permission from Seivert H, Qureshi SA, Wilson N, Hijazi ZM (eds): Percutaneous Interventions for Congenital Heart Disease. London: Informa Healthcare, 2007, Figure 59.8.)

Intraoperative stenting of pulmonary arterial branches has been used to rehabilitate severely hypoplastic or stenotic vessels during complex repairs.[133–135] Insertion of the stents under direct vision is very effective in improving the size of the pulmonary arteries, and in reducing operating time. Further interventions may be necessary to redilate the stents, or provide surgical enlargement after removal of the stents during subsequent procedures.

COMPLICATIONS OF INTERVENTIONAL CATHETERISATION

Complications of cardiac catheterisation in general such as vascular injury, bleeding, arrhythmia, thromboembolism, cardiac perforation, air embolism, infection, and death could occur during interventional catheterisation. The use of large sheaths, stiff wires, large devices, and high-pressure balloon inflations all add to the standard risk.

The use of various new devices and procedures, even in the hands of experienced operators, contribute to the problems seen during the learning curve. Appropriate training, use of simulation software modules, and peer-to-peer hands-on training have made a significant contribution towards reducing these problems.

Balloons can rupture at full inflation at a high pressure, or due to disruption against a sharp edge of calcium or a previously implanted stent. Meticulous de-airing should be carried out to prevent the risk of air embolism. A circumferential tear in the balloon material leads to risk of embolisation of the material into the circulation. The ruptured balloon, when removed from the patient, should always be thoroughly examined to confirm that no residual parts have remained in the circulation. Maintaining the guide-wire position is crucial in these circumstances. A large-bore long sheath and a snare are then used to remove the remnants.

Embolisation may occur during deployment of stents due to displacement over the balloon. Usually, the stent can be fixed over a partially inflated balloon, and parked in a vessel without compromising vascular supply to any vital organs. Expanded stents within cardiac chambers may need to be removed surgically.

Dislodged devices, and embolisation, are often treated with transcatheter techniques. The basic principles of retrieval of foreign bodies from the circulation are applied. The primary aim should be to avoid haemodynamic compromise and injury to cardiac structures during retrieval, rather than avoidance of surgery. Large sheaths and a variety of devices may have to be used.

Difficult catheter manipulations lead to risk of knotting of catheters within small cardiac chambers or blood vessels. It is important to avoid this complication by careful manipulation of catheters and wires, with screening at all times during difficult procedures.

Trouble-shooting for unanticipated but well-described complications should be part of the training of an interventional cardiologist. As the incidence of complications in well-established procedures is decreasing over time due to technical advances in catheter and technology, younger interventional cardiologists are less exposed to problem-solving on their feet. Prevention of complications still remains the best way of staying out of trouble during interventional catheterisation. Surgical back-up should always be available for a cauterisation laboratory undertaking complex intervention.

The complete reference list can be found on the companion Expert Consult web site at www.expertconsult.com.

ANNOTATED REFERENCES

- Rubio-Alvarez V, Limon R, Soni J: [Intracardiac valvulotomy by means of a catheter]. Arch Inst Cardiol Mex 1953;23:183–192.

  This was the first report of interventional catheterisation, marking the beginning of a new era.
- Rashkind WJ, Miller WW: Creation of an atrial septal defect without thoracotomy: A palliative approach to complete transposition of the great arteries. JAMA 1966;196:991–992.

  A landmark publication. The origins of interventional cardiology, which led from congenital cardiac disease to adult cardiology.
- Porstmann W, Wierny L, Warnke H: [The closure of the patent ductus arteriosus without thoractomy. (preliminary report)]. Thoraxchir Vask Chir 1967;15: 199–203.

  This publication closely followed that from Rashkind and his colleagues, and represented a further advance for those working in congenital cardiology and leading the interventional field.
- King TD, Mills NL: Nonoperative closure of atrial septal defects. Surgery 1974;75:383–388.

  Description of balloon-sizing and catheter closure of atrial septal defects.
- Lock JE, Niemi T, Einzig S, et al: Transvenous angioplasty of experimental branch pulmonary artery stenosis in newborn lambs. Circulation 1981;64:886–893.

  Elegant studies describing the results of balloon angioplasty.
- Kan JS, White RI Jr, Mitchell SE, Gardner TJ: Percutaneous balloon valvuloplasty: A new method for treating congenital pulmonary-valve stenosis. N Engl J Med 1982;307:540–542.

  The first report of treatment of valvar stenosis with balloon dilation.
- Mullins CE, O'Laughlin MP, Vick GW III, et al: Implantation of balloon-expandable intravascular grafts by catheterization in pulmonary arteries and systemic veins. Circulation 1988;77:188–199.

  This report marked the introduction of balloon-expandable stents for angioplasty in arterial and venous lesions, leading to still further new interventional techniques being introduced to congenital cardiology.
- Sharafuddin MJ, Gu X, Titus JL, et al: Experimental evaluation of a new self-expanding patent ductus arteriosus occluder in a canine model. J Vasc Interv Radiol 1996;7:877–887.

  The description of a versatile device used to occlude intracardiac and extracardiac shunts.
- Andersen HR, Knudsen LL, Hasenkam JM: Transluminal implantation of artificial heart valves: Description of a new expandable aortic valve and initial results with implantation by catheter technique in closed chest pigs. Eur Heart J 1992;13:704–708.

  The first study to describe the transcatheter implantation of cardiac valves.
- Akintuerk H, Michel-Behnke I, Valeske K, et al: Stenting of the arterial duct and banding of the pulmonary arteries: Basis for combined Norwood stage I and II repair in hypoplastic left heart. Circulation 2002;105:1099–1103.

  The evolution of catheter interventions to achieve early palliation for hypoplastic left heart syndrome.
- Hausdorf G, Schneider M, Konertz W: Surgical preconditioning and completion of total cavopulmonary connection by interventional cardiac catheterisation: A new concept. Heart 1996;75:403–409.

  Futuristic view of a hybrid approach, albeit at different stages, emphasising close collaboration between cardiac surgeons and cardiologists.
- Bonhoeffer P, Boudjemline Y, Saliba Z, et al: Percutaneous replacement of pulmonary valve in a right-ventricle to pulmonary-artery prosthetic conduit with valve dysfunction. Lancet 2000;356:1403–1405.

  The first report of percutaneous valve implantation in humans.
- Cribier A, Eltchaninoff H, Bash A, et al: Percutaneous transcatheter implantation of an aortic valve prosthesis for calcific aortic stenosis: First human case description. Circulation 2002;106:3006–3008.

  The first account of implantation of the aortic valve in humans.
- Gibbs JL, Wren C, Watterson KG, et al: Stenting of the arterial duct combined with banding of the pulmonary arteries and atrial septectomy or septostomy: A new approach to palliation for the hypoplastic left heart syndrome. Br Heart J 1993;69:551–555.

  This report introduced the concept of transcatheter palliation of hypoplastic left heart syndrome, and also introduced the hybrid concept.
- Galantowicz M, Cheatham JP: Lessons learned from the development of a new hybrid strategy for the management of hypoplastic left heart syndrome. Pediatr Cardiol 2005;26:190–199.

  The authors have refined the hybrid approach with the combined strategy in a hybrid suite, where all stages of functionally univentricular palliation can be performed.

Cross Sectional Echocardiographic and Doppler Imaging

CHAPTER 18A

LUC L. MERTENS, MICHAEL L. RIGBY, ESTELA S. HOROWITZ, and ROBERT H. ANDERSON

Since the late 1970s, perhaps the most important change in the practice of clinical paediatric cardiology has been the introduction of cross sectional echocardiography, with this advance then being facilitated by ongoing and continuous technical improvements. Echocardiography currently allows highly accurate diagnosis of nearly all morphological abnormalities, for the most part making invasive diagnostic techniques obsolete. Nowadays, cardiac catheterisation and angiography is no longer a routine investigation in most patients prior to cardiac surgery, as it used to be a few decades ago. Indeed, the main indication for such an investigation, apart from the purposes of intervention, is the display of structures beyond echocardiographic visualisation, such as peripheral pulmonary arteries, distal coronary arteries, and more rarely complex abnormalities of systemic and pulmonary venous return. For these indications, magnetic resonance and computerised tomographic imaging are progressively replacing cardiac catheterisation. All paediatric cardiologists, cardiac intensivists, and paediatric cardiac surgeons, therefore, should be familiar with echocardiographic imaging and diagnosis. The first part of this chapter is devoted to the principles of cross sectional and Doppler echocardiography as applied in clinical practice. In the subsequent parts of the chapter, our colleagues discuss some more advanced applications, such as tissue Doppler techniques, three-dimensional echocardiography, and computed tomography and magnetic resonance imaging.

PHYSICAL PRINCIPLES OF ULTRASONIC IMAGING

We begin with a limited introduction to the physical principles of ultrasound, as some background knowledge is relevant for optimization of images in clinical practice. Those interested in more details on the physics of imaging should consult more comprehensive reviews, or specialised textbooks of echocardiography.[1]

The Physical Properties of Ultrasound

An acoustic wave is a mechanical wave causing particles to be displaced from a position of equilibrium while traveling through the medium, causing local compression and rarefaction influenced by the elasticity and density of the medium. Ultrasonic waves are longitudinal sound waves with a frequency above 20 kHz, the highest frequency which can be detected by the human ear. The waves are generated and detected by a piezoelectric crystal, which deforms under the influence of an electrical field. The velocity of a sound wave is dependent upon the density and stiffness of the medium. Stiffness is the hardness or resistance of the material to compression. Density is the concentration of the matter. Increase in stiffness also increases speed, whereas an increase in density decreases speed. Transmission of such sonic waves is slow in air or gasses, but fast in solid mediums. In the tissues of the body, the velocity of sound is relatively constant, at 1540 m/sec. The frequency represents the numbers of cycles occurring in each second of time, and is expressed in hertz, with 1 hertz corresponding to one cycle per second. The wavelength corresponds to the length over space over which one cycle occurs. The amplitude reflects the strength divided by the intensity of a soundwave, and is expressed in decibels. The velocity of transmission, the frequency, and the wavelength are related by the formula $c = f \times \lambda$, where c is the speed of sound through the medium, f is the the frequency of the wave, and λ is the wavelength.

The range of frequencies used for medical applications is from 2 to 12 megahertz (mHz). Corresponding wavelengths, therefore, are in the range 0.8 to 0.13 mm. This implies an intrinsic limitation for spatial resolution, as two structures need to be separated by more than one wavelength in order to be resolved. This relationship also explains why a probe with a higher frequency has a greater spatial resolution. When sound travels through a homogeneous medium, different interactions occur, such as reflection, attenuation, refraction and scattering. Reflection occurs at a boundary or interface between two mediums having a different acoustic density. The difference in acoustic impedance, known as z, between the two tissues causes reflection of the sound wave in the direction of the transducer. Reflection from a smooth or specular interface between tissues causes the sound wave to return to the transducer. Irregular interfaces will cause scatter in different directions. The ultrasonic image is created based on the reflected waves. Refraction is the phenomenon that the ultrasound wave, which passes through the tissue, is refracted based on the incidence of the beam. The incidence is oblique when the direction of the sound beam is not at a right angle to the boundary of the two mediums. This same phenomenon explains why a straight pencil that sits in a glass of water appears to have a bend in it. Attenuation is the loss of sonic energy as sound propagates through a medium. It is produced by the absorption of the ultrasonic energy by conversion to heat, as well as by reflection and scattering. The deeper the wave travels in the body, the weaker it becomes. The amplitude and strength of the wave decreases with increasing depth. Overall attenuation is dependent upon the frequency, such that ultrasound with lower frequencies penetrates more deeply into the body than ultrasound with higher frequencies. Probes with lower frequencies produce better penetration, but as mentioned above, have lower spatial resolution. Probes with higher frequencies have lower penetration, but higher spatial resolution. Attenuation also depends on acoustic impedance, and on mismatch in impedance between adjacent structures. Since air has a very high acoustic impedance, any air between the transducer and the cardiac structures of interest results in substantial attenuation of the signal produced. This is avoided on transthoracic examinations by use of water-soluble gel to form an airless contact between the transducer and the skin. The air-filled lungs are avoided by careful positioning of the patient, and by the use of acoustic windows that allow access of the ultrasonic beam to the cardiac structures without the need to pass through intervening lung tissue. Attenuation causes decrease in amplitude as the wave passes through the tissue. In most ultrasonic systems, this is corrected for by automatic compensation. Further manual compensation in terms of gain in depth or time can be achieved by changing controls on the machine, which correct for the automated attenuation at specific depths of image.

Production of Images

Each ultrasonic pulse, encountering numerous interfaces, gives rise to a series of reflected echoes returning at time intervals corresponding to their depths. In this way, each pulse from the ultrasonic crystal demonstrates a line of information that corresponds to the structures encountered by the sound beam. The returned signal is processed so that the radiofrequency signal is converted into an image. The M-mode represents one line of information displayed on the vertical axis, with time on the horizontal axis. Its advantage is the very high temporal resolution. The frequency of repetition of the pulse producing a typical M-mode trace is approximately 1000 frames per second. The shade of grey on the M-mode recording is determined by the intensity of each reflected echo.

Conventional cross sectional echocardiography depends on the construction of an image using multiple individual lines of information. Typically 64 or 128 lines of information are required to produce one image or frame. Multiple frames are constructed in real time each second, the limiting factor being the time necessary for the echoes from each pulse to return to the transducer. At depths of 5 to 15 centimetres, it is possible to achieve frame rates of 28 to 50 per second. Modern systems are capable of manipulating the frame rates by sending out different pulses at different times, but in general increasing the frame rate will reduce the quality of the image, and hence its spatial resolution.

Quality of Images

When concerning the image, quality refers to the resolution of the imaging system. Spatial resolution refers to the capacity of the system to resolve small structures. It can be considered as the smallest distance by which the system is capable of identifying two dots as separate entities. Contrast resolution is the ability of the system to distinguish differences in the density of the soft tissues. Temporal resolution refers to the capacity of the system to resolve differences in time. There are many potential sources for artifacts in ultrasonic images that affect their quality.

Spatial Resolution

This can be defined as the combination of axial and lateral resolution. Axial, or depth, resolution is the capacity of the ultrasonic system to distinguish how close together two objects can be along the axis of the beam, yet still be distinguished as two separate objects. Wavelength affects axial resolution, and it is improved by increasing the frequency. Axial resolution is much higher compared to lateral resolution, which is the capacity of the system to resolve two adjacent objects that are perpendicular to the axis of the beam as separate entities. The width of the beam affects the lateral resolution: the wider the beam the lower the lateral resolution. This is influenced by the focal zone, which is the depth of the smallest beam width. The near field is the zone between the transducer and the focal zone, and the far field is the region beyond the focal zone. Optimising the focus at a certain depth optimizes lateral resolution. The limit using the focal zone is determined by the size and frequency of the transducer. Small transducers focus well in the near field, while large transducers perform better in the far field. The width of the beam is also influenced by the frequency of the transducer, with higher frequency probes having a better lateral resolution compared to those which have a low frequency. Probes with higher frequency, however, suffer from their limited ability to penetrate into the tissue. Line density can also be improved by decreasing the sector width, resulting in better lateral resolution, but more limited image sector.

Temporal Resolution

To image moving objects, structures such as blood and heart, the frame rate is important, and is related to the motion speed of the object. The eye generally can only see 25 frames per second, providing a temporal resolution of about 40 msec. The temporal resolution is limited by the sweep speed of the echo beam, which in turn is limited by the speed of sound, as the echo from the deepest part of the image has to return before the next pulse is sent out at a different angle in the neighboring beam. The speed of the sweep can be increased by reducing the number of beams, or increasing the beam width in the sector, by using the frame rate control, or by decreasing the width of the sector. The first option decreases the lateral resolution, while the second decreases the image field. Temporal resolution, therefore, cannot be increased without a trade-off, due to the physical limitations of echocardiography.

Ultrasonic Imaging Artifacts

There are many potential sources for artifacts in echocardiography. For interpretation of the images it is important to know and recognise them.

- Drop-out of parallel structures. When structures are parallel to the ultrasonic beam, there is very little reflection caused by the structure, resulting in drop-out. A typical example is the atrial septum when viewed from the apex.
- Acoustic shadowing. Transmission of the ultrasonic beam through the tissue is influenced by the presence of tissue with very high density. Typical examples are prosthetic valves, devices, catheters, or calcifications.

These structures can make it impossible to view structures behind them.

- Reverberations can occur with lateral spread of high-intensity echos. Bright echos can have considerable width. A lot of reverberations originate from the interaction between the transducer and the ribs.
- Mirror-imaging. This artifact appears as a display of two images, one real and one artifactual, and is due to the sound beam interacting with a strong reflector.
- Ring down or comet tail. The ring down artifact comes from gas bubble in a fluid medium. The comet tail originates from highly reflective structures, such as surgical clips.

Doppler Echocardiography

The Doppler principle is the frequency shift caused by ultrasonic waves if they are reflected by a moving reflector. The frequency of reflected waves increases as the target approaches the receiver, and decreases as it moves away from the observer. A typical example is the sound of an ambulance siren, which has a higher pitch sound when moving towards the observer, and a lower pitch sound when moving away. When initially applied to echocardiography, the Doppler technique was used to measure the velocities of blood pools. A Doppler shift is caused by interaction of the ultrasonic beam with a moving pool of red blood cells. The Doppler shift depends upon the velocity and direction of the flowing blood, the angle between the beam and the flow, and the velocity of sound within in the tissues. This is expressed in the Doppler formula:

$$F_d = \frac{2F_0V \cos \theta}{c}$$

where F_d is the observed shift in frequency, F_0 is the transmitted frequency, V is the velocity of flow of blood, θ is the angle of intercept between the beam and the direction of blood flow, and c is the velocity of sound in human tissue, which is 1540 m/sec.

The observed frequency shift is several kilohertz in magnitude, and produces an audible signal that can be electronically processed and displayed graphically. As different velocities are present within the ultrasonic beam for any given time instance during the cardiac cycle, a range of Doppler frequencies is typically detected. Thus, a spectrum of Doppler shifts are measured and displayed in the spectrogram, hence the term spectral Doppler as often encountered in the literature. The Doppler-shifted frequencies usually undergo fast-Fourier transformation, converting the original Doppler waveform into a spectral display with velocity on the vertical axis, time on the horizontal axis, and amplitude as shades of grey. Conventionally, Doppler signals from blood moving towards the transducer are displayed above the baseline. Similarly, when blood flows away from the transducer, the display is below the baseline. When the Doppler shift is known, the Doppler equation outlined above can be rearranged to

$$V = \frac{cF_d}{2F_0 \cos \theta}$$

In this way, the velocity of flow can be calculated. The main source of error is in the determination of the angle of intercept between the ultrasonic beam and the axis of flow. When the angle exceeds 20 degrees, it should be measured and included in the Doppler equation. In practice, it is difficult to measure accurately this angle. Potential problems arising from a large angle of interception, therefore, are overcome by obtaining the clearest audio signal with the highest velocity. The ultrasonic beam can then be assumed to be nearly parallel to the direction of flow. As blood velocities cause a Doppler shift in the audible range, the Doppler shift itself can be made audible to the user. A high pitch, with a large Doppler shift, corresponds to a high velocity, whereas a low pitch, with a small shift, corresponds to a low velocity.

Types of Doppler Ultrasound

There are three types of Doppler ultrasound, namely continuous wave, pulsed wave, and colour flow Doppler.

Continuous Wave Doppler

In continuous wave Doppler, one piezoelectric crystal is used for transmitting a continuous wave at a fixed frequency, and a second crystal is used continuously to record the reflected signals. Both crystals are embedded within the same transducer with a slight angle towards each other, and the Doppler shift is continuously sampled. As an ultrasonic wave is transmitted continuously, no spatial information is obtained. Indeed, all velocities occurring anywhere within the ultrasound beam, in other words on the selected ultrasound line of interrogation, will contribute to the reflected signal, and will appear in the spectrogram. As the ultrasound signal weakens with depth due to attenuation, velocities close to the transducer will intrinsically contribute more than the ones occurring further away. The major advantage of continuous wave Doppler is its ability accurately to measure high frequency shifts with no upper limit. It can be used, therefore, to measure high-velocity jets. To optimize the direction of the echobeam within the direction of the flow, cross sectional imaging and color Doppler can be combined with continuous wave Doppler from the same transducer, producing so-called Duplex scanning. This gives a visual impression of being simultaneous, but is achieved by rapid and automatic switching between Doppler and cross sectional imaging. Adding colour Doppler imaging helps optimally to align the beam of interrogation with the direction of the flow of blood.

Pulsed Wave Doppler

Pulsed wave Doppler has been developed to give spatial information on the detected velocities. The technique is not based on the Doppler principle, but provides an output in a spectral display which looks very similar to the way the continuous wave signal is represented. The Doppler shift itself, however, is not measured by the system. When using the pulsed wave system, an image line is chosen along which ultrasonic pulses are transmitted at a constant rate. This rate is the pulse repetition frequency. Instead of continuously sampling the backscattered waves, only one sample of the reflected wave is taken at a fixed time after transmitting a certain pulse. This time interval is the range gate. The range gate will determine the exact depth where velocities are measured. The transducer sends pulses, and must receive that signal back before other pulses can be transmitted. A sample volume is positioned at the area of interest. The velocity of sound in soft tissue is a given constant of 1540 m/sec, and the go and return time is used to determine the depth of the sample volume.

The velocities that can be measured are limited by the pulse repetition frequency, or the number of pulses that are emitted per second. Aliasing of the Doppler signal occurs when the pulse repetition frequency is too low, and the returning signals from one waveform are not received before the next waveform is sent. The frequency at which aliasing occurs is also called the Nyquist limit. Aliasing will result in velocities being displayed at the same time below and above the baseline. The Nyquist limit will be lower the deeper the velocity is measured, as the time for the wave to travel will be longer. The Nyquist limit depends on the frequency of the probe, with higher frequency probes having lower Nyquist limits, and lower frequency probes having higher Nyquist limits. A 2.5 mHz transducer will display velocities of twice the magnitude of those produced by a 5.0 mHz transducer. Appropriate selection of the probe, therefore, is important when performing pulsed Doppler measurements. Different options are possible further to increase the Nyquist limits. The first is to shift the baseline so that velocities are measured in only one direction. A second method is to send out a new pulse before the previous one has returned. This is called the high-repetition frequency method, and results in measuring velocities in more than one site or sample volume, thus reducing the spatial resolution but increasing the Nyquist limit. The size of the sample volume can also be adjusted. A smaller sample volume will result in a sharper velocity profile, as fewer velocities are sampled at the same time.

Colour Flow Interrogation

Colour Doppler displays the direction and flow velocities of the blood superimposed on the cross sectional image. In this technology, different pulses are sent across an image line, and the phase shift between the different signals is measured at two sampling points. This phase shift is proportional to the velocity of the reflecting object. A colour is assigned to the direction of flow according to whether it is away from or towards the transducer. In this respect, it may be helpful to remember the mnemonic BART, indicating blue away and red towards.

The velocity of flow is displayed in shades of these colors. The brighter the colour, the higher is the velocity. The colour information represents the mean velocity of flow. When the flow is disturbed, or not laminar, the pattern will show as a mosaic. This mosaic pattern is only produced if the variance is on. The variance is a colour Doppler option that is present with all the cardiac presets. It is important to appreciate that, because colour flow mapping is a form of pulsed Doppler, it is subject to the same physical principles. Increasing velocities are represented as increasingly bright forms of red or blue until they reach the Nyquist limit, when aliasing then superimposes new colours on the display. Typical Nyquist velocity limits are from 0.6 to 1 m/sec. For flows at high velocity, therefore, multiple aliasing occurs. The colour image is then useful only from a qualitative point of view, and does not permit the demonstration of directional flow. Similarly to pulsed Doppler, the Nyquist limit is dependent on transducer frequency and depth.

Colour flow Doppler provides information regarding the Doppler shift from an entire area, unlike pulsed Doppler, which samples from a specific point. More time is required, therefore, for colour Doppler to compute the lines of information onto the screen. Frame rate and line densities are reduced proportional to the time required. Keeping the colour sector small will provide a better frame rate, and produce a flicker-free image. When using colour flow, the operator is able to visualize the flow of blood in relation to the surrounding structures, which provides a method for rapid interpretation of abnormal location and direction of flow, and helps to guide Doppler interrogation of abnormal flow.

Comparison of Doppler Methods

The three types of Doppler interrogation described are complementary, each measuring the velocities of flow in different ways. For the evaluation of high velocities, the method of choice is continuous wave Doppler, since it does not give rise to aliasing. Although it does not permit gating for precise localisation of the target, a steerable cursor line, and a focused beam, allows precise alignment, thus assuring appropriate measurements of flow. Pulsed Doppler, in contrast, enables measurements of flow at a known depth, allowing more precise calculations, but is limited by the maximal measurable velocity. Colour flow Doppler is a qualitative method, but provides spatial information not obtained with other methods. By permitting visualisation of the disturbed jet, it facilitates the alignment of the continuous wave Doppler beam. The visual effect of colour flow Doppler provides a method of rapidly screening abnormal velocities within the heart, thus directing the more quantitative methods.

EQUIPMENT

M-Mode Imaging

M-mode echocardiography is derived from an M line superimposed on a cross sectional image. The M-mode trace itself shows time as the second dimension. Control of the speed of the sweep enables accurate measurements of intervals in the cardiac cycle, and the high-repetition frequency of the technique allows not only excellent temporal resolution of moving structures, but also precise measurements of mural thickness and cavitary size. In this way, the information derived is superior to that obtained from cross sections. M-mode echocardiography is still commonly used for the evaluation of left ventricular function, using short- or long-axis cuts through the left ventricle, and the timing of cardiac events such as left ventricular ejection time, using a long-axis cut through the aortic valve.

Cross Sectional Imaging

Rather than mechanically moving or tilting the ultrasound crystals, as was the case with the mechanical probes from the previous generation, modern devices make use of electronics to steer the beam. For this purpose, an array of piezoelectric crystals is used. The crystals can be organized in a linear or curved fashion, or more recently in a two-dimensional matrix. By introducing delays between the excitation of different crystals in the array, the ultrasonic wave can be directed without moving the transducer. The signal for transmission in a particular direction is the sum of the signals received by the individual elements. These individual contributions can be filtered, scaled, and time-delayed separately before summing to create the image.

This process is referred to as beam-forming. In the newest generation of matrix transducers, a large number of crystals are implanted in a two-dimensional matrix, which enables full steering of the beam in all three dimensions, and is capable of generating three-dimensional images. Currently, a high-frequency matrix transducer has been developed by Philips Medical Systems, which allows high resolution three-dimensional imaging in children. The current resolution of the three-dimensional images produced, however, is significantly when lower compared to the spatial and temporal resolution which can be obtained using the current probes available for cross sectional imaging.

When performing cross sectional imaging, the most appropriate probe must be selected to optimise the quality of the images produced. Probes with higher frequencies, as already discussed, have better spatial resolution but lower penetration, while probes with lower frequencies have a lower spatial resolution but higher penetration. In neonates and small infants high-frequency transducers from 7.5 to 12 mHz provide excellent cross sectional resolution. Older children, in contrast, are better studied with transducers of lower frequencies, from 5 to 3.5 mHz. Harmonic imaging was developed further to optimize the quality of the images, and to reduce the signal-to-noise ratio. Due to the phenomenon of distortion during propagation through the tissues, harmonic frequencies combining integer multiples of the transmitted frequency are generated. Transmitting a pulse of 1.7 mHz, for example, will result in the spontaneous generation of harmonic components of 3.4, 5.1, 6.8, 8.5 mHz, and so on. These harmonic components will grow stronger with the distance of propagation. The scanner can be set up in such a way as to receive only the second harmonic component, thus generating a second harmonic image. Such an image typically produces a better signal-to-noise ratio by avoiding the clutter noise due to reverberation artifacts, such as those produced by the ribs. Such harmonic imaging is often used in patients with poor acoustic windows. Its disadavantage is the reduction produced in axial resolution in the direction of the echobeam. In smaller patients, therefore, it rarely improves the quality of the images, but the technique can be useful in larger children with poor acoustic windows.

Blood-Pool Doppler

Optimising the Settings for Continuous Wave Doppler

The continuous wave image is an echocardiographic image that is influenced by all the parameters that affect a normal cross sectional picture. The gain control affects the ratio of the strength of the output signal to the input signal. The gain controls, therefore, should be manipulated to produce a clean uniform profile, without any blooming. The controls should be increased to over-emphasise the image, and then adjusted down. This will prevent any loss of information because of too little gain. The compress control assigns the varying amplitudes a certain shade of grey. If this control is either very low or very high, the quality of the spectral analysis graph will be affected, and this may lead to erroneous interpretation. The reject control eliminates the smaller amplitude signals that are below a certain threshold. This helps to provide a cleaner image, and may make measurements more obvious. The filter is used to reduce the noise that occurs from reflectors produced from walls and other structures that are within the range of the ultrasonic beam.The volume button should be at the appropriate level to hear the frequencies.

Optimising the Settings for Pulsed Doppler

The frequency of the probe will affect the Nyquist limit of pulsed Doppler, with probes of higher frequency having a lower Nyquist limit. The gain control, compress, and filter settings are similar to those described above for continuous wave Doppler. Shift of the baseline allows the entire display to be used to show either forward or reverse flow, a feature which is useful if the flow is only in one direction. The scale should always be optimised, and be set no higher than necessary to display the measured velocities. The size of the gate should be optimised, with an increase in the sample volume increasing the strength of the signal at the expense of a lower spatial resolution. In general, the smallest sample volume providing an adequate ratio of signal-to-noise should be used. The update function allows for simultaneous duplex imaging to optimise the location of sampling relative to the cross sectional image. Simultaneous cross sectional imaging, however, reduces the temporal resolution. All pulsed-Doppler traces, therefore, should be obtained with the cross sectional image frozen.

Optimising the Settings for Colour Doppler

This involves optimising the gain settings, the scale, and the size of the sector. The gain should be adjusted until background noise is detected in the colour image, and then reducing it so that the noise just disappears. The scale should be adapted depending on the velocities of the flows measured. When looking at flows with high velocities, the scale should be adapted so the maximal Nyquist limit is chosen. When flows of low velocity are studied, such as venous flows or those in the coronary arteries, the scale needs to be lowered. The size of the colour sector needs to be adjusted to optimise frame rates. The smallest necessary size should be used.

STORAGE AND REPORTING OF THE IMAGES CREATED

All current echocardiographic machines allow the recording and storing of images in a digital format, which can be retrieved, viewed, and further analysed on a digital viewing system and work station. This allows easy storage and retrieval of echocardiographic images and studies. More and more centres use digital systems for reporting, which can be integrated within the reviewing stations. The full digital workflow contributes to the quality and efficiency of paediatric echocardiographic laboratories.[2,3]

NORMAL CARDIAC ANATOMY

With cross sectional echocardiography, the clinician has at his or her disposal the technique to illustrate cardiac anatomy in all the detail seen by the morphologist, as described in Chapter 2. To take advantage of the material displayed, a thorough knowledge of normal and abnormal cardiac morphology is essential. It has been rare in the past, however, to find cardiac structures displayed by morphologists as they are oriented within the body. For example, the mitral valve is usually illustrated by incising the atrioventricular junction, and spreading the valvar leaflets and papillary muscles. This gives a spurious impression of the

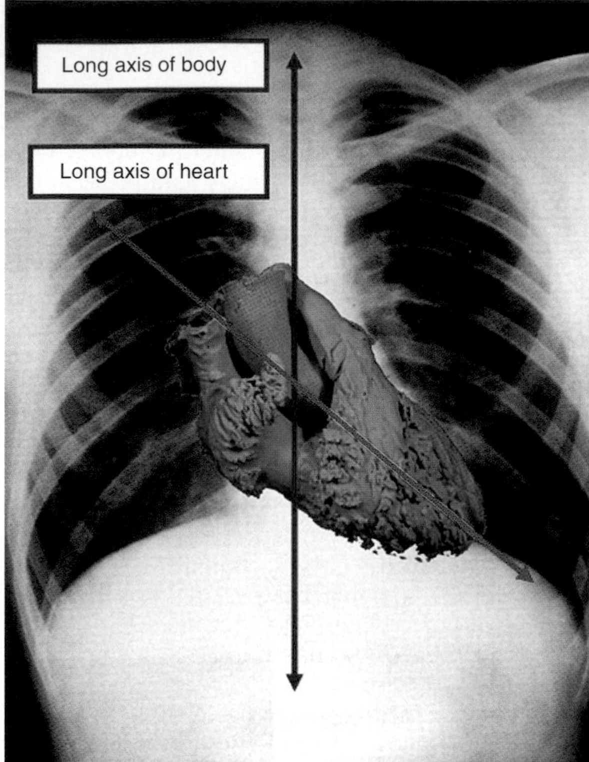

Figure 18A-1 The cartoon shows the position of the cardiac silhouette relative to the thorax, and the discrepancy in angulation of the long axis of the heart relative to the long axis of the body.

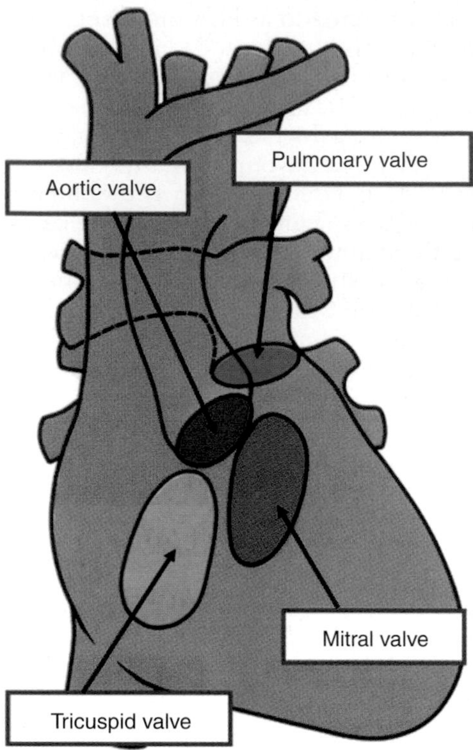

Figure 18A-2 The cartoon shows the position of the cardiac valves relative to the cardiac silhouette.

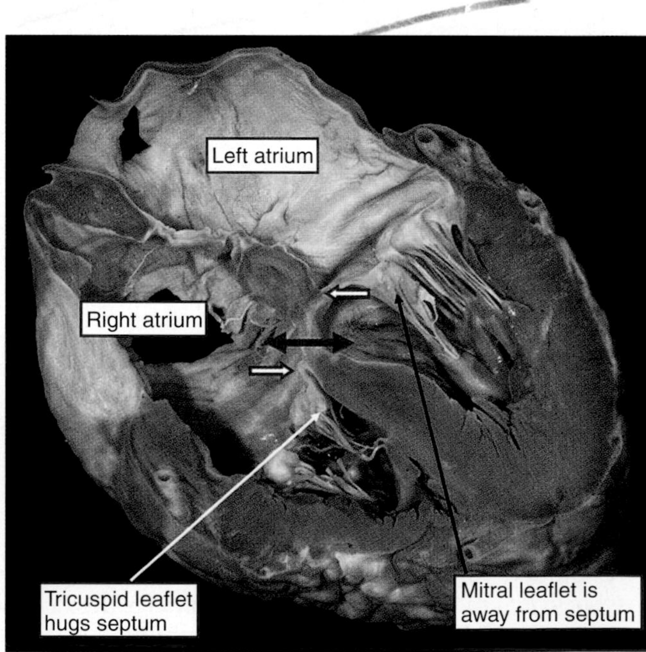

Figure 18A-3 This section through the normal heart simulates the echocardiographic four-chamber section. Note that the septal leaflet of the tricuspid valve hugs the septum, whereas there is a discrete plane of space between the septum and the leaflets of the mitral valve. The rightward border of this space is formed by the membranous part of the septum (*red double-headed arrow*) and the area of the atrioventricular muscular sandwich, which occupies the space between the offset leaflets of the atrioventricular valves (*open arrows*).

disposition of the papillary muscles. In life, they are adjacent. The echocardiographic sections display the anatomy in cross section. It is helpful, therefore, if the morphologist displays the anatomy in similar fashion. Understanding is helped further by illustrating the anatomical sections in the normal orientation of the heart as it is positioned in the body.[4] In the normal subject, the long axis of the heart is oblique, extending more or less from the left subcostal region to the right shoulder (Fig. 18A-1). The heart does not stand on its apex in St Valentine's fashion. In addition to the long axis being oblique, the cardiac chambers, particularly the ventricles, are arranged so that the morphologically right structures are anterior to their morphologically left counterparts (see Chapter 2). The left atrium is the most posterior of the cardiac chambers. Only its appendage projects to the border of the cardiac silhouette. The right ventricle lies anterior to the left ventricle. It swings across the front of the ventricular mass, reaching from the inferior and right-sided tricuspid valve to the antero-superiorly and leftwardly positioned pulmonary valve. The aortic valve is centrally located within the heart, and is related to all four chambers (Fig. 18A-2). This central position of the aortic valve, located between the tricuspid and mitral valves, is the key to the understanding of cardiac anatomy. Because of the wedged position of the aortic valve, the subaortic outflow tract lifts the leaflets of the mitral valve away from the ventricular septum. Hence, there are no direct attachments of tension apparatus to the muscular septum in the left ventricle. In contrast, the septal leaflet of the tricuspid valve hugs the septum (Fig. 18A-3), and is attached to it by tension apparatus along its length. The short-axis cuts emphasise other significant differences between the right and left sides of the normal heart. The arterial and atrioventricular valves in the right ventricle are separated by the supraventricular crest. No such muscular crest exists in the roof of the left ventricle, where the leaflets of the aortic and mitral valves

Figure 18A-4 This short-axis section of the ventricular mass is viewed from the apex looking towards the base. Note the deeply wedged position of the aortic valve between the mitral valve and the septum, with fibrous continuity between the valvar leaflets in the roof of the ventricle. In contrast, the supraventricular (SV) crest forms the roof of the right ventricle, interposing between the leaflets of the tricuspid and pulmonary valves.

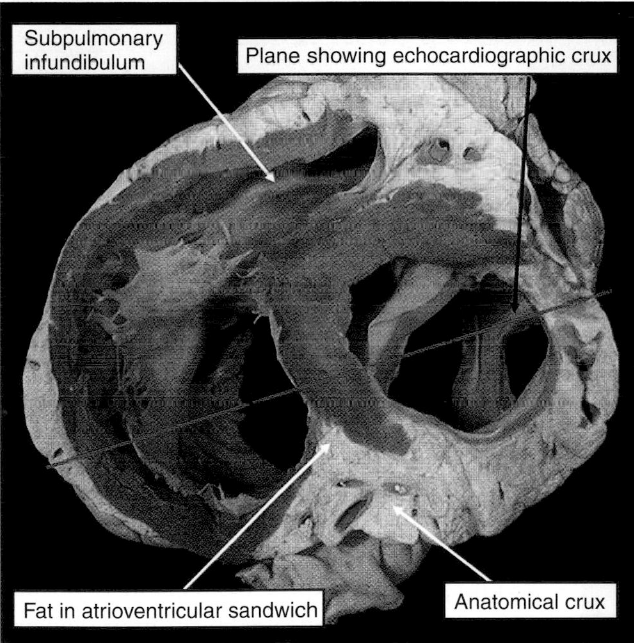

Figure 18A-5 This short-axis section is taken closer to the base than the one shown in Figure 18A-4. It shows the epicardial fat interposing between the wall of the right atrium and the crest of the ventricular septum at the anatomic crux. The echocardiographic crux is seen in so-called four-chamber planes, as shown by the *yellow* line.

are in fibrous continuity (Fig. 18A-4). The subaortic outflow tract also has important relationships to the areas of atrioventricular contiguity, these being made up of two components. The first, the atrioventricular membranous septum, is made of fibrous tissue, and is an integral part of the central fibrous body. It interposes between the medial wall of the subaortic outflow tract and the right atrium. The other area is the region of overlapping of the atrial and ventricular musculatures. It exists because the septal leaflet of the tricuspid valve is attached to the septum more towards the ventricular apex than are the leaflets of the mitral valve, producing the characteristic off-setting of the valvar leaflets. In the area between these valvar attachments, the walls of

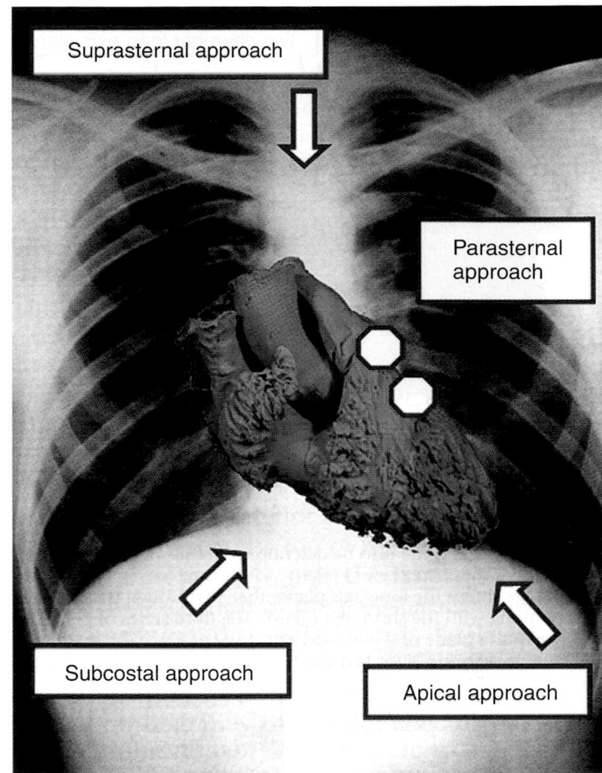

Figure 18A-6 The image shows the location of the echocardiographic windows that permit visualisation of cardiac anatomy.

the right atrium overlap the base of the ventricular mass, thus forming a muscular atrioventricular sandwich (Fig. 18A-5). The anatomist describes the location of this area as seen from the diaphragmatic surface of the heart as the cardiac crux, representing the position where the plane of the normal septal structures crosses the inferior atrioventricular groove. The echocardiographer cannot see this point on the epicardial surface of the heart, but is able to identify the so-called echocardiographic crux, the asymmetric cruciate appearance representing the off-set attachment of the atrioventricular valvar leaflets.

Anatomical Principles of Echocardiography

All of the morphological features described above are potentially amenable to dissection with the ultrasonic beam. The echocardiographic tyro will immediately become aware that the ultrasonic beam is obstructed both by bony structures and the air-filled lungs. Because of this, access from the body surface can be limited, although the heart can be viewed from many different aspects. Unobstructed views can be obtained from the cardiac apex, from alongside the sternum through the intercostal spaces, from beneath the rib cage, and from the suprasternal notch (see Fig. 18A-6). The cardiac components can also be visualised by placing a transducer within the oesophagus and stomach. From these various windows, the heart and great vessels, according to their position within the chest, can be cut in different planes. Standard echocardiographic views are well established for patients with normally located hearts. Visualisation and understanding of the congenitally malformed heart, however, is facilitated if the examiner develops

SECTION 2 Special Topics

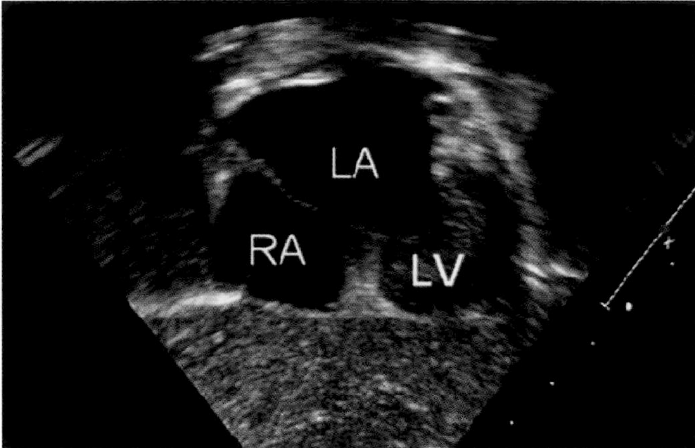

Figure 18A-12 The image shows a heart sectioned to simulate a posterior paracoronal cut obtained from the subcostal window to look at the atrial septum. The left atrium (LA) and right atrium (RA) can well be visualized. On this more posterior cut, only the left ventricle (LV) is visualized, as the right ventricle is located more anteriorly.

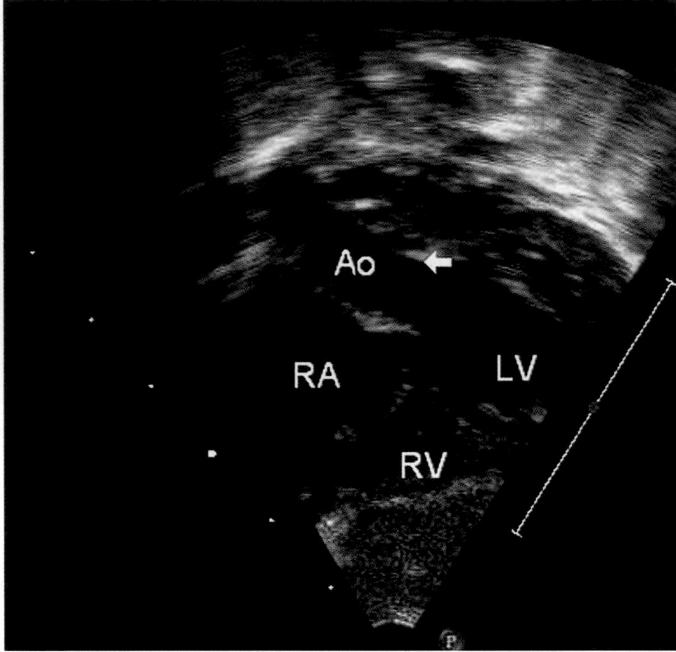

Figure 18A-13 This subcostal coronal view is tilted more anteriorly compared to Figure 18A-12. More of the right ventricle (RV) can be seen, as well as the left ventricle (LV) and the left ventricular outflow tract. The arrow points at the insertion of the aortic valve. Ao, aorta; RA, right atrium.

identity of the abdominal great vessels. Posterior coronal long-axis sections, with the transducer directed to the left of the midline, provide excellent views of the atrial septum (Fig. 18A-12). As the transducer is tilted anteriorly, the superior caval vein, the ventricles, and the left ventricular outflow tract can be imaged (Fig. 18A-13). Further anterior tilting of the probe provides views of the right ventricular ouflow tract. Counter-clockwise rotation of the transducer, with the notch in the transducer positioned inferiorly at 6 o'clock, will produce different cuts as the transducer is swept from right to left in a parasagittal plane. A cut though the atriums allows imaging of the superior and inferior caval veins and the atrial septum (Fig. 18A-14). As the transducer is moved towards the left, the subcostal short-axis section of the left ventricle and the right ventricular outflow tract can be imaged (Figs. 18A-15 and 16). In this view, the right ventricular apex and outflow tract are seen, together with the pulmonary valve and proximal pulmonary trunk (see Fig. 18A-15). By tilting the transducer further to the left, the midapical and apical portions of both ventricles can be imaged, along with the corresponding portions of the ventricular septum.

Parasternal and Apical Views

Parasternal imaging starts with obtaining a left parasternal long-axis view. This reference section shows the left ventricular outflow tract, the aortic valve, the mitral valve, the left ventricle and the left atrium (Fig. 18A-17). The fibrous continuity typically present between the leaflets of the mitral and aortic valves is easily demonstrated, and this view is useful for assessing mitral and aortic valvar motion and function. When the transducer is tilted towards the right hip, the right ventricular inflow and the tricuspid valve can be visualised (Fig. 18A-18). The orifice of the coronary

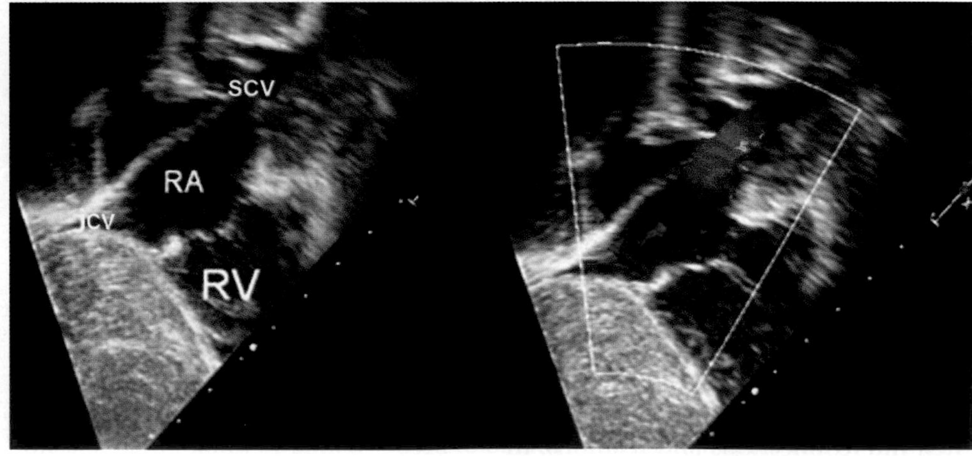

Figure 18A-14 The subcostal coronal view of the right atrium demonstrates the entrances of the superior caval vein (SCV) and the inferior caval vein (ICV) to the right atrium (RA). The tricuspid valve can be seen on this image, as well as part of the right ventricle (RV). On the colour Doppler figure on the right, the flow from the superior caval vein comes towards the probe, and is shown in red, while flow from the inferior caval vein is directed away from the probe, and is seen as blue.

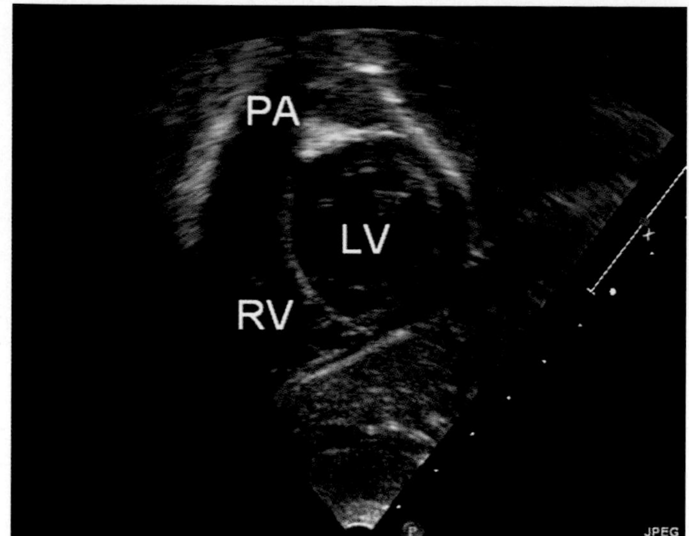

Figure 18A-15 This subcostal short-axis cut is taken at the level of the right ventricular outflow tract. Both the right ventricle (RV) and left ventricle (LV) are shown. The right ventricular outflow tract is visualized, as well as the pulmonary trunk (PA).

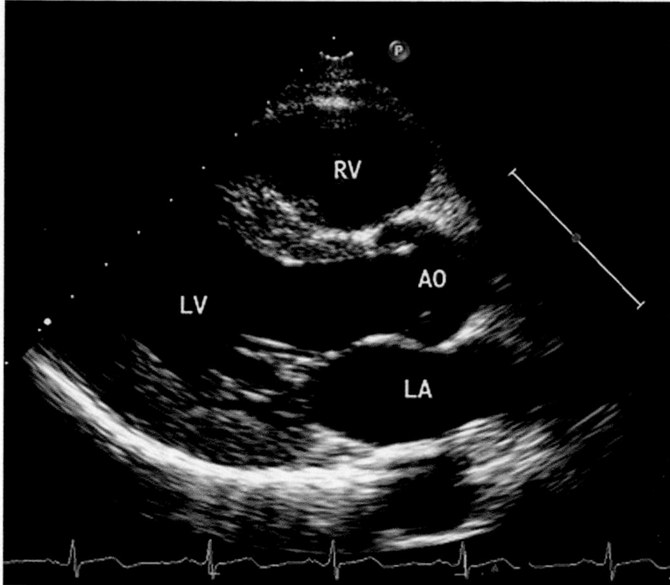

Figure 18A-17 This parasternal long-axis view shows the left atrium (LA), left ventricle (LV) and aorta (AO). Note the fibrous continuity between the leaflets of the mitral and aortic valves. The infundibulum of the right ventricle (RV) is seen antero-superiorly.

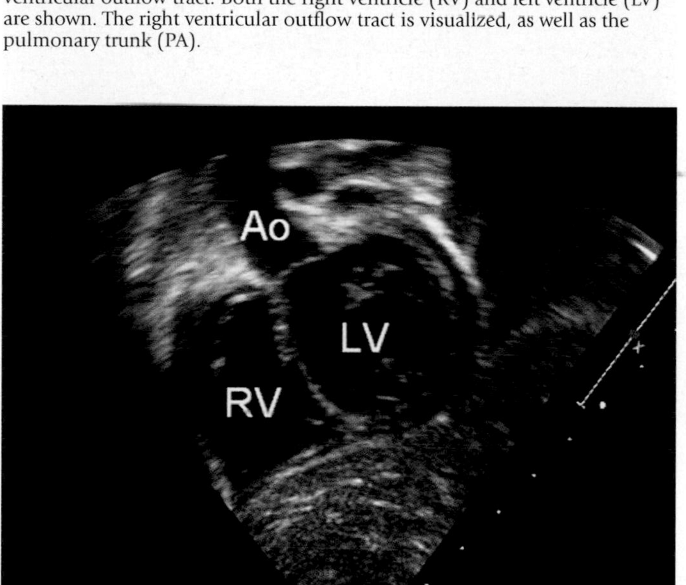

Figure 18A-16 This subcostal short-axis section, tilting more leftward showing the left ventricle (LV), shows the left ventricular outflow tract and the ascending aorta (Ao). The aortic valve is shown in a closed position. The right ventricle (RV) and the ventricular septum are also seen.

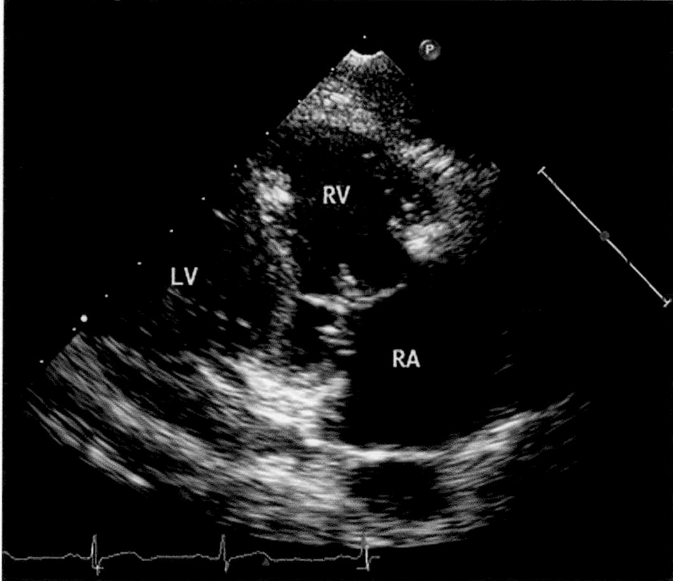

Figure 18A-18 This parasternal long-axis view shows the right ventricular inlet. The probe is tilted so the that the right atrium (RA), tricuspid valve, and right ventricle (RV) are all visualised. The left ventricle (LV) is posterior to the RV.

sinus can also be identified in this view. With anterior tilting of the transducer, the right ventricular outflow tract, the pulmonary valve and the pulmonary trunk can be visualised (Fig. 18A-19). When the transducer is rotated 90 degrees clockwise from the long-axis reference cut, a parasternal short-axis view of the base of the heart is obtained. This view can provide information on the structure of the aortic valvar leaflets (Fig. 18A-20), the right ventricular outflow tract, and the pulmonary valve (Fig. 18A-21). A short-axis sweep is then usually performed from base to apex, which visualises the ventricular septum. Short-axis cuts are obtained at the level of the leaflets of the mitral valve (Fig. 18A-22), the papillary muscles, and the left ventricular apex. The short-axis views show well the papillary muscles supporting the tendinous cords of the mitral valve (Fig. 18A-23). Although conventionally described as being postero-septal and antero-lateral, examination of short-axis sections when the heart is positioned as it lies in the body reveals that these muscles are positioned infero-anteriorly and supero-posteriorly. The short-axis views also show the origins of coronary arteries. Slight clockwise rotation from the cut showing the short axis of the aorta will demonstrate the origin of the left coronary artery, while slight counter-clockwise rotation will demonstrate the origin of the right coronary artery. The arterial duct, if patent, can be demonstrated by using a high left parasternal window

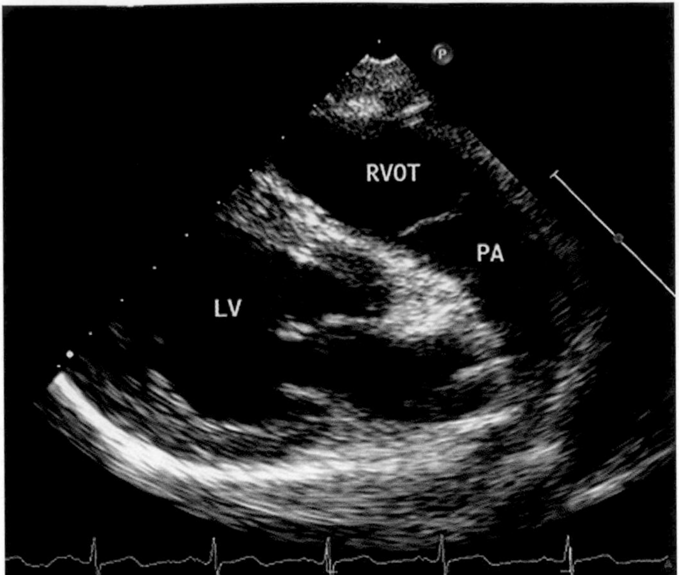

Figure 18A-19 The parasternal long-axis view shows the right ventricular outflow tract (RVOT), and is obtained by tilting the probe anteriorly. The left ventricle (LV), the infundibulum, the pulmonary valve and the pulmonary trunk (PA) are all seen in this image.

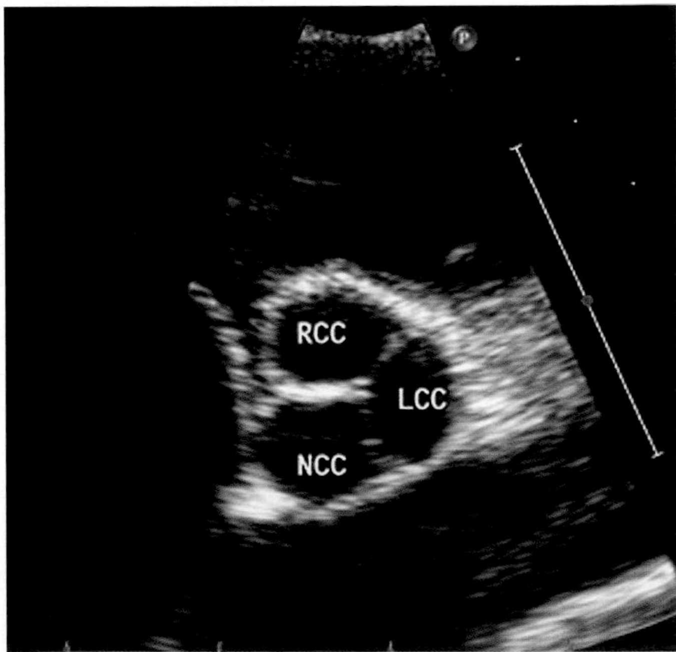

Figure 18A-20 This image shows the parasternal short-axis view of the aortic valve. Three leaflets can be seen, which are supported by left coronary (LCC), right coronary (RCC), and non-coronary (NCC) aortic sinuses.

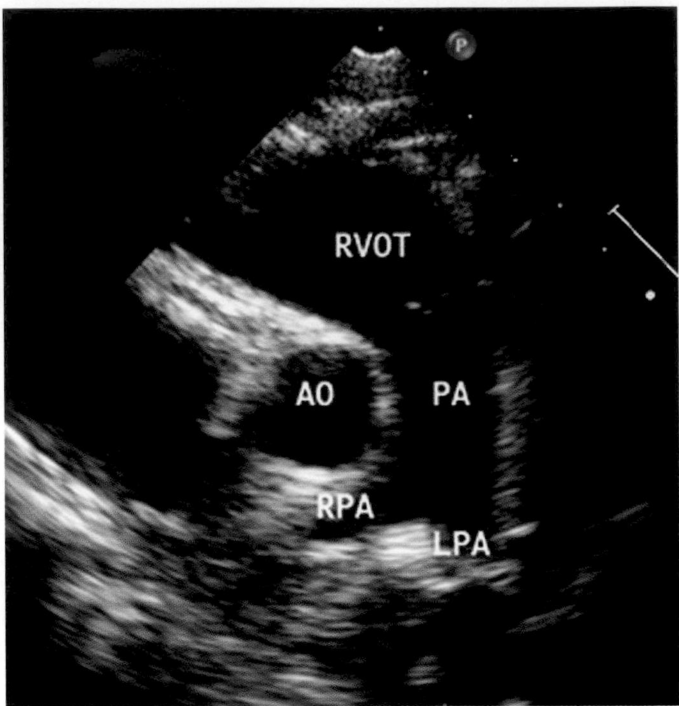

Figure 18A-21 This parasternal short-axis cut of the right ventricular outflow tract (RVOT) shows the pulmonary valve, the pulmonary trunk (PA), and the right and left pulmonary arteries (LPA, RPA). AO, aorta.

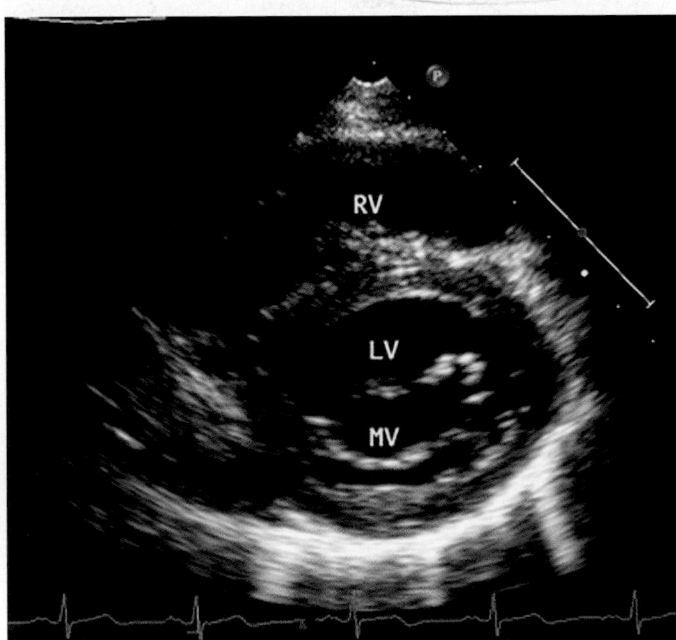

Figure 18A-22 The parasternal short-axis section of the left ventricle (LV) shows the mitral valve (MV), with its aortic and mural leaflets. The right ventricle (RV) is anterior to the left ventricle.

with the notch of the transducer at 12 o'clock. From the apical window, the apical four-chamber, three-chamber long-axis, and two-chamber views can be obtained. The apical four-chamber view allows interrogation of the atrioventricular valves and the morphology of the ventricular apical components (Fig. 18A-24). This view is particularly valuable for assessing apical displacement of the hinges of the leaflets of the tricuspid valve, as well as the septal insertions of the tendinous cords supporting the septal leaflet. Posterior tilting from the apical four-chamber view shows the coronary sinus extending through the inferior left atrioventricular groove. Antero-superior tilting provides the apical five-chamber view, which contains the left ventricular outflow tract, the aortic valve, and the ascending aorta (Fig. 18A-25). The apical long-axis view is obtained by a 60-degree counter-clockwise rotation from the cut showing the apical four-chamber view (Fig. 18A-26). This allows visualisation of the left ventricular outflow tract, as well as the

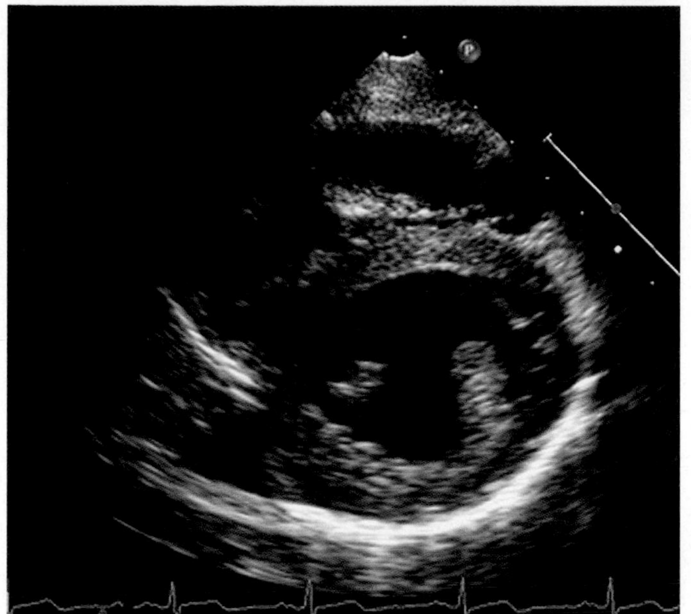

Figure 18A-23 The parasternal short-axis section of the left ventricle shows the two papillary muscles supporting the mitral valve. Note the obliquity of the papillary muscles, with the inferior muscle adjacent to the septum but anterior to its superior counterpart.

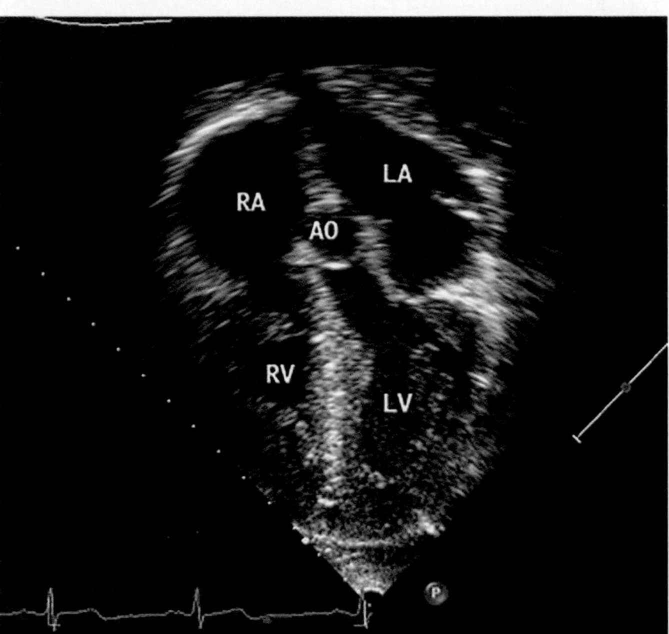

Figure 18A-25 Apical five-chamber view. Anterior tilting from the apical four-chamber view reveals the left ventricular outflow tract. In this image, the left atrium (LA), left ventricle (LV), aorta (AO), right atrium (RA) and right ventricle (RV) can all be seen.

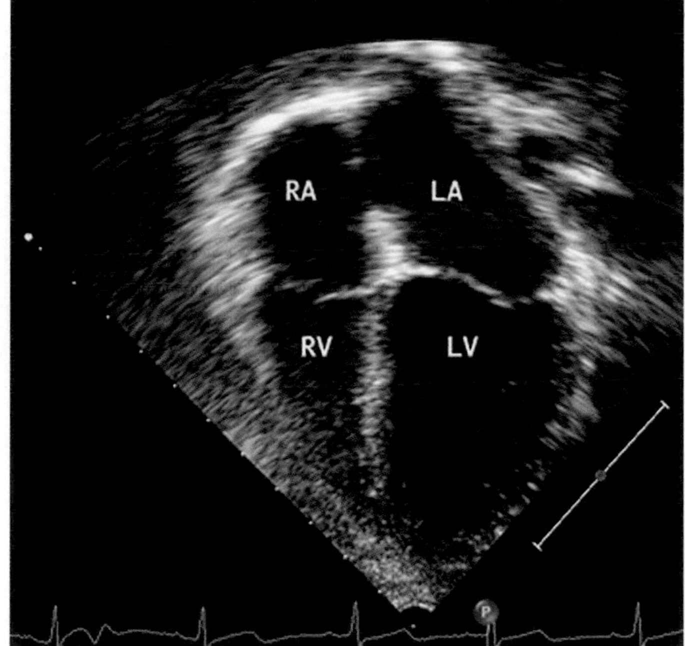

Figure 18A-24 Apical four-chamber view. On this image the right atrium (RA) and right ventricle (RV), together with the left atrium (LA) and left ventricle (LV), can be seen. Note the slight apical displacement of the tricuspid valve relative to the mitral valve on this image.

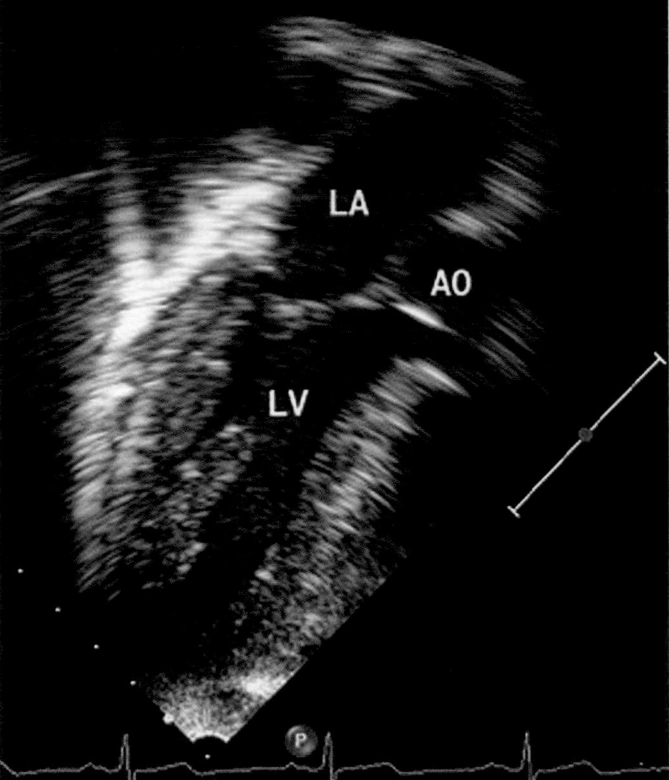

Figure 18A-26 In the apical three-chamber view, it is possible to see the left atrium (LA), left ventricle (LV) and aorta (AO).

mitral valve. The two-chamber view is obtained by further counter-clockwise rotation, and provides images of the walls necessary for assessment of left ventricular function (Fig. 18A-27).

Views from the Suprasternal Notch

When the transducer is positioned in the suprasternal notch, with the notch of the transducer itself at 3 o'clock, the standard short-axis section will demonstrate the left brachiocephalic vein, the short-axis cut of the aortic arch, the right pulmonary artery, and the left atrium (Fig. 18A-28). The four pulmonary veins can be seen entering the left atrium when the transducer is tilted more posteriorly, producing the so-called crab view. The right superior caval

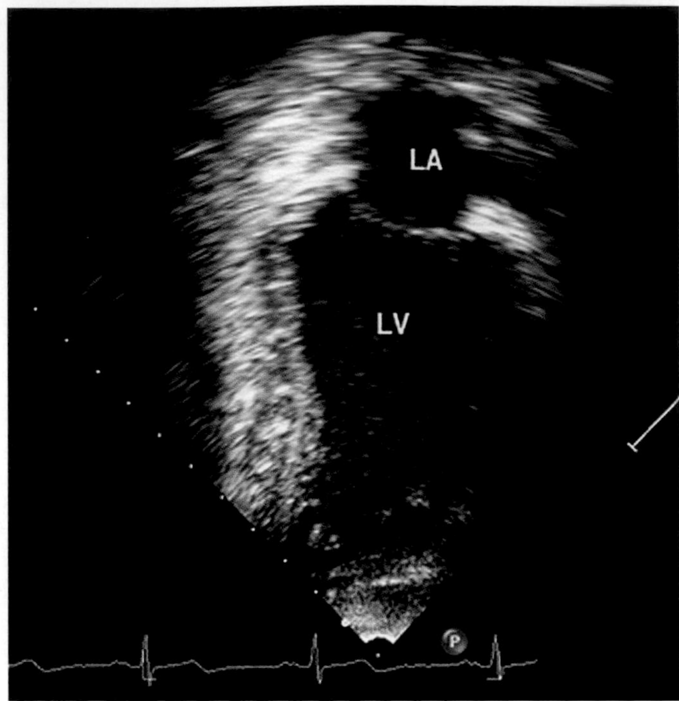

Figure 18A-27 The apical two-chamber view shows the left atrium (LA) and the left ventricle (LV), cutting the superior and inferior walls of the left ventricle. This image is important for the assessment of left ventricular function.

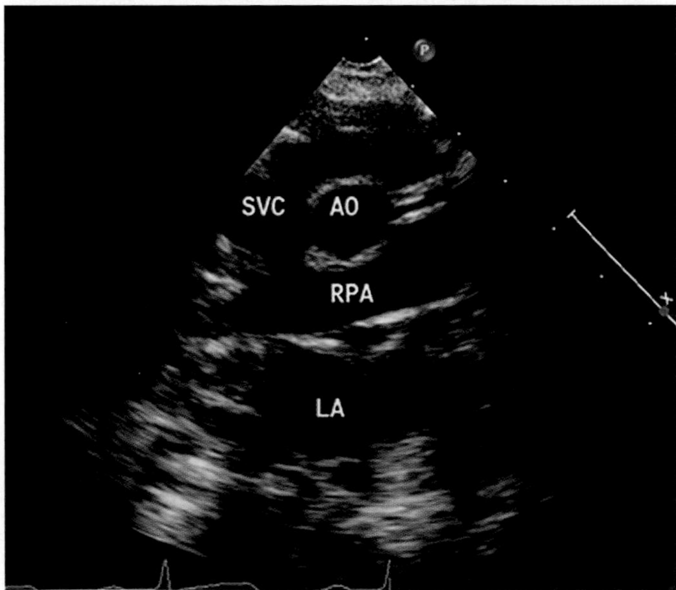

Figure 18A-28 The suprasternal short-axis view shows the superior caval vein (SCV) rightward of the aorta (AO), which is cut in its short axis. Posterior to the aorta is the right pulmonary artery (RPA), and more posterior still is the left atrium (LA). When tilted a little more posteriorly, the crab view is obtained, showing the four pulmonary veins entering the left atrium.

vein is seen to the right. A more cranial angulation of the transducer demonstrates the pattern of branching of the aorta. When the first branch of the brachiocephalic artery is directed to the right, then the aortic arch itself will be left-sided, whereas when the first branch is directed leftward, the arch will be right-sided. Should the first branch from the aortic arch not bifurcate, then an aberrant origin of the subclavian artery should be suspected. Counter-clockwise

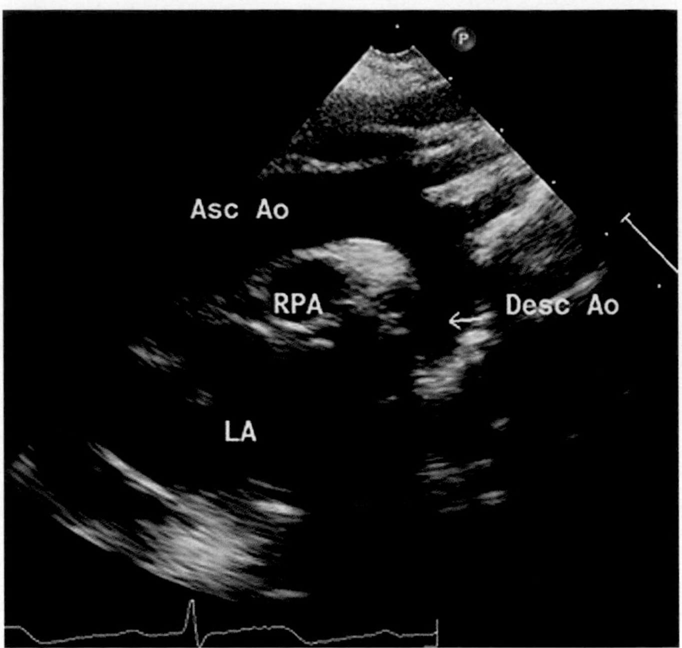

Figure 18A-29 This suprasternal long-axis view cuts through the long axis of the aortic arch, showing both the ascending and descending parts of the aorta (Asc Ao and Desc Ao). Posterior to the aorta is the right pulmonary artery (RPA), and more posterior still is the left atrium (LA).

rotation of the transducer provides a long-axis view of the aortic arch (Fig. 18A-29), with further counter-clockwise rotation and leftward angulation demonstrating the crossing of the left pulmonary artery relative to the descending aorta. Better views of the aorta are sometimes obtained with the transducer to the right of the suprasternal notch, or when it is positioned in high parasternally.

Sequential Segmental Approach to Diagnosis

Description of cardiac anatomy, be it normal or abnormal, should start with the determination of cardiac position and atrial arrangement, and then proceed with analysis of the atrioventricular and ventriculo-arterial connections. Attention is then directed at the systemic and pulmonary venous connections, abnormalities of the atriums and atrioventricular valves, anomalies of the atrioventricular septum, abnormalities of the ventricles, and anomalies of the great arteries. Attention should also be given to extracardiac structures, such as the pericardium, the thymus, and other aspects of the mediastinum.

Determination of Atrial Arrangement

Determining the arrangement of the atrial appendages, these being the most constant components of the atrial chambers themselves, is the first step in the diagnosis of any patient suspected of having heart disease (see Chapter 1). Even using current high resolution echocardiographic imaging, it remains challenging to recognise directly the morphology of the right and left atrial appendages. Instead, atrial arrangement is usually inferred from echocardiographic examination of the relationship of the abdominal great vessels as seen in the subcostal transverse view.[6] Normally the inferior caval vein is located to the right of the spine, and the aorta anterior and to the left. Demonstration of the connection of the inferior caval vein to the right atrium in the long-axis view excludes interruption of the inferior caval vein, presuming that care has been taken to ensure that more than the hepatic veins join the right atrium. If this normal abdominal arrangement of the abdominal great vessels is confirmed, it is reasonable to infer that the atrial chambers are lateralised, with the morphologically right atrium on the same side as the inferior caval vein, and the left atrium on the left side (see Fig. 18A-11). When the atrial chambers are mirror-imaged, the inferior caval vein is left-sided, and the abdominal aorta is to the right of the spine. Almost always, the hepatic veins will all drain to the inferior caval vein, entering just proximal to its junction to the right atrium. When there is isomerism of the right atrial appendages (see Chapter 22), the aorta and inferior caval vein are almost always located on the same side of the spine, either to the right or to the left, with the vein slightly anterior. At least some of the hepatic veins join the intrahepatic caval vein in this setting, although there may be partially anomalous hepatic drainage to either of the atriums. When the left atrial appendages are isomeric, there is usually a midline aorta, with a closely associated azygos vein located posterolateral to the aorta. Parasagittal sections will demonstrate that this posterolateral azygos vein does not connect with either atrium, but instead courses posteriorly to the right or left in the chest to join a superior caval vein. In left isomerism, the hepatic veins tend to drain directly to one or both of the atriums, but there can be a suprahepatic inferior caval vein, with or without anomalous hepatic venous drainage (see Chapter 22). The recognition of venous connections, however, is no more than an inferential guide to the presence of isomerism. It is much better, if possible, to identify directly the structure of the appendages.

Analysis of the Atrioventricular Junctions

The connections of atriums and ventricles across the atrioventricular junctions are determined by obtaining subcostal, parasternal, and apical four-chamber sections, as discussed above. For hearts with biventricular atrioventricular connections (see Chapter 1), the tricuspid valve, which forms an integral part of the morphologically right ventricle, typically has multiple cordal attachments to the ventricular septum. This feature is best demonstrated by the subcostal four-chamber section. In contrast, the tendinous cords from the mitral valve normally attach to two discrete left ventricular papillary muscles, and exceedingly rarely directly to the ventricular septum. In the majority of hearts with biventricular atrioventricular connections, the cordal attachments are the most reliable guide to ventricular morphology. There are, of course, other ways of determining atrioventricular valvar and ventricular morphology. In the normal heart, the medial attachments of the tricuspid valve to the ventricular septum are nearer to the ventricular apex than the corresponding leaflet of the mitral valve (see Fig. 18A-24). This is evident in any four-chamber echocardiogram, but is most striking in the apical views. There are then still other methods of identifying ventricular morphology. A parasternal short-axis section of the left ventricle will reveal the normal bifoliate mitral valve with its obliquely positioned papillary muscles. The trabecular pattern of the ventricle will appear smooth when compared with that of the right. The other characteristics of the morphologically right ventricle are the presence of a septomarginal trabeculation seen just anterior to the ventricular septum on parasternal and apical long-axis sections, an apical moderator band, best seen with parasternal four-chamber views, and a trifoliate atrioventricular valve, best identified using the subcostal short-axis section.

Having determined the structure of the junctions, it is then necessary to establish the morphology of the valves that guard them. Cross sectional echocardiography is unique in its ability to demonstrate abnormalities of the atrioventricular valves, especially in the four-chamber sections. When both atriums connect to the ventricular mass, the atrioventricular junctions may be guarded by two patent valves, by one patent and one imperforate valve, by a common valve, or by straddling or overriding valves. These different modes of atrioventricular connection can be found with concordant, discordant, biventricular and mixed, or double inlet types of connection (see Chapter 1). Overriding and straddling are distinguished by considering the junction for the former, and the tension apparatus for the latter. When there is a common valve, it is usual to find both overriding and straddling, but this is not always the case, since the common valve can guard both junctions when they connect to the same ventricle. When one atrioventricular connection is absent, of necessity there are fewer options for the modes of connection, since there is but one atrioventricular valve. This valve is usually totally committed to one ventricle, but straddling and overriding are sometimes encountered. This produces the rare findings of a uniatrial but biventricular connection. The degree of overriding of a valve will determine the categorisation of atrioventricular connections, cross sectional echocardiography readily permitting the distinction between the biventricular and univentricular arrangements.

Analysis of the Ventriculo-arterial Junctions

When assessing the junctions between the ventricles and the arterial trunks, it is necessary first to identify ventricular morphology, using the methods already described, and then to establish the arrangement of the arterial trunks. In infants and small children, the latter information is usually derived from subcostal coronal sweeps. This is generally supplemented by other echocardiographic sections, like the high parasternal short- and long-axis views. The aorta is characterised by identifying the origin of the brachiocephalic arteries from the arch. The pulmonary trunk is recognised on the basis of its bifurcation into right and left branches. A common arterial trunk is a solitary arterial trunk giving rise in its ascending part to the coronary and pulmonary arteries and the ascending aorta. Having established the connections across the ventriculo-arterial junctions, it is also important separately to determine the arrangement of the arterial valves, the relationship between the arterial trunks, and the infundibular morphology. These features are all independent of one another, and independent of the ventriculo-arterial connections. Establishing each feature separately, and describing them all, removes the potential for ambiguity (see Chapter 1).

Paediatric Transoesophageal Echocardiography

Transoesophageal echocardiography is complementary to transthoracic echocardiography in the diagnosis and monitoring of infants and children with congenitally malformed hearts. Miniaturisation of the transoesophageal probes has allowed this technique to be applied to children weighing from around 3 to 3.5 kg. Guidelines for its use have recently been updated by the American Society of

Echocardiography.[7] The technique has an important role in documenting the adequacy of surgical repair immediately after the discontinuation of bypass, and in the early post-operative period in the intensive care unit where transthoracic windows can be limited. In most centres, peri-operative transoesophageal imaging is performed during nearly every surgical intervention, and has been shown to have an important impact on the surgical results. Transoesophageal imaging is also indicated for monitoring various procedures used during interventional catheterisation. It can also be indicated for patients with inadequate transthoracic windows, although alternative imaging techniques like cardiac magnetic imaging are usually preferred in children.

Transoesophageal examinations are performed using systems offering cross sectional imaging, colour Doppler, continuous wave, and pulsed wave Doppler, as well as tissue Doppler. Multi-plane transoesophageal probes are currently available for use in children weighing from 3 to 20 kg. In smaller infants, this probe needs to be used with extreme caution. Epicardial imaging might still be a good alternative in this setting. The larger multi-planar probes designed for use in adults can be used in patients weighing more than 15 to 20 kg. Recently, an adult-sized three-dimensional transesophageal probe, which is about 2 mm thicker compared to the adult multi-planar probe, has become available, allowing real-time three-dimensional transoesophageal imaging. This probe can only be used in children above 15 kg, but it is expected to be miniaturised for future use in children. The probes should always pass easily without significant resistance. Complications are rare, but include oesophageal perforation, along with compression of vessels and airways. Because of these rare complications, nonetheless, continuous monitoring of the haemodynamic and respiratory state is always required. Transoesophageal echocardiography, therefore, requires at least two attending physicians, one to manage the airway and monitor the patient, and the other to perform the examination. For most infants and children, the studies are performed under general anaesthesia, using tracheal intubation under the supervision of an anaesthesiologist. For examination of intubated patients in the intensive care unit, and for study of adolescents, sedation is usually sufficient. Deep sedation may be adequate in an outpatient setting.

The absolute contra-indications to a transoesophaegeal examination are the presence of any pharyngeal or oesophageal lesion predisposing to laceration or perforation during manipulation of the probe. In addition, some patients with tracheomalacia may manifest a fall in systemic arterial saturation when the probe is manipulated because of tracheal compression. Although bacteraemia has been reported, the need for prophylaxis against bacterial endocarditis remains controversial. In the most recent published guidelines, the risk for bacterial endocarditis due to patients undergoing a gastrointestinal procedure was judged to be exceedingly small, not justifying the prophylactic use of antibiotics.[8]

Technique of Examination

After induction of general anaesthesia and endotracheal intubation, or following appropriate sedation, the head of the patient is positioned in the midline, or slightly to the left, the mouth opened with the jaw thrust forward, and the neck slightly extended. The unlocked tip of the probe is lubricated with a water-soluble gel, gently introduced into the hypopharynx, and advanced until an image of the heart is displayed on the screen. If there is resistance to passage of the transducer, a laryngoscope can be used to permit introduction under direct vision. Once the transducer is appropriately positioned, the head of the patient can be maintained in the midline, or placed to face the echocardiographer. The probe is then manipulated to obtain a range of transoesophageal images. A series of transgastric sections can be obtained by manipulating the tip of the probe when it has been advanced into the stomach. In contrast to transthoracic echocardiography, there is less flexibility in the imaging planes. Mulitplanar imaging allows rotation of the imaging plane between 0 and 180 degrees. Zero corresponds to a transverse view, while 90 degrees corresponds to a more longitudinal view. Use of specific angles to obtain certain images is not very useful, as the morphology might differ between individuals. The American Society of Echocardiography has issued guidelines for orientation of images, which can be used as as a reference. For those with complexly malformed hearts, unusual imaging planes might be required. Some of the standard images are further discussed.

Transoesophageal Views

Midoesophageal Four-chamber View

In a transverse plane, at around zero, it is possible to produce a four-chamber view, imaging the atrioventricular valves, the ventricles, and the atrial and ventricular septums (Fig. 18A-30). The images produced are shown with the apex down, and with the left ventricle to the right of the screen. When slightly moving the probe upwards, the atrial septum can nicely be visualised. Slight rotation to the left at atrial level allows visualisation of the left pulmonary veins, and slight rightward rotation reveals the right pulmonary veins. Adding colour Doppler with a low Nyquist limit might help to identify the pulmonary veins from this view. By very slight upward and downward motion, it is possible

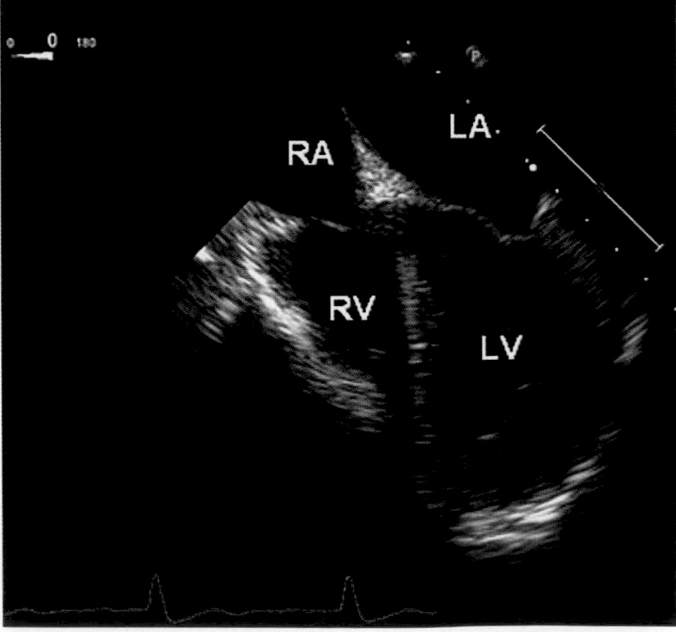

Figure 18A-30 This transoesophageal four-chamber view is obtained from a mid-oesophageal position. The left atrium (LA), left ventricle (LV), right atrium (RA) and right ventricle (RV) are all imaged in this projection.

to distinguish the upper and lower left and right pulmonary veins. The apical four-chamber view is well suited to the assessment of atrioventricular valvar function. Using color Doppler and pulsed wave Doppler, which generally can be well-aligned from this plane, it is possible to evaluate atrioventricular valvar regurgitation as well as stenosis. This view is also suited to assess the ventricular septum. A search is often made for residual ventricular septal defects using this particular imaging plane after discontinuation of cardiopulmonary bypass.

Midoesophageal Short- and Long-axis Views

From the mid-oesophageal postion, different short- and long-axis views can be obtained. By slightly advancing and flexing the probe from a standard four-chamber view, a short-axis view at the level of the atrioventricular valves can be obtained (Fig. 18A-31). This is useful for assessing the leaflets after repair of an atrioventricular septal defect. In most patients, however, the transgastric short-axis cuts are easier to obtain, and are the ones most commonly used.

From a standard apical four-chamber view, rotating the probe to between 0 and 60 degrees with slight flexion and pull-back produces an image of the aortic valvar leaflets in their short axis (Fig. 18A-32). This usually permits the distinction of trifoliate from bifoliate valves. The origins of the coronary arteries can also be assessed from this view. The left coronary artery normally originates from the left coronary aortic sinus, while the right artery originates more anteriorly from the right coronary aortic sinus. The proximal course of the coronary arteries can generally be identified. Here, it can be extremely useful to use colour Doppler with a low Nyquist limit, thus confirming normal flow in the arteries. The same view permits identification of the membranous part of the ventricular septum, and residual ventricular septal defects if present. The anterosuperior and septal leaflets of the tricuspid valves can be imaged. It is often possible obtain good alignment with a regurgitant jet across the tricuspid valve to estimate right ventricular pressures. From the same plane, the right ventricular outflow tract, the pulmonary valve, and the pulmonary trunk, can all be viewed (Fig. 18A-33). By pulling back the probe slightly, the proximal part of the right pulmonary artery, and its segment running behind the aorta, can usually be well imaged (Fig. 18A-34). Imaging the left pulmonary artery from the oesophagus can be very challenging because of the loss of the image due to interference by air as it crosses the bronchus. Slight leftward rotation might permit visualisation of the most proximal part of the artery, but this is lost as it crosses the bronchus. The distal parts can be visualised from a mid-oesophageal long-axis view, rotating the probe posteriorly to image both the descending aorta and the crossing left pulmonary artery.

When the probe is pulled back further, using the angulation between 30 and 60 degrees, a short-axis image of

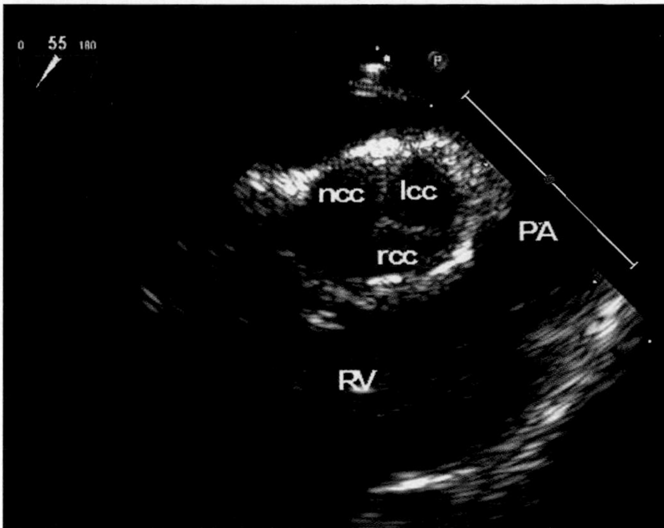

Figure 18A-32 This transoesophageal short-axis view is taken at the level of the aortic valve, showing the leaflets of the aortic valve supported by their appropriate sinuses. lcc, left coronary; ncc, non-coronary sinus; PA, pulmonary trunk; rcc, right coronary sinus; RV, right ventricle.

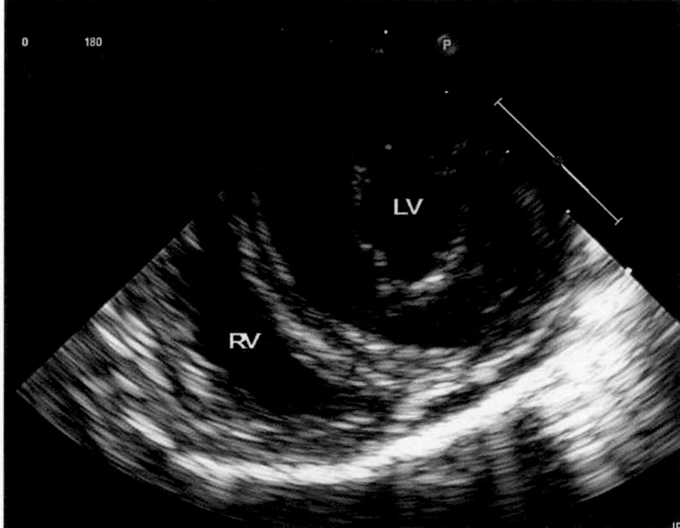

Figure 18A-31 The transoesophageal short-axis view at the level of the mitral valve shows both the left and right ventricles (LV and RV). The cut provides a nice image of the mitral valve, showing the aortic and mural leaflets seen in their open position.

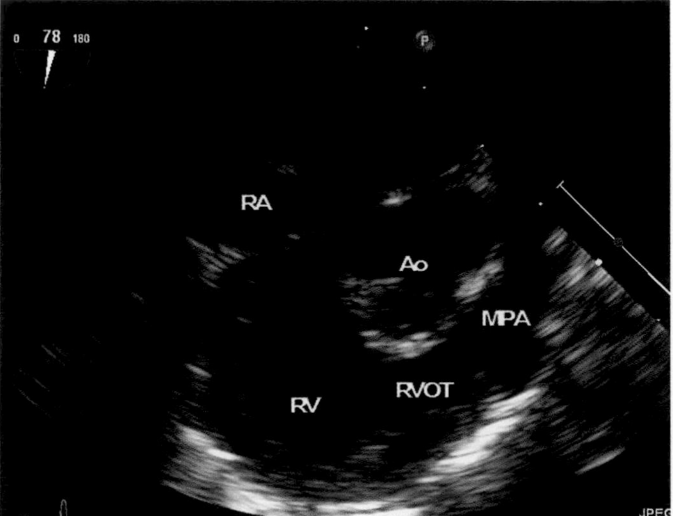

Figure 18A-33 This transoespohageal short-axis view shows the right ventricular outflow tract (RVOT), revealing the infundibulum, the pulmonary valve, and the pulmonary trunk (MPA). Ao, aorta; RA, right atrium; RV, right ventricle.

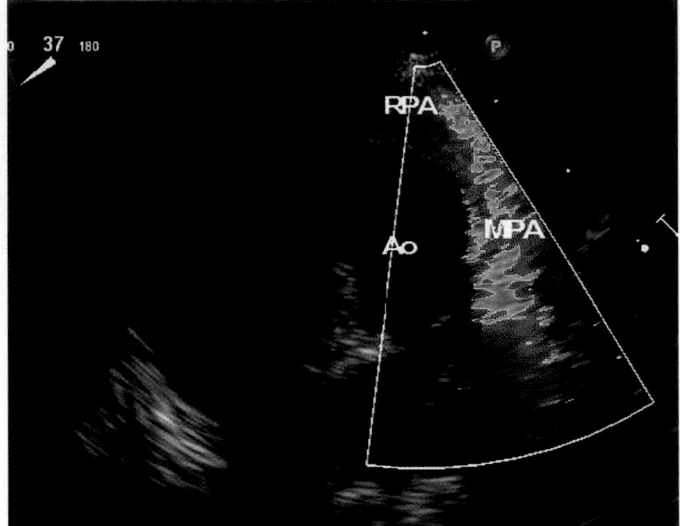

Figure 18A-34 This transoespohageal short-axis view shows the pulmonary trunk (MPA) and the right pulmonary artery (RPA). The proximal part of the right pulmonary artery runs posterior to the aorta (Ao). Note that the proximal left pulmonary artery cannot be seen on this view.

the atrial septum can be obtained. This image shows the antero-superior rim of the oval foramen, this being the region where most often the foramen is patent. The cut also shows the floor of the oval fossa, this being the location of true atrial septal defects. The view also proves very useful when monitoring the insertion of devices to close either a septal defect or a patent oval foramen, since it demonstrates well the relationship between the superior rim of the fossa and the device.

Rotating the probe to an angle between 90 and 120 degrees at mid-oesophageal level will produce a long-axis view of the left ventricle, this being the preferred view for imaging the left ventricular outflow tract, the aortic valve, and the supra-aortic region (Fig. 18A-35). Between 60 and 90 degrees, a two-chamber view is obtained, while a three-chamber long-axis view can be produced between 90 and 120 degrees. Addition of colour Doppler permits assessment of the left ventricular outflow tract, as well as aortic regurgitation. The mitral valve is well seen both on the two-chamber view and the long-axis view. This allows better evaluation of the degree of mitral regurgitation, if present, in a second plane apart from the four-chamber view. Regurgitant jets directed anteriorly or posteriorly can better be visualised, and thus can be localised in three dimensions. The same view shows well the membranous part of the ventricular septum, and helps assessment of devices inserted for closure of perimembranous ventricular septal defects, showing the relationship between the device and the leaflets of the aortic valve.

By pulling back the probe to atrial level, and angulating around 90 degrees, a long-axis view of the atrial septum and both atriums is obtained (Fig. 18A-36). This can nicely demonstrate the orifices of both caval veins. It is sometimes necessary slightly to move the probe forward and backward. This view is ideal for demonstrating the sinus venosus defects, along with anomalous connection of pulmonary veins to the superior caval vein.

Transgastric Views

Transgastric views are obtained by advancing the probe into the stomach, flexing it, and pulling it back in the flexed position until it contacts the gastric fundus. The images obtained resemble closely those obtained from subcostal position, albeit that flexibility is reduced for changing the plane of imaging when the probe is in the stomach. The transgastric images are oriented so that, when seen on the screen, the apex is down, the outflow tracts are up, and the left ventricle is on the right side of the screen, thus retaining consistency with the orientation of subcostal images. Depending on the degree of flexion, more anteriorly or posteriorly directed images are obtained.

The short-axis view is usually the first one obtained when the probe is advanced into the stomach and anteflexed to image the heart. The right and left ventricles and the intervening ventricular septum are shown, with various short-axis planes permitting analysis of the atrioventricular valves, the position of the papillary

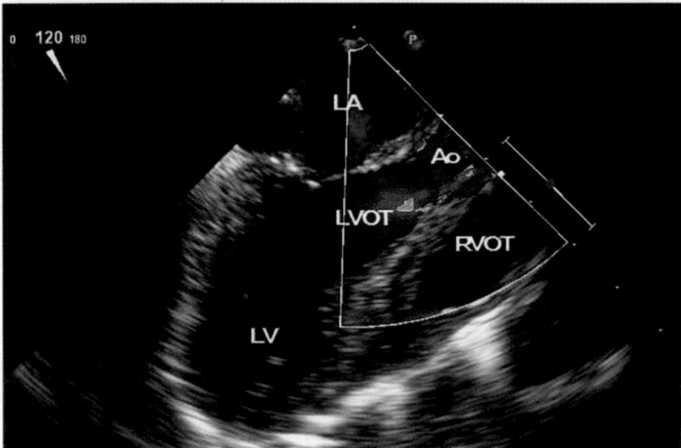

Figure 18A-35 The colour-Doppler transoesophageal long-axis view shows the left ventricle and left ventricular outflow tract (LVOT). This view is used to look for obstruction in the outflow tract and aortic insufficiency. Ao, aorta; LA, left atrium; LV, left ventricle; RVOT, right ventricular outflow tract.

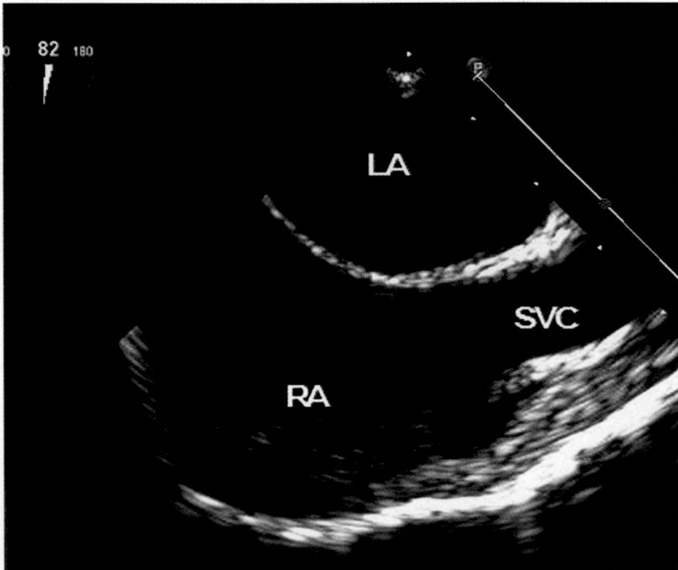

Figure 18A-36 This transoesophageal long-axis view is taken at the level of the atrial septum, showing the long axis of the atrial septum separating the left (LA) from the right atrium (RA). The superior caval vein (SVC) is seen entering the right atrium.

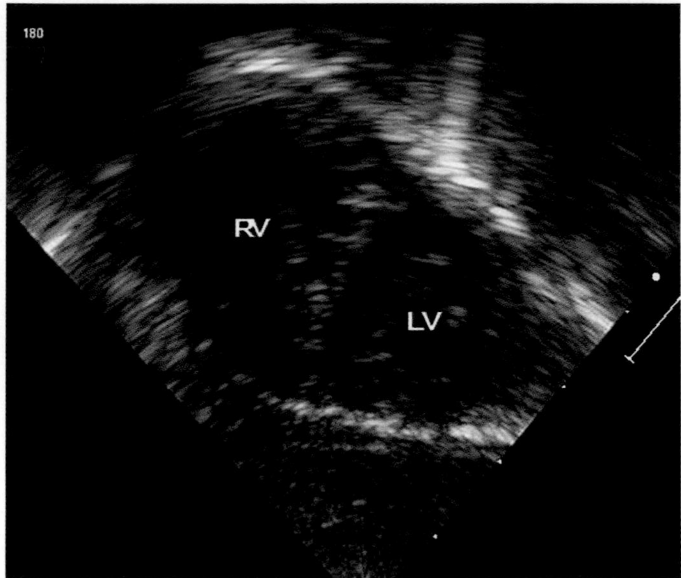

Figure 18A-37 The transgastric short-axis view cuts through both the left (LV) and the right ventricle (RV). This view is used for assessing biventricular function.

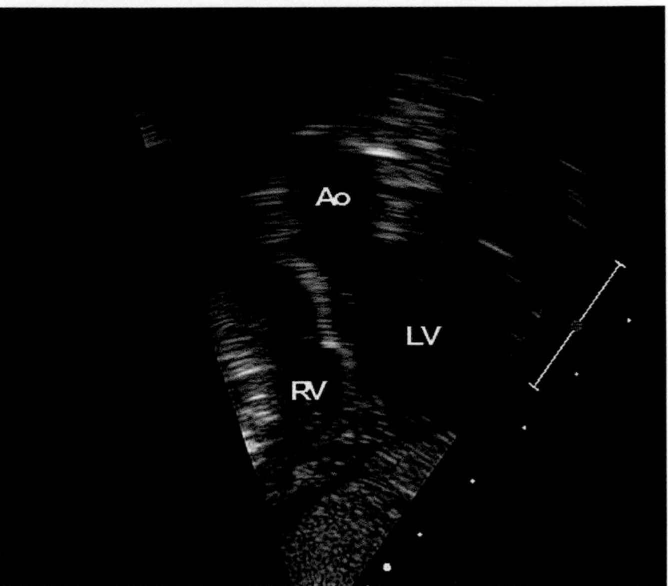

Figure 18A-39 From transgastric position, it is also possible to cut longitudinally along the left ventricular outflow tract. From this window, it is often possible to obtain good Doppler interrogation of obstructions within the outflow tract. Ao, aorta; LV, left ventricle; RV, right ventricle.

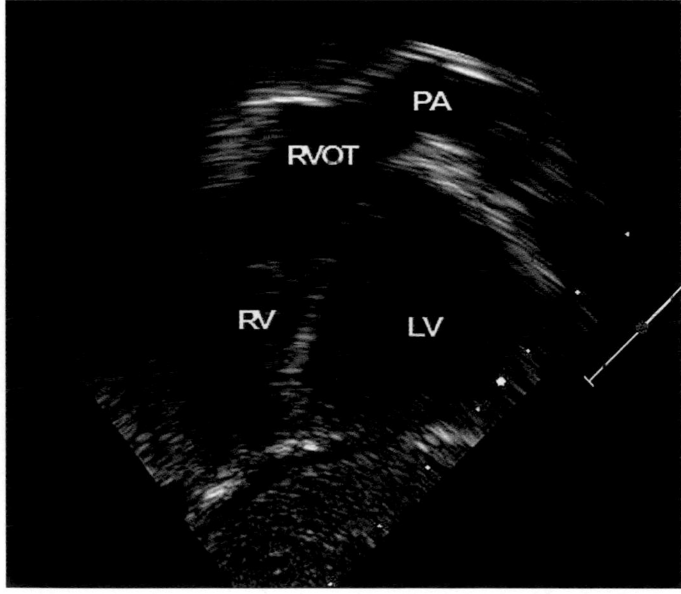

Figure 18A-38 The transgastric view provided a more longitudinal image of the right ventricular outflow tract. From this window, it is often possible to obtain good Doppler alignment to assess any obstruction within the outflow tract. LV, left ventricle; PA, pulmonary trunk; RV, right ventricle; RVOT, right ventricular outflow tract.

muscles, the pattern of the apical trabeculations, and the ventricular relationships (Fig. 18A-37). These views are also used for studying global and regional left ventricular function immediately after discontinuation of cardiopulmonary bypass. Angulating the probe in a long-axis dimension, with different degree of flexion, shows the right and left ventricular outflow tracts (Figs. 18A-38 and 18A-39). From the transgastric views, it is often possible to align a pulsed wave or continuous wave Doppler cursor in order to quantify the degree of obstruction in the outflow tracts, if present. Lack of good alignment between the signal and the flow can be an important limitation for transoesophageal echocardiography.

SPECIAL USES OF ECHOCARDIOGRAPHY

Post-operative Echocardiography

As has already been discussed extensively, transoesophageal echocardiography has now become the gold standard for post-operative monitoring. The technique plays an important role in the assessment of post-bypass ventricular function, the adequacy of the surgical repair, and detection of any residual lesion that may require immediate revision. After the patient has been transferred to the intensive care unit, echocardiographic evaluation might be required should there be unexplained haemodynamic deterioration. The windows available for imaging the patient in the intensive care unit can be extremely limited due to wound dressings, an open chest, and poor positioning. Despite these limitations, it is possible to get sufficient information in the majority of patients. Should insufficient data be gathered, repeating the transoesophageal interrogation is a good option if the patient remains intubated and ventilated. The aim of the evaluation is, first, to assess ventricular systolic function. Often this will rely on subjective evaluation. If the images are adequate, however, the biplane Simpson's method can be used to quantify ejection fraction. The second goal is to assess any haemodynamically significant residual lesion. Compared to the immediate period after discontinuation from post-bypass, important changes in preload, afterload, and contractility occur over the next 24 to 48 hours. Residual shunts, stenosis, and regurgitation all require exclusion, since these complications can be underestimated during the study performed immediately after completion of post-bypass. The third task is to evaluate ventricular filling and diastolic function. Cross sectional images permit

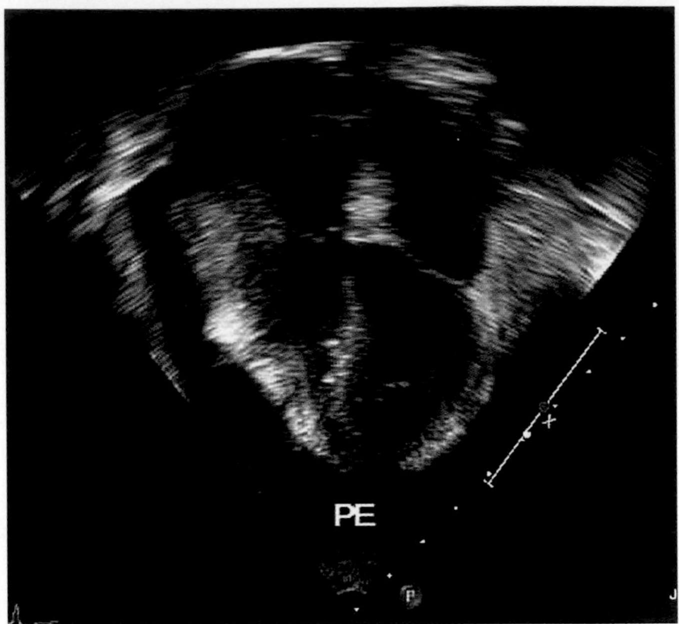

Figure 18A-40 This apical four-chamber view is taken in a patient with a large pericardial effusion, which surrounds both ventricles and extends to the left ventricular apex. PE, pericardial effusion.

Figure 18A-41 This image shows contrast echocardiography using agitated saline. The right atrium (RA) is opacified with contrast. Some bubbles pass through the atrial septum to fill the left atrium (LA). LV, left ventricle; RV, right ventricle.

assessment of the filling of the ventricular cavities. Formal assessment of diastolic function should exclude restrictive right ventricular physiology in case of right heart disease, or left ventricular diastolic dysfunction. Pericardial effusions and cardiac tamponade should also be excluded (Fig. 18A-40). Echocardiography in the intensive care unit requires good communication between the echocardiographer and the physician in charge of intensive care so that the question or clinical problem under investigation is well communicated and hopefully answered.

Contrast Echocardiography

Contrast echocardiography requires the injection of a substance that produces echocardiographic opacification of the blood, increasing the contrast between the blood and the surrounding structures. In children, this usually involves the intravenous injection of agitated saline (Fig. 18A-41). The multiple interfaces between the liquid and the air produce an increased backscatter when interacting with ultrasound. The microbubbles are filtered by the pulmonary or systemic capillary beds, and disappear very quickly from the circulation. Carbon dioxide is added to the mixture to reduce the risk of air embolisation should there be a right-to-left shunt. The carbon dioxide is quickly absorbed in the blood when the bubbles disappear. Specialised contrast agents have also been developed. They contain smaller bubbles, which are more stable compared to agitated saline. Their increased stability allows opacification of the myocardium after they have passed through the ventricular cavity, thus permitting study of myocardial perfusion. These modern agents, however, have not thus far been approved for use in children. In children, only agitated saline can be used. The main indication is the detection of right-to-left shunts not seen using colour Doppler interrogation. This can be caused by intracardiac shunts such as a patent oval foramen, or extracardiac shunts, such as arteriovenous malformations, or a left superior caval vein persisting after a bidirectional Glenn shunt.

Stress Echocardiography

Echocardiography is generally performed at rest with the patient lying in the lateral position or on the back, depending on the window used for imaging. For certain indications, like coronary arterial disease, or the evaluation of the haemodynamic significance of certain valvar lesions, studying the heart during stress provides extra information which might help subsequent treatment. Pharmacological stress and exercise echocardiography are the two common stressors used to evaluate the haemodynamic and myocardial responses. Exercise can be performed after a baseline echocardiography on a treadmill or on a bicycle, and immediately after peak exercise the echocardiographic study is repeated with the patient in a supine position. Alternatively, exercise echocardiography can be performed on a supine bicycle, which allows continuous imaging during the test. This implies that the real peak exercise can be recorded, and that the imaging is not performed during the period of recovery. Typical pharmacological stress includes the administration of dobutamine, or vasodilators such as adenosine or dipyramidole. In children, the most common indications for a stress test are the detection of vasculopathy after transplantation, or problems with the coronary arteries after operations like the arterial switch procedure or the Ross operation.

Quantitative Echocardiography

Cross sectional echocardiography allows the description of cardiac anatomy in great detail. The first prerequisite in every child is to rule out morphological abnormalities. If present, they should be fully characterized. Apart from morphological evaluation, a full echocardiographic study should also provide information on haemodynamics, specifically pressures and flows, valvar function such as the degree of stenosis and regurgitation, and ventricular systolic and diastolic function. While morphology is descriptive, functional parameters are quantititative. By combining different M-mode, cross sectional, and Doppler techniques it has become possible to gather quantitative information on the haemodynamic severity of cardiac defects.

Quantification of Echocardiographic Dimensions

Determination of the size of the heart and great vessels is essential for the diagnosis and treatment of congenital cardiac disease. One of the challenges facing the paediatric echocardiographer is the fact that cardiovascular structures grow along with the size of the body. In order to be able to compare measurements, methods need to be developed to normalise cardiac dimensions for growth. As essential as normalisation of the measurements for growth is the standardisation of cardiac measurements. The American Association for Echocardiography has published recommendations for standardisation of echocardiographic measurements, but a lot of relevant structures in children are not included in the description.[9] So, when using normative data, it is important to perform the measurement exactly the same way as the initial data was obtained. The best way to normalise measurements in children is to use z-scores.[10] The z-score of a variable corresponds to the position of an observed case relative to the mean of the distribution in the population expressed in standard deviations. The z-scores are derived from a large number of normal observations within populations in which the mean and standard deviation are derived as a function of the size of the body. Representing a measurement as a z-score immediately provides the information how the measurement is positioned relative for the mean of the population. A z-score of -4 for the annulus of the mitral valve is four standard deviations below the mean for the normal population. The z-scores can be derived from published normograms or formulas.[11,12] Ideally, each laboaratory performing paediatric echocardiography should be able to establish its own z-scores for use as a reference. The same formula should also be used to calculate body surface area as compared to the normative dataset, as different mathematical formulas have been used for these purposes.

Ventricular dimensions are still commonly measured by the M-mode technique in a large majority of paediatric echocardiographic laboratories. The high frame rate allows accurate recording of events that occur rapidly, such as mural motion, change in cavitary size, and motion of leaflets (Fig. 18A-42). Measurements can be made at precise times within the cardiac cycle. For this reason, an M-mode recording should always be accompanied by an electrocardiogram. End-diastolic measurements are typically made at the onset of the QRS-complex, while maximal mural excursion is often used for the definition of end-systole, which usually corresponds to the end of the T-wave. M-mode measurements can be made in the parasternal short-axis and long-axis cuts at the level of the leaflets of the mitral valve. Cross sectional imaging should be used to align the M-mode cursor so as to avoid oblique cuts. The M-mode measurements are then used to calculate fractional shortening on the basis of left ventricular end-diastolic dimension minus left ventricular end-systolic dimension divided by the left ventricular end-diastolic dimension. It can also

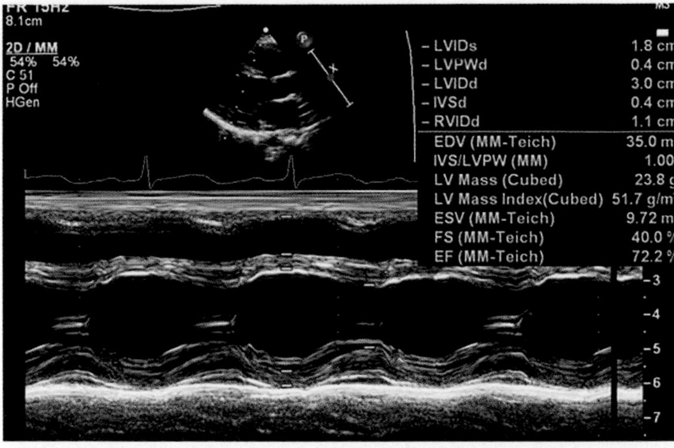

Figure 18A-42 This M-mode tracing is recorded perpendicular to the major axis of the left ventricle just distal to the mitral valve. This image is used to calculate left ventricular dimensions and fractional shortening.

be used to calculate the index of left ventricular mass. Left atrial and ascending aortic dimensions are measured with the M-line at the level of the leaflets of the aortic valve in parasternal long- or short-axis sections (see Fig. 18A-42).

Quantification of Flow, and Identification of Patterns of Flow

Normal Doppler Examination

Doppler measures the velocities of blood pools, providing both quantitative and qualitative information. When making such measurements, it is important to recognise certain patterns of flow, which are different within different parts of the circulation. It is also important to have knowledge of the different normal velocities of flow within the circulation. In this section, we discuss the qualitative and quantitative aspects of Doppler echocardiography in the normal heart. We will discuss how normal and abnormal patterns can be differentiated, emphasising the common sites used for interrogation in children with congenitally malformed hearts.

Systemic Venous Flow

The inferior caval vein can be imaged from the subcostal position using colour Doppler, ensuring a low Nyquist limit. When guided by the colour flow, the sample volume of the pulsed wave Doppler can be aligned as well as possible. Usually this will be in the paracoronal view of the inferior caval vein entering the right atrium. The scale should be lowered, and the baseline shifted upwards, as the flow is below the baseline. The superior caval vein can be imaged in subcostal or suprasternal views. From the subcostal position, flow will be towards the transducer, while from the suprasternal notch, it will be away from the transducer. Especially in larger children, it is easier to measure the flow from the suprasternal view. The normal pattern of venous flow is triphasic (Fig. 18A-43). The S wave occurs during ventricular systole, and is caused by atrial relaxation and descent of the tricuspid ring. The D wave occurs during diastole. It corresponds to ventricular filling when the tricuspid valve is open. During atrial contraction, there is a brief period during which flow is reversed in the systemic veins. This corresponds to the A wave. The S and D waves correspond, respectively, to the x and y descents of the jugular venous pulse, while the Doppler A wave corresponds to the venous A wave. There is marked respiratory variation in the velocities, with an increase in S and D velocities with

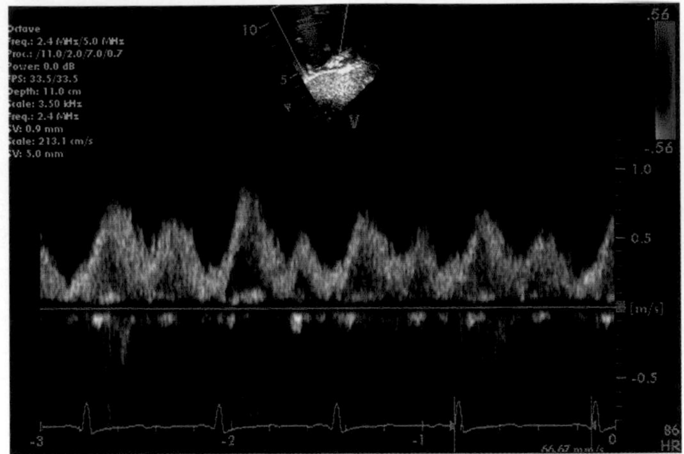

Figure 18A-43 The subcostal pulsed wave Doppler shows flow through the superior caval vein, which is in the direction of the probe. There is a systolic, as well as a diastolic component, with very limited reversal of flow during atrial contraction.

Figure 18A-44 Subcostal pulsed wave Doppler of the abdominal aortic flow. Flow is in the direction of the probe. There is a very short early diastolic reversal (*arrows*), which is normal. There is no significant diastolic flow.

inspiration. This explains why normal values have been defined during expiration. The value for the S wave is 0.70 ± 0.14 m/sec, while that for the D wave is 0.41 ± 0.09 m/sec. With high heart rates, the S and D flows may be fused and appear continuous

Abnormal patterns of flow in the caval veins can be seen in the setting of tricuspid regurgitation, which is associated with decreased S flow and increased D flow. When regurgitation is severe, there can be systolic reversal of flow. Abnormalities of right ventricular myocardial relaxation will result in decreased D flow and increased S flow. In those with restrictive right ventricles and increased right atrial pressure, the S flow is decreased, and a large A reversal is present during atrial contraction. Low flow in the hepatic veins can also be studied from the subcostal views. The Doppler waveforms are similar to those seen in the caval veins but with lower velocities.

Abdominal Aorta

From the subcostal position, it is possible to obtain a parasagittal view of the abdominal aorta. Aortic pulsatility can readily be observed using cross sectional imaging or colour Doppler (Fig. 18A-44). Pulsed wave Doppler sampling can be obtained at this site, but it is generally not possible to align the Doppler beam entirely parallel to the flow, so only quantitative information is obtained. The normal abdominal pattern shows a predominant systolic flow, with a very short early diastolic reversal and no additional diastolic flow. Continuous diastolic forward flow occurs in the context of coarctation of the aorta. In this setting, detection of diastolic anterograde flow is considered a good tool for screening. Diastolic reversal or backflow occurs in the context of severe aortic regurgitation, an aortopulmonary shunt with left-to-right shunting, such as seen in the patient with a large persistently patent arterial duct, an aortopulmonary window, aortopulmonary collateral arteries, or Blalock-Taussig or central shunts, or in case of large arteriovenous malformations in the upper part of the body. Flow in the abdominal aorta is reduced in case of low cardiac output.

Pulmonary Veins

The velocity of pulmonary venous flow can be obtained from different windows, but flow is commonly recorded in the right upper or lower pulmonary vein from the apical four-chamber view. The normal pattern is triphasic, but there can be a biphasic systolic component. The early systolic peak, S1, corresponds to atrial relaxation. The later systolic peak corresponds to systolic filling of the atrium due to systolic descent of the mitral valve. The diastolic flow corresponds to early diastolic filling, and there is atrial reversal during atrial contraction (Fig. 18A-45). Pulmonary venous flows are abnormal in the context of pulmonary venous stenosis, mitral regurgitation, and left ventricular diastolic dysfunction. Assessment of pulmonary venous flow has become an integral part of the evaluation of left ventricular diastolic function. Normal velocities of pulmonary venous flow are less influenced by respiration compared to systemic venous flow. The velocities, however, change with age, and are also dependent on heart rate.

Atrioventricular Valves

Velocities of flow through the mitral and tricuspid valves are usually best recorded from the apical four-chamber view. The cursor should be positioned at the tip of the leaflets, with the smallest possible sample volume. The flow

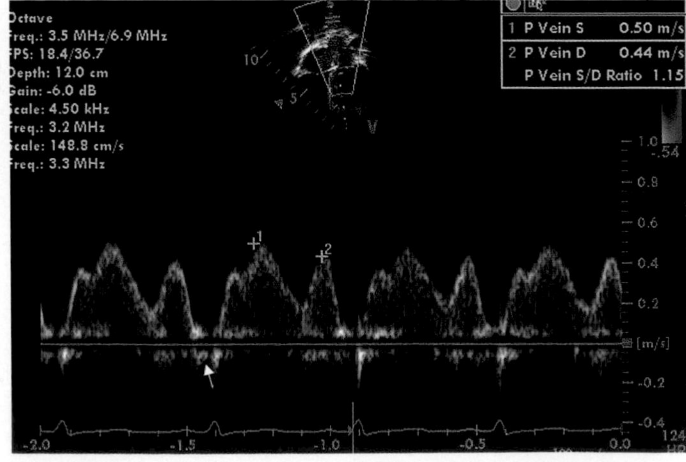

Figure 18A-45 Apical four-chamber view of a pulmonary venous tracing. Notice the biphasic pattern of systolic flow, and the monophasic diastolic flow. There is a limited reversal of flow during atrial contraction (*arrow*). The peak systolic and diastolic velocities are measured, permitting calculation of the ratio of systolic to diastolic peak velocity.

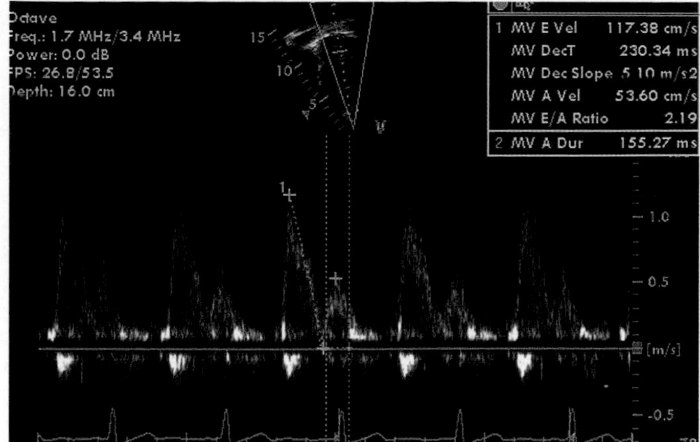

Figure 18A-46 The normal pattern of mitral inflow as imaged from the apical four-chamber view. The peak E-velocity and peak A-velocity are measured, permitting calculation of the ratio of velocities, the E to A ratio. It is also possible to measure the deceleration time of the early peak, and the duration of the A-wave.

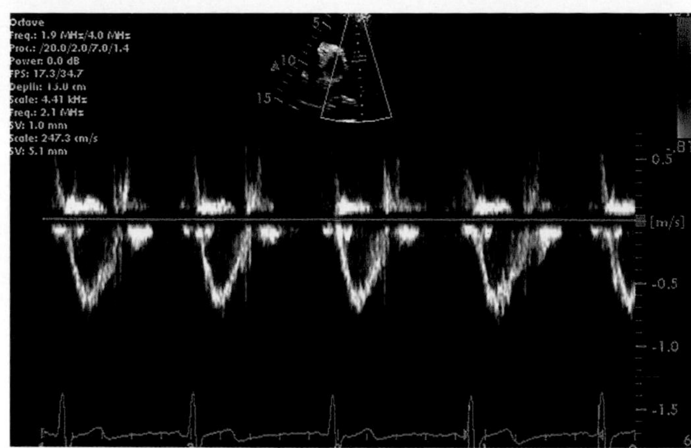

Figure 18A-47 The pulsed wave Doppler profile of normal flow in the pulmonary trunk as seen from the parasternal short-axis view. The acceleration of flow is slower compared to that seen in the left ventricular outflow tract and the aorta.

through the atrioventricular valves is towards the transducer from the apical position, and hence is displayed above the baseline. The normal pattern shows two waves. The E wave occurs during early filling after valvar opening. The A wave occurs during atrial contraction (Fig. 18A-46). In mid-diastole, there is a period of no flow, or diastasis. Typically, the velocity of the flow across the mitral valve is greater than that measured across the tricuspid valve. The tricuspid inflow, however, varies more significantly with respiration compared to the mitral inflow.

The peak velocities of the E and A waves are influenced by both age and heart rate.[13] In normal children, the mitral E velocity is larger compared to the A velocity, while in normal newborns the mitral A velocity is larger than the E velocity. This is thought to be related to immaturity of the myocardium, especially in handling of calcium metabolism, resulting in slower early relaxation, and large dependency on filling during the period of atrial contraction. The inflow velocities are used to assess diastolic function, especially of the left ventricle. This is because abnormalities of relaxation, as well as decreased compliance and increased ventricular stiffness, will affect the inflow patterns. Discussion of assessment of diastolic dysfunction, however, is beyond the scope of this chapter. Atrioventricular valvar stenosis is associated with increased velocities of flow, and continuous wave Doppler can be used to quantify the degree of stenosis, as discussed below.

Right Ventricular Outflow Tract and Pulmonary Trunk

Velocities in the right ventricular outflow tract and pulmonary trunk are best recorded from the subcostal position, or from the left parasternal short-axis views. To align better with the flow, it is useful to position the transducer one or two ribspaces lower compared to the standard parasternal position. When the transducer is tilted superiorly, flow through the outflow tract will be aligned with the Doppler beam. Flow is directed away from the transducer, and is displayed below the baseline (Fig. 18A-47). Anterograde flow occurs during systole, although some anterograde flow can occur in late diastole concomitant with atrial contraction during inspiration, as at that time pressure in the right ventricle can exceed diastolic pressure in the pulmonary arteries. This can result in late diastolic opening of the pulmonary valve, especially with inspiration when there is increased pulmonary venous return to the heart. Normally there is no flow in the pulmonary arteries during diastole, although a small amount of reversal of flow can occur early after closure of the pulmonary valve due to some backflow associated with valvar closure. The mean normal peak velocity across the pulmonary valve is 0.9 m/sec, with a range from 0.7 to 1.1 m/sec. If a left-to-right shunt is present, increased flow across the pulmonary valve at increased velocity is noted. This increased velocity needs to be distinguished from associated obstruction in the right ventricular outflow tract. In this setting, cross sectional imaging to look for muscle bundles, infundibular stenosis, pulmonary valvar motion, and to inspect changes in dimension in the supravalvar region, is an important adjunct.

Left Ventricular Outflow Tract, Ascending and Descending Aorta

Velocities in the left ventricular outflow tract are best recorded from the apical five-chamber view. The Doppler velocities recorded from this position appear as a negative systolic waveform. Flow can be recorded below or above the valve, but the peak velocities will be slightly higher above the valve. Flow in the ascending aorta can best be recorded from the suprasternal notch or a high right parasternal position. From these windows, flow will be directed towards the transducer. This view is important should supravalvar stenosis be present (Fig. 18A-48). It is also valuable in those with aortic valvar stenosis, when the jet is often directed eccentrically, and the best alignments with flow can be obtained from these positions. The non-imaging pencil probe can then be used to provide the best possible alignment with the flow. The smaller imprint on the chest allows greater flexibility in manipulation compared to the probes used for imaging. The disadvantage, of course, is that duplex scanning cannot be used to direct the probe. Flow in the left ventricular outflow tract normally occurs only during systole. In the ascending aorta, there can be a very short early diastolic reversal of flow, associated with reversal during closure of the aortic valve. A brief phase of late systolic and early diastolic reversal of flow may result from elastic recoil of the arterial system. Velocities of descending aortic flow are best recorded from the suprasternal notch. The profile is similar to that found in

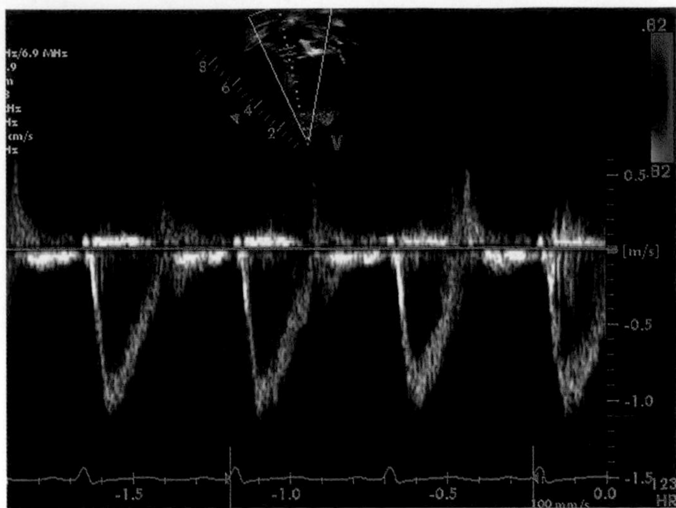

Figure 18A-48 This normal pulsed wave Doppler profile is obtained from the apical five-chamber view across the aortic valve. Notice the shorter acceleration time compared to the flow in the pulmonary trunk.

the ascending aorta, but flow is in the opposite direction, and with a slightly higher velocity (Fig. 18A-49).

Haemodynamic Measurements

Haemodynamics describe the relationship between pressure and flow. Neither of these values can be measured directly using echocardiography. Based on cross sectional imaging and Doppler, however, it has become possible to estimate flows and pressures. This has several clinical applications, explaining why the echocardiography laboratory is also a haemodynamic laboratory.

The Bernoulli equation describes the relationship between pressure and velocity in a system of laminar flow. It started from the observation that, if a flow encounters a narrowing, the velocity of the flow will increase, but there will be a drop in pressure across the narrowing. This is based on the principle of conservation of energy, where the total energy is conserved but there is an increase in kinetic energy, or speed, at the expense of potential energy, or pressure. The Bernoulli equation is $P1 - P2 = \frac{1}{2} \rho (V2^2 - V1^2)$, where P1 is pressure proximal to the obstruction, P2 is pressure distal to the obstruction, V1 is the proximal velocity, V2 is the distal velocity, and ρ is the density of the fluid. The formula can simplified as $\Delta P = 4\ V2^2$.

Despite the formula containing many simplifications, the equation can be used in Doppler echocardiography to predict differences in pressure across stenotic or regurgitant valves,[12] or across ventricular septal defects, arterial ducts, or other communications. The equation, nonetheless, remains a simplification. It has several different potential sources of error.

- Doppler techniques measure the velocity in the direction of the echobeam, so if not well aligned, they may underestimate the true velocity, which will result in an underestimation of the true gradient.
- In the equation, the proximal velocity V1 is considered to be negligible, and hence can be ignored. This is not the case if V1 is elevated. Elevated proximal velocities are found when multiple levels of obstruction occur in series, such as with discrete subaortic and valvar aortic stenosis, infundibular and valvar pulmonary stenosis, or aortic stenosis and aortic coarctation. A similar arrangement is found across a valve that is both stenotic and regurgitant, when an intracardiac shunt is associated with pulmonary stenosis, or when valvar gradients are measured during exercise.
- The formula can be used for only for discrete stenosis, since it makes abstractions from the losses of pressure related to viscous forces. These are more important in small stenotic long vessels, as for instance a Blalock-Taussig shunt. The drop in pressure associated with acceleration of flow and friction is also not negligible for orificial diameters of less than 3.5 mm. Potential errors may occur, therefore, when there is critical aortic or pulmonary stenosis.
- The Bernoulli equation should also be used with care in the setting of ventricular systolic dysfunction. In this context, the ventricle may no longer be capable of generating sufficient output, and hence produces low proximal velocities. The reduction of flow across the valve will be associated with a reduction in gradient. In case of ventricular dysfunction, Doppler gradients may be abnormally low, and should be interpreted carefully. In contrast to the adult population, this is more unusual in children.
- A final problem can be the phenomenon of recovery of pressure. As already emphasised, when flow occurs across a narrowing, potential energy is converted into kinetic energy. Distal to the narrowing, however, the vessel widens again, and kinetic energy is converted into potential energy. This phenomenon is called recovery of pressure. Because Doppler techniques do not measure such recovery, they overestimate the degree of stenosis.

Mean Pressure Gradient

The pressure gradient derived from the Bernoulli equation is the peak instantaneous pressure gradient, and not the peak-to-peak pressure gradient as measured during cardiac catheterisation (Fig. 18A-50). The peak-instantaneous gradient derived from Doppler

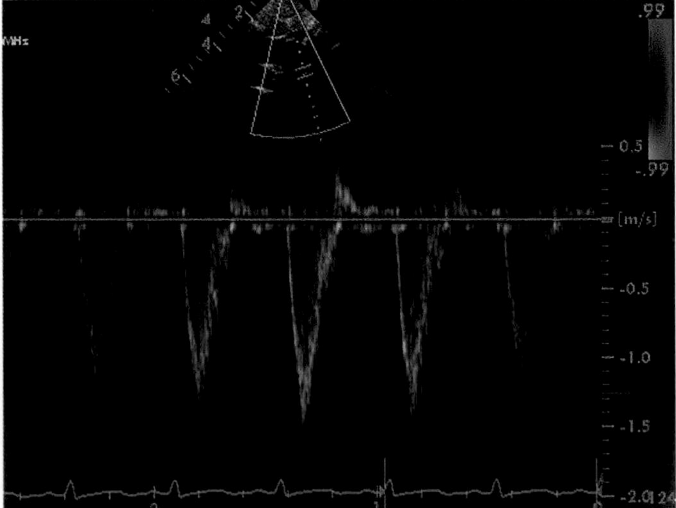

Figure 18A-49 The normal pattern of flow in the descending aorta is shown as seen from the suprasternal notch. The flow is going away from the transducer. There is no significant diastolic flow. The velocity of the flow is slightly higher than that in the ascending aorta.

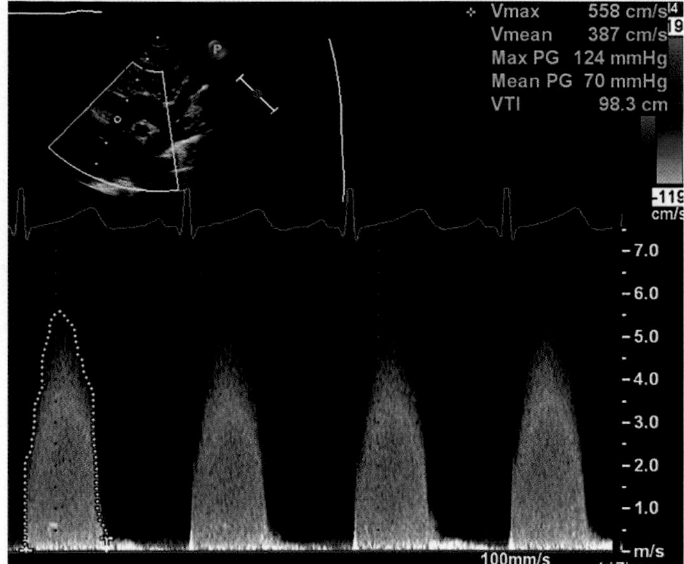

Figure 18A-50 The peak and mean gradients of flow across the aortic valve in a patient with aortic stenosis.

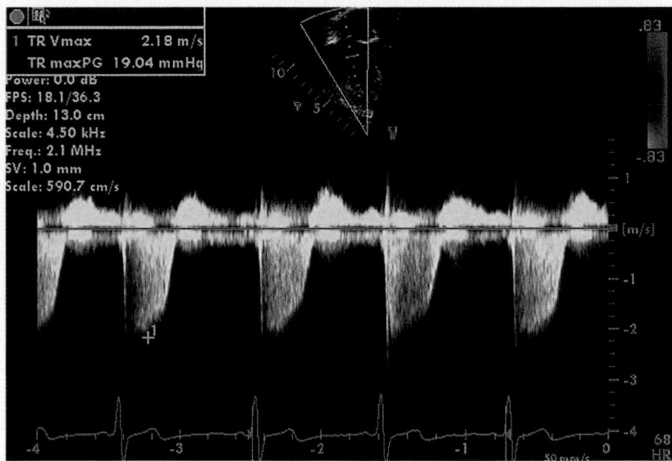

Figure 18A-51 The tricuspid regurgitant jet used to measure right ventricular systolic pressure. The peak velocity is 2.18 m/sec. This corresponds to a peak gradient of 19 mm Hg. Adding a right atrial pressure of 5 mm Hg gives a right ventricular systolic pressure of 24 mm Hg, which is normal.

measurements across a stenosis will always be higher than the peak-to-peak gradient. This means that Doppler interrogation systematically overestimates pressure gradients measured invasively. To overcome this problem, the mean pressure gradient can be calculated by integrating the velocity curve during ejection, and thus calculating the mean gradient. This is the average of all the instantaneous pressure gradients throughout ejection. This is calculated electronically by tracing the Doppler curve. Mean pressure gradients have been shown to correlate better with gradients obtained during cardiac catheterization, and are generally used to assess the severity of a stenosis. The hypertrophic response to an obstructed outflow tract, however, is related more to the peak gradient than to the mean gradient. So, in the decision-making process to judge the severity of a narrowing, both the peak as well as the mean gradient has to be taken into account, as well as the effect on the ventricular muscle.

APPLICATION OF THE BERNOULLI EQUATION IN CLINICAL PRACTICE

For the application of the Bernouilli equation in the context of valvar stenosis, reference should be made to the individual chapters devoted to valvar abnormalities in paediatric cardiac disease. In this part, we focus further on the assessment of right ventricular systolic pressure and pulmonary arterial pressures using Doppler echocardiography, as this is an important aspect in the evaluation of patients with congenitally malformed hearts, where elevated right heart pressures, as well as pulmonary hypertension, can be an important topic.

Estimation of Pressures in the Right Ventricle and Pulmonary Arteries

For the assessment of right ventricular pressures and pulmonary artery pressures, different Doppler measurements can be used. If tricuspid regurgitation is present, and at least mild, a continuous wave Doppler signal can be obtained. The four-chamber view is used most commonly, although other views can provide good alignment with the regurgitant jet. The right ventricular systolic pressure can be calculated from the peak velocity of tricuspid regurgitation using the Bernoulli equation by adding the right atrial systolic pressure, as the regurgitant jet is driven by the pressure difference between the right ventricle and the right atrium (Fig. 18A-51). If no direct or indirect measurement is present, right atrial pressure is assumed between 5 to 10 mm Hg. In the absence of right ventricular outflow tract obstruction, it can be assumed that right ventricular and pulmonary arterial systolic pressures are equal. Even in the presence of pulmonary stenosis, however, knowledge of the right ventricular pressure and the gradient across the right ventricular outflow tract will provide an estimate of pulmonary arterial systolic pressure.

If a ventricular septal defect is present, it is often possible to interrogate the flow across the defect. By measuring the peak systolic velocity, the peak instantaneous pressure difference between the left and right ventricles can then be calculated. To estimate right ventricular systolic pressure, left ventricular systolic pressure is assumed to be equal to systemic systolic arterial blood pressure. Subtracting the pressure gradient across the defect from the estimated left ventricular systolic pressure provided the right ventricular systolic pressure. This again is based on several assumptions, which can make the method unreliable. First, the assumption that arterial pressure is equal to left ventricular systolic pressure is only true is there is no left ventricular outflow tract obstruction. Second, if there is a significant delay in the build up of pressure during systole in both ventricles, as in the setting of right bundle branch block, the peak instantaeous gradient measured during systole overestimates the real gradient, potentially missing significant pulmonary hypertension. Third, it can be extremely difficult to align the cursor with the jet of the defect, potentially underestimating the gradient. It is also possible that obstruction may be present across the right ventricular outflow tract.

If the arterial duct is patent, the direction and the velocity of flow measured across the duct can be used to estimate the pulmonary arterial pressure. When the shunt is right-to-left, or bidirectional, this indicates suprasystemic or systemic pressures in the pulmonary arteries respectively. When the shunt is left-to-right, a Doppler measurement of the flow can be obtained. It can be difficult to align the cursor with the direction of the flow and obtain a reliable Doppler tracing, but in most patients it is possible to obtain a good Doppler tracing. When the duct becomes more restrictive, the flow will become continuous. It can then become difficult to define the peak gradient. In general, it is better to use the mean gradient. Subtraction of this mean ductal gradient from the mean systemic arterial blood pressure gives the mean pulmonary arterial pressure.

The majority of patients have a variable degree of pulmonary regurgitation, from which it is possible to obtain a reliable pulsed wave or continuous wave Doppler signal. This can usually be obtained from the parasternal short-axis view, or sometimes from the subcostal windows. When a good tracing is obtained, two different measurements can be performed. Of these, the peak diastolic gradient between the pulmonary artery and the right ventricle has been shown to correlate highly with the mean pulmonary arterial pressure. This relationship is coincidental, and very fortuitous for the clinical echocardiographer. As the pressure gradient reflects the pressure difference between the pulmonary artery and the right ventricle at that time, right ventricular diastolic pressure should be added to the measurement (Fig. 18A-52). An estimated right atrial pressure is also added. The pulmonary end-diastolic pressure can be estimated based on the pulmonary regurgitant jet by measuring the end-diastolic velocity P. The gradient between the pulmonary arteries and the right ventricle is then provided using the equation

$$\text{PADP} - \text{RVED} = 4V^2$$

where PADP is the pulmonary arterial end-diastolic pressure, V is the end-diastolic velocity, and RVED is the right ventricular end-diastolic pressure. Again, right atrial pressures are used as an estimate for right ventricular end-diastolic pressure but this is not always a good estimate.

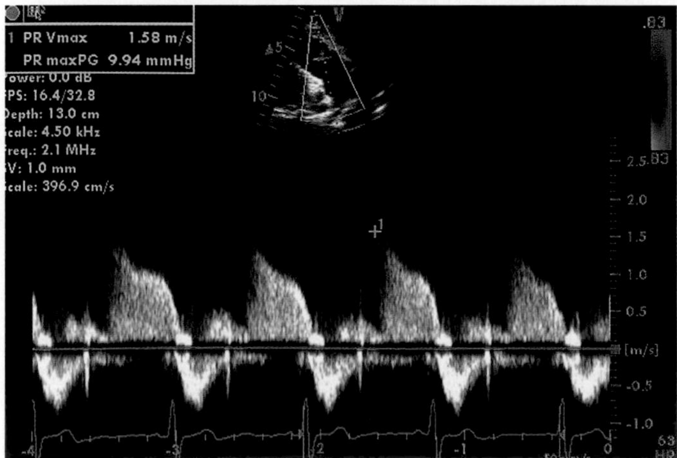

Figure 18A-52 Pulsed wave Doppler from the pulmonary regurgitant jet is obtained from a parasternal short-axis view. The maximal velocity is measured to be 1.58 m/sec, which corresponds to a gradient of 10 mm Hg. Adding a mean right atrial pressure of 5 mm Hg predicts a mean pulmonary arterial pressure of around 15 mm Hg.

When pulmonary regurgitation becomes severe, there might be significant shortening of the regurgitant jet due to fast equalization between pulmonary and right ventricular diastolic pressures related to the large regurgitant volume.

Apart from using the Bernouilli equation, there have been attempts to use different Doppler time time intervals to try to predict pulmonary arterial pressures. These intervals, however, are influenced by heart rate, contractility, and conditions of loading. When used to predict a change in afterload, the other factors are presumed to be relatively constant, and this is rarely the case. These methods, therefore, are not commonly used in clinical practice.

The Continuity Equation

A second important haemodynamic principle, which has been used in a number of Doppler applications, is the continuity equation. This is based on the principle of conservation of mass within the cardiovascular system, which predicts that the flow will be equal at various points within the circulation. The flow across all four valves within the heart will be equal in the absence of intracardiac shunts or valvar regurgitation. Flow across a fixed orifice is equal to the product of the cross sectional area of the orifice and the velocity of flow. In order to calculate velocity through an orifice, it is necessary to calculate the mean velocity across this area. This can be done by measuring the time velocity integral, which is calculated electronically by tracing the Doppler velocity signal. The stroke volume is the product of the cross sectional area and the time velocity interval. The continuity equation has been used in different echocardiographic applications.

The first is the calculation of stroke volume and cardiac output. This can be performed by obtaining a Doppler signal in the left ventricular outflow tract, usually from an apical four-chamber view, and measuring the time velocity interval. If the diameter of the left ventricular outflow tract is measured, usually from a parasternal long-axis view, the cross sectional area can be calculated as $\pi (D/2)^2$, which is equal to 0.785 D^2. Then stroke volume is the product of 0.785, the square of the diameter, and the time velocity interval. Multiplying this value by heart rate provides the cardiac output. The same can be done for the right ventricular outflow tract. If there are no intracardiac shunts, or significant valvar regurgitation, the right ventricular stroke volume should be equal to the left ventricular stroke volume. If there is an intracardiac shunt without valvar regurgitation, the ratio of right to left ventricular output should reflect the magnitude of the shunt, or the ratio of pulmonary to systemic flows. In practice, there are a lot of pitfalls associated with this method. In the first place, alignment of flow can be problematic. Second, it can be difficult to measure the diameters of the outflow tract, especially the right ventricular outflow tract, which is in the near field. The assumption that the left and right outflow tracts are circular is also not entirely true. Furthermore, in small children, a small error in measurement of diameter will result in a significant error in the calculation of output, as the error is squared in the formula. These factors explain the high variability of the measurement in children, and especially in infants.

Calculation of Valvar Area

The continuity equation can also be used to calculate the area of a stenotic or regurgitant valve. This is based on the continuity principle of conservation of mass, flow across a stenotic or regurgitant orifice being the same as an upstream flow across a known area. For instance, when considering the aortic valve, flow across the valve should be equal to flow through the left ventricular outflow tract:

$$\text{Area}_{\text{LVOT}} \times \text{TVI}_{\text{LVOT}} = \text{Area}_{\text{aortic valve}} \times \text{TVI}_{\text{aortic valve}}$$

The area of the aortic valve, therefore, can be calculated as:

$$\text{Area}_{\text{aortic valve}} = \text{Area}_{\text{LVOT}} \times (\text{TVI}_{\text{LVOT}}/\text{TVI}_{\text{aortic valve}})$$

This principle has not gained a lot of popularity in the assessment of paediatric cardiac disease for the same reasons discussed above for the continuity equation. The measurement of flow is more prone to errors than the measurement of gradients. A small error in measuring the left ventricular outflow tract, in particular, can result in significant errors when calculating the valvar area. Calculation of valvar areas, therefore, does not influence decision-making in paediatric cardiology to the same extent as in adult cardiology. There is hope that combining three-dimensional echocardiography will provide more reliable measurements of the left ventricular outflow tract and the aortic valve.

SUMMARY

Combining cross sectional echocardiography with a segmental morphological approach permits fully description of the morphology of nearly all congenitally malformed hearts. Additional imaging techniques can still be required for the assessment of extracardiac anomalies. Despite this, cross sectional echocardiography is the cornerstone for imaging in children with congenitally malformed hearts, and an indispensable tool in their subsequent management.

The complete reference list can be found on the companion Expert Consult web site at www.expertconsult.com.

ANNOTATED REFERENCES

- Lai WW, Mertens L, Cohen M, Geva T: Echocardiography in Pediatric and Congenital Heart Disease: From Fetus to Adult. New York, Wiley-Blackwell, 2009.

  A full and comprehensive textbook on paediatric echocardiography.
- Frommelt P, Gorentz J, Deatsman S, et al: Digital imaging, archiving, and structured reporting in pediatric echocardiography: Impact on laboratory efficiency and physician communication. J Am Soc Echocardiogr 2008;21:935–940.

  This paper shows that a full digital workflow in a paediatric echocardiography laboratory contributes to efficiency and improves the quality.
- Evangelista A, Flachskampf F, Lancellotti P, et al: European Association of Echocardiography recommendations for standardization of performance, digital storage and reporting of echocardiographic studies. Eur J Echocardiogr 2008;9:438–448.

  European recommendations regarding standardization of performance and reporting of echocardiographic examination in an adult echocardiography laboratory. Most of the recommendations can also be used by those working in paediatric echocardiographic laboratories.
- Cook AC, Anderson RH: Editorial: Attitudinally correct nomenclature. Heart 2002;87:503–506.

  An editorial emphasising the need for morphologists, and those now imaging the heart, to describe cardiac structures relative to the orthogonal planes of the body, rather than considering the heart in Valentine fashion.
- Lai WW, Geva T, Shirali GS, et al: Guidelines and standards for performance of a pediatric echocardiogram: A report from the Task Force of the Pediatric Council of the American Society of Echocardiography. J Am Soc Echocardiogr 2006;19:1413–1430.

  Guidelines for the performance of transthoracic paediatric echocardiography. This consensus paper provides recommendations for the different views and images that need to be obtained in a paediatric study, and tries to standardize paediatric echocardiographic imaging.
- Huhta JC, Smallhorn JF, Macartney FJ: Two-dimensional echocardiographic diagnosis of situs. Br Heart J 1982;48:97–108.

  This landmark paper set the rules for echocardiographic inference of the arrangement of the atrial chambers according to the orientation of the abdominal great vessels.
- Ayres NA, Miller-Hance W, Fyfe DA, et al: Indications and guidelines for performance of transesophageal echocardiography in the patient with pediatric acquired or congenital heart disease: Report from the task force of the Pediatric Council of the American Society of Echocardiography. J Am Soc Echocardiogr 2005;18:91–98.

  The guidelines of the American Society of Echocardiography for the performance of transoesophageal echocardiography in children.
- Wilson W, Taubert KA, Gewitz M, et al: Prevention of infective endocarditis: Guidelines from the American Heart Association: A guideline from the American Heart Association Rheumatic Fever, Endocarditis, and Kawasaki Disease Committee, Council on Cardiovascular Disease in the Young, and the Council on Clinical Cardiology, Council on Cardiovascular Surgery and Anesthesia, and the Quality of Care and Outcomes Research Interdisciplinary Working Group. Circulation 2007;116:1736–1754.

  The new guidelines for endocarditis prophylaxis provided by the American Heart Association. This recent update is less strict compared to previous versions. Transoesophageal echocardiography is not a strict indication for prophylaxis.
- Lang R, Bierig M, Devereux R, et al: Recommendations for chamber quantification. Eur J Echocardiogr 2006;7:79–108.

  This combined European and North American effort tries to standardize echocardiographic measurements. Unfortunately, the authors failed to include a lot of measurements relevant for paediatric echocardiography.
- Sluysmans T, Colan SD: Theoretical and empirical derivation of cardiovascular allometric relationships in children. J Appl Physiol 2005;99:445–457.

  This study looks for the best method for normalisation of cardiac dimensions for somatic growth. The authors show that the use of z-scores normalised for body surface area is the best method for the majority of measurements in children.
- Daubeney PE, Blackstone EH, Weintraub RG, et al: Relationship of the dimension of cardiac structures to body size: An echocardiographic study in normal infants and children. Cardiol Young 1999;9:402–410.

  Normograms and formulas for z-score for a large number of measurements in children. These data have become very popular.
- Pettersen MD, Du W, Skeens ME, Humes RA: Regression equations for calculation of z scores of cardiac structures in a large cohort of healthy infants, children, and adolescents: An echocardiographic study. J Am Soc Echocardiogr 2008;21:922–934.

  This recent publication provided normal paediatric data with the formulas for calculation of z-scores. It is very useful for those laboratories which do not have their own normal datasets.
- Baumgartner H, Hung J, Bermejo J, et al: Echocardiographic assessment of valve stenosis: EAE/ASE recommendations for clinical practice. J Am Soc Echocardiogr 2009;22:1–23.

  Recent recommendations for quantification of valvar stenosis in adults. A lot of the principles can be applied to paediatric cardiac disease.

Three-Dimensional Echocardiography

CHAPTER 18B

GIRISH S. SHIRALI

Appreciation of complex intracardiac anatomy and spatial relationships is inherent to the diagnosis of congenitally malformed hearts. Beginning over 30 years ago, and until recently, the ability of the clinician to image the heart by echocardiography was limited to cross sectional techniques displayed in two dimensions.[1] Such two-dimensional echocardiography has fundamental limitations. The very nature of a two-dimensional slice, which has no thickness, necessitates the use of multiple orthogonal sweeps. The echocardiographer then mentally reconstructs the anatomy, and uses the structure of the report to express this mentally reconstructed vision. This means that the only three-dimensional image of the heart available for diagnosis is the virtual image existing in the mind of the echocardiographer, who then translates this vision into words when preparing the report. It is not easy for an untrained, albeit interested, observer to understand the images obtained in the course of a sweep. Expert interpretation is required. Furthermore, since myocardial motion occurs in three dimensions, two-dimensional echocardiographic techniques do not lend themselves to accurate quantitation.

Recognition of these limitations of cross sectional echocardiography seen in two dimensions led to burgeoning research and clinical interest in three-dimensional echocardiography. Early reconstructive approaches were based on acquisitions of large numbers of two-dimensional images that were subsequently stacked and aligned based on the phases of the cardiac cycle, in this way producing a three-dimensional dataset.[2–4] While these approaches proved to be accurate, the need for time and offline processing equipment imposed fundamental limitations on their clinical applicability. In 1990, von Ramm and Smith published their early results with a matrix-array transducer that provided real-time images of the heart in three dimensions.[5] While this was an important breakthrough, this transducer was unable to be steered in the third dimension, which has since been termed the plane of elevation. Over the past 5 years, dramatic technological advances have facilitated the ability to perform live three-dimensional scanning, including the ability to steer the beam in three dimensions, and to render the image in real time.[6]

ADVANCES IN TECHNOLOGY

Contemporary transducers based on arrangement of elements in a matrix, piezoelectric materials, and quantitative software are the three elements that have facilitated enhancements in three-dimensional echocardiography.

Matrix-array Transducers

These transducers comprise as many elements in the elevation dimension as they do in the azimuth dimension, with more than 60 elements in each. While the elements are arranged in a two-dimensional grid, this array generates three-dimensional echocardiographic images. In order to be able to steer in the elevation plane, each element must be electrically independent from all other elements, and each element must be electrically active. The technology and electrical circuitry to insulate electrically, and connect each element, became commercially available in 2002. As a result, these transducers consist of thousands of electrically active elements, each of which independently steers a scan line left and right, as well as up and down.

Piezoelectrical Materials

The piezoelectrical material in a transducer fundamentally determines the quality of the image. Piezoelectrical elements are responsible for delivery of ultrasonic energy into the tissue that is scanned, and for converting waves of reflected ultrasound into electric signals. Their efficiency in converting electrical energy to mechanical energy, and vice versa, is a key determinant of the quality of the image, sensitivity to Doppler shifts, and the ability of transmitted ultrasound to penetrate to increasing depths. In order to create a piezoelectrical effect, these elements must be subjected to the application of an external electric field to align dipoles within polycrystalline materials. For almost 40 years, a ceramic polycrystalline material named lead-zirconate-titanate has been the piezoelectrical material that has enjoyed standard usage in medical applications. This material is a powder that is mixed with an organic binder. The resulting compound is baked into a dense polycrystalline structure. At its best, it achieves approximately 70% alignment of dipoles. This inherently constrains the efficiency of the material to achieve electromechanical coupling.

One example of new piezoelectrical material involves growing crystals from molten ceramic material, resulting in a homogenous crystal with fewer defects, lower losses, and no boundaries between grains.[7,8] When these crystals are poled at the preferred orientation or orientations, a near-perfect alignment of dipoles is achievable, resulting in dramatically enhanced electromechanical properties.

The efficiency of conversion of electrical to mechanical energy improves by as much as two-thirds to five-sixths when compared to lead-zirconate-titanate ceramics, which are otherwise currently used in ultrasonic transducers. The new piezoelectrical materials provide increased bandwidth and sensitivity, resulting in improvements in both penetration and resolution. The improved arrangement of atoms in these new piezoelectrical materials, and their superior strain energy density, has translated into advances in miniaturisation. These advances led to the availability of a high-frequency matrix three-dimensional transthoracic transducer that has dramatically enhanced the applicability of three-dimensional echocardiography for use in children.[9] Another example of emerging transducer materials consists of silicon elements. This technology is being developed at the present time.

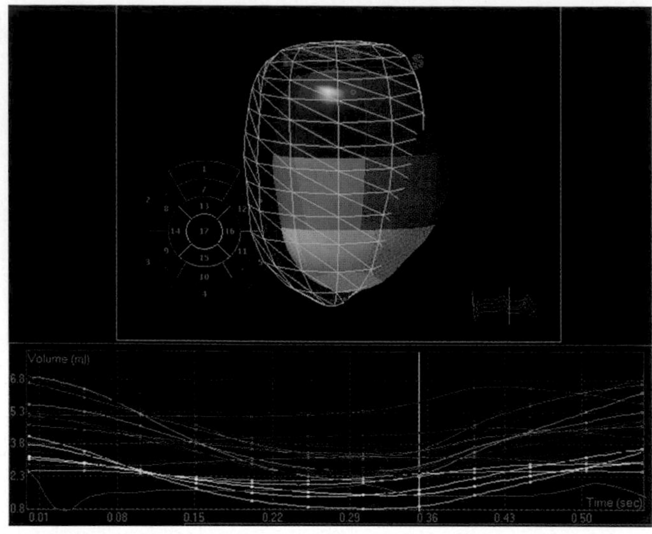

Figure 18B-1 This image demonstrates the capabilities of software that is available for quantitation of left ventricular volumes throughout the cardiac cycle, providing end-diastolic and end-systolic volumes as well as the ejection fraction. The mesh represents left ventricular volume at end-diastole. The cast of the left ventricular cavity consists of segments of varying colours, each of which represents a subvolume of the ventricular cavity based on the 16-segment model that has been standardised by the American Society of Echocardiography. The change in volume of each subvolume is represented graphically, with time on the *x*-axis and volume on the *y*-axis.

Software for Quantification

Quantification requires that the software provide the ability to separate out and segment structures of interest from the acquired data. Two-dimensional quantitative techniques are based on geometric formulas that rely on assumptions regarding the shapes of cardiac structures. These assumptions are frequently incorrect. In contrast, three-dimensional acquisitions include the entire extent of the structure, thus minimizing the possibility of foreshortening of the apex or any geometric assumptions regarding shape. Three-dimensional quantitative software has the potential to quantify cardiac structures accurately regardless of their shape. Advances in software for processing three-dimensional data sets have mirrored the rapid advances in transducer technology that have occurred over the past few years.

Three-dimensional volumetric techniques rely on definition of chamber cavities, that is, the interface between blood and endocardium. The software constructs this interface by using a process known as surface rendering, and represents it as a mesh of points and lines. This software-generated mesh is calculated for every frame of acquisition, thus providing a moving cast of the cavity of the ventricle during the cardiac cycle. Since this is digital data, it is easy to compute global and regional volumes, synchrony as well as parametric displays of endocardial excursion, and timing of contraction (Fig. 18B-1).

Tools for three-dimensional quantification of the left ventricle are more technologically advanced than for other cardiac structures. Until recently, such tools employed the method of disk summation. With improvements in computing speeds and programming, newer tools have been developed to provide instantaneous tracking of the interface between the blood pool and endocardium at each frame of acquisition. This provides a surface-rendered model that is displayed as a mesh of lines and points. These algorithms, nonetheless, are still based on some basic three-dimensional geometric assumptions regarding left ventricular shape, and therefore they cannot be applied to the right ventricle or to functionally univentricular hearts. Given the complex shape and architecture of the right ventricle, it is unsurprising that tools for quantifying its volume have been slower to mature. Until very recently, these tools utilised the method of disks for volumetrics.[10] Novel software now provides the ability instantaneously to track the interface of blood pool and endocardium at each frame of acquisition (Fig. 18B-2), yielding a surface-rendered model that is displayed as a mesh of lines and points.[11]

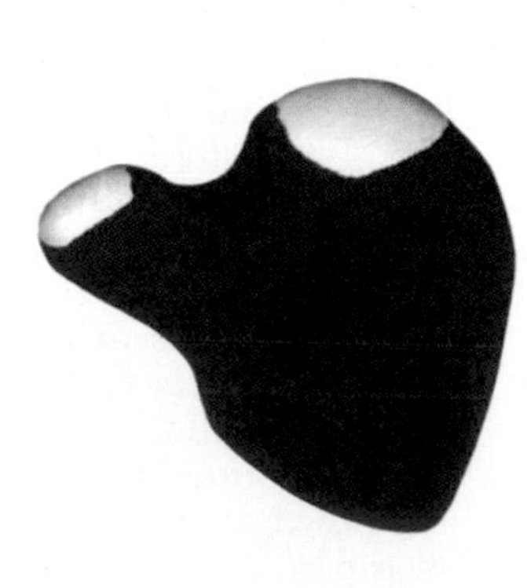

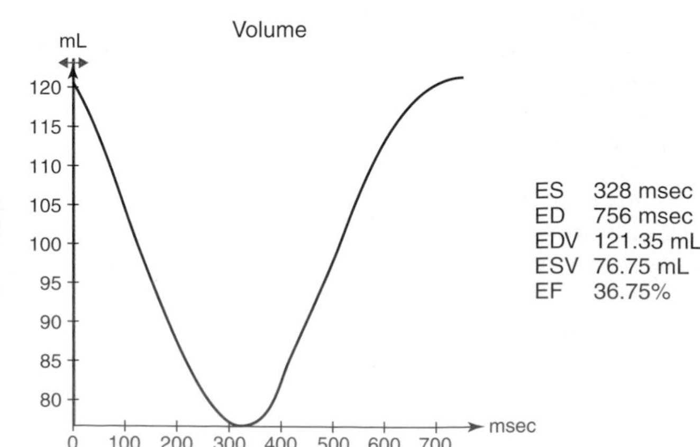

Figure 18B-2 This image demonstrates the capabilities of software that is available for quantitation of right ventricular volume throughout the cardiac cycle. This yields a surface-rendered model that is displayed as a mesh of lines and points. The change in volume of the cavity of the right ventricle is represented graphically, with time on the *x*-axis and volume on the *y*-axis. EF, ejection fraction; ED, end diastole; EDV, end diastolic volume; ES, end systole; ESV, end systolic volume.

In a recent development, quantitative software for the mitral valve has been developed. This provides the ability to perform sophisticated analyses of the nonplanar shape of the mitral valvar annulus, and to measure dimensions including annular diameters, lengths of the zone of apposition between the leaflets, and the surface areas of each leaflet.[12,13] Quantitative techniques have also been developed to provide volumetric measurements of three-dimensional colour flows using non-aliased data.[14]

CLINICAL APPLICATIONS IN PATIENTS WITH CONGENITALLY MALFORMED HEARTS

Three-dimensional echocardiographic imaging has three broad areas of clinical application among patients with congenitally malformed hearts, namely, the visualisation of morphology, the quantification of sizes of chambers and flows of blood, and the emerging area of image-guided interventions.

Visualizing Morphology

Dating from an early stage in the development of three-dimensional technology, the structural complexity that is inherent to the congenitally malformed heart has been identified as fertile substrate for exploration using three-dimensional echocardiography.[15–17]

Atrioventricular Valves

Three-dimensional echocardiography is valuable in delineating the morphology of the atrioventricular valves, with the technique being used at an early stage to delineate congenital abnormalities of the mitral valve,[18] including comprehensive assessment of double orifices.[19] The additive value of the technique, and improved quality of images, was then demonstrated in the intra-operative environment.[20] More recently, the technique was shown to be capable of delineating the morphology of the leaflets, cordal attachments, the subcordal apparatus, the mechanism and origin of regurgitation, and the geometry of the regurgitant volume.[21] In the setting of Ebstein's malformation of the tricuspid valve, the technique was shown to provide clear visualisation of the morphology of the valvar leaflets, including the extent of their formation, the level of their attachment, and their degree of coaptation.[22]

Atrioventricular Septal Defect

In patients with atrioventricular septal defect, we have found that three-dimensional echocardiographic imaging provides unparalleled views of the zone of apposition between the superior and the inferior bridging leaflets of the left component of the common atrioventricular valve (Fig. 18B-3). Our experience with a cohort of patients with atrioventricular septal defects[23] showed that gated three-dimensional echocardiographic views could be cropped to reveal the relationships of the bridging leaflets to the septal structures (Figs. 18B-4 and 18B-5). These views have been useful in determining the precise level of shunting, particularly prior to surgical repair. The technique was of particular value in patients with unbalanced defects who were being considered for biventricular repair.

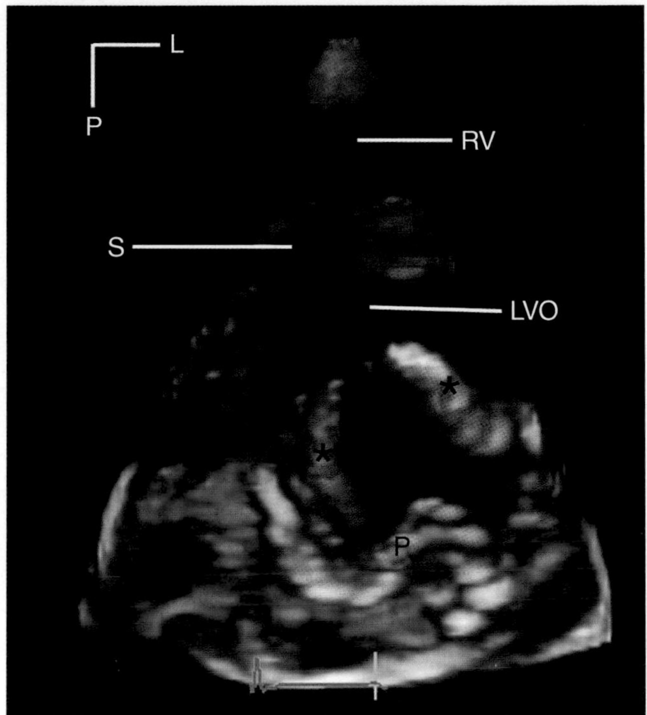

Figure 18B-3 A parasternal short-axis image of the left atrioventricular valve in a patient with atrioventricular septal defect. Asterisks mark the edges of the zone of apposition between the superior and inferior bridging leaflets. A tissue colourisation map has been applied to the image. This has the effect of colouring tissues orange in the near field, near to either the transducer or the front of the image. Tissues that are distant are coloured blue. This is a dynamic after-effect, which means that as the operator rotates, tilts, or otherwise manipulates the image, the colour effect correspondingly changes in real-time. L, left; LVO, left ventricular outflow tract; P, posterior; RV, right ventricle; S, septum.

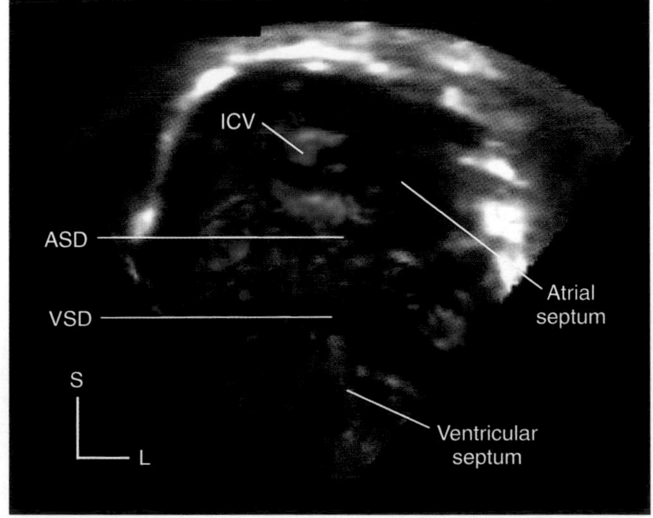

Figure 18B-4 An apical four-chamber three-dimensional echocardiogram in a patient with atrioventricular septal defect. The bridging leaflets divide the defect into an interatrial (ASD) and interventricular (VSD) component. Note the posterior location of the entrance of the inferior caval vein (ICV) relative to the septal structures. L, left; S, superior.

Atrial and Ventricular Septal Defects

Others have shown that three-dimensional echocardiography provides unique views of the surfaces of the atrial and ventricular septal structures, revealing the holes between

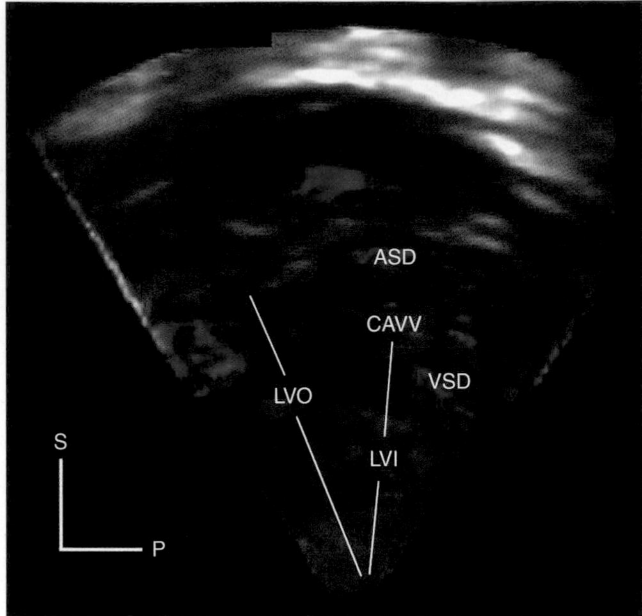

Figure 18B-5 An *en face* view of the left ventricular aspect of the ventricular septum in a patient with atrioventricular septal defect (ASD). The free walls of the left atrium and left ventricle have been cropped. The viewer is looking from left to right. This view demonstrates the disproportion between the shorter inflow (LVI) and longer outflow (LVO) dimensions that characterise the left ventricle in patients with atrioventricular septal defect. Note the crescentic inferior margin of the atrial septum, and the scooped-out edge of the interventricular septum. This view provides excellent anatomic detail regarding the relationships between the bridging leaflets of the common atrioventricular valve (CAVV) and the septal structures. P, posterior; S, superior; VSD, ventriculoseptal defect.

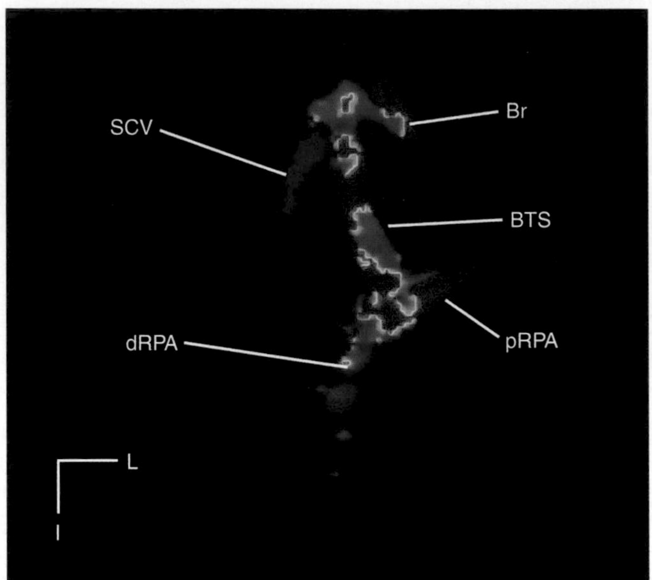

Figure 18B-6 A three-dimensional colour flow, electrocardiographically triggered, full-volume acquisition demonstrating a right sided Blalock-Taussig shunt (BTS). The gray scale image has been suppressed, thus providing an echocardiographic angiogram. The shunt is seen in its entirety from its origin from the brachiocephalic artery (Br) to its insertion. The proximal and distal right pulmonary arteries (pRPA and dRPA, respectively) are well seen. Note the proximity of the superior caval vein (SCV) to the cranial end of the shunt. This dataset can be rotated, tilted, and examined in an infinite number of planes in order to evaluate the lumen of the shunt, and to delineate the location of stenosis. I, inferior; L, left.

adjacent chambers.[24,25] The technique is of particular value in demonstrating the morphology of defects within the muscular ventricular septum,[26] and in assessing malformations of the outflow tract involving malalignment of the outlet septum.

Aortic Arch, Pulmonary Arteries, and Aortopulmonary Shunts

We have shown (Fig. 18B-6) the value of colour flow Doppler in providing echocardiographic angiograms of the patterns of flow in the obstructed aortic arch, the right and left pulmonary arteries subsequent to the Lecompte maneuver, and across Blalock-Taussig shunts.[27] In this recent experience, validation of the diagnosis made by three-dimensional echocardiography was confirmed at surgery, by cardiac catheterisation, or by magnetic resonance or computerised tomographic imaging in two-thirds of the patients.

Aortic Valve and Outflow Tract

Three-dimensional echocardiography has proved accurate in providing measurements of the orifice of the aortic valve, determining the number of valvar leaflets, and identifying sites of fusion between leaflets, as well as demonstrating nodules and excrescences characterizing dysplastic valves.[28] The technique has proved of equal value in patients with subaortic stenosis, showing abnormalities of mitral valvar leaflets or cordal attachments, abnormal ventricular muscle bands, and abnormally increased aorto-mitral separation.[29]

Characterisation of Left Ventricular Noncompaction

Three-dimensional echocardiography has enabled diagnosis, and provided detailed characterisation, of the affected myocardium, including easy visualisation of entire trabecular projections, inter-trabecular recesses, endocardial borders, and abnormalities of mural motion abnormalities.[30]

Quantification of Dimensions, Chambers, Valves, and Function

Left Ventricular Volumetrics

It is feasible to perform three-dimensional echocardiographic measurements of left ventricular end-systolic volume, end-diastolic volume, mass, stroke volume, and ejection fraction in children.[31] The measurements produced were reproducible, and comparable with those obtained from magnetic resonance imaging. The measurements of volume obtained using three-dimensional echocardiography tended mildly to underestimate those obtained using magnetic resonance imaging. Interestingly, estimates of ejection fraction were in closer agreement. In addition to evaluating the feasibility of performing left ventricular volumetrics, others have addressed the use of resources, the learning curve, and inter- and intra-observer reproducibility.[32] Observers were able to obtain, in almost all cases, three-dimensional left ventricular ejection fraction in less than 3 minutes, with the median time being less than 1.5 minutes. They demonstrated a negotiable learning curve, and excellent inter- and intra-observer reproducibility for the performance of three-dimensional echocardiographic left ventricular volumetrics.

Left Ventricular Mass

Studies in adults have validated three-dimensional echocardiography as an accurate method for measuring the mass of the left ventricle.[33,34] While studies in children have been limited in number and scope, excellent correlations have been shown between left ventricular mass measured by three-dimensional echocardiography and magnetic resonance imaging.[35]

Left Ventricular Dyssynchrony

The three-dimensional echocardiographic approach to measuring systolic dyssynchrony within the left ventricle uses the model of the left ventricle endorsed by the American Society of Echocardiography, which divides the ventricle into 16 segments.[36] The software automatically measures the time of each subvolume from maximal end-diastolic volume to minimal volume, and the standard deviation of these time intervals. The larger the standard deviation, the greater is the implied degree of left ventricular dyssynchrony. In order to control for the wide range of heart rates in children, the time intervals are represented as a percentage of heart rate. The association between left ventricular dysfunction and left ventricular dyssynchrony in children has been explored.[37] Normal children had three-dimensional echocardiographic left ventricular dyssynchrony indexes that were below 3%. Among children with dilated cardiomyopathy, there was a clearly defined threshold value of left ventricular ejection fraction, an ejection fraction below 35% being the rule for left ventricular dyssynchrony. In contrast, patients whose ejection fraction was higher than this number had indexes of dyssynchrony that did not differ from those of the normal children who were studied.

Right Ventricular Volumetrics

Until recently, the accuracy of three-dimensional echocardiographic measurement of right ventricular volume and ejection fraction had not been evaluated. This is unsurprising given the complex architecture of the right ventricle, and the technical difficulty of imaging it adequately. A large series of adults has been studied, the patients being compared in terms of volumetric measurements using magnetic resonance imaging and three-dimensional echocardiography using the method of summation of discs.[10] Right ventricular volumes have also been quantified in children with congenitally malformed hearts, using multiplanar reconstruction and tracing with semi-automated detection of borders.[11] In both adults and children, excellent correlations were obtained for both right ventricular volumes and ejection fraction. Similar comparisons between three-dimensional echocardiography and magnetic resonance imaging were made for children with functionally univentricular hearts with systemic right ventricles.[38] Calculations of diastolic volumes by three-dimensional echocardiography proved to be smaller than those made by magnetic resonance imaging, but systolic volumes and mass showed good agreement. Ejection fraction correlated less well. The intra-class correlation coefficient comparing ejection fraction was 0.64, and the measurements by three-dimensional echocardiography were lower than those obtained using magnetic resonance imaging by 6%. Inter- and intra-observer variability was below 4% for right ventricular ejection fraction, slightly below 2 mL for right ventricular end-diastolic volume, and below a seventh of a mL for right ventricular end-systolic volume. In a reflection of the speed with which technology is advancing, this study, which was published in March 2008, used a transducer that is already outdated in terms of quality of microelectronics, which translates directly into image quality and frame rates. In addition, the frequencies emitted by the transducer ranged from 2 to 4 mH. This is probably too low for optimal imaging in most of the children who were studied. Their weight ranged from under 3 kg to a little over 31 kg, with a median weight of 7 kg. It is likely that the improved spatial and temporal resolution, and higher frequency of state-of-the-art transducers and machines that is available today, will lead to further improvements in accuracy.

As these tools become more widely available, user-friendly and accurate, we anticipate the development of new paradigms in the use of quantitative echocardiographic parameters as surrogate measures of outcome in clinical trials in patients with congenitally malformed hearts.

Three-dimensional Colour Flow

Tools for multi-planar reconstruction provide the ability to not only visualise, but also to trace and measure, the area of valvar regurgitant orifices at their narrowest point. While this technique is new, and has not been validated against any gold standard for such measurements, it has been shown to be feasible, has already yielded insights into the shapes of regurgitant jets, and holds promise as a tool to enhance our ability to serially quantify valve regurgitation.[39,40]

In a series of elegant studies that began in a laboratory setting, and continued through animal models to the bedside of human beings, a technique has been developed and validated for quantifying non-aliased three-dimensional echocardiographic jets of colour flow.[41] In animal studies, measurements that were obtained by three-dimensional echocardiography were compared to those obtained from probes that were directly placed on the ascending aorta to measure flows.[14] Excellent correlation was found between the techniques. Quantification of colour flow has also been validated in adults by comparison to cardiac outputs that were obtained by thermodilution.[42] Application of this technique to pathologic states could potentially lead to more accurate measurements of regurgitant volumes and fractions.[43]

Interventions That Are Guided by Echocardiographic Imaging

The high temporal and spatial resolution of transthoracic, and particularly transoesophageal, three-dimensional echocardiography has ignited interest in the potential uses of live interrogation to guide interventions. Already this technique has been used to guide endomyocardial biopsy in children, with no complications.[44] Specifically, there were no instances of new flail tricuspid valvar leaflets, which might reflect injury or avulsion of cordal structures, or pericardial effusion, which may reflect perforation of the heart. The technique proved to be a valuable modality accurately to direct the bioptome to the desired site for biopsy within the right ventricle. With increasing familiarity, the need for fluoroscopic guidance was minimised. Three-dimensional echocardiography has also now been used to guide cardiac surgery in animals that have an open chest, but without opening the heart, and without cardiopulmonary bypass.[45–47]

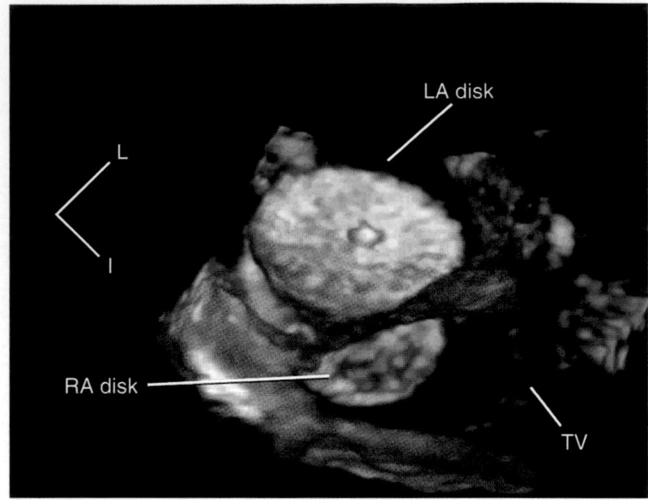

Figure 18B-7 A live three-dimensional transoesophageal echocardiographic image that was obtained immediately following closure of a fenestrated atrial septum with a cribriform Amplatzer septal occluder. The viewer is located inside the anterior portion of the left atrium, looking rightwards and posteriorly. The entire left atrial (LA) disk of the device is seen, with a central protuberance and the meshwork of metal that constitutes its frame. Part of the inferior portion of the right atrial (RA) disk, and the tricuspid valvar apparatus (TV), are also seen. I, inferior; L, left.

The three-dimensional transducer is directly placed on the heart for these procedures. This experience was validated initially by using three-dimensional echocardiography to guide the performance of common surgical tasks in the laboratory setting. More recently, small atrial septal defects have been closed in pigs. In our own recent experience, we have also been able to obtain spectacular images of cardiac chambers, septal structures, and valves, using live three-dimensional transoesophageal echocardiography to guide manipulation of catheters, puncture of the atrial septum, trans-septal procedures, and closure of atrial septal defects (Fig. 18B-7).[48]

Learning Curve

The learning curve of three-dimensional echocardiography is steep but negotiable. Our experience would suggest that successful implementation requires advocacy, and an investment of time by both echocardiographers and sonographers. The acceptance of the technique is increasing on a global level, albeit at an early stage. We have developed and implemented an interactive teaching course that utilises simulations using three-dimensional echocardiographic data sets with rehearsal and direct mentoring. This has been shown to be useful in overcoming the steep part of the learning curve.[49]

FUTURE DIRECTIONS

Advances in the arena of three-dimensional echocardiography will involve technical enhancements, such as improved speed of acquisition, improved image resolution, holographic displays, a wide range of software that has been validated for quantification, and enhancements to work flow. Refinements in technology will make high-resolution three-dimensional echocardiography available across the spectrum of sizes of patients. We anticipate a three-dimensional echocardiographic transoesophageal probe that is miniaturised for use in small children. With the growing interest in multi-modality imaging, three-dimensional volumetric and anatomic data will be able to be overlaid onto images and measurements that are obtained from other modalities.

SUMMARY

Important technological advances over the past few years have enabled three-dimensional echocardiography to emerge as a modality that provides additive value in managing patients with congenitally malformed hearts. We anticipate that, with continuing improvements in hardware and software, three-dimensional echocardiography will become, in the near future, an integral part of all standard echocardiographic examinations.

The complete reference list can be found on the companion Expert Consult web site at www.expertconsult.com.

ANNOTATED REFERENCES

- Salgo IS: Three-dimensional echocardiographic technology. Cardiol Clin 2007;25:231–239.

  This is a comprehensive review of the history and evolution of three-dimensional echocardiography. The author critically examines technological advances in several key areas that have enabled the rapid development of the field.
- Hlavacek AM, Chessa K, Crawford FA, et al: Real-time three-dimensional echocardiography is useful in the evaluation of patients with atrioventricular septal defects. Echocardiography 2006;23:225–231.

  This study of more than 50 patients describes en face *views of the atrial and ventricular septal structures using three-dimensional echocardiography and cropping techniques.*
- Hlavacek A, Lucas J, Baker H, et al: Feasibility and utility of three-dimensional colour flow echocardiography of the aortic arch: The "echocardiographic angiogram." Echocardiography 2006;23:860–864.

  This early study of three-dimensional colour flow echocardiography demonstrated the utility of the echocardiographic angiogram. This technique involves suppression of the gray scale image in order to show only the flow within the structure of interest. This technique provided new diagnostic information in more than one-third of patients who were studied.
- Baker GH, Hlavacek AM, Chessa KS, et al: Left ventricular dysfunction is associated with intraventricular dyssynchrony by three-dimensional echocardiography in children. J Am Soc Echocardiogr 2008;21:230–233.
- Soriano BD, Hoch M, Ithuralde A, et al: Matrix-array three-dimensional echocardiographic assessment of volumes, mass, and ejection fraction in young paediatric patients with a functional single ventricle: A comparison study with cardiac magnetic resonance. Circulation 2008;117:1842–1848.

  These two studies show the value and accuracy of three-dimensional echocardiography in the evaluation of ventricular function in children with congenitally malformed hearts.

CHAPTER 18C

Imaging and Functional Assessment by Novel Echocardiographic Techniques

MICHAEL C. VOGEL

Echocardiography has undergone major progress in recent years. While standard cross sectional echocardiography is still the most often used routine method for screening the anatomy of congenitally malformed hearts, and for evaluation of cardiac function, the use of echocardiography has extended to the operating theatre to review surgical results, to monitor interventions, and to evaluate ventricular function in a much more sophisticated way than conventional echocardiography. These recent developments include intracardiac echocardiography, intra-operative echocardiography using either transoesophageal or intracardiac transducers, real-time three-dimensional echocardiography, myocardial or tissue Doppler, and two-dimensional strain. In this part of our chapter devoted to imaging, I focus on myocardial Doppler and two-dimensional strain based on speckle tracing. These two techniques offer new methods for functional assessment of the heart, and are especially useful in evaluating regional and global function of both the right and left ventricle, as they allow for assessment of ventricular function irrespective of the ventricular shape.

BASIC PRINCIPLES

For myocardial Doppler, the same physical principles apply as in blood pool Doppler. The velocities of the flowing blood are high, but have low amplitude. These velocities are in the region of 1 m/sec across normal heart valves, and may increase to 6 m/sec across stenosed cardiac valves or narrowed great vessels. When blood pool sonographic Doppler was developed, special filters were used to suppress the signal having low velocity and high amplitude originating from movement of the myocardium. These myocardial velocities typically are in the range of around 10 cm/sec at rest, and may increase to 30 cm/sec under catecholamine-induced stress. It was demonstrated in 1989[1] that the myocardial velocities could be measured by pulsed Doppler sonography, and offered clinically useful information. Filters were developed, therefore, which suppress the high velocities at low amplitude originating from the flow of blood (Fig. 18C-1). After it had become evident that assessment of myocardial velocities was a useful clinical tool, colour Doppler imaging of the myocardium was also developed.[2] The velocity curves obtained from colour Doppler imaging are smoother than those from pulsed Doppler, and can be easily measured (Fig. 18C-2). Myocardial velocities, nonetheless, may be influenced by factors other than myocardial contraction alone, such as the overall motion of the heart during breathing, cardiac rotation, and motion induced by tethering to adjacent segments.[3] Some of these problems of measuring myocardial velocities can be overcome by strain and strain rate imaging,

Figure 18C-1 Pulsed Doppler myocardial velocity obtained from the base of the left ventricle. Velocities of three consecutive heartbeats are displayed. The vertical lines denote the isovolumic contraction and relaxation time. The s-wave represents the systolic myocardial velocity during shortening, the e-wave the early diastolic myocardial velocity during early relaxation of the ventricle, and the a-wave the diastolic myocardial velocity during atrial filling.

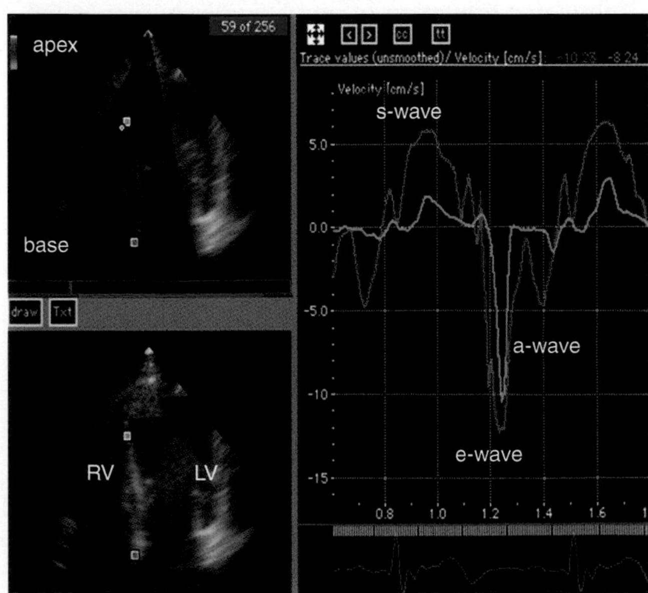

Figure 18C-2 Myocardial velocity curve obtained from colour Doppler interrogation of the interventricular septum. Myocardial velocities are recorded at base (*yellow*) and apex (*green*). s-, e-, and a-waves are named as above. LV, left ventricle; RV, right ventricle.

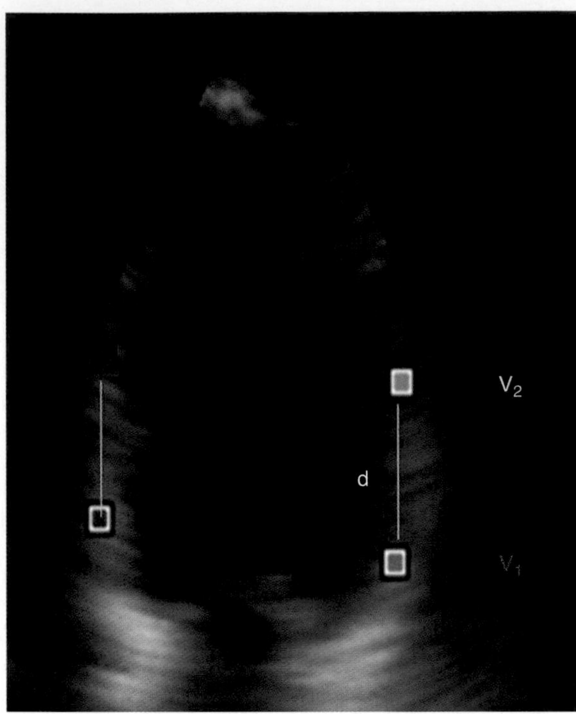

Figure 18C-3 Longitudinal strain is obtained as a gradient between velocity 1 (V_1) and velocity 2 (V_2) over a distance (d) of 1 cm. Note that both velocities are well aligned to the Doppler beam.

which is calculated as the gradient in myocardial velocities over a given distance, usually 1 cm.

Strain, notated as ε, is dimensionless, as it is calculated as a quotient of velocities (Fig. 18C-3). The first derivative of strain is strain rate. Strain provides information about the overall deformation of the myocardium, while strain rate describes how this deformation occurs over time. Both give different information, first on the degree of deformation, and second, on the time course of this deformation.

The major limitation of any Doppler measurement of myocardial velocities and its derivatives, such as strain and strain rate, is the dependency of the Doppler technique on the angulation of the insonating beam. This is a particular problem in patients with congenitally malformed hearts with abnormal chamber topography and dilated or hypertrophied ventricles, which make it very difficult to place the echocardiographic transducer correctly to align the beam with the myocardial wall.

A novel alternative method to Doppler-based measurement of strain is speckle tracking, which allows estimation of the velocity vector, rather than the velocity component, along the line of the image. This method is based on tracking patterns of radio-frequency imaging.[4] The algorithm finds the velocity vector by tracking patterns in the radio-frequency image between consecutive frames during the cardiac cycle, and thus makes it possible to find the in-plane frame-to-frame position of a pixel relative to its initial position (Fig. 18C-4). This technique requires high-quality b-mode images recorded at frame rates of at least 60 frames per second.[5] With this method, deformation can be assessed in two directions simultaneously, such as radial and longitudinal. By convention, this method has been named two-dimensional strain.

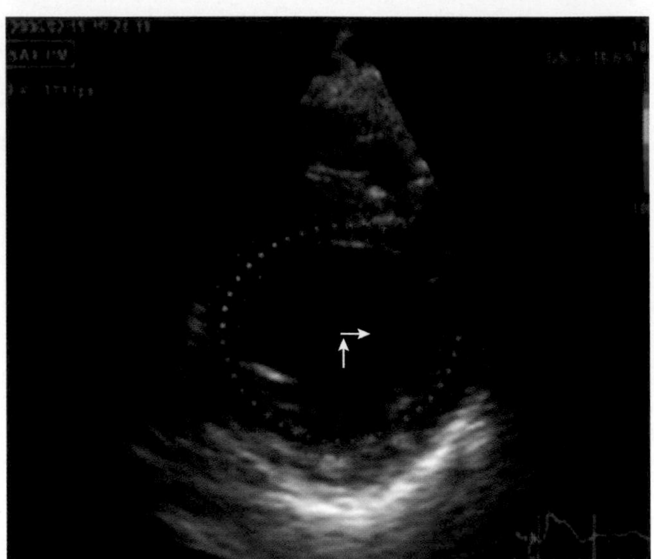

Figure 18C-4 Speckle tracking of the left ventricle in a short axis. The coloured dots show the myocardium in which the ultrasonic speckles are examined. The arrows indicate the direction of deformation in the myocardium.

EXPERIMENTAL AND CLINICAL VALIDATION OF MYOCARDIAL DOPPLER AND SPECKLE TRACKING

Measurement of myocardial velocities, assessment of longitudinal strain by estimating myocardial velocity gradients, and two-dimensional strain by speckle tracking, have all been validated experimentally.[6–8] These experimental validations were achieved by comparison of the novel echocardiographic techniques to pressure-volume loops obtained using conductance catheterisation, or using sonomicrometric crystals on the epicardium to quantify myocardial deformation.

Gorcsan et al were the first to validate colour-coded myocardial velocities for the assessment of regional and global left ventricular function.[6] Peak systolic myocardial velocities increased with dobutamine and decreased with esmolol, while simultaneously measured end-systolic elastance, by use of a conductance catheter, correlated well with these changes. Regional left ventricular peak systolic velocities mirrored changes in myocardial length as measured by the crystals placed in the respective myocardial segments. The first clinical validation of myocardial Doppler was achieved by comparing transmural myocardial biopsies obtained during coronary arterial bypass surgery with myocardial Doppler tracings.[9] The histological findings were compared to systolic and diastolic myocardial velocities measured the day before surgery, revealing significant relationships between systolic and early diastolic myocardial velocities and beta-adrenergic receptor density, and the proportion of interstitial fibrosis. The study proved that systolic and diastolic myocardial velocities in humans are dependent on the number of functioning myocytes, and the density of myocardial β-adrenergic receptors.

Doppler-derived longitudinal strain was validated experimentally using ultrasonic crystals placed near the left ventricular apex and base.[7] During ischaemia induced by occlusion of the anterior interventricular artery, the apical myocardium became dyskinetic. Doppler-derived longitudinal strain reacted the same way as the crystals. Thus, measurement of myocardial deformation by strain was shown to detect changes in regional motion affected by ischaemia. The study also demonstrated the load-dependency of myocardial velocities and Doppler-derived strain, and confirmed the techniques to be dependent on the angle of insonation, thus limiting their clinical applications.

Because of this, speckle tracking was developed and validated to assess deformation independent of the angle of insonation.[8] Again, sonomicrometric crystals were used as reference, and their changes during inotropic modulation and ischaemia were compared to changes in radial and longitudinal strain. Good agreements were obtained for measurements of both radial and longitudinal strain, and good correlations shown between ultrasonic strain as revealed by speckle tracking and deformation of the crystals.

Although these studies demonstrated the accuracy of myocardial velocities derived by Doppler and speckle tracking, as well as strain, the methods were found to be load-dependent. As such, they offered little advantage over traditional indexes, such as ejection or shortening fraction for evaluating global ventricular function.[10] Measurements of myocardial contraction during the isovolumic period are likely to be more robust. One of the commonest measured isovolumic indexes remains $dP/dt_{max,}$ which can only be assessed by invasive techniques.[11] After we had noticed that the ventricular myocardial velocity during isovolumic contraction increased more markedly than the peak systolic velocity during dobutamine stress, we used myocardial Doppler to measure the acceleration of the myocardium during isovolumic contraction, in other words isovolumic acceleration. Subsequently, we validated experimentally isovolumic acceleration as an index of contractile function, comparing it to myocardial acceleration and velocities measured during the ejection phase.[12] As the independent index of contractility for comparison of myocardial Doppler data, we used pressure-volume analysis, derived by conductance catheter, measuring in this way end-systolic and maximal elastance in both ventricles.[13,14] Our studies confirmed that small changes in contractile function during beta blockade or stimulation of beta

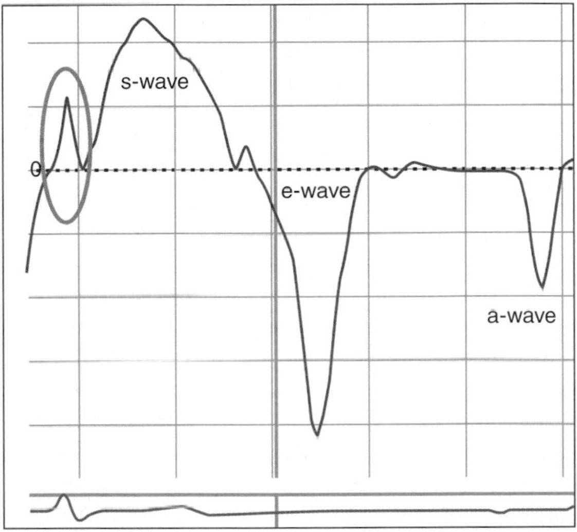

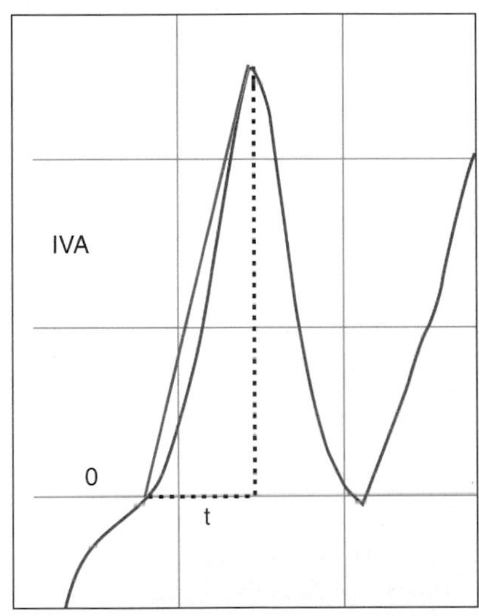

Figure 18C-5 Measurement of myocardial isovolumic acceleration (IVA). The blue circle indicates where isovolumic acceleration can be identified as the first upstroke in the velocity curve preceding the s-wave. Average acceleration is measured from the time (t) of onset of the (positive) velocity during isovolumic contraction to the point in time of the peak of this velocity. The green line indicates the line between zero and peak velocity along which the acceleration is measured.

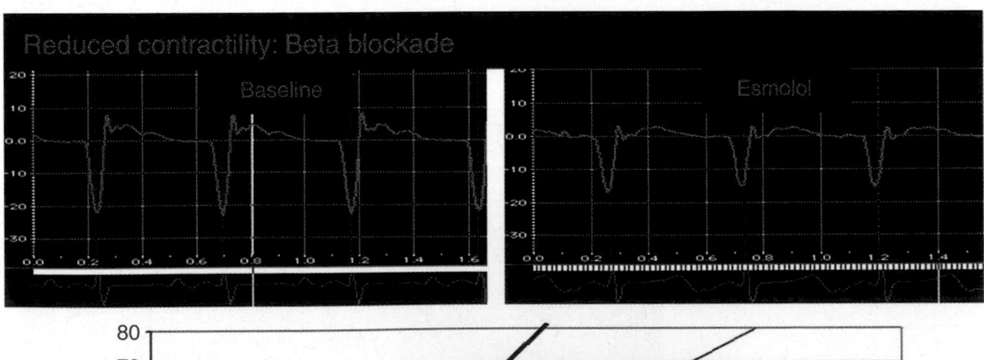

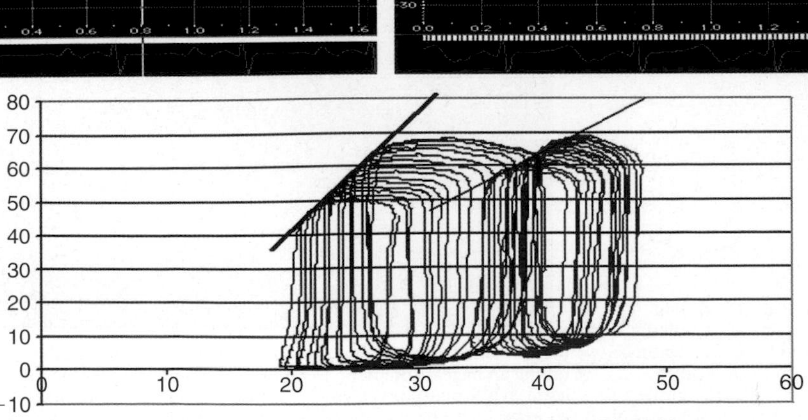

Figure 18C-6 Simultaneous velocity curves by myocardial Doppler and end-systolic pressure volume relations (Ees) obtained by conductance catheterisation at baseline and during an infusion of esmolol. Isovolumic acceleration is lower during esmolol and Ees decreases likewise.

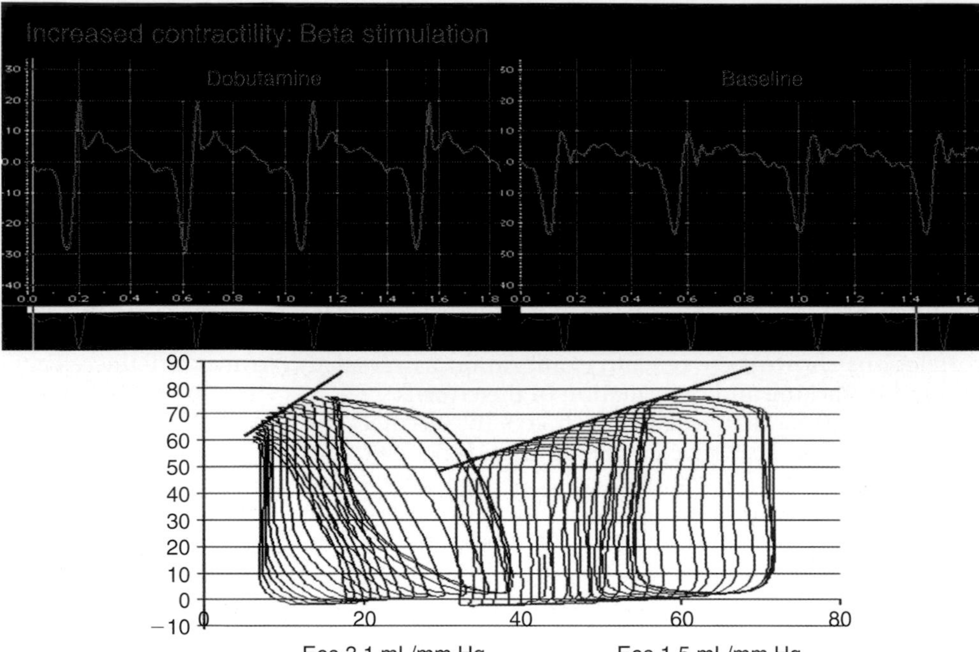

Figure 18C-7 Simultaneous velocity curves by myocardial Doppler and end-systolic pressure volume relations (Ees) obtained by conductance catheterisation at baseline and during an infusion of dobutamine to increase contractile function. During dobutamine infusion both isovolumic acceleration and Ees are significantly higher than at rest.

receptors could be detected by measuring isovolumic acceleration (Fig. 18C-5 to18C-7). Importantly, changes in pre- and after-load in a physiological range (Figs. 18C-8 and 18C-9) did not affect isovolumic acceleration, while the myocardial Doppler-derived indexes of the ejection phase were all influenced significantly by these changes. These experimental findings of the independence of measurements of isovolumic acceleration from conditions of loading were subsequently confirmed in healthy humans, as well as in patients with abnormal loading conditions.[15,16]

We also performed a clinical validation of isovolumic acceleration in patients with transposition subsequent atrial redirection procedures, in which the morphologically right ventricle continues to support the systemic circulation.[17] As some of these patients develop systemic ventricular dysfunction in the second, third, or fourth decade oflife, it is of clinical interest to assess prospectively their contractile reserve. From 80 such adults, we recruited 12 who simultaneously underwent a study using conductance catheters and myocardial Doppler. At rest, as well as during β-receptor stimulation using dobutamine, we analysed pressure-volume relations and isovolumic acceleration. Both parameters of contractile function increased significantly during β stimulation (Fig. 18C-10). This showed, first, that isovolumic acceleration can detect changes in contractile function in the human, and second, that measurement of the contractile reserve in patients with a systemic morphologically right ventricle has a clinical value. Critics have claimed that isovolumic acceleration may not be due to a ventricular event. We have demonstrated

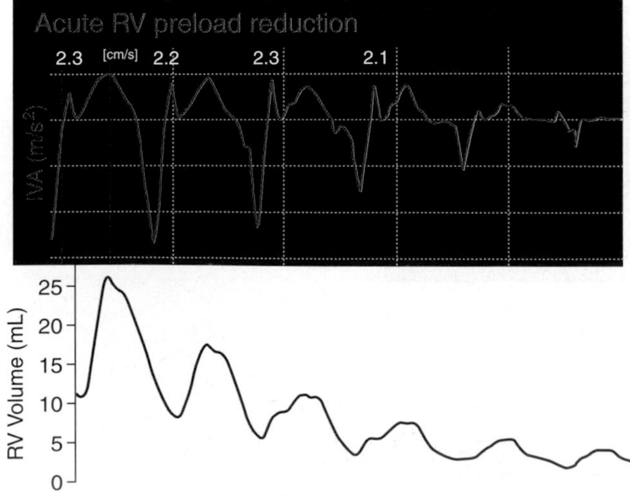

Figure 18C-8 Simultaneous myocardial velocity (*upper panel*) and right ventricular volume tracings during preload reduction produced by inflating a balloon in the inferior caval vein to reduce venous return. Up to a volume reduction of 50%, isovolumic acceleration does not change significantly, demonstrating that it is unaffected by preload changes in a physiological range. When right ventricular volumes are reduced by more than 50%, isovolumic acceleration is also affected.

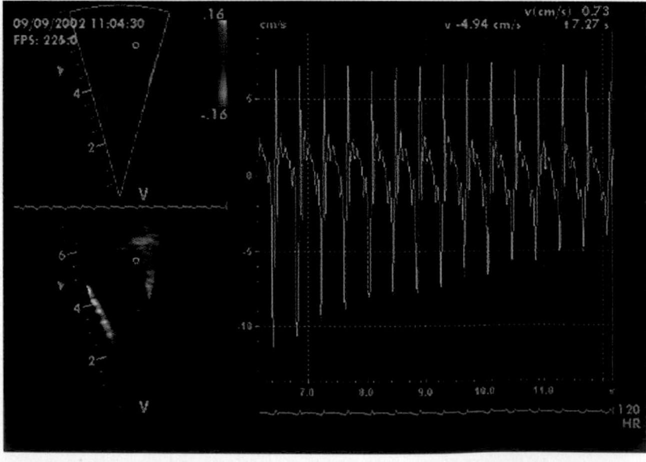

Figure 18C-9 Myocardial Doppler tracing from the base of the left ventricle during an increase in afterload produced by inflating a balloon in the ascending aorta. While diastolic velocities decrease markedly, isovolumic acceleration stays constant for 15 heartbeats. At the same time, left ventricular volume increased by 30%, and isovolumic acceleration was unaffected by this change in afterload.

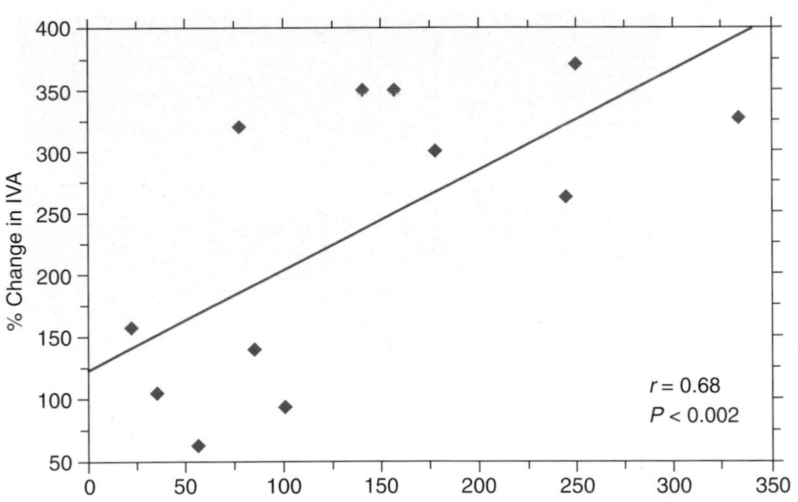

Figure 18C-10 Correlation between change in isovolumic acceleration (IVA) and change in Ees in 12 patients with transposition after a Mustard operation during a 10-minute infusion of 10 μg dobutamine/kg/min. *r* is the correlation coefficient (0.68).

experimentally, using simultaneous recordings of right ventricular pressure and myocardial Doppler, that isovolumic acceleration occurs immediately before the ventricle builds up pressure to eject blood, which may be an explanation for the relative insensitivity of isovolumic acceleration to changes in conditions of ventricular loading (Fig. 18C-11). In a patient with complete heart block, we found no signal of isovolumic acceleration during atrial contraction when we had turned off the pacemaker. Isovolumic acceleration reappeared with the first ventricular escape beat (Fig. 18C-12).

Experimental and clinical data suggests, therefore, that isovolumic acceleration provides a robust measurement of left or right ventricular contractile function, with a sensitivity approaching or exceeding those indexes traditionally measured using invasive techniques. During these experiments, we also noticed a dependency of isovolumic acceleration on the heart rate, which increased during atrial pacing. This suggested that we could non-invasively assess the force-frequency relation.[18] This force-frequency relation is a fundamental physiological parameter of myocardial function.[19] Figure 18C-13 illustrates a typical example of this ventricular phenomenon. We found that isovolumic acceleration increased significantly with heart rate during incremental pacing in both ventricles, mirroring changes in dP/dt_{max}. The normal pattern is for increasing development of force during incremental tachycardia to a point of maximal development, beyond which force then decreases with ongoing increases in heart rate.[19,20] An abnormal force-frequency relationship has been found in patients with dilated and hypertrophic cardiomyopathies, and in those with cardiac failure.[21,22] Until now, the force-frequency relation has either been assessed on the explanted myocyte, or invasively using dP/dt_{max} as a measurement of contractile force.[23,24] Subsequently the force-frequency relation could be measured non-invasively by assessing isovolumic acceleration in normal subjects, as well as patients with functionally univentricular hearts.[25]

NORMAL CARDIAC FUNCTION ASSESSED BY MYOCARDIAL DOPPLER AND TWO-DIMENSIONAL STRAIN

The myocardial Doppler-derived isovolumic acceleration, systolic velocities, and strain, as well as two-dimensional strain, change with age.[26] Thus, appropriate reference values need to be used for those of different ages.[27,28] By convention, systolic velocities, caused by shortening of

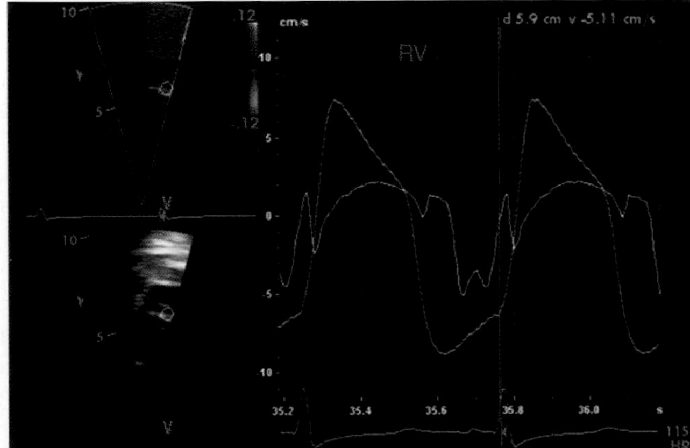

Figure 18C-11 Simultaneous recording of right ventricular pressure (*blue*), electrocardiogram (*green*), and a myocardial velocity curve (*white*) obtained from the base of the right ventricle. The pressure signal from the conductance catheter was fed into the echocardiography machine. The yellow line identifies the onset of isovolumic acceleration, which occurs simultaneously with the onset of pressure rise in the right ventricle (RV). Both isovolumic acceleration and the right ventricular pressure curve start to rise at the onset of the R-wave in the electrocardiogram.

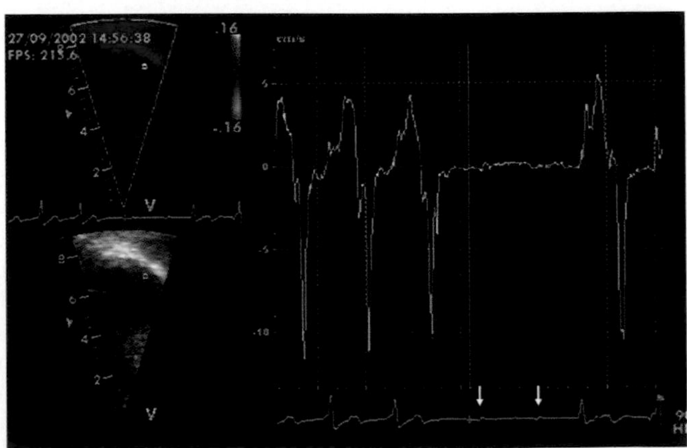

Figure 18C-12 Myocardial Doppler curve tracing (*yellow*) from the base of the left ventricle in a 12-year-old boy with complete heart block during pacemaker testing. When the pacemaker is switched off there is no QRS complex on the electrocardiographic tracings but a p-wave can be recognised. Just as the first ventricular escape beat appears, isovolumic acceleration can be seen to reappear on the myocardial Doppler velocity curve as well demonstrating the isovolumic acceleration is not related to atrial activity but is a ventricular event.

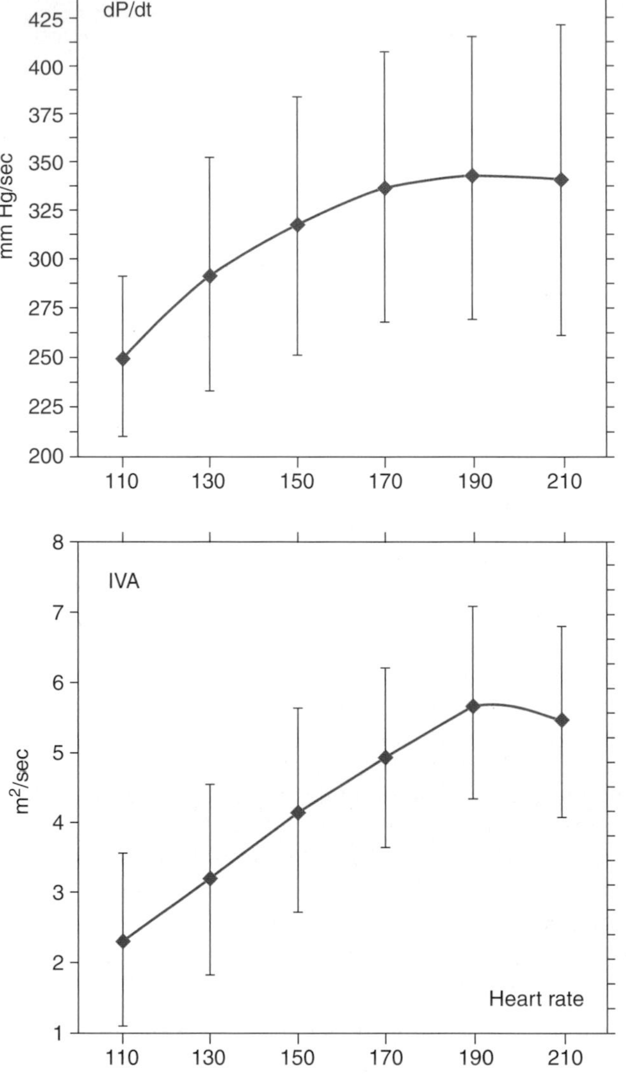

Figure 18C-13 Simultaneous force-frequency curves obtained by pressure tracings in the left ventricle to determine dp/dt and by measurement of isovolumic acceleration from the base of the left ventricle during atrial pacing in a 15-kg pig. With each increment in heart rate (by 20 beats/min), dp/dt and isovolumic acceleration increase to plateau at a rate of 180 beats/min.

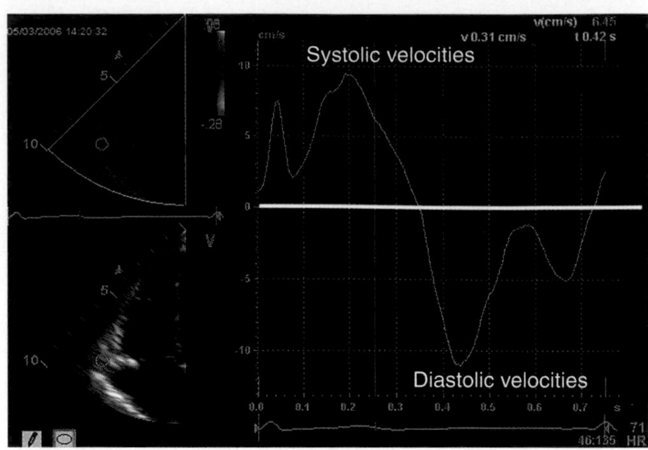

Figure 18C-14 Myocardial Doppler velocity tracing in a 10-year-old healthy boy obtained at the base of the right ventricle. Note that systolic velocities are displayed above and diastolic velocities below the zero-line.

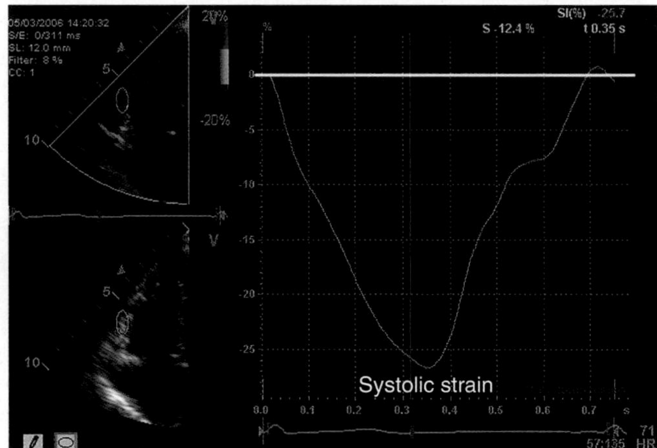

Figure 18C-15 Longitudinal strain curve obtained from myocardial velocities in the same volunteer. Note that the deformation during systole by myocardial shortening is displayed below the zero-line.

the myocytes, are displayed as positive waves above the zero line, and diastolic velocities, due to relaxation of the myocytes, are displayed as negative waves below the zero line (Fig. 18C-14). For longitudinal strain, commonly assessed in the four-chamber view, the convention is different. Deformation during systolic shortening of the myocytes is displayed as a negative curve (Fig. 18C-15) below the zero line, while deformation during diastolic lengthening is displayed as a positive curve. This is because most cardiologists imaging adults look at the heart upside down in the four-chamber view. In contrast, most cardiologists imaging congenitally malformed hearts use anatomic views in the four-chamber view. Despite this difference, the convention of displaying velocities of shortening above the zero line as positive velocities, and velocities of lengthening of myocardial fibres as negative, has been accepted by cardiologists evaluating congenitally malformed hearts.

Myocardial velocities of shortening can be displayed in a different way, which facilitates recognition of abnormalities of ventricular mural motion. The integral of myocardial velocity data displays the distance a piece of myocardium covers during movement from base to apex. Online calculation makes possible instant recognition of abnormalities of wall motion (Fig. 18C-16). The different distances are colour-coded. As only the velocities directed from base to apex are integrated, any piece of the myocardium which does not shorten from base to apex in systole remains grey. Thus, areas of abnormal motion, which paradoxically lengthen in systole when the remainder of the myocardium is contracting, can be readily identified (Fig. 18C-17).

In a normal pulsed wave Doppler, or colour Doppler, myocardial velocity tracing, it is possible to discern a positive velocity during isovolumic contraction, a positive systolic velocity, known as the s-wave, an early negative diastolic velocity, the e-wave, and a negative diastolic velocity during atrial contraction, the a-wave. In a normal morphologically right ventricle, there is no discernible isovolumic relaxation time, while a small notch can be seen in the tracing of myocardial velocity obtained from the left ventricle, the notch identifying the end of isovolumic relaxation, which begins immediately following the crossing of the zero line by the velocity of the s-wave (Figs. 18C-18 and 18C-19).

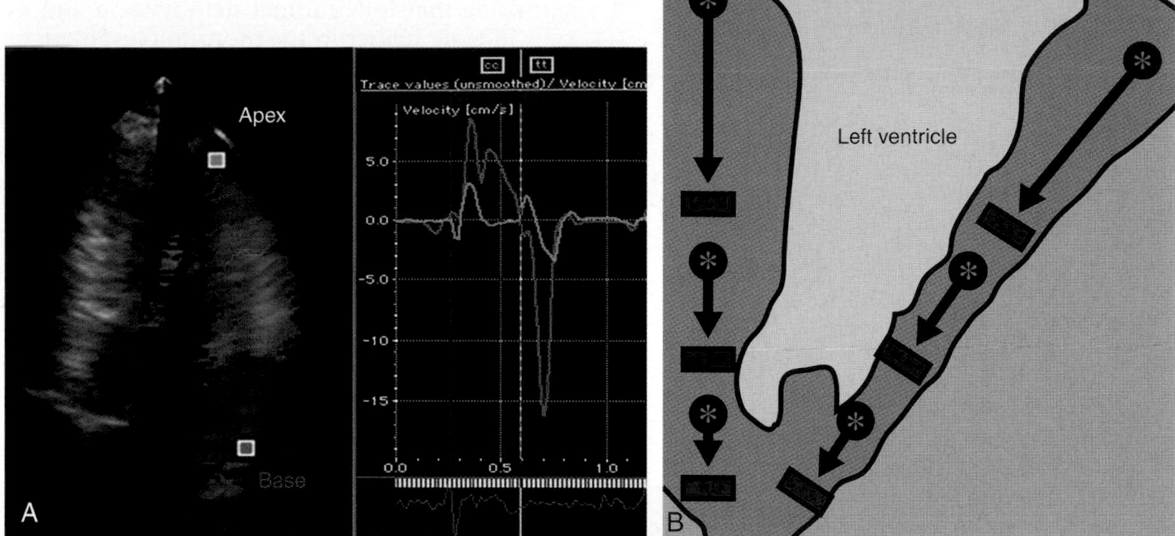

Figure 18C-16 **A,** In the middle, a standard myocardial velocity curve at the base (*yellow*) and apex (*green*) of the left ventricle is displayed. To the left of this curve, the left ventricle is displayed in a two-chamber view. The free wall is colour coded with each colour band representing the integral of the systolic myocardial velocity. This velocity integral displays a distance. **B,** On the right side, the schematic drawing illustrates the distance a piece of myocardium moves from base to apex during systole.

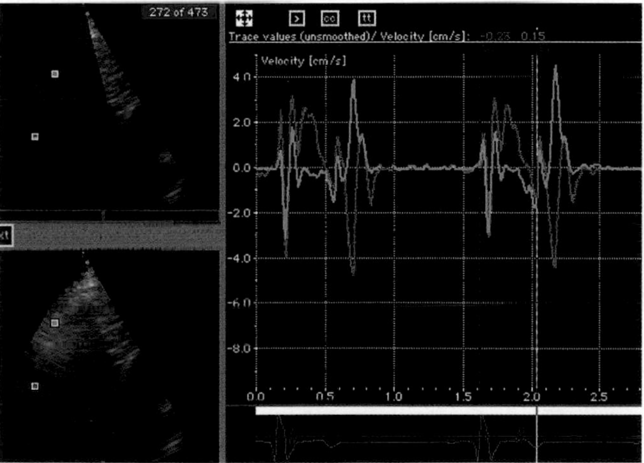

Figure 18C-17 Wall motion abnormality in the right ventricle of a 31-year-old patient with transposition who had undergone a Mustard procedure at the age of 18 months. On the right side, the myocardial velocity curve at base (*yellow*) and apex (*green*) is displayed. Note that at the apex there is a negative wave indicating lengthening at systole and a positive velocity indicating shortening during diastole in contrast to the normal myocardial velocity at the base (displayed in *yellow*). On the left hand side in the lower panel, tissue tracking demonstrates shortening at the base, which is colour encoded in yellow and red, while almost half of the free wall of the right ventricle is displayed in grey (without colour coding), indicating no shortening in systole. This corresponds to the green velocity on the right.

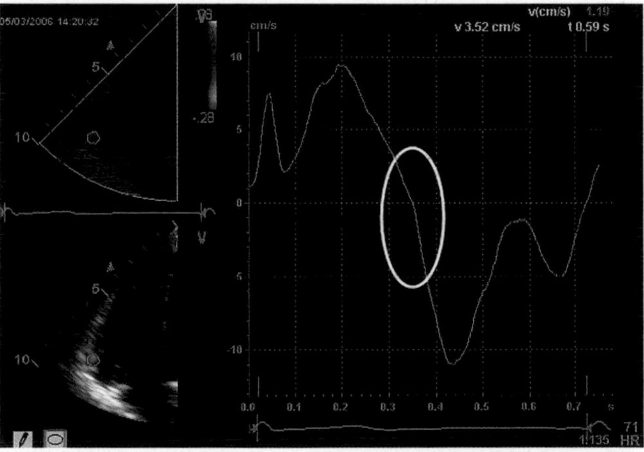

Figure 18C-18 Normal myocardial velocity curve from a 16-year-old healthy volunteer obtained at the base of the right ventricle. Note that there is no identifiable isovolumic relaxation period, which is characteristic of a right ventricle functioning normally.

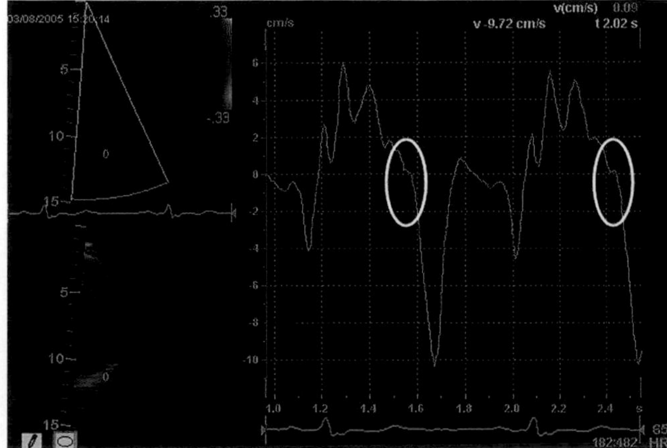

Figure 18C-19 Normal myocardial velocity curve from the same volunteer obtained at the base of the left ventricle. Note that in the myocardial velocity tracing from the left ventricle an isovolumic relaxation wave (*ellipses*) can be identified.

The normal values for isovolumic acceleration, myocardial velocities, and strain and strain rate are listed in Table 18C-1. In the normal heart, there is a gradual decrease of systolic and diastolic myocardial velocities from base to apex (Fig. 18C-20). In contrast, longitudinal strain, which represents a velocity gradient, changes little from base to apex in either ventricle (Fig. 18C-21).

Normally isovolumic acceleration, myocardial velocities, and longitudinal strain are higher in the morphologically right than in the left ventricle. This may reflect the basic physiology of the pattern of contraction of the ventricles, which is determined by the orientation of the myocytes

TABLE 18C-1

MYOCARDIAL DOPPLER STRAIN AND STRAIN RATE NORMAL VALUES

	Right Ventricle	Left Ventricle
Isovolumic acceleration, m/sec²	1.8 ± 0.4	1.0 ± 0.3
s-Wave, cm/sec	11.5 ± 0.4	8.4 ± 0.4
e-Wave, cm/sec	14 ± 0.4	12 ± 0.4
a-Wave, cm/sec	4.5 ± 0.4	4.5 ± 0.4
Longitudinal strain	45 ± 13%	25 ± 7%
Radial strain	—	57 ± 11%
Strain rate	2.8 ± 0.7	1.9 ± 0.7
Radial strain rate	—	3.7 ± 0.9

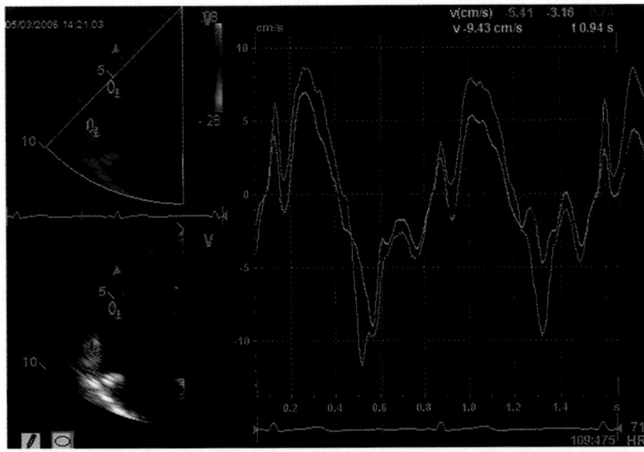

Figure 18C-20 Myocardial velocity curve from the same volunteer with myocardial velocities recorded at the base (*yellow*), middle (*green*), and near the apex (*red*) of the right ventricle demonstrating a gradual decrease of isovolumic acceleration, systolic and diastolic velocities from base to apex.

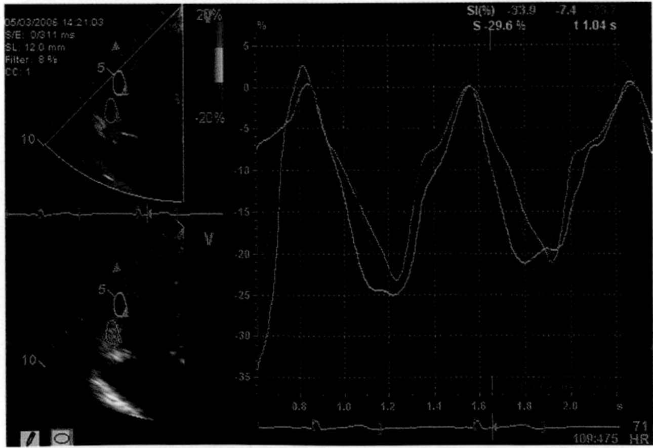

Figure 18C-21 Longitudinal strain curves of the right ventricle in the same person. Note that there is little change in maximal systolic strain between base (*yellow*), middle (*green*), and apex (*red*) of the right ventricle.

and ventricular morphology.[29] With the myocardial Doppler technique, we image longitudinal function when sampling in the four-chamber view. As the main force to eject blood from the morphologically right ventricle is longitudinal shortening of the myocytes, causing the base and the tricuspid valve to move towards the apex, it is not surprising that longitudinal deformation and myocardial velocities are higher in the morphologically right ventricle than in the left. In addition to myocardial velocities and strain, isovolumic acceleration is also higher in the right than in the left ventricle. This is in keeping with experimental data,[30] which shows that twitch velocities measured experimentally in the right ventricle exceed those of the left ventricle. In the left ventricle, only the subendocardial and subepicardial myocytes are aggregated in longitudinal fashion, with an important contribution to the ejection of blood provided by the circumferential fibres. Thus, radial function is the predominant functional component in the left ventricle, which can explain the fact that longitudinal myocardial velocities and longitudinal strain are lower in the left than in the right ventricle.

With speckle tracking, a velocity vector is tracked, which later allows for measurement of both radial and longitudinal velocities. The underlying principle of measurement of velocity by speckle tracking is different. For this reason, myocardial velocities are lower than those measured by the Doppler technique (Fig. 18C-22). As these velocities are independent of the angle of insonation, velocities in the longitudinal direction from base to apex, acquired from a standard apical four-chamber view, are not different from those acquired from a subcostal view, where the heart is imaged from a different angle (Fig. 18C-23).

ACQUISITION OF MYOCARDIAL DOPPLER AND SPECKLE TRACKING DATA FOR LATER ANALYSIS

There are some important points to consider in order to avoid pitfalls during recording of myocardial Doppler and two-dimensional strain data. For both techniques, temporal resolution is critical, and thus frame rate needs to be as high as possible. A desirable frame rate for myocardial Doppler-based isovolumic acceleration, velocity, and strain measurements is 180 frames per second, or more. This can be achieved with most commercially available echocardiographic machines by using a narrow sector of the b-mode image to image separately the free walls of the right and left ventricles and the septum (Fig. 18C-24). Typically, the heart is initially imaged in a four-chamber view to provide an overview of the anatomy. In a second step, the image sector is narrowed down just to image the structures to be analysed by myocardial Doppler. Optimal gain setting is important, focussing on a good delineation of the border between blood pool and the endocardium. The gain should be as low as possible to avoid signals from the blood pool, which potentially can interfere with the ultrasonic signal from the endo- or myocardium. This is especially important in patients with a poorly functioning ventricle and low velocity intracardiac flow, such as those with dilated cardiomyopathies.

As myocardial velocity and strain measurements are based on the Doppler principle, the most important point is to achieve an optimal angle of insonation relative to the myocardium. A deviation between the angle of the ultrasound beam and the myocardium of 15 degrees at most is acceptable. Anything larger makes measurements unreliable. In most clinical situations, these goals can be achieved using transthoracic imaging. It is generally possible also to acquire data by transoesophageal imaging,

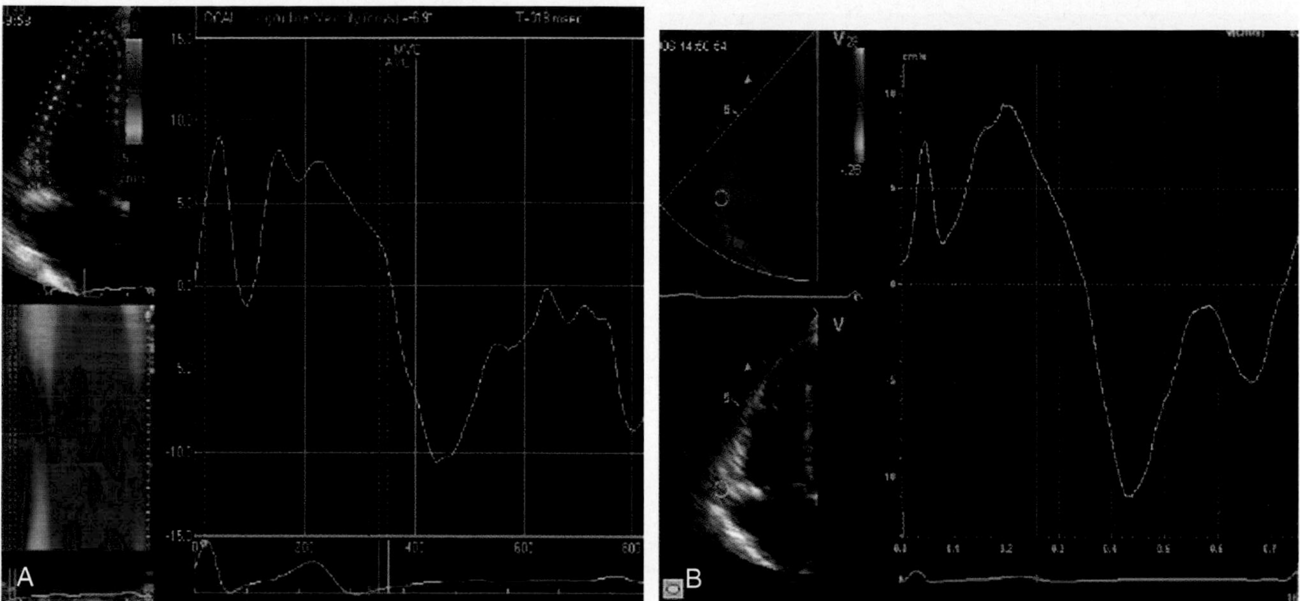

Figure 18C-22 Comparison between speckle tracking (**A**) and colour-coded myocardial Doppler-derived myocardial velocities (**B**) at the base of the right ventricle in a healthy volunteer. Note that the curves look similar while the velocities obtained from speckle tracking are generally lower in systole as well as diastole.

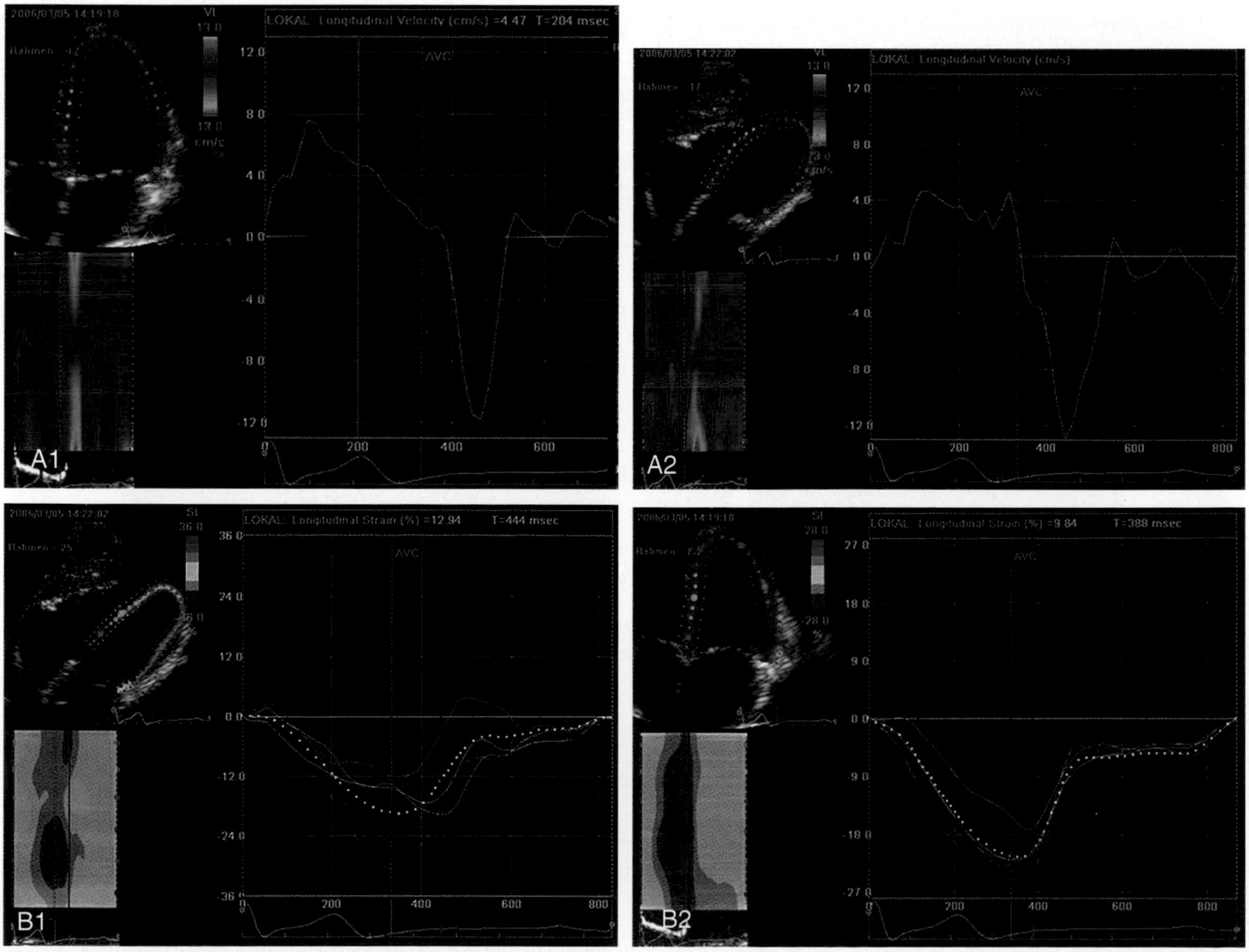

Figure 18C-23 Speckle tracking–derived myocardial velocities in the left ventricle (**A1** and **A2**) obtained from a standard apical four-chamber view (*left*) and from a subcostal view (*right*). As the velocities are independent of the angle of insonation, both velocities are similar with a small difference in peak systolic velocity and no difference in early diastolic velocity or a-wave. Similar findings are displayed in **B1** and **B2,** obtained for speckle tracking–derived myocardial strain using the same windows.

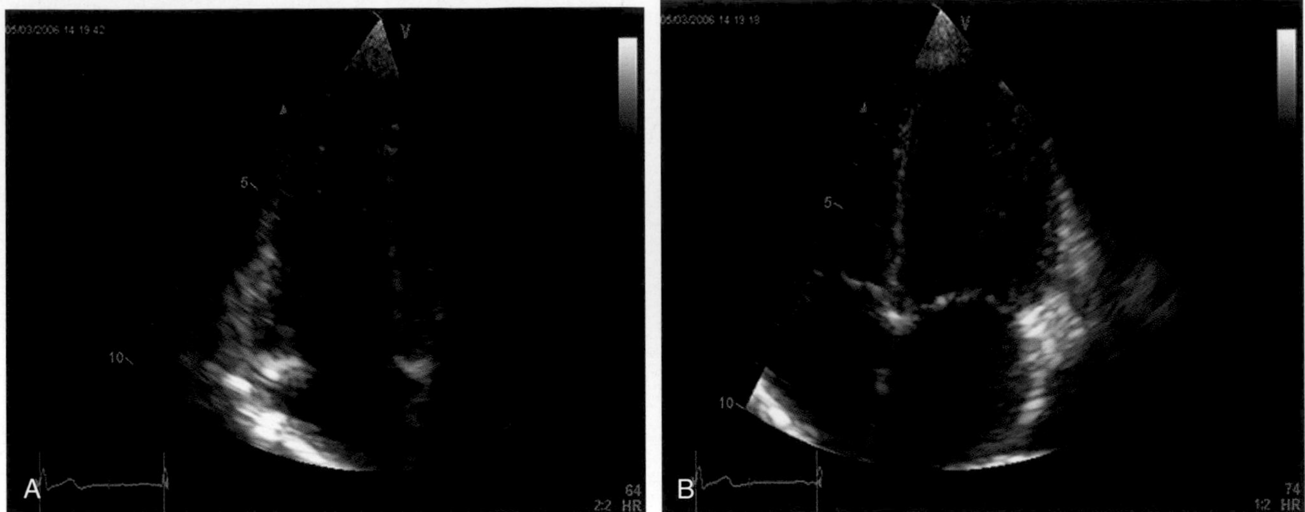

Figure 18C-24 Acquisition of data suitable for speckle tracking analysis. In order to obtain a frame rate in above 60 frames per second, the right ventricle (**A**) and the left ventricle (**B**) need to be imaged separately. Gain settings need to be optimised to have little or no blood pool signal and to delineate the endocardium.

but the measurements from this data differ from those obtained from transthoracic imaging, and different normal values have to be used for comparison.[31]

Longitudinal strain and strain rate data are derived from myocardial velocities at different locations in the myocardium, usually 1 cm apart. Ideally the angle of insonation should be the same for both velocities. If the difference in the angle between the two velocities, which are compared, becomes too large, longitudinal strain measurements may become impossible (Fig. 18C-25). The ribs can interfere with the ultrasonic signal during imaging of the ventricles, so this also needs to be avoided. An m-mode tracing can be used to identify artefacts, and distinguish these from true myocardial motion (Fig. 18C-26).

Acquiring data for two-dimensional strain analysis by speckle tracking is generally easier, as the technique is

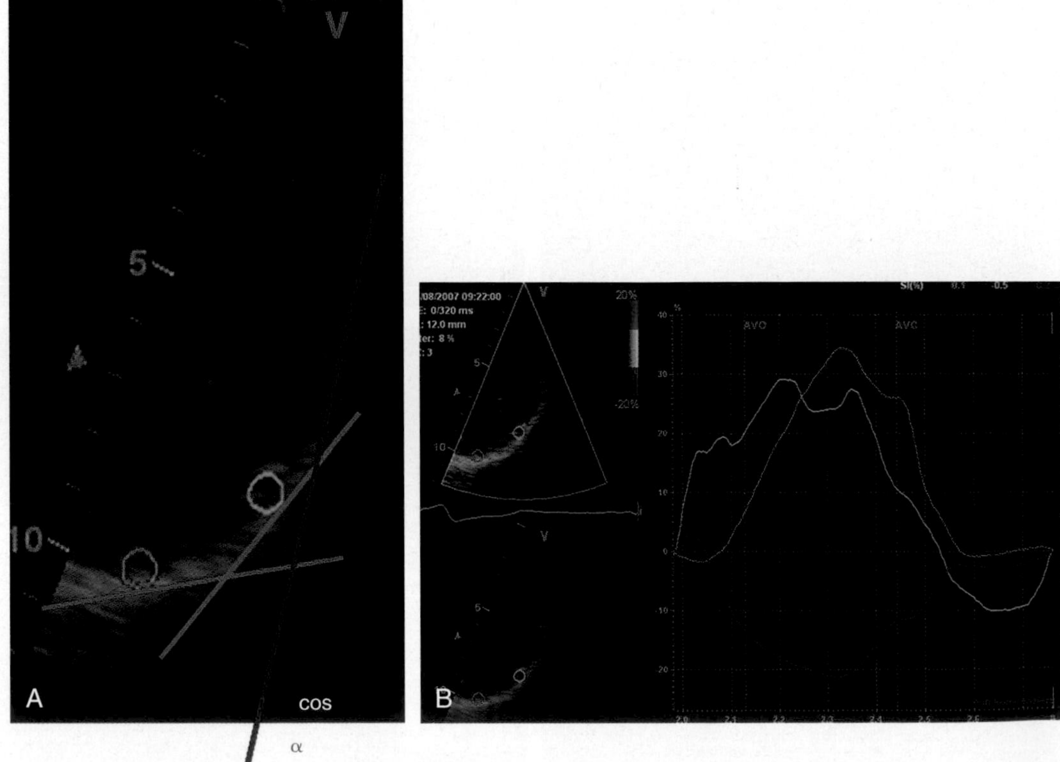

Figure 18C-25 Left ventricular strain measurement from myocardial Doppler imaging in a healthy volunteer at the base (*yellow*), middle (*green*), and near the apex (*red*). The circles in the b-mode image (**A**) represent the points where the myocardial velocities which are used to calculate the velocity gradient (strain) are sampled and the lines illustrate the angle relative to the ultrasound beam. As the ultrasound beam at the base is almost 90 degrees in relation to the sampling point the resulting strain curve (**B**) is inverted and thus (paradoxically) positive and even at an angle of about 45 degrees (*green*) the curve remains inverted. Further to the apex the sampling is done at an angle of about 15 degrees and a normal strain curve results demonstrating myocardial shortening during systole.

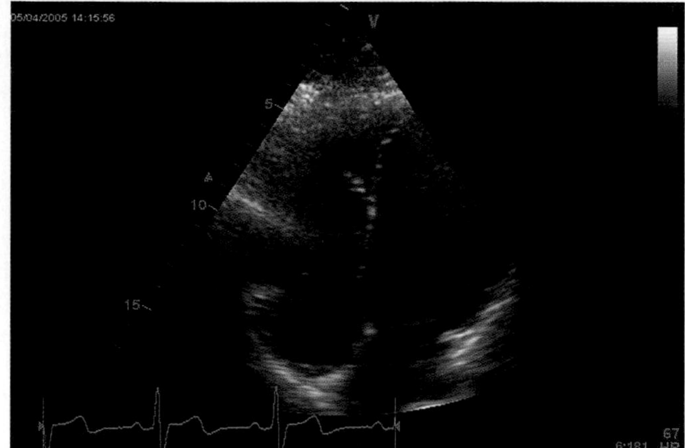

Figure 18C-26 In the b-mode image on the left an artefact most likely caused by a rib can be seen indicated by an arrow which interferes with the Doppler signal from the myocardium. Subsequently no myocardial velocity can be measured at this point.

independent from the angle of insonation, but similar principles hold true as for myocardial Doppler imaging. The frame rate of the b-mode image should be above 60 frames per second. This again can only be achieved by narrowing the sector of the heart to be imaged in most commercially available echocardiographic machines. In practise, this means that the right and left ventricle need to be imaged separately, as a recording of the entire four-chamber view is rarely possible at a high frame rate. Gain settings are as important for speckle tracking imaging as for myocardial Doppler. They should be as low as possible, with the blood pool clearly being black, allowing excellent definition of the border between blood and myocardium.

CLINICAL USE OF MYOCARDIAL DOPPLER ECHOCARDIOGRAPHY AND TWO-DIMENSIONAL STRAIN

The new myocardial Doppler and speckle tracing techniques offer information on both regional and global function. Unlike the ejection fraction, they are not dependent on geometrical assumptions, and as such are independent of the shape of the ventricle. Thus, they can be applied equally to the morphologically left and right ventricle, as well as functionally univentricular hearts. This makes them ideally suited for the assessment of patients with congenitally malformed hearts. Many such patients have undergone surgical intervention, often with production of abnormalities of ventricular mural motion. This may be due to patches used to close ventricular septal defects or enlarge outflows, scars in the myocardium, abnormal filling, or disturbances of electrical activation. While abnormal regional function has been reported in those with transposition after atrial repair using invasive techniques,[32] data obtained by non-invasive imaging has been scarce. The same holds true for analysis of regional wall motion in the setting of acquired disease, such as in those affected by Kawasaki disease.[33] Before the advent of myocardial Doppler techniques, analysis of regional function in these patients required time-consuming analysis of mural motion from b-mode images, which were semi-quantitative.[34,35]

One of the first clinical applications of myocardial Doppler in congenitally malformed hearts was in patients with tetralogy of Fallot.[36] This study not only demonstrated a high prevalence of post-operative abnormalities of right ventricular mural motion (Fig. 18C-27), but also showed for the first time an association between these mechanical abnormalities and abnormalities of electrical de- and repolarisation. Following this proof of a mechano-electrical interaction, an interesting therapeutic concept evolved. To reduce risk of sudden unexpected death,[37] and to improve

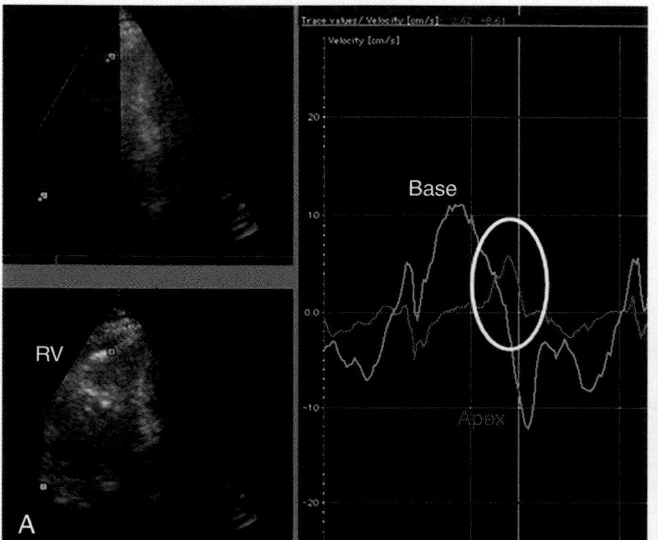

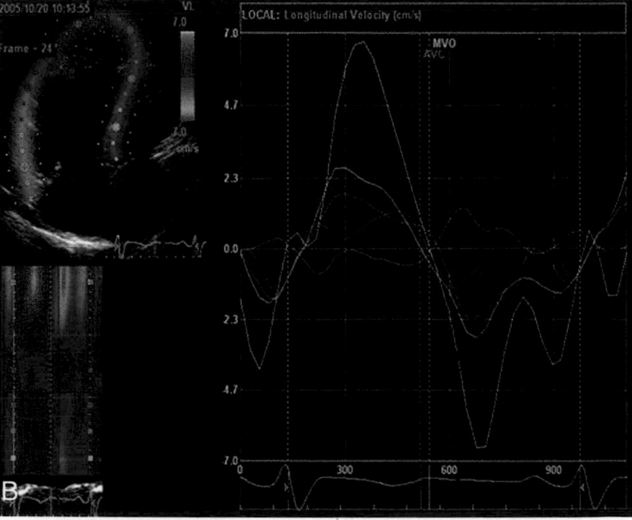

Figure 18C-27 **A,** B-mode image with colour-Doppler coded myocardium and myocardial Doppler velocity tracing (*left*) and speckle tracking with speckle-derived velocity tracing (*right*) in a 27-year-old patient who underwent surgical repair of tetralogy of Fallot with a transannular patch at age 21 months. His electrocardiogram had a right bundle branch block pattern and the maximal QRS duration was 163 ms. The myocardial velocity curve at the base (*green*) is normal, while the myocardial velocities measured near the apex (*yellow*) are inverted with a negative s-wave (indicating lengthening during systole) and a positive e-wave (indicating shortening during diastole) representing a wall motion abnormality (*ellipse*). **B,** The wall motion abnormality in the apical third of the right ventricle can be identified easily by the red colour indicating lengthening in systole and shortening in diastole. The myocardial velocities derived from the speckle tracking demonstrate again the reversed myocardial velocities in systole and diastole in the same anatomic segment of the right ventricle and the abnormal velocity distribution is identical to the abnormal distribution of the Doppler-derived myocardial velocities in **A.**

mechanical function in patients with post-operative right bundle branch block, atrioventricular pacing was successfully used in selected patients.[38] Preliminary clinical data is promising, and may offer a new option in such carefully selected patients.[39] Appropriate selection of patients who may benefit from this expensive and complex new therapy is mandatory, and can be achieved by applying the myocardial Doppler techniques.[40] Another important clinical problem in patients with tetralogy having significant post-operative pulmonary regurgitation is the optimal timing of replacement of the pulmonary valve. Previous studies using nuclear medicine or magnetic resonance imaging suggest that replacement offers little benefit if the right ventricular ejection is low, less than 40%, and right ventricular volume is in excess of 170 mL/cm^2 of body surface area.[41,42] Many patients with severe pulmonary regurgitation have a dilated right ventricle and tricuspid valve, which in turn leads also to tricuspid regurgitation. In this situation, the loading conditions of the right ventricle are markedly altered, which makes difficult the application of load-dependent indexes of right ventricular function.[43] By altering loading conditions, severe tricuspid regurgitation may mask right ventricular dysfunction. Thus, load-dependent indexes like myocardial Doppler-derived peak myocardial velocities may be normal, while load-independent isovolumic acceleration is markedly reduced, suggesting a reduced contractile function (Figs. 18C-28A and B). Indeed, in a substantial number of patients with pulmonary regurgitation, we found evidence of ventricular dysfunction when applying a relatively load-independent index of contractility.[44] Isovolumic acceleration was lower in all patients with tetralogy compared to normals, and correlated with the severity of pulmonary regurgitation, whereas the load dependent systolic velocities, strain and strain rate, which were all abnormally low, failed to correlate significantly with the severity of the regurgitation. If untreated, pulmonary regurgitation will lead to dilation of the right ventricle, which can influence left ventricular wall motion and function.[45] Besides right bundle branch block and a duration of the QRS complex in excess of 180 msec, left ventricular dysfunction has been recognised as a risk factor predisposing to sudden unexpected premature cardiac death. This may be related to left ventricular disynchrony.[45]

Abnormalities of ventricular mural motion have also been reported using invasive techniques in patients with transposition who remain with a systemic morphologically right ventricle following atrial repair.[32] Using the new myocardial Doppler methods, these abnormalities can more easily be evaluated non-invasively (Fig. 18C-29). Patients with abnormal mural motion in the systemic morphologically right ventricle also have a reduced global function, with abnormally low isovolumic acceleration. This finding is consistent with previous studies that examined excursion of the tricuspid valve using m-mode echocardiography.[46] An important contribution to the failure to augment stroke volume during exercise in these patients is the inability of the systemic venous atrium to contract and to expand, in particular in the patients following the Mustard repair.[45] The fact that the systemic and pulmonary venous atriums contribute little or nothing to ventricular filling can also be demonstrated by myocardial Doppler. The majority of patients after a Mustard procedure have no discernible a-wave (Fig. 18C-30) in the myocardial Doppler tracing, suggesting absence of active atrial contribution to ventricular filling.[47] By contrast, most patients after a Senning repair, in whom autologous tissue has been used to redirect the venous returns, have a well-identified a-wave on their ventricular myocardial Doppler tracings.

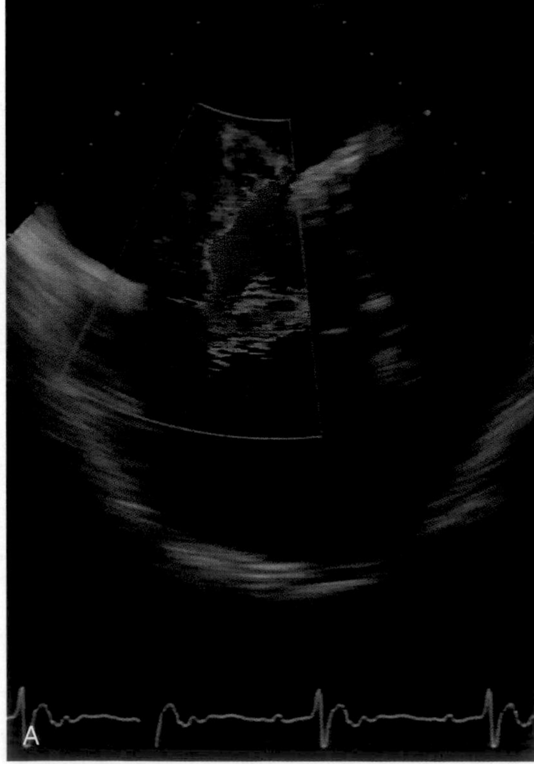

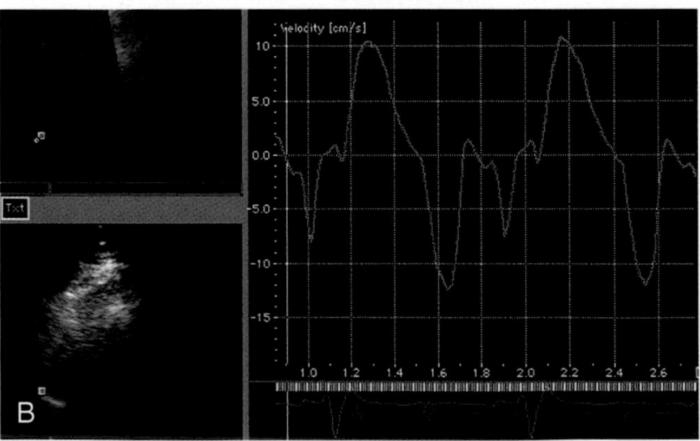

Figure 18C-28 **A,** B-mode and colour (blood-flow) Doppler obtained from a 31-year-old patient who underwent surgical repair of tetralogy of Fallot with a transjunctional patch at age 24 months. He has severe pulmonary incompetence and the blood flow colour Doppler demonstrates significant tricuspid regurgitation caused by the dilated right ventricle and tricuspid valve. **B,** The myocardial Doppler trace obtained at the base of the right ventricle demonstrates a normal systolic velocity of 10.5 cm/sec and a normal early diastolic velocity (12.3 cm/sec) but a very low isovolumic acceleration of 0.3 m/sec^2 (normal for this age range 1.6 m/sec^2), illustrating a reduced contractile function.

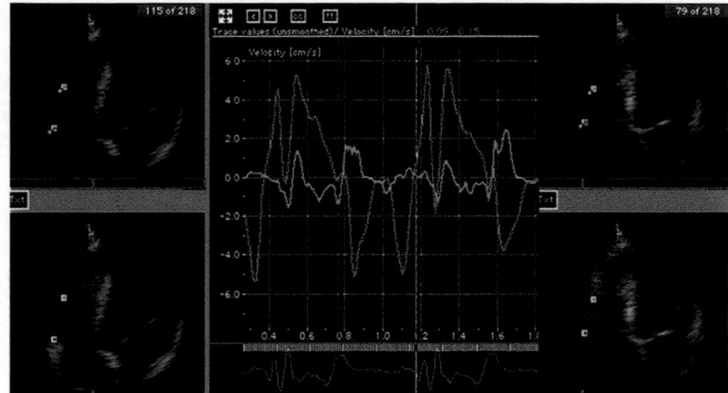

Figure 18C-29 Myocardial Doppler tracing from the right ventricle of a 29-year-old patient with transposition who had undergone a Senning procedure at the age of 19 months. The yellow velocity curve has been obtained from the base and the green one from the middle of the right ventricle. The velocity curve at the base is normal while in the middle of the ventricle the s-wave in late systole is reversed as is the early diastolic velocity. Note also that a clear a-wave can be seen at the base.

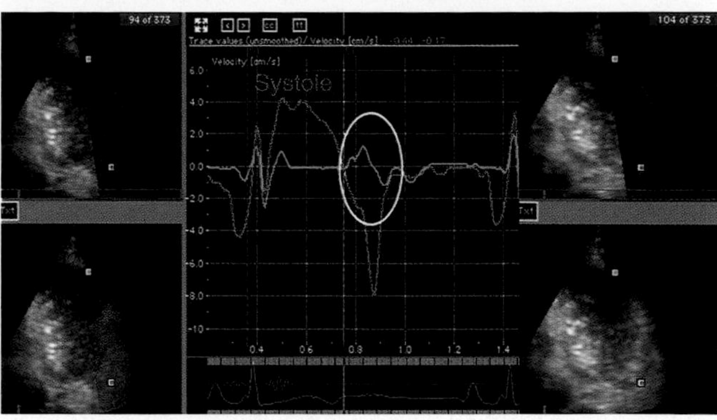

Figure 18C-31 Myocardial Doppler velocity trace and colour-coded tissue tracking of the left ventricular free wall in a 12-year-old patient with tricuspid atresia and concordant ventriculo-arterial connections who had undergone a Fontan operation at age 3.2 years. Tissue tracking on the left demonstrates no shortening near the apex, and the concomitant myocardial velocity (*green*) shows almost a flat systolic wave and a positive e-wave, indicating myocardial shortening during diastole at the apex. The ellipse highlights the area of wall motion abnormality.

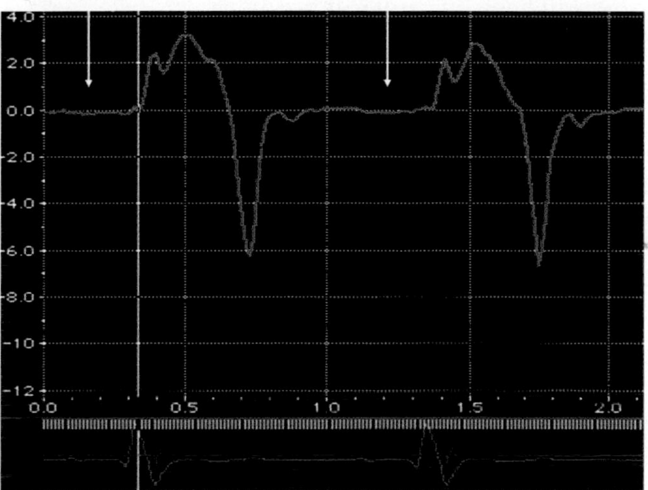

Figure 18C-30 Myocardial velocity tracing (*yellow*) obtained from the left ventricular base in a 30-year-old patient with transposition who had undergone a Mustard procedure at the age of 17 months. Note that there is no myocardial a-wave, while a p-wave can be seen in the simultaneously recorded electrocardiogram (*green*).

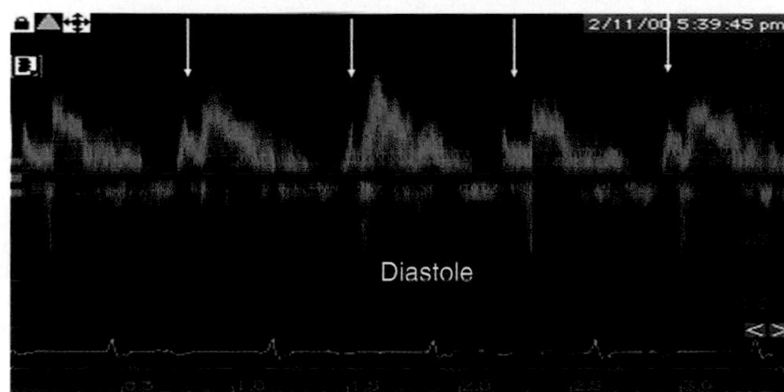

Figure 18C-32 Blood pool Doppler sampled in the left ventricle immediately below the mitral valve from the same patient as shown in Figure 18C-31, demonstrating abnormal intracardiac flow during systole (*white arrows*) preceding the flow during diastole.

A substantial number of patients with functionally univentricular hearts following conversion to the Fontan circulation have abnormalities of ventricular mural motion, with these being associated with abnormal filling of the dominant ventricle (Figs. 18C-31 and 18C-32).[48,49] Again, the new myocardial Doppler techniques allow for non-invasive diagnosis of these abnormalities,[50] and are thus much better suited to serial follow-up of these patients, who have a constant rate of attrition,[51] and in whom cardiac failure is a major cause of late death. Failure of the Fontan circulation can lead to failure of other organs, and lead to serious symptoms, such as protein-losing enteropathy.[51] Anecdotal data shows that epicardial pacing to resynchronise the dominant ventricle may improve ventricular function and abolish the protein-losing enteropathy.[52]

Congenital valvar aortic stenosis changes left ventricular afterload. Because of this, many patients with aortic stenosis have a better than average function when assessed using conventional echocardiographic parameters, such as ejection of shortening fraction. Myocardial Doppler allows for a more detailed examination of function, and revealed decreased systolic and diastolic myocardial velocities, as well as strain rate in those patients with aortic stenosis but normal shortening fraction.[53] Furthermore, the novel myocardial Doppler methods demonstrate positive effects of relief of stenosis by balloon dilation, and as such are well suited to monitor effects of treatment.[54]

Anomalous origin of the left coronary artery from the pulmonary trunk is a rare but important lesion, as it represents a clinical model of hibernating myocardium. Most patients in whom the left coronary artery can be reimplanted successfully into the aortic root may have a complete recovery of global left ventricular function, with a good long-term outcome.[55] Myocardial Doppler techniques can beautifully demonstrate the pre-operative dysfunction and the temporal evolution of recovery of myocardial function after reimplantation of the left coronary artery.[56]

Monitoring Ventricular Function in the Intensive Care Unit

The new myocardial Doppler techniques are well suited for application in the intensive care unit, where non-invasive assessment of myocardial function in particular is frequently required following surgical treatment of patients with congenitally malformed hearts. Some of these patients have poor echocardiographic windows because of artificial ventilation, drainage tubes, and dressings. Thus, an easy echocardiographic method is required, which does not depend on imaging the heart in total, but like isovolumic acceleration needs only to image the left or right ventricular free wall at the level of the atrioventricular valvar annuluses. Singular measurements of isovolumic acceleration can provide a quick overview of ventricular contractile function, but the non-invasive assessment of the force-frequency relation yields more detailed information.[25,57] Using these techniques revealed a marked variability in response to cardiopulmonary bypass, ranging from no effect in patients undergoing closure of atrial septal defects to a profound reduction in the force-frequency relation after the neonatal arterial switch operation (Fig. 18C-33).

Monitoring the Results of Cardiac Transplantation

In some patients with a failing myocardium, or very complex malformations, cardiac transplantation may be the only therapeutic option. While results of transplantation have become very good, later rejection of the transplanted heart remains a clinical problem. Non-invasive imaging techniques such as echocardiography have previously been used to monitor these patients.[58] Myocardial Doppler measurements, in particular isovolumic acceleration, are well suited to assess such patients serially.[59] We have learnt that the transplanted heart has an abnormal systolic and diastolic function, even in the absence of rejection. Thus, reference values from normal hearts cannot be used for comparison.[60] Using measurements in patients with transplanted hearts during absence of evidence for rejection, and thus using them as their own controls, showed that an acute reduction in isovolumic acceleration may be a sensitive indicator of impending rejection.[59]

Cardiomyopathies

In recent years, novel pharmacological treatments have become available for some patients with cardiomyopathies, which in turn has increased interest in their clinical monitoring. For those cardiomyopathies that cannot be treated by drugs, such as Duchenne's muscular dystrophy, echocardiography has been used to yield information on prognosis.[61] Likewise, in patients with hypertrophic cardiomyopathy for whom only symptomatic treatment is available, myocardial Doppler can identify prospectively patients with subclinical disease who may later develop the classical hypertrophy. Patients with genetic mutations known to cause hypertrophy who had no echocardiographic signs were examined by myocardial Doppler, and restudied 2 years later.[62] Those who had manifest disease at the second examination already had reduced myocardial velocities 2 years preceding manifestation of the disease.

For some having cardiomyopathies such as Pompe's and Friedreich's, new recombinant enzyme therapy has recently become available, making the diseases potentially reversible.[63] The new myocardial Doppler techniques have been successfully applied to monitor the effect of recombinant enzyme therapy on cardiac function.

Thalassaemia is another potentially reversible cardiomyopathy. Deposition of iron, which may lead to myocardial dysfunction, can be reversed by appropriate chelation therapy. Using myocardial Doppler, abnormalities of mural motion could be detected in those parts of the left ventricle in which deposits of iron were detected by magnetic resonance imaging.[64] The majority of patients had little or no clinical symptoms and normal shortening fraction on m-mode echocardiography, yet myocardial velocities were abnormally low. This is further proof that myocardial Doppler enables detection of abnormal heart function before it becomes evident clinically.

Leucaemia and other forms of childhood cancer are treated successfully with drugs, albeit potentially cardiotoxic. In many survivors of childhood cancer treated with Adriamycin, conventional m-mode based indexes of cardiac function may be normal at rest, with abnormalities only becoming evident during exercise. Myocardial Doppler-derived measurements present a sensitive tool to detect such abnormal contractile function early, without the need for further exercise testing.[65]

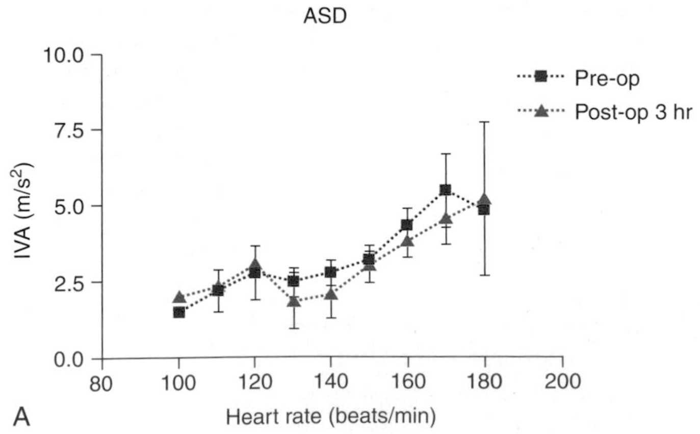

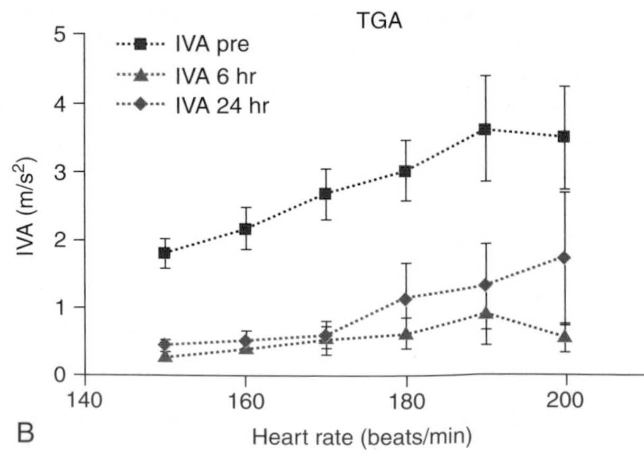

Figure 18C-33 Force frequency curves from patient after (**A**) closure of an atrial septal defect (ASD) and (**B**) transposition (TGA) following a neonatal switch operation. Note that, after closure of the atrial septal defect, there is little difference in the curve before and 3 hours following surgery, while in the neonate following the arterial switch operation the curve at 6 hours is flat with almost no increase in isovolumic acceleration (IVA) with increasing heart rate, and is still abnormally low after 24 hours, suggesting depressed contractile function following surgery.

FUTURE DEVELOPMENTS

During contraction and relaxation, the left ventricle performs a complex motion. Evaluating longitudinal and radial function alone cannot fully describe this motion, and thus is insufficient to assess function. The left ventricle also undergoes torsional deformation.[66] This can be assessed by tagged magnetic resonance imaging. Recently, myocardial Doppler techniques have also been used to assess such left ventricular torsional deformation. The torsional deformation is shown to increase from infancy to adulthood.[67] Abnormal torsion may be sign of myocardial disease. As the ventricles have a complex shape and motion during contraction and relaxation, information about these movements in three dimensions is desirable. Future developments will be directed towards techniques which enable assessment of cardiac deformation in three dimensions.[68]

The complete reference list can be found on the companion Expert Consult web site at www.expertconsult.com.

ANNOTATED REFERENCES

- Urheim S, Edvardsen T, Torp H, et al: Myocardial strain by Doppler echocardiography: Validation of a new method to quantify regional myocardial function. Circulation 2000;102:1158–1164.
- Langeland S, D'hooge J, Wouters PF, et al: Experimental validation of a new ultrasound method for the simultaneous assessment of radial and longitudinal myocardial deformation independent of insonation angle. Circulation 2005;112:2157–2162.

  These two studies validate myocardial strain Doppler echocardiography and two-dimensional strain by speckle tracking. The experimental validations were achieved by comparison of the novel echocardiographic techniques to pressure-volume loops obtained using conductance catheterisation, or by using sonomicrometric crystals on the epicardium to quantify myocardial deformation.
- Vogel M, Schmidt MR, Kristiansen SB, et al: Noninvasive assessment of left ventricular force-frequency relationships using tissue Doppler-derived isovolumic acceleration: Validation in an animal model. Circulation 2003;107:1647–1652.

  An experimental validation of the measurement of isovolumic acceleration as an index of contractile function, comparing it to myocardial acceleration and velocities measured during the ejection phase.
- Vogel M, Derrick G, Cullen S, et al: Systemic ventricular function in transposition after Mustard/Senning repair: A tissue Doppler and conductance catheter study. J Am Coll Cardiol 2004;43:100–104.
- Abd El Rahman MY, Hui W, Ygitbasi M, et al: Detection of left ventricular asynchrony in patients with right bundle branch block after repair of tetralogy of Fallot using tissue Doppler-derived strain. J Am Soc Cardiol 2005;45:915–921.

  Two examples of clinical applications of these new echocardiographic techniques in the long-term follow-up of patients with congenitally malformed hearts.

CHAPTER 18D

Magnetic Resonance Imaging and Computed Tomography

LARS GROSSE-WORTMANN, WHAL LEE, and SHI-JOON YOO

Echocardiography remains the most widely used diagnostic imaging modality in the assessment of patients with congenitally malformed hearts, owing to its portability and excellent temporal resolution, and the contrast provided by the interface between the blood and the tissues.[1] Ultrasound, however, does depend on acoustic windows, which are often limited in older patients or following surgery. Both computed tomography and magnetic resonance imaging allow imaging at all angles, and largely irrespective of surrounding structures or air. Consequently, and because they deliver multi-slice or true three-dimensional images, magnetic resonance (Table 18D-1) and computed tomography help clarify the three-dimensional morphology of the cardiovascular system and its topographic relationships to the extracardiac structures, such as the trachea and bronchuses.

The history of magnetic resonance imaging is dotted with Nobel prizes awarded in physics, chemistry, and medicine. In 1946, Felix Bloch[2] and Edward Purcell[3], in the same journal issue but independently of one another, described the behaviour of the nucleuses of certain elements of the periodic system when introduced into a magnetic field. Imaging using magnetic resonance, however, was not possible until Paul Lauterbur applied gradients spatially to encode the signal, producing the first magnetic resonance image of two tubes of water in 1971. This work was published in 1973,[4] and, in the following year, he published the first images of a living animal, a clam.[5] When Richard Ernst applied the Fourier transformation to the technique pioneered by Lauterbur, magnetic resonance imaging, as we know it today, was born.[6] The first magnetic resonance images of the heart date back to the early 1980s.[7] Major breakthroughs include electrocardiographic gating in 1984,[8] phase velocity mapping in the same year to measure the flow of blood,[9] and gadolinium-enhanced magnetic resonance angiography in 1988.[10]

Since then, improvements of the hardware, particularly stronger and faster gradients, as well as higher resolution coils, paralleled by exponential increments in the capacity to process data, have laid the foundation for an array of sequences and applications. Between the early days of cardiovascular magnetic resonance imaging in the 1980s and the present, the technique has undergone an evolution from a non-invasive anatomical tool to a powerful window towards haemodynamics and myocardial mechanics.

The technological advancement in computed tomography is moving towards faster scanning, as well as a reduction in irradiation. Both improvements have helped to establish computed tomography in the work-up of pathology of the vessels and the airways in children. We can now obtain images during spontaneous breathing, and at an acceptable level of exposure to irradiation.

In this section of the chapter devoted to imaging, we offer an overview of the information now provided by magnetic resonance and computed tomography in children with congenital and acquired cardiac disease, discussing the limitations and risks of the techniques. We hope to guide cardiologists in using the appropriate cross sectional modality for imaging their patients, and in understanding the results.

TABLE 18D-1

COMMON INDICATIONS* AT A DEDICATED PAEDIATRIC SERVICE FOR CARDIAC MAGNETIC RESONANCE IMAGING

Post-operative tetralogy of Fallot
Stenosis of the right and left pulmonary arteries
Native and repaired coarctation of the aorta
Aortic valvar insufficiency
Marfan syndrome
Partially anomalous pulmonary venous connection
Functionally univentricular circulations after the bidirectional cavopulmonary connection, or with Fontan-type anatomy
Arrhythmogenic right ventricular cardiomyopathy
Dilated and hypertrophic cardiomyopathy
Cardiac mass
Takayasu's arteritis

*Not given in order of frequency.

MAGNETIC RESONANCE IMAGING

Physical Principle

Magnetic resonance imaging utilises the varying magnetic properties of hydrogen nucleuses, or protons, in different tissues in the body.[11,12] When excited by a radio-frequency pulse, the protons, like small stab magnets, briefly change orientation before returning to their initial state. During this relaxation, the protons give off energy. This process is termed resonance, or echoing. It can be measured, and then translated mathematically into an image of grey values. The way these echoes are created and manipulated determines the shading of the resulting image, a process termed weighting. Manipulation of the echo can be achieved by applying one or more additional radio-frequency pulses following the initial pulse that change the spin of the protons. This is called spin echo. Another way to influence the echo is by alternating the orientation of the magnetic field of the scanner during proton relaxation, resulting in a gradient echo sequence.

Magnetic resonance imaging operates between the poles of the duration of the scan, its temporal and spatial resolutions, and the intensity of the signal, or its ratio to the produced noise. As a general rule, improving one of these features typically worsens the other three. The settings used, therefore, have to be composed to maximise the benefit from a particular sequence in each individual patient. A comprehensive approach to the physics is beyond the scope of this chapter, and the interested reader is directed elsewhere.[11]

Practical Considerations and Patient Safety

Cardiovascular magnetic resonance is a complex modality. Awareness of the underlying physical principles and computations is a prerequisite to its successful application to children, in whom a cookbook approach frequently fails. The field of congenital cardiac disease, on the other hand, bears its own intricacy that must be understood to best design the examination. Training in both aspects of paediatric cardiovascular magnetic resonance is essential to maximise the gain from this technique. An intimate cooperation between radiologists and cardiologists is advocated to master and help advance the fast evolving field.

It is our practice to sedate or anaesthetise most patients younger than 6 years of age. This, however, is only a rule of thumb, and varies according to the maturity of the patient, as well as to anaesthetic support, the monitoring available, and the presence of a physician. Careful preparation and guidance of the child prior to and during the scan have a beneficial effect on the quality of the images obtained. Prior to any study, absolute and relative contraindications must be addressed.[13,14] Pacemakers and other electronic implants, such as pumps for infusing drugs, are currently absolute contra-indications to magnetic resonance imaging. Controversy surrounds magnetic resonance imaging at 1.5 Tesla following implantation of metallic objects.[15] Patients with non-ferromagnetic foreign bodies can probably undergo testing immediately after implantation. For an implant or device that is weakly ferromagnetic, such as most stents, coils, and artificial valves, it is customary to wait until at least 6 weeks after implantation in order to prevent dislodging.[14] A strong magnetic field can induce an electrical current in temporary or permanent pacing wires, causing thermal injuries to surrounding structures.[16] If they are within or close to the field of view, all objects are desirably not only magnetic resonance imaging safe but also compatible, in order not to impair the information that can be obtained from the study (Fig. 18D-1).[14] If possible, dental braces should be removed. The classification into safe and compatible is currently being replaced by the terminology safe and conditional, introduced by the American Society for Testing and Materials International. According to the new terminology, a patient with an implant labeled conditional may undergo magnetic resonance testing if certain requirements pertaining to the scanner and sequences used are met. Both classifications currently co-exist and can be found on the device packaging. Gadolinium-based contrast mediums are safe, with a risk of anaphylactic reactions in the range of 0.001% to 0.01%.[14] Patients with severe renal insufficiency, expressed by a glomerular filtration rate of less than 30 mL/min/1.73 m^2, face a risk of developing nephrogenic systemic fibrosis after exposure to gadolinium, and should not receive contrast.[17] Nephrogenic systemic fibrosis was initially observed in, and thought solely to affect, the skin, but internal organs such as liver, lungs, and heart may be involved. An extensive review of the safety aspects of magnetic resonance can be found elsewhere.[14] With the exception of real-time imaging and contrast-enhanced angiography, most sequences require electrocardiographic gating to compensate for cardiac motion. Respiratory motion is countered either by breath-holding, tracking the motion of the diaphragm, or acquiring multiple sets of data to average out the effects of the inconsistent position of the thorax.

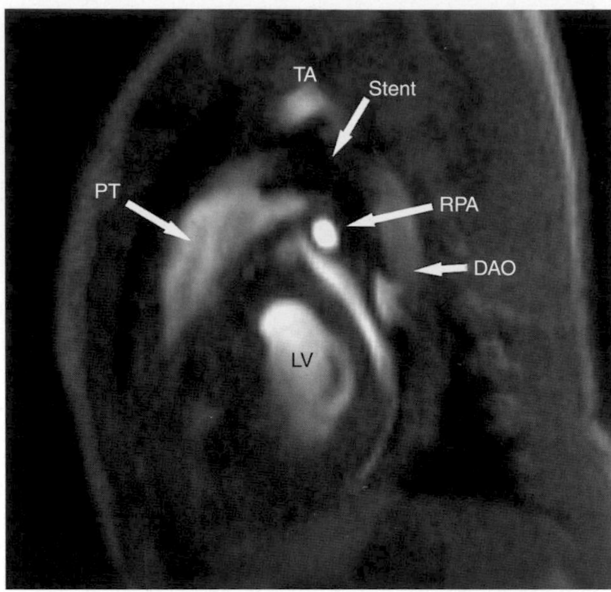

Figure 18D-1 Artifact from a vascular stent in the arterial duct following a hybrid procedure consisting of bilateral banding of the pulmonary arteries and placement of a ductal stent for hypoplastic left heart structures. DAO, descending aorta; LV, left ventricle; PT, pulmonary trunk; RPA, right pulmonary artery; TA, transverse arch.

Techniques for Imaging

Each examination begins with a series of static scout images, or localizers, of the thorax and adjacent body parts in three orthogonal body planes (Fig. 18D-2). With most

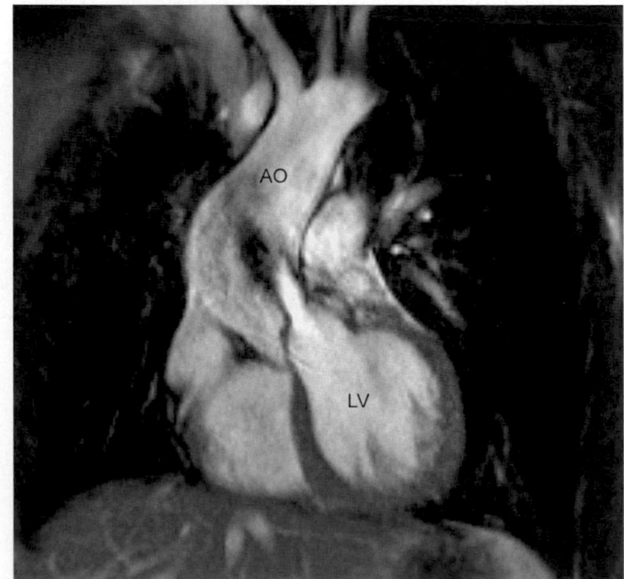

Figure 18D-2 Bright blood view of the left ventricular outflow tract in a patient with combined aortic valvar disease. The aortic valve is doming and stenotic, with post-stenotic dilation of the proximal ascending aorta. The turbulent jet causes a characteristic dephasing artifact. AO, aorta; LV, left ventricle.

recent scanners, the scout images with an acceptable spatial resolution can be obtained within 1 or 2 minutes, making most anatomical information readily available. All subsequent sequences for detailed examination are planned using this scout, as well as any subsequently obtained images, as a reference. As a principle of prescription, any imaging plane is defined unequivocally either by three points, so-called three-point planning, or by how it dissects two separate images previously obtained, the so-called double-oblique technique.

Cine Imaging

These moving images of the beating heart are the workhorse of current magnetic resonance imaging in patients with congenitally malformed hearts (Figs. 18D-3 and 18D-4; see also Fig. 18D-2). Blood is signal-intense, and contrasts well with the grey myocardium. Turbulent flow causes loss of signal from dephasing, and can be identified as dark streaks within the bright blood pool (see Fig. 18D-2). As an important difference to echocardiography, these moving images, with few exceptions, are not acquired in real time, but are assembled over many cardiac cycles, so that a temporal correlation of cardiac events with the coinciding beat-to-beat electrocardiogram is not possible. A representative work flow for cine imaging is shown in Figure 18D-3. The strategies to achieve the basic views vary between users. A stack of 10 to 12 short-axis cine images (see Figs. 18D-3 and 18D-4) are used to calculate ventricular volumes and myocardial masses (see Fig. 18D-4B). As opposed to echocardiography, this method does not rely on geometric assumptions, and is widely accepted as the gold standard tool for ventricular volumetry.

A modification of cine imaging is myocardial tagging (Fig. 18D-5): Here, selective saturation pre-pulses spoil all spins within multiple planes perpendicular to the plane of imaging, thus superimposing a grid of black lines across the field of view. The black lines persist through systole, and are deformed by myocardial contraction. From the degree of deformation, it is possible to calculate radial and circumferential strain, as well as ventricular twisting.[18–21] The assessment of cardiac function is fuelled by the expectation of better understanding of myocardial mechanics, and by the hope of detecting and treating myocardial disease in its early stages. The sensitivity of analysis of regional

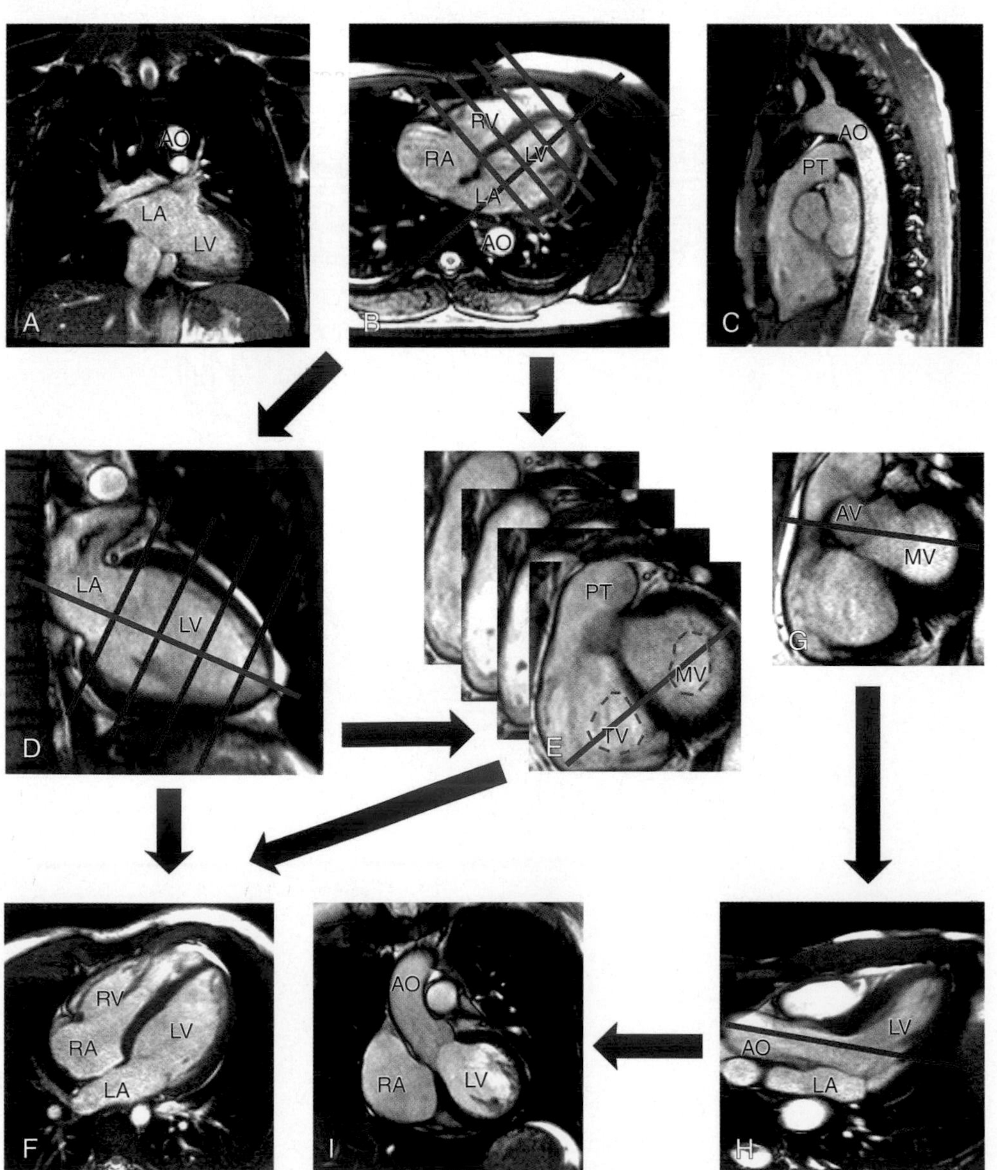

Figure 18D-3 Work flow for anatomical and cine imaging. Each scan plane is prescribed starting from two differently angled reference images, using the double oblique technique, for the four-chamber view in this figure. Following coronal (**A**), axial (**B**), and sagittal (**C**) localizer images, cine imaging begins with a vertical long-axis or pseudo-two-chamber view (**D**). From here, a set of short-axis imaging planes (**E**) is prescribed parallel to the atrioventricular groove, using the previously acquired vertical long-axis view and the axial localizer as reference images. A four-chamber view (**F**) cuts through the mitral and tricuspid valves and through the ventricular apex. If needed, a three-chamber view (**H**) of the left atrium (LA), left ventricle (LV), and proximal ascending aorta can be obtained by placing the imaging plane through the aortic and mitral valves (AV, MV) in the basal short-axis plane (**G**). Imaging perpendicular to the three-chamber view opens up the left ventricular outflow tract (**I**). AO, aorta; PT, pulmonary trunk; RA, right atrium; RV, right ventricle; TV, tricuspid valve.

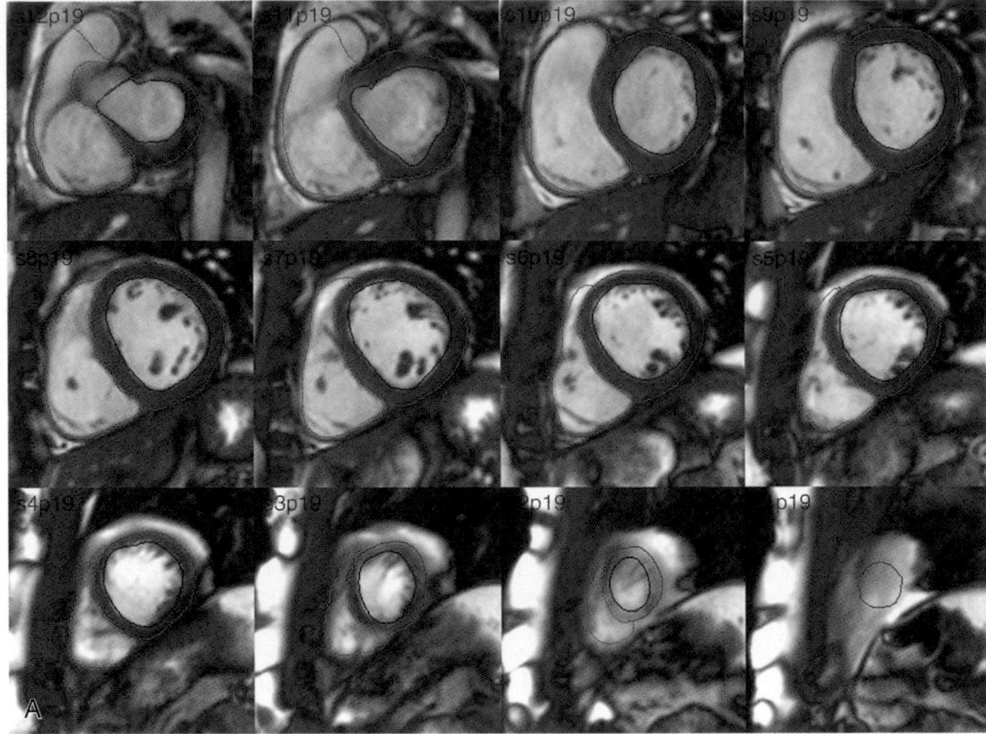

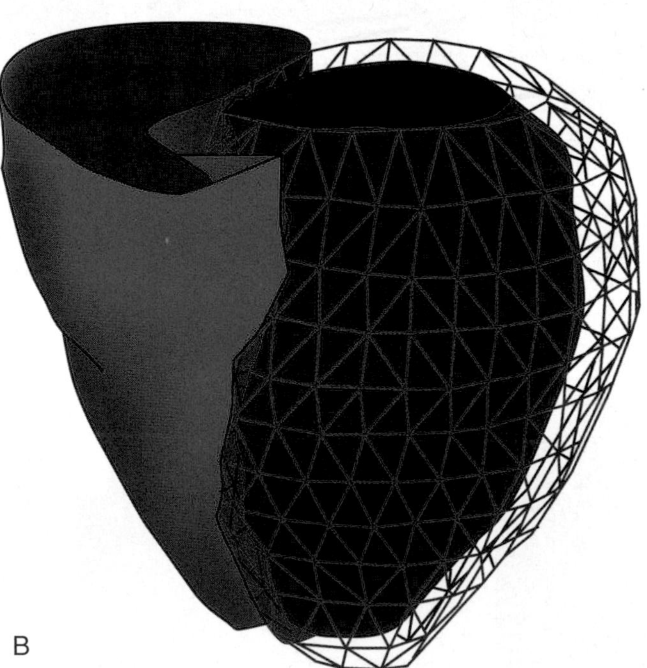

Figure 18D-4 Stack of short-axis images, parallel to the atrioventricular groove. Contours (**A**) are drawn around the left ventricular endocardium (red), epicardium (green), and right ventricular endocardium (yellow). This is repeated at end-diastole and end-systole in each slice of the short-axis stack. Using the contours in **A**, a three-dimensional model (**B**) is reconstructed. The red contours and green mesh indicate the endocardium and epicardium, respectively, of the left ventricle. The right ventricular endocardium is in yellow. The computer calculates the volumes, ejection fractions, and cardiac output. The mass is typically given only for the left ventricle, as the right ventricular trabeculations preclude accurate measurements.

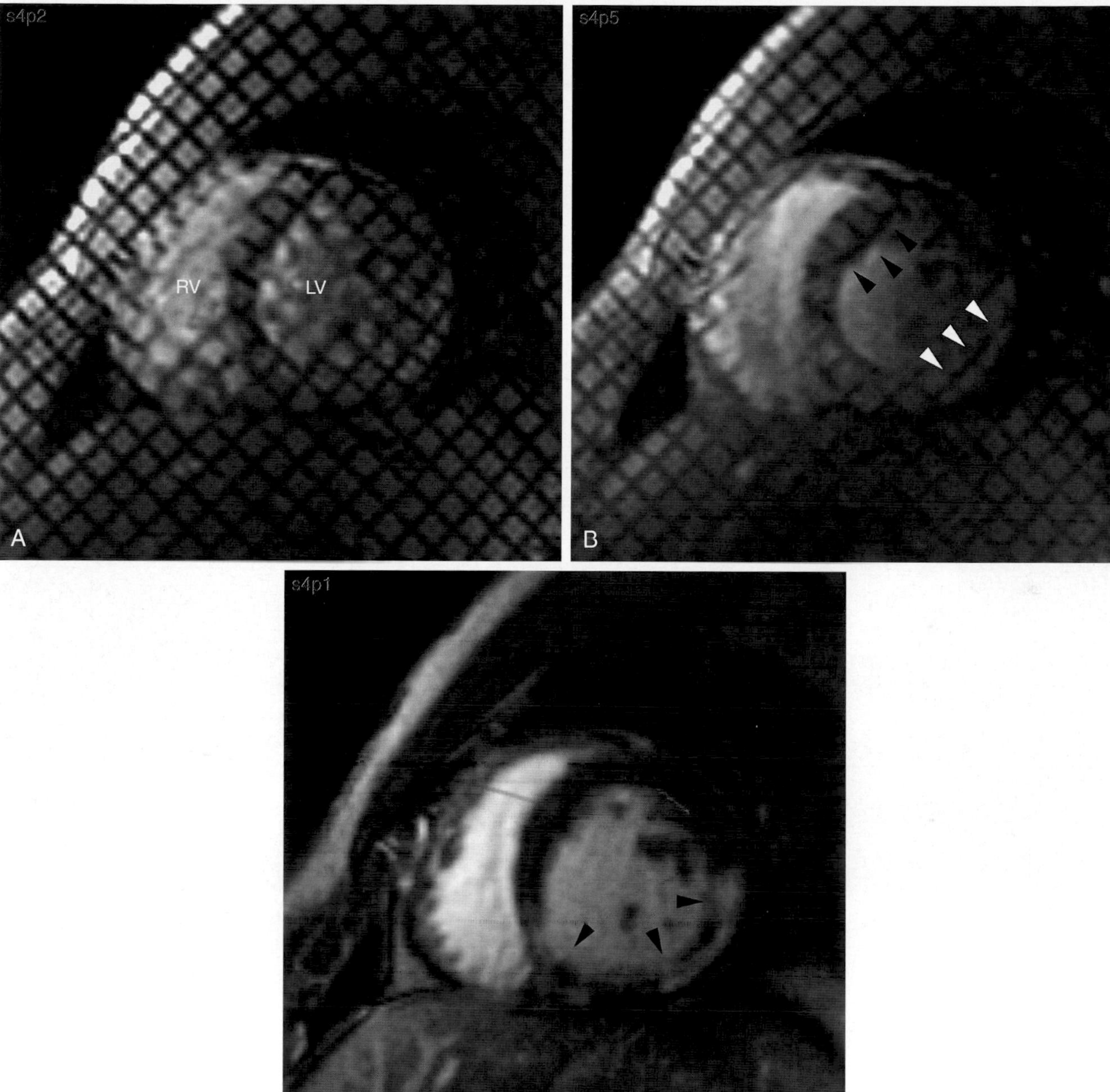

Figure 18D-5 This 17-year-old boy has myocardial infarction after Kawasaki disease as a toddler. Myocardial tagging is shown in a midventricular short-axis slice at the beginning (**A**) and end (**B**) of systole. The tagging lines change from straight to inward convex, following the myocardial motion during contraction (*black arrowheads*). The inferolateral wall of the left ventricle (LV) is akinetic (*white arrowheads*), indicated by the grid lines remaining straight. The black lines are strongest at the beginning of systole and fade during the cardiac cycle. The akinetic wall segment of the left ventricle corresponds to a zone of hyperenhancement late after gadolinium, indicating myocardial infarction (**C**; *arrowheads*). RV, right ventricle.

wall motion can be increased by protocols inducing stress, using dobutamine or magnetic resonance compatible ergometers.

Measurements of Flow

Phase contrast imaging is another key technique in the assessment of congenitally malformed hearts by magnetic resonance. It is used to quantify the velocity and volumes of flow (Fig. 18D-6).[22-24] The ability to assess the flow in all major vessels in any orientation makes this technique ideal for the assessment of congenitally malformed hearts. Data is acquired during spontaneous breathing or with the patient ventilated, as breath-holding manoeuvres can affect the flow of blood. The vessel is imaged perpendicular to its long axis, so-called through-plane imaging. In Figure 18D-7, we show the prescription of the planes to image the great vessels as well as the atrioventricular valves, using the double oblique technique. Phase contrast sequences produce a cine modulus image (see Fig. 18D-6A) of the anatomy, as well as a velocity-encoded image which contains the information pertaining to flow (see Fig. 18D-6B). Phase contrast imaging is used to

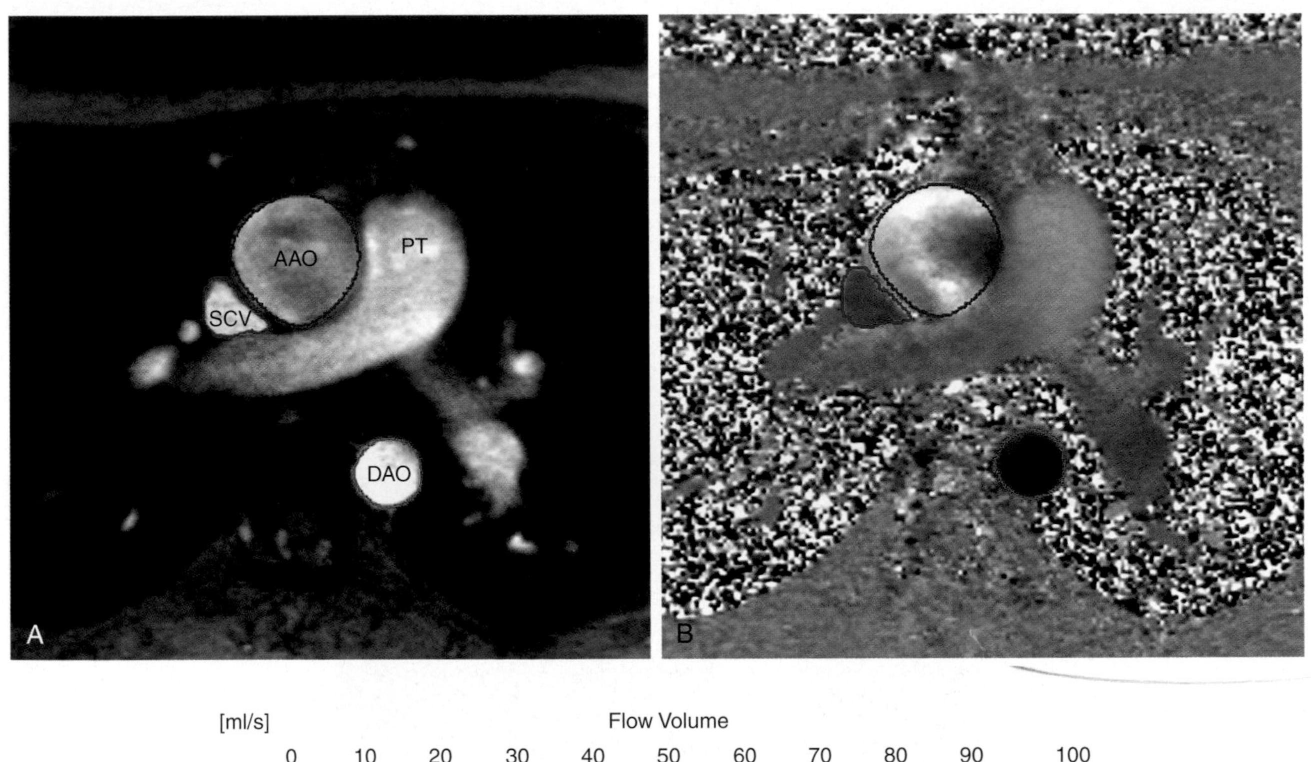

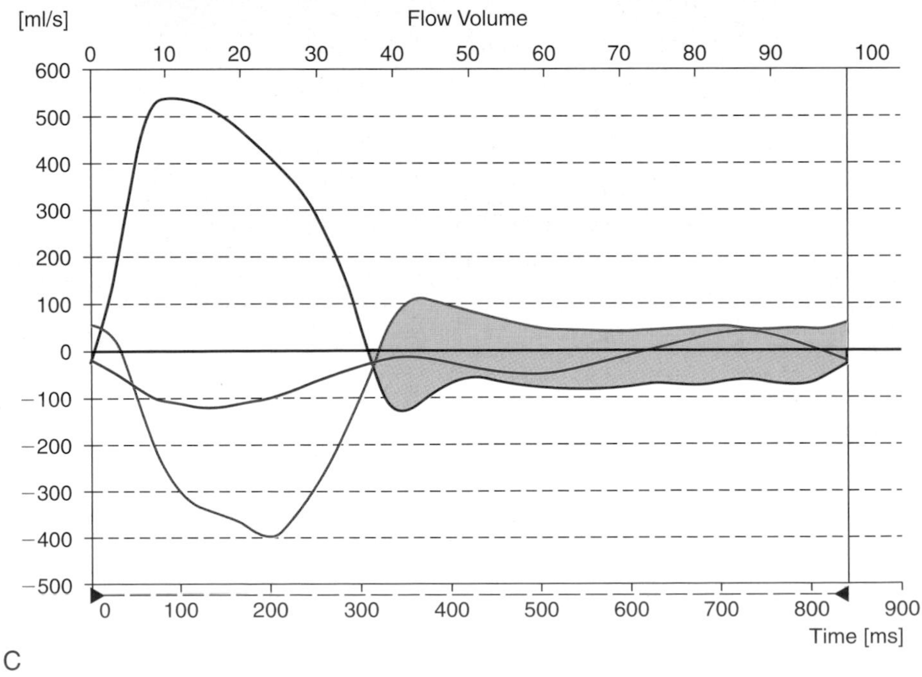

Figure 18D-6 Magnitude (A) and velocity (B) images of a phase contrast study of the ascending aorta in a patient with aortic valvar regurgitation. The resulting curves of flow volume over time (C) show flow reversal in the ascending (area shaded in red) and descending (area shaded in yellow) aorta. Flow in the superior caval vein is shown in blue. In patients without extracardiac shunts, the sum of flow volumes in the superior caval vein (SCV) and in the descending aorta (DAO) are expected to equal that in the ascending aorta (AAO) with minor discrepancies for measurement inaccuracy and blood flow into the bronchial and vertebral arteries. PT, pulmonary trunk.

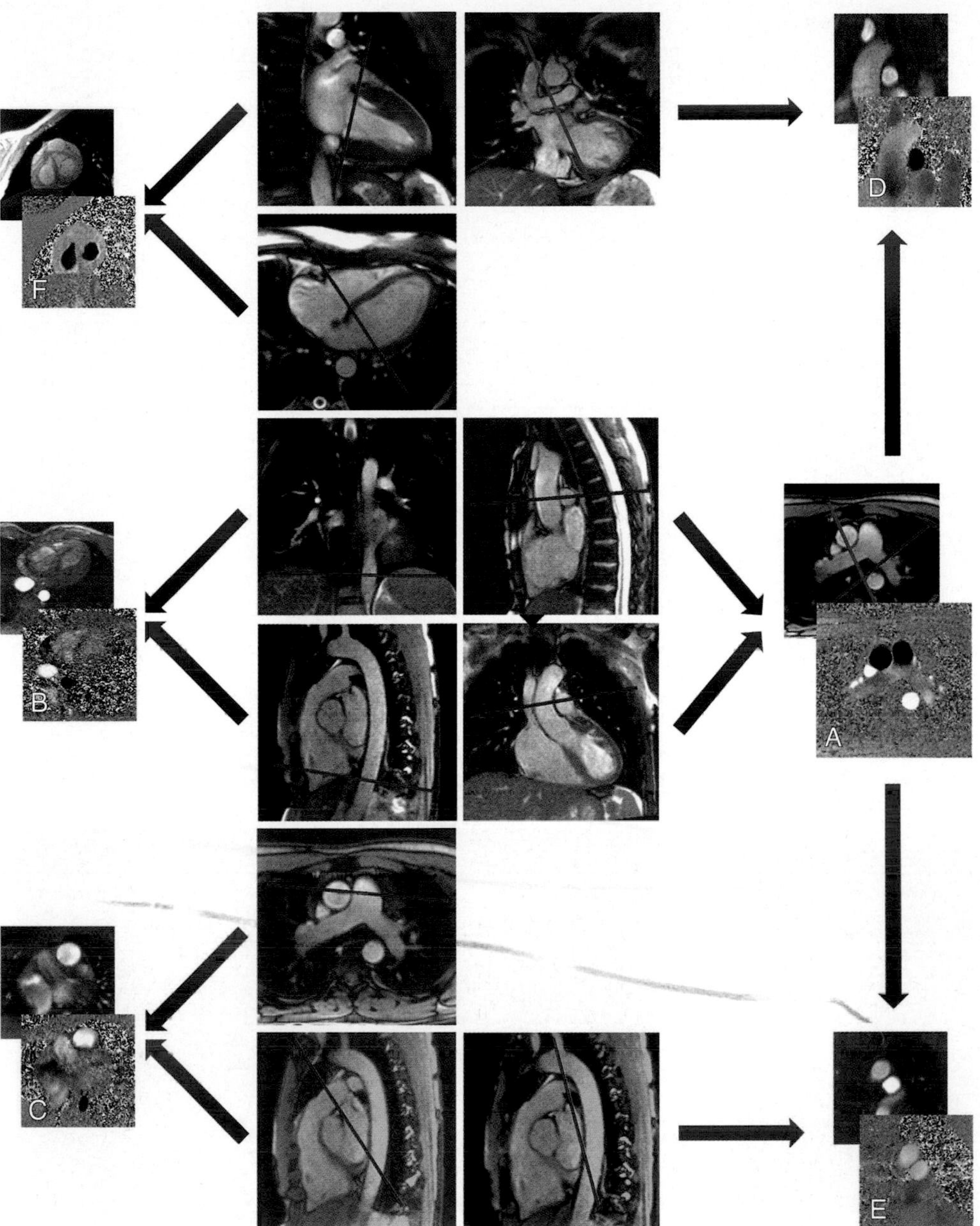

Figure 18D-7 Work flow for phase contrast imaging. The prescribed imaging planes are perpendicular to the three-dimensional course of the vessel as long as they transect the vessels on two separate images. Using the localizer images in three orthogonal planes, the cuts for the ascending aorta (**A**) at the level of the right pulmonary artery, the inferior caval vein (**B**) at the diaphragm, and the pulmonary trunk (**C**) are designed. The plane for the ascending aorta typically transects the descending aorta and superior caval vein in a near-perpendicular fashion. The plane for the descending aorta at the level of the diaphragm includes the inferior caval vein between the liver and the atrium. The right (**D**) and left (**E**) pulmonary arteries are prescribed off the ascending aorta phase contrast magnitude image and the coronal and sagittal localizers, respectively. Inflow through the atrioventricular valves (**F**) is imaged in a plane perpendicular to the atrioventricular groove in a vertical long-axis view at end-systole and an axial localizer image.

quantify valvar regurgitation. Flow can accurately be measured in the right and left pulmonary arteries, as well as in systemic vessels. By subtracting pulmonary arterial influx from venous efflux, the amount of systemic-to-pulmonary arterial collateral flow can be calculated in patients with a functionally univentricular circulation, or in those with obstructed right ventricular outflow tracts.[25–27] Flow across a patent arterial duct can be directly measured. Intracardiac shunts can be calculated by comparing flows in the ascending aorta and pulmonary trunk.[28,29] Unlike ultrasound Doppler, phase contrast imaging allows analysis of the pattern of flow in all vessels shown in the field of view, helping clarify timing of flows relative to one another. Certain conditions exhibit characteristic patterns: for example, the configuration of the velocity of flow in patients with pulmonary hypertension (Fig. 18D-8) is characterised by an early systolic peak with decreased maximum velocity; one or more secondary peaks; early cessation of systolic forward flow, with a nadir arriving before that of the ascending aortic flow; and undulation of velocities during diastole.[30] Flow trajectories and turbulence can be assessed by imaging along the vessel or jet of flow, known as in-plane imaging, and, experimentally, it is possible to produce four-dimensional phase contrast imaging (Fig. 18D-9). A number of conditions compound the accuracy of phase contrast magnetic resonance, including insufficient temporal resolution, a too high or too low limit of encoding, as well as non-laminar target flow.[23] Large translational movements of the great arteries through the fixed imaging plane, as well as turbulence and swirling in frequently dilated arterial roots hamper the quantification of regurgitation across arterial valves.[31,32]

Contrast-enhanced Magnetic Resonance Angiography

Gadolinium-based contrast agents can be used to increase the signal from the blood and reduce the time required to acquire images, thus allowing three-dimensional angiography with a submillimeter spatial resolution (Figs. 18D-10

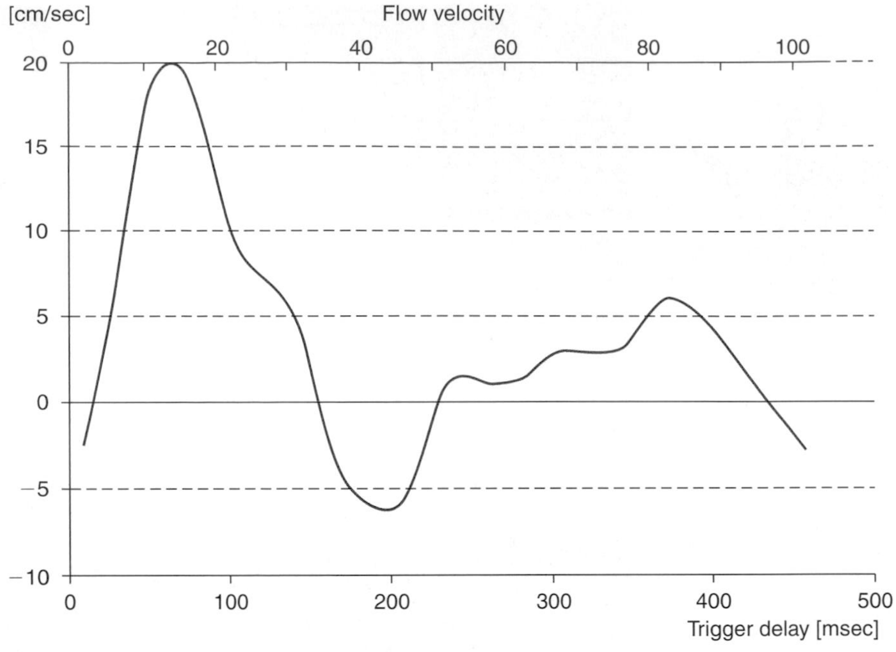

Figure 18D-8 Time-velocity flow profile in the pulmonary trunk in a patient with primary pulmonary hypertension. See text for details.

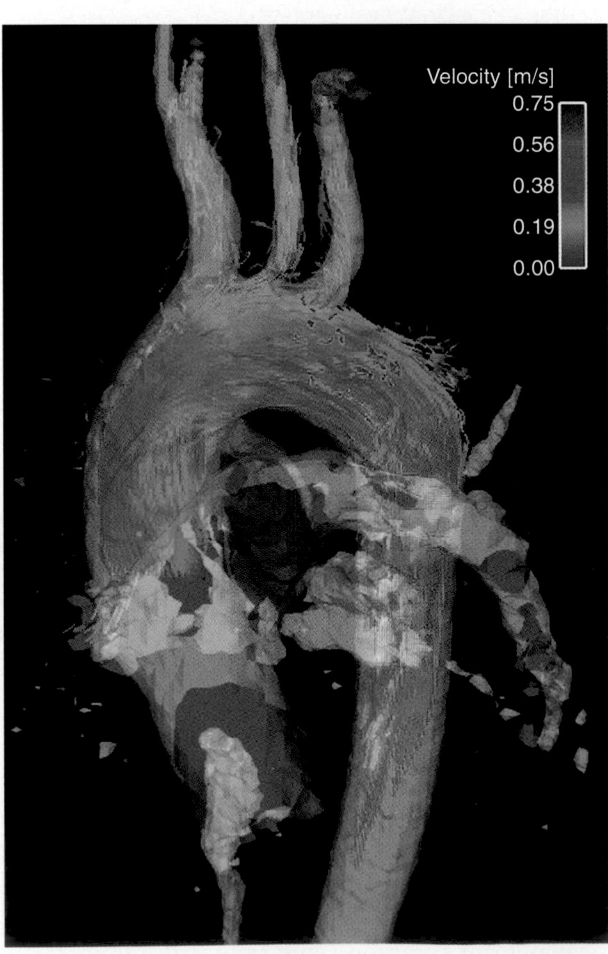

Figure 18D-9 Flow streamlines in a normal thoracic aorta, reconstructed from four-dimensional, three-directional phase contrast velocity mapping. (Courtesy of A. Frydrychowicz, Freiburg, Germany.)

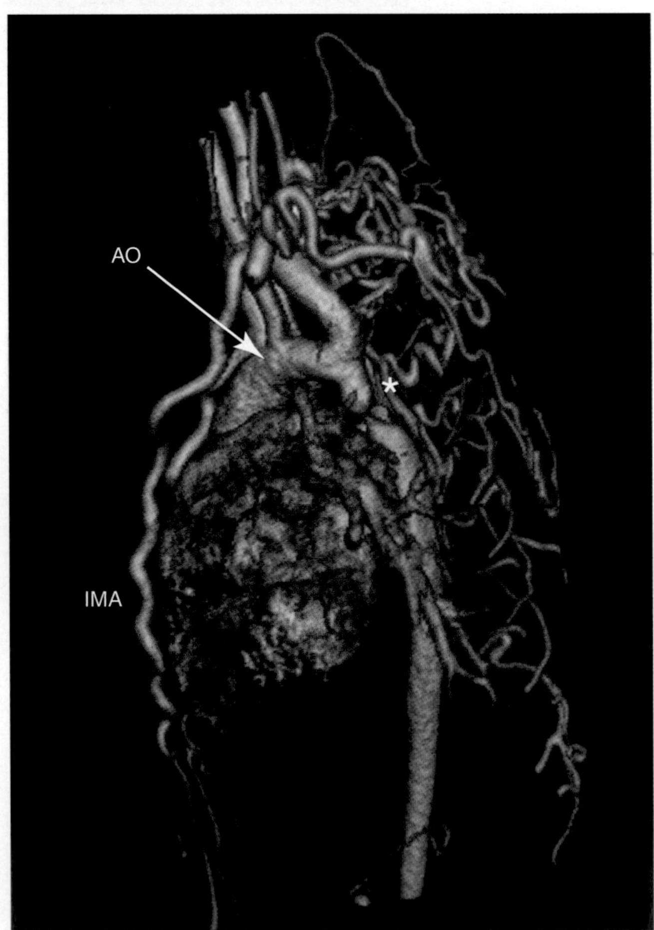

Figure 18D-10 Contrast-enhanced magnetic resonance angiography in a patient with severe native coarctation (*asterisk*) of the aorta (AO) and massive collateralisation via the internal mammary, intercostal, and vertebral arteries. IMA, internal mammary artery.

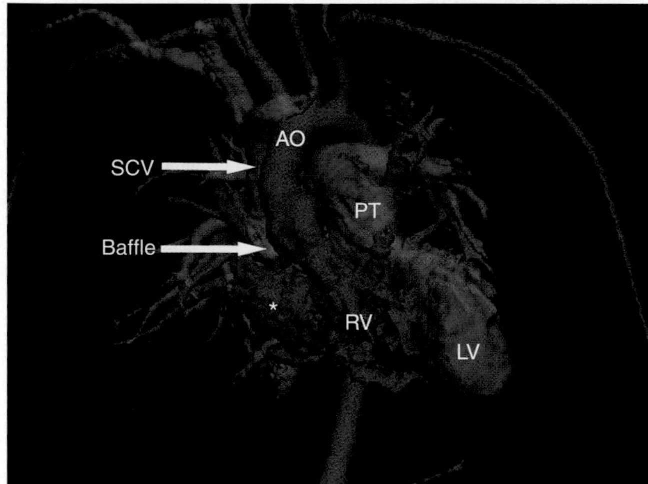

Figure 18D-11 Discordant ventriculo-arterial connections in a patient with transposition after an atrial switch procedure. The trabeculated right ventricle (RV) connects to the aorta (AO; shown in red), and the smooth-walled left ventricle (LV) gives rise to the pulmonary trunk (PT; in blue). The complex venoatrial anatomy including the baffle connecting the superior caval vein (SCV) to the mitral valve, and separating the systemic venous return from the morphological right atrium (*asterisk*) is clearly shown. (Courtesy of S. Sarikouch, Hannover, Germany.)

to 18D-12; see also Fig. 18D-9). When repeated in short intervals, four-dimensional angiography can be performed, with time added as the fourth dimension to the three-dimensional anatomy. The practical temporal resolution of four-dimensional or time-resolved magnetic resonance angiography for the pulmonary vasculature is between 0.5 and 1.0 seconds, depending on the imaging volume and the spatial resolution. The interpretation of an angiogram should always begin with a careful review of the source data. Image processing can highlight the information contained in the images, clarify topographic relationships, and facilitate demonstration of the anatomy to cardiologists and surgeons. A three-dimensional data set can be displayed either as a projection or as a volume rendered image (Fig. 18D-13; see also Figs. 18D-10 through 18D-12). Maximum intensity projections (see Figs. 18D-12A and 18D-13A), the most commonly used type of projection, resemble static images from fluoroscopic angiography. To create these images, the computer retains the brightest voxels along a virtual beam of projection. The orientation of this projection, as well as the thickness of the projected slice, is freely adjustable during post-processing. Computationally intensive volume rendered images (see Figs. 18D-10, 18D-11, 18D-12B, and 18D-13B) lend a plastic appearance to the anatomy, optionally including colour and a virtual source of light.

Tissue Characterisation

An array of types of static images are available to visualise changes within the myocardial matrix, and also to characterise cardiac or extracardiac masses. The techniques used for tissue characterisation include late gadolinium enhancement imaging, T2- as well as T1-weighted imaging. Late gadolinium enhancement (Fig. 18D-14) is based on the differences in the uptake and wash-out kinetics of contrast medium between healthy and infarcted or scarred myocardium. Acutely necrotic cells or fibrosis retain gadolinium longer than normal myocardium, thus appearing bright on a T1-weighted gradient echo image obtained 10 to 15 minutes after intravenous injection of gadolinium compound. Late gadolinium enhancement has been identified not only in coronary arterial disease,[33] but also in hypertrophic and dilated cardiomyopathy,[34] arrhythmogenic right ventricular cardiomyopathy,[35,36] sarcoidosis, and storage disorders such as Fabry's disease, and in patients after repair of tetralogy of Fallot.[37] It has also proved useful in the diagnosis of fibromas.[38]

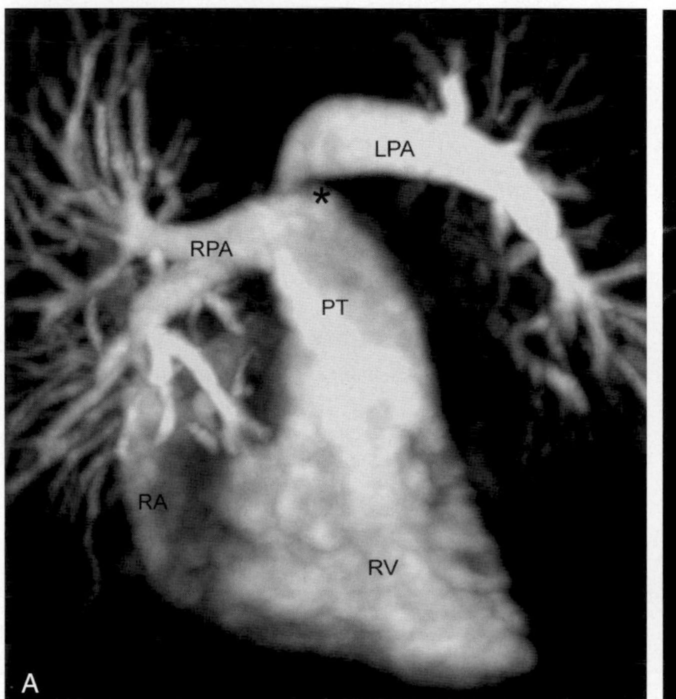

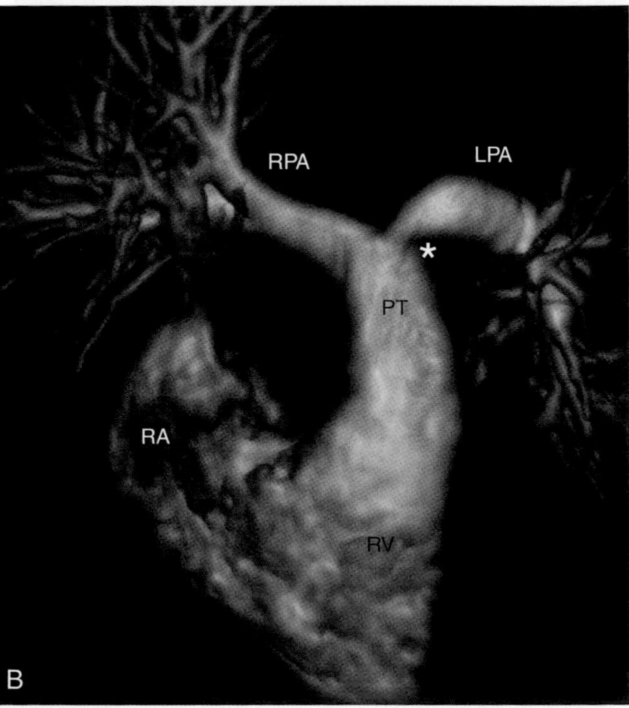

Figure 18D-12 Maximum intensity projection (A) and volume-rendered (B) images of an isolated stenosis (*asterisk*) at the origin of the left pulmonary artery (LPA). PT, pulmonary trunk; RA, right atrium; RPA, right pulmonary artery; RV, right ventricle.

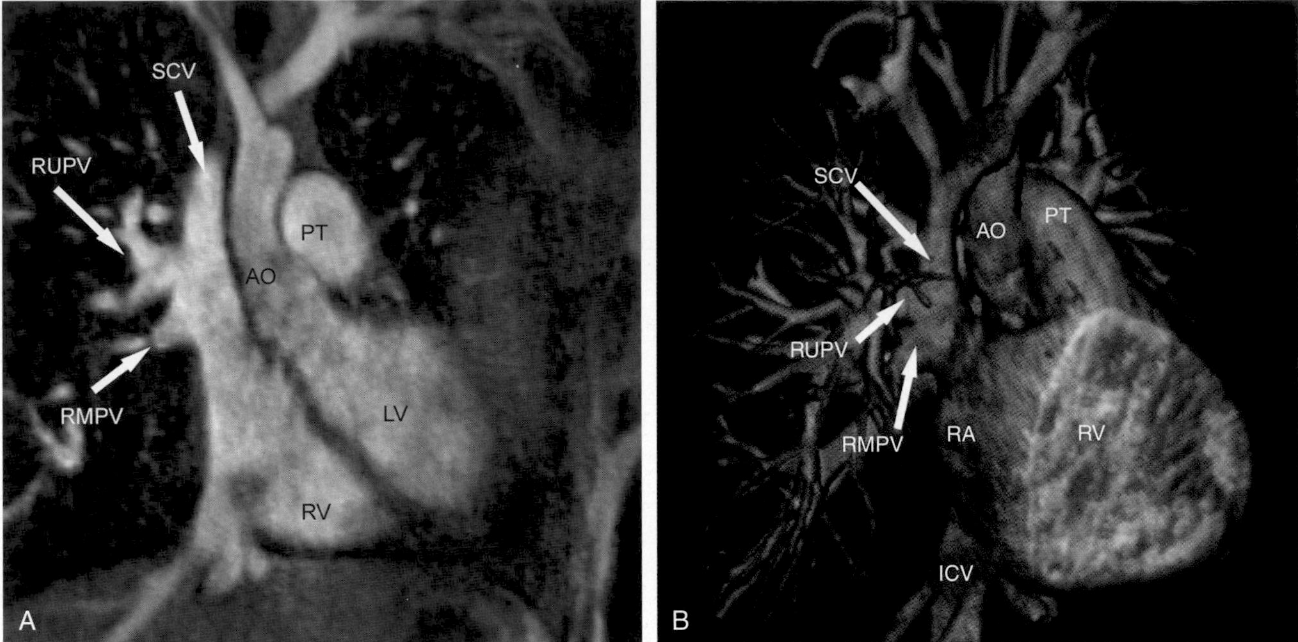

Figure 18D-13 Maximum intensity projection (A) and volume-rendered reformatting (B) of a three-dimensional magnetic resonance angiography in a patient with anomalous connection of the right upper and middle pulmonary veins to the superior caval vein (SCV). AO, aorta; ICV, inferior caval vein; PT, pulmonary trunk; RA, right atrium; RUPV, right upper pulmonary vein; RMPV, right middle pulmonary vein; RV, right ventricle.

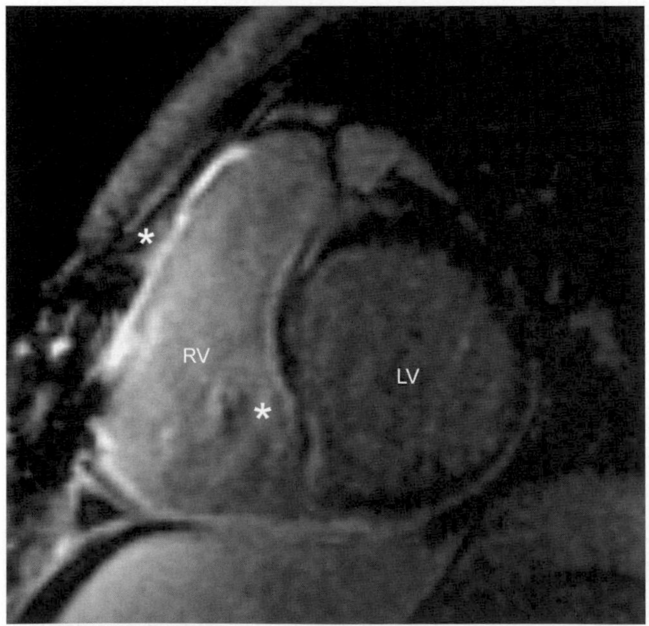

Figure 18D-14 Late enhancement imaging 10 minutes after the administration of gadolinium in a patient with right anterior myocardial infarction. The right coronary artery was severed during surgical repair of the aortic valve that had been eroded by infective endocarditis. The signal of the myocardium is nulled, whereas the anterior free wall of the right ventricle (RV) and the inferior ventricular septum are bright, indicating infarcted myocardium and scarring (*asterisks*). LV, left ventricle.

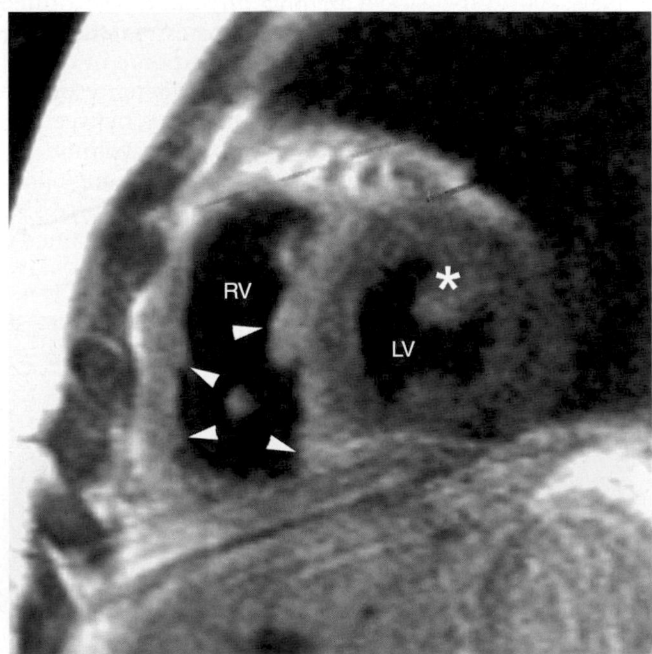

Figure 18D-15 T2-weighted image in a short-axis orientation at midventricular level in a patient 6 years after heart transplantation. The right ventricular myocardium is thickened and more signal-intense (*arrowheads*) than that of the left ventricle (LV), consistent with graft rejection. The anterolateral papillary muscle of the mitral valve (*asterisk*) is also bright. Endomyocardial biopsy one day earlier confirmed acute graft rejection. RV, right ventricle.

T2-weighted spin echo images (Fig. 18D-15) have been used to demonstrate tissue oedema based on the fact that increased amounts of free water protons give off more T2 signal than those found in normal myocardium. As myocardial oedema is found as a result of acute inflammation in myocarditis, T2-weighted imaging helps differentiate it from chronic dilated cardiomyopathy.[39] Rhabdomyomas tend to be brighter than fibromas on T2-weighted images.[38,40] A high T2 signal is a marker of acute rejection of transplanted hearts (see Fig. 18D-15).[41] T2* and T2 relaxation times correlate with overload of iron in patients with thalassaemia and are increasingly being used to guide chelation therapy.[42,43]

Fatty infiltration is a pathognomonic finding in studies of autopsied individuals with arrhythmogenic right ventricular cardiomyopathy.[44] Using a T1-weighted sequence following pre-pulses to extinguish the signal of the blood for better contrast, fat deposits in the dysplastic myocardium can be visualised experimentally as regions with high intensity of the signal, aiding in the diagnosis during life. In addition, lipomas and, occasionally, teratomas, also appear signal-intense on fat-sensitive sequences.

Imaging of the Coronary Arteries

Aneurysms of the coronary arteries may complicate Kawasaki disease. Abnormalities in origin and branching of the coronary arteries are not uncommonly found in the setting of abnormal ventriculo-arterial connections. An anomalous origin of the main stem of the left coronary artery, or its anterior interventricular branch, with an interarterial or intramyocardial course, must be ruled out in anyone with signs and symptoms of myocardial ischaemia. Imaging the coronary arteries is challenging because of their small size, tortuous course, and the extensive motion of the atrioventricular groove throughout the cardiac cycle. Non-contrast whole-heart magnetic resonance angiography (Fig. 18D-16)[45,46] uses both respiratory tracking and cardiac gating. Data is acquired only during a period of the cardiac cycle when the chamber size is relatively constant, usually diastasis, and when the diaphragm is at a defined position. Obtaining high resolution images only when the previously identified position of the heart and diaphragm coincide leads to a long scan time of, on average, 8 to 12 minutes. The three-dimensional data set can be reformatted as described above for contrast-enhanced magnetic resonance angiography (see Fig. 18D-16). Currently, however, magnetic resonance cannot rule out coronary arterial stenosis with certainty in children.

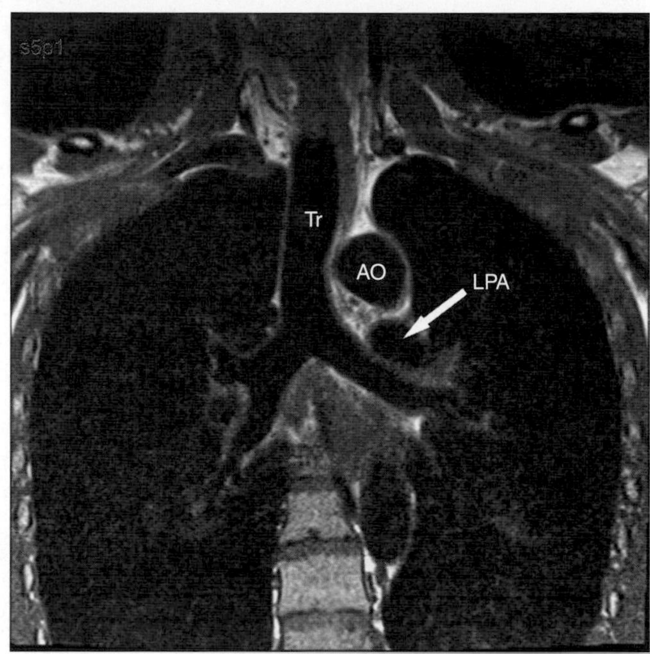

Figure 18D-17 In this T1-weighted coronal image of the thorax, the airways, lungs, as well as the vessels are shown in black. The relationships of the trachea and bronchuses to the branch pulmonary arteries and aortic arch are shown. AO, aorta; LPA, left pulmonary artery; Tr, trachea.

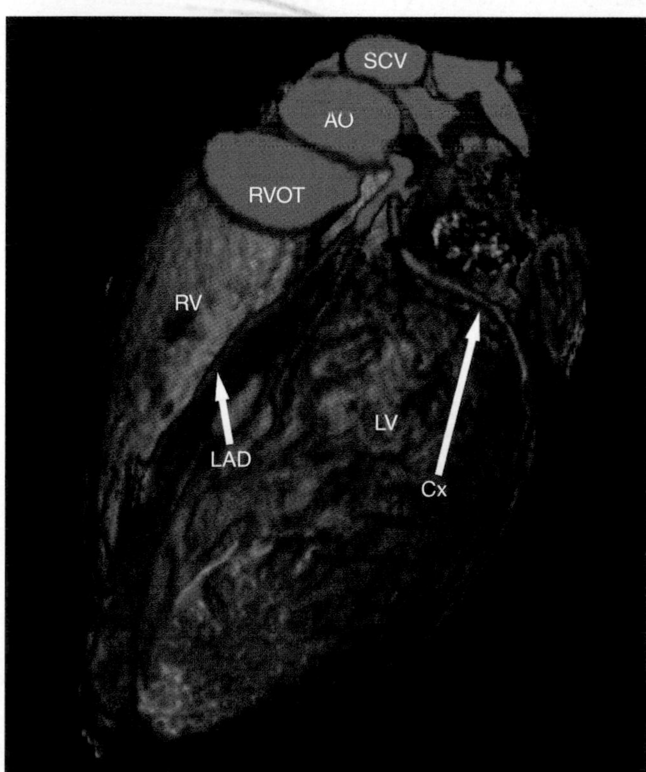

Figure 18D-16 This three-dimensional data set of the whole heart was acquired in 9 minutes without contrast, using a three-dimensional steady-state free precession technique. The left coronary artery system has a normal origin and branching patterns. There is no aneurysm and no obvious narrowing. However, stenoses cannot be ruled out with certainty. AO, aorta; Cx, circumflex artery; LAD, left anterior descending artery; LV, left ventricle; RV, right ventricle; RVOT, right ventricular outflow tract; SCV, superior caval vein.

Imaging the Airways

Magnetic resonance is suitable for depicting the tracheobronchial structures in their topographic relationship to the anomalous vascular structures in various anomalies involving the aortic arches, and in the syndrome of the pulmonary arterial sling. Air contains no signal, and the lumen of airways is shown in black in all clinically used sequences (Fig. 18D-17). Spin echo sequences are the techniques most often used for the display of tracheobronchial anatomy.[47] Cine imaging can provide useful information regarding dynamic compression of the airways throughout the cardiac cycle. Fast gradient refocused echo sequences acquire a three-dimensional data set of the entire thorax to measure lung volumes in a single breath hold. Computed tomography should be performed, nonetheless, in most patients in whom the airway is the primary object of the investigation.

COMPUTED TOMOGRAPHY

Recent Developments in Technology

The basic elements of a computed tomography scanner are the X-ray tube or tubes, and the detectors, which are housed in a gantry. The gantry spins rapidly around the patient while the tube generates X-rays, and the detectors measure the remaining irradiation after penetration of the body. The measured data is then processed to create images using a mathematical algorithm called back projection.[48] In the first two and half decades after its first clinical use in 1974, the scanners were axial scanners, and the gantry made a complete rotation to acquire an image of a slice, after which the table was advanced by an increment equal to the thickness of the slice for the next rotation, and so forth.[49] This conventional step-and-shoot technique needed a long time because of the inter-scan delays between the slices. In the late 1980s and early 1990s, spiral, or helical, scanners were introduced.[50] With this innovative technology, the gantry rotates continuously, while the table is moved at a constant speed such that the X-rays are beamed in a spiral manner to the patient. This technique allows fast and continuous acquisition of a complete set of volume data. The spiral data is then interpolated to generate axial images.[51] The speed of the scan in spiral scanning enables the complete data set to be acquired within a single breath hold. In 1998, multi-detector technology with four detector rows once again revolutionised spiral imaging technique, allowing acquisition of four imaging slices at a time with a single rotation of the gantry.[52] Since then, the number of rows of detectors has ever increased, reaching 320 in 2008.[53] Multi-detector scanners allow further improvement of the speed of scanning, and coverage of a larger volume. With a slice thickness of 0.5 mm, a single rotation of a gantry with 320 detectors covers 16 cm of the body along the z-axis. The time of rotation of the gantry is below 500 msec in most modern scanners, with the fastest rotation at 330 msec. Another innovation has been the dual-source technology, in which two sets of X-ray tubes and detectors are arranged at a right angle to each other in a gantry.[54] Dual sources increase the temporal resolution by halving the rotational travel of the gantry needed to acquire a complete image, thus allowing coverage of the whole heart without the use of medication to lower the heart rate, as well as permitting capture of the heart at any chosen time during the cardiac cycle. Coronary arterial imaging requires electrocardiographically gated scanning, in which motion artifact from cardiac pulsation is minimised by acquisition of data only during the diastatic period of the diastole, or at end-systole. Electrocardiographically gated scans have been of limited use in children because of the high doses of irradiation, but the prospective trigger gating technique now available drastically helps reduce the dose.[55]

Radiation Hazard and Reducing the Dose of Irradiation

There is a linear relationship between the excess risk of cancer and exposure to irradiation, without a threshold even in the low range of 5 to 100 milli-Sievert.[56–59] Exposure to irradiation in childhood appears to be more harmful than later in life.[60] Therefore, the prime strategy of avoiding radiation hazard is not to perform computed tomography whenever the information can be obtained with other imaging modalities that do not use irradiation. When it is obvious that computed tomography is the best option, the medical history and the available imaging findings should be carefully reviewed so that the purpose of the study is clearly defined, and scanning can be restricted to the region of interest. Routine coverage of the whole thorax simply because computed tomography is requested is obsolete (Fig. 18D-18). Pursuing quality of images without consideration of the amount of irradiation will lead to excess exposure. The state-of-the-art strategy in computed tomography is not to produce beautiful images, but to produce images of diagnostic quality with the lowest possible doses of irradiation.[60] The quality of the images tends to be better than what is required for confident diagnosis and decision making. In general, the milliamperage of the current in the tube should be the lowest possible with which quality is maintained. It has been shown

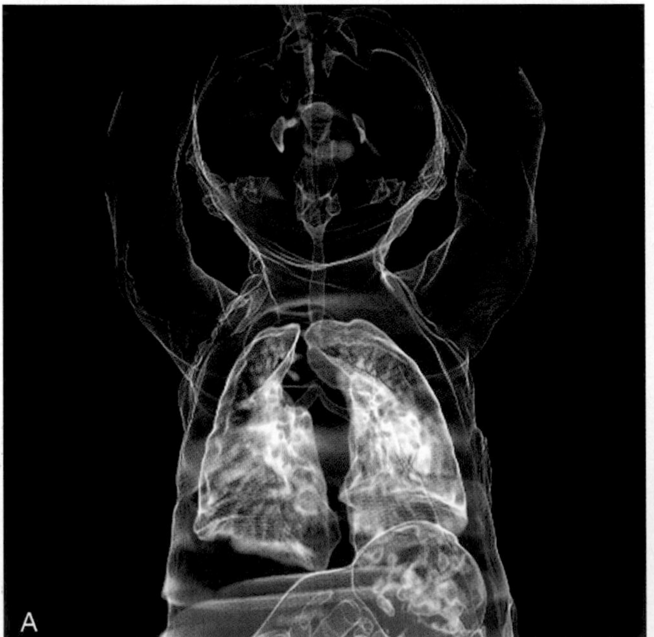

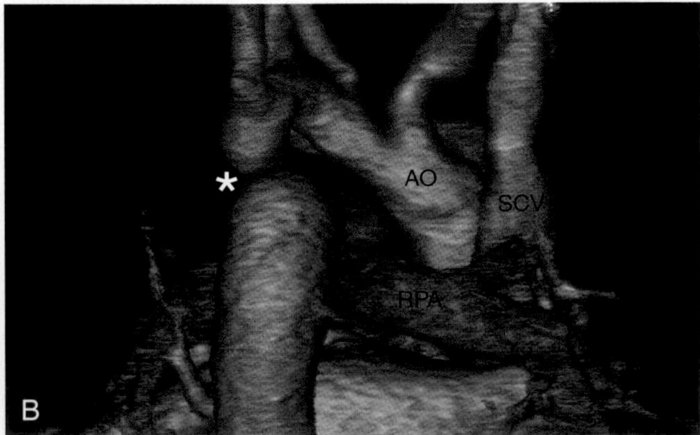

Figure 18D-18 **A,** This computed tomography was performed at an outside institution for suspected vascular pathology in a neonate. The coverage extends from the head to the abdomen, exposing the patient to an unnecessarily high amount of irradiation. The diagnosis in this case was double aortic arch (not shown). **B,** This investigation in a 2-year-old boy with complex coarctation of the aorta (*asterisk*) focused on the area of interest. It includes the aortic arch and not the intracardiac anatomy that was elucidated echocardiographically. The radiation dose was less than 0.5 milli-Sievert for this scan. AO, aorta; RPA, right pulmonary artery; SCV, superior caval vein.

that low settings of kilovoltage lead to marked reductions of the dose without sacrificing quality, especially in children.[57] In addition, the kilovoltage and current should be adjusted according to the size of the target vessels. When imaging large vessels, such as the aortic arch, a lower current can be used. If the target vessel is small, such as diminutive aortopulmonary collateral arteries, a higher current is required for proper delineation of these small structures from the background noise. The dose can be further reduced by automatic modulation, where the current is adjusted according to the thickness and density of the tissues to maintain a constant level of noise.[61] Using recent technologies, it is possible to reduce the dose in paediatric cardiovascular computed tomography to as low as less than one milli-Sievert.[62,63] Compared to other X-ray modalities, such as frontal and lateral chest radiographs, which produce about 0.1 milli-Sievert, conventional catheterisation with angiography and radioisotope studies, both using 5 to 20 milli-Sievert, or the average natural background irradiation per year, at approximately 2 to 3 milli-Sievert, the dose of computed tomography with the proper low protocol appears acceptable.[64–66] Whenever radiosensitive tissues such as breast and thyroid are within the exposed area, they should be shielded. A bismuth shield reduces the dose to the breast by approximately two-fifths.[67]

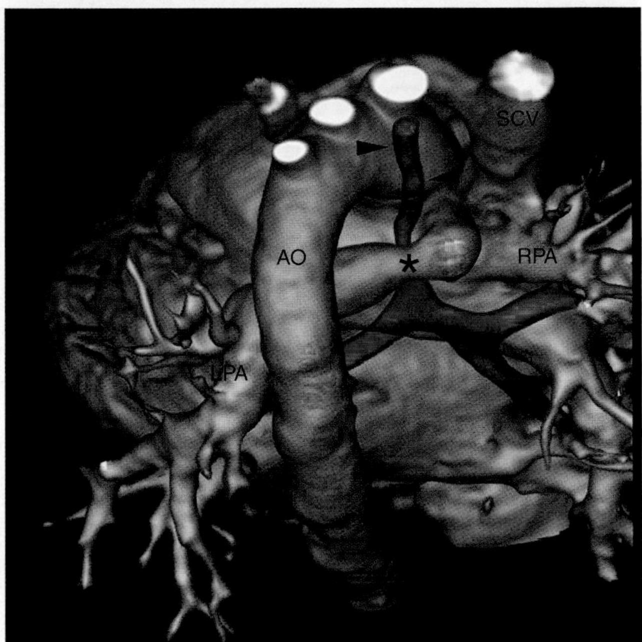

Figure 18D-19 The image is from a 5-year-old child with pulmonary arterial sling syndrome. Volume-rendered reconstruction of a computed tomography of the vascular and central airway anatomy demonstrates the origin of the left pulmonary artery (LPA) from the right pulmonary artery (RPA) and its course around the trachea. The trachea is compressed by the vascular sling (*asterisk*), but also diffusely narrowed (*arrowheads*). AO, aorta; SCV, superior caval vein.

Practical Considerations and Safety

There is no absolute contraindication for computed tomography except for a history of anaphylactic reaction to the iodine-containing contrast medium. As the time of scanning is typically less than 5 to 7 seconds, sedation or general anesthesia is rarely needed.

Vascular enhancement is usually adequate with an intravenous injection of 2 milliliters of contrast medium per kilogram of body weight, followed by a saline chaser. The rate of injection and the trigger delay after the start of injection is adjusted according to the vessels of interest and to the presence of intra- and extracardiac shunts.

Risks and side effects of contrast media are renal impairment as well as allergic reactions. In patients with renal dysfunction the dose should be reduced, or an alternative test should be sought.[68–70]

Clinical Applications and Choosing the Right Imaging Tool

Because computed tomography involves ionizing irradiation, preference should be given to magnetic resonance imaging whenever possible. Computed tomography can become the first line cross sectional imaging modality in some situations.

One of the major advantages of computed tomography over magnetic resonance imaging lies within the rapid evaluation of the airways and lung parenchyma (Fig. 18D-19; see also Fig. 18D-18). For example, computed tomography is indicated in patients with a cardiovascular malform55ation that results in compression of the airways, such as vascular rings, pulmonary arterial sling (see Fig. 18D-19), or absent pulmonary valve syndrome (Fig. 18D-20).[71]

The spatial resolution, and contrast between blood and soft tissue, provided by computed tomography are superior to that of magnetic resonance imaging.[72] The evaluation of small and tortuous vessels, such as major aortopulmonary collateral arteries, therefore, or anomalous pulmonary venous channels, is easier with computed tomography (Figs. 18D-21 and 18D-22). Post-operative complications, including mediastinal haematomas, seromas, and vascular aneurysms, are readily identified with this test. Computed tomography is the most sensitive modality for the detection of calcifications in the cardiac valves, myocardium, and stents. It is able to visualise the inside of most models of stents, which is a blind spot in magnetic resonance imaging.[71] Owing to the speed of acquisition, general anaesthesia or sedation is rarely needed, even in small infants. Unlike magnetic resonance imaging, computed tomography can be safely performed in patients with pacemakers and other metallic or electronic implants.[73,74]

FUTURE PERSPECTIVES

High-field magnets of 3 Tesla hold the promise of higher signal-to-noise ratio, higher temporal and spatial resolutions, and shorter scan times, making them especially appealing for cardiac applications in children. The problem of artifacts from field inhomogeneity at higher field strengths, however, has yet to be overcome, and the effects of peripheral nerve stimulation and body core heating must be carefully observed.

Combined imaging units set the stage for tying together the loose ends of haemodynamic measurements during cardiac catheterisation and in the magnetic resonance scanner.[75–77] Cardiac intervention guided by magnetic resonance imaging has become a reality in

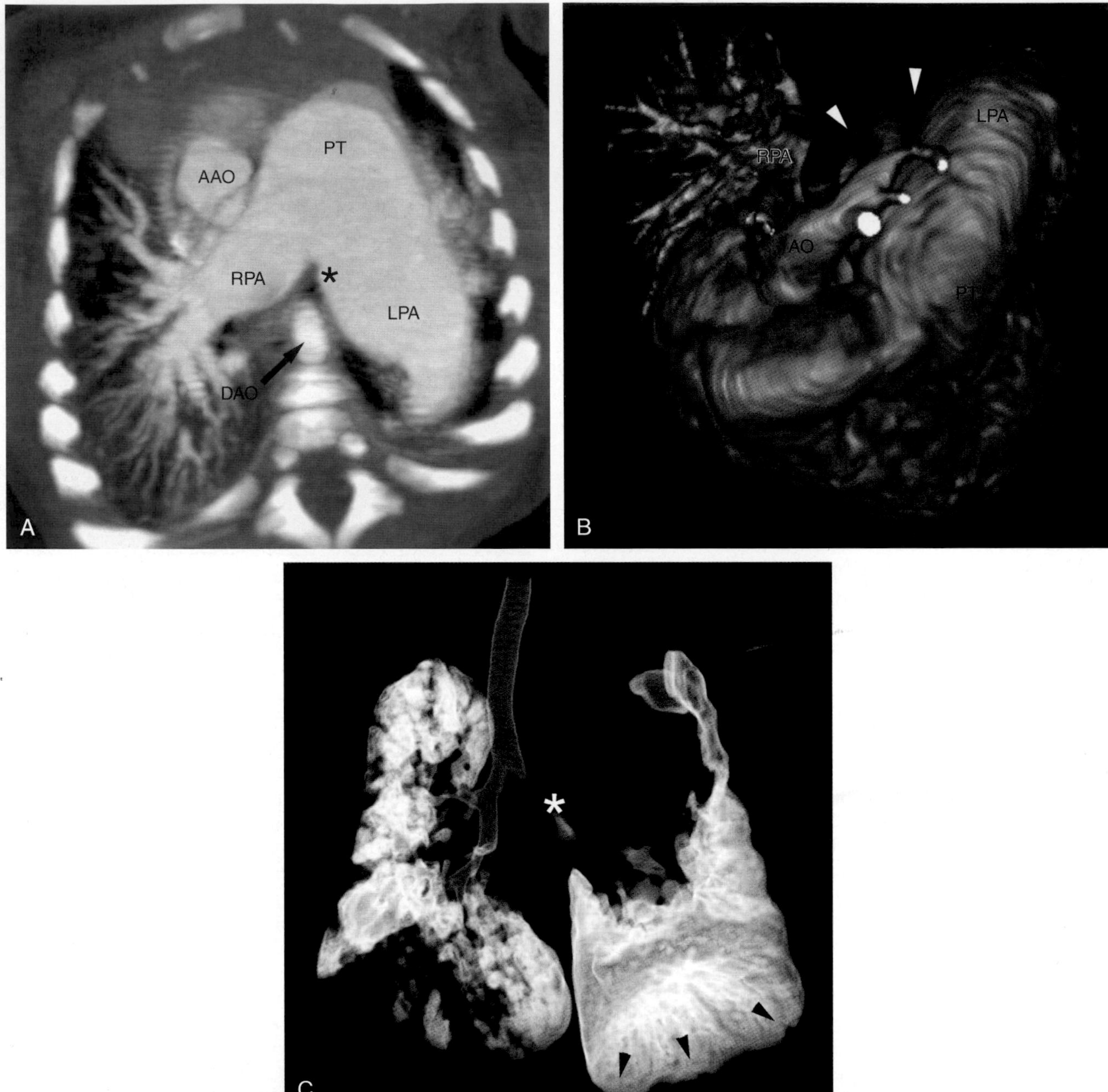

Figure 18D-20 Contrast-enhanced computed tomography angiogram in a 2-week-old patient with absent pulmonary valve syndrome. In the maximum intensity projection image (**A**), the pulmonary trunk (PT) and its branches are seen to be grossly dilated. The left main bronchus (*asterisk*) is compressed between the left pulmonary artery (LPA) and the descending aorta (DAO). This three-dimensional topographic relationship is shown more clearly in the volume-rendered reconstruction (*arrowheads along the left bronchus in* **B**). The volume-rendered image of the airways and lung (**C**) demonstrates the stenotic segment of the left main bronchus (*asterisk*). The left lung is hyperinflated (*arrowheads*). The defect in the medial and upper aspect of the left lung is due to compression of the bronchus by the dilated left pulmonary artery. AAO, ascending aorta; RPA, right pulmonary artery.

selected centers, equipped with hybrid units that incorporate both modalities. The strategies employed range from fusion of images to performing manoeuvres of the catheter and interventions guided solely by magnetic resonance imaging.

Fetal echocardiography has had a great impact on the spectrum of neonatal congenital cardiac disease that we see today. Fetal magnetic resonance imaging (Fig. 18D-23) is feasible using either very fast non-gated sequences or pseudo-gating, in which a pulsed external signal at a frequency identical to the fetal heart rate is fed into the scanner, thus allowing gated acquisitions (see Fig. 18D-23A).

Currently available contrast mediums are rapidly eliminated in the kidneys and distributed in tissues throughout the body, including the myocardium. So-called intravascular contrast agents are expected to allow acquisition of high spatial resolution three-dimensional angiographies of the arteries and veins.

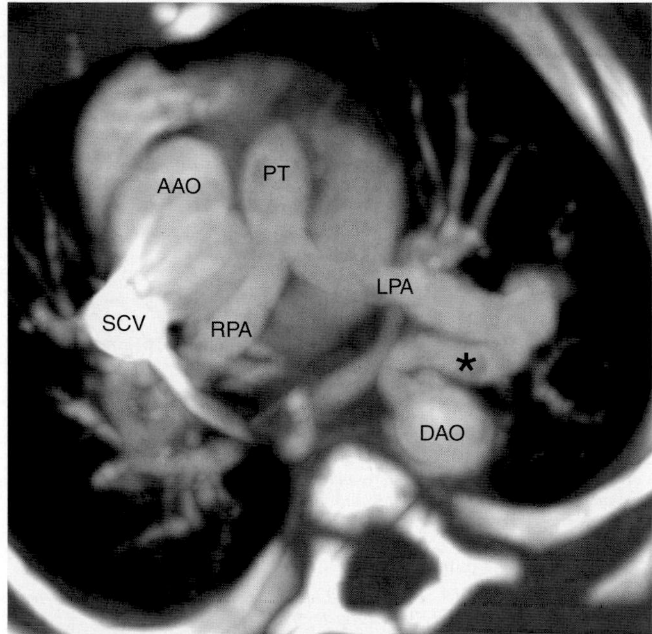

Figure 18D-21 Computed tomography in a 6-month-old patient with tetralogy of Fallot, pulmonary atresia, and major aortopulmonary collaterals. This reformatted image depicts a large direct collateral artery (*asterisk*) arising from the descending aorta (DAO) and connecting to the descending branch of the left pulmonary artery (LPA). AAO, ascending aorta; PT, pulmonary trunk; RPA, right pulmonary artery; SCV, superior caval vein.

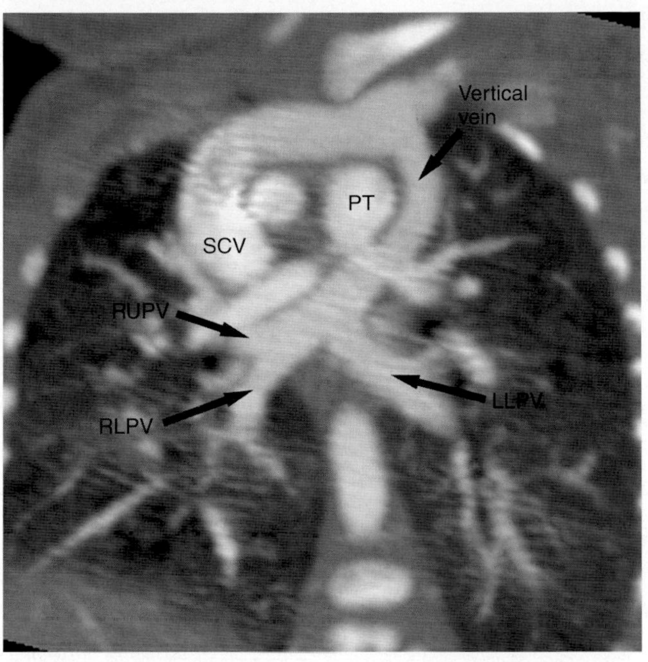

Figure 18D-22 The image shows unrepaired supracardiac totally anomalous pulmonary venous connection with a vertical vein to the left brachiocephalic vein in a 1-week-old neonate. The left upper pulmonary vein is not shown. LLPV, left lower pulmonary vein; PT, pulmonary trunk; RLPV, right lower pulmonary vein; RUPV, right upper pulmonary vein; SCV, superior caval vein.

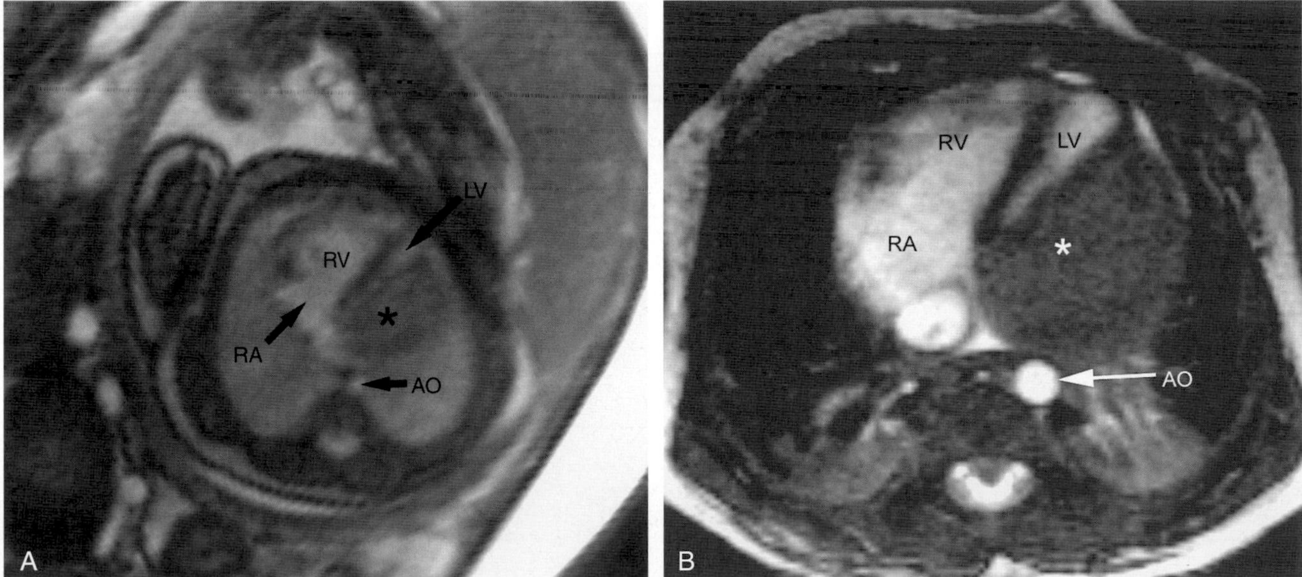

Figure 18D-23 This patient was found to have a tumour within the left ventricular mass by prenatal echocardiography. With rhabdomyoma and tuberous sclerosis as part of the differential diagnosis, a fetal magnetic resonance scan was ordered to assess for lesions of the brain and kidneys. **A,** A cardiac investigation during the same test showed the mass (*asterisk*). **B,** A postnatal scan 10 days later was conducted to assess the tissue characteristics of the tumour, as well as the ability of the left ventricle (LV) to sustain the systemic circulation. The tumour (*asterisk*) obliterates most of the left ventricle, but sufficient space for the inflow and outflow tracts was preserved (not shown). The left ventricular cavity volume was 37 mL/m^2 of body surface area. The patient is maintaining a biventricular circulation. AO, aorta; A, right atrium; RV, right ventricle.

The complete reference list can be found on the companion Expert Consult web site at www.expertconsult.com.

ANNOTATED REFERENCES

- Lauterbur PC: Image formation by induced local interactions: Examples of employing nuclear magnetic resonance. Nature 1973;242:190–191.

  Conventional nuclear magnetic resonance used uniform magnetic fields. Paul Lauterbur, as a professor in radiology and chemistry at the State University of New York, discovered that if he applied a non-uniform magnetic field, that is, magnetic gradients, he could locate where in space the signal arose. Unable to patent his idea, Lauterbur submitted it to Nature *along with magnetic resonance images of water-filled tubes. In 1977, the first commercial magnetic resonance scanner was produced based on his work.*

- Lanzer P, Botvinick EH, Schiller NB, et al: Cardiac imaging using gated magnetic resonance. Radiology 1984;150:121–127.

  Prior to this study, cardiac images produced using magnetic resonance were of poor quality as a result of the motion of the heart. The group working at the University of California in San Francisco tried three different methods of cardiac gating: plethysmography, laser Doppler, and electrocardiography. The last method produced the best results and is the current standard for all the cine images, and most static images.

- Grosse-Wortmann L, Al-Otay A, Woo GH, et al: Anatomical and functional evaluation of pulmonary veins in children by magnetic resonance imaging. J Am Coll Cardiol 2007;49:993–1002.

  Magnetic resonance imaging is ideally suited for the evaluation of pathology of the pulmonary veins. Anomalous pulmonary venous connections and their haemodynamic significance are readily demonstrated. In the setting of significant pulmonary venous stenosis, blood flow to lungs is redistributed to lung areas with unobstructed venous return.

- Kozerke S, Scheidegger MB, Pedersen EM, Boesiger P: Heart motion adapted cine phase-contrast flow measurements through the aortic valve. Magn Reson Med 1999;42:970–978.

- Kozerke S, Schwitter J, Pedersen EM, Boesiger P: Aortic and mitral regurgitation: Quantification using moving slice velocity mapping. J Magn Reson Imaging 2001;14:106–112.

  These two papers highlight the errors introduced into the quantification of valvar regurgitant volumes by translational motion of the valves perpendicular to the imaging plane. The group from Zurich presents a motion tracking technique that allows the phase contrast imaging plane to follow the valvar movements throughout the cardiac cycle. When comparing the corrected with the uncorrected method in patients with mild, moderate, and severe aortic regurgitation, they found differences of 60%, 15%, and 7%, respectively. Unfortunately, motion tracking is not commercially available.

- Fogel MA, Weinberg PM, Harris M, Rhodes L: Usefulness of magnetic resonance imaging for the diagnosis of right ventricular dysplasia in children. Am J Cardiol 2006;97:1232–1237.

  The authors analysed 81 studies in patients with either signs and symptoms of arrhythmogenic right ventricular dysplasia, or a positive family history. Only three had any magnetic resonance findings of the disease, the features being mild in two. The authors concluded that, in contrast to data in adults, cardiac magnetic resonance imaging has a low yield in children suspected of having right ventricular dysplasia, an experience that is shared by many institutions worldwide.

- Abdel-Aty H, Boye P, Zagrosek A, et al: Diagnostic performance of cardiovascular magnetic resonance in patients with suspected acute myocarditis: Comparison of different approaches. J Am Coll Cardiol 2005;45: 1815–1822.

  The authors diagnosed myocarditis using a combined approach of T2-weighted oedema imaging, and early hyperaemia and late necrosis imaging using gadolinium enhancement, achieving sensitivity of 76% and specificity of 95.5%. Their work shows the value of magnetic resonance in tissue characterisation in clinical practice.

- Razavi R, Hill D, Keevil S, et al: Cardiac catheterization guided by MRI in children and adults with congenital heart disease. Lancet 2003;362: 1877–1882.

  This work from London was the first to demonstrate the feasibility of cardiac catheterisation guided by magnetic resonance imaging in human subjects, including children. The tip of a balloon catheter was filled with carbon dioxide and maneuvered under real-time magnetic resonance imaging. The investigators applied a hybrid approach, using both X-ray and magnetic resonance guidance.

- Rees S, Firmin D, Mohiaddin R, et al: Application of flow measurements by magnetic resonance velocity mapping to congenital heart disease. Am J Cardiol 1989;64:953–956.

  Published only as a brief report, this study was the first to document the use of phase contrast imaging for the quantification of intracardiac shunting by comparing the flows in the pulmonary trunk to those in the ascending aorta. A number of subsequent studies evaluated magnetic resonance against cardiac catheterisation for the quantification of shunts. Magnetic resonance has since become the gold standard for measuring flow, especially in patients with shunts at atrial level, or extracardiac shunts, in whom the Fick method is often flawed.

- Paterson A, Frush DP: Dose reduction in paediatric MDCT: General principles. Clin Radiol 2007;62:507–517.

  This comprehensive review article explains in detail the various strategies that can be employed to reduce the amount of irradiation delivered to the patient.

- Kim YM, Yoo SJ, Kim TH, et al: Three-dimensional computed tomography in children with compression of the central airways complicating congenital heart disease. Cardiol Young 2002;12:44–50.

  Kim and colleagues assessed the quality and usefulness of computed tomography in the evaluation of compression of the airways in 49 patients, three-fifths of whom were neonates with congenitally malformed hearts. The recent development of multi-detector computed tomography can further reduce artifacts produced by motion, and the doses of irradiation, features which are not addressed in this earlier article.

CHAPTER

19 Electrophysiology, Pacing, and Devices

ELIZABETH A. STEPHENSON and ANDREW M. DAVIS

Electrophysiology is a rapidly growing and evolving discipline within both paediatric and adult cardiology. Although there is overlap in the knowledge base of the paediatric and adult electrophysiologist, there are many issues that are unique to young patients and those with congenital heart disease. The knowledge and practise of paediatric electrophysiology now requires extended training and specialised facilities. An on-site paediatric electrophysiology service has now become an essential component of major paediatric cardiac centres.

This chapter presents an overview of paediatric electrophysiology for the general paediatric cardiologist or trainee, incorporating aspects of diagnosis and treatment. Extensive references should allow the interested reader to explore topics at greater depth.

ELECTROPHYSIOLOGY AND CATHETER ABLATION

Diagnosis and Documentation of Tachycardia

When a patient presents with a tachycardia that is documented on a 12-lead electrocardiogram and with a rhythm strip, it is often straightforward to establish the diagnosis and plan the treatment. Occasionally, the diagnosis remains unclear and then the response to vagal manoeuvres or medications will often help to clarify it. Intravenous adenosine is a potent but transient inhibitor of the atrioventricular node, with lesser and variable effects on ectopic atrial or ventricular substrates. It is important to record the electrocardiogram during vagal manoeuvres or the administration of adenosine, as transient and subtle effects can be missed when observing a monitor screen. If it is still not possible to define the arrhythmia mechanism, an electrophysiological study may then be useful in establishing the diagnosis.

Suspected Arrhythmia or Unexplained Symptoms

When a patient has symptoms such as palpitations, dizzy spells, or syncope, but the rhythm is not documented, management may be less straightforward. It is always preferable to document the clinical arrhythmia, prior to undertaking a diagnostic electrophysiological study as non-clinical arrhythmias may be induced during electrophysiological testing. An aggressive protocol of stimulation, for example, those using stimulation with short coupling intervals or including an isoprenaline challenge, can produce arrhythmias in normal subjects, although these are often not sustained or specific.[1,2] Nevertheless, if an arrhythmia that does not mimic the clinical one is induced, management based on this finding may be inappropriate. Good examples are the use of antiarrhythmic medication or implantable defibrillators for induced ventricular arrhythmias without clinical correlation, or inappropriate ablation for dual atrioventricular nodal pathways with a risk of producing complete heart block. In adolescents and adults in whom electrophysiological studies can be performed with minimal sedation, it is possible to ask the patient during the procedure whether the symptoms produced by an induced arrhythmia are similar to those noticed clinically. In younger children deep sedation or general anaesthesia is often used, and thus this opportunity is not available. A recording of an arrhythmia can frequently be obtained by using the methods described below, but occasionally electrophysiological studies are necessary for better elucidation of arrhythmias that prove to be elusive.

Methods of Recording an Arrhythmia

- Documentation by paramedics or rapid presentation to an emergency department for an electrocardiogram when an infrequent arrhythmia starts. It is helpful to supply the parent with a letter stating the need for an urgent electrocardiogram and rhythm strip without waiting for triage, as arrhythmias often revert to sinus rhythm while a patient is waiting in the emergency department queue.
- Ambulatory electrocardiography (Holter monitoring) is useful to document the maximum and minimum heart rates seen during normal daytime and sleep and the presence of arrhythmias, as well as the effects of medication. In some, the patient will have a clinical arrhythmia, or short-lived asymptomatic arrhythmias, while wearing the monitor. Diagnostic clues such as intermittent pre-excitation may be documented. Repeating the test on 2 or 3 consecutive days may increase the diagnostic yield, but this is often an unrewarding investigation when symptoms are infrequent.
- Exercise electrocardiography will document the heart rate response during exercise, the exercise tolerance, and presence of ischaemia. When symptoms are related to exercise, this may also provoke the arrhythmia. Exercise tests need to be tailored to younger children who find adult protocols to be too slow and uninteresting. It is important to perform maximum, or symptom-limited, tests rather than automatically stopping the test when a preconceived maximum heart rate is achieved, as is commonly performed in adults. In addition to an exercise test based on a protocol, a shorter test in which

the treadmill is advanced manually to maximum speed over 1 minute and then to maximum elevation over 1 minute (sprint test) can be used to try to reproduce a rapid peak exercise response. Arrhythmias sensitive to catecholamines may occasionally be provoked by such a peak exercise test following a negative test based on a less aggressive protocol.

- Tilt testing is occasionally useful in establishing the cause of syncope, particularly when the symptoms are suggestive of neurally mediated (vasovagal) syncope.[3] However, the test is unpleasant for the patient, and the sensitivity and specificity of this test are mediocre, with a high rate of false positives and false negatives, and this must be taken into account when interpreting the results.[3–8]
- Event recorders are perhaps the most effective method of documenting infrequent and short-lived arrhythmias, particularly when the symptoms are vague or multiple. The patient is supplied with a small recorder that allows an electrocardiogram to be recorded when symptoms occur. Usually the recording is transmitted telephonically to a base station and then analysed. The patient can record symptoms during normal daily activities, send in any number of recordings, and keep the recorder for an extended period. There are two different types: pocket or loop monitors. The pocket monitors are carried close to the person in a pocket or handbag, and applied to the chest when the patient is symptomatic. The continuous loop recorders are of a similar size but remain attached to the chest via leads and retain a 1- to 5-minute recording that is continuously updated in memory. When a symptom occurs, the recorder is activated manually by the patient or parent and stores information from immediately before and for a programmed period after activation. The continuous recordings are more useful, albeit that constant wearing of the electrodes may cause skin irritation. Compliance can also be an issue, as it is inconvenient to reapply the monitor every day, and adolescents will frequently be quite self-conscious about wearing the monitor. Advantages include knowledge of where the device is at all times, and the ability to make recordings that include the onset of symptoms. It is also ideal for confirming symptoms caused by simple extrasystoles or other short-duration arrhythmias. Both types of recorders are also useful for confirming that symptoms, often transient and unusual, are not arrhythmic, as when numerous recordings of sinus rhythm are sent in.
- Implantable recorders are occasionally useful when recordings during the symptoms remain elusive.[9] These devices, similar in size to a small pack of chewing gum, are implanted under the skin of the chest and activated by an external unit carried by the patient when a symptom occurs. They will also automatically record any rhythms that fall outside of preset normal parameters. The recording is downloaded thereafter by telemetry, similar to pacemaker interrogation. They can function for a year or longer, until the battery is exhausted. This method is usually reserved for patients with negative non-invasive studies and continued concerning symptoms. They are particularly useful for syncope that prevents the patient from using an event recorder and for very infrequent symptoms. The invasiveness of these recorders makes them inappropriate for benign symptoms.

Life-threatening Arrhythmias

When a patient presents with an out-of-hospital cardiac arrest or a presyncopal tachycardia that reverts before diagnosis, then it is no longer safe merely to await a spontaneous recurrence to document the rhythm, and invasive electrophysiology studies may be required. In this setting, it is more likely that any arrhythmias that are found will be clinically relevant and merit appropriate treatment.

Evaluation of Effectiveness and Safety of Drug Treatment

A major early role for electrophysiological studies was to establish which medication was effective for treating an arrhythmia. This was a particularly prominent indication in adults with ventricular tachycardia and after repair of tetralogy of Fallot and in children with supraventricular tachycardia resistant to usual therapies.[10–14] Currently, there is a minimal role for such testing either for anti-arrhythmic or pro-arrhythmic effects[15–17] of drugs.

Ventricular Stimulation Testing

In adults with left ventricular dysfunction, or after myocardial infarction, electrophysiological studies have been used for assessment of the risk of sudden death. When ventricular arrhythmias are non-inducible, or become so with anti-arrhythmic medication, the prognosis may be better. Left ventricular dysfunction, however, is a powerful predictor in its own right, and in many such patients, it is not possible to find a drug that renders the arrhythmia non-inducible. While empirical treatment with amiodarone, despite leaving patients inducible, has been found in some studies to improve the prognosis, this is not a uniform finding and the trend is to use an automatic implantable cardioverter defibrillator.[18–24] The landmark sudden cardiac death in heart failure trial (SCD-HFT) showed no survival benefit in adults from the use of amiodarone as a primary prevention measure; in contrast, the implantable defibrillator conferred a 23% reduction in mortality.[25] In patients with dilated cardiomyopathy, clinical sustained monomorphic ventricular tachycardia can often be reproduced during electrophysiology study. It is important to exclude bundle branch re-entry in these patients as this arrhythmia is amenable to ablation. If the dilated cardiomyopathy patient has non-sustained ventricular tachycardia, or has presented with syncope, invasive electrophysiology study is, however, of no additional benefit in risk stratification.[26,27] While there is minimal data available, some survivors of congenital cardiac surgery with ventricular dysfunction, ventricular arrhythmias on ambulatory monitoring, or inducible arrhythmias at electrophysiological study, receive drug treatment and/or implantable defibrillators.[28,29]

Alternative approaches to ambulatory monitoring and electrophysiological studies include assessment of heart rate variability over 24 hours, as a potential predictor of sudden death. Low heart rate variability suggests a worse prognosis in adult patients with left ventricular dysfunction or after myocardial infarction, and these patients may receive antiarrhythmic treatment or undergo implantation of a defibrillator.[30] Whether it is appropriate to extrapolate this data to patients with congenital heart disease is not clear. There are significant differences related to age as well as acute effects from surgery, but few systematic studies.[31,32] Signal-averaged recordings evaluated for late ventricular potentials have also been found to be a marker of a poor prognosis in adults, and are used in the diagnosis of diffuse myocardial disease such as arrhythmogenic right ventricular dysplasia.[33] Again, even though normative data for children has been published,[34] there are few studies in children with congenital heart disease, and none as yet has demonstrated a useful role in this particular population.[35,36] (This is explored further under ventricular tachycardia, later in this chapter). Specialised exercise testing for microvolt T-wave alternans offers another non-invasive approach. In general this testing has a good negative predictive value and thus testing may be helpful in the risk stratification process. Normative data for children has been published but more paediatric follow-up data is needed.[37–39]

Evaluation of the Conduction System

Historically, invasive electrophysiology studies were used to document the level of atrioventricular block in patients with conduction system disease: block above and below the bundle of His being associated with a better and worse prognosis, respectively. Pacemaker indications are outlined in the pacing section of this chapter and no longer rely on electrophysiology study.[40,41]

Interventional Management

Overdrive pacing and programmed stimulation can be used to terminate acute arrhythmias without the need for antiarrhythmic medication or electrical cardioversion. This technique is ideal when there are already pacing leads in place, such as temporary epicardial leads after cardiac surgery or when a permanent pacemaker has been implanted. In patients with malignant recurrent arrhythmias, and/or when medication is ineffective, temporary intracardiac electrodes could be placed to avoid repeated cardioversion until a more long-term strategy is determined. A transoesophageal electrode can be used in diagnosis of arrhythmias with cryptic atrial activity on surface tracings. It can also be used to terminate atrioventricular re-entry tachycardias and atrial flutter.[42]

When antiarrhythmic medication is ineffective, poorly tolerated, or causes side effects in patients with chronic arrhythmias, then more aggressive management is required and electrophysiological testing may be performed to define the substrate for the arrhythmia and to plan treatment. Tachycardia that is reliably terminated with pace-stimulation but not amenable to ablation can be managed by implanting an anti-tachycardia pacemaker. If anti-tachycardia pacing accelerates the arrhythmia, or produces other arrhythmias, an implantable cardioverter defibrillator may be indicated. Antiarrhythmic surgery has been previously used to cure arrhythmias through excision or cryoablation of ectopic foci or accessory pathways.[43–46] Prior electrophysiological testing was usually required to confirm the anatomy of the substrate and to avoid prolonged intra-operative electrophysiological mapping. Antiarrhythmic surgery laid the foundation for transcatheter ablation therapy but is now rarely indicated for most common arrhythmias. Nonetheless, antiarrhythmic surgery is still performed, often combined with other cardiac surgery, especially Fontan revision,[47,48] and pulmonary valve replacement in patients late after repair of tetralogy of Fallot. Currently, radio-frequency ablation or cryoablation is the most common reason for undertaking an electrophysiological study in children.

RADIO-FREQUENCY ABLATION AND CRYOABLATION

Transcatheter ablation was first observed serendipitously when a patient undergoing an electrophysiological study required defibrillation. The energy from the defibrillator accidentally passed down the electrode recording from the His bundle and created complete heart block.[49] Subsequent animal studies confirmed that complete heart block could be reliably created using this technique. His bundle ablation using direct current became a useful treatment for patients with atrial arrhythmias refractory to medical therapies, especially atrial fibrillation, but it required implantation of a permanent pacemaker.[50,51] Side effects from the high energy that was required included barotrauma with ventricular dysfunction. Cardiac rupture was also described when ablation was attempted in the coronary sinus to ablate accessory pathways.[52,53] Alternative energy sources used, historically, with some success included low-energy direct current ablation, direct laser energy and indirect laser heating of the catheter tip.[54–56]

The development of radio-frequency energy as a tool for ablation was enhanced with the development of steerable electrode catheters so that discrete controlled amounts of energy could be delivered accurately to the target while avoiding damage to other structures.[57,58] Delivery of energy is gradual and steady, rather than the explosive instantaneous delivery produced by direct current ablation, and it can be applied repeatedly until effective. Unlike direct current ablation, which caused skeletal muscle contraction and pain, radio-frequency ablation is relatively painless and can be performed under local anaesthesia. While catheter ablation was initially developed to create complete heart block, this is seldom required in children, in whom radio-frequency ablation is usually used to affect a direct cure of a range of arrhythmias (Fig. 19-1).

More recently, catheter based interventions using cryoablation have become more widely used.[59,60] Using this technique, localisation of the region of interest is performed in a manner similar to radio-frequency ablations. Testing of these sites is then performed by extreme cooling, rather than heating, of the catheter tip. This temporarily inhibits tissue function (loss of pathway activity or loss of dual atrioventricular node behaviour, for example). When an appropriate site for ablation is located, the cryothermal energy is increased, freezing the tissue with a typical application time of 4 minutes, creating a permanent lesion. The typical mapping temperature is −30 °C and the typical ablation temperature is −70 to −75 °C. This technique offers the advantage of potentially reversible lesions, thus reducing the risk of permanent heart block or other undesirable tissue effects. It also offers less painful application of energy, but may be complicated by slightly higher recurrence rates.[61,62] As this remains a fairly new technology, it remains to be seen what the long-term efficacy will be, particularly once the learning curve has been completed. Many laboratories now have both radio-frequency and cryoablation available, and tailor the usage of each to the individual patient.

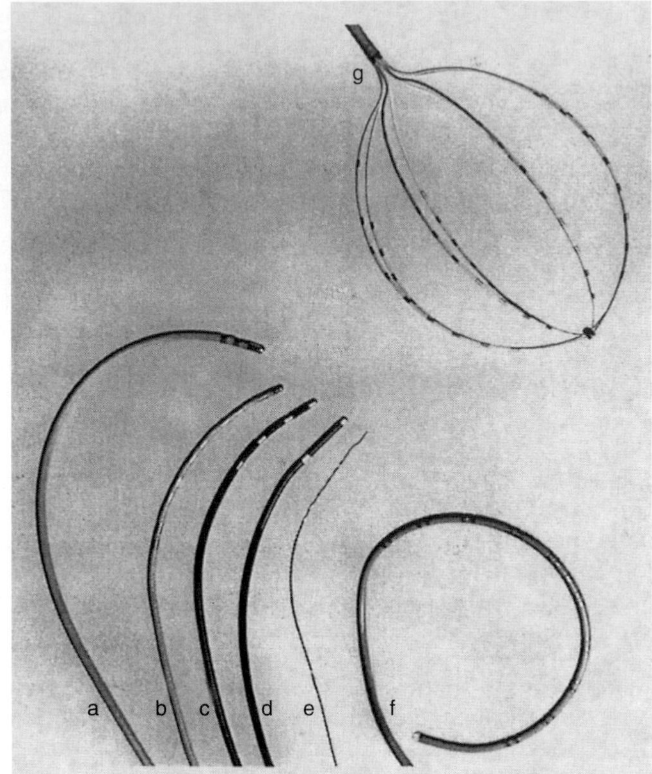

Figure 19-1 Catheter electrodes used for electrophysiology and ablation: (a) ablation catheter; (b) 6 French decapolar electrode catheter; (c) 6 French quadripolar electrode catheter, also available in 5 French; (d) 6 French bipolar electrode catheter; (e) 2 French quadripolar catheter; (f) 8 French Halo catheter; (g) basket electrode catheter.

Tissue Effects of Radio-frequency Energy

During delivery of radio-frequency energy, the tissue in contact with the ablation catheter is heated.[63] At temperatures of 50 °C and greater, there is permanent denaturation of the cell membranes and tissue dehydration. After further heating, there is coagulation necrosis of the tissue with surrounding haemorrhage and inflammation. The lesion retracts acutely because of dehydration, and the coagulation necrosis heals to form a well-demarcated fibrotic scar. The size of the lesion depends on the power of the radio-frequency energy delivered, the size of the ablation catheter, the duration of heating and the temperature achieved.[64–66] Small electrode tips result in a rapid rise in temperature with boiling at the tissue interface and charring of blood, with a rise in impedance, a decrease in heat transfer and a smaller lesion. Longer electrode tips, with less contact with tissue, have a reduced current density so that the temperature rise is curtailed. This allows use of higher powers and a longer delivery of energy without boiling and charring, and it creates deeper lesions. A standard 7 French ablation catheter with a 4-mm tip will produce lesions 5 to 6 mm in diameter and 2 to 3 mm deep. After delivery of energy is discontinued, the tissue in contact with the electrode is hotter than the surrounding tissues and continued heat transfer occurs. This thermal latency explains why lesions can continue to increase in size after cessation of delivery of energy.[67] Catheters with cooled tips allow the use of even greater power without charring and create even deeper lesions.[68] Scar tissue takes longer to heat and produces smaller lesions, thus making lesion creation in scarred regions challenging.[69]

During the healing phase, tissue on the border of the lesion may recover if permanent denaturation was not achieved. Progressive necrosis may also occur at the border of a lesion if sufficient inflammation and microvascular damage occurred during delivery of energy.[63,70,71] Therefore, it is possible for an acutely successfully ablated arrhythmia to recur, or a partially successful ablation to become completed. The latter progression is seen less often clinically. In neonatal lambs, delivery of radio-frequency energy resulted in a progressive increase in the size of lesions in the atrial and ventricular myocardium, but not in the atrioventricular groove.[72]

Procedure

Radio-frequency and Cryoablation Equipment

Radio-frequency ablation is performed using a dedicated alternating current generator coupled to an ablation catheter and an indifferent plate attached to the back of the patient. The catheters are typically 5 to 7 French, have bipolar or quadripolar tips that can be deflected, and have a steering mechanism to facilitate positioning at the appropriate site. Radio-frequency energy is delivered at cycle lengths of 300 to 750 kHz. During delivery of energy, the rhythm, temperature, and impedance at the tip of the catheter are closely monitored.

Temperatures of 60° to 70°C are required for effective ablation, while temperatures below 50°C often result in a transient effect with later recovery of conduction. Much higher temperatures can result in charring of blood at the tip of the catheter, which insulates the tip from the tissue and prevents effective heating of the tissue. Feedback control from the thermistor at the tip of the catheter to the generator is used now to limit the power, to control the rise in temperature, and to avoid excessive temperatures.[73,74]

Cryoablation can be performed with either 7 French, 6-mm tip, or 9 French, 8-mm tip, cryothermal catheters. It requires a dedicated cryoablation console. The temperature is lowered to −30°C for 60 seconds and testing can be performed to determine appropriateness of that site (cryomapping). A useful feature is the fact that the catheter adheres to the application site. Once a promising ablation site has been identified, the temperature will be decreased to −70°C for 4 minutes to complete the ablation. It is important to continuously monitor the rhythm during energy application as lesion expansion can be seen during cryoablation, even when not seen during cryomapping.[75] In some laboratories cryoablation may be performed without previous cryomapping.

Technique

Catheter ablation is usually performed immediately subsequent to diagnostic electrophysiology. It is important to discontinue antiarrhythmic medication, if at all possible, prior to the procedure as the effects may render arrhythmias non-inducible and make it impossible to find the site for ablation. In some laboratories, systemic heparinisation is used during the procedure regardless of ablation location; others only heparinise for left-sided ablations or if arterial access is required.

Once the arrhythmic substrate has been determined and mapped, an ablation catheter is advanced via an additional site of access, usually the femoral vein or artery, to the appropriate site for delivery of energy. Energy can be delivered during sinus rhythm, during tachycardia, or during atrial or ventricular pacing. In radio-frequency ablation, a short test application of 10 seconds or so, which usually does not cause irreversible changes, will be continued for 30 to 90 seconds if the test causes the desired effect, such as loss of the delta wave, termination of tachycardia, or loss of retrograde conduction.[76] Ineffective ablation may occur as a result of inexact localisation of the site, poor contact between the ablation catheter and the endocardium, or build-up of coagulum and char on the electrode tip. These problems will need to be corrected before ablation is successful. Moving the catheter to a new site guided by the electrograms is often sufficient but, if there is repeated failure, then different catheter shapes and approaches to enhance contact between catheter and endocardium should be utilized. Long sheaths with a variety of shaped tips are available to aid stability and positioning. Monitoring the impedance and temperature of a radio-frequency catheter allows delivery of the minimal energy to raise the temperature at the tip to 60° to 70°C without creating charring, which then impedes effective delivery of energy to the tissue. If necessary, the catheter is removed from the body and the char and coagulum wiped off with a saline swab. Further attempts are made until success is achieved.

Following a successful ablation, attempts are made to re-induce the tachycardia. If the ablation appears to be successful, repeat attempts to induce are made 20 to 30 minutes later, as occasionally there is recovery of the ablated area.

Placement of Electrophysiologic Catheters

Bipolar or quadripolar catheters for pacing and sensing are usually placed in the high right atrium, in the right ventricular apex, and through the antero-superior part of the tricuspid valve to record the electrical activity of the His bundle (Fig. 19-2). A multi-polar catheter is placed in the coronary sinus to record left atrial and left ventricular electrograms around the left atrioventricular groove. At least four different sheaths for venous access are required to place these electrodes. These are usually inserted through three or four sites of femoral venous puncture and/or a puncture in the subclavian or jugular vein for access to the coronary sinus. In some cases, additional electrode catheters are inserted to increase the number of sites for recording and pacing, or to serve as anatomical landmarks. Electrodes are not routinely placed in the left ventricle or left atrium unless this is indicated during the course of the study.

Programmed Stimulation and Intracardiac Recordings

The recordings of the intracardiac electrograms are used to measure the intracardiac conduction times in the baseline state. Following this, a variety of pacing protocols are used to characterise the electrophysiological properties of the atriums, ventricles, and cardiac conduction system and to induce tachyarrhythmias. The specific protocols used, and their order, will depend on the clinical indications for the study and the information emerging during the course of the study.[77,78] After any intervention, be it administration of drugs or ablation, the electrophysiological properties of the heart are re-evaluated.

Conduction Intervals

The PA interval is a measurement of the intra-atrial conduction time, the AH interval is a measurement of the atrioventricular nodal conduction time, and the HV is a measurement of the His–Purkinje conduction time (Fig. 19-3). Conduction intervals are generally measured in sinus rhythm and then during atrial pacing.

Sinus Node Function

Sinus node function can be assessed by pacing the atrium at a constant rate for 30 seconds and measuring the length of the pause after the pacing is stopped. This is the sinus node recovery time. Sinus node disease is uncommon in children unless they have had extensive atrial surgery, as in the Senning, Mustard, or Fontan operations. Clinical evaluation is usually sufficient.

Atrioventricular Conduction

Atrioventricular node conduction is assessed by measuring conduction intervals at baseline and during incremental atrial pacing until the development of atrioventricular Wenckebach, and by using atrial extrastimuli. Ventriculo-atrial, or retrograde, conduction is assessed during ventricular pacing and extrastimulation. Conduction via the atrioventricular node is distinguished from that of accessory pathways by the response to extrastimuli, as well as the location of the earliest activation. Atrioventricular nodal tissue demonstrates a decremental pattern in which conduction time increases the earlier the extrastimulus. Conduction across accessory pathways, in contrast, is non-decremental. Therefore, the conduction time remains constant with increasing prematurity of the extrastimulus until there is a sudden loss of conduction.

Incremental Pacing

Pacing is started at a low rate and gradually increased until conduction is blocked or a tachycardia is induced. This is used to assess atrioventricular conduction, to expose accessory pathways and to induce tachycardias.

Burst Pacing

Rapid atrial pacing is commenced at rates of 200 to 600 beats/min in order to induce atrial flutter and atrial fibrillation. Burst pacing is generally not performed in the ventricle, and certainly not at rapid rates, due to the risk of induction of a haemodynamically unstable rhythm.

Extrastimulus Testing

Timed extrastimuli, so-called premature beats, can be introduced during sinus rhythm or following a train of pacing, usually comprising eight beats, that stabilises the electrophysiological properties of the tissue before the extrastimulus. Successive extrastimuli are introduced with increasing prematurity. When the coupling interval between the last beat in the train and the extrastimulus is shortened sufficiently that the extrastimulus is unable to excite the tissue, then the refractory period of the tissue has been identified. This is called the effective refractory period. Atrial extrastimuli are used to measure the effective refractory period in the atrium, of the atrioventricular nodal conducting system and, when present, of accessory pathways that conduct from the atrium to the ventricle. They are also used to expose dual atrioventricular nodal pathways. Ventricular extrastimuli are used to measure the effective refractory period in the ventricle and expose concealed accessory pathways, in other words those pathways that conduct only from ventricle to atrium. Single, double, or triple extrastimuli, either in sinus rhythm or following a drive train, are introduced with increasing prematurity to induce atrial, ventricular, and atrioventricular re-entry tachycardias. Extrastimuli introduced during tachycardia can be used to help to characterise the tachycardia or to terminate it.

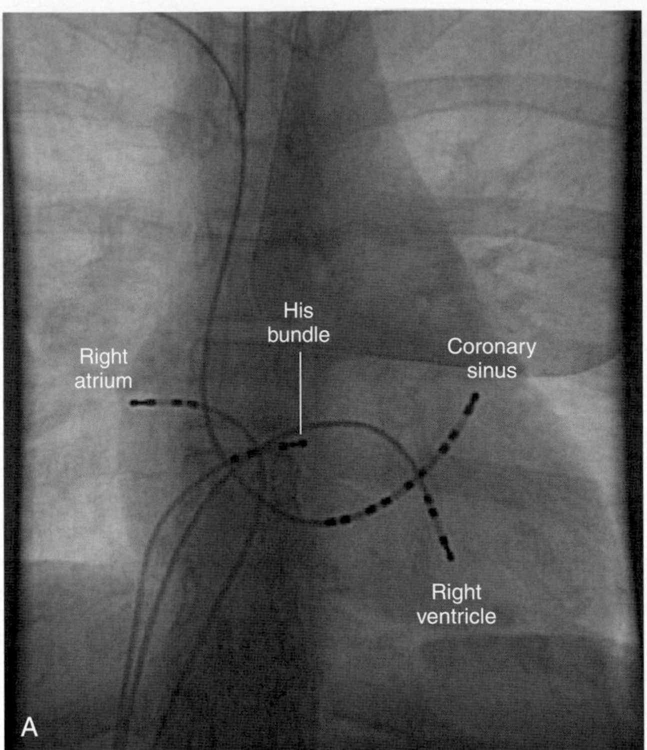

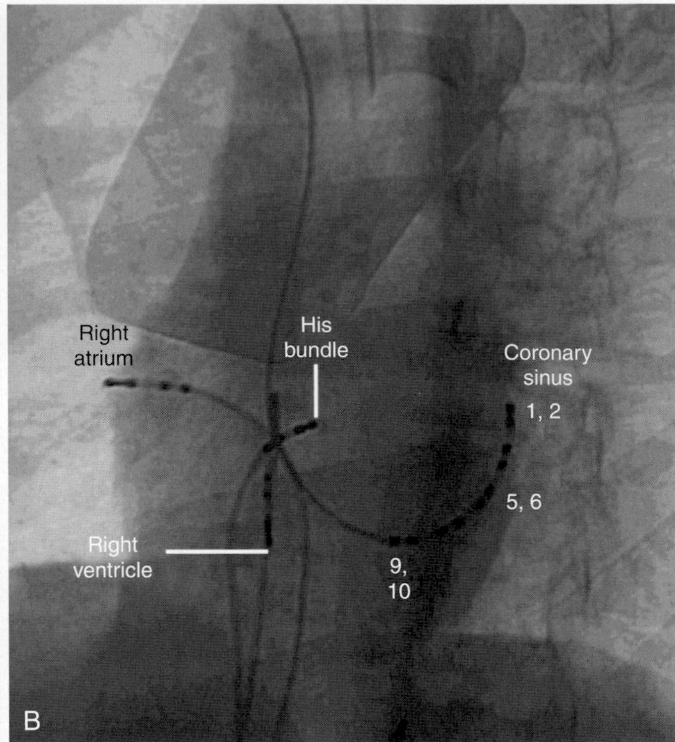

Figure 19-2 Catheter electrodes positioned in the high right atrium, right ventricular apex, site of the His bundle, and coronary sinus (poles labelled). The fluoroscopic views are frontal (**A**), left anterior (**B**), and right anterior (**C**) orientations.

Tachycardia Mapping

Mapping of the site of origin of the tachycardia, or of sites critical to maintenance of a re-entry circuit, is necessary for planning interventions to interrupt the tachycardia. One or more of the following methods are used for this purpose.

Activation Mapping

During ectopic tachycardias, an electrode catheter is moved to find an intracardiac electrogram with an onset that is earlier than that of any other intracardiac or surface electrogram. The earliest onset atrial or ventricular electrogram

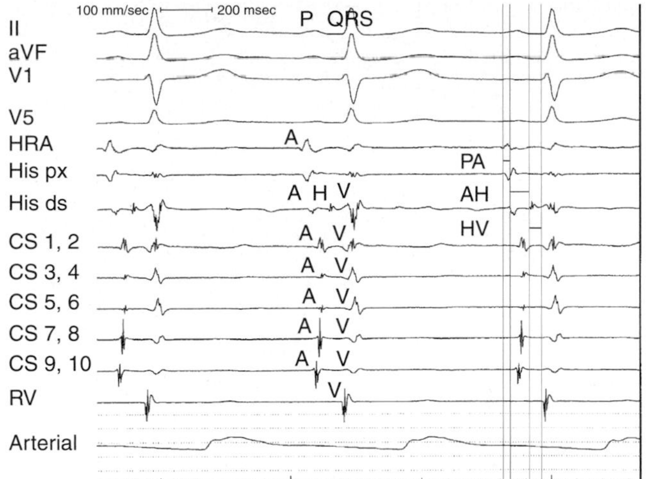

Figure 19-3 Intracardiac and surface electrograms. CS, coronary sinus poles 1–10; HRA, high right atrium; H, His (proximal and distal); RV, right ventricle.

will be found close to the site of origin of an ectopic atrial or ventricular focus. For tachycardias using an accessory pathway, the earliest onset of a retrograde atrial electrogram or antegrade ventricular electrogram on the atrioventricular groove will be at the site of the accessory pathway. It may be possible to determine this during sinus rhythm, in atrial or ventricular pacing, or during re-entry tachycardia, depending on the characteristics of the pathway.

Electroanatomic Mapping

In recent years, electroanatomic mapping systems have become more widely used, in conjunction with traditional fluoroscopy and activation mapping. These systems utilise electromagnetic fields to identify the location of a catheter in three-dimensional space. Using these systems the anatomy of the area of interest can be mapped, and location of catheters tracked. Ideally these systems will offer better definition of anatomic substrate, and reduce fluoroscopy times. Once the anatomy is defined, colour-based timing maps can be created and superimposed on the anatomical map (Fig. 19-4).

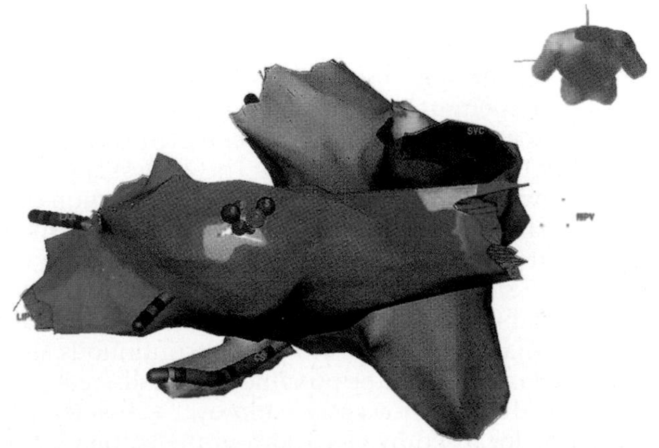

Figure 19-4 Electroanatomical map of an ectopic atrial tachycardia. The white area indicates the earliest timing at the roof of the left atrium, while colours red to purple indicate later and later timing. The yellow ball shows the site of successful ablation.

Pace Mapping

During sinus rhythm, an electrode catheter is used to pace from different sites until the paced pattern on the surface 12-lead electrocardiogram and the intracardiac electrogram are identical to that seen during the tachycardia. This method is used when an atrial or ventricular tachycardia is not sustained for sufficiently long to use activation mapping, or if a ventricular tachycardia is not sufficiently well tolerated haemodynamically.

Entrainment Mapping

Entrainment mapping is used for re-entrant circuits in the atrium or ventricle where the tachycardia is maintained by an area of slow conduction. Pacing at a rate just faster than the tachycardia will entrain the tachycardia so that the paced beat is conducted around the circuit slightly earlier than the next beat of the tachycardia circuit would have done. Manifest entrainment occurs when the pacing site is remote from the area of slow conduction of the tachycardia circuit. The intracardiac and surface leads will reveal a fusion pattern composed of the paced beat and the preceding beat that is emerging from the area of slow conduction. Concealed entrainment is inferred when the intracardiac and surface leads demonstrate identical electrograms to that of the tachycardia. This implies that the pacing electrode is close to the site of slow conduction. This site is critical for maintenance of the tachycardia and provides a target for interruption of the circuit. Observation of the events immediately after pacing is terminated also help to locate the critical site of slow conduction.[79–81]

Administration of Drugs during Catheterisation

When it is difficult to induce an arrhythmia in the basal state, sympathomimetics, such as isoprenaline (isoproterenol) given as a bolus or an infusion, are used to initiate or reduce the threshold for the arrhythmia. Further information on the mechanism of the arrhythmia may be obtained by administering drugs during pacing and/or tachycardia. Adenosine is a short-lived inhibitor of atrioventricular nodal conduction and is particularly useful. Verapamil is used to produce more sustained atrioventricular block. Atropine and propranolol are given together to produce autonomic blockade. Disopyramide is used to expose impairment of atrioventricular nodal conduction, ajmaline or procainamide to abolish conduction down an accessory pathway, and flecainide to terminate atrial fibrillation.[82,83] These antiarrhythmic agents, however, have more sustained effects than adenosine. While providing additional information, they may interfere with the remainder of the study. Some of these medications are also used in the diagnosis of inherited arrhythmias, described previously in this chapter.

Indications for Ablation

The indications for ablation have evolved since its introduction, with expansion of the arrhythmic substrates to which it is applied. This has led to a significant fall in the use of anti-tachycardia pacemakers and antiarrhythmic surgery. The threshold for intervention has also fallen, and patients who were previously well or could be controlled on medication, now undergo radio-frequency ablation in preference to chronic antiarrhythmic medication.[84] It is still not considered by many as first-line therapy in children weighing less than 15 kg, because the rate of complications is higher, and many of these children will lose the tendency to continued tachycardias with aging.[85]

ARRHYTHMIAS

Atrioventricular Re-entry Tachycardia

Atrioventricular re-entry tachycardia due to an accessory atrioventricular pathway is the commonest cause of tachyarrhythmia in the fetus, and in early childhood.[86] A minority are associated with hydrops fetalis, fetal death, or heart failure in the neonatal period. Infants presenting with supraventricular tachycardias should be evaluated for possible tachycardia-induced cardiomyopathy, as the duration of the arrhythmia is generally unknown; it is essential to confirm cardiac function prior to initiation of medications with potential negative inotropic effects, such as many of the antiarrhythmic medications. In addition echocardiography should be performed in all patients who have supraventricular tachycardia to identify structural lesions associated with accessory pathways. Some of these may be clinically silent and include Ebstein's malformation, congenitally corrected transposition, myocardial tumours, and hypertrophic and dilated cardiomyopathy.

In older children, symptomatic tachycardias are the usual presentation. Approximately one-third will have evidence of pre-excitation, with a delta wave on the surface electrocardiogram, indicating an overt accessory pathway. In the remainder the pathway is concealed. In these patients only retrograde conduction occurs, from the ventricle to the atrium, thus no change in depolarisation of the ventricle is seen in sinus rhythm. In the majority of children, the tachycardia is easily controlled with drugs. Many neonates and infants will be free from arrhythmias by the age of 1 year, without the need for medication. However, 30% to 50% do not outgrow the tendency to recurrent tachyarrhythmias, and of those who do, a small proportion have a recurrence in later childhood.[87] When tachycardias persist over the age of 5 years, about four-fifths continue to experience intermittent symptomatic tachycardias into adulthood.[88]

Arrhythmic Substrate

The accessory pathway permits retrograde conduction from the ventricle to the atrium; consequently a re-entry circuit can be established (Fig. 19-5). An early atrial extrasystole is conducted slowly down the atrioventricular node to the His–Purkinje system and ventricle; it returns to the atrium over the accessory pathway. If the atrioventricular node has recovered and is no longer refractory, then a circus movement tachycardia, also known as re-entry tachycardia or reciprocating tachycardia, can be established. A ventricular extrasystole can also trigger tachycardia in this situation, via retrograde conduction up the accessory pathway into the atrium, with the retrograde P wave then being conducted anterograde across the atrioventricular node. Following ventricular depolarisation, there is conduction back up the accessory pathway, and the tachycardia is initiated.

Histology of the accessory pathways shows that they are composed of abnormal myocardium that crosses the atrioventricular groove. They have been found around the left atrioventricular groove at the level of attachment of the mural leaflet of the mitral valve, and around the right atrioventricular groove at the level of attachment of all three tricuspid valvar leaflets. There is no atrioventricular

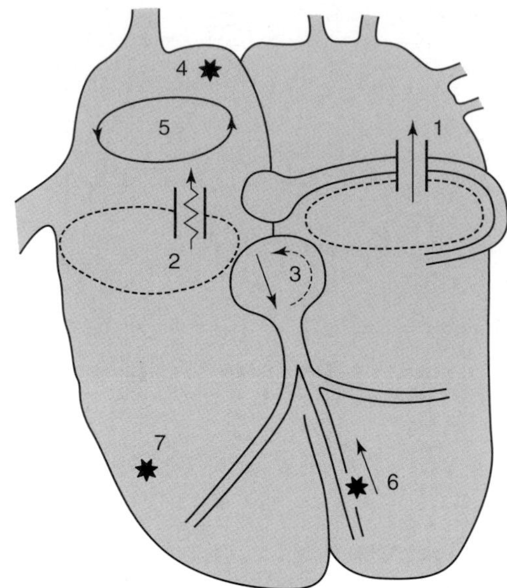

Figure 19-5 Substrates for arrhythmias that may be amenable to ablation: (1) unidirectional concealed accessory pathway; (2) slowly conducting accessory pathway, such as permanent junctional reciprocating tachycardia; (3) atrioventricular nodal re-entrant tachycardia; (4) focal atrial tachycardia; (5) intra-atrial re-entrant tachycardia; (6) fascicular tachycardia; and (7) ventricular tachycardias

junction around the aortic leaflet of the mitral valve where it joins the aortic valve. The right atrioventricular groove is thicker because of infolding of the atrial myocardium at the tricuspid valvar origin. In one-tenth of patients, there are multiple accessory pathways. Accessory pathways may be described as right-sided, left-sided, or septal, and as superior, inferior, or lateral (Fig. 19-6).[89]

Electrophysiological Findings

Atrioventricular re-entry tachycardia can be induced with atrial and ventricular extrasystoles or by pacing manoeuvres. During atrioventricular re-entry tachycardia, the earliest retrograde atrial electrogram will be detected at the atrial origin of the accessory pathway rather than at the atrioventricular node. During ventricular pacing, there may be fusion between retrograde conduction via the accessory pathway and atrioventricular node. Adenosine can be used to block the conduction through the node, thus exposing conduction via the accessory pathway, although a small percentage of accessory pathways are also adenosine sensitive. When overt pre-excitation is present, incremental atrial pacing may increase the degree of pre-excitation due to normal decrement in the atrioventricular node conduction time. Pre-excitation can also be accentuated by atrial pacing close to the accessory pathway. The earliest site of ventricular activation will be at the ventricular insertion of the accessory pathway. The ventricular electrogram frequently will be seen 10 to 30 msec prior to the onset of the delta wave on the surface electrocardiogram. At the site of the accessory pathway, there may be fusion between the atrial and ventricular electrograms to form a continuous signal. In some instances, it may be possible to see a discrete potential generated by the accessory pathway.[90] Left-sided pathways can be localised by electrodes in the coronary sinus; detailed mapping is performed using catheters moved around the atrioventricular ring. Accessory pathways that are close to the His bundle (para-Hisian pathways) may

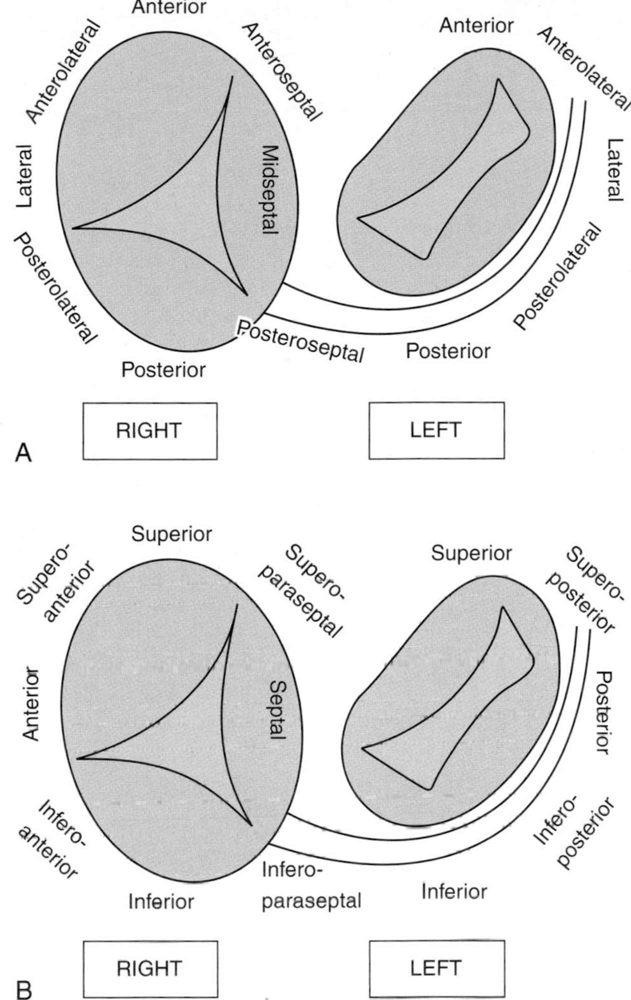

Figure 19-6 Diagram of the locations of accessory pathways comparing (A) the traditional surgical perspective and (B) an attitudinally correct nomenclature, as proposed by Cosio and colleagues.

be more difficult to differentiate from conduction via the atrioventricular node. Some accessory pathways have properties of decremental conduction and may be adenosine-sensitive, making differentiation from the atrioventricular node challenging at times.

Ablation

Left-sided pathways are accessed either via an antegrade or retrograde approach. The antegrade approach uses a patent oval foramen or requires a trans-septal puncture to place lesions on the atrial side of the atrioventricular ring. The retrograde transarterial approach requires the catheter to cross the aortic valve and be looped up under the leaflets of the mitral valve for delivery of lesions on the ventricular side of the ring. Using this route, it is also possible to cross the mitral valve and apply the lesions on the atrial side. Ablation is guided anatomically and electrographically by placing a multi-polar electrode catheter in the coronary sinus. This allows the ablation catheter to be aimed at the poles in which the earliest activation is detected (Fig. 19-7). Right-sided and septal pathways are usually approached from the inferior caval vein, though occasionally approach via the superior caval vein is required. Lesions are usually placed on the atrial side of the atrioventricular ring or in the mouth of the coronary sinus, but it may be necessary to loop the catheter in the right ventricle to ablate on the ventricular side of the atrioventricular ring. A diverticulum of the mouth of the coronary sinus is occasionally found, and an accessory pathway may run in the floor of the diverticulum, which can be identified with angiography. The ablation catheter is placed on the atrioventricular ring and moved around its circumference to identify the earliest activation. In difficult cases, where delivery of energy at the site of the earliest activation is ineffective, an intracoronary electrode catheter can be used. The catheter defines the right coronary artery, and thereby the right atrioventricular groove, and also provides electrograms so that a stable reference electrogram at the site of earliest activation can be identified to guide the ablation catheter (Fig. 19-8). The existence of additional accessory pathways that can sustain arrhythmias may only become apparent after successful ablation of the first pathway; these will also be ablated at the same procedure if possible. Mapping is always more challenging when multiple pathways are present, due to the potential for fused or figure-of-eight conduction (in which the impulse travels alternately between the two pathways, sometimes suggested by alternating tachycardia cycle length).

Ablation of left-sided pathways has a success rate of more than 90% in most centres, and the success rate increases with experience. Right-sided pathways are technically more challenging. Placement of catheters on the right atrioventricular junction is less stable and some pathways are epicardial. Nonetheless, success rates are generally above 80%. The use of long sheaths to stabilise the catheter may be helpful. Septal and paraseptal pathways can also be ablated with a high degree of success, but this does carry a risk of complete heart block owing to inadvertent damage to the atrioventricular node and bundle of His. Some centres advocate the usage of cryoablation in these situations, due to the potential reversibility of lesions. A high rate of success has also been reported in infants and neonates with intractable re-entry tachycardias, but with higher rates of complications, including major complications.[91–94] Ablation in the infant should be reserved for those with medically refractory life-threatening arrhythmias likely to respond to ablation.

Other Types of Accessory Pathways

Mahaim Fibres

Structures similar to the atrioventricular node are occasionally found in the anterolateral right atrium adjacent to the atrioventricular ring.[95–97] They usually connect to the right bundle branch, or to the right ventricle in the vicinity of the moderator band. These so-called atriofascicular accessory pathways mediate Mahaim-type physiology, conducting predominantly in an antegrade fashion, with a left bundle branch pattern in tachycardia. Retrograde conduction is through the atrioventricular node or an additional conventional accessory pathway. They demonstrate decremental conduction similar to that of the atrioventricular node, and they give rise to a Mahaim potential that is similar to a His bundle potential during atrial pacing. They are thought to arise from remnants of the ring of conduction tissue that surrounds the atrioventricular junction during early fetal development. Ablation can be performed at the

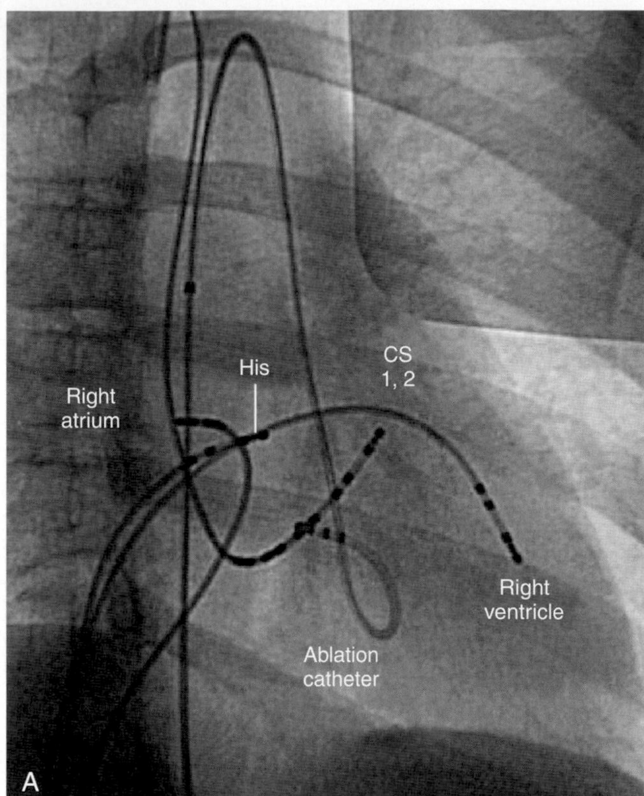

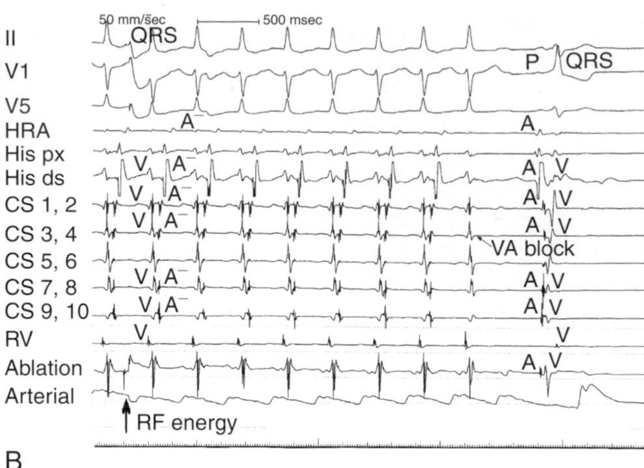

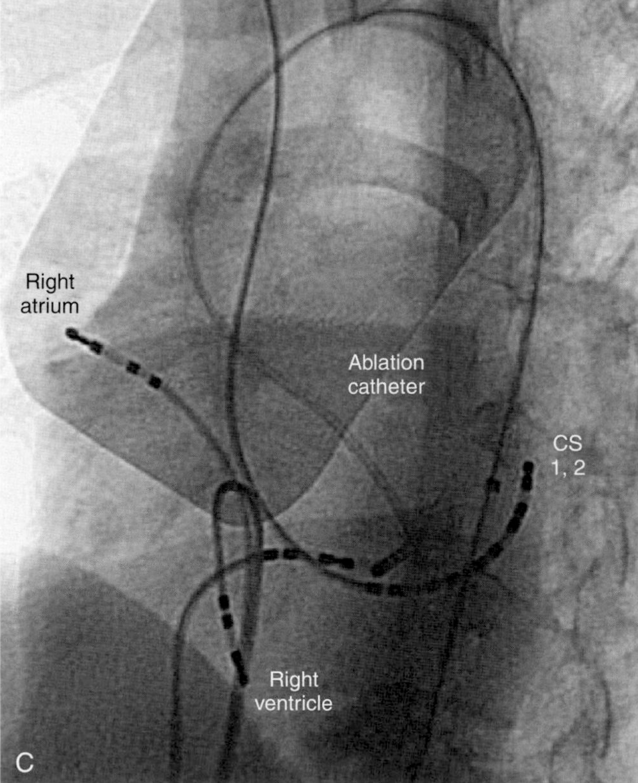

Figure 19-7 Ablation of a left-sided accessory pathway. Fluoroscopy in left anterior (**A**) and right anterior (**C**) oblique projections. **B**, Electrograms recorded during ablation with abolition of conduction across the accessory pathway. CS, coronary sinus; HRA, high right atrium; RF, radio-frequency; RV, right ventricle.

atrioventricular ring, or anywhere along the pathway up until its point of insertion within the ventricle.[98–101]

A much rarer accessory pathway is one that is acquired after surgical manoeuvres that connect the atrial myocardium to the ventricle, as in the earlier variants of the Fontan operation. These pathways between the atrial appendage and right ventricular outflow tract can also be ablated successfully.[56,102] Equally rarely, congenital muscular pathways can be found between the right atrial appendage and the supraventricular crest of the right ventricle.[103,104]

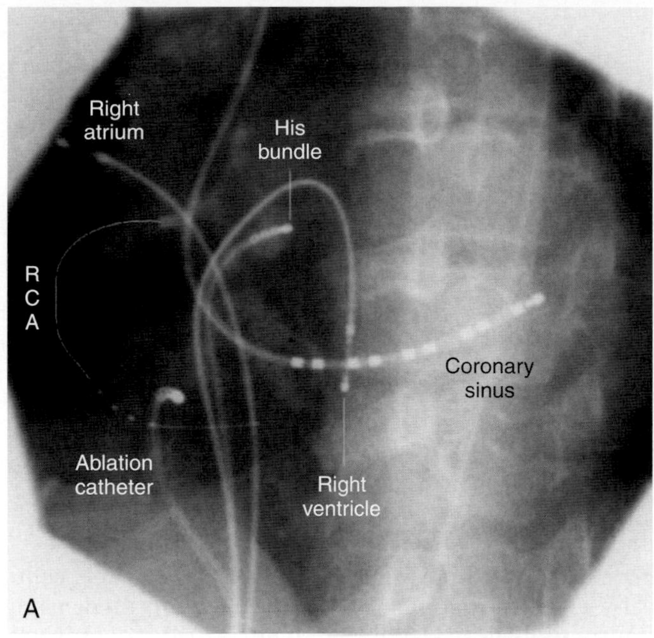

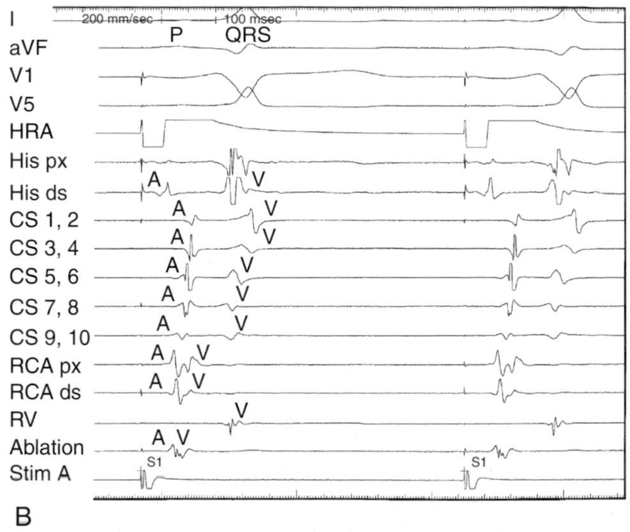

Figure 19-8 A, 2 French quadripolar electrode in the right coronary artery (RCA) through a coronary guide catheter to assist ablation of a right-sided manifest accessory pathway after a previous attempt had failed. **B**, Electrograms from surface and intracardiac leads show that the shortest atrioventricular conduction time is at the distal pair of electrodes on the catheter within the right coronary artery. The ablation catheter shows continuous atrioventricular signals at the site of successful ablation. CS, coronary sinus; HRA, high right atrium; RV, right ventricle.

Wolff–Parkinson–White Syndrome

Electrocardiographical evidence of manifest accessory atrioventricular pathways is found in up to 3 of every 1000 of the population.[105,106] The incidence is increased in family members, and in those with a congenitally malformed heart, especially Ebstein's malformation and congenitally corrected transposition.[107,108] These allow pre-excitation of parts of the ventricle before the normal impulse can arrive via the His–Purkinje system. When more myocardium is pre-excited, a wider QRS complex and more overt delta wave is seen. The pattern of the delta wave and QRS complexes can be used to identify into which portion of the ventricle the accessory pathway inserts. A number of algorithms have been developed. These algorithms correlate reasonably, though not absolutely, with the findings at electrophysiologic study.[109–112] When multiple pathways are present, or pre-excitation is only partial or intermittent, the electrocardiographic pattern can vary, making localisation from the surface recordings impossible. Right-sided pathways are more common in patients with congenital heart disease, and the algorithms are much less accurate in these patients.[113,114]

Atrioventricular re-entry tachycardia is possible because of retrograde conduction across the pathway, but not all Wolff–Parkinson–White pathways are capable of sustaining such tachycardias, due to weak or nonexistent retrograde conduction. Many patients are therefore asymptomatic, and the diagnosis is often established as an incidental finding when an electrocardiogram is performed for another reason. Patients with a delta wave and symptoms of palpitations or documented tachycardia have Wolff–Parkinson–White syndrome, while those with an asymptomatic delta wave have only the electrocardiographic phenomena of Wolff–Parkinson–White.

By definition, the manifest pathways are capable of antegrade conduction from the atrium to the ventricle. Occasionally, an antidromic circus movement tachycardia is set up with antegrade conduction down the accessory pathway and retrograde conduction via the atrioventricular node or a second accessory pathway. Pre-excitation of the ventricles in this rhythm results in a broad complex tachycardia, due to all ventricular activation occurring via the accessory pathway. Those patients who demonstrate this form of tachycardia usually also have typical orthodromic tachycardia.

Risk of Sudden Death

Wolff–Parkinson–White patients are at higher risk than the general population of developing atrial fibrillation, which may be conducted rapidly to the ventricle bypassing the atrioventricular node. This results in a broad complex irregular tachycardia. If the atrial fibrillation is conducted at a very rapid rate, then the ventricles may not be able to maintain cardiac output and even more rapid conduction can cause the ventricle to fibrillate. These patients can present with syncope or out of hospital arrest and sudden death.[115] Pre-excited atrial fibrillation or Wolff–Parkinson–White with syncope is an indication for ablation, as these patients are known to be at higher risk of ventricular fibrillation and sudden death.

Controversies in Management

There are no absolute predictors of a benign or malignant prognosis in asymptomatic patients with Wolff–Parkinson–White syndrome. Intermittent episodes, with sudden loss of the delta wave on exercise or after administration of class I antiarrhythmic drugs, suggests a benign prognosis, as pathways with this feature tend not to be able to conduct very rapidly.[82,116] The onset of symptoms, palpitations, or tachycardia suggests that the risk of sudden death is increased. When syncope is a symptom, then there is a very real risk of sudden death. Sudden death or out-of-hospital cardiac arrest can, however, be the first symptom in the previously asymptomatic patient. For this reason,

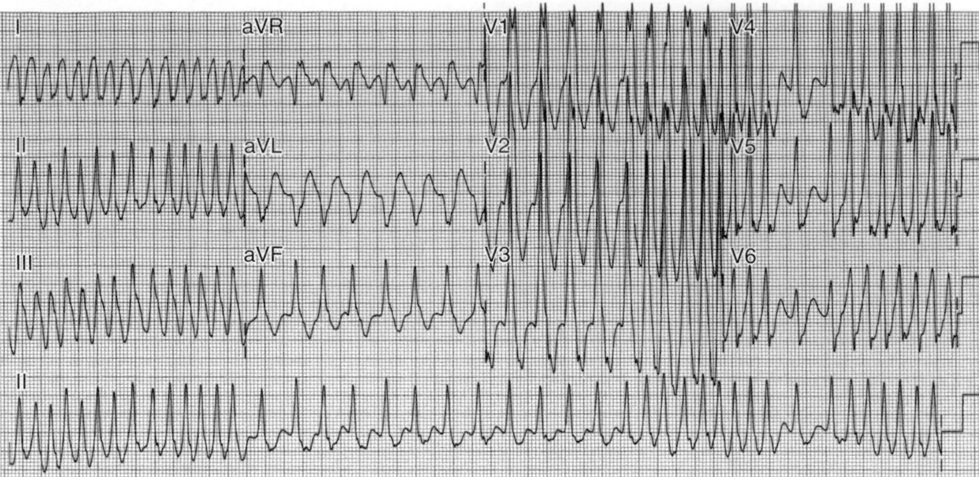

Figure 19-9 Pre-excited atrial fibrillation with extremely rapid conduction to the ventricle, consistent with a high risk Wolff–Parkinson–White accessory pathway.

attempts have been made to identify those asymptomatic patients at increased risk.

During an electrophysiological study, rapid atrial pacing is used to induce atrial fibrillation. If atrial fibrillation can be induced, the shortest interval between two pre-excited beats is measured. Intervals less than 220 msec, indicating a rate of 270 beats per minute, are defined as very rapid conduction over the pathway, thus identifying high-risk pathways. If atrial fibrillation is not able to be induced, then the antegrade effective refractory period is measured during rapid atrial pacing, though this may be less predictive than that measured during atrial fibrillation[115] (Fig. 19-9). Most patients who present with syncope or cardiac arrest demonstrate very rapid conduction over the accessory pathway. Asymptomatic patients, or those with tachycardia without syncope or cardiac arrest, may also demonstrate such rapid conduction. So, while slow conduction may identify a group at low risk, rapid conduction does not necessarily identify the patients at high risk.[116] Nevertheless, routine electrophysiological testing to distinguish between rapid and slow conductors is performed in many laboratories. Those found to have rapid conduction can be offered an ablation, accepting that not all are at high risk. It is also important to note that accessory pathway conduction rates under sedation or anaesthesia may not completely reflect those seen while awake or during exercise. When the pathway is located away from the septum, this can be performed at low risk of the complication of heart block and with a high rate of success. Ablation of pathways that are close to the septum carry a small but definite risk of complete atrioventricular block and the need for a permanent pacemaker. Pathways in the inferior paraseptal area, however, are also thought to potentially carry a greater risk of sudden death.[117]

The risk of sudden death is around 1 per 1000 patient-years of follow-up with the syndrome, while the mortality of ablation is similar (Table 19-1).[118,119] Therefore, the argument is finely balanced, and some centres do not offer electrophysiological study and ablation to asymptomatic patients. Electrophysiological study and ablation are easier to recommend in individuals undertaking extreme exertion or in those requiring a license to fly, or other occupations in which those with pre-excitation are excluded. In asymptomatic children, an electrophysiological study is often recommended in adolescence, but sudden death has also been reported in young children.[120,121] In some centres, early electrophysiological studies are performed, using a transoesophageal electrode. There is still no universally accepted policy, and the controversy remains.[122,123]

Atrioventricular Nodal Re-entry Tachycardia

Atrioventricular nodal re-entry tachycardia is an uncommon arrhythmia in the first year of life; it becomes more frequent with increasing age thereafter.

Arrhythmic Substrate

The anatomic substrate is the presence of dual atrioventricular nodal pathways, which allow a re-entry circuit to form in the atrioventricular node, for example, after an atrial

TABLE 19-1

RESULTS OF THREE LARGE MULTI-CENTRIC STUDIES OF RADIO-FREQUENCY ABLATION

	MERFS*	AMIG†	PES‡
Patients			
Age group	Adult	Adult and paediatric	Paediatric
Number of patients	4398	1050	3277
Number of procedures	n/a	1136	3653
Success Rates			
Accessory pathways	n/a	93%	91%
Nodal re-entry tachycardia	n/a	97%	96%
Complications			
Death	5 (0.11%)	3 (0.3%)	4 (0.11%)
Complete heart block	57 (1.6%)§	10 (1%)	25 (0.7%)
Tamponade or effusion	44 (1.0%)	26 (2.5%)	24 (0.7%)
Thromboembolism	28 (0.6%)	7 (0.7%)	8 (0.22%)

n/a, not available

*MERFS, Multicentre European Radiofrequency Survey.[132] Complication rates published with reference to success rates.

†AMIG, ATAKR Multicentre Investigators Group.[133]

‡PES, Pediatric Electrophysiology Society of North America.[84,85] Patients were aged below 21 years, with supraventricular tachycardia and no structural heart disease.

§Excludes 900 patients who underwent ablation of the atrioventricular node to produce complete heart block Includes a significant proportion of ablations of the fast pathway for nodal re-entry techycardia.

extrasystole. Typical nodal re-entry occurs when antegrade conduction across the atrioventricular node is blocked in a more rapid conduction region, called the fast pathway, and then conducts slowly down a region of slower conduction, called the slow pathway. By the time the impulse has crossed the atrioventricular node, the fast pathway has recovered and is no longer refractory. The impulse is then able to conduct back up the atrioventricular node retrograde to the atrium. The slow pathway has then recovered and conducts antegrade down the atrioventricular node (Fig. 19-10), and thus the tachycardia is propagated. These pathways are well defined electrophysiologically, but not so clearly histologically. The slow pathway is associated with the junction of working atrial myocardium, atrial transitional cells, and the inferior extension from the compact atrioventricular node in the area of the septal isthmus at the base of Koch's triangle.[124,125] The fast pathway is usually located more anteriorly near the apex of the triangle of Koch and is associated with transitional atrial cells in that area. The arrhythmia is usually well-tolerated haemodynamically, but can be recurrent and symptomatically poorly tolerated. Atrioventricular nodal blocking drugs, such as digoxin, beta blockers, and verapamil, will usually suppress the arrhythmia, but the ability to cure it by ablation is appealing.[126,127]

Electrophysiological Findings

At electrophysiological study, the typical finding during timed atrial extrastimulation is the presence of a jump in the atrioventricular conduction times when the fast pathway blocks and conduction occurs down the slow pathway. This is seen as a sudden extension in the atrial to His bundle electrogram interval of more than 50 msec in adults. This may then be followed by an echo beat, owing to retrograde conduction up the fast pathway to the atrium, which often sets off the tachycardia. The presence of dual atrioventricular nodal physiology is more common than re-entry and tachycardia, and at electrophysiological studies it must be confirmed that

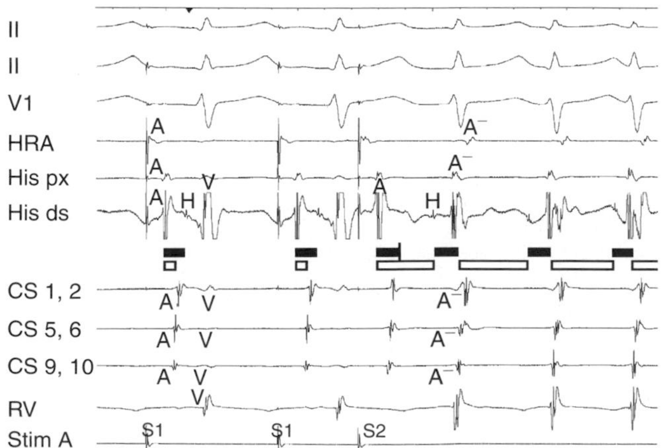

Figure 19-10 Induction of atrioventricular nodal re-entry tachycardia using a drive train (S1) and a single atrial extrastimulus (S2). The solid bar indicates conduction down the fast pathway and the hollow bar indicates conduction down the slow pathway. During the drive train, conduction form the atrium to His bundle is via the fast pathway. After the extrastimulus (S2), the fast pathway is blocked and conduction proceeds down the slow pathway to the His bundle (AH jump). At this point the fast pathway has recovered and conducts retrograde so that the A and V are superimposed in the His bundle electrode and a retrograde A is detected in the high right atrium and coronary sinus leads. Antegrade conduction is via the slow pathway and a re-entry tachycardia follows. CS, coronary sinus; HRA, high right atrium; RV, right ventricle.

the tachycardia is caused by re-entry within the node before undertaking an ablation. Dual atrioventricular nodal physiology may be present when there is another arrhythmic substrate that is responsible for the clinical tachycardia. This is particularly true in children, where dual atrioventricular nodal physiology is seen in as many as one-third of all children. Nodal re-entry may only be induced with rapid pacing or after administration of isoprenaline. The tachycardia can also occasionally be induced with ventricular extrastimulation or pacing, but much less frequently.

Ablation

Lesions are delivered into the septal isthmus at the base of the triangle of Koch to ablate the slow pathway. Some are guided by electrograms that reveal so-called slow pathway potentials, while others are guided by the anatomical landmarks alone.[128,129] During delivery of radio-frequency energy in the septal isthmus, accelerated junctional beats are a good indicator that energy is being delivered at the correct site, although this may not be essential for eventual success.[130] It is important to observe closely for any evidence of damage to atrioventricular conduction, as there is a small risk of inadvertent complete atrioventricular block. When a successful ablation has been achieved, it is no longer possible to initiate tachycardia, even though a jump and even an echo beat may remain. The procedure has an acute success rate approaching 100%, with greater than 90% long-term freedom from recurrence. In adults, persistence of the slow pathway appears to be a risk factor for recurrence.[131] There is a small risk of creating complete atrioventricular block.[84,132,133] This risk is likely significantly less if cryoablation is used; however, the recurrence rate may be higher. Some centres have chosen to use cryoablation exclusively for this diagnosis in children, while others still find the higher recurrence rate unacceptable. In small children weighing less than 15 kg, the triangle of Koch has dimensions similar to that of a single radio-frequency lesion and the margin for error is, therefore, smaller.[134] Ablation of the fast pathway carries a higher risk of inadvertent complete atrioventricular block, this complication occurring in up to one-tenth of patients even in experienced centres. Because of this, it is now rarely performed.[135]

Ectopic Atrial Tachycardia

Ectopic atrial tachycardias can arise from foci in either atrium. It may present at any age from fetal life onwards. It is a relatively uncommon arrhythmia but when incessant can cause a rate-related tachycardiomyopathy.

Arrhythmic Substrate

The arrhythmia is caused by an automatic focus in the atrium, which may be intermittent or incessant. During tachycardia, the surface P wave indicates the site of origin, with inverted P waves in inferior leads indicating a low right atrial tachycardia, while inverted P waves in lead I suggest a left atrial origin. Tachycardias that originate close to the sinus node, such as on the crista terminalis, can be extremely difficult to differentiate from sinus tachycardia. The tachycardia may be transmitted to the ventricles in a 1:1 fashion, but atrioventricular block of varying degrees is often present, or can be produced by vagal stimulation or adenosine without terminating the tachycardia. Some atrial tachycardias, however, are terminated by adenosine or may slow and then accelerate as the adenosine is metabolised.

Electrophysiological Findings

Timed atrial extrastimulation is not able to start or stop most ectopic atrial tachycardias reproducibly, as they are automatic in nature, in contrast to atrioventricular re-entrant tachycardias. Occasionally these arrhythmias can be triggered, and rapid atrial pacing may initiate such tachycardias. More frequently the rhythm is catecholamine sensitive, and an infusion of isoprenaline may be helpful for initiation. The tachycardia characteristically speeds up as it starts, and slows before termination, usually described as a warm-up and cool-down. It is frequently difficult to initiate the tachycardia under general anaesthesia, and consideration should be given to performing the procedure using sedation and local anaesthesia. Post-operative ectopic atrial tachycardia can be associated with a variety of congenital heart disease repairs, and appears to be most frequently seen in sicker cyanotic children, although the aetiology is multi-factorial. In the post-operative setting, this rhythm can be haemodynamically compromising, requiring multiple medications, but usually will resolve spontaneously.[136]

Ablation

Left-sided foci, often near the pulmonary veins, are approached via the atrial septum either using a patent oval foramen or a trans-septal puncture, while right-sided foci are generally approached from the inferior caval vein. The ablation catheter is placed at the site of the earliest activation in the atrium that occurs before any other intracardiac atrial electrograms and the surface P waves. At the site of the focus, there may be very early local activation and/or fractionation of the atrial signal. Pacing from the site of origin will produce surface P waves identical to that from the tachycardia, and identical patterns of atrial activation in the intracardiac electrodes. Radio-frequency ablation can be performed with 75% to 90% success.[137,138] The use of multi-electrode techniques may facilitate mapping in difficult cases.[139]

Chaotic Atrial Tachycardia

Chaotic atrial tachycardia is an atrial tachycardia related to abnormal impulse formation where not one, but many atrial foci fire prematurely (at least three atrial foci are required to make the diagnosis). It can be an incessant tachycardia, and thus monitoring for tachycardia-mediated cardiomyopathy is necessary. It has a different natural history than the similar multi-focal atrial tachycardia, which is an adult arrhythmia commonly in association with pulmonary disease. In children it can be seen in those with structurally normal hearts as well as those with congenital cardiac anomalies and hypertrophic cardiomyopathy. It can be a severe arrhythmia, which may be difficult to control even with multiple antiarrhythmic medications. However, following the acute phase of the disease (variable but often 1 to 2 years) spontaneous resolution can be seen in more than half the patients.[140] Ablation is not a good option, due to the multiple foci, and rate control, rather than achieving sinus rhythm, should be the goal of therapy.[78]

Permanent Junctional Reciprocating Tachycardia

An important pattern to note on the surface electrocardiogram in some supraventricular tachycardias is a long RP interval. In permanent junctional reciprocating tachycardia, the P wave is of an abnormal morphology (a retrograde P wave) and closer to the succeeding R wave than the preceding R wave. This is different from nodal re-entry tachycardia, where the P wave is buried or very close to the QRS complex, or atrioventricular re-entry tachycardia, where the P wave is closer to the preceding R wave than to the successive R wave (Fig. 19-11). The long RP pattern results from a slowly conducting concealed accessory pathway, giving the persistent form of junctional reciprocating tachycardia. The differential diagnosis of these long RP tachycardias also includes atypical nodal re-entry where antegrade conduction is down the fast pathway and retrograde conduction is via the slow pathway, or an ectopic atrial tachycardia. However, the most common mechanism in children is the persistent or permanent reciprocating tachycardia caused by a slowly conducting concealed accessory pathway with decremental properties. Such pathways are most commonly found in an inferior paraseptal position and give rise to inverted P waves in the inferior leads of the surface electrocardiogram.[141,142] Occasionally there may be multiple pathways.

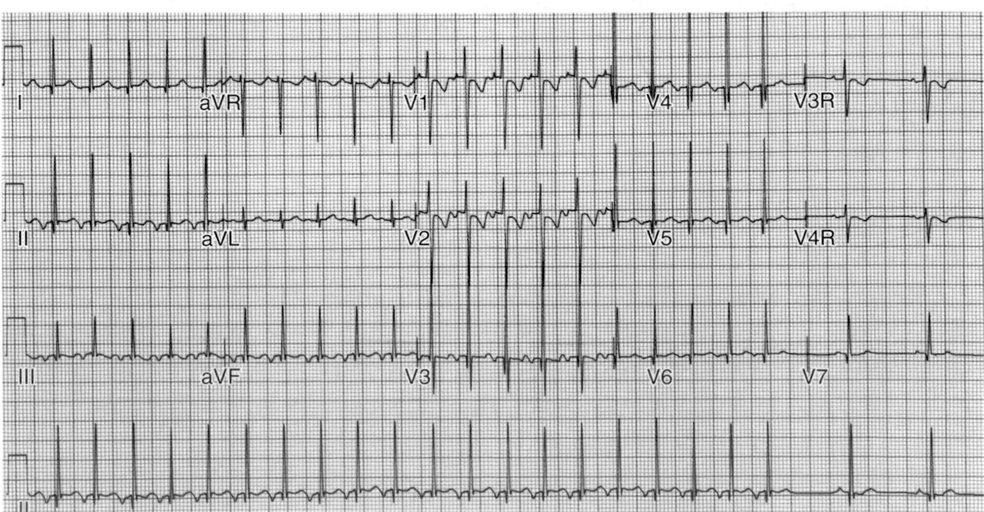

Figure 19-11 A run of permanent junctional reciprocating tachycardia with typical long RP interval and retrograde atrial activation, which breaks to sinus on the second-last beat of the tracing.

Permanent junctional reciprocating tachycardia is often incessant. When the rate is not very fast, it can be mistaken for a sinus tachycardia unless note is taken of the abnormal morphology of the P waves. The rate-related tachycardiomyopathy may then be incorrectly ascribed to myocarditis or a post-viral dilated cardiomyopathy. While antiarrhythmic medication can suppress this tachycardia, it is often difficult to control, requires multiple medications, and usually recurs after withdrawing medication. Radio-frequency ablation is especially rewarding as it effects a cure and allows cardiac function to return to normal in those patients with tachycardia-mediated cardiomyopathy.[94,143]

Atrial Flutter

Atrial flutter is an uncommon tachycardia in childhood, though it can be seen in fetal life and the newborn period. In the neonate, after return to sinus rhythm, it rarely recurs. Conversion to sinus rhythm can be accomplished via oesophageal overdrive atrial pacing, which is highly successful in the infant.[42] In rare cases it will terminate spontaneously, and even less often will require direct cardioversion. Atrial flutter can also be seen as part of the spectrum of chaotic atrial tachycardia. In older children with structurally normal hearts, atrial flutter is an unusual arrhythmia, and may be associated with sick sinus syndrome. In congenital heart disease causing right atrial dilation, it may occur either before or after surgery and can cause additional symptoms and morbidity in its own right. Atrial flutter often responds poorly to prophylactic medication.

Arrhythmic Substrate

Early experimental studies have shown that in atrial flutter there is a macro re-entrant wavefront circulating around the atria.[144] Type I flutter, with negative P waves in the inferior leads, results from a circulating wavefront that passes around the tricuspid valvar orifice and up the terminal crest in a counter-clockwise direction. The hinge of the tricuspid valve forms the anterior boundary, while the posterior border of the circuit is formed by the junction of the inferior and superior caval veins with the terminal crest.[145] Elegant entrainment studies have shown that there is often an area of slow conduction between the inferior caval vein and the tricuspid orifice, which slows conduction and prevents the wavefront from reaching a refractory portion of the circuit before it has recovered.[146] This is also anatomically the narrowest portion of the circuit and is known as cavotricuspid, or inferior, isthmus. The causes of the delay are not clear.

Ablation

Ablation can be used in this condition by creating a line of block between any of the boundaries that constrain the circulating wavefront.[147–150] Typically, a line of block created at the inferior isthmus is enough to prevent the arrhythmia. At this site, the distance between the boundaries is short and can be defined using radiographic and electrophysiological markers. In some centres, it is routine to use a halo catheter with 20 separate electrodes, which are placed in a ring around the tricuspid valve in the right atrium. This enables the activation sequence of the atrial flutter to be determined and also assists in deciding when an adequate line of block has been created. By pacing from the lower right atrium and the coronary sinus in turn, and observing the activation sequence according to the halo and coronary sinus electrodes, it is possible to detect when bidirectional block has been created, as no conduction is then possible in either direction across the isthmus. The procedure can be simplified by using a smaller 10-pole catheter extending along the anterolateral right atrium to the isthmus, which still allows determination of bidirectional block[151] If this approach is not successful, lines of block can be created between the coronary sinus and the inferior caval vein, and between the coronary sinus and the tricuspid valve. More recently, it has been shown that the necessary lines can be created with greater accuracy using an electroanatomical mapping system.[152–155]

Variants of Atrial Flutter

Atypical flutter, or type II flutter, is found when the wavefront moves in a clockwise direction. This variant may occur at a slightly faster rate, can co-exist with type I flutter in the same patient, and can also be ablated in the same fashion.[156] The results are less good when the heart is structurally abnormal and the boundaries of conduction are less clear, for example, in tricuspid atresia.

Intra-atrial Re-entry Tachycardias

Intra-atrial re-entry tachycardias are also called incisional re-entry tachycardias. They may occur when surgical scars have created areas of slow conduction and block around which the wavefronts may pass. Examples are atriotomy scars, atrial septal patches, intra-atrial patches, and baffles. There are frequently multiple circuits in patients with congenital heart disease, and therefore, successful ablation of one may not always result in clinical cure. This is particularly common after the Fontan operation with a dilated and scarred right atrium that may be under higher pressure. In this setting, more extensive electrophyslological mapping is required using multiple catheters and entrainment techniques to delineate the circuit and areas of slow conduction that might be targets for ablation. This is facilitated by using the electroanatomic mapping systems. Lines of block between two scars, or from a scar to a patch or a caval vein, are often required.[156–159] A further constraint is the fact that new circuits may emerge after a successful ablation. While in some series there have been encouraging results acutely, more extended follow-up has shown recurrence rates of up to 50% at 2 years.[153,154,159] Particularly in these patients, who may need multiple procedures, the newer non-contact balloon-mounted electrode arrays and non-fluoroscopic techniques are finding a role in improving the ability to map out the tachycardia circuit without excessive exposure to radiation. Use of irrigated catheters also appears to improve success rates.[153]

Junctional Ectopic Tachycardia

The congenital form of junctional ectopic tachycardia (previously known as His bundle tachycardia) is the least common sustained arrhythmia in childhood. If uncontrolled, it can lead to left ventricular dysfunction and a tachycardiomyopathy with heart failure. Congenital junctional ectopic tachycardia may occur in siblings of affected patients. It has been proposed that maternal anti-SSA and anti-SSB antibodies may play a role in development of congenital junctional ectopic tachycardia, suggesting a wider spectrum of AV nodal effects of maternal autoimmune disease.[160] This would also make sense, given the recognition that some patients go on to develop heart block, with or without antiarrhythmic medications. Children with the arrhythmia often require many years of medication to control the rate, although they may outgrow the tendency to arrhythmia in the second decade of life.[161] The site of the ectopic focus, at the atrioventricular node, carries a risk of complete heart block after ablation, but a number of successful reports have appeared. Indeed, this was one of the earliest arrhythmias for which radio-frequency ablation was applied in children.[162]

The more common form of junctional ectopic tachycardia is seen after cardiac surgery as a transient arrhythmia in the setting of a sick child. Although it can be seen after many congenital heart repairs, typical surgeries involve stretch or suturing close to the atrioventricular node, such as tetralogy of Fallot or perimembranous ventricular septal defect repair. It requires full supportive treatment in addition to treatment of the arrhythmia. Historically this arrhythmia was one of the causes of post-operative mortality due to haemodynamic deterioration, but with improved management this is no longer the case. Body cooling, medications (typically amiodarone or procainamide), and atrial pacing are usually able to control the arrhythmia, which does not recur once the acute post-operative phase has passed.[163]

Ventricular Tachycardia

In the setting of a structurally normal heart, ventricular tachycardia is an uncommon arrhythmia in childhood. Some cases may be a result of myocarditis or a Purkinje cell tumour, usually presenting in the first few years of life. In these types of cases, after medical control has been achieved, it is often possible to withdraw treatment some years later without a recurrence of the arrhythmia, suggesting regression of the arrhythmic substrate.[164]

Benign Ventricular Tachycardia

Arrhythmic Substrate

In the structurally normal heart, there are two common sites for an automatic focus, though they may occur at any site. Tachycardias originating in the right ventricular outflow tract are the most common and demonstrate a pattern of left bundle branch block on the surface electrocardiogram with an inferior axis. They may be sensitive to adenosine. More recently, subtle changes have been identified on resonance imaging scanning in some of these patients.[165] Left posterior fascicular tachycardias have a pattern of right bundle branch block with a superior axis. They are usually intermittent but can sometimes be incessant. Left anterior fascicular tachycardias have a pattern of right bundle branch block with an inferior axis. They are much less common. These tachycardias are often mistaken for supraventricular tachycardias and are responsive to verapamil.

Electrophysiological Findings

Timed ventricular extrastimulation may not be able to start or stop the right ventricular outflow tract tachycardia reproducibly. An infusion of isoprenaline is usually required for initiation if it is not spontaneously present. Ventricular pacing close to the site of the tachycardia origin is sometimes helpful in initiating tachycardia. Like most automatic foci, this can be challenging to induce under general anaesthesia.

Rapid atrial or ventricular pacing may be used to initiate a left fascicular tachycardia, and isoproterenol is also often helpful.

Radio-frequency Ablation

Radio-frequency ablation requires the catheter to be directed to the site of onset of the focus. Ventricular pacing at the site of origin will produce electrocardiographical recordings identical to that of the spontaneous arrhythmia. During ventricular tachycardia, an electrode catheter at the site of origin will detect ventricular activation that precedes the QRS complex in all of the surface electrocardiographical leads and any intracardiac reference electrodes (Fig. 19-12). A Purkinje potential may precede the ventricular activation at the site of a fascicular tachycardia.[166–168] Radio-frequency ablation can be performed with reasonable success.[169–171]

Post-operative Ventricular Tachycardia

Following repair of some forms of congenital heart disease, there is a small incidence of sudden death, which may occur many years after surgery. This is best recognised and studied in tetralogy of Fallot. In some patients, sustained ventricular tachycardias develop. This may be a precursor to the late complication of sudden death.[172,173] A generalised increase in fibrous tissue is present when repair is late and may explain these late arrhythmias.[174,175] In others, the origin of the tachycardia is in the subpulmonary outflow tract at the site of an infundibulotomy or transannular patch.[13,176–178] The tachycardia may be caused by a localised area of re-entry or a much larger circuit around the infundibular scar. It can be initiated and terminated by programmed stimulation.[179, 180] Mapping of these tachycardias may be difficult and require a line of block to abolish the substrate. Mapping may also be difficult because rapid ventricular tachycardia is poorly tolerated haemodynamically. In order to map the tachycardia, it may be necessary to use pace mapping until close to the site of origin, then to perform closer mapping looking for early activation and mid-diastolic potentials indicating an area of slow conduction during short periods of induced tachycardia. Alternatively, a small dose of a class I antiarrhythmic agent can be given to slow the rate of the tachycardia to improve the haemodynamics during mapping. This strategy carries the risk of making the arrhythmia subsequently non-inducible. Mapping of single or a few

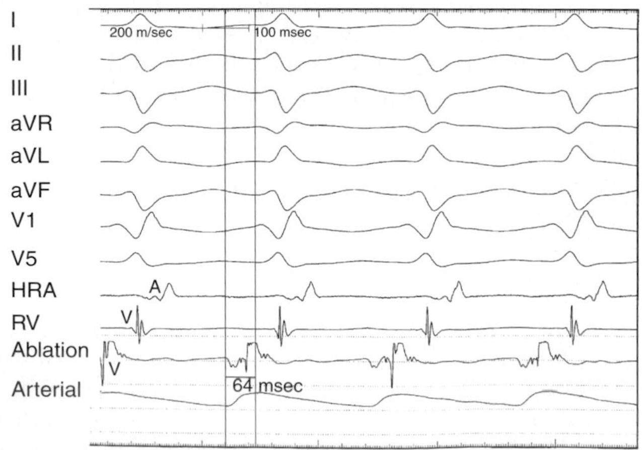

Figure 19-12 Activation mapping of a left fascicular ventricular tachycardia. The earliest activation on the ablation electrode is 64 msec ahead of the onset of the QRS complex in any of the surface ECG leads at the site of successful ablation. HRA, high right atrium; RV, right ventricle.

beats with non-contact electrode balloon arrays may minimise these problems.[181] Less commonly, other structural defects may give rise to ventricular tachycardia after surgery as a result of scarring in the right ventricular outflow tract, for example, after repair of ventricular septal defect or pulmonary stenosis.[182,183] Successful radio-frequency ablation is possible, but there are only anecdotal reports.[180] Frequently implantable defibrillators are the best choice in patients with established haemodynamically important ventricular tachycardia, if ablation is not a feasible or promising alternative.

INHERITED ARRHYTHMIA SYNDROMES

Primary electrical myopathies are frequently genetically based disorders, and thus frequently inherited. These diseases include the long QT syndromes, short QT syndrome, Brugada syndrome, arrhythmogenic right ventricular dysplasia/cardiomyopathy, familial hypertrophic cardiomyopathy (discussed elsewhere in this text), and catecholaminergic polymorphic ventricular tachycardia. Many of these diseases carry a significant risk of sudden death, as well as concomitant myocardial disease. A detailed discussion is beyond the scope of this chapter, but we briefly review the clinical syndromes.[184]

Long QT Syndromes

Resulting from abnormalities in ion channel function, there are now multiple genes associated with the long QT syndromes. Ion channel abnormalities lead to abnormal repolarisation of cardiac muscle, creating vulnerability for malignant ventricular arrhythmias and sudden death. Standard therapy includes β-blockade for most types of long QT, and if patients remain symptomatic, pacing, left cardiac sympathetic denervation, and implantable defibrillator placement may be considered.[185–187] Specific indications for device management are discussed in the pacing section of this chapter.

Brugada Syndrome

Brugada syndrome is characterised by ST segment elevation in the right precordial leads, right bundle branch block, and risk of sudden death due to malignant ventricular arrhythmias. Some patients have the Brugada QRS phenotype present on their electrocardiogram at baseline, while in others it is only evident with fever or through drug provocation with ajmaline, procainamide, or flecainide.[188] Therapy is most commonly placement of an implantable cardioverter defibrillator, although timing and risk stratification remain challenging.[189]

Arrhythmogenic Right Ventricular Dysplasia/ Cardiomyopathy

Arrhythmogenic right ventricular dysplasia, like long QT syndrome, has been shown to be caused by several different mutations, leading to desmosomal dysfunction. Clinically it is characterised by fibro-fatty replacement of the right (and in advanced disease, the left) ventricular myocardium, causing myocardial dysfunction and ventricular arrhythmias. Implantable cardioverter defibrillators are used frequently in this disease as well when life-threatening arrhythmias are seen.[190,191] The use of ventricular stimulation studies for risk stratification remains controversial.[192]

Catecholaminergic Polymorphic Ventricular Tachycardia

Catecholaminergic polymorphic ventricular tachycardia is a disease characterised by ventricular arrhythmias (typically bidirectional ventricular tachycardia which may degenerate into ventricular fibrillation) triggered by exercise or emotion. It is thought to be caused by mutations in the ryanodine receptor.[193] It is treated primarily with β-blockade, and then implantable defibrillator implantation in refractory cases.[194] Implantable defibrillator use in this population can be particularly difficult due to the possibility of electrical storm, where the pain and trauma of a shock reinduces the ventricular arrhythmia.

MISCELLANEOUS ARRHYTHMIAS

Radio-frequency ablation has also been applied to other arrhythmias, though less frequently in children.

Atrioventricular Nodal Ablation

In some patients with supraventricular arrhythmias, curative radio-frequency ablation is not possible. Good examples are some patients with atrial fibrillation, multi-focal atrial tachycardia, or multiple atrial re-entry tachycardias. In these settings, atrioventricular nodal ablation will prevent the atrial rate from being conducted to the ventricles. While this necessitates permanent pacing using either ventricular or dual chamber with mode switching, it allows a more stable ventricular rate. Although this was the original indication for ablation in adults, it has only a small role in paediatric practise. There is also an incidence of sudden death after successful catheter ablation of the atrioventricular junction despite implantation of a pacemaker. This may be because most of the patients in this group will have structural heart disease and/or ventricular dysfunction.[53] Ablation is performed from a venous approach placing the ablation catheter in a position to record a His bundle spike and then withdrawing it to increase the atrial signal. If this fails, then ablation can be performed via a transaortic approach on the left side of the septum.[195]

Atrial Fibrillation

In adults with atrial fibrillation, two approaches have been taken. In some with focal fibrillation, ablation of a focus in one of the pulmonary veins has been effective.[196] In others, long lines of block, similar to those in atrial flutter, are created in the left and right atriums, or the pulmonary veins are isolated.[197] In recent years, success rates of atrial fibrillation ablation have increased, and it usage has increased.[198] Atrial fibrillation is uncommon in children and young patients with congenital heart disease. It becomes more frequent in older patients, particularly with untreated or palliated conditions. After the Fontan operation, multiple atrial arrhythmias may be present. It is conceivable that some of the strategies being developed for atrial fibrillation will be applicable in these patients.

Ectopic Beats

There are isolated reports of ablation for frequent, symptomatic ectopic beats in both the atriums and ventricles in patients with a structurally normal heart, using similar approaches to that for sustained arrhythmias at these sites.[199] The long-term utility of these strategies is unclear.

Inappropriate Sinus Tachycardia

In some patients who are highly symptomatic, the only arrhythmia documented is an inappropriate sinus tachycardia with an excessive rate response during mild exercise. When this is unresponsive to high doses of β-blockers and/or verapamil, ablation has been used in the past to reduce the resting heart rate and rate response to mild exercise, but this is no longer accepted at some centres.[200] There is a risk of causing sinus bradycardia and the need for an atrial pacemaker, and this is a very unusual diagnosis in children. Consideration needs to be given to the important and more common differential diagnosis of postural orthostatic tachycardia syndrome, which has treatment other than ablation.[201] All efforts should be made to rule out a subtle ectopic atrial tachycardia, possibly including detailed mapping of the atrial focus.

Issues of Ablation in Congenital Heart Disease

Patients with structural congenital heart disease may present additional challenges for ablation strategies. Knowledge of the underlying anatomy, and of any previous surgery, is critical in planning and undertaking radio-frequency ablation. Despite some of the difficulties that may be encountered, it is important to consider radio-frequency ablation prior to surgery. Arrhythmias that are well tolerated pre-operatively may be less well tolerated after cardiopulmonary bypass. Inotropic support in the peri- and post-operative periods may accelerate and maintain haemodynamically unstable arrhythmias, and peri-operative atrial flutter may conduct rapidly (1:1) to the ventricle. In addition, access may be lost to relevant cardiac chambers; for example, venous access to the left atrium might be lost following completion of a Fontan. Anatomy, tissue scarring, and patient size are all sources for difficulties in ablation in congenital heart disease.[108,114,154,202–204]

Vascular Access

Even in small children, it is possible to place multiple electrode catheters using both femoral veins as well as jugular and/or subclavian veins. In those who have undergone repeated cardiac catheterisation procedures, some of the points for central venous access may have become occluded. After the Glenn or hemi-Fontan operation, use of the neck and subclavian veins is no longer possible. This may mandate use of alternative sites, for example, a transhepatic approach, or necessitate using more catheters from one site, fewer catheters overall, or a transoesophageal catheter for atrial sensing and pacing. The development of smaller catheters, which will allow more catheters from one femoral vein, is an advance. It may be necessary to recanalise occluded veins using intravascular stents prior to ablation, with the assistance of intervention catheterisation colleagues.

Venous Anatomy

Azygos continuation of an interrupted inferior caval vein is usually associated with isomerism of the left atrial appendages. This may make manipulation of catheters more difficult, if not impossible, on the venous side of the heart when approaching through the femoral vein. Use of the superior caval vein, or hepatic veins, may facilitate manipulation.[108] A left-sided superior caval vein draining to the coronary sinus is an infrequent finding in patients with a structurally normal heart, but is more common in those with congenital heart disease. The resultant coronary sinus is dilated. While this is easier to catheterise, it may not provide electrograms from as close to the left atrioventricular valve ring as normal. In addition, passage of the catheter into the terminal portion of the coronary sinus to map accessory pathways in the left lateral and supero-lateral positions is more difficult. In patients with isomerism, the coronary sinus is often absent. Indeed, this is the rule in right isomerism. This removes a useful anatomical and electrical reference. Coronary angiography may help to localise the plane of the atrioventricular ring and confirm absence of the coronary sinus. Placement of a steerable 0.018-inch electrode into the left circumflex coronary artery can delineate the left atrioventricular groove anatomically and provide electrograms to help with mapping.

Cardiac Anatomy

Certain malformations impose constraints on the procedure. In Ebstein's malformation, the septal and mural leaflets of the tricuspid valve do not arise at the atrioventricular junction. The concomitant lack of valvar tissue makes stability of the catheter at the atrioventricular ring less secure. Frequently in this setting, there are multiple accessory pathways around the right atrioventricular ring. It is usually necessary to ablate all of them to abolish the tendency to arrhythmias. Similar problems occur when Ebstein's malformation occurs in the setting of discordant atrioventricular connections. The retrograde arterial approach may be more difficult, as placing the ablation catheter below the leaflets of the left atrioventricular valve will not be close enough to the atrioventricular ring. A trans-septal approach will enhance placement of the ablation catheter on the left atrioventricular ring.[108,205] In patients with isomeric hearts, the plane of the atrioventricular ring may not fall into the usual fluoroscopy views. Transoesophageal echocardiography and angiography may help to locate the tip of the catheter and to define the plane of the atrioventricular ring.[206] Where an atrial septal defect is present, access to the left atrioventricular ring is possible from a femoral venous approach. If surgery is planned, it is appropriate to perform the ablation prior to surgery to retain the additional route to the left atrioventricular ring. Similarly, if a Fontan operation is planned, then prior ablation can be performed via the femoral venous route. After surgery, the systemic atrioventricular valve can only be approached via the retrograde arterial approach and fewer mapping catheters can be placed.

Conduction System

In order to avoid inadvertent atrioventricular block during the procedure, it is vital to know the position of the bundle of His. The His bundle catheter helps both during analysis of the arrhythmic substrate and as an anatomical marker. In patients with atrioventricular septal defects, the bundle of His is located more inferiorly than usual, towards the coronary sinus, and is more at risk when ablating inferior paraseptal accessory pathways. In patients with discordant atrioventricular connections, the bundle of His is located more anterosuperiorly, and is at risk during ablation in the superior paraseptal area. In left isomerism, there may be no discrete bundle of His, while in right isomerism there may be two atrioventricular nodes that form the substrate for twin atrioventricular re-entry tachycardias.[207]

Complications

The risks of the ablation procedure include all those seen with routine cardiac catheterisation and diagnostic electrophysiology but there are also a number of specific risks.[121,204,208,209]

Complete Heart Block

The atrioventricular node is vulnerable during ablation of dual atrioventricular nodal pathways or accessory pathways in the parahisian areas. In the Paediatric Radiofrequency Catheter Ablation Registry, which carries records of almost 2000 ablations, the incidence of atrioventricular block was 1.6% for procedures for modification of atrioventricular nodal re-entrant tachycardia, 2.7% for superior paraseptal, 10.4% for septal, and 1.0% for inferior paraseptal accessory pathways.[210] These results improved slightly in the Pediatric Prospective Ablation Registry (radio-frequency ablations only), where AV block was uncommon overall at 1.2%; occurring in 2.1% of atrioventricular nodal tachycardia ablations, and 3.0% in septal accessory pathways ablations.[208] There is a lower incidence when ablating ectopic atrial or ventricular focuses or accessory pathways in other areas unless the catheter moves during delivery of energy. When ablating in the para-Hisian areas, it is important to observe closely for any signs of atrioventricular block, either antegrade or retrograde, and to stop delivery of energy immediately when this occurs.[211] In patients with life-threatening arrhythmias or disabling symptoms, the risk of creating complete heart block may occasionally be justifiable. This is likely not acceptable in small children with atrioventricular re-entry tachycardia, or in patients with Wolff–Parkinson–White syndrome, who are asymptomatic or at low risk. While complete heart block is usually apparent immediately, it may occasionally only become evident during the few weeks after the ablation.[71,212] It is prudent to observe before proceeding directly to implantation of a permanent pacemaker in asymptomatic patients, as recovery is not uncommon in the first few days and can occur even as late as a month after the procedure.[210]

Coronary Arterial Injury

The coronary arteries can be damaged by unintended or unrecognised entry while trying to cross the aortic valve, and myocardial infarction has been reported.[84,213] A trans-septal approach will avoid these aortic complications. Delivery of energy on the atrioventricular ring may also cause heating of the wall of the coronary artery. Usually the rapid flow in the artery is able to dissipate heat and the wall is not permanently damaged, though mild stenoses have occurred in an experimental model.[214] Rarely, infarction has been recognised clinically.[215,216]

Thromboembolism

When ablating on the left side of the heart, there is a risk of the thrombosis on the ablated area embolizing. Because of this, anticoagulants should always be used during the procedure and many centres give heparin overnight following the procedure. Some of these emboli may only occur in the days or weeks after the procedure. It is a routine, therefore, to give prophylactic aspirin for 4 to 6 weeks after a procedure on the systemic side of the circulation.[213,217] There is very little data on which to base post-ablation anticoagulation, and thus a fair degree of variation in practise. On the right side of the heart, small pulmonary emboli are unlikely to be clinically apparent; in spite of this some also use heparin during the procedure and aspirin afterwards. This is mandatory when large areas are ablated, as when creating lines of block, or in patients with decreased flow, for example, after the Fontan operation.

Valvar Damage

Damage has been reported to the aortic valve and may be more common than after diagnostic catheterisation as the ablation catheter is stiffer than routine diagnostic catheters. A trans-septal approach is indicated if there is significant aortic valvar disease. The mitral valve can also be damaged during manipulation to place the ablation catheter under the valvar leaflets on the atrioventricular ring, and possibly by delivery of energy. In one echocardiographic study, mild new aortic regurgitation was reported in one-third of patients, and mitral regurgitation in one-eighth.[218] More commonly, mild valvar regurgitation occurs with a frequency of less than 2%.[219] If a patent oval foramen is present, then a trans-septal approach avoids problems of arterial access and reduces the incidence of possible valvar damage. Some have argued for routine trans-septal puncture in children to avoid the retrograde arterial approach.[220] Trans-septal puncture carries risks of its own, and air embolism during changes of catheter has been reported.[221] There have been two non-randomised comparative studies of the retrograde and anterograde approaches, with a similar incidence of complications.[222] Lower fluoroscopy times, however, were reported with the trans-septal approach.[223] In these studies, it was recognised that the two approaches could be complimentary, as failure by one route did not invalidate a successful procedure using the other route. Damage to the tricuspid valve is less common as it is rarely necessary to place the catheter below the valvar leaflets.

Cardiac Perforation and Tamponade

Tamponade due to perforation can present during or shortly after the procedure occurs.[224] Perforation can occur during delivery of energy or manipulation of catheters. Excessive temperature and repeated applications at one site are recognised risk factors. Perforation is more common when ablating in the coronary sinus than around the atrioventricular groove. The stiffer ablation catheters themselves may be responsible for perforation during intracardiac manipulation in infants, thus producing a higher incidence of pericardial effusions.[93] Percutaneous drainage is usually sufficient, but open drainage with repair of the bleeding site is sometimes required. A slow leak into the pericardial space is also possible. Because of this, many centres routinely perform an echocardiogram the following day. Late pericarditis and postpericardiotomy syndrome have also been reported.[225]

Exposure to Radiation and Non-fluoroscopic Mapping

Exposure during the earliest procedures was generally considerably longer than for routine diagnostic cardiac catheterisation, with times generally exceeding 1 hour, but not dissimilar to complex interventional catheterisation.[226] Isolated reports of radiation skin injury were associated with these early procedures using older fluoroscopy equipment, and are still seen with particularly long procedures such as atrial fibrillation ablations.[227] Early estimations were of a 0.1% per patient lifetime additional risk for a malignancy from fluoroscopy for 1 hour.[228] This is to be viewed against a 20% risk per lifetime of an individual developing a malignancy naturally. Subsequent studies suggest this additional risk is closer to 0.03%.[229] This small risk is outweighed by the benefits in avoiding a lifetime of medication, admissions to hospital, and the risks of antiarrhythmic surgery. In addition, it is highly cost effective.[230–236] Using modern fluoroscopic systems with optimised fluoroscopy settings, beam collimation, pulsed fluoroscopy, and improved procedure times, the amount of radiation has been reduced. Most procedures now require less than 1 hour of fluoroscopy.[84] It may be better to abandon a procedure and return on another day with fresh and/or additional hands and minds and different equipment than persevering when the procedure is becoming increasingly difficult. Usage of electroanatomic mapping systems may assist in decreased amount of fluoroscopy required, and may also assist with creation of improved substrate maps.[152,237–239]

Results of Radio-frequency Ablation

A number of single- and multi-centre studies have shown that the overall risk of radio-frequency ablation is low and the success rate is high. Currently, the success rate is more than 96% for nodal re-entry tachycardia, and more than 90% for accessory pathways. A learning curve of the order of 100 cases per institution has been noted. Centres that perform more procedures have a lower complication rate during shorter procedures, with shorter times required for fluoroscopy, and increased rates of success.[205,240–243] This applies to radio-frequency ablation in both adults and children.[244] Structural heart disease, a body weight of less than 15 kg, and the presence of multiple arrhythmic targets increase the risk of complications.

The multi-centre series (see Table 19-1) all have different criterions for inclusion and follow-up. In 1993, Hindricks reported the Multicentre European Radiofrequency Survey of almost 5000 adults treated up to 1992.[132] Calkins and colleagues in 1998 reported on the ATAKR Multicentre Investigators Group of just over 1000 adults and children undergoing radio-frequency ablation of supraventricular arrhythmias including ablation of the atrioventricular node.[133] The Pediatric Electrophysiology Society of North America first reported in 1994 the acute results of ablation in patients aged less than 21 years. They included those with structural heart disease and those undergoing ablation for ventricular tachycardia.[85] A later follow-up of the patients with a structurally normal heart undergoing ablation for supraventricular tachycardia was reported in 1997.[84] In these studies, the death rate was 0.1% to 0.3%, complete atrioventricular block occurred in 0.6% to 1% and pericardial tamponade or effusion in 0.7% to 2.5% (see Table 19-1). A prospective study of radio-frequency ablation of accessory pathways in children showed similar results, with overall acute success rates of 95.7%, highest for left free-wall pathways (97.8%) and slightly lower for right free-wall pathways at 90.8%.[205,208]

Although the acute rates of success and complications have been well documented, with similar results for adults and children, there have been few studies of the longer-term outcome. Calkins et al reported recurrence rates of 5% after ablation for nodal re-entry, and 8% for accessory pathways. The median time to recurrence was 35 days. Studies from individual centres have reported recurrences after successful ablation of accessory pathways in about one-tenth of patients after follow-up of about 6 months.[217,245–247] The majority occurred within the first few days of the procedure, and most patients underwent a successful second ablation. The most comprehensive follow-up study to date is from the Pediatric Electrophysiology Society.[84,205] Surprisingly, given the impressive acute results, there was a significant incidence of late recurrent arrhythmias.

ELECTROPHYSIOLOGY LABORATORY

While it is possible to perform electrophysiologic studies in a simple X-ray theatre with a single-plane image intensifier, this is less than optimal. There are many advantages to performing studies in the diagnostic and interventional catheterisation laboratory, where facilities for sedation and anaesthesia, fluoroscopy, cineangiography, haemodynamic measurements and monitoring, electrical cardioversion, defibrillation and resuscitation are all readily available.

Positioning of catheters is guided by fluoroscopy, and biplane fluoroscopy in the oblique, frontal, and lateral projections enhances their optimal positioning. Some children, especially those with complex congenital heart disease, will also undergo diagnostic cardiac catheterisation and haemodynamic evaluation and/or catheter intervention during the same procedure. Transoesophageal echocardiography may be helpful in children with malformed hearts to guide the positioning of catheters or for transseptal puncture for access to the left atrium.[206]

Personnel

The staffing requirements for paediatric electrophysiologic studies and radio-frequency ablation are similar to those required for diagnostic and interventional paediatric cardiac catheterisation (see Chapter 17). The operator and physiological measurement technician, however, will also require additional skills in planning, undertaking, and interpreting the diagnostic and therapeutic aspects of the electrophysiologic studies. In some laboratories, it is usual to have two physicians. One is then able to concentrate on the intracardiac signals and the other on manipulation of the catheter during ablative procedures. In some smaller centres, the team of physicians is composed of a dedicated electrophysiologist, usually with predominantly adult experience, and a paediatric cardiologist. More commonly, a paediatric cardiologist who is also trained in electrophysiology undertakes the procedures. There are published guidelines for both personnel and equipment.[204,248–250]

Indications for Electrophysiological Studies

Electrophysiological studies are not required in the management of all arrhythmias. When the nature of an arrhythmia is clear, symptoms are infrequent and transient, or medication is effective and well tolerated, invasive testing is not required. Some details as to appropriate indications are included with the guidelines (Table 19-2).[204]

Transoesophageal Electrophysiologic Studies

While the majority of studies are performed with intracardiac catheter electrodes, it is possible to perform limited studies of supraventricular arrhythmias via a transoesophageal electrode, which is in close proximity to the left atrium. These electrodes can be placed with minimal sedation even in small children and infants and are used for pacing and recording together with the surface electrocardiogram.[251,252] Electrodes with tip deflectors allow pacing of the ventricle from within the stomach, although ventricular capture is inconsistent.[253]

Pacemaker Lead Studies

In the post-operative period, temporary epicardial leads attached to the atrium and ventricle can be used to stimulate and record for limited electrophysiological studies.[254] In patients with certain permanent pacemakers, the pacemaker can be programmed to deliver stimuli for induction of arrhythmias and to display intracardiac electrograms, allowing limited non-invasive electrophysiological studies.

TABLE 19-2

INDICATIONS FOR RADIO-FREQUENCY CATHETER ABLATION (RFCA) PROCEDURES IN PEDIATRIC PATIENTS

Class I

1. WPW syndrome following an episode of aborted sudden cardiac death
2. The presence of WPW syndrome associated with syncope when there is a short pre-excited RR interval during atrial fibrillation (pre-excited RR interval, 250 ms) or the antegrade effective refractory period of the AP measured during programmed electrical stimulation is 250 msec
3. Chronic or recurrent SVT associated with ventricular dysfunction
4. Recurrent VT that is associated with haemodynamic compromise and is amenable to catheter ablation

Class IIa

1. Recurrent and/or symptomatic SVT refractory to conventional medical therapy and age >4 years
2. Impending congenital heart surgery when vascular or chamber access may be restricted following surgery
3. Chronic (occurring for 6–12 months following an initial event) or incessant SVT in the presence of normal ventricular function
4. Chronic or frequent recurrences of IART
5. Palpitations with inducible sustained SVT during electrophysiological testing

Class IIb

1. Asymptomatic pre-excitation (WPW pattern on ECG), age >5 years, with no recognized tachycardia, when the risks and benefits of the procedure and arrhythmia have been clearly explained
2. SVT, age >5 years, as an alternative to chronic antiarrhythmic therapy which has been effective in control of the arrhythmia
3. SVT, age <5 years (including infants) when antiarrhythmic medications, including sotalol and amiodarone, are not effective or associated with intolerable side effects
4. IART, one to three episodes per year, requiring medical intervention
5. AVN ablation and pacemaker insertion as an alternative therapy for recurrent or intractable IART
6. One episode of VT associated with haemodynamic compromise and which is amenable to catheter ablation

Class III

1. Asymptomatic WPW syndrome, age <5 years
2. SVT controlled with conventional antiarrhythmic medications, age <5 years
3. Nonsustained, paroxysmal VT which is not considered incessant (i.e., present on monitoring for hours at a time or on nearly all strips recorded during any 1-hour period of time) and where no concomitant ventricular dysfunction exists
4. Episodes of nonsustained SVT that do not require other therapy and/or are minimally symptomatic

AP, accessory pathway; AVN, atrioventricular node; ECG, electrocardiogram; IART, intra-atrial reentrant tachycardia; SVT, sustained ventricular tachycardia; VT, ventricular tachycardia; WPW, Wolff–Parkinson–White.

Equipment

Electrophysiologic Catheters

Although a limited electrophysiological study, and even catheter ablation, can be performed in some cases with a single bipolar electrode catheter that is moved to different sites in the heart, it is more usual to use between two and five multi-polar electrode catheters.[255] The simplest electrode catheters have a single bipole with spacing of 0.5 to 1 cm between the poles to enable bipolar recording and pacing. Multi-polar catheters with 4, 6, 8 or 10 poles are used to record and display multiple simultaneous electrograms and allow pacing at different sites without constantly moving the catheter. These catheters are usually of 4 to 7 French size, but recently smaller catheters have become available. More specialised catheters preshaped into a ring with 20 poles for mapping around the tricuspid annulus (halo), and 64 or more pole basket or balloon mounted electrode arrays for high-density mapping inside a cardiac chamber, are occasionally used for complex cases. High-torque steerable, 4- to 10-pole catheters, of 0.018 to 0.25 inches, have also been designed for use inside the coronary arteries and peripheral coronary veins.

Stimulating and Recording

While a complete haemodynamic assessment is possible with one or two pressure amplifiers and recording channels and a single surface electrocardiographic lead, intracardiac electrophysiology studies require considerably more sophisticated and expensive equipment. Usually there is the need for at least 3 (ideally 12) surface and 3 (ideally at least 4) intracardiac electrographic channels. The intracardiac signals are amplified and filtered to reduce noise and produce sharp deflections. Modern digital systems allow a full 12-lead surface electrocardiogram to be recorded, together with 16 or more intracardiac electrograms. The older approach of displaying the electrograms in real time on an oscilloscope, while simultaneously recording on a paper recorder and/or on magnetic tape, has been superseded by digital systems. These continuously store the electrograms and allow recall of data when required, both intracardiac electrograms and 12-lead surface electrocardiograms, from any part of the study. A programmable electrophysiology stimulator capable of pacing at rates up to 6000 beats/min is used for pacing and delivering timed extrastimuli in order to induce, terminate and modify arrhythmias. It is interfaced with a junction box into which the catheter electrodes are connected so that recording and stimulation can be performed using each electrode.

PACING AND DEVICES

Paediatrics and the History of Pacing

The early history of pacing comprises a colourful collection of intriguing stories of bravery, ingenuity, and tenacity.[256] Paediatric cardiologists should be aware that paediatric patients were at the forefront of these endeavours. The first pacemaker is attributed to Mark Lidwill, an Australian physician who demonstrated his device, which plugged in to a lighting point, in 1929 in Sydney.[257,258] One pole was soaked in a strong salt solution and applied to the skin and the other was a needle plunged into the heart. It had been used at least on one occasion to successfully resuscitate a still-born babe in whom everything else had failed.

A new era for paediatric cardiology and the whole of medicine dawned in 1954 when C. Walton Lillehei first repaired a ventricular septal defect using cross-circulation.[259] After this new surgery became established, post-operative complete heart block proved an important cause of mortality and in 1957 Lillehei first used direct myocardial stimulation from an external pacemaker powered by alternating current. After a power outage, Lillehei successfully pressed Earl Bakken to develop a portable transistorised battery-powered external pacemaker.[260]

In 1958 the first fully internal pacemaker was implanted by Swedish surgeon Ake Senning, a name well known to paediatric cardiologists.[261] The device failed within hours and was replaced by an identical model, which lasted 8 days. The 43-year-old patient had complete heart block and syncope and went on to have an additional 24 pacemakers over his lifetime. He survived a further 43 years.

Over the next 50 years, anti-bradycardia pacing became a standard therapy and pacemakers evolved well beyond simple anti-bradycardia devices. Biventricular pacemakers have revolutionised the management of heart failure and implantable cardioverter-defibrillators are a cornerstone in the prevention of sudden cardiac death. Both are increasingly used in paediatric and congenital heart disease patients.

Anti-bradycardia Pacing

The decision to place a permanent pacemaker may not be straightforward, particularly in the case of paediatric and congenital heart disease populations. Evidenced-based guidelines for prescribing anti-bradycardia permanent pacemakers are published and updated in a carefully written and thoughtful document by the American College of Cardiology (available at: www.acc.org) in conjunction with the American Heart Association (www.americanheart.org) and the Heart Rhythm Society (www.hrsonline.org).[41]

Atrioventricular Block: Definitions

First-degree atrioventricular block is PR interval prolongation greater than the upper limit of normal for age. This can be gleaned from normative paediatric electrocardiographic data.[262]

The nomenclature of second-degree atrioventricular block has a fascinating history and often causes confusion.[263] Mobitz type I second-degree atrioventricular block (Wenckebach) is usually associated with a narrow QRS complex and is generally considered benign. However, Mobitz type II second-degree block is not benign, as it is always anatomically infra-nodal and can be associated with less stable escape rhythms.

Type I block is classically characterised by progressive prolongation of the PR interval before a single non-conducted P-wave (Fig. 19-13). Type I block, however, is frequently atypical (especially in children) and can be diagnosed when the post-block PR interval is shorter than the pre-block PR interval (Fig. 19-14). In contrast, type II second-degree atrioventricular block is characterised by fixed PR intervals before and after blocked beats and is usually associated with a wide QRS complex (Fig. 19-15). When atrioventricular conduction occurs in a 2:1 pattern, block cannot be classified as type I or type II, although the width of the QRS may be suggestive (Fig. 19-16).[264]

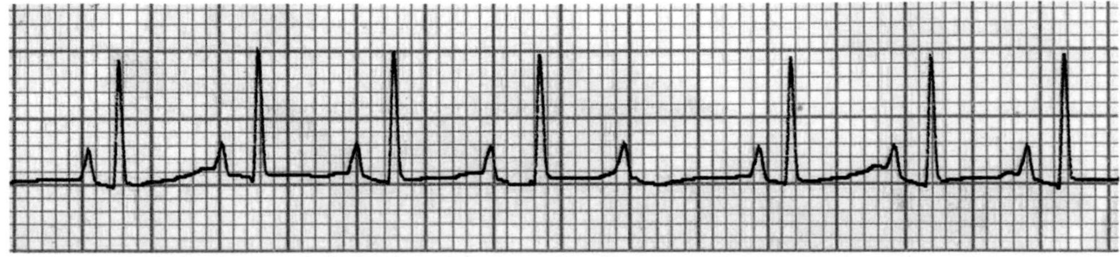

Figure 19-13 Classic type I, or Wenckebach, atrioventricular block. With each beat, there is a progressive increase in the atrioventricular interval until there is failure of atrioventricular conduction.

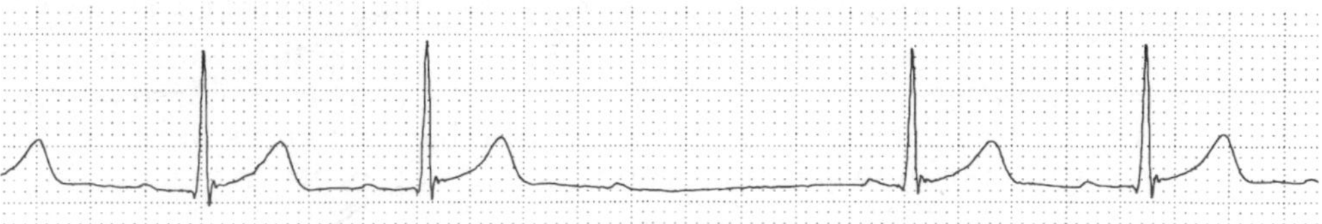

Figure 19-14 Atypical type I atrioventricular block. There is baseline first-degree atrioventricular block in this example. The PR interval after failure of atrioventricular conduction is shorter than the pre-block PR interval.

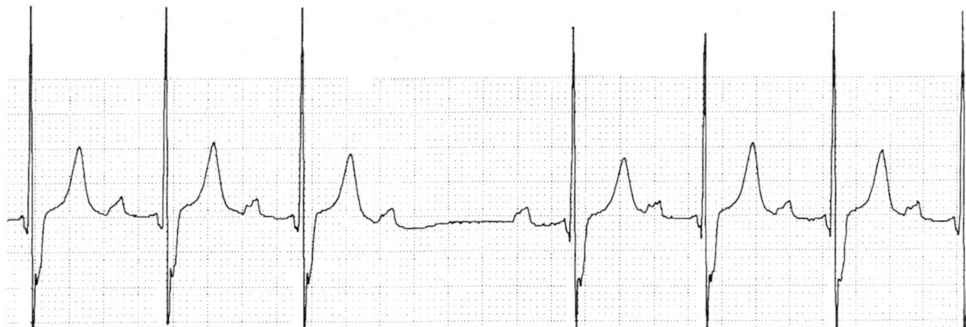

Figure 19-15 Mobitz type II atrioventricular block. There is baseline first-degree atrioventricular block and a wide QRS complex. The PR interval after failure of atrioventricular conduction is exactly the same as the pre-block PR interval. This patient had syncope in the post-operative period after implantation of a prosthetic mitral valve. A pacemaker was subsequently placed.

Advanced second-degree atrioventricular block refers to non-conduction of two or more consecutive P waves but with some conducted beats, indicating some preservation of atrioventricular conduction. Third-degree atrioventricular block (complete heart block) is absence of atrioventricular conduction and characteristically has a regular escape rhythm (Fig. 19-17).

Symptomatic Bradycardia: Definition

Sinus node dysfunction is increasingly recognised in paediatric patients, especially in those who have had surgery for congenital heart disease. It is frequently asymptomatic and in a large percentage of cases does not require pacing. Sinus node dysfunction may include sinus bradycardia, sinus pause, or sinus arrest, as well as sino-atrial block. Each of these bradycardias may occur as part of bradycardia-tachycardia syndrome.[265]

With respect to bradycardia the primary criterion for prescribing an anti-bradycardia pacemaker is the concurrent observation of symptoms. The clinical significance of bradycardia is age dependent. For example, a resting heart rate of 45 may be a normal finding in a fit adolescent, but in a neonate represents a profound bradycardia. Symptomatic bradycardia is defined as a documented bradyarrhythmia that is directly responsible for the clinical manifestations of syncope or near syncope, transient dizziness or light-headedness, or confusional states resulting from cerebral hypoperfusion. Fatigue, exercise intolerance, and congestive cardiac failure may also result from bradycardia and these may occur at rest and/or with exertion.[41]

The following guidelines for the Holter diagnosis of sinus bradycardia have been proposed based on available normative data but unfortunately most of the data does not distinguish between the asleep and awake state[265]: neonates and infants: <60 beats per minute sleeping and <80 beats per minute during waking hours; children aged 1–6 years: <60 beats per minute; children aged 7–11 years:<45 beats per minute; adolescents and young adults: <40 beats per minute; trained athletes: <30 beats per minute.

Definite correlation of symptoms with bradyarrhythmia is required prior to determining the need for permanent pacing. Caution should be exercised not to confuse physiologic sinus bradycardia (as may occur in trained athletes) with pathological bradyarrhythmias. Alternative causes need to considered and excluded as causative of the symptoms or bradycardia. These include anaemia, iron deficiency, hypothyroidism, space-occupying lesions of the central nervous system, Arnold-Chiari malformations, seizures, breath holding, apnoea, and other neurally-mediated mechanisms. On occasion, symptoms may only become apparent in retrospect after anti-bradycardia pacing.

In patients with congenital heart disease, abnormal physiology and ventricular performance can result in symptomatic bradycardia at rates that would not be symptomatic in those with more normal physiology. In these patients

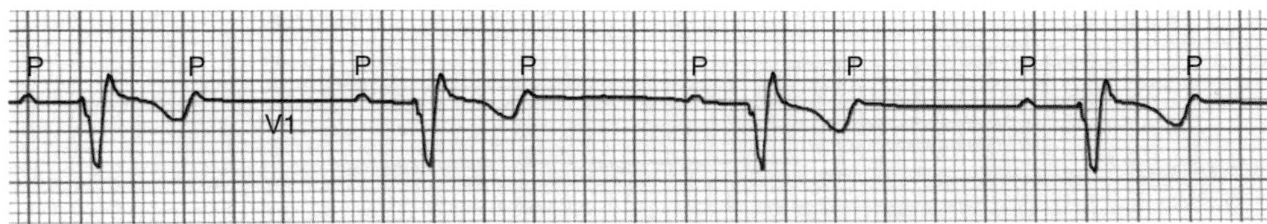

Figure 19-16 The tracing shows 2:1 atrioventricular block. This block cannot be classified as type I or type II, but the wide QRS is suggestive of infra-nodal block. Each P-wave is marked with a P; every second P is fused with the end of the T wave.

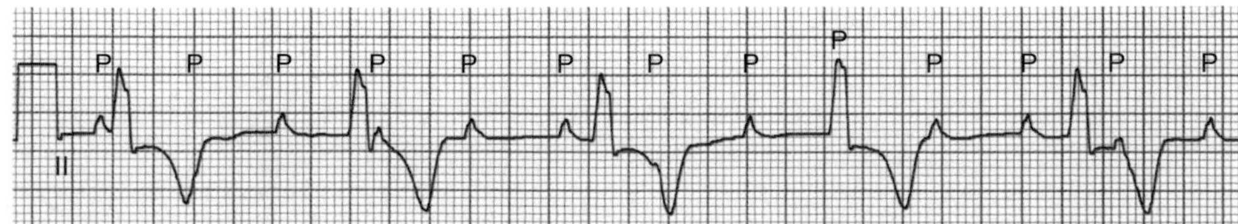

Figure 19-17 Complete atrioventricular block. The atrial rate is 135 beats per minute. The ventricular rate is 50 beats per minute. The P waves bear no relationship to the QRS complexes, which are regular. The QRS complex is wide, which in this patient with congenital complete heart block is an indication for anti-bradycardia pacing.

a lower threshold for pacing is based on the correlation of symptoms with relative bradycardia.

Implantation Guidelines

Pacemaker implantation guidelines for children, adolescents, and patients, with congenital heart disease are outlined and specific situations are discussed below.[41] Sometimes it is helpful to review adult parts of the document. With each new set of guidelines there has been a progressive trend towards less restrictive indications. Frequently individual judgements are required within the context of the document.[266]

Class I (there is evidence and/or general agreement that pacing is beneficial, useful, and effective)

1. Advanced second- or third-degree atrioventricular block associated with symptomatic bradycardia, ventricular dysfunction, or low cardiac output.
2. Sinus node dysfunction with correlation of symptoms during age-inappropriate bradycardia. The definition of bradycardia varies with the patient's age and expected heart rate.
3. Post-operative advanced second- or third-degree atrioventricular block that is not expected to resolve or persists at least 7 days after cardiac surgery.
4. Congenital third-degree atrioventricular block with a wide QRS escape rhythm, complex ventricular ectopy, or ventricular dysfunction.
5. Congenital third-degree atrioventricular block in the infant with a ventricular rate less than 50–55 beats per minute or with congenital heart disease and a ventricular rate less than 70 beats per minute.
6. Sustained pause-dependent ventricular tachycardia, with or without prolonged QT, in which the efficacy of pacing is thoroughly documented.

Class II (conditions for which there is conflicting evidence and/or a divergence of opinion)

Class IIa (weight of evidence favours pacing)

1. Bradycardia-tachycardia syndrome with the need for long-term antiarrhythmic treatment other than digitalis.
2. Congenital third-degree atrioventricular block beyond the first year of life with an average heart rate less than 50 beats per minute, abrupt pauses in ventricular rate that are two or three times the basic cycle length, or associated with symptoms due to chronotropic incompetence.
3. Long-QT syndrome with 2:1 atrioventricular or third-degree atrioventricular block.
4. Asymptomatic sinus bradycardia in the child with complex congenital heart disease with resting heart rate less than 40 beats per minute or pauses in ventricular rate more than 3 seconds.
5. Patients with congenital heart disease and impaired haemodynamics due to sinus bradycardia or loss of atrioventricular synchrony.

Class IIb (evidence for pacing is less well established)

1. Transient post-operative third-degree atrioventricular block that reverts to sinus rhythm with residual bifascicular block.
2. Congenital third-degree atrioventricular block in the asymptomatic infant, child, adolescent, or young adult with an acceptable rate, narrow QRS complex, and normal ventricular function.
3. Asymptomatic sinus bradycardia in the adolescent with congenital heart disease with resting heart rate less than 40 beats per minute or pauses in ventricular rate more than 3 seconds.
4. Neuromuscular diseases with any degree of atrioventricular block (including first-degree atrioventricular block), with or without symptoms, because there may be unpredictable progression of atrioventricular conduction disease.

Class III (pacing not indicated)

1. Transient post-operative atrioventricular block with return of normal atrioventricular conduction.
2. Asymptomatic post-operative bifascicular block with or without first-degree atrioventricular block.
3. Asymptomatic type I second-degree atrioventricular block.
4. Asymptomatic sinus bradycardia in the adolescent with longest RR interval less than 3 seconds and minimum heart rate more than 40 beats per minute.

Congenital Complete Atrioventricular Block

Congenital complete atrioventricular block is strongly associated with maternal anti-Ro and anti-La antibodies and occurs in up to 5% of fetuses whose mothers have these antibodies. The pathogenesis of block in this situation is complicated and incompletely understood.[267] Interestingly in twin pregnancies only one twin may be afflicted.[268] Diagnosis can be made antenatally and demonstration of degrees of block less than third degree remains a controversial indication for treatment with steroids to potentially avert progression (see Chapter 12). Other aetiologies include inherited conduction system diseases with diverse genetic bases.[269]

The primary reason for anti-bradycardia pacing for congenital complete heart block is to prevent syncope and sudden death.[270] In addition to alleviating symptoms, anti-bradycardia pacing may prevent ventricular dysfunction and associated mitral regurgitation.

Those with symptoms or heart failure have a class I indication for pacemaker implantation (recommendation 1). Subtle symptoms may, however, be more challenging to identify, such as long naps and nightmares.[271] Further class I indications include a wide QRS escape rhythm, complex ventricular ectopy, or ventricular dysfunction (recommendation 4). The upper limit of normal for QRS duration varies with age.[262] By adult standards a wide complex in a newborn may be narrow; for example, between days 2 and 7 of age a QRS duration of 70 msec is above the upper limit of normal. Complex ventricular ectopy is not defined in the document but can be taken to mean ventricular couplets or more.

Congenital third-degree atrioventricular block in the infant with a ventricular rate less than 50 to 55 beats per minute or with congenital heart disease and a ventricular rate less than 70 beats per minute is a class I recommendation for permanent pacing. This recommendation does not specify an awake or asleep state, and the original studies reporting these thresholds did not have 24-hour Holter data.[272,273] However, this is frequently extrapolated to mean an average heart rate over 24 hours. Many paediatric centres would undertake anti-bradycardia pacing in any child with complex congenital heart disease and congenital complete atrioventricular block.[271]

Recommendations for those with congenital complete heart block beyond the first year of life continue to use a heart rate of less than 50, but as a class IIa recommendation, leaving more room for interpretation by the physician. Of note is that in the original study, the heart rate of 50 which was used as a threshold was a mean daytime junctional rate.[274] The second part of this recommendation: abrupt pauses in ventricular rate that are two or three times the basic cycle length refer to the possibility of junctional exit block with the implication of an unstable escape mechanism. Pauses of at least 3 seconds while awake or 5 seconds while sleeping have also been used as a criterion for anti-bradycardia pacing (Fig. 19-18).[271]

Long-QT syndrome with 2:1 atrioventricular or third-degree atrioventricular block is a class IIa indication. Whether or not one considers the syndrome to be present a prolonged QTc in the setting of congenital complete atrioventricular block (Fig. 19-19) is widely considered an indication for for anti-bradycardia pacing and is alluded to in the guidelines.[41,270,271,275]

Those patients with significant bradycardia who do not undergo anti-bradycardia pacing require meticulous follow-up with serial electrocardiograms, Holter monitors, and echocardiograms. There is little data on echocardiographic monitoring; however, serial echocardiography is useful to document ventricular size and function as well as mitral valve regurgitation.[271] Ventricular dysfunction is now included in the class I recommendations, and dilatation and/or mitral regurgitation could be considered relative indications to pace.

Michaelsson has recommended that all patients with congenital complete atrioventricular block be paced by the time they reach adolescence because of a significant risk of syncope or sudden death at any time thereafter even in the absence of poor prognostic signs. This recommendation is covered in the guidelines by class IIb recommendation 2 and is becoming increasingly accepted.[270,271,276]

2:1 Atrioventricular Block

Patients with 2:1 atrioventricular block require meticulous ongoing follow-up as block may progress and the nature and rate of the escape rhythm are unpredictable. Individual consideration using the criterions for complete atrioventricular block is often helpful. For example, symptoms, a wide QRS complex, a prolonged corrected QT interval, or

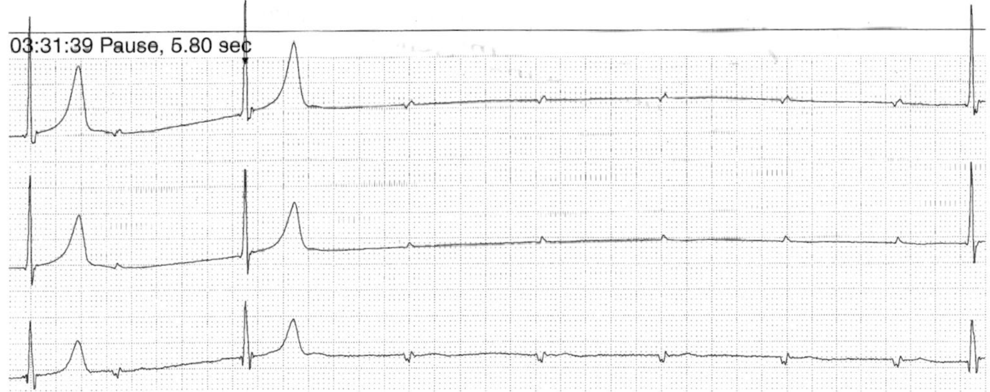

Figure 19-18 A significant pause, of 5.8 seconds, was recorded overnight in a 10-year-old patient with congenital complete heart block. The pause length is not a multiple of the previous RR interval, so it is not of the type referred to by class IIa, recommendation 2. The presence of multiple pauses like this, however, led to insertion of an anti-bradycardia pacemaker.

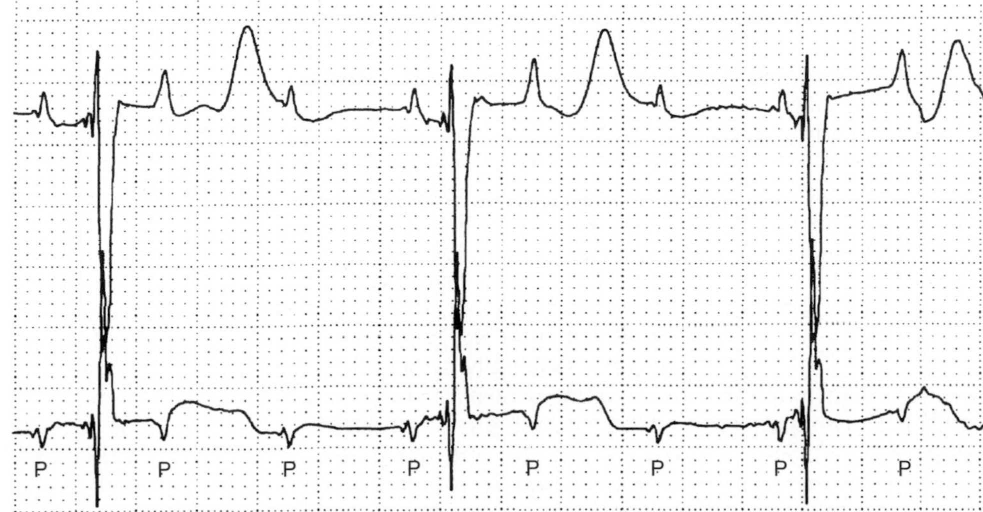

Figure 19-19 Complete heart block in a newborn. The atrial rate is 145 beats per minute, while the ventricular rate is only 50 beats per minute. The corrected QT interval is prolonged at 0.58 seconds. In addition, the QRS duration is prolonged for age at 105 msec. Both are independent indications for anti-bradycardia pacing. P, P-wave.

complex ventricular ectopy would be reasons to proceed with anti-bradycardia pacing.

Pacing for Post-operative Atrioventricular Block

Because of a high risk of sudden death, post-surgical advanced second- or third-degree atrioventricular block persisting or that is not expected to resolve or persists for at least 7 days after cardiac surgery is a class I indication for pacemaker implantation.[277] Unless the surgeon is confident of extensive damage to the conduction system, it is important to wait at least 7 to 9 post-operative days, as recovery of conduction system function is common.

Patients in whom post-operative advanced second- or third-degree atrioventricular block has resolved and in whom conduction returns to normal have a good prognosis and pacing is not indicated (class III, recommendation 1).[40] If there is incomplete recovery with new residual bifascicular block (complete right bundle branch block and left-axis deviation) uncertainty remains and this is included in class IIb as recommendation 1. Long-term instability of the conduction system has been postulated in patients with even transient post-operative heart block, and is thought to contribute to late sudden death in some patients.[278] Thus, these patients should be monitored for any recurrence of heart block or evidence of arrhythmia with regular Holter monitors.

Pacing for Bradycardia-Tachycardia Syndrome

Sinus bradycardia alternating with atrial fibrillation/flutter, intra-atrial re-entry tachycardia, or sinus node re-entry tachycardia is a common problem following surgery for congenital heart disease. Such patients warrant individual consideration of a management plan. Anti-bradycardia pacing with or without atrial anti-tachycardia pacing may be part of a management plan that includes antiarrhythmic medication. Other strategies may include catheter ablation or surgical revision with surgical creation of lines of block to prevent intra-atrial re-entry.[48,159]

Pacing for Syncope and Breath-Holding Spells

In adult practise the use of pacing for patients with neurally mediated syncope may have a role for those who have minimal or no prodrome, those who fail standard therapy, or those who have profound bradycardia or asystole during syncope.[279] For such patients, pacing may increase the time from the onset of symptoms to loss of consciousness, providing critical time for evasive action. The practise, however, is controversial with considerable evidence of a placebo effect.[280] The use of pacing for this indication in paediatrics is rare. Pacing has been used with excellent results for the rare child with severe breath-holding spells associated with profound bradycardia and major pauses.[281]

Pacing for Long QT Syndrome

Anti-bradycardia pacing with a moderately high baseline heart rate (usually a lower rate of 80–90) has been used as an adjunct to β-blocker therapy in long QT syndrome.[282] The rationale is that an increased heart rate shortens the QT together with the minimisation of pause-related QT prolongation. This use of pacing (which is not entirely protective) has diminished somewhat since the advent of the implantable cardioverter defibrillator but continues to be used. Some patients (particularly neonates) with a very long QT may have functional 2:1 block and these patients may benefit from pacing; despite pacing, however, this presentation of long QT syndrome is associated with a high risk of sudden death. Long-QT syndrome with 2:1 atrioventricular or third-degree atrioventricular block is a class IIa indication for pacing. Proven pause-dependent initiation of ventricular tachyarrhythmias with or without a long QT is a class I indication. Pacing is also used in patients with long QT and sinus bradycardia, which may be caused or exacerbated by β-blockers. Some have advocated the use of special pacing algorithms in all long QT patients to virtually eliminate pauses, as torsades de pointes may be pause dependent.[283] The use of implantable defibrillators in a subgroup of high-risk long QT patients is of proven benefit and is likely to be safer than pacing alone, despite the potential problem of a defibrillator shock causing an adrenaline surge, creating an electrical storm.[284]

Pacing for Hypertrophic Cardiomyopathy

Dual-chamber pacing can theoretically diminish left-ventricular outflow obstruction in hypertrophic cardiomyopathy by changing the activation sequence of the ventricular myocardium. When intrinsic atrioventricular conduction is intact, a short atrioventricular interval must be programmed to change the activation sequence. The response to pacing in hypertrophic cardiomyopathy is variable and it is not considered a first-line therapy. Randomised trials have failed to demonstrate benefit.[285] This treatment does not prevent sudden death and the interest in isolated dual-chamber pacing for this condition has diminished over recent years in light of important data showing the efficacy of the implantable defibrillator in decreasing sudden death.

PACEMAKER FUNCTION

Pacemaker Modes

Pacing modes (Table 19-3) are now classified by a five-position code.[286] This is often shortened to the first three positions. The first position describes the chamber(s) paced and the second the chamber(s) sensed. The third position describes the response to sensing. The fourth position indicates rate modulation, and the fifth position indicates multi-site pacing, if any.

For example, the code VVI indicates that the ventricle alone is paced and sensed and the response to sensing is to inhibit pacing. An R in position 4 would refer to the additional feature of rate response. Thus, VVIR is the same as VVI except that the rate of pacing can vary in response to in-built sensors in the device.

In DDD pacing, there is dual-chamber (atrium and ventricle) pacing and sensing and there is a dual response to sensing, depending what is sensed.[287] Other complex modes of pacing such as DDI, DVI, and VDD are less commonly used, but can occasionally be helpful in patients with atypical electrophysiology or device problems such as impaired sensing.[287]

Understanding the underlying physiology is critical to choosing the optimal mode. For example, AAIR is an appropriate mode for sinus node dysfunction with intact atrioventricular node function and VDD or DDD an appropriate mode for atrioventricular block with normal sinus

TABLE 19-3

NASPE/BPEG PACING MODE CODE*

I	II	III	IV	V
Chamber(s) Paced	Chamber(s) Sensed	Response to Sensing	Rate Modulation	Multi-site Pacing
O = None	**O** = None	**O** = None	**O** = None	**O** = None
A = Atrium	**A** = Atrium	**T** = Triggered	**R** = Rate modulation	**A** = Atrium
V = Ventricle	**V** = Ventricle	**I** = Inhibited		**V** = Ventricle
D = Dual (A+V)	**D** = Dual (A+V)	**D** = Dual (T+I)		**D** = Dual (A+V)
S = Single (A or V)	**S** = Single (A or V)			

*Five position NASPE/BPEG code for description of pacing mode. This is often shortened to the first three positions. The first position describes the chamber(s) paced and the second the chamber(s) sensed. The third position describes the response to sensing. The fourth position indicates rate modulation, and the fifth position indicates multi-site pacing, if any.
From Bernstein AD, Daubert JC, Fletcher RD, et al: The revised NASPE/BPEG generic code for antibradycardia, adaptive-rate, and multisite pacing. North American Society of Pacing and Electrophysiology/British Pacing and Electrophysiology Group. Pacing Clin Electrophysiol 2002;25:260–264.

node function. The physician must also be aware that the underlying physiology can evolve.

Pacemaker Timing Cycles and Programming

The multiple features of the current generation of pacemakers can create complex programming issues which need to be understood to interpret pacemaker electrocardiograms correctly. This is often critical in order to decide if there is any dysfunction of the pacemaker system or to allow optimisation of pacemaker settings. The task is often made easier by using diagnostic features built into the device that can provide labelling of events.

Pacemaker function is determined by a number of in-built timing cycles which are measured in milliseconds and often programmable. These include periods where sensing circuits are refractory (temporarily switch off their sensing function).[287] Some basic concepts will be covered here. In single-chamber pacing, such as VVI or AAI, each sensed or paced event is followed by a refractory period to ensure that associated depolarisation and repolarisation is not sensed as an additional event by the device.

Dual-chamber pacemakers, as expected, have a greater number of programmable intervals. The atrioventricular interval begins with a sensed or paced atrial event and ends with a sensed or paced ventricular event. Setting the atrioventricular interval and lower rate limit determines the critically important atrial escape interval, during which an intrinsic atrial event is sought to commence the next cycle or, if no sensed event from either chamber occurs, an atrial paced event occurs at the appropriate time.

The post-ventricular atrial refractory period is present to prevent sensing of P waves which have conducted retrograde and/or far-field ventricular repolarisation on the atrial channel. The aim is to prevent pacemaker-mediated tachycardia, which may occur when a retrograde or far-field signal is sensed and tracked in the ventricle. Pacemaker-mediated tachycardia is a re-entrant rhythm, with one limb of the re-entrant loop being the patient's retrograde conduction, and the other the pacemaker.

Atrial sensing is refractory during the atrioventricular interval and together the atrioventricular interval and the post-ventricular atrial refractory period constitute the total atrial refractory period which can limit the upper atrial tracking rate of the pacemaker.

A detailed understanding of timing cycles and refractory periods is required by those who programme pacemakers in paediatric patients. The default out of the box settings are based on typical adult patients, and are inappropriate for paediatric patients. Younger patients have higher heart rates than adults and attention needs to be given to the potential for pacemaker-mediated Wenckebach and even 2:1 paced atrioventricular block to occur at higher rates.

Special Features

A number of special features are available in the current generation of pacemakers and many of them are applicable to children.

Almost all pacemakers have the ability for rate-responsive (adaptive) pacing. In-built sensors are used to detect movement or physical activity and/or physiological parameters such as minute ventilation. The device can then respond to these indicators of increased physiological demand by increasing baseline heart rate. This feature is used for any loss of chronotropy, such as sinus node dysfunction or complete heart block with single-chamber ventricular pacing. It is available in either single- or dual-chamber devices, but is not appropriate until the child is able to walk. The sensitivity and responsiveness of the sensor can be adjusted to mimic normal physiology. In-built features such as heart rate graphs as well as assessment with Holter and exercise testing may be useful when optimising the settings for a patient, and some devices have automatic optimising algorithms.

Mode switching is an important feature of most dual-chamber pacemakers, designed to minimise ventricular tracking of an atrial tachycardia. For example, if a patient in DDD mode suddenly developed an intra-atrial re-entry tachycardia, the pacemaker would detect the high atrial rate and change the mode to DDIR; thus, the ventricular paced rate will be appropriate for the level of activity (sensor indicated rate) rather than inappropriately fast due to tracking of the atrial arrhythmia at the upper tracking rate (Fig. 19-20). Mode switching can add considerably to the complexity of interpreting pacemaker timing cycles, but it is essential in many patients with intermittent atrial tachycardias.[288]

Other safety and efficiency features have been developed and many have become automated. For example, some pacemakers have the ability to detect problems with the hardware, such as a significant increase in lead impedance (which could indicate a lead fracture). If such problems are detected, the device can automatically make changes to programming to ensure optimal function. Many new pacemakers have the ability to regularly check the pacing thresholds and adjust the outputs (with a programmable margin

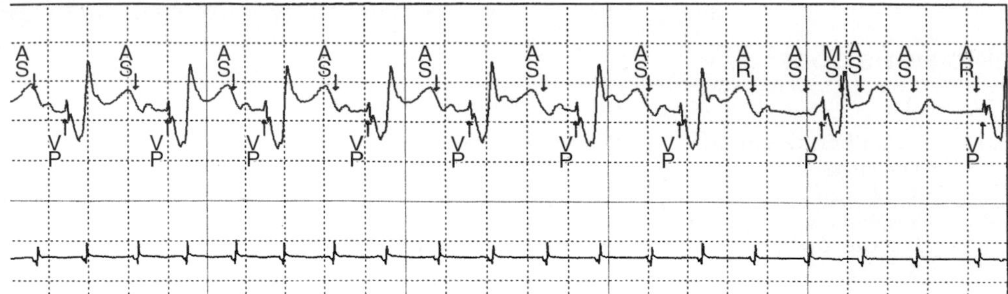

Figure 19-20 Automatic mode switching. The top part of the tracing shows an electrocardiogram with event markers. The bottom part of the tracing shows simultaneous atrial electrogram demonstrating atrial tachycardia. Each square represents 200 milliseconds. In the early part of the tracing, only every second atrial depolarisation is sensed. The other atrial depolarisation is not recognised, as it lies within the post-ventricular blanking period. An in-built algorithm intermittently seeks this situation. When the device recognises the underlying atrial tachycardia, mode switching occurs, and the paced rate slows to the sensor indicated rate. AR, atrial sensing falling within refractory period; AS, atrial sense; MS, mode switch; VP, ventricular pace.

of safety) to minimise battery usage. Such a setting would not be appropriate for children with long QT syndrome as a pause could potentially be caused (a known risk factor for torsades de pointes in some long QT patients). This feature has been designed to work with endocardial leads but it has been shown it can work successfully in children who have epicardial leads.[289] Prior to using this feature it should be tested for a period in the monitor only mode to ensure it functions well and safely in an individual child.

IMPLANTATION CONSIDERATIONS

Pacing in paediatric cardiology and congenital heart disease presents a unique set of challenges. Small patient size, patient growth, intracardiac shunts, complex anatomy, long-term venous access, surgical scarring, abnormal myocardial performance, and late post-operative arrhythmias are but a few of the issues that frequently arise in the care of this population. A good understanding of the basic principles of pacing allows individualised decisions to be made for each patient's circumstances.

Epicardial Versus Endocardial Implantation

Pacing leads are generally considered the most vulnerable and unreliable part of any pacemaker system and the majority of pacemaker system problems are directly related to lead issues. This is especially the case in paediatrics and congenital heart disease.[290] Given a likely life-long need for pacing, long-term vascular access is a critical issue. Endocardial leads in younger patients carry the risk of venous obstruction or thrombosis, making placing future pacemaker systems increasingly difficult. In the neonate and infant, most centres use an epicardial approach when pacing is needed, although controversy remains as to what the cut-off for endocardial pacing should be.

Most epicardial pacing is now performed using steroid-eluting leads which minimise inflammation at the lead-myocardial interface and have significantly better performance than the previous generation of epicardial screw-in leads. The performance of the newer leads is now competitive with endocardial leads.[291,292]

Pericardial effusion and post-pericardiotomy syndrome can occur after epicardial pacemaker implantation and also rarely after endocardial implantation, and must be considered if a patient is displaying symptoms consistent with post-pericardiotomy syndrome.[293]

Predictors for venous obstruction in children have been sought, and in one retrospective study a predictive index was created to evaluate the risk of venous obstruction.[294] In this study, the sum of the cross sectional area of all leads was indexed to body surface area at implant, a result greater than 6.6 mm^2/m^2 predicted venous obstruction with a sensitivity of 90% and a specificity of 84%. This index has been used to help determine who should receive an epicardial versus a transvenous system. However, subsequent studies have had conflicting results and the issue remains controversial.[295,296]

Each centre, depending on policy and experience has different cut-offs for deciding who should receive an epicardial versus a transvenous system. When considering using endocardial pacing in the younger child, one must take into account the child's size and anatomy, as well as the body habitus of the child.[294] Although transvenous pacing has been shown to be possible in infants, it should be avoided if possible because of the risks of pocket erosion, venous obstruction, as well as growth-related problems such as tension on the lead. The goals of pacemaker implantation must address both adequacy of pacing and long-term issues such as venous patency and potential need for future lead extractions.[297,298]

Traditionally endocardial ventricular pacing leads were placed into the right ventricular apex for stability and ease of placement. However, mounting evidence regarding the potential creation of myocardial dysfunction through ventricular dyssynchrony has led many away from this practise, and many leads are now placed on the ventricular septum.[299]

Unipolar Versus Bipolar Leads

In bipolar pacing systems the lead tip is the cathode (the negative electrode) and the closely adjacent lead ring (or in the case of epicardial electrodes a second lead button) is the anode (the positive electrode, or ground). Unipolar pacing systems use the lead tip as the cathode and the pacemaker box as the anode (ground). Sensing occurs via these same circuits. Unipolar leads have the potential disadvantage of an increased possibility of oversensing of non-cardiac signals and of unwanted skeletal muscle stimulation. Many centres prefer to use bipolar systems (due to frequently better sensing performance); however, when lead dysfunction occurs it is possible, in most devices, to reprogramme sensing, pacing, or both, to either unipolar or bipolar mode. In epicardial systems, not infrequently when bipolar pacing or sensing is inadequate, a change to unipolar will allow satisfactory pacemaker settings. This would usually occur when the lead damage has occurred in the pole that is switched off with the change for bipolar to unipolar.

Congenital Heart Diseases

Most authorities would agree that patients with intracardiac shunts should have epicardial devices. This is because patients with transvenous leads and an intracardiac shunt have a greater than two-fold risk of a systemic embolic event than those with epicardial leads.[300] Even patients with minimal, apparently pure left-to-right shunts may be at risk of embolism due to the possibility of a potentially altered haemodynamic sequence after pacing creating a brief period of right-to-left shunting.[301]

There is controversy regarding the placement of atrial pacing leads in Fontan anatomy. Some centres find the placement of endocardial atrial leads acceptable in patients without shunts, while other centres avoid placing endocardial leads within a Fontan circuit because of the potential for pulmonary emboli or systemic emboli in patients who have a fenestration. Unfortunately many patients who have had a Fontan operation have significant scarring and it can be difficult to obtain appropriate sensing and capture thresholds. When scarring precludes any possibility of appropriate pacemaker function from a traditional epicardial approach, surgically placing the lead transmurally with only its tip extending into the cardiac chamber may prove useful.[302]

Pacemaker Infection

An important potential complication of device insertion is system infection. Most centres routinely prescribe prophylactic peri-operative antibiotics. System revision and the presence of trisomy 21 have been shown to be risk factors for infection in paediatric patients.[303] Management of deep pocket infection should involve removal of the device and the leads in their entirety. The recently published American Heart Association guidelines for prevention of endocarditis do not recommend prophylaxis for patients with endocardial pacing leads.[304]

Dual- Versus Single-Chamber Pacing

In adults with structurally normal hearts the choice between single- and dual-chambered devices under various circumstances has provided the substance for much debate over the years.[305] In the adult community debate continues and practise varies widely despite a large amount of data. Although maintaining atrioventricular synchrony is intuitively appealing, there is evidence to support greater importance of minimisation of ventricular pacing.[306] In paediatrics and congenital heart disease individual consideration is made in each patient. Frequently younger, smaller children have a smaller single-chamber system as their first device, which at a future time is upgraded to a dual-chamber system when a system revision is required.

Patients with impaired haemodynamics may particularly benefit from having atrioventricular synchrony, so frequently have dual-chamber devices prescribed early in life. Some new generation devices have the capability of compound modes that give preference to intrinsic atrioventricular conduction to minimise ventricular pacing, while allowing for back-up ventricular pacing in the event of intermittent atrioventricular block.

Pacemaker Syndrome

Pacemaker syndrome comprises a constellation of symptoms resulting from loss of atrioventricular synchrony or retrograde ventriculoatrial conduction, and can occur in children.[307] When there is lack of sequential or physiological atrioventricular filling due to atrial contraction against closed atrioventricular valves during ventricular systole, transient increases in atrial pressure are caused. This may lead to symptoms including fatigue, exercise intolerance, a sensation of fullness, dyspnoea, and headache. It may also provoke vagal mediated changes associated with dizziness and syncope.[308] The syndrome most frequently occurs in patients with single-chamber ventricular pacing systems, but can also be seen with dual-chamber systems with inappropriate atrioventricular delay settings. It is less common in children than adults but may develop over time.[307] Treatment can include adjustment of atrioventricular intervals (including rate adaptive features) for those with dual-chamber systems and upgrading those with single-chamber devices to a dual-chamber system.

PACEMAKER FOLLOW-UP

All patients with any implanted rhythm devices require long-term follow-up. Monitoring for any evidence of change in device or patient status is essential, so that appropriate programming or hardware revisions can be made when necessary.

After interrogation the programmer can display important information including device warnings, estimated remaining battery life, lead impedances, and information about percentage of sensing/pacing and any tachyarrhythmias detected (sometimes including annotated electrograms of the rhythm). Heart rate graphs are commonly available. Often the type of information available is programmable.

A sudden rise in lead impedance should arouse suspicion of a lead fracture. Similarly a fall in lead impedance may represent an insulation break.

If possible the nature and rate of the underlying rhythm should be documented, by slowly reducing the pacing rate, until intrinsic rhythm emerges. If the patient displays any symptoms, the testing for intrinsic rhythm should be terminated. Most devices do not allow the rate to be turned down to less than 30 and if there is no underlying ventricular rhythm coming through the patient is classified as pacemaker dependent. Tolerable levels of short-term bradycardia vary among patients, and attention should be paid to the comfort level of the patient. It is important that pacing never be abruptly ceased, as suppression of the intrinsic rhythm is likely to be seen at physiologic pacing rates, and thus unacceptably long pauses might be seen.

Regular meticulous follow-up is mandatory to ensure that the pacemaker system is safe and set optimally and battery life is maximised. Each brand of device has its own proprietary programmer. The timing of follow-up depends on the complexity and stability of the patient and the system. Typically devices are checked the day after implantation, in 2 to 4 weeks, 3 months, and 6 months. The frequency of long-term follow-up is determined by a variety of factors related to both the device and the child. Those with pacemaker dependency, cardiac resynchronisation devices, and implantable defibrillators require more frequent follow-up.

Testing Sensing

Pacemakers are nearly always programmed to sense or to detect spontaneous cardiac depolarisations. Appropriate sensing is critical for acceptable device function. The sensing setting is the amplitude in millivolts that the device has to perceive in order that it acknowledges the presence of an intrinsic beat. Typically the device is then set with at least a two times sensing margin of safety. As an example, imagine a patient with complete heart block and a stable junctional escape rate of 55 beats per minute. For testing ventricular sensing, the ventricular rate is slowly decreased to below the rate of the intrinsic rhythm, so no pacing should occur. The ventricular sensing is set at a low level (for example, 2.0 millivolts), and then increased incrementally until appropriate sensing of the intrinsic rhythm is lost and pacing occurs. The last level at which appropriate sensing was seen is the sensing threshold.

Intrinsic atrial signals usually have a lower amplitude than ventricular signals as they are created by a smaller muscle bulk. Thus, to adequately identify the amplitude of intrinsic atrial signals one must start at very low levels, such as 0.5 millivolts.

Oversensing should also be tested for, and is most commonly seen in unipolar systems. Isometric manoeuvres involving the muscles close to the implantation site are performed during paced rhythm. If oversensing occurs, muscle noise will be picked up inappropriately as noise and pacing will not occur.

Testing Threshold

The threshold is the minimum electrical stimulus required to consistently capture the heart and trigger contraction. The stimulation threshold is a square wave, a function of both amplitude (measured in volts) and pulse width (measured in milliseconds). The threshold is tested by keeping the amplitude stable and decreasing the pulse width (or vice versa) until capture no longer occurs. In Figure 19-21 ventricular capture is demonstrated by a ventricular pacing artefact followed immediately by a wide QRS complex with a T wave in the opposite direction of depolarisation. Atrial capture is demonstrated by P wave immediately preceded by an atrial pacemaker artefact. It is important to remember that bipolar systems may not show any pacing spikes on a surface electrocardiogram, and thus electrogram morphology of the P wave and QRS must be relied upon to indicate capture of the paced chamber. Obviously when testing threshold the testing rate needs to be faster than the underlying rate (unless pacing in an asynchronous mode), or pacing will not occur. In complete heart block, atrial threshold is usually tested in DDD mode. Output should then be set at three times the pulse width or twice the amplitude to ensure an adequate safety margin, given the inherent variability of cardiac thresholds.

Many paediatric centres routinely programme pulse width with a three times pulse width threshold margin of safety in standard patients. Increasing voltage amplitude comes at a high price for battery life. The hyperbolic strength-duration curve describes the relationship between pulse duration and voltage at threshold (Fig. 19-22). At short pulse durations, an increase in pulse duration significantly lessens the voltage required but at longer pulse widths, there is little decrease in voltage for the same increment in pulse width. This must always be considered when programming. In some cases it helps to construct a strength-duration curve to optimise output settings. Some devices have testing algorithms that allow easy construction of a curve.

Pacemaker Clinic Routines

For patients with endocardial leads a regular (usually annual) chest X-ray throughout childhood is typically performed to look at lead position and the effects of growth. Some centres are decreasing the frequency of routine chest X-rays due to concerns over radiation exposure, and only performing them if there are clinical concerns or if there has been an impressive growth spurt. A regular chest X-ray for those with epicardial leads is appropriate to look for the rare but important complication of cardiac strangulation.[309] Although this has only been rarely reported, it can be fatal. Strangulation can still occur after a lead has been abandoned.

An annual Holter monitor is useful to check pacemaker function over a 24-hour period and screen for the emergence of and interaction with any tachyarrhythmias. Sometimes premature ventricular contractions are not sensed as well as intrinsic ventricular rhythm. Unless this

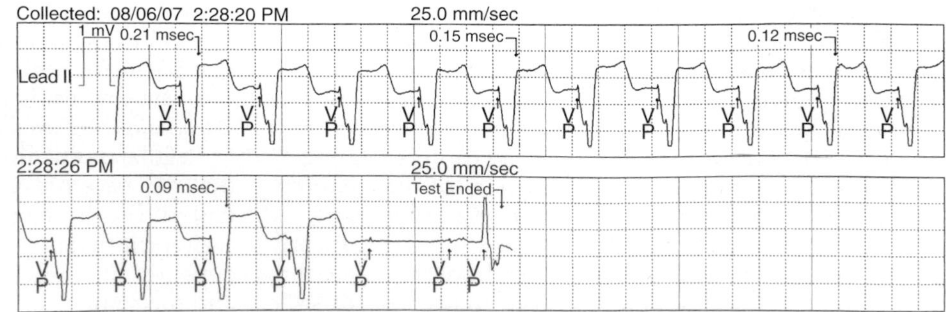

Figure 19-21 Ventricular threshold test. In this example, the amplitude is kept stable at 2.0 V and the pulse width is progressively decreased. Capture is demonstrated by a ventricular pacing artifact followed immediately by a wide QRS complex with a T wave in the opposite direction of depolarisation. At 0.12 msec, each pacemaker artefact is followed by a captured beat. At 0.09 msec, only the first beat is captured. Two further pacing artifacts are not followed by ventricular depolarisation, and later there is a ventricular escape beat. The threshold is described as 0.12 msec at 2.0 V. VP, ventricular pace.

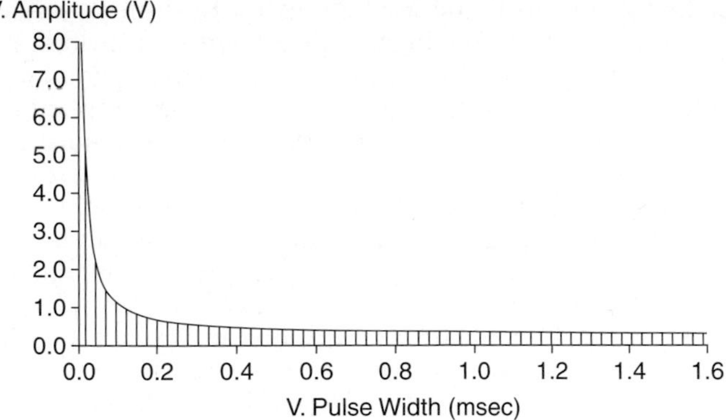

Figure 19-22 The hyperbolic strength-duration curve. This curve was estimated by a device algorithm after threshold testing. Each point on the curve describes the amplitude in volts and the pulse duration in milliseconds of various thresholds. At short pulse durations an increase in pulse duration significantly lessens the voltage required but at longer pulse widths, there is little decrease in voltage for the same increment in pulse width. This must always be considered when programming.

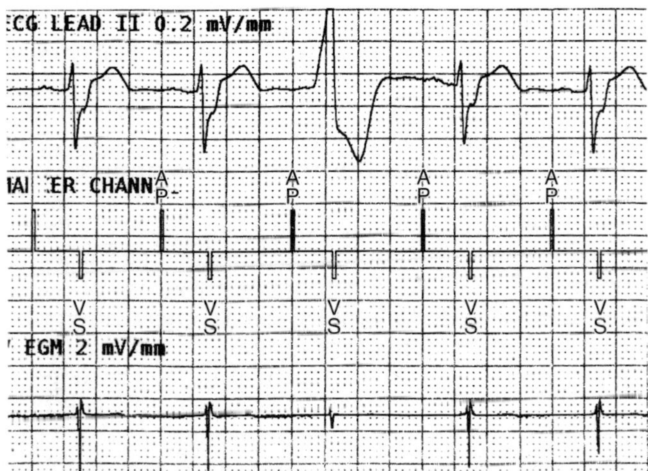

Figure 19-23 Differential sensing of premature ventricular contractions. The top panel shows the surface electrocardiogram, while the middle panel shows marker channels. The bottom panel shows an endocardial electrogram on a scale of 2 millivolts per millimeter. The middle beat is an atrial-paced event followed by a premature ventricular contraction. The amplitude of the sensed signal from the premature ventricular contraction is significantly smaller than the conducted ventricular beats. At some sensing settings, this could result in the undersensing of premature contractions. AP, atrial paced event; VS, ventricular sensed event.

is seen at a pacemaker check (Fig. 19-23), the only way to diagnose this is on Holter. There is a potential risk of ventricular arrhythmias if premature ventricular contractions are undersensed, as pacing may occur at a critical time and initiate a ventricular arrhythmia.

An annual echocardiogram is important to check ventricular function and any mechanical lead effect on valvar function (particularly tricuspid). Patients with bi-ventricular devices should have optimisation of the V-V and A-V interval under echocardiographic guidance to optimise ventricular function.

Keeping database information for all pacemaker patients is important, as from time to time there are device advisories or recalls necessitating contact and review of all patients with a particular lead or device.

Pacemaker Dependence

Patients with no underlying rhythm may collapse or die if their pacemaker loses ventricular capture. In this situation some centres set the device with broader safety margins than usual, but there is no clear data available to guide this practise. Individual decisions should be made based on apparent risk of threshold change versus cost to battery longevity. Successful use of a pacemaker with an integrated home monitoring facility that can send a message to a mobile phone–like receiver if there is a significant threshold rise has been reported in a child with no underlying rhythm.[310] Regular meticulous follow-up at more frequent intervals is appropriate.

Restrictions for Patients with Implanted Devices

All paediatric cardiologists need to encourage their patients to lead a healthy, active lifestyle. Some sporting activities with a high risk of bodily impact have the potential to damage the pacemaker system and cannot be recommended in patients who are pacemaker dependent. Depending on the underlying heart disease, the underlying rhythm, and the potential for tachyarrhythmias individual decisions need to be made regarding prescription/restriction of activity in other patients. Doctors make recommendations and then families make informed medical decisions. With respect to athletic activity restrictions, many teenagers and their families may not take heed of our advice!

Non-cardiac Surgery and Magnetic Resonance Imaging

Patients undergoing non-cardiac surgery need to have a plan made in advance about intra-operative pacing. Problems that can be encountered include diathermy signals being falsely sensed as myocardial signals resulting in inhibition of pacing. Bipolar diathermy is preferred, but still may cause some electrical interference. In some cases is it safer to change the device to a non-sensing mode (VOO or DOO) for the duration of the surgery. Electrocardiographic monitoring during the surgery is of course mandatory.[311] If no intra-operative changes are made, a pacemaker check after surgery is sensible to make sure there has been no electrical or hardware damage to the device.

In general, performing magnetic resonance imaging in patients with an implanted device is contraindicated. Death has been reported in pacemaker patients. There are a variety of mechanisms by which MR can affect pacemakers and implantable cardioverter defibrillators (ICDs). Potential interactions can involve multiple components of the device, including the leads, circuitry, reed switch, battery, and capacitors. There is now controversy about whether contraindications are absolute or relative. Device manufacturers are seeking ways to make devices magnetic resonance imaging safe.[312]

Temporary Pacemakers

Temporary pacemakers are an integral part of post-operative management following surgery for congenital heart disease. Indications for pacemaker use in these circumstances are usually

- To treat bradyarrhythmia, such as complete heart block, sinus bradycardia

- To achieve atrioventricular synchrony in the treatment of junctional ectopic tachycardia, as an adjunct to cooling and/or antiarrhythmic medication
- To overdrive re-entry tachyarrhythmias
- To use pacing manoeuvres to diagnose an arrhythmia mechanism

Sensing and pacing thresholds should be tested at least daily in any actively used temporary pacing wires, as temporary wire thresholds shift rapidly and unpredictably. With older generation pacemakers, patients with complete heart block may be at risk of losing pacing because of cross-talk. The atrial output pacemaker artefact is falsely sensed by the ventricular lead as ventricular activity and therefore no ventricular pacing ensues. Newer generation temporary pacemakers have a cross-talk sensing window to avoid this problem. All patients having temporary pacing should in addition to electrocardiogram monitoring have some form of physiological monitoring as pacing spikes without capture can be interpreted by electrocardiogram monitoring systems as a rhythm.

Future Directions for Bradycardia Pacing

A novel leadless pacemaker system is under development and has been successfully tested in animals.[313] The system comprises an ultrasound transmitter delivering energy from the chest wall to a receiver-electrode in contact with the myocardium that then converts the ultrasound energy to electrical energy sufficient to pace. If the promise of the system is fulfilled, it will revolutionise pacing and be of tremendous benefit to paediatric patients. Considerable effort, using molecular biological techniques, is also being put into the development of a biological pacemaker but many obstacles remain.[314]

IMPLANTABLE CARDIOVERTER-DEFIBRILLATORS

Ventricular arrhythmias can be seen in multiple paediatric and congenital heart disease populations, and sudden death can result from the most malignant and haemodynamically unstable of these rhythms. Implantable cardioverter-defibrillators have been shown to be effective in preventing sudden death due to arrhythmia in children and young adults with congenital heart disease or electrical myopathies.[28] There are a variety of diagnoses that may increase the likelihood of ventricular arrhythmias, including repaired congenital cardiac disease, primary electrical disease, such as the long QT syndrome, catecholaminergic ventricular tachycardia, and idiopathic ventricular fibrillation, as well as hypertrophic and dilated cardiomyopathies.[315,316] There is consensus regarding indications of use of implantable defibrillators for secondary prevention, including patients resuscitated from cardiac arrest with documented ventricular arrhythmia, and documented haemodynamically significant ventricular tachycardia requiring cardioversion or defibrillation. Other indications that may fall into this category are those that are highly suggestive of ventricular tachycardias such as unexplained syncope in the setting of repaired congenital heart disease, and repeated syncope despite adequate treatment of primary electrical disease. Primary prevention, or defibrillators placed for high-risk clinical scenarios without documentation of malignant arrhythmias, remain more difficult clinical decisions. Congenital heart disease with inducible sustained ventricular tachycardia at ventricular stimulation testing remains a controversial indication for implantable cardioverter defibrillators, although recent evidence suggests it may be clinically useful.[29] There are no paediatric randomised clinical trials looking at survival, and thus consideration of implantation of a cardioverter-defibrillator in this population must be guided by clinical judgement and extrapolation from the adult experience.

The American Heart Association and Heart Rhythm Society guidelines for cardioverter defibrillator implantation are based on adult studies, and thus do not always apply directly to the paediatric population, but can be a reasonable starting point [41] (Table 19-4).

Several retrospective studies have demonstrated a high incidence of appropriate defibrillation therapies in children, but unfortunately inappropriate shocks are common as well.[315,316] Inappropriate therapies frequently are due to supraventricular tachycardia with rapid conduction to the ventricle, sinus tachycardia, or lead failure.[315-317] Most inappropriate therapies due to supraventricular tachycardia can be prevented by programming changes such as increasing the detection threshold and discrimination algorithms, as well as usage of β-blockers. It may sometime be helpful to determine the upper intrinsic rate with exercise testing, to ensure that sinus tachycardia does not exceed the ventricular fibrillation detection threshold.[317] However, these manoeuvres do not help with the inappropriate shocks that may occur due to lead failure, which is particularly high in the paediatric population.[315] Failed high-voltage leads frequently require extraction before a new lead can be placed, due to concerns of false sensing due to interaction of two ventricular leads. Cooper et al examined laser lead extraction in the paediatric and congenital heart disease population, and found that it could be safely and effectively performed with similar complication rates to that of the general population.[298]

When cardioverter-defibrillators were first used clinically, routine defibrillation threshold testing was performed. As the technology has advanced, and technical self-diagnostics have improved, there has been a move away from routine testing. One study in the paediatric and congenital population found that the majority of routine defibrillation threshold testing did not trigger any clinical changes. However, in patients in whom there was a clinical concern (such as change on X-ray, inappropriate shocks, or a change in pace/sense values), threshold testing revealed abnormalities that led to important programming or hardware modifications.[318] Thus, routine defibrillation threshold testing may not be necessary, but any important clinical changes should lead to consideration of repeated testing.

In patients with congenitally malformed hearts, implantation of cardioverter-defibrillators may be limited due to cardiac anatomy or patient size. Epicardial patches may be used in some of these patients, but require a thoracotomy and may lead to a restrictive pericardial process. Recently, alternative configurations have been used to allow implantation in patients who are too small for traditional transvenous implantation, or those with intracardiac shunting. These alternative configurations were first published in 2001, when three centres described cases where epicardial ventricular sensing leads were utilised with a subcutaneously implanted high voltage coil, and the active generator was placed in an abdominal position.[319–321] Another configuration used a transvenous high voltage lead placed in an epicardial position, also with an abdominally positioned active generator. Both of these alternative configurations have been used successfully in children and young adults with congenital heart disease, but the patients require close monitoring and follow-up, including routine testing of the defibrillation threshold, as they are new technologies and thus are prone to unanticipated complications.[322]

CARDIAC RESYNCHRONISATION THERAPY

Cardiomyopathy affects a variety of paediatric patients, including those with idiopathic dilated cardiomyopathies, congenital heart disease, and inherited cardiomyopathies. The failing heart often has an associated intraventricular conduction delay, which may be seen as a prolonged QRS or bundle branch block. This delay may correlate with dyssynchronous, inefficient contraction of the ventricles. Using resynchronisation therapy, at least two regions of the ventricles are paced in an attempt to improve ventricular synchrony, and thus improve cardiac output. Resynchronisation therapy in adults with dilated cardiomyopathy and left bundle branch block has been shown to improve quality of life, increase exercise tolerance, and improve overall survival.[323–325] The paediatric experience with resynchronisation therapy began primarily with the congenital cardiac disease population as well as dilated cardiomyopathy. These populations, however, are very different from the population of adults in whom resynchronisation therapy was initially utilised. The vast majority of the adult patients in early trials of resynchronisation therapy had ischaemic cardiomyopathy and left bundle branch block, although more recent trials have shown similar results with non-ischaemic cardiomyopathy patients.[325] Patients with repaired congenital cardiac disease frequently have right bundle branch block, while left bundle branch block is relatively rare. The anatomy of patients with congenital heart disease is highly varied, and the regions of dyssynchrony vary similarly. Right ventricular failure, rather than

TABLE 19-4

AHA/ACC/NASPE RECOMMENDATIONS FOR ICD THERAPY

Class I (there is evidence and general agreement that placement of an implantable cardioverter defibrillator is appropriate)

1. Cardiac arrest due to VF or VT not due to a transient or reversible cause
2. Spontaneous sustained VT in association with structural heart disease
3. Syncope of undetermined origin with clinically relevant, hemodynamically significant sustained VT or VF induced at electrophysiologic study when drug therapy is ineffective, not tolerated, or not preferred
4. Nonsustained VT in patients with coronary disease, prior MI, LV dysfunction, and inducible VF, or sustained VT at electrophysiologic study that is not suppressible by a class I antiarrhythmic drug
5. Spontaneous sustained VT in patients without structural heart disease and not amenable to other treatments.

Class II (there is conflicting evidence or diverging opinion)

Class IIa (the weight of evidence favors placement)

1. Patients with left ventricular ejection fraction of less than or equal to 30% at least 1 month post-MI and 3 months post–coronary artery revascularization surgery

Class IIb (evidence is less well established)

1. Cardiac arrest presumed to be due to VF when electrophysiologic testing is precluded by other medical conditions
2. Severe symptoms (e.g., syncope) attributable to ventricular tachyarrhythmias in patients awaiting cardiac transplantation
3. Familial or inherited conditions with a high risk for life-threatening ventricular tachyarrhythmias such as long-QT syndrome or hypertrophic cardiomyopathy
4. Nonsustained VT with coronary artery disease, prior MI, LV dysfunction, and inducible sustained VT or VF at electrophysiologic study
5. Recurrent syncope of undetermined origin in the presence of ventricular dysfunction and inducible ventricular arrhythmias at electrophysiologic study when other causes of syncope have been excluded
6. Syncope of unexplained origin or family history of unexplained sudden cardiac death in association with typical or atypical right bundle-branch block and ST segment elevations (Brugada syndrome)
7. Syncope in patients with advanced structural heart disease in whom thorough invasive and noninvasive investigations have failed to define a cause

Class III (generally agreed that placement is not indicated)

1. Syncope of undetermined cause in a patient without inducible ventricular tachyarrhythmias and without structural heart disease
2. Incessant VT or VF
3. VF or VT resulting from arrhythmias amenable to surgical or catheter ablation; e.g., atrial arrhythmias associated with the Wolff–Parkinson–White syndrome, right ventricular outflow tract VT, idiopathic left ventricular tachycardia, or fascicular VT
4. Ventricular tachyarrhythmias due to a transient or reversible disorder (e.g., acute MI, electrolyte imbalance, drugs, or trauma) when correction of the disorder is considered feasible and likely to substantially reduce the risk of recurrent arrhythmia
5. Significant psychiatric illnesses that may be aggravated by device implantation or may preclude systematic follow-up
6. Terminal illnesses with projected life expectancy less than 6 months
7. Patients with coronary artery disease with LV dysfunction and prolonged QRS duration in the absence of spontaneous or inducible sustained or nonsustained VT who are undergoing coronary bypass surgery
8. NYHA class IV drug-refractory congestive heart failure in patients who are not candidates for cardiac transplantation

LV, left ventricular; MI, myocardial infarction; VF, ventricular fibrillation; VT, ventricular tachyarrhythmia.
From Gregoratos G, Abrams J, Epstein AE, et al: ACC/AHA/NASPE 2002 guideline update for implantation of cardiac pacemakers and antiarrhythmia devices: Summary article—A report of the American College of Cardiology/American Heart Association Task Force on Practice Guidelines (ACC/AHA/NASPE Committee to Update the 1998 Pacemaker Guidelines). Circulation 2002;106:2145–2161.

left, is most common, and a failing single ventricle can be of either right or left morphology. Dyssynchrony may be present with a normal QRS duration and these patients can still benefit from resynchronisation therapy.

The first studies of resynchronisation therapy in the paediatric and congenital population examined the response of patients immediately following repair of congenital heart disease.[326,327] During repair, temporary epicardial pacing leads were placed allowing pacing at multiple ventricular locations. It was found that resynchronisation therapy could increase cardiac output, could increase systolic blood pressure, and in one study could assist in weaning from bypass.[326,327] In patients with right bundle branch block, right ventricular pacing alone has also been used to resynchronise the heart.[328] In one catheterisation-based study, pacing in right ventricle was found to increase cardiac index and dP/dt.[329]

Recently, as cardiac resynchronisation therapy has been used more in paediatric and congenital heart disease patients, more literature (predominantly in the form of case reports and series) has begun to emerge. Consistently it has been found that some (but not all) in this population can benefit from this form of therapy, and predictors of response have not yet been well identified.[330–333] This difficulty has also been found in the adult population, and there is a tremendous amount of work looking now at identification of cardiac resynchronisation candidates. The largest of the paediatric studies of cardiac resynchronisation was published by Dubin and colleagues.[334] The population consisted of 103 patients from 22 centres, with a median age at the start of resynchronisation of 12.8 years and a median follow-up of 4 months. The patients predominantly had repaired congenital heart disease, with a smaller portion having cardiomyopathy. Overall the majority of the patients had decrease in their QRS duration and increase in their ejection fraction. However, 11 patients did not appear to respond, and no clear unifying characteristics of those patients could be identified, perhaps in part due to the small numbers.

ANTI-TACHYCARDIA PACING

Patients with repaired congenital heart disease have a high incidence of tachycardias, particularly intra-atrial re-entrant tachycardias. Cardioversion must sometimes be used to return these patients to sinus rhythm, but others may benefit from automated anti-tachycardia pacemakers that can pace-terminate a re-entrant rhythm. These pacemakers employ burst pacing algorithms to interrupt re-entrant tachycardias, in both the atrium and the ventricle. The current generation of implantable defibrillators have anti-tachycardia pacing capacity, and have been found to be safe and effective (and thus reduce the number of shocks) for termination of some ventricular tachycardias in the population of adults with coronary arterial disease.[335,336] Little data is available for ventricular anti-tachycardia pacing in children, but consideration should always be given to this therapy, given the possibility of reducing the incidence of shocks in this psychologically vulnerable group.[337]

Atrial arrhythmias are a frequent source of morbidity and even mortality in the population of patients with congenitally malformed hearts.[338–341] Atrial anti-tachycardia pacing has been studied in this population, and has been shown to be safe and effective in more than half of the population.[342] Due to younger, healthy atrioventricular nodes and thus frequent one-to-one atrioventricular conduction in this population, some episodes of atrial flutter were misclassified by the device as ventricular tachycardias, and thus not treated with atrial anti-tachycardia pacing. To optimise the efficacy of these systems, consideration should be given to treatment with an atrioventricular nodal blocking agent, to minimise the incidence of one-to-one conduction. Although only half of the episodes of intra-atrial re-entrant tachycardia were successfully detected and treated, these episodes could have represented multiple cardioversions for these patients, and thus even partial efficacy may offer significant improvement in quality of life.

SUMMARY

The majority of electrophysiological studies in children are currently performed with a view to proceed to radiofrequency ablation of arrhythmias. Ablation has a high rate of success, has a low incidence of complications, and is cost effective. It can now be offered as first-line treatment to children of school age when the parents or child prefer this option to medication, or when medication is not tolerated. Acceptable alternatives to ablation include observation only with no treatment (for infrequent and easily controlled tachycardias) or treatment with medication. In younger children, who may spontaneously outgrow the arrhythmic substrate and in whom the complication rate may be higher, ablation is usually restricted to life-threatening arrhythmias, to those in whom medication cannot control the arrhythmia, where medication causes severe side effects, or in advance of proposed cardiac surgery. With the continued development of equipment and advances in techniques, it is likely that the rates of success will continue to increase and more arrhythmic substrates will become amenable to curative catheter ablation.

Pacemakers and implantable defibrillators have dramatically decreased in size and increased in sophistication and programmability, allowing for much broader indications and application in the paediatric and congenital heart disease population. As survival continues to improve following congenital heart disease repair, and better understanding is gained of the risk factors for sudden death, usage of these devices will only grow in the management of children with cardiac disease.

ACKNOWLEDGEMENTS

We would like to thank our teachers, mentors and colleagues, particularly those at Boston Children's Hospital, The Hospital for Sick Children in Toronto, and The Royal Children's Hospital, Melbourne, as well as Dr. Eric Rosenthal, who wrote the previous edition of this chapter.

The complete reference list can be found on the companion Expert Consult web site at www.expertconsult.com.

ANNOTATED REFERENCES

• Gregoratos G, Gibbons RJ, Antman EM, et al: ACC/AHA/NASPE 2002 Guideline Update for Implantation of Cardiac Pacemakers and Antiarrhythmia Devices. Circulation 2002;106:2145. Updated 2008: http://content.onlinejacc.org/cgi/content/full/j.jacc.2008.02.33

These evidenced-based guidelines for prescribing anti-bradycardia permanent pacemakers are published and updated in a thoughtful document by the American College of Cardiology (www.acc.org) in conjunction with the American Heart Association (www.americanheart.org) and the Heart Rhythm Society (www.hrsonline.org). All paediatric cardiologists should regularly review the latest version of this document, which provides an excellent basis and context for decision making.

- Walsh EP, Saul JP, Triedman JK: Cardiac Arrhythmias in Children and Young Adults with Congenital Heart Disease. Philadelphia: Lippincott Williams & Wilkins, 2001.

  This recently published textbook is a thorough overview of state-of-the art paediatric and congenital electrophysiology, and an outstanding resource for any reader seeking further information on this topic.

- Kugler JD, Danford DA, Deal BJ, et al: Radiofrequency catheter ablation for tachyarrhythmias in children and adolescents. The Pediatric Electrophysiology Society. N Engl J Med 1994;330:1481–1487.

  This landmark paper documents the successes and complications of radio-frequency ablation in children, and remains one of the most thorough studies on ablation in any age group.

- Friedman RA, Fenrich AL, Kertsz NJ: Congenital complete atrioventricular block. Pacing Clin Electrophysiol 2001;11:1681–1688.

  This lovely review article from Texas Children's Hospital covers the topic of congenital complete atrioventricular block in great depth and gives an excellent perspective. It is essential reading for all paediatric cardiology trainees.

CHAPTER 20

Cardiopulmonary Stress Testing

PAUL STEPHENS, Jr, MICHAEL G. MCBRIDE, and STEPHEN M. PARIDON

Regular exercise is an important part of a healthy lifestyle. Physical activity in some westernised societies has diminished for a variety of reasons as society has trended away from outdoor activities towards other types of activities, including computer games and cable television. Healthy levels of physical fitness require regular participation in activities that generate energy expenditures significantly above the resting level.[1]

Exercise testing has become an integral part of the evaluation of children with congenital and acquired cardiovascular disease. Although children are seldom sitting or lying quietly during waking hours, most of the testing available to the cardiovascular specialist is performed in such a resting state, and sometimes in a sedated state. The evaluation of the patient in the exercise physiology laboratory allows the clinician to assess the cardiovascular system in a state that is more likely to be reflective of the normal daily physical activities.

Optimal exercise performance requires a continuous meshing of multiple systems of organs.[2] The roles of the heart and lungs are to provide adequate energy substrates to working skeletal muscle, and to remove the end products of aerobic and anaerobic metabolism during exercise. Most of the children that we encounter in the exercise physiology laboratory have, or are suspected of having, cardiac anomalies. Abnormalities of non-cardiovascular origin, however, may also play a role in limiting exercise performance in patients with surgically repaired complex congenital cardiac defects. Any malfunctioning of the muscles, bones, or nervous system will impair exercise performance. A modern laboratory for exercise physiology, therefore, must be capable of assessing all exercise-related systems, including the cardiovascular, pulmonary, neurologic, and musculoskeletal systems. Furthermore, accurate interpretation of exercise tests requires the proper equipment and personnel. This is particularly important as the cardiologist supervising the laboratory frequently evaluates children with real or suspected exercise limitations. These children seldom have any cardiovascular abnormalities, but may have involvement of other organs, such as dysfunction of the pulmonary or musculoskeletal systems. Properly performed exercise testing, and its interpretation, should also be able to identify or exclude abnormalities of extracardiac organs that normally contribute to exercise performance.

In this chapter, we review briefly basic exercise physiology as it relates to cardiopulmonary exercise testing. We discuss the equipment required for performing an exercise test, and its applications, assessing the types of data obtained from exercise testing, and their usefulness in the evaluation of the child with cardiovascular disease. We also review indications and contraindications for exercise testing in cardiovascular disease.

BASIC EXERCISE PHYSIOLOGY

Assuring proper exercise performance requires the seamless and continuous meshing of multiple systems of organs.[3,4] The classic illustration of Wasserman and colleagues (Fig. 20-1) is the widely duplicated figure that depicts the interaction of the key systems that couple internal cellular respiration to external pulmonary respiration during exercise. It shows the systems as a series of overlapping cogs, all of which must mesh seamlessly to allow exercise to occur. In such fashion, mechanical energy is produced from chemical energy at the cellular level, with subsequent delivery and removal of substrates for energy production and byproducts of muscle metabolism. All of this is accomplished while maintaining chemical and thermal homeostasis within narrow ranges.

CELLULAR METABOLISM

Adenosine triphosphate is the chief source of chemical energy for the exercising muscle. Mechanical energy is produced by the process of excitation-contraction coupling, driven by the breakdown of adenosine triphosphate and the release of inorganic phosphates and adenosine nucleotides. The stores of adenosine triphosphate and phosphocreatine in the myocytes are sufficient only for 10 to 15 seconds of activity, and so must continuously be replenished. As can be seen in Figure 20-2, adenosine triphosphate is produced in small amounts in the cytosol by anaerobic metabolism. Much larger amounts are produced aerobically in the mitochondria.[3,5]

Anaerobic and aerobic metabolic activities use glucose, which is metabolised to pyruvate. Pyruvate then has two possible fates. It may be converted into lactic acid, and excreted into the bloodstream, where it is buffered by sodium bicarbonate converting it to lactate. This reaction results in the production of carbon dioxide and water, along with small amounts of adenosine triphosphate, and the former are excreted in the lungs. The lactate molecule is taken up by the liver for resynthesis to glucose and glycogen, which can then be utilised again for energy production.

The other fate of pyruvate is aerobic metabolism. Pyruvate is converted into acetyl-coenzyme A and transported into the mitochondria where it enters the Krebs cycle, again producing carbon dioxide and water. Adenosine triphosphate is produced in large quantities via the

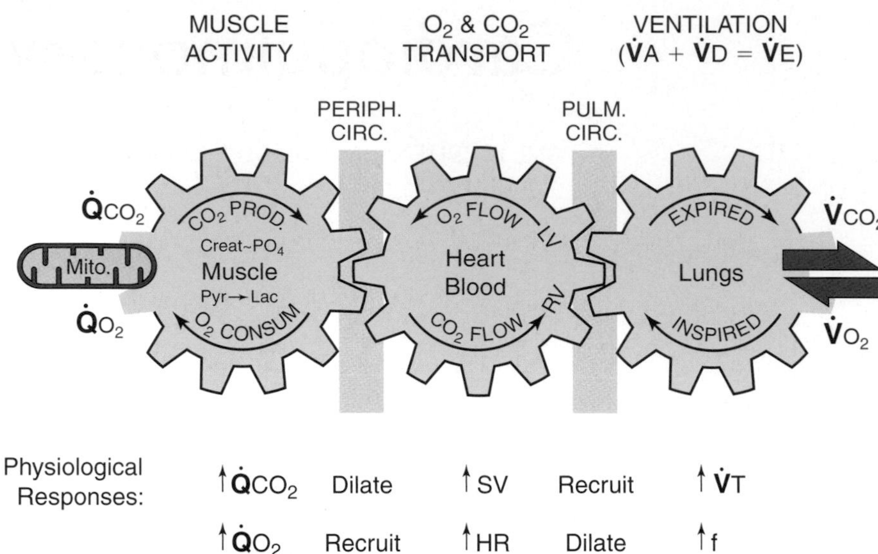

Figure 20-1 An illustration of the functional interdependence of the multiple systems of organs during exercise. The meshing gears represent the musculoskeletal and the cardiopulmonary systems, which interact to assure adequate delivery of oxygen to, and removal of byproducts from, the exercising muscles. The smooth continuous interactions of these multiple physiological systems are essential for proper function of the muscles during exercise. See the text for detailed discussion. (Reprinted with permission from Wasserman K, Hansen JE, Sue DY, et al: Exercise testing and interpretation: An overview. In Principles of Exercise Testing and Interpretation, 2nd ed, Vol 1. Philadelphia: Lea & Febiger 1994, pp 1–8.)

electron transport chain, with oxygen functioning as the terminal electron acceptor. Unlike anaerobic metabolism, fats as well as carbohydrates and proteins can undergo aerobic metabolism. Fats enter aerobic metabolism at the level of the Krebs cycle, and do not undergo anaerobic metabolism.[4,5]

During any activity, the availability and use of substrates, primarily fats or carbohydrates, will vary depending upon the type, intensity, and duration of activity. Fats are more reduced than carbohydrates, requiring more oxygen for complete oxidation compared to carbohydrates on a mole for mole basis.[4] The ratio of production of carbon dioxide to consumption of oxygen, abbreviated to Vco_2/Vo_2, is called the ratio of respiratory exchange, or if in a steady state, the respiratory quotient. In a state of high use of fat, the ratio is approximately 0.7. Conversely, during pure carbohydrate metabolism, the ratio is 1.0, reflecting the lower amount of oxygen needed to oxidise carbohydrates. The stores of glycogen in the adult body are seldom more than approximately 1500 Kcal. Some use of fat, therefore, is almost always required. As a result, the resting ratio of respiratory exchange, even in the well-fed state, will usually range from 0.8 to 0.9.

During a typical graded maximal exercise test, the work rate is gradually increased over the course of 10 to 15 minutes, as explained in our subsequent sections concerning exercise protocols. Production of adenosine triphosphate will need to increase as mechanical work increases, and at low levels of work this increase is met predominately by increased aerobic metabolism. Slow twitch muscle fibers, so-called Type 1, with high oxidative metabolism, are primarily recruited for this activity. As work rate increases, consumption of oxygen increases in a linear fashion (Fig. 20-3). Near peak work rates, consumption will tend to plateau, as maximal consumption is achieved. This phenomenon is often absent in children.[4,6,7]

As consumption of oxygen increases in response to increased work rate, there is a gradual rise in the ratio of respiratory exchange. The reason for this rise is twofold. First, there is a gradual shift in use of fats compared to carbohydrates. This shift allows for more efficient use of oxygen, as the yield of adenosine triphosphate per mole of oxygen is greater with carbohydrates. Secondly, the rise in the ratio occurs as a result of increased levels of lactate in the blood. At approximately 50% to 60% of the maximal consumption of oxygen, levels of lactate begin to rise in the serum. The point where clearance can no longer keep up with production is known as the lactate threshold. The onset of anaerobic metabolism by the exercising muscles is responsible for this production of lactate. Above the threshold, levels of lactate rise exponentially as work rate increases, necessitating increased buffering by sodium bicarbonate in order to maintain blood pH homeostasis. The byproduct of the buffering process, carbon dioxide must be removed in order to maintain levels within the normal range. This causes a significant rise in production of carbon dioxide out of proportion to the rise in consumption of oxygen, resulting in the respiratory exchange ratio increasing to greater than 1.0. The ratio in adults at peak exercise may be as high as 1.2 to 1.4, but is usually somewhat lower in children.[6–11]

The increase in production of carbon dioxide associated with the buffering of lactate allows for measurement of a non-invasive surrogate of the lactate threshold. This surrogate, known as the ventilatory anaerobic threshold, is defined as the point where production of carbon dioxide, and minute ventilation, begin to rise out of proportion to the consumption of oxygen. Like the lactate threshold, the ventilatory anaerobic threshold occurs at approximately 50% to 60% of the maximal consumption of oxygen. It may be significantly lower or higher in de-conditioned or highly trained athletes, respectively. Like maximal consumption of oxygen, the ventilatory anaerobic threshold is a physiological limit, and has been used as a marker of aerobic fitness. Unlike maximal consumption of oxygen the ventilatory anaerobic threshold has the virtue of being effort independent, is a level of exercise that can be sustained over a prolonged period of time, and is easily affected by training or sedentary behavior. Unfortunately, the ventilatory anaerobic threshold can be difficult to measure accurately in smaller children who tend to have erratic patterns of breathing.[6–11]

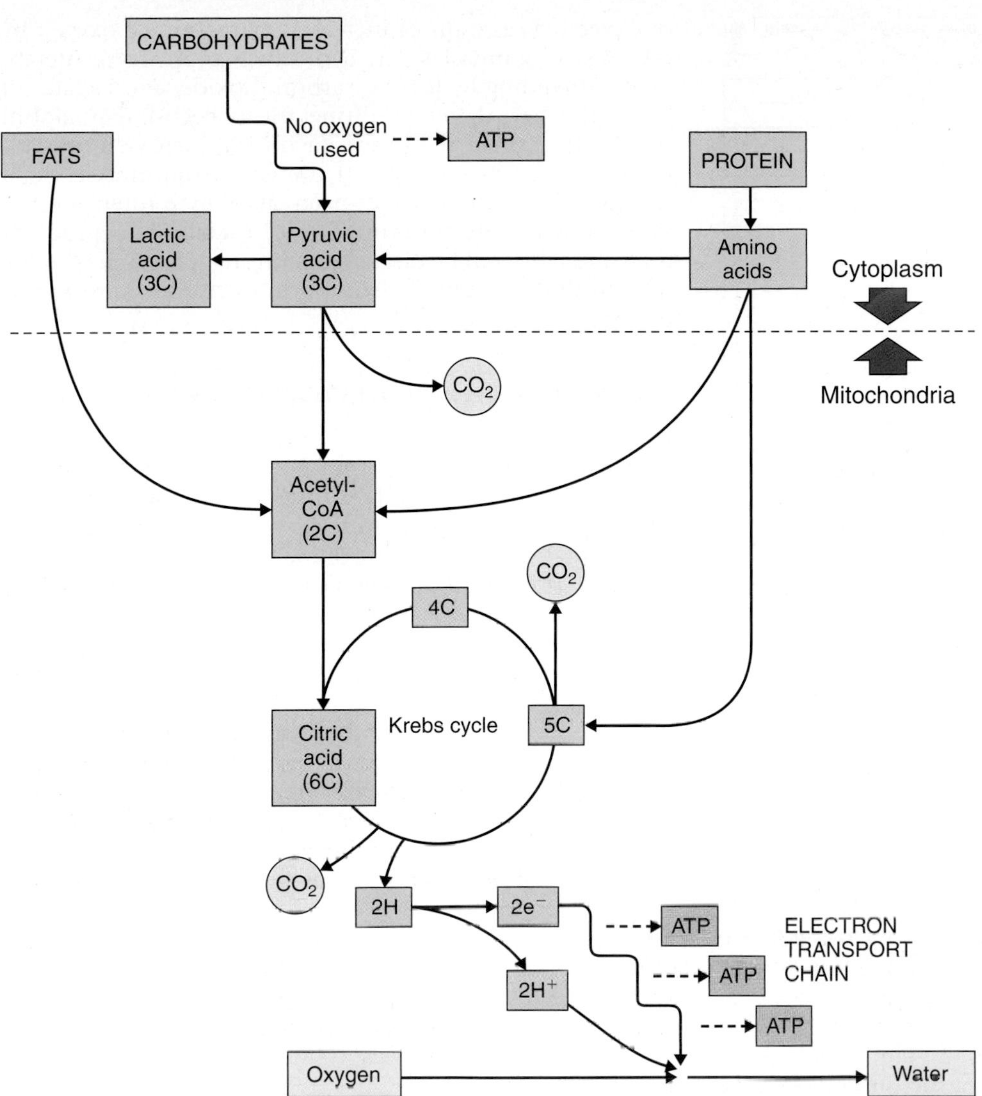

Figure 20-2 An illustration of cellular respiration, which results in the release of the energy of the terminal phosphate bond of adenosine triphosphate to fuel the contractile and related demands of the working skeletal muscle. See text for detailed discussion. (Reprinted with permission from Astrand P, Rodahl K: The Muscle and Its Contraction. Textbook of Work Physiology, Physiological Bases of Exercise, Third Edition. McGraw-Hill, Inc. 2:12–53, 1986).

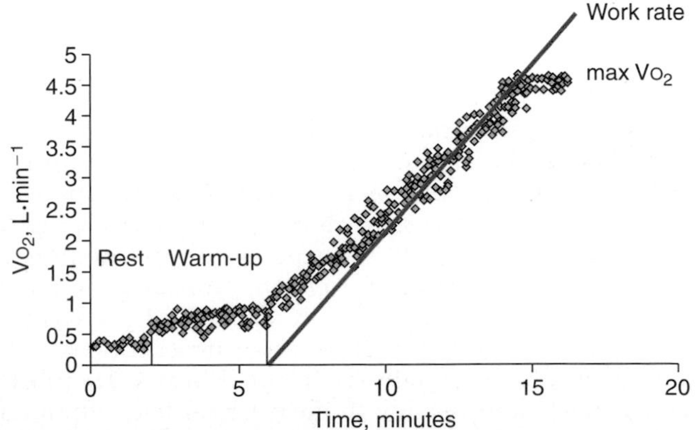

Figure 20-3 The relationship between consumption of oxygen Vo_2 and rate of work during progressive exercise in a healthy and well-conditioned adolescent. Note that, with the onset of exercise, there is an essentially linear relationship between these two features. Close to the peak of exercise, the consumption of oxygen levels off, despite the continued rise in rate of work (see text for detailed discussion).

THE HEART AND LUNG AS SERVICE ORGANS

As previously mentioned, consumption of oxygen rises in near linear response to increasing work rate. The consumption can be derived from the Fick equation as follows:

$$Vo_2 = Q \times (a - v\ O_2\ \text{diff.})$$

where Vo_2 is consumption, Q is cardiac output, and $a - v\ O_2$ diff. is the difference in content of oxygen is arterial and mixed venous blood. Q is defined as:

$$Q = SV \times HR$$

where SV is stroke volume and HR is heart rate. Rearranging the equations, we see that Vo_2 is:

$$Vo_2 = SV \times HR \times (a - v\ o_2\ \text{diff.})$$

The rise in consumption of oxygen during exercise, therefore, is dependent on the increases in stroke volume and heart rate, and widening of the difference in the content of

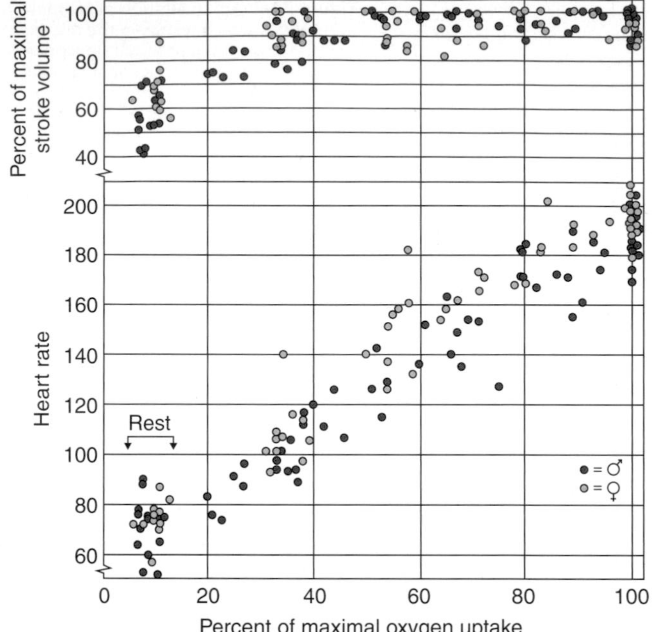

Figure 20-4 The relationship of heart rate and stroke volume to increasing consumption of oxygen during cycle ergometry in 23 male and female subjects. Note that stroke volume reaches its maximal value at approximately 30% to 40% of the maximal uptake of oxygen. Heart rate continues to rise in a linear fashion throughout exercise. (Reprinted with permission from Astrand P, Rodahl K: The Muscle and Its Contraction. Textbook of Work Physiology, Physiological Bases of Exercise, 3rd ed, Vol. 2. New York, McGraw-Hill, Inc., 1986, pp 12–53.)

oxygen in arterial and mixed venous blood. During strenuous exercise, cardiac output may rise as much as fivefold over resting levels.[5,12–15] Both stroke volume and heart rate contribute to this increase, but the relative contributions of each are different.[5] At rest, stroke volume is approximately 60% of its maximal value. At the onset of exercise, a combination of increased venous return and sympathetic tone causes stroke volume to increase. This occurs as consequence of two mechanisms. First, increased preload stretches the myocyte and increases tension, resulting in changes in the Frank–Starling forces. Second, the increase in sympathetic tone results in an increase in the inotropic state of the myocardium. This increase in inotropy improves the active tension developed for any given preload, thus further augmenting stroke volume. Most of the increase in stroke volume takes place below 30% to 40% of the maximal consumption of oxygen (Fig. 20-4). At higher heart rates diastolic filling time is decreased, which limits any further augmentation in stroke volume irrespective of any increase in the inotropic state. Therefore, at higher heart rates, and naturally at higher work loads, the relative contribution of stroke volume to the overall increase in cardiac output is small.

An increase in heart rate is the primary mechanism for the increased cardiac output at higher work rates. This is reflected in the essentially linear relationship between heart rate and consumption of oxygen as work rates increase (see Fig. 20-4). The ability to increase heart rate in a normal manner during exercise, therefore, is essential to achieving a normal aerobic workload. The difference in content of oxygen between the arterial and mixed venous blood gradually widens with increasing work rate and consumption of oxygen, as a result of increased extraction of oxygen by the exercising muscles. The byproducts of myocytic metabolism, including hydrogen, carbon dioxide, and lactate, all lower the pH, thereby shifting the oxygen-haemoglobin dissociation curve rightward, favouring increased unloading of oxygen at the level of the exercising muscle. Such unloading is more pronounced at higher intensities of exercise, when the concentration of metabolic byproducts is greater. This will be discussed in more detail below in the relationship between consumption of oxygen and cardiac output.

DISTRIBUTION OF BLOOD FLOW

For consumption of oxygen to increase during exercise, it is essential that cardiac output not only increase, but that blood flow is preferentially shunted to the exercising muscles (Fig. 20-5). At peak exercise, blood flow to exercising muscle may be 80% or more of the total cardiac output. The redistribution of blood flow is achieved by a combination of autonomic and metabolic vasoregulatory mechanisms.[16] Exercise is essentially a state of increased sympathetic nervous system tone, which is regionally overridden by metabolic vasodilation. The increase in sympathetic tone associated with exercise results in a generalised constriction of the precapillary resistance arterioles. Simultaneously, the sympathetic tone increases heart rate and cardiac contractility, resulting in increased cardiac output.[16–18] Vasodilation occurs at the level of the exercising muscle as a result of local metabolic changes. Aerobic and anaerobic metabolism, excitation-contraction coupling, and breakdown of adenosine triphosphate all result in the release of potent vasodilators into the interstitial spaces. These vasodilators include free potassium and hydrogen ions, carbon dioxide, lactate, adenosine diphosphate, and inorganic phosphate. The result is a profound vasodilation of the vascular bed in the exercising muscles.

Vasoconstriction of the splanchnic vascular bed results in either no change, or a decrease, in flow of blood to the gut and kidneys. The effect on the overall peripheral vascular resistance depends on the size of the exercising muscle groups. During dynamic exercise, which utilises large muscle groups, such as running, the net result is a significant drop in systemic vascular resistance, despite an overall increase in sympathetic tone.

SURROGATES OF CARDIAC OUTPUT

Exercise testing is frequently performed in order to assess the ability of the cardiovascular system to increase cardiac output in response to an increased workload. Measurement of cardiac output during exercise, however, is often not practical. Direct measurements are too invasive to allow adequate levels of exertion. Non-invasive methods are often technically difficult, and may be inaccurate in the pathophysiological states that are encountered in many types of congenitally malformed hearts. The obstacles accurately and reliably to measure cardiac output has lead to the use of consumption of oxygen as a surrogate of cardiac output in many clinical and research settings.[4,16,19] Over a broad range of consumption of oxygen there is a nearly linear relationship between consumption of oxygen and cardiac output (Fig. 20-6).

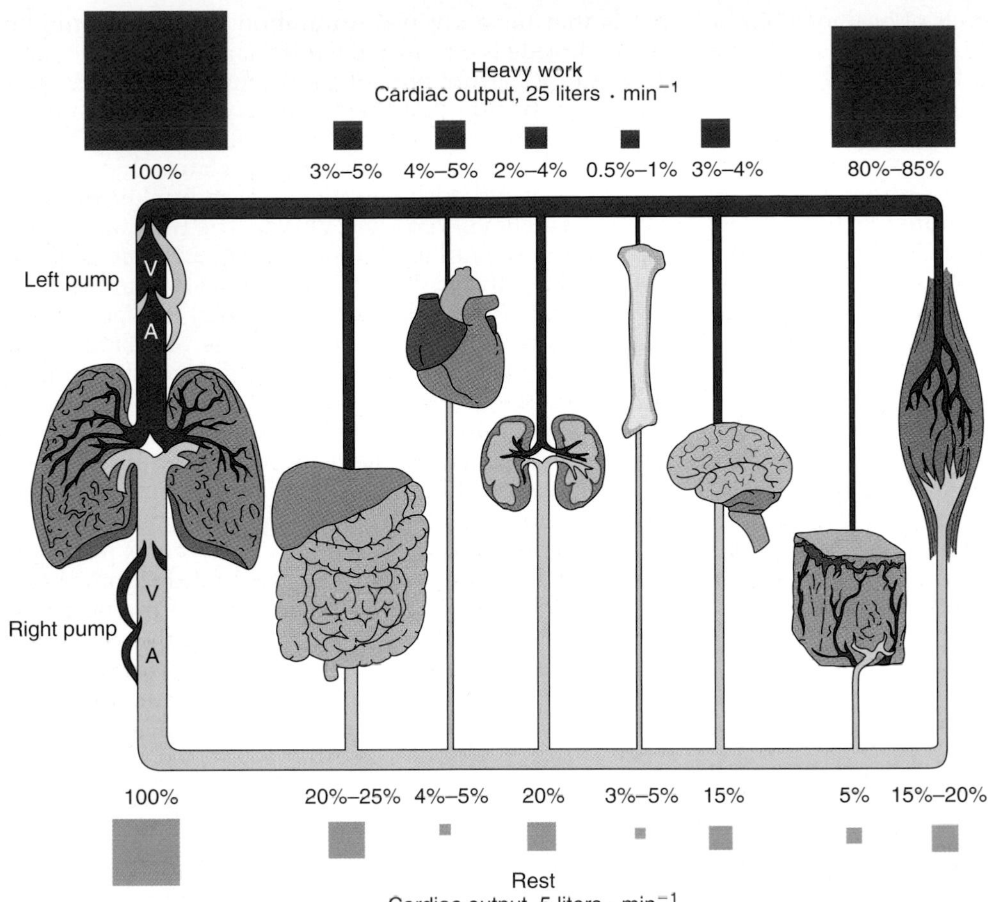

Figure 20-5 The parallel circuits of flow through the various systems of organs, both at rest and during peak exercise. Note that the cardiac output increases by approximately fivefold from rest to strenuous exercise. The relative distribution of flow to the various systems, in contrast, is significantly different from rest to peak exercise. In both states, the red squares are proportional to the percentage of cardiac output received by the particular system. Note that the flow of blood to the muscle increases from between approximately 15% to 20% of cardiac output at rest to 80% to 85% of the cardiac output at peak exercise. (Reprinted with permission from Astrand P, Rodahl K: The Muscle and Its Contraction. Textbook of Work Physiology, Physiological Bases of Exercise, 3rd ed., Vol. 2. New York: McGraw-Hill, Inc., 1986, pp 12–53.)

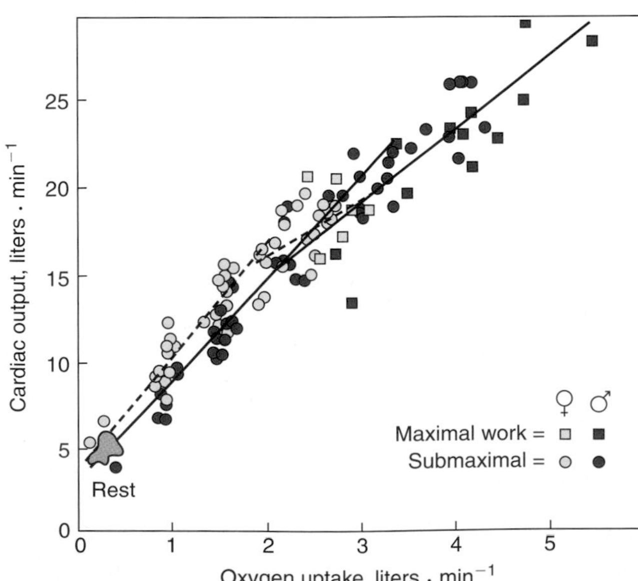

Figure 20-6 The relationship of cardiac output to consumption of oxygen measured in 23 subjects during sitting cycle ergometry. These data are from the same subjects shown in Figure 20-4. See text for discussion. (Reprinted with permission from Astrand P, Rodahl K: The Muscle and Its Contraction. Textbook of Work Physiology, Physiological Bases of Exercise, 3rd ed., Vol. 2. New York: McGraw-Hill, Inc.,1986, pp 12–53.)

Despite a plateau in cardiac output at very high work loads, consumption of oxygen continues to increase as a result of increased oxygen extraction, thereby increasing the arterial-mixed venous content of oxygen difference. Consumption of oxygen is determined by the amount of oxygen delivered in the blood that is extracted by the metabolically active tissues. During exercise, this extraction is determined by the myoglobin content of the exercising muscle, the isoenzyme characteristics of the muscle, as well as the physiological milieu in which the muscle is working.[4,16] The physiological state will have a great impact on the oxygen-haemoglobin dissociation curve. As previously stated, there are multiple byproducts of muscle metabolism which are released into the intercellular space during exercise, shifting the oxygen-haemoglobin dissociation curve to the right.[4] The local increase in muscle temperature during exercise also has the same effect. The net result is an increase in oxygen unloading to the exercising muscle particularly at high workloads. There is therefore an increase in the arterial-mixed venous content of oxygen difference, and a continued rise in consumption of oxygen, even in the presence of a flattening or plateauing of the rise in cardiac output near peak exercise.[4,16,17]

Gender differences are present in the relationship between cardiac output and consumption of oxygen (see Fig. 20-6). Females tend to have a somewhat higher cardiac output for any given consumption, as well as a lower maximal consumption.[17] These differences are likely due to the difference in content of haemoglobin between males and females. Females have lower levels of haemoglobin in the serum compared to males, and therefore have lower contents of oxygen, necessitating a higher cardiac output to deliver an equivalent consumption of oxygen. Lower values in adolescent and adult females manifest clinically in slightly higher cardiac outputs, and lower consumption of oxygen at peak exercise. It is easy to comprehend how anaemia will result in reduced consumption of oxygen and a higher ratio of cardiac output to consumption of oxygen compared to non-anaemic states. The use of consumption of oxygen as a surrogate for cardiac output, therefore, is problematic in the presence of anaemia.

OXYGEN PULSE

In a clinical setting, the practitioner is frequently interested in assessing the intrinsic inotropic state of the myocardium during exercise. As was stated earlier, this state is primarily reflected by the stroke volume of the heart. A non-invasive measurement of stroke volume is a useful tool to assess myocardial function. This has given rise to the use of oxygen pulse during exercise testing.[20]

The oxygen pulse is defined as:

$$\text{Oxygen pulse} = \text{V}O_2 \text{ in mL/min/HR}$$

Since $\text{V}O_2 = (\text{SV} \times \text{HR}) \times (\text{a} - \text{v } O_2 \text{ diff})$, the pulse also equals:

$$\text{SV} \times (\text{a} - \text{v } O_2 \text{ diff})$$

The oxygen pulse, therefore, is a value that can be measured at any given work rate or consumption of oxygen during exercise testing. A rise or fall in stroke volume will correlate with a rise or fall in the oxygen pulse. These changes can be blunted somewhat by an increase or decrease in the difference in content of oxygen between arterial and mixed venous blood, but the ability of muscles to extract oxygen usually does not significantly change except in response to prolonged training. This is particularly true at maximal exercise. The oxygen pulse is perhaps most useful in assessing changes in myocardial performance over time, or following therapeutic interventions in an individual patient. Assuming no change in the haemoglobin content, the content of oxygen of the arterial blood should be unchanged. Absent large weight changes, the consumption of oxygen required to perform a given amount of work on an ergometer for an individual patient is constant. Any increase in the oxygen pulse measured at a given work rate, therefore, would reflect a lower heart rate needed to achieve the same consumption of oxygen, and be indicative of a higher stroke volume. The converse would be true for a falling oxygen pulse. This does presume the haemoglobin content of the blood has not changed, and that the chronotropic state of the heart is also unchanged. A significant change in either of these limits the usefulness of the oxygen pulse to act as a marker of stroke volume during exercise.

PULMONARY RESPONSE TO EXERCISE

Consumption of oxygen, and removal of carbon dioxide, require that the cardiovascular and pulmonary systems work together as a single integrated unit. The ultimate goal is that for a given consumption of oxygen, minute carbon dioxide is eliminated while maintaining $\text{Pa}CO_2$ and pH within a narrow physiological range. For this reason, it is not surprising that there is a very tight relationship between minute ventilation, consumption of oxygen, and production of carbon dioxide. Such a relationship is demonstrated in ventilatory equivalents for carbon dioxide and oxygen, namely $\text{VE/V}CO_2$, and $\text{VE/V}O_2$. The typical relationship of minute ventilation to increasing work rate, and the relationship of the ventilatory equivalents for carbon dioxide and oxygen to work rate, are depicted in Figure 20-7. Note that there is a steady rise in minute ventilation with increasing work rate. Both ventilatory equivalents initially fall at the onset of exercise and then plateau. During the plateau phase, minute ventilation is increasing in proportion to both the increases in the ventilatory equivalents for carbon dioxide and oxygen. At the onset of the ventilatory anaerobic threshold, minute ventilation begins to increase out of proportion to consumption of oxygen as the respiratory drive is stimulated by increased production of carbon dioxide occurring as a consequence of the buffering of lactic acid. Note in Figure 20-7B that, at this point, the ventilatory equivalent for oxygen begins to rise while the ventilatory equivalent for carbon dioxide remains stable. At maximal exercise, production of lactic acid may rise

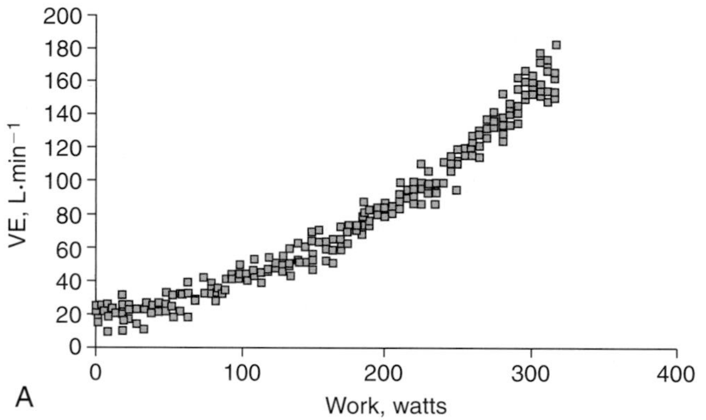

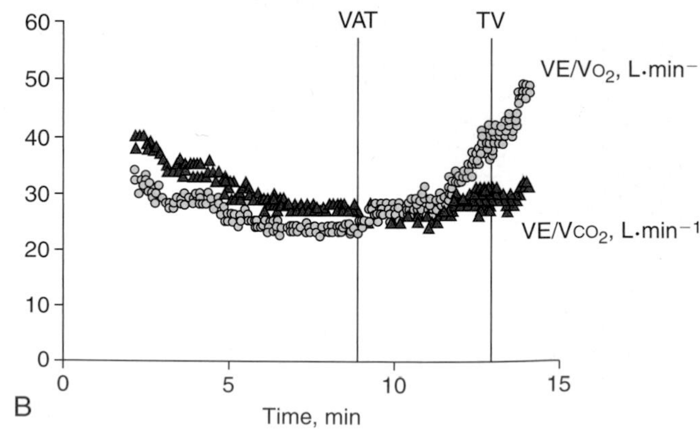

Figure 20-7 **A,** The relationship of minute ventilation (VE) to rate of work in the same subject as Figure 20-3. Note there is a steady rise in minute ventilation as rate of work increases. **B,** The ventilatory equivalents of oxygen ($\text{VE/V}O_2$) and carbon dioxide ($\text{VE/V}CO_2$) for the same subject. The onset of the ventilatory anaerobic threshold (VAT) and terminal hyperventilation (TV) are marked (see text for discussion).

to a level that can no longer be adequately buffered by sodium bicarbonate and frank metabolic acidosis ensues. The normal physiological response to acidosis is a marked hyperventilatory response referred to as terminal hyperventilation. At terminal hyperventilation, both the ventilatory equivalents for oxygen and carbon dioxide rise, resulting in a significant fall in $Paco_2$.[4,8–10]

Minute ventilation is defined as:

$$VE = V_T \times F$$

where V_T is tidal volume and F is respiratory rate.

At the onset of exercise, minute ventilation initially increases primarily by an increase in tidal volume rather than respiratory rate. Tidal volume includes both alveolar ventilation as well as the physiological dead space. Physiological dead space is made up of both anatomic components, the trachea and bronchi, as well as the functional dead space, namely the ventilation of hypoperfused or non-perfused pulmonary components. At rest the ratio of dead space to tidal volume is approximately 30% to 35% in adults and adolescents. With the increase in tidal volume at the onset of exercise, the ratio falls. This is due to a larger tidal volume relative to the fixed anatomic dead space. Additionally, there is an improvement in ventilation-to-perfusion matching as the increased negative thoracic pressure causes recruitment of additional capillary beds, resulting in a fall in the physiological dead space. At peak exercise, the ratio of dead space to tidal volume may fall to approximately 5% to 15%. Children typically have less efficient ventilation than either adolescents or adults, and tend to have a higher respiratory rate for any given minute ventilation, resulting in a higher ratio at any level of exercise.[21–25]

At higher levels of exercise, minute ventilation increases in terms of both tidal volume and respiratory rate. Much of the improvement in the ratio occurs at lower to moderate levels of work. The rapid fall in the ratio is responsible for the initial steep fall in the ventilatory equivalents for oxygen and carbon dioxide that occurs at the onset of exercise (see Fig. 20-7B). Although both consumption of oxygen and production of carbon dioxide are increasing in early exercise, this is more than compensated for by the improved efficiency of the lungs, resulting in a less than proportional rise in minute ventilation.

In healthy children and adults, ventilation is not the rate-limiting step in exercise performance.[4,20] This is because the cardiovascular system usually reaches its limit of delivery of oxygen before the pulmonary system is exhausted. At the maximal level of exercise, most subjects have not maximally stressed their pulmonary system, and there is pulmonary reserve, which is described by exercise physiologists as the breathing reserve. This is the theoretical ability to increase minute ventilation that remains untapped at maximal minute consumption of oxygen. This value is in the range of 20% to 50% in healthy children and adults.[20]

The breathing reserve is defined as:

$$(1 - \text{max VE/MVV}) \times 100$$

and is expressed as a percentage, where VE is the maximally achieved VE at peak exercise and MVV is maximal voluntary ventilation.

Maximal voluntary ventilation is obtained by having the subject hyperventilate for 10 seconds as vigorously as possible prior to exercise testing. Much longer periods of rapid and deep breathing may result in fainting, and should be avoided. The volume achieved is then multiplied by six, theoretically to give a maximally achievable minute ventilation. A low breathing reserve, of less than 20%, may indicate that primary pulmonary abnormality is limiting exercise performance. As maximal voluntary ventilation is a highly effort dependent measurement, care must be taken when interpreting breathing reserve. Other confirmatory data, such as an abnormal response of the ventilatory equivalents, or abnormal resting spirometry, should be sought to confirm pulmonary abnormalities.

LABORATORY REQUIREMENTS

Environment

Adequate space and environmental controls are important in order to assure a successful exercise test. The child should be made to feel comfortable and relaxed, which will improve exercise performance. Sufficient space is needed to accommodate the various ergometers and monitoring equipment, including emergency resuscitation equipment, while maintaining adequate space to access the patient in emergency situations. A minimum of 250 square feet of space is required, with 500 square feet or more when multiple work stations are employed.[26]

The climate of the laboratory must be well controlled to allow proper thermoregulation during the exercise test. The room should be well ventilated and temperatures should be regulated between 20° C and 23° C,[26,27] a temperature range which permits the child to be comfortable at rest but still allows for adequate dissipation of heat during exercise. Humidity should be approximately 50% to ensure free perspiration during exercise.[27]

The laboratory should be child-friendly. Television monitors with appropriate programming, and wall posters, have proven useful in minimising anxiety and/or boredom of the patients.

Safety Precautions

Exercise testing has been performed in children with very low risk, even in those who have complex cardiovascular disease.[28,29] Although significant complications of exercise testing are rare, proper safety precautions are essential. Key staff usually include at least one physician who is well trained in paediatric exercise testing. A physician does not need to be present for testing patients deemed to be at low risk or healthy,[27,30] but should be present at the testing of any child deemed to be at increased risk of a complication, such as a child with a life-threatening arrhythmia or syncope. The American Heart Association published guidelines for patients who are at low risk for exercise complications, and require a physician available, but not physically present (Table 20-1).[30] The risk for each patient must be individually assessed. Ideally, two staff members trained in exercise testing should be present for all tests. All exercise physiologists or exercise technicians should be familiar with paediatric exercise testing, and at least one of these personnel should be trained in paediatric advanced life support. A well-stocked emergency resuscitation cart,

TABLE 20-1

INDICATIONS FOR EXERCISE TESTING THAT MAY NOT REQUIRE A PHYSICIAN'S PRESENCE

1. Assessment of working capacity in healthy children for research.
2. Evaluations of chest pain of non-cardiac origin.
3. Post-operative follow-up of patients with good haemodynamics to assess working capacity or rehabilitation screen.
4. Evaluation of isolated PACs or PVCs in a healthy child with a normal QTc.
5. Routine follow-up of known arrhythmias or pacemakers.
6. Kawasaki disease or other coronary abnormalities without a known history of ischemia.
7. Asymptomatic mild aortic stenosis.
8. Evaluation of asymptomatic mild congenital or acquired cardiac malformations.

Adapted from Washington RL, Bricker JT, Alpert BS, et al: Guidelines for exercise testing in the pediatric age group. From the Committee on Atherosclerosis and Hypertension in Children, Council on Cardiovascular Disease in the Young, the American Heart Association. Circulation 1994; 90:2166–2179.

BORG SCALE
(Rating of Perceived Exertion)

6
7 Very, very light
8
9 Very light
10
11 Fairly light
12
13 Somewhat hard
14
15Hard
16
17 Very hard
18
19 Very, very hard
20

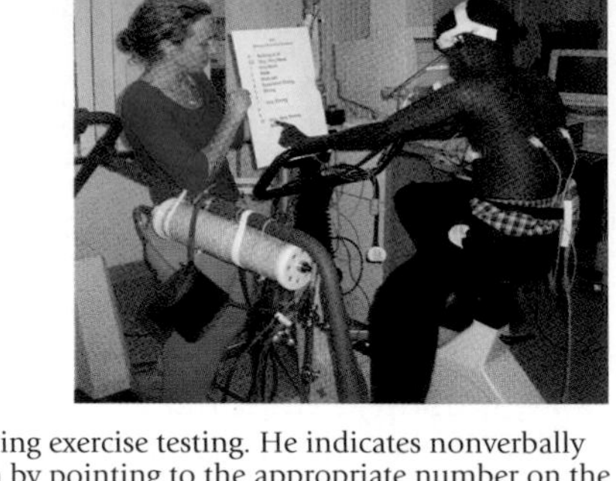

Figure 20-8 A child undergoing exercise testing. He indicates nonverbally his level of perceived exertion by pointing to the appropriate number on the Borg scale. The staff uses this information to determine the projected time to exhaustion.

defibrillator, system for delivery of oxygen, and suction apparatus are also essential.[30]

Preparation of Patients

Education and preparation of the children before and during their test are probably the most important factors in successful testing. A thorough explanation of the testing procedure results in better compliance and effort, especially in younger children. Children should avoid heavy meals for approximately 2 hours prior to the test, and wear appropriate clothing, such as shorts, T-shirts, and athletic shoes. Proper preparation of the skin helps to ensure an adequate electrocardiographic signal.[31] Superficial abrasions should be performed to remove the top layer of epidermis and enhance the electrical signal. Electrodes should be large enough to provide a good contact with the skin.

The patient should be instructed in the procedures to be used during the exercise test. These include proper use of the treadmill or cycle ergometer, and the use of hand signals to convey the level of fatigue, distress, or symptoms. Scales of perceived exertion, such as the Borg scale, can be useful in communicating with the child during the study. Such scales allow those conducting the testing to estimate when the child is likely to reach maximal effort (Fig. 20-8).[32] Special attention should be given to maneuvers, such as spirometry or inert gas rebreathing, that require proper technique and cooperation from the patient.

EQUIPMENT

Ergometers

In most paediatric exercise laboratories, testing is primarily directed toward measuring aerobic capacity. Therefore, ergometers should generate work in the large muscle groups. The two types of ergometers most commonly used are the motorised treadmill and the upright cycle ergometer. The choice of ergometer depends on the type of information desired, but there are both advantages and disadvantages to each modality (Tables 20-2 and 20-3).[33–35] It is therefore best that a laboratory be equipped to perform testing using either type of ergometer.

Treadmill

The treadmill is the most common ergometer in the paediatric exercise laboratory.

TABLE 20-2

MATCHING THE PROTOCOL WITH THE DESIRED INFORMATION

Condition or Question	Cycle Ergometry	Treadmill	Rationale
Aortic stenosis/insufficiency	Preferred		Electrocardiographic assessment for ischemia easier due to less motion artifact
Repaired transposition of great arteries	Preferred		Electrocardiographic assessment for ischemia or arrhythmia easier
Repaired tetralogy of Fallot	Preferred		Arrhythmia assessment during exercise essential
Coronary arterial anomaly (pre or post repair)	Preferred		Electrocardiographic assessment for ischemia
Single ventricle/Fontan	Either	Either	Dependent upon query
Coarctation of the aorta	Preferred		Blood pressure assessment more accurate
Exercise-induced asthma/bronchospasm/chest pain		Preferred	Running more likely than cycling to induce symptoms
Aerobic fitness		Preferred	Higher Vo_2 with treadmill compared to cycle
Arrhythmia Assessment/long QT	Preferred		Less motion artifact on ECG

TABLE 20-3

TREADMILL VERSUS CYCLE ERGOMETER

Features	Treadmill	Cycle
Patient familiarity	+	
Higher work rates and oxygen consumption	+	
Greater paediatric experience		+
Quantification of work performed		+
ECG and blood pressure artifact		+
Safety		+
Expense		+
Noise		+

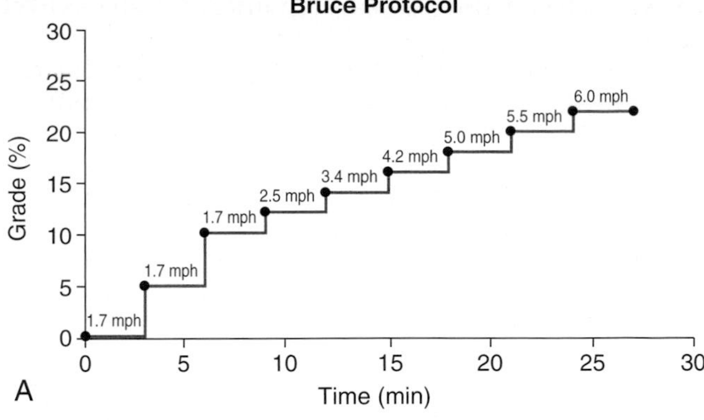

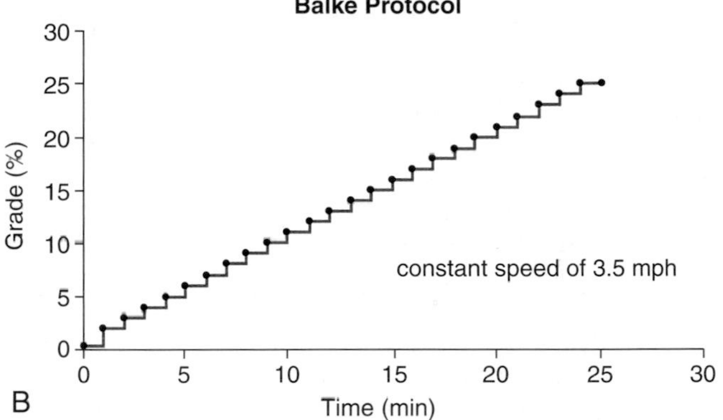

Figure 20-9 The panels show the protocols for testing using a treadmill. **A,** The Bruce protocol, which consists of 3-minute stages with an increase in both speed and grade. The first two stages are often omitted in healthy adult testing. **B,** The Balke protocol: The grade is increased from 0 to 2% after the first minute, and increased 1% in each subsequent minute. The speed of the treadmill is held constant at 3.5 mph.

The biggest advantage of the treadmill compared to the cycle ergometer is the familiarity that children have with walking or running.[35] Furthermore, more muscle groups are utilised with treadmill testing, resulting in a greater stress on the cardiovascular system and higher consumption of oxygen. Consumption of oxygen, and the oxygen pulse, are on average higher by one-tenth with treadmill testing compared to the cycle.[34]

The treadmill also has several distinct disadvantages. It is noisy, and may frighten small children. The increased movement from vigorous running results in much greater distortion of electrocardiographic and blood pressure signals compared to the cycle. The treadmill also requires more space, is not portable, and there is a danger of falling off of the moving platform. Care must be taken to ensure that the patient is closely monitored, and does not attempt to get off of the treadmill abruptly. Another disadvantage of the treadmill is the inability accurately to determine rate of work. The latter disadvantage is less of a clinical than a research concern, where an accurate measurement of rate of work is desirable (see Table 20-2).

Treadmill Protocols

The Bruce protocol and its modifications are the most commonly used protocols in the paediatric exercise laboratory.[35] This protocol consists of 3-minute stages, with an increase in both speed and grade of the treadmill at each stage. Despite its popularity, the incremental increases in work load for the Bruce protocol are large even when modified for children. This frequently makes the shift in rate of work between stages difficult for younger children. The relatively long stages also make more difficult interpretation of metabolic data from analysis of expired gases. The graphic displays of various metabolic measurements, such as consumption of oxygen versus time, are not linear but rather appear as a series of slopes followed by partial plateaus. Such non-linear graphic displays makes determination of key parameters of exercise performance, such as the onset of ventilatory anaerobic threshold, more difficult than in protocols with a continuous increase in work load.

In the last decade, the protocols with shorter stages, usually of 1 or 2 minutes, and smaller incremental increases in rates of work, have gained popularity. These protocols, such as the Balke treadmill protocol, may use a fixed speed, with increases only in grade, or may increase both speed and grade. These protocols can also be modified according to the age, size, and physical conditioning level of the child being tested, thereby allowing the total exercise time to be relatively constant for all subjects. Such a relatively constant duration of exercise is important because previous studies have demonstrated that total testing for more than approximately 12 to 15 minutes is associated with decreased aerobic performance, due to both shunting of blood to the skin for thermoregulation, and poor motivation caused by boredom. A total time of less than 10 minutes may result in poor aerobic performance, because the patient ceases exercising due to excessive muscle fatigue caused by the higher rates of work.[34] The Bruce and Balke protocols are summarised in Figure 20-9.

Cycle Ergometers

These machines have several significant advantages compared with treadmills. A distinct advantage is decreased distortion of electrocardiographic and blood pressure recordings, particularly crucial when there are concerns about arrhythmias, ischaemia, or changes in morphology of the QRS complexes. The cycle also accurately measures external work performed during the test. This requires that the rate of work be relatively independent of speed of pedalling. The ergometer should be regularly calibrated, and carefully assessed before its use, in light of signal-to-noise ratio on some cycles, which may be excessive at the low initial rates of work used in paediatric protocols. Low signal-to-noise ratios are not common problems in the newer generation of cycles, that use digital rather than analogue controllers of the rate of work. Other advantages of cycle ergometers include lower cost, portability, and increased safety. Musculoskeletal injuries are also less likely with a cycle.[34]

Disadvantages, as stated previously, include a generally lower achieved level of exertion and maximal consumption of oxygen. In addition, the current generations of cycles are frequently unable to accommodate younger children who are less than 130 cm in height. The crank arm is frequently too large for these small children. Ergometers used for testing children, therefore, should have an adjustable crank arm. Several cycle ergometers are commercially available with paediatric modifications.

Protocols

The most commonly used protocol is that devised by James, which consists of 10 stages, each lasting 3 minutes.[36] The incremental increases for each stage vary depending upon body surface area. The James protocol has been extensively validated for use in children over the last two decades,[35–37] and hence has well established normative data. Its major disadvantage is the difficulty of analysing metabolic data with its long 3-minute stages, similar to those encountered with the Bruce protocol.

Collection of expired gas is such a common occurrence that many laboratories are now using ramp cycle protocols. In this protocol, the rate of work is increased in small, frequently single-watt, increments, thus producing a smooth continuous rise throughout the test.[26,34,35] These protocols have several advantages. First, the gradual rise in rate of work avoids problems encountered with the large sudden jumps seen when using 3-minute increments. Second, the slopes of the ramps are seamlessly adjusted to accommodate a wide range of sizes, ages, and levels of physical conditioning. Third, relationships between metabolic data and rate of work are easier to appreciate with this type of protocol. The two protocols are shown in Figure 20-10.

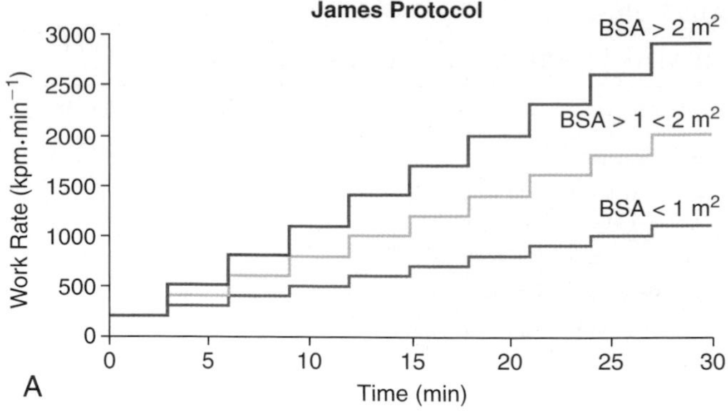

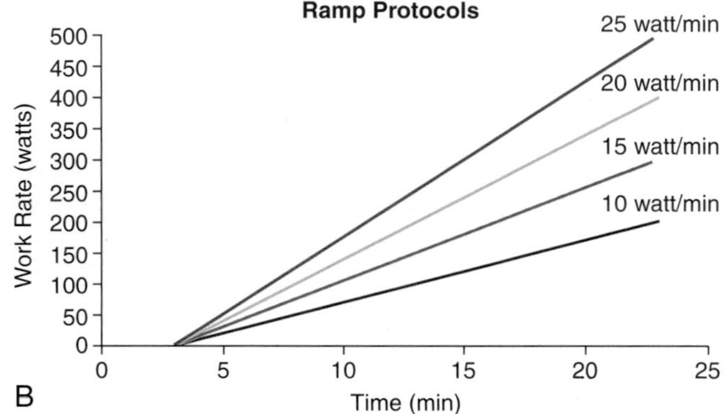

Figure 20-10 Protocols for use with an upright cycle ergometer. **A,** The James protocol. The initial rate of work is 200 kpm/min. The rate is increased every 3 minutes by different amounts, depending on the body surface area of the patient (BSA). **B,** The Ramp protocol. The patient initially pedals for 3 minutes with unloaded cycling to establish a baseline metabolic state. The rate of work is then increased continuously at a chosen level based on the physical condition, age, and size of the patient.

Electrocardiographic Recorders

Many high-quality commercial electrocardiographic recording systems are currently available. No system currently available is designed specifically for paediatric use, but all are generally acceptable without modification. Minimisation of distortion of signals is accomplished with computer digitisation of the analogue electrical signal. The printer should use a direct writer mechanism.[31]

A liquid crystal or cathode ray tube display is essential so that the rhythm, and morphology of the QRS complexes, can be monitored continuously. The display should show at least one, and ideally multiple, leads continuously. The technician obtains a complete 12-lead recording at set time intervals, usually of 1 minute, and when needed during the course of an exercise test. Ideally, all QRS complexes should be stored, either as a hard copy or digitally.[26] Automated devices are available on many recorders to detect arrhythmias, and are useful, except when there are abnormal QRS complexes, pacemaker generated complexes, or if significant motion artifact is present.

Most computerised recorders have algorithms that will average the recorded signals, thus eliminating baseline drift and background artifact, permitting easy interpretation of changes in the QRS and ST segments. It is possible that data may be lost with certain algorithms at very high heart rates, so it is important to compare the averaged to the raw data when interpreting the test.

Analysers of Exchange of Respiratory Gases

The use of these analysers has become routine in laboratories studying paediatric exercise physiology. Measurements of consumption of oxygen, production of carbon dioxide, as well as pulmonary functions such as minute ventilation, tidal volume, and respiratory rate, are easily obtainable. Several systems at reasonable prices are commercially available. In addition to measuring expired gases, these systems are frequently equipped to perform resting spirometry, and to receive input from other sources, such as an electrocardiographic recorder. This allows a single system to generate complete and final reports.

Analysers using inert gases can be used to estimate cardiac output.[38] The patient breathes room air during most of the test. During the measurements of cardiac output, ventilation is diverted via a valve into a closed system, usually through a 3-liter rebreathing bag, containing a mixture of oxygen, an inert diffusible gas, and an inert non-diffusible gas. After one to two breaths, the non-diffusible gas equilibrates between the lungs and the bag, and the final concentration of this gas can be used to calculate the volume of the lungs. The diffusible gas is removed from the system in proportion to the flow of blood to the lungs. The assumption when assessing cardiac output is that flows are equal in the pulmonary and systemic circulations,

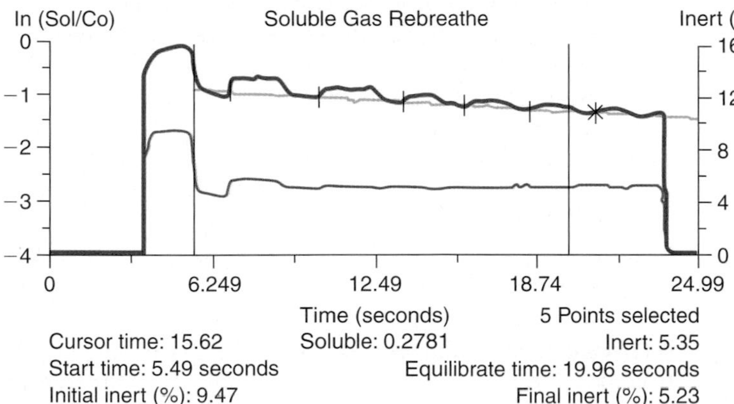

Figure 20-11 This figure displays a noninvasive measurement of cardiac output using the diffusible gas technique. Time is on the x-axis, and the natural log of the concentration of the diffusible gas, in this case acetylene, is on the y-axis. The lower curve shows the concentration of helium that equilibrates between the lungs and the rebreathing bag after several breaths. This allows calculation of the lung volume. The slope of the decay of the acetylene is calculated from the top curve, and is used to measure the flow of blood to the lungs that should equal systemic cardiac output, in this case 11.26 L/min, in the absence of pulmonary disease or intracardiac shunting.

and there is no significant intrapulmonary or intracardiac shunting. The calculated flow of blood to the lungs then reliably estimates systemic cardiac output. Unfortunately, residual pulmonary and/or intracardiac shunts frequently limit the usefulness of this measurement. Such assessment also requires cooperation from the patient, and expertise of tester in performing the rebreathing maneuvers correctly.

Acetylene and helium are commonly used inert soluble and insoluble gases, respectively. A mass spectrometer is usually required (Fig. 20-11). These systems are considerably more expensive than most commercially available metabolic carts, and are typically designed by the individual laboratories using them. Compact, commercially available, systems have come on the market in the last decade. They are less costly, and more user-friendly, than individually designed systems. Alternatively, rebreathing of car bon dioxide is commonly employed in commercially available systems. The latter system uses the indirect Fick method to estimate cardiac output. A number of assumptions are necessary in order to estimate arterial partial pressures of carbon dioxide,[38,39] which may result in significant inaccuracies in children with congenital cardiac disease. The rebreathing method also has the disadvantage of requiring steady state minute ventilation, and therefore is not suitable for protocols with frequently changing rates of work.

Methods for noninvasive measurement used less frequently with exercise testing include electrical bioimpedance and Doppler measurement of aortic blood flow.[38,39] Bioimpedance has the advantage of requiring very little cooperation from the patient, albeit that studies comparing this method with diffusible gas methods have shown poor correlation.[39] Correlations of Doppler with diffusible gas methods are superior to bioimpedance, but obtaining an adequate Doppler signal with exercise remains a cumbersome undertaking.

Spirometry

Essential measurements include basic inspiratory and expiratory flow volume loops, and assessment of maximal voluntary ventilation. Maximal voluntary ventilation is measured by the sprint method as outlined by the American Thoracic Society, wherein maximal ventilation is measured for an interval of 10 to 15 seconds, and extrapolated to 1 minute,[40] Spirometry is used to identify patterns of obstructive or restrictive pulmonary disease that could impair exercise performance. Post-exercise spirometry is useful for identifying patients with exercise-induced bronchospasm. Maximal voluntary ventilation is used in the assessment of the remaining pulmonary capacity at the end of exercise, the breathing reserve. As already discussed, this is the fraction of the capacity of the pulmonary system to increase minute ventilation at maximal exercise, with normal values ranging from 20% to 50%. In situations of testing where the maximal voluntary ventilation sprint method is not feasible, it may be estimated using any one of the following equations:

$$MVV = FEV_1 \times 35$$ [41]

$$MVV = FEV^1 \times 40$$ [42]

$$MVV = 27.7(FEV_1) + 8.8(Pred\ FEV_1)$$ [43]

where MVV is maximal voluntary ventilation, and FEV_1 is forced expiratory volume in 1 second.

Although widely accepted as accurate in healthy adults, not all of the above equations have been validated in healthy children, albeit that the first equation has been validated in healthy African-American adolescent girls. Whenever possible, therefore, maximal voluntary ventilation should be determined using the sprint method as recommended by the American Thoracic Society.

Blood Pressure Monitors

Monitoring of blood pressure has been a significant problem during exercise testing due to artifact from motion of the arm, making accurate measurements difficult to obtain.[26] This is a greater problem with treadmill than with cycle ergometry. Automated systems designed for exercise testing incorporating a sensitive microphone positioned over the brachial artery are now commonly used in many laboratories. Many of these systems simultaneously receive an electrocardiographic signal, allowing precise gating to the QRS complex while filtering background noise. These systems generally measure pressure both oscillometrically and, using head phones, by direct auscultation. Direct auscultation is the preferred method, as there is a tendency to overestimate systolic and underestimate diastolic pressures with oscillometric measurements. Several sizes of blood pressure cuffs are necessary equipment.[30] Most automated systems also have paediatric-sized cuffs, as well as oversized cuffs for large subjects.

Oximeters

Oximeters fitted for the finger or ear are used to measure arterial saturation of oxygen. The devices are frequently inaccurate, particularly at high rates of work when children are prone to grasp the cycle handlebars too tightly.[26] Therefore, ear oximetry is better for laboratories using primarily cycle ergometry. All oximeters are less accurate at higher rates of work due to excessive motion.[26]

INDICATIONS FOR EXERCISE TESTING

These depend upon symptoms, and/or the presence of cardiovascular disease. The American Heart Association issued guidelines for indications for stress testing in children (Table 20-4).[30] We will discuss some of the more common reasons.

TABLE 20-4

INDICATIONS FOR PERFORMING AN EXERCISE TEST

1. Evaluate specific symptoms or signs induced by exercise.
2. Identify abnormal adaptive responses to exercise in cardiac or non-cardiac disorders.
3. Assess the effectiveness of medical or surgical interventions.
4. Assess functional capacity for vocational, recreational, and athletic recommendations.
5. Discover prognosis for a specific disorder.
6. Evaluate overall physical fitness levels.
7. Establish baseline data for follow-up of rehabilitation programs.

Adapted from Washington RL, Bricker JT, Alpert BS, et al: Guidelines for exercise testing in the pediatric age group. From the Committee on Atherosclerosis and Hypertension in Children, Council on Cardiovascular Disease in the Young, the American Heart Association. Circulation 1994; 90:2166–2179.

Evaluation of Overall Exercise Performance in Structural Heart Disease

Evaluation of the overall performance of the cardiovascular, pulmonary, and musculoskeletal systems in children with structural heart disease may be the most common indication for testing. The goals of such evaluations primarily consist of identifying potential causes of exercise intolerance, stratification of risk for patients who have significant structural defects, and assessment of the physical capacity of postoperative patients. The data obtained may be helpful in the decision process regarding therapeutic intervention, restriction of physical activity, and programmes for rehabilitation or conditioning.

Evaluation of Rhythm

Evaluation of the heart rate response and exercise-induced arrhythmias is essential in selected patients with surgically repaired congenital defects, and in patients with known or suspected arrhythmias. Increasingly, exercise testing is used to assess the efficacy of pacemakers, and to help modify settings in order to improve exercise performance.

Evaluation of Myocardial Ischaemia

This is a common reason for referral for exercise testing, particularly with left-sided obstructive lesions, such as aortic stenosis.[31] In addition, a growing number of patients may be at risk for coronary arterial insufficiency after the arterial switch procedure.[44] Evidence of abnormal myocardial perfusion as a result of Kawasaki disease is also not a rare finding.[45] Less common anomalies, such as anomalous origin of the coronary arteries, and coronary arterial fistulas, place the subendocardium at risk.[46]

Evaluation of Exercise-Induced Symptoms of Uncertain Etiology

One of the largest groups of patients seen in the exercise physiology laboratory is children who have various exercise-induced symptoms without a clearly identifiable source. Exercise testing may be useful in identifying potential aetiologies of symptoms. Exercise-induced dyspnoea, or new onset of exercise intolerance and fatigue, may be due to non-cardiac causes, such as pulmonary, musculoskeletal, or haematological disorders. Evaluation of exercise-induced syncope or near-syncope may result in the diagnosis of cardiac arrhythmias.

Evaluation of Exercise Capacity with Chronic Illness

The treatment of certain illnesses, such as childhood cancer, requires long and sometimes debilitating therapy. The chronic effects of therapy, at times cardiotoxic as with adriamycin, are highly variable. Evaluation of the exercise capacity in these patients is valuable in identifying cardiovascular impairment, as well as for implementing rehabilitation therapy.

DATA OBTAINED DURING EXERCISE TESTING

During each exercise test, obtaining as complete a set of data as possible is essential. Occasionally, compromises are made regarding collectable data, especially in very young patients. Nevertheless, it should be possible to obtain the data listed below.

Rate of Work

The rate of work, or power, is measured in kiloponds for each meter per minute (kpm/min), or more commonly in watts.[47] The maximal rate can be measured directly on a cycle ergometer. The measurement must be inferred when a treadmill is used based on height and weight as well as the speed and grade of the treadmill. For this reason, when using a treadmill, it is often easier to use the exercise time for analysis rather than the rate of work, comparing the time to normal values based on age, height, and gender.

Normal values for maximal rate in healthy children are approximately 3.5 watts/kg in boys, and 3.0 watts/kg in girls.[35] These values appear to be relatively constant throughout the paediatric age range. In the absence of other measurements, maximal rate provides only limited information. The rate of work is reassuring if it falls within the normal range. Low values, however, do not give any information as to the cause of the limited rate. Measurements of aerobic capacity, therefore, and the ventilatory anaerobic threshold, are often more useful in the evaluation of exercise performance.

Aerobic Capacity

These values are generally presented as maximal consumption of oxygen, and the consumption of oxygen at the onset of the ventilatory anaerobic threshold. Large variations in these measures are secondary to body size. Because of this, the values are generally normalised for body weight: milliliters of oxygen consumed per minute per kilogram of body weight ($mL \cdot kg \cdot min^{-1}$).

Maximal consumption of oxygen in children varies depending on the type of protocol and ergometer used and, to a lesser extent, on the age range of the subjects.[37,48–50] As stated previously, values obtained on a treadmill are roughly one-tenth higher than with a cycle ergometer. Normal values for children using a ramp cycle protocol are shown in Table 20-5.[29]

In light of the broad range of maximal measurements of consumption of oxygen in children, it is difficult to determine if an individual value for maximal consumption represents the highest achievable Vo_2. In studies of adults, maximal consumption frequently levels off, or plateaus, at higher rates of work.[51] This finding has been useful in ensuring that achieved maximal consumption truly represents the maximal aerobic capacity. This phenomenon is less likely to occur in children,[52] hence it is necessary to use other methods to assess maximal aerobic effort. The measurement of the ratio of respiratory exchange is useful for this purpose, this ratio increasing from a normal resting value of approximately 0.8 to about 1.2 as a result of the exchange of increasing volumes of carbon dioxide. A maximal ratio of approximately 1.2 is a good indication of maximal aerobic effort.

Many children with minor structural cardiac disease, either repaired or unrepaired, will have maximal consumption of oxygen similar to that of their healthy peers.[53] Children with significant structural abnormalities, in contrast, even if completely repaired or palliated, seldom have normal aerobic capacity. It is nevertheless important to measure aerobic capacity in this group, as it may prove useful in the functional assessment of the surgical repair or palliation, particularly when compared to patients who have similar congenital defects. Values for aerobic capacity are available for most large groups of patients with different structural defects.[54–61] These latter values are frequently more useful in assessing the success of a palliation in a complex defect, such as functionally univentricular physiology, than exercise data from healthy control populations. Serial comparison of aerobic capacity in an individual is also useful in assessing changes in haemodynamic state, as well as assessing the success of any therapeutic intervention.

Ventilatory anaerobic threshold is frequently expressed relative to the maximal consumption of oxygen. This value in children is in the range of 55% to 65% of the maximally achieved consumption of oxygen (see Table 20-5).[49] The ventilatory anaerobic threshold has been used less in children as a marker of aerobic fitness compared to maximal consumption of oxygen. It does have some advantages over maximal consumption of oxygen for this purpose. First, the ventilatory anaerobic threshold is a more accurately measured and repeatable measurement because it is not as effort dependent as maximal consumption of oxygen. Second, this value may have more physiological significance than maximal consumption of oxygen. The ventilatory anaerobic threshold represents, to an extent, the maximal amount of work an individual can sustain for a prolonged period of time. It is a useful guide, therefore, in assessing the ability to perform a given task. A difficulty with using this threshold to assess aerobic fitness is that it requires accurate measurement of a stable ventilatory pattern. This may be difficult to achieve, particularly in young children. The sense of dyspnoea associated with the onset of the anaerobic threshold can often result in erratic patterns of breathing in young children. As a whole, the ventilatory anaerobic threshold may not be measurable in one-fifth of children.[62]

In studies of children with structural cardiac disease, the threshold is low when compared with healthy populations. If expressed as a percentage of the maximal consumption of oxygen, the percentage values are similar in patients with structural defects compared to the healthy population, being in the range of 55% to 65%.[63–65] The threshold can be used by the providers of healthcare to set safe work

TABLE 20-5

NORMAL VALUES FOR AEROBIC CAPACITY IN CHILDREN AND ADOLESCENTS USING CYCLE ERGOMETRY

	BOYS		GIRLS	
	≤13 Years	>13 Years	≤11 Years	>11 Years
Maximal Vo_2 ($mL \cdot kg \cdot min^{-1} \pm SD$)	42 ± 6	50 ± 8	38 ± 7	34 ± 4
Vo_2 at VAT ($mL \cdot kg \cdot min^{-1} \pm SD$)	26 ± 5	27 ± 6	23 ± 4	19 ± 3
Vo_2 at VAT/Max Vo_2 (%)	54 ± 6	55 ± 10	61 ± 7	58 ± 8

VAT, ventilatory anaerobic threshold; VO_2, minute oxygen consumption.
Adapted from Cooper DM, Weiler-Ravell D, Whipp BJ, Wasserman K: Aerobic parameters of exercise as a function of body size during growth in children. J Appl Physiol 1984;56:628–634.

loads, and to establish levels of exertion for programmes of exercise fitness. Serial measurement is probably a better indicator of changes in aerobic fitness than maximal consumption of oxygen.

Cardiac Output

Noninvasive measurement of cardiac output is an important adjunct to the assessment of aerobic capacity. In children with diminished ability to increase cardiac output, working capacity and aerobic capacity can be preserved by several mechanisms. Exercising muscles can extract a higher percentage of delivered oxygen, widening the arterio-venous gradient of oxygen. A higher amount of work can also be performed anaerobically. Assessment of the increase in cardiac output with exercise may identify these compensatory mechanisms.

Data on the response of cardiac output in healthy children is less available than that on aerobic capacity. Most healthy children increase resting cardiac output approximately fourfold during progressive exercise. The maximal cardiac output with exercise is less in preadolescents compared with adolescents and adults when normalised for body surface area,[30,38] primarily because of lower stroke volume. Noninvasive measurement of cardiac output is one of the less reliable measurements routinely made in a paediatric exercise laboratory. Variations of at least one-tenth from test to test have been found in individual subjects.[38] The reasons for such variation are multiple, and reflect inherent inaccuracies in the methodology, technical difficulties, and variation from test to test within individual patients. Normal values for exercise cardiac output are presented in Table 20-6.

Pulmonary Function

Measurements of pulmonary function with exercise are often abnormal in children with structural heart defects.[60,61,64,65] The causes of these abnormalities are not entirely clear, but are probably multi-factorial. Defects involving abnormalities of the pulmonary vasculature, such as seen in patients with tetralogy of Fallot, appear to be more commonly observed. In these patients, a restrictive pattern of breathing, with decreased forced vital capacity and tidal volume, is commonly observed on resting spirometry.[60] This results in a higher frequency of breathing during exercise in order to maintain adequate minute ventilation. Obstructive patterns occur less frequently. Multiple thoracotomies resulting in formation of scar tissue may be one cause of these findings. These patterns have also been observed in children who have had a single surgical intervention.[60] Residual lesions, such as significant pulmonary regurgitation, appear to be associated with increased ventilatory abnormalities. In some cases, there is evidence that developmental abnormalities of the airway may be an intrinsic part of this particular cardiac abnormality.[60,65]

There are age-related changes that should be considered in the assessment of the patterns of ventilation of children and adolescents. Younger children normally have more inefficient patterns, with lower tidal volumes and higher frequencies of breathing than adolescents and adults.[66] This inefficiency results in a higher ratio of physiological dead space to tidal volume, and should not be misinterpreted as evidence of a pulmonary abnormality. Most pulmonary abnormalities do not limit exercise performance in children with congenitally malformed hearts. In many cases, the pulmonary abnormalities are relatively mild, and the exercising subject compensates by changing the pattern of breathing. Also, many children with congenitally malformed hearts have impairment in their cardiovascular system that limits their exercise capacity before decreased pulmonary reserve becomes a factor in exercise performance. Occasionally, a child is limited by pulmonary performance. Treatment directed at improving their pulmonary function may then result in improved exercise performance.

TABLE 20-6

CARDIAC OUTPUT WITH EXERCISE

Age	Resting Cardiac Index	Maximal Cardiac Index
11–13 years	3.9 L/min/m^2	12.5 L/min/m^2
13–14 years	5.25 L/min/m^2	17.4 L/min/m^2

Adapted from Eriksson BO, Koch G: Cardiac output and intraarterial blood pressure at rest and during submaximal and maximal exercise in 11–13 year old boys before and after physical training. In Bar-Or O, Natanya I (eds): Pediatric Work Physiology. Netanya, Israel: Wingate Institute, 1973, pp 139–150; and Eriksson BO, Grimby G, Saltin B: Cardiac output and arterial blood gasses during exercise in pubertal boys. J Appl Physiol 1971;31:348–352.

Response of Blood Pressure

Systolic blood pressure rises during exercise. Diastolic blood pressure generally falls, or is unchanged. Age, gender, and racial differences in blood pressure are found in the general population. Using appropriate normal values is essential, therefore, when assessing the response of blood pressure response. As a general rule, it is uncommon for systolic blood pressure to exceed 200 mm Hg in healthy children. In the evaluation of children with suspected hypertension and a structurally normal heart, systolic blood pressure in excess of 250 mm Hg is usually grounds for terminating the test.[30]

Abnormal responses during exercise are seen with certain cardiac lesions. A blunted rise or fall in systolic blood pressure may indicate severe obstruction of the left ventricular outflow tract, or pulmonary hypertension.[30] Elevated systolic blood pressures have been observed with residual coarctation of the aorta, and with abnormalities of the sympathetic-adrenal axis following successful repair of coarctation.[56,67]

Electrocardiographic Data

Complete electrocardiographic data is routinely obtained during testing of patients with structural cardiac disease. Evidence of chronotropic impairment, exercise-induced arrhythmias, and changes suggestive of myocardial ischaemia, are also routinely assessed. We will discuss the latter in more detail in the subsequent section. Impairment of the response of the heart rate to exercise limits augmentation of cardiac output. Chronotropic impairment is common after surgical repairs such as the atrial switch and Fontan operations[61,63] as well as following surgical repair of tetralogy of Fallot.[60] Often, it is difficult to determine the effect that mild chronotropic impairment will have on aerobic performance. Marked impairment invariably results in decreased aerobic capacity.

Evaluations of arrhythmias include identification of the source, be it supraventricular or ventricular, and the response of the disturbance to increasing exercise effort. The occurrence of new or potentially malignant arrhythmias, such as premature ventricular depolarisations that degenerate into ventricular tachycardia during exercise, is part of the stratification of risk that should be offered by the exercise physiology laboratory.[68] Changes in the QRS complex, such as when the morphology during ventricular pre-excitation is replaced with antegrade atrioventricular nodal conduction, or changes in the QTc duration in individuals at risk, are also routinely assessed.

Evaluation of pacing includes assessment of proper function at rest, during exercise, and recovery. The electrocardiographic recording should be assessed to show that sensing and pacing are appropriate to the settings. A recent interrogation and confirmation of the settings prior to the test are helpful to the exercise physiology laboratory staff. The type of exercise protocol used may be important to such testing. Rate responsive pacemakers, which have motion detecting piezoelectric crystals, usually require a treadmill protocol in order to provide sufficient motion for a normal response of rate.[69,70] Evaluation of a rate responsive pacemaker includes assessment of the maximal heart rate, as well as the slope of the rise in heart rate versus rate of work. A slope that is too shallow or steep may impair cardiac output and aerobic capacity. Measurement of aerobic capacity becomes useful in the evaluation of pacemaker settings, especially rate responsive models. The effects of changes in settings can be more easily evaluated by serial assessment of aerobic capacity.

Evaluation of Myocardial Ischaemia

Traditional assessment for possible coronary arterial insufficiency has centered upon the classic signs and symptoms of myocardial ischaemia, such as chest discomfort and electrocardiographic changes. Unfortunately, many children with coronary arterial insufficiency do not experience the classic symptom of crushing sternal chest pain. Furthermore, coronary arterial insufficiency which occurs in a controlled setting, such as in the exercise physiology laboratory, may not be accompanied by changes in the ST segments. Most of the previously published literature regarding exercise-induced myocardial ischaemia in children is based on the assumption that the indicators of myocardial perfusion, namely electrocardiographic changes or nuclear perfusion abnormalities, are similar to those seen in adults. This may not be a valid assumption. Fortunately, significant advancements in medical diagnostics have provided the clinician with alternative methods for detecting subclinical coronary arterial insufficiency.

Electrocardiographic Changes

The electrocardiogram is the initial diagnostic tool in the evaluation of possible coronary arterial insufficiency. Dysfunctional or ischaemic myocardium depolarises abnormally, and therefore will repolarise abnormally. It is this characteristic of abnormal repolarisation which was first recognised and documented in 1918, when Guy Bousfield noted depression of the ST segments during a spontaneous anginal attack in an adult who had a history of syphilis and clinically had aortic insufficiency.[71] Electrocardiographic criterions for ischaemia in children have been extrapolated from changes noted in adults. Horizontal or downward depression of 1 mm or more for greater than 60 to 80 msec has been universally accepted as that criterion which suggests myocardial ischaemia. Historically, such changes have been observed in many disorders that are characterised as having either abnormal coronary vasculature, or increased myocardial demands for oxygen (Table 20-7). There remains controversy regarding the most accurate assessment of depression of the ST segments.[31] The two common methods for measuring changes on raw data, the PR isoelectric method and the PQ–PQ isoelectric method, are shown in Figure 20-12. Although the PQ–PQ isoelectric method is easier, assuming a flat baseline, it has a higher incidence of false positive values in healthy children.[31] With current technology, signal averaging is superior to either technique (see Fig. 25-12).

Studies of patients with congenitally malformed hearts in which coronary arterial insufficiency was assessed electrocardiographically have primarily focussed on abnormalities of the coronary arteries. Such lesions include anomalous origins or courses of the coronary arteries, coronary vasculitides such as seen in Kawasaki syndrome, and surgically reimplanted coronary arteries as encountered after the arterial switch procedure and the Ross operation.[46,54,72,73]

Neither the sensitivity nor specificity of the changes compares favourably with other tests of myocardial perfusion in children. ST segment changes and nuclear perfusion imaging have correlated poorly in such conditions as anomalous origin of the left coronary artery from the pulmonary trunk, Kawasaki disease, and after the arterial switch procedure.[44–46] Correlation with the severity of obstruction in left-sided obstructive lesions such as valvar aortic stenosis is somewhat better.[54] Correlation is poorer, nonetheless, following surgical repair of these lesions.

TABLE 20-7

DIAGNOSES ASSOCIATED WITH ST SEGMENT CHANGES DURING EXERCISE

Aortic stenosis
Anomalous left coronary artery from the pulmonary artery (ALCAPA)
Anomalous origin of a coronary artery from the opposite facing sinus of Valsalva
Kawasaki syndrome
TGA, arterial switch operation
Hypertrophic cardiomyopathy
Heart transplantation
Thromboembolic disease
Mucopolysaccharidoses
Coronary vasculitides
Systemic hypertension
Drug ingestions (e.g., cocaine)
Hyperlipidemias with premature atherosclerosis

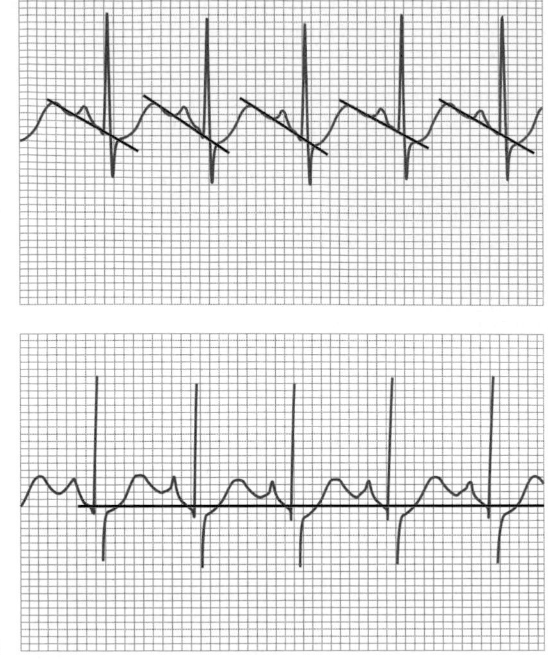

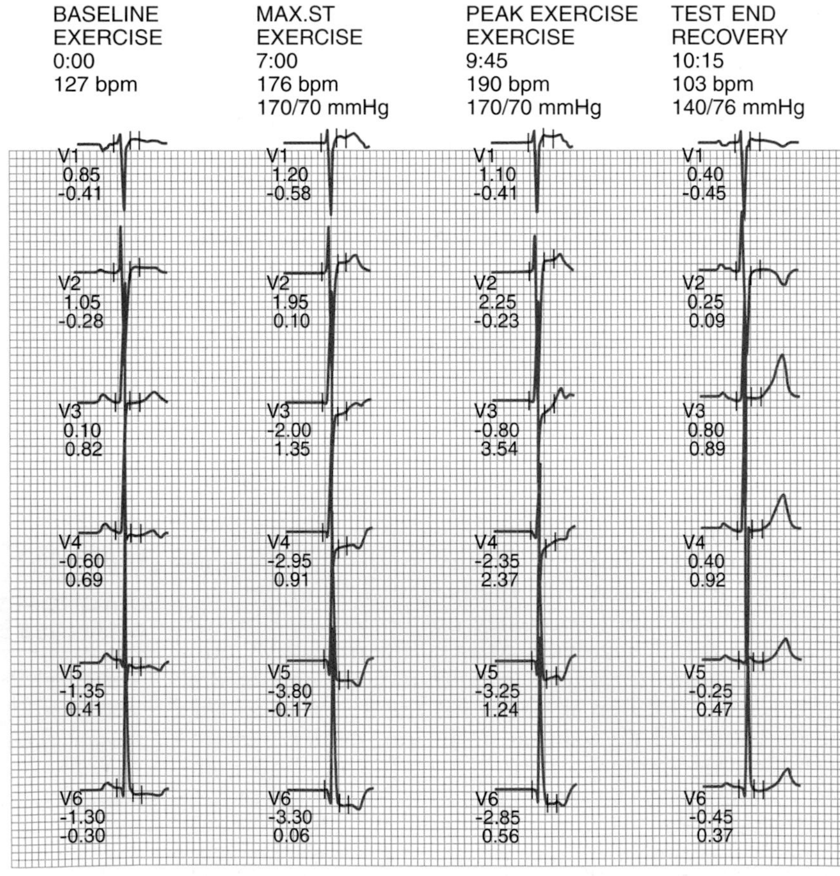

Figure 20-12 Methods of measuring changes in the electrocardiographic ST segments. **A,** The method using the PR isoelectric line (upper trace) and the method using the PQ–PQ isoelectric line (lower trace). Both methods are sensitive to artifact and baseline drift. **B,** Composite QRS beats obtained by signal averaging. The computer inserts markers at the point of initial deflection of the QRS, the J point, and 40 msec after the J point. (Top panels, reprinted with permission from Bricker JT. Pediatric exercise electrocardiography. In Rowland TW (ed): Pediatric Laboratory Exercise Testing: Clinical Guidelines. Champaign, IL: Human Kinetics Publishers, 1993.)

A number of conditions will produce a false positive test, including hyperventilation, digoxin therapy, antidepressants, oestrogen therapy, hypokalaemia, mitral valvar prolapse, or stove chest. False negative tests are also common as previously mentioned, easily comprehendible given that the changes appears to be a relatively late finding in the evolution of the ischaemic process (Fig. 20-13). Furthermore, the magnitude of the change does not always correlate with the severity of the disease. Although historically used in adults, therefore, the electrocardiogram does not appear to be the

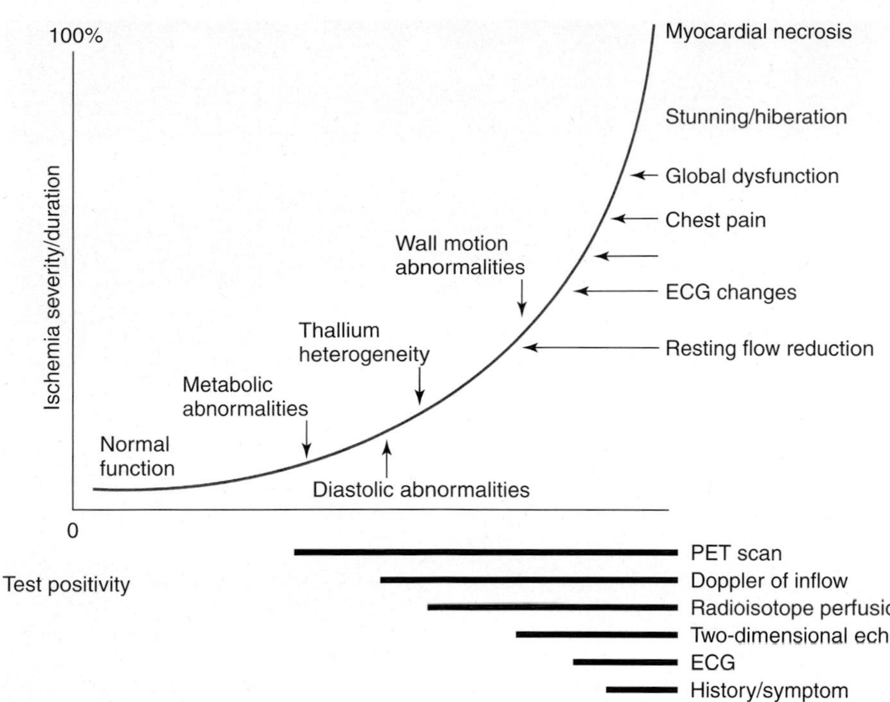

Figure 20-13 The evolution of the ischaemic process and the clinically applicable tests. (Reproduced with permission from Kimball TR: Pediatric stress echocardiography. Pediatr Cardiol 2002; 23:347–357.)

most accurate test for detecting coronary arterial insufficiency in children. Alternative methods are commonly used.

Nuclear Perfusion Imaging

Myocardial perfusion imaging has been used extensively in the assessment of myocardial ischaemia, infarction, and viability in congenital and acquired cardiac disease. Such studies are performed by injecting a radioisotope, which is a relatively unstable element that emits photons and is bound into functioning cardiac myocytes. The receptive myocytes emit a signal which can be captured by a gamma scintillation camera and processed with digital computer systems. Utilising a series of rotating head cameras that can acquire images in multi-plane slices, it is possible to generate a tomogram of the photon-emitting myocardial tissue; hence the name single photon emission computed tomography. The magnitude of the uptake of the isotope correlates with the thickness of the tissue, so that the right ventricle is not typically imaged with this modality unless there is significant hypertrophy, such as in severe pulmonary stenosis or a systemic right ventricle.[74] Injured, diseased, or dead myocardial cells do not readily take up the radioisotope, resulting in a perfusion defect on resting and/or stress images (Fig. 20-14). Typical protocols utilise studies at rest and after stress-imaging done on the same day, allotting enough time between the sessions to allow washout of the radioisotope. Comparison between the sets of images allows qualitative assessment of relative decreased perfusion in regions of the myocardium.

Two isotopes are commonly used in children. The tracer thallium-201 was once commonly used in most major paediatric centers, but has given way to technetium, a radioactive product of uranium decay. Thallium has the advantage of rapid clearance, allowing for less time between resting images and images acquired at peak exercise. Its rates of washout, however, have been quite variable in children.[75] Furthermore, there is a relatively high incidence of false positives with thallium during pharmacological testing in adults with coronary arterial disease.[76] Technetium 99m has several advantages over thallium, principally its improved radiation dosimetry, producing less gonadal absorption.[75] The disadvantage with technetium is the low hepatic clearance. Because of this, it is necessary to wait at least one hour to avoid marked hepatic activity, which can obscure results. Technetium linked to methoxy-isobutyl-isonitrile is employed in many centers.

The diagnostic accuracy of such imaging has been studied to a limited extent in patients with Kawasaki disease.[77] The sensitivity of myocardial perfusion imaging in this disorder has been good, ranging from 70% to 90%. The specificity, however, has been limited. Imaging has also been valuable in stratification of risk, as the presence of reversible defects during stress testing has been predictive of future cardiac events.[78]

The technique has also been used in patients after a successful arterial switch procedure.[44,77,80] Perfusion abnormalities appear to be common in such patients, although the correlation between perfusion defects and clinical outcome has yet to be determined.

Positron Emission Tomography

Positrons are positively charged subatomic particles, generated with the use of a medical cyclotron. Commonly employed elements such as oxygen, nitrogen, and rubidium are made unstable in medical cyclotrons, producing very short lived isotopes that are safe for medical use. When injected into the targeted tissue, the positrons from these elements combine with the electrons in surrounding tissue and annihilate each other. This annihilation reaction emits gamma ray photons, which are visible and therefore recordable with tomographic equipment. These tracers are excellent choices for myocardial blood flow studies.

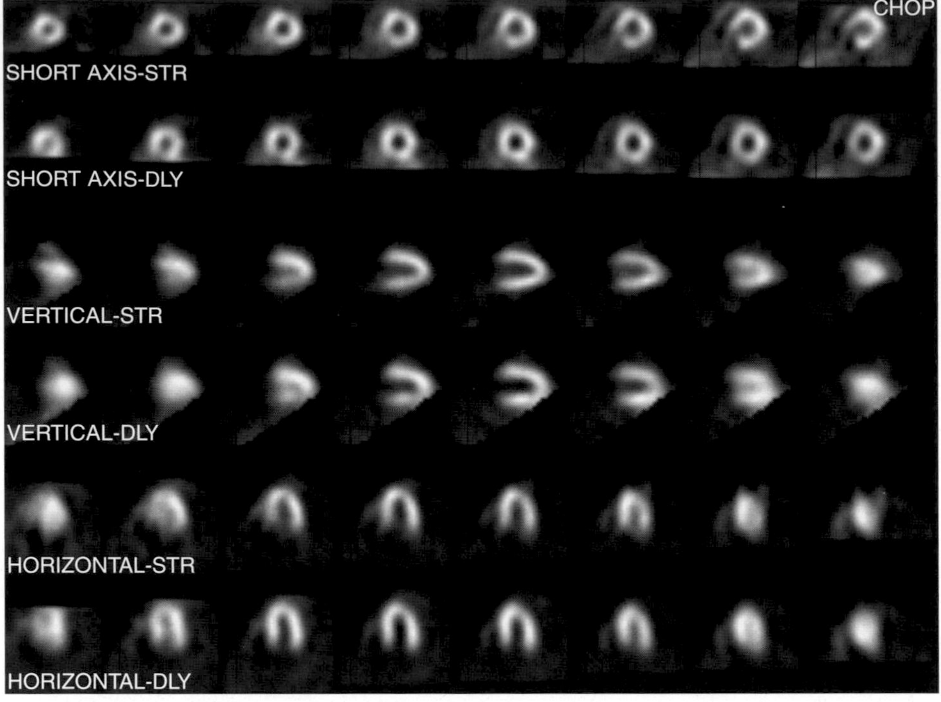

Figure 20-14 Preoperative images obtained using single photon emission computed tomography (SPECT) in an 8-year-old with anomalous origin of the right coronary from the left facing aortic coronary sinus. Note the reversible, inferior basal perfusion defect shown in the top right frames at 8 o'clock.

Advantages of this form of imaging include higher count rates, better image quality, superior attenuation correction algorithms, and greater ability to quantify myocardial flow of blood and flow reserve.[81] Its disadvantages are that the tracers are very unstable, and must be used immediately, often requiring an on-site cyclometer which increases the cost relative to imaging based on single photon emission computed tomography.

Because of the extremely short half-life of the positron-emitting isotopes, exercise testing is impractical, resulting in pharmacological stress testing as the preferred method for studies using positron emission tomography. These studies are usually performed while the patient is in the scanner in order to allow for immediate acquisition of images following completion of the protocol for intravenous infusion of the drug. The short half-life of the isotope limits the utility of imaging in circumstances where additional data regarding exercise performance such as maximal consumption of oxygen or working capacity is desired.

Despite these limitations, the technique has significant advantages over the alternative technique using single photons. Lower radiation doses of emitted photons compared to single photons permits its use in research studies on healthy adults. In addition, technology allows for quantification of regional myocardial flow of blood, resulting in absolute flows at rest and stress for all myocardial regions, and computation of coronary arterial flow reserve, this being the ratio of peak over resting flows. Studies of patients with congenitally malformed hearts utilising positron emission technology have focused on lesions in which manipulation of a coronary artery was part of the surgical repair, including the arterial switch operation and aortic valvar disease. Investigators found perfusion defects in one-third of patients when compared to controls,[82] a finding confirmed by others, albeit with the second group finding no perfusion defects in patients undergoing the Ross operation.[83] Children have also been studied with acquired coronary arterial disease, typically due to Kawasaki disease, such patients having diminished flow reserves compared to normal subjects.[84–87] All of these studies have compared regional flow to data obtained from young healthy adults. Even with extremely low-dose radiation, it has not been ethically feasible to collect data on regional myocardial blood flow in healthy children and adolescents using positron emission technology. The assumption in current studies is that the myocardial response to pharmacological vasodilation and coronary arterial flow reserve are similar in children compared to young adults. Given the lack of reliable data to substantiate this assumption, literature reporting the coronary arterial flow reserve in children must be interpreted cautiously.

Reports of exercise testing in patients with both Kawasaki disease and after the arterial switch procedure have found that a significant number of exercise-induced defects are not associated with either symptoms of ischaemia or electrocardiographic changes.[44,45] Similar findings have been reported for anomalous origin of the left coronary artery from the pulmonary trunk.[46] The reason for these discordant findings is unclear. It is possible that these perfusion defects are false positive findings caused by photon attenuation from overlying tissue. Unlike in adults, there are no normal standards to correct for attenuation in children. Lack of demonstrable lesions in the coronary arteries by cardiac catheterisation or echocardiography would support this hypothesis. Another possibility is that these defects represent microvascular disease. The latter explanation is congruent with the proposed ischaemic cascade (see Fig. 20-13), in which electrocardiographic changes and symptoms of ischaemia are relatively late findings. This may suggest a fundamentally different electrocardiographic and symptomatic response to subendocardial ischaemia in children compared with adults. Currently, the significance of exercise-induced myocardial perfusion defects observed on nuclear imaging in children remains uncertain for many lesions.

Stress Echocardiography

Kraunz and Kennedy were the first to report on mural motion after exercise using echocardiography,[88] with Berthe and colleagues[89] then describing dobutamine stress of the myocardium as assessed by echocardiography.[89] This technique has since been used in attempts to improve on changes in the ST segments alone in the assessment of exercise-induced myocardial ischaemia in certain congenital cardiac lesions.[90] In situations where the cardiovascular anatomy has been essentially restored, such as after the arterial switch procedure or repair of anomalous origin of the coronary arteries, the technique allows for the assessment of regional left ventricular wall motion both at rest and during exercise, using the same criterions established for adults with coronary arterial disease. The approach uses standardised echocardiographic views before and after stress, providing the stress either using a treadmill or cycle ergometer, or by employing pharmacological agents, such as dobutamine, adenosine, or dipyridamole. Dobutamine mimics exercise by increasing heart rate and blood pressure, while adenosine causes vasodilation of the normal coronary vasculature, which steals from the diseased segments, revealing subsequent abnormalities of mural motion. Dipyridamole inhibits cyclic nucleotide phosphodiesterase, and inhibits uptake of adenosine. Wall motion is analysed either globally or by grading 16 myocardial segments.[91] Ischaemia is manifest as either new or worsened abnormalities of motion.

There are limitations when utilising stress echocardiography that are unique to patients with congenitally malformed hearts. In those with complex defects, or those with artificial material such as patches or baffles, unusual ventricular anatomy such as a systemic morphologically right ventricle creates problems unusual ventricular anatomy such as a systemic morphologically right ventricle, in the assessment of changes in mural motion. Many postoperative patients have varying degrees of electrocardiographic abnormalities of conduction, which can also make analysis difficult, both at rest and during exercise. In patients with congenital cardiac lesions, it can also be difficult to measure mural motion immediately after exercise. Often, this is related to poor acoustical windows after surgery, and the high respiratory rates typically seen in young patients. High respiratory rate results in more lung interference, which often impairs imaging. Lack of cooperation in very young patients may also be an impediment to obtaining clear images. These problems have led to the use of pharmacological stress testing in certain subgroups of patients when performing stress echocardiography.

Pharmacological stress echocardiography, therefore, has gained favour for use in children for a variety of reasons, including the technical difficulties in providing maximal exercise. The available pharmacological agents, as discussed above, are those that increase myocardial consumption of oxygen, such as dobutamine and isoproterenol, and those that cause coronary vasodilation, such as adenosine and dipyridamole.[90] The choice of the agent to be used is based on the type of defect and the reason for the study. Coronary vasodilators are usually chosen when a stenotic coronary lesion is suspected.

Dobutamine, possessing both positive chronotropic and inotropic properties, is the most frequently used agent. In the typical test, the resting images are obtained for baseline comparison. Dobutamine is then infused usually at an initial dose of 5 μg/kg/min. The dose is then increased at a fixed time interval, often 3 minutes, to either a predetermined maximal level or until the development of symptoms. Assessment of changes in mural motion are usually made at the completion of each dosing increment.

The technique has been now been validated as an accurate diagnostic tool in patients with Kawasaki disease.[92] It has also been found to be congruent with myocardial perfusion imaging in patients after the arterial switch operation.[93–95] These studies show that stress echocardiography offers good sensitivity and specificity. Its predictive value in children, nonetheless, remains to be seen.

CONTRAINDICATIONS AND REASONS TO TERMINATE EXERCISE TESTS

Contraindications

There are both absolute and relative reasons not to perform exercise testing. Many of these reasons are listed in Table 20-8. As a rule, absolute contraindications result from an acute ongoing process affecting one or more of the major organ systems, such as myocarditis or hepatitis.[27,30]

Relative contraindications require that the physician supervising the laboratory evaluate the relative risk and benefit for exercise testing for that particular patient.[27,30] Occasionally, a relatively high risk during exercise testing may be acceptable. For example, routine exercise testing in patients with advanced pulmonary vascular obstructive disease is not appropriate because of the high risk of exercise-induced sudden death. Exercise testing, nonetheless, may be warranted as part of an evaluation to make a difficult decision concerning the timing of lung or heart-lung transplantation.

TABLE 20-8

CONTRAINDICATIONS TO EXERCISE TESTING

Contraindications
Absolute
1. Active inflammatory heart disease
2. Active hepatitis
3. Acute myocardial infarction
4. Active pneumonia
5. Severe systemic hypertension for age
6. Acute orthopedic injury to an exercise muscle group
Relative
1. Severe left ventricular outflow obstruction
2. Severe right ventricular outflow obstruction
3. Congestive heart failure
4. Pulmonary vascular obstructive disease
5. Severe mitral stenosis
6. Ischemic coronary artery disease
7. Advanced ventricular arrhythmias

Adapted from Washington RL, Bricker JT, Alpert BS, et al: Guidelines for exercise testing in the pediatric age group. From the Committee on Atherosclerosis and Hypertension in Children, Council on Cardiovascular Disease in the Young, the Ameriacn Heart Association. Circulation 1994;90:2166–2179.

TABLE 20-9

INDICATIONS TO TERMINATE AN EXERCISE TEST

1. Patient requests termination
2. Diagnostic criterions for the test are met
3. Equipment failure
4. Chest pain*
5. Dizziness, headache*
6. Syncope
7. Severe dyspnea*
8. Advanced arrhythmias or progressive atrioventricular block
9. ST segment depression greater than 3 mm
10. Systolic blood pressure greater than 250 mm Hg
11. Progressive drop in systolic blood pressure*

*Symptoms should be evaluated with all other monitored patient information to determine if the test needs to be terminated.
Adapted from Washington RL, Bricker JT, Alpert BS, et al: Guidelines for exercise testing in the pediatric age group. From the Committee on Atherosclerosis and Hypertension in Children, Council on Cardiovascular Disease in the Young, the Ameriacn Heart Association. Circulation 1994;90:2166–2179.

Reasons to Terminate an Exercise Test

There are at least four reasons to terminate an exercise test:

- The patient requests termination.
- The diagnostic criterions for performing the exercise test have been met.
- The monitoring equipment has failed and could compromise safety.
- Signs or symptoms are present that suggest the patient could be at significant risk if exercise continues.

Judging the level of fatigue of the patient using a perceived exertion scale, such as the Borg scale, is useful in anticipating when a patient is likely to refuse further exercise. Onset of dizziness, erratic respiratory patterns, or chest pain frequently indicates potential abnormalities requiring termination of testing. A significant fall in systolic blood pressure may indicate inadequate cardiac output. Likewise, an excessive rise in blood pressure greater than 250 mm Hg may be considered reason to terminate a test, although there is no evidence of significant increase in risk in an asymptomatic child who has a structurally normal heart.[30] ST segment depression of greater than 3 mm should be observed to indicate significant ventricular ischaemia, and is an indication for termination. Increasing frequency of arrhythmias, or exercise-induced atrioventricular block, will often require termination, but should be judged on an individual basis. Reasons for termination are summarised in Table 20-9. Careful preparation and monitoring are essential to successful testing. If adequate attention is given to appropriate preparation and monitoring, it is unusual that an exercise test will need to be terminated before achieving the diagnostic goals.

CONDITIONS WHERE EXERCISE TESTING IS OF VALUE

Congenital Cardiac Disease

More formal exercise studies have been performed in children with congenitally malformed hearts than any other group of children. Exercise testing in such patients can aid the decision-making process as to whether an intervention such as surgery is needed or can help in assessing the success of a previously performed intervention.

Unrepaired Congenital Cardiac Lesions

Left-sided obstructive lesions, including aortic stenosis, have been the subject of numerous studies, and are common reasons for referral of the patient for stress testing. The exercise test should evaluate for the presence of subendocardial ischaemia. A blunted rise in systolic blood pressure may occur in severe cases. Results of exercise testing alone are seldom a definitive reason for surgical intervention, but may be useful as part of an overall assessment of the severity of obstruction.

Surgically Repaired Congenital Cardiac Disease

Transposition

Atrial redirection operations were widely used during the 1960s and 1970s, with identified later sequels of atrial arrhythmias, diminished right heart function, chronotropic impairment, and reduced exercise performance.[63] Improvements in surgical technique and post-surgical management resulted in advent of the arterial switch operation in the late 1970s, still employed as the procedure of choice at the time of this writing. Both physical working and aerobic capacities are clearly superior in patients after an arterial compared to an atrial switch.[63,96] Patients who have undergone the arterial switch operation as a group have normal consumption of oxygen, and maximal cardiac indexes compared to healthy subjects, which is not the case with patients after atrial redirection.[72] The potential late-term sequels of re-implanted coronary arteries remain to be seen. Published studies to date indicate an incidence of approximately 10% in exercise-induced ischaemic changes in patients after an arterial switch.[72] Studies of myocardial perfusion imaging in this population were discussed above.

Tetralogy of Fallot

Most studies of exercise performance before 1990 in patients after surgical repair of tetralogy of Fallot found mild-to-moderate reduction of aerobic capacity compared to healthy controls.[65,97–104] More recently, a study found near normal physical working and aerobic capacities.[105] The presence of free pulmonary insufficiency and right ventricular dilation appear to be key factors in limiting aerobic capacity in this population.

Repair of Anomalous Coronary Arteries

No significant differences were found in rate of work or consumption of oxygen in patients with anomalous left coronary artery from the pulmonary trunk when repair was performed at less than 2 years of age compared to those repaired beyond infancy,[46] albeit that the clinical significance of these findings remains to be seen.[46]

Fontan Physiology

Several studies have shown that patients with the Fontan circulation uniformly have diminished physical working and aerobic capacities, chronotropic impairment, reduced stroke volume, intracardiac and intrapulmonary shunting, and abnormal pulmonary mechanics.[106–112] Important work in the field of exercise physiology has helped to influence the timing of surgical intervention. A decade ago, it was common for the Fontan procedure to be delayed until age 3 or 4 years or beyond. Following work at a number of institutions, showing that exercise capacity is higher when the systemic ventricle is volume unloaded at an earlier age,[113,114] it is now common to perform an intermediate procedure, such as a bidirectional Glenn anastomosis, within the first year of life, then complete the Fontan circuit by 2 or 3 years of age. Heart rate responses are often impaired in patients with the Fontan circulation, and rate responsive pacemakers have been implanted in order to make the response during exercise as close to normal physiology as possible, albeit that physical working and aerobic capacities do not always improve significantly.[70,115] This contrasts with results for patients with failing Fontan physiology, who demonstrate improvement in nearly all indexes of exercise performance.[113–118]

Coarctation of the Aorta

Residual coarctation is commonly observed in patients after repair of coarctation. Previous studies demonstrated that a significant residual coarctation may be unmasked during exercise testing when systolic hypertension occurs during exercise. Other investigators found significant residual lesions noted at cardiac catheterisation when the exercise study prior to the catheterisation uncovered an elevated systolic gradient between the limbs during recovery. The presence of augmented sympathetic nervous system and renal responses to exercise may contribute to the development of chronic hypertension in patients with this condition.[67]

Totally Anomalous Pulmonary Venous Connection

There is very little data regarding exercise performance in patients after repair of this lesion. Those with no residual anomalies have mildly reduced aerobic capacity, along with mild chronotropic impairment. Mild restrictive mechanics on formal pulmonary function testing has also been noted, but these do not appear to impact on performance.[64,119]

Acquired Disease

Kawasaki Syndrome

The impact that Kawasaki syndrome has on the coronary vascular bed has been the subject of much work, anticipating that this childhood illness may have late-term effect (see also Chapter 52). We routinely perform exercise studies on patients long after the acute illness has resolved in order to help with assessment of risk.[120] Others using quantitative analysis with positron emission tomography have shown that patients with Kawasaki disease without echocardiographic evidence of coronary arterial abnormalities had abnormal responses to adenosine stress testing, with evidence of reduced myocardial blood flows, reduced myocardial blood flow reserve, and higher total coronary resistance.[85] Despite these abnormal laboratory findings, maximal consumption of oxygen is normal, regardless of the state of the coronary arteries.[45]

Arrhythmias

It has been observed in patients with long QT syndrome that the QTc interval may prolong during intense work, and potentially lead to life-threatening arrhythmias. A formal exercise test, therefore, may be useful in excluding the syndrome in selected patients. We have found that exercise testing, although not always diagnostic, can be helpful when attempting to stratify risk. The morphology of the T wave at rest, during exercise and recovery, may also be of diagnostic value.[121]

Recipients after Heart Transplantation

Exercise performance is impaired following orthotopic heart transplantation compared to otherwise healthy peers.[122–124] Several factors are thought to be involved, including chronotropic impairment, musculoskeletal abnormalities, and abnormalities in systolic and diastolic function.[125–127] Studies of supervised programmes of rehabilitation have shown initial improvement, but subsequent decrease in exercise performance.[122,129] These findings suggest that exercise testing may be an additional useful noninvasive marker of early dysfunction of the graft, and if followed serially, exercise testing may serve to alert clinicians to modify the treatment and management of children subsequent to cardiac transplantation. Myocardial perfusion imaging and stress echocardiography could also be useful in evaluating the coronary arteries and abnormalities in mural motion, factors which may also contribute to progressive deterioration in exercise performance.

Non-Cardiac Illnesses

Survivors of Childhood Cancers

Anthracycline-induced cardiomyopathy, seen in children who survive childhood cancers, causes a reduction in physical working and aerobic capacities.[130] In this group of patients, working rate may improve with time, although afterload reduction did not alter the indexes of exercise performance.[131]

Systemic Hypertension

Differences in gender and race are found in responses of blood pressure to treadmill testing in healthy children.[132–134] The implication of these findings is not clear.[134,135] In most studies, systolic blood pressure rarely exceeds 240 mm Hg. These publications contain tables and figures that assist in assessing an abnormal response to graded exercise. We do not terminate testing unless the systolic blood pressure exceeds 250 mm Hg.

Most exercise physiologists agree that, despite the occurrence of systolic hypertension during exercise, there are beneficial effects of regular aerobic exercise toward lowering resting blood pressures.[1,136] There are no large studies to suggest that regular exercise is harmful to hypertensive youth. Regular exercise, therefore, should be part of the therapeutic regimen for hypertensive youth.

Exercise-Induced Asthma

Asthma and suspected exercise-induced asthma is a common reason for referral for exercise testing. The possible mechanisms by which exercise induces asthma are both physical, such as cooling and drying of the airways, and chemical, such as metabolic acidosis, these triggers initiating an abnormal physiological response which affects the bronchial smooth muscle. Complete reviews of these mechanisms are available elsewhere.[137,138]

Exercise-induced asthma occurs in up to nine-tenths of patients with persistent asthma, and in about one-tenth of the general population.[139] This condition is defined as 'transient narrowing of the airway that follows vigorous exercise'.[140] In healthy individuals, there is a fall of no more than 5% in forced expiratory volume in 1 second with exercise, but in exercise-induced asthma, the fall is between 10% and 25%.[137-143] Most clinicians consider a drop of 15% as diagnostic. The deterioration in lung function typically manifests as cough, shortness of breath, wheeze, chest pain/tightness, or inability to perform at physical activities and exercise.[139] Our protocol, which consists of rapidly increasing treadmill speed and grade such that the patient is running near their maximal capacity for approximately 6 to 8 minutes, is designed to provoke bronchospasm in pre-disposed subjects. Treadmill or free running is the preferred modality because it increases the time spent at high minute ventilation, thus decreasing the refractory time for potential bronchospasm. These features are not appreciated when using a graded or ramp protocol. Pre- and post-pulmonary function studies, and flow-volume loops obtained during the study, are analysed by pulmonologists working jointly with cardiologists. Significant exercise-provoked deterioration in pulmonary function is treated with bronchodilators, and pulmonary function studies are repeated. After appropriate treatment, children with exercise-induced asthma should be able to participate in sports and maintain normal activity.[139]

Cystic Fibrosis

This is a progressive disease that occurs in approximately 1 of every 1700 live Caucasian births. The primary organs involved in this disease, which is non-curable, are the lungs, pancreas, sweat glands, and intestinal mucosa. Striking heterogeneity in the presentation, clinical course, and prognosis of individuals with cystic fibrosis has been noted for decades.[144] Survival has now increased significantly, with many individuals living well into their fourth decade of life as a result of advances in medical therapy.[145]

Exercise capacity is directly related to the degree of pulmonary dysfunction, and is of prognostic value.[146] Patients are often under-nourished, which may affect the function of skeletal and respiratory muscles,[147] and portends higher mortality.[148] Published data has demonstrated low physical working and aerobic capacities, as well as low pulmonary reserves.[144,150] Unpublished data from our laboratory has confirmed the suspicion that there is a positive correlation between lean body mass, pulmonary function, and exercise performance. We surmise that actively supervised programmes for physical rehabilitation, and improved nutritional support, will likely be an integral part of a comprehensive approach to fostering a normal quality of life for these individuals.

The complete reference list can be found on the companion Expert Consult web site at www.expertconsult.com.

ANNOTATED REFERENCES

- Williams CL, Hayman LL, Daniels SR, et al: Cardiovascular health in childhood: A statement for health professionals from the Committee on Atherosclerosis, Hypertension, and Obesity in the Young (AHOY) of the Council on Cardiovascular Disease in the Young, American Heart Association. Circulation 2002;106:143–160.

  This scientific statement provides background, assessment, and strategies of treatment for promoting cardiovascular health in the care of children and adolescents. Background information, methods of assessment, and strategies of treatment are presented for each major area, including physical activity, obesity, insulin resistance and type II diabetes mellitus, hypertension, high blood cholesterol, and cigarette smoking. Strategies are directed toward promoting optimal cardiovascular health for all children.

- Wasserman K, Hansen JE, Sue DY, et al: Exercise testing and interpretation: An overview. In Principles of Exercise Testing and Interpretation, 2nd ed. Philadelphia: Lea & Febiger, 1994, pp 1–8.

  An introductory, yet comprehensive text illustrating the physiology of normal exercise and the pathophysiology of certain disease states. The reader will gain a wider understanding of the approach toward patients with exercise intolerance. Gas exchange, energy substrates, exercise protocols, and other topics are discussed. The final sections of the text are devoted to diagnostic case illustrations of patients with exercise intolerance using normal gas exchange parameters as frames of reference.

- Rowland TW: Response to endurance exercise: Cardiovascular system. Dev Exerc Physiol 8:117–140, 1996.

  A comprehensive text dedicated to the physiology of exercise as children become adolescents and subsequently adults. The text focuses on the process of maturation with central themes that address two functions, first the processes that support the performance of muscle, and second, the processes that assure homeostasis during the stresses of physical exercise.

- Washington RL, Bricker JT, Alpert BS, et al: Guidelines for exercise testing in the paediatric age group. From the Committee on Atherosclerosis and Hypertension in Children, Council on Cardiovascular Disease in the Young, the American Heart Association. Circulation 1994;90:4;2166–2179.

  This scientific statement from the American Heart Association describes the role of exercise testing in the evaluation of children and adolescents with known or suspected cardiovascular diseases. Included are the minimum training requirements for the exercise physiology laboratory staff, as well as a primer on accurate interpretation of tests based upon size and age-appropriate normal data.

- Cooper DM, Weiler-Ravell D, Whipp BJ, Wasserman K: Aerobic parameters of exercise as a function of body size during growth in children. J Appl Physiol Respirat Environ Exerc Physiol 1984;56:628–634.

  This research study examined metabolic and respiratory data during cycle exercise as a function of the changes in body weight during growth in 109 healthy children using ramp cycle ergometry. Results indicate that work efficiency and the mean response time for consumption of oxygen each minute are independent of age and size, but increased in a higher ordered manner with increasing size, and the onset of anaerobic metabolism during exercise occurs at a relatively constant proportion of the overall limit of gas exchange.

- Kondo C: Myocardial perfusion imaging in paediatric cardiology. Ann Nucl Med 2004;18:551–561.

  This article reviews the basics of myocardial perfusion imaging. The advantages and disadvantages of commonly employed myocardial perfusion agents are discussed, as well as the sensitivity and specificity of these agents in congenital and acquired cardiovascular disease.

- Kimball TR: Paediatric stress echocardiography. Pediatr Cardiol 2002; 23:347–357.

  This article reviews the history of stress echocardiography and its application in children. The advantages and disadvantages of physical and pharmacological stress testing are discussed, including specific pharmacological agents. Interpretation of abnormalities of motion is reviewed, and various disease states in which abnormal results from stress echocardiography occur is also discussed, as well as predictive values of results. Training guidelines for accurate performance and interpretation are reviewed.

- Vogel M, Smallhorn JF, Trusler GA, Freedom RM: Echocardiographic analysis of regional left ventricular wall motion in children after the arterial switch operation for complete transposition of the great arteries. J Am Coll Cardiol 1990;15:1417–1423.

  This study evaluated the effectiveness of echocardiographic evaluation of regional wall motion in 21 patients an average of 2 years after the arterial switch operation for transposition. A strong correlation was found between wall motion abnormalities on stress echocardiography and myocardial perfusion defects using the tracer thallium-201.

- Gewillig MH, Lundstrom UR, Bull C, et al: Exercise responses in patients with congenital heart disease after Fontan repair: Patterns and determinants of performance. J Am Coll Cardiol. 1990;15:1424–1432.

  This study evaluated the exercise responses of 42 patients with Fontan physiology to that of 28 age-matched controls during supine cycle ergometry. Results indicated that impairment in ventricular filling is more predictive of exercise performance than the heart rate responses.

- Davis JA, McBride MG, Chrisant MA, et al: Longitudinal assessment of cardiovascular exercise performance after paediatric heart transplantation. J Heart Lung Transplant 2006;25:626–633.

  Serial longitudinal exercise performance was evaluated in 28 children following cardiac transplantation. Results indicated that exercise performance is impaired, and despite an initial improvement, declines over time. The deterioration in exercise performance correlated with increasing diastolic dysfunction, a finding also frequently cited in adult studies in this population of patients.

CHAPTER 21

Description and Analysis of Data, and Critical Appraisal of the Literature

BRIAN W. McCRINDLE

The current standard of practise when faced with a clinical dilemma is to make decisions based on the use of evidence. This is broadly defined as decision-making that incorporates the best available research, together with clinical judgement, while considering also the preferences of the patient, or his or her parents. Thus, evidence based on research is brought to bear on individual and specific circumstances. Evidence based on research implies the use of data or measurements acquired in order to test a hypothesis concerning an area of uncertainty. The data itself may have been initially collected for reasons other than research, as is the case with data acquired from administrative, medical record, or observational sources, or to address specifically a research question, such as with prospective studies or clinical trials. The circumstances under which the data were collected, including their purpose, degree of measurement, rigour, and design of the study, play an important role in influencing the degree to which any conclusions or extrapolations from that data are valid or reflect the truth, in other words, whether they are free from systematic error and bias, are reliable, being free from random error, and apply to the clinical situation at hand. Data must be clearly described, relationships must be accurately and reliably determined, and the report must have sufficient detail to allow complete critical appraisal. The evaluation of presented data and analyses is a key skill for the contemporary clinician faced with increasingly complex clinical situations, and an exponentially expanding body of available literature.

MEASUREMENT AND DESCRIPTION OF DATA

Level of Measurement

Data is specific pieces of information that are defined by their level of measurement and their relationship to other data. Those pieces of information are often referred to as variables, since they may take on different values. The type of values that a variable may assume determines the level of measurement. The level of measurement determines how the values for a given variable are to be described, and how associations between variables are to be assessed and related to random error or variations. Levels of measurement can be categorical, ordinal, ratio, and interval.

Categorical variables are those for which the values fall into discrete and mutually exclusive categories. The value for a given individual or measurement can be applied to only one category. The relationship between the different categories reflects a qualitative difference. Variables with only two categories are referred to as being dichotomous or binary. Examples of dichotomous categories include yes or no, present or absent, male as opposed to female, and right versus left. Examples of variables with more than two categories include the type of connection used to create the Fontan circulation, the position of a ventricular septal defect, and medications used.

When presenting measurements related to a categorical variable, the frequency can be given either as the absolute number of measurements within that category, or as a proportion or percentage of the measurements from all of the categories. It is important to be clear about the denominator when giving percentages, and not to provide decimal places for percentages unless they will have meaning or importance. Giving the denominator is also important, since often the values for some individual measurements may be either missing, either because they were not measured or are not available, or else not applicable, in that the variable may not apply to that individual, such as the presence of amenorrhea in male subjects. The denominator should represent only those with non-missing and applicable values. The number of missing and inapplicable values should be reported separately. Alternatively, the number of non-missing and applicable values should be given. For example, 'Of 38 patients converted to the Fontan circulation, 21 (55%) were male, and chromosomal abnormalities were present in 4 (8%) of the 48 subjects tested'. For some categorical variables, an individual may have multiple values that place him or her in more than one category. A patient may be taking more than one medication. For this situation, there are two approaches. First, a category for that variable could include a specific combination of categories. For example, 'At most recent follow-up, 19 (50%) of the 38 patients with the Fontan circulation were taking anticoagulant medication, including warfarin alone in 10, aspirin alone in 8, and one patient taking both'. Second, the variable could be split into multiple categorical variables reflecting each category. In this example, the sentence would be, 'Warfarin was used in 11 patients and aspirin in 9 patients, with one patient taking both'.

A specific type of dichotomous categorical variable is the occurrence of a discrete event, such as performance of an intervention, or death. Events are almost always associated with an interval reflecting a period of time at which the risk exists. That period of time is an important aspect of that particular variable. This can be presented as the number of patients experiencing the particular event during a specified period expressed as a proportion of patients at risk for that event. For example, 'There were 5 (13%) deaths within 30 days of surgical completion, in 38 patients, of the Fontan circulation'. A frequent problem, however, is that not all individuals will have the same period of risk, given that some patients will be lost to follow-up, or something will happen, usually another event, which will cause them no longer to be at risk. The interval of risk for these individuals is said to be censored. Thus, the numerator, that is, the number of individuals free of the event, and the denominator, namely, the number of individuals remaining at risk for the event, are both decreasing over time. For this situation, techniques analyzing survival or timed events are applicable to describe the data, such as the estimates based on the technique established by Kaplan and Meier to make survival curves.

Ordinal variables reflect a specific type of categorical level of measurement whereby the categories can be ordered, such that we know that one category is more or less than another category. The exact magnitude by which one category differs from another category, however, is not known, and remains only semi-quantitative. An example would be the subjective grading of valvar regurgitation or ventricular function from echocardiography. We would know that mild regurgitation across the mitral valve is less than moderate, but more than trivial. We do not know the exact magnitude by which the so-called trivial variant differs from that labeled mild, or how the mild variant differs from the moderate grade. The categories are discrete and ordered, and the values would be presented in a manner similar to other categorical variables, that is, as frequencies, proportions, and percentages. A common mistake with ordinal variables is to assign or code them with a numerical grade, and then to present or analyse them as if they were continuous variables, erroneously implying that an equal distance or magnitude exists between each numerical category.

Quantitative or continuous variables are those whereby the difference between two values reflects a quantifiable amount. In addition, a constant difference between two values across the spectrum of possible values always represents the same amount. For some continuous variables, there is a defined zero, a point at which the quantity reaches nil, and there cannot be a negative value. This is referred to as a ratio variable. Ratio variables are common, and examples include height, weight, age, ventricular ejection fraction, and blood pressure. We know the exact meaning of the absolute difference between two values regardless of those values. The difference between 120 and 100 cm in height is the same 20 cm as the difference between 80 and 60 cm in height. With a ratio variable, however, the difference from the defined zero allows the ratio to have meaning. For example, 120 cm is 1.2 times, or 20%, greater than 100 cm. For some variables, in contrast, there is no defined zero or point of absence. These are referred to as interval variables. The relative relationships between these values cannot be quantified. For example, it is possible to consider changes in ejection fraction in response to a medication. Some individuals will show worsened ejection fraction, and have a negative value, others will stay the same, while still others might improve, and exhibit a positive response. The value recorded will reflect the quantity of the magnitude of change.

Since continuous variables can usually take on an infinite variety of values, reporting frequencies of values is meaningless, unless specific cut-points are used, or the values are grouped. Such categorisation of a continuous variable is rarely justifiable, nonetheless, since it overly simplifies the meaning and the presentation of the data, as well as diminishing statistical power. Continuous variables tend to take on a distribution, and the standard is to present some measure of the center of the values, along with the magnitude and pattern of their variation. The first step is to look at a frequency plot of the distribution of values. In general, some sort of bell-shaped curve will be observed, with a central hump tapering to the two sides. If the distribution is bell-shaped, we refer to this is as being normally distributed. This implies that the centre, and the variance, has specific definable properties or parameters. The measure of the centre would be the mean or average value, calculated as the sum of all values divided by the number of values. For the mean of a perfect normal distribution, half of the values would be less, and half would be greater than this value. The measure of variation would be the standard deviation. This is calculated as the sum of the square of each of the differences between the values and the mean divided by the number of values. The standard deviation has specific properties in defining the proportion of values represented, and is an assumption supporting probability theory, which underlies statistical or inferential testing.

The normal curve, however, can be subject to distortion. If the central hump is abnormally peaked or flat, this is referred to as kurtosis. If the tails or the sides of the distribution are unequal, then there is skewness. Important kurtosis or skewness can cause the distribution to become abnormal. The standard parameters and characteristics of mean and standard deviation then no longer apply. In this case, measures of the centre might be chosen which reflect the ranking of values, and not their interval magnitude. In ranking all of the values, the median value would be that measured value at the 50th percentile. For skewed data, the greater the amount of skewness, the greater the difference between the median value and the calculated mean. Less frequently, the most common value, referred to as the mode, is taken as the measure of the centre. Measures of variation include values at specific percentiles, such as the quartile values, presented as the measured values at the 25th and 75th percentiles, with the interquartile range presented as the difference between these two values. Alternatively, the measured values at the 5th and 95th percentiles might be presented, or the minimum and maximum values. Since these values are not dependent on the distribution being normal, they are often referred to as non-parametric distributions. The use of non-parametric statistical testing tends to be less robust and less powerful than parametric statistical testing. Hence, mathematical transformations of the measured values may be performed to create a more normal distribution. This can sometimes be accomplished by calculating and plotting the logarithm or the square root of the measured values, or applying other types of mathematical transformations. The normalised transformed variable is then used in parametric statistical analyses.

Validity, Accuracy, and Reliability

In addition to level of measurement, variables have properties reflecting the impact of how the measurements were made or determined. These properties include validity, accuracy, and reliability. Validity is the property by which the measurement used is a true reflection of the desired concept. It answers the question, 'Am I really measuring what I think I am measuring?' Accuracy is the degree to which the measurement comes close to the truth in the subjects being measured. It is a property of the measurement tool itself, and often reflects systematic bias or error. Reliability is the degree of variation in the measurement that is attributable to application of the tool. This may reflect both systematic and random bias. For example, if the purpose of my measurement is analogous to shooting a gun at a target, validity is the degree to which I am aiming at the correct target, accuracy is the degree to which I come closest to the bull's-eye, and reliability reflects how closely multiple hits are clustered together. If the hits are tightly clustered together, but always to the right of the bull's-eye, then this may reflect a problem with the sight of the gun. The error is systematic, or reflective of a component of the system. If the hits are at, or close to, the bull's-eye, but widely scattered, then this may reflect some twitchiness or poor eyesight on the part of the shooter, or subtle variations in the bullets that influence their trajectory. The error may be both random and systematic. When using or interpreting a measurement, one must be aware of these properties of validity, accuracy and reliability. This becomes more important when attempting to measure more subjective concepts, such as quality of life or cardiac failure.

Validity can be an elusive entity to achieve when the concept or phenomenon being measured is more qualitative and subjective. Rather than a gold standard or criterion, it is usual to begin with a definition, and then attempt to develop measurable aspects that reflect that definition. If we take aortic regurgitation as an example, a subjective grading is often applied when performing echocardiographic assessment, characterised by ordinal categories of none, trivial or trace, mild, moderate, or severe, with some intermediate categories. The subjective or qualitative grade is meant to reflect the overall impression of the observer, and informally takes into account many aspects related to the concept being pursued, giving more weight to some than to others. If we wished to validate our subjective system of grading, we might start by convening a panel of expert echocardiographers and asking them first to define the concept of aortic regurgitation. There may be agreement that it has something to do with the volume of blood that re-enters the left ventricle via the aortic valve during diastole. Some may argue, however, that this would represent the total volume adjusted for the size of the patient. Others may argue that it would represent the proportion or percentage of the forward stroke volume ejected through the aortic valve. The panel of experts may agree that there is no method of echocardiography permitting quantification of this volume, but that indirect measures may exist against which the subjective grade might be compared. It is agreed that no single indirect measure will suffice, and that multiple aspects may need to be considered simultaneously. These indirect measures are chosen because they have validity of content, meaning that they are judged to be related to specific aspects reflecting aortic regurgitation, and validity of construction, or construct validity, meaning that they are judged to have a plausible causal or physiological reason for having a relationship to aortic regurgitation. The panel may choose measures that reflect the state of the aortic valve in producing regurgitation, such as the width of the regurgitant jet relative to the width of the aortic outflow tract as measured using cross sectional and colour Doppler interrogation. They may choose measures that might reflect the volume of regurgitant blood, such as measurement of areas from colour Doppler mapping of flow, or even less direct measures, such as pressure half-time intervals or patterns of reversal of flow in the aorta as acquired using Doppler interrogation. They may choose measures that reflect the impact of aortic regurgitation on the ventricle, such as end-systolic and end-diastolic ventricular dimensions and volumes, as well as functional indexes such as shortening and ejection fraction. Alternatively, they may seek to measure this volume using other methods, such as with magnetic resonance imaging, or by creating an experimental model system. This process is aimed at criterion-related validity, or the degree to which the proposed measure relates to accepted existing measures. They may also seek to assess how the subjective grade relates to clinical or outcome measures, known as predictive validity. Subjective grading may be shown to relate to clinical symptoms, abnormalities of exercise capacity, ventricular dysfunction, or arrhythmias and sudden death, or to need for repair or replacement of the aortic valve.

If subjective grading of aortic regurgitation is judged, as based on content, construct, criterion-related and predictive validity, to be a valid measure of aortic regurgitation as it was conceived, then additional assessment is required regarding accuracy and reliability. Accuracy is a reflection of validity, but also includes any systematic error or bias in making the measurement. Systematic error refers to variations in the measurements that might always occur predominately in one direction. In other words, the deviation from the criterion or reference standard tends to be consistent. This may occur at the level of the tools or instruments used to make the assessment, and may represent lack of calibration. Regarding aortic regurgitation, this might reflect differences in the settings of gain or frequency of the probe used when the assessment was made. This may occur at the level of the observer, whereby the observer has a consistent bias in making the interpretation. Regarding aortic regurgitation, this might reflect the fact that some observers do not describe physiological amounts of regurgitation, and assign a subjective grade of none, and might not use intermediate grades. Alternatively, some observers may place more weight on a specific aspect when assigning a specific grade, such as areas as revealed by colour Doppler interrogation. This may also occur at the level of the subject, whereby a condition exists relative to the subject which biases the measurement. In terms of aortic regurgitation, this might reflect differing physiological conditions present in some subjects, such as concomitant mitral valvar regurgitation or aortic valvar stenosis.

Reliability or precision refers to the reproducibility of the measurement under a variety of circumstances, and relates more to random error or bias. It is the degree to which the same value is obtained when the measurement is made under the same conditions. Specific aspects of reliability should be assessed. If we again consider aortic regurgitation, we would want to know that, if two observers assess the same subject using the same methodology, they would report the same subjective grade. This is referred to as inter-observer variability. We would also want to know that, if an observer repeats the assessment in same subject using the same methodology, he or she would report the same subjective grade. This is referred to as intra-observer variability. Both of these sources of variability would be determined using measures of agreement, and not correlations or associations. Some of the random variation in measurements may be attributed to the instruments, such as variations in settings, differing equipment, or different algorithms or processing. Some of the random variation may also relate to the subject, such as variations in physiological state, medications, or the position when the assessment was made.

Ideally, the assessment should be as accurate and reliable as possible. This would minimise variation in measurements related to systematic and random error or bias, and would improve statistical power, minimising the necessary number of subjects to be studied, or observations to be made. This can be optimised by standardizing as much of the assessment as possible. Training sessions for observers can be designed whereby criterions and skills for making the assessment and interpreting the results are reviewed and practised, so that they are applied in a uniform manner. Limiting the number of observers, and having independent adjudications, also improves reliability, particularly if the review is blinded. Having protocols in place that define and standardise all aspects of the assessment also improves reliability. This would specify the equipment, calibration, and settings to ensure quality control. It would also specify the conditions under which the assessment should take place, standardizing the setting and the preparation of the subject. Taking repeated assessments, and pooling the results within subjects, also reduces random error.

There are some additional features of measurement that may need to be considered. Sensitivity refers to the degree to which the value of the assessment can detect differences. If patients with clinically important differences in the volume of aortic regurgitation are both subjectively graded as moderate, then such subjective grading might not be sufficiently sensitive. An aspect of sensitivity is responsiveness, or the degree to which the measurement reflects change related to time or an intervention. If a medication results in a clinically important reduction in the volume of aortic regurgitation, but the subjective grade remains moderate, then this means of grading might not be a sufficiently responsive measure. Measurements should also be specific, being a measurement only of the entity of interest as it was defined. Measures of ventricular function, such as shortening and ejection fraction, may not be very specific indirect measures of aortic regurgitation, and may be more influenced by many other factors. The measurement should also have a sufficient distribution of responses. If the object is to study factors associated with aortic regurgitation after repair of subaortic stenosis, yet the population studied has mainly grades of none to mild, then such subjective grading may not be a good measure to use for the assessment of aortic regurgitation. When many measures that assess different or similar aspects of an entity are available, completeness and appropriateness should be balanced with efficiency or parsimony. In a study of aortic regurgitation, all of the indirect measures could be assessed, as well as subjective echocardiographic grading, as well as some novel measures, which might include magnetic resonance imaging. This might provide the most complete assessment, but would be intensive in terms of time and resources, and might limit the recruitment of suitable subjects, as well as creating logistical issues regarding operationalisation, standardisation, and adjudication. It might also lead to inclusion of measurements that might be inappropriate to the aim of the study. It would be very complex to handle this large number of different measurements with different properties in an analysis aimed to address the question at hand. It would be preferable to focus on those measures which would give the highest level of measurement, in other words a continuous value, and which are valid, accurate, reliable, specific, sensitive or responsive, and parsimonious.

ANALYSIS OF DATA

Analysis is the method by which data or measurements are used to answer questions and generate knowledge, and then to assess the confidence in inferring those findings beyond the subjects that were studied. Analysis is often a secondary consideration when designing and implementing a study, and not considered until after the measurements have been made and the study is completed. In fact, the plan for analysis of the data is an integral part of the study protocol. It has an important relationship to the research questions being pursued, and a strong influence on the measurements to be made. Also, the chosen form of analysis can be an important tool to increase the validity of observed associations, by providing adjustment for potential sources of bias, such as confounding, or to determine more complex associations, such as interaction. The appropriate planning, strategy, execution and interpretation are essential elements to the critical appraisal of any research report.

What Is the Plan?

Research Question

Every study must begin with a well-defined question. The drafting of this question is the first step towards creating a research protocol. It is common to start with a topic of interest, or sometimes a clinical dilemma, and through consultation with experts, review of the published literature, and other sources of information, to define a discrete area of controversy to be addressed. Keeping track and documentation of this process often leads to the background section of a protocol, the reason for the study, and the introduction section of a subsequent manuscript. Often, constant revision, clarification, and specification of the question are required as part of this process. New investigators tend to be overly ambitious in their scope. The process of defining the research question often incorporates considerations of feasibility, relevance, novelty, and interest to the investigators. It is an iterative process that is not complete until a well-defined question, drafted in the form of a question, is finalised. It is not sufficient to only have objectives, aims, or purposes.

A well-defined question often suggests the design of the study, the population to be studied, the measurements to be made, and the plan for analysis of the data. It also determines whether the study is descriptive or comparative. For example, in considering the topic of hypertrophic cardiomyopathy, a descriptive research question might be, 'What are the outcomes of hypertrophic cardiomyopathy?' In appraising this question, its overt vagueness would be noted. The first step would be to determine what answers are already known regarding this question, and what areas of controversy remain. The investigator might look at the question and the background review and ask some of the following: 'What outcomes do I wish to study?', 'How will I define hypertrophic cardiomyopathy and in what subjects?', 'At what time point or over what time do I wish to examine these outcomes?' In answering these questions, the research question is revised and further specified to 'What is the subsequent risk of sudden death for children with familial hypertrophic cardiomyopathy presenting to a specialised clinic?' This question suggests an observational study of a chosen cohort. Depending on feasibility for the investigators, the study may be conducted non-concurrently from existing medical record information, or concurrently by enrolling subjects in the present, and following them forward in time. The question also suggests the population of interest, and from this the investigators would develop criterions for inclusion and exclusion with definitions, and how the subjects would be identified from the specialised clinic. The measurements are also suggested, in that baseline characteristics would need to be obtained to define the criterions, and to describe the characteristics of the included subjects. The definitions and sources of data would need to be defined regarding detection of events of interest. The plan for analysis is suggested in that the question is descriptive, and would need to describe the proportion of subjects who would have experienced sudden death over a defined period of time, or more likely a time-event type of analysis would be performed. While the primary question here is descriptive, the investigators would be missing an important opportunity if they did not have secondary questions that explored the impact of treatments or risk factors on the risk of sudden death. It is rarely justified, or necessary, to perform a study that is only descriptive in nature. A well-defined and focused research question, nonetheless, is essential before considering other aspects of the proposed study or report.

Using Variables to Answer Questions

When the question is established, the next step is generating a plan for analysis so as to select and define variables. What information will be needed to answer the defined question? In the process of defining variables, should be given to considerations of their measurement. Specifically, definitions should be defined, sources of data determined, and issues of validity and reliability of measurements considered.

Classification

Variables can be classified for statistical purposes as either dependent or independent. Dependent variables are generally the outcomes of interest, and either change in response to an intervention or are influenced by or associated with factors. Independent variables are those which influence or are associated with the dependent variable. A detailed consideration of the question should clearly identify the key dependent and independent variables. Independent variables can be further classified. Some independent variables have a direct causal or predictive relationship with the dependent variables, and are the variables in which we are most interested. Some independent variables have a direct influence on the dependent variables, but influence each other in the nature of that relationship. This is referred to as interaction. Some independent variables also have an indirect relationship with the dependent variables, primarily by their association with other independent variables that have a more direct association. This is referred to as confounding. Some dependent or outcome variables can become independent variables in their association with subsequent outcomes or dependent variables. An important step in creating a plan for analysis is to classify the available variables prior to considering how they will be described and related to one another in order to address the research question.

Outcomes or Dependent Variables

In any study, there are usually one or two primary outcomes of interest. There are often additional secondary outcomes, which are usually included to support the analysis based on the primary outcomes. If analysis of the primary outcomes is negative, conclusions from a study must be negative, regardless of those associated with the secondary outcomes. Analysis of secondary outcomes is also used for exploring or generating additional hypotheses and should not represent a definitive analysis. It should be recognised that the greater the number of outcomes examined in a study, the more likely it is that statistical significance will be reached on at least one of them. This is the challenge of multiple comparisons. With advances in management of many diseases and conditions, some outcomes have become increasingly rare, and many studies are grouping outcomes into composite outcomes. An example might be creating a composite outcome of death, myocardial infarction, or stroke in a clinical trial of cardiovascular risk factor reduction. The appropriateness of composite outcomes is questionable, and issues have been raised about their validity.[1] First, not all possible outcomes that might be included in a composite outcome have the same importance for subjects. Second, the creation of a composite outcome might obscure differences between the individual outcomes. The risk for the component outcomes may be different, as well as the impact of therapy or associated variables. Specific outcomes should be favored over composite outcomes when feasible and relevant.

Outcome variables can differ in their nature, which influences how they should be handled in an analysis plan. Some outcomes are discrete, being either present or absent, or classified into nominal categories. Some outcomes can be ordinal or continuous in nature, indicating a degree or magnitude. Some outcomes are discrete events that have a relationship with time. These outcome events may be repeated or recurrent, and subjects may be simultaneously at risk for different and mutually exclusive outcome events that may compete. Some outcomes may evolve over time, and thus have a longitudinal dimension or trend over time. Each of these features needs to be considered, as specific methods of data and statistical analysis need to be applied.

Independent Variables

Independent variables are variables for which an association with the dependent variables is sought. These variables can include subject characteristics and interventions, but sometimes outcomes that may be predictive or causal of other subsequent outcomes. The research question should define the primary independent variable, which is commonly a specific treatment or a key subject characteristic. Independent variables can be grouped according to the proposed nature of their relationship with the dependent variable, which is described in more detail in a subsequent section. We usually have some independent variables in which we are interested whether or not they have a direct predictive or causal relationship with the dependent variable. We also have some independent variables in which we are less interested, but which may act as potential confounders.

Planning the Description

The first step in the plan for analysis is to define how all of the variables are to be described. The methods by which this is done have been covered in a previous section. In describing data, the results or values of each individual variable are summarised. Description is important in detailing the characteristics of the subjects to be studied, usually at baseline, and will allow the reader of a subsequent report to determine if the results of the study might be applicable to their own clinical practice. Description of the data also can give the details of what interventions were performed, and what outcomes occurred. Additionally, we can describe data that were collected in order to establish compliance with the study protocol. This might include compliance with therapy, co-interventions, cross-over from assigned treatment, duration of follow-up and completeness of follow-up. Description is also used to determine issues that might have an impact on statistical testing, such as extreme values or outliers, missing values, categories with too few values, and skewed distributions.

Planning to Establish Relationships and Associations

This step in the plan is guided by the research question. The aim of most research questions will fall into one of three main categories. Some studies aim to answer questions about the effect of a treatment, either alone or in comparison with either no treatment or an alternative treatment. In this case, the treatment is the primary independent or predictor variable, and there can be many different outcome or dependent variables. If the study is comparative, then the characteristics of the subjects should be compared at baseline for the groups. We also need to compare additional management that might have occurred. If the treatment allocation was randomised, then comparison of baseline characteristics determines the success of equivalency between groups. If the treatment allocation was not randomised, the comparison of baseline characteristics might highlight important or relevant differences between groups that could potentially confound comparisons of outcomes, and for which statistical methods for adjustment should be used.

The second category includes those research questions aimed at determining the prognosis of subjects with a common characteristic or after a specific intervention, the risk of a particular adverse outcome, or factors that might be predictive or associated with prognosis or risk, particularly those of a potential causal nature. The dependent variable is the outcome variable of interest, and associations are explored with multiple independent variables that may include subject characteristics, interventions and other outcomes. This type of analysis plan should take into account independent variables that may serve as potential confounders, and that have a direct relationship to the outcome, but are also associated with the independent variable of interest for which we would like to infer a direct relationship with the outcome.

The third category includes those questions aimed at identifying factors that may discriminate or differentiate different groups of subjects. Some of these questions may be aimed at evaluating a diagnostic test. In this case the dependent variable is the group status of the subjects, usually as defined by application of a criterion standard, and the primary independent variable is the result of the diagnostic test. Some questions may be aimed at contrasting characteristics between two or more defined groups of subjects. Case-control studies are a classic example. In this case the primary dependent variable is the characteristic by which the cases and controls were defined, and multiple independent variables including subject characteristics, interventions and outcomes are contrasted.

Types of Relationships Between Variables

An important defining feature of variables, in addition to the level of measurement and measurement properties, is the relationship between them. Variables can be classified in terms of their relationship to one another. Independent variables are those variables which incite, influence or are associated with a response. The response variable is termed the dependent or outcome variable. Independent variables may have a direct association with the dependent variable, either through prediction or causality, or they may have an indirect or confounding association.

Causality is a desired feature of associations we wish to determine. The aim of many studies is to determine relationships that are cause leading to effect. The nature of associations and features of study designs that help to give confidence that a discovered association is cause and effect will be described later in this chapter, but include evidence of a correct temporal relationship, a strong dose-response relationship, freedom from bias, consistency, and biological or pathophysiological plausibility. When we cannot be certain that the temporal relationship is correct, that the potential causal factor was present first and led to the subsequent development of the effect or outcome, we cannot exclude that the relationship between the two variables is actually reversed. In this case the putative causal factor may actually be caused by the assumed effect or outcome. For example, in a cross sectional study of treatment with β-blockers, we note that the use of β-blockers and the presence of palpitations are significantly associated. We might erroneously conclude that β-blockers are causal of palpitations, when in fact arrhythmia causing palpitations has lead to treatment with β-blockers.

Confounding occurs when the independent variable exerts its influence or association with the dependent variable primarily through its relationship with a further independent variable that is more directly related to the dependent variable. The identification and adjustment for confounding can be a challenge in the analysis and interpretation of observational or non-experimental study data. Confounding is most likely to occur when independent variables are highly related or correlated with one another, which is referred to as colinearity. For example, a hypothetical study shows an association between increased use of systemic anticoagulation and increased risk of death after the Fontan procedure. Consideration is given to recommending against the use of routine anticoagulation. Further analysis, however, may reveal that the use of systemic anticoagulation was predominately in those patients with poor ventricular function. Poor ventricular function is then found to be causally and strongly related to mortality, and the association of anticoagulation with mortality is felt to be confounded and hence indirect because of its increased prevalence of use in patients with poor ventricular function. Stratified or multi-variate analyses are often used to explore, detect, and adjust for confounding, and to determine relationships between variables that are independent of other variables.

Interaction is a particular type of relationship between two or more independent variables and a dependent variable. The relationship between one independent variable and a dependent variable is influenced or modified by an additional independent variable. For example, in our hypothetical study, further analysis shows that the relationship between systemic anticoagulation and mortality is more complex. For patients with poor ventricular function who are treated with systemic anticoagulation, mortality is less than for those not treated. For patients without poor ventricular function, there is no difference in mortality between those treated versus those not treated with systemic anticoagulation. Thus, there is a significant interaction present between systemic anticoagulation and poor ventricular function, demonstrated by the differential association of anticoagulation with mortality as influenced by the presence of poor ventricular function. In order to be certain that the anticoagulation was the true cause of the reduction in mortality, and not attributable to some other unmeasured confounding factor, a properly designed and executed randomised clinical trial should be undertaken.

Statistical Analysis—Detecting Associations and Relationships with Confidence

Opinions about the extent of statistical knowledge of physicians vary widely. On the one hand, conducting or appraising clinical research sometimes requires knowledge of increasingly complicated statistical methodology. On the other hand, little time in medical school is available appropriately to address statistics and their use and applicability in clinical practice. A recent survey of 171 articles published in the journal *Pediatrics* found that nine-tenths of published studies used some sort of inferential statistics. The same study found that a reader who understands descriptive statistics, proportions, risk analysis, logistic regression, *t* tests, non-parametric statistics, analysis of variance, multiple linear regression and correlations could still only fully understand the analysis in just under half of the articles.[2] Despite disagreements on the extent of statistical education in clinical training, the increasing complexity of statistics reported in the medical literature clearly appeals for a standard of at least some statistical literacy among practicing clinicians and clinical researchers.

Principles of Probability and Probabilistic Distribution—The Science of Statistics

While conducting a census of every citizen of a given country, you find that the proportion of women in the population is exactly 52%, and that their average height is 152 cm. You select a random sample of 100 people from this same population and, to your surprise, 55% of your sample is composed of women and their average height is 149 centimeters. Subsequently, you decide to select a second random sample of 100 people. This time, 47% of your sample is women and the average height is 158 centimeters. The phenomenon at play here is called random effect, random error, or random variation. Each individual sample taken randomly from a larger population will have an uncertain distribution in terms of characteristics. The distribution of characteristics in each sample, nonetheless, is based on the probability of those outcomes for the entire population, which has a specific distribution of features known as parameters.

If you flip a coin, the probability of the coin landing on heads is exactly 50%. If you flip that coin 100 times you might get 50 heads, as you would expect, but owing to random effect you may get 49 or 52 heads, and on rare occasions 45 or 55. If you repeat this exercise numerous times, you will get exactly 50 heads a few times, most of the times you will get somewhere between 48 and 52 heads, and in the great majority of tries you will get between 45 and 55 heads. The outcome of each series of 100 tosses is random, but remains a function of the true probability of getting a head with each coin toss. If we were to plot the frequency of heads in our many samples, we might see a bell-shaped curve centered at or very close to 50 that slopes to the right and the left, with more extreme values occurring less frequently in the tails. This curve is called a distribution of probability. It has some specific properties about the variation that allow us to be able to predict how frequently a given outcome will be observed in an infinite number of random samples.

Inference Based on Samples from Random Distributions

When we measure something in a research study, we may find that the values from our study subjects are different from what we might note in a normal or an alternative population. We want to know if our findings represent a deviation from normal, or whether they were just due to chance or random effect. Inferential statistics uses probability distributions to tell us what the likelihood might be for our observation in our subjects, given that our subjects come from a larger population which forms the basis for the probability distribution. We can never know for certain if our subjects truly deviate from the norm, but we can infer the probability of our observation from the probability distribution. If that probability is low, we can feel confident in our conclusion. In general, we assume that if we can be 95% certain, and accept a 5% chance that our observation is really not different from normal, or the center of the probability distribution, then we state that our results are significant. The probability that the observed result may be due to chance alone represents the *P*-value of inferential statistics.

When a random sample is selected from a population, differences between the sample and population are due to the random effect, or random error. In our census, while the entire population had an average height of 152 cm, it does not mean that everyone in this population was 152 cm tall. Some were 130 cm in height, and others were 170 cm. Hence, if you select a random sample of 100 people, some will be taller and some shorter. By chance alone, it might be that a specific sample will have fewer shorter people or fewer taller people. Thus, the average height for this specific sample might be lower or higher than the average by chance alone. The key point to remember is that as long as the sample was randomly chosen, the mean of your sample should be close to the mean of the population. The larger your sample, the more precise the measurement is, and the closer you are to the true mean of 152 cm. This is because each value contributes less to the total and, as such, extreme values have less of an effect. The same is true with the example of coin tossing. Out of 10 tosses, a result of heads for 90% or 10% of tosses is rare but not impossible. If the coin toss is repeated 1000 times, the results will certainly be much closer to the 50% probability of a single coin toss. The fact that the result is different from that in the population from which the sample was taken does not necessarily imply that the subjects in your samples are inherently different from that population. This might just be due to random error.

Consider a situation in which a researcher polls a random sample of 100 paediatric cardiologists regarding their preferred therapy for failure, and found that 72% of the sample prefers using drug A over drug B. Since the sample was chosen at random, the researcher decides that it is a reasonable assumption that this group is representative of all paediatric cardiologists. A report is published entitled 'Drug A is preferred over drug B for the treatment of heart failure in children'. Had all paediatric cardiologists been polled, would 72% of them have chosen drug A over drug B? If another researcher had selected a second random sample of 100 paediatric cardiologists, would 72% of them also have chosen drug A over drug B? The answer in both cases is probably not, but if both the samples come from the same population, and were chosen randomly, the results should be close. Consider that a new study is subsequently published that reports that drug B is actually better than drug A. You then poll a new sample of 100 paediatric cardiologists and find that only 44% still prefer drug A. Is the difference between your original sample and your new sample due to random error, or did the publication of the new study have an effect on preference in regard to therapy for children in heart failure? The key to answering this question is to estimate the probability by chance alone of obtaining a sample in which 44% of respondents choose drug A when, in fact, 72% of the population from which the sample is drawn actually prefers drug A. In such a situation, inferential statistics can be used to assess the difference between the distribution in the sample as opposed to the population, and the likelihood or probability that the difference is due to chance or random error.

Relationship between Probability and Inference

A detailed explanation of the exact methods used to determine if the probability distribution of the sample is different from or similar to that of the overall or target is beyond the scope of this chapter. Suffice to say that each type of data, and each specific question, requires specific methodologies and tests, some of which will be briefly introduced later. The common point of any statistical test is that all types produce a *P*-value, which represents the probability that two distributions are similar. Statistical testing takes into account the number of subjects being tested, the observed variation in the data, the magnitude of any differences, and the underlying nature of the probability distribution, and thus the results are influenced by these features. Every statistical test comparing two groups starts with the hypothesis that both groups are equivalent. A two-tailed test tests the probability that group A is different from group B, either higher or lower, while a one-tailed test tests the probability that group A is either specifically higher or lower than group B, but not both. As a general rule, only two-tailed tests should be used in most situations, as they assess the probability of two groups being different without any presumptions about the direction of the difference between groups. There is no assumption that A is higher or lower than B, just that the two are different. One-tailed tests assume that the difference observed has a direction, for example, higher or lower, but not both. These tests should be used only in specific situations, an example being a non-inferiority trial. By convention, statistical significance is reached when the *P*-value obtained from the tests is under 0.05, meaning that the probability that both groups are equivalent, and not different, is lower than 5%. The *P*-value is an expression of the confidence we might have that the findings are true and not the result of random error. From our previous example of preferred treatment for heart failure, the *P*-value was less than 0.001 for 44% being different from 72%. This means that in a population where 72% of cardiologists prefer drug B the probability of having a random sample with 44% favoring drug B is less than 1 in 1000 trials. We can confidently conclude, therefore, that the second sample is truly different from the original sample, and that the opinion in the population of paediatric cardiologists had changed.

Relevance of *P*-values

Limitations

The threshold of $P < 0.05$ for defining statistical significance is acknowledged to have been selected somewhat arbitrarily, and is consequently a subject of debate. With this in consideration, it is important to bear in mind the implications and meaning of a *P*-value. Statistical testing takes into account the number of subjects being tested, the observed variation in the data, the magnitude of any differences, and the underlying nature of the probability distribution, and thus the results are influenced by these features. The magnitude of any difference is only one component, yet many assume that if the *P*-value is less than 0.05 then the results are important and meaningful. This is not the case, since a *P*-value only is a measure of confidence. *P*-values are highly dependent on the number of study subjects or observations. As the size of the sample increases, the precision of the estimate around the true mean increases, and thus the random error decreases. With large enough samples, the random error will be close to zero, hence very small differences or associations could meet the confidence threshold, yet be unimportant. With a sample size of 10,000, a *P*-value of 0.04 is probably of limited interest because the large size of the sample will ensure that even very small differences will be statistically significant. On the other hand, with very small samples, statistical significance at $P < 0.05$ is much less likely to occur even with large differences or associations. With small sample sizes, a non-significant *P*-value implies that we do not have sufficient confidence in the result, not that it might represent an important difference or association. *P*-values are only a measure of confidence, and the results must always be considered in light of the magnitude of the observed difference or association, the variation in the data, the number of subjects or observations, and the clinical importance of the observed results.

Clinical Relevance versus Statistical Significance

A primary consideration regarding statistical analysis in medical research is the difference between statistical significance and clinical relevance. There is no real value to an association that is highly statistically significant but clinically or biologically implausible. Likewise, studies with results that are clinically important but not statistically significant are of uncertain value. This is a key concept that is not widely acknowledged. Statistical significance does not necessarily equate to clinical relevance and, similarly, a result that is not statistically significant might be clinically important. Statistics are a tool to describe and to uncover evidence regarding the underlying mechanism of disease and impact of therapy, but it is important to know how to translate statistical knowledge into clinical knowledge.

Assessing the clinical relevance of an observed difference or association and the impact of random effect can be helped by examining the confidence interval. Confidence intervals are important tools to assess clinical relevance as they are intrinsically linked to a statistical *P*-value, but give much more information. The confidence interval is a representation of the underlying probability distribution of the observed result, based on the sample size and variation in the data. A 95% confidence interval would encompass 95% of the results from similar samples with the same sample size and variation properties, and thus represents a wider range of values over which we can be confident that the true result might lie. We can also construct a 70% confidence interval if we are willing to accept a greater chance of random error.

The confidence interval gives us the greatest information regarding the possibility that we have made an error in the interpretation of the results. The confidence interval asks two questions: first, what is the likely difference between groups, and second, what are the possible values this difference might have? For example, the randomised clinical trial testing the effect of drug B for children in cardiac failure found a reduction in mortality with drug B compared to drug A, but the *P*-value was greater than 0.05 and hence the result did not achieve statistical significance, or a sufficiently high level of confidence. Before we conclude that there was no relative benefit to drug B, we need to examine the result and the confidence interval. The trial randomised 60 patients equally to the two drugs. The mortality after 5 years was 40% with drug A and 20% with drug B, giving a 20% absolute difference in mortality after 5 years with drug B relative to drug A (–20%). We calculate a number needed to treat of 5 patients, meaning that based on this result we would need to treat only 5 patients with drug B in order to prevent one death relative to treatment with drug A. The 95% confidence interval, however, ranges from –41% to +3% and the *P*-value is 0.09. Based on the *P*-value, we might mistakenly conclude that there is no benefit to drug B. The 95% confidence interval from this sample suggests that, if the true size of the effect is –20%, 95% of random samples would have a difference in mortality ranging from a 41% reduction in mortality with drug B compared to drug A through to a 3% increased mortality with drug B compared to drug A. We are 95% confident that the truth lies somewhere between these two points, and since the interval includes the value 0%, we cannot confidently conclude that there is a difference between the two drugs. We also cannot confidently conclude that there was not an important difference between the two drugs, including a benefit as great as a 44% absolute reduction in mortality with drug B. It then becomes difficult to know what to conclude from this study. This situation most commonly arises when we have an insufficient number of study subjects or observations. We can calculate the power of this study, which is the probability of concluding that there was benefit with drug B when in truth there really was a difference. Based on the observed findings and the number of subjects studied, the power would be 0.29, meaning that if we conclude that there was a benefit of a 20% absolute reduction in mortality with drug B over drug A, we would have only a 29% chance of being correct. We might suppose that a 4% difference in mortality would be the smallest effect that we would consider to be clinically relevant and would prompt us to prefer drug B over drug A, with a number needed to treat of 25. With our observed difference of 20% and our sample size, we would have a power of 0.89 to detect this effect of 4%, meaning that we could conclude that the benefit of drug B is at least a 4% absolute reduction in mortality relative to drug A with an 89% chance of being correct.

Type I and Type II Error and Power

A study can have one of four possible conclusions. Two are desirable. We might truthfully conclude from our results that a difference or association exists or does not exist, with confidence. Alternatively, we can incorrectly conclude that a difference or association exists or does not exist, when in truth the opposite is true. Although the *P*-value is a highly useful statistical indicator, it is an imperfect one and we cannot rely on it as the sole piece of information on which to base a conclusion. Results drawn from samples and inferred to a target population are susceptible to two types of error: type I error and type II error. A type I error is one in which we conclude that a difference or association of a certain magnitude exists, when in truth it either does not or is less. From probability distributions, we can estimate the probability of making this type of error, which is referred to as alpha. We also know this entity as the *P*-value, or the probability that we have made a type I error. Such errors are evident when a *P*-value is statistically significant, but there is no true difference or association. With a *P*-value of 0.05, we are taking a 5% likelihood that our conclusion is incorrect, and the results are due to chance or random error. In a given study, we may conduct many tests of comparison and association, and each time we are willing to accept a 5% chance of a type I error. The more tests that we do, the more likely we are to make a type I error, since by definition, 5% of our tests may reach the threshold of a *P*-value less than 0.05 by chance or random error alone. This is the challenge of doing multiple tests or comparisons. In order to avoid making this error, we can lower our threshold for defining statistical significance, or we can perform adjustments that take into account the number of tests or comparisons being made. Alternatively, we can report only those comparisons or associations that are significant in multi-variable analyses.

The second error which is of concern is the so-called type II error. In this situation, we might conclude from the results in our sample that there is no difference or association, when in truth one exists. We can determine the probability of making this type of error, called beta, from the probability distribution. Beta is most strongly influenced by the number of subjects or observations in the study, with greater number of subjects giving a lower beta. We can use beta to calculate power, which is 1-beta. Power is the probability of concluding from the results in our sample that a difference or association exists when in truth it does. It is a useful calculation to make when the *P*-value of a result is non-significant, and we are not confident that the observed result is due to chance or random error. Before we conclude that there is no difference or association, we need to be sure that there was sufficient power in order to detect reliably an important difference or association. If we can be fairly certain that we can exclude the fact that we might be missing a clinically important difference or association, we can be confident in our conclusion. We calculate the power in order to determine what might be the likelihood that a difference or association truly exists based on our observed results and the number of subjects we studied. As a general rule, a study reporting a negative result needs to have a power of at least 80%. This means that we are 80% sure that the negative results from this study are not due to a failure to reject a difference, when there is actually one. We are taking a 20% chance of making a type II error.

Applying Statistical Testing

Techniques for analysis of data are used to describe characteristics and to determine associations. Statistical analysis is then used to determine the likelihood that the observed differences or associations are due to chance or random error, and gives us confidence in inferring the results from our study sample to the target population. The selection of statistical test depends on the level of measurement of the dependent and independent variables. It must be remembered that statistical analysis is strictly a mathematical operation based on both facts and assumptions, and that meaning comes from our interpretation of the variables and the results. As such, we must ensure that we are first specifying a hypothesis, performing the appropriate statistical tool, and then interpreting the result. We must avoid the situation where we have a certain result in mind, and then apply different manipulations of the variables and statistical testing to achieve an analysis that supports that result.

Comparing Two or More Groups or Categories

The most common type of plan for analysis involves the comparison of two or more groups defined by a particular characteristic or treatment. The group assignment represents the independent variable, and we seek to determine differences in characteristics and outcomes which are the dependent variables. The simplest form of comparison between two groups is the comparison of two dichotomous or binomial variables from a two-by-two cross-tabulation table using a chi-square test, which compares the variables based on the probability of obtaining a given distribution of dichotomous outcomes. The chi-square test becomes inaccurate when any cell in the cross-tabulation table has less than 5 subjects or observations, and a Fisher exact test is then used. The chi-square test can be applied if there are more than two categories for either the dependent or independent variable or both. Again, if any cell in the cross-tabulation table has less than 5 subjects or observations, the chi-square test cannot be reliably applied. Categories should then be combined in a logical manner until all cells in the table have 5 or more subjects or observations, then the chi-square test can be applied. If the categories of the dependent variable are ordinal in nature, then a Mantel Haentszel chi-square test can be an indicator of trend. Chi-square testing contrasts the difference between a distribution of values in the cells of a cross-tabulation table that would be expected if they were distributed at random, versus the observed distribution. The difference between the observed and expected result is then related to the chi-square probability distribution to determine whether the difference is sufficiently unlikely.

When the dependent variable is continuous, and the independent categorical variable has only two categories or groups, then the Student *t* test is applied. The probability of the observed difference relative to an hypothesis that there is no difference is derived from the *t* probability distribution. When there are more than two groups or levels, then an analysis of variance is applied, with use of the F distribution. If the dependent variable is a highly skewed continuous variable or an ordinal variable with many levels, then a nonparametric analysis of variance may be needed that utilises ranks rather than the actual values.

Correlations and Associations

In specific circumstances a statistical test is aimed not at comparing two groups, but at characterizing the extent to which two variables are associated with each other. Correlations estimate the extent to which change in one variable is associated with change in a second variable. Correlations are unable to assess any cause-and-effect relationship, only associations. The strength in the association is represented by the correlation coefficient r, which can range from −1 to 1. An r value of −1 represents a perfect inverse correlation, where an increase of 1 unit in a variable is exactly associated with a decrease of 1 unit in the other. Conversely, an r value of 1 is a perfect correlation, where an increase of 1 unit in a variable is exactly associated with an increase of 1 unit in the other. An r value of zero indicates that a change in one variable is not associated with a change in the other, meaning that both variables are independent of each other. Correlation coefficients are directly proportional to the strength of the association between the variables. *P*-values for correlation coefficients represent the probability that there is no association between the variables, or an r value of zero. There are many types of measures of association for assessing the relationship between two categorical variables. For two ordinal variables, Spearman rank correlation is used. For two continuous variables, Pearson correlation is used. Underlying the analysis of association between two continuous variables is a regression line, with the correlation coefficient representing the amount of variation around that line.

Matched Pairs and Measures of Agreement

Usually measurements for a study are independent of one another. For example, we may wish to compare measurements made in two groups of subjects where we know that the groups are composed of separate individuals that bear no relationship to one another. In order to reduce variation or to control for a given factor, we may create pairs of individuals matched for a common characteristic. Alternatively, the two groups may not be independent but have an individual level relationship, such as a group of subjects and a group of their siblings. The subjects and their sibling represent matched pairs. When this is the case, we must use statistical testing that takes into account the fact that the two groups are not independent. If the independent variable is categorical, we would use a McNemar chi-square test. If the independent variable is ordinal, we would use an appropriate nonparametric type of test, such as Wilcoxon signed rank test. If the independent variable is continuous, we would use a paired *t* test. Each of these tests would relate to a different and specific type of probability distribution.

Sometimes, we will make repeat measurements in the same subject but using different methodology. By their nature, it is not surprising that the measurements will correlate, since they are measuring the same thing. What we are actually interested in is the degree to which the measurements agree, or agree with a criterion standard. Agreement between two binary variables can be expressed in one of two ways, either through the raw agreement or through the chance corrected agreement. The raw agreement is merely the number of times two measures agree divided by the total number of measures. By chance, two binary variables will agree approximately half of the time. Based on this, raw agreement is of limited interest. Cohen's kappa or chance-corrected agreement is the degree of agreement between variables beyond that expected by chance alone. When continuous variables are of interest, agreement is assessed and depicted using Bland-Altman plots. A Bland-Altman plot plots the difference between two measurements in a pair on the y-axis versus the mean of those two measurements on the x-axis. If the agreement were perfect, all of the points would be at a difference of zero regardless of the value of the measurement. The plot can show the degree and limits of agreement, but also any patterns. Systematic bias can be noted, as well as changes in the magnitude of agreement as the average values get larger or smaller. A paired *t* test can be used to determine if any systematic differences exist between pairs of measures.

Linear and Logistic Regression Models

Often the relationship between two variables can be represented by a line. For continuous dependent variables, that line can be straight, in which case the analysis would be a simple linear regression. Sometimes the relationship is more complex over the range of values of the dependent variable, and may not be linear. In this case, transformations of dependent and independent variables may be used, or non-linear regression techniques can be applied. If the dependent variable is dichotomous, then the relationship is between the probability of a value of the dependent variable as a function of the independent variable. In this case, a logistic regression or log-linear technique would be used. These different regression techniques can be applied to incorporate the relationship between the dependent variable and multiple independent variables. The relationship between the dependent variable and each independent variable would then be independent of the effect of the other independent variables included in the analysis. The output is in the form of an additive mathematical equation, called a regression equation, whereby the value of each independent variable is weighted in its effect on a baseline value called the intercept. The weighting factors are called regression coefficients or parameter estimates, and take into account the level of measurement of the variable and its units of measurement. Regression equations are useful in determining the independent effect of specific variables of interest on a given dependent variable, by allowing the investigator to account for bias resulting from potential confounding factors. Statistical testing can be applied to the whole regression equation, and to the individual variables that were included. Interaction can also be explored within regression modeling by incorporating interaction terms as additional independent variables in the equation.

Survival or Timed-event Analysis

Since death is a certain event for all of us, if you follow every subject in a cohort for an infinite amount of time, your cumulative survival will eventually reach 0%. If a study reports that the survival of a cohort of subjects is 50%, the number is meaningless unless the time interval over which that survival was accrued is also reported. Additionally, we would need to be assured that all of the surviving subjects at risk are accounted for. One of the challenges of following cohorts is that subjects may be lost to follow-up or be lost to further observation before they achieve the event of interest, which is known as censoring. For estimates of survival, subjects may be dropping out of the numerator as they achieve the event of interest, but also out of the denominator as they terminate their contribution to the cohort. In order to accurately depict this phenomenon over time, we need to continuously account for these changes to the cohort. We also need to line up the subjects at a common starting point. In order to correctly assess time-related events, a time-related analysis should be used. Common events that are studied include death, intervention and repeat intervention. The events must occur at a discrete time point. Common starting points that are studied include birth, presentation, diagnosis and intervention. They must also be at a defined discrete time point. For an analysis of survival from birth, every subject is assigned an interval to either death, or to the end of the observation period at which they were last known to be alive. The proportion of subjects surviving to a given time point is continuously calculated, with subjects who die dropping out of the numerator and denominator, and subjects ending their period of observation but still alive dropping out of the denominator, representing the remaining patients alive and at risk of death at a given time point.

The most common form of survival analysis is to calculate and plot non-parametric Kaplan-Meier estimates. We can use statistical tests to determine whether independent variables have an association with time-related survival using Wilcoxon and log rank tests. We can use a particular type of regression analysis which handles time-related events as the dependent variable by using Cox's proportional hazard regression modeling. This allows us to explore the independent relationship with multiple independent variables, with the parameter estimates representing risk ratios.

If we wish to use independent variables to predict time-related survival, we can use mathematical modeling of the underlying rate or hazard at which events occur. Parametric analysis techniques are increasingly being used, and survival models can be derived which encompass three phases of time-related risk: early, constant, and late. Independent variables associated with each phase can be modeled separately. From this type of analysis, we might discover that the factors associated with early mortality are not the same as those associated with late mortality. One of the most interesting applications of parametric survival models is the creation of competing risk models. Competing risk analysis establishes the likelihood of subjects to have achieved one of two or more mutually exclusive events over time for which they are simultaneously at risk. The competing risk analysis estimates, at each time point, the likelihood of each competing event occurring against all others, based on a parametric survival model for each event. An excellent example of how this might be applied was a study of outcomes after listing for heart transplantation.[1] After listing, a patient may die without getting a transplantation, may have a transplantation, may be taken off the list if they no longer require a transplantation because they improve or because they develop complications that preclude transplantation, may have an alternative procedure, or may remain on the list surviving without having any of the previously mentioned events. A given patient is simultaneously at risk for all of these mutually exclusive events or end-states. The rate at which patients are achieving these events over time can be modeled mathematically and associated factors determined. These rates and their associated factors can then be used for prediction. We can determine the likelihood of a patient with a given set of characteristics receiving a transplantation at a given point in time, remaining on the list, being removed from the list, or dying. The advantage of competing risk analysis over multiple survival curves is that every subject is calculated once and not censored in multiple different curves.

Longitudinal or Serial Measures Analysis

The value of some variables can change over time if we measure them repeatedly, and trends can be noted. Examples might be changes in left ventricular ejection fraction or subjective grade of mitral valve regurgitation. If we measure something repeatedly in a subject, then the measures are not independent, and we need to account for this in the analysis. If the measurements occur at discrete and common time points across subjects and there is little missing data, then a repeated measures analysis of variance can be used. This is rarely the case using clinical data, since patients rarely all have measurements at the same time, some patients may have more measurements than others and may have been followed longer, and there may be variable amounts of missing data. We may also wish to determine if independent variables are associated with the measurements and with changes over time. Specific types of regression analyses have been developed and applied to handle this type of complex data. If the serial measurements are of a continuous variable, then mixed linear or non-linear regression analysis can be used. The effect of time course can be included as an independent variable, and interactions with time and other independent variables can be explored to determine associations with trends. If the variable is categorical or ordinal, then a general estimating equation type of regression analysis can be used.

Accounting for Non-random Allocation in Comparison of Therapies

Non-random allocation of patients to therapies is one of the limitations of using observational clinical data to compare therapies. Patient characteristics that influence the selection of particular therapies may also influence the outcomes of those therapies, and hence bias any comparison. This is especially true for patients receiving new and higher risk therapies, since they are often the patients with the most severe/active disease and are the ones expected to have the worst clinical outcomes. The statistical analysis should include the methodology to adjust for non-random assignment to therapy, and to equalise comparisons. One method often used is the creation of a propensity score.[3] A propensity score is the probability, based on a subject's characteristics, that the subject would have been selected for a specific therapy versus the alternative. The propensity score is derived from a logistic regression model with the treatment assignment as the dependent variable, and all known subject characteristics as independent variables. The logistic regression equation is then solved for each subject and converted to a probability, which is the propensity of that subject to have been selected to the specific therapy. The propensity score can be used in three different ways. The first method uses the propensity score to select and create pairs of subjects, one from each treatment group, that are matched according to the score. The second method recreates a blocked randomised controlled trial by dividing subjects within treatment groups into tiers, quartiles or quintiles based on their propensity score. Outcomes for each block in the treatment group are then compared against those for the corresponding block in the alternative group. These two uses of the propensity score often require a large number of patients and imply that the propensity score will be balanced and sufficiently overlapping between treatment groups, which is not always the case. When propensity scores are highly unbalanced between groups and little or no overlap exists, the score can be used as an adjustment factor or an additional independent variable in regression analysis. Using the propensity score as an independent variable in regression equations is how it is most commonly used. The use of propensity scores, and other forms of statistical adjustment for potential confounding, only adjusts for those variables that are measured. It does not replace randomisation, which randomly distributes not only measured but unmeasured factors as well, and gives the greatest likelihood of an unbiased comparison.

Seeking Statistical Expertise

One of the key elements of data and statistical analysis is to know when to seek the assistance of a statistician. There are several statistical software programmes available for performing analysis, and some are more user friendly than others. Nearly all will allow you to perform statistical analysis without knowledge of the underlying mathematics and assumptions on which the tests are based, which increases the chances for a novice to make important errors regarding inappropriate application. In general, most individuals can handle the description of data, and do some simple testing where two variables are involved. Analysis which incorporates multiple independent or dependent variables, such as most forms of regression analysis, in contrast, should be performed with the guidance of or by a statistician. Additionally, consultation should also be obtained for instances where types of nonparametric tests are needed. We might sometimes think that statisticians speak a different language, but it is important to remember that for the majority of statisticians your data is but numbers, without meaning. It is essential, therefore, when enlisting a statistician, that your data be clearly organised and defined and that you have a detailed plan of how the analysis should proceed. This should be discussed with the statistician, and any questions answered and misinterpretations clarified. The role of the statistician is to apply the most appropriate technique given the level of measurement and assumptions about the data, to report the results, and to assist in the interpretation.

CRITICAL APPRAISAL OF THE LITERATURE

It is increasingly important for clinicians to have sufficient skills in order critically to appraise the quality and relevance of studies being published, especially in an era which has seen an exponential growth in the number of scholarly journals and reports. These reports, whether they are guidelines or clinical trials, constitute the evidence that is incorporated into the practice of evidence-based clinical decision-making. The reports vary widely in their quality, which reflects the design of the study, the degree of rigour with which the research was performed, the ability of the authors to present the work in a format that enables accurate and complete appraisal, and the skills of peer reviewers and editors in appraising the submission. Readers must, therefore, develop their own skills when searching the medical literature, selecting and appraising the most appropriate reports, and incorporating the best evidence into their clinical decisions and continuing education.

Levels of Evidence

The design of the study is the primary attribute of a report that influences the quality and level of evidence provided by that report. The design is important because it has the greatest influence on reducing bias and error in the findings noted. When producing a recommendation for clinical practice, whether it is for broader dissemination or for personal practice, the appraisal and incorporation of multiple reports has an important impact on the level of evidence that is assigned to that recommendation. Several schemes have been devised with the purpose of grading the evidence (Table 21-1). A grade should be assigned to any recommendation, and should influence the strength of that recommendation.[4] Recommendations supported by high levels of evidence should carry the greatest weight in influencing clinical practice. The overall quality of evidence currently available regarding paediatric and congenital cardiac disease is somewhat low, given the paucity of randomised clinical trials, with the majority of recommendations being

TABLE 21-1

SYSTEM FOR GRADING THE QUALITY OF EVIDENCE AND STRENGTH OF RECOMMENDATIONS

EVIDENCE QUALITY FOR GRADES OF EVIDENCE	
Grade	**Evidence**
A	Well-designed randomised, controlled trials or diagnostic studies performed on a population similar to the guideline's target population
B	Randomised, controlled trials or diagnostic studies with minor limitations; genetic natural history studies; overwhelmingly consistent evidence from observational studies
C	Observational studies (case-control and cohort design)
D	Expert opinion, case reports, or reasoning from first principles (bench research or animal studies)

DEFINITIONS FOR EVIDENCE-BASED STATEMENTS		
Statement Type	**Definition**	**Implication**
Strong recommendation	The reporter(s) believe that the benefits of the recommended approach clearly exceed the harms and that the quality of the supporting evidence is excellent (grade A or B). In some clearly defined circumstances, strong recommendations may be made on the basis of lesser evidence when high-quality evidence is impossible to obtain and the anticipated benefits clearly outweigh the harms.	Clinicians should follow a strong recommendation unless a clear and compelling rationale for an alternative approach is present.
Recommendation	The reporter(s) feel that the benefits exceed the harms but the quality of the evidence is not as strong (grade B or C). In some clearly defined circumstances, strong recommendations may be made on the basis of lesser evidence when high-quality evidence is impossible to obtain and the anticipated benefits clearly outweigh the harms.	Clinicians should generally follow a recommendation but remain alert to new information and sensitive to patient preferences.
Option	Either the quality of the evidence that exists is suspect (grade D) or well-performed studies (grade A, B or C) show little clear advantage to one approach versus another.	Clinicians should be flexible in their decision-making regarding appropriate practise, although they may set boundaries on alternatives; patient preference should have a substantial influencing role.
No recommendation	There is both a lack of pertinent evidence (grade D) and an unclear balance between benefits and harms.	Clinicians should feel little constraint in their decision-making and be alert to new published evidence that clarifies the balance of benefit versus harm; patient preference should have a substantial influencing role.

Adapted from American Academy of Pediatrics, Steering Committee on Quality Improvement and Management: Classifying recommendations for clinical practice guidelines. Pediatrics 2004;114:874–877.

supported by expert or consensus opinion, themselves fraught with bias, or weak observational studies. Assigning grades to the evidence used when making recommendations, nonetheless, remains important, as it tempers their adoption, and highlights areas for further and more rigourous study.

Design of the Study

Not all types of study provide the same level of evidence, and not all studies should be evaluated in the same way.

Case Reports and Commentaries

These submissions provide the lowest level of evidence in the literature. They may be useful in identifying unique clinical observations. Case reports are often short communications, detailing either a single patient or a limited group of patients. While the literature was composed mostly of case reports in the first half of the previous century, today they account for only a small portion of all published studies. Their primary utility is potentially to highlight areas for further investigation, and increase awareness of possible rare variations and complications. They can also point to effective therapies, particularly if the patient described underwent multiple trials of a particular therapy, showing improvements when receiving the treatment, but suffering exacerbations when off the therapy.

Observational Studies

Observational studies are non-experimental in nature, whereby the phenomenon of interest is observed without imposing experimental or controlled conditions. They are highly variable regarding the quality and quantity of evidence they provide, and are fraught with potential bias and error. Carefully performed observational studies may be valuable in determining long-term outcomes and associated factors, in describing rare adverse events or rare disorders, and in determining the characteristics of diagnostic tests. Alternatively, hard-line proponents of evidence-based medicine will often reject offhand any type of observational study as inherently biased and of low validity. Previous studies have found that observational studies and randomised control trials often arrive at conflicting results about similar treatments.[5]

The designs of observational studies can be classified along several axes. First, they can be classified according to how they relate to a population. Studies using cohorts assemble a population either at risk for a given condition, or one that uniformly has a risk factor or condition. They may employ various strategies of sampling to reduce the number of subjects being studied, which ideally should be random. Case-control studies assemble a group of subjects with a given risk factor or condition, and a separate group of subjects without the risk factor or condition for the purposes of comparison. The validity of these studies rests largely on the representativeness of the chosen respective target populations. Ideally, the controls should be derived from the same general population as the cases. Second, observational studies can be classified as to the period of observation. Cross sectional studies examine subjects at a single point in time. Longitudinal studies follow subjects through time, tracking risk factors and outcomes. Third, observational studies can be classified as to the time when the measurements were made. Measurements can be made concurrently, meaning that they are made as the investigation proceeds forward in time. This provides much better data, as it gives the investigator the opportunity to standardise definitions and methodology, and to apply measures for the control of quality. Measurements can be made non-concurrently, meaning that they were made in the past, and that the investigator is relying on recorded information. Abstractions from the medical records, and other uses of secondary data, constitute non-concurrent collection of data. This data may be of poor quality, since it would have been recorded by multiple individuals in a non-standardised manner, and collected for purposes other than addressing the research question at hand. The terms are also not mutually exclusive, in that collection of data for a given study may include both concurrent and non-concurrent elements. Fourth, observational studies can be classified according to their perspective regarding risk factors and outcomes. Studies that determine the state of a population in terms of risk factors, and then follow these factors forward in time to determine the development of outcomes, are referred to as being prospective in nature. Studies that determine the outcome for a population, and then trace it back to determine risk factors, are referred to as being retrospective in nature. These terms are almost exclusively used to describe studies of cohorts. The terms do not imply whether or not the collection of the data was concurrent or non-concurrent, and may not be mutually exclusive, since some observational studies identify a cohort of patients with a given condition, and then simultaneously collect data relating to risk factors and outcomes from the medical records. Many investigators erroneously describe non-concurrent collection of data as being retrospective in nature, when this may not be the case. When appraising a given report, it is important for the reader to be able to differentiate these various aspects of design, as they have important impacts on the validity and quality of the findings.

Cohort Studies

These studies are often employed to describe characteristics, management, and outcomes for a defined population. They can be solely descriptive in nature, or they can look for associations between characteristics and outcomes. Some of the characteristics may be factors in management. Since these factors are not randomly assigned, important bias is often introduced into any comparison of strategies for treatment, since the patients themselves, and other characteristics, often influence decisions regarding the selection of the treatment, which may also influence outcomes. These studies define the prognosis after different strategies for management have been applied to different cohorts of subjects. Several types of statistical adjustments are available to help minimise bias in these comparisons, but they are not uniformly applied, provide incomplete adjustment, and only adjust for characteristics known and measured by the investigators.

The first step in designing a cohort study is to define and assemble the cohort. The cohort must be relevant to the question at hand, and representative of the target population for which the investigator wishes to be able to extrapolate the results. Baseline demographic data are required. The study may be prospective in nature. The investigator would then measure predictive and potential confounding variables, and then follow the cohort forward in time, with tracking and assessments made to identify those subjects who develop outcomes. This design has advantages in that multiple potential factors can be assessed at baseline with standardised measures, ensuring some control of quality. Risk factors can also be assessed dynamically, identifying those that are acquired over time, particularly those relating to management. In addition, multiple types of outcomes can be assessed dynamically. This type of design is useful for determining the incidence of outcomes, and for determining potential causal associations between risk factors and outcomes, albeit subject to the effects of potential confounding. The design is efficient if the prevalence of risk factors and outcomes is relatively common, and the time over which outcomes may occur is short. The design also allows the investigator to examine multiple outcomes. A prospective cohort may arise from a randomised clinical trial. After the analysis of primary and secondary outcomes related to the intervention being randomised, an analysis of the cohort may take place whereby factors associated with outcomes, other than the studied intervention, are sought. The quality of the data is usually excellent, although the problem of potential confounding still exists.

Studies of cohorts can also be retrospective in nature, in that a cohort is assembled, the outcome is determined, and then an assessment of risk factors is pursued, either in a cross sectional manner or through non-concurrent assessment of available sources of data, including recall of the subjects. These studies are useful in giving an estimate of the prevalence of outcomes and conditions. They are often more efficient than prospective studies, in that the cohort usually has been assembled and characterised in the past and the follow-up has occurred. The potential biases, however, are much greater, and the quality of the available data is suboptimal.

Cross Sectional Studies

Cross sectional studies are a type of study in which a cohort is assembled, and then all of the measurements are made at a single time in the present. They are useful for determining the prevalence of risk factors at a chosen point, and the outcomes in a population. Associations between risk factors and outcomes are sought, albeit that it is difficult to establish any causal relationships. Surveys are the most common methodology used for cross sectional studies.

Case-control Studies

Case-control studies are efficient designs for studying rare risk factors, or rare outcomes, for which study of a cohort would require an excessively large number of subjects, or an excessively long duration of follow-up. They are useful for generating hypotheses. They are most commonly retrospective in nature. A population of subjects with a given condition or outcome is assembled, and a comparison group is assembled from a much larger population known to be free of the given condition or outcomes. The two groups are then assessed for baseline characteristics and risk factors, usually from non-concurrent sources of data, sometimes including recall of the subjects. The relative frequency of risk factors is then determined in the cases compared to the controls. Since they are not population-based, these studies do not give estimates of prevalence or incidence, or relative risk.

The studies can be very efficient and cost-effective, but have many threats to their validity that are both difficult to control and detect. First, since the groups are differentiated on the basis of a single condition or outcome, this is the only outcome that can be assessed. Second, the selection of both cases and controls can be challenging, and sampling bias and non-representativeness are important threats. It is often only prevalent cases that are represented, excluding subjects who died, or those whose condition resolved without detection, or those lost, and cases usually derive from a setting of medical care, this time excluding subjects with missed or incorrect diagnoses, or those who do not present for medical care, or present elsewhere. They may over-represent subjects with more symptomatic, severe, complex, or prolonged disease. The presence of a risk factor may influence the detection and inclusion of a case, which would cause the risk factor to be over-represented. Likewise, the selection of controls can be challenging. The goal ideally is randomly to select the controls from the larger population at risk from which the cases were derived. For convenience, controls can be recruited from the same setting in medical care. The controls would then be representative of the cases derived from the same catchment area. This might work if the setting is an outpatient clinic, and the controls are selected from those presenting for routine care. Controls derived from hospital-based populations are often presenting for care of their illness, which may falsely elevate the level of risk factors or confounding conditions. Controls can be derived from population-based samples from the same general population from which the cases were derived. This has the advantage in that a large number of potential controls are available. The population is defined either by geography or the medical catchment area, and controls are selected randomly. Additionally, they can be matched regarding important confounding characteristics, commonly age and sex, with the individual cases. This is a useful strategy when a known or highly suspect confounder has the potential for being differentially represented in the cases as opposed to the controls. A final strategy would be to have two or more control groups derived using different strategies or settings. Third, the nature of the assessment of risk factors is fraught with biases, particularly with regard to the potential for differential measurement in the cases versus the controls. This becomes increasingly important with greater subjectivity of the risk factors being assessed. Cases may be more likely to have certain measurements, the measurements may be made and recorded by more qualified observers, or the cases may be more motivated to recall certain factors. The investigators may be more aggressive in the pursuit of risk factors if they know that the subject is a case. Blinding of assessments wherever possible becomes important, wherein the assessment is occurring without the knowledge of whether the subject is a case or a control.

Nested Case-control Studies

A case-controlled study can be effectively nested within a cohort study. This increases efficiency and cost-effectiveness when assessment of a risk factor might be expensive or undesirable. When sufficient subjects have developed an outcome, which is usually rare, a sample of controls is selected from the subjects free of the given outcome within the cohort. The subjects chosen as controls may be matched to those representing cases according to key potential confounding characteristics, particularly time or period of observation. This allows the risk factor to be assessed in a smaller proportion of the cohort, usually from biological samples collected at a common baseline, or from a more intensive review of records.

TABLE 21-2

CRITERIONS FOR DEFINING CAUSALITY IN RELATIONSHIPS BETWEEN INDEPENDENT VARIABLES, INCLUDING MANAGEMENT, AND DEPENDENT VARIABLES, INCLUDING OUTCOMES OR CONDITIONS

- Is the relationship biologically plausible in terms of the current state of knowledge regarding pathophysiology?
- Is the relationship strong?
- Is the temporal relationship correct, in that the risk factor precedes the development of the outcome or condition?
- Is there evidence for a dose-response relationship?
- Is the relationship specific for the risk factor and outcome of interest?
- Is the relationship consistent across variations in study populations, settings and investigators, and design?
- Is the relationship free of known and potential confounding?
- Is the relationship free of systematic and random measurement error?
- If an intervention is successful in reducing or eliminating the risk factor, does this alter the outcome in a consistent and predicted manner?

Causality from Observational Studies

While associations between risk factors and outcomes can readily be determined from observational studies, the ideal is to identify those associations that are causal in nature, and free from bias, error, and confounding. There are several criterions that must be satisfied before concluding that a relationship is causal in nature, as outlined in Table 21-2. This becomes particularly important if the factor is a form of management.

Randomised Clinical Trials

Randomised control trials remain the gold standard for evaluation of the efficacy and safety of treatments or interventions. The principle of a randomised control trial is simple. A homogenous group of subjects is randomly assigned to an experimental arm or arms, or to a comparison arm or arms. Randomisation eliminates systematic differences at baseline between the groups. Any outcomes observed during the period of follow-up, therefore, should be attributable to the treatment alone, and not to underlying differences in subjects.

Randomised clinical trials provide the highest grade of evidence, particularly regarding establishing a causal relationship between an intervention and an outcome. This is for two primary reasons. First, randomisation provides the best chance that the groups chosen for study will be equivalent at baseline regarding both measured and unmeasured characteristics. Any differences would be attributed to chance or random error. The larger the population studied, the less likely random maldistributions are to occur. Random assignment must be truly random and tamperproof. Strategies can be used to ensure equal numbers of subjects in groups, so-called block randomisation, and to ensure key characteristics are equivalent in groups, this being stratified randomisation. When assessing the success of randomisation at the end of a trial by comparing measured characteristics at baseline, it is important to note clinically meaningful differences between groups, rather than statistically significant differences, the latter being dependent on the numbers of subjects. If the sample is large, small and unimportant differences may be statistically significant. If the sample is small, large and important differences may not be statistically significant.

The second feature of randomised clinical trials that contributes to providing evidence of high quality is the fact that all clinical trials rely on concurrently collected data. Thus, there is opportunity for standardisation of definitions, methodology, measurements and reporting, and implementation of measures for control of quality, such as adjudication. An important aspect of assessment is the concept of blinding, whereby the subjects, the investigators, and study personnel, and those analyzing the data, have no knowledge of the randomised assignment of the subjects. This ensures that the protocol is implemented identically in all groups, and is particularly important for assessments or outcomes that are more subjective in nature. For example, it is often surprising the number of subjects that will report hallucinations while taking an inert placebo. Additionally, even the most well-meaning assessors may interpret subjective tests differently if they think that they know the assignment of the subject. The blinding must be tamperproof. It may not be feasible for some interventions to be blinded completely, such as a trial of surgical compared to transcatheter closure of septal defects, but as a minimum, measurements, assessments and analysis of the data can almost always remain blinded.

There are multiple phases in clinical trials depending on the amount of previous knowledge available on a specific intervention. Also, there are different types of clinical trials depending on the aim to be achieved. Clinical trials can be divided into four phases. Phase 1 trials establish the safety of the intervention, phase 2 trials establish a therapeutic effect, phase 3 trials compare the intervention to either a placebo or standard practice and establish relative benefit and risks, and phase 4 trials evaluate the long-term effects of an intervention.[6,7] Prior to performing a clinical trial, it is important to determine which phase of the intervention the trial will represent, and what evidence is needed. The first and second phases are often small trials, using under 50 patients, and aimed at establishing safety and therapeutic effect. They are rarely reported in the literature, and rarely contribute to major changes in clinical practice. The third and fourth phases strive to compare the intervention with either the standard of care or a placebo, or non-intervention. These trials are most often reported in the literature, and are the driving force behind changes in clinical practice and development of guidelines. Investigators performing clinical trials have to respect the concept of equipoise, which states that patients cannot be deprived of care by receiving a placebo when a suitable alternative exists. Most randomised control trials aim to demonstrate that the new alternative is better than current standard of care. Some clinical trials, nonetheless, are aimed at establishing equivalence between the new intervention and the previous alternative. This type of trial is often conducted for the approval of generic drugs, and is called a non-inferiority trial.

Since the methodology for designing, performing, analyzing, and reporting of clinical trials is fairly standardised, this makes them easier to appraise. In the past 10 years, many biomedical journals have adopted the CONSORT guidelines for the report of clinical trials in the scientific literature.[8]

Meta-analyses

One criterion establishing causality is consistency of results from study to study. Before large-scale changes are made in clinical practice, a high level of certainty needs to be achieved. In recent years, meta-analyses and systematic reviews have been conducted in order to pool data from multiple clinical studies. Meta-analyses identify a problem of interest and compile all studies, whether observational or randomised clinical trial, whether producing positive or negative results, and whether published or not, which have previously studied the issue at hand. Results from each study are then compiled, and a summary conclusion is achieved.[9,10] Meta-analyses have many advantages, mainly to dilute the effect of studies with limited validities which might have inconsistent results. Statistical analysis of meta-analyses is highly complex and beyond the scope of this chapter. Peer-reviewed meta-analysis is published in the Cochrane Review, a repository of meta-analyses and systematic reviews, which is a high-quality reference on which to base changes in clinical practices. Unfortunately, few such meta-analyses are possible relevant to paediatric and congenital cardiac disease, given the paucity of clinical trials that are performed.

Critical Appraisal

Critical appraisal of published reports is an important activity, whether being pursued for the purpose of continuing education, or for the practice of an evidence-based approach to a clinical dilemma. Several guides are available for assisting with critical appraisal, with specifics depending on the perspective of the report being appraised. The *British Medical Journal* published a series of articles regarding specific methodology critically to assess the quality of different types of publications.[11–18] Additionally, the *Journal of the American Medical Association* has published a series relevant to critical appraisal of the literature.[19–25]

Critical appraisal begins by identification of the underlying question being addressed and the appropriateness of the design of the study. The quality of the design and its conduct is then assessed, in order to determine if the investigation has succeeded in achieving valid findings. The next step is to examine the findings to determine if they are both clinically important and relevant, and statistically significant. Finally, the report is appraised as to its relevance to personal practice or a specific clinical situation relevant to the reader. Critical appraisal can sometimes be challenging when the investigators do not provide sufficient information regarding various aspects of their study in their report.

Therapy

The reports of greatest interest to the clinician are those that report results of specific therapies. Those therapies may be aimed at producing a beneficial effect or at preventing an adverse outcome from occurring. Some reports are observational, and include only patients who receive a specific therapy. These studies are largely descriptive in nature, and may include an analysis for factors associated with observed outcomes. As such, these reports are about prognosis after a specific therapy. Some such observational studies may include a comparison group of an alternative therapy. These studies are weakest if the comparison group is largely historical, with the subjects accrued in a previous time period. If subjects are accrued similarly into the intervention groups throughout the period of study, but were not randomly assigned, then the report is a comparison of prognosis of two or more observational cohorts. Appropriate statistical adjustment for measured factors will not completely account for differences related to the non-randomised assignment. The key feature that determines whether a report represents a valid study of therapy is random assignment of the intervention or interventions studied, as previously discussed. Critical appraisal can then proceed according the questions outlined as follows:

Was the study conducted in manner that minimised bias?

Were the subjects randomly assigned to the study interventions?

- Was the randomisation strategy appropriate and tamperproof?
- Was randomisation successful, with measured baseline characteristics being equivalent for the study groups?
- If subjects were not randomly assigned or if randomisation did not succeed in producing equivalent groups, was appropriate statistical adjustment performed for differences in measured baseline characteristics and important potential confounding factors? Critical appraisal of non-randomised comparisons should be based on the guidelines for appraisal of a study dealing with prognosis.

Of those subjects randomised, what proportion in each group completed the study according to the protocol? It is important that all subjects be accounted for and that loss to follow-up be minimised. Studies where loss to follow-up occurs more frequently in one group versus the others may reflect an unanticipated effect of the intervention and bias comparisons regarding outcomes.

- What were the reasons for failure to complete the study, especially those related to study withdrawal and cross-over to an alternative group?
- Was the primary analysis based on the assignment at randomisation of the study subjects (that is, intention to treat analysis)? This type of analysis preserves the equal distribution of both measured and unmeasured characteristics between groups achieved by randomisation, and represents the most unbiased and hence valid comparison.
- What deviations from and violations of the study protocol were apparent, particularly premature, or temporary discontinuations of interventions?
- Was there evidence that the groups were treated differently, other than the randomised interventions, such as co-interventions? Co-interventions are additional interventions that may be necessary to manage effects of the primary intervention, and they have the potential to further influence outcomes and bias comparisons.

Was blinding as to study group feasible, attempted, and achieved for subjects, care providers, personnel, data analysts and investigators?

- If episodes of unblinding occurred, what was the level of unblinding and the reasons?

Were assessments conducted, evaluated, and interpreted in a rigorous and standardised manner?

- Was independent adjudication performed for key factors and outcomes, particularly those of a more subjective nature?

Are the results reported appropriately?

Are both absolute and relative differences in outcomes reported? If the outcome is dichotomous, then the absolute difference is the difference in the proportion of subjects in each group who develop the outcome. The relative difference would be the absolute difference between the groups relative to the proportion in the comparison group.

Are confidence limits provided around differences? Confidence limits are necessary to determine whether no difference has been reliably excluded, or if no difference is noted, whether a clinically important difference has been reliably excluded.

Are benefits interpreted in light of associated risks and adverse outcomes?

Are the results of sufficient magnitude and relevant?

Is the magnitude of the difference reported clinically important?

- Is the absolute benefit sufficiently clinically important to justify a change to the evaluated intervention in terms of relative costs, resources, risk of adverse effects, or outcomes?
- Is the number needed to treat to achieve or prevent an outcome provided, or is sufficient information given that it can be calculated, that is, the number of subjects needed to be treated relative to the alternative in order to achieve relative benefit for one subject? The number needed to be treated to achieve one beneficial outcome is calculated by taking the inverse of the absolute difference between groups in the proportion of subjects developing the outcome.
- Is the number needed to treat to achieve benefit offset by the presence of adverse effects or outcomes, or increased costs or resources, or is sufficient information given that it can be calculated, that is, the number of subjects who would have an adverse effect or outcome per subject with relative benefit?

Is there inordinate emphasis given to results from analyses of subgroups? Sometimes if the primary results of the clinical trial are negative, the investigators will attempt to determine whether there was a significant treatment effect in variously defined subgroup. While this type of analysis is important, it should not be viewed as definitive, and is a means for generating further hypotheses to be tested with additional studies.

Are the findings and implications of the report applicable to my own clinical practise?

Are the characteristics of the subjects studied, that is, inclusion and exclusion criterions and baseline characteristics, similar to those in my practise? For your patients for whom you would like to apply the intervention, you would expect them to meet the criterions for inclusion, and to have no criterions for exclusion, and to have characteristics similar to those reported.

Were all clinically important outcomes, particularly those most relevant to my patients, considered and assessed? If you are interested in using an intervention to have an impact on a particular outcome, you would expect that outcome to have been assessed and a benefit noted in the report. Alternatively, studies that fail to assess all relevant outcomes may note a benefit regarding a particular outcome but fail to note an adverse effect on other relevant outcomes that were not assessed, for which the balance of benefits versus risks would be tipped away from favoring the intervention.

Can the intervention be feasibly and practically applied within my practise?

Prognosis

This is the predominant type of report in the literature relating to paediatric and congenital cardiac disease. This mainly results from the fact that the conditions are rare, and that longer follow-up is required to detect relevant outcomes. Also, innovation in the field is occurring more rapidly than studies can be designed and implemented. The predominant factors being sought for association with outcomes are management factors, although such associations may be fraught with bias given the observational study designs. The predominant design is a cohort study, whereby the subjects have a common anatomical diagnosis or condition, or have undergone a specific type of intervention. The nature of the collection of data is usually non-concurrent, with the primary source being the medical record. The better studies have been prospective in nature with concurrent collection of data, and are often multi-institutional. The critical appraisal of such studies proceeds as follows:

Was the study conducted in manner that minimised bias?

Were the subjects that were studied representative of the larger population to which the investigators wish to extrapolate their results?

Did observation of the subjects start at a uniform point in time? Commonly, this represents the time of diagnosis, or the time that a specific intervention was performed. A common mistake is to start the period of observation at birth, rather than diagnosis. We do not know anything about the subject before they present and are diagnosed, and we cannot assume that we do. We also might erroneously assume that all subjects survive from birth to achieve diagnosis or intervention, which may not be the case. The situation becomes more complex with conditions that may be associated with a long pre-clinical period or with disease progression, such as hypertrophic cardiomyopathy or Marfan syndrome. If time of diagnosis is the starting point of observation, then there may be wide variation in age at diagnosis, which may be an important prognostic factor that needs to be explored. If the starting point is a diagnosis, then careful and objective definitions of that diagnosis need to be reported.

Were the subjects followed sufficiently long for the outcomes of interest to occur with sufficient frequency? If survival after diagnosis or an intervention is achieved, it may take many years before there is recurrence of disease or important complications arise.

Were all of the subjects followed completely? Subjects may become lost to follow-up for reasons that are related to their diagnosis, intervention, or outcomes that develop. Failure to account for these subjects may bias estimates of prognosis and associated factors.

Were outcomes and potential associated factors measured uniformly, objectively, and in an unbiased manner?

In defining the prognosis or comparing the prognosis for different diagnoses or interventions, was adjustment appropriately made for potential important prognostic factors?

Are the results reported and interpreted appropriately?

Was the correct methodology used in presenting the outcomes of interest?

- For time-related outcomes or events, were appropriate methods used to account for the time-relatedness of these data? Likewise, special analytic techniques are required to handle events that may be repeated, or to handle different mutually exclusive events that may compete with one another.
- For outcomes that evolve over time, were appropriate methods used to account for serial measures within individuals and changes in magnitude?

Was the correct methodology used to determine associations between outcomes and potential associated factors? Unless the number of subjects is extraordinarily small or the outcomes are very infrequent, some sort of multi-variable analysis should be performed.

Are the results reported with confidence intervals, or at least measures of variation, particularly when differences relevant to a particular factor are being reported?

Do the associated factors change over time? Does the magnitude of the association with outcome change over time? Do new factors emerge while others become less relevant? Do the factors themselves change over time?

Are the results of sufficient magnitude and relevant?

What is the magnitude and nature of risk of the outcome? Outcomes that are frequent and of greater clinical importance are of more interest. The nature of the risk of an outcome can be particularly of interest. Does the risk of the outcome change over time, indicating high-risk periods? Are there periods of stability followed by rapid progression?

How strong are the factors associated with the outcomes? This is particularly evident if a strong dose-response relationship is noted, whereby a small increment in a factor is associated with a greatly increased likelihood of the outcome. Threshold effects should be sought.

Are the findings and implications of the report applicable to my own clinical practise?

Do my patients meet the entry criterions described in the report, and do they have similar characteristics to the study subjects?

Are the results such that they provide valid and important information regarding counseling about prognosis for my patients?

Are the results such that they would alter patient management in the presence of associated factors reported? This might lead to the pursuit of alternative therapy that might provide a better prognosis or prevent certain outcomes. It might also lead to the monitoring of selected patients more closely who have certain associated factors. Interventions might be directed specifically at treating or preventing certain associated factors if they were shown to have sufficient evidence of a causal association with the outcome.

Harm

Some reports focus on adverse effects or events related to a given exposure or intervention. These types of reports are much less common in the literature pertaining to paediatric and congenital cardiac disease. Nearly all types of study can give evidence regarding the relationship between an adverse outcome and a given factor, and critical appraisal of the report necessarily must take into account aspects of the design in the evaluation. A specific example might be a report addressing the question, 'What is the risk of congenital cardiac disease in offspring of mothers taking blockers of angiotensin receptors during pregnancy?' A randomised clinical trial could be designed to address this question, but would be difficult to perform, given concerns about feasibility and ethical issues. This would, however, give the strongest evidence in support of a causal relationship. Alternatively, a cohort study might be used whereby all pregnant mothers are enrolled shortly after conception, taking note of history of medication, and its use during pregnancy, and screening all fetuses and neonates for congenital cardiac disease. The outcomes of pregnancies of mothers taking blockers would be compared to those of pregnancies where the mothers took either no or different medications. This would necessarily have to involve huge numbers of pregnancies, since the proportion of mothers taking a blocker, and the proportion of fetuses and neonates who have a congenital cardiac defect, would both be expected to be very low. The design might work well for factors and adverse outcomes that are more prevalent and are evident after only a short period of follow-up. The key measure would be the relative risk, or the ratio of the risk of development of congenital cardiac disease for the offspring of mothers taking a blocker of angiotensin receptors versus the risk for offspring of mothers not taking any medication. In this case, the most efficient design would be a case-control study that is prospective in nature, whereby a group of pregnant mothers were enrolled who were taking a blocker and were matched on key characteristics to a group of mothers who were taking no medications. The two groups would then be followed and assessed as to the proportion of fetuses and neonates who develop congenital cardiac defects. The study would potentially have the bias inherent to the case-control study design, predominantly the adequacy of selection of both the cases and the controls. The key measure would be the odds ratio, or the ratio of the odds of development of congenital cardiac disease for the offspring of mothers taking the blocker versus the odds for offspring of mothers not taking any medication. When the exposure or risk factor is not dichotomous in nature, relative risk and odds ratios may be expressed as the increase in the ratio for a given increment increase in the magnitude of the risk factor. More complex measures of association are required when the outcome is not dichotomous, or when the outcome is a time-related event. The critical appraisal of studies of harm proceeds as follows:

Was the study conducted in manner that minimised bias?

Was a comparison group without the exposure or factor of interest clearly identified and similar regarding other important factors that might influence outcome?

Were assessments of both the exposure or factor and the relevant outcomes conducted and interpreted in an identical manner irrespective of the exposure status of the subject?

Was follow-up sufficiently long and complete in order to ensure development and ascertainment of outcomes?

Was the study design such that there was a correct temporal relationship between the exposure and subsequent development of the outcome? This is one of the criterions that contribute to assurances that the association is causal in a nature.

Is there evidence that a dose-response relationship exists between the magnitude of the exposure or factor and the subsequent development and magnitude of the outcome? Again, another criterion that implies a causal nature to the observed association.

Are the results reported and interpreted appropriately?

Are the measures of association reported appropriate for the study design and the level of measurement of the exposure or factor and the outcome?

Are confidence intervals provided for all measures of association?

Are the results of sufficient magnitude and relevant?

Is the observed association strong?

Are observed measures of association sufficiently reliable?

- Are the confidence intervals sufficiently narrow?
- Do the confidence intervals include values that would indicate no association?
- If the observed association is weak or in the wrong direction, implying a decreased risk of the outcome related to the exposure, do the confidence intervals exclude a clinically important positive association?

Are the findings and implications of the report applicable to my own clinical practise?

Do my patients meet the entry criterions described in the report, and do they have similar characteristics to the study subjects?

Are the results such that they provide valid and important information regarding counseling about prognosis for my patients should they have the exposure or factor?

Is the association of sufficient magnitude that it would alter management? This might lead to reduction or eliminations of the exposure or factor. It might also lead to monitoring selected patients more closely who have the exposure or factor. It also might lead to additional therapies aimed at neutralising causal pathways attributable to the exposure or factor if it could not be avoided.

Diagnosis

The clinical practise of those involved with paediatric and congenital cardiac disease relies heavily on diagnostic testing, primarily imaging. A good diagnostic test is valid, reliable, quick, safe, simple, associated with minimal discomfort, inexpensive and ethical. Studies about optimal and novel methods for making measurements are common, often in comparison with an accepted methodology. These studies of comparison often do not relate the methods to a standard criterion, and it is difficult to determine which method is better when the analysis shows only differences between the two methods. In addition, measures of association are often used, when in fact we are more interested in measures of agreement. Other studies aim to look at the contribution of new tests to the definition of clinical conditions and their prognosis or response to treatments, such as defining the relationship of brain natriuretic peptide levels in relation to clinical markers of heart failure. For these studies, measures of association are appropriate.

The classic study of a diagnostic test is one designed to determine the performance characteristics of a given test in making or excluding a specific diagnosis. These studies are much less prevalent. The methodology also applies to studies about screening. We are interested in the accuracy of the methods themselves, particularly if they require subjective assessment. We wish to know features such as test-retest reliability, and intra- and inter-observer variability. Test-retest reliability is the amount of variation in pairs of measurements performed in the same individuals under the same conditions by the same observers but at different times. It represents variation of the test itself together with intra-individual variation. Intra-observer variability is the amount of variation when the same observer performs or interprets the same test in the same individual at the same point in time. Inter-observer variability is the amount of variation when two or more different observers perform or interpret the same test in the same individual at the same point in time. Each of these is defined by determining the degree and pattern of agreement, not correlation or association.

In relation to defining or excluding a diagnosis, we wish to know the performance characteristics of the test itself in both subjects with and without the disease or condition of interest as defined by application of a criterion standard. Sensitivity is the ability of the test to accurately identify those subjects with the disease. It is the proportion of subjects with the disease, the denominator, who would have a positive test result and be identified, the numerator. The remaining proportion would represent those subjects with missed disease. Specificity is the ability of the test to accurately exclude the diagnosis in those who do not have the disease. It is the proportion of subjects who do not have the disease, the denominator, who would have a negative test result, the numerator. The remaining proportion would represent those subjects who would be incorrectly identified as having the disease, or false positives. These subjects would either be incorrectly labeled and managed for the condition, or may require further confirmatory testing. For tests which give a result which is a continuous measure, one can calculate the sensitivity and specificity using as cut-points all values of the variable, and plot a receiver-operating characteristic curve. This curve plots sensitivity on the y-axis and the proportion of false positives on the x-axis. A plot that results in a diagonal line running from the bottom left to the upper right corner represents a test that has no discriminatory ability. Plots that are curves towards the upper left corner show greater discrimination the closer they get to that corner. Alternatively, one can plot the area under the curve as a proportion. The closer the proportion of area under the curve is to 1, the more perfect the discrimination of the test. The test value with the sensitivity and proportion of false positives that comes closest to the upper left corner is the value that has the best discriminatory performance, and may be used as a cut-point.

Additionally, it is possible to calculate an entity called the likelihood ratio associated with a particular result. The likelihood ratio associated with a positive test result would be the ratio of the proportion of subjects with the disease who would have a positive test result, the numerator and its sensitivity, divided by the proportion of subjects without the disease who would have a positive test result, the denominator and the false positives. The likelihood ratio associated with a negative test result would be the ratio of the proportion of subjects with the disease who would have a negative test result, the numerator or missed disease, divided by the proportion of subjects without the disease who would have a negative test result, this representing the denominator and specificity. Likelihood ratios of 1 represent tests with no ability to differentiate those with versus without the disease. Increasingly larger or smaller likelihood ratios indicate increasing performance of the test. These performance characteristics can be determined from a case-control study, or from a cohort study where all members of the cohort have had their disease status defined using the standard criterion. For rare diseases, the case-control design is more efficient, but may be biased in terms of the representativeness of the cases and the controls. These characteristics are fixed, and do not change when the test is applied to different populations.

We are also interested in the performance of the test under different clinical situations when applied to cohorts of subjects, particularly where the prevalence of the disease in the cohort or the probability of disease in the individual before application of the test can be estimated. This can only be determined from cohort studies where the criterion is uniformly applied to determine the prevalence of disease. Two performance characteristics are highly influenced by the prevalence of the disease in the population being tested. Positive predictive value is the proportion of subjects who have a positive test result, the denominator, with those having the disease representing the numerator. The remaining proportion would represent false positives. Negative predictive value is the proportion of subjects with a negative test result, the denominator, with those who do not have the disease being the numerator. The remaining proportion would represent missed disease. Alternatively, likelihood ratios can be used to determine the performance of the test in different cohorts or individuals where the likelihood of disease varies. If one can estimate the likelihood of disease before applying the test, this being the pre-test probability, the likelihood ratio can be applied based on the results of the test to a nomogram (Fig. 21-1) to determine the likelihood of disease in the subject given the test result, or the post-test probability.[26]

The critical appraisal of studies of diagnosis proceeds as follows:

Was the study conducted in manner that minimised bias?

Were a criterion and the test uniformly both applied to all subjects in an independent and blinded manner? It is important that knowledge of the disease status of the subject does not influence a decision to perform the test or influence its interpretation. Likewise, all subjects should be assessed as to the state of their disease. This should occur independently of performance of the test, and without knowledge of the results.

If the design is a cohort study, does the cohort include sufficient subjects with the disease at appropriate stages for which the test might be applied for screening or diagnosis in clinical practise?

If the design is a case-control study, are the cases and controls representative of the cohort to whom the test might be applied in clinical practise?

Are the methods by which the test was performed described in sufficient detail that they can be replicated in clinical practise?

- Are the sources of variability assessed or described, such as test-retest reliability, and intra- and inter-observer variability?

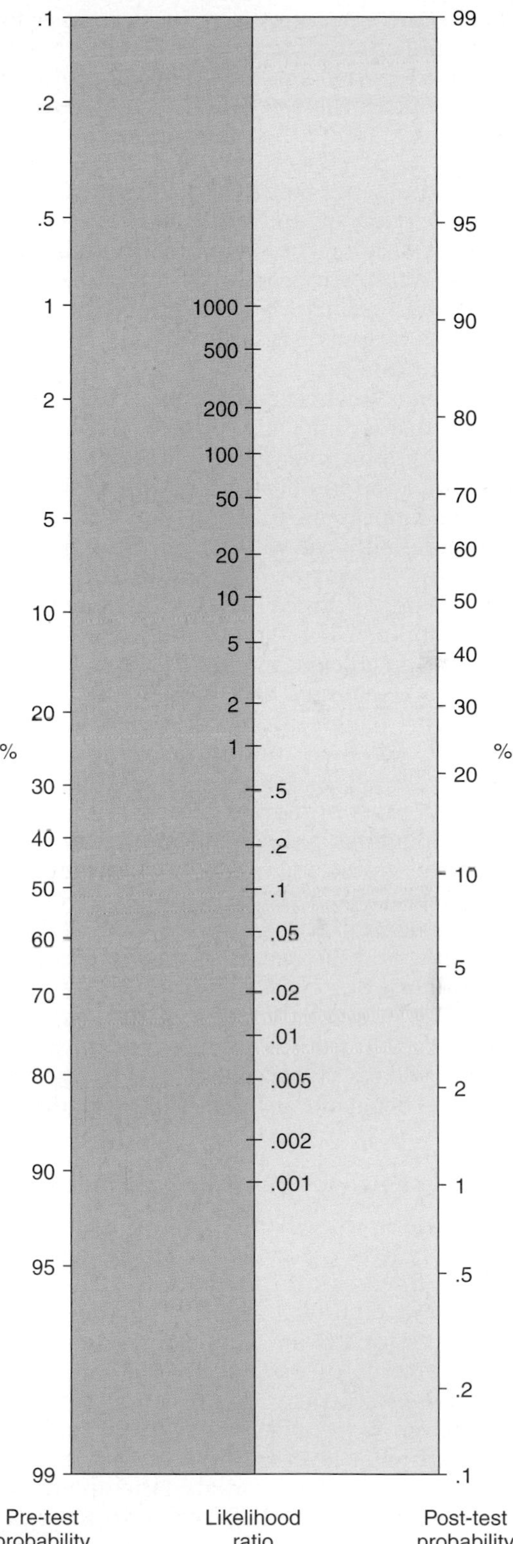

Figure 21-1 The nomogram is designed to interpret the results of diagnostic tests using likelihood ratios and incorporating the pre-test probability to determine the post-test probability of the condition or disease. To use the nomogram, locate the relevant pre-test probability on the line on the left and the likelihood ratio appropriate for the test result from the middle line. Connect these two points and extrapolate the line until it intersects the line on the right, and note the corresponding post-test probability. (From Fagan TJ: Nomogram for Bayes theorem [Letter]. N Engl J Med 1975;293:257.)

- What control measures were in place to reduce variability and ensure accuracy?

Are the results reported and interpreted appropriately?
- Are performance characteristics, such as sensitivity and specificity reported, with appropriate confidence limits?
- Are likelihood ratios reported, or are sufficient data provided that they might be calculated?

Are the results of sufficient magnitude and relevant?
- Are there performance characteristics of the test, such as sensitivity, specificity, and likelihood ratios, sufficient that both missed disease and false-positive diagnoses will be minimised?
- If the design is a cohort study, what is the magnitude of missed disease and false-positive diagnoses for this cohort, and the potential implications of such?

Are the findings and implications of the report applicable to my own clinical practise?
- Is it feasible and achievable to incorporate the testing procedure into my own clinical practice?
- Can the test be performed in my clinical practise with sufficient reliability and accuracy, and the results obtained in a timely and efficient manner?
- Are there acceptability or ethical issues which might preclude the patient from allowing the test to be performed? Are there undue discomforts or adverse effects?
- Would the results of the test be applicable to the diagnostic dilemmas and patients in my clinical practise?
- If applicable, would the results be sufficient or contribute to decisions regarding further investigation or management?
- If applied, would the results of the test be of benefit to my patients?
- Would knowledge of the state of the disease lead to interventions that would optimise outcomes?
- Would knowledge of the state of the disease contribute to beneficial behavioural changes in my patients?

Incorporating Evidence into Clinical Practise

Evidence is incorporated into clinical decision-making through the practise of evidence-based medicine. This is broadly defined as the integration of the best available research with clinical expertise taking into account the preferences for therapies and outcomes of patients. Although the roots of evidence-based medicine derive from a trend established in the early 1800s to have medicine driven by science, it has been developed and elevated to a higher level in the past few years with the increase in the number of available therapeutic options. Additional factors include the escalation in costs associated with the introduction of new technologies into routine medical practises. Before implementing widespread changes in clinical practise, especially when those changes may be associated with higher costs yet benefit fewer patients, health care managers and providers increasingly demand a much higher level of evidence regarding their relative efficacy and safety. It is clear that the era of evidence-based medicine is just starting and that the clinical practice of the future will need to be based on valid evidence, even in the absence of randomised control trials.[27]

There is a real concern among some in the medical field that the blind use of evidence-based medicine in clinical practise might lead to a cookbook approach to clinical practise. From the beginning, nonetheless, evidence-based medicine has been defined as the integration of the highest level of evidence about medicine with clinical expertise and patients' values. The practice of evidence-based medicine must consider and incorporate the beliefs, values and preferences of an individual patient, as well as consideration of the local resources, expertise and outcomes and the unique characteristics and circumstances of that patient. It does imply that clinical decisions must be based on sound science and research.

In most clinical situations, the process of evidence-based medicine is started by the building and critical appraisal of a body of evidence relevant to a specific clinical question or dilemma. Drafting of the question, specifically as a question and not as a topic or a statement, is an essential first step that will guide the search strategy for relevant and applicable research evidence. Questions that seek general knowledge about a disorder or condition are less relevant for this process than questions which relate to specific clinical dilemmas, usually arising from uncertainties in clinical decision-making around specific cases. Questions that are more specific and include more elements relevant to the clinical dilemma are desired. These specific components can then be incorporated into search terms and limits. Textbooks, unless they are research–evidence-based and updated in real time, are poor sources of evidence. Searchable databases of either evidence reviews or the medical literature are preferred. Retrieved reports can be scanned as to their relevance to the specific question at hand, and the nature and degree of rigour of the study design or evidence review. Greater weight is given to studies which are valid, reliable and accurate. It is usually necessary to include only one or two reports in the process of critical appraisal. Based on the appraisal, the decision is made as to whether the findings are sufficiently valid and important that a preliminary answer or decision may be supported. Consideration is then given as to how the answer or clinical decision supported by the evidence might be mediated by clinical expertise and patient characteristics and preferences. The process should be evaluated and recorded for future reference, and updated with the addition of new research evidence and greater clinical experience. As such, these steps integrate the process directly into clinical care (Table 21-3).

TABLE 21-3

STEPS IN THE PRACTISE OF EVIDENCE-BASED MEDICINE

- Convert information needs usually relevant to a clinical question or dilemma into answerable questions.
- Search for the best evidence usually through searchable databases of published reports with which to answer the question.
- Critically appraise the evidence for its validity, the importance and reliability of the findings and the applicability to the general clinical question or dilemma at hand.
- Evaluate, record and archive the previous steps for the purposes of future use and to allow integration of new evidence as it arises.

The complete reference list can be found on the companion Expert Consult web site at www.expertconsult.com.

ANNOTATED REFERENCES

Books

- Straus SE, Richardson WS, Glasziou P, Haynes RB: Evidence-Based Medicine: How to Practice and Teach EBM, 3rd ed. Edinburgh: Churchill Livingstone, 2005.

  This book provides clear explanations of the primary steps in the practise of evidence-based medicine, including how to ask answerable clinical questions, how to translate them into effective searches for the best evidence, how critically to appraise that evidence for its validity and importance, and how to integrate it with patients' values and preferences.

- Hall GM: How to Write a Paper, 4th ed. London: BMJ Books, 2008.

  This concise book provides clear instructions on getting reports published in biomedical journals and covers all aspects of writing each section of a structured paper, incorporating the latest information on open access, electronic publication, and submission.

- Elwood M: Critical Appraisal of Epidemiological Studies and Clinical Trials, 3rd ed. New York: Oxford University Press, 2007.

  This book presents a logical system for critical appraisal, and helps readers evaluate studies and carry out their own studies more effectively. It is applicable to a wide range of issues, and to both intervention trials and observational studies.

- Altman DG: Practical Statistics for Medical Research. London: Chapman & Hall/CRC, 1990.

  This is a problem-based textbook for those who need to use statistics but have no specialised mathematics background. It provides clear explanations of key statistical concepts, with a firm emphasis on practical aspects of designing and analysing medical research. Special attention is given to the presentation and interpretation of results and the many real problems that arise in medical research.

- Hulley SB, Cummings SR, Browner WS, et al: Designing Clinical Research, 3rd ed. Philadelphia: Lippincott Williams & Wilkins, 2006.

  This book is an excellent practical guide to planning, tabulating, formulating, and implementing clinical research, with an easy-to-read, uncomplicated presentation. The book explains how to choose well-focused research questions, and details the steps through all the elements of study design, data collection, quality assurance, and basic grant-writing.

- Norman GR, Streiner DL: Biostatistics: The Bare Essentials, 3rd ed. Toronto: BC Decker, 2008.

  Free of calculations and jargon, this book speaks so plainly that you will not need a technical dictionary. The principles of probability and statistical tests, and their use, are explained simply and clearly with a sense of humour. Throughout the guide, areas in which researchers misuse or misinterpret statistical tests are highlighted.

- Silverman WA: Where's the Evidence? Debates in Modern Medicine. New York: Oxford University Press USA, 1999.

  The author asks us to consider whether the preoccupation of institutional review boards with informed consent makes sense without a parallel requirement that the scientific design of the research be valid, and the question that it asks be worthwhile. The commentaries cover a multiplicity of topics, from observer bias to sampling and representativeness, from eugenics to euthanasia, from information overload to random assignment.

- Lang RA, Secic M (eds): How to Report Statistics in Medicine: Annotated Guidelines for Authors, Editors, and Reviewers, 2nd ed. Philadelphia: American College of Physicians, 2006.

  This book presents a comprehensive and comprehensible set of guidelines for reporting the statistical analyses and research designs and activities commonly used in biomedical research.

Internet-based Resources

- User's guide to evidence-based practice. Available at: http://www.cche.net/usersguides/main.asp.

  Complete set of Users' Guides, originally published as a series in the Journal of the American Medical Association. The Centre for Health Evidence continues to maintain the full-text pre-publication version of this series on behalf of the Evidence-Based Medicine Working Group, also available at: http://www.usersguides.org/ and with a subscription to JAMA.

- CEBM: Centre for evidence-based medicine. Available at: http://www.cebm.net/.

  This Centre for Evidence-Based Medicine is located at Oxford University, is aimed at promoting evidence-based health care, and provides resources to make use of it.

- Centre for evidence-based medicine: University Health Network. Available at: http://www.cebm.utoronto.ca/.

  This comprehensive Web site on evidence-based medicine also serves as a support to the book by Straus et al listed above.

- Statpages. Available at: http://www.statpages.org/.

  This is an excellent resource for statistical analysis, and includes links to Web pages with over 300 statistical calculators, statistical software packages, and resources for how to choose the right statistical tests and appropriate methodology.

- Cochrane database. Available at: http://www.cochrane.org/.

  This is the largest repository of systematic reviews and meta-analyses, with resources on clinical research and critical appraisal of published literature.

SECTION

3

Specific Lesions

CHAPTER 22

Isomerism of the Atrial Appendages

STEVEN A. WEBBER, HIDEKI UEMURA, and ROBERT H. ANDERSON

It has long been recognised that congenital absence of the spleen, or the presence of multiple spleens, is associated with severe congenital malformations of the heart.[1–3] Some of the most complex forms of congenital cardiac disease are associated with these splenic abnormalities, and the prognosis for many patients with these lesions remains poor, even in the modern era of congenital cardiovascular surgery. If progress is to continue in the care of these children, the cardiac abnormalities need to be determined with precision in each case, and their nature be conveyed in unambiguous fashion to the surgeon attempting correction or palliation. Description of the cardiac malformations found in association with splenic abnormalities, however, has been the cause of much confusion and controversy. It is now established that cardiac structures are best identified on the basis of their most constant components, following the so-called morphological method.[4] When considering the atriums, it is the appendage which is most constantly present (see Chapter 1). It is then the presence of isomeric atrial appendages that is the most accurate feature with which to stratify the patients previously labeled as having splenic syndromes,[5] or more recently as having visceral heterotaxy.[6–8] In the first part of this chapter, we review some of the historical landmarks in the recognition of the cardiac malformations seen in the presence of isomeric atrial appendages, and attempt to clarify some of the confusing nomenclature that has evolved over the last few decades. Subsequently, we describe in detail the morphological and clinical features of these cardiac malformations. We then focus attention on the progress made in recent years in the diagnosis and surgical treatment of these generally highly complex malformations.

HISTORICAL NOTES AND DEFINITIONS

Absence of the spleen is an obvious autopsy finding, which is unlikely to be missed, being noted as long ago as the 16th century, but very likely then as the consequence of tuberculous infection. The earliest recorded examples of congenital absence of the spleen are probably those appearing in 1826.[2] Multiple spleens occurring as a congenital malformation had been recorded more than 30 years previously.[1] These early accounts recognised not only the splenic anomalies, but also abnormal arrangements of other organs, as well as the cardiac malformations. Over the last five decades, there has been a more systematic analysis of the cardiac and extracardiac malformations seen in patients with congenital splenic anomalies. This has resulted in recognition that the entire bodily arrangement of patients, now often described as visceral heterotaxy,[6–8] differs from the usual arrangement, or situs solitus, and also from the mirror-imaged variant, typically described as situs inversus. Those observing the abnormal arrangement of the abdominal organs[3,9] had noted the association with congenital cardiac disease. They had also noted the symmetrical nature of the lungs. Ivemark, in his classical description, introduced the phrase 'asplenia, a teratologic syndrome of visceral symmetry'.[3] Putschar and Mannion,[9] with remarkable prescience, stated: 'The relationship of agenesis of the spleen to disturbed development of laterality, however, goes beyond the manifestations of obvious situs inversus. Between the normal situs, which is asymmetrical, and the situs inversus, which is the asymmetrical mirror-image of normality, a symmetrical situs sometimes exists, exhibiting symmetrical rightness or leftness on both sides'. It is hard to find any subsequent account that so well expresses the concept of biological isomerism, namely, lack of normal lateralisation leading to visceral symmetry.

Others had also emphasised this symmetry, with note taken of isomerism of the right atrial appendages and sinus nodes in patients having absence of the spleen,[10] and bilateral left-sidedness in patients with multiple spleens.[11] Despite such long-standing recognition of isomerism of the organs and atriums as the essence of these malformations, others had argued that the concept of isomerism had no scientific foundation,[12] and continued to stratify the cardiac malformations found in these settings under the headings of asplenia and polysplenia, grouping them together as situs ambiguus.[13] This approach is less than ideal at a time when most centres dealing with congenital cardiac disease use a sequential segmental approach to diagnosis, a form of analysis which must start with accurate identification of the arrangement of the atrial chambers. When the essence of the malformations is isomerism, rather than lateralisation, of the atrial appendages, there is nothing ambiguous, or uncertain, concerning the atrial morphology. In terms of the scientific rigour, it is also the case that molecular advances have made it possible to generate knock-out mice with unequivocal isomerism of the atrial appendages.[14] We urge strongly, therefore, that the term situs ambiguus be abandoned, even though a definition for the entity was suggested by the International Working Group dealing with nomenclature.[7]

We find it difficult to understand why so many authors continued to use the terms asplenia and polysplenia to characterise the congenital anomalies of this group of patients. For the cardiologist, it is hard to believe that knowledge of the state of the spleen, even recognising the risk of overwhelming sepsis in its absence, takes precedence over precise description of the complex cardiac malformations.

When the cardiac malformations were first emphasised as a feature of patients having congenital absence of the spleen, a sequential segmental approach to the description of congenitally malformed hearts had yet to be developed. At that time, a short, but limited, diagnostic label, such as asplenia syndrome, sufficed to describe a condition then considered prognostically hopeless. These labels now surely seem obsolete for the fundamental description of the complex cardiac malformations associated with abnormalities of lateralisation. Furthermore, discordance between splenic status and the arrangement of the atrial appendages is far from rare.[5] The first step in the sequential diagnosis of any patient suspected of having congenital cardiac disease is now the identification of bodily and atrial arrangement, irrespective of the state of the spleen. This should be followed by a systematic description of the cardiac malformations, using the principles of sequential segmental analysis (see Chapter 1). This approach can include description of the state of the spleen, when pertinent, and listing of other extracardiac anomalies. It simply emphasises that analysis starts within the heart, and is based on the arrangement of the atrial appendages.

As we have already discussed, the background to some of the more complex and confusing terminology used previously to describe the hearts and organs of patients with isomeric atrial appendages was reviewed in the recent report from the International Nomenclature Group.[7] In this respect, it should be noted that the term isomerism has been widely accepted as short-hand for the overall description of hearts with isomeric atrial appendages. The atriums themselves, of course, are not literally isomeric, nor are the appendages identical in all respects. Both atrial appendages, in the setting of visceral heterotaxy, nonetheless, have morphologic features characteristic of either the typical right or left structures. It is this feature that should be used to stratify the syndrome when assessing its cardiac aspects.

ANATOMY

Atrial Anatomy

Structural isomerism, strictly enantiomerism, is seen when entities are mirror-images of each other (Fig. 22-1). In this respect, the usual arrangement of the organs within the body, when compared to its mirror-imaged variant, represents biological enantiomerism (Fig. 22-2). As applied to those with visceral heterotaxy, however, the concept of isomerism implies that the mirror-imaged structures are present in

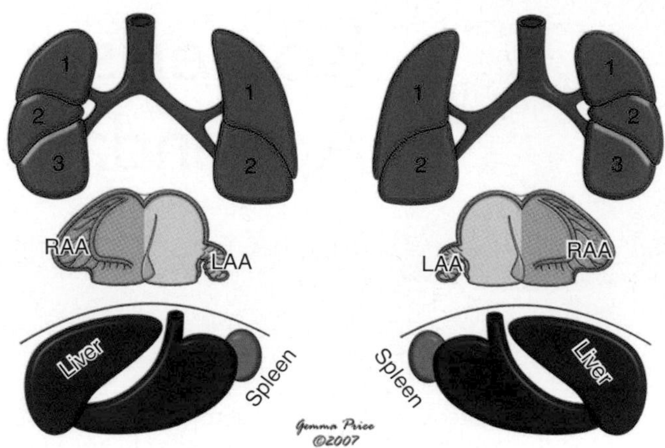

Figure 22-2 The cartoons show the essence of the usual body arrangement (left), and its mirror image (right). Individuals with these arrangements would exhibit enantiomerism relative to each other.

the same individual (Fig. 22-3). Within the heart, it is the atrial appendages, when assessed according to the extent of the pectinate muscles relative to the atrioventricular junctions,[6] which show the enantiomeric features. It should not be thought that the hearts from patients having isomeric right atrial appendages also exhibit bilateral superior and inferior caval veins, along with a coronary sinus draining to each atrium. As we will see, absence of the coronary sinus is a defining feature of those having isomeric right atrial appendages. Nor do hearts with left atrial appendages bilaterally have two normal left atriums, each receiving four pulmonary veins. The presence of isomerism within the atrial segment simply means that there is duplication of those parts of the appendages exhibiting the characteristic anatomical features of rightness or leftness. Emphasis is placed on the appendages because venous connections, vestibular morphology, and septal structure are all variable. For example, the pulmonary veins may be connected to the morphologically right atrium, or to an extracardiac site (see Chapter 24). The atrioventricular junction may be absent, as in tricuspid or mitral atresia. Although the atrial

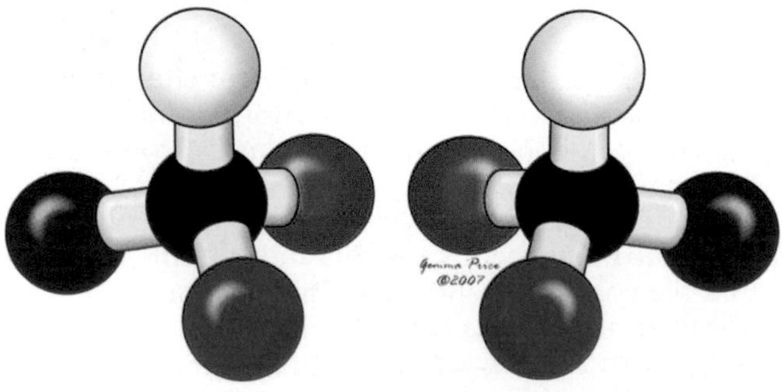

Figure 22-1 The objects shown are mirror images of each other. This is the essence of structural isomerism, properly described as enantiomerism.

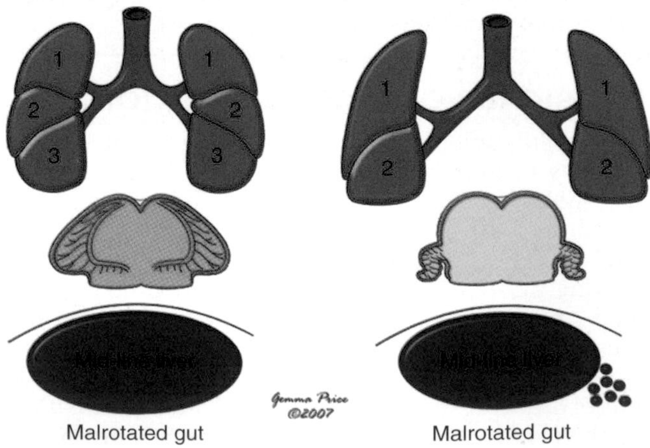

Figure 22-3 The cartoons show the typical bodily arrangements in the setting of visceral heterotaxy. In each instance, insofar as the thoracic structures are concerned and the atrial appendages, the right and left sides are mirror images of each other, hence, enantiomeric. This is the essence of bodily isomerism.

septum has typical morphologically right and morphologically left sides, it is not always there. These variable features, therefore, following the precepts established in the morphological method,[4] cannot be used as reliable indicators of morphologically rightness or leftness. Instead, the heart with right isomerism will be characterised by the presence of appendages each having the morphology of the normal right appendage. The uniformly characteristic feature of rightness is the extent of the pectinate muscles around the atrioventricular junctions, so that they meet at the crux (Fig. 22-4). In contrast, in the heart showing left isomerism, each of the appendages will have the characteristic morphology of the normal left appendage, with the pectinate muscles contained within the tubular appendages, the posterior vestibular areas being smooth on both sides, and directly confluent with the venous components (Fig. 22-5). The major morphological features of rightness of the isomeric appendages, as shown in Figure 22-4, are to be found internally. External features are also usually distinctive. In most hearts, each triangular appendage is separated along its entire border with the smooth-walled part of the atrium by an extensive groove, marked internally by a prominent terminal crest (Fig. 22-6). Although seen in most cases, this feature is not universally present. Similarly, the external shape of the appendages is usually but not constantly characteristic. Morphologically right appendages are almost always triangular, but the triangle can have a narrow base. It is the extent of the pectinate muscles which is the universal criterion for morphologically rightness on both sides of the atriums (see Fig. 22-4).

We have usually found it possible, when examining hearts from patients with left isomerism, to recognise morphologically left appendages bilaterally because of their narrow shape, along with their constricted junction with the smooth-walled atrial portions (Fig. 22-7). It is the internal characteristics which have again proved to be constant (see Fig. 22-5). Although the pectinate ridges may extend more laterally than the constricted junction of appendage and atrium, they are always significantly more limited in their extent than in the morphologically right atrium (compare Figs. 22-4 and 22-5). Using the criterion of the extent of the pectinate muscles, we have found it possible uniformly to distinguish morphologically right from left appendages, thus permitting the distinction of isomeric and lateralised arrangements, even when we studied each individual atrium in isolation.[6]

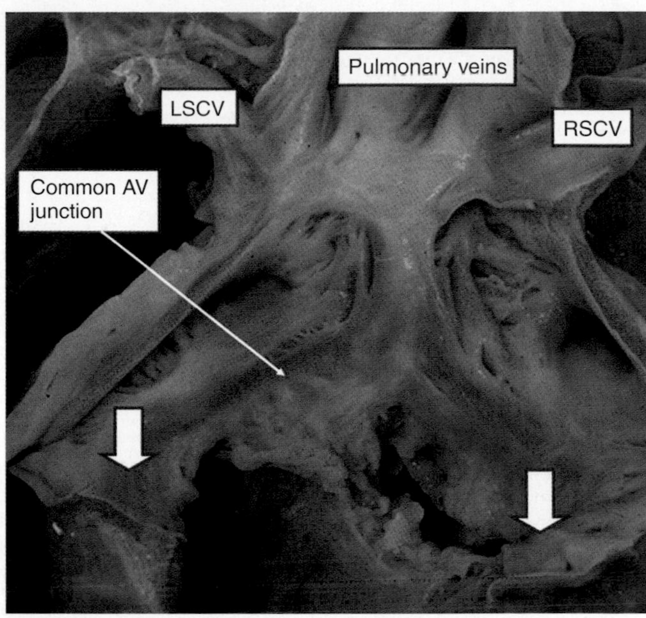

Figure 22-5 Like the heart shown in Figure 22-4, this specimen comes from a patient with visceral heterotaxy. There is again a common atrioventricular (AV) junction, and a common atrium. In this specimen, however, the pectinate muscles are confined within the tubular appendages, the vestibules being smooth at the crux on both sides (*arrows*). This is the essence of isomerism of the morphologically left appendages. LSCV, left superior caval vein; RSCV, right superior caval vein.

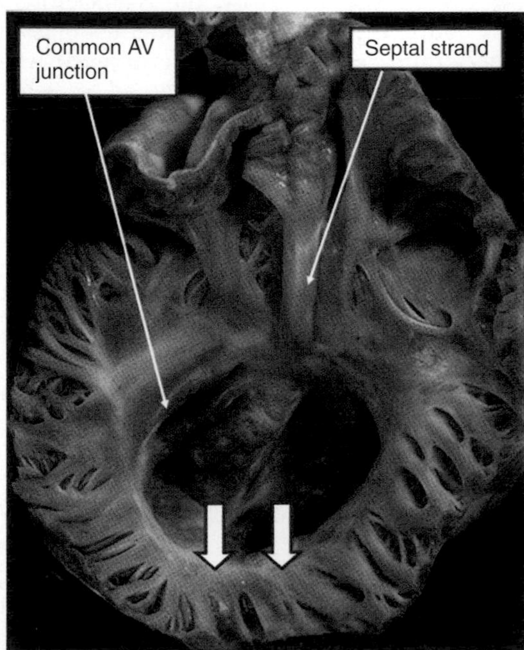

Figure 22-4 The atrial roof is reflected superiorly to show the common atrioventricular (AV) junction in this heart from a patient with visceral heterotaxy. The pectinate muscles encircle the common junction on both sides, meeting at the crux (*arrows*). This is the essence of isomerism of the right atrial appendages. Note the septal strand.

The arrangement of the appendages in patients with visceral heterotaxy is usually, but not universally, harmonious with the arrangement of the thoracic organs. Discordance between thoracic and atrial arrangement can also be found in patients with normal hearts, typically in the syndrome of biliary atresia with multiple spleens, bronchial isomerism, but usual atrial arrangement.[15,16] We discuss this discordance, and the arrangement of the other systems of organs, in greater detail in the sections that follow.

Venoatrial Connections

Anomalous venoatrial connections are the rule in patients with isomeric atrial appendages. Although a small proportion of cases have an overall pattern of drainage which can be considered usual, or mirror-imaged, even in these hearts the patterns are never morphologically normal. In each individual, any pattern must be anticipated, but certain features are sufficiently common to permit the differentiation of right and left isomerism. It is the connection of the pulmonary veins which is most reliable in permitting this distinction. In right isomerism, because the pectinate

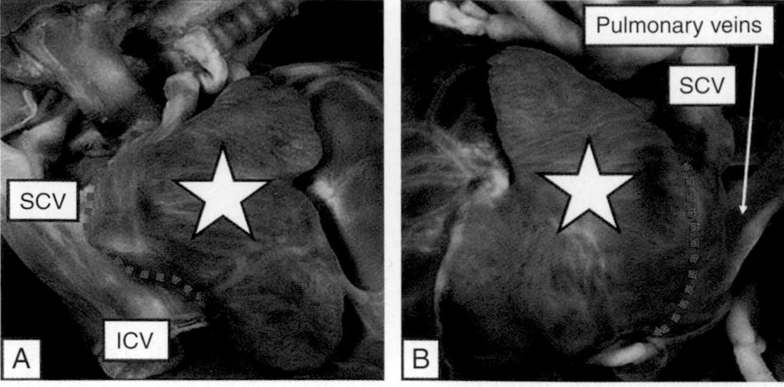

Figure 22-6 The triangular appendages (*stars*) on the right (A) and left (B) sides in a patient with right isomerism. Note the bilateral superior caval veins (SCV) and the pulmonary veins coming together in a mid-line confluence. The yellow dots show the bilateral terminal grooves. ICV, inferior caval vein.

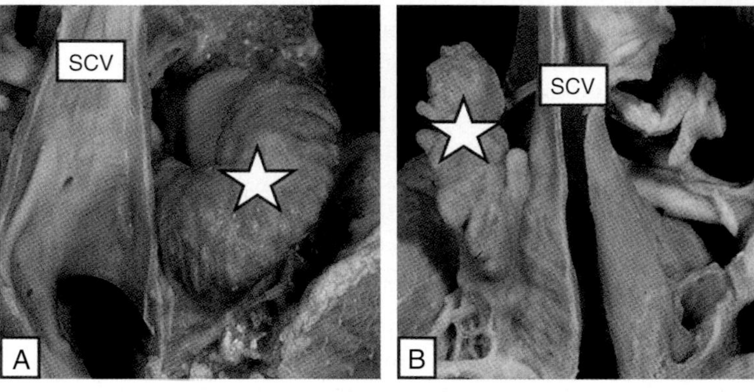

Figure 22-7 The atrial appendages (*stars*) to the right (A) and left (B) sides of a patient with visceral heterotaxy. It is easy in this instance to recognise that both are morphologically left simply from their external appearance. Note the bilateral superior caval veins (SCV).

muscles extend to the crux on both sides, the pulmonary venous connections are always anatomically abnormal. Even when all the pulmonary veins connect to one of the morphologically right atrial chambers, be the chamber right- or left-sided, the anatomy is abnormal when compared to the normal connections of the pulmonary veins to the morphologically left atrium. This is because the morphologically left atrium never exhibits pectinate muscles extending to the crux (Fig. 22-8). Most usually, if the pulmonary veins do return to the heart, they make their connection via a fibrous confluence, typically opening centrally (Fig. 22-9). When there are morphologically right appendages bilaterally, therefore, the connections of the pulmonary veins will always be anomalous anatomically, even if the atrium receiving the veins is itself left-sided.

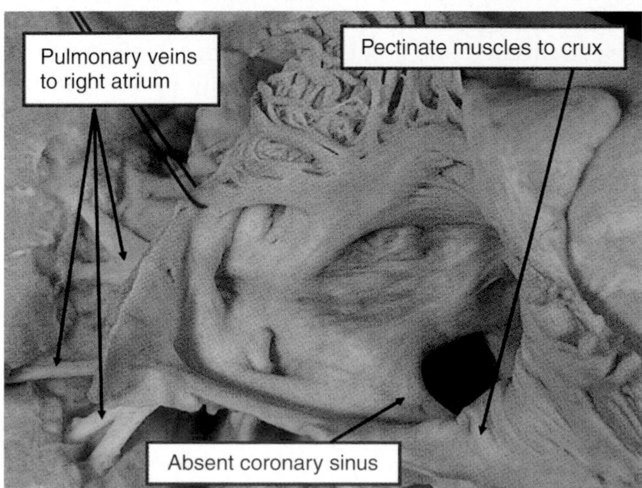

Figure 22-8 In this heart, all the pulmonary veins return to the right-sided atrium, which has an appendage of right morphology. In anatomical terms, this is totally anomalous pulmonary venous connection. Note the absence of the coronary sinus.

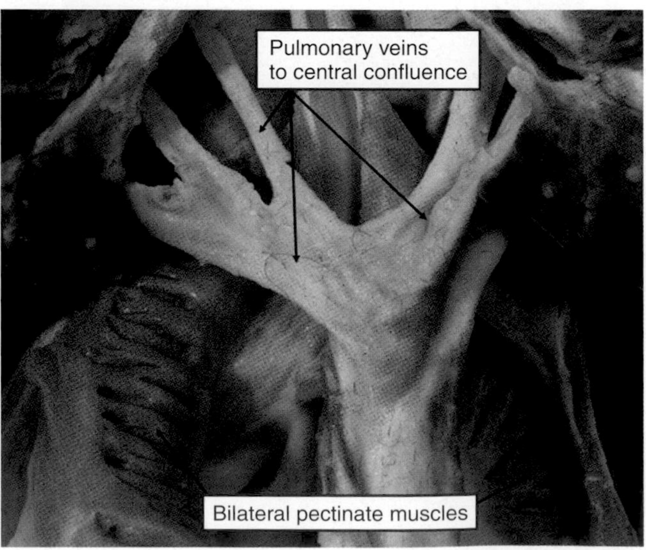

Figure 22-9 In this patient with bilateral appendages of right morphology (note the pectinate muscles extending to the crux on both sides), the pulmonary veins drain through a central fibrous confluence. This is anatomically anomalous.

In about half the patients having isomeric right appendages, such semantic pitfalls do not arise, because the pulmonary venous drainage is exclusively to an extracardiac source. The site of anomalous connection is then as varied as when totally anomalous pulmonary venous connection is seen with usual atrial arrangement (see Chapter 24). The problems of obstruction within the anomalous pulmonary venous pathway are the same. Indeed, clinical experience suggests that an obstructed supracardiac pathway is more frequent in the setting of right isomerism than in usual arrangement.[17]

The other universally constant feature of the venoatrial connections in the presence of isomeric right atrial appendages is absence of the coronary sinus, this channel being a component of the morphologically left atrioventricular junction. When the pectinate muscles extend bilaterally to the crux, there is no room to enclose the sinus within the junctions (see Fig. 22-4). It may be anticipated, nonetheless, that some patients with absence of the spleen may possess a coronary sinus, since not all patients with asplenia have isomeric right atrial appendages.

If totally anomalous pulmonary venous connection, together with absence of the coronary sinus, are the distinguishing atrial features of hearts with isomeric right atrial appendages, then it is an anomalous connection of the inferior caval vein which draws attention to the potential presence of isomeric left atrial appendages. Most frequently, the suprarenal segment of the inferior caval vein is totally absent. The abdominal segment of the caval vein continues through the azygos venous system to drain to either the right- or the left-sided superior caval vein (Fig. 22-10). In patients with left isomerism, both accessory venous systems are strictly hemiazygos, since the hemiazygos vein is a morphologically left structure. It is simpler, nonetheless, to describe communication via the azygos venous system, and then to account for the right- or left-sided location of the anomalous venous channel. Although right-sided azygos continuation has been noted in the setting of right isomerism, albeit rarely,[18] continuation through the left-sided azygos veins has been reported only in association with left isomerism, or very rarely, in patients with usual atrial arrangement or mirror-imaged arrangement. In terms of connection of the hepatic veins, a confluent suprahepatic channel was present in one-third of cases with isomeric left atrial appendages in the case material of the Children's Hospital of Pittsburgh (see Fig. 22-10). The presence of separate connection of the hepatic veins, when combined with the relationship of the abdominal great vessels relative to the spine, had been considered a reliable means of distinguishing noninvasively the presence of right and left isomerism.[19] We now know this not to be strictly accurate. It is difficult, if not impossible, to distinguish with certainty cases as having isomerism simply by studying the relationships of the abdominal great vessels to the spine. This is not to detract from the immense value of this feature when used as the initial step in the ultrasonographic assessment of sequential segmental anatomy.[19] When note is taken of the overall connections of the pulmonary veins, the inferior caval vein, and the drainage of the hepatic veins to the atriums, along with the arrangement of the coronary sinus, it should always be possible to distinguish between the right and left forms of isomerism. This is certainly not the case with the connections of the superior caval veins. Bilateral connections to the roofs of the right- and left-sided atriums are frequent in either setting. In those with isomeric left appendages, these connections are anomalous on each side. In those with isomeric right atrial appendages, in contrast, they are anatomically normal, with each caval vein appropriately related to a terminal crest, and with sinus nodes present subepicardially in the bilateral terminal grooves (Fig. 22-11).

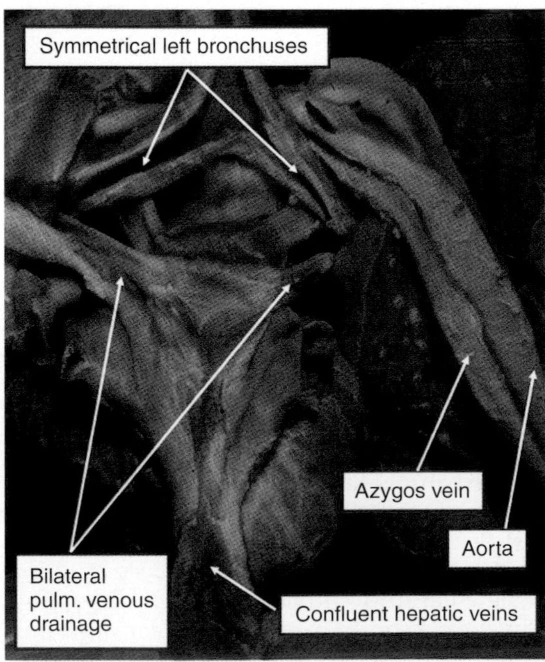

Figure 22-10 The heart and lungs from this patient with left isomerism are photographed from behind. The venous return from the abdomen, apart from that from the liver, reaches the heart through the azygos vein, which runs together with the right-sided aorta.

The drainage of the veins from the heart itself is also abnormal in both right and left isomerism. This is no more than to be expected in right isomerism since, in the universal absence of the coronary sinus, there is no transverse channel within the atrioventricular groove to collect the venous return from the heart. The variability in termination of the individual cardiac veins is surprising. The veins can terminate directly, take a crooked course for a short distance along the atrioventricular groove, or traverse the atrial wall for some distance before draining into the atrium well away from the atrioventricular groove, often adjacent to the opening of a pulmonary or systemic vein (Fig. 22-12). Such direct, crooked, or distant venous terminations are also to be found in hearts with isomeric left appendages, but a coronary sinus receiving all the coronary venous return is more frequent in cases with left isomerism.[20]

Atrial Septum

The degree of atrial septal deficiency also fails positively to discriminate between patients having isomeric right or left atrial appendages. In those with right atrial appendages bilaterally, most frequently there is simply a strand of atrial tissue which spans a common atrial cavity (see Fig. 22-4). It is rare to find the atrial septum completely lacking, but in

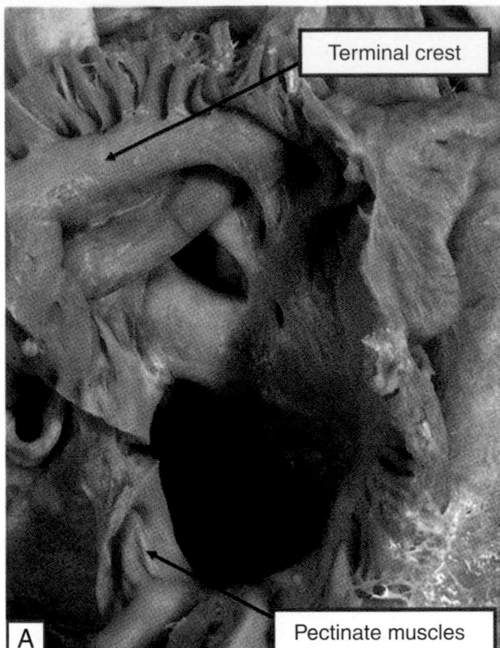

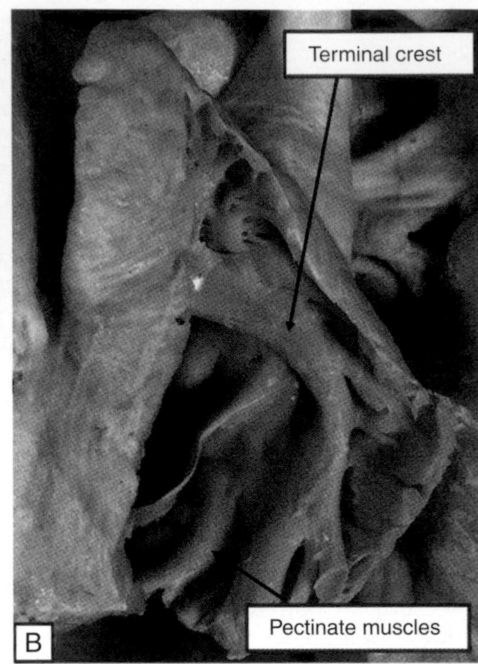

Figure 22-11 The pictures show the internal aspect of the right-sided (Panel **A**) and left-sided (Panel **B**) atrial chambers from a patient with isomeric right atrial appendages. The presence of terminal crests bilaterally is obvious.

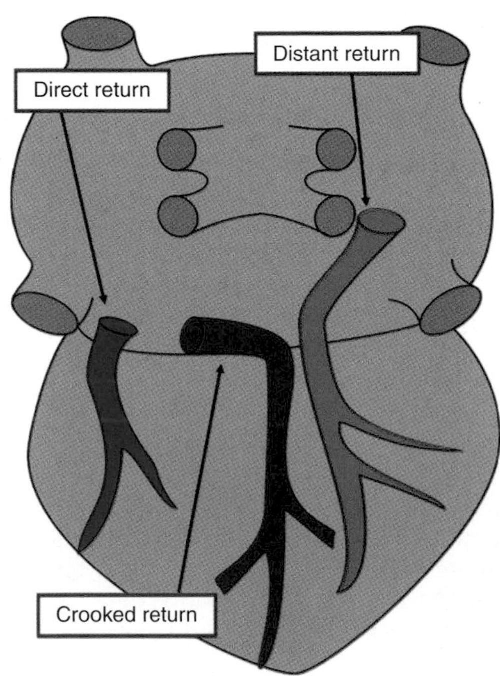

Figure 22-12 The cartoon shows the inferior surface of a heart with isomeric atrial appendages, illustrating the concept of direct, crooked, and distant return of coronary venous drainage when the coronary sinus is absent.

most cases there is, effectively, a common atrium. In about a quarter of cases, the septum is well-formed superiorly in association with an atrioventricular septal defect, while very rarely the septum can be intact, or else the oval foramen be probe patent. An effectively common atrium is to be expected in about one-half of cases with left isomerism (see Fig. 22-5). An atrioventricular septal defect is also present in nearly half, while the septum can be virtually intact in nearly one-fifth.

Atrioventricular Junctions

As with hearts in which the atrial appendages are lateralised, chambers with isomeric appendages can each be connected to their own ventricles, or else the atriums can be connected to only one ventricle. When the atrioventricular connections are biventricular, it is essential also to describe the ventricular topology. This is because there are two patterns to be found, irrespective of whether the isomeric appendages are of right or left morphology. In the first pattern, the right-sided atrium, be it associated with a morphologically right or left appendage, will be connected to the morphologically right ventricle (Fig. 22-13A), and the left-sided atrium to the morphologically left ventricle. This ventricular topology is right-handed. In the second arrangement, the right-sided atrial chamber, which again may possess either a morphologically right or left atrial appendage, will be connected to a morphologically left ventricle, and the left-sided atrium will be connected to a morphologically right ventricle. In this second pattern, the ventricular topology is left-handed (see Fig. 22-13B). When we initially defined such atrioventricular connections, we described them as ambiguous. We now recognise that it is better to describe them as biventricular and mixed (see Fig. 22-13), proceeding always to describe the ventricular topology present and, if necessary, any abnormal and unexpected ventricular relationships. Biventricular and mixed atrioventricular connections are much more frequent in the setting of isomeric left atrial appendages, and most of these patients should be anticipated to have right hand pattern ventricular topology.

Univentricular atrioventricular connections, typically with double inlet via a common atrioventricular valve, are significantly more frequent in hearts with right rather than left isomerism. In about one-third of such instances, the univentricular connection will be to a morphologically right ventricle, usually left-sided, but in some it will not be possible

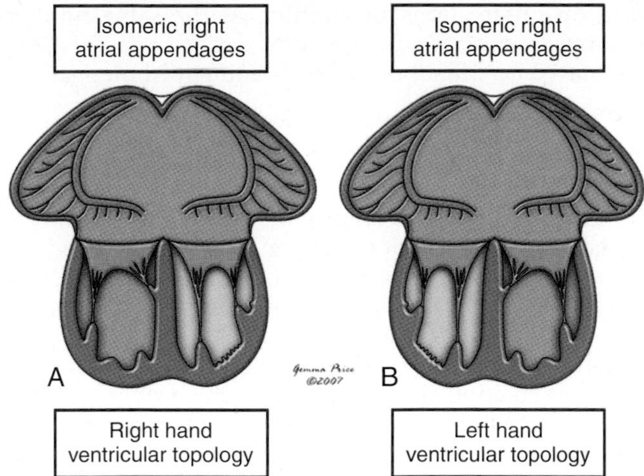

Figure 22-13 The cartoon shows the concept of biventricular and mixed atrioventricular connections. The connections would still be mixed if the appendages were of left morphology bilaterally, rather than the isomeric right variant shown.

to find a second ventricle. The majority of hearts will have double inlet to a dominant morphologically left ventricle, but solitary and indeterminate ventricles are more frequent with isomerism than in any other setting. Absence of the left-sided or right-sided atrioventricular connection is rare, but can be found with any ventricular morphology. Thus, when the atrial appendages are isomeric, any type of univentricular atrioventricular connection must be anticipated, along with any possible ventricular morphology. Fewer hearts with left isomerism have univentricular atrioventricular connections, but the same variability must be expected.

Irrespective of the presence of biventricular or univentricular atrioventricular connections, most hearts with right isomerism have a common atrioventricular junction guarded by a common valve (see Fig. 22-4). In autopsy series, the finding of normally located and unobstructed mitral and tricuspid valves is rare. In hearts with double inlet, a common valve is to be expected irrespective of the morphology of the dominant ventricle.

As would be expected, with such a high incidence of atrioventricular septal defects, the ventricular septum in the majority of hearts with biventricular atrioventricular connections is deformed in the anticipated fashion. In the very rare cases with right isomerism but without an atrioventricular septal defect, ventricular septal defects are the rule, and typically are perimembranous or muscular. In those with left isomerism, however, the ventricular septum is more frequently intact, including those having an atrioventricular septal defect with shunting exclusively at atrial level. In all hearts with univentricular atrioventricular connection, be there right or left isomerism, those with incomplete ventricles have interventricular communications as anticipated for the ventricular morphology present (see Chapter 31).

Ventriculo-arterial Junctions

Amongst the entire group of hearts with isomeric atrial appendages, there is just as much variability in type and mode of ventriculo-arterial connection, infundibular morphology, and arterial relationships as encountered in congenital cardiac disease as a whole.[21] Certain patterns occur with significantly different frequencies in hearts with isomeric right as opposed to left appendages. Pulmonary obstruction or atresia is significantly more common in association with right than with left isomerism. When there is pulmonary atresia, almost always the pulmonary supply is duct-dependent, although supply through systemic-to-pulmonary collateral arteries can sometimes be found. Obstruction of the left ventricular outflow tract, with aortic coarctation or atresia, is much commoner with left isomerism. Analysis of the ventriculo-arterial junctions as a whole shows significant differences between the two isomeric arrangements. An anterior right-sided aorta, along with subaortic or bilateral infundibulums, is commoner with right isomerism, while concordant ventriculo-arterial connections are more frequent in left isomerism.

Conduction Tissues

The morphology of the sinus node reflects the arrangement of the atrial appendages. In right isomerism, there are bilateral sinus nodes, each related to the terminal crest and the cavoatrial junction in normal fashion.[10,22] In left isomerism, in contrast, there are no terminal crests, and no right atrial appendages. The sinus node, therefore, cannot occupy its normal position. Indeed, in most hearts studied, it has not proved possible to identify with certainty the sinus node.[22] When a candidate for the sinus node is discovered, it tends to be grossly hypoplastic and located in the atrial wall adjacent to the atrioventricular junctions.

The disposition of the atrioventricular conduction axis reflects both the atrioventricular connection present and the ventricular topology.[22] When there are biventricular atrioventricular connections, the dominant feature is the ventricular topology. An atrioventricular node in its regular position, with a postero-inferior penetrating atrioventricular bundle, is found with right hand topology, the axis of conduction tissue being deviated posteriorly in presence of an atrioventricular septal defect. When there is left hand pattern ventricular topology, there is either an anterior atrioventricular node and the conduction system is found as is typical for congenitally corrected transposition, or else a sling of conduction tissue is present running along the crest of the ventricular septum, producing a connection with two atrioventricular nodes. With univentricular atrioventricular connection, ventricular morphology becomes the dominant feature. When the left ventricle is dominant, the atrioventricular node is found in anterior position, with the bundle varying its relationship to the outflow tract of the left ventricle according to the position of the incomplete right ventricle (see Chapter 31). With connection to a dominant right ventricle, the conduction system is normally situated when the incomplete left ventricle is left-sided, but an anterior node or sling may be found when the incomplete left ventricle is right-sided. The atrioventricular conduction tissues are bizarre when there is a solitary and indeterminate ventricle.[22]

Cardiac Position

An unusual position of the heart should always alert to the presence of isomerism. As reported in one extensive autopsy series[5], the heart was left-sided in three-fifths, right-sided in three-tenths, with one-tenth showing a midline arrangement. The location of the heart, and the position of its apex, however, failed to discriminate between right and left isomerism.

Arrangement of the Thoraco-abdominal Organs

Jumbled-up arrangement of the abdominal organs, or visceral heterotaxy, has long been recognised as the hallmark of the splenic syndromes. For some time, a midline liver was also considered a marker, but more recent experience shows this often not to be the case, the abdominal organs not typically being arranged in symmetrical fashion. Our own experience[5] confirms that thoracic isomerism cannot reliably be diagnosed on the basis of the disposition of the abdominal organs, particularly with regard to the morphology of the spleen. Should splenic tissue be absent, this should be documented, since this feature carries connotations for the immune state of the patient. The spleen, nonetheless, whilst expected to be absent in those with right isomerism, can also be absent in those with isomeric left atrial appendages. The arrangement of the remaining abdominal organs is also of significance. A short mesentery can lead to intestinal volvulus, and occurs in right or left isomerism.[8] The pancreas tends to be short or annular only in the presence of left isomerism.

The morphology of the thoracic organs, specifically the bronchial tree, is a much better guide to the presence of isomerism of the atrial appendages. Bilateral long and hyparterial bronchuses are indicative of left isomerism, and bilateral short and eparterial bronchuses of right isomerism, respectively. Not all cases with isomeric atrial appendages have bronchial isomerism. Thus, while examination of the penetrated chest radiograph was considered a useful step in the evaluation of the infant or child suspected of having isomeric atrial appendages, it is now rarely used as a diagnostic tool.

Visceral Symmetry without Isomeric Atrial Appendages

Whilst the focus of this chapter is on isomerism of the atrial appendages, there is increasing evidence to suggest that varying degrees of visceral symmetry may occur in the presence of usual atrial arrangement. Indeed, a symmetrical arrangement of some of the organs appears to occur with significantly greater frequency than does isomerism of the atrial appendages. Abnormal arrangement of the abdominal organs, and pulmonary isomerism, appear to be the most common abnormalities. In our reviews of the autopsy data from Children's Hospital of Pittsburgh, we noted a number of instances in which a tendency to visceral symmetry occurred with usual atrial arrangement.[16,23] In a genetic analysis of isomerism, a healthy sibling of a proband with right isomerism was noted to have left bronchial isomerism.[24] Abnormal lateralisation, with a tendency to visceral symmetry, can be found, therefore, in patients with structurally normal hearts. These observations have important implications for research into the aetiology of abnormal lateralisation, and for genetic counselling.[25] For the purposes of genetic studies, cases showing any degree of abnormal lateralisation should be distinguished from the normal. External phenotype, and cardiac morphology, is an inadequate indicator of the overall arrangement of the organs. Thus, each system of organs requires individual and specific analysis. It is best to avoid inferring the morphology of one group of organs based on observations in another. At the same time, for these purposes above all, it is necessary to stratify visceral heterotaxy into the subsets of right and left isomerism.

EXTRACARDIAC ANOMALIES

Malformations of the bodily organs, in addition to splenic anomalies and abnormal arrangements, occur with significant frequency in patients with isomeric atrial appendages.[8,9,26–28] The malformations, present in at least one-fifth of cases, included lesions involving the central nervous system, skeletal anomalies, and genitourinary anomalies. Gastrointestinal abnormalities can produce intestinal obstruction, either because of an annular pancreas or fibrous bands,[27] or subsequent to volvulus.[8] Abnormal dilated pulmonary and pleural lymphatics have been described in patients with asplenia syndrome, with the reported changes considered unrelated to any obstruction to pulmonary venous return.[29]

A wide range of anomalies is also observed in those having left isomerism. The most specific association between left isomerism, or polysplenia, and anomalies of other organ systems is biliary atresia, with or without hypoplasia or agenesis of the gallbladder. While this finding is seen in some patients with isomeric left atrial appendages, the combination of biliary atresia and multiple spleens often occurs in the setting of a structurally normal heart.[15,16] The fact that many of these patients have usual atrial arrangement does not imply the normal development of left-right asymmetry, since left bronchial and left pulmonary isomerism, intestinal malrotation, and interruption of the suprarenal portion of the inferior caval vein are frequently observed when polysplenia accompanies biliary atresia.[16] Although extracardiac anomalies are common in patients with isomeric atrial appendages, recognisable patterns of malformations that would lead to the designation of a specific syndrome or malformation sequence are rare.[27]

ISOMERISM AND CONJOINED TWINNING

There is a fascinating association between conjoined twins and disruption of normal left-right asymmetry. Complex cardiac malformations, and absence of the spleen in one of the twins, have been well described.[27,30–32] The most complex cardiac anomalies are usually, but not always, observed in the right hand twin. Features of left isomerism, in contrast, are rarely observed.

MORPHOGENESIS

Most early studies of the development of the splenic syndromes concentrated their attention upon the spleen.[3,9] While of undoubted value in terms of knowledge of splenic development, this approach does little to clarify the grossly abnormal cardiac development associated with isomerism. Here, as with the analysis of the heart itself, the significant feature is the isomeric nature of the atrial appendages. The significant point from the stance of development is that the apical parts of the ventricles, which confer morphological rightness or leftness, balloon in series from the inlet and outlet parts of the ventricular component of the primary heart tube, while the atrial appendages balloon in parallel from the atrial component (see Chapter 3). It is not surprising, therefore, that the isomeric malformation should produce duplication of the atrial appendages, without producing symmetry of the ventricles. The venous malformations are then equally well explained. With bilateral morphologically right atrial appendages, there will be no focus for incorporation of the pulmonary venous component. In normal development, this occurs by lumenisation of the pulmonary vein in the developing mediastinum, the vein using the dorsal mesocardial connection between the heart tube and the body as its entrance to the heart (see Chapter 3). These connections are grossly abnormal when both appendages develop with right morphology. The intrapulmonary venous plexuses developing in the mediastinum will, therefore, join up with suitable systemic channels to form totally anomalous connections, or else will connect directly but anomalously to the roof of the atrial chambers. Persistence of the initial bilateral symmetry of the systemic venous tributaries accounts for the usual finding of bilateral superior caval veins and absence of the coronary sinus. The bilateral formation of the terminal crests accounts for the development of bilateral sinus nodes. Since the inferior caval vein is able to drain in normal fashion to the atrial chamber, the hepatic veins will also develop normally.

When both the atrial appendages develop morphologically left characteristics, the pulmonary venous channels can be incorporated into either side of the atrium, accounting for the common finding of bilateral pulmonary venous connections. Because the terminal crest develops from the morphologically right side, the superior caval venous channels will never drain in normal fashion in hearts with left isomerism, and there will be no potential for formation of a normal sinus node. Since the ventricles develop in series, they can form in any fashion as occurs in malformations without isomerism. This is reflected in the variation seen in ventricular morphology. It is not clear why isomerism of the right appendages should more frequently be associated with a univentricular atrioventricular connection, nor with either pulmonary atresia or stenosis.

Much has now been learned concerning the genetic pathways producing these changes, with experiments confirming the reality of isomerism of the atrial appendages. Thus, it is known that cilia in the primitive node create a wave that drives molecules in one specific direction across the cells of the developing embryo, with expression of the gene *Nodal* mostly confined to the left side.[33] The wave of molecular material produced from the node that influences development of lateralised features is stopped from crossing the midline of the embryo, this process known to be under the influence of the gene *Sonic hedgehog*.[34] Because of this midline barrier, other genes, such as *Lefty*, and *Pitx2*, along with the gene *Cited2*, also known to be part of the genetic cascade,[14] have their expression confined to the left side of the body, thus producing the morphologically left characteristics (Fig. 22-14). Knocking out genes such as *Pitx2* or *Cited2* in mice then produces animals with unequivocal right isomerism (Fig. 22-15),[14,35] while knocking out *Sonic hedgehog* permits the left-forming genes to occupy the right side of the body, and produces left isomerism[34,36] (Fig. 22-16).

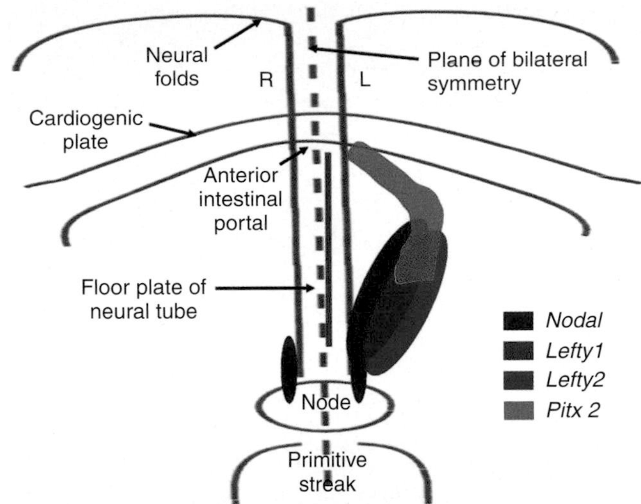

Figure 22-14 The cartoon shows the basic plan of the developing embryo at the stage of a flat disc (see Chapter 3). It shows how genes such as *Lefty* and *Pitx2* are confined to the left side (L) by virtue of a midline barrier involving the genes *Lefty-1* and *Sonic hedgehog*.

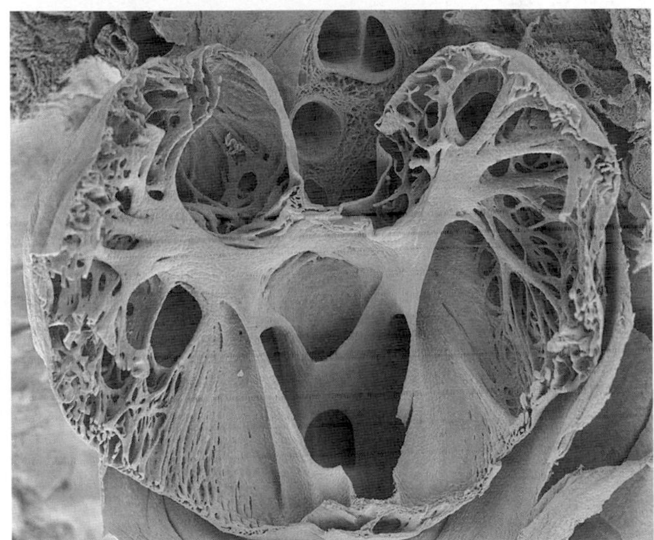

Figure 22-15 The scanning electron micrograph shows the atrial chambers of *Pitx2* knock-out mouse from the ventricular aspect. The isomeric nature of the morphologically right appendages and venous valves is unmistakable. (Courtesy of Professor Nigel Brown, St George's University, London, United Kingdom.)

INCIDENCE

It is difficult to calculate precisely the incidence of isomerism. This is because, until recently, the malformation has been described under a bewildering plethora of titles, and has been recognised most frequently at postmortem rather than during life. In the New England survey,[37] 95 of the 2251 infants presenting with congenital heart disease had visceral heterotaxy. Another study[38] estimated the incidence at around 1 in 40,000 live births. In a population-based study of all infants born with congenital asplenia in British Columbia, we calculated an incidence for right isomerism of 1 in 22,000 live births.[17] The Baltimore–Washington Infant Study[39] identified heterotaxy as representing 2.3% of congenital cardiac disease seen in infants, giving an incidence of 1 in 9158 live births. In the Active Malformation Surveillance Program at the Brigham and Women's Hospital, Boston,[40] prevalence of heterotaxy among the offspring of mothers who had planned delivery at that hospital was approximately 1 per 10,000 total births. The degree of potential underestimation of incidence and prevalence given by these studies is difficult to

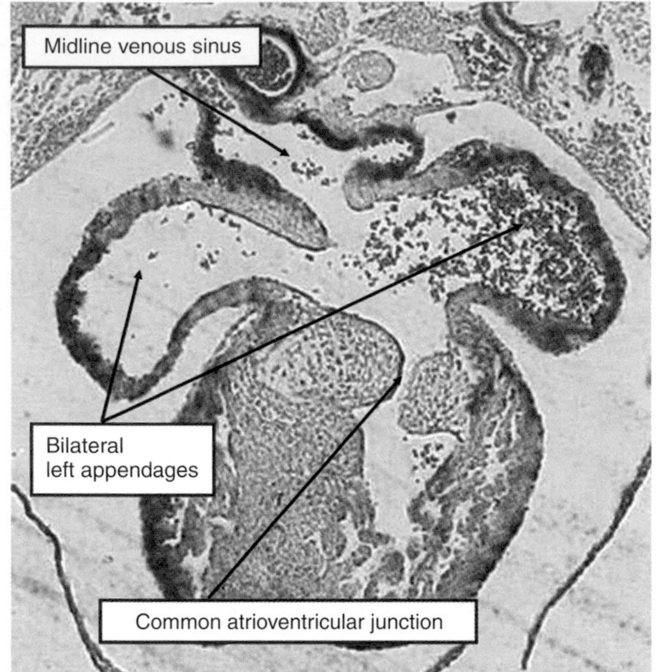

Figure 22-16 This histological section, in the frontal plane, is from a *Sonic hedgehog* knock-out mouse. Both the atrial appendages are of left morphology, with a symmetrical midline systemic venous sinus. (Courtesy of Dr Victoria Hildreth and Professor Deborah Henderson, University of Newcastle, Newcastle-upon-Tyne, United Kingdom.)

establish. It seems likely that most cases of right isomerism are recognised in infancy because of the presence of severe forms of cyanotic heart disease. Failure to recognise left isomerism is more likely because of the wider range of associated heart disease, including mild forms that may not even warrant surgical intervention. We have observed patients with isomerism of the left atrial appendages with interruption of the inferior caval vein and no other cardiac anomalies. Such patients are unlikely to be identified in life unless extracardiac anomalies, such as biliary atresia, lead to cardiac evaluation. It may be that patients with isomeric atrial appendages represent only the tip of the iceberg of the total population with abnormal lateralisation.

AETIOLOGY

There is compelling evidence that there is no single aetiology responsible for the development of abnormal lateralisation and isomerism. Evidence for causal heterogeneity comes from studies of humans and from animal models. Chromosomal anomalies are only rarely associated with visceral heterotaxy. We found no karyotypic abnormalities among infants with right isomerism and asplenia.[17] In the Baltimore–Washington Infant Study, 1 of 99 infants with heterotaxia had trisomy 13, and two other infants had unspecified chromosomal abnormalities.[39] An association between trisomy 13 and abnormalities of left-right development, nonetheless, has been noted,[41] as had a case of balanced translocation of chromosomes 12 and 13 associated with right isomerism and asplenia.[42] This latter observation suggests that a gene at break points 12q13.1 or 13p13 might be important in development of normal asymmetry. A patient with heterotaxy was also noted to have a new, apparently balanced, reciprocal translocation with breakpoints at 6q21 and 20p13.[43] Because another patient with heterotaxy was previously reported with such a new balanced translocation involving chromosome band 6q21, the authors speculated that a critical gene, or genes, in this region may be important in the development of heterotaxy. Several studies of families also suggest that hereditable single gene defects may be important aetiological factors.[44–46] Probable autosomal dominant inheritance has been described in more than one family.[47,48] Another family with heterotaxy provides clear evidence of X-linked recessive inheritance.[49] Linkage analysis in a second family with this mode of inheritance mapped the abnormal gene or genes to the region Xq24–q27.1.[50] More recently, mutations in the zinc finger transcription factor ZIC3 have been demonstrated to cause at least some cases of X-linked heterotaxy.[51] Molecular cytogenetic investigations in another patient identified a breakpoint spanning a small region on the X chromosome containing the *ZIC3* gene.[52] Although distinct anatomical differences of the heart and other organs distinguish patients with left and right isomerism, it is interesting to note that patients have been identified with both right and left isomerism, along with multiple or absent spleens, in several familial cases of visceral heterotaxy.[47,53,54] Anatomical variations, therefore, do not necessarily reflect genetic differences.

At present, we do not know the proportion of cases of human isomerism caused by inheritable single gene defects. The finding of three pairs of siblings in 60 cases of asplenia or polysplenia gives a recurrence risk of just under 5%,[38] which is much too low for simple autosomal recessive transmission, yet much higher than would be predicted from the multi-factorial threshold model. We found no familial cases among 43 examples of congenital asplenia.[17] Others calculated a risk of recurrence of 3% to 4%.[24] Despite this, the Ivemark syndrome is listed as an autosomal recessive condition.[55,56] The lower than expected risk of recurrence is explained in various ways, including causal heterogeneity, low fertility of affected patients, reduced penetrance of some recessive traits, and fetal loss. We observed only one case of right isomerism, nonetheless, amongst 5000 postmortems performed on early fetuses and stillbirths over a 21-year period in British Columbia.[17]

While the study of family kindreds may supply important information about modes of human inheritance, animal models, including knock-out and knock-in models, are a more potent tool for studying the molecular pathways that lead to abnormal lateralisation. Fortunately, several animal models of visceral heterotaxy exist, and have been studied in detail. The *iv/iv* mouse has been studied most comprehensively.[57] This recessive trait was initially considered to be a model of mirror imagery, in which homozygous animals exhibit random lateralisation, with half manifesting mirror-imaged arrangement.[58] Subsequent, more detailed anatomical studies showed that a minority of the affected animals had visceral heterotaxy, with isomerism of the atrial appendages, along with both splenic abnormalities and complex cardiac defects strongly reminiscent of human hearts with isomerism.[59] Other mutations in the mouse, the result of insertion of transgenes, have resulted in abnormalities of lateralisation. Individual *inv/inv* mice show evidence of isomerism as well as mirror imagery,[60] and the insertional mutation has been mapped to mouse chromosome 4. The *legless* mice represent another insertional mutation associated with partial deletion of chromosome 12. The genetic defect appears to involve the *iv/iv* locus. Molecular genetic studies of these models have helped bridge the gap between genetics and our understanding of the molecular pathways involved in normal and abnormal lateralisation, as discussed earlier. Abnormalities in nodal cilia and nodal flow are a common theme in several animal models of abnormal lateralisation with visceral heterotaxy, including the iv/iv and inv/inv models. For more detailed understanding of the molecular pathways involved in abnormal lateralisation, the reader is referred to several excellent reviews.[8,61,62] When the genes involved in lateralisation abnormalities have been fully localised within the mouse genome, analysis of syntenic regions on human chromosomes and studies of affected human kindreds should result in characterisation of the genes involved in human syndromes associated with isomerism and abnormal lateralisation.[63]

Other animal studies suggest that non-genetic factors may result in abnormal lateralisation. In the non-obese diabetic mouse, visceral heterotaxy and isomerism of the atrial appendages are frequently seen when diabetes develops early in pregnancy.[64] Retinoic acid has also been reported to cause heterotaxy in rat embryos,[65] and isomerism has been produced in offspring of pregnant rats kept at warm temperatures.[66] At the present time, no specific environmental factors have been implicated in the aetiology of human heterotaxy.

CLINICAL FINDINGS

Increasingly, the diagnosis of isomeric atrial appendages, and abnormal arrangements of the thoraco-abdominal organs, is being made in fetal life.[67–73] This largely reflects the more frequent use of ultrasound in the second trimester, including four-chamber cardiac screening in many centres. Even when cardiac abnormalities are not detected, the presence of abnormal arrangement of the abdominal organs frequently leads to referral for fetal echocardiography. In addition, a proportion of fetuses with left isomerism present with bradycardia, with or without non-immune hydrops.[69,74] This finding also results in referral for fetal echocardiography, which should, in turn, lead to an accurate anatomical diagnosis.[67,72] The most challenging aspect of fetal diagnosis is accurate delineation of systemic and pulmonary venous connections. The latter is of greatest clinical importance in the neonatal period, since obstruction to pulmonary venous return is common in right isomerism, and is a major predictor of postnatal survival. In general, the intracardiac structures and connections are accurately defined in experienced hands. There is a tendency for right isomerism predominantly to affect males,[17,38] but with conflicting findings for left isomerism.[38,75] Gender, therefore, cannot be used reliably to predict cardiac or splenic state in infants with suspected isomerism. Almost without exception, infants with right isomerism have obstruction of the pulmonary outflow tract, as well as common mixing, and pulmonary atresia is present in two-fifths.[76] When the pulmonary valve is patent, obstruction is generally at least moderate in nature, and presentation on the first or second day of life is usual.[17] While cyanosis is by far the most common presentation, occasional infants with right isomerism present with severe respiratory distress and cyanosis resulting from obstructed anomalous pulmonary venous connection. Several reports have drawn attention to the potential for masking of the obstructed pulmonary venous return by reduction in the flow of blood to the lungs concomitant with closure of the arterial duct. In this situation, the obstruction may be unmasked by administration of prostaglandin E_1, or by the placement of a systemic-to-pulmonary shunt, resulting in the development of pulmonary oedema.[77–80] It seems likely that there has been a bias in the literature towards reports that emphasise this clinical dilemma. This probably reflects the wish to provide a cautionary tale to other clinicians by those groups who have experienced this serious clinical problem. In our experience, most obstruction to pulmonary venous return is apparent in the neonatal period, when there is early development of pulmonary oedema and severe cyanosis.[81] On occasion, nonetheless, pulmonary venous obstruction may be mild at birth, and may progress over the first few weeks and months of life. This is most common when the anomalous venous connection is supracardiac in nature. Patients with right isomerism may occasionally present with serious extracardiac anomalies[26–28] or, more rarely, with a murmur originating from the pulmonary outflow tract when pulmonary stenosis is mild and cyanosis has gone unrecognised. In these situations, physical examination may provide clues to the presence of abnormal arrangement of organs, such as a right-sided cardiac apex or a midline liver.

The clinical findings in left isomerism are non-specific and will reflect the associated lesions. In contrast to right isomerism, the heart disease may be relatively mild. Indeed, we have observed the presence of isomerism of the left atrial appendages in association with interrupted inferior caval vein and no other cardiac or vascular abnormalities. Such patients may never be diagnosed as having isomerism unless extracardiac anomalies, such as biliary atresia or intestinal malrotation, draw attention to the abnormal arrangement of the abdominal organs. In a recent review of all patients diagnosed with isomeric left atrial appendages at the Children's Hospital of Pittsburgh, we noted that two-thirds had simpler forms of cardiac disease potentially suitable for biventricular repair. The remaining patients had complex cyanotic heart disease, frequently associated with univentricular atrioventricular connection. Although some infants with left isomerism present with cyanosis because of the combination of common mixing and obstruction of the pulmonary outflow tract, as for right isomerism, many infants with complex disease and isomeric left appendages present with cardiac failure owing to left-to-right shunting without pulmonary obstruction, and frequently with obstruction of the left ventricular outflow tract. Indeed, some will present with shock and congestive failure because of hypoplasia of the left heart, with or without signs of coarctation. These infants are frequently referred to tertiary centres with a suspected diagnosis of hypoplastic left heart syndrome. Cardiac failure may also be evident at presentation when severe regurgitation of a common atrioventricular valve, or severe bradyarrhythmia, is present at birth. The two often co-exist, and they frequently lead to fetal hydrops and intra-uterine death.[68,74,82] When such infants survive to term, they are frequently moribund at presentation and the prognosis is grave. Progression of atrioventricular block in fetal life has also been observed in patients with left isomerism.[69]

INVESTIGATIONS

The Electrocardiogram and Abnormalities of Cardiac Rhythm

The electrocardiographic findings are not specific for a diagnosis of isomerism, but once isomerism is identified, the pattern present should help differentiate most into either right or left isomerism. In right isomerism, the frontal plane P wave axis is usually inferior[83-85] but may be to the left, as with the usually arranged atrium, or to the right, as with the mirror-imaged atrium. In some instances, right- and left-sided atrial origin of the P wave is present at different times in the same patient (Fig. 22-17),[83-85] reflecting activity of bilateral sinus nodes.[86] Slow atrial rhythms, with or without junctional escape, are very rare in right isomerism. In left isomerism, true sinus rhythm is less common, as might be anticipated from the known hypoplasia of the sinus node in patients with isomeric left appendages.[86,87] About four-fifths of patients with left isomerism have a superiorly oriented axis for the P wave. This usually results from an ectopic atrial focus but is sometimes caused by junctional escape rhythm. In some patients, it is possible to find progression between these patterns (Fig. 22-18). Atrial rates below the second percentile for age have been noted in half of patients with left isomerism, being persistent in one-tenth. In many patients, progressive slowing was noted with advancing age. Despite these observations, the atrial or nodal rhythms were usually of adequate rate to prevent symptoms in childhood. Progressive slowing has been seen in adulthood, leading to the need for placement of a permanent pacemaker.[88] Atrioventricular block is

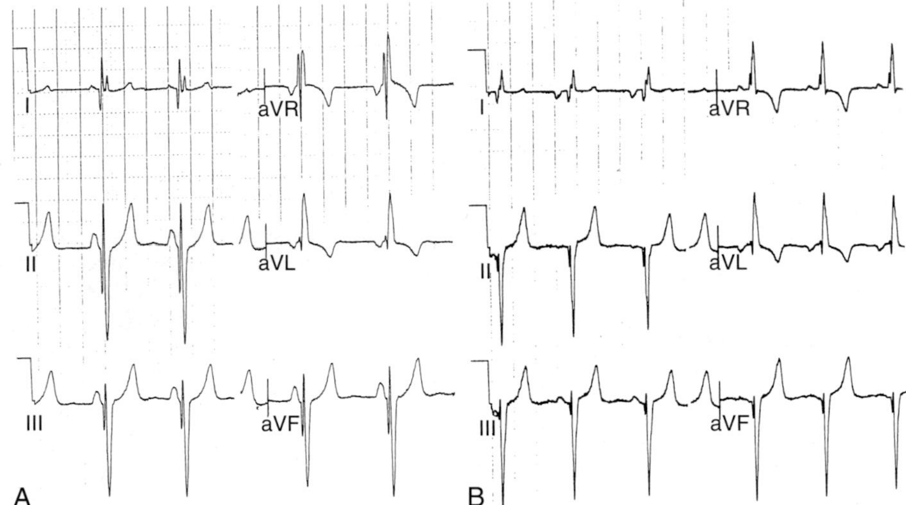

Figure 22-17 Electrocardiographic limb lead recordings taken a few weeks apart from a 12-year-old child with right isomerism. **A,** The P wave axis is normal, consistent with activation from a right-sided sinus node. **B,** Change of the axis consistent with activation from a left-sided sinus node.

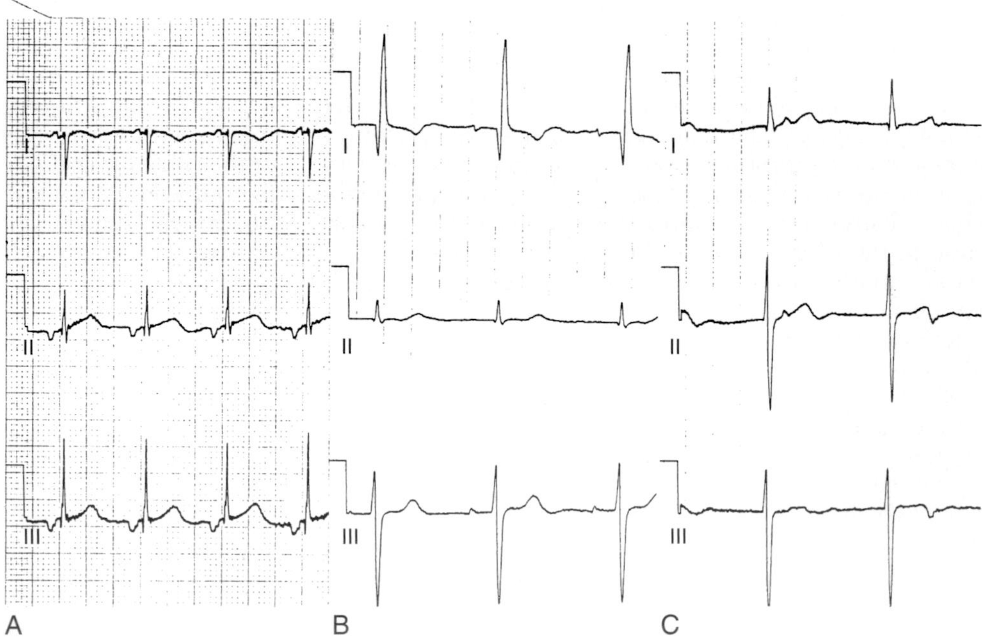

Figure 22-18 Electrocardiographic tracings from the limb leads of a child with left isomerism reveal changing patterns with age. **A,** In infancy, a low atrial rhythm with a superiorly orientated axis of the P wave is seen. **B,** Later in childhood, there was evidence of another ectopic atrial rhythm. **C,** Two years later, the patient developed permanent junctional rhythm.

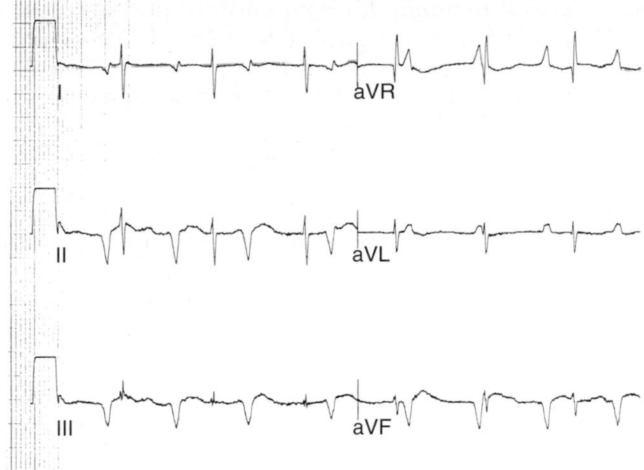

Figure 22-19 These electrocardiographic limb leads from a newborn show a superior P wave axis together with complete heart block. The combination is highly suggestive of left isomerism, which was indeed present. Note also the features of marked atrial enlargement.

exceedingly rare in right isomerism, but at least one case has been reported.[89] By contrast, varying degrees of atrioventricular block are common in left isomerism (Fig. 22-19). These findings reflect differences in the anatomy of the conduction system, as discussed earlier in this chapter. For those diagnosed in fetal life, there appears to be a higher incidence of heart block[68] than seen in those diagnosed postnatally.[84,85] Overall, complete atrioventricular block is observed in one-tenth of cases of left isomerism.[84,85] The morphology and axis of the QRS complex in hearts with isomeric appendages will reflect the ventricular morphology and the cardiac position. In view of the strong association with atrioventricular septal defect, it is not surprising that a high proportion of cases have a superiorly oriented frontal QRS axis. As is the case with the P wave, it is also the case that different QRS axes can exist in the same patient. This reflects the presence of dual atrioventricular nodes joining a ventricular sling of conduction tissue.[22] These abnormally structured atrioventricular nodes and bundles allow retrograde conduction, which can be identified by ventricular pacing. When such dual conduction pathways are present, they frequently form atrioventricular re-entry circuits. Such re-entry is an important mechanism of tachycardia, particularly in those with right isomerism. Because of the variation in QRS morphology, this situation can easily be misinterpreted as representing ventricular tachycardia. Indeed, in our experience such atrioventricular re-entrant tachycardiac is much commoner than atrial tachycardia in the setting of right isomerism. Atrial tachycardia, nonetheless, can be caused by competition between the two sinus nodes. Atrial fibrillation, in contrast, is rare in infants with right isomerism.

Chest Radiography

Evaluation of the chest radiograph can provide strong evidence for the presence of isomerism. In the neonatal period, abdominal structures are frequently included on the plain chest radiograph. Abnormal position of the stomach bubble, and a large midline liver, may provide immediate clues to the presence of visceral heterotaxy. Cardiac malposition is also often present. If umbilical venous and arterial catheters have been placed, the characteristic relationships of the aorta to the inferior systemic venous drainage will be apparent. More specifically, the presence of isomerism of the atrial appendages can be inferred, with some exceptions, from the finding of bronchial isomerism. As long ago as 1970, it was suggested that isomerism of the bronchial tree could be used as a means of diagnosing these syndromes during life.[90] Although it is sometimes possible to be confident about the diagnosis of bronchial isomerism from the plain chest radiograph, this has not proved to be consistently reliable.[91] A technique using high kilovoltages and filters provides superior images of the bronchial anatomy when compared to standard chest radiograph.[22] On the radiograph, which is exposed with rather less irradiation than a standard chest film, bone detail is effaced to a considerable degree so that the interfaces of soft tissue and gas in the mediastinum and adjacent lung are readily seen. Exposure time is very short, and breathing blur, therefore, is rarely a problem. Using this technique, adequate bronchial visualisation can be obtained in almost all infants. The position of the aortic arch, assessed from the side of tracheal indentation, is also usually apparent. These views are now rarely performed, since it has been demonstrated that cross sectional echocardiography can provide similar information about atrial arrangement, but without the need to assume bronchio-atrial concordance.

Other important information can be gleaned from the plain chest radiograph of infants with suspected isomerism. Absence of the shadow produced by the inferior caval vein on the lateral chest radiograph may suggest azygos continuation of an interrupted inferior caval vein.[92] Particular attention should also be paid to the pulmonary vasculature. This is of great importance in patients with right isomerism, where almost all infants will have pulmonary arterial obstruction and totally anomalous pulmonary venous connection. Increased vascularity in this setting should lead to the immediate suspicion of obstruction to pulmonary venous return (Fig. 22-20A). When severe cyanosis is present, even normal to mildly increased vascularity should raise this suspicion, since pulmonary oligaemia would be anticipated if pulmonary venous return were unobstructed (see Fig. 22-20C and D). With careful clinical evaluation, review of the chest radiograph, and cross sectional echocardiographic interrogation, the diagnosis should be sufficiently secure to prevent the unmasking of pulmonary venous obstruction by inappropriate placement of a systemic-to-pulmonary shunt without concomitant relief of pulmonary venous obstruction.[81] When marked discrepancies in vascularity exist between different lung segments, mixed anomalous pulmonary venous connection with varying degrees of obstruction should be suspected (see Fig. 22-20B).

Echocardiography

Cross sectional echocardiography, based on the principles of sequential segmental analysis (see Chapter 18A) can provide a complete anatomical diagnosis in almost all cases of isomerism. Some time ago,[19] it was suggested that atrial arrangement could be identified by demonstrating the characteristic relationships of the aorta to the inferior systemic

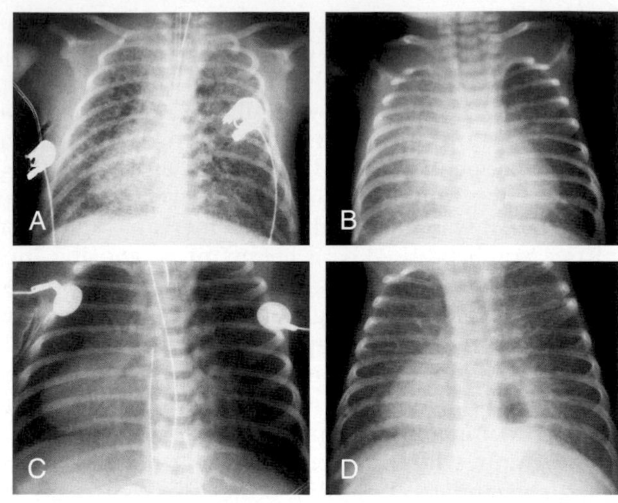

Figure 22-20 These radiographs show the spectrum of pulmonary venous obstruction seen in four newborns with right isomerism. Note also the right-sided location of the heart in three of the panels. **A**, In this child, there is severe pulmonary oedema. This can be confused with the radiographic features of parenchymal pulmonary disease, such as aspiration of meconium. **B**, In the child with a left-sided heart, the greater severity of pulmonary oedema on the right is explained by the presence of mixed totally anomalous pulmonary venous connection, with more severe obstruction of the right-sided pulmonary venous return. **C**, The increase in pulmonary vascularity is subtle but, in the presence of severe cyanosis, the absence of pulmonary oligaemia raises the suspicion of obstructed pulmonary venous return. **D**, This child has mild obstruction from totally anomalous pulmonary venous connection to a left superior caval vein.

venous drainage in short-axis sections of the abdomen taken just below the xiphisternum. This technique retains its value, but in addition, careful interrogation is required of the hepatic venous return. In the person with usual lateralised bodily arrangement, the inferior caval vein is identified to the right of the spine, with the aorta usually lying anterior and just to the left of the vertebral column (Fig. 22-21A). The venoatrial connections can then readily be demonstrated by rotating the transducer into the long axis and tracing the venous channel caudally, at the same time observing its connections with the hepatic veins. With usual atrial arrangement, the hepatic veins can be seen to join the inferior caval vein just proximal to its connection with the right atrium. The arrangement is mirror-imaged when the atrial appendages themselves show mirror-imagery (see Fig. 22-21B). In right isomerism, the aorta and the inferior caval vein are usually juxtaposed to the left or right of the spine, with the inferior caval vein found in anterolateral position (see Fig. 22-21C). The inferior caval vein receives all of the hepatic veins in the majority of patients.[6] In about one-fifth, bilateral hepatic venous drainage can be demonstrated. In patients with left isomerism, there is interruption of the inferior caval vein in approximately seven-tenths of cases. The abdominal venous return reaches the heart through the azygos or hemiazygos vein, which runs on the same side of the spine as the aorta but in a posterior position. This is easily demonstrated during short-axis scanning of the upper abdomen (see Fig. 22-21D). Hepatic venous return is markedly variable in the setting of left isomerism. The majority demonstrate a confluence to an atrium, but bilateral drainage of the hepatic veins to each atrium is also common.[6] Careful echocardiographic evaluation of the hepatic venous drainage is mandatory, therefore, in all patients suspected of having isomerism to aid in surgical planning for separation of the circulations. The precise connections cannot be inferred. Recognition of bilateral drainage will also aid in the preoperative planning of more complex cavopulmonary connections in candidates for the Fontan procedure.

More than one-half of patients with isomerism have bilateral superior caval veins.[6] When bilateral superior caval veins are found, colour flow imaging is helpful in establishing their precise point of junction with the atrium. In all patients with right isomerism, and in over half with left isomerism, bilateral superior caval venous drainage is directly to each atrial roof. In left isomerism, one superior caval vein can also drain through the coronary sinus. This finding is again readily made by cross sectional and colour flow imaging. Failure to identify bilateral drainage to the roof of each atrium will lead to severe desaturation if biventricular repair is performed without appropriate baffling of all systemic venous return to the appropriate atrium. The echocardiographic recognition of bilateral superior caval veins is also of importance for the majority of patients with isomerism in whom it is not possible to achieve biventricular repair. Increasingly, such patients undergo intermediate palliation by construction of a bidirectional superior cavopulmonary anastomosis prior to completion of the Fontan circulation.

Equally important is knowledge of pulmonary venous connections. If left isomerism is suspected, then bilateral drainage to each atrium can be anticipated in over half the hearts, with direct drainage to one or the other atrium in the remaining ones. This can usually be well demonstrated in subcostal and apical four-chamber views. The characteristic absence of obstruction to pulmonary venous return can be confirmed by colour flow and pulsed wave Doppler interrogation. In the setting of right isomerism, pulmonary venous drainage is more complex. Obstruction must be ruled out in each case irrespective of whether the pulmonary veins drain above or below the diaphragm. We have observed obstruction at the site of insertion of pulmonary veins directly to the superior caval vein, at the junction of a vertical vein to the brachiocephalic vein, and, of course, where drainage is infradiaphragmatic. Rarely, obstruction may even be observed with cardiac connection of the anomalous pulmonary venous return in right isomerism. A vertical vein can be compressed externally, and can take a retrobronchial path in right isomerism.[93] The principles of echocardiographic identification of anomalous pulmonary venous return, and recognition of its obstruction, are the same as for hearts with lateralised atriums (see Chapter 24). Despite the presence of decreased pulmonary blood flow in right isomerism, we have noted the characteristic disturbance of colour flow and pulsed Doppler in all patients that we have studied with obstructed pulmonary venous return.

In general, the evaluation of the intracardiac abnormalities poses few problems for the experienced echocardiographer. All the individual intracardiac anomalies seen in patients with isomeric atrial appendages have been observed in those with usual or mirror-imaged arrangement, and their echocardiographic features have been described in other chapters. These will not be discussed further here. It should be noted, nonetheless, that direct visualisation of the atrial appendages can still be difficult when using the transthoracic windows, albeit that it is

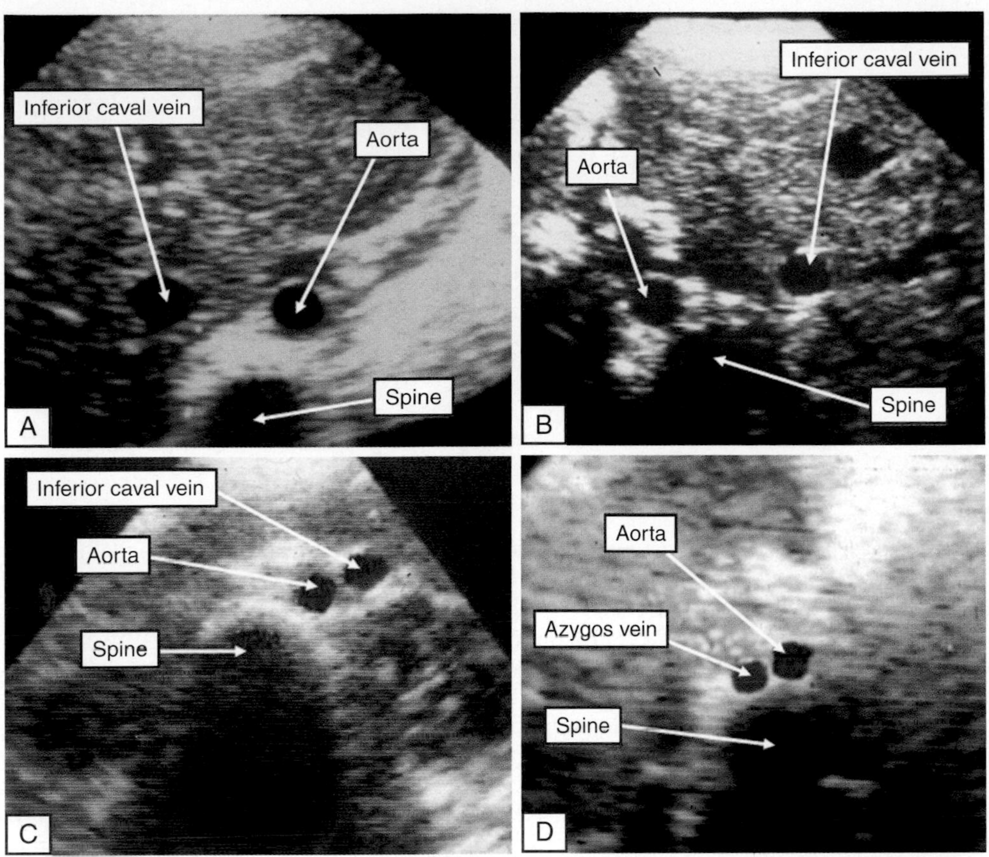

Figure 22-21 The typical arrangement of the great vessels, as seen in the echocardiographic short-axis view of the upper abdomen. **A,** The inferior caval vein is to the right (and slightly anterior) and the aorta to the left of the spine. This feature is an inferential guide to usual atrial arrangement. **B,** The opposite pattern is observed in mirror-image atrial arrangement, sometimes referred to as situs inversus. **C,** In this patient, the aorta and the inferior caval vein are both to the left of the spine, with the venous channel in anterior position. This is highly suggestive of right isomerism. **D,** The typical arrangement of the abdominal great vessels in left isomerism. The aorta and the venous channel are to the same side of the spine (compare with **C**), but now with the vein in posterior position. This is interruption of the inferior caval vein in the setting of left isomerism and the venous channel continues to the azygos venous system to the superior caval vein (see text for further discussion).

possible on occasion to recognise with certainty isomeric appendages of left morphology (Fig. 22-22). With transoesophageal echocardiography, it is possible better to visualise the atrial appendages, and to make direct assessment of their morphology, distinguishing the normal appendages one from the other (Fig. 22-23), and recognising isomeric appendages when present (Fig. 22-24). Due to its invasive nature, this is usually only performed if transthoracic echocardiography proves inadequate to make a comprehensive anatomical diagnosis. When performed, excellent visualisation of the atrial appendages is obtained from the oesophageal and gastric windows, allowing accurate determination of atrial arrangement.[94,95]

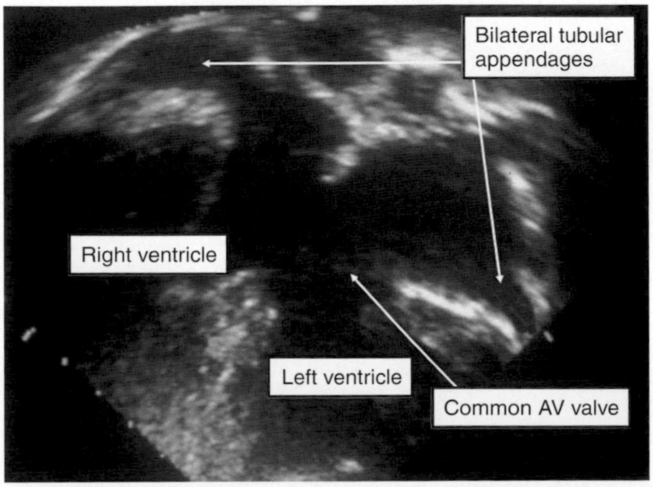

Figure 22-22 This precordial echocardiogram from a patient with atrioventricular septal defect and right hand ventricular topology reveals the presence of isomeric left atrial appendages. AV, atrioventricular.

Cardiac Catheterisation and Angiography

Echocardiography has obviated the need for cardiac catheterisation in the majority of neonates suspected as having isomerism of the atrial appendages. Cardiac catheterisation should be reserved for those rare instances in which echocardiographic interrogation has failed to provide the surgeon with sufficient information for planning of the initial palliative procedure. The operator should enter the catheterisation laboratory with specific questions in mind. It is not justified in the current era to perform a complete study on these sick infants if information sought has already been obtained by echocardiography. For example, if the source of pulmonary blood flow has not been adequately delineated in a neonate with right isomerism and pulmonary atresia, aortography will suffice to rule out systemic-to-pulmonary collateral arteries. The approach to catheterisation, therefore, will depend on the information required, and will be guided by the knowledge already obtained from the echocardiogram. In the presence of left isomerism with interrupted inferior caval vein, it may be easier to manoeuvre the catheter around the heart when access is obtained from the internal jugular vein. Access to the pulmonary arteries may be particularly awkward when catheterisation is performed from the femoral vein. This is because of the sharp angulation of the catheter as it passes from the azygos venous system to the superior

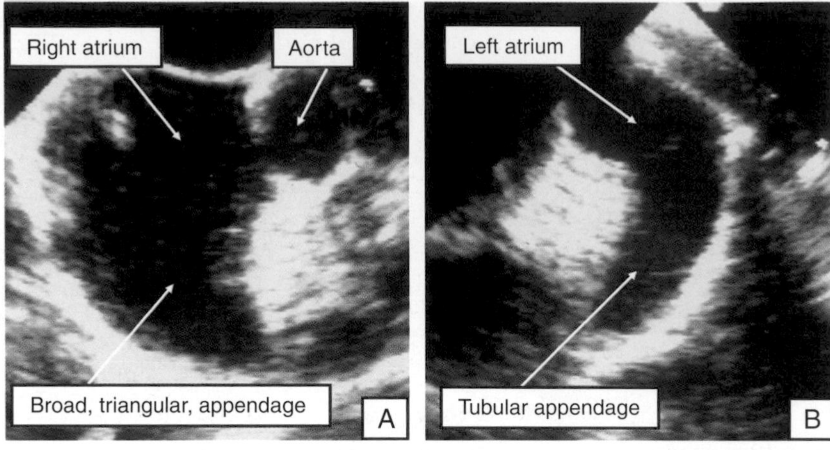

Figure 22-23 These transoesophageal images distinguish clearly the morphology of the right (A) as opposed to the left (B) atrial appendages.

caval vein and atrium (Fig. 22-25). In right isomerism, every attempt should be made to delineate the pulmonary venous connections if these have not been fully established non-invasively. This may be necessary when complex patterns of drainage are present, for example, mixed anomalous pulmonary venous connection. In practical terms, the site of drainage of pulmonary venous return is less important than the presence of obstruction in the setting of common mixing and decreased pulmonary blood flow. The initial palliation for the majority of these infants will be construction of a systemic-to-pulmonary shunt. Surgical attention to the pulmonary venous drainage will usually be required in the neonatal period only if obstruction is present. In right isomerism, the pulmonary trunk cannot usually be entered from the ventricular mass. Placement of a catheter across the arterial duct for the purposes of pulmonary arteriography is not advisable in the duct-dependent circulation. Ventriculography and aortography often provide poor visualisation of the pulmonary venous return. Whenever possible, therefore, the pulmonary venous channels should be entered directly via their site of drainage. This will allow direct angiography of the pulmonary venous pathways (Fig. 22-26). A more complete haemodynamic and angiographic evaluation of patients with isomeric atrial appendages is usually performed in preparation for further surgery sometime after the initial surgical palliation. Since many patients will be unsuitable for biventricular repair, attention will focus on those factors important for planning of partial or total cavopulmonary connections. Angiographic delineation of all systemic and pulmonary venous return should be completed at this time. In addition, selective injection of agitated saline in each pulmonary artery, combined with

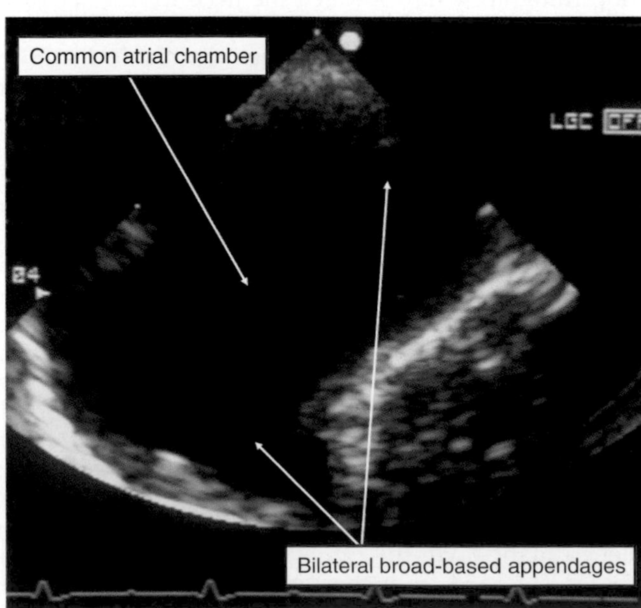

Figure 22-24 This transoesophageal image from a patient with double inlet right ventricle through a common atrioventricular valve shows broad-based morphologically right atrial appendages arising bilaterally from the common atrial chamber.

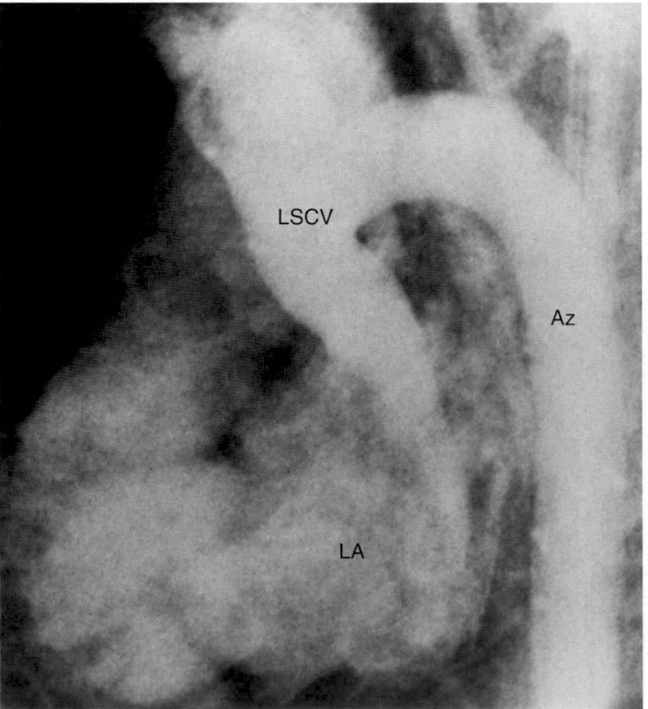

Figure 22-25 This lateral angiogram shows the characteristic features of interruption of the abdominal inferior caval vein, with continuation through the azygos (Az) venous system. The azygos vein is seen joining the left superior caval vein (LSCV), which drains to a morphological left atrium (LA).

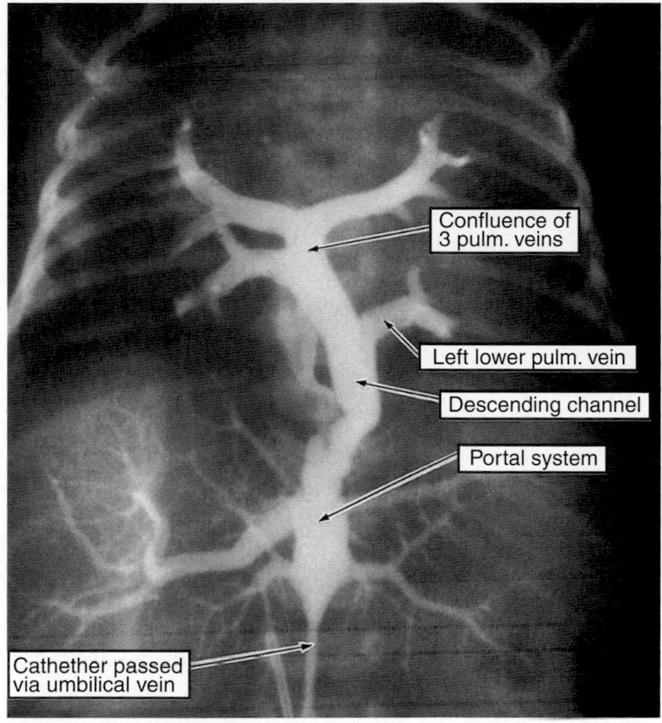

Figure 22-26 In this patient with right isomerism, it was possible to manoeuvre a catheter via the umbilical vein and the venous duct into the portal venous system to show totally anomalous infradiaphragmatic pulmonary venous connection.

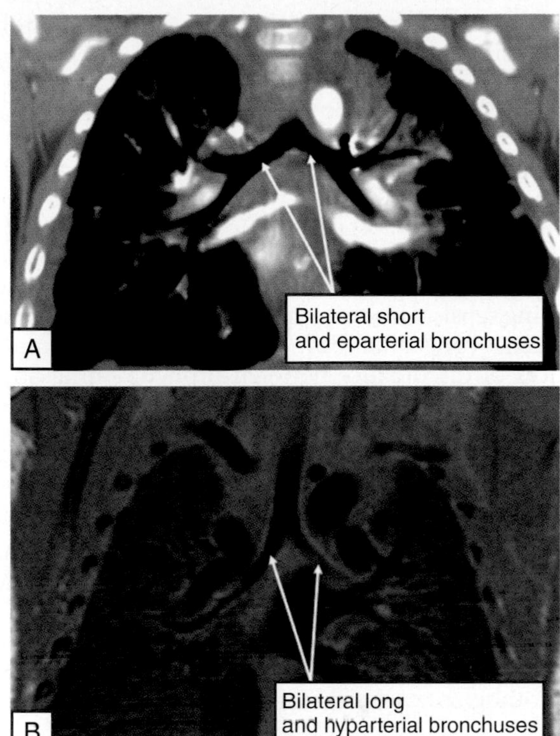

Figure 22-27 The magnetic resonance images show (**A**) the bilaterally short and eparterial bronchuses typical of right isomerism, and (**B**) the bilaterally long and hyparterial bronchuses, typical of left isomerism. (Courtesy of Dr Sameh Tadros, Children's Hospital of Pittsburgh, Pittsburgh, Pennsylvania).

cross sectional echocardiography, is prudent for all patients being staged towards cavopulmonary repair. This, along with determination of pulmonary venous oxyhaemoglobin saturation, will document the presence of pulmonary arterio-venous malformations. A detailed account of the angiographic evaluation of patients with isomerism has been provided by Freedom and colleagues.[96]

Magnetic Resonance Imaging

Resonance imaging can provide accurate delineation of the thoracic, cardiac, and vascular abnormalities seen in patients with isomeric appendages.[97–100] As might be anticipated, the technique is particularly good at demonstrating the presence of right (Fig. 22-27A) or left (see Fig. 22-27B) bronchial isomerism. It is also possible to recognise absence of the spleen (Fig. 22-28). We anticipate that the images should also reveal the presence of bilaterally symmetrical appendages of either right or left morphology, particularly when taking note of the presence or absence of venous channels within the atrioventricular junctions. As well as revealing the patterns of coronary venous return, the technique is also able to demonstrate the specific patterns of systemic and pulmonary venous return. In the setting of cyanotic disease, magnetic resonance imaging can provide details of the sources of flow of blood to the lungs, and the anatomy and size of the pulmonary arteries. Resonance imaging may be particularly useful in obviating the need for cardiac catheterisation in critically sick infants prior to initial surgical intervention.[100] It also provides confirmation of splenic morphology, if present. Serial imaging may prove very useful during long-term follow-up and prior to

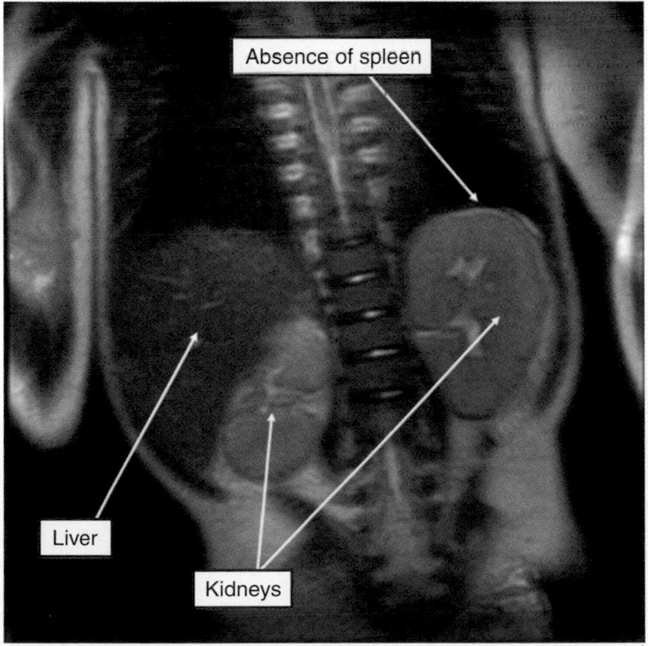

Figure 22-28 This magnetic resonance image shows absence of the spleen in a patient known to have isomeric right atrial appendages. (Courtesy of Dr Sameh Tadros, Children's Hospital of Pittsburgh, Pittsburgh, Pennsylvania.)

each planned surgical intervention. Computed tomography may also be useful in the non-invasive evaluation of children with heterotaxy syndromes.[101] The exposure to radiation is a disadvantage compared to resonance imaging, especially for serial studies and rapid heart rates complicate the acquisition of good images.

Investigation of Splenic State

The presence of multiple spleens is an anatomical curiosity of little clinical significance, and splenic function is generally preserved. The absence of the spleen (see Fig. 22-28), or severe splenic hypoplasia, in contrast, is of major clinical importance, since this results in increased risk of overwhelming sepsis. This risk appears greatest when absence of the spleen is congenital.[102] Since there are many documented instances of discordance between bronchio-atrial arrangement and splenic state, all infants with suspected isomerism should undergo evaluation for possible absence of the spleen.[103] In the absence of a spleen, Howell–Jolly bodies are usually present on a smear of peripheral blood. Their presence is highly suggestive of asplenia.[104,105] On occasion, these bodies can be found in the blood of patients with normal spleens,[106] especially in the neonatal period.[107] A variety of imaging modalities has been reported to be useful in the identification of asplenia.[103] These include cross sectional echocardiography,[107] radionuclide scintigraphy,[108] and computed tomography or magnetic resonance imaging.[100,109]

MANAGEMENT

The treatment of patients with isomerism will be determined by the nature and severity of the associated cardiac and extracardiac lesions. Some patients with left isomerism may have no additional cardiac lesions, and they will require no treatment. Patients with left isomerism in general have less severe cardiac malformations than those with right isomerism and, hence, more chance of corrective surgery. Those with right isomerism usually require palliative surgery in the neonatal period, and very few will progress to biventricular repair. Cardiac interventions, therefore, will be geared towards subsequent completion of the Fontan circulation. It is axiomatic, nonetheless, that patients are treated on their own merits.

Medical Management

Many infants with right or left isomerism will present severely ill as a result of duct-dependent congenital cardiac disease. The severely cyanotic infant will usually have right isomerism with severe obstruction in the pulmonary outflow tract. These patients are usually easily stabilised by treatment with prostaglandin E_1. When there is associated severe obstruction to pulmonary venous return, no medical therapy other than standard supportive measures will help, and early surgery is indicated. Preoperative stabilisation with extracorporeal membrane oxygenation has been recommended by some groups. Left isomerism is most likely to present in the neonatal period when there is severe obstruction of the left heart. Cardiac failure and shock are managed in the standard fashion as for severe left-sided obstruction with usual atrial arrangement. Occasionally, hydropic fetuses with left isomerism, severe bradycardia, and severe atrioventricular valvar regurgitation will survive to term. This constellation of findings is usually lethal. It is questionable whether attempts at emergency pacing are worthwhile, especially when there is associated complex cardiac disease.

Since neonates with isomerism are generally referred early in life to tertiary centres, the paediatric cardiologist often must to assume responsibility for complete evaluation of the infant. As we have stressed, isomerism is a fundamental disorder of lateralisation, and is often associated with important extracardiac abnormalities. Careful evaluation of all systems is mandatory before referral for cardiac surgery. Renal ultrasound is probably warranted on a routine basis because of the high incidence of abnormalities of the renal tracts, as is cerebral ultrasound. Routine abdominal ultrasound, with focus on the biliary tree, is warranted even in the absence of jaundice in infants with left isomerism, since early diagnosis of extrahepatic biliary atresia will strongly influence overall management of these infants. Persistent vomiting in the neonatal period should raise the suspicion of upper gastrointestinal obstruction owing to duodenal atresia or compression. All families should be told of the risk of late intestinal obstruction caused by gastrointestinal malrotation or gastric volvulus.[110–112]

As already discussed, the state of the spleen should be established in all patients. When right isomerism is diagnosed, the presence of Howell–Jolly bodies on the peripheral blood film suffices to make a presumptive diagnosis of asplenia. If Howell–Jolly bodies are not observed, absence of the spleen should still be assumed until imaging studies have confirmed its presence. When left isomerism is diagnosed, the absence of Howell–Jolly bodies on several blood films can be considered as adequate evidence of functioning splenic tissue, and routine radionuclide scintigraphy or computed tomography are not warranted. When congenital absence of the spleen is diagnosed, there is a lifelong risk of overwhelming infection. Although infection is most commonly caused by polysaccharide-encapsulated bacteria, such as *Streptococcus pneumoniae* and *Haemophilus influenzae,* infection with Gram-negative organisms may predominate in the first 6 months of life.[110] When septicaemia develops in the asplenic patient with congenital cardiac disease, the clinical course is often fulminant.[113,114] The family members of such infants should be made aware of the risk of fatal sepsis, and should seek medical attention early when fevers develop so that blood cultures can be drawn and antibiotics started if there is no clear evidence of viral illness. Prophylactic antibiotics should be given from the time of diagnosis. Amoxicillin is often recommended for the first 5 years, after which time penicillin can be substituted. This should be continued for life. Pneumococcal vaccine should be given, although its immunogenicity in this setting is unclear.[115] Conjugate vaccines for *Haemophilus influenzae* type b do appear to be effective in patients with congenital asplenia.[116] This should be given in infancy according to standard protocols.[117] Whenever possible, immunogenicity of polysaccharide vaccines should be confirmed serologically.

Surgical Management

All cardiac operative procedures for patients with isomerism are palliative in nature, since normal anatomy is never achieved, and late complications, such as disturbances of rhythm, may develop. Recent experience in Osaka, nonetheless, shows that surgical results are improving, albeit better in those with left compared to right isomerism (Fig. 22-29). In this section, we use the term corrective for those procedures that result in complete, or near complete, separation of the circulations. Approximately two-thirds of patients

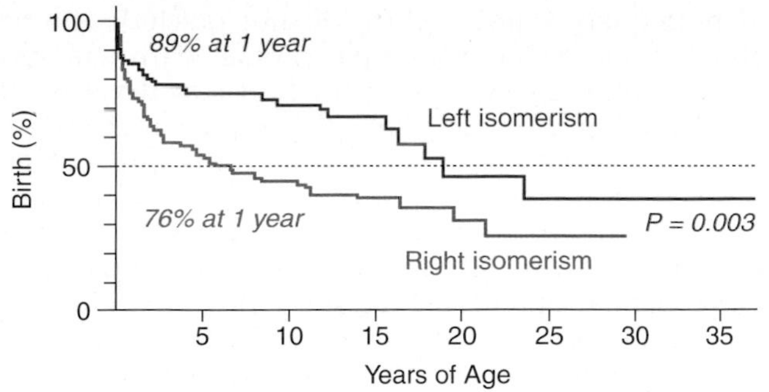

Figure 22-29 The graph shows the results of surgical treatment at the National Cardiovascular Centre, Osaka, Japan, for patients with left as compared with right isomerism.

with left isomerism have anatomy suitable for biventricular repair. Most commonly such patients have atrioventricular septal defects, with anomalies of systemic and pulmonary venous return, but with concordant ventriculo-arterial connections. Repair is achieved using standard techniques with appropriate baffling of anomalous venous return.[118,119] After biventricular repair, however, it is frequent to encounter progressive valvar regurgitation, particularly across the left atrioventricular valve. This often results in the need for reoperation, as does recurrent subaortic stenosis, which is commoner in those with left isomerism than in the setting of usual atrial arrangement. In the recent experience at Osaka, one-fifth of patients undergoing repair of atrioventricular septal defect in the setting of left isomerism required reoperation on the left atrioventricular valve, and one-sixth needed further surgery to the left ventricular outflow tract. In contrast, reoperation was necessary for 7% of those having usual atrial arrangement, and only for repair of the left atrioventricular valve. These differences were highly statistically significant, and reflect the subtle morphologic variations found in those with left isomerism.[120]

The anomalies observed in right isomerism are rarely amenable to biventricular repair, even when two well-balanced ventricles are present. Rare reports of biventricular repair of right isomerism do exist.[121–124] Almost all patients with right isomerism, and many patients with left isomerism, will require initial surgical palliation in the neonatal period or during early infancy. Corrective procedures may be possible at a later date in selected patients. Little data is available to indicate what proportion of newborn infants with isomerism will go on to achieve complete separation of the systemic and pulmonary circulations.

In right isomerism, the initial need is usually to increase the flows of blood to the lungs. Placement of a systemic-to-pulmonary shunt should only be performed when it is certain that there is no obstruction to pulmonary venous return. We believe that careful evaluation of the patient, taking note of the chest radiograph and the echocardiogram, should allow for the preoperative diagnosis of obstructed pulmonary venous return. This should avoid the high mortality that will occur when shunts are constructed in the presence of undiagnosed obstructed pulmonary venous return.[78–80] When obstruction to pulmonary venous return is present, the outcome is much less favourable, even if the diagnosis is made prior to construction of the shunt.[79] This reflects the difficult post-operative course of patients undergoing combined repair of obstructed pulmonary veins with construction of a systemic-to-pulmonary shunt under cardiopulmonary bypass. This combination was traditionally considered lethal, and many infants were not offered surgery. More recently, successful initial palliation has been achieved by creating an anastomosis between the pulmonary venous confluence and the atrium, and constructing a systemic-to-pulmonary arterial shunt.[125] There is some evidence for improving outcomes with this constellation, although long-term outcomes appear poor. Note should also be taken of the fact that, in those with right isomerism, one-tenth have mixed totally anomalous pulmonary venous connections. If unrecognised, this can also complicate the post-operative course.

The palliative procedures required for neonates and infants with left isomerism are diverse and reflect the highly variable anatomy. Some infants present with complex disease associated with subpulmonary obstruction. They are initially managed by construction of a systemic-to-pulmonary shunt as for those with right isomerism. In other patients, a univentricular atrioventricular connection may be associated with unobstructed pulmonary blood flow, and banding of the pulmonary trunk may be indicated. More commonly, complex left heart obstruction may be present. When this is associated with left ventricular hypoplasia, severe subaortic stenosis or a diminutive aorta, a neonatal Norwood approach will be required if palliation is to be attempted. This will not be feasible if there is significant regurgitation of the common atrioventricular valve.

For almost all patients with right isomerism, and for many with left isomerism, biventricular repair will not be feasible, and all palliations are then staging procedures towards a Fontan-type repair. Increasingly, patients with isomerism will be staged via one or more intermediate procedures, usually involving a superior cavopulmonary anastomosis or its physiological equivalent, the hemi-Fontan procedure. When bilateral superior caval veins are present, bilateral bidirectional superior cavopulmonary anastomoses are performed. It has been argued that bidirectional superior cavopulmonary connection, augmented by an additional small source of pulsatile flow to the lungs, may be the optimal final procedure for selected patients with isomerism, who are at high risk for completion of a total cavopulmonary connection.[126] When there is interruption of the inferior caval vein, bidirectional superior cavopulmonary anastomosis will result in all systemic venous return being diverted to the lungs except for that returning from the hepatic veins, which drains directly to the atrium. This procedure, the so-called Kawashima operation,[127] has been widely used in patients with left isomerism. In many respects, the end result is similar to completion of the fenestrated Fontan circulation incorporating a fenestration. The early clinical course is usually excellent. Important late problems, nonetheless, have been observed. First, venovenous collaterals may develop between the systemic venous system above the diaphragm, which is at relatively high pressure, and the low pressure hepatic venous system below the diaphragm. This can result in steal of desaturated blood away from the lungs to the hepatic veins, and then to the atrium. This can then result in progressive cyanosis.[128] A similar phenomenon has been observed when large venous collaterals drain from the inferior caval vein through the liver to the hepatic veins, diverting systemic venous blood to the pulmonary venous atrium, and away from the lungs.[129] Such a right-to-left shunt from the inferior caval vein can also occur in right isomerism after completion of the Fontan circuit if any hepatic vein remains draining to the low pressure pulmonary venous atrium.[130] A second cause of progressive cyanosis after the Kawashima procedure is the development of pulmonary arterio-venous malformations. Patients with multiple spleens and left isomerism seem particularly prone to this complication.[131,132] There is increasing evidence that a hepatic factor may be important in preventing this development.[133] We believe that the indications for the original Kawashima procedure require careful re-evaluation. Whenever possible, the hepatic venous return should be diverted to the pulmonary arteries via a baffle or conduit should a bidirectional superior cavopulmonary anastomosis be performed beyond infancy in patients with interruption of the inferior caval vein. Thus, it is better to achieve the Fontan circulation in one-stage primary fashion, or in two stages with a short interval between them. An alternative surgical technique, recently described, is to combine the Kawashima procedure with a direct connection of the hepatic veins to the azygos venous system.[134] Late incorporation of the hepatic venous return to the pulmonary arteries after development of pulmonary arterio-venous malformations has been shown to result in their regression, and relief of cyanosis.[135,136]

The almost universal presence of anomalies of venoatrial connections creates extra problems for complete separation of the systemic and pulmonary circulations. Cardiac surgeons, nonetheless, have risen to the challenge, and it is now technically feasible to achieve this separation in almost all cases. A variety of novel modifications of the total cavopulmonary connection have been devised to achieve this result.[137–139] Introduction of the extracardiac conduit technique for construction of the Fontan circuit has particular benefits for this group of patients with anomalies of systemic and pulmonary venous return, since the need for complex intra-atrial baffles and tunnels is obviated.[140] Initial results of the Fontan procedure in patients with isomerism were significantly inferior to those for patients with lateralised arrangement undergoing similar procedures.[141,142] In recent years, a number of groups have reported significantly improved results.[125,140,143–145] Careful pre-operative delineation of anatomy, improved selection of patients, enhanced surgical experience, newer surgical techniques, and improved post-operative care probably account for the improved outcomes.[146]

When attempting to complete the Fontan circulation by means of a total cavopulmonary connection, another compromising factor is the orientation of the ventricular apex relative to the junction between the inferior caval vein and the atrial chambers. When the apex is juxtaposed to the cavo-atrial junction, the channel to be reconstructed towards the pulmonary arteries needs to be placed so as to avoid compression by the ventricular mass. Particular care is required in design of the channel in presence of independent drainage of the hepatic veins. It is always possible successfully to complete the Fontan circulation, but surgeons must take care to avoid the various potential anatomical pitfalls.

Transplantation has also been advocated as an option for treatment for selected infants and children.[147,148] This would seem most appropriate when other palliative procedures are contraindicated. This might include infants with severe atrioventricular valvar regurgitation associated with complex cardiac disease. Complex anomalies of systemic and pulmonary venous return do not preclude the possibility of successful orthotopic cardiac transplantation, though pulmonary venous obstruction may develop after transplantation.[147] There is insufficient data at the present time to know how absence of the spleen will impact on the occurrence of rejection and infection. The main limitation to transplantation for this group of infants is the low availability of donors. Furthermore, there is growing evidence that neonatal recipients are not immune from lethal long-term complications of transplantation, in particular the development of coronary arterial disease.[149]

PROGNOSIS

It is hard to define the prognosis for infants with isomerism, since there is little longitudinal follow-up data. The natural history for patients presenting in infancy is very poor, with death occurring in the majority in the first year of life.[38] Surgical reports provide limited information about overall prognosis, since patients are preselected as suitable surgical candidates. Longitudinal population-based studies are required to assess outcome from presentation through all stages of surgical reconstruction. They must include all causes of death, whether cardiac or non-cardiac.[17]

Recent advances in medical management, and in particular the improvements in cardiac surgical skills and techniques occurring throughout the world, are likely to result in improvement in survival for these infants. Key factors limiting success at this time are the presence of moderate or greater atrioventricular valvar regurgitation, generally with a common atrioventricular valve, and the development or persistence of recurrent obstruction of a pulmonary venous confluence, or instrinsic pulmonary venous stenosis, after initial surgical palliation.[150] There is also a high incidence of atrial arrhythmias in this population, both early and late after completion of the Fontan circulation.[144,145,151] As would be expected, ongoing attrition and morbidity among these children can be anticipated late after conversion to Fontan physiology.[140–146] Encouragingly, though, the Pediatric Heart Network of the National Heart, Lung, and Blood Institute of the National Institutes of Health has recently shown that exercise performance, and functional state of health, are comparable between those surviving with the Fontan circulation irrespective of the presence or absence of heterotaxy.[152] While surgical data suggests improving outcomes, nonetheless, other findings continue to suggest an overall poor prognosis for infants with isomerism when evaluated from the time of birth.[17,153] These disorders remain one of the greatest challenges for paediatric cardiologists and congenital cardiovascular surgeons.[154]

The complete reference list can be found on the companion Expert Consult web site at www.expertconsult.com.

ANNOTATED REFERENCES

- Ivemark B: Implications of agenesis of the spleen in the pathogenesis of conotruncus anomalies in childhood: An analysis of the heart; malformations in the splenic agenesis syndrome, with 14 new cases. Acta Paediatr Scand 1955;44(Suppl 104):1–110.

  This landmark paper was one of the first to recognise the association between splenic status, complex congenital cardiac disease, and abnormal arrangement of the viscera, focusing on the tendency to symmetry, hence, his description of 'asplenia, a teratologic syndrome of visceral symmetry'.

- Putschar WGJ, Mannion WC: Congenital absence of the spleen and associated anomalies. Am J Clin Pathol 1956;26:429–470.

In the year following Ivemark's landmark study, Putschar and Mannion provided further evidence of the entities that we now call left and right isomerism. They referred to a 'symmetrical situs [that] sometimes exists, exhibiting symmetrical rightness or leftness on both sides'. Although terminology has evolved, this is probably the most eloquent description of isomerism in the historical literature.

- Van Mierop LHS, Wiglesworth FW: Isomerism of the cardiac atria in the asplenia syndrome. Lab Invest 1962;11:1303–1315.

  This study was the first carefully to describe the presence of two appendages both of right-sided morphology, along with duplication of sinus nodes. This confirmed the reality of isomerism of the atrial appendages.

- Moller JH, Nakib A, Anderson RC, Edwards JE: Congenital cardiac disease associated with polysplenia: A developmental complex of bilateral 'left-sidedness.' Circulation 1967;36:789–799.

  This report was the first to describe in a large number of patients the relationship between the presence of multiple spleens, congenital cardiac disease, and the presence of left isomerism, which they described as bilateral left-sidedness.

- Uemura H, Ho SY, Devine WA, Anderson RH: Analysis of visceral heterotaxy according to splenic status, appendage morphology, or both. Am J Cardiol 1995;76:846–849.
- Uemura H, Ho SY, Devine WA, et al: Atrial appendages and venoatrial connections in hearts from patients with visceral heterotaxy. Ann Thorac Surg 1995;60:561–569.

  These two reports are from a series of carefully performed studies that define the spectrum of morphology in hearts from patients with visceral heterotaxy. The authors emphasise that it is the arrangement and extent of the pectinate muscles that is the most constant feature of the morphology of the appendages, permitting distinction of the appendages as being of left or right morphology. The reports also provide precise details of venoatrial arrangements, and emphasise that cardiac morphology should not be inferred from splenic status.

- Layton WM, Jr: Heart malformations in mice homozygous for a gene causing situs inversus. Birth Defects Orig Artic Ser 1978;14:277–293.

  This report describes the first vertebrate animal model of abnormal lateralisation to be studied in detail. Initially it was thought to be a model of mirror-imaged arrangement, or so-called situs inversus.

- Seo J-W, Brown NA, Ho SY, Anderson RH: Abnormal laterality and congenital cardiac anomalies: Relations of visceral and cardiac morphologies in the iv/iv mouse. Circulation 1992;86:642–650.

  This was the first detailed evaluation of the cardiovascular anomalies in the iv/iv mouse model of abnormal lateralisation. Contrary to prior reports, the authors observed that some animals had clear evidence of isomeric atrial appendages, either left or right, and associated cardiac and venous abnormalities. This demonstrated that the iv/iv model is more complex than a model of usual and mirror-imaged atrial arrangement.

- Kawashima Y, Kitamura S, Matsuda H, et al: Total cavopulmonary shunt operation in complex cardiac anomalies: A new operation. J Thorac Cardiovasc Surg 1984;87:74–81.

  The initial description by Kawashima and colleagues of four patients with azygos or hemiazygos continuation of the inferior caval vein who underwent a direct superior caval-to-pulmonary artery anastomosis. This operation has been widely used in patients with left isomerism as definitive repair. Although the early results are generally very good, serious late complications include veno-venous collaterals draining from above the diaphragm to the hepatic veins, and the development of pulmonary arterio-venous malformations. Both complications have led to late severe cyanosis.

- McElhinney DB, Kreutzer J, Lang P, et al: Incorporation of the hepatic veins into the cavopulmonary circulation in patients with heterotaxy and pulmonary arteriovenous malformations after a Kawashima procedure. Ann Thorac Surg 2005;80:1597–1603.

  The largest report to date emphasising that incorporation of the hepatic veins into the cavopulmonary circulation can reverse pulmonary arteriovenous malformations after the Kawashima procedure. This provides further evidence for a hepatic factor.

- Bartz PJ, Driscoll DJ, Dearani JA, et al: Early and late results of the modified Fontan operation for heterotaxy syndrome: 30 years of experience in 142 patients. J Am Coll Cardiol 2006;48:2301–2305.

  A recent large single-centre review of outcomes after the Fontan procedure for patients with heterotaxy, emphasising improving outcomes in the modern era.

- Atz AM, Cohen MS, Sleeper LA, et al, for the Investigators of the Pediatric Heart Network: Functional state of patients with heterotaxy syndrome following the Fontan operation. Cardiol Young 2007;17(Suppl 2):44–53.

  The first study to address functional state and quality of life issues after construction of the Fontan circulation in patients with visceral heterotaxy. Atrial arrhythmias were more common in the patients with heterotaxy. Exercise performance, and results from health state questionnaires, did not differ between patients with and without heterotaxy.

- Freedom RM, Jaeggi ET, Lim JS, Anderson RH: Hearts with isomerism of the right atrial appendages—one of the worst forms of disease in 2005. Cardiol Young 2005;15:554–567.

  This review by the late Robert Freedom and his colleagues emphasises how prognosis remains very poor for patients with right isomerism, despite improved surgical outcomes in some reports. The review emphasises that outcomes are best assessed from population data, starting from the time of birth, or even from time of diagnosis in fetal life. Surgical series may distort true outcomes by analysis of highly selected populations, such as those deemed suitable for conversion to the Fontan circulation.

CHAPTER 23

Anomalous Systemic Venous Return

JEFFREY F. SMALLHORN and ROBERT H. ANDERSON

In this chapter, we deal with abnormalities of position and connection of the major systemic venous channels that drain to the heart, and also with abnormal persistence of the valves of the embryonic systemic venous sinus. Many of these anomalies are incidental findings, having little haemodynamic significance. They may, however, complicate interventional procedures, and they may be associated with other more important congenital cardiac anomalies. A consideration of the morphogenesis of the normal systemic venous system is helpful in understanding the wide variety of systemic venous anomalies that exist. We will review briefly the presumed embryology of the systemic venous system, therefore, before considering the individual anomalies and their clinical significance.

MORPHOGENESIS OF THE SYSTEMIC VENOUS SYSTEM

Normal venous development is a process of progressive appearance of a series of paired venous structures, development of anastomotic channels between them, and the eventual selective regression of certain segments. The systemic venous tributaries are initially bilaterally symmetrical. They join together on each side, opening to the developing heart tube through paired channels known as the sinus horns. When first seen joining the developing atrium (Fig. 23-1), there are no anatomical landmarks that permit distinction of a separate segment as a sinus venosus, such as exists in the hearts of lower vertebrates.[1] Initially, three major venous channels drain into each horn, namely the omphalomesenteric or vitelline veins medially, the umbilical veins in the middle, and the common cardinal veins laterally (Fig. 23-2). Each common cardinal vein is formed by the union of the superior and inferior cardinal veins, which drain the cephalic and caudal regions of the embryo, respectively. Concomitant with development of anastomotic channels between the right- and left-sided venous channels formed throughout the embryo, there is preferential flow to the right-sided structures. The left horn then rotates beneath the atrioventricular junction, moving around the fulcrum provided by the developing pulmonary vein, so as to open in the right side of the developing atrial component of the heart tube (Fig. 23-3). It is only at this stage, which is also the period of initial formation of the primary atrial septum, that it becomes possible to recognise the valvar structures marking the junction between the systemic venous tributaries and the developing morphologically right atrial chamber. These structures serve as the valves of the systemic venous sinus, and are often described simply as the venous valves (see Fig. 23-3). There then follows gradual regression of the left-sided vitelline and cardinal veins, with increasing prominence of the right sinus horn. Eventually, the entirety of the systemic venous sinus within the confines of the valves becomes incorporated as the smooth-walled venous component of the morphologically right atrium, with the opening of the right common cardinal vein becoming the orifice of the superior caval vein, and that of the right vitelline vein becoming the entrance of the inferior caval vein. The mouth of the left sinus horn then persists as the orifice of the coronary sinus (Fig. 23-4).

The initial anastomotic connection between the right and left cranial cardinal veins enlarges, and becomes the left brachiocephalic vein, often illogically termed the innominate vein. What is the purpose of having an unnamed vein? In the process of normal development, the left superior cardinal vein below this point gradually regresses, with its remnant forming the ligament and oblique vein of Marshall (Fig. 23-5). With ongoing development, there are further changes in the valves of the systemic venous sinus. The right-sided valve is prominent during embryonic life, while the left valve is less prominent, eventually fusing with the atrial septum. The right valve subsequently also regresses

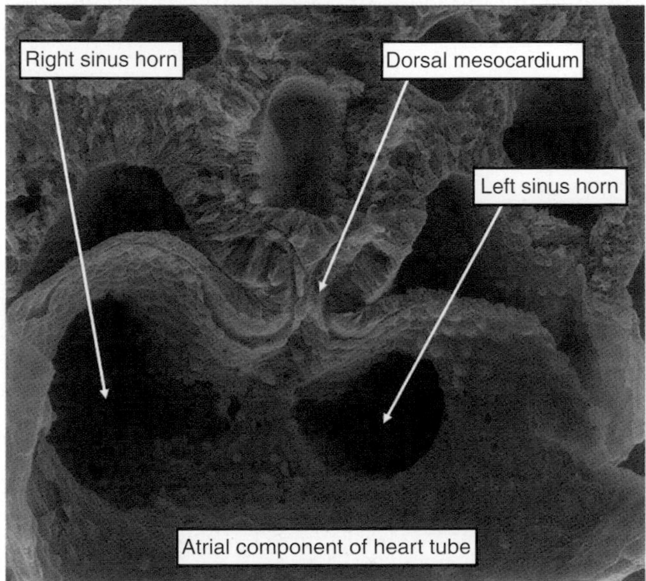

Figure 23-1 This scanning electron micrograph shows the developing atrial component of the mouse heart. Already the left sinus horn is diminished in size relative to the right horn, but no discrete structures mark the junction of the systemic venous tributaries with the heart. Note also that, as yet, there is no canalisation of the pulmonary vein within the dorsal mesocardium, nor indeed any formation of the lungs. (Courtesy of Professor Nigel Brown, St George's Medical University, London, United Kingdom.)

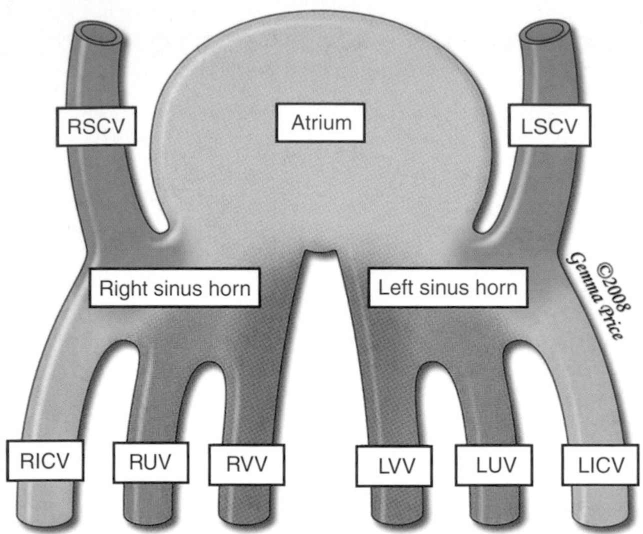

Figure 23-2 The cartoon shows the initial arrangement of the venous channels draining via the sinus horns to the atrial component of the developing heart. LICV, left inferior caval vein; LSCV, left superior caval vein; LUV, left umbilical vein; LVV, left vitelline vein; RICV, right inferior caval vein; RSCV, right superior caval vein; RUV, right umbilical vein; RVV, right vitelline vein.

for its most part, except for portions which persist as folds related to the orifices of the inferior caval vein, the Eustachian valve, and the coronary sinus, the Thebesian valve.

The development of the pulmonary venous system is also of significance, considering the occasional co-existence of anomalies of pulmonary and systemic venous drainage. The developing lungs are derived from the primitive foregut. They share their early vascular supply with the gut via a splanchic plexus.[2] This plexus initially drains the intraparenchymal pulmonary tissues to the cardinal venous system. With normal development, these connections are lost as the pulmonary vein itself canalises in the dorsal mesocardium and gains entrance to the developing morphologically left atrium.[3]

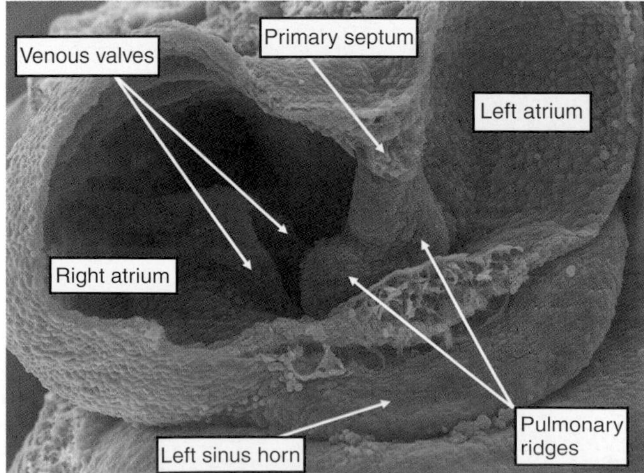

Figure 23-3 This scanning electron micrograph shows the developing right atrium subsequent to incorporation of the systemic venous sinus and formation of the venous valves. It shows the course of the left sinus horn through the developing left atrioventricular junction. The pulmonary ridges can also be seen at the base of the primary atrial septum, albeit that the opening of the solitary pulmonary vein between them is not visible. (Courtesy of Professor Nigel Brown, St George's Medical University, London, United Kingdom.)

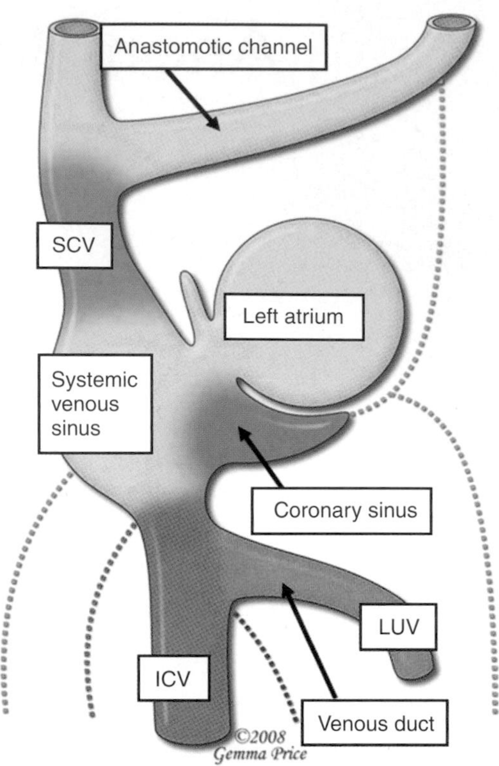

Figure 23-4 The cartoon shows the arrangement of the systemic venous tributaries subsequent to the formation of the anastomoses that permit the systemic venous sinus to become incorporated into the right side of the developing atrial component of the heart tube. ICV, inferior caval vein; LUV, left umbilical vein; SCV, superior caval vein.

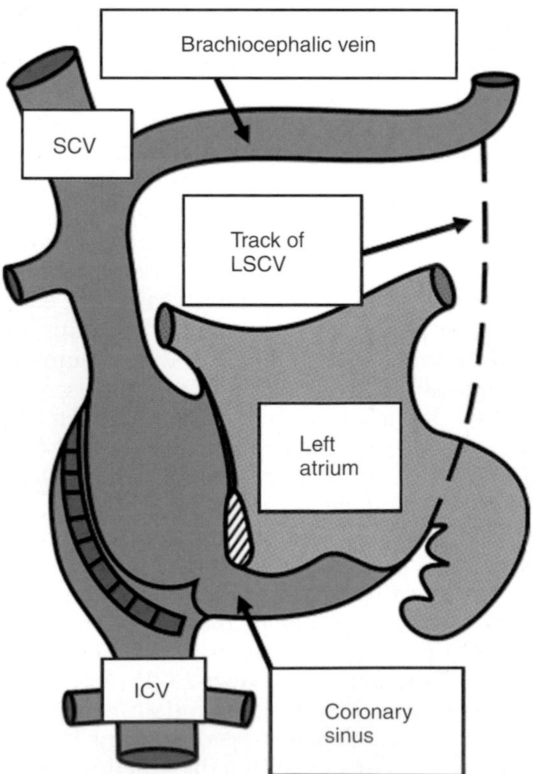

Figure 23-5 The cartoon shows the initial course of the left-sided cardinal vein draining to the left sinus horn. As shown, this channel usually regresses, but can persist as the left superior caval vein (LSCV). Its remnant in the posterior wall of the left atrium is the oblique vein and the ligament of Marshall. ICV, inferior caval vein; SCV, superior caval vein.

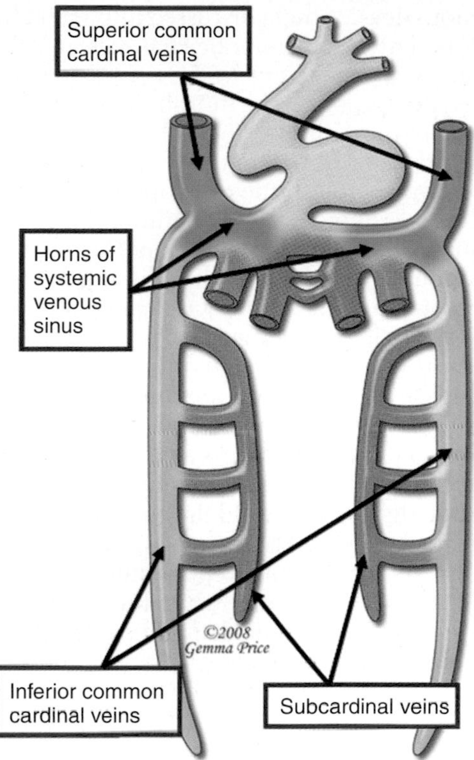

Figure 23-6 The cartoon shows the formation of the subcardinal venous system, which initially drains bilaterally into the cardinal system of veins.

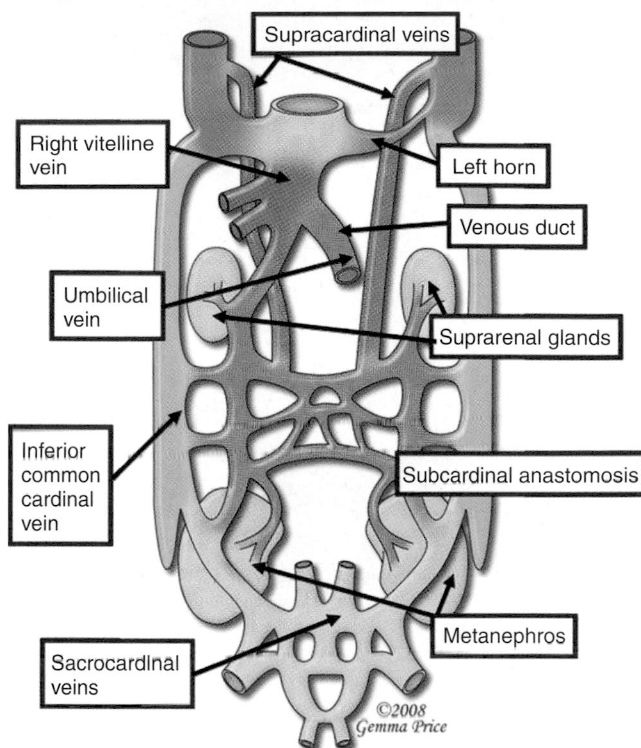

Figure 23-7 Formation of the subcardinal anastomotic channels, and the sacrocardinal plexus, which contribute to formation of the renal and suprarenal venous systems along with the abdominal inferior caval vein. Note also, however, the formation of the supracardinal venous system, which forms anastomotic channels between the subcardinal and common cardinal systems within the developing thorax.

Initially, therefore, there are three systemic venous systems developing within the embryo, namely the vitelline, umbilical, and cardinal systems (see Fig. 23-2). The vitelline system largely becomes a vascular network draining the liver. These channels are predominant on the right side of the embryo, maintaining their connection to the right side of the systemic venous sinus through structures known as the hepatocardiac channels. As we have seen, it is the right-sided vitelline vein that ultimately becomes the terminal post-hepatic portion of the inferior caval vein (see Fig. 23-4). The umbilical veins are also paired structures when first seen. They lose their connection to the venous sinus, and anastomose to the hepatic sinusoids. The right-sided umbilical vein then regresses, while the left umbilical vein enlarges to become the only channel bringing blood from the placenta to the embryo, forming an anastomosis with the hepatocardiac channel which becomes the venous duct.

Further important changes occur within the developing abdominal region of the embryo that underscore normal and anomalous formation of the inferior caval vein. By the fifth week of gestation, paired subcardinal veins arise medial to the inferior cardinal veins, serving initially to drain the forming urogenital sinuses. When traced cranially, these subcardinal veins empty into the caudal cardinal veins on both sides (Fig. 23-6). Anastomotic channels then develop between the two subcardinal veins, as well as between the right subcardinal and hepatocardiac channels. It is the right subcardinal vein that becomes predominant, developing into the infrahepatic segment of the inferior caval vein, and joining this segment to the right vitelline vein, which forms the entrance to the morphologically right atrium. With continued growth of the trunk of the embryo, yet another system of veins, the sacrocardinal veins, arises dorsal and caudal to the inferior cardinal system. Anastomotic channels between the subcardinal and sacrocardinal systems on the right side will form the renal segment of the inferior caval vein, while the distal portions of the right sacrocardinal vein enlarge and become its most inferior portion (Fig. 23-7).

Concomitant with these developments of the paracardinal systems, and apart from their most proximal portions, the inferior cardinal veins themselves gradually involute. This involution occurs concomitant with the transformation of the supracardinal venous system into the azygos and hemiazygos veins on the right and left sides, respectively, which terminate cranially in the right cardinal venous system (Fig. 23-8). The definitive inferior caval vein, therefore, has multiple embryological origins. Its terminal suprahepatic portion is derived from the right vitelline vein. The infrahepatic segment arises from the right subcardinal vein, the intermediate segment from the anastomotic channels initially developed between the subcardinal and sacrocardinal veins, and the most inferior segment from the right sacrocardinal vein. The azygos and hemiazygos veins are derived from the supracardinal system (Fig. 23-9). Should there be abnormal development of these multiple abdominal venous channels, it is possible for the supracardinal venous system to become dominant. This then results in the venous return from the lower abdomen returning through the azygos system of veins to either the right- or left-sided superior caval vein. The inferior caval vein is then itself interrupted between the abdominal and hepatic segments, the hepatic segment draining only the blood from the liver and the portal venous system back to the heart.

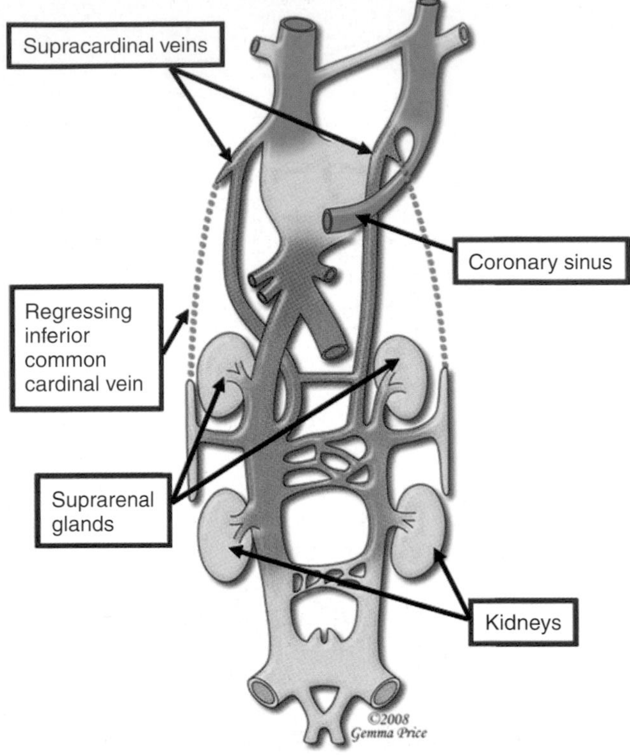

Figure 23-8 With further development of the abdominal venous system, there is regression of the cardinal veins, albeit that the supracardinal veins, which form the azygos system, use the terminations of the cardinal veins to establish their eventual connections with the superior caval venous system.

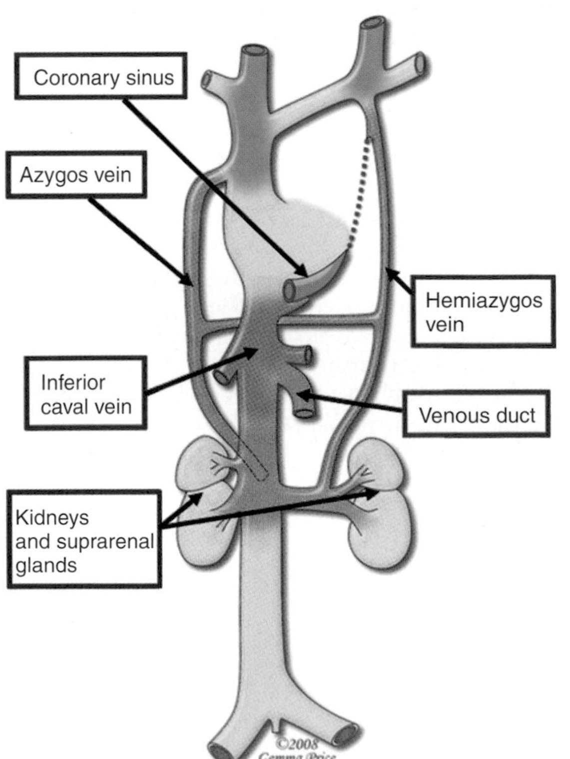

Figure 23-9 The origin of the components of the definitive inferior caval vein. Note the relationship to the azygos venous system. These connections explain how the abdominal venous return can reach the superior caval veins when the inferior caval vein itself is interrupted.

The venous development discussed thus far has presumed the development of anastomotic channels and connection of the systemic venous sinus to the right-sided atrium. It is this process that produces the morphologically right atrium, which contains the entirety of the embryonic systemic venous sinus. The left side of the initial atrial component of the heart tube, together with the developing pulmonary veins, becomes the morphologically left atrium. Concomitant with these changes, the appendages balloon from each side of the atrial component of the heart tube. The appendage growing to the right assumes its typically triangular shape, incorporating the cephalic part of the valve of the systemic venous sinus to form the terminal crest and the spurious septum. The appendage growing from the pulmonary side is much narrower. It has no relation with the valves of the systemic venous sinus, and therefore lacks a terminal crest. All of this occurs concomitant with development of anastomoses from the left to the right side. Should the anastomoses develop in right-sided to left-sided fashion, then the left-sided atrium will incorporate the systemic venous sinus and become the morphologically right atrium, while the right-sided atrium becomes the morphologically left atrium. This will produce a mirror-imaged atrial arrangement.

In certain circumstances, however, the process of lateralisation does not occur, and the systemic venous tributaries retain their bilateral symmetry. This lack of lateralisation occurs in two forms. In the one, the valves of the systemic venous sinus are incorporated bilaterally, along with bilateral right atrial appendages. This process squeezes out the anlagen of the primary pulmonary vein so that there is either no atrial site, or else a restricted anomalous site, for pulmonary venous drainage. Such right isomerism is characterised by presence bilaterally of appendages with right morphology, bilateral sinus horns together with bilateral systemic venous drainage, as well as anomalous pulmonary venous drainage. In the other pattern, there is bilateral growth of morphologically left structures. Consequently, the pulmonary venous component predominates in relation to the systemic venous tributaries. The major systemic venous channels then make anomalous connections to the atrial chambers, which have morphologically left appendages bilaterally. The common cardinal veins are more successful in this respect, tending to enter the atrial roof on each side in absence of a terminal crest. The hepatic veins also enter the atrium directly, often bilaterally. The venous return from the lower body, in contrast, usually continues through the supracardinal azygos system, draining to one or other of the superior cardinal veins to produce azygos continuation of the inferior caval vein. In those cases with isomeric left appendages in which the inferior caval vein does achieve a direct atrial connection, it tends to do so separately from the hepatic veins. Because of these developmental associations, anomalous systemic and pulmonary venous connections are part and parcel of the syndromes of isomerism and visceral heterotaxy (see Chapter 22).

CLASSIFICATION OF SYSTEMIC VENOUS ANOMALIES

Even though the account of development given above provides the background to understand their morphology, an organised classification of the multiple anomalous systemic

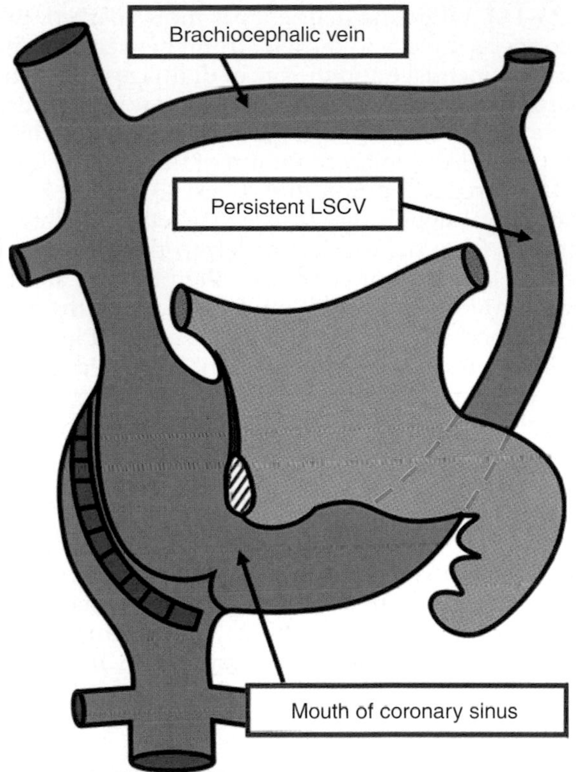

Figure 23-10 The cartoon shows the course of a left superior caval vein (LSCV) in presence of a brachiocephalic vein. Compare with Figure 23-5.

venous connections can be most easily achieved by using anatomical subdivisions. Thus, we can consider aberrations of development in the superior and inferior caval veins and the coronary sinus, as well as totally anomalous systemic venous connection, and abnormal persistence of the embryonic valves of the systemic venous sinus. Prevalence, pathophysiology, clinical and laboratory findings, and management will be discussed where appropriate for each anomaly.

Anomalies of the Superior Caval Vein

A left-sided superior caval vein draining to the coronary sinus is the most common systemic venous anomaly. The venous channel, which follows the course of the embryonic left cranial cardinal vein (see Fig. 23-5), enters the pericardial cavity to the left of the left upper pulmonary veins, and runs posterior to the dome of the left atrium, having the mouth of the left atrial appendage to its left side. The lesion has been noted in almost one in every 200 postmortems in the general population,[4] but occurs in up to one-twentieth of patients with congenitally malformed hearts.[5] The left-sided venous channel usually co-exists with a right-sided superior caval vein. A brachiocephalic vein connects these two structures in three-fifths of patients, with its size varying inversely with that of the left vein (Fig. 23-10). When present, the left vein usually is positioned anteriorly relative to both the aortic arch and the left pulmonary artery, but can pass posterior to these structures (Fig. 23-11). (See also Fig. 23-12.)

Although persistence of the left superior caval vein has no direct consequences concerning the mode of drainage of systemic venous return, its presence has recently been shown potentially to be of more concern. Thus, there is evidence that the persistent vein can impinge on the vestibule of the mitral valve, producing obstruction to left ventricular inflow which can be alleviated by surgical plication.[6] There is also an increased incidence of left-sided obstructive lesions in patients with persistent left superior caval veins.[7] Imaging of a left superior caval vein to the coronary sinus is usually achieved with cross sectional echocardiography (Fig. 23-13), but more recently magnetic resonance imaging is playing a greater role, particularly in older patients (Fig. 23-14).

Absent Right Superior Caval Vein

Complete absence of the right superior caval vein occurs occasionally in the presence of a left vein draining to the coronary sinus. In this situation, the left vein receives a right-sided brachiocephalic vein. A vestigial cord is often recognised as the remnant of the right superior caval vein when specimens are available for study.[8]

Left Superior Caval Vein with Interatrial Communication Through the Mouth of the Coronary Sinus

The known spectrum of fenestration of the coronary sinus[9] provides the understanding for an interatrial communication through the mouth of the coronary sinus.[10] A localised window in the adjacent walls of the left atrium and coronary sinus produces a limited communication between the systemic venous channel and the left atrium

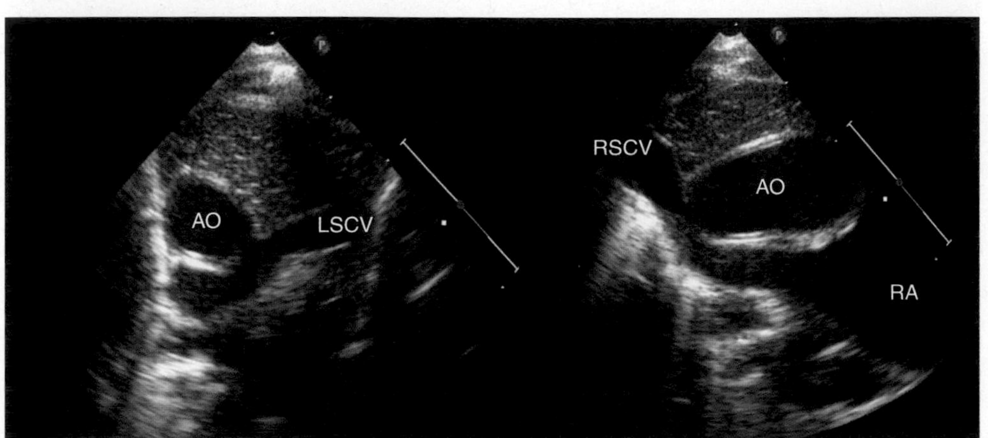

Figure 23-11 In this patient, the left superior caval vein runs beneath the aorta. As it passes inferiorly, it accepts the hemiazygos vein, descends medially into the inferior atrioventricular groove, and enters the right atrium through the enlarged mouth of the coronary sinus (Fig. 23-12). AO, aorta; LSCV, left superior caval vein; RA, right atrium; RSCV, right superior caval vein.

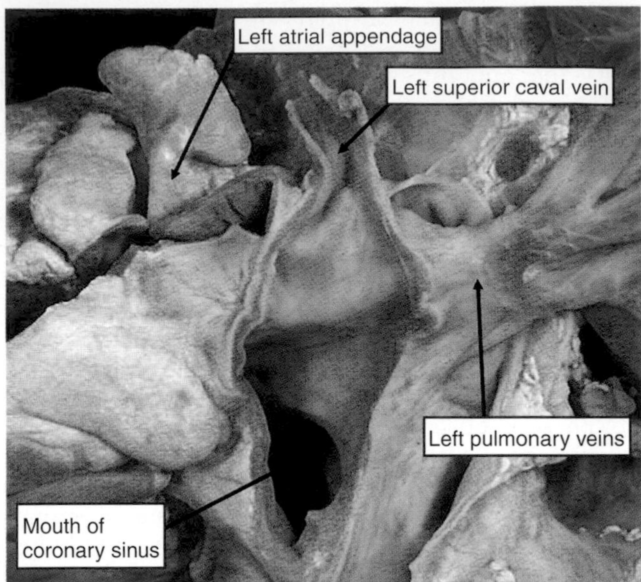

Figure 23-12 The heart is photographed from behind, showing the typical course of a persistent left superior caval vein, sandwiched between the left atrial appendage and the left pulmonary veins as it passes over the dome of the left atrium.

(Fig. 23-15). When the deficiency is more marked, the left vein connects directly to the left atrium between the mouth of the left appendage and the site of drainage of the left pulmonary veins. In the total absence of the walls that usually separate the cavities of the coronary sinus and the left atrium, this leaves the enlarged mouth of the sinus to function as an interatrial communication (Figs. 23-16 and 23-17).

The clinical significance relates to whether the interatrial shunting is from right-to-left, or left-to-right. If there is an associated left superior caval vein, then there is an obligatory right-to-left shunt, with mild cyanosis. In the absence of a left superior caval vein, there may be a net left-to-right shunt. The presence of the persistent left-sided caval vein can be confirmed by injections of saline injection into a vein in the left arm, with subsequent opacification of the left atrium. In other cases, the fenestration can be seen with cross sectional imaging (see Fig. 23-17).

Left Superior Caval Vein Draining to the Left Atrium

When there is persistence of the left superior caval vein, the venous channel is reported to connect directly to the left atrium in just less than one-tenth of cases,[11] typically in the setting of complex malformations. Thus, bilateral superior caval veins, with the left vein draining to the left-sided

Figure 23-13 The left superior caval veins as seen by echocardiography. Note the absence of a bridging brachiocephalic vein. CS, coronary sinus; LSCV, left superior caval vein; PA, pulmonary artery; RA, right atrium.

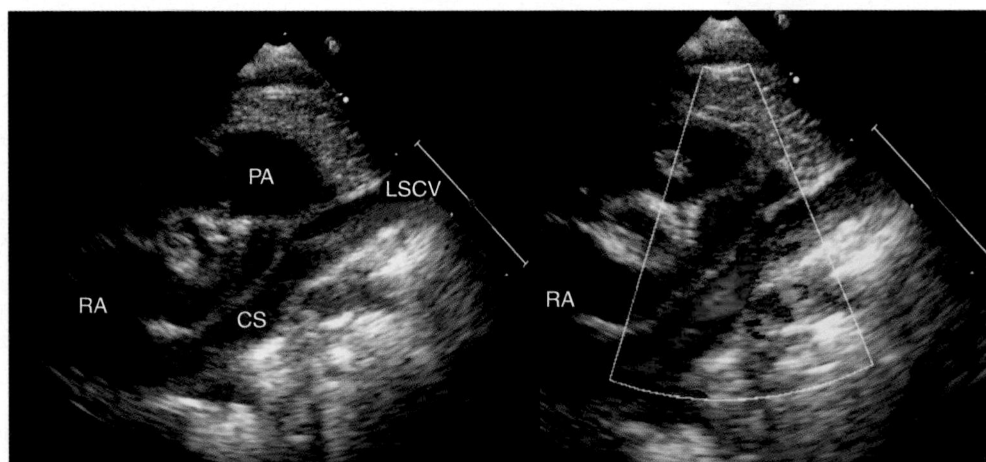

Figure 23-14 The left superior caval vein draining to the coronary sinus as revealed by magnetic resonance imaging (*arrow*). CS, coronary sinus; LA, left atrium; LV, left ventricle; RA, right atrium; RV, right ventricle.

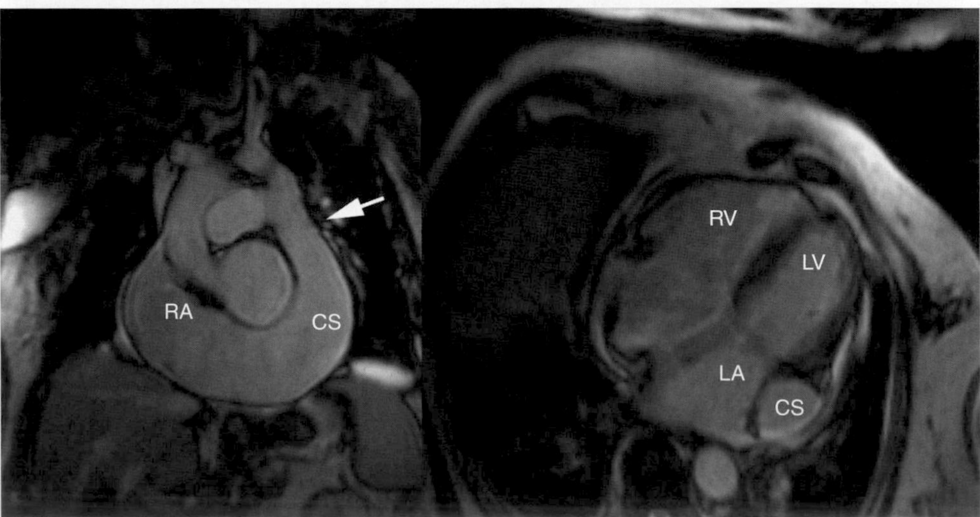

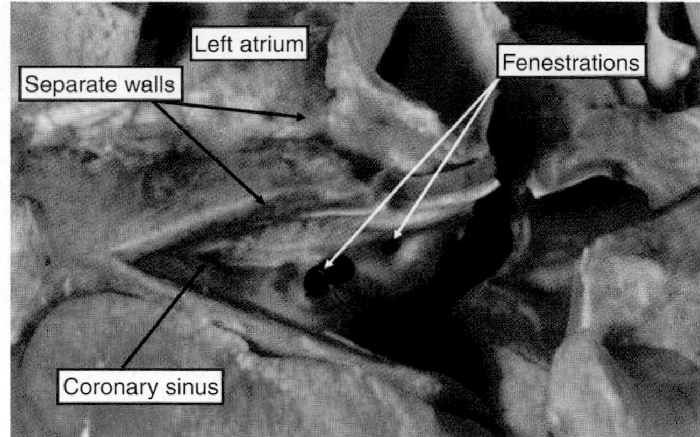

Figure 23-15 The heart is photographed from behind, showing two fenestrations between the cavity of the coronary sinus and the left atrium.

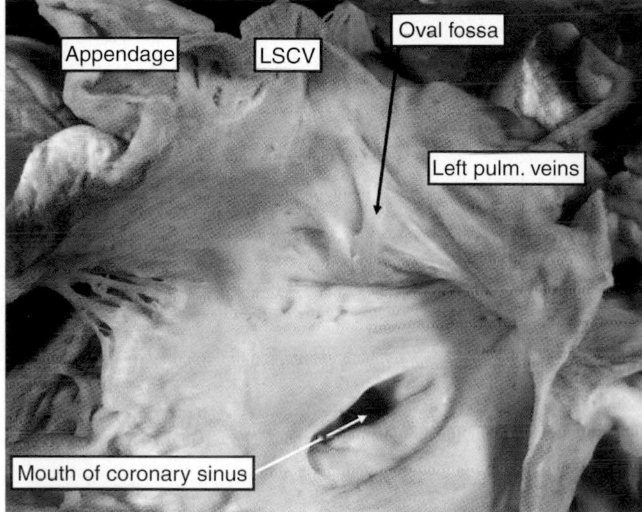

Figure 23-16 In this heart, all the walls that should normally separate the coronary sinus from the left atrium have disappeared, leaving the persistent left superior caval vein draining to the roof of the left atrium, and the mouth of the coronary sinus functioning as an interatrial communication. Note the intact oval fossa. LSCV, left superior caval vein.

atrium, are usually seen when there is isomerism of the atrial appendages. The so-called developmental complex[12] of left caval venous connection to the left atrium, with purported absence of the coronary sinus is, in reality, no more than absence of the walls normally interposed between the sinus and the left atrium (see Fig. 23-16). In this situation, it is the mouth of the coronary sinus that functions as the interatrial communication.[11] The left superior caval vein can also drain directly to the left atrium when there are no associated defects at atrial level, with either right-to-left shunting[13] or left-to-right shunting.[14]

This anomaly can be seen by both cross sectional echocardiography and magnetic resonance imaging (Figs. 23-18 and 23-19). By echocardiography it is best seen in a sagittal long-axis view in the ductal cut (Fig. 23-20). Further exploration of the dome and posterior wall of the left atrium reveals absence of the walls that normally interpose between the persistent caval vein and the atrial cavity. The anomaly should be suspected when scanning a patient with an apparent abnormality of atrial arrangement. Magnetic resonance imaging is now being used more frequently to delineate the systemic and pulmonary venous drainage in those with isomeric atrial appendages.

Laevoatrial Cardinal Vein

This channel,[15] in reality, is neither laevo, atrial, or cardinal. It provides overflow to the systemic venous circuit when there is obstruction of the outlet from the left atrium and the atrial septum is intact or closed (Fig. 23-21). It typically runs a serpentine course (Fig. 23-22). It can also decompress the left side in situations such as divided left atrium (Fig. 23-23).

Right Superior Caval Vein Draining to the Left Atrium

Anomalous drainage of the right superior caval vein into the left atrium has been reported rarely as an isolated anomaly.[16] We have never seen such a lesion in an autopsied specimen, albeit that we have recently been shown a good example revealed by three-dimensional echocardiography. Drainage of a right superior caval vein into both atriums is also described, being seen in a patient in whom the right-sided pulmonary veins drained into the superior caval vein, which then connected through separate channels into the two atriums.[17] This seems more like a variant of the

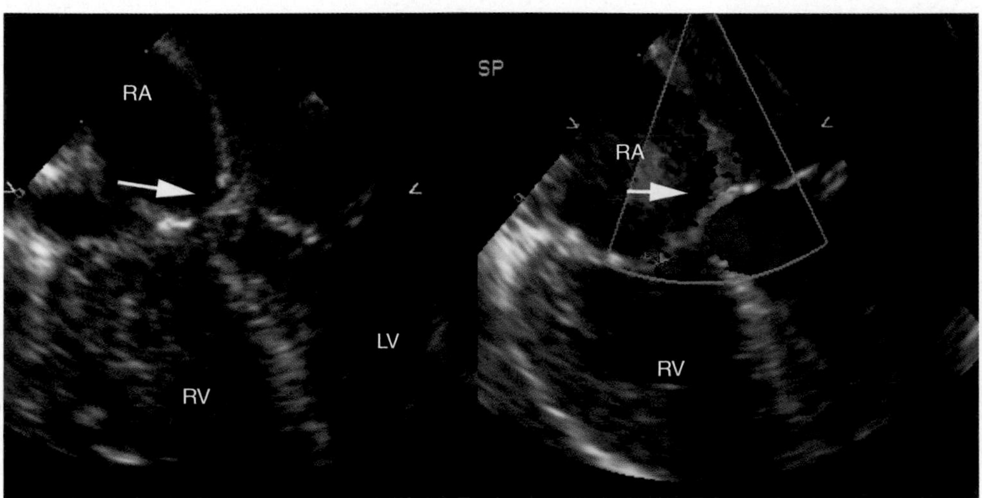

Figure 23-17 In this patient, unroofing of the coronary sinus produces a small interatrial communication at the mouth of the coronary sinus (*arrow*). LV, left ventricle; RA, right atrium; RV, right ventricle.

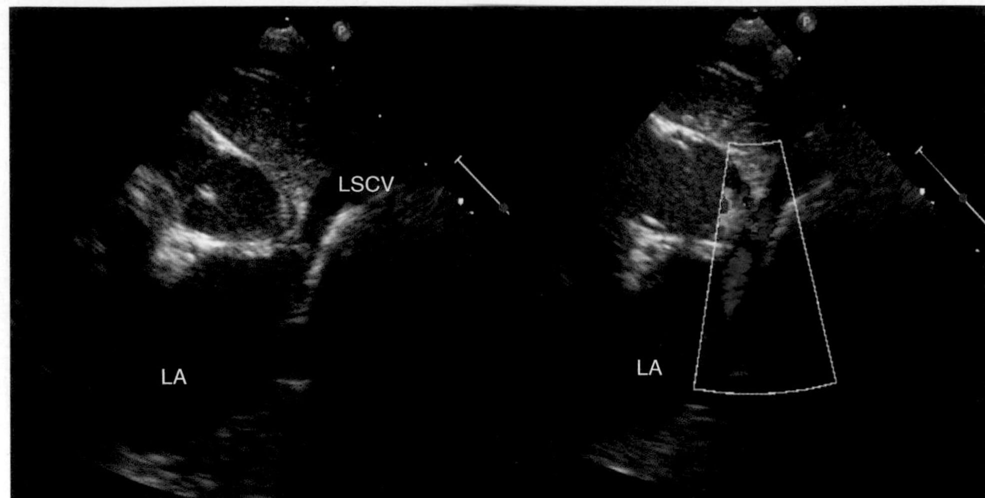

Figure 23-18 The high sagittal cut demonstrates a left superior caval vein to the roof of the left atrium. Note the complete absence of the walls that usually separate the caval vein from the cavity of the left atrium. LA, left atrium; LSCV, left superior caval vein.

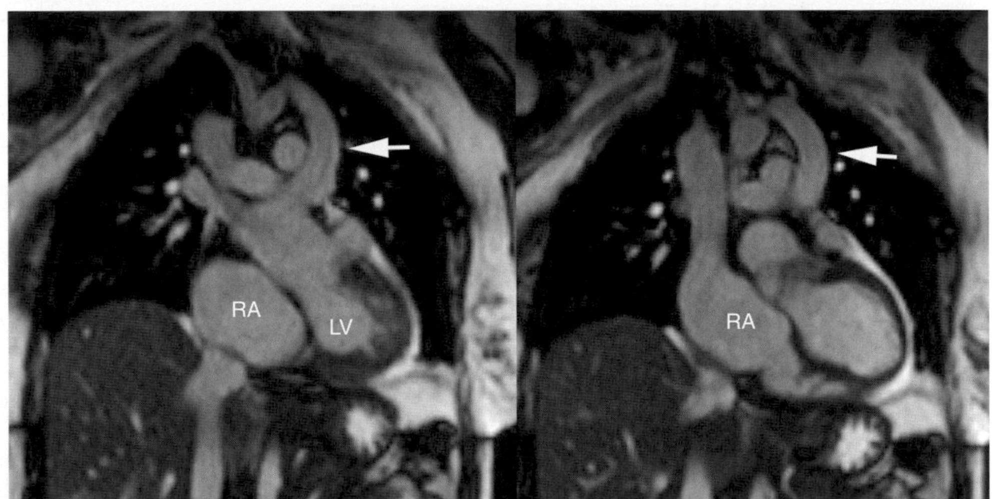

Figure 23-19 The magnetic resonance image shows a left superior caval vein draining to the roof of the left atrium (*arrows*). LV, left ventricle; RA, right atrium.

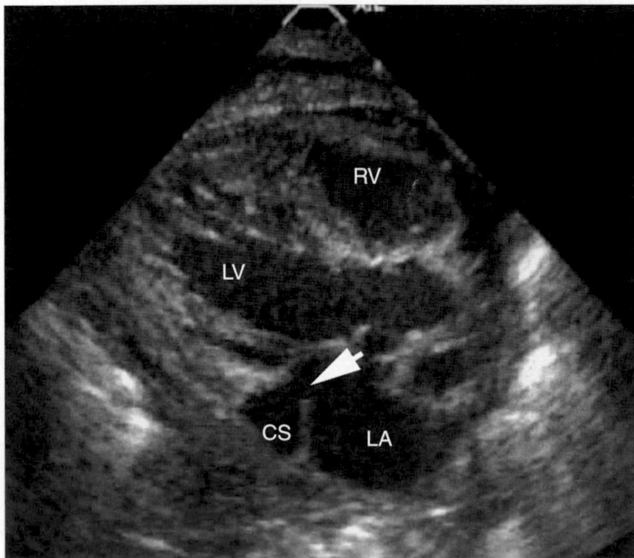

Figure 23-20 The parasternal long-axis echocardiographic cut shows a fenestration in the coronary sinus, with communication to the left atrium as indicated by the arrow. CS, coronary sinus; LA, left atrium; LV, left ventricle; RV, right ventricle.

sinus venosus interatrial communication, albeit that other cases are reported in the foreign literature.

Aneurysm of the Superior Caval Vein

Parts of the superior caval vein may become aneurysmal as isolated abnormalities in asymptomatic patients. The term aneurysm is usually reserved for arterial structures, but has been applied to such discrete dilations of the superior caval vein, and is probably more appropriate than that of varix, which implies a twisted conformation. Most of the aneurysms have been described in adults, albeit that a recent report concerned a 13-year-old boy.[18] It is presumed that these defects are of a congenital nature, and possibly reflect an inherent weakness in the structure of the venous wall. As far as we are aware, rupture of the aneurysms has yet to be reported.

Anomalies of the Inferior Caval Vein

Absence of the Hepatic Segment of the Inferior Caval Vein with Azygos Continuation

The most common venous anomaly involving the inferior caval vein is absence of its infrahepatic segment, with azygos continuation to the superior caval vein (Fig. 23-24).

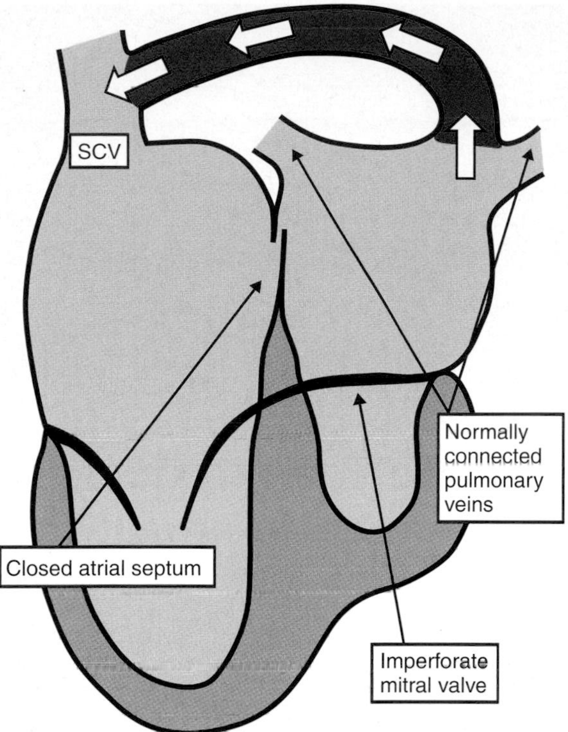

Figure 23-21 The cartoon shows the course of the so-called laevoatrial cardinal vein. The anomalous channel arises from the roof of the left atrium that receives the pulmonary veins in normal fashion, so that it provides anomalous pulmonary venous drainage in the setting of normal pulmonary venous connections. The vein then runs a variable, often serpentine, course (Fig. 23-22) before terminating in the superior caval vein (SCV).

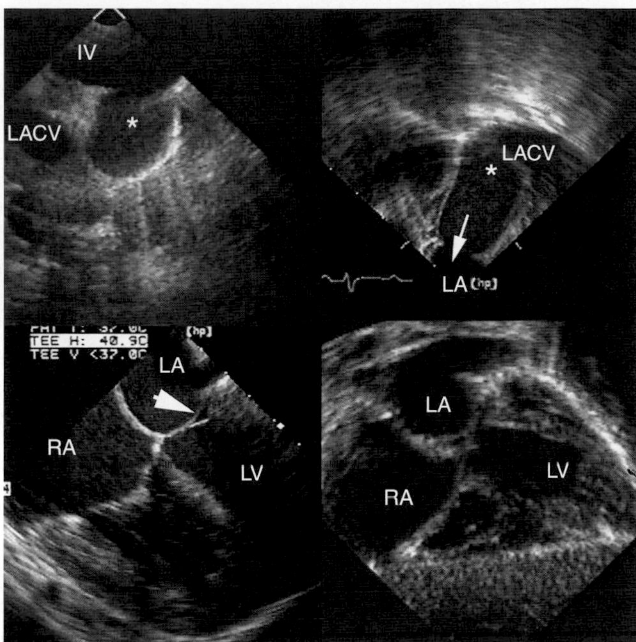

Figure 23-23 This patient had divided left atrium, with no orifice between the proximal and distal components of the left atrium, but with a decompressing lavoatrial cardinal vein indicated by the star. The upper left picture shows the connection with the brachiocephalic vein (*asterisk*), and the upper right panel shows the connection with the left atrium (*arrow*). Note the normal pulmonary venous drainage, as shown in the lower right panel. The lower left panel shows the divided left atrium. The left ventricle was not hypoplastic, as there was an associated perimembranous ventricular septal defect. IV, brachiocephalic vein, LA, left atrium; LACV, laevoatrial cardinal vein; LV, left ventricle; RA, right atrium.

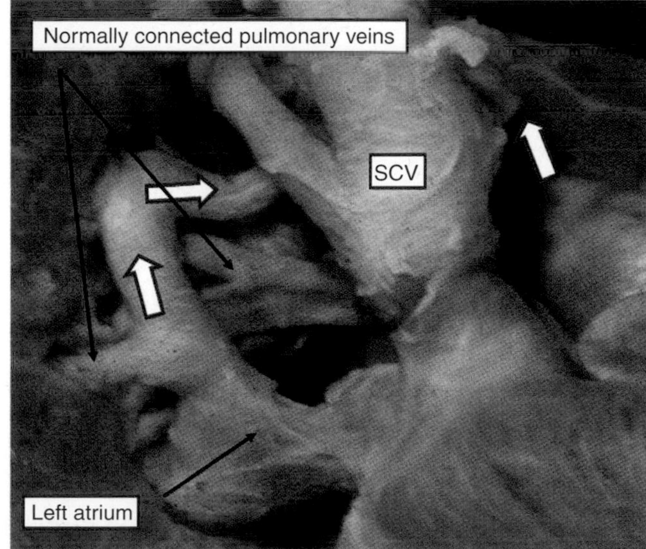

Figure 23-22 The serpentine course of the laevoatrial cardinal vein (*arrows*). In essence a pulmonary to systemic venous collateral channel, it is typically found in the setting of hypoplasia of the left heart,[15] but can exist in other settings. SCV, superior caval vein.

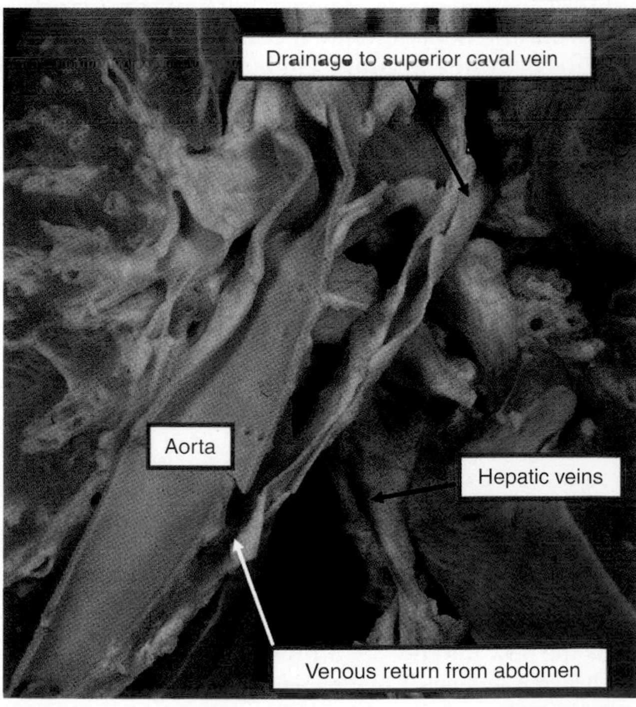

Figure 23-24 A heart-lung block photographed from behind. The venous return from the abdomen passes through a venous channel running posterior to the aorta, and terminating in the left superior caval vein. The abdominal inferior caval vein is interrupted, with only the hepatic veins draining directly to the atrium. This is interruption of the inferior caval vein with azygos continuation. This patient also had isomerism of the left atrial appendages.

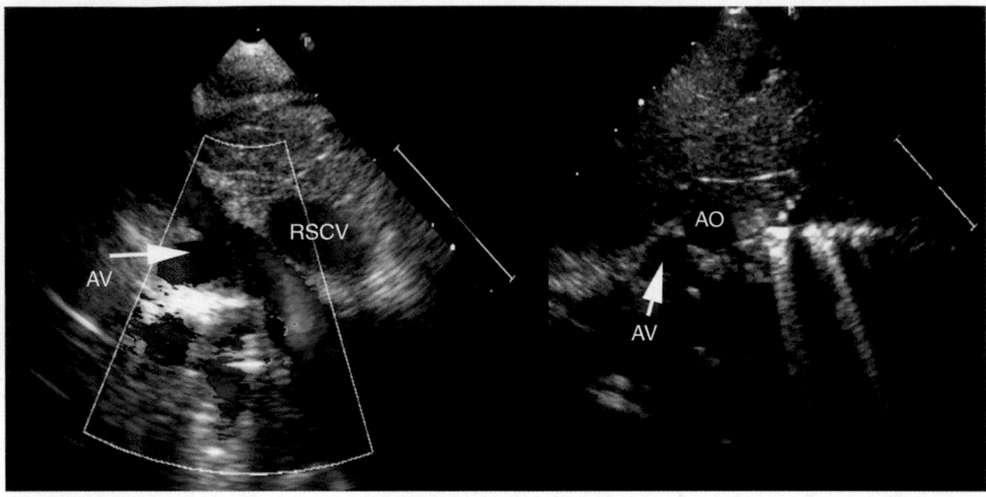

Figure 23-25 The echocardiogram shows interruption of the inferior caval vein with azygos continuation to the right superior vena caval vein (RSCV). Note that the azygos continuation (*arrow in right picture*) runs in the paravertebral gutter behind the liver. AO, descending aorta; AV, azygos vein.

The dilated azygos system serves as the major channel of systemic venous return from the lower half of the body. Only the hepatic veins continue to drain to the right atrium, albeit also carrying the portal venous return. The lesion is the consequence of abnormal development of the right subcardinal system, which fails to anastomose with the right vitelline vein. The supracardinal venous system, which normally forms the azygos system, then provides continuation of systemic venous return to the developing superior caval vein.

The malformation is said to occur in 0.6% of all patients with congenital cardiac disease.[19] When found, it should raise the suspicion of isomerism of the left atrial appendages, but certainly exists in patients with usual or mirror-imaged atrial arrangement.[20] In the setting of isomerism, the hepatic venous connections usually connect directly to the atriums, either separately or through a confluent channel. Strictly speaking, the anomalous vein in the setting of left isomerism is a hemiazygos vein, but it is convenient to term it the azygos vein. Interruption of the inferior caval vein is readily seen by cross sectional echocardiography, where the azygos vein is situated behind the liver in the paravertebral gutter. The thoracic connection with either the left or right superior caval vein can be seen in a high right or left sagittal plane (Fig. 23-25).

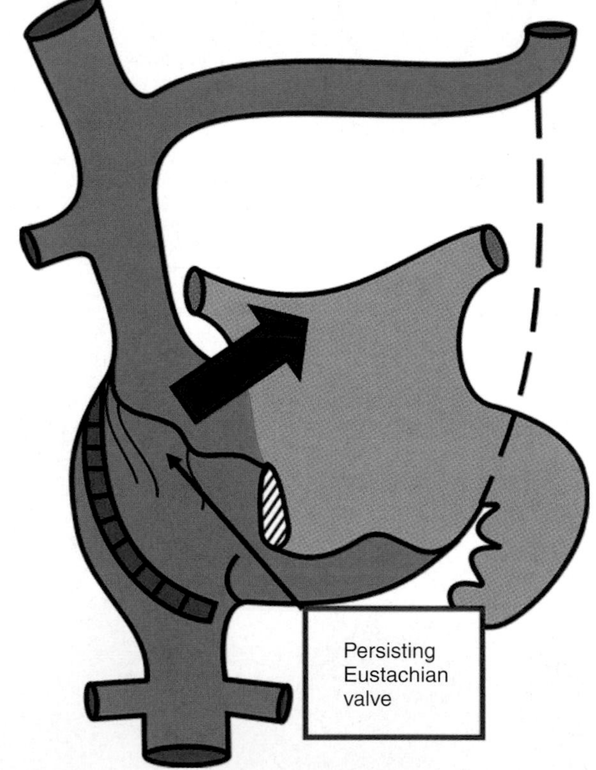

Figure 23-26 The cartoon shows a persistent Eustachian valve directing inferior venous caval flow into the left atrium. This should not be mistaken for connection of the inferior caval vein to the left atrium.

Inferior Caval Vein Connected to the Left Atrium

The inferior caval vein has been reported as connecting directly to the left atrium both with an intact atrial septum[21] and in association with an atrial septal defect.[22] In this respect, it is necessary to distinguish between direct connection to the left atrium and the arrangement in which an inferior caval vein overrides a low-lying interatrial communication and allows functional drainage of inferior caval venous flow to the left atrium. The latter situation can be exacerbated by persistence of an unduly prominent Eustachian valve that directs the flow into the left atrium (Fig. 23-26).

Miscellaneous Anomalies of the Inferior Caval Vein

A variety of minor abnormalities of the inferior caval vein have been documented in the general population. They have no definite relationship to other congenital cardiac lesions. These include duplication of the inferior caval vein below the level of the renal veins, left-sided inferior caval vein, and circumaortic renal collar. The anomalies can easily be explained by variation in the pattern of regression and anastomosis of the many embryological structures that contribute to the development of the vein (see Figs. 23-6 through 23-9). They have no haemodynamic significance, but may be of importance when surgical procedures are necessary in the retroperitoneal area. The hepatic veins normally connect to the inferior caval vein, but have been reported to connect directly to the left atrium.[23] Complete absence of the inferior caval vein, with systemic venous return from the lower extremities flowing entirely through the paravertebral

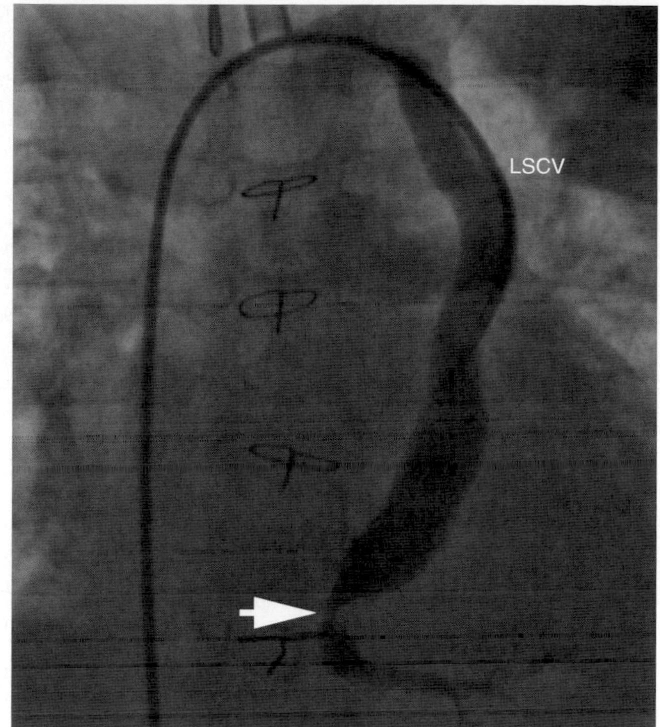

Figure 23-27 The angiogram shows atresia of the mouth of the coronary sinus atresia (*arrow*) in the setting of a left superior caval vein (LSCV).

venous plexus and the azygos and hemiazygos systems, is also reported,[24] but was probably the consequence of venous thrombosis from a prior pelvic staphylococcal infection, with development of collateral channels.

Anomalies of the Coronary Sinus

Several systemic venous anomalies that involve alterations in normal structure of the coronary sinus have already been discussed. These include the various degrees of so-called unroofing of the coronary sinus in association with a left superior caval vein connected directly to the left atrium. As we have discussed, this is better considered in terms of a spectrum of fenestration of the walls that usually separate the sinus from the cavity of the left atrium.[9,10] Varying degrees of hypoplasia have also been reported, in which some of the cardiac veins drain separately through dilated Thebesian veins directly into the atriums. The Thebesian valve can also persist in its entirety, and produce atresia of the sinusal orifice (Fig. 23-27). This is also reported with coronary venous drainage to a persistent left caval vein. Intraoperative ligation of the caval vein in this setting produced coronary ischaemia and death.[25] Other rare anomalies include connection of the hepatic veins to the coronary sinus, fistulous communication with coronary arteries, and connection of the coronary sinus to the inferior caval vein. Diverticulums of the coronary sinus (Fig. 23-28) are also known to be associated with ventricular pre-excitation.[26] It is unusual for anomalies of the coronary sinus to occur as isolated defects. Any enlargement of this structure, therefore, should raise suspicions of an anomalous systemic or pulmonary venous channel draining through it.

Totally Anomalous Systemic Venous Connection

Various cases have been reported previously with alleged totally anomalous systemic venous connections.[27] The described anatomical features, however, are all suggestive of isomerism of the left atrial appendages.

Anomalies of the Embryonic Valves of the Systemic Venous Sinus

The valves of the systemic venous sinus are prominent structures during early embryological development, when the right valve nearly divides the right atrium into two portions. With normal maturation, they usually involute. As we have already described, the cephalic portion of the right

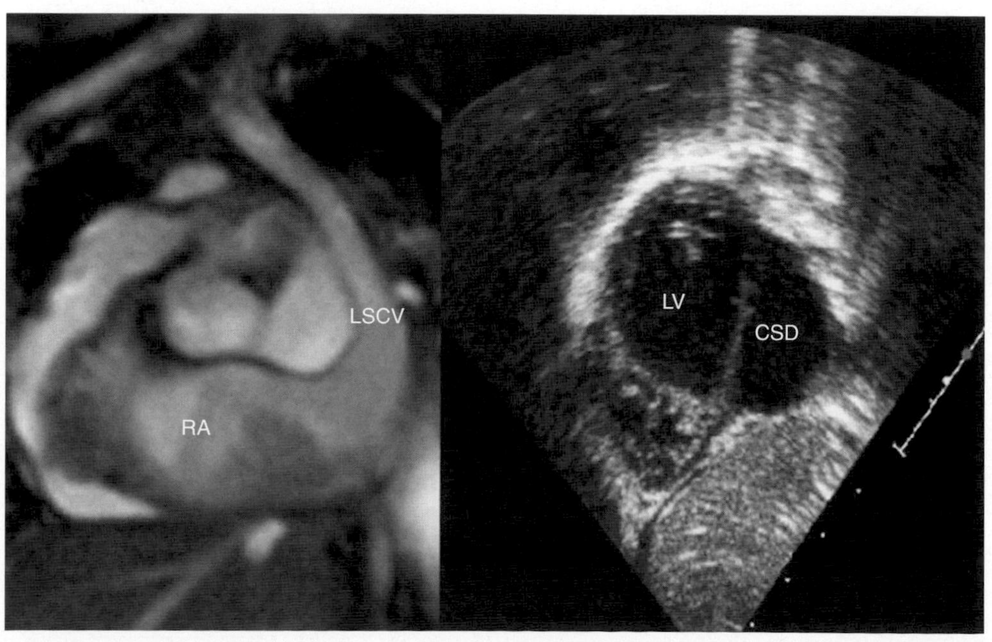

Figure 23-28 The coronary sinus, which drains a small left superior caval vein, is aneurysmal in a patient who had an associated ventricular septal defect. Note the dilated coronary sinus seen on the right-hand panel echocardiogram. CSD, dilated coronary sinus; LSCV, left superior caval vein; LV, left ventricle, RA, right atrium.

valve becomes incorporated into the terminal crest, while its caudal portion becomes the Eustachian and Thebesian valves. The left venous valve becomes incorporated into the atrial septum. The valves can persist in varied fashion, from small remnants to semilunar membranes with and without fenestrations. When seen in the form of fine or coarse fibrous strands extending across the cavity of the right atrium from the terminal crest to either the Thebesian or Eustachian valves the entity is known as a Chiari network. Such networks are usually not of haemodynamic significance, although Chiari himself attributed the death of his patient to embolisation of a thrombus formed on the network.[28] Undue persistence of the valves can produce partial or complete division of the right atrium into a venous component, accepting some or all of the systemic veins, and the remainder of the atrium, including the right atrial appendage and the vestibule of the tricuspid valve. The venous sinus is in communication with the oval foramen, which allows the potential for right-to-left shunting of systemic venous blood to the left atrium. In some instances, the dividing partition can balloon as a windsock membrane.[29] This can then extend through the tricuspid valve into the right ventricle. There is a striking association of pathological persistence of the right-sided venous valves with hypoplasia of the right ventricle and pulmonary arteries, probably because reduced flow through the tricuspid valve leads to failure of proper development of the right-sided cardiac structures. These lesions are discussed in greater detail in our chapter devoted to division of the atrial chambers (Chapter 26).

The complete reference list can be found on the companion Expert Consult web site at www.expertconsult.com.

ANNOTATED REFERENCES

- Anderson RH, Brown NA, Moorman AFM: Development and structures of the venous pole of the heart. Dev Dyn 2006;235:2–9.

  The review discusses recent findings concerning the embryological origin of the systemic venous sinus of the right at rium, and its relationship to the developing pulmonary vein.

- Cochrane AD, Marath A, Mee RB: Can a dilated coronary sinus produce left ventricular inflow obstruction? An unrecognized entity. Ann Thorac Surg 1994;58:1114–1116.
- Agnoletti G, Annechino F, Preda L, Borghi A: Persistence of the left superior caval vein: Can it potentiate obstructive lesions of the left ventricle? Cardiol Young 1999;9:285–290.

  Two investigations pointing to the role of the persistent left superior caval vein in producing obstruction to the inlet of the morphologically left ventricle.

- Rose AG, Beckman CB, Edwards JE: Communication between coronary sinus and left atrium. Br Heart J 1974;36:182–185.

  An early and important study that showed the spectrum of malformations extending from fenestrations in the walls between the coronary sinus and the left atrium to complete unroofing of the coronary sinus.

- Knauth A, McCarthy KP, Webb S, et al: Interatrial communication through the mouth of the coronary sinus. Cardiol Young 2002;12:364–372.

  This study extended the observations reported by Rose and colleagues in 1974, but showed also that, as had been reported by Chauvin and colleagues, separate walls of the coronary sinus and left atrium usually interposed between their cavities, rather than the party wall that had previously been suggested.

- Pinto CAM, Ho SY, Redington A, et al: Morphological features of the levoatriocardinal (or pulmonary-to-systemic collateral) vein. Pediatr Pathol 1993;13:751–761.

  A review of the features of this enigmatic structure, which is neither laevo, atrial, nor cardinal. As shown, it provides a pulmonary-to-systemic collateral venous channel when there is obstruction to the outflow from the left atrium.

- Debich DE, Devine WA, Anderson RH: Polysplenia with normally structured hearts. Am J Cardiol 1990;65:1274–1275.

  A significant study showing that multiple spleens are not always associated with isomerism of the left atrial appendages. They are still, however, associated with azygos return of the interrupted inferior caval vein.

- Tham EBC, Ross DB, Giuffre M, et al: Cardiac magnetic resonance of a coronary sinus diverticulum associated with congenital heart disease. Circulation 2007;116:e541–e544.

  An observation pointing to the increasing role of magnetic resonance imaging in diagnosis of systemic venous anomalies.

- Trento A, Zuberbuhler JR, Anderson RH, et al: Divided right atrium (prominence of the eustachian and thebesian valves). J Thorac Cardiovasc Surg 1988;96:457–463.

  A review of the role of undue prominence of the valves of the systemic venous sinus in producing subdivision of the morphologically right atrium. These lesions are discussed in greater detail, and illustrated, in Chapter 26.

CHAPTER 24

Pulmonary Venous Abnormalities

ANTHONY M. HLAVACEK, GIRISH S. SHIRALI, and ROBERT H. ANDERSON

In this chapter, we consider abnormalities of the pulmonary veins, in particular their anomalous connections to the systemic venous system. The variant of partially anomalous pulmonary venous connection associated with the sinus venosus interatrial communication is described in detail in the chapter that follows. The anomalous pulmonary venous connections so commonly associated with isomerism of the atrial appendages are mentioned in this chapter, but have been discussed more fully in Chapter 22, not least because of the particular problems of nomenclature that arise in the setting of isomerism. Though division of the morphologically left atrium was, in the past,[1] considered a pulmonary venous anomaly, we deal with this lesion, along with division of the morphologically right atrium, in Chapter 26.

TOTALLY ANOMALOUS PULMONARY VENOUS CONNECTION

Incidence and Aetiology

It was at the turn of the 17th century that Wilson[2] described a 'monstrous formation of the heart in which the superior caval vein was joined by a trunk formed by two large veins coming out of the lungs'. We now know that the various forms of such totally anomalous pulmonary venous connection, in the absence of isomerism of the atrial appendages, or visceral heterotaxy, accounted for one-fortieth of the patients registered in the New England Regional Infant Cardiac Program.[3] As such, the entity ranked 12th in frequency, and occurred once in 17,000 live births. In the Baltimore–Washington Infant Study, the malformation was encountered less commonly, accounting for 1.5% of all patients with a cardiovascular malformation, and being seen once in 14,700 live births.[4] Totally anomalous pulmonary venous connection is known to be part of the Holt-Oram, Klippel-Feil, phocomelia, and Schachermann syndromes.[5] It is more difficult to establish the incidence of partially anomalous pulmonary venous connection, since anomalous connection of a solitary vein (Fig. 24-1) may be unrecognised either in life or death. Such anomalies have been reported in about 1 in 200 routine postmortems.[6,7] Furthermore, in an extensive investigation based on surgical and autopsy experience, seven-tenths of all cases of anomalous pulmonary venous connection were found to be of the partial variety, albeit that this review included patients with isomerism of the atrial appendages.[8]

Earlier reports on totally anomalous pulmonary venous connection stressed the preponderance of males in the setting of infradiaphragmatic drainage,[5] with an equal mix of gender in the remaining types. In those recorded in the New England Regional Infant Cardiac Program,[3] however, two-thirds with supracardiac and cardiac connections were males, while it was the infradiaphragmatic variant that showed an equal mix of genders. As with so many lesions, there are some examples of familial clustering,[9] with one report[10] suggesting autosomal dominant inheritance. Some evidence suggesting maternal exposure during the first 3 months of pregnancy to teratogens emerged from the Baltimore–Washington Infant Study.[4] Reanalysis of that dataset in 2004[11] found the association with maternal exposures inconclusive, but identified a link between totally anomalous connection and paternal exposure to lead prior to conception.

Anatomy

Anomalous pulmonary connections take various forms, and show several important clinical features. The first important feature is the proportion of the pulmonary venous drainage that is connected to sites other than the morphologically left atrium. This can be a solitary pulmonary vein, all of the veins from one lung, or the entirety of the pulmonary venous drainage (Fig. 24-2). Combinations are also possible when all veins do not drain anomalously, so although rare, it can be possible for all of the drainage from one lung, and a solitary vein from the other lung, to

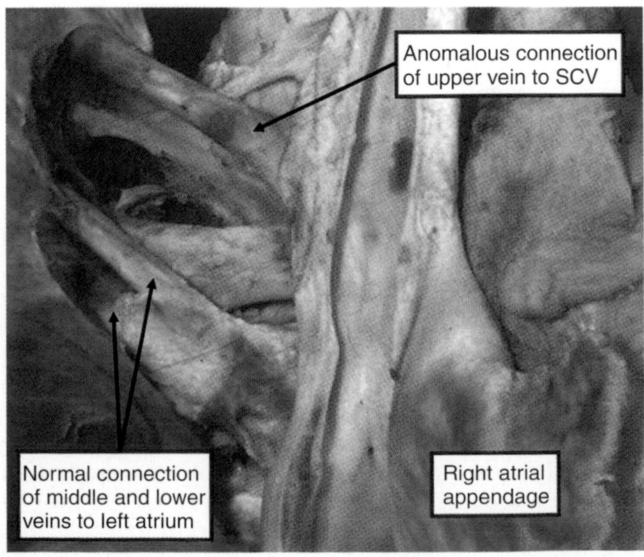

Figure 24-1 This picture shows anomalous connection of the right upper pulmonary vein to the superior caval vein (SCV). This was discovered as an incidental finding in an otherwise normal autopsy.

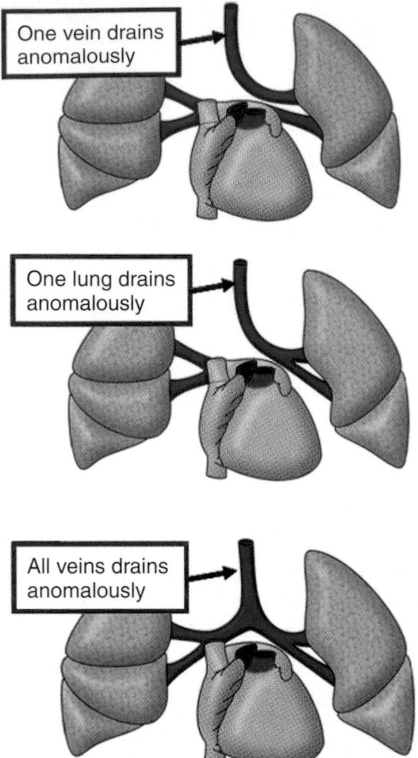

Figure 24-2 The cartoon shows the possibilities for anomalous connection of the pulmonary veins.

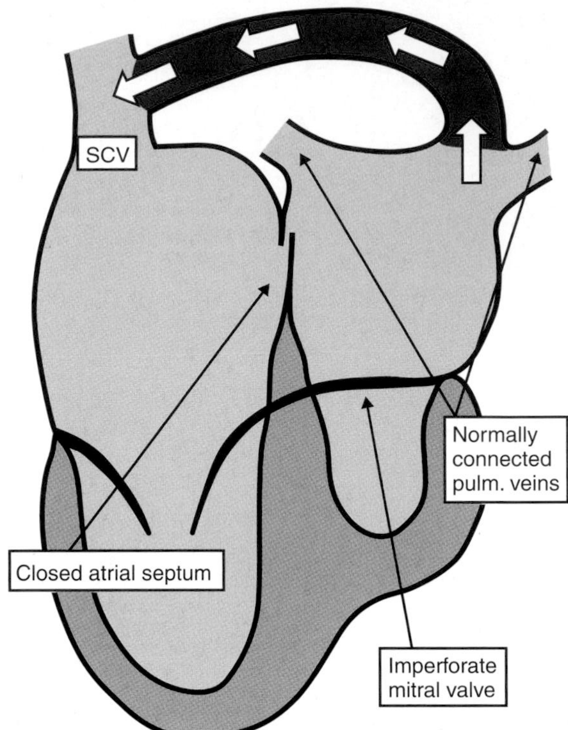

Figure 24-3 The cartoon shows an example of totally anomalous pulmonary venous drainage in the setting of normally connected pulmonary veins, in this instance because a so-called laevoatrial cardinal vein joins the left atrium to the superior caval vein (SCV) with mitral atresia and an intact atrial septum.

be connected to sites other than the morphologically left atrium. Once it has been established that a pulmonary vein, or pulmonary veins, are draining anomalously, it is equally important to determine the site of drainage, and whether all the veins drain to the same site. It is then necessary to seek stenotic areas or regions along the route of anomalous drainage. It is also necessary to establish whether the anomalous pulmonary venous connection is an isolated malformation, or part of a more complex anomaly, and whether there are associated structural malformations of the pulmonary vasculature.

Before discussing these important anatomic variables in more detail, we need to explain our use of the term anomalous pulmonary venous connection. This is because, in certain circumstances, pulmonary veins connected in normal fashion to the morphologically left atrium can drain anomalously to a systemic site, as for example when there is mitral atresia and an atrial septal defect, or fenestration to the coronary sinus, or in presence of the so-called laevoatrial cardinal vein (Fig. 24-3).

A pulmonary vein is connected anomalously only when it is attached to a site other than the morphologically left atrium. In this respect, it is also important to distinguish between the left-sided and the morphologically left atrium. In the presence of isomerism of the right atrial appendages, as we will show, all four pulmonary veins are frequently connected to the roof of an atrium with a morphologically right appendage, which can be left-sided. Because, in this setting, the atrium possesses a morphologically right appendage, this anatomical pattern is anomalous. Indeed, the pulmonary veins must be connected anomalously in the setting of right isomerism irrespective of their site of drainage. The topic of pulmonary venous connections in hearts with isometric appendages, therefore, represents a special situation. It is discussed in depth in Chapter 22. In this section, we are concerned primarily with totally anomalous connection in the setting of lateralised atrial chambers, in other words the usual and mirror-imaged arrangements, but we will make reference where appropriate to hearts with isomeric appendages.

When all the pulmonary veins are connected anomalously, then usually they drain to the same site. In some situations, nonetheless, different pulmonary veins are connected to separate anomalous sites. This is called mixed drainage. The sites of such drainage are the same as when the entirety of the pulmonary venous return reaches an extracardiac site through a confluence. These sites of anomalous connection are divided into supracardiac, cardiac, and infracardiac groups. The first two, taken together, constitute supradiaphragmatic drainage, while infracardiac drainage is at the same time infradiaphragmatic (Fig. 24-4).

Cardiac and intracardiac anomalous connections account for approximately one-quarter each of the total group. Supracardiac connection can be to the left brachiocephalic vein, directly to the right superior caval vein, to the azygos system of veins, or to the left superior caval vein, albeit that when the left vein drains to the coronary sinus this is considered cardiac drainage. In the most common pattern, the four pulmonary veins usually join in turn to a venous channel behind the left atrium. This channel is traditionally termed the confluence but the individual veins usually join the channel sequentially. From this horizontal channel, a vertical vein typically runs through the left paravertebral gutter to join the left brachiocephalic vein, which

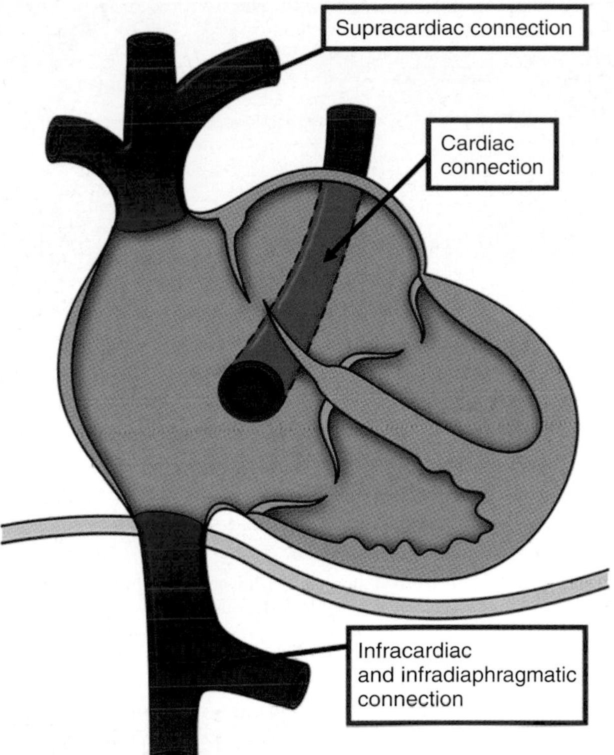

Figure 24-4 The cartoon shows the different sites of anomalous pulmonary venous connection. The commonest site for anomalous connection is supracardiac, accounting for nearly half of cases.

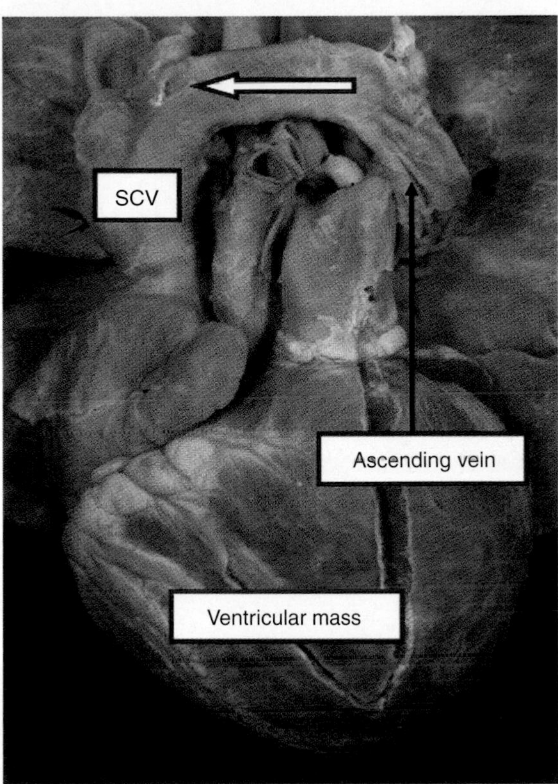

Figure 24-5 The picture shows the typical snowman pattern of supracardiac totally anomalous pulmonary venous connection to the superior caval vein (SCV). The anomalous venous pathway forms the head of the snowman, whilst the ventricular mass accounts for the body. The *arrow* shows the direction of flow of the anomalous pulmonary venous return through the brachiocephalic vein.

then terminates in the right superior caval vein (Fig. 24-5). It is the course of the vertical vein that usually determines whether or not the pathway is obstructed. If the vein passes anterior to the left pulmonary artery, then this course is not associated with obstruction. Should the vein pass between the left pulmonary artery and the left bronchus, these two structures clasp the channel in the so-called bronchopulmonary vice (Fig. 24-6). Obstruction with this snowman pattern of anomalous connection can also occur, albeit rarely, at the opening of the brachiocephalic vein into the superior caval vein. Supracardiac connection can also be found when the vertical vein joins directly with the right superior caval vein. Obstruction may then occur either at this caval venous junction, or in another vice, this time between the right pulmonary artery and the carina. When the anomalous pulmonary veins join the systemic venous system through the azygos vein, the horizontal vein usually crosses from left to right beneath the heart, again receiving the individual pulmonary veins in sequential fashion. The vertical vein then ascends in the right paravertebral gutter, joining the superior caval vein through the azygos vein (Fig. 24-7).

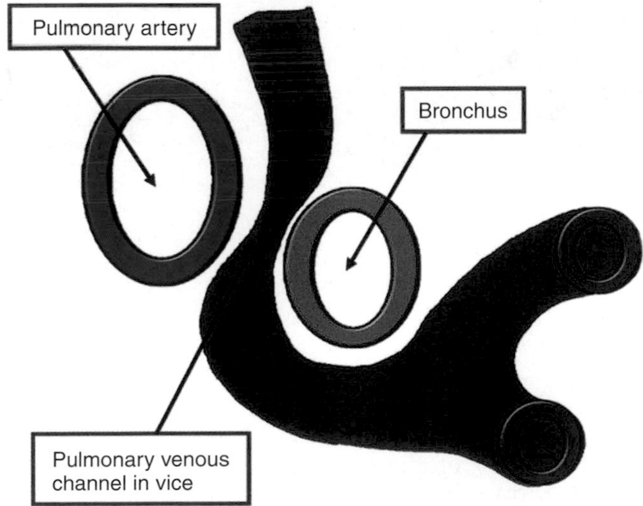

Figure 24-6 The cartoon shows the nature of the bronchopulmonary vice, which produces obstruction with supracardiac connections.

When there is usual, or mirror-imaged, atrial arrangement, then almost always the cardiac form of anomalous connection is found when the pulmonary veins join the right atrium via the coronary sinus (Fig. 24-8). It can be questioned whether this should be considered a cardiac connection, or one via the persistent left superior caval vein. Irrespective of such niceties, there is no question but that the site of return is within the heart, so cardiac connection is an apt description. The individual pulmonary veins can drain in various patterns to the coronary sinus, but the final common pathway is the sinus within the left atrioventricular groove, this typically being enlarged relative to the normal situation. Separate walls of coronary sinus and left atrium then separate the horizontal venous channel from the left atrial cavity, albeit that the walls can readily be removed surgically. Repair of the anomalous connection is then achieved simply by closing both the mouth of the coronary sinus and the interatrial communication,[12] taking care, of course, to respect the atrioventricular conduction

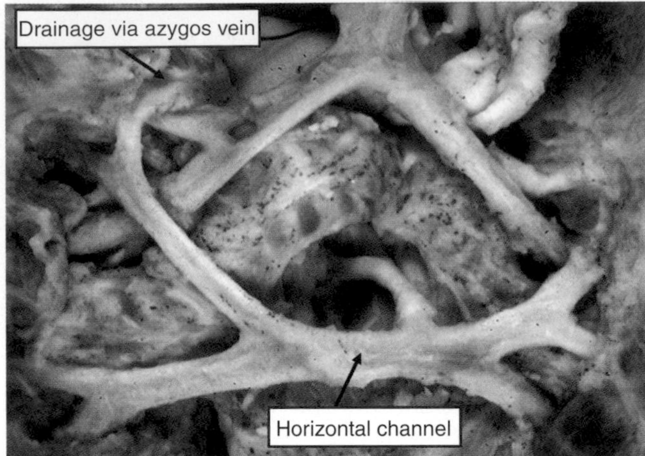

Figure 24-7 In this specimen, from a patient with isomeric right atrial appendages, the horizontal vein passes from left to right and ascends in the right paravertebral gutter, draining in supracardiac fashion through the azygos vein.

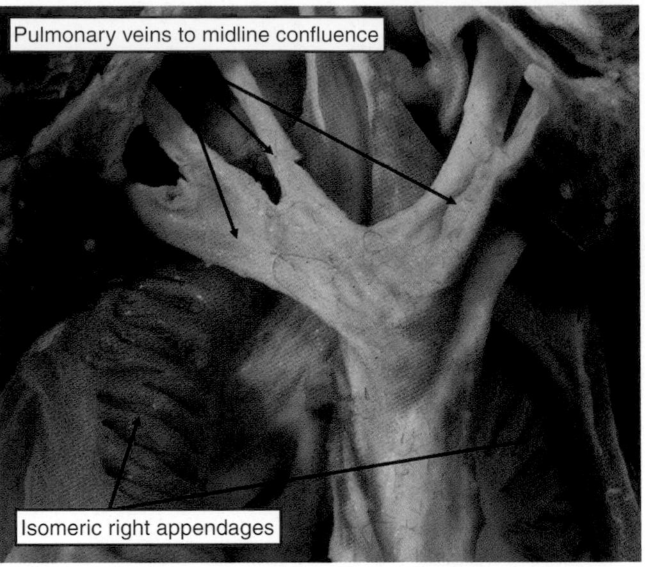

Figure 24-9 In this heart from a patient with isomeric right atrial appendages, all the pulmonary veins drain through a midline fibrous confluence.

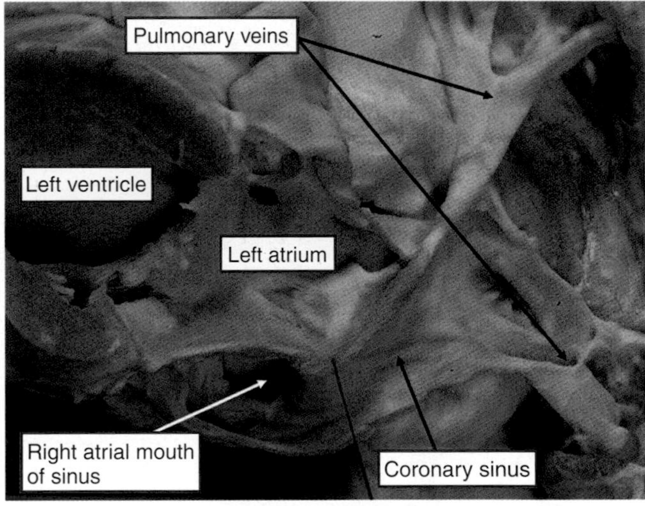

Figure 24-8 The picture shows totally anomalous pulmonary venous connection through the coronary sinus to the left atrium. The heart is photographed from behind and from the left side. If the walls separating the cavity of the sinus from the left atrium are removed, the anomaly can be corrected simply by closing the right atrial mouth of the coronary sinus.

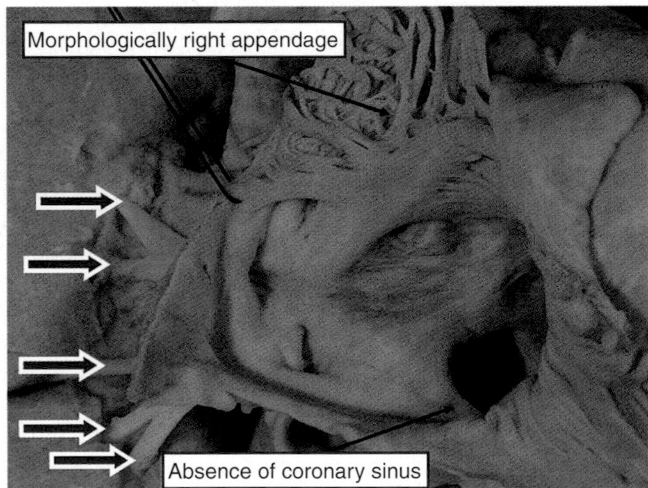

Figure 24-10 This heart is again from a patient with isomeric right atrial appendages. Note the absence of the coronary sinus. All pulmonary veins connect directly but separately to the right-sided atrium, as shown by the *arrows*.

tissues within the triangle of Koch. Obstruction is rare when the pulmonary veins drain through the coronary sinus, but can be produced by persistence of the Thebesian valve, or within the sinus when the individual veins connect in unusual fashion.

Direct connection of the pulmonary veins to the morphologically right atrium is exceedingly rare other than in the setting of isomerism of the right atrial appendages. In this setting, the coronary sinus is absent, and most usually the atrial septum is deficient, frequently virtually absent. The pulmonary veins then tend to crowd together, opening through a midline fibrous confluence in the atrial roof (Fig. 24-9). Because the confluence lacks muscle,[13] it can be obstructive. Less frequently in hearts with isomeric right appendages, the atrial septum can be much better formed, yet still the pulmonary veins connect directly to one of the atriums (Fig. 24-10). This arrangement must be anticipated in hearts with usual or mirror-imaged atrial arrangement, but we have yet to identify such a case.

The final site of anomalous connection is both infracardiac and infradiaphragmatic. In this pattern, the pulmonary veins join together, entering a descending vertical vein that passes into the abdomen through the oesophageal orifice of the diaphragm. It then usually drains to the portal vein, or to one of its tributaries (Fig. 24-11). Drainage to the inferior caval vein is very rare. When the infracardiac connection is to the portal venous system, obstruction is almost always present subsequent to closure of the venous duct. Once this component of the fetal circulation has closed, the blood must pass through the hepatic tissues to reach the systemic veins. Additional discrete stenosis can be found as the vertical vein passes through the diaphragm, while the channel can also break up into a delta of smaller channels that terminate in the tributaries of the portal vein.

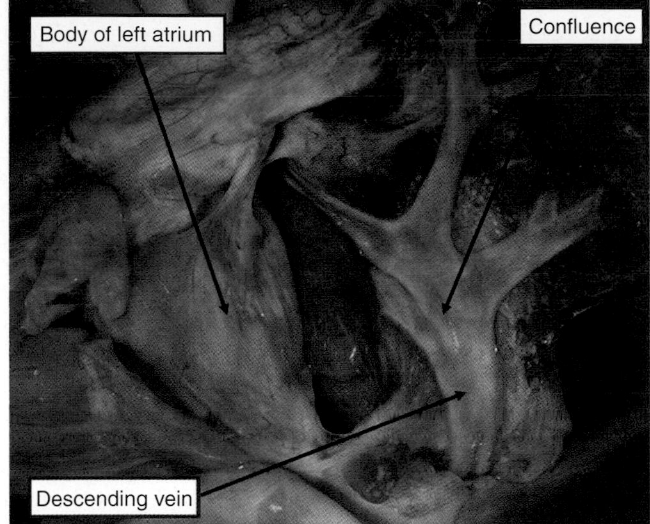

Figure 24-11 The picture shows infradiaphragmatic and infracardiac totally anomalous pulmonary venous connection. Having passed into the abdomen, the venous confluence terminates in the portal venous system.

In all the situations illustrated thus, we have shown the anomalously connecting pulmonary veins draining to the same site within the systemic system. As discussed, it is also possible for different veins to terminate in different anomalous sites. This is called mixed anomalous connection.[14] When seen, some of the veins can join together before draining to one of the multiple sites of anomalous connection, but different parts of the lung usually drain through discrete channels. In very rare situations, all of the pulmonary veins can join a common confluence, but the confluence itself then drains via separate channels, for example to both a left vertical vein and the coronary sinus.[14] With all these patterns of mixed anomalous connection, the same potentials exist for the pathways to become obstructed as when all the pulmonary veins drain anomalously to the same site, as discussed above.

Even excluding those cases of totally anomalous pulmonary venous connection associated with isomeric right atrial appendages, a large proportion of the patients have significant associated malformations. In these patients, such as those with abnormal ventriculo-arterial connections or tetralogy of Fallot, the associated abnormality is probably the major lesion. Even when the anomalous connection is isolated, there is almost always an interatrial communication present, so that venous blood is able to reach the left side of the heart. The atrial septum, nonetheless, can be intact. This then requires an alternative route for blood to reach the left side of the heart.

In any patient with totally anomalous pulmonary venous connection, the size of the left atrium and left ventricle are of obvious concern to the surgeon. At first sight, these structures seem small to the morphologist because of the disparate hyperplasia of the right atrium and right ventricle. Measurements, however, show that the left-sided structures are usually of adequate dimensions.[15] It is rare for there to be any great distance between the pulmonary venous confluence and the left atrium (see Fig. 24-11). Taken together, these features serve to facilitate surgical repair in virtually all patients. Problems, when they exist, are likely to be found in patients with mixed drainage, or in the setting of isomerism of the morphologically right atrial appendages.

Further problems can be created by changes in the pulmonary vasculature. Autopsy studies reveal changes in the veins of all patients studied, even including those dying on the first day of age, indicating that the changes themselves occur during fetal life. The veins take on arterial characteristics, while there is also an increase with age in the muscularity of the pulmonary arteries.[15–17] All these features point to the need for immediate surgical repair once the anomaly is diagnosed.

Morphogenesis

Knowledge of development of the pulmonary veins provides a good explanation for anomalous pulmonary venous connections. The developing atrium is itself initially connected to the mediastinum through the so-called dorsal mesocardium, even prior to formation of the lung buds from the trachea (see Chapter 3). As the lungs develop, the plexus of intrapulmonary veins joins with a pulmonary venous channel that canalises in the developing mediastinum. The newly formed primary pulmonary vein then uses the original connections of the dorsal mesocardium to gain access with the atrial component of the developing heart tube.[18,19] After normal fusion with the developing intrapulmonary venous plexuses, the pulmonary veins themselves are cannibalised by the atrium to form the venous components of the normal morphologically left atrium.[19] This occurs relatively late in development. Totally anomalous pulmonary venous connection is the consequence of failure of canalisation of the pulmonary venous channel in the mediastinum. Initially, since the lung buds themselves are derived from the foregut, the intrapulmonary veins also have connections to the systemic venous system.[20] Should the pulmonary venous channel fail to develop, these anastomoses between pulmonary and systemic venous systems persist and enlarge. An anastomosis with the anterior cardinal systemic venous system then results in supracardiac anomalous connection. Anastomosis with the systemic venous sinus, or the left sinus horn, produces cardiac connection, while infradiaphragmatic connection is the consequence of anastomosis with the omphalomesenteric system. In the strictest sense, these anastomoses are neither anomalous nor pulmonary.[21] If they persist, nonetheless, they certainly result in an anomalous pulmonary venous connection. Rarely, hearts may be found in which the pulmonary venous channel has formed, but has become atretic in its course between the atrium and the intrapulmonary venous plexuses.[22] Indeed, sometimes the pulmonary veins may be adjacent to the left atrium, but with musculature present between the two developmental components. An anomalous channel, analogous to the laevoatrial cardinal vein, then provides the only route for drainage of pulmonary venous blood. All of these examples, nonetheless, are readily explained using the developmental hypothesis discussed above. It should be noted that while the development of normal pulmonary venous anatomy is well studied, current thoughts about the development of anomalous pulmonary venous connections is conjectural, based on a combination of morphological observations and findings from normal development. The above discussion should, therefore, be viewed in light of that caveat.

Pathophysiology

Shunts

There is an obligatory left-to-right shunt, since pulmonary venous return is to the systemic veins or right atrium. A systemic output can only be maintained if there is a right-to-left shunt, which is almost always at atrial level. As discussed above, exceptional cases have been described in which the atrial septum was intact. In these patients, the right-to-left shunt occurred either at ventricular[21,23] or ductal level.[24]

When the right-to-left shunt is at atrial level, there is a tendency for fetal patterns of flow to be maintained by the valvar mechanism of the oval foramen.[5,25] Thus, in most patients with infradiaphragmatic connection, the oxygenated blood ascending the inferior caval vein towards the right atrium is directed towards the left atrium. Systemic arterial oxygen saturation is accordingly higher than that in the pulmonary arteries. When the anomalous venous connection is supracardiac, oxygenated blood tends to be directed down the superior caval vein and through the tricuspid valve. Consequently, in some of these patients, pulmonary arterial blood is more oxygenated than systemic arterial blood. In the others, mixing is complete. Similar patterns are found for anomalous connection to the coronary sinus. This is presumably because the orifice of the coronary sinus is directed more towards the tricuspid valve than the oval fossa.[5,26]

Obstruction to Pulmonary Venous Return

Obstruction to pulmonary venous return can occur at any of the anatomical sites documented above. Infants with evidence for borderline venous obstruction should be reevaluated, since the combination of decreasing pulmonary vascular resistance and increased flow of blood to the lungs typically seen in the postnatal period may unmask more severe obstruction.[27] When there is definable obstruction, the right ventricular pressure is usually suprasystemic.[28,29] There are many infants, particularly those with return to the coronary sinus, in whom the systolic pressure in the two ventricles is more or less equal, despite absence of any definable obstruction.[28] Indeed, in one study, no significant difference was found in systolic pressures measured in either the right ventricle or pulmonary arteries between patients with and without obstruction, and with supracardiac or intracardiac connections.[26] This suggests that the main cause of pulmonary hypertension in patients without apparent pulmonary venous obstruction is elevation of pulmonary resistance, presumably as a result of extension of muscle into peripheral arterioles and veins.[15,16] If this is the cause, the almost invariable fall to normal after successful repair indicates that the process is reversible. Alternatively, at least part of the problem may result from undetected anatomical causes of pulmonary venous obstruction.[30]

The contribution of the oval foramen to the problem is controversial. In theory, obstruction of this foramen leads to a high right atrial pressure, which impedes pulmonary venous return, thus producing pulmonary hypertension. Gathman and Nadas[5] argued on three grounds, however, that significant obstruction of pulmonary venous return at atrial level was rare. First, patients as a group had similar right atrial pressures whether they were pulmonary hypertensive or not. Second, about a third of patients with pulmonary hypertension had no pressure gradient at atrial level. Indeed, in a few, mean left atrial pressure was higher than right. Third, almost all patients with pulmonary vascular obstruction also had pulmonary venous obstruction. While these arguments are persuasive as to the insignificant role of the oval foramen in producing pulmonary hypertension, they do not rule out the possibility that a small foramen could limit systemic flow.

Consequences of Pulmonary Venous Obstruction

When pulmonary venous return is unobstructed, right ventricular diastolic pressure is low and right ventricular compliance relatively high. Blood returning to the right atrium, therefore, tends to enter the right ventricle rather than the left atrium. Flow of blood to the lungs tends greatly to exceed flow in the systemic circuit. Right ventricular end-diastolic and stroke volumes are considerably increased in consequence.[31,32] Since mixing of pulmonary and systemic venous blood is complete, apart from the minor degrees of streaming discussed above, right atrial and, therefore, systemic arterial blood is well oxygenated, with saturations of oxygen found in excess of 90%.

In the presence of pulmonary venous obstruction, in contrast, pulmonary venous pressure is raised. Pulmonary oedema is then produced if the pressure is sufficiently severe, though bronchopulmonary venous anastomoses may relieve pressure to some degree. In severe cases, nonetheless, pulmonary arterial pressure is raised even above systemic pressure, and pulmonary blood flow is reduced. The right ventricle, therefore, becomes pressure rather than volume overloaded.[31,32] Systemic arterial oxygen saturation may then fall to values of 20% to 30%. The depression of systemic arterial saturation, and possibly also output, results in tissue hypoxemia and metabolic acidosis. These effects of pulmonary venous obstruction are compounded by the changes in small pulmonary veins and arteries already described, which may further increase pulmonary vascular resistance.

In the occasional patient who survives infancy without severe pulmonary venous obstruction, late pulmonary vascular obstructive disease may develop as in those with atrial septal defect. The effects are the same as those of pulmonary venous obstruction, except that no pulmonary oedema occurs.

Presentation and Symptoms

Very occasionally, totally anomalous pulmonary venous connection can present as sudden death in the first 2 months of life.[33] As long ago as 1962, Hastreiter and colleagues[24] recognised that the main determinant of the clinical picture was the presence of pulmonary venous obstruction. Consequently, for each of the ensuing sections relating to the clinical picture, patients will be divided into those with and without pulmonary venous obstruction. Some patients with only modest obstruction fall between the two groups and exhibit features of both.

Patients with severe pulmonary venous obstruction present in the first week or two of life with obvious cyanosis and difficulties with feeding and respiration.[34]

In contrast to what is observed in the respiratory distress syndrome, grunting respiration is very rarely seen in obstructed venous return. Pointers to respiratory distress syndrome rather than totally anomalous pulmonary connection are maternal diabetes, prematurity, caesarean section, and very early onset of respiratory difficulties. Any, or all, of these can, nonetheless, be found in the setting of anomalous pulmonary venous connection. In the registry of the Extracorporeal Life Support Society, containing 4823 patients, 623 patients were thought to have persistent fetal circulation. Of these, one-tenth were shown to have congenital heart disease. About half had totally anomalous pulmonary venous connection, while one-tenth had complete transposition. This emphasises how easy it is to mistake totally anomalous pulmonary venous connection for persistent fetal circulation if echocardiography is not performed.[35] A unique mode of presentation, haematemesis, was described in one patient with infradiaphragmatic return to the left gastric vein.[36] Another unique mode was severe unconjugated hyperbilirubinemia in the setting of infradiaphragmatic return. The patient survived exchange transfusion and surgical repair.[37]

Patients without severe pulmonary venous obstruction tend to present in heart failure at 2 to 3 months of age. They have a history of difficulties with feeding and, sometimes, chest infections. Cyanosis is generally not a symptom.

Those with severe pulmonary venous obstruction are sick neonates with obvious or severe cyanosis. Skin mottling is frequent, reflecting poor peripheral perfusion and metabolic acidosis. Tachypnea is usually marked, though respiration is quiet. Hepatomegaly is occasionally considerable, particularly when drainage is to the portal vein. The peripheral pulses are often somewhat weak. The precordium is quiet. On auscultation there are usually no murmurs. If a murmur does exist, it is usually unimpressive and mid-systolic. Occasionally a venous hum is heard in the region where pulmonary venous return is obstructed, under the left clavicle, for example, in anomalous connection via a left vertical vein. The first heart sound is single and the second heart sound is described as exhibiting physiological or fixed splitting.[5] The pulmonary component is accentuated and a fourth heart sound may be heard. Rarely, the second heart sound appears single.

When seen from the end of the bed, patients without severe pulmonary venous obstruction resemble patients with large ventricular septal defect. They are scrawny and tachypneic, with retractions. The presence of cyanosis can certainly be missed if the infant is examined in a poor light. Even in a good light, it may not be detected. There is usually hepatomegaly, and rales may well be heard in the lungs.

The peripheral pulses are normal to small and the precordium overactive, but without any thrill. On auscultation, the first heart sound is normal and, usually, there is wide fixed splitting of the second sound. An ejection systolic murmur is heard in the pulmonary area owing to excessive flow through the pulmonary valve. A mid-diastolic murmur tends to be heard at the lower left sternal border, representing excessive flow through the tricuspid valve.

Patients without pulmonary venous obstruction very occasionally survive infancy without heart disease being detected. These patients present as does a typical patient with atrial septal defect, but with the added features of mild cyanosis and clubbing.

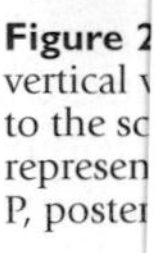

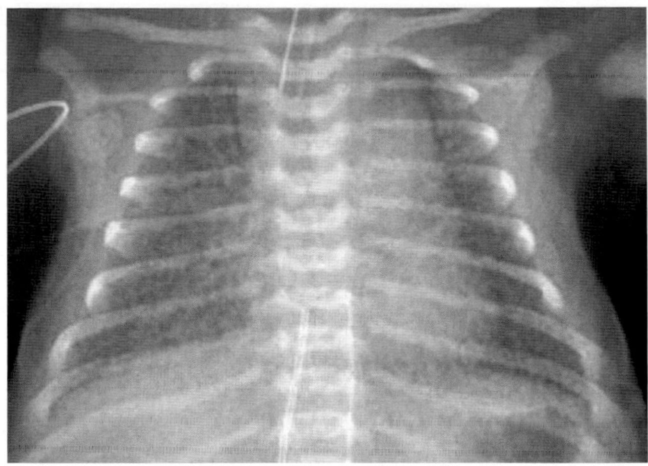

Figure 24-12 This chest radiograph is typical of obstructed totally anomalous pulmonary venous connection, showing a ground-glass appearance in both lung fields and a small cardiac shadow.

Investigations

Chest Radiography

Newborns with severe pulmonary venous obstruction have an extremely characteristic chest radiograph, with a small or normally sized heart framed by ground-glass lung fields[24,38,39] (Fig. 24-12). Kerley B lines are occasionally seen.[40] These appearances are sometimes confused with those of respiratory distress syndrome. The latter diagnosis can easily and correctly be made in most cases in which it is present because of the more patchy distribution of changes in the lung fields. Furthermore, obliteration of part or the entire cardiac silhouette and the appearance of an air bronchogram are both highly characteristic of respiratory distress syndrome and are rare in those patients with totally anomalous pulmonary venous connection.

Patients without severe pulmonary venous obstruction have enlarged hearts because of the right ventricular volume overload, together with engorged lung fields. The pulmonary trunk becomes prominent in older patients, as does the left vertical vein when this is the site of the anomalous venous connection. This gives rise to the snowman appearance, known to almost every paediatrician and also described as the W. C. Fields heart. This is now of mainly historical importance because patients usually have their defect corrected long before the snowman has time to appear, which was usually in the second year of life.[41] Less than one-third of infants with supracardiac anomalous connection exhibit the snowman.[28] Exceptionally, however, the snowman has been seen at 3 months of age.[5]

Electrocardiography

The electrocardiogram shows right-axis deviation with a clockwise frontal plane loop and right ventricular hypertrophy. V_1 usually shows an rsR′ pattern, though a qR is seen in four-fifths of patients. The latter might be thought to indicate the presence of more severe pulmonary hypertension, but there is poor correlation between the two.[5] Disturbances of conduction are rare. Under 1 month of age, only about one-twelfth of patients have right atrial hypertrophy, whereas this is seen in three-quarters between 1 and 3 months, and in nine-tenths over 3 months. Patients with pulmonary venous obstruction, who present younger,

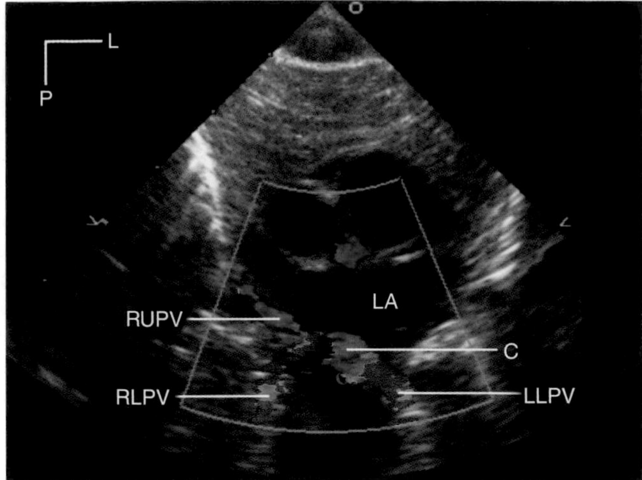

Figure 24-19 In this patient with totally anomalous pulmonary connection, a suprasternal view reveals three pulmonary veins (RUPV, RLPV, and LLPV) draining into the coronary sinus posterior to the left atrium (LA). Further imaging revealed that the left pulmonary vein drained into a separate vertical vein (see Fig. 24-30), emphasising the importance of identifying all four pulmonary venous connections. C, confluence; L, left; P, posterior.

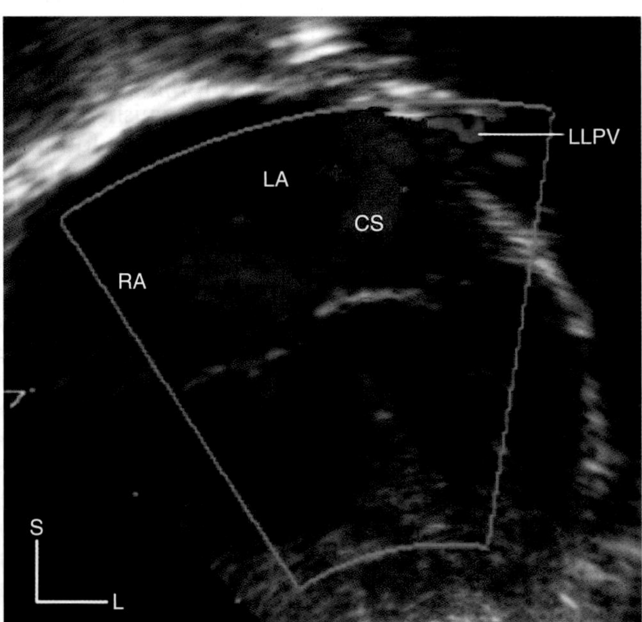

Figure 24-20 This apical four-chamber view reveals drainage of the left lower pulmonary vein (LLPV) into the coronary sinus (CS). L, left; LA, left atrium; RA, right atrium; S, superior.

should be suspected. This distinction can be confirmed by making small tilting and rotational movements of the transducer, which show the anomalously connecting pulmonary veins. Anomalous connection to the right atrium can be diagnosed if there is no ascending or descending vein, the coronary sinus is of normal size and the pulmonary veins can be followed to their site of entry to the right atrium. The echocardiographer should consider measuring the diameter of all four pulmonary veins between hilum and confluence, as the sum of these diameters is a strong and independent predictor of surgical survival.[47] Most of the late deaths in this study were the result of individual pulmonary venous stenosis at sites remote from the surgical

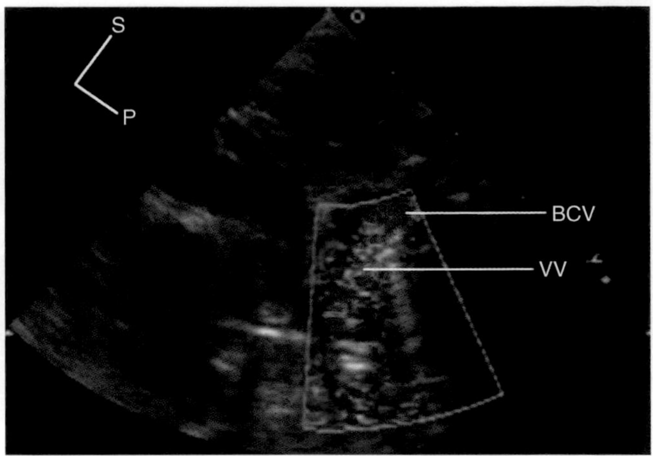

Figure 24-21 This image, taken from a suprasternal view, shows a stenotic vertical vein (VV) connecting to the left bracheocephalic vein (BCV) in a patient with obstructed supracardiac totally anomalous pulmonary venous connection. Note the aliased flow in the vertical vein. P, posterior; S, superior.

anastomosis to the left atrium. In older patients, it can be difficult to image pulmonary veins from the precordium. Under these circumstances, transoesophageal echocardiography can be most helpful.[48]

Colour Doppler is essential to diagnosis in these patients. First, it becomes impossible to confuse a left vertical vein draining to the brachiocephalic vein with a persistent left superior caval vein, except in the highly improbable association with atresia of the coronary sinus. The differences demonstrated in direction of flow apply equally to distinction between the inferior caval vein and the descending pulmonary venous pathway. Second, where there is doubt as to whether an image obtained is a genuine pulmonary vein or an artifact, the demonstration of colour within the structure indicates that it is vascular. Third, sites of obstruction along the pulmonary venous pathway can be demonstrated as points of turbulence (Fig. 24-21), or even absent flow, both pre- and post-operatively.[49–51] As is essential with colour Doppler imaging of any venous structure, care must be taken to ensure an appropriate Nyquist limit for optimal detection of pulmonary venous drainage and obstruction.

In areas where colour Doppler suggests obstruction, pulsed wave Doppler offers an objective measure. The presence of a focal increase in flow velocity with a continuous, non-phasic flow pattern distally is a characteristic finding[27] (Fig. 24-22). A sensitivity of 100% and specificity of 85% have been claimed for detection of obstruction by cross-sectional imaging and colour Doppler.[52]

It is now standard of care to diagnose and repair totally anomalous pulmonary venous connection based on echocardiography alone. In 1983, Stark and colleagues[53] first reported successful repair of totally anomalous pulmonary venous connection in six young infants without previous cardiac catheterisation. Subsequent experience confirms that skilled use of cross sectional echocardiography avoids the need for cardiac catheterisation in the majority of patients.[54] Mixed totally anomalous pulmonary venous return cannot always be recognised,[54,55] but then such arrangements are not always diagnosed by traditional angiography. As always, if the clinical and cross sectional echocardiographic findings do not fit the clinical situation, additional imaging should be performed without hesitation.

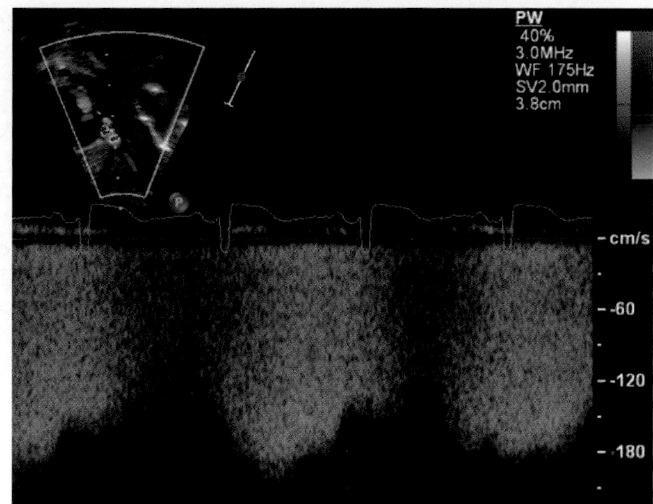

Figure 24-22 The Doppler profile that corresponds with the image in Figure 24-17. It reveals high velocity flow with a continuous, non-phasic flow pattern, which is characteristic of obstructed pulmonary venous flow.

Ultrasound technology has progressed to a degree that it is possible to diagnose totally anomalous pulmonary venous connection by fetal echocardiography, although it is often missed on screening ultrasounds in the absence of additional cardiac anomalies. The presence of a confluence behind the left atrium, a vertical vein, or a widened gap between the descending aorta and the posterior wall of the left atrium are the most consistent echocardiographic clues.[56,57] As with postnatal echocardiography, colour and spectral Doppler analysis can assist greatly in identifying venous obstruction.

Cardiac Catheterisation

Cardiac catheterisation is rarely indicated in this era. If performed, it will document the pathophysiology already indicated. The pulmonary venous anatomy can almost always be delineated non-invasively, and the clinical scenario of pulmonary venous obstruction can almost always be determined without invasive testing.[27,52] If performing catheterisation, it should be remembered that passage of a catheter across an obstruction will temporarily make it worse. Since obtaining the information demands advancing the catheter through an abnormally positioned vein, the safest approach is first to determine the site of the vein. This can be done using echocardiography, computed tomographic angiography, or magnetic resonance imaging. Vertical veins can be entered with ease using a suitably curved catheter. If necessary, a guide wire can be used, passing the catheter from below through the right atrium and via the right superior caval and brachiocephalic veins.[28] When return is to the coronary sinus, this structure may be entered in the usual fashion. Having reached the coronary sinus, it is extremely important to try and enter all pulmonary veins, in order to detect any pressure differences between pulmonary veins or confluence and coronary sinus, or else between coronary sinus and right atrium. It is usually a simple matter to enter the pulmonary confluence when it connects either to the right atrium or to the right superior or inferior caval veins. In the special case of anomalous connection to the portal vein, the umbilical vein is the approach of choice.[58] No-one has reported success in traversing the venous duct from the inferior caval vein. In any case, this structure has often closed by the time the patient is catheterised. The catheter should not be left in position for long, as pulmonary venous pressure can rise as high as 50 mm Hg if it is not removed at once.[59]

Traditional Angiography

It is not easy to demonstrate well the detailed anatomy of the route of anomalous return by traditional angiography. This is probably why relatively little was published on the subject. In theory, selective pulmonary venous injection is the method of choice. In practice, it is often a frustrating experience because of the refusal of contrast medium to reflux into pulmonary veins against the current unless there is severe pulmonary venous obstruction. The pulmonary venous injection in obstructed connection to the portal vein published by Tynan and colleagues[58] shows superb opacification of the pulmonary veins. In contrast, on injection into the coronary sinus, it is rare to see opacification of pulmonary veins even if all are connected to it. While the techniques below generally allow one to define the pulmonary venous anatomy, these findings can almost always be defined non-invasively using echocardiography, along with the occasional need for magnetic resonance imaging or computed tomographic imaging as described in the next section.

Pulmonary arteriography works well if there is just the right amount of pulmonary venous obstruction. If this is too severe, and particularly if the duct is patent, it may be impossible to demonstrate the pulmonary veins because of loss of contrast medium into the systemic circulation. This happens despite the use of large doses of rapidly injected contrast medium and filming for 20 seconds or more. Furthermore, in the absence of pulmonary venous obstruction, pulmonary blood supply may be so high that serious dilution of contrast medium prevents optimal visualisation of the pulmonary veins. Mixed anomalous connection may be missed because of inadequate definition and simultaneous opacification of all the cardiac chambers. Selective left or right pulmonary arterial injection may improve recognition of the sites of drainage in mixed return. Pulmonary arterial wedge injection may be even better.

When opacified, the appearance of the vertical vein is characteristic (Fig. 24-23). So is the typical site of obstruction halfway along its course when it is present, representing the site where the vertical vein passes through the vise between the left pulmonary artery and left main bronchus. Anomalous connection to the portal vein is also characteristic. The pulmonary venous confluence, instead of being horizontal, tends to be vertical (Fig. 24-24). This gives the picture poetically termed the tree in winter.[60] When the anomalous connection is to the azygos or right superior caval vein, the course of the common pulmonary vein is frequently tortuous. Drainage to the coronary sinus is typified by the golf-ball appearance of the dilated coronary sinus in the frontal projection.[61] Anomalous connection to the right atrium is much more difficult. The angiographic diagnosis depended on the recognition that right atrial opacification preceded that of the left atrium, but for none of the reasons listed above.[61]

Computed Tomographic Angiography and Magnetic Resonance Imaging

Technological advances in medical imaging have increased the utilisation of computed tomographic angiography and magnetic resonance imaging in the evaluation of patients

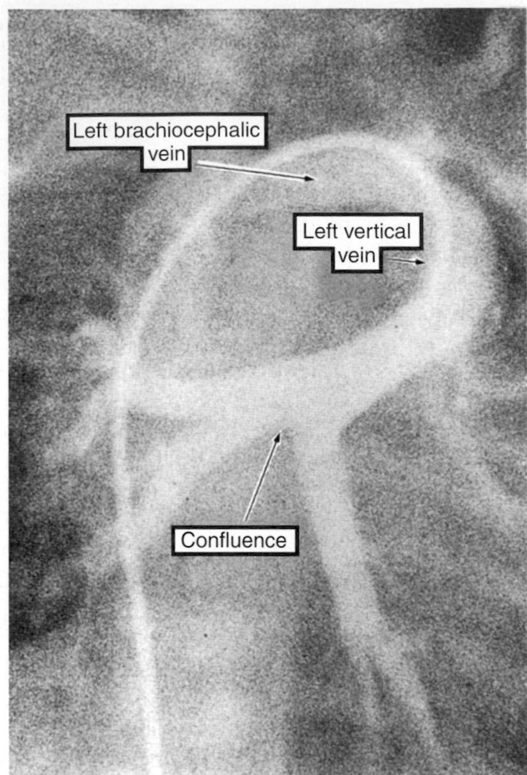

Figure 24-23 This selective injection, profiled in frontal projection, shows totally anomalous pulmonary venous connection to a left vertical vein.

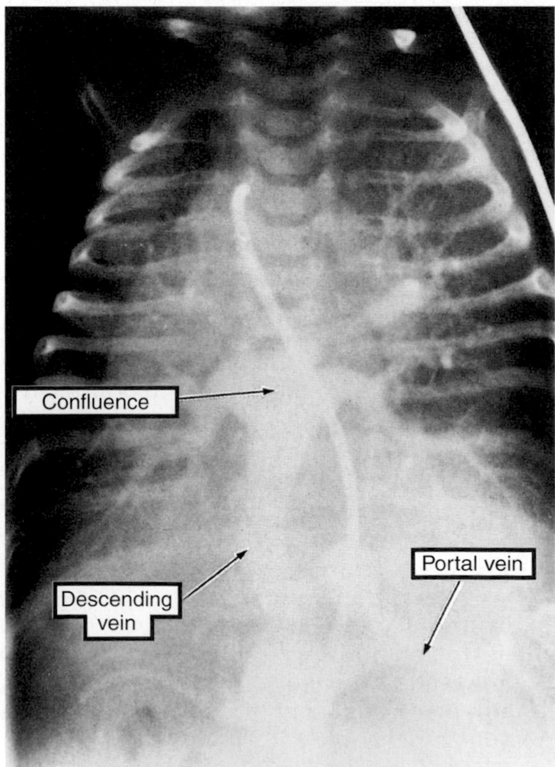

Figure 24-24 This pulmonary arteriogram shows totally anomalous pulmonary venous connection to the portal vein. The position of the catheter in the left-sided inferior caval vein, and the heart lying to the right, together with the presence of totally anomalous pulmonary venous connection, strongly suggest right isomerism, which was indeed present in this patient.

with anomalous pulmonary venous connection.[62] Given the inherent complexity involved in understanding the three-dimensional relationships in these patients, multiplanar imaging techniques such as magnetic resonance imaging and computed tomographic angiography allows one to understand the involved anatomy in more straightforward manner. Pulmonary venous connections with a particularly tortuous course, as is often seen with infracardiac connection or drainage via the azygous system, can be difficult to follow by echocardiography. These multi-planar modalities allow one to follow even the most tortuous vessels in a relatively simple fashion. As early as 1991, Masui and colleagues[63] found magnetic resonance imaging to be superior to both echocardiography and conventional angiography in patients with totally anomalous pulmonary venous connection. Since then, numerous other authors have endorsed its utility in these patients.[64–68] Magnetic resonance imaging permits imaging in virtually any plane, allowing for accurate characterisation of the course and size of all pulmonary venous connections, along with other structural anomalies. Contrast-enhanced magnetic resonance angiography allows for three-dimensional reconstructions, which has been proven to be useful in these patients.[69,70] In addition, magnetic resonance imaging allows for functional data including flow quantification and volumetric analysis. However, cardiac magnetic resonance imaging requires a combination of technical expertise and knowledge of cardiac anatomy that is not readily available in all centers, and time-consuming scanning protocols along with the need for transition to equipment suitable for use in magnetic resonance imaging limit the practicality of this imaging modality in the most critically ill infants.

High-resolution computed tomographic angiography using helical multi-detector scanners has proven to be a highly accurate alternative to conventional angiography in the diagnosis and characterisation of anomalous pulmonary venous connections.[71–75] Newer scanners have cut the scanning time to a few seconds,[76] allowing most scans to be performed without sedation. Commercial software is readily available for three-dimensional reconstruction of these datasets, along with datasets from magnetic resonance angiography, permitting those with reasonable knowledge in congenital heart disease to manipulate the anatomy in such a way that is easily understandable.[76,77] In contrast to magnetic resonance angiography, computed tomographic angiography allows for simultaneous three-dimensional reconstructions of additional thoracic structures, making it particularly useful in patients with the bronchopulmonary vise described above. In critically ill patients, computed tomographic angiography can be performed in an expeditious manner with minimal time away from the intensive care unit, without need to transition to specialised equipment. This can be useful for patients who are on extracorporeal membrane oxygenation.

Unlike what is seen with traditional angiography, magnetic resonance angiography and computed tomographic angiography will display contrast in multiple structures simultaneously. This is particularly useful when documenting mixed connections and in understanding spatial relationships in those with more complex anatomic arrangements (Figs. 24-25 and 24-26). Instead of using multiple injections and catheter courses to search for each pulmonary venous connection, all connections can

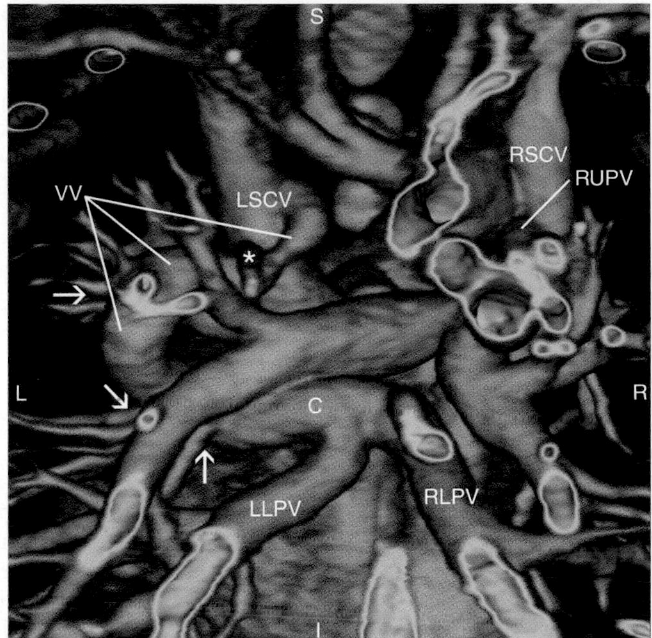

Figure 24-25 This computed tomographic angiogram reveals the complex pulmonary venous connections in a patient with mixed totally anomalous pulmonary venous connection. The right and left lower pulmonary veins (RLPV and LLPV) connect to a horizontal confluence, which leads into a vertical vein (VV). Pulmonary venous drainage from the left upper lung empties via multiple separate veins (*arrows*) as the vertical vein ascends. The vertical vein dives underneath the left azygous vein (*star*), resulting in stenosis before joining the rightward aspect of the left superior caval vein (LSCV). The right upper pulmonary vein (RUPV) connects with the leftward aspect of the right superior caval vein (RSCV). This image highlights the utility of CT angiography in evaluating complex pulmonary venous connections. I, inferior; L, left; R, right; S, superior.

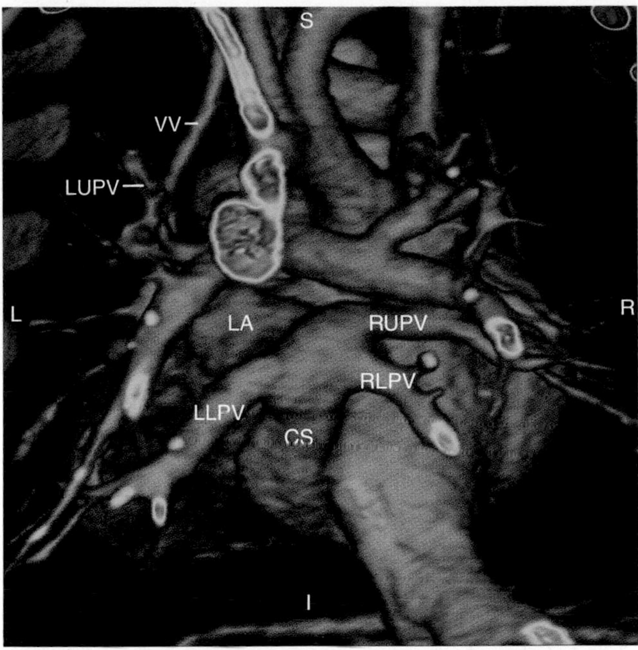

Figure 24-26 In this patient with mixed totally anomalous pulmonary venous connection, the right pulmonary veins (RUPV and RLPV) and left lower pulmonary vein (LLPV) connect with the coronary sinus (CS). The left upper pulmonary vein (LUPV), however, connects with a vertical vein (VV) that drains into the left bracheocephalic vein (not imaged here). I, inferior; L, left; LA, left atrium; R, right; S, superior.

be located on one contrast injection. On the other hand, traditional angiography is likely superior in identifying pulmonary venous drainage from areas of the lung where there is little to no pulmonary blood flow, as these newer modalities have no acceptable substitute for a pulmonary artery wedge angiogram. When imaging patients with suspected supracardiac drainage, it may be useful to inject contrast from below the heart. Assuming the scan is performed with the first pass of contrast through the heart, as is standard procedure, any contrast in a venous structure above the heart can clearly be identified as pulmonary venous in origin (Fig. 24-27). This is particularly useful when trying to differentiate a left superior caval vein from a vertical vein. The converse can be applied to infracardiac connection.

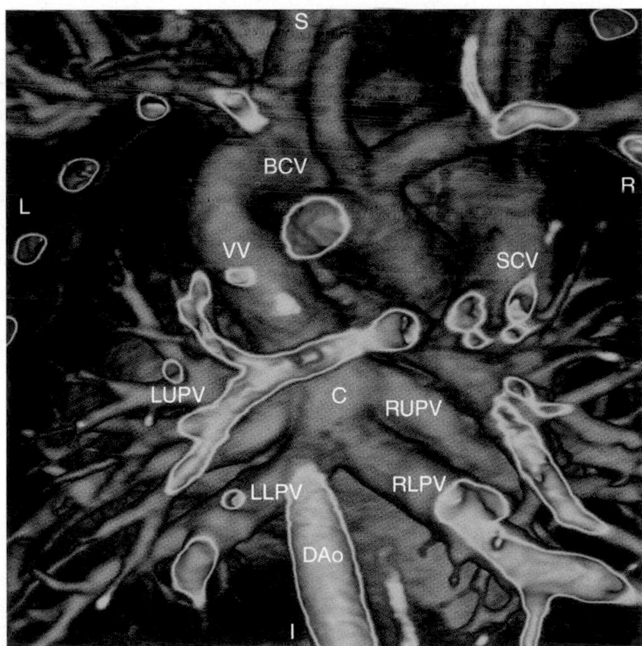

Figure 24-27 This computed tomographic angiogram reveals all four pulmonary veins (RUPV, RLPV, LUPV, LLPV) connecting to a confluence (C), which leads to a vertical vein (VV) and then on to the left bracheocephalic vein (BCV) in a patient with supracardiac totally anomalous pulmonary venous connection. DAo, descending aorta; I, inferior; L, left; R, right; S, superior; SCV, superior caval vein.

Differential Diagnosis

Much of the basis of differential diagnosis has already been discussed and will not be repeated. As we shall see, pulmonary venous atresia also presents as totally anomalous connection with severe pulmonary venous obstruction. The two conditions, however, may be indistinguishable prior to surgery if no common pulmonary vein is seen by preoperative imaging.

Unobstructed connection has to be distinguished from other conditions producing heart failure, mild cyanosis, and cardiomegaly with pulmonary plethora and right ventricular hypertrophy. The most important of these is complete transposition with large ventricular septal defect, in which the second heart sound is commonly single. Atrioventricular septal defect with common atrium is easily distinguished by the typical electrocardiogram, showing a superior counter-clockwise frontal plane QRS loop. Totally anomalous connection to the left vertical vein has to be distinguished from the laevoatrial cardinal vein found in association with mitral atresia and intact atrial septum. In both conditions, pulmonary venous blood flow is to a confluence via left vertical vein. In the case of the laevoatrial cardinal vein, the confluence is the left atrium, the pulmonary veins being normally connected.

Course and Prognosis

With medical treatment alone, three-quarters of all children with totally anomalous pulmonary venous connection uncomplicated by isomerism were dead or had undergone surgery by their first birthday.[41] It is of interest that this poor survival occurred despite the fact that less than 10% had infradiaphragmatic anomalous connection. In one study, of 25 patients with pulmonary venous obstruction treated medically, only two survived their first year.[5] In the postmortem study from central Bohemia, which relates to the time before advanced cardiac surgery, 95.8% of deaths occurred in the first year of life.[78] The only place for medical treatment, therefore, is in resuscitation of the critically ill neonate.

In the past, balloon atrial septostomy was shown to produce clinical improvement in the short term in some patients. It was impossible, however, to identify in advance those patients who would benefit from the procedure.[79,80] At the time, septostomy was recommended as a procedure to buy time so as to permit the baby to undergo surgery at a size when the immediate surgical risk was lower. Recent improvements in surgical results, even at very young ages, militate strongly against this expectant policy. Furthermore, balloon atrial septostomy is technically more difficult than in complete transposition because two methods normally used to check that the catheter is in the left atrium do not apply. The left atrial saturation is not higher than the right, and pulmonary veins cannot be entered from the left atrium. Even using biplane screening, it can be difficult to distinguish a catheter positioned in the left atrium from one in a dilated coronary sinus. Sano and colleagues[81] found that in no case did septostomy result in sufficient clinical improvement in critically ill patients to permit deferral of the operation. In patients with severely obstructed pulmonary venous return, stent placement in the area of obstruction can be considered as a temporising measure if surgery cannot be performed in a timely manner.[82,83]

Management

Medical Treatment

In the current era, medical management consists solely of supportive measures in preparation for surgical management.

Surgery

With rare exception, neonatal repair is the standard of care. Totally anomalous pulmonary venous connection was the first condition in which the necessity of open heart repair in infancy was forced upon surgeons as a result of the appalling natural history, the lack of any adequate alternative by way of palliation and the potential for excellent long-term results if immediate survival could be achieved. The early results in infancy inevitably involved a high mortality.[28,79,81,84,85] Operations at this time included those in which an anastomosis between the pulmonary venous confluence and the left atrium was created but the interatrial communication was not closed; the common pulmonary vein, if obstructed, was not ligated.[28,81,85] Though subsequent spontaneous closure of the interatrial communication was documented in some patients,[86] this staged approach is now rarely used. Surgical results have now greatly improved (Table 24-1). There used to be debate as to whether age or site of connection was the most important determinant of operative survival, but most recent studies have not shown either to be significant.[87–94] Mortality in current era[10,81,87–91,95,96] has been so low that analysis of risk factors has become challenging. Pre-operative pulmonary venous obstruction has been shown to be a risk factor in some series,[87,88,90,91,96] but this effect may have been neutralised with improved perioperative care.[87,91,92] Another study from Boston Children's found functionally univentricular physiology, as would be expected, to be a significant risk factor for hospital mortality.[90] In the series reported from the University of Alabama, the significant incremental risk factors for death were younger age, higher New York Heart Association class, higher pulmonary arterial systolic pressure, lower systolic pressure in the left ventricle, and previous balloon atrial septostomy.[97] Bando and colleagues[87] found emergency surgery, diffuse pulmonary vein stenosis, requirement of pre-operative inotropic agents, and post-operative pulmonary hypertensive events to be significant predictors of hospital mortality, while Bogers and colleagues[88] found that the use of circulatory arrest was a risk factor. In a study covering 50 years of surgical results in Toronto,[96] pulmonary venous obstruction, earlier year of repair, younger age at repair, and type of connection were all found to be significant predictors of death. Interestingly, and in contrast to other studies, the cardiac

TABLE 24-1

RESULTS OF REPAIR OF TOTALLY ANOMALOUS PULMONARY VENOUS CONNECTION IN INFANCY

Report	Date of Operation	Hospital Mortality (Number [%])
Katz et al[100]	1974–1977	4/19 (21%)
Whight et al[126]	1969–1976	3/23 (13%)
Hammon et al[31]	1969–1979	5/25 (20%)
Bove et al[138]	1971–1979	26/73 (36%)
Yee et al[221]	1975–1986	8/75 (11%)
Lamb et al[29]	1968–1985	14/80 (18%)
Lincoln et al[222]	1973–1986	12/83 (14%)
Sano et al[81]	1979–1987	1/44 (2%)
Raisher et al[10]	1983–1990	1/20 (5%)
Korbmacher et al[223]	1958–1992	18/52 (35%)
Lupinetti et al[95]	1985–1993	2/41 (5%)
Sinzobahamvya et al[91]	1977–1994	6/71 (8%)
Bando et al[87]	1966–1995	10/105 (10%)
Calderone et al[89]	1982–1996	19/126 (15%)
Bogers et al[88]	1973–1998	6/44 (14%)
Michielon et al[94]	1983–2001	11/89 (12%)
Hyde et al[92]	1988–1998	6/85 (7%)
Hancock Friesen et al[90]	1989–2000	10/84 (12%)

form of connection was associated with an increased risk of surgical mortality. Failure to monitor pulmonary arterial pressure in the post-operative period was put forward as a risk factor for operative death in another series.[98]

The inaccessibility of the pulmonary venous confluence behind the heart has meant that a bewildering variety of different surgical approaches have been employed for correction. Repair of anomalous connection to the coronary sinus involves either cutting back the mouth of the sinus into the left atrium and repairing the atrial septum in such a way as to leave the opening in the coronary sinus on its left side, or else using the technique promoted by Van Praagh and colleagues,[12] which involves removal of the muscular wall between the coronary sinus and left atrium and closing both the atrial septal defect and the mouth of the coronary sinus. Aeba and colleagues[99] described their experience over 30 years with repair of anomalous venous connection to the coronary sinus, finding favorable results with the use of autologous material rather than prosthetic material. Drainage to the right atrium or lower right superior caval vein can be repaired by shifting the atrial septum to its right side or by creating a prosthetic tunnel to lead pulmonary venous blood to the left atrium. The opening between the confluence and the right atrium may need to be enlarged. When connection is to other sites, the confluence must be reached by dislocating the cardiac apex forwards, by incising posterior pericardial attachments on the right so as to elevate the heart and caval veins and retract them to the left, by approaching through the transverse sinus or by cutting through the atrial septum and the posterior left atrial wall.[100] A confluence connected to a left vertical vein can also be approached from a left thoracotomy extended trans-sternally.[101] A superior approach between the superior caval vein and ascending aorta, occasionally necessitating transaction of the aorta, can be useful for those with supracardiac or mixed drainage.[102] Whatever the approach, the objective must be to create as wide an anastomosis as possible between the confluence and the left atrium. Given the small size of the left atrium that is commonly associated with this lesion, some surgeons chose to augment the atrium. However, this technique appears to be associated with late arrhythmias.[94]

Because the left heart may have difficulty tolerating an acute increase in pulmonary venous return after surgery, resulting in low cardiac output, many surgeons leave the vertical vein intact after surgery.[103] After repair, flow through this high resistance pathway is thought to be negligible,[100,104] although a follow-up study on these patients suggests that this vein often remains patent.[105] In 1994, a useful strategy was proposed by Stark.[106] The left atrial and systemic arterial pressures are measured after the patient is taken off bypass. The vertical vein is then snared. If occlusion of the vertical vein can be achieved without a rise in left atrial pressure and a fall in systemic pressure, then ligation of the vein is performed. Otherwise, the vein is left patent. Subsequent authors have validated the utility of this concept.[107,108] To facilitate this strategy, percutaneously adjustable devises to ligate the vertical vein are under development, and have been found to be potentially useful.[109] The post-operative course is frequently marked by pulmonary hypertensive crises. Post-operative pulmonary hypertension in this population was traditionally managed with 100% oxygen and epoprostenol (prostacyclin),[110] but nitric oxide has shown promising results over the last 10 years.[111–114] However, one should be cognisant of the rare possibility of paradoxical pulmonary hypertension with the use of nitric oxide in patients with poor left heart compliance.[115]

Results of Surgery

The late results of repair are, in general, excellent.[116,117] The hazard function for death has become similar to that of the general population within about 24 months of operation.[97] Nonetheless, late pulmonary venous obstruction is not uncommon. This serious complication is poorly understood and occurs in patients with and without obstruction prior to surgery.[92] It occurs in about 10% of all large surgical series and has remained stable over the last 30 years. Some authors have found it to be more common in patients with infracardiac or mixed drainage.[55,93] Others have noted that it is more common in patients repaired at a younger age.[117] The patient typically has undergone a reasonably smooth post-operative course and is discharged from hospital, only to be readmitted 4 to 6 weeks after operation with pulmonary oedema. It is more common in patients with a small pulmonary venous confluence and post-operative pulmonary hypertension.[87] In earlier studies, reoperation carried a high mortality and a strong chance of recurrence, whatever the nature of the obstruction. Few cases of survival beyond 1 year from the original operation were documented. In 1996, Lacour-Gayet and collegues[118,119] introduced a sutureless technique for reoperation using in situ pericardium with promising results. In this procedure, the pulmonary veins are incised from the ostia emptying into the left atrium out to the pericardial refection, usually removing scarred tissue and left atrial wall. The presence of pericardial adhesions allows for the posterior pericardial cavity to be closed to the left atrium, occasionally reinforced by securing the resected free left dorsal atrial wall to the posterior pericardium with several sutures. A vascularised flap of pericardium can also be anastamosed to the right atrial wall used to create a pouch of in situ pericardium through which the right pulmonary veins can drain into the left atrium. Mid-term results from this technique have been encouraging.[93,120–123]

Suggested pre-operative predisposing factors include hypoplasia of the pulmonary veins,[16,47] the extension of muscle from intrapulmonary to extrapulmonary veins, thickening of the pulmonary venous wall and intimal proliferation.[16] Most authors describe sclerosis or fibrosis as the substrate for progressive obstruction, though these statements are rarely supported by histology. Pre-operative pulmonary hypertension is present in most, but not all, of these patients.[29,30]

A careful reading of the literature suggests that there are three groups of patients who have post-operative venous obstruction. In the first group, accounting for a minority of patients,[84,100,124,125] post-operative pulmonary venous obstruction is clearly a consequence of a surgical error, such as construction of an insufficiently large anastomosis between the left atrium and the pulmonary venous confluence. Inadequate unroofing of the coronary sinus[126] is held by some to be preventable by using the approach suggested by Van Praagh and her colleagues.[12] In a second group, obstruction has been blamed, at least in part, on reaction of tissues either to the operation itself or to the prosthetic material employed.[30] In the third group, post-operative pulmonary venous obstruction is caused primarily by unrelieved obstruction upstream to the post-operative pulmonary venous pathway. This usually occurs in drainage to the coronary sinus, the only variety in which the surgeon has not had to create an anastomosis between the heart and the pulmonary venous confluence.

The diagnosis is most simply made by colour flow mapping and Doppler interrogation. This will demonstrate a small anastomosis (Fig. 24-28) and/or a continuous, non-phasic relatively high-velocity Doppler flow signal and an enlarged right ventricle.[54] If none of these are present, venous obstruction is almost certainly absent. Cardiac catheterisation and angiography should be reserved for those patients for whom a site of obstruction cannot be identified, those whose clinical course and echocardiographic findings do not match, and those in whom placement of stents is intended. If catheter-based intervention is not planned, consideration should be given to magnetic resonance imaging or computed tomographic angiography as the imaging modality used to clarify questionable echocardiography findings. At catheterisation, injection of contrast medium is best made into the pulmonary veins or, failing that, into a wedged pulmonary arterial catheter.[127] Magnetic resonance imaging shows high-intensity signals in obstructed veins.[128] Both magnetic resonance angiography and computed tomographic angiography can delineate the precise anatomy of the stenosis (Fig. 24-29). The poor results of surgical relief of post-operative pulmonary venous obstruction have led to placement of stents across the stenoses either percutaneously or intraoperatively, but the results have either been disappointing, or else satisfactory over a very short term.[93,129–133]

Incorporation of the pulmonary veins into the left atrium seems to have restored left atrial volume to normal in most of a small number of patients studied. Though the resting electrocardiogram is usually normal on 24-hour monitoring, supraventricular tachycardia, bradyarrhythmia and multi-form supraventricular and ventricular ectopic beats have been described.[134] Some groups have reported a high incidence of sinus note dysfunction, with three-tenths of subjects having chronotropic incompetence on exercise testing, but a very low incidence of significant arrhythmias.[135] Sudden late death 6 weeks post-operatively has been ascribed to documented sick sinus syndrome.[136] Another patient who required cardioversion post-operatively died suddenly at the age of 20.[137] These findings underscore the need for long-term follow-up for rhythm abnormalities. The chest radiograph returns to normal in 90% of patients, and 93% have a normal resting pulmonary arterial pressure. Pulmonary arterial pressure returns to normal even in patients with infradiaphragmatic connection.[138]

A recent study by Kirshbom and colleagues[139] evaluated long-term results of patients with totally anomalous pulmonary venous connection repaired between 1983 and 2005. They reported an 84% 17-year survival rate, with most deaths occurring within a few months after surgery. Over 90% of their patients reported excellent or good overall health, and school performance was average or better in 69% of subjects. Pulmonary venous obstruction prior to repair and chromosomal or other non-cardiac abnormalities were found to be predictive of poor school performance and poor overall health. Another group reported 87% survival at 18 years, rising to 92% in those without additional cardiac or non-cardiac anomalies.[94] A group from western Canada further evaluated neurodevelopmental outcomes after neonatal repair and found that that mean developmental scores for psychomotor and mental functions were in the low range of normal, with socioeconomic factors predicting mental scores and higher post-operative lactate levels predicting lower psychomotor scores.[140] A report from patients repaired at the Children's

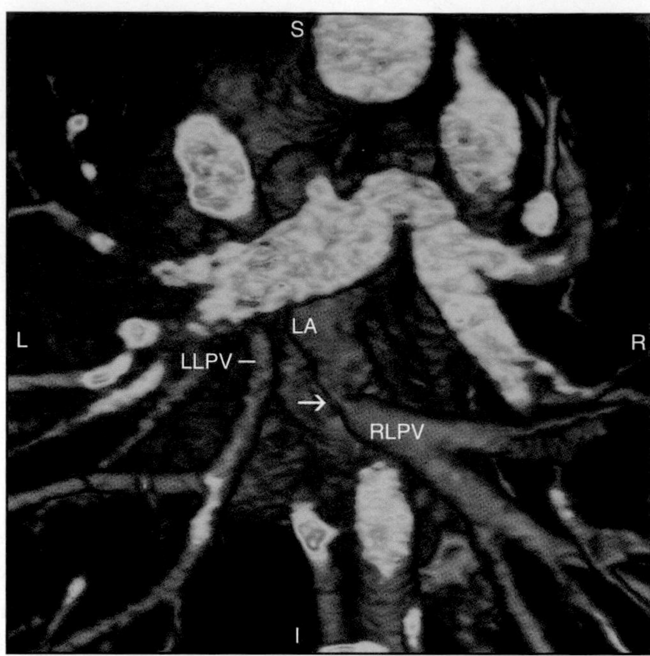

Figure 24-29 In this patient with repaired totally pulmonary venous connection, computed tomographic angiography reveals the substrate for significant obstruction (*arrow*). The right lower pulmonary vein (RLPV) is stenotic at its junction with the left atrium (LA), and the left lower pulmonary vein (LLPV) appears to no longer be connected to the left atrium. The left pulmonary veins drain via a vertical vein (not imaged here), which was left patent at surgery. I, inferior; L, left; R, right; S, superior.

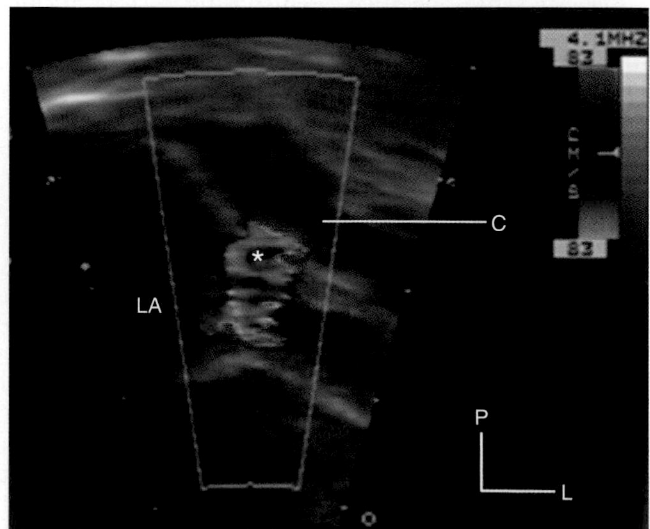

Figure 24-28 In this zoomed up apical image, angled posteriorly, turbulent flow (*star*) can be seen at the surgical anastamosis between the confluence (C) and the left atrium (LA). Note that the Nyquist limit is 83 cm/sec. Pulmonary venous flow should not alias in this setting, unless there is obstruction. L, left; P, posterior.

Hospital of Philadelphia between 1983 and 1996[141] found that exercise performance was mildly impaired, but only 13% of patients had significant impairment of aerobic capacity below the 95% confidence limit for age. Almost half of the subjects were found to have deficits in one or more of the four domains of neurological outcomes assessed in the study.

ATRESIA OF THE COMMON PULMONARY VEIN

Anatomy

As we have discussed briefly in the previous sections, the essence of atresia of the common pulmonary vein is absence of functional connection between the pulmonary veins and the morphologically left atrium.[22] The normally formed pulmonary veins converge immediately behind the left atrium to form a venous confluence that has either no outlet or a very limited outlet for pulmonary venous return. In these patients, atretic strands have been described connecting to the left atrium, right atrium, superior caval vein, along the oesophagus, and paratracheal venous plexuses[1,22] (Fig. 24-30). The embryology has been discussed in the previous section.

Pathophysiology

There is no direct route for blood to enter either the left atrium or any systemic vein and yet patients have lived for up to a month with this condition.[22] How oxygen reaches the systemic arteries is uncertain. One suggested route is via bronchopulmonary venous anastomoses to the pleurohilar bronchial veins, which drain into the azygos, hemiazygos and brachiocephalic veins. Alternatively, blood could reflux from pulmonary capillaries into pulmonary arteries, and thence pass through bronchopulmonary arterial anastomoses and bronchial arteries into the systemic circuit.[142]

The elevated pulmonary capillary pressure causes pulmonary oedema. Excess fluid may escape through dilated lymphaticocoronary sinuses, which have frequently been described in this condition.[22,142–144] They also exist in obstructed totally anomalous pulmonary venous connection.[16]

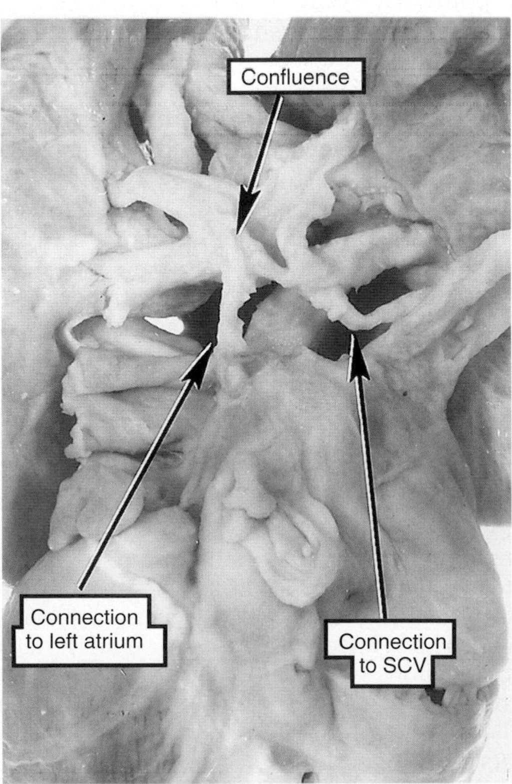

Figure 24-30 This specimen shows atresia of the common pulmonary vein between the pulmonary venous confluence and the left atrium, together with a tightly stenotic anomalous connection to the superior caval vein (SCV).

Clinical Presentation and Investigation

The age at presentation, clinical findings, electrocardiogram and chest radiograph are as for totally anomalous connection with severe pulmonary venous obstruction. There may be a specific association between early spontaneous pneumothorax and atresia of the common pulmonary vein.[145] Echocardiographic findings have not always been diagnostic. A confluence with pulmonary veins connected to it, but with no flow in the veins, has been described in three patients. In two patients in the same series, colour flow mapping was said to show four veins draining to the left atrium.[146] Consequently, the diagnosis is difficult.

Imaging

Given the often small pulmonary venous confluence and severely obstructed flow through the pulmonary veins, this diagnosis can be very challenging to make using echocardiography.[147] The presence of exclusively right-to-left flow through the oval foramen and evidence of pulmonary hypertension, along with the inability to visualise a confluence, vertical vein, or pulmonary venous entry into the left atrium should suggest this diagnosis. Computed tomographic angiography can be attempted to define the anatomy. Considering the limited amount of flow into the pulmonary veins, the pulmonary veins may not be sufficiently opacified to clearly differentiate this entity from totally anomalous pulmonary venous drainage with severe obstruction. While cardiac catheterisation with pulmonary arterial wedge angiography may be necessary to fully define the anatomy, catheterisation is often poorly tolerated.[147] Characteristically, catheterisation reveals severe pulmonary hypertension with low arterial oxygen saturations in all vessels and cardiac chambers. Pulmonary angiography often fails to show any pulmonary veins at all, though the confluence can sometimes be recognised.[142,143,146] As with computed tomographic angiography, it is very easy to confuse totally anomalous pulmonary venous connection with extreme pulmonary venous obstruction.

Management

There is no medical treatment. In the presence of a strongly supportive clinical situation, it may be necessary to pursue surgery despite the lack of a definitive anatomic diagnosis.[148] Surgical repair was often unsuccessful until the 1980s.[143,149,150] More recently, a few centers have reported success using aggressive haemodynamic stabilisation techniques, often including extracorporeal membrane oxygenation, and early surgical repair.[146,148,151] Some of these patients were placed on extracorporeal membrane oxygenation for erroneously diagnosed pulmonary disease, but rapid improvement was achieved with clearing of the chest radiograph, leading to further investigation and then surgical repair.[146]

UNILATERAL PULMONARY VENOUS ATRESIA

Unilateral pulmonary venous atresia is a very rare condition in which there is complete obliteration of luminal continuity between the pulmonary venous pathway of one lung and the left atrium. The majority of patients present within the first 3 years of life, displaying recurrent pulmonary infections, exercise intolerance, and/or haemoptysis. Less than 30 cases have been reported in the literature, with mortality approaching 40%.[152] Diagnosis is best documented using pulmonary wedge angiography, although supporting information can be obtained using pulmonary perfusion studies. The affected lung often has poor ventilation and oxygenation, resulting in a large dead space, and the arterial supply is frequently hypoplastic. Over time, collateral blood supply to the affected lung develops, and flow in the ipsilateral pulmonary artery is reversed, resulting in a left-to-right shunt. Both reparative surgery and unilateral pneumonectomy have been successfully performed, although survival appears to be superior with pneumonectomy, particularly when diagnosed in older children and adults.[152–155]

PARTIALLY ANOMALOUS PULMONARY VENOUS CONNECTION

Anatomy

The anomalous pulmonary venous connections are not always total. Partially anomalous connection exists where one or more of the pulmonary veins is connected to the morphologically left atrium, while the rest are connected to a systemic vein or the right atrium. The varieties of partial return are legion. It may be restricted to part of one lung (see Fig. 24-1). Alternatively, all of one lung may drain anomalously (see Fig. 24-2), or parts of both lungs may drain anomalously. All of one lung and part of the other may also be connected to anomalous systemic sites. The sites of anomalous connection can be to any of those discussed for totally anomalous connection. As with totally anomalous connection, depending on the extent of the malformation, all the anomalously connected veins may drain to the same site, or there may be mixed drainage. Obstructed drainage, however, has not to the best of our knowledge been described in the partial form, but it must be anticipated. By describing the amount of lung connected anomalously, the site and drainage and the presence of associated lesions, it is possible to describe clearly all the potentially bewildering complex variations.[8]

Some associations with partially anomalous pulmonary venous connection are so frequent as to warrant special consideration here, even though they are also considered in other chapters. The association between the sinus venosus interatrial communication and anomalous drainage of the right pulmonary veins is described in the next chapter. Indeed, in this setting it is the anomalous pulmonary venous connection that produces the extracardiac conduit permitting interatrial shunting. We have discussed at length the necessary association of totally anomalous connection in the setting of isomeric right atrial appendages. The pulmonary veins frequently connect bilaterally when there are isomeric left atrial appendages, but in terms of the anatomic arrangement, this is not abnormal. It does, however, produce an obvious haemodynamic problem. This situation is described and discussed in detail in Chapter 22. The other association requiring special attention is the scimitar syndrome.[156,157] In this lesion, the lower lobe of the right lung is hypoplastic, and is supplied with arterial blood from the descending aorta. Its pulmonary venous return is connected to the inferior caval vein. There are marked variations in the combination of abnormal connections, including sequestration of the abnormal lobe of the lung.[156]

Morphogenesis

Presumably the canalising pulmonary vein in patients with partially anomalous connection will have made connection only with part of the intraparenchymal pulmonary venous plexus. Anastomoses between the unconnected pulmonary segments and the systemic venous plexuses persist and develop. There is no doubt that very bizarre patterns of drainage do occur that present a challenge to the embryologist, as discussed by Blake and colleagues.[158] This re-emphasises the inadvisability of basing descriptions of congenitally malformed hearts on embryological hypotheses.

Pathophysiology

Because pulmonary venous obstruction is rarely present with partially anomalous venous connections, the haemodynamic effects are almost always the result of an obligatory left-to-right shunt through the anomalously connected segments of lung. No right-to-left shunt occurs as a result of the anomalous connection. In older patients with pulmonary vascular obstructive disease, a right-to-left shunt can occur through an associated atrial septal defect.[159]

When partially anomalous pulmonary venous connection occurs in association with an atrial septal defect, as it does more often than not,[8] it is difficult to separate the haemodynamic effects of the two. Here, we will only consider the pathophysiology of cases with an intact atrial septum.

When only one pulmonary vein is connected anomalously, as in Figure 24-1, there may be no discernable consequences of the malformation. When there is complete anomalous connection of one lung, in contrast, be it right or left, the left-to-right shunt is usually greater than 50%. In other words, more blood flows through the anomalously connected lung than would be the case if it were normally connected.[160] The reason for this is almost certainly that pulmonary venous return is to the systemic side of the circulation, which has a lower mean pressure than the left atrium. When calculations of pulmonary vascular resistance are made, correcting for the proportion of blood flow that would normally go to the anomalously connected lobe or lobes, it appears that this resistance is the same in the normally and anomalously connected regions of lung.[161] Therefore, it is not the vascular resistance that determines preferential flow to the anomalously connected lobe or lobes.

The left-to-right shunt at atrial level has the same consequences on the right heart and pulmonary circulation as does an atrial septal defect (see Chapter 25). Pulmonary hypertension is rare, except in some infants with scimitar syndrome who exhibit arterial, but not venous, muscularity in both lungs.[162]

Presentation and Symptoms

Presentation is as for an atrial septal defect (see Chapter 25), except that some asymptomatic patients may present with an unexpected abnormality on chest radiograph (see below). Presentation with heart failure occurs rarely, as with interatrial defects at the oval fossa.[160] Patients with scimitar syndrome can present with recurrent pneumonia, wheezing, or haemoptysis.

The physical signs in patients with an associated atrial septal defect are as for the atrial septal defect. In those patients with an intact atrial septum, the signs are as for atrial septal defect with left-to-right shunt of comparable size, except that the second heart sound, though widely split, often varies normally with respiration.[160,163] Sinus arrhythmia is common. This is presumably because changes in intrathoracic pressure affect the atria to different degrees, as in normal individuals. This contrasts with what happens in the presence of a large atrial septal defect. Therefore, if a patient has the pulmonary ejection systolic murmur of an atrial septal defect and yet has physiological splitting of the second heart sound, the diagnosis is highly likely to be partially anomalous connection with intact atrial septum.

Investigations

Chest Radiography

The general appearances of the heart and pulmonary vessels will be exactly as for an atrial septal defect with a comparable left-to-right shunt. But the anomalous pulmonary vein may also be evident. A snowman appearance would suggest return to the left vertical vein; in older patients with return to the inferior caval vein, the anomalous pulmonary vein is always visible.[159,160] We have already highlighted the importance of this appearance as seen in the scimitar syndrome.[157] The hypoplasia of the right lung, pulmonary sequestration, and secondary right-sided location of the heart usually accentuate the scimitar sign as seen in the frontal projection of the right lung. It is formed by the anomalous right pulmonary vein (Fig. 24-31), though rotation of the heart to the right may completely obscure the scimitar in infants.[162] Exceptionally, such a scimitar may be formed by a common right pulmonary vein that descends towards the diaphragm but ascends to connect normally to the left atrium[164–166] or to the left atrium and the inferior caval vein.[166]

Electrocardiography

When the partially anomalous connection is associated with an atrial septal defect in the oval fossa, or the atrial septum is intact and the anomalous connection is supracardiac or to the right atrium, the electrocardiogram is identical to that of an atrial septal defect. Specifically, V_1 shows an rsr′ or rsR′, or rarely a QR, or pattern in V_1. Partial, return to the inferior caval vein with intact atrial septum is characterised by a terminal s or S wave in V_1.[160]

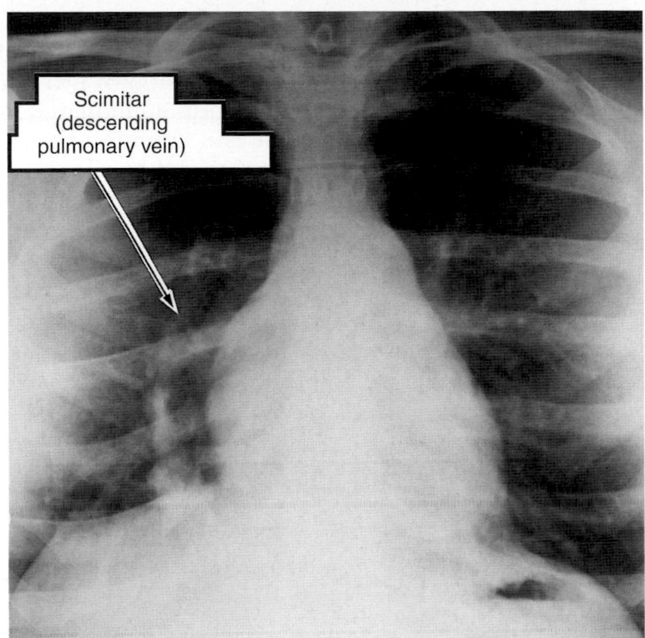

Figure 24-31 Plain chest radiograph showing the scimitar syndrome. There is only mild hypoplasia of the right lung; consequently, the bulk of the heart is still in the left chest. (Original photograph kindly supplied by the late Dr Simon Rees, National Heart Hospital, London, United Kingdom.)

Echocardiography

As with totally anomalous pulmonary venous connection, echocardiography is primary means of defining pulmonary venous anatomy in these patients. As when dealing with all patients, echocardiographers should persistently attempt to identify pulmonary venous connections from all portions of the lung into the heart. Increased or atypical flow in the superior or inferior caval veins should alert one to the possibility of partially anomalous pulmonary venous connection (Fig. 24-32). Nevertheless, partially anomalous venous connection is the Achilles heel of the echocardiographer, particularly when associated abnormalities mask

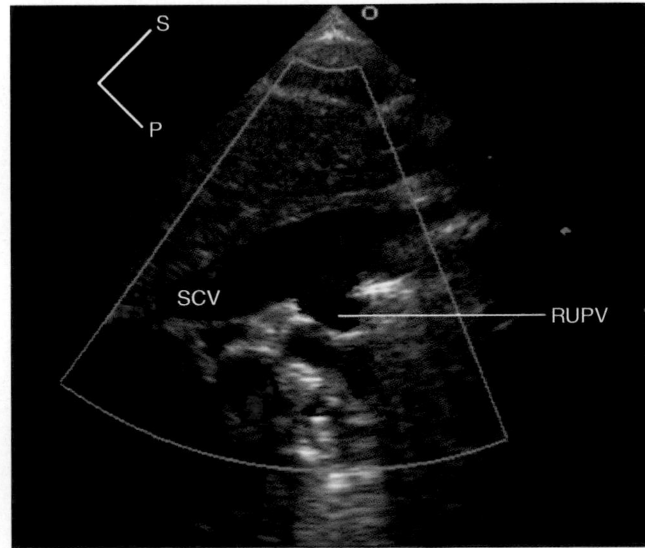

Figure 24-32 In this high right parasternal view, the right upper pulmonary vein (RUPV) can be seen entering the superior caval vein (SCV). P, posterior; S, superior.

its clinical effects. There are three problems. First, even when all four pulmonary veins are normally connected, they may not be imaged. In particular, fusion of two pulmonary veins on one side into a common pulmonary vein may not be recognised, though it is a common normal variant. Second, some patients have more than four pulmonary veins. For example, if a patient has a right middle lobe draining normally to the left atrium, but a right upper lobe draining to the superior caval vein, the echocardiographer may visualise four pulmonary veins entering the left atrium and erroneously assume completely normal pulmonary venous connections are present (Fig. 24-33). Third, the great clue to the diagnosis of totally anomalous pulmonary venous connection, namely a collecting pulmonary venous channel, or confluence, is almost invariably missing in partially anomalous connection. In short, partially anomalous venous connection can be positively and reliably diagnosed, particularly if it is via a left vertical vein, but it can rarely, if ever, be ruled out, even using colour flow mapping and transoesophageal echocardiography.[64,167] Surgeons should be aware of this caveat in diagnosis. Partially anomalous pulmonary venous connection is occasionally identified by fetal echocardiography.[56]

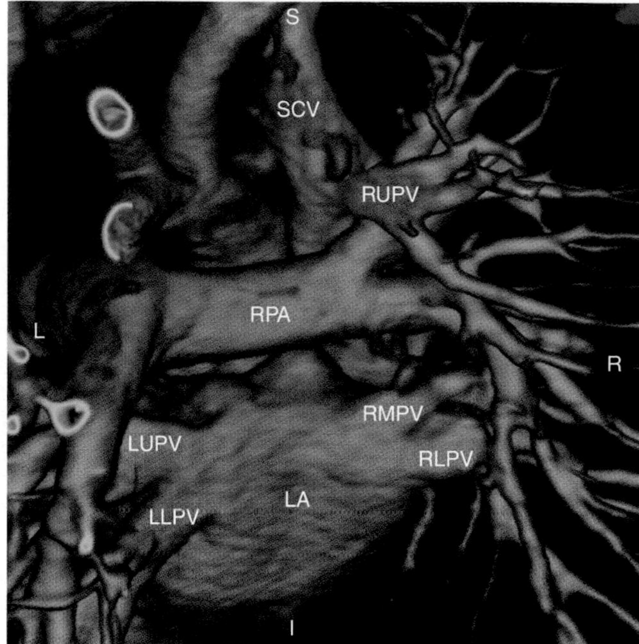

Figure 24-33 This computed tomographic angiogram shows the anomalous connection of the right upper pulmonary vein (RUPV) to the superior caval vein (SCV). Note that there are four pulmonary veins (LUPV, LLPV, RMPV, RLPV) entering the left atrium (LA). This highlights the challenge in detecting this anomaly by echocardiography. I, inferior; L, left; R, right; RPA, right pulmonary artery; S, superior.

Computed Tomographic Angiography and Magnetic Resonance Imaging

As with totally anomalous pulmonary venous connection, computed tomographic angiography[62,73,74,168,169] and magnetic resonance imaging[64,67–69] are very accurate noninvasive methods to evaluate anatomy in patients with partially anomalous pulmonary venous connection (see Fig. 24-33). Computed tomographic angiography is particularly useful for patients with scimitar syndrome, given that this modality allows for simultaneous evaluation of lung parenchyma and pulmonary venous anatomy (Fig. 24-34). Both methods are also valuable in screening for pulmonary venous anomalies in patients being assessed for Fontan-like operations.[170] Such screening is necessary because failure to recognise the presence of an anomalous vein will result in an important left-to-right shunt and elevation of systemic venous pressure.

It is important to distinguish between partially anomalous connection to a left vertical vein and persistence of the left superior caval vein.[171] Traditionally, the characteristic finding by magnetic resonance imaging was a lateral break

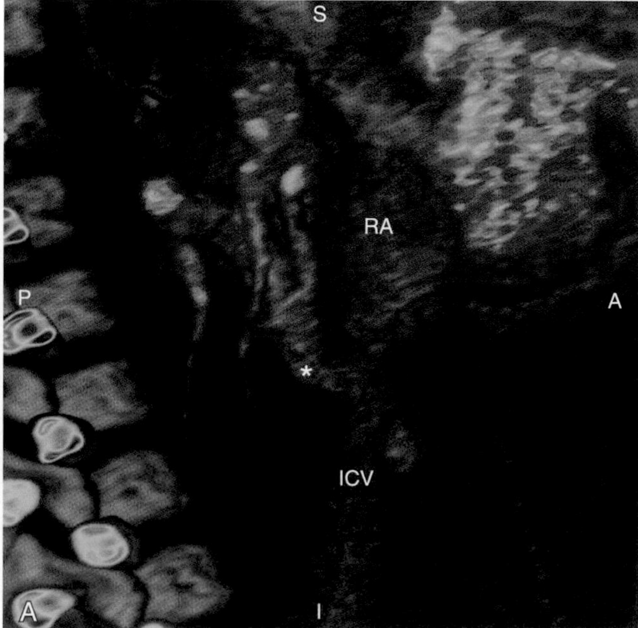

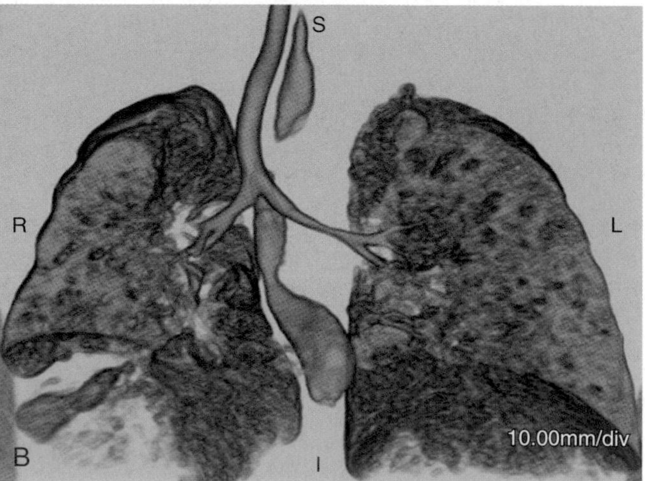

Figure 24-34 **A,** This computed tomographic angiogram on a patient with scimitar syndrome shows the right pulmonary venous confluence (*star*) draining into the junction between the right atrium (RA) and inferior caval vein (ICV). **B,** In this same study, reconstructed with settings appropriate for evaluation of the lung fields, one can see the relative hypoplasia of the right lung. A, anterior; I, inferior; L, left; P, posterior; R, right; S, superior.

in the complete ring created by fat surrounding the superior caval vein in the transverse plane.[172] Newer protocols for imaging, incorporating three-dimensional reconstructions, make this distinction much more straightforward.

Cardiac Catheterisation and Angiocardiography

Cardiac catheterisation is rarely indicated for these patients. A combination of non-invasive imaging techniques will document the pathophysiology already described. In diagnosing partially anomalous pulmonary venous connection, a step-up in oxygen saturation in the superior caval vein, the brachiocephalic vein, or the inferior caval vein is suggestive of anomalous pulmonary veins draining into the respective site.[173] Entry to the anomalous veins may be achieved as for totally anomalous connection. In patients with scimitar syndrome and a hypoplastic right lung, measurement of oxygen saturations in the anomalous right pulmonary veins could be helpful when deciding whether to pursue surgery, as repair is unlikely to be advantageous in patients with pulmonary venous desaturation.

To demonstrate drainage outside the heart, pulmonary arteriography and selective pulmonary venous angiograms may be performed as for totally anomalous connection (Fig. 24-35). It should be noted that pulmonary angiography alone may not be sufficient to fully document anomalous pulmonary venous drainage, particularly anomalous drainage from the right lower lobe.[173] In the case of the scimitar syndrome, selective injection of the systemic arterial supply to the lungs is also essential (Fig. 24-35B). Along these lines, if there is dual arterial supply (both systemic and pulmonary) to any portion of the lung, embolisation of the aorto-pulmonary collateral in the catheterisation laboratory should be considered.

Differential Diagnosis

The main differential diagnosis is an atrial septal defect in the oval fossa, which has been discussed at length already. In most cases, particularly when associated with atrial septal defect, it is not critical that the anomalous connection be diagnosed pre-operatively, since surgery can usually be adjusted accordingly. Therefore, invasive investigation of a typical atrial septal defect is not justified simply to rule out partially anomalous pulmonary venous connection. The only possible exception is connection of both left pulmonary veins to a vertical vein. This then involves a rather more complex operation than simple closure of an atrial septal defect or diversion of other forms of partially anomalous connection.

Anomalous connection of a solitary pulmonary vein may give no more than an unimpressive systolic murmur and can, therefore, be confused with a normal heart. Even if this error is made, the patient will not suffer, since the haemodynamic consequences are trivial and there is no risk of bacterial endocarditis.

Course and Prognosis

The course and prognosis for partially anomalous pulmonary venous connection are probably similar to those of an isolated atrial septal defect with a comparable left-to-right shunt. Pulmonary vascular obstructive disease is rare but undoubtedly occurs.[174,175] Prognosis for patients with scimitar syndrome is worse than other types of partially anomalous pulmonary venous drainage, particular among those who develop symptoms within the first year of life.[176]

In the particular case of anomalous connection of all the veins from one lung, there is a risk that death may result if the respiratory function of the normally connected lung is compromised. In that case, fully saturated pulmonary venous blood will only be recirculated to the lung, and relatively desaturated blood will be sent to the body.[177]

Management

Medical Treatment

Medical management is as for any atrial septal defect and is rarely necessary.

Surgery

As the repair for partially anomalous pulmonary venous connection associated with a sinus venosus defect is described in Chapter 25, the following discussion covers only those patients in which the atrial septum is intact or with only a patent oval foramen. Surgical repair is recommended if the ratio of pulmonary-to-systemic flow is greater than 2 to 1.[160,173,175,178] The techniques are broadly similar to those already described for totally anomalous connection. In the case of supracardiac or intracardiac drainage, unilateral anomalous connection of all pulmonary veins will not be associated with a collecting channel behind the left atrium. This complicates repair. When the right veins

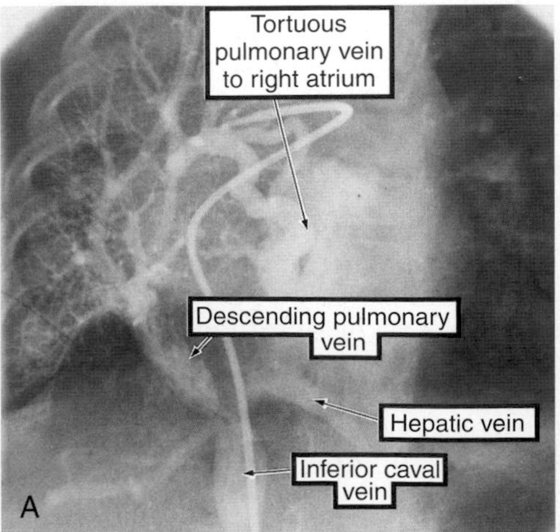

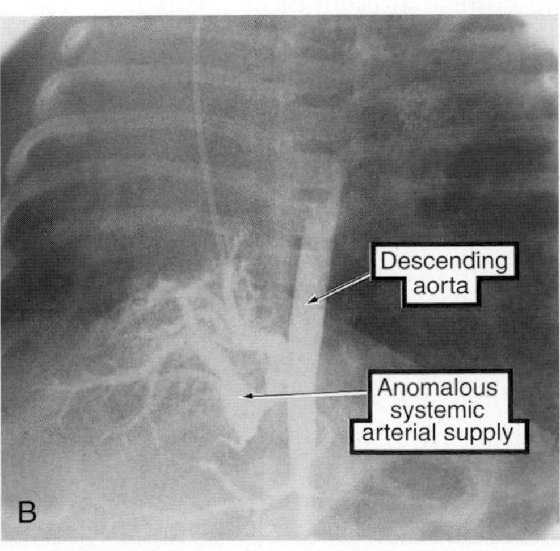

Figure 24-35 Selective angiography in the scimitar syndrome displayed in the frontal projection. **A,** The pulmonary arteriogram, filmed in its late stages, demonstrates that the pulmonary veins return by two routes to the heart: one a tortuous vein to the right atrium, and one a descending pulmonary vein to the inferior caval vein. **B,** A selective injection into a branch of the descending aorta demonstrates the anomalous systemic arterial supply.

are connected to the superior or inferior caval veins, or to a hepatic vein, it is usually possible to create a baffle within the caval vein and right atrium so as to direct blood to the left atrium.[179] Interposition grafts made of polytetrafluoroethylene have been used, in place of a baffle, to direct blood to the left atrium.[180] Direct anastomosis of the right pulmonary vein to the left atrium has also been achieved.[160,181] This approach can be performed off bypass through a right thoracotomy, and avoids the possibility of stenosis developing at the margins of the baffle.[182] Some patients with scimitar syndrome benefit from a concomitant resection of the pulmonary sequestration, if present.

The usual method of repair of unilateral connection of all the veins from the left lung to a left vertical vein is to connect the common left pulmonary vein to the amputated stump of the left atrial appendage.[183] More or less the same technique was used in one series, being accomplished without early or late death, even though the repairs were performed without cardiopulmonary bypass.[184] On the grounds that this kind of anastomosis, like all venous anastomoses, is liable to late stenosis, some[185] have advocated dividing the vertical vein and incising it longitudinally to form a cobra-head, which was then anastomosed to the left atrium between the left atrial appendage and the entrance of the right pulmonary vein. The circumference of this oblique anastomosis is clearly much larger than the circumference of the vein. Repair of partially anomalous pulmonary venous return should be carried out electively before a child goes to school. The mortality is less than 1%. The long-term results of venous anastomosis should be followed with care, but there is limited literature available documenting these results.

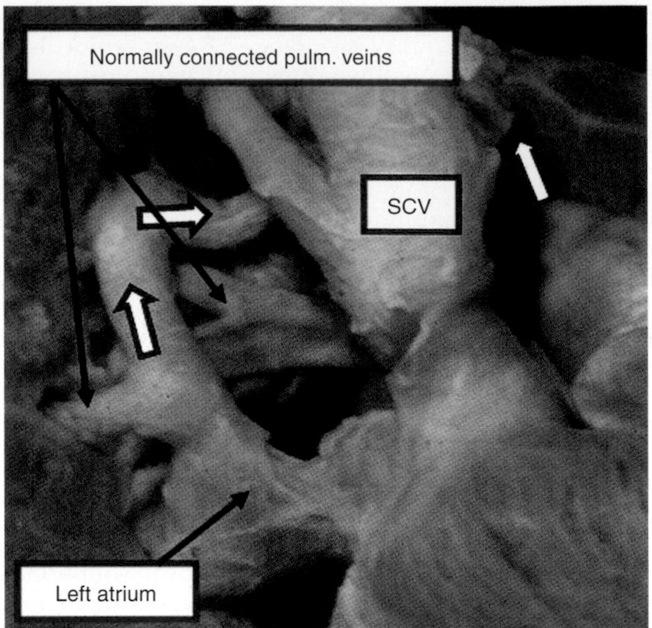

Figure 24-36 The picture shows a so-called laevoatrial cardinal vein, which originates from the roof of the left atrium and, as shown by the *arrows*, passes behind the superior caval vein (SCV) before terminating in the systemic venous channel. It is easy to mistake this for an anomalous pulmonary venous connection, but as can be seen, the pulmonary veins join in normal fashion to the left atrium.

ANOMALOUS PULMONARY-TO-SYSTEMIC COLLATERAL VEINS AND THE LAEVOATRIAL CARDINAL VEIN

Anomalous pulmonary-to-systemic collateral veins, along with the so-called laevoatrial cardinal vein (see Fig. 24-3), are frequently found in association with more serious causes of obstruction of pulmonary venous return, such as an intact atrial septum with left atrioventricular valvar atresia, aortic stenosis or aortic atresia, and divided left atrium. They act as safety valves, enabling pulmonary venous return to escape to the systemic circulation, and producing the arrangement of anomalous pulmonary venous drainage with anatomically normal pulmonary venous connections.[21] In these circumstances, the clinical presentation will be generally dominated by the lesion causing the pulmonary venous obstruction. If the laevoatrial cardinal vein is of insufficient caliber to provide unobstructed passage of pulmonary venous blood to the systemic circulation, the patient may present with profound cyanosis. Along those lines, Vance[186] reported placement of a stent in the laevoatrial cardinal vein as a bridge to surgery in a patient with severe pulmonary venous obstruction due to an intact atrial septum in the setting of mitral atresia.

The presence of the anomalous collateral channels, or the laevoatrial cardinal vein, will emerge as a chance finding on traditional angiography,[187] cross sectional echocardiography,[49] or computed tomographic angiography.[188,189] At first glance, either lesion may be mistaken for totally anomalous connection to the left vertical vein, or the right superior caval vein (Fig. 24-36). In both instances, pulmonary venous blood returns to a confluence, which then drains via a vertical vein. In anomalous connection to the left vertical vein or right superior caval vein, the confluence is distinct from the left atrium and its appendage. In these other conditions, the effective confluence is the left atrium (see Fig. 24-3). Confusion of these two entities can be disastrous. Distinction is more difficult in that hypoplasia of the left heart can be associated not only with normally connected but abnormally draining pulmonary veins, but also with totally anomalous pulmonary venous connection. Nowadays, distinction is usually possible using cross sectional echocardiography with colour flow mapping. Another lesion to be distinguished from anomalous venous connection is the fistulous channel connecting the left upper pulmonary vein to the brachiocephalic vein, or similar connections. This can occur as an isolated abnormality, giving rise to a characteristic, if exceptionally rare, clinical picture.[188,190,191] Patients present without symptoms but with a venous hum under the left clavicle. Unlike the benign systemic venous hum at the same site, no amount of movement of the head or compression of jugular veins will abolish it.

STENOSIS OR ATRESIA OF INDIVIDUAL PULMONARY VEINS

Anatomy

Individual pulmonary veins can be stenosed at their junction with the atrium (Fig. 24-37), or exhibit tubular hypoplasia over a significant intra- and extrapulmonary distance (Fig. 24-38).[1,192] It is only when several veins are involved that the condition becomes clinically manifest. Pulmonary venous stenosis can also result from acquired causes, such as constrictive pericarditis, mediastinitis, pulmonary tuberculosis or invasion by tumour.

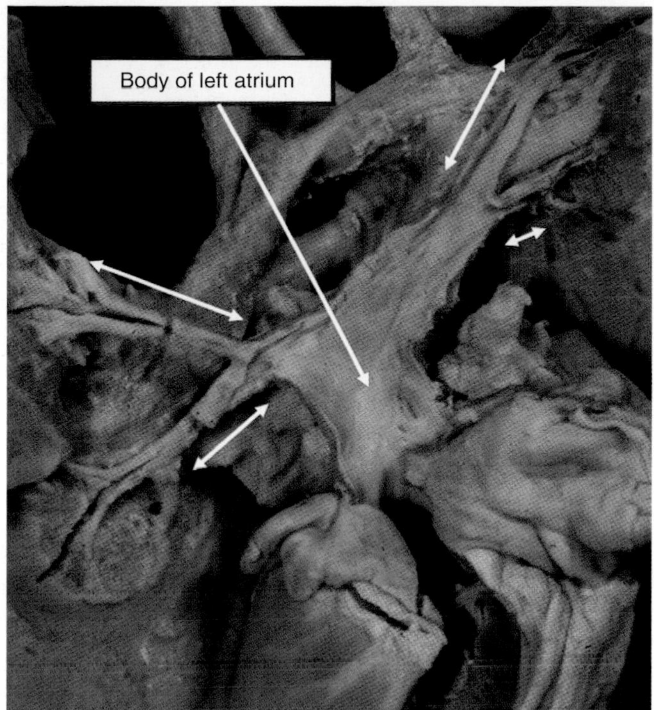

Figure 24-37 The heart from this patient, who died due to pulmonary venous stenosis, has been dissected to show the tubular hypoplasia of each of the four individual pulmonary veins (*arrows*).

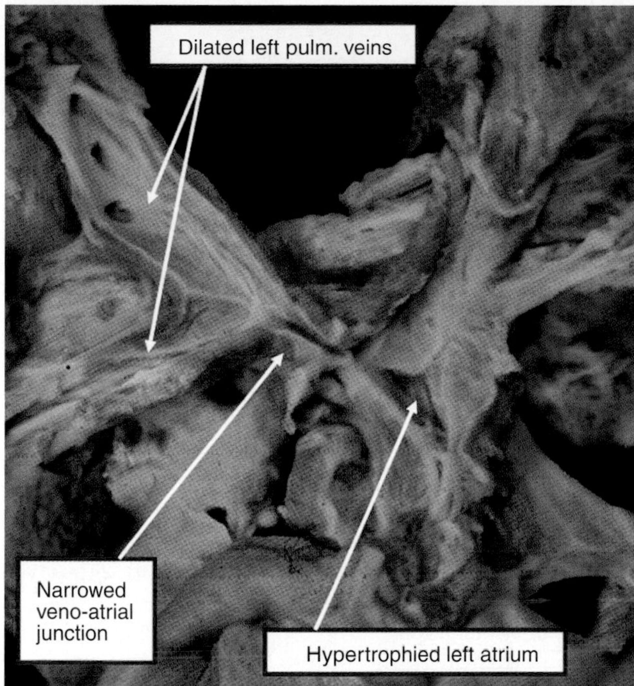

Figure 24-38 In this patient, who also suffered severe pulmonary stenosis in life, the stenotic sites are at the junctions of the individual pulmonary veins with the body of the left atrium. Note the dilated pulmonary veins, and the hypertrophied walls of the left atrium.

Pathophysiology

Stenosis or atresia of a solitary pulmonary vein unassociated with other severe cardiac anomalies has not, to our knowledge, been described. Most commonly, both pulmonary veins from one lung are affected. Just under half the patients described have had other congenital heart defects, varying from the simple to the complex.[193] Pulmonary venous pressure becomes elevated on the afflicted side as a result. Pulmonary arterial hypertension usually ensues, though patients have been described with a normal pulmonary pressure.[194] In the case of unilateral pulmonary venous atresia, or severe stenosis, pulmonary blood flow will be largely or completely diverted to the contralateral lung. The result is that the pulmonary artery on the obstructed side may be unusually small, and there will be none of the usual signs of pulmonary venous hypertension.[195,196] The greater the number of pulmonary veins obstructed, and the more severe the obstruction, the more severe will be the pulmonary hypertension. Elevation of right ventricular end-diastolic pressure may result in a right-to-left shunt through the oval foramen.[197]

Presentation and Symptoms

Lesions of a single pulmonary vein might well be asymptomatic and not produce problems. When sufficient veins are affected, patients usually present in early infancy, though sometimes presentation is delayed until early childhood. Dyspnea and repeated pulmonary infections with failure to thrive are the rule.[198] Many patients have haemoptysis and, occasionally, cyanosis.[154,155]

Patients generally look unwell, with tachypnea, retractions, and occasional cyanosis. There are frequently rales in the chest, and sometimes evidence of right heart failure.[199] One patient had signs of right pleural effusion.[196] Murmurs are usually unimpressive, and the heart sounds unremarkable apart from accentuation of pulmonary closure. Occasionally, there is a pulmonary ejection click.

Investigations

Chest Radiography

A chest radiograph is the most likely examination to suggest the diagnosis. Although the chest radiograph may be normal in the early stages,[195] marked abnormality is the rule. The heart is usually normal in size or slightly enlarged, with prominence of the pulmonary trunk. The lungs show a reticular appearance or ground-glass opacification, with or without Kerley B lines in the region of the obstructed vein or veins. There may be hypoplasia of the lung on the affected side. Therefore, the regional nature of the abnormality is the key to the diagnosis except when all the pulmonary veins are affected.[200] It is important to realise that preferential flow occurs to the contralateral lung when unilateral pulmonary venous stenosis or atresia is associated with a left-to-right shunt. If there are no specific indicants of pulmonary venous hypertension on the same side, the appearance may be misinterpreted as being caused by pulmonary arterial stenosis.

Electrocardiography

Right atrial and right ventricular hypertrophy without left-sided changes are almost invariably found by electrocardiography.[198]

Echocardiography

It is imperative that all four pulmonary veins be visualised by echocardiography in order to screen for this diagnosis. When pulmonary venous stenosis is suspected, colour and spectral Doppler of each pulmonary vein will document

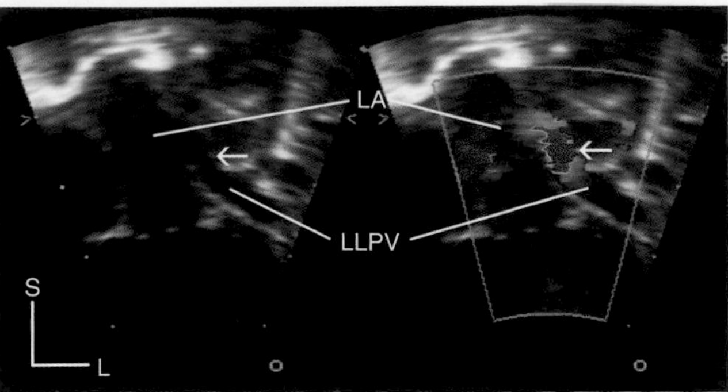

Figure 24-39 In this zoomed apical four-chamber view, shown with and without colour Doppler, an area of turbulence (*arrow*) can be seen as the left lower pulmonary vein (LLPV) enters the left atrium (LA). L, left; S, superior.

the presence or absence of stenosis.[201–203] In some patients, transoesophageal echocardiography will be required. Turbulence or a focal increase in flow velocity with a continuous, non-phasic flow pattern distally in a pulmonary vein suggests stenosis (Fig. 24-39).

Radionuclide Angiography

Nuclear perfusion lung scans, following injection of labeled technetium, show reduced or absent perfusion in the region of lung drained by the vein or veins that are obstructed.[154] In two patients, ventilation on the affected side was said to be reduced.[155,196]

Cardiac Catheterisation

Cardiac catheterisation documents the pathophysiology described. Provided that the pulmonary vein is not atretic, it is helpful to record withdrawal traces from pulmonary veins to left atrium, though care should be employed in interpreting the findings. In neonates particularly, pressure gradients may be found in normal pulmonary veins because the veins are not much larger than the catheter. If the left atrium cannot be entered, or the pulmonary veins are atretic, pulmonary capillary wedge pressures should be recorded in upper and lower regions of both lungs, preferably simultaneously with a left-ventricular end-diastolic or left atrial pressure.[204] It should be remembered that a normal wedge pressure does not necessarily exclude pulmonary venous stenosis.[205] This is because, when a catheter is wedged in a pulmonary arteriole, the capillary, venule, and vein beyond the catheter act as an extension of it; the catheter, may, therefore, reflect left atrial pressure rather than pulmonary venous pressure proximal to the stenosis.

Traditional Angiography

Pulmonary angiography will show slow clearance of contrast medium from one lung in the case of unilateral pulmonary venous stenosis. If this is sufficiently severe, or the pulmonary veins are atretic, the contrast medium may well run to-and-fro into the pulmonary artery on that side without ever opacifying the pulmonary veins.[195,196] Pulmonary arteriography is often disappointing in demonstrating the precise anatomy of pulmonary venous stenosis. Pulmonary arterial wedge angiography may well do better (Fig. 24-40).[127] Selective pulmonary venous injection, if possible, is ideal (Fig. 24-41).[193]

Computed Tomographic and Magnetic Resonance Angiography

Provided that there is more than trivial flow through the pulmonary veins, both computed tomographic and magnetic resonance angiography should be able to show the precise anatomy of the stenosis well (Fig. 24-42).

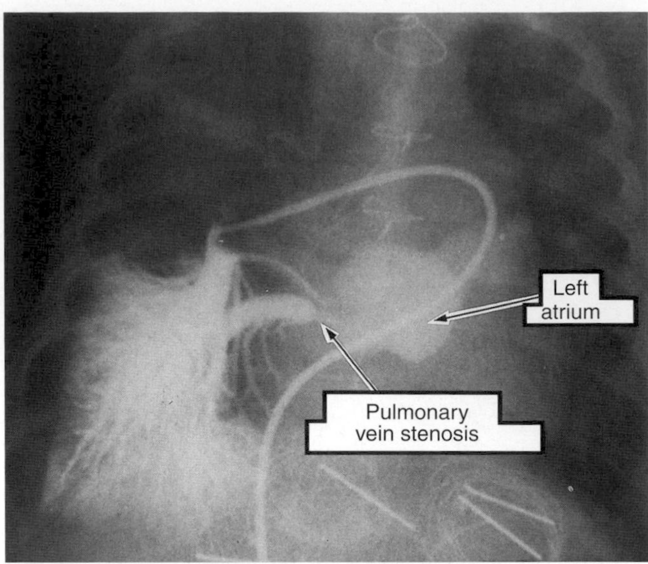

Figure 24-40 In this patient, pulmonary arterial wedge injection clearly demonstrates the right lower pulmonary vein but reveals a severe stenosis as it enters the left atrium. (Original photograph courtesy of the late Dr Robert Freedom, Hospital for Sick Children, Toronto, Ontario, Canada.)

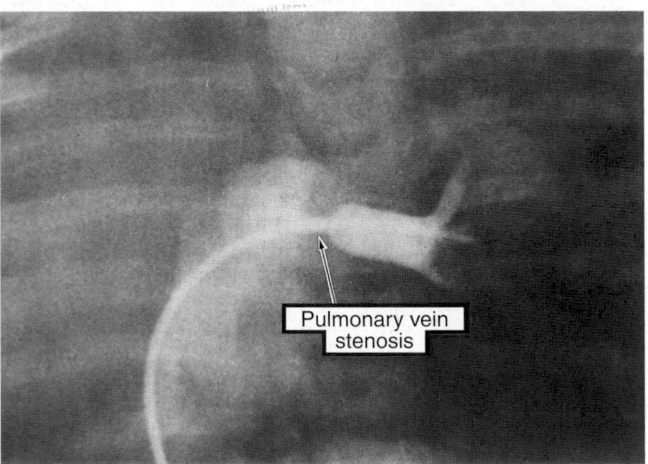

Figure 24-41 In this patient, left pulmonary venous stenosis is demonstrated by selective injection in the pulmonary vein. (Original photograph courtesy of the late Dr Robert Freedom, Hospital for Sick Children, Toronto, Ontario, Canada.)

Differential Diagnosis

Stenosis or Atresia of One or Two Pulmonary Veins

Stenosis or atresia of one or two pulmonary veins must be distinguished from pulmonary infection, which is far more common. Lack of fever, elevation of sedimentation rate, leucocytosis, and response to antibiotic should lead to the suspicion of pulmonary venous stenosis.

Stenosis or Atresia of Most or All Pulmonary Veins

Stenosis or atresia of most or all pulmonary veins must be distinguished from other causes of generalised pulmonary venous hypertension. The absence of severe cardiomegaly distinguishes pulmonary venous obstruction from left ventricular disease and mitral regurgitation. Mitral stenosis and supravalvar mitral ring almost always exhibit diastolic murmurs and are easily recognisable on echocardiography, as is divided left atrium. Totally anomalous pulmonary venous connection and atresia of the common pulmonary vein only present a problem in cyanotic patients, and

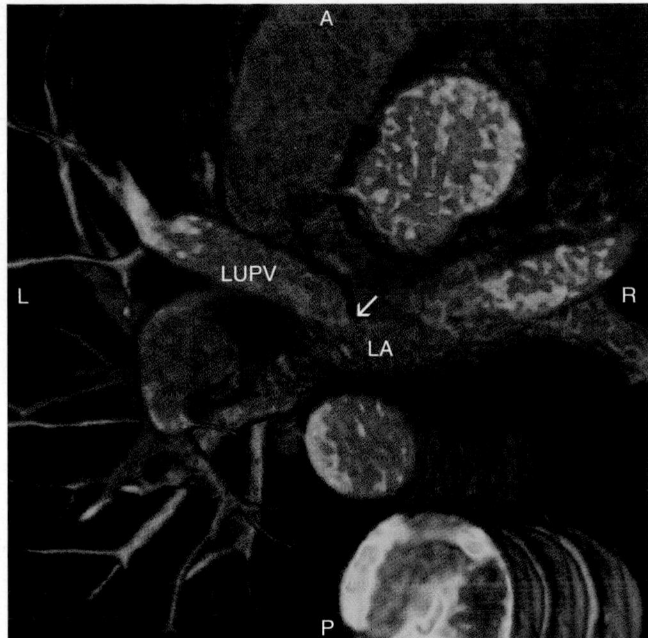

Figure 24-42 This computed tomographic angiogram shows stenosis (*arrow*) of the left upper pulmonary vein (LUPV) as it enters the left atrium (LA) in a patient after radio-frequency ablation for atrial fibrillation. A, anterior; L, left; P, posterior; R, right.

echocardiographic demonstration of a pulmonary venous confluence will rule out stenosis or atresia of individual pulmonary veins.

The most likely disease to cause confusion is pulmonary veno-occlusive disease. Here, however, the pulmonary capillary wedge pressure is usually normal, and no obstruction can be demonstrated in the pulmonary veins either by measurements of pressure or angiography. Pulmonary veno-occlusive disease is very rare in young infants.

Course and Prognosis

Without surgical treatment, most patients will die before reaching adulthood, and frequently much sooner.[154,193] An analysis using the Pediatric Cardiac Care Consortium database[206] identified 31 patients, from a total group of 98,126 patients, who had primary pulmonary venous stenosis. Of these, three-fifths either died or underwent lung transplantation. Four-fifths of those with a mean pulmonary arterial pressure higher than 33 mm Hg experienced death or lung transplantation.

Management

Medical Treatment

Standard anti-failure treatment will relieve the immediate problem, but is unlikely to be effective for long.

Surgery

Localised atresia or stenosis has been successfully treated by patch grafting,[195,202,204] side-to-end anastomosis of the vein to the left atrium,[154] excision of an obstructing membrane at the junction of the pulmonary vein with the left atrium,[207] or by the so-called sutureless technique described above for treatment of post-operative stenosis after repair of anomalous pulmonary venous connection.[121,123] Of these, the sutureless technique is currently the most promising. Not only was this technique found to have improved freedom from reoperation and death compared to traditional surgical techniques, but despite the absence of retrocardiac adhesions, operative mortality was not increased compared with that of the patients who had a sutureless repair as a reoperation.

While catheter-based interventions using stents, and cutting balloons, have been successful in adults with pulmonary venous stenosis occuring after catheter ablation for atrial fibrillation,[208-210] the long-term results for other causes of pulmonary venous stenosis have been disappointing.[131,132,193,206,211-213]

The only effective treatment for long-segment atresia or severe pulmonary venous hypoplasia is pneumonectomy, when the disease is unilateral and the objective is to cure massive haemoptysis.[196,200]

PULMONARY VARIX

Pulmonary varix is a rare anomaly, presenting as a mass in the lung on routine chest radiograph, usually between the fourth and sixth decades. It has been found in patients as young as 7 years. It is usually observed in the right upper pulmonary lobe. The differential diagnosis includes all other space-occupying lesions, but can be established by pulmonary angiography, magnetic resonance angiography, computed tomographic angiography,[214,215] or if it is related to the heart, by transoesophageal echocardiography.[216] This lesion is considered benign, and treatment is generally reserved for those who experience complications such as haemoptysis or cerebral embolic events, or for those in whom growth of the defect results in compression of surrounding structures.[217] Death caused by rupture has been reported.[218-220]

The complete reference list can be found on the companion Expert Consult web site at www.expertconsult.com.

ANNOTATED REFERENCES

- Gathman GE, Nadas AS: Total anomalous pulmonary venous connection: Clinical and physiologic observations of 75 pediatric patients. Circulation 1970;42:143–154.
- Delisle G, Ando M, Calder AL, et al: Total anomalous pulmonary venous connection: Report of 93 autopsied cases with emphasis on diagnostic and surgical considerations. Am Heart J 1976;91:99–122.

  These two seminal works are extensive case series, documenting the array of anatomical variants, physiology, and the natural history present with anomalous pulmonary venous connections.
- Van der Velde ME, Parness IA, Colan SD, et al: Two-dimensional echocardiography in the pre- and postoperative management of totally anomalous pulmonary venous connection. J Am Coll Cardiol 1991;18:1746–1751.

  This article documents the value of echocardiography in the pre- and postoperative evaluation of patients with totally anomalous pulmonary venous connection. This study was among the first to encourage the use of echocardiography alone, without catheterisation, in the management of most patients with this diagnosis.
- Hancock Friesen CL, Zurakowski D, Thiagarajan RR, et al: Total anomalous pulmonary venous connection: An analysis of current management strategies in a single institution. Ann Thorac Surg 2005;79:596–606.

  This article evaluates the results and risk factors for surgical repair of totally anomalous pulmonary venous connection at a large referral center in the current era.
- Yun TJ, Coles JG, Konstantinov IE, et al: Conventional and sutureless techniques for management of the pulmonary veins: Evolution of indications from postrepair pulmonary vein stenosis to primary pulmonary vein anomalies. J Thorac Cardiovasc Surg 2005;129:167–174.

  This article describes the current surgical management, both primary and postoperative, for pulmonary venous obstruction, with a particular emphasis on the so-called sutureless repair.

- Alton GY, Robertson CMT, Sauve R, et al: Early childhood health, growth, and neurodevelopmental outcomes after complete repair of total anomalous pulmonary venous connection at 6 weeks or younger. J Thorac Cardiovasc Surg 2007;133:905–911.e903.
- McBride MG, Kirshbom PM, Gaynor JW, et al: Late cardiopulmonary and musculoskeletal exercise performance after repair for total anomalous pulmonary venous connection during infancy. J Thorac Cardiovasc Surg 2007;133:1533–1539.e1532.

  These multi-centric studies offer an extensive evaluation into the long-term outcomes after repair of totally anomalous pulmonary venous connection.
- Baron O, Roussel JC, Videcoq M, et al: Partial anomalous pulmonary venous connection: Correction by intra-atrial baffle and cavo-atrial anastomosis. J Card Surg 2002;17:166–169.
- Brown JW, Ruzmetov M, Minnich DJ, et al: Surgical management of scimitar syndrome: An alternative approach. J Thorac Cardiovasc Surg 2003;125: 238–245.

  These articles review the surgical management of partially anomalous pulmonary venous connection in the current era.
- Holt DB, Moller JH, Larson S, Johnson MC: Primary pulmonary vein stenosis. Am J Cardiol 2007;99:568–572.

  This article describes the clinical presentation, strategies for management, and outcomes in children with primary pulmonary venous stenosis.

CHAPTER 25

Interatrial Communications

ROBERT F. ENGLISH, ROBERT H. ANDERSON, and JOSÉ A. ETTEDGUI

Holes between the atrial chambers are important congenital cardiac anomalies, both because they are relatively common, and because they are more nearly completely correctable than most other cardiac malformations, the more so in the new era of catheter intervention. It may be difficult, nonetheless, to diagnose the presence of such holes, and often there is no suspicion of organic cardiac disease during infancy and early childhood. Moreover, the anatomical arrangement, on occasion, is more complex than mere deficiency of the floor of the oval fossa. It is these anatomical features that underscore our specific description of holes between the atrial chambers, rather than the more usual reference to atrial septal defects. We will emphasise the subtle differences between true atrial septal defects and interatrial communications in our initial section devoted to morphology. It is the lack of early symptoms, nonetheless, coupled with the added subtlety of the physical findings, which delay the diagnosis, sometimes until well into adult life, or even until middle or old age. In contrast, if the left-to-right shunt is large, clinical diagnosis can still be made on the basis of a meticulous cardiac physical examination. The chest radiograph and electrocardiogram usually support such diagnosis, but echocardiography and Doppler studies are diagnostic in virtually all cases. Therapeutic intervention during childhood, after documentation of an important shunt at atrial level, should now result in a normal life expectancy, free of cardiac morbidity, and with the increasing use of devices inserted on catheters, without the need for thoracotomy.

INCIDENCE

Reports of incidence of holes between the atrial chambers have varied between the lesions accounting for one-twentieth to one-tenth of all congenital cardiac anomalies.[1–3] To a large extent, these discrepancies may depend on the definition of holes between the atriums. In the autopsy room, it may be difficult to distinguish those patients with deficiencies of the floor of the oval fossa from probe patency, in which the flap of the foramen had been competent during life, with the atrial communication being only potential. Probe patency is remarkably frequent, being discovered in up to one-third of all the hearts, irrespective of age.[4,5] With the finding that probe patency may underscore some cases of migraine,[6] diagnosis of this normal finding has achieved increased significance. Irrespective of the incidence of probe patency, the variable prevalence of defects noted in the different clinical series is related to the ages of the patients within the series. Thus, a series of infants and young children will have a relatively low prevalence of a clinically apparent interatrial communication as the primary defect, while a series of adults with congenital cardiac disease will have a high prevalence. This is due both to the attrition of patients with other severe and life-threatening defects, and to the frequent delay in diagnosis of an atrial defect until young adulthood. The prevalence also depends upon whether clinically unimportant interatrial communications accompanying more serious defects are included in the series. Prevalence of clinically significant defects, therefore, can perhaps best be judged by the relative frequency of the necessity for surgical closure. When preparing this chapter for the second edition of this book, we noted that, over a period of 25 years, more than 6000 infants and children under the age of 19 years had undergone surgery for treatment of congenital cardiac malformations at the Children's Hospital of Pittsburgh. Of these children, an interatrial communication was the sole, or most important, anomaly in one-tenth of the series. Surgical closure of a hole between the atriums had been undertaken in a further one-sixth, in conjunction with repair of other anomalies. The excellent records kept of autopsies performed at Children's Hospital in Pittsburgh also permit similar observations concerning recognition at postmortem examination. So, during that 25-year period, just over 1000 infants and children with congenital cardiac malformations had come to autopsy. Of these, none had died because of a hole between the atriums, but an interatrial communication had been observed as an incidental finding in one-sixth. The oval foramen was found to be probe patent in nearly two-fifths of the specimens. Holes between the atriums are said to be more common in females, with one report suggesting a ratio of this finding in two females to every male.[7] Others,[8] in contrast, found a slight predominance of males. The defects may be found in higher prevalence in populations residing at higher altitudes.[9]

AETIOLOGY

There are no known intra-uterine events which predispose to deficient atrial septation, and most cases occur sporadically, with no family history of congenital cardiac disease. There is a significant familial incidence when the atrial septal defect is associated with certain skeletal abnormalities of the forearm and hand, the so-called Holt-Oram syndrome.[10] This has now been shown to be due to mutations of the *Tbx5* gene, a member of the *Brachyury* family of genes.[11] When observed in families, atrial septal defects are also associated with prolongation of the PR interval.[12] There is also, occasionally, a familial incidence without these associated abnormalities of the skeleton or atrioventricular conduction. In the patients undergoing surgical closure in Pittsburgh over the period of 25 years discussed above, from one to five close relatives were recognised in nine families, giving a total of 18 familial cases.

MORPHOLOGY AND CLASSIFICATION

The accurate classification of interatrial communications is important, not because the location of the defect alters haemodynamics, but rather because of differences in the incidence of associated anomalies, differences in techniques of surgical repair, and implications for the option of interventional closure. For the surgeon, when planning repair, it is important to be aware of the anomalously connecting pulmonary veins which are the essence of the sinus venosus defect, or of the atrioventricular valvar abnormalities which are part and parcel of the ostium primums defect. This latter lesion, of course, is an atrioventricular septal defect with common atrioventricular junction, but with shunting between the chambers confined at atrial level. It will be described in a chapter to follow. As an extreme example of anatomical difficulties, nonetheless, it may be difficult to recognise a hole at the mouth of the coronary sinus as an interatrial communication, and not simply enlargement of the coronary sinus, if the diagnosis has not been established prior to attempted closure, either by surgery or interventional catheterisation.

The Normal Atrial Septum

Understanding the morphology, and classification, of interatrial communications is itself dependent on a thorough knowledge of the anatomy and extent of the atrial septum. This is because, as we will emphasise, some of the defects which permit shunting of blood at atrial level are outside the confines of the atrial septum. The septum has markedly different characteristics on its morphologically right and left sides. When the right atrium is opened through a wide incision, it seems at first sight that a large expanse of the atrial walls between the orifices of the superior and inferior caval veins and the attachment of the septal leaflet of the tricuspid valve are interposed between the right and left atriums (Fig. 25-1). Sectioning the heart shows that only a small part of this area interposes as a common wall between the atrial cavities, specifically the floor of the oval fossa and its antero-inferior muscular margins (Fig. 25-2). The superior part of the rim, often called the septum secundum, is produced because of infolding of the atrial walls between the mouth of the superior caval vein and the insertion of the right pulmonary veins to the left atrium. This is the area known to surgeons as Waterston's, or Sondergaard's, groove. A substantial cleavage plane, filled by extracardiac fat in the adult heart (Fig. 25-3), extends down to the margin of the fossa.

The internal aspect of this groove represents the prominent muscle bundle which separates the fossa from the orifice of the superior caval vein. It is described appropriately as the superior rim of the fossa, or the superior interatrial fold. More anteriorly, the rim continues as the antero-superior atrial wall overlying the aortic root. This part is well described as the aortic rim of the fossa (see Fig. 25-2). When traced rightwards as viewed in attitudinally appropriate orientation, the rim of the fossa becomes directly continuous with the wall of the inferior caval vein. It is along the antero-inferior margin of the fossa that the morphology is most complicated. This part of the rim separates the fossa from the orifice of the coronary sinus, the mouth of the coronary sinus itself being separated from the mouth of the inferior caval vein by an additional folding, called the sinus septum. The tendon of Todaro, one of the important landmarks of the triangle of Koch, runs through this area to insert into the central fibrous body (see Fig. 25-3). The remainder of the antero-inferior rim

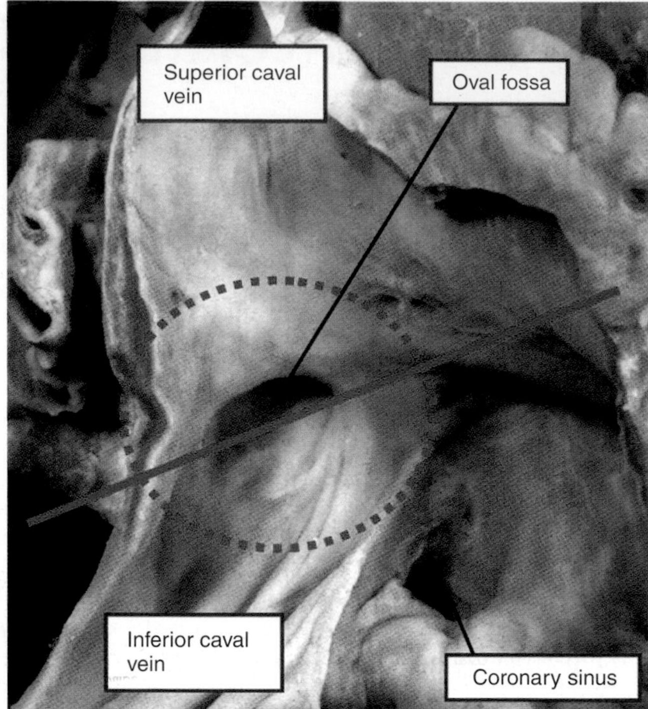

Figure 25-1 Opening the right atrium gives the impression, at first sight, that an extensive area of wall interposes between its cavity and that of the left atrium, as shown by the *dotted circle*. Sectioning along the line shows the true arrangement, as seen in Figure 25-2.

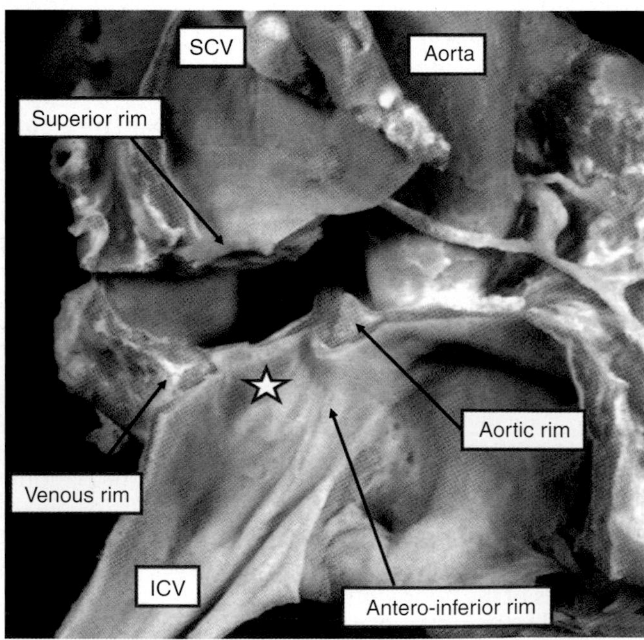

Figure 25-2 The heart shown in Figure 25-1 has been sectioned along the *yellow line* shown in that figure. As can be seen, the rims adjacent to the rightward margins of the openings into the systemic venous sinus of the superior (SCV) and inferior (ICV) caval veins and the aorta are infoldings of the walls, as is the superior rim. It is only the floor of the oval fossa (*star*), and the antero-inferior margin, that represent true septal structures (see Fig. 25-4).

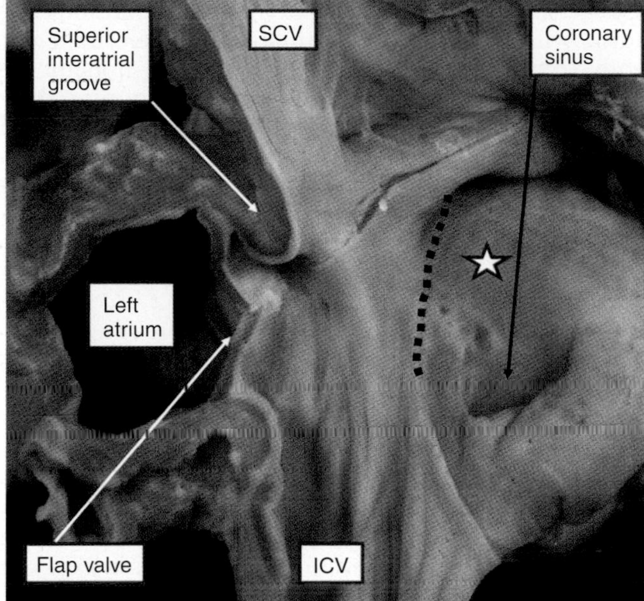

Figure 25-3 The heart shown in Figure 25-2 has been reconstituted, and sectioned through the oval fossa in four-chamber fashion, but photographed so as to show the anterior parts. Note that the alleged septum secundum is no more than an infolding between the opening of the superior caval vein (SCV) to the right atrium and the right upper pulmonary vein to the left atrium. Note also the course of the tendon of Todaro (*black dotted line*), the continuation of the Eustachian, which guards the mouth of the inferior caval vein (ICV). The atrial wall beyond the tendon (*star*) is the vestibular component of the atrioventricular muscular sandwich.

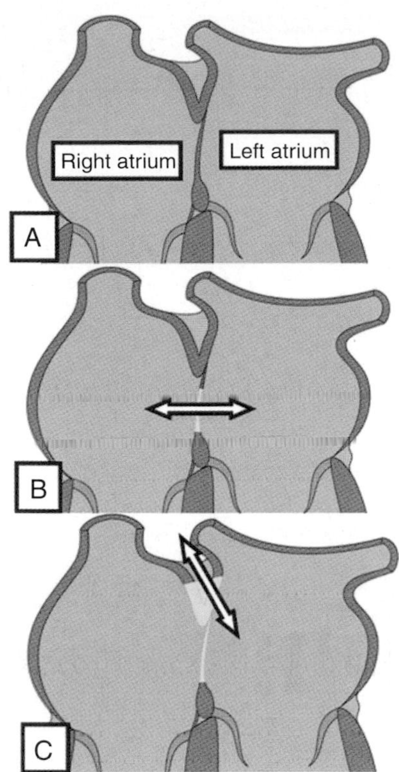

Figure 25-4 The cartoon illustrating the structure of the septal components (**A**) shows how it is possible to remove the floor of the oval fossa (**B**) and stay within the heart, whereas removing the superior rim (**C**) takes the prosector into the pericardial cavity.

is another true septal structure, produced by muscularisation of the developmental component known as the vestibular spine (see below). The right atrial wall continues beyond this septal component, inserting into the vestibule of the tricuspid valve, and forming the atrial component of the muscular atrioventricular sandwich (see Fig. 25-3; see also Chapter 27). As explained in Chapter 2, this region is a sandwich rather than a true septum. This is because an extension of the inferior atrioventricular groove produces a fibroadipose layer between the sheet of atrial musculature and the underlying ventricular mass. It is only the thin translucent floor of the oval fossa, formed from the primary atrial septum, together with the antero-inferior muscular rim of the fossa, which are true interatrial septal structures. As such, they can be removed without exiting from the cavities of the heart (Fig. 25-4). When viewed from the left atrial aspect, the morphology is less complex. The floor of the fossa is smooth, but in its anterosuperior margin it is roughened and wrinkled, forming two horns where it overlaps the infolded superior interatrial groove. In the majority of normal individuals, the flap valve and rim are fused, but as emphasised, anatomical fusion does not occur in about one-third of the population, and the heart shown in Figure 25-5 has probe patency of the oval foramen (Fig. 25-6).

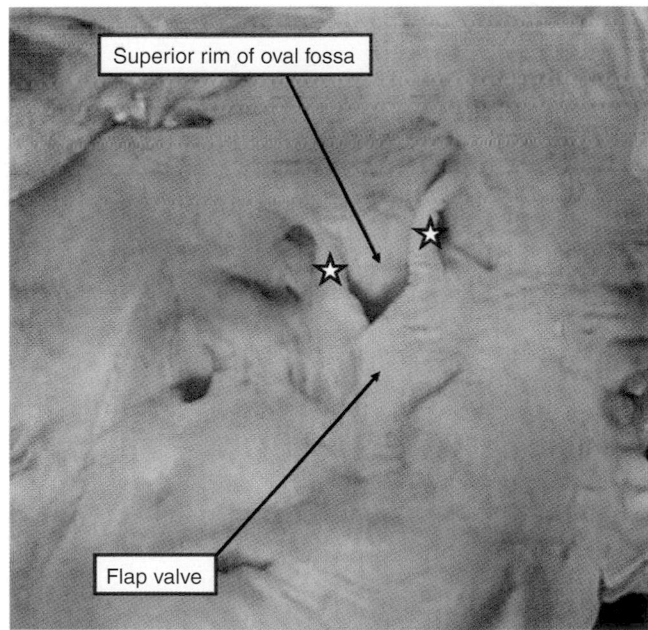

Figure 25-5 When viewed from the left atrium, the flap valve of the oval fossa in the usual situation overlaps the infolded superior rim. The *stars* show the attachment of the horns of the flap valve on the left atrial aspect of the oval fossa.

Types of Interatrial Communication

It is on the basis of this septal morphology that we should distinguish between the different anatomical types of interatrial communications, and recognise that not all are deficiencies of the septal components. Holes between the atriums can be divided into the so-called primum and secundum types, to which need to be added the sinus venosus defects, those found at the site of the mouth of the coronary sinus, and the rare vestibular defect (Fig. 25-7).

Of these various lesions, it is the alleged secundum defects that are within the confines of the oval fossa, and

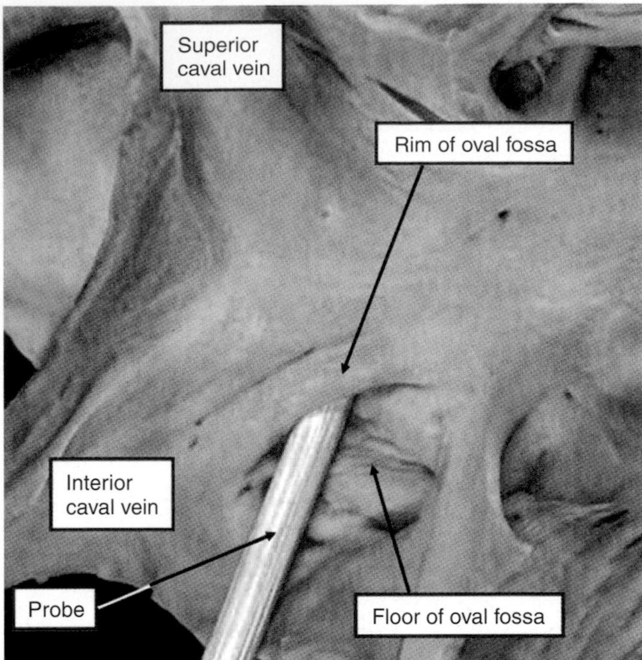

Figure 25-6 In the heart shown in Figure 25-5, as demonstrated by passing a probe up the inferior caval vein, although the floor of the fossa overlaps its rim on the left atrial aspect, the two components are not fused one to the other. This is probe patency of the oval foramen, and is found in about one-third of the normal population.

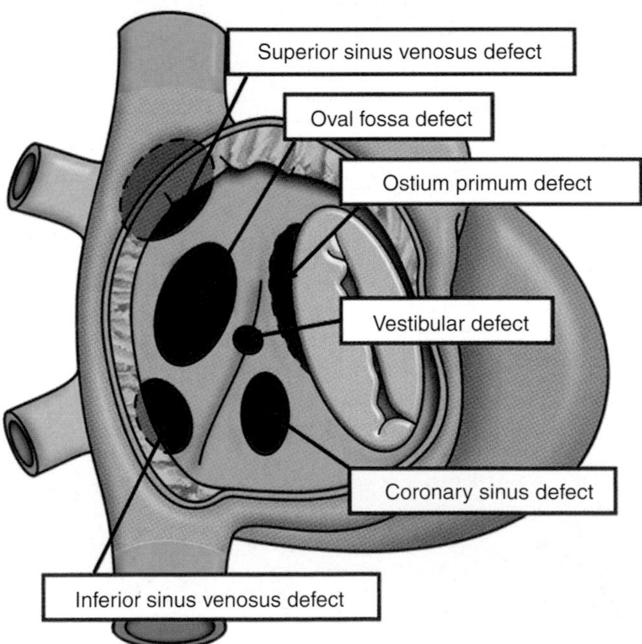

Figure 25-7 The cartoon shows the various types of interatrial communication. Only the defects within the oval fossa, and the rare vestibular defects, are produced by true deficiencies of the septal components.

hence, along with the vestibular defect,[13] those which represent true deficiencies of the atrial septum. The so-called secundum defects result from deficiency of the primary atrial septum, which forms the floor of the oval fossa. The vestibular defect occurs because of inappropriate muscularisation of the vestibular spine and the mesenchymal cap that clothes the leading edge of the primary septum during cardiac development (see Chapter 3). The other defects do unequivocally permit interatrial shunting, and so, with the exception of the primum defect, they are rightly considered in this chapter. They are, nonetheless, more accurately described as interatrial communications.

The so-called ostium primum defect is an atrioventricular septal defect found in the setting of a common atrioventricular junction, but in which the fused bridging leaflets of the common atrioventricular valve are also fused to the scooped-out crest of the ventricular septum. Because of this, shunting across the atrioventricular septal defect occurs only at atrial level. This defect is considered in Chapter 27. The sinus venosus defects are found in the mouths of the caval veins, most usually the superior caval vein, but also in the mouth of the inferior caval vein. The phenotypic feature of these defects is that the oval fossa itself is intact, or else its floor is deficient.[14-16] These defects exist because of anomalous attachment of one or other of the right pulmonary veins. The coronary sinus defect is at the mouth of the coronary sinus.[17] It permits interatrial shunting because of fenestration of the walls which normally separate the coronary sinus and the left atrium. This type of defect is almost always associated with drainage of the left superior caval vein to the roof of the left atrium. The rare vestibular defect is another true septal defect, which is found when the components forming the antero-inferior rim of the fossa do not muscularise appropriately during cardiac development.[13] On the basis of this introduction, we will now describe these defects in more detail.

Defects Within the Oval Fossa

These defects are by far the most common type of interatrial communication, and are true atrial septal defects. Although usually termed secundum defects, this term is justified only because the defect is present at the site of the secondary embryonic foramen, and not because there is inappropriate formation of the so-called septum secundum. As we have emphasised, this alleged septum is no more than a deep fold between the attachments of the superior caval vein to the right atrium, and the right pulmonary veins to the left atrium (see Fig. 25-3). The defects found within the oval fossa result from deficiency, perforation, or complete absence of its floor, which is derived from the primary embryonic septum. As we have also emphasised, the upper border of the primary septum fails to fuse with the left atrial aspect of the infolded superior rim of the oval fossa in around one-third of normal individuals, even though it overlaps the rim (see Fig. 25-6). This is probe patency of the oval foramen. As long as left atrial pressure is higher than right, which is the normal situation, such a happening does not permit interatrial shunting under ordinary circumstances. Probe patency, nonetheless, is known to be responsible for paradoxical embolism, and can be an important finding in those undertaking deep sea diving. The finding has also been implicated recently as a cause of some cases of migraine,[6] and for this reason there has been a vogue for closing such probe-patent foramens by non-surgical means. When measuring such foramens, it should be remembered that the potential hole is a tunnel between the edge of the flap valve and the infolded superior rim of the fossa, rather than being a hole with dimensions that can be measured as occurs for the true septal deficiencies. There is a spectrum of size for defects within the oval fossa, depending on the degree of deficiency of the primary septum. The least severe type of defect is found when the flap valve is minimally deficient, so that it fails to overlap entirely the left atrial margin of the rim of the fossa. With increasing deficiency of the flap valve (Fig. 25-8), the defect becomes larger. In extreme cases there may be no floor to the fossa (Fig. 25-9). Alternatively, the flap valve may be perforated, with either single or multiple perforations (Fig. 25-10). When the deficiency is marked, the hole can extend towards the mouth of the inferior caval vein, which may then straddle the persisting rim to open in part to the left atrium. In the most extreme form of septal deficiency, the hole can extend from the openings of the caval veins and coronary sinus to the septal attachment of the tricuspid valve, but still with a muscular infero-anterior rim separating the right and left atrioventricular junctions. This arrangement should be distinguished from an atrioventricular septal defect with common atrioventricular junction and virtually absent atrial septum. In addition to the small rim of antero-inferior musculature persisting when the defect is due to absence of the floor of the oval fossa, the atrioventricular valvar morphology will distinguish the two types. When the defect is within the oval fossa, the left atrioventricular valve has the characteristic morphology of the mitral valve, whereas when there is a common atrioventricular junction, it has the anticipated trifoliate arrangement (see Chapter 27).

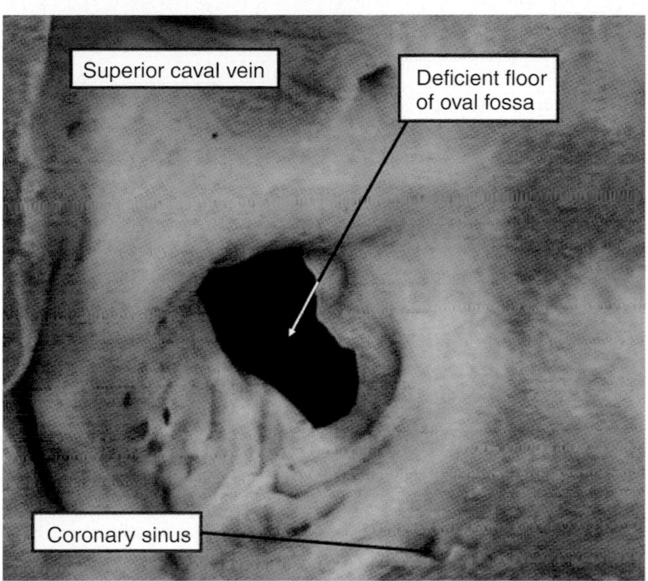

Figure 25-8 In this instance, about half of the floor of the fossa is deficient, producing a defect of significant size.

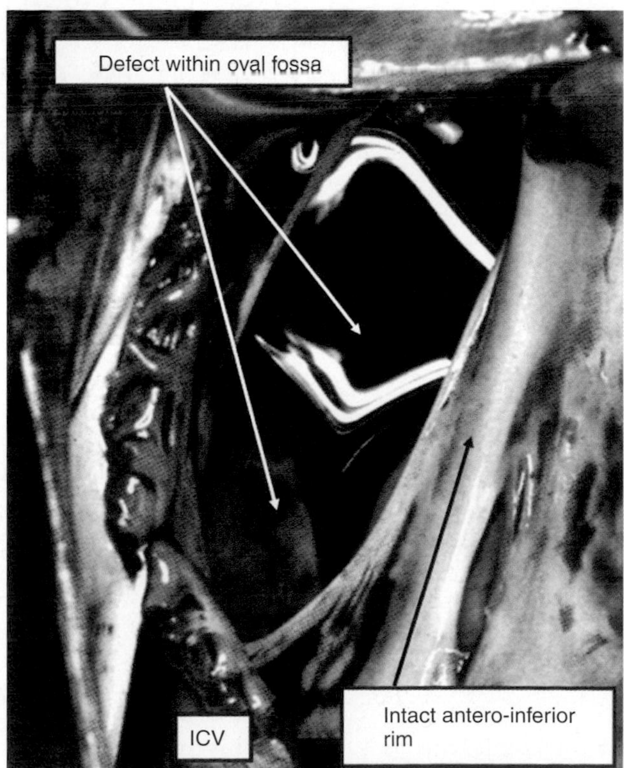

Figure 25-9 In this patient, the floor of the oval fossa is totally deficient, but there is preservation of the antero-inferior rim. Note the extension of the defect towards the inferior caval vein (ICV). (Courtesy of Dr Benson R. Wilcox, University of North Carolina, Chapel Hill.)

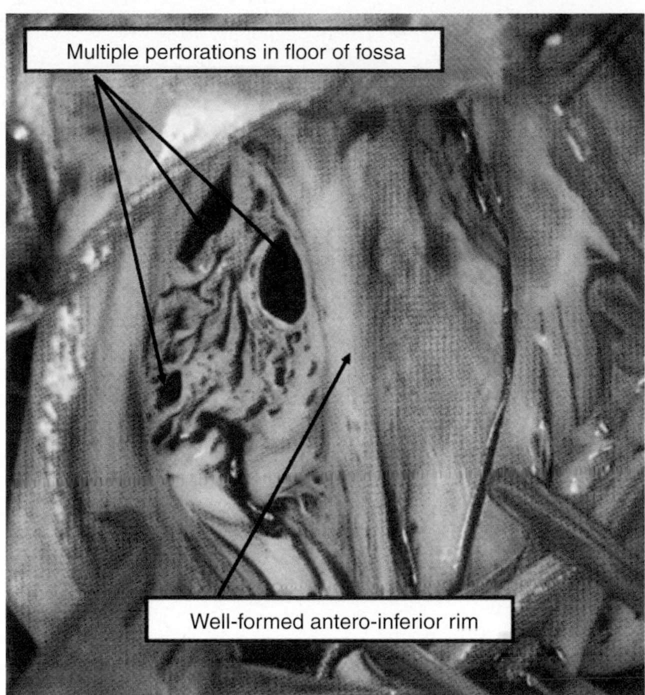

Figure 25-10 The defects in this patient are due to multiple perforations in the floor of the oval fossa. (Courtesy of Dr Benson R. Wilcox, University of North Carolina, Chapel Hill.)

When defects are present within the confines of the fossa, they do not alter the basic disposition of either the sinus or atrioventricular nodes. When the inferior rim is effaced, the node will of necessity be confined to the narrow strip of myocardium between the edge of the defect and the septal attachment of the tricuspid valve. This will still be within the triangle of Koch, readily visible in Figures 25-9 and 25-10, but the triangle itself will be narrow. Apart from this circumstance, the morphology of the atrioventricular junctional area will be normal in the presence of septal defects within the oval fossa. Although these defects may exist in isolation, they often occur in combination with many other congenital cardiac malformations.

Sinus Venosus Defects

The essence of the so-called sinus venosus defects is that they exist outside the confines of the oval fossa.[14–16] The defects are usually found in the mouth of the superior caval vein, but can also be found at the orifice of the inferior

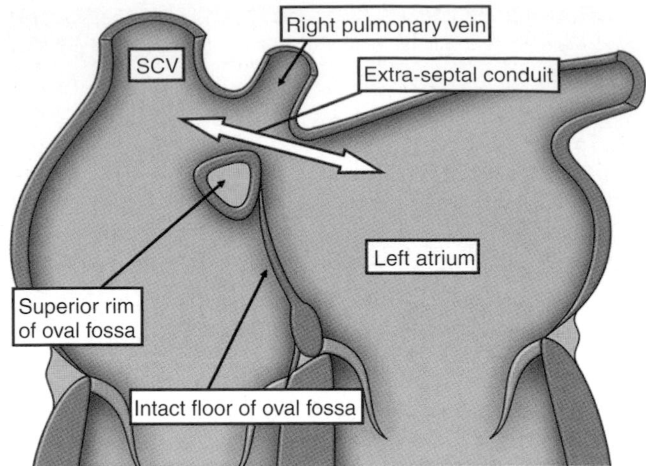

Figure 25-11 The cartoon shows the phenotypic feature of the superior sinus venosus defect, namely an extracardiac conduit created by anomalous connection of the right pulmonary veins at the superior cavoatrial junction. SCV, superior caval vein.

caval vein (see Fig. 25-7). In the case of the superior sinus venosus defect, the orifice of the superior caval vein typically overrides a defect, which has the superior rim of the fossa as its floor. The phenotypic feature of the defect is anomalous insertion of right pulmonary veins into the wall of the superior caval vein, which creates the conduit through which the blood can shunt between the atrial chambers (Fig. 25-11). Indeed, we have now encountered a heart with such a defect in which there is no overriding of the orifice of the superior caval vein. Despite the normal attachment of the caval vein to the right atrium, the anomalous attachment of the right pulmonary veins still create the interatrial communication outside the confines of the intact atrial septum (Fig. 25-12). In most instances, nonetheless, as seen in the specimen shown in Figure 25-13, the defect has a well-circumscribed inferior margin, the superior rim of the oval fossa, but does not have a roof. In these more usual circumstances, the superior caval vein is attached in part to the right atrial wall and in part to the left atrial myocardium (see Fig. 25-13). Usually, the lower right pulmonary vein inserts into the left atrial wall, the middle pulmonary lobe vein drains into the area of the defect, and the upper right pulmonary vein drains directly into the superior caval vein. In this setting, the superior rim of the fossa becomes a muscular tube enclosing a corridor of extracardiac fat. A probe can be passed from back to front through the tube without encroaching on the atrial cavities (see Fig. 25-13). The presence of a superior sinus venosus defect does not markedly affect the site of the sinus node, which is found lateral to the superior cavoatrial junction, lying immediately subepicardially within the terminal groove. Thus, a patch placed within the atrium to reconnect the caval vein to the right side should not jeopardise the sinus node. Because of the usual overriding of the superior caval vein, and the usual presence of anomalous pulmonary veins, it may not be possible to septate the defect in such a way that normal pulmonary venous return is restored without narrowing the superior caval pathway. In these circumstances, it may be difficult to widen the caval vein without putting either the sinus node or its vascular supply at risk, since the artery to the node may pass either in front of or behind the cavoatrial

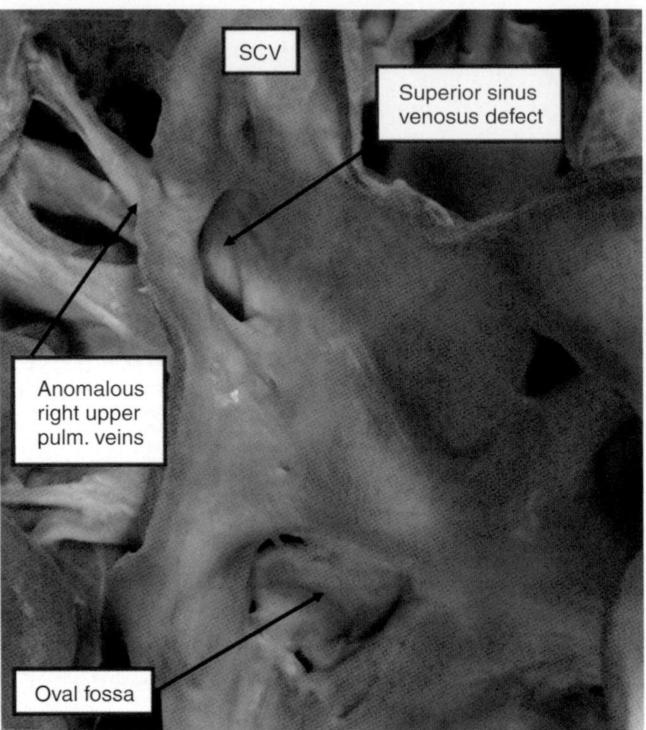

Figure 25-12 In this specimen, the superior caval vein (SCV) is normally attached within the right atrium, but the anomalous attachment of the right upper pulmonary veins creates a superior sinus venosus defect well removed from the margins of the oval fossa.

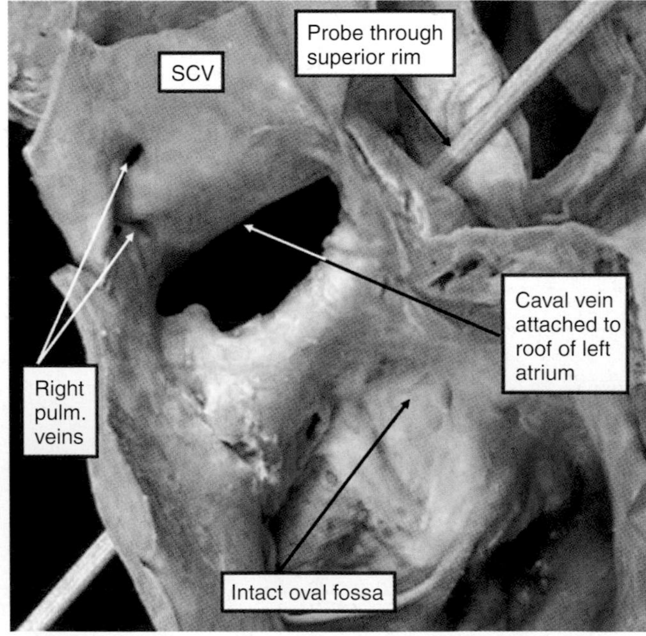

Figure 25-13 In the more usual type of superior sinus venosus defect (compare with Fig. 25-12), the mouth of the superior caval vein (SCV) overrides the intact superior rim of the oval fossa, which encloses a corridor of extracardiac fat, through which the probe has been placed from the back to the front of the heart.

junction to enter the node. Despite this caveat, most defects can be closed without jeopardising normal function of the node. Inferior sinus venosus defects are far less common.[16] They, too, are associated with an anomalous attachment of the right pulmonary veins, but in these cases, it is the

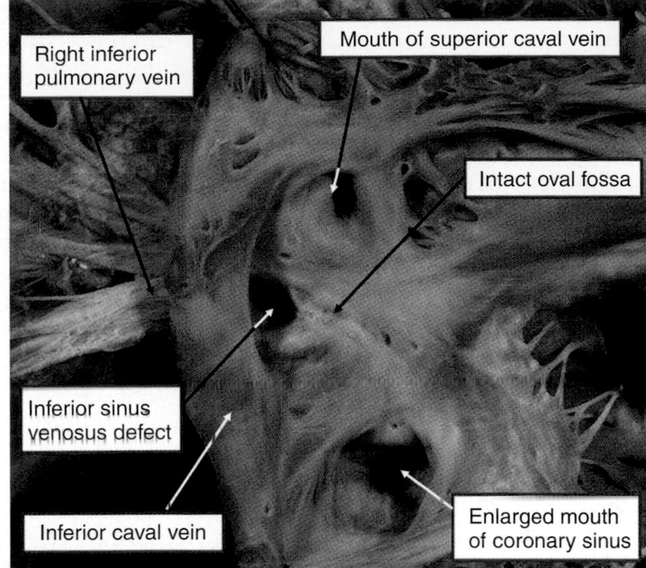

Figure 25-14 An inferior sinus venosus defect is shown from its right atrial aspect in a heart with an intact oval fossa and a persistent left superior caval vein draining through the enlarged opening of the coronary sinus. Note that the inferior caval vein is attached in normal fashion to the right atrium, with the defect produced by anomalous attachment of the right inferior pulmonary vein.

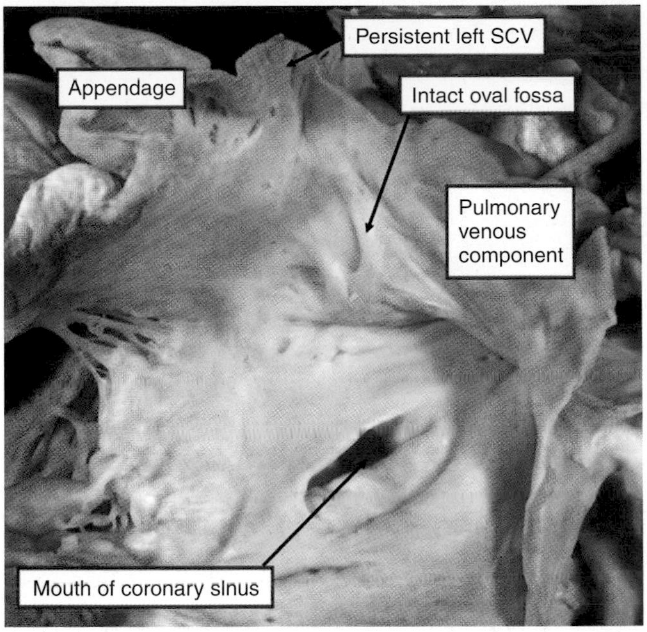

Figure 25-15 In this heart, absence of the walls that normally separate the coronary sinus from the left atrium have left the mouth of the sinus to function as an interatrial communication. SCV, superior caval vein.

anomalous attachment of the right inferior pulmonary vein that creates the extracardiac conduit (Figs. 25-14). Closure of such a defect should not jeopardise either the sinus or the atrioventricular node. Inferior sinus venosus defects must, of course, be distinguished from defects within the oval fossa which extend towards the mouth of the inferior caval vein (see Fig. 25-9).

Coronary Sinus Defects

The coronary sinus defect consists of an interatrial communication through the orifice of the coronary sinus, with absence of the usually adjacent walls of the coronary sinus and left atrium. Most times there is also connection of a persistent left superior caval vein to the left atrial roof.[17] In essence, the anomaly is the consequence of absence of the walls which normally exist between the coronary sinus and the left atrium. In their absence, the orifice of the coronary sinus becomes an interatrial communication (Fig. 25-15). In some examples of this combination, filigreed remnants of the atrial wall persist between the orifice of the coronary sinus and the termination of the left caval vein in the left atrium. More commonly, as shown in Figure 25-15, there is no tissue separating the coronary sinus, the mouth of the left caval vein, and the cavity of the left atrium. The opening of the coronary sinus is usually large. When such a defect is large, its anterior margin encroaches on the triangle of Koch, approximating the area of the atrioventricular node. Care must be taken, therefore, when the defect is closed. In this respect, unless previously diagnosed, a coronary sinus defect may be difficult to recognise as an interatrial communication in the operating room, appearing simply to be the mouth of the coronary sinus itself.

The Vestibular Defect

The heart shown in Figure 25-16 has a defect in the antero-inferior margin of the oval fossa. The fossa itself exhibits two additional defects, and the tricuspid valve is hypoplastic, since the patient also had pulmonary atresia in the setting of an intact atrial septum. This lesion is a true atrial septal defect through the septal component of the muscular margin of the oval fossa.[13]

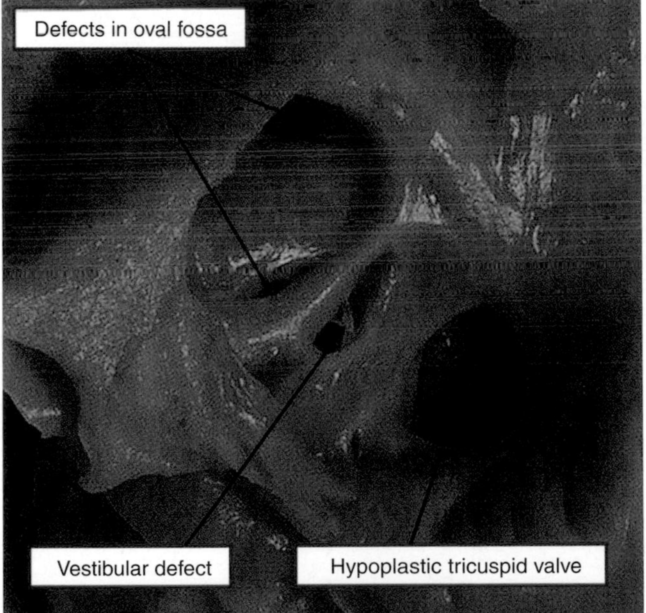

Figure 25-16 The heart has a septal deficiency in the antero-inferior margin of the oval fossa, this being the part derived by muscularisation of the vestibular spine.[13] (Courtesy of Dr Geoffrey Sharratt, Halifax, Nova Scotia, Canada.)

Morphogenesis of Interatrial Communications

During normal development, the embryonic primary septum grows down to divide the primary atrium, carrying with it a cap of mesenchymal tissue (Figs. 25-17 and 25-18, upper panels). This cap will fuse with the atrioventricular

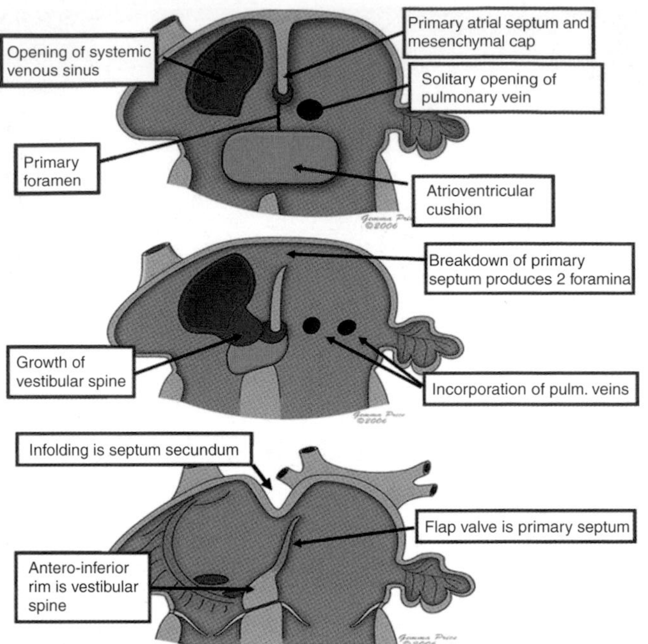

Figure 25-17 The panels show the sequence of formation of the normal atrial septum as seen in the four-chamber orientation.

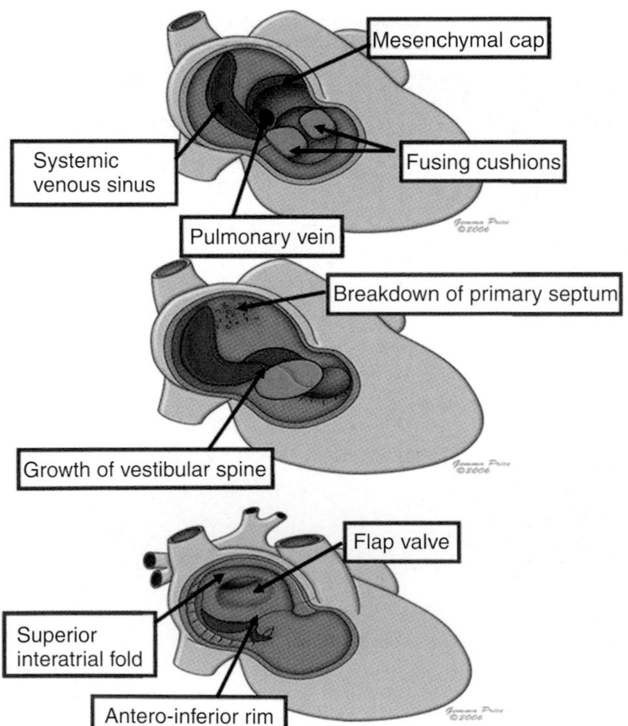

Figure 25-18 The panels show the same sequence of events as shown in Figure 25-17, but as seen from the right side.

endocardial cushions, and will then be reinforced by the vestibular spine to close the primary interatrial foramen (see Figs. 25-17 and 25-18, middle panels). As its lower edge fuses with the cushions, its top edge breaks down to form the secondary foramen (see Fig. 25-18, middle panel). The upper edge of the remaining primary atrial septum is then usually overlapped by the infolding of the atrial roof between the superior caval and pulmonary veins, this fold forming the superior rim of the oval fossa, often described as the septum secundum (see Figs. 25-17 and 25-18, lower panels).

Failure of normal development of the atrioventricular junction prevents the lower edge of the primary septum from fusing with the ventricular septum. This results in the so-called ostium primum defect, which is an atrioventricular septal defect with common atrioventricular junction, and is described further in Chapter 27. It is maldevelopment of the primary atrial septum itself, after it has fused with the ventricular septum and the endocardial cushions, which results in defects within the oval fossa. This can either be due to deficiency of its superior edge, so that it no longer overlaps the infolded superior rim, or breakdown of the septum to a greater or lesser degree, resulting in the various types of perforate or fenestrated defects within the fossa (see Fig. 25-10). In the most severe defects, the muscular rim also becomes effaced. It is possible to envisage temporary effacement of the rim of the oval fossa, since this is no more than a muscular infolding. Such effacement in the presence of volume load, with subsequent restoration of the fold once the volume load has been corrected, is a likely explanation for so-called spontaneous closure of some defects within the oval fossa during the neonatal period. Sinus venosus defects are best explained on the basis that the right pulmonary veins are abnormally attached to the wall of either the superior or inferior caval veins (see Figs. 25-12 and 25-14). Resorption of the walls normally formed between the pulmonary and caval veins will produce a defect outside the margins of the oval fossa, usually also permitting biatrial communication of the caval vein itself. The coronary sinus defect is best explained on the basis of similar resorption of the walls which usually separate the lumen of the coronary sinus from the cavity of the left atrium (see Fig. 25-15). The rare vestibular defect (see Fig. 25-16) is likely due to improper muscularisation of the antero-inferior rim of the oval fossa, this usually requiring involvement of both the vestibular spine and the mesenchymal cap carried on the leading edge of the atrial septum.[13]

Associated Anomalies

Cardiac

Certain cardiac and vascular anomalies have been reported to occur more frequently in patients with an atrial septal defect than in the general population. The atrioventricular valve is essentially a common structure in the setting of an atrioventricular septal defect with common atrioventricular junction but with shunting confined at atrial level, the so-called ostium primum defect, as considered in Chapter 27. Hence, it is inappropriate always to consider such valves as abnormal, albeit that they often show additional malformations. Such additional malformations are less common with other varieties of interatrial communication, but do occur. A prolapsing mitral valve, for instance, was found in one-sixth of one series of patients.[18] The incidence amongst the patients undergoing surgical closure in Pittsburgh was only 2.5%. The true incidence is hard to determine, since the criterions for diagnosing prolapse are different in different institutions.

Anomalous connection of the pulmonary veins is a relatively common associated finding in patients with interatrial communications. Indeed, it is the phenotypic feature of the sinus venosus variety. This feature was reported in one-sixth of the patients undergoing surgery at Pittsburgh, but was seen in five-sixths of those said to have sinus venosus defects, compared to only 1.7% of those with a defect within the oval fossa. This statistic, however, calls into question the nature of those patients allegedly having a sinus venosus defect in the absence of anomalous connection of the pulmonary veins. It is very likely that re-examination of these patients would reveal that initially they had oval fossa defects extending towards the openings of the caval veins.

An interatrial communication may co-exist with a ventricular septal defect, persistent patency of the arterial duct, or coarctation of the aorta. The true incidence is hard to determine, since each of these defects may lead to increased left atrial pressure and size, while the interatrial communication may be due to incompetence of a stretched oval foramen. Although a small gradient across the right ventricular outflow tract is common in patients with an interatrial communication, such stenosis is usually functional, and related to increased flow. Organic pulmonary stenosis requiring surgical attention was uncommon in the series of patients undergoing surgery in Pittsburgh, occurring in less than one-twentieth.

Non-cardiac

The association of Down's syndrome with ostium primum defects is well known. It occurred in three-tenths of patients undergoing surgery for such defects in Pittsburgh. The incidence of Down's syndrome was only 2.9% in those having surgery for atrial septal defect in the oval fossa. The skeletal anomalies of the Holt-Oram syndrome,[10] and electrophysiological abnormalities,[12] are examples of non-cardiac anomalies, which occur in a few patients. As with associated cardiac malformations, non-cardiac anomalies are relatively rare in patients with an atrial septal defect.

PATHOPHYSIOLOGY

The pathophysiology of an atrial septal defect is related to the magnitude and direction of shunting of blood across the interatrial communication. There is usually a substantial left-to-right shunt, resulting in a high ratio of pulmonary to systemic flow. The primary determinants of the amount of shunting are the size of the defect and the relative resistance to inflow, or the compliance, of the ventricles. The latter factor is greatly influenced by pulmonary vascular resistance. The compliance of the right and left atriums themselves may also play a role, but this has been difficult to prove. As with a ventricular septal defect, the site of the defect in the atrial septum does not influence the magnitude of flow across it, although relative contributions to the shunt from the individual pulmonary veins do vary depending on the location of the defect.

Effect of Size of the Defect

The size of the interatrial communication is an important determinant of the magnitude of the shunt. Because of the lower resistances involved, an interatrial communication tends to be larger than a ventricular defect for a shunt of similar magnitude. Most interatrial communications recognised clinically are essentially non-restrictive, and approximate the area of the mitral valvar orifice. The defect imposes no more restriction to flow across it than does the mitral valve. There is, therefore, at most a small pressure gradient between the atriums. If the defect is smaller and restrictive, the flow of blood to the lungs will be limited by the size of the defect. The ratio of flows usually will be less than 2 to 1. There is no doubt that many small defects escape clinical detection because a limited left-to-right shunt is haemodynamically well tolerated, and causes no abnormalities in the physical examination.

In some cases, the interatrial communication may result from incompetence of the valve of the oval foramen, rather than a true deficiency of the atrial septum. This incompetence can lead to considerable left-to-right shunting when there are associated abnormalities that lead to increased left atrial pressure. Mitral stenosis, a dysfunctional left ventricle, aortic stenosis, coarctation of the aorta, systemic hypertension, patency of the arterial duct, and ventricular septal defect are examples. If the primary defect leading to volume or pressure overload of the left atrium can be corrected, the valve may become competent and the atrial shunt will then disappear. Some otherwise normal infants have left-to-right atrial shunting owing to transient incompetence of the valve of the oval foramen. This phenomenon was well described,[18] and subsequently confirmed by the widespread use of Doppler echocardiography in newborns and young infants. It is likely to be caused by effacement of the superior infolded rim.

Effect of Ventricular Compliance

If the atrial defect is non-restrictive, the magnitude of the shunt will be directly related to the relative resistance to filling offered by the right and left ventricles. The inflow resistance of a ventricle, or its compliance, is related to its diastolic function and distensibility. This is largely related to its mass, but other factors may also play a role in the complex determination of diastolic function. The mass, and hence the compliance, of the right ventricle is influenced by pulmonary vascular resistance. It undergoes predictable postnatal changes. At birth, right and left ventricular compliances are approximately equal, and there is little shunting across an atrial defect in either direction. Pulmonary vascular resistance and pressure generally undergo their normal dramatic fall over the first days of life in patients with an interatrial communication. This is true even in a patient with a large defect, since the pulmonary vascular bed is never exposed to systemic arterial pressure, as it is with a large ventricular septal defect or aortopulmonary communication. It takes several months, however, before the mass of the right ventricle decreases relative to that of the left ventricle. Only then is a normal adult relationship reached between the two ventricles. Hence, a significant left-to-right shunt is not expected until several months of age. Pulmonary arterial pressure at this stage is almost always normal. Although patients with an atrial septal defect have a normal regression of pulmonary vascular resistance, they are susceptible to a secondary increase in resistance if the flow of blood to the lungs remains high for many years, usually several decades.[3,18,19] As pulmonary vascular resistance rises, the pulmonary arterial pressure also increases. This causes right ventricular hypertrophy with a concomitant decrease in compliance, which leads to less left-to-right shunting. As right ventricular compliance approaches that of the left ventricle, there is little shunting across the defect. If right ventricular compliance exceeds that of the left ventricle, there will be a right-to-left atrial shunt, since the atriums will empty preferentially into the more easily filled left ventricle. If there is associated severe pulmonary stenosis, hypertrophy of the right ventricle will occur. The resulting decreasing compliance of this chamber may eventually lead to right-to-left shunting. A right-to-left atrial shunt may also be caused by tricuspid stenosis or severe tricuspid valvar regurgitation. In addition to changes in right ventricular compliance, abnormal filling characteristics of the left ventricle can also influence the magnitude of the atrial shunt. Filling of the left ventricle is impaired by mitral stenosis, or by any abnormality that leads to increased diastolic pressures in the left ventricle. This may result in marked accentuation of the left-to-right shunt across the atrial defect.

Cardiac Response to the Interatrial Communication

The usual haemodynamic characteristics of an uncomplicated interatrial communication are a large left-to-right shunt and normal pulmonary arterial pressure. Flow across the defect is phasic, and occurs predominantly in late ventricular systole and early diastole.[20] Numerous studies have documented that most patients with a typical defect within the oval fossa have a small right-to-left shunt. It occurs mainly from streaming of a portion of the return from the inferior caval vein directly across the defect into the left atrium.[19,21] This small shunt is not detectable by oximetry, so there is no systemic desaturation, but it can be demonstrated by indicator dilution techniques,[22] contrast echocardiography,[23] and Doppler studies.[24]

The contribution of the pulmonary venous return from each lung to the total left-to-right shunt is unequal. In a typical large defect, four-fifths of the pulmonary venous return from the right lung shunts left to right. This is in contrast to between one-fifth and two-fifths of the pulmonary venous return from the left lung.[18,19,22] In a sinus venosus defect, it is the anomalously connected right pulmonary veins that provide most of the shunted blood. This preferential shunting from the right lung does not occur to any great extent with an ostium primum interatrial communication.

A large left-to-right shunt at the atrial level leads to enlargement of both the right atrium and the right ventricle.[25] The left atrium is of normal size despite the increased pulmonary venous return, since the atrial septal defect allows its decompression. Left ventricular dimensions are usually normal, although some studies have shown left ventricular end-diastolic volume to be less than normal.[26]

Systemic cardiac output is almost always normal in children. Exercise tolerance is good, probably because the cardiovascular response to exercise favours a decrease in the magnitude of the atrial shunting. The afterload on the left ventricle is decreased by the drop in systemic vascular resistance that attends exercise, tending to facilitate left ventricular filling. The increased cardiac output also augments systemic venous return, competitively filling the right atrium at the expense of shunting across the defect. In contrast to the situation in childhood, systemic cardiac output has been found to be decreased in up to half the patients with an atrial septal defect who are older than 18 years of age.[27] Numerous studies in adults have shown significant left ventricular dysfunction, which may persist even after surgical correction.[26,28,29]

Despite the greatly increased flow of blood to the lungs, pulmonary arterial pressure is rarely elevated in children, and pulmonary vascular resistance is low, frequently less than 1 Wood unit.[30] The incidence of pulmonary hypertension in children less than 20 years of age is no more than one-twentieth in most studies but increases to one-fifth of those aged from 20 to 40 years, and is found in half of the patients older than 40 years.[3,19,31,32] The incidence of elevated pulmonary vascular resistance also increases with age.[27,33] Severe elevation of resistance, and Eisenmenger's reaction, however, is unusual, occurring in only about one-twentieth of patients.[34,35] With severe elevation of pulmonary vascular resistance, right ventricular hypertrophy may increase, and compliance decrease, sufficiently that cyanosis results from reversal of the atrial shunt. This suggests slowly progressive development of pulmonary vascular disease, presumably resulting from increased flow of blood to the lungs over many years. Heath and Edwards[36] described changes in the pulmonary vascular bed consistent with this hypothesis, including a predominance of intimal fibrosis and endothelial proliferation, but with less medial muscular hypertrophy than is seen in patients with ventricular septal defects. There are many aspects of the clinical spectrum that are not explained by this simplistic scheme. On the one hand, although it is uncommon, some children with isolated atrial septal defects do have pulmonary hypertension. On the other hand, there are adults who live into their sixth and seventh decades with markedly increased flow to the lungs who have normal pulmonary vascular resistance and normal pulmonary arterial pressure.[27,37] There must, therefore, be individual variation of pulmonary vascular reactivity to various noxious stimuli such as increased pulmonary flow, increased pressure, and so on. As yet, these features are poorly understood.

The chronic right ventricular volume overload caused by an interatrial communication is generally well tolerated for many years, particularly when there is no associated elevation of pulmonary arterial pressure. Congestive heart failure rarely occurs before the fourth or fifth decades but has been reported to be present in approximately one-third of patients greater than 40 years of age.[27,33] Rarely, an isolated defect may cause congestive heart failure in infancy.[38–40] Another cardiac consequence of the long-standing left-to-right shunt is the occurrence of atrial arrhythmias, particularly atrial flutter and fibrillation. They presumably result from chronic stretching of the atriums, and occur most commonly in patients greater than 40 years of age.[37,41,42] As with the other complications associated with inter-atrial communications, atrial arrhythmias rarely occur in childhood. Electrophysiological studies, nonetheless, have demonstrated a high incidence of subclinical dysfunction of the sinus node, along with conduction disturbances, in children prior to operative intervention.[43–46]

CLINICAL FINDINGS

Presentation

Mild dyspnoea on exertion, and/or easy fatiguability, are the most common early symptoms of an interatrial communication. They are not usually present during infancy and childhood, or may be appreciated only in retrospect after a diagnosis has been made. Not infrequently, parents report increased activity and vigour after repair, even though they had considered their child to be asymptomatic prior to surgery. Infants less than 1 year of age may rarely present with congestive heart failure owing to an isolated defect. Some children have an increased number of respiratory infections. Additionally, some infants who are predisposed to respiratory compromise, such as those with bronchopulmonary dysplasia, may suffer more significant effects from the atrial shunting, and may benefit from early closure of the defect. Symptoms become much more common in the fourth or fifth decades, for reasons already discussed. Some patients, even with a large defect, may be in their sixth or seventh decades before they demonstrate dyspnoea on exertion, easy fatigue, or frank congestive heart failure. A few remain free of disabling symptoms throughout life.

Physical Examination

The general physical examination is usually normal, although there is a tendency toward a slender physique (Fig. 25-19). Associated non-cardiac abnormalities are uncommon in individuals with a defect within the oval fossa or a sinus venosus defect.[8] Skeletal anomalies of the forearm and hand do occur occasionally, and this syndrome may be inherited.[10] Non-cardiac anomalies much more commonly accompany ostium primum defects. Notable examples include Down's syndrome[47] and the visceral anomalies typically present with isomerism of the atrial appendages.[48]

The jugular venous pulse is usually normal, as are blood pressure and peripheral arterial pulses. A left parasternal lift is often present, but precordial motion is normal in some patients, especially if the left-to-right shunt is not large. Rarely, there is asymmetric development of the chest with a protuberance of the lower left aspect of the thorax. Cyanosis is not part of the clinical picture of an uncomplicated interatrial communication. It can occur under certain circumstances, for example with virtual absence of the interatrial septum or when there is anomalous systemic venous connection to the left atrium.

The heart sounds are almost always abnormal. It is difficult to entertain making the diagnosis clinically when auscultation is completely normal. The first sound at the low left sternal border is usually accentuated because of prominent closure of the tricuspid valve.[49] The increased diastolic flow across the tricuspid valve tends to keep the leaflets widely open until ventricular systole begins. The wider excursion of the leaflets prior to coaptation may, therefore, explain the loudness of the closure. Alternatively, the wide-open position of the leaflets may result in closure that is slightly late. As a result, closure occurs during the more steeply rising portion of the ventricular pressure curve and causes a more forceful coaptation. The second sound is characteristically widely and fixedly split, with little or no variation in the width of the split during the respiratory cycle. Fixed splitting may be appreciated during quiet respiration, or by listening during held expiration. The latter technique has the advantage of eliminating breath sounds during auscultation and is probably the more sensitive method. If an individual with a normal heart is asked to breathe all the way out, and then stop breathing, the second sound will be single for one to three beats. It will then become split, the splitting gradually widening over the next several beats (Fig. 25-20A). In contrast, the second sound of a patient with an atrial septal defect is split at the end of expiration. The degree of splitting then varies little or not at all during held expiration (see Fig. 25-20B).

The normal inspiratory exaggeration of splitting is supposedly related to the augmentation of systemic venous return induced by the negative intrathoracic pressure of inspiration. The increased right ventricular filling prolongs ejection, leading to a delayed closure of the pulmonary valve, which is then separated from the sound of aortic closure. Several reasons for the lack of respiratory variation in splitting in patients with an interatrial communication have been suggested. The most widely accepted explanation postulates a reciprocal relationship of changes in pulmonary and systemic venous return with respiration.[50] An alternative explanation relates the delayed closure to a separation of the right ventricular and pulmonary arterial pressure curves rather than to prolongation of ventricular systole, which rarely occurs. The pulmonary arterial curve is typically delayed, and the dip, corresponding to pulmonary valvar closure, hangs out beyond the descending ventricular pressure curve.[51] Whatever the true genesis of fixed splitting, it is a most valuable sign of a large left-to-right shunt at the atrial level.

The murmurs associated with an atrial septal defect are typically soft. They may be absent in infancy and early childhood, explaining the relative lateness of diagnosis in most individuals. It is extremely uncommon for a murmur to arise at the site of the interatrial communication itself, since there is usually little or no gradient across it. Instead, the murmurs are generated by rapid blood flow through the right heart and the pulmonary arterial bed. Almost all individuals with a clinically recognisable atrial septal defect have a crescendo–decrescendo systolic murmur at the high left sternal border. This is related to rapid flow across the pulmonary valve. The murmur is usually soft, and a murmur of greater than grade 3 to 6 should suggest the possibility of accompanying pulmonary stenosis. It is easy to overestimate the severity of obstruction within the right ventricular outflow tract. Even a loud systolic murmur may be generated at a very mildly stenotic pulmonary valve. A similar systolic murmur is usually audible in the axillas

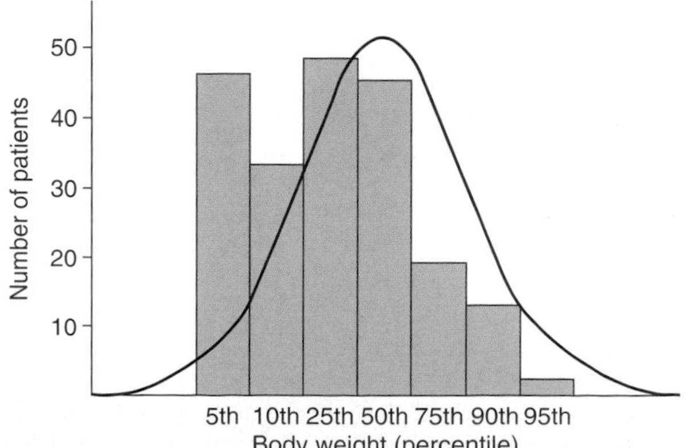

Figure 25-19 The centiles for weight of patients undergoing surgical repair of an atrial septal defect at the Children's Hospital of Pittsburgh. The normal distribution of weight is indicated by the *solid line*, and that in the patients by the *bars*. The distribution is skewed in the patients toward the lower percentiles.

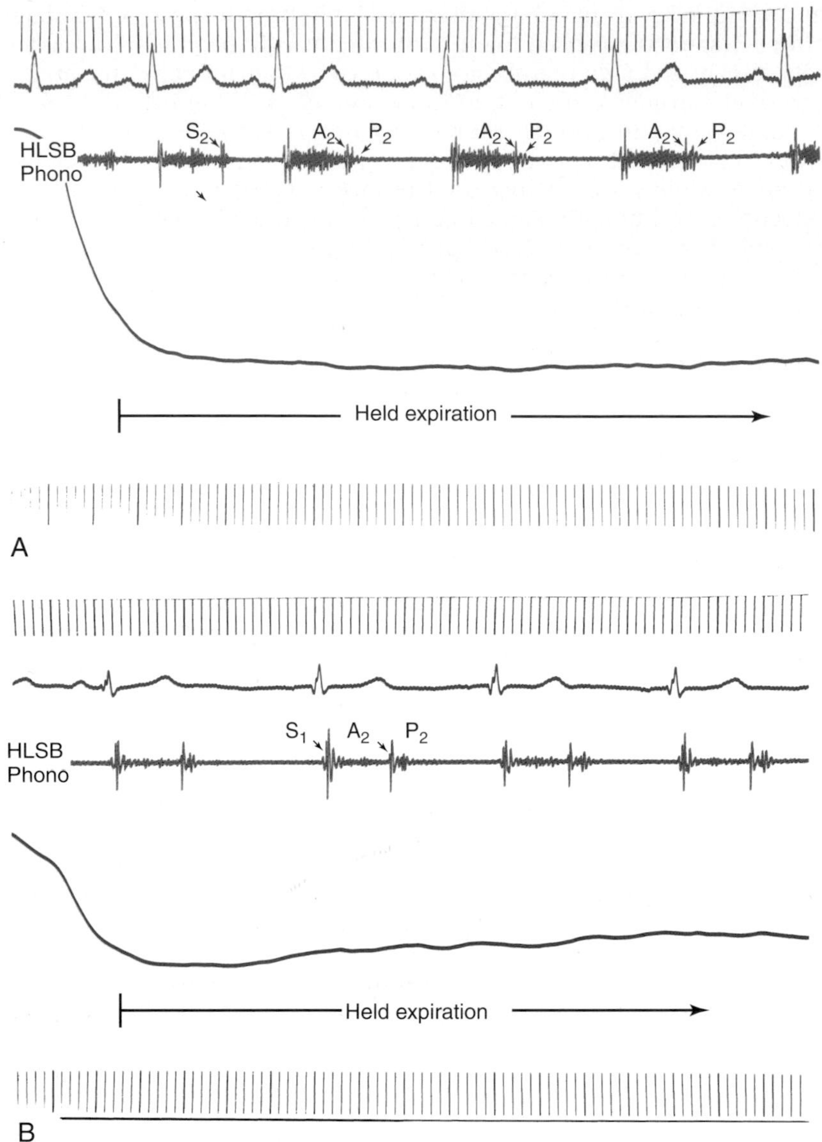

Figure 25-20 This phonocardiogram was recorded at the high left sternal border during held expiration. Respiration is indicated by the solid line. **A,** Normal splitting. The second heart sound is single on the first beat, while subsequent beats show gradually increasing splitting. **B,** Fixed splitting. The second heart sound is split on the first beat, and there is only trivial widening of the split with subsequent beats. A_2, aortic valvar closure sound; HLSB phono, high left sternal border phonocardiogram; P_2, pulmonary valvar closure sound; S_1, first heart sound; S_2, second heart sound.

and over the posterior thorax. It is generated by rapid flow of blood through the pulmonary arteries.

Most individuals with a large left-to-right shunt through an interatrial communication also have a soft mid-diastolic murmur at the low left sternal border. This murmur is always subtle and is almost never recognised unless specifically listened for. The murmur is that of relative tricuspid stenosis, and is generated by rapid flow across a normal tricuspid valve. Unlike the murmur of organic or relative mitral stenosis, the murmur is not low pitched and rumbling. Rather, it is of medium pitch and is often scratchy. There is always an audible gap between the second heart sound and the murmur. None of the murmurs associated with an interatrial communication are affected significantly by the phase of respiration or by position. Although the murmurs just described arise at a distance from the defect, under certain circumstances a murmur may be generated at the defect itself. The prerequisite is a relatively large gradient between the atriums. Such a gradient occurs only if the defect is small and restrictive and if left atrial pressure is higher than normal, usually because of mitral stenosis[52] or mitral atresia.[53] The murmur is continuous, since under these circumstances, left atrial pressure exceeds right atrial pressure throughout the cardiac cycle. The murmur is usually soft and maximal near the lower sternum. Rarely, the murmur is loud with an accompanying thrill and may have a roaring quality.

The physical findings associated with an interatrial communication are greatly altered by the appearance of pulmonary vascular disease. With an increase in right ventricular pressure, the left parasternal lift may become more pronounced. An elevation of pulmonary arterial pressure tends to close the pulmonary valve earlier as the typical loose system of an uncomplicated atrial defect becomes more tight. The interval of hang out then decreases. The elevated pulmonary arterial diastolic pressure also contributes to earlier pulmonary closure. The second heart sound, therefore, becomes narrowly split, or single, as long as right ventricular function is not severely impaired. If right ventricular contractility is sufficiently diminished, pulmonary valvar closure will be delayed by a prolonged ejection time, and the second heart sound will again become

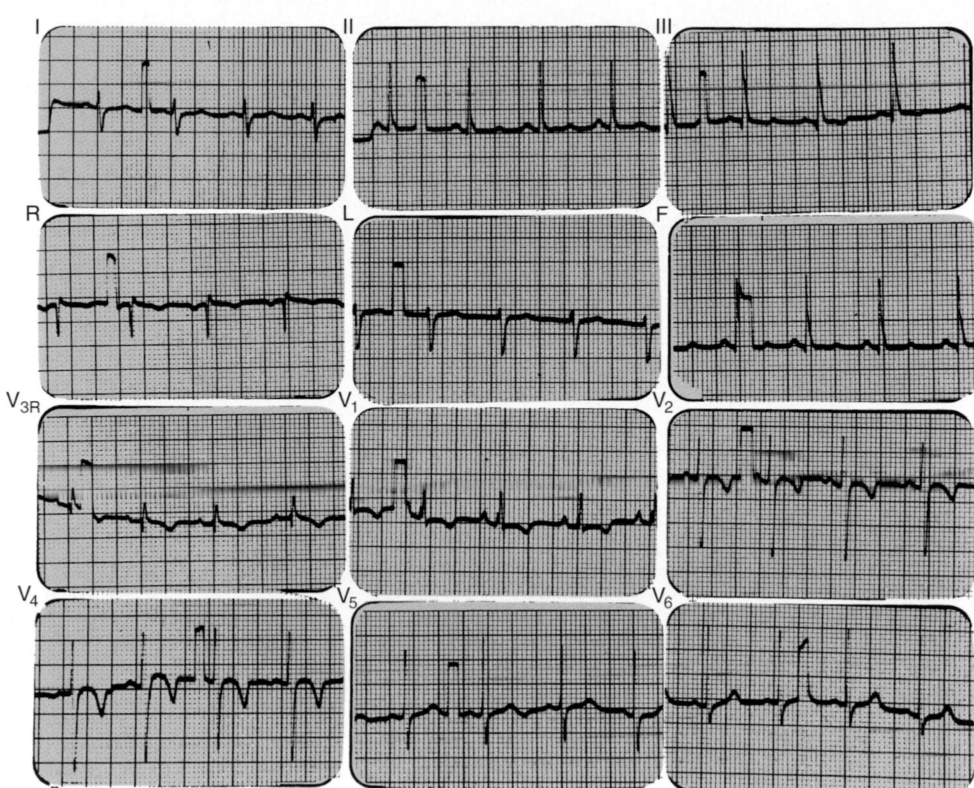

Figure 25-21 Surface electrocardiogram from a child with an atrial septal defect within the oval fossa. There is right-axis deviation and mild right ventricular hypertrophy manifested by an RSR′ pattern in the right precordial leads.

widely split. Splitting of the second heart sound in an individual with an atrial septal defect and pulmonary hypertension, therefore, depends on right ventricular function. It is narrow or absent as long as right ventricular function is normal; it is wide if right ventricular function is compromised. With an increase in pulmonary vascular resistance, there is a decrease in the flow of blood to the lungs. The systolic and diastolic murmurs associated with rapid flow of blood through the right heart and pulmonary arteries then disappear. If pulmonary hypertension is severe, new murmurs of pulmonary and tricuspid regurgitation may occur. The murmur of hypertensive pulmonary regurgitation is typically high pitched and decrescendo, being maximal at the high and mid-left sternal border. This murmur is usually clinically indistinguishable from the murmur of aortic regurgitation unless the second heart sound is widely split, and it can be appreciated that the diastolic murmur begins with the second pulmonary component. The murmur of tricuspid regurgitation is high pitched and systolic; it is usually maximal at the low left sternal border. It may be either early or pansystolic, and it may increase in intensity with inspiration, a feature known as Carvallo's sign.[54]

INVESTIGATIONS

Electrocardiography

The electrocardiographic features of an interatrial communication are stereotyped in childhood (Fig. 25-21). Similar findings may be present, nonetheless, in normal children or in individuals with other conditions that cause right ventricular volume overload. Normal sinus rhythm is the rule in childhood, but atrial flutter or fibrillation is seen with increasing frequency after 40 years of age. First-degree atrioventricular block has been reported to occur in up to one-third of patients.[3,30] In contrast to this high reported prevalence, this finding was present in only 4% of the patients with defects within the oval fossa seen at the Children's Hospital of Pittsburgh. The morphology of the P wave is normal in such defects, but one review demonstrated that, in nearly half of sinus venosus defects, the frontal plane axis of the P wave was less than 15 degrees, suggesting a low atrial focus.[55] In Pittsburgh, however, a definite ectopic atrial rhythm was seen in only 7% of patients with sinus venosus defects. In children with deficient atrial septation, the frontal plane QRS axis is almost always in the range from 90 degrees to 170 degrees, but in the adult the axis may shift leftward to the range of 70 degrees to 90 degrees. Although left-axis deviation occurring in the setting of an atrial shunt strongly suggests the presence of an ostium primum defect, approximately one-twentieth of those with oval fossa and sinus venosus defects have this axis.[30,55] Mild-to-moderate right ventricular hypertrophy is present in more than five-sixths of patients, and is usually manifested by an RSR′ pattern in the right precordial leads. The R or R′ wave rarely exceeds 15 mm unless there is significant elevation of pulmonary vascular resistance and pulmonary arterial pressure.[18,33] The QRS duration is either normal or mildly prolonged, rarely exceeding 0.11 second. Complete right bundle branch block is very rare in childhood, but occurs in nearly half of patients older than 60 years of age.[37]

Radiology

The chest radiograph shows mild-to-moderate cardiomegaly in most patients, but up to one-sixth of patients have a heart of normal size, even in the presence of a large left-to-right shunt.[33,56] Irrespective of whether or not the heart is enlarged, there is almost always an abnormal contour, with a large right atrium, right ventricle, and pulmonary trunk and a diminutive aorta (Fig, 25-22). Pulmonary vascular markings are usually increased when the ratio of pulmonary to systemic flow is 2 to 1 or greater, but the vascularity correlates poorly with the magnitude of the shunt.[57] Once pulmonary vascular disease develops, the typical findings of Eisenmenger's syndrome may be present, with aneurysmal dilation of the proximal pulmonary arteries and distal tapering of the vessels. In patients with a sinus venosus defect, there may be localised dilation of the proximal superior caval vein at the entrance of the anomalous pulmonary veins, giving the appearance of a higher than normal vascular pedicle in the right hilum. In most patients with this type of defect, however,

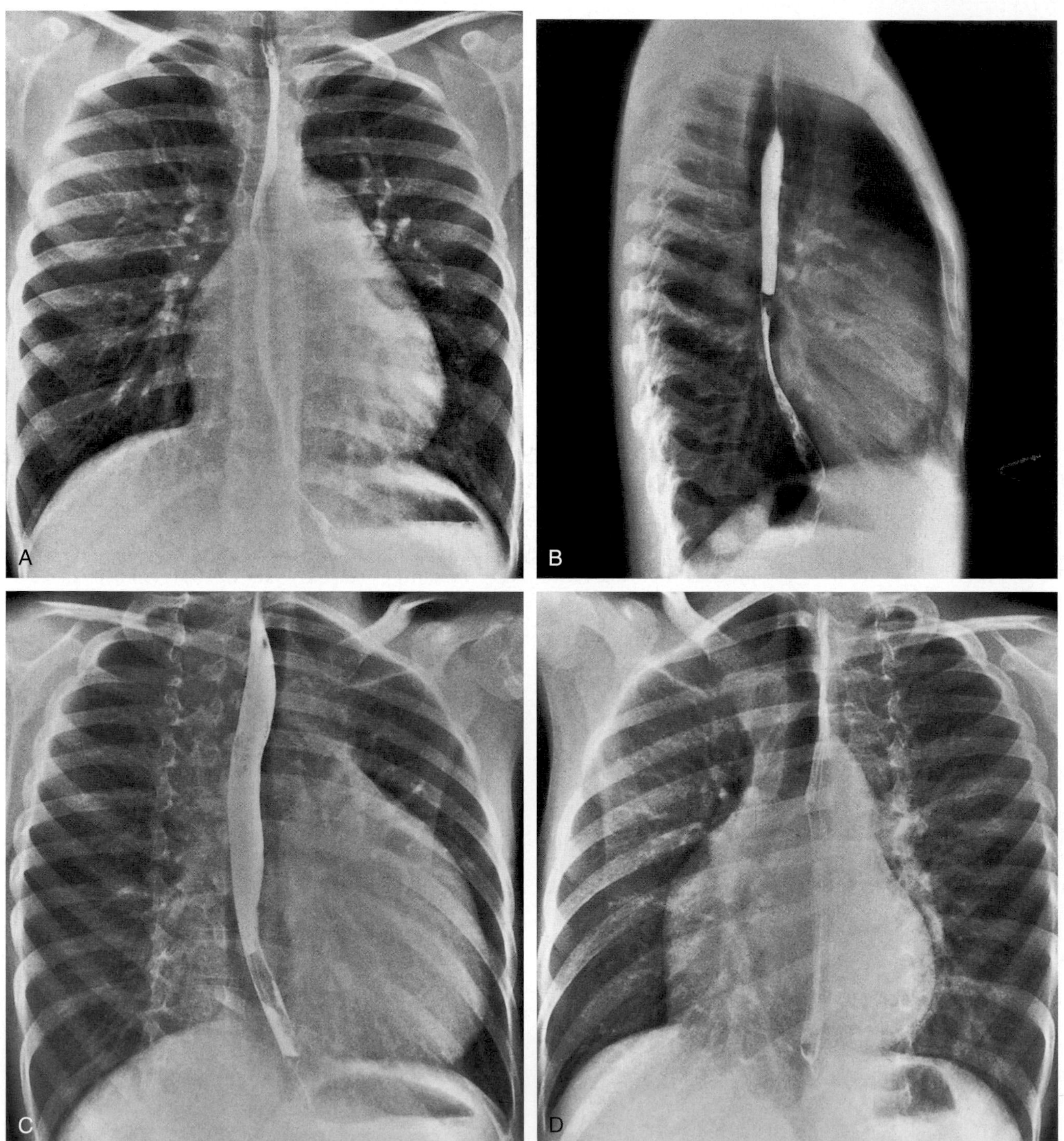

Figure 25-22 Chest radiographs and barium swallow in a patient with an atrial septal defect. **A,** Frontal view shows cardiomegaly and increased pulmonary vascular markings. The pulmonary trunk is large, and the aortic knob is not apparent. **B,** Lateral view shows that there is no oesophageal deviation to suggest left atrial enlargement. **C,** Right anterior oblique view confirms the absence of left atrial enlargement, but the cardiac shadow approaches the left thoracic wall, suggesting right ventricular enlargement. **D,** Left anterior oblique view.

the radiological findings are identical to those of a typical defect within the oval fossa.

Echocardiography

Echocardiography, particularly when combined with Doppler studies, has proved to be diagnostic in the majority of patients with interatrial communications. These techniques allow accurate assessment of the size and location of the defect, as well as the degree of right ventricular volume overload. Both the M-mode and cross sectional echocardiogram are useful in detecting the most significant haemodynamic effect of an important atrial shunt, namely right ventricular enlargement. The classic M-mode echocardiographic findings are nearly always present when there is a large left-to-right shunt. Right ventricular dimensions are increased, and there is frequently flattened or paradoxical septal motion (Fig. 25-23).[58–61] Of the parameters used to judge the degree of left-to-right shunting, the ratios between pulmonary and aortic trunks and between the right and left ventricles were the most reliable indicators of the size of the shunt.[62] A ventricular ratio greater than 0.46, and an arterial ratio greater than equity, were almost always found in patients with a ratio of pulmonary to systemic flows of greater than 1.5. The lack of increase in right ventricular size with respiration has also been shown to be useful in differentiating a haemodynamically important shunt from one that is small.[63] Other causes of right ventricular volume overload may result in similar echocardiographic findings, including partially or totally anomalous pulmonary venous connection, and pulmonary and tricuspid regurgitation.

Although M-mode echocardiography can itself be diagnostic, nowadays cross sectional echocardiography has become the diagnostic technique of choice. It provides excellent visualisation of the atrial septum in multiple planes, with the most useful being the subcostal view.[64,65] The apical four-chamber view may be unreliable in evaluation of the atrial septum, as artefactual echo dropout may simulate an atrial septal defect. The subcostal view allows imaging in a plane perpendicular to the atrial septum and can reliably define the site and approximate size of the defect. A defect of the oval fossa is seen in the central portion of the septum, while the sinus venosus and ostium primum defects are positioned superiorly and inferiorly relative to the oval fossa, respectively (Fig. 25-24). Pulmonary veins can usually be visualised and anomalous connections identified, for example in the sinus venosus defect.[66] The basic diagnostic feature of a superior sinus venosus defect, overriding of the superior caval vein and its biatrial connection, can be well demonstrated using echocardiography from the subcostal position (Fig. 25-25).[14,67] An inferior sinus venosus defect is very uncommon, accounting for less than one-fifth of all the sinus venosus defects undergoing operative repair at Pittsburgh. Although difficult, this diagnosis can also be made by echocardiography.[15] The features include a posterior and inferior location of the defect adjacent to the atrial connection of the inferior caval vein, and anomalous drainage of the right-sided pulmonary veins (Fig. 25-26). Although routine transthoracic studies are generally more than adequate for diagnosis in children, transoesophageal

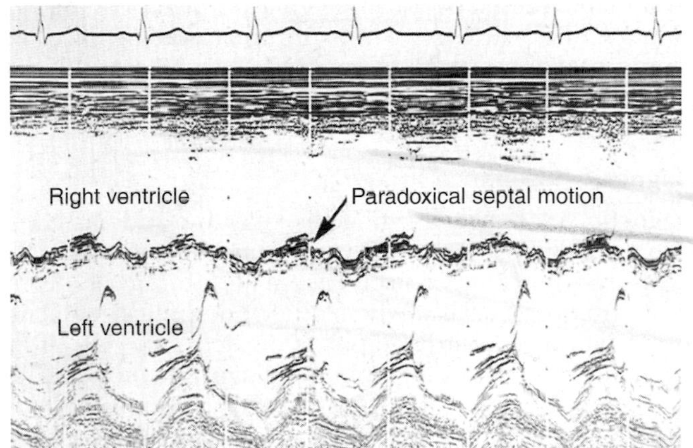

Figure 25-23 The M-mode echocardiographic tracing from a patient with a defect in the oval fossa reveals the signs of an enlarged right ventricle and paradoxical septal motion.

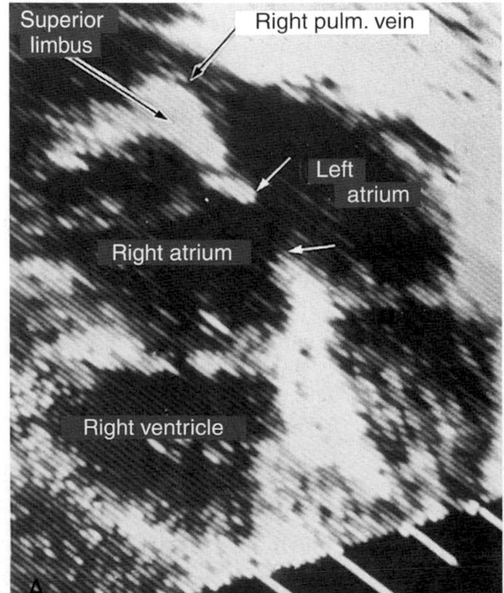

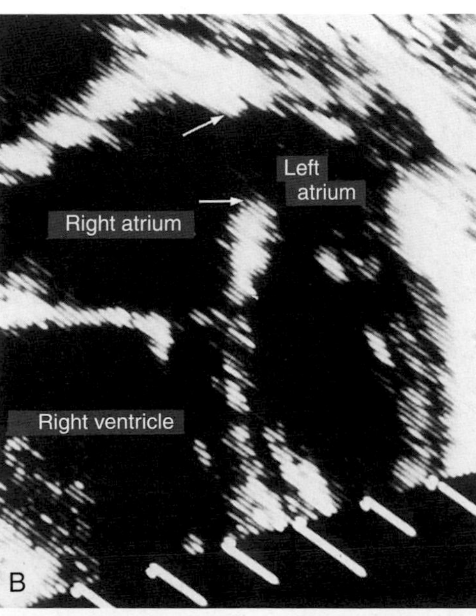

Figure 25-24 Cross sectional echocardiograms of atrial septal defects (between *arrows*) in the subcostal view. **A,** The typical location of a defect in the oval fossa. **B,** The sinus venosus defect is superior to the intact rim of the oval fossa. pulm., pulmonary.

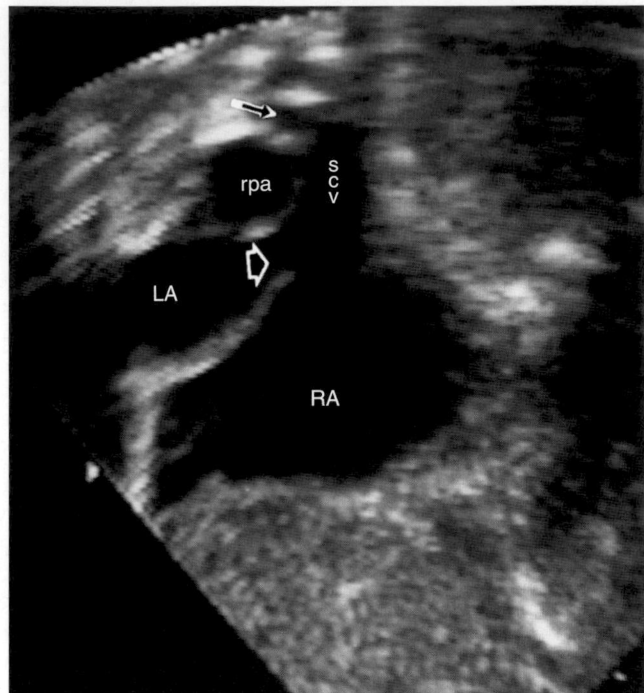

Figure 25-25 This cross sectional echocardiogram in the long-axis subcostal view shows the pathognomonic feature of a superior sinus venous defect (*open arrow*): overriding and biatrial connection of the superior caval vein (scv). Note the anomalous drainage of the right upper pulmonary vein (*small arrow*). LA, left atrium; RA, right atrium; rpa, right pulmonary artery.

echocardiography allows superb evaluation and visualisation of the atrial septum in patients with a poor standard echocardiographic window.[68,69] Contrast echocardiography may provide supplementary information,[24,70] but this is rarely necessary.

Doppler echocardiography, including pulsed wave studies and colour flow mapping, is an invaluable adjunct in the evaluation of interatrial communications (Fig. 25-27). Pulsed Doppler determination of the velocity of the transatrial shunt has been correlated with the ratio of flows of the pulmonary and systemic bloodstreams,[71] but there has been little enthusiasm for this technique in recent years. The degree of shunting can also be calculated using echocardiographic and Doppler measurements of flow across the right- and left-sided valves.[72–74]

Colour flow mapping is extremely useful in the evaluation of atrial shunts.[24] Flow across the defect can be clearly visualised, confirming that echo dropout is real rather than an artefact. The width of the flow gives some indication of the size of the defect, but we have found the reliability of colour flow in predicting size to be significantly limited by variability in gain settings and alignment of the scanning plane relative to the shunt. By combining direct echocardiographic imaging with Doppler studies, an interatrial communication can be well characterised.

An important aspect of interatrial communications has become apparent in recent years with the widespread use of echocardiographic and Doppler techniques. Small shunts in the region of the oval fossa can be demonstrated by Doppler interrogation in a high proportion of newborns and infants less than 3 months of age who have either no defect, or a very small one as judged by echocardiographic imaging.[75,76] These shunts (Fig. 25-28) are presumably caused by incompetence of the flap of the oval foramen and will close within the first year of life. They should probably not be interpreted as true defects within the oval fossa.

Magnetic Resonance Imaging

Magnetic resonance imaging, as may be anticipated, is able to demonstrate interatrial communications.[77] The technique may also be useful for determining the degree of shunting, especially when other anatomical data not discerned on echocardiography is needed.[78] In view of the excellence of echocardiography for diagnostic purposes, we have not found it necessary to use this technique. Should a device have been used to close an atrial septal defect, there may be concern as to safety should the patient be subjected to powerful magnetic fields. In a phantom study of various devices, all but one of the currently available devices were found to be safe in fields having strengths up to

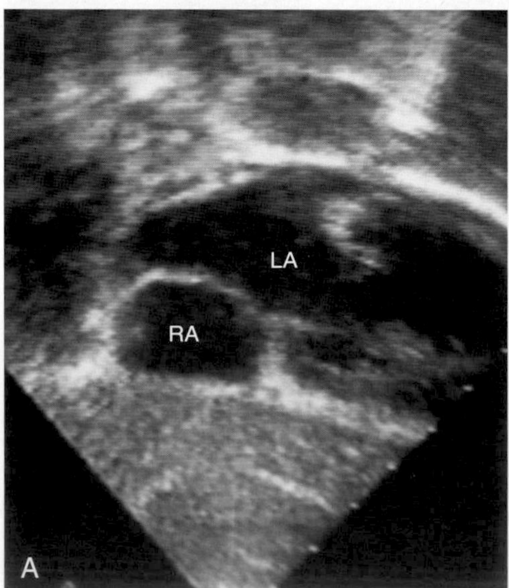

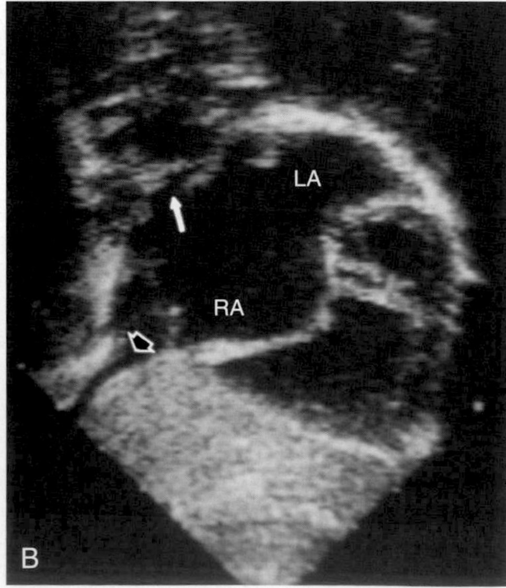

Figure 25-26 These cross sectional echocardiograms, in the subcostal view, demonstrate the features of an inferior sinus venosus defect. **A,** The oval fossa is intact when a plane is taken through the mid-portion of the septum. **B,** Scanning inferiorly reveals the large interatrial communication between the right atrium (RA) and left atrium (LA). The defect is adjacent to the mouth of the inferior caval vein (*open arrow*). The right lower pulmonary vein drains into the right atrium (*solid arrow*).

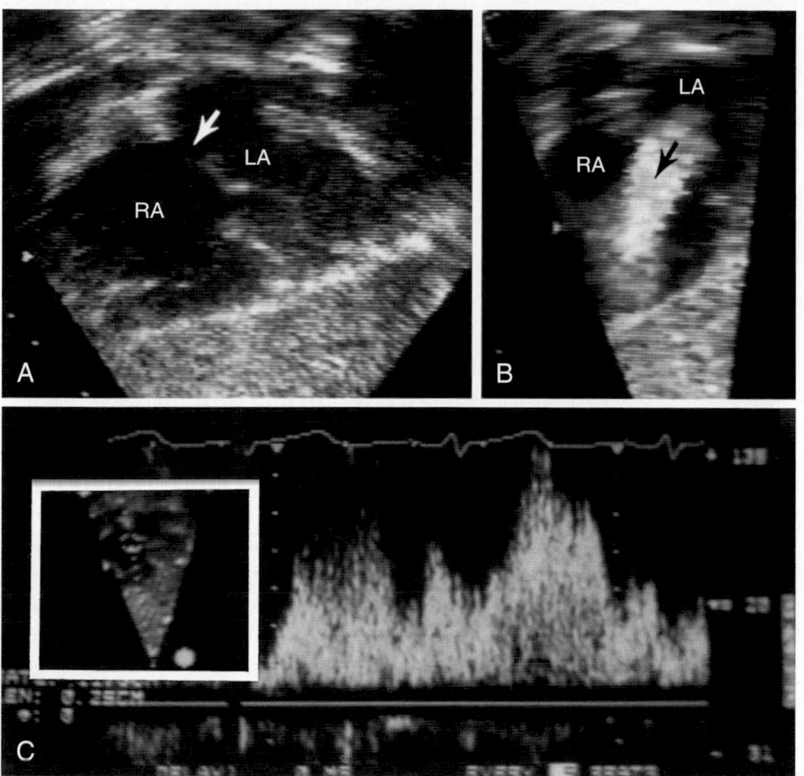

Figure 25-27 Doppler echocardiograms of an atrial septal defect in the oval fossa from subcostal view. **A,** The mid-septal location of the defect (*white arrow*) can be seen. **B,** The colour flow map demonstrates left-to-right atrial shunting (*black arrow*) across a broad front. **C,** Pulsed Doppler shows the pattern of continuous flow of an atrial shunt with late systolic and early diastolic accentuation. The insert illustrates the position of the sample volume in the right atrium (RA) adjacent to the defect. LA, left atrium.

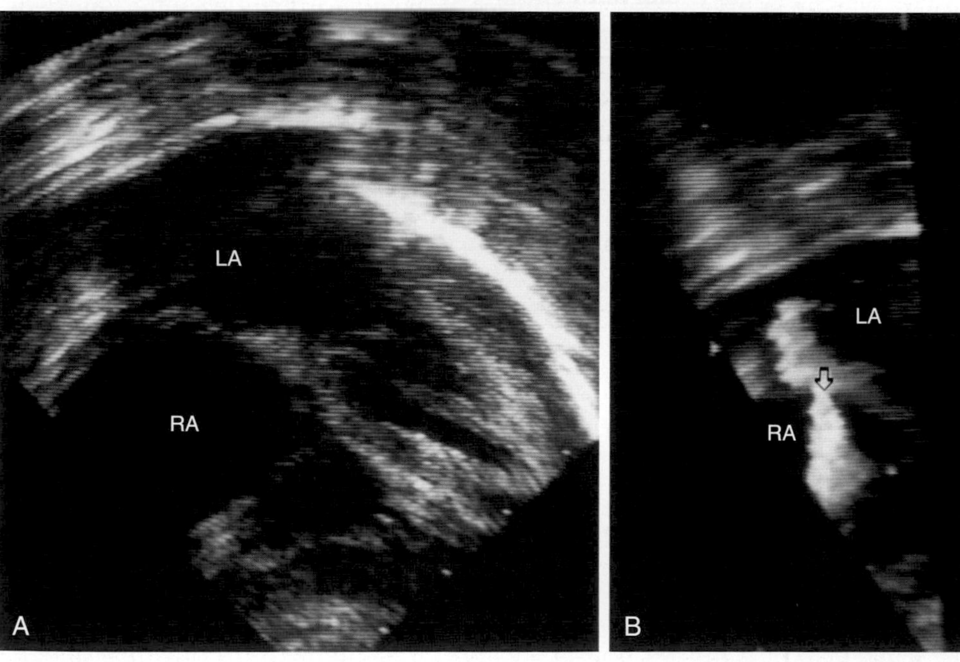

Figure 25-28 Cross sectional echocardiogram and colour flow map of a patient with a suspected defect in the oval fossa. **A,** On the initial scan, the atrial septum appears to be intact. **B,** Colour flow mapping, in contrast, demonstrates a small left-to-right jet (*arrow*) across a patent oval foramen. This is of no functional significance. LA, left atrium; RA, right atrium.

1.5 tesla, with no excessive heating noted, and minimal artifact induced in imaging.[79]

Cardiac Catheterisation

Echocardiography and Doppler studies have now largely supplanted invasive studies in patients with atrial septal defects. Cardiac catheterisation continues to be the most precise method of quantifying the left-to-right shunt, and measuring intracardiac and pulmonary arterial pressures. It is now also necessary to undertake catheterisation if interventional closure is to be attempted (see below). When the femoral venous approach is used, the catheter almost always passes easily through the mid-portion of the atrial septum into the left atrium when the defect is within the oval fossa. An attempt should be made to enter the pulmonary veins to confirm their normal connection to the left atrium.

An ostium primum defect may be recognised by a lower than usual atrial pass. It is usually easier to enter the left ventricle and more difficult to enter the pulmonary veins when this type of interatrial communication is present. A sinus venosus defect is sometimes difficult to traverse when the approach is through the inferior caval vein. Considerable probing in the region of the superior cavoatrial junction may be needed to reach the left atrium. The lateral border of the proximal superior caval vein and right atrium should be explored for possible anomalous return of the right upper or middle lobe pulmonary veins, particularly if a sinus venosus defect is suspected.

The hallmark of an atrial shunt is a step-up in saturations of oxygen of at least 5% when moving from the superior caval vein to the right atrium. If the saturation in the superior caval vein is abnormally high, greater than 85%, anomalous pulmonary venous return must be considered. Saturations should then be obtained from the left brachiocephalic, right subclavian and right internal jugular veins. Anomalies other than an atrial septal defect that result in an increased saturation of oxygen in the right atrium include isolated partially anomalous pulmonary venous return, a ventricular septal defect associated with tricuspid insufficiency, a shunt from left ventricle to right atrium, and an aneurysm of the aortic sinus of Valsalva ruptured into the right atrium. Another potential pitfall in the use of oximetry for diagnosis stems from the fact that streaming of oxygenated blood directly across the tricuspid valve can occur such that a step-up in oxygenation is not evident proximal to the right ventricle. This is much more likely to occur with an ostium primum defect. Even when there is an isolated atrial septal defect producing a step-up in oxygenation in the right atrium, there may be a further step-up in the right ventricle. Samples from the left side of the circulation are fully saturated. The ratio of pulmonary-to-systemic flow can be calculated using oximetry and the Fick principle. This ratio is 2:1 or greater in over two-thirds of patients having clinically recognised defects.[33]

Mean right atrial pressure is generally normal, but the magnitude of the V wave is usually equal to that of the A wave, with consequent loss of the normal dominance of the A wave. Phasic and mean pressures are commonly equal in the two atriums if there is a large atrial septal defect, but there may be up to a 3 torr mean gradient across the defect. Right ventricular and pulmonary arterial pressures are almost always normal in childhood, but pulmonary hypertension may develop with increasing age.[31] An occasional infant with a large atrial shunt has elevated pulmonary arterial pressure.[39] Pulmonary vascular resistance is usually normal or low, at 1 Wood unit or less, in children, but may be elevated in adults. Severe elevation of pulmonary vascular resistance with Eisenmenger's reaction is uncommon even in older patients, occurring in only about one-twentieth of individuals with an atrial septal defect.[34,35] In some patients, the large flow of blood to the lungs causes a peak systolic gradient of 10 to 30 torr across a normal pulmonary valve, and/or a systolic gradient of 10 to 15 torr between the pulmonary trunk and its branches.[18,19,30] Left atrial pressure is usually somewhat lower than normal, and left ventricular pressure is normal.

Indicator dilution studies may be useful in qualitatively and quantitatively evaluating a left-to-right shunt at the atrial level. The ratio of pulmonary to systemic flows calculated from such curves correlates well with that obtained by oximetry.[80] Selective pulmonary arterial injections of the indicator may suggest the presence of partially anomalous pulmonary venous connection by showing variable magnitudes of shunting, and/or times of appearance from various portions of the lungs. It must be emphasised that functional return to the right atrium does not imply anatomical connection to the right atrium, since there may be remarkable streaming from normally connected veins. Cardiac output may be determined by injecting indicator into the left ventricle and sampling from the aorta.

Angiocardiography

A left ventriculogram may be useful in patients with an atrial septal defect, particularly if a high-quality echocardiogram is not available. This is helpful in determining the presence of an atrioventricular septal defect, mitral valvar prolapse, mitral insufficiency, left ventricular dysfunction or a ventricular septal defect. We usually prefer the antero-posterior and lateral views if a ventricular septal defect is not suspected, as this best demonstrates the gooseneck deformity of the left ventricular outflow tract and the trifoliate left atrioventricular valve of an atrioventricular septal defect. A right ventricular or pulmonary arterial injection in the anteroposterior and lateral views defines pulmonary arterial anatomy and pulmonary venous return and allows assessment of the magnitude of the atrial shunt during the laevophase. A right ventriculogram has the advantage of demonstrating right ventricular size as well as tricuspid valvar competency and pulmonary valvar anatomy. The pulmonary arteriogram has the advantage of avoiding arrhythmia at the time of the injection; it sometimes allows better definition of the pulmonary venous return. We have found that injection into the right upper pulmonary vein filmed in the four-chamber view[81] is particularly helpful in confirming normal drainage of this vein, and may delineate the location and size of the atrial defect (Fig. 25-29). Any anomalously connecting pulmonary veins that are entered by the catheter should be selectively visualised.

DIAGNOSIS

The diagnosis of an interatrial communication can be made with virtual certainty when the classical findings of an ejection murmur at the high left sternal border, wide and fixed splitting of the second heart sound, and a medium-pitched mid-diastolic murmur at the low left sternal border are associated with typical radiographical and electrocardiographical findings. A sinus venosus defect with partially anomalous pulmonary venous return cannot usually be differentiated clinically from a defect within the oval fossa, but a low atrial rhythm, and/or an unusual shadow in the upper right hilum or the proximal superior caval vein on the chest radiograph, should lead one to suspect its presence. Left-axis deviation on the electrocardiogram, with or without a murmur at the apex suggesting insufficiency of the left atrioventricular valve, makes the diagnosis of an ostium primum defect very likely. Echocardiographic and Doppler studies are used to confirm the presence of an important left-to-right shunt with right ventricular volume overload and to characterise the size and location of the atrial defect. Several reports have shown that uncomplicated defects within the oval fossa, and sinus venosus defects, can safely be closed surgically with confirmatory non-invasive studies without routine preoperative

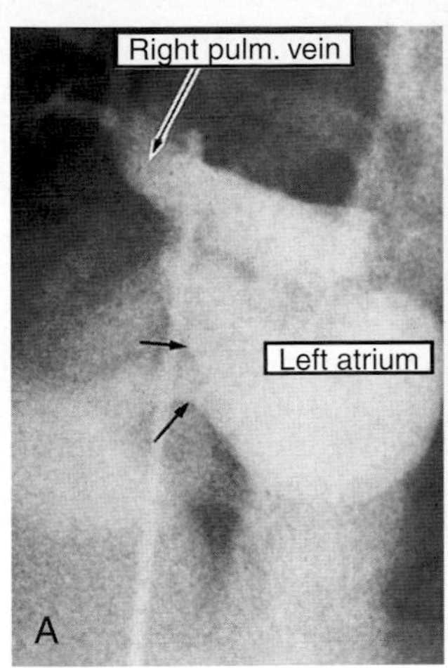

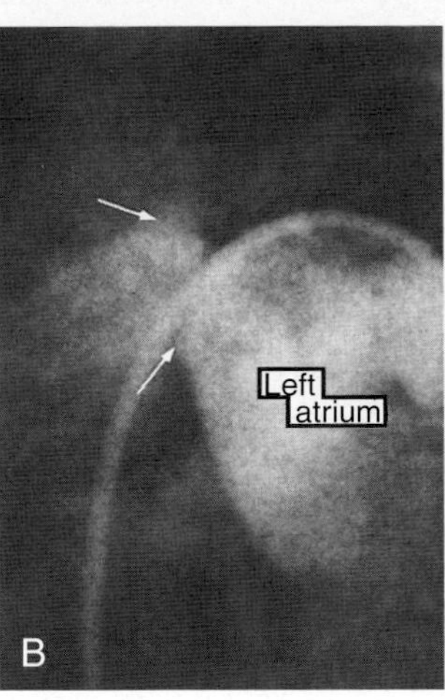

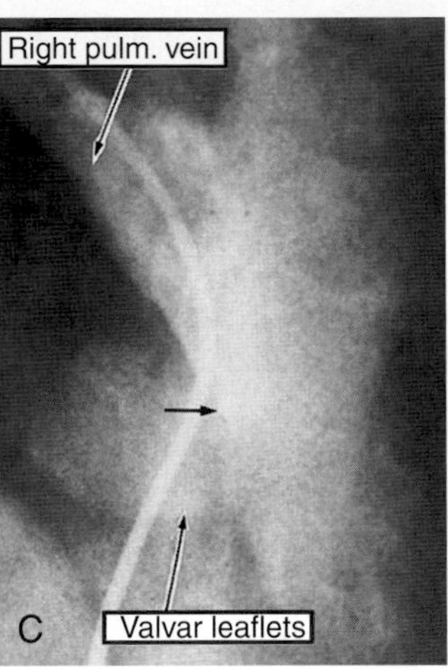

Figure 25-29 Pulmonary venous angiograms in patients with atrial septal defects. **A,** Right upper pulmonary venous angiogram in the four-chamber view reveals shunting across a defect in the oval fossa (*between black arrows*). **B,** Left upper pulmonary venous angiogram profiled in the left anterior oblique view reveals a sinus venosus defect (*between white arrows*), with shunting across the superior rim of the intact oval fossa. **C,** Right upper pulmonary venous angiogram in the four-chamber view shows shunting across an ostium primum defect (*between black arrows*). There is a common atrioventricular junction that is partitioned into separate left and right atrioventricular valvar orifices.

catheterisation.[82,83] Although partially anomalous pulmonary venous connection may be undetected, or sinus venosus defects occasionally misclassified, this has not resulted in increased morbidity during operative repair. Currently, at our institution, cardiac catheterisation is performed only on patients in whom we insert a device to close the defect, and in those patients in whom the anatomy has not been completely defined by echocardiography.

Several common conditions must be considered in the differential diagnosis of a soft systolic ejection murmur at the upper left sternal border, including a functional murmur, mild valvar pulmonary stenosis and pulmonary arterial stenosis. Mild valvar pulmonary stenosis is virtually always accompanied by an early systolic ejection sound, and the murmur becomes strikingly louder with exercise. Pulmonary arterial stenosis has very prominent radiation of the systolic murmur to the back. These latter two anomalies have normal splitting of the second heart sound, lack a diastolic murmur at the low left sternal border and usually do not have evidence of right ventricular overload on the echocardiogram. A functional murmur is distinguished by an otherwise normal cardiovascular examination. Certain other abnormalities must be considered when a systolic ejection murmur at the upper left sternal border is associated with a medium-pitched diastolic murmur at the low-left sternal border. Ebstein's malformation usually has other auscultatory abnormalities, including a widely split first sound and/or a gallop. It can be definitively diagnosed by echocardiography. Congenital pulmonary stenosis and regurgitation may prove difficult to distinguish from an atrial septal defect on clinical grounds, but the diastolic murmur is best heard higher along the left sternal border and becomes louder in the recumbent position. Congenital tricuspid stenosis produces a diastolic murmur similar to that present with a large atrial defect. This anomaly is quite rare and should be apparent on the echocardiogram. A shunt from left ventricle to right atrium is another unusual entity that may be considered in the differential diagnosis, but the systolic murmur in this condition is loud and pansystolic and quite different from the systolic ejection murmur associated with an atrial defect. Partially anomalous pulmonary venous return without an associated atrial septal defect is a rare anomaly and usually requires cardiac catheterisation for diagnosis. Totally anomalous pulmonary venous return without obstruction may at times present similar findings to a large atrial septal defect. The anomalous venous connections should be evident on the cross sectional echocardiogram, and the presence of a higher than expected haemoglobin for the age of the patient may suggest mild systemic desaturation. A common atrium may be associated with an atrioventricular septal defect and will be apparent on the echocardiogram. Occasionally, a functional mid-diastolic murmur at the left sternal border is not associated with any structural heart disease.[84] Another entity that may be confused is the straight back syndrome, with its systolic ejection murmur at the upper left sternal border and prominent pulmonary trunk on the chest radiograph. The lack of the normal thoracic kyphosis on the lateral chest radiograph is diagnostic.

COURSE AND PROGNOSIS

An isolated interatrial communication, even a large one, is usually well tolerated for many years.[32] As has been noted, symptoms are usually minimal or absent during infancy and childhood. This is because the right ventricle is well adapted to pure volume overload,[85] and secondary pulmonary hypertension is usually a late complication. In the usual patient with an interatrial communication, the appearance of a large left-to-right shunt is delayed until the right ventricular hypertrophy present at birth regresses and right ventricular compliance increases. The pulmonary vascular bed, therefore, has time to mature, and can accept a large blood flow without an increase in pressure. In the absence of pulmonary hypertension, pulmonary vascular disease either fails to develop or follows an indolent course.

Symptoms tend to occur earlier and to be more severe when there is an associated anomaly, particularly one that tends to impede left atrial emptying through the mitral valve. Examples include obstruction of the left ventricular outflow tract, coarctation of the aorta, primary left ventricular myocardial disease, and mitral stenosis. In this respect, Lutembacher's syndrome refers to the combination of an atrial septal defect and mitral stenosis. It now seems to be quite uncommon, probably because of a decreasing incidence of rheumatic heart disease, and because of early closure of atrial septal defects. Non-obstructive associated anomalies may also lead to early congestive heart failure. Infants with both interatrial and interventricular communications, or a patent arterial duct, are likely to be symptomatic because atrial shunting across even a small defect may be greatly augmented by the increased left atrial pressure caused by the associated lesion.

If impedance to left atrial emptying is markedly increased, and is present before the pulmonary vascular bed has had an opportunity to mature, the fetal pulmonary vascular pattern tends to persist, exaggerating the degree of pulmonary hypertension. Under these circumstances, signs of severe and rapidly progressive congestive heart failure may occur. An example is the infant who has both a severe aortic coarctation and an interatrial communication. The left ventricular dysfunction engendered by the coarctation raises left atrial pressure. This may produce a torrential left-to-right interatrial shunt along with severe congestive heart failure, which can be effectively treated only by correcting the coarctation.

Occasionally, infants with isolated and uncomplicated atrial septal defects may be symptomatic and experience congestive heart failure.[38–40] It is not clear how these infants differ from asymptomatic ones, although it has been postulated that an atrial septal defect is usually small in infancy and grows large enough to produce symptoms only later in life. According to this formulation, the occasional infant with a large defect is the one who has symptoms early. It is much more likely, however, that a left-to-right shunt large enough to produce symptoms during infancy results from some unrecognised increased impedance to flow into the left ventricle, such as a subtle alteration in left ventricular compliance or an abnormality of the mitral valvar apparatus.[7] Perhaps the situation is analogous to the older individual with an atrial septal defect that has been well tolerated for several decades. Such a patient develops a larger left-to-right shunt and becomes symptomatic following the appearance of left ventricular dysfunction, whether it is induced by systemic hypertension, coronary arterial disease or some primary myocardial abnormality.

Secondary pulmonary hypertension does eventually appear in some patients with an atrial septal defect. This is an important factor in the development of both the cyanosis and congestive heart failure that can complicate the course of the anomaly. The addition of a pressure load may compromise right ventricular function and lead to congestive heart failure, or to right-to-left shunting through the atrial defect even in the absence of overt failure. Cyanosis that appears only with congestive heart failure tends to disappear after treatment with diuretics or cardiotonic agents, while cyanosis occurring in the absence of failure tends to be permanent and is an important sign of irreversible pulmonary vascular disease. Pulmonary vascular obstructive disease, defined as a pulmonary vascular resistance greater than 7 index units, was found in one-twentieth of patients in one large series.[35] This finding was much more prevalent in females. Although a trivial degree of right-to-left shunting occurs in many individuals with an interatrial communication,[21] sufficient shunting to produce recognisable cyanosis is distinctly unusual in an uncomplicated atrial defect. If the atrial septum is rudimentary, or entirely absent, some right-to-left shunting is usual and there may be mild cyanosis. Anomalies of systemic venous return are not common but may be responsible for cyanosis in an occasional patient with atrial septal defect. Drainage of a persistent left superior caval vein to the left atrium can be part of a developmental complex associated with an interatrial communication at the orifice of the coronary sinus.[86] Inferior caval venous drainage may be anatomically or functionally anomalous, with flow to the left atrium or to both atriums. This most commonly occurs with an inferior type of sinus venosus defect since the inferior caval vein overrides the interatrial septum. It has also been reported with defects in the oval fossa associated with overriding of the inferior caval vein.[14]

Although spontaneous closure of an atrial septal defect is less common than spontaneous closure of a defect in the interventricular septum, numerous authors have reported such closure, with an incidence varying from 3% to 67%.[38,75,87–89] This marked variability in estimated rates of closure results from several factors. The incidence is higher when the atrial defect is detected in the first year of life, as illustrated by the closure rate of more than half in one series.[87] Another important factor is that ascertainment of atrial shunts has been dramatically increased in recent years by the remarkable sensitivity of Doppler and cross sectional echocardiography.[75] Undoubtedly, many of these atrial shunts detected in early infancy result from transient incompetence of the flap of the oval fossa and are not defects within the fossa. The former should be considered a normal variant, and can be identified when the atrial septum is virtually intact echocardiographically but there is a small atrial shunt on colour flow mapping (see Fig. 25-28).

In a review at the Children's Hospital of Pittsburgh, the overall rate of spontaneous closure was only 3%.[90] The natural history may have been affected in some patients by surgical intervention before the age of 4 years. Surprisingly, factors such as age at presentation, symptoms, magnitude of shunt, size of the defect, or degree of right ventricular volume overload did not predict which patients would undergo spontaneous closure or decrease in size of their defects. The mechanism of closure is uncertain, but has been ascribed to an atrial septal tissue flap[89] or, in some cases, to aneurysm of the oval fossa.[90,91]

Atrial arrhythmias are relatively uncommon in children with atrial septal defects, but they tend to become more common with advancing age.[32,37,41,42,92,93] Atrial flutter or fibrillation occurs frequently in older individuals, with a large left-to-right shunt and an enlarged right atrium being found in two-thirds of patients in one series.[41]

Rarely, paradoxical embolism may occur, with a clot from a pelvic or leg vein crossing the defect and entering the systemic circulation. As has been discussed above, a small right-to-left shunt is not uncommon in patients with an atrial septal defect. This may be augmented during a Valsalva manoeuvre or similar activities such as straining at stool. Other studies have shown that patency of the oval foramen, even without an atrial shunt, may be a risk factor for strokes in young adults.[94,95] Infectious endocarditis is a very rare complication of an atrial septal defect unless there is a predisposing associated anomaly.[8]

Studies of natural history in patients with atrial septal defects who have not undergone surgical correction suggest an average life expectancy between 36 and 49 years, with three-quarters of patients dying before age 50 years, and nine-tenths by 60 years.[32,41,96,97] Longevity, however, was much greater in the absence of pulmonary hypertension.[98] Although symptoms are very uncommon in the first several decades of life, dyspnoea and fatigue with exertion become more prevalent in adulthood and are experienced by the majority of patients over 50 years of age.[99] Approximately two-thirds of patients older than 40 years of age will have one or more of the complications discussed above, such as congestive heart failure, pulmonary hypertension, atrial arrhythmias or paradoxical embolisation.[3] Because the data from these studies were largely gathered in an era when associated rheumatic mitral valvar disease was more common, they probably do not accurately reflect the current life expectancy of an individual with an isolated atrial septal defect. A more benign natural history can now be predicted for asymptomatic or minimally symptomatic patients who present after 25 years of age,[100] with findings in this study equivalent to the results from a similar group of patients who underwent surgical repair.

MANAGEMENT

As has been noted, symptoms rarely occur in children with interatrial communications. An attempt at medical management with digitalis and diuretics is worthwhile in the occasional infant who presents with congestive heart failure, since several studies have shown that many of these children will have spontaneous closure of the defect or, at least, will have abatement of their symptoms.[38,39,40,87,101] Closure is clearly indicated in all children with ratios of left-to-right shunting of greater than 2 to 1 to prevent eventual pulmonary hypertension, congestive heart failure, and atrial arrhythmias. When the defect is small, and the ratio of flow is estimated to be less than 1.5 to 1, closure is probably not indicated, since late sequels are rare, and life expectancy is probably normal. The ease of closure using a device, nonetheless, combined with the increasingly recognised association between cryptogenic stroke and small atrial communications, has resulted in many interventionalists adopting a more aggressive approach in recommending closure of small defects. With borderline shunts having ratios of flow between 1.5 to 1 and 2 to 1, various features, including presence of a murmur of tricuspid flow, right ventricular enlargement, the size of the defect on the echocardiogram, and radiographic findings, should be considered when evaluating the need for closure. Our current approach is to recommend closure if there is definite evidence of right ventricular enlargement, or if there are signs of respiratory compromise, particularly in infants with a history of chronic respiratory disease. There are no data to suggest that there is any risk to the patient in delaying closure for several years in the hope that the magnitude of the shunt may decrease. The only contraindication to closure is pulmonary vascular disease, evidenced by marked elevation of pulmonary vascular resistance. When closure was achieved only by surgery, high operative mortality and decreased life expectancy were reported for patients who underwent repair in the face of pulmonary vascular disease.[98] On a more optimistic note for this group of patients, a review more reflective of the modern surgical era demonstrated a low perioperative mortality rate and improved prognosis in surgically versus medically treated patients with total pulmonary vascular resistance between 7 and 15 index units.[35]

The timing of elective closure does not seem to be crucial. As spontaneous closure becomes increasingly uncommon after 2 years of age, we recommend correction any time after this age. There is probably a psychological advantage in accomplishing repair prior to the school years. In addition, if open surgical repair is required, performing this at an older age may be done successfully without exposing the child to blood products. Earlier intervention is indicated if there is marked cardiomegaly, failure of growth, or congestive heart failure. Although significant impairment of growth is only rarely seen in childhood, a post-reparative growth spurt can be expected.[102]

Until relatively recently, there was no choice in terms of the technique for closure. Open heart repair of interatrial communications has been carried out with excellent success for many years, and the operative mortality is now expected to be zero in centres experienced in surgical correction of congenital cardiac malformations. The surgical approach to defects within the oval fossa consists of either direct suture or patch closure, depending on the size of the opening. When a sinus venosus defect is present, a patch is always necessary. It can usually be placed so as to close the interatrial communication and, at the same time, redirect anomalously draining pulmonary veins into the left atrium. Perioperative complications are rare. They include the postpericardiotomy syndrome and transient arrhythmias. Air embolisation is an uncommon but tragic complication. It is more likely when a right lateral thoracotomy is used, since this approach makes evacuation of air more difficult. Obstruction at the superior caval vein may rarely occur following repair of a superior sinus venosus defect, while a misplaced patch during the repair of an inferior defect may result in cyanosis due to shunting from the inferior caval vein to the left atrium.

The long-term results of surgery are excellent, and residual shunts are very rare. Resolution of cardiomegaly as seen on the chest radiograph, and of right ventricular hypertrophy seen on the electrocardiogram, are expected. Radiographic evidence of cardiac enlargement can persist in some patients,[56] as can right ventricular enlargement as revealed by echocardiography.[103] Actuarial survival calculated over 27 years for patients undergoing surgery at less than 24 years of age was identical to controls.[41] In contrast, a review of more than 100 patients who underwent surgery at less than 14 years of age, and were followed for an average of 14.5 years, revealed right ventricular dilation in one-quarter.[104] Numerous studies have also shown surgical intervention in adults, even those older than 60 years, to be safe and effective.[41,100,105–107]

Arrhythmias, including sinus nodal dysfunction, supraventricular tachycardia, and atrioventricular disturbances of conduction, do occasionally occur after repair of atrial septal defects.[43,56,108] Implantation of pacemakers may be required in a small number of patients.[104,108] The incidence of tachyarrhythmias, particularly atrial flutter or fibrillation, increases with age at operation.[93,109] Patients with sinus venosus defects appear to be more at risk for bradyarrhythmias than those with defects within the oval fossa.[110] We found that one-third of patients at the Children's Hospital of Pittsburgh with sinus venosus defects had persistent sinus nodal dysfunction after surgery. In contrast, less than one-sixth with defects in the oval fossa had post-operative sinus nodal dysfunction, and a pacemaker was required in only one patient. Although it has been presumed that these post-operative arrhythmias result from intra-operative damage to nodal or conduction tissue, numerous intracardiac

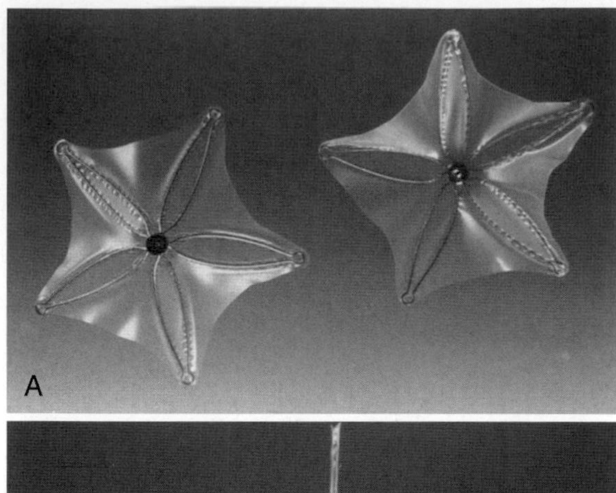

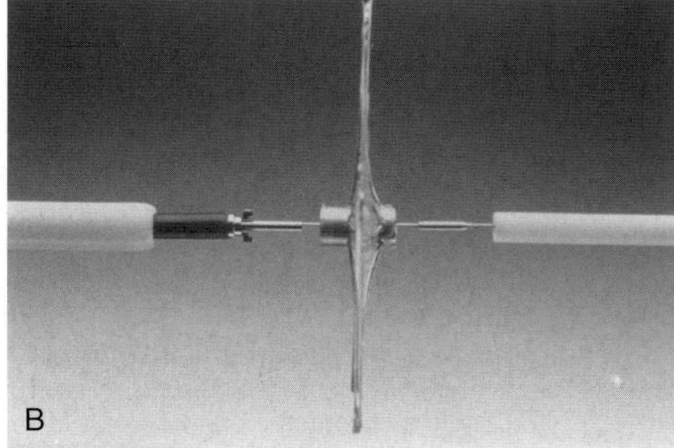

Figure 25-30 An ASDOS device, demonstrating the principle of devices that close interatrial communications by placing umbrellas to either side of the rims of the oval fossa. **A**, The umbrellas separated. **B**, The umbrellas in profile once they are connected. (Reproduced by permission of the late Professor Gerd Hausdorf and the publishers of Cardiology in the Young.)

electrophysiological studies show a high pre-operative incidence of sinus nodal and, to a lesser extent, atrioventricular nodal, dysfunction in patients with atrial septal defects in the oval fossa.[43,44,45,46] Because bacterial endocarditis is so rare with isolated secondary atrial septal defects, antibiotic prophylaxis is no longer recommended.[8,111]

As an alternative to surgical correction, patients with atrial septal defects within the oval fossa are now increasingly submitted to closure by means of interventional catheterisation. The technique was initially used some time ago,[112,113] but the devices employed were cumbersome. More recently, the double umbrella device known as the Clamshell occluder, developed by Lock and his colleagues,[114] was used successfully to close atrial defects in more than 200 patients.[115–118] Effective closure was achieved in more than nine-tenths, but clinical trials with this initial device had to be suspended because of a high incidence of fracture of its arms. At least five new devices have now been the subject of clinical trials.[119] These are CardioSEAL, the modification of the initial Clamshell device; various generations of the Sideris buttoned device[120–122]; the ASDOS occluder[123,124]; the self-centring AngelWings device[125,126]; and the nitinol Amplatzer septal occluder.[127] The first four of these devices are designed to close the defect by means of a membrane placed on one or both sides of the rims of the oval fossa (Fig. 25-30). All of these devices have arms that stabilise the membrane against the atrial wall. The Amplatzer device, in contrast, is a dumbbell-shaped nitinol plug that stents the defect, sitting like a peg within it (Fig. 25-31). As Bjornstad comments, it is unlikely that all five of these devices will survive.[119] It is also possible that the optimal device has not yet been made, though the Amplatzer septal occluder has gained wide popularity, primarily because of its ease of deployment and recapture.

Figure 25-31 The stages of deployment of the nitinol Amplatzer plug. Stage D is the first point at which centring is possible. (Reproduced by permission of Drs J. L. Wilkinson and T. H Goh, and the publishers of Cardiology in the Young.)

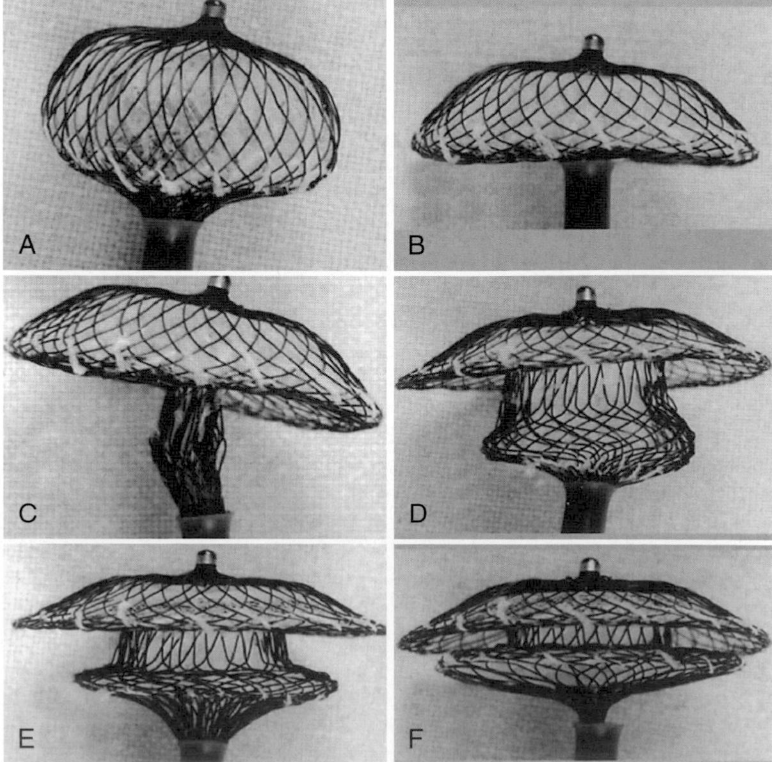

This procedure has evolved somewhat over time. Bjornstad has highlighted some of the caveats concerning the insertion of these devices, and the choices of interventional closure as opposed to surgery.[119] Not all defects within the oval fossa are suitable for closure,[128,129] so careful selection of patients is mandatory.[130,131] As discussed above, surgical closure has a low rate of complications, leaves very little residual shunting, and can now be achieved with virtually no mortality. Note has also to be taken of the more recent trend to undertake less-invasive surgical procedures, which limit the surgical incision without compromising exposure.[132–134] Interventions to close atrial septal defects produce results comparable to those obtained with these most recent surgical innovations.[135] The procedure of closure using the Amplatzer device is relatively simple and effective (Fig. 25-32), with complete closure achieved in over nine-tenths of one series as based on initial echocardiographic follow-up.[127] Closure with a device can be complicated by endocarditis. Since these initial reports, interventional closure of defects within the oval fossa has become the treatment of choice. Closure of atrial septal defects within the oval fossa, therefore, will increasingly become the province of interventionists, just as they have monopolised the therapy for valvar pulmonary stenosis and patency of the arterial duct.[119]

While the technical aspects of closure of defects within the oval fossa using a device inserted through a catheter are beyond the scope of this chapter, several key issues must be noted. Anticoagulation during the procedure and afterward is particularly critical to avoid formation of thrombus on the device, which could lead to pulmonary or systemic vascular embolism. A combination of aspirin and clopidogrel has been demonstrated to be effective in preventing such formation.[136] A second issue arises with defects which are difficult to close. On occasion, the Amplatzer device will assume a position perpendicular to the plane of the atrial septum, with the left atrial disc prolapsed into the right atrium. This can occur with large defects, with defects possessing small rims of tissue for anchoring of the device, or in younger patients with relatively smaller hearts. Various techniques have evolved to assist in closure of such defects, including use of a balloon to support the left atrial disc during deployment,[137] use of the right or left upper pulmonary vein for positioning of the delivery sheath,[138] use of a modified straight delivery sheath to facilitate angled delivery of the left atrial disc,[139] and use of a Hausdorf sheath or a Judkins right coronary guiding catheter.[140] We have found that closure of large defects, while technically more challenging, is readily accomplished, and should always be considered unless there is an absence of rims surrounding the defect, particularly along the floor or anteriorly. Additionally, our experience with closure of defects in children under 1 year of age, always undertaken due to co-existent respiratory compromise, has been favourable. In addition to the absolute size of the defect, the rims of the defect play an important role in determining the suitability for closure. Typically, the adequacy of the rims is easily assessed by transthoracic echocardiography prior to undertaking catheterisation, though a deficiency of the inferior rim may escape detection until a transoesophageal study can be performed.

An important complication, which can occur both early and late after closure, is erosion of the device along its edges into adjacent structures. Typically, such erosions occur into the aortic root, though damage to the primary septum has also been reported.[141] Erosions into the aortic root are considered due in part to oversizing of the device, and may also be more common in patients with deficiency of the superior or aortic root rims of the defect. Recommendations on how best to avoid this potentially lethal complication include avoidance of overstretching the defect during balloon-sizing, which can lead to selecting a larger device than is necessary. In general, the device implanted should not be greater than 50% larger than the unstretched diameter of the defect. Additionally, patients with deficient superior or aortic rims should be followed closely, especially if any pericardial effusion develops within 24 hours of device implantation.[142]

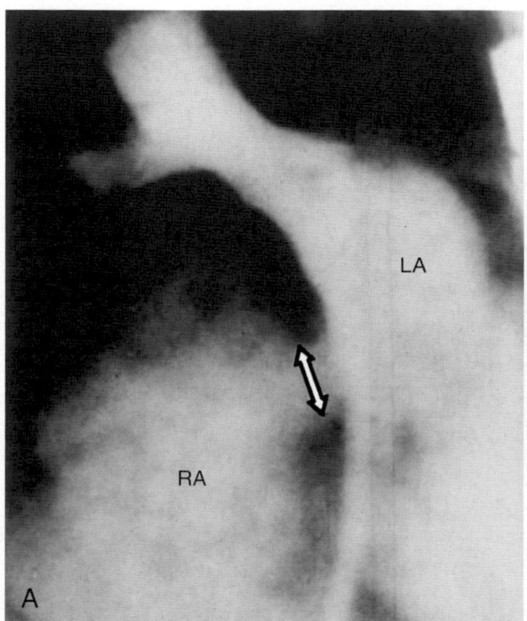

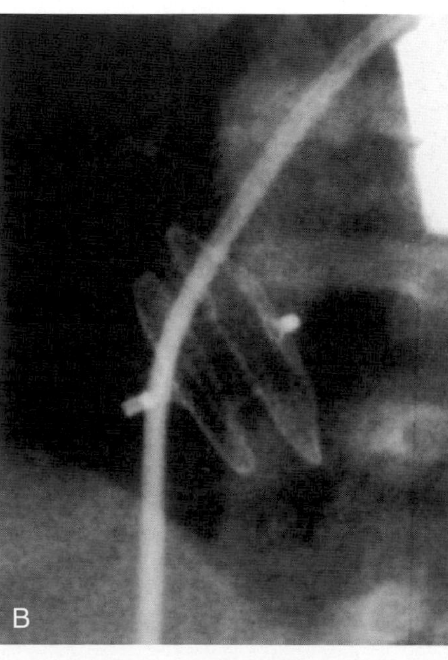

Figure 25-32 A, An atrial septal defect (*double arrow*) within the oval fossa. B, The hole has been closed by insertion of a nitinol Amplatzer plug. LA, left atrium; RA, right atrium. (Reproduced by permission of Drs J. L. Wilkinson and T. H. Goh, and the publishers of Cardiology in the Young.)

The complete reference list can be found on the companion Expert Consult web site at www.expertconsult.com.

ANNOTATED REFERENCES

- Feldt RH, Avasthey P, Yoshimasu F, et al: Incidence of congenital heart disease in children born to residents of Olmsted County, Minnesota, 1950–1969. Mayo Clin Proc 1971;46:794–799.

  The authors reported on the incidence of various forms of congenitally malformed hearts seen over a period of 20 years amongst the residents of a single county in Minnesota.

- Ettedgui JA, Siewers RD, Zuberbuhler JR, Anderson RH: Echocardiographic diagnosis of inferior sinus venosus defects. Cardiol Young 1992;2:338–341.

  The investigators described the anatomy of the inferior sinus venosus defect, emphasising the necessity for the lesion to be located outside the confines of the true atrial septum, and establishing the diagnostic findings as seen on cross sectional echocardiography.

- Knauth A, McCarthy KP, Webb S, et al: Interatrial communication through the mouth of the coronary sinus. Cardiol Young 2002;12:364–372.

  In this study, an anatomical description was provided of the defects resulting from total or partial absence of the walls normally present between the coronary sinus and the left atrium, permitting interatrial shunting through the mouth of the coronary sinus.

- Campbell M: Natural history of atrial septal defect. Br Heart J 1970;32:820–826.

  This important study permitted calculations of life expectancies for patients with unoperated defects.

- Murphy JG, Gersh BJ, McGoon MD, et al: Long-term outcome after surgical repair of isolated atrial septal defect: Follow up at 27 to 32 years. N Engl J Med 1990;323:1645–1650.

  An important long-term follow-up study of 123 patients who underwent surgical repair of an atrial septal defect. The authors emphasised that the best outcomes were achieved when surgery was perfomed before the patient reached the age of 25 years.

- Aygen MM, Braunwald E: The splitting of the second heart sound in normal subjects and in patients with congenital heart disease. Circulation 1962;25:328–345.

  The authors described the phonocardiographic findings in 350 children, including 118 with atrial septal defects. They emphasised the significance of the second heart sound.

- Ettedgui JA, Siewers RD, Anderson RH, et al: Diagnostic echocardiographic features of the sinus venosus defect. Br Heart J 1990;64:329–331.

  In this study, the authors described the anatomy of the superior sinus venosus defect, again establishing the diagnostic findings on cross sectional echocardiography. In all the patients seen, the orifice of the superior caval vein was overriding the true atrial septum.

- Freed MD, Nadas AS, Norwood WI, Castaneda AR: Is routine preoperative cardiac catheterization necessary before repair of secundum and sinus venosus atrial septal defects? J Am Coll Cardiol 1984;4:333–336.

  This study was one of the first to highlight the importance of accurate preoperative assessment using non-invasive techniques in children undergoing repair of atrial septal defects, negating the need for cardiac catheterisation.

- Ferreira SMAG, Ho SY, Anderson RH: Morphological study of defects of the atrial septum within the oval fossa: Implications for transcatheter closure of left-to-right shunt. Br Heart J 1992;67:316–320.

  The authors reviewed the anatomical details of 100 specimens, concentrating on variations in the structure of the oval fossa in the setting of deficient atrial septation, and establishing the factors which might make such defects suitable or unsuitable for closure by umbrella or clamshell devices.

- Amin Z, Hijazi ZM, Bass JL, et al: Erosion of Amplatzer septal occluder device after closure of secundum atrial septal defects: Review of registry of complications and recommendations to minimize future risk. Catheter Cardiovasc Interv 2004;63:496–502.

  The authors reviewed the cases referred to a registry, identifying the potential risk factors for erosion into the aortic root of devices inserted percutaneously so as to close defects within the oval fossa.

CHAPTER 26

Division of Atrial Chambers

ROBERT H. ANDERSON and ANDREW N. REDINGTON

Division, or partitioning, of one of the atrial chambers is a rare malformation. Severe symptoms, or even death, may ensue if it is untreated. When recognised, and treated surgically, life expectancy should be normal. Either the morphologically right, or the morphologically left, atrium can be divided by fibromuscular partitions. Division of the morphologically left atrium is by far the most common, and the most important, type. When used in isolation, the term cor triatriatum almost always refers to the divided left atrium.[1] For those who prefer classical terminology, it is more accurate to describe either cor triatriatum sinister or cor triatriatum dexter. For those who prefer the vernacular, the lesions can be described simply as divided left or right atriums. Division of one or other atrium was the rarest lesion, bar one, in the files of the Hospital for Sick Children, Toronto, when they were used for the classical textbook emanating from that institution.[2] Despite their rarity, the malformations are sufficiently well circumscribed anatomically to warrant their own chapter in our book.

DIVIDED MORPHOLOGICALLY LEFT ATRIUM

Morphology and Morphogenesis

Church[3] is usually credited as being the first to describe division of the left atrium, albeit that it was Borst[4] who coined the term cor triatriatum. Since then, there have been several classifications, not all of which are restricted to cases that represent a congenitally partitioned left atrium. James,[5] for example, included examples of totally anomalous pulmonary venous connection to the coronary sinus in his grouping, together with aneurysms of the atrial septum, neither of which would now be considered as examples of divided left atrium. Thilenius and his colleagues[6] proposed a much expanded concept, which included rare cases reported in the literature with atresia of the mouth of the coronary sinus and anomalous pulmonary venous connection to a midline additional chamber, which then drained to the morphologically right atrium. They also described a further solitary case, with mitral atresia, in which there was a midline atrial compartment that received neither systemic nor pulmonary veins. As they indicated, it is as well to be aware of these variants. There is little doubt, however, that almost all cases encountered in clinical practice will be of the classical type. It is this anomaly, typically called cor triatriatum sinister, with which we shall be concerned in the remainder of this chapter.

In the typical lesion, an obliquely orientated fibromuscular partition divides the morphologically left atrium into a proximal compartment which is connected to the pulmonary veins, and a distal portion in communication with the atrial appendage and the mitral valvar vestibule (Fig. 26-1). These components of the left atrium have been described in various ways, such as superior and inferior, upper and lower, common pulmonary venous and left atrial, and accessory and left atrial chambers. In this respect, the terms proximal and distal have themselves been used with opposite meanings, according to the fashion in which they are perceived. We agree with Thilenius and his colleagues[6] that it is sensible to name the chambers according to the direction of flow of blood.

Although all the examples falling within the characteristic pattern have the oblique dividing partition, there is still scope for considerable anatomical variability. The significant variations are the size of the communication between the proximal and distal compartments, the site of an interatrial communication, if present, and the connection of the pulmonary veins, although any other associated malformation can co-exist. The communication between the compartments can vary from being non-restrictive, which is rare, to the more usual arrangement in which there is a pinhole meatus (Fig. 26-2). Usually the communication is single, but multiple orifices can be found. The atrial septum is intact in up to half of patients. When present, a septal defect is almost always within the oval fossa. It most

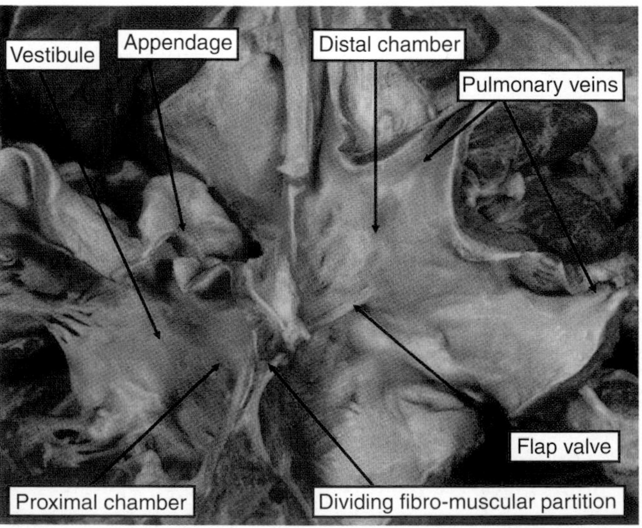

Figure 26-1 This heart with division of the left atrium is photographed from the left side. The partition divides the chamber into a distal component, which receives the pulmonary veins, and into which the oval foramen opens, and a proximal part, made up of the vestibule of the mitral valve and the left atrial appendage.

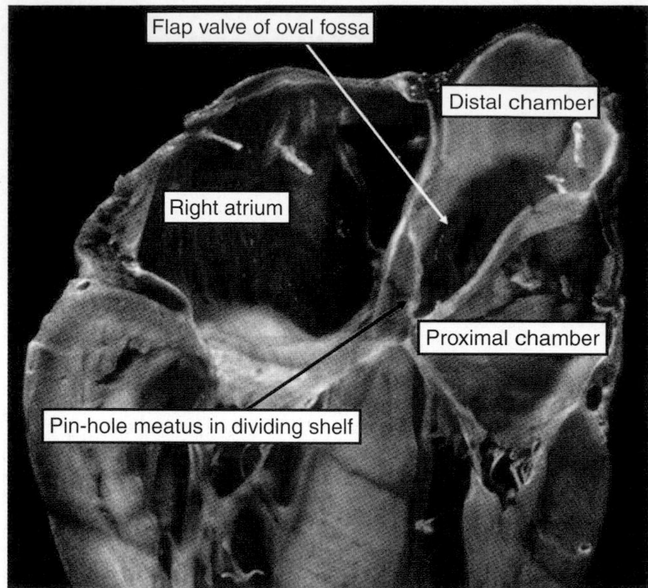

Figure 26-2 The heart shown in Figure 26-1 has been reconstituted and sectioned to replicate the echocardiographic four-chamber view. Note the oblique dividing shield, with only a pinhole meatus between the two subcomponents of the left atrium. Note also that the oval fossa opens to the distal component.

frequently communicates with the distal compartment (see Figs. 26-1 through 26-3). In the series reported by Thilenius and his colleagues,[6] nonetheless, about one-quarter of their classical cases were found with the oval fossa in communication with the proximal atrial component. Almost always the atrial communication is within the oval fossa, albeit that rare cases have been described where the communication with the distal chamber is an atrioventricular rather than an atrial septal defect.[6] One case of divided left atrium has also been found in the setting of an atrioventricular septal defect with intact septal structures.[7] Just as the morphology of the interatrial communications can vary, so can their size. While the pulmonary veins usually connect to the distal atrial compartment, many types of partially anomalous venous connection are described, and it such associations that, for the most part, account for the exceedingly complex categorisation designed by Thilenius and his colleagues.[6] We prefer to account for these uncommon associated lesions in descriptive fashion. As emphasised, any other lesion can co-exist with a divided left atrium, including such malformations as mitral atresia,[8] and discordant atrioventricular connections.[8] The dividing partition itself is made up of a double layer of myocardium, arguably giving clues as to the morphogenesis of the lesion.[9,10] The right side of the heart is usually considerably hypertrophied when the left atrium is partitioned. In keeping with this, as with other cases of obstructed pulmonary venous return, there are marked changes within the lungs,[11] with varicose dilation of the alveolar capillaries, concentric medial thickening of the pulmonary arterioles with luminal narrowing. There can also be prominent dilation of the pleural lymphatics.[12] Division of the left atrium was conventionally explained on the basis of failure of absorption of the common pulmonary vein into the left atrium. This malincorporation hypothesis was then replaced by the entrapment concept.[10] This concept was based on the belief that the primary pulmonary vein, during its development, was caught in a vice between the left sinus horn and the rest of the systemic venous sinus. The concept accounts well for the classical anomaly. It less readily explains the variant in which the atrial septal defect, unequivocally at the oval fossa, communicates with the proximal chamber. It is possible, however, to combine concepts of malseptation with the entrapment hypothesis to account for these variants. As Thilenius and his colleagues rightly commented,[6] all these theories are of necessity speculative.

Incidence and Aetiology

As already discussed, division of the left atrium represented less than 0.1% of the case load in the files of the Hospital for Sick Children, Toronto.[2] Only four examples were found in nearly 4000 catheterisations performed at the Royal Brompton Hospital from 1970 through 1982.[13] Males are affected more frequently than females.[6,14] There has been no observed aetiology for the lesion, although it is suggested[15] that the partition may be induced during development by persistence of the left superior caval vein. Although superficially attractive, it is difficult to reconcile this hypothesis with the fact that so few patients with persistent left caval veins also have a divided left atrium.

Presentation and Clinical Features

The age and mode of presentation relate to the tightness of the communication between the proximal and distal chambers. Presentation with symptoms usually implies a small communication, but symptoms will be amplified in the presence of a left to right shunt. Usually, patients then present in infancy, or early childhood, with dyspnoea and frequent respiratory infections, although presentation with congestive heart failure, unexplained pulmonary hypertension, and haemoptysis in adult life is well-described. The cases presenting earlier do so with tachypnoea with or without cyanosis, as in totally anomalous pulmonary venous connection. When cyanosis is present, this usually is the consequence of a right-to-left shunt from the right atrium through an oval foramen or atrial septal defect to the distal compartment of the divided left atrium. Partially anomalous pulmonary venous connection, when present, removes the chance of cyanosis, and may alleviate the obstructive symptoms.[16]

The clinical signs are dominated by evidence of pulmonary venous congestion and pulmonary hypertension. The child will be pale and sweating, with tachycardia, and extreme breathlessness on feeding, but usually will remain fully saturated. There is a right ventricular heave and, on auscultation, the pulmonary component of the second sound is almost always accentuated. No murmurs may be heard, although an apical diastolic murmur may simulate mitral stenosis. A soft, blowing systolic murmur may represent secondary tricuspid regurgitation in severe disease. Occasionally the apical murmur is continuous, or the early diastolic murmur of pulmonary incompetence may be heard secondary to pulmonary hypertension. The signs of congestive heart failure are found when this supervenes, including crepitations in the lungs and a palpable liver.

Investigations

The chest radiograph usually reveals cardiomegaly and shows the presence of pulmonary venous obstruction. The so-called staghorn, or butterfly wing, sign is seen because of prominent venous engorgement of the upper pulmonary veins. Pulmonary arterial hypertension is reflected by a prominent pulmonary knob.

Right ventricular hypertrophy is almost invariably present on the electrocardiogram. The frontal mean QRS axis is usually between +120 and +140 degrees. Apart from broad P waves, which are sometimes present as a consequence of right atrial hypertrophy, the rhythm and remainder of the electrocardiographic pattern are usually within normal limits.

Cross sectional echocardiography (Fig. 26-3) is the definitive investigation, permitting direct visualisation of the obstructive partition, and showing the site of interatrial defects, if present. The technique should also permit the recognition of any associated malformations. Doppler studies will then help clarify the situation. The position and size of the communication between the distal and proximal chambers are often best delineated by colour flow mapping (Fig. 26-4), while spectral Doppler studies will define the pressure difference between the two (Fig. 26-5).

It will be rare nowadays that invasive investigation is necessary for diagnosis. If performed, however, the haemodynamic findings can be highly suggestive of the usual form of divided left atrium. An elevated pulmonary arterial wedge pressure is found in the presence of normal pressure tracings in the distal left atrial chamber and left ventricle.

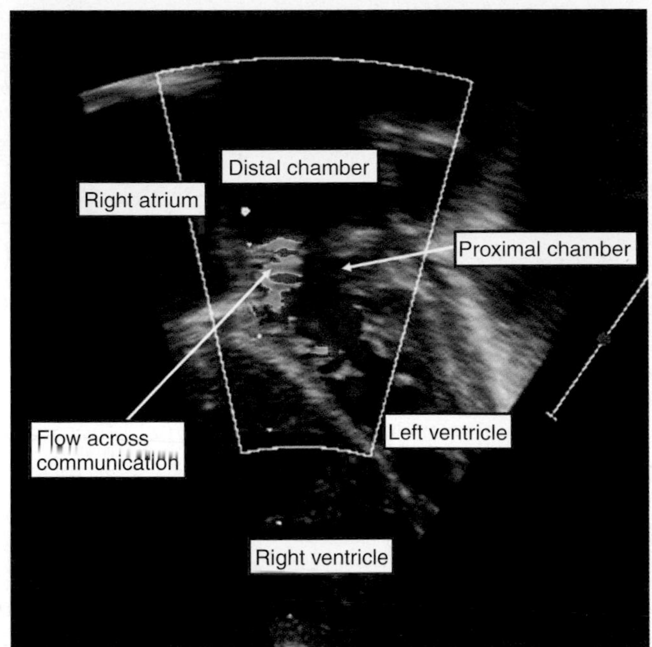

Figure 26-4 Colour flow mapping in the patient shown in Figure 26-3 reveals turbulent flow across the communication between the distal and proximal chambers.

Differential Diagnosis

In infants and children, this lesion has to be distinguished from other causes of pulmonary venous obstruction. It may be difficult to differentiate totally anomalous pulmonary venous connection from pulmonary venous obstruction, since the conditions may have similar clinical, radiological, and electrocardiographic findings. Most patients with divided left atrium will be fully saturated while breathing 100% oxygen, in contrast to most patients with totally anomalous pulmonary venous connection. The two are readily distinguished by echocardiography, even when the partitioned left atrium is itself associated with anomalous pulmonary venous connections. The other conditions to be distinguished in infancy and childhood are congenital

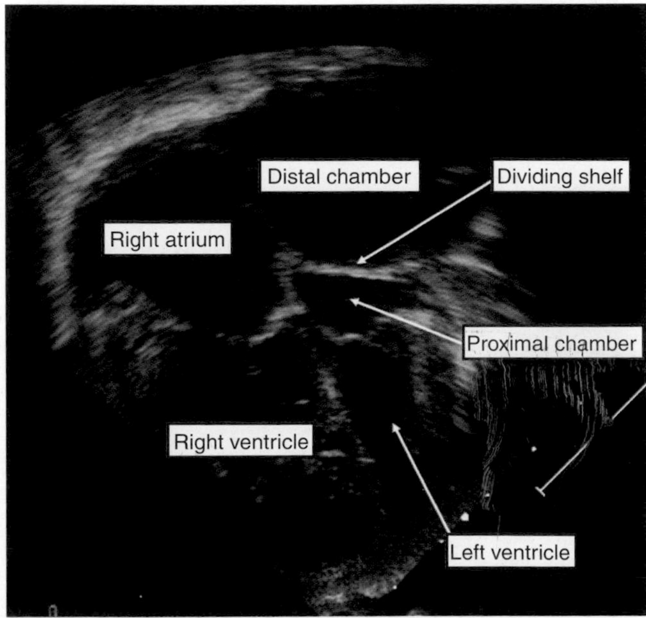

Figure 26-3 The cross sectional echocardiogram shows the features of divided left atrium.

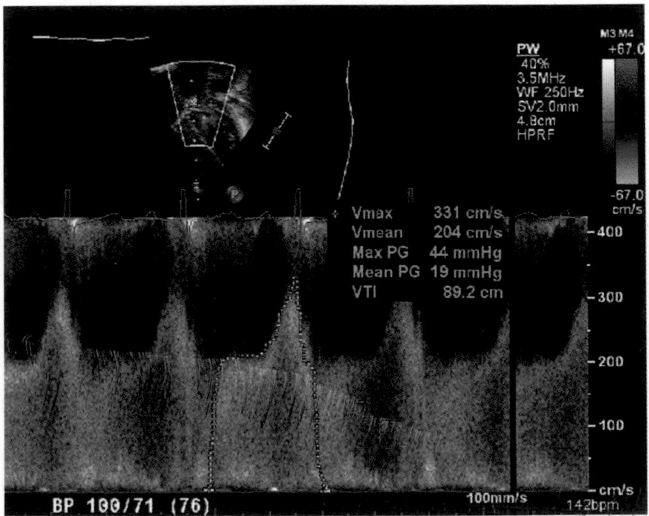

Figure 26-5 Spectral Doppler recording in the patient shown in Figures 26-3 and 26-4 reveals the velocity of flow at the communication between distal and proximal chambers of the left atrium. There is continuous flow at high velocity, suggesting severe stenosis and pulmonary venous hypertension secondary to peak and mean gradients of 44 and 19 mm Hg, respectively.

stenosis of individual pulmonary veins, atresia of the common pulmonary vein, supravalvar stenosing ring of the left atrium producing the so-called hourglass left atrium, congenital mitral stenosis, and perhaps endocardial fibroelastosis with severe aortic stenosis. In older patients, there is a quite different differential diagnosis. Rheumatic mitral stenosis, or left atrial tumour or thrombus, are then the most likely alternatives. A more important differential diagnosis is obstruction of the vestibule of the left atrium by persistence of the left superior caval vein draining to the coronary sinus. Several examples of the latter lesion have now been documented in which symptoms were relieved subsequent to surgical plication of the caval vein.[17] It should be an easy matter to distinguish the entity from divided left atrium using cross sectional echocardiography.

Treatment

The only appropriate treatment is surgical. The dividing partition is resected on cardiopulmonary bypass. This is usually achieved via a right atrial incision, visualising the partition through the oval foramen or an atrial septal defect. The shelf can also be removed via a left atrial incision. Medical treatment is indicated initially for those patients in heart failure, but only until the diagnosis is made. Surgery nowadays should carry zero mortality, and carries an excellent prognosis.

DIVIDED MORPHOLOGICALLY RIGHT ATRIUM

Division of the morphologically right atrium is considerably rarer than that of the left. It results from persistence of the valves of the embryonic systemic venous sinus.[18] The dividing partition, therefore, is placed between the systemic venous sinus and the distal part of the right atrium, made up of the vestibule and appendage. The embryonic valvar structures, whose significance during fetal life is to direct the richly oxygenated inferior caval venous blood across to the left atrium and thence to the aorta, normally regress in late fetal life and early childhood. They persist as the Eustachian and Thebesian valves, the valves of the inferior caval vein and coronary sinus, respectively. These valves can retain their fetal proportions in abnormal conditions and then divide the right atrium. The dividing partition can itself be fenestrated so as not to produce major obstruction to the flow of blood. This is termed a Chiari network, and may not produce problems (Fig. 26-6). If, in contrast, the persisting valvar structures are not fenestrated, then they can produce partitions within the right atrium. Most examples seen in postnatal life have co-existed with atresia or stenosis of the pulmonary valve, or else with tricuspid atresia (Fig. 26-7).[18]

The haemodynamic effect of the partition itself is then of little significance, since the blood is required to cross the oval fossa, and the persistent valve augments this pattern of flow, albeit that the opening of the superior caval vein may not be included within the partitioned venous sinus (see Fig. 26-7). The lesion is of more significance when the tricuspid and pulmonary valves are patent, when the persisting valve can become aneurysmal and protrude into the right ventricle like a windsock (Fig. 26-8).

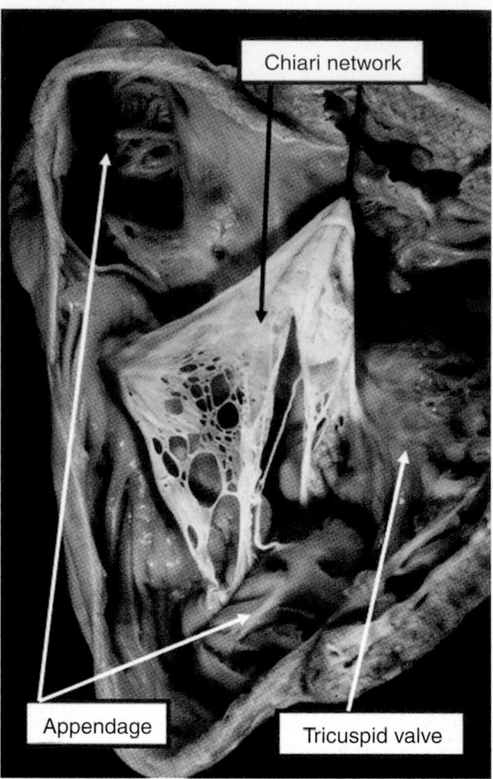

Figure 26-6 In this heart, the valves of the embryonic venous sinus have persisted in postnatal life, but have become fenestrated, producing the so-called Chiari network.

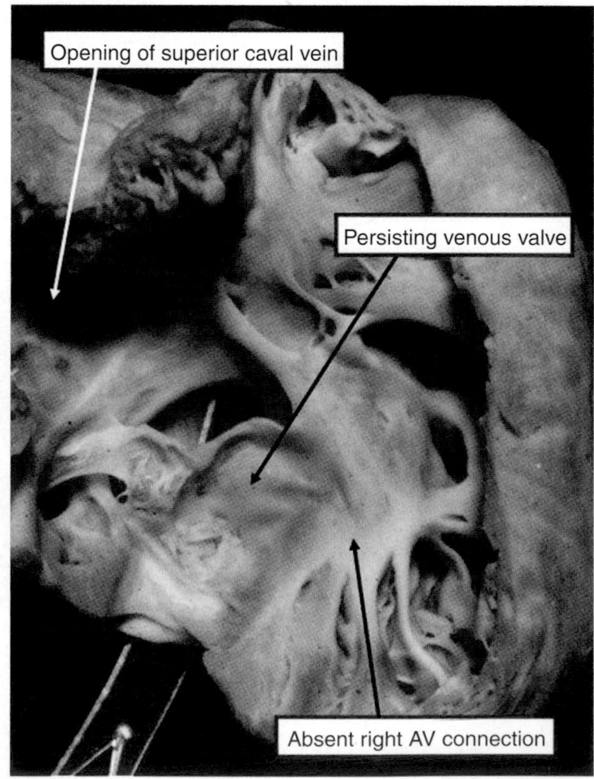

Figure 26-7 This heart also exhibits postnatal persistence of the valves of the embryonic venous sinus, but unlike the heart shown in Figure 26-6, the valves have not become fenestrated, so that they produce a partition between the systemic venous sinus and the appendage of the morphologically right atrium. In this heart, however, there is co-existing tricuspid atresia due to absence of the right atrioventricular connection, so that the partition merely exaggerates the flow of blood from the inferior caval vein to the patent oval fossa, as shown by the large piece of red tape cut in the shape of an arrow.

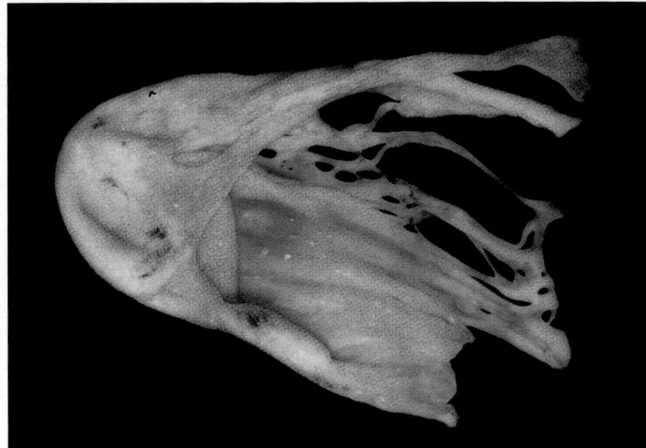

Figure 26-8 In the patient from whom this windsock was removed, the valves of the embryonic venous sinus had become aneurysmal, and herniated through the tricuspid valve, obstructing the flow of blood through the right side of the heart.

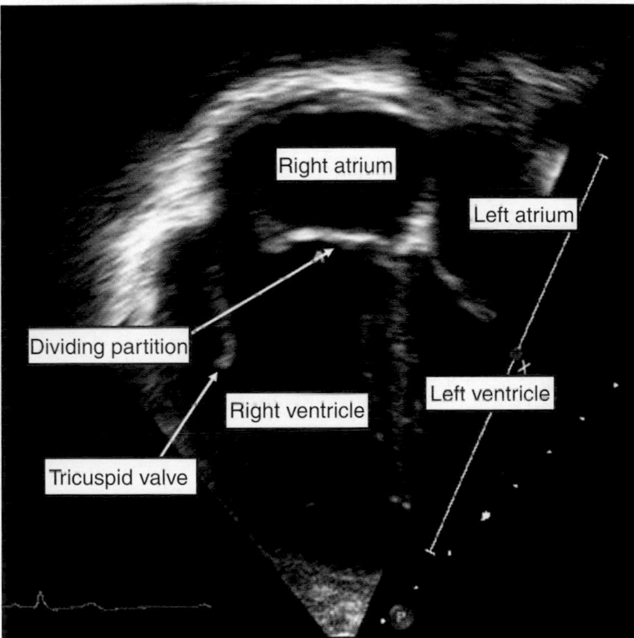

Figure 26-9 The cross sectional echocardiogram shows division of the morphologically right atrium produced by persistence of the valves of the embryonic systemic venous sinus.

Surgical removal is an easy matter once diagnosis has been made.[18] Diagnosis is now readily made using cross sectional echocardiography[19] (Fig. 26-9), albeit that the aneurysmal valve does not always produce symptoms, and can be a chance finding.[20]

The complete reference list can be found on the companion Expert Consult web site at www.expertconsult.com.

ANNOTATED REFERENCES

- Anderson RH: Editorial: Understanding the nature of congenital division of the atrial chambers. Br Heart J 1992;68:1–3.

  An editorial comment explaining the anatomic substrates producing the substrates for division of the atrial chambers, and emphasising the benefits of describing the lesions using simple language.

- Thilenius OG, Bharati S, Lev M: Subdivided left atrium: An expanded concept of cor triatriatum sinistrum. Am J Cardiol 1976;37:743–752.

  An important review of an autopsied series of hearts from the Hektoen Institute, in Chicago, with division of the left atrium, describing multiple patterns of partitioning, some of which have not subsequently been identified in clinical practise.

- Marin-Garcia J, Tandon R, Lucas RV Jr, Edwards JE: Cor triatriatum: Study of 20 cases. Am J Cardiol 1975;35:59–66.

  Another review of an extensive series of autopsied hearts with divided left atrium collected by Jesse Edwards, albeit producing a different classification from that suggested by Thilenius and colleagues.

- Van Praagh R, Corsini I: Cor triatriatum: Pathologic anatomy and a consideration of morphogenesis based on 13 postmortem cases and a study of normal development of the pulmonary vein and atrial septum in 83 human embryos. Am Heart J 1969;78:379–405.

  This publication proposed a concept for the morphogenesis of divided left atrium based on study of an extensive series of developing hearts, and also 13 hearts from the archive of Boston Children's Hospital with the classical form of divided left atrium. The outcome was the so-called entrapment hypothesis.

- Ostman-Smith I, Silverman NH, Oldershaw P, et al: Cor triatriatum sinistrum: Diagnostic features on cross sectional echocardiography. Br Heart J 1984;51:211–219.

  One of the first studies to emphasise the value of cross sectional echocardiography in diagnosing patients with divided left atriums.

- Trento A, Zuberbuhler JR, Anderson RH, et al: Divided right atrium (prominence of the Eustachian and Thebesian valves). J Thorac Cardiovasc Surg 1988;96:457–463.

  A review of the hearts from the Pittsburgh archive with persistence of the valves of the embryonic venous sinus, explaining how the valves can become aneurysmal, and then obstruct the flow of blood through the right side of the heart.

CHAPTER 27

Atrioventricular Septal Defects

TJARK EBELS, NYNKE ELZENGA, and ROBERT H. ANDERSON

There is a group of lesions unified by the anatomical hallmark of a common atrioventricular junction co-existing with deficient atrioventricular septation. The key to their differentiation from other potentially related defects is the presence of the common junction, including the arrangement of the fibrous skeleton of the heart, which is fundamentally different from the morphology found either in the normal heart, or in patients with separate right and left atrioventricular junctions. In clinical terms, it is probably the influence of this abnormal architecture of the atrioventricular valves that is the most prominent feature. In this respect, there is a common atrioventricular junction irrespective of whether there are separate atrioventricular valvar orifices for the right and left ventricles, the lesion traditionally described as the ostium primum defect, or whether the valve itself is also a common structure, often described as the complete form of the malformation. As we will show, the abnormal morphology of the ventricular mass and the atrioventricular junction is more or less constant within the overall group, thus calling into question the notion of distinguishing between partial and complete variants. Also described previously as endocardial cushion defects, or atrioventricular canal malformations, we describe the lesions here simply as atrioventricular septal defects,[1] this term slowly coming to achieve recognition as being the most accurate descriptor. Very rarely, nonetheless, hearts with deficient atrioventricular septation can exist with otherwise normal atrioventricular junctions.[2] Patients with all the stigmas to be described in this chapter can also be found, again rarely, when the septal structures are intact,[3,4] presumably due to spontaneous closure of a preexisting atrioventricular septal defect.[5] Not withstanding these potential caveats, it remains our conviction that atrioventricular septal defect is the best default option for this important group of malformations. For precision, nonetheless, it is necessary also to specify the presence of the common atrioventricular junction, and to indicate spontaneous closure in those rare instances when the septal structures are intact despite the presence of the common junction.[5]

PREVALENCE AND AETIOLOGY

Early reports of the prevalence of atrioventricular septal defects with common atrioventricular junction varied markedly.[6,7] These differences almost certainly reflect the problems inherent in most epidemiological studies due to the bias in selection. The most accurate data is that provided by study of a stable population backed up with verification at clinical study or autopsy. Using such an approach, Samanek et al[8] calculated a prevalence of 0.19 per 1000 live births, which accounted for 2.9% of the patients examined with congenitally malformed hearts. Of the cases identified in Bohemia, three-fifths had shunting confined at atrial level, the so-called ostium primum defects, while the remainder had associated ventricular shunting. A marked seasonal variation was found, with the highest incidence in March, July, and October, and the lowest in May. These differences were unlikely to be due to chance. Regional differences were also found, with most of the afflicted children being born in industrial areas, and girls just predominated in the overall numbers. The lesion was even more frequent in stillborns, accounting for 6.2% of all congenitally malformed hearts.[8]

There is a strong association of deficient atrioventricular septation with Down's syndrome (see Chapter 9). In Toronto, about one-third of patients with Down's syndrome had an atrioventricular septal defect with common valvar orifice, while only one-twentieth had the so-called ostium primum variant.[9] In the Bohemian population, half of those with deficient atrioventricular septation had Down's syndrome.[8] This close association with trisomy 21 is cited as evidence against the usual multi-factorial model put forward to explain the inheritance of congenital cardiac disease.[10] Evidence has been found of autosomal dominant inheritance, not linked to chromosome 21, in large families involving many patients with atrioventricular septal defect,[11] and there is appreciable evidence of familial recurrence.[12,13] It is possible, therefore, to discern at least three different genetic patterns, one found in association with Down's syndrome, a second emerging as an autosomal dominant trait, and the third being isolated. There is a high rate of recurrence, particularly in females. Major anatomical differences are present within the overall population of patients having atrioventricular septal defects with or without Down's syndrome, such as the atrioventricular valve being common or divided into separate left and right valvar orifices. It is intuitive to suggest that these differences must be a reflection of the different genetic mechanisms involved.[14]

ANATOMY

Basic Morphology of the Atrioventricular Junctions

It is the structure of the atrioventricular junctions which provides the phenotype for the group of lesions under discussion.[15] By atrioventricular junctions, we mean those areas of the heart where the atrial myocardium becomes contiguous with the ventricular myocardium. In the normal heart, the myocardial segments within these areas are completely

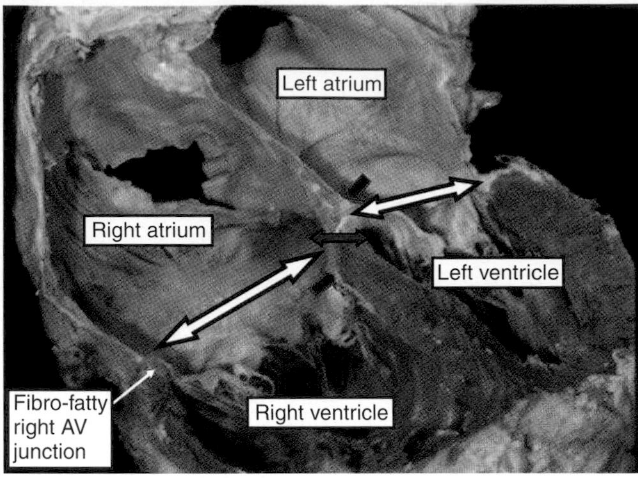

Figure 27-1 This normal heart has been sectioned in four-chamber fashion to show the separateness of the normal atrioventricular junctions, one for the tricuspid valvar orifice and the other for the mitral valve (*white double-headed arrows*). Note that, apart from at the site of the penetrating bundle (*green arrow*), the atrial myocardium is separated from the ventricular myocardium by the fibro-fatty tissues of the junctions. Note also the off-setting of the attachments of the mitral and tricuspid valves at the septum (*red arrows*). AV, atrioventricular.

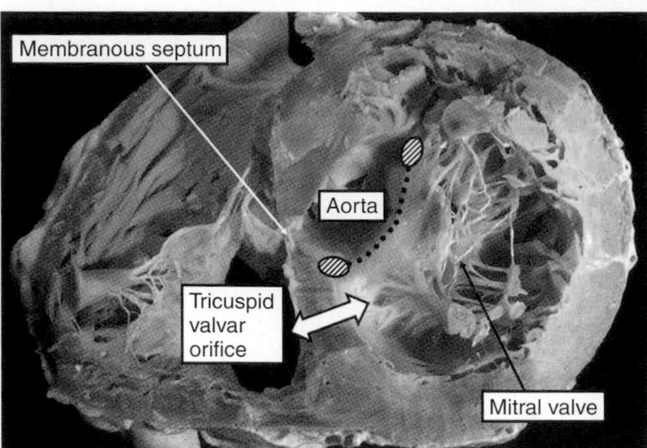

Figure 27-2 This normal heart is sectioned in its short axis, and is viewed from the apex. Note the separate nature of the right and left atrioventricular junctions, with the aorta interposing between the mitral valve and the septum. The leaflets of the aortic and mitral valve are in fibrous continuity in the roof of the left ventricle, with the area of fibrous continuity (*red dotted line*) thickened at both ends to form the right and left fibrous trigones (*cross-hatched ovals*). The right trigone is continuous with the membranous septum, forming the central fibrous body. The double-headed arrow shows the area of overlapping of the atrial and ventricular walls between the off-set hinges of the mitral and tricuspid valves (see Fig. 27-3).

separated from one another, save for the site of penetration of the muscular axis responsible for atrioventricular conduction, this being the bundle of His (Fig. 27-1). The separation within the junctions, providing the necessary electrical insulation, is produced largely by the fibro-fatty tissues of the atrioventricular grooves, which account for the greater part of the so-called valvar annuluses. These annuluses also support the attachments of the leaflets of the atrioventricular valves. In the normal heart, of course, there are two atrioventricular valves. It follows, therefore, that there are also two atrioventricular junctions, which surround the tricuspid and mitral valvar orifices.[16] There is then a complex junctional component present between these orifices, which also abuts the subaortic outflow tract. The morphology of the normal junctions is such that this septal component is relatively small. This is, in part, because the left ventricular outflow tract, incorporating the orifice of the aortic valve, is deeply wedged between the diverging antero-superior margins of the mitral and tricuspid valve (Fig. 27-2). Furthermore, over a significant part of the left atrioventricular orifice, there is not even the potential for contiguity between the atrial and ventricular myocardial masses. This is because of the extensive area of fibrous continuity that exists between the leaflets of the aortic and mitral valves. The right and left margins of this region of valvar fibrous continuity are thickened to form the right and the left fibrous trigones, respectively (see Fig. 27-2). The right trigone is itself combined with the membranous septum to form the central fibrous body. It is the arrangement of the junctional component between the valvar orifices that is most pertinent to the morphology of atrioventricular septal defects. In the apparently septal component, small as this may be, the septal leaflet of the tricuspid valve is attached at a considerably more apical level than is the corresponding leaflet of the mitral valve (see Fig. 27-1). In this area, the atrial myocardium overlaps the crest of the muscular ventricular mass, with an extension of the insulating infero-posterior fibro-fatty atrioventricular groove separating the two muscular masses. In effect, this produces a sandwich of muscular and fibro-fatty tissues that interposes between the cavities of the right atrium and the left ventricle. In the past, we thought this was a true septum,[1] but the presence of the insulating layer means that it is a sandwich, rather than a true septum (Fig. 27-3). The true septum is found antero-superior to this muscular area, and is the atrioventricular component of the fibrous membranous septum (Fig. 27-4).

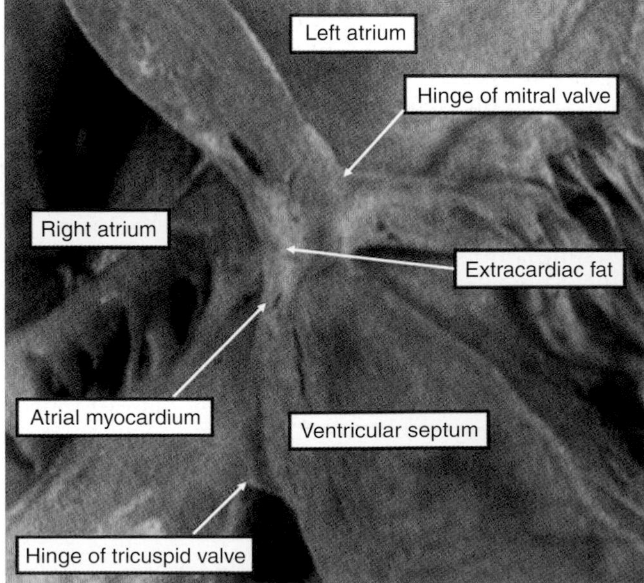

Figure 27-3 So as to provide this cut, the heart has been sectioned in four-chamber plane immediately inferior to the area where the aortic root interposes between the mitral valve and the septum. The feature of this area, which previously we suggested was an atrioventricular muscular septum, is that the right atrial wall overlaps the crest of the muscular ventricular septum between the off-set hinges of the mitral and tricuspid valves. A layer of extracardiac fat, the continuation of the inferior atrioventricular groove, and carrying the artery of the atrioventricular node, interposes between the muscular layers, so that the area represents a sandwich rather than a true septum.

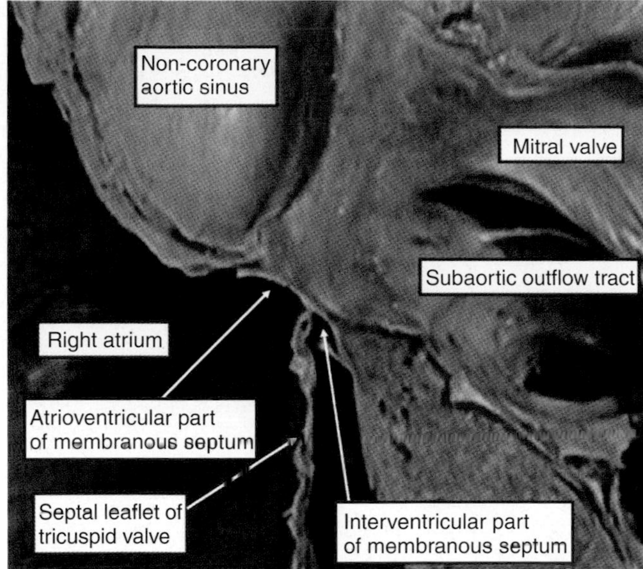

Figure 27-4 In this heart, the cut, in four-chamber plane, is through the aortic root, in the area where the root lifts the mitral valve away from the septum (see Fig. 27-2). The section, in four-chamber plane, shows how the attachment of the septal leaflet of the tricuspid valve divides the membranous septum into atrioventricular and interventricular parts. The fibrous atrioventricular part is the only true atrioventricular septal structure.

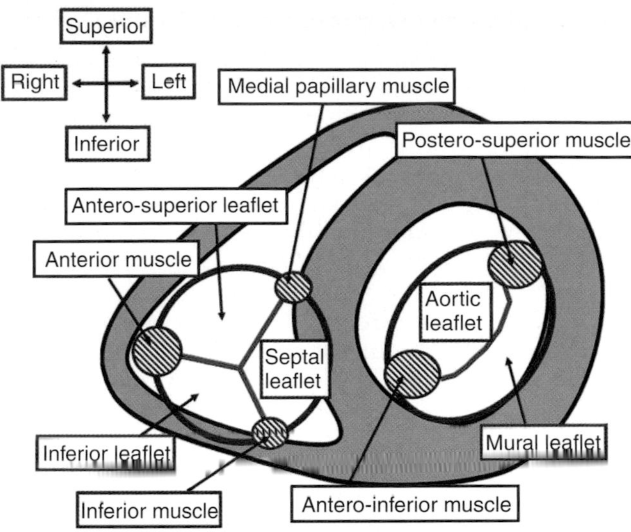

Figure 27-5 The cartoon shows the short-axis section of the ventricular mass as viewed from the cardiac apex. The silhouettes of the mitral and tricuspid valvar orifices are marked by the red rings, with the positions of the papillary muscles superimposed as cross-hatched ovals. Note that, although the muscles supporting the mitral valve are usually described as being postero-medial and antero-lateral, when described according to the coordinates of the body, they are positioned antero-inferiorly and postero-superiorly. They support the two ends of the solitary zone of apposition between the leaflets of the mitral valve.

As already emphasised, this structure, together with the interventricular membranous septum, is an integral part of the central fibrous body, and forms the rightward wall of the left ventricular outflow tract (see Fig. 27-2).[17] It interposes between the subaortic outflow tract and the chambers of the right part of the heart. Because of its wedged position, the subaortic outflow tract in the normal heart also interposes between the mitral valvar orifice and the septum. In contrast, in the inlet to the right ventricle, one of the leaflets of the tricuspid valve is adherent to the ventricular septum over a considerable area. This anatomy is pertinent to the naming of the leaflets of the normal valves. In the mitral valvar orifice, the curtain of leaflet tissue is divided by an obliquely orientated solitary line of apposition into a short and square leaflet, best termed the aortic leaflet, but often termed the anterior leaflet.[18] The other leaflet is more extensive in terms of its circumferential attachment, but shallower. This is the mural, or posterior, leaflet. This mural leaflet is usually divided into a variable number of scallops, most often three. The paired left ventricular papillary muscles supporting the solitary zone of apposition between these leaflets are positioned obliquely within the ventricle, occupying infero-posterior and supero-anterior locations (Fig. 27-5). The normal tricuspid valve has three leaflets, which are located in antero-superior, septal, and inferior or mural positions. The zone of apposition between septal and antero-superior leaflets is supported peripherally by the medial papillary muscle. From this small muscle, the extensive antero-superior leaflet, hanging from the supraventricular crest to separate the inlet and outlet portions of the right ventricle, reaches across to the large anterior papillary muscle, which in many hearts supports the middle portion of the leaflet. When the anterior muscle supports the end of the zone of apposition with the mural or inferior leaflet, the latter leaflet extends to the inferior papillary muscle, which is frequently indistinct. Then, between the inferior and the medial papillary muscles, numerous small muscles and tendinous cords anchor the septal leaflet of the tricuspid valve directly to the muscular septum. The final feature worthy of emphasis so as to provide the background for understanding the consequences of deficient atrioventricular septation in the setting of a common atrioventricular junction relates to the structure of the ventricular mass. In the normal heart, the distance from the attachment of the mitral valve at the crux to the ventricular apex, or the inlet dimension, is much the same as that from the ventricular apex to the antero-superior attachment of the leaflets of the aortic valve, this being the outlet dimension (Fig. 27-6). As we will see, there is marked inequality of these dimensions in the abnormal hearts.

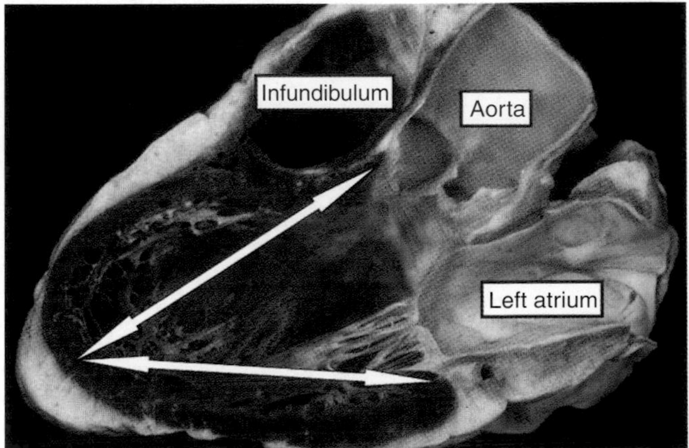

Figure 27-6 The heart in this image has been sectioned in parasternal long-axis plane, showing the dimensions of the ventricular mass (*double-headed arrows*). Note that, in the normal heart, these inlet and outlet dimensions are equal.

Basic Morphology of Atrioventricular Septal Defects

The essential morphological ingredient of the hearts we describe here as having atrioventricular septal defects is the presence of a common atrioventricular junction.[15,19] Part and parcel of this arrangement is the abnormal formation of the fibrous skeleton of the heart. The fibrous skeleton can only be seen in anatomical specimens, and cannot, as yet, be imaged clinically. The overall structure of the junctional arrangement, in contrast, can readily be identified. It is either common to all four cardiac chambers, or it is not. There are no intermediate, or transitional, arrangements. In the normal heart, as already illustrated, there are separate right and left atrioventricular junctions (see Fig. 27-1). This goes hand in hand with the presence of a normal fibrous skeleton, the essence of the normal skeleton being the fusion of the right fibrous trigone with the membranous septum to form the central fibrous body. This arrangement is, of necessity, fundamentally disturbed when there is as common atrioventricular junction (Fig. 27-7).

Because of this fundamentally different junctional architecture when compared to the normal arrangement (see Fig. 27-2), there are significant departures from normality in at least four of the features enumerated above as characteristic for hearts with separate right and left atrioventricular junctions. First, almost always, but not universally, there is a defect at the anticipated site of the structures which usually interpose between the right atrium and the left ventricle. These structures are the muscular atrioventricular sandwich and the membranous atrioventricular septum. The septal deficiency is comparable irrespective of whether there is a common valvar orifice within the common junction (Fig. 27-8), or separate atrioventricular valvar orifices for the right and left ventricles (Fig. 27-9), this latter arrangement, of course, also being known as the ostium primum defect. The septal deficiency exists because of lack of contiguity between the leading edge of the atrial septum and the crest of the muscular ventricular septum.

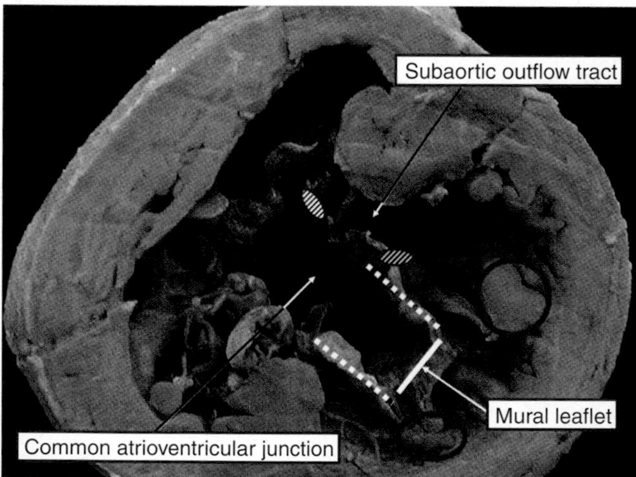

Figure 27-7 This specimen, from a patient with atrioventricular septal defect with common atrioventricular valve, has been sectioned in the short axis of the ventricular mass and photographed from the ventricular apex (compare with Fig. 27-2). Note the commonality of the atrioventricular junction, with the subaortic outflow tract now squeezed between the junction and the superior ventricular wall. The site of fibrous continuity between the aortic and common atrioventricular valves is marked (*red dotted line*), along with the positions of the fibrous trigones (*red cross-hatched areas*). There is no formation of a central fibrous body. Note also the changed location of the papillary muscles supporting the left ventricular component of the common atrioventricular valve (*red circles*). The mural leaflet of the left component of the valve guards less than one-third of the circumference of the left half of the common atrioventricular junction (*white lines*).

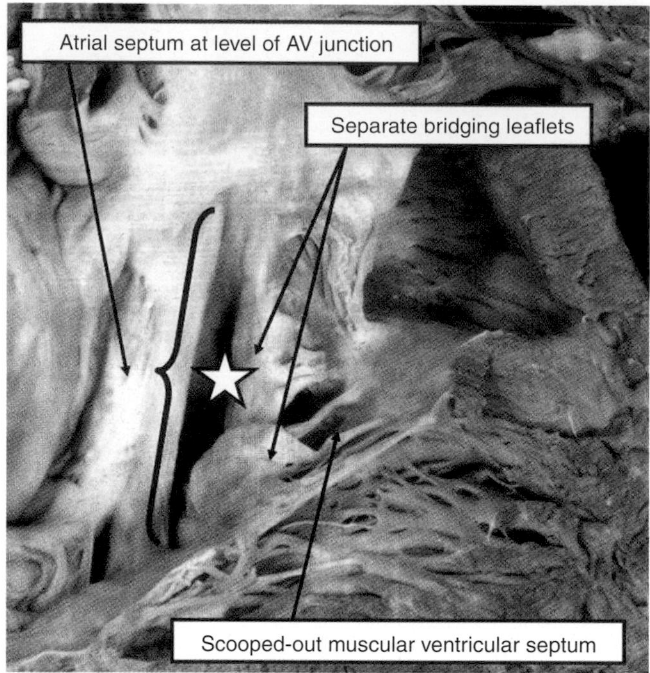

Figure 27-8 This specimen, from a patient with atrioventricular (AV) septal defect and common atrioventricular valve, is photographed from the right side. Note the common atrioventricular junction (*bracket*), and the septal defect (*star*) between the leading edge of the atrial septum and the scooped-out crest of the ventricular septum.

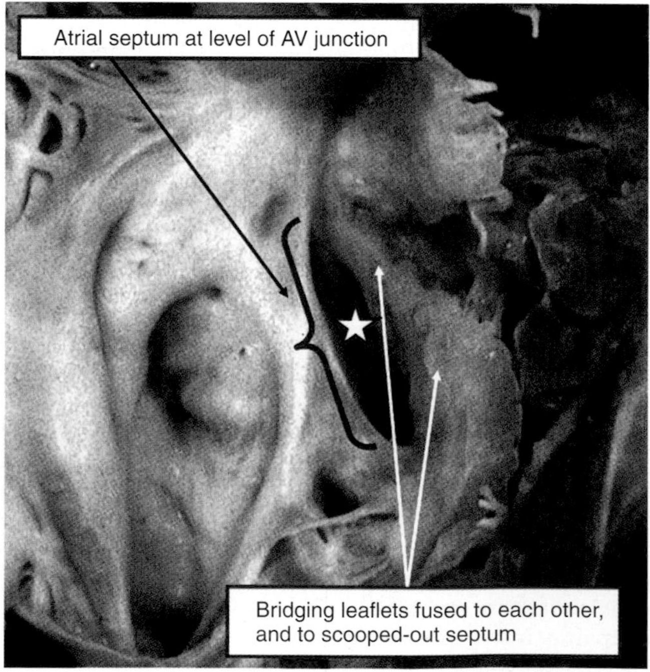

Figure 27-9 In this heart, with a so-called ostium primum defect, the septal deficiency (*star*) is again between the leading edge of the atrial septum and the scooped-out crest of the muscular ventricular septum, but in this instance because the leaflets that bridge between the ventricles are not only fused to each other, but are also fused to the crest of the muscular ventricular septum. The phenotypic feature is the common atrioventricular (AV) junction (*bracket*).

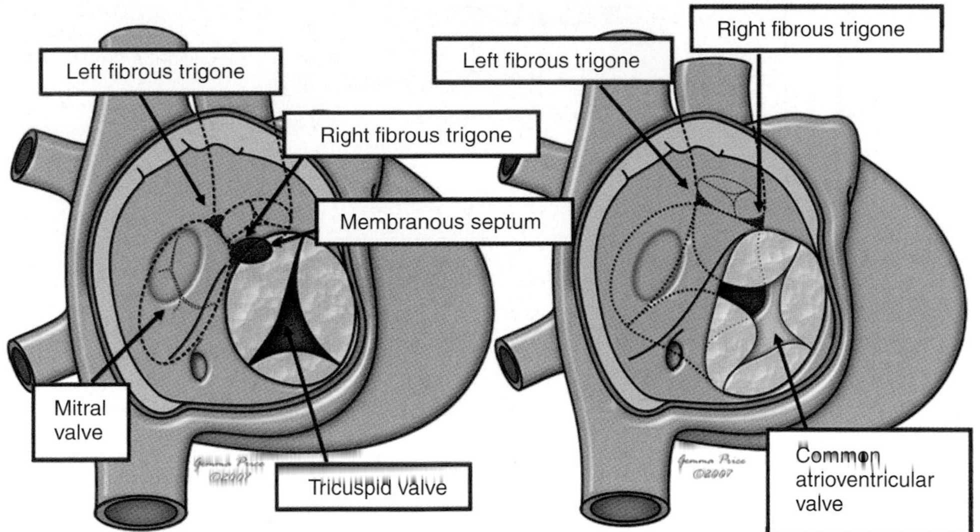

Figure 27-10 The cartoons show the difference in structure of the fibrous skeleton when there is a common atrioventricular junction (*right hand panel*), as opposed to separate right and left atrioventricular junctions (*left hand panel*; see also Figs. 27-2 and 27-7). The membranous septum is fused with the right fibrous trigone to produce the central fibrous body when there are separate junctions.

The second feature is the ovoid shape of the common atrioventricular junction. Irrespective of the number of atrioventricular valvar orifices within the junction, the left ventricular outflow tract is no longer wedged between the left and right atrioventricular orifices, as is seen in the normal heart (see Fig. 27-2). Instead, the aortic orifice is antero-superior to the common junction. Although there is still fibrous continuity between the leaflets of the aortic and atrioventricular valves, and although the ends of this area of fibrous continuity are strengthened to form left and right fibrous trigones, the morphology of the trigones cannot be compared with those found in the normal heart (compare Figs. 27-2 and 27-7). Indeed, as we have already emphasised, the entire fibrous skeleton differs fundamentally from the normal arrangement (Fig. 27-10). The right trigone may, at times, interpose between the left ventricular outflow tract and the right atrium. It may also be part of an abnormal atrioventricular fibrous septum.[20] It is in a different location, nonetheless, from the normal right trigone.

Since there is a common atrioventricular junction, and a lack of any septal atrioventricular muscular contiguity, the third feature that differs from the normal is the arrangement of the valvar leaflets that guard the common junction. These leaflets, irrespective of whether they guard a common atrioventricular orifice or separate orifices for the right and left ventricles, bear scant resemblance to the arrangement of the leaflets of the normal mitral and tricuspid valves (see Fig. 27-5). When describing the valves, and comparing them with the arrangement seen in the normal heart, it is important to state how we distinguish the boundaries of the individual leaflets. Joseph Hyrtl, the eminent Viennese anatomist of the 19th century, showed great prescience when he commented that the mitral valve came into the heart like a devil into the baptismal font.[21] To avoid the semantic problems that have complicated previous definitions, we distinguish between several significant aspects of atrioventricular valves when making our own choices. First, we assess the nature of the junction that they guard separately from the precise origin of their hinge points, since the latter are not always being concordant with the junction. We then distinguish both of these features from zones of apposition between the parts of the valve as seen in closed position. It is this latter feature we then use as the arbiter of the number of leaflets within the overall curtain of valvar tissue,[18] rather than seeking to distinguish the gaps between the leaflets on the basis of their chordal support.[22] The nature of the cordal support, of course, is also of importance, but this is yet another feature of which we take note. This feature, however, is insufficiently discrete to act as the criterion for the boundaries between the leaflets. Furthermore, the cordal arrangement is best seen when the valve is open, whereas the leaflets subserve their most important function, namely to prevent valvar regurgitation, when in their closed position. It makes most sense to us, therefore, to assess their boundaries when seen in their closed position.[23] When studied in this suggested fashion, the overall curtain of leaflet tissue in hearts having the phenotypic feature of an atrioventricular septal defect with common atrioventricular junction can be separated into five discrete components (Fig. 27-11). These five leaflets, seen to their best advantage when the common junction is guarded by a common valvar orifice (Fig. 27-12), can be arranged so as to provide separate orifices within the common junction for the inlets to the right and left ventricles. This latter pattern is achieved when a tongue of valvar tissue joins together the two leaflets of the essentially common valve that bridge the ventricular septum (Fig. 27-13). This tongue is usually attached also directly to the musculature along the length of the crest of the ventricular septum (see Fig. 27-9). It is not, therefore, analogous to the so-called annulus of the valve, which is typically part and parcel of both the atrioventricular junction and the fibrous skeleton. In the so-called ostium primum defect, the fused bridging leaflets are depressed into the ventricular cavity, and fused to the crest of the scooped-out ventricular septum (see Fig. 27-9).

A further fundamental difference from the normal situation is seen in the arrangement of the left ventricular papillary muscles. Paired muscles remain in the left ventricle but, instead of being located in antero-inferior and postero-superior positions (see Fig. 27-5), they are

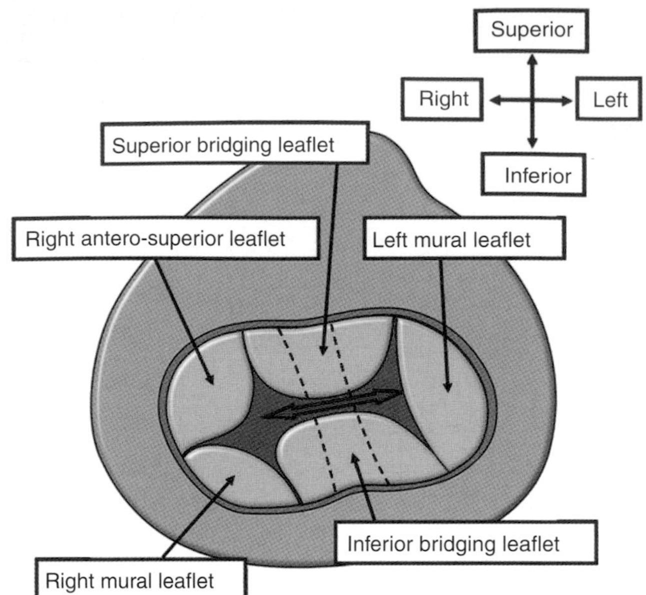

Figure 27-11 The cartoon shows the basic arrangement of the leaflets to be found in the valve guarding the common atrioventricular junction. The black dotted lines show the plane of the ventricular septum, while the double-headed arrow shows the zone of apposition between the leaflets that bridge the ventricular septum. The valve is shown as seen from the cardiac apex, looking up the barrels of the ventricles.

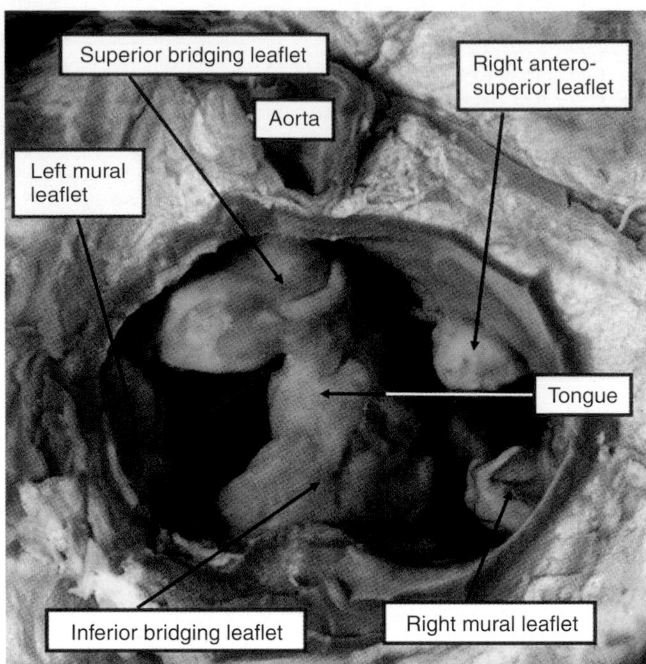

Figure 27-13 This heart, representing the ostium primum defect, is prepared in the same fashion as the one shown in Figure 27-12. Note the tongue of valvar tissue joining together the two bridging leaflets. Apart from this feature, the two specimens are directly comparable. In particular, note that the dotted line marks the zone of apposition between the left ventricular components of the two bridging leaflets.

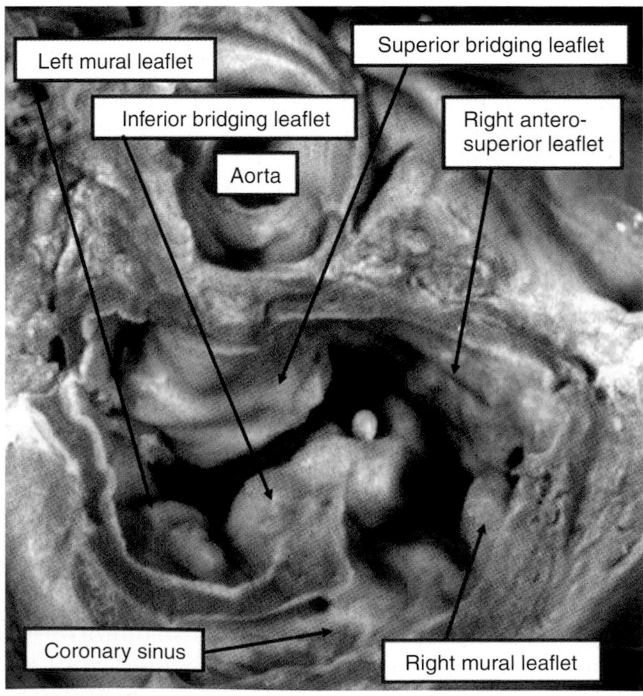

Figure 27-12 This heart with common atrioventricular valvar orifice has been prepared by removing the atrial musculature, along with the arterial trunks. It is photographed from the atrial aspect. Note the common atrioventricular junction. The dotted line marks the zone of apposition between the bridging leaflets.

positioned in more or less direct supero-inferior position (see Fig. 27-7). On occasion, they may be even more abnormally arranged. The superior muscle may be located in a manner that compromises the left ventricular outflow tract. Alternatively, many small separate papillary muscles can be present, the muscles may fuse, or one muscle may be grossly hypoplastic or absent. It is these last arrangements that are usually described as the parachute arrangement.[24] In reality, the abnormal valve looks more like a funnel, representing the spatial inverse of a parachute.[25] A parachute constructed in this way would be a lethal device! The arrangement of the right ventricular muscles is comparable with the normal heart, being in medial, anterior, and inferior positions. The position of the medial papillary muscle, nonetheless, is itself variable, this variability reflecting the extent to which the superior leaflet bridges into the right ventricle.

The basic arrangement of the curtain of leaflet tissue guarding the common atrioventricular junction, therefore, is that of a valve with five leaflets (see Fig. 27-11). Three of the leaflets are confined to one or other of the ventricles, one being in the left ventricle and two in the right ventricle. The left mural leaflet, much less extensive than the mural leaflet of the normal mitral valve,[26] is tethered between the superior and inferior papillary muscles of the left ventricle. The antero-superior leaflet and the right mural leaflet are confined to the right ventricle. These leaflets retain to greater extent the pattern as seen in the normal tricuspid valve, although the antero-superior leaflet is of variable size, being reciprocal to the extent of bridging of the superior leaflet into the right ventricle. This bridging leaflet, and its facing partner positioned inferiorly, have no counterpart in the normal heart. They are tethered so as to extend between the cavities of the left and right ventricles, being anchored across the septum, albeit in some cases to a limited extent. In many instances, they are firmly attached to the septal structures at their point of crossing. Since they extend across the ventricular septum, they can appropriately be

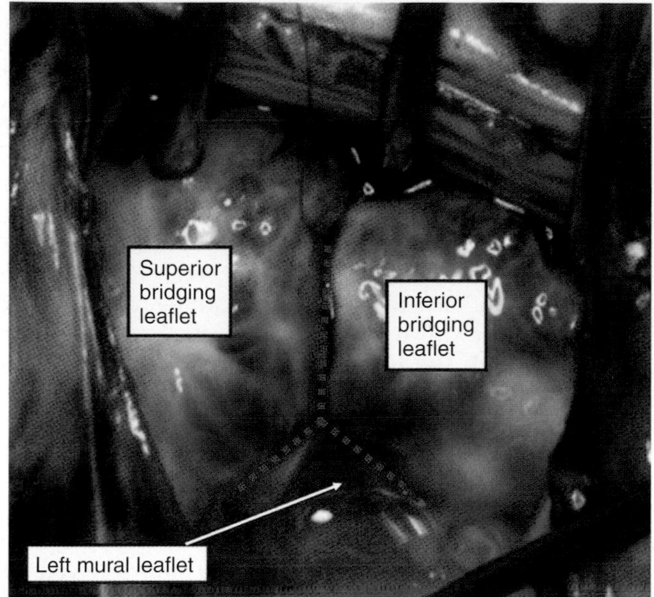

Figure 27-14 The left atrioventricular valve in this heart with common atrioventricular valvar orifice is photographed by the surgeon in the operating room, and is shown in surgical orientation. Note the trifoliate pattern of valvar closure (*dotted lines*). (Courtesy of Dr Benson R. Wilcox, University of North Carolina, Chapel Hill.)

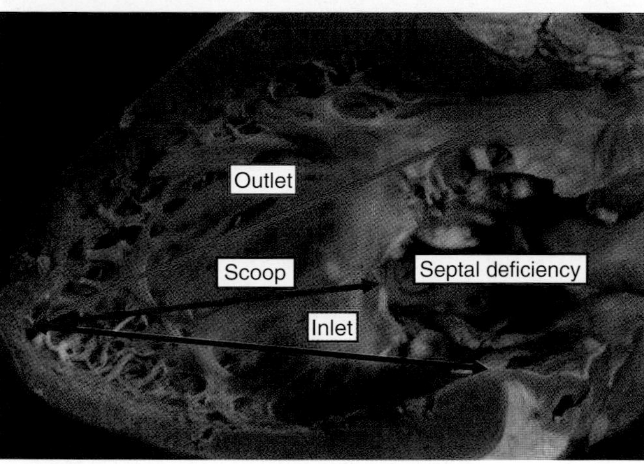

Figure 27-15 In this heart with atrioventricular septal defect and common atrioventricular junction, the valvar leaflets have been stripped away from the ventricular base. Although this reveals the extent of disproportion between the inlet and outlet dimensions of the ventricular mass, and shows the extent of scooping of the ventricular septum, there is no way of knowing whether the heart initially had a common valvar orifice, or separate valves for the right and left ventricles within the common junction. (Courtesy of Professor Anton E. Becker, University of Amsterdam, Amsterdam, The Netherlands.)

called bridging leaflets. The space between them is their zone of apposition. This zone of apposition was rightly compared to so-called commissures found in the normal mitral and tricuspid valves.[27] Describing the appositional zone as a commissure, however, can be contentious, and creates unnecessary problems with the need to distinguish this structure from a so-called cleft. Arguments about the commissural or non-commissural nature of the space between the left ventricular components of the bridging leaflets also conceal the fact that it is, unequivocally, a zone of apposition between them. Indeed, because of this, the left valve closes in trifoliate fashion (Fig. 27-14). Such closure is markedly different from the pattern of closure of the mitral valve, the two leaflets of which come together along a solitary zone of apposition. If the aortic leaflet of the normal mitral valve is cloven artificially, then the space thus created extends into the subaortic outflow tract, as do congenital clefts of the otherwise normal mitral valve (see Chapter 35). The zone of apposition between the left ventricular components of the bridging leaflets, irrespective of how it is named, is part of the orifice between left atrium and left ventricle. It has no morphological affinity with clefts seen in the aortic leaflet of the otherwise normal mitral valve (see Chapter 35). As we will discuss, almost always nowadays the surgeon will close the space as part of the operative repair, but this surgical manoeuver never produces an arrangement of leaflets for the new left atrioventricular valve that replicates the arrangement seen in the normal mitral valve (see Fig. 27-2).

The fourth difference in morphology that characterises an atrioventricular septal defect with common atrioventricular junction is found in the architecture of the ventricular mass. In the normal heart, the inlet and outlet dimensions of the left ventricle are approximately the same (see Fig. 27-6). In atrioventricular septal defects with common junction, the dimension of the outlet is considerably greater than that of the inlet (Fig. 27-15). It is of little consequence morphologically whether this is because the inlet is shorter than normal, or because the outlet is longer. Probably it is a combination of the two. Irrespective of such niceties, the disproportion between inlet and outlet dimensions is readily apparent (see Fig. 27-15). More significantly, it is within the same range be there a common orifice within the overall curtain of valvar tissue, or separate valvar orifices at the inlets to the right and left ventricles (Fig. 27-16).[26] Indeed, once the curtain of valvar leaflets is removed from the atrioventricular junctions in any individual heart, it is not possible to judge simply from examination of the ventricular mass whether there had initially been a common valvar orifice or separate right and left atrioventricular orifices (see Fig. 27-15).[1] When large numbers of hearts are studied, nonetheless, the extent of deficiency of the mid-point of the septum,

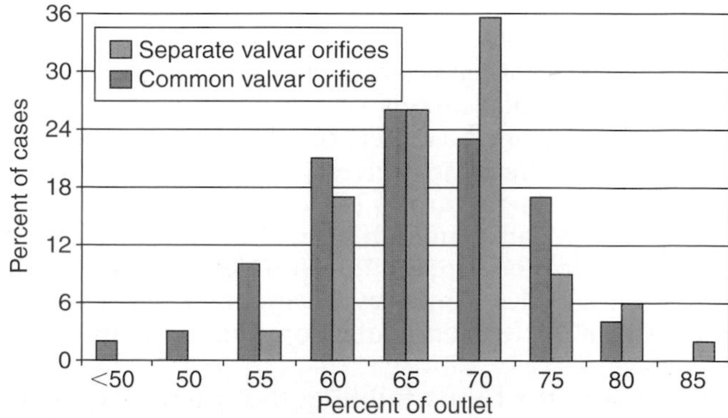

Figure 27-16 The graph shows the measurements of the ventricular inlet as a ratio of the outlet in a large series of hearts in the archive of Children's Hospital of Pittsburgh. The proportions do not vary significantly between hearts having a common valvar orifice as opposed to separate valves for the right and left ventricles, although there is a greater degree of scooping in presence of a common valvar orifice.

which we describe as the degree of scooping, is usually greater in those hearts having a common atrioventricular valvar orifice.[28]

Categories of Atrioventricular Septal Defect

All the lesions falling within the group to be discussed in this chapter are unified by presence of a common atrioventricular junction. Although the individual internal structures of the hearts unified in this fashion can differ widely, clinicians recognise two major categories, often considered to be partial and complete. There are two aspects of the underlying anatomy underscoring these differences in clinical stratification. The first is the arrangement of the individual leaflets within the overall curtain of valvar tissue guarding the common atrioventricular junction. The second is the relationship between the bridging leaflets of the common valve and the atrial and ventricular septal structures. There are problems in seeking to combine these two features so as to identify presumed complete and partial variants, since the two aspects of anatomy are mutually independent. It has been attempts to combine description of the two features to give one all-embracing categorisation that has produced the bewildering array of definitions for so-called transitional or intermediate lesions. By describing the two features separately, we avoid the need to nominate intermediate categories. Other features, nonetheless, are important in categorisation. Examples are the sharing of the common atrioventricular junction between the atrial and ventricular chambers, and the presence of associated lesions. All of these features require description.

Arrangement of the Valvar Leaflets Relative to the Atrioventricular Orifices

In all hearts having the phenotype of atrioventricular septal defect with common atrioventricular junction, the curtain of valvar tissue guarding the junction can be described in terms of five leaflets (see Fig. 27-11). On the basis of the anatomical relationship between the two bridging leaflets, all of these hearts can be placed into one of two groups, with no intermediate categories. The majority have a space between the two bridging leaflets and, hence, have a common atrioventricular valvar orifice (see Fig. 27-12). The component of this common valve committed to the left ventricle almost always closes in trifoliate pattern, with zones of apposition between the left mural leaflet and the left ventricular components of the superior and inferior bridging leaflets, and a further zone of apposition between the bridging leaflets themselves (see Fig. 27-14). Within this arrangement, the mural leaflet guards less than one-third of the left component of the common junction.[26] It is not possible for the surgeon to restore the anatomy of the normal mitral valve simply by closing the zone of apposition between the left ventricular components of the bridging leaflets.

In some of the hearts fulfilling the criterion for inclusion within the overall anatomical group, the two bridging leaflets are themselves joined to each other by a connecting tongue of valvar tissue. This divides the common atrioventricular junction into right and left components (see Fig. 27-13). In most instances, shunting across the defect in this setting is confined at atrial level, since the leaflets are also fused to the crest of the muscular ventricular septum (see Fig. 27-9). Such fusion to the ventricular septum, however, is not a universal feature of hearts in which the common junction is divided into right and left ventricular components by the union between the bridging leaflets. In some instances, the bridging leaflets can be fused to each other, thus dividing the valvar orifice, but also fused to the underside of the atrial septum so that the potential for shunting is restricted at ventricular level. Furthermore, in rare instances, the bridging leaflets can be fused so as to produce separate valvar orifices for the right and left ventricles even when the tongue of leaflet tissue joining the leaflets is well away from both the atrial and ventricular septums (Fig. 27-17). The presence of the hearts such as illustrated in Figure 27-17 shows that, in reality, the hallmark of the so-called partial defect is the presence of dual orifices within a common atrioventricular valve. When the valvar orifice is divided into separate components for the right and left ventricles, it is unusual to find a freestanding septal leaflet on the right side of the septum. Instead, in most instances, the right ventricular component of the inferior bridging leaflet is the only component that stands free, with the connecting tongue and the superior bridging leaflet usually confluent with the septal surface. When seen from the left side, these components often form a pouch that bulges to the right. In terms of the overall morphology of the curtain of valvar tissue, therefore, all hearts can be divided into those with a common atrioventricular valvar orifice guarding the common junction, and those in which the common junction is guarded by separate right and left atrioventricular valves for the right and

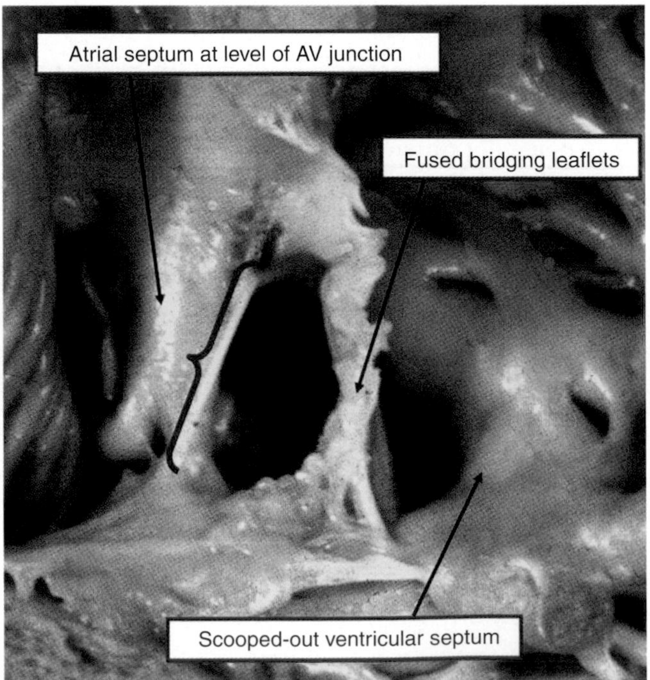

Figure 27-17 In this heart with atrioventricular (AV) septal defect and common atrioventricular junction (*bracket*), the bridging leaflets are fused to each other, producing separate valvar orifices for the right and left ventricles, but float freely within the septal defect, so that there is the potential for shunting at both atrial and ventricular levels.

left ventricles, respectively. This feature is an all-or-none phenomenon.

Potential for Shunting across the Atrioventricular Septal Defect

It is the potential for shunting across the septal defect that is probably the single most important anatomical variant that influences clinical presentation. The anatomical variability depends upon the relationship of the bridging leaflets, and of the connecting tongue, if present, on the one hand to the lower edge of the atrial septum, and on the other hand to the crest of the scooped-out ventricular septum. In most cases, the two bridging leaflets are not attached directly to either septal component as they bridge between the ventricles (Fig. 27-18B). In this arrangement, therefore, the potential exists for shunting at both atrial and ventricular levels, as it does even if fused bridging leaflets float freely within the septal defect (see Fig. 27-17). The extent of ventricular shunting then depends upon the proximity of the bridging leaflets to the ventricular septal crest. If the leaflets float freely, then there will be an extensive interventricular communication. In other cases, however, cords from the septal crest can tightly tether one or other leaflet, or both leaflets. Ventricular shunting can then be limited. Very rarely, in the presence of separate superior and inferior bridging leaflets, both leaflets may be fused to the ventricular septal crest. Shunting will then only occur at the atrial level, even though there is a common valvar orifice. The arrangement in which the bridging leaflets are attached directly to the ventricular septum (see Fig. 27-18A) is more typically seen when they are additionally attached to each other by the connecting tongue so as to produce separate valvar orifices for the right and left ventricles. As discussed already, this produces the typical ostium primum defect (see Fig. 27-9). But as also emphasised, this feature is not universal. In a proportion of patients with separate right and left atrioventricular valvar orifices, the bridging leaflets may be attached to each other by the connecting tongue, but intercordal spaces beneath the tongue, and beneath the bridging leaflets, can permit small interventricular communications. It s also the case that, in rare circumstances (see Fig. 27-13), the leaflets and connecting tongue can float freely in the space between the septal components, leaving large communications at atrial and ventricular levels. Should, however, the bridging leaflets, and a tongue if present, be firmly attached to the undersurface of the atrial septum (see Fig. 27-18C), shunting will be possible only at the ventricular level. The heart itself, of course, will still exhibit all the features of an atrioventricular septal defect with common atrioventricular junction. The most distinctive feature will be a left atrioventricular valve that closes in trifoliate fashion. We now know that the tissue of the bridging leaflets can close entirely the septal deficiency. Such spontaneous closure produces a heart with a common atrioventricular junction, but lacking the opportunity for shunting across the pre-existing atrioventricular septal defect.[3–5] In terms of overall shunting across the atrioventricular septal defect, therefore, the key feature is the relationship between the bridging leaflets and the septal structures, a feature which is independent of the arrangement of the valvar leaflets that guard the junction.

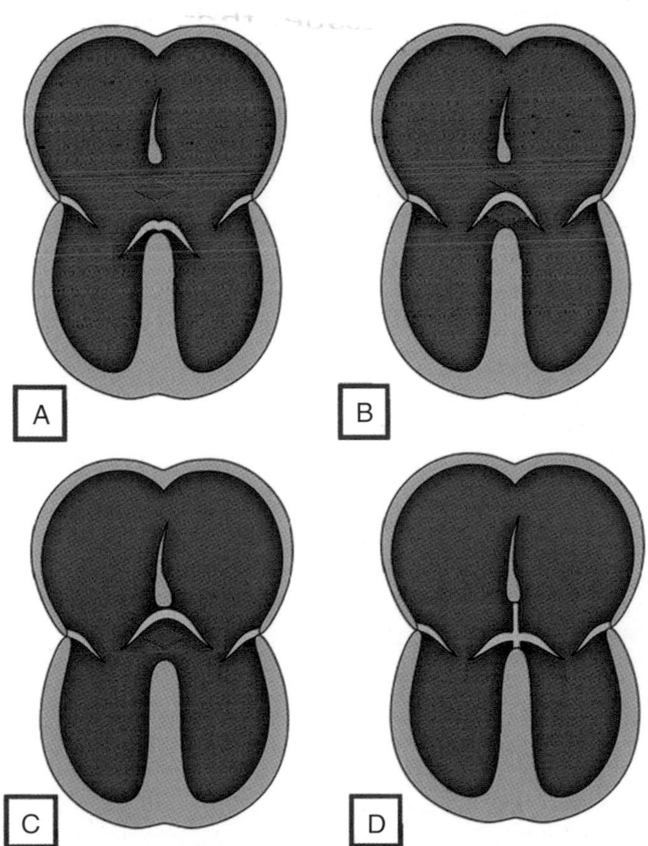

Figure 27-18 The cartoon shows how the potential for shunting across the atrioventricular septal defect (*double-headed arrows*) depends on the relationship between the bridging leaflets and the septal components. When attached to the crest of the ventricular septum (A), shunting is confined at atrial level. If the leaflets float (B), then shunting is possible at atrial and ventricular levels. If attached to the underside of the atrial septum (C), shunting can only occur at ventricular level, whereas if the bridging leaflets close the septal defect (D), then the heart has a common atrioventricular junction in the absence of the potential for shunting.

Abnormalities of the Left Atrioventricular Valve

It is, perhaps, the arrangement of the curtain of atrioventricular valvar tissue found guarding the left ventricular half of the common atrioventricular junction that is the single most obvious feature of hearts under discussion. The part of the curtain contained within the left ventricle closes in trifoliate fashion (see Fig. 27-14), with zones of apposition between mural, superior, and inferior leaflets. Apart from its residence within the morphologically left ventricle, the only anatomical affinities with the morphologically mitral valve are the fabric of the valve, and even this shows significant differences.[29] The left valve, like the mitral valve, nonetheless, is itself liable to be congenitally malformed. Presence of additional connecting tongues between the leaflets of the valve can produce dual orifices (Fig. 27-19). Rarely, such fusion of leaflets can produce a left valve with three orifices. The presence of these tongues of leaflet tissue extending between adjacent leaflets, usually between one of the bridging leaflets and the mural leaflet, and separating the orifice into subordinate compartments, can be compared to the way in which the connecting tongue itself divides the common orifice into separate right and left atrioventricular components (see Fig. 27-19). When a tongue produces dual orifices within the left valve, each orifice is usually related to one of the paired papillary muscles, which supports the

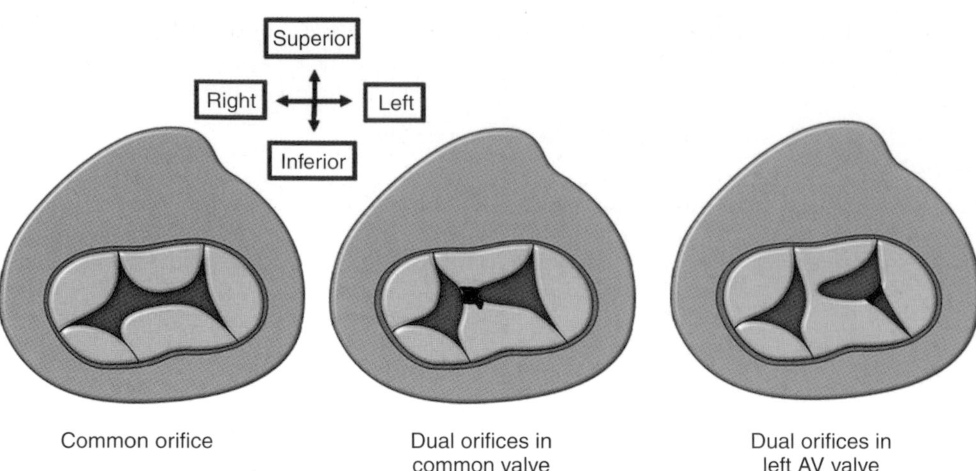

Figure 27-19 The cartoon shows how additional tongues of tissue (*red*) convert a common valve with common orifice (*left hand panel*) into a common valve with dual orifices (*middle panel*), and then into the situation in which the left atrioventricular (AV) valve has dual orifices (*right hand panel*). The tongue in the right hand panel is shown between the inferior leaflet and the mural leaflet, but tongues can also be found between the superior leaflet and the bridging leaflet, while further tongues can be found in the right component of the valve. Indeed, it is possible for the left valve to have three valvar orifices.

leaflets. Such dual orifices do not usually render the valve incompetent. The papillary muscles themselves can also be abnormal. Hypoplasia of one or other papillary muscle, or fusion of the muscles, produces an arrangement replicating a funnel, albeit usually, and misleadingly, described in terms of a parachute. In this entity, the orifice of the valve is, effectively, represented by the space between the bridging leaflets. In severe cases, the valve can take on a bifoliate configuration. Such a left valve with two leaflets remains anatomically different from the arrangement of the normal mitral valve. The superior papillary muscle can also be abnormally attached across the subaortic outflow tract and can then contribute to left ventricular outflow obstruction.

Rastelli Classification

In the past, it was conventional to subdivide atrioventricular septal defects with common valvar orifice depending on the morphology of the papillary muscle supporting the right ventricular extremity of the superior bridging leaflet. Such variability was first noted, and highlighted, by Rastelli et al.[30] They described three major types. In the first, which they dubbed type A, the bridging leaflet was mostly contained in the left ventricle, and was usually tightly tethered by tendinous cords to the crest of the ventricular septum (Fig. 27-20A). In this arrangement, the zone of apposition of the superior bridging leaflet with the anterosuperior leaflet of the right ventricle is supported by the medial papillary muscle, which arises in relatively normal fashion from the right side of the ventricular septum. In the second type, the superior bridging leaflet extends more into the right ventricle, usually being unattached to the ventricular septum as it crosses the septal crest but being supported by an anomalous right ventricular papillary muscle arising from the septomarginal trabeculation (see Fig. 27-20B). In the third type, the free-floating bridging leaflet, again unattached to the septum, extends even further into the right ventricle and is attached to an anterior papillary muscle (see Fig. 27-20C). In this spectrum, as the superior bridging leaflet becomes increasingly committed to the right ventricle, the zone of apposition with the anterosuperior leaflet of the right ventricle also moves into the right ventricle, with corresponding diminution in size of the anterosuperior leaflet. The spectrum can be extended, therefore, to include the so-called ostium primum defect. In this lesion, of course, the bridging leaflets are usually fused to the ventricular septal crest, but with minimal bridging of the superior leaflet. Variability is also found in the arrangement of the inferior bridging leaflet. This relates not so much to the extent of bridging, since almost always the leaflet extends well into both ventricles, but more to its tethering. Sometimes, the leaflet is separated into right and left ventricular components by a well-formed raphe, which is firmly attached to the ventricular septum. In other hearts, the bridging leaflet is tethered by short tendinous cords as it crosses the septum, while in still others it can float freely. Thus far, no obvious relationship has been discovered between the degree of tethering of the two bridging leaflets. With recent refinements in the surgical technique for repair of the malformations, it is the degree of tethering of the leaflets that probably has more significance, so that increasingly the Rastelli classification itself[30] becomes more of historic interest.

Left Ventricular Outflow Tract

By virtue of its anterior and unwedged position, the left ventricular outflow tract is particularly susceptible to obstruction. This is true irrespective of whether there is a common valvar orifice or separate right and left atrioventricular valves within the common junction. On anatomical examination, the tract almost always seems narrowed. The length of the outflow tract, and the extent of the apparent narrowing, is more marked, nonetheless, in defects in which the superior bridging leaflet is firmly fused to the septal crest, in other words, in ostium primum defects.[31] This apparent obstruction, however, is not reflected by pressure gradients measured prior to surgical repair. It is additional lesions compromising the already narrow channel that are responsible for haemodynamically significant obstruction or, alternatively, the effects of the surgery itself. The outflow tract, being largely muscular, has been shown to constrict during systole.[32] Indeed, a systolic murmur can be present in these patients in the absence of atrioventricular valvar regurgitation. This might well be caused by the dynamic properties of the outflow tract. Such a murmur is probably a physiological finding. Any of the lesions that produce subaortic stenosis in the normal heart can rapidly produce similar problems in the setting of atrioventricular septal defects with common

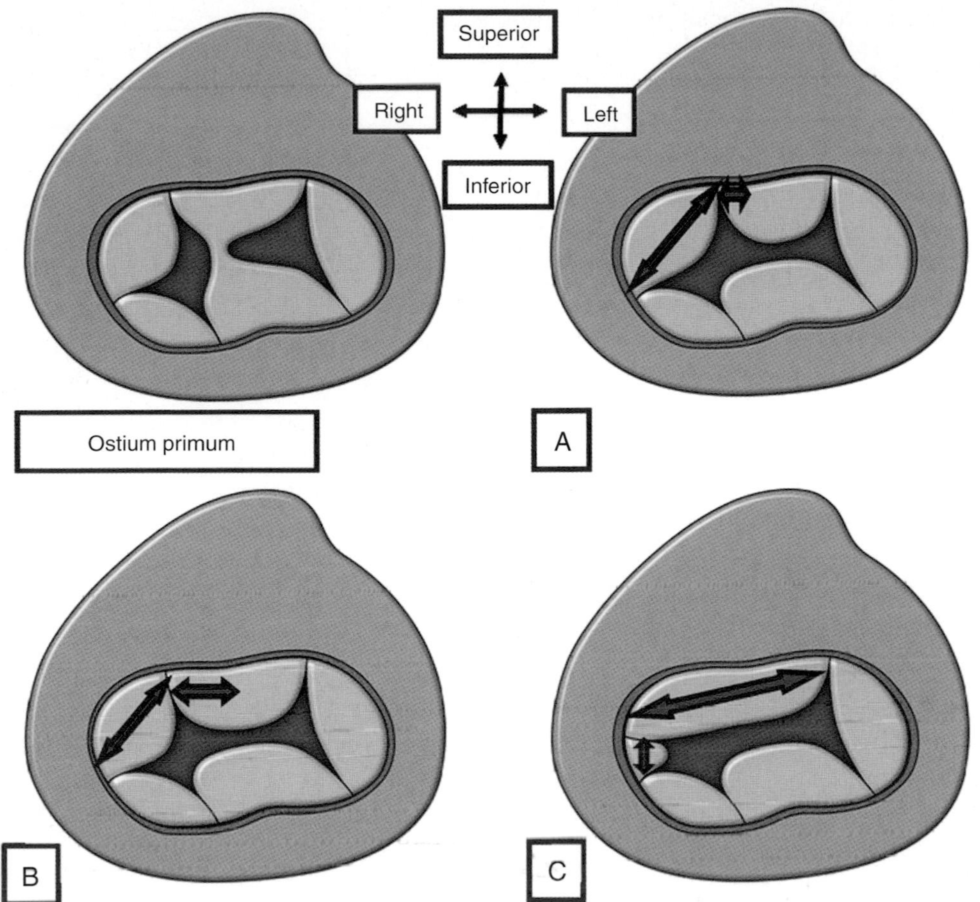

Figure 27-20 The cartoon shows the essence of the Rastelli classification of variability in the superior bridging leaflet. Although not included by Rastelli et al,[20] it is now evident that the spectrum of malformation can be extended to include the ostium primum defect (*top left hand panel*). Then, depending on the commitment of the superior bridging leaflet to the right ventricle (*broad double-headed arrow*), there is a spectrum with reciprocal diminution in size of the antero-superior leaflet of the right ventricle (*narrow double-headed arrow*), as shown in panels **A** through **C**, which represent the types designated alphabetically in the original description.

atrioventricular junction, particularly when there is tethering of the superior bridging leaflet, or separate valvar orifices for the two ventricles. These lesions are septal bulging of a fibrous subaortic shelf or tunnel, anomalous insertion of left ventricular papillary muscles, and tissue tags. The tissue tags can take origin from the partially formed interventricular membranous septum, from the superior bridging leaflet, or from anomalous fibrous tissue around the septal defect. When florid, such tags can contribute to spontaneous closure of the defect,[33] potentially producing a common atrioventricular junction in the absence of any intracardiac shunts.

Dominance of Chambers

Most usually in atrioventricular septal defects, be there separate right and left atrioventricular valvar orifices or a common valvar orifice, the right and left components of the common atrioventricular junction are of comparable circumference, and the ventricles are then of similar size. This arrangement produces the so-called balanced form of defect. The common atrioventricular junction, nonetheless, can be committed in its larger part to the right ventricle, producing right ventricular dominance, or to the left, giving a dominant left ventricle. Right ventricular dominance is usually associated with clinically significant hypoplasia or abnormality of the left ventricular and aortic structures, but most often with normal alignment between the atrial and ventricular septal structures. In the presence of left ventricular dominance, in contrast, it is the right ventricular and pulmonary arterial structures which are hypoplastic, typically in association with malalignment between the atrial and the muscular ventricular septal structures. Such hearts with atrioventricular septal malalignment then constitute part of a spectrum that extends to double inlet left ventricle, but through a common atrioventricular valve. In these variants, the ventricular septum no longer meets the atrioventricular junction at the crux, with important consequences for the disposition of the atrioventricular conduction axis.[34] A similar spectrum obviously exists when the right ventricle is dominant, with the extreme end of this spectrum being double inlet right ventricle with common atrioventricular valve. It may be difficult clinically to distinguish between the hearts with double inlet and a common valve and those with atrioventricular septal defect and right ventricular dominance. The clinical point of note will be whether the patient in question is suitable for biventricular as opposed to functionally univentricular surgical correction (see Chapter 32). It is important, therefore, to recognise the hypoplasia of one of the ventricles when the other ventricle is dominant, and to search for any malalignment of the septal structures, recognizing the implications that such malalignment has for the disposition of the atrioventricular conduction axis.[35]

The concept of chamber dominance can also be extended to include the atriums. When one of the atriums is dominant, the common atrioventricular junction is more or less equally shared by the ventricles, but is mostly connected to the dominant atrium. The only exit for the other atrium is then across the atrial component of the atrioventricular septal defect. This arrangement is often termed double outlet atrium, but this description is also applicable to hearts having absence of one atrioventricular connection and straddling of the other atrioventricular valve (see Chapter 33). This last entity, of course, should be distinguished from atrioventricular septal defect with common atrioventricular junction and imbalance of the chambers. The significant distinguishing feature is the presence of the common atrioventricular junction as opposed to the absence of one atrioventricular connection. In those with the common junction, surgical repair usually becomes feasible once the atrial septum is removed,[36] taking care, of course, to respect the landmarks to the conduction system when resecting the septum.

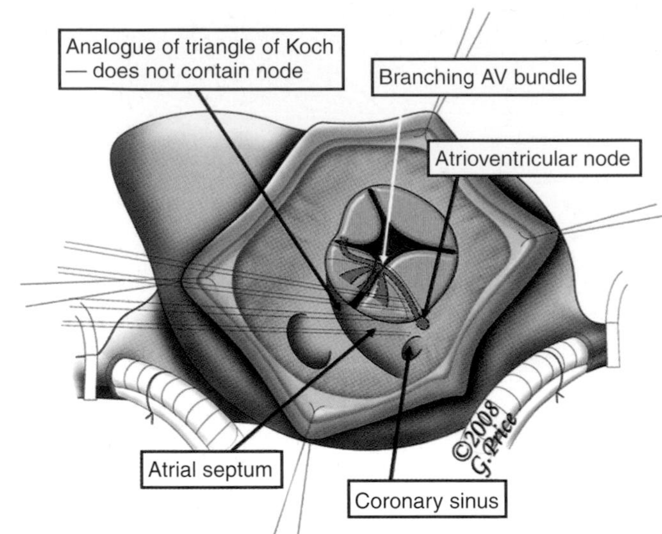

Figure 27-21 The cartoon shows the basic disposition of the atrioventricular conduction tissues in atrioventricular septal defect with common atrioventricular junction and usual alignment of the septal components.

Associated Malformations

If not ruled out by its anatomy, any lesion must be anticipated to exist in hearts having an atrioventricular septal defect with common atrioventricular junction. We have already mentioned some of the more frequent, notably, obstructions within the left ventricular outflow tract, and those affecting the left atrioventricular valve. Additional deficiencies of the atrial septum are important, and are sometimes described in terms of common atrium. Common atrioventricular valves can also be found in hearts with abnormal segmental connections, such as double inlet ventricle, and discordant or ambiguous atrioventricular connections. In these settings, the patients can have concordant ventriculo-arterial connections, but they are found, much more frequently, with other ventriculo-arterial connections. Discordant ventriculo-arterial connections are the rule in association with either double inlet left ventricle or discordant atrioventricular connections. Double outlet from the right ventricle is frequently found particularly when there is isomerism of the atrial appendages (see Chapter 22). Of the other associated lesions, tetralogy of Fallot or pulmonary stenosis is particularly important, occurring in up to one-tenth of patients with atrioventricular septal defect and common atrioventricular junction. Presence of a second muscular ventricular septal defect is also significant. In those hearts with obstruction of the left ventricular outflow tract, right ventricular dominance, along with coarctation or interruption of the aortic arch, are to be expected.

Atrioventricular Conduction Tissues

When the atrial and ventricular septal structures are appropriately aligned, the atrioventricular conduction tissues have the same basic disposition. The arrangement is different from normal, but comparable in all types of atrioventricular septal defect with common junction.[37-39] The fundamental difference from the normal arrangement reflects the lack of the atrioventricular septal structures, and the concomitant lack of a normal central fibrous body. The central fibrous body, of course, is the area of the normal heart where the atrioventricular node penetrates from the atrial musculature to become the atrioventricular bundle. In the hearts with common junction, because of the deficient atrioventricular septation, the inferior limb of the atrial septum usually makes contact with the ventricular septum only at the crux. It is at the crux, therefore, that the atrioventricular conduction axis usually penetrates (Fig. 27-21). In consequence, the entire nodal area is displaced posteriorly and inferiorly. Although a well-formed triangle can be seen at this location, this nodal triangle is not the same as the normal triangle of Koch. It does, however, continue to provide a guide to the site of penetration of the atrioventricular bundle. This area of union between the postero-inferior extremity of the ventricular septum and the atrioventricular junction is the most reliable guide to the position of the conduction axis. The insulating tissue of the atrioventricular groove is particularly well formed at the point of penetration of the conduction axis from atrium to ventricle. The landmark of union of the ventricular septum with the atrioventricular junction is to be found even when the coronary sinus is unroofed or opens to the left atrium.[34] It is also present when there is malalignment between the atrial and ventricular septal structures (Fig. 27-22).[35] Having taken origin from the atrioventricular node, either in the nodal triangle or along the inferior atrioventricular junction, the elongated non-branching bundle runs either on the crest of the muscular ventricular septum or to its left side, being covered by the inferior bridging leaflet. The bundle branches are then found more posteriorly than in the normal heart. Only the right bundle branch extends along the crest in the bare area found in the presence of a common orifice. In hearts with separate valvar orifices for the right and left ventricles, this part of the axis is covered over by the connecting tongue of leaflet tissue. This feature is of major surgical importance, since it permits sutures to be secured on the left side of the fibrous raphe, or within the bridging leaflets themselves,

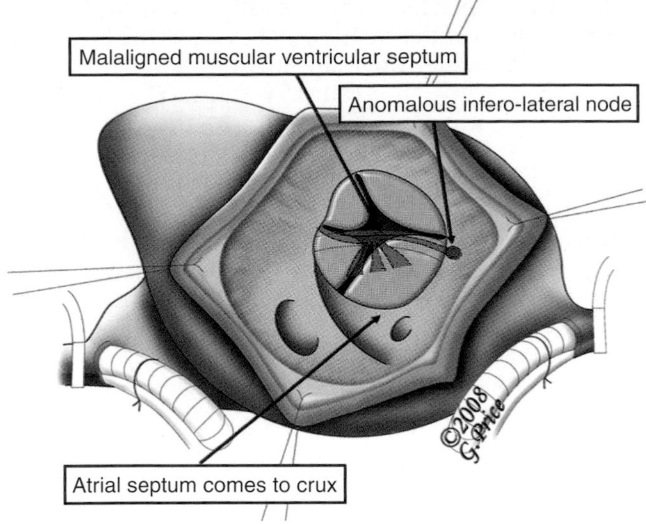

Figure 27-22 When there is malalignment of the atrial septum relative to the muscular septum, the atrioventricular node is formed at the point where the muscular ventricular septum meets the atrioventricular junction.

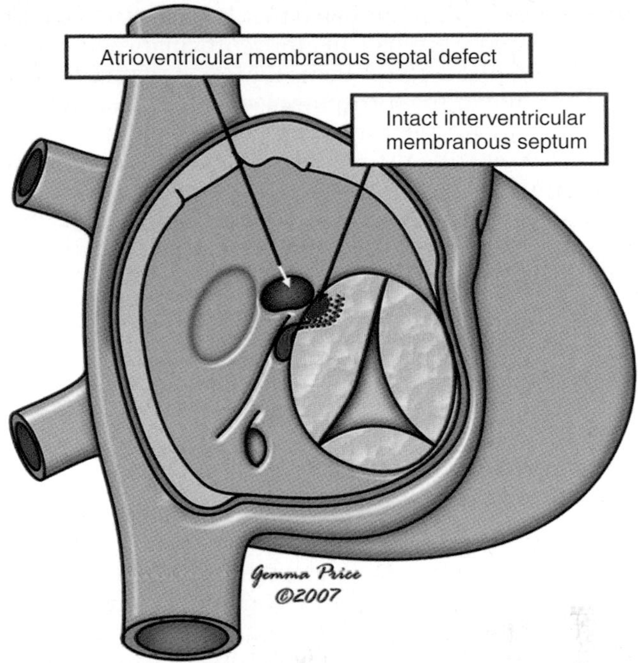

Figure 27-23 The cartoon shows the essence of the Gerbode defect, which is a deficiency of the atrioventricular component of the membranous septum, but with separate atrioventricular junctions.

without courting damage to the underlying conduction tissues. The left ventricular outflow tract, by virtue of its unwedged location, is unrelated to the conduction axis. This feature eliminates the risk of surgical damage compared with the normal heart should removal be attempted of the obstructing lesions.

Related Lesions

Having defined the anatomical hallmarks of atrioventricular septal defect with common atrioventricular junction, it is possible to highlight other lesions with some similar features, but which do not fit into the group as defined because they do not possess a common atrioventricular junction. This distinction is particularly important for the epidemiologist because, in the past, such lesions have often been described as atrioventricular canal defects. It is also important because some of the hearts described do, indeed, show evidence of deficient atrioventricular septation, albeit with separate atrioventricular junctions. The most obvious lesion falling into the category of deficient septation is the heart with a normally located subaortic outlet, but with absent or deficient atrioventricular component of the membranous septum (Fig. 27-23).[2] Such defects permit shunting from left ventricle to right atrium, but only because there are separate right and left atrioventricular junctions. They have a normally wedged subaortic outflow tract, and they are very rare.[40]

Closely related are the hearts with separate right and left atrioventricular junctions and normally wedged aorta, but with direct shunting across a perimembranous ventricular septal defect into the right atrium because of anomalous attachment of the leaflets of the tricuspid valve (Fig. 27-24).[41] It is the presence of a mitral valve guarding a discrete left atrioventricular junction that distinguishes them from atrioventricular septal defects with common atrioventricular junction. This distinction holds equally good for hearts having a perimembranous inlet ventricular septal defect and a cleft in the aortic leaflet of an otherwise normally structured mitral valve. This lesion, the so-called isolated cleft, is often considered to be directly related to atrioventricular septal defects. It may, indeed, have some developmental affinities.[42] The anatomical arrangements underscoring the two lesions, nonetheless, are quite different. The two are unequivocally distinguished when the separate right and left atrioventricular junctions are recognised in the setting of the isolated cleft.[43]

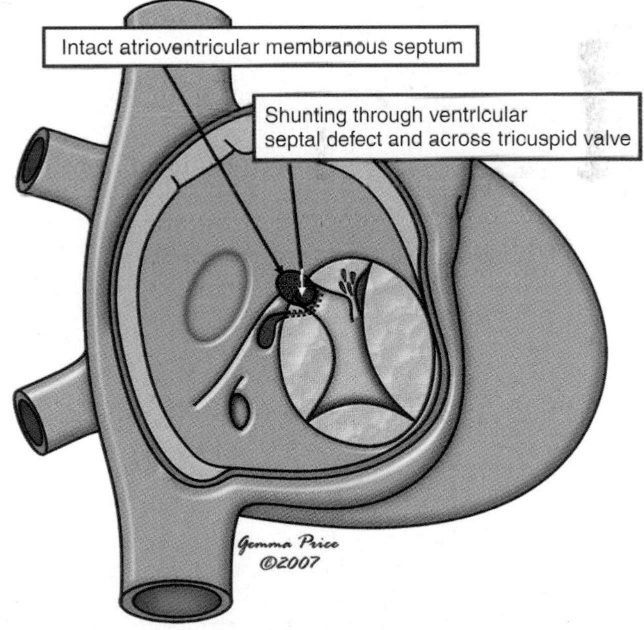

Figure 27-24 In this cartoon, we show how ventriculo-atrial shunting can also occur through a perimembranous ventricular septal defect when there is an associated deficiency of the septal leaflet of the tricuspid valve. The phenotypic feature of this lesion, however, is the presence of separate atrioventricular junctions.

It also used to be considered that hearts with straddling of the tricuspid valve had an atrioventricular canal-type of ventricular septal defect.[44] Again, the lesions with straddling and overriding of the tricuspid valve have some features in common with atrioventricular septal defect, namely, valvar leaflets that override the septum, and they do lack normal atrioventricular septal structures. The presence of separate right and left atrioventricular junctions, nonetheless, serves once more to distinguish the straddling right valve from the entity with common atrioventricular junction.

In summary, therefore, it is the presence of the common atrioventricular junction that is the anatomical hallmark of all the hearts with deficient atrioventricular septation that are to be discussed further in this chapter with regard to clinical diagnosis and treatment.

MORPHOGENESIS

In the past, the starting point when considering the morphogenesis of atrioventricular septal defects was usually the assumption that the atrioventricular endocardial cushions contributed markedly to the formation of the septal structures that are lacking in the malformed hearts, and also to the atrioventricular valvar leaflets.[45] It was because of these assumptions that endocardial cushion defect came to enjoy some popularity as a descriptive term. The concepts underscoring this approach do not bear rigorous examination, neither from the stance of embryological evidence, nor on the basis of the anatomy of the definitive lesions. It is very attractive to argue that complete failure of fusion of the endocardial cushions will result in the so-called complete defect. Partial failure of fusion could then, arguably, result in the ostium primum, or partial, defect and, in similar fashion, account for the cleft in the aortic leaflet of the mitral valve. But something much more fundamental must happen to produce the group of hearts under discussion. We have already seen how their anatomy differs from the normal state in far more respects than presence of a simple hole in the septum, coupled with a cleft in the aortic leaflet of the mitral valve. Indeed, the very fact that isolated clefts in the aortic leaflet of the mitral valve do exist, but have markedly different anatomy from the group under discussion, is additional strong evidence that the abnormal development is more than simple failure of fusion of the embryonic endocardial cushions.

It could well be that an initial failure of fusion of the cushions is the first step in the production of an atrioventricular septal defect. But the cushions do not go on to produce all the valvar leaflets together with the atrioventricular septal structures. Formation of the valvar leaflets is a very late developmental event. It occurs predominantly by undermining of ventricular myocardium, a fact well known to German embryologists and anatomists in the 19th century.[46,47] Thus, the abnormal atrioventricular valvar leaflets found in atrioventricular septal defects with common atrioventricular junction will be produced and sculpted, in part, from the grossly abnormal ventricular mass. It is the abnormal architecture of the ventricles, specifically their junction with the atriums, which is the anatomical hallmark of this lesion. When searching for the mechanism that results in the development of a common atrioventricular junction, therefore, it is necessary to direct attention to the formation of the junctional regions. This is where it is important to understand the initial function of the atrioventricular endocardial cushions. They act as the forerunner of the atrioventricular valves in early development, serving also to glue together the central point of the developing atrioventricular junctions. Only after the superior and inferior aspects of the junction have been stuck together can the aortic outflow tract be incorporated into the developing left ventricle (see Chapter 3). The leaflets of the mitral and tricuspid valves are then subsequently delaminated from the ventricular walls, or else sculpted in part from the fused cushions, but in the setting of a normally wedged subaortic outflow tract. If the endocardial cushions do not fuse together, or if there is an intrinsic abnormality in the formation of the atrioventricular junctions, this focal point for subsequent development of the ventricles is lost. The atrioventricular junctions will not grow as separate left and right components, with a septum and the subaortic outflow tract interposed between them. Instead, the superior and inferior margins of the junctions will spring apart, or else will retain their initial common appearance. The subaortic outflow tract will not then be incorporated appropriately into the developing left ventricle. It is the persistence of the initial common arrangement of the atrioventricular junction, therefore, which will produce the prototypic ventricular mass of an atrioventricular septal defect with common atrioventricular junction. The maldevelopment will also explain the presence of the basic septal defect itself. This is because, in the normal heart, the fusing cushions also provide the focal point for appropriate development and alignment of the atrial and ventricular septal structures. In the absence of such a keystone, the precise type of atrioventricular septal defect formed will then depend upon the way in which the atrioventricular valvar leaflets are delaminated, and developed, from the abnormal ventricular mass. In this respect, it should be remembered that a tongue of valvar tissue joins together the bridging leaflets in the ostium primum defect. Paradoxically, therefore, a lesion often presumed to develop because of failure of fusion of endocardial cushions has continuity of valvar tissue through the centre of the common junction. Consequently, although the initial insult resulting in an atrioventricular septal defect may well prove to be failure of fusion of the endocardial cushions, it is simplistic to suggest that the septal defect and valvar malformations all result from failure of the development of tissue derived from the atrioventricular endocardial cushions.

As yet, the tissues derived from the cushions have still to be determined with certainty. The abnormality, furthermore, involves more than the atrioventricular endocardial cushions themselves. Recent studies of developing mice show that other mesenchymal tissues around the embryonic primary atrial foramen are involved in its closure. These include a mesenchymal cap on the leading edge of the primary atrial septum, together with a mound of tissue, with its own mesenchymal covering, that grows into the heart from the posterior mediastinum. This latter structure, the vestibular spine, was discovered by His in 1880,[48] but disappeared from consideration for some considerable time before its recent resurrection.[49–52] The vestibular spine, the primary atrial septum, and the endocardial cushions themselves, are all abnormal in mice with trisomy 16, which have deficient atrioventricular septation and a common atrioventricular junction.[53] Unlike the arrangement as typically seen in humans, however, the trisomic mice have the common atrioventricular junction exclusively connected within the left ventricle, typically in association with abnormal ventriculo-arterial connections.[53] Further study of this mouse model,[51] and other abnormal mice that have deficient atrioventricular septation,[52] will undoubtedly clarify very soon the morphogenesis of atrioventricular septal defect with common atrioventricular junction. Such studies are also likely to identify the genes involved in normal and abnormal development. It will be necessary, nonetheless, to take careful note of the precise structure of the cardiac abnormalities produced in these experimental animals in order to make appropriate inferences for the situation pertaining in human maldevelopment.

PATHOPHYSIOLOGY

Atrial Shunting

There is almost always an atrial component of the defect, the so-called ostium primum defect, across which there is a left-to-right shunt. In about one-third of patients, even those with separate right and left atrioventricular valvar orifices, there is also a small right-to-left shunt. When the atrial septum is malaligned leftwards in relation to the common atrioventricular junction, a proportion of the systemic venous blood is directed into the left ventricle, and thus into the aorta. In those in whom the atrial septum is virtually absent, often described as common atrium, there is usually admixture of the systemic and pulmonary venous returns. This is largely because of the absence of a septum, but it is also, in part, because of the high incidence of anomalous venous connections, particularly in hearts from patients having isomerism of the atrial appendages. In the latter setting, with isomeric right appendages, the blood from a left-sided superior caval vein, if present, empties directly into the left upper corner of the atrium instead of flowing into the coronary sinus and thence into the right-sided atrium. The coronary sinus, of course, is absent in the setting of right isomerism, so perforce coronary venous blood must drain directly into the atrial cavities. As a result a mild degree of undersaturation is not uncommon in patients with right isomerism also having an atrioventricular septal defect.

Ventricular Shunting

If there is an unobstructed ventricular component to the defect, the direction of flow through it will depend upon resistance to outflow from the two ventricles. Subaortic stenosis, or aortic coarctation, will favour left-to-right shunting, whereas obstruction of the right ventricular outflow tract or pulmonary vascular obstructive disease will favour right-to-left shunting. When none of these complicating factors is present, the shunt is left-to-right, as in simple ventricular septal defect.

Ventriculo-atrial Shunting

Ventriculo-atrial shunting is a phenomenon that is found most typically in patients with deficient atrioventricular septation. In all those with a common atrioventricular junction, ventriculo-atrial shunting can occur during ventricular systole through the zones of apposition between the bridging leaflets, should they be regurgitant. Such shunting is seen in more than half of all patients, irrespective of the valvar morphology. Significant shunting, however, associated with regurgitation across abnormal valves, is seen in a smaller proportion, perhaps one-fifth. The ventriculo-atrial shunting, best revealed with colour flow Doppler interrogation, usually tracks from left ventricle to right atrium. Right ventricular to left atrial shunting is uncommon, but when present adds to the arterial undersaturation.

Volume Loading

A left-to-right shunt at atrial level produces right ventricular volume overload, whereas a ventricular shunt in this direction primarily overloads the left ventricle. In patients with a common valvar orifice, volume overload of both ventricles is the rule. In those with a restrictive atrial component of the defect, left ventricular volume load will predominate, whereas restriction to left ventricular inflow will lead to a predominant right ventricular volume overload.

The leaflets guarding the common atrioventricular junction are often regurgitant, particularly in older patients, be there a common valvar orifice or separate ones for the right and left ventricles.[54] Such regurgitation can occur across either the left or right sides of the effectively common atrioventricular valve, but left-sided regurgitation is more important clinically because of its effect upon the systemic ventricle. This regurgitation, when present, produces further volume overloading of the ventricles. Although it is convenient, in order better to understand the pathophysiology, to separate the septal defects from valvar regurgitation, in reality the two are inseparable. For example, the regurgitant jet through the left atrioventricular valve is frequently directed toward the right atrium, thereby having a similar haemodynamic effect as a communication from the left ventricle to the right atrium. If there were such a thing as a pure shunt from left ventricle to right atrium in a patient with an atrioventricular septal defect, it would be obligatory, since it would not depend on pulmonary vascular resistance.[55] Excessive flow through the left and right components of the common atrioventricular junction occurs both because of the left-to-right shunts and because of the valvar regurgitation.

Pressure Loading

The right ventricular pressure is most commonly elevated because of an unobstructed ventricular component of the atrioventricular septal defect. Right ventricular hypertension, however, can also reflect increased left atrial pressure and pulmonary hypertension. This can be produced, for example, by an associated partition within the left atrium, or by left-sided malalignment of the atrial relative to the ventricular septum, with an associated obstructive interatrial communication. Such right ventricular hypertension is also seen in some patients with isolated atrial shunting, when there is a large left-to-right shunt and increased flow of blood to the lungs. Included amongst these patients will be those with stenosis of or regurgitation across the left atrioventricular valve. An alternative cause for pulmonary hypertension in this setting is the presence of an obligatory shunt from left ventricle to right atrium. This also produces, effectively, a large left-to-right shunt.

A raised pulmonary arterial pressure, therefore, is a feature of patients having atrioventricular septal defects with large ventricular components. In those with shunting exclusively at atrial or ventriculo-atrial levels, it is caused by high pulmonary blood flow, or obstruction to pulmonary venous return. Elevated flow to the lungs, and increased right ventricular pressures, are instrumental in the development of obstructive pulmonary vascular disease. This develops earlier than is usually the case for those having an isolated ventricular septal defect. It is now accepted that this tendency is further accentuated in the presence of Down's syndrome because of the susceptibility of such patients to obstruction of the upper airways and associated alveolar hypoventilation. This tendency to more rapid progression of pulmonary vascular disease is one of the reasons underscoring the trend to earlier surgical intervention for those patients with a common atrioventricular valvar orifice. Most centres would now elect to operate on such patients within the first 6 months of life.

PRESENTATION AND SYMPTOMATOLOGY

In the current era of routine screening of patients deemed at high risk, such as those with Down's syndrome, and increasing likelihood of prenatal diagnosis, the full clinical picture as described in this section is encountered in an ever decreasing number of patients. Patients with large ventricular components to the septal defect, severe left atrioventricular valvar regurgitation, significant left ventricular hypoplasia, or complicating associated lesions such as aortic coarctation, present with severe cardiac failure in early infancy. If the ventricular component was the only problem, there would be a latent period of 1 to 2 months occurring after birth but prior to presentation. Those with both ventricular and atrial components tend to present earlier, due to the more rapid increase in left-to-right shunting. In a number of infants, however, pulmonary vascular resistance remains high after birth, and they may present late due to a lack of symptoms in infancy. This is a documented risk in the setting of Down's syndrome. As a result of routine screening programmes for cardiac disease in these children, development of Eisenmenger's syndrome is nowadays rare. Patients without these complicating factors, typically those with separate atrioventricular valvar orifices and the potential for shunting exclusively at atrial level, often escape detection of their cardiac disease in infancy. They then present during childhood with an incidental murmur or, in those with a common atrium, with mild cyanosis. In rare instances, they may not present until adolescence or adult life.

CLINICAL FINDINGS

In those patients with separate atrioventricular valvar orifices and shunting confined exclusively at atrial level, the clinical findings are as expected for simple interatrial communications within the oval fossa (see Chapter 25). Consequently, infants and children are usually free from symptoms, although some may have recurrent chest infections. On auscultation, wide splitting of the second heart sound is the most characteristic feature, although, in infants and younger children, the split may not be fixed. An ejection systolic murmur, of grade 2 or 3, is typically heard, being maximal at the upper left sternal edge. When there is a large right-to-left shunt, a mid-systolic rumble may also be audible at the lower left sternal edge.

In the presence of a common atrioventricular valvar orifice, or significant ventricular shunting, failure to thrive and signs of congestive heart failure are frequent during early infancy. These patients usually present within the first 3 months of life. Recurrent chest infections are also encountered. The typical findings on clinical examination are an undernourished infant with tachycardia, tachypnoea, and hepatomegaly. The praecordium is hyperactive, and a systolic thrill is sometimes palpated at the lower left sternal border. The first heart sound is accentuated, with the second sound being narrowly split, its pulmonary component having an increased intensity. Murmurs heard can vary markedly, from a short murmur graded at 2 out of 6, and a soft ejection systolic murmur at the mid-to-lower left sternal border in those with a large ventricular septal defect and elevated pulmonary vascular resistance, to a pansystolic murmur graded at 4 out of 6 due to ventricular shunting and heard at the same site. Not infrequently, a soft mid-diastolic murmur is heard at the left lower sternal edge or the apex, reflecting increased flow across the common atrioventricular valve.

These cardinal physical findings reflecting differences in the specific anatomy may then be modified by the presence of atrioventricular valvar regurgitation. This can produce symptoms of a large left-to-right shunt and congestive heart failure, even in an infant with shunting exclusively at atrial level. The valvar regurgitation will be associated with a pansystolic murmur heard maximally between the lower left sternal edge and the apex. In this setting, there may also be a prominent mid-diastolic apical murmur due to flow. Presence of associated malformations can further modify these findings. Cyanosis, for example, could reflect abnormal systemic venous drainage, common mixing at atrial level, or co-existing tetralogy of Fallot.

As indicated in the previous section, infancy is occasionally uneventful, particularly in those patients with Down's syndrome. The patient can then present later in childhood with Eisenmenger's syndrome. Such patients are cyanotic, and the systolic and diastolic murmurs noted above are usually reduced or absent. Such an absence of murmurs is less likely than in those with isolated ventricular septal defects, for example, because of the frequency of atrioventricular valvar regurgitation. Pulmonary valvar closure is even more accentuated, and the second heart sound may become single. An early diastolic murmur of pulmonary regurgitation may supervene.

In patients with very little shunting, clinical symptoms are limited to atrioventricular valvar regurgitation, which can become clinically manifest in adult life. The same goes in all probability for the very rare patients having a common atrioventricular junction but with intact septal structures.

INVESTIGATIONS

Chest Radiography

The heart and aortic arch are usually on the left. There is generalised cardiac enlargement in proportion to the volume overload of the two ventricles. Because of the frequent atrioventricular valvar regurgitation, the heart may be enlarged even in the absence of a left-to-right shunt. The heart may be enlarged, therefore, even when there is severe obstruction in the right ventricular outflow tract or pulmonary vascular obstructive disease, or when the septal structures are intact. The pulmonary trunk is prominent, and the peripheral vasculature is engorged except in the presence of obstruction within the right ventricular outflow tract. High kilovoltage filtered beam chest radiography may show left bronchial isomerism. If this is discovered, then interruption of the inferior caval vein, common atrium, or both, should be suspected.

Electrocardiography

A highly distinctive pattern of abnormalities is usually evident from the electrocardiographic tracings. The P wave is usually normal, except in the presence of isomerism of the left atrial appendages, when a superior P wave axis is usually found. Prolongation of the PR interval is found in over nine-tenths of patients with common valvar orifice, and in almost three-quarters of those with separate right and left atrioventricular valvar orifices. The superiorly orientated frontal QRS loop is manifested by dominant S waves in leads III and aVF, and prominent R waves in aVR (Fig. 27-25). When the frontal QRS loop is displayed or constructed, it is seen to run counter-clockwise. The further the frontal axis is deviated upwards and to the right, the deeper the scooping of the ventricular septum, and the more likely there is to be a common valvar orifice.[56,57] In nine-tenths of patients, the initial portion of the QRS loop is directed downward and to the right. This characteristic feature serves to distinguish patients with atrioventricular septal defects and common junction from those other lesions with a superiorly orientated and counter-clockwise frontal plane loop. Amongst this group, tricuspid atresia is easily distinguished by the lack of right ventricular forces in the precordial leads. In atrioventricular septal defects, a delay in right ventricular depolarisation is almost invariable, indicating right ventricular volume overload. A qR pattern in the right precordial leads in the presence of an otherwise typical electrocardiogram suggests left ventricular hypoplasia. This feature also occurs in one-fifth of patients with common orifice without other complicating features. The superiorly orientated frontal axis frequently prevents left ventricular hypertrophy from manifesting itself on the precordial leads. Prolongation of the QRS interval occurs in three-fifths of patients with common orifice, and in nearly two-fifths of those with separate right and left valvar orifices.

Echocardiography

Cross sectional echocardiography should provide a complete morphological diagnosis in all children with common atrioventricular junction and atrioventricular septal defect. Although the recognition of the presence of an atrioventricular septal defect is usually quite easy, even for those inexperienced in the analysis of congenitally malformed hearts, the complete delineation of all the relevant features requires considerable skill and knowledge.

The start to a successful complete morphological diagnosis is knowledge of the cardinal anatomic features.[15] Absence of the atrioventricular septum is not unique to those with atrioventricular septal defects, but some other features are. The disproportion between the inlet and outlet dimensions of the ventricular mass results in deviation of the plane of the left atrioventricular orifice and valve as seen in the views showing the ventricular short axis. As a consequence, the standard basal view through the short axis of the left ventricle will cut the left atrioventricular valve in an oblique fashion, while the standard parasternal long-axis view does not section the point of maximal opening of the valve. If the latter plane is obtained, part of the left atrioventricular valve appears to be floating in the left ventricular outflow tract.

The unwedged position of the aorta, together with the relatively elongated left ventricular outflow tract, produces

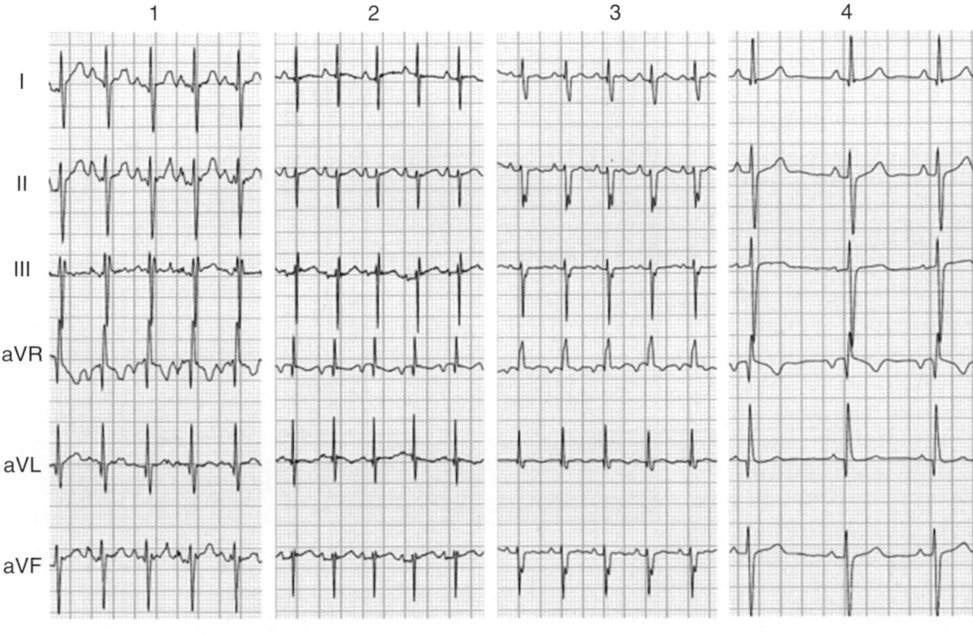

Figure 27-25 The frontal leads of these electrocardiograms display a variable leftward deviation of the frontal axis in four different patients, indicating variable depth of the scoop of the ventricular septum. The prolongation of the PR interval is also a typical feature of patients having atrioventricular septal defect with common atrioventricular junction.

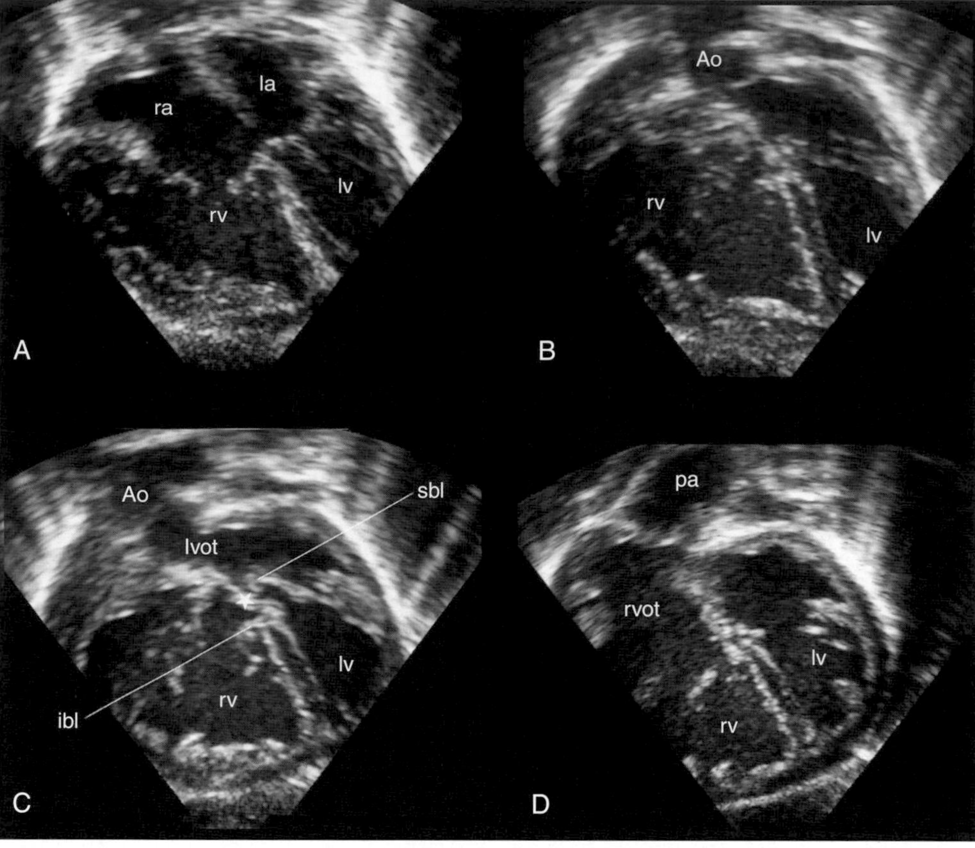

Figure 27-26 These images are from a subcostal scan from a patient with separate atrioventricular orifices. Imaging starts in a subcostal four-chamber plane (**A**) depicting the right and left atrium (ra and la) the lack of off-setting of the atrioventricular valves, and a small atrial component of the defect. The transducer is tilted to show the aortic valve, which only appears when the left atrium is no longer in the imaging plane, indicating the unwedged position of the aortic root (**B**). Slight additional tilting (**C**) shows the gooseneck deformity of the left ventricular outflow tract (lvot), the superior (sbl) and inferior (ibl) bridging leaflets, and the tongue of tissue (*star*) connecting the bridging leaflets and separating the two orifices. Additional tilting (**D**) demonstrates the right ventricular outflow tract and the pulmonary trunk. All images are taken at the end of diastole. Ao, aorta; lv, left ventricle; pa, pulmonary trunk; rv, right ventricle; rvot, right ventricular outflow tract.

the classic gooseneck appearance of the left ventricular outflow tract, which is usually apparent only in angulated subcostal paracoronal planes. A standard view showing the four chambers together with the aortic root, erroneously referred to as five-chamber view, therefore, can never be obtained in a patient with an atrioventricular septal defect and common atrioventricular junction. The left side of the atrioventricular valve is trifoliate. This is easily seen in a subcostal paracoronal plane taken a little to the right of the one displaying the gooseneck. In practise, scans rather than planes will reveal all the features necessary for the diagnosis, the subcostal approach being the most informative (Fig. 27-26).

Colour flow Doppler interrogation complements the anatomical investigation by demonstrating the sites of intracardiac shunting, and the presence or absence of atrioventricular valvar regurgitation and pulmonary hypertension, as well as pin-pointing any obstructions within the ventricular outflow tracts. Pulsed and continuous wave Doppler are used for quantitative measurements. Interventricular shunting at very low velocity readily establishes any elevation of right ventricular pressures, but pulsed or continuous wave Doppler interrogation is needed to calculate the difference in pressures between the ventricles. As in patients with isolated ventricular septal defects, it is usually possible to estimate both the flow of blood to the lungs and pulmonary vascular resistance. A regurgitant jet across the right atrioventricular valve with high velocity may be the result of left ventricular to right atrial shunting (Fig. 27-27). This type of shunting is relatively common, and although readily appreciated in the presence of a ventricular septal defect, may lead to the erroneous conclusion of right ventricular hypertension in those patients with shunting exclusively at atrial level, or after surgical closure of the defect.

Because patients with atrioventricular septal defects frequently have isomerism of the atrial appendages, it is important precisely to determine the atrial arrangement,

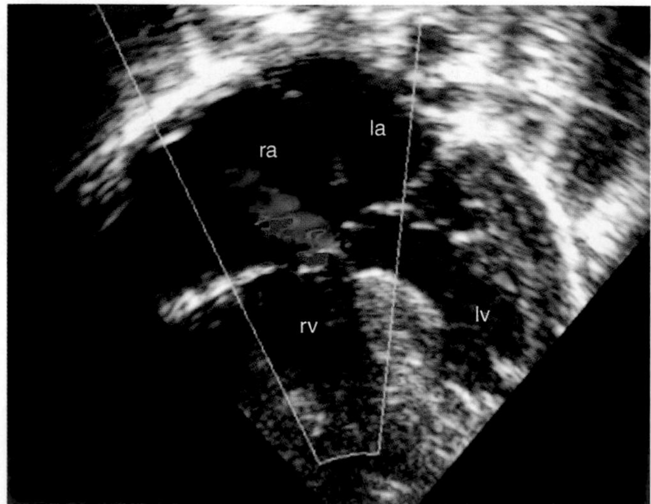

Figure 27-27 This systolic frame from a subcostal four-chamber image with colour flow mapping demonstrates shunting from left ventricle (lv) to right atrium (ra). The colour flow jet may be misinterpreted as right atrioventricular valvar incompetence. la, left atrium; rv, right ventricle.

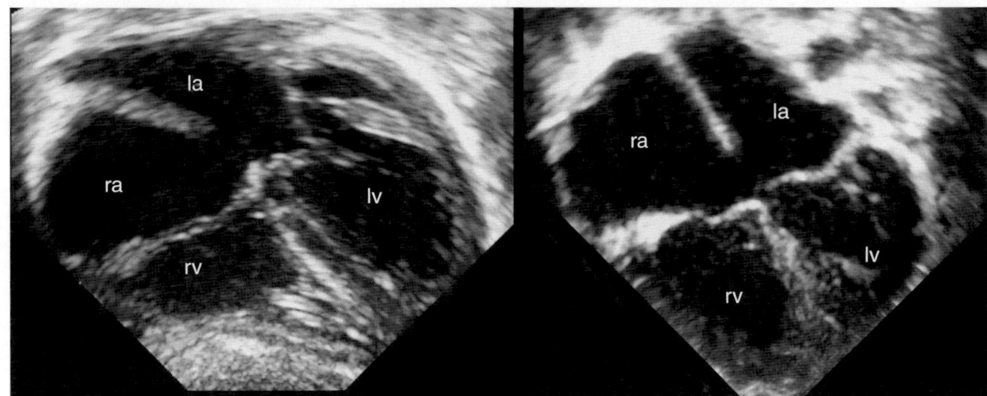

Figure 27-28 Both of these four-chamber images show the classic appearance of an atrioventricular septal defect with separate atrioventricular valvar orifices and potential for atrial shunting only, the so-called ostium primum atrial septal defect. Subcostal four-chamber image (*left*) and apical four-chamber image (*right*). Both images are taken at the end of diastole. la, left atrium; lv, left ventricle; ra, right atrium; rv, right ventricle.

as well as the ventricular topology. Elevated pulmonary vascular resistance can usually be excluded by appropriate Doppler interrogation of the flow to the lungs.

Separate Valvar Orifices

Separate valvar orifices within a common junction are the consequence of a tongue of valvar tissue joining together the facing surfaces of the bridging valvar leaflets (see Fig. 27-26). Almost always there is an interatrial communication between the leading edge of the atrial septum and the crest of the ventricular septum, to which the bridging leaflets are usually connected. Consequently, there is absence of the normal off-setting of the leaflets, and no potential for ventricular shunting. Historically, such a lesion was called an ostium primum atrial septal defect, but since the shunting is across an atrioventricular septal defect, the disadvantages of this usage are obvious.

Standard four-chamber sections readily demonstrate the atrioventricular septal defect, limited on one side by the atrioventricular valvar apparatus, and on the other side by the leading edge of the atrial septum (Fig. 27-28). The other key diagnostic features are the trifoliate configuration of the left atrioventricular valve, well seen in the subcostal or high parasternal short-axis sections of the left ventricular inlet (Fig. 27-29), and the gooseneck-like elongation of the left ventricular outflow tract. This latter feature is best seen in subcostal long-axis sections of the left ventricle (Fig. 27-30). It is more prominent in hearts with separate right and left atrioventricular valves, where the attachment of the superior bridging leaflet to the ventricular septum accentuates the nature of the body of the goose (see Fig. 27-30). The skilled echocardiographer readily distinguishes the less common variants in patients having an atrioventricular septal defect with common atrioventricular junction, but with separate atrioventricular valvar orifices. When there is complete absence of any interatrial communication, and four-chamber sections demonstrate an interventricular communication opening to the inlet of the right ventricle, it is lack of off-setting between left and right atrioventricular orifices and, again, the trifoliate arrangement of the left atrioventricular valve that give the diagnostic clues (Fig. 27-31). This feature distinguishes those with an atrioventricular septal defect from others with an isolated perimembranous ventricular septal defect opening to the inlet of the right ventricle. Occasionally, a left atrioventricular valve with three leaflets may be the only manifestation of patients having an atrioventricular

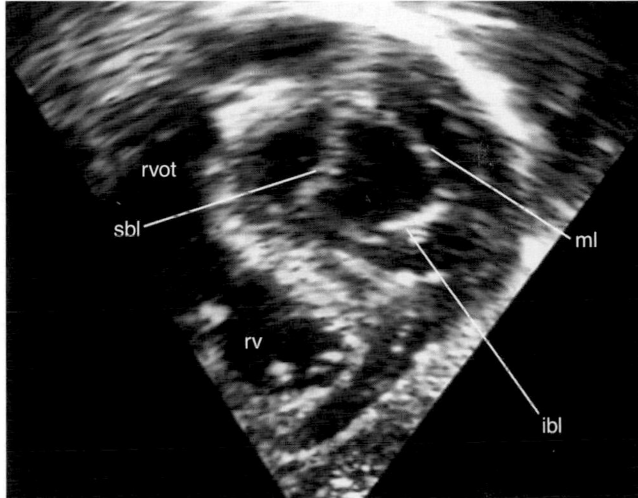

Figure 27-29 This subcostal short-axis image of the left atrioventricular valve is from a patient with an atrioventricular septal defect with common junction and separate atrioventricular valvar orifices. The three leaflets are best visualised in a slightly angulated paracoronal plane, which as in this example is usually closer to the right ventricular outflow tract (rvot) view than to the left ventricular basal short-axis view. Compare with the right image of Figure 27-31. ibl, inferior bridging leaflet; ml, mural leaflet; rv, right ventricle; sbl, superior bridging leaflet.

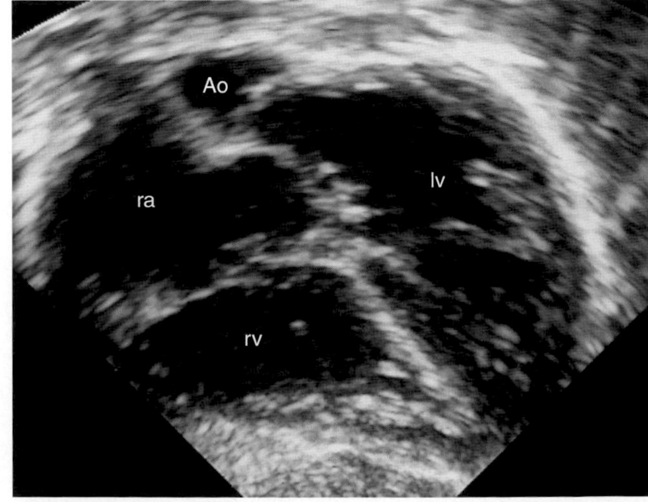

Figure 27-30 This angulated subcostal paracoronal image shows well the body of the goose. The plane is almost comparable to that shown in Figure 27-26B, but has been obtained with slight clockwise rotation. Ao, aorta; lv, left ventricle; ra, right atrium; rv, right ventricle.

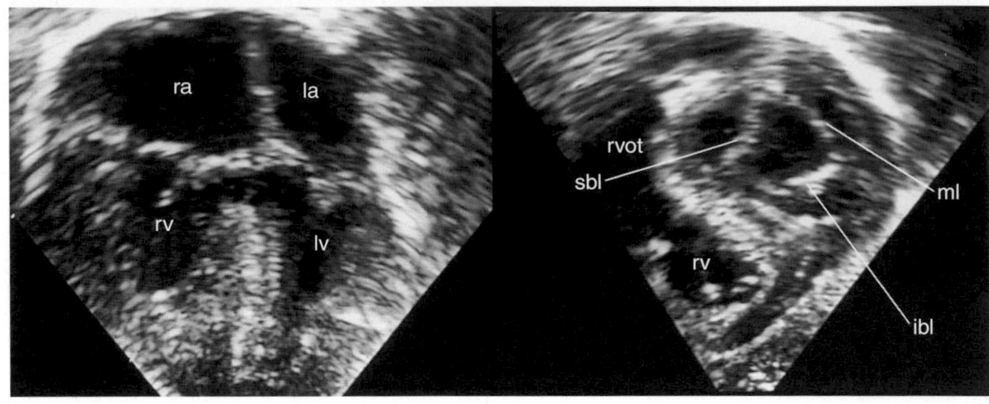

Figure 27-31 This image is from a patient with an atrioventricular septal defect with separate atrioventricular valve orifices and an intact atrial septum. There is only a potential for ventricular shunting, as is apparent from the left image, which also shows the lack of off-setting of the atrioventricular valves. The right image demonstrates the trifoliate configuration of the left atrioventricular valve in a right ventricular outflow tract (rvot) subcostal plane (see also Fig. 27-29). ibl, inferior bridging leaflet; la, left atrium; lv, left ventricle; ml, mural leaflet; ra, right atrium; rv, right ventricle; sbl, superior bridging leaflet.

septal defect with common atrioventricular junction, the atrial and ventricular septal structures being intact. Such patients may well present as having mitral regurgitation, with the true nature of their spontaneously closed atrioventricular septal defect not initially being recognised. The diagnostic echocardiographic hallmarks, however, are the same as for the other forms of atrioventricular septal defect.[58,59] Other less common variants found with separate atrioventricular valvar orifices, such as common atrium and so-called double outlet left or right atrium (Fig. 27-32), are easily recognised in a complete echocardiographic examination.

Additional abnormalities of the trifoliate left atrioventricular valve are frequently encountered in patients having an atrioventricular septal defect and separate valvar orifices. Varying degrees of valvar regurgitation may occur, and often shunting may be from left ventricle to right atrium (see Fig. 27-27). Because of the presence of an interatrial communication, significant enlargement of the left atrium is unusual, even in the presence of severe valvar regurgitation. The presence of a large interatrial communication also precludes demonstration of any gradient between the left atrium and left ventricle. The quantitative assessment of valvar stenosis, in that setting, cannot be made with Doppler echocardiography. Since stenosis usually is the result of morphologic variants such as dual orifice left atrioventricular valve, or marked hypoplasia or absence of the mural leaflet (Fig. 27-33), the recognition of these variants is of crucial importance. A dual orifice within the left valve is a well-recognised abnormality, in which colour flow Doppler may demonstrate two discrete profiles of flow across the left-sided atrioventricular junction. This diagnosis, nonetheless, can be difficult. A bifoliate arrangement can present with a single papillary muscle in the left ventricle, easily seen on the apical left ventricular short-axis section. Double orifice or bifoliate left atrioventricular valves should always be suspected in young infants presenting with marked enlargement of the right ventricle. Severe stenosis or hypoplasia of the left atrioventricular valve is associated with hypoplasia of the left ventricle. Abnormalities of the right atrioventricular valve are less

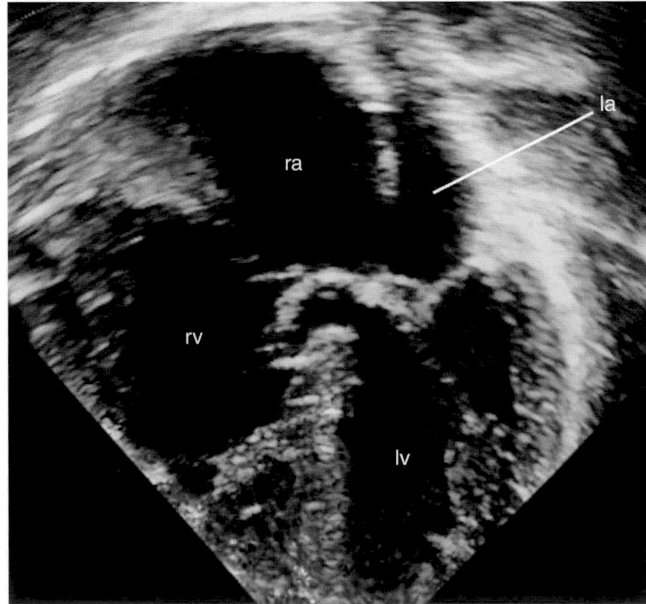

Figure 27-32 This apical four-chamber section is from a patient with separate atrioventricular orifices and so-called double outlet right atrium. This end-diastolic frame clearly shows the malalignment between the atrial septum and the muscular ventricular septum. The superior bridging leaflet is firmly attached to the right side of the ventricular septum, allowing no interventricular shunting. la, left atrium; lv, left ventricle; ra, right atrium; rv, right ventricle.

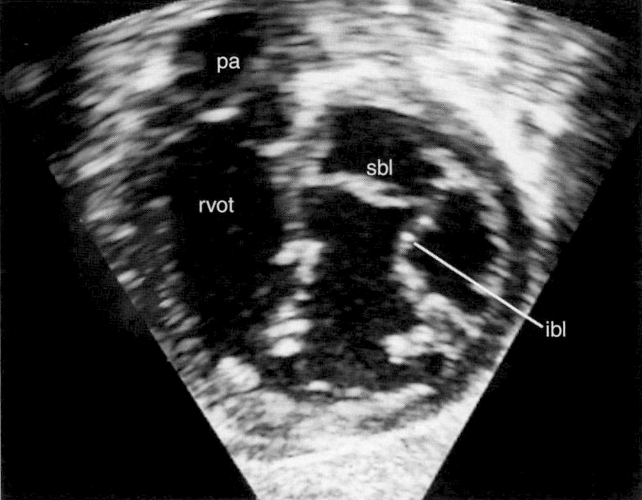

Figure 27-33 This subcostal angulated paracoronal view is from a patient with absence of the mural leaflet of the left atrioventricular valve. Although the left valve has a bifoliate appearance, it is clearly different from a normal mitral valve. This valve was supported by a single papillary muscle in the left ventricle. ibl, inferior bridging leaflet; pa, pulmonary trunk; rvot, right ventricular outflow tract; sbl, superior bridging leaflet.

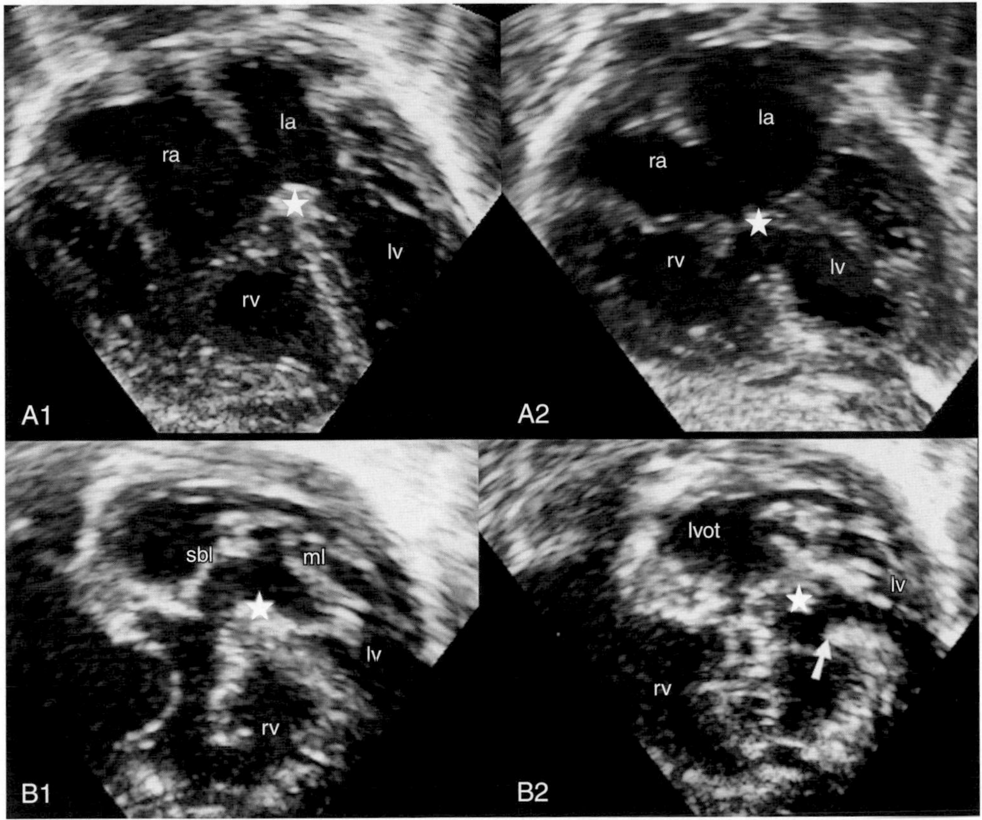

Figure 27-34 These subcostal four-chamber and paracoronal sections show the variation in size of the interventricular communication below the inferior bridging leaflet. Images **A1** and **A2** are from a case with firm attachment of the inferior bridging leaflet to the crest of the ventricular septum, allowing no interventricular shunting under this leaflet. In the case depicted in images **B1** and **B2**, a large ventricular septal defect is present beneath the inferior bridging leaflet (*star*). The *arrow* in **B2** shows the attachment of the mural leaflet in the left ventricle. la, left atrium; lv, left ventricle; lvot, left ventricular outflow tract; ml, mural leaflet; ra, right atrium; rv, right ventricle; sbl, superior bridging leaflet.

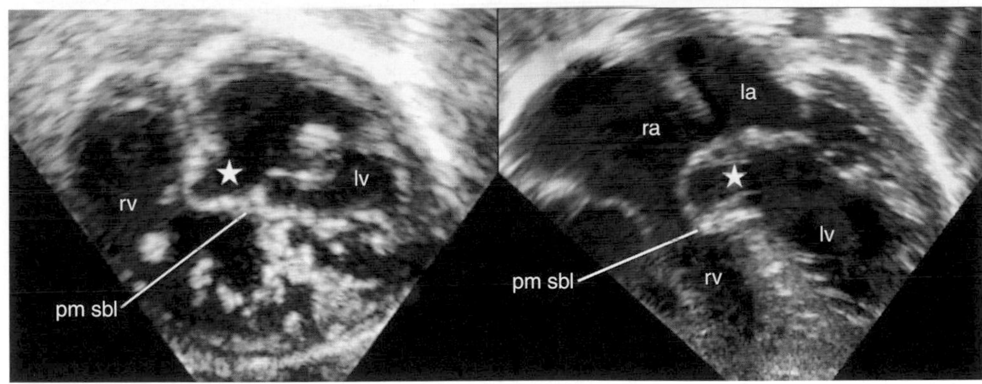

Figure 27-35 These apical four-chamber (*left*) and subcostal paracoronal (*right*) images show a patient with limited potential for shunting under the superior bridging leaflet (sbl). The superior bridging leaflet is attached to a papillary muscle (pm) on the crest of the interventricular septum, the Rastelli type A variant. In the case demonstrated here, the superior bridging leaflet is also attached by multiple cords to the crest itself. There is a slight bulging (*star*) of the leaflet towards the right ventricle at end-diastole (*left*) becoming more pronounced in systole (*right*). la, left atrium; lv, left ventricle; ra, right atrium; rv, right ventricle.

frequent, although regurgitation from the right ventricle to the right or left atrium is commonly encountered.

Common Valvar Orifice

The typical echocardiographic features of an atrioventricular septal defect with a common valvar orifice are first identified in four-chamber sections. There are usually both interatrial and interventricular communications, albeit that the sizes of the components of the defect are variable. The right ventricle is often dilated, as significant shunting at atrial level is the rule. The attachments of the bridging leaflets to the crest of the ventricular septum are variable, as is the extent of their bridging. The inferior bridging leaflet, often best visualised in the subcostal four-chamber sections, is frequently attached by a midline raphe to the crest of the ventricular septum, precluding any interventricular shunting close to the crux (Fig. 27-34). It may, however, be free-floating, and then the ventricular component will usually be evident throughout the length of the septum (see Fig. 27-34). Most variation in the size of the ventricular component, however, is seen beneath the superior bridging leaflet. This is demonstrated superiorly in subcostal paracoronal or parasternal four-chamber sections. The superior bridging leaflet may sometimes be firmly bound down to the septal crest, with no potential for shunting beneath it. This is rare. More commonly, the superior bridging leaflet is attached to a normally positioned medial papillary muscle, and is additionally attached by multiple cords to the crest of the septum (Fig. 27-35). In the four-chamber and subcostal paracoronal sections, the interventricular communication appears to be shielded by a pouch of valvar tissue, bulging towards the right ventricle during systole. There are then multiple interventricular communications through the intercordal spaces, the patterns of flow being recognised with colour flow Doppler (Fig. 27-36). This

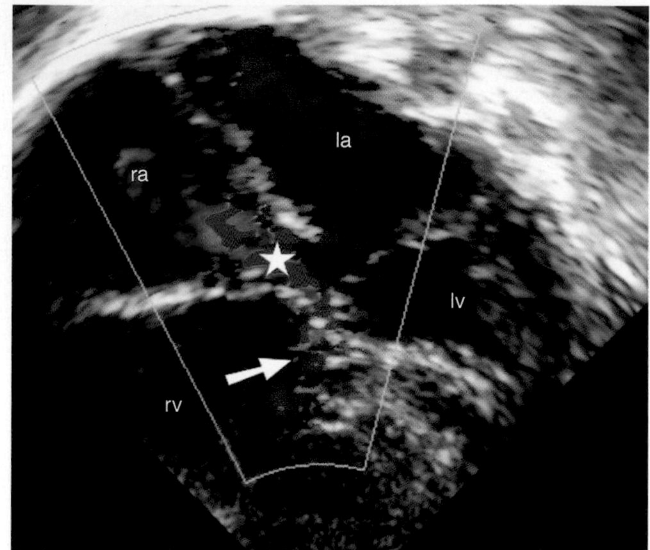

Figure 27-36 This apical four-chamber section with colour flow mapping is from a patient with limited potential for interventricular shunting under the superior bridging leaflet. The systolic frame shows a small jet of interventricular shunting (*arrow*) and a larger jet of left ventricle to right atrial shunting (*star*). (Compare also with Fig. 27-27.) la, left atrium; lv, left ventricle; ra, right atrium; rv, right ventricle.

arrangement is often dubbed the Rastelli type A lesion. Occasionally, the pouch may contain accessory valvar tissue and, as in those with isolated ventricular septal defects, such a pouch may eventually seal the defect. The so-called Rastelli type B defect, in which the papillary muscles in the right ventricle supporting the zone of apposition between the superior bridging and antero-superior leaflets is positioned in an anomalous mid-septal position, may be hard to recognise, particularly when it is associated with a very deep scoop of the muscular ventricular septum or with accessory valvar tissue. The presence of the so-called Rastelli type C defect, in which the superior leaflet is free-floating, is readily appreciated on the subcostal paracoronal planes as well as in the apical four-chamber section (Fig. 27-37). Almost always the interventricular communication is then very extensive. This pattern is always seen in association with either tetralogy of Fallot (Fig. 27-38) or double outlet right ventricle, and is also frequent in those with Down's syndrome.

The other important diagnostic feature is again the trifoliate arrangement of the left component of the common atrioventricular valve, as demonstrated in short-axis sections of the left ventricular inlet. The elongated, or gooseneck, shape of the left ventricular outflow tract is less obvious than in those with separate right and left atrioventricular valvar orifices, and in those with the Rastelli A malformation, since the superior bridging leaflet is less well attached to the septal crest (Fig. 27-39).

Possible variations in the morphology of the left part of the atrioventricular valve, albeit less common than in defects with separate atrioventricular orifices, should always be excluded. If found, they may have major implications for surgical repair. Less common variants include virtual absence of the potential for interatrial shunting when the atrial septum meets the bridging leaflets of the common valve, and absence of any ventricular component when the bridging leaflets are firmly attached to the ventricular septum. This latter variant is difficult to distinguish echocardiographically, and is clinically indistinguishable from the patients having separate atrioventricular valves and shunting confined at atrial level.

Variants Found with Either Separate Valves or a Common Valvar Orifice

An extremely important variation, usually readily recognised in four-chamber sections, is ventricular imbalance. Left ventricular hypoplasia is commonly associated with obstruction of the left ventricular outflow tract, whatever its cause, and is easily identified on four-chamber (Fig. 27-40) and long-axis sections. Right ventricular hypoplasia, by comparison is often not immediately apparent on a single image section and usually associated with atrioventricular septal malalignment, often described as double outlet atrium. This has important implications for disposition of the conduction tissues (see Fig. 27-22). Proper identification of right ventricular hypoplasia requires acquisition of image scans (Fig. 27-41). The association of tetralogy of Fallot or double outlet right ventricle does not fundamentally change the features of the common atrioventricular junction.

Isomerism of the atrial appendages is frequently found (see Chapter 22). The morphologically right ventricle may be to the right or to the left of the morphologically left ventricle, giving either right hand or left hand ventricular topology. The left hand pattern may then give the

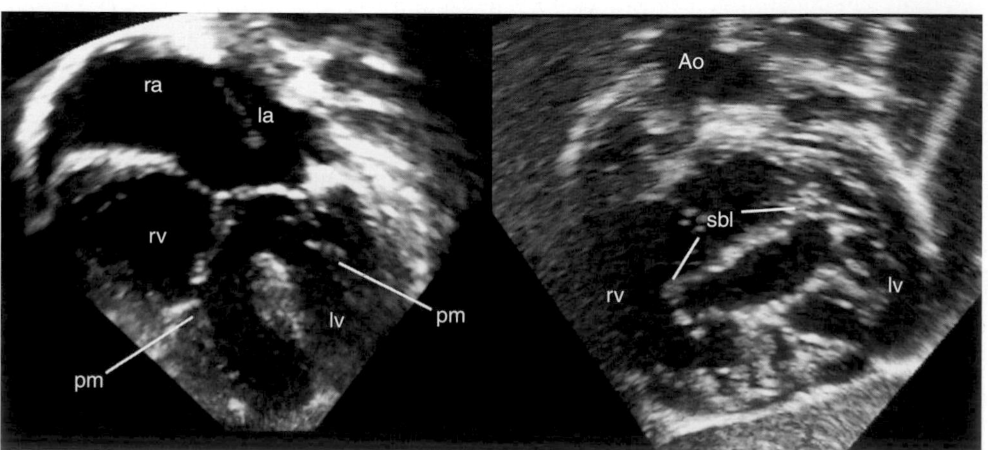

Figure 27-37 The subcostal four-chamber (*left*) and angulated paracoronal (*right*) images demonstrate a large defect under the superior bridging leaflet. The superior bridging leaflet is free floating, being attached to a papillary muscle (pm) well within the right ventricular chamber and having no connection with cords to the interventricular septum, the so-called Rastelli type C defect. (Compare with Fig. 27-38.) Ao, aorta; la, left atrium; lv, left ventricle; ra, right atrium; rv, right ventricle; sbl, superior bridging leaflet.

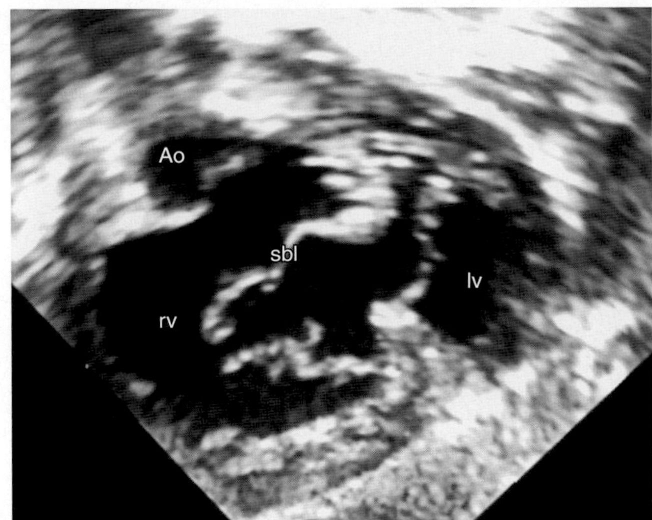

Figure 27-38 This subcostal image is from a patient with a free-floating superior bridging leaflet (Rastelli type C defect) and tetralogy of Fallot. The aorta is overriding the ventricular septal defect, which is thus limited on one side by the superior bridging leaflet and on the other side by the aortic valve. Ao, aorta; lv, left ventricle; rv, right ventricle; sbl, superior bridging leaflet.

impression of discordant atrioventricular connections (see Chapter 39). When there is isomerism of the atrial appendages co-existing with an atrioventricular septal defect, the identification of the right ventricle depends on the recognition of cords from the bridging leaflets inserting into the septum, along with the coarse apical trabeculations. In contrast, no cords insert into the left ventricular surface of the septum, and the morphologically left ventricle has paired papillary muscles.

Obstruction of the left ventricular outflow tract may or may not be associated with hypoplasia of the left ventricle. It may be caused by a particularly deep scoop of the ventricular septum, in combination with firm attachment of the superior bridging leaflet, or may be due to accessory tissue tags or fibrous ridges. The two forms can be found separately or in combination, and are identified in apical or subcostal long-axis cuts (Fig. 27-42).

Three-dimensional Echocardiography

With the rapid development of three-dimensional echocardiography, atrioventricular septal defect is among the first congenital lesions in which its value has been demonstrated.[60,61] The interest is not surprising, since many echocardiographers find the evaluation of patients with an atrioventricular septal defect extremely difficult when using cross sectional imaging. Although the obvious reason is a lack of understanding of the particular diagnostic features as described in our previous sections, three-dimensional technology does facilitate understanding. The three-dimensional representation demonstrates the common atrioventricular junction, the atrioventricular valvar leaflets, the unwedged position of the aortic valve, and the scoop of the muscular ventricular septum in a way that

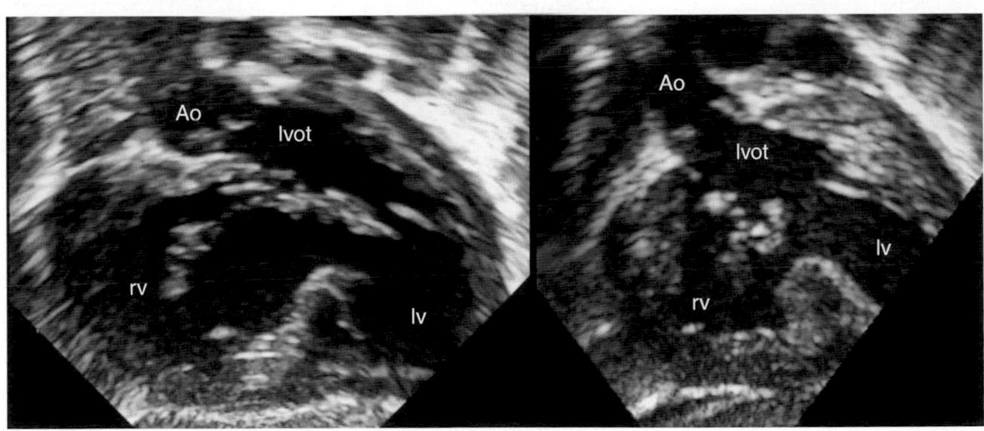

Figure 27-39 These angulated subcostal long-axis sections are taken from a patient with Rastelli type A defect (*left*). The gooseneck malformation of the left ventricular outflow tract is readily appreciated. The gooseneck is far less apparent in the right image, taken from a patient with a Rastelli type C defect. See text for further discussion. Ao, aorta; lv, left ventricle; lvot, left ventricular outflow tract; rv, right ventricle.

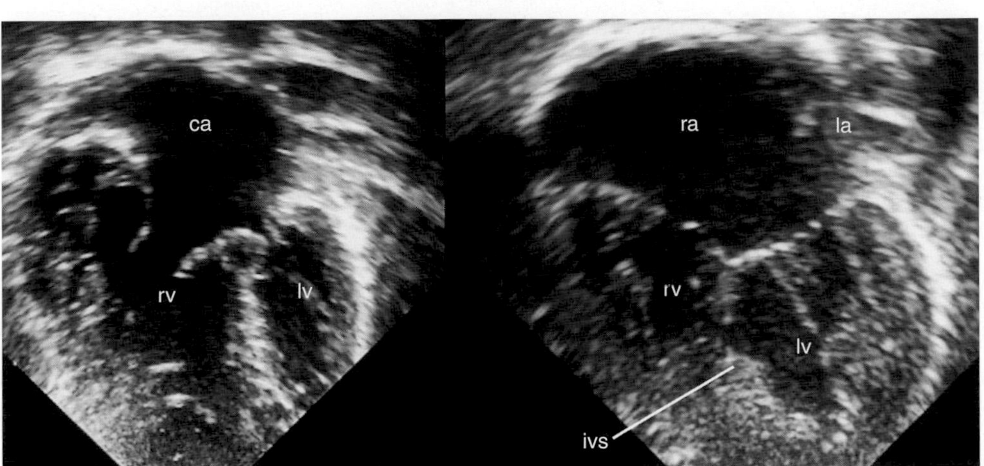

Figure 27-40 These apical four-chamber sections are from two patients with ventricular hypoplasia. The image on the left clearly shows left ventricular hypoplasia, and in addition a (surgically created) common atrium (ca). The image on the right is from a patient with right ventricular hypoplasia. This right ventricular hypoplasia, however, is hardly appreciated on this single apical four-chamber section. See Figure 27-41 for additional planes. ivs, interventricular septum; la, left atrium; lv, left ventricle; ra, right atrium; rv, right ventricle.

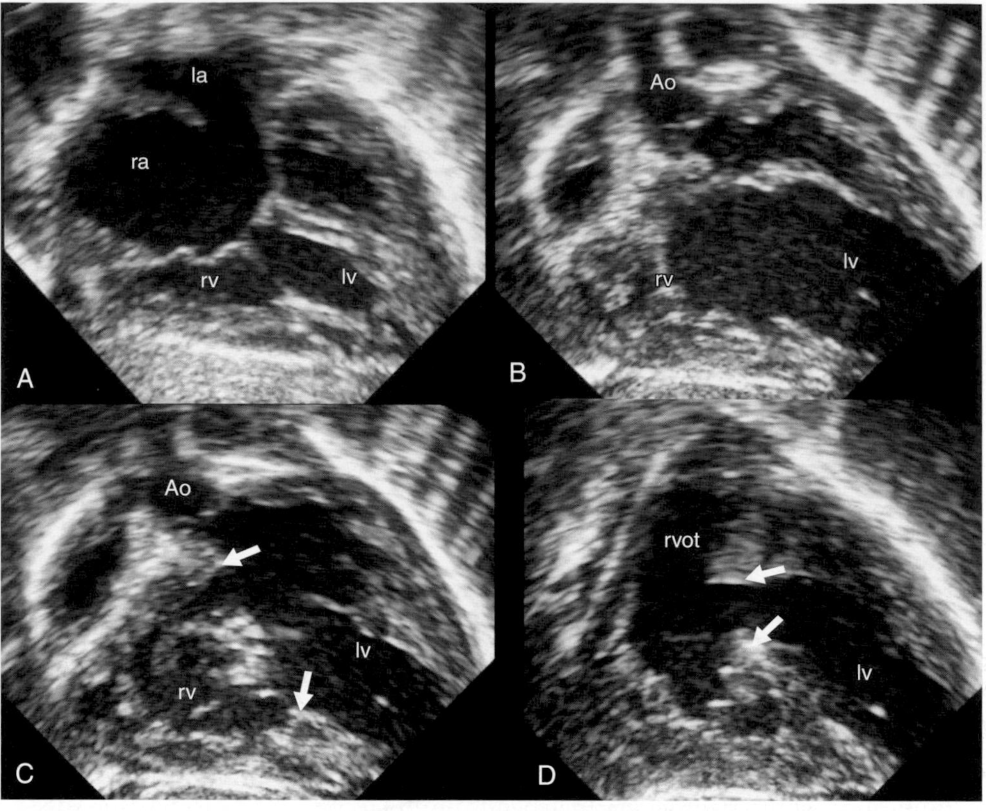

Figure 27-41 These images are from a subcostal scan in a patient with right ventricular hypoplasia. The scan starts with a subcostal four-chamber section (**A**) and continues by tilting the transducer ventrally. It is very hard to identify the interventricular septum in sections **A** and **B**, although it is very clear in the latter that the left ventricle is much larger than the right. Sections **C** and **D** show the interventricular septum (*arrows*) and the very large ventricular septal defect. The right ventricular outflow tract is the only part of the right ventricle that is well developed (**D**). Ao, aorta; la, left atrium; lv, left ventricle; ra, right atrium; rv, right ventricle; rvot, right ventricular outflow tract.

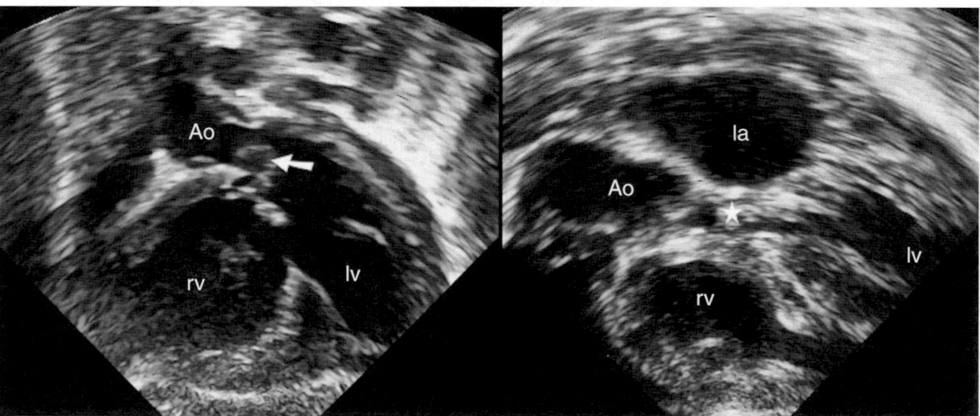

Figure 27-42 The image on the left is a subcostal long-axis section from a patient with a common atrioventricular valve orifice. It shows an obstructed left ventricular outflow tract due to a tissue tag (*arrow*). The image on the right is an apical long-axis plane from a patient with separate left and right atrioventricular valve orifices and a very deep scoop of the muscular interventricular septum. There is severe intrinsic narrowing of the elongated left ventricular outflow tract combined with abnormal connections of valvar tissue (*star*). Ao, aorta; la, left atrium; lv, left ventricle; rv, right ventricle.

cross sectional imaging in isolation cannot. The technique has huge potential, for the purposes of both diagnosis and teaching. With the present generation of echocardiographic equipment, however, maximal frame rates are limited, and the quality of the images is far inferior to those obtained using cross sectional equipment. The technique is thus not yet ready for routine use in infants and small children, although this is likely to change quickly, possibly even within the time taken for this book to proceed to production.

Doppler Interrogation

When investigating any patient with an atrioventricular septal defect, colour flow Doppler interrogation is used to demonstrate interatrial, interventricular, or ventriculo-atrial shunting. Pulsed and continuous wave Doppler interrogation can be used to measure the drop in pressure across any interventricular communication, across the left or right ventricular outflow tract, and across the right atrioventricular valve. This last measurement allows an accurate estimation of the right ventricular and pulmonary arterial systolic pressures. It is important to be aware, however, that the velocity profile in the right atrium will not allow an accurate prediction of right ventricular systolic pressure if there is shunting from left ventricle to right atrium. In addition, Doppler interrogation shows clearly any valvar regurgitation, including the specific site of regurgitation when present. This is crucial for the surgeon, enabling attention to be focused specifically at this part of the anatomy.

Regurgitation can be quantified by measuring the surface area of regurgitant jets, and by investigating the flow in the pulmonary veins. For infants and children, however, such quantification has its limitations. Measuring the surface area of regurgitant jets may be less reliable in children due to the obligatory use of different probes and settings of the machine in different age groups. Investigation of the flow in pulmonary veins is unreliable in the presence of unobstructed shunting at atrial level, where systolic backflow in the pulmonary veins is rarely encountered, even in the presence of significant regurgitation. If backflow can be demonstrated within the pulmonary veins, nonetheless, regurgitation is certainly significant.

Magnetic Resonance Imaging

Resonance imaging provides images similar to those obtained by echocardiography, but at much greater expense, often necessitating anaesthesia in infants and small children. Skilful selection of appropriate sections, nonetheless, permits original sections to be obtained, notably those in the plane of the inlet part of the ventricular septum. These show well the relationships between the bridging leaflets and the septal structures, and permit quantification of the potential for shunting at ventricular level (Fig. 27-43). Four-chamber sections also illustrate particularly well the relationship between the bridging leaflets and the septal structures (Fig. 27-44), revealing any disproportion between the ventricles (Fig. 27-45), and demonstrating malalignment between the atrial and ventricular septums when present. The short-axis sections obviously illustrate the pathognomonic feature of the common atrioventricular junction. Volumetric measurements by magnetic resonance imaging are superior to those obtained using cross sectional echocardiography in demonstrating the degree of right or left ventricular hypoplasia. Some prefer magnetic resonance imaging to evaluate all the morphological aspects of atrioventricular septal defects, stating that its potential to define the anatomy is superior.[62] Although this may be true for a selected group of adults, it is certainly not valid for infants and children.

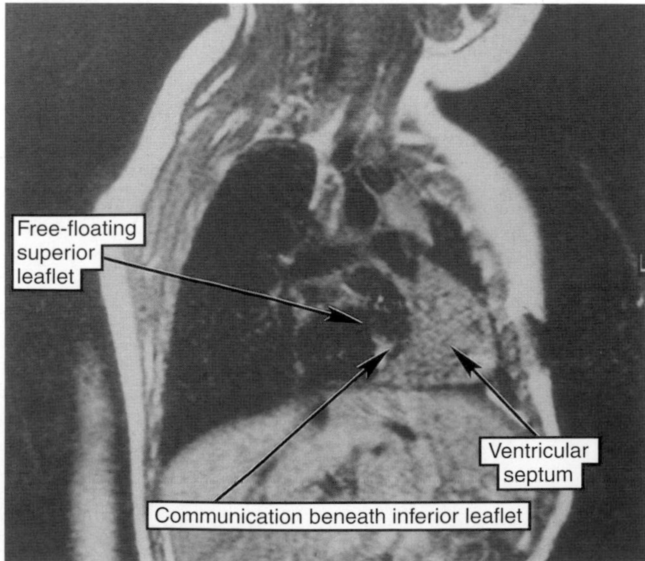

Figure 27-43 This magnetic resonance image is orientated so as to be in the plane of the ventricular septum. A common valvar orifice is clearly seen where the superior bridging leaflet is free-floating, whilst the inferior bridging leaflet is somewhat tethered to the septal crest.

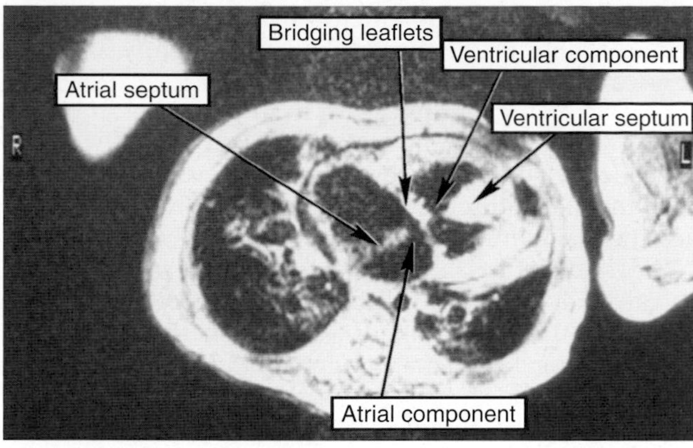

Figure 27-44 This magnetic resonance image displays a four-chamber section and shows the common atrioventricular junction with the bridging leaflets floating within the septal defect.

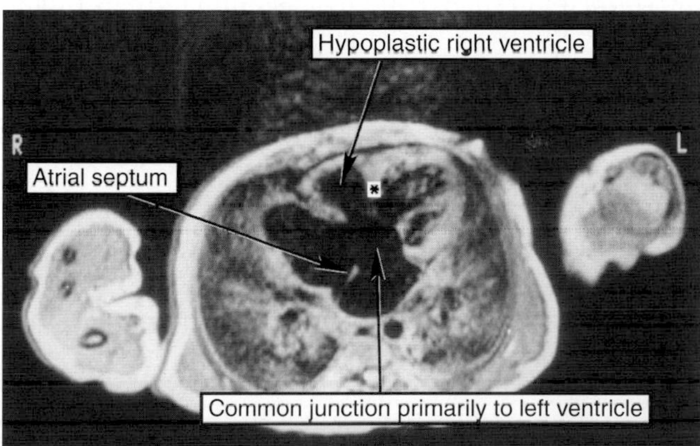

Figure 27-45 This magnetic resonance image, again producing a four-chamber section, shows malalignment between the atrial and ventricular septums. The asterisk indicates the crest of the ventricular septum. There is marked ventricular imbalance.

Magnetic resonance imaging can also be used to measure precisely the regurgitant fraction across leaking valves and to calculate effective shunting. There are two methods available for quantification of shunting using cine-imaging, namely the volumetric and the flow quantification techniques. Only the second approach, using the phase-contrast sequence, is applicable to those with atrioventricular septal defects, allowing calculation of the ratio of flows and the shunt fraction. This technique can be used as an adjunct to Doppler echocardiography. Clinical decisions can then be made based on the combination of Doppler estimates of pulmonary and systemic arterial pressure and calculation of the ratio of flows using magnetic resonance imaging.

Cardiac Catheterisation and Angiocardiography

The obvious indication for cardiac catheterisation is to measure the pulmonary vascular resistance prior to operative correction. In addition, pulmonary vascular reactivity can be tested. The haemodynamic abnormalities found will be as already documented, and will normally be indistinguishable from those of an atrial septal defect with or without an associated ventricular septal defect.

Nowadays, cross sectional echocardiography demonstrates everything that angiocardiography did in the past, and more, and complementary non-invasive imaging techniques are readily available. Consequently, in almost all circumstances, there is no indication for cardiac catheterisation or angiography prior to surgery. This applies not only to young infants but also to older patients who have no evidence for elevated pulmonary vascular resistance. Even the brief discussion of angiography that follows, therefore, is mainly of historic interest.

The best-known angiocardiographic feature was also the one that proved so difficult to interpret, namely the gooseneck malformation. It is seen on the frontal projection of the left ventriculogram, and depends primarily upon the abnormal left ventricular origin of the aorta (Fig. 27-46). The body of the goose is produced by the abnormal parietal attachment of the left component of the common atrioventricular junction. It is seen in all types of atrioventricular septal defect with common atrioventricular junction, and is characteristically smooth in outline. The scooped-out interventricular septum, initially thought to produce the body of the goose, is seen only when the bridging leaflets are firmly attached to it, or in other words in those with shunting confined at atrial level.

Should angiography be needed, most information is provided by ventricular injections profiled in left and right anterior oblique projections, usually modified by caudocranial angulation. In left anterior oblique projections, whether there is a common valvar orifice or separate right and left valvar orifices, the left atrioventricular component of the valve is seen in diastole to arise from the expanded common atrioventricular junction. In the right anterior oblique projection of the normal heart, the area of the muscular atrioventricular sandwich is seen between the mitral and tricuspid valvar orifices. In atrioventricular septal defects, its absence is manifested by the bridging leaflets hanging down superiorly and inferiorly from the common atrioventricular junction.

Interventricular communications are shown directly on the four-chamber projection. When there is a right-to-left shunt at ventricular level, these signs may be seen on both right and left ventricular angiocardiograms. Adding caudocranial tilt to the left anterior oblique view profiles the atrial septum much better, and also elongates the otherwise foreshortened muscular ventricular septum. In general, the less foreshortening of the ventricular septum the better, because this increases the chance of demonstrating a second muscular ventricular septal defect and separating it from the atrioventricular septal defect. Lengthening of the subaortic outflow tract by caudocranial tilt also improves demonstration of obstruction within the outflow tract, whether it is due to a discrete shelf, a fibromuscular tunnel, or accessory valvar tissue.

NATURAL HISTORY

When we wrote the first edition of this book, discussions of natural history were pertinent, since arguments raged as to the justification of offering surgical repair to patients with Down's syndrome. This, in turn, was because, although some good outcomes had been reported for surgical repair, on the whole the overall results for operative treatment in 1987 were less than outstanding, and often did not match the observed findings of an expectant approach.[63] This has changed in recent decades. Surgical mortality is now expected to be close to zero in the best hands. Paradoxically, because Down's syndrome and co-existing atrioventricular septal defects with common atrioventricular junction are frequently encountered by fetal scanning, many parents now elect for termination of pregnancy. The number of infants undergoing surgical repair, therefore, has declined in many developed countries. In those being considered for surgical repair, nonetheless, the major feature remaining of note in

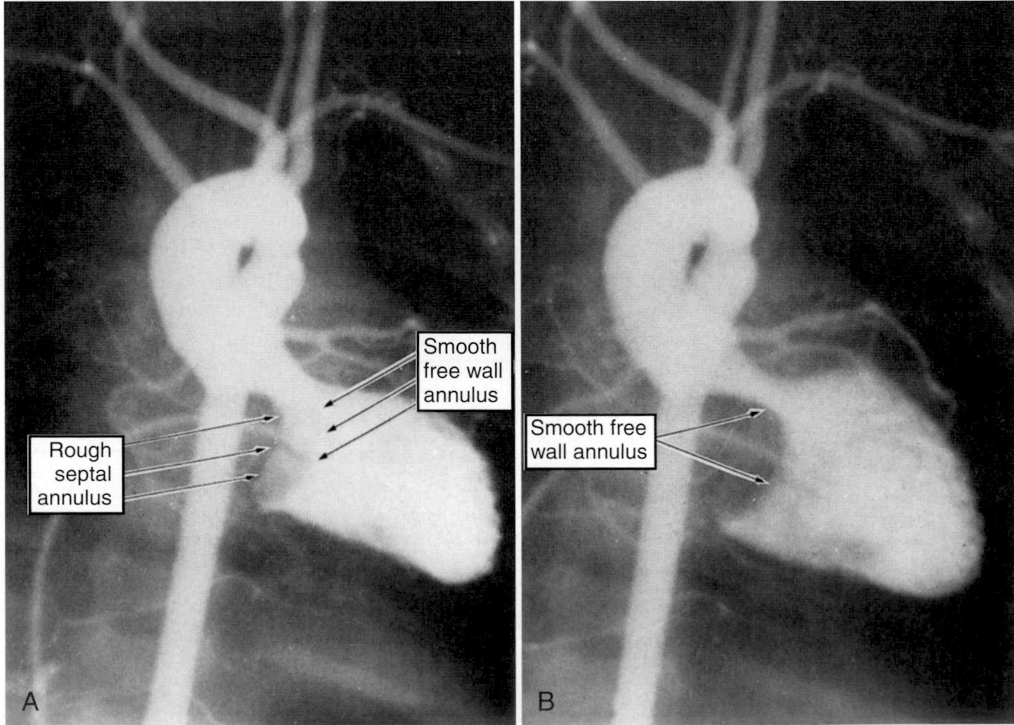

Figure 27-46 This classic left ventricular angiogram is profiled in the frontal projection. Dye fills the left ventricle, the aorta, and adjacent vessels, one of which is an aberrant left subclavian artery. The typical so-called gooseneck deformity is clearly visible. The slight difference in angulation of panels **A** and **B** shows the so-called septal annulus in **A,** produced by the attachment of the bridging leaflets to the scooped-out ventricular septum, and the parietal attachments of the leaflets of the left atrioventricular valve in **B**.

terms of natural history is the rapid onset of pulmonary vascular disease. Because of this, most centres opt for surgical repair in patients with common atrioventricular valvar orifice before the age of 6 months, with a tendency in some centres to undertake surgery within the first 3 to 4 months of life.

In patients with shunting only at atrial level, the natural history is similar to that observed in the setting of atrial septal defect. The history can, however, be made worse by atrioventricular valvar regurgitation, or less commonly stenosis, of the left atrioventricular valve. This feature necessitates earlier surgical repair, often during the first year of life. In uncomplicated cases, elective surgical repair is undertaken around 4 years of age, before the patients begin school. The only feature that might prompt earlier repair is the occurrence of frequent respiratory infections, or failure to thrive. A small cohort of patients, with exclusively atrial shunting, may escape detection until adolescence or adult life. For these patients, studies of natural history show that very few are well at the age of 40 years, usually because of the development of arrhythmias.[64]

TREATMENT

Medical Treatment

Heart failure and associated respiratory infections need the usual pharmacological treatment (see Chapter 14). Acute administration of beta-blockers and inhibitors of angiotensin-converting enzyme has been shown to reduce the left-to-right shunt in the majority of infants, but there have been no reports of chronic use of such treatment. Infants who do not respond to medical therapy require surgical treatment. The argument for a prolonged trial of medical treatment before undertaking surgery is less strong than in isolated ventricular septal defect, since there is a strictly limited chance of spontaneous cure or reduction in the significance of the atrioventricular septal defect.

Surgical Treatment

Indications for Operation

With the exception of those rare patients with small septal defects and competent atrioventricular valves, the treatment for all patients with an atrioventricular septal defect will be surgical correction. Medical therapy with digoxin and diuretics serves to stabilise the patients with a large shunt and cardiac failure during early infancy. Feeding by gastric tube is sometimes necessary to provide adequate caloric intake. The only aim of medical therapy is to postpone surgery in symptomatic infants, preferably until the age of 6 months. In young infants with a very high pulmonary vascular resistance, oxygen is occasionally given continuously during the last weeks prior to surgery in an attempt to reduce the incidence of post-operative pulmonary hypertensive crises. As discussed, pre-operative assessment can now generally be achieved by echocardiography alone. Catheterisation is indicated only when there is strong echo-based evidence of severe pulmonary hypertension.

The age at which to perform surgical repair has tended to become lower over recent years, which is in keeping with the general tendency in paediatric cardiac surgery. There are no systematic studies, however, investigating the matter of timing thoroughly. Normally, in the absence of congenital cardiac disease, pulmonary vascular resistance drops, and remains fairly constant after 1 month of age. In the presence of atrioventricular septal defect with interventricular shunting, resistance may increase in the year following the initial drop. In some infants, resistance may even never show the anticipated initial drop. This rise in pulmonary vascular resistance has served as a strong incentive to operate earlier in life. Recent cohort studies indicate generally that repair below a body weight of 5 kg, or an age of 6 months, is only possible at the cost of more complications and a higher rate of reoperation.[65] Severely symptomatic patients may benefit from earlier operative repair because of failure to thrive, and to prevent secondary changes accompanying a large shunt and/or severe atrioventricular valvar regurgitation. In these patients, the atrioventricular anulus may dilate as the result of the large shunt, and valvar tissue may fibrose at the site of regurgitation, factors that may well complicate a repair postponed too long.

Objectives of Surgical Correction

Surgical correction aims at closure of all septal defects in order to abolish shunting and subsequent pulmonary congestion. Evolving insight dictates closure of the zone of apposition between superior and inferior bridging leaflets at all times, unless specifically contraindicated. The policy not to close the zone when the valve is competent has resulted in large numbers of reoperations for valvar regurgitation. The most frequent contraindication to closing the zone of apposition is absence or hypoplasia of the left mural leaflet, whence closure of the zone would render the valve stenotic. When striving to achieve these primary goals, care should be taken to avoid two complications, namely damage to the atrioventricular conduction system, and obstruction within the left ventricular outflow tract.

Closure of the Septal Defect

The manner in which the defect is closed can have a profound effect on the subsequent architecture of the atrioventricular valvar complex, because defect and valve are inseparable parts of the three-dimensional anomaly of the abnormal common atrioventricular junction. The shape of the patch or patches, and the technique used for insertion of sutures, therefore, are of utmost importance not only for septal closure but also for post-operative valvar function (Fig. 27-47).

Methods of repair can be categorised classically as use of one or two patches for closure of the entire defect, presuming there are atrial and ventricular components to close. A further categorisation is whether or not bridging valvar

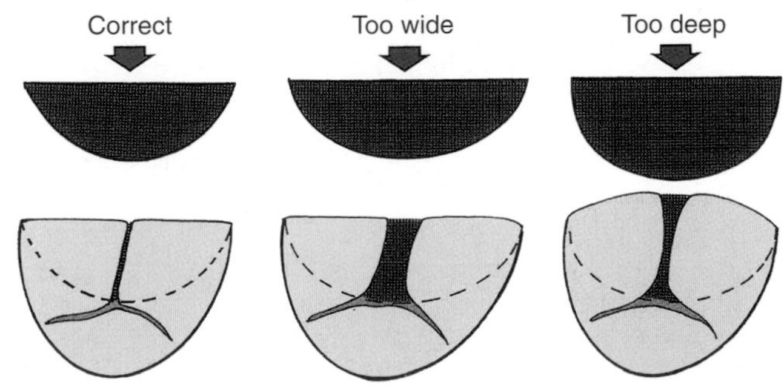

Figure 27-47 So as to avoid distortion of the valvar leaflets during surgical correction, the size and shape of the interventricular patch must be tailored to fit the defect precisely. Use of patches of inappropriate shape, shown as too wide or too deep, will distort the anatomy, which in these cases widens the zone of apposition of the bridging leaflets.

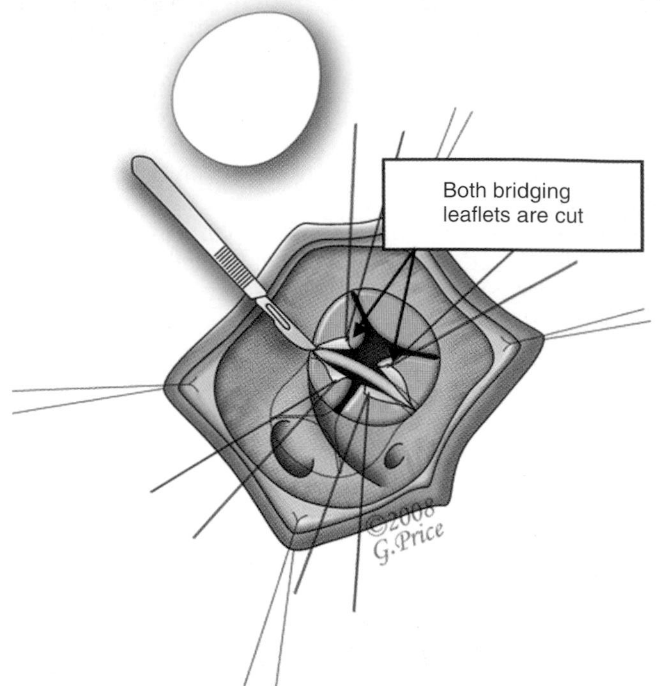

Figure 27-48 The cartoon shows the essence of the classic technique for surgical repair, whereby both bridging leaflets are cut in the plane of the ventricular septum, so as to expose its crest. The single patch is sutured to the right side of the ventricular septum, and thereafter the cut edges of the bridging leaflets are sutured together, sandwiching the patch between them.

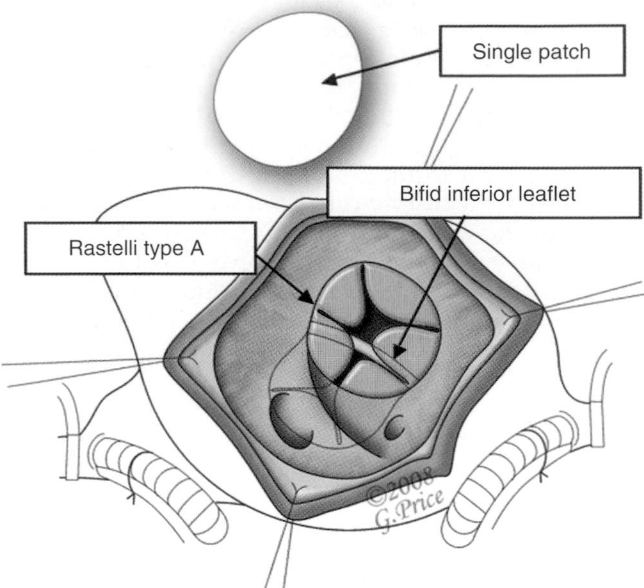

Figure 27-49 The cartoon illustrates the situation where the septal crest is exposed naturally, because of a Rastelli A configuration of the superior bridging leaflet, whilst in this case the inferior bridging leaflet is bifid. The single patch can then be attached to the right side of the ventricular septum, following which the adjacent leaflets, or parts of them, are sutured together, sandwiching the patch between them.

leaflets are cut in order to expose the atrioventricular valvar annulus at the ventricular septal junction. The cutting of bridging leaflets can be applied to both the superior and inferior bridging leaflet, depending on their extent of bridging. A further variable is the provided by the possibility of attaching one or both bridging leaflets directly to the septal crest. Permutation of these strategies results in at least eight possible combinations of techniques:

- Using one patch, and cutting the bridging leaflets[66,67] (Fig. 27-48).
- Using one patch, but leaving the bridging leaflets intact. This is only possible with minimal bridging of both bridging leaflets, and constitutes a numerically minor subset (Fig. 27-49).
- Using one patch in which a cut is made to accommodate one of the bridging leaflets. This is applicable should one of the bridging leaflets bridge minimally, as in the Rastelli A malformation (Fig. 27-50).
- Using one patch, having sutured the bridging leaflets directly to the ventricular septal crest[68,69] (Fig. 27-51).
- Using two patches, and attaching the inferior bridging leaflet to the ventricular septal crest, while inserting a patch between the septal crest and the superior bridging leaflet, which is left intact[70] (Fig. 27-52).
- Using two patches, attaching the inferior bridging leaflet to the ventricular septal crest, while cutting the superior bridging leaflet (Fig. 27-53).
- Using two patches, and cutting the bridging leaflets[71] (Fig. 27-54).
- Using two patches, leaving the bridging leaflets intact (Fig. 27-55).

All techniques have protagonists, and publications on all techniques exist. No systematic trial has been carried

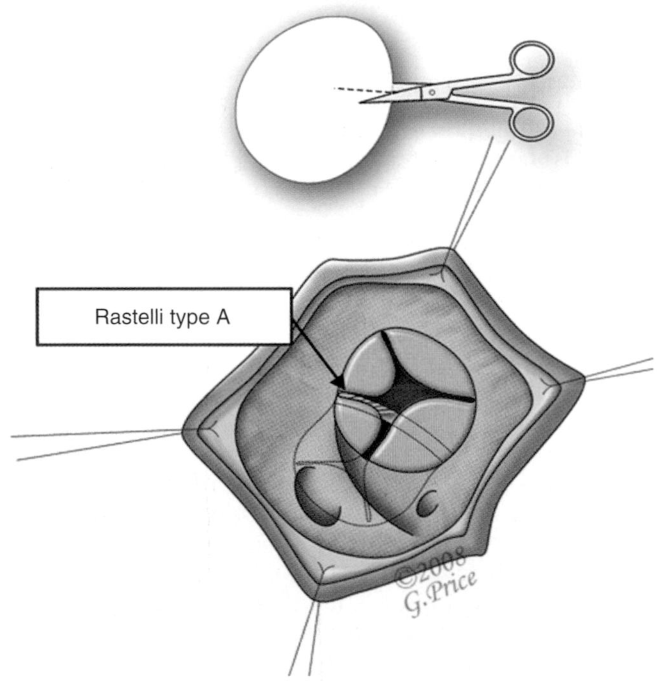

Figure 27-50 The cartoon shows the situation where the inferior bridging leaflet bridges extensively and is not bifid. A cut is made into a single patch, to accommodate the inferior leaflet, while the minimally bridging superior leaflet can be sutured to the single patch. The superior part of the patch is then sandwiched between the superior and the antero-superior leaflet.

out so as to draw conclusions on their merits. Publication bias has it that usually only desirable results are published (Table 27-1). The major advantage of the technique using only one patch is the excellent exposure of the entire ventricular septal crest, so that suturing of the ventricular patch is made much easier. The major disadvantage is the valvar

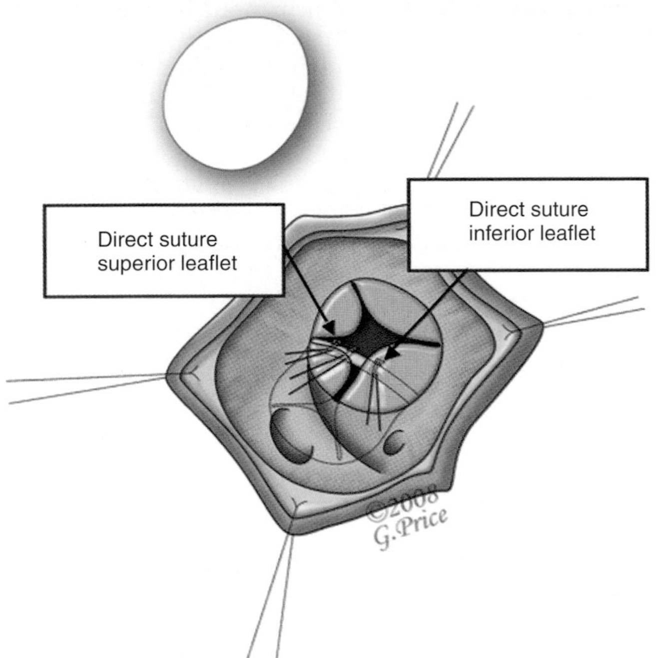

Figure 27-51 The cartoon shows the method of suturing the bridging leaflets to the septal crest directly, in this case with pledgeted sutures. The single patch is then confined to the interatrial part of the defect.

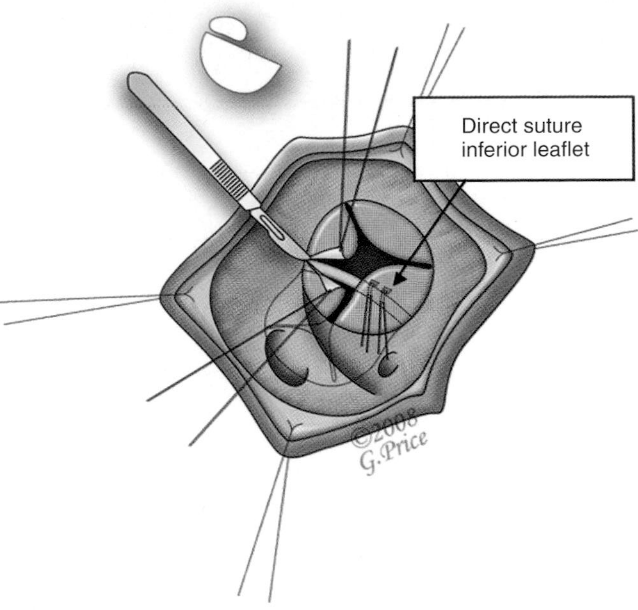

Figure 27-53 The cartoon shows the situation where the inferior bridging leaflet is sutured to the septal crest directly, in this case with pledgeted sutures. The superior bridging leaflet is cut so as to expose the superior part of the septal crest. A smaller patch is inserted between the septal crest and the cut edges of the superior leaflet. The patch is sandwiched between the two parts of the superior leaflet.

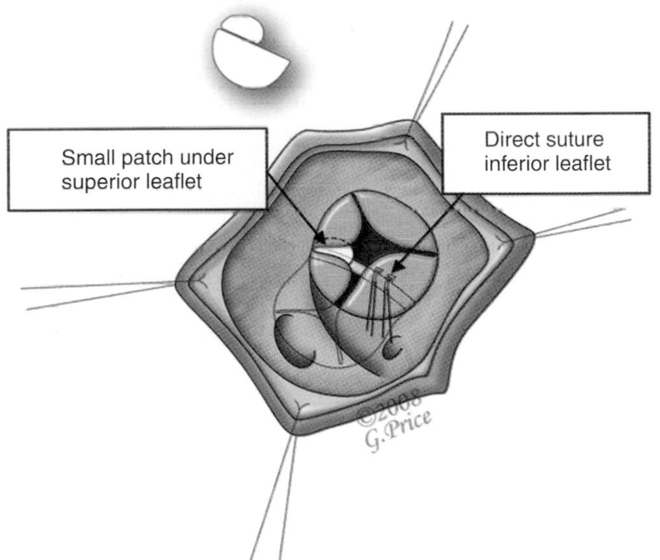

Figure 27-52 In this cartoon, the situation is shown where the inferior bridging leaflet is sutured to the septal crest directly, in this case with pledgeted sutures. A smaller patch is inserted between the septal crest and the superior bridging leaflet, so as to avoid obstruction of the left ventricular outflow tract, and/or distortion of the valvar leaflets.

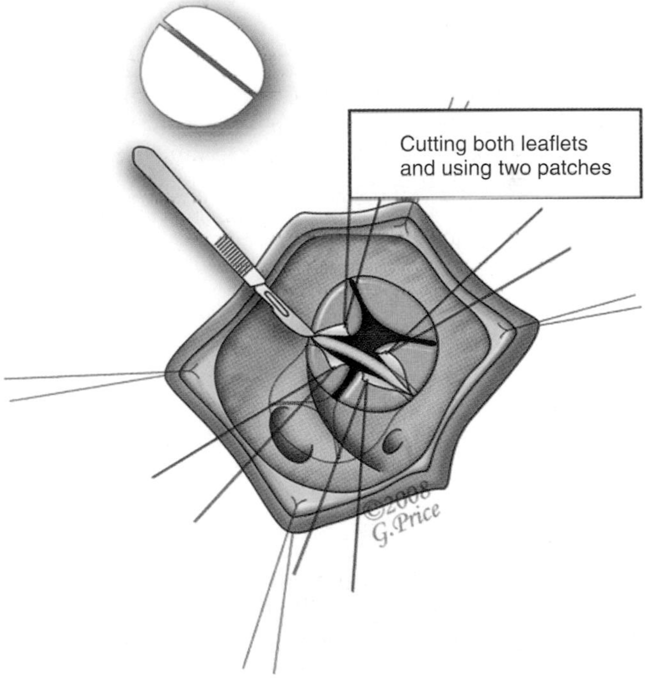

Figure 27-54 In this cartoon, we show the technique whereby both bridging leaflets are cut so as to expose the ventricular septal crest fully. Two patches are used, of which the ventricular patch is attached to the right side of the ventricular septum, whilst the valvar side of the patch is sandwiched between the cut edges of the bridging leaflets. The atrial patch then is attached to the latter suture line.

suture line. Where friable valvar tissue might tear, the suture line takes up tissue, promoting the possibility of disruption, particularly in the setting of post-operative endocarditis. Good exposure of the ventricular septal crest may counterbalance these drawbacks.

The attraction of suturing the bridging leaflets directly to the ventricular septal crest is the obvious simplicity of the procedure, because placement of the more difficult of the two patches is eliminated entirely.[72] The potential drawbacks are, first, the possibility of narrowing of the left ventricular outflow tract superiorly, and second, distortion of the valvar apparatus, particularly if the septal defect has depth, in which situation the leaflets have to be brought down considerably to reach the septal crest. Personal

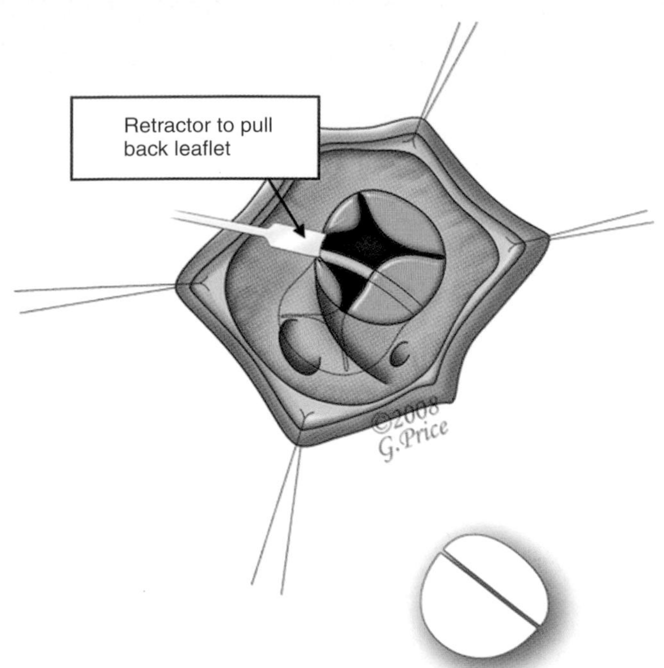

Figure 27-55 The cartoon shows the technique in which neither of the bridging leaflets is cut, nor are they sutured directly to the ventricular septal crest. An interventricular patch is inserted and attached to the right side of the septal crest, which is exposed by gently retracting the bridging leaflets one at a time with a retractor. The bridging leaflets are sandwiched between the interatrial and interventricular patches.

communication from Benson Wilcox, who was the first to advocate this policy, makes it clear that he only employed this technique if the ventricular defect was not too deep.

The tissues of the valvar leaflets are rarely normal, and are often deficient. It is illogical in our opinion, therefore, further to reduce the amount of tissue available for repair. Above all, we feel it to be unnecessary, unless bridging of one or both leaflets is minimal, when these leaflets can easily by sutured to the patch without having to be cut. Whether a single patch or two patches are to be used, therefore, should in our opinion depend on the anatomy of the individual bridging leaflets. Only when both inferior and superior leaflets bridge the septum extensively, seen most often in patients with Down's syndrome, is a two-patch technique warranted. In all other anatomical variants, when one or both of the superior and inferior leaflets do not bridge the septum extensively, a single patch can be used. This single patch then has to be incised to accommodate any leaflet that bridges extensively (see Fig. 27-50). So, instead of employing one or two patches dogmatically, our approach is not to cut leaflets unless it proves impossible to visualise the location of intended stitches, which is a highly unusual circumstance.

Patches can be fashioned from synthetic material, or from autologous or xenologous pericardium. Synthetic fabric is sturdy, but any rough texture to its surface can lead to haemolysis should it be impinged upon by a regurgitant jet. Even in the absence of clinically significant regurgitation, haemolysis can be so severe as to necessitate reoperation. Pericardium is always smooth and does not lead to haemolysis, so is preferable in our opinion. Above all, autologous pericardium is cheap, supple, and easy to use. Its use minimises distortion of the delicate valvar tissues. Autologous pericardium should be treated for 5 minutes in 0.2% glutaraldehyde in order to prevent distension and aneurysmal widening, specifically of the interventricular patch.[73] Our favourite operative technique is illustrated in Figures 27-56 to 27-63.

The size, and semilunar shape, of the interventricular patch are of the utmost importance in determining the future function of the left atrioventricular valve. This is because, subsequent to correction, the leading edge of the patch will constitute part of the hinge of both atrioventricular valves. When the patch is either too broad or too deep, the valve is likely to become regurgitant (see Fig. 27-47).[74,75] The interventricular patch is ideally always slightly shorter than measured. The bridging leaflets are then brought

TABLE 27-1

RESULTS OF SURGICAL CORRECTION IN SELECTED SERIES

First Author	Publication Year	Defect Type	Period of Inclusion	Maximum Follow-up (Years)	Number of Operated Patients	Survival at 5 Years	Survival at 10 Years	Survival at 20 Years	Survival at 40 Years
Welke*	2007	All operated partial defects	1958–2000	43	133	90	88	86	78
Frid†	2004	All operated defects	1973–1997	28	502	79	77	61	—
Murashita‡	2004	All operated partial defects	1983–2002	21	61	94	91	91	—
El-Nadjawi§	2000	All operated partial defects	1955–1995	40	334	94	93	87	76
Guenther‖	1998	All operated complete defects	1974–1995	20	320	80	78	78	—

*Welke KF, Morris CD, King E, et al: Population-based perspective of long-term outcomes after repair of partial atrioventricular septal defect. Ann Thorac Surg 2007;84:624–629.
†Frid C, Björkhem G, Jonzon A, et al: Long-term survival in children with atrioventricular septal defect and common atrioventricular orifice in Sweden. Cardiol Young 2004;14:24–31.
‡Murashita T, Kubota T, Oba J, et al: Left atrioventricular valve regurgitation after repair of incomplete atrioventricular septal defect. Ann Thorac Surg 2004;77:2157–2162.
§El-Nadjawi EK, Driscoll DJ, Puga FJ, et al: Operation for partial atrioventricular septal defect: A forty-year review. J Thorac Cardiovasc Surg 2000;119:880–890.
‖Guenther T, Mazzitelli D, Haehnel CJ, et al: Long-term results of complete atrioventricular septal defects: Analysis of risk factors. Ann Thorac Surg 1998;65:754–760.

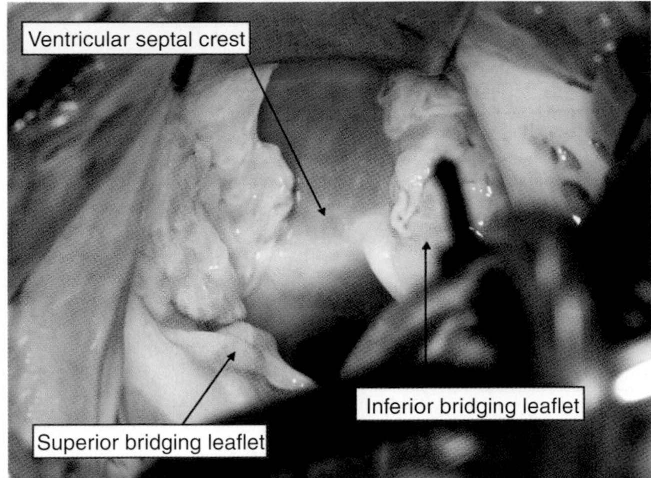

Figure 27-56 This operative picture, and those which follow (through Fig. 27-63), are from a patient aged 6 months, weighing 7.1 kg, and having a body surface area of 0.38 m^2, with Down's syndrome, elevated pulmonary vascular resistance, and additional obstruction in the left ventricular outflow tract produced by accessory valvar tissue. The series shows the view of the atrioventricular junction obtained by the surgeon working through the opened right atrium. A retractor is elevating the right ventricular lateral aspect of the common atrioventricular valve. In this heart, being empty due to the use of cardioplegia, the valvar leaflets are flaccidly lying in the junction. The left ventricle is on the small side, the diameter of the left part of the atrioventricular valve is 14 mm, which is the norm for the size of the patient. The mural leaflet, in keeping with the smallish left ventricle, is also very small with an angular annular size of around 45 degrees. The superior bridging leaflet crosses the ventricular septum only minimally, typical of the so-called Rastelli A configuration. The ventricular septal crest is bare.

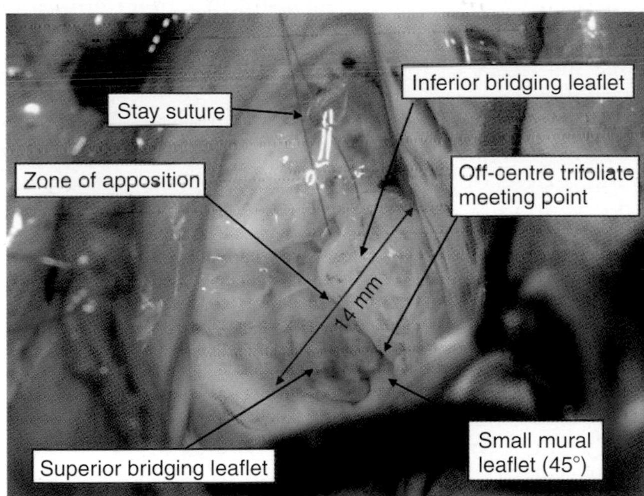

Figure 27-57 The view obtained of the common atrioventricular valve. The ventricles have been instilled with saline so as to test for valvar competence. The zone of apposition between superior and inferior bridging leaflets does not leak in this situation. A stay suture indicates where these two leaflets could be sutured together.

together, a manoeuvre that almost always abolishes regurgitation. As discussed, when surgeons use only a single patch for closure of both atrial and ventricular parts of the defect, it may be necessary to incise the leaflets, depending on the extent of their bridging. Success then depends on the technique of suturing.[76] In skilled hands, nonetheless, use of a single patch can produce results that are equally as good as those achieved using two patches. We conclude, therefore, that it is probably less the technique, but rather

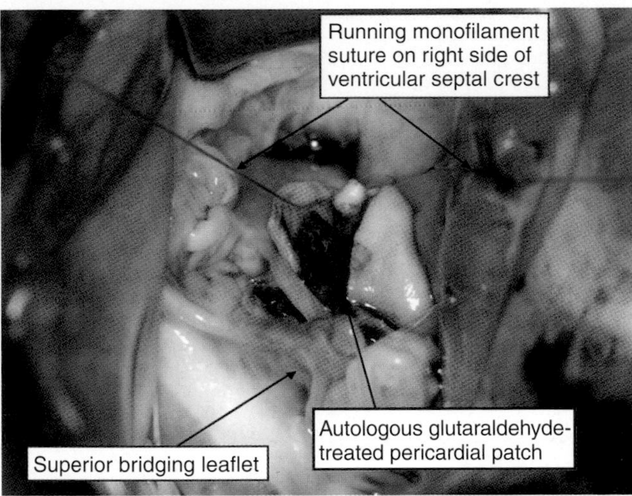

Figure 27-58 The autologous glutaraldehyde-treated patch is being sutured to the right side of the ventricular septum with a running monofilament suture. Staying on the right side of the ventricular septum avoids the conduction tissues. Cords from the right ventricle should remain on the right side of the patch.

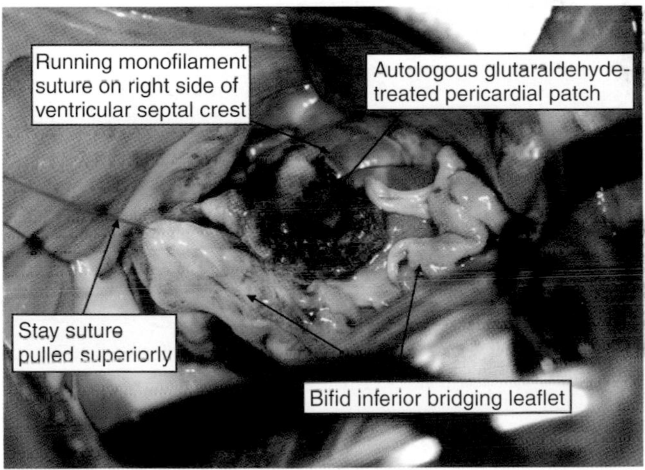

Figure 27-59 The stay suture pulls the bridging leaflets superiorly, exposing the inferior part of the ventricular septum. The suture line is being carried towards the crux, which is facilitated in this particular case by the bifid nature of the inferior bridging leaflet.

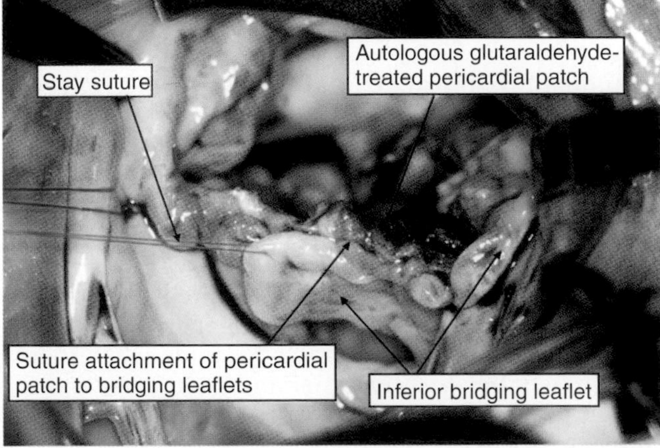

Figure 27-60 The insertion and attachment by running suture of autologous glutaraldehyde-treated pericardial patch has been completed. A running monofilament mattress suture attaches the pericardial patch to the bridging leaflets.

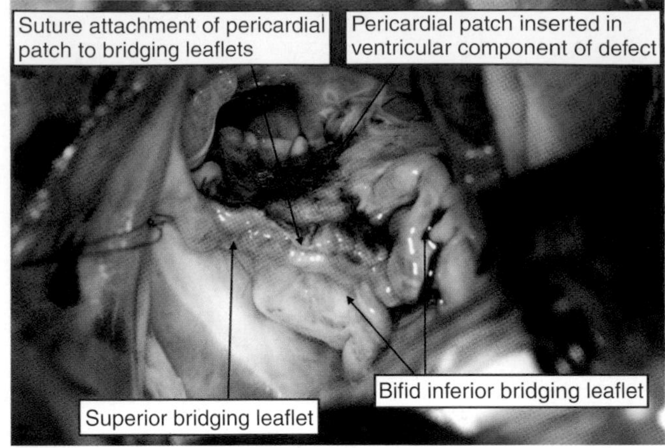

Figure 27-61 The stay suture has now been knotted to attach the bridging leaflets together at the site of the patch. The position of the ventricular patch can be seen clearly. The zone of apposition has not been sutured in this case, because this would make the valve stenotic, due to the very small size of the mural leaflet. The size of the left atrioventricular valve is now 13 mm, which is only 1 mm too small for the size of the patient. This was tolerated well, without physiologic stenosis.

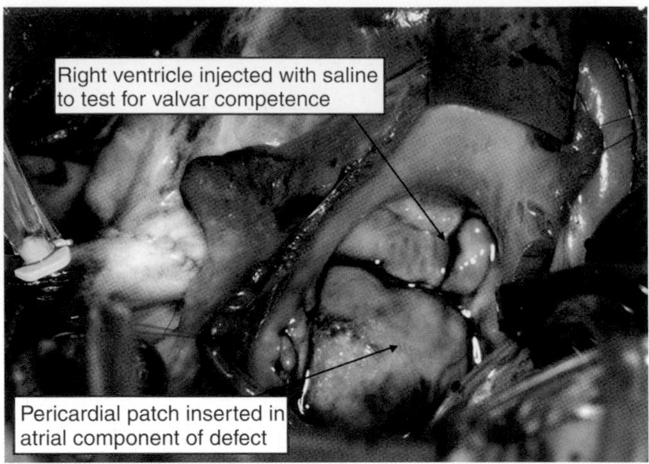

Figure 27-63 Injection of saline into the right ventricle shows that there is no leakage of the right atrioventricular valve. Post-operatively, this patient required ventilation with nitric oxide and delivery of sildenafil to decrease pulmonary vascular resistance. The patient was monitored by means of lines to measure left atrial and pulmonary arterial pressures.

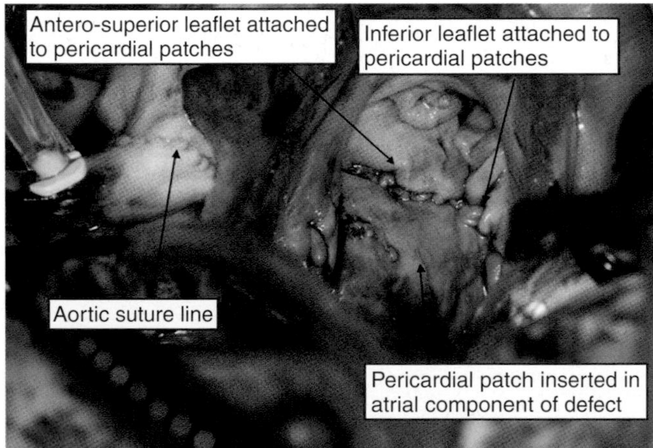

Figure 27-62 The atrial pericardial patch has now been inserted, also with running monofilament sutures. The antero-superior leaflet and the right half of the bifid inferior bridging leaflet have both been attached to the suture line joining the ventricular and atrial patches. The slight bulging of the atrial patch shows that the left atrium is being filled by pulmonary venous blood. Absence of leakage into the right ventricle indicates absence of any residual interventricular communication. The aortic suture line indicates removal of the obstructing tissues in the left ventricular outflow tract through the aortic valve.

the familiarity of the surgeon with it, which determines the result.

Avoidance of Conduction Tissues

It is the course of the suture line relative to the ventricular septum and the coronary sinus that is the critical factor in avoidance of the conduction tissues. On the inferior side, the septal aspect of the mouth of the coronary sinus is a useful surgical landmark with which to predict the position of the atrioventricular node and the penetrating bundle[39] (Fig. 27-64), albeit that this loses its value when there is malalignment between the atrial and ventricular septums, or when the coronary sinus opens within the left atrium. As we have discussed, the triangle of Koch as such does not exist in atrioventricular septal defect, so only the coronary sinus and the cardiac crux point to the position of the atrioventricular node. Indeed, as emphasised, should there be malalignment rightward of the ventricular septum, then it is the point of union between the ventricular septum and the atrioventricular junction that marks the location of the atrioventricular node (see Fig. 27-22).

There are two possible placements of surgical suture lines that permit avoidance of the conduction tissues. The first is to stay on the right side of the ventricular septum, and the coronary sinus, leaving the sinus to drain into the left atrium (see Fig. 27-64). The resulting small right-to-left shunt is clinically irrelevant. This suture line takes a wide curve around the site of the atrioventricular node, permitting relatively wide margins for stitches. As this suture line takes an inferior route around the coronary sinus, the atrial patch has to be of a shape and size so as to accommodate for that extension. The alternative line is on the left side of the ventricular septum and the atrioventricular node, calling for shallow bites so as not to impinge upon the non-branching bundle, particularly beneath the inferior bridging leaflet, or the connecting tongue in those with separate valvar orifices. When using this suture line, a somewhat smaller atrial patch can be inserted, because the coronary sinus stays on the right side. When the septal crest is devoid of fibrous tissues that can serve as safe points for anchorage of sutures, this route places the branching bundle and its left fascicles in greater danger, so that those using this approach should take great care that their sutures do not impinge on the crest of the muscular ventricular septum.

On the superior side, the superior half of the ventricular septal crest is devoid of conduction tissue. The bundle branches take off on their course on the endocardial septal surface, more or less in the middle of the septum. The suture line on the right side, out of necessity crosses the right bundle branch. A right bundle branch block pattern in the pre-operative electrocardiogram, however, is a standard feature in this anomaly. Probably, therefore, no change is apparent on the post-operative tracings indicative of damage to the right bundle branch. The absence of conduction tissues in the superior half of the septum also means that the left ventricular outflow tract and aortic valve are safe areas for surgical manoeuvres, unlike the situation in the normal heart.

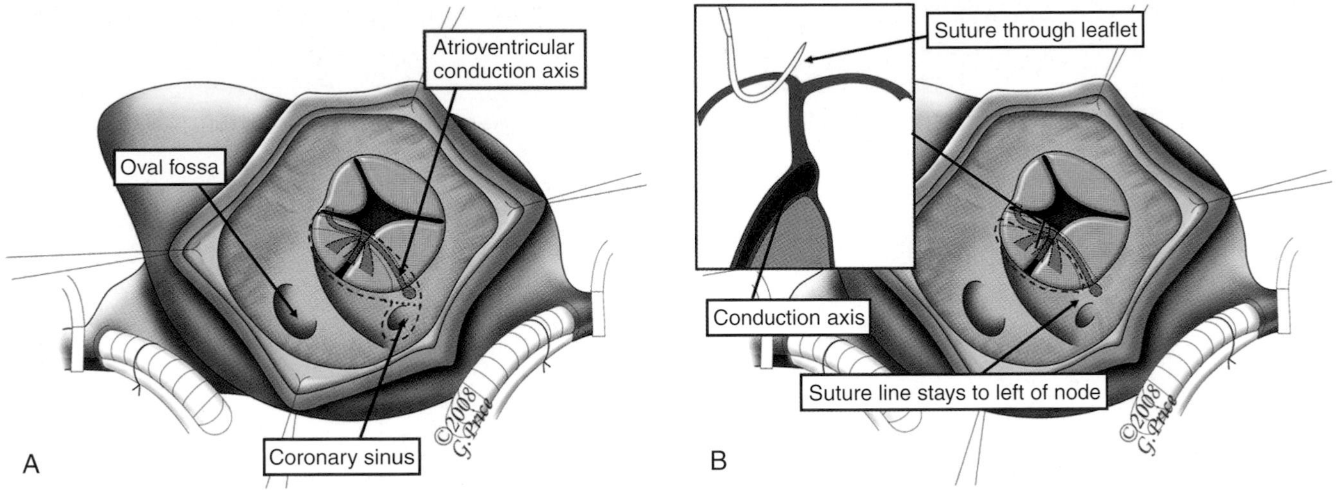

Figure 27-64 The cartoon shows the two suture lines that can be used to close the septal defect. In panel **A**, the line stays on the right side of the ventricular septal crest, crossing only the right bundle branch. The suture line leaves the mouth of the coronary sinus draining into the left atrium and thus goes widely around the atrioventricular node. Superior to the coronary sinus, the suture line follows the leading edge of the atrial septum. Panel **B** shows how the suture line can stay on the left side of the conduction axis. Care has to be taken to confine suture bites to the fibrous tissue of the bridging leaflets, or a connecting tongue between them, in the region of the crest of the muscular septum, lest there be damage to the left bundle branches. If care is taken to ensure that the sutures avoid the muscular septum, then it is possible to avoid the conduction tissues, but this is probably more dangerous than using the option shown in panel **A**.

The suture line to be used is again a matter of personal preference. Excellent results have been published using either one of the described strategies. We are of the opinion that it is probably wise to stick with the technique with which one is accustomed, and that produces the desired results.

Atrioventricular block is not the only, albeit the most devastating, result of surgical damage to the conduction tissues. The gravity of condemning patients to life-long artificial pacemaking is a sequel often not sufficiently appreciated. As well as atrioventricular block, other arrhythmias can also be produced by the placement of stitches. In the directly post-operative period, junctional ectopic tachycardias can be life-threatening, calling for core cooling of the patient. Proximity of stitches to conduction tissues, with consequent localised haematoma and oedema, can elicit these tachycardias. Fortunately, with time, these tachycardias tend to extinguish spontaneously, albeit gradually. As far as we are aware, there have been no studies or reports comparing the described two different suture lines with regard to complications of the conduction system.

When a left superior caval vein drains to the coronary sinus, it is impossible to leave the sinus draining into the left atrium. If this were the case, the resulting right-to-left shunt would be sizable, causing cyanosis. When there is a persisting left superior caval vein, however, the margin for safety between the orifice of the coronary sinus and the leading edge of the atrial septum is significantly smaller, thus rendering the conduction tissues more vulnerable.[77] The likely course for the suture line in these cases is widely around, and to the right, of the excessively wide mouth of the coronary sinus, unless, of course, the line itself has been brought along the left side of the ventricular septum. Sometimes, nonetheless, the superior caval vein drains into the left atrium, is absent or malformed, or else there is malalignment between the atrial and ventricular septums. In the latter situation, as already discussed, the best guide to the location of the node is the point at which the ventricular septum approaches the atrioventricular junction[78] (see Fig. 27-22).

Repair of the Left Atrioventricular Valve

Two schools of approach had evolved in past decades for repair of the left atrioventricular valve. Some argued that, since the left atrioventricular valve is trifoliate rather than bifoliate, it should be treated as such. The normal mitral valve, of course, has two leaflets, and takes its name from the Episcopal mitre. Thus, those espousing the trifoliate approach argued that the basic arrangement of three leaflets should be respected during surgery. Valvar repair, in these circumstances, was then said to be indicated only in the presence of regurgitation.[79,80] The alternative view was that a cleft exists in an, albeit abnormal, mitral valve. Those taking this stance argued that closure of the purported cleft was essential, irrespective of absence or presence of regurgitation, to restore the structure of the valve.[81–85] Protagonists of both schools had been driven to assume polarised stances, whilst it was claimed by each school that acceptable results could be obtained using their approach. As has been shown since our previous edition, good and particularly sobering evidence has emerged that the approach involving closure of the zone of apposition between the bridging leaflets, irrespective of the true nature of the so-called cleft, produces superior long lasting results, particularly concerning the competence of the left atrioventricular valve. It must be admitted, nonetheless, that there is also rare evidence for the contrary, the reasons for which escape us.[86] A landmark paper, coupled with rich personal experience with reoperations for leaking valves, has convinced us that it is, indeed, mandatory to close the zone of apposition between the bridging leaflets.[87] The paradox is that, although the zone is not a cleft in an otherwise normal mitral valvar leaflet, it should be closed to prevent future regurgitation. The morphologic reason for this course of events is probably the fact that the zone is often not well supported by cords, leading to later regurgitation should it be left alone.[88]

A uniform technique for suturing the zone of apposition is essential in producing a lasting effect, and calls for four indispensable considerations. First, the zone should be closed from the septal aspect to the leading edge at which

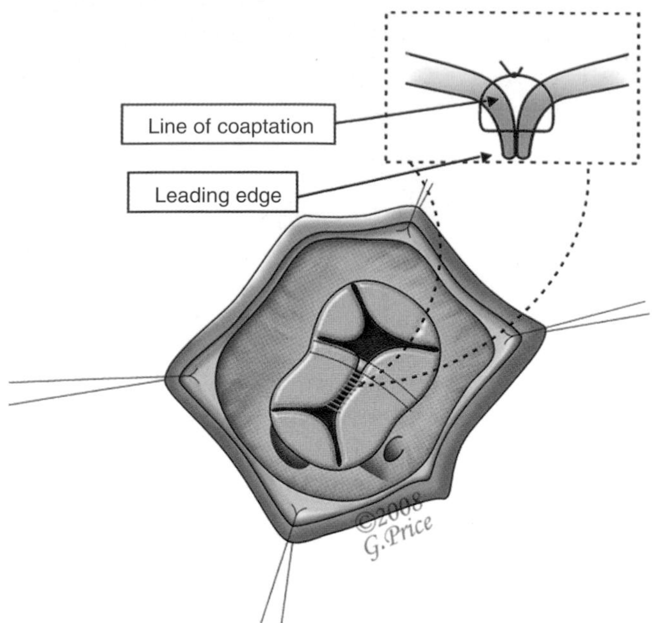

Figure 27-65 The zone of apposition between the left ventricular components of the bridging leaflets should be closed carefully, using interrupted sutures so as to avoid shrinkage of tissue leading to central regurgitation. Braided non-absorbable suture material is advisable to prevent rupture. The zone should be closed at the line of coaptation, which is different from the leading edge.

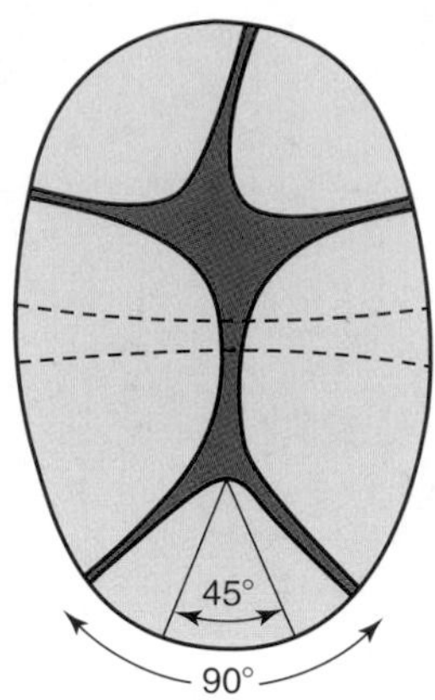

Figure 27-66 The cartoon shows the technique for measurement of the angular size of the valvar leaflets. Extremely small mural leaflets, guarding less than 45 degrees, are usually associated with a single papillary muscle. In these situations, care should be taken not to produce stenosis by closing the zone of apposition between the left ventricular components of the bridging leaflets.

the major cords are attached. Second, the ridge where the two leaflets coapt should be sutured, not the physical edge of the leaflet, in order to prevent distortion of the leaflets. Third, single sutures should be used so as not to reef inadvertently the suture line, this happening producing central leakage. Fourth, a braided nonabsorbable suture material should be used, since the repetitive forces predispose to rupture (Fig. 27-65).

Post-operative stenosis when the mural leaflet is small or absent has been documented after closure of the zone of apposition. An absent mural leaflet is usually accompanied by a single papillary muscle. Small or absent mural leaflets are usually seen guarding the entrance of small left ventricles, in other words in the setting of right ventricular dominance. Such hypoplastic left valves, being already small for body size, become stenotic when the zone of apposition is sutured completely. This is understandable, because it would be the equivalent of closing half of an otherwise normal mitral valve. The surgical problem posed by these valvar dispositions can then be impossible to solve perfectly. The choice can well be between leaving some stenosis and some regurgitation. The anatomical variability in the sizes of the leaflets can be quantified intra-operatively using a device that measures the angular size of the leaflets, presuming the basic shape of the left atrioventricular valve to be a circle (Fig. 27-66). The size of leaflets, obviously, is a combination of the valvar diameter, the angular size of the leaflets, and the anatomical centre of the valve (see Fig. 27-57). Unusually large, as well as small, mural leaflets can be part of anatomical proportions making for a difficult repair.[89]

If regurgitation is still present when saline is instilled in the left ventricle, the specific site of regurgitation must be defined. If regurgitation is located at either one of the juxtamural commissures, annuloplasty of that specific section is performed. If regurgitation is located at the zone of apposition between inferior and superior bridging leaflets, these leaflets are sewn together, starting at the pericardial patch and continuing until regurgitation is abolished. If no regurgitation is present, no further surgery is warranted, and the atrial part of the septal defect is then closed with the patch.

Repair by creating a double orifice is a technique that has merit when no other conventional technique seems to result in competence (Fig. 27-67). This method was first described in a patient with atrioventricular septal defect, remarkably in a patient with a double-orifice left atrioventricular valve.[90] Thereafter, this method was used in patients with anatomically otherwise normal but regurgitating mitral valves, where it became known as the edge-to-edge repair. Further results of this technique in atrioventricular septal defect have been described,[91,92] and we have a personal experience of 13 patients. In the short- to medium-term,

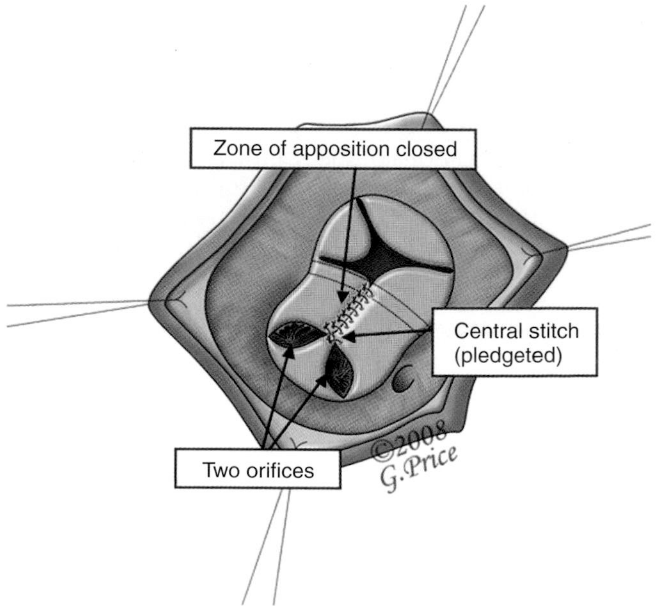

Figure 27-67 The cartoon shows the creation of dual orifices within the left atrioventricular valve using a central pledgeted stitch. The apex of the mural leaflet is sutured to the end of the zone of apposition between the left ventricular components of the bridging leaflets. The two orifices should be measured, and their combined area should not be less than Z–2 for body surface area.

the technique seems to work well, its major drawback being the potential for creating stenosis. We hypothesised that the joint surface area of the two orifices should be as large as the area of the orifice of the normal mitral valve for a patient of comparable body surface area but without an atrioventricular septal defect (Fig. 27-68). This hypothesis results in a formula and a nomogram that can be used in the operating theatre so as to avoid stenosis. Long-term results, however, are lacking.

Reoperative surgery for left atrioventricular valvar regurgitation, or rarely stenosis, differs in its possibilities and risks as compared to reoperations on the mitral valve. The possibilities for repair are somewhat larger in that the zone of apposition that is not closed fully can easily be sutured so as to abolish regurgitation. The edges are usually extremely fibrosed, which facilitates closure. Tissue advancement can alleviate central shortage of valvar tissues.[93] If repair fails, and the valve has to be replaced, care has to be taken not to create obstruction within the left ventricular outflow tract. It is wise then to resect the inferior wall of the outflow tract with the aid of a dental mirror so as to abolish any possible obstruction, whilst at the same time avoiding damage to the aortic valve.[31]

Surgery for Dual Orifices in the Left Atrioventricular Valve

Dual orifices in the left or right ventricular components of the atrioventricular valve occur in about one-twentieth of patients, more often in the setting of separate left and right valvar orifices.[94] Although recognition is difficult, such valves with dual orifices can be suspected using pre-operative echocardiography.[95] It is an abnormal and incomplete connection between two of the leaflets that forms the anatomical basis for the extra orifice, which in the setting of the left valve is usually committed to a inferomural or superomural papillary muscle and, most significantly, is usually not regurgitant. Should the abnormal connection between leaflets be severed, joining together the two orifices, catastrophic regurgitation is certain to ensue. Consequently, the possibilities for surgical repair of these valves are limited. Any annuloplasty will reduce even further the effective area of the valvar orifice. The need to replace these valves, therefore, is substantially greater than for the usual trifoliate left valve with a single orifice. If possible, these extra orifices are best left alone.

Association with Tetralogy of Fallot

The relative paucity of papers on clinical results describing the repair of the combination of atrioventricular septal defect and tetralogy of Fallot is not in keeping with the reported incidence of this combination, said to be present in about one-twentieth of all patients with atrioventricular septal defect. Papers of substance describe experience in extremely small series, although some larger series have appeared.[96,97] This paucity of reports might be explained by publication bias, or by selection of patients. Publication bias could play a role when the results are so bad that clinicians feel disinclined to publish. Notably, case reports on failures are singularly absent. Selection of patients could also play a role when operation is deemed unsuitable because of natural palliation, with the pulmonary stenosis counterbalancing the potential shunt in the setting of fairly well functioning atrioventricular valves. Down's syndrome is present in about three-quarters of these patients, which to some clinicians is a further argument against repair. Such patients can be only mildly symptomatic. Previously, the generally accepted policy for treatment was to palliate first

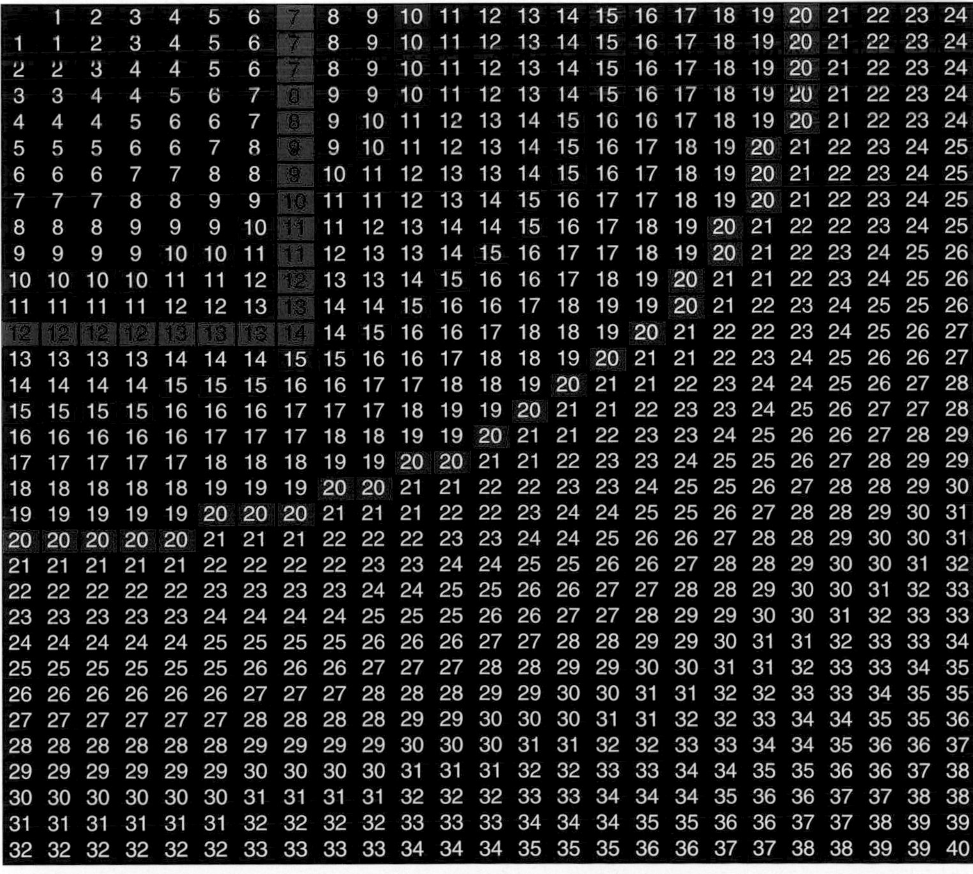

	1	2	3	4	5	6	7	8	9	10	11	12	13	14	15	16	17	18	19	20	21	22	23	24
1	1	2	3	4	5	6	7	8	9	10	11	12	13	14	15	16	17	18	19	20	21	22	23	24
2	2	3	4	4	5	6	7	8	9	10	11	12	13	14	15	16	17	18	19	20	21	22	23	24
3	3	4	4	5	6	7	8	9	9	10	11	12	13	14	15	16	17	18	19	20	21	22	23	24
4	4	4	5	6	6	7	8	9	10	11	12	13	14	15	16	16	17	18	19	20	21	22	23	24
5	5	5	6	6	7	8	9	9	10	11	12	13	14	15	16	17	18	19	20	21	22	23	24	25
6	6	6	7	7	8	8	9	10	11	12	13	13	14	15	16	17	18	19	20	21	22	23	24	25
7	7	7	8	8	9	9	10	11	11	12	13	14	15	16	17	17	18	19	20	21	22	23	24	25
8	8	8	9	9	9	10	11	11	12	13	14	14	15	16	17	18	19	20	21	22	22	23	24	25
9	9	9	9	10	10	11	11	12	13	13	14	15	16	17	17	18	19	20	21	22	23	24	25	26
10	10	10	10	11	11	12	12	13	13	14	15	16	16	17	18	19	20	21	21	22	23	24	25	26
11	11	11	11	12	12	13	13	14	14	15	16	16	17	18	19	19	20	21	22	23	24	25	25	26
12	12	12	12	13	13	13	14	14	15	16	16	17	18	18	19	20	21	22	22	23	24	25	26	27
13	13	13	13	14	14	14	15	15	16	16	17	18	18	19	20	21	21	22	23	24	25	26	26	27
14	14	14	14	15	15	15	16	16	17	17	18	18	19	20	21	21	22	23	24	24	25	26	27	28
15	15	15	15	16	16	16	17	17	17	18	19	19	20	21	21	22	23	23	24	25	26	27	27	28
16	16	16	16	16	17	17	17	18	18	19	19	20	21	21	22	23	23	24	25	26	26	27	28	29
17	17	17	17	17	18	18	18	19	19	20	20	21	21	22	23	23	24	25	25	26	27	28	29	29
18	18	18	18	18	19	19	19	20	20	21	21	22	22	23	23	24	25	25	26	27	28	28	29	30
19	19	19	19	19	20	20	20	21	21	21	22	22	23	24	24	25	25	26	27	28	28	29	30	31
20	20	20	20	20	21	21	21	22	22	22	23	23	24	24	25	26	26	27	28	28	29	30	30	31
21	21	21	21	21	22	22	22	22	23	23	24	24	25	25	26	26	27	28	28	29	30	30	31	32
22	22	22	22	22	23	23	23	23	24	24	25	25	26	26	27	27	28	28	29	30	30	31	32	33
23	23	23	23	23	24	24	24	24	25	25	25	26	26	27	27	28	29	29	30	30	31	32	33	33
24	24	24	24	24	25	25	25	25	26	26	26	27	27	28	28	29	29	30	31	31	32	33	33	34
25	25	25	25	25	25	26	26	26	27	27	27	28	28	29	29	30	30	31	31	32	33	33	34	35
26	26	26	26	26	26	27	27	27	28	28	28	29	29	30	30	31	31	32	32	33	33	34	35	35
27	27	27	27	27	27	28	28	28	28	29	29	30	30	30	31	31	32	32	33	34	34	35	35	36
28	28	28	28	28	28	29	29	29	29	30	30	30	31	31	32	32	33	33	34	34	35	36	36	37
29	29	29	29	29	29	30	30	30	30	31	31	31	32	32	33	33	34	34	35	35	36	36	37	38
30	30	30	30	30	30	31	31	31	31	32	32	32	33	33	34	34	34	35	36	36	37	37	38	38
31	31	31	31	31	31	32	32	32	32	33	33	33	34	34	34	35	35	36	36	37	37	38	39	39
32	32	32	32	32	32	33	33	33	33	34	34	34	35	35	35	36	36	37	37	38	38	39	39	40

Figure 27-68 The table shows how the diameters of two separate orifices can be converted to the equivalent diameter of a single orifice. When the diameter of one orifice is indicated in the leading column and the diameter of the other orifice in the leading row, their combined orifice area can be found at the intersection of column and row.

with an arteriopulmonary shunt, and undertake surgical repair only after the age of 4 years. Evidence now favours primary repair.

Intraoperative Echocardiography

Intraoperative epicardial or transoesophageal echocardiography has become standard practise in surgical correction of atrioventricular septal defect. Pre-bypass evaluation is sometimes indicated. Obtaining additional information concerning the morphology of the left ventricular part of the atrioventricular valve is most essential. The function of this left atrioventricular valve is further assessed in detail by colour-coded Doppler imaging. An image of the left ventricular outflow tract is also obtained in order positively to exclude obstruction.

The imaging procedure is then repeated at the completion of the operative procedure. Not only can the resulting anatomy be reassessed, but also colour-coded Doppler imaging will visualise residual shunts after correction and, most notably, reveal any valvar regurgitation. The location of regurgitation, or of a residual shunt, can then be visualised, indicating the possible need for further repair and facilitating its execution. Residual interventricular shunting should not be accepted, because such shunting is unlikely to disappear spontaneously. When significant, it may lead to post-operative annular dilatation and progressive left atrioventricular valvar regurgitation. Quantification of residual regurgitation, however, is notoriously difficult and disappointing, since its degree often seems to increase in the days immediately after operation. Epicardial echocardiography is more versatile, and usually permits the recording of images of better quality in small infants. A potential problem is that use of expanded polytetrafluoroethylene for the patch creates echo dropout, blinding the area behind the patch to echocardiographic interrogation. It is in this precise position, unfortunately, that the usual planes of epicardial imaging reveal the left atrioventricular valve. Although use of tanned autologous pericardium for the patch gives fewer problems during epicardial imaging, transoesophageal echocardiography is generally recommended for larger infants and children.

Post-operative Management

After the operation, the patient is kept intubated and ventilated until the haemodynamic situation is stable. Because of the known tendency of these post-operative patients to develop pulmonary hypertensive crises, it is wise to prevent acidosis, and to avoid other precipitating factors, such as overly vigorous intratracheal suction. Monitoring of pulmonary arterial pressure is advantageous in patients known to have pulmonary hypertension. Ventilation with nitric oxide has a tremendously advantageous effect in post-operative care for patients suffering from pulmonary hypertensive crises. It may be necessary to prolong such inhalation of nitric oxide until pulmonary vascular resistance drops.[84,98,99]

Monitoring of left atrial pressure has now become standard practise after surgical repair. The presence of a conspicuous left atrial v wave, both before and after the procedure, is a good indication for regurgitation. The absence of a v wave, unfortunately, is not a foolproof indicator that the valve will be competent immediately after repair, possibly because of the altered haemodynamics due to anaesthesia, or through the damping effect of a large atrium. Presence of substantial v waves, nonetheless, is an indication for further investigation and, usually, further attempts at repair of the valve. Even in the absence of problems with repair of the left atrioventricular valve, monitoring of the left atrial pressure facilitates post-operative management, particularly in control of the fluid balance and treatment of pulmonary hypertensive crises. Monitoring of pulmonary arterial pressure, in contrast, is not routinely necessary. It is prudent, nonetheless, to monitor this value when it is known to be strongly elevated, since the evidence obtained facilitates management of pulmonary hypertensive crises with inhalation of nitric oxide or intravenous substances.

Results of Surgical Repair

Categorisation of lesions does demand a special word of caution. It has been a long-standing custom to categorise as intermediate all those patients who do not have either exclusively atrial shunting, or else a significant ventricular shunt in the setting of a common valvar orifice. Usually, these so-called intermediate types are associated with a higher mortality subsequent to operative correction. If such cases are excluded from the overall series then, by default, the results will improve for those in the stereotypic complete and partial categories. Furthermore, many different definitions exist for categorisation of the presumed intermediate variants, thus confounding comparison of results. Another source of serious problems in comparing results reflects the differences in criterions used to select patients for operative repair. These differ markedly among surgeons but are seldom mentioned in surgical reports. It makes a lot of difference, for example, if one either accepts or rejects for surgical repair children with markedly elevated pulmonary hypertension, those with ventricular imbalance, and those with serious atrioventricular valvar deficiencies. Criterions for exclusion, therefore, should be mentioned explicitly when reporting the results of surgical correction, and journal editors should make it their policy to insist on such descriptions. Ideally, any report of surgical correction should also include the results of medical treatment for those children who, for whatever reason, were not submitted to repair. The necessary prerequisite for such an ideal study, namely, a stable community provided with a comprehensive system of health care, is, sadly, not uniformly present. With the information available, it seems currently that the function of the left atrioventricular valve, ventricular imbalance, and pulmonary hypertension are the sole incremental surgical risk factors for death.

Results of surgical repair have improved steadily over the decades, concomitant with developments in medical therapy, more appropriate criterions for selection, and improvements in myocardial preservation, surgical skill, and post-operative care. The difference in mortality when repair of defects with shunting at ventricular level is compared with repair for those with exclusively atrial shunting has largely disappeared. The function of the left atrioventricular valve has determined the operative result, in both the short and the long term. Late reoperations for left atrioventricular valvar dysfunction have been a source of considerable morbidity, and indeed also mortality. It is the results over the long term, obviously, that matter most, but current analysis of such results reflects the techniques and practises used in previous eras. It is not so easy, at the same time, to estimate the long-term efficacy of modern techniques, because good short-term results do not preclude problems over the long term.

The results published to date include the follow-up over a period of 43 years of a surgical correction between 1958 and 2000 of 133 patients with shunting exclusively at atrial level. Actuarial survival was 78%.[100] Operative methods employed during this period reflect contemporaneous knowledge and fashions. Mortality at 30 days was about 7%, which currently could be expected to be no more than 1%. Extrapolating from this premise would make predicted actuarial survival for current patients about 84%. Survival of an age- and era-matched population without any congenital cardiac anomaly was about 90%. Subtraction of these two figures leads us to predict an excess mortality of just 6% 43 years after the surgical correction. Similar results have been reported elsewhere,[101,102] but it is impossible to predict with total accuracy the outcomes for correction at the present time, albeit that results are anticipated to be excellent for those with shunting exclusively at atrial level, presuming it is possible to create a competent left atrioventricular valve.

Long-term results for repair of those having a common atrioventricular valve are well documented in analysis of 801 children in Sweden born alive between 1973 and 1997.[103] Mortality at 30 days for the 502 patients undergoing surgical correction over the last 5 years of the study was 1%. The actuarial survival curve flattens off after 1 or 2 years, and shows a loss of lives of about 10% in 30 years. How this compares to an age- and era-matched population is not known. Although similar results have been published, there are not many papers on results over the long term[104] (see Table 27-1).

Down's Syndrome

Discussion of surgical treatment of atrioventricular septal defect cannot be concluded without consideration of the problems created by co-existing Down's syndrome. Three principle issues are at stake. First, it is often claimed that children with Down's syndrome have a higher incidence of pulmonary hypertension. Second, the anatomical spectrum is different in children with Down's syndrome when compared with their chromosomally normal peers. Third, there has been some controversy on the perceived benefit of surgical repair. Pulmonary hypertension is about 10 times more prevalent in patients with Down's syndrome, and has an earlier onset.[105] Those patients with Down's syndrome, therefore, must undergo surgery at a very young age, preferably before 6 months,[106] while some argue for even earlier repair.[107] Pulmonary hypertension has been reported to be more prevalent in those having the Rastelli A configuration.[108]

Obstruction to left ventricular inflow and outflow, in contrast, is said to be far less frequent in the setting of Down's syndrome.[109] This probably reflects the more frequent existence of common valvar orifice in association with trisomy 21. Extensive bridging of both inferior and superior leaflets, rather than one or both leaflets being committed primarily to the left ventricle, is more usual in children with trisomy 21. Accordingly, the angle of the zone of apposition between the inferior and superior leaflets is usually perpendicular to the ventricular septum in children with Down's syndrome, while this angle is often crooked, and deviated from perpendicular, in those with normal chromosomes. Recently published series show that Down's syndrome is not a risk factor for surgical repair. If anything, anatomy is more favourable in those with trisomy 21. It is pulmonary vascular resistance, itself related to age, and other associated problems, that determine the risk for these patients.[110]

The complete reference list can be found on the companion Expert Consult web site at www.expertconsult.com.

ANNOTATED REFERENCES

- Becker AE, Anderson RH: Atrioventricular septal defects: What's in a name? J Thorac Cardiovasc Surg 1982;83:461–469.

  In this important review, it was the common morphologic features that were promoted as the best denominator for naming these defects so as also to understand the anatomy. Older names implying presumed developmental mechanisms, such as atrioventricular canal and endocardial cushion defect were rejected as being non-descriptive and embryologically speculative.

- Ebels T, Anderson RH, Devine WA, et al: Anomalies of the left atrioventricular valve and related ventricular septal morphology in atrioventricular septal defects. J Thorac Cardiovasc Surg 1990;99:299–307.

  This review of the large series of specimens in the Pittsburgh archive permitted documentation of the anatomical variability in sizes and presence of left valvar leaflets, these then being put into a logical sequence. This variability was related to left ventricular size, to the morphology of the ventricular septum, and to the size of the atrioventricular septal defect.

- Thiene G, Wenink ACG, Frescura C, et al: Surgical anatomy and pathology of the conduction tissues in atrioventricular septal defects. J Thorac Cardiovasc Surg 1981;82:928–937.

  The anatomy of the conduction system in atrioventricular septal defect was reviewed, and put into context of previous studies, providing the anatomical basis for its avoidance during surgery.

- Anderson RH, Ho SY, Becker AE: Anatomy of the human atrioventricular junctions revisited. Anat Rec 2000;260:81–91.

  The atrioventricular junction being common to both ventricles is essential in understanding atrioventricular septal defect. In this paper, the authors review the structure of the normal atrioventricular junctions. The state of the junctions is unrelated to the presence of a septal defect permitting a shunt. This concept increases our understanding the paradox of atrioventricular septal defect with intact septal structures.

- Kaski JP, Wolfenden J, Josen M, et al: Can atrioventricular septal defect exist with intact septal structures? Heart 2006;92:832–835.

  After isolated reports of hearts displaying all features of atrioventricular septal defect with paradoxically intact septal structures, this was the first paper to address this phenomenon from the clinical stance. Many more of these patients must exist, albeit being unrecognised as such, possibly displaying only some degree of left valvar regurgitation. Some of these patients may also have hearts without any functional defect.

- Wetter J, Sinzobahamvya N, Blaschczok C, et al: Closure of the zone of apposition at correction of complete atrioventricular septal defect improves outcome. Eur J Cardiothorac Surg 2000;17:146–153.

  Closure of the zone of apposition during surgical correction of atrioventricular septal defect had been contentious for nearly two decades. Those choosing not to close the zone argued that the trifoliate nature of the valve had to be maintained. The results of this important study showed that non-closure resulted in a substantial proportion of patients needing reoperation for secondary closure of the leaking valve. The paradox is that, while the zone of apposition cannot be compared to a cleft in an otherwise normal leaflet, it must still be closed.

- Mahle WT, Shirali GD, Anderson RH: Echo-morphological correlates in patients with atrioventricular septal defect and common atrioventricular junction. Cardiol Young 2006;16(Suppl 3):43–51.

  The paper describes well how the anatomy of atrioventricular septal defect can be visualised by various echocardiographic planes, emphasizing their limitations. It also introduces the potential value of three-dimensional echocardiography.

- Najm HK, Van Arsdell GS, Watzka S, et al: Primary repair is superior to initial palliation in children with atrioventricular septal defect and tetralogy of Fallot. J Thorac Cardiovasc Surg 1998;116:905–913.

  The group from Toronto presents an analysis of the largest series of patients with the combination of atrioventricular septal defect and tetralogy of Fallot. Their evidence shows that primary repair is the preferred surgical option.

- Frid C, Björkhem G, Jonzon A, et al: Long-term survival in children with atrioventricular septal defect and common atrioventricular orifice in Sweden. Cardiol Young 2004;14:24–31.

  With a maximum follow-up of 28 years, this is the longest comprehensive follow-up of a series of patients undergoing surgery for all forms of atrioventricular septal defect. The 20-year survival of 61% obviously reflects older surgical and medical techniques, but the decreasing slope of the survival curve is a comforting observation.

- Kogon BE, Butler H, McConnell M, et al: What is the optimal time to repair atrioventricular septal defect and common atrioventricular valvar orifice? Cardiol Young 2007;17:356–359.

  The issue of timing of operation for atrioventricular septal defect with unrestricted ventricular shunt is addressed well in this paper. The authors convincingly demonstrate that operation before the age of 6 months is now possible with low mortality, albeit at the cost of higher morbidity and a higher incidence of complications.

CHAPTER 28

Ventricular Septal Defects

LEE N. BENSON, SHI-JOON YOO, FAHAD AL HABSHAN, and ROBERT H. ANDERSON

Holes between the ventricles can occur as isolated anomalies, but are also seen in association with many other defects. For example, they are found as integral parts of entities such as the tetralogy of Fallot, double-outlet ventricles, and most cases of common arterial trunk. They occur as a component of atrioventricular septal defects with common atrioventricular junction, and are frequently encountered in association with transposition and congenitally corrected transposition. They are an integral part of the functionally univentricular circulation. Taken together, they unequivocally make up the commonest congenital cardiac malformation. In this chapter, we consider only the so-called isolated examples, albeit that we discuss the complications produced by other minor associations. Although holes between the ventricles have a long pedigree, it is with the name of Henri Roger[1] that the anomaly is historically linked. It was Roger who recognised that an isolated ventricular septal defect produced a typical murmur, and could be consistent with prolonged life and good health.

PREVALENCE

If we exclude aortic valves having two leaflets, and also exclude prolapse of the mitral valve,[2] then isolated ventricular septal defect is the most common congenital cardiac malformation. It is difficult to obtain an accurate assessment of prevalence, since most individuals with an isolated defect, being asymptomatic, are not candidates for cardiac catheterisation and angiography. In the past, therefore, there frequently was no objective proof of the presence of a defect. It was the advent of cross sectional echocardiography, and colour flow Doppler, that changed all that. The known high rate of spontaneous closure[3] meant that postmortem data certainly underestimated the incidence of the defect. In series depending heavily on clinical observation, the estimated prevalence has varied markedly. The incidence has been shown to be higher in fetuses dying prenatally, and there is some variation depending on the time of fetal death. Hoffman[4] summarised the literature addressing the proportional distribution of congenital cardiac defects from 22 series, showing that the median distribution for ventricular septal defect was 31%. The most accurate clinical data comes from the prospective Bohemia survival study,[5] which revealed a prevalence of 2.56 per 1000 live births, accounting for two-fifths of all cardiac malformations, similar to the data from Merseyside in the United Kingdom, where the figure was 2.74 per 1000 births.[6] A study from Malta, in contrast, revealed a figure of 3.94, a significant difference.[7] This reflects the increased use of echocardiography in diagnosis. This trend is confirmed by data from the Baltimore–Washington Infant Study,[8] which also used echocardiographic techniques, and showed a remarkable increase in the diagnosis of muscular defects, with a tenfold increase in prevalence. Ventricular septal defects accounted for one-third of the lesions identified in the infants of this study, and made up over two-fifths of the malformations encountered in Malta. A particularly high prevalence of muscular defects has also been reported by those who scanned populations of neonates using colour flow imaging, noting subsequent spontaneous closure of many of the defects.[9–12] None of these studies, however, were population based.[13] Ventricular septal defects are more common in premature infants, and those born with low weight. Incidence, however, is not related significantly to race, sex, maternal age, birth order, or socioeconomic state.

While there does not appear to be a genetic bias towards the incidence of ventricular septal defects, genetics do influence the specific type of defect. The doubly committed subarterial, or juxta-arterial, defect is more common in Asian populations, whereas muscular and multiple defects are less common in the same population. According to Wilkinson,[14] the frequency of the doubly-committed subarterial or juxta-arterial defect requiring repair accounts for at least 30% in an Asian population, compared with the incidence of about 5% of Occidental patients requiring surgery in Western societies. Wilkinson[14] also noted that, while muscular defects account for about three-tenths of defects requiring closure in the Western world, they are uncommon in the Asian population referred for surgical closure, where multiple ventricular septal defects are very rare. Such multiple muscular defects account for one-tenth of operative closures in the west.

MORPHOLOGY AND MORPHOGENESIS

Categorisation of Defects

It is, perhaps, surprising that, as we start the 21st century, there is still no consensus concerning the best way to categorise and describe holes between the ventricles. The lesion, however, is not always as simple as it first appears. For example, when the hole between the ventricles is overridden by an arterial valve, it is open to debate as to which plane in space represents the defect.[15] This is because the septum that interposes between the outflow tracts is no longer an interventricular structure. This fact, in itself, negates the possibility of defining a ventricular septal defect as a simple hole in the substance of the ventricular septum. This situation is magnified in the setting of double-outlet right ventricle. In this setting, the hole in

TABLE 28-1

CRITERIONS FOR CLASSIFICATION OF A VENTRICULAR SEPTAL DEFECT

Define the plane of the defect
Define the boundaries of the defect
Account for the anatomical features:
- The relation of the defect to the atrioventricular conduction axis
- The relation of the defect to the atrioventricular valves
- The relation of the defect to the arterial valves
- The position of the defect within the ventricular septum: opening to the inlet, apical trabecular, or outlet parts of the right ventricle
- The size of the defect

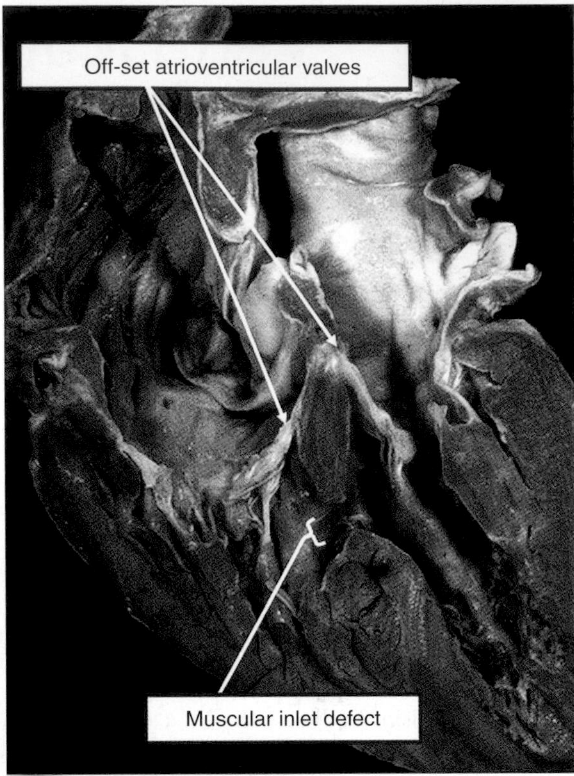

Figure 28-1 The hole in this heart (*bracket*) is enclosed within the muscular septum. None would have difficulty in establishing the margins of the defect, and recognising that it opens between the ventricular inlets.

the ventricular septum, or the interventricular communication, functions as the outlet from the left ventricle. Surgical correction of patients with double outlet right ventricle, therefore, is based on the concept of tunneling this hole to one or other of the ventricular outflow tracts. In this setting, closure of the hole between the ventricles would wall off the left ventricle from both arterial trunks. Because of these subtle differences in the potential definition of septal defects, different investigators have chosen different features on which to base their criterions for classification. It is hardly surprising, therefore, that currently there is lack of concensus on the best options for categorisation. Indeed, as yet there is no agreement on what defines a ventricular septal defect. Our proposal for definition and classification is based upon several principles (Table 28-1).

First, it is necessary to define clearly and unambiguously the plane of space chosen to represent the defect. Having defined this plane, the second principle is to account for all its various anatomical features. Most important of these are its boundaries. As we will show, it is the structure of the boundaries that permits phenotypic categorisation. Having established the phenotype of the defect, it is then necessary to describe the position of the hole relative to the landmarks and components of the ventricular septum, including the surgically significant atrioventricular conduction axis. If present, it is also necessary to take account of valvar overriding. When either an atrioventricular or an arterial valve overrides the crest of the muscular ventricular septum, then of necessity there is malalignment between the different septal components. Attention must also be given to the size of the hole chosen to represent the defect. The system, to be used throughout our volume, and forming the basis for the categorisation used in the European Paediatric Cardiac Code,[16] caters for all these features. As we will subsequently show, this system is applicable not only to isolated defects to be described in this chapter, but for those in all the various settings described elsewhere in these pages.

What Is the Defect?

When there is a simple hole, punched as it were into the substance of the muscular ventricular septum, then there is no problem in defining its margins, nor in agreeing that the margins are exclusively muscular (Fig. 28-1). Many holes, however, have the crest of the muscular ventricular septum as one of their margins, but abut directly upon the hingepoints of the leaflets of either the atrioventricular or the arterial valves (Fig. 28-2), or on occasion the attachments of both the arterial and atrioventricular valvar leaflets. Some of these lesions are associated with marked overriding of an arterial or atrioventricular valvar orifice. An example of overriding of the arterial valve is demonstrated in Figure 28-3. In this particular circumstance, it is much harder to define the precise borders and margins of hole between the ventricles. This is because an inverted cone of space, with an elongated base, extends from the attachments of the leaflets of the overriding arterial valve to the crest of the muscular ventricular septum (Fig. 28-4). Within this inverted cone, any of a number of planes can justifiably be nominated to represent the defect. When viewed in a single section, as seen by the echocardiographer, then at least three of these planes are important (see Fig. 28-4). One is the continuation of the long axis of the ventricular septum to the underside of the overriding valvar leaflets, the green oval as shown in Figure 28-4. This particular choice for defining the defect, which without question represents the plane of the superior continuation of the muscular ventricular septum, exists only when the valvar leaflets are closed. Even though this plane represents the geometric interventricular communication, it is never the locus for placement of a patch by the surgeon during operative repair of an isolated defect. Indeed, when the arterial valvar leaflets open during ventricular systole, the superior margin of this hole is the underside of the aortic arch! The second plane, shown by the yellow oval in Figure 28-4, marks the boundary between the cone of space subtended beneath the overriding valve and the left ventricle. This plane is the opening from the left ventricle to the subaortic outflow tract, presuming that it is the aortic valve which is

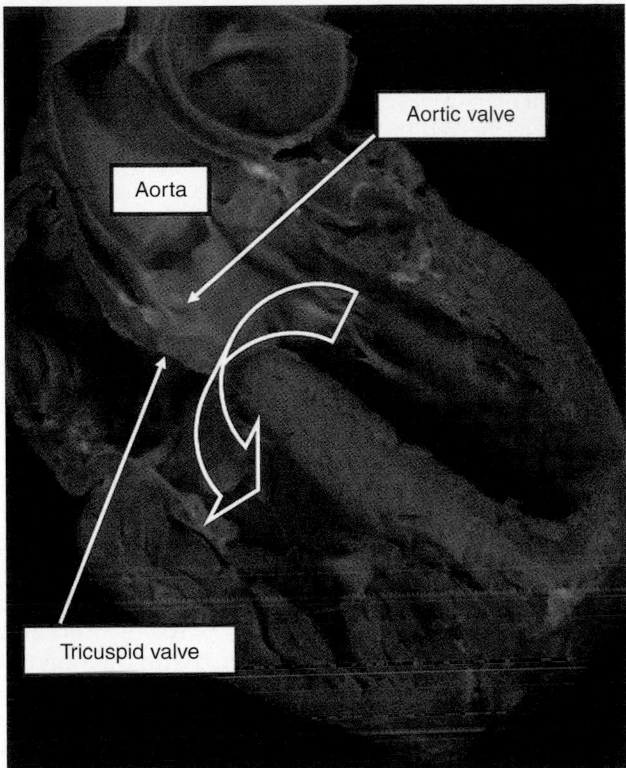

Figure 28-2 It is much more difficult to identify the precise plane of the defect (*open arrow*) in this heart, sectioned to replicate the parasternal long-axis oblique plane incorporating the aortic root. The aorta is overriding the crest of the ventricular septum, and the superior margin of the defect is formed by fibrous continuity between the leaflets of the aortic and tricuspid valves (see Fig. 28-3).

overriding the septal crest. Although unequivocally important, this plane is also unlikely to be chosen as the septal defect. The third plane, shown as the red oval in Figure 28-4, has features in common with the second, in that it marks a ventricular border of the inverted cone of space. This plane, to our eyes, is of greatest practical importance, since it is the border around which the surgeon will insert sutures to secure a patch placed to prevent shunting between the ventricles. It is also the position where the interventionist will place a device with the same goal in mind. It is this third plane, therefore, that we choose to define as the ventricular septal defect, considering the hole as the plane of space that must be closed so as to restore septal integrity. It is the difference in the anatomical make-up of the margins of this hole, as viewed from the morphologically right ventricle, which provide the phenotypic features of the different types of defect. This also is the view obtained by the surgeon when restoring septal integrity in the operating room. In many instances, the hole closed by the surgeon to restore septal integrity is also the obvious hole within the ventricular septum (Fig. 28-5). In these situations, therefore, the septal defect and the interventricular communication are one and the same. In the situation of double outlet right ventricle, this is obviously not the case (Fig. 28-6). When both arterial trunks arise from the right ventricle, the hole closed so as to restore septal integrity is the plane from the crest of the muscular ventricular septum to the underside of the right ventricular outlet septum. This hole is now markedly different from the interventricular communication, which is the outlet for the left ventricle. In the setting of double outlet right ventricle, therefore, as already discussed, it would be a disaster if the

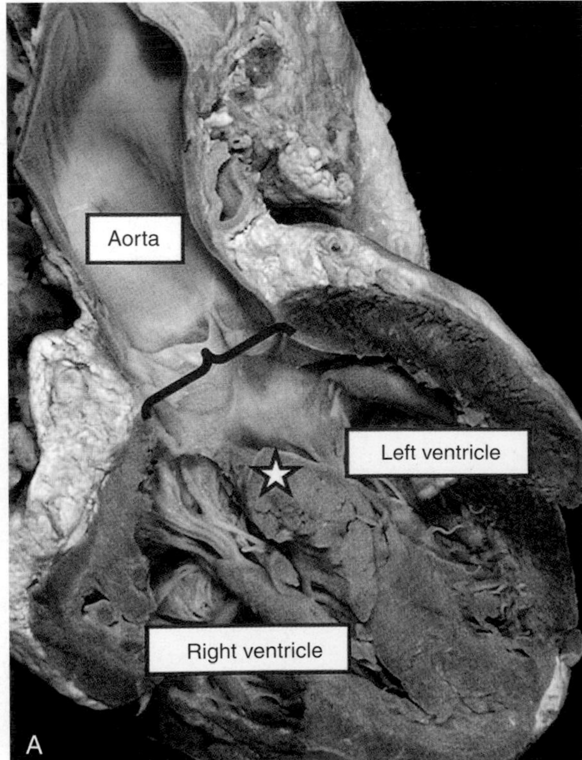

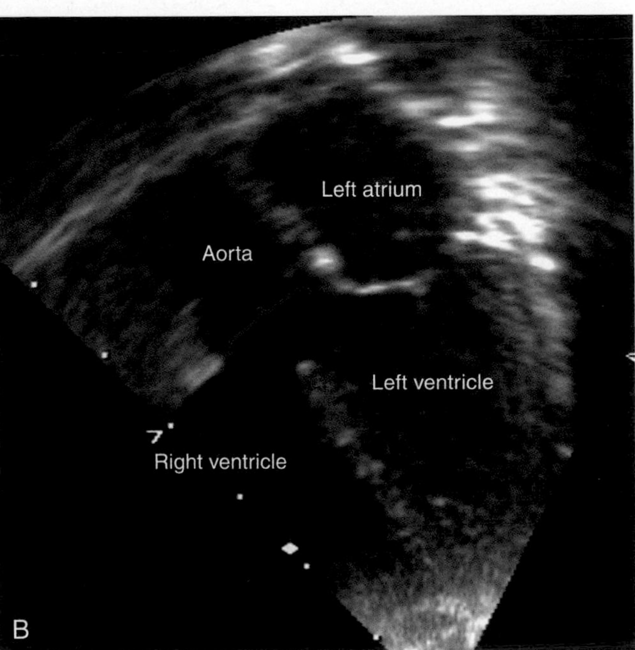

Figure 28-3 In this example (A), with its equivalent echocardiogram (B), the degree of aortic valvar overriding is more obvious. There is now an inverted cone of space that extends from the attachments of the valvar leaflets (*bracket*) to the crest of the ventricular septum (*star*). It is reasonable to nominate any plane within this cone as a ventricular septal defect, but three particular planes are of special importance (see Fig. 28-4).

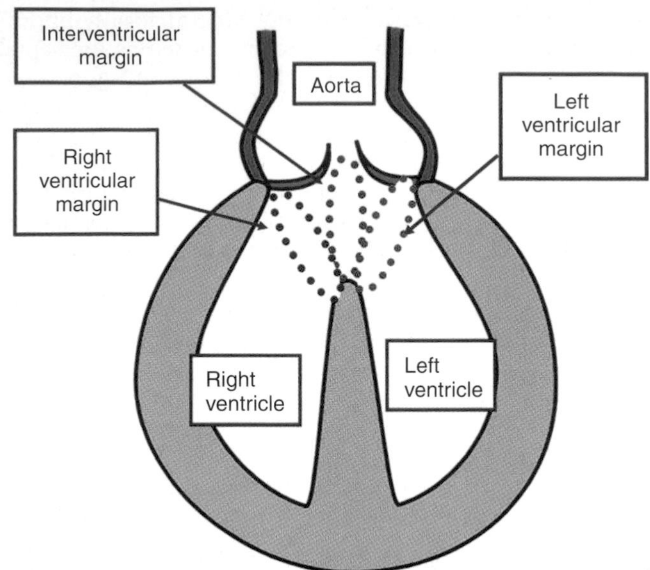

Figure 28-4 Within the cone as illustrated in Figure 28-3, at least three planes are particularly important. They are the right ventricular margin (*red oval*), the plane of the interventricular communication marked by the upward continuation of the ventricular septum (*green oval*), and the left ventricular margin (*yellow oval*). When categorising the hole between the ventricles, we use the features of the right ventricular margin, this being the space closed by the surgeon to restore septal integrity.

surgeon chose to close the interventricular communication, as opposed to the hole which, when closed, restores septal integrity (see Fig. 28-6).

Features Requiring Description

As shown, the holes to be closed so as to restore septal integrity are either found within the muscular septum, or else at its margins. The holes at the margins of the muscular septum can be related directly to the hinges of the leaflets of the atrioventricular, or those of the arterial valves, or in some circumstances to the leaflets of both arterial and atrioventricular valves. It is an appreciation of these relationships, as viewed from the right ventricle, which we use as the primary criterion for description. When considered from this stance, all defects can be placed into one of four groups, namely those which are muscular, those which are perimembranous, those which are juxtatricuspid (and non-perimembranous), and those which are both doubly committed and juxta-arterial (Fig. 28-7 and Table 28-2).

Muscular Defects

Those holes within the substance of the septum of necessity have exclusively muscular rims, and hence are described as muscular defects (Fig. 28-8).

Perimembranous Defects

The second group of holes are those related to the aortic root, opening into the right ventricle in the area where the subpulmonary outflow tract turns superiorly relative to the atrioventricular junction. We describe this area as the inner curvature of the right side of the heart (Fig. 28-9). When the ventricular septum is intact, this is the area occupied by the membranous part of the septum, with the supraventricular crest separating the area from the leaflets of the pulmonary valve (see Chapter 2). The membranous septum, on its left ventricular aspect, is directly continuous with the area of fibrous continuity between the leaflets of the aortic and mitral valves. The right end of this zone of continuity is called the right fibrous trigone. It is fusion of this trigone with the membranous septum that produces the central fibrous body (Figs. 28-10 and 28-11).

This entire area is then part of the fibrous root of the aorta, and is itself continuous with the triangle of fibrous tissue which ascends to occupy the space between the non-coronary and right coronary leaflets of the aortic valve. On the right side, the membranous septum itself is

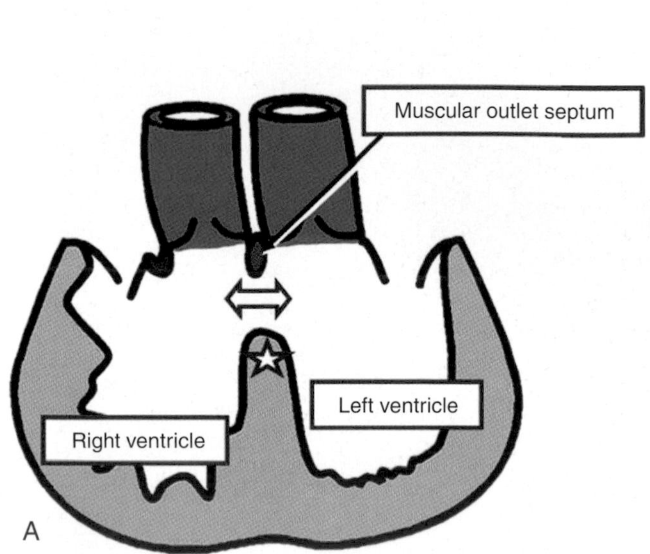

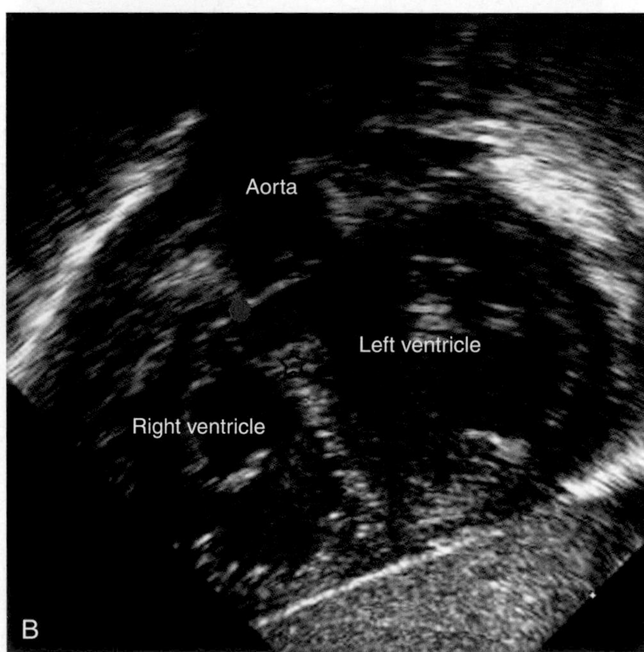

Figure 28-5 The cartoon (**A**), along with an equivalent echocardiogram (**B**), shows the arrangement in which there is a simple hole within the muscular ventricular septum (*double-headed arrow*). This is the interventricular communication, and is located between the crest of the muscular ventricular septum (*star*) and the underside of the muscular outlet septum (*green oval*). This is the hole closed so as to restore septal integrity. In this situation, there is no problem in defining the interventricular communication as being the ventricular septal defect.

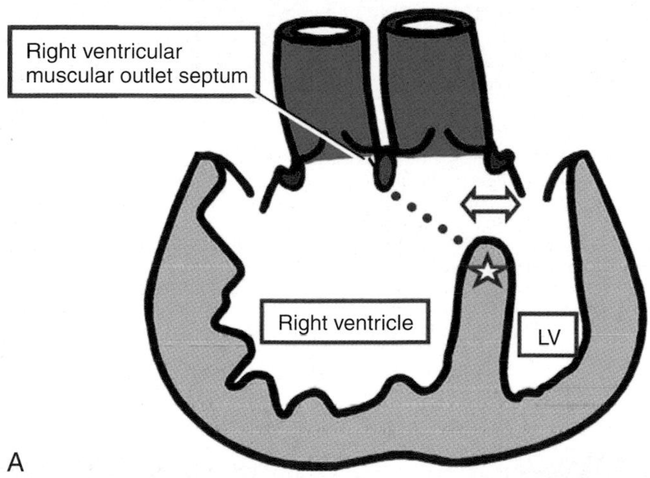

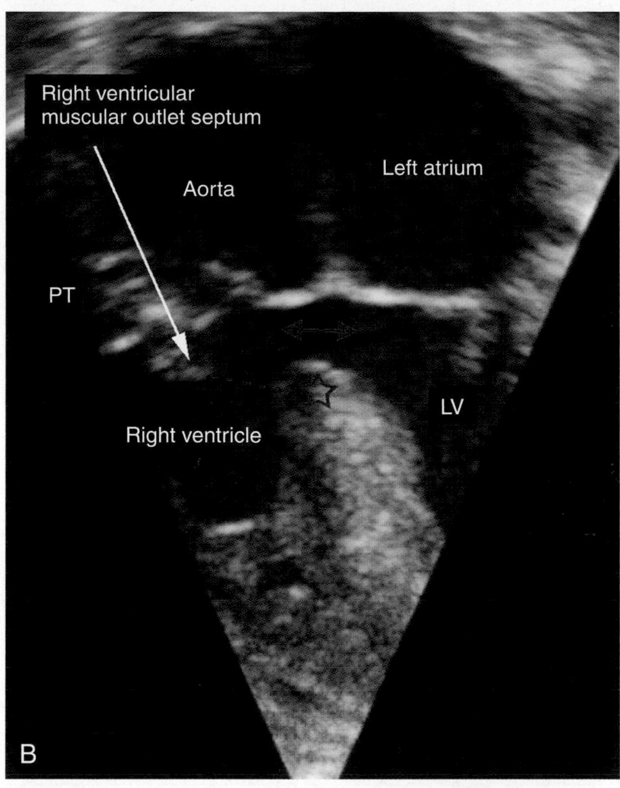

Figure 28-6 The cartoon (A), together with an equivalent echocardiogram (B), shows the arrangement in which both arterial trunks arise in their entirety from the morphologically right ventricle. The muscular outlet septum (*green oval*) is now a right ventricular rather than an interventricular structure. The plane closed so as to restore septal integrity (*red dotted line*) is now within the cavity of the right ventricle. It is no longer the interventricular communication (*double-headed arrow*). Indeed, in this situation it would be a disaster to close the interventricular communication. The ventricular septal defect, therefore, or the red dotted line, is no longer the same thing as the interventricular communication. The *star* shows the crest of the muscular ventricular septum. LV, left ventricle; PT, pulmonary trunk.

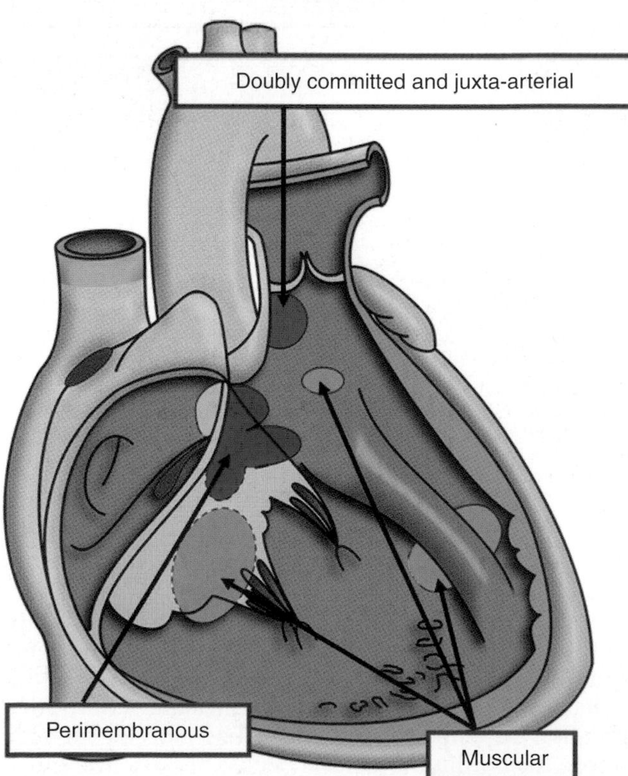

Figure 28-7 The cartoon shows the locations of the various phenotypic types of holes permitting shunting between the ventricles as seen from the right ventricle.

crossed by the hinge of the septal leaflet of the tricuspid valve, dividing it into atrioventricular and interventricular components. The axis of atrioventricular conduction tissue penetrates through this septum from the apex of the triangle of Koch (see Chapter 2). Having penetrated, when

TABLE 28-2

CLASSIFICATION OF THE BORDERS OF VENTRICULAR SEPTAL DEFECTS

Defects abutting on area of continuity between atrioventricular and arterial valves (perimembranous)
Opening into inlet of right ventricle
Opening into outlet of right ventricle
Confluent defects
Defects encased within musculature of ventricular septum (muscular)
Opening to the inlet of the right ventricle
Opening between the apical components
Opening to the subpulmonary outlet
Multiple
Co-existing with perimembranous defect
Defects roofed by arterial valves in fibrous continuity (doubly committed and juxta-arterial)
With muscular postero-inferior rim
Extending to become perimembranous
Defects roofed by the tricuspid valve, with an intact membranous septum

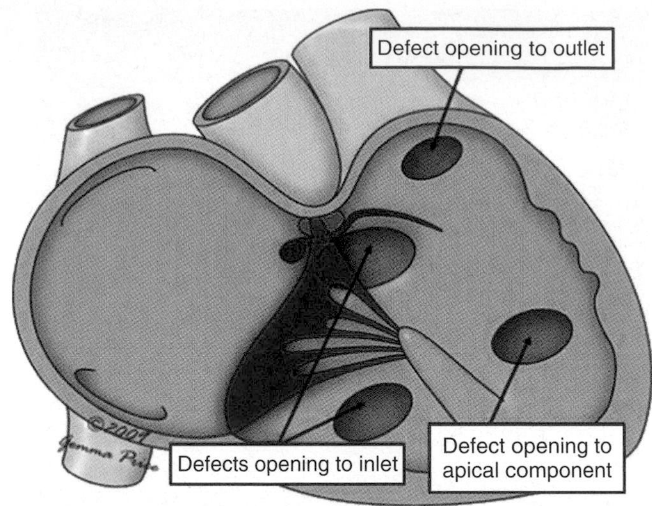

Figure 28-8 Holes with exclusively muscular borders, as seen from the right side, can permit shunting to the inlet, to the apical component, or to the outlet of the right ventricle. Depending on their location, they will bear different relationships to the atrioventricular conduction axis, shown in red. The membranous septum, perforated by the conduction axis, is shown in yellow.

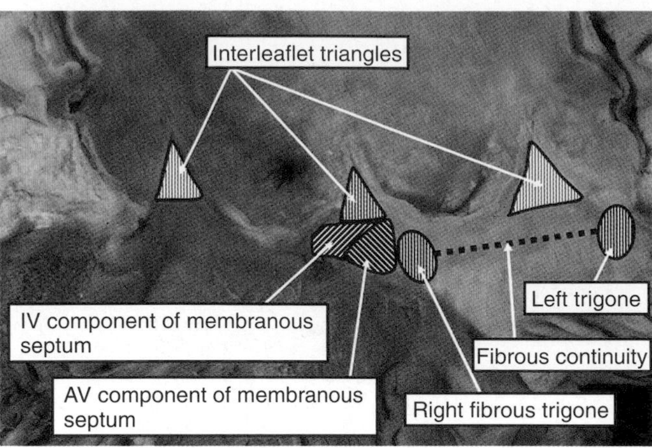

Figure 28-10 The aortic outflow tract of the normal heart is shown having removed the leaflets of the aortic valve. Note that the membranous septum (outlined by *blue cross-hatching*) is continuous with the right fibrous trigone (*red cross-hatching*) and the interleaflet triangle between the right coronary and non-coronary sinuses of the aortic valve (*blue vertical hatching*). When the septum comes apart, as it does in the setting of perimembranous defects, it does so between the crest of the muscular ventricular septum and the components of the membranous septum. The interventricular (IV) component of the membranous septum often persists as a flap in the postero-inferior margin of the defect. AV, atrioventricular.

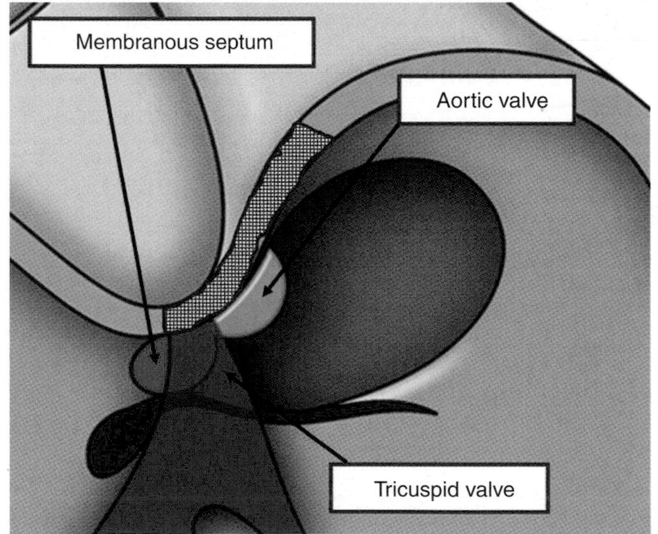

Figure 28-9 When a hole between the ventricles is at the borders of the muscular septum, and opens into the right ventricle in the area between the membranous septum and the subpulmonary infundibulum, the area we call the inner curvature (*cross-hatched area*), it is formed postero-inferiorly by fibrous continuity between the leaflets of the superiorly located aortic and posteriorly located tricuspid valves (see also Fig. 28-10). The membranous septum is then an integral part of this fibrous continuity, albeit usually shielded from view by the septal leaflet of the tricuspid valve. The conduction axis, as it penetrates from atrium to ventricle, is directly related to this postero-inferior border (see Fig. 28-15). We describe any defect possessing this phenotypic feature as perimembranous.

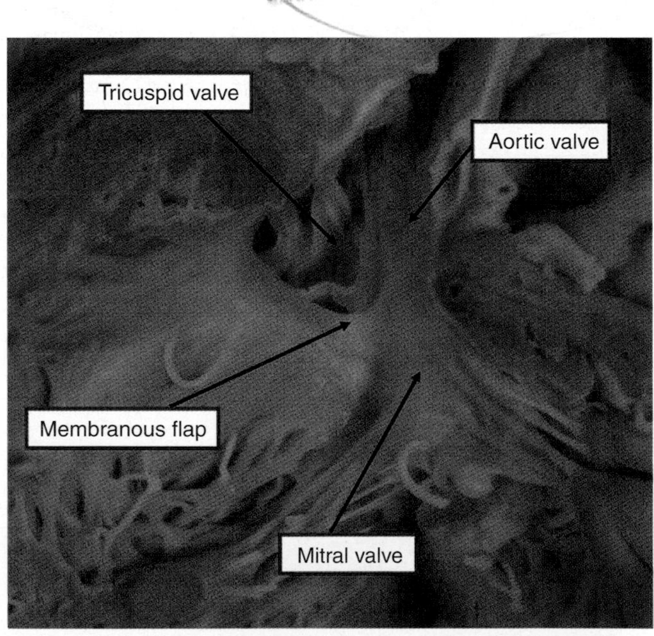

Figure 28-11 This specimen is photographed from the left side, showing that the posterior margin of a defect we categorise as being perimembranous is formed by fibrous continuity between the leaflets of the mitral, aortic, and tricuspid valves. Note the small remnant of the interventricular component of the membranous septum, which is part of the central fibrous body.

the septum is intact, the conduction bundle runs on the crest of the muscular septum, being sandwiched between the fibrous and muscular septal components, along the postero-inferior margin of the interventricular part of the membranous septum. When the ventricular septum is deficient in this area, it springs apart between these two septal components. In consequence, the postero-inferior margin of the defects opening from the aortic root is formed by fibrous continuity between the leaflets of the aortic and tricuspid valves (see Fig. 28-9). In the past, such defects were often called membranous defects, since it was presumed that they existed because of a deficiency in the membranous septum. It was pointed out long since[17] that this is unlikely, since the defects are always larger than the normal dimensions of the membranous septum. Furthermore, the membranous septum is not divided into its interventricular and atrioventricular components until after the embryonic septum has closed.[18] It seems far more likely that the defects persist because the muscular ventricular septum is deficient in the environs of the developing membranous septum. Taking account of this fact, we suggested that the defects should be considered perimembranous.[19] Their anatomical hallmark in the otherwise normally constituted heart is the presence, as seen from the right side, of fibrous continuity between the leaflets of the aortic and tricuspid valves (see Fig. 28-9). When viewed from the left side, the continuity is seen to include also the aortic leaflet of the mitral valve (see Fig. 28-11). Some of these defects, because of associated anomalies of tricuspid valve, such as clefts or perforations of the septal leaflet, or deformity or adherence of valvar tissue to the margins of the septal defect and widening of the anteroseptal commissure,[20] produce the potential for ventriculo-atrial shunting. Defects of this type are the commonest examples of so-called Gerbode defects.[21] Ventriculo-atrial shunting can also be produced when there is deficiency of the atrioventricular component of the membranous septum, producing a true atrioventricular septal defect with separate right and left atrioventricular junctions, but these lesions are exceedingly rare (see Chapter 27). They form the rarer variant of the Gerbode defect.[21]

Doubly Committed and Juxta-arterial Defects

There is then a third group of defects that is discrete from the first two groups. The feature of these defects is that they occupy the region in the normal heart formed by the free-standing component of the muscular subpulmonary infundibulum. The infundibulum is the sleeve of free-standing muscle that lifts the leaflets of the pulmonary valve away from the base of the heart. In our initial description,[19] we interpreted this part of the infundibulum as being formed by the muscular outlet septum. We now know this to be incorrect, since as emphasised above, the leaflets of the pulmonary valve, in the normal heart, are supported by a complete sleeve of free-standing infundibular musculature. Defects of this third type, therefore, which are both doubly committed and juxta-arterial, and characterised by fibrous continuity in their roof between the leaflets of the aortic and pulmonary valves (Fig. 28-12), cannot exist in hearts in which the free-standing muscular subpulmonary infundibulum has developed in normal fashion. In other words, the presence of this type of defect implies abnormal formation of the subpulmonary infundibulum in such a way as to permit a hole to exist directly beneath the arterial roots. When viewed from the right ventricle, most defects of this type are seen to have a muscular postero-inferior rim separating the leaflets of the aortic and tricuspid valves. They are, therefore, described as doubly committed and juxta-arterial (see Fig. 28-12, upper panel). On occasion, nonetheless, they can extend so that the postero-inferior margin is formed by fibrous continuity between the aortic and tricuspid valvar leaflets, the roof continuing to be made up of aortic to pulmonary valvar continuity. Defects with such margins are both doubly committed and juxta-arterial and, at the same time, perimembranous (see Fig. 28-12, lower panel).

Juxta-tricuspid and Non-perimembranous Defects

The juxta-tricuspid, and non-perimembranous, defect is very rare. The hole between the ventricles is roofed by fibrous continuity between the leaflets of the tricuspid and mitral valves, but is separated from the area of the membranous septum.[22] The atrioventricular valvar leaflets are then in direct contact through the posterior margin of the defect. In contrast to perimembranous defects, the tricuspid valve is not in direct contact with the aortic valve. It was defined on the basis of the four-chamber echocardiographic cut, and its angiographic equivalent.[22] Those describing the defect commented that it may be difficult to distinquish from a perimembranous defect, and indeed, one of us (RHA) has never encountered an autopised specimen with such a defect. The conduction axis will be located at the anterior aspect of the defect, coursing along the postero-inferior margin of the intact membranous septum.

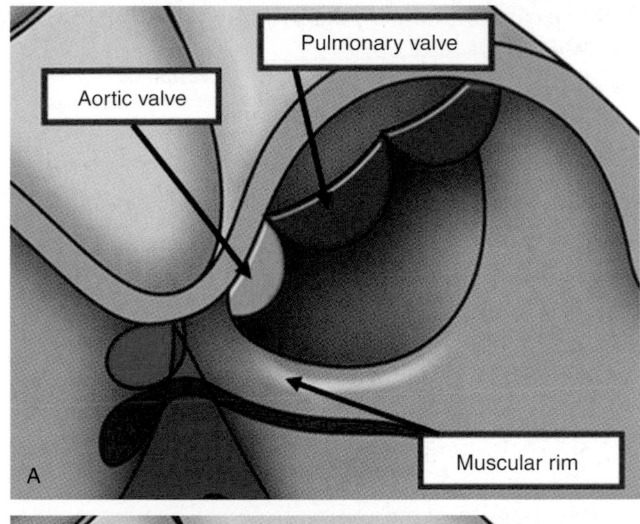

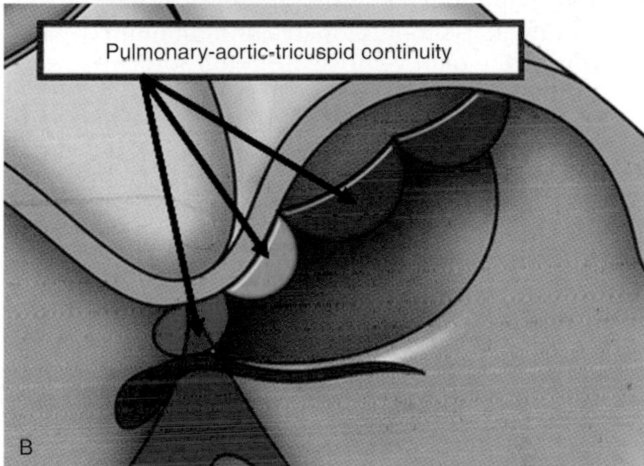

Figure 28-12 There is a third phenotypic variant for holes between the ventricles, which we describe as being doubly committed and juxta-arterial. As shown in the cartoon, holes fulfilling the criterion for inclusion in this group are characterised by fibrous continuity between the leaflets of the aortic and pulmonary valves. **A**, most hearts of this type have a muscular postero-inferior rim that protects the conduction axis (*red*). This arrangement makes the defect as shown in the upper panel both doubly committed and juxta-arterial, but not perimembranous. **B**, On the other hand, these defects can also extend so that there is continuity also with the leaflets of the tricuspid valve. The defects are then both doubly committed and juxta-arterial, and perimembranous.

Position of Defects

Having accounted for the margins of the various defects, as viewed from the right side, and having used this as our primary criterion for definition, we then describe the position of the defect relative to the landmarks and components of the right ventricle. For the muscular defects, this creates no problems, since these holes are punched within the substance of the muscular septum so as to open directly to the inlet, the outlet, or the apical parts of the right ventricle.

For the perimembranous defects, the situation is more complicated.

Relation of Perimembranous Defects to Components of the Right Ventricle

In our initial account,[19] we described perimembranous defects as excavating into the inlet, outlet, or apical trabecular components of the septum. This is incorrect. Although much of the septum, when viewed from the right side, seems to be positioned to separate the inlet of the right from the inlet of the left ventricle, this is not the case. Because of the deeply wedged location of the normal subaortic outflow tract, the majority of the septum as viewed from the right side in relation to the septal leaflet of the tricuspid valve separates the inlet of the right from the outlet of the left ventricle. As discussed, it is also the case that, in the normal heart, the seemingly septal surface of the right ventricular outflow tract is formed by the free-standing muscular subpulmonary infundibulum. The posterior wall of this muscular subpulmonary infundibulum separates the cavity of the right ventricle from the aortic root, rather than forming a septum between the cavities of the right and left ventricles. Indeed, in the normal heart it is not possible to recognise the boundaries of a discrete muscular outlet septum (see Chapter 2). When perimembranous defects open anteriorly towards the pulmonary valve, they do not excavate directly into the free-standing muscular subpulmonary infundibulum. Instead, the presence of the defect now makes it possible to recognise a discrete muscular outlet septum, which forms the superior margin of the hole between the ventricles. This true outlet septum, located within the right ventricle, can be extensively malaligned relative to the remainder of the muscular septum. The arrangement permits shunting between the subaortic and subpulmonary outlets (Fig. 28-13). Because of the close relationship of the aortic valve to the tricuspid valve, some of the shunting will still be directed towards the inlet of the right ventricle. Large perimembranous defects, therefore, can be considered confluent, shunting to all parts of the right ventricle.

Valvar Overriding and Septal Malalignment

The third important feature that requires description, when present, is valvar overriding, along with its associated feature of malalignment of septal components. Malalignment can involve the muscular outlet septum, as discussed above. In the situation illustrated thus far (see Fig. 28-13), the outlet septum is a right ventricular structure, as is also the case in tetralogy of Fallot (see Chapter 36). The outlet septum can be deviated posteriorly to become a left ventricular structure, then obstructing the outflow tract of the left ventricle (Fig. 28-14). There can also be malalignment between the muscular ventricular septum and the atrial septum. This is the phenotypic feature of hearts with overriding of the orifice of the tricuspid valve and straddling of its tendinous cords (Fig. 28-15).

Size and Shape of the Defect

Size is obviously important in determining the haemodynamic consequences of the various types of defects, and also in determining those defects most likely to diminish in size or close spontaneously. Size can be described according to taste, either using subjective adjectives such as large, medium or small, or by relating the different dimensions of the plane of space measured as the defect to the diameter

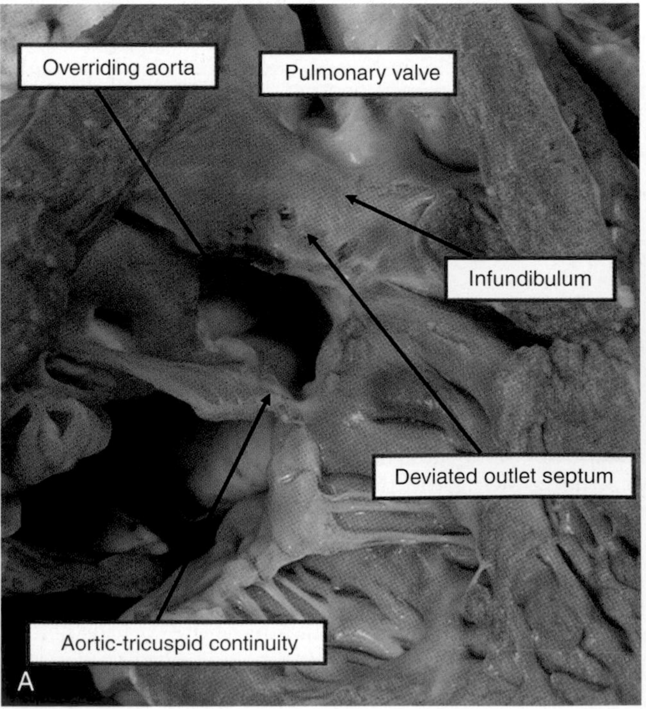

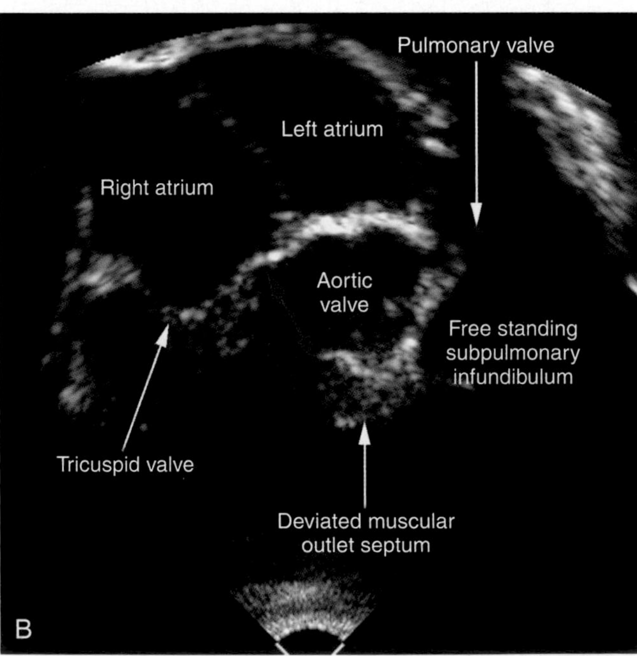

Figure 28-13 These perimembranous defects, shown in the specimen (A) and the subcostal short-axis echocardiogram (B), open into the outlet of the right ventricle. In the specimen, a significant proportion of the aortic leaflets attached to right ventricular, rather than left ventricular, structure. When viewed along the long axis of the ventricular septum, the aortic valvar orifice overrides the crest of the ventricular septum (see also Fig. 28-20). The muscular outlet septum can now be recognised as a discrete structure, located exclusively in the right ventricle, separating the subaortic and subpulmonary outflow tracts, and supporting the free-standing muscular subpulmonary infundibulum. The *double-headed red arrow* on echocardiogram indicates the defect through which the aortic and tricuspid valves are in direct contact.

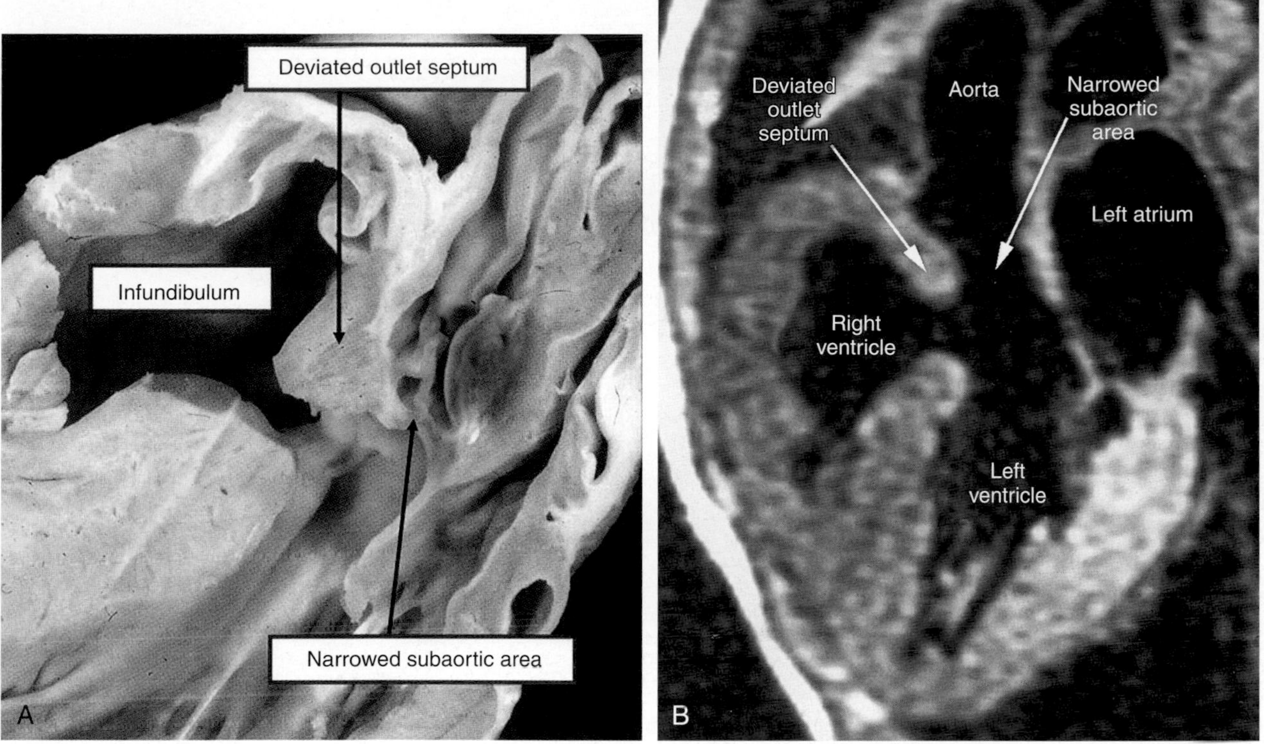

Figure 28-14 This specimen (A), and corresponding magnetic resonance image sectioned in parasternal long axis plane (B), show how the muscular outlet septum is deviated posteriorly to obstruct the subaortic outlet.

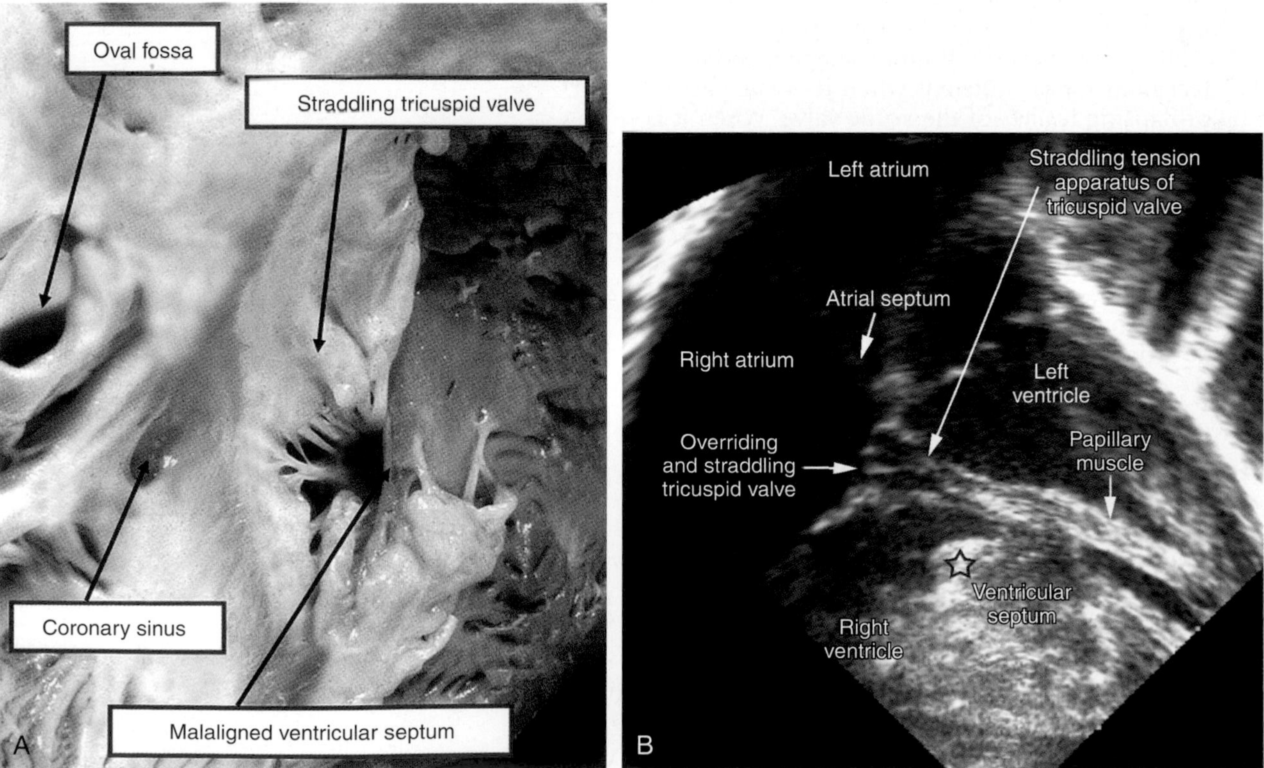

Figure 28-15 **A**, In this heart, even though the hole between the ventricles is perimembranous, there is malalignment between the atrial septum and the crest of the muscular ventricular septum, the inferior part of the muscular ventricular septum being deviated anteriorly and superiorly into the right ventricle. This permits straddling and overriding of the tricuspid valve. **B**, A corresponding subcostal echocardiogram shows malalignment between the atrial and ventricular septum. The tension apparatus of the tricuspid valve inserts to the papillary muscle in the left ventricle through the defect above the crest of the malaligned ventricular septum (*star*).

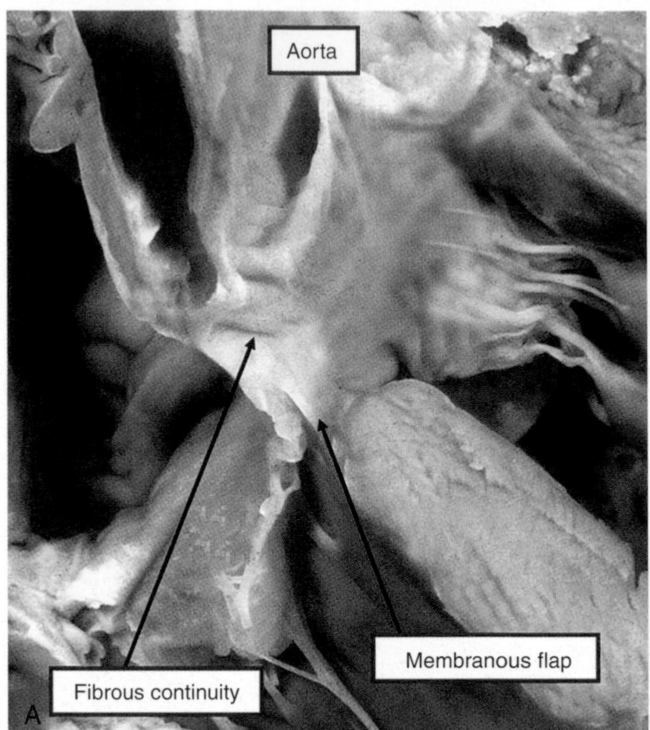

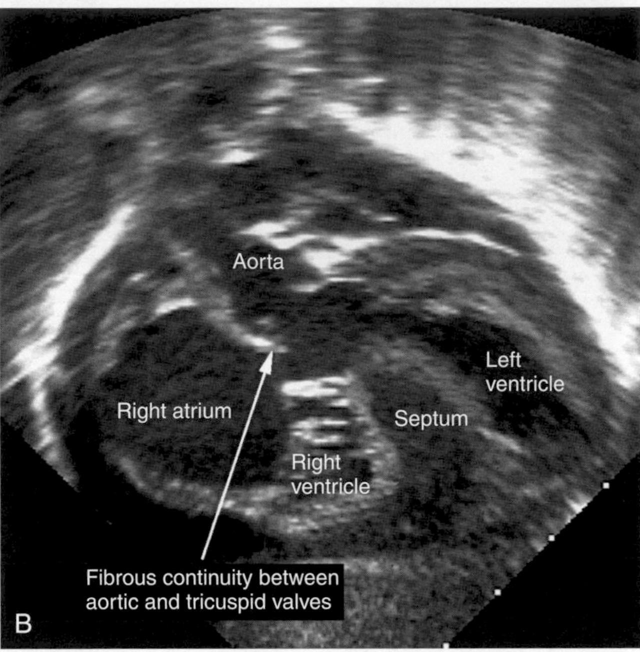

Figure 28-16 When viewed in the subcostal long-axis oblique cut of the left ventricular outflow (**A**), it can be seen that the postero-inferior margin of the perimembranous defect is formed by fibrous continuity between the leaflets of the aortic and tricuspid valves. Note the remnant of the membranous septum in the specimen, forming a membranous flap, which reinforces an area of fibrous continuity between the tricuspid and mitral valves. Panel **B** shows a comparable echocardiographic section.

of the aortic root. The shape of the defect may also vary; muscular defects are typically round or oval when seen from the right ventricle, although they can be crescentic or cashew-like. Defects that are bordered by atrioventricular or arterial valves are typically half-moon shaped. The shape of the defect may appear different when it is encroached upon by prolapsing leaflets of the aortic valve. When it is not round, the defect may appear larger on one plane than on another as seen using cross sectional and angiographic imaging.

Having discussed the general principles of categorisation, and the system by which we describe ventricular septal defects, we will now consider each of four morphological types of defects in more detail, emphasising their relationships to the atrioventricular conduction axis.

Perimembranous Ventricular Septal Defects

Perimembranous defects are those opening in the region of the inner curvature of the right ventricle, having as their diagnostic feature continuity between the leaflets of the tricuspid and aortic valves, this continuity incorporating also the central fibrous body. In this situation, the crucial postero-inferior part of the margin of the defect as seen from the right ventricle is formed by the area of fibrous continuity (Fig. 28-16). When such defects open to the inlet of the right ventricle, and are viewed from their right side, the crucial distinguishing part is often curtained from view by the leaflets of the tricuspid valve (Fig. 28-17). On occasion, a defect opening between the ventricular inlets can be part of a heart having a common atrioventricular junction (Figs. 28-18 and 28-19). In this setting, the left atrioventricular valve will have three leaflets, and the heart

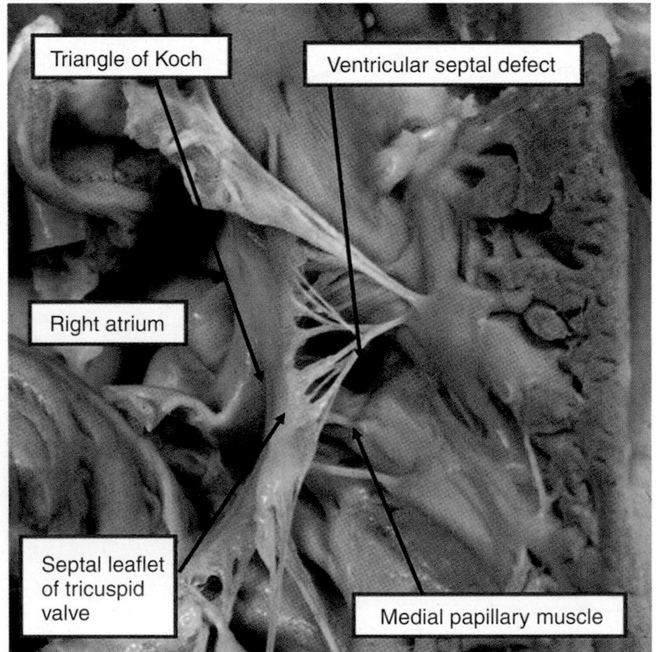

Figure 28-17 When viewed from the right side, the postero-inferior margin of this perimembranous defect, which opens to the inlet of the right ventricle, is obscured by the septal leaflet of the tricuspid valve. It is still possible to recognise, nonetheless, the landmarks to the location of the atrioventricular conduction axis, these being the apex of the triangle of Koch and the medial papillary muscle.

will show all the other features of an atrioventricular septal defect with common atrioventricular junction (see Chapter 27), albeit with shunting occurring only at the ventricular level because the bridging leaflets of the valve guarding the common junction are firmly attached to the under surface

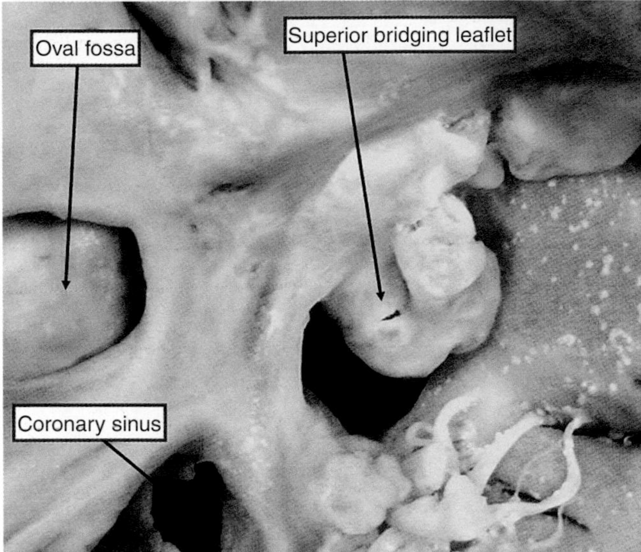

Figure 28-18 This defect also opens between the ventricular inlets, but on closer inspection it can be seen that the leaflets of the atrioventricular valve bridge through the ventricular septum. The phenotypic feature of this heart is the presence of a common atrioventricular junction, so that the defect is not simply a perimembranous defect opening to the inlet of the right ventricle, as shown in Figure 28-17.

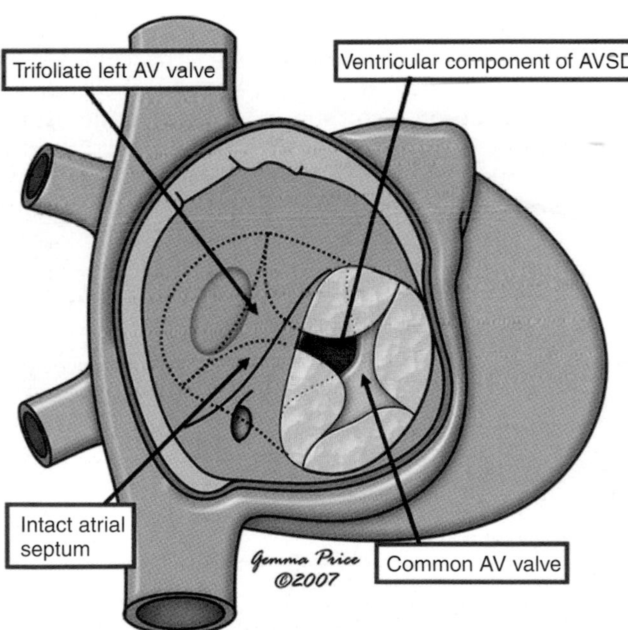

Figure 28-19 The cartoon shows how, in the defect shown in Figure 28-18, the leaflets of the right atrioventricular (AV) valve bridge into the left ventricle, since there is a common atrioventricular junction, but with only shunting at ventricular level through the atrioventricular septal defect (AVSD) because the bridging leaflets are firmly attached to the underside of the atrial septum. Note that the left component of the valve, shown in dotted lines as seen through the intact atrial septum, is trifoliate.

of the atrial septum. Such defects should be distinguished from perimembranous ones opening to the inlet of the right ventricle. Irrespective of their size, the latter defects have separate atrioventricular junctions, with a mitral valve guarding the left junction, even when it is cleft.[23] The hearts already discussed with atrioventricular septal malalignment, and with the tricuspid valve straddling and overriding a defect between the ventricular inlets (see Fig. 28-15),

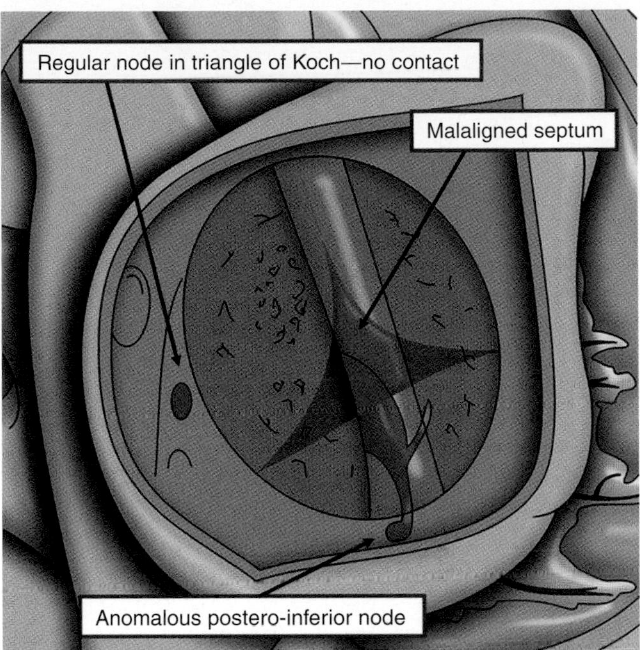

Figure 28-20 When there is malalignment between the atrial septum and the muscular ventricular septum, seen in the setting of straddling tricuspid valve, then it is no longer possible for the conduction axis, carried on the crest of the ventricular septum, to take origin of the regular atrioventricular node positioned at the apex of the triangle of Koch. Instead, the bundle takes origin from an anomalous node formed at the point where the malaligned ventricular septum meets the right atrioventricular junction.

should also be distinguished from hearts with atrioventricular septal defect and common atrioventricular junction. The ones with overriding of the tricuspid valve constitute a particular subset of perimembranous defect, since they still possess the phenotypic feature of aortic–tricuspid valvar fibrous continuity. The septal malalignment, however, predicates that there will be an anomalous location of the atrioventricular conduction axis (Fig. 28-20). Similar septal malalignment can also be found in the setting of a common atrioventricular junction (see Chapter 27). When perimembranous defects permit shunting primarily to the inlet of the right ventricle, the septal leaflet of the tricuspid valve is frequently divided or deficient. If the two components of the abnormal leaflet are at all bound down to the margins, then shunting can occur from left ventricle to right atrium. Such shunting is frequently held to be caused by absence of the atrioventricular membranous septum, but this is very unusual. Deficiency of the atrioventricular component of the membranous septum can occur, very rarely, in the setting of separate right and left atrioventricular junctions (Fig. 28-21). More usually when there is ventriculo-atrial shunting, this is first across a perimembranous defect, and only subsequently to the right atrium (Fig. 28-22). As already discussed, the two defects permitting ventriculo-atrial shunting are also decribed as Gerbode defects.[21]

The other frequent type of perimembranous defect is the one that extends so as to open primarily beneath the ventricular outlets. The outlet compoment of the ventricular septum is not normally in the same plane as the remainder of the muscular septum. Defects involving the junction of the inlet and outlet components of the ventricular septum, therefore, are characterised by a degree of overriding of the aortic valve. The feature of these defects, as shown in

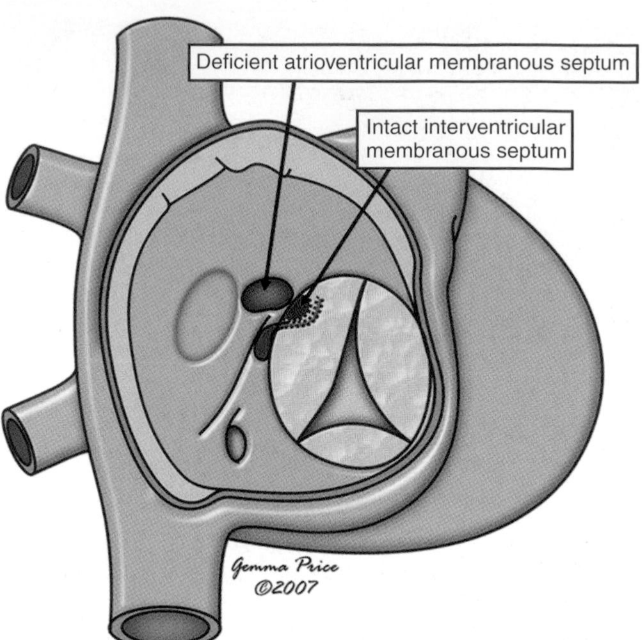

Figure 28-21 The cartoon shows shunting through a deficient atrioventricular component of the membranous septum—the so-called Gerbode defect. This is a true atrioventricular septal defect with separate atrioventricular junctions.

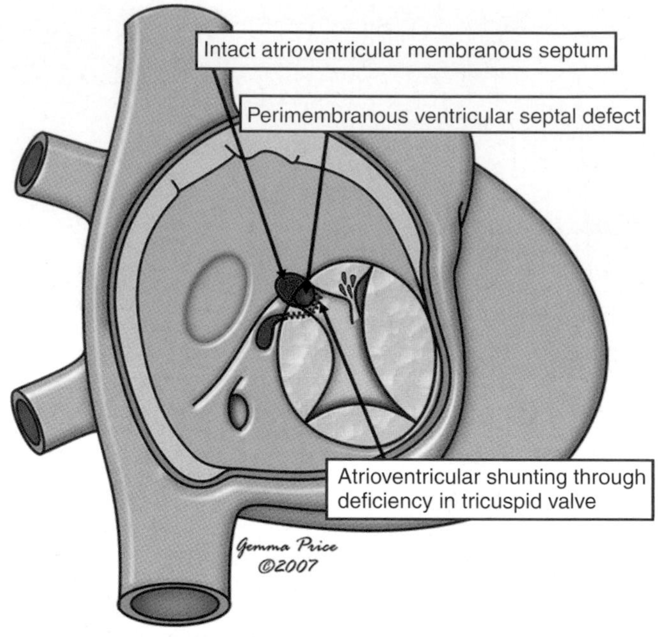

Figure 28-22 More usually, shunting from left ventricle to right atrium in hearts with separate atrioventricular junctions occurs initially through a perimembranous defect, as shown here, with further shunting across a deficiency of the tricuspid valve. Compare with Figure 28-21.

Figure 28-13, is that the muscular outlet septum, supporting the free-standing muscular subpulmonary infundibulum, becomes recognisable as a discrete entity, being malaligned relative to the rest of the muscular septum, and most usually occupying a position exclusively within the right ventricle, although the outlet septum can also be deviated into the left ventricle. In these settings, the orifice of the aortic valve overrides the muscular ventricular septum (Fig. 28-23). Such defects opening between the outlets in the presence of aortic overriding and with the outlet septum deviated into the right ventricle are closely related to tetralogy of Fallot (see Chapter 36). The distinction between the two entities depends upon the presence or absence of muscular infundibular stenosis. The lesion with valvar overriding

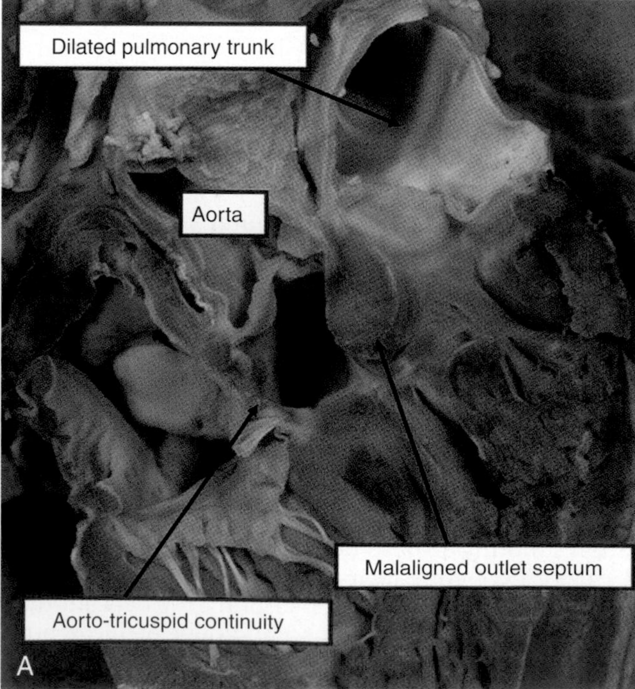

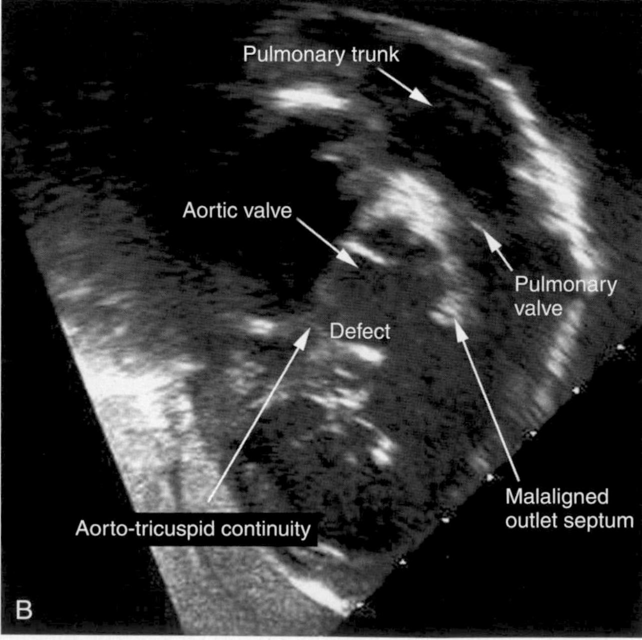

Figure 28-23 The heart shown previously in Figure 28-13 has been sectioned to simulate the subcostal right oblique echocardiogram in B. The outlet septum is malaligned into the right ventricle. The cut has also passed through the aortic root, confirming that a good part of the aortic valve is supported in the right ventricle, and confirming the presence of overriding of the aortic valve. Note the unobstructed subpulmonary outlet. This is an example of the so-called Eisenmenger ventricular septal defect.

in the absence of obstruction to pulmonary flow is often described as the Eisenmenger ventricular septal defect.

As we have also discussed, the outlet septum can be deviated posteriorly into the left ventricular outflow tract. This usually produces subaortic obstruction (see Fig. 28-14), and is almost always associated with obstructive lesions of the aortic arch, either severe tubular hypoplasia or interruption. It would seem that the pulmonary valvar orifice should override the muscular ventricular septum in such defects. Because of the length of the free-standing muscular subpulmonary infundibulum, however, valvar overriding is rare, usually being seen only when the defect is doubly committed and juxta-arterial.[24]

Irrespective of whether a perimembranous defect extends to open between the inlet or outlet ventricular components, or is large enough to open to all parts of the ventricle, a situation described as being confluent, the basic distribution of the axis for atrioventricular conduction is the same. In the normal heart, the penetrating component of the atrioventricular conduction axis passes through the central fibrous body, and branches on the crest of the muscular ventricular septum. Since the central fibrous body forms the postero-inferior margin of perimembranous defects, this will be the site of penetration of the axis. The landmark of the atrioventricular node, as in the normal heart, is the apex of the triangle of Koch. When the defect opens to the right ventricular inlet, the triangle may itself be displaced posteriorly, but its apex still serves as the guide to the site penetration of the conducting bundle. When the axis has penetrated through the central fibrous body, it is related to the postero-inferior rim of perimembranous defects. The precise relationship of its non-branching component to the septal crest depends upon the location of the defect. It is much closer to the crest when a defect opens to the inlet, becoming more remote as the defect extends to open between the outlets.

Because perimembranous defects are closely related to the septal leaflet of the tricuspid valve, there is always the possibility that they may be closed by plastering down of the leaflet across the defect, with small ones being those most likely to close. Defects between the outlet components, particularly when complicated by malalignment, are unlikely to close by this mechanism. Neither are extensive inlet defects. A more frequent, and closely related, mechanism of closure is aneurysmal enlargement of fibrous tissue in the environs of the defect. Although often described as aneurysms of the membranous septum, it is unusual for the remnant of the membranous septum itself to be involved. In most cases, the grape-like lesions are sculpted from the underside of the leaflets of the tricuspid valve. On occasion, the tags can be more extensive hammock-like lesions, with cordal attachments to the septum (Fig. 28-24). The presence of tissue tags is an indication that defects may close spontaneously, and hence that there will be less necessity for surgical closure. On rare occasions, however, the tags can become sufficiently large as to balloon into the right ventricular outflow tract and produce subpulmonary obstruction.

Aneurysmal prolapse of the right coronary leaflet of the aortic valve can be found in the setting of perimembranous defects, particularly those opening between the outlets, when the outlet septum is markedly deficient. Sometimes the non-coronary aortic leaflet, and rarely the left, can also prolapse through the defect. Rarely, such valvar prolapse may produce partial or complete plugging of the defect, and result in spontaneous closure or a false sense of security that the defect is small when, in reality, it is a large defect. The prolapse can also result in aortic regurgitation.

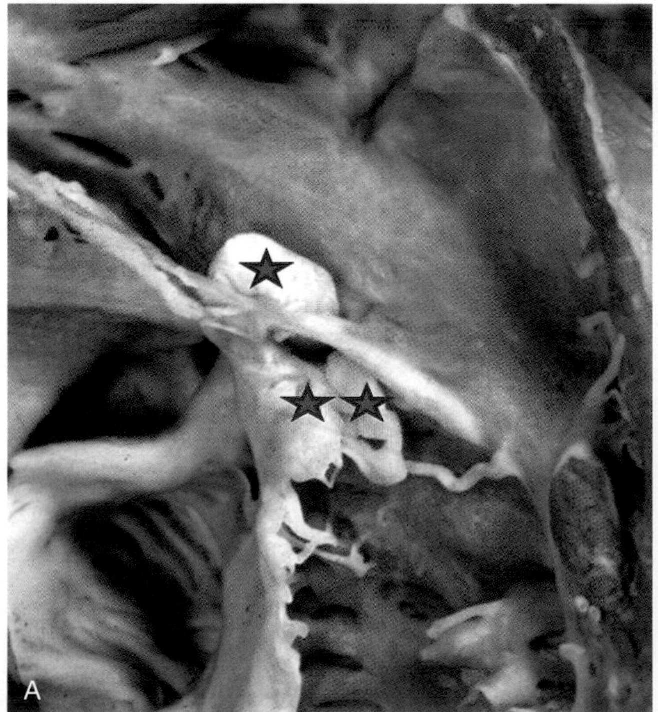

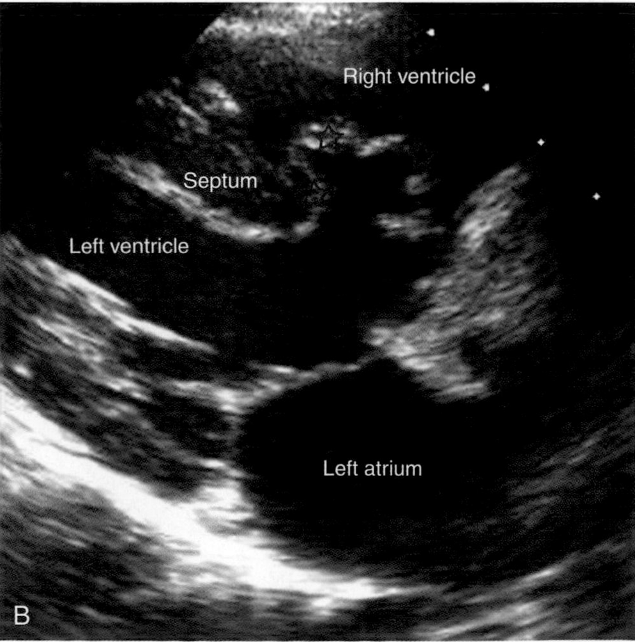

Figure 28-24 A, This perimembranous defect, opening to the inlet of the right ventricle had been almost closed by the tissue tags (*stars*) derived from the leaflets of the tricuspid valve. Note the cordal attachments to the septum. **B**, The parasternal long-axis echocardiogram from a different patient shows the corresponding anatomy.

In all of these possible mechanisms of closure or diminution in size, contraction and fibrosis around the edges of the defect are additional contributory factors.

Muscular Defects

Defects with entirely muscular rims are also distinguished according to whether they open mostly to the inlet, mostly to the apical trabecular component, or mostly to the subpulmonary outlet as seen from the right ventricular side. Such defects can be multiple, particularly when in the apical trabecular septum, or can co-exist with perimembranous or juxta-arterial defects. Those opening to the right ventricular inlet will be covered to some extent by the septal leaflet of the tricuspid valve, and can then be difficult to distinguish from perimembranous defects opening to the inlet. For the defect to be muscular, a bar of muscle, which may be quite small, must interpose between the defect and the hingepoints of the leaflets of the mitral and tricuspid valves (see Fig. 28-1). When a defect is perimembranous, or juxta-tricuspid and non-perimembranous, the leaflets of the mitral and tricuspid valves are in fibrous continuity in its postero-inferior margin (see Fig. 28-16). When the defect is muscular, or juxta-tricuspid and non-perimembarnous, the atrioventricular conduction axis passes above, or anterosuperior, and will be to the left hand when viewed by the surgeon in the operating room. The bundle is always located postero-inferiorly when the defect is perimembranous, and hence will be to the right hand as viewed by the surgeon (Fig. 28-25).

Muscular defects in the apical trabecular septum are frequently large holes that tend to be found to one or other side of the septomarginal trabeculation. Not infrequently, a single opening, as viewed from the left ventricular aspect, is crossed by trabeculations to produce two, or more, openings when viewed from the right ventricle (Fig. 28-26). Multiple smaller muscular defects give the so-called Swiss-cheese septum. These may be particularly difficult to define, even in the postmortem specimen. Although the atrioventricular conduction axis is itself unrelated to muscular defects in the apical septum, the distal bundle branches may pass through the muscular septum between holes, producing pseudobifurcations.

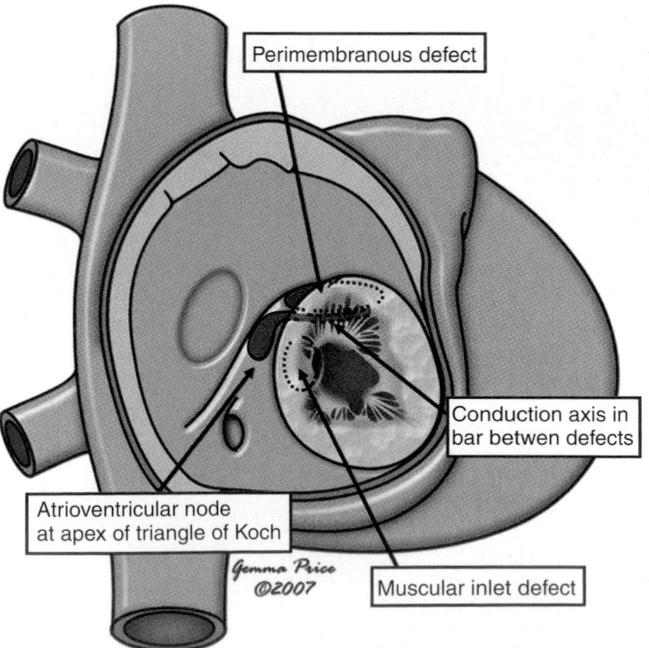

Figure 28-25 The cartoon shows the crucial difference in disposition of the atrioventricular conduction axis when perimembranous as opposed to muscular defects open to the inlet of the right ventricle.

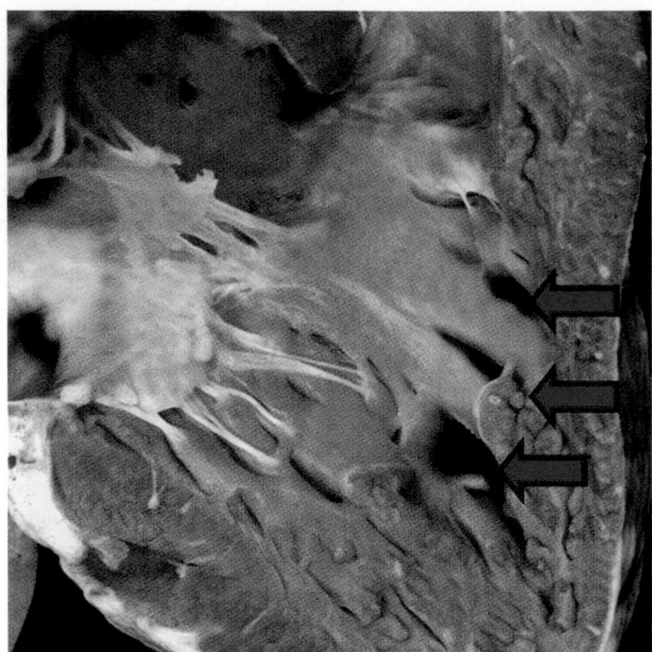

Figure 28-26 There seem to be three muscular defects opening to the anterior apical part of the right ventricle (*arrows*). In reality, this is but a single hole crossed by two septoparietal trabeculations.

Outlet, or infundibular, muscular defects are small and usually single, although they can be larger (Fig. 28-27). The superior rim of such outlet defects is the outlet septum, often attenuated, along with the sleeve of free-standing subpulmonary infundibulum, while the inferior muscular rim, which separates the defect from the membranous septum, is formed by fusion of the posterior limb of the septomarginal trabeculation with the ventriculo-infundibular fold. This muscular tissue separates the conduction tissue axis from the crest of the septum, thus providing protection from surgical damage by sutures placed in the postero-inferior edges of the defect. Small muscular defects close spontaneously simply by growth of the muscular structures surrounding them. As already discussed, they are almost certainly the most common defects undergoing spontaneous closure.[9–12]

Doubly Committed Juxta-arterial Defects

The defect is termed juxta-arterial because it is directly related to both aortic and pulmonary valves (see Fig. 28-12), this feature underscoring echocardiographic recognition (Fig. 28-28). It is also because of this feature that both arterial valves frequently override the septum, giving a progressive spectrum of anomalies the end-point of which is double outlet left ventricle. Such hearts have also been termed double outlet both ventricles.[25] Prolapse of the aortic valvar leaflets is frequent with the juxta-arterial defect, albeit that, as already discussed, such prolapse can also lead to valvar insufficiency when a defect is perimembranous. The relationship of the atrioventricular conduction axis to

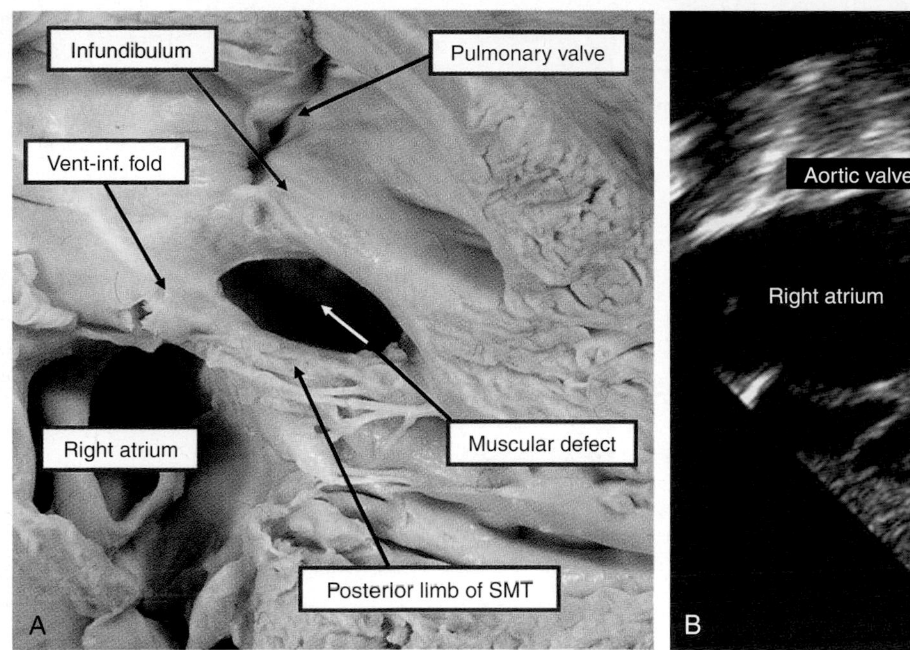

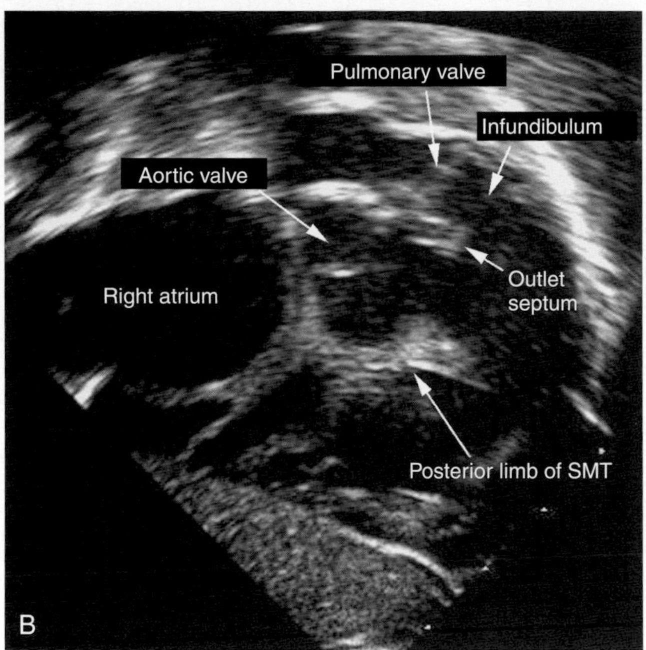

Figure 28-27 A, This defect opening to the outlet of the right ventricle has exclusively muscular rims. The superior rim is the muscular outlet septum, supporting the free-standing sleeve of infundibular musculature, whilst the postero-inferior muscular rim is formed by fusion of the posterior limb of the septomarginal trabeculation (SMT) with the ventriculo-infundibular (vent-inf.) fold. B, The subcostal echocardiogram through the right ventricle from a different patient shows the corresponding anatomy.

the doubly committed defect depends on the morphology of its postero-inferior margin. A well-formed muscular rim (Fig. 28-29) separates the conduction axis from the postero-inferior margin of the defect. In contrast, the atrioventricular bundle is more at risk when the doubly committed defect is also perimembranous (Fig. 28-30).

Juxta-tricuspid and Non-perimembranous Defects

This rarest type of ventricular septal defect involves the inlet muscular septum along the tricuspid annulus but does not reach the membranous septum and therefore the aortic valve.[22] In a four-chamber view, the defect may not show any features different from a perimembranous defect extending toward the inlet along the tricuspid valvar annulus. The tricuspid and mitral valves are in direct contact above the defect in a four-chamber view. The major distinguishing feature of the juxta-tricuspid and non-perimembranous defect from the perimembranous variety is seen in a parasternal long axis cut, which shows that the defect is some distance from the aortic valve. As discussed, the conduction axis is located at the anterior aspect of the defect along the postero-inferior margin of the intact membranous septum.

Morphogenesis

It is impossible to achieve normal closure of the embryonic interventricular communication until the right atrioventricular junction is connected to the right ventricle, and the subaortic outflow tract transferred to the left ventricle. Thereafter, the persisting interventricular communication is closed by tissue derived from various sources (see Chapter 3 for details). It is not closed specifically, however, by the interventricular membranous septum. When the interventricular communication is closed, the septal leaflet of the tricuspid valve has yet to be delaminated from the muscular septum.[18] There cannot, therefore, at this stage, be an interventricular component to the membranous septum. Perimembranous defects cannot be explained simply on the basis of failure of closure of the embryonic interventricular communication by the interventricular component of the membranous septum. It is more likely that the muscular septum is deficient in the environs of the closing plug of tissue, which is a consequence of insufficient area or volume. Deficiency of the different parts of the muscular septum then accounts for the diversity in position and orientation of perimembranous defects.

The formation of muscular defects is more easily explained. It is now established that, at least in the chick,[26] the muscular septum is produced by coalescence of embryonic trabeculations. Muscular defects, therefore, likely result from failure of the trabeculations to coalesce. This notion is now supported by the fact that, increasingly, such an arrangement is seen in association with ventricular noncompaction. When extensive, and involving the septum, such noncompaction produces the Swiss-cheese septum. Alternatively, there may be failure of fusion of the muscular septum with the free-standing septal component of the subpulmonary infundibulum, derived by muscularisation of the outflow cushions. Such failure of fusion of the infundibulum with the muscular septum and the septomarginal trabeculation gives a good explanation for the muscular defect opening between the outlets.

The doubly committed juxta-arterial defect is well explained simply on the basis of failure of muscularisation of proximal outflow cushions during division of the embryonic outflow tract. Because of the failure of formation of the muscular subpulmonary infundibulum, the defect is

Figure 28-28 The specimen (A) and corresponding echocardiogram (B) sectioned through a doubly committed and juxta-arterial defect in long-axis oblique plane reveals the fibrous continuity between the leaflets of the aortic and pulmonary valves that is the key to diagnosis of this type of defect. The star shows the crest of the muscular ventricular septum. The echocardiogram shows the prolapsed aortic valve, with the colour flow showing aortic regurgitation.

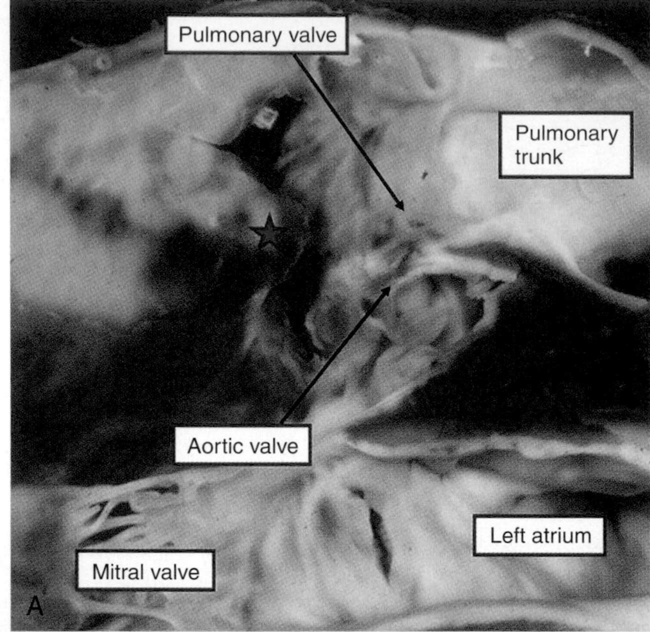

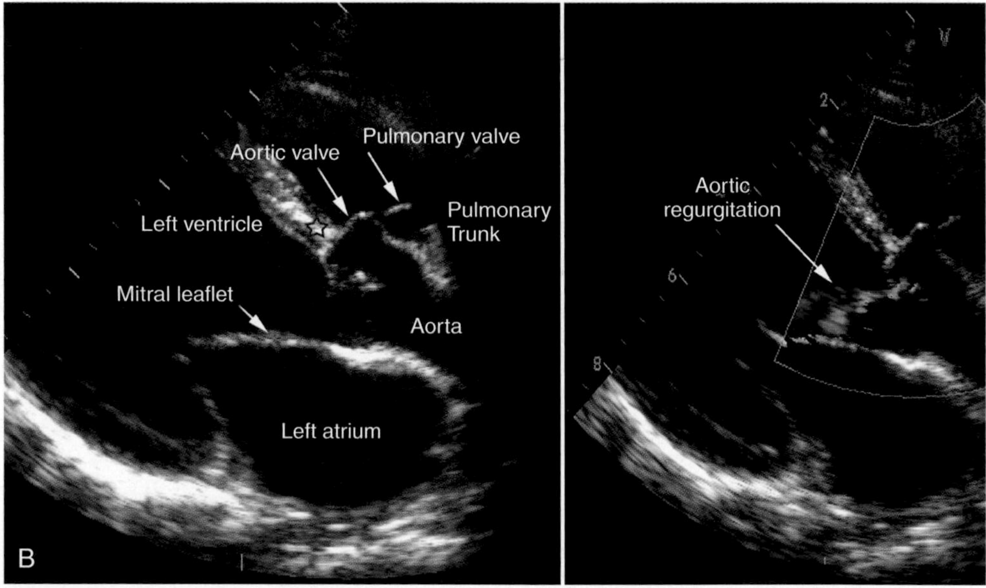

closely related developmentally to common arterial trunk (see Chapter 41).

PATHOPHYSIOLOGY

The pathophysiology of ventricular septal defect is determined by the size of the defect and the state of the pulmonary vascular resistance. The site of the hole between the ventricles has little influence. Between them, size and resistance govern the direction and magnitude of flow through the defect, and thus the clinical features and symptomatology.

Effect of Size

The size of the defect is crucial. Below a critical size, the defect itself presents a resistance to flow through it, which controls the magnitude but not the direction of the shunt. Above this critical size, there is no appreciable resistance to flow. Both magnitude and direction of flow are then determined by the level of pulmonary vascular resistance. There is little data concerning this critical size. Some authorities have argued, unsupported by scientific investigation, that defects smaller than the aortic orifice are restrictive. Others[27] attempted to quantify the critical size by comparing the diameter of the defect with body surface area, suggesting that the key value was a diameter of 1 cm/m^2 body surface area, corresponding to an orificial area of approximately 0.8 cm^2/m^2 body surface area. Defects having ratios smaller than this were restrictive, and produced minor or no haemodynamic changes. This suggests that the critical size is smaller than the aortic orifice, since a normal aortic valvar orifice is calculated to be approximately 2.0 cm^2/m^2 body surface area. In practise, the judgement of the size of a defect is generally made on haemodynamic

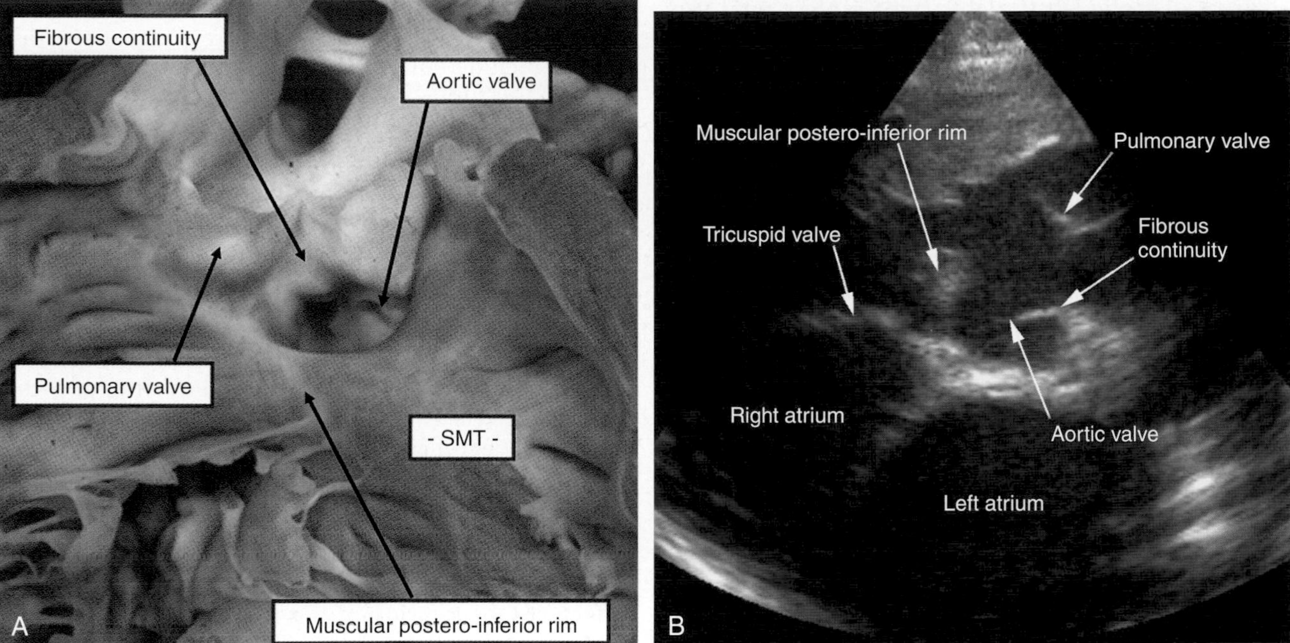

Figure 28-29 A, In this doubly committed and juxta-arterial defect, there is an extensive muscular postero-inferior rim separating the margin of the defect from the tricuspid valve. Though the conduction axis is related to the postero-inferior margin of the defect, this muscular bar separates the atrioventricular conduction axis from the edge of the defect, thereby protecting it from injury when sutures are placed in the margin of the defect. **B**, In the corresponding echocardiogram obtained along the short-axis plane of the aortic valve, the leaflet of the aortic valve is in direct fibrous continuity with the leaflet of the pulmonary valve. Muscle separates the tricuspid and aortic valves along the postero-inferior rim of the defect. SMT, septomarginal trabeculation.

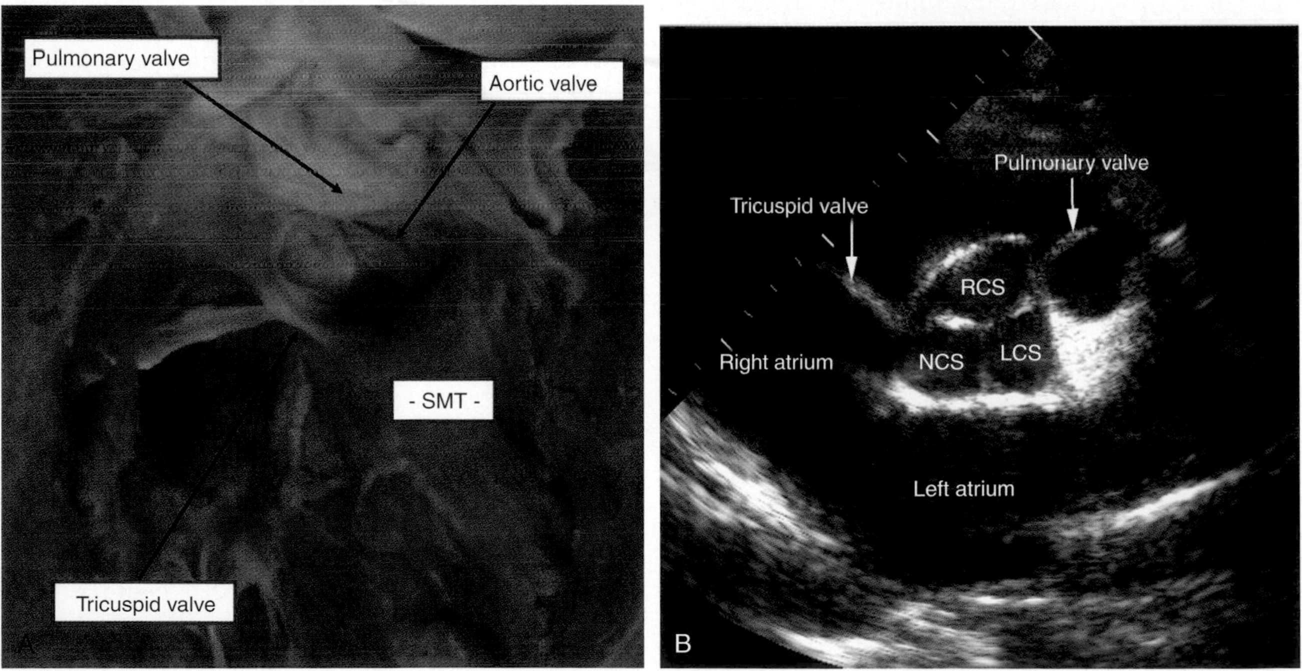

Figure 28-30 A, In this doubly committed and juxta-arterial defect (compare with Fig. 28-29), the hole extends postero-inferiorly so that there is fibrous continuity between the leaflets of the aortic and tricuspid valve, making the defect perimembranous. This means that the conduction bundle will be at potential surgical risk in the postero-inferior margin of the defect. **B**, In the corresponding echocardiogram obtained along the short-axis plane of the aortic valve, the right coronary sinus (RCS) of the aortic valve is entirely devoid of muscular support from the right ventricle. The leaflet of the right coronary sinus is in direct fibrous continuity (*red star*) with the leaflet of the pulmonary valve, and the leaflet of the non-coronary sinus (NCS) is in direct fibrous continuity (*green star*) with the leaflet of the tricuspid valve. LCS indicates the left coronary sinus.

grounds. When there is a left-to-right shunt, and no other associated anomalies such as pulmonary stenosis, a large defect is one that permits equalisation of systolic pressures in the two ventricles, and the defect is also unrestrictive. Since the right and left ventricles do not contract exactly simultaneously, there is always some inequality in the ventricular pressures. Consequently, throughout the greater part of systole, the pressure difference will promote left-to-right shunting. During isovolumic relaxation, additional right-to-left shunting occurs, which is then cleared by the subsequent diastolic left-to-right shunt, unless right ventricular ejection is obstructed.[28]

A restrictive defect, therefore, is one in which right ventricular and pulmonary arterial systolic pressures are lower than those in the left ventricle and aorta. The size of such defects may vary from those that are just restrictive, allowing some elevation of right-sided pressures, to small defects in which the right-sided pressures are normal. In effect, defects can be considered either restrictive or unrestrictive. In those that are restrictive, there is then a continuum of size between those large enough to allow a serious haemodynamic disturbance, and those so small that there is only a small left-to-right shunt, with normal right-sided pressures.

Effects of Pulmonary Vascular Resistance

The effect of pulmonary vascular resistance on the flow through restrictive defects is always secondary to the size of the hole. The smaller the defect, the lower the flow through it. When defects are unrestricted, the pulmonary vascular resistance, and, to a lesser extent, systemic vascular resistance, is the controlling factor. When the pulmonary vascular resistance is low, the flow through the defect, and the flow of blood to the lungs, will be high. Such a high flow is not present at birth. It takes a finite time for the pulmonary resistance to fall from the high intrauterine to the normal postnatal levels, usually accomplished in the normal infant within the first 2 weeks of life.

This fall may be delayed and limited in its extent in infants with a large ventricular septal defect. Contributory structural factors include limited postnatal growth of the lungs, and limitation of the number of intra-acinar blood vessels. In addition, there is hypertrophy of the muscular coat of the intra-acinar arteries and veins (see Chapter 7). It is not entirely clear why growth of the lungs, and proliferation of pulmonary vessels, is limited. Muscular hypertrophy of the walls of the vessels is probably secondary to the increased pulmonary flow. Such high flow to the lungs leads to increased left atrial pressure, which is known to cause pulmonary vasoconstriction in experimental animals. If the vasoconstriction is maintained, vascular muscular hypertrophy will presumably occur. This delay in the fall of the pulmonary resistance means that the maximal haemodynamic effects of an unrestrictive defect may not be reached for some weeks after birth. The time and course, and the extent of the fall in pulmonary resistance, are all variable. The maximal flow through the defect is usually achieved between 1 and 6 weeks of age. This is usually enough to allow a very high pulmonary flow, but the fall in pulmonary vascular resistance may be so limited that little flow occurs through the defect. Such patients may escape detection until the effects of severe pulmonary vascular disease have become apparent.

Once it has fallen to its lowest value, pulmonary vascular resistance may increase again with the development of the pathological changes of pulmonary vascular disease.[29,30] This usually occurs only in patients in whom the pulmonary arterial pressure is high from birth. In consequence, it is almost entirely confined to those with an unrestrictive defect. As the resistance rises, flow across the defect decreases. When pulmonary vascular resistance exceeds that in the systemic circuit, the flow through the defect will change from left to right to a flow from right to left. Thus, the level of resistance determines the direction of flow. Secondary effects of severe pulmonary vascular disease include enlargement of the right ventricle and the pulmonary trunk, and dilation of the infundibular attachments of the leaflets of the pulmonary valve. These may cause detectable, but usually haemodynamically insignificant, pulmonary regurgitation.

When defects are restrictive, there is wide spectrum of restrictiveness. In many, the defect is so small that the pulmonary vascular resistance has little or no effect on the magnitude of flow through it. In others, the defect is restrictive, not allowing equalisation of pressures between the two ventricles, but is big enough to permit a significant elevation of right ventricular and pulmonary arterial pressures. In these defects, the level of pulmonary vascular resistance will play a significant, albeit subordinate, role in controlling the magnitude of flow of blood to the lungs. Between the two extremes of restrictive defects, there is a continuum of size and, therefore, of pathophysiological effects.

Effect of Obstruction of the Pulmonary Outflow Tract

All our discussion thus far has presumed an unobstructed pulmonary outflow tract. If there is co-existing obstruction within the right ventricular outflow tract, either valvar or subvalvar, then the resistance to ejection from the right ventricle will have a similar effect to elevation of the pulmonary vascular resistance. The flow through an unrestrictive defect, and thence flow to the lungs, will be limited in proportion to the severity of the obstruction. In restrictive defects, obstruction to the right ventricular outflow will result in elevation of right ventricular pressure, again in proportion to the severity of obstruction. The right ventricular pressure, in extreme cases, may come to exceed that in the left ventricle. As in unrestrictive defects, obstruction of the pulmonary outflow tract in the larger of the restrictive defects will also have a limiting effect on the magnitude of flow. There will be a reversal in the direction of the shunt in all cases where right ventricular pressure exceeds that in the left ventricle. Although pulmonary valvar obstruction may be present unequivocally from birth, subvalvar obstruction can be acquired.

Response of the Heart to Flow between the Ventricles

The cardiac effects of a ventricular septal defect depend initially on the magnitude of flow to the lungs. With florid pulmonary flow, usually in the setting of unrestrictive defects, left atrial and left ventricular end-diastolic volumes are increased, and left ventricular muscle mass is also increased. Studies of pressure and volume in the left ventricle demonstrate the marked increase in left ventricular work imposed by a large defect. This necessitates left ventricular hypertrophy as a compensatory mechanism. With extreme pulmonary flow, there is also an increase in right ventricular dimensions. Because of the elevated right ventricular pressure, there will be an even more marked increase in right ventricular work. This results in additional right ventricular hypertrophy. This may be one mechanism for the development of subvalvar pulmonary stenosis.

Left ventricular work is increased by restrictive defects in relation to the flow to the lungs, but the right ventricle is relatively spared. Consequently, there is left ventricular hypertrophy, but little increase in right ventricular size or muscle mass. With elevation of pulmonary vascular resistance, or with development of right ventricular outflow obstruction, left ventricular work is diminished because of the decrease in left-to-right shunting and pulmonary flow. The elevation of right ventricular pressure then results in right ventricular hypertrophy, which dominates the picture.

The pathophysiological effects of a ventricular septal defect can, in three situations, result in congestive cardiac failure. The first is an unrestrictive defect with high pulmonary flow, when the compensatory mechanisms are insufficient to provide an adequate systemic flow. These compensatory mechanisms include recruitment of sarcomeres to operate at an optimal end-diastolic length, muscular hypertrophy of right and left ventricles, and increased catecholamine drive to the ventricles. Those circumstances are usually reached before the age of 6 months. The second situation occurs much later. It is encountered when the right ventricular myocardium has undergone degenerative changes as a consequence of long-term ejection against high resistance. This is found with pulmonary vascular disease, and with prolonged and severe obstruction to the right ventricular outflow tract. The third situation is when a ventricular septal defect is complicated by aortic regurgitation, imposing a further volume load on the left ventricle, outstriping the compensatory mechanisms as discussed above. It is most frequently seen in older children and adults.

CLINICAL FEATURES

Presentation

The typical murmur of a ventricular septal defect is rarely heard at birth, since it takes time for the pulmonary vascular resistance to fall from the high levels of fetal life, which are sufficiently high to limit the flow through even an unrestrictive defect to levels insufficient to provide an audible murmur. The diagnosis can now be made during fetal life by means of echocardiographic screening. Even when cases are diagnosed during fetal life, it is necessary to exercise caution, since many subsequently close spontaneously. Very few, if any, of those diagnosed during fetal life will have the full clinical picture at birth. If diagnosis is made in the neonatal nursery, it is almost invariably during examination of the baby just prior to maternal discharge. At the end of the first week of life, when many murmurs are detected, it is rare for the pulmonary vascular resistance to have fallen sufficiently for the child to be symptomatic. Symptoms, when they occur, are related to the high flow of blood to the lungs, diminished pulmonary compliance, and elevation of the left atrial pressure as a result of the high pulmonary flow. This initially causes tachypnoea, which progresses with the onset of congestive cardiac failure to give dyspnoea on effort, most obvious when the baby feeds. In a baby with a typical unrestrictive or large restrictive defect, the parents are likely to complain that feeds take progressively longer over the first month or two of life, and lead to rapid exhaustion of the baby. Not only is the feeding prolonged, but it does not provide sufficient caloric intake for weight gain. With the development of severe cardiac failure, the baby will become obviously dyspnoeic even at rest. Intercostal, subcostal, and supraclavicular recession are then readily seen. This increased work of respiration imposes an increased requirement for energy, which is not satisfied because of the difficulty of feeding, a vicious circle resulting in failure to thrive. Failure to thrive is, indeed, an alternative mode of presentation in infancy. It occurs in those babies with defects large enough to allow high pulmonary flow, but in whom the size of the defect, or the level of pulmonary vascular resistance, prevents the development of intractable congestive cardiac failure. Another association with high pulmonary flow is an increased susceptibility to respiratory infection. The parents may complain that their baby has frequent chesty colds. It may be during such an episode that a murmur is noted, and that cardiac failure is precipitated.

A small and restrictive defect may be detected at any age by the discovery of a murmur. But such a defect will rarely, if ever, cause symptoms. When a defect is found in this fashion after the age of 1 year, it is highly unlikely that, in itself, it will ever cause congestive cardiac failure. No such assurance can be given when discovery occurs in early infancy. There is a further small group of patients with ventricular septal defect who escape detection in infancy. They present with diminished effort tolerance and cyanosis during middle childhood or adolescence. These patients usually have severe pulmonary vascular disease. Even careful history-taking fails to elicit evidence of symptoms during infancy. It is probable that at no stage did their pulmonary vascular resistance fall to levels that permitted sufficient left-to-right shunting to allow recognition of the defect.

Another alternative, and rare, presentation is with respiratory symptoms from bronchial compression caused by grossly enlarged pulmonary arteries. Typically, the right middle lobe bronchus is compressed, but the left main and upper lobe bronchuses may also be involved. This presentation is most frequently seen in patients with severe pulmonary vascular disease, or in those with so-called absent leaflets of the pulmonary valve.

Infants with holes between the ventricles, therefore, rarely present in the first days of life. In those with small restrictive defects, presentation is by the incidental discovery of a murmur, the child remaining asymptomatic. In those with large but restrictive defects, and with unrestrictive defects, the initial finding may be a murmur, but symptoms rapidly ensue. It may be the symptoms of dyspnoea and failure to thrive that call attention to the heart. Presentation occurs only at the point of recognition of a right-to-left shunt in those rare patients with irreversible vascular disease, who may also present because of respiratory problems.

Physical Examination

The appearance of the patient is again dependent on the magnitude of flow through the defect. Those with small and restrictive defects are generally entirely normal. With large restrictive defects, but without frank congestive cardiac failure, patients tend to be small and thin for their age, with evidence of dyspnoea such as intercostal recession. Chronicity is suggested by a depression at the insertion of the diaphragm. This depression is at the site described by Harrison, a general practitioner working in the English county of Lincolnshire over the turn of the nineteenth century, as a late effect of rickets.[31] There will also be bulging of the left chest, indicating cardiomegaly. In presence of large unrestrictive defects, similar appearance of more severe degree will be seen without the evidence of chronicity. Cyanosis will not be seen except in those older patients with severe pulmonary vascular disease or in those with severe obstruction within the right ventricular outflow tract.

A systolic thrill is felt in almost all patients, except those with tiny muscular or perimembranous defects. When a thrill is present, it is localised to the second, third, and fourth intercostal spaces at the left sternal border. If the thrill is maximal in the first intercostal space or higher, and yet the auscultatory features are otherwise typical of a ventricular septal defect, the likelihood is that the defect is doubly committed and juxta-arterial.[32] There are usually no other palpable abnormalities in the presence of small restrictive defects. When the defect is large, with a high flow, the cardiac impulse will be hyperdynamic and the thrill may be more widespread. In presence of severe pulmonary vascular disease, the striking features are a localised left parasternal heave of right ventricular type and a palpable second sound. The peripheral pulses are normal. Abnormalities such as a pulse with high volume or absence of the femoral pulse should suggest an associated arterial duct or coarctation, respectively.

The most typical auscultatory finding, a loud pansystolic murmur localised to the second and third left intercostal spaces, was not accepted as being caused by a hole between the ventricles when Roger gave his initial presentation to the Académie de Médicine.[1] This murmur is typical of many ventricular septal defects with a left-to-right shunt, even when they are small and restrictive. The murmur starts with the first sound, and continues up to the second sound. If the murmur starts with the first heart sound but stops short of the second, the defect is likely to be a small muscular one closing in late systole. Large unrestrictive defects in infants sometimes give rise to a shortened ejection systolic murmur that is not accompanied by a thrill. It is said that a pansystolic murmur may continue past the aortic component of the second heart sound. This is rarely appreciated by the ear. Similarly, the ear usually does not detect any variation in the intensity of the murmur, although phonocardiography does show that the murmur is loudest during mid-systole. When flow to the lungs is limited by pulmonary resistance, the systolic murmur is abbreviated, and may be completely absent. In such cases, an early diastolic murmur of pulmonary regurgitation may be heard, as well as a pulmonary click. In patients who have excessive flow to the lungs, the flow through the mitral valve is sufficient to produce a mid-diastolic murmur at the apex. The presence of this murmur is taken to indicate that pulmonary flow is more than twice the systemic flow. In patients with no other signs of pulmonary vascular disease, the appearance of a high-pitched early diastolic murmur is highly suggestive of the onset of aortic regurgitation.

In the absence of pulmonary vascular disease, the heart sounds are normal. It is claimed that the second heart sound is widely split, with delay of its pulmonary component.[33] In our experience, this is rarely appreciated on auscultation, although it is seen on phonocardiography. The pulmonary second sound is louder in patients with pulmonary hypertension. In those with severe pulmonary hypertension, the increased intensity is easy to detect. In less severe cases, the fact that the second heart sound is audibly split at the apex indicates that the pulmonary component is louder than normal. Development of this finding during follow-up should alert to the possibility of development of pulmonary vascular disease. The second heart sound becomes single once severe pulmonary vascular disease has developed.[34]

INVESTIGATIONS

Electrocardiography

The electrocardiographic features are not specific for ventricular septal defect. As may be expected, they do reflect the haemodynamic state. In patients with large unrestrictive defects presenting with a high pulmonary blood flow in infancy, there will be a normal sinus rhythm, probably with tachycardia, a frontal QRS axis within the normal range for age, and biventricular hypertrophy. Finding a superior axis suggests multiple defects,[35] that the lesion is the ventricular component of an atrioventricular septal defect, or that an isolated perimembranous defect with separate atrioventricular junctions excavates extensively to open to the right ventricular inlet. Tall upright T waves over the right praecordial leads in infancy strongly suggest that the right ventricular pressure is at systemic levels. Cardiac rhythm and the QRS axis are usually normal in those with large restrictive defects after the first few months of life. The QRS pattern is that of left ventricular dominance, with deep Q waves over the left chest leads indicating left ventricular volume overload. The electrocardiogram may be normal in patients with small restrictive defects.

Serial electrocardiograms provide more prognostic information in the early months of life than does a single tracing. Large and unrestrictive defects maintain the biventricular QRS morphology, while the smaller defects show the normal diminution of right ventricular forces with age. At any age, the presence of pulmonary vascular disease, or severe obstruction to the right ventricular outflow tract, is reflected by right without left ventricular hypertrophy, and by right-axis deviation. Should aortic regurgitation complicate a small defect or, alternatively, occur in a patient with established obstruction of the right ventricular outflow tract, then the changes of left ventricular volume overload will come to dominate the picture.

Radiology

Once more, radiological findings reflect the haemodynamic state. The chest radiograph is usually normal in the first days of life. With the development of left-to-right shunting, the lung vascularity becomes plethoric. When flow to the lungs is large, as in unrestrictive defects, cardiomegaly is noted and pulmonary plethora is marked (Fig. 28-31). The cardiac contour in such infants has no specific features. The lungs tend to be hyperinflated with flattened diaphragmatic contours. Subsegmental or segmental collapse of the lower lobes, particularly the left lower lobe, is often seen. A markedly enlarged heart may compress the left main bronchus, causing collapse of the left lower lobe. When defects are restrictive, with only mild elevation of the pulmonary flow, the chest radiograph may appear normal.

The development and progression of pulmonary vascular disease are reflected in diminution of the peripheral pulmonary vascular shadows, leading to the classical pruning of the peripheral pulmonary arteries, seen best in older children and adults. This is accompanied by progressive overall reduction in cardiac size as the flow of blood to the lungs falls, but with characteristic enlargement of the pulmonary knob. When obstruction develops in the right

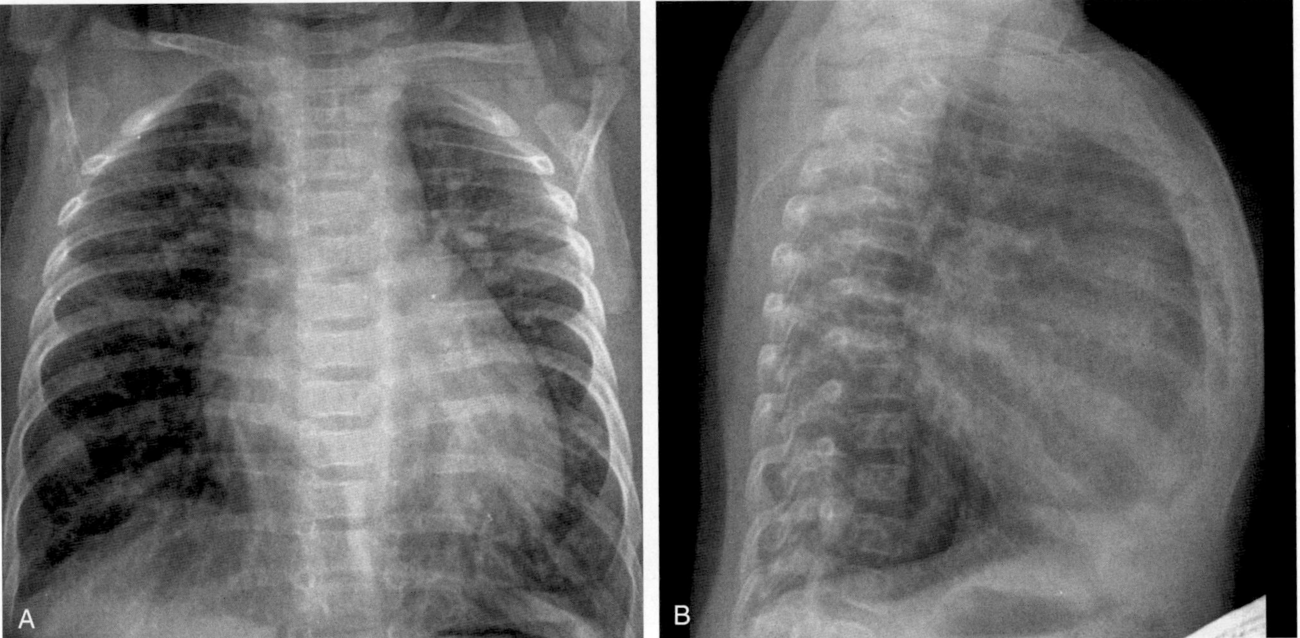

Figure 28-31 Frontal (A) and lateral (B) chest radiographs of a 13-week-old infant with a large ventricular defect. Note the increased pulmonary vascularity and nonspecific enlargement of the cardiac silhouette. The lungs are hyperinflated.

ventricular outflow tract, there is reduction in both central and peripheral pulmonary arterial shadowing, but enlargement of the pulmonary trunk is rare. When complicated by aortic regurgitation, there will be progressive enlargement of the heart, with the cardiac contour suggesting left ventricular dominance. As the prolapsed leaflet or leaflets of the aortic valve reduce the size of the defect, or may close the defect, there will be a progressive reduction in the prominence of pulmonary vascular markings.

Echocardiography

Cross sectional echocardiographic examination[36-40] is now recognised as the technique of choice for diagnosis.[41] Not only does the technique show the presence of a defect, it also permits its accurate localisation. Furthermore, because the defect should be identified in more than one plane, its size can be estimated. Perimembranous defects are recognised in long-axis, four-chamber and short-axis views, with fibrous continuity between the leaflets of the tricuspid and mitral or aortic valves being the pathognomic feature. Perimembranous defects opening to the inlet of the right ventricle are recognised by cuts through the ventricular inlets (Fig. 28-32). The four-chamber sections will demonstrate continuity between the leaflets of the tricuspid to mitral valves via the central fibrous body, with loss of the usual off-setting of the hingepoints of the leaflets. A gentle sweep of the transducer from a four-chamber cut to a long axis cut will demonstrate the continuity of the leaflets of the tricuspid and aortic valves through the central fibrous body. In the so-called juxta-tricuspid and non-perimembranous defect,[22] the defect is described as being at some distance from the aortic valve because it does not reach the central fibrous body. We initially believed that we had identified such a defect echocardiographically (Fig. 28-33). When the surgeon closed the defect, however, he discovered a muscular ridge separating the hinges of the tricuspid and mitral valves in the roof of the defect. Hence, the defect

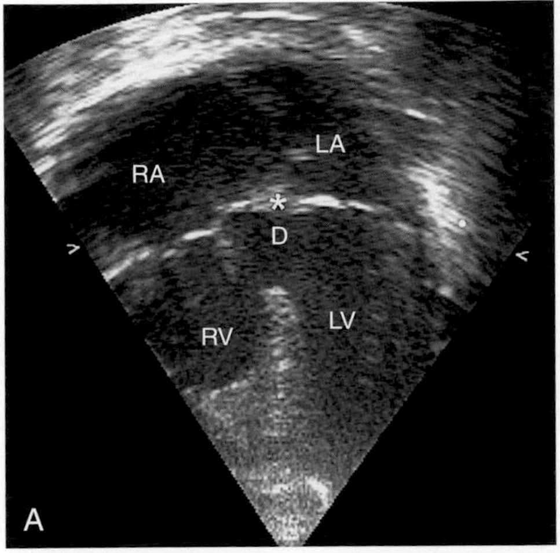

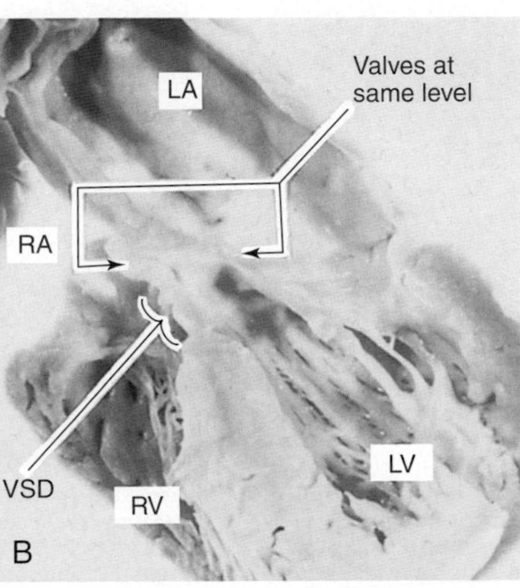

Figure 28-32 This cross sectional echocardiogram (A), with a comparable specimen (B), shows the features of a perimembranous defect (D) opening to the inlet of the right ventricle. The tricuspid and mitral valves are attached to the septum at the same level (*asterisk*). LA, left atrium; LV, left ventricle; RA, right atrium; RV, right ventricle; VSD, ventricular septal defect.

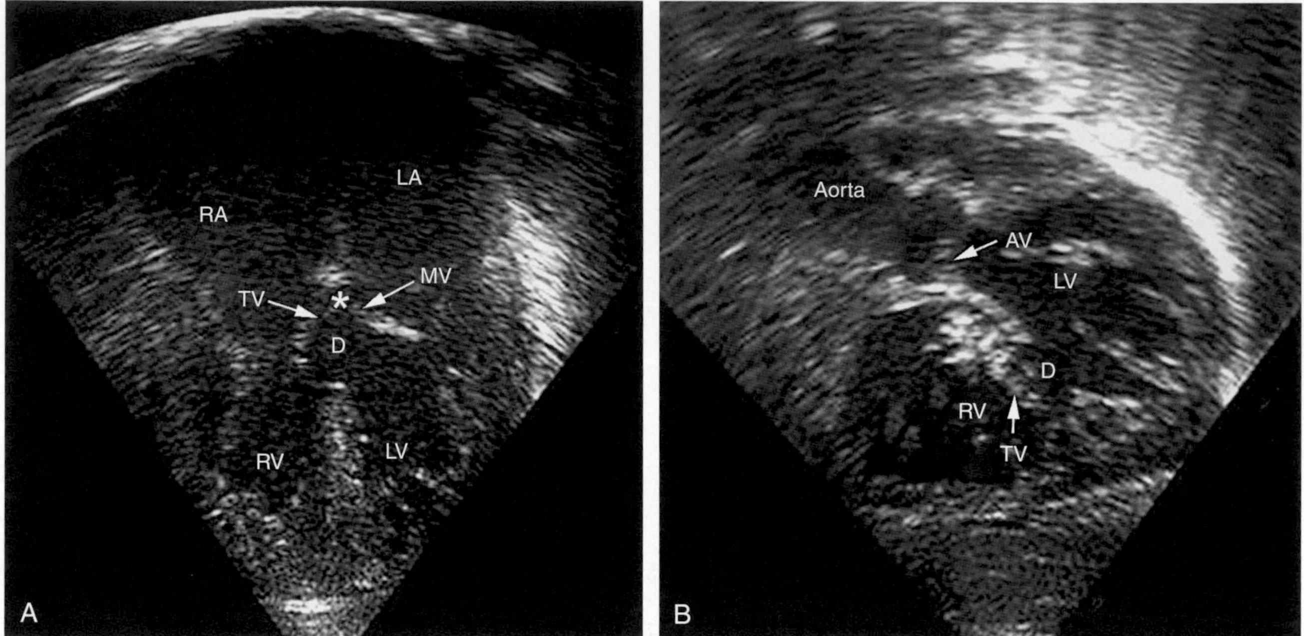

Figure 28-33 Echocardiograms in apical four-chamber (**A**) and subcostal left ventricular outflow tract cut (**B**) show a defect (D). The defect is demarcated by the tricuspid and mitral valves that are in direct contact (*asterisk*). However, the defect is at some distance from the aortic valve annulus. It was considered a juxta-tricuspid non-perimembranous defect. At surgery, a thin muscle tissue was found between the defect and the tricuspid valve annulus, and the defect was a muscular inlet defect by definition. AV, aortic valve; LA, left atrium; LV, left ventricle; MV, mitral valve; RA, right atrium; RV, right ventricle; TV, tricuspid valve.

was surrounded by muscle, and opened to the inlet of the right ventricle—in other words a muscular inlet defect. It remains the fact, therefore, that we have still to identify a patient with a juxta-tricuspid and non-perimembranous defect, either in the clinical setting or at autopsy. Defects opening between the outlets are best identified in the subcostal right oblique section, which shows the muscular outlet septum as an interventricular structure immediately beneath the subpulmonary infundibulum (Fig. 28-34; see also Figs. 28-13 and 28-23). This is evidence of the biventricular aortic connection.[42]

The parasternal short-axis cut at the level of the aortic valve will similarly show this discrete outlet septum (see Fig. 28-34). When this feature is present, the parasternal long-axis section will usually demonstrate overriding of the leaflets of the aortic valve (Fig. 28-35). For those defects opening between the outlets, and associated with posterior longitudinal deviation of the outlet septum, usually in the

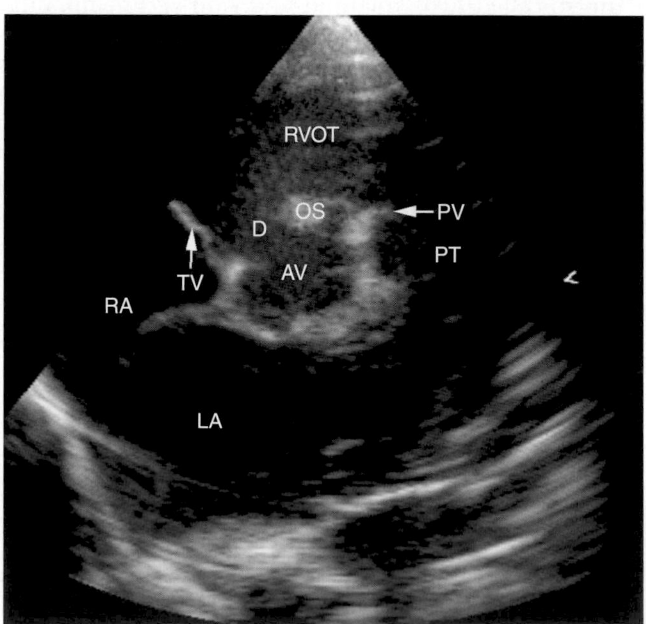

Figure 28-34 This echocardiogram in a short-axis plane through the aortic valve (AV) shows a perimembranous defect opening to the outlet of the right ventricle (RVOT). Note that the aortic valve is in direct contact with the tricuspid valve (TV) through the defect. The outlet septum separates the aortic valve from the pulmonary valve (PV). OS, outlet septum. Other abbreviations as in Figure 28-33.

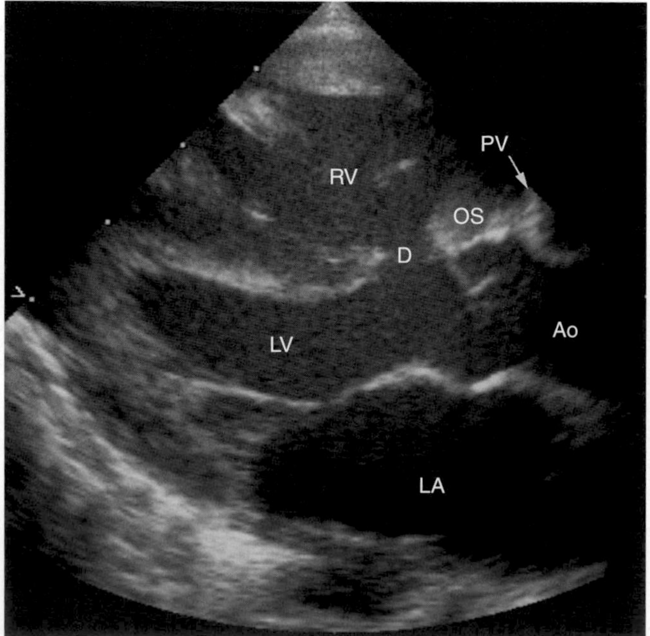

Figure 28-35 This echocardiogram in a parasternal long-axis plane shows the features of a perimembranous defect (D). The aortic valve shows a mild degree of overriding. Ao, aorta; LA, left atrium; LV, left ventricle; OS, outlet septum; PV, pulmonary valve; RV, right ventricle.

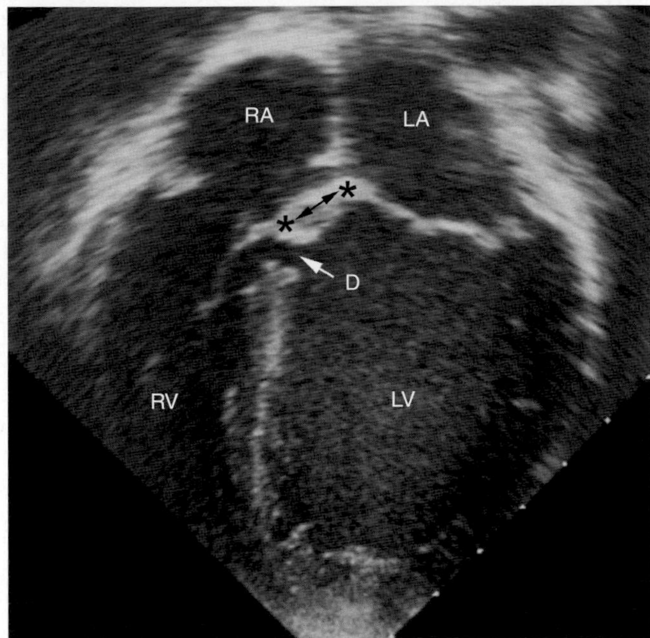

Figure 28-36 This echocardiogram is taken in an apical four-chamber cut, showing the features of a muscular inlet defect (D). The hinges of the atrioventricular valves (*asterisks*) retain their normal off-set (*double-headed arrow*). Abbreviations as in Figure 28-32.

Figure 28-37 This echocardiogram, taken in an apical four-chamber plane, shows the features of a muscular defect (D) opening between the trabecular parts of the ventricles. The hinges of the atrioventricular valves (*asterisks*) retain their normal off-set. Abbreviations as in Figure 28-32.

setting of aortic coarctation or interruption, the parasternal long-axis section will be the optimal plane for diagnosis. Muscular defects opening to the right ventricular inlet are best seen in the four-chamber view, but retain the feature of atrioventricular valvar off-setting (Fig. 28-36). Large defects within the apical trabecular septum are identified in four-chamber and short-axis planes (Fig. 28-37), while muscular defects opening to the subpulmonary outlet are identified in short-axis or right anterior oblique planes from parasternal or subcostal approaches. The best view with which to distinguish perimembranous from muscular outlet defects is the high-parasternal short-axis section. This cut demonstrates the presence or absence of continuity between the leaflets of the tricuspid and aortic valves. Small or multiple muscular defects in the apical muscular septum are those least likely to be visualised without the aid of colour flow mapping. Doubly committed juxta-arterial defects are recognised because of the continuity of the leaflets of the aortic and pulmonary valves in the roof of the defect, with absence of much of the subpulmonary

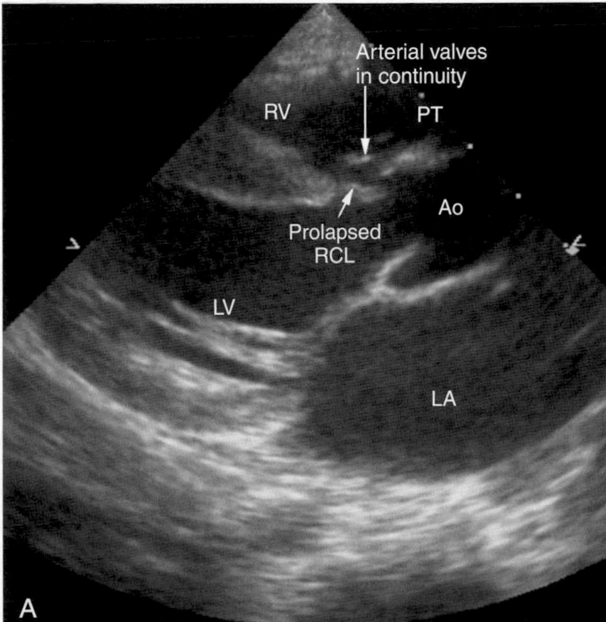

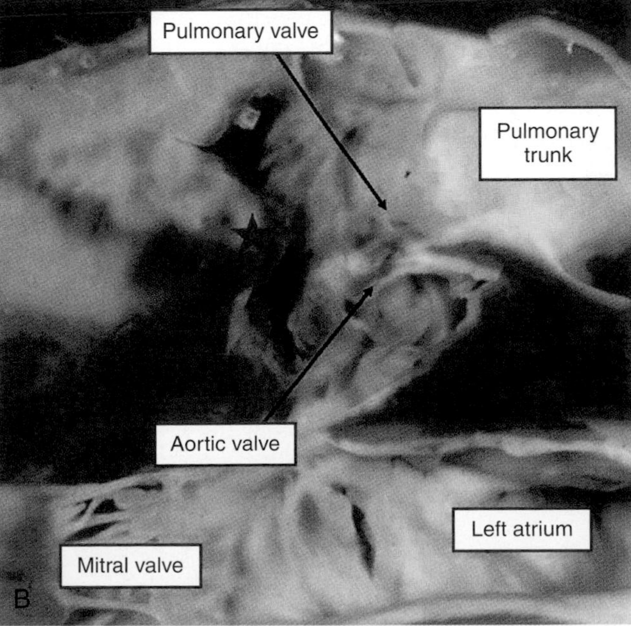

Figure 28-38 A doubly committed juxta-arterial defect seen in a parasternal long axis cut (**A**) with a comparable section in a heart from a different patient (**B**). In the echocardiogram, the defect is partly closed by the prolapsed right coronary leaflet (RCL) of the aortic valve. Note that the aortic and pulmonary valves are in direct contact through the defect. The *star* shows the crest of the muscular ventricular septum. PT, pulmonary trunk. Other abbreviations as in Figure 28-33.

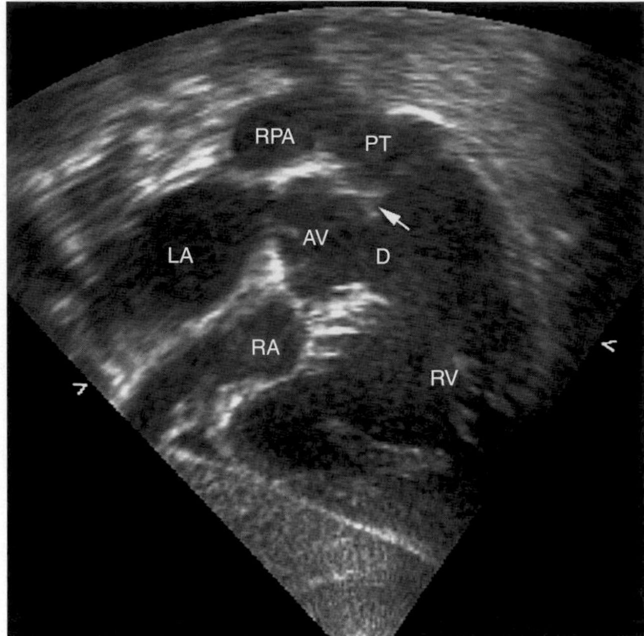

Figure 28-39 A doubly committed juxta-arterial defect (D) seen in subcostal right anterior section. The aortic and pulmonary valves are seen in fibrous continuity (*arrow*). AV, aortic valve; LA, left atrium; PT, pulmonary trunk; RA, right atrium; RPA, right pulmonary artery; RV, right ventricle.

infundibulum. These features are seen in long-axis (Fig. 28-38; see also Fig. 28-28), short-axis (see Fig. 28-29), and subcostal right oblique views (Fig. 28-39). If present, prolapse of the aortic valvar leaflets will be visualised (Fig. 28-40; see also Figs. 28-28 and 28-38). By rotating the transducer to focus on the leaflets of the tricuspid valve, it is also possible to show whether a doubly committed juxta-arterial defect is perimembranous, or is separated from the central fibrous body by a muscular rim. This feature will best be appreciated from the parasternal short-axis section across the aortic valve. Cross sectional echocardiography also demonstrates the proximity of the defect to structures that may close it, such as aneurysmal formation of tricuspid tissue tags (Fig. 28-41; see also Fig. 28-24), or plastering of the tricuspid valvar leaflet tissue across the defect. Although transoesophageal echocardiography is not usually necessary in the delineation of ventricular septal defect in childhood, it may provide crucial information when there is straddling or overriding of the tricuspid valve (see Chapter 33). Identification of the site of the ventricular septal defect at initial examination will also provide hard evidence on the rate of spontaneous closure for different types of defects in different sites.[3]

In addition to these specific diagnostic findings, the echocardiogram also reflects the haemodynamic state. Left atrial and left ventricular dilation are easily seen in infants with a high pulmonary blood flow, the left ventricle being hyperdynamic. With large unrestrictive defects, there will be a concomitant increase in right ventricular dimensions, while in small restrictive defects the ventricular size and performance may be normal. Further insight into the physiological state is obtained by studying the motion of the leaflets of the pulmonary valve. With high flow to the lungs, but low pulmonary vascular resistance, the motion is normal. When there is a high pulmonary vascular resistance, the closure line of the leaflets is flattened, and the a-dip disappears. The onset of aortic regurgitation is indicated by the appearance of diastolic vibration of the mitral valve, well appreciated in earlier times on the M-mode tracing, but now visualised directly with colour flow mapping. In this case, the cross sectional echocardiogram should show the abnormalities of the aortic valve responsible for the regurgitation. For example, a prolapsing aortic valvar leaflet may be demonstrated (see Figs. 28-28 and 28-40). Alternatively, perforations and vegetations associated with infective endocarditis may be identified. As might be expected, all the advantages of cross sectional echocardiography in diagnosis are accentuated when enhanced by three-dimensional reconstruction. Such techniques, while not yet generally available, have immense potential, as shown by the reports describing their value.[43,44]

Doppler Interrogation

The complete evaluation of a ventricular septal defect includes not only an assessment of the size, site and number of defects, but also an estimate of the haemodynamic consequences. By using continuous wave Doppler ultrasound, it is possible to measure the velocity of flow across any ventricular septal defect. Then, by invoking the

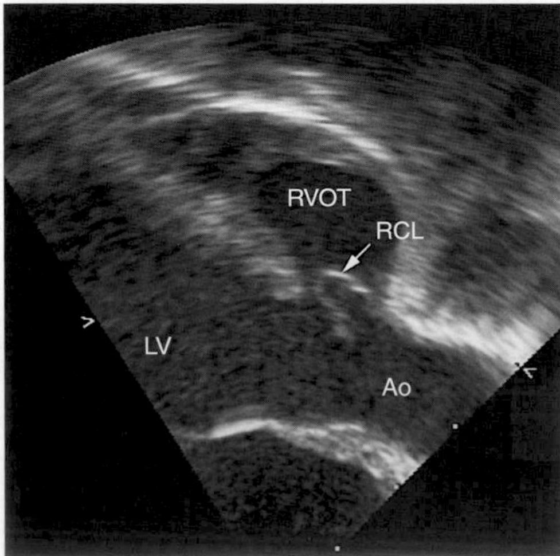

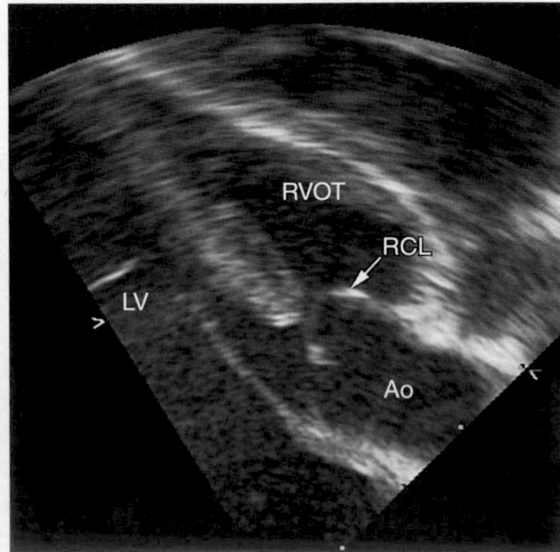

Figure 28-40 The long-axis views (systole and diastole) of a doubly committed juxta-arterial defect from a transoesophageal echocardiogram shows prolapse of the right coronary leaflet (*arrow*) of the aortic (Ao) valve into the right ventricular outflow tract (RVOT). LV, left ventricle; RCL, right coronary leaflet.

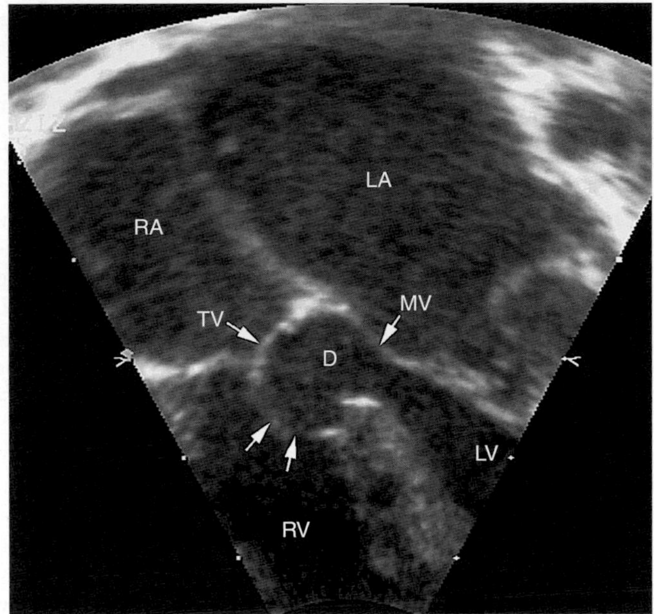

Figure 28-41 This four-chamber cut shows a fibrous tissue tag (*arrows*) from the tricuspid valve (TV) partially closing a perimembranous ventricular septal defect (D). MV, mitral valve. Other abbreviations as in Figure 28-32.

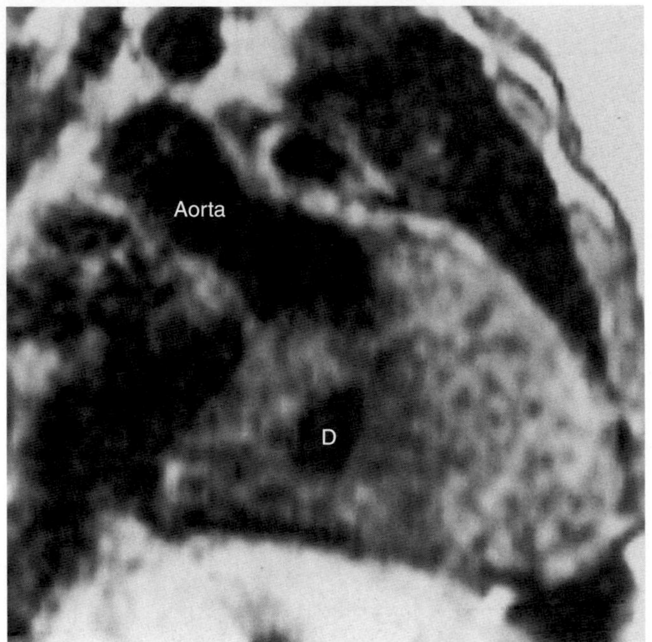

Figure 28-42 This resonance image, taken so as to be in the plane of the muscular ventricular septum, shows a muscular inlet ventricular septal defect (D).

principles of the Bernoulli equation, it is possible to calculate the instantaneous peak systolic pressure drop between the ventricles. Assuming that the left ventricular peak systolic pressure is the same as the systolic blood pressure, the right ventricular systolic pressure can then be estimated. In the absence of any obstruction within the right ventricular outflow tract, this can be presumed to be equal to the pulmonary arterial systolic pressure.

Infants and children with congenital cardiac defects, including those with a ventricular septal defect, frequently have mild tricuspid insufficiency. In this situation, it is possible to estimate the pressure drop across the tricuspid valve and, therefore, to estimate the right ventricular and pulmonary arterial systolic pressures. A potential source of error arises when there is a shunt from left ventricle to right atrium through the defect via a deficiency in the septal leaflet of the tricuspid valve. In this situation, the regurgitant jet reflects the pressure drop between the left ventricle and right atrium.

Colour flow mapping has greatly facilitated the echocardiographic diagnosis of ventricular septal defect.[45] Its most important uses include accurate alignment of the Doppler beam with the flow of blood, thus enhancing accurate quantification of velocity, the detection of multiple ventricular septal defects, and the demonstration of shunting from left ventricle to right atrium. Colour flow mapping also plays a role in distinguishing innocent murmurs from those caused by very small ventricular septal defects.

Transoesophageal Echocardiography

Precordial cross sectional echocardiography detects the vast majority of even small ventricular septal defects. In a small number of patients, especially older children, adolescents, and adults, transoesophageal echocardiography may be required for complete assessment. This technique may also be of particular value during the peri-operative period in the operating theatre and intensive care unit, especially to evaluate residual shunts. An important further use of transoesophageal echocardiography is to distinguish between a ruptured sinus of Valsalva and a perimembranous ventricular septal defect associated with aortic insufficiency. The technique is also indispensible when attempting closure of ventricular septal defects by interventional catheterisation because it allows precise positioning of the retention discs on either side of the defect. On-line three-dimensional echocardiography, at present, represents a growing area and is now being introduced as a routine clinical tool. Reconstruction achieved in this fashion can provide additional information about the morphological features of a ventricular septal defect.[46]

Magnetic Resonance Imaging

As may be anticipated, magnetic resonance imaging clearly shows the location and structure of defects (Figs. 28-42 and 28-43; see also Fig. 28-14). Hardly ever is there a clinical indication for pre-operative morphological investigation of the defect unless echocardiography fails to visualise pertinent anatomical features of the defect. Phase-contrast velocity mapping, an accurate tool for the assessment of volumes of flow of blood, can be used to quantify pulmonary and systemic flows and the calculation of the left-to-right shunt. In addition, magnetic resonance imaging can be used for post-operative assessment of the ventricular volumes and function.

Computed Tomography

Computed tomography is indicated when the ventricular septal defect is complicated by or associated with the abnormalities of the airway or lungs, such as bronchial compression, atelectasis, or pneumonia. Contrast-enhanced computed

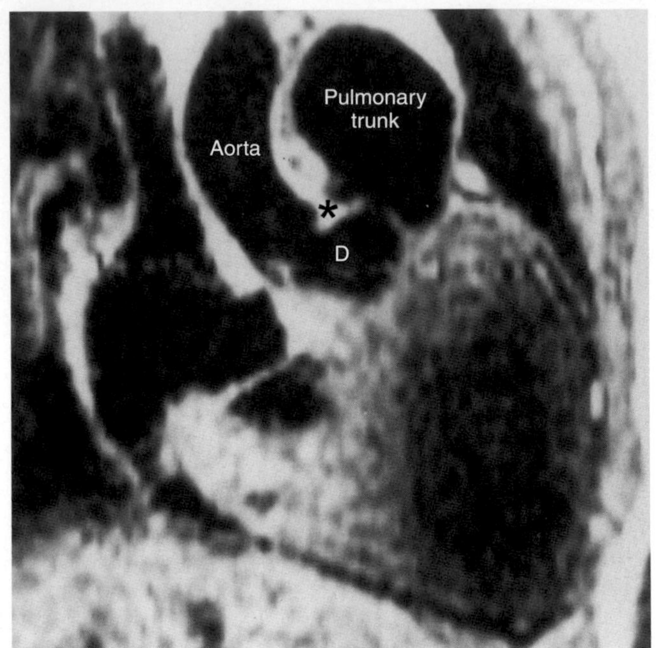

Figure 28-43 The features of a doubly committed juxta-arterial defect (D) are seen in this magnetic resonance image taken through the outlet of the ventricular septum. The aortic and pulmonary valves are in direct contact above the defect (*asterisk*).

tomography can also be useful when obstruction of the aortic arch is suspected, but the echocardiographic findings are inconclusive.

Nuclear Angiography

First-pass studies in nuclear angiography demonstrate the presence of either a left-to-right or a right-to-left shunt, and permit quantification of the ratios of systemic to pulmonary flows.[47,48] Gated blood-pool scans allow assessment of left ventricular size and performance, but do not differentiate the different sites or type of defect. These techniques are largely replaced by magnetic resonance imaging, but can be of value in long-term post-operative assessment, particularly when performed in association with an exercise or stress-testing protocol.

Cardiac Catheterisation

Prior to the advances made in cross sectional echocardiography, catheterisation was an essential part of the assessment of patients having large restrictive and unrestrictive defects. It made possible the measurement of intracardiac pressures, particularly the pulmonary arterial pressure, along with quantification of the flow of blood to the lungs. This information made it possible to calculate the pulmonary vascular resistance. In addition, the technique provides confirmation of the interventricular location of the defect by the detection of a step-up in saturation of oxygen at ventricular level, or by visualisation of the passage of the catheter from right to left ventricle or to the aorta. If the defect is modified by abnormal attachments of the leaflets of the tricuspid valve, such that the shunt is from left ventricle to right atrium, then the step-up in saturation of oxygen is detected in the right atrium. This is also found when a ventricular septal defect co-exists with an atrial septal defect, or when there is an atrioventricular septal defect. Cardiac catheterisation provides further information about the associated defects. Passage of the catheter from the pulmonary trunk to the descending aorta, for example, indicates the presence of a communication between these two arteries, usually an arterial duct.

The findings at catheterisation reflect the pathophysiology. Unrestrictive defects with a high pulmonary blood flow have similar pressures in right and left ventricles. With an unobstructed right ventricular outflow tract, and a low pulmonary vascular resistance, the pulmonary arterial systolic pressure will be similar to that in the aorta. The diastolic and mean pulmonary arterial pressures will be lower than aortic pressures. In such cases, a high flow to the lungs will be measured oximetrically, or in the past by dye dilution curves. In large but restrictive defects, the right ventricular and pulmonary arterial pressures will be lower than those in the left ventricle and aorta. The main current indication for cardiac catheterisation other than for interventional closure of the defect is to establish, beyond doubt, that patients suspected to have pulmonary vascular disease do have an elevation of pulmonary vascular resistance so great as to render them inoperable.

Angiocardiography

Although a case can still be made for performing catheterisation in order to take measurements and calculate shunts and pressures, it is now rarely necessary to perform angiography. In the past, the technique was directed to anatomical delineation of the defect itself, and to the diagnosis or exclusion of associated abnormalities. Left ventricular angiocardiograms were best for anatomical diagnosis. If still performed, it is best to choose an axial oblique projection.[49–52] The long-axis view is the best for demonstration of the different types of perimembranous defect (Fig. 28-44).[53] Doubly committed juxta-arterial defects will also be shown on this view, but demonstration of the lack of infundibular musculature separating the defect from the hingepoints of the leaflets of the pulmonary valve requires a right anterior oblique projection (Fig. 28-45). The long-axis view is again best for demonstrating muscular defects in the apical trabecular septum (Fig. 28-46). A muscular defect between the inlets is clearly demonstrated in the four-chamber view, while a muscular defect between the outlets is profiled in long axial or right anterior oblique projection (Fig. 28-47). If there is doubt about the site of the defect, the long-axis view is helpful, because defects opening to the right ventricular inlet appear behind the line of the anterior portion of the muscular septum. If performed, careful examination of the angiocardiograms should always be undertaken to exclude mitral regurgitation. In patients with pulmonary hypertension, a persistent arterial duct must always be excluded. This is frequently possible on the axial oblique left ventricular injection. When this is not the case, and echocardiography has not resolved the issues, aortography must be performed. A similar approach may also be necessary to exclude associated aortic coarctation. Retrograde aortography is important when aortic regurgitation is suspected. Right ventricular angiography is indicated when obstruction in the right ventricular outflow tract is

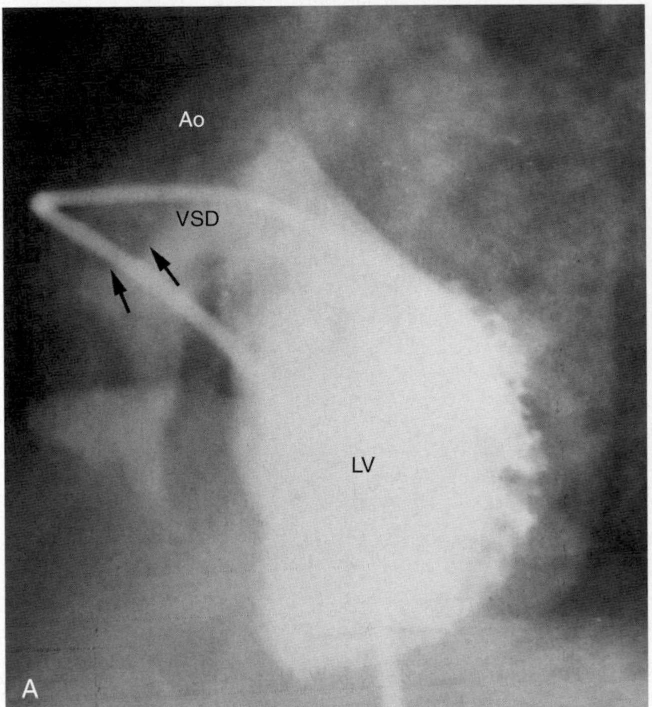

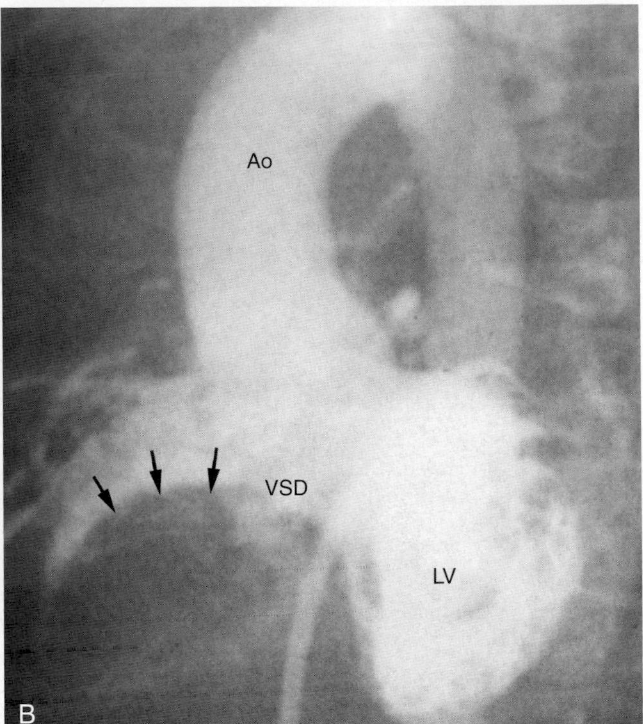

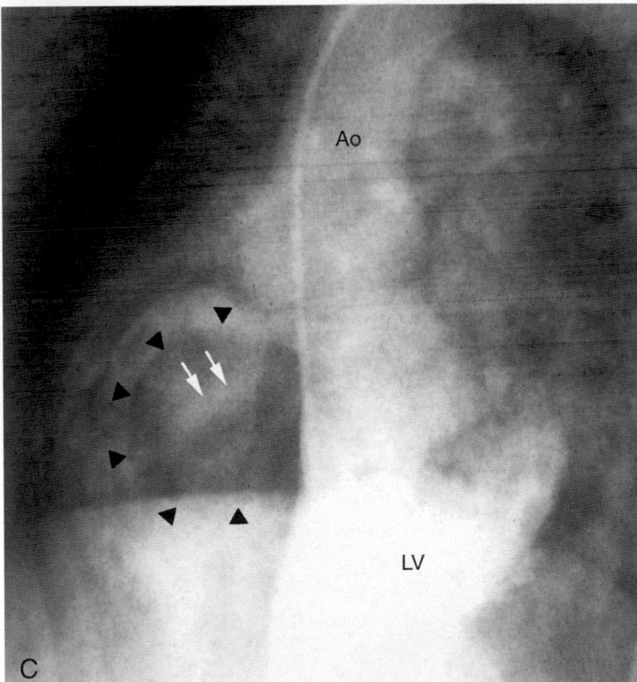

Figure 28-44 The different types of perimembranous defects seen in the long-axial oblique views. **A**, A defect opening to the inlet of the right ventricle (*arrows* delineate the septal leaflet of the tricuspid valve). **B**, A defect extending toward the inlet of the right ventricle (*arrows* delineate the anterior leaflet of the tricuspid valve). **C**, A defect extending toward the trabecular part of the right ventricle. Shunt flow (*arrows*) does not delineate the tricuspid valve orifice, which is denoted by *arrowheads*. Ao, aorta; LV, left ventricle; VSD, ventricular septal defect. (Reproduced with permission from Freedom RM, Mawson JB, Yoo S-J, Benson LN: Congenital Heart Disease: Textbook of Angiocardiography. Armonk, NY: Futura, 1997.)

found on cardiac catheterisation. This is best performed in the 45-degree head-up position using antero-posterior and lateral projections.

Left ventricular angiograms can be used for quantitative assessment of left ventricular function. Left ventricular end-diastolic volume is usually increased, and the ejection fraction is normal or increased. These indexes have prognostic significance but rarely, if ever, will the decision whether or not to opt for closure be influenced by these findings. Nowadays, it is rarely necessary to perform invasive studies in infants with ventricular septal defects. All the necessary information required to determine the need for surgical treatment is provided by non-invasive tests.

DIAGNOSIS

The definitive diagnosis of isolated ventricular septal defect no longer depends upon cardiac catheterisation and angiocardiography but, as discussed above, is made with certainty in the majority of patients using cross sectional echocardiography. In many instances, nonetheless, the diagnosis can also be made from purely clinical

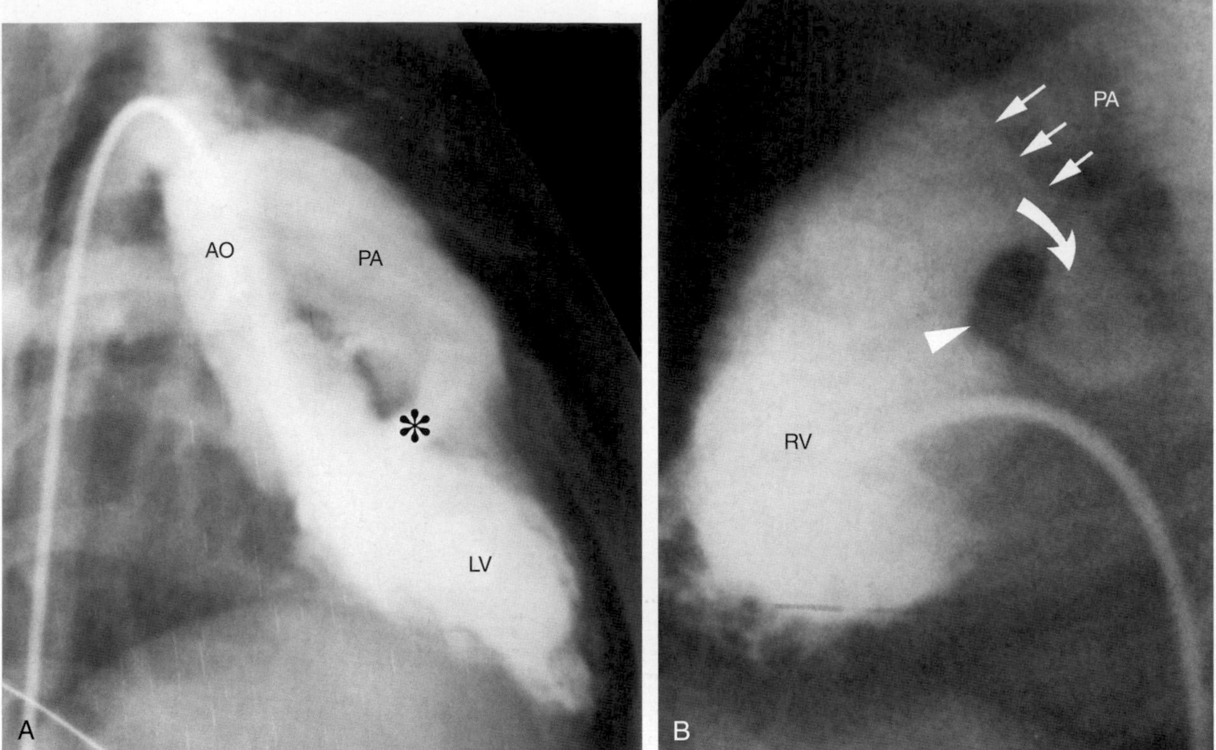

Figure 28-45 A doubly committed juxta-arterial defect in the right anterior (**A**) and lateral (**B**) views. The defect (*asterisk*) is in the outlet septum. The pulmonary and aortic valves are seen in direct contact above the defect. The initial shunt flow delineates the pulmonary valve in part **A**, while part **B** shows a different patient with pulmonary hypertension and a right-to-left shunt flow immediately below the pulmonary valve (*arrows*) and well above the tricuspid valve (*arrowheads*). AO, aorta; LV, left ventricle; PA, pulmonary trunk; RV, right ventricle. (Reproduced with permission from Freedom RM, Mawson JB, Yoo S-J, Benson LN: Congenital Heart Disease: Textbook of Angiocardiography. Armonk, NY: Futura, 1997.)

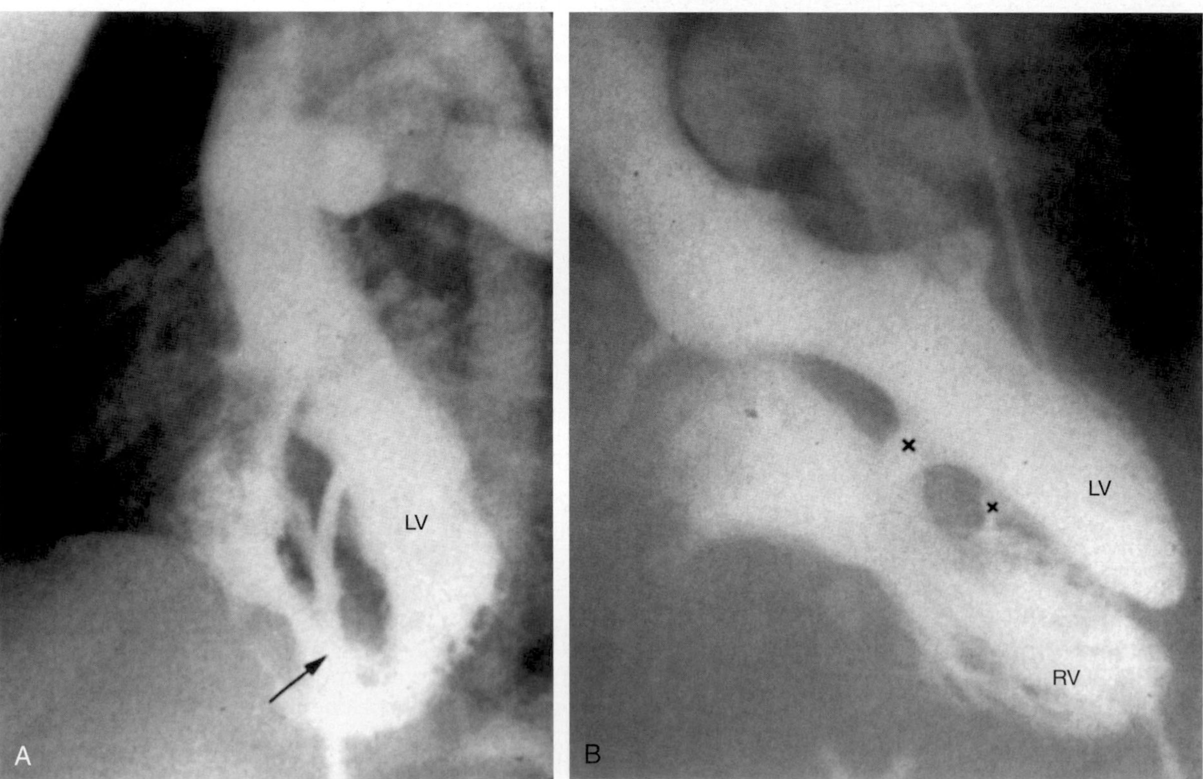

Figure 28-46 Long-axis projections of left ventricular injections showing a solitary (*arrow* in part **A**) and multiple (*X* in part **B**) muscular defects of the apical trabecular septum. LV, left ventricle; RV, right ventricle.

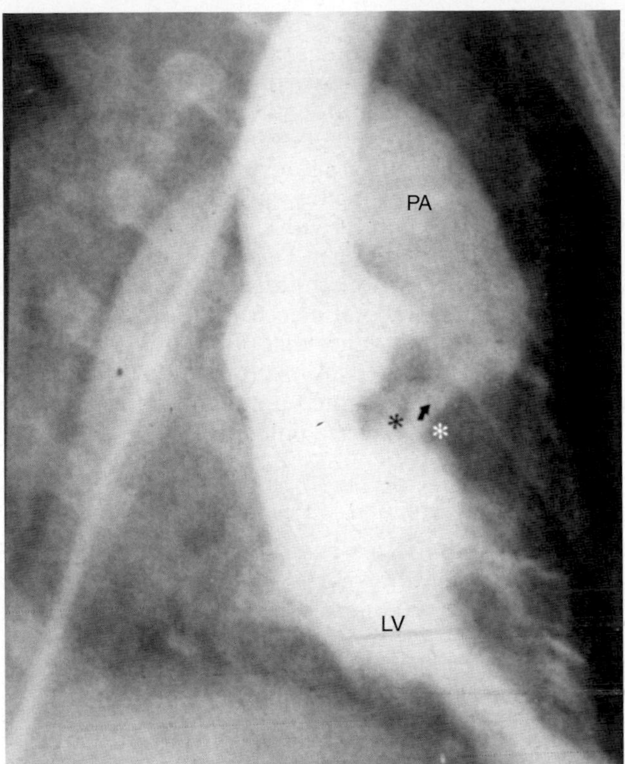

Figure 28-47 Left ventricular injection profiled in the right anterior oblique view reveals a shunt flow (*arrow*) through an outlet muscular defect (*between asterisks*). LV, left ventricle; PA, pulmonary artery.

evidence, supported by the electrocardiogram and the chest radiograph. Thus, in an asymptomatic child over the age of 1 year, the typical physical signs, taken together with the chest radiograph and electrocardiogram, permit a confident diagnosis. This is not the case in infancy, particularly during early infancy. In this setting, a ventricular septal defect is frequently a component of a more complex lesion. It may also be difficult, on clinical grounds alone, to be certain whether the defect is isolated. For example, when a ventricular septal defect occurs in the setting of transposition, the flow to the lungs may be so high that cyanosis is not clinically apparent. Yet the thrill and murmur, and the radiographic and electrocardiographic features, may be compatible with an isolated lesion. In such patients, the response of blood gases to inhalation of 100% oxygen may indicate that the malformation is a complex one. Occasionally this test is misleading, particularly when the ventricular septal defect is found in the setting of a common arterial trunk. Echocardiography is crucial in differentiating isolated defects from more complex anomalies and should, therefore, be performed in all infants suspected of having a ventricular septal defect.[54] Although the clinical features may leave the diagnosis of isolated ventricular septal defect in doubt, the investigations when expertly performed leave little possibility of an alternative diagnosis. The only possible area of confusion is a ventricular septal defect so large that only a rim of septal tissue can be identified separating apical portions of the ventricles with distinctive right and left patterns. This condition is frequently misdiagnosed as double inlet to a solitary indeterminate ventricle. Although it may be suspected on angiocardiographic or echocardiographic grounds that a rim of ventricular septum is present, this can only be confirmed by direct inspection (see Chapter 31).

COURSE AND PROGNOSIS

The majority of patients live normal lives.[55,56] It is difficult, if not impossible, to give accurate figures for the proportion of defects that close spontaneously. A wide range of estimates have been reported. Studies from the 1970s cite closure in up to three-fifths of cases.[57,58] Even when patients present in congestive cardiac failure, the size of the defect in some can diminish over the first year, either anatomically or to the point where it is restrictive and pulmonary arterial pressures are normal. When account is taken of smaller defects now diagnosed echocardiographically, the proportion is almost certainly higher, with perhaps up to nine-tenths closing.[3] This is of little clinical relevance, since many of these represent trival defects. In practical terms, among those with clinically significant defects, closure occurs in about one-quarter of patients, mostly in those with small muscular and perimembranous defects. Occasionally, even a large unrestrictive defect associated with clinical symptoms may close spontaneously. Closure usually happens during the first 2 years of life, but can occur at any age. Indeed, many defects close during fetal life.[59] As the defect becomes smaller, the murmur is said to lose its pansystolic nature, becoming shorter and decrescendo. These changes have value in predicting those defects that are about to close.[60] Even in the group of patients whose defects persist, most lead normal active lives with very little risk of a cardiac death before the age of 40 years.[58] In adults with small defects, with ratios of flow of less than 2 to 1, normal pulmonary arterial pressures, and no element of left ventricular hypertrophy, the outcome is reported to be excellent.[61] In this series, the majority of patients remained free of any symptoms. Aortic regurgitation and endocarditis were infrequent, and arrhythmias, if occurring, were benign.

The longest follow-up is that provided by the First and Second Joint Studies on the Natural History of Congenital Heart Defects.[55,62] For this entire group, the probability of survival at 20 years was 87%. Survival for those with trivial or small defects was equivalent to the general population. For those with moderate or large defects, irrespective of whether the defect has been closed, 89% and 67%, respectively, survived. Of those children admitted with a diagnosis of pulmonary vascular disease, just over half were alive 20 years later. Risk factors for death were related to the size of the defect, and the presence or absence of pulmonary arterial hypertension on admission to the study. Follow-up data underscored the importance of surgical closure during infancy if the ventricular defect remained unrestricted and pulmonary hypertension persisted.[63]

Some children may develop infundibular stenosis, limiting the shunt, and eventually become cyanotic. They require management as for the child with tetralogy of Fallot (see Chapter 36). A few children may develop mid-right ventricular obstruction, creating a two-chambered right ventricle.

Up to one-sixth of infants develop congestive cardiac failure requiring medical treatment.[64] This almost always occurs during the first 6 months of life. Many of these children will not survive longer than 6 months unless the defect is closed. Some are adequately controlled on medical treatment, and do not require closure as a life-saving procedure. Such infants frequently have pulmonary hypertension as a consequence of their large defects, and are at risk for the development of pulmonary vascular disease. They form the only reliably identifiable group of the 3% to 6% of all patients who develop this complication. Any infant with pulmonary hypertension persisting through the early months of life is likely to develop pulmonary vascular disease. This becomes established and irreversible in the majority before the age of 2 years.[63] Patients who have experienced little or no fall in pulmonary vascular resistance after birth form the remainder of the subjects at high risk. Tragically, this latter group may escape detection until cyanosis supervenes. It is important, therefore, to recognise that irreversible and progressive pulmonary vascular disease is present in the affected patients long before they become cyanosed. The prognosis of patients with ventricular septal defect and pulmonary vascular disease is poor, but survival into adult life is common. Death usually occurs before 40 years of age. In females with pulmonary vascular disease, pregnancy poses a particular risk. This is because loss of blood of even moderate degree, as may occur at delivery, can precipitate an irreversible state of low output. Women with this condition should be advised to avoid pregnancy. If they do not heed this advice, a difficult choice is necessary, since termination of pregnancy also carries a significant risk. On balance, unwanted pregnancies should be terminated. If the patient strongly wishes to continue the pregnancy, many can deliver safely with careful supervision,[65–67] although the maternal mortality may be as high as 50%.

There are two other complications of isolated ventricular septal defect that may cause death before the age of 40 years. The first is development of aortic regurgitation.[68] This is reported to occur in up to one-twentieth of patients, albeit that others report a much lower incidence.[60,69] It occurs most usually either when the defect is doubly committed and juxta-arterial, when more than seven-tenths may be affected,[70] or when the defect is perimembranous.[71] It can also occur in the presence of muscular outlet defects when the muscular outlet septum is hypoplastic.[72] Almost always it is the right coronary aortic leaflet that prolapses through the defect. In perimembranous defects, the non-coronary leaflet, and rarely the left, may also be involved. It is often recommended that surgical treatment be offered as soon as significant aortic regurgitation is recognised.[73] It is now known that the condition is well tolerated during childhood in the majority of patients. It can occasionally precipitate cardiac failure refractory to medical treatment during childhood, but this complication is more frequently encountered during adult life.

The second complication is infective endocarditis. The incidence is approximately 1 to 2 per 1000 patient-years.[64,74–76] This represents a risk of approximately 1 in 10 of developing infective endocarditis before the age of 70 years.[65] It is more likely that infective endocarditis will be contracted after the age of 20 years, rather than in childhood or adolescence. The size of defect has no influence on its incidence.[75] Most patients who develop infective endocarditis nowadays are successfully treated. The lifetime risk of dying of infective endocarditis as a complication in the setting of isolated ventricular septal defect has been computed to be of the order of 2% to 3%.[64] Closure of the defects does not eliminate the chance of contracting this infection. Indeed, it may initiate it.[64,75] Avoidance of infective endocarditis cannot, therefore, be proposed as an indication for the closure of ventricular septal defects.[77] The problem also continues into adult life, with one-tenth of one series of patients having episodes of bacterial endocarditis.[78] These were adults with small defects. Recent data, summarised by the American Heart Association,[79] recommended that, as in previous guidleines, those with isolated acyanotic ventricular septal defects did not require antibiotic coverage, citing evidence that prior antibiotic coverage in this situation, was not universally effective, and that prophylaxis was only reasonable for patients with the highest risk of developing an adverse outcome.

MANAGEMENT

When presentation occurs in early infancy, the outcome is always in doubt until a precise diagnosis has been made by echocardiography. For example, an asymptomatic infant presenting with a murmur at 1 month of age may be in intractable heart failure by the age of 3 months. Similarly, spontaneous closure of ventricular septal defect may occur even when the defect has been large enough to cause cardiac failure in infancy. The prognosis must always, therefore, be guarded during the first few months of life. Asymptomatic infants should be closely followed using echocardiography to assess the anatomy and the gradient from the left to the right ventricle. Those who remain asymptomatic, with no signs or investigations suggesting pulmonary hypertension, require no treatment, including no measures against infective endocarditis. These infants have small restrictive defects. Infants with congestive cardiac failure should be treated medically. If the cardiac failure is intractable to medical treatment, then surgical intervention is indicated. These infants usually have unrestrictive defects. Intractability of the cardiac failure can be deemed to be present when, despite maximal medical treatment with diuretics and afterload reduction, the infant fails to thrive despite agressive feeding regimes, including nasogastric tube feeding. Subsequent to closure, improvement in growth is almost universal.[80]

Infants responding to medical treatment may have unrestrictive defects, but they usually have large and restrictive ones. In either event, the pulmonary arterial pressure will be elevated in early infancy but may fall to normal by 6 months of age should the defect become smaller. Closure is indicated in these patients if Doppler echocardiography fails to show a fall in right ventricular pressure to less than 60% of the left ventricular pressure by 5 to 6 months of age, and the baby is failing adequately to grow. This is because such babies are at risk for the development of irreversible pulmonary vascular disease. If the Doppler velocity indicates a lower right ventricular pressure, conservative management should be continued. A basic assumption behind this policy is that pulmonary vascular disease can be prevented or reversed in its early stages. It is not certain that this is possible in all cases. The above recommendations give the best chance of achieving this aim at present.[81] It must be borne in mind that, in some patients, this policy will carry attendant risks for closing defects that would have closed spontaneously.[82] At present, the balance of the risks between corrective and expectant management appears to favour correction.[83] If, and when, more precise ways of predicting reversibility and irreversibility of pulmonary vascular disease are developed, this policy will be modified accordingly.

It is rare for closure to be required for a patient with an isolated defect after the age of 1 year. Occasional patients who have escaped detection, and who have a large left-to-right shunt and an enlarged heart, may need closure in childhood. Recently this conservative policy has been questioned in the light of excellent surgical results, particularly with the prospect of possibly preventing aortic regurgitation.[85] The question posed was, should all defects be closed? Despite cogent arguments of this type, most paediatric cardiologists and surgeons favour a conservative approach.

Aortic regurgitation, when it occurs, may be sufficiently severe to cause cardiomegaly or heart failure. In the latter instance, surgery should be performed at any age. If frank cardiac failure is not present, it is best, if possible, to defer surgery until adolescence or adult life, since it may be necessary to replace the aortic valve, or to perform a Ross operation. Such delay is not advisable in the setting of significant left ventricular dilation. In this situation, we would recommend operation on the basis of echocardiographic measurements. If the end-systolic dimension is greater than 50 to 55 mm in adults, and greater than 29 mm/m^2 body surface area in children, surgery is indicated even in the absence of symptoms.[84] Severe obstruction of the right ventricular outflow tract develops in up to one-tenth of patients.[85,86] It always requires surgical treatment. If possible, corrective surgery should be performed. The best results are probably obtained if this complication is treated as soon as it is recognised.

Surgical and Catheter-based Management

When surgery is required as a life-saving procedure in early infancy, there are two options. The first is to band the pulmonary trunk, followed by correction at a later age. The second is to perform primary closure. Banding of the pulmonary trunk is a safe and effective palliative procedure.[87] When assessing the approaches, account must be taken of the cumulative risk of palliation and subsequent correction. In the best hands, this was shown some time ago to be below 10%,[88–90] but this figure is now much too high when set against the excellent results of primary closure. Banding, furthermore, has its own complications, particularly the development of subvalvar pulmonary obstruction. This may contribute to the development of cyanosis with its attendant risks, which will make definitive surgery an even more complex undertaking. It is, therefore, advisable that the corrective operation should not be delayed beyond the second year of life. Patients with ventricular septal defect who have had banding of the pulmonary trunk also have an unduly high incidence of subaortic stenosis.[91] It is not quite clear whether this is because the presence of the subaortic stenosis meant that banding was more likely to be needed, or because banding has a tendency to cause subaortic stenosis. In most centres nowadays, nonetheless, banding is reserved for small infants with multiple ventricular septal defects, and those with inlet defects where primary closure would carry a significant risk of damage to the atrioventricular valvar tension apparatus or the conduction axis. Banding is rarely, if ever, indicated nowadays in patients beyond the age of 6 months.[92,93]

Closure of an isolated ventricular septal defect can now be performed within the first 6 months of life, and results in the best centres now approach zero mortality.[94] This is clearly superior to the best results of a two-stage approach. The operation can be performed using a ventriculotomy or by a transatrial approach. The applicability of the transatrial approach depends upon the site of the defect. Doubly committed juxta-arterial defects, and multiple defects, present particular difficulties. Nothing is lost, even in these patients, by carrying out an initial transatrial exploration, since this allows accurate placement and, therefore, limits the extent, of the necessary ventricular incision.[95] Multiple defects present a particular challenge. Apical left ventriculotomy has been proposed as the best approach.[96,97] An alternative is to use a large Dacron patch covering all the muscular defects.[98] Even with this approach, left ventriculotomy is not always avoidable, with a reported hospital mortality of 7.7%. The way forward is likely to be the combined use of surgery and catheter intervention.

More recently, catheter-based approaches, either using periventricular[99] or primary percutaneous techniques,[100,101] have supplanted in many instances the traditional surgical approach requiring cardiopulmonary bypass. A variety of devices have been employed, beginning with the clamshell double umbrella device.[102] Structural problems plagued this, and other, devices,[103] until the introduction of a nitinol wire mesh plug with retention discs, the so-called Amplatzer Muscular VSD Occluder (AGA Medical Corp) (Fig. 28-48). Data from the United States registry of patients with muscular ventricular septal defect undergoing closure with a device[104] shows that successful percutaneous implantation occurred in 87% of patients, including those requiring multiple deployments, with a rate of closure of 97% at 12 months. Complications occurred in 11% of patients, including two patients who died, giving a worrisome mortality of 3%. An individual experience in 50 patients with muscular defects reported no procedural

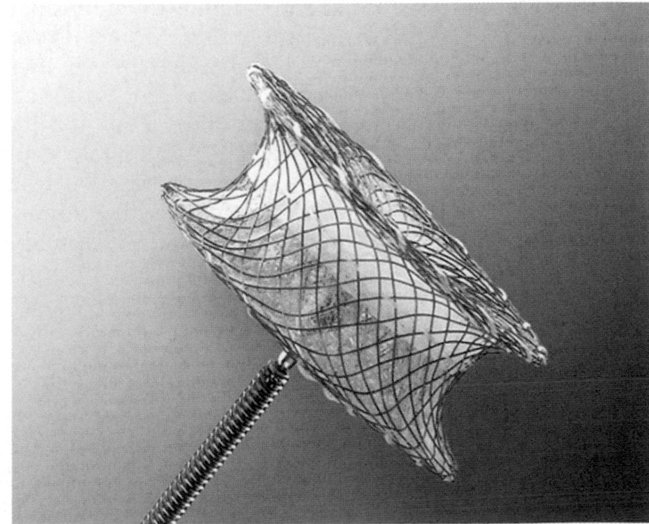

Figure 28-48 An Amplatzer Muscular VSD Occluder (AGA Medical Corporation). Note the two retention discs that support the central plug, which stabilises the implant across the ventricular septum.

complications.[105] A number of devices designed for other cardiac and intracardiac applications have been used to close perimembranous defects,[103,106] but with an undue incidence of complications and residual shunting. The Amplatzer Membranous VSD Occluder was specifically designed to address anatomical concerns, particularly the possiblity of causing aortic insufficiency. This self-expanding double-disc device, also made of a nitinol mesh, has been implantated successfully with great success, and provides a high rate of closure without producing significant aortic valvar dysfunction. Such implantation, however, has been associated with an unacceptable incidence of complete heart block, both acutely and in longer term follow-up.[107,108] It may well be that devices designed specifically for closure of perimembranous defects may have a role in future, although it is difficult to see how such devices could avoid impinging on the atrioventricular conduction axis. We cannot recommend this procedure, therefore, for those with perimembranous defects except in truly exceptional circumstances.

Elective surgery for those having ventricular septal defects should aim to be corrective. Patients surviving the first 6 months of life with persisting pulmonary hypertension should have primary closure of the defect before the age of 1 year. Pulmonary vascular disease is rare before the first birthday. Its incidence increases thereafter,[109] and is more common in those with multiple defects, or when associated with a patent arterial duct. With early surgery, the incidence of pulmonary vascular disease should approch zero, which it has, for all practical purposes. The possible routes for closure are either transatrial, transaortic, or apical approaches.[110] Similarly, those with a large left-to-right shunt who have escaped detection, or for other reasons have survived the first year of life, should be corrected at the first opportunity. In all patients, the only direct contra-indication to surgery is the presence of established and severe pulmonary vascular disease. The initial assessment of pulmonary vascular disease is made from the haemodynamic data. Patients with a calculated pulmonary vascular resistance greater than 8 Wood units/m^2 body surface area are generally considered inoperable. In those with calculated resistances of between 4 and 8 Wood units/m^2 body surface area, it is not possible to say whether the pulmonary vascular disease has become irreversible. More information must be provided to permit rational decisions in these patients. The administration of 100% oxygen during cardiac catheterisation nearly always produces a fall in calculated pulmonary vascular resistance. The greatest fall occurs in the patients with the highest pulmonary vascular resistance. When breathing room air, patients with undoubtedly severe pulmonary vascular disease retain measurable reactivity in their pulmonary vasculature.[111] In the presence of severe pulmonary vascular disease, therefore, the demonstration of reactivity is not necessarily an index of operability. This casts doubt on the value of this test in the assessment of operability in patients with less severe elevation of pulmonary vascular resistance. Administration of 100% oxygen may be helpful in patients with pulmonary venous desaturation, since it should reverse the transient hypoxic vasoconstrictor response. Indeed, if such patients have a restrictive ventricular septal defect, administration of 100% oxygen can cause a prompt drop in pulmonary arterial pressure from systemic levels. Inhalation of nitric oxide has been shown to cause a fall in pulmonary vascular resistance in patients with pulmonary hypertension of various causes, and it has become a useful test in differentiating those who are operable from those who are not.[112,113] In doubtful situations, a lung biopsy may provide useful information.[30] In practise, perhaps because of the small and possibly unrepresentative sample, biopsy is prone to give misleading information. It is rarely used nowadays for clinical decision-making.

Elective surgery is also required when subvalvar pulmonary stenosis is present. Resection of the obstructing muscle will be necessary at the time of closure. The presence of aortic regurgitation poses greater problems. It has been suggested that closure of the defect in itself may limit the valvar regurgitation, this being most effective in doubly committed juxta-arterial defects.[68] Indeed, there is a case to be made for closing all doubly committed juxta-arterial defects as soon as they are diagnosed, even in those rare instances where there is neither congestive cardiac failure nor high pulmonary arterial pressure. Once aortic regurgitation has developed, it is rarely possible in our experience to avoid a direct attack upon the aortic valve. Initially this may be conservative, and good results have been reported in the short and longer term.[114,115] Replacement of the aortic valve has been recommended as the best initial form of treatment, particularly when the valvar leaflets are deformed.[116] The balance of the evidence leads us to recommend an initial conservative approach wherever possible, with replacement only where this has failed or is impossible.

Course after Surgery

Subsequent to correction, the majority of patients live virtually normal lives and have normal exercise capacity.[117] The clinical condition of almost nine-tenths of the patients is graded as good or excellent on follow-up examination. Of the remaining patients, very few are still classified as poor, whereas such a classification is frequent prior to surgery.[55,56,80] A significant cause of morbidity and mortality is pulmonary vascular disease. When this is established, it usually progresses inexorably despite a corrective operation. This complication is avoided by early corrective surgery.[117] Late post-operative exercise testing confirms the improvement after correction, again pointing to the advantage of early surgery.[117]

Disturbances of cardiac rhythm occur in perhaps one-twentieth of patients following corrective surgery,[55,62,63] with some still suffering complete heart block. Even with precise knowledge of the conduction tissues, surgical heart block does still occur, although today it is extremely rare, with less than 1% of children affected. Should the complication occur, it requires the insertion of an artificial pacemaker, with its attendant morbidity.[118] Permanent pacing should certainly be provided if the patient remains in congestive cardiac failure with a slow heart rate. When Stokes–Adams attacks occur, or if 24-hour monitoring of the electrocardiogram demonstrates prolonged period of asystole, episodes of ventricular tachycardia, or ventricular fibrillation, then even if the patient is asymptomatic, it is probably best to insert a pacemaker. In practise, a slow heart rate of 30 to 40 beats per minute at any time of the day is frequently used as a relative indicator for pacing. Transient heart block after surgery may predispose to late sudden death.[77]

The Second Natural History Study showed a higher prevalence of both serious arrhythmias and sudden death in this setting.[62] It follows that 24-hour tape monitoring is mandatory in all patients with heart block following surgery for ventricular septal defect, even when this resolves spontaneously. This investigation should be repeated periodically during follow-up. In the absence of symptoms, it should be performed at yearly or 6-monthly intervals. Monitoring should also be performed in patients with post-operative ventricular ectopic beats. There is some suggestive evidence that these, by triggering a life-threatening ventricular arrhythmia, may be responsible for sudden death.[119,120]

Intraventricular conduction disturbances are seen in the majority of patients who have had open heart surgery. Right bundle branch block is certainly seen following repair of ventricular septal defect, be this performed transatrially or by the ventricular route.[95,121] When this is an isolated phenomenon, it is not a prognostic sign. When it is associated with left-axis deviation and a prolonged PR interval (see Chapter 19), it may well be a precursor of late complete heart block, particularly when the post-operative period has been complicated by a period of transient complete heart block.[122] In these patients, and in those where the right bundle branch block and left-axis deviation are not associated with a prolonged PR interval, intracardiac electrophysiological studies may assist in predicting the outcome.[121] The prognostic significance of all these changes for the occurrence of sudden unexpected death remains uncertain.[120] Close surveillance with 24-hour tape monitoring is a wise precaution. As with complete heart block, there are no generally accepted criteria for the insertion prophylactically of a pacemaker.

Crucial to the long-term outcome in patients with intraventricular conduction disturbances is the site of interference with the conduction tissues. If this is central, that is, within the atrioventricular bundle, the risk of complete heart block is greater than if the damage is solely within the peripheral bundle branches. While intracardiac electrophysiological studies (see Chapter 19) have been suggested as being helpful, this is not always the case.[120] Atrial arrhythmias may occur if there is damage to the sinus node, for instance, during cannulation, but these are a rare occurrence nowadays following surgery for correction of ventricular septal defect.

The other common complication is a residual ventricular septal defect.[55,110] In general, such residual defects are of little haemodynamic significance.[117] Occasionally they will be large enough to permit a considerable residual left-to-right shunt. When this results in congestive, or persistent, cardiac failure, closure is indicated. Frequently this may be addressed with catheter-based approaches.[123] In the presence of a residual ventricular septal defect, lifelong prophylactic measures against infective endocarditis are still recommended.[79] These measures should be continued even when the operation appears to have been totally successful.

Patients undergoing surgery for ventricular septal defect are at risk for all the complications associated with open heart surgery performed for any reason, including cerebral damage, renal damage, postpericardotomy syndrome, pulmonary complications, and so on. The majority of patients, however, suffer no ill-effects, are improved and go on to lead normal lives. This they should be encouraged to do. Although it is too early to predict the ultimate lifespan of such patients, organisations such as the armed services and the police force can be prevailed upon to accept recruits who have undergone closure of a ventricular septal defect. It is also the case that those who survive into adulthood without the need for closure can continue to pose a problem, albeit at low risk.[61,63] In one cohort of adult patients,[78] although half had no complications over many years, and spontaneous closure occurred in one-tenth, serious complications were encountered in one-quarter. The malformation, therefore, is not entirely benign.

The complete reference list can be found on the companion Expert Consult web site at www.expertconsult.com.

ANNOTATED REFERENCES

- Soto B, Becker AE, Moulaert AJ, et al: Classification of ventricular septal defects. Br Heart J 1980;43:332–343.

  This classification with obvious clinical relevance was based on study of hearts with concordant atrioventricular and ventriculoarterial connections. The ventricular septum itself was viewed as having muscular and membranous portions, the muscular septum itself being divided into inlet, trabecular, and outlet components. Defects observed in the area of the membranous septum were termed perimembranous, distinguishing them from muscular defects and those in the area of septum subjacent to the arterial valves, termed subarterial infundibular defects. Perimembranous defects could be found extending towards the inlet, apical, or outlet components of the right ventricle. Muscular defects were found opening to the inlet, apical trabecular, and outlet components of the right ventricle. These observations form the basis of classifying such defects in clinical practise.

- Soto B, Ceballos R, Kirklin JW: Ventricular septal defects: A surgical viewpoint. J Am Coll Cardiol 1989;14:1291–1297.

  This anatomical study categorised ventricular septal defects from a surgical viewpoint. The defects were classified as being conoventricular, in the right ventricular outlet, in the inlet septum, or in the trabecular septum, with each category having several subcategories. Emphasis was placed on the relations of the defects to the left ventricular outflow tract. The borders of the ventricular septal defects were described in detail, with use of the prefix juxta- to indicate the immediate adjacency of the defect to a structure such as the tricuspid valve. Taken together with the classification discussed above, this provides the foundation of the terminology used today.

- Cheatham JP, Latson LA, Gutgesell HP: Ventricular septal defect in infancy: Detection with two dimensional echocardiography. Am J Cardiol 1981;47:85–89.
- van Mill GJ, Moulaert A, Harinck E: Two-dimensional echocardiographic localisation of isolated ventricular septal defects. In Hunter S, Hall R, eds: Echocardiography I. Edinburgh: Churchill Livingstone, 1981, pp. 249–265.
- Sutherland GR, Godman MJ, Smallhorn JF, et al: Ventricular septal defects: Two dimensional echocardiographic and morphologic correlations. Br Heart J 1982;47:316–328.
- Capelli H, Andrade JL, Somerville J: Classification of the site of ventricular septal defect by 2-dimensional echocardiography. Am J Cardiol 1983;51:1474–1480.

  These studies utilised cross sectional echocardiography to identify and classify ventricular septal defects. Multiple precordial and subcostal echocardiographic planes are described. Defects visualised were classified on the basis of the structures which formed their margins, and correlations made angiographically, surgically, and pathologically. Echocardiography was reliable in identifying subaortic, inlet, small, moderate, and large subtricuspid, large subpulmonary, and large central and apical muscular ventricular septal defects. These studies describe the initial views used today in routine clinical practise to image and classify ventricular defects.

- Chen FL, Hsiung MC, Nanda N, et al: Real time three-dimensional echocardiography in assessing ventricular septal defects: An echocardiographic-surgical correlative study. Echocardiography 2006;23:562–568.

  This study examines the potential value of real time three-dimensional echocardiography in accurately and quantitatively estimating the size of ventricular septal defects, correlating observations with surgical findings. The technology offered intra-operative visualisation of ventricular defects to generate a virtual sense of depth. From left ventricular en face projections, the position, size, and shape of the defects could accurately be determined to permit quantitative examination of dynamics. This study underscores this as a potentially valuable clinical tool to provide imaging for surgical and catheter-based interventions.

- Bargeron LM, Elliott LP, Soto B, et al: Axial cineangiography in congenital heart disease. Section I. Concept, technical and anatomical considerations. Circulation 1977;56:1075–1083.
- Elliott LP, Bargeron LM, Bream PR, et al: Atrial cineangiography in congenital heart disease. Section II. Specific lesions. Circulation 1977;56:1084–1093.
- Santamaria H, Soto B, Ceballos R, et al: Angiographic differentiation of types of ventricular septal defects. Am J Radiol 1983;141:273–281.

These studies represent a must read for any paediatric cardiologist interested in the anatomy of the congenitally malformed heart. They set the stage for the detailed understanding, definition and characterisation of ventricular septal defects.

- Kidd L, Driscoll DJ, Gersony WM, et al: Second natural history study of congenital heart defects: Results of treatment of patients with ventricular septal defect. Supplement: Report from the Second Joint Study on the Natural History of Congenital Heart Defects (NHS-2). Circulation 1993;87:38–51.

  The Natural History of Congenital Heart Defects studies were the first significant multicentric investigations of outcomes for a variety of congenital cardiac lesions commonly seen in practise. These studies set the goal posts for the definition of severity, and the impact at the time of medical and surgical therapies. They became, and to a large extent remain, the basis for the decisions we make as paediatric cardiologists.

- Gersony WM: Natural history and decision-making in patients with ventricular septal defects. Progr Pediatr Cardiol 2001;14:125–132.

  Welton Gersony is an experienced paediatric cardiologist who has contributed significantly to our understanding of the clinical course of many congential cardiac lesions. In this paper, he provides a sensible approach to management, based on data from the previous natural history studies. The section presenting various questions in management, and providing their answers, is particularly useful for the young cardiologist.

- Yeager SB, Freed MD, Keane JF, et al: Primary surgical closure of ventricular septal defect in the first year of life: Results in 128 infants. J Am Coll Cardiol 1984;3:1269–1276.
- Chen JM, Mosca RS: Surgical management of ventricular septal defects. Progr Pediatr Cardiol 2001;14:187–197.

  These excellent studies review the outcomes of primary surgical management of the infant with a ventricular septal defect.

- Van Hare GF, Soffer LJ, Sivakoff MC, Liebman J: Twenty-five-year experience with ventricular septal defect in infants and children. Am Heart J 1987;114:606–614.
- Gabriel HM, Heger M, Innerhofer P, et al: Long-term outcome of patients with ventricular septal defect considered not to require surgical closure during childhood. J Am Coll Cardiol 2002;39:1066–1071.
- Neumayer U, Stone S, Somerville J: Small ventricular septal defects in adults. Eur Heart J 1998:19:1573–1582.
- Meijboom F, Szatmari A, Utens E, et al: Long-term follow-up after surgical closure of ventricular septal defect in infancy and childhood. J Am Coll Cardiol 1994;24:1358–1364.

  Long-term outcomes are summarised for those patients with a ventricular septal defect requiring surgical correction and those needing medical management alone. Outcomes are good in childhood through adulthood. We learn however, that the lesion in a small minority of adults does cause disability, cardiac failure, disturbances of rhythm, and endocarditis.

- Wilson W, Taubert KA, Gewitz M, et al: Prevention of infective endocarditis: Guidelines from the American Heart Association—A guideline from the American Heart Association Rheumatic Fever, Endocarditis, and Kawasaki Disease Committee, Council on Cardiovascular Disease in the Young, and the Council on Clinical Cardiology, Council on Cardiovascular Surgery and Anesthesia, and the Quality of Care and Outcomes Research Interdisciplinary Working Group. Circulation 2007:116:1736–1754. Erratum in Circulation 2007:116(15):e376–377.

  The American Heart Association has recently changed it recommendations for prevention of endocarditis. These recommendations are very different from what has been applied in clinical practise for the last 3 decades. The reasons for these changes are presented. Note is made that the risk of endocarditis in any individual patient has not changed, just as its prevention with so-called endocarditis prophylaxis has not been effective. This should now be limited to those at the highest risk.

- Diab KA, Cao QL, Hijazi ZM: Device closure of congenital ventricular septal defects. Congenit Heart Dis 2007;2:92–103.
- Holzer R, Balzer D, Cao QL, et al: Device closure of muscular ventricular septal defects using the Amplatzer muscular ventricular septal defect occluder: Immediate and mid-term results of a U.S. registry. J Am Coll Cardiol 2004;43:1257–1263.
- Arora R, Trehan V, Thakur AK, et al: Transcatheter closure of congenital muscular ventricular septal defect. J Interv Cardiol 2004;17:109–115.
- Carminati M, Butera G, Chessa M, et al: Transcatheter closure of congenital ventricular septal defects: Results of the European Registry. Eur Heart J 2007;28:2361–2368.

  This series of papers summarises the applications of interventional techniques in the management of ventricular septal defects. Periventicular closure avoiding cardiopulmonary bypass, catheter laboratory based closure for native or unoperated defects, and the management of residual defects after surgery are presented. Technical success in the muscular defect is well over 90%, with excellent medium-term outcomes. The management of the perimembranous defect, however, eludes the interventionalist. While it can be closed, conduction complications make it less attractive at present.

CHAPTER 29

Hypoplasia of the Left Heart

GIL WERNOVSKY, TROY E. DOMINGUEZ, PETER J. GRUBER, and ROBERT H. ANDERSON

Rather than being a single lesion, the entity usually described as hypoplastic left heart syndrome is a group of conditions with characteristic anatomical, physiological, and clinical properties. The earliest grouping of these features was made by Lev,[1] but he described the syndrome as hypoplasia of the aortic tract. Hypoplasia of the left heart is not always the same as aortic atresia or hypoplasia, since the aortic lesions can exist with a left ventricle of normal size, particularly when the aorta takes its origin from the morphologically right ventricle. As far as we are aware, it was Noonan and Nadas[2] who first used the term hypoplastic left heart syndrome. This is the term now generally accepted for description, despite the concerns that some have with regard to the definition of a syndrome. Geneticists define a syndrome as involving organs of several systems. Patients with the classical picture of hypoplasia of the left heart rarely have syndromic problems elsewhere in their bodies. If we wish to be specific, therefore, it is better to use hypoplasia of the left heart to describe the anatomical features of the entity to be discussed in this chapter. It is most unlikely, nonetheless, that those who diagnose and treat the entity will call it anything other than hypoplastic left heart syndrome, so we anticipate that the classical term will retain its currency.[3]

Although the combinations of anatomical lesions that constitute the syndrome are variable, the features when seen together are unmistakable. Thus, the syndrome includes the majority of cases of aortic atresia, and most cases of atresia of the left atrioventricular valve. Aortic atresia, nonetheless, when associated with deficient ventricular septation, can be found with a left ventricle of normal size. In these cases, the aorta may be in potential connection with the morphologically left ventricle. The atretic aorta may also be connected potentially to the morphologically right ventricle when the ventriculo-arterial connections are essentially discordant. In the latter setting, of course, the morphologically left ventricle is dominant rather than hypoplastic. In most of the cases of left atrioventricular valvar atresia with right hand ventricular topology, it is the left ventricle which is hypoplastic. Patients with hearts of this type fall within the group of classic cases when the ventricular septum is intact. When both arteries take their origin from the morphologically right ventricle in this setting, the aorta may be of good size despite the left ventricular hypoplasia. Furthermore, should the ventriculo-arterial connections be discordant, the left ventricle can again be hypoplastic. With such discordant ventriculo-arterial connections, the small left ventricle is in potential communication with the pulmonary trunk rather than the aorta. In the rare instances of this combination existing with an intact ventricular septum, the combination will present clinically as pulmonary atresia, although the ventricular morphology is more representative of hypoplasia of the left heart. The left ventricle, aortic valve, and ascending aorta may all also be hypoplastic in the context of atrioventricular septal defect with common atrioventricular junction when there is right ventricular dominance. Patients with this combination are discussed in Chapter 36. In most of the cases initially studied by Noonan and Nadas,[2] aortic coarctation was the major anatomical feature, although the left ventricle was described as being hypoplastic. It is questionable whether such cases would nowadays be considered as examples of hypoplastic left heart syndrome, albeit that examples of the classical syndrome are held to exist with mitral and aortic valves of normal dimensions relative to the co-existing hypoplasia of the left ventricle. Some, therefore, describe these cases as a complex rather than a syndrome, and maintain that biventricular repair is possible following simple relief of any obstruction within the aortic arch and descending aorta.[4]

It follows from all the above discussion relating to different morphological patterns that there are major difficulties in providing an all-encompassing anatomical definition for hypoplasia of the left heart. It is more realistic, therefore, to analyze the unifying haemodynamic features. In physiological and clinical terms, hypoplasia of the left heart can be defined as the situation in which the systemic circulation is dependent on the morphologically right ventricle in the setting of atresia or severe hypoplasia of the aortic valve.[5] For the purposes of this chapter, we will follow this definition, dealing exclusively with those lesions having a small morphologically left ventricle, an intact ventricular septum, and either atresia or critical stenosis of the aortic valve.

EPIDEMIOLOGY

Before fetal echocardiography routinely became a part of antenatal screening, the reported incidence of the hypoplastic left heart syndrome ranged from 0.16 to 0.36 per 1000 live births.[6,7] In many countries, screening to establish normality of the four cardiac chambers is now routinely performed during antenatal ultrasonography, and the diagnosis of hypoplasia of the left heart is often made by non-cardiologists. Some parents, learning of the diagnosis prior to 20 weeks of gestation, will opt for termination of the pregnancy. This contributed, in some areas of the world, to a decline in the number of neonates born with the syndrome.[8] In this respect, although the syndrome is not a common form of congenital cardiac disease, in the past it generated a large proportion of the cardiovascular mortality occurring in the first month of life, since prior to the late 1980s, there was no treatment for the condition. It remains to be seen, with the improvements in surgical treatment to be discussed in this chapter, whether the observed decline in incidence because of termination of pregnancy will continue. In support of this speculation, a recent report from the United Kingdom demonstrated a reduction in the rate of termination of pregnancy of 50%.[9]

Of those surviving to term, two-thirds are male. It has been estimated that the risk of recurrence in siblings is 0.5%, with a risk of 2.2% for the occurrence of other congenitally malformed hearts.[10] The syndrome can occur in the setting of Turner's syndrome, or its mosaic variant. It can also accompany Noonan's syndrome, microdeletion of chromosome 22q11, Holt–Oram syndrome, Edward's syndrome, and Jacobsen syndrome, and can be found with other chromosomal abnormalities, including trisomy 13, trisomy 18, and deletions of chromosomes 4q, 4p, 11q, and 18p. It has also been associated with different mendelian syndromes, but without a robust genetic association. With the advent of fetal echocardiography, it has become evident that recurrence of obstructive lesions in the left heart is particularly high in mothers referred with a family history of congenital cardiac disease. Such observations support a genetic predisposition to the development of such lesions. Epidemiological evidence in favour of this notion was provided by the Baltimore–Washington infant study.[11] It is also increasingly recognised that first-degree relatives of probands with hypoplasia of the left heart are at increased risk of less severe abnormalities of the left heart. In two recent reports from the United States, a bicuspid aortic valve was identified in 5% to 11% of first-degree relatives of affected probands.[12,13]

AETIOLOGY

The aetiology of hypoplasia of the left heart is unknown in most instances. Associations with chromosomal or extracardiac defects are inconsistent, but more common than with many other forms of congenital cardiac malformations. Thus far, they have failed to refine our understanding of the genetic precursor of the disease, although recent work suggests that the basic helix-loop-helix transcription factors may play a role.[14] Most current theories on the aetiology of hypoplastic left heart syndrome are based on autopsy findings, along with echocardiography, particularly fetal echocardiography. It is examination of the heart during the latter trimesters of gestation that has better enabled us to define its normal and abnormal development. In those eventually developing the syndrome, evidence of impaired growth of the left ventricle has been associated with diminished inflow or obstruction to outflow, although this does not become obvious until after 20 weeks of gestation.[15]

Experiments using chick embryos showed that hypoplasia of the left ventricle could be produced following intervention to occlude the mitral valve.[16] This is unlikely to underscore development of the syndrome in humans, as mitral stenosis occurring as a primary lesion results in enlargement, rather than hypoplasia, of the left atrium. Displacement of the primary atrial septum has been noted in autopsied specimens,[17] and has been presumed potentially to reduce flow through the inferior caval vein via the oval foramen to the left atrium and left ventricle, resulting in left ventricular hypoplasia. The displaced septum could equally be the consequence of the ordered flow. Indeed, studies of flow during fetal life suggest that it is likely that the ventricular problem occurs first.[18] Obstruction to the outflow from the left ventricle is always present, and it, too, has been implicated as an aetiological factor.[19] Ventricular endocardial fibro-elastosis is prominent when the mitral valve is patent. In these patients, there can be little doubt that the high left ventricular pressure, particularly in diastole, is an important additional aetiological factor in the development of the endocardial ischaemia and scarring. In the light of the varied anatomical findings to be described below when the left ventricle is hypoplastic, it is unlikely that a solitary aetiological factor unifies their development. The familial occurrence of obstructive lesions in the left ventricular outflow tract and aortic arch, nonetheless, suggests that ongoing genetic advances will provide additional aetiological insights.

ANATOMY

Overall Structure

Hypoplasia of the left heart is usually found in the setting of usual atrial arrangement with concordant atrioventricular and ventriculo-arterial connections (Fig. 29-1), with absence of the left atrioventricular connection in some instances (Fig. 29-2). The combination should be anticipated to exist in the mirror-imaged format. There is usually obstruction to the left ventricular inflow and outflow, but this is variable. At the extreme, the left ventricular cavity may be no more than a slit in the postero-inferior wall of the ventricular mass (see Fig. 29-2).

While the anatomist can discover small ventricles by dissecting between the delimiting coronary arteries, it is almost impossible to determine morphologically when the left ventricle is to be considered hypoplastic in patients

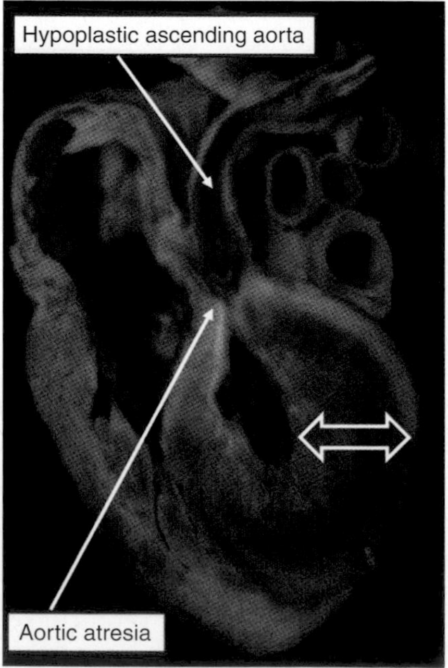

Figure 29-1 The classic form of hypoplasia of the left heart, with marked left ventricular mural hypertrophy (*arrow*).

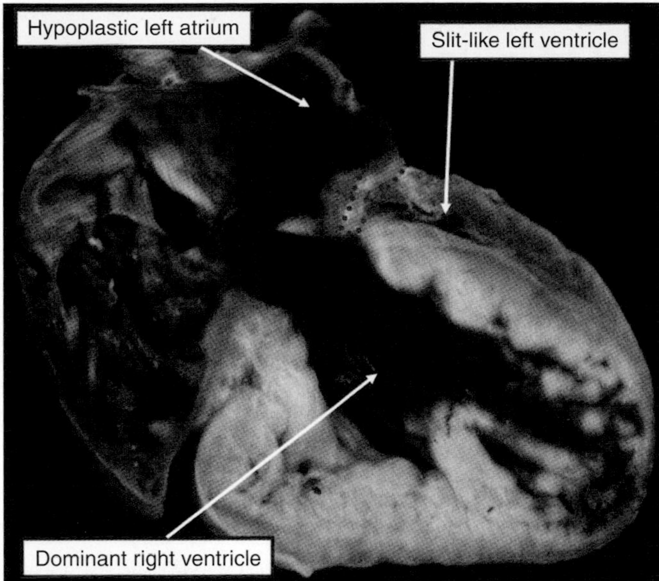

Figure 29-2 In this heart, which also had aortic atresia, there is absence of the left atrioventricular connection (*green dotted lines*). The left ventricle is no more than a slit in the postero-inferior margin of the ventricular mass.

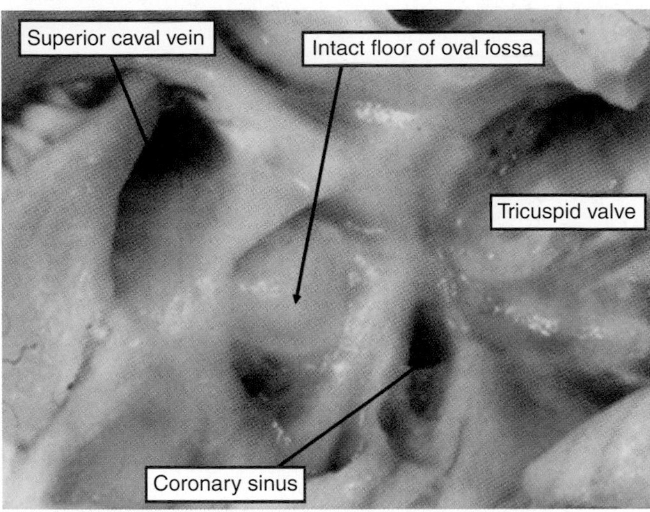

Figure 29-4 This picture shows the atrial septum in a heart with hypoplasia of the left ventricle. The atrial septum is intact, the flap valve being fused with the left atrial aspect of the rims of the oval fossa.

with aortic valvar stenosis rather than atresia. Some of these hearts show obvious fibro-elastosis in the small ventricle and certainly fulfill the anatomical criterions for the syndrome (Fig. 29-3).

Under other circumstances, the ventricle may seem hypoplastic, but the morphologist will be unable to judge its ability to maintain an effective systemic circulation during life. It is the existence of such small left ventricles, in which the dimensions of the aortic and mitral valves are in keeping with the dimensions of the ventricle itself, which

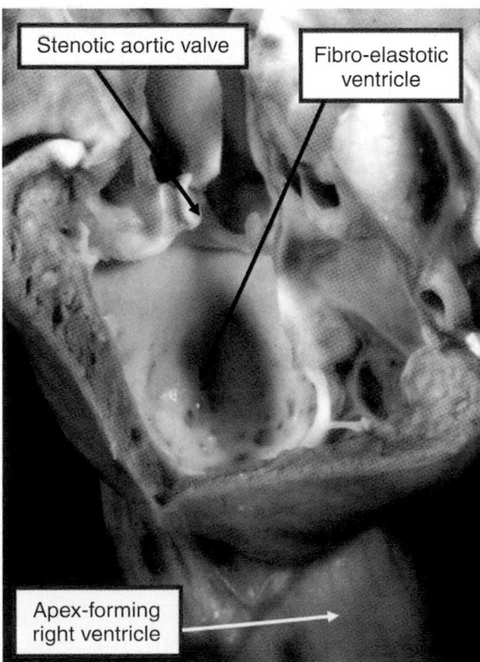

Figure 29-3 In this heart from a patient with critical aortic stenosis, the right ventricle is apex-forming, and the hypoplastic left ventricle has an obvious fibro-elastotic lining. This is an example of hypoplastic left heart syndrome.

underscore the suggestion that some forms of the syndrome can be corrected in biventricular fashion without the need for surgery on either valve, hence the description of the so-called hypoplastic left heart complex.[4]

Typically, the left ventricular walls are hypertrophied (see Fig. 29-1). Indeed, the mass of the left ventricle may rarely be increased rather than decreased, despite the cavitary hypoplasia. The left atrium is usually small (see Fig. 29-2). In typical cases, there can be hypertrophy of the left atrial walls, and some patients can be seen with an enlarged atrium, particularly the appendage. Left atrial endocardial fibro-elastosis is rare. In up to one-tenth of patients, the atrial septum will be intact (Fig. 29-4). In some of these patients with an intact floor to the oval fossa, while the pulmonary venous connections are normal, the pulmonary venous drainage can be abnormal because of the presence of a so-called levo-atrial cardinal vein, or because of fenestration of the walls that usually separate the left atrium from the cavity of the coronary sinus. This provides an overflow for the left atrial return. In other circumstances, however, there is no such overflow when the atrial septum is intact. The resulting increase in left atrial pressure then produces increased left atrial hypertrophy, along with changes in the lungs, including arterialisation of the pulmonary veins (Fig. 29-5) and lymphangiectasia, with a cobblestone appearance of the pulmonary surfaces seen at autopsy (Fig. 29-6). This is a bad prognostic feature. In most instances, however, the oval foramen is patent and does not obstruct flow from left to right, albeit that the primary atrial septum is frequently deviated into the left atrium (Fig. 29-7).[17] Anomalous pulmonary venous connections are seen in a small proportion of patients, with supracardiac drainage being most often encountered.

Obstruction of Inflow to, and Outflow from, the Left Ventricle

In almost all cases, the mitral valve is either stenosed or atretic. In the presence of mitral stenosis, all components of the valve contribute to the obstruction (Fig. 29-8). When atretic, the mitral valve may be imperforate, or absent

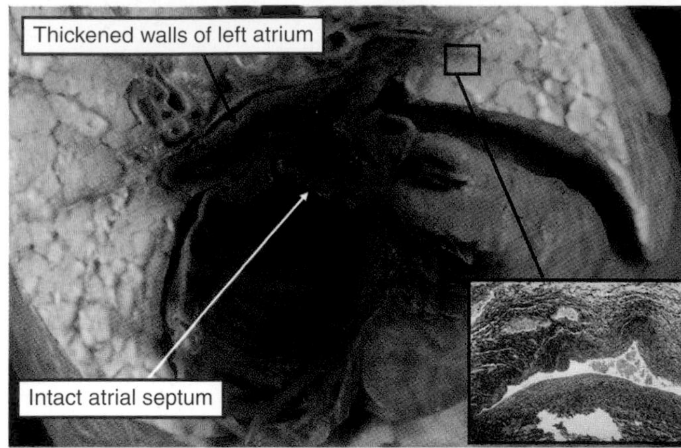

Figure 29-5 In this heart from a patient with hypoplastic left heart syndrome, the atrial septum is intact. Note the hypertrophied walls of the left atrium. As shown in the inset, histology revealed arterialisation of the pulmonary veins. (Courtesy of Dr Andrew Cook, Great Ormond Street Hospital, London, United Kingdom.)

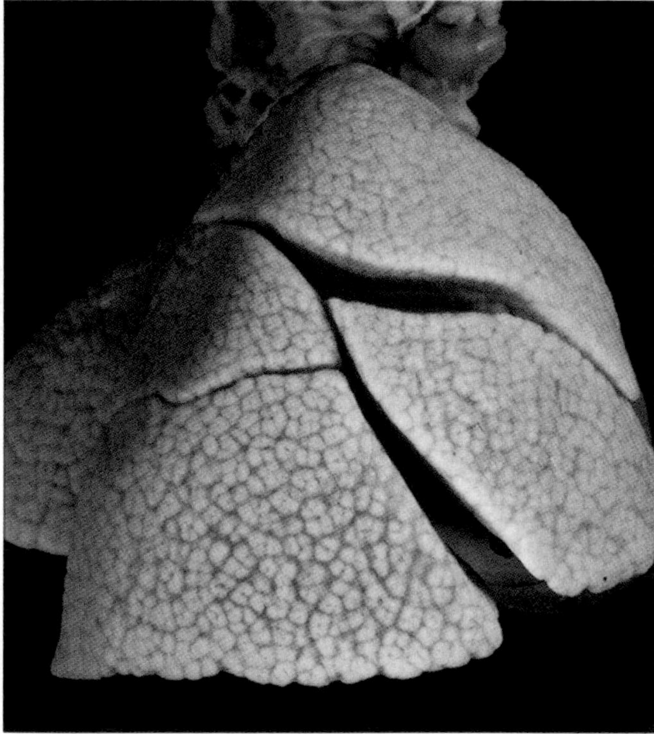

Figure 29-6 This image shows the right lung from the patient whose heart is shown in Figure 21-5. There is an obvious cobblestone appearance of the pulmonary surface, which is due to marked lymphangiectasia. This is a bad prognostic feature. (Courtesy of Dr Andrew Cook, Great Ormond Street Hospital, London, United Kingdom.)

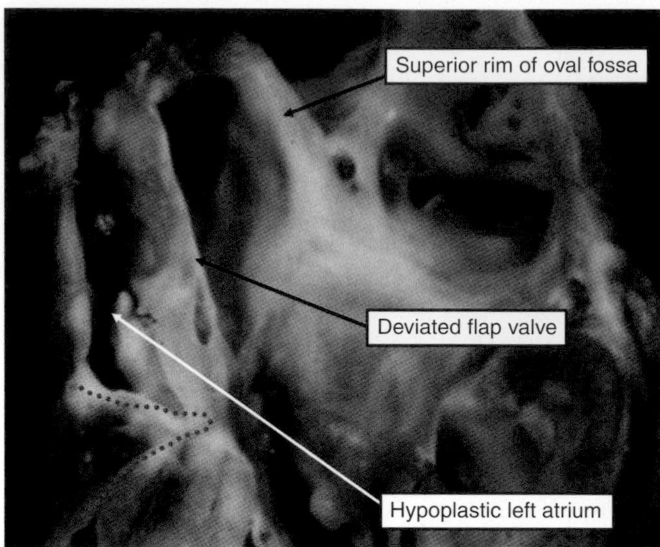

Figure 29-7 This heart with hypoplasia of the left ventricle and absence of the left atrioventricular connection (*green dotted lines*) has been sectioned in four-chamber fashion, and is photographed from behind. Note the deviation of the flap valve of the atrial septum away from the infolded superior rim of the oval fossa, further diminishing the volume of the hypoplastic left atrium.

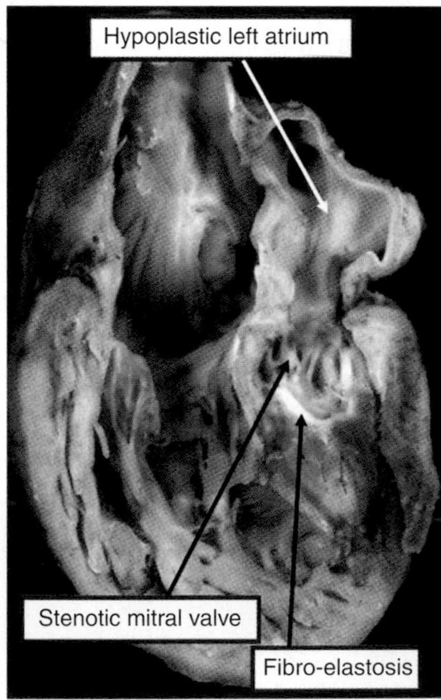

Figure 29-8 In this example of hypoplasia of the left heart, sectioned in four-chamber fashion, the mitral valve is stenotic, with shortened cords and dysplastic leaflets. Note the fibro-elastotic lining of the hypoplastic left ventricle.

together with the left atrioventricular connection (see Figs. 29-2 and 29-7). Left ventricular endocardial fibro-elastosis is seen only when the mitral valve is perforate (see Figs. 29-3 and 29-8). Obstruction of the left ventricular outflow tract is an invariable feature. Aortic atresia, as with mitral atresia, can result from an imperforate valve, but more usually there is no evidence of persisting leaflets at the ventriculo arterial junction, fibromuscular tissue interposing between the ventricular cavity and the blind-ending aortic root (see Fig. 29-1). The aortic root itself is usually markedly hypoplastic, with the ascending aorta serving only as a conduit to feed the coronary arteries. The components of the arch itself are variably hypoplastic, including the ascending component.[20] When the outflow tract is patent, the aortic leaflets are thickened and dysplastic (see Fig. 29-3). Rarely, they may be absent, with a stenosing ring seen at the ventriculo-arterial junction, similar to that observed in so-called absent pulmonary valve syndrome.[21] Further distally, aortic coarctation is common, occurring in more than four-fifths of patients. The obstructive shelf is typically in preductal location (Fig. 29-9) but can be found paraductally (Fig. 29-10). Ductal tissue is not only incorporated into the stenosing shelf, but also

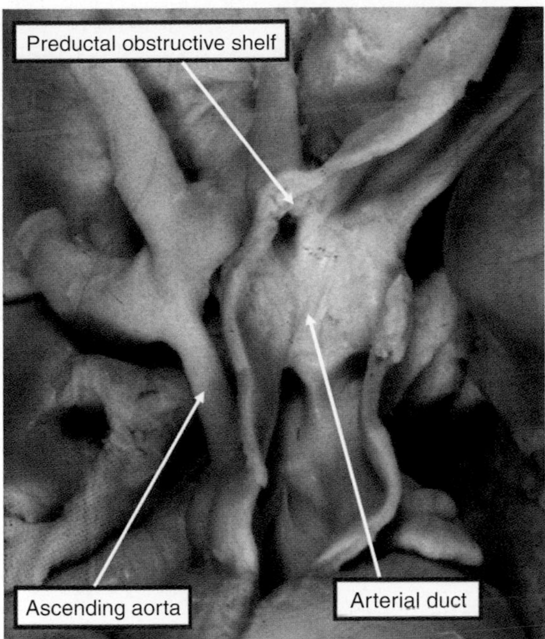

Figure 29-9 In this heart from a patient with hypoplastic left heart syndrome, the tissue of the arterial duct surrounds the orifice of the isthmus of the aortic arch, producing a preductal coarctation.

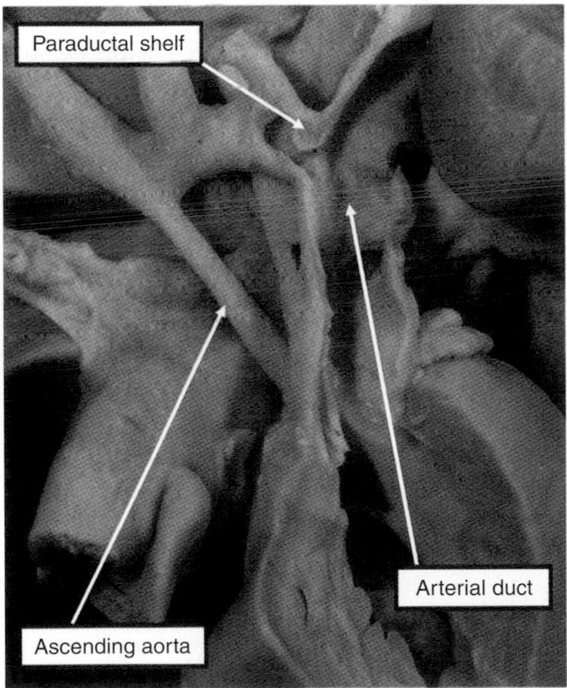

Figure 29-10 In this heart, again from a patient with hypoplastic left heart syndrome, the coarctation shelf is in paraductal position, with direct flow possible from the duct into the aortic isthmus.

may extend proximally and distally,[22] an important point for those undertaking surgical palliation of these patients.

The Coronary Arteries and Conduction Tissues

Abnormalities of the coronary arteries, such as ventriculo-coronary fistulas and abnormal tortuosity, are more common in the subgroup of patients with mitral stenosis and aortic atresia, but not nearly as frequent as in pulmonary atresia with intact ventricular septum (see Chapter 30). Coronary arterial fistulas, if present, are not necessarily associated with abnormalities of the right ventricular myocardium, but can produce an increased risk of mortality at the first stage of Norwood reconstruction.[23] The conduction tissues are in their expected location, albeit with miniaturisation of the left bundle branch in keeping with the size of the left ventricle.

NATURAL HISTORY

The two most significant advances in altering the natural history in infants with hypoplasia of the left heart are the widespread availability of antenatal ultrasonography and prostaglandin E_1. As mentioned above, in the current era the majority of neonates who survive to term have already been diagnosed antenatally by ultrasonography. It is increasingly rare for neonates to present with critical congenital cardiac disease with shock, acidosis, and hypoxemia.[24] Antenatal diagnosis allows the neonate to be delivered at or near a tertiary care centre for therapy, stabilisation with prostaglandin, and the ability to plan intervention on a semi-elective basis, with a decreased likelihood of cerebral injury, as well as hepatic, renal, or cardiac dysfunction. Prior to the availability of prostaglandin E_1, virtually all children died in early infancy, nine-tenths within the first 30 days of life.[25]

Atresia, or significant hypoplasia, of the mitral valve results in a physiological state where there is complete mixing of the systemic and pulmonary venous circulations in the right atrium. The mixed venous blood then passes across the tricuspid valve to the dominant right ventricle. Thereafter, the right ventricular output must be divided between the pulmonary and systemic arterial circuits, which are in parallel. In this situation the saturations of oxygen in the pulmonary artery and the aorta are equal, and the ventricular output is the sum of the flow of blood to the lungs and to the systemic circulation. The proportion of the ventricular output that goes to either of these vascular beds is determined by the relative resistance to flow into the two circuits. Tricuspid regurgitation may further add to the volume work of the dominant right ventricle.

THE TRANSITIONAL CIRCULATION

In the neonate with hypoplasia of the left heart, the normal fall in pulmonary vascular resistance over the first few hours to days of life, in the absence of a significant obstruction to flow into the lungs, results gradually in increased pulmonary flow. The right ventricle becomes progressively volume overloaded, with mildly elevated end-diastolic and atrial pressures. Expected physiological responses include oliguria, with an increase in retention of salt and water, an increase in ventricular stroke volume, tachycardia, and tachypnea. If the saturation of oxygen in the pulmonary veins is assumed to be from 95% to 100%, and that in the systemic veins is between 60% and 65%, with equal distributions of pulmonary and systemic flows, and hence venous returns, the saturation of oxygen in the aorta will be approximately 80%. This has been termed the so-called balanced circulation.

With a continued decrease in the pulmonary vascular resistance, there is an increase in flow to the lungs, and the neonate may show signs of respiratory distress. The greater proportion of pulmonary venous return in the mixed ventricular blood results in an elevated saturation of oxygen in the systemic circulation, to approximately 90% or higher, and visible cyanosis may be mild or absent. Prior to surgical intervention, a number of manoeuvres may be employed to balance the circulation, in attempts to maximise delivery of oxygen and systemic flow. These include sedation, neuromuscular blockade, tracheal intubation and mechanical ventilation with precise control of pH and alveolar pressures of carbon dioxide, addition of inspired gases such as nitrogen or carbon dioxide, and transfusion to increase the viscosity of the blood. Manoeuvres that lower systemic vascular resistance, such as the use of intravenous vasodilators, despite reducing pulmonary flow, may compromise systemic flow. The goal of management prior to surgery, therefore, should not be to seek to balance the circulations by equalizing pulmonary and systemic flows, but rather to provide adequate delivery of oxygen to the tissues. In usual practise, this correlates more or less with equal pulmonary and systemic flows. Many patients, nonetheless, will have adequate delivery of oxygen with minimal symptoms despite significantly increased flow to the lungs, a situation frequently dubbed pulmonary over-circulation. Such pulmonary over-circulation, nonetheless, does not cause a problem unless accompanied by systemic undercirculation. In practise, most patients tolerate the transitional circulation well for a number of days or longer, and most invasive interventions can and should be avoided. In most of these patients, an escalation in ventilation and pharmacological management only temporises the need for surgical intervention, and increases the potential for iatrogenic complications. Patients with unbalanced functionally univentricular physiology may be considered in a spectrum of two physiological extremes, namely, inadequate flow to the lungs, which results in hypoxemia, and excessive flow, which results in congestive cardiac failure.

Inadequate Flow

The newborn with hypoplasia of the left heart and an inadequate arterial saturation of oxygen, below 65%, may have limited flow of blood to the lungs due to elevated pulmonary vascular resistance. More commonly, however, the cause is obstruction to pulmonary venous outflow, most commonly due to a restrictive intra-atrial communication. Alternatively, the hypoxaemic newborn may have adequate flow to the lungs, but this will be hypoxaemia due to pulmonary disease, the latter causing intrapulmonary right-to-left shunting.

Excessive Flow

A more common situation in patients with hypoplasia of the left heart who have not undergone surgical intervention is progressively increasing flow to the lungs at the expense of systemic flow. When severe, this results in systemic hypoperfusion, metabolic acidosis, and shock. Once persistent patency of the arterial duct has been confirmed, manoeuvers should be instituted to minimise systemic and maximise pulmonary vascular resistance. Hypotensive patients with a relatively high arterial oxygen saturation, greater than 95%, generally have a severe steal by the pulmonary vascular circuit from the combined ventricular output. In these over-circulated patients, excessive inotropic support, particularly at alpha-doses, should be minimised. Reduction of afterload using agents such as sodium nitroprusside or milrinone may be especially helpful in patients with elevated systemic vascular resistance and an adequate blood pressure.

Patients with hypoplasia of the left heart and high arterial saturations, nonetheless, may suffer decreased delivery of oxygen to the tissues. The increased content of oxygen comes at the expense of a relative reduction of systemic flow, which results in inadequate perfusion, metabolic acidosis, and low cardiac output. In addition, ventricular mural tension and consumption of oxygen are increased in the dilated, volume-overloaded, dominant right ventricle, potentially contributing to myocardial dysfunction and atrioventricular valvar regurgitation. Progressive metabolic acidosis is a worrisome sign in these patients and requires prompt evaluation and, in many cases, surgical intervention.

Manoeuvres to increase pulmonary vascular resistance have been shown clinically to be effective in reducing excessive flow to the lungs. Provision of supplemental inspired nitrogen or carbon dioxide may elevate pulmonary vascular resistance by inducing alveolar hypoxia. The haematocrit should be maintained at greater than 40% to 45%, as the increased viscosity may also serve to elevate the pulmonary vascular resistance. Intubation and mechanical ventilation with sedation, paralysis, and permissive hypoventilation can be used to elevate the partial pressures of carbon dioxide into the range from 40 to 50 torr.

As already discussed, patients with marked over-circulation and systemic hypoperfusion should not undergo a lengthy period of medical management of their unstable physiology prior to surgical intervention. If a patient requires intubation and sedation to maintain adequate systemic flow, early surgical intervention is indicated to achieve more favourable physiology.

CLINICAL PRESENTATION AND PRE-OPERATIVE STABILISATION

Neonates tend to present in one of three mutually exclusive ways. If the diagnosis has been made prenatally, an expectant team of caregivers manages a metabolically stable neonate. Neonates can also present with symptoms of mild congestive heart failure, with or without a cardiac murmur and no dysfunction of the end-organs, or with profound circulatory collapse and failure of organs in multiple systems. In this last group, a sudden deterioration takes place, with rapidly progressive congestive cardiac failure and shock occurring concurrent with constriction of the arterial duct. There is decreased systemic perfusion, and greatly increased flow to the lungs, largely independent of the level of pulmonary vascular resistance. The peripheral pulses are weak to absent. Renal, hepatic, coronary, and central nervous system perfusions are compromised, possibly resulting in acute tubular necrosis, necrotizing enterocolitis, or cerebral infarction or haemorrhage. A vicious cycle may also result from inadequate retrograde perfusion of the ascending aorta and coronary arterial supply, with further myocardial dysfunction and continued compromise of flow to the coronary arteries. The ratio of pulmonary-to-systemic flows approaches infinity as systemic flow nears zero. Thus, one has the paradoxical presentation of a profound metabolic acidosis in the face of a relatively high partial pressure of oxygen, in the region of 70 to 100 mm Hg. At the initial presentation, sepsis is frequently suspected before the cardiac diagnosis is made.

Analysis of arterial blood gases is typically a commonly employed indicator of haemodynamic stability and adequacy of systemic delivery of oxygen. While a low arterial saturation of oxygen, in the region from 75% to 80%, with a normal pH and partial pressures of carbon dioxide, indicates an acceptable balance of systemic and pulmonary flows with adequate peripheral perfusion, elevated saturations of greater than 95%, when associated with acidosis, represent significantly increased pulmonary and decreased systemic flows, with probable myocardial dysfunction and secondary effects on other organ systems.

Oxygen

In general, supplemental oxygen should be avoided preoperatively in the infant with hypoplasia of the left heart. Oxygen will act as a pulmonary vasodilator, increasing the flow of blood to the lungs at the expense of systemic flow. The presence of pulmonary pathology, such as atelectasis, meconium aspiration, or pneumonia, or a restrictive interatrial communication, may result in a requirement for supplemental oxygen. In the absence of these features, most neonates with hypoplasia of the left heart have increased pulmonary flow prior to surgery, with saturations of oxygen in room air from 88% to 95%, representing partial pressures of oxygen from 45 to 50 mm Hg or greater. Patients with a mildly restrictive interatrial communication and/or elevated pulmonary vascular resistance will have saturations of oxygen in the high 70s to low 80s. Although the temptation is to increase the inspired oxygen, if the low saturation represents the best balance between pulmonary and systemic flows, increasing the supplemental oxygen may paradoxically decrease delivery of oxygen to the tissues.

When to Treat a High Saturation of Oxygen

The clinically stable infant may tolerate significantly increased pulmonary flow in the pre-operative period without significant intervention or obvious untoward effects. When the diagnosis is made early, before significant constriction of the arterial duct and development of a state of low flow, acidosis is usually avoided. Infants in this setting often have a mild degree of restriction across the interatrial communication, with left atrial hypertension elevating pulmonary vascular resistance, and limiting to some extent the flow to the lungs. Although tachypnoeic, with respiratory rates from 60 to 80 per minute, and with an arterial oxygen saturation of 90% or higher, they remain clinically stable with minimal intervention. This group of patients maintains adequate systemic flow despite increased pulmonary flow. Further interventions designed to achieve an arbitrary partial pressure of oxygen, such as intubation and/or supplemental provision of inspired gases, may not stabilise the patient, but rather increase the potential for iatrogenic complications. In short, the neonate without significant symptoms of congestive heart failure, acidosis, or progressive respiratory distress should not necessarily require significant therapy to treat high partial pressures of oxygen. Only two subsets of infants require aggressive pre-operative management of the balance between their pulmonary and systemic blood flow. The first group is made up of those who are diagnosed late, following constriction of the arterial duct and circulatory collapse. The second group is composed of those with clinically significant pulmonary over-circulation and systemic undercirculation, independent of the timing of diagnosis.

Presentation in Shock

Infants presenting with inadequate systemic cardiac output, either due to ductal constriction or pulmonary over-circulation, often have depressed cardiac function with significant tricuspid insufficiency, profound metabolic acidosis, usually some hepatic and renal failure, and occasionally bowel ischaemia or disseminated intravascular coagulopathy. These infants require rapid and aggressive resuscitation. Prostaglandin E_1 must be given, the dose being adjusted according to the degree of patency of the arterial duct as revealed echocardiographically. Intravenous infusions of catecholamines, such as dopamine or adrenaline, will help augment overall cardiac output. Sedation, paralysis, and endotracheal intubation will allow for controlled ventilation and minimise systemic consumption of oxygen. If a patient continues to have inadequate delivery of systemic oxygen despite controlled ventilation with 21% oxygen, the addition of inspired carbon dioxide has been shown to improve systemic delivery of oxygen (see below). Most commonly, infants with hypoplasia of the left heart presenting in shock benefit from recovery of end-organ function before proceeding to the operating room for surgical reconstruction or transplantation. Importantly, infants with persistent metabolic acidosis despite resuscitative efforts should be evaluated by echocardiography to establish adequate patency of the arterial duct. Rarely, a pre-operative infant with hypoplasia of the left heart persists with medically refractory pulmonary over-circulation and may require urgent construction of the initial stage of the Norwood sequence.

Hypotension

Although mild pre-operative hypotension is common, and frequently thought to be caused by increased pulmonary flow at the expense of systemic flow, alternative aetiologies also play a role. Prostaglandins are potent pulmonary and systemic vasodilators, and adequate fluids are needed following their administration. Neonatal myocardium is particularly sensitive to intracellular calcium and glucose, so the levels of both agents in the serum should be monitored periodically. Myocardial dysfunction may co-exist, and although small-to-moderate doses of inotropic agents are frequently beneficial, large doses may have a deleterious effect, depending on the relative effects on the systemic and pulmonary vascular circulations. Preferential selective elevations of systemic vascular tone will secondarily increase pulmonary flow, and careful monitoring of mean arterial blood pressure and arterial saturations of oxygen is warranted. Tricuspid regurgitation from an anatomically abnormal valve, or secondary to ventricular dysfunction, may also contribute. Low doses of inhibitors of phosphodiesterase, such as milrinone, which may seem counter-intuitive for the mildly hypotensive patient, may improve overall perfusion and delivery of oxygen. Patients with hypotension that remains refractory despite all of the above interventions should undergo echocardiographic evaluation to ensure that the arterial duct remains widely patent and non-restrictive.

Inadvertent or unrecognised problems in the administration of prostaglandin E_1 can constrict the arterial duct.

Inspired Gases

The use of mixtures of inspired gases to balance the pulmonary and systemic flows prior to surgical intervention remains controversial.[26–28] Until recently, prospective, controlled data comparing hypoxia to hypercarbia was limited to studies in shunt-dependent animal models of the functionally univentricular circulation.[29] Use of both induced alveolar hypoxia and increased inspired carbon dioxide produced a significant decrease in the ratio of pulmonary to systemic flows compared to baseline. In a prospective crossover study measuring saturations of oxygen in the superior caval vein and aorta while estimating saturations of oxygen in the brain using near infrared spectroscopy, however, it was shown that hypoxia induced by nitrogen and hypercarbia by carbon dioxide both decreased the ratio of pulmonary to systemic flows. Importantly, only hypercarbia increased cardiac output and cerebral oxygenation.[27]

In our practise at The Children's Hospital of Philadelphia, therefore, we tend not to use inspired gases pre-operatively. Surgery is undertaken as soon as is medically and logistically possible. For the neonate presenting with circulatory collapse and pulmonary over-circulation, and already intubated and mechanically ventilated, nonetheless, we give inspired carbon dioxide until surgery is undertaken. For patients in whom surgery must be delayed, and there is clinically significant pulmonary over-circulation with low systemic flow, nitrogen is inspired to the spontaneously breathing patient, and carbon dioxide reserved for the mechanically ventilated patient until surgery is undertaken.

Restrictive Atrial Septum

A severely restrictive atrial septum limits outflow from the pulmonary veins. If coupled with mitral atresia, this results in profound obstruction to left atrial egress, producing pulmonary venous hypertension and hypoxaemia following birth. Newborns with this combination are extremely unstable, and difficult to manage immediately following birth. Recent strategies to improve the dismal prognosis have been met with limited, albeit encouraging, success, including prenatal intervention with static atrial septal dilation with or without placement of a stent, and/or planned delivery by cesarean section at a centre equipped to provide surgical or catheter intervention within a very short time frame. Following birth, if inadequate flow to the lungs and systemic oxygenation are confirmed, the infant should be intubated, umbilical access obtained, and prostaglandin E_1 given in the delivery room, followed by direct transportation to the operating room or catheterisation lab where the planned septectomy or catheter intervention may be performed. In the absence of a prenatal diagnosis, the clinical presentation is identical to obstructed totally anomalous pulmonary venous return, or severe pulmonary disease. From the stance of management, intubation, positive end expiratory pressure, and supplemental oxygen are needed to maintain a saturation of oxygen in the aorta of around 80%, coupled with umbilical access, inotropic support, and other supportive strategies.

Unfortunately, the association of a severely restrictive or intact atrial septum with hypoplasia of the left heart has a significantly worse prognosis over the short and long term compared with other forms of left heart hypoplasia[30,31] mainly due to the secondary changes that occur in the pulmonary vascular bed from fetal obstruction to pulmonary venous outflow (see Fig. 29-5). The pulmonary vascular tree is abnormal in all patients with hypoplasia of the left heart, with an increase in the number of arteries per unit area of lung, the arteries themselves having a considerable increase in muscularity. Increased medial arterial thickness is present, as well as extension of muscle into smaller and more peripheral arteries than is normal. This may explain the predilection towards extreme sensitivity of the pulmonary vascular bed to vasoactive agents. The pulmonary veins are typically dilated with thickened walls. The degree of restriction at the atrial level influences the pathological findings within the pulmonary vascular tree. Increased arterial tortuosity and arteriopathy have been noted, along with arterialisation of the pulmonary veins.[30] These pulmonary venous abnormalities further contribute to the pathophysiology once these infants are born, and may explain why most continue to do poorly with high mortality despite creation of a large and effective interatrial communication at birth.

PRE-OPERATIVE EVALUATION

Newborns with hypoplasia of the left heart require a thorough evaluation of cardiac and non-cardiac issues upon admission to the intensive care unit. Vascular access should be secured, prostaglandin administered, and evaluation of acid-base status undertaken. The physical examination should assess adequacy of systemic perfusion, and carefully evaluate for additional congenital anomalies and dysmorphic features. A complete echocardiogram is usually sufficient to plan surgical intervention. In particular, care should be taken to establish the presence or absence of bilateral superior caval veins; the number of, and patterns of flow in, the pulmonary veins; the state of the atrial septum and ventricular myocardium; the anatomy and function of the tricuspid and pulmonary valves; the size of the ascending aorta; and the presence of any abnormal patterns of branching of the brachiocephalic arteries. Representative examples of important aspects of the anatomy are shown in Figures 29-11 to 29-13. The patency and characteristics of flow through the arterial duct are crucial to maintaining the stability of the patient and understanding the physiology, and may be utilised to estimate the ratio of pulmonary to systemic flows[32] (Fig. 29-14). Coronary arterial sinusoids may be identified in some patients in the setting of aortic atresia and mitral stenosis. These are particularly important to identify as they have been recently shown to be risk factors for mortality following surgical intervention.[33,34] Should there be evidence of retardation of growth or additional congenital anomalies, the remaining systems such as the brain, kidneys, liver, and gastrointestinal tract should be evaluated. Consultation with a clinical geneticist may be helpful.

THERAPEUTIC OPTIONS AND POST-OPERATIVE CARE

There are currently four options available for the neonate with hypoplasia of the left heart. The first is to abstain from intervention. The second alternative is that of

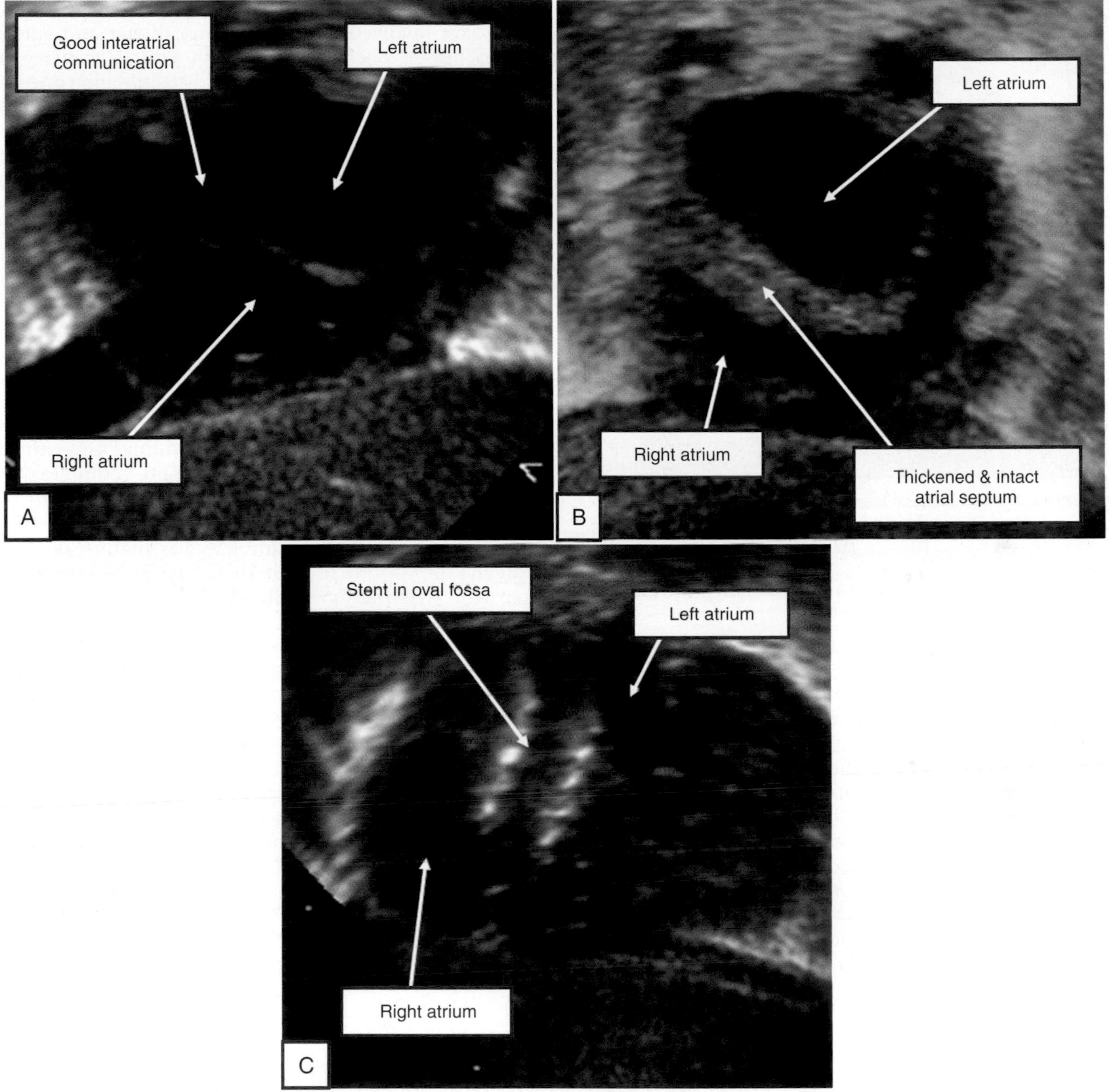

Figure 29-11 These subcostal echocardiographic images show the atrial septum, and the right and left atriums. In panel **A**, there is a defect of adequate size in the atrial septum, allowing pulmonary venous egress to the right atrium, right ventricle, and systemic circulation. Panel **B** shows a thickened and intact atrial septum. The patient from whom the image in panel **A** was obtained was asymptomatic, with an acceptable saturation of oxygen. The patient from whom we obtained the image shown in panel **B** was profoundly ill, hypoxaemic, and required mechanical ventilation, with urgent placement of a stent in the atrial septum, as shown in panel C. Placement of the stent produced marked improvement in oxygenation. (Courtesy of Dr Michael Quartermain, Children's Hospital of Philadelphia.)

staged reconstruction, beginning with the first stage of the Norwood protocol and culminating in construction of the Fontan circulation. The third option is to opt for primary cardiac transplation. The fourth involves a hybrid approach, stenting the arterial duct, banding the pulmonary arteries, and opening the interatrial communication if necessary.

The option of declining to intervene is now controversial.[26,35,36] Most centres currently active in cardiac surgery for neonates and infants do not actively offer non-intervention,[26] although non-intervention might be adopted by many providers of health care if personally faced with the situation.[35] It is beyond the scope of this chapter to review the ethical issues, tenets of informed consent, and changing landscape of this controversial topic.

EVOLUTION OF SURGICAL THERAPY

Surgical palliation for a patient with hypoplasia of the left heart was first attempted in 1961,[37] and the first survivors were reported in the early 1970s.[38,39] Alternative innovative approaches were then reported in the later part of the 1970s, indicating that staged reconstruction would be needed successfully to achieve the Fontan circulation.[40]

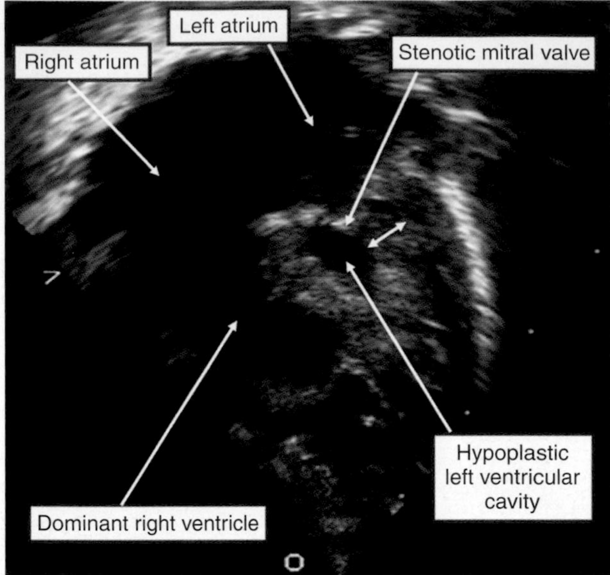

Figure 29-12 The apical echocardiographic image of a newborn shows the typical findings of hypoplasia of the left heart, in this instance produced by mitral stenosis and aortic atresia. Note the diminutive cavity of the hypoplastic left ventricle, with hypertrophy of the left ventricular myocardium (*double-headed arrow*) when compared to the normal thickness of the right ventricular wall. (Courtesy of Dr Michael Quartermain, Children Hospital of Philadelphia, Philadelphia, pennsylvania.)

Such a staged approach was formulated by Norwood during the early 1980s.[41] Even in experienced centres, however, initial survival remained poor. Shortly thereafter, primary cardiac transplantation was shown to be achievable in the neonate.[42] While the initial surgical mortality was superior to staged reconstruction, and the possibility of a biventricular circulation was appealing, the approach was limited by the availability of suitable donors, with many patients dying in the waiting period prior to transplantation. The introduction of ABO-incompatible cardiac transplantation increased the availability of donors,[43] albeit that such an approach has not universally been adopted as primary therapy at many centres.[26] The most recent major innovations have involved combined transcatheter and surgical approaches.[44,45] Such palliation with a ductal stenting and banding of the pulmonary arteries was initially conceived as a bridge to cardiac transplantation, but more recently has been used prior to a simultaneous reconstruction of the aortic arch and construction of a superior cavopulmonary connection, dubbed the comprehensive second stage. The ideal surgical strategy, therefore, remains controversial. Most likely it will eventually be tailored to fit the risk factors of the specific patient. Results from all currently available strategies, nonetheless, have vastly improved the outlook for infants born with hypoplasia of the left heart.

FIRST STAGE OF RECONSTRUCTION

There are three main principles underscoring the first stage of palliation. First, it is essential to establish an unobstructed intra-atrial communication, providing unobstructed pulmonary venous inflow. The second requirement is unobstructed systemic outflow, while the third is to provide a reliable source of flow of blood to the lungs, allowing development of the pulmonary vasculature as well as reducing the volume load on the ventricle. Nearly all children with hypoplastic left heart syndrome are candidates for surgery. The first stage of palliation, nonetheless, carries considerable risk, and parents should be counselled appropriately. Chromosomal abnormalities or extracardiac malformations are frequently associated with higher risk, and may be considered to represent relative contraindications, depending on their severity. Patients with severe tricuspid valvar regurgitation or right ventricular dysfunction also have an increased risk of mortality.

The first stage of reconstruction using the classic Norwood operation is typically performed through a median sternotomy, and involves construction of a modified Blalock-Taussig shunt. Recently, there has been interest in creation of the shunt from the right ventricular infundibulum to the central pulmonary arteries.[46] The theoretical advantages of a shunt from the right ventricle to the pulmonary arteries

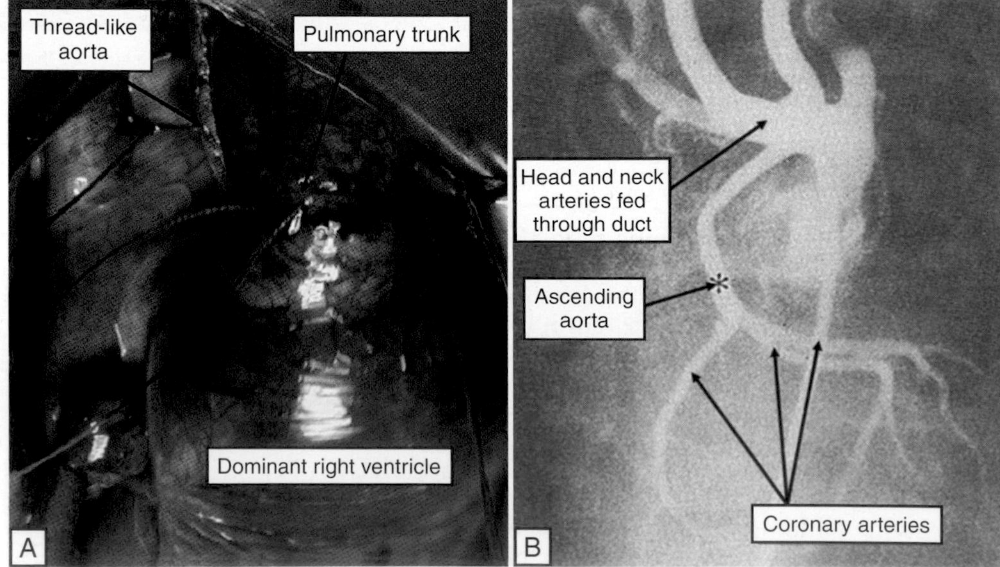

Figure 29-13 Panel A shows an intra-operative image following sternotomy in a patient with aortic atresia. Note the diminutive ascending aorta, which measured 2 millimeters, compared to the pulmonary trunk. The angiographic image shown in panel **B** is from a different patient with aortic atresia. Note the filling of the arteries to the head and neck through the arterial duct, with continuation of retrograde flow to fill the diminutive ascending aorta and the coronary arteries.

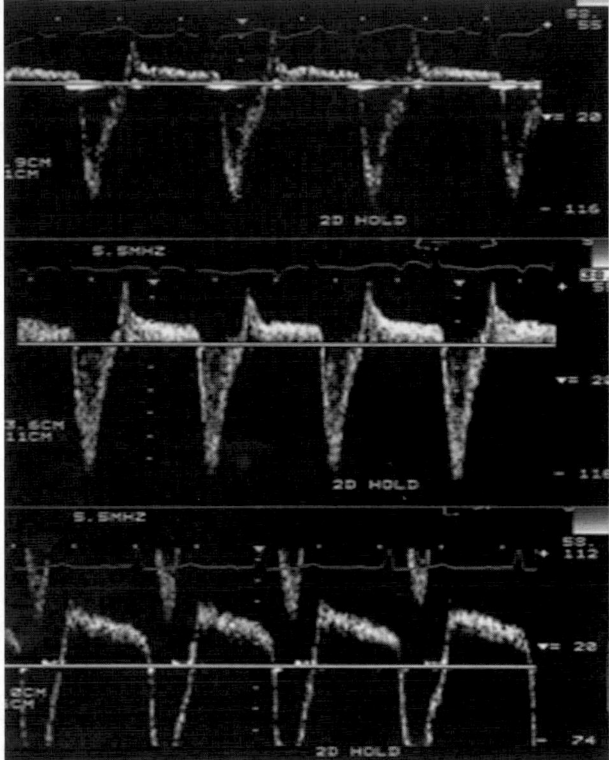

Figure 29-14 The Doppler spectral display shows the waveforms generated when sampling in the descending aorta after first stage of reconstruction for hypoplasia of the left heart. Flow below the baseline represents antegrade flow in systole; flow above the baseline represents retrograde flow in diastole. A ratio is calculated by measuring the velocity-time integral of retrograde and antegrade flow done by using planimetrics for the area under each curve and dividing the former by the latter. Three patients are exhibited. The top panel demonstrates a small amount of flow reversal, indicating relatively low amounts of flow to the pulmonary artery; the middle panel demonstrates a moderate amount of flow reversal into the pulmonary artery; and the lower panel demonstrates a large degree of reversal, indicating a large amount of flow into the pulmonary artery in a retrograde fashion from the descending aorta. (Reproduced with permission from Rychik J, Bush DM, Spray TL, et al: Assessment of pulmonary/systemic blood flow ratio after first-stage palliation for hypoplastic left heart syndrome: Development of a new index with the use of Doppler echocardiography. J Thorac Cardiovasc Surg 2000;120:83.)

are a higher post-operative diastolic pressure,[47] improved coronary arterial flow, pulsatile end-organ perfusion, and improved growth of the central pulmonary arteries.[48] This technical modification, however, employs a small incision in the systemic right ventricle, and the long-term effects on ventricular function and/or arrhythmia are unknown. Follow-up studies examining the theoretical advantages of the suggested modification are currently under way, but short term in duration. Decades of follow-up are likely to be necessary to determine the better overall surgical strategy to be used in the neonatal period.

The technical aspects of the operation vary among centres, and controversy exists regarding the best strategy for intra-operative support, especially with regard to that given during reconstruction of the aortic arch (see Chapter 13). At the Children's Hospital of Philadelphia, and other centres, circulatory arrest is used. The arterial duct is ligated on the side of the pulmonary artery and divided on the aortic side. The atrial septum is completely excised, and the pulmonary trunk divided close to its bifucation, the resulting defect being closed with a patch of homograft tissue. At a point beginning immediately adjacent to the divided trunk, the diminutive aorta is incised inferiorly along the transverse arch through the site of ductal insertion. All redundant ductal tissue is excised, and the ascending aorta is anastomosed to the pulmonary trunk, the aortic arch being reconstructed using a homograft patch. The distal end of the Blalock-Taussig shunt is then connected to the right pulmonary artery, or else the shunt is placed from the right ventricle, thus completing the palliative procedures.

The surgical results of the first stage of reconstruction have progressively improved after the initial successes reported in the early 1980s.[41] In the current era, it is increasingly recognised that there are patients having standard as opposed to higher risk for the first stage of palliation. Those with increased risk have the need for mechanical ventilation prior to surgery, low weight at birth, typically less than 2.5 kg, and the association of other cardiac or associated genetic anomalies.[49,50] Up to 1 in 10 patients with the standard risk have a chance of dying after surgery, whereas those with additional risk factors have an incrementally increased risk.[49] There is then another risk of up to 1 in 10 patients dying prior to the second stage of palliation,[51] albeit that recent success with home monitoring programmes may reduce this risk.[52] The expected operative mortality risks for the second stage, involving construction of a superior cavopulmonary connection (Fig. 29-15), and subsequent completion of the Fontan circuit, are currently in the range of no more than 1% to 2%. Thus, the greatest risk of death for newborns with hypoplastic left heart syndrome undergoing surgical reconstruction is concentrated

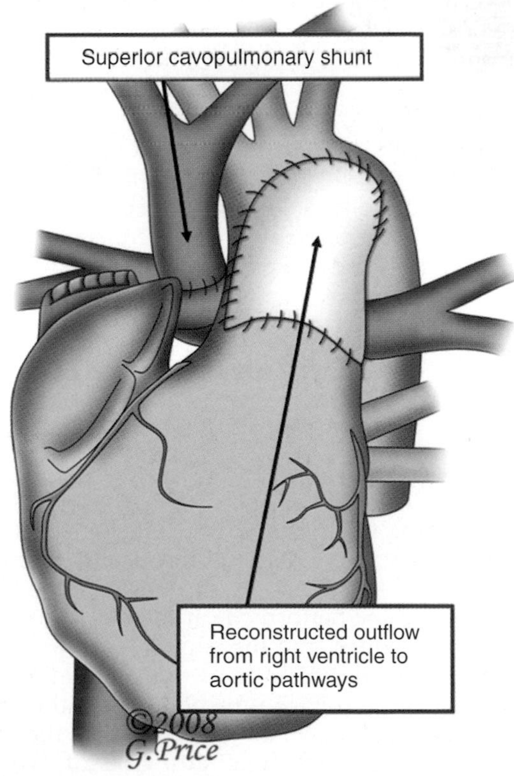

Figure 29-15 The cartoon shows the second stage of the Norwood sequence of palliative surgery for hypoplasia of the left heart. The outflow tract from the right ventricle has been reconstructed to supply the systemic circulation, while a superior cavopulmonary anastomosis supplies systemic venous blood to the lungs.

in the periods of neonatal and early infant life through the second stage of palliation.

INFANT CARDIAC TRANSPLANTATION

In recent years, survival following cardiac transplantation in the neonate has improved, and this remains an important surgical option for patients with acquired and congenital cardiac disease in whom medical and surgical treatment schemes are exhausted.[53] In neonates, hypoplastic left heart syndrome remains the most common indication for transplantation, either as initial therapy or as a treatment for those failing attempted staged reconstruction. The overall survival for cardiac transplantation in children worldwide is 73% at 1 year, and 70% at 4 years after transplantation.[54] The biggest drawback to the routine use of transplantation as primary therapy for neonates with hypoplastic left heart syndrome remains the lack of available organs. Even with most centres in North America performing staged reconstruction as primary therapy, thus limiting the number of babies with hypoplastic left heart syndrome waiting for an organ at any given time, up to one-third of listed children never receive a transplant because of the limited supply of organs. Risk factors for early mortality after transplantation in children, for any underlying cause, include congenital cardiac disease, use of a ventricular assist device prior to transplantation, younger age, presence in an intensive care unit, retransplantation, and transplantation in centres with low volume. The surgical technique is conceptually straightforward, with the primary technical consideration being reconstruction of the aortic arch. The procedure is more technically demanding if staged reconstruction has already been performed. Because of the need to reconstruct the aortic arch, residual coarctation or stenosis can develop at the anastomotic site, and may be successfully treated with balloon angioplasty. Rejection of the graft can occur at anytime, and up to three-quarters of children will have at least one episode of rejection. Infectious complications are common, occurring most often in the immediate period after transplantation. They are a major cause of early morbidity and mortality, especially in the first year after transplantation. Longer-term sequels include lymphoproliferative disease and graft vasculopathy, both affecting up to one-tenth of recipients.

TRANSPLANTATION VERSUS STAGED RECONSTRUCTION

As already discussed, there is no consensus concerning the optimal surgical management of hypoplastic left heart syndrome. At the present time, the overall risks of death are similar presuming the availability of organs continues at the current rate, and there is no significant shift in the numbers of centres adopting one or another strategy. If transplantation were to be performed on the basis of intention to treat at more centres, and the supply of donors did not change, the rate of death prior to transplantation would inevitably increase. Primary transplantation, therefore, is not a reasonable strategy for all patients. Thus, the optimal strategy depends upon the long-term risks of dying, and the morbidity associated with each strategy. Organs should be allocated to those patients for whom no reasonable reconstructive strategy exists. These include patients with a poorly functioning right ventricle with severe tricuspid regurgitation. Patients who have failed the first stage of reconstructive palliation despite optimal medical managementshould also be considered for transplantation. There are certain morbidities inherent in transplantation, such as immunosuppression, lymphoproliferative disease, and graft vasculopathy, and others inherent in staged reconstruction culminating in construction of the Fontan operation circuit, such as arrhythmias, protein-losing enteropathy, and thromboembolism. There are also a number of morbidities that are nearly identical with either strategy, including retardation of growth, limitation of exercise, need for chronic medication, developmental delay, and psychological factors produced by a chronic disease. Further research is necessary, therefore, to determine which strategy is ideal for individual patients and their families.[54]

COMBINED SURGICAL AND TRANSCATHETER, OR HYBRID, PALLIATION

The combined transcatheter and surgical approach was pioneered by Schranz and colleagues in Geissen, Germany.[44] Initially, palliation with a ductal stent and banding of the pulmonary arteries was conceived as a bridge to cardiac transplantation. More recently, the approach has evolved with the collaborative modifications of Galantowicz and Cheatham in Columbus, Ohio, with modifications of the Geissen technique performed prior to a planned comprehensive second stage, involving surgical reconstruction of the aortic arch combined with a superior cavopulmonary connection. Initial palliation is performed by intraoperative, off-pump, placement of bands on both pulmonary arteries, followed by a stent in the arterial duct placed through a sheath in the pulmonary trunk (Fig. 29-16). Alternatively, the entire palliative procedure may be performed with transvascular catheterisation, with placement of a stent in the arterial duct and flow-restricting devices in the proximal portions of the right and left pulmonary arteries. When necessary, transcatheter enlargement of an atrial septal defect is performed as a separate procedure. Occasionally, a stent is placed within the oval fossa to create a durable interatrial communication (Fig. 29-17). At the age of 3 to 6 months, a comprehensive second stage, incorporating the elements of the traditional first and second stages, is performed, with a plan to complete the Fontan circulation using transcatheter techniques. During the comprehensive second stage, the bands on the pulmonary arteries and the ductal stent are removed, the pulmonary arteries are repaired, the aorta is enlarged and anastomosed to the pulmonary trunk as in the traditional first stage of palliation in the Norwood sequence, atrial septectomy is performed with removal of any atrial stent, and the operation is completed by construction of a modified hemi-Fontan connection. This modification includes anastomosing the transected distal end of the superior caval vein in an open fashion to the right pulmonary artery, and then excluding it with a pericardial patch within the right atrium. This provides a rim of tissue below the right pulmonary artery to anchor an eventual stent placed during transcatheter completion of the Fontan circulation. In addition, a ring cut from a Gore-Tex tube graft attached to a radio-opaque marker is placed around the inferior caval vein between the diaphragm and right atrium to facilitate

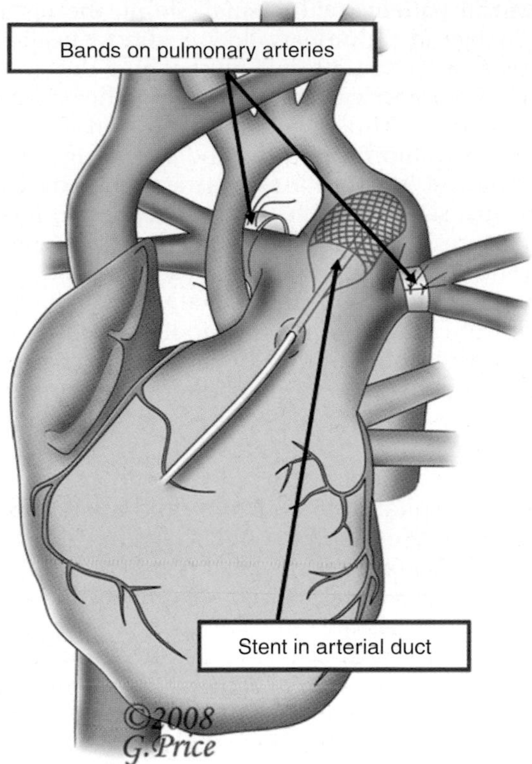

Figure 29-16 The cartoon shows the initial steps of the hybrid procedure for hypoplastic left heart syndrome. Bands are placed surgically round the right and left pulmonary arteries, and a stent is placed in the arterial duct.

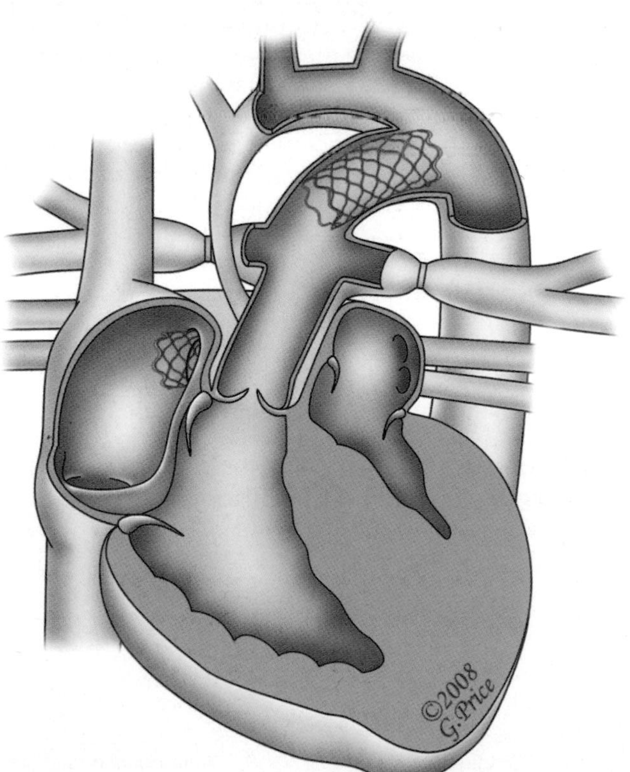

Figure 29-17 The cartoon shows the conclusion of the hybrid palliative strategy for hypoplasia of the left heart. The stent in the arterial duct provides unobstructed flow to the distal aorta, and the bands placed on the right and left pulmonary arteries restrict the flow of blood to the lungs. A catheter-based atrial septectomy is augmented by implantation of a stent across the atrial septum, assuring adequate egress of pulmonary venous blood to the right atrium.

precise placement, and to serve as an anchor for the inferior margin of the stent. At approximately 2 years of age, the Fontan circulation is completed by placement of a covered stent. With this strategy, there is but one exposure to cardiopulmonary bypass, aortic cross-clamping, and circulatory arrest, although there is a significant learning curve. Although promising, it is not yet clear whether this hybrid strategy will yield better outcomes over the long term.[45]

ROUTINE ACUTE POST-OPERATIVE MANAGEMENT

Post-operative Management in the Operating Room

Post-operative management begins in the operating room with separation from cardiopulmonary bypass. Most of the monitoring techniques that we employ in the post-operative period are initiated in the operating room, either at the outset or completion of surgery. We prefer to place umbilical arterial and venous catheters pre-operatively, and to maintain patients with spontaneous ventilation prior to surgery. An indwelling catheter is inserted into the urinary bladder, and a peripheral arterial catheter is inserted if an umbilical arterial catheter is not in place.

Following a loading dose of milrinone while on cardiopulmonary bypass, modified ultrafiltration is then performed to achieve haemoconcentration and reduction of total body water, following which the patient is separated from extracorporeal circulation. Upon decannulation, two or three transthoracic right atrial catheters are placed through the right atrial appendage. Inotropic support is initiated and the patient is weaned from cardiopulmonary support, with adjustment of inotropic support as necessary. Mechanical ventilatory support is then resumed. Prior to closure of the sternum and the median sternotomy, temporary epicardial atrial and ventricular pacing wires are placed. In selected patients with excessive myocardial oedema, cardiopulmonary instability, or mediastinal bleeding, or in rare cases in which post-operative mechanical circulatory support is required, the chest can be left open, with a patch of silicone elastomer sutured to the skin for coverage of the incision.[55,56] With our current protocol, this is performed in approximately one-twentieth of patients. After haemodynamic stabilisation and closure of the chest, the patient is transported to the intensive care unit.

Acute Post-operative Management in the Intensive Care Unit

Early post-operative management following the first stage of palliation is based on the pathophysiological conditions typically present (Table 29-1).

Cardiovascular Pathophysiology in the Early Post-operative Period

The most important physiological consideration after the first stage of palliative reconstruction is maximizing the ratio of delivery to extraction of oxygen. This is fundamentally a function of systemic requirement for oxygen, systemic blood flow, and the systemic arterial content of oxygen, which depends on the haematocrit and the percent of oxyhaemoglobin (Fig. 29-18). In the patient with circulation in series, the items listed above are essentially the sole variables determining effective delivery of oxygen. In patients with a functionally univentricular circulation, in

TABLE 29-1

EARLY MANAGEMENT AFTER THE FIRST STAGE OF RECONSTRUCTION

Optimize cardiac output
Inotropic support
Lusitropic support
Anticipation and management of common postoperative problems
Minimize potential complications of intensive care
Avoid unnecessary interventions
Remove invasive catheters as soon as possible
Optimize nutritional support
Initiate parental nutrition on the first postoperative day
Nasogastric feeding following extubation, gradually introducing oral intake

contrast, the parallel delivery of pulmonary to systemic flows, as well as the regurgitant fraction, are potentially confounding variables in optimizing effective delivery. In the post-operative patient with a systemic-to-pulmonary arterial shunt, the ratio of flows is particularly important. In keeping with the potential significance of this variable, there have been several theoretical and clinical studies aimed at determining the ideal ratio.[57–61] Although some mathematical studies have predicted that optimal availability will occur with a ratio of less than 1,[58] models that incorporate the non-linear function of extractability,[60] as well as more complex computational methods[57] and animal studies,[61] suggest that optimal delivery occurs at a ratio of approximately 1. Calculation of this ratio, however, is an estimate at best, as there is no truly mixed venous blood, the pulmonary venous saturation is frequently estimated,[32,62] and the possibility of a significant regurgitant fraction across the tricuspid valve is frequently overlooked.

Historically, the ratio of flows has been a vexing and frequently critical variable after the initial stage of palliative reconstruction. Regarding the regulation of pulmonary flow, the resistance provided by the systemic-to-pulmonary arterial shunt, which is directly proportional to its length and inversely proportional to its radius to the fourth power, is perhaps the most important of the variables that can be controlled. In the physiological range of cardiac output, manipulation of the diameter, length, and location of the shunt has a substantially greater impact on pulmonary flow than does pharmacological or ventilatory manipulation of intrinsic pulmonary vascular resistance. While changes in intrinsic resistance will still have an effect on pulmonary flow even in patients with a small shunt, the magnitude of the change in pulmonary flow is almost negligible in comparison with that affected by changing the size of the systemic-to-pulmonary arterial shunt and the systemic vascular resistance.[57] Thus, while the ratio of flows can be a useful means of monitoring and understanding the circulatory and metabolic conditions in patients who have undergone the first stage of reconstruction, moderate changes in pulmonary resistance are of minor practical importance when a shunt of appropriate size is used.

With the routine application of an intermediate palliation prior to completion of the modified Fontan circulation, such as construction of the hemi-Fontan procedure or a bidirectional superior cavopulmonary connection at approximately 4 to 6 months of age, it is no longer important to place a shunt of adequate size to accommodate pulmonary flow sufficient for an older infant. Accordingly, at Children's Hospital of Philadelphia and many other centres, the shunt typically has a diameter from 3.5 to 4 mm if arising from the brachiocephalic artery, and 5 mm if arising from the right ventricle. A shunt of this size provides sufficient resistance to flow to prevent pulmonary steal in the early post-operative period, but also allows adequate flow to maintain acceptable systemic arterial oxygenation for up to 6 months of age, when the next stage of palliation is typically performed. Moreover, with the shunt taking origin from the base of the right subclavian artery, which is typically smaller in diameter than a 3.5-mm shunt,[63] pulmonary flow is further limited in the neonate, and will be able to increase to a modest extent with growth of the subclavian artery. Thus, when a shunt of appropriate size is used to provide flow to the lungs, increased pulmonary at the expense of systemic flow becomes a minor variable in managing systemic delivery of oxygen.

In the majority of cases, total cardiac output and systemic extraction of oxygen are the most important, most variable, and most manageable determinants of systemic delivery of oxygen in the acute post-operative period following the initial stage of reconstruction. Importantly, the systemic resistance, ratio of flows, and consumption of oxygen may be more easily manipulated than pulmonary resistance. The typical haemodynamic profile following cardiac surgery with cardiopulmonary bypass in neonates and infants has been well characterised,[64] with a general pattern, with a decrease in cardiac output reflected by a widening difference in systemic arterial and venous oxygen saturations, demonstrated in multiple

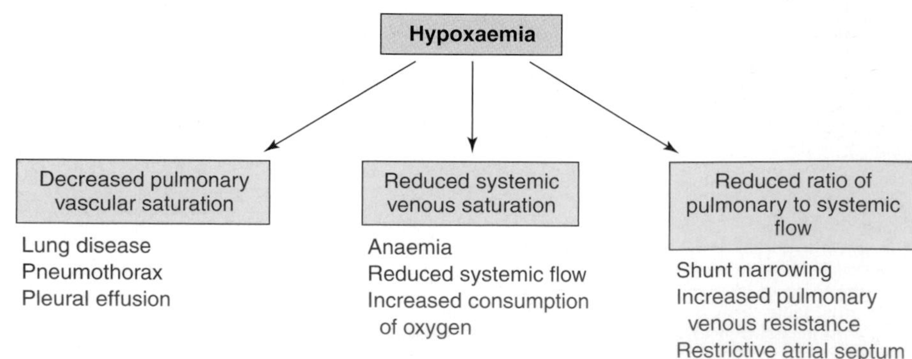

Figure 29-18 Factors causing arterial hypoxaemia may be divided into three main categories: those that reduce the saturation of oxygen in the pulmonary venous blood, those that reduce the saturation of oxygen in the systemic venous blood, and those that reduce the amount of blood flow to the lungs. (Modified from Wernovsky G, McElhinney D, Tabbutt S: Stage I postoperative management. In Rychik J, Wernovsky G [eds]: Hypoplastic Left Heart Syndrome. Boston: Kluwer, 2003.)

studies in the setting of both biventricular and univentricular circulations.[64–68]

Monitoring and Evaluation in the Acute Post-operative Period

Haemodynamic, metabolic, and oximetric monitoring is helpful in the post-operative management after the first stage of palliation (Table 29-2). All patients are monitored with standard functional parameters. Continuous invasive monitoring of systemic venous oxygen saturation is employed at some centres.[66] While this been shown to be an effective strategy, it requires placement of a special intracardiac oximetric catheter directly into the superior caval vein. In selected cases, we have found that a transthoracic catheter placed in the superior caval vein under direct vision through the right atrium is useful for assessment of saturations, and avoids the potential complications associated with an additional intravascular catheter. We have a low threshold for performing bedside echocardiography to assess ventricular and valvar function, pericardial effusion, shunt patency, and to estimate the ratio of flows.[32] Recently, there has been increased utilisation of non-invasive monitoring of cerebral and somatic oxygen saturations, estimated by near infrared spectroscopy.[26] There are on-going studies to assess the specificity and sensitivity of this new monitoring strategy, as well as the impact on perioperative and longer term outcomes.

Management Strategies during the Acute Post-operative Period

Given the expected fall in combined cardiac output, the expected increase in systemic resistance, and the marginal myocardial reserve early after cardiac surgery, it is advantageous both to maximise effective delivery of oxygen to the myocardium and other vital organs, and to minimise myocardial and systemic demand for oxygen. An important means of achieving the latter objective is to prevent excessive and the often inefficient metabolic activity and neurohormonal stress response that typically occur in the acute post-operative period. Neuromuscular blockade and sedation are components of this strategy (see Table 29-2), and should be considered in children with marginal delivery of oxygen.

TABLE 29-2

TYPICAL POSTOPERATIVE PARAMETERS EARLY AFTER THE FIRST STAGE OF RECONSTRUCTION

Continuous Monitoring
Surface electrocardiogram
Pulse oximetry
Central venous pressure
Near infrared spectroscopy (in some centers)
Intermittent Monitoring
Arterial blood gas analysis
Co-oximetry in superior caval vein
Echocardiography
Mechanical Ventilation
Pressure-regulated, volume controlled; ~15 mL/kg
Intermittent mandatory breaths; ~18/min
Positive end-expiratory pressure; ~3–5 mm Hg
Medications
Dopamine and/or adrenaline
Milrinone
Fentanyl

Paralysis interrupts neuromuscular activity that may be induced by the thermoregulatory axis, spontaneous respiratory drive, and agitation, as well as neurovascular stimulation that can directly affect haemodynamic parameters. For sedation, we prefer to use fentanyl, a potent agonist of opioid receptors that also acts to block the stress response that occurs in response to cardiac surgery and endotracheal intubation.[69] Fentanyl does not induce histamine release or significantly affect systemic or pulmonary haemodynamics.[69]

Full mechanical ventilation removes the burden of respiration from the patient, and accordingly eliminates the metabolic demand that spontaneous respiratory function imposes. We prefer to ventilate paralyzed post-operative patients with the pressure-regulated volume-controlled mode of ventilation (see Table 29-2). Positive end-expiratory pressure has been shown have salutary effects on lung mechanics and pulmonary venous oxygen saturation,[62,70] and pressures in the range that we use do not have a deleterious impact of effective pulmonary flow.[61] Cardiovascular pharmacotherapy is focused on optimisation of the ratio of delivery and extraction of systemic oxygen, which depends on providing adequate systemic blood flow, adequate but not excessive pulmonary flow, and sufficient oxygen-carrying capacity, as well as minimizing systemic consumption of oxygen (Fig. 29-19). For most levels of consumption of oxygen, systemic delivery is best ensured if the systemic cardiac index is maintained above 2 liters per minute per meter squared. Excessive end-diastolic ventricular volume or pressure increase ventricular wall tension and, hence, myocardial demand for oxygen. Right atrial pressure is thus usually maintained in the range of 6 to 10 mm Hg. Systemic afterload reduction is achieved with milrinone.[71] The other important determinant of cardiac index is heart rate. Bradycardia results in a significant decrease in cardiac output, but tachycardia may result in increased myocardial oxygen consumption without a concomitant increase in cardiac index. The typical target following the first stage of palliation is from 140 to 180 beats per minute. Oxygen-carrying capacity is optimised by keeping the haematocrit in the range of 40% to 50%.

In the early post-operative period, neonates with palliated heart defects have significantly elevated metabolic needs and may be in an energy deficit even prior to surgery. Moreover, cardiac surgery with cardiopulmonary bypass has significant effects on resting energy expenditure and metabolism of nutritional substrate.[72] Thus, optimisation of nutrition in the early post-operative period is imperative for the facilitation of healing and ensuring the best possible metabolic reserve. Because we tend to initiate enteral nutrition relatively slowly after first-stage palliation, total parenteral nutrition through a central venous catheter, usually the umbilical venous or right atrial catheter, is initiated on the first day after surgery. It is continued until an adequate enteral feeding regime has been established.

Minimisation of Complications in the Intensive Care Unit and Physiological Stress

An important means of optimizing outcome in the greatest number of patients is to avoid intensive care unit complications. We aim to achieve this end by minimizing elective procedures that have the potential for complications, removing invasive catheters, and discontinuing mechanical ventilation and intravenous infusions as expeditiously as is safely possible. Although strategies and interventions such as open sternotomy with delayed sternal

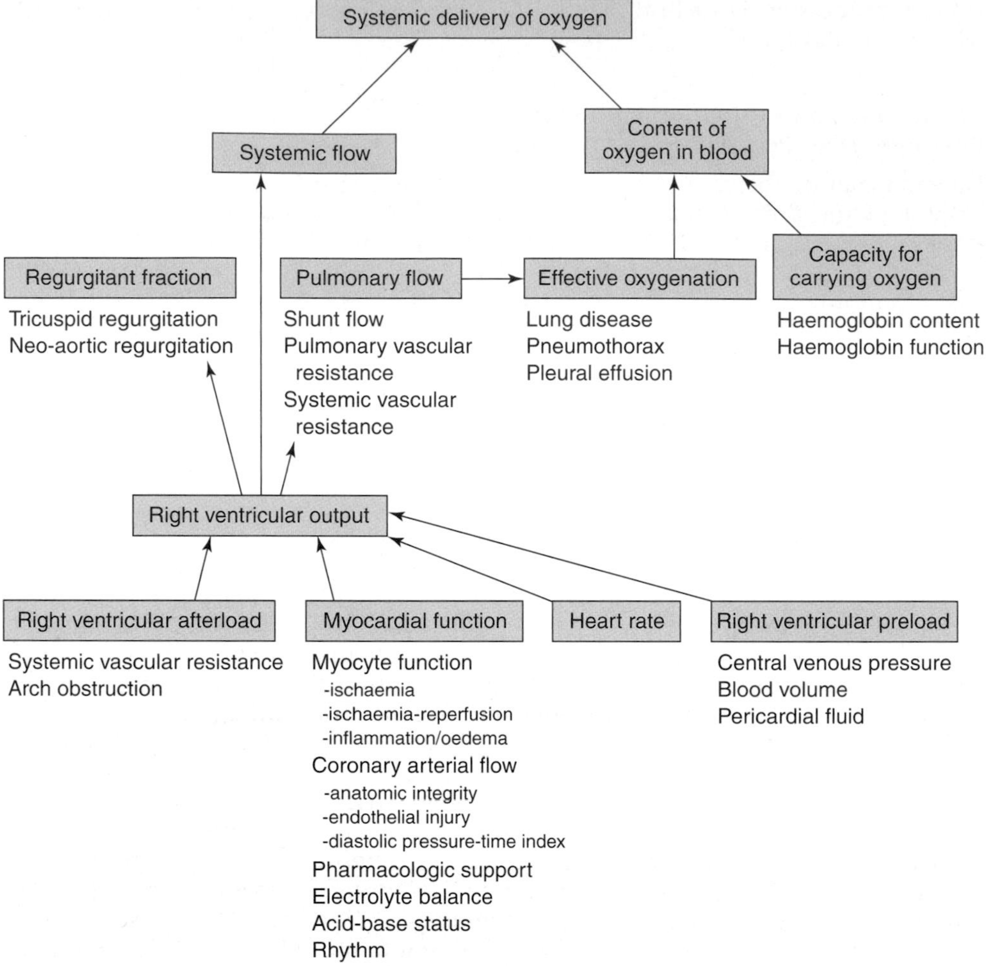

Figure 29-19 Schematic representation of the protean factors affecting delivery of oxygen to the tissues. (Modified from Wernovsky G, McElhinney D, Tabbutt S: Stage I postoperative management. In Rychik J, Wernovsky G [eds]: Hypoplastic Left Heart Syndrome. Boston: Kluwer, 2003.)

closure, peritoneal dialysis, and intracardiac catheters do not frequently cause complications,[55,56,73,74] we employ them only in selected patients, rather than routinely.

Physiological stress, which can cause increased consumption of oxygen and reactivity of the pulmonary and systemic vascular beds, is minimised as much as possible during the first 12 to 24 hours post-operatively. Suctioning of the endotracheal tube is performed only as necessary, as determined by increased inspiratory pressures, and falling systemic arterial oxygen saturation. Similarly, laboratory tests are drawn from indwelling catheters to avoid the stress of venipuncture, and other potentially painful procedures are avoided if possible.

IDENTIFICATION AND MANAGEMENT OF COMMON PROBLEMS

The most common problems encountered early after the first stage of palliation are low cardiac output and hypoxaemia. While is it not always possible to avoid the development of such problems, rapid recognition and prompt management may have a dramatic effect on outcome when they do occur.[75]

Low Cardiac Output

Low cardiac output is one of the most important predictors of poor outcome after surgery for congenital heart defects.[76] Patients are at high risk for poor systemic perfusion for a variety of reasons, which can be divided into two principle and overlapping categories, namely, compromised myocardial function, and normal ventricular output but with maldistribution of flow.

Myocardial Dysfunction

Impaired myocardial performance is essentially a universal phenomenon after the first stage of reconstruction. It is due to a combination of factors, some of which are intrinsic to this population, while others are a consequence of cardiac surgery in general. Among the manifold implications of these alterations are increased capillary leakage, perturbation of the normal vasoactive feedback pathways, a systemic inflammatory response, and disturbances in fluid-electrolyte and metabolic homeostasis. As already discussed, combined cardiac output is expected to fall by up to two-fifths during the first night after surgery. A longer duration of cardiopulmonary bypass is known to be a risk factor for low systemic venous oxygen saturation and an increased disparity in systemic arterial and venous oxygen saturations,[66] and in our experience it has been associated with increased risk of mortality following the first stage of reconstruction.[77] Cardiac afterload is also affected by changes in systemic resistance which typically occur after cardiopulmonary bypass.[64] Taken together, these factors may have a substantial impact on myocardial function and ventricular-vascular coupling, and effectively narrow the buffer zone of myocardial reserve. Occasionally, patients with persistent bleeding or other complicating factors, such as infection, may have an absolute or relative hypovolemia that magnifies that state of low cardiac output from ventricular dysfunction.

There are a number of factors specific to patients with hypoplasia of the left heart that may act in concert with post-bypass myocardial dysfunction to predispose to states of low cardiac output. Anatomically, the patients have a functionally single morphologically right ventricle. The structure of the right ventricle differs from that of the left ventricle in several respects, which may place it at a mechanical disadvantage with respect to pumping blood across the higher resistance systemic circulation. Similarly, because there is but a single functional ventricle, ventricular mechanics do not benefit from the right-left ventricular interaction that occurs in the presence of two normally proportioned ventricles.[78,79] Moreover, the co-existence of a small left ventricle with a hypertrophied and low-compliance left ventricular mass that does not provide substantial systolic ejection may impair right ventricular diastolic function,[80] though recent work from Wisler and colleagues has suggested that the negative impact of a rudimentary left ventricle is most important just prior to the Fontan procedure, rather than after the first stage of reconstruction.[81]

Another anatomical issue that may affect ventricular function is impairment of coronary arterial flow.[82] While this is in part a result of the anastomosis, there is little reserve diameter in the severely hypoplastic ascending aorta in some of these patients. In addition, patients with aortic atresia and mitral stenosis may have an intrinsically abnormal coronary arterial circulation,[33,34,83] similar to the pattern in patients with pulmonary atresia and an intact ventricular septum.

Myocardial ischaemia during aortic crossclamping and circulatory arrest further contributes to impaired post-operative ventricular function.[82] Myocardial ischaemia in the pre-operative period, more likely in patients with aortic atresia where coronary arterial flow is completely dependent upon patency of the arterial duct, and a late presentation, have an impact in the post-operative period, as coagulation necrosis and myocyte dropout evolve. This is compounded by intraoperative myocardial ischaemia, which may occur despite efforts at myocardial protection.

Maldistribution of Blood Flow

The other major category of factors that may contribute to low systemic perfusion is maldistribution of ventricular output. There are two primary situations in which this may occur: pulmonary over-circulation and valvar regurgitation. When a relatively large systemic-pulmonary arterial shunt is used, pulmonary over-circulation may be a significant problem. As already discussed, pulmonary over-circulation is less of a concern when a smaller shunt is placed, with its origin from the proximal subclavian artery or right ventricle. Although a mild degree of tricuspid or neo-aortic regurgitation is common, significant tricuspid or arterial valvar regurgitation is relatively rare.[84] The tricuspid valve, which serves as the systemic atrioventricular valve, is morphologically abnormal in as many as one-third of patients,[85] which may predispose to regurgitation. In addition, functional impairment of the valve may occur, especially in patients with marked ventricular dysfunction and dilation. For example, patients who experience significant metabolic acidosis in the pre-operative period frequently have tricuspid regurgitation,[86] which may carry over into the post-operative period.

Evaluation of Low Cardiac Output

In the first 24 to 36 hours after surgery, patients are monitored closely for evidence of decreasing cardiac output and hypoxemia (Fig. 29-20). Haemodynamic parameters are monitored continuously, and the acid-base state and level of lactate in the serum are followed periodically to assess for hypoxaemia and inadequate delivery of oxygen. The difference in systemic arterial and venous saturations of oxygen, along with the ratio of systemic delivery to systemic consumption of oxygen, are useful measures to determine the adequacy of effective delivery. Also, as stated above, there is increasing interest in assessing systemic oxygen delivery non-invasively using near infrared spectroscopy. These parameters may become abnormal before indexes such as the level of lactate in the serum and the arterial base deficit.[57,59] The arterial-venous difference is probably a more useful indicator in the setting of a functionally univentricular circulation,[57] though the validity of the systemic saturation in the superior caval vein as truly mixed venous blood is difficult to confirm.[67] The anaerobic threshold after first-stage palliation has been estimated to correlate with a systemic venous oxygen saturation of approximately 35%.[87] Electrocardiographic evidence of myocardial ischaemia or echocardiographic signs of depressed ventricular function may also indicate compromised myocardial blood flow before metabolic and oximetric measures. When it becomes apparent that systemic blood flow is decreased, supportive therapy is initiated and a specific cause is sought.

Echocardiography is performed to determine whether there is a specific anatomical cause of the decreased cardiac output. Features assessed include the quality of ventricular function, the competence of the tricuspid and arterial valves, the presence of a pericardial effusion, the appearance of the systemic-to-pulmonary arterial shunt and the interatrial septum, the aortic arch, and the native pathways to the ascending aorta and coronary arteries. If these anatomical features are all essentially normal, the ratio of flows is calculated with a combination of oximetric calculations and the Doppler echocardiographically derived index described above.[32] Simultaneous with these investigations, laboratory studies are performed in order to ensure normal electrolytes, haematocrit, and acid-base state.

Management of Low Cardiac Output

Low cardiac output is managed according to the underlying cause (see Fig. 29-20). In most cases, this involves primarily support of cardiac function with positive inotropic agents and normalisation of blood pH, reduction of ventricular work by means of afterload-reduction, and minimisation of systemic demand for oxygen. The oxygen-carrying capacity of the blood is optimised by transfusion of packed red blood cells if the haematocrit is less than 40%.

In patients who develop acute decompensation due to potentially reversible myocardial dysfunction resulting from factors such as arrhythmia, discrete impairment of

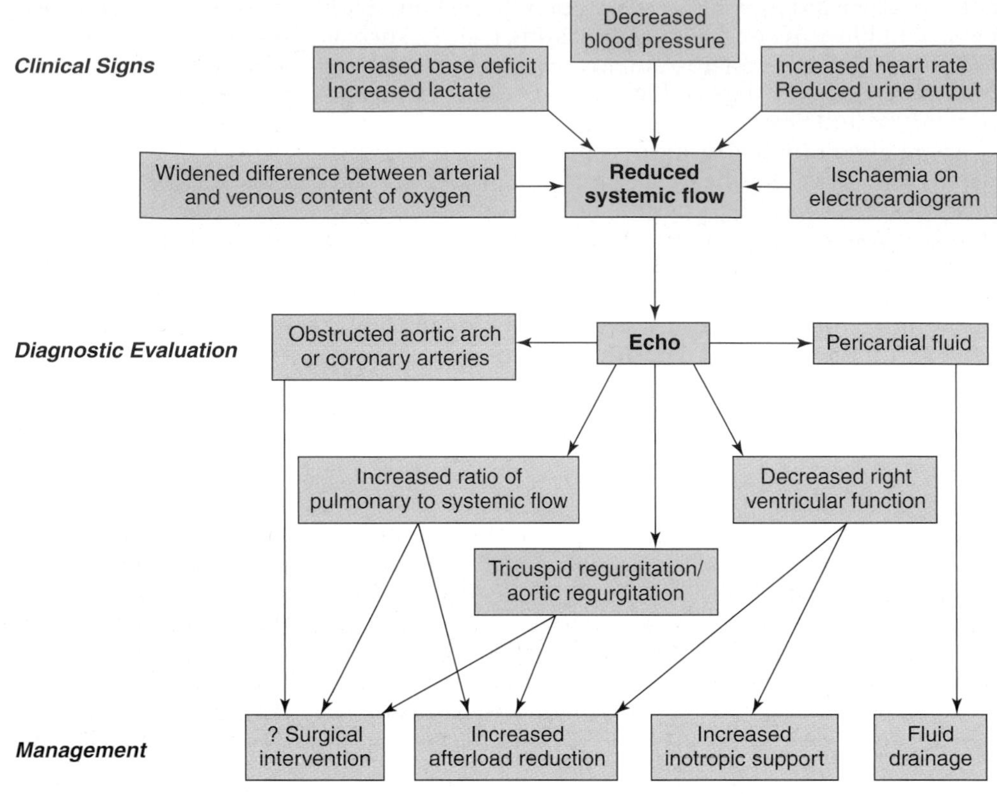

Figure 29-20 Clinical presentation, diagnostic studies, and management algorithms for the child with evidence of low cardiac output following the first stage of reconstruction. (Modified from Wernovsky G, McElhinney D, Tabbutt S: Stage I postoperative management. In Rychik J, Wernovsky G [eds]: Hypoplastic Left Heart Syndrome. Boston: Kluwer, 2003.)

coronary arterial perfusion, or compromise of the systemic-pulmonary arterial shunt, mechanical circulatory support may be indicated. With prompt initiation in appropriately selected patients, extracorporeal membrane oxygenation has been shown beneficial.[88] If systemic perfusion is impaired as a result of increased volume load, systemic afterload reduction is increased by raising the dose of milrinone and/or initiating a continuous infusion of nitroprusside. If a correctable anatomical cause is identified, the appropriate invasive intervention is performed. If a pericardial effusion is detected, the chest is usually opened and the fluid drained, the patient is taken to the operating room or the chest opened at the bedside, depending on the urgency of the situation, in order to drain the fluid and identify and control the site of bleeding. If there is evidence of significant tricuspid or arterial valvar regurgitation, or of obstruction in the aortic arch (Fig. 29-21), the appropriate surgical intervention is performed.

As we have discussed, pulmonary over-circulation is uncommon after the initial stage of reconstruction when a restrictive systemic-to-pulmonary arterial shunt is used. In small patients, however, such a shunt may occasionally produce excessive flow to the lungs, as may a shunt of 4 mm diameter in larger neonates. In such circumstances, low systemic flow is managed initially by reducing systemic resistance by increasing the dose of milrinone, and/or by adding an infusion of nitroprusside infusion. Pulmonary resistance can be increased by using positive end-expiratory pressure, hypoxia, or hypercarbia.[27] Surgical revision of the shunt may also be considered.

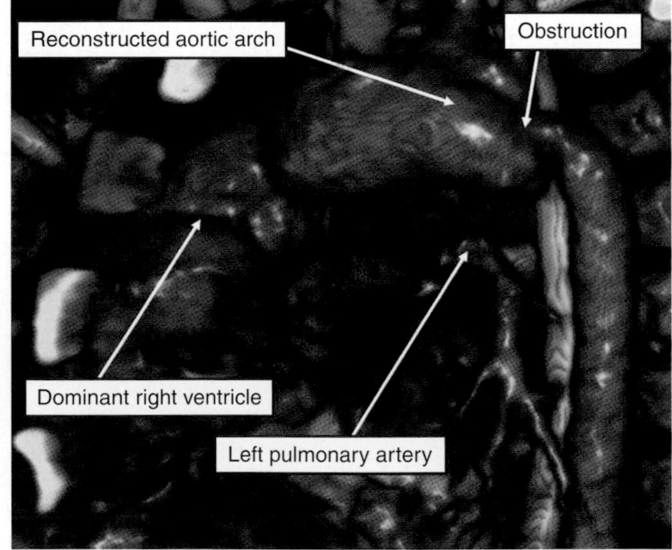

Figure 29-21 This reconstructed computerised tomographic image shows a surgically reconstructed aortic arch. Note the discrepancy in size between the patch used to augment the ascending aorta, and the distal descending aorta. A moderate degree of obstruction is seen at the most distal end of the homograft patch, which was successfully relieved by balloon angiography. (Courtesy of Dr Jeffrey Hellinger, Children's Hospital of Philadelphia, Philadelphia, Pennsylvania.)

Hypoxaemia

Pathophysiology of Post-operative Hypoxaemia

As summarised in Figure 21-19, systemic arterial oxygenation in patients with complete intracardiac mixing of blood is determined by three basic factors, namely, the content of oxygen in the pulmonary veins, the systemic venous oxygen content, and the ratio of these two measures. When any of these is abnormally low, regardless of the state of the others, hypoxaemia may result. Not unexpectedly, therefore, hypoxaemia in the early post-operative period after the initial stage of palliation in neonates can be traced to conditions affecting one or more of these factors.

A decreased content of oxygen in the pulmonary veins results from suboptimal oxygenation of the blood leaving the lungs, and is relatively common.[62] Potential causes of such poor oxygenation include intrapulmonary shunting, impaired exchange of gases due to pulmonary disease or oedema, and reduced effective lung volume resulting from pneumothorax or a pleural effusion, all of which may occur in the early post-operative period. Pulmonary venous desaturation without an identifiable cause may also be seen.[62]

Systemic venous deoxygenation is most commonly due to low systemic flow and low cardiac output, as already discussed, but may also result from an abnormally low capacity to carry oxygen, or high systemic consumption of oxygen. Anaemia is the most common cause of decreased carrying capacity, while high consumption can be the result of inadequate sedation or paralysis, thermoregulatory drive, seizures, infection, or an accelerated catabolic state.

The commonest causes of decreased flow to the lungs are globally low cardiac output, which also affects the mixed venous saturation of oxygen, and technical problems with the systemic-to-pulmonary arterial shunt. Pulmonary vascular resistance typically fluctuates in the early post-operative period following neonatal repair, especially in the context of anomalies with high pre-operative pulmonary flow or obstructed pulmonary venous outflow. This is due to pulmonary vascular hyperreactivity, which is a complex phenomenon influenced by pulmonary endothelial dysfunction, itself resulting from high pre-operative and altered post-operative shear stress in the pulmonary circulation, as well as the pulmonary vascular effects of cardiopulmonary bypass and its adjunctive measures.[64] In order for endogenous pulmonary resistance to exert a substantial effect on the flow of blood to the lungs in patients with a restrictive systemic-to-pulmonary arterial shunt, it must be elevated well beyond the physiological range. Thus, increased resistance is rarely the sole factor responsible for significant hypoxaemia in this setting. It is more likely that problems with the systemic-to-pulmonary arterial shunt, rather than an elevated pulmonary resistance, will be responsible for reductions in flow that result in hypoxaemia. If elevated resistance is considered to be a factor in a patient with severe hypoxaemia, a trial of inhaled nitric oxide can be considered. In patients with labile pulmonary resistance, nitric oxide will improve systemic oxygenation. Lack of any response suggests a technical problem with the shunt, which may be compromised by constriction at either of the anastomotic sites, kinking, or partial or complete thrombosis, or simply because it is of insufficient diameter or excessive length to accommodate the necessary pulmonary flow in a given patient.

Evaluation of Post-operative Hypoxaemia

The cause of hypoxaemia can generally be distinguished by a combination of physical examination, chest radiography, pulse oximetry, and measurements of arterial blood gases, combined with echocardiography with Doppler analysis of flows. Pulmonary causes of inefficient oxygenation are investigated with a combination of chest radiography, monitoring of ventilatory pressures and flow-volume relations, assessment of the function and pattern of drainage from the thoracostomy, and ultrasound, which can be an efficient means of evaluating a pleural effusion.

Decreased systemic venous oxygenation is determined by a combination of measurement of the haematocrit, venous co-oximetry, confirmation of paralysis and sedation, and exclusion of seizures or infectious causes of increased consumption of oxygen. If the patient is not anaemic, demonstrates no evidence of seizure activity or infection, and is adequately sedated and paralysed, the cause of decreased oxygenation is most likely poor ventricular function and/or cardiac tamponade, which is investigated and managed as described above.

Management of Post-operative Hypoxaemia

Management is tailored to the underlying cause. In patients with pulmonary venous desaturation due to extrinsic pulmonary compression, such as a pleural effusion or pneumothorax, the pleural fluid or air is drained with a small pleural catheter, which is left in place as necessary. Pulmonary parenchymal disease is treated with a combination of ventilatory manipulations and appropriate pharmacological therapy if indicated. Increased positive end-expiratory pressure can recruit atelectatic segments of lung, and facilitate improved ventilation-perfusion matching. It is effective at reducing pulmonary oedema.[62] Increasing the fraction of inspired oxygen may also be effective at improving pulmonary venous desaturation.[62]

Hypoxaemia due to decreased systemic venous saturation in association with low systemic flow is managed according to the principles discussed earlier. In patients with normal cardiac output but increased consumption of oxygen due to agitation, pain, and so on, pharmacological minimisation of systemic demand for oxygen, as with sedation and paralysis, is initiated or augmented. In patients with increased consumption due to infection, fever, or seizures, the underlying cause is treated with the appropriate measures.

Anatomical problems with the shunt causing inadequate flow to the lungs are managed with the appropriate intervention. Delivery of oxygen is generally optimised in patients with an obstructed shunt by administering volume, keeping the systemic arterial pressure high, ensuring adequate sedation, and providing supplemental oxygen. If the shunt is obstructed, management is with surgery or interventional catheterisation in most cases. If acute deterioration occurs, resuscitation with extracorporeal oxygenation may be necessary.

Summary

The goals of the first 24 hours of post-operative care include supporting combined cardiac output with inotropes and reduction of systemic afterload, minimizing the demand for oxygen with sedation and occasionally neuromuscular blockade; minimizing stressful procedures that increase such demand, taking note of pulmonary and systemic vascular resistances; treating pain; and anticipating common complications, and managing them promptly. The cost of this strategy is the need for indwelling invasive catheters, mechanical ventilation, and medications with potentially important toxicities. Equally important in optimizing recovery following the first stage of palliation is appropriate management of the second phase of post-operative care, when myocardial function has returned to baseline and vascular resistances have stabilised. This requires the prompt removal of invasive catheters and tubes, and the weaning of pharmacological support, in other words, de-intensification.

SUBACUTE/STEPDOWN MANAGEMENT

De-intensification

In the patient with an uncomplicated acute post-operative course, we begin preparing for step-down management approximately 16 to 20 hours after surgery, a strategy that is based on the typical post-operative haemodynamic profile as discussed above. Although myocardial function and cardiac output may not have fully normalised by this point, the trend is towards improved cardiac function. De-intensification can then be initiated in anticipation of normalised haemodynamics. This strategy decreases the likelihood of iatrogenic complications without sacrificing optimal care during the critical acute post-operative period.

If utilised, neuromuscular blocking agents are generally discontinued within 12 to 18 hours after the operation, with return of spontaneous breathing within the next 12 to 24 hours, depending on the renal function and drug clearance. The level of mechanical ventilatory support is gradually decreased, and the patient extubated 1 or 2 days after surgery. Following extubation, intravenous inotropic and afterload-reducing medications are weaned, as diuretic medications, and occasionally digoxin, are continued. Once inotropic agents and afterload-reducing medications are discontinued, the umbilical and urinary catheters are removed. Right atrial catheters are typically maintained to provide parenteral nutrition until full enteral feeds are tolerated. Routine laboratory studies are decreased in frequency and scope during the course of de-intensification, and usually obtained only once a day following removal of the indwelling vascular catheters. Enteral feeding is initiated once inotropic support has been weaned and the umbilical arterial catheter has been removed. The goal is to complete the process within 4 to 5 days of admission to the intensive care unit following surgery.

Feeding and Necrotizing Enterocolitis

Enteral nutrition is usually initiated with continuous nasogastric feeds, with a steady increase in the rate until gastrointestinal tolerance has been amply demonstrated. Most patients are also maintained on ranitidine. Parenteral nutrition is gradually decreased in accordance with the advance in feeding, and discontinued once the patient is tolerating enteral feeds sufficiently to meet the full nutritional requirement. The transition is then made to intermittent nasogastric feeds, and oral feeds are introduced gradually. Neonates frequently have difficultly resuming normal oromotor and pharyngeal coordination after the first stage of palliation, and feeding is often impaired.[89] Evaluation of the left vocal cord should also be considered in patients who demonstrate coughing or respiratory distress with oral feeds. Although patients are given every opportunity to meet their nutritional needs with oral feeding, approximately two-fifths of those undergoing the first stage of palliation at our centre are ultimately discharged on a regime of supplemental nasogastric feeding, or have a gastrostomy tube placed. All patients with congenitally malformed hearts are a population at nutritional risk,[90,91] and supplemental tube feeding has been demonstrated to benefit such infants.[92]

One of the most important considerations in resuming enteral feeds after the initial stage of reconstruction is the possibility of necrotizing enterocolitis. Over a 4-year period, almost one–twenty-fifth of neonates with congenitally malformed hearts admitted to our cardiac intensive care unit developed this complication, with those having hypoplasia of the left heart being at significantly increased risk.[93]

Intermediate Outcomes Following First-stage Reconstruction

Following hospital discharge, infants who have undergone the first stage of reconstruction remain at risk for haemodynamic compromise, as mentioned above. Residual or recurrent obstruction to systemic blood flow may occur in up to 1 in 10 infants, requiring balloon angioplasty[94] or surgical revision. Following the second stage of reconstruction, later mortality is rare, on-going monitoring is rarely necessary, and growth and development improve. In the 25 years since the first successful reports of palliation for hypoplasia of the left heart, infants and children have been shown to have a similarly low risk of later mortality compared with other children with functionally univentricular hearts who have undergone staged reconstruction culminating in a Fontan procedure. Surgical mortality for the second- and third-stage procedures are less than 5% in most reported series, and late death has been rare.[95–97]

The protean cardiovascular and non-cardiovascular morbidities following the Fontan procedure have been well documented.[54,98,99] At the current time, most of these important morbidities, including arrhythmias, hypercoagulability and thrombosis, protein-losing enteropathy, plastic bronchitis, and a reduced ability to exercise, occur in similar frequencies in children with hypoplasia of the left heart and those with other forms of functionally univentricular hearts. The only two exceptions to this generalisation are the potential for dilation of the neo-aortic root, and the increased frequency of impairment to the central nervous system, as discussed in Chapter 64.

Progressive dilation of the anatomical pulmonary valve and root has been reported,[100] with progressive regurgitation of the neo-aortic valve in some children, including isolated case reports of replacement of the neo-aortic valve in children and adolescents with hypoplasia of the left heart following staged reconstruction. It is likely that the frequency of this complication will increase with increasing duration of follow-up, as has been seen following the arterial switch and Ross operations. Finally, children with hypoplasia of the left heart are more likely than others with congenital cardiac malformations to have microcephaly at birth, other structural abnormalities of the brain at birth, and genetic syndromes. School-age children with hypoplasia of the left heart have an increased prevalence of attention, behavioural, and learning disorders compared to the normal population, as well as to other children who have undergone the Fontan procedure with other forms of functionally univentricular heart.

The complete reference list can be found on the companion Expert Consult web site at www.expertconsult.com.

ANNOTATED REFERENCES

- Tchervenkov CI, Jacobs JP, Weinberg PM, et al: The nomenclature, definition and classification of hypoplastic left heart syndrome. Cardiol Young 2006;16:339–368.

  This extensive review was prepared by the International Working Group for Mapping and Coding of Nomenclatures for Paediatric and Congenital Heart Disease. They discuss the evolution of nomenclature and surgical treatment for the spectrum of lesions making up the hypoplastic left heart syndrome and related malformations. Associated codes for diagnoses and procedures are also established.

- Ilbawi AM, Spicer DE, Bharati S, et al: Morphologic study of the ascending aorta and aortic arch in hypoplastic left hearts: Surgical implications. J Thorac Cardiovasc Surg 2007;134:99–105.

  This study evaluated 96 autopsy specimens to identify important areas of obstruction in the ascending aorta in patients with hypoplasia of the left heart. The pathogenesis and importance of the findings in relation to the optimum surgical approach also are discussed. The authors suggest incorporating the ascending aorta into the aortic reconstruction at the time of initial palliation given their results.

- Rychik J, Rome JJ, Collins MH, et al: The hypoplastic left heart syndrome with intact atrial septum: Atrial morphology, pulmonary vascular histopathology and outcome. J Am Coll Cardiol 1999;34:554–560.

  This paper describes the problematic, high-risk group of patients with intact atrial septum. The authors review the atrial morphology and pulmonary vascular histopathology associated with outcome. Only 6 of the 17 patients survived, and all the survivors had an unobstructed decompressing pathway. There were three additional deaths in this group after second-stage palliation. Patients with an obstructed or no decompressing pathway had severely dilated lymphatics and arterialisation of the pulmonary veins.

- Norwood WI, Lang P, Hansen DD: Physiologic repair of aortic atresia–hypoplastic left heart syndrome. N Engl J Med 1983;308:23–26.

  This report described the first successful physiological repair of aortic atresia with hypoplastic left heart syndrome. The repair was achieved with two separate operations, consisting of the Norwood procedure itself followed by the modified Fontan procedure. It was this account that established the principle of staged palliation.

- Akintuerk H, Michel-Behnke I, Valeske K, et al: Stenting of the arterial duct and banding of the pulmonary arteries: Basis for combined Norwood stage I and II repair in hypoplastic left heart. Circulation 2002;105:1099–1103.

  Using a previous technique reported to be successful by Gibbs and colleagues, a series of patients with hypoplasia of the left heart underwent stenting of the arterial duct and banding of the pulmonary arteries in Geissen, Germany. Of the patients, one died 4 months after the procedure whilst awaiting cardiac transplantation. A second death occurred in a patient after the second stage of palliation, consisting of reconstruction of the aortic arch and a superior cavopulmonary anastomosis. These improved outcomes promoted further interest in this strategy.

- Sano S, Ishino K, Kawada M, et al: Right ventricle–pulmonary artery shunt in first-stage palliation of hypoplastic left heart syndrome. J Thorac Cardiovasc Surg 2003;126:504–509.

  This report established the concept of placing a conduit from the right ventricle to the pulmonary arteries as the source of pulmonary flow in infants who undergo the modified Norwood procedure. In the hands of the authors, this approach improved early survival to 89%, in comparison to previous survival of no more than 50% using the standard Norwood procedure. They describe their surgical technique in detail.

- Ghanayem NS, Hoffman GM, Mussatto KA, et al: Home surveillance program prevents interstage mortality after the Norwood procedure. J Thorac Cardiovasc Surg 2003;126:1367–1377.

  With improvement in outcomes over time, interstage mortality between initial and subsequent palliative surgeries was identified to be important, with deaths between stages approaching surgical mortality for the initial palliation. In this study, the group from Milwaukee describes a methodology for improving interstage mortality using a programme of home surveillance. Additionally, the authors suggest not delaying the second-stage palliation beyond 5 to 6 months, since a plateau in weight gain was identified at this age.

- Wernovsky G, Chrisant MR: Long-term follow-up after staged reconstruction or transplantation for patients with functionally univentricular heart. Cardiol Young 2004;14(Suppl 1):115–126.

  This article reviews the literature and nicely summarises important aspects for long-term survivors with functionally univentricular hearts who have undergone staged palliation or cardiac transplantation. Important issues such as medical and functional state are covered.

- Migliavacca F, Pennati G, Dubini G, et al: Modeling of the Norwood circulation: Effects of shunt size, vascular resistances, and heart rate. Am J Physiol Heart Circ Physiol 2001;280:H2076–H2086.

  This article presents a mathematical model of the circulation after a Norwood procedure, and examines the effect of three significant variables. The results have important clinical implications with regard to monitoring and post-operative therapies in the intensive care unit.

- Tweddell JS, Hoffman GM, Fedderly RT, et al: Patients at risk for low systemic oxygen delivery after the Norwood procedure. Ann Thorac Surg 2000;69:1893–1899.

  This paper highlights the importance of systemic delivery of oxygen in the post-operative period after the Norwood procedure. This is one of a series of papers from this group, suggesting a change in style of management from focusing on balancing the pulmonary and systemic circulation to focusing on the systemic circulation. The authors identify lower mixed venous saturations of oxygen in the groups of patients with a high risk of death.

- Bartram U, Grunenfelder J, Van Praagh R: Causes of death after the modified Norwood procedure: A study of 122 postmortem cases. Ann Thorac Surg 1997;64:1795–1802.

  Identifying the causes of death after the Norwood procedure may help in treating or evaluating sick patients. This study reviews the causes of death in 122 patients after the Norwood procedure at Boston Children's Hospital. The authors identify that over one-half the deaths were related to surgical technical issues, or with perfusion of the lungs or myocardium.

- Skinner ML, Halstead LA, Rubinstein CS, et al: Laryngopharyngeal dysfunction after the Norwood procedure. J Thorac Cardiovasc Surg 2005;130:1293–1301.

  A significant portion of inpatient stay after the Norwood procedure often relates to issues relating to feeding or the airways. In this investigation, the authors identified a high rate of feeding issues, including abnormal swallowing in one-half the patients and aspiration in one-quarter, with paralysis of the vocal cords in one-tenth. They also discuss the natural history of these problems.

- Zeltser I, Menteer J, Gaynor JW, et al: Impact of re-coarctation following the Norwood operation on survival in the balloon angioplasty era. J Am Coll Cardiol 2005;45:1844–1848.

  The investigators review the important complication of re-coarctation in a large series of patients who underwent the Norwood procedure. Re-coarctation occurred in one-tenth of the cohort, and recurred in one-fifth of these patients. Balloon angioplasty proved successful as treatment for the majority of these patients, and was achieved with low morbidity.

CHAPTER 30

Hypoplasia of the Right Ventricle

PIERS E.F. DAUBENEY

The right ventricle can be hypoplastic in various settings. It can be small in the presence of deficient ventricular or atrioventricular septation, producing so-called left ventricular dominance. The chamber can also be small and incomplete in the setting of univentricular atrioventricular connections such as double inlet left ventricle or tricuspid atresia. The ventricle can be hypoplastic when the ventricular septum is intact and there is so-called critical stenosis of the pulmonary valve. All of these entities are dealt with elsewhere in this book. In this chapter, we are concerned with pulmonary atresia in the setting of an intact ventricular septum (Fig. 30-1), and have included the situation in which the cavity of the right ventricle is dilated, as well as hypoplastic. Almost invariably the heart is left-sided, with concordant atrioventricular and ventriculo-arterial connections, but rarely pulmonary atresia can be found in the setting of an intact ventricular septum when the ventriculo-arterial connections are discordant. In these cases, of course, it is left ventricular hypoplasia which dominates the picture, typically with the ventricle having a fibroelastotic lining as is the case in hypoplasia of the left heart with usual segmental combinations (see Chapter 29). Pulmonary atresia itself can also occur in various additional settings, such as when the intracardiac anatomy is that of tetralogy of Fallot, and in conjunction with other complex lesions such as atrioventricular septal defect, isomeric atrial appendages, or discordant ventriculo-arterial connections. In all of these situations, however, ventricular septation is deficient. When seen with an intact ventricular septum, there is considerable diversity of the morphology of the tricuspid valve, the right ventricle, and the pulmonary arteries, as well as frequent coronary arterial abnormalities. In two of the final encyclopaedic reviews led by Freedom,[1,2] attention was directed to the huge problems produced by lesions of the coronary arteries or tricuspid valve in this setting, making it one of the most lethal of current congenital cardiac malformations. It was not without reason that Freedom[3] had previously commented, in one of his many perceptive reviews of this lesion, 'How can something so small cause so much grief?' I will deal with all of these aspects in the sections that follow.

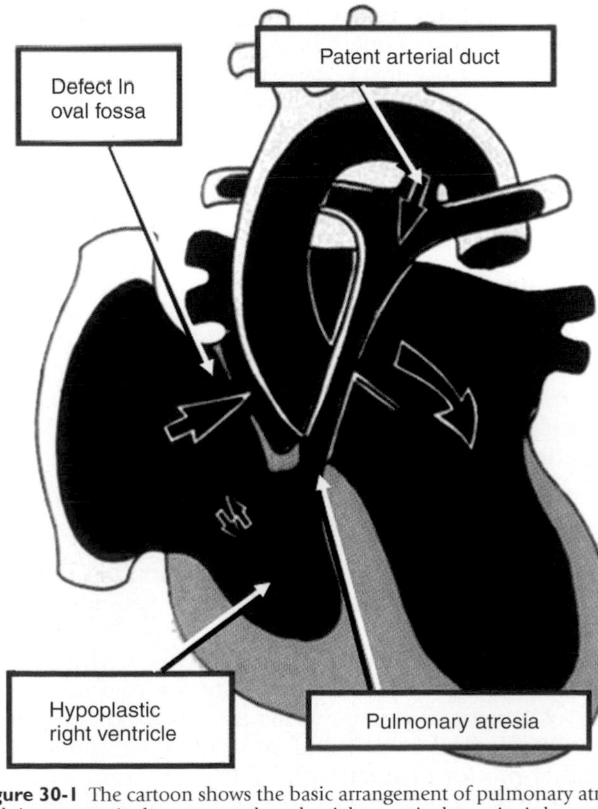

Figure 30-1 The cartoon shows the basic arrangement of pulmonary atresia with intact ventricular septum when the right ventricular cavity is hypoplastic rather than dilated.

GENETICS, EMBRYOGENESIS AND INCIDENCE

Pulmonary atresia with intact ventricular septum is a relatively uncommon disease accounting for about 3% of serious congenital heart disease at birth.[4] It is the third most common type of cyanotic congenital cardiac malformation in neonates, coming after transposition and tetralogy of Fallot with pulmonary atresia.[5] The distribution according to gender was 1.5 males to 1 female in the population-based study carried out in the United Kingdom and Eire from 1991 through 1999, with figures of 1.3:1 in the Swedish based study.[6] The estimated prevalence at birth from the various epidemiological studies varies from 4.2 to 8.5 per 100,000 live births.[6–12]

These data, of course, reflect the prevalence of the disease at birth. The advent of fetal echocardiography has shown that there may be significant spontaneous death prior to this during fetal life. In particular, those fetuses with severe tricuspid regurgitation seem to have a poor outcome, often developing hugely dilated atriums, hypoplasia of the lungs, atrial arrhythmias, ascites, and pleural and pericardial effusions.[13–18] It was predicted that fetal echocardiography would lead to a substantial reduction in the prevalence of complex congenitally malformed hearts seen at birth because of selected termination of pregnancy.[19] This was confirmed in the collaborative study performed in the United Kingdom and Eire,[9] with only about one-third of those diagnosed during life surviving to become live births.[9]

The prevalence at birth in mainland Britain was estimated to have fallen by 26% because of fetal diagnosis.

MORPHOGENESIS AND AETIOLOGY

Morphogenesis

As for many types of congenital heart disease, the morphogenesis of the lesion is unclear, although the morphology dictates that the insult producing the atresia must have occurred after the completion of ventricular septation. There is some evidence as to the timing of this developmental insult. Several groups have examined various morphological features, including the size and morphology of the pulmonary valve, and the topology of the arterial duct.[20–22] The angle subtended by the duct to the postductal descending aorta may be an indicator of whether the pulmonary arterial pathways became atretic earlier or later in gestation. In normal hearts, the duct runs almost parallel with the transverse arch, forming an obtuse angle with the postductal aorta (Fig. 30-2). In pulmonary atresia in the setting of deficient ventricular septation, the duct may originate more proximally on the aortic arch than normal, is usually sigmoid in shape, and subtends an acute angle to the postductal aorta. This led to the hardly surprising suggestion that the atresia develops early in these lesions during cardiac morphogenesis, at or shortly after partitioning of the outlets of the developing heart, but before closure of the embryonic interventricular communication.[21]

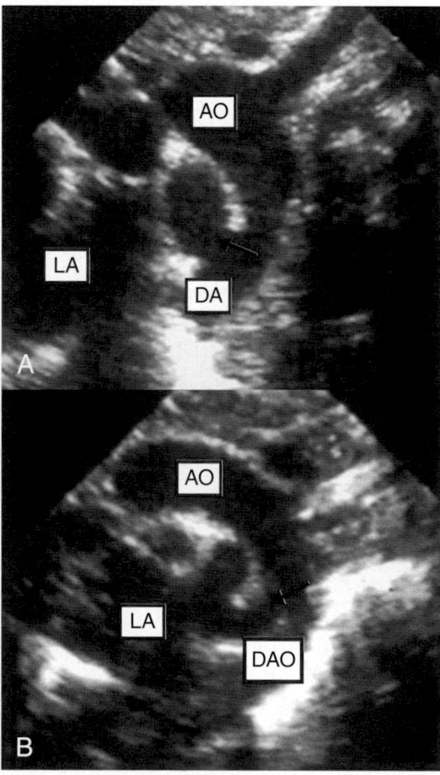

Figure 30-2 These echocardiograms show the variation in ductal angle. **A,** A normal angle between the arterial duct and the descending aorta (DAO), of greater than 90 degrees, in a patient with a tripartite right ventricle and an imperforate pulmonary valve. **B,** An acute angle, of less than 90 degrees, in a patient with unipartite right ventricle and muscular atresia. The *arrows* superimposed on these echocardiograms show the variation in ductal angle. AO, aorta; LA, left atrium. (From Daubeney PE, Delany DJ, Anderson RH, et al: Pulmonary atresia with intact ventricular septum: Range of morphology in a population-based study. J Am Coll Cardiol 2002;39:1670-1679.)

In those in whom the ventricular septum is intact, the duct subtends a highly variable angle to the postductal aorta. Patients with better developed right ventricular cavities tend to have ducts subtending normal angles, whilst in those with severely hypertrophied ventricles, and ventricular-to-coronary fistulous connections, it tends to be acute[23] (see Fig. 30-2), supporting the notion that those with smaller and hypertrophied right ventricles suffered their developmental insult earlier in gestation than did those with ventricles having better developed cavities.[24] This notion has now been supported by evidence from fetal echocardiography, where progression from pulmonary stenosis to atresia has been documented during later pregnancy.[9,17]

Previously, it was assumed that atresia of the pulmonary valve was the primary morphogenetic event, leading to right ventricular hypertension, and development of the fistulous communication with the coronary arteries. More recently, several groups have suggested that, at least in those with fistulous connections, the primary disease may be one of persistence of these communications,[25] or abnormal morphogenesis of the right ventricle,[26] rather than the pulmonary valve itself. As fistulous communications have been identified from 13 weeks gestation onwards, and as it is known that the embryonic interventricular communication closes in the ninth week, Chaoui and colleagues have doubted that this leaves enough time for right ventricular hypertension to cause the development of fistulas.[25] Their argument goes on to state that, as prenatal afterload is higher in the right ventricle compared to the left,[27,28] blood would preferentially pass through the fistulous communications, rather than the pulmonary valve, leading to pulmonary stenosis and atresia. As an alternative they suggested that there may be a primary insult at right ventricular level, leading to both pulmonary atresia and to persistence of the communications from the right ventricle to the coronary arteries,[25] a concept also supported by Bonnet and colleagues.[26] The concept has now been further extended by Gittenberger-de Groot and her colleagues,[29,30] who refute the suggestion that the pulmonary valve is the site of the primary abnormality. Her group propose that the primary anomaly in this subset of patients is lack of ingrowth of the developing coronary arteries even prior to development of pulmonary atresia, since the coronary vasculature develops from the epicardium, and not from the intertrabecular spaces.[31,32] They also highlighted the role of cells migrating from the neural crest in this process of vascular development.[30] The likely morphogenesis has been summarised neatly by Bonnet and colleagues as a 'primitive alteration of a mechanogenic transduction pathway, crucial for right myocardial remodelling during embryogenesis'.[26]

Aetiology

The underlying abnormality in this condition has not been elucidated. Both congenital and acquired aetiologies have been proposed.[21,33] Some thought that the coronary arterial pathology seen represented an endarteritis,[34] while others proposed that a prenatal inflammatory disorder may cause the development of atresia.[21] This has not been supported by any histological evidence of an acute or subacute disorder, either pre- or postnatally.[2,15,17] There is some evidence showing that the lesion can be acquired during fetal life in association with twin-to-twin transfusion.[35] Twinning studies have also demonstrated an excess of congenitally malformed hearts in monozygotic twins, often in only one of the set of twins,[36] leading to the suggestion that the twinning process itself may lead to increased congenital cardiac malformations, possibly due to loss of laterality in one twin. Furthermore, siblings have been described, both having the lesion, suggesting an autosomal recessive trait, with doubt being expressed as to whether the disease can really be acquired.[37] It seems likely, therefore, that the morphological entity represents a common endpoint for a range of underlying disorders, both hereditary and acquired during fetal life.

MORPHOLOGY

The lesion is a global condition affecting the entirety of the right ventricle.[38–40] The extent of morphological heterogeneity is illustrated by the frequency in which each anatomical feature occurs within the United Kingdom and Eire population-based study[23] (Table 30-1) This can then serve a reference to ensure that future studies are reflective of the population as a whole.

Tricuspid Valve

Almost invariably, the right ventricular inlet valve is abnormal.[38,41–47] Abnormalities can include dysplasia, Ebsteinoid displacement, and a wide range of annular size, ranging from tiny to hugely dilated. Often the valve shows all three abnormalities to a variable degree. At a functional level, there is a continuum from severely stenotic to freely regurgitant.

Tricuspid stenosis at its most severe may be due to an obstructed muscularised annulus with dysplasia of the valvar leaflets and their supporting tension apparatus.[45] The free edges of the leaflets may be thickened and nodular, the cords reduced in number, and shortened with fibrous thickening. The papillary muscles can be underdeveloped with abnormal attachments.[47] Even the most severely stenotic tricuspid valve is likely also to have a degree of regurgitation.[45]

Tricuspid regurgitation at its most severe may be accompanied by a grossly dilated annulus, with displacement and severe dysplasia of the tricuspid valvar leaflets (Table 30-2).[23,37] At its extreme, the tricuspid valve may be devoid of all leaflet tissue, leaving an unguarded tricuspid valvar orifice, and leading to a hugely dilated and thin-walled right ventricle.[47–50] Ebstein's malformation is seen in about one-tenth of cases[23,49] (see Table 30-1), and can be found with both hypoplasia (Fig. 30-3) and dilation of the right ventricular cavity. In the setting of a dilated cavity, there is sail-like enlargement of the anterosuperior leaflet, whereas when the ventricle is hypoplastic, the changes are confined to downward displacement of an often dysplastic septal leaflet.[47] Whereas Ebstein's malformation usually leads to a regurgitant valve, the displaced valve may also be virtually imperforate when the cavity is hypoplastic.[44]

Severe tricuspid regurgitation, whether due to dysplasia or Ebstein's malformation, can lead to functional pulmonary atresia.[51–53] This occurs when the right ventricle is unable to generate sufficient pressure to open an anatomically normal pulmonary valve. Distinguishing functional from true atresia can be difficult. It normally relies on the fact that there is a degree of diastolic regurgitation through the pulmonary valve that can be seen echocardiographically[54–56] or angiographically.[57]

The size of the tricuspid valve correlates well with the size of the right ventricular cavity[23,38,43,44,47,58–60] (see Table 30-2), unlike the situation in critical pulmonary stenosis.[61] This correlation, and the importance of the right ventricular inlet in surgical repair, has led to several groups advocating use of the dimensions of the tricuspid valve as a guide to surgical management.[60,62–74] This is usually based on the *z* score, the number of standard deviations a measurement departs from the mean normal. Several nomograms are available for these derivations.[75,76] Caution must be adopted, nonetheless, in interpreting these *z* scores, as they are not always comparable. Some depend on normal data obtained from echocardiographic studies,[75] while others come from postmortem studies of formalin-fixed hearts.[77]

TABLE 30-1

SUMMARY OF PRINCIPAL MORPHOLOGIC FINDINGS IN THE POPULATION-BASED STUDY CARRIED OUT IN THE UNITED KINGDOM AND EIRE FROM 1991 THROUGH 1995

Morphologic Feature	Type	Number
Type of pulmonary atresia	Membranous	130/174 (74.7%)
	Muscular	44/174 (25.3%)
Partite state of the RV	Tripartite	84/143 (58.7%)
	Bipartite	48/143 (33.6%)
	Unipartite	11/143 (7.7%)
Coronary arterial abnormalities	RV-to-coronary fistulas	60/132 (45.5%)
	Coronary arterial stenoses, interruption and ectasia	10/132 (7.6%)
Ebstein's malformation		18/183 (9.8%)
Significant RV dilatation		8/183 (4.4%)
Size of tricuspid valve	Median *z* score: echo*	−5.2 (range: −18.3 to 9.4)
	Median *z* score: autopsy†	−1.6 (range: −2.9 to −0.4)
Size of RV inlet	Median *z* score*	−5.1 (range: −16.0 to 3.5)

*z scores calculated from echocardiographically-derived normal values,[7] rather than †postmortem-derived normal values.[77] In all, 15 abnormalities of the left ventricle were documented, including 4 with extreme septal hypertrophy with bulging into the left ventricular outflow.

RV, right ventricle.

From Daubeney PE, Delany DJ, Anderson RH, et al: Pulmonary atresia with intact ventricular septum: Range of morphology in a population-based study. J Am Coll Cardiol 2002;39:1670–1679

TABLE 30-2

INTER-RELATIONS OF MORPHOLOGIC VARIABLES AT PRESENTATION FROM THE UNITED KINGDOM AND EIRE POPULATION-BASED STUDY

	RV Inlet *z* Score (Increased Inlet Length)	Ductal Angle (Normal)	Fistulae (Absence)	Type of Atresia (Membranous)	Partite (Tripart)	Stenoses (Absence)	Tricuspid Regurg. (Increased)	RV pressure (Lower)
TV *z* score (increased valve size)	$P < 0.0001$ $R = 0.45$	$P = 0.0120$	$P < 0.0001$	$P < 0.0001$	$P < 0.0001$	$P = 0.1763$	$P = 0.0050$	$P = 0.0011$ $R = 0.402$
RV inlet *z* score (increased inlet length)		$P = 0.3304$	$P = 0.0011$	$P = 0.0131$	$P < 0.0001$	$P = 0.5755$	$P = 0.0052$	$P = 0.7459$ $R = 0.041$
Ductal angle (normal)			$P = 0.0095$	$P < 0.0001$	$P < 0.0001$	$P = 0.0852$	$P = 0.0743$	$P = 0.3077$
Fistulas (absence)				$P < 0.0001$	$P < 0.0001$		$P = 0.0055$	$P = 0.0321$
Type of atresia (membranous)					$P < 0.0001$	$P > 0.9999$	$P = 0.0140$	$P = 0.1938$
Partite (tripartite)						$P = 0.8409$	$P = 0.0022$	$P = 0.9720$
Stenoses (absence)							$P = 0.2090$	$P = 0.0008$
Tricuspid regurgitation (increased)								$P = 0.0143$

There is considerable covariance of morphologic features: for example a small right ventricle will tend to have muscular atresia and a small tricuspid valve. Such covariance is shown in this table. This table shows, for a population of patients with pulmonary atresia with intact ventricular septum at presentation, the *p* value for the presence, absence (or other denoted state) of key morphologic features co-existing in the same heart.

RV, right ventricle; TV, tricuspid valve.

From Daubeney PE, Delany DJ, Anderson RH, et al: Pulmonary atresia with intact ventricular septum: Range of morphology in a population-based study. J Am Coll Cardiol 2002;39:1670–1679

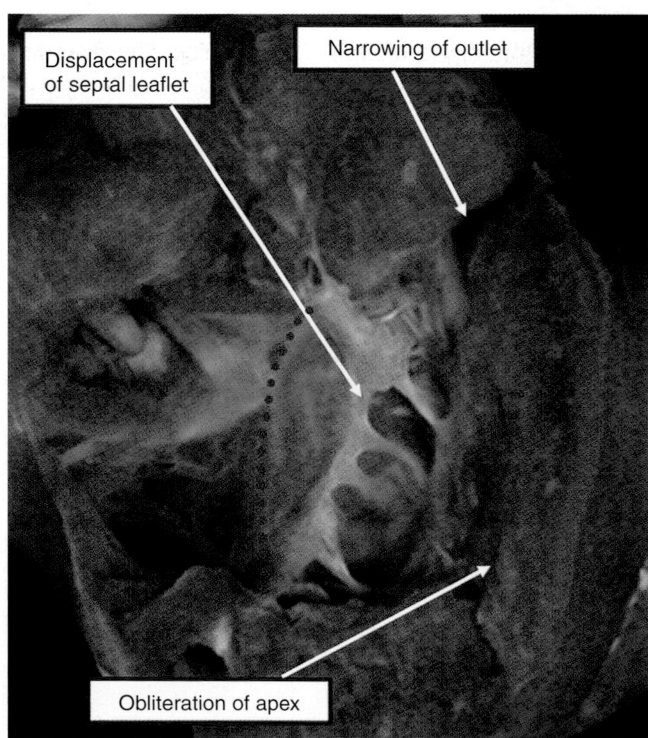

Figure 30-3 In this heart with obliteration of the apical component, and hypoplasia of the outlet component, the tricuspid valve shows evidence of Ebstein's malformation, with the septal leaflet hinged away from the atrioventricular junction *(yellow dotted line)*.

Right Ventricle

Although the initial classification of the right ventricle was into small as opposed to normal or dilated categories,[78] this concept has now been refined to acknowledge the continuum in right ventricular size.[44,79] When the right ventricle is said to be hypoplastic, it is not the ventricle itself that is hypoplastic, but rather the ventricular cavity that is obliterated by the severe muscular hypertrophy. Using the observations of Goor and Lillehei, that normal right ventricle has three parts,[80] Bull and colleagues proposed the tripartite approach to categorisation of pulmonary atresia with intact ventricular septum, and this was subsequently used as the basis for surgical decision-making.[63,81] Patients were categorised as to the degree of mural hypertrophy present, giving the following options:

- All three portions of the right ventricle cavity being well-formed, with minimal mural hypertrophy (Fig. 30-4).
- Muscular overgrowth of the apical trabecular portion. The cavity in this setting is effectively formed by the inlet and outlet components, with the infundibulum still extending to the undersurface of the imperforate valve, but through a very narrow channel. The inlet component also becomes hypoplastic, with the tricuspid valve usually tethered by short cords to the margins of the obliterated apical component (Fig. 30-5). Although the cavity effectively has only two components, all three initial parts of the morphologically right ventricle are readily identified.
- Muscular overgrowth of both apical and outlet portions. It is this process that produces the severest examples of the lesion, with the cavity in this setting effectively represented only by the hypoplastic inlet component (Fig. 30-6). Even with this arrangement, nonetheless, all three portions of the right ventricle are present, with the cavities of the apical trabecular and outlet parts being obliterated.

Management of these patients, be it by surgical or interventional catheterisation techniques, requires selection of

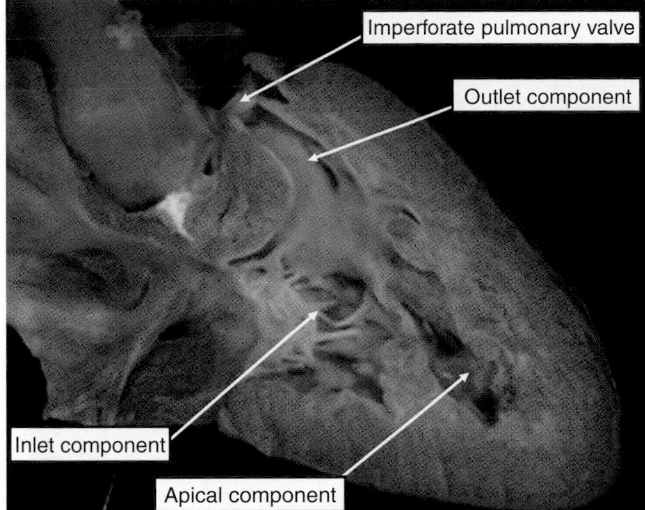

Figure 30-4 In this heart, the pulmonary valve is imperforate, but all three parts of the ventricular cavity are well-formed. Note the relatively normal tricuspid valve.

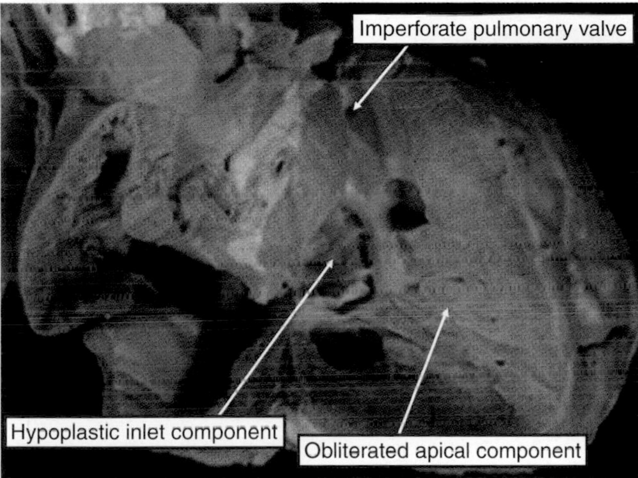

Figure 30-5 In this heart, mural hypertrophy has obliterated the apical component of the right ventricle, the cavity being represented by the hypoplastic outlet and inlet components. Note the abnormalities of the tricuspid valve.

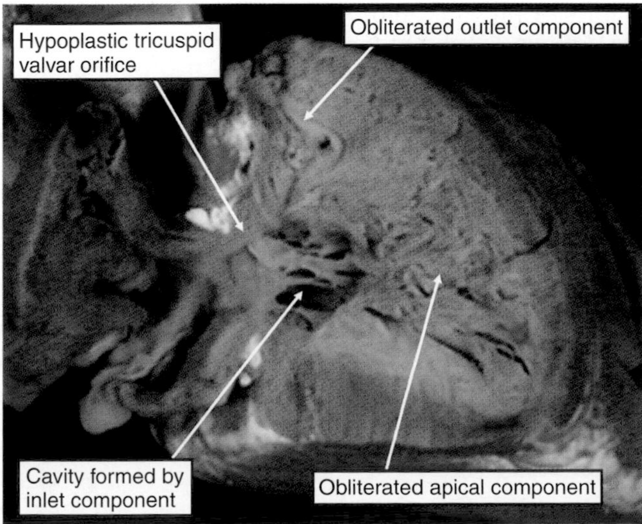

Figure 30-6 Mural hypertrophy in this heart has squeezed out the apical and outlet components, leaving the ventricular cavity represented only by the inlet.

patients with suitably sized right ventricles in early life. Numerous attempts have been made to assess the adequacy of the right ventricle in order to guide the optimal strategies for management.[6,38,60,62,65,71,72,81–94] Owing to the fact that the walls of the right ventricle are usually severely hypertrophied, with sometimes bizarrely irregular cavities, quantification of size may be inaccurate, particularly when assessed using methodologies designed for the left ventricle.[38,95] The advantage of the tripartite approach to classification[38] is that, following angiography, the ventricles can be relatively easily grouped into subtypes. This may be more clinically relevant than estimations of volume. Thus, about three-fifths of cases have the so-called tripartite arrangement, about three-tenths have bipartite cavities, and just under one-tenth have the unipartite form.[23] The disadvantage of this classification is that it is qualitative, and perhaps over-simplistic.[40] Deciding how much muscular overgrowth of the apical region of the right ventricle is needed to make a right ventricle bipartite as opposed to tripartite is very subjective. Furthermore, there is a great deal of variability in size within a subtype. So-called tripartite right ventricles can range from having severely hypoplastic to hugely dilated cavities. It has also been observed that the degree of muscular hypertrophy can increase over time, both pre- and postnatally.[17,39] Despite these limitations, the partite classification is of considerable use. Its ultimate utility may be as one of several morphological markers for the state of the right ventricle, that can be used in combination as independent risk factors for analysis of procedural outcomes.

Dilation of the right heart occurs in just under one-twentieth of cases,[23] and is caused by a tricuspid valve with either severe Ebstein's malformation (Fig. 30-7), or significant tricuspid valvar dysplasia,[15] both these lesions leading to severe tricuspid regurgitation. The dilation of the cavity occurs during fetal life, so that, at birth, the heart fills the entirety of the thoracic cavity, producing the so-called wall-to-wall arrangement[1] (see Fig. 30-7). The right ventricle is still tripartite because none of its portions are overgrown with muscle. It is also very thin-walled, particularly the atrialised portion if there is tricuspid valvar displacement.[95] These hearts may have minimal inlet and trabecular myocardium, superficially resembling hearts with Uhl's anomaly.[96,97] They should not, however, be described in this fashion, since the changes are the consequence of right ventricular dilation, whereas the anomaly described by Uhl is due to congenital absence of the right ventricular parietal musculature. The dilated ventricles seen with pulmonary atresia have low pressures, and hence do not develop right ventricular to coronary arterial fistulous connections (see Table 30-2). The consequence of the gross dilation of the heart is that the lungs become squeezed during fetal life, and do not develop properly. All the component parts are present, but they are unable to expand in appropriate fashion because almost all the space within the thorax is occupied by the heart.[15]

When the right ventricle is very hypertrophied, often in conjunction with tricuspid stenosis, there may be suprasystemic right ventricular pressure, assuming insignificant tricuspid regurgitation (see Table 30-2). It is these hearts that typically are associated with numerous fistulous communications between the ventricular cavity and the coronary arteries, and which can exhibit a right ventricular dependent coronary arterial circulation.

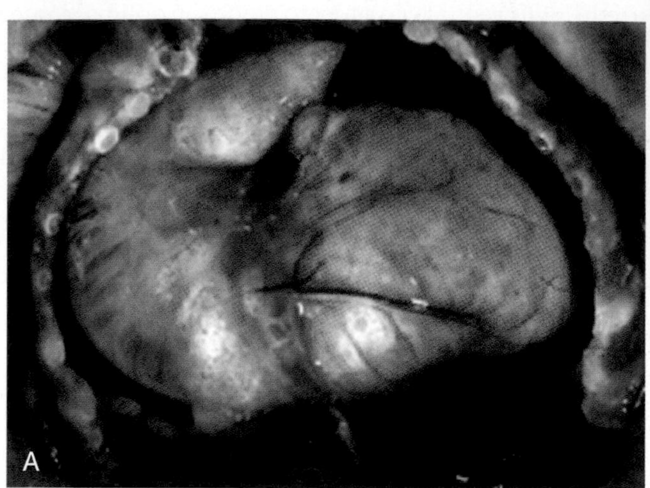

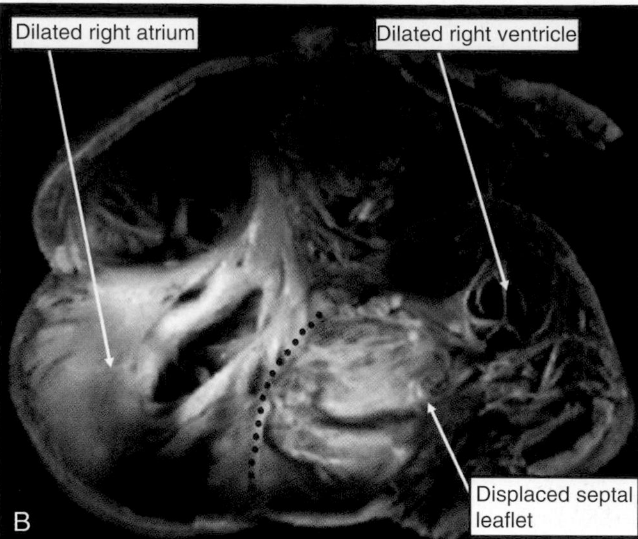

Figure 30-7 A, A typical wall-to-wall heart. The lungs are not seen, being squeezed out by the huge size of the dilated right-sided chambers of the heart. B, Opening the heart shows marked displacement of the hingelines of the leaflets of the tricuspid valve away from the atrioventricular junction (*red dotted line*), the hallmark of Ebstein's malformation.

At a histological level, a wide range of abnormalities of the right ventricle have been found, including subendocardial and transmural ischaemia, fibrosis, infarction, so-called spongy myocardium, myocardial disarray, and endocardial fibroelastosis.[1,2,29,39,44,46,95,98–106] There is an inverse relationship between endocardial fibroelastosis and the presence of fistulous coronary arterial connections, albeit that the reason for this is unknown. It may be that the endocardial fibroelastosis blocks the communications during their development, or alternatively that the communications may decompress the right ventricle, hence preventing the development of endocardial fibroelastosis.[103,107] Ischaemic changes to the right ventricle can be seen even in the absence of fistulous connections.[104]

At a functional level, it is not surprising that the right ventricle shows disorders of both systolic and diastolic function.[105,108,109] Even after complete biventricular repair, diastolic abnormalities have been documented, with antegrade diastolic flow occasionally being found in the pulmonary trunk.[109]

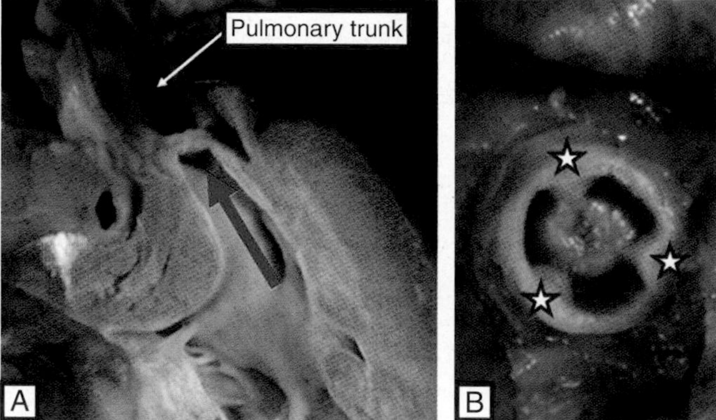

Figure 30-8 A, An infundibulum (*arrow*) that is patent to the level of an imperforate valve. B, When viewed from the arterial aspect there is evidence that the valve initially possessed three leaflets, the sites of attachment to the sinutubular junction being readily apparent (*stars*).

The Right Ventricular Infundibulum

As with the tricuspid valve and the right ventricle, there is a wide spectrum of morphology of the infundibulum. This can range from a patent infundibulum of normal size extending to an atretic valvar membrane[110] (Fig. 30-8), to its complete obliteration by muscular hypertrophy (see Figs. 30-6 and 30-9). The latter arrangement produces the so-called unipartite arrangement of the ventricular cavity[38] (see Tables 30-1 and 30-2). Membranous atresia is found in three-quarters of cases, and muscular in the remainder.[23] In the cases with a well-formed infundibulum, the pulmonary valvar remnant shows evidence of the initial three leaflets, fused along their zones of apposition into a fibrous plate,[44,58,110–112] with raphes showing the sites of fusion (Fig. 30-8B), albeit on occasion the zones of fusion can suggest an initial bifoliate, or even a quadrifoliate valve.

When the outlet component is also obliterated, it is not possible to trace a patent infundibulum to the ventriculo-arterial junction, although evidence of the channel initially present can be seen in dissected hearts (see Fig. 30-6). When examined from the arterial aspect, it can be seen that the pulmonary trunk retains its origin from the right ventricle (see Fig. 30-9), so that the ventriculo-arterial connections remain effectively concordant. The blind-ending pulmonary trunk originates above the triradiating sinuses, with remnants centrally showing that, initially, the root did support valvar tissue (see Fig. 30-9). Assessment of the size of the right ventricular outflow is of great importance when contemplating either surgical or catheter manoeuvres to enlarge the outlet component. Indeed, several groups have advocated taking the size of the outflow tract as a means of determining the best strategy for management.[38,63,81,83,85,86,88,91,113]

Pulmonary Arteries

The pulmonary arteries are usually confluent, and supplied by a left-sided arterial duct.[37] Should systemic-to-pulmonary arteries be encountered, then suspicion should be raised

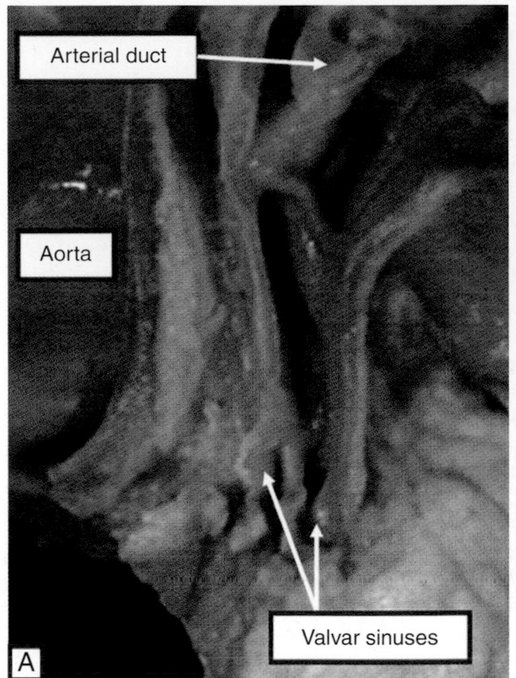

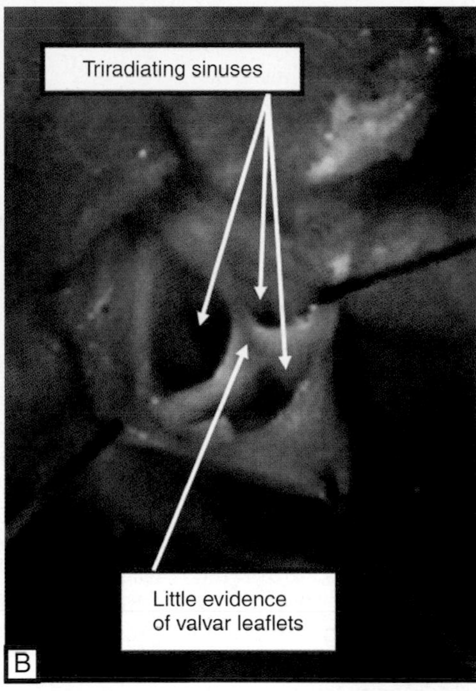

Figure 30-9 In these images, from patients with muscular atresia and unipartite ventricle, the pulmonary trunk has been dissected to show the evidence of sinuses of Valsalva, but absence of any leaflets of the pulmonary valve (**A**) and minimal formation of the leaflets (**B**).

that, initially, there was an interventricular communication, but that the hole between the ventricles closed during fetal life. The pulmonary trunk is usually mildly hypoplastic or of normal size (Fig. 30-10A), although it may, rarely, be small or even no more than a thread-like solid cord (Fig. 30-10B). The dimensions of the pulmonary trunk and arteries may be unrelated to the size of the right ventricular cavity.[44,111] Even those with a tiny right ventricle can have a pulmonary trunk of near-normal size. When the right ventricle is excessively dilated, the pulmonary arteries tend to be severely hypoplastic, with greatly reduced volumes of the pulmonary parenchyma.

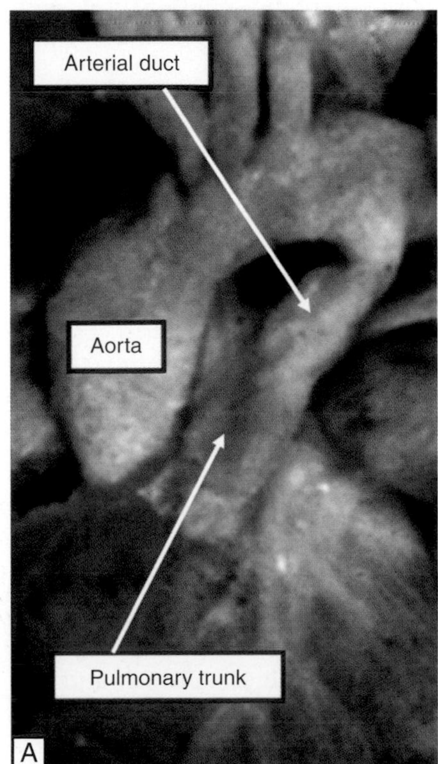

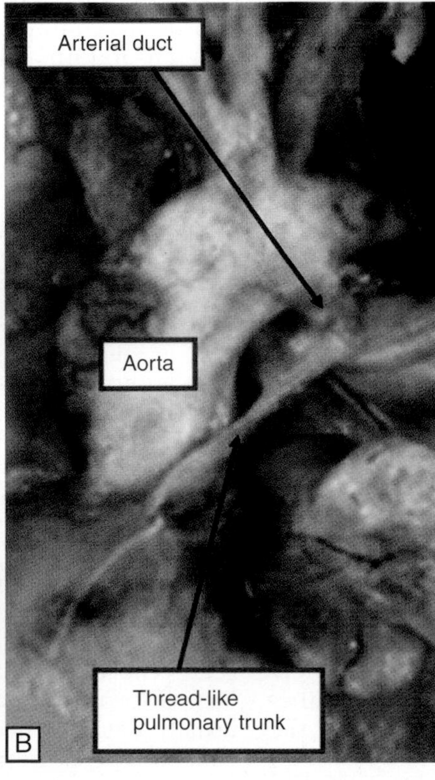

Figure 30-10 The figures show the variability in dimensions of the pulmonary trunk. Usually it is no more than mildly hypoplastic (**A**), but it can rarely be a solid cord (**B**). Note that in both instances pulmonary arterial supply is through the persistently patent arterial duct.

Left Ventricle and Mitral Valve

The mitral valve is usually normal, but dysplasia has been documented.[112,114] The left ventricle is often dilated, with a degree of mural hypertrophy,[112,114] and may exhibit disorders of systolic and diastolic function.[105,108,115–118] With a severely hypertensive right ventricle, the ventricular septum may bulge into the left ventricular outflow tract, thus providing the substrate for subaortic obstruction,[44,112,114] particularly after the Fontan procedure,[119] but only rarely before.[23,120]

At a histological level, abnormalities of the left ventricle may comprise myocardial disarray, non-compacted myocardium, and endocardial fibroelastosis.[44,101,105] An increase in collagen in the subendocardial layer has been implicated as suggesting chronic ischaemia, indicating that the left ventricle may be the limiting factor for long-lasting intervention.[114] Abnormalities of contractility and efficiency noted in patients after the bidirectional Glenn and total cavopulmonary procedures, unrelated to fistulous connections, have also been related to the impact of the high-pressure residual right ventricle impairing left ventricular performance.[118] Abnormalities of the aortic valve have been reported, even critical aortic stenosis.[121] They are rare, but if severe, presage a poor outcome.[112,122–124]

Coronary Arterial Circulation

What sets this lesion apart from most other congenital cardiac disorders is the high incidence of coronary arterial abnormalities.[23,60] These changes were first described in 1926, in a 14-month-old who had intermuscular spaces with free communications between the right ventricular cavity and the coronary arteries.[125] Over the next 50 years, appreciation of their significance changed from innocent bystanders to a major potential cause of myocardial ischaemia.[126] The abnormalities involve disorders of origin and distribution of the coronary arteries, fistulous connections to the right ventricle, absence of proximal connections to the aorta, stenoses or interruption, and hugely dilated ectatic segments. Although some use the term ventriculo-coronary connections synonymously with coronary artery fistulas, a distinction should be drawn between blind-ending sinusoids that may connect to the myocardial capillary bed, but not the coronary arteries, and those connections which are direct communications to the coronary arteries.[30,103] Only in the latter setting is it expected to find histological abnormalities of the coronary arteries themselves.

The ventriculo-coronary fistulous connections can be single or multiple, and tend to communicate with the anterior interventricular or the right coronary arteries, less commonly to the circumflex artery.[23,127] There is a wide spectrum of histopathological changes, found in both the intra- and extramural coronary arteries. These range from mild degrees of intimal and medial thickening, known as myointimal hyperplasia, to loss of normal morphology, with replacement of the arterial wall by fibrocellular tissue.[37] The process can cause severe distortion of the arterial structure, leading to endothelial irregularity, severe stenosis, or obliteration of the lumen.

Right Ventricular Dependent Coronary Arterial Circulation

As awareness of ventriculo-coronary arterial connections developed, so did an appreciation that surgical outcomes could be influenced by their presence and extent. Thus became established the concept of the right ventricular dependent coronary arterial circulation. In the normal situation, flow through the coronary arteries is mediated by the aortic diastolic pressure. Where there are ventriculo-coronary fistulous connections, exposure of the coronary arterial system to the high right ventricular pressures can result in stenoses and distortions, such that the aortic diastolic pressure is insufficient to drive flow into the arteries. The territory distal to the stenosis is then perfused retrogradely in systole by the right ventricle. Thus, the coronary arterial circulation is, at least, in part dependent on the right ventricle. Continued exposure of the arteries to the high pressures generated by the right ventricle then leads to further damage, thus compounding the problem. The consequence is that any intervention, resulting in decompression of the right ventricle, whether surgical or catheter, will lead to loss of coronary arterial perfusion, myocardial ischaemia, infarction, and possibly even death.[2] As summarised by Freedom and colleagues in their excellent review,[2] and listed in decreasing order of severity, the problems include:

- Atresia of the aortic orifices of both coronary arteries[128–132]
- Atresia of the aortic orifice of the left coronary artery[133]
- Proximal interruption or occlusion of the main stem of the left coronary artery, its anterior interventricular or circumflex branches, or the right coronary artery (Fig. 30-11), combined with fistulous communications from the right ventricle
- Important stenosis of the main stem of the left coronary artery, its anterior interventricular or circumflex branches, or the right coronary artery, in combination with fistulous communications from the right ventricle. Less severe abnormalities could also progress with time.
- Presence of a huge fistulous communication from the right ventricle to a coronary artery (Fig. 30-12). Although this situation is rare, decompression of the right ventricle in this setting would result in a massive steal, and hence result in coronary arterial insufficiency.

In two large series, the frequency of such a circulation has been documented at one-twentieth and one-tenth.[23,60,72] Other studies have documented higher frequencies,[92,93,127] but this may partly reflect the degree to which its presence is sought. There is also controversy as to how much myocardium must be jeopardised before the arrangement is termed a right ventricular dependent coronary arterial circulation.[60,134–136] If it is to be of clinical value, of course, the right ventricular dependent coronary arterial circulation must be predicted prior to any attempted decompression.

CLINICAL DIAGNOSIS

Prenatal Diagnosis

Fetal echocardiography is now well-established, and has proved to be effective at detecting the lesion.[17] Cases are usually detected because of an abnormal four-chamber view on echocardiography, but prenatal identification

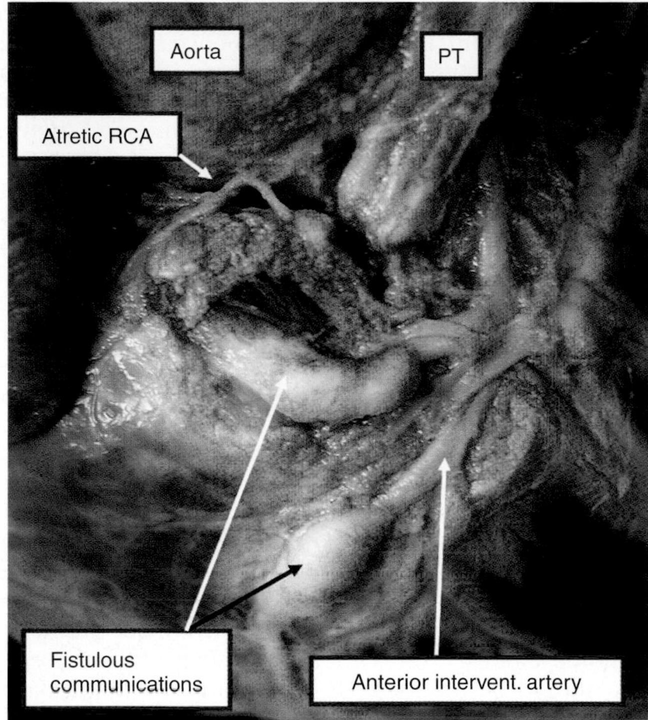

Figure 30-11 This image shows a magnification of the base of the heart. Note that the right coronary artery (RCA) is atretic at its origin from the aorta. The territory of the anterior interventricular (intervent.) artery is fed primarily from the right ventricle by two prominent and ectatic fistulous communications. The pulmonary trunk (PT) is also grossly hypoplastic.

of tricuspid regurgitation, and even recognition of coronary arterial abnormalities, is now feasible.[17,137–142] In the mainland of the United Kingdom, even by the early 1990s, two-fifths of all cases were diagnosed during fetal life.[9] The proportion must now be even higher. This has changed the natural history of the disease, leading at least in the United Kingdom to selective termination of pregnancy, fetal intervention, and planned delivery.

Postnatal Diagnosis

After birth, infants present with cyanosis in the neonatal period. The arterial duct is the sole source of flow of blood to the lungs, although this channel rarely remains widely patent for more than a few days. Very rarely, patients may be found with systemic-to-pulmonary collateral arteries,[23,143–146] but usually, as soon as the duct narrows, arterial desaturation increases, and deep cyanosis results. Closure of the duct may be intermittent at first, and cyanosis may wax and wane. Infants with severe tricuspid regurgitation may also show signs of congestive heart failure.

PHYSICAL FINDINGS

The usual physical findings can be explained by the abnormal morphology. Cyanosis has already been discussed. Pulses and blood pressure are normal, since cardiac output is not impaired. The jugular venous pulse is hard to evaluate in newborns, and is not a useful diagnostic sign. Praecordial motion is normal, since a pure pressure overload of the right ventricle does not usually result in an exaggerated left parasternal lift. The second heart sound at the high left sternal border is soft and single, or is inaudible. The first heart sound is normal, and an ejection sound is not present. Several murmurs may be heard. The most common is a soft high-pitched continuous murmur at the high left sternal border. This murmur originates in the duct, and is usually quite subtle. Occasionally, it may be heard only intermittently, disappearing when the duct narrows and cyanosis deepens, and appearing again as the duct opens and cyanosis lightens. Some infants with pulmonary atresia have a soft high-pitched systolic murmur of tricuspid regurgitation at the low left sternal border. The presence of

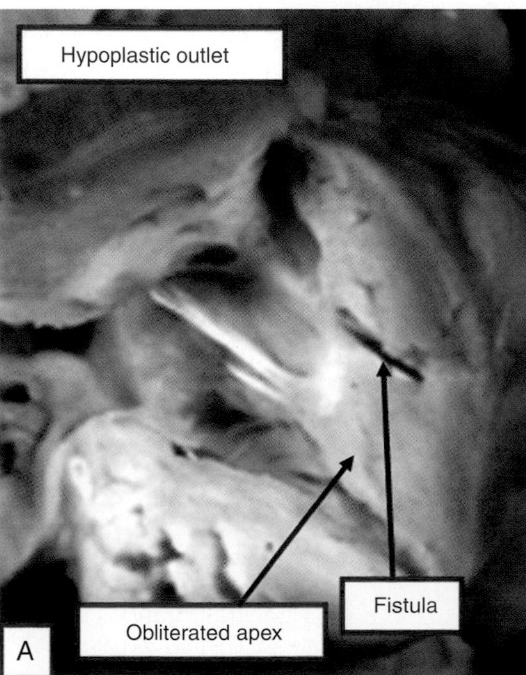

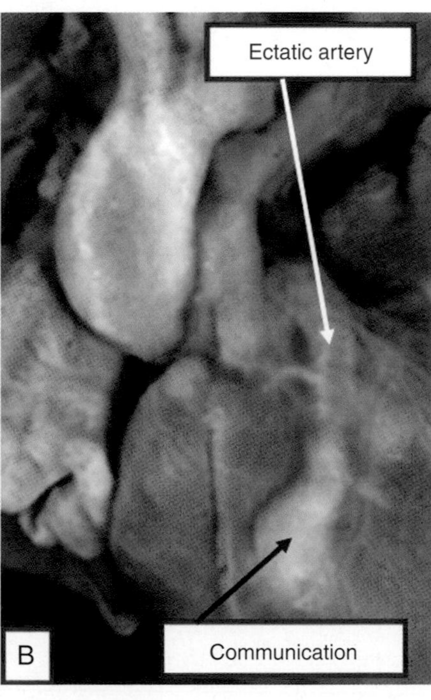

Figure 30-12 In this heart, mural hypertrophy has obliterated the apex and narrowed significantly the outlet component. **A,** A fistulous communication is present in the anterior wall of the right ventricle. **B,** This feeds the ectatic anterior interventricular artery.

this murmur correlates strongly with a relatively large right ventricle,[147] but lack of a murmur of tricuspid regurgitation does not rule out a right ventricle of normal size. When there is severe tricuspid regurgitation, there is often a soft, medium-pitched, mid-diastolic murmur at the low left sternal border, representing increased tricuspid flow. Such a murmur is not heard in those with severe tricuspid stenosis alone, since there is little or no flow across such a valve in the presence of pulmonary atresia. Some infants with pulmonary atresia have no murmur. In this situation, the only indication of congenital cardiac disease on physical examination is the severe cyanosis.

INVESTIGATIONS

Electrocardiography

The electrocardiogram is usually abnormal, and reflects the abnormal morphology. The frontal plane axis is less rightward than normal, usually between 30 and 90 degrees. Most newborns have an adult praecordial pattern, rather than the usual right ventricular hypertrophy (Fig. 30-13). Less commonly, the pattern of right ventricular hypertrophy is present. It must be noted that the electrocardiographic patterns of right ventricular hypertrophy, or of left ventricular predominance, do not reliably predict right ventricular size. ST–T wave changes suggestive of myocardial ischaemia are occasionally present and may be related to the abnormal coronary arteries.[126] The tall peaked P waves of right atrial enlargement may be present.

Chest Radiography

There is no characteristic radiographic appearance. The abdominal organs are normally positioned, and the heart is left-sided. The bronchi are normally lateralised, and the aortic arch is left sided. Pulmonary vascular markings are not increased, but the distinction between normal and decreased markings is difficult at best in the neonatal period, which is when most infants with pulmonary atresia present. The cardiac contour is not distinctive, and there is a wide range of cardiac size, from normal to wall-to-wall (Fig. 30-14). Although the very largest hearts occur when there is severe tricuspid regurgitation, the size of the heart is not a reliable predictor of the size of the right ventricular cavity.

Echocardiography

Cross sectional echocardiography is the diagnostic investigation of choice. As well as confirming the diagnosis, it is important also to document all the morphological features systematically, and then use the findings to determine the optimal strategy for treatment. In the first instance, the atrial arrangement should be confirmed. The right atrium will often be dilated. Any prominent venous valves should be noted. The oval foramen is usually widely patent before, but not always after, construction of a systemic-to-pulmonary shunt.[148] Next, the morphology of the tricuspid valve should be assessed, documenting any dysplasia or displacement of the leaflets (Fig. 30-15). The degree and velocity of regurgitation should be recorded (Fig. 30-16). The diameter of the valvar orifice should be measured, and converted to a *z* score using published nomograms.[75,76] The measured orifice may not represent the effective orifice, particularly where there is limited opening due to tethering or raised filling pressures.

The right ventricle should be assessed to determine its overall size, and the degree of mural overgrowth (Fig. 30-17). A judgement should be made as to whether the cavity possesses all three of its components, or only one

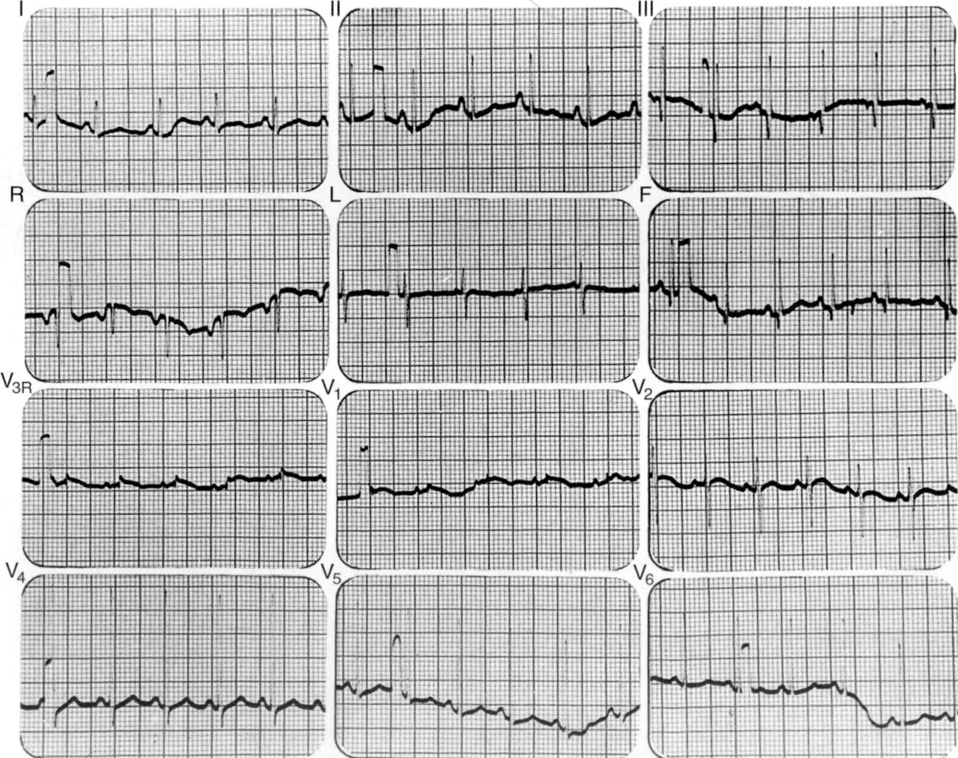

Figure 30-13 Electrocardiogram demonstrating right atrial enlargement and left ventricular predominance that is abnormal for a term newborn infant.

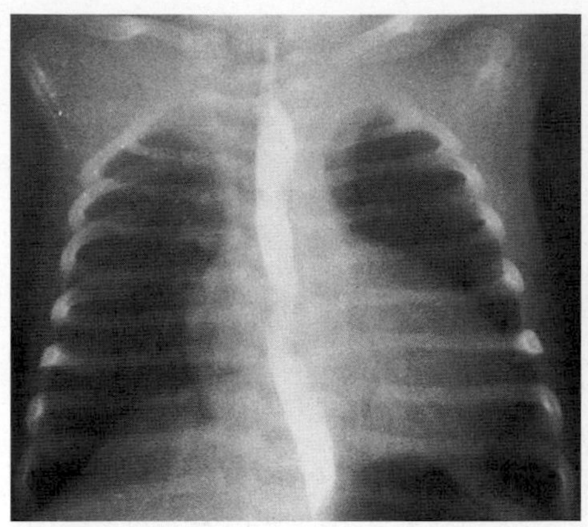

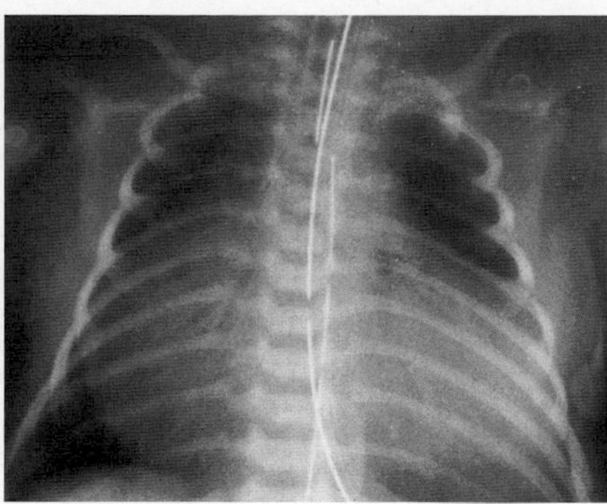

Figure 30-14 Chest radiographs in two patients with pulmonary atresia and intact ventricular septum. **A,** Moderate cardiomegaly, right atrial enlargement, and decreased pulmonary vascular markings. **B,** Marked cardiomegaly in an infant with Ebstein's malformation of the tricuspid valve and severe tricuspid regurgitation.

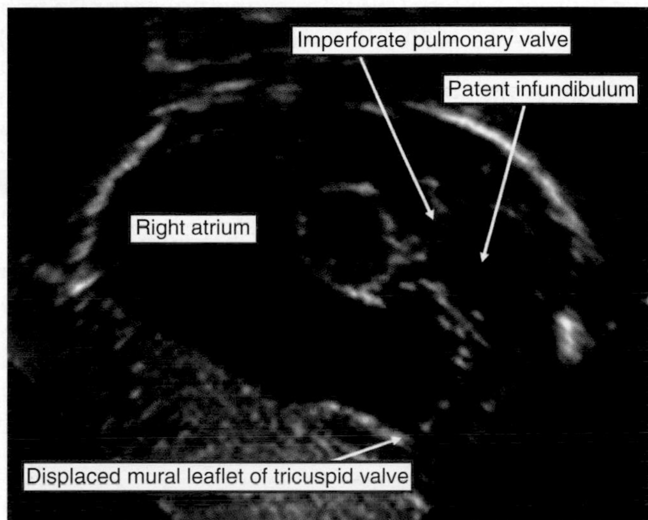

Figure 30-15 This subcostal para-oblique view reveals a tripartite right ventricle with an imperforate pulmonary valve. There is minimal mural hypertrophy, but there is Ebstein's malformation of the tricuspid valve.

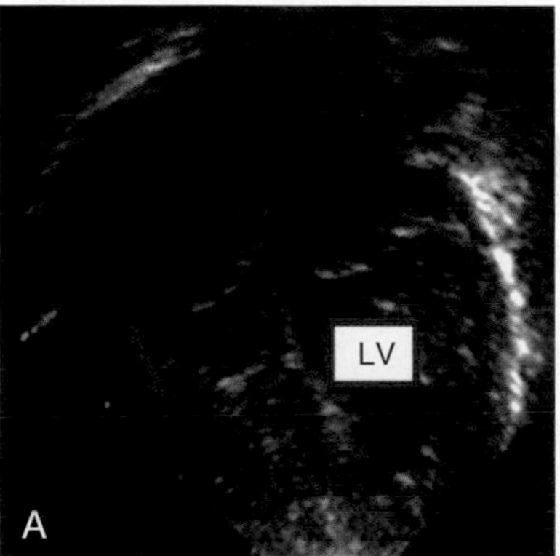

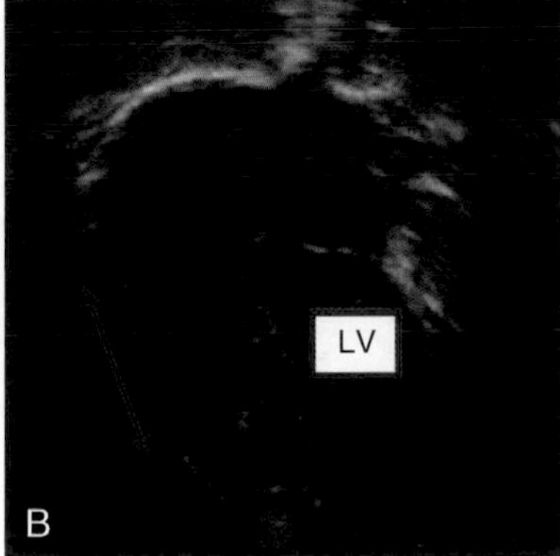

Figure 30-17 These two echocardiograms, both showing the four-chamber, illustrate the range in size of the right ventricular cavity. The upper panel shows a unipartite right ventricle, with considerable mural hypertrophy and obliteration of the cavity *(arrow)*. The lower panel shows a tripartite right ventricle of near-normal size *(arrow)*, with minimal mural hypertrophy. LV, left ventricle.

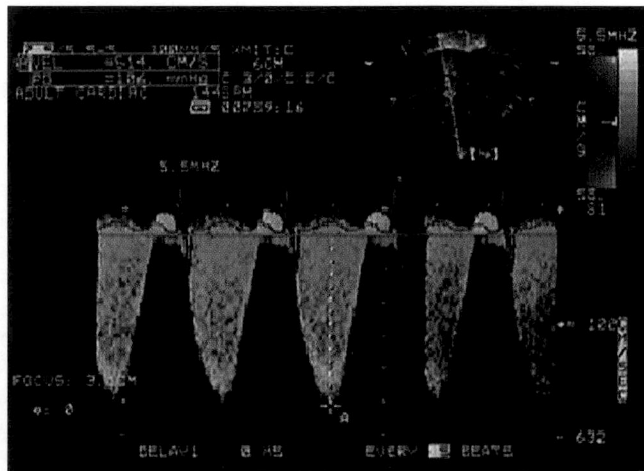

Figure 30-16 The image shows the continuous Doppler trace through the tricuspid valve of a baby with pulmonary atresia and intact ventricular septum. There is high velocity tricuspid regurgitation, with a peak velocity of more than 5 m/s, indicative of supra-systemic right ventricular pressures.

or two. In our experience, the right ventricular cavity may seem smaller echocardiographically than it appears angiographically, largely because the apical trabecular zone may seem completely obliterated when, in reality, there are intertrabecular spaces. The presence of tiny ventricular septal defects should be noted. An assessment of the patency of the infundibulum should be made, particularly from the subcostal para-oblique view. The atresia may be membranous (Fig. 30-18) or muscular depending on the extent of muscular mural hypertrophy. The presence of any forward or retrograde flow across the pulmonary valve should be assessed to exclude critical pulmonary stenosis

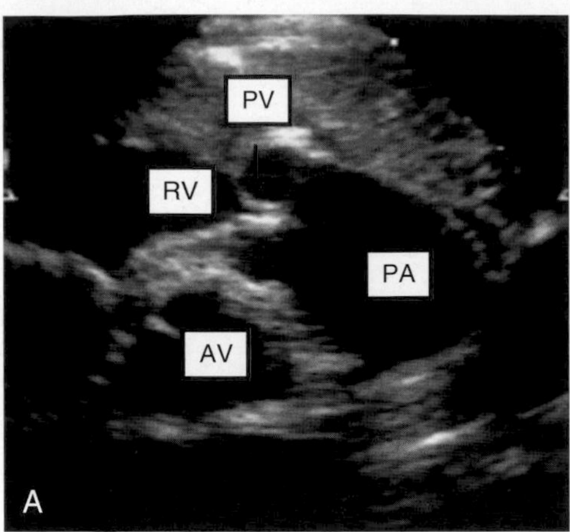

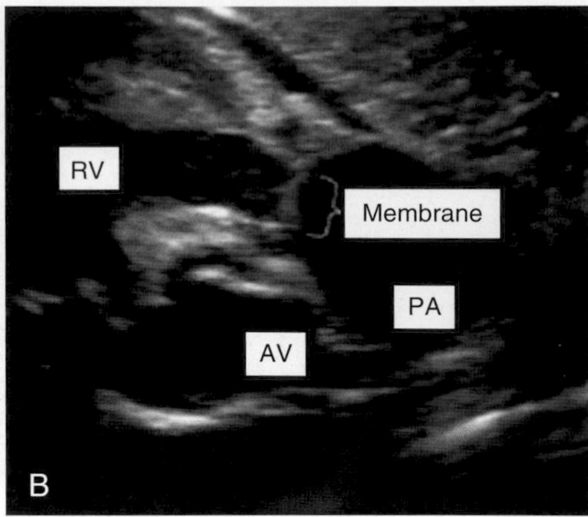

Figure 30-18 These images show an imperforate pulmonary valve suitable for balloon perforation. The left hand panel, seen from the parasternal short-axis view in ventricular diastole, demonstrates a normal appearance of the valve leaflets. The right hand panel shows the imperforate valve in systole, with excursion of the fused valvar leaflets. AV, aortic valve; PA, pulmonary trunk; PV, pulmonary valve; RV, right ventricle. (Reproduced with permission from Abrams DJR, Rigby ML, Daubeney PEF: Membranous pulmonary atresia treated by radiofrequency-assisted balloon pulmonary valvotomy. Circulation 2003; 107:e98–e99.)

or functional atresia. The presence of any fistulous communication to the coronary arteries should be sought.

The pulmonary trunk and branches should be measured to ascertain their size, and the source of flow of blood to the lungs determined. Normal pulmonary venous return should be confirmed. Structure and function of the left ventricle should be assessed, including regional abnormalities of mural motion.

Following such investigations, it should be possible to decide whether the long-term strategy is for biventricular as opposed to univentricular repair, and to plan the initial intervention.

Cardiac Catheterisation and Angiography

Despite the increased role of echocardiography, cardiac catheterisation and angiography may still be helpful in the evaluation of an infant with this lesion, particularly to assess the size of the right ventricle, and the presence and severity of fistulous communications. The usual approach is via the femoral vein, as it can be difficult to enter the right ventricle from the umbilical vein.[149] The latter approach can be used, however, for balloon atrial septostomy. Oximetry is not particularly helpful, except to show right-to-left shunting at atrial level. A step-up from right atrium to ventricle of more than 6% is said to be indicative of retrograde flow into the right ventricle from coronary arterial fistulous connections.[149] Mean right atrial pressure is usually slightly higher than left atrial, but a large gradient is not expected, since the oval foramen is usually large and widely patent. Right ventricular pressure is usually suprasystemic, although right ventricular pressure is low if tricuspid regurgitation is very severe (see Table 30-2). If the right ventricle is small, it may be entered only after repeated probing with an end-hole catheter.

The diagnosis will usually have already been made by echocardiography, but it can be confirmed by the right ventriculogram. Assessment of right ventricular size is far from simple in often bizarrely shaped right ventricles[150,151] (Fig. 30-19). Stenosis or atresia of the infundibulum can be diagnosed. If an imperforate pulmonary valve is present, it may be seen moving to and fro at the top of a patent infundibulum. Tricuspid regurgitation can be roughly quantified, since catheter-induced regurgitation is usually mild. Coronary arterial fistulous connections are also well-demonstrated by right ventriculography (see Fig. 30-19). Stenoses in, or interruption of, both right and left coronary arteries should be sought. If there is doubt about the coronary arterial anatomy or distribution after the right ventriculogram, then an injection should be performed in the aortic root. A left ventriculogram should also be performed, both for judging the relative right ventricular size, and to visualise the duct and the pulmonary trunk. Simultaneous injection into the aorta and into the right ventricle may show the extent of the gap between the right ventricular cavity and the pulmonary trunk in the presence of muscular atresia.[126] Cardiac catheterisation nowadays can be the prelude to an interventional approach to management.

Other Imaging Modalities

There has been rapid development of cardiac magnetic resonance and computerised tomographic imaging over the past decade. Both offer non-invasive alternatives to cardiac catheterisation and angiography, and may ultimately supplant such invasive techniques.[152] They both provide excellent three-dimensional anatomical imaging of the cardiovascular system. Magnetic resonance provides assessment of flows, and does not require ionising radiation, but usually requires anaesthesia in the newborn. Computerised tomography offers fast acquisition, and perhaps better resolution, but does require ionising radiation.

HAEMODYNAMICS AND PHYSIOLOGY

Systemic venous return to the right atrium is normal (see Fig. 30-1). The flow prenatally was to the left atrium through a patent oval foramen, and to the left heart, continuing retrogradely via the arterial duct into the pulmonary arteries. This continues after birth until closure of the duct. The increased pulmonary venous return to the left atrium may reduce the size of the foramen, which is particularly important after construction of a systemic-to-pulmonary arterial shunt, since the restrictive foramen may need to be enlarged using balloon atrial septostomy.[148]

When the tricuspid valve is hypoplastic, its opening may be limited anatomically, but also functionally by high filling pressures. The right ventricular pressure will then be

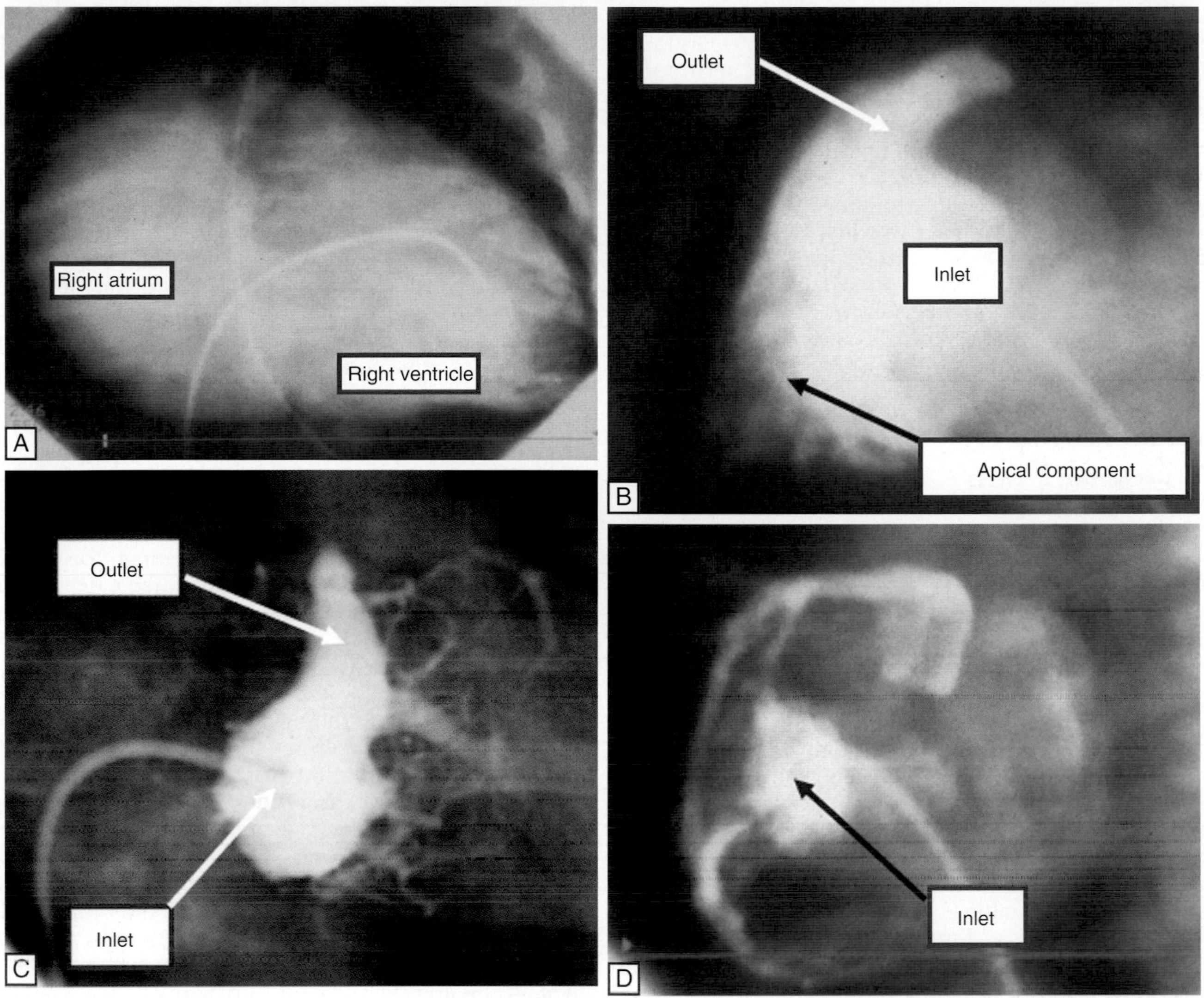

Figure 30-19 The angiograms show the range of morphology to be seen in pulmonary atresia with intact ventricular septum. **A,** Right ventricular angiogram showing a dilated and thin-walled right ventricle and atrium, with severe tricuspid regurgitation, in the setting of an imperforate pulmonary valve, seen in the frontal projection. **B,** A so-called tripartite right ventricle, seen in lateral view. **C,** Frontal projection showing the so-called bipartite arrangement, in this instance with an imperforate pulmonary valve and some fistulous connections with the coronary arteries. **D,** Lateral projection showing the tiny, so-called unipartite, arrangement with muscular atresia and fistulous communications filling the coronary arteries.

supra-systemic. Egress of blood from the right ventricle is via low volume, but high velocity, tricuspid regurgitation and/or ventriculo-coronary arterial connections into the aorta during systole. There can be retrograde filling of the right ventricle from the coronary arteries during diastole. Right ventricular systolic pressures can cause high shear stress to the coronary arterial walls, leading to stenoses and the right ventricular dependent coronary arterial circulation. In these circumstances, alteration of the balance of right ventricular and aortic diastolic pressures can lead to myocardial infarction. Hence, right ventricular decompression should be avoided whenever there is a right ventricular dependent coronary arterial circulation. Caution should be undertaken when creating a systemic-to-pulmonary arterial shunt, taking care to ligate the arterial duct so as to prevent any disastrous falls in the diastolic blood pressures.[153]

Left ventricular function can also be affected,[44,112,114] and it has been suggested that the left ventricle may ultimately be the limiting factor in this disease.[114] Long-term haemodynamic effects usually reflect residual lesions. Biventricular circulation may be complicated by the long-term effects of residual pulmonary stenosis, regurgitation, and tricuspid regurgitation. The functionally univentricular circulation may be complicated by the long-term effects of high venous pressure, right atrial dilation, and coronary arterial stenoses. Incompletely separated circulations may suffer the additional long-term effects of cyanosis.[152]

THERAPEUTIC OPTIONS

Historical Perspective

Already by the mid 1950s, pulmonary valvotomy had been proposed as an appropriate treatment when the right ventricle was of good size.[78,154] It was also suggested that a systemic-to-pulmonary arterial shunt be performed when the right ventricle was small.[155] The first reports of successful surgery came from the Mayo Clinic, the University of Minnesota, and the Henry Ford Hospital.[155–157]

The combination of repair of the right ventricular outflow tract and construction of a systemic-to-pulmonary arterial shunt was first reported in 1971.[158] These techniques are still the mainstay of surgical interventions today, but the indications for each have been considerably refined as our knowledge of the morphological complexities have grown.

Successful percutaneous perforation of the atretic pulmonary valve with a catheter was first reported in 1991, using either a guide-wire,[159] laser energy,[160,161] or radiofrequency energy.[162,163] This approach has now become the treatment of choice in many centres for those patients with a good-sized right ventricle and an atretic valvar membrane.

Contemporary Approaches

Fetal Intervention

Fetal intervention is now a reality, although its rate of success at present is low, and it must still be considered an experimental technique.[164–167] Its role in management is still being explored.

Postnatal Intervention

Since the lesion is duct-dependent, an infusion of prostaglandin is commenced after diagnosis, and the baby transferred to a cardiac unit. The investigations discussed above are performed to identify the unique constellation of morphological features. The long-term goal of intervention is to separate the pulmonary and systemic circulations. The investigations, therefore, are directed to ascertain whether this can be achieved by creating either biventricular or functionally univentricular circulations. Different strategies are adopted depending on whether it is deemed likely that one or other repair is possible (Table 30-3).

For patients with a diminutive right ventricle, which would never support the pulmonary circulation, the ultimate aim would be a modified Fontan-type circulation in which systemic venous return was directly to the pulmonary arteries. This strategy would commence initially with consideration of a balloon atrial septostomy. Unless the oval foramen is substantial, a septostomy is recommended, the more so since, after construction of a systemic-to-pulmonary arterial shunt, the foramen can become restrictive, either immediately or over time, with disastrous outcome.[148] Following septostomy, the shunt is constructed,[155] usually a left- or right-sided modified Blalock-Taussig shunt. The next procedure, performed at the age of 3 to 24 months, would be a bidirectional cavopulmonary anastomosis. The Fontan circulation would then be completed at the age of 24 to 60 months.

Surgical management of the right ventricle of good size is aimed at achieving a biventricular circulation, in which the right ventricle can pump blood to the lungs (see Table 30-3). This needs consideration of the size and function of the tricuspid valve and right ventricle. Where there is a good-sized right ventricle and infundibulum, then a pulmonary valvotomy or valvectomy can be performed,[78] with or without cardiopulmonary bypass, and with or without creation of a systemic-to-pulmonary arterial shunt as an adjuvant to pulmonary flow. Where there is a less substantial infundibulum, a transjunctional patch can be performed with a limited ventriculotomy, or alternatively a pulmonary homograft inserted. Where there is doubt about whether the right ventricle alone can provide enough forward flow to the pulmonary arteries, a transjunctional patch could be combined with a systemic-to-pulmonary arterial shunt.[168] Ultimately, as the right ventricular hypertrophy regresses and compliance improves, the shunt can be closed. In those in whom this initial approach failed to lead to growth of the right ventricle, the right ventricular hypertrophy can be debulked, combined with repair of the tricuspid and pulmonary valves as required.[169]

Where forward flow through a repaired right ventricular outflow is insufficient to prevent cyanosis, a bidirectional cavopulmonary anastomosis can also be created. This has been termed the one and a half ventricle repair, and may be a suitable long-term palliation for some bipartite right ventricles.[170] Variations of the above strategies have been described, whereby continuity is maintained between the right atrium and the superior caval vein.[171]

For patients with a right ventricular dependent coronary arterial circulation, other procedures have been proposed, such as closure of the tricuspid valve at the same time as concurrent procedures,[172–174] or construction of a conduit from the aorta to the right ventricle.[175–177] More recently, it has been shown that a successful outcome can be achieved

TABLE 30-3

OPTIONS FOR MANAGEMENT FOR EACH INITIAL STRATEGY

Initial Strategy		Procedures			
Biventricular repair		Catheter	Wire perforation + balloon dilation Laser perforation + balloon dilation Radio-frequency perforation + balloon dilation		
		Surgery	Pulmonary valvotomy Pulmonary valvectomy Transjunctional patch Monocusp homograft		
	Any of above with systemic to pulmonary shunt				
Univentricular repair	Balloon atrial septostomy	Surgery	Systemic-to-pulmonary shunt	Superior cavopulmonary anastomosis	Total cavopulmonary connection

From Daubeney PEF: Pulmonary atresia with intact ventricular septum. In Gatzoulis MA, Webb GD, Daubeney PEF (eds): Diagnosis and Management of Adult Congenital Heart Disease. London: Churchill Livingstone, 2003, pp 339–347 by following a staged palliation directed towards completion of a fenestrated Fontan circulation.[178]

Various controversies still remain. Whether a procedure on the right ventricular outflow tract should be performed in all cases, even when the right ventricle is diminutive, excepting cases of right ventricular dependence, is unresolved. Whether all such procedures should also be accompanied by construction of a systemic-to-pulmonary arterial shunt is also not clear. The need for a transjunctional patch needs clarification. Lastly, it needs to be resolved whether an early procedure on the right ventricular outflow tract is required to optimise right ventricular growth.

Catheter Management

The majority of patients have membranous rather than muscular atresia, with a patent infundibulum, and often a well-developed right ventricular cavity (see Fig. 30-18). Diverse surgical strategies have been recommended for this group, such as neonatal valvotomy, valvectomy, and transjunctional patching with or without concomitant placement of a systemic-to-pulmonary shunt. Since the early 1990s, there has been an increasing trend toward perforation of the atretic pulmonary valve as the primary procedure.[67,68,74,148,159–163,179–191] In some cases, the arterial duct is also stented.[188] As technical success in perforating the atretic valve has increased, the place of this technique in the management of those with good-sized right ventricles has been hotly debated. This issue remains unanswered, but from a pragmatic stance, the choice of surgical versus catheter valvotomy in an individual institution should be determined on the basis of the technique which causes the least mortality and morbidity.

Outcomes of Intervention

After hypoplastic left heart syndrome, this lesion has proved to be one of the most disappointing to treat. Improvement in outcome over the past 20 years has been extremely slow (Table 30-4), with occasion exceptions.[90] In Figure 30-20, survival curves are shown as drawn from the population-based study conducted in the United Kingdom and Eire, stratified for initial procedure and the partite state of the right ventricle.[9,148]

Why this lesion should have such a poor outcome is not well-identified, and optimal strategies for treatment remain to be elucidated. The largest four studies have identified risk factors for poor outcome. These include factors relating to the small size of the right ventricle, dilated right ventricular size, low birth weight and prematurity, presence of right ventricular-to-coronary artery fistulous connections, and a right ventricular dependent coronary arterial circulation.[60,66,72,84,92,148] As more is learnt about adverse risk factors, clinicians are tailoring their approach, for example by not decompressing right ventricles where there is thought to be a right ventricular dependent arterial circulation. Freedom and colleagues stated in 2005 that 'ventriculo-coronary connections, and a right ventricular dependent coronary circulation, an important risk factor in our (their) earlier surgical experience,[84,192] therefore, had been effectively neutralised by the introduction of the functionally univentricular palliation'.[2]

Catheter perforation of the imperforate pulmonary valve is now a well-established technique for primary intervention. It accounted for three-fifths of all valvotomies performed without concomitant construction of a shunt in the study carried out in the United Kingdom and Eire.[148] When analysed on the basis of intention to treat, survival was similar between those treated at catheterisation or surgically. A recent report notes ongoing technical improvement, with a mortality of only 10%.[188] Successful perforation of the atretic pulmonary valve is not guaranteed, but rates of success recently published range from 85 to 90%.[185–187]

LONG-TERM OUTCOME

Survivors are now reaching adulthood, but their numbers are small due to the rarity of the disease, and high mortality in previous eras. Little data is available about long-term survival and functional state. Mortality tends to occur in the first 6 months of life and the survival curves then flatten (see Fig. 30-20).[60,148,193] One study documented survival after 14 years following biventricular repair of 86%.[193] Of the patients, one-fifth had late arrhythmias, and right atrial dilation was found in all patients. At the current time, prediction of longer-term outcome for a biventricular repair can only be made by drawing parallels with other diseases, such as those who have undergone definitive repair of pulmonary stenosis and tetralogy of Fallot (see Chapters 43 and 36).

For those embarking down the route toward construction of the Fontan circulation, mortality tends to occur early in childhood, often within a few months of the initial procedure.[60,194] There is an ongoing mortality hazard but the early data available indicates that the influence of coronary arterial abnormalities may be less than predicted.[194,195]

TABLE 30-4

COMPARATIVE MORTALITY FROM THE LARGEST FIVE STUDIES OF PULMONARY ATRESIA WITH INTACT VENTRICULAR SEPTUM

Name of Study/Centre	Years	Study Number	Survival at 1 Year	Survival at 5 Years	Reference
Great Ormond Street	1976–1989*	135	72%†	49%†	Bull et al[66]
UK and Ireland population-based	1991–1995	183	71%‡	64%‡	Daubeney et al[9]
Congenital Heart Surgeons	1987–1997	408	68%	60%	Ashburn et al[72]
Toronto	1992–1998*	210	75%	67%	Dyamenahalli et al[92]
UCLA, Los Angeles	1982–2001	106	88%†	86%	Odim et al[93]

*Uses most recent era data from the study.
†Estimate of mortality at 1 and 5 years.
‡Survival of those who underwent a procedure.

Figure 30-20 The graphs show the Kaplan-Meier survival curves for subgroups of patients with pulmonary atresia and intact ventricular septum. (Data from the UK and Ireland population-based study.[148])

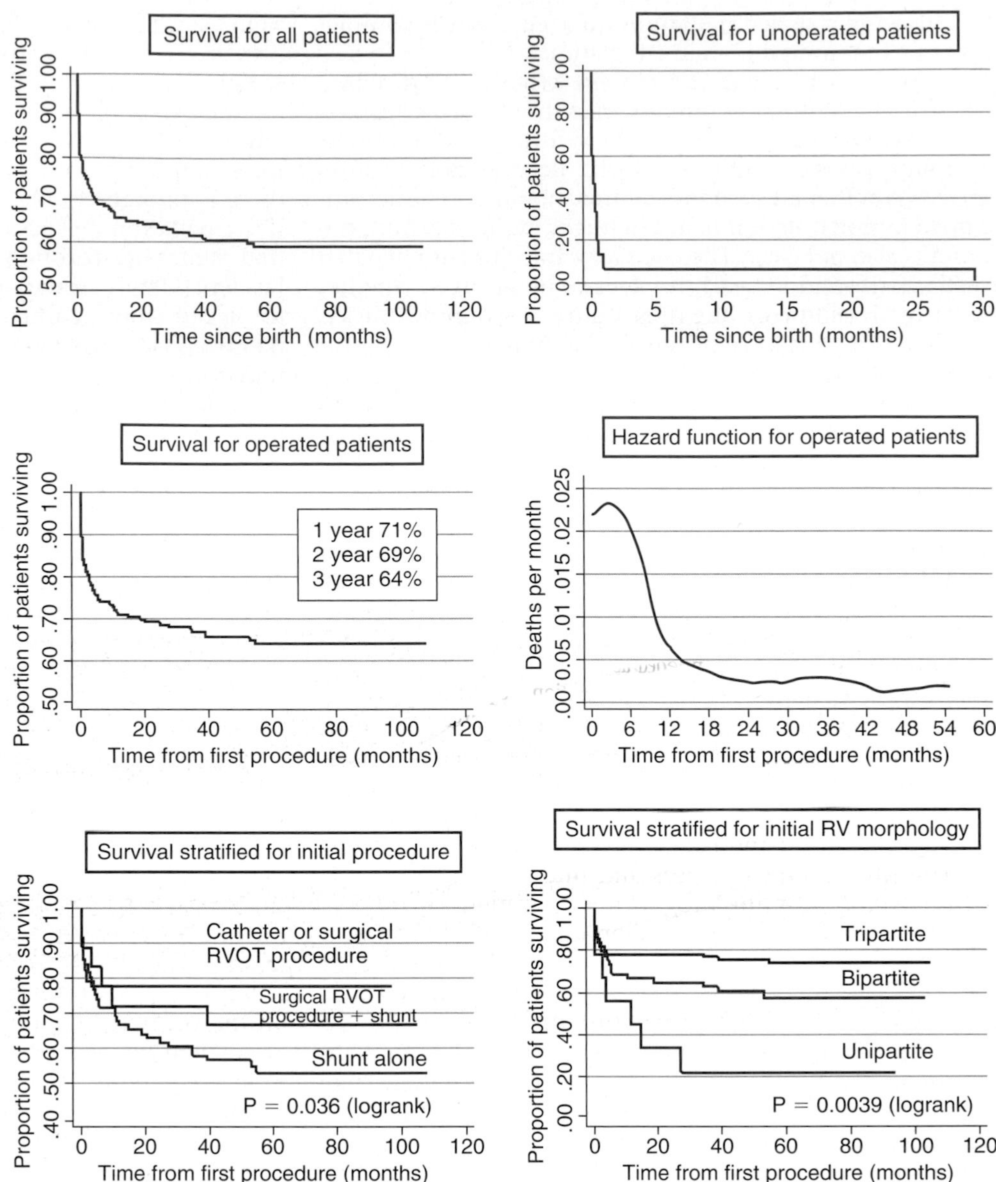

In the future it will be interesting to discover how persisting right ventricular hypertension, and coronary arterial fistulous connections, influence long-term outcome.

Recommendations for Long-term Follow-up

For those with a biventricular repair and minimal residual haemodynamic lesions, patients should be seen every 1 to 3 years by a cardiologist. Where there are significant residual lesions, follow-up should be yearly by an adult congenital cardiologist. Similarly, patients with mixed or functionally univentricular circulations warrant follow-up in a tertiary centre. For patients with venous shunts, or the Fontan circulation, strong consideration should be given to full anticoagulation, particularly if there is suspicion of coronary arterial abnormalities.

Exercise limitations need to be reviewed on an individual basis, depending on type of surgical route followed, the underlying haemodynamics, and the overall state of the patient. Endocarditis prophylaxis is not required but high levels of dental hygiene are recommended.

At each visit, it is essential to assess residual morphological lesions. Following a biventricular repair, the patient should be pink, with normal volume pulses, albeit that the jugular venous pulse may be elevated, and the right ventricular impulse increased. There will usually be a normal first heart sound with single second, which may be split if a homograft has been inserted. Murmurs of residual pulmonary stenosis, regurgitation, and tricuspid regurgitation may be evident. Hepatomegaly may be present. Indeed, if tricuspid regurgitation is severe, the liver may be pulsatile. Patients are prone to atrial arrhythmia.

Following a Fontan procedure, the patient should be pink, with saturations in the 90s, brachial pulses may be absent following previous arterial shunt procedures, the jugular venous pulse will be greatly elevated, and may only be visible on sitting up. There will be a single heart second. There may be a murmur from tricuspid regurgitation or a systolic murmur caused by blood flow from a high pressured right ventricle into a coronary arterial fistula. Hepatic congestion may be evident.

For patients with a mixed circulation, the patient will be cyanosed with clubbing, erythrocytosis, possible continuous murmurs due to patent systemic shunts, and may have features of either circulation described above.

Chest radiography will often show an increased cardiothoracic ratio with, in particular, a dilated right atrial contour. In patients with severe tricuspid regurgitation, the right ventricle may also be dilated. In those with a mixed circulation, there may be pulmonary oligaemia.

The electrocardiogram may show the presence of arrhythmias, atrial or ventricular. There is often P pulmonale due to right atrial dilatation. The QRS axis usually shows left ventricular dominance.

Echocardiography should be used to document systematically and sequentially all the morphological features discussed at the beginning of this chapter. Residual lesions such as atrial septal defects and patent systemic shunts should be sought. For those with a biventricular circulation, the presence and degree of tricuspid regurgitation, pulmonary regurgitation, and stenosis should be documented. The size and z score of the tricuspid valve should be documented. For those with a Fontan circulation, careful assessment of the anastomoses is needed as well as assessment of left ventricular function, mitral regurgitation and the presence of right atrial thrombus. Imaging of the coronary artery origins and their size may suggest significant fistulous communications.

Cardiac catheterisation may be required to assess the haemodynamics of the Fontan circuit. Coronary arteriography is essential as stenoses and interruptions may play a significant part in the prognosis. Assessment of the pulmonary arterial anatomy is important, as the patient may have had a systemic-to-pulmonary arterial shunt in the past, with pulmonary arterial distortion. In contrast to pulmonary atresia with tetralogy of Fallot, native stenoses or hypoplasia of the pulmonary arteries are relatively uncommon. Baffle leaks should be sought in those with a Fontan circulation.

Cardiac magnetic imaging and computer tomography may supplant catheterisation as a means of non-invasive assessment of the range of morphological lesions found in this condition. They give excellent anatomic and, in the case of magnetic imaging, excellent functional information.

Nuclear imaging conveys important information about myocardial perfusion and ischaemia, particularly for those patients with significant coronary artery lesions although abnormal anatomy imposes technical challenges.

Implications in Adult Life

Physiological

Many patients with this condition are reaching adulthood. Their well-being in adult life depends on the cumulative effect of complications throughout their life, be they cardiac and non-cardiac, reasonable cardiac function, and avoidance of residual lesions.[152]

For those with biventricular or one and a half ventricle repairs, residual lesions comprise pulmonary stenosis, regurgitation, and tricuspid regurgitation. These can lead to atrial and ventricular arrhythmias, syncope, sudden death, reduced exercise tolerance, fatigability, and angina. For those with a functionally univentricular repair, such as a total cavopulmonary connection or Fontan-type circulation, residual lesions comprise right atrial dilation, coronary arterial stenoses, high systemic venous pressures, and systemic-to-pulmonary arterial and venous collateralisation. These can lead to atrial and ventricular arrhythmias, sudden death, thrombo-embolism, right pulmonary venous occlusion, angina, left ventricular dysfunction, protein-losing enteropathy, hepatic dysfunction and cyanosis. For those with incompletely separated circulations, there is common mixing of systemic and pulmonary circulations leading to cyanosis, erythrocytosis, thrombo-embolism, fatigability, and arrhythmias.

Contraception and Pregnancy

Pre-pregnancy counseling is essential. This should include contraceptive advice tailored to the individual cardiac structure and function. Those with a good biventricular repair should be suitable for all forms of contraception. Those with ongoing cyanosis or a Fontan-type circulation should avoid the combined contraceptive pill. Detailed advice is beyond the scope of this book but is thoroughly covered elsewhere.[196]

Biventricular Repair with Residual Pulmonary Stenosis or Regurgitation

The increased haemodynamic load of pregnancy may precipitate right heart failure, atrial arrhythmias, or tricuspid regurgitation. Balloon dilation can be performed during pregnancy, preferably after organogenesis, although it is better to treat before conception.

Functionally Univentricular Circulation

There are increased risks of systemic venous congestion, deterioration in ventricular function, atrial arrhythmias, thrombo-embolism, and paradoxical embolisation if there is a fenestration in the atrial baffle. Successful pregnancy is possible, however, with meticulous cardiac and obstetric planning and supervision. If anticoagulation is required additional risks to the fetus are involved.

Mixed Circulations with Cyanosis

There is an increased risk of maternal cardiovascular complications, prematurity and fetal death, particularly when baseline maternal resting saturations are less than 85%.

All patients should have cardiological counselling prior to conception, and follow-up by an adult congenital cardiologist and a high-risk obstetrician during pregnancy and the peripartum. Fetal echocardiography is recommended.

Insurance and Employment

This will depend on the original diagnosis and residual lesions. There may not be specific stratification of risk for this particular lesion, and parallels from other lesions, such as pulmonary stenosis, tetralogy of Fallot, and patients with Fontan-type circulations, may have to be taken. Employability will depend on exercise ability, avoidance of complications, and ongoing particularly neurological morbidity. Employment would need to be tailored to individual needs. Detailed discussion of these topics is beyond the scope of this chapter, albeit that they are thoroughly covered elsewhere.[197]

The complete reference list can be found on the companion Expert Consult web site at www.expertconsult.com.

ANNOTATED REFERENCES

- Freedom RM (ed): Pulmonary Atresia with Intact Ventricular Septum. Mount Kisco, NY: Futura Publishing Company, 1989.

  A superb monograph of all facets of this disease. Although the outcome data is dated this is an excellent resource for those wishing further insight into this disease.

- Freedom RM, Anderson RH, Perrin D: The significance of ventriculo-coronary arterial connections in the setting of pulmonary atresia with an intact ventricular septum. Cardiol Young 2005;15:447–468.

  An encyclopaedic review ostensibly of the role of fistulas in this condition but containing a wide-ranging review of historical perspective, morphology, pathology, fetal diagnosis and outcome.
- Freedom RM, Jaeggi E, Perrin D, et al: The "wall-to-wall" heart in the patient with pulmonary atresia and intact ventricular septum. Cardiol Young 2006;16:18–29.

  A further in-depth review focussing on the dilated right ventricle in this condition. A definitive review containing historical perspective, morphology, fetal diagnosis, and outcome.
- Hanley FL, Sade RM, Blackstone EH, et al: Outcomes in neonatal pulmonary atresia with intact ventricular septum. J Thorac Cardiovasc Surg 1993;105:406–427.
- Ashburn MD, Blackstone EH, Wells WJ, et al: Determinants of mortality and type of repair in neonates with pulmonary atresia and intact ventricular septum. J Thorac Cardiovasc Surg 2004;127:1000–1008.

  The early and mid-term results from the Congenital Heart Surgeons Study of pulmonary atresia with intact ventricular septum in North America. This is the largest study of the disease to date with 408 patients. There is excellent statistical analysis (parametric modelling of time-related death) particularly of optimal initial procedure relating to the size of the tricuspid valve, and factors influencing achievement of definitive repair.
- Daubeney PEF, Sharland GK, Cook AC, et al: Pulmonary atresia with intact ventricular septum: Impact of fetal echocardiography on incidence at birth and postnatal outcome. Circulation 1998;98:562–566.
- Daubeney PE, Delany DJ, Anderson RH, et al: Pulmonary atresia with intact ventricular septum: Range of morphology in a population-based study. J Am Coll Cardiol 2002;39:1670–1679.
- Daubeney PEF, Wang D, Delany DJ, et al: Pulmonary atresia with intact ventricular septum: Predictors of early and medium-term outcome in a population-based study. J Thorac Cardiovasc Surg 2005;130:1071.

  The results from the collaborative study performed in the United Kingdom and Eire. This is the largest population-based study of this disease containing all 183 patients born in a fixed geographical area in a fixed time-frame. There is detailed data about fetal diagnosis and its effects. The range of morphology is described in a population-based setting, which can serve as a reference to ensure future interventional studies reflect the population at large. Outcome data is given and risk factors influencing poor outcome. There were a high proportion of primary catheter interventions in this study.
- Dyamenahalli U, McCrindle BW, McDonald C, et al: Pulmonary atresia with intact ventricular septum: Management of, and outcomes for, a cohort of 210 consecutive patients. Cardiol Young 2004;14:299–308.

  The results from Hospital for Sick Children, Toronto. This excellent study details range of morphology, outcome and risk factors for poor outcome from 1965–1998. It is the largest and most comprehensive single institutional study to date. Similar statistical methods to the Congenital Heart Surgeons Study.
- Odim J, Laks H, Plunkett MD, Tung TC: Successful management of patients with pulmonary atresia with intact ventricular septum using a three tier grading system for right ventricular hypoplasia. Ann Thorac Surg 2006;81: 678–684.

  Large series from University of California at Los Angeles, where eventual outcome is predicted by presenting right ventricular hypoplasia. Excellent long-term surgical outcome.
- Daubeney PEF: Pulmonary atresia with intact ventricular septum. In Gatzoulis MA, Webb GD, Daubeney PEF (eds): Diagnosis and Management of Adult Congenital Heart Disease. London: Churchill Livingstone, 2003, pp 339–347.

  Very good review of the disease in adult life including outcome, complications, and outpatient assessment and management.

CHAPTER 31

Other Forms of Functionally Univentricular Hearts

DANIEL J. PENNY and ROBERT H. ANDERSON

The terms univentricular and single have proven to be amongst the most controversial adjectives used to describe some of the most complex congenital malformations of the heart. Since the mid-1990s, light has begun to emerge at the end of the tunnel for those who have attempted to provide a logical framework for the description of these complex conditions. This has stemmed from the realisation by clinicians that the decision underscoring the eventual presence or absence of a functionally univentricular arrangement is whether treatment of the individual patient is to proceed towards creation of biventricular circulations, or rather to establish the Fontan circuit, which of necessity produces circulatory patterns supported by only one ventricle, even if two chambers are unequivocally present within the ventricular mass.[1] For example, in a patient with critical aortic stenosis, the clinician will seek to determine whether the best option for the patient is to seek to achieve biventricular repair or opt for univentricular palliation, recognising that such a patient possesses both morphologically right and left ventricles. There are many patients, therefore, including those with hypoplastic left heart syndrome, those having pulmonary atresia with intact ventricular septum, as well as some with straddling of the atrioventricular valves or double outlet ventricle, for whom the clinician may choose a mode of treatment culminating in production of a functionally univentricular heart. All these conditions have either already been considered in other chapters—hypoplasia of the left heart in Chapter 29 and pulmonary atresia with intact septum in Chapter 30, or will be considered in chapters to follow, specifically straddling atrioventricular valves in Chapter 40 and double outlet ventricles in Chapter 33. In this chapter, we are concerned with describing the underlying morphology, and clinical diagnosis, of the lesions that produced most controversy previously in the definition of single ventricles or univentricular hearts, namely, double inlet ventricle and atrioventricular valvar atresia. In the next chapter, having established the principles for analysis of these problematic lesions, we will discuss the long-term options for all those patients having the functionally univentricular arrangements.

PHILOSOPHICAL CONSIDERATIONS

When considered from the stance of cardiac morphology, hearts having a solitary chamber within the ventricular mass, and hence truly being univentricular, are extremely rare. They do exist, and when found, they most usually exhibit double inlet to a chamber having indeterminate apical trabeculations, and in which the only septal structure present is the muscular outlet septum (Fig. 31-1). The essence of such hearts is that the atrial chambers are joined to the solitary ventricle. It is possible, of course, that such an arrangement, with the atrial chambers connected exclusively to a solitary ventricle of indeterminate morphology, can be found when either the right- or left-sided atrioventricular connection is absent, but such hearts are exceedingly rare. It was recognition of the significance of such a univentricular arrangement of the atrioventricular junctions, nonetheless, than clarified the polemics underscoring the previous disagreements.[2,3] Thus, subsequent to the important study that had appeared in 1964,[4] it had become accepted[5] that the criterion for definition of a single ventricle was the presence of double inlet. Those accepting this concept, however, ignored that fact that, when the morphology of the small ventricle in patients with tricuspid atresia was compared to that of the same chamber in those with double inlet left ventricle, the comparison being made in the setting of lesions with the same ventriculo-arterial connections, then the small ventricles were essentially indistinguishable[6] (compare Figs. 31-2 and 31-3). This is because, in the setting of either the commonest form of tricuspid atresia or in those with double inlet left ventricle, the big ventricle is of left ventricular morphology, while the small ventricle is an incomplete right ventricle, lacking totally its inlet component (Figs. 31-4 and 31-5). Recognition of this feature led to the realisation that, in both these anomalies, it was the atrioventricular

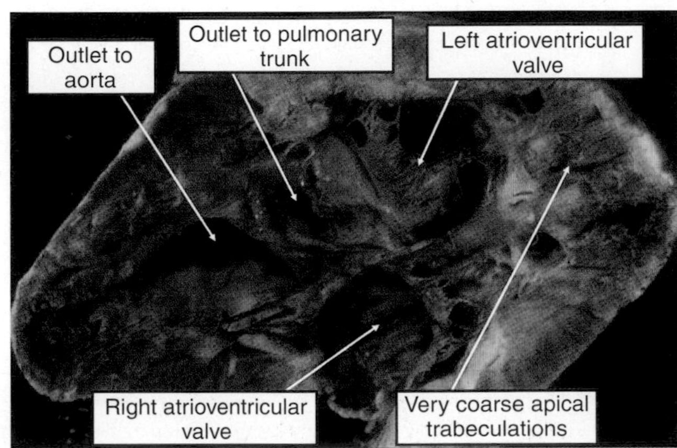

Figure 31-1 This heart has a truly solitary ventricle, with exceedingly coarse apical trabeculations of indeterminate morphology. There is double inlet to, and double outlet from, the solitary ventricle. This is the anatomical univentricular heart.

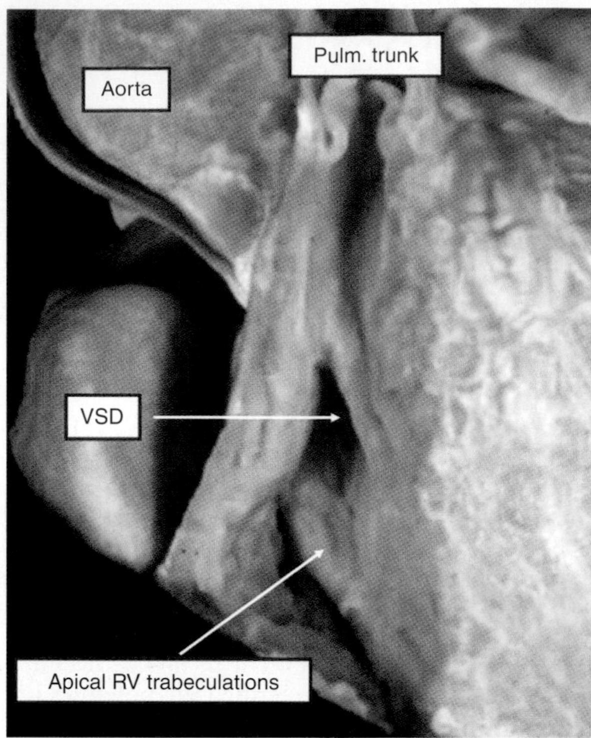

Figure 31-2 The heart is photographed from the front to show the morphology of the antero-superior ventricular chamber, which lacks its inlet, but has an apical component of right ventricular (RV) morphology. The ventricle gives rise to the pulmonary trunk, whilst the aorta arises from the dominant ventricle, which also receives both atrioventricular valves. This is an example of the so-called Holmes heart. VSD, ventricular septal defect.

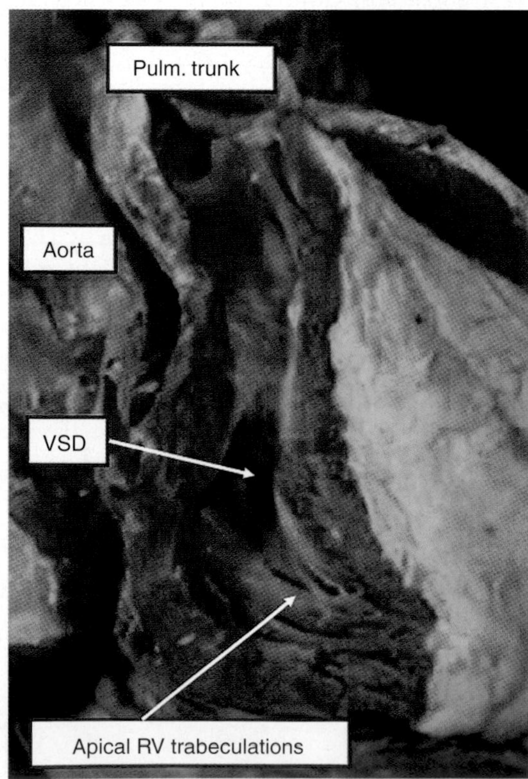

Figure 31-3 This heart is photographed in comparable fashion to the one shown in Figure 31-2. In this instance, however, there is tricuspid atresia due to absence of the right atrioventricular connection. There is no fundamental difference in the structure of the morphologically right ventricle (RV) from that shown in Figure 31-2. Both ventricles are incomplete because they lack their inlet components. VSD, ventral septal defect.

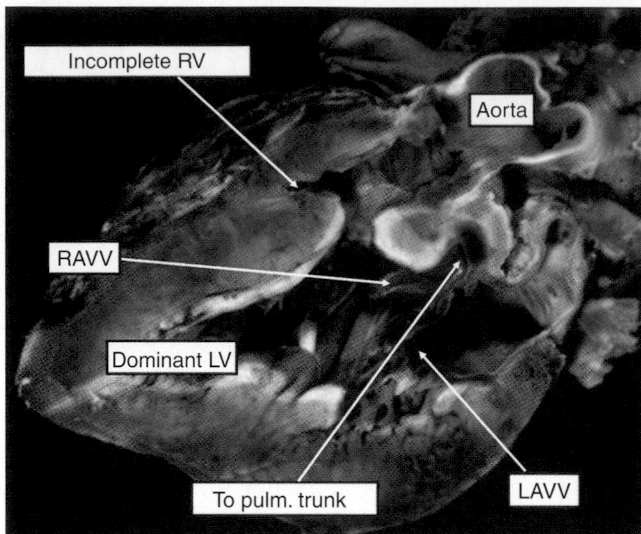

Figure 31-4 The heart is sectioned to replicate the parasternal long-axis section. It shows the structure of double inlet left ventricle (LV) with discordant ventriculo-arterial connections. Note the dominant left ventricle and the antero-superiorly located incomplete right ventricle (RV). LAVV, left atrioventricular valve; RAVV, right atrioventricular valve.

connection, rather than the ventricular mass, which was univentricular.[2,3] This, in turn, led to the realisation that all patients with congenitally malformed hearts, with one small exception, could be divided into those with biventricular atrioventricular connections, this group made up of those with concordant, discordant, and ambiguous and mixed atrioventricular connections, and those unified because the atriums are joined to only one ventricle, either because both atriums are committed to the same ventricle, in other words those with double inlet ventricle, or because one of the connections between the atriums and the ventricular mass is completely absent, producing the commonest form of atrioventricular valvar atresia. The very small third group of patients is made up of those with absent atrioventricular connection and straddling and overriding of the solitary atrioventricular valve,[7] this combination producing a uniatrial but biventricular connection (Fig. 31-6). In all those with univentricular atrioventricular connections (Fig. 31-7), apart from the very small minority having solitary and indeterminate ventricles, there is a second ventricle within the ventricular mass that, of necessity, is incomplete and rudimentary. Among these patients, three additional groups stand out as requiring separate description, namely, those with double inlet, those with absence of the right atrioventricular connection, and those with absence of the left atrioventricular connection. It is patients with hearts of this type we describe in this chapter, along with their close cousins with imperforate atrioventricular valves, the latter also producing unequivocal atrioventricular valvar atresia.

MORPHOLOGY

As we have already explained in Chapter 1, there are three possible junctional arrangements producing anatomical univentricular atrioventricular connections (see Fig. 32-7). The first is when the cavities of right- and left-sided atrial chambers are connected directly to the same ventricle. This

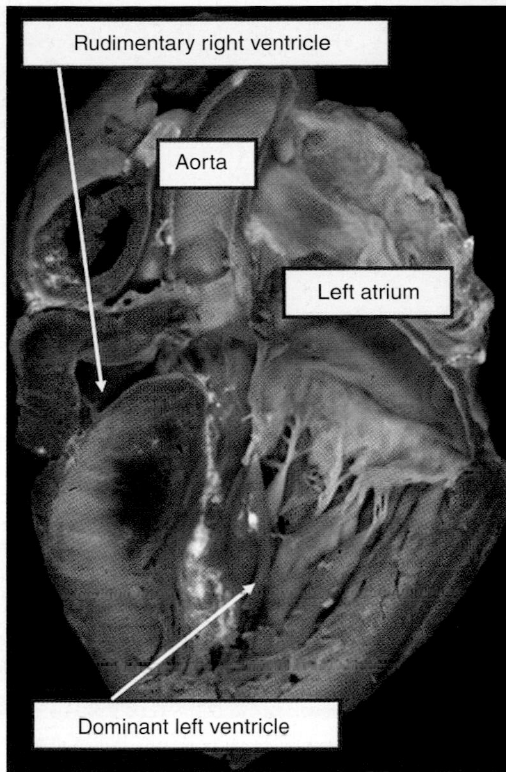

Figure 31-5 This example of tricuspid atresia is sectioned to replicate the parasternal long-axis section. As with the heart shown in Figure 31-4 with double inlet left ventricle, there is a dominant left ventricle, and an incomplete right ventricle located antero-superiorly.

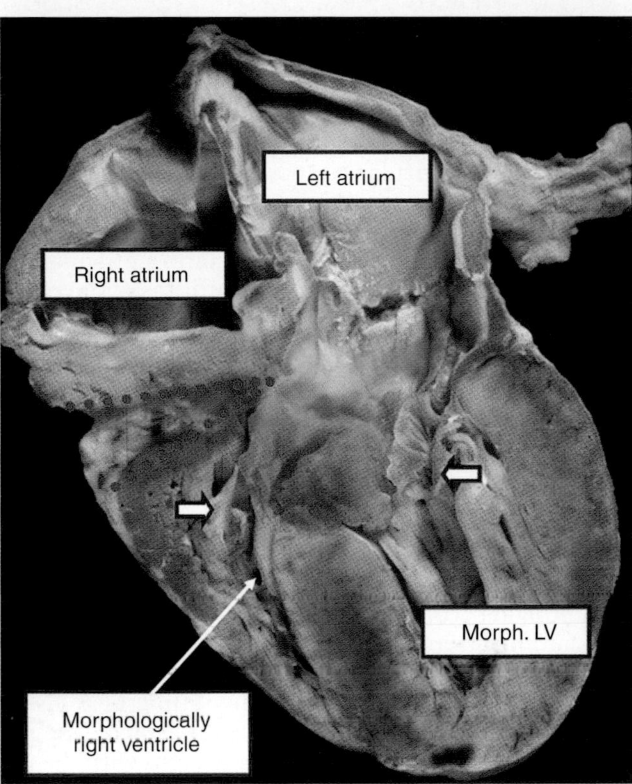

Figure 31-6 The heart illustrated shows a rare variant of tricuspid atresia due to absence of the right atrioventricular connection (*yellow dotted lines*), but with straddling and overriding of the left atrioventricular valve (*arrows*). Because the valve is supported by both ventricles but takes its origin only from the left atrium, the resulting atrioventricular connection is uniatrial but biventricular. Morph. LV, morphologically left ventricle.

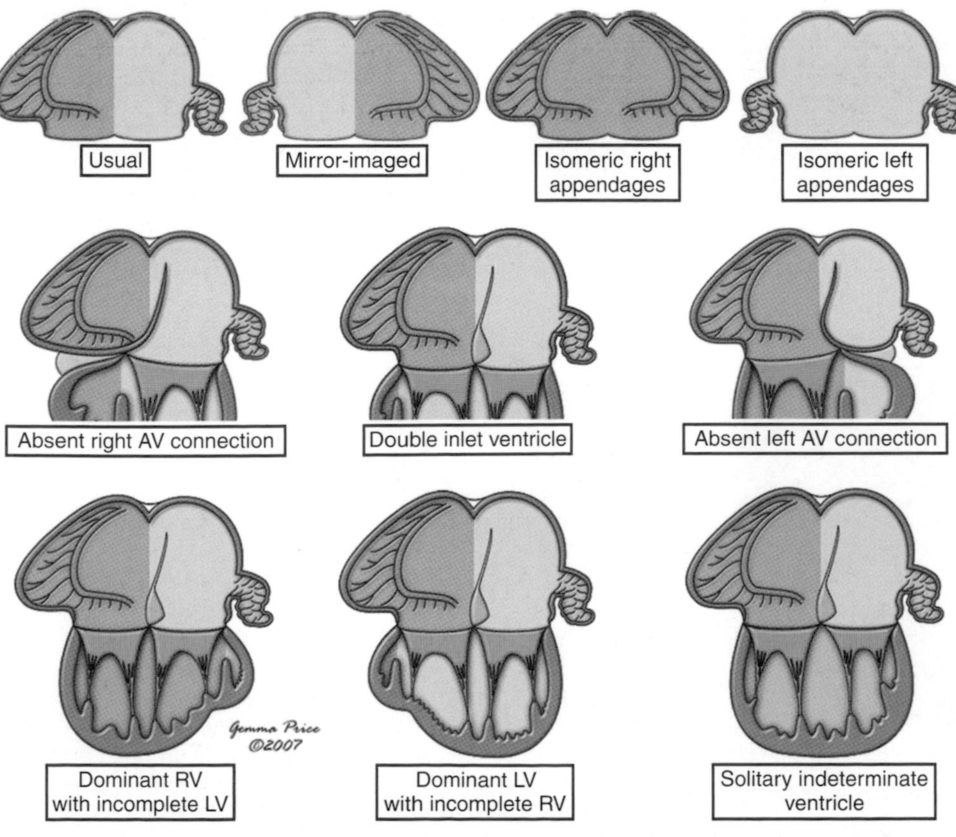

Figure 31-7 The cartoon shows the segmental combinations producing a univentricular atrioventricular connection. The middle row shows the possible connections, which can co-exist with any atrial arrangement, as shown in the top row. Any of the atrioventricular connections can also exist with any of the three ventricular morphologies shown in the bottom row, although they are illustrated only with double inlet ventricle. Further variations are possible at the ventriculo-arterial level, and because of associated malformations.

is called double inlet atrioventricular connection, irrespective of whether the atrioventricular junctions are guarded by two atrioventricular valves or a common valve. The other two arrangements exist when one atrioventricular connection is absent, giving absence of the right-sided and left-sided atrioventricular connections, respectively. All of these patterns at the atrioventricular junction can be found in patients having usually arranged, mirror-imaged or isomeric atrial appendages. Each type of atrioventricular connection can also be found with the atriums connected to a dominant right ventricle, a dominant left ventricle, or rarely, to a solitary and morphologically indeterminate ventricle (see Fig. 32-1).

Atrioventricular Connections

The feature underpinning the anatomy of absent right atrioventricular connection is emphasised when patients having an imperforate tricuspid valve (Fig. 31-8) are compared with those having complete absence of the right atrioventricular connection (Fig. 31-9). Although these two anatomical entities produce the same physiological effect, their morphology is totally different. An imperforate valve can only be formed in the setting of a discrete atrioventricular junction. With this arrangement, the parietal myocardium of the atrium is continuous with the parietal ventricular wall. Hence, the cavities of the atrium and the underlying ventricle are in potential communication. When the atrioventricular connection is absent, this is not the case. The parietal walls of the right atrium and of the ventricle have no direct continuity, but instead they meet at the central fibrous body, with the fibro-fatty tissues of the atrioventricular groove filling the space between the adjacent layers of atrial and ventricular myocardium. The atrium has a complete muscular floor, which is the lateral wall of the appendage. A muscular dimple is frequently seen antero-superior to the orifice of the coronary sinus. This is often, incorrectly, presumed to represent the site of the right atrioventricular orifice. Sectioning through the dimple shows that it overlies the atrioventricular membranous component of the central fibrous body, and points to the outflow tract of the morphologically left ventricle (Fig. 31-10). A similar distinction needs to be made between

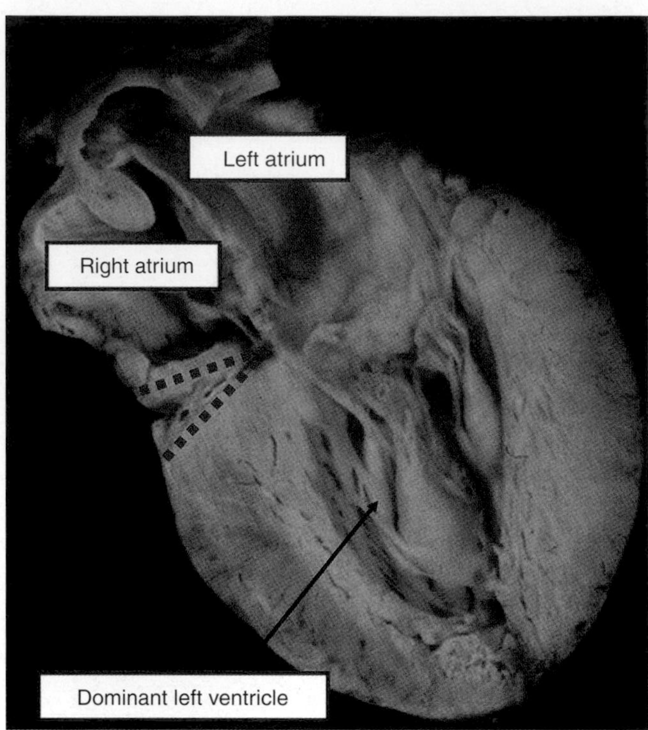

Figure 31-9 This heart, to be compared with the one shown in Figure 31-8, and also sectioned to replicate the echocardiographic four-chamber cut, shows that the essence of classical tricuspid atresia is complete absence of the right atrioventricular connection (*green dotted lines*).

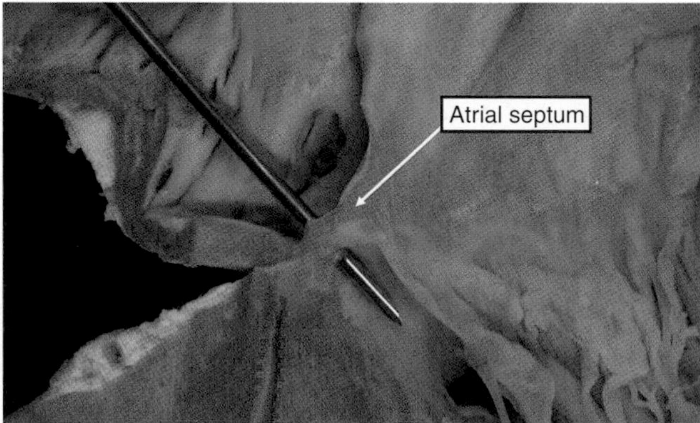

Figure 31-10 The image is a close-up of a section through the dimple in a heart with classical tricuspid atresia. The green dotted lines show the cavity of the incomplete right ventricle. As shown by the probe, the dimple points into the cavity of the dominant left ventricle. It is the atrioventricular component of the membranous septum.

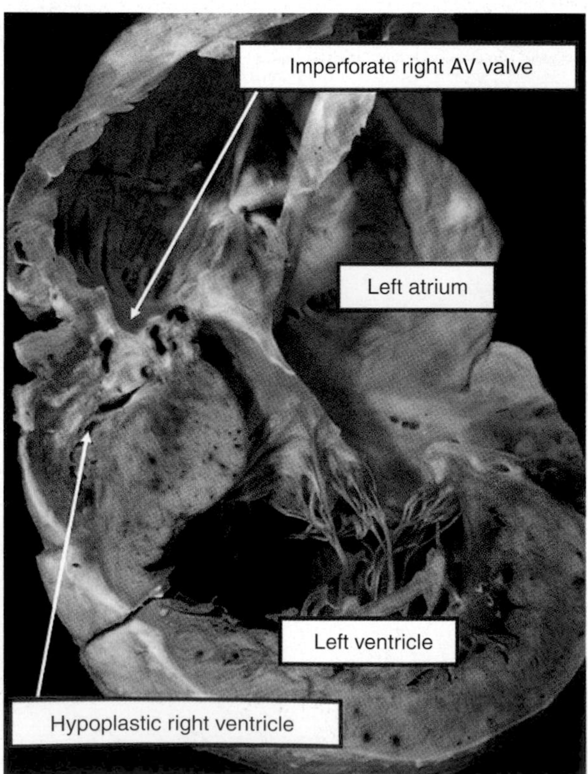

Figure 31-8 The heart, with imperforate right atrioventricular valve producing tricuspid atresia, has concordant atrioventricular connections. This is a rare variant of tricuspid atresia, in this instance co-existing with pulmonary atresia in the setting of intact ventricular septum.

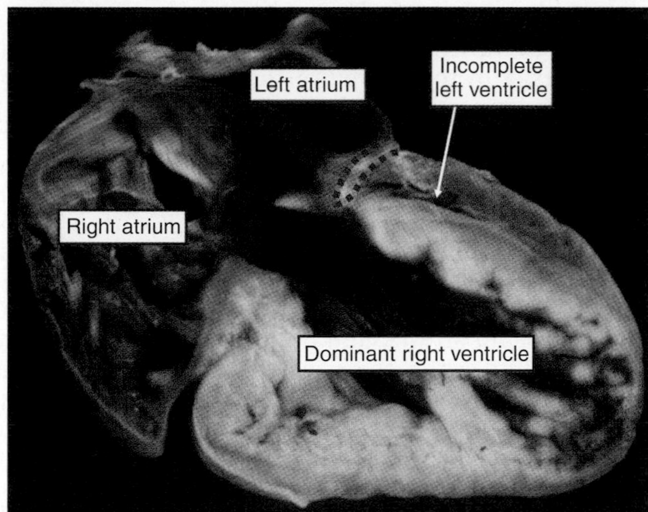

Figure 31-11 This heart, a variant of hypoplastic left heart syndrome, has been sectioned in four-chamber fashion. It shows complete absence of the left atrioventricular connection (*green dotted lines*), with the incomplete left ventricle in inferior and left-sided position.

absence of the left atrioventricular connection and biventricular atrioventricular connections with an imperforate mitral valve. When the left connection is absent, the fibro-fatty tissue of the left atrioventricular groove separates completely the muscular floor of the left atrium from the underlying ventricular myocardium (Fig. 31-11).

When analyzing the morphology of the atrioventricular junctions in hearts with double inlet ventricle, it should be noted that double inlet exists because both atrial vestibules connect to the same ventricle, irrespective of whether the right- and left-sided atrioventricular junctions are guarded by two separate atrioventricular valves or a common valve (Figs. 31-12 and 31-13). And, as we have already shown in Figure 31-7, double inlet ventricle can occur with any atrial arrangement. The usual arrangement is the most common, but isomerism of the right atrial appendages is by no means rare, particularly when there is double inlet right ventricle. Common atrioventricular valves are also particularly frequent when there is right isomerism.

Abnormalities of the atrioventricular valves are frequent, in particular in hearts with double inlet left ventricle. In this setting, when there are separate right and left atrioventricular valves, both usually resemble mitral valves, lacking any tethering to the antero-superiorly located ventricular septum. They are also usually supported by separate papillary muscles, but often separated on the inferior ventricular wall by a prominent ridge. The two valves can also share papillary muscles, with no plane of cleavage between them, this feature ruling out the potential for ventricular septation. Where one or the other arterial valve is connected to the left ventricle, both atrioventricular valves are usually in continuity with it, although either, or rarely both, may be separated from it by persistence of the ventriculo-infundibular fold. Either the right or the left atrioventricular valve may be imperforate or stenotic, or may straddle or override the ventricular septum. In the setting of overriding and straddling atrioventricular valves, as we will explain in greater detail in Chapter 33, providing more than half of the vestibule of the overriding

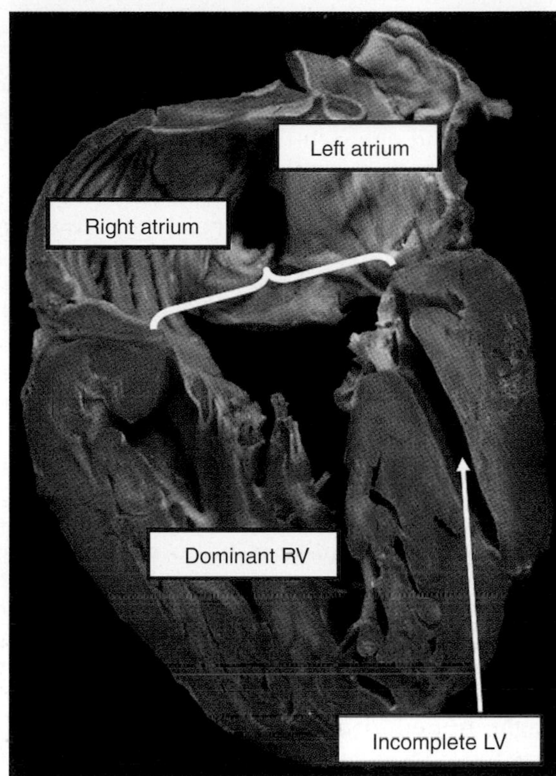

Figure 31-12 This heart has double inlet right ventricle (RV), with the right and left-sided atrioventricular junctions guarded by a common atrioventricular valve (*bracket*). Note that the incomplete left ventricle (LV) is positioned inferiorly and to the left, but with the ventricular septum extending to the crux.

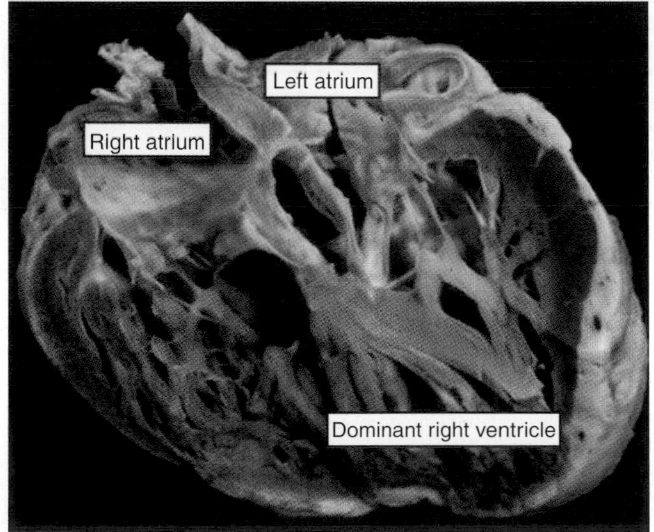

Figure 31-13 This heart, sectioned to replicate the four-chamber section, shows double inlet to a dominant right ventricle with separate right and left atrioventricular valves. The incomplete left ventricle, not seen, is positioned inferiorly and to the left.

junction is connected to the dominant ventricle, we continue to categorise the connection as double inlet. In patients with absence of either the right or left atrioventricular connection, the remaining atrioventricular valve may straddle, producing the rare uniatrial and biventricular connection (see Fig. 31-6).

The Ventricles

In almost all hearts in which there is a univentricular atrioventricular connection, there are complementary ventricles present of left and right ventricular morphology, separated by the apical muscular ventricular septum (see Figs. 31-4 and 31-12). In the majority of patients with absent right atrioventricular connection, this being the arrangement producing classical tricuspid atresia, the left atrium is connected to a dominant left ventricle (see Fig. 31-9). In these hearts, and indeed in all those having a dominant left ventricle, the incomplete right ventricle is carried on the antero-superior shoulder of the ventricular mass, almost always with its trabecular component to the right. In hearts with double inlet left ventricle, when the incomplete right ventricle is again found in an antero-superior position, the apical trabecular component can be either right- or left-sided, or directly anterior. In all situations in which the left ventricle is dominant, unlike in hearts with biventricular atrioventricular connections, the hypoplastic apical muscular ventricular septum does not extend to the crux.

When it is the right ventricle which is dominant, the incomplete left ventricle is located in postero-inferior position, usually to the left of the dominant ventricle, but rarely to the right. In both of these settings, the hypoplastic ventricular septum does extend to the crux. Absence of the left atrioventricular connection with the right atrium connected to a dominant right ventricle produces one of the frequent variants of hypoplastic left heart syndrome (see Fig. 31-11). Absence of the right atrioventricular connection can also rarely be found when the left atrium is connected to a dominant right ventricle, and again the incomplete left ventricle will usually be located postero-inferiorly, this arrangement being found most frequently in association with straddling and overriding of the left atrioventricular valve (Fig. 31-14).

Ventriculo-arterial Connections

Any type of ventriculo-arterial connection must be anticipated to exist in the setting of the univentricular atrioventricular connection, as long as they are anatomically feasible. Should there be a solitary ventricle of indeterminate morphology, however, the only possibilities are double outlet from the solitary ventricle (see Fig. 31-1), or one of the variants of single outlet, usually pulmonary or aortic atresia rather than common arterial trunk. When the left ventricle is dominant, then concordant ventriculo-arterial connections are the rule in the setting of tricuspid atresia, and discordant connections are typically found when there is double inlet. When it is the left atrioventricular connection which is absent, then it is most usual to find aortic atresia with origin of the pulmonary trunk from the right ventricle, this being one of the frequent variants of hypoplastic left heart syndrome (see Fig. 31-11 and Chapter 29). As emphasised, however, any connection must be anticipated to exist, and concordant ventriculo-arterial connections are by no means rare when there is double inlet left ventricle, this combination producing the so-called Holmes heart (see Fig. 31-2). Should there be double inlet to, and double outlet from, the dominant left ventricle, then the incomplete right ventricle is represented only by its apical trabecular component, which continues to be positioned antero-superiorly, albeit either to the right or the left. When it is the right ventricle that is dominant, then most usually there is also double outlet from the right ventricle. The incomplete left ventricle is then represented only by its apical trabecular component, positioned postero-inferiorly, and usually to the left. Concordant ventriculo-arterial connections can be found, most usually when there is a common atrioventricular valve, but other connections are rare.

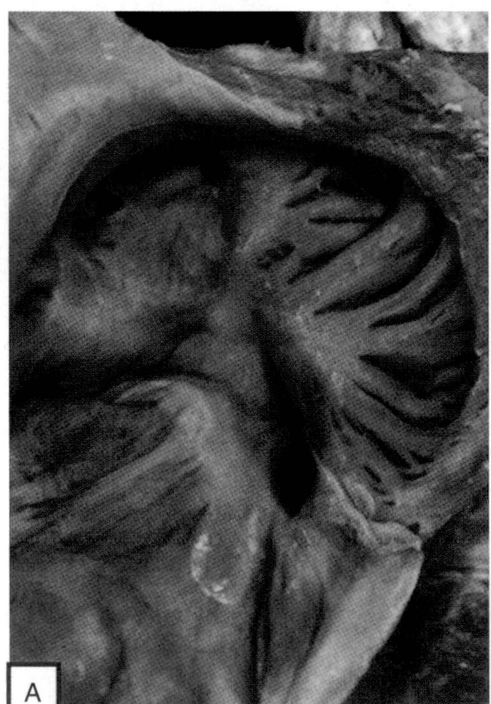

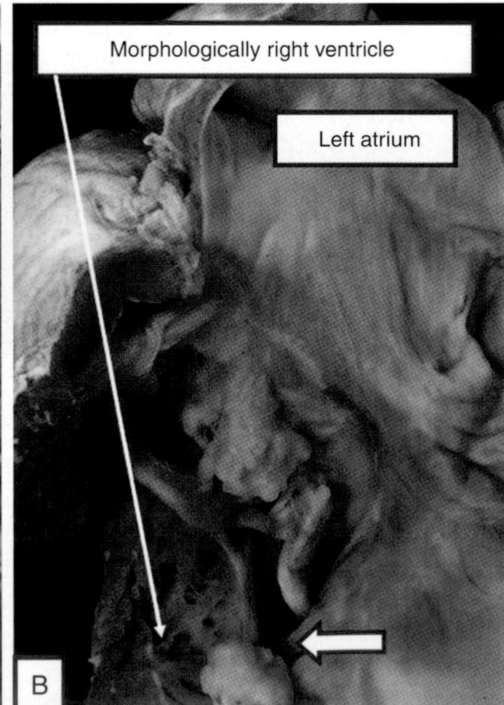

Figure 31-14 These images show a heart with absence of the right atrioventricular connection (**A**), but with straddling and overriding of the left atrioventricular valve, viewed from the left atrium and from behind in panel **B**. As with the heart shown in Figure 31-6, this produces a uniatrial but biventricular connection, but unlike the heart shown in Figure 31-6, in this heart there is left hand ventricular topology. The morphologically left ventricle is positioned inferiorly and to the right (*arrow* in **B**).

Interventricular Communication

In patients with a dominant left ventricle, irrespective of the precise atrioventricular connection, the hole between the ventricles is almost always completely surrounded by muscle, being located between the apical and outlet components of the ventricular septum. This hole has been described in various ways over the years, being called a bulboventricular foramen, an outlet foramen, or a ventricular septal defect. It is an integral part of one of the circulations when the ventriculo-arterial connections are concordant or discordant. It has a tendency to become obstructive with time (see Figs. 31-2 and 31-3). In the setting of discordant ventriculo-arterial connections, such a reduction in the size produces subaortic obstruction (Fig. 31-15), but results in subpulmonary obstruction when it is the pulmonary trunk which arises from the incomplete right ventricle. It is well established that the defect can decrease markedly in size, albeit that a purported causal association with banding of the pulmonary trunk[8] remains to be proved.

The interventricular communication in hearts with dominant right ventricles is usually perimembranous, since the hypoplastic septum extends to the crux in this setting, and the defect is directly related to the atrioventricular valve or valves. In most instances when the right ventricle is dominant, both arterial trunks also arise from the dominant right ventricle, and the left ventricle is represented only by its apical trabecular component, albeit often in association with minimal straddling of the left atrioventricular valve (Fig. 31-16). In this situation, the interventricular communication is not an integral part of the circulation to one or other outflow tract, as it usually is when the left ventricle is dominant, and hence the morphology of the interventricular communication is of less clinical significance.

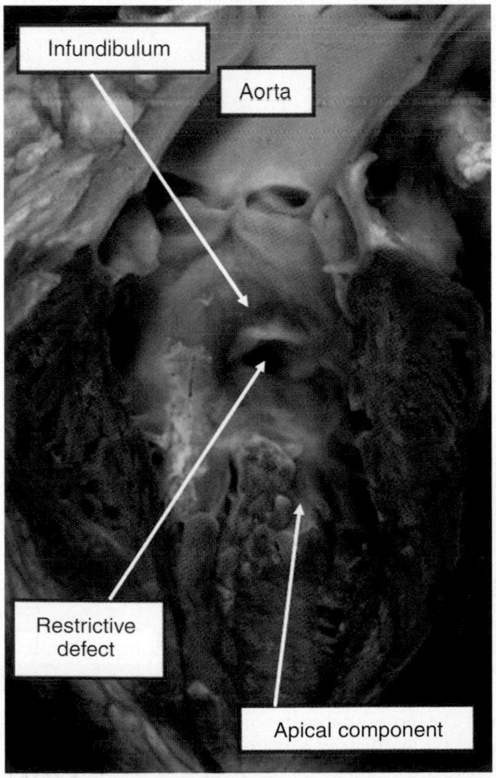

Figure 31-15 This picture, taken from the front, shows the small right ventricle in the setting of double inlet left ventricle, but with a restrictive interventricular communication, producing subaortic obstruction in this instance, since the aorta arises from the small right ventricle. Note that the defect has exclusively muscular borders, opening to the right ventricle between the outlet and apical trabecular components of the chamber.

Associated Malformations

The interventricular communication is part and parcel of the morphology of hearts having dominant right or left ventricles, and does not exist in those with solitary and indeterminate ventricles. In those with dominant left ventricles, it is the size of the interventricular communication that is the major determinant of clinical presentation, recognising that this feature is, of course, also dependent on the ventriculo-arterial connections. The presence of other associated malformations can then further modify the clinical presentation. Any lesion that can feasibly exist must be anticipated to be present in some patient at some time. Some lesions, nonetheless, are particularly frequent, such as deficiencies of the floor of the oval foramen, producing an interatrial communication. An intact atrial septum can also produce problems in the setting of absence of the left atrioventricular connection. Persistent patency of the arterial duct is frequent, this being an important part of the circulation when there is pulmonary stenosis or atresia, or aortic coarctation or interruption. It is the obstructive lesions in one or the other of the outflow tracts, nonetheless, which are probably the most important associated lesions. In the setting of a dominant left ventricle, deviation of the muscular outlet septum can produce either subpulmonary or subaortic obstruction, depending on whether the ventriculo-arterial connections are concordant or discordant. A deviated outlet septum can also produce either subpulmonary or subaortic obstruction in the setting of double outlet ventricle. Subarterial obstruction can also be produced by tissue tags, or by anomalous attachment of the tension apparatus of the atrioventricular valves. Other lesions of the pulmonary pathways must be anticipated, such as discontinuous pulmonary arteries, whilst anomalies of venous connection are by no means infrequent, particularly when there is isomerism of the atrial appendages. And the atrial appendages themselves can be juxtaposed. In short, a multitude of associated malformations can be found in patients having

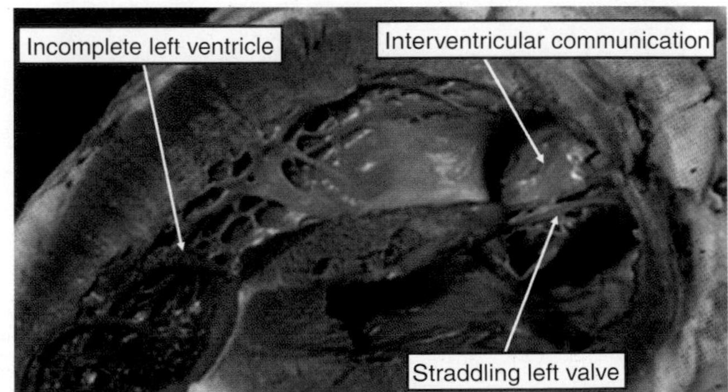

Figure 31-16 The picture shows the postero-inferior incomplete left ventricle, in left-sided position, from the heart also shown in Figure 31-13. The interventricular communication is perimembranous, being roofed by fibrous continuity between the leaflets of the straddling left atrioventricular valve and the right atrioventricular valve.

either double inlet ventricle or absence of one atrioventricular connection.

Conduction Axis

An understanding of the structure of hearts with univentricular atrioventricular connection, as described above, provides the information needed to determine the location of the atrioventricular conduction axis. This is because the ventricular components of the conduction axis are carried on the crest of the apical muscular ventricular septum, and the atrioventricular node, or in some instances nodes, is formed at the point, or points, of union of the apical septum with the atrioventricular junctions.

When the left ventricle is dominant, the atrioventricular conduction axis is grossly abnormal.[9,10] The pattern is dictated by the lack of any ventricular septum at the crux. Because of this, the regular atrioventricular node in the atrial septum is unable to make contact with the atrioventricular conduction tissues positioned astride the apical ventricular septum. Instead, an anomalous atrioventricular node is found in the superior quadrant of the right atrioventricular orifice (Fig. 31-17). From this node, the conduction axis penetrates the atrioventricular fibrous plane, the precise course of the non-branching bundle then depending on the position of the incomplete right ventricle. When the right ventricle is right sided, the bundle is able to descend directly onto the septum, and is unrelated to the pulmonary outflow tract. When the incomplete ventricle is left sided, the bundle extends antero-superiorly around the pulmonary valvar orifice to reach the septum. Irrespective of the position of the right ventricle, the relation of conduction tissue and the interventricular communication is the same when viewed from the right ventricular aspect (Fig. 31-18). The conduction axis branches on the left ventricular aspect of the septum, and is well below the septal crest. Only the right bundle branch extends upwards, piercing the septum to ramify in the apical component of the incomplete right ventricle. The basic disposition of the axis, therefore, is always the same, being dictated by the orientation of the ventricular septum. The septum joins the atrioventricular junction more parietally when there is straddling and overriding of the right atrioventricular valve. Because of this, the node and penetrating bundle are formed postero-laterally in the right atrioventricular orifice (see Chapter 33). The position of the conduction axis relative to the interventricular communication is the same be there absence of the right or left atrioventricular connection. One important variation is found, however, should there be an apical muscular interventricular communication in addition to the usual defect between the outlet and apical components of the muscular septum. In the presence of two defects, the conduction axis courses within the muscular bar separating the holes (Fig. 31-19). A further variation is found in the setting of tricuspid atresia due to absence of the right atrioventricular connection. Because there is no right atrioventricular valvar orifice, the atrioventricular node is found adjacent to the dimple, with the apex of the triangle of Koch now serving as a guide to the location of the node (Fig. 31-20).

When the right ventricle is dominant, the disposition of the conduction axis is determined in part by the septal orientation, and in part by ventricular topology. Hearts with left-sided incomplete left ventricles have a right-handed pattern of ventricular topology. Then, because the septum extends to the crux, the connecting node is in its anticipated regular position. The atrioventricular bundle penetrates postero-inferiorly, and branches astride the apical muscular

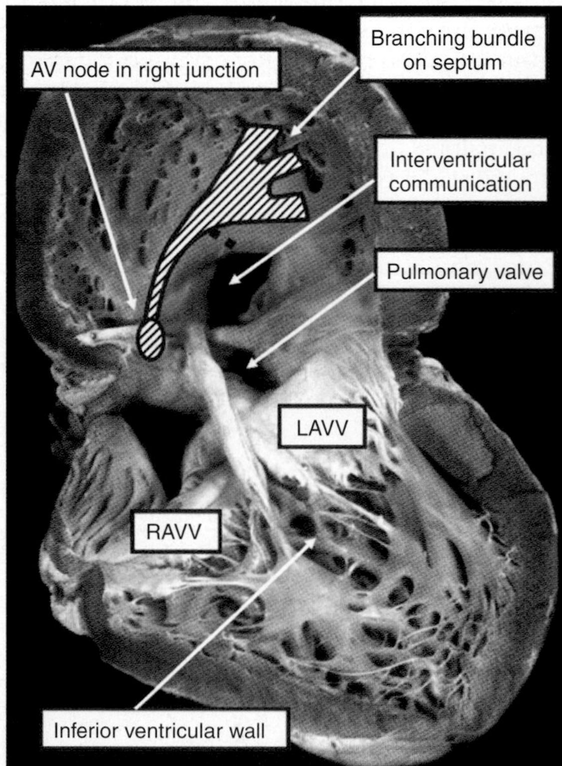

Figure 31-17 This specimen with double inlet left ventricle and discordant ventriculo-arterial connections has been opened in clam-like fashion, and the superior wall reflected upward to show the double inlet through two atrioventricular valves (RAVV, LAVV). The course of the atrioventricular conduction axis has been superimposed using red cross-hatching. The branching bundle is on the crest of the hypoplastic ventricular septum, with the right bundle branch shown in dashes. The atrioventricular node is placed superiorly in the right atrioventricular junction, with the bundle joining these two components (see text for further discussion).

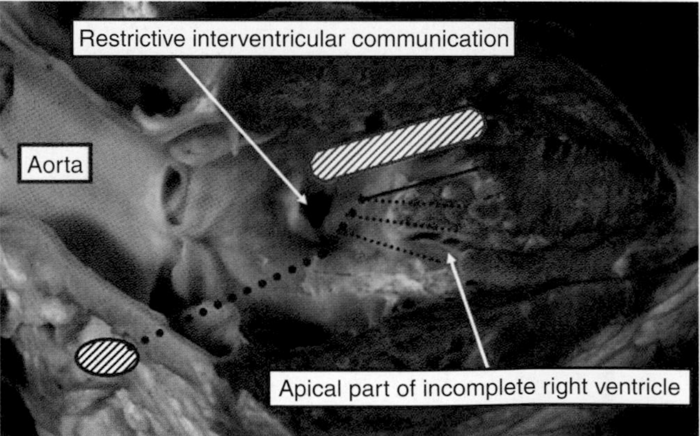

Figure 31-18 The incomplete right ventricle shown in Figure 31-15 has been reoriented to show the view that might be obtained by the surgeon working within this chamber. The head of the patient would be to the left hand. The red oval shows the site of the atrioventricular node in the superior quadrant of the right atrioventricular junction (see Fig. 31-17). The course of the axis within the dominant left ventricle is shown by the large red dotted line. The smaller red dotted lines show the location of the left bundle branch in the dominant ventricle, with the right bundle branch shown by the solid red line. The green area is the part of the septum that can safely be resected if there is need, as there would be in this heart, to enlarge the interventricular communication.

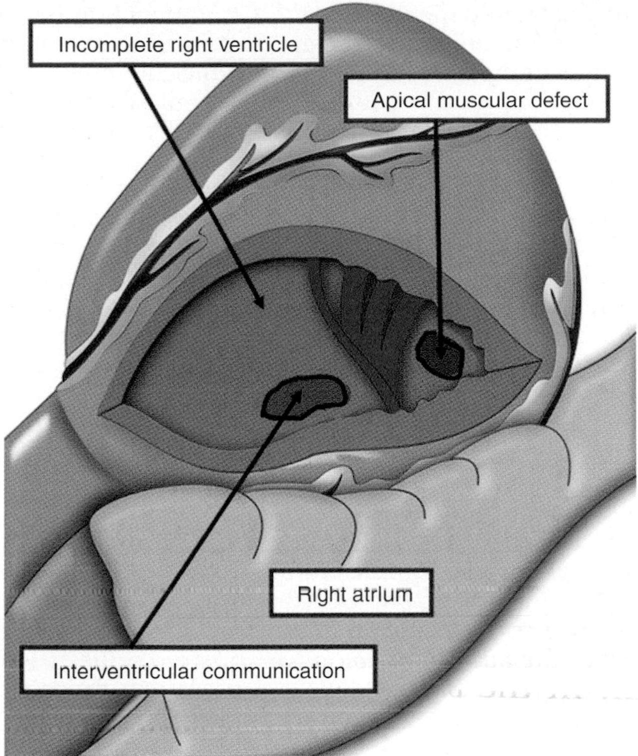

Figure 31-19 The cartoon shows the interior of the incomplete right ventricle as it might be viewed by the surgeon in a patient with tricuspid atresia, and a muscular apical defect in addition to the regular muscular interventricular communication. As is shown, the atrioventricular conduction axis would run in the muscular bar between the holes. (Modified from the original prepared for *Surgical Anatomy of the Heart,* with permission of Gemma Price, Andrew Cook, and Benson Wilcox.)

septum.[11] When the left ventricle is right sided, the ventricular topology is left-handed. This is then the dominant feature in determining the location of the conduction tissue, over and above the fact that the septum reaches to the crux. In the only heart of this type we studied histologically, there was a sling of conduction tissue between anterior and regular nodes. The ventricular conduction tissue descended on a trabeculation within the right ventricle.[12] We anticipate that the same rules will apply when either the right or left atrioventricular connection is absent in association with univentricular connection to a dominant right ventricle.

When there is a solitary and indeterminate ventricle, then because there is no apical trabecular septum, there cannot be a normal conduction system. Most frequently, in our experience,[13] there has been an anterior node with the bundle descending onto a free-standing muscle bar. The bundle can also descend in the parietal ventricular wall or else drop from a regular node. Slings of conduction tissue have been found in the postero-inferior ventricular wall in patients with right isomerism.[14]

Huge Ventricular Septal Defects

Hearts also exist in which most of the ventricular septum is absent, but an apical muscular rim persists, dividing the ventricular mass into right ventricular and left ventricular components (Fig. 31-21). Because of the presence of the apical remnant of the ventricular septum, the ventricular inlets in this setting are committed to recognisably separate

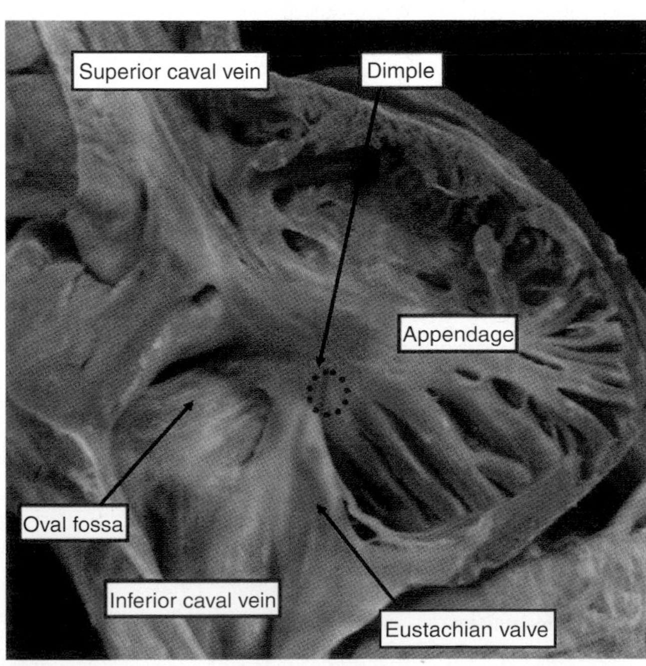

Figure 31-20 The image shows the right atrium in the heart from a patient with classical tricuspid atresia. The red dots show the site of the atrioventricular node, adjacent to the dimple, where there is absence of the right atrioventricular connection.

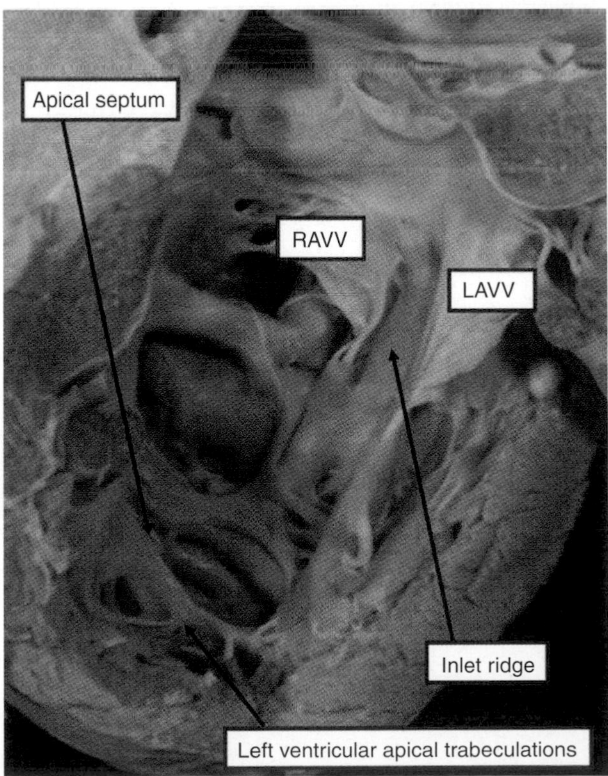

Figure 31-21 This heart is from a patient with a huge interventricular communication. The apical septum, which separates the apical trabecular components of the right and left ventricles, each receiving a separate atrioventricular valve (RAVV, LAVV), continues between the valves as an inlet ridge, which carries the atrioventricular conduction axis from the atrioventricular node at the apex of the triangle of Koch.

apical ventricular components. More importantly, in most cases but not all, it is usual to find a rim of septum extending from the apical septum to the crux. In our experience, this rim has always carried the non-branching bundle from a regularly positioned node. Morphologically, therefore, the hearts are readily distinguished from those with double inlet atrioventricular connection. We categorise them as huge ventricular septal defects, diagnosing the atrioventricular connections according to the union of the atrial chambers with the apical ventricular components.

Morphogenesis

The problems arising from morphogenesis relate as much to terminology of the embryonic heart tube as they do to positive disagreements. When considering the occurrence of double inlet connection, therefore, we should remember that, initially, the orifice of the atrioventricular canal was supported almost exclusively above the inlet part of the primary heart tube, with the presumptive arterial pedicles supported by the outlet component (Fig. 31-22). As described in Chapter 3, the apical component of the developing left ventricle balloons from the inlet component of the ventricular loop, while that of the developing right ventricle balloons from the outlet part. The ballooning of the two apical ventricular components occurs concomitant with development of the apical muscular septum. If the two pouches did not grow separately, but rather there was formation of a general apical component from the primary heart tube, then the end result would be a solitary ventricle of indeterminate morphology (see Fig. 31-22, left hand panel). Whether the atrioventricular junctions are guarded by two valves, or a common atrioventricular valve, depends on the partitioning of the atrioventricular junction. Should the pouches form in normal fashion, but the atrioventricular junction remain connected only to the inlet part of the ventricular loop, then the end result would be double inlet left ventricle. The hypoplastic trabecular component derived from the outlet part of the loop would form the basis of the incomplete right ventricle (see Fig. 31-22, lower right hand panel). Again, the arrangement of the atrioventricular valves would depend upon the mode of development of the atrioventricular junction. The ventriculo-arterial connections present would depend on the development of the outlet portions. The position of the incomplete right ventricle would probably be determined by the initial looping of the primary tube, but equally it could be influenced by rotation of the entire heart.

Double inlet right ventricle results from transfer of the entire inlet part of the primary heart tube to the apical component derived from the outlet, this process occurring subsequent to formation of the apical component of the left ventricle (see Fig. 31-22, upper right hand panel). This apical component will then form the basis of the postero-inferiorly located incomplete left ventricle. Valvar morphology, and ventriculo-arterial connections, will again depend on the development of the other parts of the heart tube. The position of the incomplete ventricle will depend on the initial direction of ventricular looping. Rightward looping will give a left-sided rudimentary left ventricle, while leftward looping will result in a right-sided left ventricle. The morphogenesis of straddling and overriding valves is discussed in Chapter 33.

Absence of an atrioventricular connection is much harder to explain. Any offered hypothesis must account for the known anatomical facts, namely, that in the setting of absence of the right connection, the left atrium can be connected to a morphologically left, right or indeterminate

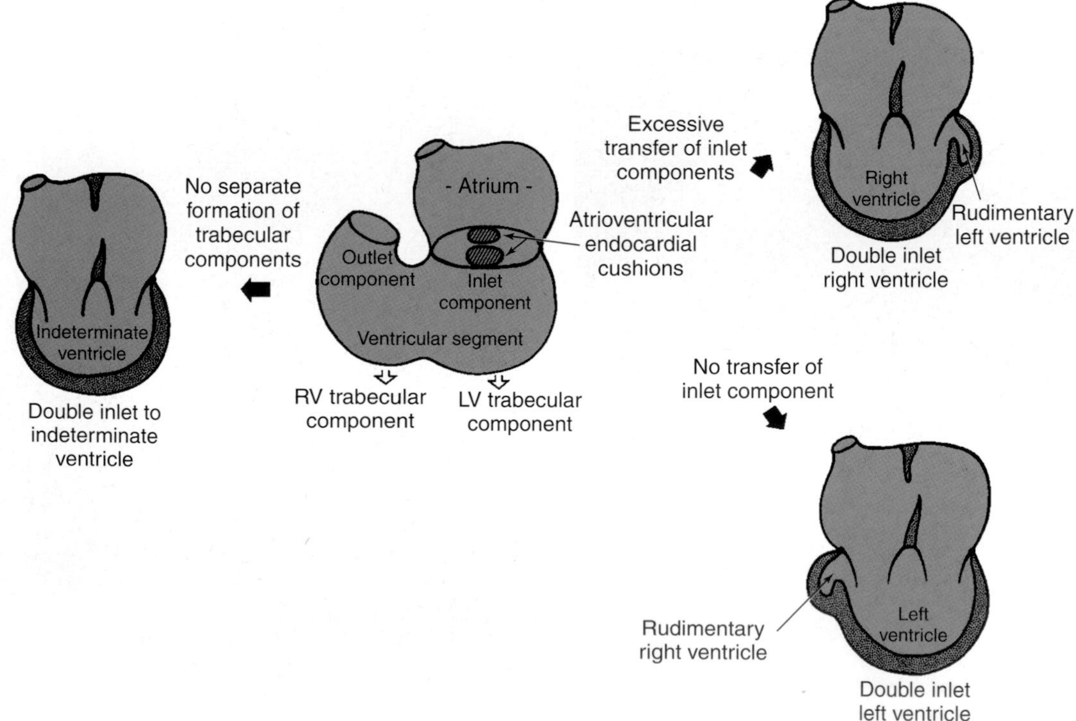

Figure 31-22 The cartoon shows the hypothetical steps that could produce the various form of double inlet ventricle.

ventricle. In each of these circumstances, the right atrial anatomy is indistinguishable, as is the left atrial anatomy in the setting of absence of the left connection, irrespective of whether the right atrium is connected to a morphologically right, left or indeterminate ventricle. The most likely explanation, therefore, is that atrioventricular junctions developed as though to produce double inlet connection, but for some reason the right, or left, atrioventricular orifice failed to develop. Indeed, examination of the developing human heart has shown that a stage exists early in its formation which is remarkably similar to absence of the right atrioventricular connection, albeit prior to formation of the atrial septum.[15]

EPIDEMIOLOGY

Double inlet ventricle occurred in 1.5% of patients with congenitally malformed hearts seen at the Hospital for Sick Children, Toronto, between 1950 and 1973. The ratio of males to females was 1.25 to 1,[16] although difficulties in diagnosis, particularly in the days before cross sectional echocardiography, cast some doubt on the reliability of this figure. In 378 siblings of patients with double inlet ventricle, the overall incidence of congenital heart disease was 2.8%.[17] Although numbers were small, malformations were more frequent in the siblings of patients with isomerism of the left atrial appendages. When characteristics of infants with double inlet ventricle and their parents were compared with randomly selected controls,[18] paternal consumption of alcohol, smoking, and use of marijuana were associated with increased risk of double inlet ventricle in the offspring, particularly when associated with isomerism. Around 1% of a cohort of more than 1 million infants born in Atlanta between 1968 and 2000 were found to have tricuspid atresia,[19] with advanced maternal age associated with an increased incidence. Tricuspid atresia, along with transposition and common arterial trunk, was also found more frequently in offspring of women with diabetes mellitus.[20]

PATHOPHYSIOLOGY

Mixing of Blood

The major consequence of the univentricular atrioventricular connection is obligatory mixing of the pulmonary and systemic venous streams in the dominant ventricle, irrespective of its morphology. This mixing will, in general, be complete in most patients in whom an atrioventricular connection is absent, albeit in only a third of those with double inlet ventricle. In the latter setting, of course, it is guaranteed to be complete only if one cardiac valve is imperforate. In those with double inlet left ventricle, preferential streaming does not appear to be affected by obstruction of the subpulmonary outflow, but it is strongly influenced by the position of the incomplete ventricle. Consequently, patients with usual atrial arrangement and a right-sided incomplete right ventricle tend to have favourable streaming in the presence of concordant ventriculo-arterial connections, and unfavourable streaming when the ventriculo-arterial connections are discordant. This is because the systemic venous blood preferentially enters the incomplete right ventricle. In contrast, if the right ventricle is to the left, and connected to the aorta, it is closer to the left atrioventricular valve and, therefore, preferentially receives pulmonary venous blood.

Atrial Septal Defect

Where there is absence of an atrioventricular connection, the predominant egress of blood from the affected atrium is through an atrial septal defect, although in some in whom there is absence of the left atrioventricular connection, a laevoatrial cardinal vein may contribute. Significant obstruction to the atrial septal defect is manifest in the patient with absent right atrioventricular connection in the form of hepatic enlargement and a reduced cardiac output, while the patient with absent left atrioventricular connection will demonstrate evidence of pulmonary venous congestion and hypoxaemia. Significant obstruction across the atrial septal defect may be important in the patient with double inlet ventricle in one of two settings. The first is when there is stenosis of one of the atrioventricular valves, and the second is where streaming is unfavourable. In the latter situation, an atrial septostomy may reduce the effects of unfavourable streaming and enhance systemic oxygenation.

Pulmonary and Systemic Flows

Clinical presentation is independent of ventricular morphology, but strongly related to the presence of associated lesions. As discussed above, patients with restriction to the pulmonary venous return tend to present in early infancy with pulmonary congestion and hypoxaemia. In patients with absent right atrioventricular connection, restriction of the interatrial communication may result in hepatic congestion. Apart from this, the mode of presentation is almost entirely dependent on the degree of restriction to the pulmonary or systemic circulations. At one extreme are patients with pulmonary atresia, who present with severe cyanosis shortly after birth. If no pulmonary stenosis is present, infants present in the first month or two of life with signs of increased pulmonary flow, often without clinically evident cyanosis. This is exacerbated by the co-existence of interruption of the aortic arch or coarctation, which has been reported in about one-third of autopsied cases where the aorta arises from the incomplete right ventricle, frequently in association with obstruction at a subaortic interventricular communication. It is much rarer if the aorta arises from the dominant ventricle. In the latter situation, it is related to postero-caudal deviation of the outlet septum into the subaortic region. In between the Scylla of severe cyanosis, and the Charybdis of flooded lungs, lies just the right amount of pulmonary stenosis. Patients in this favourable category may present as asymptomatic children, or even as adults with murmurs detected at routine physical examination.

CLINICAL FINDINGS

Although the majority of patients present in the neonatal period or early infancy, the timing and exact clinical presentation will always be dictated by the associated anomalies and their severity. When there is severe obstruction of flow to the lungs, presentation is usually in the neonatal period with a duct-dependent pulmonary circulation. Cyanosis will be present at birth, and will become more severe with impending closure of the arterial duct. There will be a single second heart sound, a short ejection systolic murmur of pulmonary stenosis at the upper left sternal edge, and sometimes a soft continuous ductal murmur. When there is pulmonary atresia, there will be a single second heart sound, and frequently a continuous murmur from the arterial duct. In contrast, an infant with aortic coarctation will exhibit weak or absent femoral pulses, mild central cyanosis, and symptoms of high pulmonary blood flow, including tachypnoea, enlargement of the liver, and difficulties with feeding. When there is severe aortic coarctation, or aortic interruption, presentation may be with shock during the early neonatal period. Similarly, although the infant with a large interventricular communication will usually be symptom free at birth, the pulmonary vascular resistance will have fallen sufficiently by the beginning of the second month of life for the symptoms and signs of increased pulmonary flow to have become evident. In contrast, the infant with balanced systemic and pulmonary flows because of moderate pulmonary stenosis will be well, with mild central cyanosis and a systolic murmur heard best at the lower left sternal edge. Should the degree of obstruction to pulmonary flow increase, cyanosis will become more obvious, and cyanotic spells might occur.

INVESTIGATIONS

Electrocardiography

In theory, electrocardiography should be very useful in these patients, given the abnormal position of the conduction system and the abnormal size of the ventricles. Correlation might be expected between the direction of the initial QRS vector and the orientation of the ventricular septum, and between the progression of the R wave across the precordium with the relative positions of the dominant and incomplete ventricles.

The standard surface electrocardiogram reveals a leftward superior axis in more than four-fifths of patients in whom the right atrioventricular connection is absent. An electrical axis between 0 and +90 degrees occurs in approximately one-tenth of patients, occurring more frequently, but not exclusively, when the ventriculo-arterial connections are discordant. In the majority of patients in whom the left atrioventricular connection is absent, the frontal QRS axis is between +90 and +180 degrees. The frontal QRS axis can be highly variable in patients with double inlet ventricle. Vectorcardiograms, for example, did not usefully distinguish patients with double inlet ventricle from those with large interventricular communications and comparable ventriculo-arterial connections.[21]

In patients with tricuspid atresia, a pattern of left ventricular dominance is seen in the majority, while right ventricular hypertrophy is associated with unusual anatomical arrangements, including that in which the left atrium connects to a dominant right ventricle. In those in whom the left atrioventricular connection is absent, the typical pattern of the ventricular forces tends to indicate right ventricular dominance. In patients with double inlet left ventricle, a pattern of left ventricular dominance occurs more commonly in those with right-sided incomplete right ventricles, while a pattern of right ventricular dominance is found in most having double inlet right ventricle. It is possible to make sense of the electrocardiogram, therefore, when the diagnosis is known. Making the diagnosis from the electrocardiogram, in contrast, is much more difficult.

Chest Radiography

There is no particular configuration of the cardiac outline that typifies the patient with a univentricular atrioventricular connection. Abnormalities present on plain chest radiography are the consequence of malposition of the heart, the relatively high incidence of isomerism, and the high incidence of discordant ventriculo-arterial connections or abnormally related great arteries. Left-sided incomplete right ventricles occasionally protrude from the left border of the heart in a characteristic fashion in those with double inlet left ventricle. A prominent right heart border, reflecting right atrial distension, may suggest a restrictive interatrial communication in a patient with tricuspid atresia.

There is a close correlation between the size of the heart and the volume of flow to the lungs. With diminished pulmonary flow, the size of the heart remains normal, although in the absence of pulmonary stenosis, when pulmonary flow is increased, cardiomegaly is the rule. If the pulmonary vascularity is increased, and the heart is greatly enlarged, and yet the child is markedly cyanotic, the inference can be drawn for markedly unfavourable streaming of blood within the heart, or possibly obstruction to pulmonary venous return.

Transthoracic Echocardiography

M-mode Tracings

Considerable attention was directed to the inferential echocardiographic diagnosis of a univentricular atrioventricular connection using M-mode techniques. These studies remain of historical interest, but since the advent of cross sectional techniques are no longer useful in the anatomical delineation of these hearts.

Cross Sectional Echocardiography

As in any congenital cardiac lesion, accurate echocardiographic diagnosis is facilitated by use of the segmental approach. Given the complexity of these hearts, a systematic approach is of particular importance. Having determined the atrial arrangement, the examination proceeds to the delineation of the atrioventricular connections. The key to the diagnosis of double inlet ventricle lies in the demonstration of two atrioventricular valves, one of which may be imperforate, or a common valve, opening into one ventricle. In hearts with absent atrioventricular connection, the prominent atrioventricular groove, which may contain fibro-fatty tissue, will be seen interposing between the floor of the atrium and the ventricular mass. These appearances are best demonstrated from the subcostal (Figs. 31-23 and 31-24) or apical windows (Fig. 31-25), with the transducer oriented so as to demonstrate both atriums and both atrioventricular valves (Fig. 31-26). This is the cut that would normally produce a four-chamber section. In patients with double inlet ventricle, it is sometimes difficult to see both junctions in the same plane, particularly from the subcostal position, but slight rocking of the transducer from side to side so as to bring first one valve and then the other into view, while recording continuously, will normally produce the necessary information. In patients with double inlet ventricle, the relations between the atrioventricular junction and the ventricular septum should be assessed for overriding. If this exists, biventricular connections must

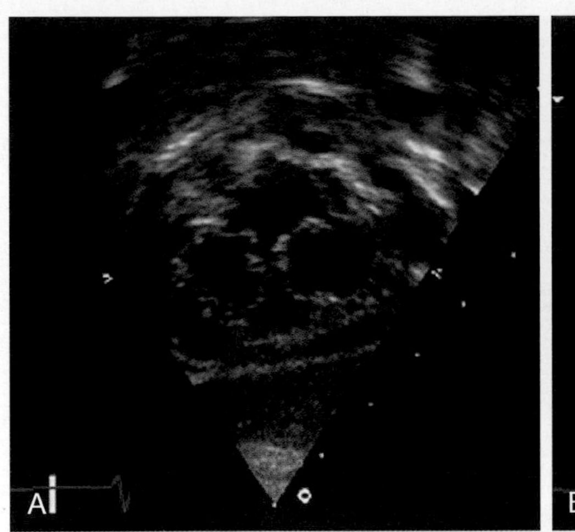

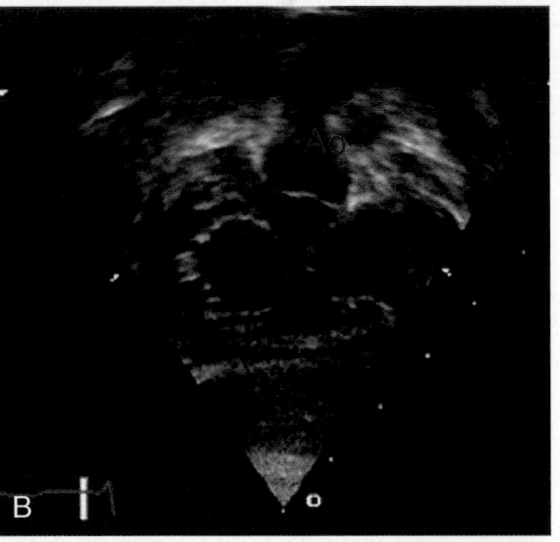

Figure 31-23 These images obtained from a subcostal window demonstrate double inlet left ventricle via two atrioventricular valves. Panel **A** demonstrates the size of the atrioventricular valves (*arrows*), while slight anterior angulation (**B**) demonstrates the aorta (Ao) which arises from the dominant ventricle.

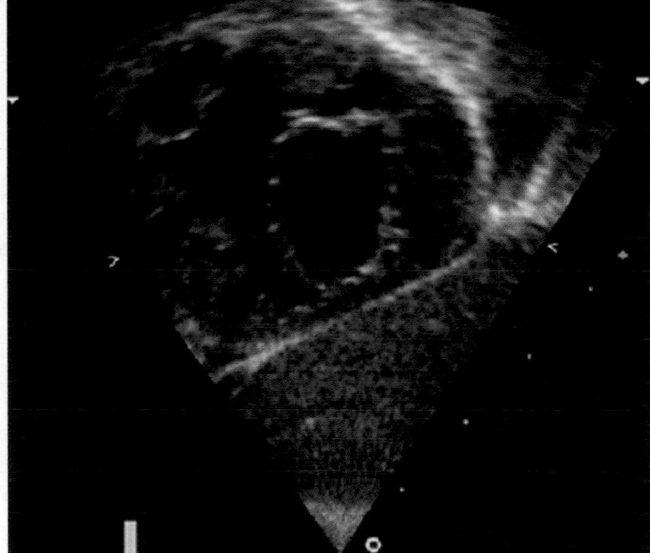

Figure 31-24 In this image, obtained from a subcostal window, in a patient with isomerism of the right atrial appendages, it can be seen that both atrial chambers connect to the dominant ventricle through a common atrioventricular valve.

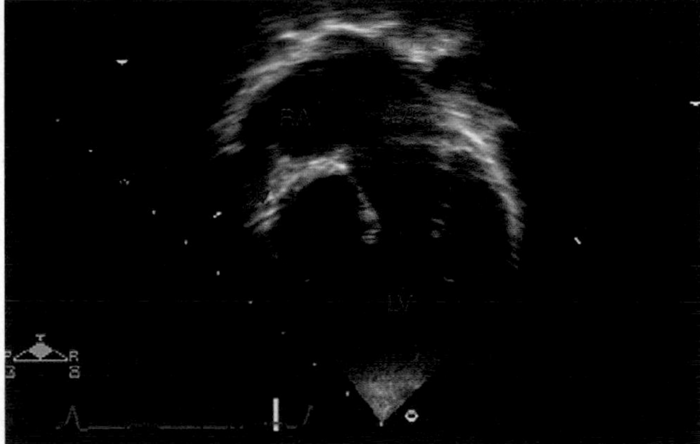

Figure 31-25 The image is obtained from an apical window in a patient with tricuspid atresia. The fibro-fatty tissue within the atrioventricular groove (*arrow*) is seen separating the right atrium (RA) from the ventricular mass. This is the consequence of absence of the right atrioventricular connection. LA, left atrium; LV, left ventricle.

be distinguished from the univentricular connection by applying the 50% rule. Precordial short-axis cuts, on occasion, can demonstrate well the double inlet connection.

Should an imperforate valve exist in the setting of double inlet ventricle, it is seen as a thin mobile echo between one or the other atrium and the dominant ventricle, sometimes with tension apparatus inserting into it. If this is suspected, it is important to scan from front to back of the heart to ensure that it is not the valvar annulus that is being misinterpreted as an imperforate valve. A common valve appears quite different from a single valve to the experienced observer, resembling closely the common atrioventricular orifice of atrioventricular septal defects. The easiest way to recognise a common atrioventricular junction is to identify the so-called ostium primum defect, which has always been present in cases described so far. In patients in whom one of the atrioventricular connections is absent, care should be taken to document abnormalities of the solitary atrioventricular valve, which are common.[22]

In hearts with one big and one small ventricle, short- and long-axis scans from subcostal or precordial windows demonstrate the malaligned and hypoplastic muscular ventricular septum. Such cuts also demonstrate well the relation of the incomplete and dominant ventricles. These spatial relationships as seen in the long- and short-axis planes are most useful in determining the morphology of the ventricles. In hearts in which the left ventricle is dominant, the incomplete right ventricle is always carried on its antero-superior shoulder. In contrast, in hearts with dominant right ventricles, the incomplete left ventricle occupies a postero-inferior position. If a second ventricle is not identified, the ventricular morphology is presumed to be indeterminate. Once the existence and morphology of any incomplete ventricle has been determined, the ventriculo-arterial connections can be established by tracing the arterial roots in subcostal or precordial long-axis cuts until they can be identified as either aorta or pulmonary trunk. Similar cuts will also demonstrate the nature of any subvalvar obstruction.

Having established the basic anatomy, using the sequential approach, other features must be considered. Abnormalities of systemic (Fig. 31-27) and pulmonary venous return (Fig. 31-28) can usually be readily identified from

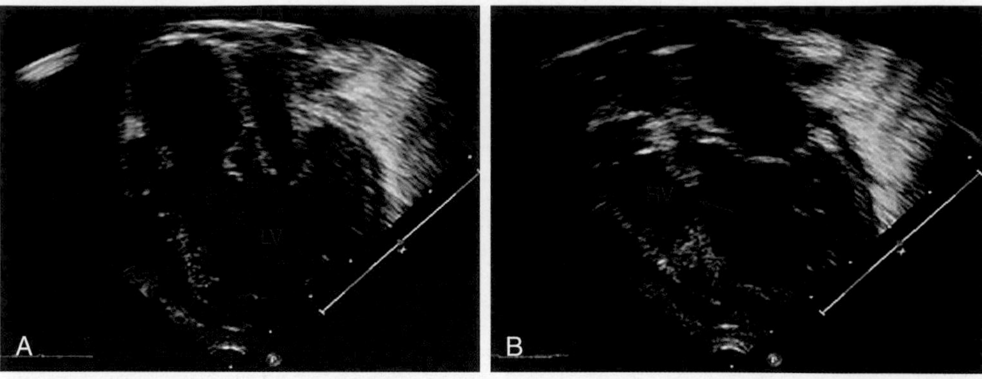

Figure 31-26 These images are obtained from an apical window in a patient with double inlet left ventricle via two atrioventricular valves (**A**). Slight anterior angulation of the transducer (**B**) demonstrates an unrestrictive communication (*arrow*) between the dominant left ventricle and the incomplete right ventricle (RV), which gives rise to the aorta.

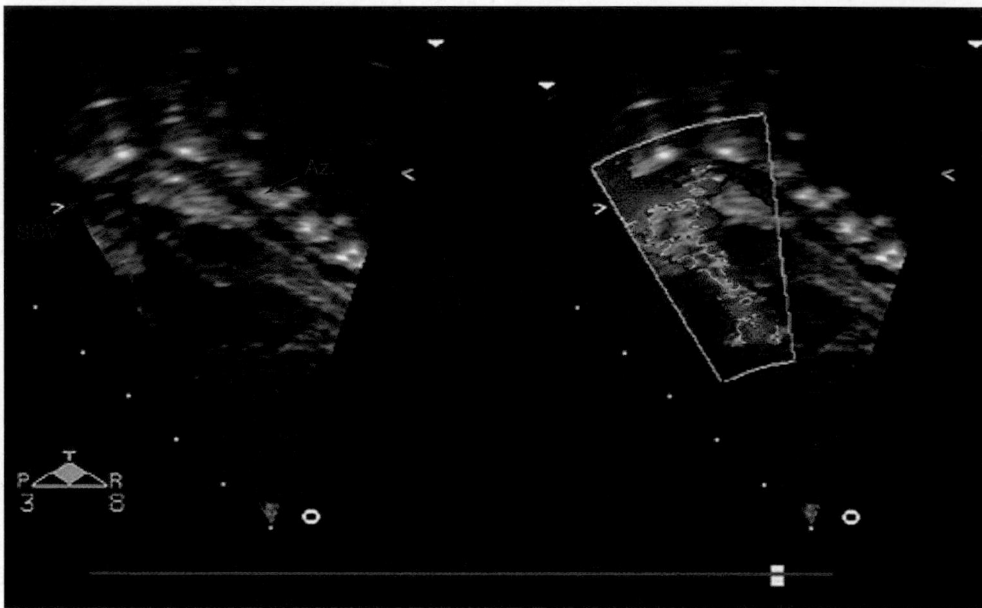

Figure 31-27 These images, obtained from a subcostal window in a patient with isomerism of the left atrial appendages, show azygos (Az.) continuation of the abdominal venous return to the superior caval vein (SCV). The colour flow seen in the right panel shows the flow from the superior caval vein into the heart.

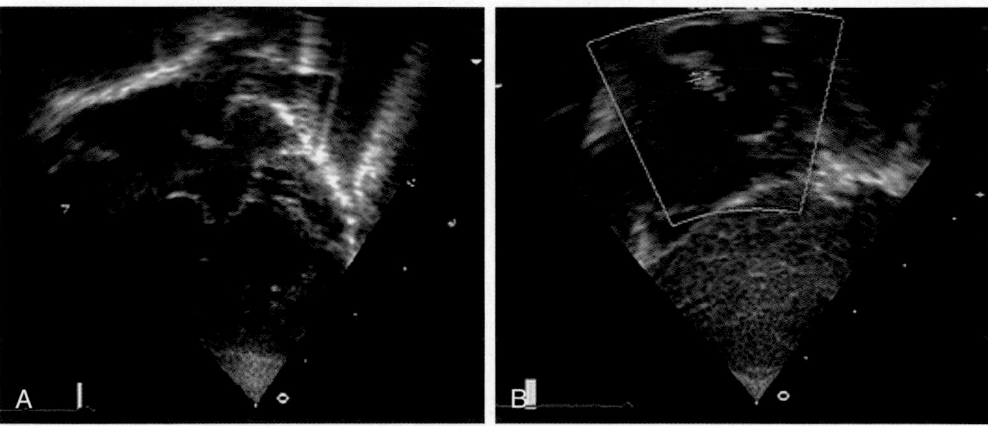

Figure 31-28 These images are obtained from a subcostal window in a patient with isomerism of the right atrial appendages and double inlet ventricle. The pulmonary veins drain to a confluence (C). There is restrictive egress from the confluence (**A**), which results in distension of the pulmonary veins (*arrows* in **B**).

subcostal, parasternal, and suprasternal views. Identification of bilateral superior caval veins will assume greater importance in planning cavopulmonary shunts. Considerable attention should be directed to the assessment of the interventricular communication (Fig. 31-29). The muscular, perimembranous, doubly committed or multiple nature of such defects can readily be identified. Measurements of the interventricular communication should be performed in two planes, usually taking the maximal diameters in both the short- and long-axis projections. These measurements can be used to calculate the area of the interventricular communication using the formula for a regular ellipse, which can be indexed either to body surface area[23] or to the cross sectional area of the aorta. When available,

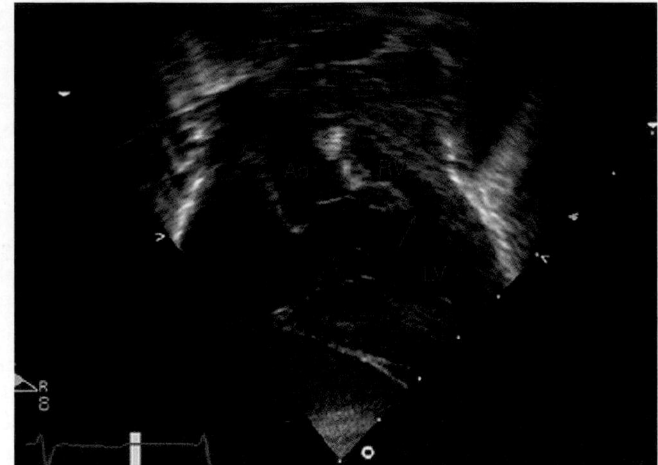

Figure 31-29 This image is again obtained from a subcostal window in a patient with double inlet ventricle. The interventricular communication (*arrow*) and the incomplete and small right ventricle (RV) can be seen. The aorta (Ao) arises from the dominant left ventricle (LV).

three-dimensional echocardiography may be useful. It has been shown to provide accurate measurements of the size of the interventricular communication in cardiac specimens, and in a small group of patients.[24] Careful attention must be paid to the aortic arch to exclude either interruption or coarctation, particularly in those in whom the aorta arises from the incomplete ventricle (Figs. 31-30 and 31-31). Because abnormalities of the atrioventricular valves are frequent, particular attention should be paid to their size and tension apparatus, using multiple cuts as necessary. Colour mapping and Doppler interrogation is of value in detecting valvar regurgitation, although it may be misleading in the assessment of stenosis in patients with double inlet ventricle in the presence of an interatrial communication. The examination is modified accordingly when the heart is in the middle or to the right of the chest, but the basic principles of diagnosis remain the same.

Fetal Echocardiography

Fetal ultrasonic scanning is now a routine part of antenatal care in many countries, and consequently increasing numbers of cardiac anomalies are being detected prior to birth. Data from the 12 registries included in the Eurocat study revealed that, between 1990 and 1994, half of those with double inlet ventricle, and more than two-fifths of those with tricuspid atresia, were diagnosed in this fashion.[25] Nuchal thickening is an established marker for the presence of congenital cardiac disease in fetal life. Using this feature, one study[26] found one-sixth of patients with congenitally malformed hearts and normal chromosomes to have tricuspid atresia. In a series of patients diagnosed prenatally with tricuspid atresia, almost three-tenths were either terminated or died prior to birth. Of those surviving to active management, the probability of survival was 91% at 1 month, 87% at 6 months, and 83% at 1 year. Multi-variate analysis revealed that the presence of a chromosomal anomaly or syndrome, and the requirement for

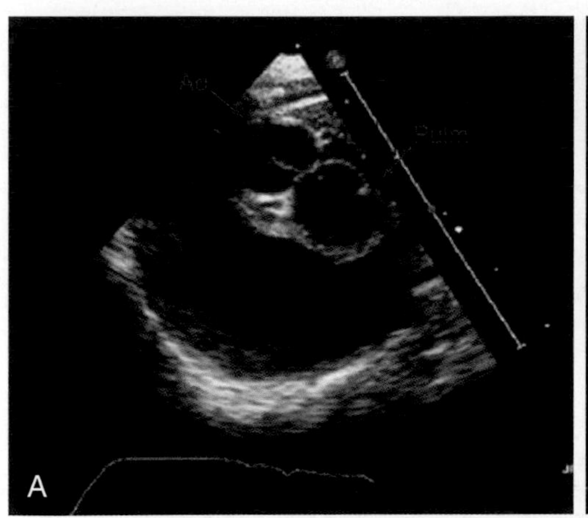

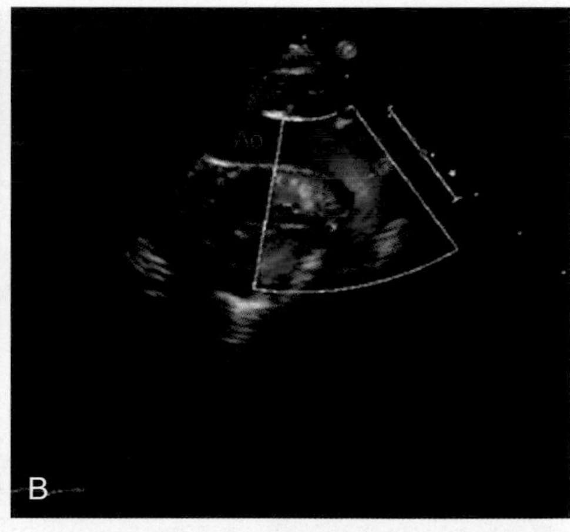

Figure 31-30 These images are obtained from high parasternal and suprasternal windows in a patient with double inlet left ventricle and discordant ventriculo-arterial connections. The size of the aortic valve is similar to that of the pulmonary valve (Pulm in **A**), and the aortic arch is unobstructed (**B**). Parasternal images had revealed a large interventricular communication. Ao, aorta.

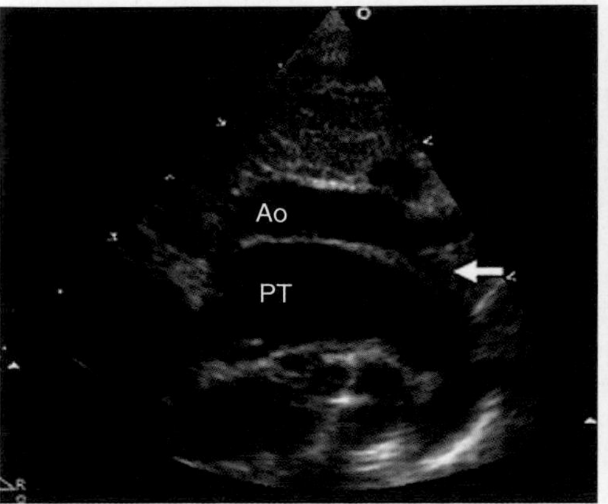

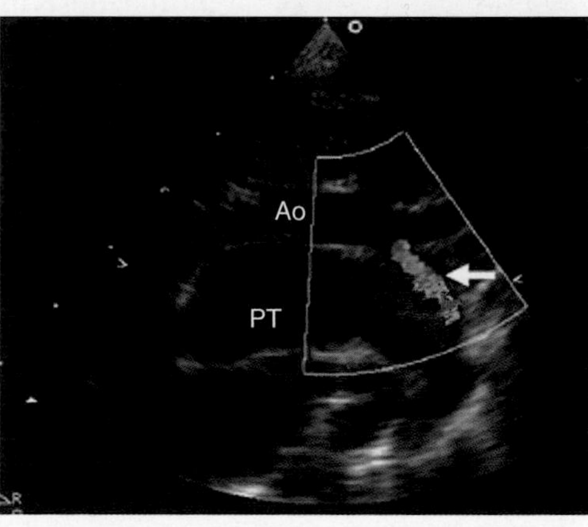

Figure 31-31 These images are obtained from a suprasternal window in a patient with double inlet left ventricle and discordant ventriculo-arterial connections. The aortic valve is considerably smaller than the pulmonary valve. The distal portion of the aortic arch is hypoplastic and obstructed (*arrow*). Parasternal imaging had demonstrated a restrictive interventricular communication, resulting in subaortic obstruction. Ao, aorta; PT, pulmonary trunk.

extracorporeal membrane oxygenation, were independent risk factors for death.[27] An important potential benefit of antenatal diagnosis overall is that it permits transfer of fetuses with potentially duct-dependent systemic or pulmonary circulations for delivery and treatment in specialist centres, resulting in improved survival. Such benefits have yet to be proven, nonetheless, for fetuses known to have either double inlet ventricle or tricuspid atresia. In a study of patients with isomeric atrial appendages, with over half diagnosed antenatally, diagnosis during fetal life did not improve survival.[28]

Nuclear Imaging

Nuclear imaging is of little value in the diagnosis of patients with univentricular atrioventricular connection.

Magnetic Resonance Imaging

The recent widespread use of magnetic resonance imaging has provided exciting new insights into the anatomy and pathophysiology of those having univentricular atrioventricular connections.[29] Magnetic resonance imaging can provide a complete sequential diagnosis in most patients (Fig. 31-32). It is of particular value in those in whom echocardiographic images are suboptimal. Its ability to demonstrate the distal portions of the pulmonary arteries, and the function of the morphologically abnormal ventricles, may be of particular interest. In some centres, magnetic resonance imaging has established a central role in planning for intermediate palliation,[30] making cardiac catheterisation unnecessary. It is unlikely, however, that the technique will, in the near future, entirely replace cardiac catheterisation in the assessment of the patient prior to definitive palliation.

Cardiac Catheterisation

It has been suggested that, in many patients, advances in non-invasive investigative techniques may make cardiac catheterisation unnecessary prior to definitive palliation.[31,32] In our centre, nonetheless, at least for now, we continue to recommend cardiac catheterisation in all such patients. This is principally because of the necessity to measure the flow of blood to the lungs, along with pulmonary resistance, but also because of the difficulty in recognising mild degrees of subaortic obstruction, which occurs most commonly in patients in whom the left ventricle is dominant, and the aorta arises from the incomplete right ventricle.[33]

Cardiac catheterisation is almost always performed using a femoral approach, although, in patients after a bidirectional cavopulmonary anastomosis, cannulation of the internal jugular vein also is necessary if the cavopulmonary anastomosis is the only source of flow to the lungs. The dominant ventricle is usually entered with ease, although difficulties may be encountered entering the artery supported by it. Use of a flow-directed balloon catheter may be helpful. If not, retrograde arterial catheterisation almost always succeeds when the catheter is passed through the aortic valve and looped in the dominant ventricle. Entry into the dominant left ventricle from a retrograde arterial approach, nonetheless, must be performed with extreme caution in the patient with double inlet left ventricle and discordant ventriculoarterial connections, as it may result in subaortic obstruction or damage to the aortic valve. Careful withdrawals across the interventricular communication should be recorded to document any obstruction at that site.

The pulmonary arteries must always be entered in order to assess pulmonary vascular anatomy and physiology. When it is not possible to enter the pulmonary arteries, it has been suggested that measurements of a pulmonary venous wedge pressure may provide an estimate of pressure in the pulmonary arteries. Such measurements provided a relatively accurate estimate of the pressure in the pulmonary arteries when this was less than 18 mm Hg.[34] In patients in whom the aorta arises from the incomplete right ventricle, an intravenous infusion of isoprenaline can be used to provoke a gradient across the interventricular communication while simultaneously measuring left ventricular and ascending aortic pressures. Careful withdrawal around the aortic arch will aid in the exclusion of obstruction within the arch (Fig. 31-33).

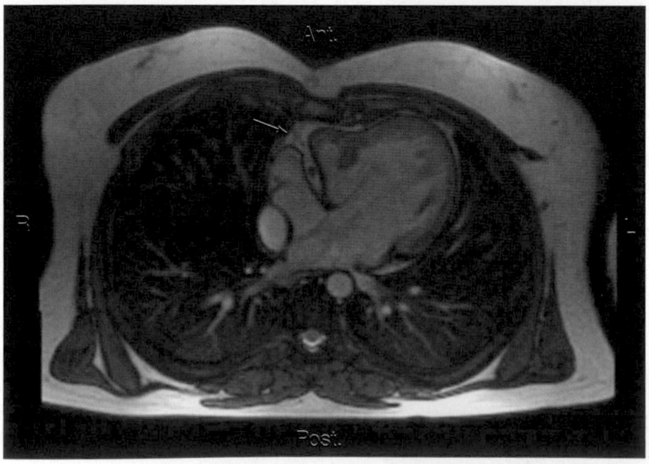

Figure 31-32 This magnetic resonance image is profiled in four-chamber projection and obtained in a patient with tricuspid atresia. The fibrofatty tissue within the atrioventricular groove (*arrow*) is shown separating the right atrium from the ventricular mass. Ant., anterior; L, left; post., posterior; R, right.

Angiocardiography

The investigator who can produce high-quality angiocardiograms in patients with a functionally single ventricle will have no difficulty in any other field of angiocardiography. Although a detailed angiographic approach to establishing the diagnosis in patients with a univentricular atrioventricular connection has been described, advances in non-invasive imaging have now rendered this approach obsolete.

If performed, injections into the dominant ventricle show the interventricular communication (Fig. 31-34), demonstrate the relationships between the two ventricles, serve to exclude incompetence of the atrioventricular valves (Fig. 31-35), and function to opacify the systemic and pulmonary outflow tracts. Opacification of the volume-overloaded dominant ventricle usually requires injection of 1.8 to 2 mL/kg of contrast medium. Biplane cineangiography is recommended, with one intensifier providing a lateral projection. Information obtained from the transthoracic echocardiogram may help in planning the optimal position of the second intensifier. In patients

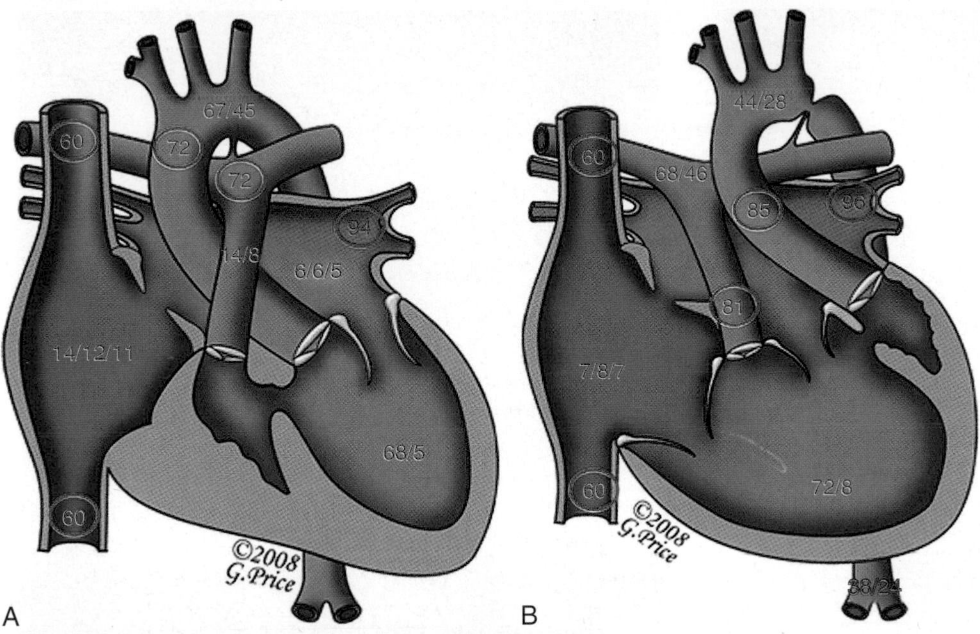

Figure 31-33 Illustrative haemodynamic and oximetric data from a patient with tricuspid atresia and concordant ventriculo-arterial connections (**A**), and double inlet left ventricle with discordant ventriculo-arterial connections (**B**). Panel **A** shows the situation with restricted pulmonary flow, so that the pulmonary arterial pressure is lower than systemic. The saturation of oxygen in the aorta is 72%, because of the low pulmonary flow. The atrial septal defect is restrictive, resulting in a drop in pressure across the atrial septum. In panel **B**, there is a drop in pressure between the left ventricle and the aorta, which reflects restriction at the level of the interventricular communication and a further drop in pressure across the aortic arch, reflecting the presence of aortic coarctation. The saturation of oxygen in the aorta is slightly higher than that in the pulmonary arteries because of a minor degree of streaming.

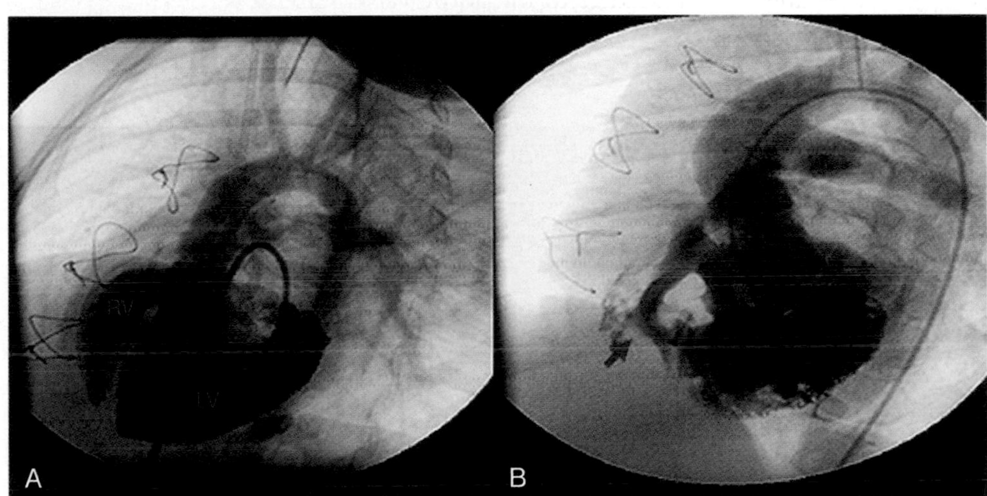

Figure 31-34 These ventriculograms were performed in the dominant left ventricle in a patient with a solitary interventricu (LV) lar communication (**A**), and one with multiple interventricular communications (*arrows* in **B**). RV, right ventricle.

with a dominant right ventricle, or a dominant left ventricle with a left-sided incomplete right ventricle, an antero-posterior projection is chosen. These projections also serve to identify the solitary and indeterminate ventricle when the apical trabeculations are coarse and it is not possible to identify a second ventricle. In patients with a dominant left ventricle and a right-sided right ventricle, a long-axial projection is usually best in profiling the ventricular septum. This demonstrates well the ventriculo-arterial connections, and also reveals the presence of a common valve. Injections into the small ventricle can provide further imaging of the interventricular communication, and demonstrate obstruction within the cavity of the small ventricle itself.

Pulmonary angiography should be performed in all patients prior to definitive palliation. The size of the pulmonary arteries can be measured and indexed to either the surface area of the body or to the aorta. Distortion of the pulmonary arteries, or pulmonary arterial stenoses, can be demonstrated, and the pattern of pulmonary venous return delineated. In patients after staged palliation with either systemic-to-pulmonary arterial or cavopulmonary shunts, further angiograms are required to verify patency of the shunt (Fig. 31-36), while in others, caval venous injections (Fig. 31-37), and/or angiography of the aortic arch (Fig. 31-38), will be necessary.

Biopsy of the Lung

Given the importance of the pulmonary vasculature in determining outcomes after definitive palliation, biopsies of the lung were formerly frequent in assessing potentially high-risk patients. Although biopsies are now rarely performed, a recent study analysed biopsies from patients who were considered to be good candidates for definitive palliation, to determine whether pulmonary histology could predict failure. Specimens were abnormal in almost half of patients with low pulmonary arterial pressure. While there was no relationship between preoperative pulmonary arterial pressure and outcome, extension of muscle into peripheral arteries was always present in cases of failure of

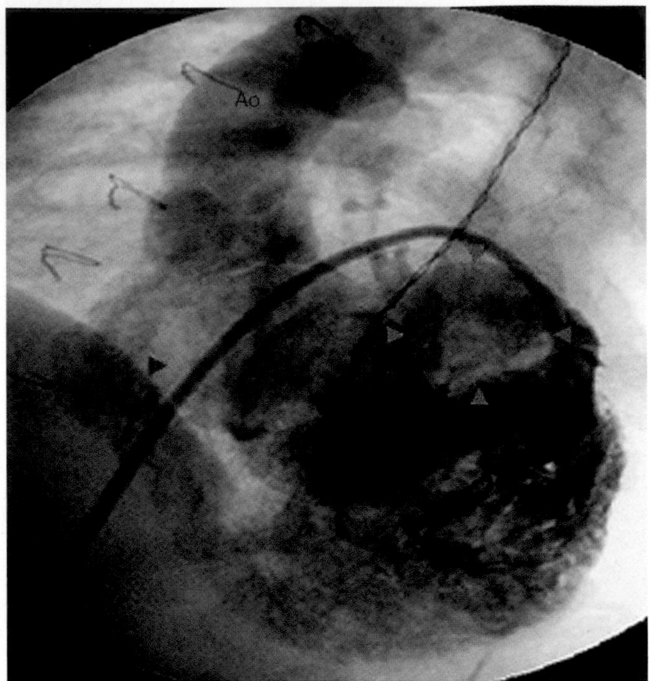

Figure 31-35 This ventriculogram was performed in the dominant ventricle of a patient with double inlet left ventricle via two atrioventricular valves. The atrioventricular valves can be seen *en face* with the *reds arrowheads* showing the orifice of the right atrioventricular valve, and the *yellow arrowheads* the orifice of the left valve. Ao, aorta.

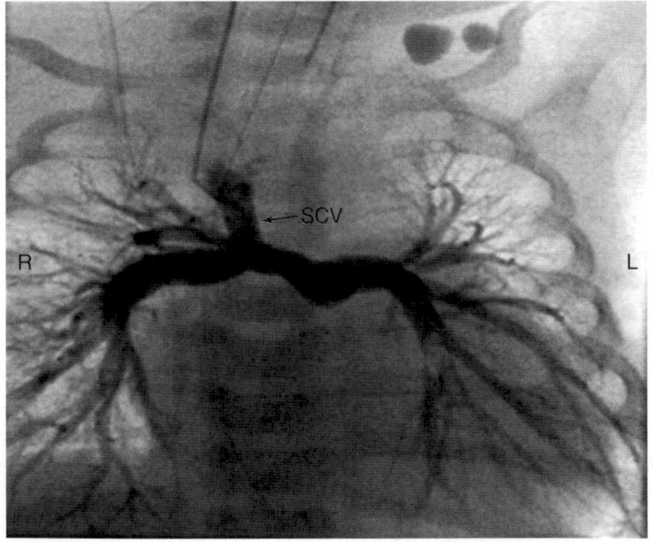

Figure 31-36 The angiogram was performed in the superior caval vein (SCV) in a patient in whom a bidirectional cavopulmonary shunt has been completed. The shunt is widely patent, and the right and left pulmonary arteries can be easily seen. L, left; R, right.

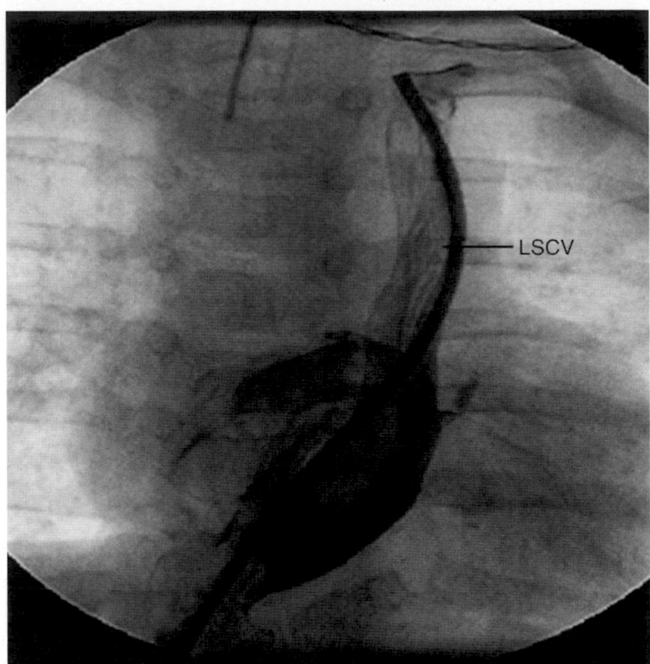

Figure 31-37 In this patient with tricuspid atresia and a left superior caval vein (LSCV) connected to the coronary sinus, a catheter has been passed from the femoral vein through the coronary sinus to the left superior caval vein, and an angiogram has been performed.

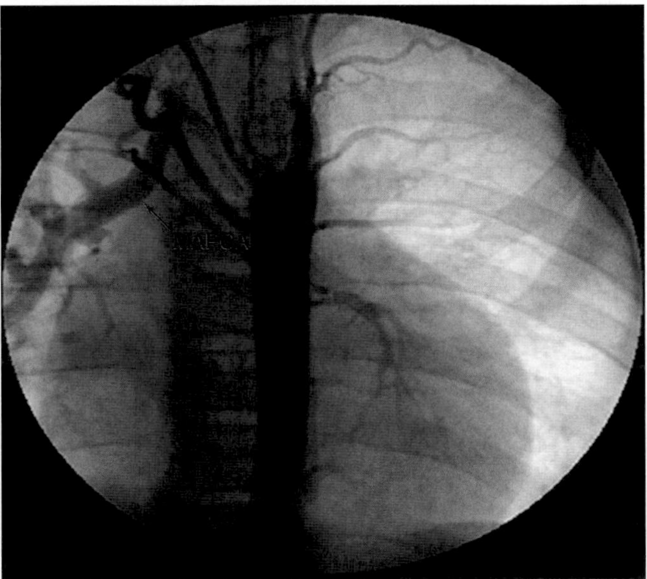

Figure 31-38 An aortogram in this patient with double inlet left ventricle and diminutive pulmonary arteries revealed a major aortopulmonary collateral artery (MAPCA), which perfused the right lung.

the Fontan procedure. It was concluded that histomorphometric examination of pulmonary biopsies may still be a useful adjunct to the usual criterions for selection of therapeutic options in some patients.[35]

MANAGEMENT

Medical Management

Neonates with cyanosis and duct-dependent pulmonary flow usually improve rapidly once ductal patency is re-established by intravenous infusion of prostaglandin E. A poor response to prostaglandin, particularly in the setting of right isomerism, may indicate obstructed pulmonary venous return. In these patients, supportive care, with mechanical ventilation and correction of acidosis, may provide temporary stability while awaiting urgent surgery. Patients with obstructed systemic circulation and duct-dependent systemic blood flow may be in critical condition, with poor peripheral pulses, acidosis, and oliguria. Again, infusion of prostaglandin E, combined with manoeuvres to augment pulmonary vascular resistance, may be life saving.

Once ductal patency is established in those with duct-dependent circulations, medical management is directed to optimizing the delicate balance between systemic and pulmonary flows. This is achieved by gentle reduction of systemic afterload, combined with manoeuvres to augment pulmonary vascular resistance, including positive pressure ventilation with a fraction of inspired oxygen between 0.21 and 0.25.

Surgical Management

Initial Palliative Surgery

Initial surgical palliation is performed in order to allow survival in the short term, and to set the scene for definitive palliation at low risk. This is achieved, first, by ensuring that there is adequate, although not excessive, flow at low pressure through a low-resistance, non-distorted pulmonary vascular bed. The second prerequisite is to optimise systemic outflow in those with subaortic or aortic arch obstruction. The third is to ensure that systemic and pulmonary venous return is unobstructed. In a large cohort of patients with functionally univentricular hearts treated between 1988 and 2000, just under two-fifths were initially palliated using only a systemic-to-pulmonary arterial shunt, one-fifth by banding the pulmonary trunk, one-sixth by construction of a bidirectional cavopulmonary shunt, another fifth by conversion to the Fontan circulation, and the remaining one-twentieth by a Norwood operation. Almost one-quarter of the patients died before definitive palliation could be achieved by means of a Fontan operation.[36] In another cohort with tricuspid atresia and concordant ventriculo-arterial connections, presenting prior to 2004, antegrade flow in the pulmonary arteries was absent in one-fifth, restricted in half, and unrestricted in three-tenths. Initial palliation included a systemic-to-pulmonary arterial shunt in one-third, banding of the pulmonary trunk in one-tenth, and construction of a cavopulmonary anastomosis in one-quarter. By the age of 2 years, nine-tenths had undergone a cavopulmonary connection, 6% were dead, and 4% remained alive without a cavopulmonary connection. Risk factors for death without a cavopulmonary anastomosis included the presence of mitral regurgitation and the use of systemic-to-pulmonary arterial shunts which did not originate from the brachiocephalic artery. Of those who underwent a cavopulmonary anastomosis, three-quarters had undergone a Fontan operation within 3 years. Overall, after 5 years, 86% of the patients were still alive.[37]

Patients with Excessive Pulmonary Flow

Banding of the pulmonary trunk is performed to reduce the volume load to the dominant ventricle, to reduce the flow of blood to the lungs and pulmonary arterial pressure, and to prevent the development of pulmonary vascular disease. The role of banding has been controversial in patients in whom the left ventricle is dominant because of a statistical association between this procedure and the development of acquired subaortic obstruction. It remains unclear, however, whether this relationship is a causal one, or just reflects the evolution over time in the size of the muscular interventricular communication.

Banding of the pulmonary trunk may be performed through a left thoracotomy or through a median sternotomy, making limited dissections between the aorta and pulmonary trunk so as to reduce the risk of distal migration of the band producing stenosis of the pulmonary arterial branches. The size of the band can be predicted according to published formulas, although fine-tuning of the size is usually performed according to systemic and pulmonary arterial pressures and systemic arterial saturations of oxygen. The difficulties in the intra-operative assessment of the adequacy of the band have resulted in the development of a number of novel techniques that permit percutaneous adjustment in the post-operative period.[38,39] These newer approaches may well reduce mortality and adverse events early after surgery.[38]

A recent study[40] has examined outcomes for patients with functionally univentricular circulations undergoing banding of the pulmonary trunk as a primary surgical procedure. In almost half, aortic coarctation or interruption had been repaired at the same procedure, while in almost one-quarter a subsequent procedure was required to relieve subaortic obstruction. Death occurred during the procedure in one-twentieth of the cohort, with additional late deaths bringing the rate of mortality to almost 25%. Overall survival was 84% at 1 year, and 76% at 5 and 15 years. Citing the aforementioned difficulties with banding, nonetheless, it has been suggested[41] that division of the pulmonary trunk and placement of a systemic-to-pulmonary arterial shunt provide an alternative surgical option for patients with excessive flow to the lungs. Using this strategy, the group encountered no operative deaths, and only 1 of their 22 patients died at a later stage. All the patients subsequently underwent a bidirectional cavopulmonary shunt, and almost one-quarter have now been converted to the Fontan circulation, with no additional mortality.

Patients with Inadequate Pulmonary Flow

The modified Blalock–Taussig shunt, in which a graft is interposed between the subclavian or brachiocephalic and the pulmonary arteries, is the procedure of choice. Alternative anastomoses, such as those pioneered by Potts and Waterston, are no longer performed because of their tendency to produce pulmonary arterial distortion and excessive flow to the lungs. Although traditionally the interposition graft has been placed through a thoracotomy, recently some groups have advocated use of a median sternotomy. Potential advantages of this approach are, first, that the shunt can be placed more centrally, facilitating access during further procedures through the midline, and second, that entry to the pleural space is avoided. It has been suggested that shunting into the pulmonary trunk may provide more uniform growth of the pulmonary arteries, compared to when the shunt is inserted directly into them.[42] In some patients with so-called pulmonary coarctation, it has been suggested that concomitant surgical angioplasty of the pulmonary artery involved by the coarctation lesion may enhance growth of the pulmonary artery on the other side.

The syndrome of a reduced systemic output may complicate the post-operative course of patients after construction of a systemic-to-pulmonary arterial shunt. While most patients will respond to optimisation of ventilation, or to infusions of inotropes or vasodilators at low rates, it has been controversial as to whether patients who do not respond to these therapies should be considered for extracorporeal membrane oxygenation. A review of such patients supported in this fashion between 1996 and 2005 showed that almost half survived to be discharged from hospital.[43] The strongest predictor of outcome was the indication for support, with four-fifths of patients cannulated for hypoxaemia, but only three-tenths of those cannulated for hypotension, surviving to discharge. Those requiring support because of obstruction to flow through the shunt showed the greatest survival, at 83%. Thus, the presence of a systemic-to-pulmonary arterial shunt in the setting of a functionally univentricular circulation should not be considered a contra-indication to extracorporeal membrane oxygenation.

In some patients with obstruction to pulmonary flow, the intrapericardial pulmonary arteries may be diminutive, with most flow to the lungs derived through major systemic-to-pulmonary collateral arteries. In these circumstances, unifocalisation of the pulmonary vasculature can facilitate construction of a cavopulmonary circulation, albeit with nearly half of such patients suffering either early or late mortality.[44] Of those surviving, nonetheless, a bidirectional cavopulmonary shunt was constructed in all but one, and half of these were converted to the Fontan circulation.

Subaortic Obstruction

In patients with a dominant left ventricle, the development of subaortic obstruction is a major indicator of poor prognosis. In some, subaortic obstruction is overt at birth, when it is often associated with obstruction in the aortic arch and duct-dependent systemic circulation. In others, progressive restriction may develop during postnatal life. While some of these children will have undergone banding of the pulmonary trunk in early infancy, as we have already discussed, a causal relationship between this procedure and the development of subaortic obstruction remains unproven. Progressive subaortic obstruction has certainly been described in patients who have not undergone banding. Indeed, it has been suggested that banding, by keeping the patient alive, allows the interventricular communication to manifest its natural tendency towards a reduction in size.

A number of surgical approaches to this problem have been described, suggesting that none is ideal. Direct relief has been achieved by enlargement of the interventricular communication, combined with enlargement of the cavity of the incomplete right ventricle. This procedure can be performed through the aortic valve or directly through the rudimentary ventricle. In one large series employing this approach, almost half of the patients were younger than 1 year of age.[45] Previous banding of the pulmonary trunk had been undertaken in over four-fifths of the cohort, and half of these required repair of aortic coarctation. A patch to enlarge the incomplete right ventricle was inserted in all bar one. Of the group, one-fifth died in the early postoperative period, but complete heart block requiring insertion of a pacemaker occurred in only two patients (8%). The overall survival at 1 and 3 years was 73%, and at 5 and 10 years was 68% and 60%, respectively.

An alternative approach used to alleviate subaortic obstruction in the neonate is to perform the arterial switch operation, leaving the restrictive interventricular communication to limit the flow of blood to the lungs. Because of differences in sizes of the arterial outflow tracts, the arterial switch is technically difficult in this setting. Furthermore, even minor degrees of pulmonary arterial distortion secondary to the arterial switch operation may assume greater significance in the patient in whom the eventual treatment requires conversion to the Fontan circulation. We have treated 12 neonates with univentricular atrioventricular connection in this fashion, undertaking concomitant repair of the aortic arch in all but one. Of the group, one-third died either early or later. In the survivors, however, we observed neither recurrence of subaortic obstruction nor aortic valvar incompetence, albeit that we needed to create a modified Blalock–Taussig shunt in two-thirds because of increasing restriction at the level of the interventricular communication. All but one of survivors in the medium term, nonetheless, have now progressed to more definitive palliation by means of cavopulmonary shunting procedures.

It is the creation of an anastomosis between the proximal pulmonary trunk and the ascending aorta, the so-called Damus-Stansel-Kaye procedure, which has been used most frequently as a means of alleviating subaortic obstruction in these patients. Flow of blood to the lungs is ensured by placing an interposition graft between the systemic and pulmonary arteries. In the older infant, it is possible to achieve a cavopulmonary connection,[46] achieving operative results comparable to those undergoing the Damus-Kaye-Stansel procedure beyond the neonatal period, or those having subaortic resection. Overall mortality, nonetheless, remains high irrespective of the chosen therapeutic option.

Anomalies of Pulmonary Venous Return

Anomalies of pulmonary venous return significantly complicate the care of patients with functionally univentricular circulations at all stages of their care, whether during primary palliation, creation of the bidirectional Glenn shunt, or conversion to the Fontan circulation. These anomalies are most frequent in patients with isomeric atrial appendages.[47] Obstruction to flow is common in those with totally anomalous pulmonary venous connections, with this feature present in almost one-third of the patients in one large series.[48] In almost half, repair of the anomalous pulmonary venous return was performed as part of the initial palliative procedure. Although survival was improved in patients undergoing surgery after 1997, only half of the cohort survived to reach the age of 5 years.

Atrial Septectomy

Atrial septectomy may be necessary to improve mixing, or for palliation in patients with associated stenosis of the left atrioventricular valve.

Intermediate Palliation Using a Bidirectional Cavopulmonary Shunt

In recent years, the classic Glenn shunt, which sacrifices the continuity between the right and left pulmonary arteries, has been replaced by the bidirectional cavopulmonary shunt, in which an end-to-side anastomosis is constructed between the superior caval vein and the undivided right pulmonary artery. The bidirectional shunt has now become widely used as a palliative procedure for all patients with univentricular atrioventricular connections. It is well established that the procedure can be performed with low operative risk, and it has been suggested that use of this shunt may reduce the risk of subsequent conversion to the Fontan circulation.[49] Its physiological advantage as a palliative procedure is that the volume load on the dominant ventricle is reduced, and often regurgitation of the atrioventricular valves is alleviated. The operation is usually performed through a median sternotomy, using cardiopulmonary bypass, although it can be performed without cardiopulmonary bypass.[50] In some centres, a physiologically similar operation, the so-called hemi-Fontan procedure, is performed, which more completely prepares the patient for subsequent conversion to the Fontan circulation.[51,52]

It remains controversial whether accessory sources of flow of blood to the lungs should be left in place when constructing a bidirectional cavopulmonary shunt. The systemic arterial saturations of oxygen may be higher in patients in whom there is an alternative source of pulmonary flow. It has also been suggested that such an additional source of pulmonary flow may enhance growth of the pulmonary arteries, which is commonly impaired after a bidirectional cavopulmonary shunt.[53] Others have shown, nonetheless, that such an accessory source of pulmonary flow fails to confer additional benefits in terms of outcome, either after the bidirectional cavopulmonary shunt itself or after subsequent conversion to the Fontan circulation.[54] Although, traditionally, the tendency has been to avoid use of this shunt in young infants, recent data has shown an overall mortality of only 4.8% in patients who underwent this procedure before the age of 6 months.[55] In this series, however, creation of the shunt in the neonatal period proved to be a risk factor for death, prompting the suggestion that the procedure be deferred until after the age of 2 months. Another large series of over 300 patients was collected with early mortality of less than 1%, albeit with 22 later deaths in patients who had not undergone conversion to the Fontan circulation. At the time of follow-up, two-thirds of the cohort had been converted to the Fontan circulation, with mortality of less than 2%. Overall survival at 10 years was 89.8%. Elevated pulmonary arterial pressures, and the presence of isomerism, emerged as independent risk factors for death, takedown, or unsuitability for definitive palliation.[56] In another large series, freedom from death or transplantation was 96% at 1 year, and 89% at 5 years. In this series, atrioventricular valvar regurgitation proved to be an independent risk factor for death or transplantation.[57]

Definitive Palliation

The ultimate aim of initial and intermediate palliation is to prepare the patient for definitive palliation by conversion to the Fontan circulation. The operation and our understanding of its physiology have developed since the original description of Fontan and Baudet.[58] The most notable of these developments have been by de Leval and coworkers,[59] which resulted in the development of the total cavopulmonary shunt, the introduction of fenestration, popularised by the Boston group,[60] and more recently, the introduction of the extracardiac conduit.[61] The considerations and outcomes related to this procedure are detailed in Chapter 32, and so will not be considered here.

An alternative approach to definitive palliation is to septate the dominant ventricle, which will maintain pulsatile flow in the pulmonary circulation. Ventricular septation for double inlet ventricle was first accomplished in the mid 1950s, with results from reasonably large series published in the 1970s and early 1980s. The major problems with early attempts were the need for ventriculotomy, the development of obstruction to ventricular outflow due to billowing of the non-contractile patch, and a high incidence of surgically induced heart block. The incidence of these problems was subsequently reduced by the development of transatrial approaches and staging. Imai and coworkers[62] employed a transatrial approach to septation in a series of 19 patients, many of whom had contraindications to the Fontan approach. Of the patients, one died within 30 days of surgery, while three developed permanent and complete heart block at the time of operation. There were three further deaths within 100 days of surgery. Neither pre-operative mean pulmonary arterial pressure, nor pulmonary vascular resistance, emerged as risk factors, but significant predictors of death were the presence of a high pressure gradient between the dominant ventricle and pulmonary arteries, a high peak systolic pressure, an elevated left ventricular end-diastolic pressure, and a higher body surface area. Based on their experience, Imai and colleagues suggested that septation should only be considered in patients in whom the combined volumes of the right and left ventricles at end-diastole exceeded approximately two and one-half times the expected normal left ventricular end-diastolic volume.[63] In a subsequent analysis, the same group observed that ventricular hypertrophy was also a risk factor. Despite the intuitive appeal of achieving a biventricular circulation subsequent to septation, most centres nowadays still recommend the Fontan operation as the definitive palliative procedure in patients with a functionally univentricular circulation.

The complete reference list can be found on the companion Expert Consult web site at www.expertconsult.com.

ANNOTATED REFERENCES

- Jacobs ML, Anderson RH: Nomenclature of the functionally univentricular heart. Cardiol Young 2006;16(Suppl 1):3–8.

  A review of the problems that have existed in providing a logical description of the ventricular mass in patients having one big and one small ventricle. The necessary logic is provided when it is appreciated that very few of these patients have solitary ventricles, but that all have a functionally univentricular circulation.

- Anderson RH, Macartney FJ, Tynan M, et al: Univentricular atrioventricular connexion—the single ventricle trap unsprung. Pediatr Cardiol 1983;4:273–280.

  The key publication emphasising that, in patients with double inlet ventricle and absence of one atrioventricular connection, it is exceedingly rare to find a solitary chamber within the ventricular mass. Hence, although possible on rare occasions, the ventricle itself is not solitary, and the heart is not univentricular. Since, however, the atrial chambers in both these situations are joined to only one ventricle, the atrioventricular connection is univentricular. The hearts are unified because they possess a univentricular atrioventricular connection, but they would be described on the basis of the specific connection present.

- Kiraly L, Hubay M, Cook AC, et al: Morphologic features of the uniatrial but biventricular atrioventricular connection. J Thorac Cardiovasc Surg 2007;133:229–234.

  A review of a series of hearts having absence of one atrioventricular connection, but with straddling and overriding of the solitary atrioventricular valve. It is explained that this produces a uniatrial but biventricular connection. Such hearts can exist with absence of either the right or left atrioventricular connection, and with right or left hand ventricular topology. This lesion is one variant of double outlet atrium.

- Anderson RH, Ho SY, Becker AE: The surgical anatomy of the conduction tissues. Thorax 1983;38:408–420.

  A review of the disposition of the conduction tissues in many congenitally malformed hearts, explaining in particular the arrangement in functionally univentricular hearts.

- Festa P, Ait Ali L, Bernabei M, De Marchi D: The role of magnetic resonance imaging in the evaluation of the functionally single ventricle before and after conversion to the Fontan circulation. Cardiol Young 2005;15(Suppl 3):51–56.

  This useful review summarises the contribution of magnetic resonance imaging to the care of patients with a univentricular atrioventricular connection at all stages of their palliation.

- Fogel MA: Is routine cardiac catheterization necessary in the management of patients with single ventricles across the staged Fontan reconstruction? No! Pediatr Cardiol 2005;26:154–158.
- Ro PS, Rychik J, Cohen MS, et al: Diagnostic assessment before Fontan operation in patients with bidirectional cavopulmonary anastomosis: Are noninvasive methods sufficient? J Am Coll Cardiol 2004;44:184–187.
- Nakanishi T: Cardiac catheterization is necessary before bidirectional Glenn and Fontan procedures in single ventricle physiology. Pediatr Cardiol 2005;26:159–161.

  The necessity for routine cardiac catheterisation before definitive palliation of the patient with a univentricular atrioventricular connection is a topic of current debate. These three important articles summarise some of the key issues in the discussion.
- Karamlou T, Ashnurn DA, Caldarone CA, et al, Members of the Congenital Heart Surgeons Society: Matching procedure to morphology improves outcomes in neonates with tricuspid atresia. J Thorac Cardiovasc Surg 2005;130:1503–1510.

  This important study, on behalf of the Congenital Heart Surgeons society examined outcomes for 150 babies with tricuspid atresia. Antegrade pulmonary blood was absent in 19%, restricted in 54%, and unrestricted in 28%. Overall survival at 5 years was 86%. Initial palliation included systemic-to-pulmonary arterial shunt in 64%, banding of the pulmonary trunk in 11%, and cavopulmonary anastomosis in 24%. Risk factors for death without cavopulmonary anastomosis included the presence of mitral regurgitation and palliation with systemic-to-pulmonary arterial shunts which did not originate from the brachiocephalic artery. Factors associated with decreased transition rate to cavopulmonary connection included variables related to the patient (younger age at admission and the presence of noncardiac anomalies) and variables related to procedures (use of a larger systemic-to-pulmonary arterial shunt diameter). Of patients undergoing cavopulmonary anastomosis, 75% had undergone a Fontan operation within 3 years. The authors concluded that outcomes can be improved by placing smaller shunts from the brachiocephalic artery, especially in patients with regurgitation of the left atrioventricular valve.

CHAPTER 32

The Principles of Management, and Outcomes for, Patients with Functionally Univentricular Hearts

DAMIAN HUTTER and ANDREW N. REDINGTON

In 1699, Chemineau[1] described a human fetus having an allegedly univentricular heart. Since then, the patients characterised as possessing functionally univentricular hearts have held a unique position among all congenital cardiac malformations, not only because of the challenges of describing their diverse morphology, but also because of the continuing difficulties associated with their staged palliative repair, and the uncertainties of their outcomes in the long term. The evolution of thought concerning classification has been described at length in the previous chapter, along with discussions as to the nature of rudimentary, dominant, or incomplete ventricles,[2–4] and we will not reiterate the arguments here. Suffice it to say that recognition that patients with either biventricular or univentricular atrioventricular connections can exhibit the functionally univentricular arrangement, in which the driving force to both the systemic and pulmonary circulations is provided by but one ventricle, albeit that in most situations a second ventricular chamber is usually to be found within the ventricle mass.[5]

A thorough understanding of the anatomical substrate is necessary fully to understand the resulting physiology, and therapeutic options, in the individual patient. Specific therapeutic algorithms, particularly in terms of decision-making early in life, are also discussed in detail in the preceding chapter (Chapter 31), and those concerned with hypoplasia of either the right or left ventricles (Chapters 29 and 30), these being the major lesions producing the functionally univentricular arrangement. In this chapter, we will endeavor to provide a more generic approach to the understanding of the complexities of the physiology of the circulations produced by the functionally univentricular arrangement, and discuss the late outcomes of repair. No matter what the anatomic diagnosis, the restoration of a normal preload, and optimisation of afterload, to the dominant ventricle represents an overarching physiologic principle, albeit not always achieved, which underscores the current tripartite approach to management. The three stages are early neonatal palliation, followed by construction of a bidirectional cavopulmonary anastomosis, and completed with the creation of the Fontan circulation.

NATURAL HISTORY OF PATIENTS WITH FUNCTIONALLY UNIVENTRICULAR HEARTS

Long-term Survival without Surgical Intervention

Based on analysis of a large cohort of unselected patients having functionally univentricular hearts without surgical intervention,[6] we know that about seven-tenths of those with a dominant left ventricle died before they reached the age of 16 years, and only half of those with a dominant right ventricle survived for 4 years after diagnosis. Congestive cardiac failure, arrhythmias, and unexplained sudden death were the leading causes for mortality in both groups. Subsequent to this, the poor outcome for these patients if not undergoing surgical palliation was confirmed by lesion specific reviews, such as that emanating from the United Kingdom.[7] Indeed, the predicted outcome was worse than that reported from the Mayo Clinic.[6] Some natural survivors, nonetheless, survive to adulthood, most of whom have naturally occurring lesions that balance their systemic and pulmonary circulations.[8–10] Analysis of series of patients showed that those with such balanced circulations, providing there is good ventricular function, might survive to their seventh decade.[11]

Long-term Management of Patients with Previous Surgery

Patients coming to attention without previous surgery usually have the balanced circulation discussed above, either because of pulmonary stenosis or some degree of pulmonary vascular disease, but necessarily are subject to the effects of chronic cyanosis, and circulations in parallel rather than series. Assuming that they are unsuitable for palliation prior to transplantation, management should be directed at minimising the repercussions in the multiple systems of the body, which we discuss briefly below.

Haematological Disorders

Erythrocytosis, iron deficiency, thromboembolism, and bleeding diatheses are all well described phenomenons in adults with congenitally malformed hearts.[12,13] The management of erythrocytosis and hyperviscosity syndrome will be discussed in detail in Chapter 61. In patients who have not had surgical palliation of their functionally univentricular heart, however, there may be physiological options to improve effective flow of blood to the lungs by judicious use of interventional techniques, such as partially relieving pulmonary stenosis, or stenting of a persistently patent arterial duct, or surgical creation of either venopulmonary anastomoses or arterial shunts, thereby reducing the stimulus to erythrocytosis. Surgery in these patients is often more complicated than expected, not only because of the tenuous circulation, and multi-system effects of chronic hypoxaemia, but also because of co-existing bleeding diatheses. These bleeding disorders include altered levels of coagulation factors in the plasma, platelet dysfunction, and idiopathic thrombocytopaenia. The latter might be related to the degree of right-to-left shunting, and the consequent physiological exclusion of the lungs from the circulation. Subsequently, the normal fragmentation in the lungs of megakaryocytes into platelets is reduced, lowering the numbers of circulating platelets.[14]

Neurological Complications

The unrepaired functionally univentricular circulation of necessity produces intra- and extracardiac shunting, which exposes patients to a higher risk of paradoxical systemic and cerebral thromboembolism and abscess. This mandates the use of air filters, and vigilant attention to the presence of venous thrombosis and infection, when central or peripheral cannulation is required. Similarly, treatment of cutaneous or deep bacterial sepsis requires early aggressive antibiotic treatment.[15]

Gastrointestinal Complications

Hepatic, intestinal, and renal dysfunction are all common sequels of chronic cyanotic cardiac disease. Membranous glomerulosclerosis is well documented and, because of the lack of adequate resorption of uric acid, hyperuricaemia may lead to nephrolithiasis and urate nephropathy. Furthermore, hyperuricaemia is linked to rheumatological disorders, such as hypertrophic osteoarthropathy, which may be seen in up to three-tenths of patients.[16] In addition, cholelithiasis is a very common finding on routine abdominal ultrasonic surveillance, with acute cholecystitis being the leading cause of non-cardiac surgical procedures in patients with Eisenmenger's syndrome.[17]

Non-cardiac Surgery

Non-cardiac surgery carries an increased risk in patients with unrepaired functionally univentricular hearts. Although no specific data relating to outcome is reported in the literature, those with a low pulmonary blood flow, but normal pulmonary arterial pressure, are likely to tolerate anaesthesia better than those with raised pulmonary vascular resistance. In the latter group, mortality is probably comparable with other patients having the Eisenmenger syndrome, which varies between 7% and 30%.[17,18]

Cardiac Surgery Late in the Natural History

Survival without intervention, or only partial palliation, is well reported,[19] but does not obviate the possibility of a Fontan procedure. Remarkably, the early mortality in this series of patients undergoing completion of the Fontan circulation in adulthood was just 6%, while at this time the reported overall mortality for all patients undergoing completion of the Fontan circulation at the same institution was 17%.[19] A more recent study[20] showed similar high late mortality for adults with functionally univentricular hearts undergoing completion of the Fontan circuit to another cohort of patients with functionally univentricular hearts palliated with either an aortopulmonary shunt or a superior cavopulmonary connection. In those undergoing palliation, construction of a superior cavopulmonary shunt produced the worst outcomes. This group[20] concluded that completion of the Fontan circuit in adulthood, despite the lack of significant better long-term outcomes, may offer better preservation of functional state and ventricular function, and more freedom from arrhythmia, than palliation alone. Earlier reports[21] had reported late mortality in one-fifth of patients with functionally univentricular physiology definitively palliated by construction of a cavopulmonary shunt alone, while experience from Texas Children's Hospital[22] reveals that construction of the Fontan circuit in adulthood in patients not previously undergoing a cavopulmonary shunt procedure improved the functional state of all but one of the patients. Age alone, therefore, is not a significant risk factor for poor outcomes in the contemporary era, providing that the pre-operative haemodynamics are ideal.

EARLY PALLIATIVE APPROACHES—THE PRE-FONTAN ERA

Prior to the development of the Fontan procedure, patients with functionally univenticulaqr hearts were managed with a variety of manoeuvres to increase or reduce the flow of blood to the lungs, and to optimise systemic cardiac output. Many of these strategies are now incorporated into contemporary algorithms, but we provide a brief historical review, concentrating on the adverse consequences of long-term partial palliation.

Aortopulmonary Shunts

The advent of the Blalock-Taussig shunt revolutionised the management of patients with cyanotic cardiac disease, and those with functionally univentricular heart were no exception. Indeed, long-term survival into adult life with shunting alone is well described.[23] More recently, aortopulmonary shunts have been reserved for short-term neonatal palliation, prior to conversion to a bidirectional cavopulmonary shunt at 3 to 6 months of age. In the past, nonetheless, patients have been exposed to the whole range of arterial shunts, with all their benefits and disadvantages (Table 32-1).

Given the specific complications outlined in Table 32-1, and the generic disadvantages of a chronic volume load on the systemic ventricle, with consequent predisposition to arrhythmia, atrioventricular valvar regurgitation, and myocardial failure, few would now consider construction of a systemic-to-pulmonary arterial shunt in isolation as viable palliation for these patients. The group working at Hôpital Enfants-Malades in Paris,[24] nonetheless, have recently proposed a delayed strategy, not involving conversion to the Fontan circulation, but rather combining a superior cavopulmonary anastomosis with a systemic-to-pulmonary arterial shunt as definitive palliation for these patients. While the early results have been interesting, and the functional outcomes comparable to conversion to the Fontan circulation, the late results must be more uncertain. This strategy has not been widely adopted.

Banding of the Pulmonary Trunk

In patients with anatomical variants that permit unrestricted or excessive flow of blood to the lungs, progressive symptoms of congestive cardiac failure can be expected as the pulmonary vascular resistance falls in the first weeks of life. While banding of the pulmonary trunk will both protect the pulmonary vascular bed against progressive pulmonary vascular disease, and relieve the ventricle from

TABLE 32-1

SYSTEMIC ARTERIAL-TO-PULMONARY SHUNTS

Shunt Type	Anatomy	Advantage	Disadvantage
Classic Blalock-Taussig shunt	Subclavian artery to pulmonary artery on the same side	Growth of pulmonary vascular bed Increased flow commensurate with somatic growth	Frequent stenosis at level of anastomosis Poorer outcomes when performed on the same side as aortic arch
Modified Blalock Taussig shunt	Subclavian artery to pulmonary artery on the same side	Calibrated shunt appropriate for body size	Thrombosis Pulmonary arterial stenosis Reduced effective flow with somatic growth
Potts' anastomosis	Descending aorta to left pulmonary artery	Easy to accomplish	Left pulmonary arterial stenosis Risk for pulmonary over-circulation
Waterston shunt	Ascending aorta to right pulmonary artery	Easy to accomplish	Right pulmonary arterial stenosis Risk for pulmonary over-circulation

excessive volume load, it should be remembered that these patients often have co-existing anatomy that adversely affects systemic blood flow, such as a restrictive ventricular septal defect in the setting of double inlet left ventricle and discordant ventriculo-arterial connections. Under such circumstances, the effect of banding is frequently adverse in the long term, because of the development of ventricular hypertrophy, feeding a vicious cycle of an ever more restrictive obstruction to the systemic outflow tract.[25] Prior to the now almost uniform application of the Norwood strategy to such patients as neonates, those developing systemic obstruction subsequent to banding were treated by either direct enlargement of the interventricular communication[26] or a direct aortopulmonary connection.[27] In the rare case where banding alone was sufficient throughout infancy, there was almost inevitable progressive hypoxaemia with somatic growth. In such cases, addition of an arterial shunt or shunts, or in some institutions the construction of a classical Glenn anastomosis, was often associated with excellent outcomes in the mid-term.

The Classical Glenn Shunt

The classical Glenn shunt[28] is a direct anastomosis between the transected distal end of the right pulmonary artery and the superior caval vein, in either end-to-end, or end-to-side fashion, with ligation of the distal end of the caval vein. Despite excellent early results, results in the mid and late term have been disappointing, and the operation is now rarely performed. Significant numbers of patients survive, nonetheless, to require care in clinics dealing with adults having congenitally malformed hearts.

The commonest complication is the development of progressive hypoxaemia, resulting from intrapulmonary shunting as a result of the development of pulmonary arterio-venous malformations. Their exact prevalence varies depending on the mode of investigation, but they are found in between one-quarter and three-fifths of patients. Their cause remains fully to be elucidated, but clearly is related in some way to the lack of direct exposure of the lungs to an unknown hepatic factor. Restoration of hepatic flow to the lungs, by either aortopulmonary shunting or completion of the Fontan circuit, has widely been reported to reduce intrapulmonary shunting, and improve cyanosis, within a few weeks of the procedure. Alternative strategies include embolic occlusion, but this is appropriate only for those with focal abnormalities, a relative rarity. Although many patients have been successfully palliated for many years by the classical Glenn anastomosis, the introduction of the bidirectional superior cavopulmonary anastomosis has largely obviated its use.

FROM GLENN TO FONTAN, AND CONTEMPORARY STRATEGIES FOR MANAGEMENT

The success of the classical Glenn procedure described previously was a tantalising stimulus to complete exclusion of a ventricle on the right side of the circulation.[29] Various iterations of veno- and atriopulmonary anastomoses were tried, and often failed, prior to the seminal work published in 1971.[30] While early animal experiments had shown good tolerance when the right atrium was anastomosed to the pulmonary artery with closure of the pulmonary valve, the results where uniformly fatal when the right ventricle was completely disconnected. The scene was set for complete exclusion of the right side of the heart; long-term survival was achieved in animals with the superior caval vein anastomosed to the right upper pulmonary artery, later combined with connection of the inferior caval vein to the left atrium.[29]

The Fontan Procedure

The original report of the Fontan circulation was based on total exclusion of the right side of the heart in three patients, aged 12, 36 and 23 years respectively.[30] Although Fontan and his colleagues initially placed homograft aortic valves into the atriopulmonary connection, and into the inferior caval vein, it rapidly became apparent that this was an unnecessary addition to the procedure.[31] Indeed, following the initial report, there was a remarkably rapid evolution of operative variants (Table 32-2),[32-40] criterions for exclusion, and haemodynamic requirements, the essence of which we outline next.

Modifications of the Fontan Procedure

Despite all the modifications described above, the generic term Fontan circulation remains as a unifying description of

TABLE 32-2

MILESTONES IN THE DEVELOPMENT OF THE FONTAN PROCEDURE

Early Animal Experiments		
Anastomosis of systemic venous return and pulmonary arteries	1951	Carlon
Shunt between azygos vein and pulmonary arteries	1954	Glenn
Complete disconnection of the right ventricle	1966	Robicsek
Superior Cavopulmonary Anastomosis		
Anastomosis between superior caval vein and pulmonary arteries	1956	Meshalkin
End-to-end anastomosis between SCV and distal right PA	1958	Glenn
Fontan Procedure		
Complete disconnection of the right ventricle with direct drainage of systemic venous return into the pulmonary vascular bed	1971	Fontan
Kreutzer Modifications		
Removal of homologous valves	1973	Kreutzer
Atriopulmonary anastomosis	1982	Kreutzer
Björk Modification		
Anastomosis of right atrium to right ventricle	1983	Björk
Bidirectional Cavopulmonary Anastomosis		
Introduction of the bidirectional cavopulmonary anastomosis	1985	Hopkins
Total Intracardiac Cavopulmonary Anastomosis		
Total intracardiac cavopulmonary anastomosis	1988	De Leval
Lateral Tunnel and Tunnel Fenestration		
Tunnel fenestration for patients with increased surgical risk	1990	Bridges
Staged Fontan Procedure		
Introduction of the staged Fontan procedure	1993	Norwood
Total Extracardiac Cavopulmonary Anastomosis		
Extracardiac Fontan procedure	1995	Black

PA, pulmonary artery; SCV, superior caval vein.

those patients in whom circulations have been established in series without the inclusion of a subpulmonary ventricle. Each iteration has been associated with its own advantages and disadvantages, and the results of each variant, in terms of specific complications and outcomes, should be assessed separately. All of these efforts have culminated in a staged strategy of palliation, often starting with aggressive management of potentially adverse haemodynamics in the early neonatal period.

Contemporary Strategies and Outcomes

The contemporary strategy for managing patients with functionally univentricular hearts is a staged process designed to obviate obstruction to systemic outflow, and minimise the amount and duration of volume loading of the systemic ventricle. The type of early neonatal palliation will vary depending on the underlying anatomy, but the aim is to optimise haemodynamics towards the construction of a bidirectional cavopulmonary anastomosis at the age of from 3 to 6 months, and completion of a total cavopulmonary anastomosis in the second or third year of life. This strategy has resulted in far superior results compared with those achieved even a decade previously, and the benefits have clearly been multi-factorial. Improved early palliation, particularly for those with hypoplastic left-sided heart syndrome, which is now the commonest anatomical subtype progressing to palliation with the Fontan circuit, and the introduction of the bidirectional cavopulmonary anastomosis as an interim step prior to completion of a Fontan circulation, must represent two of the most important advances in the field since the original successful clinical application.[30]

Long-term Outcomes of the Completed Fontan Circulation

The results of the allegedly perfect Fontan procedure were analysed in a large series of patients.[41] Most of these patients, however, had undergone surgery prior to routine interim staging using a bidirectional superior cavopulmonary anastomosis. The investigators predicted survival under optimal conditions of 92%, 89%, 88%, 86%, 81% and 73% at the age of 1 month, 6 months and 1, 5, 10 and 15 years, respectively, highlighting the late attrition that appears inevitable with this flawed circulation. With improved strategies, however, come improved results. Thus, survival of 91% at 10 years is now reported in patients with lateral tunnels,[42] and overall mortality rate of 2.8% for one cohort of patients.[43] Overall early mortality rate was

2.8%. Others[44] have reported overall survival rate of 85% at 15 years, albeit with an incidence of major co-morbidities, such as arrhythmias in one-tenth, and other complications, such as obstruction of the extracardiac conduit or left pulmonary artery, ventricular failure, and protein losing enteropathy bringing the onset of problems in up to almost one-quarter of the patients. A further analysis[45] of over 300 patients showed an overall survival at 24 years of 84%. Survival was lower for those with an atriopulmonary connection compared to a lateral tunnel. Arrhythmias and failure were also less frequent in those having a lateral tunnel. Since the introduction of extracardiac conduits in 1990, mortality has been zero in this group, and there have been no sustained arrhythmias or failure. The authors[45] concluded that, with improvement of surgical techniques, and careful selection of patients, the hospital mortality, as well as the rates of complications, will be lower, or at least deferred, in those operated in the modern era.[46] Even so, the Fontan circulation, and its physiological consequences remain as a unique experiment that remains to be fully understood, both in terms of its optimal performance, and its modes of failure.

THE PHYSIOLOGY OF THE FONTAN CIRCULATION AND ITS FAILURE

Basic Principles

Regardless of the exact nature of the connections, the completed circulation is often described as one having a single energy source, namely the dominant ventricle driving the systemic circulation. This energy is dissipated through a series of resistors. The first is in the ventricle itself, and is related to diastolic function, with others provided by the systemic vascular bed, the systemic venous bed, and the pulmonary vascular bed. It is now apparent that there are additional sources of energy, and potentially additional sources of dissipation of energy. All of these are modified by time. Each element of the Fontan circulation is abnormal and while the circulation must be considered as a whole, we analyse here the contribution and adverse effects of each.

The Ventricle

Debate continues as to whether ventricular morphology has a significant impact on the efficiency and outcomes of the Fontan circulation. This is increasingly pertinent given the improved survival of patients with hypoplastic left-sided heart syndromes. There can be no doubt that there are inherent differences between the architecture, atrioventricular valvar morphology, and functional responses when either the left or right ventricle is dominant in these patients, and virtually no attention has been paid to the truly univentricular arrangement. If the dominant left ventricle is compared between patients having tricuspid atresia and double inlet left ventricle,[47] differences between the groups are difficult to discern in terms of early geometric adaptation and outcomes of the Fontan operation. Similarly, little evidence exists to differentiate between those with dominant right or left ventricles. Indeed, in one large study, a systemic right ventricle was shown not to influence early outcomes,[48] and in another, those with dominant right ventricles had superior survival to, albeit more complex, patients with a dominant left ventricle.[49]

At the time of the bidirectional Glenn procedure, or at the time of completion of the Fontan circuit if no bidirectional Glenn procedure has been performed previously, there is usually a marked decrease in the preload to the dominant ventricle. The degree of reduction primarily depends on the prior ratio of pulmonary-to-systemic flows, which often exceeds 2:1. It is, of course, the reduction of preload, and hence ventricular dilation and work, which provides much of the reason for undertaking the operations themselves. While few would disagree that reduction of systemic ventricular volume load is generally beneficial, it does come at a price when completing the Fontan circulation.

Prior to construction of the Fontan circuit, abnormal systolic ventricular performance is rarely a major problem, and is sustained or improved in most after completion of the circuit. In an elegant study from Boston's Children's Hospital,[50] it was shown that restoration of normal systolic ventricular mural stress was achieved in most individuals undergoing a Fontan procedure prior to the age of 10 years, an important feature when examining the potential effects of volume unloading of the systemic ventricle. The law of preservation of mass predicts that, given a marked reduction in ventricular preload, preserved shortening and constant mural mass, there must be a resulting increase in mural thickness. This was shown experimentally,[51] and demonstrated clinically in children undergoing the Fontan operation in the 1990s.[52] The implications of this increased mural thickness are, perhaps, not intuitive. It might be reasonable to think that this increased thickness would modify the properties of end-diastolic compliance, and hence mural stiffness. There is very little evidence for this. Rather, the evidence points to abnormalities of early relaxation as being the major result. We have shown that prolongation of the time constant of early relaxation, known as tau, and the isovolumic relaxation time, are both inversely related to the characteristically reduced early rapid filling.[52,53] Consequently, much of diastolic filling is dependent on atrial systole. Very recently, this early diastolic dysfunction, also demonstrable after bidirectional Glenn procedures, was shown to impact negatively on recovery after subsequent conversion to the Fontan circuit,[54] and may also be important in the late follow-up of these patients (see later discussion).

This incoordinate relaxation is a feature of hearts affected by hypertrophy, ischaemia, and abnormal mural motion, all of which may exist in the ventricular myocardium of patients converted to the Fontan circulation. It is the adverse effect of abnormalities of mural motion, nonetheless, that appears to predominate. Using both direct angiographic analysis,[55] and surrogate measurements by Doppler echocardiography,[56] we have been able to show that abnormalities in base-to-apex mural motion are mirrored by abnormal flow from base to apex during isovolumic relaxation of these ventricles. These abnormalities persist at mid-term follow-up, but interestingly, late diastolic abnormalities, characteristic of worsening ventricular compliance, also become apparent at this time.[57] The combination of persistently abnormal early relaxation with worsening ventricular compliance is particularly malignant, markedly reducing the ability of these ventricles to fill, potentially reducing the flow of blood to the lungs, or at least leading to elevated pulmonary arterial pressure. The changes may also account for some of the late failure seen in these patients. There is little that can be done therapeutically to avoid the early diastolic abnormalities, and they may indeed worsen naturally with age, as in the normal heart.[58] Avoidance of those factors known to lead to worsening compliance, nonetheless, such as persistent obstruction of the left ventricular outflow tract or hypertension, is of fundamental importance.

While diastolic abnormalities predominate early-on, there is no doubt that systolic failure also becomes apparent in some patients late after the procedure. This may be a reflection of abnormal vascular properties, of ventricular vascular interactions (see below), or maybe intrinsic to the previously stressed or damaged myocardium itself. We,[59] and others,[60] have recently shown abnormal myocardial force frequency relationships in these patients, probably reflecting abnormal handling of calcium by the myocardium. Although abnormal, the changes seen are not at the level seen in adults with end-stage cardiac failure secondary to dilated cardiomyopathy.[61] Although a similar degree of physical incapacity may exist, with similar degrees of elevation of neurohormonal markers,[62] the successful response to pharmacological interventions noted in those with dilated cardiomyopathy remains to be adequately addressed in patients with the Fontan circulation. As will be demonstrated later, sometimes the response of those with the Fontan circulation is counter-intuitive to the concepts established in cardiac failure due to other causes.

Although difficult to prove, it is likely that staged transition to the Fontan circulation has contributed significantly to the overall improvements in outcome for these patients. Avoidance of excessive early volume loading, avoidance of excessive myocardial hypertrophy, and therefore avoidance of the major geometric changes discussed previously, would all seem conceptually beneficial. For the long-term outcome of these patients, avoidance of the age-related naturally occurring changes in late diastolic performance, particularly in relation to the changes in compliance seen with ageing, hypertension, and so on, may be the next frontier for maintenance of myocardial performance.

The Systemic Vascular Bed, and Ventricular–Vascular Coupling

Elevated systemic vascular resistance is well recognised after conversion to the Fontan circulation.[63,64] How much of this is related primarily to the intrinsically low resting cardiac output, and how much is secondary to circulating vasoconstrictors, and so on, has not been fully elucidated. The impact of this elevation of systemic vascular resistance on ventricular–vascular coupling also remains fully to be elucidated. When control patients, and others with a Blalock-Taussig shunt, were compared to those with the Fontan circuit, the relationship between cardiac index and vascular impedance, at baseline and with dobutamine, was highly abnormal in the Fontan group.[64] Careful analysis of this data, with the relationship between cardiac index and impedance being almost flat in those with a Fontan circuit, suggests that simply changing impedance may not necessarily lead to an improved cardiac index. This is crucial when considering the potential role for vasodilation in these patients.

It would appear intuitive that, in these patients with markedly elevated systemic vascular resistance and abnormal ventricular–vascular coupling, vasodilation would improve their circulatory performance. This would only be the case if the abnormal vascular characteristics were of primary importance, rather than a secondary phenomenon. Randomised double-blind, placebo-controlled studies of therapeutic intervention in the setting of congenital cardiac disease are a rarity, but such data is available for the inhibition of angiotensin converting enzyme in patients with the Fontan circulation.[65] Enalapril or placebo was given in crossover fashion. Overall, there was no change in Doppler echo characteristics, and a tendency to worse exercise performance. Indeed, there was reduced incremental cardiac index during exercise in the patients receiving enalapril. Despite this data, many physicians continue to give drugs to inhibit the angiotensin converting enzyme, presumably in the hope of a beneficial effect when given chronically. It is possible, but unproven, that there are subgroups, such as those with severe systolic dysfunction or atrioventricular valvar regurgitation, that may benefit. It is also possible to put forward theoretical arguments for the use of inhibitors with tissue-inhibitory properties, such as quinapril or ramapril, in order to avoid the adverse remodelling described above. Irrespective of the attraction of the theories, there is presently no evidence for this therapy being beneficial in these patients.

The Veno-pulmonary Circuit

There has been a major evolution in the design of the haemodynamics in the Fontan circuit since its inception. As already discussed, the initial connection from right atrium to pulmonary arteries has been abandoned in favor of more streamlined versions. The benefits of such modifications have been confirmed experimentally and clinically. When comparing contemporaneously treated patients undergoing either an atriopulmonary connection or construction of a lateral tunnel,[66] no difference was noted between the groups at rest, although cardiac output in both was significantly lower than in normal controls. Cardiac output was higher, however, in those with a lateral tunnel at low and moderate workloads, as was the rate of respiration. Despite a similar production of carbon dioxide, and similar minute ventilation, those with a lateral tunnel were taking more frequent, smaller, breaths during exercise. We speculated that these patients were harnessing the beneficial effects of the work of breathing on the pulmonary circulation, this being a particularly prominent feature in patients with veno-pulmonary connections.

Indeed, the work of breathing is a significant additional source of energy for the circulation in these patients. Normal inspiration at negative pressures has been shown to increase the flow of blood to the lungs after the Kawashima operation,[67] those with an atriopulmonary connection,[68] and in patients after the total cavopulmonary connection.[67] Using magnetic resonance imaging to measure flow, it has been shown that approximately one-third of the cardiac output can be directly attributed to the work of breathing in patients after a total cavopulmonary connection.[69] Regional properties of subdiaphragmatic venous flow are fascinating in these patients.[70] While portal venous flow is markedly abnormal after the Fontan operation, the respiratory influence is relatively limited. Inferior caval venous flow does vary with respiration, but in a relatively normal fashion. It is the hepatic venous flow that differentiates these patients from their normal counterparts. There is a very marked influence of respiration on total hepatic venous flow. Inspiration, presumably by a dual effect on venous pressure and compression of the liver by diaphragmatic descent, markedly augments hepatic venous contribution to the total venous return. The liver appears to act as a sump of blood, which can be drawn upon during inspiration.

The converse is true when considering positive pressure ventilation. It has long been known that increasing levels of positive end-expiratory pressure, during positive pressure ventilation, has adverse effects on the Fontan circulation.[71] We have learnt over the years that early post-operative restoration of normal negative pressure ventilation can be beneficial in these patients. We investigated this experimentally in children after the Fontan operation, comparing the effects of a negative pressure cuirass device with standard positive pressure ventilation.[72] By mimicking the normal action of breathing, negative pressure ventilation, when compared to positive pressure, led to an average increase in cardiac index of approximately two-fifths. While not advocated as a routine clinical tool, although sometimes very useful therapeutically, this data heightens our awareness of the relationship between mean airway pressure and cardiac index in these patients. The available data suggests an approximately linear relationship between the two. Thus, the higher the mean airway pressure, the lower is the cardiac index. Management of these patients, therefore, should be directed towards minimising mean airway pressure when they are being ventilated for cardiac and non-cardiac procedures. This can be achieved by minimising plateau pressures, end-expiratory pressures, and rate of rise of pressure. The patients should be maintained with the minimum mean airway pressure compatible with normal oxygenation, avoiding any collapse of the airway or similar complication, and achieving adequate alveolar ventilation to ensure normal partial pressures of carbon dioxide.

The Pulmonary Vascular Bed

A low pulmonary vascular resistance is a prerequisite for early success after completion of the Fontan circuit. The lower the total pulmonary resistance, which incorporates the pulmonary vascular resistance, pulmonary venous resistance and left atrial resistance, the better the end result. We have already discussed the influence of abnormal ventricular responses to potentially raised left atrial pressure, and therefore left atrial resistance. Structural pulmonary venous abnormalities are also important. Naturally occurring pulmonary venous stenosis may occur in many of the disease substrates that necessitate the Fontan circulation, such as those with isomerism of the right atrial appendages, or may evolve as a result of abnormal haemodynamics after, for example, an atriopulmonary anastomosis. In the latter case, gross enlargement of the right atrium may compress the adjacent pulmonary veins as they return to the left atrium.[73] This complication should always be excluded in patients with worsening functional performance late after these operations. Less well characterised is the chronic effect of the Fontan circulation on pulmonary arterial resistance. Pulmonary thrombo-embolism is not infrequent,[74] may be covert,[75] and clearly will lead to adverse changes in vascular resistance. Abnormalities of arteriolar resistance adversely influence early outcome, in terms of both morbidity and mortality,[76,77] but there is little data available regarding the long-term effects of the Fontan circulation on the pulmonary vascular bed.

COMPLICATIONS OF THE FONTAN CIRCULATION AND THEIR MANAGEMENT

Although there is ample evidence for improved mid-term results as a result of improvements in early palliation, operative techniques, and in the design of the Fontan circuit itself, as we have discussed, the nature of Fontan physiology is intrinsically flawed, and the circuit is likely to fail earlier than its normal biventricular counterpart. Furthermore, there are large numbers of patients surviving into adult life having been treated in an earlier era with less advantageous surgical algorithms. Because of the increasing survival of patients with the hypoplastic left heart syndrome, management of the late complications of the Fontan circulation, and ultimately its failure, is likely to become a larger issue, rather than a diminishing burden, to those specialising in the future in the treatment of those with congenitally malformed hearts. Although often forming a constellation of inter-related co-morbidities, it is convenient to discuss separately the modes of failure.

Arrhythmias

Sinus nodal dysfunction occurs in up to one-sixth of patients after conversion to the Fontan circuit, and increases with time of follow-up.[78] Among other reported arrhythmias, re-entry atrial tachyarrhythmias are the commonest, and are often associated with haemodynamic deterioration, either causally or as a result.[79] All patients with new arrhythmias should undergo full haemodynamic assessment in order to exclude important anatomical or functional substrates for the abnormal rhythms. If present, haemodynamic abnormalities should be treated aggressively. Specific treatment of the arrhythmias remains challenging. They are difficult to control pharmacologically, and although contemporary three-dimensional mapping systems and catheter ablation may provide immediate relief in up to four-fifths, persistent arrhythmias,[80] or recurrent or new atrial arrhythmias are frequent. For that reason, those with persistent or recurrent atrial arrhythmia may be candidates for a conversion of the circuit combined with arrhythmic surgery,[81] as we discuss later.

Hepatic Dysfunction and Thrombo-embolic Events

The patients are at high risk for thrombo-embolic events. In addition to the obvious risk from sustained atrial arrhythmias, the low flow in the distended pathways, abnormal ventricular anatomy, the use of intravascular prosthetic material, and impaired hepatic function all contribute to the elevated risk for thrombo-embolism. Abnormal coagulative factors have been shown before and after completion of the Fontan circuit.[82] Optimal management of such changes, also reported by others, remains to be defined. Although anatomical and haemodynamic abnormalities are clearly responsible for some events, the effect of co-existing hepatic dysfunction cannot be ignored. Increased activity of platelets,[83] as well as persistent thrombocytopenia,[84] has also been reported. The cause of hepatic dysfunction, and even frank cirrhotic changes, remains poorly understood, but presumably relates in some way to chronic elevation of hepatic venous and portal venous pressures. As with atrial arrhythmias, new onset thrombo-embolic symptoms require full haemodynamic re-evaluation to exclude, and potentially treat, any anatomical and functional substrates. Most would consider anti-coagulation to be indicated in those with a documented and clinically significant thrombo-embolic event, but the use of prophylactic anti-coagulation or anti-platelet therapy remains a subject of continuing debate.[85–88] Those reviewing thrombo-embolic outomes[89] found a high incidence of thrombo-embolic events within the first year after surgery, and then again with a second peak beyond 10 years, with the lowest incidence in those receiving coumadin. A similar study, however, showed no differences between patients receiving no medication, aspirin, or coumadin.[90] Furthermore, the overall incidence of thrombo-embolic events was remarkably lower in the latter study, leading the authors to speculate that ethnic differences may exist in regard to this complication. These data are far from definitive, and therapeutic policies vary from unit to unit, and even within units! This issue will not be resolved in the absence of a long-term randomised clinical trial.

Cyanosis

Most patients, in the absence of a fenestration, will have arterial saturations in excess of 90%. Unexpected desaturation, either at rest or on exercise, should prompt surveillance for abnormal systemic venous connections to the left heart, or the development of pulmonary arterio-venous fistulas. The question as to whether, in the long term, the presence of a fenestration might reduce the incidence of complications associated with venous hypertension, at the cost of chronic cyanosis and right-to-left shunting, remains unanswered. In one study of patients followed for 10 years after closure of their fenestration, there was improved oxygenation, reduced need for anti-congestive medication, and improved somatic growth, with minimal instances of death or haemodynamic decompensation.[91] Thus, most would consider persistent resting desaturation below 90% to 95% as an indication for investigation and treatment, if the haemodynamics allow.

Exercise Intolerance

Abnormalities of exercise function are ubiquitous. Their cause and effect, however, is less well understood. Overall, the patients demonstrate reduced responses to workload and cardiac output, increased ventilation, and decreased anaerobic threshold and consumption of oxygen, in addition to chronotropic incompetence. Those with atriopulmonary connections fare less well than those with intra- or extracardiac conduits, but multiple additional factors, such as era of operation, ventricular function, number of operations, and so on, contribute to ultimate performance. There also appear to be significant non-physical constraints. We recently reported reduced levels of the physical activity in patients having an overly protective social environment, consequent upon adverse perception by both the patients and their parents of the risks and benefits of exercise. Exercise testing, nonetheless, is useful for longitudinal follow-up. Any significant deterioration should be a stimulus for detailed anatomical and functional surveillance to establish for possible causes of circulatory impairment.

Protein Losing Enteropathy

One of the most severe manifestations of the failing Fontan circulation is protein losing enteropathy. Chronic loss of protein into the gastrointestinal tract leads to hypoalbuminaemia, effusions, ascites, oedema, and ultimately muscle wasting and cachexia. The underlying pathogenesis remains to be fully explained, but its development in the absence of a major, treatable, haemodynamic disturbance carries an extremely poor prognosis. Only half the patients with generalised oedema are alive after 5 years.[92] The reported incidence varies depending on era and cohort, but in one review it was present in 4% of patients at an average of 6.9 years after completion of the Fontan circuit.[93] Diagnosis relies on the demonstration of hypoalbuminaemia in the presence of increased faecal loss of protein. The latter is usually measured as increased levels of α_1–antitrypsin in the faeces, but it should be remembered that elevated levels may occur in the absence of overt loss of protein. As with all other late complications of the Fontan circulation, diagnosis of the complication should prompt a vigilant anatomical and haemodynamic evaluation for correctible abnormalities.

In the absence of an overtly treatable cause, careful attention to diet, fluid balance, and the judicious use of diuretics and infusions of protein may all provide symptomatic relief. Although there are many reports of individual patients, and small case series, purporting to show benefit from various therapeutic strategies, no single intervention can be considered to be of uniformly proven benefit. Apparent improvement has been described in those receiving steroids, high molecular weight heparin treatment, sildenafil, octreotide, atrioventricular synchronous and biventricular pacing, and after fenestration of the circuit. Successful reversal following revision of the circuit has also been described,[94] particularly if attempted in an early stage.[92,95,96] As we discuss later, resolution is almost invariable in survivors after cardiac transplantation.

Plastic Bronchitis

Plastic bronchitis is a rare and potentially fatal complication after completion of the Fontan circulation.[97,98] It manifests clinically by expectoration of long, branching, bronchial casts with recurrent life-threatening obstruction of the airways (Fig. 32-1). Its pathogenesis is still not entirely clear, but elevated pulmonary and central venous pressures have been implicated, along with endobronchial lymphatic leakage. The complication can occur in the early post-surgical period after creation of the Fontan circuit, or as a late complication in the patient with a failing Fontan circulation, often together with protein losing enteropathy.[99] Symptoms of acute respiratory distress, and cough producing pearly white bronchial casts, without signs of acute inflammation or acute cardiac failure, should suggest the diagnosis.

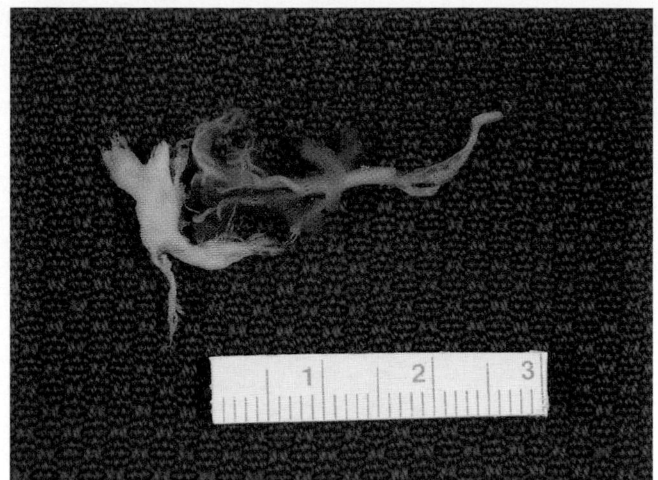

Figure 32-1 Bronchial cast.

The standard treatment involves strategies designed for both the short and long term. Immediate treatment is targeted at resolving the obstruction in the airways. Chest physiotherapy, mucolytics and in severe cases bronchoscopy are accepted options to remove the casts. Aerosolised urokinase, or r-TPA, are other medical options, but should be used carefully in the early post-surgical course.[100,101]

Treatment over the long term aims to lower the pulmonary and central venous pressures. In patients in the early period, enlargement or reopening of a fenestration, or creation of a fenestration,[102] should be considered. Atrial and ventricular arrhythmias need to be ruled out,[103] along with failure of the systemic ventricle due to the increased volume load. Successful use of drugs to reverse pulmonary hypertension, such as treatment with sildenafil or an endothelin-1 antagonists,[104,105] has been reported. In patients with a generalised failure of their Fontan circulation, management is based on the severity of the presentation and the existence of additional clinical features, such as protein losing enteropathy. It might, therefore, additionally involve the various medical approaches already discussed,[99,106,107] as well as the surgical options to be reviewed in the sections that follow.[108]

Surgical Management of the Failing Patient

Revision of the Circuit

The aims of conversion of the circuit are to improve haemodynamic efficiency, address atrial arrhythmias, and improve functional capacity. To that end, those with either an atriopulmonary connection or a lateral tunnel have it replaced by an extracardiac conduit, and right- and left-sided Maze procedures are performed, usually with coincident insertion of an epicardial, anti-tachycardia, pacemaker in patients with atrial flutter or fibrillation.[81,109] A right atrial maze is usually incorporated irrespective of symptoms, but in patients free of documented atrial arrhythmias, the left-sided Maze procedure is not recommended owing to the longer ischaemic time required for the combined procedure.

A group from Children's Memorial Hospital in Chicago has championed revision of the circuit as a therapy for late failure.[110] Mortality in a series of over 100 patients was only 0.9%, a quite remarkable achievement, not consistently reproduced in other series. The overall incidence of recurrent arrhythmia was 12.8% during a mean period of follow-up of almost 5 years. They concluded that conversion combined with arrhythmic surgery is a procedure with low surgical risk, and relatively low risk of recurrence of tachycardia, and which provides marked improvement in the functional state of most patients. Selection, and stratification of risk, of the patients, however, is not well defined. It remains the case that for some patients with late failure, cardiac transplantation may be the only viable therapeutic option.

Cardiac Transplantation after Fontan Palliation

Despite the excellent results reported for conversion of the circuit, not all patients are suitable, and others continue to experience significant symptoms, or deteriorate, after conversion. Cardiac transplantation may be the only option for such patients. Earlier reports suggested a prohibitively high mortality, but more recent series report rates of death from 2.4% to 6.7%.[81,111] Symptomatic improvement is almost uniformly observed in survivors.[112]

Based on their experience, the group from Padova[112] recommended that cardiac transplantation should be considered in the decision-making process for adult patients at high risk as an alternative to completion of the Fontan circuit. This is supported by two additional recent studies.[113,114] Of particular note was the complete resolution of protein losing enteropathy in the survivors, with the group as a whole having marked improvement in symptoms and functional capacity.[114]

CONCLUSIONS

The understanding of the functionally univentricular circulation and its management has improved markedly over the past three decades. Although improved early palliative strategies have led to improved early and mid-term results, failure of the circuit is the likely outcome for most patients at some stage in their late follow-up. Strategies to avoid, defer, and treat such failure continue to be developed.

The complete reference list can be found on the companion Expert Consult web site at www.expertconsult.com.

ANNOTATED REFERENCES

- Franklin RC, Spiegelhalter DJ, Anderson RH, et al: Double-inlet ventricle presenting in infancy. I. Survival without definitive repair. J Thorac Cardiovasc Surg 1991;101:767–776.

  An important early paper analysing the outcomes of patients with functionally univentricular heart. Early and late survival was stratified according to anatomical subtype, and underlying physiology.

- Fontan F, Baudet E: Surgical repair of tricuspid atresia. Thorax 1971;26: 240–248.

  This article presents the seminal description of Fontan's initial experience.

- Leval MR de, Kilner P, Gewillig M, et al: Total cavopulmonary connection: A logical alternative to atriopulmonary connection for complex Fontan operations. Experimental studies and early clinical experience. J Thorac Cardiovasc Surg 1988;96:682–695.

  This article is an experimental and clinical description of the reasons underscoring a streamlined Fontan circulation, introducing the concept of the lateral wall Fontan circuit.

- Fontan F, Kirklin JW, Fernandez G, et al: Outcome of the perfect Fontan operation. Circulation 1990;81:1520–1536.

  This statistical analysis of survivors of the Fontan procedure highlights the attrition that can be expected as a result of the intrinsic limitations of the Fontan circulation itself. While the late outcomes have improved, in terms of mortality rate and age at failure, this paper reminded us that the Fontan circulation is palliative rather than curative.

• Penny DJ, Lincoln C, Shore DF, et al: The early response of the systemic ventricle during transition to the Fontan circulation: An acute hypertrophic cardiomyopathy? Cardiol Young 1992;2:78–84.

This study described the acute adaptation of the ventricle to transition to the Fontan circulation. Using peri-operative echocardiography, and micromanometer catheters placed in the ventricle during surgery, the geometric adaptation of the ventricle during acute preload was described, and the resultant abnormalities of diastolic function were emphasised.

• Kouatli AA, Garcia JA, Zellers TM, et al: Enalapril does not enhance exercise capacity in patients after Fontan procedure. Circulation 1997:96:1507–1512.

This randomised, blinded, placebo-controlled cross-over study failed to demonstrate any benefit from Ramipril after the Fontan procedure. Indeed, some of the parameters of exercise performance were worse during treatment compared with placebo.

• Deal BJ, Mavroudis C, Backer CL: Arrhythmia management in the Fontan patient. Pediatr Cardiol 2007;28:448–456.

This article offers the most recent update of the outstanding work of the Chicago group concerning conversion of the Fontan circuit. The mid-term outcomes for 117 patients are described. In carefully selected patients there can be low early and later mortality, and excellent functional improvement with this strategy.

• Bernstein D, Naftel D, Chin C, et al: Outcome of listing for cardiac transplantation for failed Fontan: A multi-institutional study. Circulation 2006;114:273–280.

This article is an excellent review of contemporary outcomes of heart transplantation as ultimate palliation of the failing Fontan circulation. Resolution of protein-losing enteropathy, and improved functional performance, was uniform in those who survived the early post-operative period.

CHAPTER 33

Straddling Atrioventricular Valves

MICHAEL L. RIGBY and ROBERT H. ANDERSON

The entities to be considered in this chapter differ from all those others considered in this section of our book devoted to specific lesions. This is because hearts with straddling and overriding atrioventricular valves represent a series of anatomical stages between the extremes of double inlet and biventricular atrioventricular connections. As such, therefore, straddling and overriding can involve the right or left atrioventricular valve, or a common atrioventricular valve, in the setting of either double inlet right or double inlet left ventricle. The other end of these various spectrums will then depend upon the particular valve involved, and on the topological arrangement of the ventricular mass. The structure of the individual heart itself will reflect the precise degree of straddling, as opposed to overriding of the valvar structures. Because of this, it is not possible to approach the lesions in the same fashion as all others discussed in this section of our book. The clinical features will not only reflect the variations already discussed above, but will also differ markedly according to the specific ventriculo-arterial connections present, and the associated malformations. The understanding of the malformations, and their correct diagnosis, depends on a thorough appreciation of their anatomical features. In this chapter, therefore, we describe the different patterns on the basis of their structure. This in itself requires that we define precisely our understanding of the nature of straddling and overriding, since the definition of these features, and the way in which they are described, has varied markedly.

DEFINITIONS

In the normally structured heart, each ventricle, which functions as the muscular pump driving its circulation, has competent valves guarding its inlet and its outlet. The functional components of these valves are the leaflets. Of necessity, if the heart is normal, these leaflets are attached exclusively within their own ventricle. There are subtle differences between the nature of the valvar attachments which are not strictly relevant to this chapter, but worthy of emphasis. Thus, the leaflets of the atrioventricular valves are normally attached in annular fashion, and their line of attachment is coincident with the anatomical atrioventricular junction (Fig. 33-1). The leaflets of the arterial valves, in contrast, are attached in semilunar fashion, with their line of attachment crossing the anatomical ventriculo-arterial junction (Fig. 33-2). Much more significant from the stance of our definitions for straddling and overriding is the nature of the free edge of the valvar leaflets. The atrioventricular valves close against the full force of ventricular systole. So as to retain valvar competence, therefore, the free edges of the leaflets are furnished with tension apparatus (see Fig. 33-1). In the normal ventricles, the entire tension apparatus for each valve, like the attachments of the leaflets at the atrioventricular junctions, is exclusively contained within its own ventricle. The arterial valves, in contrast, close in ventricular diastole. It is the force of the column of blood supported by the leaflets which ensures their competence. Arterial valves, therefore, lack any tension apparatus.

When hearts are congenitally malformed, either the atrioventricular or the ventriculo-arterial junctions, or on occasion both junctions, can be shared between the ventricles. It is the sharing of an atrioventricular junction between the ventricles that is usually the essential feature of the entities to be discussed in this chapter. In the abnormal hearts to be discussed, it is also the case that, in the majority of cases, the tension apparatus is attached not in one, but in both of the ventricles. In order to distinguish between the sharing of the junctions, and the abnormal location of the tension apparatus, and to produce a terminology which is applicable to both atrioventricular and ventriculo-arterial valves, we define separately the nature of these two independent features.[1]

Overriding, therefore, describes the situation in which a junction, either atrioventricular (Fig. 33-3) or ventriculo-arterial (Fig. 33-4), is shared between the ventricles. This permits us to reserve straddling to describe the arrangement in which the valvar tension apparatus is attached to either

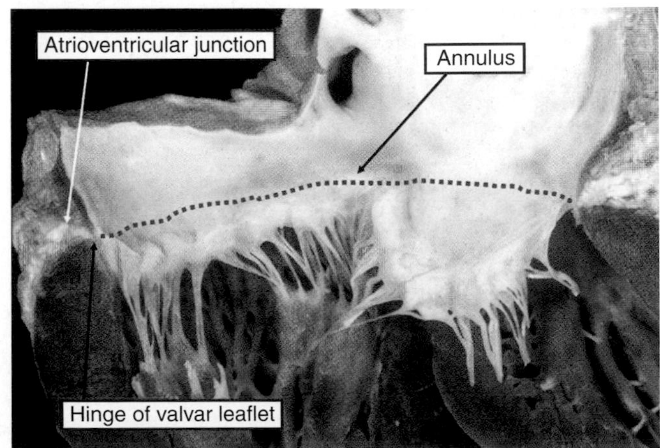

Figure 33-1 The left atrioventricular junction of a normal heart has been opened inferiorly by a cut parallel to the atrial septum, and the junction spread to show the attachments of the leaflets of the mitral valve. The hinges of the leaflets are arranged in annular fashion (*purple dotted line*), and along the mural leaflet the line corresponds to the atrioventricular junction. Note that the free edges of the leaflets are tethered by the tendinous cords to the papillary muscles within the left ventricle.

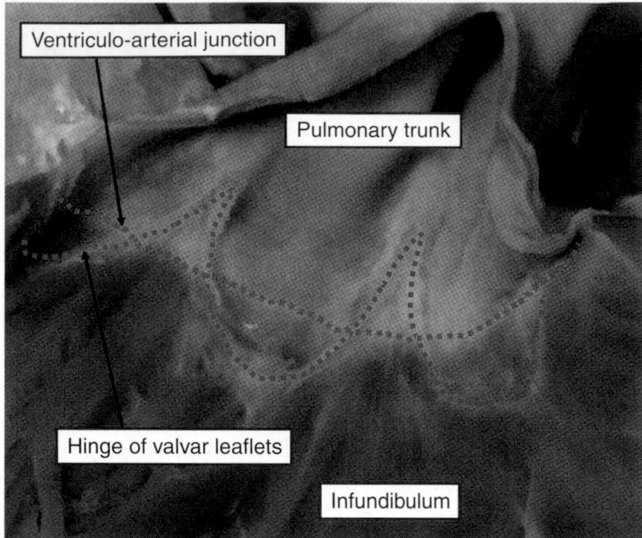

Figure 33-2 The ventriculo-pulmonary junction of a normal heart has been opened anteriorly, and the junction spread to reveal the arrangement of attachment of the leaflets of the pulmonary valve, the leaflets themselves having been removed. The hinges of the leaflets are semilunar (*purple dotted line*), and cross the anatomical ventriculo-arterial junction between the muscular infundibulum and the fibrocollagenous wall of the pulmonary trunk (*yellow dotted line*). Unlike the atrioventricular valves, the arterial valves lack tension apparatus.

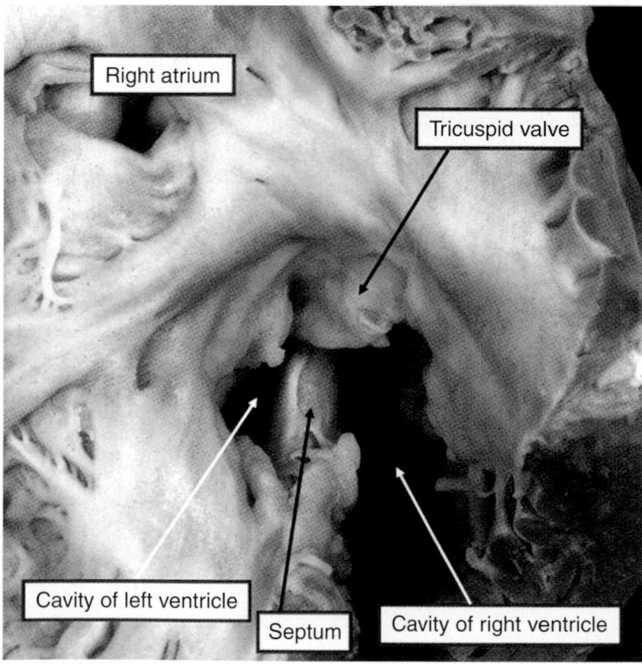

Figure 33-3 The picture of a straddling tricuspid valve in a patient with concordant atrioventricular connections shows how, almost always in this situation, the atrioventricular junction is shared between the ventricles, the right atrium connecting directly with the left and the right ventricular chambers.

side of the ventricular septum and, hence, tethers the valvar leaflets in both ventricles (Fig. 33-5). Using these definitions, it follows that an atrioventricular valve can straddle and override. Such an arrangement (Fig. 33-6) is by far the commonest encountered. But it is also possible for an atrioventricular valve to straddle without overriding (Fig. 33-7), or to override in the absence of straddling of the tensor apparatus (Fig. 33-8). It also follows that, within our definitions, it is possible for an arterial valve to override,

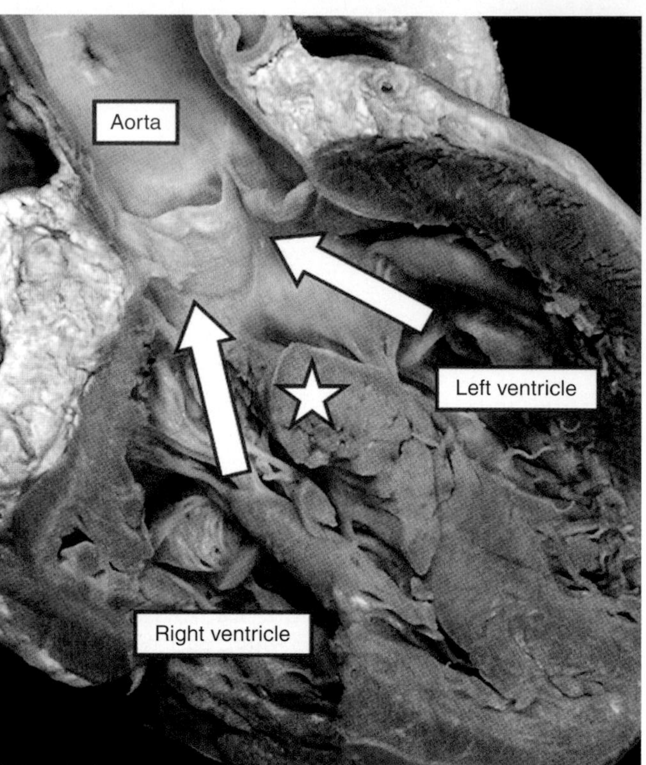

Figure 33-4 The picture shows a simulated four-chamber echocardiographic section in a heart with tetralogy of Fallot. The orifice of the aortic valve overrides the crest of the ventricular septum (*star*) so that both the right and left ventricles communicate directly with the aorta (*arrows*).

but not to straddle, since arterial valves lack any tension apparatus.

These chosen definitions have major implications for the description of other features of the hearts that are malformed because they contain straddling and overriding atrioventricular valves. The degree of overriding of the abnormal valve determines the precise atrioventricular connections, which can vary from double inlet to concordant or discordant. A spectrum exists between these extremes. There are two ways of coping with this situation. One way is to consider straddling in itself as a special case. The second approach is to emphasise the effect of the degree of override on the atrioventricular connection, dividing the spectrum at its midpoint when categorising the segmental arrangement (see Chapter 1). Thus, considering as an example the spectrum of straddling of the tricuspid valve, as illustrated in Figure 33-3, the hearts containing the straddling valve can be categorised as exhibiting either double inlet ventricle or concordant atrioventricular connections, depending of the proportion of the overriding junction supported within the right as opposed to the left ventricles. This is the principle used throughout this chapter. In the past, it was much easier to divide this spectrum in theory than it was in practise. The development of tomographic diagnostic techniques, and the ability to reconstruct individual anatomy in three dimensions, now means that it is possible also to make these distinctions in the clinical setting.

It was also the case that, when we first used this 50% rule for the purpose of assigning patients with straddling valves as having double inlet or biventricular atrioventricular connections, we had problems in moving from 49% to 51%. This was because, depending on our decision, a

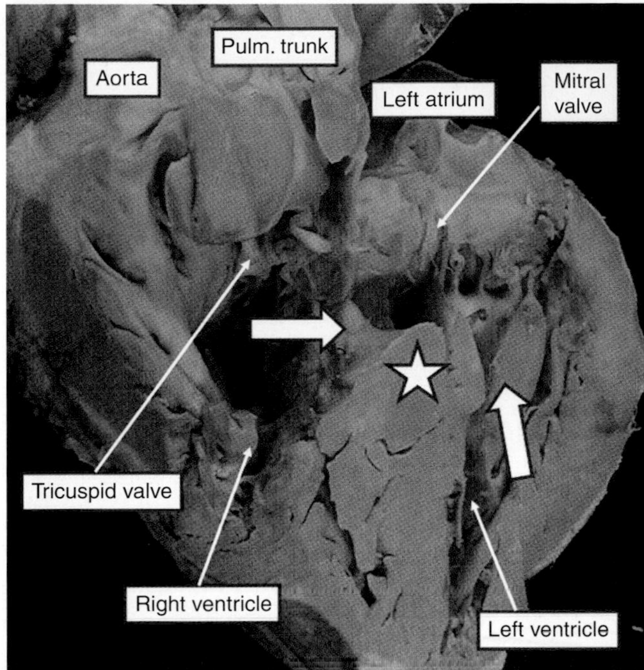

Figure 33-5 This simulated four-chamber echocardiographic section is from a patient with double outlet right ventricle and straddling mitral valve. It shows how, in addition to overriding of the left atrioventricular junction, the tension apparatus of the mitral valve (*arrows*) is attached to both the right and left ventricular sides of the ventricular septum (*star*). It is the abnormal attachment of the tension apparatus that we describe as straddling.

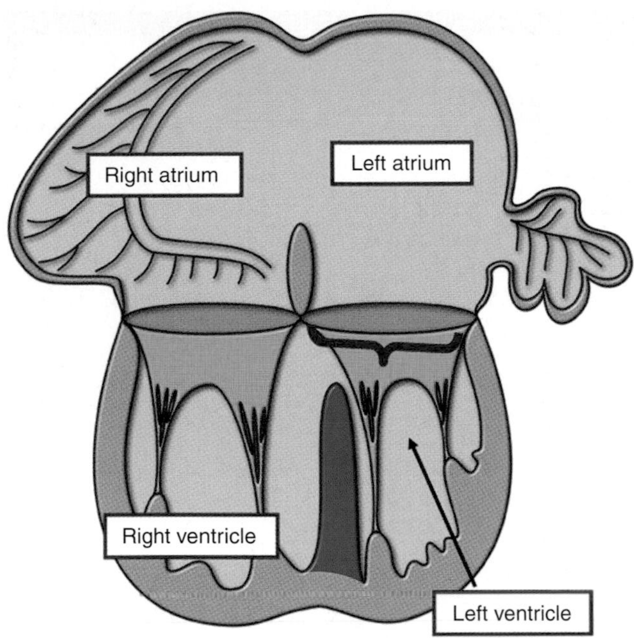

Figure 33-7 The cartoon, again illustrating the mitral valve, shows overriding, with the valvar orifice supported within both ventricles (*bracket*), but no straddling, all the tension apparatus being contained within the left ventricle.

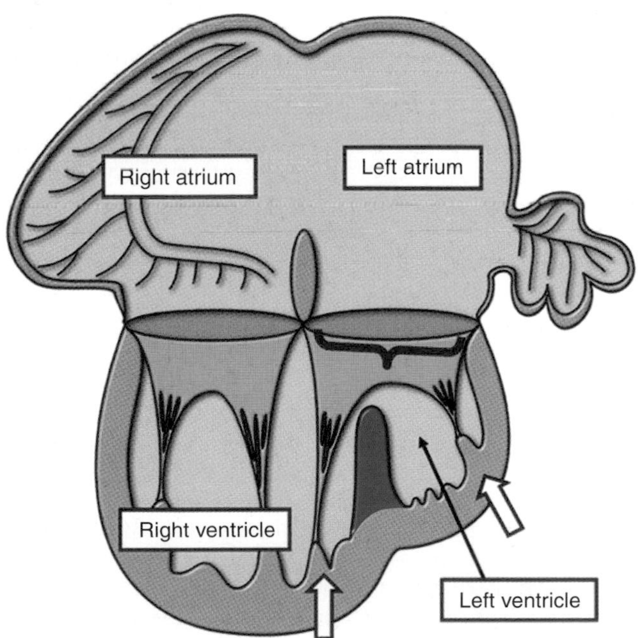

Figure 33-6 The cartoon illustrates overriding of the mitral valvar annulus (*red bracket*) and straddling of the tension apparatus (*arrows*) relative to the muscular ventricular septum (*purple*).

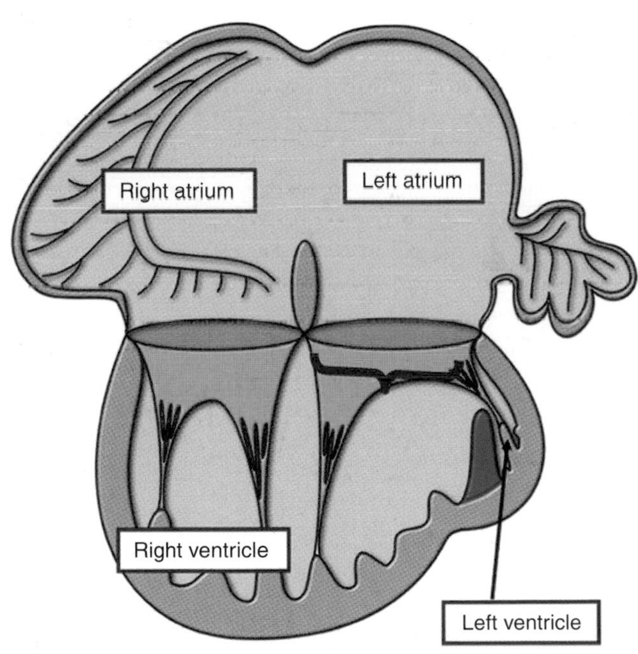

Figure 33-8 This cartoon (compare with Figs. 33-6 and 33-7) shows straddling of the mitral valve, but no overriding, all of the orifice of the valve being supported within the right ventricle (*bracket*).

patient considered to have a biventricular heart in the setting of biventricular connections would suddenly possess a univentricular heart if we designated the connection as double inlet. At that time, we were also promoting the concept of univentricular hearts as discrete from hearts with two ventricles, illogically disqualifying as ventricles all those chambers which lacked an inlet component or, more specifically, half an inlet component.[2] Once the lack of logic in this approach was identified,[3] and we realised that it was the atrioventricular connection, rather than the ventricular mass, which was effectively biventricular or univentricular, then the semantic problems disappeared.[4] The procedural problems, nonetheless, remain. It is still difficult precisely to adjudicate between 49% and 51% of overriding of an atrioventricular junction. Since the decision will no longer affect the description of the ventricles, the distinction loses much of its force. As we will see, in clinical practise it is more important in this setting to describe

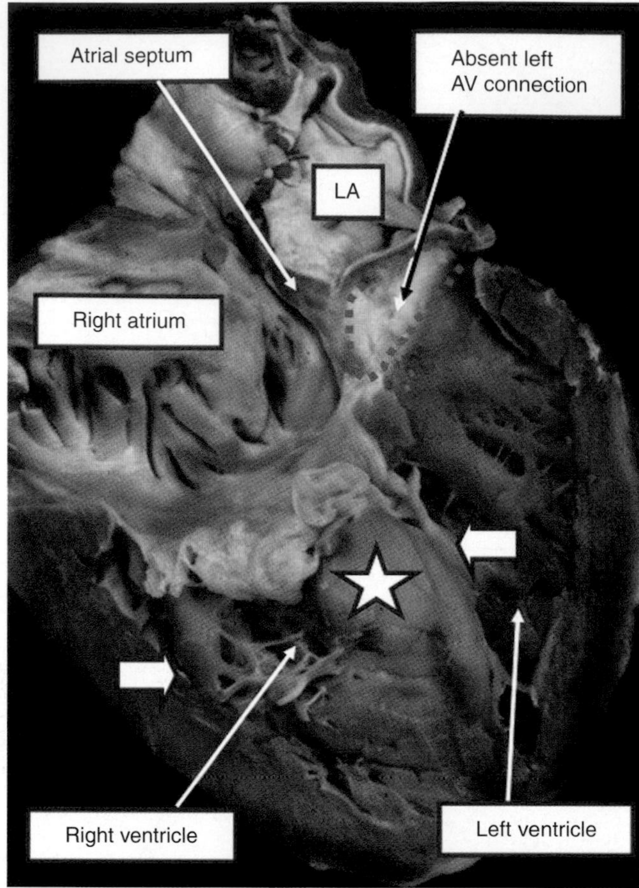

Figure 33-9 This anatomical section, in four-chamber plane, shows the essence of a uniatrial but biventricular atrioventricular connection (AV), here due to absence of the left atrioventricular connection (*green dotted lines*) and straddling of the crest of the ventricular septum (*star*) by the right atrioventricular valve (*arrows*) in the setting of right hand ventricular topology. Note that the atrial septum walls off the left atrium from the atrioventricular junction.

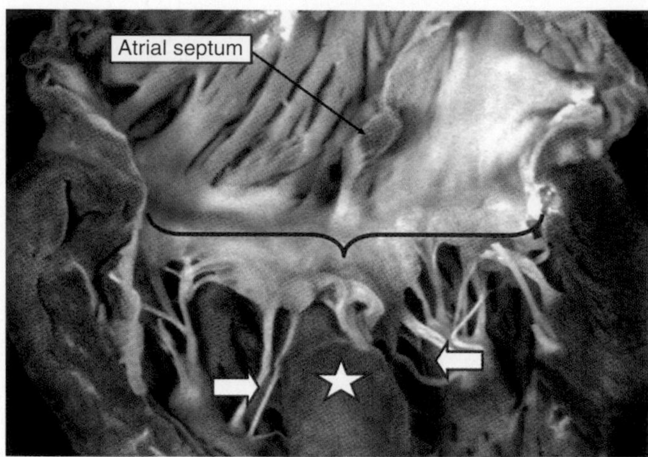

Figure 33-10 This four-chamber section, to be compared with Figure 33-9, shows how, in atrioventricular septal defect with common atrioventricular junction (*bracket*), the junction is shared more or less equally between the four chambers, and there is a septal defect between the leading edge of the atrial septum and the crest of the ventricular septum (*star*). Note also, however, that the inferior leaflet of the common atrioventricular valve straddles the ventricular septum (*arrows*).

the size of the ventricles. While this, to some extent, reflects the precise atrioventricular connection, it is certainly not the only determining feature. The degree of override, therefore, is determined with as much accuracy as is possible, dividing the spectrum on the basis of the proportion of the overriding junction attached within the two ventricles relative to the location of the ventricular septum (see Fig. 33-3).

There is then a second major point to consider in terms of definitions. This is when the valve which straddles and overrides is guarding a common atrioventricular junction, rather than a separate right or left atrioventricular junction. The first problem here is in defining a common atrioventricular junction, and distinguishing the common junction from the arrangement seen when one atrioventricular connection is absent and the other junction is itself straddling and overriding (Fig. 33-9). We use the atrial septum as our defining feature. We define a common atrioventricular junction as one which is common to both atriums and both ventricles, although the sharing of this junction does not have to be uniform between the four chambers. The exemplar of hearts with such a common junction is the entity usually described simply as an atrioventricular septal defect (see Chapter 27). In these hearts, the presence of the septal defect between the leading edge of the atrial septum, and the crest of the ventricular septum (Fig. 33-10), serves to emphasise the common nature of the junction. In all hearts having such an atrioventricular septal defect and common atrioventricular junction, the common atrioventricular valve of necessity both straddles and overrides. According to conventional wisdom,[5] such hearts are not discussed under the heading of straddling and overriding. There is no morphological reason why they should not be thus described, since the feature of leaflets being tethered in both ventricles is found in both settings. Other hearts, nonetheless, can have a common atrioventricular junction guarded by a common atrioventricular valve, and not usually be described in terms of atrioventricular septal defects. These are the hearts with double inlet ventricle, but with both atrioventricular junctions guarded by a common atrioventricular valve. In these hearts (Fig. 33-11), the common atrioventricular valve does not straddle and override. In between these extremes, there are further spectrums of malformations that reflect the precise degree of override of the common valve. These series of anomalies parallel the spectrums of overriding of the right or left valves, to be described in the body of this chapter. In such hearts with eccentric commitment of the common atrioventricular valve, it is again hard to make the distinction between double inlet and biventricular atrioventricular connections. Here, the decision reached probably will affect clinical decision-making, since it will determine whether to proceed to univentricular as opposed to biventricular repair. From the morphological stance, the decision is also harder to make than when either the right or left valve is straddling, since it requires the use of a 75% rather than a 50% rule. In clinical terms, it is almost certainly the size of the ventricle which is most important in determining the feasibility of biventricular versus univentricular repair. The precise atrioventricular connection, however, is by no means insignificant. This is again made, therefore, on the basis of the perceived attachments of the overriding junction, using the best information available to reach this decision. We will not consider further in this chapter those hearts with common valve which are intermediate between the extremes of atrioventricular septal defect and double inlet

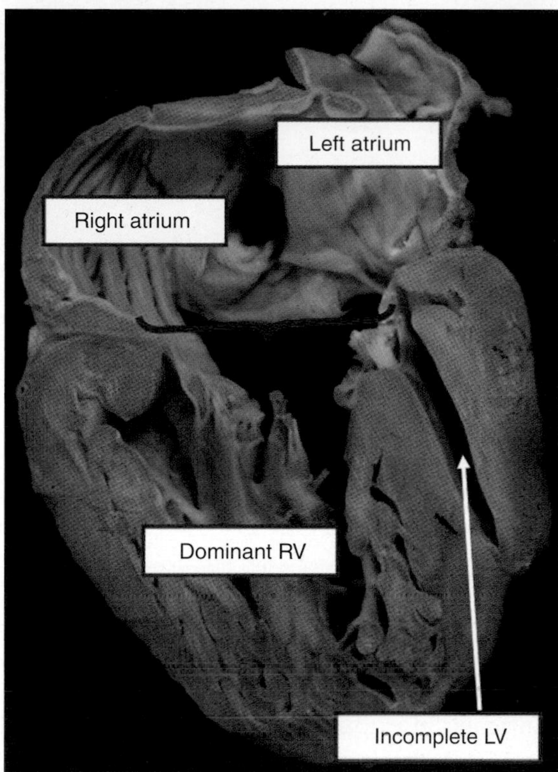

Figure 33-11 The four-chamber section of this heart shows that not all hearts with common atrioventricular junction and valve (*bracket*) have straddling of the leaflets. In this case, the common valve is exclusively connected to the right ventricle (RV) because of double inlet atrioventricular connection (compare with Fig. 33-10). LV, left ventricle.

ventricle, but they exist in the same patterns of right hand and left hand ventricular topology which will be discussed for straddling and overriding of those having separate right and left atrioventricular valves.

Before leaving the topic of definitions, we should address the problems of distinguishing a common valve from a straddling solitary valve associated with absence of one atrioventricular connection (see Fig. 33-9). We use the arrangement of the atrial septum as our arbiter. In almost all hearts in which one atrioventricular connection is absent, the atrial septum fuses with the parietal atrial wall so as to separate the blind-ending atrial chamber from the patent atrioventricular junction. This arrangement is seen even when the valve guarding the right or left atrioventricular junction is itself straddling and overriding between the ventricles (see Fig. 33-9). This morphological pattern serves to distinguish these hearts in which one atrium is connected to both ventricles, in other words, those with a uniatrial but biventricular atrioventricular connection, from other hearts with comparable connection of one atrium to both ventricles, so-called double outlet atrium, but in the setting of a common atrioventricular junction. In these latter hearts, which unequivocally have straddling and overriding of an atrioventricular valve, the valve itself is common to both the atriums because the atrial septum has failed to fuse with the parietal atrioventricular junction. The overall lesion, in the setting of common atrioventricular junction, is the consequence of malalignment between the atrial and ventricular septums, but with retention of the septal deficiency. This space, between the malaligned atrial septum in these hearts and the atrioventricular junction, is the so-called ostium primum defect. It can be argued that, on morphogenetic terms, this interatrial communication can become gradually smaller until it disappears, and therefore that the entities should be grouped together. From the stance of strict morphology, nonetheless, the junction remains a common structure until the primary foramen, or the ostium primum, has closed. The hearts with common atrioventricular valves and double outlet atrium are discussed further in Chapter 27. Those with a uniatrial but biventricular atrioventricular connection[6] will receive further attention in this chapter, and are also discussed in Chapter 31.

INCIDENCE AND AETIOLOGY

In that all atrioventricular septal defects with common orifice have a straddling valve as here defined, they should strictly be included in statistics concerning incidence. Because of problems of this kind, and because recognition of straddling and overriding is a recent event, it is difficult, if not impossible, to give precise figures. In our experience, straddling valves are recognised with more frequency now that they are specifically sought, particularly in anomalies such as congenitally corrected transposition (see Chapter 39), hearts with double inlet ventricle (see Chapter 31), and in double outlet right ventricle with subpulmonary ventricular septal defect (see Chapter 40 and Fig. 33-5). Clinical recognition of straddling, as opposed to overriding, of atrioventricular valves was not possible prior to the advent of cross sectional echocardiography. Until recently, straddling tended to be inferred when angiography demonstrated that the valvar orifice was overriding the ventricular septum. As overriding or straddling can exist in isolation, there were obvious diagnostic limitations. Straddling valves in the context of the congenitally malformed heart, therefore, should be considered relatively rare, but highly significant, malformations. In terms of aetiology, straddling mitral and tricuspid valves have been produced experimentally in rat fetuses exposed to teratogens,[7] while straddling tricuspid valve was produced by preventing expansion of the right atrioventricular junction.[8]

MORPHOLOGY AND DIAGNOSIS

Although straddling right or left atrioventricular valves can be found with any segmental combination,[1,6,9] description and diagnosis are simplified if they are considered in five series of malformations. In four of these series, either the right or left atrioventricular valve is straddling and overriding in the setting of right hand or left hand ventricular topology, respectively. As we have discussed, a common valve can also straddle and override with either right hand or left hand ventricular topology, and can show all the extremes between double inlet and biventricular atrioventricular connections. As explained, these variants with common valve will not be further discussed in this chapter, although it would be entirely appropriate to include such details. The fifth series is the uniatrial but biventricular atrioventricular connection.[6,9] As we will see, there are also several morphological variants to be found within this prototype, depending on ventricular topology and the side of absence of the atrioventricular connection. First, we

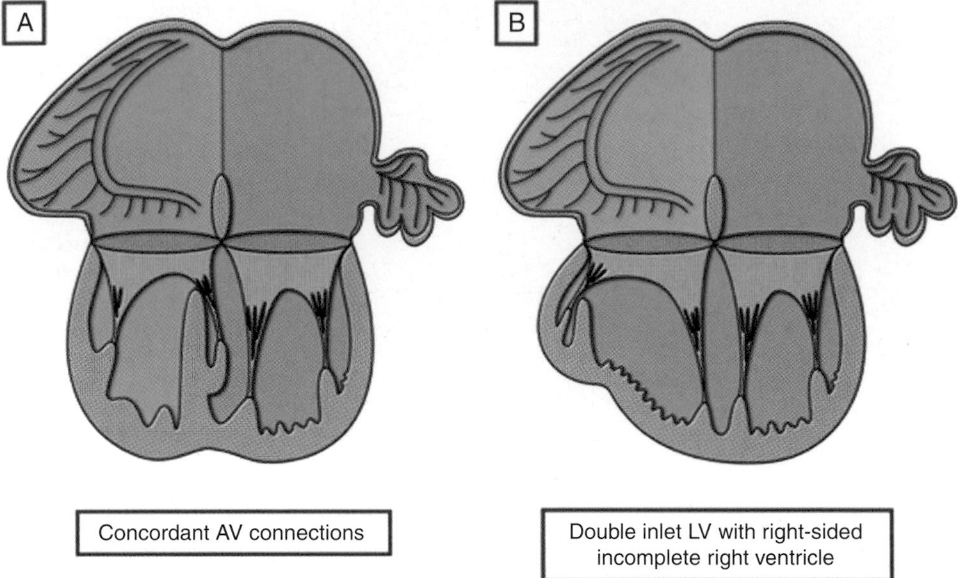

Figure 33-12 The cartoon shows the extremes of the series of malformations, extending from concordant atrioventricular connections (**A**) to double inlet left ventricle (**B**), found when the right atrioventricular (AV) valve, morphologically tricuspid, straddles and overrides in the setting of right hand ventricular topology.

account for the four patterns in which either the right or left atrioventricular valve is straddling.

While it might appear self-evident that straddling of an atrioventricular valve implies the presence of a ventricular septal defect, hearts are found in which an overriding atrioventricular valve straddles the septum, but the valvar leaflets are firmly adherent to the septal crest as they straddle. In such cases, a bridging tongue between the straddling leaflets usually creates two orifices within the overriding valve, with one valvar orifice then opening into each ventricle. This situation is comparable to atrioventricular septal defect with common atrioventricular junction guarded by separate right and left atrioventricular valves (see Chapter 27).

Straddling Morphologically Tricuspid Valve in the Setting of Right Hand Ventricular Topology

As is shown in Figure 33-12, the extremes of this spectrum are concordant atrioventricular connections (see Fig. 33-12A) and double inlet left ventricle with right-sided incomplete right ventricle (see Fig. 33-12B). The essence of this series is that the valve usually overrides the postero-inferior part of a malaligned ventricular septum which does not extend to the crux (see Fig. 33-3). When the atrioventricular connections are concordant, the septum joins the atrioventricular junction in its postero-inferior quadrant, whereas when the connection is basically double inlet, the septum joins the junction more or less at the acute margin. When the degree of override is approximately equal, the septum joins the junction halfway between the crux and the acute margin (Fig. 33-13). Irrespective of the precise atrioventricular connection, the septum does not reach the crux, and is malaligned relative to the atrial septum. Because of this, there is an abnormal atrioventricular conduction system (Fig. 33-14). The atrioventricular node is formed at the site where the ventricular septum joins the atrioventricular junction, the bundle branches being disposed astride the postero-inferior part of the septum. We have, on one occasion, seen straddling of the tricuspid valve through a muscular inlet defect, in the absence of override of the atrioventricular junction. In this setting, the atrioventricular connections were concordant, and the atrioventricular bundle arose from a regular atrioventricular node located in the atrial septum at the apex of the triangle of Koch.

The size and morphology of the right ventricle depend in part on the degree of override. When the valve is connected mostly to the right ventricle, the ventricle tends to be of more or less normal morphology. When the degree of override is such as to produce effective double inlet left ventricle, the morphology of the chamber can be virtually identical to the incomplete right ventricle typically seen in double inlet left ventricle. The ventriculo-arterial connections can be concordant or discordant. When the connections are concordant, the defect straddled by the valve has often been described as being of atrioventricular

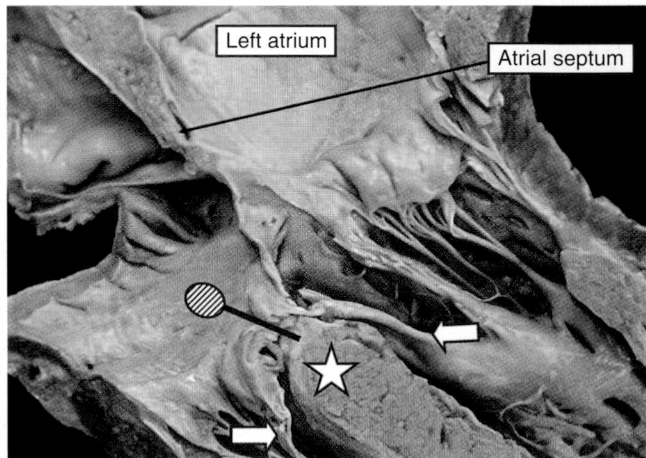

Figure 33-13 Close-up of the right atrioventricular junction from a heart with straddling tricuspid valve (*arrows*) sectioned to replicate the four-chamber echocardiographic cut shows the essence of the malformation. The ventricular septum (*star*) is malaligned relative to the atrial septum, the latter structure supporting the leaflets of the atrioventricular valves at the same level. Because of the malalignment, the atrioventricular bundle (*red line*) takes origin from a node (*cross-hatched oval*) in the postero-inferior part of the atrioventricular junction.

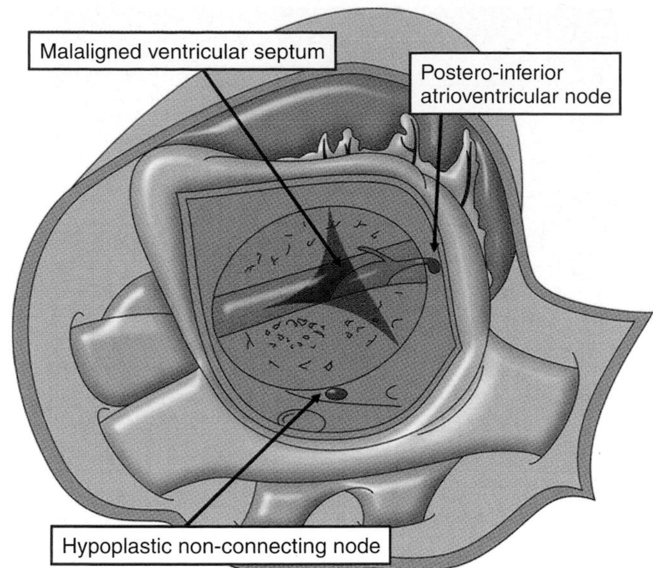

Figure 33-14 The cartoon shows the course of the conduction system in a situation comparable to that shown in Figure 33-13, but as might be viewed by the surgeon in the operating room. The atrioventricular node is formed at the point of union between the malaligned ventricular septum and the right atrioventricular junction. A node is present at the apex of the triangle of Koch, but is unable to make contact with ventricular conduction tissues. (Modified from the original prepared by Gemma Price for *Surgical Anatomy of the Heart* and reproduced with her permission.)

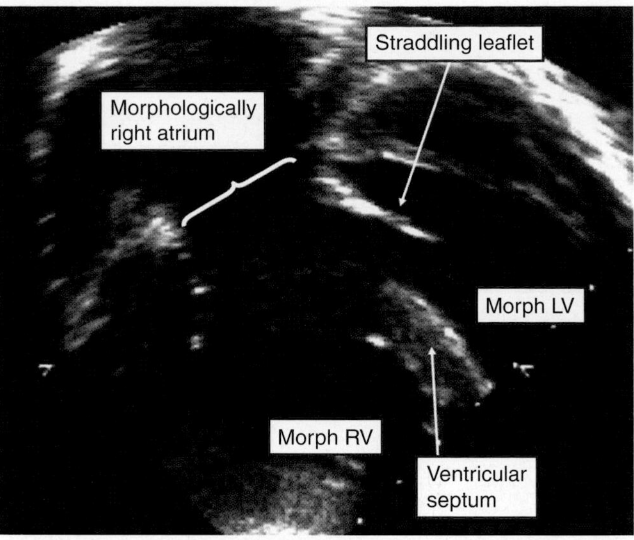

Figure 33-15 The cross sectional echocardiographic image, in four-chamber format, shows straddling of the leaflets of the tricuspid valve with effectively concordant atrioventricular connections. The overriding valvar orifice (*bracket*) is mostly supported by the morphologically (Morph) right ventricle (RV). LV, left ventricle.

canal type.[10,11] This is an inappropriate description, since the essence of the atrioventricular canal malformation is a common atrioventricular junction. The straddling tricuspid valve arises from a separate right atrioventricular junction, and hence cannot be associated with an atrioventricular canal. Rarely, nonetheless, a common valve can override in a fashion analogous to the straddling tricuspid valve. This is when there is marked malalignment between the atrial and ventricular septal structures, and the common atrioventricular junction is connected predominantly within the dominant left ventricle. The atrioventricular conduction tissues are then disposed in similar anomalous fashion (see Fig. 27-24).[12] Double outlet right ventricle, and Fallot's tetralogy, can also be complicated by straddling of the tricuspid valve.

Straddling and overriding of the tricuspid valve are readily identified using cross sectional echocardiography (Fig. 33-15), and it is also usually possible to recognise the pathognomonic malalignment between the atrial and ventricular septal structures (Fig. 33-16). Such examinations show the precise morphology present, particularly when conducted via the transoesophageal portal. In the setting of straddling and overriding, the leaflets of both atrioventricular valves are attached to the atrial septum at the same level (see Fig. 33-16). In the rare instances of straddling without overriding, however, the integrity of the atrioventricular septum will produce normal off-setting of the leaflets of the atrioventricular valves (Fig. 33-17). The degree of overriding, and hence the precise atrioventricular connection, is determined by assessing the point of attachment of the malaligned ventricular septum to the right atrioventricular junction. This is best done in a cut in which the overriding junction and the ventricular septum are visualised without showing the orifice of the mitral valve. A normal four-chamber cut may be too anterior to detect

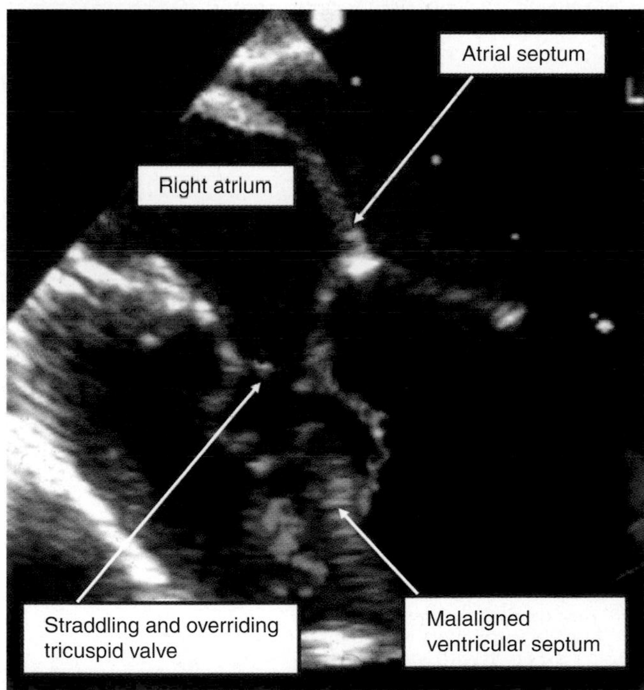

Figure 33-16 This cross sectional echocardiographic image, again in four-chamber format, shows the pathognomonic feature for straddling tricuspid valve of malalignment between the atrial septum and the muscular ventricular septum. Note that the leaflets of the mitral and tricuspid valves are attached to the underside of the atrial septum at the same level.

the displacement of the postero-inferior extent of the ventricular septum. A straddling tricuspid valve should always be suspected when the right ventricle is found to be unexpectedly hypoplastic. This feature was of great value in the past, when angiography was the technique used for diagnosis (Fig. 33-18). The accuracy of echocardiographic diagnosis now obviates the need for angiography, particularly when accompanied by flow mapping, or when performed from the transoesophageal or transgastric windows.

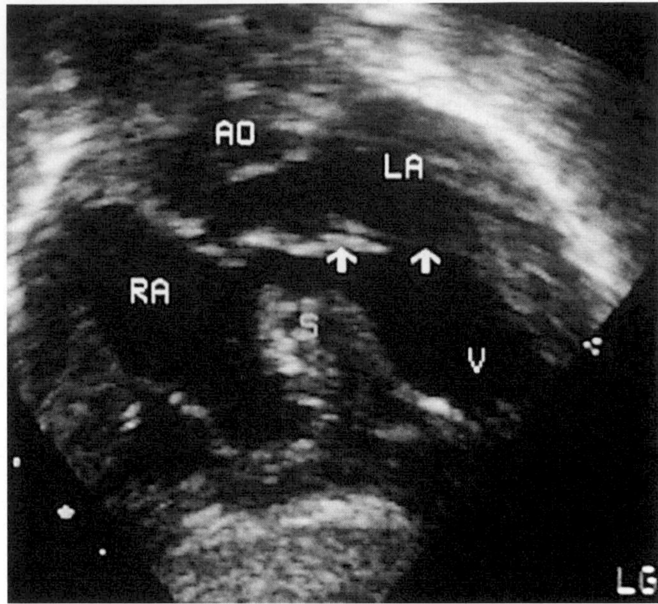

Figure 33-17 This transthoracic subcostal echocardiogram shows straddling of the tension apparatus of the tricuspid valve (*arrows*) in the absence of junctional overriding. The atrioventricular septal structures were intact in this patient; note the normal wedged position of the aorta (AO). LA, left atrium; RA, right atrium; S, septum; V, left ventricle.

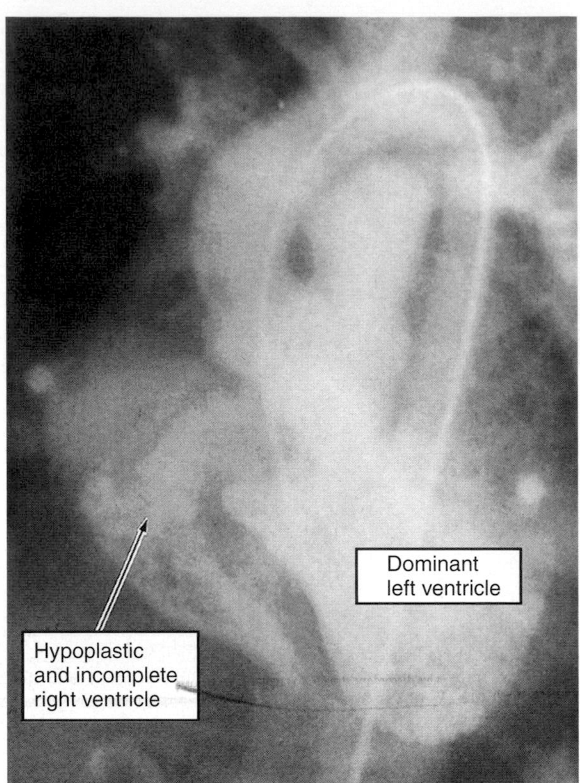

Figure 33-18 The right ventricle is shown to be hypoplastic by angiocardiography in this patient with straddling tricuspid valve. The part of the right junction committed to the left ventricle is shown by unopacified blood. (Courtesy of the late Dr R. M. Freedom, Hospital for Sick Children, Toronto, Ontario, Canada.)

Straddling Morphologically Mitral Valve in the Setting of Left Hand Ventricular Topology

In the second series of malformations, the spectrum is between discordant atrioventricular connections (Fig. 33-19A) and double inlet right ventricle with right-sided incomplete left ventricle (see Fig. 33-19B). In this series, the right-sided morphologically mitral valve straddles the anterior part of a ventricular septum which does extend to the crux (Fig. 33-20).[13] When the overriding atrioventricular junction is connected mostly to the left-sided morphologically right ventricle, then the atrioventricular connection is effectively double inlet right ventricle. The right-sided morphologically left ventricle may than be no more than a postero-inferior slit, particularly as the ventriculo-arterial connection is almost always double outlet from the dominant right ventricle. Double outlet right ventricle is also the expected ventriculo-arterial connection when the atrioventricular connections are discordant rather than double inlet (see Fig. 33-20). Alternatively, there may be single outlet with pulmonary atresia, the aorta arising from the right ventricle. Discordant

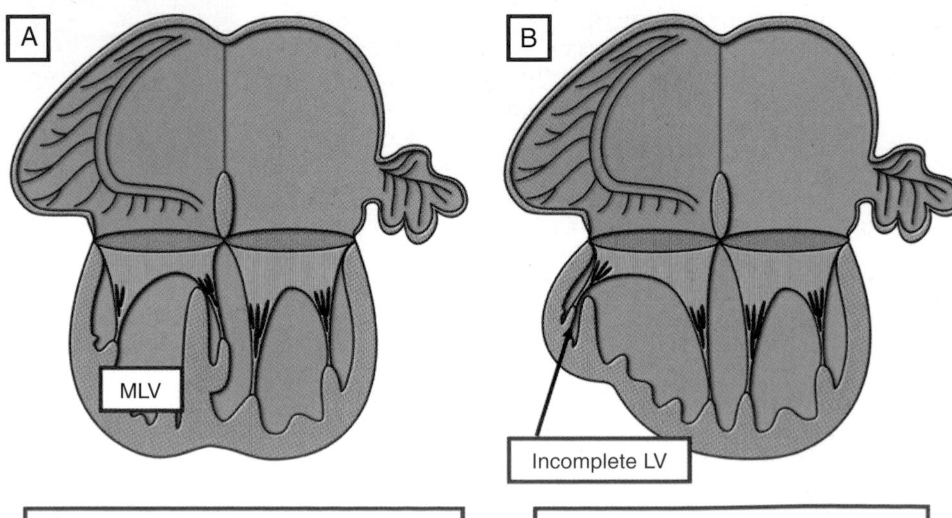

Figure 33-19 The cartoon shows the extremes of the series of malformations found when the right atrioventricular valve, in this instance morphologically mitral because of the presence of left hand ventricular topology, straddles and overrides. This combination produces discordant atrioventricular connections on the one hand (**A**), but double inlet right ventricle with right-sided incomplete left ventricle on the other hand (**B**). Compare with Figure 33-12. MLV, morphological left ventricle.

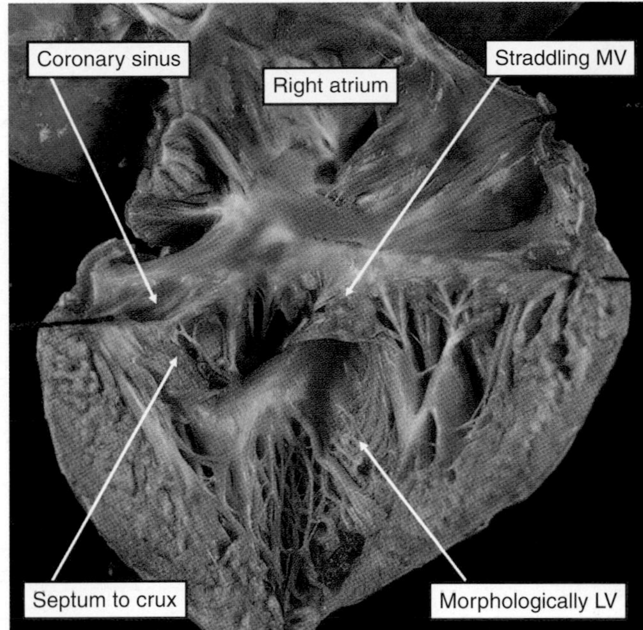

Figure 33-20 This heart has discordant atrioventricular connections and double outlet from the left-sided morphologically right ventricle (not seen in the photograph). The image shows straddling and overriding of the right-sided morphologically mitral valve (MV). Note that the septum extends to the crux (compare with Fig. 33-3). (Courtesy of Mr Don Perrin, Hospital for Sick Children, Toronto, Ontario, Canada.)

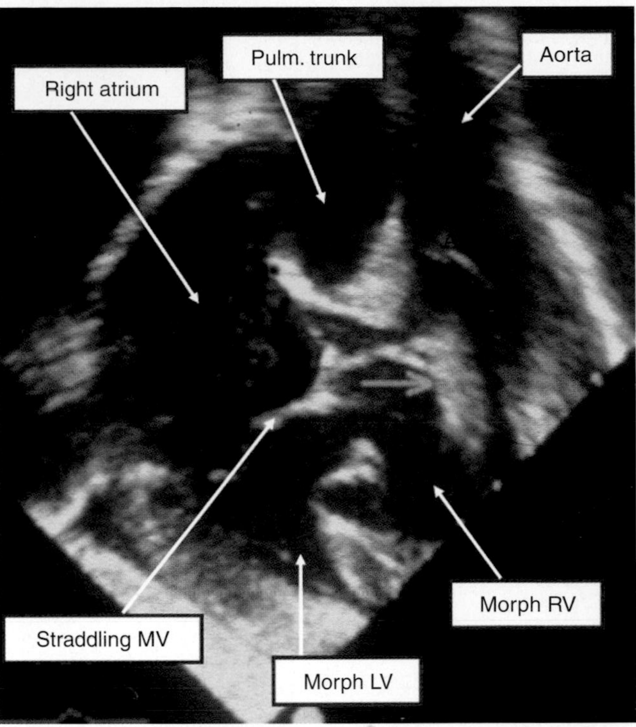

Figure 33-21 This cross sectional echocardiogram, taken subcostally, shows straddling of the tension apparatus of the morphologically mitral valve (MV) in a patient with left hand ventricular topology and effectively discordant atrioventricular connections. The pulmonary (Pulm.) trunk was arising, together with the aorta, from the morphologically right ventricle (Morph RV). Morph LV, right sided morphologically left ventricle.

ventriculo-arterial connections are rare, and concordant connections even rarer. The disposition of the conduction tissues is dictated by the left hand pattern of ventricular topology.[13] When the ventriculo-arterial connection is double outlet from the right ventricle, it is possible for both an anterior and a postero-inferior atrioventricular node to make contact with the ventricular conduction tissues, producing the so-called Monckeberg sling.[14,15] This arrangement is in contrast to the expected situation in congenitally corrected transposition, where typically only the anterior node makes contact with the ventricular conduction tissues.[16] A heart with congenitally corrected transposition and straddling mitral valve has been described, nonetheless, in which the only atrioventricular node was regularly positioned within the atrial septum.[17] Both the presence of a sling, and the existence of a regular node, reflect the better alignment of the atrial and muscular ventricular septums in the presence of double outlet right ventricle.

The presence of straddling of the mitral valve should always be suspected when clinical investigation suggests discordant atrioventricular connections, but the morphologically left ventricle is small. Cross sectional echocardiography is again the diagnostic technique of choice (Fig. 33-21). Angiography in the past was able to show the division of the stream of blood leaving the right atrium, and it was thought that ventricular angiograms, taken in the appropriate projection, would illustrate the degree of override of the atrioventricular junction. All of these features are now better quantified using echocardiography, particularly with the increasing availability of the three-dimensional format. If necessary, tomographic techniques such as magnetic resonance imaging or computerised tomography will confirm the findings.

Straddling Left-sided Morphologically Mitral Valve in the Setting of Right Hand Ventricular Topology

In this series of malformations, the extremes of the spectrum are concordant atrioventricular connections (Fig. 33-22A), and double inlet right ventricle with left-sided incomplete left ventricle (see Fig. 33-22B). This variant of straddling mitral valve,[18,19] as with the lesion seen with effectively discordant atrioventricular connections, is again encountered most frequently in association with double outlet right ventricle, be the atrioventricular connections concordant or double inlet right ventricle. The essence of the anomaly is that the mitral valve straddles and overrides the antero-superior part of the muscular ventricular septum (see Fig. 33-4). With this arrangement, again as in the setting of discordant atrioventricular connections (see Fig. 33-20), the postero-inferior part of the septum does extend to the crux (Fig. 33-23). Because of this, the conduction tissues are located in their usual position for the normal heart irrespective of the atrioventricular connection.[1] The leaflet of the mitral valve which straddles into the right ventricle is itself frequently cleft.[20]

Diagnosis of the anomaly using cross sectional techniques (Fig. 33-24), particularly combined with flow mapping and use of the transoesophageal window, is remarkably accurate. Though ventricular hypoplasia, when it occurs, usually affects the left-sided morphologically left ventricle, a small series of right-sided hearts have been described[21] with usual arrangement and straddling mitral valve with concordant atrioventricular connections and double outlet right ventricle. In these patients, diagnosed using cross sectional echocardiography, it was the right

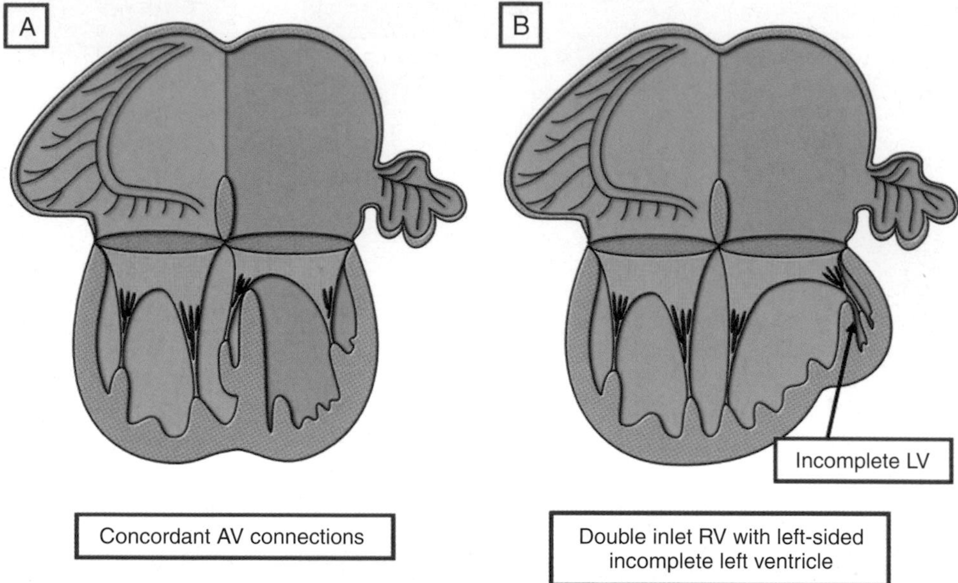

Figure 33-22 The cartoon shows the extremes of the series of malformations found when the left atrioventricular valve, in this instance morphologically mitral because of the presence of right hand ventricular topology, straddles and overrides. This combination produces concordant atrioventricular (AV) connections on the one hand (**A**), but double inlet right ventricle (RV) with left-sided incomplete left ventricle (LV) on the other hand (**B**). Compare with Figure 33-12.

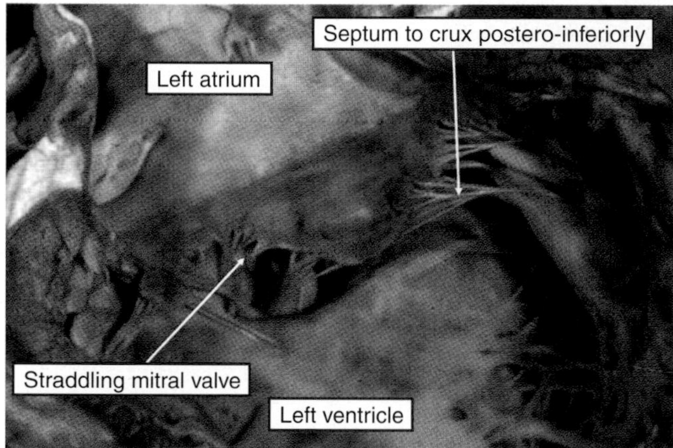

Figure 33-23 The picture shows straddling of a left-sided morphologically mitral valve as seen from the left ventricular aspect in the setting of usual atrial arrangement and right hand–pattern ventricular topology. In this instance, the atrioventricular connections are concordant, and there is double outlet right ventricle. The other end of the spectrum is double inlet right ventricle. Note that the valve straddles the outlet part of a septum, which continues postero-inferiorly to reach to the crux.

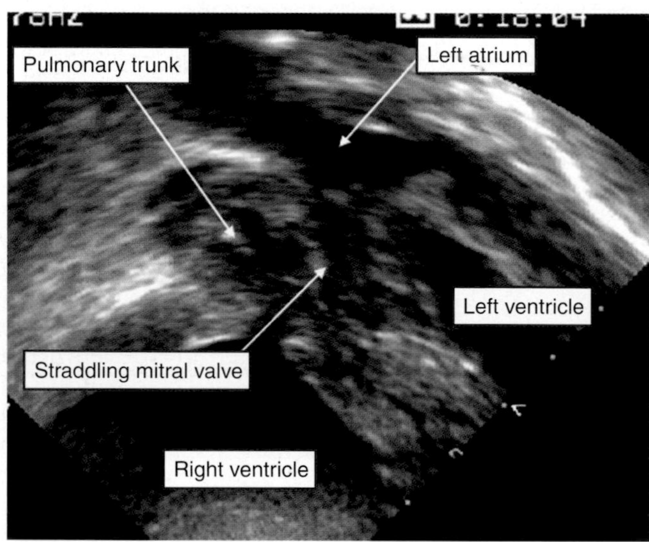

Figure 33-24 This four-chamber echocardiographic cut, taken subcostally, shows straddling and overriding of the left-sided morphologically mitral valve in the setting of usual atrial arrangement, effectively concordant atrioventricular connections, and right hand ventricular topology. Both the pulmonary trunk and the aorta were originating from the morphologically right ventricle. Note that the straddling tension apparatus of the mitral valve produces marked subpulmonary obstruction.

ventricle which was hypoplastic. There was associated tricuspid stenosis and hypoplasia, a large right ventricular outflow tract, an antero-superior interventricular communication, and criss-cross atrioventricular relations. It proved possible to diagnose this pattern angiographically, either directly following left atrial injection, or by observing the flow of contrast-free blood through the annulus following a ventricular injection in the four-chamber projection.[20] As with the other entities discussed in this chapter, nonetheless, the need for angiographic investigation has now been obviated by the accuracy of cross sectional echocardiography.

Straddling Left-sided Morphologically Tricuspid Valve in the Setting of Left Hand Ventricular Topology

In the final series of malformations with biatrial connections, the spectrum extends from discordant atrioventricular connections (Fig. 33-25A) to double inlet left ventricle with left-sided incomplete right ventricle (see Fig. 33-25B). The straddling valve overrides the postero-inferior part of the muscular ventricular septum, which does not extend to the crux (Fig. 33-26). The ventriculo-arterial connections in either type are usually discordant, but other connections must be anticipated. Whatever the atrioventricular connections, the ventricular conduction tissues arise from an anterolateral node in the right atrioventricular junction. A long non-branching bundle encircles the pulmonary valvar orifice to reach and branch on the antero-superior part of the muscular ventricular septum (Fig. 33-27).[1]

As with all the other variants, the diagnosis is readily made nowadays using cross sectional echocardiography (Fig. 33-28). This shows both the degree of override of the valvar

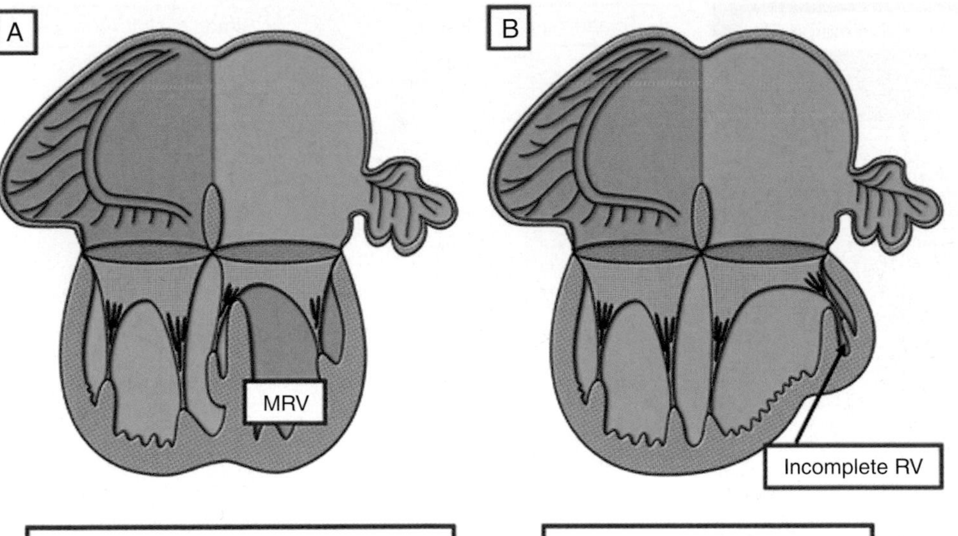

Figure 33-25 The cartoon shows the extremes of the series of malformations found when the left atrioventricular valve, in this instance morphologically tricuspid because of the presence of left hand ventricular topology, straddles and overrides. This combination produces discordant atrioventricular connections on the one hand (**A**), but double inlet left ventricle (LV) with left-sided incomplete morphologically right ventricle (MRV) on the other hand (**B**). Compare with Figure 33-22.

annulus, and the precise attachments of the tension apparatus of the straddling valve.[22] The entity should be suspected whenever the morphologically right ventricle is unexpectedly small in patients thought to have congenitally corrected transposition, or unusually large when the working diagnosis is double inlet left ventricle with left-sided incomplete right ventricle. Angiography as a diagnostic tool has been rendered obsolete by the excellence of cross sectional echocardiography, particularly when interrogation is carried out from the transoesophageal portal. The diagnostic yield will improve still further as three-dimensional techniques become better established.

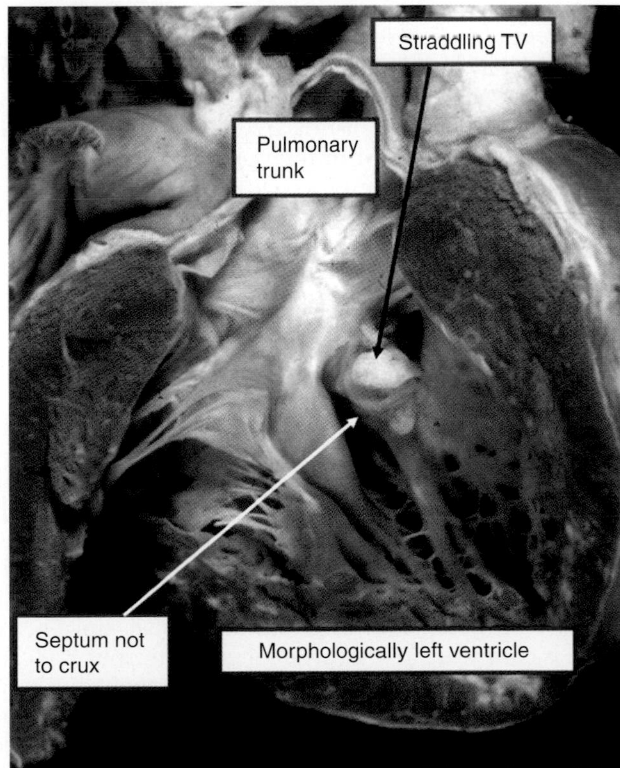

Figure 33-26 The image shows the morphologically left ventricle from a patient with congenitally corrected transposition and usual atrial arrangement. There is minimal overriding and straddling of the left-sided morphologically tricuspid valve (TV). Note that the ventricular septum does not extend to the crux.

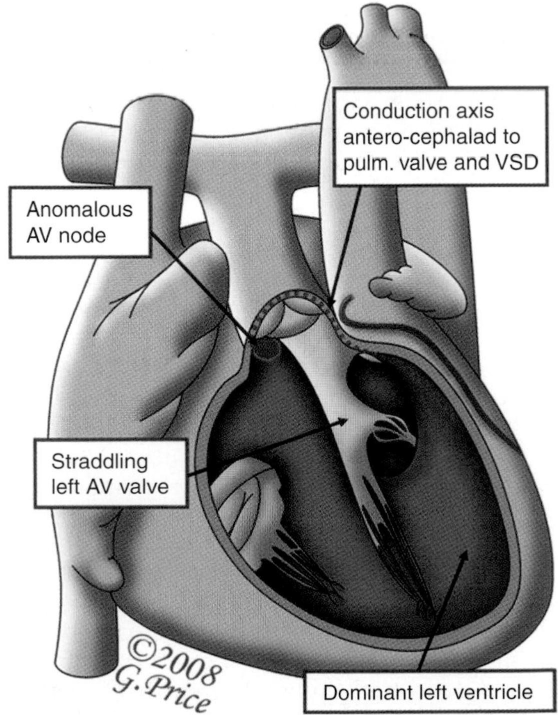

Figure 33-27 The cartoon shows the disposition of the conduction tissues as would be seen through the right-sided morphologically left ventricle in a patient with congenitally corrected transposition and usual atrial arrangement with straddling of the left-sided morphologically tricuspid valve (left AV valve). Note that the bundle (*dashed green line*) runs cephalad to the ventricular septal defect (VSD) and the pulmonary (pulm.) valve. Compare with Figure 33-26.

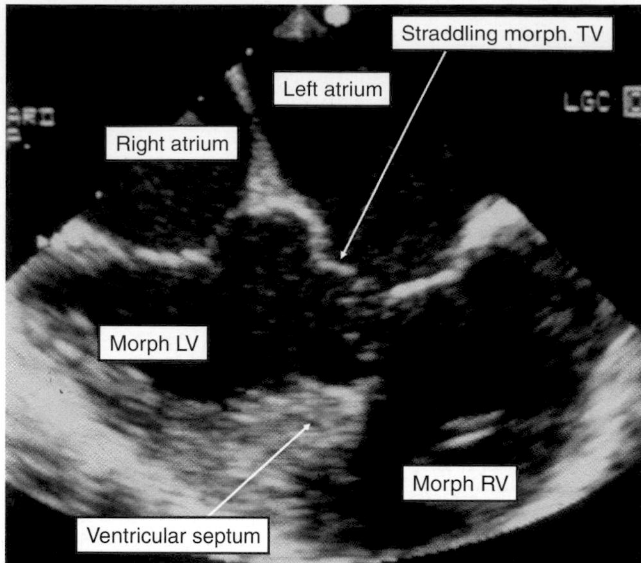

Figure 33-28 This echocardiogram, taken in a patient with effectively discordant atrioventricular connections, shows the tension apparatus of the left-sided morphologically tricuspid valve (morph. TV) overriding the ventricular septum, which does not reach to the crux. The tension apparatus of the valve was also straddling. Morph LV, right-sided morphologically left ventricle; Morph RV, left-sided morphologically right ventricle.

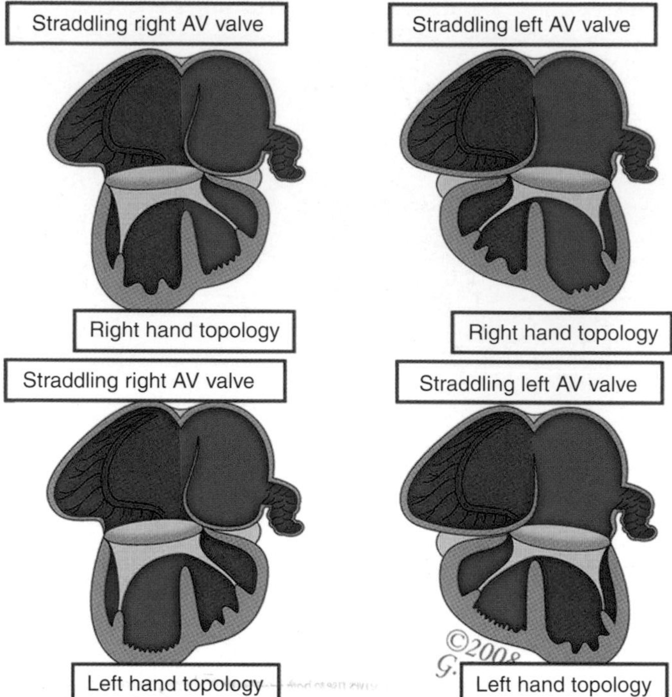

Figure 33-29 The cartoon shows how, when there is absence of either the right or the left atrioventricular connection, the solitary atrioventricular (AV) valve, which will be right-sided (*left hand panels*) or left-sided (*right hand panels*), can straddle and override in patients with usual atrial arrangement when there is either right hand (*upper panels*) or left hand (*lower panels*) ventricular topology. Further variability is then seen in terms of the dominance of the ventricles, different ventriculo-arterial connection, and so on.

Straddling Valves with Absent Atrioventricular Connection

The final group of hearts to be discussed in this chapter are those in which one atrioventricular connection is absent, but in which the solitary atrioventricular valve straddles and overrides the ventricular septum (see Fig. 33-9). Such hearts, which have a uniatrial but biventricular connection, are extremely rare and exceedingly complex anatomically.[6,9] They are important for understanding the range of morphology to be found in congenitally malformed hearts, and they emphasise the value of sequential segmental analysis. Examples exist of absence of either the right or left atrioventricular connections, and of either right hand or left hand ventricular topology (Fig. 33-29). Furthermore, for each prototypic heart shown in Figure 33-29, there are two examples, depending on which ventricle is dominant. This means that there are at least eight possible arrangements, and most have now been well documented. [6,9,22,23]

Ventricular topology has proved to be of great significance when categorising these hearts,[6,9] the disposition of the conduction system in particular depending on this feature. Studies carried out in two patients revealed unexpected findings.[9] In one, when the right atrioventricular connection was absent and the left valve was straddling in the setting of left hand ventricular topology, a sling of conduction tissue was encountered, with the posterior node formed in the left sided atrioventricular junction (Fig. 33-30). This finding points again to the crucial feature of the junction between the muscular ventricular septum and the atrioventricular junction in determining the location of the atrioventricular node, along with the equally important facet of ventricular topology. Also, irrespective of how the heart is imaged, the result will be heavily dependent on the ventricular topology, even in hearts in which the blood goes round the same way physiologically. And, from an embryological point of view, there is all the difference in the world between a heart with absent right connection in left hand and right hand topology, just as there is a great difference between straddling mitral and straddling tricuspid valve. It is usually, but not always, possible to predict the valvar morphology from the ventricular topology, and vice versa.[9] Hence, it is best to establish both the morphology of the straddling valve and the ventricular topology. On occasion, nonetheless, in some hearts it may prove impossible to determine the topology of the ventricular mass.[24] Should that prove to be the case, clear and unambiguous description is essential.

In the hearts having a uniatrial but biventricular connection, the clinical picture will be dominated by the side of the absent connection, and by other associated anomalies, such as those that reduce the flow of blood to the lungs. The finding of unexpected ventricular morphology should alert to the possibility of the lesion, and echocardiography readily demonstrates the combination of a straddling valve with absence of one atrioventricular connection (Fig. 33-31). During echocardiographic examination, it is important to assess the competence of the straddling valve, since regurgitation is common, at least when it is the morphologically tricuspid valve which is straddling.[22] Although, on some occasions, the ventricles are of comparable size, offering the theoretical option of surgical septation should the ventriculo-arterial connections be favourable, the morphology is so complex that the operative options are unlikely ever to extend beyond either palliation or construction of the Fontan circulation.

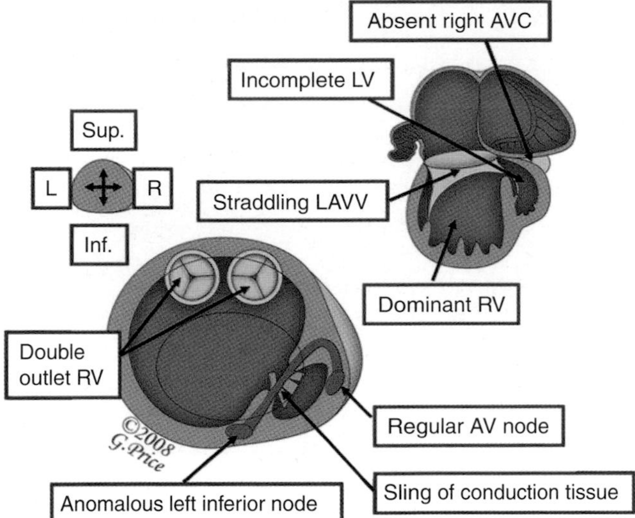

Figure 33-30 The cartoon shows the location of a sling of conduction tissue, viewed from the atrial aspect and shown relative to the ventricular mass in the main left hand and lower panel, in a heart with absent right atrioventricular connection (AVC) and straddling left atrioventricular valve (LAVV) as seen in the setting of left hand ventricular topology, shown in the upper right hand panel as seen in four-chamber projection from behind. There is a dominant left-sided right ventricle (RV) which gives rise to both arterial trunks, with the incomplete left ventricle (LV) in right-sided and inferior position. The compass in the upper left quadiant of the cartoon shows the orientation of the ventricular mass as seen in the lower part of the panel. Inf., inferior; Sup., superior.

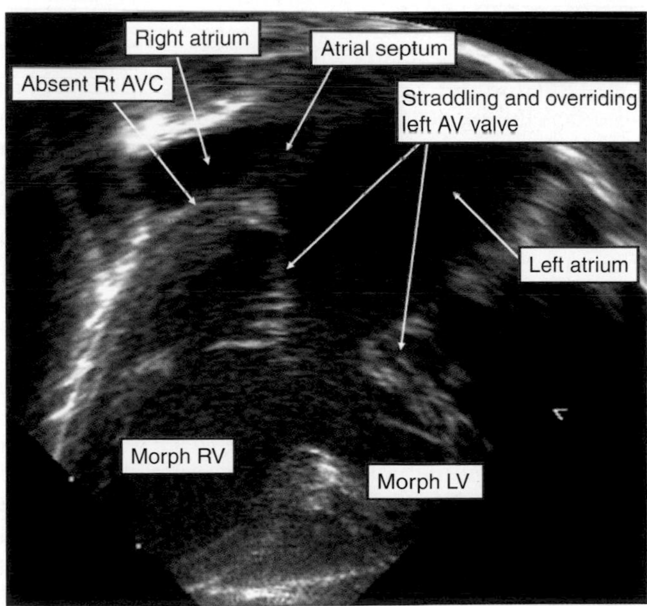

Figure 33-31 This cross sectional echocardiogram, obtained from the subcostal window, shows absence of the right atrioventricular connection (Absent Rt AVC), with straddling and overriding of the solitary left atrioventricular (AV) valve into a ventricular mass with right hand topology. Note that the atrial septum fuses with the atrioventricular junction, meaning that the straddling valve is left-sided rather than common. Morph LV, morphologically left ventricle; Morph RV, morphologically right ventricle.

THERAPEUTIC OPTIONS

In determining the options for treatment, which will be surgical once the diagnosis has been made, it will be necessary to take note of the precise connections of the overriding junction and the arrangement of the straddling tension apparatus, together with the morphology and size of the dominant and incomplete ventricles.[24] In the past, purely palliative options often offered the best chance of success, although increasing experience with conversion to the Fontan circulation (see Chapter 32) now suggests this will be the alternative should biventricular repair be deemed impossible. Palliative procedures may still be needed even if the decision is made to proceed eventually to conversion to the Fontan circulation. These have included redirection of the circulations at either atrial or arterial levels, banding of the pulmonary trunk or release of a previously placed band, and construction of systemic-to-pulmonary arterial shunts. In extreme cases, the regurgitant straddling valve has been replaced, with a conduit placed to the pulmonary trunk so as to bypass pulmonary stenosis.[25] Nowadays, construction of a bidirectional cavopulmonary connection is the most likely palliative option. Biventricular repair can be achieved in those with the most favourable anatomy. This is particularly the case when valvar overriding exists in the absence of straddling. This presents only a minor problem to the surgeon, since any patch placed to close a ventricular septal defect can be deviated to the plane which passes between the atrioventricular valves. By contrast, straddling of the valvar tension apparatus, occasionally with the apparatus from both valves straddling, presents major problems. In these instances, many will opt for functionally univentricular repair. If one atrioventricular connection is absent, then biventricular repair is virtually impossible, although it may theoretically be possible to resect the atrial septum and divide the overriding valve if each ventricle is of substantial size, and the ventriculo-arterial connections are appropriately arranged.

Should the decision be made to proceed with biventricular repair, then if the straddling tension apparatus inserts within 1 cm of the crest of the ventricular septum, the septal defect can be closed in such a way as to leave the cords initially on the wrong side of the ventricular septum on the correct side of the patch.[25] This is relatively straightforward if the cords are straddling towards the ventricle containing the greater part of the overriding valve, as would be the case in concordant atrioventricular connections with straddling mitral valve.[24] It is not so simple when the straddling cords insert on the far side of the ventricular septum from the surgeon, as is the case with straddling tricuspid valve and right hand ventricular topology. The technical challenge of securing the patch on the wrong side of the septum is then comparable with the technique used to avoid the conduction tissues in patients with discordant atrioventricular connections uncomplicated by straddling.[26] Sometimes it may be necessary to enlarge the defect so as to bring the straddling cords nearer its margin.[25,27] Further possibilities include division of tendinous cords attached to a limited amount of atrioventricular valvar tissue. Alternatively, the cords may be passed through a slot in the patch.[28] The slot is then sutured to create the smallest possible residual defect consistent with free movement of the cord. When the straddling tension apparatus is attached only to one papillary muscle, or to an area of the muscular ventricular septum in the inappropriate ventricle, then

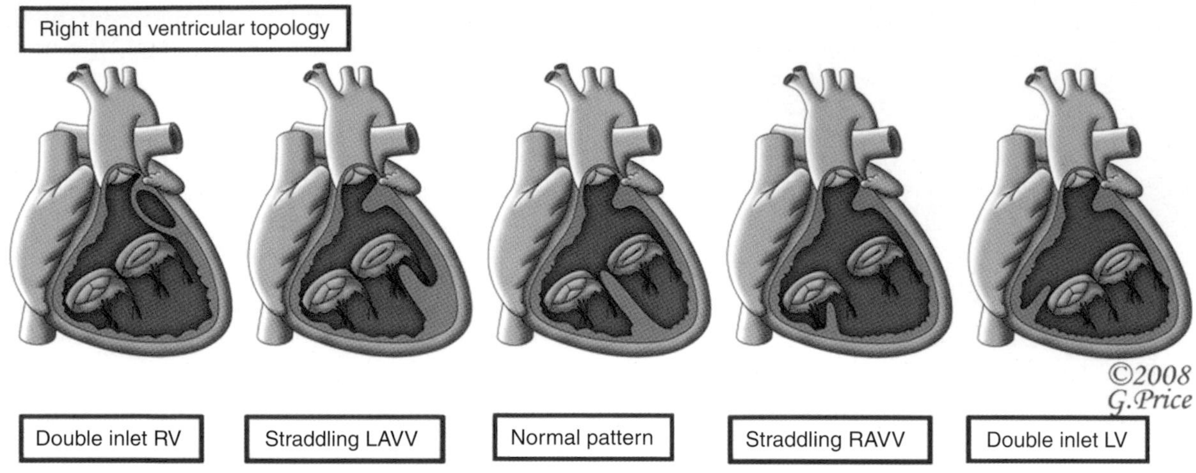

Figure 33-32 The cartoon shows the suggested morphogenetic sequences which link straddling of the right and left valves in the setting of right hand topology. The middle panel shows the normal heart. Straddling of the left-sided morphologically mitral valve produces a spectrum leading to double inlet right ventricle (RV) with left-sided and inferior incomplete left ventricle (LV), while straddling of the right-sided morphologically tricuspid valve produces a similar spectrum with double inlet left ventricle and right-sided incomplete right ventricle as the end point. The ventriculo-arterial connections will vary depending on the precise ventricular morphology. LAVV, left atrioventricular valve; RAVV, right atrioventricular valve.

that muscle may be sectioned at its base if it has no other cordal attachments. The septal defect can then be closed and the papillary muscle reattached to the patch or the intraventricular tunnel thus created.[29]

There is also the problem of avoiding the conduction tissues when attempting to close the ventricular septal defect, or achieving septation, in hearts with straddling atrioventricular valves. As we have described, the arrangement is frequently abnormal, even in hearts with straddling tricuspid valve and concordant atrioventricular connections. Indeed, in many reported series, surgically induced atrioventricular dissociation has been a major complication.[28] In the past, this was presumably because the ventricular conduction tissues were presumed to arise from the regular atrioventricular node located in the triangle of Koch.[30] As we have emphasised, in this entity the node is formed at the point where the muscular ventricular septum makes contact with the atrioventricular junction. Success can be achieved in avoiding heart block, nonetheless, simply by the expedient of placing very fine sutures in the crest of the ventricular septum.[26] It would seem more prudent, nonetheless, for surgeons to attempt to avoid the known site of the atrioventricular node. This is always abnormal when the tricuspid valve straddles in the setting of right hand topology, in the group of hearts with straddling left valve in the setting of left hand ventricular topology, and usually deviates from the normal when the right valve straddles in this setting. These arrangements are already well recognised in patients with congenitally corrected transposition (see Chapter 39). All things considered, surgical repair of straddling valves is a daunting prospect. When straddling is minimal, and the patient is larger, closure of the defect by deviating the patch is to be recommended. This may also be done in infancy when there is no valvar regurgitation. Excellent results reported by some groups point to the potential advantages of this approach.[26,29] When the morphology precludes deviation of the patch, it is still possible to replace the straddling valve and close the ventricular septal defect once the patients have reached a suitable age. In these latter situations, nonetheless, many would consider construction of the Fontan circulation a safer approach, despite its long-term uncertainties (see Chapter 32).

MORPHOGENESIS

The various series of hearts with straddling valves are readily explained on the basis of abnormalities of connection of the developing atrioventricular junctions to the ventricles.[30–33] During normal development with rightward ventricular looping (Fig. 33-32), the atrioventricular canal is initially committed exclusively to the developing left ventricle. With rightward expansion, and division, of the atrioventricular canal, the right atrium becomes connected to the developing right ventricle.[34] Incomplete connection of various degrees produces straddling of the right atrioventricular valve, while exaggerated commitment of the newly formed left atrioventricular junction to the developing right ventricle accounts for straddling and overriding of the left atrioventricular valve. The extreme of such exaggerated rightward commitment then explains pure double inlet right ventricle, the left ventricle remaining as the incomplete left-sided chamber. Exactly the same processes can occur with left hand ventricular looping, thus producing the other series of straddling valves (Fig. 33-33). Similar events, but with eccentric development of the atrial septum and fusion with the atrioventricular junction, will produce all the variants of straddling valve with absent atrioventricular connection. As we have discussed, straddling of an atrioventricular valve in the setting of absent atrioventricular connection produces one variant of double outlet atrium. The other variant is found in the setting of a common atrioventricular junction with gross malalignment of the atrial septum.[35] This is well explained on the basis of eccentric formation of the atrial septum, but retention of a common atrioventricular junction. As we have emphasised, it is the morphology of the atrial septum which serves to distinguish these lesions.

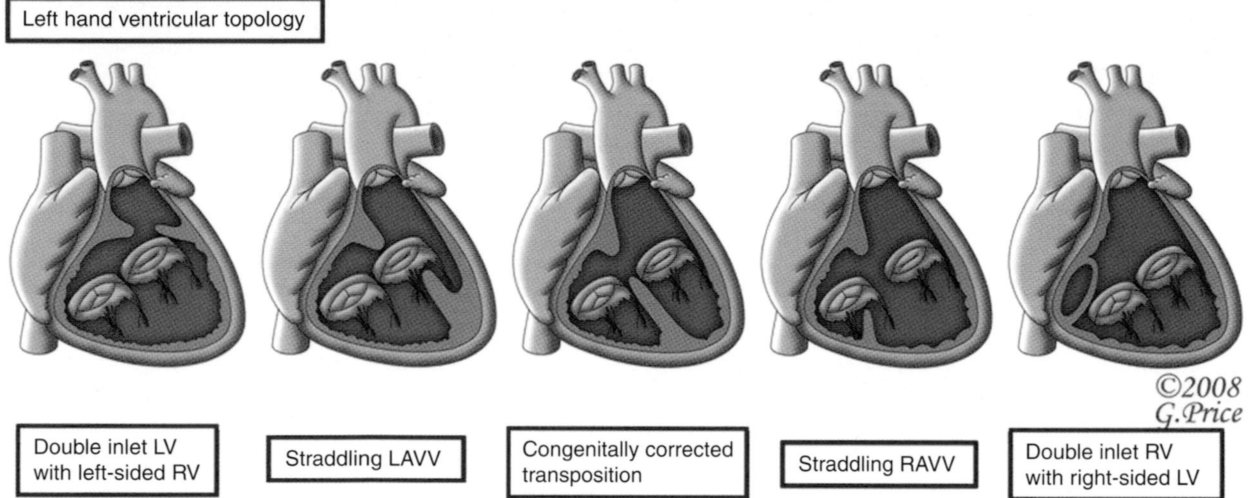

Figure 33-33 The cartoon shows the suggested morphogenetic sequences which link straddling of the right and left valves in the setting of left hand topology. The middle panel shows congenitally corrected transposition. Straddling of the left-sided morphologically tricuspid valve produces a spectrum leading to double inlet left ventricle (LV) with left-sided and superior incomplete right ventricle (RV), while straddling of the right-sided morphologically mitral valve produces a similar spectrum with double inlet right ventricle and right-sided and inferior incomplete left ventricle as the end point. As with the spectrums shown in Figure 33-32, the ventriculo-arterial connections will vary depending on the precise ventricular morphology. LAVV, left atrioventricular valve; RAVV, right atrioventricular valve.

The complete reference list can be found on the companion Expert Consult web site at www.expertconsult.com.

ANNOTATED REFERENCES

- Milo S, Ho SY, Macartney FJ, et al: Straddling and overriding atrioventricular valves: Morphology and classification. Am J Cardiol 1979;44:1122–1134.

  This study established the difference between straddling, defined on the basis of the tension apparatus, and overriding, defined according to the support of the atrioventricular junction within ventricles. It also established the anatomical differences between straddling of the morphologically mitral and tricuspid valves.

- Ho SY, Milo S, Anderson RH, et al: Straddling atrioventricular valve with absent atrioventricular connection: Report of 10 cases. Br Heart J 1982;47:344–352.
- Kiraly L, Hubay M, Cook AC, et al: Morphologic features of the uniatrial but biventricular atrioventricular connection. J Thorac Cardiovasc Surg 2007;133:229–234.

  These investigations established the morphological heterogeneity to be found when the solitary atrioventricular valve straddles when there is absence of either the right- or left-sided atrioventricular connection. The latter study extended the findings of the earlier investigation, emphasising that such hearts exhibit uniatrial but biventricular atrioventricular connections.

- Aziz KU, Paul MH, Muster AJ, Idriss FS: Positional abnormalities of atrioventricular valves in transposition of the great arteries including double-outlet right ventricle, atrioventricular valve straddling and malattachment. Am J Cardiol 1979;45:1135–1145.

  This important early study showed the frequent association of straddling and overriding of the mitral valve through an antero-superior ventricular septal defect in hearts either with double outlet right ventricle and subpulmonary defect or discordant ventriculo-arterial connections, the so-called Taussig-Bing malformation.

- Soto B, Ceballos R, Nath PH, et al: Overriding atrioventricular valves: An angiographic-anatomical correlate. Int J Cardiol 1985;9:327–340.

  This investigation, importantly at the time, showed that it was possible accurately to diagnose overriding of the orifice of straddling atrioventricular valves using angiography. The authors also emphasised that the straddling mitral valve seen in the setting of the Taussig-Bing malformation was often additionally cleft.

- Rice MJ, Seward JB, Edwards WD, et al: Straddling atrioventricular valve: Two-dimensional echocardiographic diagnosis, classification, and surgical implication. Am J Cardiol 1985;55:505–513.

  This important study established cross sectional echocardiography as the technique of choice for identification of straddling and overriding atrioventricular valves. The principles described in the paper still hold good. The authors emphasised the surgical significance of the attachments of the straddling tension apparatus within the opposite ventricle.

- Tabry IF, McGoon DC, Danielson GK, et al: Surgical management of straddling atrioventricular valve. J Thorac Cardiovasc Surg 1979;77:191–200.

  This important early study set the ground rules for surgical treatment of patients with the various forms of straddling atrioventricular valves.

- Serraf A, Nakamura T, Lacour-Gayet F, et al: Surgical approaches for double-outlet right ventricle or transposition of the great arteries associated with straddling atrioventricular valves. J Thorac Cardiovasc Surg 1996;111:527–535.
- Reddy VM, Liddicoat JR, McElhinney DB, et al: Biventricular repair of lesions with straddling tricuspid valves using techniques of cordal translocation and realignment. Cardiol Young 1997;7:147–152.

  These reports of surgical experience, one from Paris and the other from San Francisco, emphasised the potential for biventricular repair in many patients with straddling atrioventricular valves.

- Aiello V, Ho SY, Anderson RH: Absence of one atrioventricular connection associated with straddling atrioventricular valve: Distinction of a solitary from a common valve and further considerations on the diagnosis of ventricular topology. Am J Cardiovasc Pathol 1990;3:107–113.

  Although describing a solitary case, this report summarises the arguments concerning the morphology of so-called double outlet atrium, emphasising that the entity can exist either with a common atrioventricular valve, or with straddling of a solitary atrioventricular valve. The authors also discuss the potential problems of diagnosing ventricular topology in these situations.

- de la Cruz MV, Miller BL: Double-inlet left ventricle: Two pathological specimens with comments on the embryology and on the relation to single ventricle. Circulation 1968;37;249–260.
- Quero-Jimenez M, Martinez VMP, Azcarate MJM, et al: Exaggerated displacement of the atrioventricular canal towards the bulbus cordis (rightward displacement of the mitral valve). Br Heart J 1973;35:65–74.

  These investigations, based on examination of autopsied specimens, discussed how the lesions were best explained on the basis of incomplete transfer of the atrioventricular canal to produce straddling tricuspid valve, or exaggerated displacement to produce straddling mitral valve. The findings from the developing heart over the past decade have shown the accuracy of the speculations.

CHAPTER 34

Diseases of the Tricuspid Valve

PATRICK W. O'LEARY, JOSEPH A. DEARANI, and ROBERT H. ANDERSON

The most common congenital malformations afflicting the tricuspid valve are Ebstein's malformation and tricuspid valvar dysplasia. We will primarily consider Ebstein's malfor mation in this chapter. Isolated dysplasia of the tricuspid valvar leaflets, and other right ventricular abnormalities frequently mistaken for Ebstein's malformation, will be briefly described. Tricuspid valvar abnormalities or abnormalities of the morphologically right atrioventricular valve are also often associated with atrioventricular septal defects with common atrioventricular junction (Chapter 27), ventricular septal defect with straddling valve (Chapter 33), or pulmonary atresia with intact septum (Chapter 30). These lesions are described in detail in the appropriate chapters of our book.

NAMING OF THE TRICUSPID VALVAR APPARATUS

We have chosen to adopt an anatomically unambiguous system of names to describe the components of the tricuspid valvar apparatus. This will create some differences between the descriptions contained within this chapter and many previous publications. It seems best concretely to define this system to avoid potential confusion. The three valvar leaflets will be referred to as the anterosuperior, the septal, and the mural leaflets. The designation of the septal leaflet is already clear. The anterosuperior leaflet has most commonly been referred to as the anterior leaflet. The mural leaflet has often been called the posterior leaflet. This designation is anatomically incorrect. The mural leaflet is positioned inferiorly within the ventricular cavity, lying adjacent to the diaphragm in the normal heart. We recognise that abnormal valves often display rotation of their components away from the normal position. We prefer, therefore, to refer to this leaflet as mural, since it will invariably be more closely associated with the ventricular free wall than its counterparts.

EBSTEIN'S MALFORMATION

Ebstein's malformation has an extremely variable natural history depending on the degree of abnormality of the right ventricle and the tricuspid valvar apparatus, which may range from mild to severe. If the deformity of the tricuspid valve is severe, it may result in profound congestive heart failure in the neonatal period, or even in intrauterine death. At the other end of the spectrum, patients with mild degrees of displacement and dysfunction may remain asymptomatic until late adult life or may remain symptomless throughout life.

Ebstein's own description[1] of the malformation in 1866, with illustrations by Dr Weiss (Fig. 34-1), was based upon the anatomical findings relating to the heart of Joseph Prescher, a 19-year-old labourer with cyanosis, who had been troubled with dyspnoea and palpitations since childhood. The premortem diagnosis had been congenital cardiac defect. The first case described in the English literature was not published until 1900.[2] It was not until 1951 that the diagnosis was made during life, using angiocardiography.[3] In the 1950s, successful surgical palliation was achieved, and the association with Wolff-Parkinson-White syndrome had been recognised. In the 1960s came the first attempts at corrective surgery, including valvar replacement[4] and repair.[5] The malformation accounts for no more than 0.3% to 0.5% of congenital heart disease.[6,7] Equal numbers of male and female patients with Ebstein's malformation are usually observed.[8,9]

With the advent of cross sectional echocardiography,[10] it became much easier to make the diagnosis, even in fetal life.[8] The malformation is now known to be more common

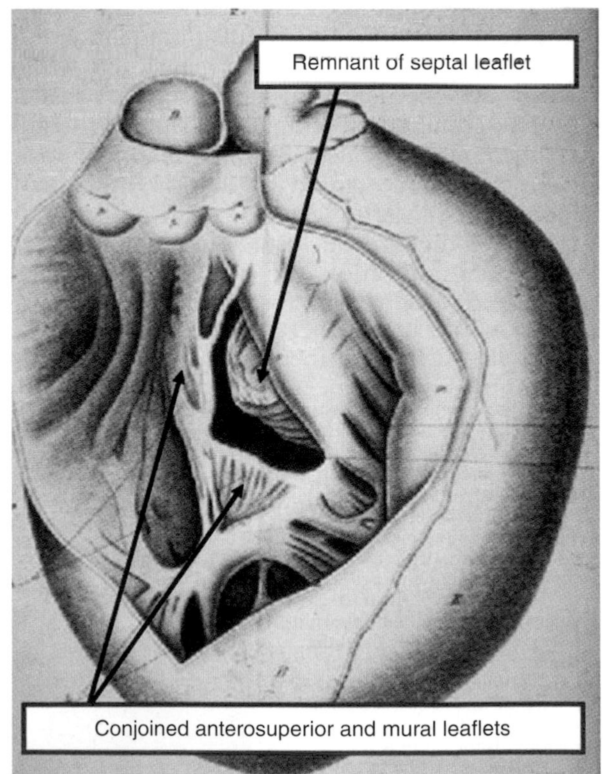

Figure 34-1 The illustration of the heart of Joseph Prescher as seen from the ventricular aspect, and as illustrated for Wilhelm Ebstein by Dr Weiss. Note how the leaflets of the deformed valve close in bifoliate fashion, forming a keyhole orifice that opens towards the outlet component of the right ventricle.

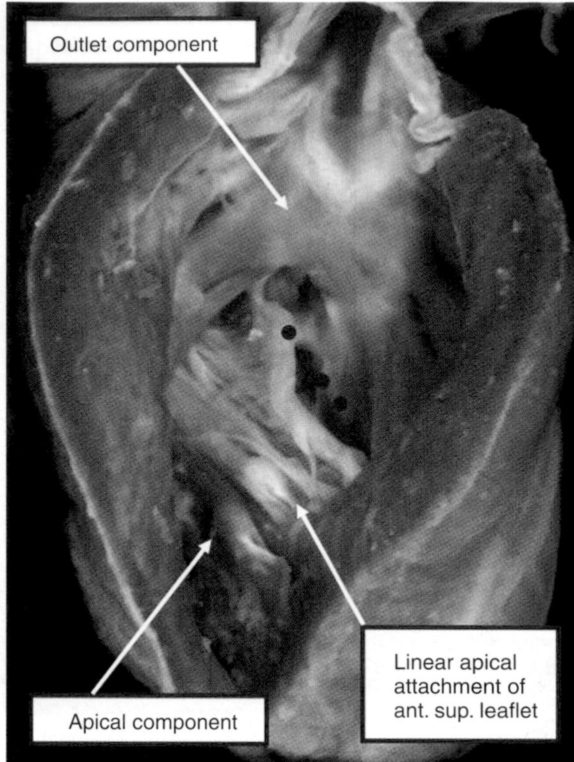

Figure 34-6 This view of the ventricular aspect of the deformed valve, from a different heart than that shown in Figure 34-5, shows the bifoliate pattern of closure between the anterosuperior leaflet and the deviated septal leaflet (*red dotted line*). The abnormal valve opens towards the outlet of the functional right ventricle, made up of the outlet and apical ventricular components. Compare this heart with the original specimen described by Ebstein himself (Fig. 34-1).

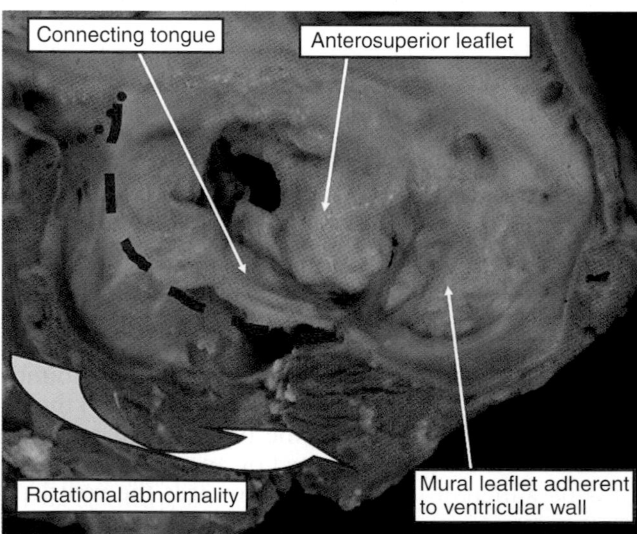

Figure 34-7 This view of the atrial aspect of a typically deformed valve shows the rotational displacement of the hinges of the septal and mural leaflets (*dashed line*) away from the atrioventricular junction (*dotted line*). Note the connecting tongue with the anterosuperior leaflet, the latter retaining its normal attachment at the atrioventricular junction. The resulting valvar orifice points towards the right ventricular infundibulum.

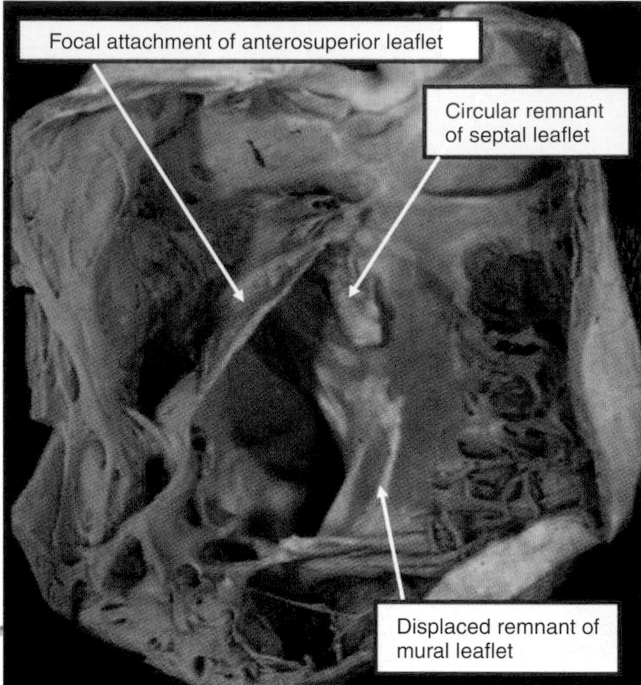

Figure 34-8 In this specimen, the septal leaflet is represented by a circular remnant, as in the initial case described by Ebstein. Note the focal attachments distally of the anterosuperior leaflet.

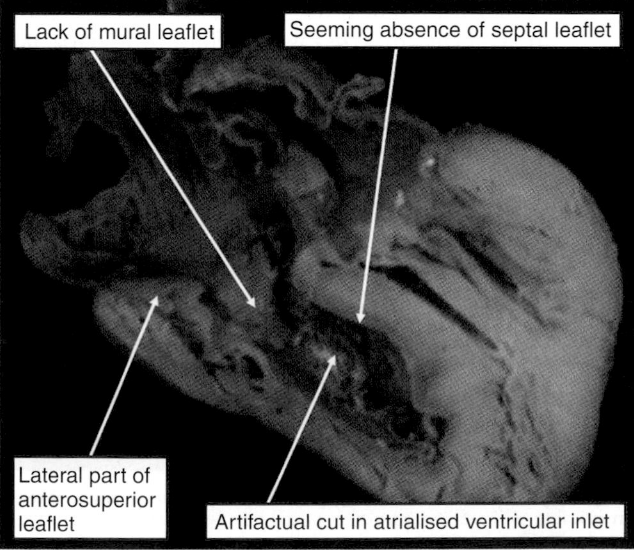

Figure 34-9 This specimen was prepared by making a simulated four-chamber section, having repaired a cut initially made into the wall of the inlet component. The section shows that the atrioventricular junction, as seen in this section, is essentially unguarded, the valvar leaflets being rotated towards the ventricular apex (see Fig. 34-10).

the mural and anterosuperior leaflets themselves tend to be combined as an abnormal curtain, which forms the parietal part of the abnormal bifoliate valve (see Fig. 34-5). The part formed by the anterosuperior leaflet usually retains its normal hinge from the atrioventricular junction along the supraventricular crest, but the hinges of the valve move increasingly away from the junction as attention is directed to the attachments along the diaphragmatic surface of the ventricular mass. When seen in the postmortem room, this arrangement can give the impression of forming a potentially competent valve. In other cases, nonetheless, the valvar mechanism is clearly seen to be incompetent, due to either inadequate leaflet size, mobility, or fenestrations in the body of the leaflet itself (Fig. 34-11). Relative to the

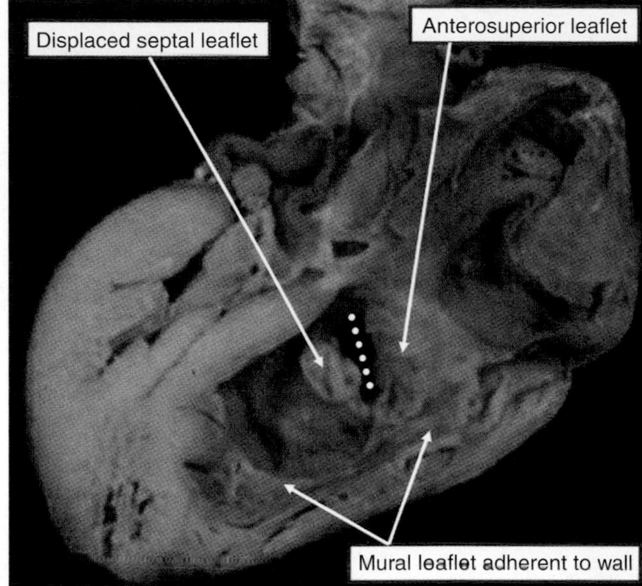

Figure 34-10 This image shows the anterior part of the four-chamber section also illustrated in Figure 34-9 but now photographed from the posterior aspect. It shows how the valvar leaflets guard the junction between the atrialised inlet and the functional right ventricle, forming a bifoliate valvar mechanism (*dotted line*).

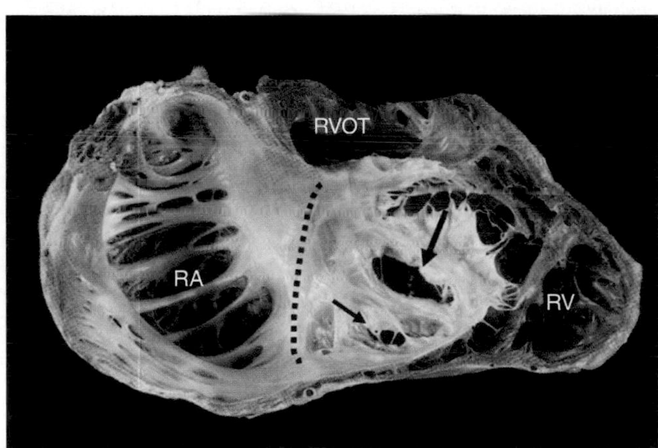

Figure 34-11 This image shows the lateral and anterior portions of the right atrium and ventricle. The anatomic atrioventricular junction is marked by the dotted line. There are multiple points of tethering and failed delamination. In addition, there are two large fenestrations (*arrows*) in the sail-like anterosuperior leaflet of the tricuspid valve. In cases like this, tricuspid regurgitation originates not only from the functional orifice of the displaced valve, out of the plane of this image, but also from these fenestrations, complicating attempts at surgical repair. RA, right atrium; RV, right ventricle; RVOT, right ventricle outflow trait.

mass of the atrialised right ventricle, the functional valvar orifice is frequently judged to be stenotic. In this setting, the upstream components of the right side of the heart, both the atrium and the right ventricular inlet, are dilated and thin walled. This produces anatomic atrialisation.

Further variation is then seen in the nature of the distal attachments of the mural and anterosuperior components of the valvar curtain, which are almost always additionally dysplastic.[20] In some cases, the anterosuperior leaflet retains its focal attachment to the medial and anterior papillary muscles (see Fig. 34-8). In the most florid cases, the entire leading edge of the anterosuperior leaflet is attached

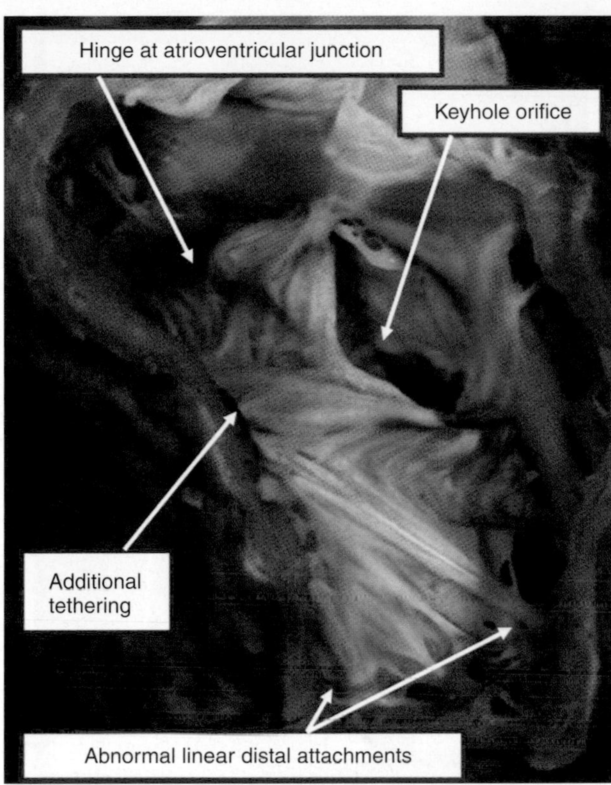

Figure 34-12 In this heart, the anterosuperior leaflet and the connecting tongue with the septal leaflet have a linear attachment at the ventricular apex. Note the additional tethering of the ventricular aspect of the leaflet and the keyhole orifice pointing towards the ventricular outlet.

linearly to a muscular shelf formed between the inlet and apical trabecular components of the ventricle (Fig. 34-12). Between these extremes are found hearts in which the edge of the leaflet is attached in hyphenated fashion along the muscular shelf (Fig. 34-13). Further abnormal tetherings can be found between the ventricular aspect of the abnormal leaflets and the parietal ventricular wall (Fig. 34-14). Such tetherings serve to constrain still further the motion of the abnormal sail produced by the combined mural and anterosuperior leaflets.[21,22] When the valvar mechanism is arranged as a bifoliate structure, then its opening is adjacent to the septum and is directed towards the ventricular outlet component. This keyhole can become increasingly restricted and stenotic. Should the leaflets fuse along the edges of the keyhole, the result is tricuspid atresia in the setting of Ebstein's malformation (Fig. 34-15).

The essence of symptomatic Ebstein's malformation, therefore, is formation of an abnormal bifoliate valvar mechanism, with septal and parietal components, at the junction between the atrialised inlet part of the right ventricle and the functional right ventricle, the latter comprising the apical and outlet components. Although the annular attachments of the septal leaflet of the valve are displaced from the atrioventricular junction, the triangle of Koch continues to be the landmark for the atrial components of the atrioventricular conduction tissue axis. Right bundle branch block is commonly found and may be caused by fibrosis in the distal conduction tissue. The frequent presence of accessory muscular pathways across the atrioventricular junctions results in a high incidence of preexcitation, this feature being found in up to one quarter

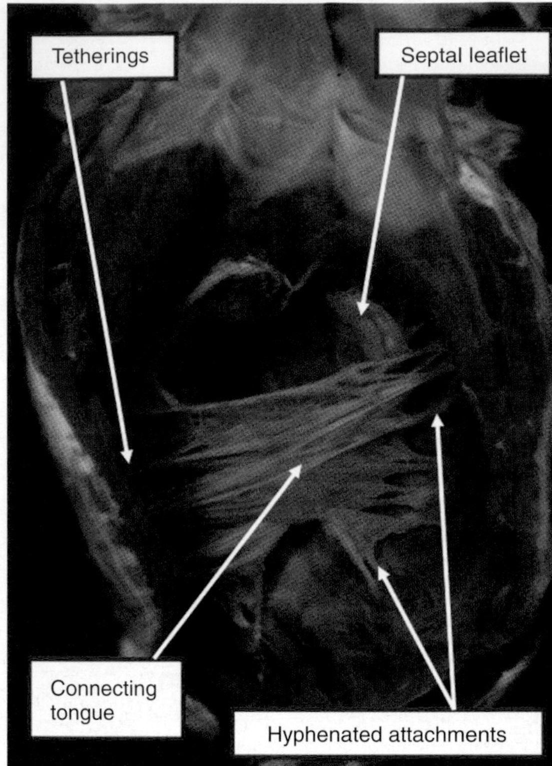

Figure 34-13 In this heart, the connecting tongue has hyphenated attachments at the ventricular apex, again with additional tethering to the parietal ventricular wall.

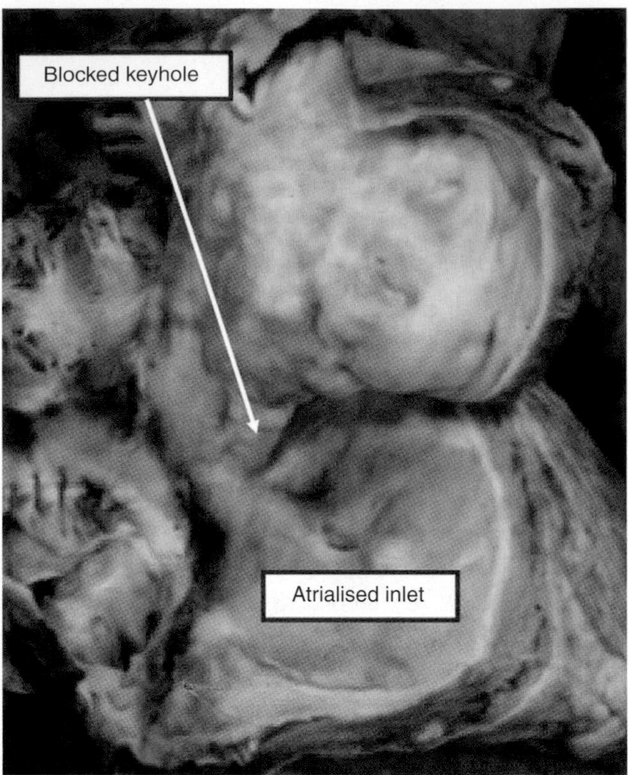

Figure 34-15 In this specimen, the keyhole orifice is blocked by fusion of the valvar leaflets, producing tricuspid atresia in the setting of Ebstein's malformation.

of patients.[7] The accessory pathways are often multiple and are usually found to the right of the inferior paraseptal space or in the parietal part of the junction.[23] When found laterally, they frequently arise from a remnant of atrioventricular ring tissue and produce the so-called Mahaim variant of pre-excitation.[24]

As we have already discussed, the abnormally located line of attachment of the valvar leaflets divides the right

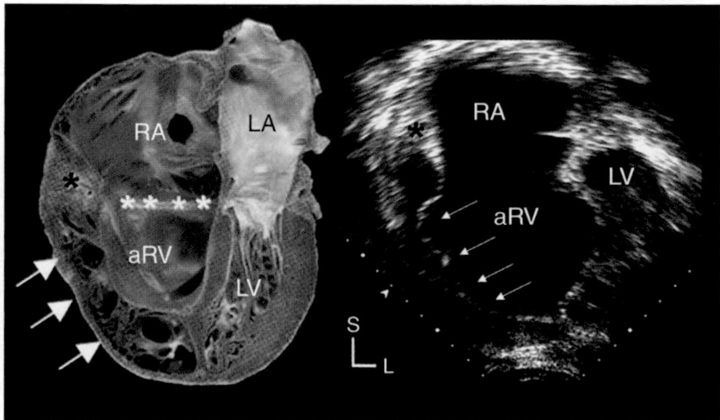

Figure 34-14 The anatomic specimen on the left and the echocardiographic four-chamber image to the right, demonstrate extremely severe examples of Ebstein's malformation. No remnants of the septal leaflet are present within the inlet. Even the anterosuperior leaflets have failed to fully delaminate in these hearts, being firmly adherent to the underlying right ventricular myocardium (*arrows*). The anterosuperior leaflet in the echocardiographic example has a small segment that retains its junctional hinge (*black asterisk*). The anatomic specimen displays the rare situation in which even the hinge of anterosuperior leaflet is displaced into the ventricular cavity (anterior to the plane shown in this photograph). The anatomic atrioventricular junction is outlined by the *white asterisks* in the anatomic specimen. aRV, anterior right ventricle; LA, left atrium; LV, left ventricle; RA, right atrium.

ventricle into proximal atrialised and distal functional portions. The proximal portion lies between the atrioventricular junction and the displaced attachments of the leaflets. This atrialised portion has walls of ventricular myocardium but in severely affected patients tends to be smooth, thin-walled, and dilated, with a high content of fibrous tissue. When very thin, it moves paradoxically during ventricular systole, and it may also expand during atrial systole. Its electrical potentials are ventricular, but its pressure pulse shows an atrial waveform.

The cavitary portion of the functional right ventricle is usually smaller than the normal ventricle. This feature, however, may be modified by dilation, which is a frequent finding. The functional portion consists of the infundibulum, the apical trabecular component, and that portion of the ventricle beneath the distal attachments of the combined mural and anterosuperior leaflets. The walls of this functional ventricle, particularly when dilated, are also usually thinner than normal. They contain fewer than normal myocytes and more fibrous tissue.[25] Left ventricular abnormalities are frequent. They can sometimes simply be the consequence of the gross dilation of the right-sided chambers. In severe cases, the left ventricular free wall also has an abnormally high content of fibrous tissue, although its thickness is usually normal.[25] The mitral valve is frequently nodular and thickened, and prolapse of the leaflets is common.

Associated cardiac defects are also common, particularly in the patients diagnosed in fetal or neonatal life. Almost all patients have a co-existing interatrial communication at the oval fossa, usually a patent foramen. Any type of communication, nonetheless, may be present, including atrioventricular septal defects in the setting of a common atrioventricular junction. A large spectrum of other lesions has been described in addition to atrioventricular septal defects, including ventricular septal defects, tetralogy of Fallot, aortic coarctation, and persistent patency of the arterial duct. The most common associated defect is pulmonary stenosis or atresia, which is found in up to one third of those presenting in infancy.[26] Obstruction of the right ventricular outflow tract is commonly associated with Ebstein's malformation when diagnosed in fetal life.[8] In this setting, it may be difficult to distinguish structural from functional pulmonary atresia using echocardiography, especially in the presence of severe tricuspid regurgitation. In either case, the pulmonary valvar abnormality is probably secondary to the malformation of the tricuspid valve, with hypoplasia of the outflow tract resulting from low anterograde flow through the right heart. When severe Ebstein's malformation is associated with fetal and neonatal distress or death, both lungs are usually hypoplastic but otherwise normal. The hypoplasia is secondary to the gross cardiomegaly, itself caused by dilation of the right heart.[27]

In the setting of gross dilation of the heart because of severe tricuspid valvar incompetence, whether the consequence of Ebstein's malformation or dysplasia of the valvar leaflets, the overall ventricular myocardium can become particularly thin. This should not be described as Uhl's malformation. In the lesion described by Uhl,[28] the tricuspid and pulmonary valves were both normal. The essence of Uhl's malformation is congenital absence of the parietal myocardium, histological analysis showing that the epicardial and endocardial layers of the wall lie edge-to-edge.[29] It is also a mistake to correlate fibro-fatty replacement of the right ventricular parietal walls with either Ebstein's malformation or Uhl's malformation. Fibro-fatty replacement is the essence of arrhythmogenic right ventricular cardiomyopathy, now recognised as a cardiomyopathy in its own right, with various genetic causes (see Chapter 54). While dysplasia of the valvar leaflets is often an integral part of Ebstein's malformation, dysplastic leaflets can also be found when retaining their normal hinges at the atrioventricular junction (Fig. 34-16). Such dysplasia of normally hinged leaflets can produce just as much valvar incompetence as Ebstein's malformation. Isolated dysplasia can produce the same wall-to-wall heart,[30] with the same consequences for pulmonary problems in the neonatal period.[27]

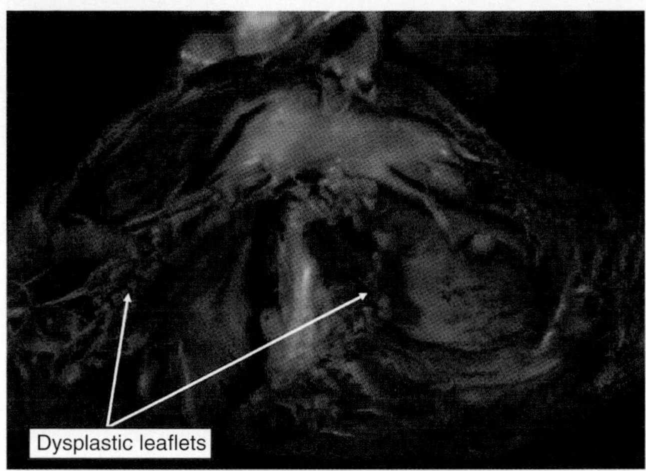

Figure 34-16 This specimen has unequivocal dysplasia of the leaflets of the tricuspid valve but does not exhibit Ebstein's malformation, the leaflets retaining their normal hinges from the atrioventricular junction.

Causation and Genetics

No specific cause has been consistently associated with Ebstein's malformation. Based on retrospective case reporting, treatment with lithium during the first trimester of pregnancy was thought to be strongly associated, producing a 400 fold relative risk, with the occurrence of Ebstein's malformation in the fetus.[31] More recent cohort and case-control epidemiologic studies have not confirmed these initial findings.[32] In contrast, these more rigorous studies found that, while the frequency of all congenital malformations was increased with gestational exposure to lithium, the relative risk for any malformation, not only cardiac, was only two to three times that of non-treated mothers. More importantly, although the frequency of all congenital cardiac malformations was greater in pregnancies exposed to lithium, there was no increase in the frequency of Ebstein's malformation relative to controls. Given the rarity of Ebstein's malformation, these studies did not have the power completely to exclude a connection between lithium and the development of Ebstein's malformation. They do conclusively demonstrate that the relative risk of treatment with lithium during pregnancy is much less than was originally estimated from the retrospective case reports. The decision to continue or discontinue such treatment during pregnancy must now be made by weighing the relative risk of teratogenicity against the risks of relapse of manic/depressive disease in the mother.[32] The majority of cases of Ebstein's malformation are sporadic, but some familial cases have been reported. There continues to be a difference of opinion as to whether there is a major hereditary basis for transgenerational transmission in Ebstein's malformation.[33,34]

PATHOPHYSIOLOGY AND CLINICAL ASPECTS OF EBSTEIN'S MALFORMATION

The broad range of anatomic severity seen in Ebstein's malformation, combined with the variable myopathy, produce a wide spectrum of clinical and haemodynamic manifestations. The pathophysiologic changes are related to several factors. These include the functional state of the tricuspid valve in terms of the degree of regurgitation or more rarely, stenosis, the presence, or absence, and size of the interatrial communication or other congenital cardiovascular malformations, the degree of right ventricular dysfunction, and the amount of left ventricular dysfunction. To a lesser degree, the pathologic substrates predisposing to tachyarrhythmias produce an additional dimension contributing to the pathophysiology.

The dysfunctional nature of the right ventricular myocardium, and the co-existing abnormalities of the tricuspid valve, impair flow through the right heart and the pulmonary circulation. The interaction between the dilated right atrium and the atrialised segment of the right ventricle are perhaps just as important in the creation of ineffective patterns of flow within the right heart. During ventricular systole, the atrialised right ventricular myocardium is contracting. There is no valvar tissue separating this area from the true atrial chamber and the great veins. This results in increased venous pressure, and effectively increases resistance to forward flow. This decreases the ability of the great veins to empty into the anatomic right atrium while its myocytes are relaxed. The increase in resistance to flow out of the atrium will also augment the amount of right-to-left shunting through any co-existing interatrial communication.

When the atrialised portion of the right ventricle relaxes, it will expand, and can even balloon outwards during true atrial contraction. This creates a reservoir for venous blood, and decreases the amount of effective forward flow that crosses the abnormal tricuspid valve. This to and fro flow pattern between the right atrium and the atrialised right ventricle not only decreases effective output from the right heart, but also provides an ongoing stimulus for atrial dilation and atrial arrhythmias, even when there is little transvalvar regurgitation. The degree of functional impairment experienced by patients with Ebstein's malformation has been directly related to these anatomic and physiologic abnormalities. Shiina and colleagues[10] found that a small functional right ventricle and large atrialised right ventricle, extreme displacement or absence of the septal leaflet, the degree of displacement or tethering of the anterosuperior leaflet, and the aneurysmal dilation of the right ventricular outflow tract were all associated with reduced functional state as measured using the categorisation prepared by the New York Heart Association.

Although the primary focus in patients with Ebstein's malformation has been on right-sided structures, there have been an increasing number of reports of left-sided abnormalities, specifically in left ventricular size, shape, and function.[35-37] In the past, these have been attributed to the degree of enlargement of the right heart compromising the left ventricle, and to leftward diastolic bowing of the interventricular septum. Radionuclide scans and cineangiograms have shown impaired left ventricular function at rest in unoperated patients. During formal exercise testing, most unoperated patients show an appropriate increase in left ventricular ejection fraction due to a reduced end-systolic volume and unchanged end-diastolic volume.[37] Recently, however, Attenhofer and colleagues[13,38] reported that one-fifth of their cohort of patients with Ebstein's malformation had a markedly abnormal echocardiographic appearance of the left ventricular myocardium. These patients displayed segments of left ventricular myocardium with multiple layers and deep intratrabecular recesses, consistent with myocardial noncompaction. An additional one-tenth had hypertrabeculated segments of left ventricular myocardium reminiscent, but not diagnostic, of noncompacted myocardium. Although most patients had satisfactory left ventricular function, a small percentage showed severe systolic and diastolic dysfunction, even contributing to the need for transplantation in one young patient.[38] These left-sided myocardial abnormalities, although seen in only a fraction of patients, support the concept that Ebstein malformation is actually a global myocardial disorder that primarily manifests itself within the right ventricle and its derivative, the tricuspid valve.

The infant with Ebstein's malformation poses an especially difficult clinical problem. Pulmonary vascular resistance is always high immediately after birth, and usually decreases fairly rapidly in the first days of life. The infant with severe Ebstein's malformation is poorly prepared to deal with the transition to the neonatal circulation. The combination of right ventricular myopathy, tricuspid regurgitation, and elevated pulmonary resistance can lead to poor pulmonary perfusion when the arterial duct constricts or closes. Venous pressures rise, leading to right-heart failure and cyanosis due to right-to-left shunting across the oval foramen. Until the pulmonary resistance decreases, and the pulmonary flow increases, these infants present a diagnostic and therapeutic dilemma. Patency of the pulmonary outflow tract and valve must be confirmed. This can be done by demonstrating opening of the pulmonary valvar leaflets by cross sectional echocardiographic scans, or by documenting either forward, or more commonly regurgitant, flow across the valve using Doppler techniques.

In the rare case where echocardiographic findings are inconclusive, an angiogram demonstrating pulmonary regurgitation following injection of contrast into the arterial duct, or the ability to advance a catheter across the valvar orifice, are other methods that can confirm patency of the right ventricular outflow tract. When the outflow tract is open, infusions of prostaglandin to maintain ductal patency, with or without mechanical ventilation, will often allow the baby to transition to the postnatal circulation without the need for palliative surgery.

Clinical Presentation

Patients with Ebstein's malformation may present at any age. The most severe cases present prenatally, or as newborns. Prenatal diagnosis is dependent upon ultrasonic screening examinations. Fetal presentation is accompanied by increased heart size, a significant incidence of fetal hydrops and, in the most severe cases, pulmonary parenchymal hypoplasia secondary to marked cardiac enlargement. Prenatal arrhythmia is not common. Newborns most often present with cyanosis, while slightly older infants present with a combination of desaturation and symptoms of cardiac failure. Murmurs and arrhythmias are more frequently encountered as presenting complaints in older patients. Although some patients remain asymptomatic, most will have some cardiovascular symptoms. Beyond infancy, the majority will display abnormal fatigueability, dyspneoa, or cyanosis with exertion or palpitations. Palpitations in a cyanotic child should raise the possibility of Ebstein's malformation (Table 34-1).[9,39,40]

Ultrasonic technology has significantly influenced the age at which most patients with Ebstein's malformation are diagnosed. In 1979, Guiliani and colleagues found that just under one-third of patients were diagnosed before 4 years of age. Another two-fifths were diagnosed before the age of 19, with the remainder presenting in adulthood, some at 80 years of age.[40,41] In contrast, in the experience reported by Celermajer and colleagues in 1994[9] (see Table 34-1), three-fifths came to clinical attention before the age of 1 year, with half diagnosed prenatally or as newborns. One-tenth presented between 1 and 12 months of age, with only three-tenths presenting as children or adolescents. Despite the increased availability of ultrasonic examination

TABLE 34-1

MAJOR FEATURES OF EBSTEIN'S MALFORMATION IN 220 SUBJECTS AT PRESENTATION

	Prenatal (N = 21)	Neonate (N = 88)	Infant (N = 23)	Child (N = 50)	Adolescent (N = 15)	Adult (N = 23)	All (%)
Cyanosis	0	65	8	7	2	1	83 (38)
Heart failure	0	9	10	4	2	6	31 (14)
Murmur	0	8	3	33	5	3	52 (24)
Arrhythmia	1	5	1	6	6	10	29 (13)
Abnormal prenatal ultrasound	18	0	0	0	0	0	18 (8)

Neonate = 0–1 month; infant = 1 month–2 years; child = 2–10 years; adolescent = 10–18 years; adult = >18 years.
Adapted from Celermajer DS, Bull C, Till JA, et al: Ebstein's anomaly: Presentation and outcome from fetus to adult. J Am Coll Cardiol 1994;23:170–176.

in this more recent cohort, one-tenth remained undiagnosed until adulthood.[9]

Physical Findings

Growth and development are generally normal. Inspection reveals cyanosis and digital clubbing in patients with an associated right-to-left shunt. Many have an unusual facial coloration, described as violaceous hue, flushed, florid, red-cheeked, or malar flush.[40] Usually these patients have an associated mild polycythemia. Prominence or asymmetry of the chest is a frequent finding secondary to the dilated nature of the right heart. Arterial and venous pulsations are usually normal, even in the presence of tricuspid insufficiency. The jugular venous pulsations may not have a large V wave because of poor transmission of the venous pulse wave in the presence of a dilated and compliant right atrium. The praecordium is usually not overactive.

After the neonatal period, it is auscultation that often alerts the physician to the diagnosis of Ebstein's malformation. Many patients have multiple sounds and murmurs present, especially those with mobile anterosuperior valvar leaflets. These multiple sounds are so characteristic as to stand out even to the untrained ear. Occasionally, the heart sounds are soft, but usually they are of normal intensity. The first heart sound is widely split because of increased excursion of the anterosuperior leaflet and the subsequent delayed closure of the abnormal tricuspid valve. The second heart sound is also widely and persistently split owing to late closure of the pulmonary valve, believed to be due to right bundle branch block. Ventricular filling sounds are common contributors to the multiplicity of heart sounds. In the presence of so many heart sounds, there is frequently a gallop or quadruple rhythm, or cadence quality, which is fairly easily recognised. A holosystolic murmur, typically graded at 2 to 4 out of 6, is found along the left sternal border in those with an organised jet of tricuspid regurgitation. Low-intensity diastolic murmurs can be appreciated in the same location as a result of anterograde flow across the tricuspid valve. All murmurs tend to vary with respiration, increasing during inspiration. There may be few murmurs present in patients with very little functional tricuspid valvar tissue, since the flows between right atrium and the ventricle are essentially unrestricted and not turbulent. The first heart sound is single in these cases.

Electrocardiography

The electrocardiogram is usually abnormal and helps to confirm the clinical diagnosis[40] (Fig. 34-17). Although sinus rhythm is usually present at the time of initial diagnosis, atrioventricular dissociation or atrial fibrillation can be found in a few patients. In large series, one-third to one-half of the patients have prolonged PR intervals, and one-fourth to three-fourths meet the criterions for right atrial enlargement, showing so-called Himalayan P waves.[40] The QRS axis in the frontal plane occasionally shows right-axis deviation. Most patients have right bundle branch block, and many have low-voltage QRS complexes in the right praecordial leads. Findings consistent with right ventricular hypertrophy are extremely uncommon.

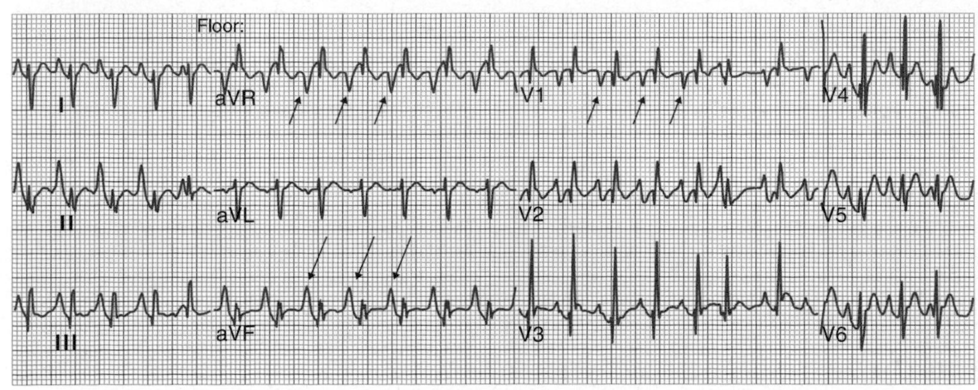

Figure 34-17 This electrocardiogram comes from an infant with Ebstein's malformation. The QRS axis is shifted to the right (175 degrees), and there is evidence of prominent atrial enlargement with large P waves that exceed the voltage achieved by the ventricular QRS complexed in some leads (P waves in leads aVR, aVF, and V1 are indicated by the series of three *arrows*). The rhythm is slightly irregular due to occasional premature contractions.

Up to one-quarter of patients with Ebstein's malformation have the Wolff-Parkinson-White pattern on their electrocardiogram.[40,42] This is due to the presence of accessory myocardial atrioventricular connections across the insulating plane of the atrioventricular junction. Several resting or exercise electrocardiograms or 24-hour ambulatory electrocardiograms may have to be examined to find the characteristic pattern. Occasionally, the pattern is transient or intermittent.[43–45] In addition, concealed accessory pathways, without manifest delta waves, are not uncommon. Absence of anterograde preexcitation, therefore, indicates neither that the accessory connection is no longer present, nor that the patient is no longer susceptible to tachycardia. The patient may still have retrograde conduction, which allows for atrioventricular reciprocating tachycardia. Patients with Ebstein's malformation may still have Wolff-Parkinson-White syndrome, a manifest delta wave, and a paradoxically normal PR interval. In these patients, the PR interval is artificially lengthened by delayed conduction through the large right atrium. The presence of left axis deviation in a patient with Ebstein's malformation suggests the presence of the Mahaim variant of preexcitation, produced by atriofascicular tracts.[46]

Arrhythmias in the non-neonatal, unoperated patient with Ebstein's malformation are common.[47] Almost four-fifths of preoperative patients in this series either had documented arrhythmias, or histories of palpitations, near-syncope, or syncope. In those with documented arrhythmias, half had paroxysmal supraventricular tachycardia, one-quarter had paroxysmal atrial fibrillation or flutter, another quarter had ventricular arrhythmias, either with frequent ventricular premature complexes or nonsustained ventricular tachycardia, and one-tenth had some form of atrioventricular block. Of those with ventricular arrhythmias, one-third also had paroxysmal supraventricular tachycardia, another third had paroxysmal atrial fibrillation or flutter, and one had complete heart block. The patients with arrhythmias or symptoms compatible with arrhythmia were significantly older than those without symptoms or arrhythmias.

Even prior to the widespread application of complex surgical antiarrhythmic procedures, surgical intervention appeared to decrease the frequency of arrhythmias, at least in early, short-term follow-up. Review of a large series of patients treated at the Mayo Clinic, as yet unpublished, before and after definitive repair of Ebstein's malformation has revealed arrhythmias in just over two-fifths after operative repair compared with three-fifths preoperatively. Supraventricular tachycardias decreased from one-half to one-quarter postoperatively. In one-sixth of the cohort, an accessory pathway was ablated at the time of repair or replacement of the tricuspid valve and closure of the interatrial communication, with no evidence of postoperative complete heart block. Despite the overall reduction in arrhythmias, when arrhythmias were observed early during postoperative recovery, these patients had an increased risk of late sudden death.

Introduction of more extensive antiarrhythmic surgery seems to improve results even further. Greason and colleagues[48] reported their results using the right atrial maze procedure for atrial arrhythmias in patients with congenitally malformed hearts, and seven-tenths of their cohort had Ebstein's malformation. Only one patient, with severe anatomic disease and multiple arrhythmias, did not survive the operation. Of the overall group, five-sixths remained in sinus rhythm at a mean of 17 months postoperatively. Only 6% had recurrent atrial fibrillation or flutter, albeit that 8% were in junctional rhythm, but only one patient required long-term pacing.

Chest Radiography

The cardiac size may vary from near normal to extreme cardiomegaly. When the heart is severely dilated, it takes on a globular shape that is similar to that seen with large pericardial effusions or severe dilated cardiomyopathy (Fig. 34-18A). There may be a dramatic change from preoperative to postoperative radiographs (Fig. 34-18B). The dilated right atrium is responsible for most of the enlarged cardiac silhouette. In the frontal view, the right atrium produces a significant convexity of the right heart border, and in the lateral view, the right atrium may fill the entire retrosternal space. The convex left border is primarily due to dilation of the right ventricular outflow tract. The convexities of both left and right heart borders produce the characteristic globular cardiac silhouette. In cyanotic

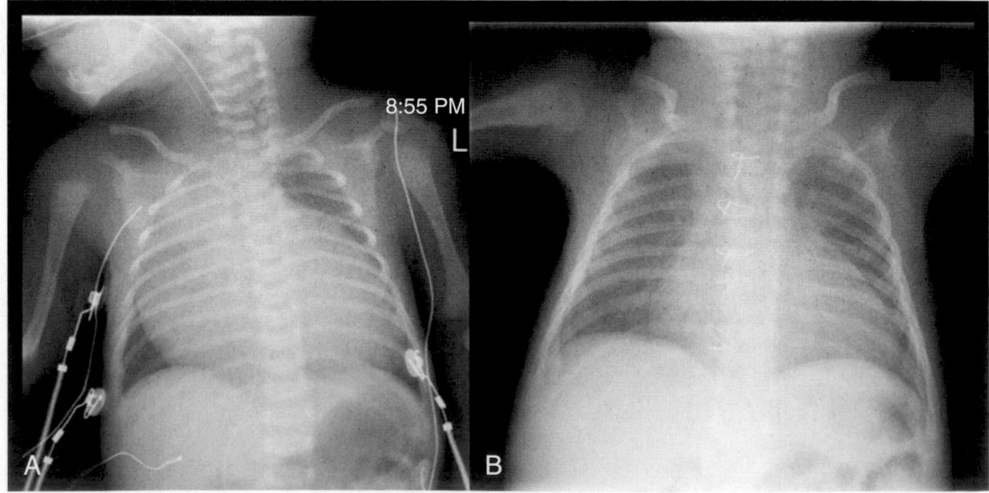

Figure 34-18 These two chest X-rays were taken from the same infant with severe Ebstein's malformation before (**A**) and after (**B**) repair of the tricuspid valve, right atrial reduction, closure of arterial duct, and partial closure of the atrial septal defect. Preoperatively, the heart nearly fills the chest on this frontal view, with the globular appearance reminiscent of a large pericardial effusion. Although the heart is still significantly enlarged after surgery, the cardiac volume has been markedly decreased, allowing improvement in both cardiac and lung function.

patients with a right-to-left shunt, the pulmonary vascularity is decreased. Otherwise, it is usually normal. In the asymptomatic patient, it is not unusual for the heart to have a normal size and shape. This may confuse the clinical diagnosis.

Echocardiography

Echocardiography has become the procedure of choice for both the diagnosis and long-term assessment of patients with Ebstein's malformation. In the 1980s, cross sectional echocardiography replaced M-mode as the clinical standard.[49–51] As early as 1984, cross sectional imaging was considered sufficiently comprehensive that angiography was no longer necessary to diagnose Ebstein's malformation.[10] Imaging of the internal cardiac crux, the components of the abnormal tricuspid valve, and the right ventricular myocardium reveal several features that are reliably used to identify patients with Ebstein's malformation. The single most sensitive and specific diagnostic feature is the displacement of the annular hinge of the septal leaflet. This displacement is most easily appreciated by comparison to the annular hinge of the mitral leaflet as seen in the apical four-chamber view. Even the septal leaflet of the normal tricuspid valve inserts at a position that is slightly apical to the insertion of the mitral valve. In patients with Ebstein's malformation, this displacement is exaggerated. The distance between the valvar hinge points can easily be measured (see Fig. 34-4). This distance, when divided by the body surface area in square meters, is known as the displacement index. In a heart with evidence of failed delamination, an index value greater than 8 mm/m^2 reliably distinguishes those with Ebstein's malformation from both normals and from patients with other disorders associated with enlargement of the right ventricle.[10,49]

Occasionally, it can be difficult to assess the off-set between the valvar hinges at the internal crux. Other echocardiographic features can then help in diagnosis, including elongation of the anterosuperior leaflet, tethering of any of the leaflets to the underlying myocardium, shortened cordal support, attachment of the leading edge of the anterosuperior leaflet to the right ventricular myocardium, displacement of the annular attachment of the anterosuperior leaflet, absence of the septal or mural leaflets, congenital fenestration of the leaflets, and enlargement of the valvar annulus.

Echocardiography is also used to define suitability for valvar repair, associated cardiovascular abnormalities, and myocardial function. There are several anatomic features of the valvar apparatus that indicate good candidacy for monoleaflet repair, to be discussed at length later in this chapter. The most important determinant of a durable monoleaflet repair is a freely mobile anterosuperior leaflet, especially its leading edge. The mobile leaflet tissue should be visualised within the right ventricular inflow tract, and this assessment must be made in the apical four-chamber view (Fig. 34-19). Extensive adherence of more than half of the anterosuperior leaflet to the ventricular myocardium (see Fig. 34-14) makes a successful repair unlikely. A single central jet of regurgitation is more easily eliminated than are multiple regurgitant orifices (Fig. 34-20). Even when there is a significant amount of leaflet tissue present, direct muscular insertions from the ventricular free wall into the body of the anterosuperior leaflet can make repair impossible (Fig. 34-21).

The functional impact of the malformation of the right ventricle and tricuspid valve should be determined. Anatomic and functional severities are usually similar, but they are not always the same. For example, a patient can have a severe anatomic displacement with Ebstein's malformation but only mild functional impairment. This can occur if the interatrial communication is small, the displaced valve is relatively competent, and the myocardium is only mildly dysfunctional. Both aspects of severity play an important role in determining functional state, prognosis, and reparability of the tricuspid valve.[10] The degree of right atrial and ventricular enlargement and functional state of the right ventricular myocardium should also be defined.[50] Other important features include the degree of dilation of the right ventricular outflow tract, the presence and size of any atrial septal defect, and the degree of transvalvar regurgitation.[10,51] The left ventricular myocardium has also been described as being abnormal in a significant fraction of the patients with

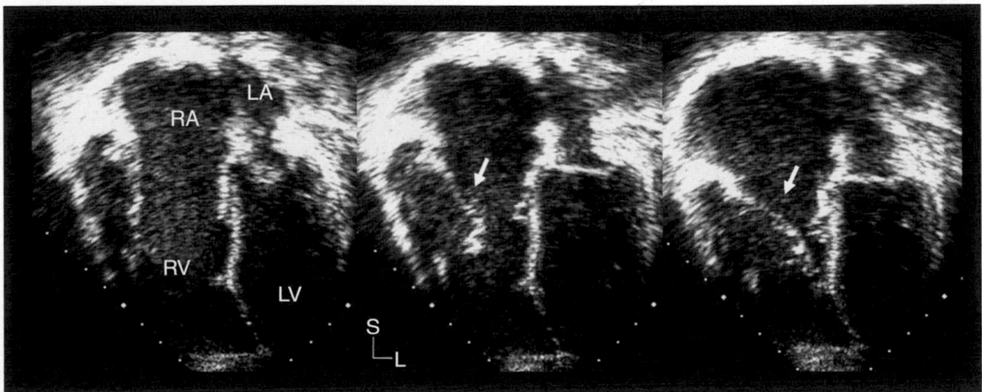

Figure 34-19 The three panels of this figure are all apical four-chamber inflow images of the same patient with Ebstein's malformation. The left frame is from mid-diastole. The middle and right frames are from mid- and end-systole, respectively. Features that suggest favorable anatomy for monoleaflet repair are that the anterosuperior leaflet in this patient is freely mobile, including its leading edge (*arrows*). There are no muscular insertions that limit or distort the motion of the valve. The regurgitant jet originated only from the gap in coaptation seen between the anterosuperior leaflet and the remnant of the septal leaflet. The leading edge of the valve reaches a point near enough to the septum that, given the degree of annular dilation, an annuloplasty can advance it to a point where it will coapt with the septum and the vestiges of the septal leaflet. LA, left atrium; LV, left ventricle; RA, right atrium; RV, right ventricle. (Modified from Cetta F, Edwards WD, Seward JB, et al: Congenital heart disease. In Vannan MA, Lang RM, Rakowski H, Tajik AJ [eds]: Atlas of Echocardiography. Philadelphia: Current Medicine LLC, 2005.)

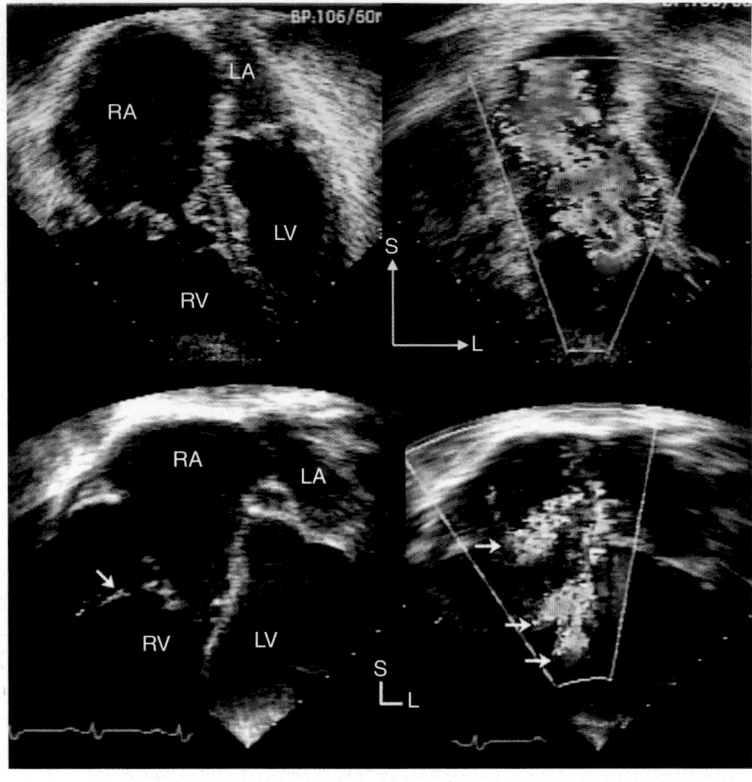

Figure 34-20 These apical four-chamber images show two patients with Ebstein's malformation. The case illustrated in the upper panels shows a valve that is freely mobile (*upper left panel*) and colour flow mapping (*upper right panel*) revealed that there was only a single, central jet of regurgitation. This patient subsequently had a successful valve repair with only mild residual tricuspid regurgitation and no stenosis. The case shown in the lower panels displays a large muscular insertion to the middle of the anterosuperior leaflet (*lower left*) and multiple fenestrations and sites of regurgitation. The tethering and multiple origins of regurgitant flow dramatically decrease the chance for successful repair. LA, left atrium; LV, left ventricle; RA, right atrium; RV, right ventricle. (Modified from Cetta F, Edwards WD, Seward JB, et al: Congenital heart disease. In Vannan MA, Lang RM, Rakowski H, Tajik AJ [eds]: Atlas of Echocardiography. Philadelphia: Current Medicine LLC, 2005.)

Ebstein's malformation.[26,35,52,53] Quantitative evaluation of left ventricular performance, therefore, should also be a routine component of the echocardiographic evaluation of the patient with Ebstein's malformation. Defects such as ventricular septal defects and pulmonary stenosis may also be found in association with Ebstein's malformation. Doppler and colour flow echocardiographic assessment can help determine haemodynamic alterations such as valvar regurgitation and intracardiac shunting. Additional experience with, and follow up after, the cone reconstruction[49] of the tricuspid valve is needed before we can confidently define the anatomic features associated with favourable results from this procedure.

Echocardiography also plays an important role intraoperatively and postoperatively in assessing adequacy of tricuspid valvar repair or replacement.[50,51] The most important use of intraoperative echocardiography is the immediate evaluation of the repaired valve. A repair that is not functioning can be revised, or else the valve can be replaced without a repeat operation. The post-operative examination can also be used to assess prosthetic valvar function and changes in right and left ventricular function and to exclude significant residual atrial level shunting. Similarly, post-operative echocardiography is important not only to assess the adequacy of the surgical repair, but also to exclude post-operative complications, including pericardial or pleural effusion, mediastinal haematoma, and intracardiac thrombus. The degree of residual tricuspid regurgitation or tricuspid stenosis should be determined. Assessment of ventricular function and regional abnormalities of wall motion plays an important role. Rarely, flow can be compromised in the right coronary artery because

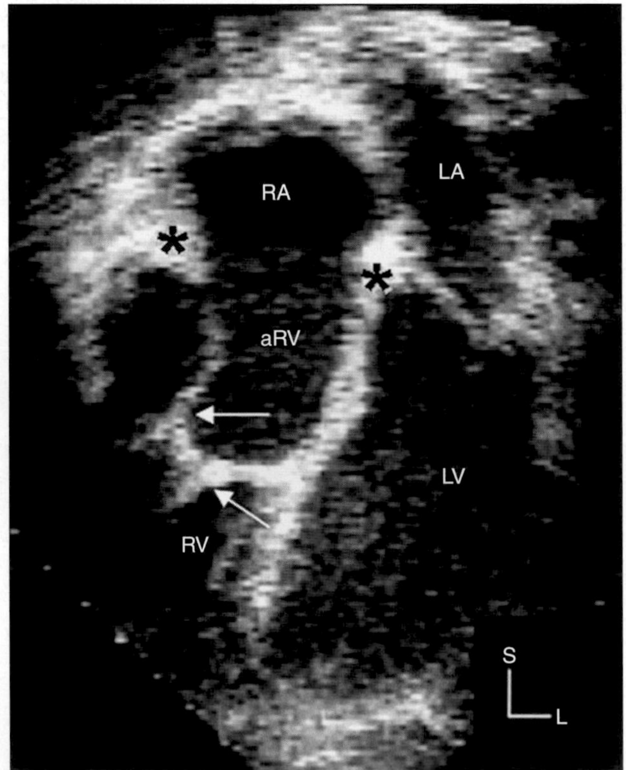

Figure 34-21 The arrows in this apical four-chamber image point to significant, direct muscular insertions from the right ventricular free wall into the midsection of the anterosuperior leaflet of the tricuspid valve. Even though this valve leaflet has separated from the underlying myocardium, its mobility was quite limited by these attachments to the ventricular free wall. aVR, anterior right ventricle; LA, left atrium; LV, left ventricle; RA, right atrium; RV, right ventricle.

of its proximity to the plicated portion of the atrialised right ventricle.

Prenatal Detection of Ebstein's Malformation

Echocardiography can accurately define the features of Ebstein's malformation in the fetus. Characteristics that have been identified with early neonatal mortality include marked enlargement of the right heart, severe tethering of the anterosuperior leaflet, left ventricular compression, and associated lesions such as pulmonary atresia.[52] Pulmonary hypoplasia develops secondary to severe cardiomegaly and hydrops with pleural and pericardial effusions. Detection of disturbances of rhythm, such as supraventricular tachycardia, should be attempted at the time of fetal echocardiography because they can contribute to the development of hydrops. Finding the ratio of the combined right atrial and atrialised ventricular area compared to the combined area of the functional right ventricle and left heart to be greater then 1 was shown to be associated with very poor fetal or neonatal outcome.[53] Other fetal or neonatal findings that were associated with increased risk of mortality were a larger atrial septal defect, functional or anatomic pulmonary atresia, or reduced left ventricular function.

Exercise Testing

Exercise testing has become one of the routine noninvasive studies used to evaluate patients with Ebstein's malformation, both before and after surgical intervention. Studies performed before and after surgery have revealed several interesting findings.[54–56] In the largest of these series,[56] unoperated patients had significantly reduced indexes of exercise tolerance for work, duration, and maximal oxygen uptake. In post-operative patients, these indexes all increased and approached the lower limits of normal. Arterial saturations of oxygen both at rest and during exercise were significantly lower in unoperated than in post-operative patients, undoubtedly due to closure of the atrial septal defect. In the unoperated patient, progressively lower saturations at rest and at maximum exercise were associated with progressively reduced exercise tolerance. Surgical intervention improved exercise tolerance. Most post-operative patients had resting and exercise cardiac outputs that were similar to the normal population. Patients with an atrial septal defect and right-to-left shunting demonstrated excessive ventilation at rest and during exercise. In these patients, a right-to-left shunt is a strong stimulus to increased ventilation.

Cardiac Catheterisation and Haemodynamics

In the early days of intracardiac investigation, it became evident that patients with Ebstein's malformation were at increased risk during catheterisation. Concerns about the safety of cardiac catheterisation in these patients have now been dispelled by modern techniques of monitoring the haemodynamic state during the study, more flexible catheter materials, and the availability of effective treatment for arrhythmias provoked by manipulation of the catheter. Even though patients with Ebstein's malformation can now be safely studied, the need to do so arises infrequently, such as when there are clinical questions regarding pulmonary arterial resistance.

There is usually moderate elevation of the right atrial pressure, often with a dominant V wave and steep Y descent. When the right atrium is massively dilated, the atrial pressure may be normal in spite of severe tricuspid regurgitation. Most often, the right ventricular pressures are normal, but in some the end-diastolic pressure may be elevated. Generally, the pulmonary arterial pressure is normal, but it may be decreased in those with severe tricuspid regurgitation and right-to-left shunting. In those with an atrial septal defect, right-to-left shunting will result in systemic arterial desaturation. Historically significant is a technique of simultaneously recording the intracavitary pressure and intracardiac electrogram tracing. When a catheter with an end hole and an electrode at the tip was positioned in the atrialised portion of the right ventricle, the pressure tracing recorded was atrial, but the electrogram showed ventricular activity. This was one of the earliest methods used confidently to make a diagnosis of Ebstein's malformation.

Angiocardiography

Except in its mildest forms, right ventricular angiocardiography is usually diagnostic of Ebstein's malformation. In the frontal plane, injection of contrast medium in the right ventricle will demonstrate tricuspid regurgitation, a large sail-like anterosuperior leaflet, and frequently a distinct notch at the inferior cardiac border to the left of the spine. The notch is created by the displaced tricuspid valve, and marks the point of division between the atrialised and functional zones of the right ventricle. Frequently, a trilobed appearance occurs as a result of contrast medium outlining the enlarged right atrium, atrialised ventricle, and the outflow portion of the functional ventricle. The presence of the associated defects can be demonstrated by angiocardiography. Injection of contrast medium into the right ventricle of a cyanotic newborn with Ebstein's malformation may show tricuspid regurgitation and little or no contrast medium in the pulmonary arteries. This same finding may occur in the absence of anatomic obstruction if the pulmonary resistance is elevated. Patency of the right ventricular outflow tract should be established by other techniques, such as advancement of the catheter through a patent pulmonary valve, or injection of contrast medium in the arterial duct to show contrast medium filling the pulmonary trunk and regurgitating into the right ventricle.

Invasive Electrophysiology

Echocardiographic evaluation of anatomy is so accurate that diagnosis of Ebstein's malformation no longer depends on catheterisation and angiocardiography. Invasive electrophysiologic testing and catheter ablation, however, maintain their importance. The Pediatric Electrophysiology Society reported 65 patients with Ebstein's malformation that had invasive studies and attempted radio-frequency ablations.[57] Tachycardia mediated via an accessory pathway was very common, with only one-tenth having other mechanisms for their tachyarrhythmias. The pathways were right-sided or septal in the majority of patients with re-entrant arrhythmias, with only 4% being left-sided. In three-tenths, the patients had multiple pathways. Radio-frequency ablation was able temporarily to eliminate the tachycardia in almost nine-tenths of cases, depending on its mechanism, albeit that recurrence was common. Long-term success was achieved in only one-third in this early series.

More specific delineation of the anatomy of accessory conduction pathways in Ebstein's malformation has been provided by Olson and colleagues.[58,59] In their series, the pathways were localised to the right inferolateral free wall in 11 patients, to the inferior paraseptal area in 9, and to both the septum and right free wall in 4. One patient had a right anterolateral connection. The mechanisms of arrhythmia included orthodromic reciprocating tachycardia in 15 patients, both orthodromic and antidromic reciprocating tachycardia in 4, inducible atrial flutter or fibrillation in 7, atrioventricular nodal re-entry in 2, and ventricular tachycardia in 1. All of these patients had surgical pathway ablations. None had recurrence of a tachycardia mediated through an accessory pathway during follow-up lasting for 4 years. Early results of the right-sided atrial maze procedure have also been encouraging in patients with Ebstein's malformation.[45,60,61]

Clinical Course and Treatment of Patients with Ebstein's Malformation

Natural History, Pregnancy and Risks of Recurrence

The outcome of Ebstein's malformation depends a great deal on the age of the patient at presentation, the severity of the lesion, and the presence of associated defects, these features being inter-related. Severely affected fetuses or neonates can easily be detected with echocardiography. As a result of their severe disease, they generally have a poor outcome.[9] In one series, all neonates died when the combined area of the right atrium and atrialised right ventricle was greater than the combined area of the functional right ventricle, left atrium, and left ventricle.[62] Mild disease in neonates and young children has a relatively good outcome, depending primarily on the presence of associated lesions.

The natural history of Ebstein's malformation was first reviewed by Watson in 1974.[7] In this international cooperative study, 505 patients were collected from 61 centers in 28 countries. Only 35 patients were less than 1 year old, 403 were between 1 and 25 years, and 67 were over 25 years. Cardiac failure was present in almost three-quarters of infants. In contrast, four-fifths of the patients presenting at older ages were said to have had normal growth and development during infancy. Also, almost three-quarters of the patients aged from 1 to 25 years and three-fifths of those older than 25 years had little or no disability at the time of diagnosis and were placed in the first or second categories of the classification of the New York Heart Association. Catheterisations had been undertaken on 363 patients, with 13 deaths and 6 cardiac arrests that were treated successfully. Paroxysmal tachycardia occurred during the catheterisation in 90 patients. Of the overall cohort, 77 (15.2%) died secondary to medical complications of the disease. After an initial higher risk of death in the neonatal period, the hazard for death was similar among all those aged greater than 1 year. Of the 403 patients aged between 1 and 25 years, 50 (12.4%) died of the disease. Half of the deaths were due to cardiac failure, with one-fifth dying suddenly, presumably due to an arrhythmia. In those over 25 years, 11 of 67 patients (16.4%) died of natural causes, 2 from congestive cardiac failure and 2 suddenly.

In 1994, Celermajer and colleagues described 220 cases of Ebstein's malformation presenting from fetus to adulthood (see Table 34-1).[9] The median age at time of presentation had decreased to less than 1 year, emphasising the role echocardiography now plays in early diagnosis. Neonatal mortality was due to cardiac failure and pulmonary hypoplasia, secondary to cardiomegaly. Associated cardiac defects were more common in patients who presented early. Those newborns with the isolated form of the malformation usually showed spontaneous improvement as the pulmonary vascular resistance decreased. Patients diagnosed later in childhood tended to present with a cardiac murmur discovered incidentally. Arrhythmias and progressive desaturation due to right-to-left shunting were more common in the older child and adult.

Women with Ebstein's malformation can tolerate pregnancy, particularly when their functional state is good prior to commencement of the pregnancy.[63–65] As a group, nonetheless, there is an increased risk of fetal demise and prematurity in mothers who had more significant disease.[66–68] In 1994, Connolly and Warnes reported a comprehensive review of pregnancy outcome in patients with Ebstein's malformation, analyzing histories of pregnancies in 72 couples in which one member, 44 women and 28 men, had Ebstein's malformation.[69] Pregnancy seemed well tolerated by the affected mothers but was associated with an increased risk of prematurity, fetal loss, and congenital cardiac disease in the offspring. The rates of miscarriage and fetal loss were 18%, slightly higher than the expected age-matched rates of 10% to 15%. Infants born to cyanotic women had significantly lower birth weights than did those born to noncyanotic mothers. Congenital cardiac disease was found in 6% of the offspring of the women with Ebstein's malformation but was found in only 1 of the 75 children (1.3%) born to couples in whom the man had the malformation. The incidence of Ebstein's malformation in the offspring was 0.6%, occurring in only 1 of the 158 children born to the couples. There were no significant maternal complications or death, suggesting that women with Ebstein's malformation tolerate pregnancy well. Maternal arrhythmias and cyanosis, of course, warrant close observation during the pregnancy.

Medical Therapy

Patients with Ebstein's malformation display a wide spectrum of haemodynamic abnormalities and arrhythmias that can occur at a variety of ages. Because of this, no dogmatic recommendations can be applied. It is possible to assemble general guidelines for treatment. At one end of the spectrum are patients with mild anatomic abnormalities, relatively normal haemodynamics, and no symptoms. These patients require only observation and normal precautions to prevent bacterial endocarditis. Beyond this, the anatomic and haemodynamic abnormalities may become important enough to cause symptoms and significantly alter lifestyle. For these patients, surgical therapy is often the most effective treatment.

Treatment of the critically ill neonate with Ebstein's malformation involves use of prostaglandin E_1 to maintain patency of the arterial duct, and the use of pulmonary vasodilators. High levels of inspired oxygen, nitric oxide and occasionally sildenafil, epoprostenol, or tolazoline, are also used. Many babies improve spontaneously as the pulmonary vascular resistance falls, with consequent improvement in forward flow through the tricuspid valve and right ventricular outflow, and reduced right-to-left shunting at atrial level. Intensive support, including ventilation, may be required during the first few days to weeks. If cyanosis is caused by associated structural obstruction of the right ventricular outflow tract, palliative surgery is indicated.

Many older children and adults are asymptomatic and can be managed conservatively. Exceptions include those with symptomatic arrhythmias, poor exercise tolerance, significant resting or exertional cyanosis, or symptoms of cardiac failure. Arrhythmias in general are difficult to treat. Accurate diagnosis should be obtained by 12-lead or ambulatory electrocardiographic monitoring, or home telemetry devices if necessary. Drug-refractory patients, or those with syncope, should have detailed electrophysiological studies. Over half the patients require a trial of two or more antiarrhythmic agents to obtain reasonable symptomatic control with medications.[70] Digoxin is useful for controlling the rate of response of the ventricles in those with atrial fibrillation, but is relatively contraindicated in patients with pre-excitation. Radio-frequency ablation may prove an effective alternative for those with accessory atrioventricular connections, although the procedure may be complicated by the presence of multiple pathways, the enlarged right atrium and the distorted anatomy of the tricuspid valve.

Cardiac failure may be treated with diuretics, and afterload reduction is appropriate for those with known left ventricular dysfunction. Oral anticoagulation is advisable for any patient with paroxysmal or chronic atrial fibrillation or flutter, except in those with a bleeding diathesis or other contraindication.

Most patients in the first or second functional classes, with mild or no cardiomegaly, can be managed medically. Operative correction is generally reserved for those with progressing symptoms, increasing cyanosis, or intractable arrhythmias requiring surgical elimination, or if paradoxical embolism occurs. Operation should also be considered if there is objective evidence of deterioration, such as decreasing exercise performance by exercise testing, progressive increase in the size of the heart on the chest radiograph, progressive right ventricular dilation, or reduction of systolic function, by echocardiography, or inadequate control of atrial or ventricular arrhythmias. In borderline situations, echocardiographic images demonstrating features favourable for valvar repair make the decision to proceed with operation easier.

Once symptoms develop and progress such that the patient is in the third or fourth functional classes, medical management has little to offer. Operation then becomes the only chance for improvement. A biventricular repair is usually possible, but in some circumstances, such as when significant left ventricular dysfunction has developed, cardiac transplantation may be the best option.

Surgery for Ebstein's Malformation

Palliative operations, such as construction of a systemic-to-pulmonary arterial shunt, a bidirectional Glenn anastomosis, or pulmonary valvotomy, may be required for neonates and infants with persistent cyanosis associated with structural pulmonary stenosis or atresia. In general, these procedures can be performed with low risk.[71] Open heart surgery for the symptomatic neonate usually consists of either a biventricular repair[72] or a functionally univentricular strategy.[11] The neonatal biventricular repair typically consists of repair of the tricuspid valve with subtotal closure of the atrial septal defect. The functionally univentricular strategy consists of an initial operation to close the tricuspid valve with a patch, atrial septectomy, and construction of a systemic-to-pulmonary arterial shunt. The second stage includes construction of a bidirectional Glenn anastamosis at 3 to 6 months of age and conversion to the Fontan circulation at 2 to 4 years of age. Occasionally, surgery for repair of associated defects is indicated in isolation, such as closure of an atrial septal defect in the setting of left-to-right shunting, closure of an associated ventricular septal defect, or isolated surgery to cure arrhythmias.

Indications for surgery include symptoms, cyanosis, decreased exercise tolerance, poor growth, the presence of an atrial septal defect, paradoxical embolism, increasing cardiomegaly, and onset or progression of atrial tachyarrhythmias. Operation is considered in asymptomatic patients who have anatomy that would have high probability of successful repair. Early[11,73,74] and intermediate[49,75–78] results have produced good to excellent outcomes.

The anatomy of the valve that is ideal for monoleaflet repair includes greater than half of the anterosuperior leaflet being free from tethering to the ventricular wall, and the leaflet possessing a free and mobile leading edge. The presence of leaflet tissue adjacent to the pulmonary valve in a short-axis view indicates severe displacement, and makes successful repair less likely (Fig. 34-22). Additional delamination of the septal and/or mural leaflets provides a more promising situation for successful repair. In complex cases, replacement of the valve may be required.

The optimal technique for valvar reconstruction has yet to be established since the first report by Hardy in 1964. Contemporary techniques commonly used include those of Danielson,[73,77,79–81] and most recently Da Silva.[49]

Each method of repair typically incorporates selective plication or resection of the atrialised right ventricle, especially when it is thin-walled and moves paradoxically. A current technique has been proposed that moves the tricuspid valve to an anatomic position, the so-called cone reconstruction.[49] The surgeons from the Deutches Herzzentrum have long used the monoleaflet approach, but without resorting to plication of the atrialised inlet component.[82] Results of these procedures have been good for selected older children and adults, with an early mortality rate of 5%. Good results, with slightly higher mortality rates of 10%, have also been reported for the repair devised by Carpentier and colleagues,[81] which involves longitudinal plication of the atrialised right ventricle and tricuspid annuloplasty, with or without placement of an annuloplasty ring.[22] A similar approach has been used by Quaegebeur and colleagues,[83] and more recently by Chen and colleagues.[76] Most survivors of repair achieve good functional state, and have improved exercise performance.[84,85] In a proportion of patients who come to surgery, the morphology or immobility of the anterosuperior leaflet is deemed to prevent repair, and replacement is required.[71] The number of such patients often reflects the skill of the surgeons in reparative procedures, with less than 3% of those patients referred to Hôpital Broussais requiring valvar replacement.[22] When replacement is necessary, the abnormal leaflet tissue in the right ventricular outflow tract is excised in order to prevent obstruction. In addition, care is made to preserve the membranous septum and conduction tissue. Whether the

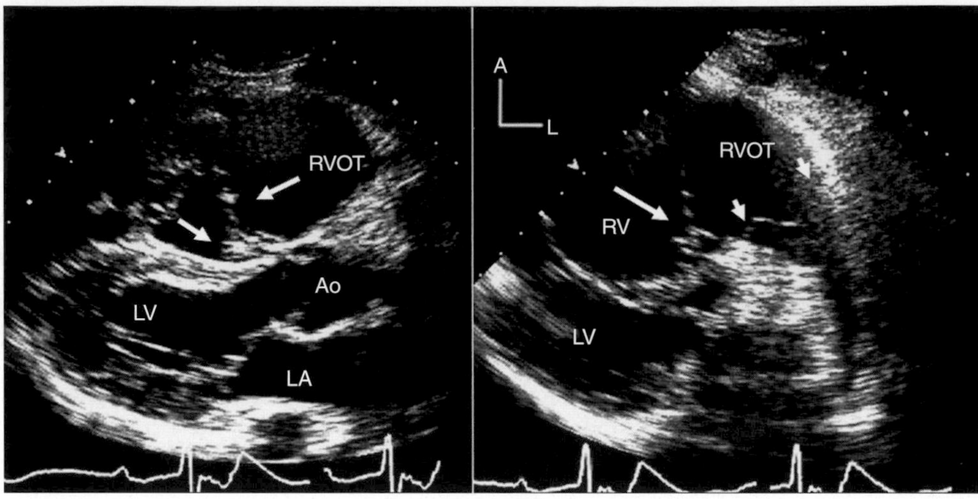

Figure 34-22 These two parasternal echocardiographic images (long axis to the left and an oblique view of the right ventricular outflow tract to the right) demonstrate extreme displacement of the tricuspid valve apparatus into the right ventricular outflow tract or infundibulum (*long arrows*). The short arrows show the septal hinge point of the pulmonary valve. When the tricuspid valve is so severely displaced, only the infundibulum is downstream from the displaced functional orifice. Successful valve repair would be difficult in this case. Ao, aorta; LA, left atrium; LV, left ventricle; RV, right ventricle; RVOT, right ventricular outflow tract.

coronary sinus is left to drain above or below the prosthesis is determined by its proximity to the conduction tissue.[78] Many types of prostheses have been used, including Dacron-mounted allograft pulmonary valves,[71] dura mater prostheses,[86] large heterograft valves, or mechanical prostheses in adults.[87] In the current era, it is our practice to utilise a porcine bioprosthesis when we need to replace the valve because of good durability,[78] and the lack of a need for warfarin anticoagulation. Reoperation, however, is inevitable in these patients. Although some have reported peri-operative mortality rates in these patients of up to 15% to 20%,[71] in our experience it has been less than 5%. We have reserved replacement with a mechanical prosthesis for rare circumstances, specifically the presence of a left-sided mechanical prosthesis. Caution should be exercised with the use of a mechanical valve when there is significant right ventricular dysfunction, since the motion of the disc may be abnormal, and the risk of thrombosis may be increased, even in the presence of warfarin anticoagulation.

Another factor that has recently received much attention is the role of the bidirectional Glenn anastamosis as part of the so-called one and a half ventricle repair for Ebstein's malformation. While some have proposed routine use of the Glenn anastomosis,[88] we have utilised it only in selective circumstances. In patients with Ebstein's malformation and impaired right ventricular function, the bidirectional Glenn may facilitate operation by unloading the enlarged and dysfunctional right ventricle, and provide preload to the left ventricle.[74] In addition, if the size of the functional right ventricle is felt to be small, which is rarely the case, or the tricuspid repair results in a small valvar orifice, then a bidirectional Glenn anastamosis becomes an option. Rarely is a Fontan-type operation required when the first operation is beyond the neonatal period.

Atrial tachyarrhythmias commonly co-exist. A concomitant maze procedure is then recommended at the time of repair of the Ebstein's malformation.[45,60] Accessory conduction pathways producing the Wolff-Parkinson-White syndrome are present in approximately one-sixth of patients with Ebstein's malformation. In the current era, electrophysiologic study and ablation in the catheterisation laboratory are the norm. Intraoperative mapping and ablation are reserved for an unsuccessful percutaneous approach. Less common arrhythmias, such as atrioventricular nodal re-entry tachycardia, are also treated in the catheterisation laboratory. Surgical treatment is indicated only when transcatheter treatment has been unsuccessful. In some circumstances, surgical treatment has been performed when operation for Ebstein's malformation is required anyway.

In our experience, we have been able to perform a biventricular or one and a half ventricle repair for most of our patients, with an operative mortality of less than 5%. It is very rare for orthotopic cardiac transplantation to be necessary as the first method of treatment. Circumstances when it may be considered include the presence of severe biventricular dysfunction.[12,74]

OTHER TRICUSPID VALVAR ABNORMALITIES

Tricuspid Valvar Dysplasia

While dysplasia of the valvar leaflets is often an integral part of Ebstein's malformation, dysplastic leaflets can also be found when retaining their normal hinges at the atrioventricular junction (see Fig. 34-16). Such dysplasia of normally hinged leaflets can produce just as much valvar incompetence as Ebstein's malformation (Fig. 34-23).

In contrast to Ebstein's malformation, the myocardium in these hearts is usually normal, at least early in life. As a result, ventricular function is better preserved, and outcomes are more favorable. Isolated dysplasia can produce the same wall-to-wall heart,[30] with the same consequences for pulmonary problems in the neonatal period.[27]

Other Abnormalities

Lesions associated with severe right ventricular enlargement, but having anatomically normal tricuspid valves, should not be mistaken for Ebstein's malformation or tricuspid valvar dysplasia. Traumatic rupture of the cordal support of the valve (Fig. 34-24), Uhl's malformation, and arrhythmogenic right ventricular cardiomyopathy have been misidentified as Ebstein's malformation in the past. Traumatic rupture of tricuspid cords can produce abnormal motion of the leaflets, severe regurgitation, and chamber enlargement. The leaflets, however, are not adherent to the myocardium, and the junctional hinges are normally

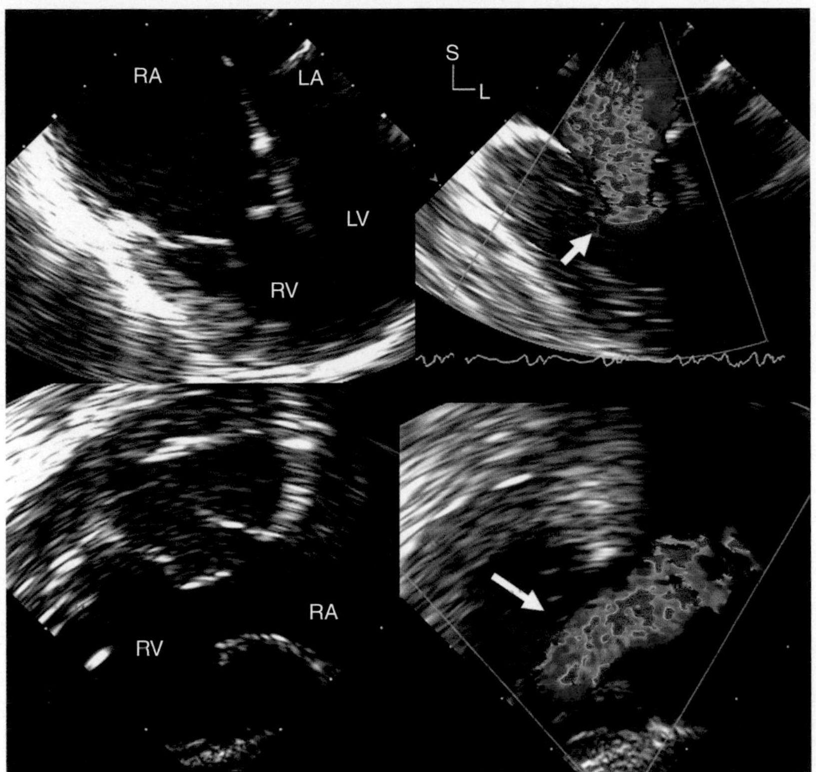

Figure 34-23 These echocardiographic images display a case of tricuspid valvar dysplasia. The upper panels are apical four-chamber images from a transoesophageal exam. The lower panels are parasagittal transgastric images of the right ventricular inlet. The tricuspid leaflets are thick and demonstrate reduced systolic motion. The leaflets cannot fully coapt in systole, and there is a large central jet of tricuspid regurgitation seen in both right hand panels (*arrows*). All segments of this valve have delaminated from the underlying myocardium. All of the annular hinge points are in their normal positions at the atrioventricular junction. LA, left atrium; LV, left ventricle; RA, right atrium; RV, right ventricle.

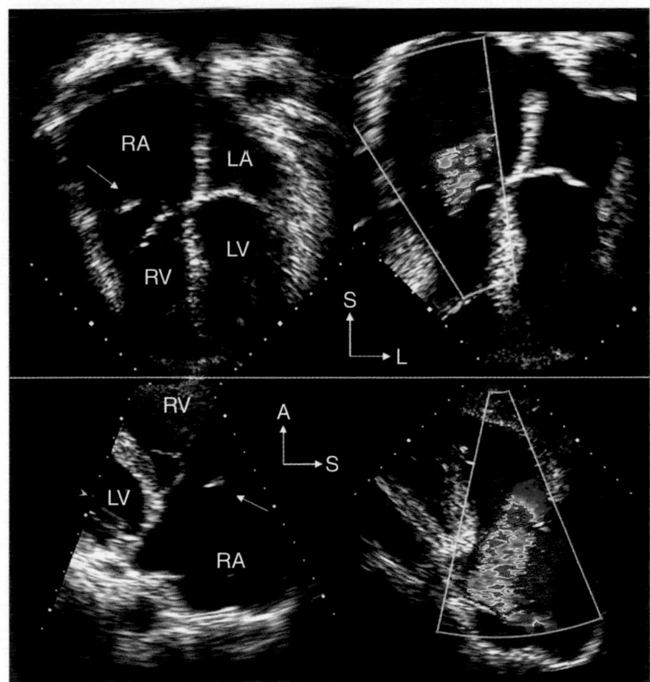

Figure 34-24 These echocardiographic images demonstrate traumatic rupture of the cordal supports to the anterosuperior leaflet of an otherwise normal tricuspid valve. The patient was involved in a serious motor vehicle accident 20 years prior to this examination. The cause of his tricuspid regurgitation had been previously misidentified as Ebstein's malformation. The upper panels are apical four-chamber images, and the lower panels are parasternal images aligned with the right ventricular inlet. Both the anterosuperior and septal leaflets are fully delaminated, and their junctional hinges retain a normal position at the atrioventricular groove. The arrows highlight the flail nature of the anterosuperior leaflet. The leaflet abnormality correlates well with the severe regurgitation displayed in the corresponding color flow images to the right. LA, left atrium; LV, left ventricle; RA, right atrium; RV, right ventricle.

positioned. In the lesion described by Uhl,[28] the tricuspid and pulmonary valves were both normal. The essence of the malformation is congenital absence of the parietal myocardium, histological analysis showing that the epicardial and endocardial layers of the wall lie edge-to-edge.[29] It is also a mistake to correlate fibro-fatty replacement of the right ventricular parietal walls with either Ebstein's malformation or Uhl's malformation. Fibro-fatty replacement is the essence of arrhythmogenic right ventricular cardiomyopathy, now recognised as a cardiomyopathy in its own right, with various genetic causes.

ACKNOWLEDGEMENTS

The authors gratefully acknowledge David S. Celermajer and John E. Deanfield for their efforts in preparation of the previous editions of this chapter, which we have relied on for guidance. We appreciate the assistance of Kim Feils and Sharon Long in the preparation of this chapter and the unique input of William D. Edwards for his anatomic insights and generosity in sharing his photographic examples. Lastly, we owe a tremendous debt to the contributions of Gordon K. Danielson to our understanding of the anatomy, pathophysiology and care of the patient with Ebstein's malformation.

The complete reference list can be found on the companion Expert Consult web site at www.expertconsult.com.

ANNOTATED REFERENCES

- Watson H: Natural history of Ebstein's anomaly of tricuspid valve in childhood and adolescence: An international co-operative study of 505 cases. Br Heart J 1974;36:417–427.

  An early review of a large number of patients with Ebstein's malformation and their natural history. Unique for details of the problems created by the malformation with less influence from modern medical and surgical treatments. This review lacks a perspective on the neonate with Ebstein's malformation because of its early date and therefore the lack of prenatal and neonatal cases.

- Celermajer D, Bull C, Till J: Ebstein's anomaly: Presentation and outcome from fetus to adult. J Am Coll Cardiol 1994;23:170–176.

A more modern perspective on the presentations and clinical courses seen in patients with Ebstein's malformation. Provides a better assessment of the differences between the very young (fetus and neonate) and the older patient with Ebstein's malformation.

- Attenhofer Jost C, Connolly H, O'Leary P, et al: Occurence of left ventricular myocardial dysplasia/noncompaction in patients with Ebstein's anomaly. Mayo Clinic Proc 2005;80:361–368.

  A large series outlining the myocardial abnormality that is the central component of Ebstein's malformation. This series primarily focuses on the left ventricular involvement that is seen in up to one-fifth of patients with the malformation.

- Schrieber C, Cook A, Ho S, et al: Morphology of Ebstein's malformation: Revisitation relative to surgical repair. J Thorac Cardiovasc Surg1999;117: 148–155.

  A complete anatomic description of the displacement of the tricuspid valvar hinges and leaflets. This paper highlights the rotational nature of the displacement in three dimensions, resulting in a functional tricuspid valvar orifice that is spirally displaced, both anterosuperiorly and apically, from its normal position. The malformed orifice is usually postioned at the junction of the atrialised inlet and functional ventricular components of the right ventricle.

- Celermajer D, Cullen S, Sullivan I, et al: Outcome in neonates with Ebstein's anomaly. J Am Coll Cardiol 1992;19:1041–1046.

  An excellent description of the presentation and clinical course of the neonate afflicted with Ebstein's malformation. This manuscript presented the concept of comparing the combined four-chamber view areas of the true right atrium and atrialised right ventricle to the combined areas of the functional right ventricle, left atrium, and left ventricle as a prognostic tool. No survivors were observed when the combined area of the true right atrium and atrialised right ventricle exceeded the area of the remaining cardiac chambers in this view.

- Cohen L, Friedman J, Jefferson J, et al: A reevaluation of risk of in utero exposure to lithium. JAMA 1994;271:146–150.

  This study reevaluated the frequency with which gestational exposure to lithium therapy was associated with development of Ebstein's malformation. Although the risk of any congenital malformation, not only cardiac, was two to three times that seen in nontreated mothers, there was no increase in the frequency of Ebstein's malformation relative to controls. This demonstrated that the relative risk of treatment with lithium during pregnancy is much less than was originally estimated from the retrospective case reports. The decision as to whether or not to continue such treatment during pregnancy must now be made by weighing the relative risk of teratogenicity against the risks of relapse of manic/depressive disease in the mother.

- Da Silva J, Baumgratz J, da Fonseca L, et al: The cone reconstruction of the tricuspid valve in Ebstein's anomaly. The operation: Early and midterm results. J Thorac Cardiovasc Surg 2007;133:215–223.

  Description and results of an innovative valvar repair for Ebstein's malformation that shifts the valvar apparatus into closer proximity to the anatomic atrioventricular junction.

- Greason K, Dearani J, Theodore D, et al: Surgical managment of atrial tachyarrhythmias associated with congenital cardiac anomalies: Mayo Clinic experience. Semin Thorac Cardiovasc Surg Pediatr Card Surg Annu 2003;6:59–71.

  A comprehensive description of techniques and results of surgical treatment for arrhythmia in congential cardiac malformations that includes an extensive experience with Ebstein's malformation.

- Connolly H, Warnes C: Ebstein's anomaly: Outcome of pregnancy. J Am Coll Cardiol 1994;23:1194–1198.

  A comprehensive review of the challenges that pregnancy poses to the patient with congenital heart disease. This paper includes a large experience with Ebstein's malformation. Pregnancy seemed well tolerated by the affected mothers, although it must be remembered that these pregnancies were followed closely by an experienced group of cardiologists and maternal fetal medicine specialists. There was an increased risk of prematurity, fetal loss, and congenital cardiac disease in the offspring of mothers with Ebstein's malformation. Mothers who remained cyanotic during gestation gave birth to infants with lower birth weights than did mothers with Ebstein's malformation and normal oxygen saturations.

- Knott-Craig C, Goldberg S: Management of neonatal Ebstein's anomaly. Semin Thorac Cardiovasc Surg Pediatr Card Surg Annu 2007:112–116.
- Quinonez L, Dearani J, Puga F, et al: Results of 1.5-ventricle repair for Ebstein anomaly and the failing right ventricle. J Thorac Cardiovasc Surg 2007;133:1303–1310.
- Dearani JD, GK: Surgical management of Ebstein's anomaly in the adult. Sem Thorac Cardiovasc Surg 2005;17:148–154.
- Dearani J, O'Leary P, Danielson G: Surgical treatment of Ebstein's malformation: State of the art in 2006. Cardiol Young 2006;16(suppl 3):4–11.

  Taken together, the last four articles provide a comprehensive summary of the issues surrounding the surgical treatment of the patient with Ebstein's malformation. They cover indications for intervention, factors influencing the choice of surgical procedure, technical descriptions of reparative manuvers as well as summaries of results.

Anomalies of the Morphologically Mitral Valve

JEFFREY F. SMALLHORN and ROBERT H. ANDERSON

In this chapter, we discuss those lesions than afflict the morphologically mitral valve, the likeness to the episcopal mitre of this valve in the normal heart first being emphasised by Andreas Vesalius, the Belgian morphologist, who worked in Padova, the birthplace of cardiac morphology, in the 15th century. As with the episcopal headwear, the feature of the normally constructed mitral valve is the solitary zone of apposition between its component parts, the leaflets, this feature producing a bifoliate pattern of closure. The pattern of closure, in turn, distinguishes the normally structured left valve from the left half of the common valve seen in the setting of atrioventricular septal defect with common atrioventricular junction. Although similar lesions can affect the left-sided heart when there are separate or common atrioventricular junctions, the anomalies involving the left half of the common valve will be discussed in Chapter 27. We also reserve discussion of anomalies of the left-sided valves in hearts with double inlet ventricle for Chapter 31, despite the fact that, when there is double inlet to a dominant left ventricle, it is usual for both atrioventricular valves to resemble the morphologically mitral valve. Either the right-sided or left-sided valve, nonetheless, can be deformed in this setting. In this chapter, therefore, we confine our attention to the valve guarding the inlet to the morphologically left ventricle in hearts with separate right and left atrioventricular junctions. The lesions to be described that involve the morphologically mitral valve, therefore, can also involve this valve when both the atrioventricular and ventriculo-arterial connections are discordant. The latter malformation, best described as congenitally corrected transposition, will receive its own coverage in Chapter 39.

MORPHOLOGY

It is convenient, albeit not always entirely accurate, to describe the abnormal morphology in terms of malformation of the various components of the mitral valve, remembering that, in functional terms, such derangement can result in stenosis, incompetence, or both.[1-3] In terms of anatomy, we will discuss anomalies of the leaflets, the tension apparatus, and the papillary muscles, all of these components working in harmony when the valve is normal (Fig. 35-1). The leaflets are hinged from the annulus, but this is far from a constant structure in the mitral valve. Furthermore, as far as we are aware, there are no specific congenital lesions that afflict only the annulus. The hinges of the aortic and mural leaflets are markedly different in their structure. The hinge, or annulus, of the anterior leaflet of the valve is the area of its fibrous continuity with the leaflets of the aortic valve, hence our preference to describe this leaflet of the valve as being aortic. The two ends of the region of fibrous continuity between the leaflets of the atrioventricular and arterial valves are themselves thickened as the right and left fibrous trigones. It is the anchorage of these trigones to the basal surface of the ventricular mass that secures the combined unit of the inlet and outlet valves within the left ventricle (Fig. 35-2). The part of the mitral valvar circumference formed by the aortic leaflet, therefore, is strong. It is much less likely to dilate under abnormal circumstances than the remaining part of the valve. This second part of the valve, the mural or posterior leaflet, is anchored along the parietal part of the left atrioventricular junction. There is marked variation in the arrangement of the mural annulus itself.[4] In places, it is a firm fibrous cord that fits well with the notion of a ring (Fig. 35-3). It is unusual, nonetheless, for such a fibrous ring to support the entirety of the leaflet throughout the mural part of the valvar perimeter. In places, the cord is replaced by a longer fibrous sheet, or else the fibrous tissue becomes deficient, with the atrial and ventricular musculatures separated by fibroadipose tissue rather than a true annulus.[4] Because of this variation, and the frequent lack of a complete fibrous ring, it is this part of the valvar circumference that dilates in

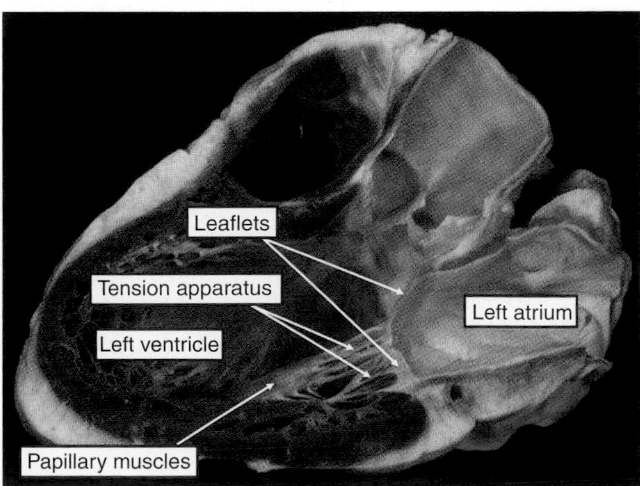

Figure 35-1 The long-axis section through the left ventricle, showing the parasternal echocardiographic view, illustrates the components of the mitral valvar complex that work in harmony when the valve is normal. The specimen was prepared subsequent to injection of fixative under pressure in the left ventricle, maintaining the systolic configuration of the leaflets.

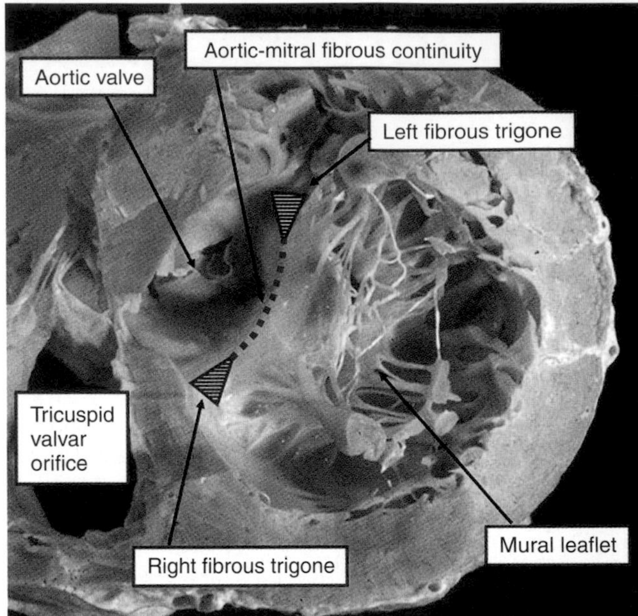

Figure 35-2 The normal heart has been sectioned to replicate the echocardiographic short axis of the left ventricle. Note the thickening of the two ends of fibrous continuity between the leaflets of the aortic and mitral valves (*purple dotted line*) to form the fibrous trigones (*red triangles*). The fibrous continuity is the annulus of the aortic leaflet of the mitral valve, the mural leaflet being hinged along the parietal atrioventricular junction (see Fig. 35-3).

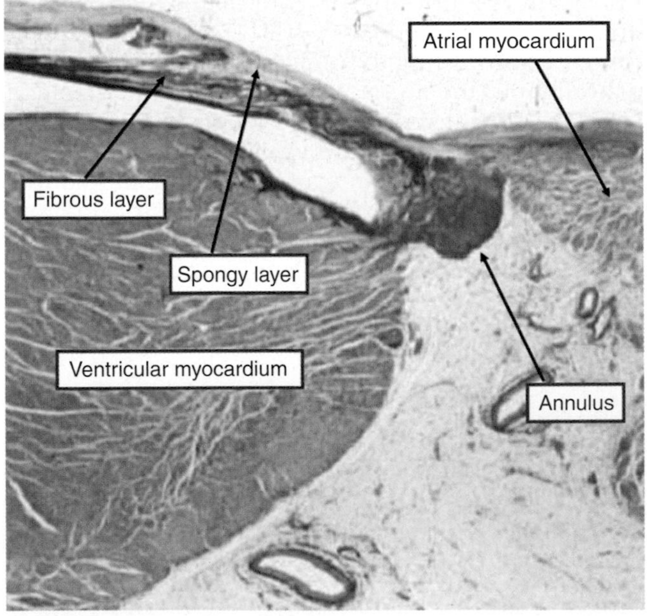

Figure 35-3 This section through the parietal part of the left atrioventricular junction shows how, in some instances, the mural leaflet of the mitral valve is hinged from a firm fibrous ring. The section is stained with Van Gieson's reagent, which shows the fibrous tissue, including the fibrous ventricular layer of the valvar leaflet. Note the thin layer on the atrial aspect of the leaflet, known as the spongy layer.

the setting of valvar disease. In such cases of acquired change, it is often the case that all parts of the valve are abnormal. We commence our account of morphology, therefore, by considering anomalies of the entire valvar apparatus.

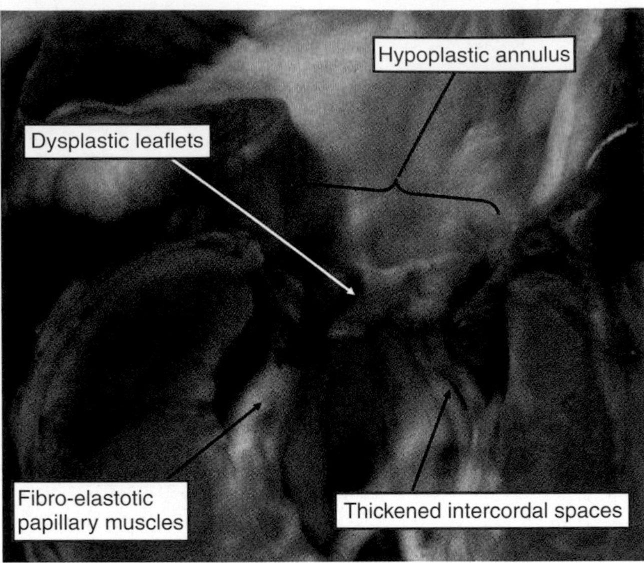

Figure 35-4 This valve is from a patient with hypoplasia of the left heart. The entire valvar complex is miniaturised, and the leaflets are dysplastic.

Mitral Valvar Dysplasia and Hypoplasia

All components of the complex are malformed when the valve is dysplastic and hypoplastic. The leaflets are thickened, the intercordal spaces often obliterated and the papillary muscles deformed, the last frequently extending as muscular strands directly into the leaflets. Usually such a valve shows global hypoplasia, and is the most common lesion underscoring congenital mitral stenosis, be this isolated or as seen most frequently in the setting of hypoplasia of the left heart (Fig. 35-4).

When the free edges of the dysplastic valve leaflets are thickened and rolled, the valve may be incompetent as well as stenotic. Occasionally, mitral stenosis may be produced when the valve is hypoplastic and dysplastic.

Anomalies of the Leaflets

The most extreme anomaly involving the leaflets is an imperforate valve (Fig. 35-5). Such imperforate valves are seen most frequently in combination with aortic atresia, when they form part an integral part of the hypoplastic left ventricle syndrome (see Chapter 29). In this setting, from the stance of anatomy, the imperforate valve is distinguished from absence of the left atrioventricular connection (Fig. 35-6), since both produce atrioventricular valvar atresia. In the setting of left heart hypoplasia, of course, this morphological distinction is rarely, if ever, of clinical significance. In hypoplasia of the left heart, when the left atrioventricular connection is absent, the right atrium is connected to a dominant right ventricle. The left atrioventricular connection can also be absent when the right atrium is connected to a dominant left ventricle (Fig. 35-7). This lesion is best considered in the setting of the functionally univentricular heart (see Chapter 31). Imperforate mitral valves, of course, can also be found without aortic atresia (see Fig. 35-5), and are then part of the combination termed mitral atresia with patent aortic root.[5] The ventriculo-arterial connection is often double outlet from

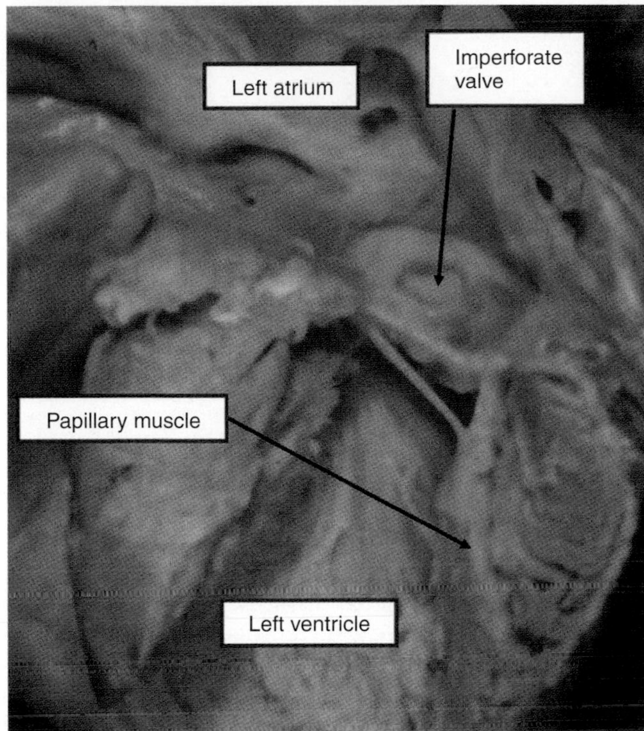

Figure 35-5 The leaflets of the mitral valve are formed, but fused to form an imperforate shelf. Note the papillary muscles supporting the ventricular aspect.

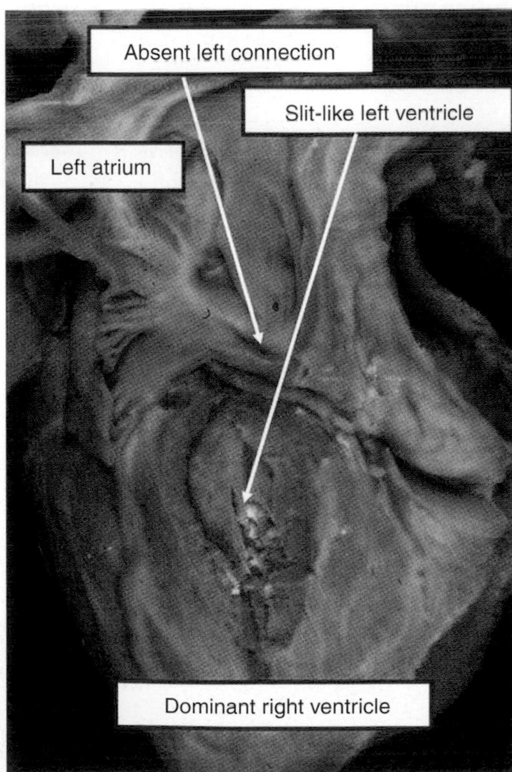

Figure 35-6 This dissection of the heart from a patient with hypoplastic left heart syndrome shows complete absence of the left atrioventricular connection. The right atrium is connected to a dominant right ventricle. Note the left coronary artery interposed between the blind-ending floor of the left atrium and the incomplete left ventricle.

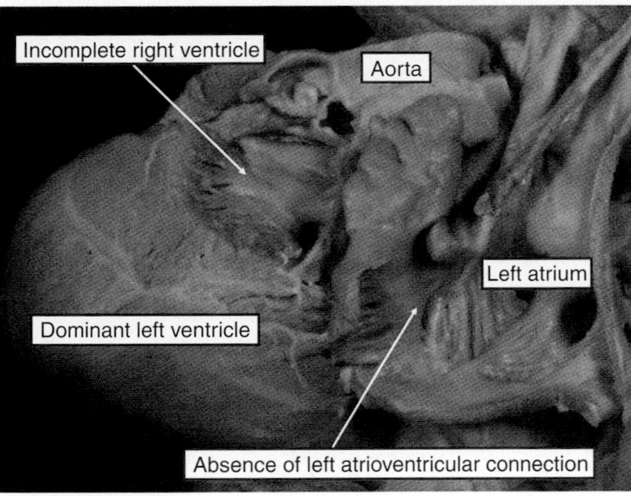

Figure 35-7 This dissection, comparable to the one shown in Figure 35-6, shows absence of the left atrioventricular connection in the setting of the right atrium connected to a dominant left ventricle. It is now the right ventricle, positioned on the left shoulder of the ventricular mass, which is incomplete. Note that the right ventricle gives rise to the aorta, the ventriculo-arterial connections being discordant.

the right ventricle, but in a significant number of cases, the patent aorta arises from a good-sized left ventricle. The ventricle is then filled through a ventricular septal defect.

Ebstein's malformation can rarely affect the morphologically mitral valve.[6] When this is the case, the mural leaflet is plastered down onto the ventricular wall, with its hinge below the atrioventricular junction (Fig. 35-8, left panel). In this setting, there is no thinning of the atrialised inlet portion, as is usually seen when it is the morphologically tricuspid valve that is deformed in the setting of concordant atrioventricular connections (Fig. 35-8, middle panel). Such lack of morphologic atrialisation is also a feature of Ebstein's malformation of the left-sided atrioventricular valve in the setting of congenitally corrected transposition, but then, of course, the valve itself is of tricuspid morphology (Fig. 35-8, right panel; see Chapter 39).

The isolated cleft is another anomaly confined to the leaflet, usually involving the leaflet in fibrous continuity with the leaflets of the aortic valve (Fig. 35-9). Well explained on the basis of failure of fusion between the left ventricular components of the superior and inferior atrioventricular cushions,[7] the space between the cleft components of the leaflet creates the substrate for valvar incompetence. Both parts of the cleft leaflet tend to be dysplastic, and the edges are usually rolled and thickened (see Fig. 35-9). The cleft valve often co-exists with deficient ventricular septation, and the edges of the cleft are then frequently tethered to the crest of the ventricular septum by tendinous cords. The essence of these so-called isolated clefts of the aortic leaflet is that they are found in hearts with separate atrioventricular junction.[8,9] The space between the edges of the cleft then points towards the subaortic outflow tract (Fig. 35-10), or to the antero-superiorly located interventricular communication when seen in the setting of the Taussig-Bing malformation. The lesion must be distinguished from the so-called cleft found in the left half of the atrioventricular valve of patients having atrioventricular septal defects with common atrioventricular junction (see Chapter 27). In the setting of the common junction,

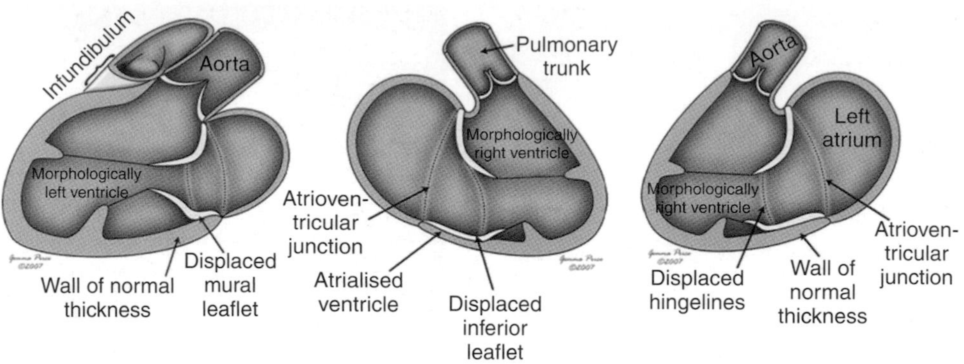

Figure 35-8 The cartoon shows how, when Ebstein's malformation afflicts the morphologically mitral valve (*left panel*), it is the mural leaflet that is involved, and it is rare to find thinning of the atrialised ventricular inlet. When afflicting the morphologically tricuspid valve, the atrialised ventricular component usually shows marked thinning (*middle panel*), but such thinning is usually absent when the left-sided morphologically tricuspid valve shows Ebstein's malformation in the setting of discordant atrioventricular connections (*right panel*).

the so-called cleft is the zone of apposition between the left ventricular components of the leaflets that bridge the ventricular septum. This space points at the ventricular septum. Although the space between the leaflets is nowadays readily reconstituted by suture of its edges in both settings, it is only when there is a separate left atrioventricular junction that the surgical maneuver restores the morphology of a relatively normal mitral valve.

Another isolated anomaly of the valvar leaflets is the so-called funnel-shaped valve.[10] This entity is characterised by thickening and retraction of the leaflets, with fused tendinous cords, but in the presence of normal papillary muscles. The funnel produces mitral stenosis. It is rare in postmortem collections. More common are valves with dual orifices. The dual orifices are produced by a tongue of valvar tissue that extends between the mural and aortic leaflets, dividing the valvar orifice into two components, with each orifice then supported by one of the papillary muscles (Fig. 35-11). Dual orifices are more common within the left half of the atrioventricular valve of patients having atrioventricular septal defects with common atrioventricular junction (Chapter 27). As with the so-called cleft, these malformations should again be distinguished from those afflicting the bifoliate and otherwise normally structured mitral valve.

A rarer abnormality that can result in congenital mitral valvar regurgitation is hypoplasia of the mural leaflet, such that the valve leaflets cannot coapt normally during systole.[11] More frequent is straddling and overriding of the valvar leaflets. These anomalies can affect either the tricuspid or the mitral valve. Bridging of leaflets is also, of course,

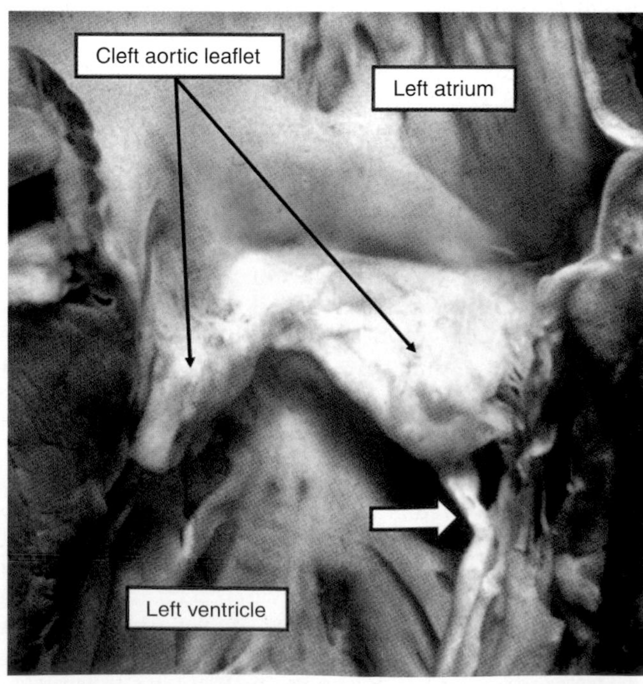

Figure 35-9 There is a congenital cleft in the aortic leaflet of the mitral valve. Note that both parts of the cleft leaflet are dysplastic, and there is thickening of the tendinous cords (*arrow*).

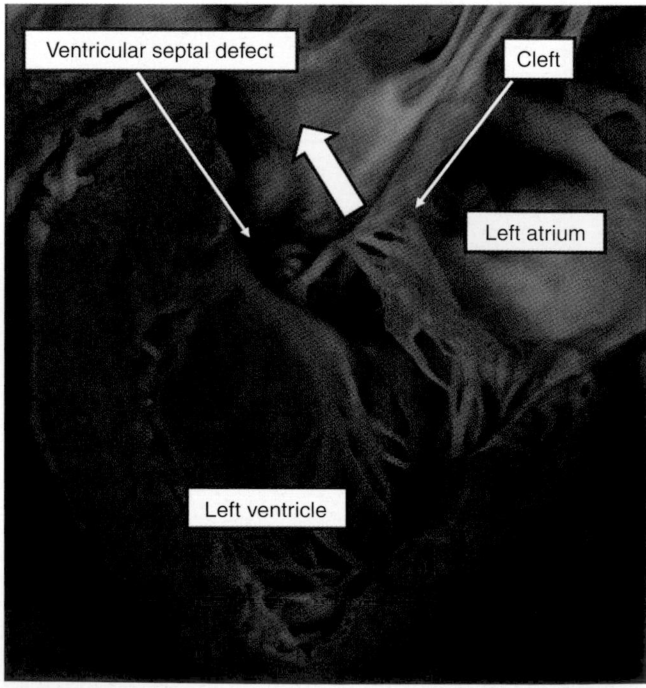

Figure 35-10 In this heart with a cleft of the aortic leaflet of the mitral valve, there is also a perimembranous ventricular septal defect. Note that the edges of the cleft leaflet are attached by tendinous cords to the crest of the ventricular septum, and that the cleft itself points towards the aorta (*arrow*).

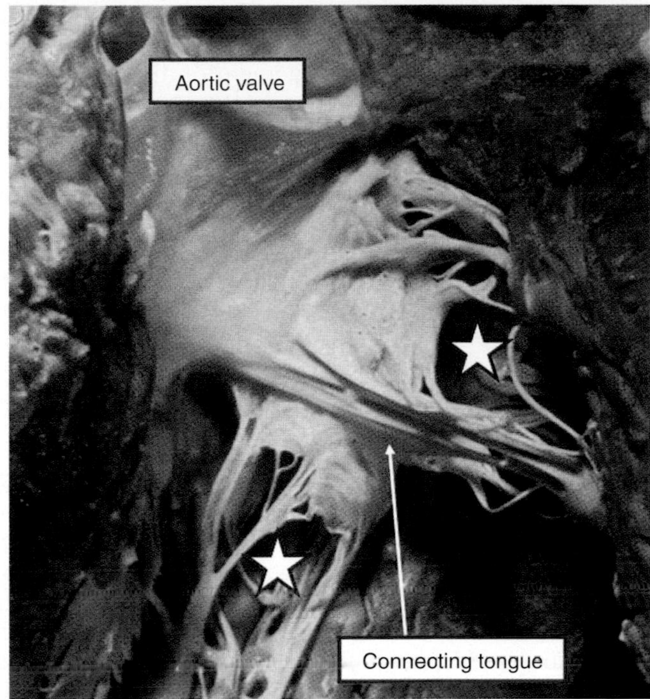

Figure 35-11 In this heart, a tongue of valvar tissue has joined together the aortic and mural leaflets of the mitral valve, producing dual valvar orifices (*stars*). Note that each orifice is supported by one of the paired papillary muscles of the valve.

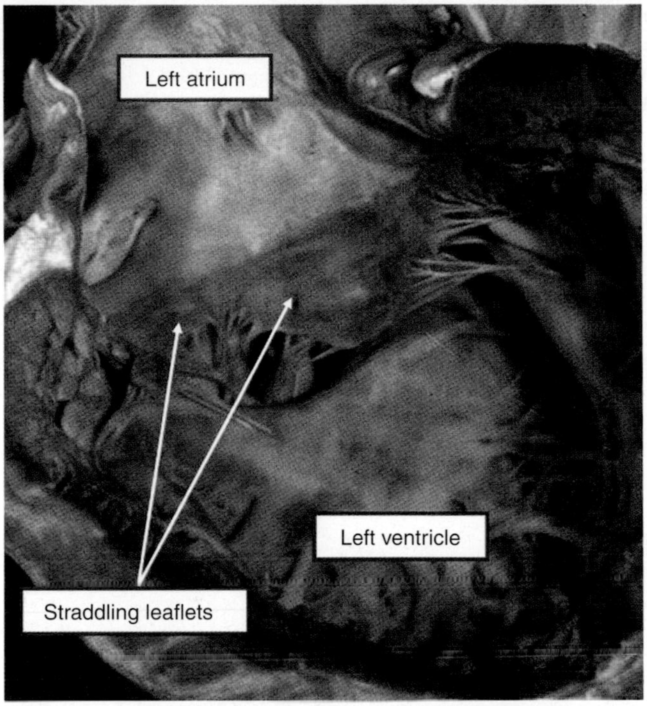

Figure 35-12 In this heart with double outlet right ventricle and subpulmonary interventricular communication, the so-called Taussig-Bing malformation, there is straddling and overriding of the supero-anterior end of the zone of apposition between the aortic and mural leaflets, the papillary muscle being attached in the right ventricle.

a common feature of the common atrioventricular valve, albeit that a common valve can be exclusively connected to one or other of the ventricles. It is the spectrum between the commitment of straddling valves to one or other ventricle, underscoring the difference between functionally univentricular and biventricular arrangements, which forms the focus of our chapter devoted specifically to straddling and overriding (see Chapter 33). When the morphologically mitral valve straddles and overrides, the valve always straddles through an antero-superior interventricular communication and is found with either discordant or double outlet ventriculo-arterial connections—the so-called Taussig-Bing malformation (Fig. 35-12).

When discussing malformations of the leaflets, we should also pay attention to a fibrous ridge that anchors together the aortic and mural components, narrowing the valvar orifice. Although usually described as a supravalvar structure, the abnormal fibrous shelf is an integral part of the atrial surface of the leaflets,[12] and can readily be removed at surgery. Shelves can, indeed, exist within the left atrium, and produce true supravalvar rings, but these are much rarer than the variant attached to the atrial aspect of the leaflets (Fig. 35-13).

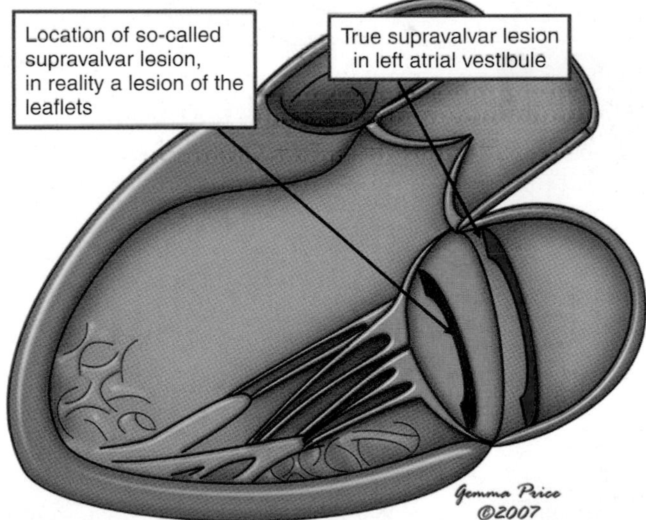

Figure 35-13 The cartoon, illustrating the parasternal long-axis section, shows the fundamental anatomic difference between a true supravalvar left atrial ring and the so-called supravalvar stenosing ring. The latter lesion is attached to the atrial surface of the valvar leaflets and should be considered an abnormality of the leaflets.

Without question, the commonest lesion afflicting the leaflets of the mitral valve is prolapse. The problems concerning the pathology of prolapse of the mitral valve, however, are as numerous as those concerning its clinical features. There is no unanimity concerning nomenclature or aetiology and, perhaps more important, no standard definition of what precisely constitutes prolapse of the leaflets. The morphologist is under considerable constraint in this respect, since of necessity, in autopsy studies, the valve is viewed only in its fixed state. The morphologist can only speculate on what might have happened as the valvar leaflets moved from their open diastolic position to the closed systolic pattern, unless the heart is fixed with pressure in the left ventricle so that the leaflets assume their systolic position (see Fig. 35-1). Much can be learnt concerning the mechanics of prolapse, nonetheless, by comparing the morphology of the prolapsing valve with the normal arrangement. The pathologist usually describes the prolapsing variant as being floppy. Several pathological processes can produce a prolapsed leaflet as their end-point, such as ruptured tendinous cords secondary to ischaemic heart disease. The particular process producing the floppy valve is the one associated with the so-called click/murmur syndrome, this being the essence of the commonest form of mitral valvar prolapse. It is the mural leaflet that is most usually involved when the valve is floppy. The lesion may affect only one of its scallops (Fig. 35-14), but in severe cases the aortic leaflet may also be involved (Fig. 35-15).

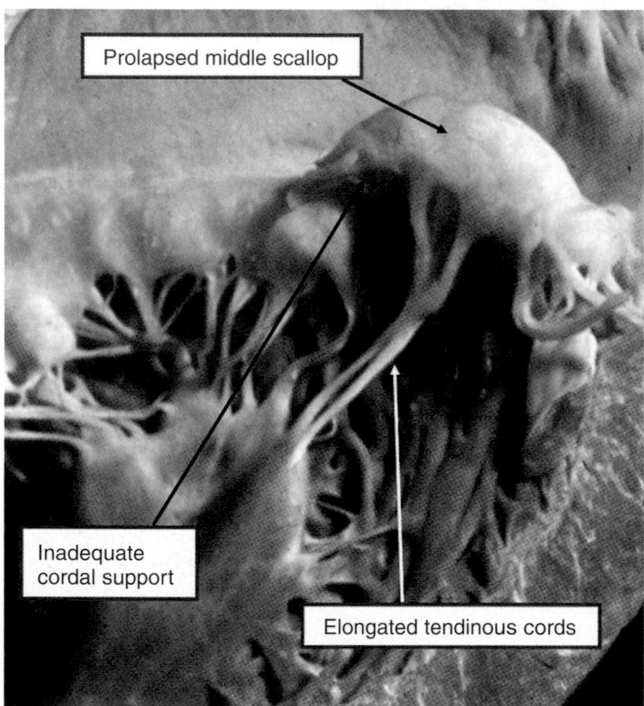

Figure 35-14 In this heart, only the middle scallop of the mural leaflet of the mitral valve is prolapsing. Note the lack of cordal support to much of the scallop and the elongation of the persisting cords.

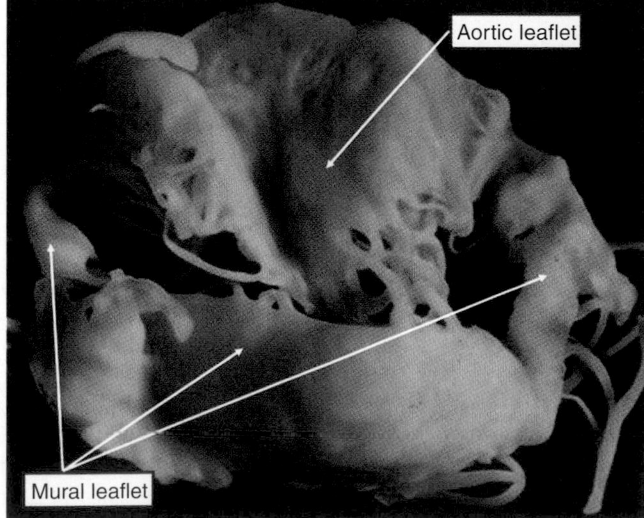

Figure 35-15 In this valve, removed at surgery, all parts of both leaflets are abnormal, and were prolapsing, albeit that the disease process afflicts the middle scallop of the mural leaflet most severely. Note the similarity of the valve to a parachute.

The affected leaflets are hooded, with their convexity to the left atrium. When the whole leaflet is involved, as is seen mostly in adults, the arrangement of the domed leaflets with their elongated cords takes on a parachute-like appearance, particularly when surgically removed (see Fig. 35-15). Pathologists dealing with disease of the adult population have described the valve in this fashion, but the choice of parachute is perhaps unfortunate in the setting of congenital cardiac malformations, since as we will see, the term is more usually used to described malformations of the papillary muscles. Irrespective of the descriptions, when the leaflets are grossly prolapsed, there is little difficulty in recognition. Most floppy valves, nonetheless, are seen in adult patients, and in this setting it can be difficult to distinguish minimal prolapse from the normal arrangement. This may well be significant, since Becker and de Wit[13] have pointed out that, in some normal valves, parts of the leading edge of the mural leaflet are less well supported by tendinous cords than other parts. They suggested that such an arrangement might predispose to prolapse, and subsequent observations confirmed that prolapsed segments of an affected leaflet are, indeed, less well supported than the non-prolapsed parts.[14] The affected leaflets are markedly thickened, with myxomatous transformation of their atrial aspect. When the prolapse is marked, there is also dilation of the annulus, involving the attachment of the mural rather than the aortic leaflet. Part and parcel of the myxomatous proliferation of the spongy layer of the leaflet is an increased proliferation of acid mucopolysaccharides. These then impinge on the fibrous layer, with focal interruption. The end result is destruction of the fibrous core of the valve, some considering this to be the essence of the lesion.[15,16] Histological studies of the abnormal leaflets, however, reveal no appreciable inflammatory reaction. It is the accumulation of acid mucopolysaccharides, with weakening of the fibrous core of the valve, along with the inequality of cordal support to the free edge of the affected valvar leaflet, therefore, which most probably account for the pathogenesis of prolapse. A myocardial factor has been proposed by many authors but is probably not of significance. The accumulation of acid mucopolysaccharide with weakening of the fibrous tissue and impaired collagen formation is seen typically in Marfan's syndrome, and it is no coincidence that prolapsed valvar leaflets are a well-recognised feature of this syndrome. Indeed, it has been suggested that isolated prolapse is an atypical form of Marfan's syndrome.[17] As with so many controversies, the truth may well prove to lie between the two extremes, with disorders of both biochemical make-up and cordal support contributing to production of the floppy leaflets.

Anomalies of the Tension Apparatus

Anomalies of the tension apparatus include the lesions variously referred to as mitral arcade[18] or hammock[10] valve. These terms likely describe the same lesion, in which the papillary muscles extend directly to the edges of the leaflets (Fig. 35-16). In the most severe form, the muscles fuse on the leading edge of the aortic leaflet, forming the muscular arcade observed by the pathologist. When viewed from the atrial aspect, with the valve intact as seen by the surgeon, the intermixing of cords attached to the enlarged papillary muscle gives the appearance of a hammock. The abnormal

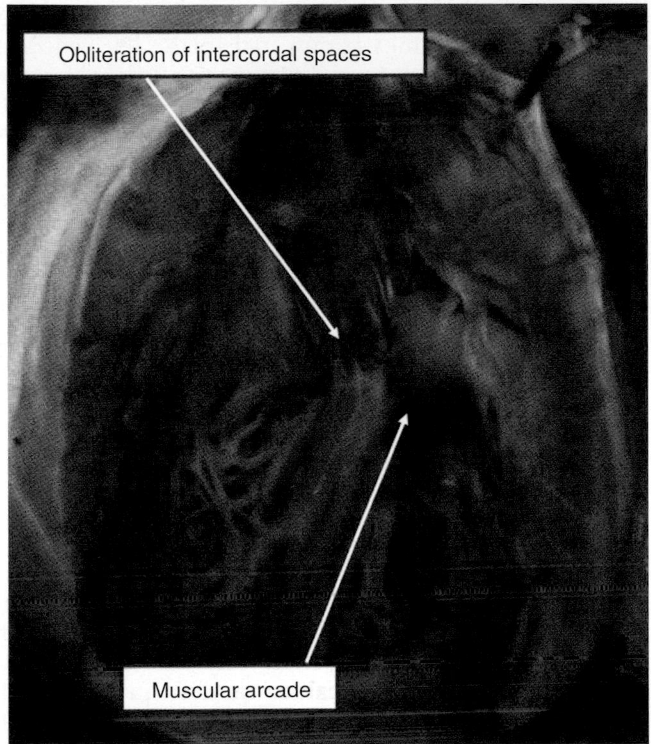

Figure 35-16 In this heart, the papillary muscles supporting the leaflets fuse along the leading edge of the aortic leaflet, producing a muscular arcade. Note also the obliteration of the intercordal spaces, which would have rendered the valve stenotic.

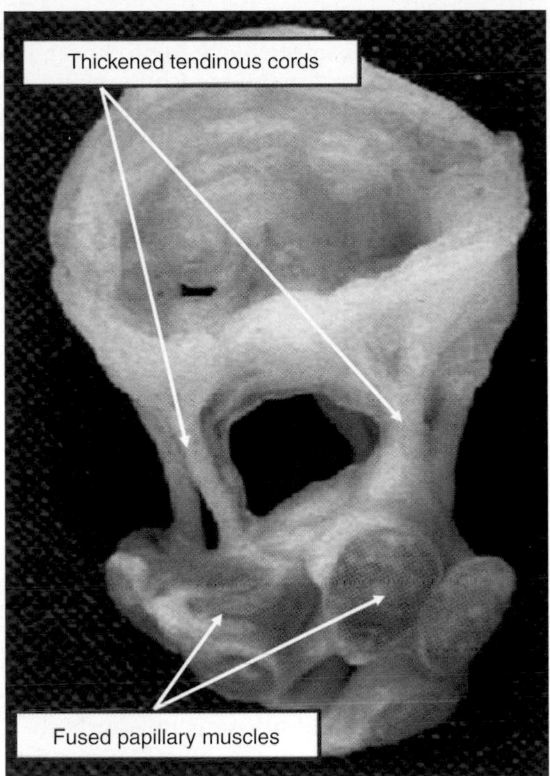

Figure 35-17 This abnormal mitral valve was removed at surgery. The papillary muscles are fused, and the tendinous cords are thickened. The arrangement of the papillary muscles bears some resemblance to a parachutist, but the open cavity of leaflets would be a lethal device!

attachments produce mitral valvar insufficiency, but the morphologic appearance suggests that the valve would also be stenotic.

Anomalies of the Papillary Muscles

It is anomalies of the papillary muscles that produce the lesion most usually described by paediatric cardiologists and surgeons as being the parachute lesion, although it must be admitted that the valve malformed in this fashion bears appreciably less similarity to a parachute than the prolapsing valve (compare Figs. 35-17 and 35-15). There is also lack of agreement as to what produces the parachute malformation when the term is applied to the papillary muscles. The situation most closely resembling the parachute is seen when the two muscles are fused to produce a solitary mass (see Fig. 35-17). The alternative arrangement that has been likened to the parachute is seen when one papillary muscle, usually the anterolateral muscle, is grossly reduced in size or even, on occasions, totally absent. The tension apparatus then has a grossly eccentric appearance, effectively inserting into a solitary papillary muscle (Fig. 35-18). It was the latter arrangement, with a solitary papillary muscle, which was illustrated by Shone and colleagues[19] when they introduced the term parachute mitral valve. This confusing situation was highlighted by Rosenquist,[20] who preferred to use the term to account for the arrangement with fused muscles. Furthermore, Carpentier and colleagues[10] described fused papillary muscles as producing parachute valves. In the detailed study of Ruckman and Van Praagh,[21] however, such cases were specifically excluded, since they did not fit the original illustration of

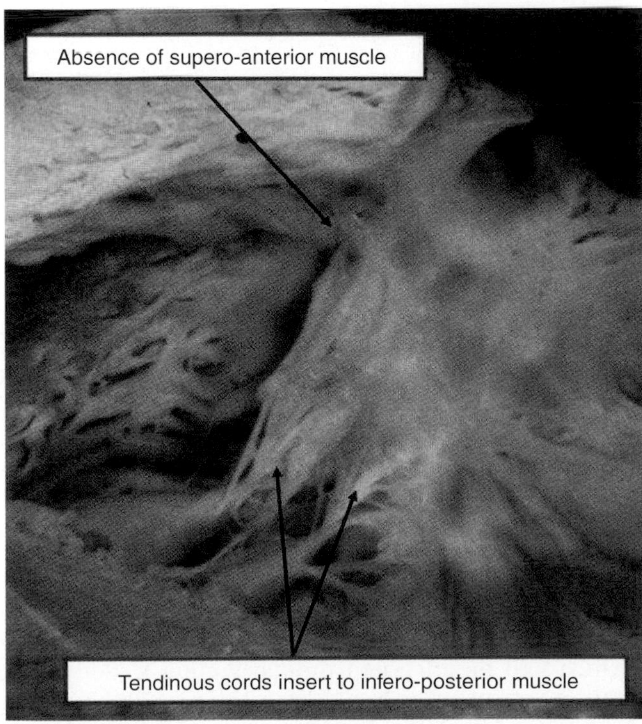

Figure 35-18 In this malformed valve, from a patient with tricuspid atresia, all the tendinous cords insert to the infero-posterior papillary muscle of the mitral valve. Some describe this arrangement as the parachute malformation.

Shone and his colleagues.[19] The form with fused papillary muscles, nonetheless, is more likely to be chosen by clinicians as their paradigm for the parachute malformation. For the morphologist, an absent or hypoplastic papillary muscle is readily recognised and described as such. Similar precision can also be provided by cross sectional echocardiography.[22] So as to remove any confusion, when we speak of parachute valves, we will specify whether we are discussing the variant produced by fusion of the papillary muscles into a solid mass, often additionally dysplastic, or whether there is hypoplasia or absence of one or other of the papillary muscles.

Stenosis versus Incompetence

It is often difficult for the morphologist to predict from a specimen whether the observed pathology would have produced stenosis or incompetence. A much better appreciation is obtained by the surgeon.[2,3,10] When insufficiency is the primary lesion, then this is most frequently the consequence of problems with the leaflets, exacerbated by dilation of the annulus. Alternatively, insufficiency as a primary feature can be caused by subvalvar problems, such as cordal retraction or elongation, or hypoplasia or agenesis of the papillary muscles. Prolapse is obviously the major substrate for many patients with mitral valvar problems. When stenosis is the major problem, this is likely to be a result of fusion along the ends of the zone of apposition between the leaflets of a dysplastic valve, a hammock lesion, a parachute deformity, or a funnel-shaped valve. Combined stenosis and insufficiency are related to fusion of the ends of the zone of apposition between the leaflets, a hammock valve, a parachute deformity, or papillary muscular hypertrophy.

Effect on the Heart

Valvar pathology always affects the cardiac pump and, despite compensatory mechanisms, may lead to serious side effects in the myocardium and endocardium. It should always be remembered that valvar pathology can also affect the pulmonary vascular bed, with pulmonary hypertension as a possible consequence.[23]

DEVELOPMENT OF THE MORPHOLOGICALLY MITRAL VALVE

The atrioventricular junction comes into prominence following the rightward looping of the heart tube after the 25th day of gestation.[7] By the end of the fifth week, the developing apical parts of the ventricles are visible, with the future left ventricle supporting the larger part of the circumference of the atrioventricular canal. The lumen of the atrioventricular canal is occupied by the inferior and superior endocardial cushions. Initially separate and discrete, these cushions eventually fuse during the sixth week, producing the right and left atrioventricular junctions, to which will be anchored the developing leaflets of the mitral and tricuspid valves. Parts of these fused cushions remain to the left side of the crest of the muscular ventricular septum, forming the scaffold of the aortic leaflet of the mitral valve.

Formation of the normal mitral valve can proceed only when the aorta becomes committed to the left ventricle, permitting the development of fibrous continuity between one of the leaflets of the mitral valve and two of the leaflets of the aortic valve, hence the name of aortic leaflet for the mitral component, which distinguishes it from its mural counterpart. Initially, there is still a cleft at the parietal margins of the site of fusion of the superior and inferior cushions within the left ventricle. The mural leaflet of the mitral valve is formed by protrusion and growth of a sheet of atrioventricular myocardium into the ventricular lumen, with subsequent formation of valvar mesenchyme on its surface, rather than by delamination of the lateral cushion from the ventricular myocardium, as was previously thought. The myocardial layer is then removed by apoptosis.[24] The aortic leaflet of the mitral valve, along with parts of the septal leaflet of the tricuspid valve, develops from mesenchyme of the superior and inferior atrioventricular cushions. Whereas the septal leaflet of the tricuspid valve delaminates from the ventricular myocardium, the aortic leaflet is never attached to, or supported, by the myocardium, except at its cranial and caudal margins, which develop with cordal and papillary muscular attachments to the left ventricular wall. Expansion of the inferior quadrants of the left atrioventricular junction involves growth of the parietal wall of the left ventricle, with comparable growth of the lateral cushion. This eventually results in the lateral cushion occupying two-thirds of the circumference of the developing mitral valvar orifice.

This expanded crescent is associated with compacting columns in the trabecular layer of the ventricular muscle, which eventually form the papillary muscles. Excessive or abnormal compaction of this trabecular layer of the developing ventricular myocardium is responsible for the parachute mitral valve. Failure of the formation of the tendinous chords from the myocardial primordiums results in the mitral arcade lesion, with muscle extending from the tips of the leaflets to the papillary muscles. When Ebstein's malformation of the mitral valve occurs, it is the mural leaflet that is involved, as this is the leaflet that excavates from the parietal ventricular wall.

Reciprocal signaling between the endocardial and myocardial cell layers in the cushion is mediated in part by members of the TGF-β family, and induces a transformation of endocardial cells into mesenchymal cells. Sox 9 is activated when myocardial cells undergo mesenchymal transformation. Sox 9 deficient mesenchymal cells fail to express ErbB3, which is required for proliferation of the cells within the endocardial cushions. The mesenchymal cells migrate into the cushions, and differentiate into the fibrous tissue of the valves. Several genes play a role in formation of the valvar leaflets, including calcineurin, with signalling and downstream activation dependent on the NFAT family of transcription factors. Absence of any of these genes results in fatal defects of valvar formation.[25]

INCIDENCE AND AETIOLOGY

Congenital deformities of the mitral valve are rare, if those involving the left valve in hearts with common atrioventricular junction are excluded, with mitral stenosis occurring in 0.6% of postmortems and in 0.21% to 0.42% of clinical series.[26] Congenital mitral incompetence is even rarer.

There is a male to female ratio of around 1.5 to 1 to 2.2 to 1.[26,27] Congenital mitral valvar anomalies are rarely isolated. The fully developed syndrome of so-called parachute mitral valve,[19] for example, includes four obstructions within the left heart, namely the valvar lesion itself, supravalvar mitral ring, subaortic stenosis and aortic coarctation. Any of these obstructions may co-exist with any congenital lesion afflicting the mitral valve, particularly coarctation. In a clinical series of patients with congenital mitral stenosis, excluding hypoplasia of the left heart, almost three-quarters had additional anomalies.[26] It is tempting to imagine that development of one abnormality upstream may, during morphogenesis, result in a series of more distal abnormalities owing to disturbance in the patterns of flow. Annular hypoplasia of the mitral valve is almost always associated with hypoplasia of the left ventricle and aortic stenosis or atresia. Ventricular septal defect is quite common in this setting, and double outlet right ventricle and tetralogy of Fallot occasionally occur. When the mitral valve is imperforate, left ventricular hypoplasia is inevitable unless there is an associated ventricular septal defect.[21]

PATHOPHYSIOLOGY

Supravalvar mitral ring and congenital mitral stenosis are, by and large, indistinguishable in their effects. Unless specific differences are mentioned, they may be assumed to behave in the same way. Pure mitral stenosis, or imperforate mitral valve, results in a diastolic pressure difference between the left atrium and left ventricle with a consequent elevation of left atrial pressure. Patients in sinus rhythm, the great majority, have a tall a wave in the left atrial trace. Co-existence of an interatrial communication results in decompression of the left atrium. This may be so profound as to obscure or eliminate the transmitral pressure difference, even when the mitral valve is imperforate. By contrast, excessive flow through the mitral valve, as may result from an associated ventricular septal defect, will exaggerate the transmitral diastolic pressure difference. Elevation of the left atrial pressure usually results in reflex pulmonary vasoconstriction, particularly if the development of pulmonary oedema results in mismatch between ventilation and perfusion, and pulmonary venous hypoxaemia. The combined effect is to produce pulmonary hypertension. In the presence of associated patency of the arterial duct, or a ventricular septal defect, this can result in right-to-left shunting at an earlier age than would be expected were mitral obstruction not present. The rise in pulmonary vascular resistance, and consequent fall in pulmonary blood flow, means that, on sequential cardiac catheterisations in individuals with mitral stenosis, the gradient is frequently found to fall. This finding is similar to medical intervention using nitric oxide in patients with congenital mitral stenosis,[28] where it was observed that the pulmonary vasoreactivity was greater than previously reported in adults. In the absence of pulmonary stenosis, and without any communication at great arterial or ventricular level, the pulmonary arterial systolic pressure may exceed systemic pressure. Right heart failure may then ensue. By contrast, severe pulmonary stenosis in the setting of a ventricular septal defect may mask entirely the effects of the valvar obstruction by reducing the flow of blood to the lungs. Left atrial pressure is bound to be lower than pulmonary arterial pressure, irrespective of the severity of the mitral obstruction. Pure mitral insufficiency may cause left atrial hypertension with all the consequences already described. More commonly, considerable left atrial dilation occurs, with the result that left atrial hypertension is modest or non-existent. Cardiac output is maintained with a normal left ventricular ejection fraction by a modest increase in left ventricular end-systolic volume and a marked increase in left ventricular end-diastolic volume. This is not as striking as the increase in left atrial volume. The regurgitant fraction may be as high as 83%. Associated obstructive lesions downstream obviously increase the severity of the mitral regurgitation. In contrast to rheumatic mitral disease, the congenitally malformed mitral valve is usually either obstructed or regurgitant. An intermediate situation is produced in the rare case of mixed stenosis and incompetence.

CLINICAL PRESENTATION AND SYMPTOMATOLOGY

Congenital disease of the mitral valve usually presents as a result of the associated abnormalities, such as coarctation or ventricular septal defect. In these lesions, the symptoms are exacerbated by the presence of the mitral valvar problem, but this may be too subtle to detect. As already mentioned, the effects of the valvar anomaly are more or less neutralised by pulmonary stenosis and an interventricular communication. So, whatever the associated anomaly, the result tends to be that mitral disease is masked, and will not be recognised unless specially looked for. The presentation of isolated mitral valvar disease is largely determined by the height of the left atrial pressure. If this is normal, there are usually no symptoms at all. At most, there will be fatigue after severe exertion. A high left atrial pressure is likely to result in poor feeding, sweating in infancy, and failure to thrive. Patients with severe obstruction are likely to present in intractable cardiac failure in the first month or so of life. Orthopnoea is extremely rare, but patients frequently complain of a dry nocturnal cough. Wheezing and respiratory infections are frequent. Syncope, haemoptysis, or aphonia owing to compression of the recurrent laryngeal nerve by an enlarged left atrium, have occasionally been described. Pure mitral stenosis is characterised by poor nourishment, tachypnoea, and intercostal recession. There are normal-to-small peripheral arterial pulses, and the jugular venous pulse is also usually normal. If pulmonary hypertension is severe, a prominent a wave will reflect the raised right ventricular end-diastolic pressure. A systolic wave will demonstrate secondary tricuspid incompetence. Palpation of the heart will reveal either a normal impulse or right ventricular hypertrophy, and there may be an apical diastolic thrill. Pulmonary valvar closure will be palpable if pulmonary hypertension is severe. The first heart sound is either normal or loud and, in contrast to rheumatic mitral stenosis, an opening snap is only occasionally audible. Closure of the pulmonary valve is accentuated in patients with pulmonary hypertension. There is a loud low-pitched mid-diastolic murmur at the apex, usually with presystolic accentuation. Occasionally, no diastolic murmur is heard. In severe untreated disease, an early diastolic murmur of pulmonary incompetence and a pan-systolic murmur of tricuspid incompetence may be heard, both resulting from pulmonary hypertension. Crepitations may be heard in the lung fields, but these are usually clear. Cyanosis is not seen unless there is severe pulmonary venous desaturation, or a right-to-left shunt through an associated defect.

PURE MITRAL INSUFFICIENCY

Most children are well nourished and in no distress. The peripheral pulses are usually normal, though sometimes jerky because of the predominant ejection of blood in early, rather than late, systole. The jugular venous pulse is normally not elevated. On palpation of the heart, left rather than right hypertrophy is usually discovered. On auscultation, the first and second heart sounds are usually normal, except in the relatively rare case of pulmonary hypertension. There is a blowing pan-systolic murmur at the apex. The pan-systolic murmur of ventricular septal defect is much rougher, is maximal at the left sternal border, and does not radiate to the axilla. If mitral regurgitation is more than mild to moderate, an apical third heart sound will be heard, followed in severe cases by a diastolic flow murmur. This diastolic murmur, particularly if it is accompanied by a third sound, does not necessarily indicate stenosis. When congenital mitral anomalies are associated with other cardiac defects, the physical signs are usually dominated by the other lesions. In particular, an imperforate mitral valve generates no direct physical signs, though evidence of pulmonary hypertension is almost invariable. The main clue to the presence of mitral stenosis in association with other defects is an inappropriately prominent mid-diastolic murmur. A typical example would be that of a 6-month-old child who, in earlier life, had typical signs of ventricular septal defect and yet who now has all the signs of Eisenmenger's syndrome except an unexpected loud mid-diastolic murmur, often with presystolic accentuation. Care has to be taken with many children with aortic coarctation, and a few with discrete subaortic stenosis. Such patients may have short apical mid-diastolic murmurs, which, for reasons that are not obvious, disappear after resection of the obstruction.

INVESTIGATIONS

Electrocardiography

Sinus rhythm is the rule in children, though first-degree heart block is common, particularly when the left atrium is greatly enlarged. Left atrial hypertrophy occurs in about nine-tenths of patients, and right atrial hypertrophy is the rule in patients with pulmonary hypertension. In mitral stenosis, the mean frontal QRS axis is usually normal, or to the right and inferior, whereas it is generally normal in mitral incompetence. The pattern of ventricular hypertrophy reflects the underlying haemodynamics. Consequently, patients with mitral stenosis tend to have right ventricular hypertrophy, while those with mitral incompetence have left ventricular hypertrophy. All of these findings are modified by associated abnormalities. In patients with the physical signs of mitral regurgitation, the electrocardiogram provides important clues to the presence of atrioventricular septal defects with common atrioventricular junction, when there is a superior counter-clockwise QRS loop, and discordant atrioventricular connections, characterised by Q waves in the right and inferior precordial leads. Mitral regurgitation secondary to anomalous origin of the left coronary artery from the pulmonary trunk is suggested by a pattern of anterolateral infarction.

Chest Radiography

Whatever the nature of the mitral abnormality, cardiac enlargement tends to be considerable. Splaying of the bronchuses by the enlarged left atrium is particularly prominent. Infants with imperforate mitral valve, or severe mitral stenosis, very occasionally show the ground-glass appearance of pulmonary oedema. More commonly, left atrial hypertension is manifested in older children by Kerley B lines and diversion of blood to the upper lobes. In infants, the pulmonary trunk and left atrial appendage do not form discrete bulges on the upper left cardiac border, which is consequently straighter than normal. In older children, prominence of the left atrial appendage is the rule and, in patients with pulmonary hypertension, the pulmonary trunk is prominent. These appearances may be profoundly modified by associated abnormalities. If the ascending aorta is seen on the left upper cardiac border and the patient has clinical features of mitral incompetence, then congenitally corrected transposition with tricuspid rather than mitral incompetence is the most likely diagnosis.

Echocardiography

M-mode echocardiography provides non-specific evidence as to enlargement of the left ventricle, left atrium, and right ventricle. It is unhelpful in diagnosing mitral incompetence. A number of features are suggestive of mitral stenosis, but none of them is invariably present. These include anterior movement of the mural leaflet in diastole, a prolonged time to reach one-fifth of the peak rate in change of left ventricular dimensions, and a reduced peak rate of these changes in dimension.[29] A flattening of the E-F slope is again suggestive, but difficult to recognise in infants with tachycardia (Fig. 35-19). The time from closure of the aortic to opening of the mitral valve, and from left ventricular minimum dimension to mitral opening, have proved unhelpful as indicators of congenital mitral stenosis,[30] though they are useful in assessment of acquired mitral valvar disease.

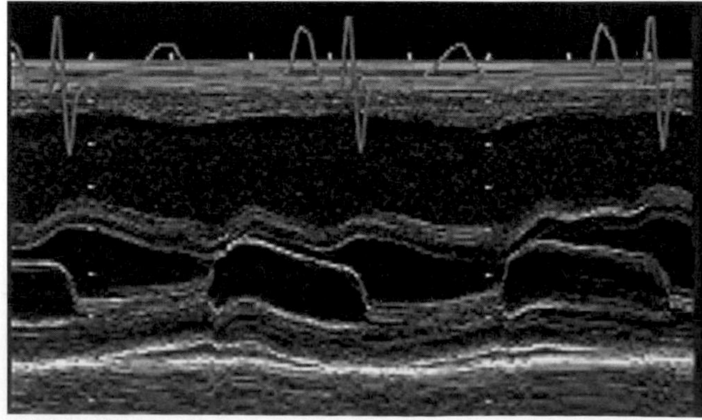

Figure 35-19 This M-mode echocardiogram is from a patient with mitral valvar stenosis. Note the prolonged E-F slope, and the anterior motion of the mural leaflet.

Cross Sectional Echocardiography

The advent of this modality made a major difference to the non-invasive understanding of pathology.[28] Assessment usually consists of short-axis scans from the apex of the left ventricle to the base, carried out from both subcostal and precordial windows. In such scans, the papillary muscles normally appear at 3 and 8 o'clock in the parasternal short-axis view.[29] In the parachute valve, the two muscles are usually fused into one. The alternative arrangement, with hypoplasia or absence of one papillary muscle, may also be observed, particularly in patients with associated coarctation.[29] The paired papillary muscles are frequently closer together (Fig. 35-20) in cases with coarctation of the aorta.[31] As the beam is moved towards the base, so the mitral orifice appears. This is normally symmetrical but is frequently eccentric in patients with congenital mitral stenosis; consequently, standard cuts give little idea of the severity of stenosis. This view is also of value for recognising the anomalous mitral arcade.[32] The most striking and important abnormality recognised in these short-axis sections is the isolated cleft of the aortic, or anterior, leaflet. This appears as a splitting of the leaflet into two during diastole. The cleft points to the left ventricular outflow tract, not the septum,[33] and is seen in normal short-axis planes,[34] not the horizontal precordial plane, which best demonstrates the zone of apposition between the left ventricular components of the bridging leaflets in atrioventricular septal defect with common atrioventricular junction (Figs. 35-21 and 35-22). When it is the mitral valve that is involved, the orientation of the papillary muscles is also normal in the majority of cases.[35] Cordal attachments from the edges of the cleft aortic leaflet are frequently observed. In hearts with discordant ventriculo-arterial connections, or double outlet right ventricle with subpulmonary ventricular septal defect,[36] particularly in the presence of a straddling mitral valve (Fig. 35-23), we have observed that the cleft appears to be more asymmetrical, pointing towards the anterolateral aspect of the left ventricle. This, in turn, is often associated with medial rotation of the supero-posterior papillary muscle. It has been questioned on embryological premises whether this represents a true cleft in the mitral valve as opposed to a commissure.[37] In functional terms, however, the space is not a usual zone of apposition between valvar leaflets, and it requires closure at surgery.

The short-axis view also provides an excellent means for identifying dual orifices in the mitral valve (Fig. 35-24), particularly when each orifice is supported by its own papillary muscle.[38,39] Parasternal long-axis sections permit further assessment of texture and mobility of the leaflets. They frequently demonstrate crowding of the subvalvar apparatus, with difficulty in differentiating between the leaflet and the tension apparatus to which it is fused. This is particularly valuable for detecting a so-called supramitral ring, which is usually associated with both valvar and subvalvar pathology (Fig. 35-25). As has been emphasised, the ring is usually related intimately to the valvar leaflets.[12] The ring,

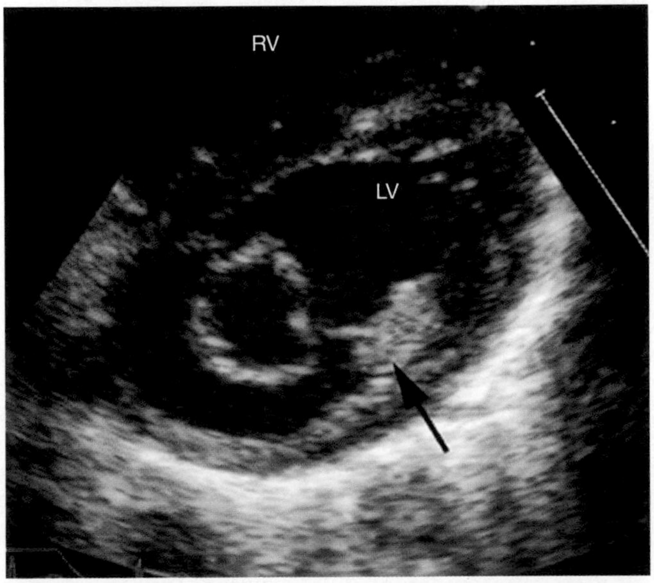

Figure 35-20 This short-axis echocardiographic view shows a patient with a dominant anterolateral papillary muscle (*arrow*). Note that most of the mitral valve is inserted into this dominant muscle. LV, left ventricle; RV, right ventricle.

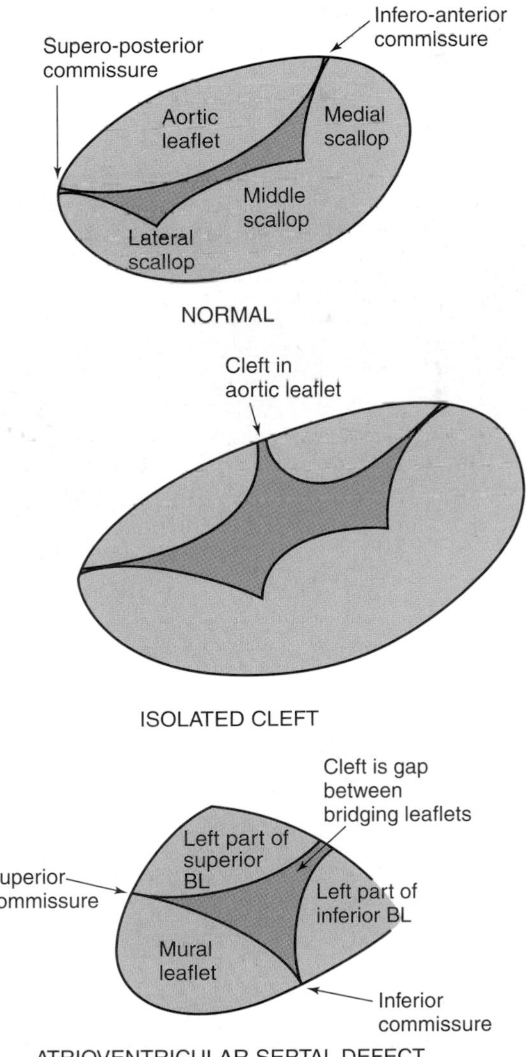

Figure 35-21 The diagram shows the difference between an isolated cleft in the aortic leaflet of the mitral valve, and the zone of apposition between the left ventricular components of the bridging leaflets (BL) seen in atrioventricular septal defect with common atrioventricular junction. Note that the isolated cleft of the aortic leaflet points to the left ventricular outflow tract, while the zone of apposition between the bridging leaflets is directed towards the ventricular septum.

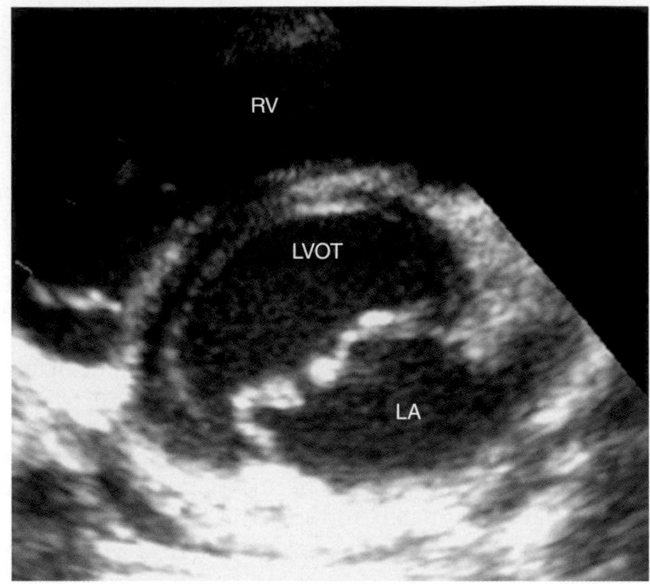

Figure 35-22 This precordial short-axis view demonstrates an isolated cleft in the aortic leaflet of the otherwise normal mitral valve. Note the thickened edges of the cleft. LA, left atrium; LVOT, left ventricular outflow tract; RV, right ventricle.

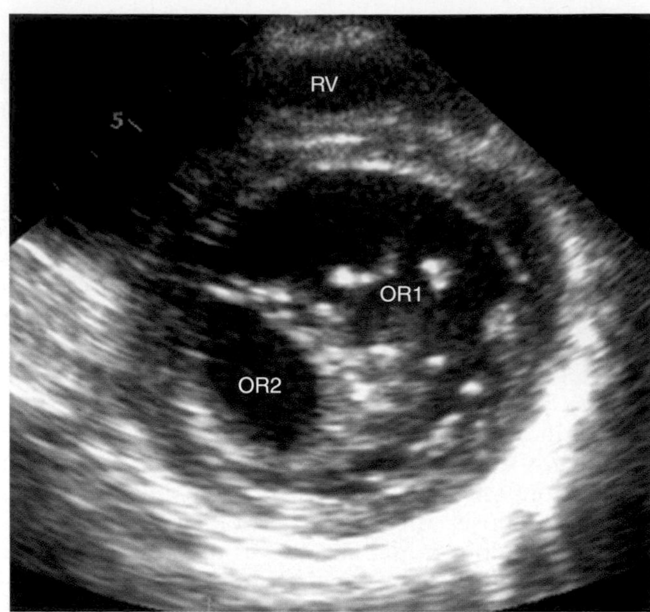

Figure 35-24 The precordial short-axis view demonstrates a double orifice in the mitral valve. Note that one orifice is smaller than its counterpart. OR1, orifice 1; OR2, orifice 2; RV, right ventricle.

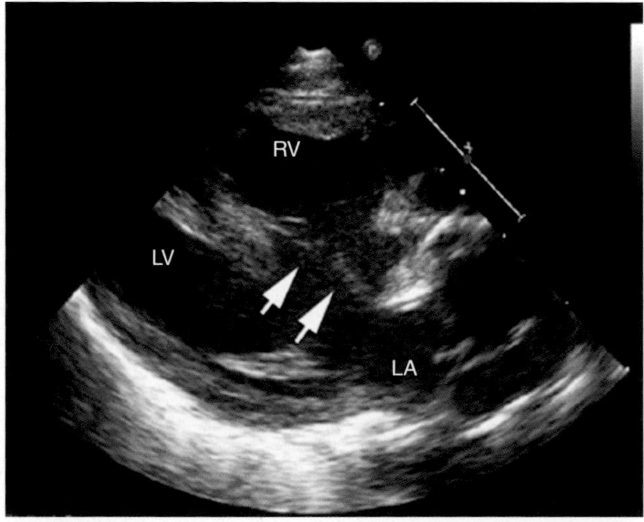

Figure 35-23 The parasternal long-axis view demonstrates straddling of the aortic leaflet of the mitral valve (*arrow*). Note that it attaches to the right side of the upper margin of the ventricular septum. LA, left atrium, LV, left ventricle; RV, right ventricle.

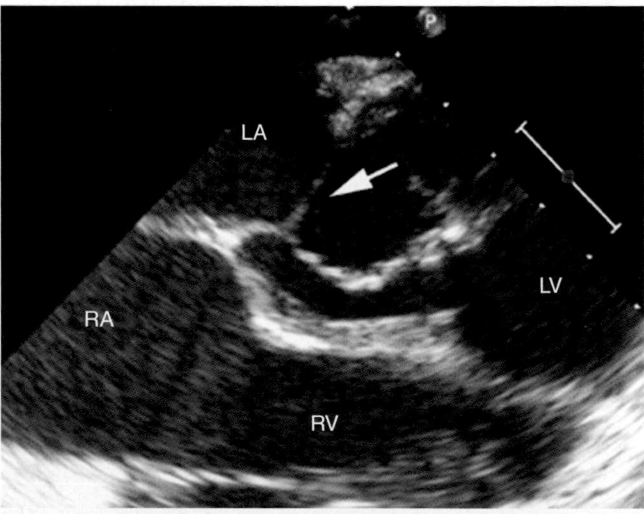

Figure 35-25 This transoesophageal echocardiogram shows a so-called supramitral ring (*arrow*), with attachments to the aortic leaflet of the valve. Note that the fibrous ring is attached within the funnel of the valvar leaflets. Also note the abnormal thickening of the valvar leaflets. LA, left atrium; LV, left ventricle; RA, right atrium; RV, right ventricle.

which starts at the annulus, extends downwards onto the valve leaflets, such that at first glance the echocardiographer has the impression that it is an intravalvar structure.

Normal values have been published for mitral annular dimensions as seen in parasternal long-axis and apical four-chamber views.[40] In the great majority of patients with congenital mitral stenosis, these values are normal. Occasionally, particularly in the presence of a ventricular septal defect, annular hypoplasia can be the main component of the mitral stenosis. Four-chamber sections, either from the apical or subcostal approach, complete the morphological picture, with the former providing the best location for Doppler assessment of any valvar gradient. As in the parasternal long-axis view, the valve appears to be thickened, with evidence of doming during the cardiac cycle (Fig. 35-26). The presence of a supramitral ring is also appreciated in this position. This position is also suitable for diagnosing the rare finding of Ebstein's malformation of the mitral valve, and for assessing left atrial size. In this condition, the aortic leaflet of the mitral valve originates normally with respect to the tricuspid valve, but the mural leaflet is displaced downwards.[6] Mitral regurgitation secondary to myocardial dysfunction is suggested by poor myocardial contractility and/or dyskinesis.

It is essential to demonstrate origin of the left coronary artery from the aortic root in all patients with the clinical picture of pure mitral regurgitation, bearing in mind

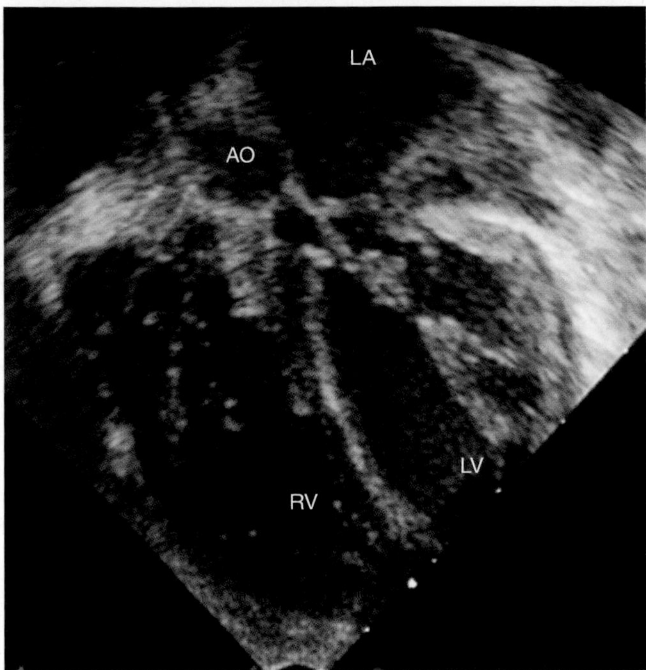

Figure 35-26 The four-chamber view shows dysplastic mitral valvar stenosis. Note the thickened leaflets, shortened cords, and an associated so-called supramitral ring. AO, aorta; LA, left atrium; LV, left ventricle, RV, right ventricle.

that, in patients with a pericardial effusion, the transverse sinus of the pericardium may be mistaken for the left coronary artery by the inexperienced observer. If not diligently sought, anomalous origin or atresia of the left coronary artery may well be missed. With the advent of colour flow Doppler, in conjunction with a measurement of the right coronary artery,[41,42] it is now rare to miss the diagnosis. Imperforate mitral valve may be recognised as a thin, sometimes mobile, membrane between the left atrium and left ventricle, which can usually, but not invariably, be distinguished from the thick wedge produced by the atrioventricular groove when the left atrioventricular connection is absent. In other cases, the mitral valvar regurgitation can be caused by dysplastic leaflets that are relatively immobile, thus preventing full coaptation during systole (Fig. 35-27). From personal experience, the mural leaflet seems to be involved more frequently in this process.[11]

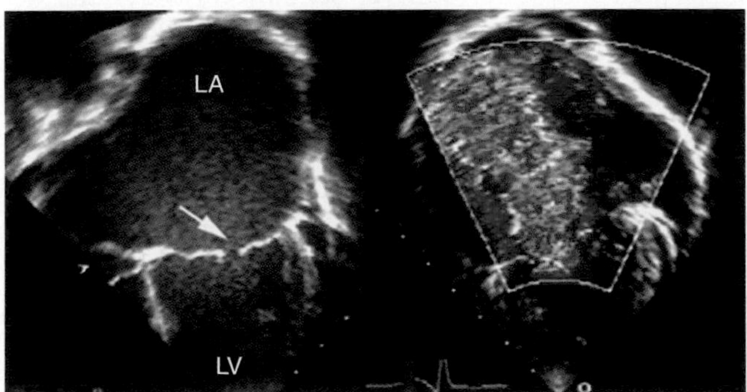

Figure 35-27 The cross sectional image, and colour Doppler display, in a patient with dysplastic mitral valvar regurgitation. There is poor coaptation of the leaflets (*arrow*), with a large central jet of regurgitation. LA, left atrium; LV, left ventricle.

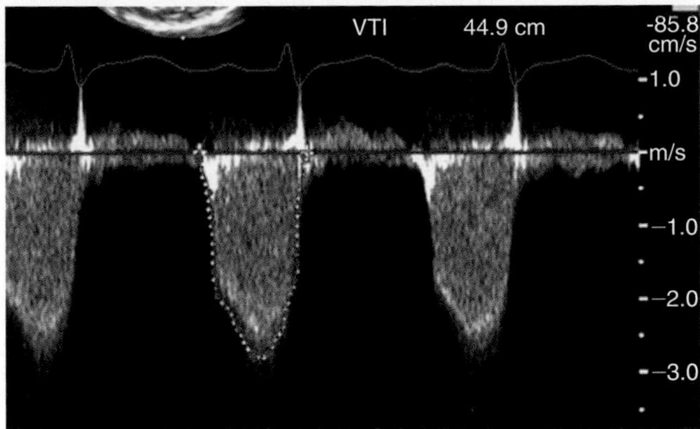

Figure 35-28 The continuous wave tracing shows the flows across a stenotic mitral valve. Using this trace, it is possible to calculate the mean gradient across the valve (see Chapter 18A).

Pulsed and Continuous Wave Doppler Echocardiography

Doppler echocardiography has had a major impact on the evaluation of mitral valvar disease, in the areas of both stenosis and regurgitation. With mitral valvar stenosis, a turbulent inflow jet is seen, both by pulsed and continuous wave Doppler. The latter modality can be used to calculate the gradient across the valve, and also its area. In adults and older patients, the pressure half-time provides an accurate assessment of area, independent of cardiac output. This same technique can be applied to children, although absolute areas calculated in this way are of little value because of the wide variation in body surface area.[43] Mean gradients across the valve, as assessed using colour flow images, have traditionally been used in assessment of congenitally malformed hearts (Fig. 35-28), despite the limitation of their dependency on cardiac output.[43] In our laboratory, we use a combination of pressure half-time, mean mitral gradient, and left atrial size to assess the severity of congenital mitral valvar stenosis. This, in conjunction with an assessment of pulmonary arterial pressure, either resulting from tricuspid regurgitation or pulmonary insufficiency, completes the haemodynamic evaluation.

While pulsed Doppler flow mapping has fallen from grace in assessing the severity of mitral regurgitation, it still plays a small semiquantitative role through the use of pulmonary venous sampling. In general, reversed systolic flow is seen in hearts with more severe regurgitation.[44] A quantitative measurement of regurgitant volume and fraction can be obtained using pulsed Doppler techniques. This is achieved by calculating the difference between forward stroke volume through the aorta and that measured through the mitral valve, the latter consisting of normal pulmonary venous return plus the regurgitant volume.[45]

The contribution of colour flow Doppler in this lesion is twofold. First, it excludes or establishes associated regurgitation and, second, it pinpoints the site of obstruction and the pattern of flow through the valve (Fig. 35-29). In patients with an associated supramitral ring, the variance starts just above the annulus. In the other forms, it starts below the level of the annulus. This technique also provides valuable clues about the site of exit of the blood. In a parachute valve, for example, there appears to be a conical jet of blood, whereas in those with two papillary muscles, the jet is more dispersed. Assessment of mitral valvar regurgitation is well suited to the technology of colour flow Doppler. This

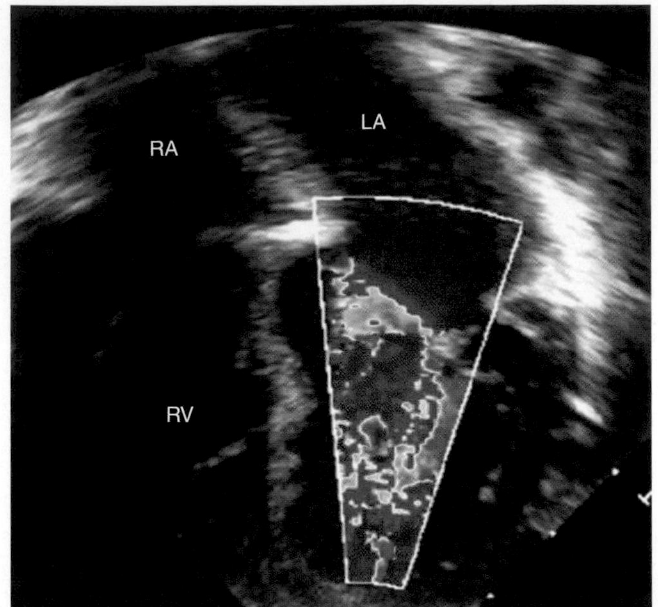

Figure 35-29 The colour flow tracing comes from the same patient as shown in Figure 35-28. Note that there is aliasing just beyond the annulus, with variance distal to that. LA, left atrium; RA, right atrium; RV, right ventricle.

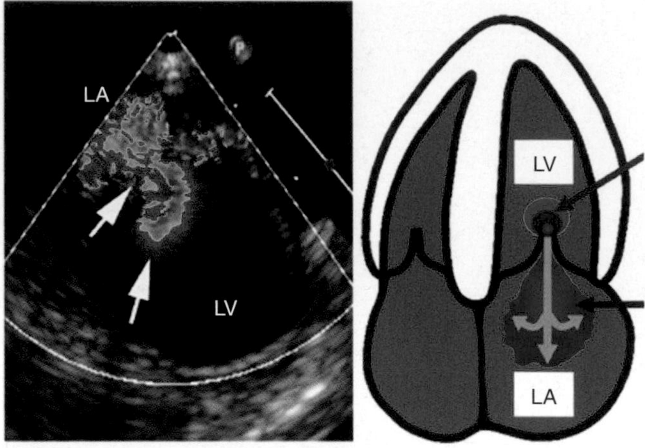

Figure 35-30 The anatomy of a regurgitant jet as revealed by colour Doppler interrogation. The *red arrow* represents the aliasing velocities, the so-called PISA, while the *black arrow* shows the regurgitant jet in the left atrium. The *upper white arrow* in the left hand picture is pointing at the so-called vena contracta, while the *lower white arrow* shows the PISA. LA, left atrium; LV, left ventricle.

technique permits an accurate assessment of the site of the regurgitant jet, for example from the edges of a cleft mitral valve or at the site of prolapse in those with floppy leaflets. It also provides information regarding the direction of the jet, along with the extent to which the velocity signal can be observed in the left atrium. One of the major problems, however, is that mapping of flow provides only a semiquantitative assessment of the severity of the regurgitation, as the echocardiographer measures velocity not volume. Despite this limitation, a reasonably reliable assessment of severity is possible, particularly if more than one plane is used. Limitations relate to depth, position of the jet in relationship to the atrial wall, gain settings, driving pressure, and transmitted frequency.[46,47] Similarly, in large populations of apparently normal subjects, physiological mitral regurgitation is encountered in up to around two-fifths of individuals.[48]

More recently, attempts have been made to assess the volume of flow by using other techniques, such as calculations of the proximal isovelocity surface area, or PISA, by cross sectional echocardiography (Fig. 35-30), and the width of the jet.[49–52] These are, potentially, the key to an accurate assessment of volume of flow, which can then be related to changes in left ventricular dimension. The problem with calculation of the proximal isovelocity surface area is that it does not account for varying shapes of the regurgitant orifice. A recent study comparing use of this feature in the calculation of regurgitant volume, to that measured by real-time three-dimensional echocardiography, showed that the former method significantly underestimated the true volume.[52]

The problem, at present, is that it is not clear whether an increase in the size of a ventricle represents a deterioration in ventricular function, or just an alteration to accommodate an increase in regurgitant volume.[53] As a result of problems in calculating absolute regurgitant volumes reproducibly by Doppler echocardiography, the role of this method in children has still to be established. It is probably safer to extrapolate from data obtained in adults using an indexed end-systolic diameter of greater than 4.5 cm, or an ejection fraction by volumetric assessment of less than 60%, as echocardiographic indications of the need for valvar surgery.[54,55]

The more recent advent of transoesophageal echocardiography has provided an additional tool for the evaluation of the congenitally abnormal mitral valve. Fortunately, apart form the older child or obese patient, this technique is unnecessary in most children. It is also apparent that transoesophageal colour flow mapping appears to be more sensitive than transthoracic assessment. Systematic overestimation of the severity of regurgitation is found when it is compared with standard transthoracic assessment.[56,57] Despite this difference, both techniques provide a good correlation with angiography and surgery.[57,58]

Three-Dimensional Echocardiography

Until recently, adequate three-dimensional echocardiographic images of the mitral valve were possible only using the transoesophageal rotational system, which could be used only in children weighing more than 13 to 14 kg. The technique also usually required intubation, which resulted in minimal practical application for children. Likewise, due to the rotational nature of the collection of data, little information was typically obtained regarding the subvalvar apparatus. With the recent advent of the matrix array real-time three-dimensional echocardiographic system, a whole new world has opened up to the echocardiographer. More recently, a higher frequency matrix array transthoracic probe has become available which permits imaging in neonates and infants. Importantly, this permits the echocardiographer to image not only the leaflets, but also the subvalvar apparatus (Figs. 35-31 and 35-32). The data can be displayed so as to provide a surgical view, thus permitting the surgeon finally to understand the presented echocardiographic images. Another important view is that seen from the left ventricular aspect. This permits a more detailed assessment of the zones of apposition between the edges of the leaflets. The leaflets billow naturally in systole, which

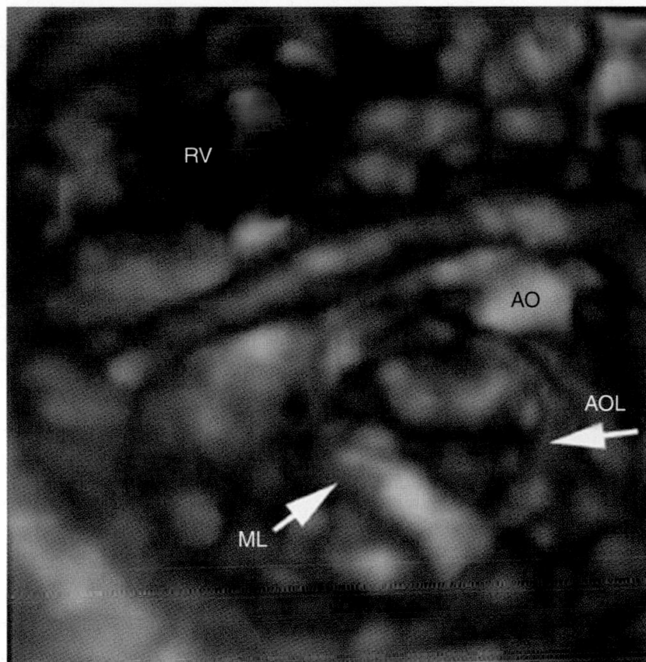

Figure 35-31 The three-dimensional echocardiographic image shows a dysplastic mitral valve with associated stenosis. Note the thickened aortic and mural leaflets. There is some tethering of the mural leaflet, seen near the end of the zone of apposition between the leaflets. AO, aorta; AOL, aortic leaflet; ML, mural leaflet; RV, right ventricle.

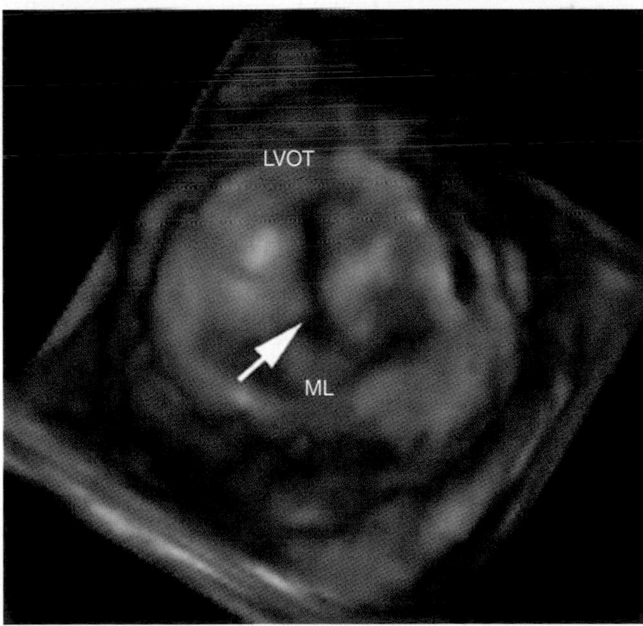

Figure 35-32 This three-dimensional echocardiographic image shows a cleft (*arrow*) in the aortic leaflet of the mitral valve, as seen from the left ventricle. The cleft points towards the left ventricular outflow tract. LVOT, left ventricular outflow tract; ML, mural leaflet.

makes assessment of their zone of apposition difficult in some cases when viewed in surgical fashion. This can, in part, be overcome by cropping just below the annulus of the mitral valve when seen in this view. It is also possible to combine real-time three-dimensional colour Doppler imaging, which helps provide an improved understanding of regurgitant jets. This technique also provides details regarding regurgitation through the zone of apposition, which has previously been difficult to demonstrate using standard cross sectional imaging. There is already data emerging to show the additional benefit of three-dimensional echocardiography in adults with mitral valvar pathology.[59–62] At present, there is some data acquired in children showing the benefit of the technique in evaluating left atrioventricular valves, particularly with regards to abnormalities of the zones of apposition between the leaflets.[63,64]

Magnetic Resonance Imaging

This technique is currently finding its role in the routine investigation of the child with a congenitally malformed heart. So far, its strengths have revolved around the evaluation of the extracardiac anatomy, in particular the aortic arch and pulmonary arteries, where detailed structural information is available. The technique is equally suited to the evaluation of intracardiac structures, both static and dynamic. The mitral valve can be imaged in several planes, along with its supporting papillary muscles. Few data is available at present with regards to detailed anatomical descriptions of congenital anomalies. While this would be interesting, it is probably in the area of functional assessment that the technique holds the greatest promise. The ability to assess mass and volume with a high degree of accuracy, in conjunction with the determination of regurgitant volumes, is of great potential for the evaluation of the chronically regurgitant mitral valve. This is achieved by phase shift velocity mapping, which permits the assessment of mean velocities. These can then be integrated over time and, when multiplied by area, yield volume flow. Using this technique, a very good correlation has been found between measured and calculated regurgitant volumes, with a correlation coefficient of 0.99.[65] As well, it provides more reliable data with regards to mitral annular diameter when compared to cross sectional echocardiography.[65] Of note, with the introduction of three-dimensional echocardiography, this limitation of the cross sectional modality should be overcome.

Cardiac Catheterisation

The final arbiter of mitral obstruction is demonstration of a difference in diastolic pressures between the left atrium and ventricle. Murphy's law dictates that, when you most need to know the left atrial pressure, it is most difficult to obtain. The high left atrial pressure seems to seal the valvar mechanism of the oval foramen with remarkable effectiveness. Entry to the left atrium from the right, therefore, often demands trans-septal puncture. While this technique is remarkably safe, particularly in the hands of experts who practise it constantly, it is not to be recommended to the occasional operator. Retrograde passage of the catheter through the mitral valve is an alternative but is more difficult if the valve is stenotic. Before any of these techniques are used, efforts should be made to obtain a satisfactory pulmonary capillary wedge pressure simultaneous with the left ventricular pressure. The wedge pressure can be regarded as a reliable reflection of left atrial pressure if the wave form is undamped, fully saturated blood can be aspirated through the catheter and repeated measurements in different sites give the same pressure. Routine measurement of wedge pressures during cardiac catheterisation goes a long way towards detecting otherwise masked mitral stenosis. The documentation of a pressure gradient between the pulmonary capillary wedge pressure and the left ventricular diastolic pressure only proves the existence of mitral stenosis or supravalvar ring if the pulmonary veins are normally connected to the left atrium and there is no partition, tumour or thrombus within it. All of these can be excluded by cross sectional echocardiography.

Angiocardiography

In general, angiocardiography has been relegated to the history books for the evaluation of mitral valve pathology and function. It is rarely used in this era to diagnose lesions responsible for mitral valve regurgitation or stenosis, nor is it utilised to quantify the severity of a regurgitant valve. Although certain pathological entities can be determined by this technique, these represent an indirect evaluation, rather than the true pathology as seen by either two- or three-dimensional echocardiography.

DIFFERENTIAL DIAGNOSIS

As already emphasised, the main problem lies in recognising that a mitral valvar anomaly is present when associated defects dominate the clinical picture. Careful clinical examination and echocardiography, coupled with a high index of suspicion in patients with other left-sided obstructive lesions, provides the best means of making the diagnosis. In secondary mitral regurgitation, left ventricular dysfunction usually dominates the clinical picture, whereas left ventricular function is usually normal in primary regurgitation. The possibility of silent mitral stenosis always haunts the clinician confronted with the patient with apparently severe and irreversible pulmonary vascular disease. Currently cross sectional, three-dimensional echocardiography, and Doppler examination can rule out significant obstruction in all cases, making catheterisation is unnecessary for diagnostic purposes in patients where high-quality non-invasive investigation is possible.

COURSE AND PROGNOSIS

In this current era, patients with severe obstruction to left ventricular inflow, and relative left ventricular hypoplasia, are frequently managed along protocols involving an initial Norwood procedure, followed by a construction of cavopulmonary shunt prior to conversion to the Fontan circulation. Many of these are diagnosed prenatally, with the neonates in consequence being in a more stable condition, usually because of infusion of prostaglandins. Mitral stenosis with an adequate size left ventricle has a slightly better, but still poor, prognosis. In one series,[26] actuarial survival was shown to be 40% at 10 years of age when patients were treated medically, and 56% at the same age for surgically treated patients. At the age of 18 years, survival was 18% in both groups. Although the prognosis has improved in the current era, it still carries a higher mortality and morbidity than those presenting at a later age. Mitral incompetence has the best prognosis. Even when associated with coarctation, most patients survive childhood. The degree of mitral regurgitation may remain static, or even decrease once the coarctation is resected. Prolonged and significant mitral regurgitation will eventually depress left ventricular function, though it is unclear whether it does so at a similar rate as in adults.

MANAGEMENT

Medical Management and Timing of Intervention

For patients with congenital stenosis, medical management is frequently dictated by the nature and severity of the associated lesions. In those patients where the valvar lesion is isolated, treatment with diuretics may buy some time. Although surgical repair is possible, the long-term results are disappointing. Unfortunately, pulmonary hypertension is frequently encountered in these patients, thus forcing the hand of the cardiologist and surgeon. Until recently, surgery was the only option, but in both adults and children, angioplasty has now become the treatment of choice for those with rheumatic valvar disease, with acceptable results published in the short term.[66,67] There is little data for balloon angioplasty performed in the setting of congenital mitral valvar stenosis, albeit that encouraging results have now been reported from a single center with many years experience, the results being comparable to those provided by surgical intervention.[67] In this series, those with a supramitral ring, prior mitral valvar regurgitation, and being younger at the time of intervention, all suffered a poorer outcome after dilation. For those who did not have these adverse risk factors, there was a good initial reduction in gradient, albeit a high risk of recurrent stenosis, and with over a quarter developing significant valvar regurgitation. Regurgitation is generally managed medically until there is evidence of clinical symptoms that are not improved by standard therapeutic regimens combined with a trial of afterload reduction. With the introduction of inhibitors of angiotensin converting enzyme, which reduce the afterload on the left ventricle, morbidity and mortality have both been shown to improve in adults with left ventricular dysfunction.[68,69] Thus far, however, no studies have demonstrated that such treatment in isolation prolongs the time from diagnosis to eventual repair, or replacement in cases where regurgitation is the primary lesion, and is not secondary to left ventricular dysfunction. Indeed, in one investigation using an animal model of chronic mitral regurgitation, inhibition of angiotensin converting enzyme decreased the end-diastolic pressure in the left ventricle, along with the pulmonary capillary wedge pressure, but did not increase the forward stroke volume, nor the contractility.[70] The addition of β-blockade to the inhibition of the angiotensin converting enzyme had similar affects, although β-blockade also increased forward stroke volume and contractility.

Surgical Management

Patients with severe mitral valvar stenosis who present in the neonatal period, and frequently have some degree of left ventricular hypoplasia and aortic valvar stenosis, now tend to be managed by following the Norwood sequence of operations. This includes creating an aortopulmonary anastomosis, performing an open atrial septectomy, and constructing a shunt from the aorta to the pulmonary arteries, either centrally or peripherally, or more recently placing a conduit from the right ventricle to the pulmonary arteries. It is also possible to perform the so-called hybrid procedure, which involves banding of the right and left pulmonary arteries, stenting the persistently patent arterial duct, and in some cases, stenting the interatrial communication. The hybrid procedure, when performed, is a prelude to construction of a cavopulmonary shunt and aortic reconstruction at 4 to 5 months of age.

Outside the neonatal period, if balloon valvoplasty is not available, the best option is to attempt to repair the valve, as valvar replacement in children is still fraught with problems. The presence of intractable heart failure, severe pulmonary hypertension, or pulmonary oedema, means that the need for operation in infancy or early childhood is forced upon the management team. In contrast, in congenital mitral incompetence, the generally good prognosis with medical management means that operation can usually be postponed for as long as is possible. The exception to this conservative approach is that for the isolated cleft of the aortic, or anterior, leaflet of the valve, where the results of repair are so good as to justify surgery at any age if there is significant cardiomegaly.[71]

Reconstructive surgery currently has acceptable results with regards to mortality and morbidity over the medium term. Both a younger age at presentation and the association with additional intracardiac lesions are associated with a poorer outcome. In general, survival over the medium term is close to 90%, with a freedom from reoperation of approximately 76% over the variously reported periods of follow-up.[72–74] There are multiple surgical techniques that are tailored to the specific pathology at the levels of the annulus, leaflets, and supporting tension apparatus. Frequently, due to the complex nature of the valvar pathology, one or more of these has to be applied to an individual patient. For regurgitant valves, it is possible to perform annuloplasty, or insert mitral rings, with the latter currently being designed so as to fit the normal saddle-shape of the mitral valvar annulus. For those with dysplastic leaflets, augmentation has been employed with some success. Occasionally, it is necessary to place a stitch between the leaflets so as to create double orifices within the valve. For stenotic lesions, it is possible to resect supramitral ring, split the papillary muscles in those with the parachute malformation, enlarge the zone of apposition between the leaflets, or resect accessory valvar tissue.[75] It is also possible to shorten or transfer the tendinous cords, as well as insert synthetic cords.

Replacement of the valve is considered only after all other surgical options have been exhausted. Even in this current era, the results of valvar replacement are still somewhat disappointing, particularly in the very young child. The initial experience gained with insertion of homograft valves was disappointing, with reoperation needed in two-fifths at 5 years, and three-fifths by 7 years. As a result, this technique is rarely used in this current era. Mechanical valves are the treatment of choice, with the valves inserted usually being bileaflet and having a low profile. From several series that followed patients from 10 to 15 years, overall survival was in the mid-1960s, with freedom from the need to insert a second valve varying between 54% and 66%.[76–78] With improved management of anticoagulation, the incidences of thrombosis and infection are low, occurring in less than one-tenth. It is the need for valvar replacement, and the size of the initial prosthesis, that stratifies the patients. In many younger patients, where stenosis is the predominant lesion, there is associated annular hypoplasia that limits the size of the prosthesis which can be inserted during the initial operation. Indeed, in some cases the annulus is deemed too small, and the prosthesis has to be positioned in the supra-annular position. Although there has been some limited experience with this approach, it is not without complications.[79] To overcome this problem, some groups have used a pulmonary autograft in the so-called Ross-2 procedure. The pulmonary valve removed from the patient is sewn into a Dacron tube, which is then inserted into the mitral annulus. Although experience is limited with this technique, the initial results seem encouraging, with a low mortality, albeit that as yet there is no data over the long term.[80]

MITRAL VALVAR PROLAPSE

Incidence

Suggestions were made, based on M-mode evaluation, that prolapse could afflict up to one-third of the otherwise normal population. When cross sectional echocardiography was introduced, the incidence was still high, despite its improved spatial resolution. This was due, in part, to a lack of understanding of the anatomy of the mitral valvar annulus. This was initially believed to be planar, and hence the diagnosis of prolapse was made using both long-axis and four-chamber views. The advent of three-dimensional echocardiography has pointed to the incorrectness of these approaches, since the normal valvar annulus has high and low points, appearing like a saddle.[81] It is the anterior and posterior aspects that represent the high points, while the medial and lateral parts are the low points. Taking into account this morphology, prolapse of the leaflets should only be consistently diagnosed when using the parasternal long-axis view. Using this criterion, a report from the Framingham study demonstrated an incidence of 2.4%.[82] Such improved accuracy of diagnosis will have a profound effect on future genetic studies.

The diagnosis is rarely made in young children and indeed is exceptionally rare in neonates outside those patients having Marfan's syndrome and presenting in the neonatal period. With an improved understanding of the structure of the mitral valve, and its potential genetic implications, the lack of diagnosis in childhood points to the need for many years of stress on a potentially abnormal valve before the leaflets begin to prolapse.

Genetics

Non-syndromal prolapse is probably an autosomal dominant disorder, with variable penetrance, as there is clinical heterogeneity in families. It is well recognised that prolapsing leaflets of the mitral valve are found in patients with Marfan's syndrome, Ehlers-Danlos syndrome, osteogenesis imperfecta, dominant cutis laxa, and pseudoxanthoma elasticum. Prior studies had failed to link the familial and non-syndromal disease with fibrillar or other collagen genes. The recent ability to understand the three-dimensional nature of the mitral valve has provided greater diagnostic specificity, and this has provided an improved understanding of the genetics of the nonsyndromal variant. Based on this new understanding, myxomatous prolapse has been linked to chromosome 16 in some families with an autosomal dominant form, while in others linkages have been found with chromosome 11p15.4 and 13q31.3–q32.1. Some of the studies have identified a prodromal form, with no true prolapse, but rather with anterior shifted of the zone of coaptation, indicating elongation of the mural leaflet. Others have studied an X-linked valvar dystrophy with mutations of so-called filament A. Overall, therefore, the genetic background to mitral valvar prolapse may be similar to that found for hypertrophic cardiomyopathy, with multiple genetic abnormalities responsible for a common phenotype.[25]

That prolapse is due to a structural abnormality of the proteins has little support outside the mutations of collagen found in Ehlers-Danlos syndrome. The picture appears to be more complex than a simple mutation in fibrillin. Indeed, recent work has demonstrated that the picture is more complex. Mice with a fibrillin-1 mutation can be rescued by perinatal administration of neutralising antibodies to TGFβ, a growth factor that stimulates activity and matrix formation by the valvar interstitial cells. Fibrillin is, therefore, an important regulator of the interplay between growth factors made by interstitial cells and the cells themselves. The current theory is that fibrillin stabilises the TGFβ complex so that a mutation results in overexpression of TGFβ.

Presentation, Symptomatology, and Pathophysiology

An understanding that prolapse of the leaflets of the mitral valve represents an increase in area and length of the tissues that happens over many decades helps to explain why the lesion is uncommon in childhood and adolescence, outside of those patients with co-existing disease of the connective tissues. The leaflets billow back and cross the line of coaptation, which normally is in close proximity to the plane of the superior part of the mitral annulus. Eventually, regurgitation ensues in some patients, which progresses to resultant heart failure, and its associated symptoms. In children, therefore, the majority of patients have no symptoms at all. They present with murmurs found on routine examination, usually in late adolescence or adulthood. Early presentation should raise the suspicion of Marfan's syndrome. The intensity of the murmur is critically dependent on posture. A large minority of patients have other symptoms. The most common is chest pain, usually unrelated to activity, that is ill-defined, located to the praecordial area, is sharp and fleeting, or more prolonged. Other symptoms include dyspnoea, fatigue, light-headedness, and palpitations.

Physical Signs

It is frequent to find associated skeletal abnormalities, such as a flat chest, a straight back, or a pigeon chest. Peripheral arterial and venous pulses are normal. Palpation of the heart is usually normal, unless a honk is present. This is usually accompanied by a thrill. Careful palpation with the patient lying in left lateral position may permit detection of mid-systolic retraction. Auscultation at the apex reveals a mid-systolic click, which may be multiple; a late systolic murmur; or both.

The murmur must be heard to reach the second heart sound, if necessary by inching the stethoscope from the apex to the base. Clicks are sometimes heard only with the patient upright, or lying in the left lateral position (Fig. 35-33). As long as the murmur remains late systolic, the heart sounds can be normal. When the murmur is holosystolic, then a loud first heart sound indicates early prolapse. A soft first heart sound indicates flail leaflets. Manoeuvres that decrease left ventricular end-diastolic volume, or increase the rate of left ventricular contraction, such as sitting or standing from the supine position, the strain phase of a Valsalva manoeuvre, tachycardia, or administration of vasodilators such as amyl nitrate, all move the click and murmur closer to the first heart sound. Squatting, the release phase of the Valsalva manoeuvre, bradycardia, and administration of vasoconstrictors, in contrast, all move the click and murmur towards the second heart sound, and often make the murmur become fainter or disappear. Pregnancy also may cause disappearance of the murmur.

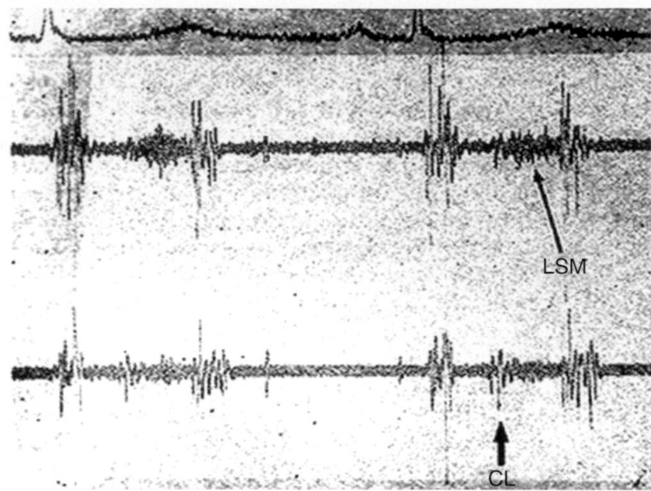

Figure 35-33 The phonocardiogram shows a mid systolic click and late systolic murmur in a patient with a floppy mitral valve. CL, click; LSM, late systolic murmur.

With prolonged follow-up, the murmur does become pan-systolic in some adults. This finding is rare in children unless they have Marfan's syndrome. An early diastolic sound or, less often, an early diastolic murmur, is occasionally heard or recorded by phonocardiography. This has been ascribed to recoaptation of the prolapsing leaflets, but could also be caused by prolapse of the leaflets of the aortic valve.

Investigations

Chest Radiography

Chest radiography usually gives normal results, apart from the skeletal abnormalities already noted. If mitral valvar regurgitation is severe, there will be an increase in the cardiothoracic ratio and the size of the left atrium.

Electrocardiography

About one-fifth of children with the auscultatory syndrome have inverted T waves in leads II, III, and aVF and rather less commonly in leads V_5 and V_6. These abnormalities may not be constant. Prolongation of the Q–Tc interval occurs in up to one-sixth of all patients.[83,84] Although brief runs of ventricular and supraventricular tachycardia have been described, many of these findings are also seen in normal individuals.[85]

Echocardiography

When the cross sectional echocardiographic appearances of prolapsing leaflets are appreciated, it becomes easier to understand how pseudo-prolapse may be produced using M-mode interrogation. Cross sectional echocardiography, and particularly the three-dimensional format, enhances the diagnosis of prolapse by enhancing the spatial configuration of the valvar leaflets.[86] During diastole, the leaflets of the normal valve lie widely open and are more-or-less parallel, as seen in parasternal long-axis sections. With the onset of systole, the two leaflets, moving in opposite directions, coapt to give a funnel-shaped appearance. As systole continues, the line of coaptation moves anteriorly and lags behind the aortic root. The entire valvar apparatus then moves anteriorly and inferiorly. Both leaflets frequently arch slightly towards each other and become more horizontal, but no part of the leaflets appears above the plane of the atrioventricular junction. In prolapsing valves, the mural or, less often, the aortic leaflet, or sometimes both, arch towards each other to an excessive degree, passing above the plane of the atrioventricular junction into the left atrium. The line of coaptation between the leaflets is displaced superiorly and posteriorly. M-mode criterions for the floppy valve syndrome are mid-systolic buckling and pan-systole hammocking. Despite these observations, there was a tremendous over-diagnosis of mitral valve prolapse by M-mode echocardiography, so much so that it is rarely used in this current era.

Cross sectional echocardiography has provided improved spatial resolution, but initially, as already explained, was just as guilty in misleading the clinician and echocardiographer. It is the observation that the valvar annulus is not perfectly circular, but rather possesses a saddle-shape, with one dimension being in a different plane to the other,[87,88] which provides an explanation for the discrepancy between findings obtained using the parasternal long-axis and four-chamber views. It has been suggested,[86] therefore, that fairly reliable signs of mitral valvar prolapse include late systolic bulging as seen on M-mode tracings, displacement of the leaflets into the left atrium by more than 2 mm as seen in the parasternal long-axis view, along with thickening of the leaflets (Fig. 35-34). Regurgitation in the setting of prolapsing leaflets is best assessed by colour flow Doppler interrogation. Care must be taken if attempts are made to quantify the severity by using the phenomenon of the proximal isovelocity surface area, since the amount of regurgitation is not constant throughout systole.[89]

Transoesophageal multi-plane echocardiography is useful in identify the specific components of the leaflets that are prolapsing. At 20 degrees interrogation, it is the medial component of the aortic leaflet, along with the lateral scallop of the mural leaflet. At 60 degrees, it is the medial and lateral scallops of the mural leaflet, along with the middle part of the aortic leaflet. Interrogation at 90 degrees shows the medial scallop of the mural leaflet, along with the lateral part of the aortic leaflet, while using scans from 120 to 160 degrees shows the middle parts of both leaflets.[58] Even though this has been helpful to the cardiologist and surgeon, such interrogation is now being replaced by three-dimensional echocardiography to aid in the diagnosis and surgical planning of patients with prolapse. Indeed, views showing the structure of the valve as seen by the surgeon in the operating room can be obtained from either the transthoracic approach using either real-time three-dimensional echocardiography or, until recently by transoesophageal echocardiography using a rotational device. There is good evidence emerging that the three-dimensional technique is superior to either transthoracic and transoesophageal cross sectional echocardiography with regards to identification of specific pathology of different parts of the leaflets, as well as abnormalities along their zone of apposition (Fig. 35-35). As this book is being prepared for publication, the transoesophageal real-time three-dimensional echocardiographic

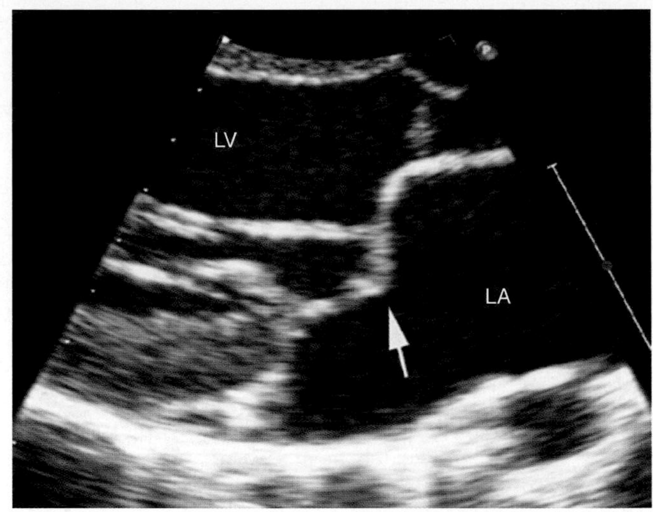

Figure 35-34 The cross sectional parasternal long-axis view in a patient with prolapsing mitral valve. Although the prolapse is seen (*arrow*) it is difficult to pinpoint which component of the aortic leaflet is involved. LA, left atrium; LV, left ventricle.

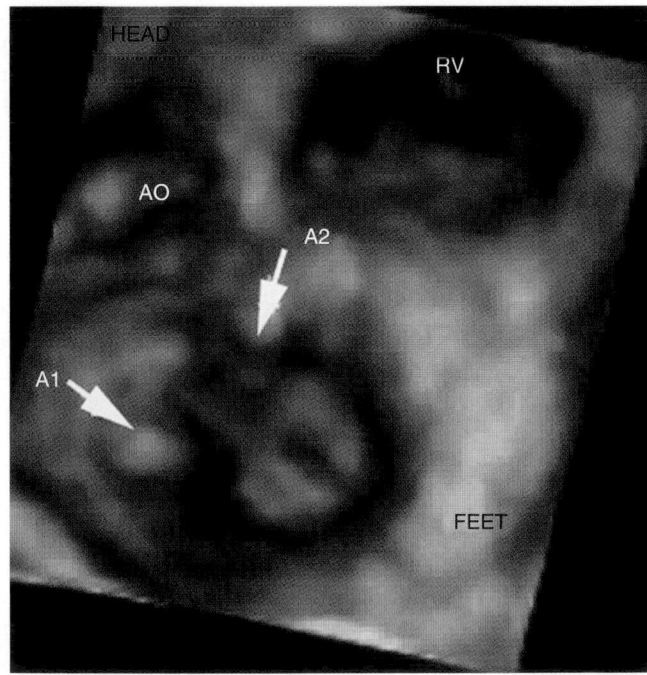

Figure 35-35 The prolapsing valve seen in Figure 35-34 as revealed by three-dimensional echocardiography, prepared so as to show the valve as seen by the surgeon in the operating room. Note that the prolapse involves the lateral part of the aortic leaflet of the mitral valve. AO, aortic valve; RV, right ventricle. A1, A2, portions of the aortic leaflet of the mitral valve facing the scallops of the mural leaflet usually described as P1 and P2.

probe is about to be released, which should further enhance the role of three-dimensional echocardiography.

Cardiac Catheterisation and Angiocardiography

In this current era, cardiac catheterisation, and angiography, is not used to make the diagnosis of, nor to assess, a patient with prolapsing leaflets of the mitral valve.

Course and Prognosis

Floppy mitral valve syndrome is an entirely benign condition in the great majority of patients. This is particularly so in children, where associated significant valvar regurgitation is rarely seen, outside those having a co-existing disorder of connective tissues. Looking beyond the paediatric age range into adulthood, patients are stratified according to whether they have risk factors such as significant valvar regurgitation, left ventricular dysfunction, left atrial dilation, a flail leaflet, or atrial fibrillation.[90,91] Progressive regurgitation occurs in approximately one-sixth of adults over a period of 10 to 15 years.[92] Such patients usually have thick and redundant leaflets and are usually male and over 50 years of age. Although infective endocarditis occurs more frequently in the setting of the regurgitant valve,[93] the current guidelines from the American Heart Association do not ask for antibiotic prophylaxis.

Sudden death has been reported in those with prolapsing valves, albeit that the cause and effect is unclear. At the best, it could be stated that those cases with severe valvar regurgitation, or complex arrhythmias, are at a higher risk of sudden events.

Management

For children with normal T waves and QT interval, no evidence of Marfan's syndrome, and with only a valvar click, review over periods of 5 years is suitable treatment. It is not necessary to prescribe prophylaxis against bacterial endocarditis, even if there is evidence of valvar regurgitation. Children with inversion of the T waves in leads II, III, aVF, V_5 or V_6, or prolongation of the QTc interval, and those with a family history of premature sudden death and the click/murmur syndrome, should undergo 24-hour electrocardiographic monitoring, which must be compared against standards for normal individuals of their age. If this shows ventricular tachycardia or fibrillation, or if there are significant symptoms and an abnormally high incidence of premature ventricular contractions, then it is sensible to begin antiarrhythmic therapy. The frequency of follow-up should be adjusted according to the response. If the 24-hour electrocardiogram is within normal limits, annual follow-up is sufficient, repeating the 24-hour monitoring only if indicated by symptoms such as dizziness or syncope, or if the incidence of arrhythmias increases as seen in the standard electrocardiogram.

Parents of children with a persistent late systolic murmur should be advised of the small chance of progressive mitral regurgitation, which might necessitate surgery in adulthood. These patients should be followed on an annual basis, performing an echocardiogram to reassess the severity of regurgitation, as well as left ventricular function and left atrial size.

Surgical management for those with significant valvar regurgitation is similar to that for adults. Prolapse of the mural leaflet, or one of its scallops, presages a better outcome than evidence of prolapse of the aortic leaflet. Quadrangular resection of the involved segment of the mural leaflets is undertaken, with or without a sliding plasty. For those with prolapse of the aortic leaflet, it is possible to perform a triangular resection, as well as shortening and transfer of the tendinous cords. As well as resection of parts of the leaflets, it may be necessary to perform annuloplasty or insert an annular ring. Although the results of surgical repair are very good, recurrent regurgitation occurs in a subset of patients, necessitating replacement of the valve.

The complete reference list can be found on the companion Expert Consult web site at www.expertconsult.com.

ANNOTATED REFERENCES

- Carpentier AL: Cardiac valve surgery: The French correction. J Thorac Cardiovasc Surg 1983;86:323–337.
- Chauvaud SM, Milhaileanu SA, Gaer JAR, Carpentier AC: Surgical treatment of congenital mitral valvar insufficiency: 'The Hopital Broussais' experience. Cardiol Young 1997;7:5–14.
- Chauvaud SM, Milhaileanu SA, Gaer JAR, Carpentier AC: Surgical treatment of congenital mitral valvar stenosis: 'The Hopital Broussais' experience. Cardiol Young 1997;7:15–21.

  These three reviews encapsulate the approach to classification and surgical treatment of congenital malformations of the mitral valve evolved by Alain Carpentier over his considerable lifetime experience, emphasising the importance of taking the function of the malformed valvar components into consideration, as well as their anatomy.

- Kanani M, Moorman AFM, Cook AC, et al: Development of the atrioventricular valves: Clinicomorphologic correlations. Ann Thorac Surg 2005;79:1797–1804.
- de Lange FJ, Moorman AFM, Anderson RH, et al: Lineage and morphogenetic analysis of the cardiac valves. Circ Res 2004;95:645–654.

  An overview of recent morphological considerations relating to the development of the various components of the atrioventricular valves, and a study of the lineage of the tissues contributing to them. The first review emphasises the developmental, as well as the anatomic, differences between the valve guarding the separate left atrioventricular junction, and the left half of a common atrioventricular junction.

- Becker AE, de Wit APM: Mitral valve apparatus: A spectrum of normality relevant to mitral valve prolapse. Br Heart J 1979;42:680–689.
- Van der Bel Kahn J, Duren DR, Becker AE: Isolated mitral valve prolapse: Chordal architecture as an anatomic basis in older patients. J Am Coll Cardiol 1985;5:1335–1340.

  Two important studies showing how prolapse of the leaflets may reflect abnormal and minor deviations in cordal support of the leaflets of the valve.

- Shone JD, Sellers RD, Anderson RC, et al: The developmental complex of 'parachute mitral valve', supravalvular ring of left atrium, subaortic stenosis, and coarctation of aorta. Am J Cardiol 1963;11:714–725.

  The original study that established the fact that malformations on the left side of the heart are rarely isolated lesions and set the scene for the future description of Shone's syndrome.

- Atz AM, Adatia I, Jonas RA, Wessel DL: Inhaled nitric oxide in children with pulmonary hypertension and congenital mitral stenosis. Am J Cardiol 1996;77:316–319.

  One of the first studies to show the importance of inhaled nitric oxide in the management of patients with mitral valvar disease.

- Asante-Korang A, O'Leary PO, Anderson RH: Anatomy and echo of the normal and abnormal mitral valve. Cardiol Young 2006;16:27–34.
- Smallhorn J, Tommasini G, Deanfield J, et al: Congenital mitral stenosis: Anatomical and functional assessment by echocardiography. Br Heart J 1981;45:527–534.

  The study by Smallhorn and colleagues was one of the very first studies to show the value of cross sectional echocardiography in the assessment of malformations of the mitral valve, while the more recent review by Asante-Korang and associates and a more recent review encapsulates the evolution of the echocardiographic approach.

- Mele D, Soukhomovskaia O, Pacchioni E, et al: Proximal flow convergence region as assessed by real-time 3-dimensional echocardiography: Challenging the hemispheric assumption. J Am Soc Echocardiograph 2007;20:389–396.

  A recent study from the group who initially put forward the so-called PISA as a means of evaluating mitral valvar function, but now questioning the validity of their earlier findings on the basis of three-dimensional interrogation.

- Anwar AM, Soliman OII, ten Cate FJ, et al: True mitral annulus diameter is underestimated by 2d echocardiography as evidenced by real time 3d echocardiography and magnetic resonance imaging. Int J Cardiovasc Imaging 2006;23:541–547.

  An important work emphasising the saddle-shape of the mitral valvar annulus and showing how diagnosis based using cross sectional interrogation in the four-chamber plane can lead to overdiagnosis of the malformation.

- McElhinney DB, Sherwood MC, Keane JF, et al: Current management of severe congenital mitral stenosis, outcomes of transcatheter and surgical therapy in 108 infants and children. Circulation 2005;112:707–714.

  A recent study comparing the results of catheter intervention and surgery in the treatment of congenital mitral valvar stenosis.

- Wood AE, Healy DG, Nolke L, et al: Mitral valve reconstruction in a pediatric population: Late clinical results and predictors of long-term outcome. J Thorac Cardiovasc Surg 2005;130:66–73.

  A recent review of surgical results from a single centre, showing the difficulties still encountered in treating surgically congenital malformations of the mitral valve during childhood.

Tetralogy of Fallot with Pulmonary Stenosis

CHRISTIAN APITZ, ROBERT H. ANDERSON, and ANDREW N. REDINGTON

Even though, as stated by Lev and Eckner,[1] no two cases are exactly the same, it is the characteristic anatomy that permits the instant recognition of the tetralogy of Fallot. As was emphasised by Arthur Louis Etienne Fallot, as long ago as 1888, all cases have an interventricular communication, biventricular origin of the aorta, muscular obstruction within the right ventricular outflow tract, and right ventricular hypertrophy (Fig. 36-1). There is no question but that hearts with this phenotypic morphology had been described long before Fallot emphasised the constellation of lesions that now bears his name. Thus, according to Marquis,[2] the malformation was first described in 1673 by the Danish monk, Nicholas Steno, in an ectopic heart from a fetus. Fallot deserves his eponym, nonetheless, since it was he who first observed that the combination of lesions accounted for the majority of cases of la maladie bleue, or cyanosis, which he encountered at autopsy. Abbott,[3] in her classic *Atlas of Congenital Cardiac Disease*, emphasised the observations of Fallot,[3] and the eponym has continued to retain favour since her own descriptions of permanent cyanosis. Arguments have continued, however, as to the essence of the malformation, and which variants should be described with the eponym. Thus, when obstruction within the right ventricular outflow tract is minimal, it can be hard to distinguish tetralogy from the variant of ventricular septal defect with aortic overriding known as the Eisenmenger defect,[4] even using anatomic criterions.[5] When obstruction is complete, the condition unequivocally represents the commonest variant of pulmonary atresia with ventricular septal defect, although not all accept that this form should be described as tetralogy with pulmonary atresia. The phenotypic feature that underscores the existence of the tetralogy is anterior and cephalad deviation of the septal insertion of the outlet septum relative to the septomarginal trabeculation, combined with an arrangement of the septoparietal trabeculations that produces an annular obstruction at the mouth of the infundibulum. Within the collection of hearts unified in this fashion, there is ample room for significant individual variation, as emphasised by Lev and Eckner.[1] It is this variation that will be the focus of our anatomic discussions in this chapter, with emphasis placed on the major differences from the normal heart.

Figure 36-1 The photograph, taken from the apex of the morphologically right ventricle looking towards the base, shows the phenotypic features of tetralogy of Fallot. Note that the muscular outlet septum, separating the overriding component of the aortic outlet from the subpulmonary (subpulm.) infundibulum, is inserted to the antero-cephalad limb of the septomarginal trabeculation (*yellow Y*).

INCIDENCE, PREVALENCE, AND AETIOLOGY

Of infants born with congenital heart disease, approximately 3.5% will have tetralogy of Fallot, giving a figure of 0.28 per 1,000, or 1 in 3,600, live births.[6] Males and females are equally affected. According to existing statistics, the frequency increases with age when compared with other forms of cyanotic congenital cardiac malformations. This is largely because, in the past, infants with more lethal cardiac anomalies tended to die, whereas many with tetralogy of Fallot survive beyond infancy even without treatment. This could well change in the current era.

As with so many congenital cardiac anomalies, precise aetiology is unknown. The majority of cases are sporadic. According to Nora and colleagues,[7] the risk of recurrence in siblings is about 3% if there are no other affected first-degree relatives. Rubella in the first trimester of pregnancy has been implicated in a small number of cases,[8] while viruses have been isolated from cases with severe pulmonary arterial hypoplasia.[9] Keeshond dogs were bred to produce a spectrum of inherited malformations of the ventricular outflow tracts, which included anomalies similar to tetralogy of Fallot.[10] The findings indicated a polygenic model of inheritance, in which the genes act additively to produce the spectrum of maldevelopment. The lesion is also known to be linked with abnormal migration of cells from the neural crest. Dosage of rats with bis-diamine, known to inhibit migration from the neural crest, produces the phenotypic features of tetralogy when given at critical periods of development, including cases with pulmonary atresia rather than stenosis.[11,12] In a significant proportion of cases, it is possible to find microdeletions of the q11 region of chromosome 22, such deletions being known to produce Di George syndrome and the velocardiofacial syndrome, also known as the conotruncal anomaly face syndrome.[13] In some series,[14] microdeletion was found in up to a quarter of cases, suggesting that investigation using fluorescent in situ hybridisation should be undertaken in all patients with the phenotypic features of tetralogy.

Almost all those born with tetralogy of Fallot in all its variants can now expect to survive surgical correction, and reach adult life. Female patients may well ask the question 'Is it safe for me to become pregnant?', while both women and men will wish to know the risks of their progeny inheriting the condition. It has been known for some time that the incidence of congenital cardiac disease is higher in children born to women with congenitally malformed hearts than in the normal population,[15] albeit that, with respect to tetralogy, no differences are found in the incidence of affected children according to whether it is the mother or father who had the lesion initially. According to some, the risk is approximately one-tenth for the offspring being affected. This risk is as for any congenital cardiac malformation, including minor lesions not requiring intervention.[16] The risk is much higher, at above two-fifths, however, if the affected parent has a sibling with the same or a similar cardiac anomaly. Identification of those patients having microdeletion of chromosome 22q11 could well allow refinement of these calculations for risk of recurrence.

ANATOMY AND MORPHOGENESIS

Phenotypic Features

The phenotypic feature of the lesion is antero-cephalad deviation of the insertion of the muscular outlet septum relative to the limbs of the septomarginal trabeculation, coupled with an arrangement of the septoparietal trabeculations which produces a squeeze at the mouth of the infundibulum[17] (Fig. 36-2). In the normal heart, the muscular outlet septum is an insignificant structure, inserted and buried between the limbs of the prominent septomarginal trabeculation. Indeed, it is so fully incorporated into the septum (Fig. 36-3) that it is not possible to distinguish an anatomically discrete outlet septal component from the dominant part of the supraventricular crest, which is the ventriculo-infundibular fold, itself supporting the free-standing subpulmonary infundibulum (Fig. 36-4). In tetralogy, these components of the supraventricular crest are divorced one from the other, with the right ventricular muscular outlet septum, rather than the ventriculo-infundibular fold, now supporting the narrowed free-standing subpulmonary infundibulum (Fig. 36-5).

Because of the abnormal position of the outlet septum, which is exclusively a right ventricular structure in tetralogy, the interventricular communication is situated between the limbs of the septomarginal trabeculation, whilst the right ventricular origin of the overriding aortic valve is supported by the ventriculo-infundibular fold (see Fig. 36-1). These three anatomic features of the tetralogy, therefore, all reflect the abnormal location of the outlet septum.

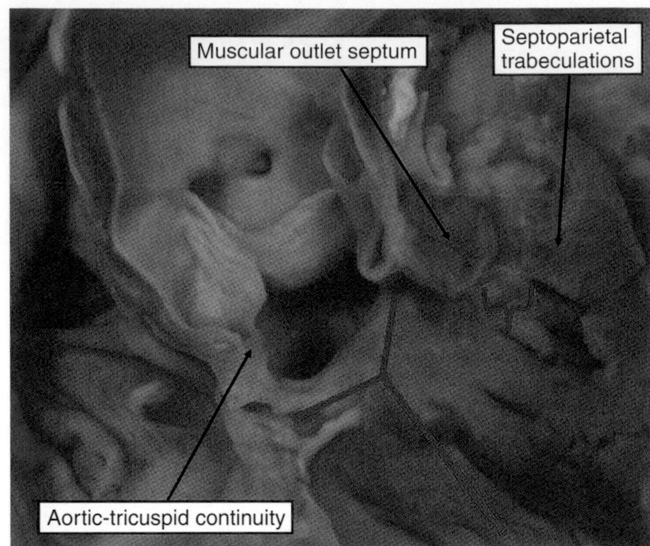

Figure 36-2 The heart has been sectioned to replicate the oblique subcostal echocardiographic cut, and shows the phenotypic feature of tetralogy, namely insertion of the muscular outlet septum antero-cephalad relative to the limbs of the septomarginal trabeculation (*yellow Y*), together with an abnormal arrangement of the septoparietal trabeculations. The abnormalities combine to produce an annular obstruction at the mouth of the subpulmonary infundibulum (*yellow bracket*).

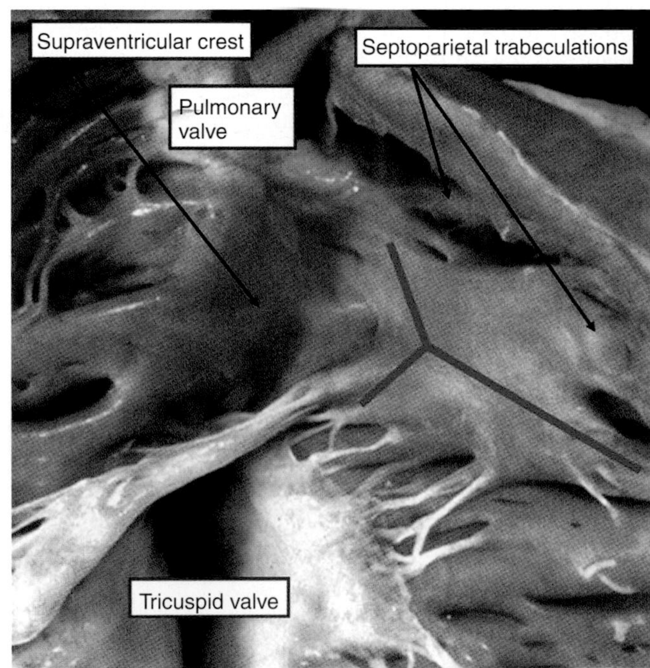

Figure 36-3 The subpulmonary outflow tract of the normal heart is opened to show how the supraventricular crest, the muscular fold separating the attachments of the tricuspid and pulmonary valves, is inserted between the limbs of the septomarginal trabeculation (*yellow Y*). Note the location of the septoparietal trabeculations.

This particular phenotypic combination, nonetheless, cannot be produced in the absence of the squeeze produced together with the septoparietal trabeculations, which are themselves often hypertrophied, particularly in hearts from older patients. The outlet septum, nonetheless, can be markedly deviated in antero-cephalad direction without there being subpulmonary stenosis, despite the presence

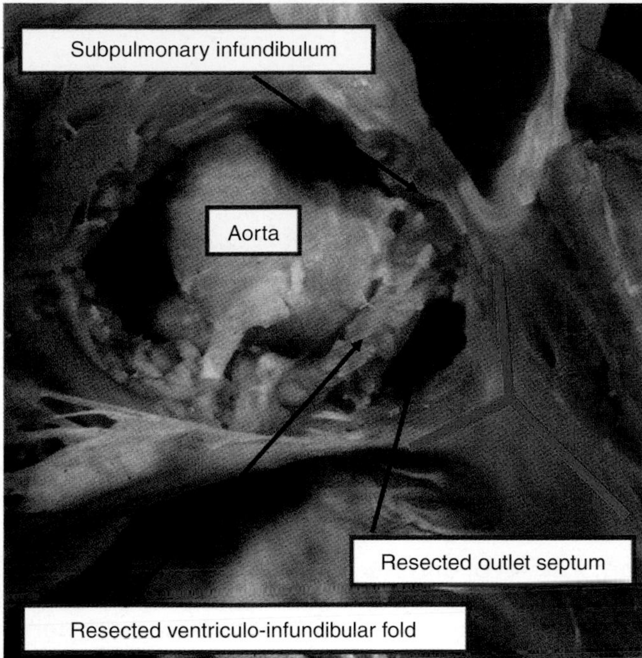

Figure 36-4 Another normal heart has been dissected to show that the greater part of the supraventricular crest is the ventriculo-infundibular fold, or inner heart curvature, supporting the free-standing subpulmonary infundibulum. A small part of the septum can be resected to gain entrance to the left ventricle, but there are no anatomic landmarks delineating this from the inner heart curvature. The *yellow Y* shows the septomarginal trabeculation.

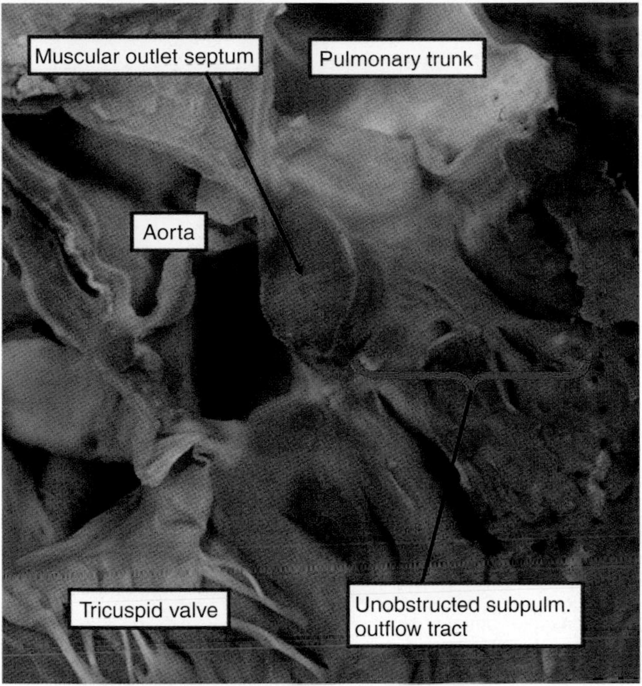

Figure 36-6 This heart has been sectioned in the same plane as that shown in Figure 36-2. There is again antero-cephalad deviation of the insertion of the muscular outlet septum, but in this instance without producing muscular subpulmonary (subpulm.) obstruction. This is the Eisenmenger defect, but not an example of tetralogy of Fallot.

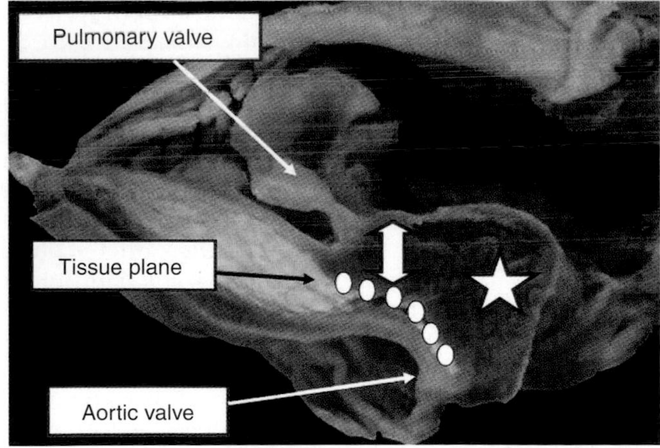

Figure 36-5 The adjacent parts of the subaortic and subpulmonary outlets have been removed from a heart with tetralogy of Fallot. The section shows how the narrowed subpulmonary infundibulum is made up of the outlet septum (*star*) and the free-standing infundibular sleeve (*double-headed arrow*). Note the tissue plane (*dots*) between the infundibulum and the aortic root.

of hypertrophied septoparietal trabeculations, as in the so-called Eisenmenger complex (Fig. 36-6).

Although the divorce of outlet septum, ventriculo-infundibular fold, and septomarginal trabeculation are the essence of tetralogy when combined with the annular muscular obstruction at the mouth of the subpulmonary infundibulum, and despite the fact that each can be recognised anatomically in its own right, there has been significant previous confusion and controversy in description of the abnormal outflow tracts. This is because each of these three structures, at various times and in various places, had been nominated as a component of the so-called crista. Consequently, when alleged parts of the crista were described in the setting of tetralogy, it was difficult to be sure which of the different structures was being described. Because of these problems, we suggested quite some time ago[18] that the term crista, or its translation as supraventricular crest, be reserved for description of the muscular structure separating the attachments of the leaflets of the tricuspid and pulmonary valves in the normal right ventricular outflow tract (Fig. 36-7). In situations where the muscular structures are separated one from the other, as is the case in tetralogy, we suggested that each structure be accounted for in its own right, using descriptive and mutually exclusive terms (Fig. 36-8). This suggestion has since stood well the test of time. Thus, the outlet septum is any muscular or fibrous structure that interposes between the subpulmonary and subaortic outflow tracts. This septum has septal and parietal insertions, and is contiguous with the sleeve of free-standing subpulmonary infundibular musculature, albeit that the infundibulum itself is absent when the outlet septum is exclusively a fibrous structure. The ventriculo-infundibular fold, being part of the muscular inner heart curvature, is any muscular structure that separates the leaflets of an arterial from an atrioventricular valve. It is the extensive trabeculation reinforcing the septal surface of the morphologically right ventricle that is nominated as the septomarginal trabeculation, or septal band. It has a body, together with anterior-cephalad and postero-caudal limbs, the latter components usually supporting the inferior margin of the interventricular communication, not only in tetralogy, but also in other lesions such as double outlet right ventricle and common arterial trunk. The moderator band arises apically from its body, and crosses to the free ventricular wall. The moderator

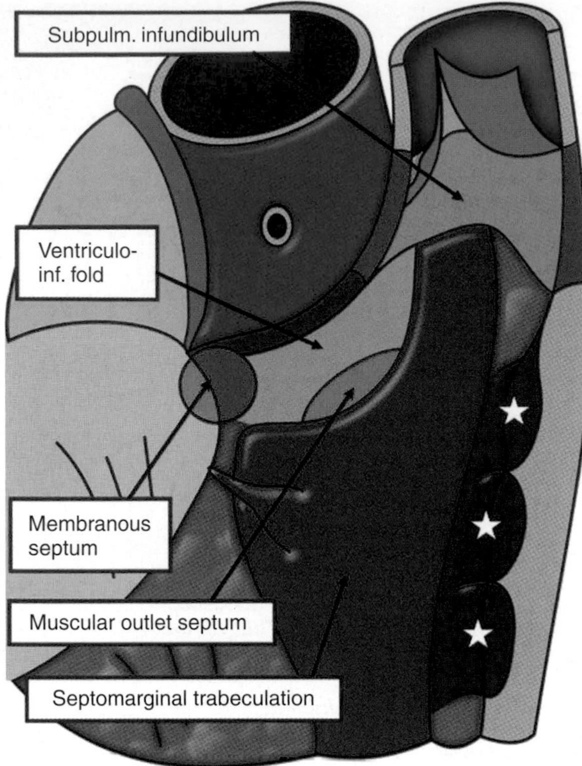

Figure 36-7 The cartoon shows the building blocks of the outflow tract of the normal right ventricle. Note, however, that it is impossible to distinguish between the outlet septum and the ventriculo-infundibular fold in the normal situation without resorting to dissection (see Figs. 36-3 and 36-4). The *stars* show the location of the septoparietal trabeculations.

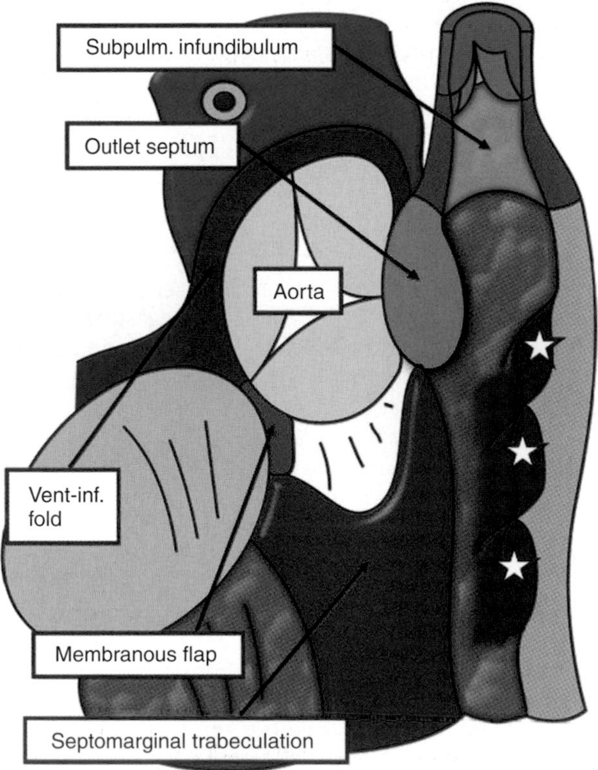

Figure 36-8 The cartoon shows how the building blocks of the normal outflow tract (see Fig. 36-7) come apart one from the other in the setting of tetralogy of Fallot. The subpulmonary (subpulm.) obstruction is produced by a squeeze between the muscular outlet septum and the most distal of the septoparietal trabeculations. As in Figure 36-7, the *stars* show the septoparietal trabeculations.

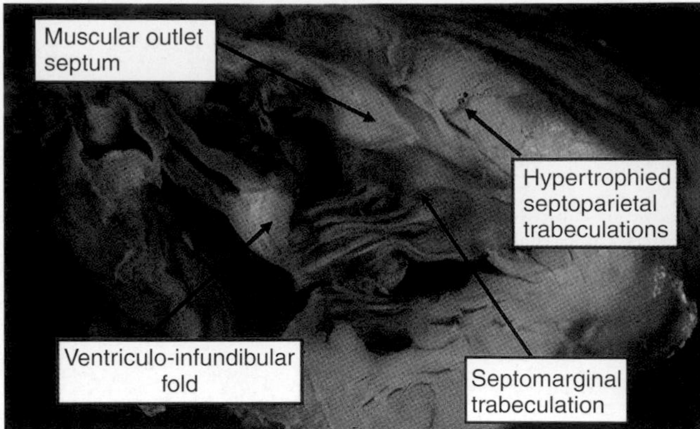

Figure 36-9 This specimen with tetralogy of Fallot has been sectioned to replicate the oblique subcostal echocardiographic cut. It shows how the building blocks of the outflow tract can readily be distinguished and described.

band is, however, only one of a series of muscle bars which extend to the parietal wall. The others are the septoparietal trabeculations, an integral component of the normal heart, but forming an integral part of the obstruction to the pulmonary pathways seen in tetralogy. Use of these terms makes it a simple matter to describe and differentiate the muscular structures forming the outflow tracts in tetralogy of Fallot (Fig. 36-9).

Variability in the Margins of the Ventricular Septal Defect

The hole between the ventricles is directly beneath the overriding aortic valvar orifice. It can thus be considered an outlet defect. The muscular outlet septum itself, however, is usually well-formed, albeit malaligned relative to the rest of the muscular septum. Indeed, as already discussed, part of the essence of tetralogy is antero-cephalad deviation of the septal insertion of the outlet septum such that it becomes a right ventricular rather than an interventricular structure, this deviation co-existing with the abnormal arrangement of the most distal septomarginal trabeculation (see Figs. 36-2 and 36-9). It is the outlet septum, therefore, and its fusion with the antero-cephalad limb of the septomarginal trabeculation, which forms the anterior margins of the defect. The crest of the muscular ventricular septum, reinforced by the limbs of the septomarginal trabeculation, forms the floor of the defect. Because of the septal malalignment, the roof of the defect is formed by the attachments of the leaflets of the overriding aortic valve to the ventriculo-infundibular fold. Indeed, because of the overriding of the aortic orifice, problems exist in defining specifically the nature of the ventricular septal defect. Any one of a host of planes within the cone of space subtended from the valvar leaflets to the crest of the septum can be nominated as a septal defect (Fig. 36-10).

When describing the boundaries of these planes, we concentrate on the margins of the cone as viewed from the right ventricle,[19] since this is the locus along which the surgeon will attach the patch used to repair the malformation so as to reconstitute the ventricular septum (see Fig. 36-10). When the ventricular septal defect is defined in this fashion, it is the postero-inferior quadrant that shows most anatomic variability. In about four-fifths of cases, this margin is formed by fibrous continuity between the leaflets of the aortic, mitral and tricuspid valves (Fig. 36-11).

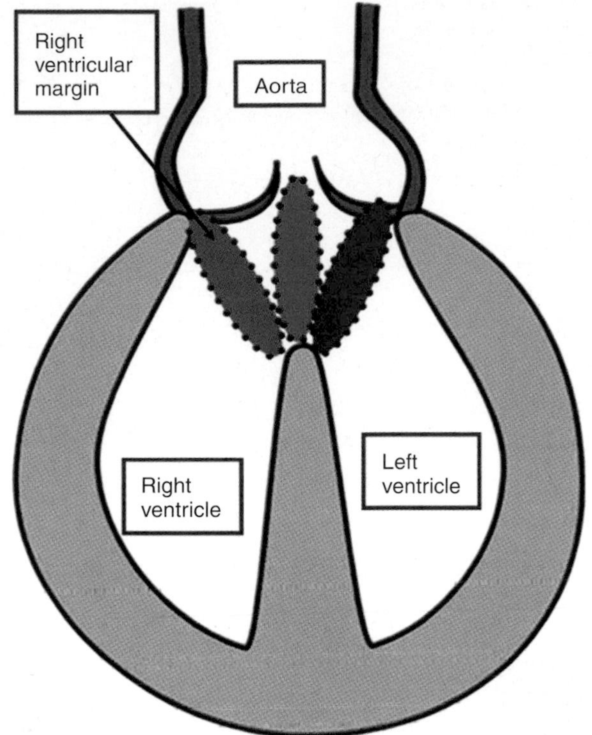

Figure 36-10 The cartoon shows three planes within the cone of space subtended from the crest of the ventricular septum to the attachments of the overriding aortic valve that could be defined as the ventricular septal defect. The *red disc* is the outlet from the left ventricle, whilst the *yellow disc* represents the continuation of the muscular ventricular septum. It is the *green disc*, however, that we describe as the ventricular septal defect, since this is the locus along which the surgeon will place the patch to reconstitute the ventricular septum.

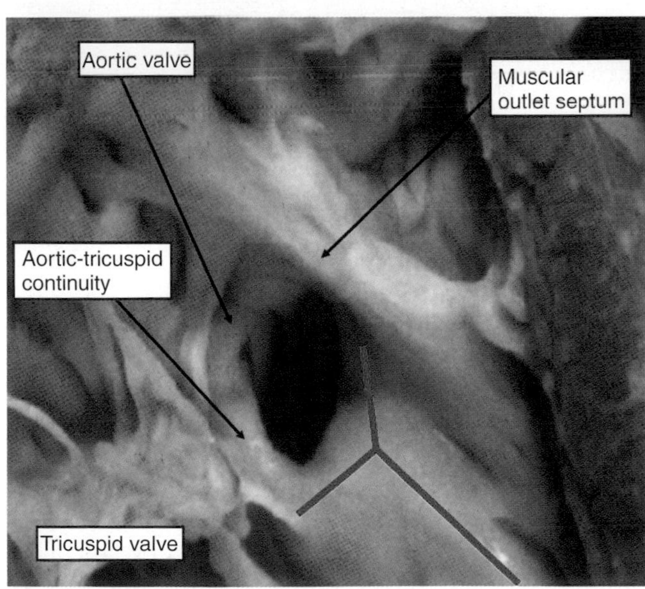

Figure 36-11 The illustration shows the morphology of the commonest type of interventricular communication found in the setting of tetralogy of Fallot. There is fibrous continuity between the leaflets of the aortic and tricuspid valves in the postero-inferior margin of the defect, making it perimembranous. The yellow Y shows the septomarginal trabeculation.

In this respect, the defect is directly comparable to typical perimembranous defects opening to the outlet of the right ventricle in the absence of subpulmonary obstruction. In our view, it is unnecessary to consider the defect in tetralogy as a separate entity should it co-exist with malalignment of the outlet septum. In that the postero-inferior margin is an area of fibrous continuity between the leaflets of the aortic and tricuspid valves, the defect is unequivocally perimembranous. These anatomic features are reflected in the distribution of the atrioventricular conduction tissues. As in all other hearts with concordant atrioventricular connections, the guides to the location of the atrioventricular node are the landmarks of the triangle of Koch. The penetrating bundle perforates the central fibrous body through the area of valvar continuity (Fig. 36-12). Here, the bundle is frequently overlaid by a remnant of the interventricular membranous septum, which may on occasions become aneurysmal. The septal remnant itself, called the membranous flap,[20] is safe tissue for anchorage of sutures when such stitches are placed with care.[21] It is positioned, however, directly superficial to the penetrating bundle.[22] Sutures placed deeply in this area are liable to produce complete heart block. It is safer, therefore, to place sutures through the leaflet of the tricuspid valve, which usually overlaps the membranous flap in this area of the defect. Having perforated, the nonbranching atrioventricular bundle enters the left ventricular part of the aortic outflow tract, and almost always then veers away from the septal crest, the branching atrioventricular bundle being carried on the left ventricular

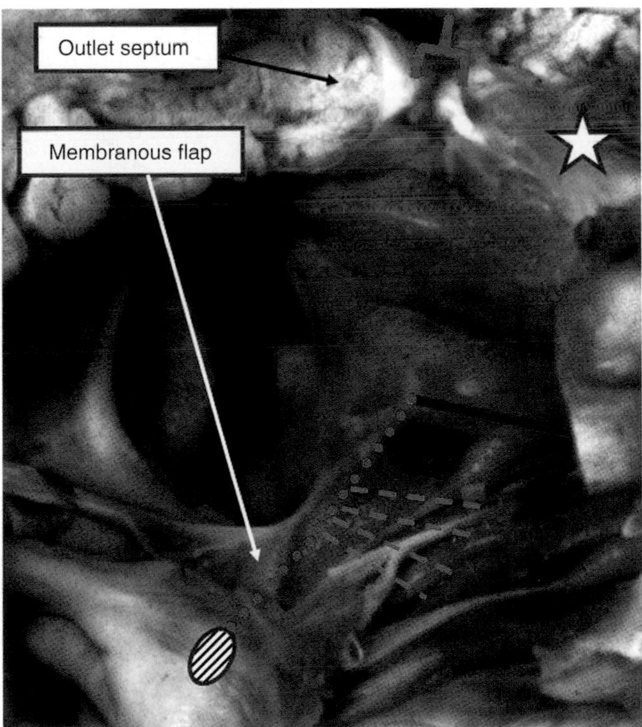

Figure 36-12 The heart illustrated has been prepared by removing the septal leaflet of the tricuspid valve, revealing the crest of the muscular ventricular septum, reinforced by the limbs of the septomarginal trabeculation. Note the mouth of the infundibulum (*yellow bracket*), squeezed between the deviated outlet septum and the hypertrophied septoparietal trabeculation (*star*). The location of the atrioventricular conduction axis has been superimposed on the image, showing the atrioventricular node at the apex of the triangle of Koch (*cross-hatched red oval*), the penetrating, non-branching and branching components of the axis (*yellow dotted line*). The left bundle branch, taking origin below the crest of the septum, is shown in the *blue-green dashed lines*. The axis then penetrates back through the septum (*continuation of yellow dotted line beyond the green dashed lines*), before surfacing beneath the medial papillary muscle and continuing as the right bundle branch within the body of the septomarginal trabeculation (*red line*).

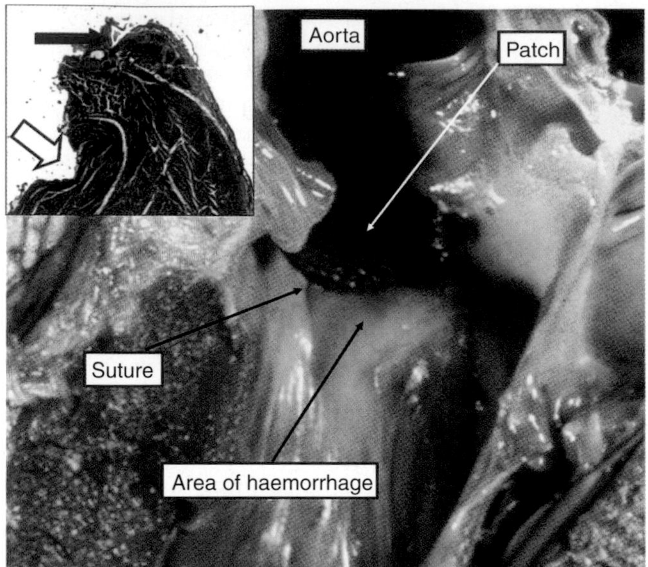

Figure 36-13 In this patient with tetralogy of Fallot and a perimembranous septal defect, the surgeon placed the stitches to secure the patch through the crest of the ventricular septum, as was recommended at that time. As can be seen, one of the stitches has produced an area of haemorrhage on the left ventricular aspect of the septal crest, and as shown by the histological section, the haemorrhage is contained within the non-branching atrioventricular bundle (*red arrow in inset*). The *open arrow* in the inset shows the bite of the suture through the septal crest.

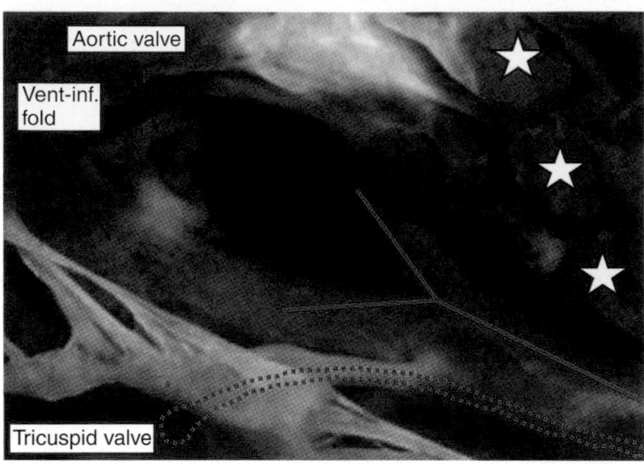

Figure 36-14 In this heart from a patient with tetralogy of Fallot, the postero-caudal limb of the septomarginal trabeculation (*yellow Y*) fuses with the ventriculo-infundibular fold (vent-inf. fold) in the postero-inferior margin of the defect. This protects the conduction axis (*yellow dotted lines*). Note the hypertrophied septoparietal trabeculations (*stars*).

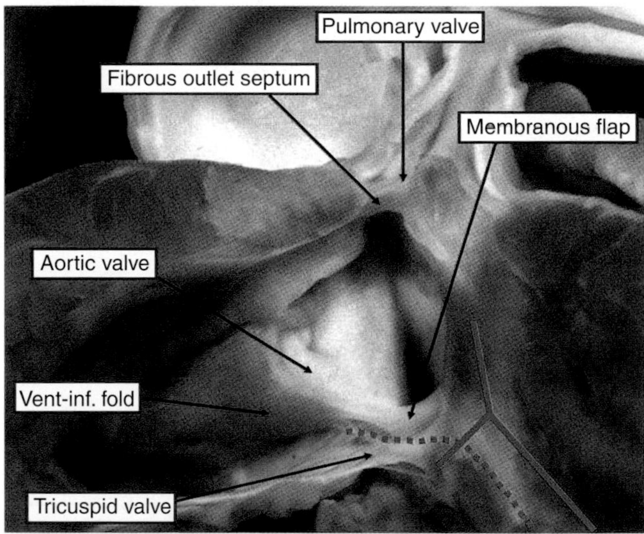

Figure 36-15 In this heart from patient with tetralogy of Fallot, the interventricular communication is roofed by fibrous continuity between the leaflets of the arterial valves, making it doubly committed, and also extends to an area of fibrous continuity between the aortic and tricuspid valves, the ventriculo-infundibular fold (vent-inf. fold) stopping short of the postero-caudal limb of the septomarginal trabeculation (*yellow Y*). Because the defect extends to become perimembranous, the conduction axis is at potential risk in its postero-inferior margin (*yellow dotted line*). Note the remnant of the interventricular membranous septum, which forms the so-called membranous flap. Note also the deviated fibrous outlet septum in the roof of the defect.

aspect of the septum and staying remote from the septal crest. In a minority of hearts, nonetheless, the bundle may branch directly astride the septum. Such an arrangement places the bundle at risk should sutures be placed into the crest of the septum (Fig. 36-13). Irrespective of these differences, the right bundle branch penetrates back through the septum, emerging within the postero-caudal limb of the septomarginal trabeculation and then descending within its substance towards the apex.

The second most common pattern, occurring in about one-fifth of cases, is characterised by interruption of the area of fibrous continuity between the aortic and tricuspid valves by a muscular fold.[17,19] When viewed from its right ventricular aspect, therefore, the septal defect has exclusively muscular rims. The fold itself is formed by fusion of the postero-caudal limb of the septomarginal trabeculation with the ventriculo-infundibular fold. An intact membranous septum is found between the muscular fold and the remaining atrioventricular septal structures. Since the atrioventricular conduction axis runs postero-inferior to the membranous septum, the muscular fold, together with the membranous septum itself, separates the conduction tissues from the crest of the ventricular septum (Fig. 36-14). When the muscular fold is of good dimensions, as is usually the case, the entire muscular margins of the defect are suitable for anchorage of sutures, provided that the stitches are not placed too deeply.

There is then yet a third variety of defect, characterised by presence of a fibrous rather than a muscular outlet septum, and absence of the free-standing subpulmonary infundibular sleeve.[17,19] This is the doubly committed and juxta-arterial defect, by far the least common in the Western World, but commoner in the Far East and South America. The defect is both subaortic and subpulmonary as a consequence of failure of formation of the muscular subpulmonary infundibulum. Such defects can also be found with fibrous continuity between the leaflets of the aortic and tricuspid valves, making them perimembranous (Fig. 36-15), but more usually there is a muscular postero-inferior rim, comparable to the muscular structure seen in Figure 36-14. If present, the muscular structure will protect the atrioventricular conduction axis, but in the heart shown in Figure 36-15, the conduction axis will be at direct risk in the postero-inferior margin of the defect.

Patients with tetralogy, of course, all possess defects as described above, which open between the outflow tracts. They can also be encountered with additional defects elsewhere in the septum. Inlet defects are particularly important, be they muscular inlet defects, defects associated with straddling and overriding of the tricuspid valve, or the ventricular component of an atrioventricular septal defect associated with common atrioventricular junction. The combination of tetralogy and an atrioventricular septal defect with common atrioventricular junction, in the past, was considered to pose significant additional problems to the surgeon, but these difficulties have now been overcome in most centres of excellence. Almost always in tetralogy, the ventricular septal defect is large, approximating in size the diameter of the aortic root. Rarely, it may be restrictive due to the presence of accessory fibrous tissue tags formed at the margins of the defect. Such tags may be derived in part from the tricuspid valve, or extend from attachment of the tension apparatus of the mitral valve across the left ventricular aspect of the defect.

Narrowing of the Subpulmonary Infundibulum

The subpulmonary stenosis, which is an essential part of tetralogy, is due to the squeeze between the antero-cephalad deviation of the outlet septum and the abnormal arrangement of the distal septoparietal trabeculations, this being the phenotypic feature of the lesion (see Figs. 36-2 and 36-9). The antero-cephalad component of the obstruction, therefore, is produced by the septoparietal trabeculations, often additionally hypertrophied, which extend onto the ventricular free wall. These muscular bundles can be removed by the surgeon without fear of causing damage to significant structures. The maximal area of stenosis, when viewed from the apex of the right ventricle, produces an obvious mouth to the subpulmonary infundibulum, the so-called os infundibulum (Fig. 36-16).

Additional stenosis can then be found more proximally within the ventricle, produced either by hypertrophy of the moderator band, which is one of the septoparietal trabeculations, or by prominent apical trabeculations. This gives the arrangement often described as two-chambered right ventricle. The subpulmonary infundibulum itself, distal to the squeeze between outlet septum and septoparietal trabeculations, varies markedly in length. In some instances, when the ventricular septal defect is doubly committed, the infundibulum is no longer an exclusively muscular structure (see Fig. 36-15). In other instances, the narrowed infundibular chamber has considerable length (see Fig. 36-16). There is a spectrum between these extremes, but measurements of series of hearts from patients with tetralogy,[23] when compared to measurements of normal hearts, show that the infundibulum is longer in the setting of the malformation (Fig. 36-17). In addition to the muscular stenosis, it is also usual to find obstruction at valvar level, with the valve itself often possessing two rather than three leaflets. Further stenotic lesions can then be found within the pulmonary arterial pathways.

Overriding of the Aortic Valve

In the normal heart, although the right aortic sinus of the aortic valve overrides spatially the crest of the muscular ventricular septum, the leaflets of the valve are attached exclusively within the left ventricle. Whenever the ventricular septum is deficient, however, part of the circumference of the aortic valvar orifice of necessity becomes attached to, and supported by, right ventricular structures.[24] Such aortic overriding becomes more obvious when the outlet septum is deviated so as to become exclusively a right ventricular structure, as in tetralogy of Fallot (see Fig. 36-1) or the Eisenmenger ventricular septal defect (see Fig. 36-6). The precise degree of override, in other words the proportion of the aortic valvar circumference supported by right as opposed to left ventricular structures, can therefore vary between 5% and 100%. This feature has obvious surgical

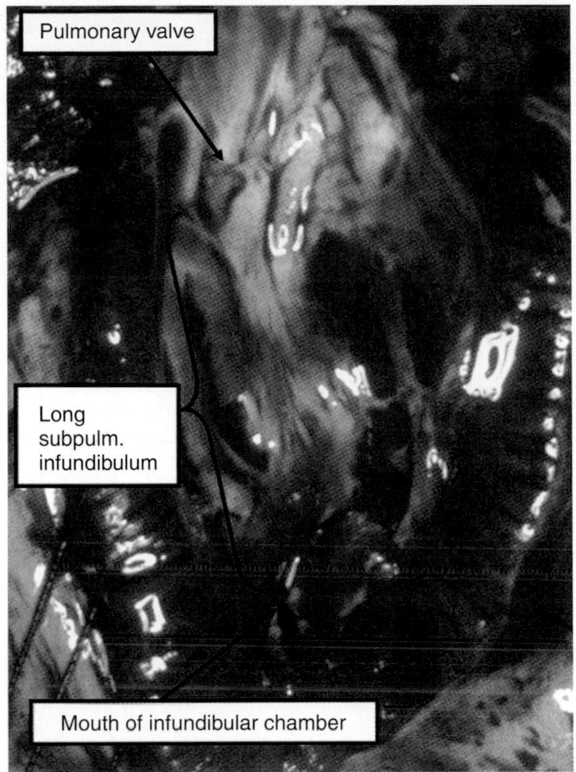

Figure 36-16 This picture was taken in the operating room during surgical correction of a patient with tetralogy of Fallot. The photograph has been reorientated in attitudinally appropriate fashion. It shows the narrow mouth of the subpulmonary infundibulum in this patient, the infundibulum itself having significant length. (Courtesy of Dr Benson Wilcox, University of North Carolina, Chapel Hill.)

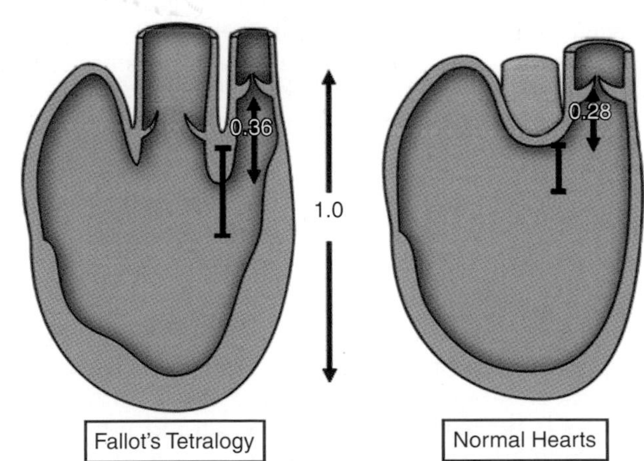

Figure 36-17 Measurements of the length of the subpulmonary infundibulum in 16 patients with tetralogy of Fallot, and 14 normal hearts, taking the length of the right ventricle as unity. The difference in the lengths, in favour of the patients with tetralogy, was highly significant statistically. Values taken from Becker and colleagues.[23]

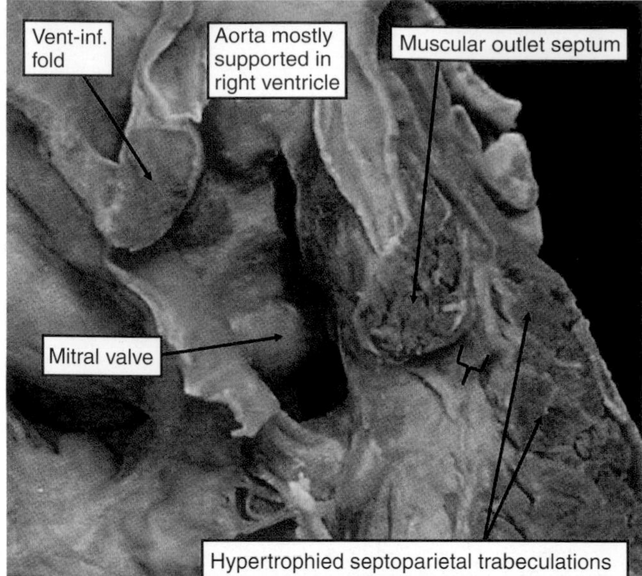

Figure 36-18 In this heart with the phenotypic features of tetralogy of Fallot, the *bracket* showing the squeeze at the mouth of the infundibulum between the outlet septum and the septoparietal trabeculations, the overriding aorta is supported almost exclusively in the right ventricle. The patient, therefore, has double outlet ventriculo-arterial connections. Note that in this particular heart, the ventriculo-infundibular fold has persisted between the leaflets of the aortic and mitral valves, so the patient also has a completely muscular subaortic infundibulum, albeit that the ventricular septal defect is perimembranous because of fibrous continuity between the leaflets of the mitral and tricuspid valves.

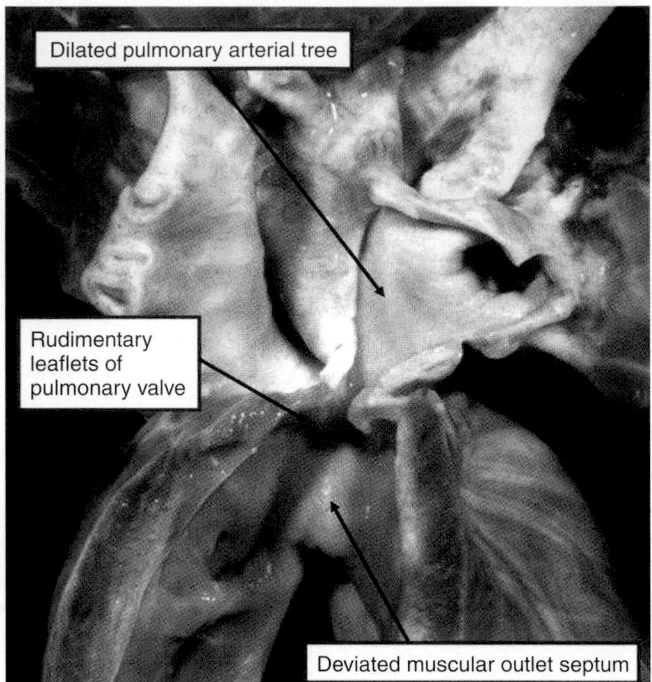

Figure 36-19 The illustration shows tetralogy of Fallot with so-called absence of the leaflets of the pulmonary valve. In reality, the leaflets form an annular rudimentary array at the ventriculo-arterial junction. Note the dilation of the pulmonary trunk and its branches, albeit that the ventriculo-arterial junction itself is narrowed.

significance. A much larger patch will be required to reconstitute the ventricular septum, and connect the aorta to the left ventricle, when the larger part of its circumference is supported by the right ventricle. Care must be taken to be sure that the patch is not placed so tightly as to obstruct the newly created left ventricular outflow tract.

This feature also has implications for nomenclature, albeit that the importance has been somewhat exaggerated. As has been explained in Chapter 1, we describe the situation in which more than half of the circumferences of both great arterial valves are connected in the same ventricle as double outlet ventriculo-arterial connection. In the context of tetralogy of Fallot, in which the entirety of the pulmonary valve is supported by the right ventricular subpulmonary infundibulum, if more than half of the leaflets of the aortic valve are hinged from right ventricular structures, we describe the situation as tetralogy of Fallot co-existing with the ventriculo-arterial connection of double outlet ventricle. There is no reason why the two should not co-exist. Double outlet is simply one particular ventriculo-arterial connection. Tetralogy of Fallot is defined on the basis of its phenotypic feature, namely antero-cephalad deviation of the outlet septum combined with hypertrophy of the septoparietal trabeculations. These two features, self-evidently, are not mutually exclusive (Fig. 36-18).

Other Lesions of the Pulmonary Circulation

Although the subpulmonary infundibulum is usually the narrowest part of the pulmonary outflow tract, other lesions are to be found elsewhere in the outflow tracts and the pulmonary arteries. Pulmonary valvar stenosis is a frequent accompaniment. This is sometimes due to domed stenosis, more frequently to stenosis of a bicuspid valve or to stenosis of a valve with three leaflets. The valvar lesion is rarely the major cause of obstruction, albeit that in some young infants it can be the predominant finding. The valve can also become imperforate as an acquired change. So-called absence of the leaflets of the pulmonary valve is another important lesion. Most usually, the valve is represented by an annular array of fibrous rudiments, usually found with dilation of the pulmonary trunk and its branches (Fig. 36-19).

Stenoses within the pulmonary arteries themselves are of major surgical significance, and usually occur at branching sites from the bifurcation outwards. Lack of origin of one pulmonary artery, typically the left, from the pulmonary trunk is by no means infrequent. The isolated pulmonary artery is almost always present, usually being connected by the arterial duct, or ligament, to some part of the system of aortic arches. Rarely, one pulmonary artery may arise directly from the ascending aorta, but then it tends to be the right one which is anomalously connected. Major systemic-to-pulmonary collateral arteries are sometimes present in association with tetralogy and pulmonary stenosis, but in association with normal right and left pulmonary arteries. Such arteries can be the sole source of pulmonary arterial flow when tetralogy co-exists with pulmonary atresia (see Chapter 37).

Associated Anomalies

Many other lesions can co-exist with tetralogy. Patency of the oval foramen is common, and a deficiency of the floor of the oval fossa is far from infrequent. In addition to a second inlet muscular ventricular septal defect, straddling of the tricuspid valve, or presence of a common atrioventricular valve, features already emphasised, the most important associated lesion from the stance of the surgeon is probably anomalous origin of the anterior interventricular coronary artery from the right coronary artery. A right aortic arch, though not of functional importance, is also common. When detected, it alerts to the diagnosis of tetralogy. Aortic incompetence is commoner in older patients.

Morphogenesis

The notion that tetralogy of Fallot reflects malseptation of the arterial segment of the developing heart has a long pedigree, and is supported by observations concerning naturally occurring infundibular lesions in Keeshond dogs.[10] These animals show a spectrum of malformations, ranging from absence of the medial papillary muscle, through presence of a ventricular septal defect, to a constellation of anomalies similar to tetralogy. Study of embryos, in which developmental stages of these malformations were observed, showed that the factory for production of the lesions was within the ventricular outflow tracts. Specifically, abnormalities were found in the formation and position of the endocardial cushions which normally fuse to septate the ventricular outlets. These observations have now been confirmed in rats dosed with bis-diamine,[11,12] while the concept of muscularisation of the proximal outflow cushions to form the subpulmonary infundibulum of the normal heart has been confirmed by observations in the developing human heart (Figs. 36-20 and 36-21).

The findings in patients with deletion of chromosome 22q11 also support the existence of malseptation of the outflow tracts in humans, and point to this being due to problems in migration of cells from the neural crest. Based on the anatomic findings, therefore, it can be said with some degree of certainty that there is malseptation of the ventricular outlets and the arterial pole of the heart at the expense of the pulmonary trunk, together with failure of normal incorporation of the aortic outflow tract into the morphologically left ventricle. As discussed, the abnormal attachment of the muscular outlet septum is sufficient to account for the presence of the interventricular communication and the biventricular connection of the aorta, but production of subpulmonary muscular stenosis requires an additional abnormality involving the septoparietal trabeculations. The right ventricular hypertrophy is simply a haemodynamic consequence of the anatomic lesions.

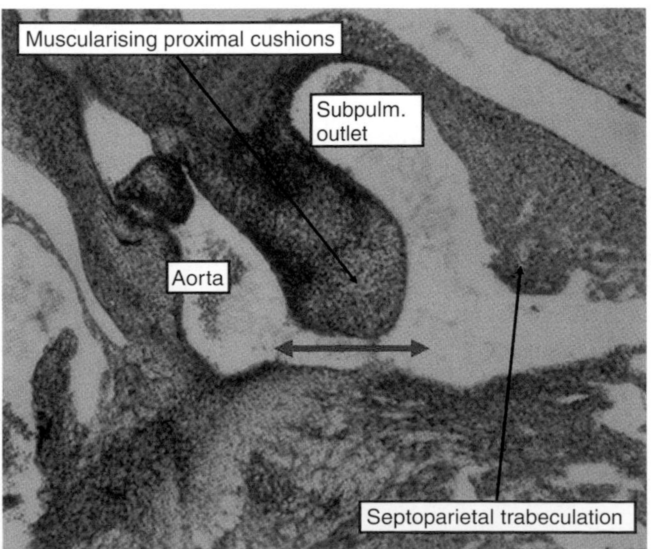

Figure 36-20 This section, from a human embryo just prior to closure of the embryonic interventricular communication *(double-headed arrow)* shows muscularisation of the proximal outflow cushions, which are about to fuse with the muscular interventricular septum so as to wall the aorta into the left ventricle.

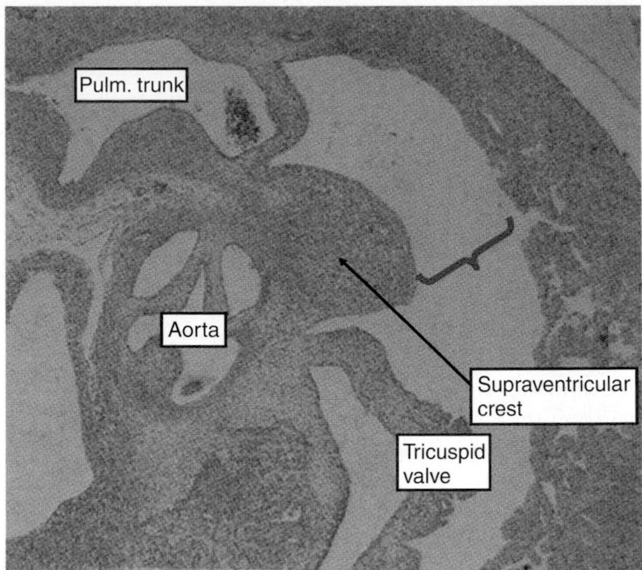

Figure 36-21 This section comes from another human embryo, just after the completion of ventricular septation. It shows how the muscularised outflow cushions, with normal development, form the supraventricular crest of the right ventricle. After normal development, the outflow to the pulmonary trunk is unobstructed *(yellow bracket)*. It is easy to see how, with malseptation of the outflow tracts, the cushions will form the muscular outlet septum and with hypertrophy of the septoparietal trabeculations produce the phenotypic morphology of tetralogy of Fallot.

Clinical Diagnosis

The clinical presentation is dominated by the degree of muscular obstruction of the right ventricular outflow tract.[25] This is sometimes modified by associated anomalies, such as persistent patency of the arterial duct, or presence of large systemic-to-pulmonary collateral arteries.

Presentation When Subpulmonary Obstruction Is Severe from Birth

When the obstruction of the right ventricular outflow tract is severe at birth, presentation is in the neonatal period. Persistent cyanosis becomes apparent within the first few hours or days of life. With severe arterial desaturation, a metabolic acidosis develops that is compensated by an increased respiratory rate. The concomitant fall in arterial content of carbon dioxide gives rise to a compensatory respiratory alkalosis. Intercostal or subcostal recession, however, is unusual. Cyanosis, which dominates the clinical picture, increases with crying, feeding, or other activities. At least initially, the baby does not appear unduly distressed. Sometimes the pulmonary circulation is duct-dependent. In this setting, the degree of subpulmonary obstruction is so great that there is inadequate antegrade flow, and virtually all pulmonary blood flow is derived from a left-to-right shunt via the arterial duct. Under such circumstances, spontaneous closure of the duct results in death. Maintenance of ductal patency, usually by infusion of prostaglandin E, is crucial.

Presentation When Subpulmonary Obstruction Is Moderate at Birth

The majority of children with tetralogy of Fallot are acyanotic at birth. Consequently, they often present because a systolic murmur is detected during routine examination. The development of cyanosis is dependent on increasing infundibular stenosis, and not on the degree of aortic override.[26] This is usually noted within the first few weeks of life, but development of cyanosis may rarely be delayed to late childhood. The systolic murmur, present in all patients other than those with very severe stenosis or acquired atresia, originates at the site of subpulmonary obstruction, and not because of flow across the ventricular septal defect.[27] At this stage, infants or children are usually asymptomatic. Later, hypercyanotic spells or squatting on exercise may all occur. With improved medical surveillance, all of these symptoms are now less often encountered than even a decade ago.

Presentation When Subpulmonary Obstruction Is Minimal at Birth

Some infants with tetralogy may uncommonly present at the age of 4 to 6 weeks with features indistinguishable from those of a large ventricular septal defect (see Chapter 28). These babies are breathless, feed poorly, gain weight poorly, and are not cyanosed. With increasing right ventricular hypertrophy, the subpulmonary obstruction becomes more marked and, as the shunt is reversed, the patients exhibit the signs and progression as described for the group with moderate obstruction.

Presentation with Absent Pulmonary Valve

When tetralogy is complicated by so-called absence of the leaflets of the pulmonary valve, which are usually present in rudimentary form (see Fig. 36-19), the presentation is characteristic yet different from the previously described groups. The majority with this complication present in infancy with respiratory symptoms of inspiratory and expiratory stridor, dyspnoea caused by lobar collapse or, at times, lobar emphysema. These features reflect compression of the bronchial tree by the grossly dilated proximal pulmonary arteries. While bronchial obstruction may lead to lobar collapse, and subsequent infection, partial obstruction may produce a ball-valve effect, resulting in emphysema. Because there is stenosis at the site of the rudimentary leaflets of the pulmonary valve, symptoms directly related to abnormal haemodynamics are unusual.

Squatting

Squatting, along with other postures, may alleviate the degree of cyanosis, dyspnoea or feeling of faintness induced by exercise. The means by which squatting alleviates the symptoms of cyanosis and dyspnoea have caused considerable debate. Irrespective of the precise mechanisms, there is little doubt that squatting causes an abrupt increase in systemic venous return and a rise in systemic vascular resistance. Right-to-left shunting is decreased by an increase in systemic vascular resistance. This means that the volume of blood passing through the right ventricle to the lungs is proportionally increased, with immediate improvement in effective pulmonary flow, and hence arterial saturations of oxygen.

Hypercyanotic Attacks

An important, and often dramatic, feature of patients with tetralogy is the occurrence of unprovoked severe cyanosis, which may lead to reduced cardiac output, and be accompanied by transient loss of consciousness.[28] These episodes, which are most common between 6 months and 2 years of age,[29] are potentially dangerous, as they may lead to cerebral damage or even death.[28] The majority last between 15 and 60 minutes, but an individual spell may be of shorter duration, or can last for several hours. Initial presentation of infants or children may be with a history of episodic loss of consciousness, or convulsions, episodes of going floppy or pale, transient vacant episodes, or episodes of becoming deeply cyanosed followed by loss of consciousness or sleep. Another striking feature of these spells may be episodes of very rapid deep respiration or hyperpnoea, or a high-pitched abnormal cry. The episodes are usually sufficiently dramatic or unusual for parents to volunteer information, but specific questioning concerning their presence should be part of every outpatient assessment. It was Wood (1958) who postulated that the spells resulted from infundibular spasm or shutdown.[28] Many now believe the concept of infundibular spasm, as a primary phenomenon, to be unsupported by the anatomy or physiology of the subpulmonary infundibulum, and suggest that the shutdown is secondary to other primary physiologic influences, such as dehydration, or tachycardia-induced reduction in right ventricular preload, systemic vasodilation in response to fever, or other sympathetic activity. Irrespective of their aetiology, their occurrence should lead to prompt treatment with continuous β-blockade, and referral for surgery or interventional catheterisation as dictated by the institutional protocols.

Physical Examination

The essential abnormal cardiac findings in the neonate with severe tetralogy of Fallot are cyanosis and, on auscultation, a systolic ejection murmur with a single second heart sound. Overt clubbing of fingers and toes is typically not detected until 2 or 3 months of age. The baby may be normally grown, although a higher proportion weighs less than would be expected by chance. Some degree of facial dysmorphism is quite common, and typical features of associated syndromes may be obvious, such as the DiGeorge, Goldenhauer, or Down syndromes. All patients should now undergo chromosomal analysis on presentation, with specific fluorescent in situ hybridisation for 22q11 deletion. Pulses are almost always normal in all limbs, aortic coarctation being exceedingly rare in symptomatic neonates with tetralogy of Fallot. The cardiac impulse may be normal, or the parasternal right ventricular impulse may be increased. The first heart sound is normal, but the second is characteristically single. In contrast to patients having pulmonary stenosis with an intact ventricular septum, pulmonary ejection sounds in the second or third intercostal space, or third and fourth heart sounds, are virtually never found in children with tetralogy. An aortic ejection click may sometimes be heard at the lower left sternal edge or at the apex. The duration of the systolic ejection murmur will vary depending on the degree of infundibular stenosis. The shorter the murmur, the tighter will be the stenosis and, in turn, the greater the cyanosis. Co-existing rudimentary formation of the leaflets of the pulmonary valve is characterised by an additional long loud early diastolic decrescendo murmur from pulmonary regurgitation, which should be easily distinguishable from a continuous murmur. When a loud continuous murmur is heard in the neonatal period, and clinical features are otherwise compatible with the diagnosis of tetralogy, it is more likely to originate from flow through large major systemic-to-pulmonary collateral arteries than the arterial duct. The patient is then likely to have co-existing pulmonary atresia. In these patients, cyanosis may not be so marked, since pulmonary blood flow is more adequately maintained through the collateral arteries.

Children with tetralogy in whom subpulmonary obstruction is minimal or absent at birth exhibit tachypnoea, dyspnoea, and intercostal or subcostal recession. This group has a large left-to-right shunt, with an increased flow of blood to the lungs. A prominent parasternal impulse, and hepatomegaly, may be present. On auscultation, the second sound is split, possibly with an accentuated pulmonary component.

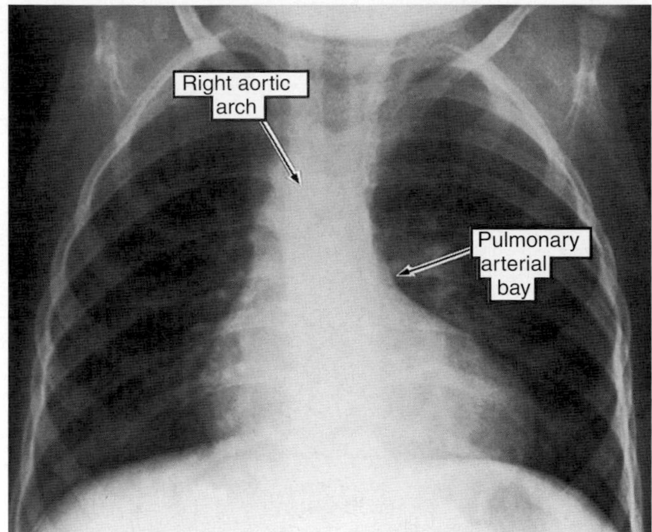

Figure 36-22 The chest radiograph of this young infant presents the typical features of a patient with tetralogy of Fallot. The trachea is slightly compressed by the aorta arching to its right side. Instead of the normal convexity produced by the pulmonary trunk, a concavity, or pulmonary arterial bay, is present.

Investigations

While the diagnosis of tetralogy of Fallot is usually made from clinical assessment, confirmation is now provided largely by cross sectional echocardiography. Before describing the typical echocardiographic features, however, we will discuss the plain chest radiograph and the electrocardiogram, as these are usually carried out as part of the general cardiac assessment of a child.

Chest Radiograph

In the acyanotic patient with tetralogy, the plain chest radiograph may be normal. Most patients have the usual arrangement of thoracic and abdominal organs, together with a left-sided heart, but tetralogy may occur with mirror-imaged arrangement, when the heart is usually right-sided. With usual atrial arrangement, up to one-third of patients with tetralogy have a right aortic arch. Of all subjects with a right aortic arch, three-quarters have tetralogy of Fallot with or without pulmonary atresia. The diagnosis is even more likely if there are reduced pulmonary vascular markings. Pulmonary vascular markings will usually be reduced in cyanotic patients, the lung fields being strikingly oligaemic in neonates when subpulmonary obstruction is severe. In contrast, vascular markings will be normal when infundibular stenosis is moderate. When subpulmonary obstruction is minimal, there will be pulmonary plethora, reflecting the left-to-right shunt. The heart is usually of normal size, but the upper right cardiac border may be prominent owing to displacement of the superior caval vein by a right aortic arch. A pulmonary bay, or concavity at the upper left heart border, reflects a small pulmonary trunk (Fig. 36-22). The apex of the heart may be upturned, probably because the hypertrophied right ventricle forms the apex in the postero-anterior projection. Post-operatively, the heart size can be used as a reasonable surrogate of right ventricular dilation, although other methods are clearly more accurate, and appropriate, for detailed assessment.

Electrocardiography

There is usually sinus rhythm, a normal or rightward QRS axis and overt right ventricular hypertrophy. After surgery, right bundle branch block with prolongation of the QRS duration is frequent.

Echocardiography

Transthoracic cross sectional echocardiography usually allows clear demonstration of all the intracardiac anatomy. As always, a sequential approach is used. The subcostal paracoronal view shows the narrowed subpulmonary outflow tract, with malalignment of the anteriorly displaced muscular outlet septum (Fig. 36-23). Parasternal long-axis

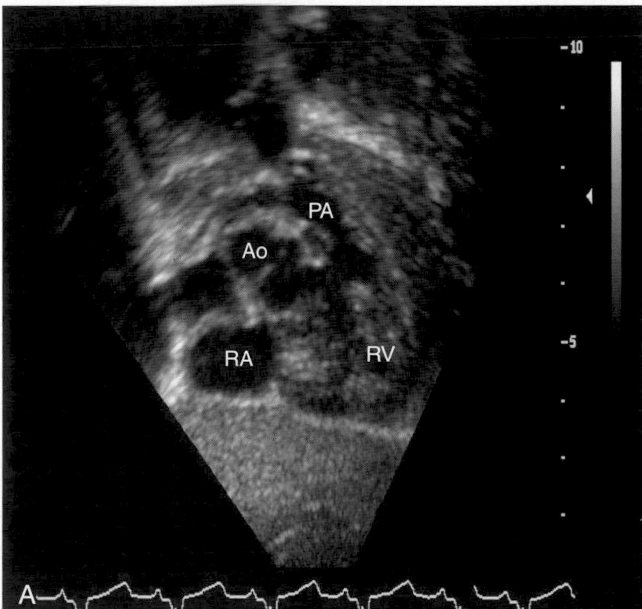

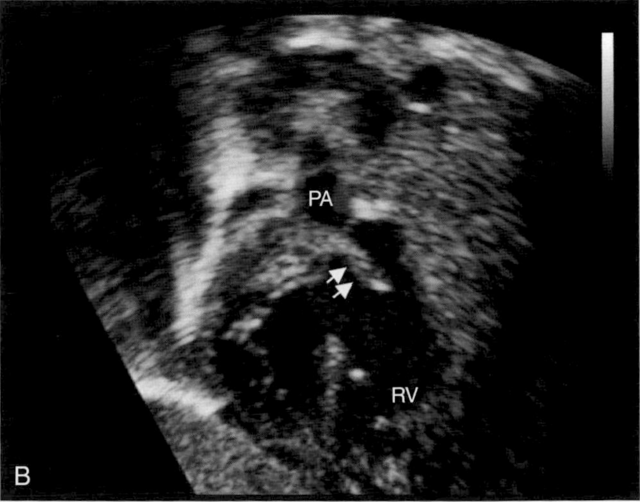

Figure 36-23 This echocardiogram shows a subcostal right anterior oblique view which presents an excellent overview of all the salient features of tetralogy. Panel **A** shows the classical subcostal right anterior oblique view and demonstrates marked trabeculations of the right ventricle (RV), antero-cephalad deviation of the outlet septum and narrowing of the right ventricular outflow tract. Panel **B** is a modified right anterior oblique view showing different anatomy in this case. The outlet septum (*arrows*) is elongated with lengthening of the subpulmonary infundibulum. Ao, overriding aorta; PA, pulmonary trunk; RA, right atrium.

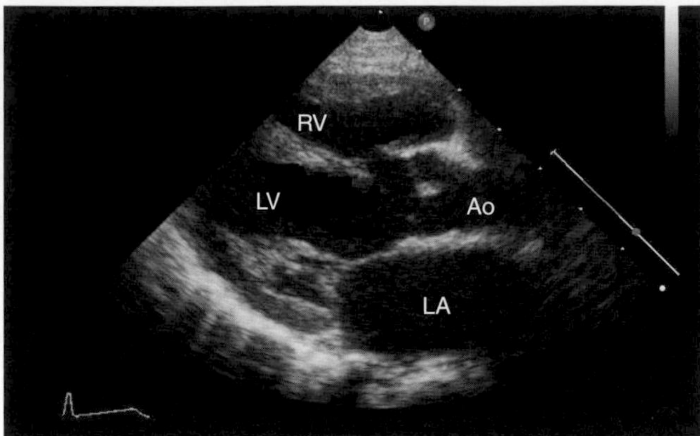

Figure 36-24 The parasternal long-axis view demonstrates the aortic valve (Ao) overriding the crest of the muscular ventricular septum and marked hypertrophy of the right ventricular myocardium. LA, left atrium; LV, left ventricle; RV, right ventricle.

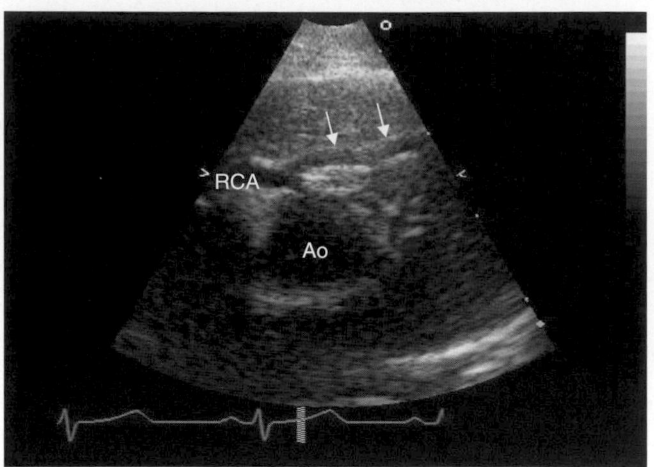

Figure 36-26 This short-axis echocardiogram shows an anomalous artery (*arrows*) arising from the right coronary artery (RCA) and crossing the subpulmonary infundibulum. Ao, aorta.

views demonstrate the aortic override (Fig. 36-24). Biventricular connection is seen also in the anteriorly tilted four-chamber view, but this is less reliable at defining the degree of override. If present, a straddling or overriding tricuspid valve is also seen in the four-chamber view, as is the common atrioventricular junction in hearts with deficient atrioventricular septation. These views, together with a parasternal short-axis view, allow the margins of the ventricular septal defect to be identified. The defect is usually perimembranous, but may have a muscular postero-inferior rim. The defect can also extend to become doubly committed and juxta-arterial when the outlet septum is fibrous and there is absence of the free-standing subpulmonary infundibulum. When the pulmonary trunk is traced to its bifurcation, it is possible to determine the size of the pulmonary arteries (Fig. 36-25) to the level of their first bifurcation, but not the more distal pattern of branching. Views of the aortic arch show the pattern of branching of the brachiocephalic arteries, a right brachiocephalic artery usually being found when the aortic arch is left-sided. When the first branch from the arch itself divides into left carotid and subclavian arteries, then it can be inferred that this vessel is the brachiocephalic artery, and that the arch itself is right-sided. These views will also show a persistent arterial duct, if present, while colour flow Doppler can confirm patency of previous palliative shunts, and may show collateral arteries. As with the echocardiographic assessment of all anomalies, it is essential to confirm normal systemic and pulmonary venous connections. Anomalous pulmonary venous connections in particular, if present, must be identified. Associated anomalies, such as rudimentary formation of the leaflets of the pulmonary valve, and dilation of the pulmonary trunk, are readily identified (see Fig. 36-25). In most patients, the origins of the right and left coronary arteries from the aorta can also be visualised, as can branching of the left artery into the circumflex and anterior interventricular arteries. Anomalous arteries can be identified crossing the subpulmonary infundibulum (Fig. 36-26), and their precise origin now determined. Similarly, the post-operative assessment of the early surgical result, the presence of residual lesions, and their haemodynamic sequels, are all well demonstrated by transthoracic echocardiography. The assessment of pulmonary regurgitation and its secondary effects on right ventricular performance can be assessed qualitatively, but for clinical decision making, there is an increasing reliance on magnetic resonance imaging, particularly in the teenager and adult.

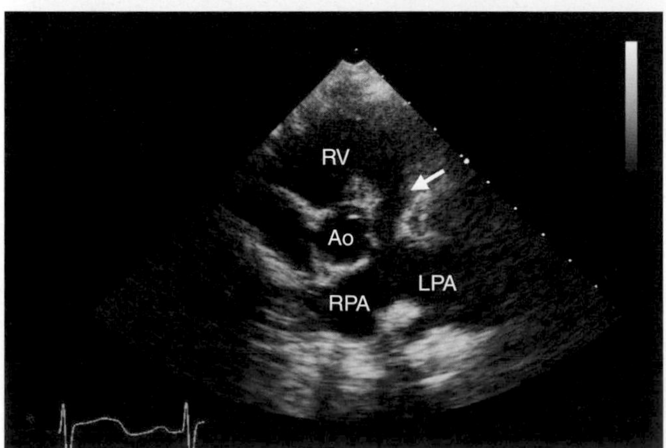

Figure 36-25 This echocardiogram in short-axis view shows the rudimentary nature of the leaflets of the pulmonary valve and narrowing of the pulmonary trunk (*arrow*) as well as markedly dilated left and right pulmonary arteries in a patient with so-called absent pulmonary valve.

Magnetic Resonance Imaging

With the exception of those with major aortopulmonary collaterals, there is rarely an indication for pre-operative cardiac studies using magnetic resonance imaging. Conversely, post-operative evaluation and decision-making are increasingly reliant on measurements obtained using this technique. Indeed, magnetic resonance imaging has rapidly become the gold standard for quantitative assessment of right ventricular volume, mass, and function, regardless of the position of the heart in the thorax.[30,31] Spin echo, or black blood, sequences are used for exploration of anatomy, and gradient echo, or white blood, sequences are employed for assessment of right ventricular function (Fig. 36-27). Magnetic resonance imaging may give an unrestrictive view of the right ventricular outflow tract, and if present, any aneurysmal enlargement can be demonstrated

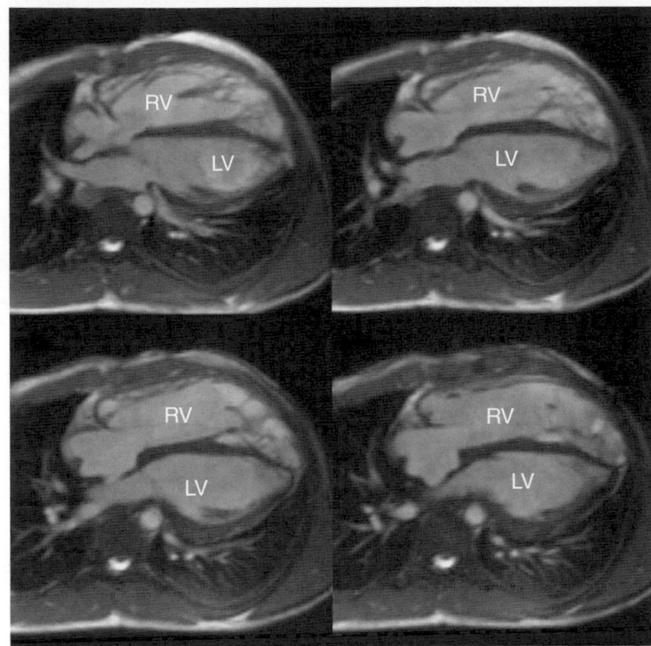

Figure 36-27 Magnetic resonance imaging in a patient with tetralogy of Fallot late after surgical correction. Cine-still-frame images of a four-chamber view show markedly dilated right ventricle (RV) and moderately dilated left ventricle (LV).

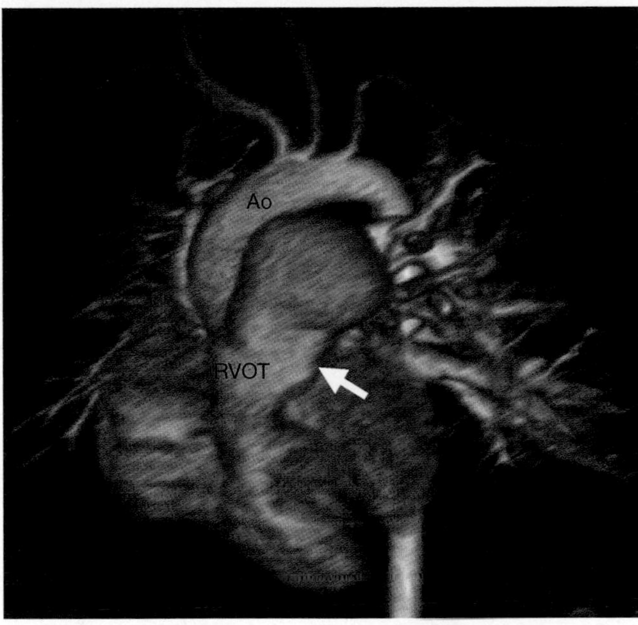

Figure 36-29 Magnetic resonance three-dimensional rendition in the late postoperative follow-up of a patient with tetralogy of Fallot demonstrates an aneurysmal right ventricular outflow tract (RVOT) (*arrow*) and left aortic arch (Ao).

(Figs. 36-28 and 36-29). Volumetric analysis of the right ventricle is performed by manually drawing endocardial contours at end-diastole and end-systole (Fig. 36-30A). Ejection fraction is then calculated by dividing stroke volume, represented by the difference between end-diastolic and end-systolic volumes, by the end-diastolic volume.

By using velocity mapping, quantification of the flow of blood to the lungs allows for accurate calculation of the pulmonary regurgitant volume and fraction (Fig. 36-30B). The latter is less reliable as an index of right ventricular preload, although is often considered, incorrectly in some patients, to be proportional to severity. Resonance imaging also permits measurements to be made with precision. The diameter of the aortic root, and any aortic insufficiency, can be quantified, while the peripheral pulmonary arteries can be demonstrated with unsurpassed clarity (see Fig. 36-28). The distribution of flow between the right and left pulmonary arteries can be assessed, and the influence of arterial size and discrete stenoses, if present, can be quantified. Imaging of delayed enhancement using gadolinium can show any scarring or fibrosis of the ventricles, these lesions potentially contributing to an increased propensity for arrhythmias, or formation of aneurysms in the right ventricular outflow tract.

Cardiac Catheterisation and Angiography

In most large units, diagnostic cardiac catheterisation is now rarely performed prior to palliative or corrective surgery (Fig. 36-31). Those with multiple aortopulmonary collateral arteries are a frequent exception to this rule (see Chapter 37), but increasingly magnetic resonance imaging is used rather than angiography to delineate their anatomy and distribution. The role of cardiac catheterisation in such patients, therefore, is to assess the haemodynamics within, and

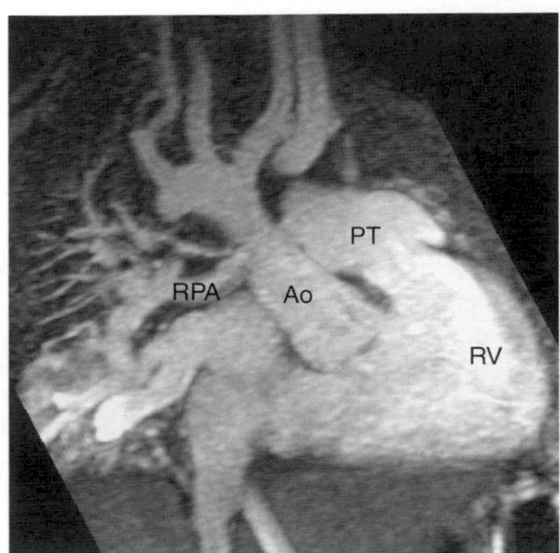

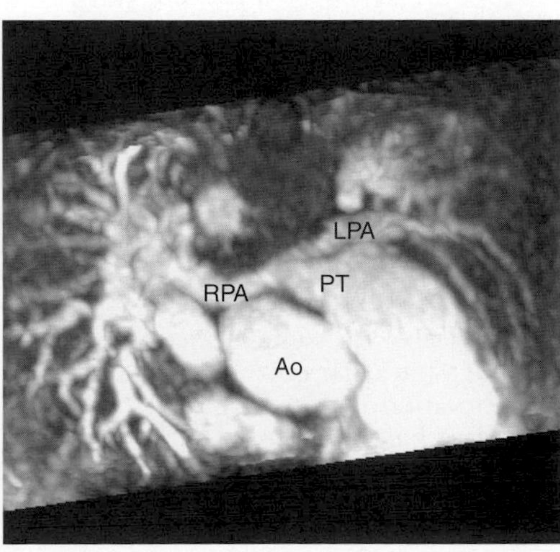

Figure 36-28 Magnetic resonance angiography and volume-rendered image shows hypoplasia of the right and left pulmonary arteries in a patient after repair of tetralogy of Fallot with additional distal arborisation abnormalities. Ao, Aorta; LPA, left pulmonary trunk; PT, pulmonary trunk; RPA, right pulmonary artery; RV, right ventricle.

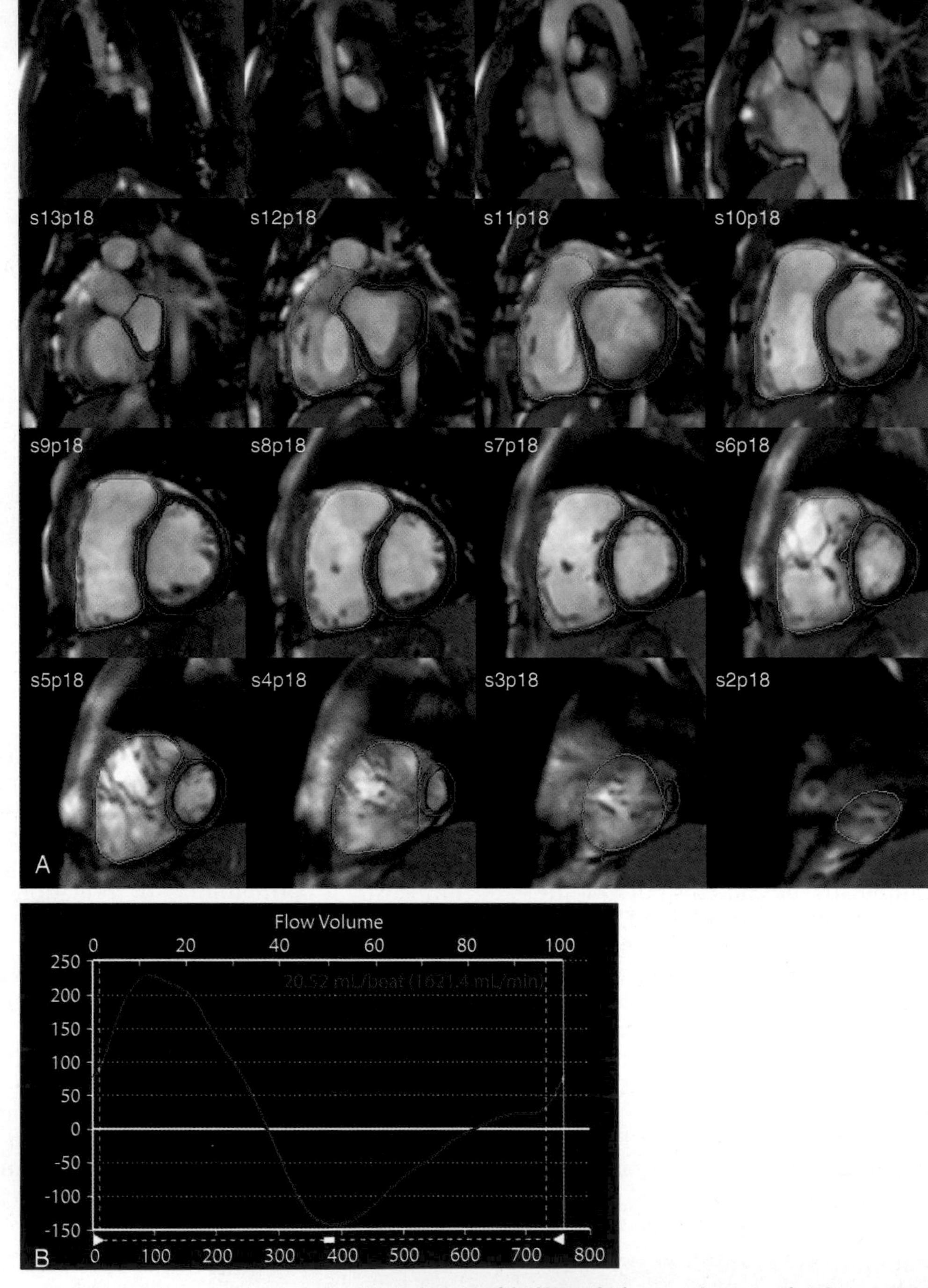

Figure 36-30 Panel A shows multiple short-axis cines from the apex to the base of the heart which are used to quantify right ventricular and left ventricular volumes by epicardial and endocardial tracing. The *yellow lines* show the tracing of the endocardial surface of the right ventricle, while the *green* and *red lines*, respectively, show the epicardial and endocardial surfaces of the left ventricle. In this patient with dilated right ventricle following correction of tetralogy of Fallot, the indexed end-diastolic volume was calculated to be 275 mL/m^2 body surface area (BSA) and the indexed left ventricular volume was 140 mL/m^2 BSA. Panel B demonstrates a flow profile, acquired with velocity mapping of the pulmonary trunk, that can be created by outlining the pulmonary artery in all phases of a heart circle. Pulmonary regurgitation and late diastolic forward flow are clearly shown.

connections between, the individual vessels when necessary. Interventional catheterisation remains applicable for some patients. Dilation and stenting of the right ventricular outflow tract, with prior radio-frequency perforation if atretic, have a role in some. Similarly, pre-operative balloon dilation of the pulmonary arteries, stenting of the arterial duct, and interventions on the aortopulmonary collateral arteries, may be part of a combined surgical and medical programme of management, often with the need for additional post-operative interventions in the more challenging cases.

Haemodynamics and Physiology

The haemodynamic consequences of the lesion are dominated by the severity of obstruction within the subpulmonary right ventricular outflow tract, superimposed

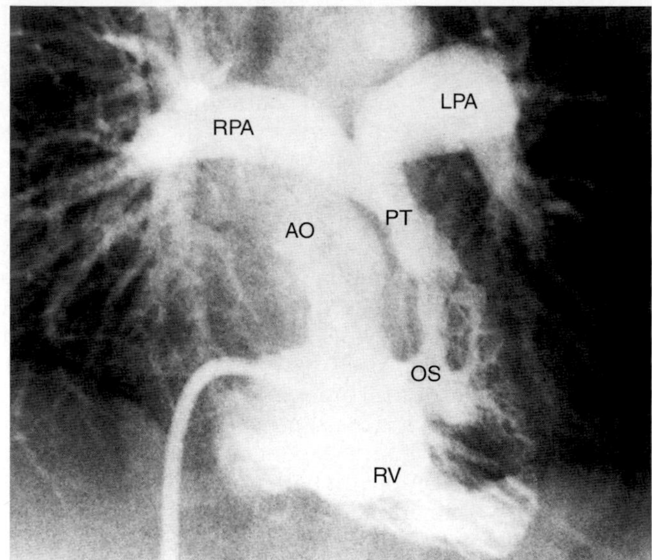

Figure 36-31 Angiography of the right ventricle performed in right anterior oblique projection. The outlet (infundibular) septum (OS), profiled in cross-section, together with hypertrophied septoparietal trabeculations of the right ventricular free wall produce muscular subvalvar stenosis. The pulmonary trunk (PT) is seen, together with the size of the right and left pulmonary arteries (RPA, LPA, respectively). The aorta (AO) has been opacified by contrast passing through the ventricular septal defect. RV, right ventricle.

upon the presence of a large ventricular septal defect. In almost all patients, the interventricular communication is large and non-limiting. This results in equalisation of right and left ventricular systolic pressure, regardless of the severity of pulmonary stenosis. The relative flows in the pulmonary and systemic circuits depend on the relative resistances, or impedances, to emptying of the right and left ventricles. When right ventricular outflow obstruction is minimal, and the pulmonary vascular resistance is normal, the flow of blood to the lungs will exceed that in the systemic circuit. There will then be a dominant left-to-right shunt, and the clinical picture will resemble closely that of a ventricular septal defect. Under these circumstances, resting cyanosis may be absent. When obstruction to right ventricular emptying is similar to that provided by the systemic vascular resistance, a balanced situation exists. There will be no overall shunting in either direction, although transient small right-to-left and left-to-right shunts occur during each cardiac cycle. Pulmonary and systemic flows, at least at rest, will be equal. On exercise, however, a fall in systemic vascular resistance, with or without an increase in infundibular stenosis, will result in a right-to-left shunt with cyanosis. The systemic flow will then exceed the pulmonary flow. With increasing degrees of obstruction in the subpulmonary right ventricular outflow tract, a dominant right-to-left shunt develops. Cyanosis then becomes a constant feature. Such severe obstruction may be present from birth. More usually, increasing infundibular stenosis develops coincidentally with progressive right ventricular hypertrophy. Cyanosis is dependent on the degree of pulmonary stenosis but is unrelated to the degree of aortic override.

Typically, the mean pulmonary arterial pressure is lower than normal, consequent upon the reduced flow of blood to the lungs. The pulmonary arterial systolic pressure, though lower than that in the right ventricle, may be higher than normal in the group with mild stenosis and increased pulmonary flow. The right ventricular systolic pressure rises with systemic hypertension, or on administration of pressor agents such as phenylephrine. But it falls in the presence of a vasodilator agent. The right ventricular pressure may also fall, along with aortic pressure, during, or particularly after, exercise when the systemic vascular resistance is decreased. As already indicated, a fall in systemic resistance, with no change in resistance to right ventricular emptying, will result in an increased right-to-left shunt.

Therapeutic Options

In many centres, primary complete correction is now the treatment of choice, almost no matter what the age or size of the patient. Precise timing may depend on the experience of the particular unit; there is a role for interventional catheterisation in some. Otherwise, the medical management of a symptomatic child is devoted principally to preparation for surgery.

Medical Management

When called to a child undergoing a hypercyanotic crisis, the first actions should be to place the child in the knee-chest position and administer oxygen by face mask. If the child is extremely restless, an intravenous line should be inserted, and a small dose of morphine sulphate, at 0.1 mg per kg, may be all that is required to abort the crisis. If this fails, treatment with a β-blocking agent such as propranolol will reduce tachycardia and increase systemic resistance. It may also have an effect to reduce hypercontractility in response to endogenous release of catecholamine, but there is no evidence for a specific effect to reduce infundibular muscular spasm. The drug should be administered intravenously. Half of this should be given rapidly, and the remaining half more slowly over the next few minutes. If this fails to lead to prompt improvement, then arterial blood gases should be assessed. Accompanying metabolic acidosis should be corrected. Intubation and ventilation may be required in extreme cases, and at this stage an intravenous vasoconstrictor, such as phenylephrine, is often effective. Exceptionally, it will be necessary to construct an emergency systemic-to-pulmonary shunt. In any case, the patient should immediately be referred for definitive intervention, with treating orally with propranolol during the interim.

Surgical Management

The symptomatic infant or child requires surgery, and there is little controversy regarding those over a few months of age. For neonates and young infants, some centres continue to offer surgical palliation for that age group, temporising by construction of a systemic-to-pulmonary arterial shunt. In recent years, there has been a resurgence in transcatheter palliation, including balloon dilation and stenting of the right ventricular outflow tract,[32] and stenting of the arterial duct. The role of these interventions, usually reserved for the smaller patient or those with additional anomalies, remains uncertain.

Palliative Procedures

It was in patients with tetralogy that Taussig noted that persistent patency of the arterial duct often prevented the onset of cyanosis. From this, together with Blalock, she developed the idea that it would be beneficial to use the subclavian artery to create an artificial duct. The procedure is traditionally performed on the side opposite to that of the aortic arch. On this side, the subclavian artery arises from the brachiocephalic artery rather than directly from the aorta. Because of this, kinking is less likely to occur at its origin when it is turned down to become a shunt. When the arch is right sided, therefore, a left-sided shunt is normally performed. Nowadays, modification of the classical shunt by placement of interposition grafts has achieved such excellent results, with negligible mortality and adequate patency, that the modified shunt has become the procedure of choice. While several alternatives were used in the 1950s and 1960s, they were never as popular, or consistently effective, as the Blalock-Taussig shunt. The modified version is now frequently performed through a median sternotomy, rather than the classical thoracotomy approach. Following creation of such interposition shunts in small infants, most units choose to treat the patient with heparin in the initial post-operative period, followed by aspirin until the time of corrective surgery. Studies are underway to examine the potential role of more powerful anti-platelet agents. Acute thrombosis of the shunt, nonetheless, is now rare, but remains an important co-morbid feature, in addition to concerns regarding stenosis of the pulmonary artery, potential damage to the recurrent laryngeal or phrenic nerves, and adverse physiologic effects such as increased flow of blood to the lungs, systemic steal syndrome, and so on. For these reasons, the modified Blalock-Taussig shunt is becoming less frequently used.

Definitive Repair

Intracardiac repair involves reconstituting the ventricular septum, and relieving subpulmonary obstruction. The operation is now rarely performed via a large ventriculotomy, with transatrial closure of the septal defect now almost universal. Any ventriculotomy, even when involving a transjunctional incision to relieve obstruction in the subpulmonary outlet, is minimised, given the late results now being observed in survivors of correction as they reach adulthood.

The hypertrophied outlet septum, together with its parietal and septal extensions, is excised as indicated. In the past, the decision as to whether a transjunctional patch would be necessary was often made based on measurements made on pre-operative angiograms to determine the sizes of the pulmonary arteries relative to the aorta. The need for a patch can also be determined during the operation by using Hegar dilators to measure the narrowest part of the pulmonary outflow tract. Free pulmonary incompetence is inevitable when a patch is placed across the ventriculo-pulmonary junction, often considered transannular, although of course the arterial valvar leaflets are not supported in annular fashion. A unicusp aortic homograft was inserted by some in attempts to avoid this complication, but no evidence has accrued to show that the late results of this strategy are superior to use of a non-valved patch. The ventricular septal defect is closed using a patch of knitted Dacron, Teflon, or pericardium secured with either continuous or interrupted sutures.

Surgery should, ideally, result in normal right ventricular pressures, absence of any gradient in pressures between the right ventricle and the pulmonary arteries, and a competent pulmonary valve. Unfortunately, the nature of the subpulmonary obstruction rarely allows this ideal result. The last decade has seen a shift away from the obsession with complete relief of obstruction, towards attempts to preserve the pulmonary valve, even at the expense of a modest degree of residual stenosis. The belief is that this will minimise the adverse late effects of pulmonary incompetence, and retain the integrity of the outflow tract, avoiding late dilation and formation of aneurysms. The success of such an approach, or course, remains to be seen. The timing of definitive repair must be based on the results in the institution offering treatment. While the literature is replete with excellent results, even when performed routinely in the neonatal period, such outcomes are of little relevance to a unit that cannot provide the same level of intra-operative and post-operative care. The experience at the Hospital for Sick Children in Toronto with palliative shunting for tetralogy of Fallot was reviewed for the period between 1990 and 1994. The analysis revealed a relatively high rate of shunt-related complications, and worse overall survival than in patients who had not undergone palliation. Those undergoing palliation who had a shunt placed in the neonatal period experienced more problems with pulmonary arterial distortion and poor pulmonary arterial growth, and required more reinterventions, than did patients palliated at an older age.[33] For that reason, primary definitive repair for those suffering symptoms, even in newborns, is now the rule in Toronto. Exceptions may be made, nonetheless, for those with small pulmonary arteries, for small or premature infants, and for those with additional cardiac or extracardiac anomalies that might significantly modify the outcome. If palliation is to be undertaken, nonetheless, it is done by the transcatheter route.[32]

Early Outcomes

The outcomes for corrective surgery continue to evolve and improve. In an earlier period, and excluding the influence of pulmonary atresia, several factors were identified that introduced a significant increment of risk.[34] While historical, they remain as interesting discussion points, and retain their validity today. The first feature was the presence of diffusely small pulmonary arteries, the effect of which is to increase the ratio between the peak ventricular pressures subsequent to repair. The detrimental effect of this feature is neutralised by not attempting primary repair when the ratio of the combined diameter of the right and left pulmonary arteries, measured just before their first bifurcation, to that of the descending aorta is less than 1.5 to 1.[35]

The second factor relates to abnormalities of the pulmonary arteries, such as anomalous origin of one artery, or stenosis of either artery at its origin. These can all be alleviated by appropriate reconstructive procedures. Additional peripheral stenoses can now be dealt with by balloon dilation at later cardiac catheterisation,[36,37] particularly when using high-pressure balloons.[38] The third risk factor is a small pulmonary valvar orifice, producing a high right ventricular pressure subsequent to repair if the obstruction is unrelieved. The necessary relief is usually achieved by insertion of a patch across the ventriculo-pulmonary junction. This, in and of itself, is no longer a risk factor for early mortality, but it is clearly a risk factor for morbidity in the long term. The use of a valved conduit was another factor identified in this earlier experience. This is now almost certainly of historical interest, since few would now place a conduit in patients with tetralogy and pulmonary stenosis. The exception, of course, might be when there is anomalous origin of the anterior descending artery from the right coronary artery. A transatrial–transpulmonary approach can also be used in this setting, nonetheless, thus avoiding the need for a conduit.

The final risk factor identified in this historical series remains the most contentious, namely age at repair. Both old and young age appeared as incremental risks in the initial analysis. Old age introduced risks for hospital death, poor post-operative exercise capacity, and impaired left ventricular function. Old age at that stage seemed to be more than 5 years, way beyond any contemporary protocol. But how early should primary correction be recommended? In contrast to surgery for ventricular or atrioventricular septal defects, young age had still remained an incremental risk for repair of tetralogy in some earlier series, but certainly not all. For example, one group reported repair of 100 infants with symptomatic tetralogy undergoing surgery consecutively at under 1 year of age with only 3 patients dying.[39] Another group corrected 56 infants under 6 months, with 41 undergoing primary repair, and suffered only one death.[40] Still another group gave details of 30 neonates, 11 with associated pulmonary atresia and 5 with non-confluent pulmonary arteries, and reported no mortality prior to discharge from hospital, albeit with significant late morbidity and mortality.[41] These exceptional surgical results showed what could be achieved, and set the scene for the philosophical change towards definitive repair being performed, at any age, in the symptomatic neonate and infant. There remain, nonetheless, important questions as to what, in the long term, is optimal. For example, in these latter series, over half of the infants required patches across the ventriculo-pulmonary junction. We will discuss the inevitable adverse influence of the resulting pulmonary incompetence below.

Early Post-operative Complications

Problems can occur both in the immediate and late post-operative periods. Apart from the usual complications of cardiac surgery, such as bleeding, a low cardiac output may occur because of inadequate relief of subpulmonary obstruction, or an obstructed or restrictive pulmonary vascular bed. More usually, however, the low cardiac output syndrome occurs in the face of an apparently adequate repair, with preserved ventricular systolic function. In such patients, echocardiographic Doppler studies show evidence of what has now been termed restrictive right ventricular physiology.[42] There is antegrade diastolic flow in the pulmonary arteries, coinciding with atrial systole throughout the respiratory cycle. As the pulmonary vascular resistance is low, atrial contraction causes flow to be transmitted through a poorly compliant right ventricle into the pulmonary arteries in such a way that, if pulmonary incompetence is present, its duration is shortened (Fig. 36-32). Not only does atrial constriction cause antegrade diastolic flow in the pulmonary arteries, but retrograde flow can also be detected in the superior caval vein, again reflecting a poorly compliant right ventricle.[43] The occurrence of restrictive physiology does not appear to be related to age at operation, but is more common on follow-up of patients in whom a patch had been inserted across the ventriculo-pulmonary junction.[44] Management consists of maintenance of sinus rhythm and right ventricular preload, keeping the central venous pressure at 12 to 15 mm Hg, early drainage of resulting effusions, and early extubation. If this is not possible, ventilation should be continued using the lowest possible mean pressure in the airways. Careful use of inotropic or inodilator support is required, as these may make things worse and are rarely required, as systolic function is usually preserved. Indeed, a stronger case can be made for the use of vasoconstrictors to maintain pressures of perfusion. Early post-operative restriction is a transient phenomenon, usually resolving within 72 hours, although reappearance in the later postoperative follow-up period may occur.[44] Paradoxically, if encountered, it is associated with superior functional performance.

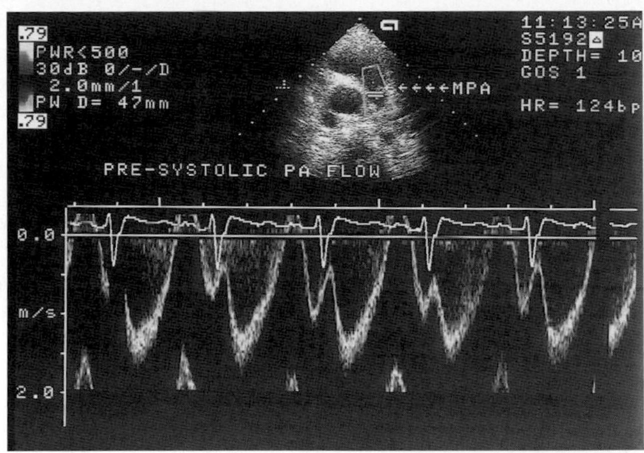

Figure 36-32 Doppler echocardiography of pulmonary arterial flow in the early post-operative course following corrective surgery in tetralogy of Fallot shows antegrade flow occurring in diastole coincident with atrial systole, thus shortening the duration of pulmonary regurgitation. This pattern is considered the hallmark of isolated right ventricular restriction. (Reproduced with permission of Dr Seamus Cullen and GMM Publishers, from *The Right Heart in Congenital Heart Disease* edited by Redington et al, 1998.)

Late Outcomes of Intervention

An important paper was published in 1993, which reviewed the late survival and outcomes of surgical repair of tetralogy of Fallot.[45] Actuarial survival was overall at 86% among patients surviving 30 days after complete repair, compared with 96% in the control population. Further analysis showed rates of survival after 30 years of 90%, 93%, and 91%, in patients undergoing surgery below the age of 5 years, from 5 to 7 years, and at 8 to 11 years, respectively. Of patients who were 12 years or older at the time of operation, only 76% were alive, compared with 93% in controls. Although reflecting a success story, in terms of modification of the natural history of the disease, it became clear, and is increasingly the case, that the late mortality after definitive repair will far exceed the early post-operative risk. Consequently, the last decade or so has seen a shift towards improved understanding of the determinants of late outcomes, with concentration on the adverse effects of pulmonary incompetence, previously considered to be a benign side-effect of relief of the obstructed right ventricular outflow tract.

Physical Response to Correction

Following successful repair, almost all children rapidly catch up in terms of their height and weight. They grow faster than their peers, and height and weight are normal 5 years after repair. Murmurs frequently persist after operation, usually but not always related to mild residual subpulmonary obstruction, or to acquired pulmonary incompetence. The typical auscultatory findings on follow-up are a single second sound, an ejection systolic murmur in the second or third left intercostal space, and a slightly delayed diastolic decrescendo murmur. If the pulmonary valve has been preserved, the second sound may be split. If subvalvar obstruction is completely relieved without a patch across the ventriculo-pulmonary junction, there may be no murmurs.

Presence of an ejection systolic murmur may complicate assessment of other problems, such as a residual ventricular septal defect, although cross sectional echocardiography with Doppler studies easily allows quantification of residual intracardiac anomalies. In patients who have undergone a staged surgical approach, with a preceding systemic-to-pulmonary anastomosis, reappearance of a continuous systolic-diastolic murmur may be first symptom of a recanalised anastomosis. Those patients have a high risk for acquiring endocarditis, so elective closure in the catheter laboratory is recommended.[46]

Apart from a right aortic arch, when present, the chest radiograph may return to normal, but some will have a bulge over the upper left heart border as a consequence of patching the outflow tract. Cardiomegaly evolves with longer duration of follow-up, and largely reflects right-sided dilation. The electrocardiogram will often show right bundle branch block, with the duration of the QRS complex lengthening in response to dilation of the right heart.

Pulmonary incompetence is found by echo-Doppler examination in between three-fifths and nine-tenths of patients post-operatively. Pulmonary insufficiency is well-tolerated for the first few years, but may result in a chronically dilated right ventricle. Patients with isolated congenital pulmonary regurgitation are known to remain asymptomatic for up to 20 years, but thereafter freedom from symptoms declines rapidly with time.[47] Symptoms include effort intolerance, right-sided failure, arrhythmias, and sudden death. Chronic pulmonary regurgitation may also adversely affect exercise performance and right ventricular function. One of the difficulties hitherto has been lack of a technique to assess quantitatively the amount of pulmonary regurgitation. By using pressure–volume loops derived from simultaneous intraventricular pressure recordings during angiography, it has now become possible to achieve this goal.[48] Using this technique, exercise ability using a standard Bruce protocol has been combined with measurements of maximal consumption of oxygen and exchange of metabolic gases using respiratory mass spectrometry.[49] Maximal heart rate and total duration of exercise were less in those with pulmonary incompetence than in matched controls, and impairment of exercise capacity was shown to be directly related to the degree of pulmonary regurgitation. Those with more severe regurgitation had both reduced exercise performance, and reduced lung compliance. A higher incidence of exercise-induced ventricular arrhythmias was also noted in patients with the most severe pulmonary regurgitation.

Nowadays, pulmonary incompetence can also be measured directly and accurately by cardiac magnetic resonance. Results using this approach have reinforced the earlier data regarding the adverse effects of pulmonary incompetence on functional performance and disturbances of conduction. Before dwelling in more detail on the arrhythmic problems and their relationship to haemodynamic disturbances, it is of note that, in the long term, the consequences of chronic pulmonary regurgitation may be modified by the diastolic properties of the right ventricle.[50] Restrictive right ventricular physiology, found in some patients early after operation (see Fig. 36-32), is correlated with beneficial rather than adverse haemodynamic consequences when found on long-term follow-up. Exercise tolerance is enhanced, the heart does not enlarge despite pulmonary regurgitation, and intraventricular conduction disturbances, as reflected by the QRS prolongation, may be less.[50] In this respect, it should also be noted that the presence of peripheral pulmonary stenosis will increase the amount of pulmonary incompetence following surgery.[51] In the context of the mechanical dysfunction of the right ventricle, it is increasingly appreciated that additional left ventricular dysfunction seems to co-exist in many patients with tetralogy. The right ventricle is anatomically integrated with the left ventricle through subepicardial bundle of aggregated myocytes that run from the free wall of the right ventricle to the anterior wall of the left ventricle. Moreover, the ventricles share the septum, and are enclosed in the same pericardial cavity. The interaction of the two ventricles results in alterations of both diastolic and systolic function.[52] Experimental work demonstrated that part of the external mechanical work generated by the right ventricle is a direct consequence of left ventricular contraction, or contraction of shared myocytes.[53] Patients late after repair show a reasonably strong linear relationship between right and left ventricular ejection fractions.[54] Left ventricular dysfunction is also known to be a risk factor for sudden death late after repair of tetralogy,[55] with experimental work showing that acute dilation of the right heart can modify left ventricular performance by a direct effect on load-independent indexes of systolic performance.[56] Thus, right ventricular dilation may significantly impact on left ventricular systolic function.[57] In addition, progressive right ventricular enlargement, and worsening right bundle branch block, may result in increasing ventricular dyssynchrony. Indeed, patients with the longest delay between the onsets of contraction of the two ventricles had worse exercise performance, and a higher incidence of ventricular arrhythmia.[58] Pacing the right ventricle may also improve synchronicity of right ventricular contraction,[59] and biventricular resychronisation produces a significant increase in cardiac output.[57] This method, therefore, may be an effective strategy for patients with biventricular dysfunction who do not respond adequately to replacement of the pulmonary valve. While most attention has been directed towards assessment of problems in the right heart, there are other important late anatomic problems. For example, aortic dilation and valvar incompetence is recognised increasingly with duration of follow-up,[60] and the risk of endocarditis is significant. Nonetheless, the issues of pulmonary incompetence and the resulting secondary functional and conduction disturbances dominate the clinical picture in most patients.

Post-operative Conduction Disturbances and Arrhythmias

Complete right bundle branch block is frequently produced following surgical correction of tetralogy, and is primarily benign. The duration of the QRS complex in this setting appears to be loosely related to the size of the right ventricle, and in turn, related to the risk of late ventricular arrhythmia. As such, its documentation and intermittent assessment is important in the late follow-up of these patients.

While heart block can be a cause of death at or soon after surgery, and may cause some late sudden deaths, it is unlikely to account for the majority of deaths. Multiple ventricular premature beats may be a harbinger of more serious ventricular arrhythmias. Ventricular arrhythmias, rather than conduction defects, are more likely to be the basis for sudden death.[61] In this light, the use of ambulatory monitoring has greatly increased the detection of arrhythmias after surgical correction of congenitally malformed hearts, bringing with it many dilemmas in management.[62]

Disturbances of rhythm, such as frequent unifocal ventricular extrasystoles, more complex couplets, multi-focal extrasystoles, and even asymptomatic non-sustained ventricular tachycardia, were reported in two-fifths or more of patients undergoing 24-hour monitoring on medium-term follow-up.[63] Attempts were made in these, and other, series to correlate arrhythmias with residual haemodynamic disorders, such as poorly-relieved subpulmonary obstruction, but the results were conflicting. What has emerged is that frequency of arrhythmias correlates well with age at operation.[62]

One possible explanation for this finding is the presence with older age of increasing amounts of fibrosis in the right but not the left ventricle.[64,65] Not only age, but more extensive surgery,[66] and the extent of the ventriculotomy,[67] are associated with an increase in ventricular arrhythmias. Whether asymptomatic arrhythmias predict the risk of sudden death is a different matter. Sudden death occurs in about 6% of patients over the long term,[45] or 4.5 per 100 patients-years,[68] but can it be predicted? As discussed previously, poor right ventricular systolic or diastolic function, residual subpulmonary obstruction, or a residual ventricular septal defect have been associated with a poor prognosis, possibly owing to arrhythmias. The presence in asymptomatic patients of complex ventricular arrhythmias on 24-hour tape recordings, nonetheless, did not identify a group at risk.[69]

Perhaps the most important recent development in the ability to predict sudden death over the long term in patients with corrected tetralogy of Fallot comes from the establishment of a relationship between QRS prolongation, right ventricular dilation, sustained ventricular arrhythmias, and late sudden death.[50] Prolongation of the QRS complex of 180 msec or more was shown to predict a 95% probability of near-miss sudden death from sustained ventricular arrhythmias. Conversely, no patient with sustained ventricular tachycardia dying suddenly had a duration less than 180 msec. Prolongation of the QRS complex was associated with right ventricular dilation, and often associated with pulmonary regurgitation, although this was not quantified in the study. When restrictive right ventricular physiology was identified on late follow-up, duration of the QRS complex was always less than 180 msec. In these patients, the right ventricle has a limited end-diastolic volume, since antegrade diastolic pulmonary flow owing to atrial systole limits the amount of pulmonary regurgitation. The myocardial structure that prevents right ventricular dilation even in the presence of pulmonary regurgitation is not currently known, but it appears to be protective in the long term against sudden death and sustained ventricular arrhythmias.

What emerges from these studies is that a mechanoelectrical interaction in the right ventricle, namely ventricular dilation and stretch, may underlie ventricular electrical instability. Such mechanisms have already been established for the left ventricle.[70,71] Of particular interest is that a decrease in right ventricular volume, caused by a Valsalva manoeuvre, can terminate ventricular tachycardia in some patients.[72] Electrophysiological studies have indicated a re-entry mechanism for sustained ventricular arrhythmias in this setting, which requires areas of slow conduction.[73] Further support to the notion that inhomogeneity in depolarisation and repolarisation may form the substrate for malignant ventricular arrhythmias late after repair of tetralogy of Fallot comes from the finding that, in patients with a duration of the QRS complex greater than 180 msec, there are increased dispersions of the QT, QRS, and JT intervals in those with, but not those without, episodes of ventricular tachycardia.[74]

Fragmented electrograms indicative of localised areas of slowed conduction, however, have also been recorded from the inflow region,[75] the outflow tract,[76] and throughout the right ventricle in the absence of sustained ventricular tachycardia.[77] It could be, therefore, that the mechanisms for non-sustained and sustained ventricular arrhythmias are different. This is an important consideration when we consider management of arrhythmias or disorders of conduction during follow-up. It must also not be forgotten that atrial arrhythmias, albeit less dramatic in their effects, are equally as prevalent as ventricular arrhythmia in these patients, and are a significant cause of late morbidity.

Treatment of Arrhythmias and Conduction Disturbances at Follow-Up

The aims of treatment are relief of symptoms and prevention of sudden death. Non-sustained ventricular tachycardia is present in two-fifths or more of asymptomatic patients on follow-up, but the incidence of late sudden death is low, and cannot be predicted from analysis of 24-hour tape recordings. For this reason, routine treatment of asymptomatic patients with non-sustained tachycardia is not currently indicated.[62] Those with symptomatic ventricular arrhythmia require intervention. If not associated with significant right ventricular remodeling, then insertion of an implantable defibrillator may be indicated.[78] In many, there will be associated severe pulmonary incompetence, and surgical repair or replacement of the pulmonary valve, often with coincident arrhythmic surgery, and sometimes with insertion of an implantable defibrillator, will usually be performed. Atrial arrhythmias usually respond to medical therapies in the first instance, but increasingly catheter-based ablation of pathways is performed, and is increasingly successful in the early-mid term. Many will also fulfil criterions for surgery to the pulmonary valve, and an additional maze procedure may be indicated.

Treatment of Pulmonary Valvar Incompetence

For years, surgical replacement of the pulmonary valve in symptomatic patients has been the treatment of choice.[79] When it was shown that right ventricular function did not always recover after valvar replacement, especially if right ventricular ejection fraction was substantially decreased, an earlier intervention was advocated.[80] This is now one of the most discussed questions in the long-term follow-up of patients with tetralogy of Fallot. Optimal timing of pulmonary valvar replacement is important to preserve right

CHAPTER 37

Tetralogy of Fallot with Pulmonary Atresia

EDWARD J. BAKER and ROBERT H. ANDERSON

In this chapter, we deal with one of the most complex, and difficult to treat surgically, of all congenital cardiac malformations. It is still frequent to find the lesion described as pulmonary atresia with ventricular septal defect. Here, we have chosen to call it tetralogy of Fallot with pulmonary atresia. Why should we consider this anomaly part of the spectrum of tetralogy? It is certainly the case that all the patients to be discussed have pulmonary atresia in the setting of a deficient ventricular septum. But other patients with diverse morphologies also have variants of pulmonary atresia with ventricular septal defect, and they will not be discussed. For example, patients with discordant ventriculo-arterial connections as their primary feature, or those with isomeric atrial appendages, or double inlet ventricle, or atrioventricular valvar atresia, can all have pulmonary atresia associated with a hole between the ventricles. In those patients, almost always, the pulmonary arteries are confluent, and are fed by a patent arterial duct. They do not demonstrate the complexity of pulmonary arterial supply that produces the problems encountered so frequently in the setting of systemic-to-pulmonary collateral arteries. We use the heading of tetralogy with pulmonary atresia for this chapter, therefore, because almost without exception, the intracardiac anatomy is that of tetralogy of Fallot when the pulmonary arterial supply is derived from systemic-to-pulmonary collateral arteries.

PREVALENCE AND AETIOLOGY

Because there is no uniformity in how to classify the patients to be described, it is difficult to provide precise incidence for those having tetralogy with pulmonary atresia. Patients with tetralogy of Fallot, considered as a group, made up almost 4% of those with congenitally malformed hearts in the series reported from Liverpool.[1] It is likely that up to one-tenth of these patients will have had pulmonary atresia rather than pulmonary stenosis. In many, the intracardiac anatomy suggests that the pulmonary outflow tract was initially patent, but became atretic during fetal life. In others, particularly in those with systemic-to-pulmonary collateral arteries, the atresia was probably part and parcel of the initial developmental abnormality.[2] Tetralogy of Fallot with pulmonary atresia is known to be associated with deletions of chromosome 22q11,[3,4] such deletions also now established as the cause of the velo-cardiofacial syndrome, which typically consists of tetralogy of Fallot along with facial and aural anomalies, cleft palate, and developmental delay.[5]

MORPHOLOGY

Pulmonary atresia exists when there is either complete obstruction, or absence, of the communication normally present between the cavities of the ventricular mass and the pulmonary arteries. In the setting of tetralogy of Fallot (Fig. 37-1), the obstructive form can sometimes be produced

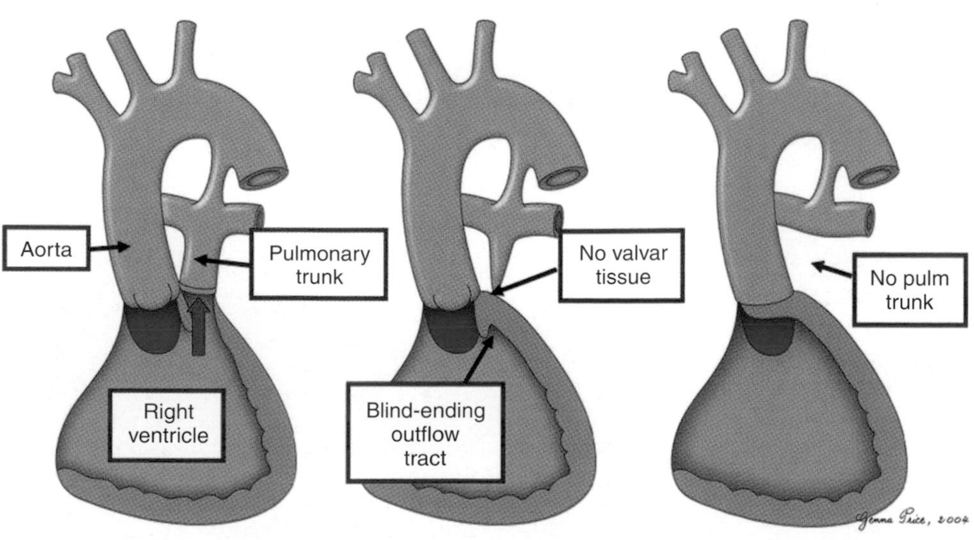

Figure 37-1 The cartoon shows the variants of obstruction within, or absence of, the pulmonary arterial pathways. The left hand drawing shows an imperforate pulmonary valve (*yellow arrow*), the middle drawing shows muscular obstruction, whilst the right hand drawing shows the solitary arterial trunk.

by an imperforate pulmonary valve. More usually, the blockage of the pathway is muscular, either at the entrance to, or at the distal end of, the subpulmonary infundibulum. The connection is lacking when there is absence of the pulmonary trunk, with the extreme form represented by absence of all the intrapericardial pulmonary arteries. Just as tetralogy of Fallot with pulmonary stenosis can be found with marked variability in intracardiac morphology, so can tetralogy with pulmonary atresia. Before discussing the crucial variations in pulmonary arterial anatomy, therefore, we will discuss the variations in morphology within the heart.

Intracardiac Structure

Significant variations are to be found in the morphology of the ventricular outflow tracts, in the morphology of the interventricular communication, and in the precise connection of the aorta to the ventricular mass, as well as in the associated malformations. Apart from the associated malformations, these features are interrelated. To fulfill the basic diagnosis as tetralogy of Fallot, the aorta must be connected to the ventricles in posterior position relative to the atretic pulmonary outflow tract. The aortic valvar orifice then overrides the crest of the muscular ventricular septum, albeit to varying degree. The phenotypic feature of tetralogy is seen in the structure of the subpulmonary outflow tract, with the muscular outlet septum, or its fibrous remnant, being displaced anteriorly and cephalad relative to the limbs of the septomarginal trabeculation (Fig. 37-2).

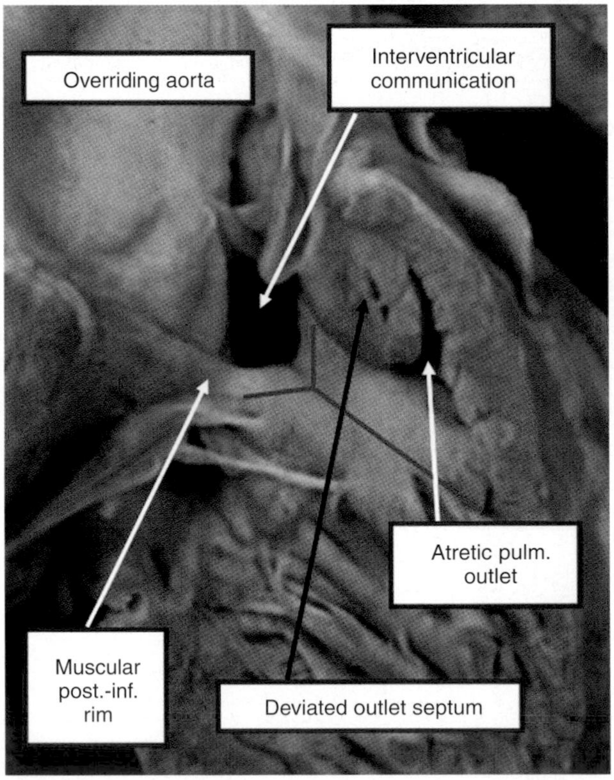

Figure 37-2 The specimen shows the phenotypic features of tetralogy of Fallot, in that the deviated outlet septum is attached antero-cephalad relative to the limbs of the septo-marginal trabeculation (*yellow Y*). In this heart, however, there is muscular subpulmonary (pulm.) atresia, rather than pulmonary stenosis. Note also the muscular postero-inferior (post.-inf.) rim to the interventricular communication.

In a small number of cases, the atresia is found at the mouth of the muscular infundibulum, and the pulmonary valve itself may then be patent. Alternatively, there can be an imperforate pulmonary valve (Fig. 37-3). In the most common pattern, the muscular outlet septum fuses directly with the parietal musculature of the right ventricle, thus obliterating the ventriculo-pulmonary junction. There is then a muscular wall between the cavities of the right ventricle and the pulmonary trunk. Occasionally, the subpulmonary outflow tract is completely absent, so that the leaflets of the aortic valve are attached directly to the parietal ventricular wall (Fig. 37-4). This arrangement is reminiscent of common arterial trunk. In the example shown in Figure 37-4, however, the atretic pulmonary trunk takes its origin from the right ventricular musculature, confirming that the patent arterial trunk is an aorta. Should the intrapericardial pulmonary arteries also be absent, it would be impossible to be sure whether the patent trunk had, initially, been an aorta, and not a common structure. Thus, the arrangement with absence of the pulmonary trunk is best described as a solitary arterial trunk, albeit that clinical presentation is as for tetralogy with pulmonary atresia. In other cases, a fibrous remnant of the outlet septum interposes between the leaflets of the aortic valve and an imperforate pulmonary valve (Fig. 37-5). This arrangement represents tetralogy of Fallot with pulmonary atresia in the setting of a doubly committed and juxta-arterial ventricular septal defect.

The interventricular communication, roofed by the overriding aorta, usually has a fibrous postero-inferior border, made up of continuity between the leaflets of the aortic and tricuspid valves, and often reinforced by

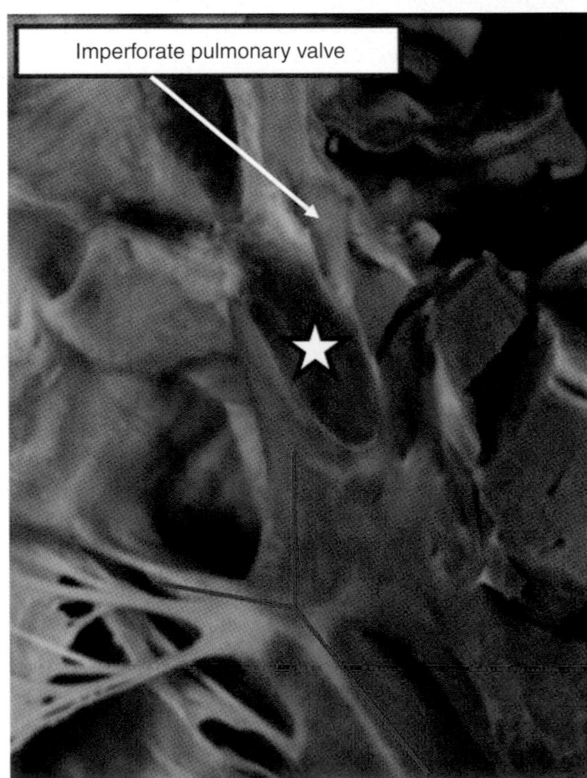

Figure 37-3 In this example, the atresia is produced by an imperforate pulmonary valve. Note again the abnormal insertion of the outlet septum (*star*) relative to the septo-marginal trabeculation (*yellow Y*).

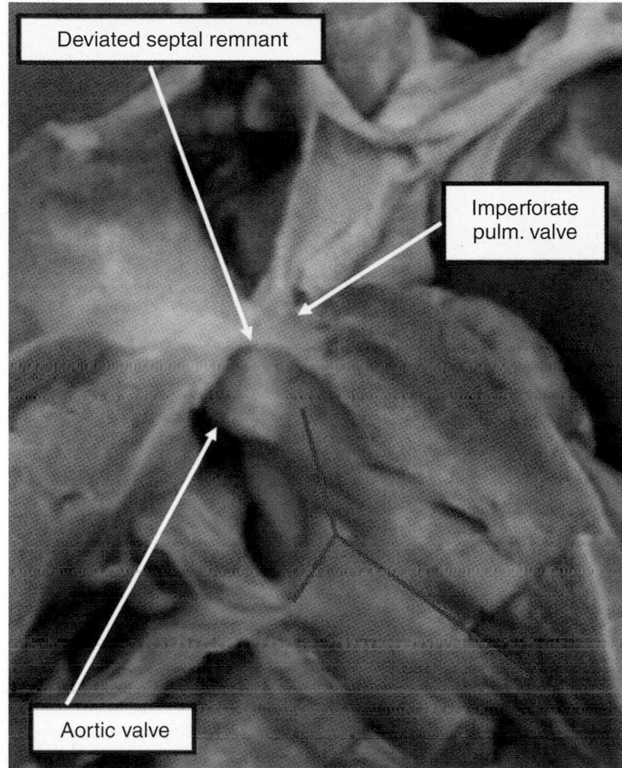

Figure 37-4 In this heart, the pulmonary trunk is represented by a fibrous strand, but the strand takes its origin from the right ventricle. The aortic valve is attached directly to the parietal ventricular wall, with no evidence of the subpulmonary infundibulum. The *yellow* Y shows the septo-marginal trabeculation.

a membranous flap. This arrangement makes the defect perimembranous (Fig. 37-6). Cases can also be found, as in tetralogy with pulmonary stenosis, when the postero-inferior limb of the septo-marginal trabeculation fuses with the ventriculo-infundibular fold. In this setting, the defect has exclusively muscular borders when viewed from its right side (see Fig. 37-2). This muscular rim, when present, serves to protect the ventricular conduction tissues, separating them from the crest of the septum. As discussed previously, the defect can also extend to become doubly committed and juxta-arterial (see Fig. 37-5). Such doubly committed defects can themselves extend to become perimembranous, but more usually have a muscular postero-inferior rim. Rarely, the ventricular septal defect may be restrictive, or even completely blocked, due to tissue tags derived from the leaflets of the tricuspid valve. In this latter setting, the overall anatomy of the heart is more like pulmonary atresia with intact ventricular septum, usually with a thick-walled right ventricle and a reduced cavity.

The precise connection of the leaflets of the aortic valve, as in tetralogy with pulmonary stenosis, can vary markedly. In most instances, the leaflets of the aortic valve are connected largely within the left ventricle. Hearts can also be found with predominant, or even total, commitment of the aorta to the right ventricle. This latter combination produces tetralogy of Fallot with pulmonary atresia, but with the ventriculo-arterial connection of double outlet ventricle.

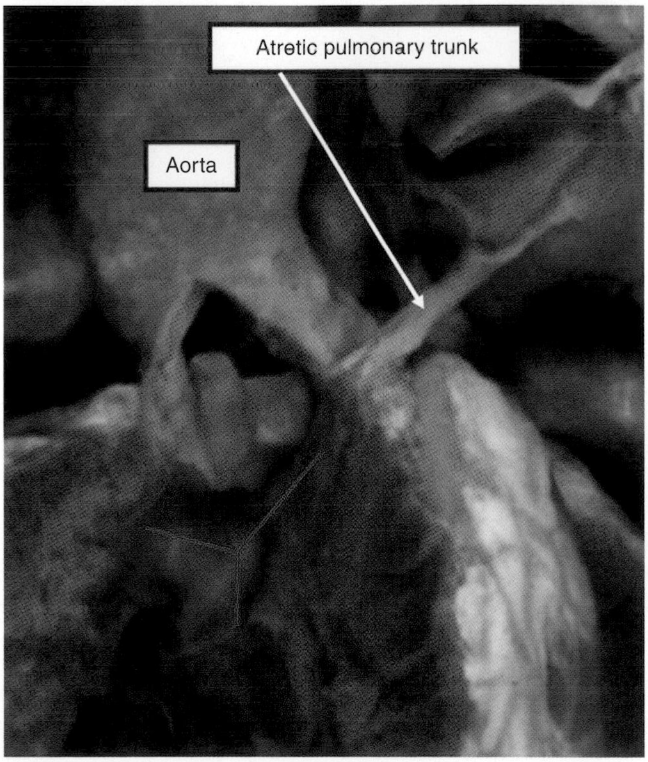

Figure 37-5 In this example, the deviated outlet septum is no more than a fibrous raphe, and there is an imperforate pulmonary valve. This is tetralogy of Fallot with pulmonary atresia in the setting of a doubly committed and juxta-arterial interventricular communication. Note the position of the septo-marginal trabeculation (*yellow* Y).

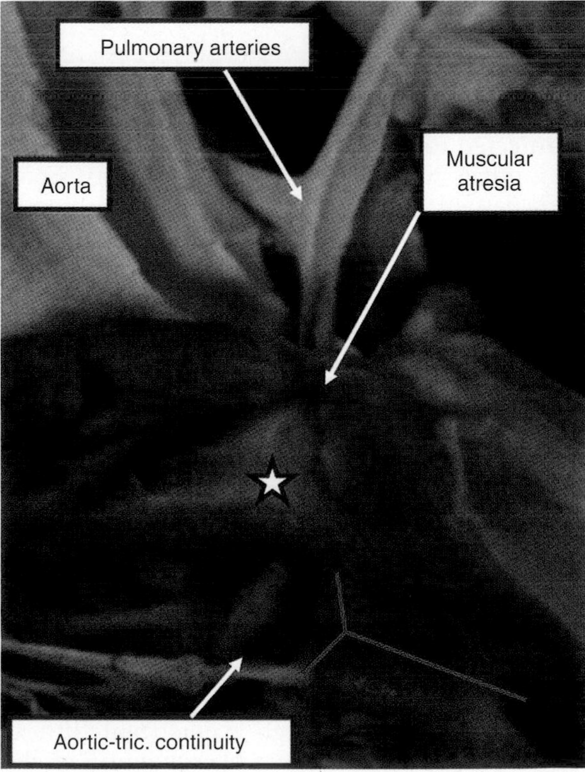

Figure 37-6 In this heart, there is obvious deviation of the outlet septum (*star*) relative to the septo-marginal trabeculation (*yellow* Y), with muscular pulmonary atresia, and a perimembranous interventricular communication. Note the fibrous continuity between the leaflets of the aortic and tricuspid (tric.) valves, and the seagull configuration of the pulmonary arteries.

Morphology of the Intrapericardial Pulmonary Arteries

When the pulmonary valve is imperforate, the pulmonary trunk is present, and patent, to the level of the ventriculo-pulmonary junction (see Fig. 37-3). Even in this setting, the trunk itself may supply only one pulmonary artery, the other either having no connection with the pulmonary trunk, or else being completely absent. In many other cases, the pulmonary trunk itself is atretic (see Fig. 37-5). In extreme cases, it is recognisable only as a fibrous strand running between the ventricular outflow tract and the pulmonary arterial confluence, or else joining to one or other of the pulmonary arteries. When the right and left pulmonary arteries are present, usually they are confluent. The confluence itself, usually tethered by either a patent or atretic pulmonary trunk to the ventricular mass, has the characteristic angiographic appearance of a flying seagull. It can vary markedly in size, usually dependent on its source of arterial supply.

The right and left pulmonary arteries can be non-confluent, but one of them usually retains its connection to the remnant of the pulmonary trunk. Non-confluent pulmonary arteries can rarely be found in the absence the pulmonary trunk. Each can then either be supplied by one of bilateral arterial ducts, or one lung can be supplied by systemic-to-pulmonary collateral arteries, with the other fed by a duct through the persisting extrapericardial pulmonary artery. In the most severe examples, the entire intrapericardial arterial tree can be lacking, with supply to the lungs exclusively through systemic-to-pulmonary collateral arteries.

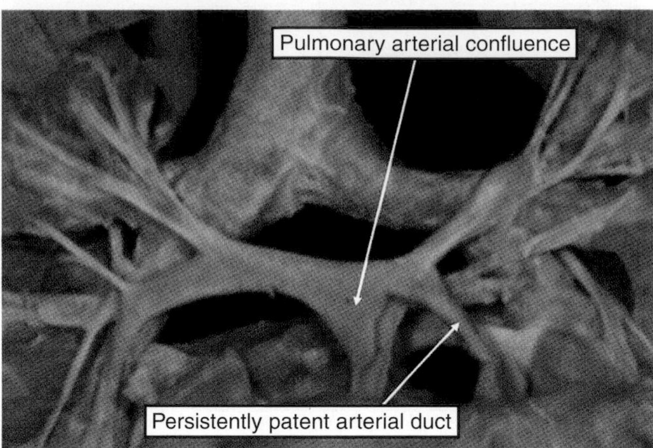

Figure 37-7 This image shows the confluent pulmonary arteries in a patient with tetralogy with pulmonary atresia in which the arterial supply is derived through a persistently patent arterial duct.

Morphology of Pulmonary Arterial Supply

The final common pathway of pulmonary supply is the capillaries supplying the air sacks of the lungs. These capillaries are connected to an intrapulmonary plexus of arteries, which ramifies within the bronchopulmonary segments. Different parts of the plexus can be supplied with blood from different systemic sources. If all intrapulmonary arteries are connected to unobstructed and confluent intrapericardial pulmonary arteries, the confluence typically supplies all of both lungs, and pulmonary arterial supply is said to be unifocal. When different parts of one lung are supplied from more than one source, the supply is said to be multi-focal.

Unifocal Pulmonary Blood Supply

It is usually the persistently patent arterial duct that provides unifocal pulmonary arterial supply (Fig. 37-7). It is exceedingly rare for confluent pulmonary arteries feeding all of both lungs to be supplied by a solitary systemic-to-pulmonary collateral artery. In rare cases, however, the confluent pulmonary arteries can be fed in unifocal fashion through an aortopulmonary window, or via a fistula from the coronary arteries. In the past, it has also been suggested that the pulmonary arteries can be fed unifocally through a persistent fifth aortic arch.[6] A fifth arch has never been identified during embryological development, so this explanation seems unlikely. Almost certainly the structures described as the fifth arch represent a malpositioned arterial duct (Fig. 37-8).

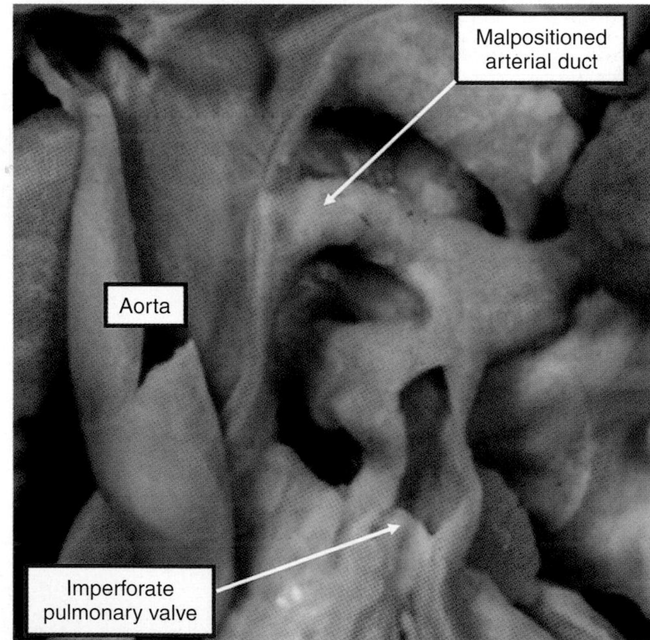

Figure 37-8 In this specimen, the vessel feeding the pulmonary arteries was initially interpreted as a fifth aortic arch. No such structure, however, exists during embryological development. The vessel is a malpositioned arterial duct. Note that the atresia is produced by an imperforate pulmonary valve, and the pulmonary arteries are of good size.

Multifocal Pulmonary Blood Supply

It is the presence of multifocal pulmonary arterial supply that creates the clinical complexity in tetralogy with pulmonary atresia. The multiple vessels feeding the pulmonary parenchyma are systemic-to-pulmonary collateral arteries (Fig. 37-9). Such arteries hardly ever feed a lung that also receives supply via the arterial duct. It is a useful working rule, therefore, to assume that an arterial duct will not be present when a lung is supplied by systemic-to-pulmonary collateral arteries. Although the systemic-to-pulmonary collateral arteries hardly ever co-exist in the same lung with an arterial duct, they do usually co-exist with confluent

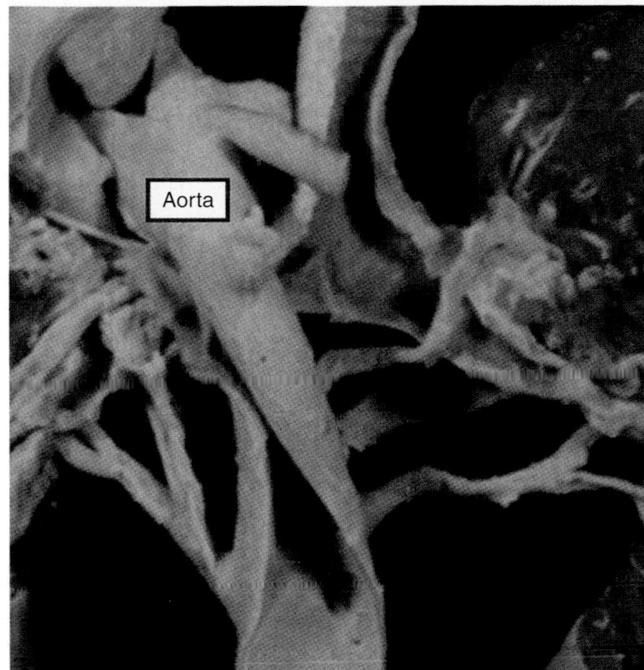

Figure 37-9 The block is photographed from behind in this patient having tetralogy with pulmonary atresia. Note the multiple systemic-to-pulmonary collateral arteries extending from the descending aorta to feed the intrapulmonary arterial tree.

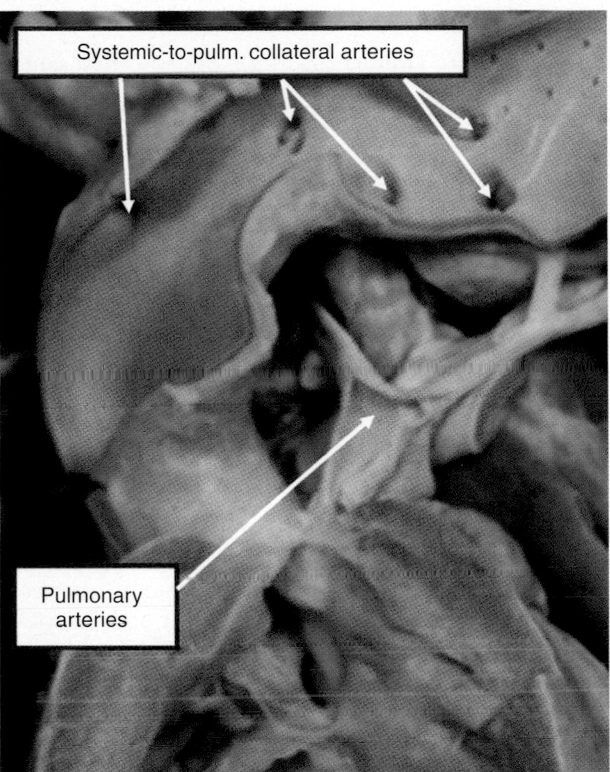

Figure 37-10 The same block as shown in Figure 37-9 is shown from the front. The systemic-to-pulmonary collateral arteries co-exist with good-sized intrapericardial pulmonary arteries. The heart also has a doubly committed interventricular communication, as shown in Figure 37-4.

intrapericardial pulmonary arteries (Fig. 37-10). In such circumstances, the confluent pulmonary arteries are hardly, if ever, connected to all of the bronchopulmonary segments of both lungs. Instead, it is the rule for different arteries to supply different segments of the two lungs. The confluence of intrapericardial pulmonary arteries, itself fed by one or more major systemic-to-pulmonary collateral arteries, is connected to only part of the lungs, while the remainder of the pulmonary parenchyma is supplied directly by a variable number of major systemic-to-pulmonary collateral arteries. These individual collateral arteries feed individual intrapulmonary segments, or groups of segments (Fig. 37-11). They can also communicate with the confluent intrapericardial pulmonary arterial tree (see Fig. 37-10). When both intrapericardial and systemic-to-pulmonary collateral arteries feed different parts of the pulmonary parenchyma, it is essential to determine the proportions supplied by each of the pathways, remembering that in the extreme form of the anomaly, the entirety of both lungs is fed exclusively by systemic-to-pulmonary arteries.

Another variety of multifocal supply is found when the pulmonary arteries are present but non-confluent. The different parts of the lungs may then be supplied by systemic-to-pulmonary collateral arteries, by a duct, by a coronary arterial fistula or aorto-pulmonary window, or by a combination of these. Alternatively, the intrapulmonary arteries may not be supplied either via an arterial duct or by major systemic-to-pulmonary collateral arteries. Blood can then reach them only at precapillary level through acquired collateral arteries. These may either enter the lungs centrifugally through the bronchial arteries, or centripetally via the intercostal or coronary arteries. These acquired collateral arteries can co-exist with the other varieties of arterial supply.

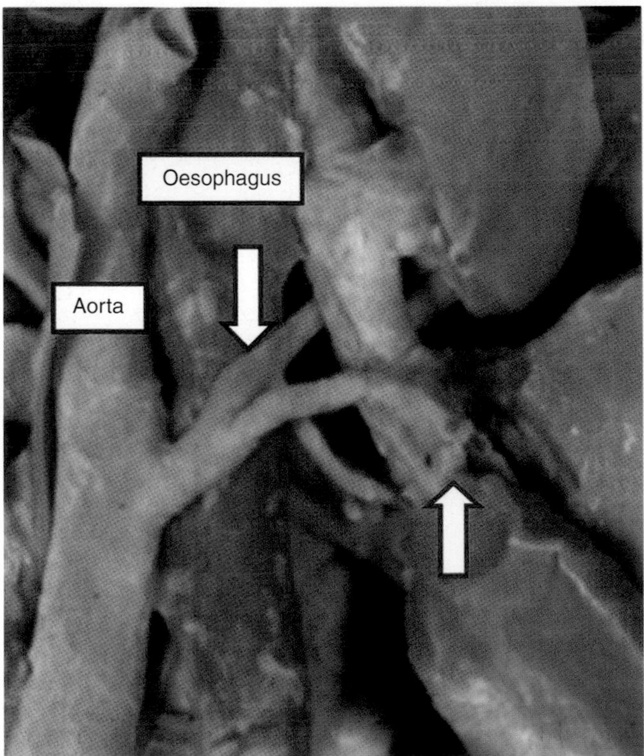

Figure 37-11 This image, taken from behind, shows a systemic-to-pulmonary collateral artery dividing, with one branch passing in front of (*red arrow*), and the other behind (*green arrow*), the oesophagus. The branch passing posteriorly supplies directly a small part of the lung, without anastomosing with the intrapericardial pulmonary arteries.

Major Systemic-to-Pulmonary Collateral Arteries

These arteries are characteristic for the so-called complex variant of tetralogy of Fallot with pulmonary atresia. Their relationship to the bronchial arteries has yet to be fully established. Some of the major collateral arteries have no independent course within the lung parenchyma, extending only from a systemic artery, usually the aorta, to the origin of the intrapulmonary arteries at or near the hilum (Fig. 37-12). Arteries with this morphology are simple conduits. In other circumstances, the collateral arteries extend into the lung along the bronchial tree, branching in the pattern of a bronchial artery, and supplying also the bronchial wall (Fig. 37-13).

A common embryological origin of these vessels with the bronchial arteries cannot be excluded.[7] It is still recommended, nonetheless, to describe these vessels as systemic-to-pulmonary collateral arteries. The arteries, typically two to six in number, usually arise from the anterior wall of the aorta opposite the origin of the intercostal arteries (see Fig. 37-9). Individual collateral arteries can also take origin from the brachiocephalic arteries, or even from the coronary arteries. When arising from the aorta, the arteries frequently run a retro-oesophageal course (see Fig. 37-11). Usually they can be distinguished from a duct by their histological structure. They can also be distinguished anatomically in most cases, since the arterial duct originates only from a given point within the aortic arch, albeit masquerading sometimes as a purported fifth aortic arch (see Fig. 37-10). Typically, even when branching from a non-dominant aortic arch, the duct originates more or less opposite the take-off of a brachiocephalic or subclavian artery.

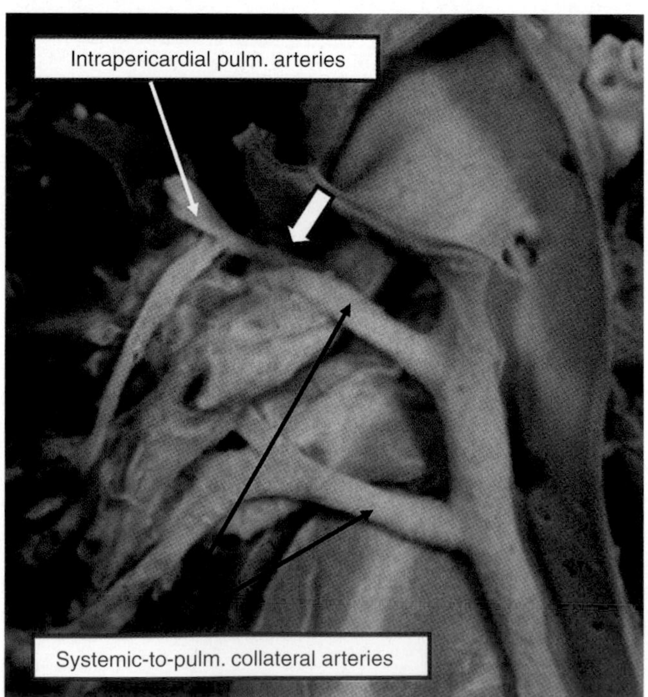

Figure 37-12 Another picture of the heart and lungs shown in Figures 37-4, 37-9 and 37-10. This shows the anastomosis at the hilum of the left lung (*arrow*) between a systemic-to-pulmonary collateral artery and the intrapericardial pulmonary arteries.

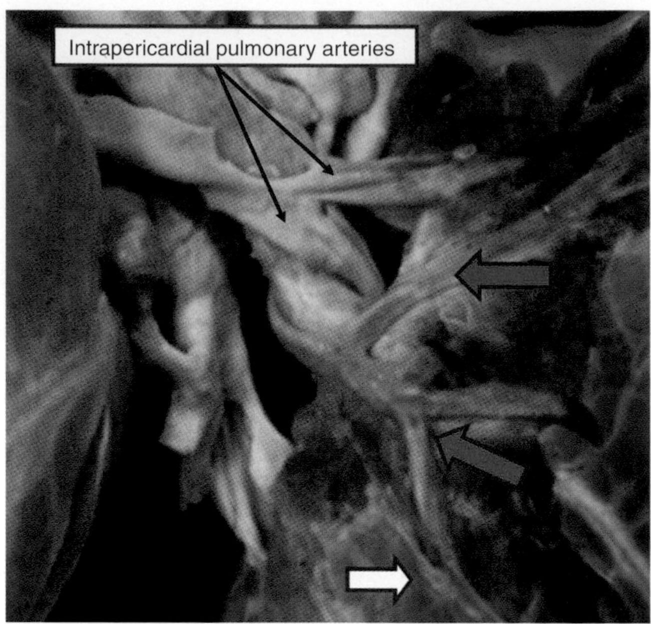

Figure 37-13 In this heart-lung preparation, the systemic-to-pulmonary collateral artery highlighted by the yellow arrows branches in concert with the bronchial tree, and is reminiscent of a bronchial artery. The white arrow shows an anastomosis at segmental level between the artery and a branch of the intrapericardial arterial tree.

Characteristic Patterns of Pulmonary Arterial Supply

The potentially complex situation can be simplified by recognition of three major patterns of pulmonary arterial supply. The most favourable arrangement is that in which the right and left pulmonary arteries are confluent, and are supplied by an arterial duct (see Fig. 37-7). With this pattern, the pulmonary arteries themselves are usually distributed in normal fashion to all the bronchopulmonary segments. Such pulmonary arterial supply is unifocal.

In the second major pattern, the intrapericardial pulmonary arteries are confluent, but co-exist with systemic-to-pulmonary collateral arteries (Fig. 37-14). The distribution of the confluent pulmonary arteries themselves is then variable, but hardly ever supplies all the bronchopulmonary segments, with blood passing through the confluence often supplying two-thirds or less of the pulmonary parenchyma. Even in this setting, the ultimate supply to the pulmonary arteries is via the collateral arteries, with anastomoses with the intrapericardial network being possible at hilar, lobar, or segmental levels (Fig. 37-15). The confluence of the pulmonary arteries itself also varies markedly in size, reflecting the number of the bronchopulmonary segments supplied. In this setting, those parts of the lung not supplied by the intrapericardial pulmonary arteries are fed directly by systemic-to-pulmonary collateral arteries, with further variation in the number of arteries present, and the amount of lung supplied by each artery. In most cases, the peripheral supplies of central pulmonary arteries and the collateral arteries do not overlap, but in a proportion of segments two sets of arterial ramifications intermingle (Fig. 37-16).[7,8]

The third typical pattern of arterial supply (Fig. 37-17) is encountered when there is absence of the intrapericardial pulmonary arteries. In such circumstances, all the bronchopulmonary segments are supplied by multiple

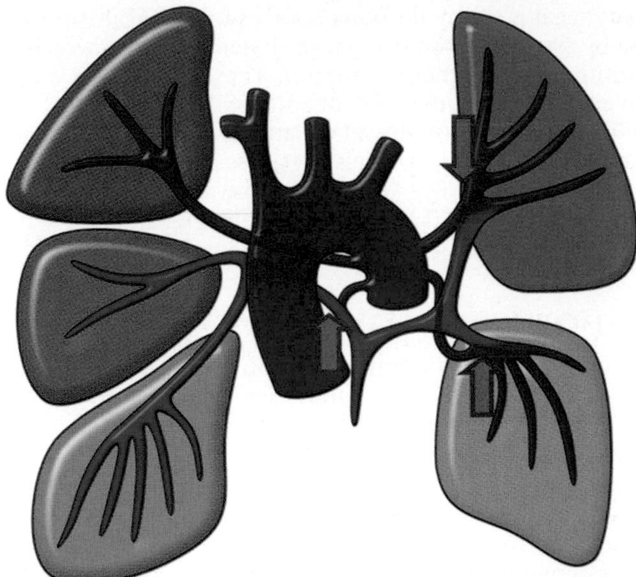

Figure 37-14 The cartoon shows a hypothetical example of multifocal supply. Four collateral arteries are illustrated, shown in red arising from the descending aorta. The right upper artery supplies exclusively the right upper lobe in direct fashion. The right lower artery feeds the middle and lower lobes of the right lung through an anastomosis with the intrapericardial arterial tree, shown in blue, at hilar level (*left hand yellow arrow*). The left sided collateral arteries are shown feeding the left lung (*right hand yellow arrows*) through anastomoses at segmental level (see Fig. 37-15). This cartoon takes no cognisance of dual supply (see Fig. 37-16).

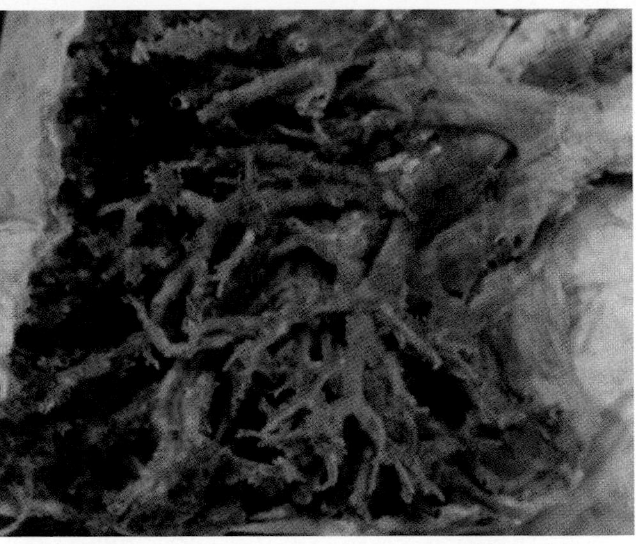

Figure 37-16 A part of the lung has been dissected in which the same bronchopulmonary segment is fed both by systemic-to-pulmonary collateral arteries (*red*) and intrapericardial pulmonary arteries (*blue*). Note the overlap of the circulations.

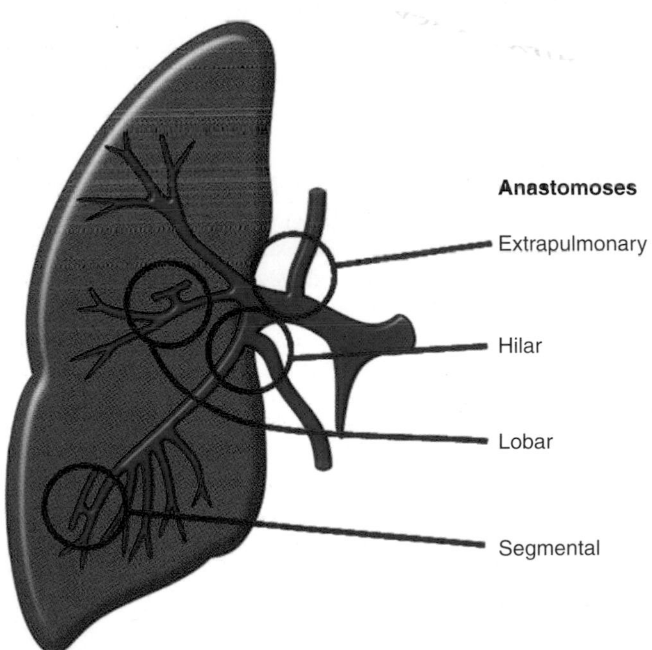

Figure 37-15 The cartoon shows the level of anastomoses between the collateral arteries and the intrapericardial pulmonary arteries.

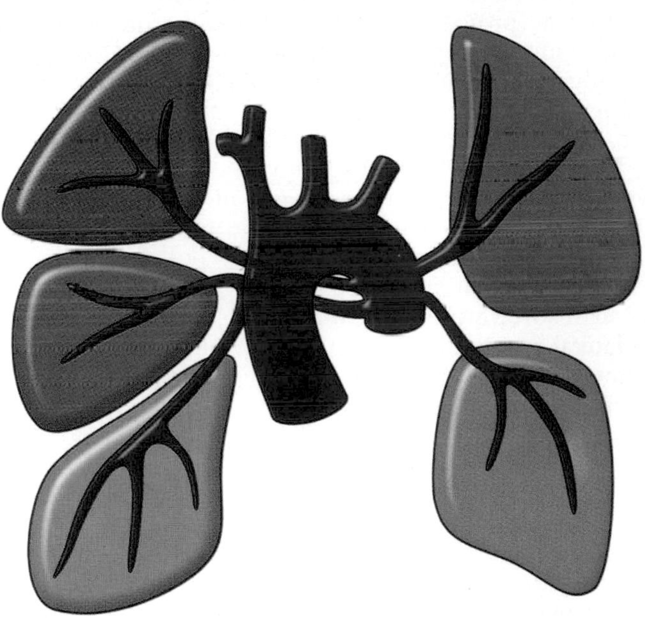

Figure 37-17 The cartoon shows the situation in which there is absence of all the intrapericardial pulmonary arteries. The pulmonary parenchyma receives its arterial supply exclusively through systemic-to-pulmonary collateral arteries.

systemic-to-pulmonary collateral arteries. In the presence of systemic-to-pulmonary collateral arteries, therefore, the key to complete clinical diagnosis is to establish the course of each artery, to establish whether it runs directly into the lung or makes connections with intrapericardial and central pulmonary arteries, and to identify with precision the sites of these anastomoses.

MORPHOGENESIS

Much has been written about the morphogenesis of both the ventricular and pulmonary arterial features of tetralogy of Fallot with pulmonary atresia, albeit derived from speculative embryological concepts, and arguably not improving our understanding. From the stance of ventricular morphology, nonetheless, the anomaly is readily explained in terms of end-stage tetralogy of Fallot, with variation depending upon the specific morphology of the subarterial outlets. Some cases, in contrast, can be interpreted as representing common arterial trunk with absence of the intrapericardial pulmonary arteries, such as those in which a solitary trunk is connected to the ventricular mass in absence of central pulmonary arteries. This anomaly was initially classified along with other variants of common arterial trunk.[9] On re-examination of these specimens, doubt was raised as to whether the central pulmonary arteries were indeed absent, or instead were severely hypoplastic.[10] Examples do exist, nonetheless, with unequivocal absence of the intrapericardial pulmonary arteries absent, and with no evidence within the right ventricle of the subpulmonary infundibulum. The argument of common trunk versus tetralogy then depends upon whether the absent pulmonary arteries, had they been present, would have taken origin from an arterial trunk or directly from the right ventricle. The argument is no longer hypothetical, since hearts have now been found with an atretic pulmonary trunk arising from an arterial trunk, showing that the trunk itself had initially been a common structure.[11] Experimental studies of rats dosed with bisdiamine have also shown that some fetuses develop classical tetralogy of Fallot, while others exhibit common arterial trunk with pulmonary atresia.[2] From the standpoint of anatomy, this conundrum is easily resolved simply by describing the ascending great artery found in absence of the pulmonary trunk as a solitary arterial trunk rather than an aorta. Summarising the overall morphogenesis of tetralogy of Fallot with pulmonary atresia, the anatomical prototypes can readily be interpreted, on the basis of morphology, as developing in the setting of typical tetralogy, in the setting of tetralogy with doubly committed ventricular septal defects or, very rarely, in the setting of common arterial trunk.

Embryology has also been invoked to account for the typical patterns of pulmonary arterial supply.[12] Thus, the lungs in tetralogy with pulmonary atresia are supplied either through the confluence of the pulmonary arteries fed by the arterial duct, itself derived from the embryological sixth aortic arch, or else through systemic-to-pulmonary collateral arteries. Initially, it is known that the developing intrapulmonary arterial plexus is connected to the primitive intersegmental arteries, which in turn are connected to the aortic arch system, eventually via the fourth arch.[13] The concept advanced to explain the arrangement seen in the abnormal hearts is that, when the intrapulmonary plexus eventually achieves its connection to the sixth arch, it loses its connections with the fourth arch and the systemic arterial system. The systemic-to-pulmonary collateral arteries are then explained on the basis of persistence of the primitive intersegmental arteries, some of which also become bronchial arteries. It is argued that these collateral arteries persist only in absence of the duct, which is the critical connection between the structures derived from the sixth arch and the aortic sac. This concept accounts adequately for the majority of cases, and offers an excellent working hypothesis. It is undermined by those occasional instances when systemic-to-pulmonary collateral arteries co-exist with the duct, and both supply the intrapulmonary plexus in the same lung.

In the majority of cases, nonetheless, embryology aids greatly in understanding the complexity of the pulmonary arterial supply. In essence, the intrapulmonary arteries develop along with the lung. They are the final common pathway supplying arterial blood to the pulmonary air sacs. This common pathway can be supplied at the hilum, either by the intrapericardial pulmonary arteries fed through the arterial duct, the derivative of the artery to the sixth pharyngeal arch, by the rarer sources of unifocal supply, or else by systemic-to-pulmonary collateral arteries, which are primitive intersegmental arteries. These sources of supply can anastomose with different parts of the lungs in the same patient, although usually all the arteries in one lung are supplied either by the duct, or else by the systemic-to-pulmonary collateral arteries. The common pathway can subsequently be further enhanced by acquired collateral arteries, which then reinforce the acinar supply at precapillary level.

PATHOPHYSIOLOGY

The interventricular communication is almost always large and non-restrictive, only rarely being small and obstructive. In a few cases, obstruction may be encountered between the right ventricle and the aorta, producing suprasystemic right ventricular pressures. There is complete mixing of pulmonary and systemic venous blood in the aorta. Hence, distribution of blood to the body as opposed to the lungs depends on the relative resistances offered by the two circulations. The systemic vascular resistance is no different from that in any other cyanotic condition. The complicated pattern of pulmonary arterial supply, however, means that the pulmonary vascular resistance is both complex and variable. Some parts of the lung may be under-perfused and some over-perfused in the same patient. This adds to the difficulties of assessment during life.

Pulmonary Vascular Resistance

The pulmonary vascular resistance results from obstruction at various sites between the aorta and the pulmonary capillaries. These are as follows.

Obstruction at the Aorto-pulmonary Connection

It is rare for there to be a direct connection between the aorta and pulmonary arteries. Examples are an aortopulmonary window along with now rarely performed direct surgical anastomoses. Another direct aortopulmonary connection that can be obstructed, albeit rarely, is a pulmonary artery arising anomalously from the ascending aorta. The connection between the aorta and pulmonary circulations more commonly is a vessel or surgical conduit between the aorta and either the central or intrapulmonary arteries, or the junction between the two. The same principles concerning haemodynamics apply to natural communications, such as a duct or major systemic-to-pulmonary collateral arteries or the rarer coronary-to-pulmonary arterial fistulas, and to surgically created shunts or conduits inserted between the aorta or subclavian arteries and the pulmonary arteries. The difference in pressure between the aorta and the pulmonary arteries is not usually a gradual change in pressure over the whole length of the conduit or vessel. Instead, there is usually an abrupt drop at the pulmonary end. This may be no more than a reflection of the Venturi effect, but there may also be an anatomical obstruction at the pulmonary arterial end of the conduit. This is particularly true in the case of surgical shunts created in early infancy. It is also true of a duct, which tends to become constricted at its pulmonary rather than its aortic end. Localised obstructions and pressure gradients also occur within major systemic-to-pulmonary collateral arteries. In many cases, these obstructions can become more stenotic with time.[14]

Obstruction Within the Pulmonary Arteries

If the central pulmonary arteries lie in the pathway of blood between the aorta and one lung, stenoses may be important, though their inaccessibility makes this difficult to establish. For example, in cases where the entire pulmonary blood flow is derived from a left duct, a stenosis of the central right pulmonary artery would be one factor limiting flow to the right lung. Pressure gradients may also occasionally be demonstrated in intrapulmonary arteries, whether or not these are connected to confluent intrapericardial pulmonary arteries.

Obstruction at Arteriolar Level

Pulmonary vascular disease may develop in parts of the lungs. It can occur in pulmonary segments perfused at high pressure by unobstructed major systemic-to-pulmonary collateral arteries. Changes due to hypoperfusion may also affect pulmonary vascular resistance. In particular, intimal proliferation in an acquired collateral circulation appears to extend into the pulmonary arteries within the acinus, at least in experimental animals.[15] This is likely to raise pulmonary vascular resistance in affected segments.

The combination of all these obstructions is sufficient to reduce the flow of blood to the lungs to below systemic levels in most patients, though a few may show a marked increase in the total pulmonary flow. Since pulmonary and systemic blood becomes completely mixed, systemic arterial hypoxaemia is most severe in patients with a low pulmonary and high systemic flows. Total pulmonary resistance is, therefore, usually high. But this, as outlined above, is the result of obstruction at a number of different levels. From the point of view of surgical repair, what matters is the resistance relative to the vessel to which the right ventricle is to be connected. Normally this is a central pulmonary artery.

When the supply of blood to the lungs is unifocal, all intrapulmonary arteries are connected to a single source of pressure, usually the pulmonary trunk or the confluence between the right and left pulmonary arteries. Under these circumstances, pulmonary vascular resistance can be calculated, provided that mean arterial pressure at that point is known. When pulmonary blood supply is multifocal, in contrast, different intrapulmonary arteries are supplied from different sources. Since the different parts of the lung will then most probably be at different pressures, it is impossible to calculate the overall pulmonary vascular resistance. In fact, all the evidence indicates that regional flow is extremely variable throughout the lungs. Hyperperfused and hypoperfused segments of lungs may be immediately adjacent.

Acquired Collateral Circulation to the Lungs

Collateral arterial supply to the lungs may develop in any cyanotic cardiac condition. These collateral arteries, therefore, can develop in tetralogy with pulmonary atresia, but they are distinct from the major systemic-to-pulmonary collateral arteries that are typical of the condition. From the pathophysiological point of view, the most important distinction lies in the site of the anastomosis with the pulmonary circulation. Acquired collateral arteries, with rare exceptions, join the pulmonary circulation at immediately precapillary level. Major systemic-to-pulmonary collateral arteries join at the hilum, or at segmental level. Both types of collateral artery provide an effective supply of blood to the lungs. Since acquired collateral circulation never produces cardiac failure, there must be a high resistance to flow between the aorta and the pulmonary arteries.

PRESENTATION

Fetuses with tetralogy and pulmonary atresia can be diagnosed with a high degree of accuracy before birth.[16] The postnatal clinical presentation is almost entirely dependent on the amount of flow to the lungs. If such supply depends on patency of a duct, then patients are liable to present as neonates with severe cyanosis when the duct narrows or closes. Major systemic-to-pulmonary collateral arteries, by comparison, form a relatively stable source of pulmonary arterial supply. In these patients, therefore, the onset of clinically detectable cyanosis may be delayed well beyond the neonatal period. Indeed, of patients with major systemic-to-pulmonary collateral arteries, a small proportion has excessive pulmonary flow, and presents in cardiac failure.

The patients usually present with the combination of cyanosis and exertional dyspnoea. Failure to thrive is often present. Many patients, however, have a balanced flow to the lungs, with few, if any, symptoms and occasionally may demonstrate normal growth. Patients may initially present with non-cardiac clinical features of chromosome 22q11 deletion, such as difficulties with feeding and developmental delay. Occasionally, they may present with evidence of immunodeficiency or hypocalcaemia as part of the picture of the DiGeorge syndrome.

CLINICAL FINDINGS

Most, but by no means all, patients are clinically cyanosed from birth. In the minority with increased flow of blood to the lungs, cyanosis may escape detection until the patient is a few months, or even years, old. Respiration is quiet unless pulmonary flow is excessive. Since there is run-off from the aorta, the peripheral pulses are equal and jerky in proportion to the pulmonary flow. The praecordium is characteristically quiet, since there are no thrills, and the degree of right ventricular hypertension is not usually sufficient to give a right ventricular lift. Only in infants with excessive pulmonary flow is the praecordium active. It may be possible to feel both the ejection click and the second heart sound.

The first heart sound may be followed by a loud aortic ejection click in all but young infants, this being due to the dilation of the aortic root. The second heart sound is single. Blowing and continuous murmurs are frequently audible. A localised continuous murmur may suggest persistent patency of the arterial duct, while widespread continuous murmurs are more characteristic of major systemic-to-pulmonary collateral arteries. There is no systolic ejection murmur such as would arise from infundibular stenosis. The continuous murmurs may obscure the early diastolic murmur of aortic regurgitation that often develops beyond the age of 8 years or so as a result of dilation of the aortic root or infective endocarditis.

Continuous murmurs may not be heard if the pulmonary flow is too low to generate audible turbulence. This is the case in about half of severely cyanotic newborns with this condition. Such newborns are nearly always duct dependent. Severe pulmonary vascular obstructive disease in older children with unobstructed major systemic-to-pulmonary collateral arteries, however, may also prevent generation of a continuous murmur.

DIAGNOSIS

There is, in general, little difficulty with the diagnosis of tetralogy with pulmonary atresia. In older patients with surgical shunts, nonetheless, it may be impossible to distinguish between congenital and acquired pulmonary atresia. In all cases, other clinical features of the velo-cardiofacial and DiGeorge syndromes should be sought, and chromosomal analysis performed to establish 22q11 deletion.

INVESTIGATIONS

Chest Radiography

The so-called coeur-en-sabot heart of tetralogy of Fallot is most often found when there is pulmonary atresia. This is because when hypoplasia of the pulmonary trunk is more severe, the hollowness of the pulmonary bay is more pronounced. A right aortic arch is twice as common as in tetralogy with pulmonary stenosis. These findings occur in almost half of all patients with tetralogy and pulmonary atresia. The lung markings are characteristically uneven in size and hence patchy, abnormal linear shadows indicating the position and course of collateral arteries. The unevenness exists because, in the presence of major systemic-to-pulmonary collateral arteries, some parts of the lung may be under-perfused while others are over-perfused. Furthermore, in older patients, particularly those who have had previous thoracotomies, the extensive acquired collateral circulation may produce rather granular lung fields.

Electrocardiography

The electrocardiogram usually shows right atrial hypertrophy, and almost always right ventricular hypertrophy. This feature easily distinguishes the condition from pulmonary atresia with an intact ventricular septum in newborns, who usually have a conspicuous lack of right ventricular forces. The mean frontal QRS axis is downward and to the right, usually between +100 degrees and +180 degrees.

Echocardiography

The diagnosis of the intracardiac arrangement will be confirmed echocardiographically, but in most cases echocardiography will not be able to demonstrate all aspects of the complex pulmonary arterial supply. Colour Doppler imaging, nonetheless, can exclude significant major collateral arteries in many cases.[17]

The parasternal long-axis view shows a large aortic valve overriding the crest of the muscular ventricular septum. The atretic right ventricular outflow tract may be seen in short-axis parasternal cuts. Hypoplasia of the pulmonary trunk frequently permits the left lung to intrude between it and a transducer placed in praecordial position, thus obscuring the pulmonary valve and trunk. This can be overcome by moving the transducer into a high praecordial, or even suprasternal, position and obtaining a ductal cut. This shows the left pulmonary artery, the pulmonary trunk, and the right ventricular outflow tract in their long axis. The same cut will image a left duct in the presence of a left aortic arch. From these, and subcostal cuts, the origin of the left and the proximal right pulmonary artery may be seen, as may their confluence when it is present.

From the subcostal view, the overriding aorta can be seen when the transducer is depressed and angled anteriorly from the four-chamber view. With clockwise rotation from this point, it is usually possible to demonstrate the blind-ending right ventricular infundibulum when present, and thereby rule out common arterial trunk in most cases. Subcostal imaging can also demonstrate those rare cases in which the pulmonary arterial supply is derived through an aortopulmonary window.

Instances of an imperforate pulmonary valve can often only be differentiated from severe tetralogy by means of Doppler colour flow imaging. In both, the hypoplastic pulmonary trunk continues beyond the dense immobile echo immediately distal to the right ventricular outflow tract, which is either the imperforate or a severely stenotic pulmonary valve.

Suprasternal imaging of the right pulmonary artery is almost always possible when it is present, even if it is hypoplastic, although care must be taken not to confuse this structure with collateral arteries in the mediastinum. In terms of size of the arteries, there is a good correlation between echocardiographic imaging and angiocardiographic investigation, though the lumen imaged echocardiographically is always slightly smaller than the true lumen.[18] Having found the right pulmonary artery, the operator should rotate the transducer while keeping the artery in view so as to demonstrate its continuity with the left pulmonary artery. As continuity is most reproducibly assessed in a single cut, it is a good idea to move the transducer a little down from the suprasternal notch. The confluence will then appear as an inverted V. As the transducer is rotated counterclockwise from suprasternally, a left aortic arch is normally seen. If this does not happen, the counter-clockwise rotation should be continued, for then it is likely that the bifurcation of a left brachiocephalic artery will be seen, indicating the presence of a right aortic arch. The region of the bifurcation should be scanned with colour Doppler imaging to search for an arterial duct. Then the transducer should be returned to its neutral position used for imaging the right pulmonary artery, and then rotated clockwise. If there is indeed a right aortic arch, the round or elliptical section of the aorta seen above the right pulmonary artery will elongate as this rotation occurs, and the tight curve of a right arch will emerge. In the presence of a left arch, similar clockwise rotation will ultimately demonstrate the bifurcation of a right brachiocephalic artery, which should again be scrutinised for a duct.

Suprasternal views will also demonstrate anomalous origin of one pulmonary artery from the ascending aorta, the appearances usually being very similar to those of a common arterial trunk. The key to the differentiation between common trunk and tetralogy with pulmonary atresia in this situation is the presence of a blind right ventricular outflow tract and pulmonary trunk in those patients with tetralogy. If neither of these is seen, it may be impossible to distinguish echocardiographically between these two conditions in the presence of anomalous origin of one pulmonary artery. Colour Doppler usually allows the origins of major systemic-to-pulmonary collateral arteries to be established. The lungs themselves, however, obscure the intrapulmonary arteries. As a result, it is often not possible to establish the connections between the collateral arteries and the pulmonary arteries. As part of the echocardiographic study, the function of the patent cardiac valves should be studied. In particular, aortic regurgitation must be ruled out in adolescents or adults.

Magnetic Resonance Imaging

Cardiac magnetic resonance imaging with three-dimensional reconstruction is excellent at demonstrating the anatomy of the central pulmonary arteries.[19] It can often demonstrate these arteries when other techniques, including angiography, have failed.[20] It can also show the presence and origin of major collateral arteries[21] (Fig. 37-18). For these reasons, if it is available, it should be used prior to angiography to help in planning invasive studies. Fast imaging combined with breath-holds allows imaging of the peripheral distribution of the pulmonary and major collateral arteries (Fig. 37-19).

Computerised Tomographic Imaging

Where magnetic resonance imaging is not available, contrast computerised tomographic angiography can provide similar anatomical information.[22] The exposure to irradiation involved precludes the repeated imaging of the pulmonary vasculature in children with this anomaly, and magnetic resonance imaging is generally preferred.

Cardiac Catheterisation and Angiography

Complete investigation of the pulmonary arterial supply is essential in a patient with tetralogy and pulmonary atresia. It is best undertaken early in life, or as soon after presentation as possible. The intracardiac anatomy is usually clearly shown by echocardiography. The source, or sources, of pulmonary perfusion, and the presence and size of central pulmonary arteries, should be established echocardiographically, by magnetic resonance, computerised tomographic imaging, or by angiography. The details of the distribution of pulmonary perfusion, nonetheless, can often only be ascertained by selective catheterisation and angiography (Figs. 37-20 to 37-22).

It is usually best to make injections of contrast in the upper part of the descending aorta as the first stage of an angiographic investigation. This will demonstrate patency of any normally positioned duct, as well as the origin of the majority of major systemic-to-pulmonary collateral arteries. A similar angiogram can be obtained if a balloon catheter is floated through the heart and aorta to lie in the lower descending thoracic aorta. During transitory occlusion of the aorta with the inflated balloon, contrast medium is injected through side holes proximal to the balloon.

Angiography in the aortic root is necessary if non-invasive imaging has indicated that there is a more proximal source of pulmonary perfusion, such as a fistula between the coronary and pulmonary arteries, an aortopulmonary window, an anomalous origin of one pulmonary artery, a duct that arises from the brachiocephalic artery, or major collateral arteries arising from the brachiocephalic arteries. Postero-anterior and lateral projections with craniocaudal tilt are preferred. These are particularly helpful in showing small confluent pulmonary arteries, since the craniocaudal angulation elongates the V-shaped confluence in the postero-anterior projection. The craniocaudal tilt will also help separate the anterior pulmonary confluence from more posteriorly placed major systemic-to-pulmonary collateral arteries.

Selective Catheterisation

Selective catheterisation can be achieved in major systemic-to-pulmonary collateral arteries, surgical shunts, and central pulmonary arteries. It is best to enter the central intrapericardial pulmonary arteries whenever possible. This is particularly valuable when the arterial supply to the lungs is unifocal, since pulmonary vascular resistance can then be estimated. Catheters should be passed as far distal into any collateral artery as is possible in order to detect pressure gradients.

Selective angiography should address three questions. First, how does blood reach each part of the lungs? Second, are the central pulmonary arteries and the sources of pulmonary blood supply interconnected? Finally, are there any obstructions to the pulmonary blood flow? Manipulation of catheters from a transvenous route through the heart into the aorta enables most of the necessary selective angiograms to be carried out. It is usually best, nonetheless, to use the retrograde arterial route. Precurved catheters, with end holes so a guidewire can be used, are ideal for this. The long curve of the neck of the catheter keeps the tip pressed against the wall of the aorta, and it is often difficult to avoid entering collateral arteries originating from the descending aorta. The tight curve at the tip is valuable for crossing surgical shunts. In the case of shunts between the subclavian and pulmonary arteries, the tip, once engaged in the shunt, then directs the guidewire down it.

If a central pulmonary artery can be entered, a pulmonary arteriogram is best taken in the right and left anterior oblique projections, since this permits assessment of which segments of the two lungs are connected to the central pulmonary arteries. The disadvantage of frontal and lateral projections in this case is the overlapping between the two lungs in the lateral projection. Injection of contrast medium by hand is usually adequate for demonstration of smaller major systemic-to-pulmonary collateral arteries, but power injections are preferable for larger arteries. Otherwise, the large flow will excessively dilute the contrast medium.

During manipulation to enter major systemic-to-pulmonary collateral arteries originating from the descending aorta, intercostal arteries are frequently entered, particularly when they are enlarged as a result of supplying acquired collateral circulation to the lungs. Entry to

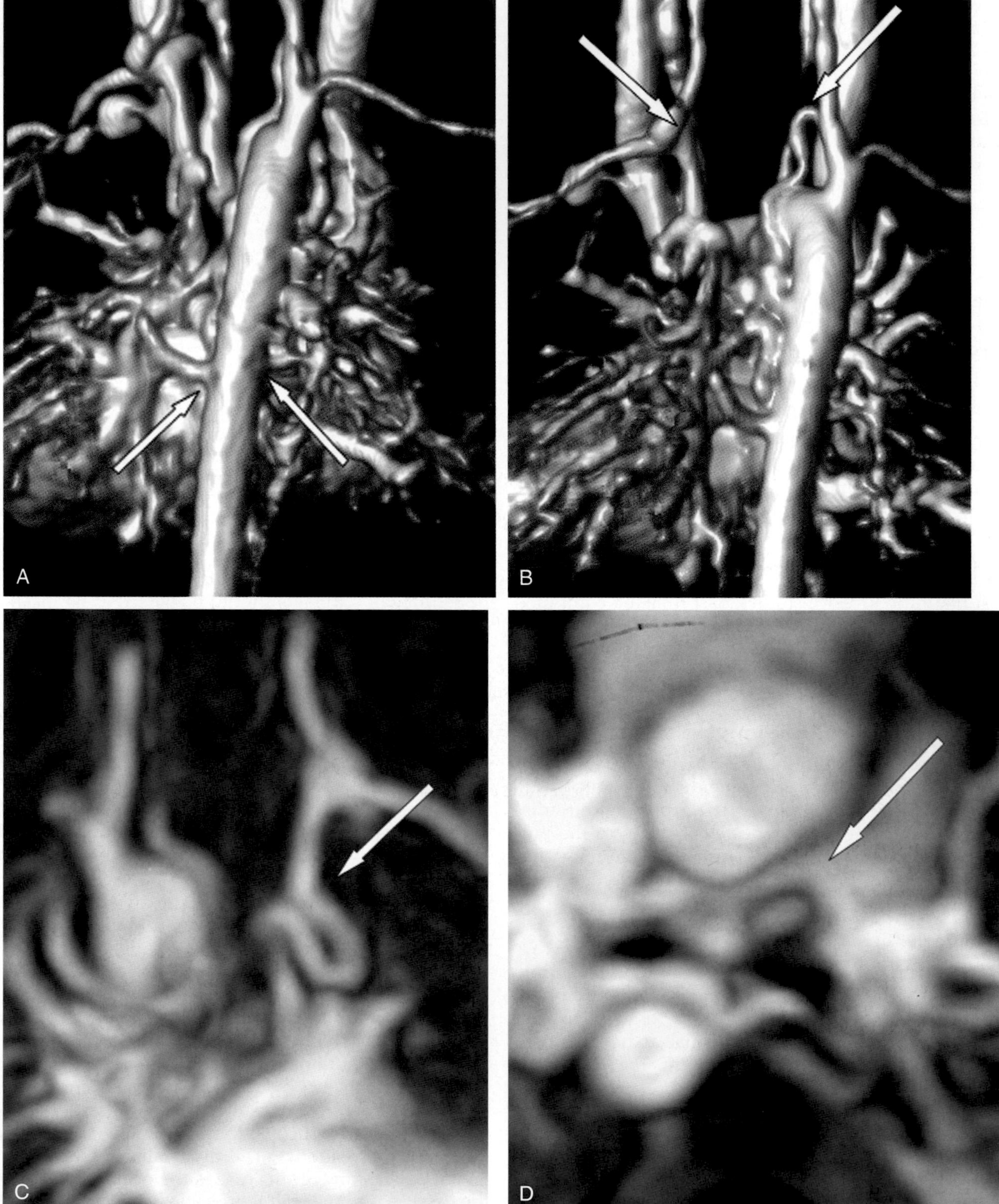

Figure 37-18 These magnetic resonance images, from the same patient, show the morphology of the pulmonary arterial supply. **A**, A three-dimensional rendering from behind. Two large systemic-to-pulmonary collateral arteries are seen emerging from the descending aorta (*arrows*). **B**, A slightly rotated view compared to panel **A** shows two additional major systemic-to-pulmonary collateral arteries arising from the left subclavian artery and the right common carotid artery (*arrows*). The reformatted planar images (**C** and **D**) allow the course of these arteries to be followed. **C**, The collateral artery arises from the left subclavian artery as it descends into the left lung (*arrow*). **D**, A horizontal planar slice demonstrates the presence of hypoplastic, confluent pulmonary arteries (*arrow*).

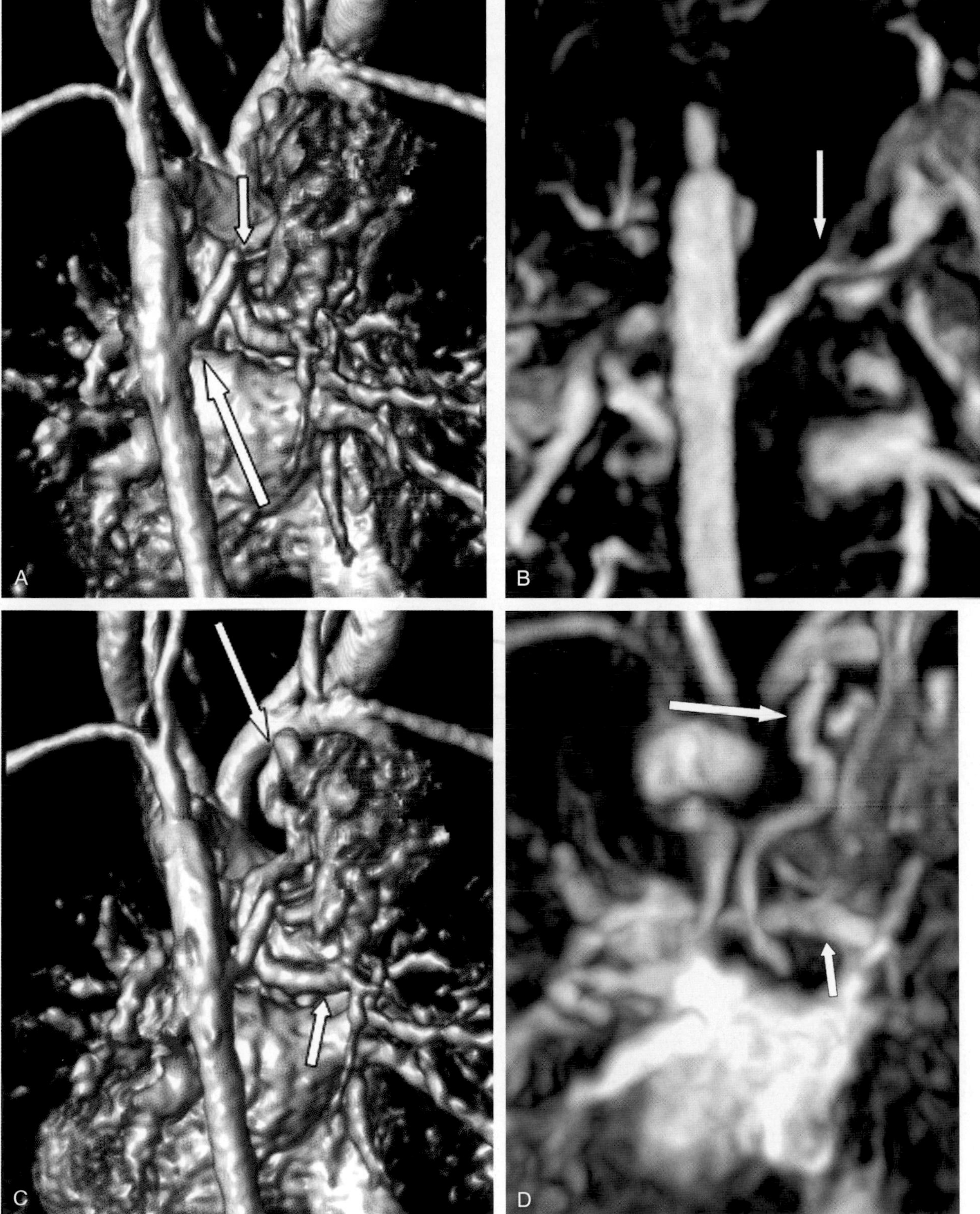

Figure 37-19 These magnetic resonance images are again from the same patient. As in Figure 37-18A, panel **A** shows a three-dimensional rendering from behind. In this patient, a large systemic-to-pulmonary collateral artery arises from the descending aorta (*larger arrow*). It passes to the right, and there is a severe narrowing before it enters the vasculature of the upper lobe of the right lung (*smaller arrow*). **B**, A reformatted planar image of the collateral artery permits the area of narrowing to be examined in greater detail (*arrow*). **C**, Another systemic-to pulmonary collateral artery, taking its origin from the right subclavian artery (*larger arrow*), extends to supply the lower part of the right lung. Its tortuous course can be followed until it divides to supply a large part of the lung (*smaller arrow*). **D**, This collateral artery in planar view (*larger arrow*), which shows at the same time the hypoplastic intrapericardial pulmonary arteries (*smaller arrow*).

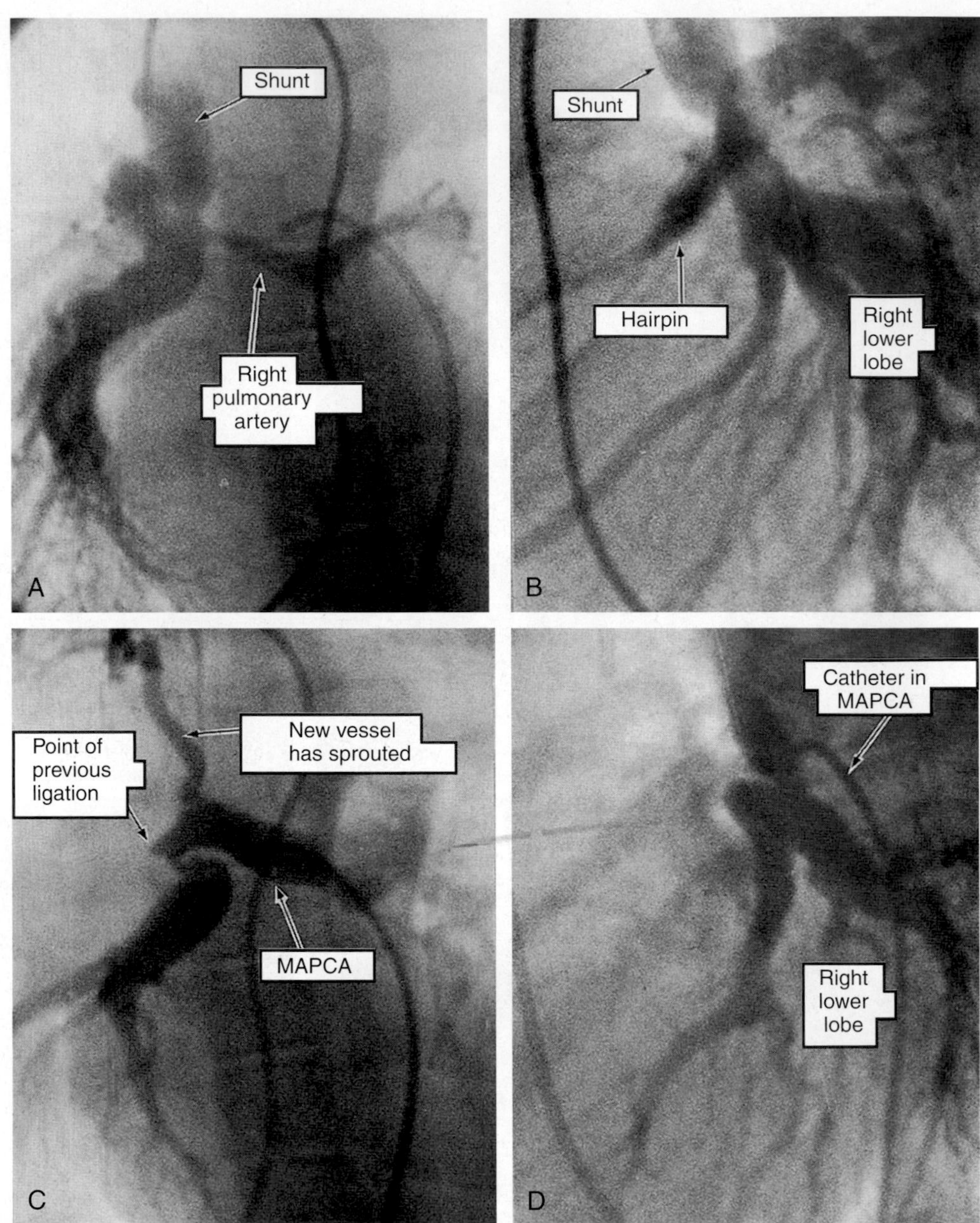

Figure 37-20 These frames, together with those shown in Figures 37-21 and 37-22, are all from the same patient. They show how it is possible to build up a composite picture of the blood supply to the lungs. Panels **A** and **C** are frontal plane projections, while panels **B** and **D** are the corresponding lateral projections. The collateral artery shown in **C** was not present on a previous angiocardiogram. It is possible to infer the segmental distribution of the pulmonary arteries, as for example the supply to the right lower lobe as shown in **D**, by summing the information available in the frontal and lateral projections. Note the obstruction at the end of the shunt in **A**. The intrapericardial pulmonary arteries are seen as a hairpin configuration in the lateral projection. MAPCA, major aorto-pulmonary collateral arteries.

an intercostal artery may be suspected from the posterior course of the catheter from the aorta toward the paravertebral gutter, in contrast to the anterior course of major systemic-to-pulmonary collateral arteries toward the hilum.

Other varieties of preformed catheters may occasionally prove helpful, for example, coronary arterial catheters when the supply to the lungs, be it acquired or congenital, is derived from the coronary arteries.

Pulmonary Venous Wedge Angiography

With good non-invasive imaging, and selective angiography of the major systemic-to-pulmonary collateral arteries, the anatomy of the pulmonary arteries should have been demonstrated. Only occasionally will it be necessary to use pulmonary venous wedge angiography. Indeed, a pulmonary venous wedge angiogram may fail to demonstrate central pulmonary arteries even when they are present. Either the pressure in the artery may be too high to permit contrast medium to be forced back to the hilum, or the vessel opacified may not be connected to the central pulmonary artery. Confident exclusion of the presence of central pulmonary arteries may, therefore, require pulmonary venous wedge angiography in several sites (Fig. 37-23).

FEATURES OF SOURCES OF PULMONARY ARTERIAL SUPPLY

Major Systemic-to-Pulmonary Collateral Arteries

The major systemic-to-pulmonary collateral arteries appear as large tortuous arteries, originating usually from the descending aorta, but occasionally from the brachiocephalic arteries and, exceptionally, from coronary arteries. They anastomose with intrapulmonary arteries in the

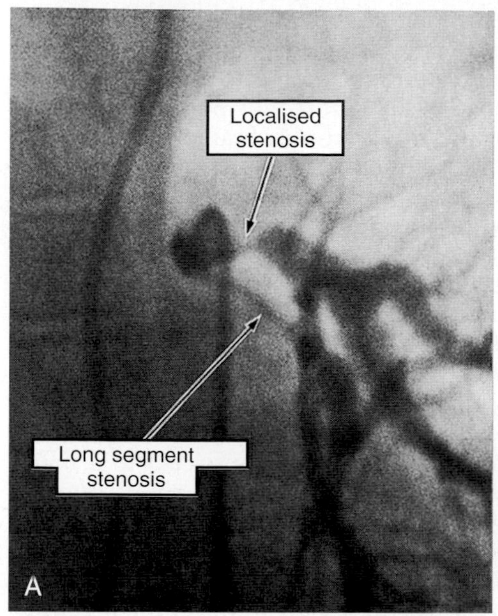

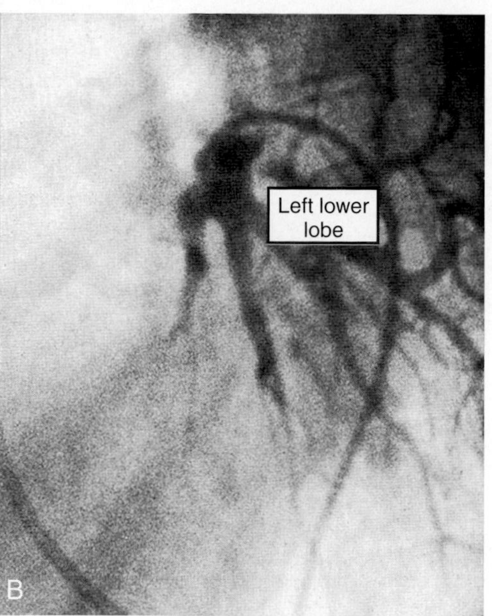

Figure 37-21 Panels A and B, in frontal and lateral projections, respectively, are selective injections into one of the systemic-to-pulmonary collateral arteries found in the patient illustrated also in Figures 37-20 and 37-22. Note the obstruction in the collateral artery.

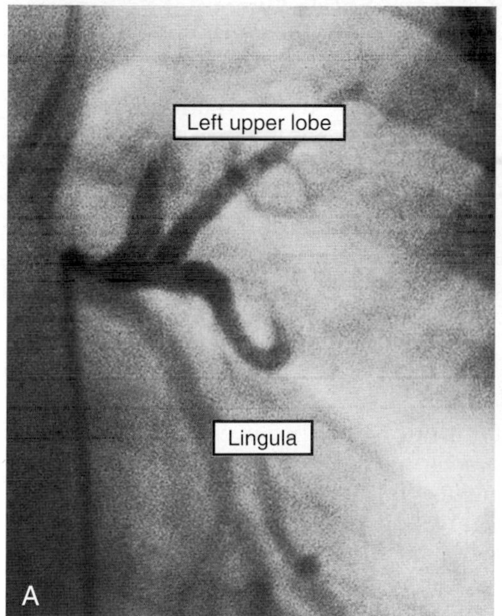

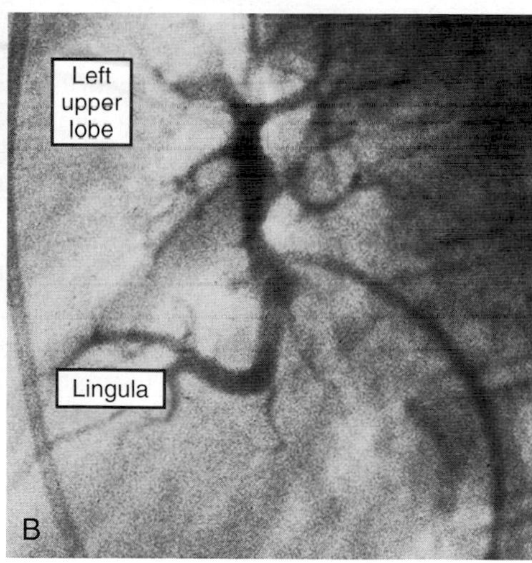

Figure 37-22 This selective injection, shown in frontal (A) and lateral (B) projections, was made into another of the major systemic-to-pulmonary collateral arteries found in the patient illustrated in Figures 37-20 and 37-21.

region of the hilum and are never connected to intercostal arteries. They accompany bronchuses, but only rarely form a plexus around them. In essence, they are no different in appearance in the neonatal period from later life.

Arterial Ducts

When a duct originates on the side opposite to the aortic arch, it is likely to arise close to the bifurcation of the brachiocephalic artery and pass to the intrapericardial pulmonary artery on that side, usually taking a straight course, but sometimes showing a wandering track. Rarely, the duct may originate from an anomalous retro-oesophageal subclavian artery arising as the last branch from the aorta. Exceptionally, bilateral ducts may be present.

Intrapericardial Pulmonary Arteries

Central pulmonary arteries are most easily recognised when they are confluent, as they usually are. The confluent pulmonary arteries, together with the abbreviated pulmonary trunk, appear like a seagull in flight when seen in the frontal projection. This resemblance is heightened by craniocaudal tilt, this procedure elongating the pulmonary trunk. The confluent central pulmonary arteries appear in the lateral projection like a hairpin, extending anteriorly to the trachea. Where there is doubt as to the identity of an artery

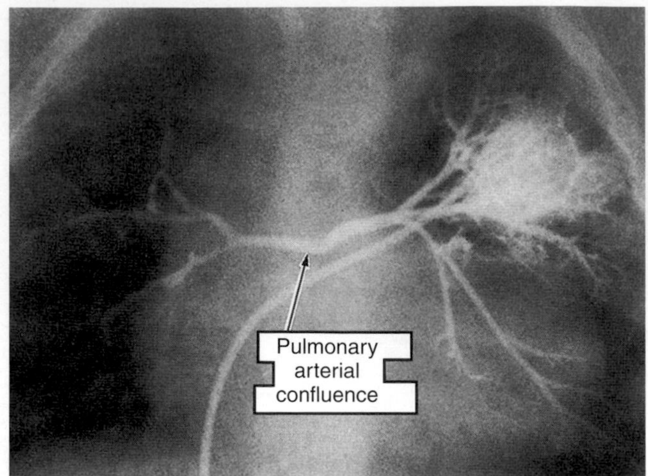

Figure 37-23 The confluence of the intrapericardial pulmonary arteries in this patient is illustrated by means of a pulmonary venous wedge injection. (The original picture was supplied by the late Dr Robert Freedom, Hospital for Sick Children, Toronto, Canada, for the second edition of this book, and was reproduced with his permission.)

in the mediastinum, a particular problem when the central pulmonary arteries are not confluent, the fact that the pulmonary trunk is usually attached to the heart, if only by a fibrous cord, is helpful. Because of this, on a cineangiogram viewed in motion, the intrapericardial pulmonary arteries are seen to move with the heart, whereas other mediastinal arteries move, if at all, with the lungs.

Interconnections Between Major Systemic-to-Pulmonary Collateral Arteries, Central Pulmonary Arteries, and Intrapulmonary Arteries

The intraparenchymal pulmonary arteries in tetralogy with pulmonary atresia are essentially normal. In particular, with rare exceptions, their distribution is that of normal pulmonary arteries. If they are hypoperfused at low pressure, they appear narrow, with deficient peripheral branching. By comparison, if they are hyperperfused, and at high pressure, they appear large and tortuous, with increased background haze. If pulmonary vascular obstructive disease supervenes, the background haze diminishes, but the arteries remain tortuous.

The abnormalities of the intrapulmonary arteries occur mainly at the hilum. Instead of fusing into a single hilar artery, as they normally do, they may remain separate. As a result, the pulmonary arterial supply to an entire lobe, segment, or even part of a segment may be completely isolated from the remainder of the lung. The segmental or lobar arteries can be connected proximally to a central pulmonary artery, to a major systemic-to-pulmonary collateral artery, or to both. The usual result is that supply of blood is compartmentalised, with each major collateral artery being the sole arterial blood supply to part of the lungs. Injection of contrast medium into that artery will then opacify only that region of lung. Occasionally, on viewing a selective injection of contrast medium into a major collateral artery on a moving cineangiogram, wash-out of contrast medium may be seen as a result of non-opacified blood entering the intrapulmonary artery. This may be because more than one major systemic-to-pulmonary collateral artery is supplying the same region of lung, and hence there is a duplicate pulmonary arterial supply. When a surgical shunt has been created to augment pulmonary arterial supply, and contrast medium is injected into the pulmonary artery by some route other than the shunt, wash-out of contrast medium is to be expected at the point of anastomosis of the shunt to the pulmonary artery.

By combining the information obtained from all the selective injections into major systemic-to-pulmonary collateral arteries, shunts, and intrapericardial pulmonary arteries, it should be possible to determine the supply to each pulmonary segment. Most importantly, it should also be possible to establish how much of the parenchyma of each lung is connected to each pulmonary artery. In making this assessment, it is important to recognise duplicate supply when it exists. For example, if the left upper lobe is connected to a major systemic-to-pulmonary collateral artery and to the central left pulmonary artery, whereas the left lower lobe appears only to be connected to a major systemic-to-pulmonary collateral artery, a shunt into the central left pulmonary artery will, on the face of it, only increase blood supply to the left lower lobe. If careful inspection reveals wash-out from one lobe to the other, then this would increase the supply to the entire left lung.

Obstructions Within the Entire System of Pulmonary Arterial Supply

As has been described, obstructions and stenoses can occur at many levels in the pulmonary circulation. Haemodynamic pressure gradients are sometimes documented at sites where no angiocardiographic stenosis is seen. Usually, obstructions are angiocardiographically obvious. Craniocaudal tilt during injection into a central pulmonary artery increases the likelihood of detection of proximal stenosis of the central right or left pulmonary artery.

Acquired Collateral Arteries

An acquired collateral circulation is a rare finding in the first 3 months of life, but it develops over time, particularly after surgical thoracotomies, when adhesion of the visceral and parietal pleural layers permits the development of centripetal collateral circulation from the chest wall to the lungs. Acquired collateral circulation appears on aortography as myriads of tiny vessels, which may originate from any artery in the thorax. Bronchial arteries are recognised by their relation to the trachea and bronchial tree, and the way in which they form a nutritive plexus in the bronchial walls. The result is that the bronchial tree lights up in the course of the aortogram because of the contrast between the air in the lumen and the contrast medium in the walls.

NATURAL HISTORY

It is difficult to be sure of the natural history of patients having tetralogy with pulmonary atresia, since before cardiac surgery was available, the condition was frequently confused with either tetralogy of Fallot or common arterial trunk. The prognosis without treatment is extremely poor for patients with duct-dependent pulmonary supply. At the other end of the scale, patients with increased, but not excessive, pulmonary arterial supply can survive into the third and fourth decade of life without surgical treatment. Adults with the condition eventually develop left ventricular dysfunction, often compounded by aortic regurgitation.[23] Systemic arterial saturations of oxygen fall slowly with increasing age. These two examples represent the two ends of the spectrum of prognosis. Overall, the majority of patients with tetralogy of Fallot and pulmonary atresia will not survive more than a few years without surgical treatment.

MANAGEMENT

Neonates with duct-dependent pulmonary blood supply should be treated with parenteral prostaglandins E_1 or E_2 while waiting for surgical palliation. Treatment may be required to combat heart failure for patients with excessive pulmonary blood flow through major systemic-to-pulmonary collateral arteries.

Definitive Repair

When confluent pulmonary arteries are present, definitive repair consists of closing the ventricular septal defect and connecting the right ventricle to the pulmonary trunk or pulmonary arterial confluence. This was first reported by Rastelli and colleagues, who used a valveless conduit.[24] The long-term results using aortic or pulmonary homografts are better, as obstruction appears to be rare in this type of conduit. These are now the preferred surgical conduit. If there is continuity between the right ventricle and pulmonary trunk, correction can often be achieved with a patch reconstruction, similar to the technique for tetralogy with pulmonary stenosis.

Results for radical correction in suitable patients were reported some time ago[25] with an overall mortality of 14%. Just over half the patients required a valved conduit to restore continuity from the right ventricle to the pulmonary arteries. In the remainder, it proved possible to reconstruct the right ventricular outflow tract with a patch. It was subsequently demonstrated that there was a strong positive correlation between the probability of hospital death and the ratio between the right and left ventricular systolic pressures after bypass.[26–28] The risk of post-operative death rises steeply if the ratio of these pressures at the end of the repair is equal to or greater than one. The causes of a high ratio are residual gradients in the right ventricular outflow, residual major systemic-to-pulmonary collateral arteries, and hypoplasia and incompleteness of arborisation of the intrapericardial pulmonary arteries. Definitive repair is possible if 15 of the 18 bronchopulmonary segments are connected to confluent pulmonary arteries. Repair can also be achieved if 11 or more segments are connected to the central pulmonary arteries, but when the number is between 11 and 14, there is an increased risk of a high post-operative pressure ratio and an increased surgical mortality.[29,30] Other risk factors are related to the number of segments fed by the central pulmonary arteries. These are small size of the proximal right and left pulmonary arteries, non-confluent pulmonary arteries, and a high number of systemic-to-pulmonary collateral arteries. There is also some evidence that very young age, or age greater than 8 years, adds to the risk of definitive repair.[30] More recent analysis of a large cohort of patients treated over almost 30 years, with around one-third having major systemic-to-pulmonary collateral arteries, showed that results had improved with time, but the number of broncho-pulmonary segments supplied by the native pulmonary arteries remained a significant determinant of achieving complete repair.[31]

The key to achieving satisfactory results is careful selection of patients, attempting repair only in those who are predicted to have a low probability of severe post-operative right ventricular hypertension. Recent surgical reports have supported this view, with most authors favouring a staged approach to repair. In patients unsuitable for primary repair, palliative procedures are undertaken to encourage growth of hypoplastic pulmonary arteries. Systemic-to-pulmonary collateral arteries are ligated or occluded, or else anastomosed to the central pulmonary arteries.[32–34]

An alternative approach has been advocated by Reddy and colleagues.[35] They argue that systemic-to-pulmonary collateral arteries are not a reliable source of flow of blood to the lungs. The flow may be too high, leading to pulmonary vascular disease, or the collateral artery may become progressively stenosed, leading to distal arterial hypoplasia. Either way, segments of lung may be lost to the pulmonary circulation, and the proportion of patients eventually suitable for definitive repair reduced. They reported their experience of one-stage complete unifocalisation, with repair where possible, in 85 patients ranging in age from 10 days to 37 years. In one-sixth of this cohort, the central pulmonary arteries were absent. Complete unifocalisation with repair was achieved in 56 patients, unifocalisation without closure of the ventricular septal defect in 23, and multi-stage sequential unifocalisation, involving the anastomosis of all the collateral arteries to the central pulmonary arteries or to a central conduit, in 6. The decision to proceed to complete repair with closure of the ventricular septal defect was taken intra-operatively, guided by a study of flow to gauge the resistance of the newly unifocalised pulmonary vascular bed. In those patients in whom it proved possible to achieve complete repair, the pressure post-operatively in the right ventricle was between 25% and 80% of that measured in the left ventricle. There were nine early, and seven late, deaths, these fatalities occurring mostly in younger patients, and those undergoing complete repair. Survival at 4 years was 74%, but three-fifths of the patients required reintervention for residual pulmonary arterial problems in the first 5 years.

Palliative Procedures

Palliative procedures may be necessary to increase, or occasionally to decrease, the flow to the lungs. The long-term goal is definitive repair, so palliative procedures have a dual purpose: first, to improve the management of the immediate clinical problem, and second, to make the patient suitable for definitive surgical repair. Preparation for definitive repair needs to address two problems: enlargement of hypoplastic central pulmonary arteries and unifocalisation of pulmonary perfusion.

Management of Hypoplastic Central Pulmonary Arteries

Early intervention to increase the flow in diminutive central pulmonary arteries has long been advocated. There is good evidence that it can improve the eventual outcome,[32,33,36] even though the enlargement achieved may not affect uniformly the entire pulmonary arterial tree. The choice is between a shunt, and reconstruction of the right ventricular outflow tract using a patch or conduit while leaving open the ventricular septal defect. There is no clear consensus about which choice is preferred. There is evidence that early connection of the right ventricle to the pulmonary arteries promotes more pulmonary arterial growth than does a shunt.[37] Reconstruction of the right ventricular outflow also has the advantage of allowing direct access to the pulmonary arteries so that interventional procedures can be undertaken to address stenosis of the pulmonary arteries.

Since enlargement of the pulmonary arteries is not uniform, areas of pulmonary arterial stenosis may well remain following palliation. A combined surgical and interventional approach to the pulmonary arteries is now widely advocated. Balloon angioplasty, and the deployment of intravascular stents, are used after reconstruction of the right ventricular outflow tract to promote unobstructed flow to the maximum number of bronchopulmonary segments.[20,33]

One disadvantage of early reconstruction of the right ventricular outflow tract is that it needs cardiopulmonary bypass, and carries a higher risk than does placement of a shunt. It is also recognised that reconstruction using a patch can lead to stenosis of the pulmonary arteries, especially the left, and that the patch can dilate in aneurysmal fashion. These considerations have led some surgeons to prefer a shunt as an initial procedure.[27,32] Peripheral shunts have fallen from favour, since they can lead to distortion of the pulmonary arteries. Central shunts, either constructed of a Gore-Tex tube or by disconnecting the pulmonary trunk and anastomosing it end-to-side to the ascending aorta,[38] are now preferred.

Unifocalisation

There are two options for dealing with the major systemic-to-pulmonary collateral arteries. The first is to obliterate them, either by surgical ligation or by embolisation using coils, while the second is surgical unifocalisation. If there is a dual blood supply to pulmonary segments, and obliteration is combined with, or follows, construction of a shunt or reconstruction of the right ventricular tract, this combination will encourage flow, and hence growth and development of the central pulmonary arteries. If the collateral artery is the sole supply to an area of lung, ligation has been advocated in the hope that hypoplasia of that region of the lung will result, with compensatory hypertrophy of those regions connected to the central pulmonary arteries. Necrosis of the region of lung supplied by the ligated collateral artery is unlikely, but has been reported in exceptional cases. In practise, this approach has not been successful.

A better approach to collateral arteries that are the sole supply to parts of the lung is surgical unifocalisation. The aim of this approach is to maximise the number of bronchopulmonary segments perfused from the central pulmonary arteries. Technically this is not easy, as the collateral arteries are located posteriorly in the mediastinum, while the pulmonary arteries are anterior. Early results were disappointing, but better results have now been achieved. Depending on the precise anatomy found, a number of techniques have been used, including direct and prosthetic anastomosis, division of a collateral artery with end-to-side anastomosis of its distal end to a pulmonary artery, and insertion of xenograft pericardial tubes.[32,34] Such operations rarely achieve unifocalisation at a stroke, since it is often difficult to connect together all intrapulmonary arteries on one side, let alone both. The procedures can be carried out at the same time as construction of a shunt or surgical relief of pulmonary arterial stenosis, but not in combination with reconstruction of the right ventricular outflow tract. Where the central pulmonary arteries are non-confluent, completely absent, or judged to be too hypoplastic to be amenable to the staging approach, an artificial confluence can be created using a prosthetic or xenograft pericardial tube. The confluence is connected to a shunt, and the collateral arteries unifocalised by connection to the confluence.[34,39,40] Collateral arteries can be embolised with coils after definitive repair, and when there is still a large left-to-right shunt through unligated arteries. It is preferable to embolise such collateral arteries prior to definitive repair if this is undertaken as part of a combined interventional and surgical strategy.[20,33]

Obstructions in major systemic-to-pulmonary collateral arteries can lead to a progressive reduction in overall pulmonary perfusion, or to hypoperfusion of a significant part of the pulmonary parenchyma. There is little in the literature about balloon angioplasty and stenting of these obstructions as purely palliative measures to improve systemic oxygenation or as a prelude to unifocalisation. The interventional approach may have a limited role in some circumstances, but some of these stenoses cannot be successfully dilated even with high-pressure balloons.[41]

Strategies for Management

In this complex and varied condition, generalisations about regimes for treatment are unwise. Each patient requires detailed investigation, and an individual strategy for treatment must be devised by a clinical team that has extensive experience in management. Earlier in this chapter, we identified three characteristic patterns for pulmonary perfusion. These were confluent pulmonary arteries with a unifocal supply, confluent but hypoplastic central pulmonary arteries with major systemic-to-pulmonary collateral arteries, and complete absence of the central pulmonary arteries with the pulmonary perfusion solely from major collateral arteries.

The first of these patterns is the easiest with which to deal. The pulmonary arteries are generally of a good size, and are connected to all of the bronchopulmonary segments. The management is comparable to that for tetralogy of Fallot with pulmonary stenosis. Definitive repair can be carried out as a primary procedure,[42] or a shunt is constructed in the neonatal period and definitive repair carried out in the first few years of life. The decision between the two will depend upon the size of the pulmonary arteries and the experience of the surgeon.

In patients with hypoplastic pulmonary arteries, it is essential to intervene early in life to encourage growth. This involves either reconstruction of the right ventricular outflow tract, with a patch or valveless conduit, or placement of a central aortopulmonary shunt. Major collateral arteries that form a dual supply to part of the lung with the central pulmonary arteries are ligated or embolised as part of the same procedure, or more commonly as a second staging procedure. Collateral arteries providing the sole supply to part of the lung are anastomosed to the central pulmonary arteries, ideally directly, but if necessary using a prosthetic graft. The aim is to connect the central pulmonary arterial confluence to as much of the pulmonary parenchyma as possible, and to achieve unobstructed flow of blood. Balloon angioplasty, or stenting, of the pulmonary arteries may be necessary to deal with localised obstructions. Using this approach, approximately half of these patients will eventually have central pulmonary arteries of sufficient size, and supplying sufficient arterial supply to the lungs, to make them suitable for definitive repair.

The third pattern is the most difficult to treat. Operations to create a central pulmonary confluence using grafts have been described.[34,39,40] The long-term success of this approach, however, is not established. In patients with a stable and well-balanced pulmonary perfusion, conservative management has been advocated, with the eventual aim of offering them transplantation of the heart and lungs.[30,43]

Results of Surgery

The majority of patients require multiple surgical interventions. Results of individual operations, therefore, are not as important as the results of the overall programme of treatment. The results can be difficult to ascertain from published surgical series. What is clear is that the results are much worse when tetralogy is associated with pulmonary atresia rather than stenosis. The early mortality of definitive repair reported in published series varies between 4% and 15%.[14,20,27,32,33,34,38] Many patients, despite palliative staging procedures, are never candidates for definitive repair. The proportion of patients that can be converted from being inoperable to operable by staging procedures is difficult to determine from the published series, but overall it seems to be little more than half. The staging procedures themselves carry a significant risk, with a reported mortality of at least 10% in most series. There does seem to be some evidence that the chances of achieving operability from staging operations are improved by starting early in life.[36]

Recent studies have shown that the mortality for either primary or staged repair has improved,[35,44,45] but there is limited information about the long-term outcome for survivors of surgery. One large series[46] showed a significant late mortality and rate of reintervention, while others[27] found that there was a low, but constant, risk of dying in survivors of surgery.[27] Survival was 82%, 69%, and 58% at 1, 10, and 20 years, respectively. Taking into account the attrition rate before surgery, it is clear that, despite the many advances in recent years, the overall results of treatment for this condition remain disappointing.

The complete reference list can be found on the companion Expert Consult web site at www.expertconsult.com.

ANNOTATED REFERENCES

- Kirklin JW, Blackstone EH, Shimazaki Y, et al: Survival, functional status, and reoperations after repair of tetralogy of Fallot with pulmonary atresia. J Thorac Cardiovasc Surg 1988;96:102–116.
- Cho JM, Puga FJ, Danielson GK, et al: Early and long-term results of surgical treatment of tetralogy of Fallot with pulmonary atresia, with or without major aortopulmonary collateral arteries. J Thorac Cardiovasc Surg 2002;124:70–81.

  These reports are long-term studies of outcome for surgical repair of tetralogy and pulmonary atresia. For those patients who achieve definitive repair, survival after 10 years is reported as 69% and 86%. A significant proportion of patients require reoperation.
- Reddy VM, McElhinney DB, Amin Z, et al: Early and intermediate outcomes after repair of pulmonary atresia with ventricular septal defect and major aortopulmonary collateral arteries: Experience with 85 patients. Circulation 2000;101:1826–1832.

  The report described experience of early unifocalisation and definitive repair for a large series of patients, mostly infants, with tetralogy with pulmonary atresia and major collateral arteries. Early unifocalisation was achieved in more than nine-tenths of the patients, with complete repair achieved in one procedure in two-thirds. Survival was 80% at 3 years.
- Amark KM, Karamlou T, O'Carroll A, et al: Independent factors associated with mortality, reintervention and achievement of complete repair in children with pulmonary atresia with ventricular septal defect. J Am Coll Cardiol 2006;47:1448–1456.
- Duncan BW, Mee RBB, Prieto LR, et al: Staged repair of tetralogy of Fallot with pulmonary atresia and major aortopulmonary collateral arteries. J Thorac Cardiovasc Surg 2003;126:694–702.
- Marshall AC, Love BA, Lang P, et al: Staged repair of tetralogy of Fallot and diminutive pulmonary arteries with a fenestrated ventricular septal defect patch. J Thorac Cardiovasc Surg 2003:126:1427–1433.

  These three recent surgical series demonstrate the outcomes currently achievable by experienced clinical teams. Despite the progress made, and the lower operative mortality, the outcomes remain mixed, with many patients not achieving definitive repair. These series show a variety of approaches to staged repair of patients with different morphologies, including those with very small intrapericardial pulmonary arteries.
- Brown SC, Eyskens B, Mertens L, et al: Percutaneous treatment of stenosed major aortopulmonary collaterals with balloon dilatation and stenting: What can be achieved? Heart 1998;79:24–28.

  This report describes the use of interventional balloon dilation and implantation of stents to palliate patients with complex pulmonary arterial supplies. The results are mixed.
- Boechat MI, Ratib O, Williams PL, et al: Cardiac MR imaging and MR angiography for assessment of complex tetralogy of Fallot and pulmonary atresia. Radiographics 2005;25:1535–1546.

  This review addresses the imaging of the pulmonary circulation in patients with tetralogy and pulmonary atresia, demonstrating the value of magnetic resonance imaging and three-dimensional reconstruction.

Transposition

CANER SALIH, CHRISTIAN BRIZARD, DANIEL J. PENNY, and ROBERT H. ANDERSON

The congenital malformation characterised by origin of the arterial trunks from morphologically inappropriate ventricles has probably been the source of as much confusion and controversy as any other single topic in paediatric cardiology. When Matthew Baillie described the first case,[1] he had no problems with nomenclature, describing the entity in accurate fashion as a singular malformation (Fig. 38-1).

His choice of terminology was echoed in the description of the second case by Mr Langstaff,[2] albeit that this gentleman did not even give his readers the pleasure of knowing his initials! Since then, the entity most usually described simply as transposition has been defined in many different ways, and has been used to describe many different types of congenital cardiac malformations. The term, however, has not always been employed with the accuracy displayed by Matthew Baillie. Perhaps because of this, the malformation has been the source of several polemics within the last decades. The arguments have centred on whether the morphological arrangement of the arterial trunks should be defined primarily according to their ventricular origin,[3] or on the basis of an anterior location of the aorta relative to the pulmonary trunk.[4] The disagreements have been non-productive. The problems are readily circumvented by distinguishing between these features, and then by describing both, rather than nominating one in isolation as the basis of diagnosis.[5] There is little doubt, however, that in the clinical setting it is the origin of the arterial trunks from the ventricles which is paramount. It is this feature that determines the patterns of flow of blood through the heart, irrespective of the relationships of the arterial trunks. It is the combinations of segmental connections that produces the variations still described in terms of transposition. We will describe the combination to be discussed in this chapter simply as transposition, including only those patients having the specific combination of concordant atrioventricular and discordant ventriculo-arterial connections (Fig. 38-2). In this way, we distinguish the group of patients with this particular variant of discordant ventriculo-arterial connections from those associated also with discordant connections at the atrioventricular junction. This second combination is best described as congenitally corrected transposition (see Chapter 39). Both these variants are then distinguished from discordant ventriculo-arterial connections seen in combination with isomeric atrial appendages (described in Chapter 22), and those found with functionally univentricular atrioventricular connections (described in Chapter 31). Relationships of the aorta relative to the pulmonary trunk are described separately as also, when necessary, is the specific infundibular morphology.

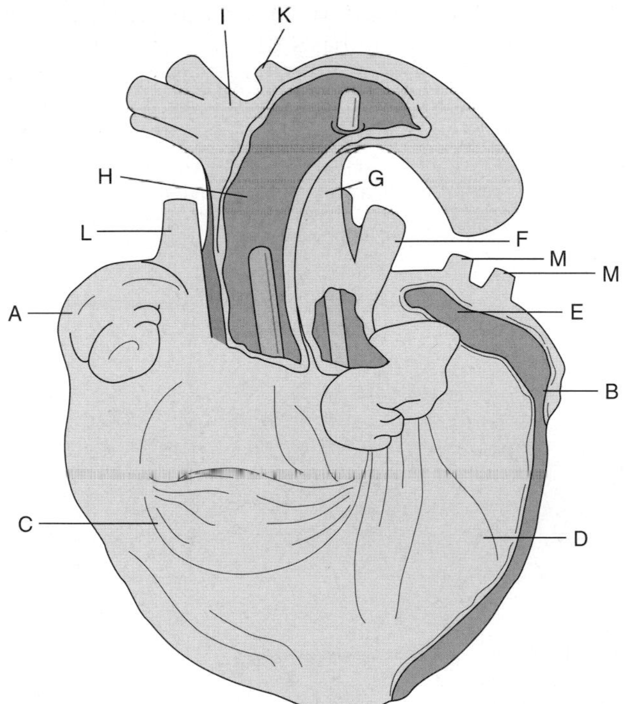

Figure 38-1 The illustration used by Matthew Baillie to show the essence of his singular anomaly. Note the anterior and right-sided location of the aorta. The crow quill inserted from the left ventricle passes through the pulmonary trunk, and then through a persistently patent arterial duct so as to emerge in the aorta. The alphabetic notation used by Baillie is as follows: A shows the right atrial, and B the left atrial appendages. C and D are the morphologically right and left ventricles, respectively. E is the cavity of the left atrium, and F is the left pulmonary artery. G shows the persistently patent arterial duct, while H is the aorta arising from the right ventricle. J and K are brachiocephalic arteries, and M shows the pulmonary veins. Baillie seems to have ignored J!

HISTORICAL BACKGROUND

Before we describe the specific morphology of hearts showing the combination of concordant atrioventricular and discordant ventriculo-arterial connections, it is pertinent to review briefly the controversies that underscored the disagreements discussed above. To the best of our knowledge, it was John Farre[6] who first used the term transposition in the context of a cardiac malformation. He undoubtedly used it to describe the origin of the great arterial trunks from morphologically inappropriate ventricles. Since then, however, there was a period during which it became the norm to define the entity in terms of the anterior location of the aorta.[7] During this period, it was also considered that the anterior location of the aortic valve should be combined with support from a muscular infundibulum.[8] If transposition is defined on the basis of an anterior aorta, and this feature

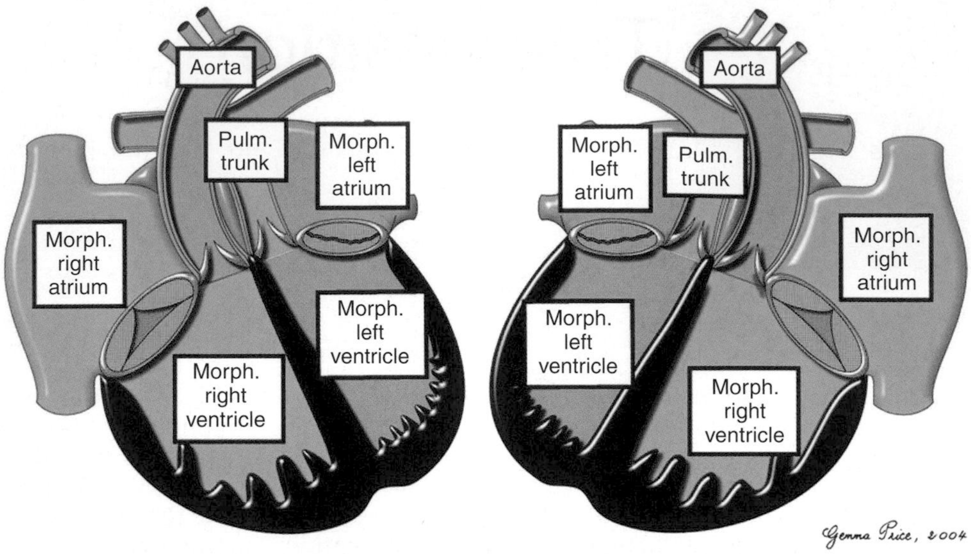

Figure 38-2 The cartoon shows the segmental combinations producing the lesion described as transposition, namely, concordant atrioventricular and discordant ventriculo-arterial connections. As shown, the lesion can exist with either usual atrial arrangement (left hand) or in the mirror-imaged variant (right hand). Note that the aorta is usually left-sided with the mirror-imaged variant. Morph, morphologically.

is then combined with considerations of segmental connections at the atrioventricular and ventriculo-arterial junctions, it is possible to define eight basic patterns in which each arterial trunk arises from its own ventricle (Fig. 38-3).

It is the use of the concept encapsulated in Figure 38-3 that has underscored the use of the qualifier congenitally corrected as frequently applied to transposition. Amongst the variants shown in the figure, some produce physiological correction of the circulatory patterns, such that the systemic venous blood reaches the lungs despite being pumped by the morphologically inappropriate ventricle. In two of these variants, however, there is also anatomical correction, in that the aorta takes its origin from the morphologically left ventricle despite its anterior position. In two of the other variants, the circulations are in parallel rather than in series, despite the fact that the aorta arises in concordant fashion from the morphologically left ventricle. It was the use of corrected in an anatomical sense, being dependent upon the definition of transposition as an anterior aorta, that produced the potential for confusion. Still further problems arose when it was suggested that the aorta also required to be supported by a muscular infundibulum if it was to be considered corrected in terms of its morphological origin.[9] In reality, it makes little sense when considering clinical presentation to describe a patient with an anterior aorta arising from the left ventricle as having transposition when the atrioventricular connections are also concordant. Thus, over recent years, there has been an increasing groundswell of opinion in favour of defining transposition on the basis of the origin of the great arterial trunks from morphologically inappropriate ventricles. Such a definition, in addition to removing the confusion of an anterior aorta arising from the left ventricle being considered as transposed when the atrioventricular connections are concordant, also proves its value when considering those rare cases in which the arterial trunks

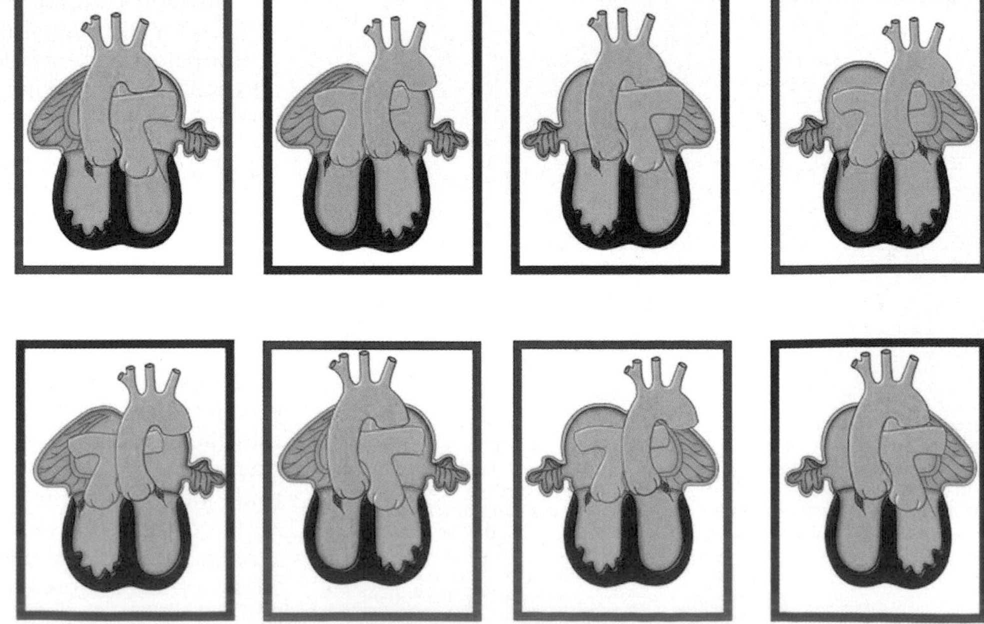

Figure 38-3 The cartoon shows the eight variations that can be constructed by combining usual and mirror-imaged atrial arrangements (morphologically right atrium in teal, morphologically left atrium in pink); right hand and left hand ventricular topology (morphologically right ventricle with a teal cavity; morphologically left ventricle with a pink cavity), and an anterior right-sided or left-sided aorta (aorta in pink; pulmonary trunk in teal). The upper four panels show the arterial trunks arising in discordant fashion, while they are concordantly connected in the lower four panels. The combinations in blue squares have the circulations in parallel, whilst those shown in red squares have circulations in series. The orange commas show infundibular musculature supporting an arterial valve.

are connected to morphologically inappropriate ventricles, but with the aorta in posterior position, and with fibrous continuity between the leaflets of the aortic and mitral valves.[10] The pattern of arterial relationships and infundibular morphology seen in this setting[10] is the one more usually encountered in the normal heart. Such abnormal hearts, with an aorta located posteriorly and rightward but arising from the morphologically right ventricle, obviously cannot be described as transposition by those who insist upon an anterior position for the aorta as the essential criterion for definition.[4] Such an approach to nomenclature, based primarily upon relationships of the arterial trunks, can be internally consistent. It is inappropriate, therefore, to insist that the users of an internally consistent system simply abandon it, and adopt another system that may itself have deficiencies. The system that we now use, therefore, is a compromise, basing the use of transposition on the combination of specific atrioventricular and ventriculo-arterial connections. This is also the solution adopted by the International Working Group on Nomenclature, and that advocated by the consensus statement prepared on behalf of the Society of Thoracic Surgeons.[11] The approach is based on the paramountcy of segmental connections, but recognises the need also to describe, when appropriate, both arterial relationships and infundibular morphology, albeit using mutually exclusive terms. In this way, all potentials for confusion are avoided.[5]

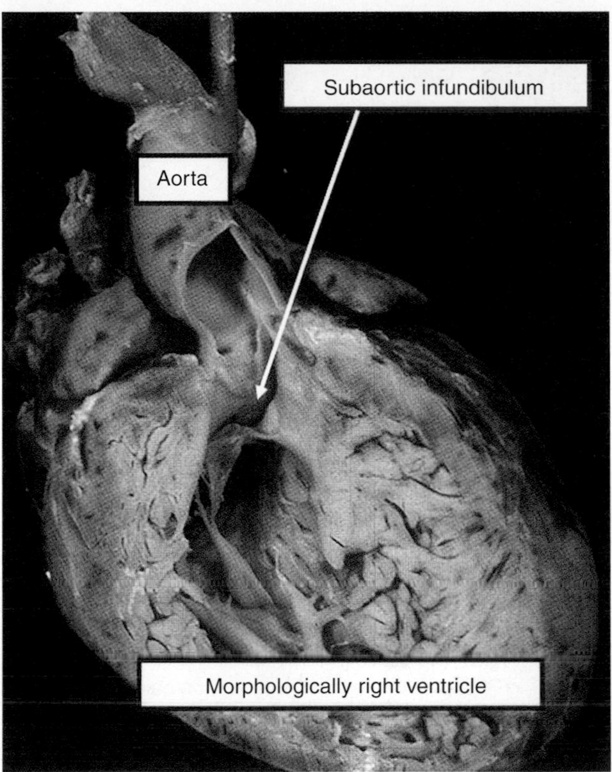

Figure 38-4 The morphologically right ventricle in this heart, connected by the tricuspid valve to the morphologically right atrium, supports the aorta above a muscular infundibulum. This, together with the arrangement shown in Figure 38-5, is the essence of transposition, in this case with an intact ventricular septum.

PREVALENCE AND AETIOLOGY

Although a rare malformation, accounting for only about one-twentieth of all congenital cardiac malformations, transposition was responsible for up to one-fifth of cardiac deaths in infancy prior to the era of surgical correction. Boys are affected two to three times as frequently as girls. Although no definite aetiological factors have been identified, the condition is held to be more frequent in infants of diabetic mothers.[12] Maternal intake of alcohol,[13] poor nutrition[14] or a stressful life event[15] during pregnancy may increase the risk of transposition in the offspring, while addition of folic acid to the maternal diet may result in a modest reduction in risk.[16]

ANATOMY AND MORPHOGENESIS

Anatomy

It is the basic combinations of concordant atrioventricular and discordant ventriculo-arterial connections that produce the entity we call transposition (see Fig. 38-2). The anatomical situation can be complicated by the presence of a ventricular septal defect, an obstruction within the left ventricular outflow tract, both of these malformations, or by other associated malformations.[17] It has become customary, nonetheless, to describe cases as being simple when hearts have an intact interventricular septum and no obstruction of the left ventricular outflow tract, even if they are complicated by other lesions such as persistent patency of the arterial duct.

Basic Segmental Combinations

The essence of transposition is the presence of a morphologically right atrium joined to a morphologically right ventricle that gives rise to the aorta (Fig. 38-4), together with a morphologically left atrium connected to a morphologically left ventricle that supports the pulmonary trunk (Fig. 38-5).

This combination of connections can be found with either usual or mirror-imaged atrial arrangements (see Fig. 38-2). It cannot exist when there is isomerism of the atrial appendages. Hearts with isomeric atrial appendages can, of course, have biventricular atrioventricular connections, right hand topology, and discordant ventriculo-arterial connections. Such hearts are closely related to transposition as it is defined for the purposes of this chapter, but those with isomeric atrial appendages have grossly abnormal venoatrial connections as their major feature (see Chapter 22).

The internal anatomy of the atriums is basically normal, although most frequently the oval foramen is patent, or there is a deficiency of the floor of the oval fossa. Even if the flap valve overlaps the rim of the oval fossa, it is flimsy and can be ruptured easily by balloon septostomy. In keeping with this normal atrial anatomy, the sinus and atrioventricular nodes are in their anticipated position. There are no histologically specialised tracts of conduction tissue between the nodes. This is not to deny the importance of the prominent muscle bundles in the right atrium in conduction of the sinus impulse. These bundles, such as the terminal crest or the superior rim of the oval fossa, are, however, composed of ordinary working myocardium.

Unlike the atrial chambers, ventricular morphology is subtly different from normal. The ventricular septum is much straighter than usual, not showing the multiple curves so typical of the normal heart. The pulmonary valve

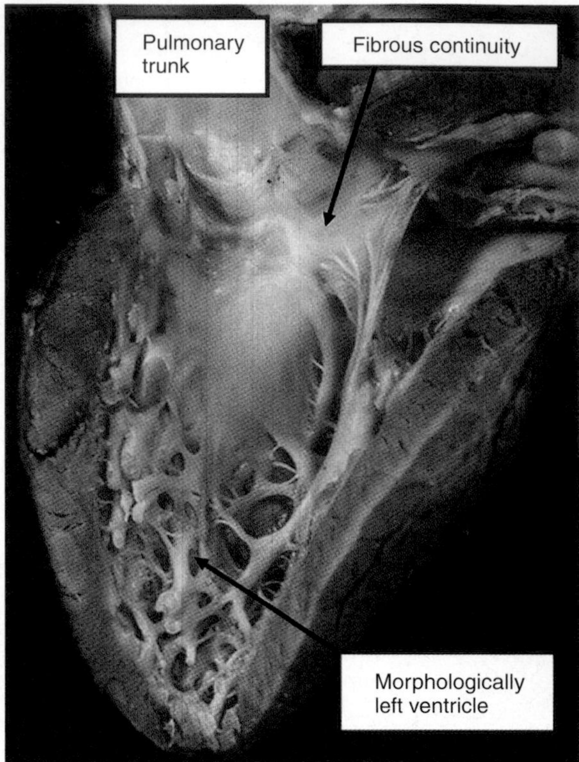

Figure 38-5 The other half of the heart shown in Figure 38-4. The morphologically left ventricle, connected to the morphologically left atrium through a mitral valve, gives rise to the pulmonary trunk. Note the fibrous continuity between the leaflets of the pulmonary and mitral valves.

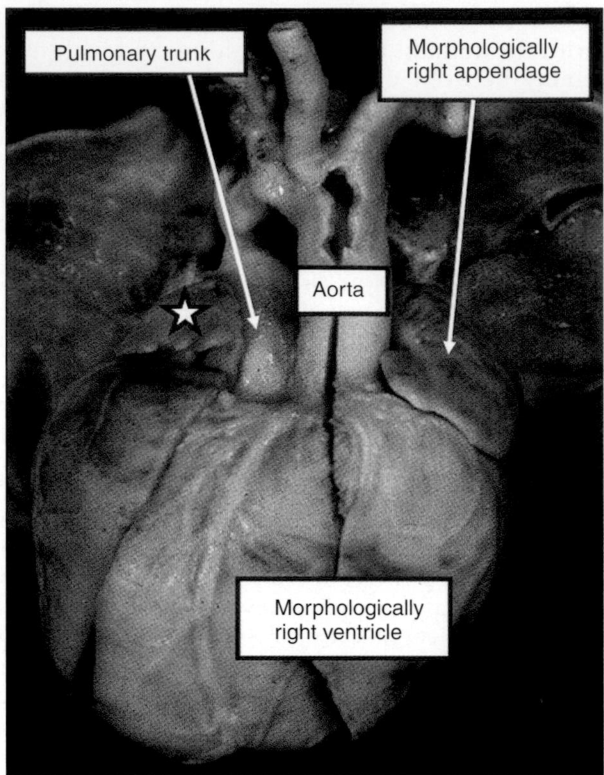

Figure 38-6 This heart is from a patient with mirror-imaged atrial appendages. The star shows the right-sided morphologically left appendage. There is left hand ventricular topology, with the morphologically right ventricle being left-sided, and discordant ventriculo-arterial connections. As is usual for this combination, the anterior aorta is left-sided.

is not wedged as deeply between the mitral and tricuspid valves as is the aortic valve in the normal heart. This, in turn, means that the area of off-setting of the leaflets of the atrioventricular valves is much less marked, as is the area occupied by the membranous septum. Indeed, in over half the hearts with intact septum, it is not possible to find a fibrous component of the ventricular septum. Another consequence of this abnormal arrangement is that the ratio of the dimensions of the inlet and outlet components of the ventricular mass are abnormal in favour of the outlet dimension, although not to the extent seen in atrioventricular septal defects (see Chapter 27). At birth, the walls of the morphologically left ventricular wall are marginally thicker than those of the right ventricle. The right ventricular mural thickness then rapidly increases in the first 2 years of life, becoming much thicker than that of the left ventricle.

The most obvious external abnormality is the relationship of the aorta to the pulmonary trunk. In the majority of patients with an intact ventricular septum, the aortic root is to the right of the pulmonary trunk in hearts in the setting of usual atrial arrangement (see Fig. 38-4), and to the left in the mirror-imaged variant (Fig. 38-6). This is by no means the rule, and patients are found with usual atrial arrangement and intact ventricular septum when the aorta is to the left (Fig. 38-7). Rarely, the aorta may be right-sided and posterior (Fig. 38-8), even when the ventricular septum is intact.

Infundibular Morphology

When the ventricular septum is intact, the aorta almost always has a complete muscular infundibulum, while the leaflets of the pulmonary valve are in fibrous continuity

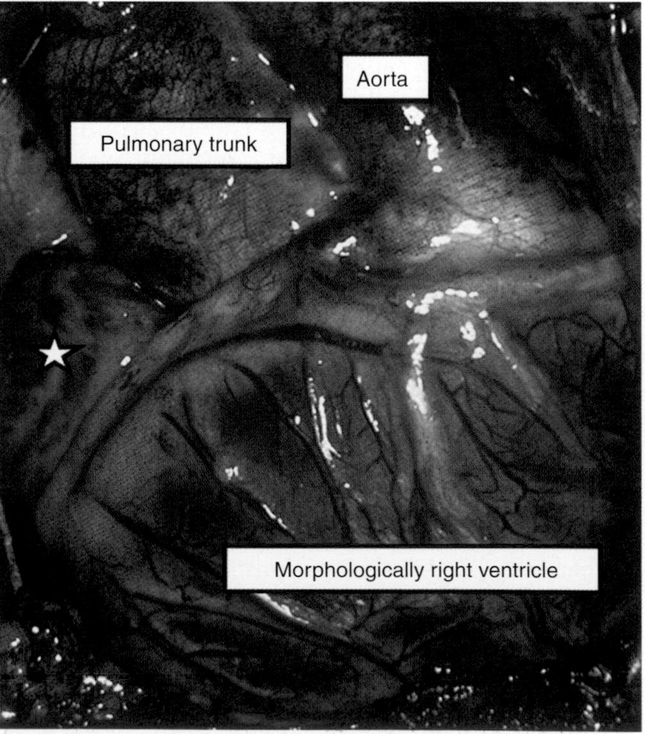

Figure 38-7 In this patient, the atrioventricular connections are concordant with usual atrial arrangement. The star shows the right-sided morphologically right atrial appendage. The discordantly connected aorta is to the left of the pulmonary trunk. The image has been reoriented so as to show the heart in attitudinally appropriate fashion. (Courtesy of Dr Benson R. Wilcox, University of North Carolina, Chapel Hill.)

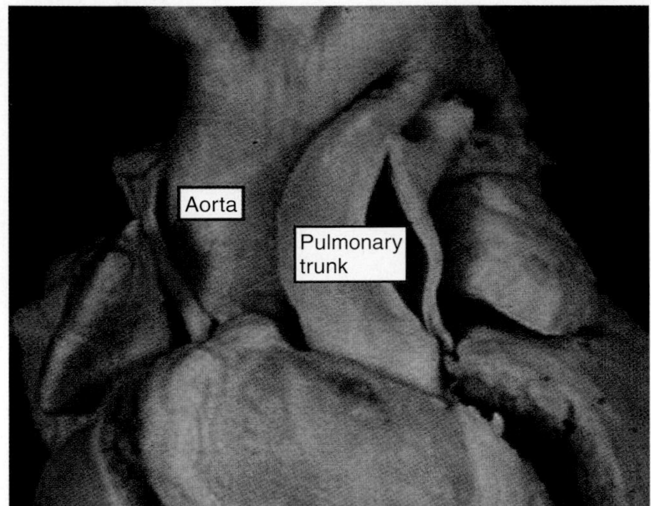

Figure 38-8 In this heart from a patient with usual atrial arrangement, concordant atrioventricular connections, and discordant ventriculo-arterial connections, the aorta is posterior and to the right of the pulmonary trunk. There is also fibrous continuity between the leaflets of the aortic and mitral valves in the roof of a co-existing ventricular septal defect.

with the mitral valve (see Figs. 38-4 and 38-5). Variations in this infundibular morphology, for example, the presence of bilaterally complete muscular infundibulums, are not seen nearly as frequently when the ventricular septum is intact as when there is a ventricular septal defect.

Coronary Arteries

Whenever the position of the aortic root is abnormal, the origins of the coronary arteries deviate from those found in the normal heart. The arteries, however, continue to arise from one or the other, or both, of those aortic sinuses that face, or are adjacent to, the pulmonary trunk (Fig. 38-9). The epicardial course of the arteries arising from these adjacent sinuses is much less predictable. Attempts to account for all these patterns in alphabetic fashion, or even worse, alpha-numeric fashion, have led either to systems that do not account for all patterns,[18] or else to truly formidable codifications that placed immense demands on the memory.[19] When describing the coronary arterial arrangement, therefore, it is best to use a descriptive approach, accounting separately for the origins of the three major coronary arteries from the aortic sinuses, describing their course relative to the vascular pedicle, noting any intramural course, with attention paid to the location of the artery supplying the sinus node.[20]

Although the coronary arteries always arise from one or both of the aortic sinuses which are adjacent to the pulmonary trunk, the position of these sinuses in space can vary according to the relationship of the arterial trunks (Fig. 38-10). To account for this variability, it is necessary to have a system of description that is independent of spatial relationships. This can be achieved by considering the aortic sinuses as they would be visualised, figuratively speaking, by an observer standing in the non-adjacent aortic sinus and looking towards the pulmonary trunk (see Fig. 38-10). The sinuses supporting the coronary arteries are then located to the right and left hands of the observer. The sinus to the right hand has now become universally known as sinus 1, while that to the left hand is distinguished as sinus 2.[21] All patterns are then accounted for according to whether the right, circumflex, and anterior interventricular arteries arise from sinus 1 or from sinus 2.[20] The system accounts for any and all departures from the normal situation

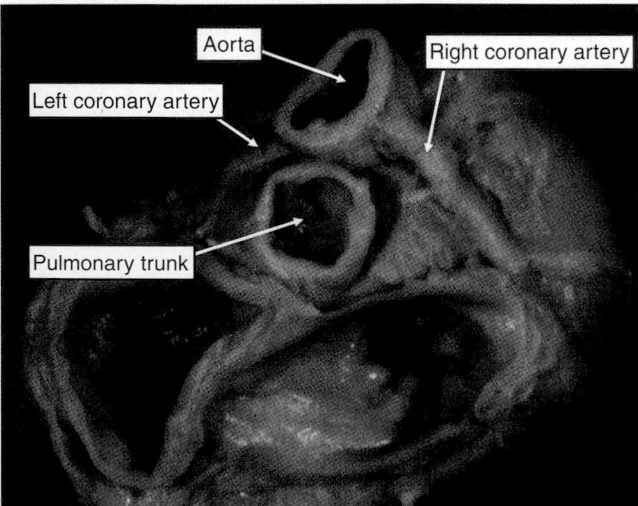

Figure 38-9 The heart was prepared by removing the atrial chambers and the arterial trunks, and is photographed from the atrial aspect. Note the anterior and right-sided location of the discordantly connected aorta. As is always the case in transposition, the coronary arteries arise from the aortic sinuses adjacent to the pulmonary trunk, in this instance with one coronary artery arising from each sinus.

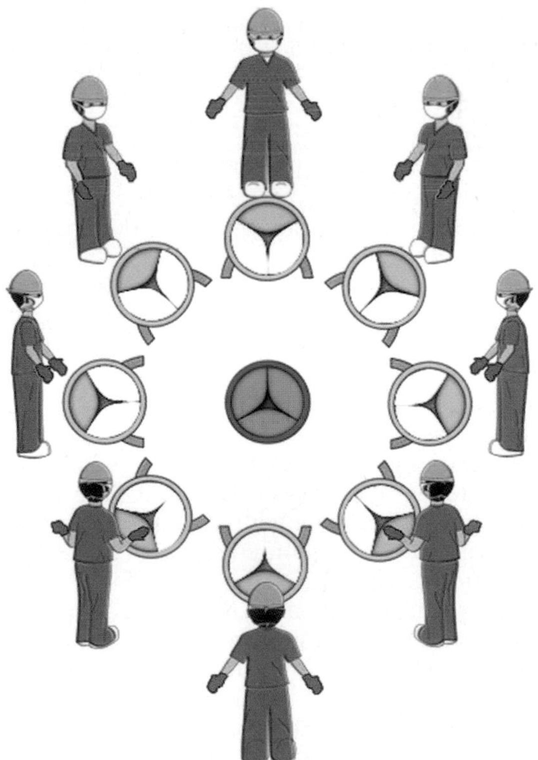

Figure 38-10 The cartoon shows the potential variability of the aorta relative to the pulmonary trunk in congenitally malformed hearts. With this degree of variability, it is not possible to account for the location of the aortic sinuses in terms of right or left, or anterior or posterior, coordinates without describing each heart separately. Always, however, the coronary arteries arise from the sinuses closest to the pulmonary trunk, and always these sinuses can be distinguished as being to the right hand of the observer standing in the non-adjacent sinus and looking towards the pulmonary trunk, this sinus distinguished as sinus 1, or to the left hand, this sinus then named sinus 2.

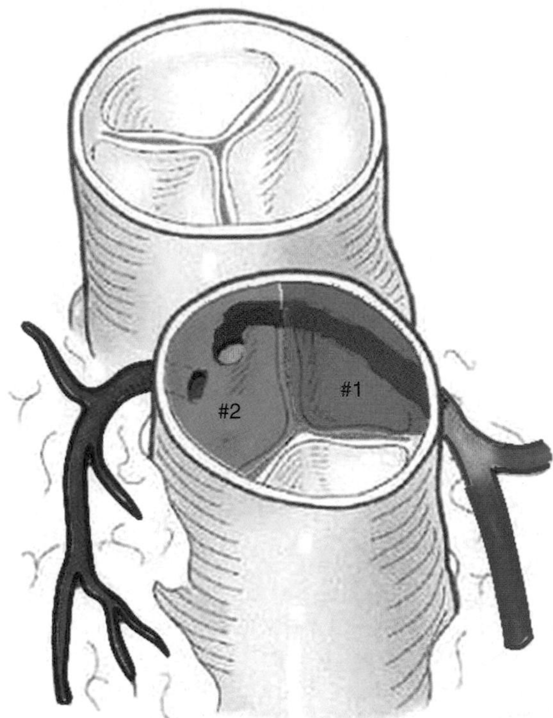

Figure 38-11 The cartoon shows the usual arrangement of the coronary arteries in patients with transposition, found in two-thirds of cases. The right coronary artery (*red*) arises from sinus 2, while the main stem of the left coronary artery (*green*) arises from sinus 1 before branching into the circumflex (*blue*) and anterior interventricular (*purple*) arteries. All variations are described simply by accounting for origin of the three arteries from either sinus 1 (*pink*) or sinus 2 (*yellow*), irrespective of the relationship of the arterial trunks themselves. (Original cartoon prepared by Dr Francois Lacour-Gayet, Children's Hospital, Denver, Colorado, and modified and reproduced with permission.)

anticipated for transposition (Fig. 38-11), abnormalities in origins of the coronary arteries in the past representing one of the major risk factors during the arterial switch procedure.

When considering the sinusal origin of the major coronary arteries, it is also necessary to note their radial, vertical, and tangential origin relative to the sinuses themselves. Most usually, the arteries arise within the sinus or at the level of the sinotubular junction, albeit usually eccentrically placed within the sinus. Significant problems can be created for the surgeon during the arterial switch procedure when the arteries take a high origin above the sinotubular junction, or if they have tangential origin through the aortic wall, crossing the attachments of the valvar leaflets at the junction (Fig. 38-12).

These arrangements are associated with an initial course of the artery running obliquely through the aortic wall, so-called intramural origin.[22] In addition to sinusal origin, epicardial course is also important, in particular retropulmonary or antero-aortic position of any of the three major coronary arteries.[20] The artery to the sinus node is of further significance. It can arise from the initial course of either the right or the circumflex coronary arteries, or it can take a direct origin from one or other of the facing aortic sinuses. Its most important variation, however, is when it crosses the lateral margin of the right atrial appendage (Fig. 38-13). In such lateral position, it is at surgical risk during a standard atriotomy.

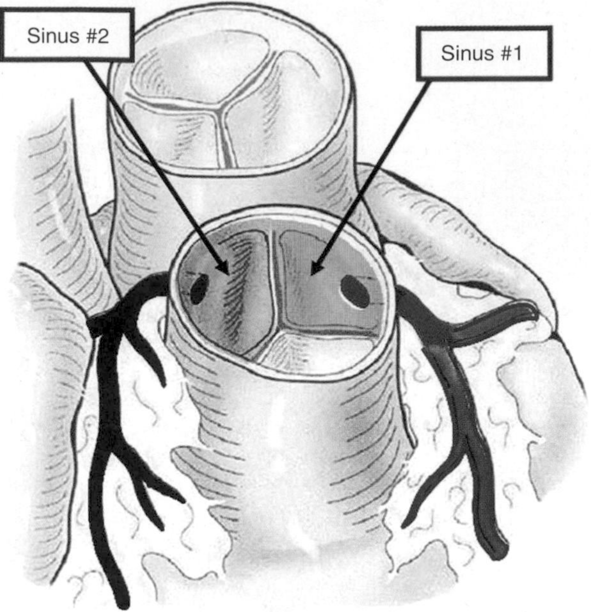

Figure 38-12 The cartoon shows an intramural origin of the left coronary artery (compare with Fig. 38-11). At first sight, the arrangement seems the usual one. Closer inspection shows that the main stem of the left coronary artery extends across the zone of apposition of the aortic valvar leaflets, and takes its origin from sinus 2, which also gives rise to the right coronary artery. Colourings as for Figure 38-11. (Original cartoon prepared by Dr Francois Lacour-Gayet, Children's Hospital, Denver, Colorado, and modified and reproduced with permission.)

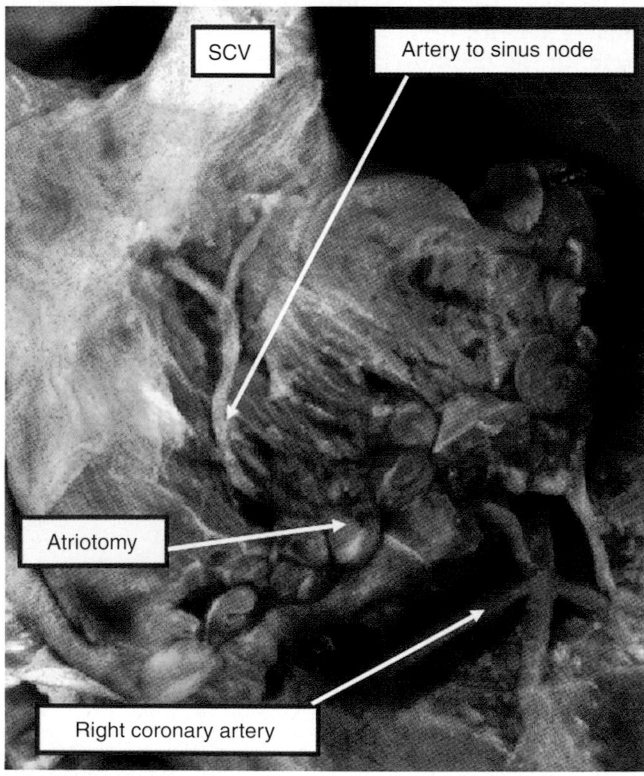

Figure 38-13 In this heart, the artery to the sinus node arises from the right coronary artery, and crosses the atrial appendage to reach the node located in the terminal groove. It was transected by the standard atriotomy. SCV, superior caval vein.

Ventricular Septal Defect

The most significant, and frequently occurring, associated lesion in complete transposition is a ventricular septal defect.[17] As with isolated defects, these may be small, large

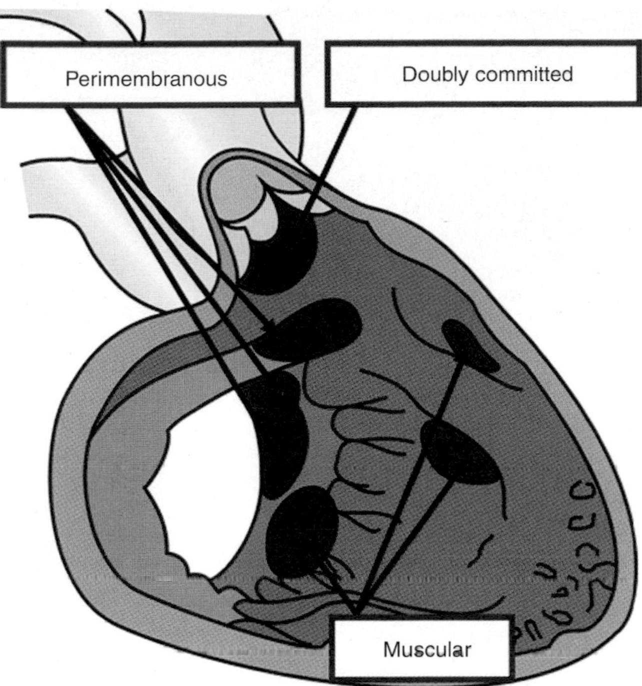

Figure 38-14 As with interventricular communications in the otherwise normal heart, those in patients with transposition can be characterised as being muscular, perimembranous, or doubly committed.

or multiple, and they can be located within any part of the ventricular septum (Fig. 38-14). The most characteristic defects are those that open beneath the ventricular outlets, with the muscular outlet septum being malaligned relative to the rest of the ventricular septum, and located within the right ventricle (Fig. 38-15).

Such defects, which occupy a subpulmonary position when seen from the left ventricle, may have a muscular postero-inferior rim, as shown in Figure 38-15, or may extend to become perimembranous. Frequently, such defects are crossed by the tension apparatus of the tricuspid valve, which often inserts to a papillary muscle arising from the outlet septum. The superior and inferior margins, formed by the outlet and apical components of the muscular septum, diverge towards the parietal wall of the right ventricle. The outlet septum can also be malaligned into the left ventricle. This then narrows the left ventricular outflow tract, producing pulmonary stenosis in association with overriding and biventricular connection of the aortic valve (Fig. 38-16).

In the more common malalignment defects as shown in Figure 38-15, in which the outlet septum is positioned within the right ventricle, it is the pulmonary valve that overrides the septum. With ever greater degrees of overriding, and increasing connection of the leaflets of the pulmonary valve within the right ventricle, a spectrum of anomalies is seen culminating in double outlet from the right ventricle with subpulmonary ventricular septal defect. This whole series is often called the Taussig–Bing complex. We divide the series at its midpoint, including only those with less than half the circumference of the overriding pulmonary valve connected within the right ventricle as examples of discordant ventriculo-arterial connections.

Equally significant from the surgical standpoint are those defects that extend to open to the inlet of the right ventricle. These are hidden beneath the septal leaflet of the tricuspid valve, complicating their surgical repair. When the defect extends to open into the right ventricular inlet, there is the potential for straddling and overriding of the tricuspid valve. In this setting, the muscular ventricular septum no longer extends to the crux, and the atrioventricular conduction axis takes origin from an anomalous postero-inferior atrioventricular node (see Chapter 33).

Apart from in the presence of overriding of the tricuspid valve, the conduction tissue is carried on the left ventricular aspect of the septum, and the postero-caudal rim of the defect is most vulnerable during surgical correction. As with isolated defects, the conduction axis is better protected when the posterior limb of the septomarginal trabeculation fuses with the ventriculo-infundibular fold. Should a muscular defect open to the inlet, however, the axis of conduction tissue will be found in antero-cephalad position.

Other types of defect can be found, such as multiple muscular defects, solitary apical muscular defects, or doubly committed defects roofed by the conjoined leaflets of

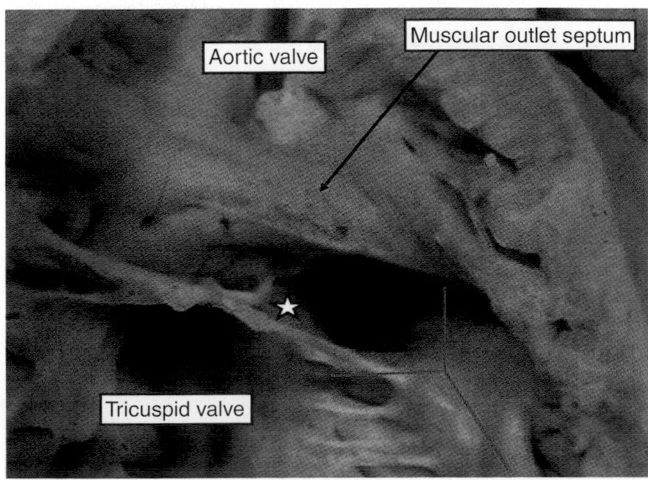

Figure 38-15 There is a malalignment defect between the outlet septum and the septomarginal trabeculation (*yellow Y*). Note the muscular postero-inferior rim to the defect (*star*).

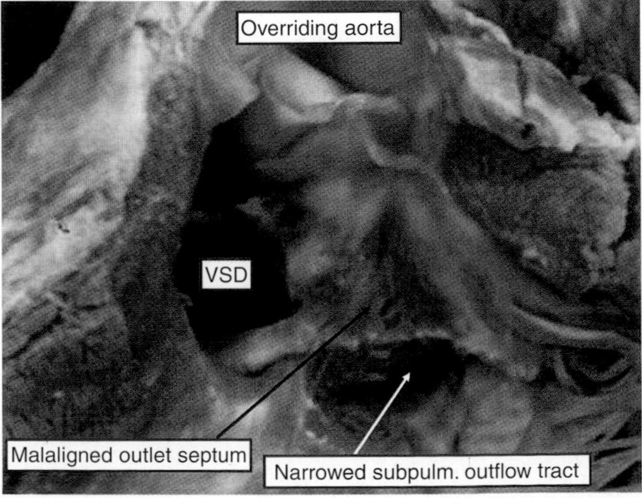

Figure 38-16 In this heart, the outlet septum is malaligned posteriorly into the left ventricle, and obstructs the subpulmonary outflow tract. VSD, ventricular septal defect.

the aortic and pulmonary valves. They are less common. The aorta is also occasionally found posteriorly and to the right in the presence of a ventricular septal defect. With this arrangement, there is usually aortic–mitral valvar continuity through the roof of the defect. Bilateral infundibulums are also seen more frequently in association with a defective ventricular septum, again most frequently when the arterial trunks are side by side. Other anomalies are also more frequent in association with ventricular septal defect, including juxtaposition of the atrial appendages, aortic stenosis, and aortic coarctation.

Obstruction of the Left Ventricular Outflow Tract

Any lesions that produce obstruction to the outflow tract of the morphologically left ventricle, and which in the normal heart produce aortic obstruction, will produce subpulmonary obstruction in the setting of transposition.[17] Such lesions can be found at valvar or subvalvar level (Fig. 38-17).

Isolated valvar obstruction is rare, being more common in combination with subvalvar obstruction, which may be dynamic, fixed or both. Dynamic obstruction is produced by bulging of the ventricular septum. In its most severe form, this is reminiscent of hypertrophic obstructive cardiomyopathy. When septal bulging itself is less severe, obstruction of the left ventricular outflow tract is frequently exacerbated by a fibrous ridge located on the septal bulge. This can progress to form a complete subvalvar shelf, the ridge extending onto the facing surface of the mitral valvar leaflet (Fig. 38-18). The extent of fibrous stenosis can also be more elongated, giving a tunnel lesion. Other rarer forms of stenosis are produced by anomalous attachment of the tension apparatus of the mitral valve across the outflow tract, or by aneurysms of fibrous tissue tags bulging into the outflow tract (Fig. 38-19). All can exist with an intact ventricular septum, or in association with a ventricular septal defect. When there is a septal defect, however, there is another most significant type of stenosis, namely, malalignment and deviation of the muscular outlet septum into the left ventricle that narrows the subpulmonary outflow tract in association with overriding of the aortic valve (see Fig. 38-16). Most of these fixed stenoses present major problems in surgical removal, either because of their own intrinsic morphology, for example a papillary muscle, or because of their proximity to vital structures, such as the left ventricular conduction tissues or the left coronary artery in the transverse sinus. If removal is attempted, the safest area for resection is the area occupied by the muscular outlet septum.

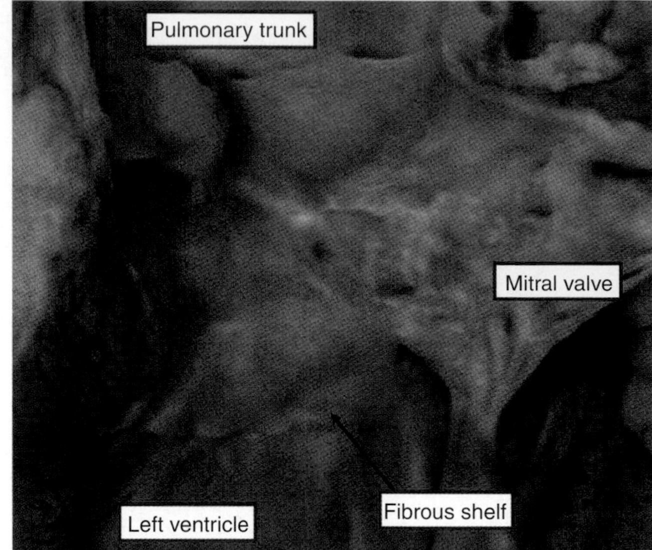

Figure 38-18 In this heart, a fibrous shelf extends from the septum onto the leaflet of the mitral valve. The extent of fibrous stenosis can also be more elongated, giving a tunnel lesion.

Associated Malformations

Other malformations can co-exist either when the ventricular septum is intact, or in association with a ventricular septal defect or obstruction of the left ventricular outflow

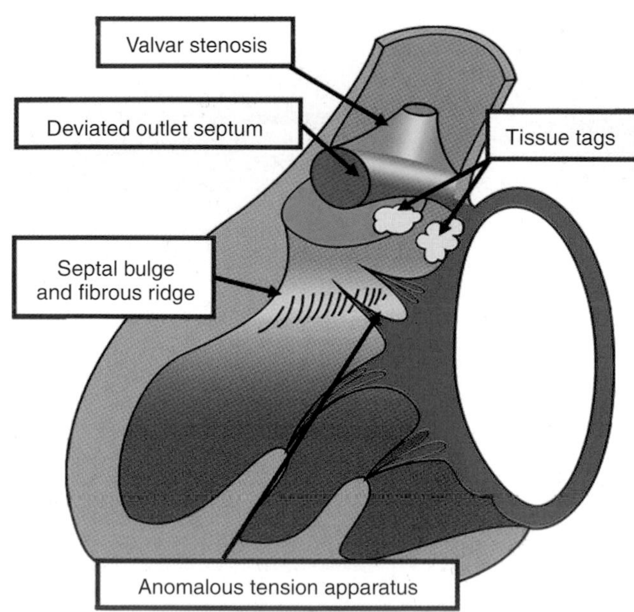

Figure 38-17 The substrates producing subpulmonary stenosis in transposition are the same as those that produce subaortic stenosis when the ventriculo-arterial connections are concordant.

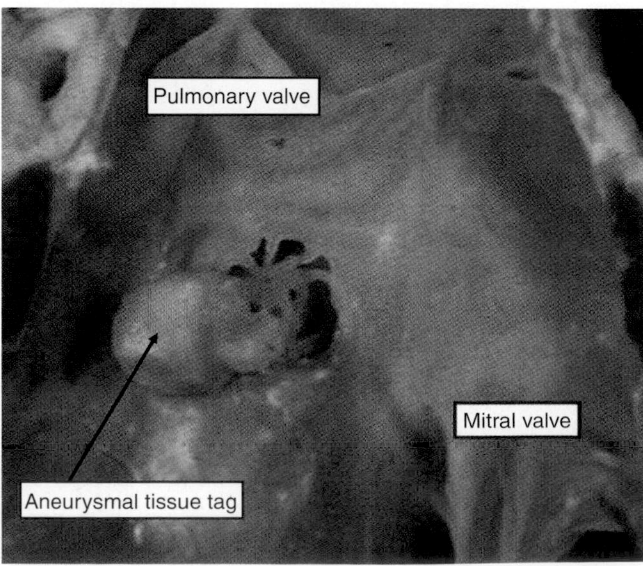

Figure 38-19 A tissue tag originating from the tricuspid valve in the right ventricle has herniated through a co-existing ventricular septal defect to produces subpulmonary obstruction.

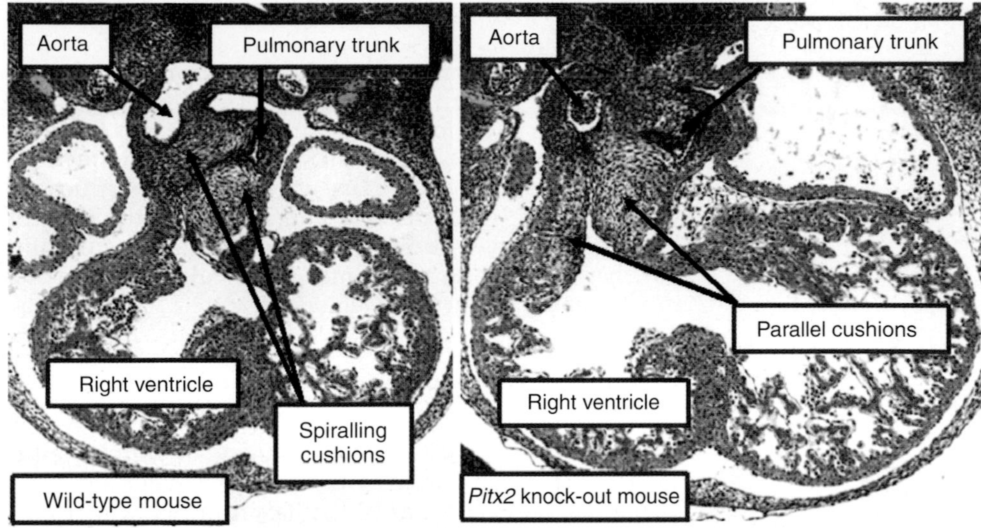

Figure 38-20 These frontal sections are from a wild-type mouse (*left hand panel*) and a *Pitx2* knock-out mouse (*right hand panel*) at comparable stages of development. They illustrate the markedly different orientation of the cushions in the developing outflow tract. The knock-out mice proceed to develop either discordant ventriculo-arterial connections or double outlet right ventricle with subpulmonary interventricular communication. (Courtesy of Professor Nigel Brown, St George's Medical University, London, United Kingdom.)

tract. Persistent patency of the arterial duct is particularly significant because it loads the left ventricle, producing a thicker wall. Other significant anomalies are infrequent, but can occur. They include stenosis of the subaortic outflow tract, aortic coarctation, or anomalous pulmonary venous connections.

Morphogenesis

The morphogenesis of transposition is almost as contentious as the definition itself. There are two basic concepts. The first suggests that the anomaly is the consequence of inappropriate separation of the arterial pole of the heart. As a result, the sixth aortic arches, destined to supply the pulmonary arteries, are connected to the morphologically left ventricle, while the fourth aortic arches take their origin from the morphologically right ventricle, the process occurring because the ridges septating the arterial segment of the heart tube fuse in straight rather than in their normal spiral fashion.[23] The second theory puts the seat of maldevelopment not in the arterial trunks, but in the ventricular outflow tracts. This hypothesis suggests that, rather than the subaortic outflow portion of the right ventricle becoming connected to the left ventricle, as occurs in normal development, it is the subpulmonary outflow component, together with the pulmonary trunk, which is thus connected. This concept was first proposed by Keith,[24] who invoked differential absorption of the infundibular structures as the causative mechanism. The concept was revitalised under the guise of differential conal growth.[3] It now seems that, to explain all the known variants of transposition, including the arrangement in which the aorta arises posteriorly and to the right, it is necessary to invoke maldevelopment within both the outflow tracts and the arterial segment.[25] The elucidation of the various theories will require more detailed studies of experimental animal models, such as the Perlecan knock-out mouse.[26] Initial evidence from other animal models showing discordant ventriculo-arterial connections, such as the *Pitx2* knock-out mouse, do reveal an abnormal location of the outflow cushions during early development (Fig. 38-20).

PATHOPHYSIOLOGY

Circulatory Physiology

The predominant physiological abnormality in transposition is that the systemic venous return is recirculated to the body via the right ventricle and the aorta, whilst the pulmonary venous return is recirculated to the lungs via the left ventricle and pulmonary trunk. Thus, whereas in the normal heart the systemic and pulmonary circulations are in series, in transposition they function as two separate and parallel circuits. In the fetus, this arrangement results in more desaturation of the upper body than is usual, but is not associated with other significant circulatory instability. After birth, the oxygenated pulmonary venous blood does not reach the systemic circuit, and the systemic venous return does not circulate to the lungs. This results in severe systemic arterial desaturation. In the absence of any communication between the pulmonary and systemic circulations, this is incompatible with life.

In infants, early neonatal survival depends upon persistence of the arterial duct, and an interatrial communication. The arterial duct allows blood to flow from the aorta to the pulmonary vascular bed and increases left atrial filling. Patency of the oval foramen, or a native atrial septal defect, permits mixing at atrial level. During this period, the total flow to the lungs is the sum of the effective and the recirculated pulmonary flows. Likewise, the total systemic flow is the sum of the effective and the recirculated systemic flows. A less obvious, but important, consequence of the separation of the two circulations is that the absolute flows in the systemic and pulmonary circuits may differ markedly one from the other (Fig. 38-21).

Determinants of Systemic Arterial Oxygenation and Mixing

When the ventricular septum is intact, the level of systemic arterial saturation is determined by the effective systemic flow, which is proportionate to the degree of circulatory mixing. The dynamics of intercirculatory mixing are complex.

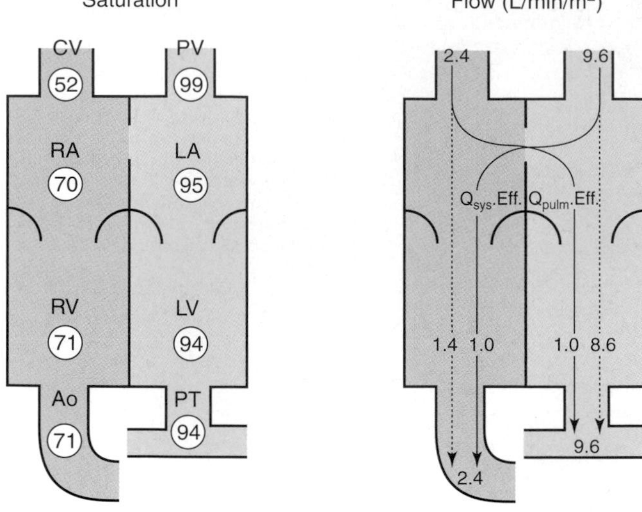

Figure 38-21 Saturations (*left hand panel*) and flows (*right hand panel*) within the heart of a patient with transposition of the great arteries and atrial mixing. Effective pulmonary (Q_{pulm}.Eff.) and systemic (Q_{sys}.Eff.) flows are equal (1 L/min/m²), resulting from the bidirectional shunt at atrial level. However, total systemic (2.4 L/min/m²) and total pulmonary (9.6 L/min/m²) differ considerably such that the pulmonary-to-systemic ratio is 4 to 1. Ao, aorta; CV, caval veins; LA, left atrium; LV, left ventricle; PT, pulmonary trunk; PV, pulmonary veins; RA, right atrium; RV, right ventricle.

The magnitude of the atrial shunt is primarily determined by size of the interatrial communication, the volume and compliance of the atriums and ventricles, and the resistances of the systemic and pulmonary vascular beds. A low-resistance pulmonary circuit combined with a compliant left ventricle results in right-to-left interatrial shunting during ventricular diastole. This leads to increased flow of blood through the left heart to the lungs, which in turn increases pulmonary venous return to the left atrium, and left-to-right interatrial shunting during ventricular systole.[27] Conversely, a poorly compliant left ventricle results in reduced right-to-left shunting during diastole, decreased pulmonary flow, and less left-to-right shunting in systole. As a result, the effective systemic flow is reduced, and the arterial saturation is lower.

At the level of the arterial duct, the direction of shunting largely depends upon the pulmonary vascular resistance, and is also determined by the interatrial communication. If the pulmonary vascular resistance is low, and the interatrial communication is non-restrictive, then the ductal shunt is from aorta to the pulmonary arteries, and predominantly from left to right atrium. If the pulmonary resistance is elevated such that the pulmonary arterial pressure exceeds the pressure in the aorta, then the ductal shunt may be reversed, from the pulmonary arteries to the aorta. This results in an important clinical observation whereby the post-ductal blood is more highly saturated than preductal blood. This life-threatening situation is commonly associated with a restrictive interatrial communication, and requires urgent decompression with an atrial septostomy.

Ventricular Septal Defect

The presence of a ventricular septal defect can have a variable influence on the circulation. This in part depends on the size of the defect, as well as on the presence of interatrial mixing, and the pulmonary vascular resistance. A large interventricular communication may provide good circulatory mixing, but as for infants with concordant ventriculo-arterial connections, the presence of unrestricted flow to the lungs may result in symptomatic heart failure. If surgery is not performed during infancy, then this can predispose to early pulmonary vascular disease, which is generally evident by 6 to 12 months of age.[28-30] The presence of additional pulmonary, or subpulmonary obstruction, modifies these relationships, and may limit the flow of blood to the lungs. These infants are generally asymptomatic, having a protected pulmonary circulation, adequate mixing, and a well-trained left ventricle.

Growth and Development during Fetal Life and Infancy

Most newborns with transposition are of normal birth weight.[31] They have been noted to have smaller occipito-frontal circumferences at birth than controls, which may reflect the abnormal haemodynamics and relative desaturation during fetal development of the blood circulating to the brain and upper body.[32,33] Their growth tends to be restricted in the early post-operative period, but this is followed by an acceleration so that the majority of children have caught up with their unaffected peers by 2 years of age.[34]

CLINICAL DIAGNOSIS

Presentation

The rates of detection prior to birth are variable, and are discussed elsewhere. If made, antenatal diagnosis allows clinicians to assess the full anatomy in detail, with particular attention to the interatrial communication. The clinical team are then able to organise delivery of the infant in a specialist centre, with immediate postnatal initiation of prostaglandins to maintain ductal patency. Moreover, this enables early transfer to a cardiac centre for full assessment and further intervention with a septostomy. Prenatal diagnosis, therefore, facilitates pre-emptive care and offers early therapeutic intervention, with the intention of preventing haemodynamic instability.

Infants without an antenatal diagnosis present with cyanosis, with or without clinical evidence of circulatory insufficiency. The state of the circulation itself depends on the extent of mixing at ductal and intracardiac levels. In the extreme, some infants may present shortly after birth with cyanosis and circulatory collapse, which is most often related to restriction of the interatrial communication. This situation requires definitive management with an urgent balloon atrial septostomy.[35] Infants with a widely patent arterial duct, and a large unrestrictive ventricular septal defect, may present with only minimal cyanosis, but symptomatic pulmonary over-circulation.

Clinical examination during infancy reveals a variable degree of cyanosis, which is unresponsive to inspired oxygen. The adequacy of the peripheral pulses generally reflects the overall circulatory state. Infants with real or pending circulatory collapse will tend to be profoundly desaturated, with globally reduced peripheral perfusion and weak pulses. The presence of pulses in the legs of reduced volume should alert the clinician to an associated coarctation or interruption of the aorta. Cardiac auscultation typically reveals a single second heart sound, and there may also be an audible continuous murmur from the arterial duct, or a systolic murmur related to a ventricular septal defect.

Chest Radiography

The chest radiograph may be unremarkable or abnormal. Cardiac size is often normal, while the pulmonary vascular markings may be reduced, normal, or increased reflecting the volume of flow to the lungs or a restrictive interatrial communication. In around one-third of neonates, the mediastinum is narrow, reflecting the antero-posterior relationship of the arterial trunks.

Electrocardiography

In most newborns, the electrocardiogram is normal. During early infancy prior to surgical intervention, the electrocardiogram may begin to reflect right ventricular hypertrophy, and later demonstrate right-axis deviation. A superior axis in the neonatal period suggests associated abnormalities of the tricuspid valve, particularly straddling or overriding.

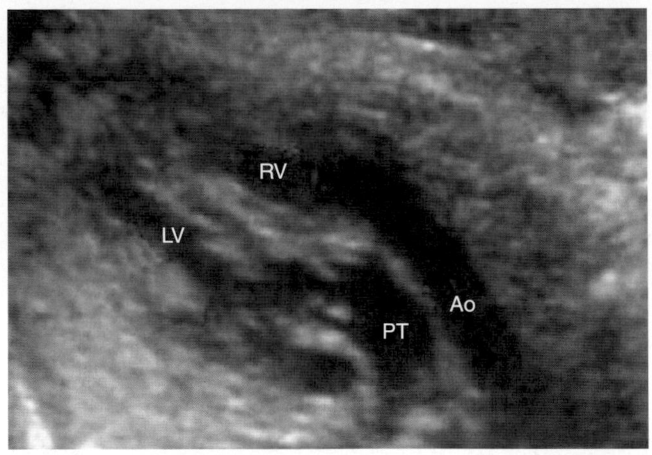

Figure 38-22 Fetal echocardiogram, demonstrating the origin of the aorta (Ao) from the anterior right ventricle (RV) and the pulmonary trunk (PT) from the left ventricle (LV).

Fetal Echocardiography

Significant progress has been made in the screening of fetuses for cardiac malformations.[36,37] The efficacy of fetal screening is based on the premise that high rates of detection will provide opportunities for parental choice, along with optimal neonatal care and pre-operative management. An improvement in mortality and morbidity for neonates diagnosed prenatally as having transposition has already been demonstrated,[35] albeit largely related to improved survival prior to surgical intervention subsequent to antenatal diagnosis rather than to any impact on surgical outcome.[35] Nowadays, the patients at highest risk are those with a restrictive interatrial communication, and prenatal diagnosis does not have an impact on this important factor.

Rates of antenatal detection of transposition are very variable, and clearly suboptimal in some regions.[38] In mothers referred for comprehensive fetal echocardiography performed by specialist sonographers, the lesion can be detected with high levels of accuracy (Fig. 38-22). A systematic segmental approach is recommended, just as for postnatal studies.[39] Regular and detailed assessment of the adequacy of intracardiac mixing, particular at the atrial level, is also useful. Although such restriction at atrial level is a highly specific predictor of the need for emergency neonatal care, its sensitivity is too low to permit detection in all fetuses.[40] Of recent interest is the advent of four-dimensional fetal echocardiography.[41] A particular advantage of this technique may be that it provides an en face view of the four cardiac valves, thus enhancing definition of the spatial relationships of the great arteries and, in turn, the likelihood of abnormal distribution of the coronary arteries.[42]

Postnatal Echocardiography

Echocardiography of the neonate with transposition requires confirmation of the basic diagnosis, along with a full assessment of the cardiac anatomy, including the adequacy of intracardiac and ductal mixing, and the likely ability of the left ventricle to support the systemic circulation. The echocardiographic confirmation requires demonstration of concordant atrioventricular and discordant ventriculo-arterial connections. The diagnosis may be suggested by the parallel relationship of the great vessels, but cannot be based on these alone, as this arrangement is also seen in other congenital cardiac malformations, including

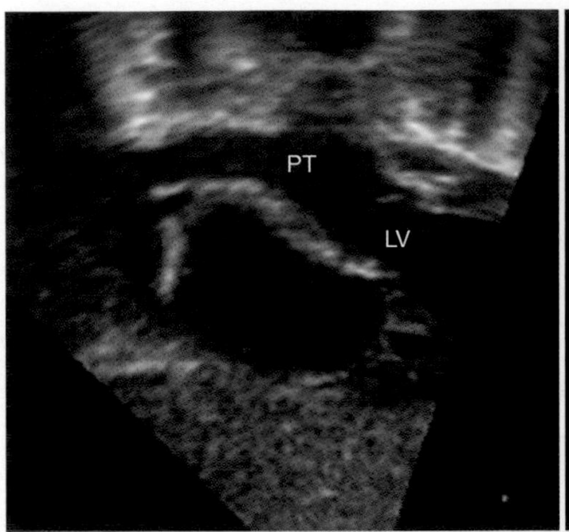

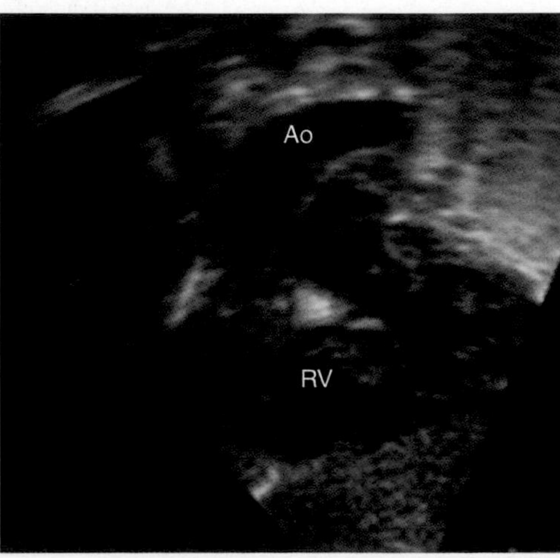

Figure 38-23 Cross sectional images obtained from a subcostal window in a patient with transposition. Anterior angulation demonstrates the bifurcating pulmonary trunk (PT) arising from the left ventricle (LV; *left hand panel*). Further angulation demonstrates the aorta arising from the right ventricle (RV; *right hand panel*). In this patient, the aortic valve is anterior and to the right of the pulmonary valve.

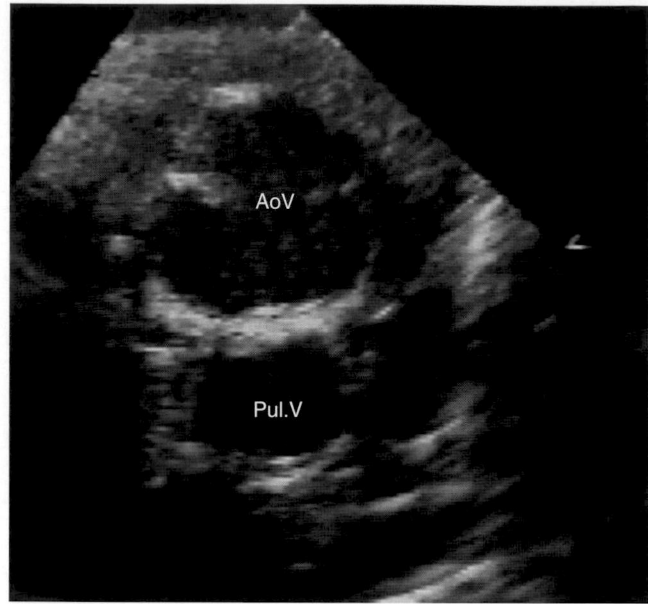

Figure 38-24 Cross sectional image obtained from a high parasternal window, demonstrating the antero-posterior relationship of the aortic (AoV) and pulmonary (Pul.V) valves.

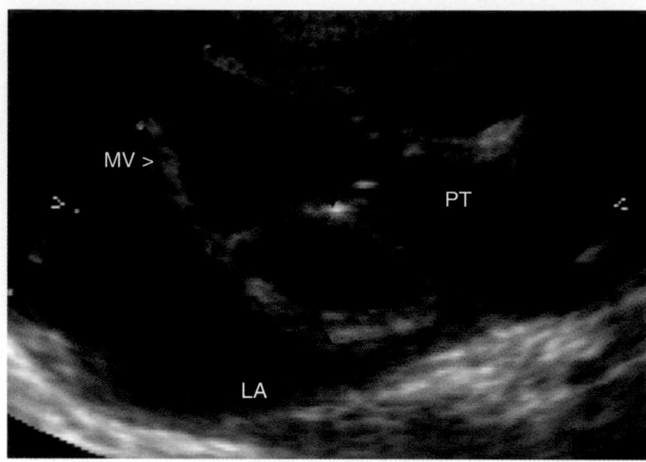

Figure 38-25 Image obtained from a parasternal window in a patient with left juxtaposition of the atrial appendages. The right atrial appendage (outlined by arrows) is seen interposed between the pulmonary trunk (PT) and left atrium (LA). MV, mitral valve.

double outlet right ventricle, or double inlet ventricle with discordant ventriculo-arterial connections.

The atrioventricular connections can readily be determined using subcostal and apical four-chamber cuts. Anterior angulation then confirms the discordant ventriculo-arterial connections. Specifically, the bifurcating pulmonary trunk can be demonstrated originating from the morphologically left ventricle, and the aorta, which is usually anterior, from the morphologically right ventricle (Fig. 38-23). Parasternal imaging reveals the relationships of the arterial trunks. Typically, the aortic valve is positioned anterior and to the right of the pulmonary valve (Fig. 38-24). Parasternal imaging will also reveal the characteristic appearances of juxtaposed atrial appendages (Fig. 38-25).

Additional subxiphoid, apical, and parasternal views, combined with the use of colour Doppler interrogation, should be used to confirm or exclude ventricular septal defects, and demonstrate the direction of associated shunting. The left ventricular outflow tract should always be carefully examined to exclude any obstruction, and the atrioventricular valves should be assessed carefully to identify any abnormal attachments of the tendinous cords. Detailed examination of the pulmonary valve and the sub pulmonary region are an essential part of the pre-operative assessment, as any significant obstruction to the left ventricular outflow may influence surgical management.

Detailed echocardiographic assessment of the origin and course of the coronary arteries should routinely be performed prior to surgical intervention.[43,44] This requires subcostal views of the outflow tract, as well as parasternal short-axis views of the arterial trunks (Fig. 38-26). The aortic arch should always be assessed in detail in order to exclude coarctation or interruption. As it is difficult to exclude coarctation in the presence of a widely patent arterial duct, further echocardiograms should be performed to reassess the arch after prostaglandin is discontinued.

The atrial septum, and flow between the atriums, are best visualised in the subcostal four-chamber view. Deviation of the atrial septum towards the right atrium, with a reduction in the colour flow signal, and increased velocity on pulsed wave Doppler, should immediately suggest the presence of restriction at the interatrial communication. Patency of the arterial duct, and the direction of ductal shunting, should also be confirmed. These features are best visualised from the suprasternal view.

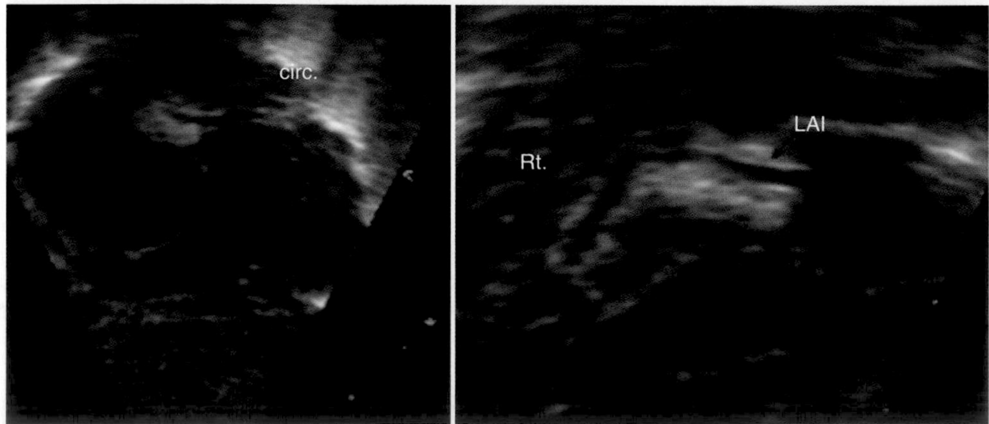

Figure 38-26 Images obtained from a subcostal window demonstrating the coronary arteries. Anterior angulation demonstrates the course of the circumflex artery (circ.; *left hand panel*). Further angulation demonstrates the right (Rt.) and left anterior interventricular arteries (LAI) originating from a common origin.

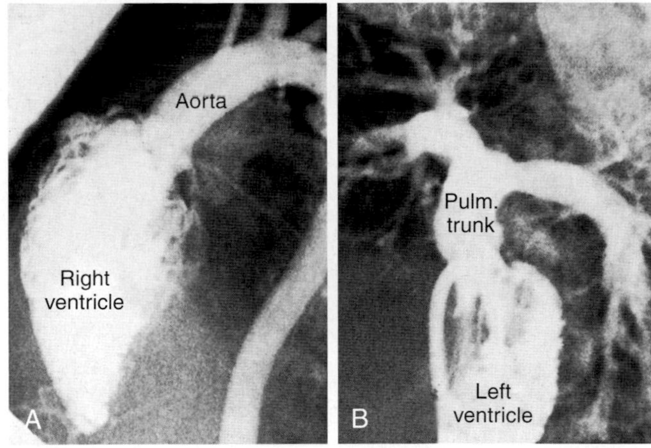

Figure 38-27 Angiocardiograms revealing discordant ventriculoarterial connections in a patient with complete transposition. (Courtesy of Dr B.L. Soto, University of Alabama, Birmingham.)

Cardiac Catheterisation

Cardiac catheterisation is no longer routinely performed; all necessary anatomical information should be obtained from cross sectional echocardiography. There is still an occasional role for cardiac catheterisation in the assessment of the pulmonary vascular resistance (Fig. 38-27) of patients in whom there is a clinical suspicion of pulmonary vascular disease. The course and distribution of the coronary arteries can be demonstrated by angiography, particularly when using the laid-back view,[45] although the important features will usually have been visualised with echocardiography.

Magnetic Resonance Imaging

Pre-operative magnetic resonance imaging may provide useful complementary information in the assessment of the anatomy (Fig. 38-28). It is particularly useful in the assessment of the mass of the left ventricle in the infant presenting late (Fig. 38-29). This may assist involved clinicians in assessing the suitability of an individual patient for an arterial switch operation. Post-operative magnetic resonance imaging after the arterial switch operation provides excellent assessment of the reconstructed arterial trunks (Fig. 38-30), and can also be used to image the origins of the reimplanted coronary arteries (Fig. 38-31). In the patient after an atrial redirection procedure, in whom conversion to an anatomical repair is being contemplated, magnetic resonance imaging can provide detailed assessment of the function of both the systemic morphologically right ventricle and the morphologically left ventricle.[46]

MEDICAL MANAGEMENT OF NEONATES

Postnatal Stabilisation

The most recent report from the Congenital Heart Surgeons Society identified a mortality rate of 2.5% prior to the arterial switch operation.[47] Even higher rates have been described.[35,48] This important pre-operative mortality, in a congenital cardiac malformation which is now associated with excellent post-operative survival, underpins the importance of fetal diagnosis and targeted perinatal care. Neonates diagnosed antenatally should ideally be delivered in a high-risk obstetric unit, with rapid access to cardiac care.[42] Venous access should be obtained immediately after delivery, and an intravenous infusion of prostaglandin E should then be commenced. Patients with severe acidosis or hypoxaemia may require an immediate balloon atrial septostomy.[35] In others, septostomy is generally performed if there is inadequate intracardiac mixing, and significant cyanosis. At our institution, the presence of adequate intracardiac mixing, be it native or after septostomy, is the usual indication to discontinue prostaglandin.

Atrial Septostomy

Following its introduction by Rashkind and Miller in 1966,[49] atrial septostomy has become well accepted in pre-operative management. The procedure requires passage of a balloon-tipped catheter from the right to left atrium, crossing the oval foramen. The balloon is then inflated with saline and, with a quick, short motion, is pulled into the right atrium. While a femoral venous

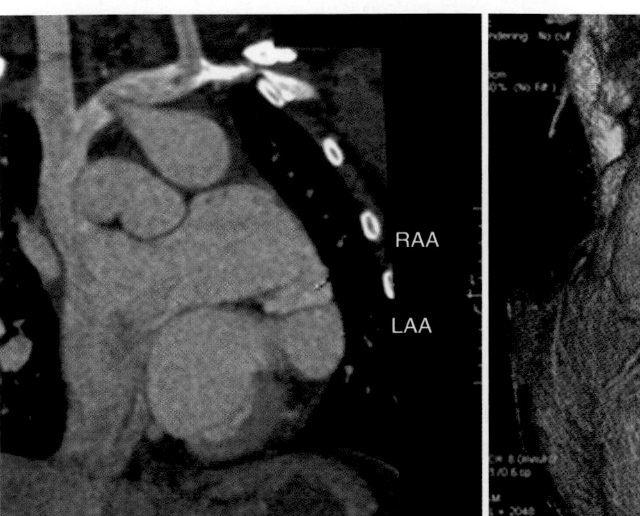

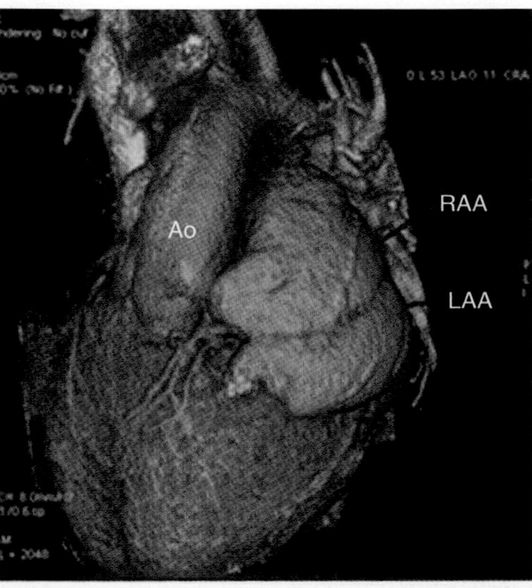

Figure 38-28 Magnetic resonance image in a patient with left juxtaposition of the atrial appendages. The aorta (Ao) can be seen arising from the anterior surface of the heart. The right atrial appendage (RAA) can been seen crossing to the left and is superior to the left appendage (LAA).

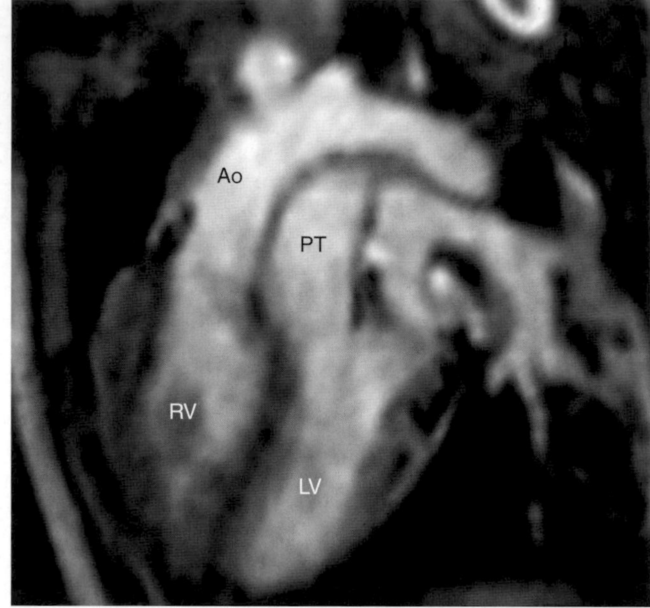

Figure 38-29 Magnetic resonance angiogram in a 9-month-old patient who presented from a developing country with an intact ventricular septum. The aorta (Ao) can been seen arising from the right ventricle (RV) and the pulmonary trunk (PT) from the left ventricle (LV).

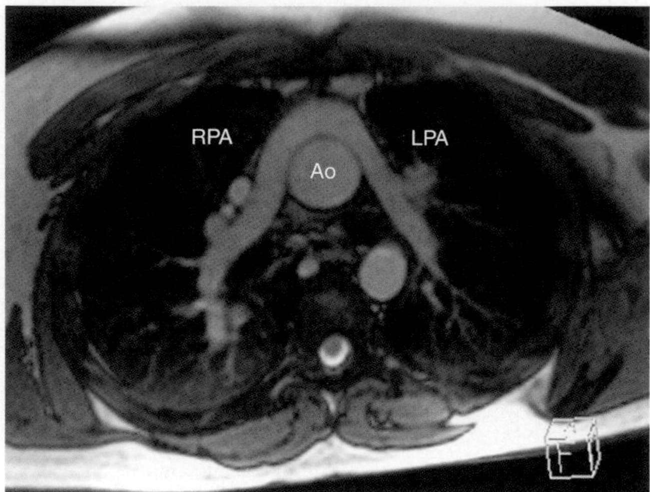

Figure 38-30 Magnetic resonance image from a patient after the arterial switch operation. The relationships between the great vessels can be easily identified. The pulmonary arteries (RPA and LPA) straddle the aorta (Ao), typical of the Lecompte manoeuvre. The pulmonary arteries are widely patent.

approach was routine, it is now common to use the umbilical vein to enter the heart through the venous duct. Fluoroscopic screening was previously used to guide the procedure (Fig. 38-32), but has largely been replaced by cross sectional echocardiography (Fig. 38-33). This provides a simple and reliable method for monitoring the position of the balloon, as well as assessing the success of the septostomy. It also allows the procedure to be performed, if required, on the intensive care unit. Recently, the routine use of septostomy has come under scrutiny following the observation, in one institutional series, of an association between septostomy and abnormal findings on pre-operative cranial magnetic resonance studies.[50] These observations have provoked caution in the application of septostomy although their significance will be a matter for debate and further investigation in the future.

SURGICAL MANAGEMENT

Historical Perspective

Some of the earliest procedures described for prospective surgical treatment were aimed at achieving anatomical correction. Considering the hurdles existing at the time, which included limited pre-operative assessment of ventricular function and imaging of the coronary arteries, inadequate microvascular surgical techniques, and primitive cardiopulmonary bypass circuits, it is hardly surprising that these attempts were uniformly fatal. Furthermore, many babies with poor intracardiac mixing tended to be extremely unwell at the time of surgery. Even with the advent of the palliative surgical atrial septectomy, morbidity and mortality remained significant.[51] The improved survival in infancy after surgical intervention can largely be ascribed to the advent of the balloon atrial septostomy. This relatively simple procedure, which did not require sternotomy or opening of the pericardium, provided rapid circulatory stabilisation, and afforded a relatively uncomplicated period of growth and nutrition prior to definitive surgery.

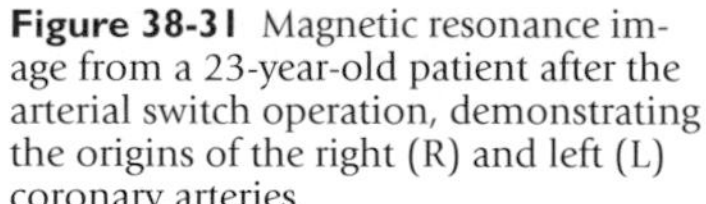

Figure 38-31 Magnetic resonance image from a 23-year-old patient after the arterial switch operation, demonstrating the origins of the right (R) and left (L) coronary arteries.

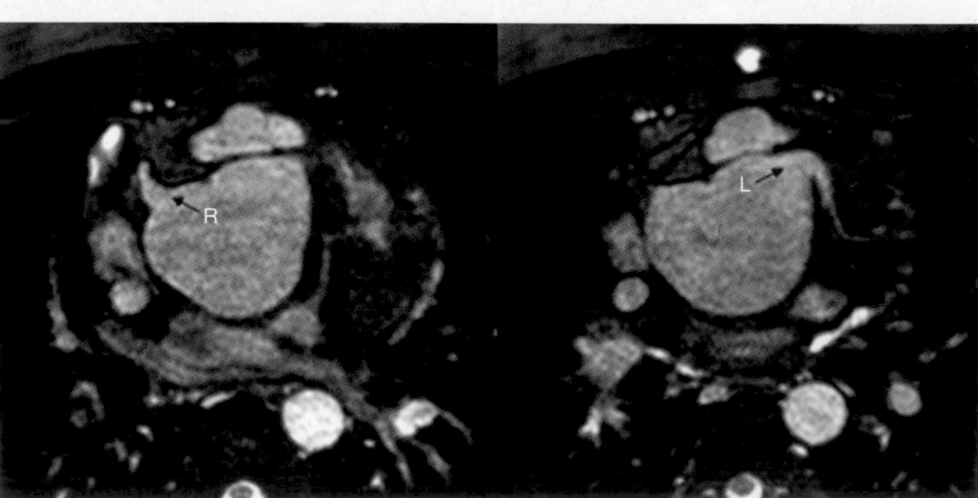

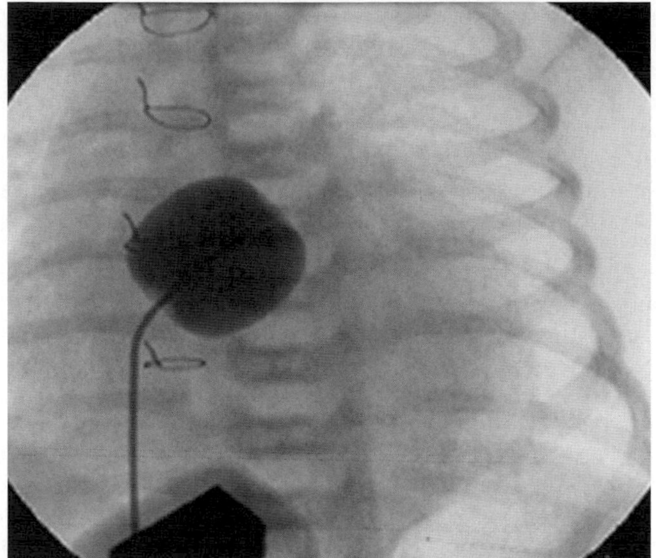

Figure 38-32 Images obtained by fluoroscopy in a patient undergoing an atrial septostomy. While the balloon is clearly visible, its precise relationships with important structures including the mitral valve and the pulmonary veins are difficult to discern.

Atrial Redirection Procedures

The ability to achieve stabilisation of the patient by means of the atrial septostomy before surgery set the scene for important surgical advances in the early 1970s. Atrial redirection surgery, however, provided physiological correction, in contrast to the anatomical correction more recently offered by the arterial switch operation. Nowadays, therefore, the Mustard and Senning procedures are rarely, if ever, performed as primary procedures, and will only be briefly discussed here.[52–55] Their greatest relevance in current practise relates to the significant population of adolescents and young adults that are developing late complications, such as baffle obstruction, arrhythmias, ventricular dysfunction, and end-stage heart failure.

Mustard and Senning Procedures

These procedures involve removal of the atrial septum, and redirection of the systemic venous pathways to the sub pulmonary morphologically left ventricle, and pulmonary venous blood to the systemic morphologically right ventricle. In the Senning operation, the rerouting of systemic venous blood was achieved by means of infolding of the atrial walls, whereas in the Mustard operation this was achieved using synthetic or pericardial tissue. One of the most popular modifications of the Mustard operation involved creation of a trouser-shaped baffle, with the legs anastomosed to the superior and inferior caval venous inflows.[56] By the 1980s, such atrial redirection procedures were associated with early post-operative survival exceeding 95%.[57]

Arterial Switch Operation

An important impediment to the earlier success of anatomical correction was the requirement also to relocate the coronary arteries, which in turn demanded advanced microvascular techniques, unavailable at those times. The advent of coronary arterial surgery in adults in the late 1960s changed the potential scope of surgery for neonates with transposition. Alongside these new techniques in adults, coronary arterial translocation, and hence anatomical correction, became a realistic possibility for affected infants. The first successful arterial switch operation was reported by Jatene and colleagues in 1975,[58] in an older infant with an associated ventricular septal defect. Others around the world quickly followed suit, and within a matter of months there were reports of similar successes.

It became clear rapidly that an important determinant of early outcome was the condition of the morphologically left ventricle prior to surgery, which determined its ability to support the systemic circulation afterwards. Hence the introduction of two-stage repair for patients with a deconditioned left ventricle, with banding of the pulmonary trunk and, if required, placement of a systemic-to-pulmonary arterial shunt. These first-stage procedures trained the left ventricle, permitting the arterial switch itself to be performed some months later.[59]

Another important modification to the arterial switch was then introduced in 1981. This procedure, known as the Lecompte manoeuvre, involved the forward looping of the bifurcation of the pulmonary arteries over the divided aorta, leaving the neo-aorta lying posteriorly. Following the manoeuvre, the pulmonary trunk itself was positioned anteriorly, and could be anastomosed to the original aortic root without creating anatomical distortion.[60] This procedure is

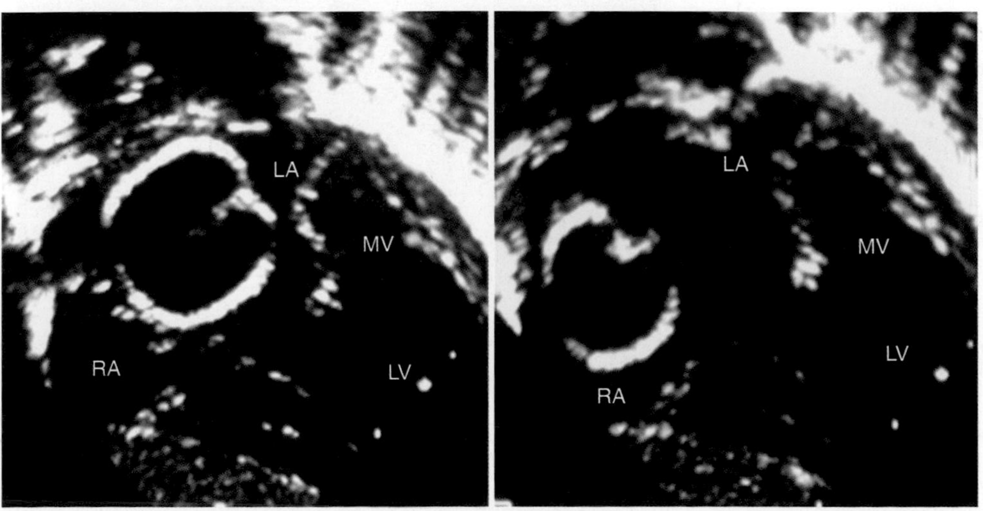

Figure 38-33 Images obtained during an atrial septostomy using echocardiography. The balloon can be seen inflated within the left atrium (LA), and its relationship to the mitral valve (MV) can be seen (*left hand panel*). After the balloon is pulled across the atrial septum, its location in the right atrium (RA) can be seen (*right hand panel*). LV, left ventricle.

still incorporated by most surgeons performing the arterial switch operation. During the first decade of anatomical correction, the pioneers of the arterial switch undertook the operation in infants with associated ventricular septal defects, which were generally beyond the early neonatal period. The first report of successful correction of a neonate with an intact ventricular septum appeared in 1984.[61]

The procedure as currently performed involves the transection of the aorta and the pulmonary trunk. The coronary arteries are then detached from the aorta, along with a cuff of aortic tissue, and transferred to the proximal end of the divided pulmonary trunk, thus forming the new aortic root, or the neoaorta. The defects in the original aortic root left subsequent to detachment of the coronary arteries are repaired with pericardium. The distal end of the divided aorta is then anastomosed to the neo-aorta, thereby connecting the morphologically left ventricle to the systemic circulation. The Lecompte manoeuvre is performed, and the anastomosis of the pulmonary outflow tract is completed (Fig. 38-34).

The arterial switch is now the procedure of choice for almost all neonates. In the current era, the overall mortality is very low, although the early surgical experience demonstrated a significant learning curve.[62] Whereas, in earlier reports, additional anatomical factors, such as a ventricular septal defect, the coronary arterial pattern, or obstruction within the aortic arch, had an impact on mortality, more recent reports have shown that these effects have decreased over time.[63,64]

Timing of the Arterial Switch Operation

In most newborns diagnosed in timely fashion with an intact ventricular septum, the arterial switch is undertaken towards the end of the first week of life. The principal reason for carrying out surgery early in the neonatal period in such infants is to avoid the deconditioning of the morphologically left ventricle. The left ventricular mass begins to regress within a few days of birth, and if this continues, the left ventricle gradually loses its ability to support the systemic circulation subsequent to the arterial switch. Deconditioning may be arrested, or slowed, by the presence of a ventricular septal defect, a large patent arterial duct, or obstruction to the left ventricular outflow tract.

The interval beyond which a primary arterial switch operation cannot safely be undertaken is ill defined. A multi-institutional study carried out by the Congenital Heart Surgeons Society in 1988 suggested that, for neonates with an intact interventricular septum, and without any native pulmonary obstruction, this interval was only 14 days.[65] No more than one decade later, it has been shown that primary repair can be undertaken at up to 2 months of age without increased mortality, irrespective of the pre-operative echocardiographic appearance.[66] In recent years, the arterial switch has been reported in infants at even up to 6 months of age, but this account highlighted the potential need for temporary mechanical support in these patients considered to be at high risk.[67]

While our readiness to perform the arterial switch as a primary procedure beyond the first 2 weeks of life has increased substantially over the past decade, our ability to assess the state of the morphologically left ventricle in the pre-operative setting remains limited. The position of the interventricular septum as determined echocardiographically has traditionally been used to assess the readiness of the left ventricle to support the systemic circulation (Fig. 38-35). The compression of the ventricle to a banana shape, however, was shown not to be predictive of the duration of post-operative ventilation, the subsequent need for extracorporeal support, or mortality in patients undergoing an arterial switch operation at greater than 3 weeks of age.[67] Several quantitative criterions have subsequently been proposed to identify the patient in whom training of the left ventricle may be required, though none appear

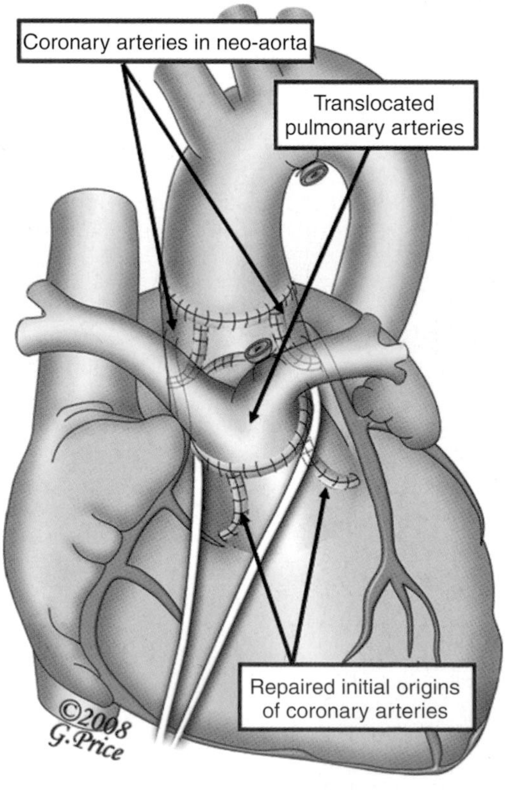

Coronary arteries in neo-aorta
Translocated pulmonary arteries
Repaired initial origins of coronary arteries
©2008 G.Price

Figure 38-34 The cartoon shows the typical postoperative appearance as seen by the surgeon after completion of the arterial switch operation.

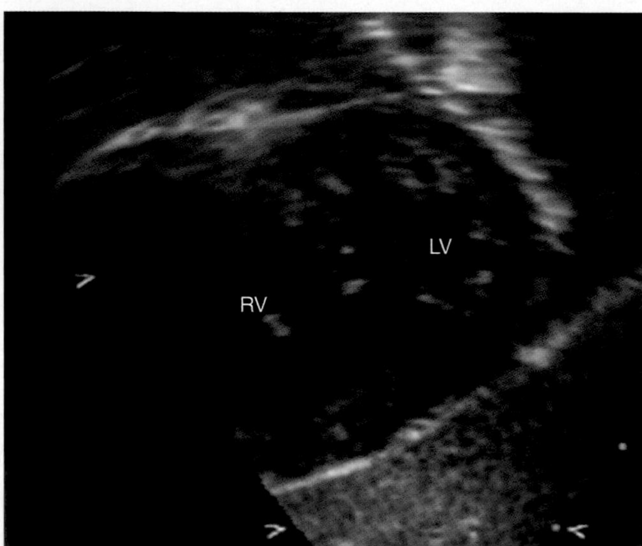

Figure 38-35 Echocardiographic image from a patient with an intact ventricular septum. The ventricular septum can be seen bulging into the left ventricle (LV). The patient was aged 9 months at the time of presentation to a specialist centre. RV, right ventricle.

to be robust. These include a left ventricular end-diastolic volume of less than 90% of predicted, a left ventricular ejection fraction of less than 0.5, a left ventricular mural thickness at end-diastole of less than 4 mm, a predicted left ventricular mural stress of less than 120×10^3 dynes/cm^2,[68] a left ventricular mass of less than 60% of predicted[69] or, when indexed to the surface area of the body, of less than 35 G/m^2.[70]

Ventricular Training

An important determinant of the likely success of the arterial switch operation for an individual patient is the potential for the left ventricle to support the systemic circulation. When first introduced, the two-stage approach involved an interval of between 5 and 8 months between the stages. It has since become clear that the immature ventricle has the capacity for rapid hypertrophy,[71] and adequate preparation can instead be achieved within days. Thus, the group at Boston Children's Hospital developed the rapid two-stage approach, in which the arterial switch itself was performed within one week of banding.[72] This strategy, nonetheless, carries significant risks, including volume overload of the right ventricle secondary to the shunt, and an acute increase in impedance to the left ventricle. Taken together, these may contribute to a significant risk of a ventricular dysfunction, and a state of low cardiac output in the early period after banding.[73,74] In the longer term, abnormal function of the left ventricle, associated with reduced myocardial contractility,[75] and unexplained increases in ventricular volume, have also been observed after the two-stage procedure.[76,77]

Considering the potential hazards of preparatory banding, and the ability of the left ventricle rapidly to become conditioned, our institutional preference for patients deemed to be at high risk is to undertake the arterial switch as the primary procedure, with the elective use of a left ventricular assist device immediately after cardiopulmonary bypass.[78]

Coronary Arterial Anatomy

Almost a decade before the arterial switch became routine, Yacoub and Radley-Smith[18] described their classification of the most common coronary arterial patterns, as well as methods for their transfer. Once the arterial switch had become routine in Melbourne, Brawn and Mee described a variety of techniques for coronary arterial transfer in those patients with more complex arrangements.[79] In an analysis of the outcomes for a large cohort, it was shown that an arrangement in which one or both of the major coronary arteries passed between the arterial trunks was associated with an increased risk of mortality.[80] An extensive multi-institutional analysis undertaken by the Congenital Heart Surgeons Society has been reviewed on a regular basis. Although earlier reviews[65,81] suggested that the arrangement of the coronary arteries did not impact on outcome, in retrospect, the relatively high overall mortality at this time may have masked the subtle contribution of coronary arterial anatomy. In a later analysis,[82] which included more than 500 patients, the anatomy of the coronary arteries was shown to be a risk factor. In this series, there were a number of arrangements which were associated with reduced survival. These included the main stem of the left coronary artery, the left anterior interventricular or the circumflex artery arising from sinus 2, or the presence of an intramural coronary artery. A recent meta-analysis,[83] which included almost 2000 patients, showed that mortality for those with any variant coronary arterial pattern (Fig. 38-36) was almost twice that seen in patients with the usual pattern. In this review, a single origin of the coronary arteries, and intramural patterns, were associated with death.

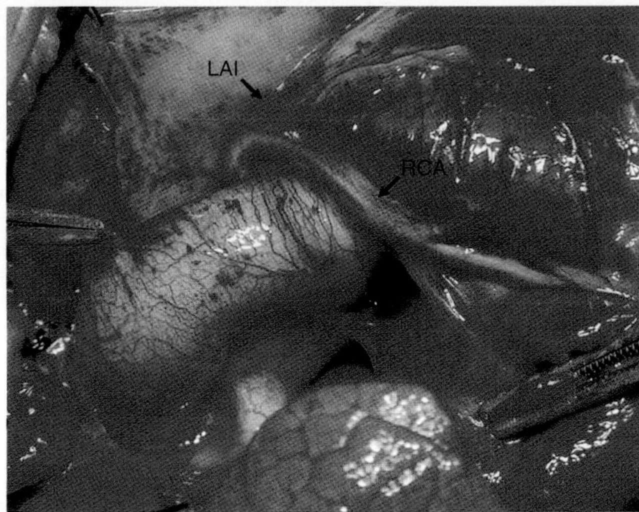

Figure 38-36 Intra-operative image demonstrating an anomaly of the coronary arteries. The right coronary artery (RCA) and left anterior interventricular artery (LAI) can be seen to share a common origin. The right coronary artery sweeps anterior to the arterial pedicle.

Surgery for Complex Transposition

Transposition with a Ventricular Septal Defect

The presence of a ventricular septal defect was previously an important risk factor for increased surgical mortality, although this is less so in the current era. Thus, in a review of European centres, the mortality for the arterial switch in the presence of a ventricular septal defect was found to be 13%, compared to 3% when the ventricular septum was intact. The presence of the interventricular communication was found to be significant on univariate but not on multivariate analysis.[64] Similarly, in a recent review of the experience in Michigan,[63] it was observed that the presence of a ventricular septal defect did not affect the outcome for the arterial switch operation.

Surgery in Infants with Significant Pulmonary Hypertension

Pulmonary vascular disease develops rapidly in the presence of a ventricular septal defect, or when an arterial duct is sufficiently large to cause pulmonary hypertension. When pulmonary vascular disease is established, patients are no longer candidates for corrective surgery. As a guide, a pulmonary vascular resistance of greater than 8 Wood units is considered to indicate unsuitability. If the saturation in the pulmonary arteries is higher than the aorta, an atrial redirection procedure, leaving the interventricular communication open, the so-called palliative atrial redirection, will improve streaming and improve systemic oxygenation. The concept of leaving the interventricular communication open is based on the premise that it will act as a route for decompression of the left ventricle if the pulmonary vascular resistance suddenly rises. Applying the same principles, a palliative arterial switch has been employed.[84] Given the progressive nature of the pulmonary vascular disease, morbidity and mortality remain high.

Transposition with Coarctation of the Aorta or Interruption of the Aortic Arch

Obstruction of the aortic arch is rare when the ventricular septum is intact. It is more common in those with a ventricular septal defect, when it is often associated with anterior deviation of the outlet septum. Thus, the detection of hypoplasia, interruption, or coarctation of the aorta should alert the cardiologist to examine even more carefully the right ventricular outflow tract, the size of the right ventricle, and the tricuspid valve. If the right ventricle or tricuspid valve is small, a conventional repair may not be appropriate. It is generally accepted that a single-stage operation should be performed for repair of transposition associated with obstruction of the aortic arch. Although not the first to describe this as a single operation, Planché and coworkers were the first to demonstrate the superiority of this over a staged approach.[85,86] The surgical technique for the aortic anastomosis does not require significant modification, as the Lecompte manoeuvre generally allows a direct repair of the coarctation with minimal tension on the anastomosis, though augmentation with a patch may occasionally be required.[87] A recent analysis of the arterial switch procedure in European centres did not demonstrate any additional risk of death in patients with an abnormality of the aortic arch.[64]

Surgical Options in the Presence of Obstruction to the Left Ventricular Outflow Tract

Obstruction to left ventricular outflow, or pulmonary obstruction, is most commonly associated with a ventricular septal defect. Minor degrees of obstruction may be resected at the time of the arterial switch itself, and do not necessarily contraindicate this operation. Where the obstruction is severe or complex, it may be more appropriate to consider an alternative procedure. A number of approaches have been described:

Rastelli Procedure

The principle of this procedure is shown in Figure 38-37. It involves patching the interventricular communication so that the output of the left ventricle is directed to the aorta.

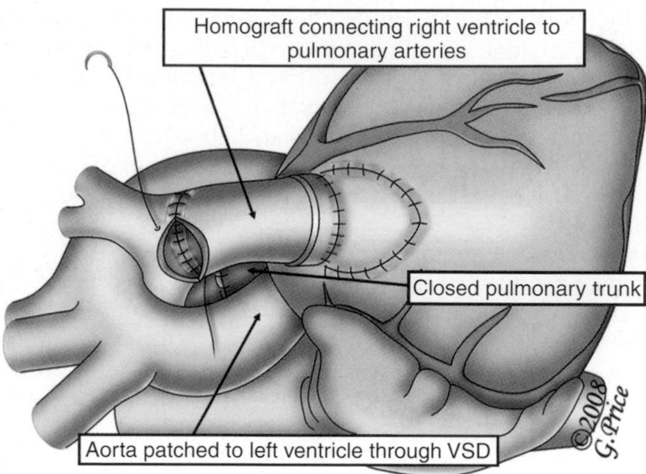

Figure 38-38 The cartoon shows the end result of the Rastelli procedure, with a conduit from the morphologically right ventricle to the pulmonary arteries.

The pulmonary valve is oversewn, the pulmonary trunk divided or ligated, and continuity between the pulmonary artery and the right ventricle is established by a conduit (Fig. 38-38). The main drawback of this procedure is the high likelihood of the need for replacement of the conduit during later childhood.

Réparation à l'Etage Ventriculaire, or REV Procedure

This operation involves extensive resection of the outlet septum, and the use of a patch to baffle oxygenated blood from the left ventricle to the aorta.[88] The Lecompte manoeuvre is then performed, as for the arterial switch, and the pulmonary outflow tract is reconstructed by directly suturing the posterior rim of the pulmonary trunk to a right ventriculotomy (Fig. 38-39). Excellent rates of survival have been reported after the REV procedure, albeit with post-operative obstruction to the right ventricular outflow in one-quarter of patients, possibly related to the anterior location of the pulmonary arteries subsequent to the procedure.[89] To combat this problem, the technique

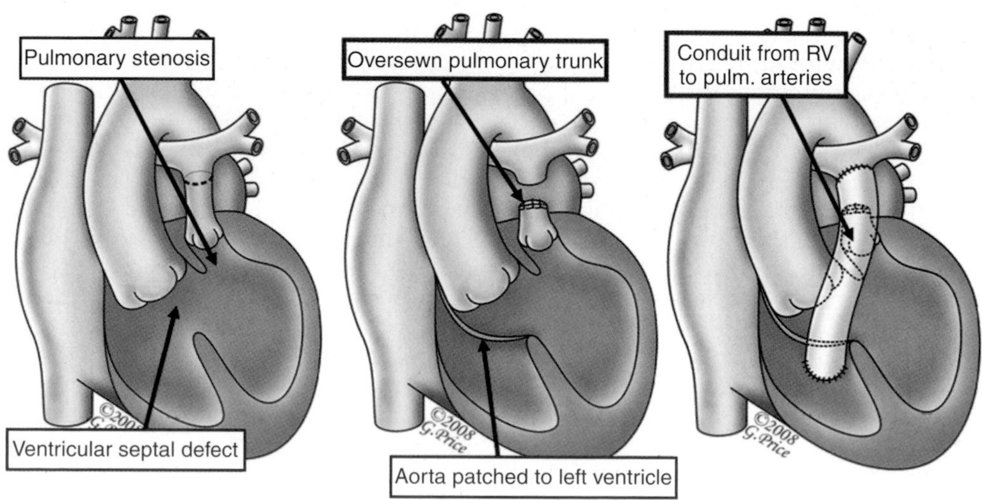

Figure 38-37 The cartoon shows the principles underscoring the Rastelli procedure used for anatomical correction of patients with transposition, a ventricular septal defect, and deviation of the muscular outlet septum (*left hand panel*). A patch is placed to create an intraventricular tunnel (*middle panel*), and an extra cardiac conduit is placed between the right ventricle (RV) and the pulmonary arteries (*right hand panel*). The pulmonary arteries are connected to the right ventricle using a homograft conduit.

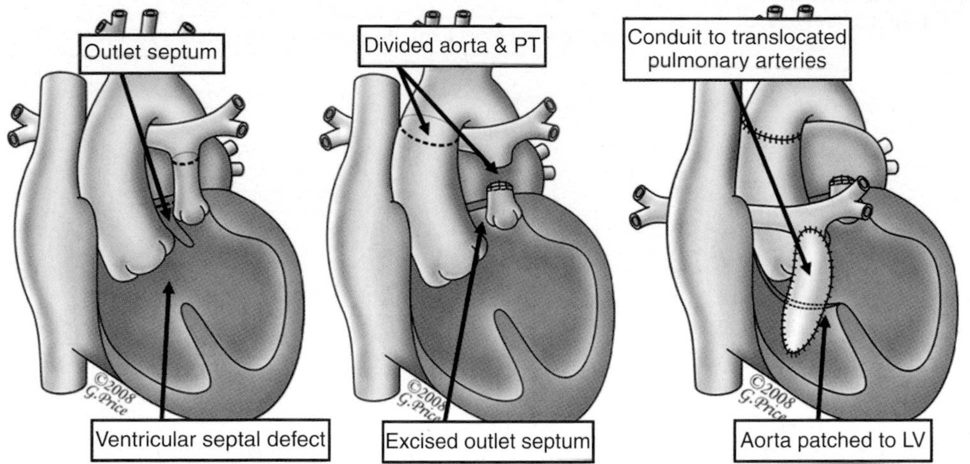

Figure 38-39 This cartoon shows the principles of the REV operation. As with the Rastelli operation, the procedure is employed for correction of patients with a ventricular septal defect and subpulmonary obstruction produced by posterior deviation of the outlet septum (*left hand panel*). The muscular outlet septum is resected and the aorta and the pulmonary trunk are divided (*middle panel*). The left ventricle (LV) is then patched to the aorta through the ventricular septal defect and, using the Lecompte manoeuvre to bring the pulmonary arteries anterior to the newly reconstructed aorta, the distal component of the divided pulmonary trunk (PT) is anastomosed to a right ventriculotomy, the anterior aspect of the pulmonary outflow being restored using a pericardial patch (*right hand panel*).

has been modified using a segment of aortic autograft to reconstruct the right ventricular outflow tract, keeping the pulmonary arteries in their anatomical position posterior to the aorta.[90]

Nikaidoh Procedure, or Aortic Translocation

This procedure represents a very useful technique in patients with obstruction to left ventricular outflow, and offers a sound option to patients with anatomical variants that may render them unsuitable for the Rastelli or REV procedure.[91] This includes patients with a small right ventricle, those with an inlet or restrictive ventricular septal defect, those with straddling or overriding of the atrioventricular valves, and those with a large coronary artery crossing the right ventricular outflow tract. The procedure (Fig. 39-40) involves harvesting the aortic root, along with the attached coronary arteries, from the right ventricle. The stenosed pulmonary valve is excised, and the outlet septum divided. The aortic root is then translocated posteriorly to lie over the left ventricle. The interventricular communication is closed, and the right ventricular outflow tract is reconstructed with pericardium. The pulmonary arteries, remaining posterior to the aorta, are connected to the right ventricle with a homograft. The Lecompte manoeuvre may be required, and sometimes the coronary arteries have to be detached and reimplanted to minimise rotational or longitudinal tension during translocation. The most intuitive advantage of the Nikaidoh over the REV, and particularly the Rastelli, operations, is that systemic outflow is not directed through an intraventricular baffle, and therefore the procedure carries a lower risk of obstruction developing later within the left ventricular outflow tract. Results from this procedure have been promising,[92] although more extended follow-up is needed to assess any potential advantages over other procedures.

SURGICAL OUTCOMES

Atrial Redirection Procedures

The late outcome after atrial redirection is well understood, since the operation has been performed for nearly five decades. Long-term outcome has generally been very good, with survival after 27 years of greater than 90%, nine-tenths of these not requiring reoperation.[93] When needed, the main indications for late surgery were obstruction of the venous baffles, failure of the systemic right ventricle, regurgitation of the tricuspid valve, and acquired obstruction to the left ventricular outflow tract (Fig. 38-41).[93] Obstruction to systemic venous return can be managed with transcatheter or surgical intervention. Balloon dilation tends to provide only temporary relief, whereas transcatheter stenting is more reliable and long-lasting.[94] An alternative option is reoperation, with the aim of either revising the baffle, or more complex surgery with conversion to the arterial switch. Others have reported the need for reoperation in only one-twentieth of almost 500 patients after a mean follow-up of 11.6 years for those undergoing the Mustard operation.[95]

Late dysfunction of the systemic right ventricle is a frequent concern after an atrial redirection procedure, and is commonly associated with regurgitation of the systemic morphologically tricuspid valve. Medical treatment remains empirical, and is based on principles developed for the treatment of patients with left ventricular dysfunction in the setting of myocardial ischaemia. Thus, inhibitors of angiotensin-converting enzyme and β-blockers are commonly used, although data are lacking as to whether they improve either functional state or survival in patients after atrial redirection. The high incidence of ventricular dyssynchrony indicates that some patients may benefit from cardiac resynchronisation.[96] When failure of the morphologically right ventricle is more severe, the only options available may be cardiac transplantation or takedown of the atrial baffle and an arterial switch operation. The latter procedure is usually preceded by banding of the pulmonary trunk, in order to prepare the left ventricle, although patients with co-existing obstruction to the left ventricular outflow may be suitable for a single-stage procedure.

In a series of 39 patients who were entered into a programme for conversion to an anatomical repair at The Royal Children's Hospital, Melbourne, and The Cleveland Clinic Foundation, 4 underwent conversion as a single-stage

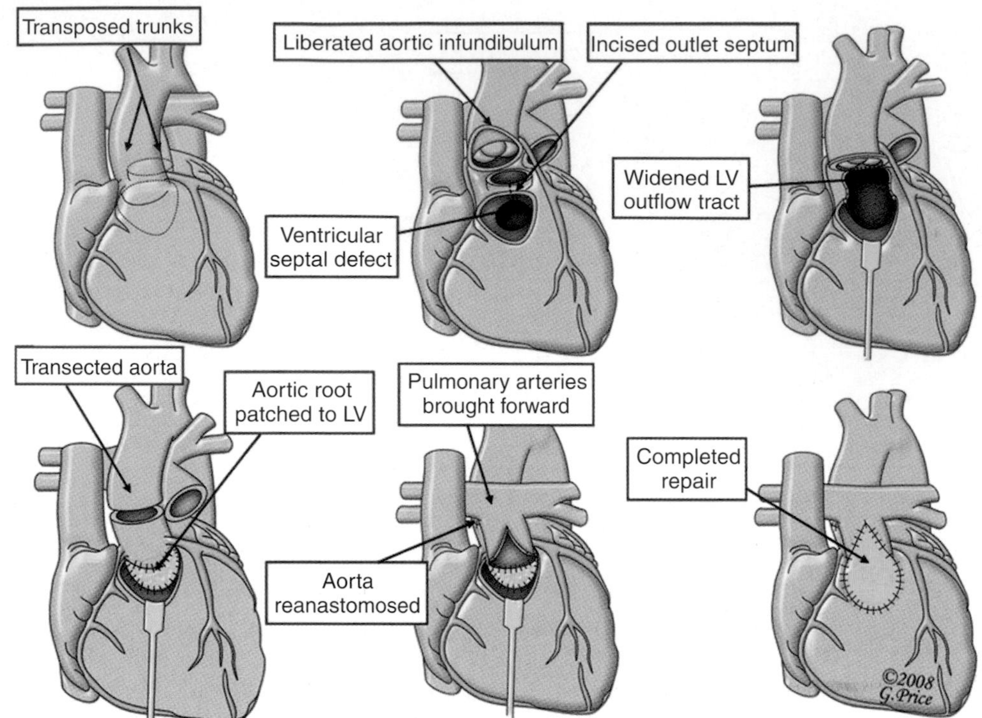

Figure 38-40 The cartoon shows the steps involved in the Nikaidoh procedure. This operation is also used for correction in patients with a ventricular septal defect and obstruction to outflow from the left ventricle into the pulmonary trunk. The upper left hand panel shows the original situation, with the dotted lines showing the incisions for division of the transposed arterial trunks, and the opening to the subaortic infundibulum. The middle panel of the upper row shows how the aortic root is liberated from the right ventricle, taking with it the coronary arteries, and an incision made through the outlet septum into the pulmonary root. The right hand panel of the upper row then shows how the anterior aspect of the pulmonary root is excised to widen the outflow from the left ventricle. The left hand panel of the lower row shows how the aortic root is translocated posteriorly and sutured into the outflow tract from the left ventricle, attaching the root to the ventricular septum with a patch so that the left ventricle ejects into the aorta. The aorta itself is then divided. The middle panel of the lower row shows how the separated pulmonary arteries are translocated between the components of the divided aorta, and the posterior aspect of the pulmonary trunk is attached to the superior aspect of the patch used to close the ventricular septal defect, the aorta having been reanastomosed behind the pulmonary trunk. The right hand panel of the lower row shows how the procedure is then completed by use of a patch to reconstruct the outflow tract from the right ventricle to the pulmonary arteries.

procedure, and 35 underwent preparatory banding of the pulmonary trunk.[97] Of those undergoing banding, three-fifths subsequently underwent anatomical repair, but the other two-fifths did not, as left ventricular training was not achieved. Of those that underwent anatomical repair, almost two-thirds either died or required transplantation. This series highlights the complex decision-making, and difficulty with predicting suitability for definitive surgery, in this high-risk group. In this cohort, banding was associated with an improvement in the severity of tricuspid regurgitation and functional state. This observation supports the concept that banding may be used as a palliative measure, even if conversion to an arterial switch cannot be performed.[98]

Both atrial bradyarrhythmias and tachyarrhythmias are recognised complications of atrial redirection. Dysfunction of the sinus node is common, and is thought to be related to either damage to the sinus node or its blood supply at the time of surgery. Although the criterions for pacemaker insertion are equivocal, most would agree that if a patient is symptomatic, or if monitoring reveals long pauses, severe bradycardia, or tachyarrhythmia in the presence of bradycardia, then a pacemaker is justified, although implantation may be difficult because of the complex anatomy. Atrial tachyarrhythmias, including flutter, may precipitate deteriorations in ventricular function and may indicate an increased risk of sudden death. Antiarrhythmic therapies must be closely monitored because of the risk of atrioventricular block, while radio-frequency ablation may be technically difficult because of the complexities of the anatomy, the presence of the baffle and atrial scarring.

Late Outcome after the Arterial Switch Procedure

General Health, Quality of Life, and Neurodevelopmental Outcome

The majority of children and adolescents who have undergone the arterial switch operation experience good overall health and quality of life that is not significantly different from their peers. Although they may undertake less exercise than controls,[99] their exercise capacity is usually excellent.[100] The intelligence quotient of most children late after the arterial switch operation is within normal limits. More detailed neurodevelopmental and neuropsychological assessment reveals that, while they achieve normal scores in many domains, they frequently perform below expectation in a number of aspects, including academic achievement, fine motor function, visual-spatial skills, and sustained attention.[101,102] It will be important to determine not only which factors contribute to these deficits, but whether they can be alleviated by early neuropsychological interventions.

Fate of the Coronary Arteries

Translocation of the coronary arteries is a critical element of the arterial switch operation, and its success contributes to both early and late survival. In a review of late outcome in more than 1000 patients after the arterial switch operation, coronary arterial problems were reported in almost one-tenth, and these problems contributed to nearly one-third

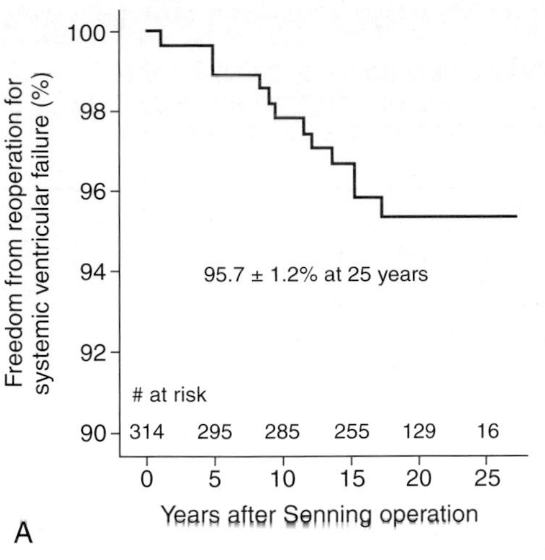

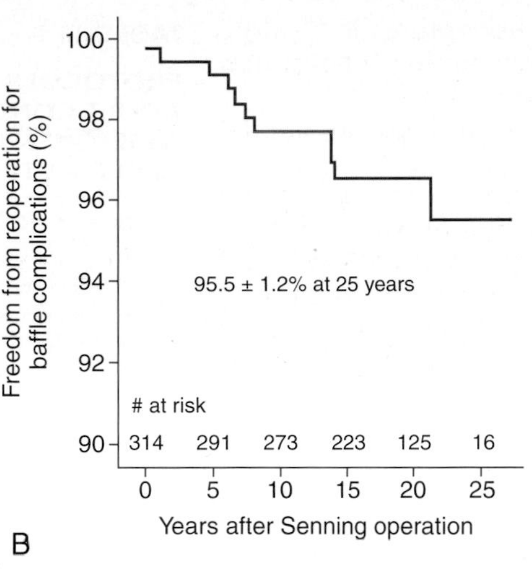

Figure 38-41 Freedom from reoperation for failure of the systemic ventricle (A) and complications related to the baffle (B) for patients after a Senning operation. (From Horer J, Karl E, Theodoratou G, et al: Incidence and results of reoperations following the Senning operation: 27 years of follow-up in 314 patients at a single center. Eur J Cardiothorac Surg 2008;33:1061–1068.)

of late deaths.[103] There are a number of potential mechanisms for late problems after coronary arterial translocation, which include anatomical distortion, extrinsic compression, stretching, and intimal proliferation. There are a number of modalities for the diagnosis and investigation of coronary abnormalities. Currently, direct coronary angiography remains the gold standard investigation, although this can be technically challenging after reimplantation. A number of alternative, or complementary, investigational modalities are now in use. These include myocardial perfusion techniques with technetium and thallium-201[104] and positive emission tomography.[105] Perfusion techniques have demonstrated that coronary arterial reserve may be decreased after the arterial switch, even in the absence of ischaemic symptoms. This concern is borne out by a study which confirmed a low, but significant, rate of coronary arterial occlusion or stenosis in nearly 8% of children at a median of 7 years after surgery. Importantly the

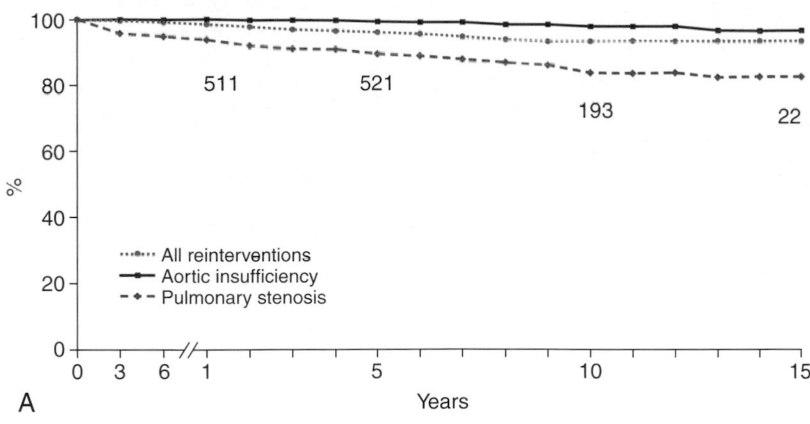

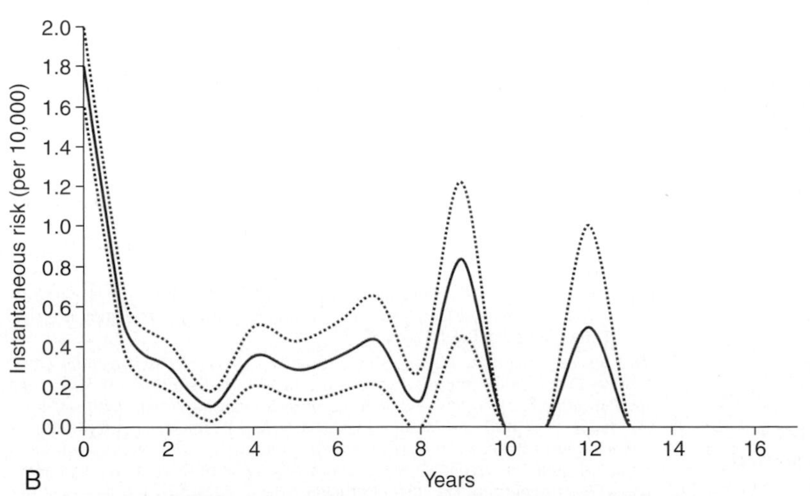

Figure 38-42 Survival free of reoperation for survivors of the arterial switch operation (A) and hazard functions for reoperation (B). Dotted lines indicate 70% CI. (Used with permission from Losay J, Touchot A, Serraf A, et al: Late outcome after arterial switch operation for transposition of the great arteries. Circulation 2001;104[Suppl I]:I-121–I-126.)

majority of these patients were asymptomatic.[106] More recently, coronary arterial lesions requiring intervention were identified in 5% of a cohort of 755 patients.[107]

Innovative methods for detection of coronary arterial abnormalities have recently been reported. Multi-slice computed tomography[108] and magnetic resonance imaging may have a role in detecting ostial and proximal obstruction.[109] Intravascular ultrasound has also been used, and may specifically examine the lumen and intima of the coronary arteries.[110] The exact implications of many of these findings are currently uncertain, but clearly are a potential concern, and reinforce the need for careful follow-up and regular reassessment.

Fate of the Neo-aortic Root and Valve

After the arterial switch operation, the native pulmonary valve must assume the function of the systemic arterial valve. In addition to the general concern that the pulmonary valve is not appropriately structured to fulfill this role, despite its semilunar arrangement, two of its three sinuses will have been incised at the time of original surgery in order to accommodate the coronary arterial buttons. These factors, combined with the recognised complication of dilation of the newly reconstructed aorta, place the patient at risk of neo-aortic incompetence. Such regurgitation across the neo-aortic valve was discovered in two-fifths of patients corrected with the arterial switch procedure after a mean follow-up of 20 months,[111] and after 10 years, only half are likely to be free of regurgitation.[112] Typically, regurgitation is associated with dilation of the ascending aorta, which may, in turn, reflect decreased distensibility and augmented reflection of waves within it, as well as abnormal angulation of the aortic arch after the arterial switch.[113,114]

Pulmonary Arteries

Obstruction within the pulmonary outflow tract is the most frequent residual anatomical problem after the arterial switch operation, and is the most frequent indication for reoperation (Fig. 38-42). The obstruction can occur at multiple levels. Diffuse hypoplasia of the pulmonary trunk commonly results from inadequate mobilisation of the pulmonary arteries, leading to tension on, and flattening of, the reconstructed pulmonary channel. Circumferential narrowing at the anastomotic margins can cause discrete narrowing, while the right or left pulmonary arteries can themselves be stenotic. Such obstruction in the pulmonary outflow tract accounted for more than two-fifths of all reoperations reported in a recent series from Paris.[103] The majority of initial reoperations for pulmonary obstruction are required relatively early, within the first year after the arterial switch operation. This then commonly heralds the need for repeated reintervention.

RECOMMENDATIONS FOR LONG-TERM FOLLOW-UP

Guidelines from both North America and Europe suggest that, after surgery, patients should be followed indefinitely in a specialist centre dealing with adults having congenitally malformed hearts.[115,116] The Canadian Adult Congenital Heart Network recommends regular detailed assessment, as outlined in Table 38-1.[117]

TABLE 38-1

PROTOCOLS DEVELOPED BY THE CANADIAN ADULT CONGENITAL HEART NETWORK FOR THE ASSESSMENT OF ADULTS WITH TRANSPOSED ARTERIAL TRUNKS

All patients should have at a minimum

- A thorough clinical assessment
- An electrocardiogram
- A chest radiograph
- Oximetry at rest and possibly with exercise

Patients who have had an atrial redirection procedure also require

- An echocardiogram to detect baffle obstruction or leak, to detect regurgitation of the atrioventricular valve, to assess the function of the systemic ventricle, and to detect subpulmonary obstruction
- A Holter monitor because of the high prevalence of sick sinus syndrome and atrial arrhythmias and possible ventricular arrhythmias in older patients

and may require

- A transoesophageal echocardiogram if there is inadequate visualisation of the intra-atrial baffle on the transthoracic study
- Radionuclide assessment of myocardial perfusion (if ischaemia is suspected), or of ventricular function
- Magnetic resonance imaging to evaluate the baffle for obstruction or leak and ventricular volumes, shapes, and function
- Cardiac catheterisation including coronary angiography if there are doubts about additional lesions, and if surgical reintervention is planned, or if adequate assessment of the haemodynamics is not obtained by non-invasive means
- Exercise testing to evaluate functional capacity, including heart rate and blood pressure measurement, and to assess whether arrhythmias may be provoked

Patients who have had an arterial switch operation also require

- An echocardiogram to assess obstruction to the right ventricular outflow tract, ventricular function, neo-aortic root dilation, and regurgitation of the aortic valve and the coronary arterial orifices
- Exercise testing for possible coronary ischaemia

and may require

- Holter monitoring if arrhythmia is suspected
- Nuclear assessment of myocardial perfusion periodically
- Coronary arteriography if ischaemia is documented on non-invasive testing
- Cardiac catheterisation if adequate assessment of the haemodynamics is not obtained by non-invasive means or additional lesions are suspected
- Magnetic resonance imaging to exclude obstruction of the right ventricular outflow tract

Modified from Canadian Adult Congenital Heart Network: Complete transposition. Available at: www.cachnet.org.

The complete reference list can be found on the companion Expert Consult web site at www.expertconsult.com.

ANNOTATED REFERENCES

- Anderson RH, Weinberg PM: The clinical anatomy of transposition. Cardiol Young 2005;15(Suppl 1):76–87.

  This review article provides a useful and current review of the clinical anatomy of transposition.

- Jaggers JJ, Cameron DE, Herlong JR, Ungerleider RM: Congenital Heart Surgery Nomenclature and Database Project: Transposition of the great arteries. Ann Thorac Surg 2000;69:S205–S235.

  This report summarises the attempts by members of The STS-Congenital Heart Surgery Database Committee and representatives from the European Association for Cardiothoracic Surgery to establish a unified reporting system with respect to the diagnosis of transposition of the great arteries. A number of categories were defined, which included: transposition with intact ventricular septum, transposition with ventricular septal defect, and transposition with ventricular septal defect and left ventricular outflow tract obstruction.

- Soongswang J, Adatia I, Newman C, et al: Mortality in potential arterial switch candidates with transposition of the great arteries. J Am Coll Cardiol 1998;32:753–757.
- Bonnet D, Coltri A, Butera G, et al: Detection of transposition of the great arteries in fetuses reduces neonatal morbidity and mortality. Circulation 1999;99:916–918.
- Jouannic J-M, Gavard L, Fermont L, et al: Sensitivity and specificity of prenatal features of physiological shunts to predict neonatal clinical status in transposition of the great arteries. Circulation 2004;110:1743–1746.

  These three articles highlight the important pre-operative morbidity and mortality in neonates with transposition and examine the extent to which antenatal diagnosis can predict and prevent these problems.
- McQuillen PS, Hamrick SE, Perez MJ, et al: Balloon atrial septostomy is associated with preoperative stroke in neonates with transposition of the great arteries. Circulation 2006;113:280–285.

  This important article initiated the discussion of the potential problems with the almost routine use of atrial septostomy in neonates with transposition. It will be a source for considerable debate and study in the years ahead.
- Kang N, de Leval MR, Elliott M, et al: Extending the boundaries of the primary arterial switch operation in patients with transposition of the great arteries and intact ventricular septum. Circulation 2004;110(11 Suppl 1): II123–II127.

  This important article provides an excellent consideration of the issues related to the limits of the arterial switch operation in patients who present late to specialist centres.
- Bull C, Yates R, Sarkar D, et al: Scientific, ethical and logistical considerations in introducing a new operation: A retrospective cohort study from paediatric cardiac surgery. BMJ 2000;320:1168–1173.

  This article is compulsory reading for all practitioners in a developing specialty. While specifically related to the introduction of the arterial switch problems, it highlights some of the ethical and logistical issues related to the introduction of any innovative treatment in medicine or surgery.
- Horer J, Karl E, Theodoratou G, et al: Incidence and results of reoperations following the Senning operation: 27 years of follow-up in 314 patients at a single center. Eur J Cardiothorac Surg 2008;33:1061–1068.

  This important article provides an excellent analysis of the long-term medical and surgical problems facing patients after the Senning operation.
- Qamar, ZA, Goldberg CS, Devaney EJ, et al: Current risk factors and outcomes for the arterial switch operation. Ann Thorac Surg 2007;84:871–878.
- Losay J, Touchot A, Serraf A, et al: Late outcome after arterial switch operation for transposition of the great arteries. Circulation 2001;104 (Suppl I): I-121–I-126.

  These two articles provide excellent discussions of the medium-term surgical and medical issues in patients after the arterial switch operation.
- Hovels-Gurich HH, Segahaye MC, Schnitker R, et al: Long-term neurodevelopmental outcomes in school-aged children after neonatal arterial switch operation. J Thorac Cardiovasc Surg 2002;124:448–458.
- Bellinger DC, Wypij D, duPlessis AJ, et al: Neurodevelopmental status at eight years in children with dextro-transposition of the great arteries: The Boston Circulatory Arrest Trial. J Thorac Cardiovasc Surg 2003;126:1385–1396.

  These articles provide an excellent reminder that, while the majority of children after the arterial switch operation have an excellent quality of life and outcome, a significant proportion demonstrate neurodevelopmental deficiencies. These articles will act as a stimulus for more detailed assessment of outcome and follow-up, as well as intervention studies.

CHAPTER 39

Congenitally Corrected Transposition

WILLIAM J. BRAWN, TIMOTHY J.J. JONES, ROBERT H. ANDERSON, and DAVID J. BARRON

The essence of congenitally corrected transposition is the presence of discordant connections at both atrioventricular and ventriculo-arterial junctions. This segmental combination, like transposition itself (see Chapter 38), can be found in patients with either usual or mirror-imaged atrial arrangement (Fig. 39-1), but not in the presence of isomeric atrial appendages. Strictly speaking, congenitally correct transposition exists only when the ventriculo-arterial connections are also discordant. Discordant connections across the atrioventricular junctions, nonetheless, can also be found with double outlet from either ventricle, usually the morphologically right, with pulmonary or aortic atresia, and rarely with concordant ventriculo-arterial connections. These entities, therefore, are close cousins of the main malformation, and we will discuss their diagnosis and treatment in this chapter. The combination of discordant atrioventricular with concordant ventriculo-arterial connections, of course, produces the clinical picture of transposition, since the circulations are corrected only when there is double discordance. Even with double discordance, however, the purportedly corrected pattern of the circulation is usually perturbed by the associated anomalies, of which an interventricular communication, obstruction of the outflow tract from the morphologically left ventricle, and abnormalities of the morphologically tricuspid valve are sufficiently frequent to be considered part and parcel of the malformation.[1,2] The other complication occurring with sufficient frequency to be considered as almost part of the malformation is problems with the atrioventricular conduction axis.[3] We will discuss all of these anatomical combinations, emphasising their clinical significance.

ANATOMY AND MORPHOGENESIS

Basic Morphology

As far as we are aware, the lesion was first described by the Baron Von Rokitansky.[4] It was with great prescience that he provided an exquisite illustration of the morphology as seen by the echocardiographer cutting the heart in the short axis of the ventricular mass (Fig. 39-2). When the atrial chambers are in their usual position, which is typically the situation, with only about one-tenth of all cases exhibiting mirror-imaged atrial arrangement, then by virtue of the discordant atrioventricular connections, the right-sided morphologically right atrium is connected to the right-sided morphologically left ventricle through a mitral valve, while the left atrium is joined to the left-sided morphologically right ventricle through a tricuspid valve. When the ventricular septum is intact, there is reversed off-setting of the septal attachments of the leaflets of the atrioventricular valves (Fig. 39-3). The morphologically left ventricle then gives rise to the pulmonary trunk, and almost always

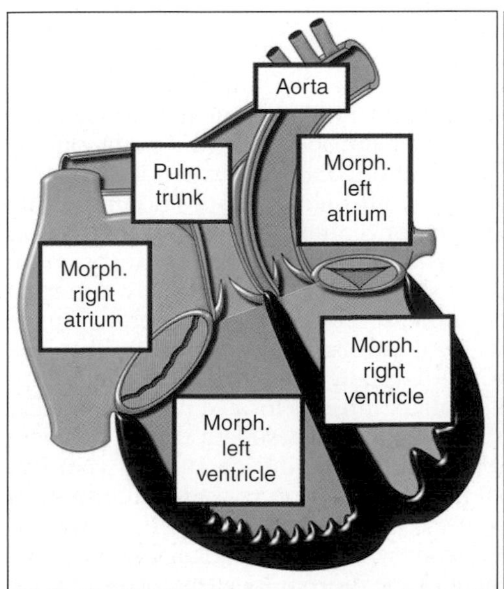

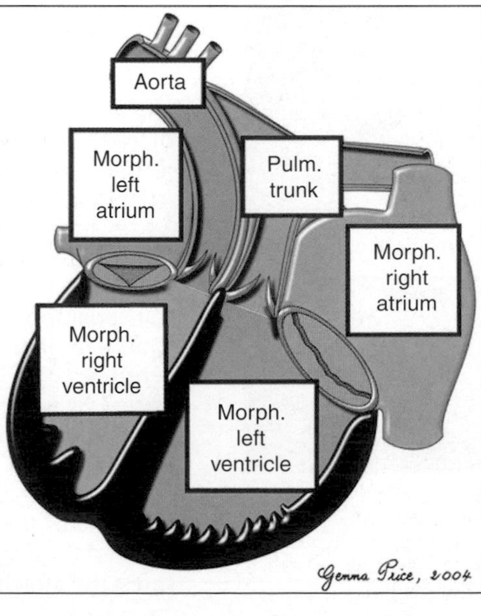

Figure 39-1 Congenitally corrected transposition is the combination of discordant connections at both the atrioventricular and ventriculo-arterial junctions, and hence produces double discordance. It can exist in either usual (*left*) or mirror-imaged (*right*) arrangement, but not in patients with isomeric atrial appendages. Morph., morphologically; Pulm., pulmonary.

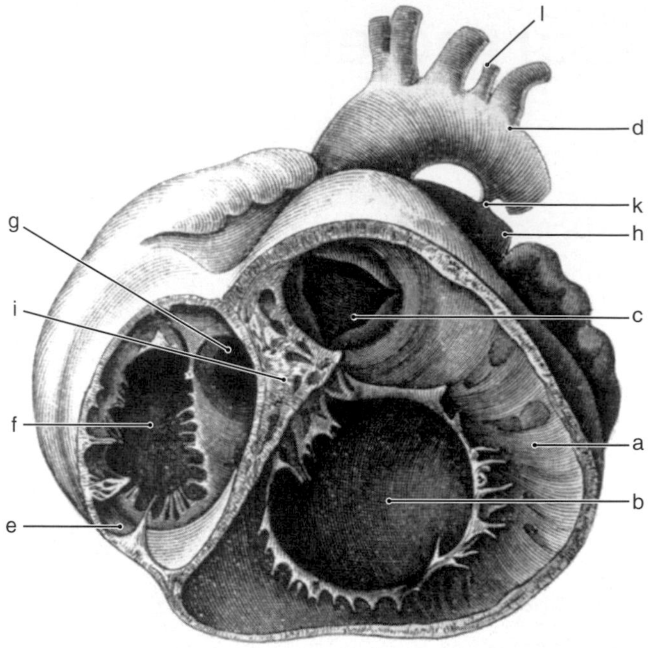

Figure 39-2 This illustration from the atlas of the Baron von Rokitansky[4] shows the short axis of the ventricular mass viewed from the ventricular aspect in a specimen with congenitally corrected transposition with usual atrial arrangement. Note the fibrous continuity between the leaflets of the right-sided mitral (f) and pulmonary (g) valves, and the muscular infundibulum supporting the leaflets of the left-sided and anterior aortic valve (c).

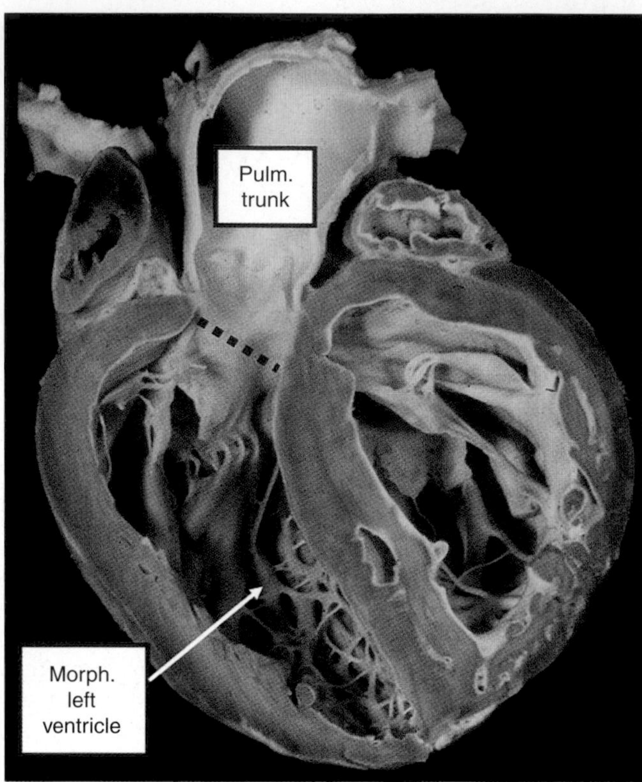

Figure 39-4 A section taken slightly anterior and superior to the one shown in Figure 39-3 reveals the outflow tract from the right-sided morphologically left ventricle, which gives rise to the pulmonary trunk. Note the fibrous continuity between the leaflets of the pulmonary and mitral valves (*dotted red line*), and note how the outflow tract is wedged between the mitral valve and the septum. Morph., morphologically; Pulm., pulmonary.

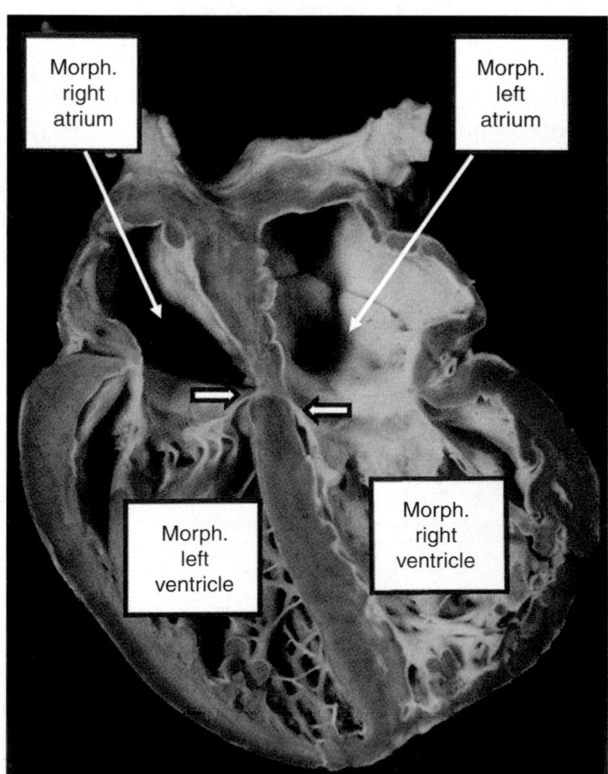

Figure 39-3 This four-chamber section through a heart with congenitally corrected transposition and usual atrial arrangement shows the discordant atrioventricular connections. Note the reversed off-setting, albeit minimal, of the septal attachments of the atrioventricular valves (*arrows*) in this specimen with an intact ventricular septum. Morph., morphologically.

there is fibrous continuity between the leaflets of the pulmonary and mitral valves (Fig. 39-4). The wedging of the pulmonary valve between the septum and the mitral valve deviates the atrial septum away from the ventricular septum, this having crucial significance for the disposition of the atrioventricular conduction axis.[4] The morphologically right ventricle, receiving the pulmonary venous return, empties into the aorta, which almost always in those with usual atrial arrangement is supported by a complete muscular infundibulum, the aortic valve typically being anterior and to the left relative to the pulmonary trunk (Figs. 39-5 and 39-6).

In a small proportion of hearts from patients with usually arranged atriums, and with the segmental arrangement of congenitally corrected transposition, the aorta can be found in right-sided position, or directly anterior to the pulmonary trunk. Anterior and right-sided positioning of the aorta is the rule when congenitally corrected transposition is found in the mirror-imaged arrangement. L-transposition, therefore, is not the same thing as congenitally corrected transposition, the more so since left-sided aortas can be found in patients with regular transposition. Within the ventricles, the morphologically mitral valve is usually supported by paired papillary muscles located in infero-medial and supero-lateral positions. The supero-lateral papillary muscle is potentially vulnerable during surgical ventriculotomy, albeit that in most instances nowadays the surgeon approaches the ventricles either through an atrioventricular or arterial valve. In hearts with intact ventricular septal structures, the attachment of the morphologically tricuspid valve

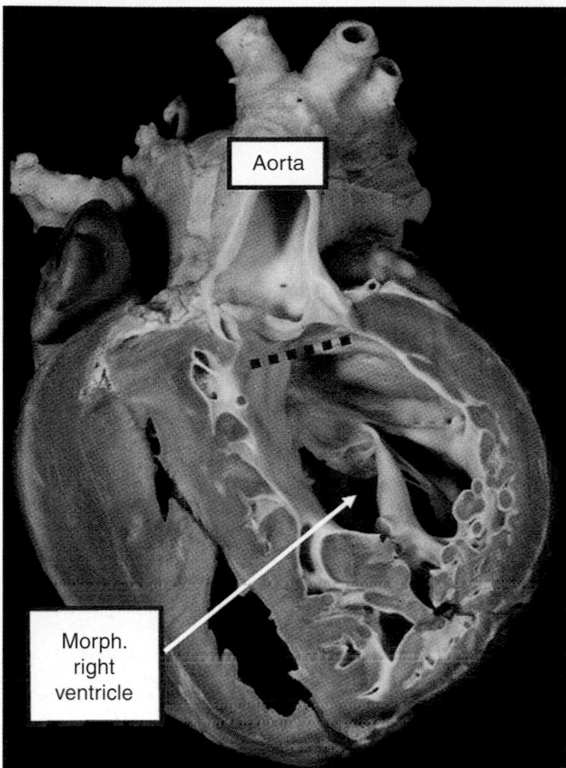

Figure 39-5 A third section through the heart illustrated in Figures 39-3 and 39-4, taken still further anteriorly and superiorly, shows the origin of the aorta from the left-sided morphologically right ventricle. Note the complete muscular infundibulum supporting the leaflets of the aortic valve (*red dotted line*). Morph., morphologically.

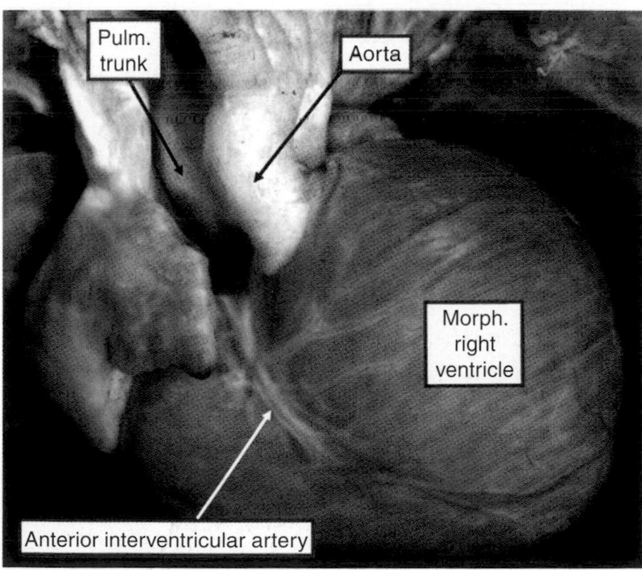

Figure 39-6 In most instances when congenitally corrected transposition is found with usual atrial arrangement, the aorta, as in this heart, is positioned anteriorly and to the left relative to the pulmonary trunk. Morph., morphologically; Pulm., pulmonary.

to the extensive membranous septum creates an interventricular part, as in hearts with concordant atrioventricular connections, along with an atrioventricular portion. Unlike the normal situation, the atrioventricular part of the membranous septum separates the morphologically left atrium from the morphologically left ventricle, the latter chamber being right-sided in the setting of usual atrial arrangement. There is also a prominent recess seen antero-superiorly within the morphologically left ventricle. This was a useful feature for recognition of the abnormality in the days when diagnosis depended on angiography.

In the past, it was frequently the practise to describe the ventricles as being inverted in the setting of usual atrial arrangement. In that they are not upside down, this is a less than accurate description of the ventricular arrangement. In terms of topology, nonetheless, the ventricular mass is the mirror image of the usual arrangement, exhibiting a left hand pattern when the atrial appendages are usually arranged, but showing right hand topology when the atrial chambers are mirror-imaged. Even with right hand topology, the ventricular mass is not the same as is seen in the normal heart, nor does the left hand topological arrangement show perfect mirror-imagery of the normal arrangement. This is largely due to the fact that the outflow tracts are parallel to each other, rather than crossing, as in the normal situation. The ventricles, therefore, tend to be side by side, often with an added supero-inferior obliquity. It is also possible to find rotational abnormalities. It is marked abnormal rotation that produces the additional malformations known as criss-cross relationships,[5,6] while excessive tilting produces supero-inferior ventricles.[6] In addition to the ventricles occupying a side-by-side relationship, it is also frequent for the entire ventricular mass to be abnormally located within the thorax, and for the apex of the ventricular mass to point in unexpected directions. Finding the heart abnormally positioned, therefore, or an unusual orientation of the apex should always raise the suspicion of the congenitally corrected transposition.

As is always the case, the coronary arteries originate from the two aortic sinuses which are adjacent to the pulmonary trunk. It is usually the case that the right coronary artery arises from one of the adjacent sinuses, and the main stem of the left coronary artery from the other adjacent sinus, but sometimes both of the arteries arise from one or the other sinus, often with the arteries having a common stem.[7] Their precise position relative to the heart will vary according to the precise position of the aortic root, but the specific arrangement is well described by taking note of their origin from either sinus #1 or #2 (Fig. 39-7). Origin of all three main coronary arteries from one or the other sinus is a frequent finding, often with the arteries having a common stem. The epicardial distribution of the arteries is reasonably constant, and is determined by the ventricular topology. Thus, in persons with atrial chambers in their expected position, the overall pattern is mirror-imaged relative to the arrangement seen in the normal heart. The right-sided coronary artery exhibits the pattern of a morphologically left coronary artery, with its short main stem dividing into anterior interventricular and circumflex branches (Fig. 39-8). The circumflex artery encircles the mitral orifice, which is right-sided when there is usual atrial arrangement. The position of the anterior interventricular artery is an excellent guide to the location of the ventricular septum. The left-sided coronary artery in the setting of usual atrial arrangement is a morphologically right coronary artery. It gives off infundibular and marginal branches while encircling the left-sided tricuspid orifice. In most instances, the inferior interventricular branch arises

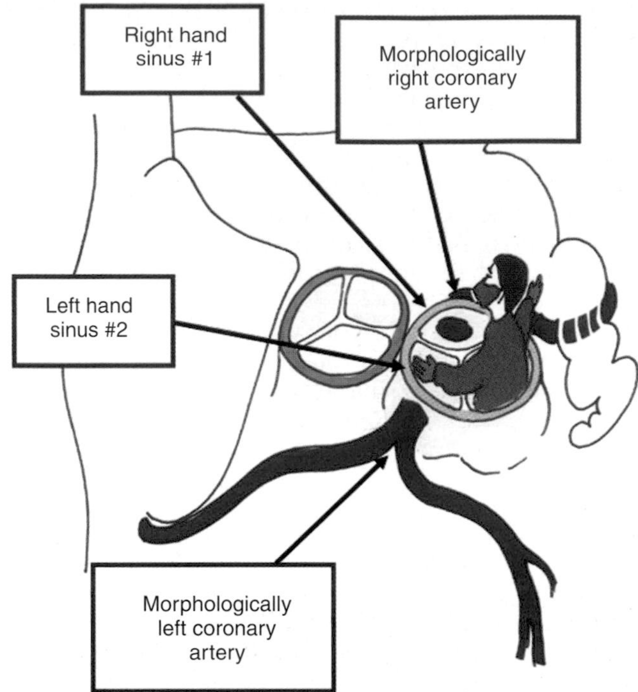

Figure 39-7 As is the case for regular transposition, sinusal origin of the coronary arteries is best described by accounting for the origin of the arteries from either the right-handed sinus (#1) or the left-handed sinus (#2) as viewed by the observer standing in the non-adjacent aortic sinus and looking towards the pulmonary trunk. In most instances with usual atrial arrangement, as shown in the cartoon, it is the left-sided morphologically right coronary artery that arises from sinus #1, and the main stem of the morphologically left coronary artery from sinus #2.

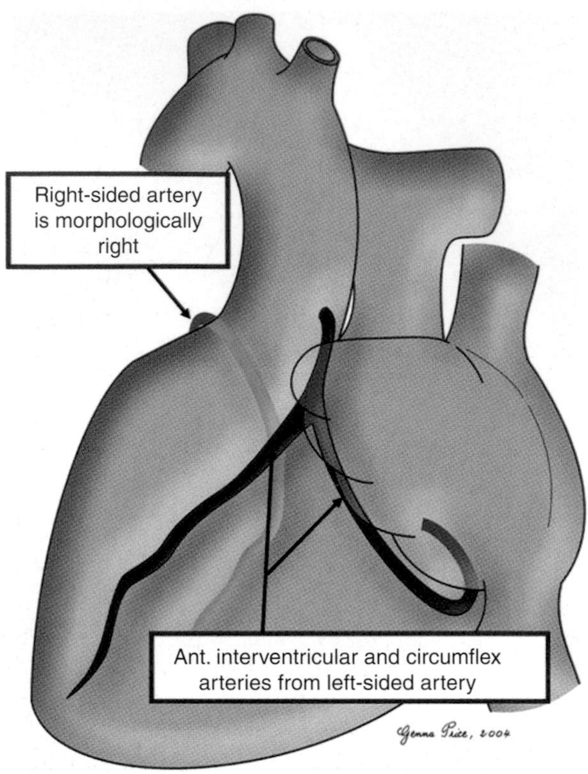

Figure 39-9 When congenitally corrected transposition is found in the mirror-imaged variant, then the ventricular topology is almost always of right hand pattern. The epicardial arrangement of the coronary arteries, therefore, is anticipated for the normal heart. Ant., anterior.

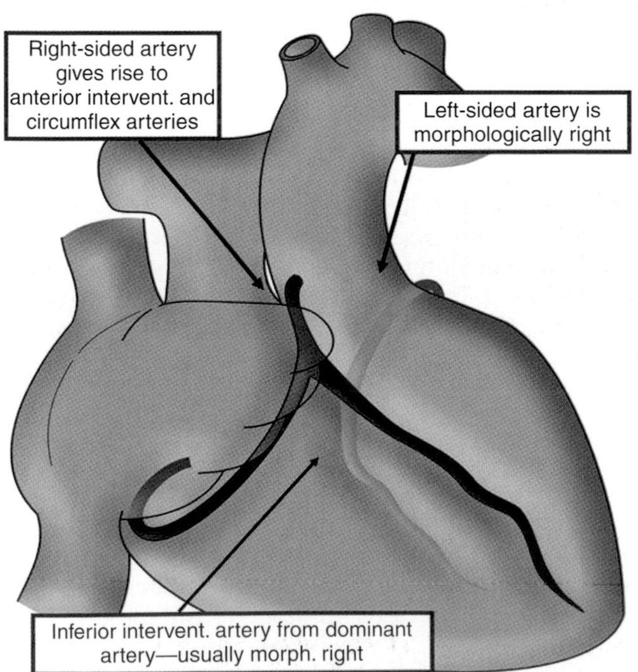

Figure 39-8 The cartoon shows the usual arrangement of the coronary arteries in the setting of usual atrial arrangement, the arterial pattern dictated by the left hand ventricular topology almost always found in this setting. intervent., interventricular morph., morphologically.

from this artery. These relationships are all mirror-imaged when the atrial chambers themselves are mirror-imaged, since this arrangement is associated with right hand ventricular topology so as to produce congenitally corrected transposition. The epicardial pattern of the coronary arteries, therefore, resembles that expected for the normal heart (Fig. 39-9).

As we have already emphasised, because of the wedged position of the subpulmonary outflow tract in the morphologically left ventricle, there is gross malalignment between the atrial septum and the inlet part of the ventricular septum (Fig. 39-10). When the septal structures are intact, the septal aspect of the malalignment gap is filled by the extensive membranous septum. Not surprisingly, deficiency of this structure is common, producing a perimembranous ventricular septal defect. Because of the gross septal malalignment, it is impossible for the penetrating atrioventricular bundle to take its origin from the regular atrioventricular node, located at the apex of the triangle of Koch in the base of the atrial septum. Instead, the atrioventricular conduction axis originates from a second anomalously located atrioventricular node, located beneath the opening of the right atrial appendage at the lateral margin of the area of pulmonary-to-mitral valvar fibrous continuity (Fig. 39-11). The atrioventricular conduction axis, having penetrated through the fibrous trigone, comes to lie immediately underneath the pulmonary valvar leaflets. An extensive non-branching bundle then runs superficially underneath the right anterior facing leaflet of the pulmonary valve, descends for some distance down the anterior septal surface of the subpulmonary outflow tract,

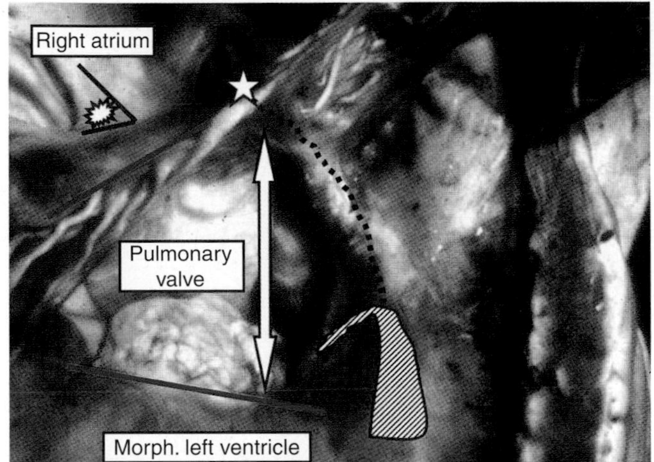

Figure 39-10 In this heart with congenitally corrected transposition, the ventricular septum was intact. The image, taken from the apex of the right-sided morphologically (morph.) left ventricle, shows the malalignment gap (*double-headed arrow*) between the planes of the atrial septum (*green line*) and the ventricular septum (*blue line*). Because of the malalignment, the regular atrioventricular node at the apex of the triangle of Koch (*squiggly symbol*) is unable to make contact with the ventricular conduction axis (*red cross-hatched area*). Instead, the connecting bundle (*red dotted line*) runs antero-cephalad to the pulmonary valve, having taken origin from an anterior atrioventricular node (*star*).

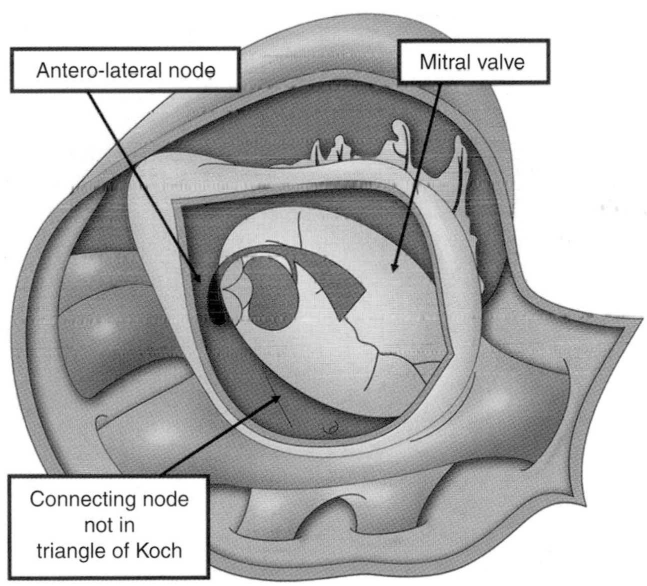

Figure 39-11 The cartoon shows the location of the atrioventricular node as found most frequently in congenitally corrected transposition with usual atrial arrangement as seen by the surgeon looking through an incision in the morphologically right atrium. In the situation illustrated, we have shown a co-existing ventricular septal defect. Note that the conduction axis runs antero-cephalad relative to the defect (see Fig. 39-12).

and branches into a cord-like right bundle branch, which extends leftwards to reach the morphologically right ventricle, and a fan-like left bundle branch, which cascades down the smooth left ventricular septal surface.

The precise anatomy of the atrioventricular conduction axis has far-reaching surgical significance in the presence of associated malformations. The close relationship between the non-branching bundle and the pulmonary valvar orifice complicates both closure of ventricular septal defects and relief of obstruction within the morphologically left ventricular outflow tract. Thus, in patients with perimembranous ventricular septal defects, the bundle has a grossly abnormal position when compared to the regular position of the conduction axis in hearts with ventricular septal defects in the setting of concordant atrioventricular connections. When viewed by the surgeon, it is to the right hand side (Fig. 39-12) rather than to the left hand side as anticipated in a heart with normal junctional anatomy.

In hearts with less malalignment between the atrial and ventricular septums, the regular node may be positioned so as to make contact posteriorly with the ventricular septum. This is produced by such lesions as double outlet from the right ventricle[8] and severe pulmonary stenosis or atresia.[9] In the past, it was often stated that the frequent origin of the conduction axis from a regular node in the setting of mirror-imaged atrial arrangement was because of the right-handed ventricular topology. As was shown by Hosseinpour and colleagues,[9] all cases described with this pattern had better septal alignment because of the presence of severe pulmonary stenosis or pulmonary atresia. Thus, the same rules apply for prediction of the location of the conduction axis in congenitally corrected transposition irrespective of whether there is usual or mirror-imaged atrial arrangement. The key is the extent of septal malalignment. When there is good septal alignment, then both the regular and the anterior nodes can give rise to penetrating bundles, both of which can join with the branching bundle. Should there be a ventricular septal defect, which is usually the case, this can produce a sling of conduction tissues, as initially described by Monkeberg.[10] The vulnerable position of the long non-branching bundle almost certainly explains why heart block remains a frequent complication after surgical closure of associated malformations. Atrioventricular dissociation, nonetheless, may sometimes be present at birth. More frequently, there is progressive acquired atrioventricular dissociation, often culminating in complete heart block.[4]

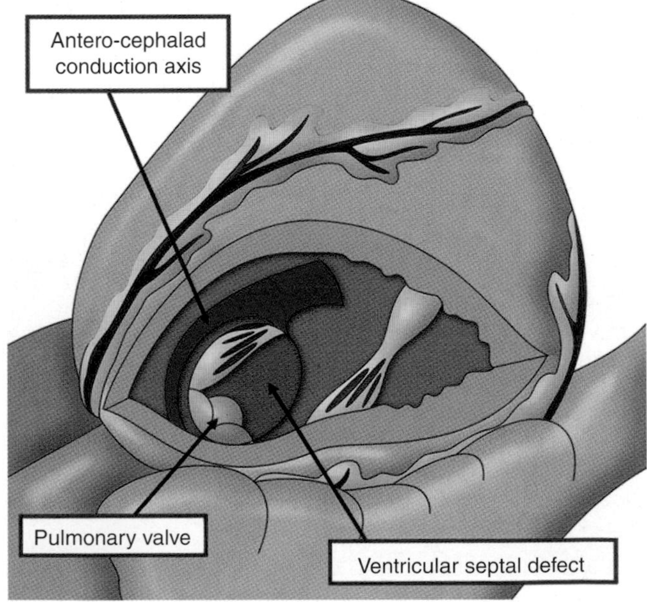

Figure 39-12 The cartoon shows the view of a perimembranous ventricular septal defect in congenitally corrected transposition through a generous ventriculotomy. In the expected situation, the conduction axis, because of the malalignment gap (see Fig. 39-10) runs antero-cephalad relative to the defect.

Associated Malformations

In the majority of cases encountered clinically, the potential correction of the circulatory pattern produced by the double discordance is uncorrected by the presence of one or more associated malformations. Of these, three are so typical as to be considered almost part of the segmental combination, namely, an interventricular communication, obstruction of the subpulmonary outflow tract, and anomalies of the morphologically tricuspid valve.[1,2] The morphology of each of these lesions can be variable.

Ventricular Septal Defect

An interventricular communication, if present, and such holes are expected in at least half the patients, is usually perimembranous. It occupies a subpulmonary position, with the diagnostic feature being fibrous continuity between the leaflets of the pulmonary valve and, in usual arrangement, the left-sided tricuspid valve (Fig. 39-13). Such perimembranous defects typically extend posteriorly and inferiorly towards the crux of the heart, opening primarily into the inlet of the morphologically left ventricle. The posterior margin of the defect is then formed by an extensive area of fibrous continuity between the leaflets of the pulmonary, mitral, and tricuspid valves (see Fig. 39-13), with this feature removing the anticipated reversed offsetting of the attachments of the atrioventricular valves. As already explained, the atrioventricular conduction axis runs antero-superiorly relative to these defects (see Fig. 39-13), the opposite of that expected for perimembranous defects in hearts with concordant atrioventricular connections. In rare instances, the defect can be subpulmonary but with exclusively muscular rims. In this setting, the atrioventricular conduction axis will continue to run antero-superiorly. Muscular defects, however, can be found in any other part of the ventricular septum. Should a muscular defect open between the outlets, then the bundle may occupy a postero-inferior position (Fig. 39-14). Defects can also be found in doubly committed and juxta-arterial position, roofed by continuity between the leaflets of the aortic and pulmonary valves, with absence of the septal component of the infundibulum. These defects are particularly common in Asian populations.[11]

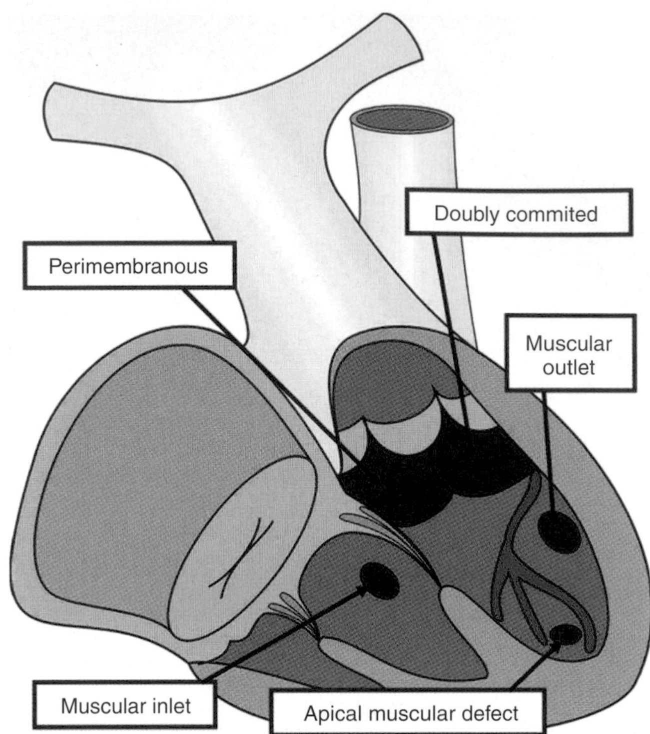

Figure 39-14 The cartoon shows how all types of ventricular septal defect can be found in congenitally corrected transposition. The location of the conduction axis is shown in yellow.

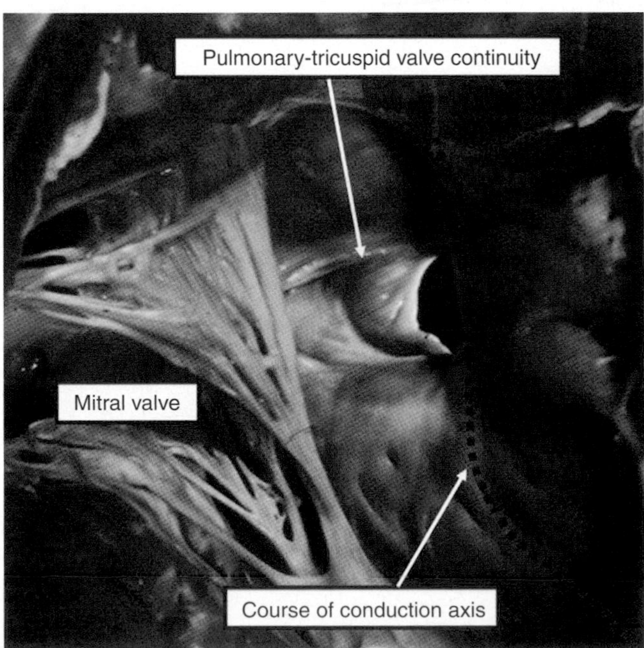

Figure 39-13 The image shows the typical perimembranous ventricular septal defect found in hearts with congenitally corrected transposition, as viewed from the morphologically left ventricle. Note the fibrous continuity between the leaflets of the pulmonary and left-sided morphologically tricuspid valves. The antero-cephalad position of the conduction axis is marked.

Obstruction of the Morphologically Left Ventricular Outflow Tract

Excluding hearts with pulmonary atresia, stenosis of the outflow tract from the morphologically left ventricle occurs in approximately one-third to one-half of patients with usual atrial arrangement. The stenosis is isolated in less than one-fifth of these cases, being combined in about four-fifths with a ventricular septal defect, and in about one-third also with abnormalities of the morphologically tricuspid valve. The anatomical nature of the stenosis varies.[12] Valvar stenosis is usually accompanied by one or another variety of subpulmonary obstruction. The latter may take the form of muscular hypertrophy of the septum and the ventricular free wall, a fibrous diaphragm, or else an aneurysmal dilation of fibrous tissue derived from the interventricular component of the membranous septum (Fig. 39-15). More rarely, tags may originate from either of the atrioventricular valves, or even from the leaflets of the pulmonary valve.[12] Subvalvar pulmonary obstructions, when present, are intimately related to the non-branching atrioventricular bundle (Fig. 39-16).

Lesions of the Morphologically Tricuspid Valve

There is a marked discrepancy between the incidence of such changes found at autopsy and those recognised during life. Examination of autopsied cases reveals anomalies

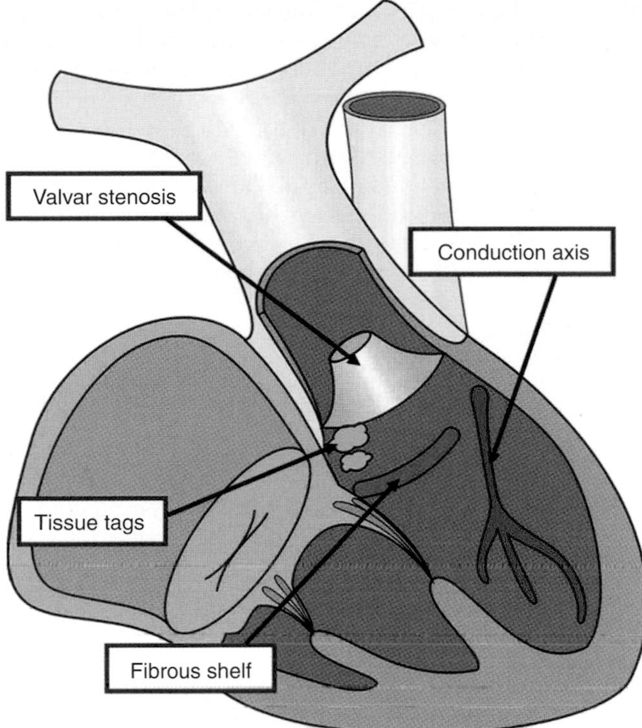

Figure 39-15 The cartoon shows the anatomical substrates for obstruction of the outflow tract from the morphologically left ventricle.

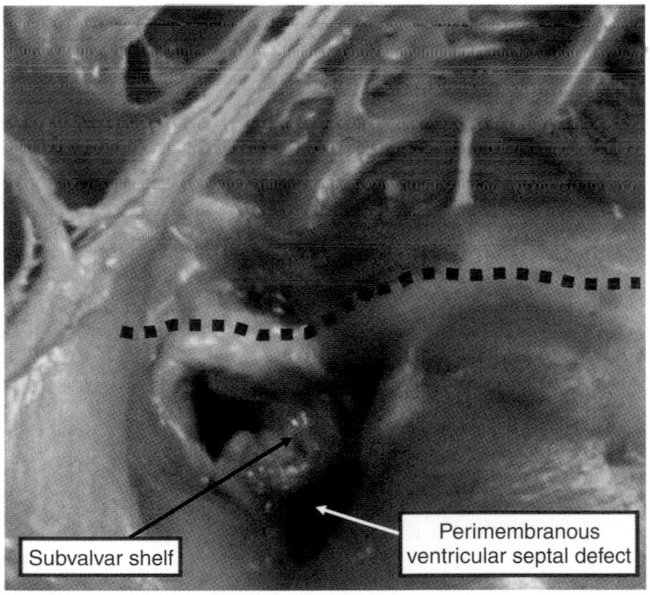

Figure 39-16 The image shows a subvalvar fibrous shelf seen from the apex of the morphologically left ventricle in a heart also exhibiting a perimembranous ventricular septal defect. Note the intimate relationship between the shelf and the conduction axis (*red dotted line*).

of the tricuspid valve in almost nine-tenths of cases, whereas only one in three patients has haemodynamic alterations due to such abnormalities. The commonest underlying pathology is valvar dysplasia, with or without apical displacement of the septal and mural leaflets, the latter of course being the essence of Ebstein's malformation. Unlike the situation in hearts with concordant atrioventricular connections, atrialisation and thinning of the inlet portion of the morphologically right ventricle, as commonly seen in Ebstein's malformation with concordant atrioventricular connections, are not always found in the setting of congenitally corrected transposition (Fig. 39-17).

In about three-quarters of the cases, the valvar anomalies are combined with a ventricular septal defect. The tricuspid valve can also override and straddle in the setting of congenitally corrected transposition, with hypoplasia of the morphologically right ventricle increasing concomitant with the proportion of the overriding atrioventricular junction connected to the dominant left ventricle (Fig. 39-18). The end-point of this spectrum of overriding is double inlet left ventricle with left-sided incomplete right ventricle, with double inlet being diagnosed when more than half of the overriding junction is connected in the left ventricle. The morphologically mitral valve can also override and straddle, often in combination with double outlet from the right ventricle.[8] As with overriding of the tricuspid valve, mitral valvar overriding is part of a spectrum of malformation, with the endpoint in this instance being double inlet right ventricle with right-sided incomplete left ventricle. The relationships of dominant and incomplete ventricles in these spectrums, of course, are reversed when congenitally corrected transposition is found in its mirror-imaged variant. The mitral valve can also prolapse with some frequency in the setting of congenitally corrected transposition.[13]

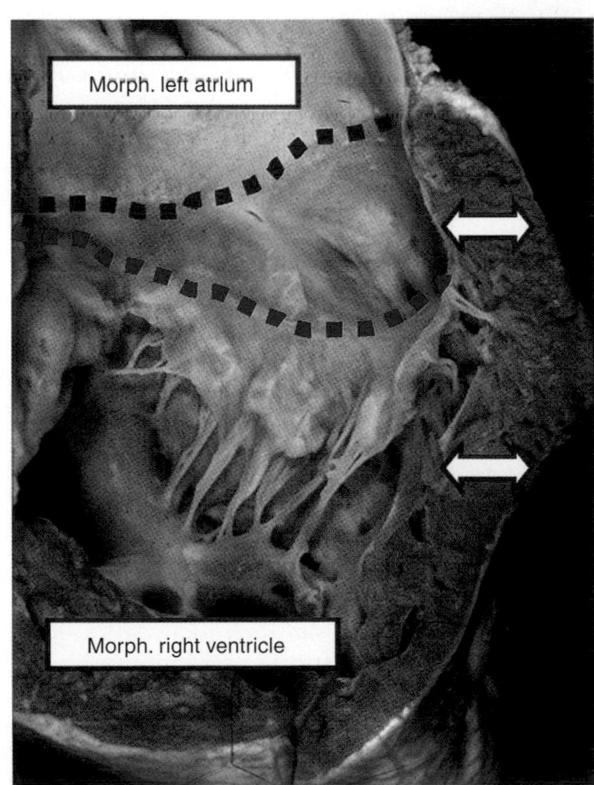

Figure 39-17 The image shows the typical appearance of Ebstein's malformation of the morphologically (morph.) tricuspid valve. The valvar hinge line (*blue dotted line*) is displaced relative to the left atrioventricular junction (*red dotted line*), but the mural thickness is the same in the inlet as in the apical trabecular component (*arrows*).

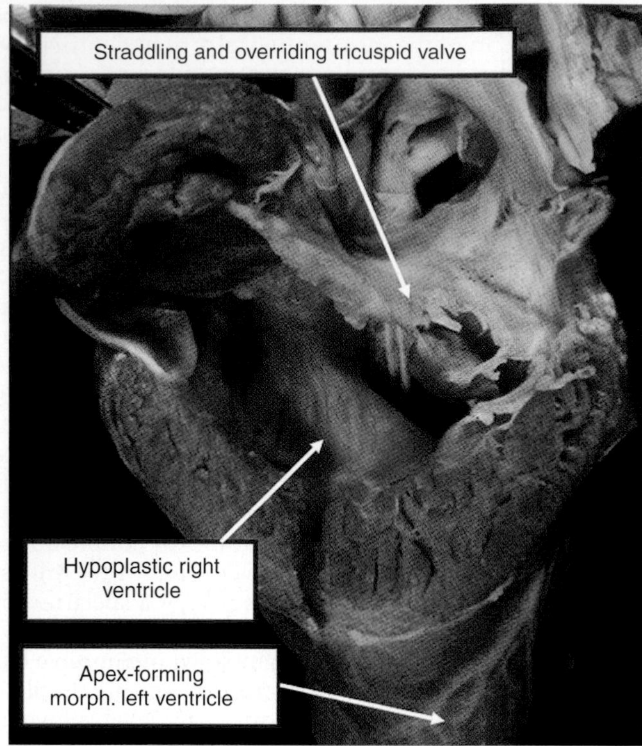

Figure 39-18 Hypoplasia of the morphologically (morph.) right ventricle, with apex-forming morphologically left ventricle in the setting of straddling and overriding of the left-sided morphologically tricuspid valve.

Disharmonious Segmental Arrangements

In almost all instances, when congenitally corrected transposition is found with usual atrial arrangement, there is left hand ventricular topology, whereas right hand ventricular topology is found when discordant atrioventricular connections are found with mirror-imaged atrial arrangement. On exceedingly rare occasions, the atrioventricular connections can be discordant when there is usual atrial arrangement and right hand ventricular topology.[14] The hearts typically show multiple associated malformations, with rotational abnormalities of the ventricular mass, straddling valves, and juxtaposition of the atrial appendages. Providing the usual rules are followed for determining the morphology of the chambers, there should be no problems these days in diagnosing the malformations, despite their complexity.

Other Ventriculo-arterial Connections

In strict terms, those patients having other ventriculo-arterial connections in combination with discordant atrioventricular connections do not have congenitally corrected transposition. It is convenient, nonetheless, to discuss them in this chapter, since it is the discordant atrioventricular connections which are the most important morphological features. The commonest variant in terms of the ventriculo-arterial connections is single outlet from the heart. In this respect, there are three possibilities: a common arterial trunk, a single pulmonary trunk with aortic atresia, and a single aortic trunk with pulmonary atresia. Of these, the first two are rare.[15,16] With pulmonary atresia, there is usually a large ventricular septal defect in the subaortic position. This lends itself to tunnelling to the aorta as part of anatomical correction. The conduction tissue should be anticipated to be antero-superiorly located relative to this defect, arising from an anterior atrioventricular node, so extreme care is needed if enlargement of the defect is attempted as part of an anatomical correction. The problem is then magnified, since it is cases such as these with pulmonary atresia that should be anticipated also to have a regular node, or else a sling of conduction tissue. Thus, the entire ventricular borders of the defect are likely to be occupied by the conduction tissue axis.[9] Pulmonary atresia can also be found when the ventricular septum is intact.[17,18] In these cases, the atretic pulmonary artery can usually be traced to the morphologically left ventricle, so it is appropriate to describe these patients as having congenitally corrected transposition with pulmonary atresia. The arrangement of the morphologically left ventricle itself, however, is reminiscent of hypoplastic left heart syndrome, and these patients will be candidates only for functionally univentricular repair.

The rare but important combination of discordant atrioventricular connections with concordant atrioventricular connections can be found either with usual atrial arrangement or in the setting of mirror-imaged atriums. Several purported examples of this rare combination have been in patients with isomeric atrial appendages, but in this combination the atrioventricular connections will be biventricular and mixed rather than discordant (see Chapter 1). In some cases, the aorta is posterior and to the right of the pulmonary trunk, albeit with a parallel rather than a spiral arrangement of the arterial trunks. The combination has been described as isolated ventricular inversion, not that this nomenclature contributes much to understanding.[19] The important feature is that, when discordant connections at atrioventricular level are combined with concordant ventriculo-arterial connections, the combination produces the haemodynamics of transposition irrespective of the infundibular morphology. Such patients are ideal candidates for surgical correction by atrial redirection procedures,[20] since this provides both anatomical and physiological correction of the circulations, restoring the morphologically left ventricle to its systemic role.

Many of the patients having discordant atrioventricular connections combined with double outlet right ventricle have right-sided hearts and pulmonary stenosis.[21] It was in a heart such as this that Mönckeberg[10] first described the unusual formation of paired atrioventricular nodes joining to a common atrioventricular bundle, the so-called Mönckeberg sling. The heart described by Mönckeberg[10] was positioned in the right side of the chest, but the segmental combination can exist with any cardiac position. The ventricular septal defect is usually in subpulmonary position, but subaortic, doubly committed, and non-committed defects have all been described. All kinds of relations between the great arterial trunks can also be present. The rarest ventriculo-arterial connection is that of double outlet left ventricle. This must also be anticipated to exist with various arterial relationships, and with the interventricular communication related in varying fashion to the arterial trunks, and with the typical complicating lesions.

Morphogenesis

As we have described in Chapter 3, the definitive chambers of the heart are produced by ballooning from the primary heart tube, with atrial appendages ballooning in parallel from the atrial component of the tube, while the apical components of the ventricles balloon in series from the inlet and outlet parts of the ventricular loop. If development proceeds in normal fashion, the primary heart tube bends to the right during early development.[22] This leaves the atrioventricular canal connected primarily to the part of the loop from which will develop the morphologically left ventricle. Expansion of the canal to the right then permits the right atrium to connect directly with the developing morphologically right ventricle, which itself is positioned rightward relative to the morphologically left ventricle. In certain circumstances, instead of bending to the right during development, the heart tube turns leftward. Such leftward looping places the outlet component of the primary tube, from which will develop the morphologically right ventricle, to the left of the morphologically left ventricle. In this setting, so as to permit the atrioventricular canal to open directly to both ventricles, it must expand leftward rather than rightward, at the same time placing the developing morphologically left atrium in communication with the morphologically right ventricle, and leaving the morphologically right atrium connecting to the morphologically left ventricle. This process, therefore, produces discordant atrioventricular connections. It is not yet known why such disharmonious looping should be associated so frequently also with discordant ventriculo-arterial connections, nor why the presence of discordant atrioventricular connections should be associated so frequently with the typical associated malformations.

INCIDENCE AND AETIOLOGY

Analysis of the patients entered into the New England regional infant cardiac programme identified only 16 infants with congenitally corrected transposition.[23] Patients with congenitally corrected transposition, however, accounted for 0.6% of those with congenitally malformed hearts seen at the Boston Children's Hospital during the period from 1972 to 1987.[24] This correlates well with the incidence for congenital corrected transposition of 0.5% calculated by the Baltimore–Washington infant study group.[25] The variant with mirror-imaged atrial chambers is said to be very rare, with less than 100 well-documented cases recorded in one review,[26] albeit that increasing clinical experience suggests that this may be an underestimate.

The commonest associated cardiac abnormality is a ventricular septal defect, found in just over two-thirds of cases.[27] In up to half, there is stenosis in the outflow tract of the subpulmonary morphologically left ventricle.[27,28] The morphologically tricuspid valve is abnormal in almost all cases seen at autopsy, with varying degrees of displacement into the ventricular cavity and Ebstein-like abnormalities. Rarely the valve can exhibit a double orifice. Coarctation of the aorta and interruption of the aortic arch are rare complications. Tricuspid valvar regurgitation develops with great frequency over the lifetime of most patients, as does complete heart block. The aetiology of the condition is unknown, and is considered multi-factorial. Familial incidence is rare, with but one publication noting its occurrence.[29] The ratio of gender in those with usually arranged atrial chambers is about 1.6 to 1, with males predominating.

CLINICAL PRESENTATION

The clinical presentation is influenced by the presence of the associated cardiac anomalies. Those with a large ventricular septal defect in the absence of obstruction to the morphologically left ventricular outflow tract obstruction will present with cardiac failure. Cardiac failure will also be seen in those with morphologically tricuspid valvar incompetence due to dysplasia of the valvar leaflets, often associated with marked displacement of the septal and mural leaflets into the morphologically right ventricular cavity, in other words producing Ebstein's malformation. Where there is severe pulmonary stenosis or atresia of the morphologically left ventricular outflow tract, the infant will be cyanosed, often having a ductal-dependent pulmonary circulation. Occasionally, there may be signs of complete heart block, either antenatally or in the immediate postnatal period, which can cause cardiac failure. When there is a large left-to-right shunt or severe tricuspid valvar regurgitation, sometimes together with complete heart block, then an infant may present with cardiomegaly in the first few days of life with cardiac failure, and may require inotropic and ventilatory support.[28,30] The development of tricuspid regurgitation and morphologically right ventricular failure, however, may not occur until later in life.[31] Those with a ventricular septal defect can also exhibit a moderate degree of obstruction within the morphologically left ventricular outflow tract. This combination provides balanced pulmonary and systemic circulations, with saturations of oxygen in the mid 80s, without cardiac failure. Rarely, those without associated cardiac anomalies can exhibit no clinical problems. In this setting, the abnormal segmental combinations can present as an incidental finding in an older patient, often with the development of complete atrioventricular dissociation. In some circumstances, the condition is brought to light when a right-sided heart is noted incidentally on a chest radiograph.

The physical findings are also determined by the nature of the associated cardiac abnormalities. Thus, there may be signs of cardiac failure, with failure to thrive, in those cases presenting in early infancy and requiring medical or surgical treatment. The cyanosed neonate will require construction of a systemic-to-pulmonary arterial shunt in the first few days of life. Signs of increasing tricuspid valvar regurgitation may be somewhat insidious, occurring over the first few years of life with the gradual onset of right ventricular dysfunction, and only then does cardiac failure become evident.[32] Examination of patients of all ages will reveal the signs of either congestive cardiac failure or cyanosis.

INVESTIGATIONS

Electrocardiography

In those with usual atrial arrangement, the ventricular conduction system is disposed in mirror-imaged fashion. Thus, the activation of the ventricular septum is from right to left in a superior and anterior direction. This results in presence of Q waves in the right precordial leads, and absence of T waves in the left precordial leads, along with a reversal of the normal precordial pattern of the Q wave pattern (Fig. 39-19).[33] This pattern of electrical activation of the myocardium is

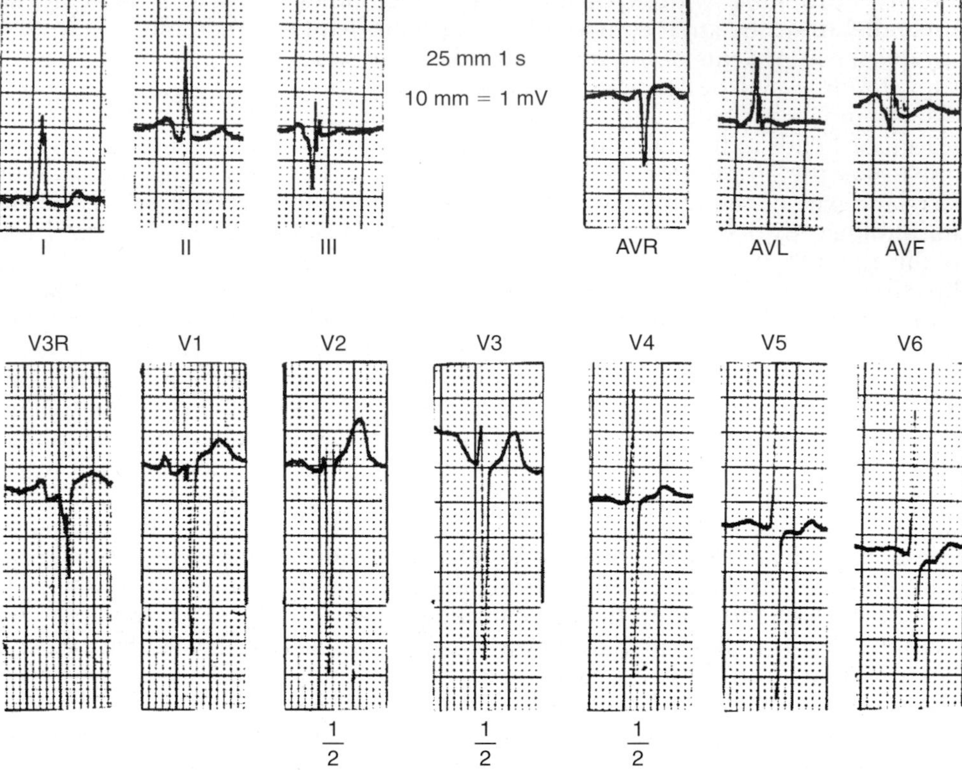

Figure 39-19 This electrocardiogram is from a boy aged 4 years, with usual atrial arrangement, a left-sided heart, moderate insufficiency of the left-sided atrioventricular valve, and mild pulmonary hypertension. Note the reversal of the pattern of the Q waves in the precordial leads, with positive T waves throughout these leads.

present in some three-quarters of patients.[34] The presence of conduction abnormalities and complete heart block is also frequent. The typical electrocardiographic pattern in those with usual atrial arrangement, therefore, can be summarised as left-axis deviation, reversal of the precordial progression of the Q waves, and prominence of the Q waves in leads III and AVF. QS complexes are seen in leads III and AVF, and over the right precordium.[35] These patterns will change when there is volume overloading or pressure overloading of either the right or left ventricle, and are mirror-imaged in those having mirror-imaged atrial arrangement.[36,37]

Chest Radiography

Detailed evaluation of the chest X-ray has been superseded by non-invasive evaluation of the cardiac morphology by echocardiography. The plain chest X-ray, nonetheless, may reveal congestion of the lung fields, or plethora suggesting cardiac failure. Cardiomegaly may either be an indication of volume loading of the heart or of cardiac failure. The heart itself is often positioned in the middle or right side of the chest, with the apex pointing directly down or to the right. In those with mirror-imaged atrial arrangement, the heart is frequently found in the left side of the chest, with the apex pointing to the left. An unusual location of the heart is a further clue to the presence of congenitally corrected transposition.[38-40] This finding, of course, is not a diagnosis in itself, but rather an indication for further investigation.

Echocardiography

Patients with congenitally corrected transposition are diagnosed nowadays echocardiographically, both antenatally and postnatally. Until very recently, the cross sectional approach was standard, but three-dimensional echocardiography is now available for detailed cardiac analysis. This permits very accurate assessment of the cardiac morphology, without the need to make recourse to further investigations.[41-43] Detailed sequential segmental analysis is the pivotal investigation. This will show that the systemic veins drain to the morphologically right atrium, which is joined to the morphologically left ventricle. The connection of the morphologically left ventricle is then to the pulmonary trunk. The pulmonary veins will be identified joining the morphologically left atrium, which is connected to the morphologically right ventricle and thence to the aorta (Fig. 39-20). The morphologic nature of the left ventricle is identified on the basis of its smooth walls, and the presence of paired papillary muscles supporting the morphologically mitral valve. The morphologically right ventricle will be recognised on the basis of its coarse apical trabeculations, the presence of the moderator band, and attachments of the septal leaflet of the morphologically tricuspid valve directly to the septum. Associated lesions, such as ventricular septal defects (Fig. 39-21), different types of obstruction within the outflow tract of the morphologically left ventricle such as tissue tags or fibrous shelves (Fig. 39-22), and pulmonary valvar stenosis or atresia will clearly be seen. The morphology of the morphologically tricuspid valve must be studied with care. This can be markedly dysplastic, with displacement of the septal and inferior leaflets into the morphologically right ventricular cavity in those with associated Ebstein's malformation (Fig. 39-23). When there is marked dysplasia of the valvar leaflets, it is usual to see moderate-to-severe tricuspid valvar regurgitation on colour flow mapping (Fig. 39-24). Straddling and overriding of either the right- or left-sided atrioventricular valves should be identified if

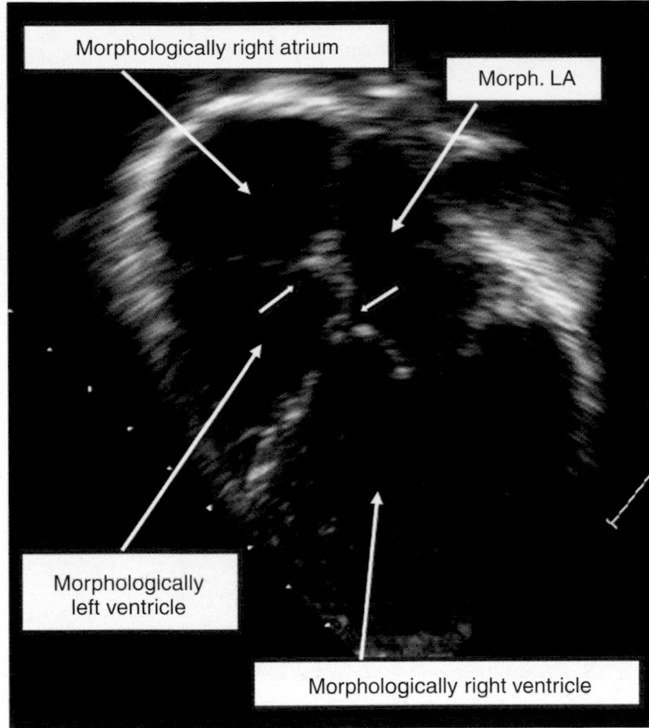

Figure 39-20 The cross sectional echocardiogram, in four-chamber projection, shows the essential features of discordant atrioventricular connections. Note the reversed off-setting of the leaflets of the right-sided mitral and left-sided tricuspid valves (*arrows*). Morph. LA, morphologically left atrium.

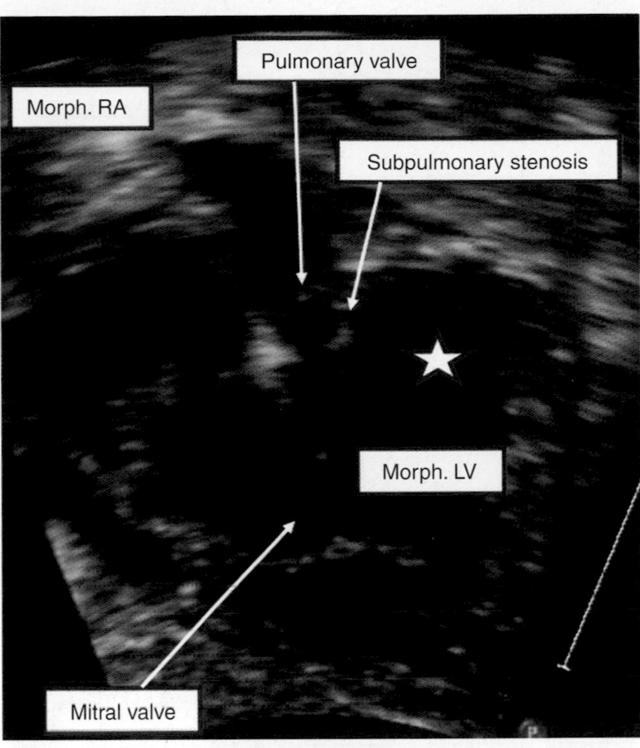

Figure 39-22 The subcostal oblique cross sectional echocardiogram shows subpulmonary stenosis produced by a fibrous shelf. The star shows the anterior recess of the left ventricle. LV, left ventricle; Morph, morphologically; RA, right atrium.

present, taking care to exclude hypoplasia of either ventricle sufficient to militate against biventricular surgical repair. Sequential segmental analysis will also serve to identify rarer combinations found in some patients with discordant atrioventricular connections, such as those with double outlet right or left ventricles, or concordant ventriculo-arterial connections. The latter combination is of particular significance, since although the patients present with the features of transposition, the segmental combinations mean that an atrial redirection procedure is the corrective procedure of choice, placing the morphologically left ventricle as the pump to the systemic circulation.[20]

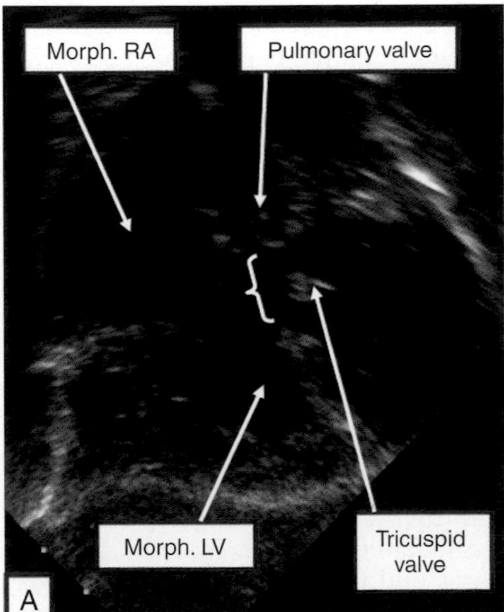

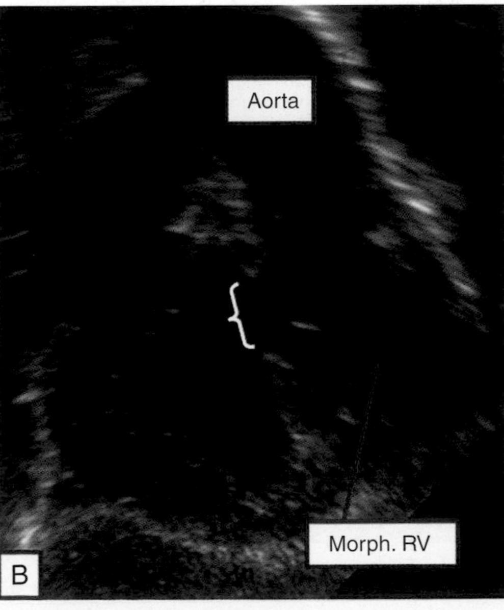

Figure 39-21 The cross sectional echocardiograms, in four-chamber section, show a perimembranous ventricular septal defect (*bracket*) in the setting of discordant atrioventricular connections. Panel **A** shows the fibrous continuity between the leaflets of the pulmonary and left-sided tricuspid valves, while panel **B** shows the anterior and left-sided location of the aorta. LV, left ventricle; Morph, morphologically; RA, right atrium; RV, right ventricle.

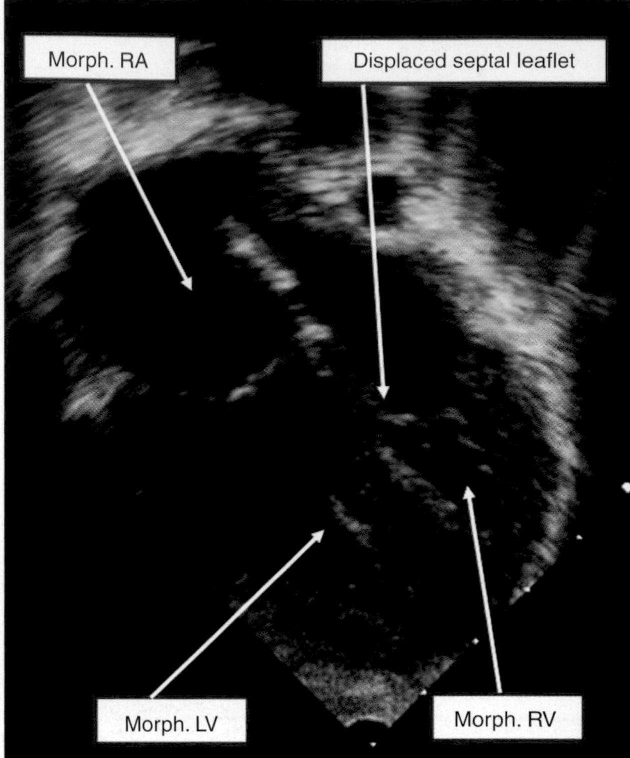

Figure 39-23 The cross sectional echocardiogram, in four-chamber projection, shows the essence of Ebstein's malformation in the setting of discordant atrioventricular connections. Note the downward displacement of the hinge of the septal leaflet of the left-sided morphologically (morph.) tricuspid valve. LV, left ventricle; RA, right atrium; RV, right ventricle.

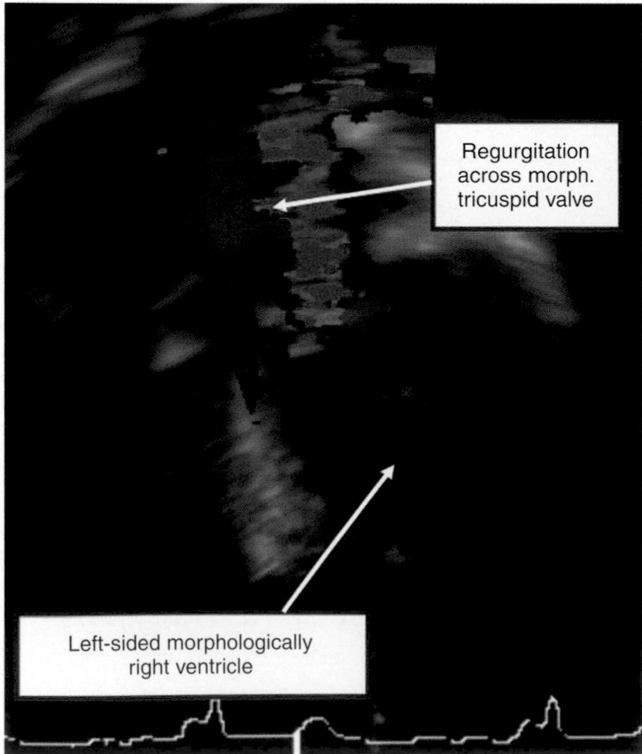

Figure 39-24 Colour flow mapping shows severe regurgitation across the morphologically (morph.) tricuspid valve.

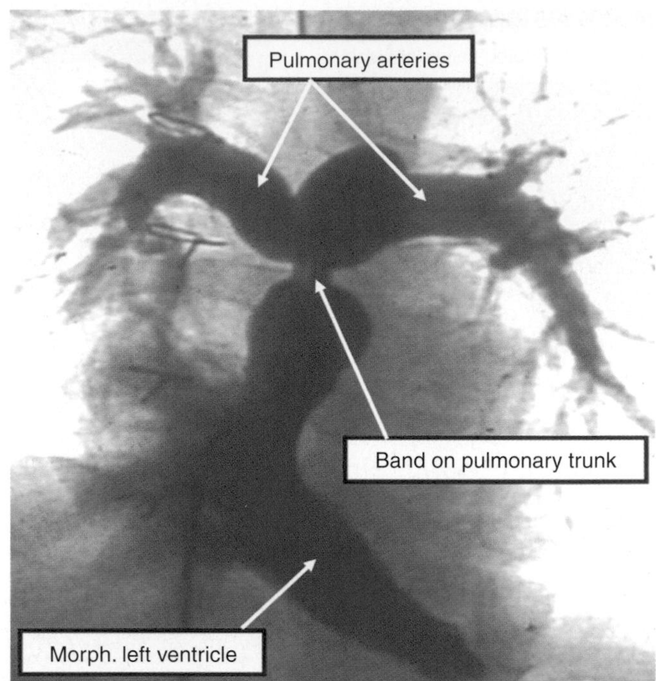

Figure 39-25 The angiogram shows a banded pulmonary trunk, the band having been placed to train the morphologically (morph.) left ventricle.

Cardiac Catheterisation and Angiography

These modes of investigation have become almost obsolete in the current management of either infants or older patients. They may be necessary in situations where there are multiple ventricular septal defects, which cannot clearly be seen using echocardiography. The investigation of pulmonary hypertension in older patients, and the evaluation and measurement of pulmonary vascular resistance, may be necessary to establish operability. Rarely, in those with pulmonary atresia, major aortopulmonary collateral arteries supply most of the blood to the lungs. The origin and course of these arteries can more clearly be shown with angiography. When anatomical repair is planned, such as the double-switch procedure, coronary angiography may be helpful in delineating the anatomy of the coronary arteries. When there has been prior construction of a systemic-to-pulmonary arterial shunt, or the pulmonary trunk has been banded to reduce the flow of blood to the lungs or to train the morphologically left ventricle (Fig. 39-25), haemodynamic and angiographic data is required to demonstrate the anatomy of the pulmonary arteries and to show whether the morphologically left ventricle has been adequately trained so that it can support the systemic circulation.[44]

Computerised Axial Tomography and Magnetic Resonance Imaging

These modalities are now available non-invasively to evaluate the morphology and haemodynamics of patients with congenitally corrected transposition. To a large extent, their use depends on their availability at individual centres. In infants and small children, a general anaesthetic is usually necessary if these scans are to provide accurate data, but more modern systems, and faster computing power, may well provide accurate data without the requirement for

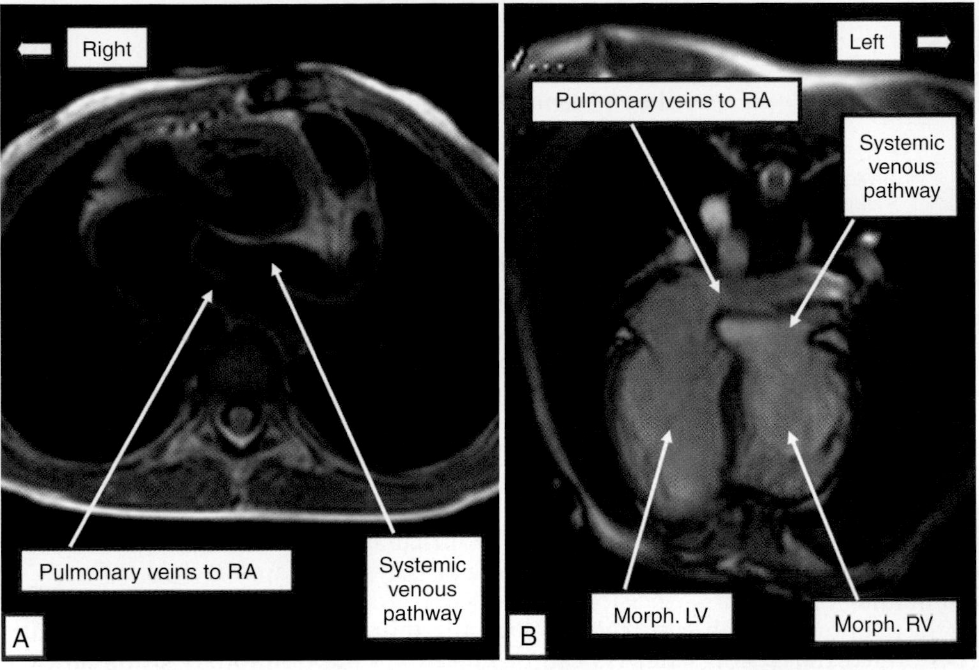

Figure 39-26 The magnetic resonance images show the results of the Senning operation as performed to redirect the atrial venous returns as part of anatomical correction. Panel **A** shows a short-axis cut and panel **B** an angulated cut producing a four-chamber section. Morph, morphologically; LV, left ventricle; RA, right atrium; RV, right ventricle.

anaesthesia. Magnetic resonance imaging is also of value in the post-operative situation to check the patency of the venous (Fig. 39-26) and arterial pathways subsequent to reconstructive surgery. The bedrock for evaluation of patients with congenitally corrected transposition of all ages, nonetheless, is echocardiography, with other modalities being used to fine-tune the diagnosis and haemodynamics.

Differential Diagnosis

It should now be always possible in all patients to make a clear diagnosis of congenitally corrected transposition and to identify all associated lesions. Some other lesions may still provide a problem. Distinction from corrected transposition can sometimes be difficult in those with discordant atrioventricular connections associated with other ventriculo-arterial connections, in those having left-handed ventricular topology in the setting of isomeric atrial appendages, in those having anterior and left-sided ascending aortas with normal atrial arrangement, and in those with anterior and right-sided aortas in the mirror-imaged situation. Appropriate echocardiographic interrogation, nonetheless, should identify these variations in morphology.

MANAGEMENT

The Morphologically Right Ventricle and Tricuspid Valve in the Systemic Circulation

The management of patients with congenitally corrected transposition would be relatively easy were it not for the morphologically right ventricle being responsible for pumping the systemic circulation. Physiological restoration of normal circulatory patterns can be restored by closing ventricular septal defects, if present, relieving any obstruction in the outflow tract to the pulmonary arteries, and repairing or replacing the morphologically tricuspid valve, while disturbances of atrioventricular conduction can be treated by placement of a pacemaker. If these procedures are undertaken leaving the morphologically right ventricle pumping the systemic circulation, however, the ventricle may show signs of severe failure in infancy or later in life. On some occasions, the ventricle may sustain normal cardiac haemodynamics until the patient is well into old age, only then to fail. The causation of such morphologically right ventricular failure is poorly understood. Various explanations can be offered, such as volume loading or increasing tricuspid regurgitation, but it as yet not known why some patients develop this problem and others do not.

In some neonates and infants, there is marked dysplasia of the leaflets of the morphologically tricuspid valve. The severe, or increasingly severe, tricuspid regurgitation thus produced creates a volume load on the morphologically right ventricle, which is then exacerbated by dilation of the valvar annulus and, hence, worsening cardiac failure. This produces a vicious circle. The strain on the morphologically right ventricle may be further exacerbated by the presence of volume-loading caused by deficient ventricular septation (Fig. 39-27). The morphologically tricuspid valve may itself initially be competent, but over the years can become regurgitant, this becoming worse with volume-loading and right ventricular dilation. It is unclear which patients might develop this complication. It seems fairly certain that, with severe dysplasia and displacement of the leaflets of the tricuspid valve towards the apex of the morphologically right ventricle, this creates a setting for tricuspid valvar regurgitation and ensuing cardiac failure. Increasing tricuspid regurgitation, nonetheless, can occur over time in patients who have a normally structured tricuspid valve. Since many patients tolerate well the tricuspid regurgitation for significant periods, along with a degree of morphologically right ventricular dysfunction, and can remain stable with medical management, it can be difficult to decide when to intervene surgically. Should surgical intervention with repair or replacement of the tricuspid valve be left too late, there is little chance of right ventricular functional recovery, with associated high operative risks. Thus, the timing

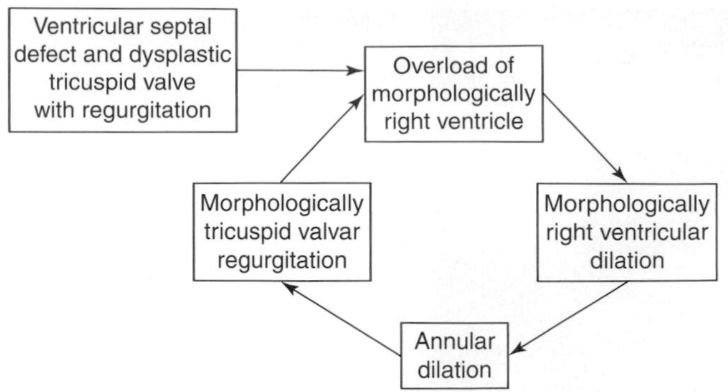

Figure 39-27 The chart shows the vicious circle of morphologically right ventricular failure, exacerbated in presence of a ventricular septal defect.

of intervention to achieve a good outcome is difficult in the group of patients who are relatively stable clinically.[32,45–50]

It was shown in those with transposition and concordant atrioventricular connections that training of the morphologically left ventricle by banding the pulmonary trunk permitted a safe arterial switch to be performed, thus restoring the left ventricle to its role of pumping the systemic circulation.[51] The same procedure has now been applied successfully in patients with congenitally corrected transposition (see Fig. 39-25), usually those having a degree of morphologically right ventricular failure and tricuspid valvar regurgitation. It has also been shown that banding the pulmonary trunk can sometimes reduce the amount of tricuspid valvar regurgitation by realigning the ventricular septum, pushing the septal leaflet of the tricuspid valve back into the right ventricle so that it apposes the other valvar leaflets and reduces the amount of valvar regurgitation. This reduction in valvar regurgitation reduces the volume loading of the morphologically right ventricle, helping to break into the vicious circle (see Fig. 39-27). Thus, banding in itself may be a therapeutic option, although more usually it is used to prepare the morphologically left ventricle for subsequent anatomical repair.[52–54]

Medical Management

Medical management involves the usual modalities for cardiac failure, such as inhibition of angiotensin-converting enzymes, diuretics, and control of arrhythmias with pacing to raise the heart rate when necessary.

Surgical Palliation

Procedures to increase the flow of blood to the lungs, such as construction of systemic-to-pulmonary arterial shunts, either centrally or by the modified Blalock-Taussig option, or banding of the pulmonary trunk to reduce flow in those with ventricular septal defects and cardiac failure, can be used to stabilise patients until they are bigger and able to undergo more complex surgical correction.

Corrective Surgery

It is increasingly apparent that curative surgery is probably not possible. It is certainly possible to provide corrective surgery, either physiologically or anatomically, but the patients always require careful follow-up, and often require other procedures, such as changes of valved conduits, repair of cardiac valves, and insertion of cardiac pacemakers should complete heart block develop. The reconstructed venous pathways may also become obstructed and require relief, after the atrial switch procedure.

Physiological Repair

Associated cardiac anomalies can be repaired with this approach, albeit that the morphologically right ventricle remains as the pump to the systemic circulation. As already discussed, ventricular septal defects, if present, can be closed, obstruction within the left ventricular outflow tract can be relieved by either resection or placement of a valved conduit, and the tricuspid valve, if leaking, can be repaired or replaced.

Usually the ventricular septal defect is perimembranous in position. It is typically approached through an incision in the right atrium, and then closed through the morphologically mitral valve. Some muscular outlet defects can be closed via the pulmonary trunk and the pulmonary valve. The conduction system passes in anterocephalad fashion around the pulmonary outflow tract. To avoid damaging the conduction system, either continuous or interrupted sutures are placed on the morphologically right ventricular margin of the defect superiorly, and from the morphologically left ventricular side of the margin inferiorly.[55]

Relief of stenosis within the morphologically left ventricular outflow tract may require careful resection of accessory tissue, or open pulmonary valvotomy, but in general a valved conduit is placed from the morphologically left ventricle to the pulmonary arteries so as to relieve the obstruction. Incisions placed across the attachments of the pulmonary valvar leaflets, because of the disposition of the conduction system, will cause heart block. In order to avoid the conduction system, and the papillary muscle of the mitral valve, the ventriculotomy is placed towards the apex of the ventricle. Valved conduits will not last forever, and most will need to be changed. It is wise, therefore, to close the pericardium with a membrane to protect the heart during sternal re-entry at reoperations. Repair or replacement of the morphologically tricuspid valve sometimes has to be done as part of physiological repairs when there is severe tricuspid valvar regurgitation. It is fraught with problems of continuing cardiac failure, since often the morphologically right ventricle is failing by the time such surgery is entertained. In addition, particularly in younger patients where there is marked dysplasia of the valvar leaflets, repair can be extremely difficult, if not impossible. Under these circumstances, replacement may well be necessary.

Problems Associated with Physiological Repair

Many centres throughout the world have highlighted the problem of right ventricular failure following physiological repair. This deterioration in right ventricular function is usually associated with the development of tricuspid valvar regurgitation, which can occur within a few months of repair, or develop more insidiously over several years.[32,45–50] It was such uncertainty regarding the longer-term outcome of physiological repair that led to the idea of restoring the morphologically left ventricle to the systemic circulation, so-called anatomical repair.

Anatomical Correction

In this approach, the morphologically left ventricle is restored to pumping the systemic circulation either by combining atrial and arterial switch procedures, or else by performing the atrial switch along with ventricular rerouting. Where the pulmonary and systemic outflow tracts are unobstructed and possess competent and non-stenotic valves, the atrial switch is combined with an arterial switch procedure, the so-called double-switch operation (Fig. 39-28). Where there is pulmonary stenosis or atresia, usually in association with a large ventricular septal defect, the atrial switch is combined with tunnelling of the morphologically left ventricle to the aorta. A valved conduit is then placed from the morphologically right ventricle to the pulmonary arteries (Fig. 39-29).[53,56–58]

In our unit, the double switch is performed under hypothermic cardiopulmonary bypass, with periods of low flow or circulatory arrest as necessary to achieve a clear operative field.[53] Other methods of cardiopulmonary bypass and cardioplegic techniques are equally applicable, and are used by other centres performing this type of surgery. Irrespective of the method used, it is important to ensure reliable myocardial protection. The procedures are long, with long myocardial ischaemic times. When performing the atrial switch, our preference is for the Senning procedure (see Fig. 39-27), sometimes with supplementation of the pulmonary venous atrium by incorporation of heterologous or homologous materials.[59,60] The Mustard operation is equally applicable. Associated lesions are dealt with in appropriate fashion, and then the arterial trunks are switched, together with the coronary arteries. Relocation of the pulmonary trunk may be achieved by transposing the pulmonary arteries anterior to the reconstructed aorta, or they may be left in posterior position. In general, if the aorta is more or less anterior to the pulmonary trunk, then the pulmonary arteries are relocated anteriorly. If the arterial trunks are more side-by-side, then we leave the pulmonary arteries behind the newly reconstructed aorta. At the end of the procedure, it is important to check on the reconstruction using transoesphageal or epicardial echocardiography, confirming the patency of the venous and arterial pathways as well as ensuring adequate ventricular function.

Ventricular Rerouting Combined with Atrial Redirection

The atrial switch is performed in the same manor as for the double-switch procedure. In most instances, in those suitable for ventricular rerouting, there is marked rightward rotation of the heart in those with usual atrial arrangement, and leftward rotation in those with mirror-imaged atrial arrangement, so that the ventricles come to lie anterior to the atrial chambers. This makes access to the atrial chambers more difficult when baffling the systemic venous pathways to the morphologically tricuspid valve, and the pulmonary veins to the mitral valve (see Fig. 39-27). Access to the morphologically tricuspid valve should reparative surgery be necessary can also be very difficult. An incision is made in the morphologically right ventricle, permitting creation of an intraventricular tunnel between the ventricular septal defect and the aorta. In creating this tunnel, care has to be taken to avoid any subaortic stenosis. The repair is completed by placing a valved conduit from the right ventriculotomy to the pulmonary arteries (see Fig. 39-29).[56,61] Once the reconstruction has been performed,

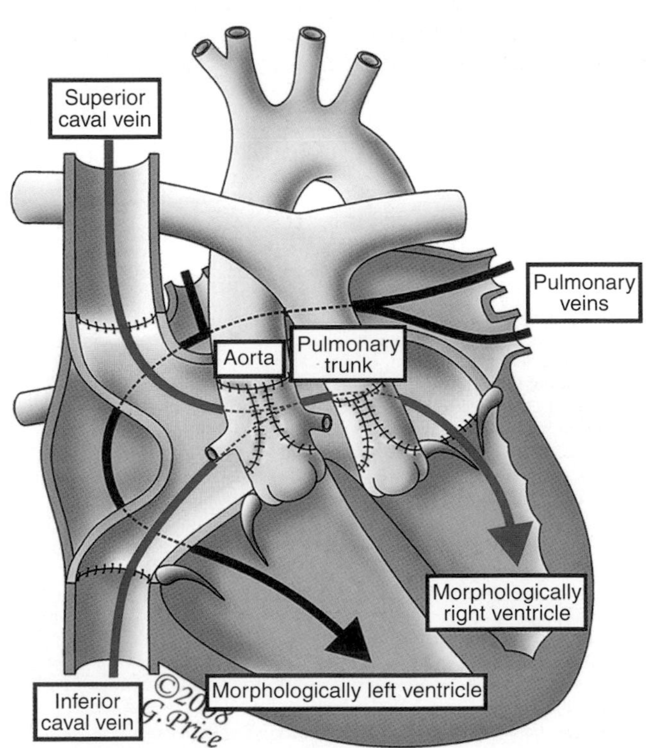

Figure 39-28 The cartoon shows the steps involved in the so-called double-switch procedure.

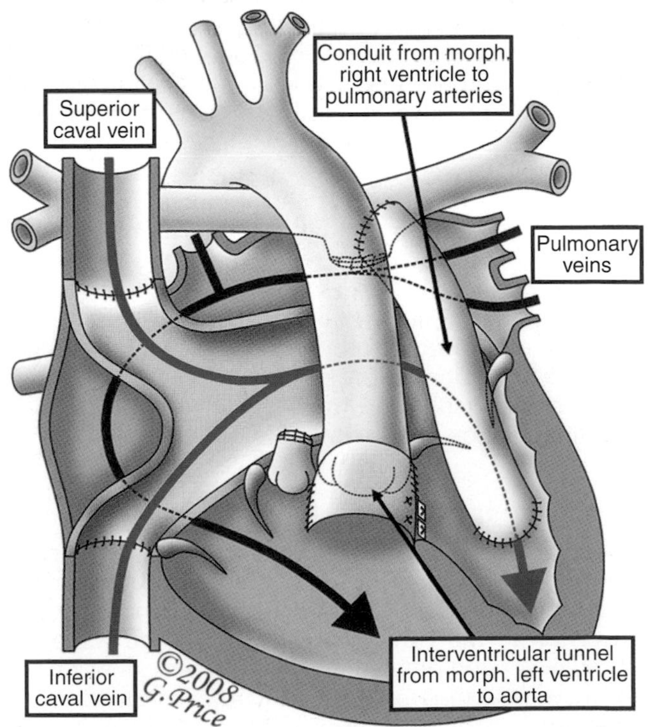

Figure 39-29 The cartoon shows the end-result after an atrial redirection procedure combined with intraventricular rerouting of the ventricular septal defect to the aorta, and placement of a conduit from the morphologically (morph.) right ventricle to the pulmonary arteries.

echocardiographic evaluation in the operating room is again important to ensure that all the reconstructed pathways are unobstructed. We would strongly advise closure of the pericardium using a membrane, facilitating reentry when the conduit needs to be changed.

Post-operative Management

The operative procedures are long. The median times of cardiopulmonary bypass in our unit have been around 2½ hours, with aortic cross-clamping lasting for more than 2 hours, and circulatory arrest lasting for almost three-quarters of an hour. It is often our practice not to close the sternum until 24 to 48 hours after completion of the operation, using inotropic support as necessary to maintain cardiac output. On occasion, extracorporeal bypass has been required for a few days to support the recovering myocardium.

Problems with Anatomical Correction

Perhaps surprisingly, infants in severe cardiac failure, with large ventricular septal defects and tricuspid regurgitation, have done well in our hands following the double-switch procedure, with none of these patients dying. Overall, in our own series of 54 patients, early mortality for anatomical repair was 5.6%, with 7 patients developing post-operative complete heart block. We have also lost two further patients thus far during follow-up. Regurgitation across the morphologically tricuspid valve has decreased in all those patients following anatomical repair in whom it was present prior to the operation. Such regurgitation has not arisen as a new problem during the period of follow-up. This is almost certainly due to the morphologically right ventricle working at lower pressures in the pulmonary circuit subsequent to repair. When anatomical correction is achieved using intraventricular rerouting, it is necessary, at some time, to change the conduit placed from the right ventricle to the pulmonary arteries, but despite the position of the conduit behind the sternum, such changes can be performed safely. Neoaortic valvar regurgitation has been reported in other series, and in a small proportion of cases, it has been necessary to replace the aortic valve. Surgically induced complete heart block can be a problem, as in one-eighth of our patients, but can be managed by placement of a pacemaker.[53,57] We have noted that the retrained morphologically left ventricle has a greater tendency to fail than the morphologically left ventricle that has been maintained at systemic pressures from birth.[62] This is of concern, and emphasises the need for continuing surveillance of these patients. It seems likely that, over time, anatomical repair will prove a better option for the majority of patients. It is not possible, as yet, to select out patients who might better be managed with physiological as opposed to anatomical repair.

Alternative Approaches

In situations in which there is hypoplasia of the left or right ventricles, or overriding or straddling of the atrioventricular valves, it may not be possible to achieve biventricular repair. Conversion to the Fontan circulation is then warranted, and can have good outcomes.[50] Conversion can be divided into two stages, with initial construction of a superior cavopulmonary bidirectional shunt, followed by completion of the Fontan circulation after a delay of 1 or 2 years, usually with placement of an external non-valved conduit from the inferior caval vein to the pulmonary arteries. The results of this approach thus far have been entirely satisfactory. Another alternative to the complex repairs may well be to maintain the pressure in the morphologically left ventricle at approximately half systemic pressure, preserving in this way the alignment of the ventricular septum, and ensuring that tricuspid regurgitation does not become a post-operative problem. This can be achieved by making limited resections of obstructions within the morphologically left ventricular outflow tract, or by placing valved conduits of smaller diameter from the morphologically left ventricle to the pulmonary arteries. When associated with construction of a bidirectional cavopulmonary shunt, this may prove a worthwhile approach, particularly when it is impossible to tunnel the ventricular septal defect to the aorta.[63]

Conclusions

Over the long term, physiological repair of patients having congenitally corrected transposition or discordant atrioventricular connections, with repair of the associated cardiac anomalies, has proved an unsatisfactory strategy for management. Over the last 20 years, therefore, use of an anatomical repair, either by the double-switch procedure or by ventricular rerouting combined with atrial redirection, has become more popular. Although more complex in technical terms, this strategy has the advantage of being applicable with good outcomes to very sick patients, who are in marked cardiac failure with severe tricuspid regurgitation. The disadvantages are the need for continuing surveillance, valvar replacement or repair, and change of conduits. There is also a concern about ventricular failure, particularly in those patients that have undergone retraining of the morphologically left ventricle. It is unlikely at this time that we can see a way forward to providing a surgical cure for patients with congenitally corrected transposition. Whilst surgical intervention will hopefully prolong life, continuing problems almost certainly will arise which require reintervention and further surgery.

The complete reference list can be found on the companion Expert Consult web site at www.expertconsult.com.

ANNOTATED REFERENCES

- Allwork SP, Bentall HH, Becker AE, et al: Congenitally corrected transposition of the great arteries: Morphologic study of 32 cases. Am J Cardiol 1976;38:910–923.

  A review of the morphological findings in the hearts from a large series of patients, describing the essence of the combination of discordant atrioventricular and ventriculo-arterial connections, and discussing the importance of the associated malformations.

- Anderson RH, Becker AE, Arnold R, Wilkinson JL: The conducting tissues in congenitally corrected transposition. Circulation 1974;50:911–923.

  This is the investigation that rediscovered the antero-cephalad location of the ventricular conduction tissues relative to the ventricular septal defect and pulmonary outflow tract in patients with discordant atrioventricular connections.

- De Leval MR, Basto P, Stark J, et al: Surgical technique to reduce the risks of heart block following closure of ventricular septal defect in atrioventricular discordance. J Thorac Cardiovasc Surg 1979;78:515–526.

  This paper describes the surgical technique of closing the ventricular septal defect to avoid the conduction system, and suggests that anatomical repair maybe possible in those patients with a large ventricular septal defect.

- Mee RBB: Severe right ventricular failure after Mustard or Senning operation two stage repair: Pulmonary artery banding and switch. J Thorac Cardiovasc Surg 1986;92:385–390.

  This paper from Melbourne describes the training of the left ventricle in transposition with concordant atrioventricular connections followed by an arterial switch procedure. This was the first paper to describe this technique, giving details of banding of the pulmonary trunk.

- Quinn D, McGuirk SP, Metha C, et al: The morphologic left ventricle that requires training by means of pulmonary artery banding before the double-switch procedure for congenitally corrected transposition of the great arteries is at risk of late dysfunction. J Thorac Cardiovasc Surg 2008;135:1137–1144.

  The morphologically left ventricle that requires training by means of pulmonary arterial banding before the double-switch procedure is at risk of late dysfunction. This paper highlights the possible problems of ventricular failure occurring more commonly in patients who have had retraining in order to relocate the left ventricle to the systemic circulation. Possibly the retrained left ventricle is not so strong in the longer term as the normal left ventricle.
- Langley SM, Winlaw DS, Stumper O, et al: Midterm results after restoration of the morphologically left ventricle to the systemic circulation in patients with congenitally corrected transposition of the great arteries. J Thorac Cardiovasc Surg 2003;125:1229–1241.
- Ilbawi MN, Deleon SY, Backer CL, et al: An alternative approach to the surgical management of physiologically corrected transposition with ventricular septal defect and pulmonary stenosis or atresia. J Thorac Cardiovasc Surg 1990;100:410–415.
- Imamura M, Drummond-Webb JJ, Murphy DJ, Jr, et al: Results of the double switch operations in the current era. Ann Thorac Surg 2000;70:100–105.
- Reddy VM, McElhinney DB, Silverman NH, Hanley FL: The double switch procedure for anatomical repair of congenitally corrected transposition of the great arteries in infants and children. Eur Heart J 1997;18:1470–1477.

  These four papers from centres performing large numbers of anatomical corrections highlight the indications, techniques and outcomes for these complex procedures. Only early- and medium-term survival is reported.
- Sano T, Riesenfeld T, Karl TR, Wilkinson JL: Intermediate-term outcome after intracardiac repair of associated cardiac defects in patients with atrioventricular and ventriculoarterial discordance. Circulation 1995;92 (9 Suppl): II272–278.
- Van Son JA, Danielson GK, Huhta JC, et al: Late results of systemic atrioventricular valve replacement in corrected transposition. J Thorac Cardiovasc Surg 1995;109:642–653.
- Yeh TJ, Connelly MS, Coles JG, et al: Atrioventricular discordance: Results of repair in 127 patients. J Thorac Cardiovasc Surg 1999;117:1190–1203.
- Piran S, Veldtman G, Siu S, et al: Heart failure and ventricular dysfunction in patients with single or systemic right ventricles. Circulation 2002;105: 1189–1194.
- Connelly M, Liu PP, Williams WG, et al: Congenitally corrected transposition of the great arteries in the adult: Functional status and complications. J Am Coll Cardiol 1996;27:1238–1243.
- Termignon JL, Leca F, Vouhé PR, et al: "Classic" repair of congenitally corrected transposition and ventricular septal defect. Ann Thorac Surg 1996;62:199–206.
- Hraska V, Duncan BW, Mayer JE, et al: Long-term outcome of surgically treated patients with corrected transposition of the great arteries. J Thorac Cardiovasc Surg 2005;129:182–191.

  These seven papers provide detailed follow-up of the outcomes for patients with uncorrected congenitally corrected transposition or who have undergone physiological repairs. They highlight the problems of tricuspid valvar regurgitation and morphologically right ventricular failure developing either as part of the natural history or in the post-operative period. They provide a body of evidence against physiological repair, giving comparison for the anatomical repair in the long term.
- Mavroudis C, Backer CL: Physiologic versus anatomic repair of congenitally corrected transposition of the great arteries. Semin Thorac Cardiovasc Surg Pediatr Card Surg Annu 2003;6:16–26.

  This thoughtful paper analyses physiological vesus anatomical repair in patients with congenitally corrected transposition, and suggests ways of maintaining right ventricular function by maintaining left ventricular pressures and alignment of the ventricular septum in order to avoid late tricuspid valvar regurgitation by displacement of the septal leaflet.

CHAPTER 40

Double Outlet Ventricle

JAMES L. WILKINSON, LUCAS J. EASTAUGH, and ROBERT H. ANDERSON

The concept of double outlet as a ventriculo-arterial connection has been well accepted for several decades. This is described elsewhere in this textbook (see Chapter 1). It may occur with each atrial arrangement, with any atrioventricular connection, and with all possible variations of ventricular morphology. The morphologic arrangement can then be further complicated by the presence of a host of associated defects, some common and some rare. The clinical picture is as inconstant as the anatomical permutations and associations would suggest. In this chapter, we review the combinations in which the outflow tracts arise from only one ventricle, but in the setting of hearts with two ventricles, and in which each ventricle possesses its own atrioventricular connection, in other words, those with biventricular atrioventricular connections. Origin of both arterial trunks from the same ventricle, of course, can also be found in the setting of univentricular atrioventricular connections, but these lesions are considered in the chapters of the book concentrating on the functionally univentricular arrangements (Chapters 31 and 32).

HISTORY

The first example of double outlet right ventricle known to us was described in 1793, by Mr Abernethy of St Bartholomew's Hospital, who commented that 'both ventricles, the left by means of an opening in the upper part of the septum ventriculorum, projected their blood into the aorta'.[1] Farre[2] regarded this case as being, in most respects, similar anatomically, and in its clinical history, to a number of other cases which were undoubtedly examples of what we would now describe as tetralogy of Fallot, albeit that Farre drew particular attention to the right ventricular origin of the aorta in the case described by Abernethy. The term double outlet right ventricle, however, did not appear until 1957.[3] Prior to that, examples of hearts with both arterial trunks arising from the right ventricle were described as partial transposition since only the aorta was considered to be placed across the ventricular septum.[4] Other hearts which would now be designated thus were included in the collections of Peacock,[5] Von Rokitansky,[6] Spitzer,[7] and Abbott,[4] generally under the terms partial transposition or complete dextroposition of the aorta.[4] It is inappropriate at this point to revisit the tortuous semantic debate that has continued over the past century, and more, with regard to the use of the term transposition, particularly in relation to hearts with both great arteries arising from the right ventricle. Suffice it to say that, for our purposes, we consider discordant ventriculo-arterial connections to be the essence of transposition (see Chapter 38). Transposition as thus defined, therefore, is mutually exclusive from double outlet right ventricle.

An equally tortured debate has surrounded the relationship between double outlet right ventricle and tetralogy of Fallot. It is a fact that the extent of right ventricular origin of the aorta is markedly variable in hearts having the phenotypic morphology of tetralogy of Fallot (see Chapter 36). In a proportion of such cases, therefore, the aortic valve will be supported predominantly by right ventricular structures. Indeed, cases of this type were included by Fallot himself in his original description of the lesion that now bears his name.[8] As we have explained, however, we consider double outlet right ventricle to represent one form of ventriculo-arterial connection, rather than a malformation defined on the basis of phenotypic anatomy. There is also no question but that, in some hearts having the phenotypic morphology of tetralogy of Fallot, the larger part of the overriding subaortic outlet is supported within the right ventricle.[9,10] Patients having such hearts will be described within this chapter. For quite some time, however, it was suggested that presence of complete muscular infundibulums supporting the entirety of the leaflets of both arterial valves was an essential part of the the diagnosis of double outlet right ventricle.[11] It was subsequently established that one of the most important principles of description of congenitally malformed hearts was that structures should be defined in their own right, and not on the basis of another feature which is itself variable.[12] On the basis of this principle, known as the morphological method, it is inappropriate to define double outlet ventricle, a specific form of ventriculo-arterial connection, on the basis of infundibular morphology, this latter feature being but one of the many variables complicating the morphology of the various entities grouped together because both arterial trunks arise in larger part from the same ventricle.

Double outlet right ventricle itself is but one part of the overall group of hearts to be described in this chapter. The other part, namely double outlet left ventricle, is very much rarer. Indeed, for quite some time distinguished morphologists and embryologists went on record as stating that double outlet from a morphologically left ventricle was an embryological impossibility.[13] Description of a heart with both arterial trunks arising from the left ventricle in the setting of an intact ventricular septum proved beyond doubt that the entity existed.[14] Since then, cases have tended to be described in isolation, rather than in large series, from either the pathological or clinical viewpoints.

PREVALENCE

Double outlet right ventricle is a rare cardiac malformation, accounting for fewer than 1% of all congenital cardiac defects. Although infrequent overall, it is sufficiently common for a number of authors to have accumulated large numbers of pathological, clinical or surgical cases. The more frequent variants of the anomaly are well documented, and present a familiar enough problem to the paediatric cardiologist and surgeon.

Double outlet left ventricle is a very much rarer malformation, albeit that the total number of published cases is now substantial. Indeed, it may be more frequent than has previously been recognised. It probably accounts for fewer than 5% of all hearts with double outlet ventriculo-arterial and biventricular atrioventricular connections. This would correspond to an incidence of fewer than 1 in 200,000 births.

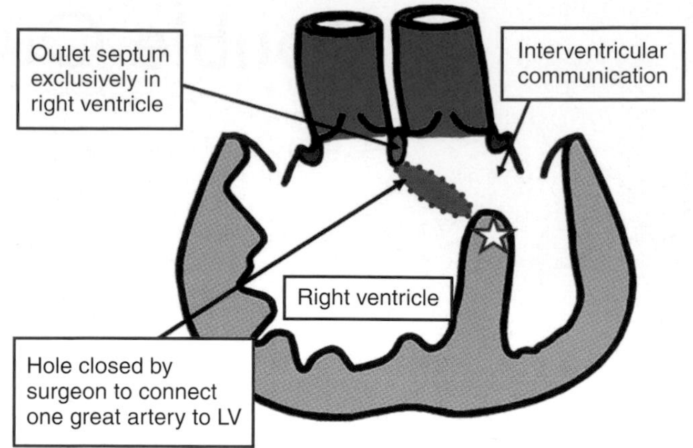

Figure 40-1 The cartoon shows the essential difference, when both arterial trunks arise from the same ventricle, in this case the right ventricle, between the interventricular communication and the hole closed by the surgeon so as to reconstitute the ventricular septum (*green oval*). Note that the muscular outlet septum is exclusively a right ventricular structure. The *star* indicates the crest of muscular septum.

MORPHOLOGY AND CLASSIFICATION

The literature relating to hearts in which both arteries arise in their greater part from the same ventricle is extensive, and includes descriptions of a bewildering variety of anatomic variations. So as to avoid confusion, in our review we focus attention, first, on the categorisation of the various malformations, and only then on the details of morphology, concentrating on the commoner, and more important, malformations.

Categorisation

A logical and step-by-step approach to diagnosis and classification proves of immense value when describing the hearts unified because both arterial trunks arise, in their greater part, from the same ventricle. Analysis, be it in the clinical or pathological situation, follows the same careful sequence that has been outlined in Chapter 1 (Table 40-1). Thus, as with any congenitally malformed heart, analysis starts with ascertainment of atrial arrangement and venous connections. Thereafter, the atrioventricular connections must be established with certainty. At the ventricular level, it is the anatomy of the connection between ventricular mass and great arteries that is the diagnostic feature, albeit that note is taken of the inter-relationships of the arterial trunks, the specific infundibular morphology, and the nature and severity of any obstructive problems in the subaortic and subpulmonary outflow tracts. The size, site, and morphology of the interventricular communication, which is categorised in the same way as any other hole between the ventricles (see Chapter 28), are also of great importance. In this respect, however, when both arterial trunks arise from the same ventricle (Fig. 40-1), the hole between the ventricles serves as the outlet for the other ventricle. Its most important feature, therefore, is its relationship with the subarterial ventricular outlets (Tables 40-2 and 40-3). Attention must also be paid to the integrity and function of the atrioventricular valves, especially the mitral valve, and to the presence of other associated cardiac defects, which are frequent (Table 40-4). It is neither practical nor desirable to use a rigid type of classification for the various malformations united simply because both arterial trunks arise, in their greater part, from the same ventricle. In our view, the categorisation of each case should be individualised, just as the medical and surgical management need to be tailored to cater to the particular problems of the individual patient. Certain anatomic variants in which both arterial trunks arise from the right ventricle, nonetheless, do occur with sufficient frequency to merit separate discussion. We commence our account, therefore, with definition and discussion of the commoner variants, as has

TABLE 40-1

ESSENTIAL ANATOMICAL INFORMATION IN ANALYSIS OF HEARTS WITH DOUBLE OUTLET VENTRICLE

Atrial arrangement
Atrioventricular connections
Atrioventricular valvar morphology
Ventriculo-arterial connection (including information about arterial overriding)
Morphology and relations of interventricular communication(s)
Morphology of outflow tracts (especially obstructive lesions)
Relationships of arterial trunks
Associated defects

TABLE 40-2

SITES OF THE INTERVENTRICULAR COMMUNICATION IN RELATION TO ARTERIAL OUTLETS IN 84 SPECIMENS OF DOUBLE OUTLET RIGHT VENTRICLE WITH USUAL ATRIAL ARRANGEMENT AND CONCORDANT ATRIOVENTRICULAR CONNECTION

Site of Defect	Percentage (of 88 defects)
Subaortic	52
Subpulmonary	24
Non-committed	14
Doubly committed	10

After Wilkinson JL, Wilcox BR, Anderson RH: The anatomy of double outlet right ventricle. In Anderson RH, Macartney FJ, Shinebourne EA, Tynan M (eds): Paediatric Cardiology, vol 5. Edinburgh: Churchill Livingstone, 1981, pp 397-407.

TABLE 40-3

TYPE OF INTERVENTRICULAR COMMUNICATION AND RELATIONSHIP TO ARTERIAL OUTLETS IN 88 SPECIMENS OF DOUBLE OUTLET RIGHT VENTRICLE WITH USUAL ATRIAL ARRANGEMENT AND CONCORDANT ATRIOVENTRICULAR CONNECTIONS

Type of Defect	Subaortic	Subpulmonary	Non-committed	Doubly Committed	Total
Perimembranous	36	13	7	5	61
Muscular	9	9	5	4	27
Total	**45**	**22**	**12**	**9**	**88**

After Wilkinson JL, Wilcox BR, Anderson RH: The anatomy of double outlet right ventricle. In Anderson RH, Macartney FJ, Shinebourne EA, Tynan M (eds): Paediatric Cardiology, Vol 5. Edinburgh: Churchill Livingstone, 1981, pp 397–407.

TABLE 40-4

ASSOCIATED DEFECTS IN 84 SPECIMENS OF DOUBLE OUTLET RIGHT VENTRICLE WITH USUAL ATRIAL ARRANGEMENT AND CONCORDANT ATRIOVENTRICULAR CONNECTIONS

Defect	No.	%
Pulmonary stenosis	31	37
Atrial septal defect	19	23
Coarctation	16	19
Mitral stenosis	7	8
Straddling mitral valve	6	7
Hypoplastic left ventricle	5	6
Aortic stenosis (valvar or subvalvar)	4	5
Restrictive ventricular septal defect	4	5
Juxtaposition of atrial appendages	4	5
Interrupted aortic arch	3	4
Common atrioventricular valve	3	4
Hypoplastic right ventricle	2	2
Criss-cross atrioventricular connection	2	2
Imperforate mitral valve	1	1
Imperforate tricuspid valve	1	1
Parachute mitral valve	1	1
Cleft mitral valve	1	1
Cleft tricuspid valve	1	1
Totally anomalous pulmonary venous connection	1	1

After Wilkinson JL, Wilcox BR, Anderson RH: The anatomy of double outlet right ventricle. In Anderson RH, Macartney FJ, Shinebourne EA, Tynan M (eds): Paediatric Cardiology, Vol 5. Edinburgh: Churchill Livingstone, 1981, pp 397–407.

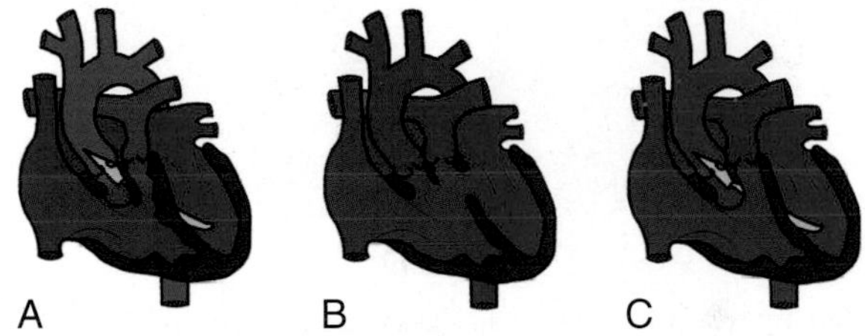

Figure 40-2 The cartoons show the commoner variants of double outlet right ventricle. **A,** The variant with a subaortic defect, infundibular pulmonary stenosis, and the aorta to the right of pulmonary trunk, a variant also known as the Fallot type. **B,** The variant with a subpulmonary defect and parallel arterial trunks, also known as the Taussig-Bing type. **C,** The variant with a subaortic defect, and with the aorta to the right of the pulmonary trunk, but without pulmonary stenosis. The *arrow* indicates the path of blood from the left ventricle to the aorta with a subaortic defect.

also been discussed in a review of double outlet right ventricle nomenclature as part of the Congenital Heart Surgery Nomenclature and Database Project.[15]

Double Outlet Right Ventricle

The commoner variants, in approximate order of frequency, are:

- Those with the interventricular communication in subaortic position, with the aorta spiralling from right to left relative to the pulmonary trunk, along with pulmonary stenosis, the so-called Fallot variant (see Fig. 40-2A)
- Those with the interventricular communication in subpulmonary position, with the aorta to the right of, and parallel to, the pulmonary trunk, the so-called Taussig-Bing variant (see Fig. 40-2B)
- Those with the interventricular communication in subaortic position, and with the aorta spiralling from right to left relative to the pulmonary trunk, but in the absence of pulmonary stenosis (see Fig. 40-2C)

Less common variants are:

- Those with the interventricular communication uncommitted, often described as non-committed, to either subarterial outlet, and with the aorta to the right of the pulmonary trunk, with either spiralling or parallel arterial trunks (Fig. 40-3A)
- Those with the interventricular communication in doubly committed position, with the aorta to the right of the pulmonary trunk, and with spiralling arterial trunks
- Those with the interventricular communication in subaortic position, but with the aorta to the left of the pulmonary trunk with parallel arterial trunks (Fig. 40-3B)
- Those with usual atrial arrangement and discordant atrioventricular connections, usually with the aorta parallel to and to the left of the pulmonary trunk (Fig. 40-3C) (see Chapter 39)
- Those with mirror-imaged atrial arrangement (Fig. 40-3D). Any of the previously mentioned variations may occur.
- Those with isomeric atrial appendages and, hence, mixed and biventricular atrioventricular connections (see Chapter 22)

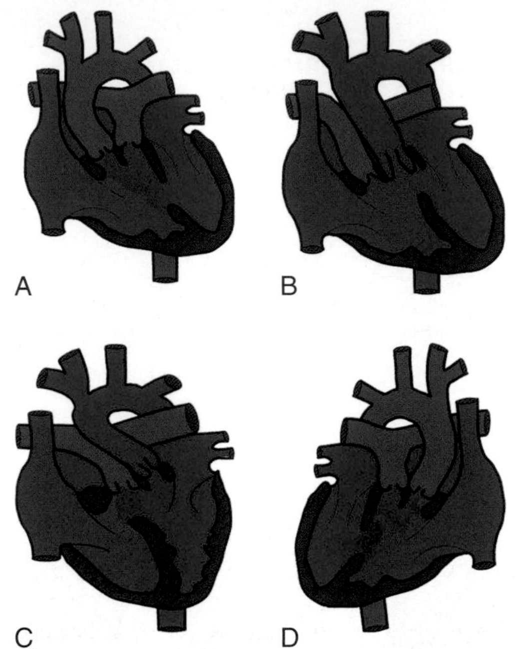

Figure 40-3 The cartoons show other, less common variants of double outlet right ventricle. **A,** The variant with a non-committed defect. **B,** The variant with the aorta to left of pulmonary trunk, parallel arterial trunks, and pulmonary stenosis. **C,** The variant with discordant atrioventricular connections and usual atrial arrangement. **D,** The variant with mirror-imaged atrial arrangement and concordant atrioventricular connections.

Specific Anatomy of the Commoner Variants

Subaortic Interventricular Communication, Aorta to Right of Pulmonary Trunk, Spiralling Arterial Trunks, and Pulmonary Stenosis

There can be a complete muscular infundibulum supporting each arterial valve in this variant (Fig. 40-4), although fibrous continuity between the aortic and atrioventricular valves is found in a high proportion of cases (Fig. 40-5). The subpulmonary outflow tract is narrowed, with or without hypoplasia of the infundibulum (see Figs. 40-4 and 40-5). Often the valve is additionally involved. The obstructive lesions are similar to those seen in Fallot's tetralogy. The interventricular communication, cradled within the limbs of the septomarginal trabeculation, is perimembranous in four-fifths (see Figs. 40-4 and 40-5), having a muscular postero-inferior rim in the remainder. This feature has major surgical significance, since the atrioventricular conduction axis is not directly related to the margins of the defect in the presence of the muscular postero-inferior rim, being posterior to it, and hence less vulnerable at operation. In many cases, the aortic valve retains part of its connection within the left ventricle, but as long as most of the aorta is supported by the right ventricle, it is appropriate to diagnose the ventriculo-arterial connection as being double outlet (Fig. 40-6). Important associated lesions may include a restrictive interventricular communication, which in essence represents obstruction of the left ventricular outlet, this occurring in up to one-tenth of cases,[10] and mitral stenosis.

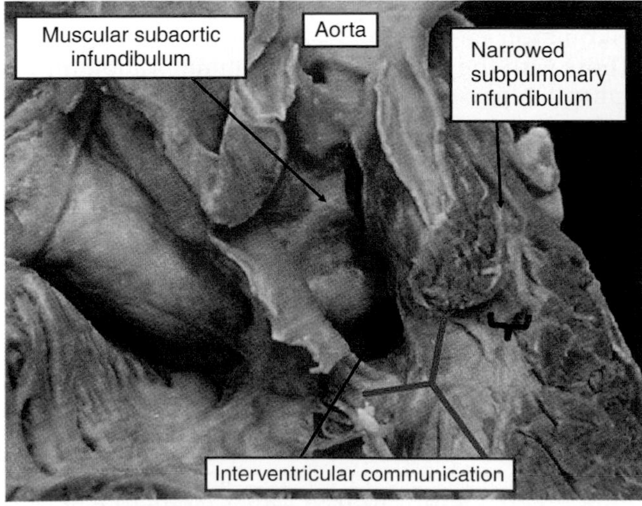

Figure 40-4 In this specimen, both arterial trunks arise from the right ventricle, with each arterial valve supported in its entirety by a complete muscular infundibulum. There is pulmonary stenosis produced by a squeeze (*red bracket*) between the deviated outlet septum and anomalous septoparietal trabeculations, the hallmark of tetralogy of Fallot, but in this instance in combination with double outlet right ventricle. The *yellow Y* shows the septomarginal trabeculation.

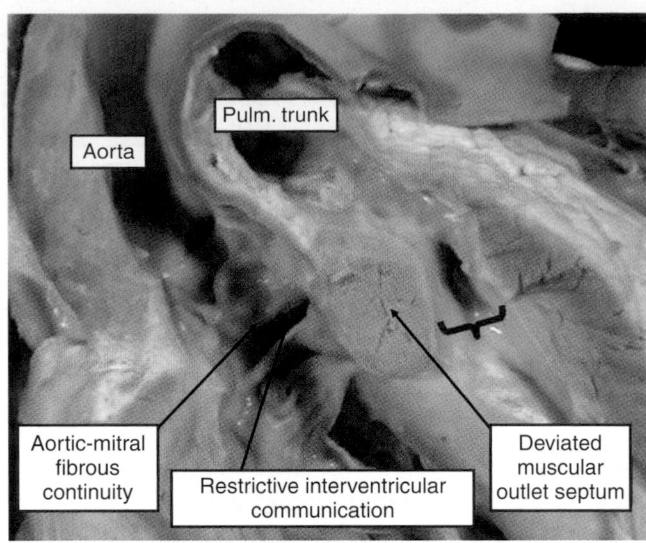

Figure 40-5 This heart also has unequivocal double outlet right ventricle in association with tetralogy of Fallot, the *red bracket* showing the narrowed subpulmonary outflow tract, but in this instance with fibrous continuity between the leaflets of the aortic and mitral valves in the roof of the interventricular communication.

With Subpulmonary Interventricular Communication

These hearts are usually described as the Taussig-Bing malformation, recognising the description of the index case in which the pulmonary trunk, which was unobstructed, lay to the left of the aorta and overrode an interventricular communication.[16] In this initial heart, both arterial valves were supported by complete muscular infundibulums. There has subsequently been much discussion as to the most appropriate use of the term Taussig-Bing anomaly,[11] but in our opinion[17] the term is best used for the spectrum of overriding of the pulmonary trunk in the setting of parallel arterial trunks, with the ends of the spectrum being either double outlet right ventricle (Fig. 40-7) or discordant ventriculo-arterial connections (see Chapter 38). The interventricular communication, again cradled within the limbs of the septomarginal trabeculation, opens beneath the pulmonary trunk because the muscular outlet septum is attached to the ventriculo-infundibular fold. A muscular postero-inferior rim, formed by union of trabeculation and

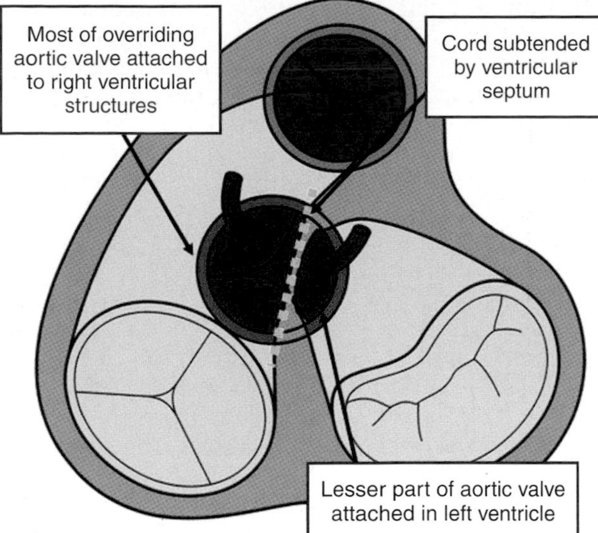

Figure 40-6 The cartoon shows how overriding valves are assigned to one or other ventricle. The short axis is viewed from the cardiac apex. According to the cord subtended by the plane of the ventricular septum relative to the overriding valvar orifice, it can be seen that the greater part of the aortic circumference (*green surround of red circle*) is supported by the right ventricle, with the lesser part (*yellow surround*) remaining in the left ventricle. The effective ventriculo-arterial connection is double outlet right ventricle.

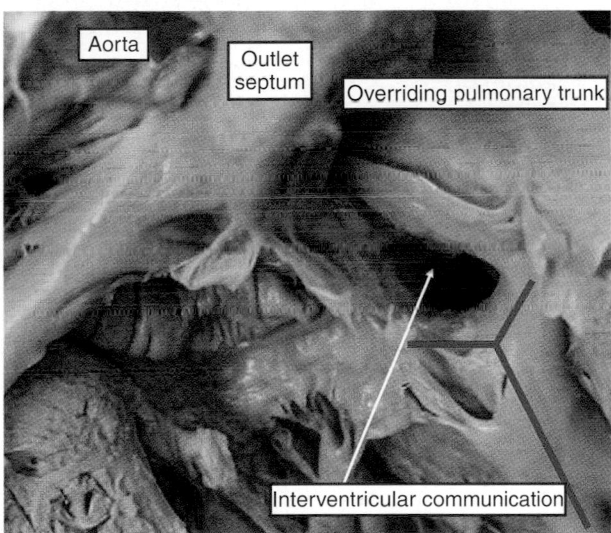

Figure 40-7 This is an example of the so-called Taussig-Bing malformation, with double outlet ventriculo-arterial connections and with an interventricular communication which opens in a subpulmonary position. It is between the limbs of the septomarginal trabeculation (*yellow Y*) because the muscular outlet septum inserts to the ventriculo-infundibular fold. Note that the fold also fuses with the postero-caudal limb of the septomarginal trabeculation, producing a muscular postero-inferior rim to the interventricular communication which protects the atrioventricular conduction axis. In this heart, however, there is fibrous continuity between the leaflets of the mitral and pulmonary valves in the roof of the interventricular communication.

fold in two-fifths of cases, often separates the rim of the defect itself it from the membranous septum (see Fig. 40-7). In three-fifths of cases, nonetheless, the defect extends posteriorly, becoming perimembranous (Fig. 40-8).

Double Outlet Right Ventricle with Subaortic Defect and No Pulmonary Stenosis

This malformation is similar in many anatomical respects to the anomaly with subaortic defect and pulmonary stenosis (compare Figs. 40-9, 40-4, and 40-5). As in the situation

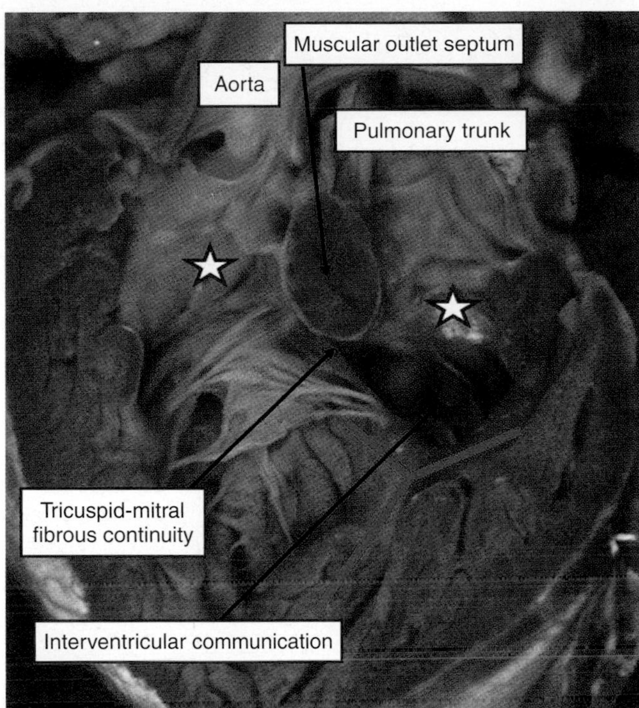

Figure 40-8 In this example of a Taussig-Bing heart with double outlet right ventricle, the interventricular communication extends to become perimembranous. In this example, there are bilateral infundibulums supporting the leaflets of both arterial valves (*stars*). Note again that the interventricular communication is cradled within the limbs of the septomarginal trabeculation (*yellow Y*). This variant of double outlet is seldom associated with pulmonary stenosis. Aortic coarctation, in contrast, is a frequent association, and in autopsied cases is often seen in association with straddling of the mitral valve. The mitral valve can itself also be stenotic, but restriction of the interventricular communication producing left ventricular outlet obstruction is very infrequent.

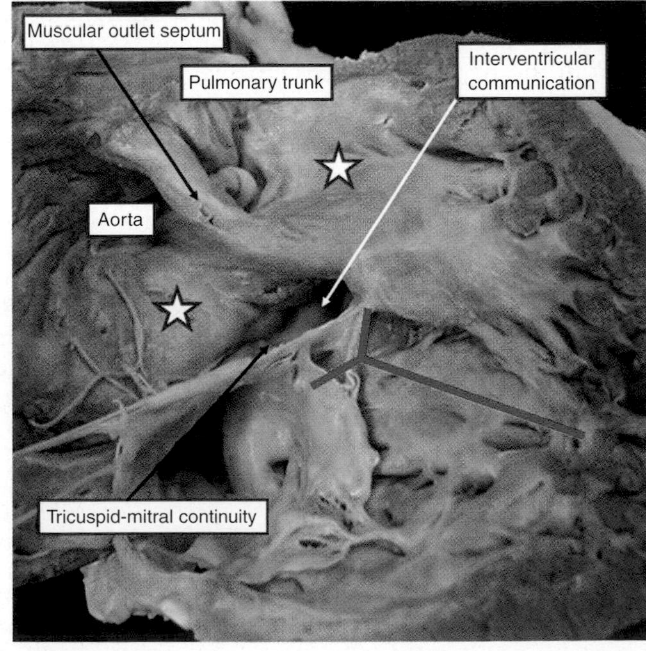

Figure 40-9 This heart has double outlet right ventricle with subaortic interventricular communication, but without subpulmonary stenosis. Note that, despite the presence of bilateral infundibulums (*stars*), the interventricular communication is perimembranous because of the fibrous continuity between the leaflets of the mitral and tricuspid valves. The *yellow Y* shows the septomarginal trabeculation.

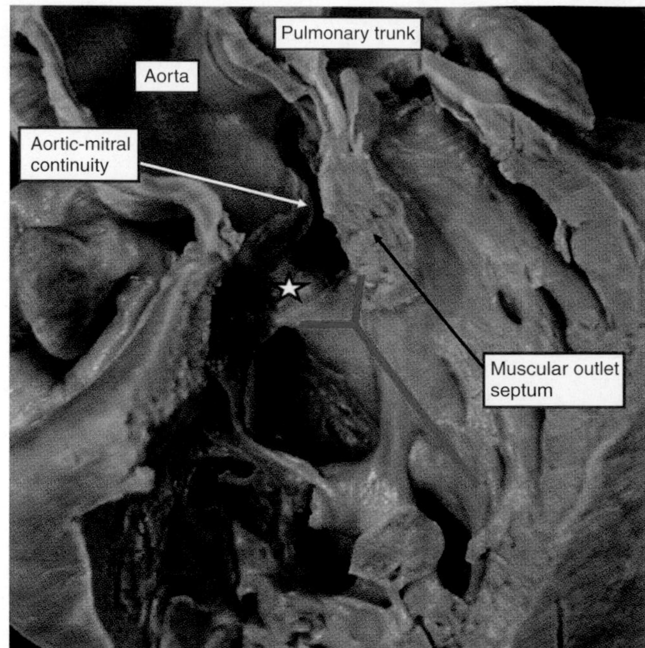

Figure 40-10 The heart again has double outlet with subaortic interventricular communication, but this time with fibrous continuity between the leaflets of the aortic and mitral valves in the roof of the interventricular communication. Note that in this heart there is a muscular postero-inferior rim to the interventricular communication (*star*). The defect itself remains within the limbs of the septomarginal trabeculation (*yellow Y*). Note that part of the aortic valve is attached within the left ventricle.

with a stenotic subpulmonary outlet, there can be bilateral infundibulums (see Fig. 40-9) or fibrous continuity between the leaflets of the aortic and mitral valves. When there are bilateral infundibulums, the arterial valves are usually side by side (see Fig. 40-9), but with fibrous continuity in the roof of the interventricular communication, the aortic valve is typically posterior and to the right of the pulmonary valve. The arterial trunks typically spiral as they exit from the heart. The interventricular communication is usually perimembranous (see Fig. 40-9), though it may have a muscular posterior margin (Fig. 40-10). When there is continuity between the leaflets of the aortic and mitral valves, the aortic root usually retains part of its connection with the left ventricle (see Fig. 40-10). In such instances, assignment of the overriding valve is made on the basis of the short axis of the root, not the long axis of the ventricular septum (see Fig. 40-6). Whilst the ventricular septal defect is often large in this group of cases, restrictive defects may be seen, which effectively produces obstruction to the outflow from the left ventricle, an important clinical consideration.

Other Anatomical Variations

As can be seen in the figures provided thus far, there is much individual variability within the malformations already described. This relates to the site, size and detailed morphology of the interventricular communication, the relationships of the arterial outlets to one another and to the septal defect, and to the frequent presence of additional malformations (see Tables 40-2, 40-3, and 40-4). With regard to the interventricular communication, although it usually extends to become perimembranous, irrespective of the infundibular morphology, a muscular postero-inferior rim is present in a substantial minority of instances (see Table 40-3). Perimembranous defects may extend variably to open towards the inlet and trabecular portions of the right ventricle, as well as opening directly into one or other outlet. Restrictive defects, which produce obstruction to the outlet from the left ventricle, are uncommon, but when present are of obvious clinical and surgical importance. Multiple interventricular communications can be found on occasion.

Abnormalities of the atrioventricular valves are found in up to one-quarter of the hearts seen in autopsied series, and include mitral stenosis and straddling mitral valve. Obstruction to one or other of the arterial outlets occurs frequently. Pulmonary stenosis, when present, is similar to that seen in Fallot's tetralogy, but is infrequent in the setting of the Taussig-Bing heart. Obstruction of the systemic outlet is much more frequent in the latter setting, with interruption of the aortic arch in a significant proportion of these cases. Other major associated malformations include juxtaposition of the atrial appendages, totally anomalous pulmonary venous connection, and criss-cross atrioventricular connections. The frequent variations in coronary arterial anatomy are particularly important in the setting of the Taussig-Bing hearts, since these are now corrected surgically using the arterial switch procedure. Interatrial communications within the oval fossa are also frequent.

Less Common Variants

Non-Committed Interventricular Communication

In about one-tenth of cases seen in autopsied series, the interventricular communication is not directly committed to either arterial outlet. Such defects are usually perimembranous, and open primarily to the inlet of the right ventricle, often in the presence of a common atrioventricular valve (Fig. 40-11). Isolated muscular interventricular communications can also open directly to the inlet or apical parts of the right ventricle, and then also be non-committed (Fig. 40-12). Such non-committed defects are particularly important surgically, and require careful delineation of the relationships of the defect to the arterial outlets and to other structures within the right ventricle, especially abnormal leaflet tissue derived from the tricuspid valve which may interpose between the defect and the arterial outlets.[18]

Doubly Committed Interventricular Communication

In another one-tenth of cases seen in autopsied series, the interventricular communication is positioned so as to open directly into both arterial outlets (Fig. 40-13). As with the majority of the hearts already described, the interventricular communication is cradled between the limbs of the septomarginal trabeculation and is usually perimembranous, although it can have a muscular postero-inferior rim. If the muscular rim is present, it will protect the atrioventricular conduction axis. The essence of these hearts, however, is absence of a muscular outlet septum, with only a fibrous raphe interposing between the leaflets of the arterial valves. This means that both outflow tracts tend to override the crest of the muscular ventricular septum, and a spectrum exists between these hearts and double outlet from the left ventricle. Indeed, the hearts can be considered as showing double outlet from both ventricles (Fig. 40-14).[19]

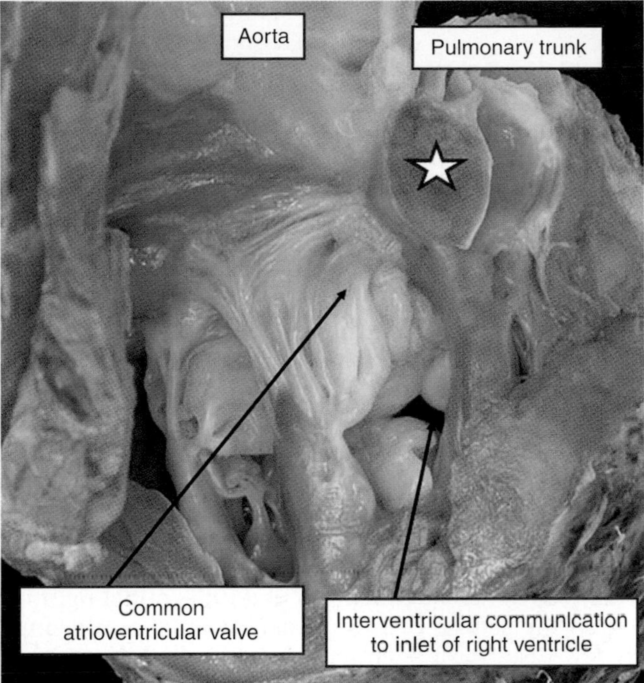

Figure 40-11 The interventricular communication in this heart opens to the inlet of the right ventricle, and hence is non-committed, albeit that a track could be established surgically between the defect and the subaortic infundibulum, which in this instance is a complete muscular tube. There is a common atrioventricular junction. The *star* shows the muscular outlet septum. (Courtesy of Diane Debich-Spicer, All Children's Hopsital, St Petersburg, Florida.)

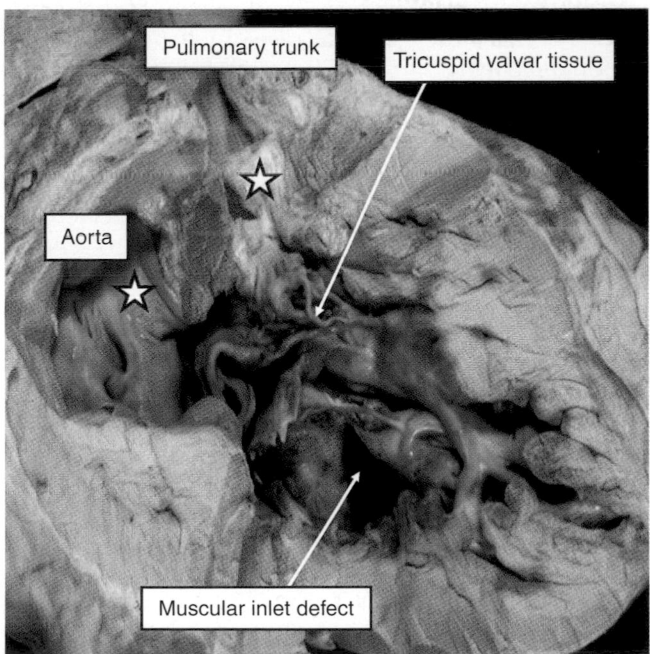

Figure 40-12 The interventricular communication is again non-committed in this heart with double outlet right ventricle and bilateral infundibulums (*stars*), but in this instance because it is a muscular inlet defect. Note that, in this heart, the tension apparatus of the tricuspid valve interposes between the defect and both arterial outlets.

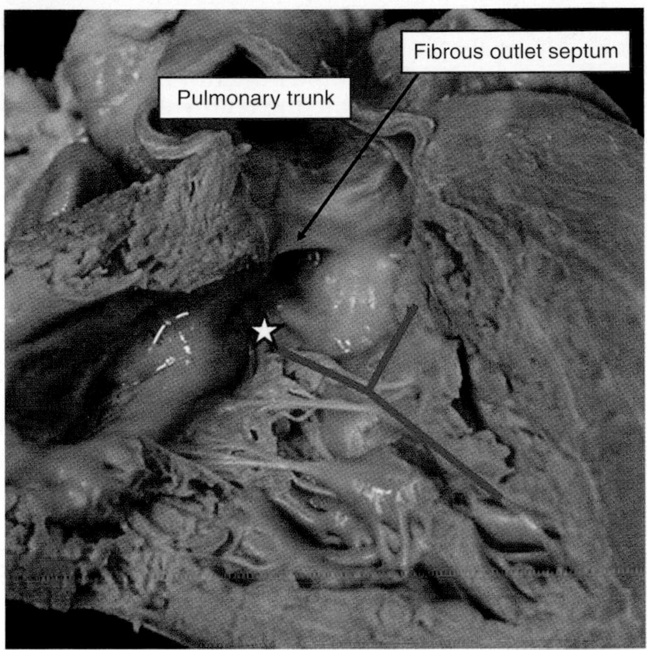

Figure 40-13 In this heart, the outlet septum is fibrous rather than muscular, and produces continuity between the leaflets of the aortic and pulmonary valves. In consequence, the interventricular communication, still between the limbs of the septomarginal trabeculation (*yellow Y*), and with a muscular postero-inferior rim (*star*), opens beneath both arterial outlets.

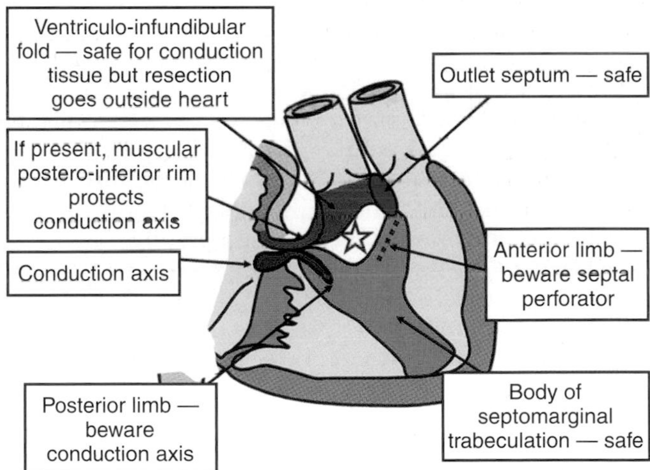

Figure 40-14 The cartoon shows how identification of the muscular structures surrounding the interventricular communication (*star*) in hearts with double outlet right ventricle identifies the potential danger areas during surgical correction.

Consistent Variations in Morphology of the Overall Group

When previous accounts of the structure of the variants of double outlet are examined, the impression is often gained that, when the interventricular communication is in subaortic rather than subpulmonary position, it has moved relative to the muscular ventricular septum. To a certain extent, this must be the case, but when examined relative to the overall landmarks of the muscular ventricular septum, its location is remarkably constant.[20,21] Thus, when the defect opens to the outlet of the right ventricle, be it subaortic subpulmonary, or doubly committed, then always it is found between the limbs of the septomarginal trabeculation. The variation in morphology depends upon the connection of the muscular outlet septum relative to the septomarginal trabeculation. When the septal defect is subaortic (see Fig. 40-4), then the muscular outlet septum is fused with the anterior limb of the trabeculation, as in tetralogy of Fallot. This fusion walls off the subpulmonary outlet from the ventricular septal defect. When the defect is in subpulmonary position, in contrast, the muscular outlet septum is fused either to the posterior limb of the septomarginal trabeculation, or to the ventriculo-infundibular fold (see Fig. 40-7). This walls off the aorta from the septal defect and, almost always, produces a complete muscular subaortic infundibulum. The degree of squeeze between the musuclar outlet septum and the ventriculo-infundibular fold determines the extent of subaortic obstruction. The smaller the subaortic muscular area, the more likely it is that there will be aortic coarctation or interruption. The characteristics of the doubly committed defect (see Fig. 40-13) are that, almost always, the outlet septum is fibrous rather than muscular, and the adjacent portions of the subaortic and subpulmonary infundibulums are absent. Such absence of the outlet septum, and incomplete formation of the subpulmonary infundibulum, is also a characteristic feature of the doubly committed and juxta-arterial ventricular septal defect found with concordant ventriculo-arterial connections (see Chapter 28). The interrelationships of the muscular structures around the interventricular communication (see Fig. 40-12) condition other important anatomic features of double outlet. Thus, the size of the ventriculo-infundibular folds determines the extent of the subarterial infundibulums. When the folds are extensive, then long infundibulums are found supporting both arterial valves (see Fig. 40-9). In contrast, when the fold is attenuated beneath each arterial valve, then there is atrioventricular-arterial valvar fibrous continuity (see Fig. 40-10), but still with double outlet ventriculo-arterial connection. It is then the relationship between the posterior limb of the septomarginal trabeculation and the ventriculo-infundibular fold which determines whether the ventricular septal defect is perimembranous (see Fig. 40-9) or has a muscular postero-inferior rim (see Fig. 40-10). All of these anatomical details are, nowadays, readily demonstrated using cross sectional echocardiography.

Double Outlet Right Ventricle with Intact Ventricular Septum

When the ventricular septum is intact, which can occur rarely in a patient with double outlet right ventricle, the left ventricle has no direct outlet, and in these circumstances is usually severely hypoplastic.

Subaortic Interventricular Communication with Left-Sided Aorta

The key point in diagnosing this variant is that, despite the aorta being left sided, the heart exhibits usual atrial arrangement with concordant atrioventricular connections. The lesions were of more significance when arguments raged concerning the significance of the so-called loop rule, left-sided aortas being presumed only to exist with left hand ventricular topology when there was the usual atrial arrangement. Nowadays there is no problem in defining with precision the atrial arrangement and the atrioventricular connections, and in recognising the left-sided location of the aorta. The interventricular communication is typically subaortic, although it can be subpulmonary or doubly committed. Infundibular morphology is also variable. The usual subaortic location of the interventricular communication makes surgical repair relatively easy,[22] although the presence of a coronary artery passing anteriorly relative to the subpulmonary outlet can complicate the situation in the presence of pulmonary stenosis, which may be both valvar and subvalvar. When encountered, left juxtaposition of the atrial appendages is frequent, as is straddling mitral valve.[22,23]

Double Outlet Right Ventricle with Discordant Atrioventricular Connections

This complex malformation has been described in association with both usual and mirror-image atrial arrangements. When seen, many patients with usual atrial arrangement have their hearts placed in the right chest, while those with mirror-imaged atriums have left-sided hearts. Pulmonary stenosis was present in four-fifths of the largest reported series,[24] with the interventricular communication being subpulmonary more frequently than subaortic. Despite the discordant atrioventricular connections, there was marked variability in the relationships of the great arteries, with the aorta to the left of the pulmonary trunk in only two-thirds of cases. This variant of double outlet right ventricle has much in common with congenitally corrected transposition, and is discussed further in Chapter 39.

Double Outlet Right Ventricle with Either Mirror-Imaged Atrial Arrangement or Isomeric Atrial Appendages

We have already made mention of double outlet right ventricle in the setting of mirror-imaged atrial arrangement. Very few cases have been reported, but the same variability must be anticipated as for double outlet right ventricle when found with usual atrial arrangement. Double outlet right ventricle is much more frequent in the presence of isomeric atrial appendages, being particularly common in the overall group of patients having isomeric right appendages. In the syndromes of isomerism, of course, variability occurs at all levels of the heart (see Chapter 22). This means that the complexity and multiplicity of the malformations seen in the presence of isomerism with double outlet right ventricle may be expected to be extreme. One combination in particular deserves mention, that of biventricular and mixed atrioventricular connections and a common atrioventricular orifice.[25] This combination is found with both right and left isomerism, and with either right hand or left hand ventricular topologies. The interventricular communication opens to the inlet of the right ventricle, and usually there are bilateral infundibulums. As shown in Figure 40-11, nonetheless, it is often possible to construct a tunnel between the interventricular communication and the subaortic outlet, so providing the associated malformations are not too severe, biventricular repair remains a possibility.

Double Outlet Left Ventricle

Because of the rarity of this malformation, pathological, clinical, or surgical series of any size have rarely been reported from individual institutions. Moreover, reviews of the subject, and reports of individual cases, have frequently included material relating to functionally univentricular hearts.[26–28] The largest review of which we are aware collected a total of 100 cases, with biventricular atrioventricular connections in four-fifths. The reviews reveal that, as might be expected, double outlet left ventricle most commonly occurs in hearts with usual atrial arrangement and concordant atrioventricular connections, making up nine-tenths of the series. Discordant atrioventricular connections with usual atrial arrangement were noted in one-twentieth of cases, and mirror-imaged atrial chambers were reported in the remaining cases, albeit that no mention was made of isomeric atrial appendages. Variability, as with double outlet right ventricle, depends on the site of the interventricular communication, its relationship to the subarterial outlets, and the relationships of the arterial trunks. Infundibular morphology has also varied dramatically, albeit that bilaterally deficient infundibulums are more frequently found with double outlet left ventricle than in any other situation. This arrangement, nonetheless, does not occur in the majority of cases, the commonest finding being a subpulmonary infundibulum with fibrous continuity between the leaflets of the aortic and mitral valves. Associated abnormalities are the rule rather than the exception. A particularly high frequency of obstruction in the pulmonary outflow tract is found when the interventricular communication is subaortic. Those with a subpulmonary defect have a high incidence of systemic obstruction, usually coarctation, with about half the reported cases being thus affected. As might be expected, there is a low incidence of pulmonary obstruction when the defect is subpulmonary. Anomalies of the atrioventricular valves occur in up to one-third of cases, and include hypoplasia, stenosis, straddling and Ebstein-like malformations. The tricuspid valve is more often abnormal than the mitral. Hypoplasia of the right ventricle is also a frequent finding. As with double outlet right ventricle, therefore, extreme heterogeneity exists. It is doubtful whether it is justifiable to seek to make groupings or categories. Each reported type is individually extremely rare, and is subject to a host of associated defects and problems. It is these features that dominate the clinical picture, and determine the surgical options.

In each case, therefore, the problem should be analysed in the same logical sequence required for any complex defect. Investigation and categorisation need to be individualised, with each patient having his or her defects systematically documented in terms of atrial arrangement, atrioventricular connection, morphology of the interventricular communication and its relationship to the outlets, arterial relations, obstruction to the ventricular outlets, atrioventricular valvar abnormalities, and other associated malformations.

MORPHOGENESIS

During early embryonic development, the outflow tract of the heart arises exclusively from the developing right ventricle. For the embryo, therefore, double outlet right ventricle can be considered the default option. Only as the ventricular septum closes does the subaortic outflow tract become connected to the left ventricle (see Chapter 3). In order for this process to occur normally, it is necessary that certain earlier cardiac developmental processes have taken place in their correct sequence. These include formation of the ventricular loop and the development, in appropriate orientation, of the primordiums of the components of the ventricular septum. Errors in these, and other, phases of early cardiac development may profoundly affect subsequent morphogenesis involving the orientation and calibre of the outflow tracts and the ventriculo-arterial connections.

In hearts with double outlet right ventricle, the only universal feature is failure of complete incorporation of either of the arterial outflow tracts into the left ventricle. In many cases, an additional feature is the persistence of a muscular infundibulum in both subarterial outlets, associated with lack of attenuation of the ventriculo-infundibular fold in the area between the atrioventricular and arterial valvar leaflets. In these cases, atrioventricular-arterial valvar fibrous continuity is not found. In addition, the muscular outlet septum remains an exclusively right ventricular structure, being malaligned, to a greater or lesser degree, relative to the apical part of the muscular septum.

The fundamental cause of the embryological error or errors leading to double outlet right ventricle remains unclear. In the experimental situation, double outlet right ventricle has been created in chick embryos by placing a loop around the infundibulum prior to its septation, thus preventing it from migrating and attenuating in the normal sequence.[29] The relevance of these experimental data, however, to the naturally occurring malformation remains uncertain. It has now transpired that many genetically modified mice develop double outlet right ventricle, or else common arterial trunk arising exclusively from the right ventricle. It is also the case that examples are now encountered with the interventricular communication in both subaortic and subpulmonary positions.

This achieves significance, since it has long been recognised that, in terms of their pathological features, many hearts with double outlet right ventricle are very similar to specimens of Fallot's tetralogy, while others bear a strong resemblance to those having discordant ventriculo-arterial connections with ventricular septal defect. It was Lev and his colleagues[30] who first proposed the presence of a pathological continuum from, on the one hand, Fallot's tetralogy to double outlet right ventricle with subaortic defect and, on the other hand, from double outlet right ventricle with subpulmonary defect to discordant ventriculo-arterial connections with ventricular septal defect, a concept then supported by others who studied congenitally malformed hearts.[31,32] All these workers took the view that these malformations were related to maldevelopment of the infundibulums, the experimental work now providing validation of this concept.

In double outlet left ventricle, both outflow tracts are incorporated into the left ventricle. This is associated with exaggerated leftward shift of the arterial valves in relation to the ventricular septum. While this is sometimes associated with attenuation of the infundibular muscle below each arterial valve, producing bilaterally deficient infundibulums, this is by no means the rule. Leftward shift of the arterial valves relative to the ventricular septum, therefore, is not dependent on absorption and shortening of the infundibulums.

PATHOPHYSIOLOGY

The pathophysiology of double outlet ventricle is complex, being determined by the site of the interventricular communication relative to the arterial outlets, the presence of obstruction to either the pulmonary or systemic outlet, the pulmonary vascular resistance, and the presence of other associated cardiac defects.

The overall effect is largely determined by the flow of blood to the lungs, the presence or absence of pulmonary hypertension, and the effect of streaming within the ventricle supporting the arterial trunks. An additional important factor may be the presence of associated aortic coarctation, which, as well as producing an increase in systemic afterload, is liable to lead to hypoperfusion of the lower systemic segment after ductal closure, resulting in renal impairment and acute retention of fluids. This usually leads to severe symptoms and rapidly progressive cardiac failure in the neonatal period.

Flow of Blood to the Lungs

Pulmonary flow is related to the presence and severity of pulmonary stenosis, be it valvar or subvalvar, and to the level of pulmonary resistance. Pulmonary arterial pressure and resistance are frequently normal or low in the presence of significant stenosis. Pulmonary flow is then also restricted, sometimes to markedly subnormal levels. Diminished flow is inevitably associated with reduced arterial saturation of oxygen, though the degree of systemic hypoxia is also dependent on the effects of streaming. In the absence of pulmonary stenosis, the systolic pressure in the pulmonary trunk is usually equal to systemic pressure. Flow is then dependent on the level of pulmonary vascular resistance. The behaviour of the pulmonary vasculature, in the presence of pulmonary hypertension, is similar to that observed in the presence of other congenital cardiac defects. In the early months of life pulmonary resistance drops at a variable, though reduced, rate from the neonatal level. During this period, the flow of blood to the lungs increases progressively. Subsequently, sustained pulmonary hypertension leads to the development of obliterative pulmonary vascular disease,[33,34] with rising pulmonary vascular resistance, until eventually flow may fall to subnormal levels. Increased flow tends to be associated with less severe systemic hypoxia though, again, the effects of streaming are important in determining the arterial tensions and saturations of oxygen.

Effects of Streaming

In the presence of a subaortic interventricular communication, left ventricular blood tends to be directed predominantly to the aorta when both trunks arise from the right ventricle. This results physiologically in a situation resembling that seen with a simple ventricular septal defect with concordant ventriculo-arterial connections. In the absence of pulmonary stenosis, little or no right-to-left shunting may be seen, with the blood in the aorta being almost fully saturated in many patients. When pulmonary stenosis co-exists, some right-to-left shunting is almost always found and the extent of this, and of the associated systemic hypoxia, is related closely to the degree of obstruction. The physiology, as also the morphology, in this situation tends often to resemble closely that found in Fallot's tetralogy. In a minority of patients with a subaortic defect, these effects of streaming are not seen, and in some the reverse may be the case, with lower saturation of oxygen in the aorta than in the pulmonary trunk.[25,35]

When the interventricular communication is subpulmonary, the aorta is perfused preferentially with deoxygenated systemic venous blood. The physiology resembles that of transposition and, as in that condition, the degree of systemic hypoxia is dependent on the adequacy of mixing between blood in the systemic and pulmonary circuits. As the situation with double outlet tends to be associated with fairly good mixing in most cases, hypoxia may not be severe and the high flow of blood to the lungs seen in most patients also militates against the development of severe hypoxia.

Streaming can be variable when the interventricular communication is either non-committed or doubly committed. In such cases, some degree of systemic hypoxia is almost invariable, and the main determinant of its severity is the degree of pulmonary stenosis.

Influence of Other Associated Defects

Mention has already been made of the serious effects which aortic coarctation may have on the pathophysiology. Many of the common associated defects may also affect the situation to a variable extent. Common atrioventricular orifice, and straddling mitral valve, probably reduce the effects of streaming, which are otherwise often seen. Hypoplasia, stenosis, or atresia of an atrioventricular valve may produce dramatic haemodynamic consequences, though mitral stenosis may produce surprisingly little effect if pulmonary blood flow is low due to associated pulmonary stenosis. A restrictive interventricular communication produces pressure loading of the left ventricle, which consequently becomes hypertrophied, but apart from elevated left ventricular pressure the haemodynamics are usually not greatly affected, unless the obstruction to flow from the left ventricle results in left atrial hypertension, with resulting pulmonary venous congestion and so on.

CLINICAL FINDINGS

Presentation

The clinical features of infants with double outlet ventriculo-arterial connection are extremely variable and may mimic those of many other defects. Those patients with double outlet right ventricle, subaortic defect, and pulmonary stenosis usually present a clinical picture which resembles that of Fallot's tetralogy. A systolic murmur is sometimes noted in the neonatal period, but the onset of cyanosis may be delayed for several months. Patients with double outlet right ventricle and subpulmonary defect, on the other hand, usually develop cyanosis in the neonatal period, though the cyanosis may not be severe. Cardiac failure, developing later in the first month of life or subsequently, with tachypnoea, dyspnoea, and failure to feed and thrive, compounds the picture. The appearance of severe cyanosis in the neonatal period is usually a reflection of the presence of severe pulmonary stenosis or atresia with very low flow to the lungs. Such a presentation is sometimes seen in those patients with the Fallot-type of double outlet, but is also seen in more complex defects, especially those with isomerism. Onset of symptoms of cardiac failure, but without cyanosis, at the end of the first month or in the second and third months of life, is typical of those cases with a subaortic defect and no pulmonary stenosis. This clinical picture resembles that of a large isolated ventricular septal defect.

Early onset of cardiac failure is particularly a feature of those cases with associated aortic coarctation or interruption of the aortic arch. A small proportion of patients do not present in early infancy, but are detected later in the first year of life, or rarely even later in childhood. Whilst some such patients may have features similar to a late presenting Fallot's tetralogy, others have evidence of severe pulmonary hypertension. They resemble more the child with a large ventricular septal defect, pulmonary hypertension, and elevated pulmonary resistance who has survived without developing cardiac failure in infancy. Data from the Hospital for Sick Children in Toronto showed that the majority of patients with double outlet right ventricle in all categories presented in the first two months of life, except for those with a subaortic defect and pulmonary stenosis, who usually presented later.[36]

The presenting features of double outlet left ventricle are similarly extremely variable. They do not permit distinction from double outlet right ventricle, or many other defects, on purely clinical grounds.

Physical Signs

The physical signs in double outlet ventricle vary with the clinical presentation and underlying pathology. Manifestations of cardiac failure in early infancy, with or without cyanosis, are usually indicative of high pulmonary flow and pulmonary hypertension. When such features appear in the first week or two of life, they are usually associated with major, or often multiple, associated defects such as aortic coarctation. Such infants usually have a hyperdynamic cardiac impulse with a parasternal systolic murmur of moderate amplitude, which often radiates fairly widely, particularly to the pulmonary area and the back. The second heart sound is usually loud, though this is often due to the aortic component, which, as in those with transposition, may be accentuated.

In the absence of cardiac failure an ejection systolic murmur varying between grades 2 and 4 of 6 may be audible along the left sternal border and in the pulmonary area, with radiation to the back. This is usually related to infundibular and/or valvar pulmonary stenosis. As in Fallot's tetralogy, the pulmonary component of the second sound is often inaudible. Cyanosis is variable, and may not appear for several months. An apical mid-diastolic murmur is occasionally heard and may reflect high pulmonary flow or associated mitral stenosis. A restrictive interventricular communication is associated with a harsh parasternal systolic murmur and a forceful apical impulse, on palpation, due to left ventricular hypertrophy. The murmur from a restrictive defect may be masked if there is associated infundibular stenosis.

Electrocardiography

Early reports[37–39] of the electrocardiogram in double outlet right ventricle suggested that certain features were of predictive diagnostic value. These included a superior frontal plane QRS axis with a counterclockwise vector loop in the presence of right ventricular hypertrophy. This pattern was said to be particularly frequent in cases with a subaortic defect but without pulmonary stenosis. Delay of atrioventricular conduction, especially first-degree block, was found to be very common, and intraventricular disturbances of conduction, especially right bundle branch block, were also frequent. Some degree of left ventricular hypertrophy in the presence of severe right ventricular hypertrophy was also found in a high proportion of cases, and was right atrial hypertrophy.[39] Subsequent investigators,[40] however, were unable to confirm that these electrocardiographic features were of any great diagnostic value.

The most consistent electrocardiographic features in the commoner types of double outlet right ventricle are the presence of right ventricular hypertrophy, right-axis deviation, and the presence of an rR′, qR, or rsR′ pattern in right chest leads. The duration of the QRS complex is normal in most patients. Right atrial hypertrophy is common, and bi-atrial or pure left atrial hypertrophy is seen in a minority of cases. The presence of left atrial hypertrophy or left ventricular hypertrophy has not been shown to correlate well with the haemodynamics.[40] In two cases of our own, however, left atrial hypertrophy and diminished R waves in right chest leads were present in association with a restrictive ventricular septal defect and mitral valvar abnormalities.

Chest Radiography

Radiological features in double outlet right ventricle depend mainly on the associated malformations and are seldom of any diagnostic value. Atrial arrangement, as indicated by bronchial morphology on a penetrated or filter film, is usual in most instances. Cardiac position is variable, though the approximately nine-tenths of patients with the more common types have left-sided hearts. A right aortic arch was seen in up to one-third of cases with a subaortic defect and pulmonary stenosis,[36] and is occasionally present in other types.

Cardiomegaly of significant degree is, in general, associated with increased pulmonary flow. It is, therefore, an almost universal feature of cases with an unobstructed pulmonary outflow tract. Patients with pulmonary stenosis, on the other hand, frequently have little or no increase in cardiac diameter. Pulmonary oligaemia or plethora are again related to the presence or absence of significant pulmonary stenosis. The cardiac contour may mimic Fallot's tetralogy, large ventricular septal defect, or transposition with ventricular septal defect. No diagnostic characteristics are demonstrable. A straight right heart border is seen in some patients with left juxtaposition of the atrial appendages. The site and size of the interventricular communication have little influence on the radiological appearances.

Echocardiography

M-mode echocardiography[41] was used in the early era of cardiac ultrasound to assess mitral-arterial valvar discontinuity and the degree of overriding of the arterial valve over the septum. Since such echocardiographic discontinuity can occur in a variety of other situations, including left ventricular dilation,[42,43] and the exact connection of the arteries to the right or left ventricle is impossible to assess accurately, the inference that double outlet right ventricle might be present was frequently incorrect.

Cross sectional echocardiography has a vitally important role in the comprehensive investigation of the patient with double outlet right ventricle. Not only may the diagnosis of double outlet be made with a high degree of certainty, but the relationship of the interventricular communication to the arterial outlets, the presence of arterial outlet narrowing or obstruction, and the co-existence of important associated defects, especially those of the atrioventricular valves, such as common atrioventricular orifice or straddling mitral valve, may all be documented.

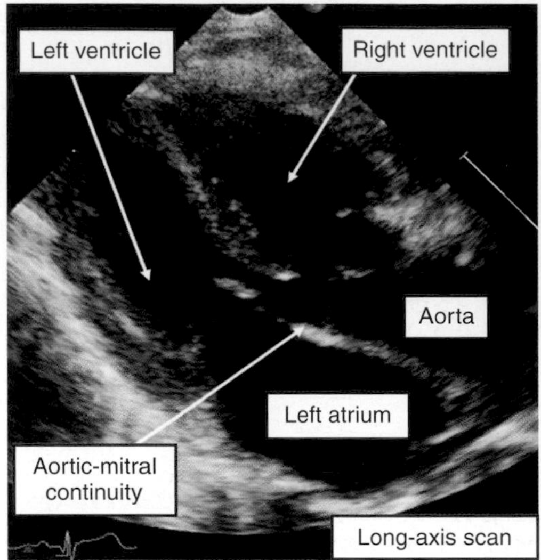

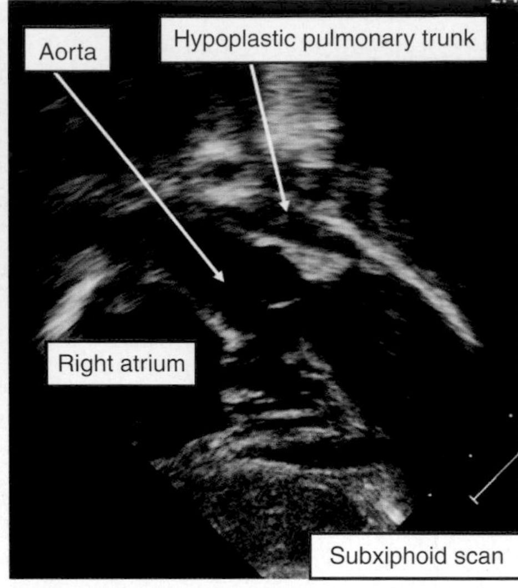

Figure 40-15 The echocardiogram in the long-axis view (*left panel*) is from a patient with the tetralogy type of double outlet right ventricle, with the subxiphoid view shown in the right panel. The aorta arises predominantly from the right ventricle, though the degree of overriding appears greater in the long-axis view. There is mitral-aortic fibrous continuity shown in long-axis view.

The diagnosis has been made on fetal echocardiography in an increasing number of cases in the last few years and is often fairly straightfoward using views which permit assessment of the arterial outlets.[44] Using such techniques, accurate planning of surgical management and appropriate counselling of parents is often possible prior to delivery.

In the postnatal period, the diagnosis of double outlet right ventricle may be suspected in the long-axis view by demonstrating that both great arteries arise predominantly or entirely from the right ventricle, and that the only exit for the left ventricle is a ventricular septal defect.[45,46] Assignment of the ventricular origin of each artery requires assessment in several different cuts, and the long-axis view can be misleading if used in isolation (Fig. 40-15). Discontinuity between the septal leaflet of the mitral valve and the leaflets of the arterial valves may be seen when present, but does not, in itself, establish the diagnosis, as it may be present in other malformations. Moreover mitral-arterial valvar continuity is characteristically present in Fallot's tetralogy, even when the aorta arises predominantly from the right ventricle. The degree of overriding of one or both great arteries over the ventricular septal crest can be assessed, using a combination of long-axis, short-axis, apical and subcostal views. In most cases, the ventricular origin of each arterial trunk can be established with a high degree of accuracy, and true distinguished from spurious overriding. A combination of long-axis and serial short-axis views is also helpful,[45,47] and subcostal short and long-axis scans (Fig. 40-16) have been used extensively.[48] Subcostal views are also helpful in analysing the relationships of the atrioventricular valves and their tension apparatus to the defect. Of particular importance in this respect, and particularly common, are abnormalities of insertion of the tricuspid valvar tension apparatus such that the pathway from the interventricular communication to one or both outflow tracts is impeded. This information may be of crucial importance to the surgeon. The views which give this information, however, may be misleading in assessing the extent of overriding of a great artery. This feature is probably better judged using parasternal long- and short-axis cuts.

The interrelationship of the great arteries and their relative sizes is usually readily demonstrable, as is the presence of valvar or subvalvar obstruction (Figs. 40-16 and 40-17). Particular questions which are of surgical relevance, and which can be answered by cross sectional echocardiography,

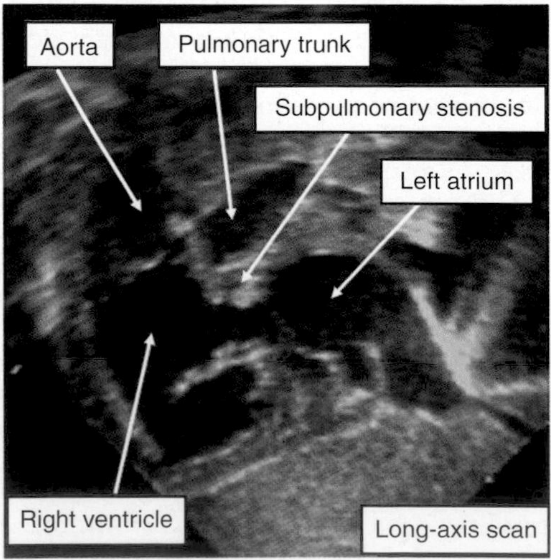

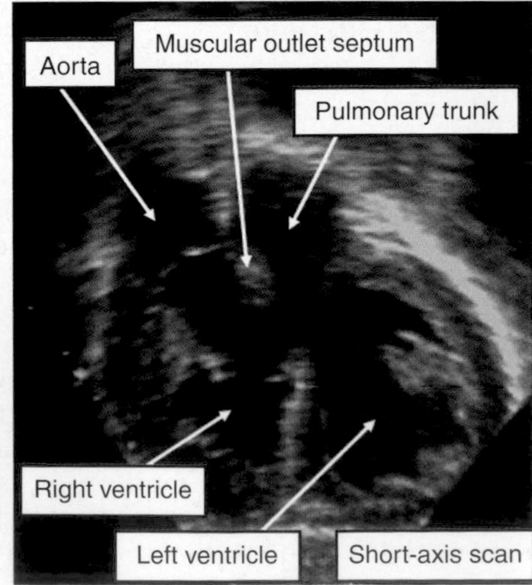

Figure 40-16 The echocardiograms show subxiphoid views in two patients with double outlet right ventricle with subpulmonary interventricular communications. The left panel shows a long-axis scan and demonstrates subpulmonary stenosis. In the right panel (short axis), the anatomy is that of the Taussig-Bing anomaly, with an overriding pulmonary valve and no obstruction to pulmonary flow, but mild subaortic stenosis.

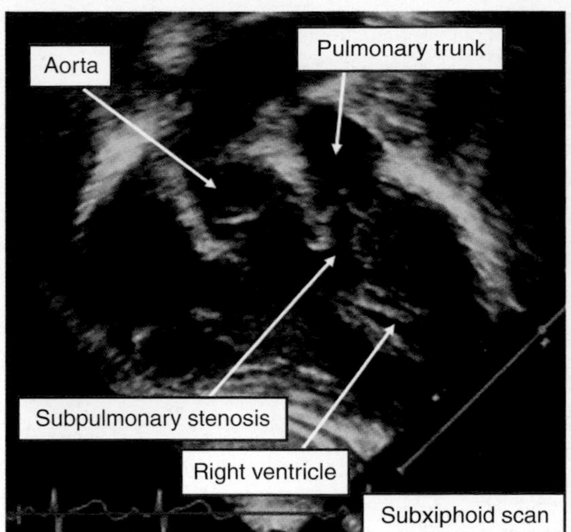

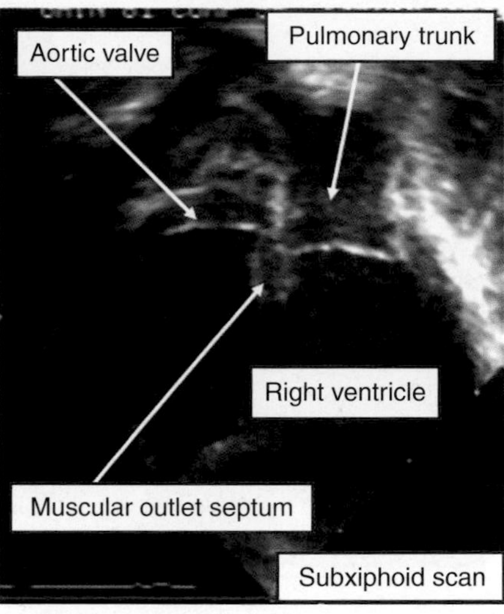

Figure 40-17 The echocardiograms show short-axis subxiphoid views in two patients with double outlet right ventricle with side-by-side arteries. The left panel demonstrates subpulmonary stenosis, while in the right panel there is no obstruction.

include the anatomy of the outlet septum, the anatomy of the roof of the interventricular communication, the relationships of atrioventricular valvar tension apparatus to the septal defect, and demonstration of which arterial outlet is most closely adjacent to the defect.[48] In addition to these features, which may be difficult to define by other means such as angiocardiography, echocardiography is of particular value in establishing the presence of major atrioventricular valvar abnormalities, such as a common atrioventricular orifice or straddling of the mitral or tricuspid valve across the septum.[46] Other associated malformations, such as hypoplasia of the left or right ventricle, juxtaposition of the atrial appendages, coarctation of the aorta and interruption of the aortic arch, may also be demonstrable echocardiographically. Doppler echocardiography is primarily of value in assessing obstructive lesions and atrioventricular valvar regurgitation. Colour flow mapping is especially helpful in regard to the latter problem.

Cardiac Catheterisation and Angiocardiography

Cardiac catheterisation and angiography were, in the past, the mainstay of diagnosis of these malformations. With improvements in non-invasive imaging, especially echocardiography, the role of cardiac catheterisation has diminished, and many patients will now be referred for surgery without catheterisation. When catheterisation is performed, the investigator must keep in mind two particular objectives. The first is the anatomy of the ventriculo-arterial connection, along with the relationships of the interventricular communication. The second is to assess all surgically important aspects of the malformation. In most cases, if appropriate preliminary investigations have been performed, the atrial arrangement, atrioventricular connections and ventriculo-arterial connection will all be known prior to catheterisation. The bulk of the data required from cardiac catheterisation, therefore, relates to the surgically important aspects of the defect. In obtaining haemodynamic data, special attention must be paid to assessing any systolic pressure gradient between left and right ventricles, which would suggest a restrictive septal defect, or any diastolic pressure gradient across the mitral valve. It is essential to gain access to the left side of the heart, either via the interventricular communication or at the atrial level, using trans-septal puncture if necessary.

Information concerning the relationship of the interventricular communication to the arterial outlets may be provided by the behaviour of the catheter, such as easy passage of a retrograde aortic catheter to the left ventricle suggesting a subaortic defect, or from an assessment of streaming. Haemodynamics resembling those of a large ventricular septal defect, or of Fallot's tetralogy, in both of which aortic saturation exceeds that in the pulmonary trunk, suggest a subaortic defect. By contrast, a higher saturation in the pulmonary trunk than in the aorta is usually indicative of a subpulmonary defect.

Measurement of pulmonary arterial pressure, and calculation of the flow and resistance, is mandatory in patients outside of infancy. The presence of pulmonary hypertension at systemic level, indicating absence of obstruction to the subpulmonary outlet, should always raise the suspicion of obstruction to the systemic outlet. A careful search should then be made for subaortic or aortic stenosis, and for aortic coarctation or interruption. The presence of pulmonary stenosis, on the other hand, makes it unlikely that any obstruction to the systemic outlet will be present.

Angiocardiography should include selective left and right ventriculograms (Fig. 40-18). The left ventriculogram should be carried out in a view designed to profile the ventricular septum, such as 45 degrees left anterior oblique inclination, with some craniocaudal tilt. The precise orientation must be assessed individually, and depends on the cardiac position and preliminary echocardiographic evidence. This view is intended to show the site and size of the interventricular communication or communications, and its relationship to the arterial outlets (Fig. 40-19). The presence of a common atrioventricular orifice, or overriding mitral valve, may also be demonstrated. The presence of mitral regurgitation may be assessed in the complementary right anterior oblique plane if biplane angiography is used.

Right ventriculography may be performed in a similar oblique projection, although frontal and lateral views may also be useful. This will normally demonstrate the relationship of the arterial outlets to one another, and the presence and nature of obstructive lesions in either outflow tract (see Fig. 40-18). The separation of the aortic valve from the

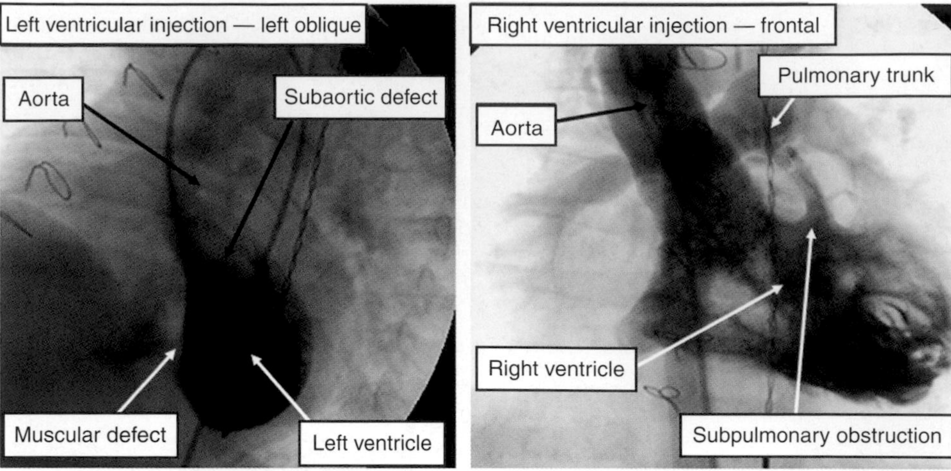

Figure 40-18 The left ventricular angiogram in left oblique projection (*left panel*) shows a muscular interventricular communication in addition to the subaortic defect. The right ventricular angiogram from the same patient, seen in antero-posterior projection (*right panel*), demonstrates infundibular stenosis of the tetralogy type.

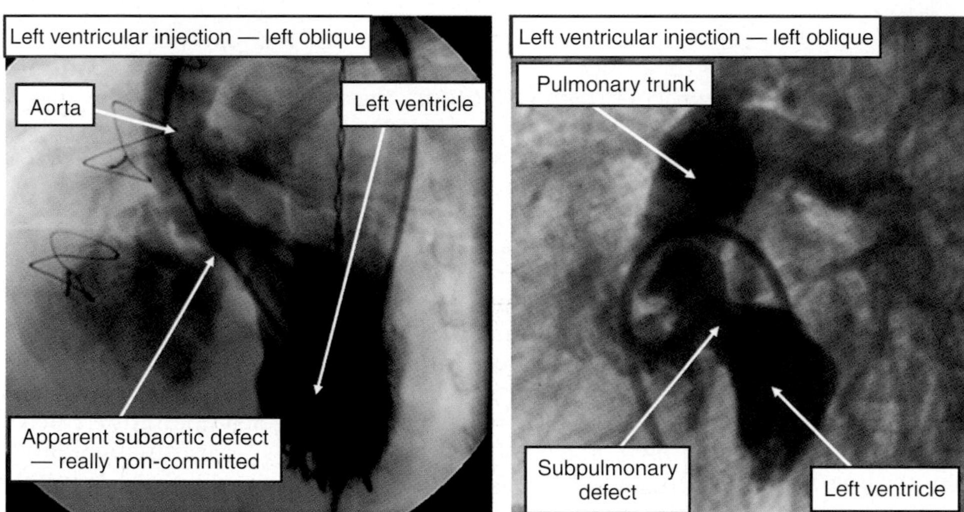

Figure 40-19 The left ventricular angiogram in left oblique prjection (*left panel*) shows an interventricular communication which appears to be subaortic, but which in reality is non-committed. The right panel shows a subpulmonary interventricular communication with streaming of left ventricular flow to the pulmonary trunk. The aorta fills very faintly in this angiogram.

mitral valve may also be assessed, usually using a left ventricular angiogram in oblique projections with appropriate cranio-caudal angulation (Fig. 40-20).

In patients with unobstructed pulmonary flow, a selective aortogram is often desirable, profiled in frontal and lateral projections, to demonstrate or confirm the presence of aortic coarctation or interruption. Those with pulmonary stenosis may require selective pulmonary arteriography with 30 degrees craniocaudal tilt in the frontal projection to define the anatomy of the pulmonary trunk and its bifurcation. In all cases, the investigator must bear in mind the high frequency of associated malformations, and take whatever steps are necessary to define them or exclude them. In cases where radical reconstruction of the pulmonary outflow tract, with or without a conduit, or an arterial switch operation is contemplated, it may be desirable to define the coronary arterial anatomy by aortography, or by selective coronary arteriograms.

Computed Tomography and Magnetic Resonance Imaging

Even with conventional angiography and echocardiography, it may be difficult to determine the precise relationship of the great arteries to the interventricular communication. Recent work with computed tomography and magnetic resonance imaging suggests that these modalities of investigation may provide useful additional information. The ability to generate cross sectional images in almost any spatial plane may be of considerable assistance in clarifying the anatomy of these complex hearts.[49,50] Unfortunately intracardiac anatomy remains more difficult to assess in detail with these methods, and echocardiography, including the burgeoning three-dimensional modality, may continue to provide the most reliable means of assessment, at least in the short-term future.

DIFFERENTIAL DIAGNOSIS

As will be apparent from the foregoing description, the clinical picture, along with the radiographic and electrocardiographic features, are very variable and non-specific. Double outlet may mimic many cardiac lesions. Those forms that do not include pulmonary stenosis may, when acyanotic, closely resemble a large isolated ventricular septal defect. In the presence of cyanosis, the picture may simulate that of transposition with a ventricular septal defect, or other cyanotic defects with high pulmonary flow. Co-existing coarctation may lead to the early development of cardiac failure, producing a clinical picture which resembles other

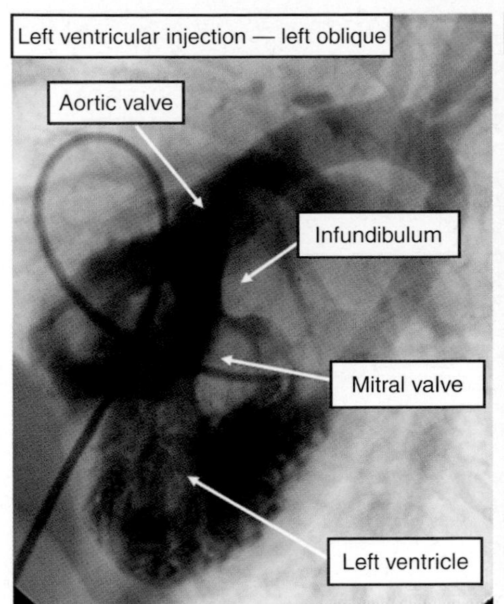

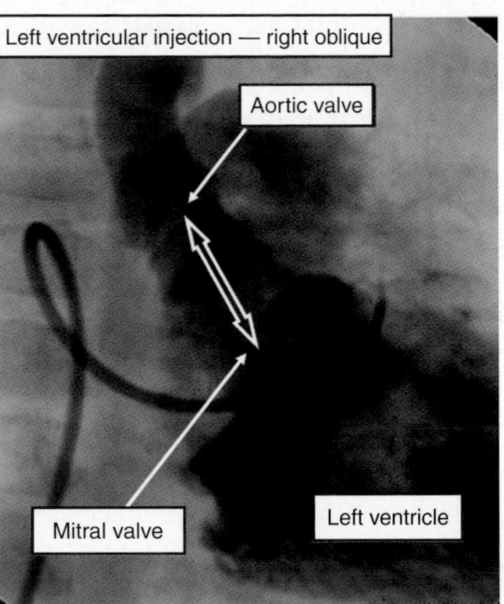

Figure 40-20 The left ventricular angiogram, shown in left oblique projection in the left panel, and right oblique in the right panel, reveals mitral-aortic valvar separation.

variants of coarctation or hypoplastic left heart syndromes. The presence of pulmonary stenosis, on the other hand, is more often associated with presentation at a later age, and gives features similar to those of Fallot's tetralogy. In all cases, the differentiation depends on careful echocardiographic and angiographic delineation of the connections and relationship of the great arteries to the ventricles.

MANAGEMENT

Treatment of double outlet ventriculo-arterial connection is essentially surgical, including the palliative procedures which may be necessary after initial diagnosis. Other then for supportive measures, there is no place for medical treatment, although interventional catheterisation may have a role in the treatment of complications of surgical palliation or repair.

SURGERY

The surgery of double outlet right ventricle has posed a great challenge to the ingenuity and skill of cardiac surgeons the world over. In the early years of cardiac surgery, the nature of the malformation was not always recognised preoperatively or intraoperatively. In this setting, closure of the interventricular communication, without redirection of left ventricular blood to the aorta, led to some operative tragedies.[51] Successful correction was first achieved in 1957.[52] Since that time, a large number of surgical reports have appeared.[24,52–64]

The surgical approach to the individual patient depends on the anatomic features present, and especially on the presence of complicating additional abnormalities. In more complex cases, corrective surgery may not be feasible. In those patients deemed unsuitable for correction, conversion to the Fontan circulation, or other palliative procedures, may be the preferred option. In the majority of patients, however, a biventricular repair is feasible. In our analysis of the series of patients undergoing surgery in Melbourne from 1978 to 1993,[64] we categorised the patients into complex and non-complex groups. Complex patients had one or more isomeric appendages, discordant ventriculo-arterial connections, multiple interventricular communications, unbalanced ventricles, straddling or hypoplasia of an atrioventricular valve, a common atrioventricular valve, pulmonary atresia or other major pulmonary arterial anomalies. Those without any of these features made up the non-complex group.

In the early weeks of life, palliation may be required prior to subsequent correction. Patients with a subpulmonary defect, in whom the physiology resembles transposition, may benefit from balloon atrial septostomy. This is also worthwhile in those infants with severe left-sided obstructive lesions, such as mitral stenosis or atresia. Infants with severe pulmonary hypertension and congestive failure may require palliation with banding of the pulmonary trunk if primary correction is likely to carry high risks (see below). Conversely, infants with restricted pulmonary flow due to pulmonary stenosis may need construction of a systemic-to-pulmonary arterial shunt if primary correction is not considered either feasible or a satisfactory option at this age. Those infants with aortic coarctation or interruption will usually require urgent surgical relief of the obstructive lesion in the neonatal period, with or without simultaneous intracardiac repair. Banding of the pulmonary trunk may be considered desirable during the same procedure if early complete intracardiac repair is not possible.

Primary repair for those cases with a subaortic defect involves the placement of an intraventricular tunnel from the defect to the aorta, attaching the patch to the right ventricular outlet septum to restore septal integrity. Subpulmonary or valvar pulmonary stenosis may be relieved by infundibulectomy, valvotomy or enlargement of the outflow tract with a gusset. An external conduit may be used in cases where these methods are not appropriate. In such cases, operative mortality, in the modern era, is generally low.[65] Among 94 such non-complex patients having biventricular repairs in Melbourne since 1978, 4 died (4.2% mortality). Others[59–62] have reported a generally favourable experience with this subgroup of patients. Risks of total correction were initially considered to be significantly higher at younger age, but this was not found to be the case in one recent analysis.[65]

By reason of concern on this score, nonetheless, some surgeons have preferred early palliation with banding of the pulmonary trunk or creation of systemic-to-pulmonary arterial shunts.[60] Other surgeons, however, report a low mortality except possibly in infants under 3 months of age. They recommend primary correction even in infancy.[59] This has been our preferred approach, as also in Boston.[63,64] More complex anatomy in some patients with subaortic defects may complicate repair and increase the risks of operation. In the experience in Melbourne, a range of such complicating features were encountered (Table 40-5). Among 41 such complex patients, the hospital mortality rate after biventricular repair was 26.8%. This has led to our considering conversion to the Fontan circulation, or construction of cavopulmonary shunts, in these more complex patients, providing the haemodynamics are suitable.

In patients with subpulmonary septal defects, surgical results in the past were less good. In selected cases, it proved possible to construct an intraventricular conduit from the left ventricle to the aorta.[66–68] In most, however, it is necessary to close the defect so that left ventricular blood is directed to the pulmonary trunk. This then necessitates an additional arterial switch procedure, or an atrial redirection operation. Atrial redirection in most instances was found to carry a high mortality.[59] For this reason, in the modern era, an arterial switch is preferable in almost all cases. It has been suggested that cases in which the great arteries are in an antero-posterior relationship are particularly suitable for the repair incorporating an arterial switch, whilst those with side-by-side arterial relationships may be more suitable for intraventricular repair.[69,70] Others have employed an arterial switch procedure in both situations.[71] Still other procedures have been attempted in some more complex cases. One such approach, the so-called REV procedure, involves sacrificing the pulmonary outflow tract in order to route an intraventricular baffle from the interventricular communication to the aorta. The pulmonary bifurcation is then brought in front of the ascending aorta using a Lecompte manoeuvre, and is sutured directly to the upper edge of the ventriculotomy incision, using a pericardial patch or monocusp gusset to complete the anterior wall of the new outflow tract to the pulmonary arteries.[72,73] This operation may be worth considering for patients with a subpulmonary defect with co-existing pulmonary stenosis, a combination which precludes an arterial switch repair. Another option in this situation is the use of a Rastelli-type repair incorporating insertion of an external valved conduit between the right ventricle and the pulmonary trunk.[74] We summarise the experience in Melbourne with subpulmonary defects in Table 40-6. The presence of associated pulmonary stenosis, and a range of other complicating factors, may prejudice a satisfactory biventricular repair but, in the absence of these complicating problems, most patients are suitable for an arterial switch procedure. The hospital mortality rate in non-complex patients submitted to biventricular repair was 3.1%, with 1 of 31 patients dying. This is no different from that experienced in non-complex patients with subaortic defects. Moreover, the presence of aortic coarctation or interruption did not impact on mortality at the time of repair, despite the fact that the arch was repaired at the same time as intracardiac repair in most cases. Over this period, we converted 10 children with subpulmonary defects to the Fontan circulation, and constructed bidirectional cavopulmonary shunts in 5, all these being considered unsuitable for biventricular repair. All survived. We palliated a further four infants with shunts, repair of coarctation, or other procedures. Of these, two died without leaving hospital, and the other two died subsequently, without reaching definitive surgery.

TABLE 40-5

SURGERY PERFORMED ON 154 PATIENTS WITH SUBAORTIC DEFECTS (60 BEING COMPLEX), FROM A COHORT OF 352 INFANTS OR CHILDREN WITH DOUBLE OUTLET RIGHT VENTRICLE, HAVING THEIR INITIAL PALLIATION OR REPAIR BETWEEN 1978 AND 2007 AT THE ROYAL CHILDREN'S HOSPITAL, MELBOURNE

BIVENTRICULAR REPAIR: NON-COMPLEX FORMS		
Additional Lesion	Number	Hospital Deaths
Pulmonary stenosis (other than Fallot's)	5	1
Tetralogy anatomy	66	1
Coarctation/arch hypoplasia	4	2
Other additional abnormality(s)	8	0
No additional abnormality	11	0
Total	**94**	**4 (4.2%)**

BIVENTRICULAR REPAIR: COMPLEX FORMS		
Complicating Lesion	Number	Hospital Deaths
Multiple interventricular communications	16	2
Pulmonary atresia	6	0
Left isomerism	5	0
Right isomerism	1	1
Criss-cross heart	1	0
Double chambered RV (superior/inferior relationship)	1	0
Restrictive ventricular septal defect	3	0
Atrioventricular septal defect	5	0
Hypoplastic left ventricle	3	3
Hypoplastic right ventricle	1	1
Straddling mitral valve	1	1
Straddling tricuspid valve	1	0
Severe ascending aorta hypoplasia and coarctation	3	1
Anomalous origin of one pulmonary artery	1	0
Pulmonary arterial sling	1	1
Aorto-pulmonary window	1	0
Exteriorized heart	1	1
Total patients	**41**	**11 (26.83%)**

(Note: Some patients had multiple complicating lesions.)

OTHER SURGERY: COMPLEX CASES		
Procedure	Number	Hospital Deaths
BCPS/Fontan	8	0
Palliation (band/shunt/coarctation repair)	11	4
Total	**19**	**4 (21%)**

TABLE 40-6

SURGERY PERFORMED ON 66 PATIENTS WITH SUBPULMONARY DEFECTS, INCLUDING 28 DEEMED COMPLEX, FROM A COHORT OF 352 INFANTS OR CHILDREN WITH DOUBLE OUTLET RIGHT VENTRICLE, HAVING THEIR INITIAL PALLIATION OR REPAIR BETWEEN 1978 AND 2007 AT THE ROYAL CHILDREN'S HOSPITAL, MELBOURNE

BIVENTRICULAR REPAIR: ANATOMIC VARIATIONS		
Complicating Lesion	**Number**	**Hospital Deaths**
Multiple interventricular communications	10	4
Coarctation	12	
Interrupted aortic arch	4	
Pulmonary stenosis	3	1
Pulmonary atresia	1	1
Small right ventricle	1	
Small left ventricle	2	2
Other additional abnormality(s)	15	
No additional abnormality	10	1
Total patients	**44**	**5 (11.4%)**

(Note: some patients had multiple complicating lesions.)

BIVENTRICULAR REPAIR: SURGICAL PROCEDURE		
Type of Operation	**Number**	**Hospital Deaths**
Senning + baffling of defect	2	
Senning + closure of defect, later converted to switch	4	
Attempted repair > later Fontan	1	1
Primary arterial switch + baffling of defect	31	2
Intraventricular repair	4	2
Intraventricular baffle + conduit	2	
Total	**44**	**5 (11.4%)**

OTHER SURGICAL PROCEDURES		
Procedure	**Number**	**Hospital Deaths**
BCPS/Fontan	15	
Palliation (coarctation/band/shunt)	4	2
Palliative senning	3	
Total patients	**22**	**2 (9.1%)**

Patients with doubly committed ventricular septal defects are usually suitable for intraventricular repair, except when other major complicating issues are present. In our overall series of 352 patients, only 8 non-complex patients had this anatomy, and all could be corrected in biventricular fashion using an intraventricular patch (Table 40-7). There were two other complex patients, one with discordant atrioventricular connections and the other with a severely hypoplastic left ventricle. This type of defect was not identified as being a risk factor for death by Kirklin and colleagues,[65] and is probably as favourable as the subaortic defect for biventricular repair, though problems with subaortic outlet obstruction have occurred occasionally.[75]

TABLE 40-7

SURGERY PERFORMED ON 10 PATIENTS WITH DOUBLY COMMITTED DEFECTS, INCLUDING 2 COMPLEX PATIENTS, FROM A COHORT OF 352 INFANTS OR CHILDREN WITH DOUBLE OUTLET RIGHT VENTRICLE, HAVING THEIR INITIAL PALLIATION OR REPAIR BETWEEN 1978 AND 2007 AT THE ROYAL CHILDREN'S HOSPITAL, MELBOURNE

Type of Surgery	Number	Hospital Deaths
DOUBLY COMMITTED INTERVENTRICULAR COMMUNICATION NON-COMPLEX REPAIR		
Intraventricular repair	8	1
Total patients	**8**	**1 (12.5%)**
OTHER SURGERY (COMPLEX)		
Fontan (complex)	1	
Palliative (complex)	1	1
Total patients	**2**	**1 (50%)**

Non-committed defects, in contrast, may present difficulties. Selection of patients for biventricular repair as opposed to conversion to the Fontan circuit or cavopulmonary shunting depends on careful assessment of the interventricular communication and its relationship to the arterial outlets, as well as any associated problems. Of 80 such patients seen in Melbourne, 37 were submitted to biventricular repair using either an intraventricular baffle in 30, or in combination with an arterial switch procedure in the other 7. Of these, 4 patients died in hospital (10.8% mortality). We created the Fontan circuit or bidirectional cavopulmonary shunts in 33 patients, with 1 dying. The remaining 10 children were submitted only to palliative procedures, albeit with 7 deaths (Table 40-8).

Other options include the use of a tubular internal conduit from the left ventricle to the aorta, accompanied by insertion of a valved external conduit from the right ventricle to the pulmonary trunk,[76] or use of double external conduits.[77]

TABLE 40-8

SURGERY PERFORMED ON 80 PATIENTS, 44 DEEMED TO BE COMPLEX, WITH NON-COMMITTED INTERVENTRICULAR COMMUNICATIONS, FROM A COHORT OF 352 INFANTS OR CHILDREN WITH DOUBLE OUTLET RIGHT VENTRICLE, HAVING THEIR INITIAL PALLIATION OR REPAIR BETWEEN 1978 AND 2007 AT THE ROYAL CHILDREN'S HOSPITAL, MELBOURNE

NON-COMMITTED INTERVENTRICULAR COMMUNICATION		
Type of Surgery	**Number**	**Hospital Deaths**
Intraventricular baffle	30	3
Arterial switch repair	7	1
Fontan procedure	24	
Bidirectional cavopulmonary shunt	9	1
Palliation (band or shunt, etc.)	10	7
Total	**80**	**12 (15%)**

Additional risk factors identified by those undertaking surgical treatment of double outlet right ventricle have included atrioventricular valvar abnormalities such as straddling or a common atrioventricular orifice.[61] The situation is further complicated for many with a common atrioventricular valve by the presence of right isomerism. This is itself associated with a wide range of other complicating anomalies which adversely affect the outcome (see Chapter 22). On the other hand, when isomeric atrial appendages are not present, an atrioventricular septal defect is usually amenable to repair with little increase in hospital mortality, but an increased risk of reintervention.[78] Patients with severe mitral or left ventricular hypoplasia, and those with supero-inferior ventricles with an inlet septal defect, have been regarded as inoperable.[59] This becomes less important if such patients are suitable for conversion to the Fontan circulation. Subpulmonary and non-committed defects were initially regarded as risk factors,[65] but this has become less significant in the current era. The need for placement of a transjunctional patch, or for an external valved conduit, have also been regarded as risk factors. Hence, the presence of pulmonary stenosis in itself may be an independent risk factor.

Multi-variate analysis of the earlier cohort of 193 patients treated in Melbourne[64] showed that the most significant anatomic features adversely affecting mortality were multiple interventricular communications and aortic interruption or coarctation. Multiple septal defects were particularly significant for those patients who had a biventricular repair. The site of a solitary interventricular communication did not have any significant effect on mortality in the series as a whole. Neither did the presence of pulmonary stenosis, an atrioventricular septal defect with common atrioventricular junction, or pulmonary atresia. Early age at the time of definitive surgery was associated with increased mortality, but only in the age group below 1 month. Those patients undergoing surgery prior to 1985 were also at greater risk, this effect being independent of the other identifiable variables. Analysis of the expanded series, now including 352 patients undergoing surgery between 1978 and 2007, no longer shows multiple septal defects as a risk factor, but this appears to reflect the fact that patients who are classified as complex are usually converted to the Fontan circulation rather than attempting biventricular repair. Our experience is in keeping with the other findings,[63,65] showing that mortality has improved substantially in the recent era. Details of the subgroups of patients treated in Melbourne with common atrioventricular valves and with multiple ventricular septal defects are summarised in Tables 40-9 and 40-10, respectively.

Apart from early mortality, late problems may also be significant, with a mortality rate of 21% reported by some[60] amongst patients with a subaortic septal defect. Most of these late deaths were related to arrhythmias. Residual haemodynamic problems have included residual defects, subpulmonary stenosis, and subaortic obstruction. Actuarial freedom from reoperation was less than 50% at 8 years for patients with non-committed defects and for those with subpulmonary defects.[63] By contrast, those with subaortic defects had a rate of freedom from reoperation better than 90% at 8 years. In those undergoing surgery in Melbourne,[64] site of the defect was not a variable which influenced the need for reoperation. In that data, freedom from either death or reoperation was 65% at 10 years from the time of definitive operation. Apart from these problems, quality of life following repair has, in most cases, been excellent.

TABLE 40-9

SURGERY PERFORMED ON 39 PATIENTS WITH COMMON ATRIOVENTRICULAR VALVE, 26 HAVING ISOMERIC ATRIAL APPENDAGES, IN A COHORT OF 352 INFANTS OR CHILDREN WITH DOUBLE OUTLET RIGHT VENTRICLE, HAVING THEIR INITIAL PALLIATION OR REPAIR BETWEEN 1978 AND 2007 AT THE ROYAL CHILDREN'S HOSPITAL, MELBOURNE

COMMON ATRIOVENTRICULAR VALVE		
Type of Surgery	Number	Hospital Deaths
Intraventricular repair	8	1
Fontan procedure	12	
Bidirectional cavopulmonary shunt	10	2
Palliation (shunt, band, TAPVD rep)	9	8
Total	**39**	**11 (28.3%)**

TABLE 40-10

SURGERY PERFORMED ON 59 PATIENTS WITH MULTIPLE INTERVENTRICULAR COMMUNICATIONS, ALL CONSIDERED COMPLEX, IN A COHORT OF 352 INFANTS OR CHILDREN WITH DOUBLE OUTLET RIGHT VENTRICLE, HAVING THEIR INITIAL PALLIATION OR REPAIR BETWEEN 1978 AND 2007 AT THE ROYAL CHILDREN'S HOSPITAL, MELBOURNE

MULTIPLE INTERVENTRICULAR COMMUNICATIONS		
Type of Surgery	Number	Hospital Deaths
Intraventricular patch	31	5
Arterial switch repair	5	1
Fontan procedure	10	
Bidirectional cavopulmonary shunt	7	1
Palliation (arch/shunt/band, etc.)	6	1
Total	**59**	**8 (13.6%)**

Additional Problems in the Surgery of Double Outlet Ventricles

In patients with restrictive interventricular communications, intraventricular repair must be accompanied by surgical enlargement of the defect. Alternatively, an extracardiac conduit can be placed from the left ventricle to the aorta, permitting the interventricular communication to be closed. The presence of complicating intracardiac anomalies, such as mitral stenosis, straddling of an atrioventricular valve, or a common atrioventricular orifice, may necessitate more extensive surgery involving valvar repair or replacement and so on.[79]

Double outlet right ventricle with discordant atrioventricular connections is amenable to correction in some cases either by construction of an intraventricular tunnel to connect the morphologically left ventricle to the pulmonary trunk, or by use of an external valved conduit inserted from the left ventricle to the pulmonary trunk combined with closure of the interventricular communication.[24] In the current era, use of the arterial switch procedure, combined with a Senning or Mustard operation, or, in the presence of pulmonary stenosis, a Rastelli type repair, also coupled with a Senning or Mustard repair, has been employed with success.[80] Whether this is a better approach than to proceed using the Fontan approach, or bidirectional cavopulmonary shunting, is debatable. Unfortunately, as with congenitally corrected transposition, there is a high incidence of heart block following surgical repair. This is almost certainly related to the abnormal disposition of the conduction system in patients with discordant atrioventricular connections.[81]

In our series of patients treated in Melbourne, 16 patients had discordant atrioventricular connections, one of whom was submitted to a biventricular repair. We adopted the Fontan route for 12, with no mortality, and 2 further children have been palliated with a bidirectional cavopulmonary shunt. In one additional patient, with complex anatomy, we proceeded with an aortic valvotomy and implantation of a pacemaker, but the patient died suddenly 2 years later. The other 15 patients are all alive.

Isomerism of atrial appendages was present in 39 patients, with 21 having right and 18 left isomerism. In this group, 26 had common atrioventricular valves, 8 underwent biventricular repair, and 23 were tracked towards Fontan palliation. Definitive surgery was not possible in 8. Overall, the presence of isomerism was a significant risk factor for early death, including those who reached definitive surgery.

Probability of Long-term Survival

Actuarial probability of survival following biventricular repair was estimated by one group[63] as being 81% at 8 years, which is similar to the earlier experience in Melbourne,[64] in which the probability was 81% at 10 years. Overall probability of survival, from the time of initial surgery be it palliative or corrective, in the entire cohort undergoing surgery in Melbourne for this earlier period was calculated as being 76% at 13 years. It is noteworthy that those patients who were considered to be unsuitable for biventricular repair, and who were managed by a Fontan or cavopulmonary shunt procedure, have had a better record of survival in the short term, with a probability of 92% survival at 6 years. This earlier experience is now borne out by a review of our enlarged cohort of 352 patients (Figs. 40-21, 40-22, and 40-23). Those converted to the Fontan circuit had a 94% probablity of survival at 10 years, compared with survival at 10 years after biventricular repair of 86%. This is amplified when comparing the complex patients who achieved definitive surgery, in whom survival probability was 78% at 10 years for those undergoing biventricular repair as compared with 94% for those who were converted to the Fontan circulation. Whilst the confidence intervals are not sufficiently tight, at 10 years, to show a clear difference, the actuarial analysis suggests that this difference increases with follow-up out to 20 years, though obviously late morbidity and mortality after the Fontan procedure may tend to reduce or reverse this difference in longer-term follow-up. Significantly the actuarial analysis of freedom from death or reoperation for all patients is much less optimistic, with only 28% of those undergoing biventricular repair being alive and free of the need for further operation at 20 years, as opposed to 60% of those converted to the Fontan circulation, although confidence intervals are wide in this analysis, and as yet do not demonstrate a significant difference (see Fig. 40-23).

Repair of Double Outlet Left Ventricle

Surgical repair of double outlet left ventricle follows similar lines to that for double outlet right ventricle.[82,83] Cases with pulmonary stenosis are usually best dealt with by insertion of an external valved conduit from the right ventricle to the

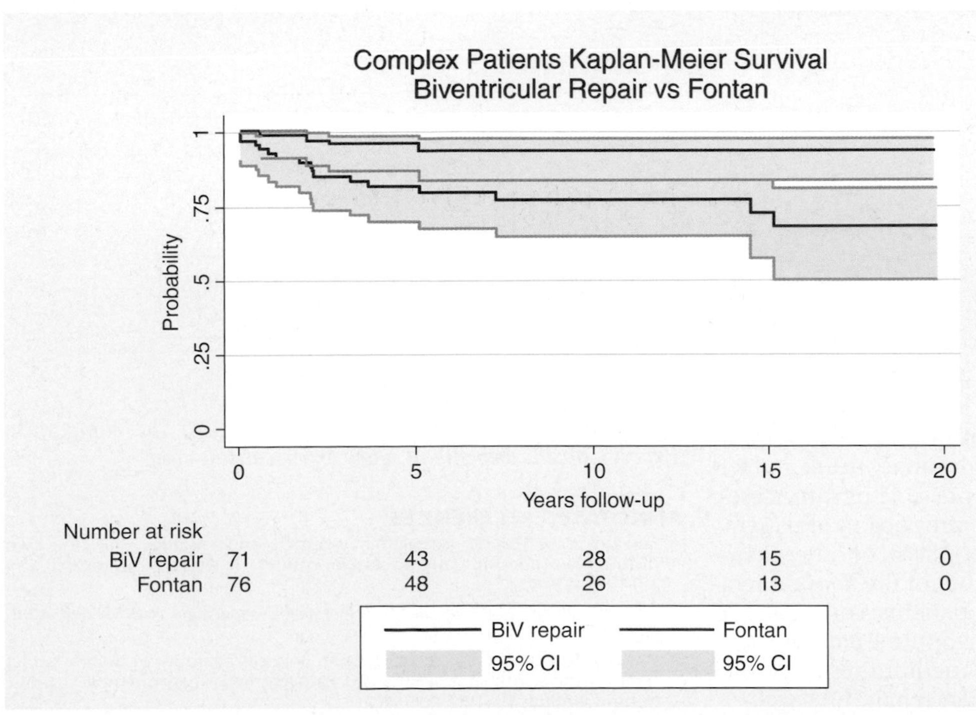

Figure 40-21 The graph shows the survival of complex patients undergoing surgery in Melbourne after biventricular repair or conversion to the Fontan circuit, indicating better long-term survival for those managed with the Fontan procedure.

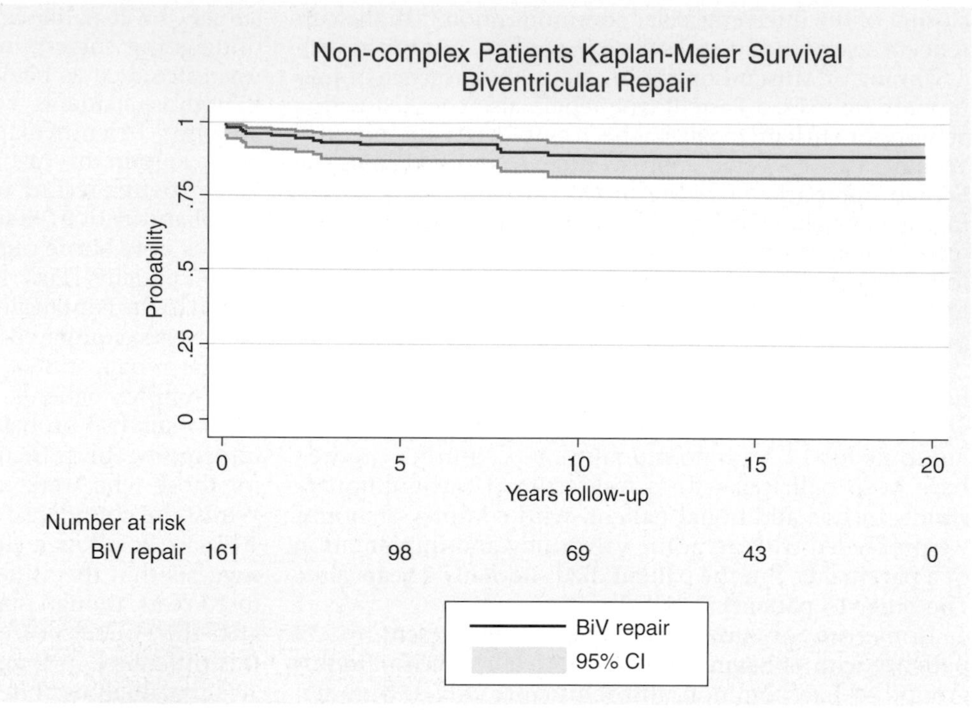

Figure 40-22 The graph shows survival for non-complex patients undergoing surgery in Melbourne who achieved biventricular repair.

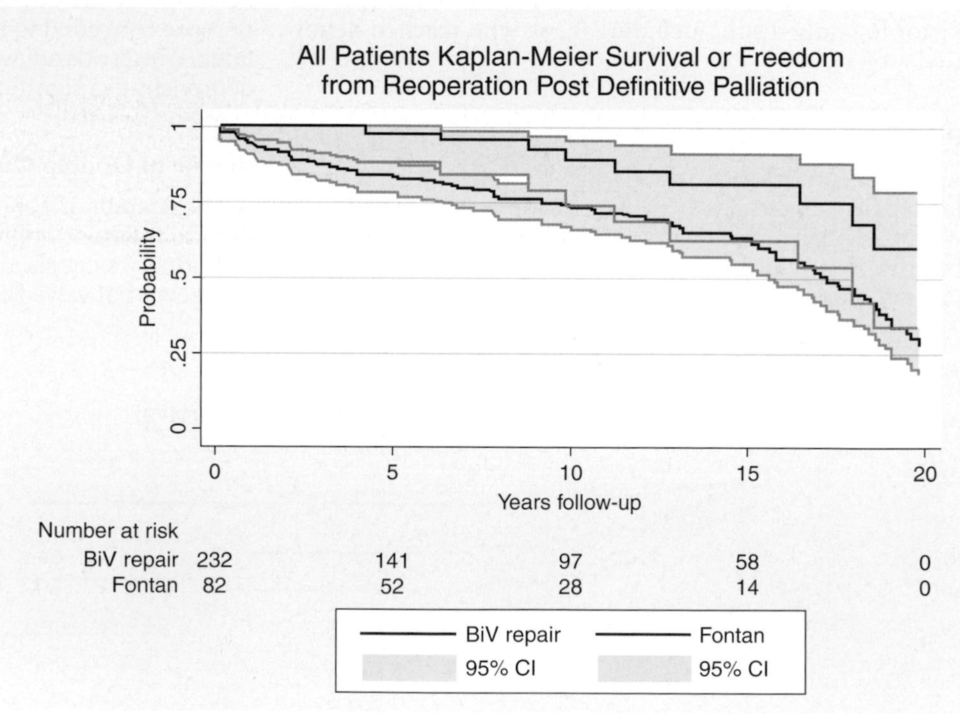

Figure 40-23 The graph shows survival, and freedom from reoperation, for all patients undergoing surgery in Melbourne who either achieved biventricular repair or were converted to the Fontan circulation. Overall, freedom from reoperation appears superior in those with the Fontan circuit, but this barely achieves significance, as the 95% confidence intervals continue to overlap out to 20 years.

pulmonary trunk. Placement of an intraventricular patch to direct right ventricular flow to the pulmonary trunk and left ventricular flow to the aorta may be possible in some cases. Unfortunately, it appears that a high proportion of patients have significant right ventricular hypoplasia, or other major complicating anomalies, making either of the above operations difficult or impossible. In such patients, conversion to the Fontan circuit, or creation of a cavopulmonary shunt, is likely to produce higher earlier and medium-term survival than an heroic attempt at biventricular repair.[26,84]

The complete reference list can be found on the companion Expert Consult web site at www.expertconsult.com.

ANNOTATED REFERENCES

- Edwards WD: Double outlet right ventricle and tetralogy of Fallot: Two distinct but not mutually exclusive entities. J Thorac Cardiovasc Surg 1981;82:418–422.

  A useful discussion of the relationship of double outlet right ventricle and tetralogy of Fallot.

- Wilcox BR, Ho SY, Macartney FJ, et al: Surgical anatomy of double outlet right ventricle with situs solitus and atrioventricular concordance. J Thorac Cardiovasc Surg 1981;82:405–417.

A review of the morphologic variability of double outlet right ventricle from a surgical perspective.

- Van Praagh R: What is the Taussig Bing malformation? Circulation 1968;38:445–449.

  This disussion covers the anatomy of the heart originally described by Taussig and Bing and the ways in which the term has been used subsequently.
- Van Praagh R, David I, Wright GB, Van Praagh S: Large RV plus small LV is not single RV. Circulation 1980;61:1057–1058.

  This crucial concept, stated in a letter to the editor, pointed out that it was philosophically unsound to base definitions of a given structure on one of its parts that was variable. Instead, they established the crucial principle of the morphological method, stating that the structures be identified on the basis of their most constant components.
- Van Mierop LH, Wiglesworth FW: Pathogenesis of transposition complexes: II. Anomalies due to faulty transfer of the posterior great artery. Am J Cardiol 1963;12:226–232.

  An early discussion of the morphogenesis of double outlet right ventricle, which claims that double outlet left ventricle is an embryological impossibility!
- Otero Coto E, Quero Jimenez M, Anderson RH, et al: Double outlet left ventricle and univentricular heart of left ventricular type. In Anderson RH, Shinebourne EA, Macartney FJ, Tynan M (eds): Paediatric Cardiology, vol 5. Edinburgh: Churchill Livingstone, 1981.

  A review of most of the published cases of double outlet left ventricle up to 1980.
- Goor DA, Edwards JE: The spectrum of transposition of the great arteries—with special reference to developmental anatomy of the conus. Circulation 1973;48:406–415.

  This article from the 1970s discusses some of the fundamental aspects of the morphogenesis of double outlet right ventricle and other defects, illustrating a spectrum of anomalies that relate to transposition and double outlet right ventricle.
- Aoki M, Forbess JM, Jonas RA, et al: Result of biventricular repair for double-outlet right ventricle. J Thorac Cardiovasc Surg 1994;107:338–350.
- Kleinert S, Sano T, Weintraub RG, et al: Anatomic features and surgical strategies in double-outlet right ventricle. Circulation 1997;96:1233–1239.

  These reviews provide a useful overview of the results of surgery for double outlet right ventricle in the modern era.

CHAPTER 41

Common Arterial Trunk

DANIEL J. PENNY and ROBERT H. ANDERSON

Common arterial trunk is a rare congenital malformation of the heart. As its name implies, its essential anatomical feature is the presence of an arterial trunk, which arises from the ventricular mass through a common ventriculo-arterial junction, giving rise directly to the systemic, pulmonary and coronary circulations. In most centres, surgical treatment, the only appropriate current therapeutic approach, is now performed routinely following only non-invasive preoperative investigations in early infancy. Operative mortality is now low, although it may be increased in patients in whom there are associated abnormalities, for example, interruption of the aortic arch, or stenosis or regurgitation of the truncal valve. In most cases, the technique used for surgical correction includes placement of a conduit as part of the reconstructed pulmonary outflow tract. Because of this, after this form of surgery patients must be followed indefinitely in a centre which specialises in the care of those having congenital cardiac disease, as most will require procedures to address stenosis of the conduit in later life.

INCIDENCE

Common arterial trunk is a rare anomaly, occurring in 0.03 per 1000 live births according to data assembled from the New England Regional Infant Cardiac Program.[1] Among 906,646 live-born infants collected in the Baltimore-Washington Study, 4390 had congenitally malformed hearts, with 51 having common arterial trunk, so that this malformation occurred in 0.056 of every 1000 live births, and represented just over 1% of all instances of congenital cardiac disease.[2] A recent study showed that surgical treatment of common arterial trunk accounted for almost 1% of open heart procedures performed at the Royal Liverpool Children's Hospital between 1993 and 2005. The incidence of congenital malformations of the heart is known to be increased in the offspring of patients with common arterial trunk, being 6.6% in the offspring of those with uncomplicated lesions, and 13.6% of those with complex forms of the condition.[4]

ANATOMY

Of all the congenital lesions that benefit from being described in straightforward fashion, common arterial trunk is the most obvious. When described in terms of truncus, or various expansions of this term that implicate persistence of an embryonic condition, it is always necessary to provide a definition of the lesion as seen in the postnatal heart. Describing the entity as a common arterial trunk negates the need for further definition. A common trunk is one that arises from the ventricular mass through a common ventriculo-arterial junction, and gives rise directly to the systemic, pulmonary and coronary circulations (Fig. 41-1).

Almost without exception, the common ventriculo-arterial junction is guarded by a common arterial valve,[4] but by analogy to atrioventricular septal defect with common junction (see Chapter 27), it might be anticipated that the arterial valvar leaflets could be divided into separate orifices for the right and left ventricles, whilst still guarding a common junction The latter situation is seen in the setting of the doubly committed and juxta-arterial ventricular septal defect (see Chapter 28), but such patients do not possess common arterial trunks. The pattern of branching of the common trunk itself can be complicated by various arrangements of the individual arteries within the systemic, pulmonary, and coronary arterial circulations. The presence of the common trunk, nonetheless, distinguishes the entity not only from those with doubly committed ventricular

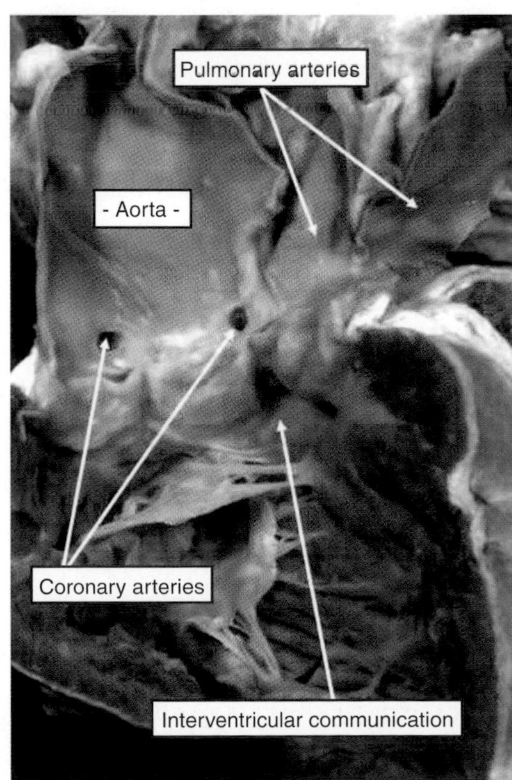

Figure 41-1 This specimen is dissected to show the typical features of a common arterial trunk, exiting from the ventricular mass through a common ventriculo-arterial junction guarded by a common arterial valve, and supplying directly the coronary, systemic and pulmonary circulations. Note the dysplastic nature of the truncal valve.

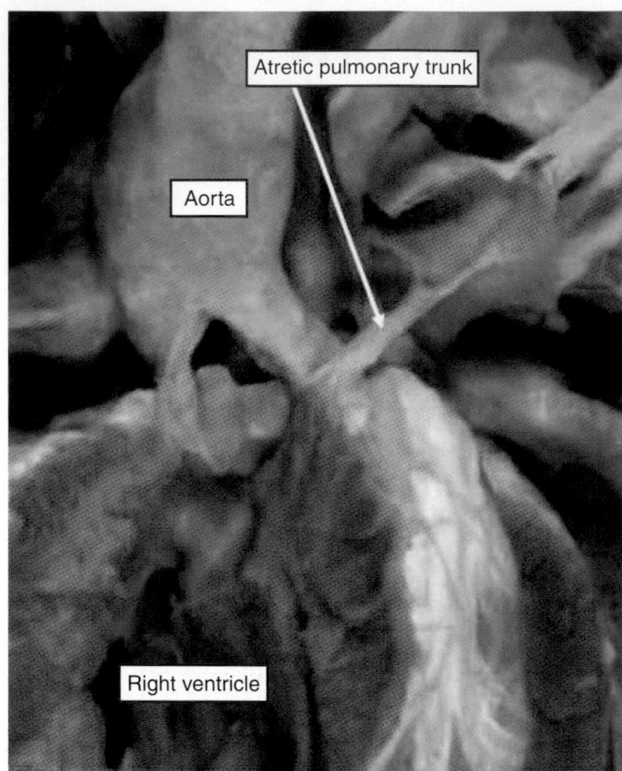

Figure 41-2 In this specimen, the atretic and thread-like pulmonary trunk can be traced back to the ventricular mass. This specimen, therefore, has a solitary aorta with pulmonary atresia, rather than common arterial trunk.

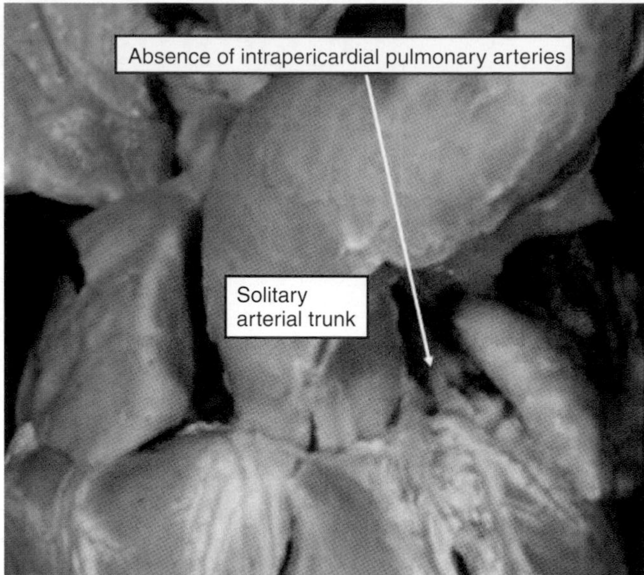

Figure 41-3 Unlike the specimen shown in Figure 41-2, in this heart there are no intrapericardial pulmonary arteries. The trunk arising from the heart, therefore, is best described as a solitary arterial trunk, since it cannot be determined with certainty whether the trunk was initially an aorta or a common trunk (see Fig. 41-4).

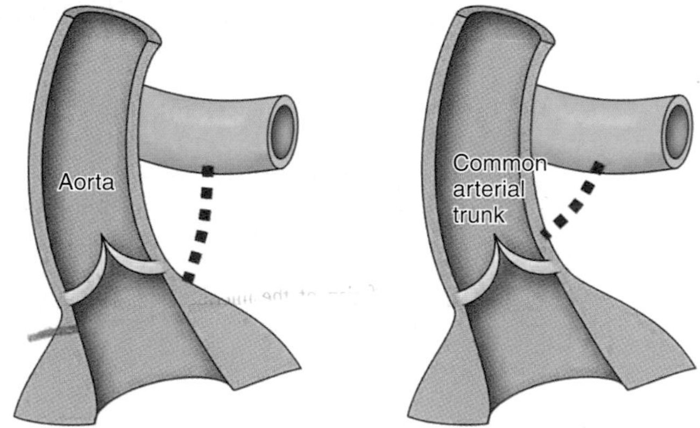

Figure 41-4 The cartoon shows that, had the pulmonary arteries been present in the heart illustrated in Figure 41-3, they could have arisen either from the heart, or from the arterial trunk itself (*dotted lines*). There is no way of knowing, therefore, whether the trunk was destined to become an aorta or a common trunk. Because of this uncertainty, it is best described as a solitary trunk. Patients with this arrangement, nonetheless, are best considered as a subset of those with tetralogy and pulmonary atresia.

septal defects with separate aortic and pulmonary valves, but also from the close cousins in which there is a window between the intrapericardial components of the aorta and pulmonary trunk, and also those patients in which a large patent trunk leaves the base of the heart in company with an atretic trunk, which can also be traced from its origin at the ventricular mass (Fig. 41-2).

One variant that can still give problems in terms of description, however, is when there is complete absence of the intrapericardial pulmonary arteries. In their time-honoured classification, Collett and Edwards[5] included this variant as the type IV within their overall grouping. The trunk arising from the ventricular mass in this setting (Fig. 41-3), however, is best described as a solitary, rather than a common, trunk. This is because there is no way of knowing, had they been present, whether the intrapericardial pulmonary arteries would have originated from the arterial trunk or from the right ventricular outflow tract (Fig. 41-4). In terms of clinical presentation and treatment, such patients with a solitary arterial trunk have more affinities with tetralogy and pulmonary atresia (see Chapter 37) than with common arterial trunk.

A common arterial trunk, as we have defined it, is one form of single outlet from the heart. As a malformation involving the ventriculo-arterial junctions, it must be anticipated to co-exist with all possible segmental combinations. In almost all instances, nonetheless, there will be usual atrial arrangement, with concordant atrioventricular connections. Examples can be found in combination with discordant atrioventricular connections, or with absence of the right atrioventricular connection.[6] While the atrioventricular junctions themselves are usually separate, and guarded by mitral and tricuspid valves, a common trunk can rarely be found in association with an atrioventricular septal defect and a common atrioventricular valve.[7]

In the presence of the common trunk, almost always the truncal valve is connected across the ventriculo-arterial junctions with both ventricles, the valvar orifice overriding the ventricular septal crest, and typically with its leaflets in fibrous continuity with the mitral valve in the left ventricle (Fig. 41-5). Such a biventricular connection necessitates the presence of a juxta-arterial interventricular communication. The defect is generally large. Its floor is the crest of the ventricular septum, reinforced on the right ventricular aspect by the limbs of the septomarginal trabeculation, or septal band, and its roof is the leaflets of the truncal valve. The cone of space subtended by the truncal valve has right and left ventricular margins, but it is usually the right ventricular margin that is considered to represent the

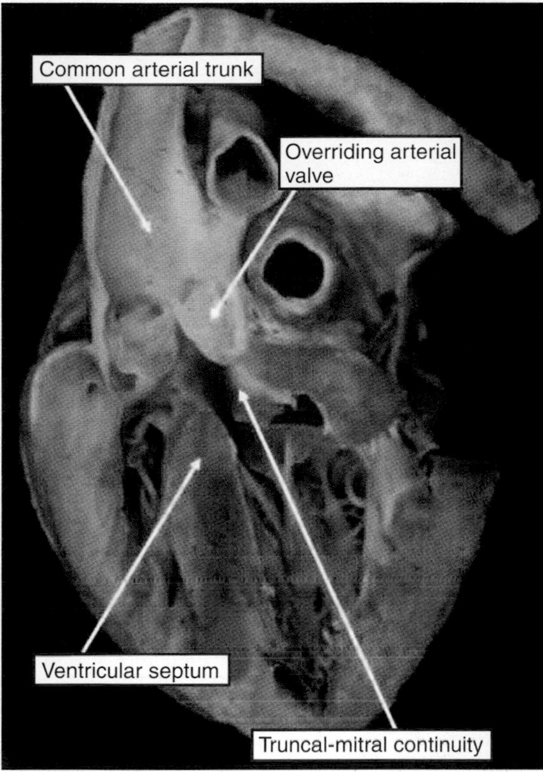

Figure 41-5 This long-axis section shows the truncal valve overriding the crest of the muscular ventricular septum with the valvar leaflets supported in both ventricles, but typically, as shown, in fibrous continuity with the leaflet of the mitral valve.

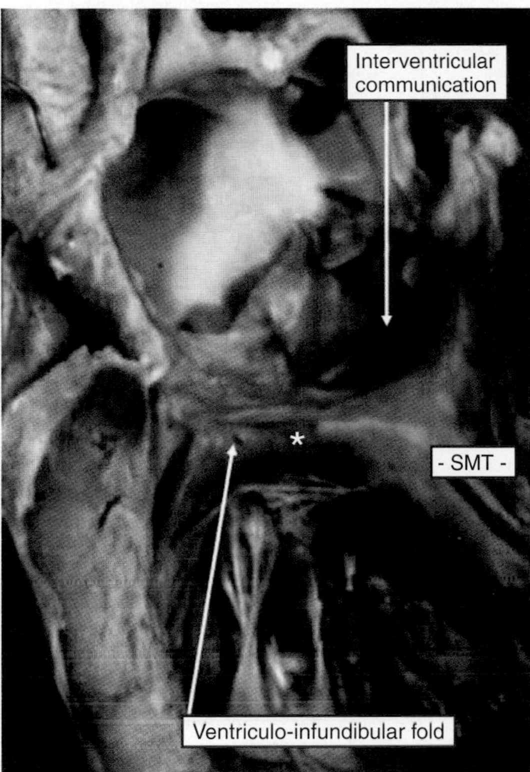

Figure 41-6 The presence or absence of a muscular rim along the postero-inferior margin of the ventricular septal defect determines whether or not the defect is considered to be perimembranous. In this specimen, the ventriculo-infundibular fold fuses with the postero-inferior limb of the septomarginal trabeculation (SMT). The muscular bar thus formed (*white asterisk*) protects the atrioventricular conduction axis during surgical correction.

ventricular septal defect, and it is this space which is closed by the surgeon during repair.

In the majority of cases, fusion of the inferior limb of the septomarginal trabeculation with the ventriculo-infundibular fold along this right ventricular margin produces muscular discontinuity between the leaflets of the tricuspid and the truncal valves (Fig. 41-6).

In the absence of such fusion, there is continuity between the leaflets of the tricuspid and truncal valves, making the ventricular septal defect perimembranous (Fig. 41-7). When present, this muscular bar in the postero-inferior margin protects the specialised axis responsible for atrioventricular conduction. In most instances, there is a large distance between the coapting arterial valvar leaflets and the crest of the septum during ventricular diastole when the leaflets are closed. This space, however, may sometimes be reduced, or the leaflets may close directly on the septal crest (Fig. 41-8).

Some have described this latter arrangement as representing an intact ventricular septum.[8] This is somewhat misleading because, even in this arrangement, a septal deficiency is seen at ventricular level when the truncal valve opens during ventricular systole. Furthermore, hearts are found when the ventricular septum is truly intact, the common trunk then arising in most instances exclusively from the right ventricle (Fig. 41-9). The ventricular septal defect can also be restrictive when the common trunk takes an exclusive origin from one or other ventricle. Such a restrictive ventricular septal defect is more likely to produce problems when the trunk arises exclusively from the right ventricle (Fig. 41-10).

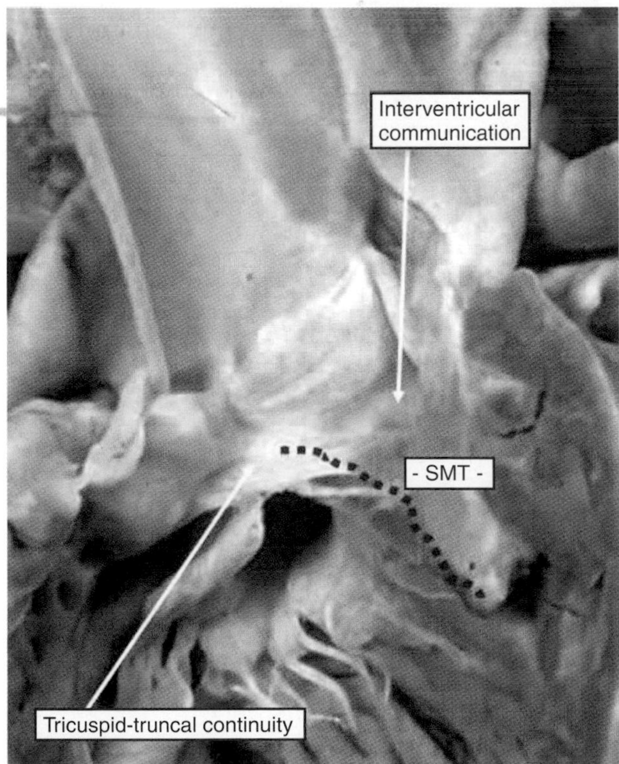

Figure 41-7 Unlike the heart shown in Figure 41-6, in this specimen the ventriculo-infundibular fold does not fuse with the postero-inferior limb of the septomarginal trabeculation. Instead, the postero-inferior margin of the defect is made up of fibrous continuity between the leaflets of the tricuspid and truncal valves, making the defect perimembranous, and putting at risk the atrioventricular conduction axis during surgical correction (*red dotted line*).

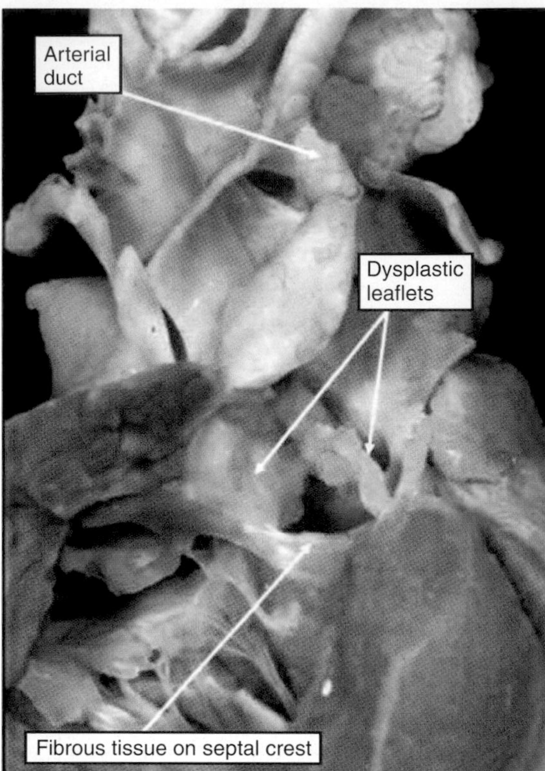

Figure 41-8 In this specimen, the dysplastic leaflets of the common truncal valve closed on the crest of the ventricular septum during ventricular diastole, the crest itself being thickened by fibrous tissue. An interventricular communication remains, nonetheless, during ventricular systole. Note the persistently patent arterial duct.

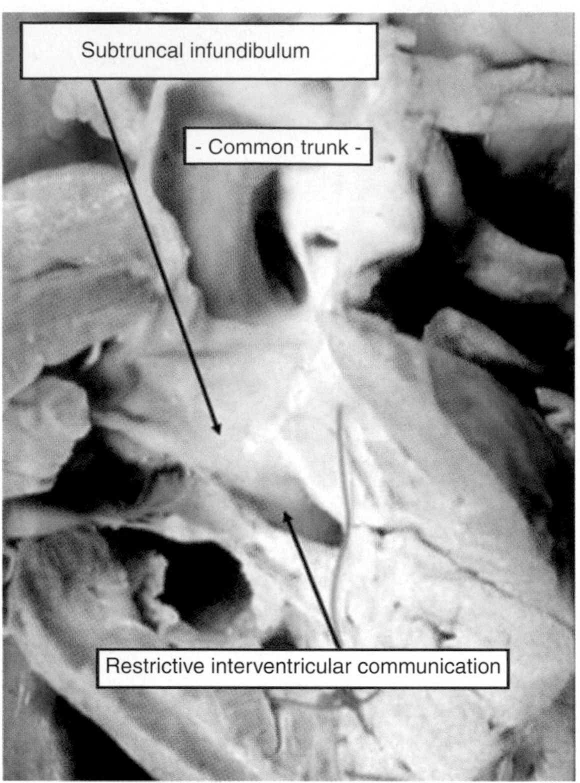

Figure 41-10 Although usually the truncal valve overrides the ventricular septal crest, as shown in Figure 41-4, occasionally the trunk can arise exclusively from one or other ventricle, here from the right ventricle. Note the completely muscular subtruncal infundibulum, and the potentially restrictive ventricular septal defect.

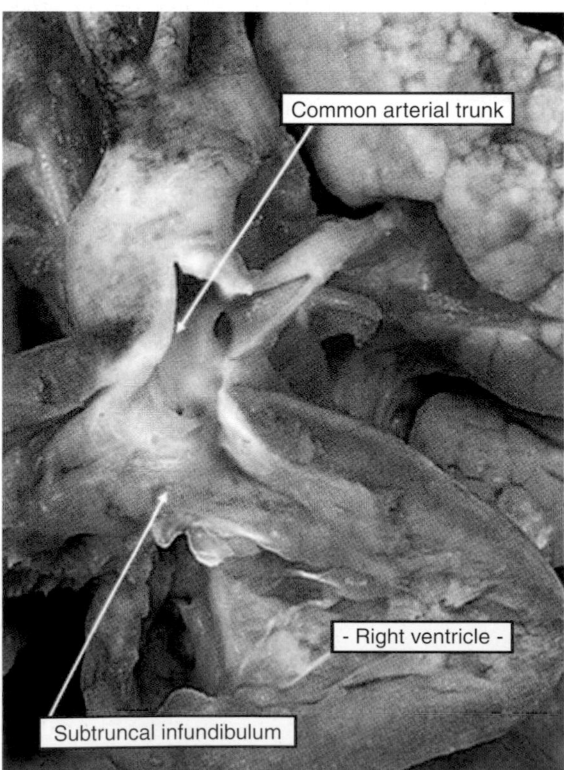

Figure 41-9 In this heart, in which there was absence of the left atrioventricular connection and hypoplasia of the incomplete left ventricle, a common arterial trunk arises from the dominant right ventricle, and the ventricular septum is intact. (Courtesy of Dr Andrew Cook, Institute of Child Health, University College, London, United Kingdom.)

The truncal valve has three leaflets in approximately two-thirds of patients. In most of the remaining patients, either two or four leaflets are seen guarding the common arterial orifice. The leaflets are almost always in fibrous continuity with the antero-superior leaflet of the mitral valve (see Fig. 41-5), but there can be a completely muscular subtruncal infundibulum, particularly when the common trunk arises exclusively from the right ventricle (see Fig. 41-10). Insufficiency of the truncal valve is not uncommon, and can be caused by thickened and dysplastic leaflets, or by prolapse of unsupported leaflets as a result of dilation of the ventriculo-arterial junction. Truncal valvar stenosis is relatively uncommon. When present, it is usually because the valvar leaflets are dysplastic.

The greatest anatomic variability is found in the pattern of the branching of the common trunk. The presence of a right-sided aortic arch, with mirror-imaged branching of the brachiocephalic arteries, is associated more often with common trunk, occurring in up to one-third of patients, than with any other congenital cardiac malformation.[4,9] Hypoplasia of the aortic arch, with or without coarctation, is a particularly important associated finding, but is less frequent than complete interruption of the arch (Fig. 41-11).

Such interruption is one of the major subgroups recognised in the alpha-numeric system that was suggested for classification.[10] When the arch is interrupted, the persistently patent arterial duct feeds the descending thoracic aorta and part of the brachiocephalic circulation, the precise proportion depending on the site of interruption. As with other forms of interruption of the aortic arch (see Chapter 46),

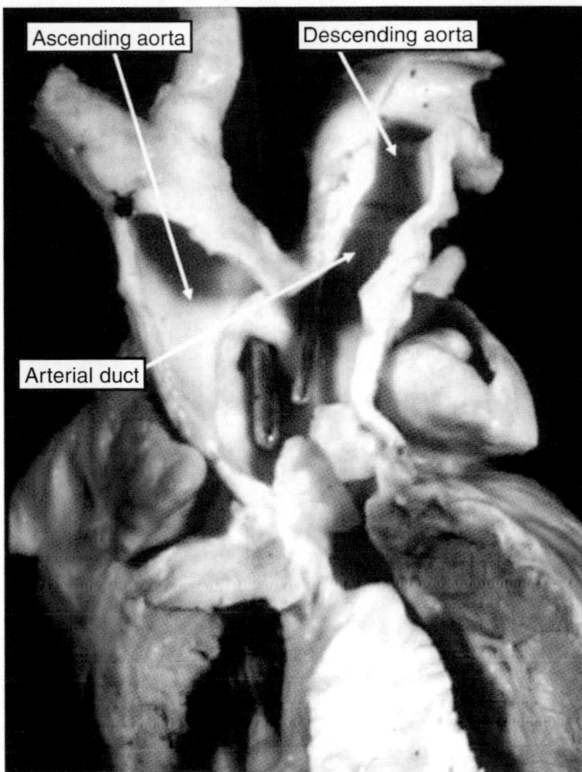

Figure 41-11 In this specimen, the systemic pathways are interrupted between the left common carotid and left subclavian arteries. The arterial duct feeds the descending aorta and the left subclavian artery. The probes are placed in the pulmonary arteries, which arise from the back of the common trunk. Note that the trunk itself arises almost exclusively from the left ventricle.

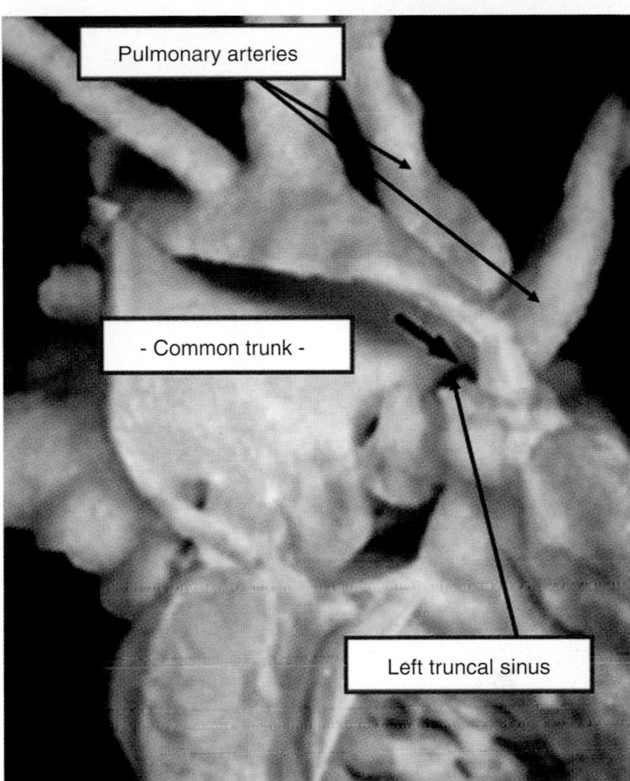

Figure 41-12 In this rare example of common arterial trunk, the pulmonary arteries arise directly from the left-sided truncal arterial sinus. (Image prepared and photographed by Dr Siew Yen Ho, Royal Brompton Hospital, London, and reproduced with her permission.)

retro-oesophageal origin of the right subclavian artery is frequently seen. Apart from those hearts with severe coarctation or interruption, or in which the pulmonary arteries are discontinuous, and one is fed through a patent duct, it is rare to find ductal patency co-existing with common arterial trunk, although it does exist (see Fig. 41-9).[11] While the state of the aortic arch is possibly the most significant clinical associated malformation, it has been the arrangement of origin of the pulmonary arteries, following the system proposed by Collett and Edwards[5] that was traditionally used most frequently for numeric classification. The pulmonary arteries typically arise from the left posterolateral aspect of the common trunk, taking origin a short distance above the truncal valve, albeit that very rarely they can take their origin directly from a truncal arterial valvar sinus (Fig. 41-12).

In the more usual situation, it is the presence of a short confluent arterial segment that produces the type I identified by Collett and Edwards (Fig. 41-13). Alternatively, the right and left arteries can take separate origin from the posterior aspect of the trunk, producing the type II variant (Fig. 41-14), or very rarely from the right and left sides of the posterior aspect of the intrapericardial segment of the common trunk, this being the type III variant. In most instances, however, the morphology is intermediate, and many have suggested that this pattern should be recognised as type 1½. It is also possible to find examples in which only one pulmonary artery arises from the common trunk, the other being supplied initially through a duct that became ligamentous. In the clinical setting, this can present as

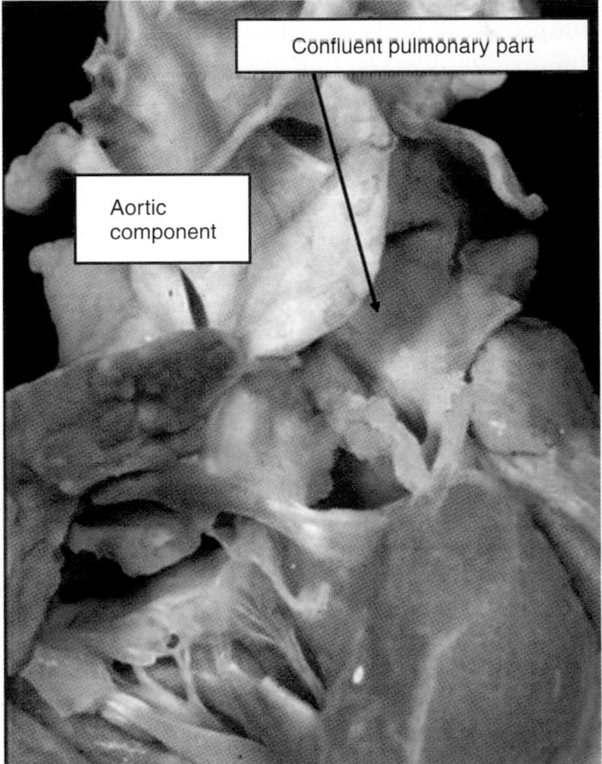

Figure 41-13 In this specimen, a short confluent pulmonary arterial segment interposes between the common trunk and the origin of the right and left pulmonary arteries. This is the so-called type I variant described by Collett and Edwards.

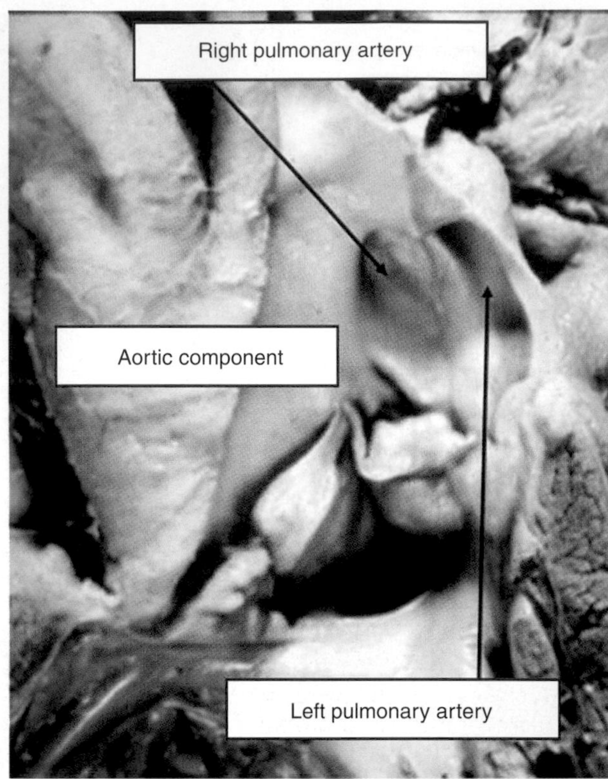

Figure 41-14 In this specimen, the right and left pulmonary arteries take separate origin from the leftward and posterior aspect of the common trunk. This is the so-called type II variant described by Collett and Edwards.

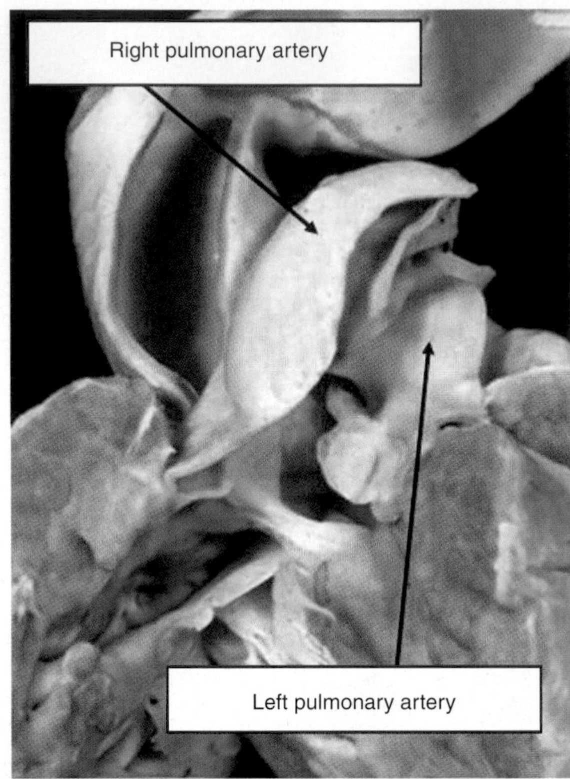

Figure 41-15 In this specimen, with a short confluent pulmonary arterial segment interposed between the common trunk and the origin of the right and left pulmonary arteries, the right pulmonary artery arises to the left of the origin of the left pulmonary artery. This is crossed pulmonary arteries.

unilateral absence of one pulmonary artery, but almost always the artery presumed to be absent is identified within the hilum of the lung. When this arrangement is found with common trunk, the discontinuous pulmonary artery initially fed by the duct is most frequently on the same side as the aortic arch. This is in contrast to the finding in patients with tetralogy of Fallot when one pulmonary artery is seemingly absent, since in this setting, the discontinuous artery is more frequently on the side opposite the aortic arch.

In some circumstances, the pulmonary artery feeding the right lung is to the left at its origin from the common trunk relative to the artery running to the left lung (Fig. 41-15). The two arteries then spiral as they extend to the pulmonary hilums. This entity is called crossed pulmonary arteries. As we have already discussed, in the original categorisation of Collett and Edwards[5] there was also a type IV variant, which exists when the intrapericardial pulmonary arteries are completely absent. As we have described (see Fig. 41-2), this arrangement is better described as a solitary arterial trunk, since in the absence of the intrapericardial pulmonary arteries, it cannot be determined whether, had they been present, they would have arisen from the heart, giving solitary aortic trunk with pulmonary atresia, or from the arterial trunk itself, producing common trunk with pulmonary atresia. Irrespective of such speculative considerations, in clinical terms patients with absence of the intrapericardial pulmonary arteries present as a subset of those with tetralogy of Fallot with pulmonary atresia, rather than common arterial trunk. It is also possible for one pulmonary artery to arise directly from the ascending aorta, while the other takes its origin from the right ventricle. Some call this malformation hemitruncus. This is incorrect since, of necessity, the hearts have separate ventriculo-arterial junctions guarded by separate aortic and pulmonary arterial valves. They cannot, therefore, be examples of common arterial trunk.

Anomalies of the origin and distribution of the coronary arteries are frequent.[10] Unlike the situation when there are separate aortic and pulmonary valves, in which virtually without exception the coronary arteries arise from one or other of the aortic valvar sinuses adjacent to the pulmonary trunk, and usually both sinuses, there is no constant pattern of sinusal origin in the presence of a common ventricular outflow tract. Instead, the coronary arteries can arise from any of the truncal valvar sinuses, albeit that in most instances there are still two coronary arteries, with the left artery giving rise to anterior interventricular and circumflex branches. The arteries often arise close to a zone of apposition between the valvar leaflets, and origin above the sinutubular junction is quite common (Fig. 41-16). This can produce potential difficulties during surgical correction should the high origin be adjacent to the origin of the pulmonary arteries.

Knowledge of location of the atrioventricular conduction axis is also important when planning surgical repair. The sinus node and the atrioventricular node are normal in their location and structure. Having taken origin from the atrioventricular node, the penetrating atrioventricular bundle pierces through the central fibrous body, and the left bundle branch originates along the left ventricular septal endocardium (see Chapter 28). The right bundle branch travels within the myocardium of the ventricular septal crest, attaining a subendocardial course at the level

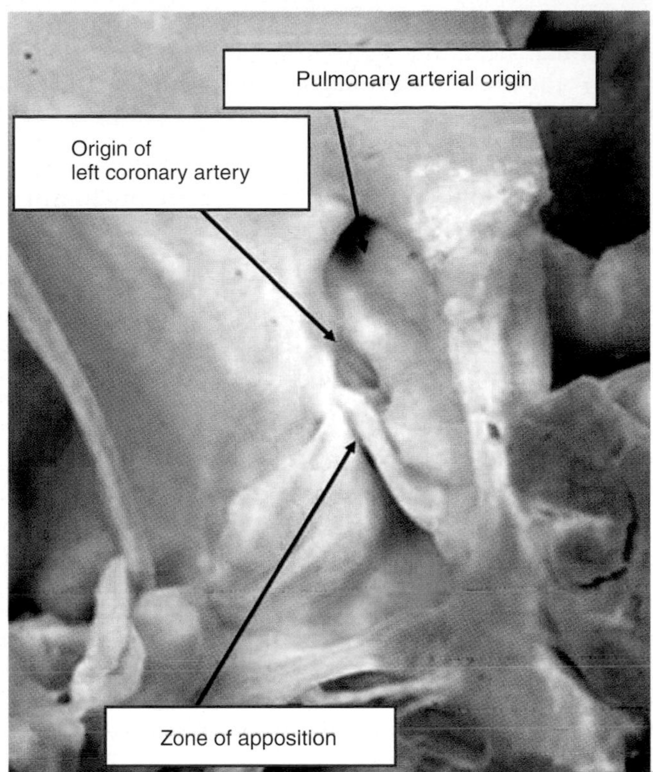

Figure 41-16 Note the origin of the left coronary artery above the zone of apposition of two of the leaflets of the truncal valve, but very close to the origin of the pulmonary arteries. The surgeon seeking to correct this specimen would need to take care not to damage the coronary arteries when removing the pulmonary arteries from the common trunk.

of the moderator band. In those hearts in which a muscular bar interposes between the attachments of the truncal and tricuspid valves in the postero-inferior margin of the septal defect, the membranous septum is intact behind the muscular tissue, and the atrioventricular conduction tissues are somewhat distant from the rim of the defect (see Fig. 41-5). In patients in whom the ventricular septal defect is perimembranous, in contrast, the conduction tissue passes directly along the left aspect of the fibrous postero-inferior rim of the defect (see Fig. 41-6). It is then at greater surgical risk. We have already mentioned most of the common associated cardiovascular anomalies found in the setting of common arterial trunk, including a right aortic arch, interrupted aortic arch, patency of the arterial duct, discontinuity of one pulmonary artery, coronary arterial anomalies, and incompetent truncal valve. A defect within the oval fossa has been noted in up to one-fifth of patients, persistence of the left superior caval vein draining to the coronary sinus in up to one-tenth, and an aberrant subclavian artery in between one-tenth and one-twentieth.[12] Partially anomalous pulmonary venous connection has also been reported.[13]

AETIOLOGY AND MORPHOGENESIS

Over the past decade, the evidence has accumulated that many cases of common arterial trunk result from a genetic defect. The evidence comes from interpretation of morphology, experiments in animals, studies on the role of cells migrating from the neural crest in the development of the outlet components of the heart and the arterial trunks,[14] and the discovery of deletions in chromosome 22q11 in patients with malformations involving the outflow tracts, often described as so-called conotruncal defects.[15,16]

The morphology of common arterial trunk supports very strongly the notion that, during development, there has been failure of septation of the ventricular outlets and the outflow segment of the heart tube. It had been suggested that the entity represents failure of formation of the subpulmonary infundibulum, with the common arterial trunk in essence representing the aorta.[12] No evidence has accrued over the last decades to support this latter notion, but much has appeared to contradict it. From the morphological stance, specimens with common arterial trunk show no evidence of a blind-ending subpulmonary outflow tract, such as is seen in tetralogy with pulmonary atresia. It is this latter entity that provides the paradigm for underdevelopment of the subpulmonary outflow tract. In such hearts with tetralogy and pulmonary atresia, four-fifths of specimens have perimembranous ventricular septal defects. In contrast, in the setting of common arterial trunk, four-fifths of hearts have a muscular postero-inferior rim to the ventricular septal defect. Additionally, if the arterial root truly represented the aorta, then coronary arteries would be anticipated to arise in patterns comparable to those seen in the normal heart. This is rarely the case in the setting of common arterial trunk, where the origins and course of the coronary arteries are frequently bizarre.[11]

Direct studies of cardiac development, on both normal and abnormal hearts, have always shown that the initially common ventricular outflow tract is separated by endocardial cushions, or ridges, to produce the intrapericardial arterial trunks, along with the arterial valvar leaflets and sinuses and their supporting ventricular outflow tracts.[17] Failure of such separation during embryological development was demonstrated conclusively as producing common arterial trunk in an elegant study using Keeshond dogs published as long ago as 1978. This study[18] showed that the cushions which normally divided the outflow segment of the heart failed to fuse in the setting of common arterial trunk, the concept subsequently being endorsed by further studies carried out by Bartelings and colleagues.[19] Much work over the past 15 years has provided further evidence of the importance of the outflow cushions in dividing the initially common ventricular outflow tract, and has demonstrated an important role for cells migrating from the neural crest in populating these cushions (Fig. 41-17).

Other studies have shown that, when the migration of the cells from the neural crest is perturbed, the cushions do not develop properly, and one of the lesions produced is common arterial trunk.[20] This is in keeping with the results of selective inbreeding of the Keeshond dogs, which were used to study normal development.[18] Using the same colony of inbred animals, a similar spectrum of malformations to that obtained subsequent to perturbation of the neural crest was observed.[21] Many animals had common arterial trunk, but others had ventricular septal defects, or tetralogy of Fallot. Significantly, the pattern of inheritance was consistent with a defect at a single autosomal locus. The genetic basis for such malformations is further supported by observations made in the homozygous mutant Splotch mouse,

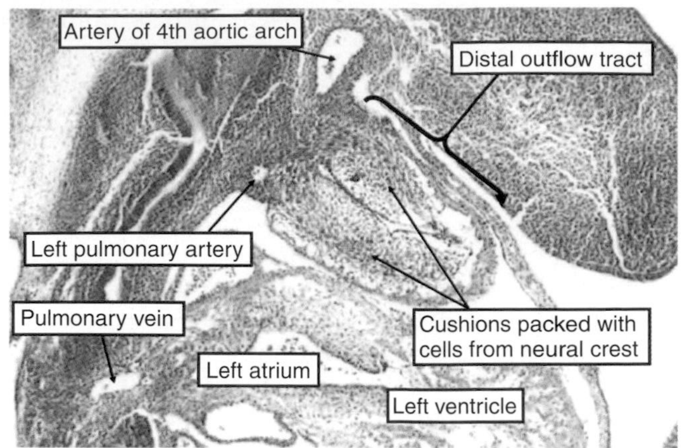

Figure 41-17 This section comes from a mouse in which the cells migrating from the neural crest are marked by a construct revealing the *Wnt1* gene, which is revealed by the blue colouration. The cells occupy both cushions, which are separating the distal outflow tract into the aortic and pulmonary channels. (Courtesy of Dr Sandra Webb, St George's Hospital Medical School, London, United Kingdom.)

in which a common arterial trunk arises exclusively from the right ventricle in many of the malformed embryos.[20] Common arterial trunk has been produced when there is deficiency of *sox4*, a gene which also normally populates the endocardial cushions of the developing outflow tracts.[22,23] Some of the afflicted embryos in these experiments, however, had doubly committed ventricular septal defects rather than common arterial trunk. This is of particular interest, since as we have already discussed, the morphology of the outflow tracts is almost identical in the setting of a common arterial trunk (see Fig. 41-17) and in doubly committed defects, apart from the finding of separate aortic and pulmonary valvar orifices in the latter malformations. All of this is pertinent to findings in humans with microdeletions of chromosome 22q11.

The initial report of a family with a chromosomal translocation resulting in partial trisomy for chromosome 20 and partial monosomy for chromosome 22, with all patients having DiGeorge syndrome, and one having common arterial trunk, led to searching for microdeletions in the 22q11 region, first by high resolution banding,[24,25] and then by fluorescent in situ hybridisation.[26] These investigations revealed that a majority of patients with DiGeorge syndrome have 22q11 deletions. As yet, however, no single gene has been found to be responsible for all cases, although the *Tuple* gene has been implicated in some cases. It has been shown, nonetheless, that the DiGeorge syndrome is best considered as the severe end of a clinical spectrum. For a while, it was referred to as CATCH 22, with reference to the novel by Joseph Heller, and reflecting cardiac defects, abnormal facies, thymic hypoplasia, cleft palate, and hypocalcaemia produced by deletions of 22q11. Experience showed that such usage was interpreted in pejorative fashion, and the term is now frowned upon. Be that as it may, nearly one-third of patients with non-syndromic defects involving the ventricular outflow tracts, and one-third of those with common arterial trunk, have been shown to have microdeletions in the DiGeorge critical region.[27] An association between common arterial trunk, and other anomalies of the outflow tracts, and CHARGE syndrome (coloboma, heart disease, choanal atresia, retardation [mental and physical] genital hypoplasia, and ear anomalies) has also long been recognised. The anomalies of the outflow tracts found with CHARGE syndrome are much the same as in DiGeorge syndrome, except that tetralogy of Fallot and double outlet right ventricle predominate in the former, whereas, in the latter, common arterial trunk and interruption of the aortic arch proximal to the left subclavian artery are more common. It seems likely therefore, that chromosomal damage leads to deletions of 22q11, which, in some way, interferes with the migration of cells from the neural crest, and thereby causes damage to the third and fourth pharyngeal pouches. We have come a long way in understanding the morphogenesis of these lesions since the late lamented Robert Freedom and his colleagues[28] drew the attention of paediatric cardiologists to the association between anomalies of these pharyngeal pouches and congenital cardiac malformations.

It should not be thought, however, that all is now resolved. One-fifth of patients with terminal deletions of the long arm of chromosome 7 have been reported to have cardiac anomalies, including common arterial trunk.[29] In patients identified in the Baltimore-Washington Infant Study,[2] those with malformations of the outflow tracts showed no recurrences from 109 parents or siblings, in keeping with the findings of Nora and Nora,[30] who suggested a lower than usual recurrence rate of 1% for common arterial trunk, although subsequent studies were less convincing in this respect.[31] Other studies have suggested an autosomal recessive pattern of inheritance.[32] There are also other reliably documented reports of common arterial trunk in siblings,[31,33,34] while two sets of three siblings have been documented with the lesion.[35,36] Dizygotic twins concordant for common arterial trunk have also been described.[37] Patients with common arterial trunk, therefore, continue to be a fertile population in which to study the genetic background of congenital cardiac malformations.

DIAGNOSTIC FEATURES

Antenatal Diagnosis

It might be expect that common arterial trunk would be detected during the mid-trimester scan for fetal anomalies, which is routine in many countries. In practice, population-based studies demonstrate that the diagnosis may often be missed,[38,39] presumably because the four-chamber view of the heart may appear to be normal on superficial examination. More detailed echocardiographic examination of the fetal heart, nonetheless, should reveal a ventricular septal defect. An arterial trunk that overrides the defect is the only outlet which arises from the ventricular mass.[40] Under ideal circumstances it will be possible to document the degree of regurgitation or stenosis of the truncal valve, and the course and integrity of the aortic arch can be delineated[40] (Table 41-1).

There are now a number of reports which document the outcomes for fetuses after such antenatal detection. Despite what we might now consider to be excellent outcomes from surgical repair, a significant proportion of parents will choose to terminate the pregnancy.[40,41] A significant proportion of

TABLE 41-1

KEY DIAGNOSTIC FEATURES IN COMMON ARTERIAL TRUNK

Fetal echocardiogram	Four-chamber view	Ventricular septal defect with truncal override (may appear normal)
	Great vessels	Single arterial trunk Truncal regurgitation
	Aortic arch	Interruption
Clinical examination	Inspection	(?)Mild cyanosis Failure to thrive Tachypnoea
	Palpation	Bounding pulses Liver enlargement
	Auscultation	Normal first heart sound May have a single second sound (although not always) Ejection click Ejection systolic murmur (?) Diastolic murmur of truncal regurgitation
Electrocardiogram		Non-specific usually combined ventricular hypertrophy
Chest radiograph		Cardiomegaly Increased pulmonary vascular markings Narrow arterial pedicle
Echocardiogram	Parasternal long axis	Truncal origin Ventricular size and mural thickness Ventricular septal defect Velocity of interventricular shunting Truncal regurgitation
	Parasternal short axis	Morphology of truncal valve Mechanism of truncal regurgitation Origin of pulmonary arteries Stenosis of pulmonary arteries Origin of coronary arteries
	Apical four chamber	Ventricular origin of trunk Truncal regurgitation Truncal stenosis Function of atrioventricular valves
	High parasternal	Aortic arch Arterial duct Interruption of aortic arch
Cardiac catheterisation	Haemodynamics	Pressure measurement in right and left pulmonary arteries Pressure drop across truncal valve
	Oximetry	Pulmonary-to-systemic blood flow ratio
	Pulmonary vasodilator	To assess pulmonary vascular responsiveness
	Angiocardiography	Truncal injection to examine the degree of regurgitation Selective pulmonary angiogram Left ventriculogram to evaluate the size and location of septal defects

fetuses will have associated non-cardiac anomalies,[41] with or without a deletion within chromosome 22.[42]

Neonatal Presentation

The typical patient with common arterial trunk will present during the neonatal period, or in early infancy, with mild central cyanosis, a hyperactive precordium, and signs of increasing congestive cardiac failure. There will be difficulties in feeding, failure to thrive, often extreme tachypnoea, and hepatic enlargement. A wide pulse pressure, with bounding pulses, is to be anticipated. While a minor degree of hypoxaemia is common, obvious cyanosis is a feature of either raised pulmonary vascular resistance, or pulmonary stenosis. Once cardiac failure is established, the chest may bulge in consequence of the cardiomegaly.

At auscultation, the first heart sound is usually normal, while the second sound is accentuated. It might be anticipated that the second sound would always be single in the presence of a common arterial valve. This is not the case. In approximately one half of infants, there is close splitting of the second sound, documented by phonocardiography as well as by auscultation.[43] Possible explanations for this finding are asynchronous closure of the valvar leaflets, or production of a duplicate sound by vibrations within the arterial trunk. In most infants, there will also be a loud systolic ejection click, heard best at the apex, which coincides with the opening of the truncal valve. A systolic murmur is almost always heard, but can be of varying intensity and duration. Other findings often include an ejection systolic murmur of grade II or III heard maximally at the mid-to-upper left sternal border, or a harsh pansystolic murmur of grade III or IV heard maximally at the lower left sternal border. Less common murmurs include the apical mid-diastolic one, which results from flow, and an early diastolic murmur heard maximally along the left sternal edge, indicating truncal valvar insufficiency. Rarely, the murmur may be continuous and heard not only over the precordium but also the back. This is indicative of pulmonary stenosis. Surprisingly, in perhaps one tenth of patients, no murmur is heard at all at the time of presentation. This indicates an absence of turbulence within the ventricles or their outflow tracts.

ELECTROCARDIOGRAPHY

Normal sinus rhythm is the rule, and conduction through the heart is similarly normal. The QRS axis as seen in the frontal plane is extremely variable and non-specific but is almost always directed inferiorly. The distribution of ventricular forces is also variable, reflecting the variability encountered in ventricular hypertrophy. The majority of patients showed evidence of combined ventricular hypertrophy, with isolated right ventricular hypertrophy also a frequent finding.[44] It is unusual to find evidence of isolated left ventricular hypertrophy, or a normal pattern. There are, therefore, no specific electrocardiographic features for patients with common arterial trunk, except perhaps that inversion of the T waves is seen with frequency in the left precordial leads, probably reflecting the impaired coronary arterial diastolic flow.

RADIOLOGIC FEATURES

The chest radiograph shows significant cardiomegaly, together with an increase in pulmonary vascular markings (Fig. 41-18). The aortic arch is right sided in approximately one-third of patients. This finding, in association with increased pulmonary vascularity, is strongly suggestive of common trunk. It may be possible to see an unusually high origin of the left pulmonary artery with no intervening confluent pulmonary arterial segment. Although the truncal root itself is dilated, the arterial pedicle tends to appear narrow simply because of its commonality. When flow of blood to the lungs is decreased, the heart is less enlarged, and the pulmonary vascular markings are closer to normal. Pronounced discrepancy between the vascular markings on the two sides suggests unilateral atresia, or absence, of one pulmonary artery. As with the electrocardiogram, there are no specific findings, but the association of right arch and plethora is highly suggestive of the diagnosis.

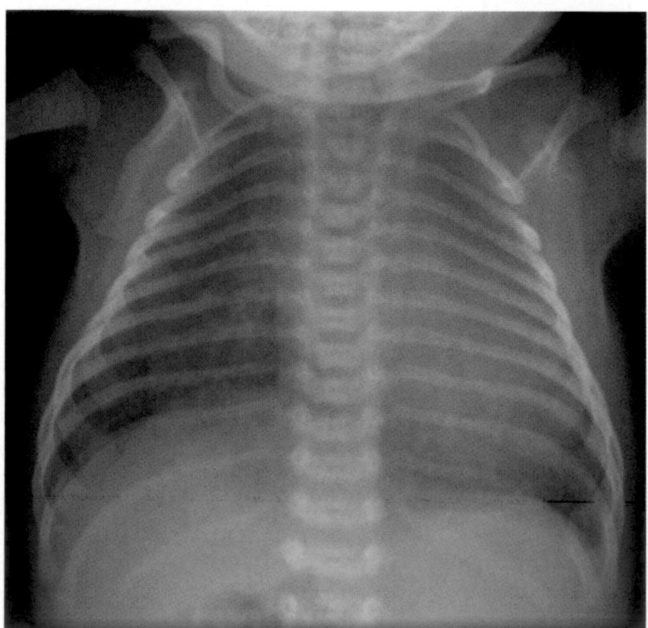

Figure 41-18 Chest radiograph obtained from a four-week-old infant with common arterial trunk, demonstrating increased pulmonary vascular markings.

ECHOCARDIOGRAPHY

It is now possible in most instances to evaluate neonates and infants having common arterial trunk with such precision that only cross sectional echocardiography is required prior to corrective surgery.[45] The goals of echocardiography are to define the ventricular origin and pattern of branching of the common arterial trunk, to determine the morphology and any functional abnormalities of the truncal valve, to exclude any stenosis at the origins of the pulmonary arteries, to distinguish a perimembranous ventricular septal defect from one with a muscular postero-inferior rim, to exclude any abnormalities of the aorta, and to define all other associated lesions. In the majority of patients, transthoracic echocardiography will provide all of the diagnostic information.

The parasternal long-axis section of the left ventricle will usually show the common arterial trunk overriding the ventricular septum, with its valve forming the superior border of the ventricular septal defect (Fig. 41-19). This feature, of course, is lacking when the trunk has a univentricular origin. If the pulmonary arteries have a confluent segment, it will be seen arising posteriorly from the common trunk in this view. The leaflets of the truncal valve are frequently dysplastic and, occasionally, can prolapse, causing the ventricular septal defect to be restrictive. Indeed, as shown morphologically, the leaflets may occasionally coapt directly on the crest of the ventricular septum. Colour flow Doppler interrogation will demonstrate flow to the aorta from both the right and left ventricle, and will document any truncal valvar insufficiency, which can be predominantly or exclusively to either

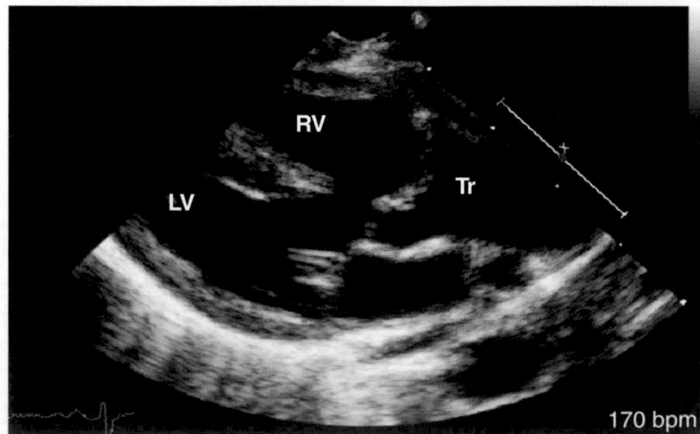

Figure 41-19 Echocardiographic image from a parasternal window, demonstrating the long axis of the heart. There is a common arterial trunk (Tr) which overrides the crest of the muscular ventricular septum. LV, left ventricle, RV, right ventricle.

the right or the left ventricle. When the valve is stenotic, there is limited excursion of the leaflets. Turbulent flow distal to the truncal valve will then be evident on colour flow or continuous wave interrogation. The parasternal long-axis sections will demonstrate the expected fibrous continuity between the leaflets of the truncal valve and the truncal leaflet of the mitral valve (see Fig. 41-19), the degree of dilation of the left ventricle and the extent of biventricular hypertrophy. Restriction of the ventricular septal defect will be seen in this view. Continuous wave Doppler interrogation will then record a drop in pressure across the defect, which may either be from left to right or from right to left, depending upon the ventricular origin of the common trunk.

The parasternal short-axis section taken just above the level of the truncal valve demonstrates the pulmonary arteries as they arise from the common trunk. In the so-called type I variant of common trunk, a short pulmonary arterial segment arises from the left lateral aspect of the common trunk, and then divides into right and left pulmonary arteries (Fig. 41-20). Stenosis at the origin of the right or left pulmonary arteries, or pulmonary arterial hypoplasia, will be evident in this section. In the so-called type II pattern, the right and left pulmonary arteries arise from the posterior wall of the common trunk through separate but adjacent orifices (Fig. 41-21). In practice, it is often difficult to distinguish these patterns, even in postmortem specimens.

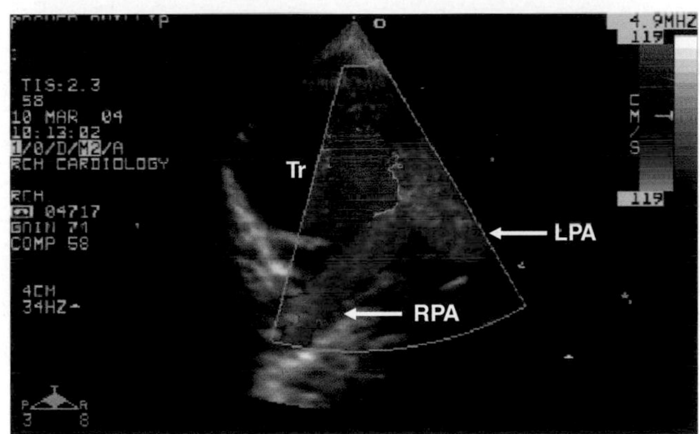

Figure 41-20 Echocardiographic image demonstrating the short axis of the arterial trunk (Tr). The right (RPA) and left (LPA) pulmonary arteries arise from a short common artery. There is laminar flow in both pulmonary arteries which are of normal calibre.

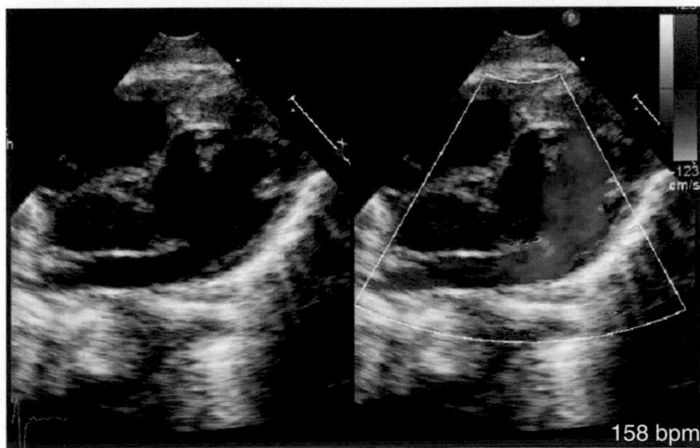

Figure 41-21 Echocardiographic image taken from a parasternal window demonstrating the separate origin of the right pulmonary artery (RPA). There is laminar flow within the pulmonary artery which is of normal calibre.

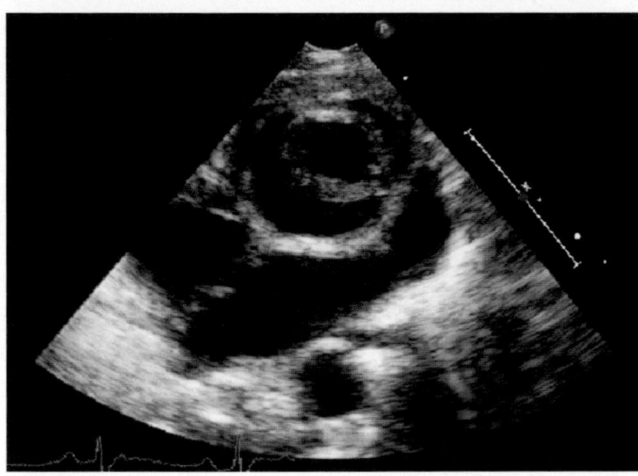

Figure 41-22 Image of the truncal valve, imaged from a parasternal window. In this patient the valve was functionally bicuspid.

In contrast, the type III variant is easily distinguished, the right and left pulmonary arteries arising from the common trunk via two widely separated orifices. Other rarer origins of the pulmonary arteries must be anticipated, including atresia or even absence of one pulmonary artery. The parasternal short-axis section will also identify the number of truncal valvar leaflets (Fig. 41-22). Discontinuity between the tricuspid and truncal valvar leaflets will be seen in this cut when there is a muscular postero-inferior rim to the ventricular septal defect, expected in four-fifths of patients.

The apical and parasternal four-chamber sections also demonstrate the large subarterial ventricular septal defect and the overriding of the truncal valve. Colour flow Doppler interrogation will usually demonstrate biventricular shunting across the defect. Any truncal valvar insufficiency will be evident in this view, while duplex scanning with continuous wave Doppler documents any systolic gradient should the truncal valve be stenotic. The diastolic drop in pressure between the common trunk and the ventricular mass can be demonstrated when there is valvar insufficiency. The drop in pressure identified across a stenotic truncal valve, however, will exaggerate the severity of stenosis. This is because the increased flow of blood to the lungs gives rise to a large left ventricular output. Gradients of up to 60 mm Hg as estimated with Doppler, therefore, will become insignificant after corrective surgery.

Although the parasternal long- and short-axis sections will demonstrate the pulmonary arteries arising posteriorly from the common trunk, the subcostal long-axis sections are unique in their ability to display most of the morphological features of common arterial trunk. The subcostal paracoronal sections demonstrate the ventricular septal defect, the nature of its postero-inferior rim, the overriding of the common trunk (Fig. 41-23), and the origin of both the ascending aorta and the pulmonary arteries (Figs. 41-24 and 41-25). Oblique sections may reveal not only the origins of the pulmonary arteries, but also the integrity of the aortic arch (Fig. 41-26). A right oblique section identifies the entirety of the proximal right pulmonary artery, whereas leftward rotation can be used to demonstrate the features of the left pulmonary artery. These sections also permit identification of any stenosis at the origins of the left and right pulmonary arteries, and will

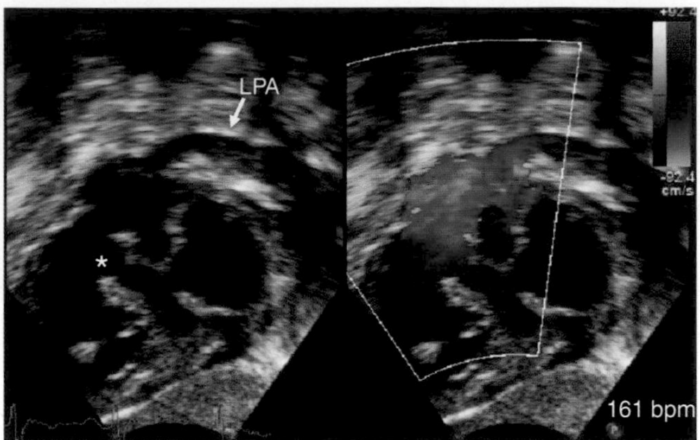

Figure 41-23 Oblique image of the heart taken from a subcostal window, demonstrating the truncal valve overriding a ventricular septal defect (*asterisk*) and the origin of the left pulmonary artery (LPA).

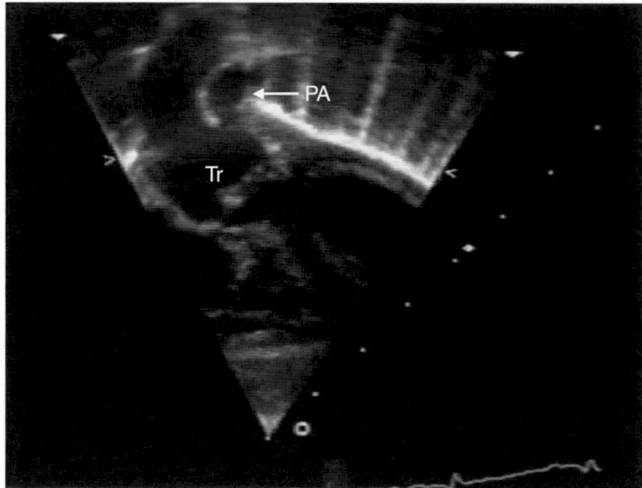

Figure 41-24 Oblique image of the heart taken from a subcostal window, demonstrating the truncal valve and the origin of the common pulmonary artery (PA), in a patient with common arterial trunk (Tr) of the so-called type I variety.

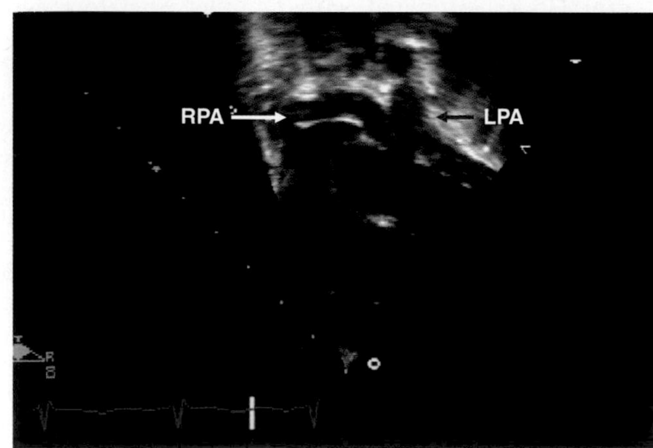

Figure 41-25 Oblique image of the heart taken from a subcostal window, demonstrating the right (RPA) and left (LPA) pulmonary arteries. It was considered that in this patient there may have been a short segment of common pulmonary artery.

reveal rare findings such as crossed origins of the pulmonary arteries.[46] Duplex scanning can be used to measure the drop in pressure across any identified stenoses. Anterior angulation demonstrates the morphology of the truncal valve, while colour mapping reveals the severity of truncal regurgitation (Fig. 41-27). Characteristically, interrogation using continuous wave Doppler identifies both systolic and diastolic flow immediately distal to the site of stenosis. Suprasternal sections can also be used to identify the origin of the pulmonary arteries from the common trunk. These cuts, in addition, will demonstrate any interruption of the aortic arch, the side of the aortic arch, and additional anomalies such as presence of an arterial duct or aortic coarctation. Retrograde diastolic flow is observed quite frequently in the aortic arch, reflecting the low diastolic pressure in the pulmonary arteries.

It is not unusual for interruption of the aortic arch to be associated with common arterial trunk, often in combination with significant dysplasia of the truncal valvar leaflets producing insufficiency and/or stenosis. Almost always the ascending aorta is relatively hypoplastic, being smaller than the proximal pulmonary arteries. The interruption can occur at any of the classical sites. At the time

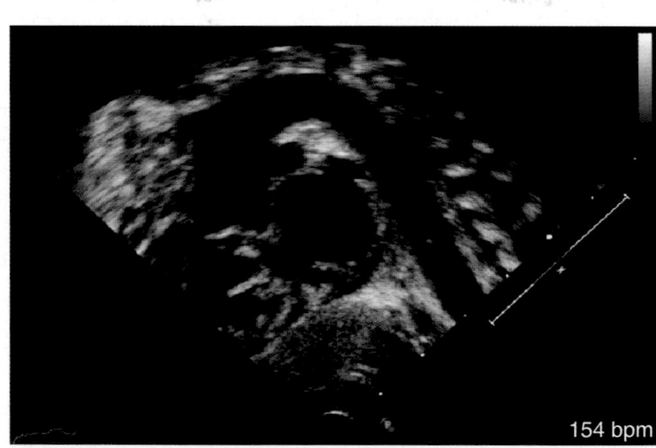

Figure 41-26 Oblique image of the heart taken from a subcostal window, demonstrating the arterial trunk, the origin of the pulmonary artery from it and the integrity of the aortic arch.

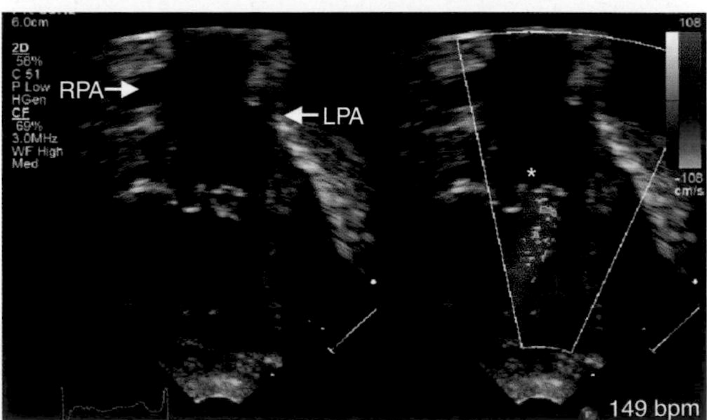

Figure 41-27 Image of the heart taken from a subcostal window, with anterior angulation of the transducer. The origins of the right (RPA) and left (LPA) pulmonary arteries are widely separated and the origin of the left pulmonary artery is hypoplastic. Colour mapping demonstrates mild regurgitation of the truncal valve (*asterisk*).

of echocardiographic investigation, most neonates will already be receiving prostaglandins intravenously. Consequently, the arterial duct will be relatively large. While the presence of a patent arterial duct would lead one to suspect the presence of interruption of the aortic arch, ductal patency may rarely be present in association with a normal arch.[47] The high left parasternal echocardiographic section demonstrates the duct, and colour flow will then usually demonstrate the flow through it to be bidirectional. Pulsed Doppler interrogation reveals that systolic flow is from the pulmonary arteries to the descending aorta, albeit that, provided that the pulmonary vascular resistance is low, there will be reversal of flow during diastole. The suprasternal parasagittal sections will reveal the site of aortic interruption, if present, relative to the origin of the brachiocephalic, left common carotid and left subclavian arteries.

CARDIAC MAGNETIC RESONANCE IMAGING

Cardiac magnetic resonance imaging is rarely used in the investigation of patients with common arterial trunk before surgery, as in most instances, cross sectional echocardiography provides adequate diagnostic information. Nonetheless, there may be some instances, for example in the examination of complex problems of the aortic arch or anomalies of the drainage of the pulmonary veins, where magnetic resonance may make a contribution to the preoperative investigation. Such imaging makes a more significant contribution to the investigations of patients after surgery, when it permits the quantitative assessment of not only the performance of the right and left ventricles, but also of the severity of regurgitation of the neo-aortic and pulmonary valves, along with measurement of residual intracardiac shunts and imaging of the aortic arch.[48]

CARDIAC CATHETERISATION AND ANGIOCARDIOGRAPHY

It is now possible to refer patients with typical non-invasive findings directly for corrective surgery. Should there be any doubt about any aspect of the presentation, however, cardiac catheterisation should be performed, particularly if there is any suggestion of pulmonary vascular obstructive disease.[49]

If catheterisation is to be performed, separate catheters should ideally be placed in each pulmonary artery, a systemic artery, the superior caval vein, and at least one pulmonary vein. Consumption of oxygen should be measured while the catheter in the superior caval vein is withdrawn to the inferior caval vein to obtain a second measurement of systemic venous oxygen. Then, with further manipulation, more values should be obtained to determine pulmonary venous saturation. The effect of administration of 100% oxygen, or pulmonary vasodilators, should be measured. Entry to the pulmonary arteries is achieved most readily by retrograde arterial catheterisation, looping the catheter in the truncal root so that it can then pass upwards into the pulmonary arteries.

Oximetry will reveal an increase in the saturation of oxygen in the pulmonary arteries, compared to the caval veins, indicative of a net left-to-right shunt (Fig. 41-28). Commonly, the saturation of oxygen in the pulmonary arteries may be lower than in the aorta, reflecting the streaming of blood preferentially from right ventricle to pulmonary arteries, and from the left ventricle to the aorta.[9,13] Pulmonary venous saturations of oxygen cannot be assumed, because pulmonary oedema or chest infection can result in pulmonary venous desaturation.

Measurements of pressure will reveal, in the typical case, similar pressures in the right and left ventricles. There may be minor differences between the measurements in the two pulmonary arteries, and between the pulmonary arteries and the aorta, which may reflect streaming. Pressure differences may also reflect obstruction at the point of origin of pulmonary arteries from the aorta, or in one pulmonary artery. Such differences in pressure between the aorta and the pulmonary arteries were found in almost half of the patients studied by Calder and colleagues.[9] Any differences in systolic pressure should be noted across the truncal valve. These were reported to occur in one third of the patients investigated by Calder and colleagues[9] and varied from 10 to 60 mm Hg. Minor differences in pressure, nonetheless, are common and reflect excessive flow, rather than truncal stenosis.

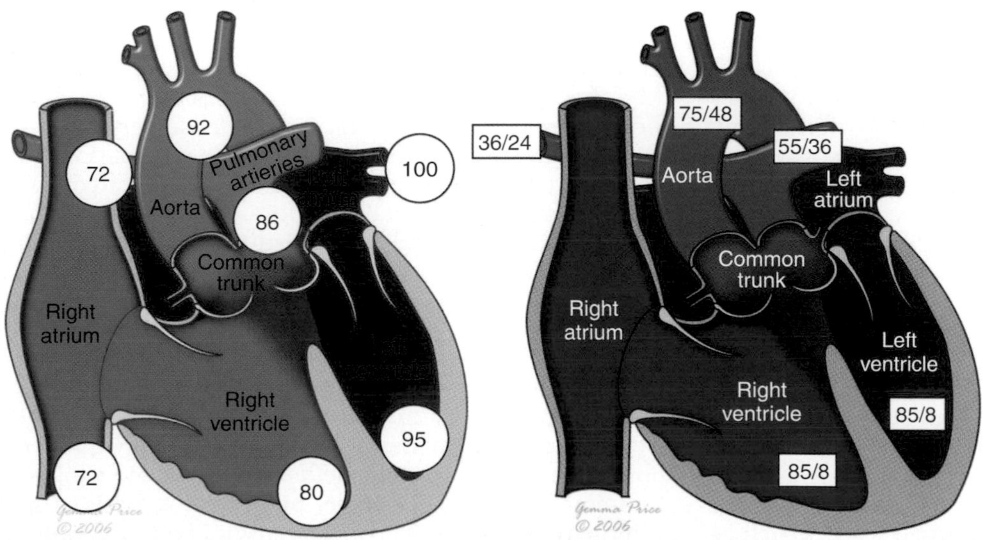

Figure 41-28 Representative measurements of oxygen saturations (*left hand panel*, in percent) and pressures (*right hand panel*, in mmHg) obtained during cardiac catheterisation in a patient with common arterial trunk. There is evidence of a substantial left-to-right shunt, with the oxygen saturation in the pulmonary arteries, exceeding that in the caval veins. Nonetheless, the oxygen saturation in the aorta exceeds that in the pulmonary arteries, because of streaming. Pressures in the right and left ventricles are equal and there is no evidence of stenosis of the truncal valve. The pressure which was measured in the left pulmonary artery is slightly less and that in the right pulmonary artery and significantly less than that in the aorta, reflecting a stenosis of the origin of the right pulmonary artery.

Selective angiocardiography should consist, first, of injecting contrast medium into the truncal root, filming in frontal and lateral projections. Elongated right anterior oblique views show well the division of the aortic and pulmonary pathways from the trunk.[50] Rapid injections are necessary to avoid excessive dilution of the contrast medium by the torrential flow. Such an injection should demonstrate the anterior tilt of the truncal root,[9] the origin of one or both pulmonary arteries from the ascending trunk, and the degree of truncal regurgitation. Exceptionally, the pulmonary arteries may be seen arising from the underside of the aortic arch,[51] albeit that it is questionable in this setting whether the trunk itself is a common rather than a solitary structure. The arteries can also arise from other unusual sites, such as one of the truncal sinuses. An injection in the truncal root will usually demonstrate any interruption of the aortic arch, and should also reveal any unilateral absence of one pulmonary artery, an association found in between one-tenth and one-sixth of patients.[9,13,52] If suspected, then a further descending aortogram, and selective injection(s) into collateral arteries, or even pulmonary venous wedge injections on the side of the absent pulmonary artery, should clarify whether the artery really is absent, or whether it originally derived its blood supply from an arterial duct. Abnormalities of the origins of the coronary arteries have been identified as a risk factor in one large surgical series of infants.[53] Although it was suggested that such abnormalities should be identified by coronary arteriography, or by echocardiography prior to surgery, there is no evidence as yet that such findings have reduced surgical mortality.

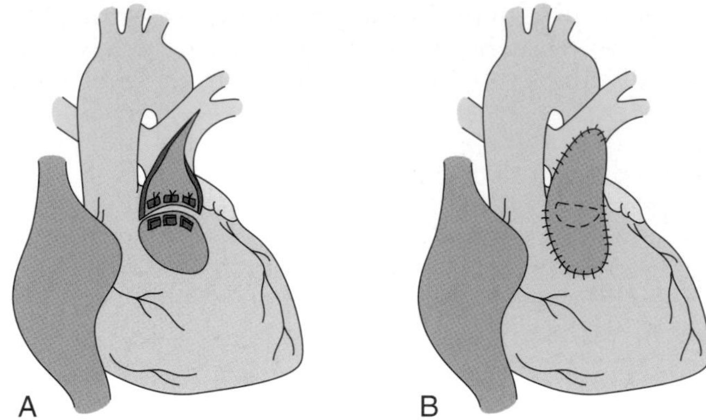

Figure 41-29 Repair of common arterial trunk, without a conduit. **A,** The pulmonary trunk is anastomosed to the right ventricle. **B,** The anterior aspect of the anastomosis and pulmonary trunk is augmented with a monocusp.

SURGICAL TREATMENT

Early attempts at surgical palliation involved banding the pulmonary arteries, either at the level of a confluent pulmonary arterial segment or separately for the right and left arteries. This procedure has now been almost completely abandoned, in favour of complete surgical repair. The first such complete repair of common arterial trunk, using a valved conduit to restore continuity from the right ventricle to the pulmonary arteries, was achieved at the Mayo Clinic in September 1967.[54]

The operation begins with dissecting both pulmonary arteries down to their points of branching in the hilums of both lungs. The aorta is fully mobilised. The surgery is performed under hypothermic cardiopulmonary bypass. The degree of truncal incompetence is carefully assessed. Significant regurgitation may interfere with myocardial protection, irrespective of whether that is carried out by intermittent crossclamping or cardioplegia, which may make it necessary to inject cardioplegic solution into the coronary arteries or coronary sinus to achieve adequate protection. The pulmonary arteries are detached from the common trunk, taking care to avoid any coronary arterial origins. The defect in the aorta may be closed by direct suture, or with a small patch of polyester (Dacron) or polytetrafluoroethylene (Gore-Tex). If there is no confluent pulmonary arterial segment, access is improved by transecting the ascending component of the common trunk. The separate pulmonary arteries are excised with the interposed portion of trunk as a single button, and the ascending aorta is reconstructed as an end-to-end anastomosis. The ventricular septal defect is then closed with a patch in such a way as to connect the remaining aortic component of the trunk with the left ventricle. Continuity between the pulmonary arteries and the right ventricle can often be established with the aorta crossclamped while the patient is being rewarmed. With adequate mobilisation of the pulmonary arteries, it should be possible to anastomose a homograft directly onto the right ventriculotomy without any prosthetic interposition.

As the availability of homografts may be limited, and in order to avoid the long-term problems of homograft stenosis, modifications to the procedure have been described which avoid their use. In one such modification, continuity between the right ventricle and pulmonary arteries is achieved without use of a conduit. This operation, originally described by Reid and colleagues,[55] and popularised by Barbero-Marcial and his colleagues,[56] involved a direct anastomosis between the pulmonary arteries and the right ventricle, with the anterior aspect of the anastomosis being augmented with a monocusp or pericardial patch (Fig. 41-29).The Brazilian series as initially reported involved seven infants aged from 2 to 9 months. Of these patients, one died early, but no late deaths were reported. The monocusp valve seemed to function well, as judged echocardiographically, but was frequently regurgitant. This novel approach was then used by others, albeit with limited success.[57,58] More recent reports suggest that, in the longer term, the requirement for surgical revision of the pulmonary outflow tract may be reduced in some patients when this approach is used.[59] Thus, the actuarial freedom from either late death or need for further surgery in those patients who survived the early postoperative period was approximately 90% at 10 years. In a series[60] reported from Birmingham, in the United Kingdom, it was observed that mortality, both early and in the medium term, was similar in patients who underwent repair using a direct anastomosis, compared to those in whom a valved conduit had been used. The freedom from reintervention to the right ventricular outflow tract, however, was greater in those having direct anastomosis, being 89% at 10 years, compared to those in whom a conduit had been used, with only 56% requiring no further intervention. Thus, while this approach may have some benefits in terms of reducing the requirement for further surgery because of stenosis of the pulmonary outflow tract, further studies will be required to examine the impact of the pulmonary regurgitation, which is common after this type of modification.

An alternative solution to overcome the limited supply of homografts has been to use alternative types of conduit. Although a number of different types of conduit have been used, there has been considerable recent interest in the Contegra conduit (Medtronic, Inc, Minneapolis, Minnesota), a heterologous bovine jugular venous graft which contains a trileaflet venous valve. It is available in sizes as small as 12 mm, making it potentially ideal for reconstructing the right ventricular outflow tract in neonates and infants. There have been recent concerns, nonetheless, with respect to the development of accelerated stenosis in the distal part of the conduit, particularly when small sizes are used. Thus, in one series, 15 of 21 conduits with a diameter of 16 mm or less were noted to be significantly stenosed within 1 year of implantation.[61]

Regurgitation of the truncal valve remains a significant challenge. In general regurgitation of even a moderate severity should be dealt with conservatively. Where severe regurgitation exists, often resulting from prolapse of a rudimentary leaflet of the truncal valve, the valve needs to be repaired, or rarely replaced.[58]

Successful surgical correction can also be achieved when the aortic arch is interrupted. The original successful repair, described by Gomes and McGoon,[60] left the duct in place to supply blood to the descending aorta. This, of course, can only be done after the age of a year or so, when there is no chance of ductal closure. Because of this, this technique is now rarely used. In younger patients, the duct and all ductal tissue must be excised. The entire thoracic aorta, the pulmonary arteries, the head and neck vessels, and the duct must then be thoroughly mobilised, so that the ascending and descending parts of the aorta can be joined. Surgery is performed using profound hypothermia and circulatory arrest, with snaring of the head vessels, or alternatively by utilising the technique of continuous cerebral perfusion.[60] It has been suggested that, if the arch can be advanced and the anastomosis performed without using a patch to augment it, the requirement for reintervention may be reduced.[62]

OUTCOMES AFTER SURGERY

Historically, surgical repair of common arterial trunk has been associated with high mortality. Thus, the Pediatric Cardiac Care Consortium reported a mortality rate of 44% for patients who underwent surgery between 1985 and 1993.[63] More recent population-based audits continue to report significant mortality in this group of patients. The publication from the Centers for Disease Control[64] reported an early mortality rate of 20.5%. The mean stay in hospital for these patients was 28.9 days, with an average cost to the hospital of approximately US$57,000.

Recent publications from single institutions, in contrast, demonstrate that surgical repair can be undertaken with low perioperative risk. Brown and coworkers[65] reported an early mortality rate of 17% for patients undergoing surgery between the years 1978 and 2000. The median age at the time of surgery was 76 days. This report highlighted the contribution of associated cardiac anomalies, such as interruption of the aortic arch, or stenosis of the truncal valve, to perioperative mortality. These anomalies were

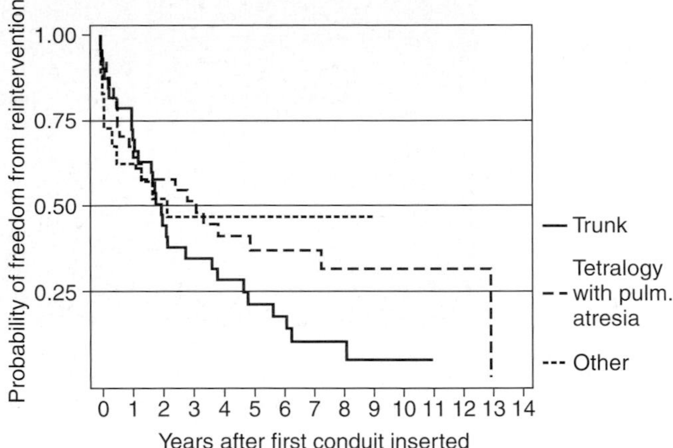

Figure 41-30 Probability of freedom from reintervention for patients (n = 142) who underwent insertion of right ventricular-to-pulmonary artery conduit between January 1990 and December 2000 at The Royal Children's Hospital Melbourne. For the 53 patients with common arterial trunk, the actuarial freedom from reintervention was 21 ± 7% and 11 ± 6% at 5 and 8 years after surgery respectively.

associated with a perioperative mortality of 29%, compared to 9% for patients without these complicating factors. The main problem in the medium term related to the conduit placed between the right ventricle and pulmonary arteries, such that by 7 years, the freedom from reoperation was only 64%.[66] A series of patients who underwent surgery at a median age of 10 days between 1992 and 1999 has recently been reported.[67] Early mortality was 5%, and 92% survived at one year and beyond. The risk of death was higher in patients who weighed less than 2.5 kg. Again, the main reason for further surgery in the medium term was stenosis of the conduit, which needed to be replaced in almost half of all patients by the age of 3 years. Very similar outcomes were reported for patients undergoing surgery at a median age of 28 days from 1995 and 2000, for whom mortality early after surgery was 3.4%, and freedom from reintervention for conduit stenosis was 50% at 6 years.[3] For patients who underwent surgery for common arterial trunk at the Royal Children's Hospital in Melbourne,[68] the freedom from reintervention was only 21% at 5 years after surgery (Fig. 41-30).

Although replacement of the conduit between the right ventricle and the pulmonary arteries has become the definitive method to relieve obstruction, transcatheter angioplasty has been reported in a number of series, with variable outcomes (Fig. 41-31). Of the 142 patients who underwent cardiac surgery which incorporated a conduit between the right ventricle and the pulmonary arteries at the Royal Children's Hospital at Melbourne between January 1990, and December 2000, transcatheter dilation of the conduit was undertaken in 15 patients. Of these, the procedure was deemed to be successful in only 4 (27%). Of the 9 patients with common arterial trunk in whom the intervention was performed between 1.1 and 8.2 years after surgery, it was considered to be successful in only 1.[69] There are a number of reports, nonetheless, which suggest that percutaneous implantation of stents may result in significant immediate haemodynamic improvement, and in some patients may prolong the lifespan of the conduit by several years.[70] Stents have been placed successfully in one recent series of patients.[71] Of these patients, 8 remained free

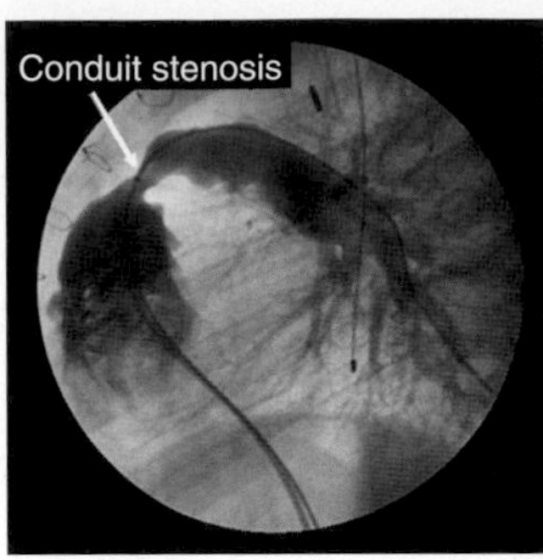

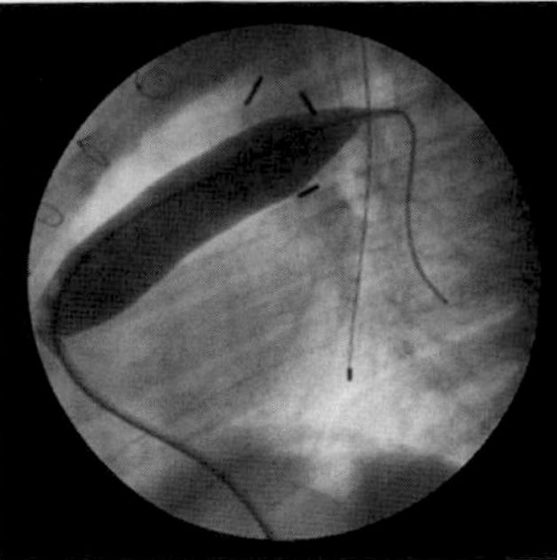
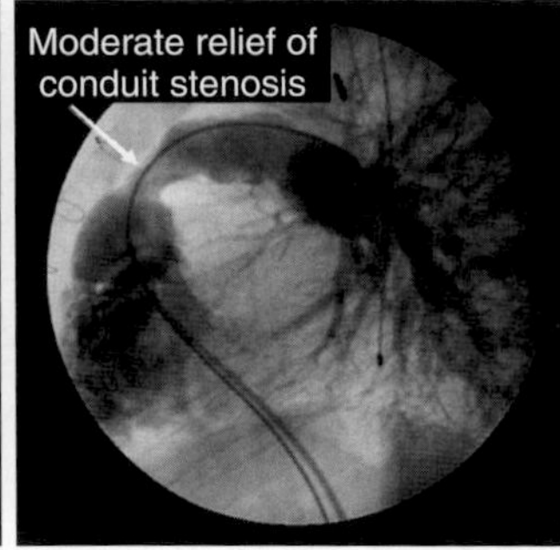

Figure 41-31 Transcatheter dilation of conduit stenosis. **Left panel,** A right ventriculogram demonstrates a significant stenosis of the conduit. **Middle panel,** Inflation of the balloon revealed a waist at the site of the stenosis was relieved by further inflation. **Right panel,** At the end of the procedure, a repeat ventriculogram demonstrated partial relief of the stenosis.

from a second intervention, although 20 required a further procedure between 6 and 44 months after the initial insertion of a stent. The authors suggested that implantation of stents is likely the procedure of choice for patients with a discrete stenosis of the conduit placed from the right ventricle to the pulmonary arteries. The recent development of the valved stent by Bonhoeffer and coworkers from Great Ormond Street Hospital in London may be particularly useful in this group of patients.

As emphasised, interruption of the aortic arch is an important risk factor in patients with common arterial trunk. Reports of small numbers of patients from single centres demonstrate excellent surgical outcomes. A recent report from the Congenital Heart Surgeons Society demonstrated survival rates of only 44% at 6 months after surgery for those patients with associated interruption of the aortic arch.[70] Patients in whom repair of the aortic arch had been undertaken as an initial and isolated procedure had a particularly high mortality. There was an additional late phase of hazard, with survival rates at 10 years being only 31%. In addition, there was an ongoing requirement for further surgery to either the aortic arch or the right ventricular outflow tract. Regurgitation of the truncal valve occurred in almost half of all patients.

RECOMMENDATIONS FOR LONG-TERM FOLLOW-UP

Common arterial trunk is a condition for which continued follow-up is recommended by those having special expertise in the care of adults with congenital cardiac disease.[72,73] The main issue of significance in the care of the adult after surgery for common arterial trunk relates to the fate of the conduit which has been interposed between the right ventricle and the pulmonary circulation. Untreated, significant obstruction to the conduit may result in problems in right ventricular performance, exercise tolerance, and arrhythmia, and may place the patient at risk of cardiac failure. Although it has been recommended that contact sports are avoided, there should be no other restriction to exercise if haemodynamics are good.[74] In general, pregnancy is tolerated well,[74] although it is likely that the presence of right ventricular dysfunction increases maternal risk.[74] As discussed earlier, there is a risk of recurrence in offspring, in particular when there is known deletion within chromosome 22.

The complete reference list can be found on the companion Expert Consult web site at www.expertconsult.com.

ANNOTATED REFERENCES

- Collett RW, Edwards JE: Persistent truncus arteriosus: A classification according to anatomic types. Surg Clin North Am 1949;29:1245–1269.

  Although in general we avoid alpha-numeric classifications of congenital malformations of the heart, this classic paper has provided the foundations for much of our understanding of the anatomy of this lesion. There are few papers in the literature related to common arterial trunk which do not cite this paper.

- Brown CB, Baldwin HS: Neural crest contribution to the cardiovascular system. Adv Exp Med Biol 2006;589:134–151.
- Hutson MR, Kirby ML: Model systems for the study of heart development and disease: Cardiac neural crest and conotruncal malformations. Sem Cell Dev Biol 2007;18:101–110.

  These two excellent articles summarise the development of our knowledge related to the role of the neural crest in the regulation of cardiac development. They provide an excellent introduction to the contributions now being made by those studying embryology to the understanding of cardiac anatomy.

- Carey AH, Kelly D, Halford S, et al: Molecular genetic study of the frequency of monosomy 22q11 in DiGeorge syndrome. Am J Hum Genet 1992;51:964–970.
- Goldmuntz E, Clark BJ, Mitchell LE, et al: Frequency of 22q11 deletions in patients with conotruncal defects. J Am Coll Cardiol 1998;32:492–498.
- Momma K: Cardiovascular anomalies associated with chromosome 22q11.2 deletion. J Cardiol 2007;114:147–149.

  The first of these three articles is one of the early studies which used probes for deoxyribonucleic acid to identify abnormalities of chromosome 22 in patients with DiGeorge syndrome. The second was one of the first large prospective studies of the frequency of 22q11 deletions in patients with so-called conotruncal defects. In this study, approximately one-third of patients with common arterial trunk had co-existing abnormalities of chromosome 22. The third article provides an excellent short review of the clinical studies which have examined the relationship between abnormalities of chromosome 22 and congenital cardiovascular malformations.

- Barbero-Marcial M, Riso A, Atik E, Jatene A: A technique for correction of truncus arteriosus types I and II without extracardiac conduits. J Thorac Cardiovasc Surg 1990;99:364–369.
- Danton MH, Barron DJ, Stumper O, et al: Repair of truncus arteriosus: A considered approach to right ventricular outflow tract reconstruction. Eur J Cardiothorac Surg 2001;20:95–103; discussion 103–104.

  The first of these articles popularised the use of the direct anastomosis procedure for common arterial trunk, albeit that the procedure had been performed earlier by Reid, from Edinburgh. The second provides an excellent comparison between this approach and the more classical procedures in a centre of excellence.

- Konstantinov IE, Karamlou T, Blackstone EH, et al: Truncus arteriosus associated with interrupted aortic arch in 50 neonates: A Congenital Heart Surgeons Society study. Ann Thorac Surg 2006;81:214–222.

  This recent publication from the Congenital Heart Surgeons Society examines the difficulties in the treatment of interruption of the aortic arch in association with common arterial trunk.

CHAPTER 42

The Arterial Duct: Its Persistence and Its Patency

LEE N. BENSON

'All these arrangements are marvellous, without any question. But we have to consider that it exceeds all expectations how soon the occlusion of all these openings takes place'.

HISTORICAL CONSIDERATIONS

When Siegal[1] re-examined the original Greek text, he pointed out that Galen was familiar with many aspects of the fetal circulation, even though he did not realise that blood circulated. Galen understood that fetal blood was aerated in the placenta, and that blood was diverted away from the liver by a short vessel connecting the portal to the inferior caval vein. He also knew that blood passed through the oval foramen to bypass the right ventricle, and reach the left side of the heart directly. He realised, nonetheless, that some blood still entered the right ventricle and pulmonary trunk, from whence it was shunted into the aorta through a special fetal channel, thereby bypassing the lungs. The quotation at the head of the chapter, taken from Siegal,[1] provides a clear indication of Galen's understanding of the dramatic readjustment of the circulation at birth.

It is Botallo, nonetheless, with whose name we usually associate the persistently patent arterial duct. In fact, Botallo described postnatal patency of the oval foramen! It was by a series of misinterpretations, and careless translations, that his name became, quite unjustifiably, attached to the arterial duct.[2] William Harvey, who was a pupil of Fabrizi d'Acquapendente in Padova for 2 years, synthesised previous detailed descriptions of fetal cardiac anatomy from his mentor in his own writings. His genius resided in proposing the concept of active circulation of the blood. He was well aware of the large size of the arterial duct prior to birth, and the fact that blood flowed through it from right to left during fetal life.[3] Harvey[3] was incorrect only in his belief that flow of blood to the lungs was completely lacking in the fetus. Subsequently, Highmore, a friend of Harvey, described closure of both the oval foramen and the arterial duct as occurring with the onset of respiration, believing the arterial duct to collapse as a consequence of blood being diverted to the lungs.[4] Since then, several ingenious theories have been put forward to explain closure of the duct, all being based on postmortem appearances, and all invoking mechanical factors.[5] It was Virchow[6] who first suggested that the closure results from contraction of its mural smooth muscle, while Gerard[7] introduced the concept of two-stage closure, in which functional constriction is followed by anatomical obliteration. Thanks to Huggett,[8] we came to understand the role of oxygen in effecting functional closure by muscular contraction.

As early as 1907, in an address to the Philadelphia Academy of Surgery, John Munro had suggested surgical ligation of the persistently patent arterial duct.[9] After an interval of 31 years, the first attempt at surgical closure was made in a 22-year-old woman with bacterial endocarditis.[10] Unfortunately, although the patient survived the surgery, she died a few days later from complications of the infection. As a result, it was Robert Gross, of Boston, who first successfully ligated a patent duct, in a 7-year-old child with intractable heart failure.[11] He thereby introduced an amazing era of progress in the surgery of congenital malformations of the heart. No historical review of the arterial duct, however brief, would be complete without recognising the importance of Gibson's exquisite description of the murmur that typifies its persistence,[12] notwithstanding the fashion in which Gibson's initial account has subsequently been misquoted.[13]

NOMENCLATURE

From time to time, authors have argued that the terms patent and persistent are redundancies that should be avoided when describing the arterial duct. In my view, this oversimplifies the situation, and both terms retain their value. Persistence implies that the duct is present after the time of its expected closure and, therefore, distinguishes a pathological from a physiological state. The concept of patency remains useful in the perinatal period, especially in the premature infant in whom the term can be used to signify a duct that is functionally open, as opposed to one that is functionally closed, but retains the potential to reopen.

THE NORMAL FETAL CIRCULATION

About two-thirds of the fetal cardiac output originates from the right ventricle, with only 5% to 10% passing through the lungs.[14,15] As such, the majority of right ventricular output passes through the arterial duct into the descending aorta, and its presence is essential for normal fetal development, permitting right ventricular output to be diverted away from the high-resistance pulmonary circulation. Premature constriction or closure may lead to right heart failure, resulting in fetal hydrops.[16]

EMBRYOLOGY AND PATHOGENESIS

During early fetal development, five arterial arches link the aortic sac with the paired dorsal aortas, although all arches are never present simultaneously (Fig. 42-1).

The arches are numbered 1 through 6, albeit that there is no evidence to support the existence of the purported fifth

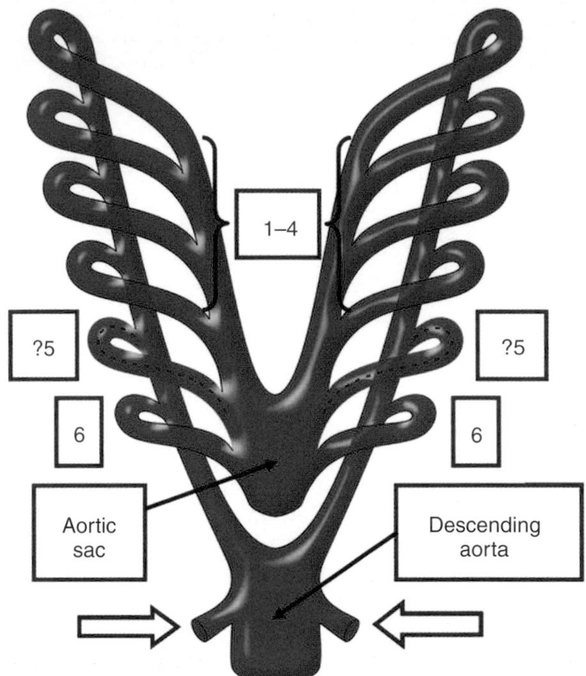

Figure 42-1 The cartoon shows the presumed arrangement of the arteries percolating the pharyngeal arches of the developing embryo. They are numbered 1 through 6, and are bilaterally symmetrical, although the purported fifth arch has never been recognised in normal embryos. They take their origin from the aortic sac, and come together in bilateral dorsal aortas, which join together to form the descending aorta. The subclavian arteries (*arrows*) are derived from the seventh intersegmental arteries, and initially arise distally from the dorsal aorta, needing to migrate cranially to reach their definitive positions.

arch, even though some congenital malformations are interpreted on the basis of its persistence. The initial symmetrical arrangement does, however, provide the basis for the pattern of the hypothetical double arch proposed by Edwards[17] to explain vascular rings and slings. This bilaterally symmetrical arrangement, with paired brachiocephalic arteries and arterial ducts (Fig. 42-2), is usually transformed to the configuration seen in postnatal life by the disappearance of some arterial segments, and realignment of others (Fig. 42-3).[18]

The normal duct develops from the dorsal portion of the left sixth arch. From their inception, the sixth arches are associated with the developing lungs. The arteries feeding the developing lungs develop within the anterior wall of the mediastinum, and take their origin of the floor of the aortic sac, which initially feeds also the bilateral arteries of the sixth arches (Fig. 42-4).

When the developing arterial segment is divided to form the intrapericardial components of the aorta and pulmonary trunk, the sixth arches, originating from the caudal part of the aortic sac, are placed in continuity with the pulmonary channel. A significant event in the appropriate connection of the pulmonary arteries with the intrapericardial pulmonary trunk is the obliteration and disappearance of the right sixth arch. On the left side, the arch persists as the arterial duct, with the pulmonary arteries left in continuity with the channel from the pulmonary trunk to the left sixth arch (Fig. 42-5).

The hypothetical double arch system devised by Edwards[17] is able to explain all developmental anomalies of the aortic arch, including those associated with an abnormally situated duct, be the duct patent or represented by the arterial ligament. The various possibilities are discussed in Chapter 47, including those in which there is persistence of both sixth

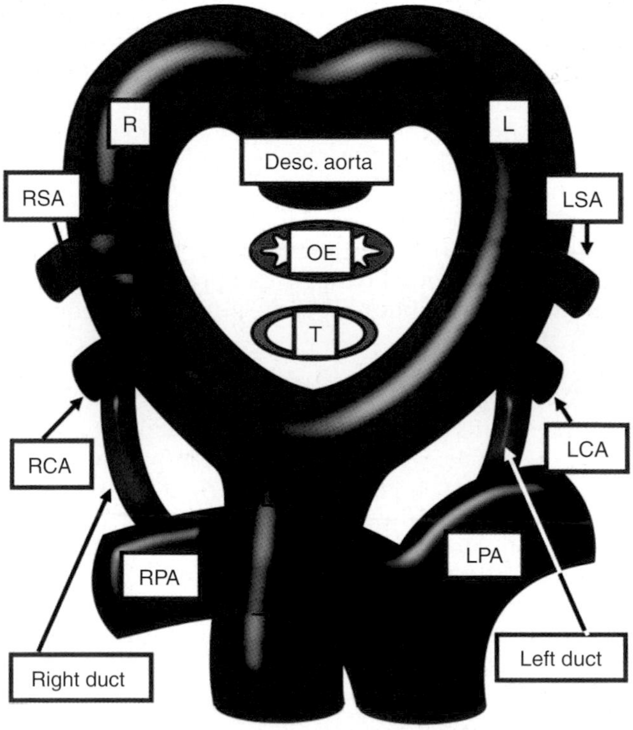

Figure 42-2 The cartoon shows the primitive system of double arches proposed by Edwards to explain vascular rings and slings. The arches persist on both the right (R) and left (L) sides, uniting posteriorly to form a neutral descending (desc.) aorta. Each arch gives rise to subclavian (SA) and common carotid (CA) arteries, along with an arterial duct, which joins the appropriate pulmonary artery (PA). The aortic sac and outflow tract have divided to form the aorta and the pulmonary trunk (PT). The double arch surrounds the tracheo-oesophageal pedicle (OE, T).

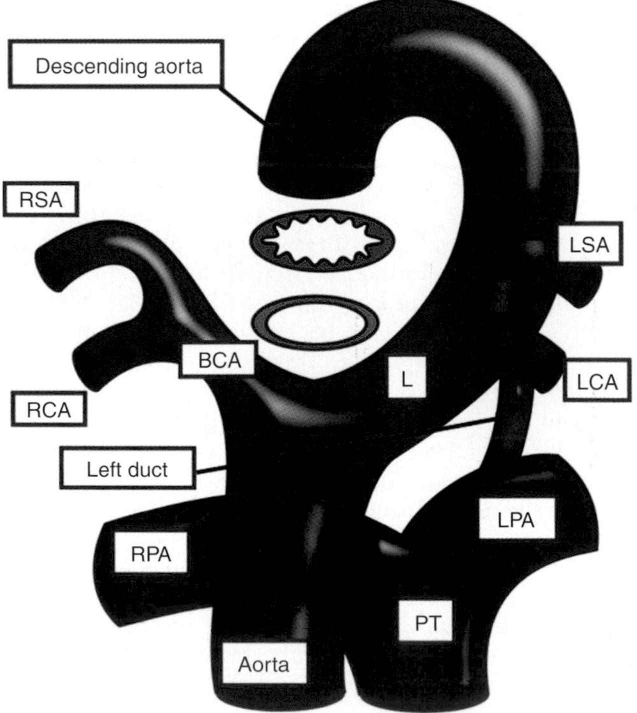

Figure 42-3 With normal development, the right arch and right duct regress, leaving a left arch feeding the descending aorta, an arterial duct on the left side, and the brachiocephalic artery (BCA) giving rise to the right common carotid and subclavian arteries. Abbreviations as for Figure 42-2.

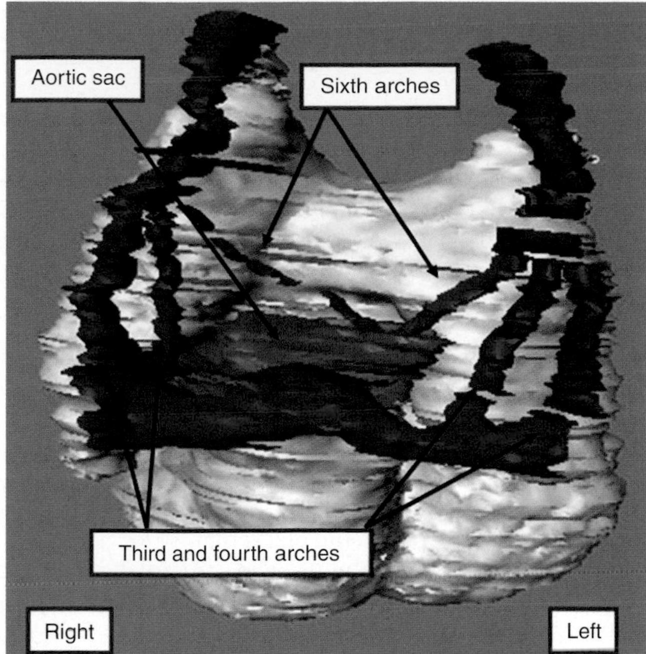

Figure 42-4 The image shows a reconstruction of the developing arteries of the pharyngeal arches in a mouse on the 12th day of development. It is viewed from above, looking down on the arterial pole of the heart, with the aortic sac and the developing intrapericardial arterial trunks shown in *green*. The pulmonary arteries are not seen, but already the right sixth arch is beginning to regress. (Courtesy of Dr Sandra Webb, St George's Medical University, London, United Kingdom.)

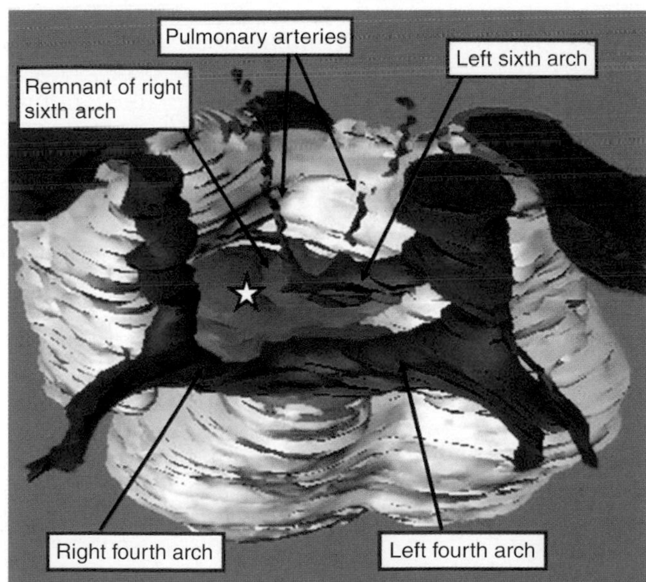

Figure 42-5 This reconstruction shows the appearance of the arteries percolating through the pharyngeal arches on the 13th day of development in the mouse. The pulmonary arteries are now seen originating from the floor of the aortic sac (*green*), which feeds the left sixth arch. The right sixth arch has already regressed (*star*), although its remnant is still visible. (Courtesy of Dr Sandra Webb, St George's Medical University, London, United Kingdom.)

arches, producing bilateral arterial ducts. Such circumstances are rare, and are always associated with intracardiac anomalies. Typically the ducts supply discontinuous pulmonary arteries in the setting of tetralogy of Fallot with pulmonary atresia, albeit that bilateral ducts can also be found in association with isolation of a subclavian artery.[19] The arterial duct does not always persist on one side. Its absence was first described as a postmortem finding in 1671, being seen in a grossly malformed infant with an extrathoracic heart and tetralogy of Fallot described by Nicolas Steno.[20] Absence of the duct is a typical finding in the syndrome of tetralogy of Fallot with so-called absent pulmonary valve and dilated pulmonary arteries.[21] It was thought that absence of the duct, and hence absence of any overflow, explained the dilated pulmonary arteries, but the pulmonary arteries can be dilated even when the duct is present and patent (see Chapter 36). The duct is also absent in approximately three-quarters of patients with a common arterial trunk. Absence of significant flow through the duct in the presence of a larger aortopulmonary connection permits the duct to disappear early in fetal life. In more complex varieties of common arterial trunk, however, such as those with so-called absence of one pulmonary artery, or those patients with an associated interruption or atresia of the aortic arch, patency of the duct is essential to maintain both the systemic and pulmonary circulations (see Chapter 41).

A number of teratogens are known to influence the development of the duct, including rubella, alcohol, amphetamines, and the anticonvulsant hydantoin, with the duct being most sensitive from 18 to 60 days of gestation.[22] Absence of the duct has been induced experimentally in chick embryos by the administration of agonists of β-adrenoceptors, leading to the suggestion that the teratogenesis is mediated by cyclic AMP.[23]

ANATOMY

The Arterial Duct and Its Normal Closure

In the fetus, and in the neonate prior to its closure, the arterial duct is a short and wide vessel of variable length. It connects the pulmonary arteries to the lesser curve of the arch of the aorta, terminating at the point of transition from the isthmus to the descending aorta, distal to the origin of the left subclavian artery (Fig. 42-6).

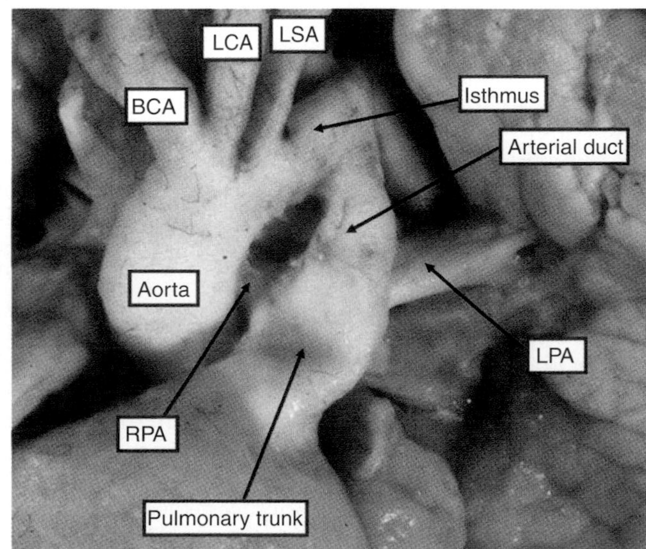

Figure 42-6 The image shows the arrangement of the arterial trunks at the time of birth. The duct is the direct continuation of the pulmonary trunk, and is larger than the right and left pulmonary arteries (RPA, LPA). The duct joins with the isthmus of the aortic arch, with both pathways continuing as the descending aorta. The aorta gives rise to the brachiocephalic (BCA), left common carotid (LCA), and left subclavian (LSA) arteries.

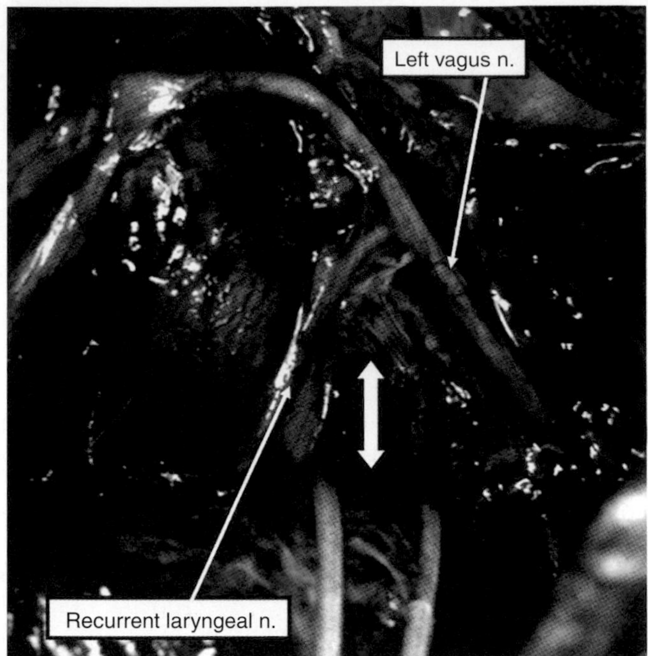

Figure 42-7 This view through a left thoracotomy shows the relationship of the left recurrent laryngeal nerve to the persistently patent arterial duct (*arrow*). The pulmonary arterial end of the vessel is covered by a reflection of the pericardium. (Courtesy of Dr Benson R. Wilcox, University of North Carolina, Chapel Hill.)

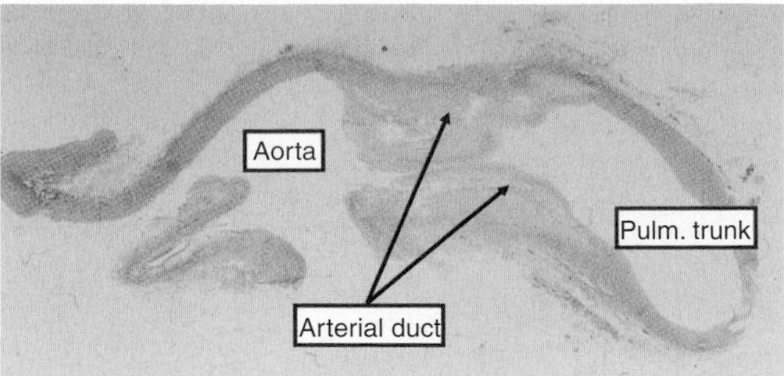

Figure 42-8 The microscopic section, stained using the trichrome technique, shows the markedly different aspect of the muscular walls of the arterial duct compared to the fibroelastic walls of the aorta and pulmonary trunk. Note the intimal mounds within the ductal lumen.

Patency is maintained by the relatively low fetal oxygen tension[24] and cyclooxygenase-mediated products of arachidonic acid metabolism, primarily prostaglandin and prostacyclin,[25] whose levels are high because of production by the placenta and decreased metabolism in the fetal lungs. Produced both locally, in ductal tissue, and circulating, these mediators cause vasodilation through interaction with prostanoid receptors.

Prior to birth, the duct is very much the direct continuation of the pulmonary trunk, with the left and right pulmonary arteries taking origin as smaller branches from the trunk. Posteriorly, the duct is related to the left main bronchus, while anteriorly it is crossed by the vagus nerve. This gives off the left recurrent laryngeal nerve, which encircles the duct before ascending behind the aortic arch into the neck (Fig. 42-7). In terms of its microscopic structure, the duct is a muscular artery endowed with an intima, media and adventitia, differing markedly from the adjacent pulmonary trunk and aorta (Fig. 42-8). While the media of the aorta is composed mainly of circumferentially arranged elastic fibers, the media of the duct consists largely of spirally arranged smooth muscle cells, some with circular and others with longitudinal orientation,[26] with an increased content of hyaluronic acid. The intimal layers are thicker than those of the adjoining vessels, and contain increased amounts of mucoid substance.[27] In the newborn, the tissues are rather loosely arranged, with a well-defined internal elastic lamina that may be single or focally duplicated, with small interruptions encountered regularly. No collagen is seen in the media by light microscopy, but abundant material that stains positively for acid mucopolysaccharides is observed between the muscle and elastic laminas. Electron microscopy reveals fine collagen fibrils lying between adjacent lamellas of smooth muscle cells and elastin. During the second half of gestation, the smooth muscle cells show decreasing evidence of secretory activity, and increasing maturation of their contractile elements.

It is known that vessels cannot close by isolated contraction of circularly arranged muscle,[28] so coincident shortening of the less abundant longitudinally arranged muscle fibres is critical to effective closure. The duct is innervated mostly by adrenergic fibres, supplying largely the adventitia and outer media, with cholinergic fibres being extremely sparse or totally absent.[29] Vessels are also found in its walls that may have a role in fuelling contraction at birth.[26] Some degree of hyperaemia of these vessels is common in newborn infants.

There is controversy with regard to the structure of the intimal layers during fetal life. Eccentrically placed intimal cushions, or mounds composed of smooth muscle and elastic tissue, have been described by many authors, with suggestions made that the formation of these mounds precedes normal ductal closure subsequent to birth. It is questionable, however, whether the intimal cushions are produced during normal fetal maturation. When account is taken of the high flow of blood through the fetal duct, it is difficult to conceive that prominent protrusions of intima into the lumen could exist without inducing turbulent flow and a bruit. No such bruit is heard in the undisturbed ducts of fetal lambs at term. Furthermore, in many of the studies suggesting the presence of intimal cushions, the tissues have usually been subjected to one or more perturbations, such as relatively slow fixation, mechanical stimulation, or cessation of circulation with loss of intraluminal distending pressure. On this basis, the existence of intimal cushions as prenatal structures has been challenged. In a series of experiments,[30–34] Hornblad and colleagues showed that, independent of the degree of closure, the lumen of the duct remained round, was without deformation, and showed no evidence of formation of mounds. Mural thickness increased at the time of closure, while the internal elastic lamina became corrugated, especially in the mid-portion of the vessels. A decrease in the lumen was associated with accumulation of endothelial cells within the lumen. They concluded that closure was aided by passive central displacement of endothelial and inner medial cells, but that no part of the medial layer was prepared prenatally for this process.[30–34] These findings endorsed earlier studies in the human, which suggested that the cushions appeared as a normal reparative reaction to distending forces during fetal life.[35]

At birth, the vessel unequivocally constricts with the abrupt increase in oxygen tension inhibiting ductal smooth muscle voltage-dependent potassium channels, resulting in an influx of calcium and ductal constriction.[36] Levels of prostaglandin and prostacyclin fall because of metabolism in the functioning lungs, and elimination of the placenta. The intimal thickenings, or cushions, become irregular ridges protruding into the lumen, running mainly lengthwise. By their extrusion, they exert traction on the media, causing disorganisation and formation of mucoid lakes (see Fig. 42-8). Anatomical obliteration follows functional closure. The process begins with necrosis of the inner wall, followed by the formation of dense fibrous tissue. The lumen is progressively obliterated by a process of fibrosis, probably representing organisation of mural or occlusive thrombus. Eventually, the duct becomes converted into a fibrous strand, the arterial ligament, which may become calcified. Anatomical obliteration may take several weeks to complete. About two-thirds of ducts are normally obliterated by the age of 2 weeks,[37] and almost all by 1 year.

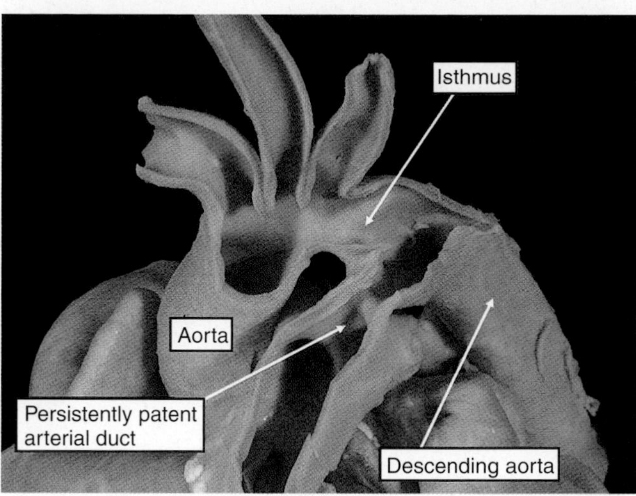

Figure 42-10 The dissection shows the course of a persistently patent arterial duct. As expected, it follows the course of the channel seen at birth (see Fig. 42-6).

The Persistently Patent Arterial Duct

As stated above, in normal circumstances all ducts should be converted to an arterial ligament within the first year of life, with two-thirds closing in the initial 2 weeks. Some ducts, however, never close. These are the channels best described as showing persistent patency. Gittenberger-de Groot[38] found the internal elastic lamina to be intact in some, but not all, of persistently patent ducts studied histologically, along with a sparsity of intimal cushions (Fig. 42-9). Bakker[35] had noted similar findings, describing them in terms of aortification. The duct, if persisting as a patent structure, joins the pulmonary arteries to the descending aorta in the fashion seen in the neonate (Fig. 42-10). The channel itself can vary markedly in its width (compare Figs. 42-11 and 42-12). The duct can also vary considerably in its shape. Study of a large number of angiograms from patients with persistently patent ducts undergoing interventional closure at the Hospital for Sick Children, Toronto[39] showed that the most frequent pattern was to find a constriction at the pulmonary end of the duct. This pattern was seen in two-thirds of cases. In just under one-fifth, a constriction was found at the aortic end of the duct, and in just under one-tenth, the lumen was unrestricted. In just under one-twentieth, there was a constriction at both ends, whilst the remaining patients showed bizarre patterns not lending themselves to classification (Fig. 42-13).

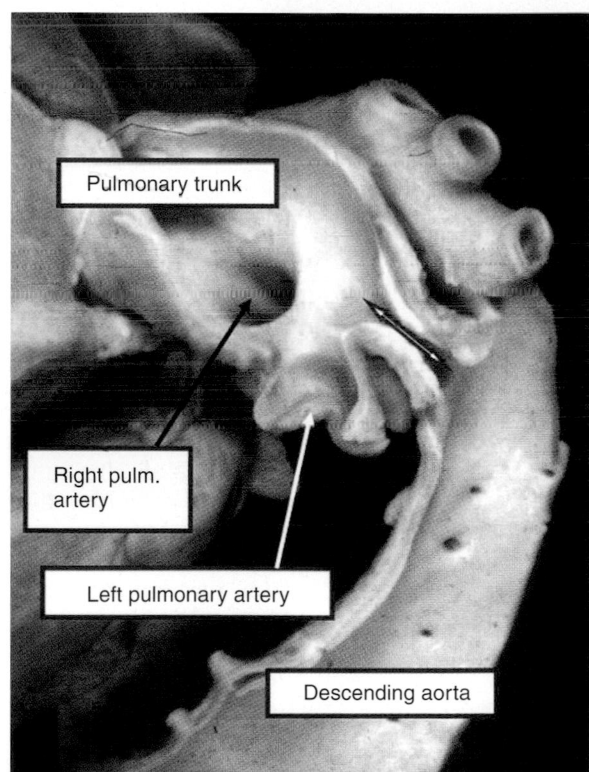

Figure 42-11 In this persistently patent arterial duct, the lumen of the channel is relatively narrow (*arrow*).

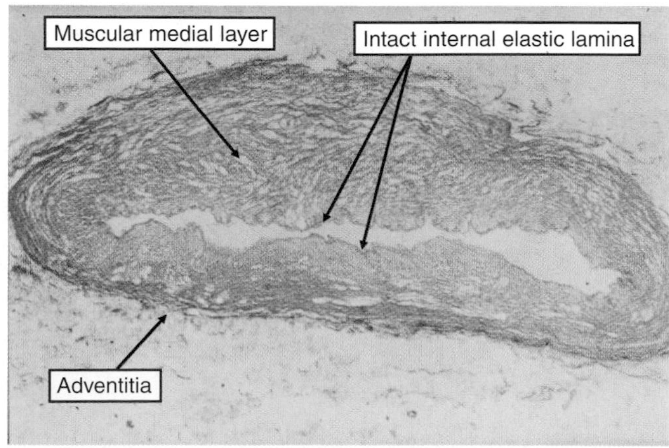

Figure 42-9 This histological section is through the walls of a persistently patent arterial duct. Note the intact internal elastic lamina, and lack of intimal mounds. (Courtesy of Dr Siew Yen Ho, Imperial College, London, United Kingdom.)

In the past, persistently patent arterial ducts were often the nidus for infectious endocarditis, but this complication is now extremely rare in developed countries. Ducts could also become aneurysmal and elongated (Figs. 42-14

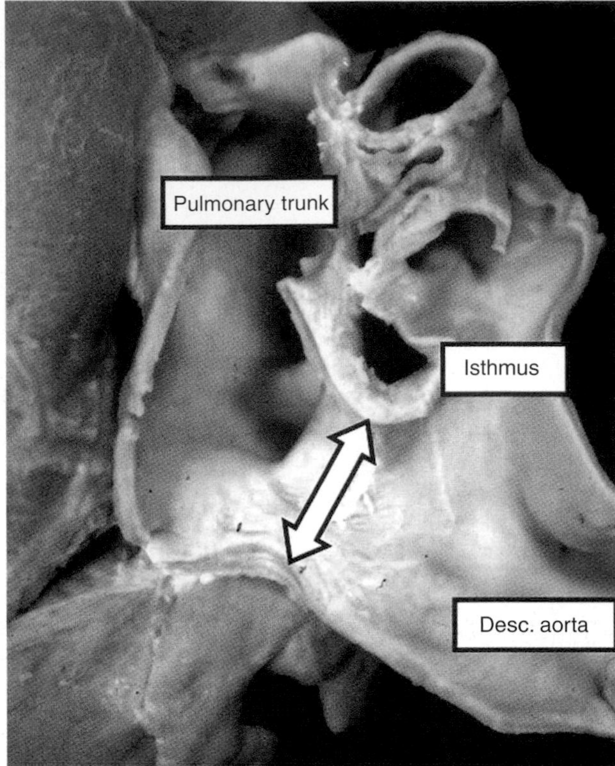

Figure 42-12 In this persistently patent duct, the lumen of the anomalous channel is wide (*arrow*). (Compare with Fig. 42-11.)

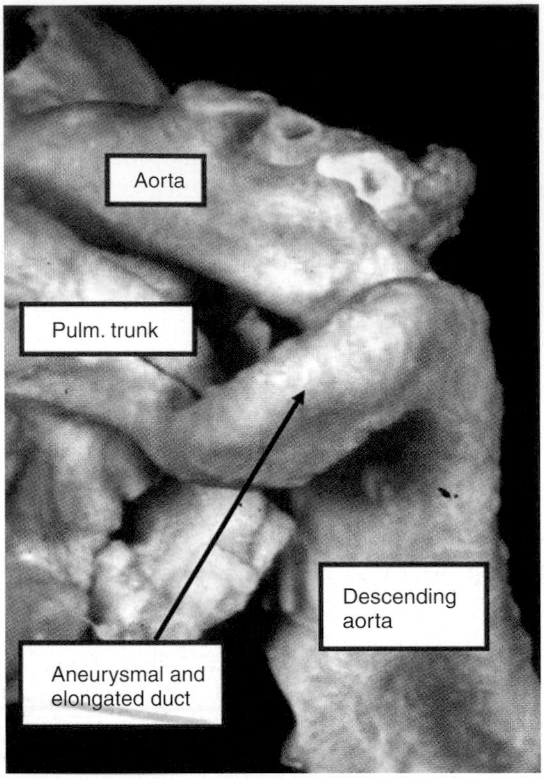

Figure 42-14 This duct has become elongated and aneurysmal.

and 42-15), but this is also now a rare finding, as is ductal rupture.

EPIDEMIOLOGY

The factors responsible for persistent ductal patency beyond the first days of life are not fully understood. An increased incidence is seen in the premature neonate due to physiological factors more related to prematurity rather than an inherent abnormality of the duct.[40] In infants born at term, persistent patency occurs sporadically, but there is increasing evidence that genetic factors, or prenatal infection, play a role in many children. The estimated incidence lies between 1 in 2000 and 1 in 5000 live births.[41–43] Persistent patency of the duct accounts for about one-eighth of all congenital cardiac malformations. The most extensive study from a relatively homogeneous population was that performed by Carlgren,[43] when he charted the incidence of congenital cardiac disease to children born in the Swedish City of Gothenburg. Persistent ductal patency was the third most common lesion identified, representing about 0.04% of live births. If children with the so-called silent duct are included, found incidentally by echocardiography performed for another reason, the incidence may be as high as 1 in 500.[44] A significantly higher incidence of ductal patency is also seen in infants born with low weight, patency being found in almost half of infants weighing less than 1750 g at birth, and up to four-fifths of those weighing less than 1200 g (see also Chapter 11).

Genetic Factors

Unlike premature infants as noted above, in whom persistent ductal patency is more often due to developmental immaturity, in the infant born at term there is likely a structural abnormality. There is also an increased frequency in several genetic syndromes, such as those with defined chromosomal aberrations, examples being trisomy 21, 14q- and 4p- syndrome, single-gene mutations such as Carpenter's syndrome and Holt-Oram syndrome, and

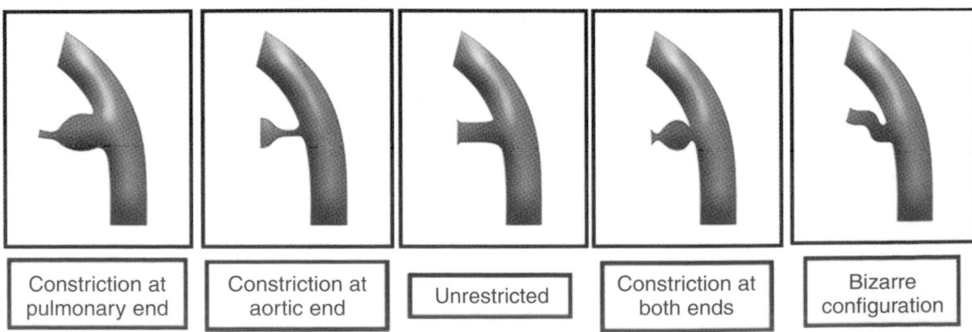

Figure 42-13 The variation in morphology of the arterial duct noted from angiograms taken prior to interventional closure at the Hospital for Sick Children, Toronto.[33]

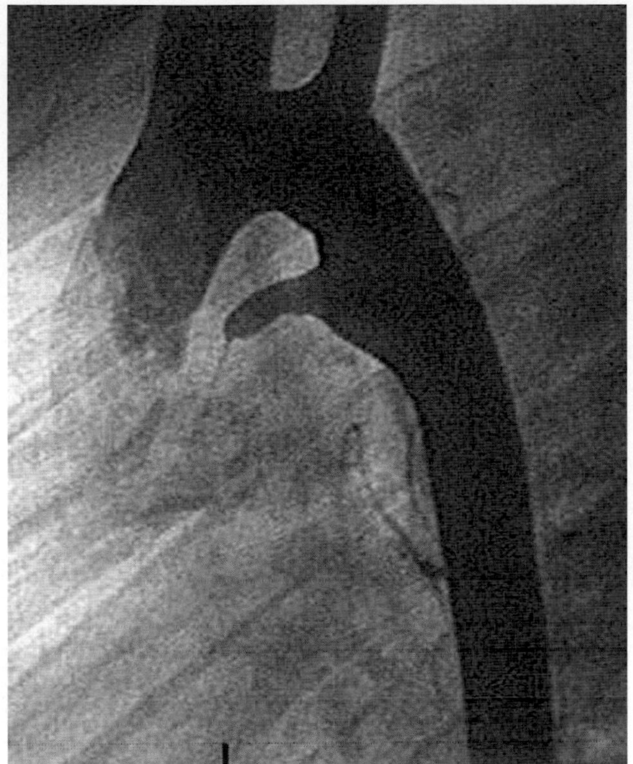

Figure 42-15 A lateral angiogram of a child with an elongated aneurysmal duct taken before transcatheter occlusion.

X-linked mutations such as incontinentia pigmenti. Although most cases of persistent patency are sporadic, many are also believed to be due to a multi-factorial inheritance pattern, with a genetic predisposition and an environmental trigger that occurs at a vulnerable time.[45] Females predominate in a ratio of greater then 2:1. The mode of inheritance appears to be autosomal recessive with incomplete penetrance.[46] In a family having one sibling with a patent duct, there is about a 3% chance of a persistent duct in a subsequent offspring,[45] and a higher risk to the offspring given one affected parent, some 45 times greater than the that for the general population. The risk to further children in sibships where two children have been affected is probably in the order of 10% and increases with each affected child.

Infection and Environmental Factors

Maternal rubella during the first trimester of pregnancy, particularly in the first 4 weeks, is associated with a high incidence of a persistently patent arterial duct.[49-50] The histology resembles that of a very immature duct, with an extensive subendothelial elastic lamina, thought to retard anatomic sealing.[51] Additional environmental factors have been reported associated with persistence, such as in fetal valproate syndrome,[52] or after thalidomide.[53] A patent arterial duct may be more likely to be found in infants born at high altitude.[54]

PATHOPHYSIOLOGY

Persistent patency results in shunting of blood from one side of the circulation to the other, the volume of flow depending on the length and internal diameter of the duct, and on the systemic and pulmonary vascular resistances. As pulmonary resistance is usually much lower than systemic, the flow is from the aorta to the pulmonary trunk. Hence, flow to the lungs is increased, and results in left atrial and left ventricular overload. If the duct is widely patent, flow depends entirely on the ratio of resistances. Right ventricular failure may occur in the presence of a large duct with pulmonary hypertension or pulmonary oedema, and an elevated left atrial pressure. In most patients, the duct is partially constricted, and the major factor limiting flow. Under these conditions, pulmonary arterial pressure is normal or only mildly elevated. Symptoms and clinical findings are largely determined by the magnitude of the shunt.

Clinical Features

Most patients are asymptomatic, the lesion recognised with detection of the characteristic murmur. Occasionally, there may be a history of prematurity or asphyxia during birth. Children with large shunts may fail to thrive, experience difficulty with feeding during infancy, and frequently suffer recurrent infections of the upper respiratory tract. Occasionally, congestive heart failure develops.

Physical Examination

There is retarded growth in about one-third of children. They are acyanotic in the absence of complicating factors. The peripheral pulses are easily palpable, with a rapid upstroke and decay. There is a widened pulse pressure, with lowering of the diastolic component. Arterial pulsation in the neck may be prominent in those with large shunts. Precordial examination reveals an active cardiac impulse, with the forceful cardiac apex displaced to the left. When the shunt is small, the only abnormal finding may be the murmur. The continuous, or machinery, murmur of the uncomplicated persistent duct is best heard in the left infraclavicular area, although it is occasionally maximal at the third left interspace. Gibson's[12] description of the murmur is quoted by Tynan[13]: 'It begins quite obviously after the commencement of the first sound. It is continued during the latter part of that sound and the whole of the short pause. It persists throughout the second sound and dies away gradually during the long pause. The murmur is distinctly rough and thrilling in its character. It begins, however, somewhat softly, and increases in intensity to reach its acme just about, or immediately after, the incidence of the second sound, and from that point wanes until its termination. The second sound can be heard to be loud and clanging and when carefully analysed it is the pulmonary part of that sound which is accentuated'. Turbulent flow through the duct itself causes the murmur. Additional murmurs may be present due to increased flow across the aortic valve, producing an ejection systolic sound, and across the mitral valve, giving a diastolic murmur with loud onset. The systolic component of the continuous murmur may be transmitted into the neck, may be associated with a thrill in the second left intercostal space, or may increase in intensity during inspiration due to a fall in pulmonary vascular resistance. Many patients with loud continuous murmurs also have multiple clanging sounds. These are relatively localised to the pulmonary area, and are most frequent in the second half of systole, corresponding to the period of peak flow within the duct. Neill and Mounsey[53] attributed these sounds to the turbulence caused by the head-on collision of opposed flow from the duct and the right ventricle, and named them eddy sounds. These auscultatory findings are only for an uncomplicated persistent duct in a child. It should be remembered that these features may differ in infancy, or be altered by the development of complications.

Investigations

Electrocardiogram

Patients with an isolated persistent arterial duct usually have some electrocardiographic evidence of left atrial and ventricular hypertrophy, reflecting volume overload of the left heart. Occasionally, the electrocardiogram may show combined ventricular hypertrophy, or, if the duct is small, be entirely normal. The electrical axis is usually normal, and deviation to the right, with right atrial and/or right ventricular hypertrophy, suggests the presence of additional defects or pulmonary hypertension. The electrocardiographic changes are less predictable in infants and clinically less helpful.[54] Prolongation of the PR interval, which disappears or decreases after closure, has been observed in about one-fifth of cases.[55] Atrial fibrillation may develop in adult life.[56,57] When the shunt is large enough to equalise the systemic and pulmonary arterial pressures, biventricular hypertrophy is likely to develop. With the onset of pulmonary vascular disease, the predominant findings will be those of right ventricular hypertrophy.

Chest Radiography

The chest film may be normal in patients with a small shunt. Cardiomegaly is present in those in whom flow to the lungs is close to twice systemic flow or greater. Increased pulmonary vascular markings are seen, with an obvious bulge of the pulmonary trunk at the left border of the cardiac silhouette. The aorta is also prominent. Both it and the pulmonary trunk tend to enlarge with age. Enlargement of the left atrium is usually present, and reflects increased pulmonary venous return due to the left-to-right shunt. Increased pulmonary vascularity may be more marked on the right, as is often seen with other left-to-right shunts (Fig. 42-16). The duct may calcify, although this complication is more common when the vessel is closed rather than patent. The aortic end of the duct, the ductal ampulla, may be seen on the chest radiograph, and can be demonstrated angiographically during the first week of life. These findings may be modified, especially if pulmonary vascular disease develops.

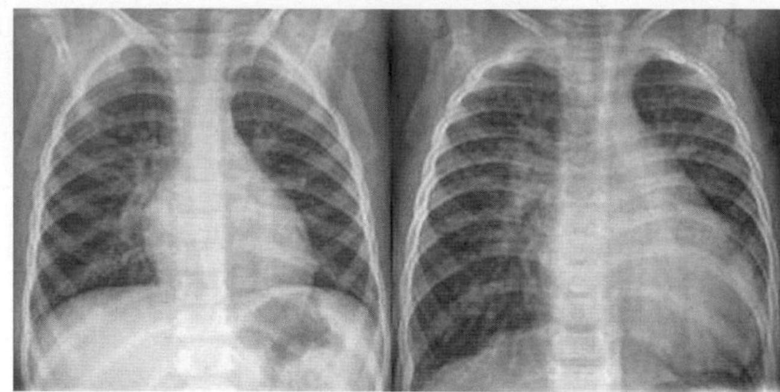

Figure 42-16 The left panel is a chest radiograph from a patient with small ducts. Note the minimally increased pulmonary vascularity. The right panel shows another child with a larger ductal communication. There is increased pulmonary vascularity and cardiomegaly.

Echocardiography

Persistent patency beyond the neonatal period is readily diagnosed from the characteristic clinical features. Cross sectional echocardiography will help rule out other structural cardiac malformations. The duct can be imaged throughout its length using a high left parasternal view,[58,59] allowing evaluation of ductal size, and the presence of tissue within the lumen, indicating imminent closure. In preterm infants, imaging may be difficult due to emphysematous lungs from high ventilatory pressures. A subxiphoid view can then be used. Characteristic diastolic flow in the pulmonary trunk identified by Doppler interrogation increases the confidence of diagnosing ductal shunting.

Flow through the duct can be quantified by analysis of Doppler tracings of diastolic flow in either the left pulmonary artery or the descending aorta. Colour flow Doppler techniques have been more useful in revealing ductal patency. This is, at present, the most sensitive method for detecting and semi-quantifying ductal flow[60] (Fig. 42-17). Qualitatively, the presence of bidirectional, or pure right-to-left, shunting is specific for elevated pulmonary arterial pressures.[61,62] In children with high pulmonary vascular resistance, with a low-velocity Doppler signal or right-to-left flow, the duct may be very difficult to demonstrate by colour flow imaging, even if it is large. Associated findings such as septal flattening, unexplained right ventricular hypertrophy, or high-velocity pulmonary regurgitation should prompt an investigation for a patent duct. Contrast echocardiography may also be helpful in this setting, identifying microbubbles in the descending aorta in

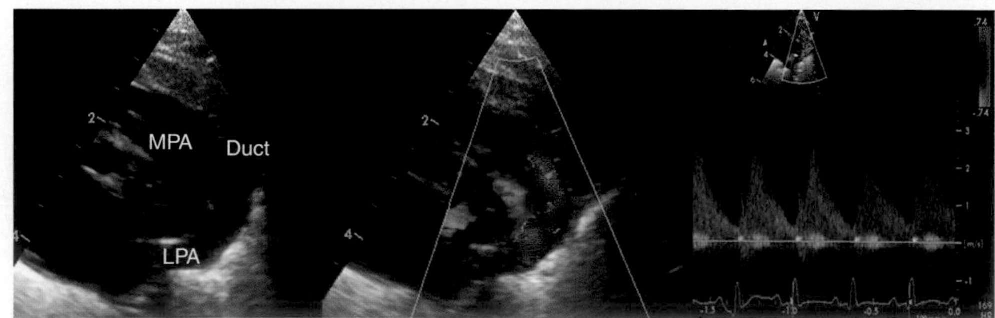

Figure 42-17 The echocardiogram (high left parasternal view) shows a large duct in a newborn (left panel). Note the proximity to the left pulmonary artery. The middle panel shows colour flow Doppler mapping, with mild turbulence confirming the presence of flow (*orange colour*) entering the pulmonary trunk (*orange coloured pattern*). The right panel is a spectral Doppler trace showing the direction, timing, and velocity of flow in the duct. MPA, main pulmonary artery; LPA, left pulmonary artery.

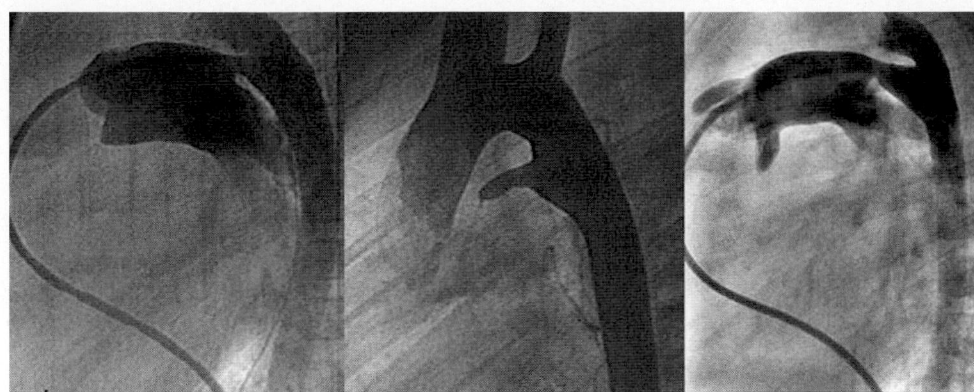

Figure 42-18 Lateral arteriograms outlining various ductal anatomies.

consequence of ductal right-to-left shunting, but not in the ascending aorta. Additionally, using colour flow mapping, Doppler measurements of velocity can be used to estimate pulmonary arterial pressure.[63–65] M-mode studies provide an assessment of left atrial and ventricular size, which gives some idea of the magnitude of the shunt. In children with a small duct, the chambers are usually of normal size, although mild left atrial and/or left ventricular enlargement may be seen. In children with a moderate or large duct, the left atrium and ventricle are enlarged. Echocardiography is probably most valuable in the diagnosis of ductal patency in the premature infant. It will be discussed further in that section.

Recent echocardiographic studies using colour flow Doppler have further identified the presence of small ductal communications in the absence of any typical murmur of patency, this degree of shunting giving uncharacteristic soft vibratory systolic murmur or no murmur at all.[44,66,67] These findings have a significant impact on estimates of the incidence of ductal patency and the risk of endocarditis.

Cardiac Catheterisation and Angiography

Most cardiologists would not consider catheterisation a necessary diagnostic procedure for children with typical clinical findings. If it is undertaken, it is usually possible to probe the duct from the pulmonary trunk, and to pass a catheter through the vessel and down the aorta. When the catheter apparently crosses a duct, but then turns in a headward direction, the alert investigator should consider the presence of an aortopulmonary window. The size of the shunt may be difficult to quantify by oximetry because it is difficult to obtain a truly representative sample distal to the site of shunting. Pulmonary arterial pressure is usually normal or slightly elevated. The duct can be visualised by selective aortography with injection of contrast media in the last part of the aortic arch (Fig. 42-18).

Therapeutic catheterisation, however, is currently the treatment of choice for most children and adults with a patent duct. In this regard, complete haemodynamic assessment is important prior to attempting closure, particularly in the adult. In patients with an elevated pulmonary arterial pressure, assessment of pulmonary vascular resistance and its response to vasodilating agents may be helpful in determining suitability of closure. Assessment of haemodynamics during temporary test occlusion with a balloon catheter may also be a helpful manoeuvre in assessing advisability of closure in marginal cases.

Angiography defines the anatomy. Such detailed assessment is essential before attempting closure so that the proper device and size can be chosen. Important features include the minimal diameter, usually at the pulmonary arterial end; the largest diameter, usually at the aortic ampulla; the length of the duct; and its relationship to the anterior border of the tracheal shadow, the latter helping to guide positioning of the device.[39] Other imaging modalities are available to confirm the presence of ductal patency. Radionuclide scanning can be used to detect the presence of shunting, but anatomic localisation is lacking. Magnetic resonance imaging provides anatomic detail,[67] and is particularly useful in the setting of unusual ductal geometry, and in those with associated abnormalities of the aortic arch (Fig. 42-19).[68,69] Examples include the patient with a ductal aneurysm

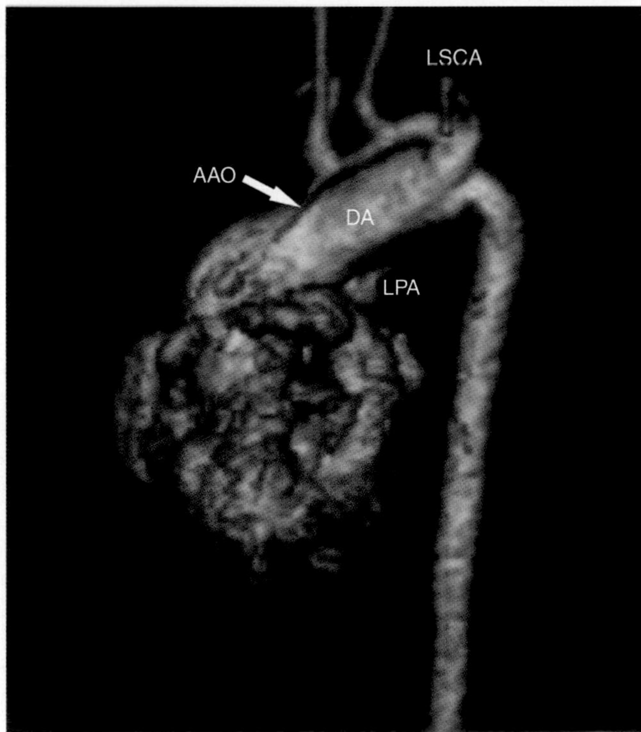

Figure 42-19 Volume rendered magnetic resonance image showing the anatomy of the aortic arch in an infant with hypoplastic left heart syndrome. Ductal anatomy (duct = DA), and its relationship to the ascending aorta (AAO, *arrow*) and left subclavian artery (LSCA) are clearly understood. LPA, left pulmonary artery.

presenting as a mass in the chest, the duct associated with a vascular ring, a right aortic arch, or cervical arch. With velocity encoding of cinemagnetic resonance signals, patterns of shunting can be detected.[70,71] In the adult, computed tomography can assess the degree of calcification, an important feature if surgical closure is considered. In general, however, the simpler technique of cross sectional echocardiography with colour flow Doppler provides sufficient anatomic and haemodynamic detail to define the anatomy and its variations, and points the way to proper management.

Diagnostic Problems

Other causes of a continuous murmur may create confusion. The venous hum often causes difficulty to the inexperienced auscultator. This noise, which can be loud, is usually best heard in the supraclavicular fossa, and while audible bilaterally, it is usually louder on the right. A venous hum, when loud, may be transmitted below the clavicle, and may be misdiagnosed as being from a patent duct. This error can be avoided by exerting pressure over the root of the neck, turning the head to the side, or laying the child down. These manoeuvres readily obliterate the venous hum, while having no effect on the murmur generated by ductal flow. An aortopulmonary window rarely causes a continuous murmur similar to that of persistent ductal patency. More typically, however, the communication is large, and does not cause a continuous murmur. Even with careful aortography, this condition may be misdiagnosed. Echocardiography should now help to avoid this error. Major aortopulmonary collateral arteries, pulmonary arteriovenous fistulas, and collateral arteries associated with coarctation, all cause continuous murmurs. These seldom cause diagnostic problems because of the general clinical picture and the location of the murmur. Other causes of continuous murmurs heard in the chest include ruptured sinus of Valsalva, peripheral pulmonary arterial stenosis, common arterial trunk, coronary artery fistulas, the supracardiac form of totally anomalous pulmonary venous connection, mitral atresia, surgically created systemic-to-pulmonary arterial shunts, and rarely anomalous origin of the left coronary artery from the pulmonary trunk. Prolapse of an aortic valvar leaflet into a ventricular septal defect may also simulate persistent patency of the duct. Most, if not all, of these potential pitfalls can be avoided by careful clinical evaluation and good echocardiography.

NATURAL HISTORY

Like most congenital cardiac malformations, reliable information about the natural history of untreated patients with a persistently patent duct is non-existent. Available data stems from the short period of time which elapses between the condition being diagnosed with any frequency and to its being relieved by an operation. Campbell[72] attempted an overview of the natural history, based on his own extensive clinical experience and on the literature. Inevitably, such calculations tend to over-emphasise the number of patients who experience events, be they favourable or adverse, and underestimate the number of patients with an asymptomatic and undetected duct.

Spontaneous Closure

By definition, a persistent duct is one that remains open beyond 3 months in an infant born at full-term. Delayed closure in premature infants, or that occurring within the first 3 months, is therefore excluded from consideration in this section. Campbell[72] analysed four series of patients in which 11 examples of spontaneous closure occurred over 1842 patient-years, giving a rate of 0.6% per annum. Several of the examples, however, were based on quite tenuous clinical impressions. In none was catheterisation performed before and after the event. The figure calculated by Campbell is almost certainly an overestimate. He did not suggest that surgery should be delayed except, perhaps, in patients with small shunts and signs that the duct was already closing. Few cardiologists would now agree even with these exceptions.

Effect on Life Expectancy

By combining four series, consisting mainly of unselected schoolchildren with a persistent duct, Campbell deduced a mortality rate of 0.42% per annum during the first two decades. Thereafter, he calculated mortality rates per year as 1% to 1.5% in the third decade, 2% to 2.5% in the fourth, and 4% for each subsequent year. These calculations indicate that one-third of patients with a persistent duct die by the age of 40, in contrast to less than one-twentieth of the normal population. Many of the figures are based on data obtained in the era before antibiotics were available. As infective endocarditis is a major cause of death, the impact of antibiotics must also be taken into account. These figures agree fairly well with age at death as reported in necropsy series. Abbott,[73] for example, found the mean age at death, having excluded those who died in infancy, to be 30 years, and in another series, the mean age was 36.5 years.[74] Despite this agreement, the fact remains that calculations from autopsy series, and from clinical series, are extrapolations from rather small numbers. They undoubtedly exaggerate the adverse aspects of the natural history.

COMPLICATIONS

The important complications of persistent patency of the duct include congestive heart failure, infective endarteritis, pulmonary vascular disease, aneurysmal formation, thromboembolism, and calcification.

Congestive Heart Failure

Congestive heart failure resulting from an isolated persistent duct develops either in infancy or during adult life. Infective endarteritis may rarely precipitate heart failure during childhood. Heart failure in infancy usually has its onset before the age of 3 months. A delayed normal fall in pulmonary vascular resistance may cause the left-to-right flow to increase progressively. The clinical picture is initially that of left heart failure, with tachypnoea and pulmonary oedema. Ultimately, signs of right heart failure appear with hepatomegaly. Although initially there may be a good response to diuretics, this is seldom maintained and closure is advisable. Infants born at term do not respond to indomethacin when over 3 months of age. The occasional occurrence of sudden death in infants treated medically further encourages a policy of early intervention. Amongst adults, there used to be a group with cardiomegaly and features of left ventricular overload and strain. Such patients now are rare in countries with well-developed systems of health care, as it is unlikely their lesion would have escaped detection. Congestive heart failure may also occur as a terminal event in patients in whom severe pulmonary vascular disease complicates a persistently patent duct. If so, transcatheter closure appears to be the treatment of choice.

Infective Endarteritis

Infective endarteritis in a patient with an uncomplicated persistent duct is uncommon in childhood, and appears to be prevented by surgery or catheter-based embolisation. In the era preceding antibiotics, and interventional or surgical treatment, it was a major cause of death, accounting for almost half of all deaths in several pooled autopsy series.[73–75] Campbell[72] calculated an infection rate of between 0.45% and 1.0% per annum for patients after the first decade. The first line of treatment should be with antibiotics, following the recommendations as established by the American Heart Association, with surgery or embolisation delayed until sterilisation is completed. Occasionally, this proves impossible, in which case surgery or occlusion should be performed under continuing antibiotic therapy.[76] Vegetations are usually found at the pulmonary arterial end of the duct, and may give rise to recurrent pulmonary embolisation, with the clinical picture suggesting recurrent pneumonia. In developing nations with limited access to health care, infective endarteritis associated with the persistently patent duct continues to be a significant health issue.[77] Infection may cause some examples of ductal aneurysms, especially those occurring postoperatively. While two cases of endarteritis on a clinically silent and non-hypertensive duct have been reported, the anticipated high incidence of the silent duct has little implications for treatment.[44,78,79]

Pulmonary Hypertension and the Persistent Duct

Although the pulmonary arterial pressure is usually normal, or only slightly elevated, in patients with persistently patent ducts, occasionally it is raised sufficiently to modify the physical findings. The implications of pulmonary hypertension secondary to an increased flow, as opposed to that caused by increased resistance are markedly different and the two situations should be clearly differentiated.

When the duct is widely patent, and pulmonary vascular resistance is low, systolic pulmonary arterial pressure equals systemic systolic pressure, and blood flow to the lungs is several times greater than that in the systemic circuit. The pulmonary arterial diastolic pressure may equal or be slightly lower than that in the aorta. These patients usually experience severe congestive heart failure, with failure to thrive and recurrent respiratory infections. Their electrocardiogram shows combined ventricular hypertrophy, while the chest radiograph reveals cardiomegaly with marked pulmonary plethora. The echocardiogram will reveal enlargement of the left heart chambers. Such patients respond poorly to medical therapy, and the correct management is to eliminate the shunt. Successful ligation or catheter occlusion usually restores pulmonary arterial pressure to normal. There appears to be little risk of subsequent pulmonary vascular changes in this group of patients.

Some individuals respond to pulmonary venous distension, and to the left atrial enlargement secondary to high pulmonary blood flow with reflex pulmonary vasoconstriction partially protecting themselves against the full effects of unrestricted ductal flow. If studied haemodynamically, these patients will be found to have a moderate left-to-right shunt, with pressure in the pulmonary circulation at systemic levels, with or without a high pulmonary capillary wedge pressure. Pulmonary arterial pressure usually falls with administration of oxygen, or in response to pulmonary vasodilators. Successful elimination of the shunt usually restores pulmonary arterial pressure to normal. Fixed and high pulmonary vascular resistance may result from progressive structural changes in patients who originally had large left-to-right shunts and normal pulmonary vessels. Alternatively, it may exist from birth.[80,81] Civen and Edwards[82] suggested that patients in this category represent a form of persistence of the fetal pulmonary circulation. As yet, there is poor understanding of the factors which initiate and maintain the progressive pulmonary vascular damage.

It is instructive to follow the clinical changes that accompany the rise in pulmonary vascular resistance. Initially, the pulmonary diastolic pressure approaches systemic levels, decreasing diastolic flow across the duct. As flow diminishes, the diastolic component of the continuous murmur becomes attenuated and eventually disappears. At this stage, the patient has a pansystolic murmur. With a further increase in resistance, systolic pressures begin to equalise, systolic flow diminishes, the systolic murmur shortens, and eventually it also disappears. Concurrent with these changes, the second sound becomes closely split or even single, and there is accentuation of the pulmonary component. The clinical findings become those of severe pulmonary hypertension, with marked right ventricular hypertrophy and a loud, often palpable second pulmonary sound; a pulmonary ejection click is almost always audible. The second sound is loud and difficult to split. A high-pitched early diastolic murmur, the Graham Steel murmur of pulmonary regurgitation, may be added to these sounds, as may a pansystolic murmur of tricuspid regurgitation when right heart failure supervenes. Equalisation of pressures with balanced resistances also brings reversal of the direction of flow through the duct, the magnitude of the flow increases concomitant with the rise in pulmonary vascular resistance. In some patients, it is possible to recognise differential cyanosis, the blue discolouration being confined to the lower body, and with clubbing of the toes but not the fingers. Unless there is differential cyanosis, it is not possible to recognise a duct clinically in patients with severe pulmonary hypertension and high pulmonary vascular resistance. The diagnosis will depend on cardiac catheterisation and angiography, or cross sectional echocardiography and colour flow Doppler studies.

Until heart failure develops, the chest radiograph shows at most mild cardiomegaly, with marked prominence of the pulmonary arterial segment (see Fig. 42-16B). Right-axis deviation, right atrial hypertrophy, and right ventricular enlargement are usually evident in the electrocardiogram. In some cases, however, a picture of combined, or even left, ventricular hypertrophy may still be seen. It is impossible to calculate accurately the risk of progressive pulmonary vascular disease in patients with a large persistent duct. Surgical treatment has been available almost as long as clinical recognition. The information in terms of natural history necessary to answer the question is not available, nor would such a study now be feasible. Campbell[72] did not address this problem in his calculations, although there are several reports in the literature concerning this complication.[83–85] These are based, however, on selected groups of patients and overemphasise the frequency of the problem. Nor do they all distinguish adequately between pulmonary hypertension with high flow and true pulmonary vascular disease. The presence of pulmonary hypertension secondary to structural changes within the pulmonary vasculature increases the risk of closure, especially once there is right-to-left shunting, with a reported mortality in more than half of a small group of such patients.[83] The complication should be largely avoided by early recognition and treatment of the hypertensive duct. In patients with pulmonary vascular resistance greater then 8 Woods units per meter square, lung biopsy has been recommended to determine candidacy for closure, but unfortunately it may not be fully predictive of outcome.[86] Such patients may be haemodynamically worse after closure with the development of suprasystemic pulmonary arterial pressure, low cardiac output, and right ventricular failure. Patients have been described, nonetheless, with severe histological changes consistent with irreversible pulmonary vascular disease, which resolves completely after closure of the duct.[87] In the occasional patient who escapes early detection, cardiac catheterisation with a vasodilator challenge may be useful in determining the extent of pulmonary vascular changes, and their potential for reversal.

Aneurysm of the Duct

True aneurysm of the duct is rare. It manifests in two distinct forms. The first presents at or shortly after birth,[88,89] the so-called spontaneous aneurysm of infancy[90] (Fig. 42-20). The second form presents in childhood or later life.[91,92] Recent studies suggest that the incidence may be as high as 8%.[93] The true incidence remains unknown, as the definition is not precise, and many aneurysms detected by fetal or neonatal echocardiography resolve spontaneously, without clinically apparent sequels. About one-quarter of patients will have an underlying disorder, such as trisomy 21 or 13, Smith-Lemli-Opitz syndrome, type IV Ehlers-Danlos syndrome, or Marfan's syndrome.[90] Ductal closure usually begins at the pulmonary arterial end of the vessel, and if closure at the aortic end fails to occur, it becomes in effect an aortic diverticulum under systemic pressure. While formation of such a diverticulum is common, it is less clear why this occasionally progresses to aneurysmal formation. Structural abnormalities are possibly present in the aortic, but not the pulmonary end of the duct, such as those associated with collagen vascular disorders. Sepsis may be involved in the pathogenesis of some cases in infancy. A diverticulum arising from the pulmonary trunk is also common. Usually, the type found in infancy is asymptomatic, and may not be uncovered until autopsy for death from other causes. It presents as a tumour-like left-sided mediastinal mass. In one-fifth of cases, rupture or embolism leads to death. Dissection and infection may also occur. Regression can occur, presumably due to thrombosis and organisation, but progressive enlargement, or the onset of hoarseness because of damage to the recurrent laryngeal nerve or left bronchial obstruction, is an indication for surgical excision. In view of the frequency of life-threatening complications, prompt surgical removal is advisable. Percutaneous occlusion of the aneurysm has not been established, but a potential approach is placement of a covered stent in the aorta to exclude the aneurysm and occlude the duct[94] Aneurysm of the duct is even more uncommon in adults.[95] The duct may be patent at both ends, but is usually closed at the pulmonary arterial end.[69–98] Possible pathogenic mechanisms include arrested closure, with persistence of an aortic diverticulum, delayed spontaneous closure of the pulmonary arterial end, infective arteritis and external trauma in a patient with a persistent duct,[99] or even coil occlusion of a preexisting patent duct.[100] Aneurysm of the duct should be considered in the differential diagnosis of adult with unexplained mediastinal masses seen on chest radiography. The diagnosis can be confirmed by aortography or by computerised tomography.[101,102] Like the pattern seen in infancy, the high incidence of rupture, embolisation, and effects of pressure suggest that surgical excision is advisable. Surgical ligation may itself be followed by aneurysmal formation,[95,103] often associated with recanalisation.

Thromboembolism

Thrombosis of the duct as a source of neonatal embolus was first described in 1859.[104] Several cases, mostly fatal, have since been noted.[105,106] Early diagnosis can provide an

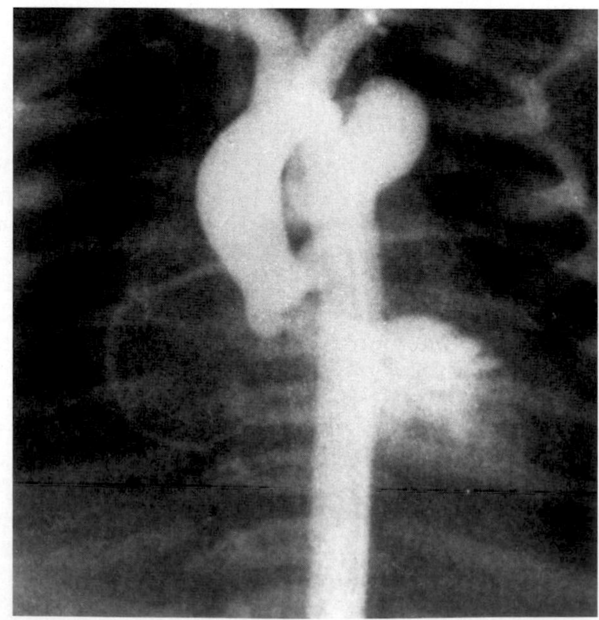

Figure 42-20 The antero-posterior retrograde aortogram shows a ductal aneurysm. Note the associated moderate aortic insufficiency.

opportunity for successful intervention, which may include thrombectomy, heparin, and resection of infarcted tissue.

TREATMENT

Once the diagnosis of uncomplicated persistent patency of the arterial duct is established, elimination of the shunt should be recommended by catheter occlusion or surgery, even when the shunt is small. The justification for closure of small communications resides in the prevention of infective endoarteritis, coupled with an extremely low procedural morbidity and mortality. As noted above, in the setting of the so-called silent duct, there is little clinical evidence to justify any intervention or recommendation to prescribe coverage against subacute bacterial endocarditis. In the occasional patient who develops congestive heart failure, excluding those patients to be discussed below in the context of prematurity, drugs should be administered to combat the failure, but only until intervention can conveniently be arranged.

Surgical Intervention

In 1939, Robert Gross performed the first successful ligation of a persistent arterial duct in a 7-year-old girl.[11,107] The duct is usually approached through a left posterolateral incision, using the third interspace in infants, and the fourth space in children over 1 year. Uncommonly, the duct is on the right side, especially in the presence of a right aortic arch. It must then be approached from the right. The duct may be ligated or divided. The relative merits of each procedure continue to be hotly debated by surgeons. Excellent results have been reported using both procedures. The incidence of clinically apparent recanalisation with ligation is about 1%,[108–111] albeit that echo-Doppler studies have detected flow after ligation in clinically silent ducts, suggesting the incidence of residual flow to be higher.[112] Large ducts exceeding 7 to 10 mm in diameter, or those associated with pulmonary hypertension, are generally divided. Mortality reported from a large experience extending over 25 years for closure of the uncomplicated duct was no more than 0.2%,[113] with a figure of 0.5% cited in another series.[114] Once the safety of the operation was established in older children and adults, it was natural for surgeons to attempt closure in infancy,[115] with Mustard already in 1951 reporting successful ligation in 4 infants.[116] Many surgeons then demonstrated the ease with which the duct could be ligated, even in those born prematurely.[117] In most units, surgical ligation is now reserved for those premature infants who have failed an adequate course of indomethacin, or when there are contraindications to its administration (see below). Such surgical ligation can be done at bedside. The need for accurate anatomical definition prior to intervention in the premature infant must be underscored.[118]

Complications are uncommon. Injury to the laryngeal nerve injury can occur occasionally, but is usually temporary,[119] although it can be permanent. Rarely, a false aneurysm may develop, prompting urgent surgical reoperation after ligation.[120] Damage to the phrenic nerve has also been reported, occurring most frequently in the premature infant. Chylothorax can also occur. Inadvertent ligation of the distal left pulmonary artery occurs infrequently. This is a hazard when the duct is large and the recurrent laryngeal nerve has an unusual course. Ligation of the descending aorta can occur, especially when the duct is approached from a median sternotomy. Signs of aortic coarctation may also be unmasked after ductal ligation.[121] This is a constant hazard in the premature infant. Abnormal findings after ductal ligation, such as decreased femoral pulses or declining urinary output, should prompt rapid re-evaluation.

Video-assisted thoracoscopic closure without thoracotomy has been a recent innovation, first reported by Laborde and his colleagues.[122] Clinical evidence of successful closure was found in all, although two attempts were necessary in two patients. Damage to the recurrent laryngeal nerve occurred in one, while four suffered pneumothorax. Increasing experience with the procedure has reduced the incidence of complications. Continued experience has shown this approach to shorten hospital stay, and to provide a cost-effective, safe and rapid technique compared to open thoracotomy.[123] Results are comparable to transcatheter closure.[124,125] Recently developed for the neonate and infant, a transaxillary muscle sparing thoracotomy provides excellent exposure for ductal division, produces less postoperative pain, and achieves an acceptable cosmetic result.[126]

Closure in the Catheterisation Laboratory

The percutaneous methods for closure were pioneered by Portsmann and colleagues,[127] who reported use of a conical Ivalon plug in 1967, with an umbrella-type device subsequently being used in 1979 by Rashkind and Cuaso.[128] Both these implants required large sheaths for introduction, and were often associated with residual shunting. In 1992, the use of spring coils was reported,[129] and due to the technical simplicity of insertion, this has became a widely used technique for closure for small-to-moderate sized ducts. In the ensuing years, a number devices and techniques have been developed to close larger ducts.

As a result, transcatheter closure has become the treatment of choice for most children and adults with patent ducts. In particular, percutaneous techniques offer considerable advantages over surgical closure for patients with a calcified ductal wall, with or without increased pulmonary vascular resistance, since the latter often necessitates cardiopulmonary bypass.

The essentials of the technique, regardless of the implant used, are to place a catheter or delivery sheath across the duct from either the pulmonary artery or the aorta, and position the implant in the duct. Several techniques have been developed to stabilise the coils during delivery, as non-detachable Gianturco coils could migrate or assume unacceptable configurations or positions.[130–133] Varieties of detachable coils are now available, which allow control of positioning prior to their release (Fig. 42-21).

The Nit-Occlud (Produkte für die Medizin AG, Koln, Germany) is a spring coil specifically designed for ductal embolisation.[133] The design is biconical, in contrast to the cylindrical Gianturco coil (Fig. 22-22). The Amplatzer Duct Occluder (AGA Medical, Plymouth, MN) is a plug-like design made of Nitinol wire woven into a mesh in the shape of a mushroom (Fig. 22-23). This device can be

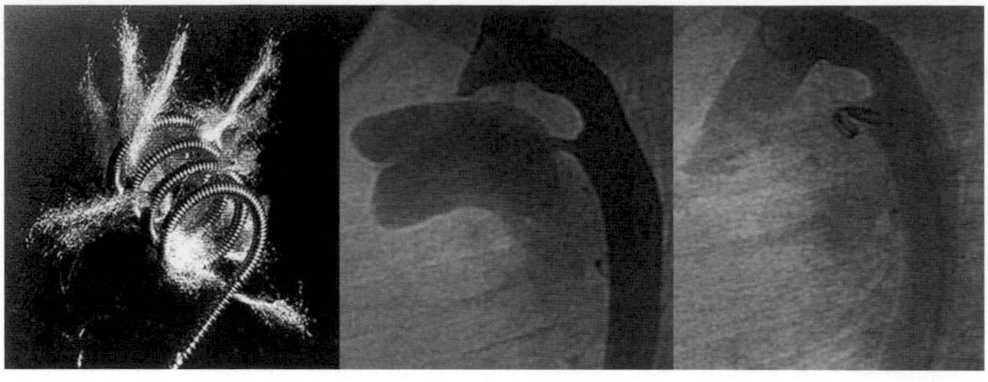

Figure 42-21 The left panel shows a detachable Gianturco coil used for ductal occlusion. Note the Dacron fibers, which promote thrombosis, along its length. The other panels show retrograde lateral aortograms before and after occlusion with such a spring coil.

effective in larger ducts.[134] The device has a detachable cable allowing repositioning or retrieval as necessary. A modified Amplatzer Duct Occluder designed so that the retention skirt has an angle and concavity to fit the aortic end has now been used in clinical practise, and a double retention disc design is now available for clinical use.[135] Other devices currently in use, or under investigation, include a modified buttoned device, and the wireless patch developed by Sideris and associates.[136] Given the variety of ductal configurations and sizes, it is apparent that no individual device will be optimal for closure in all patients. The availability of a variety of implants enhances the capability to close the majority of lesions.

The results of transcatheter occlusion have been excellent. Complete closure rates at follow-up exceed 90% to 95% in most studies.[137] Because of modifications in design, development of new techniques, and increased skill of operators, rates of complete closure have improved significantly over time.[138] Serious complications of transcatheter closure are rare. The most common complication is embolisation of the device, which was relatively common early in the experience with coils. Embolised coils can be retrieved, but even when they cannot, adverse consequences are rare. Other potentially important complications are disturbance to flow in the proximal left pulmonary artery or descending aorta from a protruding device, haemolysis from high-velocity residual shunting, femoral arterial or venous thrombosis related to vascular access, and infection.

Regardless of technique of closure, the clinical diagnosis should be confirmed non-invasively prior to catheterisation by colour Doppler echocardiography, with particular emphasis placed on the presence of associated lesions which could complicate the procedure, such as azygous continuation of the inferior caval vein, presence of an additional lesion which requires surgical intervention, or the presence of pulmonary vascular disease. Special attention should also be directed to the transverse arch and isthmic region to exclude unsuspected coarctation. The procedure is ideally suited for patients weighing more than 6 kg. In smaller infants because of the risk of the size of the implant and difficulties in positioning, left pulmonary

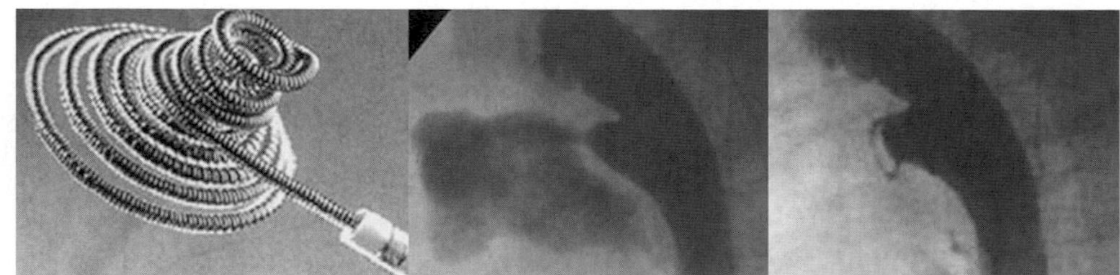

Figure 42-22 Pictured in the left panel is the Nit-Occlud PDA occlusion device, with its biconical configuration. Note the reversed winding on the proximal end. The middle and left panels show lateral aortograms before and after occlusion with the device. (Modified from Schneider DJ, Moore JW: Patent ductus arteriosus. Circulation 2006;114:1873–1882).

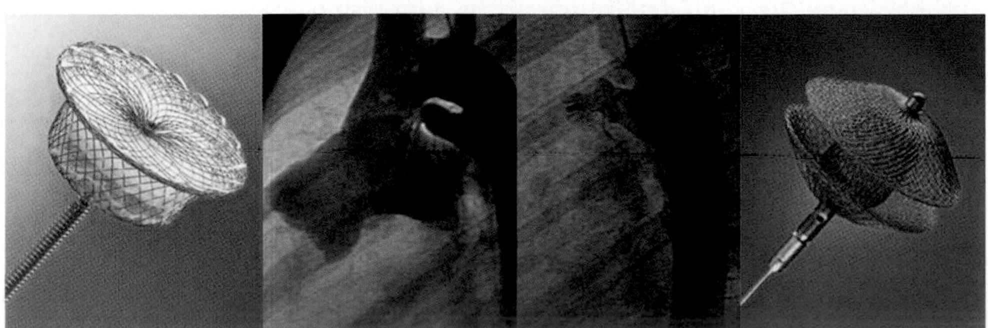

Figure 42-23 The Amplatzer Duct Occluder is shown in leftmost panel. Note the mesh-like weave retention disc that is placed in the aortic end of the duct, as shown in the middle two panels, and the control cable. The right panel shows the newest design (Duct Occluder II, AGA Medical Corporation), with two retention discs, designed to avoid embolisation.

arterial stenosis or aortic obstruction may occur. There is considerable variation in procedural details as practiced amongst centers, such as the use of coincident arterial cannulation, the number and type of angiograms, and so on. The majority of procedures, however, can be performed in an outpatient setting, with discharge on the afternoon of insertion.

PATENCY OF THE ARTERIAL DUCT IN THE PREMATURE INFANT

During the last four decades, there has been a marked increase in premature delivery in many, but not all, developed countries. While the reasons for this are obscure, the increase has been met by the development of neonatal intensive care units and, more recently, units for pregnancies considered to be at high risk. The art and science of caring for the extremely premature infant have developed to the point where survival of infants weighing no more than 500 g is not uncommon.

Pathophysiology

There are several factors which tend to prevent closure of the arterial duct in the immature infant, as both the sensitivity to oxygen and the action of prostaglandin are age dependent,[139] and the relaxant mechanism of prostaglandin is more active in the immature duct.[140,141] The type and duration of ventilatory support, drug therapy, phototherapy, blood transfusions and diuretics undoubtedly account for the wide variations in incidence reported from different institutions.

The pulmonary vascular resistance is lower in the premature than the full-term child due to the rapid increase in number of muscularised pulmonary vessels. The vessels of the immature lung also constrict less for a given stimulus than at term. Constrictive stimuli include hypoxia, acidaemia, and possibly circulating vasoactive peptides and prostaglandins, frequent co-morbidities in the respiratory distress syndromes. These factors render the immature infant especially liable to develop left-to-right shunting when the duct remains patent. Systemic vasoconstriction, so often a feature of the sick premature infant, may further encourage the shunt and exacerbate the respiratory distress syndrome.[142] The immature infant is further handicapped by its reduced cardiac reserve. The increased volume overload secondary to a left-to-right shunt produces an inordinate rise in left ventricular end-diastolic pressure, and a concomitant rise in pulmonary venous pressure. With a large left-to-right shunt through the duct, systemic diastolic pressure falls, compromising the flow through the coronary arteries, which, combined with a shortened diastole because of tachycardia and raised ventricular end-diastolic pressures, predisposes to subendocardial ischaemia. Systemic hypoxia secondary to pulmonary problems, combined with a reduced capacity to carry and deliver oxygen due to anaemia and fetal haemoglobin, further impairs myocardial function, and both are reflected in ischaemic changes in the electrocardiogram frequently seen in the sick premature infant. Other important circulations, such as those of the gut, kidneys, and brain, may be compromised by the haemodynamic changes related in part to the diastolic runoff from the aorta into the pulmonary arteries, with the duct an aetiological factor in necrotising enterocolitis, and cerebral haemorrhage.

Clinical Features

The clinical picture of patency of the duct in the premature infant depends on the size of the left-to-right shunt, on the maturity of the heart and lungs to adjust to the increased volume load, and on the presence of other pathologies, which may obscure the more typical findings. As many premature infants have respiratory distress syndrome, the use of surfactant will modify the clinical expression of ductal shunting by influencing pulmonary vascular resistance. The presence of a significant duct can often be difficult to recognise even by experienced clinicians, and echocardiography is of great value. Three distinct patterns of clinical presentation may be observed.[143]

Absence of Pulmonary Disease

These infants generally have birth weights exceeding 1500 g. Smaller infants may be encountered, nonetheless, whose mothers may have received steroids, or themselves received surfactant. Sometime a systolic murmur is detected in the first week of life. This becomes louder and longer as pulmonary vascular resistance falls, and eventually spills into early diastole. The murmur is best heard in the second and third left interspaces. It is associated with accentuation of pulmonary closure, with the typical continuous murmur as heard in older children usually not being present. If the shunt becomes large, the precordium becomes hyperactive, the pulse pressure wide, and the peripheral pulses bounding. An apical third sound may also occur associated with a diastolic flow murmur. If the left ventricle fails, tachycardia and tachypnoea develop, and moist sounds can be heard in the chest. Apnoea and bradycardia may complicate severe left ventricular failure. Hepatomegaly may only develop late. Most infants in this group do not develop massive shunts, and can be managed by simple medical means. The duct closes spontaneously in the majority at an age approximating to full-term. These older infants tend to respond less well to indomethacin than more immature infants do.

Infants Recovering from Lung Disease

Left-to-right ductal shunting may develop in infants recovering from respiratory distress syndrome. Usually they weigh between 1000 and 1500 g. Most probably the duct is patent from birth, and left-to-right shunting only develops during recovery when pulmonary vascular resistance falls. At this time, increased administration of fluids may further aggravate the loading effects of the shunt on left ventricular function. Many of these infants are still maintained on mechanical ventilators, or continuous positive airway pressure, when shunting first develops. Because of this, the initial systolic murmur may be difficult to detect. Often the clinical findings are quite labile. If the shunt increases, the murmur becomes more obvious. Like the first group, it may eventually spill into diastole. Other signs of a large shunt may be present, including bounding pulses, a hyperdynamic precordium, and tachycardia. This group of patients tends to be more immature, and to develop left ventricular failure with relatively smaller shunts. Ventilatory status may deteriorate so that higher concentrations of oxygen and increased pressure or rate settings are required to counter a deteriorating status of the blood gases. Apnoeic episodes and bradycardia are common.

Infants with Lung Disease

This group tends to include the most immature infants with birth weights below 1000 g. These patients are usually ventilator-dependent, and the development of a left-to-right ductal shunt in these patients is associated with increasing requirement for ventilator support and deterioration of the status of the blood gases. Murmurs may be difficult to hear, and occasionally a very large duct may be silent. Signs of a large left-to-right shunt may occur, but left ventricular failure is often difficult to differentiate from signs due to pulmonary disease or sepsis.

Investigations

Neither the electrocardiogram nor the chest radiograph is particularly helpful in making the diagnosis of a significant duct in premature infants. The electrocardiogram may show left ventricular hypertrophy in the group without lung disease, especially if the shunt is substantial and has been present for some time. In the other two groups, right ventricular predominance is more usual. As mentioned, ischemic changes may also be present. The chest radiograph may show cardiomegaly with increased pulmonary blood flow. Often the heart is not obviously enlarged, and pulmonary changes due to flow or failure are difficult to differentiate from those due to primary pulmonary problems.

Echocardiography

Persistent patency of the duct after the neonatal period is readily diagnosed by its characteristic clinical features. In premature infants, however, especially those with respiratory distress syndrome, the recognition of significant shunting across a patent duct can be difficult. Cross sectional echocardiography and Doppler flow studies are invaluable in determining the presence of a duct, its shunting pattern, size and response to therapy. Additionally, it is essential in ruling out other structural malformations prior to intervention. Indeed, patients with severe ventilator-dependent respiratory distress syndrome may have a large ductal shunt, which may be entirely silent due to lack of turbulent flow within the vessel. Cardiomegaly may also be absent, especially in infants who are fluid-restricted.

Management

Because many ducts will eventually close in premature infants, there has been an understandable reluctance to advise aggressive intervention as soon as a significant left-to-right shunt is recognised. The presence of a ductal shunt, however, has been implicated in the pathogenesis of bronchopulmonary dysplasia, and as a factor in the duration of ventilator support. This increased risk of chronic lung disease has led many to advocate early and effective treatment. Early experience with surgical ligation demonstrated that congestive heart failure could quickly be controlled, although mortality and morbidity from the respiratory distress syndrome remained high. With further surgical experience, mortality directly due to the operation has been reduced to less than 1%. Some centers have advocated, and successfully performed, surgery in the nursery, thereby avoiding the hazards of transport to and from the operating room.

Once the role of E-type prostaglandins in maintaining ductal patency during fetal life was established, pharmacologically induced closure using indomethacin was soon reported in the premature infant.[144,145] Transient renal insufficiency and mild gastrointestinal bleeding are the main side effects. Despite its widespread usage, questions remain concerning proper dosage, duration of treatment, and optimal timing of administration. The major determinants of success are gestational and postnatal age. In general, initial management includes maintenance of an appropriate level of haemoglobin, ventilatory support, diuretic therapy, and restriction of fluids. The trend is to earlier closure, either by medical or surgical means. In ventilated infants weighing less than 1000 g, administration of indomethacin has been associated with improved outcomes,[146–148] even in the absence of large left-to-right shunts. In contrast, in infants weighing more than 1000 g, outcomes are unaltered, and treatment with indomethacin should be restricted to those with signs of a significant shunt.[144-149] Once the problem is recognised, intake of fluid should be restricted, and furosemide given in a dose of 1 mg/kg. Digoxin is of dubious benefit in this situation. If the shunt remains large after 24 hours, indomethacin should be given, preferably intravenously although nasogastric administration can be successful. Extreme prematurity, very low birth weight, and advanced conceptional or postnatal age are all factors, which reduce the chances of successful closure using indomethacin. Renal and/or hepatic insufficiency, serious hyperbilirubinemia, or problems with coagulation are contraindications to its use. If the duct persists or recurs, a second course of indomethacin should be administered. Dosages are largely selected on an empiric basis. The initial dose is 0.2 mg/kg, while subsequent dosages depend on age at time of initial treatment. If the patient is less than 48 hours of age, the subsequent two doses are 0.1 mg/kg; if the patient is aged from 2 to 7 days of age, 0.2 mg/kg; and if the patient is greater than 7 days, 0.25 mg/kg. The rate of reopening is highest in the very premature, occurring in one-third of those weighing less than 1000 g and in less than one-tenth of those weighing 1500 g. If there is no response to indomethacin, surgical ligation should be undertaken.[149,150]

Indomethacin-induced closure of the duct is followed by immediate and progressive clinical improvement, with a decrease in requirements for oxygen and in mean airway inflation pressure during mechanical ventilation. Lung compliance has been shown to improve after both surgical ligation and medical closure with duration of ventilation, length of hospitalisation, and the costs of medical care reduced by early treatment.[151–153] The use of prophylactic indomethacin in infants without a duct may decrease the incidence of intracerebral complications but its use in this setting is controversial.[154] Such therapy has not been shown to reduce length of stay, oxygen need, or mechanical ventilatory duration nor the incidence of bronchopulmonary dysplasia.[147,155,156] Reversal of indomethacin-induced ductal closure by administration of prostaglandin, in the presence of ductal-dependent cardiac malformations, has been possible.[157]

Surgical ligation of the persistent duct in premature infants was first reported in 1963.[158] As with indomethacin, surgery has been associated with a decreased need for ventilatory support, and reduced hospital stay,[157,159] particularly in infants weighing less than 1500 g.[150,161] Surgery can be safely carried out in the neonatal intensive care unit to avoid the stress of transportation to the operating theater. While ligation has been the traditional approach, recently video-assisted thoracoscopic techniques have been proved successful.[162,163]

Overall mortality remains high, but more often is related to continuing respiratory distress, intracranial haemorrhage, necrotising enterocolitis, or coagulopathy, rather than the therapies themselves.[152] Many questions remain unanswered concerning the true impact of a large left-to-right ductal shunt on the course and outcome of prematurity and respiratory distress syndrome. In a large multi-centre trial, one-third of infants with a significant duct had spontaneous closure, while indomethacin induced closure in seven-tenths of infants treated. There was no difference in the rate of closure if indomethacin was given immediately on diagnosis, or after 48 hours of intensive medical therapy. Rates of death were identical in patients treated with indomethacin early, with indomethacin given late, or with surgery, being about 13% overall in each group.[162-164]

Infiltration of Formalin, Balloon Dilation, Implantation of Stents, and Bioengineering of the Arterial Duct

Rudolph and colleagues[165] described a technique of subadventitial formalin infiltration of the wall of the duct designed to maintain long-term patency of the vessel in patients with duct-dependent cardiac malformations in whom surgery was either inadequate or not feasible. It was shown, however, that infiltration of formalin did not ensure ductal patency even for a short time.[166] The technique was abandoned in favor of infusion of prostaglandin E_1.

Percutaneous balloon dilation has also been proposed as a method to maintain ductal patency.[167] Temporary patency can be achieved, but abrupt closure, thrombosis, or rupture can occur, making this a less reliable means of assuring patency. Except for special instances, this technique has not been pursued clinically.

To provide a mechanical scaffold for the ductal wall, resistant to the constrictive forces of ductal closure, Coe and Olley[165-168] proposed the implantation of endovascular stents. This approach, using either self- or balloon expandable stents, has had expanding clinical application. The implantation in anatomically uncomplicated ducts, such as in pulmonary atresia, critical pulmonary stenosis or the hypoplastic left heart syndrome (Fig. 42-24), has been encouraging.[169–172] Use in more complex situations, such as occur in tetralogy with pulmonary atresia, however, can be technically difficult.[173] With innovative approaches to deliver the implant, such as cut-down of the carotid arteries, transvenous through a ventricular septal defect, or after radio-frequency–assisted balloon dilation of an atretic pulmonary valve, the procedure can be performed even in ducts which originate from the undersurface of the aorta or are tortuous. Largely, application has been advanced through improved design of the stents, such as flexible balloon platforms or systems with lower profiles, or taking advantage of the potential of drug-eluting implants to alter the vessel reactivity, thus reducing in-stent stenosis. Recently, at the Hospital for Sick Children in Toronto, Lee and colleagues investigated the use of rapamycin-coated stents implanted into the ducts of small newborn pigs (unpublished data). The mean luminal diameter of bare metal implants compared with the drug-eluting stents was smaller by 32% and 42% at 4 and 6 weeks, respectively, by inhibition of neointimal formation (Fig. 42-25). While the role of stents in the management of infants with complex ductal dependent lesions has yet to be fully defined, such studies are very promising.

Bioengineering of the Arterial Duct for Therapeutic Gain

Novel methodology is emerging for maintaining ductal patency into the postnatal period to sustain life and allow surgical intervention of duct-dependent cardiac malformations. Very recently, maintenance of ductal patency was described through surgical transfection of fetal lambs.[173] By targeting the ductal smooth muscle cells with an expression vector encoding a decoy mRNA of the fibronectin message, it proved possible to sequester the protein which binds, thereby preventing upregulation of fibronectin and arresting intimal cushions. This approach both emphasises the importance of fibronectin to the process of ductal closure and identifies a new therapeutic modality and target. While fet surgery is likely not feasible in the clinical setting, an alternative approach of targeting chemotherapeutic agents given by systemic infusion to different vascular beds by unique peptide zip codes, may offer bright therapeutic avenues.[174] Recently at the Hospital for Sick Children in

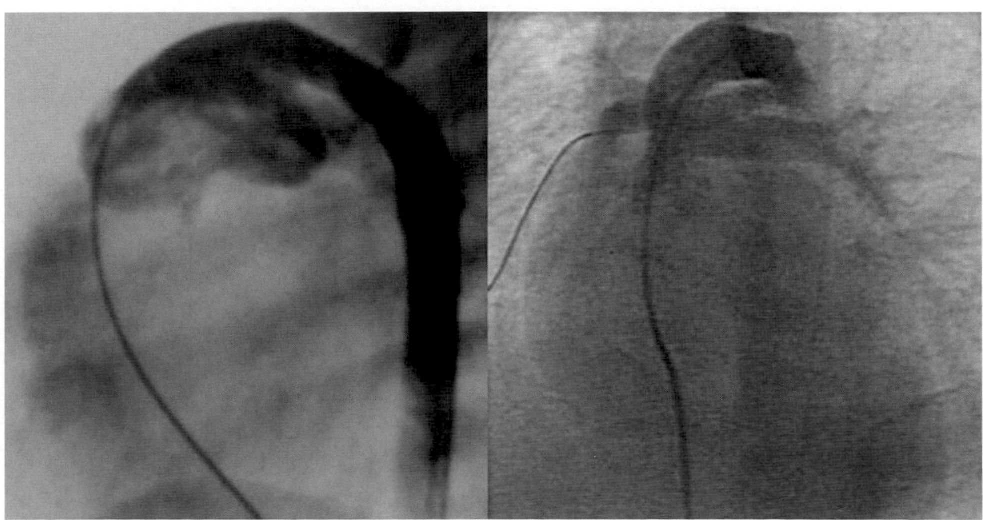

Figure 42-24 The left panel shows an infant with hypoplastic left heart syndrome awaiting cardiac transplantation. The duct became stenotic and unresponsive to prostaglandin. Here, a pulmonary arterial angiogram depicts a stent placed transvenously across the duct to relieve the stenosis. In the right panel, an aortogram is seen after implantation of a stent in an infant with pulmonary atresia and intact septum who was prostaglandin dependent.

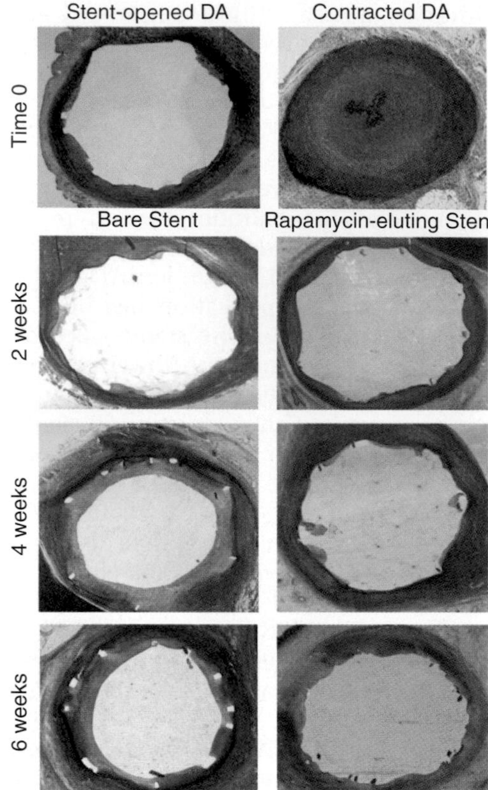

Figure 42-25 Movat pentachrome staining of the arterial duct (×400 magnification). The upper right panel shows the spontaneously contracted duct in seven-day-old piglet. The upper left panel shows the duct, stented with a bare metal stent and immediately harvested. The lower six panels show examples of stented ducts representative of the bare and drug-eluting stent groups. Note that there is negligible difference in lumen patency between the drug-eluting stent and bare metal stent at 2 weeks but increased luminal compromise in the bare metal stent group at 4 and 6 weeks compared with the drug-eluting stent.

Toronto, Humpl and colleagues investigated percutaneous postnatal transfection of a vector containing the gene for prostaglandin into ductal tissue, resulting in prolonged patency.[175]

These studies identifying and characterising the cellular and molecular mechanisms involved in ductal patency and closure have advanced our understanding of this developmentally programmed fetal vessel. The impact of these advances extends beyond the scope of ductal remodeling, as they have provided insight into the pathogenesis of occlusive vascular disease processes, which utilise similar pathways. This work has also positioned the field towards further advances associated with the development of safe therapeutic measures to maintain ductal patency for infants with cyanotic congenital heart disease, ultimately translating into improved care and clinical outcome.

The complete reference list can be found on the companion Expert Consult web site at www.expertconsult.com.

ANNOTATED REFERENCES

- Gross RE, Hubbard JP: Surgical ligation of a patent ductus arteriosus: A report of first successful case. JAMA 1939;112:729–731.

  This landmark report ushered in the era of corrective surgery for congenital heart lesions. An interesting irony is that it was management of the arterial duct by transcatheter approaches that also established minimally invasive management of congenital heart lesions.

- Tynan M: The murmur of the persistently patent arterial duct, or "The Colonel is going to a dance." Cardiol Young 2003;13:559–562.

  Michael Tynan reminds us of the history of the clinical recognition of the arterial duct by Gibson and the importance of confirming our sources!

- Coceani F, Olley PM: The response of the ductus arteriosus to prostaglandins. Can J Physiol Pharmacol 1973;51:220–225.

  A landmark paper, it was first to describe the actions of prostaglandins on the arterial duct. While the original hypothesis was that prostaglandin led to ductal constriction, these investigators' experimental findings became the underpinning for the understanding of the biological control of the duct.

- Krichenko A, Benson LN, Burrows P, et al: Angiographic classification of the isolated, persistently patent ductus arteriosus and implications for percutaneous catheter occlusion. Am J Cardiol 1989;63:877–880.

  Interested in a categorisation scheme for ductal geometry, these authors proposed an easy classification which allows retrospective data analysis.

- Smallhorn JF, Huhta JC, Anderson RH, Macartney FJ: Suprasternal cross-sectional echocardiography in assessment of patent ductus arteriosus. Br Heart J 1982;48:321–330.

  The first study defining the technique for imaging the duct by two-dimensional echocardiography.

- Lloyd TR, Beekman RH III: Clinically silent patent ductus arteriosus. Am Heart J 1994;127:1664–1665.
- Salazar J, Olivan P, Ibarra F, et al: Silent uncomplicated patent ductus arteriosus in children: Diagnosis with echo-Doppler [Spanish]. Serv Esp Cardiol 1990;43:410–412.
- Houston AB, Gnanapragasam JP, Lim MK, et al: Doppler ultrasound and the silent ductus arteriosus. Br Heart J 1991;65:97–99.
- Balzer DT, Spray TL, McMufflin D, et al: Endarteritis associated with a clinically silent patent ductus arteriosus. Am Heart J 1993;125:1192–1193.
- Parthenakis FI, Kanakaraki MK, Vardas PE: Silent patent ductus arteriosus endarteritis. Heart 2000;84:619.

  These five articles established the existence of the so-called silent (non-hypertensive) duct, and the specter of its potential risk for endarteritis.

- Campbell M: Natural history of persistent ductus arteriosus. Br Heart J 1968;30:4–13.

  Campbell analysed four series of patients in which 11 examples of spontaneous closure occurred over 1842 patient-years, giving a rate of 0.6% per annum. Several of the examples, however, were based on quite tenuous clinical impressions. In none was catheterisation performed before and after the event. The figure calculated by Campbell is almost certainly an overestimate. He did not suggest that surgery should be delayed except, perhaps, in patients with small shunts and signs that the duct was already closing. Few cardiologists would now agree even with these exceptions.

- Jacobs JP, Giroud JM, Quintessenza JA, et al: The modern approach to patent ductus arteriosus treatment: Complementary roles of video-assisted thoracoscopic surgery and interventional cardiology coil occlusion. Ann Thorac Surg 2003;76:1421–1427.

  An excellent review of the application of thorascopic surgery and percutaneous coil embolisation. Both techniques are complementary, and a rationale for selection of the appropriate treatment modality can be based upon the size and age of the patient and the size and morphology of the duct.

- Portsmann W, Wierny L, Warnke H: Closure of persistent ductus arteriosus without thoracotomy. Ger Med Monthly 1967;12:259–261.
- Rashkind WJ, Cuaso CC: Transcatheter closure of a patent ductus arteriosus: Successful use in a 3.5-kg infant. Pediatr Cardiol 1979;1:3–7.
- Cambier PA, Kirby WC, Wortham DC, Moore JW: Percutaneous closure of the small (<2.5 mm) patent ductus arteriosus using coil embolization. Am J Cardiol 1992;69:815–816

  These three reports report the first percutaneous techniques for ductal closure. While only coil embolisation is still applied today, the studies by Portsmann and colleagues and Rashkind and colleagues form the foundation for all the interventional approaches used today.

- Galal MO, Hussain A, Arfi AM: Do we need the surgeon to close the persistently patent arterial duct? Cardiol Young 2006;16:522–536.

  An excellent review of contemporary interventional techniques in transcatheter management of the patent arterial duct.

- Friedman WF: Studies of the response of the ductus arteriosus. In Heymann MA, Rudolph AM (eds): The Ductus Arteriosus: Proceedings of the Seventy-fifth Ross Conference on Pediatric Research. Columbus, OH, 1978, pp 35–43.
- Gersony WM, Peckham GJ, Ellison RC, et al: Effects of indomethacin on premature infants with patent ductus arteriosus: Results of a national collaborative study. J Pediatr 1983;102:895–860.

  These two reports review the humeral control mechanism of ductal patency and closure, and document the application of that understanding to management of the premature with a clinically significant ductal patency.

- Coe JY, Olley PM: A novel method to maintain ductus arteriosus patency. J Am Coll Cardiol 1991;18:837–841.
- Gewillig M, Boshoff DE, Dens J, et al: Stenting the neonatal arterial duct in duct-dependent pulmonary circulation: New techniques, better results. J Am Coll Cardiol. 2004;43:107–112.

- Alwi M, Choo KK, Latiff HA, et al: Initial results and medium-term follow-up of stent implantation of patent ductus arteriosus in duct-dependent pulmonary circulation. J Am Coll Cardiol 2004;44:438–445.

  Techniques non-pharmacological methods to maintain ductal patency have attained prominence in treatment strategies for the infant with ductal dependent pulmonary or systemic blood flow. These reports discuss the implantation of endovascular stents to palliate such lesions.

- Mason CA, Bigras JL, O'Blenes SB, et al: Gene transfer in utero biologically engineers a patent ductus arteriosus in lambs by arresting fibronectin-dependent neointimal formation. Nat Med 1991;5:176–182.

- Humpl T, Zaidi SH, Coe JY, et al: Gene transfer of prostaglandin synthase maintains patency of the newborn lamb arterial duct. Pediatr Res 2005;58:976–980.

  These two reports apply molecular methods, developed from an understanding of ductal vascular biology to maintain ductal patency. While neither has attended clinical application, research following these approaches will improve our methods to control ductal patency.

CHAPTER

43

Pulmonary Stenosis

GRAHAM DERRICK, PHILIPP BONHOEFFER, and ROBERT H. ANDERSON

This chapter will discuss pulmonary stenosis, where it exists as an isolated finding. Where pulmonary stenosis exists as part of a more complex anomaly, such as tetralogy of Fallot, the reader is directed to the complete descriptions found in the relevant chapters.

GENETICS, EMBRYOGENESIS AND INCIDENCE

Genetics

The first descriptions of pulmonary stenosis were recorded by Giovanni Baptista Morgagni, of Padova in Italy, in 1761.[1] This lesion is now known to be common, and comprises about one-tenth of all congenital cardiac malformations.

The incidence of pulmonary stenosis in the United Kingdom or North America is about 0.4%. The rate of familial recurrence, however, is considerably higher, at up to 4%, suggesting that a proportion of cases at least are linked to a genetic basis. Further investigations within families have supported this hypothesis, suggesting that pulmonary stenosis can be caused by a single gene defect with or without additional abnormalities within the phenotype. Clearly there are a number of genetic abnormalities involved. At the time of writing, a search on the Online database for Mendelian Inheritance in Man[2] for variants of pulmonary or pulmonic, stenosis, or valve stenosis, revealed 92 reports for conditions including pulmonary stenosis where Mendelian inheritance is suspected. Of these, the locus for a genetic abnormality, be it a point gene mutation, deletion or aneuploidy, were confirmed in two-thirds of the results, whilst the remaining third of the reports were of cases with Mendelian or suspected Mendelian inheritance. Perhaps the most frequently presenting patients with a genetic basis for their pulmonary stenosis are patients with Noonan's or Williams' syndromes.

Non-genetic factors have also been implicated. For instance, the congenital rubella syndrome, now very rarely seen because of adequate immunisation and prenatal maternal screening, includes severe peripheral pulmonary arterial stenosis.

Embryology

The precise embryology of the development of the pulmonary valve in the human, indeed both ventricular outflow tracts, is not fully understood. Because of the obvious constraints of studying human embryological development, other species of embryo have formed the basis of the understanding of embryology. The most common models have been proposed based on sequential sections and stains of the developing chick embryo or chick-quail chimera. Difficulties also exist because of differing nomenclature used between the groups studying the lesions.

As we have explained in Chapter 3, the heart develops as a tubular structure with a solitary lumen when the embryo is 20 days old, differentiating into a sequential pulsatile pump by 28 days. By 30 days, partial separation has occurred, creating a chambered structure with interatrial and interventricular communications. Remodelling of the outflow tract produces two vessels, each with its own arterial valve. The tissues of the outflow tract are derived from different sources. The cardiac mesenchyme contributes to the myocardium and some of the endothelium, with other endothelial contributions from migrating cells of the non-cardiogenic regions of the lateral plate and head mesenchyme. Initial septation is produced by ingrowth of mesenchyme, derived from the neural crest, into the cushions developing throughout the outflow tract. These cushions then fuse with each other, and also with the back wall of the aortic sac between the origins of the arteries supplying the fourth and sixth aortic arches. This process achieves separation of the intrapericardial components of the aorta and the pulmonary trunk. The proximal part of the outflow tract remains encased in a sleeve of outflow myocardium. It is division of the distal part of this persisting muscular outflow tract, again by the cushions packed with cells from the neural crest, which produces the primordiums of the developing aortic and pulmonary valves. It is the outflow cushions themselves, by a process of cavitation, that are remodelled at their distal ends to produce the leaflets and sinuses of the valves. The role of cells derived from the neural crest is demonstrated by ablation of the neural crest itself, which results in failure of septation, and a persistent common arterial trunk. Tissue derived from sources other than the neural crest also plays a role in differentiation and separation of the ventricular outflow tracts, and the origin of this tissue is still not known.[3] The reader is directed to a complete review of the literature and discussion of the role of tissues derived from the cardiac neural crest in the development of the cardiac outflow tracts provided by Waldo and colleagues.[4]

The proximal portions of the left and right pulmonary artery branches derive from the caudal portion of the aortic sac, which also feeds the arteries of the sixth pharyngeal pouches. The distal portion of the right sixth branchial arch regresses completely, while the distal portion of the left branchial arch persists as the arterial duct, and latterly the ligament of the arterial duct. The peripheral pulmonary vasculature, distal to the origin of the branches of the pulmonary trunk, derives from the postbranchial pulmonary vascular plexus, which develops in close relationship with and alongside the developing lung buds.

Incidence

Pulmonary stenosis is the second most common congenital cardiac malformation. In a large prospective study of all live born infants, including also data from autopsies of stillborn infants,[5] the total incidence of congenitally malformed hearts was 6.6 per 1000 live births. Of these, pulmonary stenosis accounted for 5.8%. Half of all congenitally malformed hearts include pulmonary stenosis as a component of the defect.

MORPHOLOGY

As far as stenosis within the pulmonary outflow tract is concerned, obstruction at valvar level is by far the most common lesion. Understanding completely the mechanisms responsible for stenosis mandates a clear appreciation of normal valvar anatomy.[6] At present, such understanding is constrained by varying use of the term annulus to describe the structure of the normal valve. Paradoxically, it is only when the valve is stenotic that the attachments of the leaflets approximate to an annular arrangement.

The Normal Pulmonary Valve

The essence of normal valvar anatomy at the ventriculo-arterial junction is the suspension of the leaflets in semilunar fashion within the sinuses of the pulmonary trunk. The key feature is that the hinges of the leaflets cross the anatomic ventriculo-arterial junction. The arrangement is best seen when the normal outflow tract is spread open, having already removed the leaflets (Fig. 43-1). The dissection shows that each leaflet is attached at its two extremities at the sinutubular junction, whilst the basal attachment is supported by the musculature of the subpulmonary infundibulum. True anatomical rings can then be identified at the level of the sinutubular junction, and also at the anatomic ventriculo-arterial junction, this latter structure being the locus over which the fibroelastic walls of the pulmonary trunk are supported by the muscular subpulmonary infundibulum. A third ring can then be constructed by joining together the basal attachments of the leaflets, but this latter ring is a geometric construction, rather than an anatomic reality. The semilunar line of attachment of each of the leaflets, which marks the haemodynamic ventriculo-arterial junction, crosses the anatomical junction between the muscular infundibulum and the pulmonary trunk in two places. Because of this, crescents of muscular infundibulum are incorporated at the base of each pulmonary sinus, while three tapering triangles of fibrous pulmonary truncal wall extend beyond the anatomical ventriculo-arterial junction as parts of the ventricular outflow tract, reaching to the level of the sinutubular junction (Fig. 43-2).

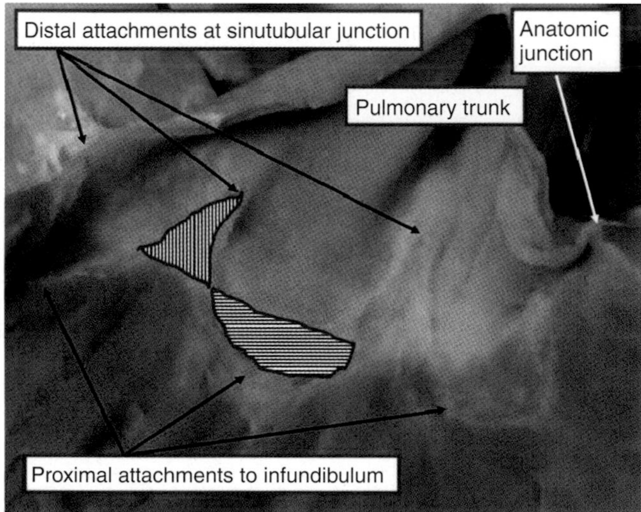

Figure 43-1 The normal pulmonary outflow tract has been opened and spread to show its full width, the leaflets of the pulmonary valve having been removed. The dissection shows how each leaflet is attached distally at the sinutubular junction, but proximally to the muscular infundibulum. The semilunar line of attachment of each leaflet, marking the haemodynamic ventriculo-arterial junction, crosses twice the anatomic junction between the wall of the pulmonary trunk and the muscular infundibulum, leaving triangles of fibrous wall (*vertical hatching*) as part of the ventricle, but sequestrating crescents of musculature (*horizontal hatching*) as parts of the valvar sinuses.

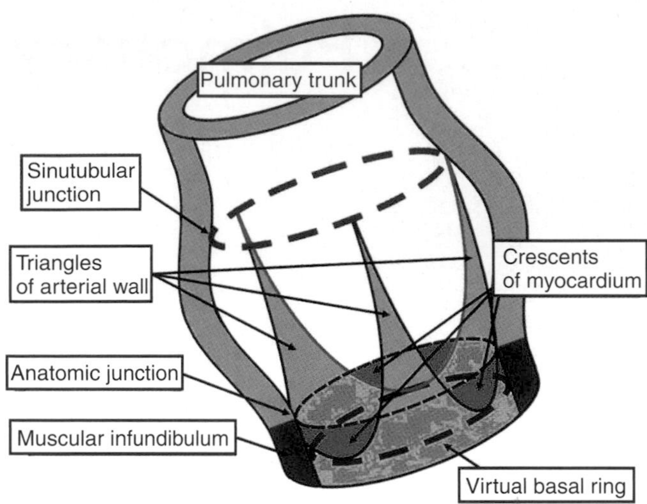

Figure 43-2 The cartoon shows the effect of the hingeline of the valvar leaflets (one shown in *purple*) crossing the anatomic ventriculo-arterial junction. Triangles of arterial wall are incorporated into the ventricular outflow tract to the level of the sinutubular junction, while crescents of muscular infundibulum are sequestrated at the base of each valvar sinus.

In this normal arrangement, the free edge of each leaflet is appreciably longer than the cord of the sinus that supports it, thus permitting the three leaflets to fit snugly together when closed so as to produce a competent valvar orifice. It is the semilunar nature of suspension of the leaflets, therefore, that permits competent closure and unobstructed opening of the valve, with the zones of apposition between the adjacent leaflets extending in triradiate fashion from the centroid of the valvar orifice to the sinutubular junction at its periphery (Fig. 43-3).

Pulmonary Stenosis

It is fusion of the adjacent leaflets along their commissures, or zones of apposition, which is the essence of valvar stenosis. The fusion along the zones of apposition is typically uniform. It begins peripherally, so that the valvar orifice is narrowed to a central opening. The more the fusion extends towards the centre of the valve, the narrower will be the central opening, and the more severe will be the valvar stenosis.

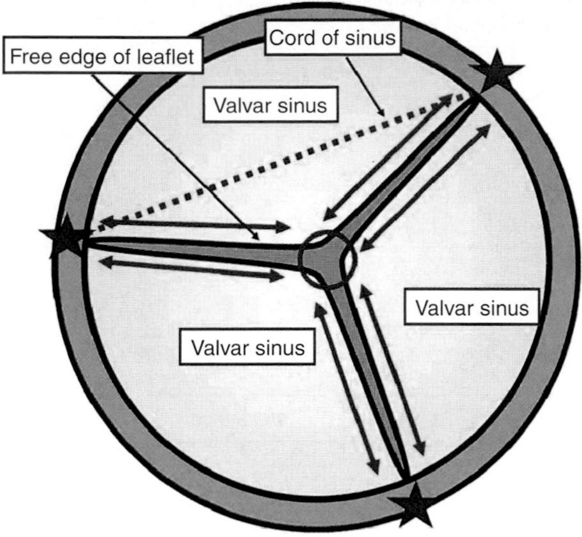

Figure 43-3 The cartoon shows the idealised arrangement of the pulmonary valvar leaflets seen from the arterial aspect. The free edge of each leaflet is longer than the cord of the sinus supporting it (*red dotted line*), permitting the leaflets to close together snugly along their zones of apposition (*red arrows*), which are attached peripherally at the sinutubular junction (*stars*), and meet at the valvar centroid (*red circle*).

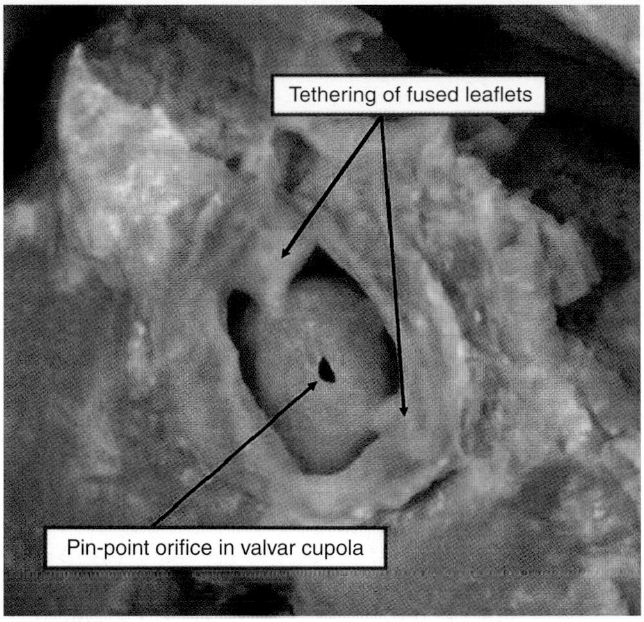

Figure 43-5 In this critically stenotic valve, the valvar dome is smooth, with evidence of the fused zones of apposition seen only at the margins of the valve.

When stenosis of a trifoliate valve is mild to moderate, the opening has a triangular configuration (Fig. 43-4).

In contrast, in the most severe forms which produce typical neonatal critical stenosis, the extent of fusion is sufficient to leave only a central pin-prick opening. In this so-called domed stenosis, the central part of the dome tends to be smooth, with evidence of the fused zones of apposition seen to varying degrees as peripheral raphes with tethering at the sinutubular junction (Fig. 43-5).

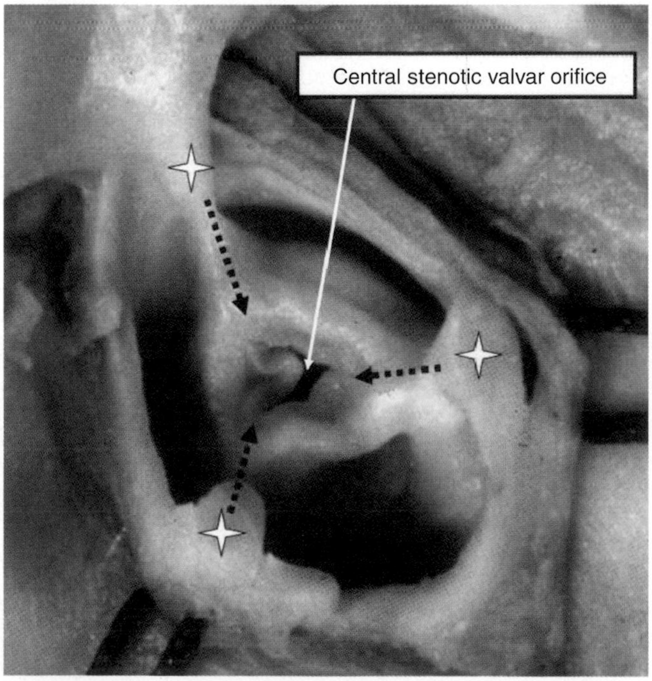

When the critically stenotic valve is opened, then because of the obliteration of the zones of apposition between the leaflets, there is also a reduction in the extent of their semilunar hingeing, so that the line of attachment within the pulmonary root achieves a more circular configuration (Fig. 43-6). This is the annular paradox, where ring-like attachments become evident only when the valve is malformed. In this respect, it should also be noted that, although it is frequent to describe the orifice of the normal pulmonary valve in terms of the annulus, the diameter usually measured in this fashion by the echocardiographer is at the level of the virtual basal ring (Fig. 43-7).

As we have already demonstrated, when such a normal valve is opened, it is the semilunar attachments of the leaflets which dominate the picture. An attachment approximating to a ring is never seen unless the valve is stenotic (see Fig. 43-6).

In some instances, it is possible to identify four raphes, suggesting that the valve itself initially had four leaflets. Indeed, quadrifoliate non-stenosed pulmonary valves are by no means unusual, and were discovered as incidental benign lesions once in each 250 postmortems by Becker.[7] The incidence of a bifoliate, or biscuspid, and stenosed pulmonary valve is reported to be between 7% and 17%, diagnosed with echocardiography or by the surgeon. Archives of autopsied hearts, including our own, have not replicated such a high incidence.[7–10]

The typical lesion producing pulmonary valvar stenosis, therefore, is uniform fusion of the peripheral zones of apposition of a trifoliate valve, leaving a central aperture. Usually this arrangement is associated with some degree of thickening at the union of the zones of apposition with the sinutubular junction, this arrangement being described surgically as tethering (see Fig. 43-4). Accentuation of such tethering can produce marked narrowing at the sinutubular

Figure 43-4 This moderately stenotic valve is shown having removed the pulmonary trunk and photographing the specimen from the arterial aspect. The zones of apposition of the leaflets are fused from their peripheral attachments (*stars*) towards the centroid of the valvar orifice (*red arrows*). This produces a narrowed central orifice. Note the tethering of the leaflets at the sinutubular junction.

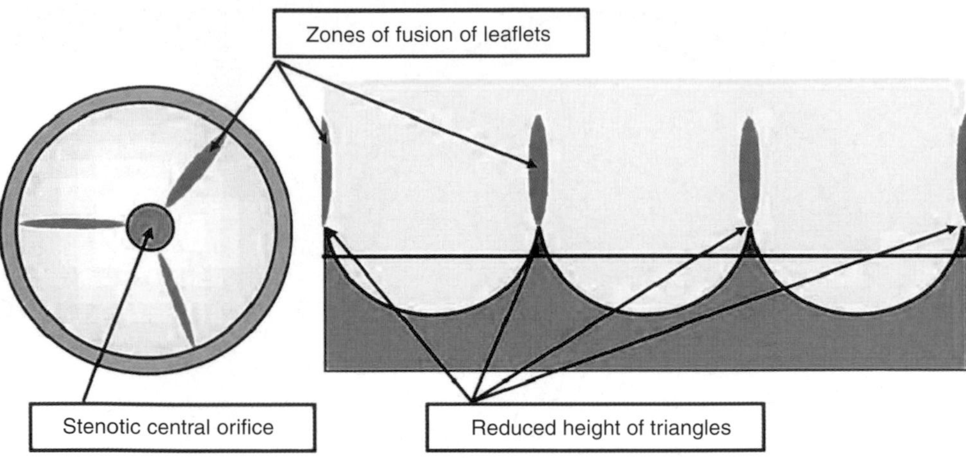

Figure 43-6 The cartoon shows the arterial view of a valve such as shown in Figure 43-5 to the left hand, and the arrangement of the opened root to the right hand. The fusion of the leaflets produces a more circular attachment within the root: the annular paradox.

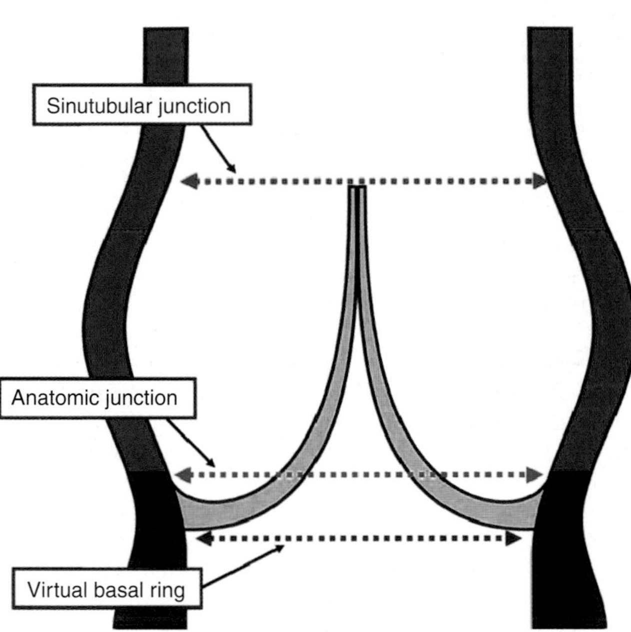

Figure 43-7 The cartoon shows a section across the pulmonary root. The measurement usually taken by the echocardiographer as the annulus (*red line*) is at the level of the basal attachment of the leaflets. As we have shown, this is a virtual ring. The true anatomic rings in the root (*blue and green lines*) are rarely measured by the echocardiographer.

junction, giving an hourglass appearance that is often described as supravalvar. In reality, the sinutubular junction is an integral part of the valvar complex. In some instances, valvar stenosis is the consequence of dysplasia of the leaflets, making them thick and mucoid. Such thickening is sufficient to produce obstruction of the valvar orifice, even should the leaflets themselves not be fused along their zones of apposition. Clinical experience indicates, however, that such thickened leaflets usually co-exist with a narrowed sinutubular junction. Most of the patients with Ullrich-Noonan's syndrome have this type of stenosis.[11]

Although pulmonary valvar stenosis may be considered a simple lesion, it is rare for the lesion to be totally isolated. Almost always there is hypertrophy of the right ventricular wall. In the neonate with critical valvar stenosis, such hypertrophy may be severe, with accompanying fibrosis of the endocardium and thickening of the tension apparatus of the tricuspid valve. The right ventricle then resembles the situation seen at the better end of the spectrum of pulmonary atresia with intact septum (see Chapter 30). The findings of areas of subendocardial right ventricular infarction in the absence of coronary arterial disease,[12] coupled with discovery of extensive areas of disarray in the myocardial and arterial walls in hearts from patients aged 6 days to 9 years,[13] point to the disease being more generalised than would be expected from a simple valvar lesion producing direct haemodynamic effects. When the right ventricular wall is hypertrophied, the size of the ventricular cavity is usually relatively reduced, and this can be the consequence of overgrowth and obliteration of the apical trabecular component, again as seen in pulmonary atresia with intact septum (see Chapter 30).

An interatrial communication, be it a probe patent oval foramen or a true septal deficiency, is more frequently seen in patients with pulmonary stenosis, occurring in up to three-quarters of cases. Indeed the presence of a left-to-right shunt at atrial level may serve to accentuate the physical signs of pulmonary stenosis, which could otherwise be mild. This combination of pulmonary stenosis, atrial septal defect, and right ventricular hypertrophy was originally described by French investigators as the trilogy of Fallots,[14] recalling the initial description of Fallot,[15] when he identified such a combination as an alternative cause of *la maladie bleue,* and distinguished it from the tetralogy. Despite this excellent historical pedigree, there now seems little justification for retaining the notion of a trilogy.

In days gone by,[16] it was also the case that cardiac cirrhosis was noted in adults dying with pulmonary stenosis, but such hepatic changes are unlikely to be encountered now. Early fibrotic changes in the livers from two children dying at the age of 6 and 7 years, nonetheless, have been reported.[17]

Infundibular Stenosis

Pure narrowing of the muscular subpulmonary infundibulum is rare in the setting of an intact ventricular septum, or with an apical ventricular septal defect. Of the cases seen at the Hospital for Sick Children, Toronto, over a period of almost 25 years, only 2.7% had this type of stenosis.[17] It is probable that many of the cases described as having isolated infundibular stenosis have previously also had a ventricular septal defect that closed spontaneously.

Combined Valvar and Infundibular Stenosis

Hypertrophy of the subpulmonary infundibulum occurs along with hypertrophy of the rest of the right ventricle in response to valvar stenosis. This reduces the infundibular diameter, and endocardial fibroelastosis may be seen along with the hypertrophy. Fixed stenosis of the infundibulum co-existing with valvar stenosis is exceedingly rare.[17] The reactive stenosis, however, is an important component to be noted when judging the results of balloon valvoplasty, since time is needed for its regression.

Other Types of Stenosis Occurring Within the Right Ventricle

These are very rare when the ventricular septum is intact, but they must be considered as possible causes of pulmonary stenosis. Hypertrophy of the body of the septomarginal trabeculation, which in its severest form produces the typical two-chambered right ventricle, is usually found with a ventricular septal defect.[18] It has been described, nonetheless, with an intact septum.[19] In other patients, the valve of the embryonic venous sinus can persist, and become so expanded and aneurysmal that it can pass through the tricuspid valve and obstruct the pulmonary outflow tract (see Chapter 26). This is described as the spinnaker syndrome.[20] A similar case has been described in which a huge aneurysm of the membranous septum produced subpulmonary stenosis.[21] More rarely, tumours can cause subvalvar right ventricular obstruction,[22] as may aneurysm of the right coronary sinus of the aorta.[23] Hypertrophic cardiomyopathy can also afflict the right ventricle, particularly in the setting of lentiginosis, although left ventricular obstruction usually dominates.

Pulmonary Arterial Stenosis

Stenoses of the pulmonary arterial tree are frequent in association with complex malformations such as tetralogy of Fallot or transposition. They can also complicate more simple lesions such as pulmonary valvar stenosis or ventricular septal defect. Stenoses in the pulmonary arteries can also occur in isolation, and in various parts of the pulmonary arterial tree. Thus, the stenosis may be localised and central, within the pulmonary trunk or its right and left branches, localised and peripheral at the sites of branching of major intrapulmonary arteries, or more extensive, then existing as a hypoplastic arterial segment commencing either at the end of the right or left pulmonary artery or a major intrapulmonary branchpoint. When found peripherally, such stenoses may be unilateral. Reported cases were well summarised by Rowe,[24] who suggested that an anomaly of medial elastic tissue, together with intimal proliferations, could be the cause. It is likely that the process of disease will not be limited to the pulmonary arteries, but will involve also the systemic vessels.[25] In this respect, it is noteworthy that the pulmonary arteries are also involved in the so-called Macaroni syndrome, a condition that primarily narrows the ascending aorta.

Pathogenesis

It is now well recognised that dome-shaped stenosis of the pulmonary valve develops as an acquired condition during intra-uterine life,[26] often progressing to produce pulmonary valvar atresia with an intact ventricular septum (see the extensive discussion of this topic in Chapter 30). The degree of severity seen at birth depends upon the extent of the process during gestation. Peripheral pulmonary arterial stenoses may be caused by congenital rubella,[27] and they are seen in recognisable syndromes of malformation such as Alagille's syndrome[28] and Williams' syndrome.[29–31] Alagille's syndrome, also known as arteriohepatic dysplasia, has been linked to several genetic malformations, such as *Jag1*[32,33] and *NOTCH2*,[34] and often includes severe intrapulmonary arterial stenoses associated with other abnormalities, including problems of the liver, eyes, and spine. Indeed, the hepatic malformation may appear to be more severe than the pulmonary arterial pathology, although experience has shown that aggressive management, such as hepatic transplantation, can be complicated by the pre-existing pulmonary arterial pathology and intracardiac abnormalities.[35] Williams' syndrome, a deficiency of elastin with a gene located on 7q22,[30] is associated with peripheral pulmonary stenosis, supravalvar aortic stenosis, and descending aortic hypoplasia.[29,36]

Pulmonary Arterial Disconnection

An important group of patients have an apparent disconnection of one pulmonary artery from the pulmonary trunk.[37,38] The disconnected pulmonary artery may have originally been connected by the arterial duct to the aorta or the subclavian artery, and is therefore a true embryological failure, with luminal and adventitial discontinuity from the pulmonary trunk, though sometimes a vestigial duct is still demonstrable (Fig. 43-8). Alternatively, the disconnection may have been acquired as a process of coarctation, where ductal tissue has constricted the lumen of the pulmonary artery to the point of obliteration. In this case, of course, there is still adventitial continuity between the pulmonary trunk and the disconnected pulmonary artery. These considerations are important when surgical reconstruction of the connection is considered, as is the size of the disconnected pulmonary artery at the hilum. Demonstrating the size and integrity of the native vessel when no arterial or ductal connection exists can be difficult. Echocardiography, computerised tomography and magnetic resonance scanning may not be helpful. Cardiac catheterisation and wedge intubation of the pulmonary vein on the side of the disconnected artery for a careful retrograde

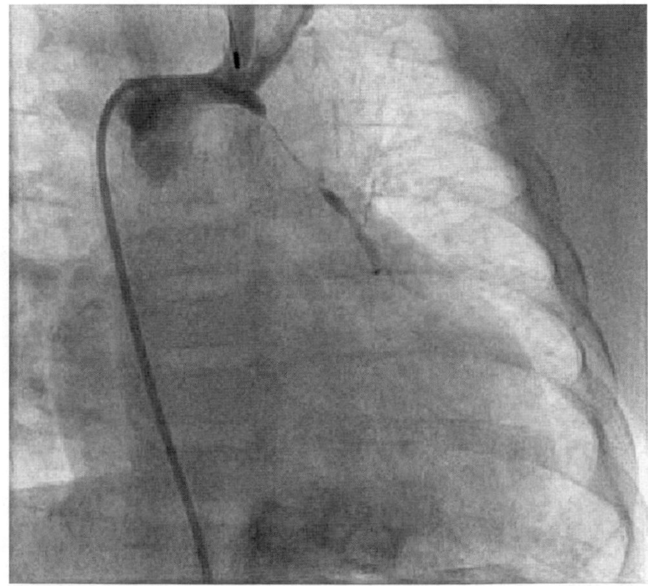

Figure 43-8 In this patient with disconnection of the left pulmonary artery, an injection of contrast into a vestigial ductal remnant in the left subclavian artery reveals a left pulmonary artery at the hilum.

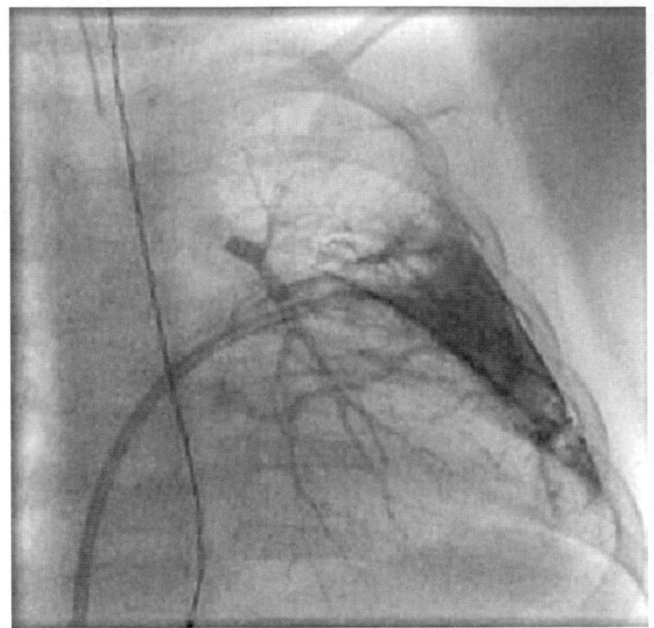

Figure 43-9 In this patient, also with disconnection of the left pulmonary artery, a retrograde pulmonary venous wedge injection demonstrates the native left pulmonary artery.

injection of contrast, may be the only helpful investigation[39] (Fig. 43-9). Where no interatrial communication exists, transarterial retrograde intubation of the pulmonary vein,[40] or needle puncture of the atrial septum permitting a trans-septal approach, will be required.

CLINICAL DIAGNOSIS

Presentation

The presentation of pulmonary stenosis depends on age and severity. In the neonate, critical pulmonary stenosis presents with life-threatening cyanosis, with a right-to-left shunt at atrial level producing cyanosis. The differential diagnosis would include other forms of neonatal cyanosis, including transposition, and the various forms of pulmonary atresia. Such patients are likely to depend on their arterial duct to provide the flow of blood to the lungs. Hence, palliation in the short term, by maintaining ductal patency with intravenous infusions of prostaglandin, is life-saving, until a more definitive diagnosis can be made and an appropriate intervention planned.

Outside of the neonatal period, mild or moderate pulmonary stenosis is not likely to cause major symptoms, unless there are associated lesions or other factors. For example, patients with the typical phenotype of Noonan's syndrome may have difficulty with feeding and gaining weight, separate in most cases to the severity of the pulmonary stenosis. Discovery of disease of mild or moderate severity is most likely when physical signs are detected during consultations for separate matters, when most commonly a cardiac murmur is heard. In patients with more severe pulmonary stenosis, the onset of symptoms can still be delayed into late childhood or early adult life. In a small proportion of patients with pulmonary stenosis, cyanosis can be present, especially on exercise. This is a late physical sign because the cyanotic shunt is at atrial level, depending firstly on an interatrial communication, and secondly on the diastolic properties of the right ventricle. With severe right ventricular hypertrophy and poor right ventricular diastolic compliance, the passage of unoxygenated blood across an interatrial communication into the left atrium is facilitated. Reported symptoms include exercise intolerance, or dyspnoea. Chest pain of an ischaemic nature, possibly due to subendocardial ischaemia of the right ventricle, syncope, and severe dyspnoea on minimal exertion, are late findings and should prompt rapid intervention.

Physical Examination

The physical examination findings are summarised in Table 43-1. There may be a thrill at the second left intercostal space, which is not felt over the carotid arteries, differentiating the cause of the thrill from aortic stenosis. Palpating for a thrill in the suprasternal notch should be avoided, since thrills here can be due to either aortic or pulmonary stenosis.

Widened splitting of the second heart sound, and an ejection systolic murmur, is maximally heard here, with radiation into the back. It is the delayed closure of the valvar leaflets that causes the widened splitting. This is not due to electrical prolongation of systole, but rather to continued flow through the pulmonary valve even after right ventricular pressures have fallen to levels that would usually have resulted in valvar closure. This is likely to be

TABLE 43-1

PHYSICAL SIGNS THAT CAN BE ELICITED IN VALVAR PULMONARY STENOSIS

	SEVERITY OF PULMONARY STENOSIS		
Physical Sign	Mild	Moderate	Severe
Cyanosis	Absent	Absent	Possible, if interatrial septal defect
Jugular venous pulse	Normal	Normal	Possibly elevated, prominent a-wave
Praecordial thrill	Absent	Probable	Pronounced
Right ventricular heave	Absent	Probable	Pronounced
Systolic ejection click	Present	Expiratory	Probably absent
Ejection systolic murmur	Mid systolic, ejection	Long ejection systolic	Long, ejection systolic, past aortic closure sound
Second heart sound	Normal	Wide, variable	Absent pulmonary closure sound

a ventriculo-arterial interaction, favoured by a normal or increased impedance of the pulmonary vascular bed. It can be termed pulmonary hangout.

In most cases of valvar pulmonary stenosis, a systolic ejection click precedes the onset of the systolic murmur. The click is usually heard loudest separate from the area of maximal intensity of the cardiac murmur, nearer the apex, or at the left lower sternal edge. The systolic ejection click originates from the rapid deceleration of the pulmonary valvar mechanism, as the fusion along their zones of apposition prevents the valvar leaflets from reaching their intended positions against the walls of the valvar sinuses. Presence of the click also depends on the timing of opening of the pulmonary valve. In mild disease, without right ventricular hypertrophy, the pulmonary valve opens in ventricular systole with the emission of an ejection click. In severe disease, with right ventricular hypertrophy and impaired diastolic compliance, the valve opens in atrial systole, without the rapid deceleration cause by ventricular systole. Thus, no click is heard. In moderate pulmonary stenosis, inspiration augments systemic venous flow, and atrial filling. The augmented atrial pressure allows atrial systole to open the pulmonary valve. Hence, the systolic ejection click is heard only in expiration. In some patients with pulmonary stenosis and tricuspid regurgitation, the right ventricular pressure is high enough to cause a pansystolic murmur at the left lower sternal edge.

The physical findings in patients with supravalvar stenosis are similar, except for the absence of the ejection click. Stenosis further out into the pulmonary arterial tree can be heard as long systolic or continuous murmurs in the axillas, or over the lung fields at the back. Careful general phenotypic assessment may show the signs or syndromic diagnosis, such as Noonan's syndrome, Alagille's syndrome, or Williams' syndrome.

Basic Investigations

Basic investigations are directed towards assessing the effects and the severity of the pulmonary stenosis (Table 43-2).

The Electrocardiogram

Electrocardiography may be normal, or reveal the degree of right ventricular hypertrophy, or indeed right atrial enlargement, which will be seen only in the more severe cases. There are no features of the electrocardiogram that are unique to the site of pulmonary stenosis, although the severity of stenosis is reflected in the degree of right ventricular hypertrophy and strain. A full right bundle branch block pattern is rare, but an RSR pattern can be seen, and reflects a lesser degree of right ventricular hypertrophy than the equivalent exclusive R wave complex in V_1.[41,42] Rudolf proposed that, in children, the voltage of a pure R-wave recorded at V_1 correlates with approximately one fifth of the right ventricular pressure.[43] It turns out that the QRS axis may be a more reliable indicator of right ventricular pressure.[44] Indeed the prediction of right ventricular pressure gradient is optimised by use of a number of variables in addition to the measurements of voltage on the electrocardiogram, as proposed by Ellison and colleagues,[45] as follows:

$$\Delta P = RV_1 + 1.5 \cdot (SV_6) + 15 \cdot (\text{murmur}[\textit{grade } 0-6]) + \text{Clinical Score} - 30$$

The clinical score included presence of cyanosis, worth + 25; the pulmonary component of the second sound, if diminished worth 15, or 25 if inaudible; a QRS axis of greater than 90 degrees, worth 10; and negative T waves in aVF and V1, worth 35, and with RV1 above 10 mm worth 15.

This complex formula has been superseded by the quicker, more accurate, and more reliable use of Doppler echocardiography.

The Chest X-Ray

The investigation shows the features of right ventricular hypertrophy, and if present, post-stenotic dilation of the pulmonary trunk. Right ventricular hypertrophy is sees as an upturned cardiac apex. The dilated pulmonary trunk is seen as a prominence of the left upper heart border, inferior to the aortic knuckle (Fig. 43-10). Right atrial enlargement causes a more pronounced convexity of the right lower heart border.

Echocardiography

The gold standard investigation for the assessment of the morphology of pulmonary stenosis is cross sectional echocardiography, coupled with Doppler analysis of the flow in the right ventricular outflow tract and pulmonary arteries.

TABLE 43-2

SEVERITY OF PULMONARY STENOSIS

	Mild	Moderate	Severe
Electrical axis	Normal	90–130 degrees	110–150 degrees
R:S ratio	Normal	Up to 4:1 in V_1	Inverted in left leads also
V_1 R amplitude	Normal	10–20 mV	>28 mV
Right atrial enlargement	Normal	Possible	Present

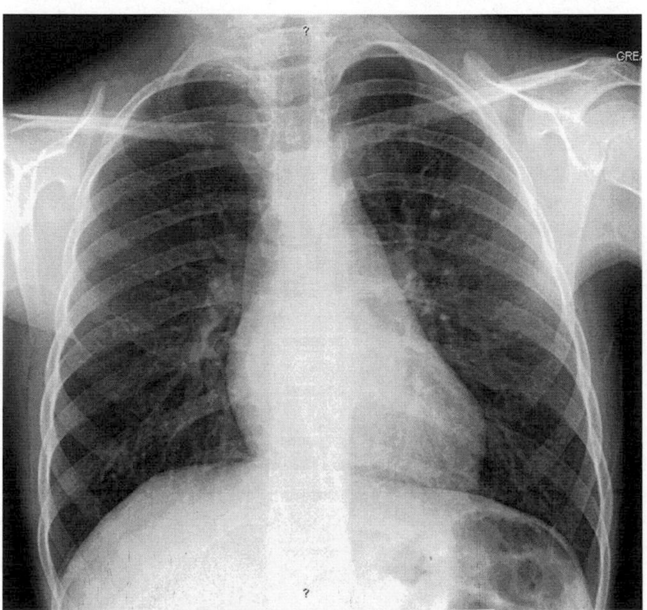

Figure 43-10 The frontal chest X-ray of mild pulmonary stenosis shows a prominent pulmonary trunk, without features of right ventricular hypertrophy.

M-mode echocardiography no longer has a part to play in the diagnostic process, although many echocardiographers will still employ M-mode to analyse timing of pulmonary valvar motion.

Cross sectional echocardiography will define whether the obstruction is at the level of the valvar leaflets (Fig. 43-11), or is subvalvar (Fig. 43-12) or supravalvar (Fig. 43-13). The presence and severity of restricted motion of the leaflets, and dysplasia, can readily be assessed, along with any post-stenotic dilation of the pulmonary trunk (Fig. 43-14). The diameter of the pulmonary valve, at the haemodynamic ventriculo-arterial junction, can be measured accurately (Fig. 43-15), facilitating the planning of intervention.

Distal to the valve, it is possible to identify stenosis within the proximal pulmonary arterial tree, although other forms of imaging are necessary to assess pulmonary arterial pathology distal to the bifurcation. The presence of additional abnormalities, such as atrial septal defects, can be recorded.

Previously, electrocardiography was the mainstay of non-invasive assessment of severity of pulmonary stenosis, although electrocardiographic correlates of right ventricular hypertrophy are relatively weak. Since the advent of Doppler echocardiography, assessment is greatly simplified. Colour flow shows turbulent blood originating at the

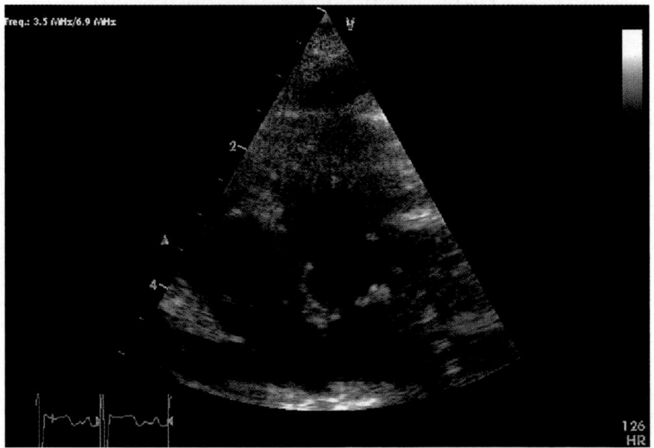

Figure 43-11 Echocardiographic assessment of pulmonary valvar stenosis.

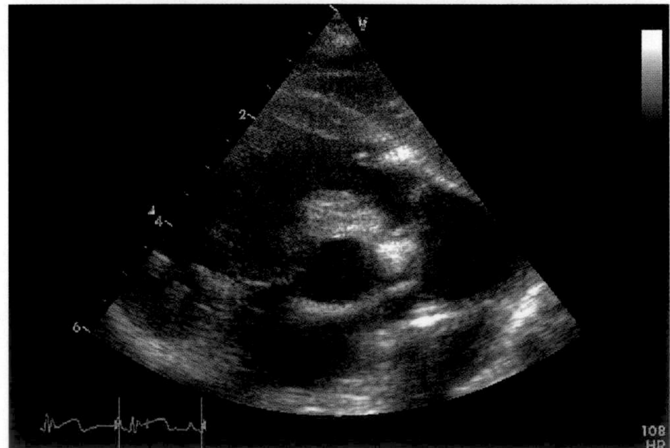

Figure 43-12 The image shows subvalvar pulmonary stenosis.

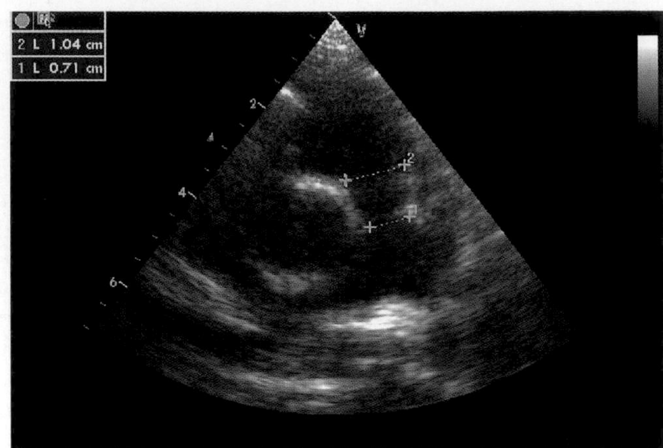

Figure 43-13 In this image, the stenosis is at the supravalvar level.

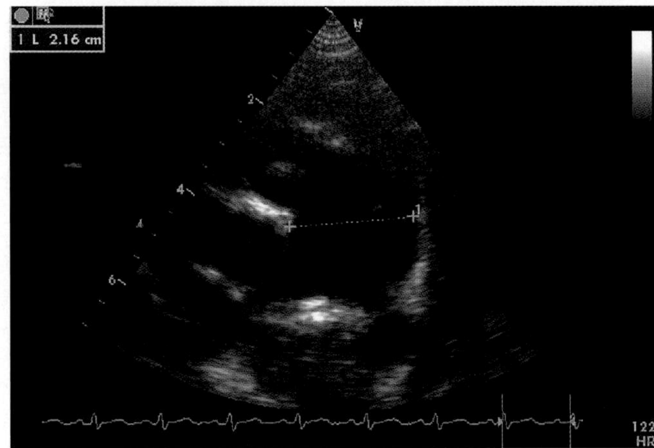

Figure 43-14 The echo shows post-stenotic dilation of the pulmonary trunk.

point of stenosis (Fig. 43-16). Both pulsed and continuous wave interrogations permit measurement of the maximal velocity of the flow across the stenosis (Fig. 43-17). The pressure gradient can be estimated more accurately using the modified and simplified Bernoulli equation, where the valvar pressure gradient, expressed in millimetres of mercury, or ΔP, is calculated from the maximal Doppler velocity at metres per second, or V, across the pulmonary valve:

$$\Delta P = 4 \cdot V^2$$

Similarly, the right ventricular pressure can also be estimated by the velocity of the jet of tricuspid valvar incompetence, where present, added to the estimated right atrial pressure (Fig. 43-18).

Calculations of estimated pressure gradients derived from Doppler measurements of velocity are now an automatic part of all commercially available systems for cardiac ultrasonic investigation.

Magnetic Resonance Imaging and Computerised Tomography

Cross sectional techniques, such as magnetic resonance angiography (Fig. 43-19), or computerised multi-slice spiral tomography, are considered to be less invasive than cardiac catheterisation, but advantages in small children may still be off-set by the need for general anaesthesia in order to allow

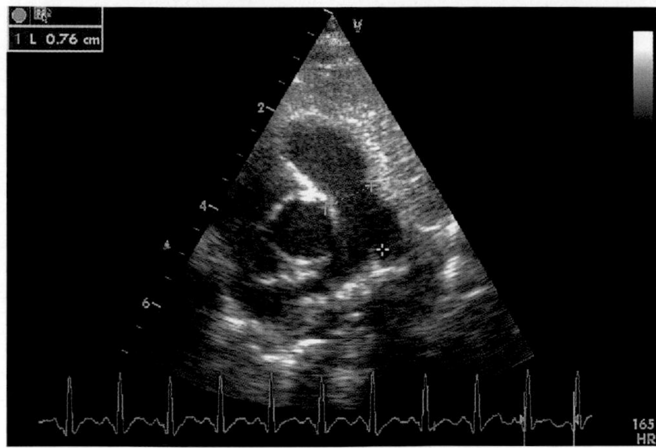

Figure 43-15 The diameter of the pulmonary valve, at the haemodynamic ventriculo-arterial junction, can be measured accurately with echocardiography, to aid planning of intervention.

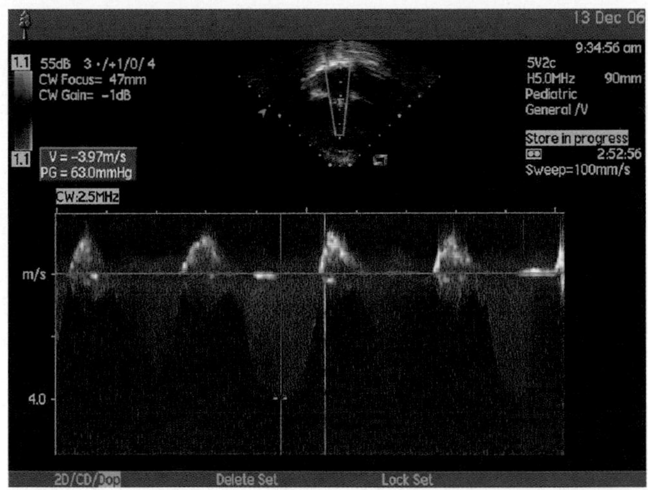

Figure 43-18 Continuous wave Doppler assessment of the jet of tricuspid incompetence, permitting the estimation of right ventricular pressure.

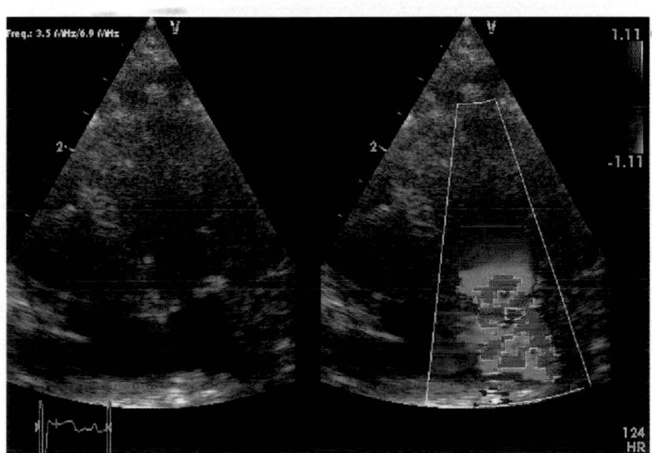

Figure 43-16 Colour flow Doppler shows the development of turbulent blood flow at the stenosed pulmonary valve.

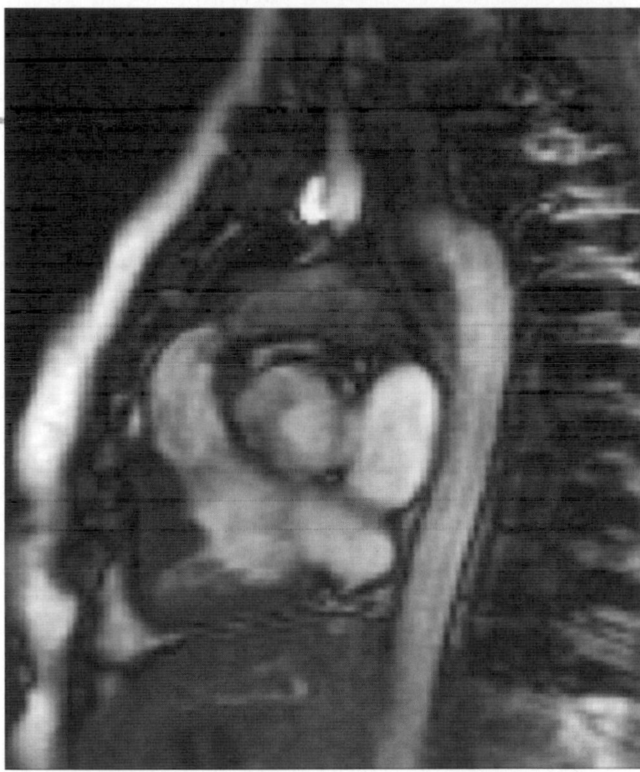

Figure 43-19 Oblique sagittal balanced steady state free precession magnetic resonance images of the right ventricular outflow tract, showing stenosis of the pulmonary trunk. (Courtesy of Andrew Taylor, Consultant Cardiac Radiologist, Great Ormond Street Hospital for Children, London, United Kingdom.)

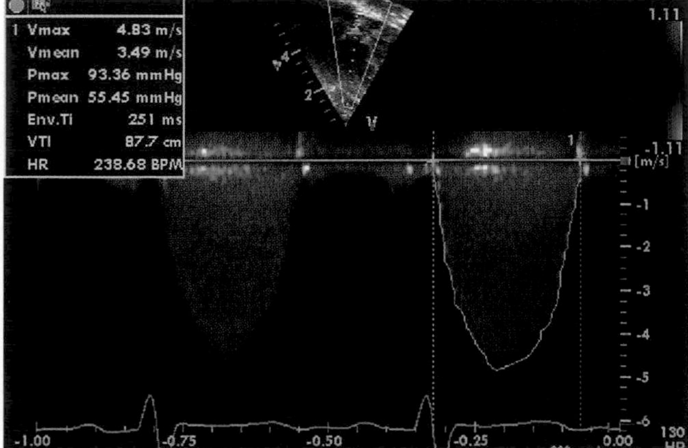

Figure 43-17 Continuous wave spectral Doppler across the pulmonary valve demonstrates a high velocity of flow, and calculated peak instantaneous and mean gradients across the valve.

compliance with respiratory manoeuvres, such as breath-holding. More recent advances in the acquisition of magnetic resonance images, using free breathing techniques, and thus obviating the need for breath-holding, may improve applicability to smaller children without anaesthesia (V. Muthurangu, personal communication, January 1, 2007). The techniques, particularly three-dimensional reconstructions (Fig. 43-20), are helpful when assessing the pulmonary trunk and its branches, particularly in relation to surrounding structures, but with present technology are less helpful for assessment of the pulmonary valve. Future technological

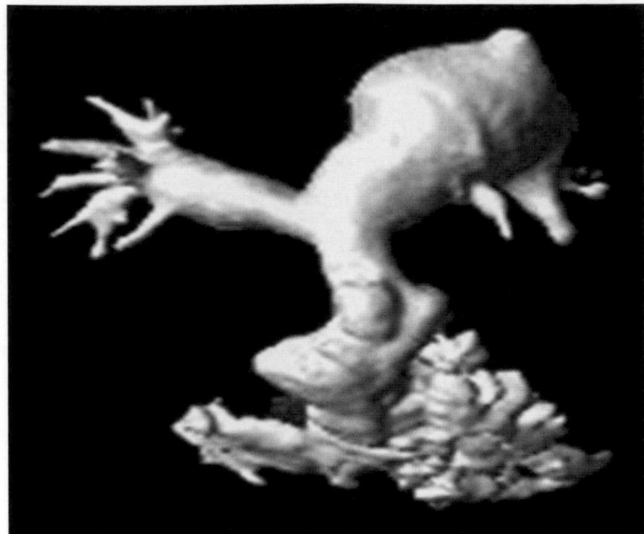

Figure 43-20 Three-dimensional volume rendered reconstructions of the right ventricular outflow tract. Images acquired with contrast-enhanced magnetic resonance angiography. Note the narrowing of the pulmonary trunk, and gross dilation of the left pulmonary artery. (Courtesy of Andrew Taylor, Consultant Cardiac Radiologist, Great Ormond Street Hospital for Children, London, United Kingdom.)

advances in speed of acquisition of images, electrocardiograph gating, and post-processing may bring these techniques into the forefront for investJ16igation of pulmonary stenosis. Presently, it is likely that more information about the morphology of the pulmonary valve, and the immediate supravalvar region, is available with echocardiography.

Cardiac Catherisation and Angiography

Diagnostic cardiac catheterisation has become almost completely superseded by less invasive techniques, such as echocardiography, for the assessment of pulmonary valvar stenosis, and is now undertaken only to perform catheter interventions.

For assessment of more distal stenosis, such as stenoses in the right or left pulmonary arteries or intrapulmonary arterial stenosis, or when access to high quality magnetic resonance or computerised tomographic techniques is not available, cardiac catheterisation and angiography can still play a useful role. Indeed, demonstration of intrapulmonary arterial stenosis, or stenoses at multiple levels, may still best be performed by conventional pulmonary arteriography. Where either the right or left pulmonary artery is thought to be interrupted from the pulmonary trunk, intubation of a pulmonary vein on the same side, and wedge injection of contrast, may be the only way to demonstrate the presence of the proximal pulmonary artery (see Fig. 43-9).

The one advantage of cardiac catheterisation over the other imaging techniques is the accurate measurement of ventricular and pulmonary arterial pressures. Using end-hole or monorail catheters, any gradient across a stenosis can be recorded. The gradient cannot be completely compared to that estimated with echocardiography because of differences in the techniques. Doppler echocardiography estimates peak instantaneous differences in pressure by application of the Bernoulli equation to the measured maximal velocity across the stenosis (see Fig. 43-17). Gradients measure using catheters show a peak-to-peak difference in pressure between the sites of measurement (Fig. 43-21).

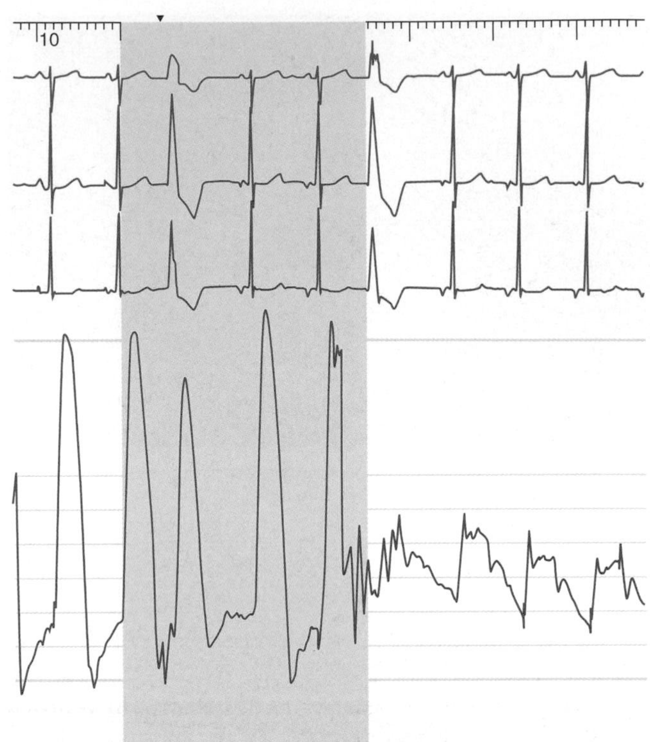

Figure 43-21 Peak-to-peak pullback gradient measured at cardiac catheterisation.

Key Diagnostic Features

The key features are summarised in Box 43-1.

HAEMODYNAMICS AND PHYSIOLOGY

The consequence of obstruction at the right ventricular outflow necessitates an increase in right ventricular pressure in order to force blood through the stenosed valve. The right ventricular pressure developed is usually proportional to the degree of obstruction present. If stenosis develops early in fetal or neonatal life, right ventricular mass increases by ventricular myocytic hyperplasia, as well as hyperplasia of the supporting apparatus, such as

BOX 43-1

Key Diagnostic Features of Pulmonary Valve Stenosis

PHYSICAL EXAMINATION

- Physical signs of right ventricular hypertrophy
- Systolic ejection click, unless severe
- Ejection systolic murmur, second left intercostal space, and back
- Associated thrill in most

INVESTIGATIONS

- Right ventricular hypertrophy on electrocardiogram
- Echocardiographic evidence of turbulence and flow acceleration at pulmonary valve

the capillaries supplying blood to the myocytes, such that the density of capillaries remains normal. In this way, in newborns or neonates, the capacity for the right ventricle to generate high pressures and tolerate moderate stenosis is high. Where pulmonary stenosis develops later in life, after the neonatal period, the capacity for hyperplasia is lost, and the increase in ventricular bulk is due to a hypertrophic response. There is a compensatory increase in capillary supply, but this does not compensate for the increase in ventricular myocardial mass, and there is a reduction in capillary density. Thus, the capacity for the ventricle to sustain high pressures, and tolerate stenosis, is less than in the newborn. In the fetus, severe forms of pulmonary stenosis may result in a circulation that resembles pulmonary atresia, and right ventricular development may be impaired, resulting in the development of a hypertrophic right ventricle with a hypoplastic cavity.

When right ventricular dilation is severe, interventricular interaction may occur, such that the left ventricle is constrained within the pericardium, impairing its ability to fill, and contributing to the compromised circulation. Central cyanosis can occur in neonates when there is a duct-dependent pulmonary circulation, or when right ventricular diastolic dysfunction allows right atrial pressure to exceed left atrial pressure, producing a cyanotic shunt across a defect in the atrial septum.

NATURAL HISTORY

Mild pulmonary valvar stenosis, with a gradient of less than 40 mm Hg, seen after the first 6 months of life is, in general, a benign condition. The severity of the disease may even improve as the child grows,[46-49] certainly with a very low incidence of deterioration to the point of requiring an intervention. In children with moderate, or even severe, pulmonary stenosis, right ventricular function seems to be maintained.[50] When first seen in infancy, however, even mild pulmonary stenosis can deteriorate.[51] Using Doppler echocardiography monitoring, one-quarter of infants with mild pulmonary stenosis in the neonatal period were shown to develop further significant stenosis,[47] and up to half of these patients require intervention.[46] Thus, it is important to monitor infants carefully, especially when the diagnosis is made in the neonatal period, regardless of their severity of pulmonary stenosis. The appearance of the valve, in terms of the thickness and mobility of the leaflets, is only weakly predictive of future deterioration.[47]

In patients with deteriorating pulmonary stenosis and intact ventricular septum, over time, right ventricular pressure may exceed left ventricular pressure. The ventricular pressure waveform changes, from a broad based triangular shape with early peak maximal pressure (Fig. 43-22), to a tall peaked waveform with the point of maximal pressure delayed to close to the end of systole (Fig. 43-23). Compensation for fixed severe stenosis with right ventricular hypertrophy can fail as the patient grows and further demands are made on the ventricle. At this stage, the right ventricle may decompensate by dilating and the onset of heart failure occurs. Further compensatory mechanisms for low cardiac output include increased extraction of oxygen. During exercise, even this compensatory mechanism is insufficient, and exercise intolerance is noted, often with the presence of peripheral cyanosis.

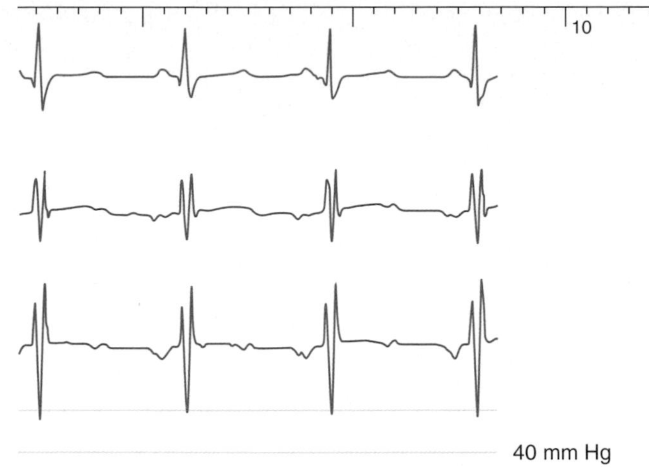

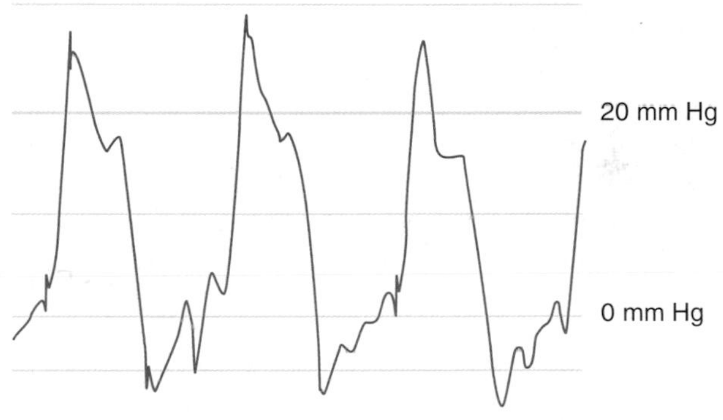

Figure 43-22 Normal low-pressure right ventricular waveform showing a broad-based triangular-shaped waveform with an early point of maximal pressure.

THERAPEUTIC OPTIONS

Historical Perspective

Though pulmonary stenosis has been recognised as a pathological entity since 1761, management of this disease has only been possible in the past 60 years or so. The first reported attempt, unsuccessful, was published in 1913.[52] The first successful pulmonary valvotomy was performed in London, by Holmes Sellors,[53] in December of 1947. The patient had tetralogy of Fallot, and although the intention had been to perform a Blalock-Taussig shunt, a stenosed pulmonary valve was palpable. A trans-infundibular approach was made to incise the stenosed pulmonary valve in two directions, resulting in immediate relief of cyanosis. Perversely, this operation was reported two weeks after the report by Brock of his own three successful operations, performed later in 1948.[54] Brock continued along the theme of direct relief of pulmonary stenosis and tetralogy of Fallot, and designed a complimentary series of instruments, comprising a valvulotome to cut the stenosed valve, an expanding dilator to split the valve, and an infundibular punch to resect the thickened infundibular muscle (Figs. 43-24 and 43-25). He reported

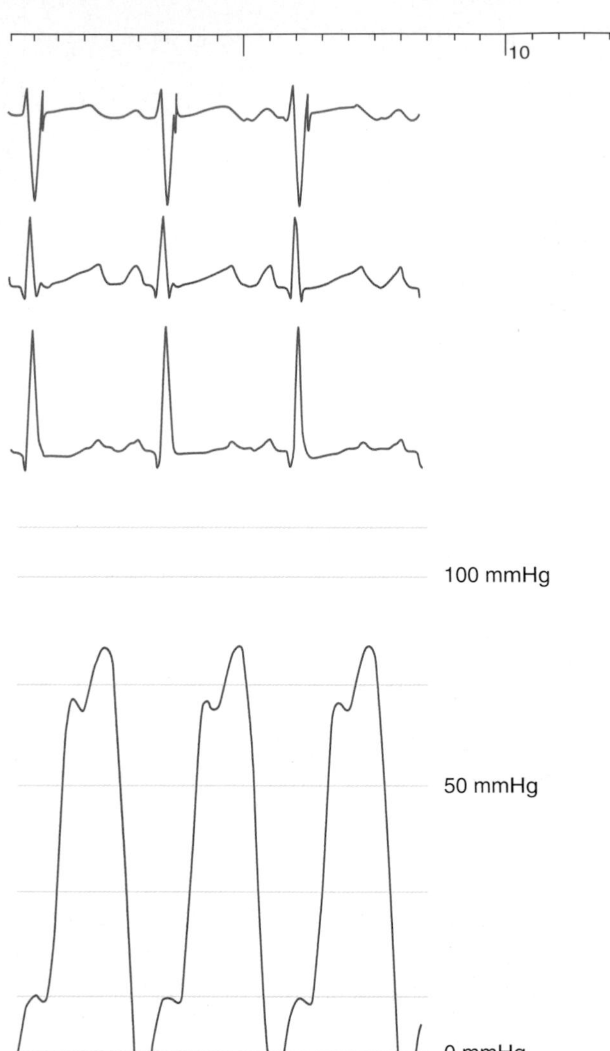

Figure 43-23 The waveform in severe pulmonary stenosis shows a taller, squarer waveform with a delayed point of maximal pressure close to the end of systole.

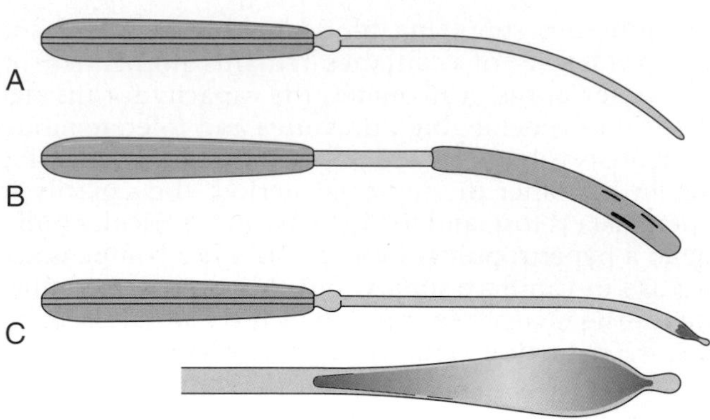

Figure 43-24 Line diagrams of the instruments invented for the first series of closed pulmonary valvotomies. **A,** Curved probe. **B,** Curved bougie. **C,** Valvulotome. (Reproduced with permission from Brock RC: Pulmonary valvulotomy for relief of congenital pulmonary stenosis: Report of three cases. BMJ 1948;1:1121–1126.)

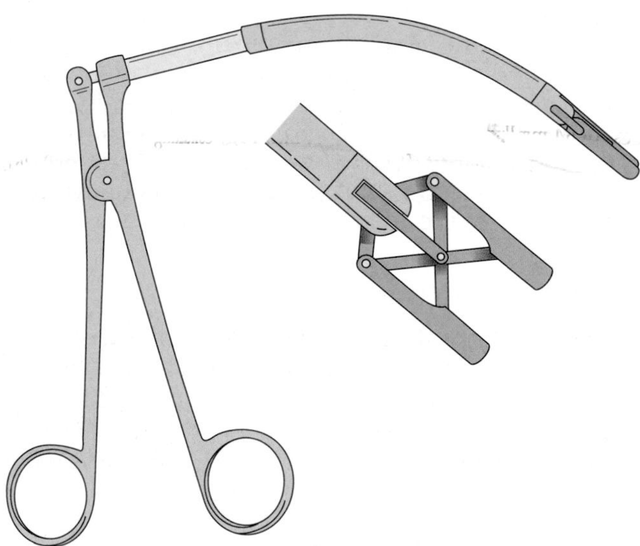

Figure 43-25 Line diagrams of the instruments invented for the first series of closed pulmonary valvotomies. The dilating instrument. (Reproduced with permission from Brock RC: Pulmonary valvulotomy for relief of congenital pulmonary stenosis: Report of three cases. BMJ 1948;1:1121–1126.)

the successful use of these instruments in 1950,[55] and described a miraculous transformation in his subjects. The Brock procedure for tetralogy of Fallot was immediately adopted for patients with pulmonary stenosis and an intact interventricular septum. The introduction of inflow occlusion,[56,57] inflow occlusion and hypothermia,[58] and subsequently extracorporeal circulation[59] in the mid 1950s, changed the surgical approach to a more precise operation involving splitting of the fused zones of apposition of the leaflets or valvectomy.

Interventional Catheterisation

The swing to an interventional approach to the treatment of pulmonary valvar stenosis resulted from a partnership between cardiologists and radiologists. The first reported catheter intervention for pulmonary valvar stenosis was performed in 1953.[60] A ureteric catheter modified with a wire was introduced through the pulmonary valve, the wire being tensioned to form a bow-shaped device which was used to incise the stenosed valve.[60] Later, the same technique was used for the stenosed tricuspid valve.[61] The use of a standard angiographic balloon to disrupt the pulmonary valve was described in 1979.[62] The technique involved a rapid pullback, in septostomy fashion, of the balloon catheter from the pulmonary trunk to the right ventricular outflow tract. Meanwhile, graded dilation was being developed for atherosclerotic vessels,[63] including important technical developments in guide-wires and catheters.[64,65] Further refinements allowed the techniques to be applied to smaller vessels, including the coronary arteries,[66–69] using a double lumen balloon catheter designed to be used over a guide-wire. It is not commonly known that the first successful static balloon dilation of the pulmonary valve, as we now know the technique, was performed in an English bulldog in 1980,[70] prior to the first report of the successful procedure in 1982 in a child.[71] Since it was first performed, the technique has rapidly become the treatment of choice for pulmonary valvar stenosis. Apart from improvements in the design of balloon angioplasty catheters and guide-wires, to improve the profile and tracking ability of the products, only one other interventional technique was reported to treat pulmonary stenosis. This involved an endovascular device with an extendable double blade, designed to be extended in the pulmonary trunk, and drawn back through the pulmonary valve to disrupt the stenosed leaflets.[72] After the first report of three children treated in Shanghai, no further report has been published in the literature.

Contemporary Approaches

Indications for intervention in children are widely discussed in the literature, with equally wide variability in the criterions for selection. The indications for catheter intervention should be similar to the indications for a surgical approach, although because of the less invasive, expensive, and time-consuming advantages of catheter intervention, this technique remains the first choice in all centres. Most groups will intervene if the echocardiographically derived peak instantaneous gradient across the pulmonary valve is in excess of 64 mm Hg, correlating to a Doppler velocity of more than 4 msec^{-1}. Some groups recommend a threshold of a peak instantaneous pressure gradient of greater than 50 mm Hg[73] when cardiac output is normal. In patients in acute or chronic heart failure, the capacity of the ventricle to generate higher pressures is impaired, cardiac output reduced and a lower threshold for intervention must be applied. Whilst attention has been paid to intervention in more mild cases, the evidence for progression of mild stenosis is lacking,[48] and follow-up can easily determine the cases that do progress, with the option to plan an intervention still available even up until adult life.[74-78] In adults with moderate to severe stenosis, persistent exercise intolerance, pressure overload, and the risk of right ventricular fibrosis provide good indications for intervention,[73] despite the usual lack of symptoms.

Infants presenting in the neonatal period with moderate or severe stenosis, especially those presenting with a duct-dependent pulmonary circulation, should be treated urgently.[79-82]

Technique

Full physical and echocardiographic assessment should precede any intervention. Informed consent is necessary, especially since the long-term effects of intervention are not completely known. The dimension of the ventriculo-arterial junction should carefully be assessed. If resuscitation is necessary, especially in infants who may need prostaglandin to stabilise the patent arterial duct, this should precede the intervention.

Cardiac catheterisation should be performed under general anaesthesia, or local anaesthesia with intravenous sedation. Facilities for management of the airway must be nearby if a full general anaesthetic is not employed. Preparation for the catheter must proceed in standard fashion, with attention as usual to sterility of the operative fields, the equipment trolley, and the operators. In addition, we recommend antibiotic prophylactic measures.

Access to the circulation is most commonly through a femoral venous puncture. In patients with problems of vascular access due to venous thrombosis, other techniques can be employed, including the jugular,[83] axillary[84] or hepatic[85] veins. A curved end-hole catheter, either a right coronary catheter or one that is Cobra shaped, or a balloon tipped angiographic catheter such as the Berman, is manipulated into the right ventricle. It is important to cross the tricuspid valve in a fashion to intubate the major aperture of the valve, rather than allowing the catheter to pass between tendinous cords, since the latter can cause avulsion of the tricuspid valve when the denatured balloon catheter is withdrawn after the dilation procedure.[86] With end-hole catheters, this can best be accomplished by catching the tip of the catheter in the hepatic vein or right atrial wall to create a curve in the tip of the catheter. The tricuspid valve can be crossed with the curved tip by rotating leftwards and anteriorly from a position in the right atrium.

Right ventricular pressure can be measured and compared to left ventricular pressure. A right ventricular angiogram can most easily be performed in the neonate by a gentle injection by hand of contrast into the ventricular outflow tract below the stenosed pulmonary valve, or in older children by using a right ventricular power injection (Fig. 43-26). Care must be taken not to infiltrate contrast into the myocardium of the right ventricular outflow tract. Such an event can be poorly tolerated. The lateral projection of the right ventricular angiogram is useful to confirm the echocardiographic measurements of the ventriculo-arterial junction, and the orientation of the domed orifice of the stenosed valve. This allows the catheter to be manipulated into the pulmonary trunk with the aid of a guide-wire, into the left or right lower pulmonary artery, or even in neonates into the descending aorta through the arterial duct.[87] The choice of guide-wire is dependent on the

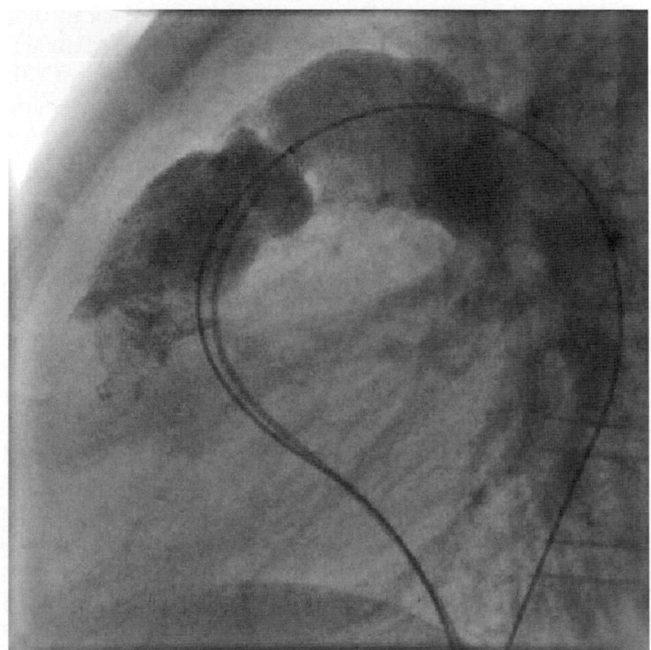

Figure 43-26 Right ventricular outflow tract angiogram, demonstrating the domed and stenosed pulmonary valve, and allowing measurement of the ventriculo-arterial junction.

operator, and on the age of the patient. In older patients, if stable during the procedure, our group would use a hydrophilic wire to gain a distal position in the pulmonary artery, exchanging it for a stiff exchange wire, over which a monorail multi-track catheter can be advanced and withdrawn for an accurate measurement of pressure gradient without losing position. In newborns, or if there is instability during the procedure, measurement of the pressure gradient can be abandoned in favour of a more rapid procedure. In neonates, a coronary angioplasty wire can be passed through the valve and used to deliver the angioplasty catheter.

The choice of dimension of the balloon has been the source of much discussion. It is clear that the balloon must be oversized in relation to the dimension of the pulmonary valve, but there is evidence that sizes in excess of 120% to 125% of the pulmonary valve are no more efficacious at reducing the severity of pulmonary stenosis, yet create more problems in terms of subsequent pulmonary incompetence or other complications.[88,89] An exception could be argued in cases where the valve is markedly dysplastic and stenosed. There is no evidence to select the length of the balloon to choose. Shorter balloons may be more difficult to stabilise centrally over the pulmonary valve. Longer balloons carry more risk of damage to the tricuspid valve,[86] atrioventricular node,[90] or distal pulmonary arteries. Simple and intuitive choices are a balloon of 20 mm for neonates and infants, one of 30 mm for children, and one of 40 mm for adolescents and adults.[73]

In most cases, therefore, a non-compliant coaxial construction angioplasty balloon of the appropriate size is selected and tracked over the guide-wire to the pulmonary valve. If the balloon fails to track through the right ventricle, then there is a good chance that the catheter has passed behind some tension apparatus of the tricuspid valve. It is better to withdraw the catheter and guide-wire, and recross the tricuspid valve so as to obtain a better position. To force the angioplasty balloon onwards is disadvantageous, because the balloon would be drawn in a denatured form back through the tricuspid valve, with the potential for serious damage.[86] When it is difficult to cross the pulmonary valve with the chosen dimension of balloon, it is often better to exchange the balloon angioplasty catheter for a smaller one, even as small as a 3-mm coronary angioplasty balloon, in order to pre-dilate the valve before returning with the original.[91]

The angioplasty balloon should be de-aired carefully and connected to a syringe containing a weak solution of about 20% to 25% contrast medium in saline. The balloon is inflated by hand or with an inflation device. An inflation device is usually recommended by the manufacturers of the balloon angioplasty catheter, yet in most cases, inflation at high pressure is not necessary, and hand inflation is sufficient. Whilst watching the hourglass impression of the pulmonary valve on the balloon during inflation (Fig. 43-27), the balloon might prolapse forwards or backwards, and manipulation of the balloon and the guide-wire can be required. Our group has not found it necessary to use high-frequency ventricular pacing or intravenous adenosine, and with attention to applying or relieving tension on the guide-wire, a stable position is usually maintained during inflation. The balloon is inflated until its walls are seen on fluoroscopy to be parallel. Application of higher pressure does not serve any useful purpose beyond the point at which parallel walls of the balloon have been reached, and carries a greater risk of rupture. If there is still a residual hourglass impression on the balloon during inflation, then the ventriculo-arterial junction itself may be hypoplastic and the procedure will have limited benefit.

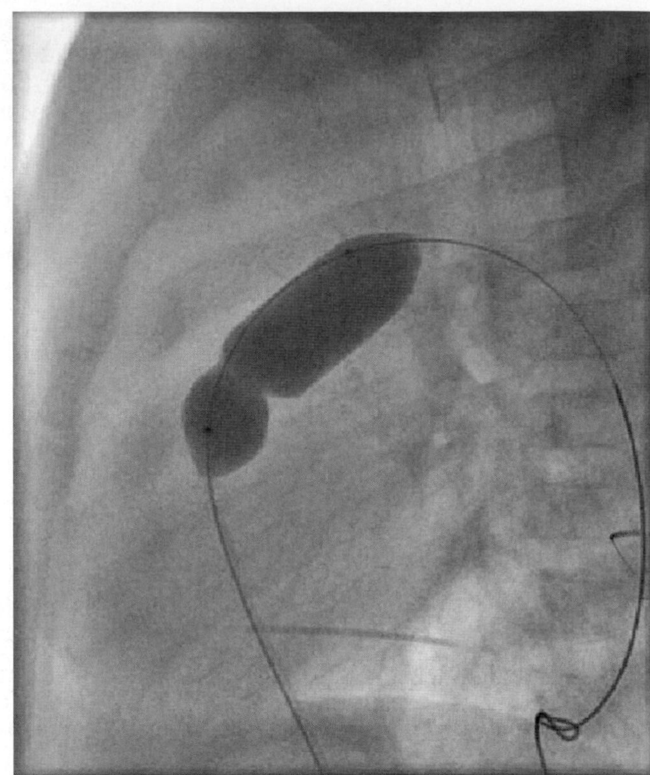

Figure 43-27 Lateral projection showing an angioplasty balloon partially inflated across the pulmonary valve, with the characteristic hourglass impression imposed on the balloon by the stenosed pulmonary valve leaflets.

Following the first inflation, most operators inflate one or more times, and study the way that the balloon inflates and deflates to determine whether an hourglass impression is still caused by the pulmonary valve. After inflation and withdrawal, the pressure in the right ventricle and the gradient across the pulmonary valve can be recorded. The position of the wire can be preserved using a monorail catheter or an end-hole catheter and a TuohyBorst adaptor. Careful pullback will show whether any residual gradient is confined to the pulmonary valve, or indeed present in the subvalvar right ventricular outflow tract. If there is significant valvar gradient, the decision to reattempt dilation with a larger balloon can be made. The presence of a significant subvalvar gradient is a well-described phenomenon after dilation of the pulmonary valve, and can have serious consequences with a low cardiac output state. This is the so-called suicide right ventricle. Careful attention to anaesthesia, the preoperative state of hydration, and use of β-blockade will usually be sufficient to deal with the acute right ventricular outflow tract reactivity.[92] Residual right ventricular subvalvar narrowing will usually settle over time.

If the procedure is successful in terms of right ventricular pressure and trans-valvar gradient, then our group will terminate the procedure without performing a follow-up right ventricular angiogram. The investigations prior to discharge are completed with echocardiography to assess the result

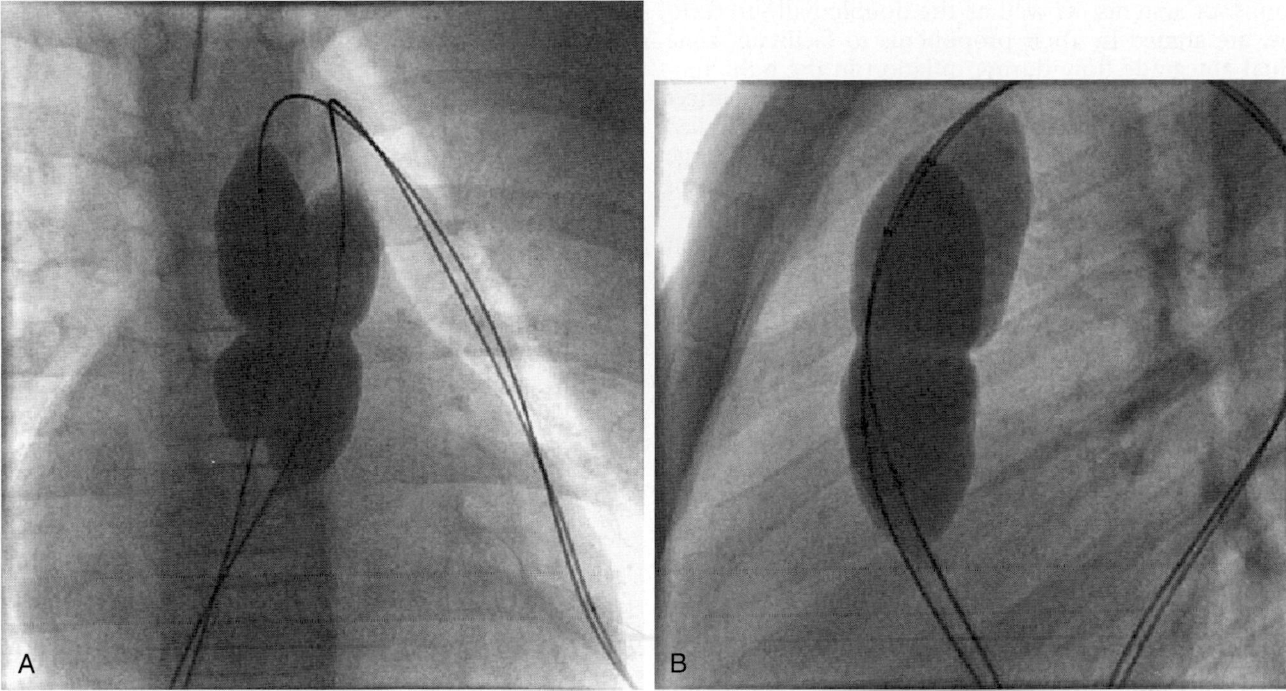

Figure 43-28 The double balloon technique for pulmonary balloon dilation, shown (A) in frontal projection, and (B) in lateral projection.

of balloon dilation, the degree of pulmonary incompetence, and the integrity of the tricuspid valve. Outside of the neonatal period, it is usually possible to perform these procedures as day cases.

Severe or Critical Neonatal Pulmonary Stenosis

The presentation and management of pulmonary stenosis in the neonatal period deserve special discussion. Infants may present in a critically ill state, with cyanosis as result of right-to-left shunting across the atrial septum, being dependent on patency of the arterial duct for survival. The efficacy of balloon dilation of the pulmonary valve depends not just on the result of the valvotomy, but also on the size and compliance of the right ventricle, tricuspid valve, and the ventriculo-arterial junction.[93] Thus the size of the structures in the right heart needs to be evaluated as part of the management. Relative hypoplasia is not a contraindication for balloon dilation of the pulmonary valve, and indeed follow-up studies have shown that the rate of growth of the right heart can exceed the rate of somatic growth after successful balloon dilation.[93–95] Immediately following balloon dilation, despite adequate opening of the pulmonary valve, it may still be difficult to separate infants from infusions of prostaglandin. This is most likely as a result of hypertrophy and diastolic dysfunction of the right ventricle, favouring a cyanotic shunt across the atrial septum. Persistent hypoxaemia may settle over a few days as the right ventricle recovers. Should hypoxaemia persist, it may be necessary to establish an alternative source of supply of blood to the lungs, such as a systemic-to-pulmonary arterial shunt, or stenting of the arterial duct. A detailed analysis of the morphology of the right heart structures may help predict whether an alternative source of such flow is going to be required. A diameter of the tricuspid valvar orifice of greater than 11 mm, right ventricular volumes of greater than 30 mL/m^2, and dimension of the pulmonary valve of greater than 7 mm, appear to stratify patients who are less likely to require an intervention to increase pulmonary flow.[96]

Multiple Balloon Techniques

Using the recommended sizing of balloons of 120% to 125% of the dimension of the pulmonary valve, it is clear that large balloons will be required for adolescents and adults. Such balloons may be difficult to source, and the frequency of use might make it impracticable to keep these items in stock in the paediatric catheter laboratory. Techniques using an additional balloon angioplasty catheter through an additional venous puncture, and over an additional guide-wire, have been reported (Fig. 43-28).[74,97–99] The effective dimension of the double balloon technique is calculated thus[100]:

$$\text{Total Diameter (mm)} = \frac{D1 + D2 + \pi\left(\frac{D1}{2} + \frac{D2}{2}\right)}{\pi}$$

The use of the multi-track double balloon mitral commissurotomy system, using two complementary angioplasty catheters designed to track along the same guide-wire, has been reported in adults with pulmonary stenosis.[101] Whilst this technique offers an easier approach, and one less venous puncture, than the conventional double balloon technique, again the technique only offers an advantage if a single balloon of appropriate dimension is not available. Similarly, angioplasty catheters with multiple balloons, bifoil and trefoil, mounted in parallel on one shaft, have been described,[102] as well as a technique using three separate angioplasty balloons, with a complicated formula described for their overall dimensions.[103] Such balloons, or systems, as well as the double balloon technique, are argued by their proponents to facilitate some residual antegrade flow during inflation in the right ventricular outflow tract. This seems unlikely when the correct oversized dimension is chosen. In addition, they are bulky, and have largely been superseded by more modern large single balloons with lower profiles which can be introduced through smaller sheaths.

Whilst the results all of these techniques have been highly effective, and well sustained, it has since been shown that, where a single balloon is available for the appropriate dimension, no advantage is conferred using multiple balloons.[104] It is important, nonetheless, that all operators have an understanding of these techniques, as well as knowledge of the equipment that is available in their own local laboratory, because the final decision may be made on supply and demand of equipment.

Complications

Acute complications of balloon dilation of the pulmonary valve are summarised in Box 43-2. Balloon dilation has proved to be very successful, and has yielded minimal immediate complications. Out of 822 procedures entered into the VACA Registry, including cases of critical pulmonary stenosis, the death rate was reported as 0.24%, and the major complication rate was only 0.35%.[105] In a smaller multi-centric series of 172 patients, excluding critical pulmonary stenosis, there was no mortality, with emergency surgery required in only one patient (0.58%), who suffered perforation of the right ventricular outflow tract.[106]

During inflation of the balloon, transient bradycardia and hypotension may be observed. This effect recovers quickly after deflation of the balloon. A patent oval foramen, or an atrial septal defect, helps to preserve systemic ventricular output during occlusion of the pulmonary arteries. So as to minimise these effects, inflation of the balloon should not be maintained for more than a second or two.

With modern design of sheaths and catheters, and improved techniques, loss of blood is minimal. Manipulation of the catheter or wire in the right heart can provoke arrhythmia, right bundle branch block, and even transient or permanent complete heart block. Other complications include stroke or seizures due to embolic complications in the context of a potential right-to-left atrial shunt.

Rupture of the balloon at high pressures of inflation, pulmonary arterial tears, perforation of the right ventricular outflow tract,[106] and rupture of tricuspid valvar papillary muscles have all been reported.[86] Failure of technical equipment, such as failure of the balloon to deflate, or rupture and embolisation of fragments, require an innovative use of troubleshooting techniques.[107–109]

Late Complications

Patients after dilation of the pulmonary valve are generally well, and enjoying a good quality of life. Femoral venous occlusion related to the intervention is well described, and may be demonstrated in over one-fifth of patients requiring further venous access.[110] Recurrence of pulmonary stenosis is reported in up to one-tenth.[111] Perhaps more topical is the early and progressive development of pulmonary incompetence in the early cohort of treated patients. The ratio of the balloon to the pulmonary valve has been discussed already, and moving away from the use of oversized balloons may reduce this trend. Indeed, late pulmonary incompetence is usually very well tolerated.[112] Nevertheless, consideration of replacement of the valve may be necessary when right ventricular dilation, right ventricular dysfunction, or symptoms develop late after dilation. Aside from these long-term complications, and allowing for anecdotal case reports, such as spontaneous pulmonary arterial dissection late after dilation,[113] the long-term follow-up is remarkably good.

BOX 43-2

Complications of Balloon Pulmonary Dilation

ACCESS
- Haemorrhage from access points

CATHETER/WIRE MANIPULATION
- Arrhythmia and hypotension
- Atrioventricular conduction block
- Embolic complications

BALLOON INFLATION
- Pulmonary arterial tear
- Tricuspid valvar papillary muscle rupture
- Cardiac perforation and tamponade

AFTER INFLATION
- Severe reactive infundibular stenosis

LATE COMPLICATIONS
- Femoral venous stenosis or occlusion
- Recurrence of pulmonary stenosis
- Pulmonary incompetence

OUTCOMES OF INTERVENTION

Surgical Valvotomy

The first description of surgical valvotomy included 33 patients in whom 18 had pure pulmonary valvar stenosis. Of those 18 patients who underwent the landmark Brock procedure,[54] 7 patients died, although many of these patients were adult, and were severely ill at the time of the procedure. In addition, an effect of the era was identified, with the mortality improving for the whole series from 50% to 18% after the first 11 patients. The survivors were followed up, and the outcome in the medium term was good. The authors recommended that the technique was best applied to patients less than 10 years of age.

The Second Natural History Study[114] identified a cohort of 592 patients with pulmonary stenosis. Of the patients who had had valvotomy, only 4% required a second operation. Patients enjoyed a quality of life similar to that of the normal population. Similar results were found in survivors followed up to 17 years after the procedure.[115] The long-term follow-up of a group of 191 consecutive patients who underwent surgery for isolated pulmonary valve stenosis at the Mayo Clinic has been excellent. The survival curve is shown in Figure 43-29. The long-term survival of patients surviving operation before 21 years of age is similar to that of an age- and sex-matched control population.[116] In the patients who had operations at a later age, there was some late attrition, possibly due to the sequels of long-standing right ventricular hypertrophy.

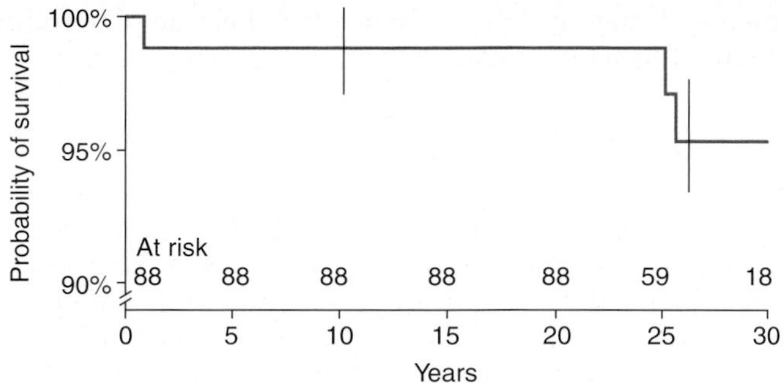

Figure 43-29 Post-discharge survival after surgery for pulmonary stenosis. Kaplan-Mayer survival curve of the 88 patients who were discharged after surgery between 1968 and 1980. (Reproduced with permission from Roos-Hesselink JW, Meijboom FJ, Spitaels SEC, et al: Long-term outcome after surgery for pulmonary stenosis [a longitudinal study of 22–33 years]. Eur Heart J 2006;27:482–488.)

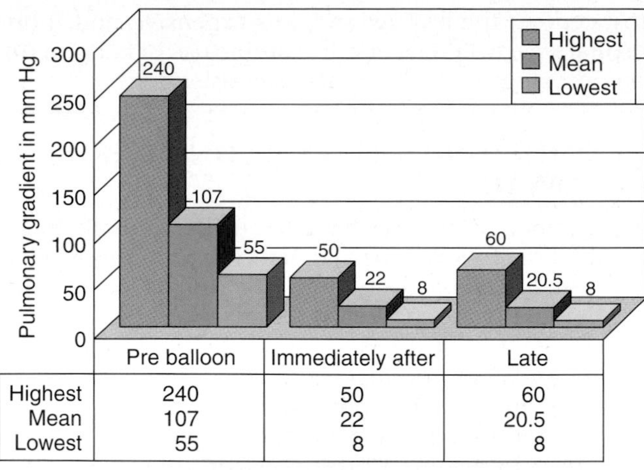

	Pre balloon	Immediately after	Late
Highest	240	50	60
Mean	107	22	20.5
Lowest	55	8	8

Figure 43-31 Pulmonary valvar gradients before, immediately after, and late after balloon pulmonary valvoplasty. (Reproduced with permission from Sadr-Ameli MA, Sheikholeslami F, Firoozi I, Azarnik H: Late results of balloon pulmonary valvuloplasty in adults. Am J Cardiol 1998;82:398–400.)

The longest study reported describes up to 33 years follow up after surgical valvotomy.[117] Survival at 25 years was 93%. Quality of life was good with 67% of patients falling into the first class of the categorisation of the New York Heart Association, and a measured exercise capacity of 90% predicted. One-sixth required surgical reintervention, but this particular cohort reflects the developing understanding of the effects of pulmonary incompetence and the need for intervention, a point that had not been appreciated in previous reports. A risk factor for reintervention included the use of a transvalvar patch.

Balloon Dilation

Long-term results of balloon dilation during childhood are excellent.[112] Figure 43-30 shows the freedom from reintervention in a large series of patients who were discharged after surgery for pulmonary stenosis between 1968 and 1980. Although late pulmonary incompetence commonly occurs, it appears well tolerated in the first decade after intervention. For those children with severe pulmonary incompetence, longer follow-up is necessary to determine if they develop or can be predicted to develop right ventricular decompensation and require replacement of the valve. Life-long follow-up is essential in children who have balloon dilation where pulmonary incompetence is present.

In adults, balloon dilation is similarly feasible.[75,97,118] Long-term follow up has again been excellent, with minimal recurrence of pulmonary stenosis.[77,119] Observed infundibular hypertrophy and tricuspid incompetence resolves over time.[76,120] In a large study of 127 adults who underwent balloon dilation, immediate relief of pulmonary stenosis was achieved, with further reduction in the measured gradient from 6 to 8 years later (Fig. 43-31).[77]

Surgery as Opposed to Balloon Dilation

In a large series of 170 patients in a single Dutch centre, direct comparison between surgical valvotomy and balloon dilation was possible.[121] Surgical relief of pulmonary stenosis yielded lower long-term gradients and a longer freedom from reintervention (Fig. 43-32). Nevertheless, in

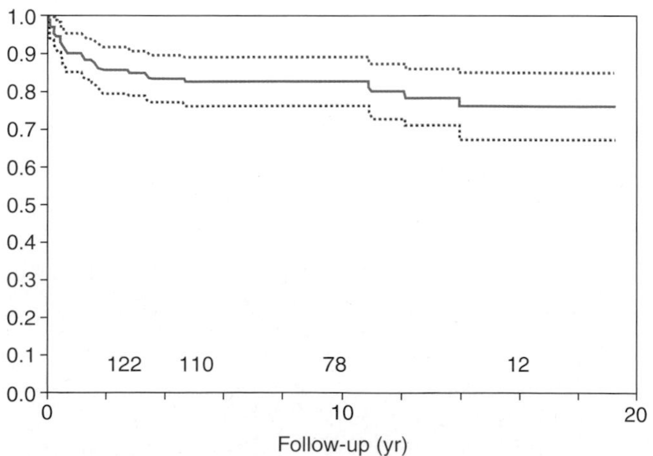

Figure 43-30 Freedom from reintervention after balloon dilation of the stenosed pulmonary valve. Ninety-five percent confidence intervals are indicated by the dotted lines. Numbers above the x-axis indicate children at risk. (Reproduced with permission from Garty Y, Veldtman G, Lee K, Benson L: Late outcomes after pulmonary valve balloon dilatation in neonates, infants and children. J Invasive Cardiol 2005;17:318–322.)

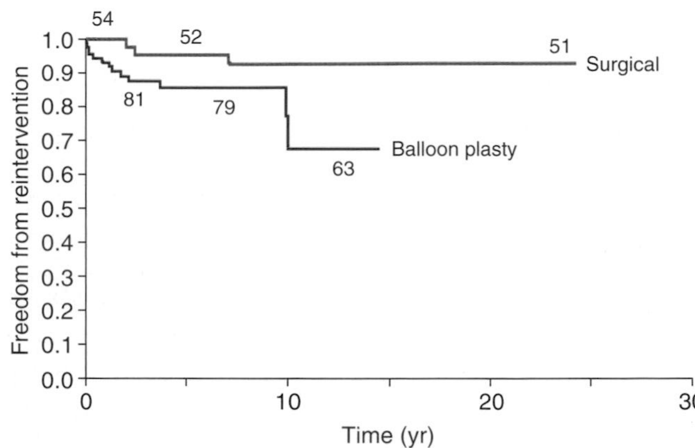

Figure 43-32 Kaplan-Meier curves illustrating freedom from reintervention in isolated pulmonary valve stenosis managed by surgery in 54 patients or balloon dilation in 92 patients. (Reproduced with permission from Peterson C, Schilthuis JJ, Dodge-Khatami A, et al: Comparative long-term results of surgery versus balloon valvuloplasty for pulmonary valve stenosis in infants and children. Ann Thorac Surg 2003;76:1078–1082.)

most centres, the less invasive, less expensive, and shorter hospital stay, would favour the routine use of balloon dilation over surgery for pulmonary stenosis.

RECOMMENDATIONS FOR LONG-TERM FOLLOW-UP

Once pulmonary stenosis has been treated, usually by balloon dilation, follow-up is mandatory. Many units will have their own protocols for follow up, laid down by senior members of the department. Without guidelines for follow-up however, it is likely that patients will be seen too often, and an unnecessary burden made on bookings. Algorithms for follow-up of many congenital cardiac malformations have been published,[122] and are still relevant to current practice, subject to the up-to-date knowledge of the conditions described. In the case of pulmonary stenosis, the natural and unnatural history has been analysed in detail, and stratification of pathways for follow-up can be made based on physiological and anatomical considerations. For instance, Figure 43-33 presents an algorithm for follow-up of patients after treatment of pulmonary stenosis. This particular algorithm must be considered also with the emerging understanding that reintervention is prompted by the effects of pulmonary incompetence, and investigations to assess this must also be performed. In our own unit we would perform serial interval cardiac magnetic resonance imaging and cardiopulmonary exercise testing, to assess the effects of pulmonary incompetence on the anatomy, physiology and functional state of the patient, and help to determine whether further interventions will be necessary.

Prophylaxis Against Endocarditis

Recent changes in the guidelines for the use of antibiotics to prevent infective endocarditis have been published.[123] Pulmonary stenosis is no longer considered to be a condition at high risk for endocarditis, either before or after balloon dilation. The current guidelines published by the American Heart Association recommend that repaired malformations with residual defects at the site of a prosthetic patch or prosthetic device, which may inhibit endothelialisation, be considered an indication for prophylaxis. The National Institute for Health and Clinical Excellence (NICE) of the United Kingdom has concluded that bacterial endocarditis prophylaxis is no longer indicated at all, unless there is existing infection at the operation site.

Recommendations for Exercise

Prior to Intervention

The recommendations for participation in exercise by patients with pulmonary stenosis is based on analysis of the known features of this disease by a taskforce of experts.[124] For these recommendations, the classification of exercise intensity is also important (Fig. 43-34).[125]

Asymptomatic patients with untreated pulmonary stenosis with peak Doppler systolic gradients of less than

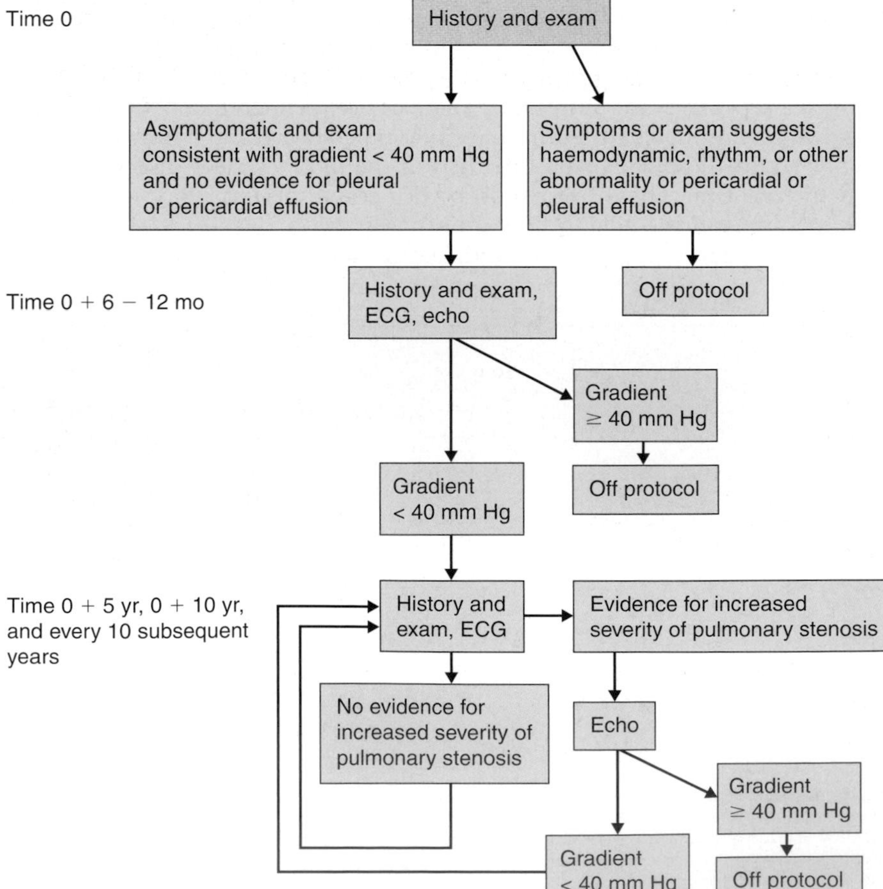

Figure 43-33 Algorithm for postoperative or post-balloon valvoplasty for pulmonary valvar stenosis. (Reproduced with permission from Driscoll D, Allen HD, Atkins DL, et al: Guidelines for evaluation and management of common congenital cardiac problems in infants, children, and adolescents: A statement for healthcare professionals from the Committee on Congenital Cardiac Defects of the Council on Cardiovascular Disease in the Young, American Heart Association. Circulation 1994;90:2180–2188.)

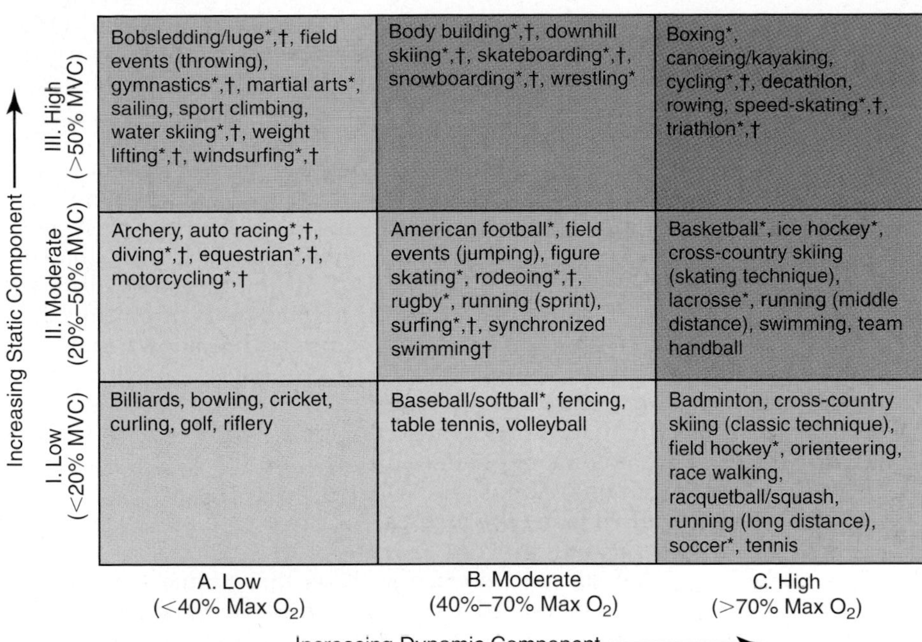

Figure 43-34 The Bethesda Classification of sports. The lowest total cardiovascular demands (cardiac output and blood pressure) are shown in *green* and the highest in *red*. *Blue*, *yellow*, and *orange* depict low moderate, moderate, and high moderate total cardiovascular demands, respectively. *Danger of bodily collision. †Increased risk if syncope occurs. (Reproduced with permission from Mitchell JH, Haskell W, Snell P, Van Camp SP: Task Force 8: Classification of sports. J Am Coll Cardiol 2005;45:1364–1367.)

40 mm Hg are encouraged to live a normal life, including any competitive sports. Patients with gradients greater than 40 mm Hg can participate in low-intensity competition, but would usually be considered for intervention.

After Intervention for Pulmonary Stenosis

Following balloon dilation, the return to all competitive sports can be counselled in patients with no or mild residual stenosis, 2 to 4 weeks after the procedure. A longer interval of about 3 months is recommended after surgical relief. Those with residual moderate pulmonary stenosis, with a gradient of greater than 40 mm Hg, should follow the same recommendations as patients before interventions. Patients with severe pulmonary incompetence and right ventricular enlargement are recommended only to participate in exercise intensities to the first classes. Care to avoid blows to the chest would be prudent.[124]

IMPLICATIONS IN ADULT LIFE

In previous years, and indeed in the present in countries with a less well developed system for healthcare, patients with pulmonary stenosis could survive without intervention into adult life. In a retrospective study of 20 years in a developing country, pulmonary stenosis accounted for 6% of unoperated adults presenting with congenitally malformed hearts.[126] Whilst there is little data in the literature, persistent and slowly progressive obstruction of the right ventricular outflow tract has led to anecdotal reports of severely debilitated patients with low cardiac output and right heart failure, particularly in developing countries. The same anecdotal reports show that, despite catastrophic existing morbidity, a successful intervention to relieve pulmonary stenosis can yield rapid and impressive improvements in clinical state.

Contraception

All advice concerning family planning and genetic counselling should be offered to patients on an individual basis, based on their primary diagnosis, interventions and sequels.[127–129] The patient will normally choose her own method of contraceptive, but the cardiologist may need to provide informed advice. In pulmonary stenosis, before or after intervention, the combined oral contraceptive pill is effective and well tolerated, for family planning and also for management of menstrual disorders. The risk of thromboembolism is low, but where a potential for right-to-left shunting exists at atrial level, the combined contraceptive pill is contra-indicated unless supplanted by anticoagulation. Progesterone-only pills, depot injections and implants are recommended where the combined oral contraceptive pill is contra-indicated. Preparations of progesterone alone are less effective, less convenient because they must be taken during a short daily time window, and may provoke depression, retention of fluid, or menstrual irregularities.

Intra-uterine devices have historically been associated with pelvic inflammatory disease, and have therefore generally been contra-indicated, especially in treated patients who need to observe precautions against endocarditis. The risk of endocarditis in patients with intra-uterine devices, nonetheless, is extremely low, and indeed an intra-uterine device releasing levonorgestrel has been approved for patients who have experienced pregnancy and remain at risk of endocarditis.[130] This device has similar efficacy to the oral combined contraceptive pill. Its local release of progesterone reduces the bleeding that is associated with other devices, albeit that more frequent replacement is necessary. The use of barrier methods remains extremely effective, especially in couples over 35 years old.

Pregnancy

Women with isolated pulmonary stenosis have been shown to tolerate pregnancy well, despite the gestational volume load as an additive effect to a potentially hypertensive right ventricle.[131–135] Vaginal delivery is tolerated well.[133] No deaths attributable to pulmonary stenosis have been reported. A meta-analysis of 2491 pregnancies over a 20-year period from 1985 in patients with congenital heart disease identified up to 127 women with pulmonary stenosis.[136] The rate of miscarriage was equivalent to that of the normal population. There were no reported cases of arrhythmia, heart failure, or endocarditis. The rates of premature delivery and stillbirth were comparable to the expected, and the babies were not growth retarded. Interestingly, there is an increased risk of non-cardiac maternal complications, such as hypertension, suffered by pregnant women with pulmonary stenosis.[132]

Whilst pregnancy is usually well tolerated in women with pulmonary stenosis, symptomatic pulmonary valvar stenosis has been reported in pregnancy.[135,137,138] Interventions during pregnancy, either surgical or by catheter intervention, were reported from as early as 1955.[137,138]

Life Insurance, Mortgage Application and Employment

Pulmonary stenosis is a survivable lesion, and children with pulmonary stenosis are destined to reach adult life. The results of the second natural history study[114] showed that 95.7% of the original cohort of 592 patients with pulmonary stenosis survived to 25 years. Almost none of the patients with mild pulmonary stenosis, that is a peak systolic gradient less than 25 mm Hg, required an operation at an older age, and the results of surgery for 283 patients with more severe disease were excellent. The employment record of these young adults was similar to that of the general population, with approximately 93% practising a profession, holding a job, or engaged in full-time education. It appears from these data that children with pulmonary stenosis develop into productive adults leading a high quality of life, becoming well educated and achieving employment. It is difficult to see how these patients can be classed as a burden to the health care or welfare systems.

Despite this, the impact of a congenitally malformed heart on an adult looking for life or health insurance has been the subject of a number of papers.[139–144] Adult patients with pulmonary stenosis are represented in this group, although the total numbers are small. In general, for patients with congenitally malformed hearts, barriers are frequently encountered, mostly based on the diagnostic code of the patient from the point of view of the insurance company, rather than on a careful functional assessment and risk stratification by the cardiologist.[140] Indeed, a simple functional classification of the severity of disease into grades of mild, significant, or complex appears to have no effect on the success of life insurance or mortgage application outcomes.

A questionnaire-based study[139] addressed to providers of mortgages and insurance showed that normal premiums applied to patients with mitral prolapse without regurgitation, postoperative patients with a closed but previously patent arterial duct, and perhaps surprisingly, subsequent to repair of coarctation. Other lesions, repaired or otherwise, including pulmonary stenosis, attracted a larger premium, or else were refused.[139] Some insurance companies allowed for cover to be arranged with exclusion of benefit for disorders relating to the congenital cardiac disease. Just over two-fifths of patients with congenitally malformed hearts who were initially refused an application for life insurance were successful in subsequent applications.[140] This may be explained by the applicants learning to place a different emphasis on their medical history, and submitting their applications to a different company. It is known that there are inconsistencies between companies offering insurance, which could be of benefit to adults with congenitally malformed hearts who are shopping around. There are no data published, however, on the rate of successful insurance claims, and whether such claims can be jeopardised when the medical history is de-emphasised in the application process.

Whilst the evidence suggests that pulmonary stenosis should be considered to be a mild, or certainly an easily treatable, disease, in practice these patients can be denied insurance, the facility to arrange a mortgage, or may only be accepted for insurance at an inflated rate. Inconsistencies found in insurance and job policies may be due to lack of knowledge or appropriate guidelines for the outcome of young adults with corrected and uncorrected congenital cardiac disease. A more evidence-based approach is emerging from insurance and mortgaging companies as long-term follow-up data becomes available, and a recent publication described three modern insurance companies which identified the risk for mortality in adults with pulmonary stenosis to be approximately equal to that of the general population.[144]

Practical strategies may be of help to patients seeking insurance, or applying for mortgages or employment. Declined patients, or patients offered high premium rate insurance can approach different companies. The local Adult Congenital Heart Disease Patients Association may have information about insurers who have a track record of covering patients with congenitally malformed hearts. Group insurance policies available through employers or professional associations often do not require individual evaluation, and even adult patients with complex congenital heart disease may therefore obtain insurance benefits by this route. The avoidance of smoking, and the adoption of good health practices, will lower overall risk and further increase the chances of insurability. Patients who are followed up in a specialist adult congenital clinic, where management of congenital heart disease and its late complications are routinely practised, may receive a more favourable response from provider companies. Cardiologists in the field of adult congenital heart disease are in a position to make recommendations for individual patients with pulmonary stenosis, by presenting the history, supporting investigations, and furnishing insurers with up-to-date information on long-term follow-up where necessary.

The complete reference list can be found on the companion Expert Consult web site at www.expertconsult.com.

ANNOTATED REFERENCES

- Stamm C, Anderson RH, Ho SY: Clinical anatomy of the normal pulmonary root compared with that in isolated pulmonary valvular stenosis. J Am Coll Cardiol 1998;31:1420–1425.

  This comprehensive morphological study of the stenosed pulmonary valve identifies the mechanism, and describes the anatomy of pulmonary stenosis. The concept of the pulmonary valve annulus is refuted, since there is no identified fibrous rings-like structure in the normal pulmonary valve. The annular paradox is described, where such a fibrous structure exists only in a stenosed valve.

- Sellors T: Surgery of Pulmonary stenosis: A case in which the pulmonary valve was successfully divided. Lancet 1948;254:988–989.
- Brock RC: Pulmonary valvulotomy for relief of congenital pulmonary stenosis: Report of three cases. BMJ 1948;1:1121–1126.

  With these two articles, the pioneering history of surgery to the pulmonary valve was elegantly described.

- Rubio-Alvarez V, Limon-Lason R, Soni J: Valvulotomias intracardiacas por medio de un cateter [Intracardiac valvulotomy by means of a catheter]. Arch Inst Cardiol Mex 1953;23:183–192.
- Semb BK, Tjonneland S, Stake G, Aabyholm G: "Balloon valvulotomy" of congenital pulmonary valve stenosis with tricuspid valve insufficiency. Cardiovasc Radiol 1979;2:239–241.

  The above two articles described the developments in interventional cardiology, leading to the present status of affairs where balloon pulmonary valvotomy is the treatment of choice for pulmonary stenosis.

- Tynan M, Jones O, Joseph MC, et al: Relief of pulmonary valve stenosis in first week of life by percutaneous balloon valvuloplasty. Lancet 1984;1:273.

  In the above article, Tynan and his colleagues described, for the first time, the application of balloon dilation for the treatment of pulmonary stenosis in a six-day-old infant.

- Rao PS: Percutaneous balloon pulmonary valvuloplasty: State of the art. Cathet Cardiovasc Intervent 2007;69:747–763.
- Rao PS: Further observations on the effect of balloon size on the short term and intermediate term results of balloon dilatation of the pulmonary valve. Br Heart J 1988;60:507–511.

  P. Syamasundar Rao has made a very detailed study of pulmonary stenosis in childhood and adult life. In these two articles, the techniques and refinements of balloon pulmonary valve dilation are discussed, specifically regarding the avoidance of long-term complications of pulmonary regurgitation.

- Fedderly RT, Lloyd TR, Mendelsohn AM, Beekman RH: Determinants of successful balloon valvotomy in infants with critical pulmonary stenosis or membranous pulmonary atresia with intact ventricular septum. J Am Coll Cardiol 1995;25:460–465.

  Severe forms of pulmonary stenosis, or pulmonary atresia, are associated with a hypoplastic right ventricle. Yet there is evidence that the structures will grow if obstruction is relieved. The above article investigates the predictors of successful outcome to biventricular repair in patients with borderline right ventricles.

- Roos-Hesselink JW, Meijboom FJ, Spitaels SEC, et al: Long-term outcome after surgery for pulmonary stenosis (a longitudinal study of 22–33 years). Eur Heart J 2006;27:482–488.
- Peterson C, Schilthuis JJ, Dodge-Khatami A, et al: Comparative long-term results of surgery versus balloon valvuloplasty for pulmonary valve stenosis in infants and children. Ann Thorac Surg 2003;76:1078–1082.

  These articles summarise the emerging long-term results of surgical and interventional treatments for pulmonary stenosis. At present, the freedom from intervention and maintenance of the relief of obstruction appears to be slightly better with surgical techniques. Balloon dilation of the pulmonary valve, however, is quicker, less invasive, and cheaper, and requires a shorter hospital stay. For this reason, balloon dilation remains the treatment of choice where the facility is available.

CHAPTER 44

Congenital Anomalies of the Aortic Valve and Left Ventricular Outflow Tract

JEFFREY F. SMALLHORN, ANDREW N. REDINGTON, and ROBERT H. ANDERSON

Abnormalities of the left ventricular outflow tract may occur at the subvalvar level, valvar, supravalvar, or a combination thereof. These abnormalities commonly co-exist with other left-sided lesions, such as aortic coarctation or anomalies of the mitral valve, as well as forming an important component of the pathophysiology of more complex lesions, such as atrioventricular septal defect with common atrioventricular junction, or discordant ventriculo-arterial connections. The latter lesions will be discussed in detail in the relevant chapters, while in this chapter we will deal predominantly with anomalies of the left ventricular outflow tract as seen in the setting of concordant connections.

Within the whole overall group, three-quarters of patients have valvar stenosis, just under one-quarter have discrete subaortic stenosis, and the remaining small proportion have isolated supravalvar obstruction. Congenital aortic valvar stenosis itself accounts for 5% of all cardiac abnormalities.[1] If all those with bifoliate aortic valves are included, then this may be the commonest of all congenital abnormalities.[2,3] It is difficult to know the true incidence, however, as congenitally abnormal aortic valves may not be recognised in childhood. Isolated stenosis as a presenting feature is more common than regurgitation, albeit that mixed lesions tend to occur over time, providing a challenge in management for the cardiologist.

MORPHOLOGY

The Normal Aortic Root

To understand the mechanisms of obstruction at any level within the left ventricular outflow tract, it is necessary first to understand the normal arrangement. Most accounts remain based on the concept of an aortic annulus, albeit this enigmatic feature is rarely described in consistent and satisfactory fashion.[4] An annulus, if defined literally, is no more than a little ring. There are several rings within the normal aortic root, but none of them support the leaflets of the aortic valve. The essence of normality is that the leaflets are hinged within the arterial root in semilunar fashion (Fig. 44-1). The root itself is formed by interlocking of the aortic valvar sinuses and the supporting ventricular structures. Because of the interlocking, there is a marked discrepancy between the locus of the haemodynamic as opposed to the anatomic ventriculo-arterial junctions.[5] The anatomical ventriculo-arterial junction is the line over which the fibroelastic walls of the aortic sinuses are supported by the base of the left ventricle. This line does form a ring, with parts supported by the musculature of the ventricular septum and the parietal left ventricular wall and the remainder integrated within the fibrous curtain formed by the continuity between the leaflets of the aortic valve and the aortic, or anterior, leaflet of the mitral valve. The rightward extent of this area of fibrous continuity also incorporates the membranous part of the ventricular septum (see Fig. 44-1). The haemodynamic junction is marked by the semilunar lines of attachment of the aortic valvar leaflets (see Fig. 44-1). These semilunar hinges cross the ring at six points. As a result, three crescents of ventricular tissue, two muscular and one fibrous, are incorporated into the bases of the three aortic sinuses of Valsalva, while three fibrous triangles are incorporated at the distal extent of the ventricular outflow tract (Fig. 44-2).

The triangles extend distally to the level of the most distal attachment of the leaflets at the sinutubular junction. This structure is also an obvious ring, marking the line over which the expanded aortic sinuses become continuous

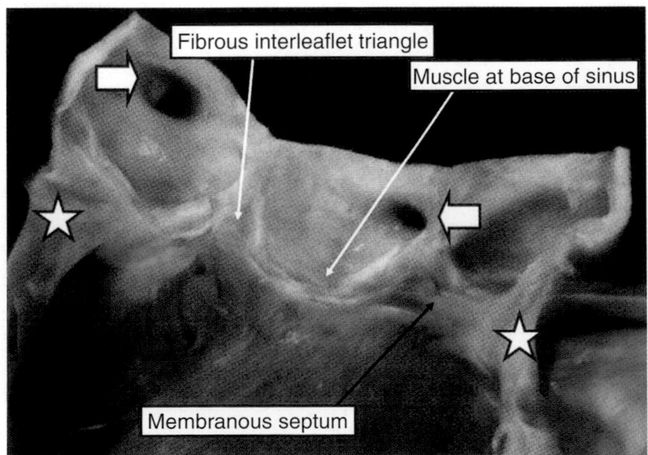

Figure 44-1 The normal aortic root has been opened through an incision in the aortic leaflet of the mitral valve (*stars*), and the leaflets of the aortic valve have been removed, showing the semilunar attachments of the three leaflets. The arrangement is such to incorporate crescents of ventricular myocardium at the base of the two leaflets attached within the coronary arterial sinuses (*arrows*). Triangles of fibrous tissue are incorporated into the outflow tract beneath the zones of apposition of the leaflets, with the membranous septum continuous with the triangle found beneath the zone of apposition between the right coronary and non-coronary leaflets of the valve.

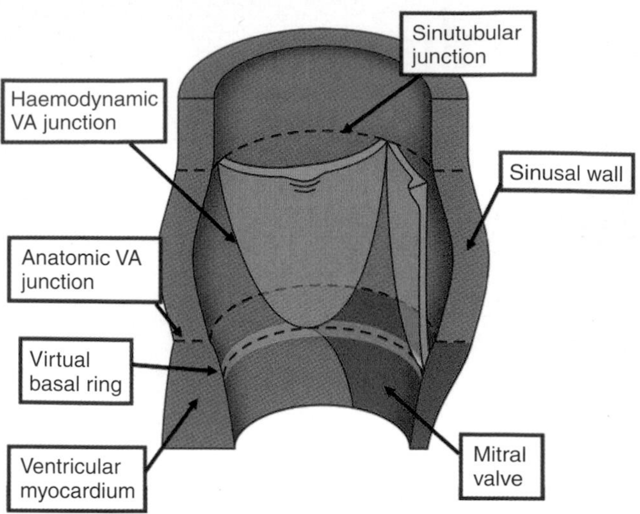

Figure 44-2 The cartoon shows an idealised view of the bisected aortic root. Note how the semilunar attachments of the valvar leaflets, marking the haemodynamic ventriculo-arterial (VA) junction, cross the anatomic junction. See text for discussion.

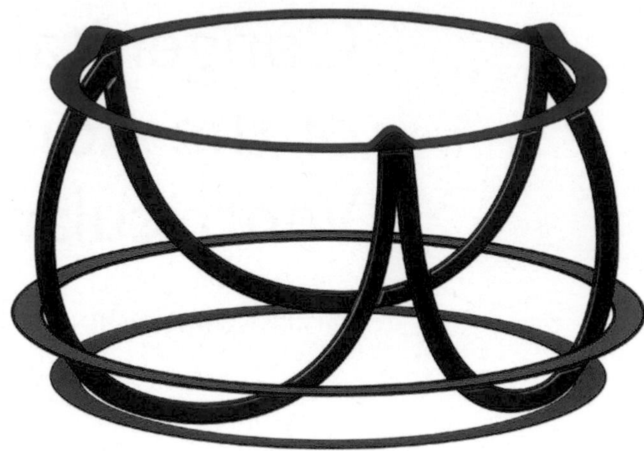

Figure 44-4 The cartoon shows the crown-like arrangement of the semilunar attachments of the leaflets of the aortic valve (*red line*), and how these extend from the sinutubular junction (*blue ring*) to the virtual basal ring (*green ring*) constructed by joining together the most proximal attachments of the leaflets within the left ventricle. Note that the semilunar attachments cross the anatomic ventriculo-arterial junction (*yellow ring*) six times.

with the tubular aorta. It marks the distal extent of the aortic root. Since it is unequivocally part of the root, and valvar competence depends on its integrity, it is somewhat illogical to describe stenosis at this level as being supravalvar. It is also illogical to consider only the peripheral attachment of the valvar leaflets to the sinutubular junction as the commissures, as is currently the usual practise. Defined literally, a commissure is a zone of apposition. The zones of apposition between the normal valvar leaflets extend from the centre to the periphery of the valve (Fig. 44-3). All parts of these zones need to open without hindrance if the valve is to function properly. There is then one further ring within the outflow tract. This ring is constructed by joining together

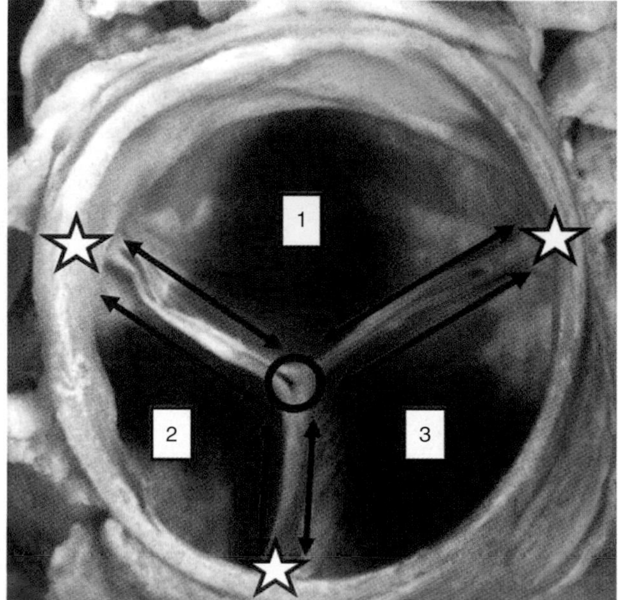

Figure 44-3 The closed normal aortic valve has been photographed from its arterial aspect. Note that the zones of apposition (*arrows*) between the three leaflets, numbered 1 to 3, extend from their attachments at the sinutubular junction (*stars*) to the centre of the valvar orifice (*circle*). It is the entirety of these zones which represents the commissures although traditionally it is only the peripheral attachments that are credited with this title.

the most proximal attachments of the three valvar leaflets within the left ventricle. This third ring, therefore, is a virtual structure (see Fig. 44-2), whereas the sinutubular junction and the anatomic ventriculo-arterial junctions are true anatomic entities. The entirety of the root, considered in three dimensions, takes the form of a crown (Fig. 44-4).

Annulus, therefore, does not seem the most obvious word the arrangement of the valvar leaflets within the root. The overall anatomic arrangement should also be taken into account when measurements are made of the outflow tract. When diagrams are made to illustrate the concept of measurement of the annulus, they often show a line drawn between proximal points of attachment of the leaflets (Fig. 44-5). Such diagrams must involve a degree of poetic licence on behalf of the observer, since the section illustrated can never cut the full diameter of the arterial root (Fig. 44-6).

All of this normal anatomy is of relevance when considering the structure of stenotic lesions within the outflow tract, particularly the fact that so-called supravalvar stenosis involves tethering of the valvar leaflets at the level of the sinutubular junction.

Valvar Stenosis

The stenotic aortic valve is traditionally considered as showing unicuspid, bicuspid, or tricuspid patterns. Strictly speaking, a cusp is a point or elevation. Despite its popularity, it is not the ideal adjective to use when accounting for lesions of the abnormal valve. Our preference is to describe unifoliate, bifoliate, or trifoliate valves, according to the number of leaflets present. When making such descriptions, note should also be taken of the number of sinuses present, since almost always, even when the curtain of leaflet tissue is compartmented to produce less than three component parts, the curtain is still suspended within three obvious sinuses. In the presence, for example, of the so-called unifoliate and unicommissural valve (Fig. 44-7), with examination from the arterial aspect showing a solitary slit-like opening within the valvar curtain, examination from the ventricular side typically reveals three interleaflet triangles, albeit with two of them being vestigial.[6]

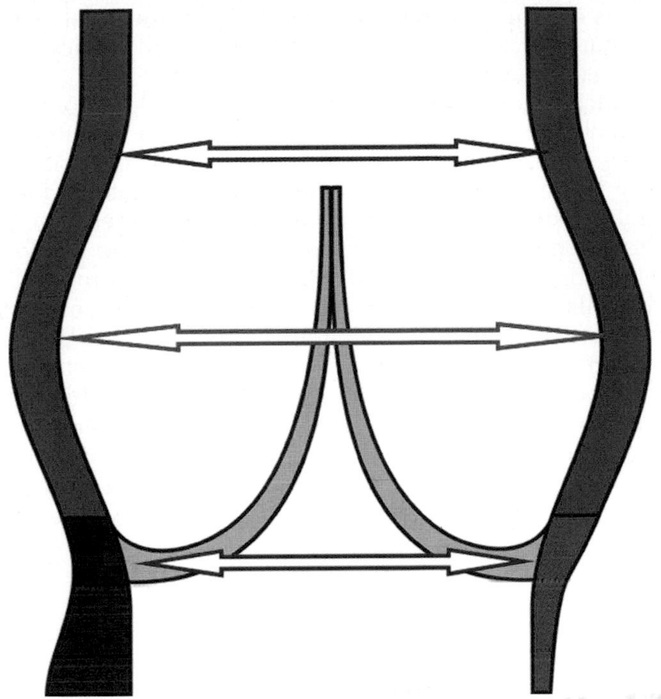

Figure 44-5 The cartoon shows an idealised arrangement of the aortic root, as frequently illustrated when demonstrating measurements for the aortic annulus. The dimension usually taken is the basal one, between the attachments of opposing leaflets (*blue double-headed arrow*). As shown in Figure 44-6, this dimension does not represent the widest diameter of the root. It is also important to take note of the dimensions at mid-sinusal level (*green double-headed arrow*), and at the sinutubular junction (*red double-headed arrow*).

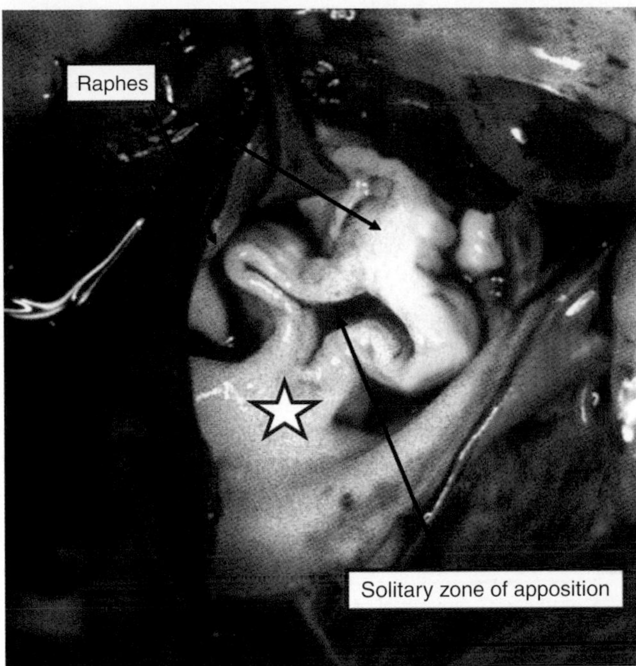

Figure 44-7 This photograph shows a unifoliate and unicommissural aortic valve. If examined from the ventricular aspect, vestigial interleaflet triangles would be found beneath the raphes in the apparently unifoliate valvar curtain. Note the tethering of the solitary zone of apposition at the sinutubular junction (*star*). (Courtesy of Dr Benson R. Wilcox, University of North Carolina, Chapel Hill.)

Similarly, examination of the majority of the valves showing a bifoliate pattern of the leaflets (Fig. 44-8) reveals that they are formed within a trisinuate prototype.[7,8] In the unifoliate, or unicommissural, valve, typically seen in infants with so-called critical stenosis, the keyhole opening within the valvar curtain represents the only properly developed zone of apposition (see Fig. 44-7). This is usually formed between the left and non-coronary aortic leaflets, and points towards the mitral valve. The other leaflets are abnormally attached in annular fashion to the ventricular wall because of the vestigial nature of the putative zones of apposition between the other leaflets (Fig. 44-9). It is paradoxical, therefore, that valvar leaflets attached more closely in annular fashion are likely to be stenotic or regurgitant.

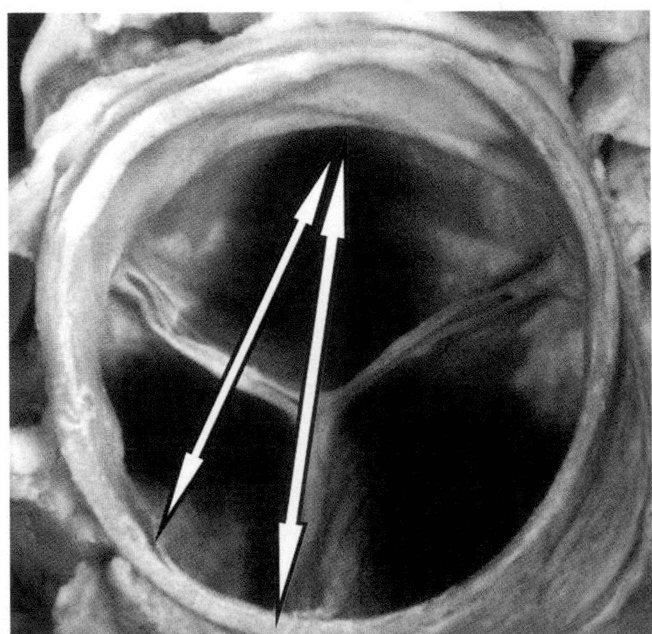

Figure 44-6 The aortic valve shown in Figure 44-3 has been relabelled to show how measurements from the basal attachment of one leaflet to the most basal attachment of an adjacent leaflet can never cut the widest diameter of the valvar orifice (*red arrow*). The widest diameter would be represented by a measurement from the basal attachment of one leaflet to the opposite interleaflet triangle (*blue arrow*).

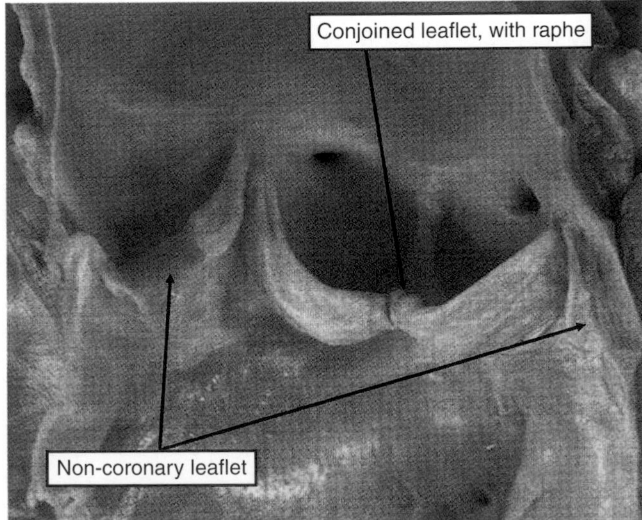

Figure 44-8 This picture shows a typical bifoliate aortic valve, with a raphe between the conjoined leaflet guarding the two aortic sinuses. Note the failure of formation of the interleaflet triangle beneath the raphe.

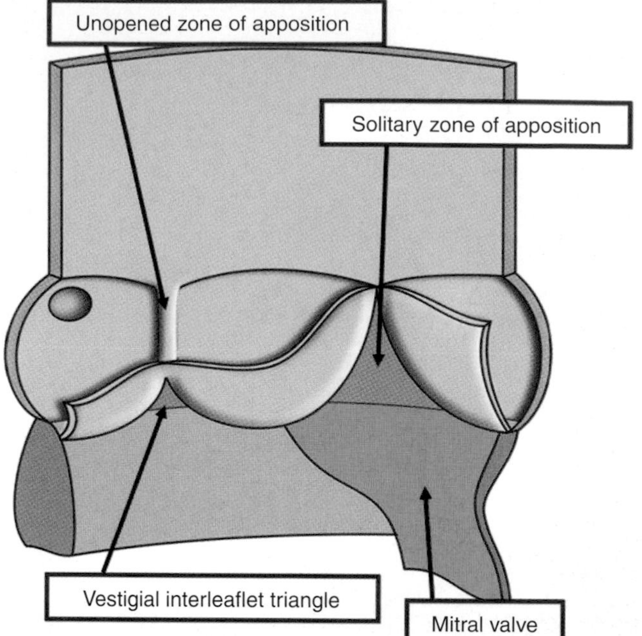

Figure 44-9 The cartoon shows the mechanism of formation of bifoliate or unifoliate aortic valves. There is failure of formation of the zone of apposition between the normal three leaflets of the valve, with failure of formation of the interleaflet triangles. In the bifoliate valve, it is one such zone of apposition that fails to form, but there is failure of formation of two zones when the valve is unifoliate and unicommisural.

Balloon dilation of such valves can do little more than open further the solitary zone of apposition, which is often tethered to the sinutubular junction (see Fig. 44-7). To produce a functioning trifoliate arrangement, it is necessary to create new triangles at the sites of the vestigial zones of apposition, with appropriate extension of the rudimentary and malformed leaflets. When seen in pathological archives, such valves are usually housed in small fibroelastic left ventricles, the heart itself often fulfilling many of the anatomic criterions for inclusion within the hypoplastic left heart syndrome (see Chapter 29).

The bifoliate aortic valve is also often described in association with critical aortic stenosis, albeit again formed on a trisinuate prototype,[8] but is also found in asymptomatic individuals. The leaflets themselves guard markedly dissimilar parts of the valvar orifice, with the larger leaflet formed by fusion of two putative leaflets, typically with a raphe showing the line of non-separation between them (see Fig. 44-8). The conjoined leaflet usually represents either fusion of the two coronary leaflets, or fusion of the right and non-coronary leaflets.[7] Truly bisinuate and bifoliate valves do exist, but are rare, as are trisinuate but bifoliate valves without evidence of a raphe between the presumed conjoined leaflets. Stenosis, when it occurs, is the result of fusion of the ends of the zone of apposition between the two leaflets. Bifoliate valves can also produce problems when they become incompetent due to prolapse, or if they provide a nidus for endocarditis. This is more likely to occur in adult life,[9] and is rarely seen in childhood.

Stenosis producing problems in childhood can also be seen in the setting of a trifoliate valve, but more usually such valves are the seat of senile aortic calcification.[10] When seen in childhood, the trifoliate valve, with dysplastic leaflets, is encountered most frequently in infants. A stenotic trifoliate valve is rare in older children and adolescents unless they have undergone previous surgery.

Calcification of the aortic valve can develop from the third decade in all patients with mildly stenotic or bifoliate valves. It may start as early as the second decade, particularly if the valves are dysplastic and myxomatous. Most patients, however, present in later life with severe calcific aortic stenosis in what was initially no more than a mildly stenosed valve, or a valve with leaflets initially of markedly dissimilar size.[10] The changes are more common in males than females. Patients with familial hypocholesterolaemia, progeria, and rickets develop calcification earlier, even if the aortic valve is only mildly abnormal. Patients with bifoliate valves producing minimal stenosis usually do not develop calcific stenosis until the sixth or seventh decade, but presence of moderate or severe stenosis in childhood can lead to quite heavy calcification in the third and fourth decades.

Subvalvar Stenosis

A variety of lesions can obstruct the subaortic outflow tract, with or without a co-existing ventricular septal defect. When there is an interventricular communication, then postero-caudal deviation of the muscular outlet septum is usually the most important lesion.[11] We discuss this lesion in the chapters devoted to ventricular septal defect and interruption of the aortic arch. Obstruction can also be produced by hypertrophy of the ventricular septum, as seen in hypertrophic cardiomyopathy (see Chapter 54), by anomalous tissue tags derived from the membranous septum or the leaflets of the atrioventricular valves, or by anomalous attachment of the tension apparatus of the left atrioventricular valve (Fig. 44-10). The last two lesions are also more likely to be found when there is a ventricular septal defect, or in the setting of common atrioventricular junction and deficient atrioventricular septation.

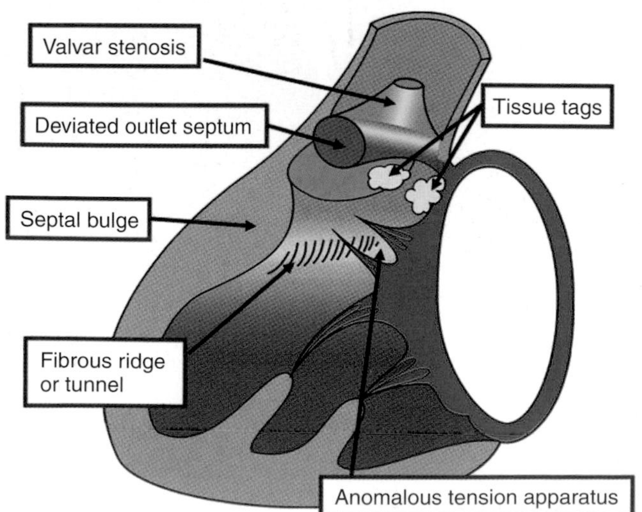

Figure 44-10 The cartoon shows the lesion producing obstruction of the morphologically left ventricular outflow tract. They produce aortic obstruction when the ventriculo-arterial connections are concordant, but subpulmonary obstruction in the setting of discordant ventriculo-arterial connections.

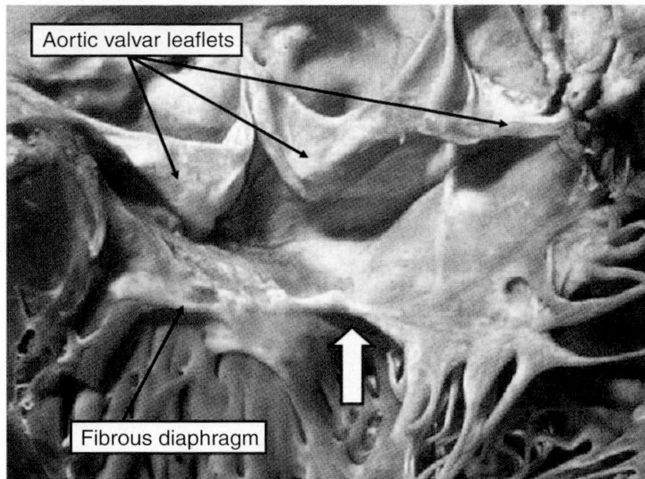

Figure 44-11 The aortic outflow tract has been opened to reveal a fibrous subaortic diaphragm. Note that the shelf-like lesion is also attached the aortic leaflet of the mitral valve (*arrow*). The aortic valve in this instance is normal.

When the ventricular septum is intact, the most significant lesion is the subvalvar fibrous ridge, or diaphragm (Fig. 44-11). This lesion has been described in many ways. Although often termed membranous, almost always the lesion is a firm fibrous shelf that encircles the outflow tract, often extending to be attached also to the aortic valvar leaflets. The septal component of the obstructive lesion overlies the left bundle branch as it crosses the ventricular septum. A discrete plane of cleavage almost always exists between the shelf and the musculature. Because of this, it can readily be stripped away by surgery (Fig. 44-12). Since the lesion is acquired, there is always the likelihood of recurrence. The position can vary with regard to its proximity to the valvar leaflets. If extensive, it can produce so-called tunnel stenosis. In florid cases, there is a marked abnormality in the alignment between the plane of the aortic root and the ventricular septum. This has been promoted as a potential cause of the malformation.[11]

Supravalvar Aortic Stenosis

Supravalvar stenosis accounts for only 1% to 2% of cases of aortic stenosis seen in childhood. The condition may be familial, or may be associated with disorders of calcium metabolism, the so-called Williams syndrome.[12] The original description included failure to thrive, gastrointestinal upset, and mental retardation.[13] The stenosis typically lies above the aortic sinuses and the coronary orifices, but incorporates the sinutubular junction (Fig. 44-13). The aortic sinuses themselves are enlarged and bulge laterally, while the aortic leaflets are often slightly thickened, and are disproportionately long in relation to the portion of sinutubular junction to which they are related. The coronary arteries, which take origin below the obstruction, are typically dilated, thick walled and ectatic. The possibility of orificial stenosis must be considered in these patients, nonetheless, as hoods, entrapment by leaflet tissue, and slit-like orificies may all lead to myocardial ischaemia. The nature of the narrowing is variable.[14] The most common form is the hourglass variety with dilation of the distal aorta (see Fig. 44-13). There are also diffuse or tubular varieties, and, very rarely, a diaphragmatic or localised form. Irrespective of the type, the ascending aorta is usually grossly abnormal, with a thickened wall and disorganisation of the media. The narrowing and scarring are not exclusive to the aorta, and may be found in the iliac arteries, and in the abdominal and renal vessels.

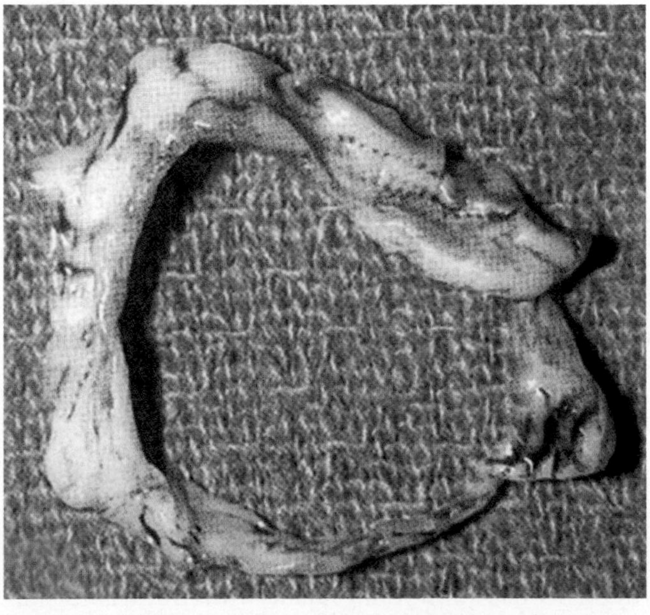

Figure 44-12 This fibrous diaphragm has been stripped away from the subaortic area by blunt dissection in a patient with discrete subaortic stenosis. (Courtesy of Dr Benson R. Wilcox, University of North Carolina, Chapel Hill.)

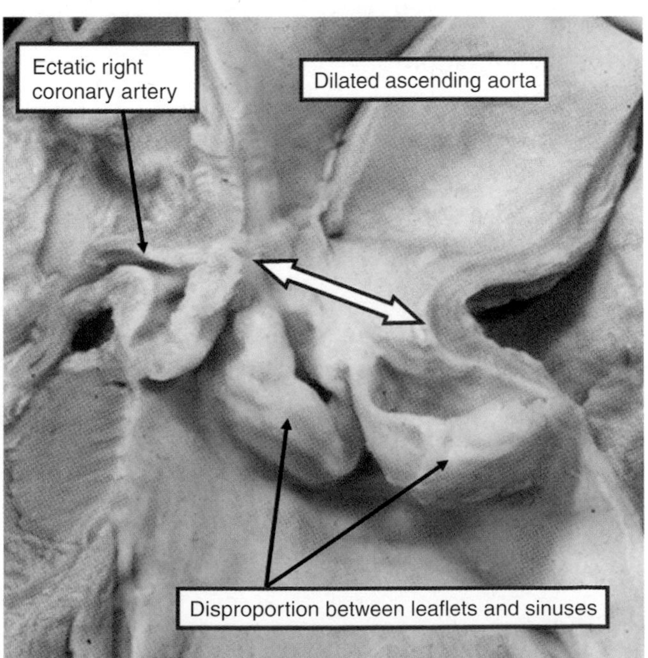

Figure 44-13 The illustration shows the typical hourglass variant of so-called supravalvar aortic stenosis. As can be seen, the stenosis is at the level of the sinutubular junction (*double-headed arrow*), and involves the peripheral attachments of the zones of apposition between the valvar leaflets. Note the disproportionate length of the free edge of the leaflets relative to their supporting sinuses.

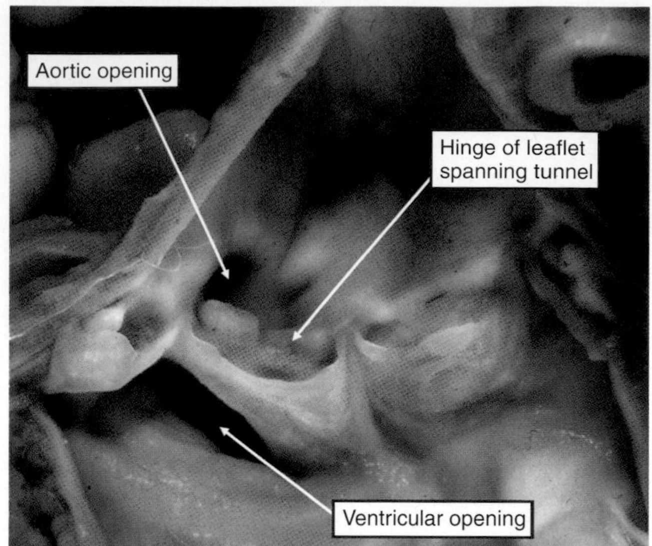

Figure 44-14 This specimen demonstrates an aorto–left ventricular tunnel. Note that the right coronary leaflet is suspended across the tunnel, and is also dysplastic.

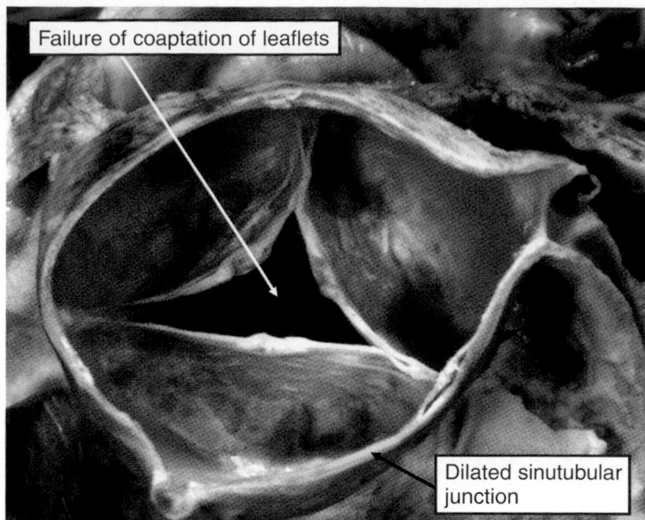

Figure 44-15 In this heart, there has been acquired dilation of the sinutubular junction. This makes it impossible for the valvar leaflets to coapt during ventricular diastole, and results in gross aortic regurgitation.

Stenosis of the origin of the carotid and subclavian arteries, and less frequently the renal and mesenteric arteries, occurs in up to half the patients. The pulmonary circulation is also affected. In one-fifth of patients, there are multiple pulmonary arterial stenoses. These are mostly peripheral, being seen where the major vessels enter the lung. Consequently, supravalvar aortic stenosis in most, but not all, patients is part of a more widespread abnormality of the cardiovascular system involving the major conducting arteries. Histological findings away from the site of the obstruction in the aorta show irregular thickening and branching of medial elastic fibres. This appearance has been dubbed a mosaic pattern,[9] or higgledy-piggledy arteriopathy.[15]

Aortic Regurgitation

The stenotic aortic valve can also be regurgitant if the lesions producing stenosis also prevent the valvar leaflets coapting snugly during ventricular diastole. Isolated aortic regurgitation is much rarer than stenosis. If seen as an isolated finding in the neonatal period, then reflux through an aorto–left ventricular tunnel should be excluded. In this entity, one of the valvar leaflets is suspended across the ventriculo-arterial junction, so that blood is able to flow around the part that should be attached within the aortic root (Fig. 44-14). Regurgitation can also be produced by abnormalities of the leaflets, such as perforations produced by infectious endocarditis, or iatrogenic damage subsequent to balloon dilation. Dilation of the sinutubular junction will also prevent the valvar leaflets coapting, but this is an acquired rather than a congenital malformation (Fig. 44-15).

VALVAR AORTIC STENOSIS

Genetics

A bicuspid or bifoliate aortic valve occurs with a frequency of 1% to 2%, with a ratio of two males to each female. Familial clustering is recognised, as well as a common association with other left-sided obstructive lesions, such as aortic coarctation. Studies assessing first-degree relatives by echocardiography have demonstrated an incidence of associated bicuspid or bifoliate aortic valve from 4.7% to 24%, with a higher incidence of other left-sided lesions in these families.[15–19]

Critical Stenosis in the Neonate and Young Infant

Aortic stenosis is an important cause of heart failure in the neonate and young infant. It is being identified more frequently in the prenatal period and indeed, intervention has now been attempted in a group of fetuses with the lesion, with varying degrees of success.[20,21] The main issue at this stage, as well as for those presenting in the newborn period, relates to the adequacy of the left ventricle to support the systemic circulation. Although many attempts have been made to address this problem, it still remains controversial as to when a left ventricle is too small, such that a biventricular repair is abandoned in favor of the Norwood protocol or cardiac transplantation.[22,23] The problem is magnified by the fact that many patients have associated endocardial fibro-elastosis, mitral valvar abnormalities, or coarctation of the aorta in addition to the stenosis of the aortic valve. Hypoplasia of the aortic root and ascending aorta may also be seen, usually in those patients having borderline left ventricles. The pathogenesis is still poorly understood, but it most likely involves a primary left-sided insult, with secondary failure of growth of the left ventricle. This theory is supported by observation that left ventricular growth is seen following relief of the obstruction, even in those with borderline left ventricular volume at the time of first presentation.[21] What is also clear is that the associated left-sided lesions have an ongoing impact on morbidity, even in those patients undergoing adequate relief of the obstruction.[21]

Pathophysiology in the Newborn Period

Why do neonates and young infants with critical aortic valve stenosis present in heart failure? In those patients with a left ventricle having borderline volume, there is associated right ventricular hypertension in addition to left ventricular failure. The right ventricular dilation associated with the pulmonary hypertension has a further negative effect on left ventricular output, due to interactions between the ventricles. The ventricular septum bows into the left ventricle, further reducing its volume, and compounding the underlying problem. Tricuspid valvar regurgitation, if present, may also result in further dilation of the right ventricle. In other cases, where the left ventricular volume is adequate, failure is most likely due to a sudden increase in left ventricular afterload after birth as a result of reduced mass necessary to normalise mural myocardial stress.

Clinical Presentation and Physical Findings in the Neonate and Young Infant

The newborn or young infant presents in one of three ways. The first is with a picture similar to other forms of left-sided obstructive disease, such as aortic coarctation, interruption of the aortic arch, or hypoplastic left heart syndrome. These patients usually have a left ventricle with borderline volume, and become profoundly unwell subsequent to closure of the arterial duct. Clinically, they are in cardiac failure, or else present with cardiovascular collapse once they become acidotic. These neonates and young infants are tachypnoeic, tachycardic, and often cyanosed, due to the combination of pulmonary venous congestion and right-to-left shunting across the duct. Of note, the shunting through the oval foramen is from left to right. The physical examination reveals hepatomegaly, right ventricular enlargement, diffusely weak pulses, and frequently no murmur to suggest aortic valvar stenosis. An ejection click is uncommon. If they have right ventricular hypertension and failure, they may have a systolic murmur of tricuspid valvar regurgitation with an associated gallop. The second heart sound is invariably single. The patients are differentiated from those with aortic coarctation or interruption in that all the pulses are weak, as opposed to the right brachial and temporal pulses being palpable when the obstruction is within the aortic arch. The neonates with problems at valvar level are best described as having critical stenosis, since they are dependent on the patency of the arterial duct to sustain systemic cardiac output.

The second mode of presentation is seen in neonates or young infants with left-sided cardiac failure, but in the absence of acidosis, in other words, without ductal dependency. In this setting, the patients are tachypnoeic, have pulses that are usually low volume, and exhibit significantly less hepatomegaly. Auscultatory findings may reveal an ejection click heard along the lower left sternal border and at the apex, with a systolic ejection murmur that is heard in the same area, with radiation towards the upper right clavicular region. An associated systolic thrill is uncommon, as is the clinical detection of associated aortic regurgitation. While these patients usually have severe valvar stenosis, they are differentiated from those with the critical form by their lack of ductal dependency, and are often somewhat older at presentation. Consequently, as we will discuss, their outcomes tend to be better.

In the third situation, some patients are referred as neonates, or during the early period of infancy, for the evaluation of a systolic murmur. These patients do not have severe stenosis. They are more likely to have an ejection click, with an associated systolic murmur, but no signs of congestive cardiac failure. Of note, the pulses are usually of normal volume.

Investigations in the Newborn and Young Infant

The Electrocardiogram

The tracings at this age may look very similar to those seen in aortic coarctation or interruption, or hypoplastic left heart syndrome. There is right ventricular dominance, with upright T waves in lead V1, and a paucity of left-sided forces. Of note, there may also be diffuse changes in the S-T/T waves related to diffuse subendocardial ischaemia. In other cases with a larger left ventricle there is still right ventricular dominance, but with better left-sided forces. In those without pulmonary hypertension, there is evidence of left ventricular hypertrophy with associated strain.

Chest Radiograph

This may demonstrate cardiomegaly, with evidence of right ventricular enlargement and associated pulmonary oedema.

Echocardiography

The echocardiographer is presented with a challenge, particularly in those cases where the left ventricle is relatively hypoplastic (Fig. 44-16). There is usually right ventricular dilation due to the associated pulmonary hypertension, as well as associated left ventricular dysfunction. The left atrium is dilated, and there is usually left-to-right shunting at high velocity across the oval foramen. Of note, this mean gradient can be used to obtain an indirect assessment of left atrial pressure, by adding the estimated mean right atrial pressure. Usually, if the inferior caval vein is non-pulsatile, then the mean right atrial pressure is greater than 10 mm Hg. An estimated systolic right ventricular pressure can be obtained from associated tricuspid valvar regurgitation, and the mean pulmonary arterial pressure via the arterial

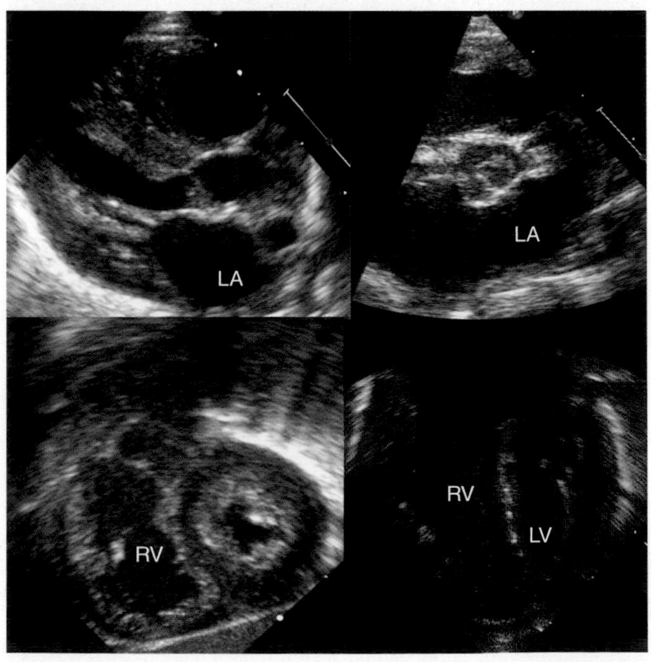

Figure 44-16 This patient has critical aortic stenosis, produced by the so-called unicommissural valve. There is borderline left ventricular volume. LA, left atrium; LV, left ventricle; RV, right ventricle.

duct. There is usually some degree of hypoplasia of the left ventricle and aortic root. Although it is possible to measure the left ventricular volume by using the calculations in the biplane Simpson approach, this is probably an underestimation of the true volume, since the left ventricle has an abnormal shape due to the associated septal shift in cases with systemic right ventricular pressures. With newer three-dimensional echocardiographic techniques, or with magnetic resonance imaging, this limitation should be overcome. In some patients, nonetheless, the true left ventricular volume remains unknown until the stenosis is relieved.

The aortic valve is more likely to be unifoliate and unicommissural in those presenting with critical aortic valve stenosis (see Fig. 44-16). In some cases, the valve appears to be so dysplastic that the precise nature of the morphology of the leaflets is difficult to determine.

Associated supravalvar and subvalvar stenosis is uncommon, albeit that endocardial fibroelastosis, and pathology involving the mitral valve, are common associations. When the endocardial fibroelastosis is extensive, this is seen as a bright layer covering the entire endocardium. When it is more patchy, it may be difficult to detect by echocardiography, which is not a good method for assessing the character of the insonated tissues. Assessing the severity of any associated mitral valvar pathology may also be difficult upon presentation due to poor left ventricular function, which in itself results in immobility of the leaflets (Fig. 44-17). Similarly, Doppler echocardiography is of limited value in determining the severity of the stenosis in the presence of a dilated ventricle with poor function. Despite this, if there is turbulence across the valve, then it most likely represents stenosis, rather than a dilated cardiomyopathy with an associated abnormality of the aortic valve, or more commonly aortic coarctation associated with a bifoliate aortic valve. Problems are created in the patients with moderate aortic valvar stenosis, coarctation of the aorta, and poor left ventricular function. In this setting, it usual first to deal with the coarctation, followed by reassessment of the aortic valve.

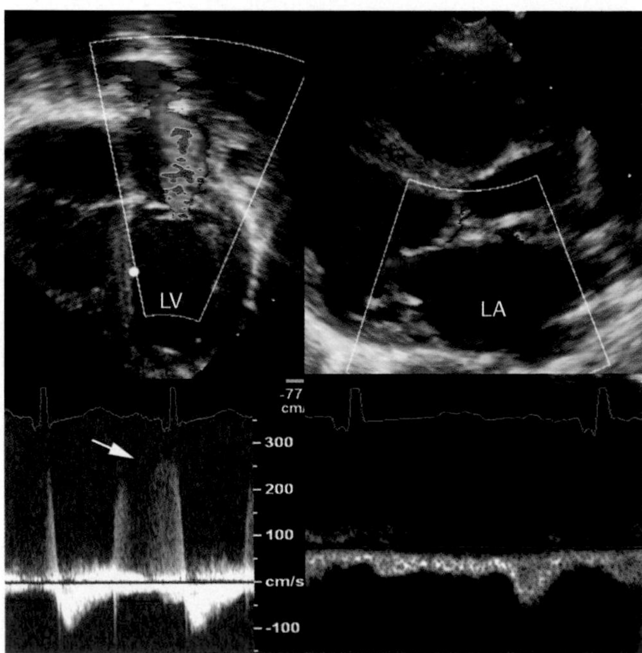

Figure 44-17 In this patient with critical aortic stenosis, there is also significant mitral valvar regurgitation. Note the adequate size of the left ventricle. Doppler interrogation of the pulmonary valvar regurgitation demonstrates high pulmonary arterial pressure. In addition, the Doppler trace of the pulmonary venous flow shows a reduced S wave (*arrow*), indicating a high left atrial pressure. LA, left atrium; LV, left ventricle.

Magnetic Resonance Imaging

More recently this technique has been employed by some to gain a more reliable assessment of left ventricular volume, though whether such measurements are accurate remains unclear.

Management of Critical Aortic Valvar Stenosis

In this current era, management starts in the prenatal period. There has been an interest in intervening prenatally in the fetus with aortic valvar stenosis, in an attempt to promote left ventricular growth. Although first described more than 10 years ago, more recently this approach has been extensively examined by the group working at Boston Children's Hospital, who now have significant experience with this technique.[20,21] The procedure involves paralysing the fetus, and then either directly via the maternal abdomen, or through the exposed uterus, an attempt is made percutaneously to dilate the aortic valve with a balloon. The results have been variable, but biventricular repair has been achieved in some who previously would have been destined to undergo functionally univentricular palliation. There is, however, mortality and morbidity associated with the procedure. It remains a matter of debate as to whether the long-term outcome of the borderline biventricular repair is better than the alternative palliation culminating in conversion to the Fontan circulation.

For the neonate or young infant where the left ventricle is deemed adequate to support the systemic circulation, balloon dilation of the left ventricular outflow tract has become the mainstay of initial therapy. With follow-up it is clear that the early results are comparable to earlier surgical outcomes, though there appears to be a higher incidence of aortic regurgitation when the valve is dilated with a balloon.[24–28] In the majority of patients, such regurgitation is well tolerated, at least for the first few years of life. Interventional cardiologists are very cautious not to oversize the balloon, since this introduces a greater chance of producing substantial regurgitation, which itself then requires further intervention. Should regurgitation ensue, then a neonatal Ross procedure is the treatment of choice.[29–31]. In general, this approach has a high rate of success, with the results in the early and medium terms being encouraging.

Those patients who present during the neonatal period or early infancy without cardiac failure present another challenge. In comparison to their older counterparts, the modest gradient seen across the valve in the early phase may progress fairly rapidly during the first one to two years of life, necessitating closer follow-up in this population.[32–35] If faced with this dilemma, it is advisable to repeat the echocardiogram every 2 to 3 months, until reassured that the rise in gradient is not rapidly progressive. A similar issue arises in those cases with combined aortic valvar stenosis and coarctation of the aorta. In this setting, the downstream obstruction results in an underestimation of the severity of the valvar stenosis, even in the presence of reasonable left ventricular function.

Again, close follow-up is warranted once the coarctation has been addressed.

Outlook in the Longer Term

Presentation during the neonatal period represents the severe end of the spectrum of this disease, with those presenting earliest usually having the most severe lesions. When the predominant lesion is stenosis, these children are likely to require further intervention in the future, in the form of further balloon dilation, while those with significant regurgitation will likely require replacement of the valve. Associated lesions such as endocardial fibroelastosis and mitral valvar disease, add to the morbidity in this group. The presence of significant endocardial fibroelastosis results in diastolic dysfunction and left atrial hypertension. To address this, some groups have attempted surgically to remove the thick peel of endocardial fibroelastosis, attempting to improve both left ventricular growth and diastolic function. The results of this strategy over the long term remain to be seen, and it has not yet been widely adopted.

AORTIC VALVAR DISEASE IN THE OLDER CHILD

Isolated Bifoliate, or Bicuspid, Aortic Valve

These children are asymptomatic. They typically present when the lesion is detected during routine evaluation, or after an episode of bacterial endocarditis. The findings at clinical examination consist of a high pitched ejection click that is heard at the lower left sternal border and at the apex, with some increase in intensity during expiration. The second heart sound is usually normal. An evaluation of the femoral pulses is essential to exclude associated aortic coarctation. Investigations reveal a normal electrocardiogram, chest radiograph, with the diagnosis being confirmed on echocardiography. Even though echocardiography is unnecessary to make the diagnosis, it is an essential part of the management in those cases with an asymptomatic and isolated bifoliate aortic valve (Figs. 44-18 and 44-19).

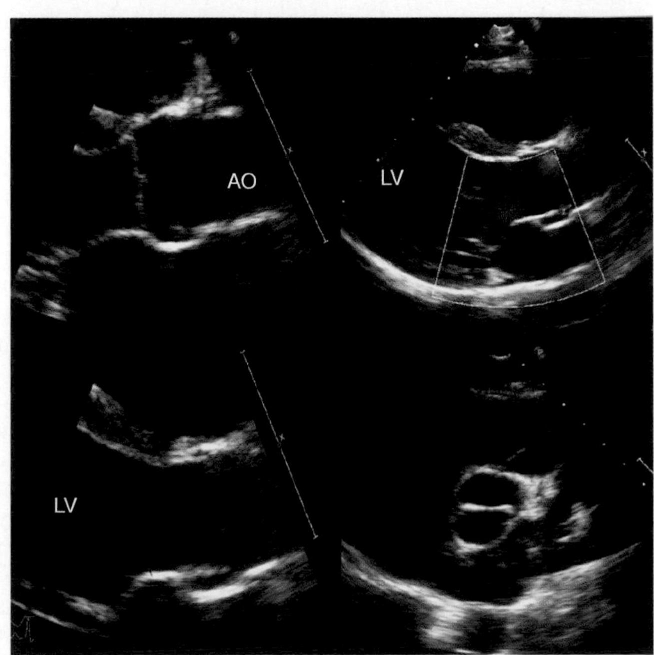

Figure 44-18 This image shows a bifoliate, or bicuspid, aortic valve with no associated aortic regurgitation. Note the thin leaflets and the horizontal line of closure. AO, aorta, LV, left ventricle.

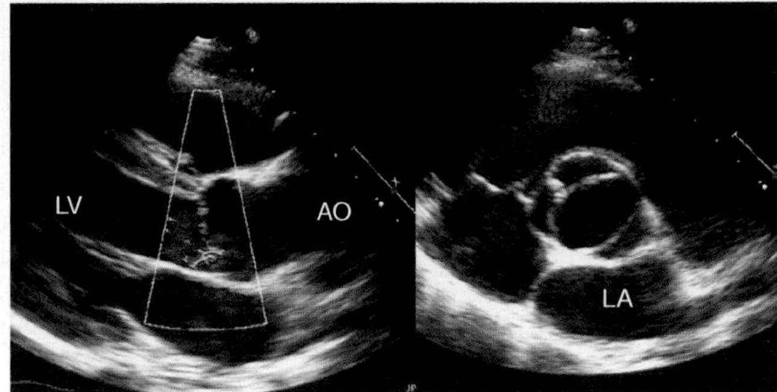

Figure 44-19 This bifoliate aortic valve is mildly regurgitant. Note the vestigial interleaflet triangle. AO, aorta; LA, left atrium; LV, left ventricle.

This relates to the fact that dilation of the aortic root can be seen in patients who do not develop stenosis or regurgitation early on in life. It is now recognised that these individuals have structural abnormalities of their aortic wall, which places them at higher risk for ongoing dilation of the aortic root, and eventual dissection.[36,37] Whether this can be prevented or delayed by β-blockade is still unclear. Because of this, these individuals should have an echocardiogram every couple of years to track the dimensions of their aortic roots, comparing the results to age-matched controls. This follow-up should continue into adult life.

Cases with Clinical Evidence of Aortic Valvar Stenosis

In this setting, the patient is usually referred for the evaluation of a heart murmur. It is important to distinguish murmurs emanating from the aortic valve from those produced by pulmonary valvar stenosis, which may be confusing to the untrained ear. The patients with aortic lesions are usually asymptomatic, as they have preserved left ventricular systolic function, the diastolic abnormalities not being of sufficient severity to cause symptoms. Congestive cardiac failure is rare, as with time the patients are able to stabilise their left ventricular mural stress by increasing mass. The physical examination depends on the severity of the stenosis. The peripheral pulses are usually normal in those patients with mild, and even moderate, stenosis. Those with significant stenosis have low volume, or plateau pulses. In some patients, the right carotid and brachial pulses have a rapid upstroke when compared to the left-sided pulses. This is due to transmission of the impulse towards the brachiocephalic artery. A systolic thrill may be felt in the right infraclavicular region, along the left sternal border in some, as well as over the carotid artery or suprasternal notch. The first heart sound is normal, and is frequently followed by a high pitched ejection click, which is best heard at the lower left sternal border, and may be maximal at the apex. This latter finding differentiates it from a click produced by the pulmonary valve, which is often lower pitched, and heard along the upper left sternal border. The second heart sound is usually normal, and the narrowly split, single or reversed splitting that may be identified in adults is uncommon in children. The reversed splitting occurs due to the significant inspiratory delay in the opening of the aortic valve in those with reduced left ventricular function. Clinical cardiomegaly is uncommon in the absence of associated aortic regurgitation, as the left ventricular internal dimension is not increased.

Although sudden death is more common in aortic stenosis than in other forms of congenital cardiac disease, the risk is small.[38] The danger of sudden death is confined to those with severe stenosis. The exact cause of the sudden death is uncertain, but ventricular arrhythmias following myocardial ischaemia may be the underlying problem.

Although syncope may occur after extreme effort with mild or moderate obstruction, it is usually found only in those with severe stenosis. It results from the inability of the left ventricle to increase its output appropriately with exercise. Auscultation reveals the click, and a long ejection systolic murmur with maximum intensity late in systole. Diastolic murmurs are heard if there is associated aortic regurgitation.

Investigations

Electrocardiogram

This shows a variable degree of left ventricular hypertrophy depending on the degree of severity.[39] Left ventricular voltages increases, with upright T waves which, with increased severity, many invert with associated depression of the ST segment in the infero-lateral leads. The presence of Q waves in the left ventricular leads is uncommon, and may suggest associated lesions. The electrical axis is usually normal.

Chest Radiograph

In the current era, it is probably unnecessary to request this investigation in a newly diagnosed case of aortic valvar stenosis. Dilations of the aortic root, and calcification in later years, however, are the features that might be identified if the procedure is performed.

Exercise Testing

The role and advisability of exercise testing remain a subject of debate. In those with mild and moderate stenosis, it is safe, but the interpretation of abnormalities is difficult, and they rarely guide treatment. The role of new depression of the ST segments on exercise is also uncertain.[40] While usually associated with higher resting gradients, and presumably reflecting a degree of exercise-induced subendocardial ischaemia, its relevance to decision-making remains poorly defined.

Echocardiography

This is currently the mainstay for the process of decision-making in children. The valvar morphology is best seen from the parasternal short-axis view (see Fig. 44-18), where the number of leaflets and their zones of apposition can be seen.[41] The parasternal long-axis view is currently favoured for measurement of the aortic root, from its left ventricular origin to the sinutubular junction (see Fig. 44-19). From a slightly more rightward location, the more distal ascending aorta can be imaged and measured. Unlike our adult counterparts, assessment of the absolute gradient is used as the basis for the timing of intervention, rather than the area of the orifice of the stenotic valve. This is for two reasons. First, outside the neonatal period and early infancy, the majority of children and adolescents have preserved, and even supernormal, left ventricular systolic function. This differs from adults, who may have mixed aortic valvar disease, with associated left ventricular dysfunction which invalidates the assessment of the pure gradient. In this setting, calculation of the area of the aortic valvar orifice is more reliable, using a modified Gorlin formula. Direct measurement of the area of the stenotic orifice by planimetry from the cross sectional echocardiogram is difficult because of its eccentric nature and the thickening of the leaflets. The continuity equation offers a theoretically satisfying method for measuring valvar area using echocardiography and Doppler.[42] Stroke volume in the left ventricular outflow tract is the same as that across the aortic valvar orifice. Consequently, the area of the valvar orifice can be calculated from:

$$A2 = \frac{A1V1}{V2}$$

where A2 is the area of the aortic value, A1 is the subaortic area, V2 is the aortic valvar velocity time integral, and V1 is the subaortic velocity time integral. Although its protagonists stress the usefulness of this method, it has inherent practical problems, and is not of proven clinical value in children.

The major source of error in using the continuity theorem lies in the difficulty in measuring accurately the left ventricular outflow tract. Doppler ultrasound seems to provide a workable method for assessing severity of stenosis. This is of particular importance in children, where the left ventricular outflow tract is smaller than in the adult, thus increasing the error, as the measurement has to be squared in the calculation. The other more practical issue is that, in the previous studies of natural history, calculations were based on peak-to-peak gradients derived at catheterisation, and not on valvar area. In general, for fully grown adolescents and adults, an area of the stenotic orifice of less than 1 cm^2 indicates significant stenosis, whereas for children this would vary considerably, due to the different ages and body surface area.

Measurement of the gradient across the aortic valve using continuous wave Doppler, therefore, is the current mainstay of timing for intervention, in conjunction with the presence of left ventricular hypertrophy. The peak instantaneous gradient across the left ventricular outflow tract, obtained from a combination of apical, suprasternal, and right parasternal locations, is also frequently used. The problem with this approach is that there is a poor correlation between the maximal instantaneous gradient and the peak-to-peak gradient as derived from catheterisation at lower gradients. This relates to the time difference between these events, with the peak-to-peak gradient occurring later than the maximal peak instantaneous gradient (Fig. 44-20).

Of note, the peak-to-peak gradient as assessed by haemodynamics is a non-physiological event, whereas the peak instantaneous gradient is physiological (Fig. 44-21). The other issue that compounds the problem is the concept of recovery of pressure. When stenosis is discrete, a jet rapidly looses its momentum, just distal to the obstruction, with some recovery of pressure downstream.[43] Doppler techniques measure the instantaneous drop in pressure across the valve, while at catheterisation the end of the catheter is invariably more distal to the obstruction. At that more distal location, there has already been some recovery of pressure, thus reducing the calculated gradient in pressure

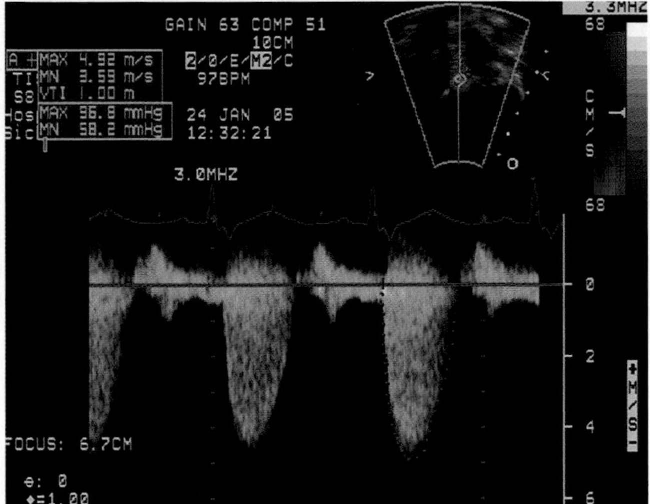

Figure 44-20 The tracing shows a gradient across the outflow tract demonstrated by continuous wave Doppler interrogation. This provides a combination of peak instantaneous and mean Doppler gradients.

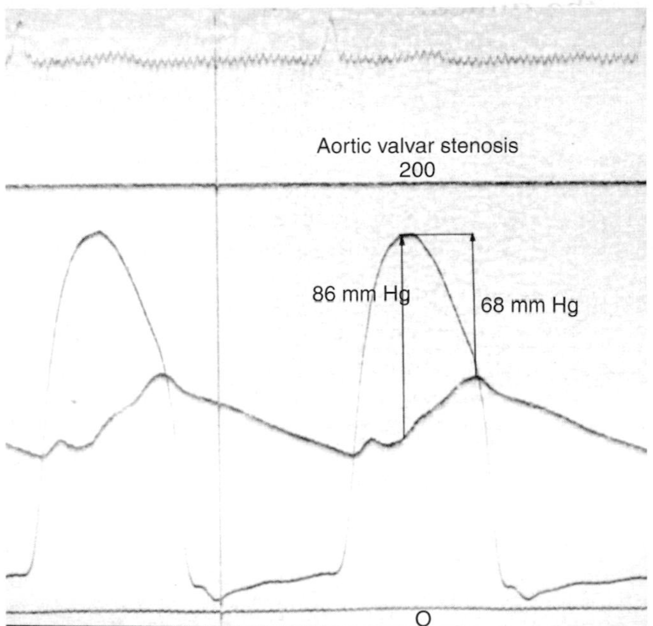

Figure 44-21 This pressure trace shows the difference between peak-to-peak and peak instantaneous measurements of pressure by catheterisation. Note that the peak-to-peak gradient is lower.

from immediately beyond the valve to the more distal site. As the stenosis becomes more severe, the aortic pressure trace shows a greater plateau, which results in an improved correlation between peak-to-peak and peak instantaneous gradients. To help overcome some of these limitations, it is possible to determine the mean aortic valvar gradient by planimetry of the Doppler spectral trace, with excellent correlation with results derived at catheterisation.

Other authors have provided regression equations that calculate a peak-to-peak gradient from the mean Doppler gradient in conjunction with the pulse pressure.[44] This is attractive, since it helps to accommodate those patients with mixed stenosis and regurgitation. A wide pulse pressure from aortic regurgitation, for example, reduces the calculated peak-to-peak gradients.

How does the clinician decide on the timing for intervention? In this current era, intervention for isolated aortic stenosis in children is invariably by balloon dilation. The timing varies from centre to centre, depending on the criterions used. It would be fair to state that intervention now takes place much earlier than was the case when cardiac catheterisation alone was used to establish the severity of the stenosis. In general, if there is a peak instantaneous gradient of more than 60 to 70 mm Hg, in the presence of left ventricular hypertrophy, then intervention is justified.

Cardiac Catheterisation

This is usually no longer performed to make the diagnosis, or to guide decision-making, but rather as an intervention when the decision has been made to treat.[45,46] The procedure may be performed antegradely in some infants, but more usually retrogradely. In older children, stripping of the balloon back and forth across the valve in diastole and systole is thought to contribute to valvar damage, and can be avoided by rapid ventricular pacing via a temporary wire placed in the right ventricle, thus lowering cardiac output and stroke volume. Oversizing of the balloon is avoided, as this results in a higher incidence of post-procedural valvar regurgitation. With current catheters having low profiles, the incidence of femoral arterial trauma is less common, though is still an ongoing morbidity, particularly in smaller children. In general, the decision to dilate the valve is made prior to commencing the catheterisation, as the estimated peak-to-peak gradient is always lower under general anaesthesia.

Surgical Intervention

In the more recent era, surgical aortic valvotomy is rarely used as the primary mode of treatment in children and young adolescents with aortic valvar stenosis. Although the results of surgical intervention are comparable to those achieved by balloon dilation, the latter technique can be performed as an outpatient with a relatively low morbidity, even in the neonatal period.[24–29]

AORTIC REGURGITATION

Pathophysiology

There is an increase in both preload and afterload when the aortic valve is regurgitant. While the cause of the increased preload is obvious, the change in afterload is related to the law of Laplace, which states that mural tension is related to the product of pressure and dimension divided by mural thickness. This is the basis of the equation that is used to calculate mural stress or afterload. As the left ventricular dimension increases with aortic regurgitation, so does the mural thickness in an attempt to normalise mural stress or afterload. With increasing severity of aortic regurgitation, the left ventricular hypertrophy cannot keep up with the dilation, resulting in an increase in left ventricular afterload. In general the left ventricular filling pressures are usually normal, as the left ventricle acts as a very compliant pump. The degree of regurgitation decreases with exercise as the heart rate increases and the peripheral resistance falls. As a result, there is an increase in cardiac output without a significant increase in end-diastolic pressure or volume.

Clinical Features

Symptomatic aortic regurgitation is very uncommon during infancy and childhood. Despite this, asymptomatic aortic regurgitation is encountered in those with a congenitally abnormal aortic valve, or as an acquired lesion in patients with associated subaortic stenosis, ventricular septal defect and aortic valvar prolapse, or as a result of infective endocarditis. Symptoms from chronic regurgitation result from left ventricular dysfunction, with exertional dyspnoea, pulmonary oedema, and occasionally heart failure. Angina is uncommon unless there is an abnormality of the coronary arterial orifices.

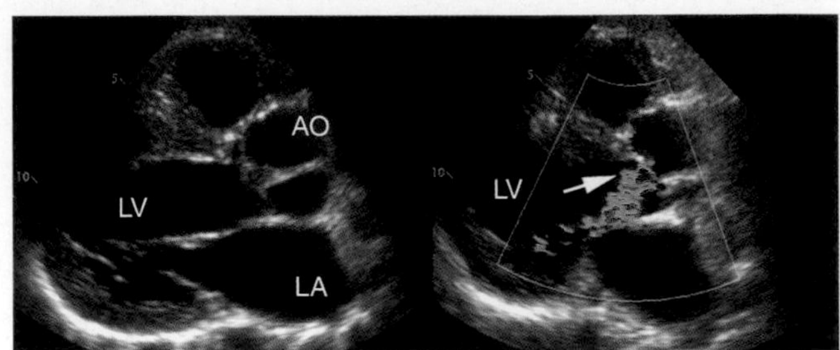

Figure 44-22 The parasternal long-axis view demonstrates thickened leaflets of the regurgitant aortic valve. The *arrow* points to the site for measurement of the ratio of width of the jet to the aorta. AO, aorta, LA, left atrium; LV, left ventricle.

Physical Examination

Except in the presence of cardiac failure, the pulse pressure reflects the degree of aortic regurgitation. The carotid arterial pulsations are usually easily visible in those with severe regurgitation. The head of the patient may nod in time with systole, a feature called the sign of de Musset, who in this instance was the patient. The pulses have an abrupt upstroke with rapid collapse, the water hammer pulse of Watson, or Corrigan's pulse. The praecordial examination is normal in mild regurgitation, albeit that as the severity increases, and the left ventricle dilates, there is evidence of a hyperdynamic and laterally displaced apical impulse. In cases with a dilated aortic root, a diastolic thrill may be present, while those with significant regurgitation may have a systolic thrill due to the increased stroke volume.

Auscultation reveals an early diastolic murmur, which is heard along the upper left sternal border, being accentuated when the patient is sitting up. As well, interventions that increase the systolic pressure, such as squatting, also accentuate the murmur of aortic insufficiency. A systolic ejection murmur can also be heard, and is related to the increased stroke volume across the left ventricular outflow tract. A mid-diastolic murmur at the apex, the Austin–Flint murmur, may be heard. It is related to the narrowing of the mitral orifice due to a sudden rise in the left ventricular end-diastolic pressure. In cases with left ventricular dysfunction, it may also be possible to hear a third sound.

Investigations

Electrocardiogram

The electrocardiographic changes depend on severity and duration of regurgitation. Voltages in the left ventricular leads increase, with deep S waves in leads V1, and R waves in leads I, AVL, V5 and V6. The T waves usually remain tall and upright until left ventricular dysfunction has occurred, when depression and inversion of the ST segment is present. Unless there is disease of the aortic root involving the coronary arterial orifices, Q waves due to dilation of the cavity precede the tall R waves in the left ventricular leads. Once regurgitation is severe and long established, so-called P mitrale is sometimes seen on the electrocardiogram.

The Chest Radiograph

The chest radiograph shows cardiomegaly, with left atrial dilation and prominence of the ascending aorta and aortic knuckle. The mildest lesions are associated with a normal chest radiograph.

Echocardiography

This technique is used to detect the presence and severity of aortic regurgitation, in conjunction with an evaluation of left ventricular function. The morphology of the aortic valve can be assessed in the praecordial short-axis view, as well as the relationship of the leaflets to the coronary arterial orifices. The presence of associated left-sided pathology can be determined, as well as an associated ventricular septal defect when this is the mechanism for regurgitation.

The severity of the aortic regurgitation is best assessed by Doppler echocardiography. Colour flow Doppler is useful for providing a semiquantitative measurement of degree, as the size of the jet (Fig. 44-22) just distal to the leaflets has a reasonable correlation with regurgitant volume.[47,48] Other measurements to be made are the pressure half-time of aortic regurgitation, and the degree of reversal of diastolic flow in the descending aorta at the level of the diaphragm. The shorter the pressure half-time, the more significant is the regurgitation. The problem in children is that any measurement of time is related to the heart rate, which limits its usefulness. As well, if there is associated aortic regurgitation and left ventricular diastolic dysfunction, the pressure half-time may be short due to the raised end-diastolic pressure. Reversal of aortic holodiastolic flow at the level of the diaphragm is consistent with significant regurgitation, but cannot be used in isolation to assess severity (Fig. 44-23). Quantitative methods to assess true regurgitant volume, or the effective area of the regurgitant orifice, can be used in adolescents,[47] but in small children the standard error is probably too great for this technique to be of practical value.

An assessment of left ventricular size and function is best achieved through the use of M-mode and cross sectional echocardiography. M-mode echocardiography is very good for assessing end-diastolic and end-systolic dimensions, but not for ejection fraction. Fractional shortening, along with Vcf and Vcfc, can be used to follow left ventricular function, as they are not so dependent on shape. For an accurate calculation of ejection fraction, either the biplane Simpson's rule, or three-dimensional echocardiographic assessment of left ventricular function, can be used. These methods allow for the changes in shape that occur with left ventricular dilation.

Magnetic Resonance Imaging

Although this technique is used less frequently in the evaluation of aortic regurgitation, it provides quantitative measurement of the regurgitant fraction that is comparable to echocardiographic data.[49] As well, this technique would be advantageous in those individuals with a poor ultrasound window.

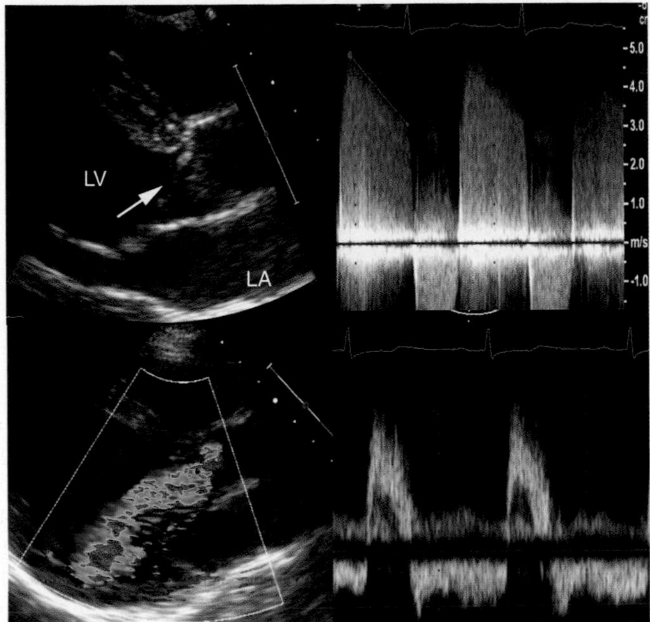

Figure 44-23 This group of images is from a patient with combined valvar and subvalvar stenosis (*arrow*) and associated significant aortic regurgitation. Note the holodiastolic reversal of flow in the abdominal aorta, shown in lower right image, and the short pressure half time seen in the upper right panel. The lower left panel shows the anatomy of the regurgitant jet, revealing the PISA, the vena contracta, and the proximal and distal jets. LA, left atrium; LV, left ventricle.

Cardiac Catheterisation

Cardiac catheterisation and angiocardiography play a very small role in the evaluation of the patient with aortic regurgitation, particularly as associated coronary arterial disease is exceedingly rare in this population. Angiographic grading of regurgitation is subjective at best, and left ventricular function is better evaluated by either echocardiography or magnetic resonance imaging.

Timing of Intervention

This is a difficult enough problem in adults, so it presents even more of a challenge in the younger population. In adults, if there is evidence of left ventricular dysfunction with an ejection fraction of less than 55%, then replacement of the valve is indicated.[50–52] The problem is more challenging in patients with preserved left ventricular ejection fraction. Part of the problem is that left ventricular ejection fraction is significantly dependent on afterload, being somewhat less influenced by preload. As a result, exercise assessment of left ventricular function, as well as tests that take end-systolic stress into consideration, has been proposed. When using resting measurements, a left ventricular internal dimension in systole equal to or greater than 55 mm, or 25 mm/m,[2] has been proposed to identify those patients who have improved survival after valvar replacement. At present, comparable data is not available for children. Consequently, many rely on the presence of symptoms, or the development of signs of uncompensated left ventricular dilation, such as a rising end-systolic volume index or worsening ejection fraction, as indications for intervention in children and adolescents.

Medical Treatment

Although afterload reduction has been disappointing in patients with mitral valvar regurgitation, there have been some encouraging results in patients with aortic valvar regurgitation. The theory behind this has been to reduce left ventricular volume, regurgitant volume and afterload, in an attempt to preserve left ventricular function and reduce left ventricular mass. Despite these encouraging results, some recent data has disputed this approach, failing to demonstrate any benefit in the long term with regards to delaying time to surgical intervention.[53]

Surgical Intervention

Once the decision has been made to treat a patient with aortic regurgitation, the decision must be made as to whether to replace the valve with a mechanical prosthesis, or to proceed to the Ross procedure. The former approach is challenging in young patients, due to problems with mismatch between the aortic root and the available prostheses, so the Ross procedure has been favoured in this population.[30,31] This latter approach also has the added advantage of not requiring anticoagulation, which is a significant issue in the active child and adolescent. The recent results of the Ross procedure are encouraging even for the smallest patient, albeit that follow-up in the medium term has identified the problem of progressive aortic root dilation and regurgitation, particularly in those having bifoliate aortic valves.[54,55] Although repair using pericardial extension of the leaflets has been used, the results are still somewhat disappointing.[56,57] The exception to this has been in stenotic valves that have been torn following balloon dilation, where the results of subsequent surgical repair are encouraging.[58]

AORTIC–LEFT VENTRICULAR TUNNEL

Although described as a tunnel, implying that it has length and two openings, this lesion is more correctly described as a defect. The defect is produced by unhinging of the leaflet guarding the right coronary aortic sinus (see Fig. 44-14), and is usually separate from the right coronary arterial orifice,[59] although the artery can take origin from the aortic end of the defect. Free reflux occurs from the aorta to the left ventricle, producing aneurysmal dilation of the right aortic sinus, dilation of the left ventricle, and widening of the ascending aorta. In time, the whole aortic root becomes dilated, with secondary valvar regurgitation. The lesion may be associated with aortic valvar stenosis, or abnormalities of the origins of the coronary arteries. It should be considered as a differential diagnosis in any child who presents with severe aortic regurgitation in infancy or in the newborn period. The tunnel can produce cardiac failure in the infant, but more often the patient presents with well-compensated and impressive aortic regurgitation and dilation, with hypertrophy of the left ventricle. The physical signs suggest severe aortic regurgitation, with loud aortic valvar closure and a systolic thrill at the left and right sternal edges, but the murmur tends to be continuous. The dilated ascending aorta may be palpable on the right side of the chest. On the chest radiograph, the dilated right aortic sinus may protrude on to the left heart border, and the aorta is enlarged. Diagnosis can be made by cross sectional

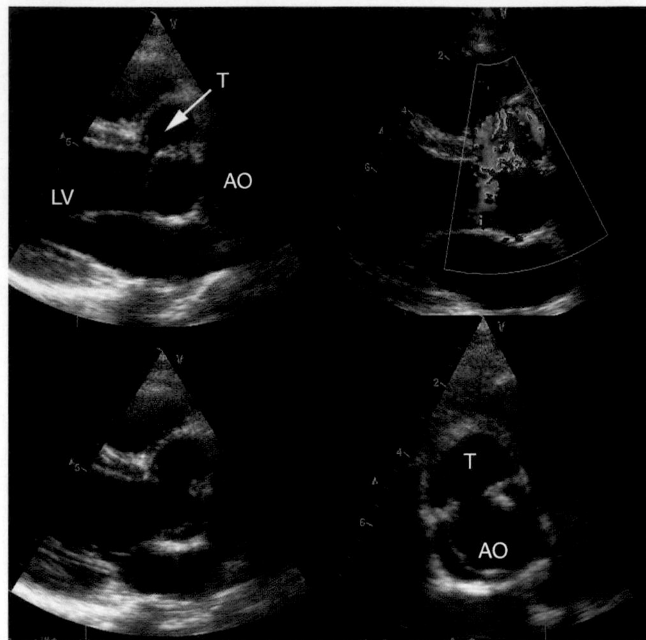

Figure 44-24 These echocardiographic images show an aortic-left ventricular tunnel. Note the aortic regurgitation arising above the valvar leaflets. AO, aorta; LV, left ventricle; T, tunnel.

echocardiography, and in the majority of cases angiocardiography is unnecessary. In the older child, it is easy to confuse the abnormality with rupture of the sinus of Valsalva (Fig. 44-24). Surgical repair is carried out as soon as the diagnosis is made in the hope of preventing valvar regurgitation. Usually, however, the regurgitation persists despite closure, and replacement of the aortic valve may be necessary.

SUPRAVALVAR AORTIC STENOSIS

Patients with isolated supravalvar stenosis rarely present in the neonatal period. More usually, infants and children present in a similar way to those with valvar stenosis, and indeed some degree of supravalvar stenosis may be present in those with predominantly valvar stenosis. Particularly when associated with familial forms, or overt Williams syndrome, supravalvar stenosis may be rapidly progressive, and careful follow-up is required in all such patients. The physical signs are also similar to those encountered with valvar stenosis as described above, with the exception that an ejection click is rarely heard on auscultation. In those with Williams syndrome, there will be the typical facial appearance, but careful examination of the entire vascular system should be performed to exclude significant stenosis of the thoracic or abdominal aorta or their branches. Careful evaluation of blood pressures in the limbs, and auscultation of the abdomen, is an essential part of the clinical examination.

Investigations

Electrocardiogram

This will show left ventricular hypertrophy with or without strain. As mentioned earlier, stenosis of the coronary arterial orifices is not uncommon, and repolarisation abnormalities, such as inversion of the T waves or changes in the ST segments out of proportion to the degree of stenosis, should raise the suspicion of impaired coronary arterial perfusion.

Chest Radiograph

This is rarely diagnostic. Unlike valvar stenosis, however, the ascending aorta is never dilated.

Echocardiography

This is the diagnostic test of choice, but the sonographer must be alert to the possibility, otherwise a spurious diagnosis of valvar stenosis is easily made. The aortic valvar leaflets are usually thin and mobile, but are tethered at the sinutubular junction, exaggerating the usual difference in calibre between the sinuses and the diameter of the junction itself. Consequently, Doppler studies will demonstrate accelerated flow and turbulence beginning at this level (Fig. 44-25). Because the diameter of the ascending aorta is often also small, there is a tendency for spectral Doppler to overestimate the gradient measured invasively, and decision-making on the basis of Doppler-derived gradients is difficult. As meXntioned above, no examination is complete without detailed assessment of the anatomy of the coronary arterial orifices and flow, as well as examination of all the branches of the aortic arch and abdominal vessels, the latter usually requiring specialist abdominal ultrasonic studies.

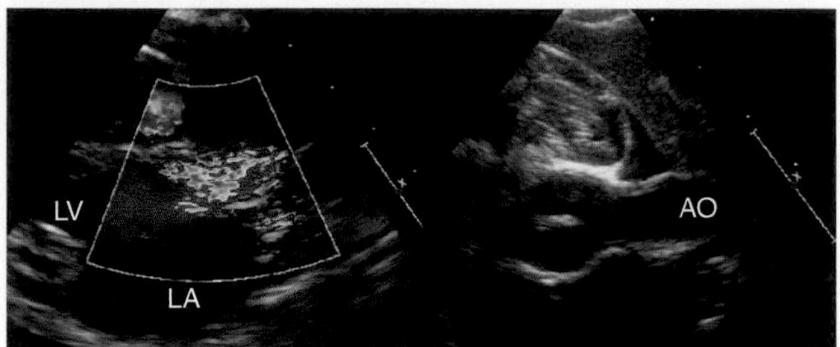

Figure 44-25 This panel demonstrates supravalvar aortic stenosis, in association with hypoplasia or the ascending aorta. Note the colour Doppler turbulence starts in the supravalvar region. AO, aorta; LA, left atrium; LV, left ventricle.

Treatment

There is no role for transcatheter intervention in the treatment of the supravalvar stenosis itself, although treatment of thoracic and abdominal aortic stenosis and stenosis of the branches may be amenable to balloon dilation and stenting. Thus, surgical repair is the mainstay of treatment, and usually involves insertion of a patch or patches across the sinutubular junction, with variable extension into the ascending aorta and aortic arch. The results are good, and reoperation is rare.

SUBVALVAR AORTIC STENOSIS

As described in our section devoted to morphology, a variety of lesions can obstruct the subaortic outflow tract, with or without a co-existing ventricular septal defect. When there is an interventricular communication, then postero-cephalad deviation of the muscular outlet septum is usually the most important lesion. This is considered in Chapter 28. Obstruction can also be

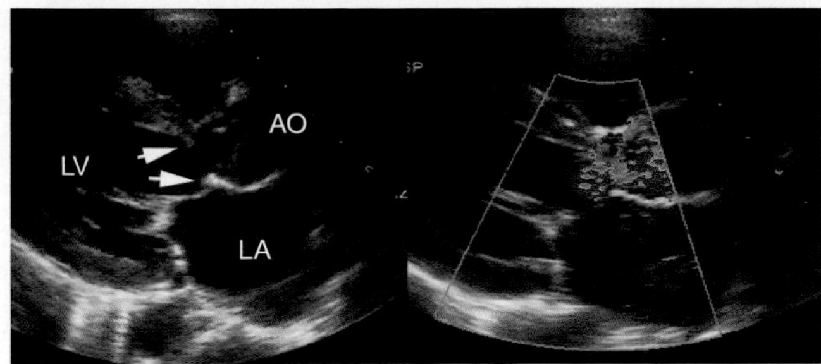

Figure 44-26 The image shows fibromuscular subaortic stenosis (*arrows*). Note the distance of the fibromuscular ridge from the leaflets of the valve. There is extension of the shelf onto the aortic leaflet of the mitral leaflet. The colour Doppler trace shows that the turbulence start at the level of the subaortic obstruction. AO, aorta; LA, left atrium; LV, left ventricle.

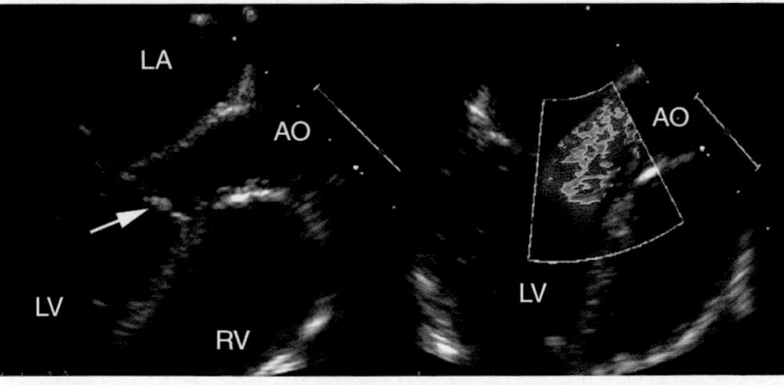

Figure 44-27 This transoesophageal echocardiogram is from a patient with subaortic stenosis produced by accessory leaflet tissue derived from the mitral valve (*arrow*). AO, aorta; LA, left atrium; LV, left ventricle; RV, right ventricle.

produced by hypertrophy of the ventricular septum, as seen in hypertrophic cardiomyopathy (see Chapter 54), by anomalous tissue tags derived from the membranous septum or the leaflets of the atrioventricular valves, or by anomalous attachment of the tension apparatus of the left atrioventricular valve (see Fig. 44-10). The last two are more likely to be found when there is also a ventricular septal defect, or in the setting of common atrioventricular junction and deficient atrioventricular septation.

When the ventricular septum is intact, the most significant lesion is the so-called subvalvar ridge (Fig. 44-26). This lesion has been described in many ways, and has been the subject of multiple investigations. Although often termed membranous, almost always the lesion is a firm fibrous and muscular shelf that encircles the outflow tract in diaphragmatic fashion (see Figs. 44-11 and 44-26). The ridge often extends to be attached to the aortic valvar leaflets themselves, and overlies the left bundle branch as it crosses the ventricular septum. The position of the shelf can vary with regard to its proximity to the valvar leaflets. If extensive, it can produce so-called tunnel stenosis. In florid cases, there is a marked abnormality in the alignment between the plane of the aortic root and the ventricular septum. This has been promoted as a potential cause of the malformation, although whether this is cause or effect is far from clear. Nonetheless, subaortic ridges are not congenital in that the vast majority are acquired after birth, albeit sometimes in the setting of other congenital cardiac defects.

Clinical Features

Symptoms are uncommon with this subvalvar stenosis, even when the narrowing is severe. Occasionally, however, syncope and presyncope may occur. If undiagnosed and presenting in middle life, congestive cardiac failure, dyspnoea and syncope have been described.

The physical signs are similar to aortic valvar stenosis with a carotid thrill, a displaced and forceful left ventricular apical impulse, and an aortic ejection systolic murmur maximal in the aortic area and down the left sternal edge, conducted to the carotid arteries. As with supravalvar stenosis, an ejection click will not be heard, and further clinical differentiation may be possible by finding the murmur to be maximal at the lower left sternal edge. There may be an early diastolic murmur if complicated by significant aortic regurgitation.

Investigations

Electrocardiogram

This will show varying degrees of left ventricular hypertrophy, normally without a Q wave. Interestingly, upright T waves are preserved even with quite severe obstruction, and other abnormalities of repolarisation are rare.

Chest Radiograph

This is often normal, although enlargement of left ventricle and left atrium may be present.

Echocardiography

Cross sectional examination in the parasternal long axis shows the characteristic ridge in the outflow tract (see Fig. 44-26). The full extent of the ridge may be difficult to assess from this approach. In older children and adults, transoesophageal interrogation demonstrates this lesion more fully (Fig. 44-27), and is probably a better way to identify associated lesions of the mitral and aortic valves. Increasingly, three-dimensional echocardiography is being used to demonstrate the nature of the lesion. In those with good transthoracic windows (Fig. 44-28), Doppler ultrasound is used to assess the extent of aortic regurgitation and the degree of obstruction within the left ventricular outflow tract. As in those with aortic valvar stenosis, peak velocities in the ascending aorta are the most reliable indicators of severity, although significant aortic regurgitation and obstruction over long segments may invalidate the Bernoulli equation, as already described for supravalvar lesions.

Assessment and Treatment

Because of the progressive nature of the disorder, and the frequent development of a regurgitant aortic valve, surgery is usually advised at gradients lower than those used to determine intervention for valvar stenosis. Indeed, the presence of more than mild regurgitation is often used as justification, irrespective of gradient. In the absence of significant regurgitation, a mean gradient of 30 mm Hg is a reasonable cut-off, particularly if a documented evolution is available. There was a trend towards surgery with much lower gradients, in the hope that this would avoid regurgitation, and perhaps obviate the need for reoperation. This did not, however, prove to be the case.[60]

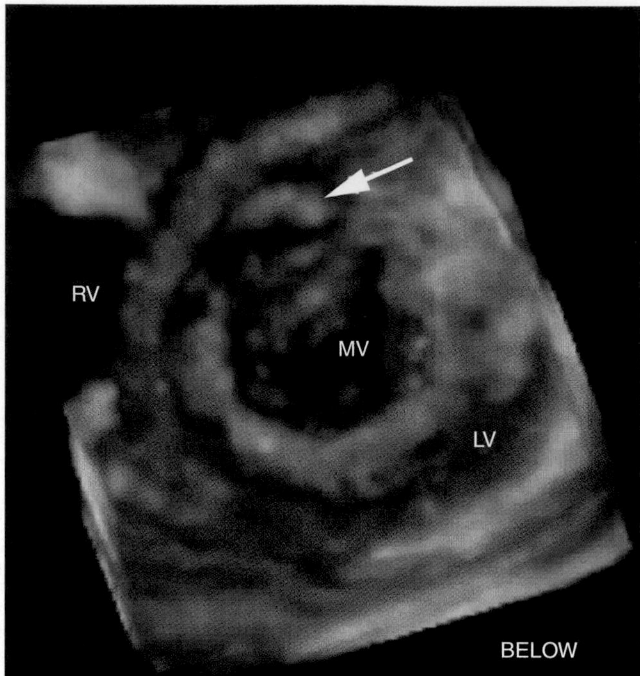

Figure 44-28 The three-dimensional echocardiogram shows fibromuscular subaortic stenosis (*arrow*), as seen from below the left ventricular outflow tract. Note that in comparison to the cross sectional counterpart, shown in Figure 44-26, the three-dimensional reconstruction reveals the full extent of the obstruction. LV, left ventricle; MV, mitral valve; RV, right ventricle.

Recurrence of the fixed obstruction may be a problem in as many as one-third of patients, but more recent reports, usually describing more extensive associated septal myectomy, suggest this risk is closer to 5% to 10%. Those with a tunnel obstruction are at particular risk, and ultimately many will require enlargement of the aortic root using the Konno procedure, with or without replacement of the valve.

The complete reference list can be found on the companion Expert Consult web site at www.expertconsult.com.

ANNOTATED REFERENCES

- Anderson RH: Demystifying the anatomic arrangement of the aortic valve: Editorial comment. Eur J Cardiothorac Surg 2006;29:1006–1007.

  The latest of a series of publications showing that the leaflets of the aortic valve are suspended in semilunar fashion within the aortic root, making it difficult to describe any part of the root consistently in terms of an annulus.

- McKay R, Smith A, Leung MP, et al: Morphology of the ventriculoaortic junction in critical aortic stenosis: Implications for haemodynamic function and clinical management. J Thorac Cardiovasc Surg 1992;104:434–442.
- Angelini A, Ho SY, Anderson RH, et al: The morphology of the normal aortic valve as compared with the aortic valve having two leaflets. J Thorac Cardiovasc Surg 1989;98:362–367.
- Leung MP, McKay R, Smith A, et al: Critical aortic stenosis in early infancy: Anatomic and echocardiographic substrates of successful open valvotomy. J Thorac Cardiovasc Surg 1991;101:526–535.

  A series of morphological investigations showing that the anatomy of the malformed valves is best determined by examining them from beneath, identifying the interleaflet triangles beneath the peripheral attachments of the zones of apposition between the leaflets, these being vestigial in the setting of so-called bicuspid and unicuspid and unicommissural valves.

- Gewilling M, Daenen W, Dumoulin M, vans der Hauwaert T: Rheologic genesis of discrete subvalvular aortic stenosis: A Doppler echocardiographic study. Ann Thorac Surg 1992;19:818–824.

  An important early study showing the influence of abnormal flow in promoting the formation of the obstructive subaortic shelf.

- McBride KL, Pignatelli R, Lewin M, et al: Inheritance analysis of congenital left ventricular outflow tract obstruction malformations: Segregation, multiplex relative risk, and heritability. Am J Med Genet 2005;134A:180–186.

  One of the recent series of papers establishing the genetic background to the occurrence of obstructive lesions within the left ventricular outflow tract.

- Mäkikallio K, McElhinney DB, Levine JC, et al: Fetal aortic valve stenosis and the evolution of hypoplastic left heart syndrome. Circulation 2006;113:1401–1405.
- Selamet Tierney ES, Wald RM, McElhinney DB, et al: Changes in left heart hemodynamics after technically successful in-utero aortic valvuloplasty. Ultrasond Obstet Gynecol 2007;30:715–720.

  The papers describe the ongoing experience obtained at Boston Children's Hospital in fetal intervention for aortic valvar stenosis.

- Lofland GK, McCrindle BW, Williams WG, et al: Critical aortic stenosis in the neonate: A multi-institutional study of management, outcomes, and risk factors. Congenital Heart Surgeons Society. J Thorac Cardiovasc Surg 2001;121:10–27.
- McCrindle BW, Blackstone EH, Williams WG, et al: Are outcomes of surgical versus transcatheter balloon valvotomy equivalent in neonatal critical aortic stenosis? Circulation 2001;104:1-152–1-158.

  Important results emanating from analysis of the large series of cases collected on the basis of the cooperative efforts of the Congenital Heart Surgeons Society.

- Hraska V, Krajci M, Haun CH, et al: Ross and Ross-Konno procedure in children and adolescents: Mid-term results. Eur J Cardiothorac Surg 2004;25:742–747.

  Results reported from a single centre showing the excellent outcomes that now can be obtained by using the Ross procedure in young children with aortic valvar disease.

- Weidman WH, Blount SG Jr, Dushane JW, et al: Clinical course in aortic stenosis. Circulation 1997;56:1-47–1-56.

  The important follow-up of the initial study done to establish the natural history of aortic valvar stenosis.

- Asante-Korang A, Anderson RH: Echocardiographic assessment of the aortic valve and left ventricular outflow tract. Cardiol Young 2005;15(suppl 1):27–36.

  A recent review emphasising the significance of echocardiography in the assessment of the stenotic left ventricular outflow tract.

- Pedra CAC, Sidhu R, McCrindle BW, et al: Outcomes after balloon dilation of congenital aortic stenosis in children and adolescents. Cardiol Young 2004;14:315–321.

  A review of the extensive experience at the Hospital for Sick Children in Toronto, emphasising the excellence of results now obtainable using balloon dilation of the congenitally stenotic aortic valve.

- Ho SY, Muriago M, Cook AC, et al: Surgical anatomy of aorto-left ventricular tunnel. Ann Thorac Surg 1998;65:509–514.

  A morphologic study describing the true nature of the so-called aorto-left ventricular tunnel, in reality a defect due to dehiscence of the attachement of the aortic valvar leaflet from its supporting valvar sinus.

CHAPTER 45

Congenital Anomalies of the Coronary Arteries

ALAN H. FRIEDMAN and NORMAN H. SILVERMAN

In this chapter, we will address the various congenital coronary arterial anomalies that may be found in the otherwise structurally normal heart. The coronary arterial circulations found specifically with major cardiac structural anomalies will be discussed in the respective chapters elsewhere in this textbook. Similarly, those abnormalities of the coronary arteries that are acquired or associated with diseases will be discussed separately in their respective chapters.

INCIDENCE AND PREVALENCE

Anomalies of the coronary arteries are rare, occurring in 0.3% to 1.3% of one autopsy series.[1] The prevalence, however, is extremely difficult to estimate, as this depends upon accurate recognition and specific identification. This task is complicated by the occurrence of coronary arterial anomalies that, in many individuals, do not lead to symptoms, morbidity, or mortality. In fact, precise diagnosis may escape notice both during life and postmortem.

MORPHOLOGY

The normal coronary arterial anatomy was well described by James[2] (Fig. 45-1). Two arterial orifices are placed, usually relatively centrally, in the right and left sinuses of Valsalva. The right coronary artery arises from the right sinus of Valsalva. Having entered the atrioventricular groove, it sends an infundibular branch anteriorly, and then courses backward and inferiorly, terminating in the majority of hearts in the inferior interventricular groove. In approximately 50% of people, there is a separate origin of the infundibular branch.[3] The main stem of the left coronary artery arises from the left sinus of Valsalva, emerging perpendicularly for a few millimetres. It then bifurcates into anterior interventricular and circumflex branches. The former courses in the anterior interventricular groove toward the cardiac apex, while the latter courses around the left atrioventricular groove and, in one-tenth of individuals, gives rise to the inferior interventricular artery, often then continuing to supply the diaphragmatic surface of the right ventricle. In 1% of people, there are separate origins of the circumflex and anterior interventricular arteries from the left sinus.[3]

When both right and circumflex coronary arteries supply a branch to the inferior interventricular groove, the system is said to be balanced. More usually, in 90% of individuals, it is the right coronary artery that supplies one large or two smaller branches to this groove, with no contribution from the circumflex artery. This is called right coronary arterial dominance. In the left dominant system, as already described, the converse is true. All three variations of coronary arterial supply to the inferior interventricular groove and the diaphragmatic surface of the hearts are considered to be normal (Fig. 45-2).

The left and right coronary arteries provide branches superiorly to the atriums, and inferiorly to the ventricles. The major branches remain superficial, and are visible through the epicardium until they terminate in broom-like arborisations that penetrate the myocardium. Over the left ventricle, these penetrating arteries proceed perpendicularly through the wall, being occluded by ventricular contraction. In consequence, the left ventricular myocardium is perfused predominately during diastole.

MORPHOGENESIS

The normal development of the coronary arteries is well proven, and provides the context in which the various anomalies and abnormalities can be understood. When myocardial cells are first observed to contract, there is no defined coronary circulation. The cells are loosely assembled, being bathed in the blood which they pump. The walls of the heart condense in gradual fashion, initially with persistence of an extensive trabeculated luminal meshwork.

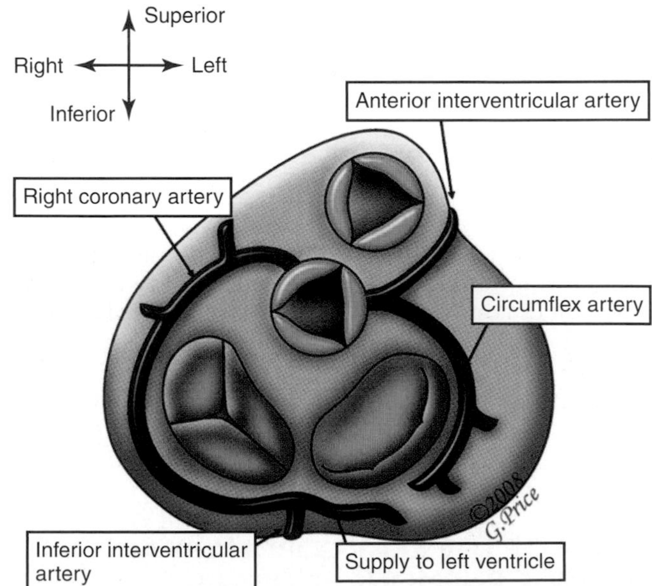

Figure 45-1 The cartoon shows the course of the normal coronary arteries as would be seen relative to the cardiac short axis as viewed from the cardiac apex. In the example shown, the inferior interventricular artery is taking origin from the right coronary artery, which then continues to supply the diaphragmatic surface of the left ventricle. This is the so-called right dominant arrangement.

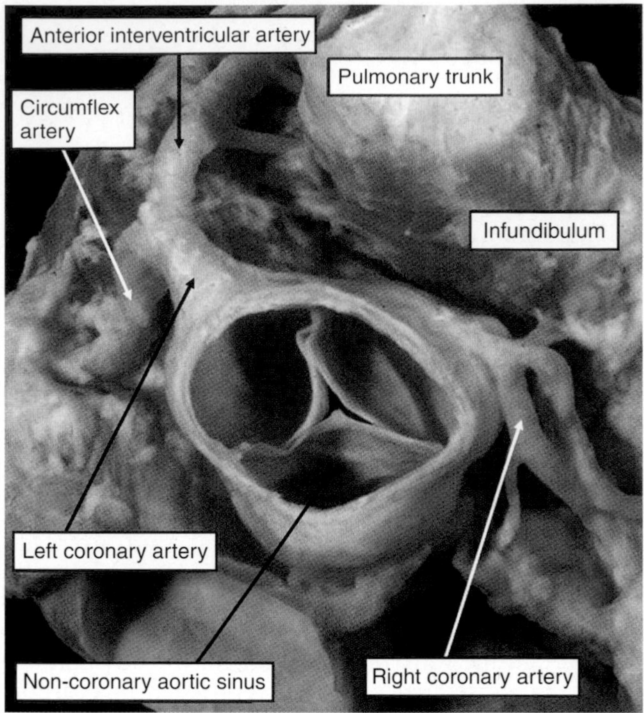

Figure 45-2 The dissection shows the normal origin of the coronary arteries from the aortic root, the heart positioned with the diaphragmatic surface inferior, and with the dissection viewed from the atrial aspect. Note that the coronary arteries arise from the aortic sinuses that are adjacent to the pulmonary trunk.

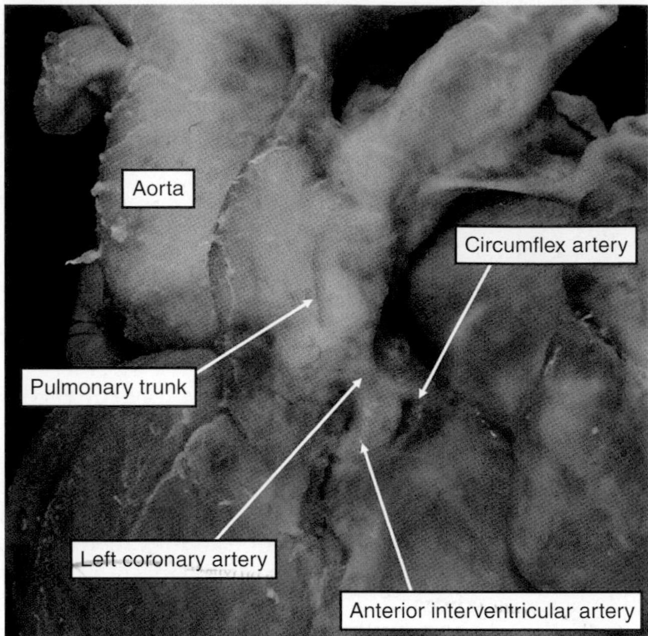

Figure 45-3 In this specimen, the left coronary artery takes its origin from one of the sinuses of the pulmonary trunk, and then branches to give rise to the anterior interventricular and circumflex arteries in normal fashion.

Early studies[4] had suggested that the coronary arteries themselves appeared as buds from the developing roots of both the aorta and the pulmonary trunk. It was subsequently shown that the coronary arteries originate specifically from the sinuses adjacent to the pulmonary trunk, which have a particular spatial configuration such that there is a positive transverse and a negative longitudinal curvature.[5] This has an effect on the wall tension whereby it is increased, perhaps acting as a stimulus for coronary bud development. The distal coronary arteries develop from a network of capillaries originating in the epicardium, with this system then sending major branches into the aortic sinuses.[6]

The numerous anomalies of the coronary arteries can then be well explained on the basis of abnormal patterns of morphogenesis. For example, there can be rudimentary persistence of an embryological coronary arterial structure, failure of normal coronary arterial development, failure of the normal atrophic process of development, or misplacement of connection of an otherwise normal coronary artery.[7] As a result, anomalies include abnormal origin, abnormal course, abnormal number, abnormal orifices, and abnormal connections or communications. It is these variations, along with their associated pathophysiology, diagnosis and management, which we discuss in the paragraphs which follow.

ORIGIN OF THE LEFT CORONARY ARTERY FROM THE PULMONARY TRUNK

Incidence

Origin of the left coronary artery from the pulmonary trunk (Fig. 45-3) is one of the more common coronary arterial abnormalities encountered in children. Also referred to as anomalous left coronary artery from the pulmonary artery, this variation occurs in from 1 in 250 to 1 in 400 of all congenitally malformed hearts, with an overall incidence of approximately 1 in 300,000 children.[8] This anomaly is seen with greater frequency in boys than it is in girls, with the ratio being 2.3 to 1.[9]

Pathophysiology

In the fetus with the origin of the left coronary artery from the pulmonary trunk, the myocardium, valves, and vessels otherwise develop quite normally. The perfusion pressure for the coronary arteries is the arterial pressure in the arterial trunk supplying these vessels minus the pressure of the chamber receiving the coronary venous flow. As the myocardium is contracting during systole, most flow occurs during diastole. Thus, in the normal situation, the coronary perfusion pressure is the aortic diastolic pressure minus the pressure in the right atrium. During fetal development, the diastolic pressure is nearly identical in the pulmonary arteries and the aorta. Thus, the coronary arterial perfusion in the fetus with the origin of the left coronary artery from the pulmonary trunk is virtually the same as in the normal fetus.

After birth, as long as the pulmonary arterial pressure remains at or near systemic levels, the left ventricular myocardium supplied by the anomalous artery remains well perfused. As the pulmonary vascular resistance, and subsequently the pressure, in the pulmonary trunk falls postnatally, the perfusion of the left ventricle becomes vulnerable, the period during which pressure in the left coronary artery exceeds intramural left ventricular pressure becoming shorter. This circulatory handicap reduces left ventricular function, and raises left ventricular end-diastolic pressure. In time, there may be a reversal of flow through the left coronary artery should the pressure in the pulmonary arteries fall below that of the left ventricle. This reverse flow leads to the phenomenon referred to as coronary arterial steal, which can lead to further ischaemia of the ventricular myocardium. When the left coronary artery originates from the pulmonary trunk, it is, of course, also perfused with pulmonary blood, which after birth has a much lower content of oxygen than does the blood in the aorta. In some cases, the ischaemic myocardium can be perfused increasingly by a set of developing collateral connections from the right coronary artery, which arises normally (Fig. 45-4). Ideally, a superb set of perfectly distributed collateral arteries could be developed before the pulmonary arterial pressure has fallen sufficiently to result in significant ischaemic damage to the left ventricle. In many circumstances, however, the collateral connections may develop, but be poorly distributed. In consequence, some portions of the left ventricle may be well perfused, while others become ischaemic.

In another pattern of abnormal distribution of the collateral arteries, there are large interconnections proximal to the branches supplying contracting myocardium that act as left-to-right, or aortopulmonary, arterial shunts, requiring extra work from the left ventricle while deviating blood supply from its myocardium. This malformation presents a picture postnatally that may vary enormously from patient to patient, and also from time to time in a given patient.[10] The end result is best evaluated in terms of time of onset of clinically observable myocardial ischaemia. At one extreme, this may never occur, while, at the other, there is disastrous damage to the myocardium in the first weeks of infancy (Fig. 45-5).

Typically, the right coronary artery enlarges at its origin, while the left tends to be small, and relatively thin-walled. The collateral circulation between the right and left systems may be diffusely large, and well distributed. As a result, the left ventricle may remain quite well perfused, allowing the heart to retain its essentially normal form and function. When the collateral connections are poorly developed, the left ventricle becomes ischaemic, dilated, infarcted and fibrosed (see Fig. 45-5). Often the fibrosis extends into the papillary muscles and the mitral valve itself. Mitral valvar competence may be compromised by these changes, as well as by dilation caused by ischaemia, resulting in stretching of the annulus. The right ventricle, and parts of the left, which are perfused by the right coronary artery, continue to contract well. The left atrium tends to enlarge, as a result of the increasing left ventricular filling pressure, the mitral regurgitation, or both. This will lead to passive congestion of the lungs, an increase in the pulmonary arterial pressure, and subsequently an increase in the pressures in the right heart.

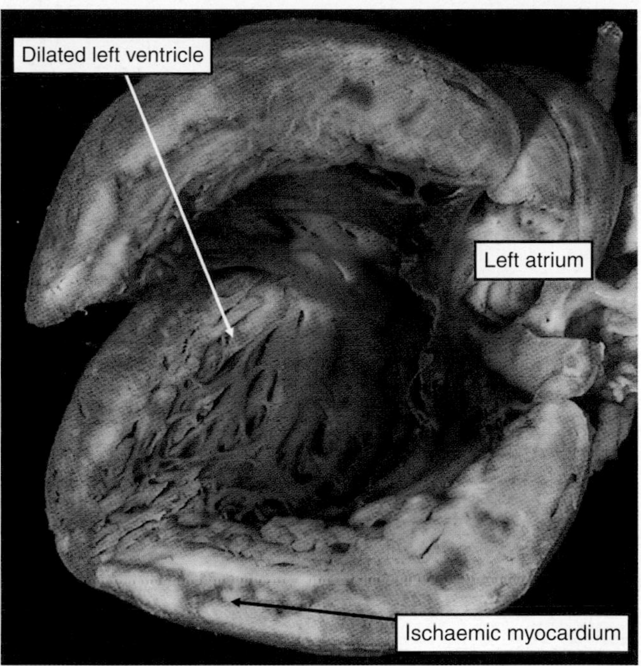

Figure 45-5 The heart, from a patient with origin of the left coronary artery from the pulmonary trunk, has been opened to show the left ventricle. Note the marked ischaemic changes to the myocardium of the inferior wall, and the dilation of the cavity. It is easy to see how such changes could be mistaken during life for dilated cardiomyopathy.

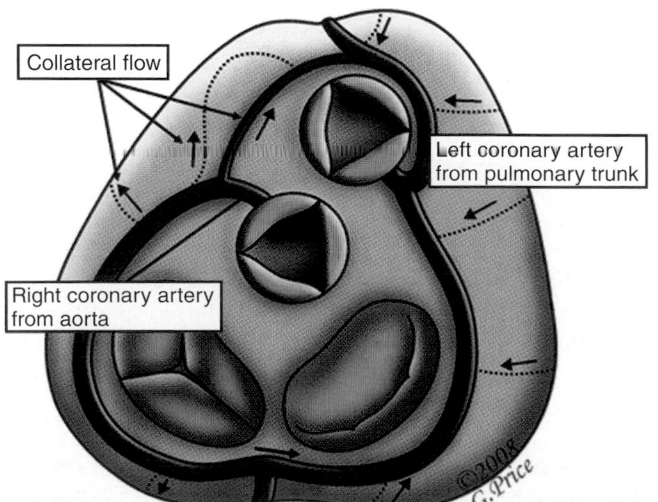

Figure 45-4 The cartoon shows the arrangement when the left coronary artery takes anomalous origin from the pulmonary trunk. The arrows show the direction of collateral circulation from branches of the right coronary artery to those of the left. The dotted lines indicate enlarged collateral connections.

Presentation

The majority of those with origin of the left coronary artery from the pulmonary trunk present during infancy. The infant with myocardial ischaemia tends to have both the classic signs and symptoms of congestive heart failure. Some affected infants will demonstrate a particular type of anginal attack. Brought on usually by the stress of feeding or defaecation, these are episodes in which the infant suddenly appears to be in severe distress, grunting or crying in short gasps, and is dyspnoeic, grey and sweaty. The child who has escaped myocardial ischaemia in infancy may present rather innocuously on a routine examination with an unexplained heart murmur, mild cardiomegaly or an abnormal electrocardiogram. Myocardial ischaemia may first present in adolescence or young adult life when, under the stress of maximally motivated exertion, either anginal pain or arrhythmia may occur. The latter may produce sudden unexplained death, or so-called near-miss death. The patient also may present with progressive mitral regurgitation, which may or may not be accompanied by electrocardiographic signs of ischaemia. All neonates and infants who present with mitral regurgitation should be evaluated thoroughly for the possibility of origin of the left coronary artery from the pulmonary trunk.

The sick infant may have the general appearance of a baby in chronic congestive heart failure, may have the episodes described above, or may have both. The heart is usually large, and the praecordial impulse is often hyperdynamic. The first heart sound may be loud, normal, or faint, with the second heart sound being loud, and third and fourth heart sounds often present. An apical holosystolic murmur of mitral regurgitation may be heard, and there may be an apical diastolic rumble. The older child with adequate collateral coronary circulation may have completely normal cardiac findings. Sometimes a continuous murmur is heard, resulting from the retrograde flow of blood from the anomalously connected artery into the pulmonary artery. In such patients, the clinical diagnosis may be a small patent arterial duct. In the child with origin of the left coronary artery from the pulmonary trunk, however, there may also be apical murmurs in systole and diastole, resulting from mitral regurgitation and relative mitral stenosis.

Course and Prognosis

It is the extent of collateral vascularisation that dictates the clinical course. Those, likely the minority, with well-developed collateral coronary arteries may have a mild, or even sub-clinical, course with spontaneous improvement. They may present later in childhood, adolescence, or adulthood with progressive mitral regurgitation, congestive heart failure, or myocardial ischaemia with exertion. The overall outlook for the group left untreated, however, is poor. Death may occur suddenly, owing to arrhythmia or to cardiogenic shock from further infarction. In the review of Wesselhoeft and colleagues,[10] almost nine-tenths of the infants with angina and/or failure died. Early and accurate diagnosis to guide surgical treatment, therefore, should be the focus of evaluation.

Management

The treatment is surgical, with several approaches being used over recent years. Surgical treatment has evolved dramatically as the transplantation of small coronary arteries during the arterial switch procedure has become commonplace. The specific aim of therapy is to preserve as much myocardium as possible.[11] The preferred surgical technique in most cases is surgical reimplantation of the left coronary artery into the aorta, thus re-establishing antegrade flow of oxygenated blood.[12] When technical considerations make this operation difficult or impossible, such as when the orifice of the artery is in an unfavourable position, a transpulmonary baffle can be constructed.[13] Bypass grafting using the carotid and internal mammary arteries, or saphenous venous grafts, is now performed much less frequently. The procedure of ligating the left coronary artery has, quite correctly, been abandoned, this decision being supported by long-term studies of outcome.[12] In the small subset of patients in whom the cardiac function is profoundly depressed, transplantation may be a more desirable option. Modern surgical techniques make it possible to support the circulation further by means of devices that assist the left ventricle or provide extracorporeal membrane oxygenation.

ORIGIN OF THE RIGHT CORONARY ARTERY FROM THE PULMONARY TRUNK

This is a far less common anomaly. Though it may occur in isolation, it is associated with other forms of congenital heart disease in up to two-thirds of cases, such as aortopulmonary window, tetralogy of Fallot, or double outlet right ventricle. Like the origin of the left coronary artery from the pulmonary trunk, the anomaly may produce myocardial ischaemia, but often those affected are asymptomatic.[14] Diagnosis is usually made by detailed echocardiography, and may be confirmed by other high-resolution imaging, such as magnetic resonance imaging or computed tomography. The approach to treatment is difficult, since the natural history remains unclear in the asymptomatic patient. In those patients with any evidence of myocardial ischaemia, surgery with re-implantation of the right coronary artery into the aorta is the preferred approach.[15]

ANOMALOUS ORIGIN OF A CORONARY ARTERY FROM THE OPPOSITE SINUS OF VALSALVA

Either the right or the left coronary artery can arise from the opposite sinus of Valsalva. Such an anomalous connection may or may not be associated with any symptoms or problems. If the anomalous artery takes an intramural course, or an interarterial course between the pulmonary trunk and the aorta, then significant clinical symptoms may occur. Sudden death may occur, frequently during or soon after competitive sporting events or strenuous exercise. Unfortunately, such sudden death may be the initial presenting event. Although a mechanism for sudden death has not been definitively established, conjecture is that coronary arterial flow is compromised by compression of the coronary artery, so-called interarterial entrapment, restriction at the site of its orifice from the sinus of Valsalva, kinking of the coronary artery itself, or arterial stenosis resulting from the intramural course.[16]

Anomalous origin of the left coronary artery from the right aortic sinus carries a higher risk of sudden death than does the anomalous origin of the right coronary artery from the left coronary aortic sinus.[17] The prevalence of the lesion has been estimated at 0.17%.[18] In nine-tenths of cases, there is also an intramural course of the coronary artery.[16] Although the incidence of sudden death in these individuals is unknown, the annual risk of death for the overall population is reported to be 0.24 per 100,000 person-years.[19] Surgical repair is the preferred treatment for symptomatic individuals.[16] There remains, however, considerable discussion as to the best approach to the asymptomatic child known to have this lesion.[7]

OTHER ANOMALIES AND VARIATIONS OF ORIGIN AND COURSE OF THE CORONARY ARTERIES

Most anomalies are extremely rare, and may not present in childhood. They may become important in adolescence and early adult life, when extremes of physical exertion may cause significant intolerance of malfunction previously well tolerated. They may also become significant with aging, when the additional effects of atherosclerotic changes typically manifest. These malformations are increasingly recognised, albeit still very rarely, in the investigation of syncopal episodes or near-miss sudden death.

Stenosis or Atresia of the Main Stem of the Left Coronary Artery

This lesion has variable presentation, but may be lethal in infancy. The origin, and sometimes a short length of the artery, either fails to canalise or else involutes after formation (Fig. 45-6). Much as when the left coronary artery arises from the pulmonary trunk, the circulation on the left side depends upon collateral blood flow from the branches of the right coronary artery. The severity of symptoms, signs, and laboratory findings are related inversely to the size and distribution of the collateral vessels.[20] Some of those affected can survive without symptoms for many years. Infants who present with evidence of myocardial ischaemia are urgently in need of correct diagnosis and treatment. Results obtained by angiography during catheterisation in these infants may be confused with those occurring with origin of the left coronary artery from the pulmonary trunk. Typically, aortic angiography will reveal a large right coronary artery that fills the distribution of the left coronary artery via multiple connections from collateral branches. No contrast material will be seen entering the pulmonary trunk. There may be a slight filling of the left coronary artery from the aorta. There will certainly be no filling of the left coronary circuit from the pulmonary trunk on pulmonary arteriography, thereby excluding the origin of the left coronary artery from the pulmonary trunk as the diagnosis. Cross sectional echocardiography will demonstrate the left coronary artery in its normal location, but it will be diminutive or atretic for a few millimetres. Surgical treatment should be undertaken in these symptomatic patients.

Other Abnormalities of Coronary Arterial Origin

The orifices of the arteries may be ovoid instead of round. They may be located eccentrically in the sinus of Valsalva, or just above or totally remote from the sinus. In this regard, it should be noted that a significant proportion of the normal population, up to one-fifth, have the coronary arteries arising at or above the level of the sinutubular junction.[21] In extremely rare circumstances, a coronary artery may originate from an artery other than the aorta or the pulmonary trunk, such as an intercostal or internal thoracic artery. Two orifices within a single sinus usually occur along with anomalous proximal arterial segments.

Anomalies of the Proximal Segments of the Coronary Arteries

A very common normal variation in the proximal segments is a second small orifice in the right sinus of Valsalva that gives rise directly to the infundibular artery (Fig. 45-7). Instead of originating from the main stem, the circumflex artery may arise as a branch of the right coronary artery (Fig. 45-8), or from a separate orifice in the right aortic sinus. It may pass between the front of the aorta and the free-standing subpulmonary infundibulum in such a way as to be compressed between them in systole. Partial intramural course of such arteries through the wall of the aortic sinus has been shown to be significant as a cause of sudden death in juveniles.[22]

The Single Coronary Artery

Solitary coronary arteries, whether arising from the right (Fig. 45-9) or the left (Fig. 45-10) sinuses of Valsalva, are large vessels that pass completely around the heart, giving off all the usual normal branches. Such anomalies account

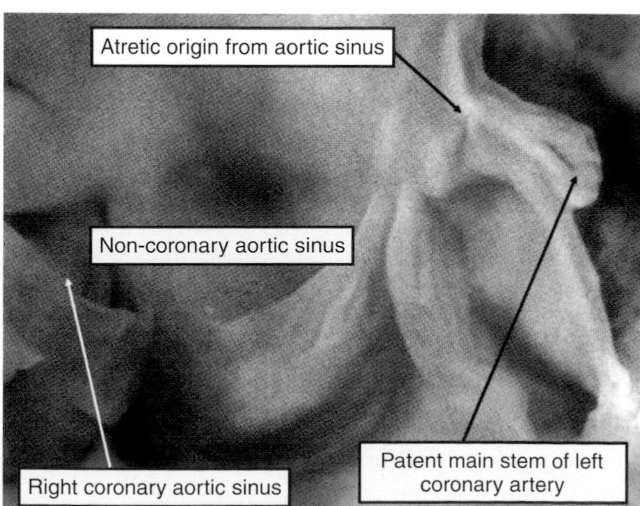

Figure 45-6 In this specimen, the origin of the left main stem of the left coronary artery from the aortic sinus is atretic. Although the orifice of the artery is atretic, the main stem of the left coronary artery is patent. The specimen was obtained from a young adult who died suddenly.

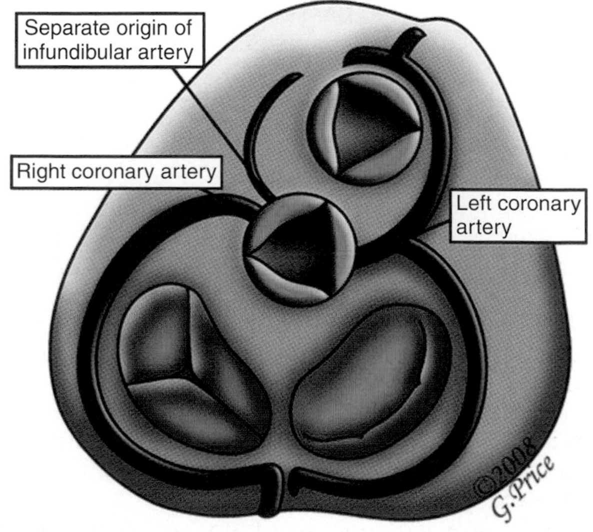

Figure 45-7 The cartoon shows the arrangement of the arteries when the infundibular, or conal, artery takes its origin from an accessory orifice in the right coronary aortic sinus of Valsalva.

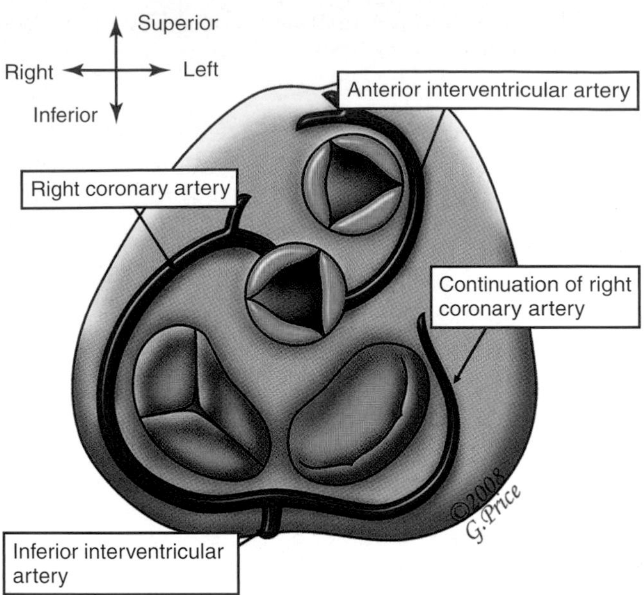

Figure 45-8 The cartoon shows the circumflex artery arising as a terminal extension of the right coronary artery. The image is drawn as seen from the cardiac apex looking towards the base (see compass).

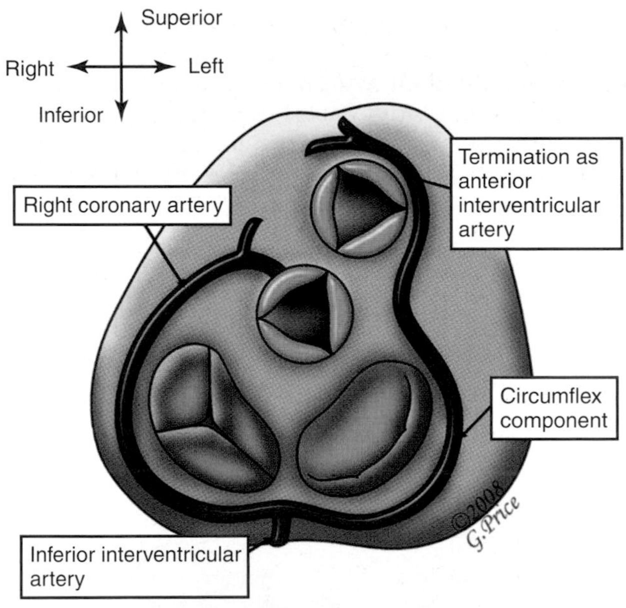

Figure 45-9 The cartoon shows the arrangement in which a single coronary artery arises from the right coronary aortic sinus of Valsalva. The image is drawn as seen from the cardiac apex looking towards the base (see compass).

for approximately one-tenth of the total number of coronary arterial anomalies. Such solitary arteries have no pathological implications except in the setting of atherosclerosis, when they take an anomalous course resulting in compression, or when there is an intramural component of the vessel.[22] There may, or may not, be an atrophic relic of the opposite artery. This lesion differs from stenosis or atresia of the orifice, in that flow to the side without the orifice is directly through the large single coronary artery with normal branches, as opposed to collateral flow through branches of the arterial bed.

Either a solitary coronary artery, or both coronary arteries arising from the right sinus of Valsalva, achieve pathological significance when the branch or artery that

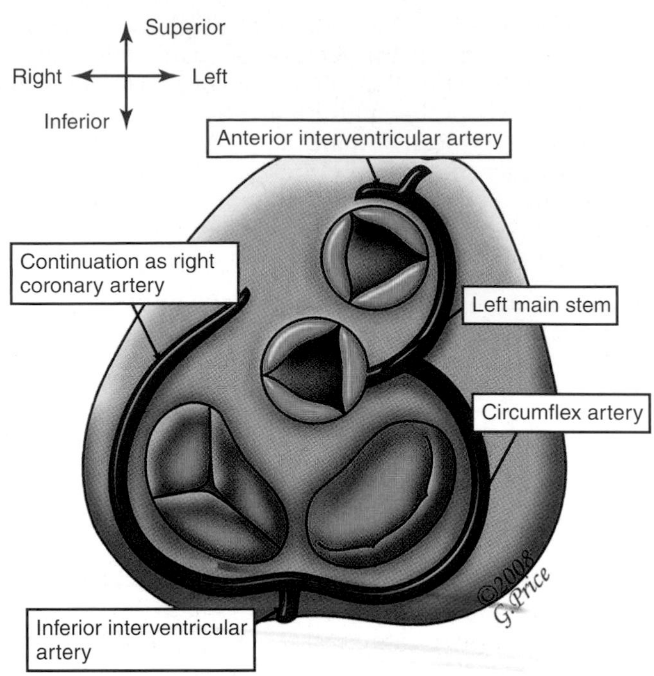

Figure 45-10 In this cartoon, a solitary coronary artery is shown arising from the left coronary aortic sinus of Valsalva. The image is drawn as seen from the cardiac apex looking towards the base (see compass).

supplies the left coronary arterial distribution courses leftward between the aorta and pulmonary trunk, then being subject to compression.[17] These features are harbingers of sudden unexplained death in adolescents and young adults, and carry a strong relation to death produced by heavy exertion.[17]

The single coronary artery from the right sinus of Valsalva can be identified on transthoracic echocardiography performed at the bedside. When found, it is imperative to determine any intramural course. Doppler colour flow confirms the direction of the flow within the coronary artery. In contrast, when the single artery arises from the left sinus of Valsalva (see Fig. 45-10), or both coronary arteries arise from separate orifices in that sinus, with the right coronary artery coursing between aorta and subpulmonary infundibulum, compression can occur, but sudden death may not, probably because of the low perfusion pressure required for the right ventricle.[23]

Myocardial Bridges

Rather than running on the surface of the heart, part of any of the epicardial coronary arteries can dip into the muscle, creating a myocardial bridge over the coronary artery. This occurs most frequently in the proximal half of the left coronary artery (Fig. 45-11). Most are not significant, but occasionally longer and thicker bridges can cause ischaemia.[24] Although this anomaly is congenital, those affected by it typically do not present with problems during childhood. It can, however, cause myocardial ischaemia, infarction and ventricular dysfunction. The diagnosis is typically made at coronary angiography, but may also be made by high resolution computerised tomographic scanning.[25]

Coronary Arterial Fistulas

The most distal malformations in the coronary arterial tree are communications between branches of the coronary

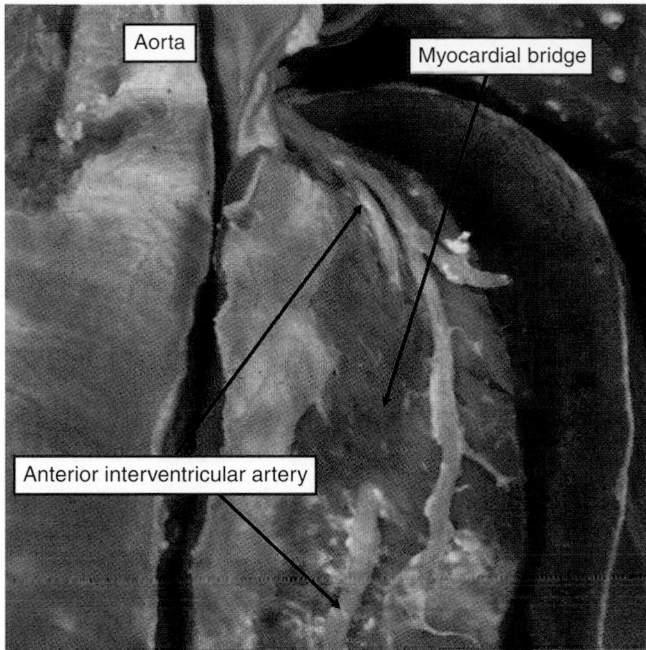

Figure 45-11 The specimen has been dissected to show an extensive myocardial bridge across the anterior interventricular artery.

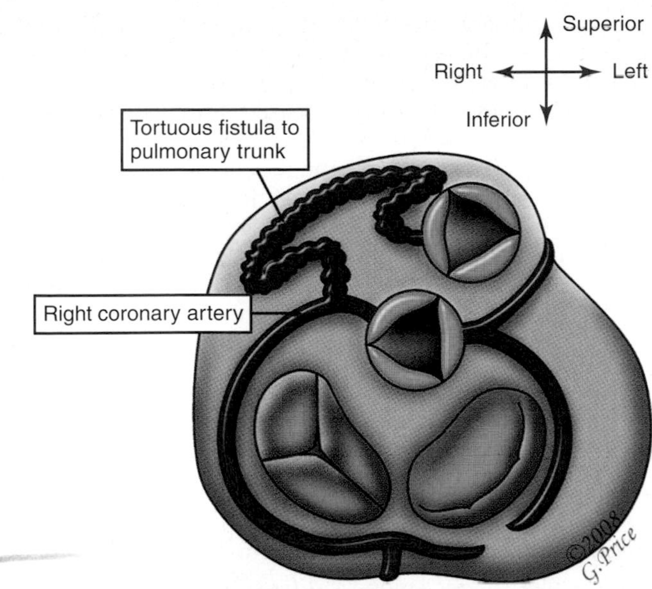

Figure 45-13 In this cartoon, a complex and circuitous fistula is shown running from a coronary artery to the pulmonary trunk, a large portion of which is aneurysmal. The image is drawn as seen from the cardiac apex looking towards the base (see compass).

arteries and another large vessel or cardiac chamber.[26] The source is most often the right coronary artery, with the left being much less frequently involved, and both coronary arteries less frequently still. The sink may be in any one or several of the superior caval vein, the coronary sinus, the right atrium, the right ventricle, the pulmonary trunk, a pulmonary vein, the left atrium or the left ventricle. Embryologically, these fistulas seem to represent persistent junctions of primordial epicardial vessel with the intramyocardial circulation. They vary from simple direct connections of a coronary artery with the lumen of a chamber or large vessel (Fig. 45-12) to complex, worm-like aneurysmal cavities in which blood may stagnate, clot and calcify (Fig. 45-13). They are as varied pathophysiologically as they are anatomically. In the simple direct connections with large communicating orifices, there may be appreciable

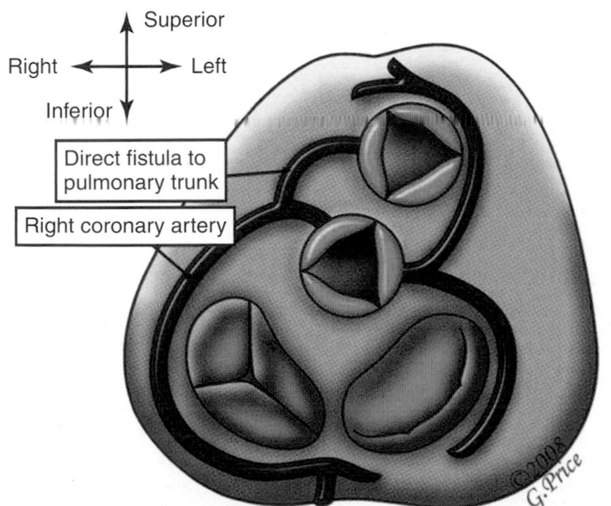

Figure 45-12 The cartoon shows a short, direct, fistula from a coronary artery to the pulmonary trunk. The image is drawn as seen from the cardiac apex looking towards the base (see compass).

shunts. The increased volume loading begins with the aorta and left ventricle in all cases, and, depending upon where the fistula drains, is reflected farther back into left atrium, pulmonary vascular bed, right ventricle, right atrium or caval veins. The largest shunts tend to be in those that connect to the right side of the heart rather than the left. This is probably because of the greater period of systolic narrowing when the orifice of communication is into the left ventricle, as well as because of the lesser pressure gradient between aorta and left ventricle. Even in those communications ending in the right side of the heart, and contributing to the flow of blood to the lungs, rarely is the ratio between pulmonary and systemic flows greater than 3 to 1.

Some fistulas have been found to be large in the newborn. Further postnatal enlargement does occur. The aneurysmal sections of the fistula, in particular, may gradually dilate over time. If striking cardiac enlargement is noted, it is more likely to be caused by a dilated complex fistula on the surface of the heart than by functional enlargement of the heart from volume overload. Dilation of a complex fistula tends to occur slowly, stretching the pericardium and compressing softer cardiac structures, potentially producing arrhythmias and obstructing veins entering the right or left side of the heart. Other effects and complications include fistulous steal from the neighbouring myocardium, with ischaemia, atherosclerotic changes at points of stress, thrombosis and embolisation, rupture and infective endocarditis.

Over half of patients are clinically asymptomatic with normal exercise tolerance, despite their moderate volume overloads. Symptoms of congestive heart failure may occur, especially when the anomaly presents in infancy. Other symptoms include exercise intolerance with dyspnoea and angina, and occasionally arrhythmia. The presenting physical finding that brings many such patients to the cardiologist is a continuous murmur over the heart. This murmur may resemble that from an arterial duct, except that it is often heard maximally in unusual locations, and may peak in diastole rather than during systolic ejection.

Electrocardiographically, there is no characteristic finding. Radiologically, the heart may be normal in size and shape and moderately enlarged. It may be overactive when there is a short, rapidly flowing, fistula. It may be very large but not overactive when there is a huge cavernous slow-flowing fistula. The cross sectional echocardiogram, especially with Doppler colour flow imaging, has permitted the display of the site of entry of these fistulas.[27] The use of Doppler colour flow, accompanied by cross sectional imaging, allows for the recognition of the site of origin, course and site of entry of the fistula. Pulsed and continuous wave Doppler ultrasound confirm the nature of the fistulous flow at the site of entry in most patients, particularly when guided by the colour flow map. Haemodynamic measurements, as well as volume loading of the receiving chamber, can be made with routine echocardiography. Ultimately, however, cardiac catheterisation with aortography provides the definitive diagnosis.

Treatment is now typically accomplished in the catheterisation laboratory. Transoesophageal echocardiography plays an important role in monitoring the success of this procedure.[28] Not much is known about the course of these lesions without surgery, because surgical treatment was already available during the years in which accurate diagnosis was feasible. The mortality has been low since the earliest period of surgical treatment, and the tendency has been practically universal to proceed in these patients in order to prevent complications. A small group of patients has been studied prospectively,[29] albeit some time ago, with little change noted, and some tendency for spontaneous resolution by thrombosis. The other side of the coin is represented by patients who have come to attention because of infective endocarditis, aggravated atherosclerotic complications, or thrombotic complications. It is rare that embolisation of the fistula with a coil, after appropriate testing for distal ischaemia, cannot be performed at catheterisation. In rare instances when interventional techniques are not successful, surgical treatment may be undertaken. In our discussion, we have purposely avoided reference to the fistulous communications seen in patients with pulmonary or aortic atresia with intact ventricular septum. These are discussed in the appropriate chapters (see Chapters 29 and 30).

Evaluation of Coronary Arterial Structure and Function

All patients with a possible anomaly of the coronary arteries should receive an electrocardiogram as part of their initial evaluation. Beyond that, specific imaging of the coronary arterial circulation may be pursued. In fact, the field of cardiac imaging in children continues to evolve at a remarkable pace. Numerous modalities that are currently available provide detailed anatomical imaging of the coronary arterial structure, course, and in some cases, function. Among these are echocardiography, computed tomographic scanning, magnetic resonance imaging and angiography, positron emission tomographic scanning, and cardiac catheterisation with angiography. The choice of the modality used for imaging should include an analysis based on the availability of expertise for interpretation, the amount of exposure to ionising radiation, and the degree of cooperation, sedation or anaesthesia required to allow for the proper examination. It is the thoughtful and careful selection of the diagnostic testing that allows for the most accurate and safest diagnosis of the anomalies of the coronary arteries. A detailed explanation of the diagnostic modalities is presented elsewhere in this text, but we provide a brief description here.

Electrocardiography

Those who present with a coronary arterial anomaly that leads to ischaemia or infarction in portions of the ventricular myocardium will almost always have sinus tachycardia in an attempt to maintain cardiac output in the face of diminished myocardial function, and thus decreased stroke volume. Rarely there may be premature ventricular contractions or ventricular tachycardia, pathological Q waves, and abnormalities of the QRS and ST-T segments, compatible with anterior, antero-septal or antero-lateral infarction.[10] Q waves may be present in leads I and aVL in patients with the origin of the left coronary artery from the pulmonary trunk. Alternatively, electrocardiographic changes may be progressive as infarcts evolve. While the electrocardiogram is not likely to be normal in the patient with a coronary artery arising from the pulmonary trunk, it may not show the classic findings for ischaemia or infarction. There are occasions in this disease, therefore, when the electrocardiogram is not diagnostic. The QRS horizontal plane typically reveals a counterclockwise loop pattern, though there is considerable variability. The older child with origin of the left coronary artery from the pulmonary trunk who has survived without symptoms may very well have a normal electrocardiogram.

Echocardiography

In the infant who is suffering from inadequate coronary arterial perfusion, echocardiography demonstrates left atrial and left ventricular enlargement, and depressed ventricular function. Mitral regurgitation is almost invariably present, and brightness of the endocardium may be observed, often associated with endocardial fibroelastosis.[30] Definitive imaging of abnormal origin of the left coronary artery from the pulmonary trunk can be achieved using the echocardiographic cut in the sagittal plane (Fig. 45-14). Color flow Doppler mapping is often of great utility. With relatively low Nyquist limits applied to the aorta and the pulmonary trunk in the parasternal short-axis view, the flow in the left coronary artery can be imaged (Fig. 45-15), as can the steal from the coronary circulation into the pulmonary arteries. Pulsed wave Doppler can be used to confirm the flow patterns.

Electrocardiography and echocardiography offer the great advantage of portability, allowing the physician to examine the patient at the bedside. There are now a number of other sophisticated imaging techniques which can provide important information about coronary arterial structure, as well as the viability of the affected myocardium in the patient with coronary arterial anomalies. Magnetic resonance imaging offers concise imaging of the coronary arterial origins (Figure 45-16), and can provide information about myocardial function and scarring. Cardiac computed tomography can also be used to evaluate the origins and course of the coronary arteries in all dimensions, and with gating to the cardiac cycle, also in time. Three-dimensional reconstruction can be performed to further delineate the precise nature of

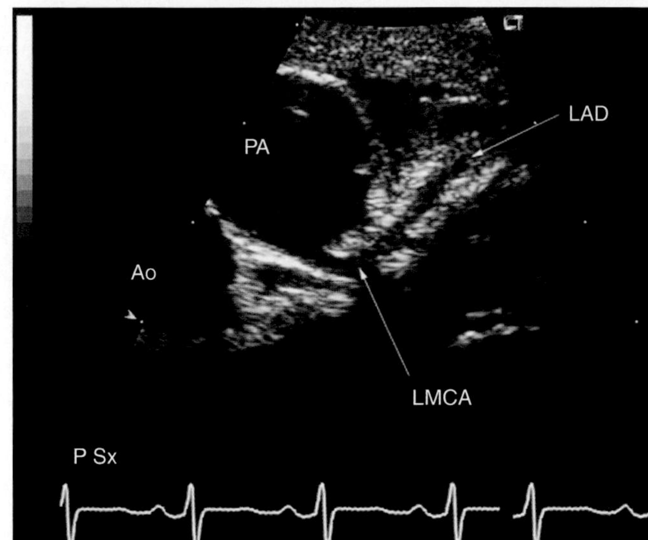

Figure 45-14 The echocardiogram shows origin of the main stem of the left coronary artery from the pulmonary trunk, with branching to supply the anterior interventricular and circumflex arteries. Ao, aorta; LAD anterior interventricular artery; LMCA, main stem of the left coronary artery; PA, pulmonary trunk; P Sx, parasternal short-axis section.

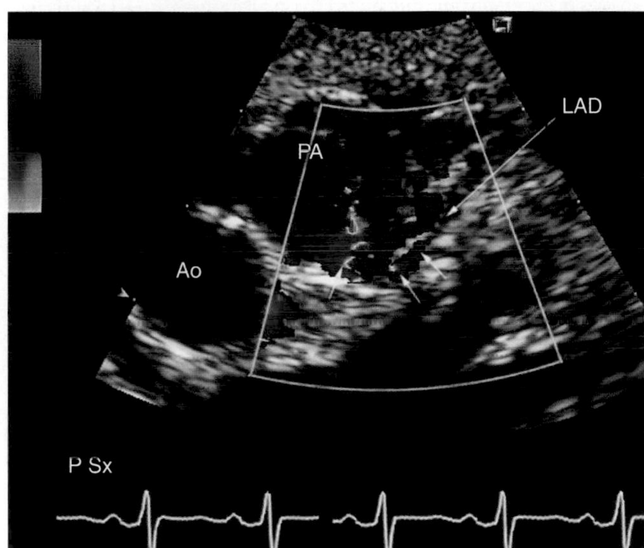

Figure 45-15 Colour flow Doppler interrogation demonstrates the abnormal patterns of flow (*arrows*) in a left coronary artery arising from the pulmonary trunk (PA). Ao, aorta; LAD, anterior interventricular artery; P Sx, parasternal short-axis section.

the coronary artery anomalies (Figs. 45-17 to 45-19). The high resolution of this technique allows for extremely precise diagnosis, albeit consideration must be given to the dose of ionizing radiation. Thallium-201 scintigraphy can yield a cold area in the affected portion of the left ventricle, albeit the same effect has been seen in some patients with cardiomyopathy. More recently, technetium has become the preferred isotope to be used in children, as it has better dosimetry with less gonadal absorption.[31] Positron emission tomographic scanning may also prove to be useful, particularly in the determination of myocardial viability relative to myocardial perfusion in the patient with the origin of the left coronary artery from the pulmonary trunk.

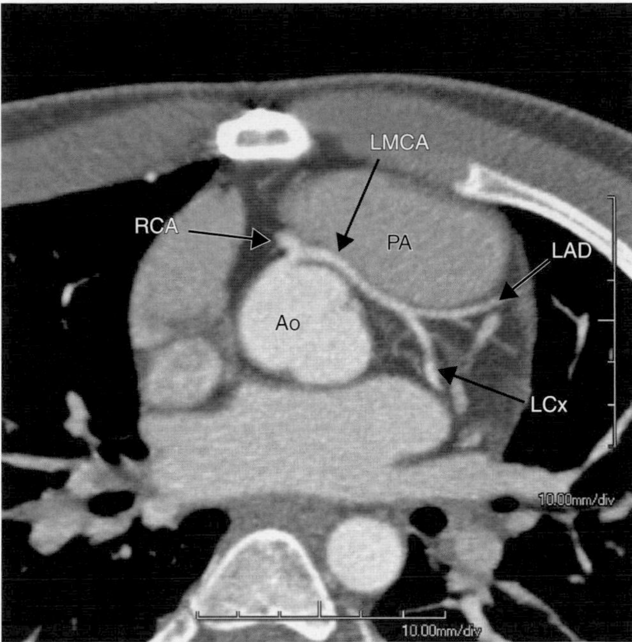

Figure 45-16 The magnetic resonance image shows the main stem of the left coronary artery (LMCA) arising from the right coronary artery (RCA) and taking a course between the aorta (Ao) and the pulmonary trunk (PA), before branching into the anterior interventricular (LAD) and circumflex (LCx) branches. (Courtesy of Dr. Francis Chan, Lucile Packard Children's Hospital, Division of Radiology and Stanford University, Palo Alto, California.)

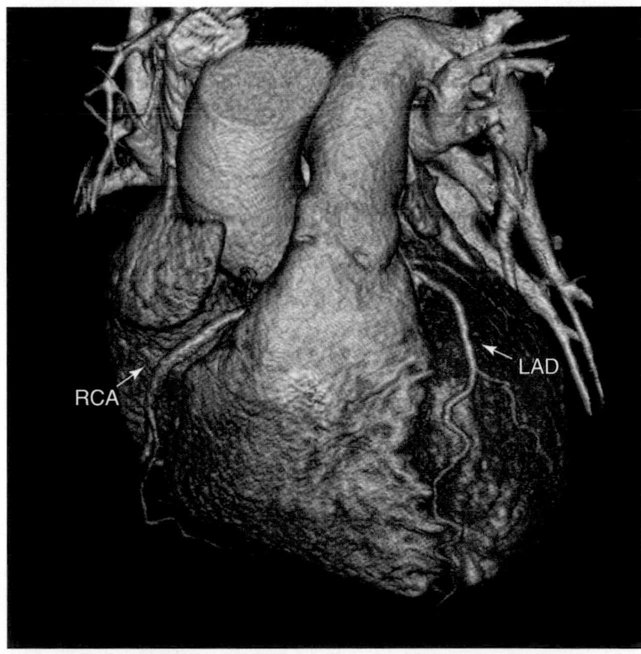

Figure 45-17 The computerised tomographic scan shows the course of the normal coronary arteries as seen from the anterior aspect of the heart. Note the location of the right coronary artery (RCA), which courses in the right atrioventricular groove, and the anterior interventricular artery (LAD), which courses in the anterior interventricular groove. (Courtesy of Dr. Francis Chan, Lucile Packard Children's Hospital, Division of Radiology and Stanford University, Palo Alto, California.)

Cardiac Catheterisation

As described previously, any child with an unexplained congestive cardiomyopathy should have detailed echocardiographic imaging, with Doppler colour flow interrogation of the left coronary arterial system. If there is any

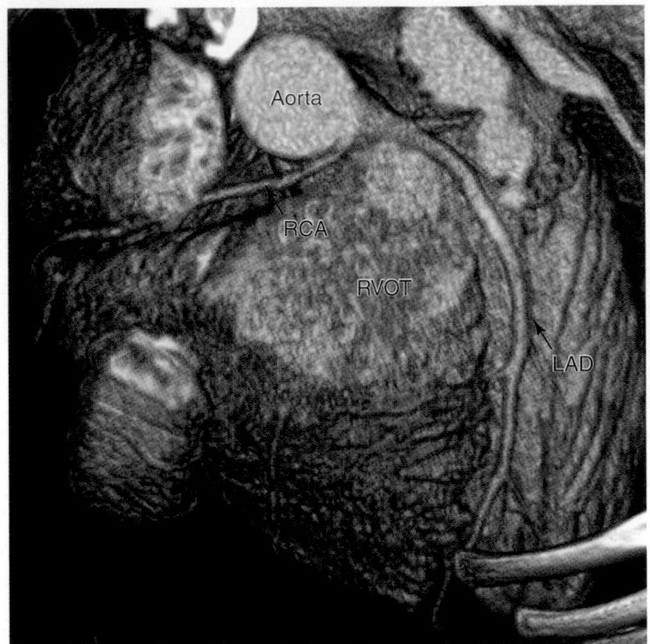

Figure 45-18 The computerised tomographic scan shows the right coronary artery (RCA) arising from the left coronary aortic sinus of the aorta, and coursing between the aorta and the pulmonary trunk, posterior to the right ventricular outflow tract (RVOT), to reach the right atrioventricular groove. The left coronary artery, also arising from the left coronary aortic sinus, branches normally into the circumflex and anterior interventricular (LAD) arteries. (Courtesy of Dr. Francis Chan, Lucile Packard Children's Hospital, Division of Radiology and Stanford University, Palo Alto, California.)

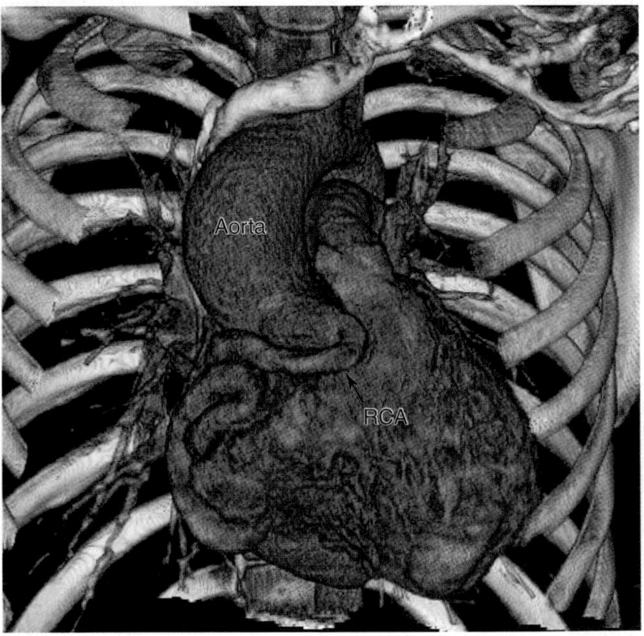

Figure 45-19 The computerised tomographic scan shows a large and tortuous coronary arterial fistula, with aneurysmal dilation of the right coronary arterial (RCA) system. (Courtesy of Dr. Francis Chan, Lucile Packard Children's Hospital, Division of Radiology and Stanford University, Palo Alto, California.)

doubt about the origins, patency, course or structure of the coronary arteries, the patient should be given the benefit of angiography.

Cardiac catheterisation is performed to measure cardiac output, left ventricular end-diastolic pressure, and pulmonary arterial pressure. The objective of angiocardiography is to establish the integrity and the source of the coronary arteries. In a very sick infant, the less done the better within the limits of adequate diagnosis. When the left coronary artery arises from the pulmonary trunk, an aortic root injection may be sufficient to show clearly the early filling of the right coronary artery and the delayed passage via collateral vessels into the left coronary arterial distribution and, finally, the pulmonary trunk. If the pulmonary trunk never clearly opacifies, it is desirable next to inject the pulmonary trunk, looking very carefully for small, usually diastolic, phasic filling of the main stem of the left coronary artery and its branches. The finding of coronary arterial filling from the pulmonary trunk should rule out ligation of the main stem of the left coronary artery at its origin as a form of treatment for the patient. Should adequate injections of both the aortic root and the pulmonary trunk still leave no clue as to the origin of the left coronary artery, selective injection of the right coronary artery should be considered.

The complete reference list can be found on the companion Expert Consult web site at www.expertconsult.com.

ANNOTATED REFERENCES

- Hutchins GM, Kessler-Hanna A, Moore GW. Development of the coronary arteries in the embryonic human heart. Circulation 1988;77:1250–1257.

  This elegant study sought to elucidate the mechanism by which the normal coronary arteries develop their connections with the right and left aortic sinuses of Valsalva. Serial sections through embryonic hearts demonstrated that the left and right aortic sinuses develop a positive transverse curvature and a negative longitudinal curvature. The other four sinuses of the great arteries develop positive transverse curvatures and also develop a positive longitudinal curvature. These differences in mural tension may explain the normal connection between the coronary arteries and the sinuses.

- Friedman AH, Fogel MA, Stephens P, et al: Identification, imaging, functional assessment and management of congenital coronary arterial abnormalities in children. Cardiol Young 2007;17(suppl 2):56–67.

  This review article provides a comprehensive overview of the current clinical science describing coronary arterial anomalies. It provides the reasoning for the imaging studies used to diagnose congenital coronary arterial anomalies, including a discussion of the functional assessment of the coronary arteries in children. The article also outlines strategies for management, including some surgical controversies, for children with coronary arterial anomalies.

- Backer CL, Stout MJ, Zales VR, et al: Anomalous origin of the left coronary artery. A twenty-year review of surgical management. J Thorac Cardiovasc Surg. 1992;103:1049–1057.

  Backer and his colleagues, from Children's Memorial Hospital in Chicago, provide a retrospective analysis of the surgical approaches to the anomalous origin of the left coronary artery from the pulmonary trunk. An analysis of outcome years after surgery is provided. They recommend that patients should undergo a direct re-implantation to the aorta at the time of diagnosis.

- Smith A, Arnold R, Anderson RH, et al: Anomalous origin of the left coronary artery from the pulmonary trunk. Anatomic findings in relation to pathophysiology and surgical repair. J Thorac Cardiovasc Surg 1989;98:16–24.

  The authors of this comprehensive discussion of anomalous origin of the left coronary artery from the pulmonary trunk characterise the primary anatomical findings by study of a series of autopsied specimens. They present the secondary pathological findings in this anomaly, and suggest that a reconstruction of a two coronary arterial system supplied from the aorta is advantageous to most patients afflicted with this condition.

- Williams IA, Gersony WM, Hellenbrand WE: Anomalous right coronary artery arising from the pulmonary artery: A report of 7 cases and a review of the literature. Am Heart J 2006;152:1004–1010.

  This article provides a detailed review of the literature on the rare, but clinically important, anomalous origin of the right coronary artery from the pulmonary trunk. The authors supplement this with their experience in seven cases from their institution. They showed that, unlike anomalous origin of the left coronary artery from the pulmonary trunk, this entity rarely leads to sudden death.

- Frommelt PC, Frommelt MA, Tweddell JS, Jaquiss RD: Prospective echocardiographic diagnosis and surgical repair of anomalous origin of a coronary artery from the opposite sinus with an interarterial course. J Am Coll Cardiol 2003;42:148–154.

  This study describes the mode of presentation, the anatomical features, the methods of diagnosis and surgical outcome for patients who have anomalous origin of a coronary artery from an opposite aortic sinus, and discuss the significance of a subsequent interarterial course. The results of 10 patients from one center are presented. Patients were noted to have frequent intramural course of the coronary artery with the anomalous origin. Surgical repair using an unroofing technique without cardiopulmonary bypass was used in these patients.

- Davis JA, Cecchin F, Jones TK, Portman MA: Major coronary artery anomalies in a pediatric population: Incidence and clinical importance. J Am Coll Cardiol 2001;37:593–597.

  This prospective study sought to determine the incidence and clinical significance of the major coronary arteries in children by the use of routine, transthoracic echocardiography. Nearly 2400 patients were evaluated, and four were found to have an anomaly of coronary arterial origin. Ischaemia was found to have occurred in those with and without symptoms, and surgical management and close clinical follow-up are recommended.

- Muriago M, Sheppard MN, Ho SY, Anderson RH: The location of the coronary arterial orifices in the normal heart. Clin Anat 1997;10:297–302.

  In this study, the authors evaluated 23 normal hearts at autopsy to determine the coronary artery orifices in relation to the aortic valve. They determined the position of the zones of apposition between the leaflets, the size of the aortic valvar leaflets, the number, shape and position of the coronary arterial orifices, and their relative position to the sinutubular junction. It was not uncommon for an accessory coronary orifice to be found in the anterior sinus. The coronary arterial orifices were frequently noted to have a non-central position, but were usually below the sinutubular junction.

- Canyigit M, Hazirolan T, Karcaaltincaba M, et al: Myocardial bridging as evaluated by 16 row MDCT. Eur J Radiol 2007; 69:156–164.

  Using non-invasive advanced computed tomography scanning, this study defines the prevalence and appearance of myocardial bridging and provides a correlation to the clinical presentation. The authors found that this non-invasive technique allowed for the direct visualisation of the myocardial bridge, and could be used to differentiate between complete and incomplete patterns of bridging. They suggest that the technique could be used to avoid invasive, higher risk procedures to image coronary arteries in situations of suspected bridging.

- Velvis H, Schmidt KG, Silverman NH, Turley K: Diagnosis of coronary artery fistula by two-dimensional echocardiography, pulsed Doppler ultrasound and color flow imaging. J Am Coll Cardiol 1989;14:968–976.

  The authors described the diagnosis and findings using echocardiography with colour flow Doppler mapping in 10 young children with a coronary arterial fistula. Bedside echocardiography accurately describes the origin, course and site of drainage of the coronary arterial fistula, and all anatomical information needed for surgical treatment was consistently obtained by echocardiograhy with colour flow Doppler mapping.

CHAPTER 46

Aortic Coarctation and Interrupted Aortic Arch

J. ANDREAS HOSCHTITZKY, ROBERT H. ANDERSON, and MARTIN J. ELLIOTT

Coarctation derives from the Latin term *coartatio*, which translated literally means a drawing together. Aortic coarctation, therefore, indicates a narrowing at some point along the course of the aorta. When used in the context of the congenitally malformed heart, coarctation most usually described an area of narrowing of the thoracic aorta in the region of the insertion of the arterial duct, with or without additional abnormalities of the aortic arch. Obstructive lesions can be found more proximally, involving the ascending aorta. These are considered, along with lesions of the aortic valve, in Chapter 44. Those distal to the thoracic aorta, together with acquired lesions, are beyond the remit of this chapter. Within this chapter, however, we will include consideration of patients with interruption of the aortic arch. This condition exists when there is discontinuity between two adjacent segments of the aortic arch, and in haemodynamic terms includes cases with a fibrous cord between the discontinuous segments. In this respect, interruption can be interpreted as the extreme end of the spectrum of obstruction of the aorta (Fig. 46-1).

HISTORICAL CONSIDERATIONS

The first description of aortic coarctation is generally attributed to Johann Freidrich Meckel, the famous Prussian anatomist, who presented the case of an 18-year-old female to the Royal Academy of Sciences of Berlin in 1750. At postmortem, she was found to have an aorta that was 'so narrow that its diameter was smaller by half than that of the pulmonary artery, which it should have exceeded or at least have equalled in calibre'. Some argue, however, that it was Morgagni who should be given priority.[1] As pointed out by Craigie,[2] nonetheless, a more recognisable description was published in Desault's *Journal de Chirurgie* in 1791. According to Craigie, Monsieur Paris, the Prosector of the Amphitheatre at the Hotel-Dieu described, in the winter of 1789, the postmortem of 'a very emaciated woman about 50 years old'. As well as recognising that the thoracic arteries were thicker and more tortuous than normal, he gave the following description: 'The part of the aorta which is beyond the arch, between the ligamentum arteriosum and the first inferior intercostal, was so greatly narrowed that it had at most the thickness of a goosequill. Hence in taking apart its walls, which had not decreased in this place, there remained only a small lumen. The part of the vessel which was above the constriction was slightly dilated; the distal part was of normal calibre. The most careful dissection did not reveal either in the aorta or in its vicinity any cause to which this extraordinary condition could be attributed'. With regard to interruption of the aortic arch, as discussed above, this can be considered as the severest end of the spectrum of aortic coarctation (see Fig. 46-1). It was Celoria and Patton[3] who classified this lesion into types A, B and C (Fig. 46-2). Interruption at the aortic isthmus had been the first pattern described, being recognised in 1778 by Stiedele in Vienna.[4] The more common variety, with interruption between the left common carotid and left subclavian arteries, was described some 40 years later by Siedel.[5] The least frequent variant, with interruption between the brachiocephalic and left common carotid arteries, was not seen until 1948.[6]

PREVALENCE AND AETIOLOGY

Aortic coarctation accounts for 7% of liveborn children with congenitally malformed hearts,[7] with a higher incidence in stillborn infants.[8] The overall incidence is in the region of 1 in 12,000, with a slight increased occurrence in males.[9] Coarctation is generally said to show multi-factorial inheritance, although genetic factors are clearly important in certain groups. The lesion was found in one-tenth of a large Danish series of patients with Turner's syndrome, albeit with a lower incidence in patients with mosaicism, or those with structural anomalies of the X chromosome.[10] Inheritance has also been reported as an autosomal dominant trait.[11] It is now known that cells migrating from the neural crest populate the aortic arches, and 22q11 deletion is well recognised as being associated with interruption between the left common carotid and subclavian arteries.[12] The finding of coarctation in an infant with this deletion, therefore, prompted suggestions of a similar association.[13] There is a reported seasonal incidence, with paucity of males born between April and August, but without any identification of an exogenous aetiological agent.[14]

Interruption of the aortic arch accounts for just over 1% of cases of so-called critical congenital cardiac disease.[9] As already emphasised, there is a known association between deletion of chromosome 22q11, or Di George syndrome, and interruption between the left common carotid and subclavian arteries. This is known to be due to abnormal migration of cells from the neural crest.[12] As many as one third of those with Di George phenotype have interruption of this type, and, conversely, two-thirds of those with interruption between the left common carotid and subclavian arteries have Di George syndrome.[15] Taking those with interruption as a group, interruption between the left common carotid and subclavian arteries is held to account for between half and three-quarters of cases, interruption at the isthmus for two-fifth, and interruption between the carotid arteries is rare.[16,17] Interruption as an isolated lesion

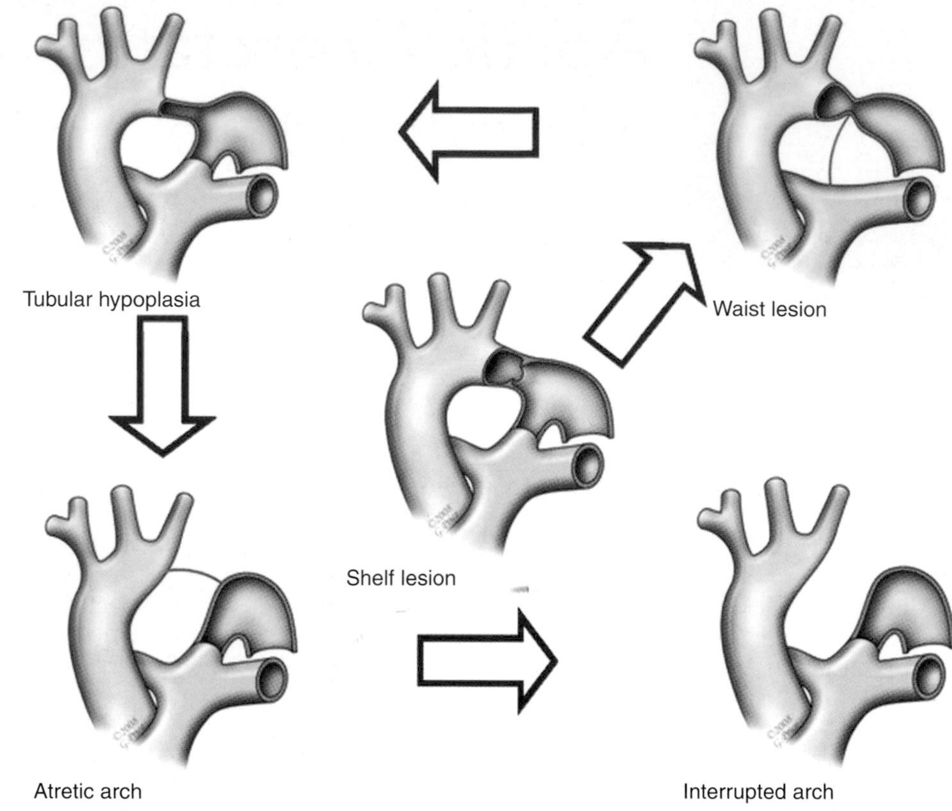

Figure 46-1 The morphological spectrum of obstruction in the aortic arch.

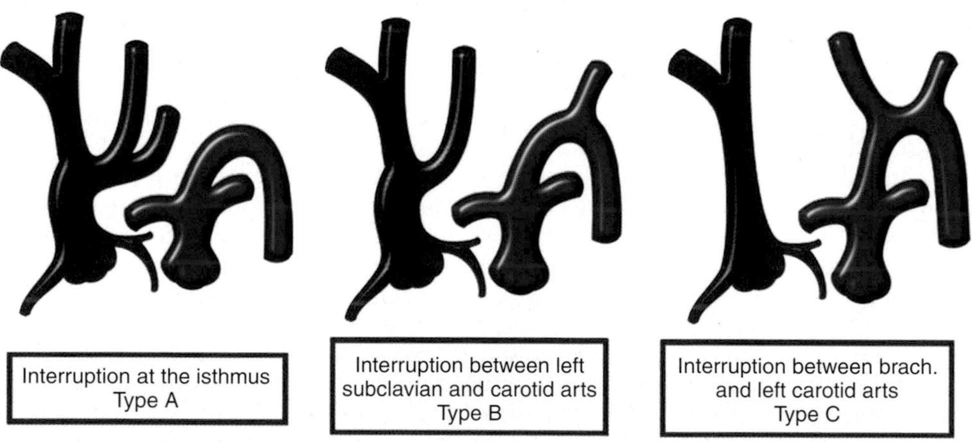

Figure 46-2 The categorisation of interruption of the aortic arch introduced by Celoria and Patton. The descending component of the aortic arch is supplied through the persistently patent arterial duct.

is also rare.[18] The combination of congenital absence of the aortic isthmus, patency of the arterial duct, and ventricular septal defect is very common and reported to occur in three-quarters of patients with interruption.[19] The incidence is equal between the genders.[16]

MORPHOLOGY

The lesions to be considered in this chapter all occur in proximity to the junction of the aortic arch and the arterial duct. This junction is clearly of fundamental importance to their evolution and morphology, although isolated coarctation can also exist proximal to the brachiocephalic arteries, or in the descending thoracic aorta. Aortic coarctation, however, is not a uniform entity. Rather, it represents a spectrum of lesions, generally encompassing variable degrees of hypoplasia, along with additionally stenotic areas, within the aortic arch. The extreme end of the spectrum is interruption of the aortic arch (see Fig. 46-1). Less severe is the presence of a fibrous cord between the interrupted segments of the arch, so that there is haemodynamic interruption but anatomic continuity. This is also known as atresia of the arch (Fig. 46-3). Tubular hypoplasia is present when there is a uniform narrowing of part of the arch (Fig. 46-4), whereas discrete coarctation is produced by a localised shelf-like lesion within the lumen of the arch, often with a degree of proximal tapering of the arch itself towards the obstructive shelf (Fig. 46-5).

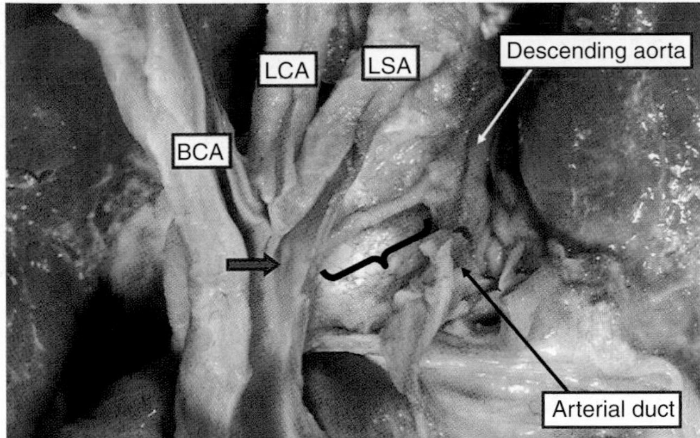

Figure 46-3 In this specimen, the segment of aortic arch between the origin of the left subclavian artery (LSA) and the descending aorta is represented by a fibrous cord (*bracket*). A dimple can be seen in the lumen of the ascending aorta (*arrow*), which shows that the arch itself was initially patent. The ascending aorta also supplies the brachiocephalic (BCA) and left common carotid (LCA) arteries, while the patent arterial duct supplies the descending aorta.

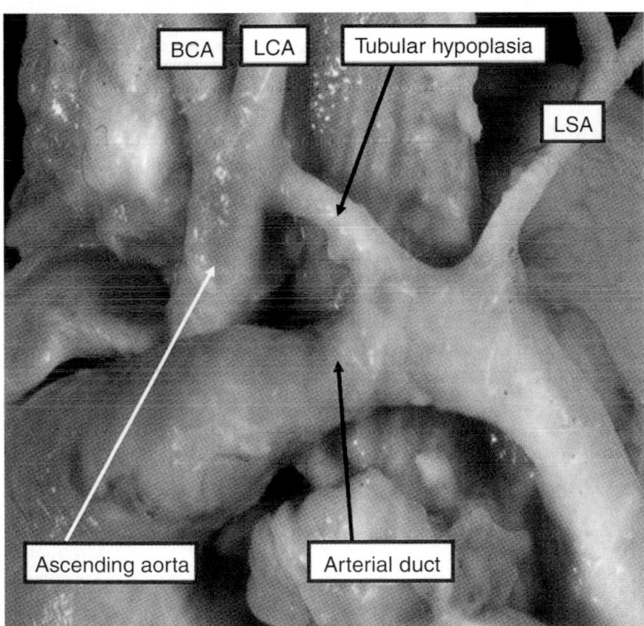

Figure 46-4 In this specimen, the segment of arch between the left common carotid artery (LCA) and the descending aorta is uniformly narrow, the anatomic feature described as tubular hypoplasia. Note the origin of the left subclavian artery (LSA) from the descending aorta. BCA, brachiocephalic artery.

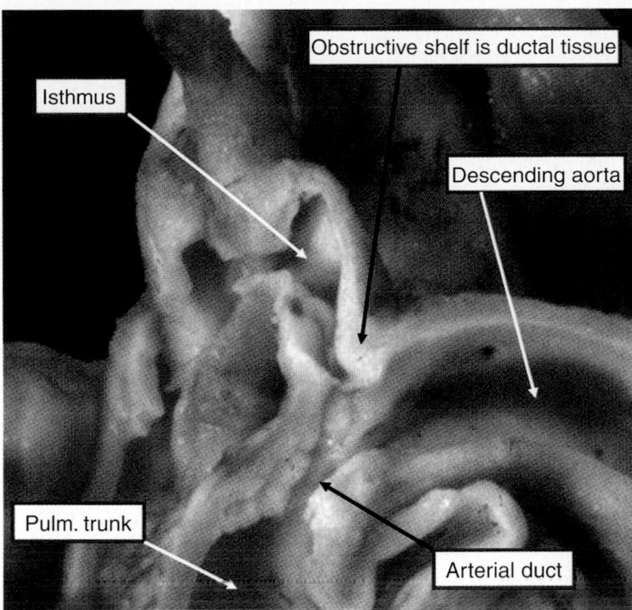

Figure 46-5 This image shows the typical features of discrete coarctation as seen in the neonatal heart. The duct is persistently patent, but the ductal tissue surrounds the mouth of the isthmus, with the shelf of ductal tissue producing the major obstruction to flow through the isthmus, albeit with some tapering of the isthmic segment.

The Obstructive Lesions

Presence of a discrete obstructive shelf within the lumen of the arch is much commoner than tubular hypoplasia, and has been the subject of manifold classifications. The most systematic approach was suggested by Edwards,[20] who emphasised the need to describe precisely the site of coarctation, irrespective of whether the arterial duct is patent, closed or ligamentous, and irrespective of the presence of additional anomalies. These other features, of course, also require description. In terms of location, nonetheless, when the arterial duct is patent, then the obstructing lesion can be preductal, paraductal, or postductal (Fig. 46-6). The most common site for discrete coarctation is at the junction of the aortic isthmus, the arterial duct or ligament, and the descending aorta. When the duct is open, there is usually a degree of isthmal hypoplasia, with the isthmus tapering down towards the junction with the duct, and the obstruction is preductal (Fig. 46-7). The obstructive lesion itself takes the form of a discrete waist, associated with infolding of the aortic wall (Fig. 46-8). In the majority of cases, the shelf is formed by ductal tissue, which completely encircles the lumen of the isthmus (see Fig. 46-5). The ductal shelf produces the major obstruction to flow, being the most important factor in coarctation. The waisting of the aortic wall usually accompanies the ductal shelf, but can occur in isolation.[21] When the arterial duct is closed, then the ductal shelf becomes converted to a fibrous diaphragm, often with a pinhole meatus (Fig. 46-9). Paraductal coarctation occurs directly opposite the mouth of the duct at its insertion to the aorta, and is found in one-tenth of cases (Fig. 46-10). Postductal obstruction is seen distal to the aortic origin of the arterial duct, and again accounts for about one-tenth of cases seen in infancy. The most important consequence of this variant is the lack of improvement of such critically ill infants despite maintenance of ductal patency with prostaglandin. Such postductal coarctation is the norm in adults, although then occurring in postligamental, rather than postductal, position.

Tubular hypoplasia, describing the presence of a uniformly narrow segment of the aortic arch, frequently coexists with discrete coarctation, but can exist in isolation (see Fig. 46-4). It is distinct from the gradual tapering of the isthmus characteristically seen with discrete coarctation (see Fig. 46-7). Histologically, the wall of an affected segment is normal, in contrast to the ductal and fibrous nature of discrete coarctation. The most frequent sites for tubular hypoplasia are either at the isthmus, or between the common carotid and the left subclavian arteries (see Fig. 46-4). It is rare for the segment between the brachiocephalic

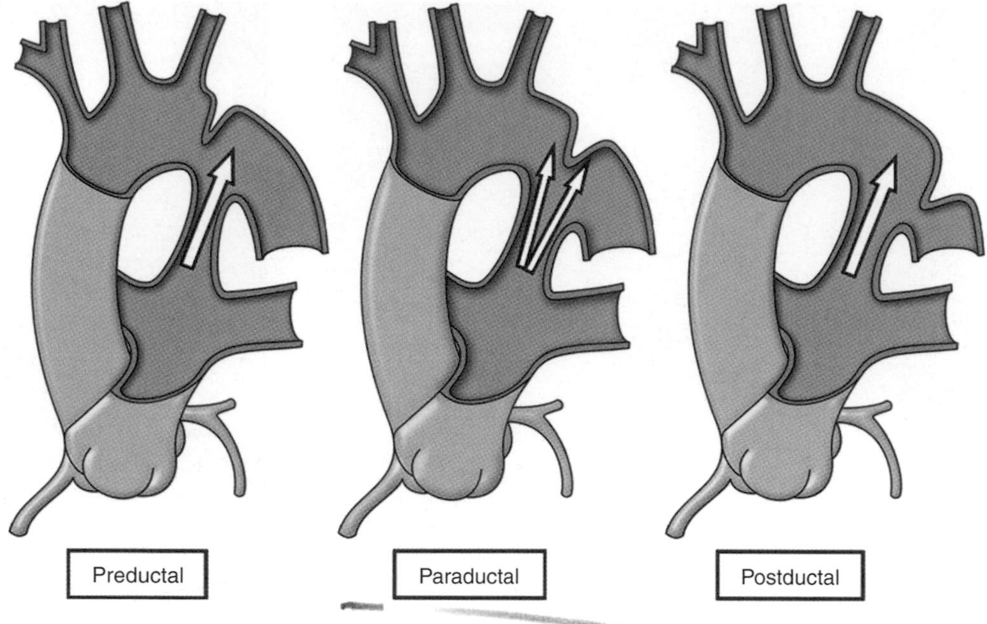

Figure 46-6 The cartoon shows how the obstructive lesion within the aortic arch can best be described as occupying preductal, paraductal, or postductal positions. The distinctions are harder to make when the duct is closed and ligamentous. The *arrows* show the preferential direction of flow through the arterial duct.

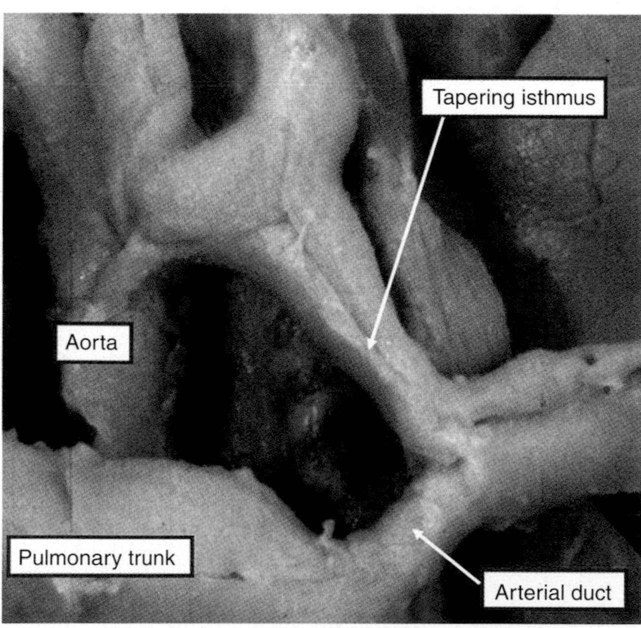

Figure 46-7 The picture shows the external view of a preductal coarctation lesion. Note the tapering of the isthmus, and the direct pathway from the duct to the descending aorta.

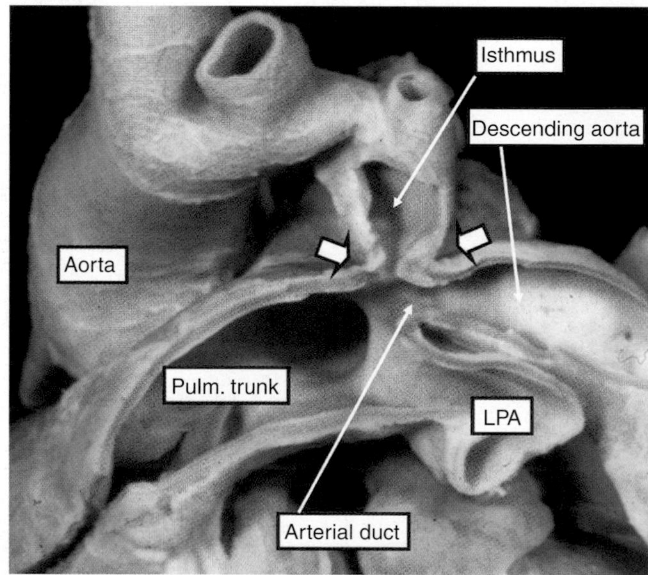

Figure 46-8 In this specimen, the junction of isthmus, duct, and descending aorta has been opened to show the shelf-like coarctation lesion, along with the waisting of the arterial walls (*arrows*). LPA, left pulmonary artery.

and left common carotid arteries to be affected. Atresia of the aortic arch exists when the arch itself is anatomically continuous, but there is no patency within one of its segments. The commonest site for such atresia is the aortic isthmus (see Fig. 46-3), but atresia can also be found between brachiocephalic and left common carotid arteries. Interruption exists when there is anatomic, as well as haemodynamic, discontinuity between segments of the aortic arch (see Fig. 46-2). The commonest site for interruption, accounting for about three-quarters of cases, is between the left common carotid and subclavian arteries (Fig. 46-11), the so-called Type B pattern of Celoria and Patton.[3] Most of the remaining cases show interruption at the isthmus, the so-called Type A (Fig. 46-12). As we have already emphasised, interruption between the brachiocephalic and left common carotid arteries, so-called Type C, is extremely rare.

Associated Malformations

The presence of associated cardiovascular lesions was one of the criterions commonly used to differentiate coarctation found in patients presenting in infancy from those presenting, often in isolation, in later childhood and adulthood. In this respect, the association of aortic coarctation, hypoplasia of the isthmus, patency of the arterial duct, and the presence of an interatrial communication or patency of the oval foramen, is so common as to be referred to sometimes as part of a coarctation complex in neonates. The typical

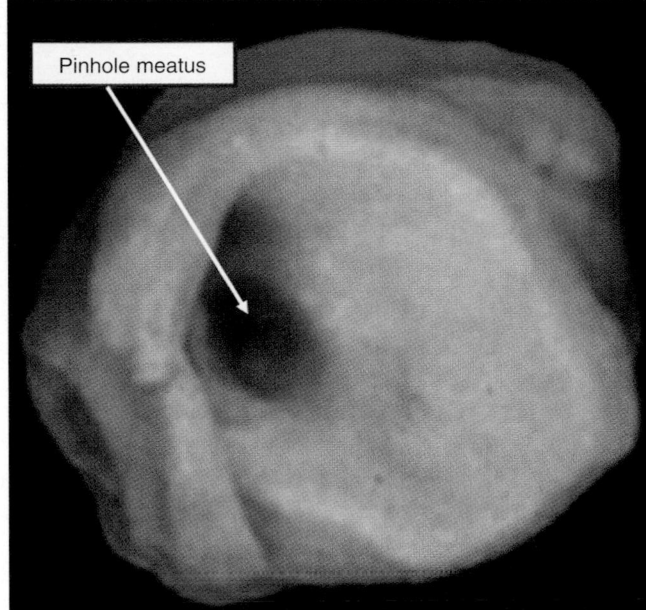

Figure 46-9 This is the specimen resected by the surgeon prior to an end-to-end anastomosis. It shows the pinhole meatus in the obstructive shelf as typically seen when the arterial duct has become ligamentous.

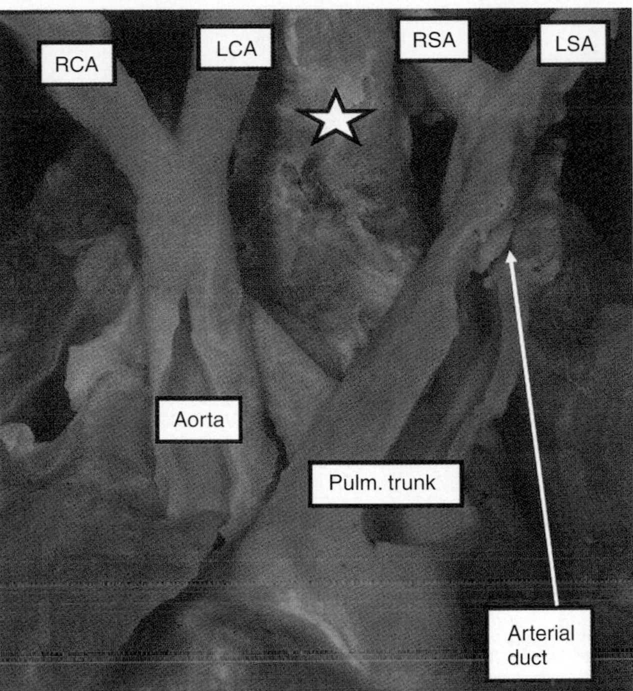

Figure 46-11 In this heart, there is interruption of the aortic arch (*star*) between the left common carotid artery (LCA) and the left subclavian artery (LSA). The right subclavian artery (RSA) has an anomalous retro-oesophageal course, so the ascending aorta gives rise to the right (RCA) and left common carotid arteries.

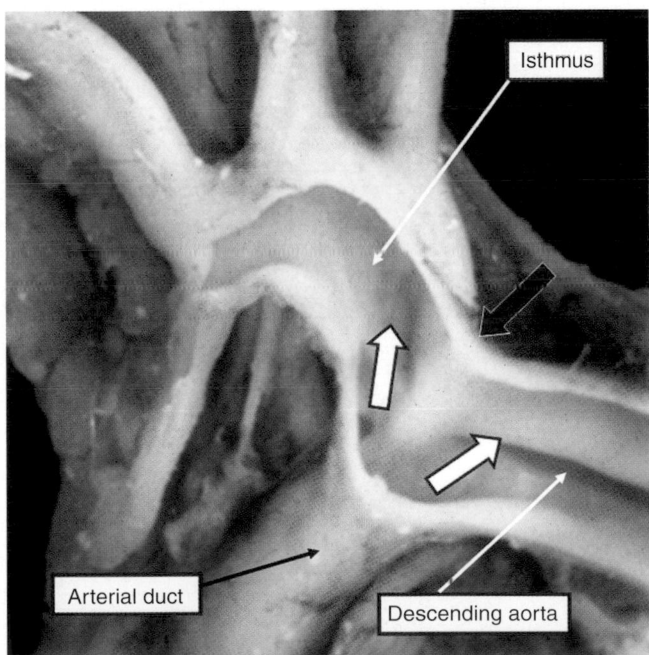

Figure 46-10 In this heart, the obstructive shelf (*red arrow*) is in paraductal position, with flow through the open duct possible to both ascending and descending segments of the aorta (*white arrows*).

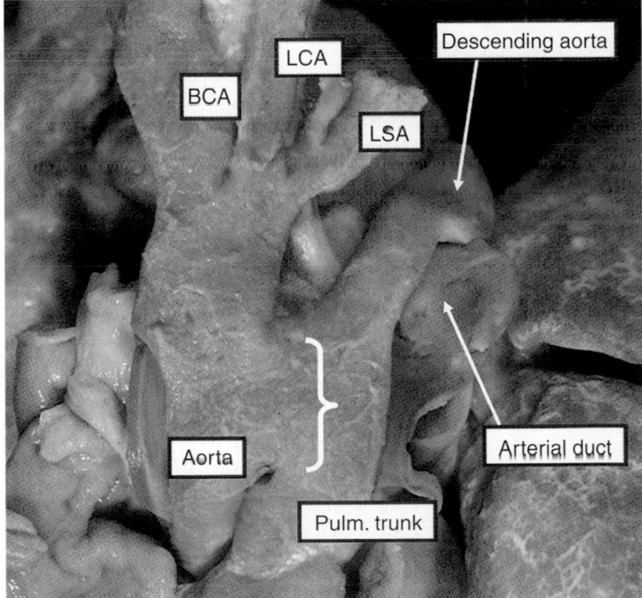

Figure 46-12 In this heart, the interruption is at the isthmus, between the left subclavian artery (LSA), which together with the left common carotid (LCA) and brachiocephalic (BCA) arteries arises from the ascending aorta, and the descending aorta, which is fed through the persistently patent duct. Note that in this heart there is also an aortopulmonary window (*bracket*).

associated anomalies are those that tend preferentially to potentiate flow to the pulmonary rather then systemic arterial pathway. Such lesions lead to reduced flow through the aortic isthmus in fetal life. This can be produced first by defects that produce left-to-right flow at either the level of the ventricles or the great arteries. The most common of these lesions is a ventricular septal defect. When found in the presence of coarctation, the ventricular septal defect is similar to the archetypical pattern found in hearts from patients with interruption of the aortic arch, with posterior deviation of the muscular outlet septum, or its fibrous remnant, into the subaortic area, the deviation leading to subaortic obstruction[22] (Figs. 46-13 and 46-14). In the setting of coarctation, however, the defects are more frequently perimembranous, and associated with postero-inferior

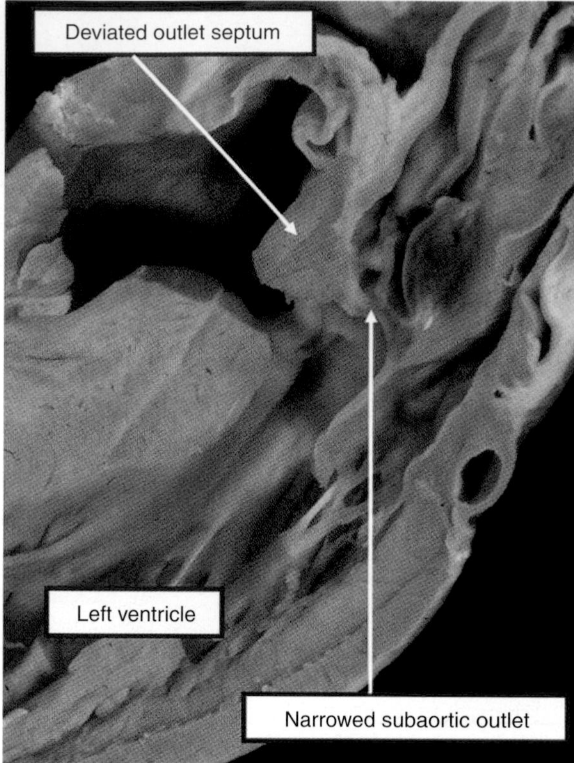

Figure 46-13 The heart has been sectioned in parasternal long-axis fashion, showing the morphology of the defect typically associated with interruption of the aortic arch, and with some cases of coarctation. There is posterior deviation of the muscular outlet septum, narrowing the subaortic outflow tract.

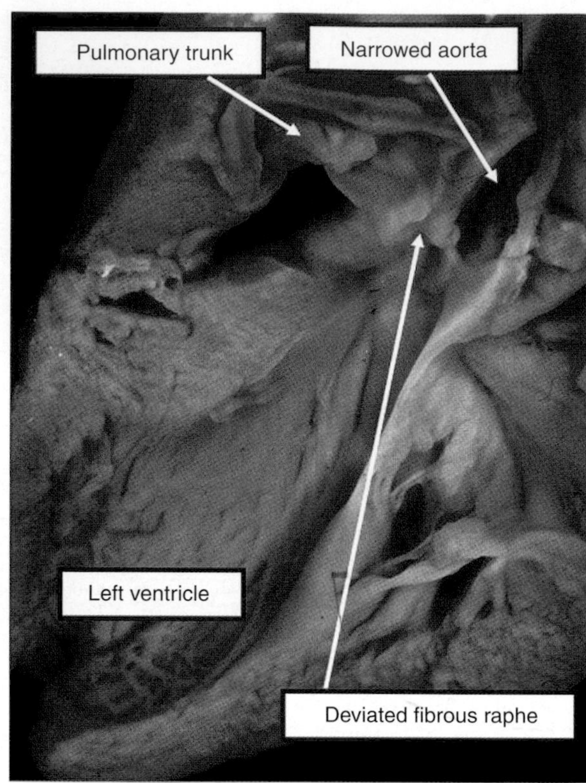

Figure 46-14 In this heart, also sectioned in parasternal long-axis fashion, there is a variation on the morphology shown in Figure 46-13. In this heart, the outlet septum is represented by its fibrous remnant, so that the defect is doubly committed and juxta-arterial. The deviated fibrous raphe, nonetheless, still obstructs the subaortic outflow from the left ventricle.

overriding of the aortic valve[22] (Fig. 46-15). Interruption of the aortic arch can be found with an aortopulmonary window rather than a ventricular septal defect (see Fig. 46-12). It, and coarctation, of course, can be found in the setting of discordant ventriculo-arterial connections, or double outlet ventricle, or common arterial trunk. The coarctation or interruption is then considered the associated lesion, and these are dealt with in the appropriate chapters of our book. Very rarely, interruption can be found in the absence of associated lesions, and with a closed arterial duct.[18,22] The supply to the lower half of the body is then dependent on collateral circulation.

The second mechanism underscoring the existence of associated lesions is one producing obstruction to the outflow from the left ventricle both pre- and postnatally. Lesions falling into this second category include valvar and subvalvar aortic stenosis, and potentially the aortic valve with two leaflets. Congenital stenotic lesions of the mitral valve will also lead to decreased flow through the aortic arch, as will supravalvar mitral shelf, stenosing left atrial ring, and divided left atrium. The presence of several such lesions in combination presents a particularly poor prognosis, with the heart itself in such settings overlapping with the hypoplastic left heart syndrome. The best known combination involves co-existence of parachute mitral valve, supravalvar left atrial ring, subaortic stenosis, and aortic coarctation. It is known as Shone's syndrome.[23]

The aortic valve with two leaflets is usually haemodynamically insignificant in early postnatal life. It is, nonetheless, a common finding in patients with aortic coarctation. In later life, the malformation of the aortic valve predisposes to calcific stenosis, regurgitation, and infective endocarditis. When found in association with coarctation, however, the morphology of the bifoliate valve is significantly different from that seen as an isolated lesion.[20] When found

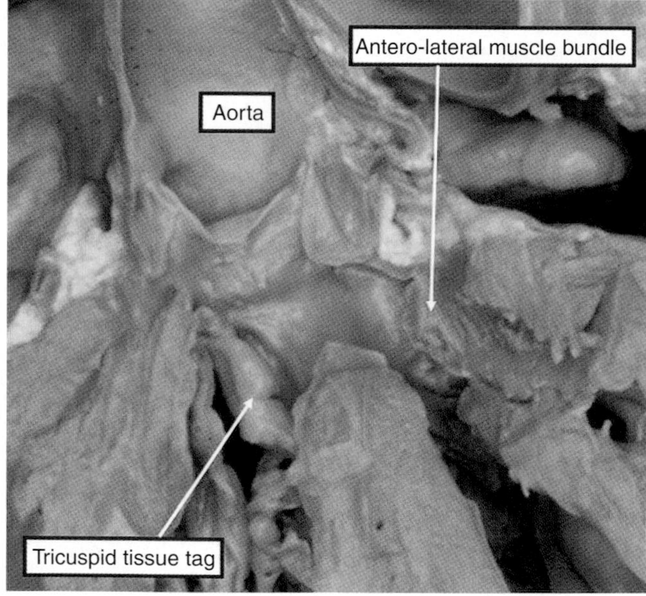

Figure 46-15 The ventricular septal defect in this heart associated with aortic coarctation is perimembranous, and overridden by the aortic valve. The entrance to the aorta from the left ventricle is narrowed by hypertrophy of the antero-lateral muscle bundle of the left ventricle, while tissue tags narrow the right ventricular origin of the aorta. These lesions presumably reduced aortic flow during fetal life.

in patients with coarctation, the valve typically has two equally sized leaflets, whereas bifoliate aortic valves seen in isolation usually have leaflets of unequal size. Irrespective of the valvar morphology, there is a known association between the bifoliate valve and weakness in the aortic wall, this accounting for the long-term incidence of dilation, and subsequent dissection of the aortic root and ascending aorta.[24] Whether this association will produce problems in the long-term follow-up of patients with coarctation has still to be established.

Anomalies of the subclavian arteries can accompany either discrete coarctation or interruption of the aortic arch. They are important both clinically and surgically, being seen more frequently in association with interruption. The most common anomaly is origin of the right subclavian from the aorta distal to the site of the ductal insertion (see Fig. 46-11). The anomalous artery then pursues a retro-oesophageal course, often arising from the expanded segment of aorta called the diverticulum of Kommerrell. The left subclavian artery can also be anomalous, arising paraductally (see Fig. 46-4). In this setting, the isthmus itself is exceedingly short or non-existent. The mouth of the subclavian artery can be incorporated in the ductal sling, and has a tendency to be stenosed at its origin.

As might be anticipated, coarctation, atresia, or interruption can also occur when the aortic arch is right sided. Coarctation can also be found in the setting of a double aortic arch, while interruption of part or parts of the hypothetical double aortic arch is an essential part of the understanding of vascular rings (see Chapter 47). Abnormal ventriculo-arterial connections are also described with interruption, including discordant ones, double outlet right ventricle with subpulmonary defect, or the Taussig–Bing malformation,[25] aortopulmonary window with intact septum,[26,27] and congenitally corrected transposition.[28]

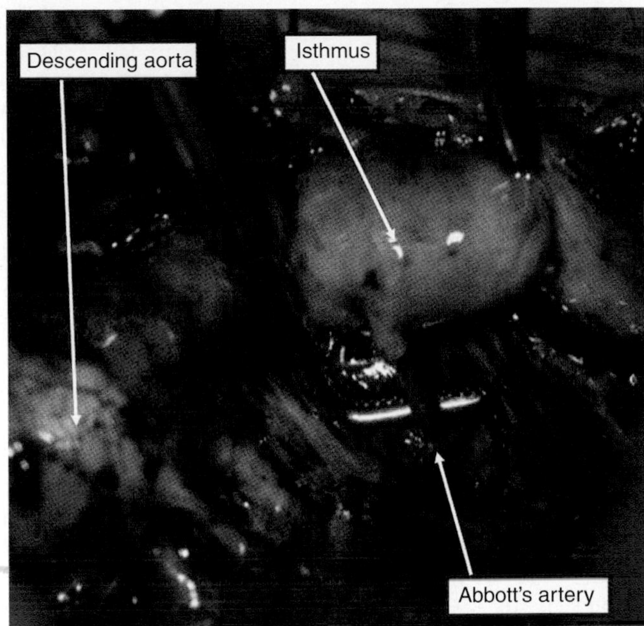

Figure 46-16 This photograph shows Abbott's artery arising from the posterior aspect of the aortic isthmus. Photograph taken in the operating room through a left thoracotomy in a patient with aortic coarctation. (Courtesy of Dr Benson R. Wilcox, University of North Carolina, Chapel Hill.)

Collateral Circulation

Although rarely present in infants, collateral circulation gradually develops throughout childhood in those with subcritical coarctation. Such collateral arteries bypass the obstruction and augment perfusion to the lower body. The most common pattern involves a large aberrant artery arising from the right subclavian artery, and supplying the aorta below the coarctation, together with various branches of the left subclavian artery, including the thyrocervical trunk, the left intercostal arteries via the left internal thoracic artery, this leading to notching of the ribs, and the anterior spinal artery through the left vertebral artery. One particular vessel in this circulation has achieved recognition as the artery of Abbott. This anomalous vessel (Fig. 46-16) arises from the posterior aspect of the isthmus, and passes medially behind the carotid artery and transverse arch.[29]

Secondary Pathology

Secondary pathology can be divided into local effects, effects on the myocardium and distant effects, the last in general caused by hypertension. The local changes tend to be characteristic. In older children and adults, fibrous intimal thickening is superimposed on the site of coarctation. The thickened layer is composed of concentric layers of collagen, with varying degrees of elastin and smooth muscle cells. The characteristic depletion and disarray of elastic tissue seen with cystic medial necrosis have also been observed.[30] The intimal proliferation, together with superimposed thrombus, can lead to near or complete obliteration of the lumen. In such instances, all distal perfusion becomes dependent on the collateral circulation. The distal aortic wall often shows post-stenotic dilatation and is somewhat thinner than normal. The abdominal aorta may, however, be somewhat hypoplastic owing to diminished flow. The combination of these local changes accounts for the occasional development of aortic dissection in patients with advanced disease without treatment. Pregnancy imposes an increased haemodynamic strain on the aortic wall owing to the physiological changes that occur, particularly in the last trimester and peripartum. Aortic dissection, and even rupture, can initially be misdiagnosed as pre-eclampsia. Such complications can also follow an apparently successful repair. Whether earlier surgical intervention decreases the occurrence of the changes in the aortic wall is not yet known.

The direct effect on the myocardium of obstruction to the left ventricular ejection depends on the rapidity of the onset, as well as the degree of the increase in afterload, the left ventricle having numerous compensatory mechanisms. In the neonate undergoing rapid decompensation with ductal closure, left ventricular systolic and diastolic dysfunction rapidly lead to congestive hear failure. Diastolic flow in the coronary arteries decreases as left ventricular wall stress increases. This leads to ischaemia, especially of the subendocardium. The resultant decrease in cardiac output causes, and then perpetuates, a metabolic acidosis, which further depresses the left ventricular contractility. In part, in infancy, this is a consequence of the inability of the myocardium to mount the usual adaptive responses to increased impedance to outflow. These will be discussed below under pathophysiology. Unless intervention is performed, death can be rapid. Of those who survive the initial insult, some develop marked subendocardial fibrosis. If the onset of obstruction is less abrupt, compensatory adaptations can occur, primarily in the form of left ventricular hypertrophy. Ischaemic heart disease eventually occurs in many, even in the absence of proximal coronary arterial occlusion. Distant complications include the well-recognised and classic berry, or saccular, aneurysm of the circle of Willis. All the organs in the upper body can sustain pathology secondary to hypertension. These changes are not entirely ameliorated by the initial relief of obstruction. This will also be discussed at greater length in the sections to follow.

Morphogenesis

There are three main aberrations in embryological development proposed to explain abnormalities of the aortic arch. The first, abnormal embryogenesis of the vessels of the arch, and the second, abnormal development of the arterial duct, are closely interlinked. The third implicates changes in the ratio of flow between the pulmonary and systemic arterial pathways.

In the usual situation, with a left-sided arch, it is the left fourth branchial arch that becomes the definitive aortic arch. The arterial duct is the persisting artery of the left sixth branchial arch, connecting to the dorsal aorta. The left subclavian artery, in contrast, forms from the seventh segmental artery. This must undergo a cephalad migration through differential growth before it assumes its definitive position proximal to the aortic isthmus. In its migration, it must cross many structures. Derangements in this process are suggested to be of importance in the pathogenesis of coarctation. The hypothesis implicating the arterial duct is based on the presence of the ductal sling around the entire circumference of the aortic isthmus in the setting of coarctation. Unequivocal evidence of such a ductal sling (Fig. 46-17) was provided initially by Wielenga and Dankmeijer,[31] and subsequently confirmed by others.[32,33]

The third proposal is that the patterns of flow of blood in the fetal circulation influences embryogenesis, specifically that a reduction in the volume of blood passing through the ascending aorta in fetal life leads postnatally to the development of coarctation.[34] Such a hypothesis is strongly supported by the common association of coarctation with other obstructive lesions in the left side of the heart, along with those malformations that result in decreased flow in the fetal ascending aorta.

No single hypothesis can explain the morphogenesis of all obstructive lesions in the aortic arch. It is most likely that there is interplay between the various mechanisms. It is highly likely, for example, that decreased flow to the aorta in some way influences the distribution of ductal tissue in the aortic arch. These basis mechanisms certainly help in the understanding of the clinical presentation, early management, and even successful treatment of the various obstructive lesions to be described below.

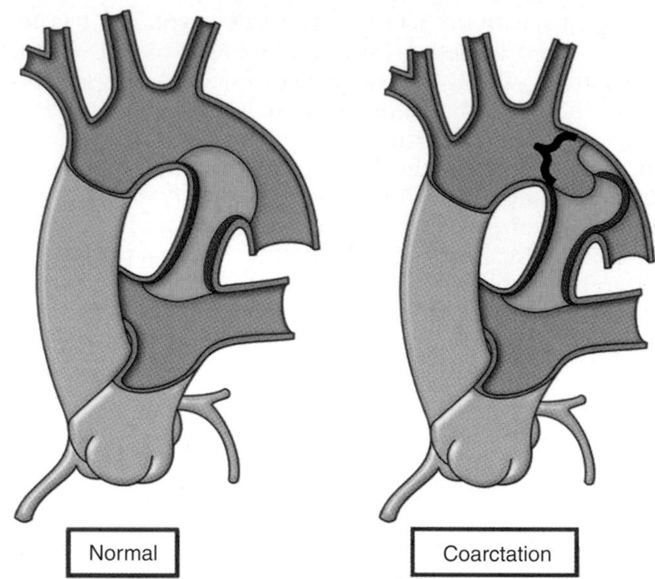

Figure 46-17 The cartoons show the differing extent of ductal tissue (*yellow*) relative to the aortic arch in the normal situation, and in the setting of aortic coarctation. The ductal tissue lassos the lumen of the isthmus (*bracket*) when there is coarctation.

Presentation and Clinical Symptomatology

Neonates and Infants

Most infants with coarctation or interruption present with varying degrees of heart failure in infancy. When seen immediately, this is manifested by collapse, or later by poor feeding, sweating, breathlessness and failure to thrive. The group that survives infancy without symptoms will be discussed below. The onset of cardiac failure is commonly within the first 3 months of life, but a significant number present within the first week of life, who uniformly will have critical narrowing of the aorta. They present when the supplementary effect of blood flow through the duct from the right ventricle to the descending aorta is interrupted by its closure, critically limiting the blood flow to the lower body. The situation, therefore, is often described as a duct-dependent systemic circulation. This process causes them to become acutely unwell with metabolic acidosis, shock, renal failure and necrotising enterocolitis. Similarly, interrupted aortic arch tends to present with cardiac heart failure of acute onset occurring simultaneously with closure of the arterial duct within the first few days of life. Four-fifths are admitted to a specialist hospital within 2 weeks.[35]

The secondary effects of acidosis on the myocardium, will then lead to additional global reduction in cardiac output. The coarctation itself may only be recognised as the infant is resuscitated. With the introduction of prostaglandin E_1 in the 1970s, it was possible to temporarily maintain ductal patency, and this revolutionised the management of these infants. This will be discussed below.

In the most common situation, where interruption is associated with a patent arterial duct and ventricular septal defect, the infant will initially be well because the pulmonary vascular resistance is high and blood will, therefore, pass through the arterial duct to the systemic circulation. One of two events will precipitate collapse in these infants. First, ductal closure will lead to a critical reduction in lower body perfusion and rapid development of acidosis and shock. Second, a falling pulmonary vascular resistance in the presence of a widely patent duct will lead to preferential flow of blood to the pulmonary circulation to the detriment of the systemic circulation. More slowly progressive, but potentially equally important, tissue acidosis leading to collapse may also occur. In those with the rarer variant of interruption occurring in isolation, there must be a collateral circulation, usually via the head and neck vessels, which can develop very rapidly.[36]

Physical Findings

The signs on presentation in infancy include tachypnea, with intercostal recession. If markedly low cardiac output is present, they will often show profound skin mottling, slow capillary refill, and peripheral cyanosis. Central cyanosis will occur only in the presence of an associated cyanotic congenital cardiac lesion, or when there is persistence of the fetal circulation. The presence of palpable femoral pulses in the first day or two of life does not exclude the diagnosis of coarctation or interruption, since flow of blood to the lower body may be maintained antegradely through the persistently patent arterial duct. Once symptoms occur, the femoral pulses are usually weaker, or absent. If the patient has severe low output and no pulses are felt, resuscitation usually causes the pulses in the right arm to return. The praecordium is often active, unless myocardial function is depressed. On auscultation, there is usually a summation gallop rhythm. There is often a systolic murmur found along the left sternal edge, from the site of coarctation, and this may also be audible posteriorly. The continuous murmur classically ascribed to coarctation is unusual in infancy. Associated cardiac or central vascular defects, such as the persistently patent arterial duct, can produce additional murmurs. An ejection systolic murmur may indicate an associated bicuspid aortic valve. Signs of congestive heart failure, such as hepatomegaly and crepitations on auscultation, are commonly found. Auscultation in patients with interrupted aortic arch is usually unhelpful. Often a gallop rhythm is present, and the heart sounds are usually easily audible, the second being split. An ejection click may indicate the presence of associated bicuspid aortic valve, but this is non-specific. If a murmur is present, it is often pan- or mid-systolic and of low intensity, indicating the non-restrictive nature of the ventricular septal defect.

Measurements of the blood pressure in all four limbs reveal a gradient between the upper and lower limbs irrespective of the method used to measure it, although Doppler appears preferable.[37] It should be remembered that differences in pressure of up to 20 mm Hg may be revealed by Doppler interrogation in the normal neonate, presumably owing to the isthmal narrowing that is normal at this stage.[38] It is sometimes necessary to measure blood pressures serially if the diagnosis remains unclear. Paradoxically, the diagnosis of coarctation can be made more difficult by the administration of prostaglandin. Although greatly improving the physical condition, the manoeuvre leads to the pressure difference between the arms and legs becoming significantly diminished, making the clinical diagnostic process less clear. Indeed, in the presence of a marked run-off between the right subclavian and the iliac arteries as occurs with a large arterial duct or a cerebral arteriovenous malformation, for example, it may be possible to detect a large difference between systolic blood pressures measured in the arms and legs and yet the femoral pulses will remain easily palpable. The combination of weak or absent femoral pulses together with a gradient in pressure between the limbs is therefore virtually pathognomonic of aortic coarctation.

Older Children and Adults

Frequently patients with coarctation go beyond infancy without detection, either because initially the coarctation was not severe enough to become critical following closure of the arterial duct, or because of a significant early collateral circulation. The diagnosis then usually follows a routine medical examination, where the murmur is discovered, femoral pulses are found to be weak, or unexplained systemic hypertension is found. Headaches, nosebleeds, cold feet, or calf pain on exercise are often experienced.[39] Sometimes patients present with end-stage systemic hypertensive disease, such as subarachnoid haemorrhage or hypertensive retinopathy. Very occasionally, the lesion is detected during investigations for coronary arterial disease in later life.

Physical Findings

The physical findings in older patients usually rest upon the appreciation of diminished or delayed femoral pulses compared with the pulses in either arm. The femoral pulse is normally fractionally earlier than the radial, with a similar character, waveform and volume. If this is not the case, then the patient should be further investigated. More reliable than the delay of the femoral pulse to exclude coarctation is measurement of blood pressures in all limbs.[40] Further signs include a normal jugular venous pressure, and normal sized liver. Indirect signs of left ventricular hypertrophy, such as a displaced apical beat and heave, are often found on palpation of the praecordium. On auscultation, the first and second heart sounds are usually normal, but may be accompanied by an apical fourth heart sound if the left ventricle is becoming non-compliant. The murmur of coarctation is best heard in the left infraclavicular fossa and radiates to the back over the left scapula. It is continuous, peaks late in systole, and continues into early diastole, corresponding with the diastolic tail seen on Doppler echocardiography. Additional continuous murmurs may be generated by larger collateral arteries, which can restore adequate flow of blood to the lower body, resulting in palpable femoral pulses, albeit usually reduced and delayed. If surgery is considered, this feature will be crucial, as it determines if partial cardiopulmonary bypass is required or not to maintain adequate perfusion of the lower body and spinal cord whilst the coarcted segment is excluded with clamps for the repair. In the patients beyond infancy, the physical findings of associated abnormalities, such as an ejection click with bicuspid aortic valve, or a murmur owing to a small ventricular septal defect, will be typical of those lesions. A search for disease caused by hypertension is often unrewarding in childhood, although fundoscopic changes with a unique corkscrew appearance to the retinal arteries has been described. These changes are different from the usual hypertensive change.[41]

Investigations

Chest Radiography

In infants, cardiomegaly and increased pulmonary vascular markings can be seen on the radiograph. In older children, the heart size is often normal, but if cardiomegaly is present, it is usually caused by left ventricular enlargement. There are two pathognomonic signs on the plain chest radiograph in older children. The first is the figure 3 sign, which appears to the left of the mediastinum and is caused by pre- and post-stenotic dilation of the aorta (Fig. 46-18). The second sign is rib notching, which is usually not seen until 4 years of age, although appearance in the first year has been described.[42] By adulthood, around three-quarters of untreated patients have rib notching. It is best seen posteriorly in the medial third of the lower borders of the fourth to eighth ribs, where the intercostal artery crosses the rib (see Fig. 46-18). The notching in coarctation is classically bilateral, to be differentiated from the unilateral notching seen after a classical Blalock–Taussig shunt, although unilateral notching can also occur with coarctation when a subclavian artery arises aberrantly distal to the site of obstruction.

In those with interruption the heart is usually left sided with normal abdominal and bronchial arrangement. Cardiomegaly, particularly enlargement of the left atrium, is present in nine-tenths of neonates.[43] Increased pulmonary vascular markings with pulmonary oedema are also the norm. In the rare patients who survive infancy untreated, more specific signs can be seen,[44] including absence of the aortic knob, a midline trachea, absence of an aortic impression on the barium swallow, and termination of the descending aorta at the level of the pulmonary trunk. Rib notching can also be seen on the side of the subclavian arteries arising from the ascending aorta in the presence of a restrictive or closed arterial duct. A narrow mediastinum may suggest absence of the thymus gland, a feature of Di George syndrome.

Electrocardiography

The majority of young infants presenting with coarctation will have normal right ventricular dominance, with extreme right-axis deviation. Later, left ventricular hypertrophy supervenes. There are early electrocardiographic signs of left ventricular dominance and strain in some infants. This has been linked to subendocardial ischaemia[45] or co-existing aortic stenosis. There are no specific features that are diagnostic for interruption. As with coarctation the findings are strongly influenced by associated abnormalities, the tracings may show any combination of ventricular hypertrophy, right, left or both, or they may be normal. Occasionally, a prolonged QT interval may be seen secondary to the hypocalcaemia of Di George syndrome.

Magnetic Resonance Imaging

Although echocardiography is a superior modality for the diagnosis of congenital cardiac disease in infants and young children, and magnetic resonance imaging is limited in smaller children because of the need for sedation or anaesthesia, the latter technique combined with phase velocity mapping can be used as a complete diagnostic tool in obtaining both morphological and physiological information in coarctation.[46] It is also an excellent tool in the assessment of postoperative repair. It can reveal not only the primary pathology and the collateral flow, but also assess secondary pathology, for example, the aortic root for dilation if a bicuspid aortic valve is present, aortic valvar incompetence and stenosis, and provide details of left ventricular mass and function. Magnetic resonance, therefore, is rapidly establishing itself as the method of choice in the evaluation of treatment and complications of aortic coarctation, most notably of aortic gradients and recoarctation. The gradient in blood pressure between the arms and legs is not a reliable indicator of haemodynamic significance of restenosis in patients with prior repair of coarctation. Direct visualisation of collateral vessels by magnetic resonance angiography, and proportional increases in flow from proximal to distal descending thoracic aorta, in contrast, are reliable indicators of haemodynamic significance.[47] Changes in the collateral circulation after stenting of coarctation segments have also been successfully demonstrated using phase-contrast magnetic resonance.[48] The combination of anatomic and flow data obtained by magnetic resonance provides a sensitive and specific test for predicting catheterisation gradient greater than 20 mm Hg in native and recurrent coarctations.[49] Contrast-enhanced magnetic resonance angiography provides additional diagnostic information compared to fast-spin echo magnetic resonance.[50]

When magnetic resonance, magnetic resonance angiography, and Doppler echocardiography are compared in relation to surgical repair of coarctation, it has been shown that magnetic resonance is superior to Doppler echocardiography in the evaluation of the aorta, and that the internal measurement of the narrowing does not correspond to the external aspect of the surgical narrowing.[51] Helical computer tomography and magnetic resonance do not

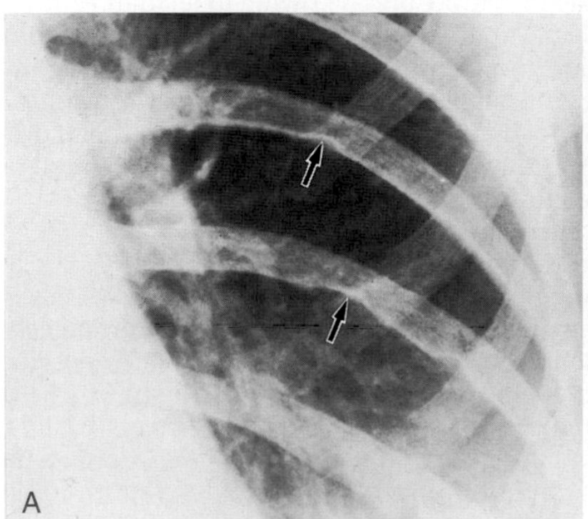

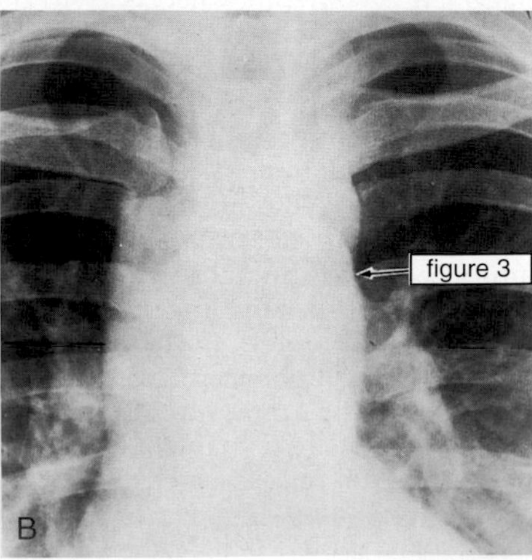

Figure 46-18 These chest radiographs show evidence of coarctation, with (**A**) rib notching (*arrows*) and (**B**) the figure 3 sign.

seem to differ when used for follow-up assessment of adults with treated coarctations. There can be a substantial variation in two subsequent measurements, without an overall substantial bias towards larger diameter in one of the two methods.[52] In those with interruption of the arch, magnetic resonance can also be a useful tool to assess the length of the interruption and any associated anomalies, most notably with three-dimensional gadolinium-enhanced magnetic resonance angiography.[53]

Echocardiography

Echocardiography has become the diagnostic method of choice in infancy. The aortic arch is best visualised from the suprasternal notch in the superior paracoronal view, revealing details of the entire arch (Fig. 46-19). In those with coarctation, there is most commonly a short narrowed segment just distal to the left subclavian artery caused by the obstructive shelf projecting into the aorta posteriorly. More rarely, there is a longer segment of narrowing involving the isthmus (Fig. 46-20). It must be remembered that the apparent anterior shelf often seen on the anterior wall of the aorta is not part of the coarctation, but the overlapping point of entry of the duct.[54] It is important, especially in infants, to assess the size of the transverse aortic arch. It can often be hypoplastic (Fig. 46-21) or stenotic, and can result in residual obstruction after distal repair. In the absence of an arterial duct, the haemodynamic severity of coarctation can readily be assessed by Doppler echocardiography.

The spectral recording shows an extension of antegrade flow, and a persisting gradient into diastole, the so-called diastolic tail. There is rarely any doubt to its significance, but if uncertainty does exist, the spectral recording can be analysed further[55] according to the peak velocity and the half-time of diastolic velocity decay. This predicts accurately the severity of anatomical coarctation (Fig. 46-22). Another useful feature is the carotid-subclavian arterial index, which is the ratio of the diameter of the aortic arch at the left subclavian artery to the distance between the left carotid artery and the left subclavian artery, with a ratio of less than 1.5 being both sensitive and specific for coarctation in infants and neonates.[56] In neonates with a patent arterial duct, measurements of ratio of diameters of the isthmus and descending aorta, along with the delineation of the posterior shelf and a discrepancy in blood pressure between the limbs, has been shown satisfactorily to identify those with coarctation.[57] In isolated coarctation, the peak instantaneous pressure drop across the obstruction can be calculated from the peak velocity of the jet by using the simplified Bernoulli equation. In the presence of

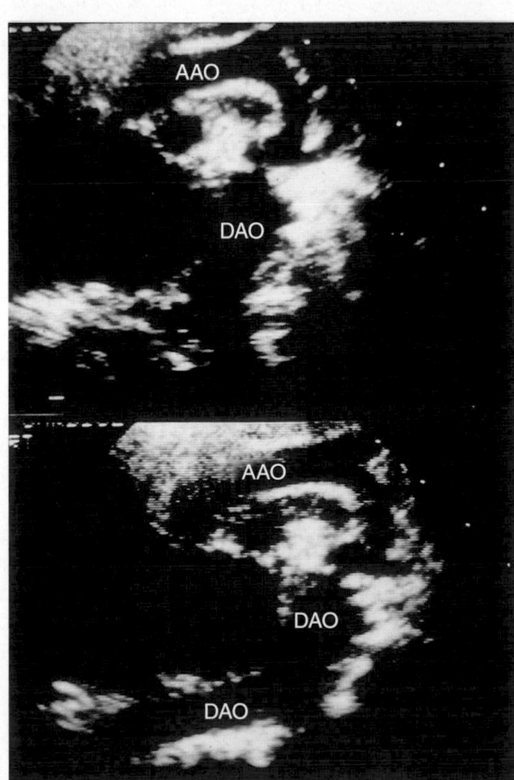

Figure 46-19 These echocardiographic images obtained from the suprasternal approach show severe discrete coarctation in a neonate. AAO, ascending aorta; DAO, descending aorta.

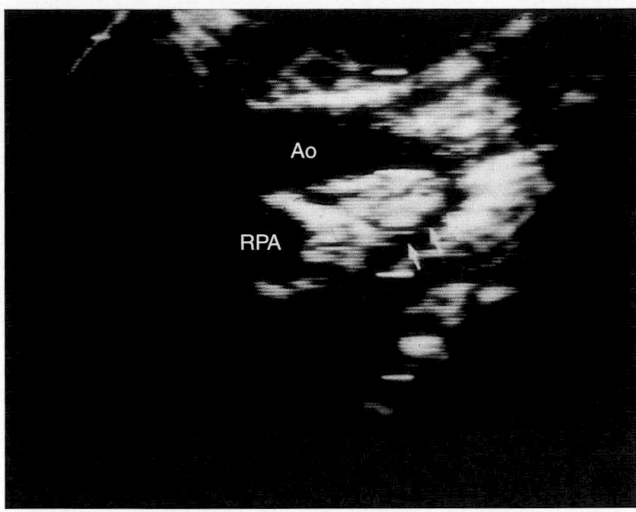

Figure 46-20 This suprasternal paracoronal section shows long segment isthmal tubular hypoplasia (*arrows*). Ao, aorta; RPA, right pulmonary artery.

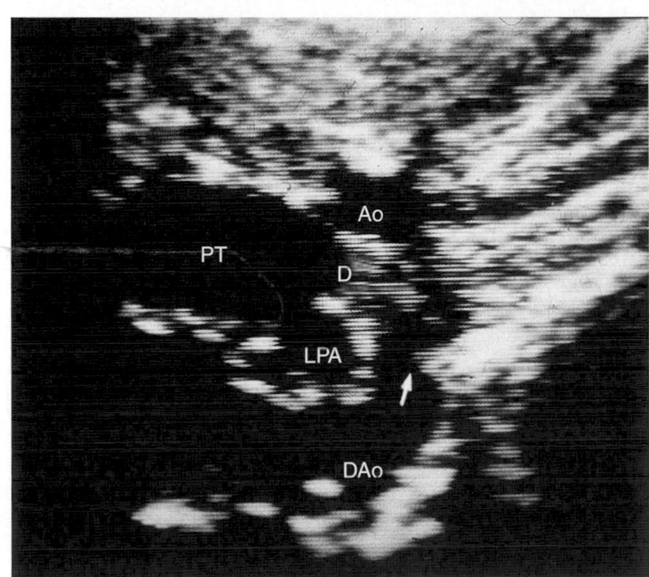

Figure 46-21 This image shows hypoplasia of the transverse arch, which is tortuous and small, with relative sparing of the isthmus (*arrow*). Ao, aorta; DAo, descending aorta; D, duct; LPA, left pulmonary artery; PT, pulmonary trunk.

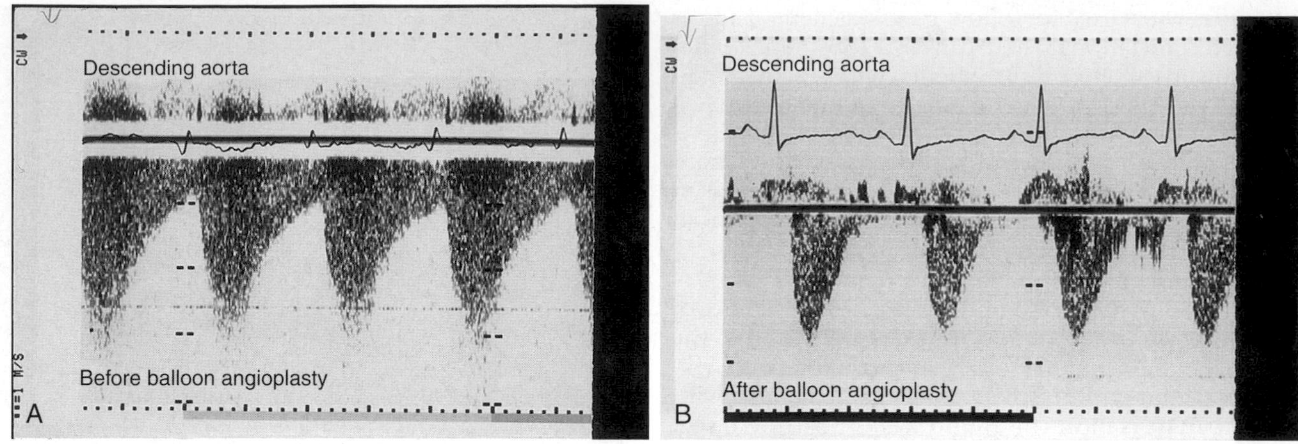

Figure 46-22 The image shows typical spectral Doppler recordings from a patient with severe aortic coarctation before (**A**) and after (**B**) balloon angioplasty. The peak velocity is 3 m/sec, but more importantly there is a prolonged diastolic tail, which is abolished immediately after balloon angioplasty.

a significant associated obstructive lesion in the left heart, it is necessary to quantify the peak velocity of the jet proximal to the site of coarctation. This can often be significantly raised and, if not taken into account by using the expanded Bernoulli equation, there can be a significant overestimation of the gradient.[58] The remaining examination must be focused on the potential associated malformations, with care taken to assess the mitral and aortic valves accurately. Left ventricular mass should be measured and an M-mode assessment of left ventricular shortening fraction should be made. It must always be remembered that, in the presence of coarctation severe enough to cause low cardiac output, the severity of associated obstructive lesions in the left heart can be underestimated. All of these observations must be modified in the presence of an arterial duct. When large, any gradient across the site of coarctation will be obviated, and the pattern of flow altered. Under these circumstances, much more reliance is placed upon adequate imaging of the stenotic area. In experienced hands, the diagnosis of coarctation using echo Doppler can be made with 95% sensitivity and 99% specificity.[59]

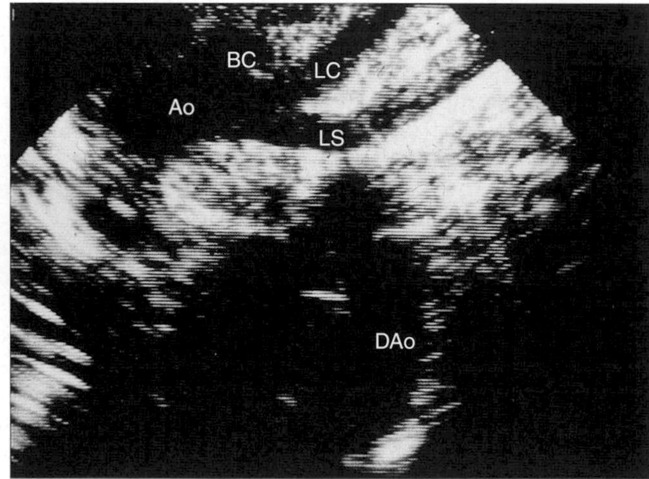

Figure 46-23 This suprasternal echocardiographic section shows the typical appearances of interruption of the aortic arch distal to the subclavian artery. Ao, aorta; BC, brachiocephalic artery; DAo, descending aorta; LC, left carotid artery; LS, left subclavian artery.

When the arch is interrupted in patients with Di George syndrome, echocardiography is more difficult because of absence of the thymic window. The examination must focus on the intracardiac anatomy, as well as on the aortic arch. Subcostal views will demonstrate the discrepancy in size between aorta and pulmonary arteries. Suprasternally, a relatively small ascending aortic arch is seen to follow an obviously straight course, leading to at least one arterial branch, while the much larger pulmonary trunk leads, via the arterial duct, to the proximal end of a much larger descending aorta.[60] If approached in this fashion, it is possible to show the entirety of the aorta, despite the interruption, permitting accurate diagnosis in almost all neonates (Fig. 46-23). The parasternal long-axis view will demonstrate the ventricular septal defect, along with the degree of obstruction of the left ventricular outflow tract. Particular care is needed to exclude an aberrant right subclavian artery, or right-sided arterial duct, in the usual setting of a left-sided aortic arch.

Fetal Echocardiography

Significant advantages accrue when congenitally malformed hearts are diagnosed accurately during fetal life, especially those lesions that can be deemed duct dependent, as intervention electively with prostaglandin can prevent shock and acidosis. For those with coarctation, antenatal diagnosis has been shown to permit presentation in a better condition, with less consequent mortality.[61] There are difficulties, nonetheless, in prenatal diagnosis of coarctation. Although a certain combination of features is strongly suggestive of abnormalities in the aortic arch, there is a significant rate of false-positive diagnosis, particularly in late pregnancy.[62,63] Severe coarctation is certainly associated with relative hypoplasia of the components of the left heart when compared with the right, and this is visible in early pregnancy, but this can also be a feature of the normal fetus later in pregnancy. Milder forms of coarctation, furthermore, are compatible with an entirely normal fetal echocardiogram, especially in the last trimester.

Cardiac Catheterisation and Angiography

In most cases, sufficient information can be obtained from clinical and non-invasive examination to decide on an appropriate plan for management. Cardiac catheterisation is of limited value in delineating further the anatomy in the neonate, and it is associated with significant

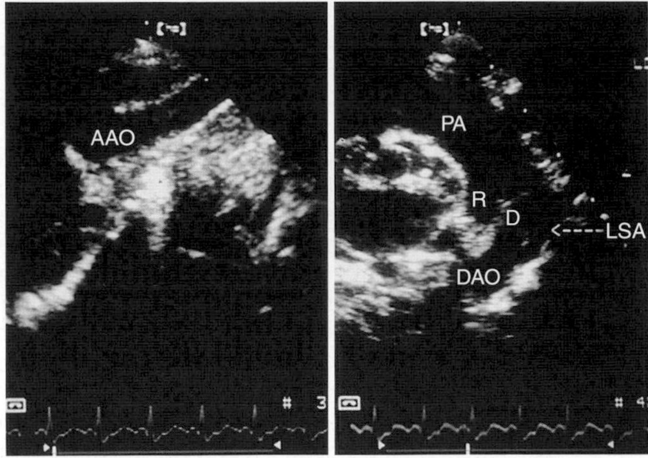

Figure 46-24 The echocardiographic images show interruption of the aortic arch between the left carotid artery and left subclavian artery (LSA), the latter arising from the descending aorta (DAO), opposite the arterial duct (D). AAO, ascending aorta; PA, pulmonary trunk; R, right pulmonary artery.

morbidity. It is rarely necessary for the assessment of associated anomalies. Indeed, even if significant mitral obstruction, mitral regurgitation or aortic stenosis is present, the baby is often better assessed after repair of the coarctation, when cardiac output, the effects of the arterial duct and other abnormalities of ventricular performance, have resolved. One potential indication for invasive assessment, nonetheless, is for intervention in the setting of coarctation. Controversy has surrounded the use of balloon angioplasty as the primary treatment for patients of various ages with coarctation since its first use in 1982.[64] This will be discussed in more detail below.

On the rare occasion that aortography is performed in the setting of interrupted arch, an injection into the ascending aorta will demonstrate, in three-fifths of cases, the classic V sign as seen in the frontal projection of the brachiocephalic and left common carotid arteries, as also seen in the echocardiogram (Fig. 46-24).[43] Occasionally, the V more resembles a U or W if all three arteries take origin proximal to the interruption. The appearance is still characteristic in that the aortic arch continues smoothly into its most distal branch proximal to the interruption, regardless of whether this is the brachiocephalic, left common carotid, or subclavian artery. If the aortic arch continues beyond its last branch, and appears to taper down to apparent complete obstruction, the diagnosis is either aortic atresia, or else severe coarctation with distal wash-in from the arterial duct and not interruption.[65]

COURSE AND PROGNOSIS

The quoted mean length of survival is 31 years for those with coarctation surviving the first year without an operation, three-quarters being dead by the age of 46 years. This information was derived from clinical records and postmortem studies.[66] In a natural history study in which infants who died in their first year of life were excluded,[66] it was suggested that those presenting with congestive heart failure might have had a survival rate at 1 year as low as 16%, this figure taking no account of associated lesions. In older patients, the cause of death was often related to systemic hypertension, the two most common findings being congestive cardiac failure and aortic dissection or rupture. Bacterial endocarditis was also common. An additional significant group died as a result of ruptured berry or saccular aneurysms causing intracranial bleeding, a feature more commonly found in coarctation.[67] Hypertension secondary to coarctation is not, however, thought to be the only pathogenetic factor. Abnormalities of the vessel wall are important, certainly in intracerebral catastrophes, but also with the other causes of death such as aortic dissection or rupture. Cystic medial necrosis and new structural abnormalities are seen in areas remote from the coarcted segment itself and may be unrelated to the type and age at surgery.

When considering interruption of the arch, the natural history is poor. Without surgery, three-quarters die in the first month of life, the majority in the first 10 days. Less than one-tenth survive without correction beyond the first year of life if there is co-existing ductal patency.[16,68,69] With the evolution of prostaglandin therapy and surgical intervention over the past decades, the impact of the associated cardiac and extracardiac defects has become of greater relevance in interruption, although little long-term follow up is available.

The mortality from bacterial endocarditis has fallen markedly in recent years through improved diagnostic techniques, especially cross sectional echocardiography, and aggressive early treatment with antibiotics. If present, the site of endocarditis is often in the aorta, distal to the site of coarctation or interruption, or on an associated bicuspid aortic valve. At present, nonetheless, it is usually recommended that children with coarctation or interruption receive prophylactic antibiotics against endocarditis, even after definitive surgical repair, during dental, colonic and genitourinary procedures.

MANAGEMENT

Stabilisation of Neonates and Infants

Clinical management of infants with coarctation and interruption was dramatically changed in the 1980s by the advent of pharmacological means to maintain patency and reopen the arterial duct. This now enables the majority of infants with either preductal coarctation or interruption, who present with heart failure, shock and deteriorating renal function, to perfuse their lower body, albeit with systemic venous blood. This will, nonetheless, reverse the tissue ischaemia as long as ductal patency and flow is maintained. The beneficial effects of prostaglandin E_1 in maintaining ductal patency under both aerobic and anaerobic conditions[70] did not lead immediately to its use, but a decade later it was commonly used in patients with obstructive lesions such as coarctation and interruption.[71] Prostaglandin E_1 is given initially at a dose of 0.05 to 0.1 μg/min/kg body weight. This can be increased to 0.4 μg/min/kg if required, although lower initial doses have been shown to be equally therapeutic and less likely to cause apnoea.[72] The maximal response occurs between 15 minutes and 4 hours.[73] Occasional improvement has been documented in infants as old as 5 weeks, but treatment is generally less impressive in older neonates, and in those whose ducts are closed at presentation.[73,74] Positive effects have also been found on the diameter of the coarcted segment of the aorta without any reopening of the arterial duct, suggesting the presence of reactive ductal tissue in the aorta.[75,76] Side effects can include a decreased respiratory drive leading to apnoea, occasionally requiring ventilation. There can also be hypotension with cutaneous vasodilation; jitteriness, which can lead to seizures; fever; susceptibility to infections; diarrhoea; and, more rarely, coagulopathy. For the neonates, management depends on timing of diagnosis. If the diagnosis has been made, or is strongly suspected, antenatally, then there is little to be lost from starting prostaglandin E_1 at birth. Certain centres advocate antenatal transfer and delivery in or close to the cardiac centre. If a neonate is found to have weak or absent femoral pulses, and remains well, it is justifiable to arrange transfer to a tertiary centre, having commenced prostaglandin E_1 to avoid the catastrophe of an acute closure of the duct during transfer.

In any infant becoming shocked within the first few weeks of life in the absence of pulses in the lower limbs, it should be mandatory to start prostaglandin along with the normal resuscitatory manoeuvres while expert assistance is sought. Ventilation with positive pressure will reduce the systemic demand for oxygen, and may improve cardiac failure. During ventilation, manoeuvres to increase pulmonary vascular resistance, and hence reduce the ratio of pulmonary to systemic blood flow, will lead to increased right-to-left flow through the arterial duct, thus improving perfusion of the lower body. The management is similar to that adopted in the pre- and post-operative care of the infant with hypoplastic left heart syndrome (see Chapter 29). This will include minimising the fraction of inspired oxygen, maintaining arterial partial pressure of carbon dioxide at 6 kPa or more, and the judicious use of volume and ionotropes. The outcome in these children with multi-organ failure is much more favourable if time is taken medically to stabilise them before carrying out definitive intervention.[77] If prostaglandin E_1 produces no effect of augmenting distal aortic flow, which occurs in a small proportion of patients, then immediate definitive treatment is required.[78]

During the preoperative workup, patients require chromosomal analysis for 22q11 deletion using fluorescent in situ hybridisation. Levels of calcium need to be measured to exclude hypocalcaemia, and to anticipate it before clinical sequels, such as convulsions, develop. Infusions of calcium are useful in the acute phase. Subsequently, the management is identical to that of isolated hypoparathyroidism, involving oral supplementation of calcium and administration of vitamin D. Documentation of decreased levels of parathormone in the setting of low levels of calcium are diagnostically important before embarking on treatment, which should ideally be conducted with advice from a paediatric endocrinologist. Abnormalities can occur in the function of the T cells, and it is important to assay their number and function. In the acute phase, infants with interruption should be presumed to have defects of the T cells. Transfusion, including cardiopulmonary bypass, should be performed using irradiated blood to avoid the possibility of transfused lymphocytes causing graft-versus-host disease. Later on, the susceptibility to infection may lead to the need for rotational antibiotics or other immune manipulation. These children often have developmental delay and problems with feeding, both of which need a significant amount of medical input after repair.

Definitive Treatment

As yet, there is no single cost-effective technique with clearly demonstrable superior outcomes in the short-term and long-term, and without significant side-effects, for all types of coarctation and interruption. The pursuit of a single ideal form of therapy for all forms of coarctation is almost certainly misguided, as the obstructive lesions show great variability in their morphology, even before ductal patency and associated intracardiac lesions are considered.[79] Furthermore, a significant proportion of the literature is now of only historical value, as over the past 50 years both surgical and cardiological techniques and medical resuscitation have improved greatly, and prostaglandin has been introduced. Many studies exist, but are based on different groups of patients from different periods of time, and treated with different techniques.[79] Large multi-centric randomised controlled trials of the various forms of surgical and interventional cardiological techniques for various types of coarctation, therefore, are long overdue.

Non-elective Surgical Repair

The majority of infants with duct-dependent circulations can be stabilised medically, and will benefit from an interlude before definitive treatment while metabolic derangements are corrected. These infants, nonetheless, will need relief of their aortic obstruction within 1 or 2 days of presentation. There have been reports that minimally symptomatic infants with isolated coarctation can be managed medically for a period of time.[80,81] Nowadays, even those born with coarctation and very low weight, less than 2 kg, can undergo corrective surgery with a low mortality, but will be at a higher risk of recoarctation.[82] The majority of symptomatic infants undergo surgery with little delay. There is a subgroup of patients who present in cardiogenic shock and cannot easily be stabilised medically. Timely intervention, with the therapeutic strategy individualised to the anatomy, has been shown to give excellent outcomes in neonates with coarctation.[83] There is ongoing debate, nonetheless, about the procedure of choice, and whether the associated defects should be addressed at the same time as resection of the coarctation, or at a second procedure.

The major concern remains the significant incidence of recoarctation. Difficulties arise in the interpretation of the data, as some papers cite residual gradients from arm to leg, others measure differences between the arms, whereas still others measure the difference in the pressure between the arms and legs as exposed by exercise. Furthermore, many cases that are termed recoarctation represent residual coarctations. In order to try to standardise these features, four patterns of gradients have been described between the arms and legs after initial surgery.[84] The first pattern results in complete and permanent abolition of the gradient after surgery, the second leads to an initial abolition followed by late recurrence. The third group has initial residual obstruction followed by late resolution, whereas the last group has persistent residual obstruction. Defining rates of recoarctation as the percentage of patients undergoing surgery who are known to have recoarctation at the time of reporting, is very dependent on the period over which progress has been monitored, and therefore actuarial rates of recoarctation should be used.[85,86]

Management of Associated Lesions in Infancy

The management of associated lesions is tailored according to clinical needs and pathology. An arterial duct, if patent, should be ligated during surgery. Controversy surrounds the management of concomitant ventricular septal defects when treating coarctation in neonates and infants. Some opt for repair of the coarctation through a lateral thoracotomy, with subsequent assessment of progress. In this approach, inability to wean from the ventilator, or failure to thrive, would indicate the need for surgical closure of the ventricular septal defect. Its advantages include allowing improvement in ventricular performance, pulmonary oedema, and the general condition of the infant. It may even buy time for spontaneous closure of small defects. More frequently, especially if there is a single defect and the child is not small, the option nowadays is to proceed with complete repair in one stage. This involves closing the defect, together with repair of coarctation, via a midline sternotomy. In earlier times, this was associated with higher mortalities, but contemporary reviews suggest this is no longer the case.[87] Another alternative is to use only one operation, but to repair the coarctation through a left thoracotomy, using a subsequent sternotomy to correct the intracardiac defect.[88] This approach has the downside of multiple incisions but will lead to shorter periods on bypass, and avoids any circulatory arrest. It also reportedly decreases the time spent in both intensive care and hospital.[88] The least fashionable option nowadays is to repair the coarctation and band the pulmonary trunk. This option remains valid for those with multiple ventricular septal defects, or for those in whom the defects are judged inaccessible. It is rarely recommended for the management of single large defects. The presence of a left-to-right shunt prior to repair of the coarctation, and extension of the defect into the right ventricular inlet or outlet, nonetheless, are two situations in which the ventricular septal defect is less likely to close spontaneously.[89] In addition more complicated associated defects, such as transposition, double outlet right ventricle, tricuspid atresia or double inlet ventricle, also need to be taken into consideration and addressed at the time of repair of coarctation.

In those infants at the extreme end of the spectrum with multiple obstructive lesions in the left heart, such as Shone's complex, the prognosis is more guarded with a significant early mortality, although there possibly is some benefit from aggressive reconstructive surgery with early attention paid to the mitral valve.[90,91] The late functional outcome can be favourable compared with more conservative approaches.[91]

Elective Repair

There has also been much debate regarding optimal age for surgical treatment in asymptomatic patients with coarctation. Various issues need to be considered. Generally, overall operative mortality is greatest in those under 1 year of age for most conditions, although this has improved greatly in recent years through a combination of improved medical and intensive care management and better surgical techniques. Furthermore, the likelihood of recoarctation is related not only to the type of repair, but also to the timing of repair, being more common in those undergoing surgery under 1 year of age.[92,93] Age at operation is also important with regard to the incidence of late hypertension. This was reported in one-tenth of patients after neonatal and early repair, but increased mortality was found in children undergoing repair over the age of 5 years.[92] It had already been demonstrated that patients undergoing repair of coarctation in their late teens had an excessively high mortality from cardiovascular causes in later life.[94] There is an age, therefore, beyond which operative repair may not change the natural history of the disease.[94] These findings were subsequently confirmed by others, who also showed that residual hypertension was a poor prognostic factor.[95] Still others have since shown that hypertension can occur late after repair,[96] while a much higher incidence of permanent hypertension not caused by recoarctation is found in patients undergoing surgery above 4 years of age.[97] The break-point in another cohort was 1 year of age, with this group making recommendation some time ago for elective repair during the second 6 months of life.[98] Since then, scattered reports have appeared of permanent hypertension occurring in patients undergoing repair of coarctation in infancy, or even the neonatal period.[99–101] The problem should, nonetheless, be kept in perspective, since one analysis found no patient with permanent hypertension without recoarctation among 118 survivors of repair of coarctation in infancy.[102] In young asymptomatic children without duct dependent circulations, a more recent report has suggested that the timing of surgical repair does not seem to be a predictor of morbidity or mortality. It also does not predict residual hypertension, any residual gradient, persistent cardiomegaly, post-operative neurological sequels, the requirement for a second surgery, or the need for balloon dilation for residual post-operative coarctation and the need for antihypertensive medications within five years after surgery within a follow-up of up to 20 years.[103] In hypertensive adults with coarctation, the hypertension was abolished without requirement for medication in two-thirds of the patients, although one-third of these were hypertensive on exercise.[104] Most adults with significant coarctation that has not been treated die before the age of 50 years from cardiovascular complications. A subset of patients can survive beyond this age, and for these the benefits of surgery are unclear. Surgery for such hypertensive patients can be undertaken with low morbidity and mortality, and most are symptomatically improved, with some normotensive at rest, although a majority remains hypertensive on exercise.[105] Some patients are found, nonetheless, in whom permanent hypertension will ensue irrespective of the age of repair. To some extent, all of this discussion has become irrelevant to contemporary management. Elective surgery is performed nowadays in most centres at, or shortly after, presentation at any age. The above discussion serves as a reminder of the potential long-term implications for those with the disease, no matter when, or how, it is repaired.

The risk of paraplegia is important. Pre-operative evaluation by magnetic resonance imaging to show the presence or absence of collateral circulation is now considered to be valuable in identifying the need for pre-emptive protective actions. Options include using a temporary bypass with a polytetrafluoroethylene tube from the ascending to the descending aorta,[106] or partial bypass from the left atrium to the descending aorta.[107]

STRATEGIES FOR SURGICAL TREATMENT

Resection and End-to-End Repair

The era of repair of coarctation started during the second world war, when Blalock performed the first experimental repairs using either the turned-down left subclavian artery or the carotid artery to bypass the induced stenosis.[108] Gross, in Boston, had also demonstrated experimentally that resection with end-to-end anastomosis was feasible.[109] The first operation to resect congenital coarctation was performed by Crafoord in Stockholm.[110] The coarctation was resected, and the aortic segments were anastomosed in end-to-end fashion. To this day, this remains the most common surgical procedure in older patients with discrete narrowing. Modifications of the technique have been suggested, including the combination of resection and end-to-end repair with a subclavian flap angioplasty. Recent reports suggest this to be a safe technique when used in infants, producing no mortality and very good resolution of the gradients.[111]

As discussed earlier, there are, as yet, no proper randomised controlled trials comparing the many techniques used for surgical repair. Because of this, retrospective studies are used to provide the evidence required to guide optimal treatment. One such study compared end-to-end anastomosis to use of a subclavian flap for repair in infants younger than 3 months of age.[112] The outcomes were similar, with a similar risk of recoarctation, albeit due to different mechanisms. The expertise of the surgeon was deemed to be the primary determinant of outcome.

Interposition Grafts

Although the first use of a graft[113] ended in failure, Gross a year later interposed an aortic homograft across the coarcted segment.[114] For a time, this was considered the treatment of choice for infants with coarctation, with successful repairs being reported in a 10-week-old infant,[115] and in a neonate.[116] A similar approach, but using prosthetic conduits, was introduced later.[117] This remained useful in older patients with aneurysms, in those with complex anatomy, or for those in whom approximation of the cut ends could not be accomplished during attempted end-to-end anastomoses.[118] Disadvantages include use of prosthetic material, and hence increased risk of infection, lack of potential for growth, and obviously the need for two anastomoses.

Extra-anatomical Bypass Grafts

The extra-anatomical bypass of complex coarctation through a sternotomy, used mainly in adults, has been promoted as a safe alternative to the alternative approach through a thoracotomy.[119] The technique yielded good results in the mid to long term, with no graft-related deaths or complications, and significant decrease of systolic blood pressures. The technique can be accomplished without the use of cardiopulmonary bypass when using a heart-lifting device.[120,121]

Patch Aortoplasty

Because of initially poor results using end-to-end anastomosis, with recoarctation reported in up to three-fifths of patients,[122,123,124] different mechanisms of repair were sought. Plasty of the aortic isthmus had already been introduced in 1957,[125] and from this developed the technique of patch aortoplasty. An elliptical patch of Dacron, or polytetrafluoroethylene, was placed over the site of coarctation opposite the site of ductal insertion, with claims made for reduction in rates of recoarctation.[126] Differences in pressure between arms and legs induced by exercise were also shown by two independent groups to be less after patch angioplasty than after resection followed by end-to-end anastomosis.[127,128] The very high frequency of true aneurysms (Fig. 46-25) developing late and opposite the site of repair, nonetheless, has now led many centres to use this technique only if no alternative is available. The pathogenesis of aneurysms is not fully elucidated. It has been suggested that excessive resection of the ductal shelf weakens the aortic media.[129] Others have implicated deviations in haemodynamic patterns caused by differing tensile strength between the prosthetic patch and the posterior aortic wall,[130] with intensification of the pulse wave at the native wall. Use of polytetrafluoroethylene as material for the patch, but without resection of ductal tissue, promised improved results.[131] A further retrospective comparison of end-to-end anastomosis with polytetrafluoroethylene patch aortoplasty accompanied by resection of the coarctation shelf revealed a similar rate of recoarctation for the two techniques, but with development of aneurysms after patch repair, and more late hypertension.[132] This technique, therefore, is nowadays rarely used.

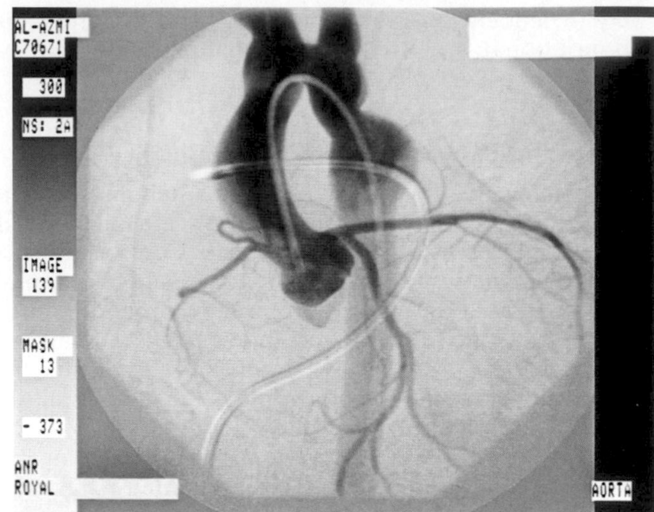

Figure 46-25 The post-operative ascending aortogram shows obvious aneurysmal dilatation of the aorta at the site of previous patch aortoplasty.

Subclavian Flap Repair

The initially reported high incidence of recoarctation with the techniques available for repair caused surgeons to develop still other approaches, amongst which was subclavian flap aortoplasty.[133] This technique (Fig. 46-26) consists of mobilisation of the subclavian artery through a standard left thoracotomy, and ligation of the subclavian artery at its first branch, attempting to preserve the thyrocervical trunk and the internal thoracic artery in order to improve perfusion to the left arm.[134] A longitudinal incision is made across the coarctation from the subclavian artery to the

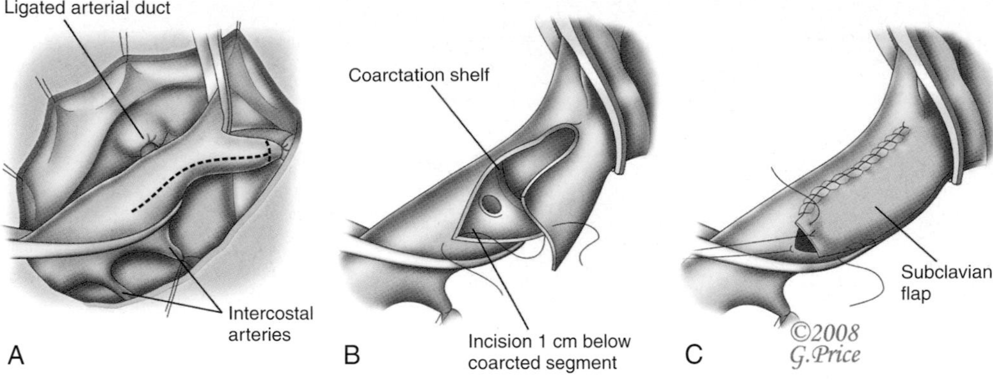

Figure 46-26 The cartoon shows the technique of subclavian flap aortoplasty. The *dotted lines* show the site of the initial surgical incisions into the narrowed arterial pathways.

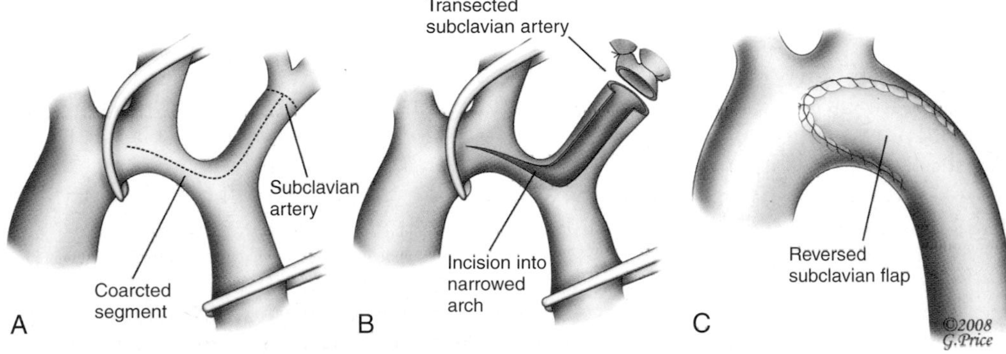

Figure 46-27 This cartoon shows the technique of reversed subclavian flap aortoplasty. The *dotted lines* show the site of the initial surgical incisions into the narrowed arterial pathways.

area of post-stenotic dilation. The proximal stump of the subclavian artery is then opened anteriorly, turned down over the incision, and the edges closed. The vertebral artery is ligated to prevent any subsequent subclavian steal leading to cerebral ischaemia. The reported benefits using this technique over others include the use of exclusively native material, with consequent decreased risk of infection, and improved potential for growth,[134] no circumferential anastomosis, less extensive dissection, and less tension on the suture lines compared with the end-to-end repair. The obvious disadvantage is the loss of the main arterial supply to the left arm, and deleterious effects on growth of the arm have been reported. These range from mild discrepancy in length of the arm, similar to that following a Blalock–Taussig shunt, to rare reports of gangrene.[135,136,137] Aneurysms have also been described,[138] but are less common than after patch aortoplasty.

Despite early studies suggesting a much lower incidence of recoarctation compared with other types of repair, some centres have moved away again from this technique after reports of unfavourable or equivocal results.[137,139–143] Other centres have continued to use subclavian flap angioplasty as their preferred technique in infants and neonates, producing an acceptable incidence of recoarctation, varying between 3% and 13% depending on the age, low early morbidity and mortality, and an overall low incidence of late hypertension.[144,145] A direct comparison between end-to-end resection and repair using a subclavian flap revealed a similar risk of recoarctation between the techniques, and as already emphasised, highlighted the experience of the surgeon as the major determinant of outcome.[112] Modifications of the subclavian flap technique itself have also been described. The most commonly used is the reversed subclavian flap for obstructive lesions proximal to the left subclavian artery,[133,146] or coarctations associated with tubular hypoplasia of the aortic arch,[147] where the reversal of the flap produces excellent relief of hypoplastic arches, and low rates of recoarctation (Fig. 46-27).

Attempts have also been made to address the loss of the subclavian artery, using techniques involving reimplantation[148,149] or by using the internal thoracic artery to preserve the arterial supply to the arm.[150] Further variants have been described to deal with rare anatomical variants, such as anomalous origin of the right subclavian artery, involvement of the left subclavian artery in the obstructive lesion, and hypoplasia of the arch.[151–153] The last technique consists of side-to-side transverse aortic anastomosis at the level of the coarctation, widening the coarctation segment and shortening the isthmus, pulling the distal end of the aortotomy more proximal, thus allowing creation of a tension-free aortoplasty. This is reported to provide very low rates of recoarctation, less than 5%, along with low morbidity and mortality even when used in neonates and infants.

Extended End-to-End Repair

The frequent finding of recoarctation by those using the subclavian flap for repair, particularly in very young infants, led to the introduction of the extended end-to-end repair.[154] Many now use this technique, or one of its modifications, electively, especially if there is associated tubular hypoplasia of the transverse arch or isthmus (Fig. 46-28). Whether tubular hypoplasia needs to be so specifically addressed is itself a contentious point. Proponents of the use of the subclavian flap argue that, in most patients, subsequent

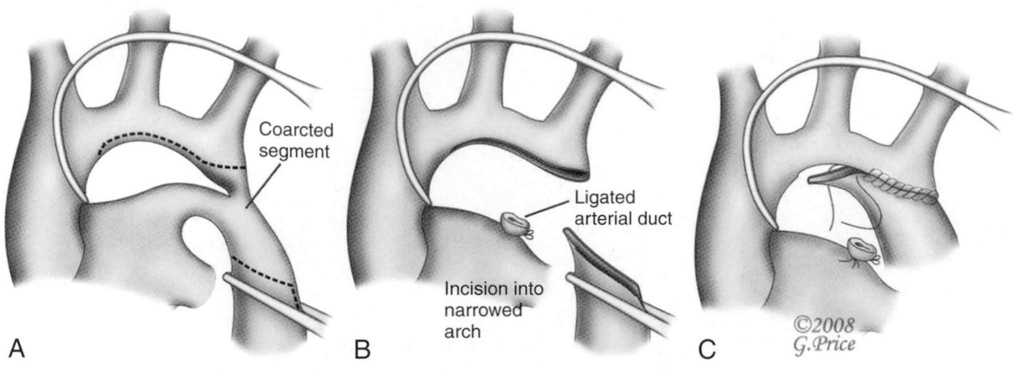

Figure 46-28 The cartoon shows the technique of extended end-to-end repair of coarctation with or without associated arch hypoplasia.

growth of the arch is sufficient once the obstruction has been relieved.[155] They suggest that recoarctation is related to the original ductal shelf,[156] and not to hypoplasia of the arch. Some evidence certainly suggests that the hypoplastic arch does have significant potential for growth after repair.[157] Correction, nonetheless, must address hypoplasia of the isthmus and distal arch. Various modifications of the original procedure were therefore introduced, varying the position of the proximal clamp. The position of the distal clamp has not changed. Initially it was placed just proximal to the left subclavian artery, with the site of proximal anastomosis being the longitudinally cut underside of the aortic arch, the distal end being the obliquely cut descending aorta. The technique was modified further by moving the proximal clamp further proximally and being more aggressive with dissection of the aortic branches and the mobilisation of the arch.[158,159] This allowed the surgeon better to address hypoplasia of the arch, placing the proximal clamp across the left subclavian, left common carotid and part of the brachiocephalic arteries, the tip being well down the left wall of the ascending aorta. This has reportedly led to a reduction in recoarctation,[159–161] but consensus is lacking due to variations in the reported experience of different surgeons.

Surgical Management of Interrupted Aortic Arch

Since the first repair of an interrupted arch using an end-to-end anastomosis was reported in 1955,[162] various techniques have emerged, from repair using a flap combined with banding of the pulmonary trunk,[163] to eventual repair in one stage in 1972.[164] The first repair using direct anastomosis was reported 5 years later.[165] The introduction of prostaglandin revolutionised the preoperative management of these critically ill children. Furthermore, in recent years it has become more common place to perform the repair using one rather than two procedures.[166–168] An area of debate has remained the material used to restore continuity of the aortic arch, either by end-to-side direct anastomosis, or by interposition of a tube graft, the latter being less favourable because of anatomical distortion and somatic outgrowth of the graft. Our current policy, mirroring practice in most large centres, is to avoid insertion of prosthetic material whenever possible, and to perform an end-to-side anastomosis of the distal segment to the ascending aorta in the same procedure as used to close the ventricular septal defect[169–171] (Fig. 46-29). Analysis of large cohorts has demonstrated that risk factors for death include low weight at birth, younger age, interruption between the left common carotid and subclavian arteries, and presence of major associated cardiac anomalies.[172,173] In the largest series, however, one-third of the patients had died after 16 years follow-up, and a repeated intervention on the arch had been needed in three-tenths.[172] In a smaller series, nonetheless, survival of 83% had been reported at 5 years.[174] Reinterventions are more likely in those patients who did not have a direct anastomosis with patch augmentation. Patients with initial associated procedures to relieve obstruction in the left ventricular outflow tract had similar rates of survival and reintervention at 16 years. Reoperation for left ventricular obstruction is often related to development of new and discrete subaortic shelves or valvar stenosis.[175]

Should the anatomy not be suitable for a biventricular strategy, such as with substantial subaortic obstruction and hypoplastic left heart syndrome, then reconstruction is feasible following the Norwood protocol.[27] This approach is indicated if the subaortic diameter measures less than 3 mm.[176,177] It is also possible to baffle the left ventricular

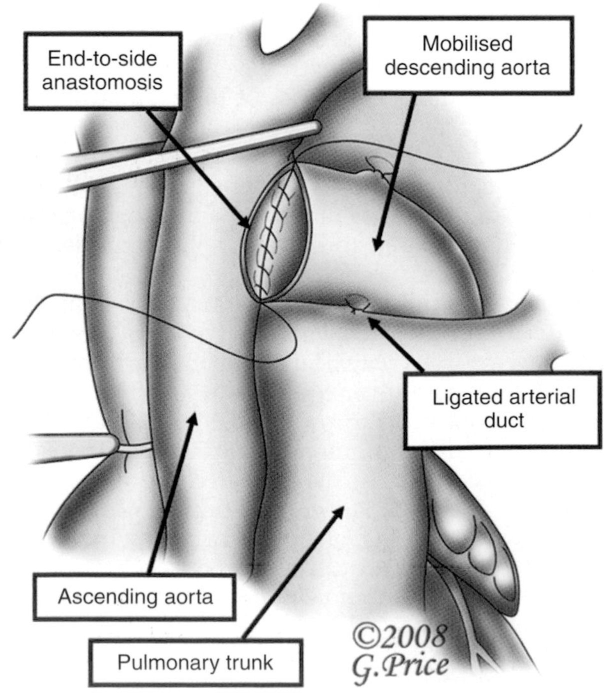

Figure 46-29 This cartoon shows the technique of end-to-side anastomosis as used in repair of interruption of the aortic arch.

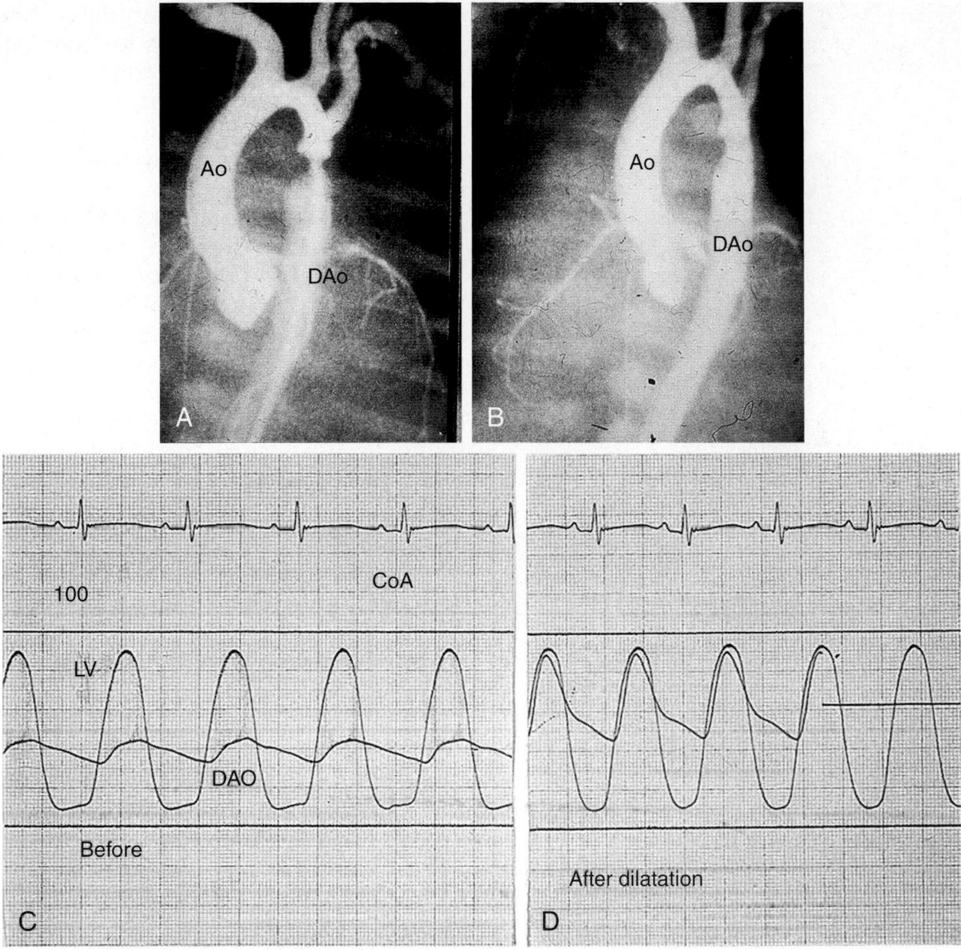

Figure 46-30 These ascending aortic angiograms are from a neonate before (**A**) and after (**B**) balloon dilation. The Doppler tracings show the initial gradient (**C**) across the narrowed aorta (Ao) and confirm (**D**) the excellent early haemodynamic result, showing abolition of the initial gradient. Severe recoarctation, however, occurred within 4 weeks. CoA, aortic coarctation; DAo, descending aorta; LV left ventricle.

outflow to the pulmonary trunk through the ventricular septal defect, creating a Damus-Kaye-Stansel anastomosis, and placing a conduit between the right ventricle and the pulmonary arteries.[178] Whenever possible, nonetheless, it is preferable to perform an anatomical correction, with resection of the subaortic lesions.[179,180]

Balloon and Stent Angioplasty

A percutaneous approach to coarctation (Fig. 46-30) was initiated clinically because surgical treatment of recoarctation carried increased morbidity and mortality.[181–184] Balloon angioplasty had been assessed in animal studies[185,186] and at a postmortem in a neonate who had died with a coarctation.[187] Initial results with balloon dilation of native coarctation were disappointing.[183] Of particular concern was the occasional incidence of aneurysms developing at the site of dilation (Fig. 46-31),[188–190] comparing unfavourably in neonates and infants at the time with contemporary results of surgical repair. Rates of recoarctation of 83% for the former, and 40% for the latter, with complications involving the femoral artery in 20% and 10%, respectively, have been quoted by the most ardent proponents of angioplasty for native coarctation.[191] These poor outcomes need to be placed in the context of continually improving surgical results, and this is supported by prospective randomised studies and non-randomised studies.[192,193] A small randomised study, for example, showed that balloon angioplasty, when used to treat children with coarctation, was associated with a higher incidence of formation of aneurysms and iliofemoral arterial injury than surgery.[194] The results of balloon angioplasty for native coarctation in selected older children and adults, nonetheless, are excellent in the mid term.[195,196] Longer-term data, albeit from non-randomised studies, is also now becoming available to suggest that primary balloon dilation for discrete coarctation in adolescents and young adults has excellent results.[197,198] This has to be placed in the light of surgery for a similar subset of patients, which also achieves a very high rate of success without the need for further pharmacological control of blood pressure.[199]

Balloon angioplasty can be performed retrogradely via a femoral or umbilical arterial catheter,[200,201] or antegradely via a patent oval fossa, the left ventricle and ascending aorta.[202,203] Although no consensus exists regarding the size of the balloon, most choose a balloon that does not exceed the diameter of any part of the aorta outside the coarcted segment, which includes areas of associated tubular hypoplasia. Angiography should be repeated after dilation to assess the degree of damage to the arterial wall.

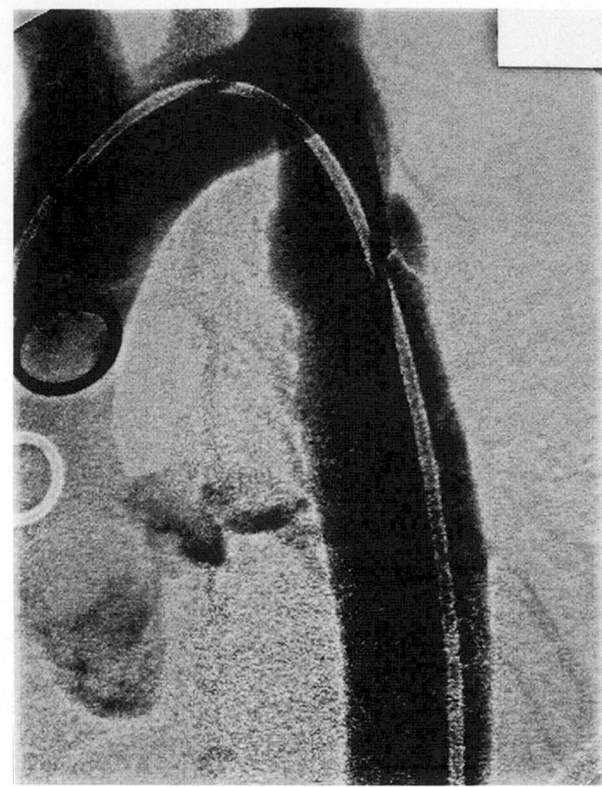

Figure 46-31 The ascending aortic angiogram is taken immediately after balloon dilation of severe aortic coarctation. There is early aneurysmal formation, with an obvious intimal flap posteriorly.

The recently dilated site should not be crossed with catheter tips or guide-wires to minimise the risk of aortic dissection, or even rupture.[182] A successful balloon angioplasty requires tearing of the intimal and medial walls of the aorta,[186,204] the extent of dissection produced being well illustrated by intravascular ultrasound, be the lesion native or residual.[205] Even though the majority of the tears remain clinically unimportant, dissection requiring surgical intervention has been reported.[206–208] Local problems include residual coarctation and development of aneurysms. Other serious complications occur at the site of vascular access. It is worth noting that balloon dilation is not entirely free from neurological sequels, particularly if associated with anomalies in cerebral vasculature.[209]

Stent angioplasty can also produce good and safe results in children with native and recurrent coarctation, with excellent relief of the gradient in children, even in patients below 20 kg.[210–213] Stenting has also been used in infants who could not undergo surgery for various reasons, as a bridge to a later definitive operation.[214] In older children and adults with native coarctation, balloon angioplasty with stenting has been shown to result in sustained reduction in gradients at early- and intermediate-term follow-up,[215–219] but aortic aneurysm was detected in almost one-fifth of patients in one of these series. In selected adults, covered stents are useful, but aneurysms can still occur in patients with markers of aortic mural weakness. Refinements in the technique of deployment and design of the stent are needed to eliminate this risk.[220] The stents can be deployed using magnetic resonance guidance.[221] A recent controversial paper by Wong and colleagues,[222] and its accompanying editorial,[223] highlighted again that, when it comes to comparing results of treatments for coarctation, we have little good quality head-to-head comparative evidence on which to base our decisions. Less robust evidence, and the preference of the individual physician, is used to formulate some of these decisions, and may bias inappropriately the process of informed consent.

Recurrent coarctations are now frequently being treated with success in children by angioplasty and stenting.[195,210,224–227] Hypoplasia of the transverse arch appears to be the primary predictor for the need to reintervene. Generally, the results of balloon angioplasty are more successful for recurrent as opposed to native coarctation, with a lower incidence of formation of aneurysms,[228,229] perhaps because of the surrounding scar tissue. In one analysis of results from a registry, nonetheless, acute angioplasty for native coarctation proved marginally superior to the same technique used for recurrent coarctation.[230] Stenting of mild gradients, less than 20 mm Hg, has also shown to benefit some patients in sofar that a proportion of them will not require medication for persistent hypertension.[231]

EARLY COMPLICATIONS

Coarctation

Local complications after surgery can result from the lateral thoracotomy, or dissection of tissues around the coarcted site, or from cardiopulmonary bypass should there have been the need to repair associated defects. Severe complications after surgery include significant bleeding from suture lines, suggested by significant losses from the chest drains or worsening haemodynamics. This should prompt immediate re-exploration. Concomitant paradoxical hypertension, often seen after coarctectomy, should be aggressively controlled in order to take away pressure on suture lines. Patients with Turner's syndrome are at significant risk for this complication, possibly due to their abnormal connective tissue.[232] Damage to the thoracic duct can result in persistent chylous effusions.

Neurological complications are occasionally seen, including palsy of the recurrent laryngeal nerve or phrenic nerves, and Horner's syndrome. The most feared surgical complication is injury to the spinal cord with subsequent paraplegia. The risk for this complication is higher if there has been poor formation of collateral arteries around the site of coarctation, and low distal pressure of perfusion.[233] Suggested interventions to minimise these risks have included minimising the period of aortic clamping, and pharmacological intervention when the pressure in the distal arch falls below 50 mm Hg in older patients.[234,235] Other less frequently employed techniques include measuring somatosensory potentials,[236] and drainage of cerebrospinal fluid.[237] The distal pressure of perfusion is particularly important. If this drops too much, a temporary extra-anatomical shunt[238,239] or partial bypass of the left heart, can be used to increase the distal perfusion, a technique that improves the margins of safety and maintains adequate perfusion of the anterior spinal artery.[240] Occasionally, subclavian steal from the circle of Willis can result if the vertebral artery is left open during subclavian flap aortoplasty. It is also important to recognise an aberrant right subclabvian originating from below the site of coarctation, as theoretically this can reduce the supply of blood to the spinal artery.[241]

As already discussed, paradoxical hypertension is commonly seen after repair of coarctation, and tends to occur in two periods of time. The initial period is caused by a noradrenergic storm due to reduced stretch of the baroreceptors in the aortic arch and carotid arteries,[242,243] and tends to subside after 24 to 72 hours. The second period produces the so-called post-coarctectomy syndrome, and occurs around the second or third postoperative day. It is associated with pan-arteritis distal to the site of repair, and is possibly due to sudden exposure of the distal vascular bed to much higher pressures after repair, causing intense arterial vasospasm and subsequent endothelial ischaemia.[243] Renin has also been implicated, with normal levels found in the plasma prior to surgery, and paradoxically elevated levels afterwards.[244–247] This post-coarctectomy syndrome can be abated by pharmacological manipulation, which includes smooth muscular relaxation, inhibition of angiotensin-converting enzyme, and β-blockade. The latter, if started prior to surgery, reduces both post-operative blood pressures and activity of rennin without affecting the usual rise in post-operative concentrations of noradrenaline in the plasma, suggesting a major role for the sympathetic nervous system.[248] No clear relationship has yet emerged between these transient changes in blood pressure and long-term hypertension.[249,250]

Interrupted Aortic Arch

Apart from the above mentioned complications, all of which can also occur after repair of an interrupted arch, it is important to exclude residual gradients across the repair, and incomplete resolution of intracardiac pathology, such as residual intracardiac shunts or stenosis of the outflow tracts. This should be achieved whilst the patient remains in the operating room, or if any deviation is noted from a routine post-operative recovery. This is most commonly achieved with echocardiography

LATE COMPLICATIONS

Coarctation

As we have discussed, there remains confusion regarding the definition of recoarctation. Most symptomatic patients require an intervention. Gradients measured using echo-Doppler assessment, and measurement of blood pressure in the limbs, tend to be reliable only in younger children, and magnetic resonance imaging with reconstruction and assessment of collateral flow is rapidly becoming the investigation of choice in most centres for assessment of recoarctation in older children and adults.[251] It has proven to be useful in assessing local and cardiac anatomy, particularly for assessing aneurysmal change, and estimation of gradients and severity of stenosis.[252–254] As far as medium-term follow-up after repair of coarctation is concerned, it is evident that, left untreated, almost half the patients will develop hypoplasia of the aortic arch. Such hypoplasia, therefore, should be addressed at the same time as the coarctation itself.[255] Very long-term data on survival and morbidity is sparse, but it appears that with the early techniques used to repair coarctation, there is an excess cardiovascular mortality and morbidity, and often a need for reintervention.[256] These patients, therefore, need careful long-term follow-up.

Abnormal physiological responses after repair are found even in infancy. In the long term, these patients have also been shown to have impaired function of the conduit arteries, with abnormal responses to flow and nitroglycerin, and increased vascular stiffness in the precoarctation vascular bed.[257] The elastic properties can be preserved with an early repair, but the reduced reactivity will remain. Cardiovascular complications secondary to hypertension have been shown to lead to reduced life expectancy, even after anatomically relieved obstruction in late childhood.[258,259] In pre-school children after initial return to normotension and normal exercise capacity and function, a tendency develops for later abnormal physiological responses to exercise,[260] with the appearance of upper body hypertension, and sometimes gradients across the vascular bed. Upper body hypertension is also seen without resting gradients across the repair, suggesting that pre-operative hypertension causes irreversible changes in the arteriolar walls with chronic baroreceptor dysfunction.[261,262] This finding is underpinned by abnormal endothelial responses in the precoarctation vascular bed in adults after otherwise successful surgical repair in childhood.[263] The exercise-induced hypertension appears unrelated to anatomical narrowing, but rather due to interaction between an enhanced sympathetic nervous system and structural and functional abnormalities of the precoarctation vessels.[264] Another factor that may play in the aetiology is the shape of the arch after the repair, with an angulated gothic arch independently associated with abnormal responses of blood pressure, highlighting a subgroup of patients at risk for development of hypertension in young adult life.[265] Long-term follow-up of patients after surgical correction shows that, despite a minority having a gradient greater than 20 mm Hg, a significant proportion have hypertension.[266]

These children also have abnormal left ventricular mass and diastolic dysfunction, thought to be due by some to occult gradients.[267,268,269] The beneficial effects of relieving the burden of long-term cardiovascular complications by pharmacological intervention remains to be proven when the gradient does not produce symptoms. When comparing the use of a subclavian flap to end-to-end anastomosis, patients were shown to have a higher incidence of late hypertension, both during exercise and ambulatory monitoring, after the former procedure.[270] Furthermore, there appeared to be lower residual aortic stiffness after an end-to-end anastomosis. These children can be encouraged to participate in sports 6 months after intervention if any residual gradient at rest is less than 20 mm Hg, and systolic pressure is normal on exercise. Should there be evidence of aortic dilation, mural thinning, or formation of aneurysms, participation should be restricted to low-impact sports.[271]

Interrupted Aortic Arch

The anastomosis requires close observation. Those in whom a patch or conduit was used will, at some stage, require replacement due to somatic outgrowth. If a gradient develops across a direct anastomosis, then balloon dilation can successfully be used to provide relief.[180,272,273] Intracardiac anatomy also requires repeated analysis, as ongoing obstruction in the left ventricular outflow tract may require surgical intervention.[273,274] The size of the outflow tract, the site of interruption, and an aberrant course of the right subclavian artery have been shown to be significant risk factors for future obstruction in the outflow tract.[275]

The outcome of repair of interrupted aortic arch is, to a large degree, dependent on the pre-operative state of the infant, this determining late neurological outcome in these children.[276] Thus, neurodevelopmental delay has been found in those patients who have 22q11 deletion.[277] Furthermore, pre-operative renal function, intracerebral haemorrhages, the number of cardioplegic injections, and age at operation all play an important role in outcome,[171] but the overall survival, of around 70% at 5 years, is mostly determined by the associated lesions.[171,272,278,279]

The complete reference list can be found on the companion Expert Consult web site at www.expertconsult.com.

ANNOTATED REFERENCES

- Walters HL, Ionan CE, Thomas RL, Delius RE: Single-stage versus 2-stage repair of coarctation of the aorta with ventricular septal defect. J Thorac Cardiovasc Surg 2008;135:754–761.

  This retrospective study compares two different strategies within one institution over the past decade, demonstrating that completion of repair is achieved at an earlier age, with fewer operations and fewer incisions, when using single staged repair. This does not result in any increase in complications or in-hospital mortality.

- Kanter KR, Mahle WT, Kogon BE, Kirshbom PM: What is the optimal management of infants with coarctation and ventricular septal defect? Ann Thorac Surg 2007;84:612–618.

  This important retrospective study compares various strategies and outcomes in a single high-volume institution of treatment of patients with either single-stage, two incisions but single-stage, or two-stage approach to coarctation and ventricular septal defect. It demonstrates that primary repair using a one-stage approach through separate incisions affords excellent clinical results, avoiding prolonged aortic cross-clamping, cardiopulmonary bypass and circulatory arrest. Furthermore, in comparison with a single-stage sternotomy-only approach, intensive care and hospital stay were significantly decreased.

- Cobanoglu A, Thyagarajan GK, Dobbs JL: Surgery for coarctation of the aorta in infants younger than 3 months: End-to-end repair versus subclavian flap angioplasty: Is either operation better? Eur J Cardiothorac Surg 1998;14:19–25.

  This retrospective single centre study compared the end-to-end resection versus the subclavian flap technique, in the same centre in infants younger than 3 months of age. It reported a similar incidence of late recoarctation in both techniques, demonstrating that outcomes are mostly determined by a surgeon's expertise at the procedure.

- Kanter KR, Vincent RN, Fyfe DA: Reverse subclavian flap repair of hypoplastic transverse aorta in infancy. Ann Thorac Surg 2001;71:1530–1536.

  Dealing with arch hypoplasia in the setting of coarctation can be challenging, and this study demonstrates nicely how a reversed subclavian flap offers excellent relief of arch hypoplasia and coarctation in infants with low rates of recoarctation, and acceptable operative and intermediate results, without the need for foreign material or cardiopulmonary bypass.

- Elliott MJ: Coarctation of the aorta with arch hypoplasia: Improvements on a new technique. Ann Thorac Surg 1987;44:321–323.

  This modification of the extended end-to-end anastomosis for coarctation in the setting of arch hypoplasia, with extensive aortic arch branch dissection and decending aortic dissection up to the diaphragm, allows for a wide open anastomosis with low residual gradients.

- Jonas RA, Quaegebeur JM, Kirklin JW, et al: Outcomes in patients with interrupted aortic arch and ventricular septal defect: A multiinstitutional study. Congenital Heart Surgeons Society. J Thorac Cardiovasc Surg 1994;107:1099–1109.

  This large multi-institutional study from the Congenital Heart Surgeons Society in North America looked at a large cohort of patients with interrupted aortic arch and ventricular septal defect. Risk factors for death included low birth weight, younger age at repair, interrupted arch type B, outlet and trabecular ventricular septal defects, smaller size of the ventricular septal defect, and subaortic narrowing.

- McCrindle BW, Tchervenkov CI, Konstantinov IE, et al: Risk factors associated with mortality and interventions in 472 neonates with interrupted aortic arch: A Congenital Heart Surgeons Society study. J Thorac Cardiovasc Surg 2005;129:343–350.

  This further study, also originating from the Congenital Heart Surgeons Society, and incorporating a few more years of this large cohort of patients and a long follow-up time up to 16 years, showed that after 16 years 33% of the patients had died and 28% had required reintervention on the aortic arch. A reintervention was more likely for those who had repair of common arterial trunk, repair of the interrupted arch by a method other than direct anastomosis with patch augmentation, and the use of polytetrafluoroethylene as either an interposition graft or a patch. Among those who had undergone an initial left ventricular outflow tract procedure, after 16 years 37% had died and 28% had undergone a second procedure.

- Cowley CG, Orsmond GS, Feola P, et al: Long-term, randomized comparison of balloon angioplasty and surgery for native coarctation of the aorta in childhood. Circulation 2005;111:3453–3456.

  This important paper is a randomised study of balloon angioplasty and surgery for native coarctation in children between the ages of 3 to 10 years. Blood pressure, residual aortic obstruction, and exercise performance were evaluated. Median follow-up time was between 10 and 11 years after the initial intervention. There was no difference in resting blood pressure, coarctation gradient, exercise performance, magnetic resonance analysis of the aortic arch, or need for repeat interventions. There was a much higher incidence of early and late formation of aneurysms in patients undergoing balloon angioplasty.

- Rodés-Cabau J, Miró J, Dancea A, et al: Comparison of surgical and transcatheter treatment for native coarctation of the aorta in patients > or = 1 year old: The Quebec Native Coarctation of the Aorta study. Am Heart J 2007;154:186–192.

  This is a contemporary multi-centric non-randomised series of children older than 1 year of age with native coarctation treated either with balloon, balloon and stenting or surgery, demonstrating again a comparable immediate haemodynamic result to surgery, and less morbidity and length of stay in hospital with angioplasty. Angioplasty was associated with a higher rate of reintervention and aneurysmal formation at a mean follow-up of 3 years.

- Hager A, Kanz S, Kaemmerer H, et al: Coarctation Long-term Assessment (COALA): Significance of arterial hypertension in a cohort of 404 patients up to 27 years after surgical repair of isolated coarctation of the aorta, even in the absence of restenosis and prosthetic material. J Thorac Cardiovasc Surg 2007;134:738–745.

  This large cohort study with long-term follow-up up to 27 years after repair of coarctation demonstrates that a large proportion of patients remain hypertensive at long-term follow-up, but this is only caused in a small proportion by recoarctation. Even in those without prosthetic material or minimal-grade restenosis, there is a substantial incidence of arterial hypertension.

CHAPTER 47

Vascular Rings, Pulmonary Arterial Sling, and Related Conditions

SHI-JOON YOO and TIMOTHY J. BRADLEY

The aortic arch, the arterial duct, and the right and left pulmonary arteries have close spatial relationships with the major airways and the oesophagus. Due to this close proximity, abnormalities in the size, position, and/or pattern of branching pattern of these structures may cause obstruction to the trachea, the bronchuses, or the oesophagus. Many of the abnormalities of position and branching, along with the so-called pulmonary arterial sling, are characterised by a complete or partial encirclement of the trachea and oesophagus, or the trachea in isolation, by a composite vascular structure. Although the terms ring and sling have been used somewhat loosely, we use vascular ring to denote a complete encirclement, and vascular sling an encirclement which is incomplete. Vascular rings and slings are the classic anomalies that cause symptoms and signs of obstruction to the airways and oesophageal compression. Not all rings and slings, however, result in clinically recognisable symptoms and signs. Conversely, there are other vascular abnormalities that do not form a ring or sling, and yet may produce significant obstruction of the airways and oesophagus. In this chapter, we discuss these various anomalies of the aortic arch and pulmonary arteries that may cause obstruction to the central airways.

ANOMALIES OF THE AORTIC ARCH

In this section, we discuss the abnormalities in position and/or branching of the aortic arch. The obstructive lesions within the arch, such as coarctation or interruption, are not generally included in this category. They are addressed in Chapter 46. Insight into the mode of development of the arterial trunks, and their pattern in the fetal circulation, is tremendously helpful in understanding the prenatal and postnatal features of the various malformations which involve the aortic arch.

Hypothetical Model of the Double Aortic Arch

The normal and abnormal development of the components of the aortic arch can best be understood by making reference to the model introduced by the pioneer pathologist, Jesse E. Edwards, in 1948 (Fig. 47-1).[1,2] The model illustrates a relatively late stage of development, in that the distal intrapericardial outflow tract has been divided into the ascending aorta and pulmonary arterial trunk, and the descending aorta occupies a neutral position. The earlier stages of development will not be discussed here, in part because the precise morphogenesis of the outflow tracts has still to be clarified, but also because most of the congenital malformations involving the aortic arch can be understood without knowledge of these earlier events, which are reviewed in Chapter 3.

In the hypothetical model, symmetrical aortic arches connect the ascending and descending aorta on each side, forming a complete vascular ring around the trachea and oesophagus. Each aortic arch gives rise superiorly to a common carotid artery and a subclavian artery. On each side, right-sided and left-sided arterial ducts pass between the pulmonary arteries and the distal part of the aortic arches, forming an additional vascular ring around the trachea and oesophagus. The hypothetical model, therefore, is made up of two vascular rings joined together at the descending aorta.

With normal development, it is the left aortic arch and left-sided arterial duct which persist, while the right aortic arch distal to the origin of the right subclavian artery, along with the right-sided arterial duct, regress (Fig. 47-2). As a result, the proximal part of the embryological right aortic arch remains as the brachiocephalic artery, which bifurcates into the right common carotid and right subclavian arteries. The brachiocephalic artery, of course, is also known as the

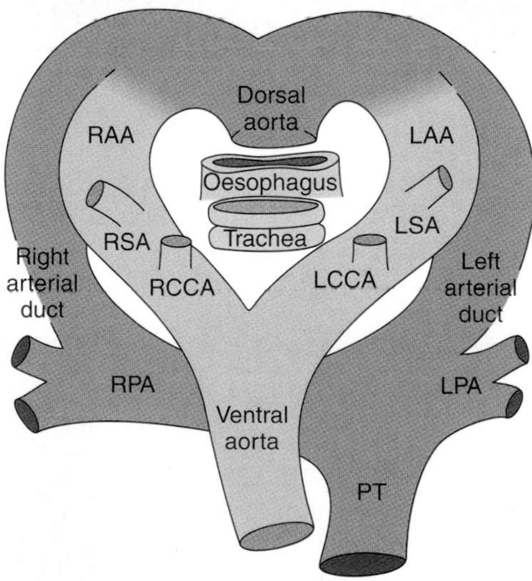

Figure 47-1 The hypothetical model for the perfect double aortic arch proposed by Jesse E. Edwards. As we will show, all malformations involving the arch can be understood on the basis of this model. LAA, left aortic arch; LCCA, left common carotid artery; LPA, left pulmonary artery; LSA, left subclavian artery; PT, pulmonary trunk; RAA, right aortic arch; RCCA, right common carotid artery; RPA, right pulmonary artery; RSA, right subclavian artery. (Modified from Edwards JE: Anomalies of the derivatives of the aortic arch system. Med Clin N Am 1948;32:925–948; and Edwards JE: Vascular rings and slings. In Moller JH, Neal AN [eds]: Fetal, Neonatal, and Infant Cardiac Disease. Norwalk, CT: Appleton & Lange, 1990, pp 745–754.)

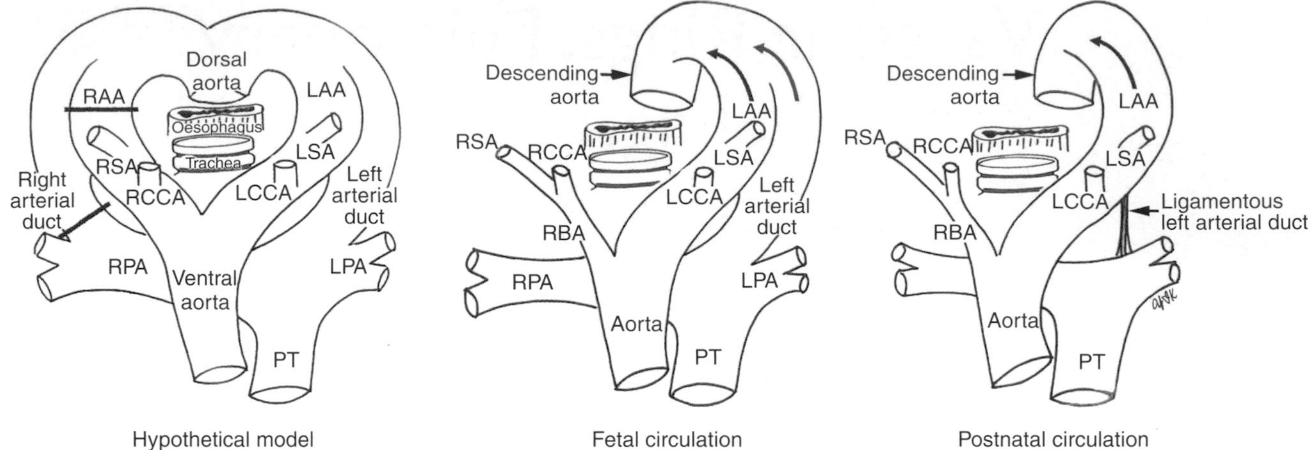

Figure 47-2 This panel of cartoons illustrates the steps involved in normal formation of a left-sided aortic arch, with a left arterial duct. In the model of the hypothetical double arch as shown in the left hand diagram, the *red bars* indicate the segments that regress. In the normal left-sided aortic arch, shown in the right hand diagram, this results in disappearance of the right aortic arch distal to the origin of the right subclavian artery (RSA), along with right-sided arterial ducts. In the fetal circulation, as shown in the middle diagram, the aortic arch (*red arrow*), and the left arterial duct (*blue arrow*), make a V-shaped confluence at the descending aorta. In the postnatal circulation, the left arterial duct closes, becoming the arterial ligament, or as we will describe it, the ligamentous arterial duct. LAA, left aortic arch; LCCA, left common carotid artery; LPA, left pulmonary artery; LSA, left subclavian artery; PT, pulmonary trunk; RAA, right aortic arch; RBA, right brachiocephalic artery; RCCA, right common carotid artery; RPA, right pulmonary artery. The red and blue arrows are used in comparable fashion in Figures 47-6, 47-9, 47-11, 47-13, 47-14, and 47-16.

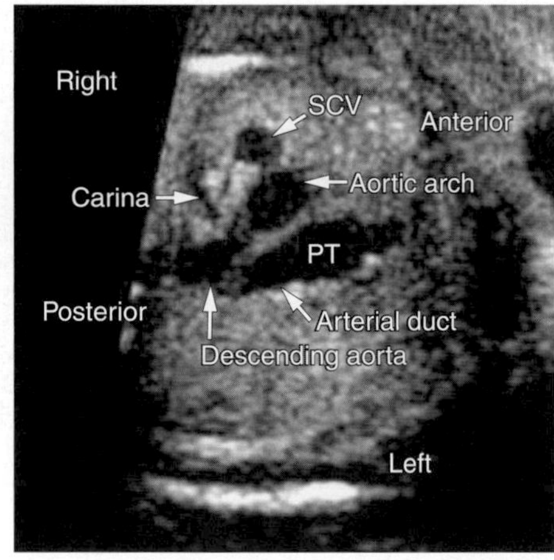

Figure 47-3 The fetal echocardiogram across the upper mediastinum shows the normal left aortic arch and left-sided arterial duct, forming a V-shaped confluence at their union to form the descending aorta. PT, pulmonary trunk; SCV, superior caval vein.

innominate artery. It seems particularly perverse, however, to continue to designate an artery supplying vessels to the head and arms as being unnamed! The left-sided aortic arch, in sequence, gives rise to the brachiocephalic, left common carotid, and left subclavian arteries (Figs. 47-3 and 47-4). Anomalies can be positional, or reflect abnormal branching due to persistence of part or parts of the double arch that normally should have regressed. In exceptional cases, nonetheless, it still remains difficult to predict the embryological mechanism, even using the concept of the double arch.

Classification

Anomalies can be classified into four groups, depending on the position of the aortic arch relative to the trachea, and the pattern of branching of the brachiocephalic arteries:

- Left aortic arch with aberrant right subclavian or brachiocephalic artery
- Right aortic arch with aberrant left subclavian or brachiocephalic artery
- Right aortic arch with mirror-image branching
- Double aortic arch

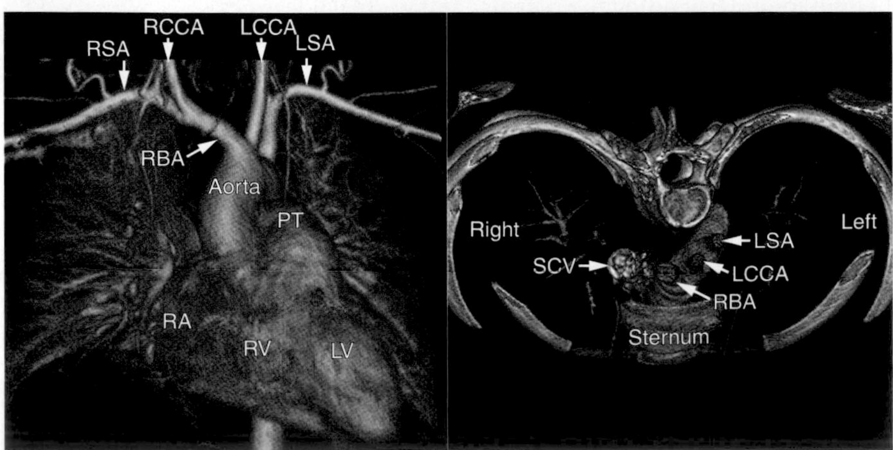

Figure 47-4 The volume rendered magnetic resonance angiogram seen from the front (*left panel*), and the computed tomographic angiogram seen from above (*right panel*), show the normal arrangement of the left-sided aortic arch, which gives rise sequentially to the brachiocephalic, left common carotid, and left subclavian arteries (LCCA, LSA). LV, left ventricle; PT, pulmonary trunk; RA, right atrium; RBA, right brachiocephalic artery; RCCA, right common carotid artery; RV, right ventricle; SCV, superior caval vein.

Most of the major anomalies produce a vascular ring, or else a sling, around the trachea and oesophagus. The only exception is the classic form of right aortic arch with mirror-image branching. Aberrant origin of a subclavian or brachiocephalic branch of the aortic arch produces encirclement of the trachea and oesophagus, since the anomalous artery takes a retro-oesophageal course. The arterial duct, regardless of whether it is patent or ligamentous, may also contribute to encirclement of the trachea and oesophagus. Occasionally the distal aortic arch itself has a retro-oesophageal course that causes oesphageal and tracheal compression. The assessment and description of the anomalies, therefore, should include description of:

- The position of the aortic arch relative to the trachea
- The location of the most proximal part of the descending aorta in relation to the spine
- The presence or absence of an aberrant branch
- The origin and insertion of the patent or ligamentous arterial duct, or rarely ducts

The anomalies producing a vascular ring or sling around the trachea and oesophagus are:

- Aortic arch anomalies forming a vascular ring:
  - Double aortic arch
  - Right aortic arch with aberrant left subclavian or brachiocephalic artery and left-sided arterial duct
  - Left aortic arch with aberrant right subclavian or brachiocephalic artery and right-sided arterial duct
  - Right aortic arch with mirror-image branching and retro-oesophageal left arterial duct between right-sided descending aorta and left pulmonary artery
  - Circumflex retro-oesophageal aortic arch
- Aortic arch anomalies forming a vascular sling or incomplete ring:
  - Left aortic arch with aberrant right subclavian or brachiocephalic artery and left-sided arterial duct
  - Right aortic arch with aberrant left subclavian or brachiocephalic artery and right-sided arterial duct
  - Circumflex retro-oesophageal aortic arch

Other anomalies that may have clinical significance include the cervical aortic arch, isolated origin of the left or right subclavian artery from a pulmonary artery, and double-barreled, or double lumen, aortic arch.

Morphology and Morphogenesis of Individual Anomalies

Double aortic arch is the tightest and most commonly recognised form of vascular ring.[1–10] It refers to the presence of two aortic arches, one on each side of the trachea and oesophagus (Fig. 47-5). Both the left and right aortic arches of the hypothetical model persist, without regression of any segment. An arterial duct, more frequently the left than the right, persists, although cases with bilateral ducts have rarely been described.[11] During fetal life, when the arterial duct is patent, the composite arrangement of the two arches and a patent arterial duct produces a figure of 9 or 6 configuration at fetal echocardiography.[12,13] Each aortic arch gives rise to common carotid and subclavian arteries. In the majority of the cases with double aortic arch, both arches are patent. Usually the right arch is larger than the left arch, or less commonly the two arches are equally sized. The left arch is dominant in less than one-fifth of cases. In general, the apex of the larger arch is higher than the smaller arch. Occasionally, a segment of one arch may be atretic, mostly on the left. The atretic segment is almost always distal to the subclavian artery, although an atretic strand may also be found between the common carotid and subclavian arteries. The atretic segment cannot be visualised by any imaging modality. It is difficult, therefore, to differentiate a double aortic arch with an atretic segment distal to the origin of the left subclavian artery from a right aortic arch with mirror-image branching. Similarly, the double aortic arch with an atretic segment between the origins of the left common carotid and left subclavian arteries is difficult to differentiate from the right aortic arch with aberrant left subclavian artery and left arterial duct. In the setting of a double aortic arch, the subclavian and common carotid arteries that arise from the patent and atretic arches almost always show a symmetrical arrangement.[14] The patent part of the atretic left aortic arch tends to have a more posterior position than the left brachiocephalic artery arising from the right aortic arch. An inferior kink of the

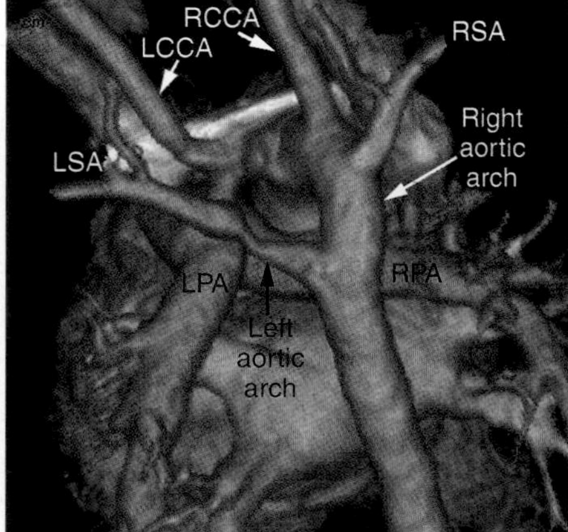

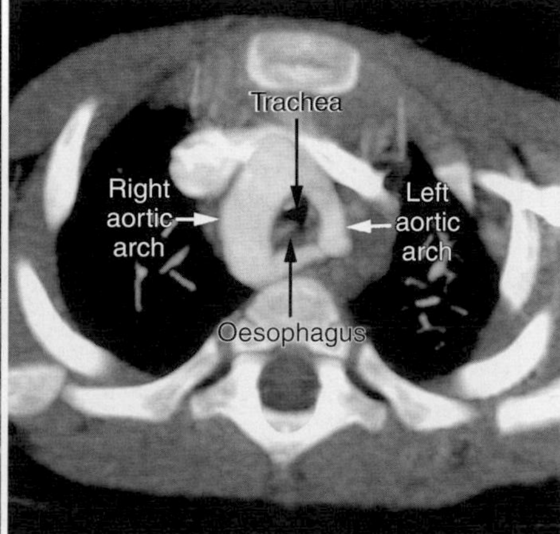

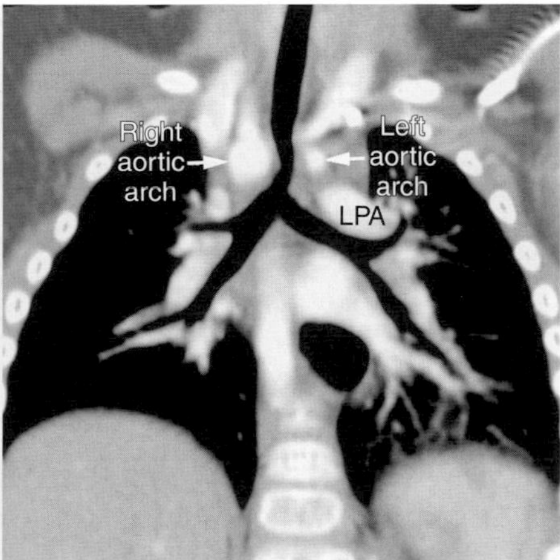

Figure 47-5 These computed tomograms, showing a complete double arch, are seen from behind and above (*left panel*), and from below (*middle panel*). The double arch encircles the trachea and oesophagus, with the right arch dominant. The reformatted image in the coronal plane (*right panel*) shows narrowing of the trachea due to compression by the dominant right aortic arch. The trachea is slightly bent to the left. LCCA, left common carotid artery; LPA, left pulmonary artery; LSA, left subclavian artery; RCCA, right common carotid artery; RPA, right pulmonary artery; RSA, right subclavian artery.

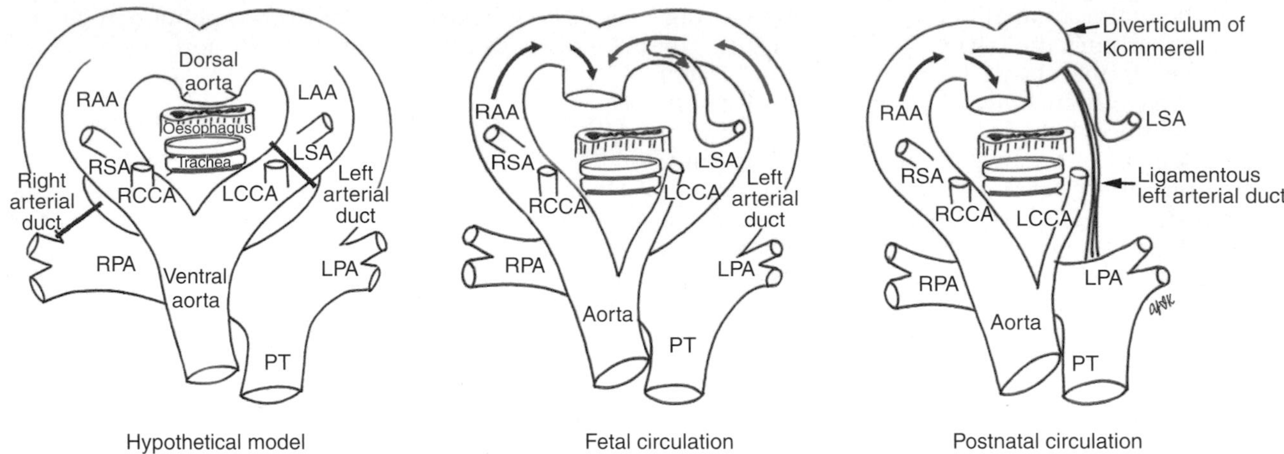

Figure 47-6 The cartoons show the mode of formation of a right aortic arch with aberrant origin of the left subclavian artery (LSA) and a left-sided arterial duct. In this, and the subsequent panels formatted in this fashion, the hypothetical model of the double arch is shown in the left hand diagram, with the *red bars* indicating the segments that will regress. The middle diagram shows the situation in the fetal circulation. In this variant, the right aortic arch (RAA), along with the remnant of the distal left aortic arch (LAA), the left-sided arterial duct, and the pulmonary trunk (PT), produce a U-shaped vascular loop around the trachea and oesophagus. As the two limbs of the U-shaped loop are attached to the heart, this produces a complete vascular ring. In the postnatal circulation, shown in the right hand panel, consequent to closure of the arterial duct, the proximal part of the aberrant LSA, representing the distal remnant of the left aortic arch usually persists as the so-called diverticulum of Kommerell. Note that the flow of blood in this distal remnant of the left aortic arch reverses direction after birth. LCCA, left common carotid artery; LPA, left pulmonary artery; RCCA, right common carotid artery; RPA, right pulmonary artery; RSA, right subclavian artery.

proximal part of the common trunk for the subclavian and common carotid arteries in the presence of a diverticular outpouching from the descending aorta is a telltale sign of the presence of an atretic segment between the kink and the apex of the diverticulum.[15] The proximal descending aorta is left-sided in just over two-thirds of patients with double aortic arch, being right-sided in almost all the rest, and only rarely occupying a neutral midline position.

Right aortic arch with aberrant left subclavian artery results from abnormal persistence of the right aortic arch, and abnormal regression of the left arch between the origins of the left common carotid and left subclavian arteries, the left subclavian artery taking its origin from the distal part of the left aortic arch (see Figs. 47-6 through 47-10). The distal remnant of the left aortic arch, along with the aberrant left subclavian artery, produces the retro-oesophageal component of the ring. It has previously been described that the aberrant artery may course either between the trachea and oesophagus, or in front of the aorta.[1] It is now usually believed that arteries that do not take a retro-oesophageal course are collateral arteries.[2] The persistent arterial duct is usually left-sided, connecting the left pulmonary artery to the distal remnant of the left aortic arch (Fig. 47-6).[1–7,10,16] This combination is the second commonest type of ring reported in most series. During fetal life, when the arterial duct is widely patent, this combination is characterised by a U-shaped vascular loop that encircles the trachea and oesophagus from behind (Figs. 47-6 and 47-7).[12,17–20] This U-shaped loop consists of the ascending aorta, the right aortic arch, the distal remnant of the left aortic arch, the left-sided arterial duct, and the pulmonary trunk. Although the vascular loop looks open anteriorly, a vascular ring is completed by the underlying heart. This configuration changes dramatically with closure of the arterial duct after birth. The left limb of the U-shaped loop disappears with ductal closure, while the distal remnant of the left aortic arch persists as a diverticular outpouching, with the left subclavian artery arising from its apex. The diverticular outpouching is called the diverticulum of Kommerell (Figs. 47-7 and 47-8).[21–24] Flow through this distal remnant, is from the left-sided arterial duct into the descending aorta in the fetal circulation, but switches its direction with ductal closure so that the aberrant left subclavian artery is supplied from the descending aorta in postnatal circulation (see Fig. 47-6, right panel). Postnatally, therefore, the presence

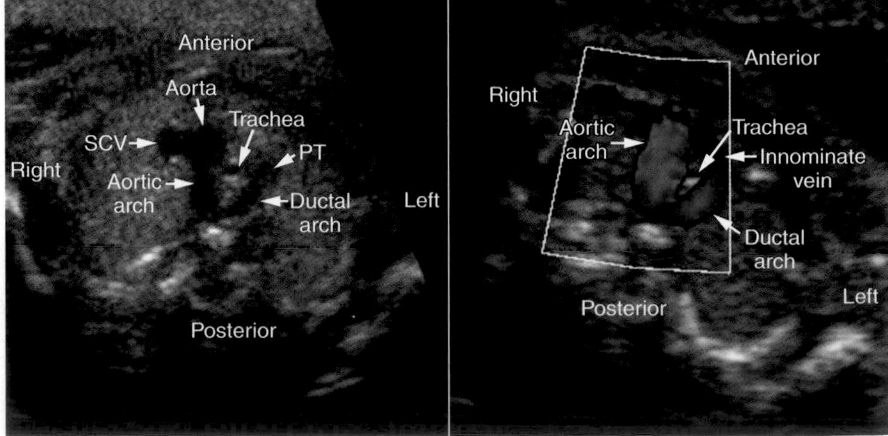

Figure 47-7 These fetal echocardiograms illustrating the situation diagrammed in Figure 47-6 show a U-shaped vascular loop around the trachea. Note the extent of the gap between the ascending aorta and the pulmonary trunk (PT). SCV, superior caval vein.

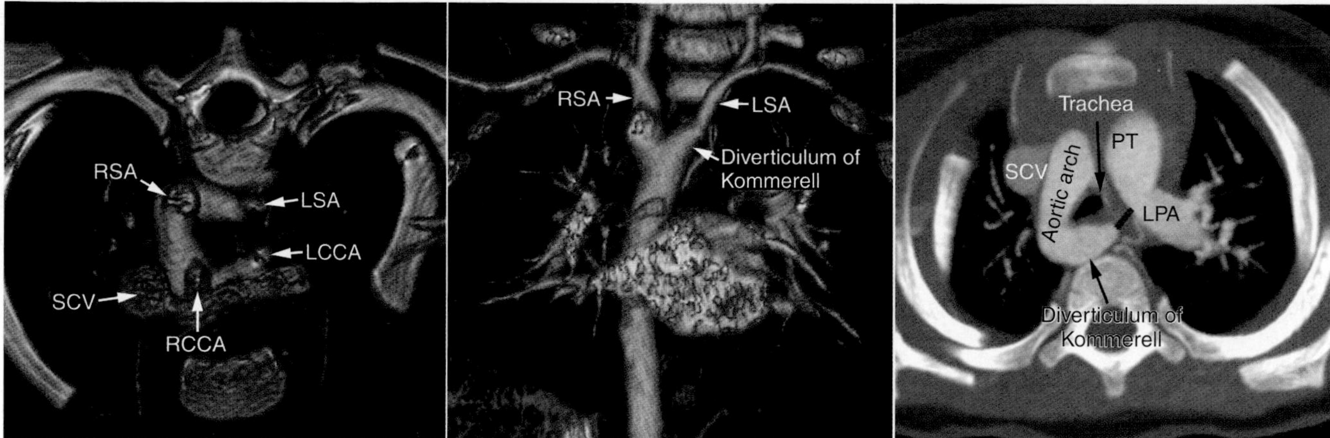

Figure 47-8 These computed tomograms, from a different patient than the image shown in Figure 47-7, but illustrating the same anomaly, show a right aortic arch with an aberrant left subclavian artery (LSA) arising from a diverticulum of Kommerell. In the right panel, the expected location of the ligamentous arterial duct is marked with a *red bar*. Note the mild compression of the distal trachea. LCCA, left common carotid artery; LPA, left pulmonary artery; PT, pulmonary trunk; RCCA, right common carotid artery; RSA, right subclavian artery; SCV, superior caval vein.

of a diverticulum of Kommerell is indicative of presence of an arterial ligament between the apex of the diverticulum and the left pulmonary artery. This vascular ring is usually not as tight as that produced by the double aortic arch. The severity of the oesophageal and, to a certain extent, the tracheal, compression varies with the size of the diverticulum. When this type of anomaly is associated with significant obstruction of the pulmonary outflow tract, as in tetralogy of Fallot, the diverticulum of Kommerell may be absent or inconspicuous (Figs. 47-9 and 47-10). This is because the flow of blood through the left arterial duct was reduced, or even reversed, during fetal life. The distal remnant of the left aortic arch, therefore, does not persist as a diverticular outpouching after ductal closure.[12] Postnatally, an arterial

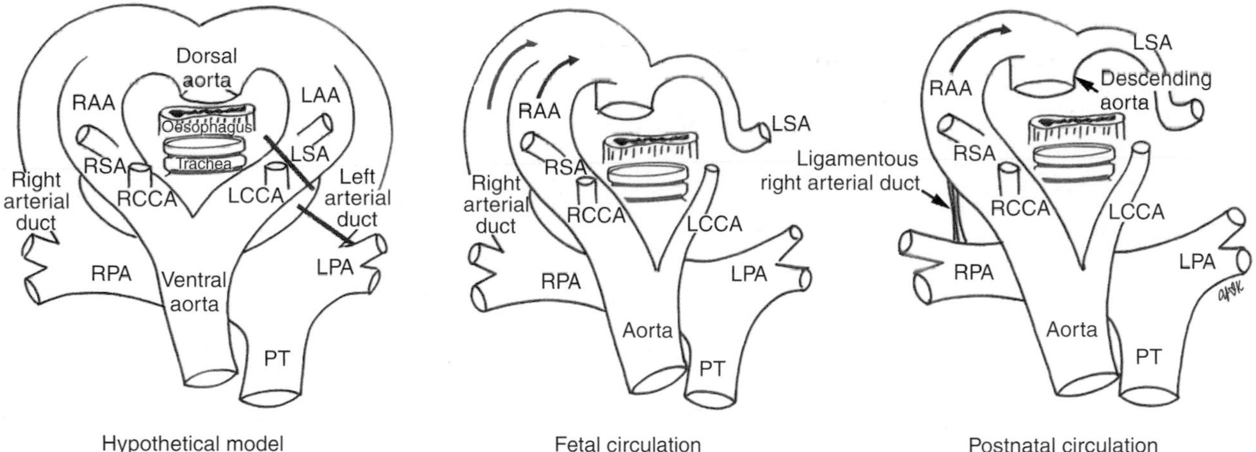

Figure 47-9 The cartoons show the mode of formation of the right aortic arch (RAA) with aberrant left subclavian artery (LSA) and right-sided arterial duct, the pattern following the same format as for Figures 47-2 and 47-6. In the fetal and postnatal circulations, this arrangement produces a vascular sling on the right side of the trachea and oesophagus. This is a rare combination. LAA, left aortic arch; LCCA, left common carotid artery; LPA, left pulmonary artery; PT, pulmonary trunk; RCCA, right common carotid artery; RPA, right pulmonary artery; RSA, right subclavian artery.

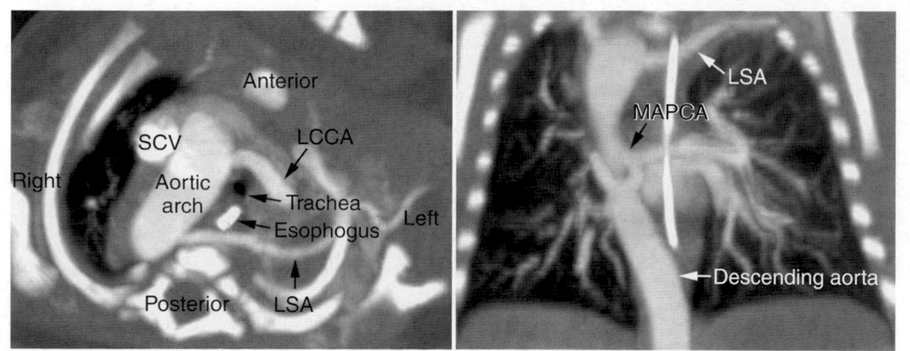

Figure 47-10 These computed tomograms show a right aortic arch with aberrant origin of the left subclavian artery (LSA), but no arterial duct, in a newborn with tetralogy of Fallot and pulmonary atresia. The computed tomograms in axial and coronal planes show that the right aortic arch gives rise to the aberrant left subclavian artery with no intervening diverticulum of Kommerell. The pulmonary arteries were non-confluent, with the pulmonary circulation supplied by major aortopulmonary collateral arteries (MAPCA), with congenital absence of both arterial ducts. LCCA, left common carotid artery; SCV, superior caval vein.

ligament is suspected when the proximal left subclavian artery is tethered inferiorly toward the left pulmonary artery. The right-sided aortic arch with aberrant origin of the left subclavian artery is occasionally associated with persistence of the right arterial duct, or even absence of arterial ducts bilaterally (see Fig. 47-9). The latter combination is typically seen in tetralogy of Fallot with pulmonary atresia and pulmonary arterial supply via major aortopulmonary collateral arteries (see Fig. 47-10). This combination forms an incomplete encirclement or a vascular sling around the right side of the trachea and oesophagus. The right aortic arch with aberrant origin of the left brachiocephalic artery is rare.[25,26] It results from abnormal regression of the left aortic arch proximal to the origin of the left common carotid artery. The persisting arterial duct is usually left-sided, completing a vascular ring.

Left aortic arch with aberrant right subclavian artery is the most common anomaly involving the aortic arch, but is usually asymptomatic.[1,2,24,27,28] It results from abnormal regression of the right arch between the origins of the right common carotid and right subclavian arteries, leaving the right subclavian artery attached to the distal remnant of the right-sided aortic arch (Figs. 47-11 to 47-13). As a consequence, the distal remnant of the right aortic arch and the right subclavian artery together constitute the aberrant segments. In most cases, it is the left arterial duct which persists. This combination forms a vascular sling around the left side of the trachea and oesophagus (see Fig. 47-12). Typically the aberrant left subclavian artery courses behind the oesophagus, but has been described to course between the trachea and oesophagus, although again these vessels may have been collateral arteries.[1,2] When there is a right-sided arterial duct between the aberrant artery and the right pulmonary artery, there is a complete vascular ring (see Fig. 47-13). The ring consists of the ascending aorta, the left aortic arch, the descending aorta, the distal remnant of the right aortic arch, the right arterial duct, the right pulmonary artery, and the pulmonary trunk, with the heart itself completing the ring. In fetal life, when the arterial duct is a wide channel that connects the pulmonary artery to the descending aorta (see Fig. 47-13, middle panel), an ℓ-shaped loop is formed around the trachea and oesophagus. With closure of the right-sided arterial duct after birth,

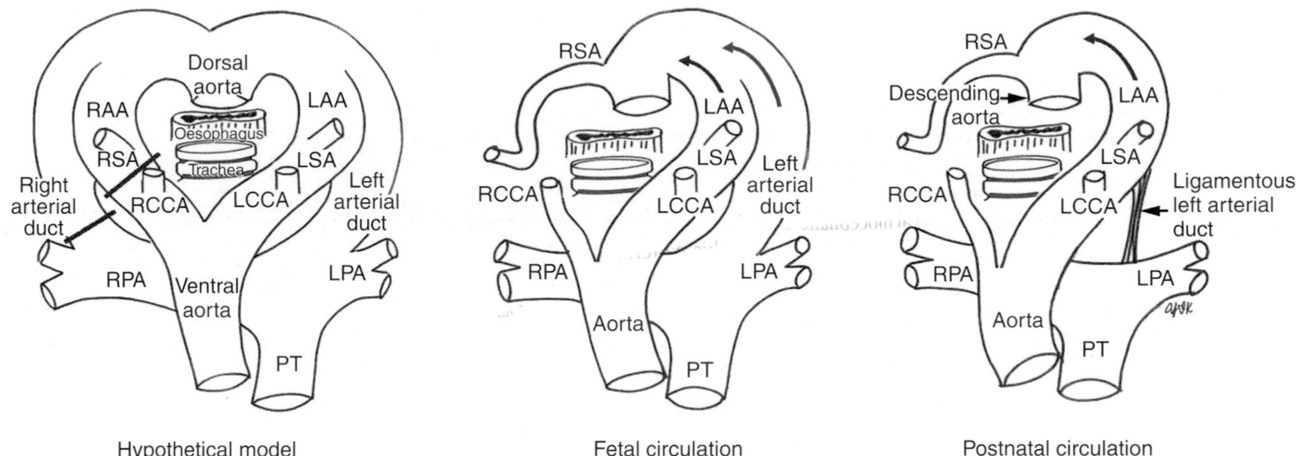

Figure 47-11 The cartoons show the morphogenesis (*left panel*), fetal arrangement (*middle panel*), and postnatal structure of left aortic arch (LAA) with aberrant origin of the right subclavian artery (RSA) and left-sided arterial duct. In the hypothetical model, the *red bars* again indicate the segments that regress. In the fetal and postnatal circulations, a vascular sling is formed on the left side of the trachea and oesophagus. LCCA, left common carotid artery; LPA, left pulmonary artery; LSA, left subclavian artery; PT, pulmonary trunk; RAA, right aortic arch; RCCA, right common carotid artery; RPA, right pulmonary artery.

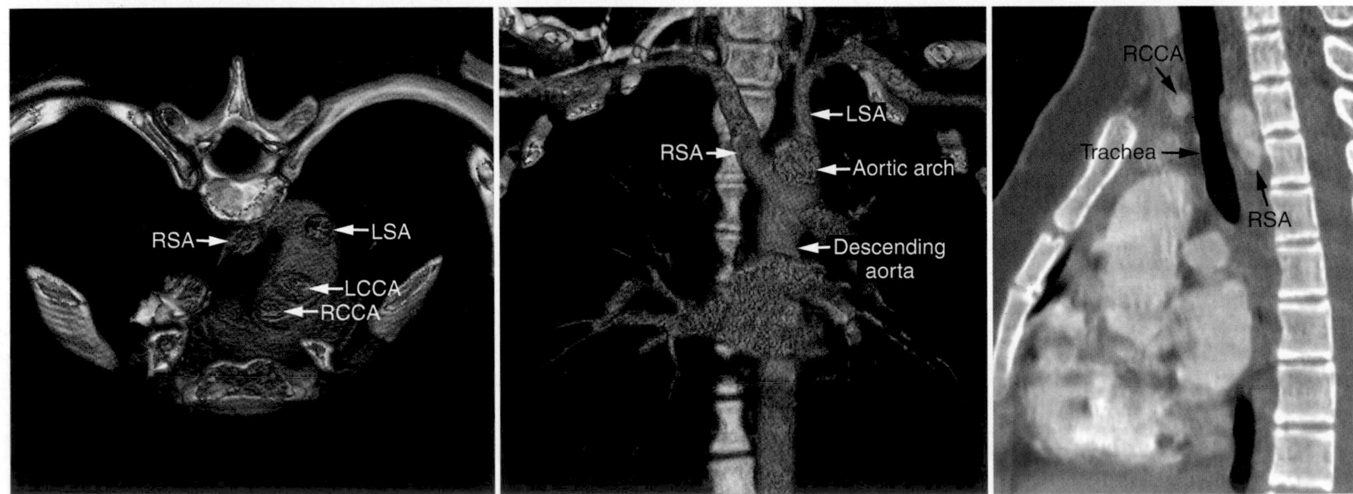

Figure 47-12 The computed tomograms show a left aortic arch (LAA) and aberrant right subclavian artery (RSA) arising from the descending aorta, with no intervening diverticulum of Kommerell. The posterior wall of the trachea shows a shallow indentation from the aberrant right subclavian artery (*right panel*). LCCA, left common carotid artery; LSA, left subclavian artery; RCCA, right common carotid artery.

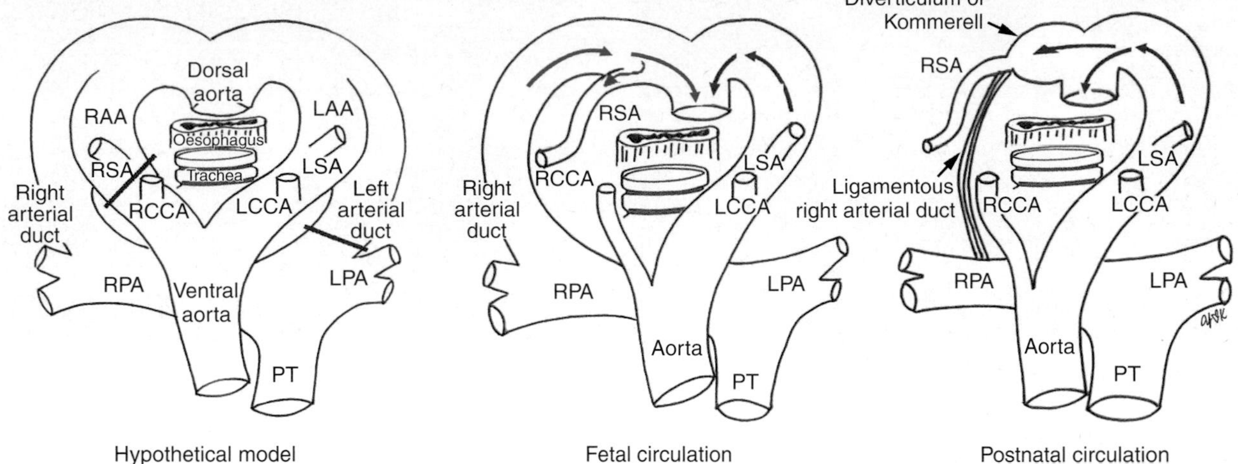

Figure 47-13 These cartoons, as with previous ones, show the derivation and structures of left aortic arch (LAA) with aberrant right subclavian artery (RSA) when the arterial duct is right-sided. In the hypothetical model, the red bars again indicate the segments that regress. In the fetal circulation (*middle panel*), the left aortic arch, the distal remnant of the right aortic arch (RAA), the right-sided arterial duct, and the pulmonary trunk (PT) produce an ℓ-shaped vascular loop around the trachea and oesophagus. As the two limbs of the ℓ-shaped loop are attached to the heart, there is a complete vascular ring. In the postnatal circulation (*right panel*), subsequent to closure of the arterial duct, the proximal part of the aberrant right subclavian artery, representing the distal remnant of the right aortic arch; persists as a diverticulum of Kommerell. Note that, as with the previous situation (see Fig. 47-6), the flow in the distal remnant of the right aortic arch switches its direction after birth. LCCA, left common carotid artery; LPA, left pulmonary artery; LSA, left subclavian artery; RCCA, right common carotid artery; RPA, right pulmonary artery.

the distal remnant of the right aortic arch persists as the diverticulum of Kommerell (see Fig. 47-13, right panel). It is theoretically possible for a left-sided aortic arch to be associated with aberrant origin of the right brachiocephalic artery, but thus far, as far as we are aware, this has not been reported. Aberrant subclavian or brachiocephalic arteries co-existing with either right-sided or left-sided aortic arches are often associated with other anomalies, including a common carotid arterial trunk, anomalous origin of the vertebral artery from the common carotid artery on the same side, anomalous point of entrance of the vertebral artery into the cervical spine, and an abnormal drainage site of the thoracic duct.[16] Although these anomalies are clinically silent, they may be of practical importance to the surgeon.

A right-sided aortic arch with a mirror-image branching results from abnormal regression of the left aortic arch distal to the origin of the left subclavian artery (Figs. 47-14 and 47-15). This is the only anomaly of the aortic arch that does not constitute a vascular ring or sling, regardless of the presence of a left-sided or right-sided arterial duct. In this pattern, the persisting arterial duct is usually on the left, connecting the base of the left brachiocephalic artery to the left pulmonary artery.[29] Less commonly, the arterial duct is either on the right, or bilateral. Rarely, the arterial duct arises from the descending aorta on the right side, and takes a retro-oesophageal course to connect to the left pulmonary artery (Fig. 47-16).[3,6,29–32] This is the only combination that constitutes a complete vascular ring in the presence of mirror-image branching. The anomaly results

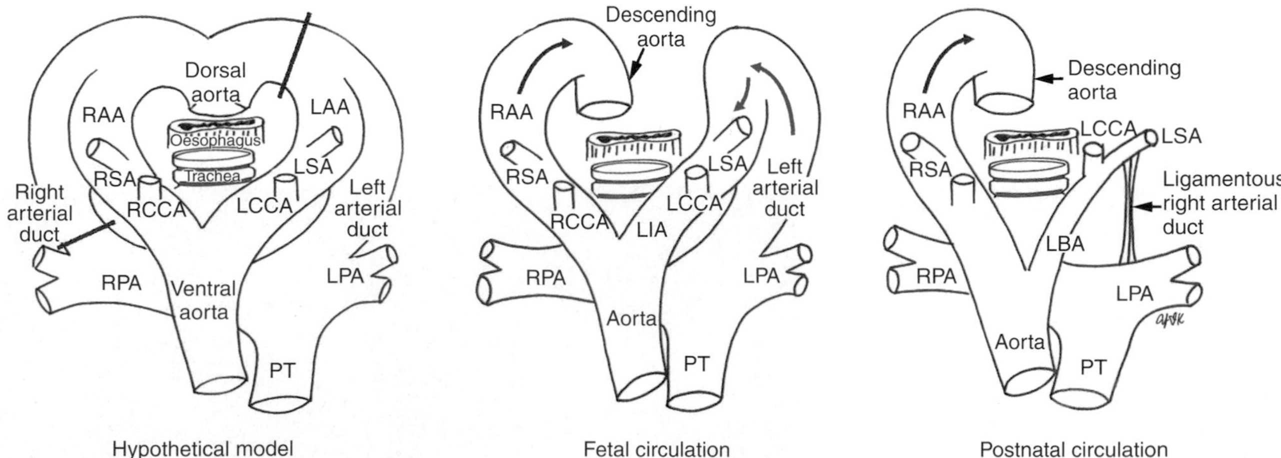

Figure 47-14 The cartoons show the morphogenesis, fetal arrangement, and postnatal structure of a right aortic arch (RAA) with mirror-image branching, the *red bars* in the hypothetical model indicating the segments that regress. In the majority of cases, it is the arterial duct on the left side that persists, with regression of the left aortic arch (LAA) distal to the origins of the left subclavian artery (LSA) and the left arterial duct, along with the right-sided arterial duct. In the postnatal circulation, the left-sided arterial ligament connects the base of the left brachiocephalic or subclavian artery to the left pulmonary artery (LPA). Persistence of the right-sided arterial duct is uncommon. LCCA, left common carotid artery; PT, pulmonary trunk; RCCA, right common carotid artery; RPA, right pulmonary artery; RSA, right subclavian artery.

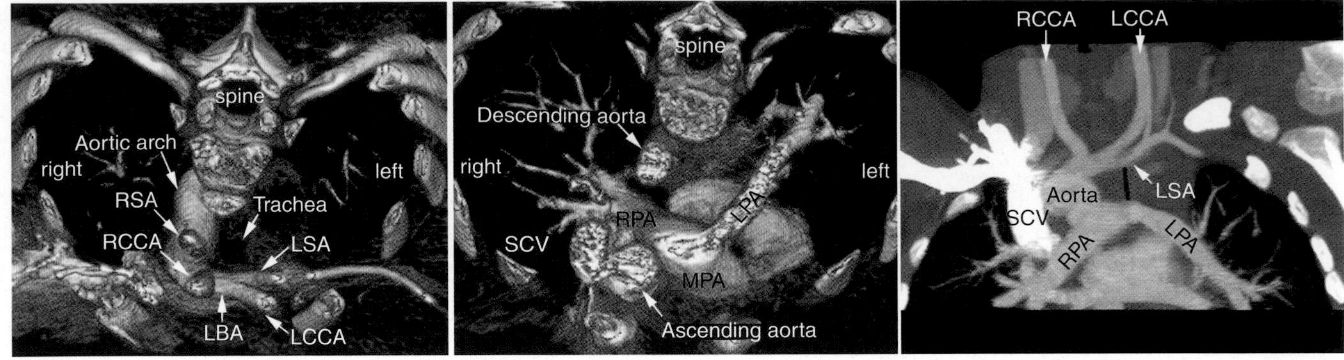

Figure 47-15 The computed tomograms, seen from above and the front, show the aortic arch on the right side of trachea. The aortic arch gives rise to the left brachiocephalic artery (LBA), the right common carotid artery (RCCA), and the right subclavian artery (RSA) in sequence. The expected location of the ligamentous arterial duct is marked by a *red bar* (*right panel*). Note that the left subclavian artery (LSA) kinks inferiorly, and the left pulmonary artery (LPA) is mildly stenotic, both highly suggestive of the presence of a left-sided arterial ligament. LCCA, left common carotid artery; MPA, pulmonary trunk; RPA, right pulmonary artery; SCV, superior caval vein.

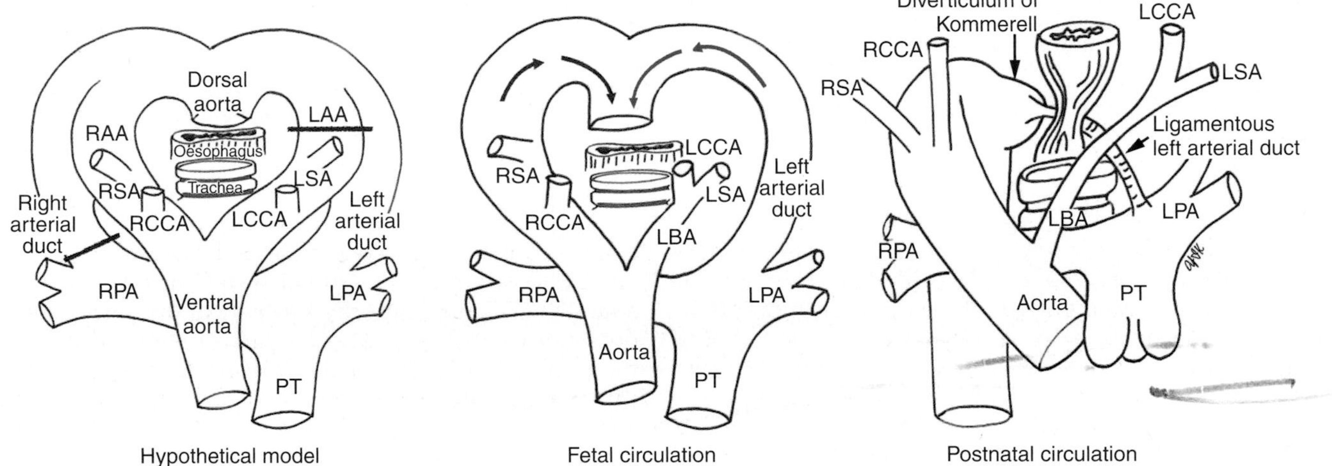

Figure 47-16 The cartoons show the mode of formation of a right aortic arch (RAA) with mirror-image branching, and retro-oesophageal course of the left-sided arterial duct between the right-sided descending aorta and the left pulmonary artery (LPA). In the hypothetical model (*left panel*), the *red bars* indicate the regression of the left aortic arch (LAA) between the origins of the left subclavian artery (LSA) and the left arterial duct, along with the right arterial duct. In the fetal circulation (*middle panel*), a U-shaped vascular loop is formed around the posterior aspect of the trachea and oesophagus. In postnatal circulation (*right panel*), the left-sided arterial duct arises from the right-sided descending aorta via a diverticulum of Kommerell, extending to the LPA, to produce a complete vascular ring in this rare anomaly. LBA, left brachiocephalic artery; LCCA, left common carotid artery; PT, pulmonary trunk; RCCA, right common carotid artery; RPA, right pulmonary artery; RSA, right subclavian artery.

from abnormal regression of the left aortic arch distal to the origin of the left subclavian artery and proximal to the insertion of the persisting left arterial duct, with regression of the right arterial duct. The distal left aortic arch remnant persists as a diverticulum of Kommerell.

Circumflex retro-oesophageal aortic arch is a rare form of aortic arch anomaly in which the aortic arch and the proximal descending aorta are placed on opposite sides of the spine (Figs. 47-17 to 47-19).[33,34] This combination requires the aortic arch to make an additional arc to the

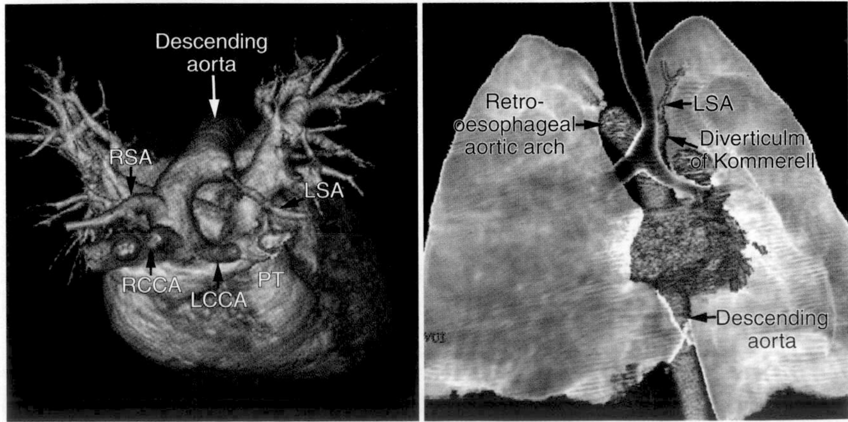

Figure 47-17 The computed tomograms show a circumflex and retro-oesophageal right-sided aortic arch. The aortic arch is located on the right side of the trachea, and makes a sharp oblique leftward and downward turn to course behind the oesophagus so as to connect to the left-sided descending aorta. The left subclavian artery (LSA) arises from the top of the descending aorta, with the presence of a diverticulum suggesting that a left-sided arterial ligament is present between the apex of the diverticulum and the proximal left pulmonary artery. LCCA, left common carotid artery; PT, pulmonary trunk; RCCA, right common carotid artery; RSA, right subclavian artery.

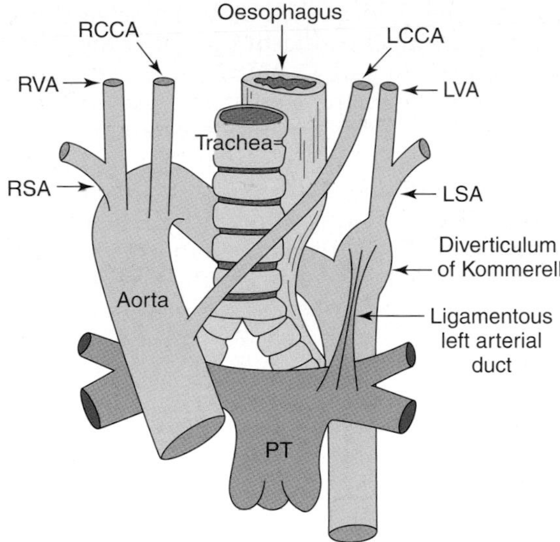

Figure 47-18 The cartoon shows the situation illustrated in Figure 47-17. LCCA, left common carotid artery; LSA, left subclavian artery, LVA, left vertebral artery; PT, pulmonary trunk; RCCA, right common carotid artery; RSA, right subclavian artery; RVA, right vertebral artery.

other side behind the trachea and oesophagus, thus reaching the descending aorta on the opposite side. The patterns of branching of the brachiocephalic arteries are variable. It is hard to explain this rare malformation. It occurs much more frequently with a right-sided than with a left aortic arch. When it occurs with a right aortic arch, the arch gives rise to the left common carotid, right common carotid and right subclavian artery from its segment on the right side of the trachea (see Fig. 47-17, left panel). Then the aortic arch makes a sharp oblique leftward and usually downward turn to connect to the left-sided descending aorta. The left subclavian artery arises from the transitional point of the retro-oesophageal part of the arch to the descending aorta. It can be named as an aberrant artery in the sense that it is the last, instead of the first, branch of the right aortic arch. It is not retro-oesophageal in location, but the aortic arch itself is behind the oesophagus. In most cases, the left subclavian artery arises from the aorta through a diverticulum of Kommerell. The apex of the diverticulum connects to the left pulmonary artery through a left arterial ligament, thus forming a complete vascular ring around the trachea and oesophagus. A circumflex retro-oesophageal aortic arch is rarely seen without aberrant origin of a subclavian artery, but does exist (see Fig. 47-19).[29] Hypoplasia of the retro-oesophageal segment of the aortic arch is common.[34]

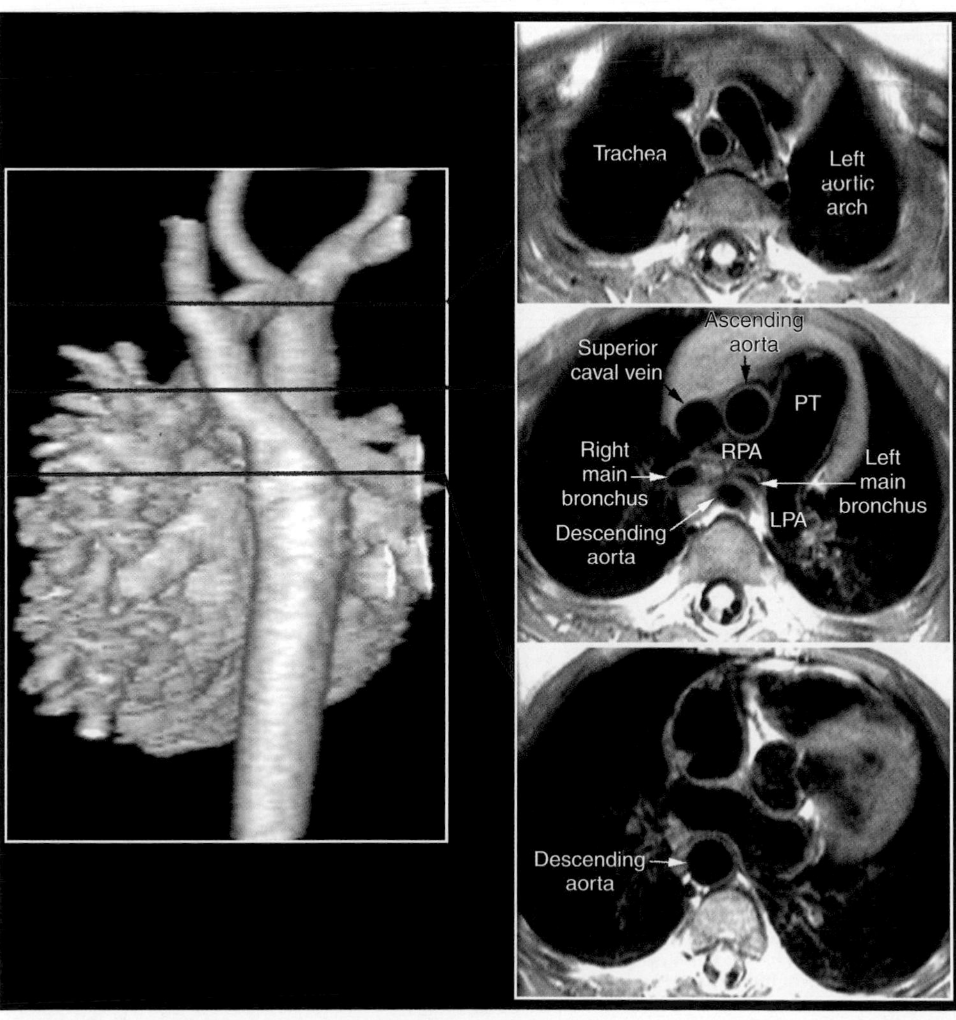

Figure 47-19 The magnetic resonance angiogram seen from behind (*left panel*) shows a normal left aortic arch with normal brachiocephalic branching, but the descending aorta takes an unusual oblique course to the right side. The transverse axial T1-weighted images (*right panel*) obtained at the levels marked on the angiogram clearly show the normal left aortic arch, but illustrate that the left main bronchus is compressed between the descending aorta and the right pulmonary artery (RPA) as the former takes its oblique retro-oesophageal course. LPA, left pulmonary artery; PT, pulmonary trunk.

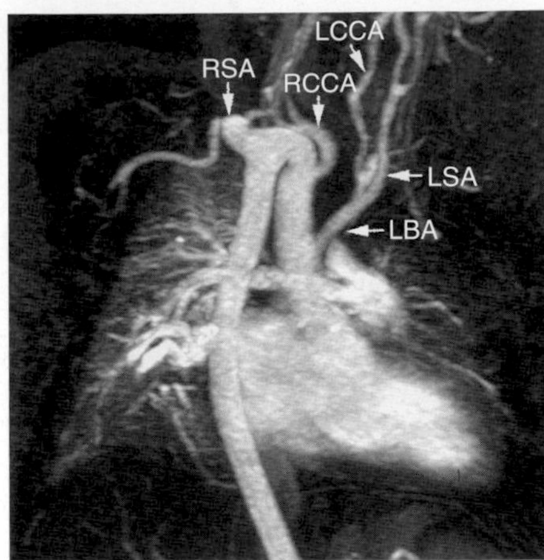

Figure 47-20 The magnetic resonance angiogram shows a so-called cervical right aortic arch, which reaches to the apex of the right lung, where it makes a hair-pin turn. It shows mirror-image branching, but the branches are tortuous, and the origin of the right subclavian artery (RSA) is aneurysmally dilated. LBA, left brachiocephalic artery; LCCA, left common carotid artery; LSA, left subclavian artery; RCCA, right common carotid artery.

The aortic arch is described as being cervical when its apex reaches the upper mediastinum above the level of the clavicles (Figs. 47-20 and 47-21).[35-37] It may be recognised as a pulsatile mass in the supraclavicular fossa or lower neck. A cervical arch is slightly more common on the right, often taking a circumflex retro-oesophageal course to form a vascular ring. A double aortic arch can also adopt a cervical position. The branching of the brachiocephalic arteries is abnormal in the majority of cases. In addition, it is common to find unusual tortuosity, obstruction and aneurysm of the aortic arch, and obstruction of a brachiocephalic branch or branches (see Figs. 47-20 and 47-21). A cervical aortic arch is often associated with tracheal obstruction because of crowding of vascular structures and airway in a confined small space of the upper mediastinum, especially when the aortic arch is right-sided and takes a hairpin turn.[38]

Isolated origin of the subclavian artery from the pulmonary artery through the arterial duct is a rare type of anomaly in which the subclavian artery is disconnected from the aorta, instead taking its origin from the pulmonary artery

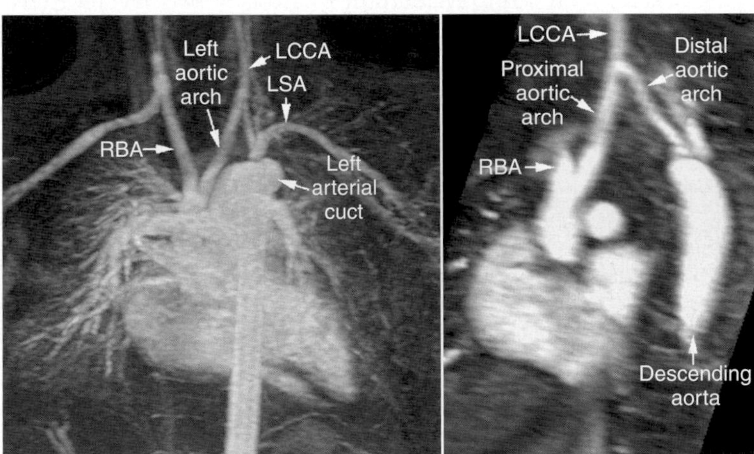

Figure 47-21 These magnetic resonance angiograms show that the severely hypoplastic cervical aortic arch, left-sided in this instance, reaches to the lower neck. It shows normal branching. Interrupted of the aortic arch has been suspected in this patient. LCCA, left common carotid artery; LSA, left subclavian artery; RBA, right brachiocephalic artery.

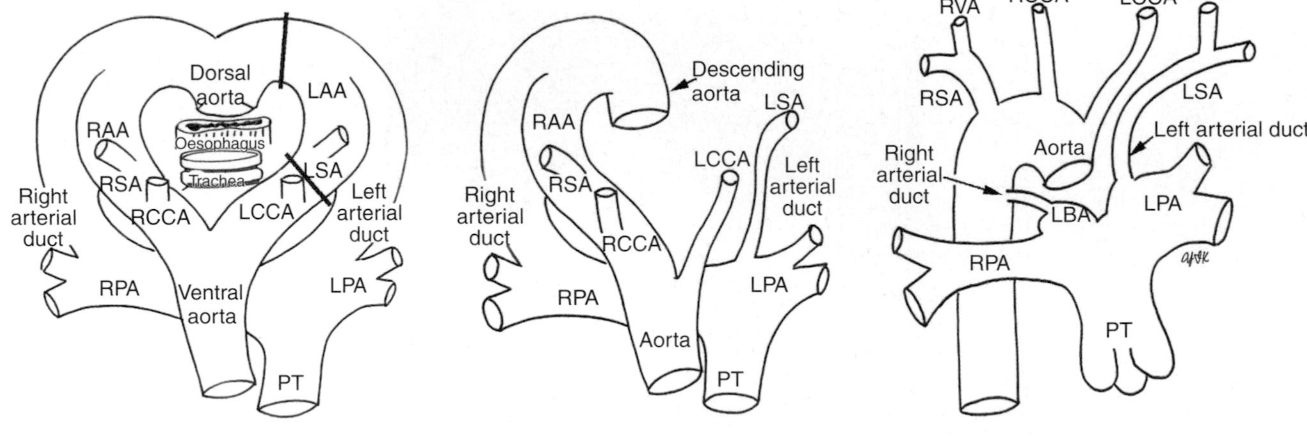

Figure 47-22 The hypothetical model for the double arch is used to explain isolated origin of the left subclavian artery (LSA) from the left pulmonary artery (LPA) through the left arterial duct (*left panel*). The *red bars* show regression of the left aortic arch (LAA) in two locations, both proximal and distal to the origin of the left subclavian artery. As the distal interruption is distal to the insertion of the left arterial duct, the LSA becomes isolated from the aortic arch, instead retaining its connection with the left pulmonary artery. The right arterial duct also persists. The middle and right panels show the arrangements in the fetal and postnatal circulations. LBA, left brachiocephalic artery; LCCA, left common carotid artery; PT, pulmonary trunk; RAA, right aortic arch; RCCA, right common carotid artery; RPA, right pulmonary artery; RSA, right subclavian artery.

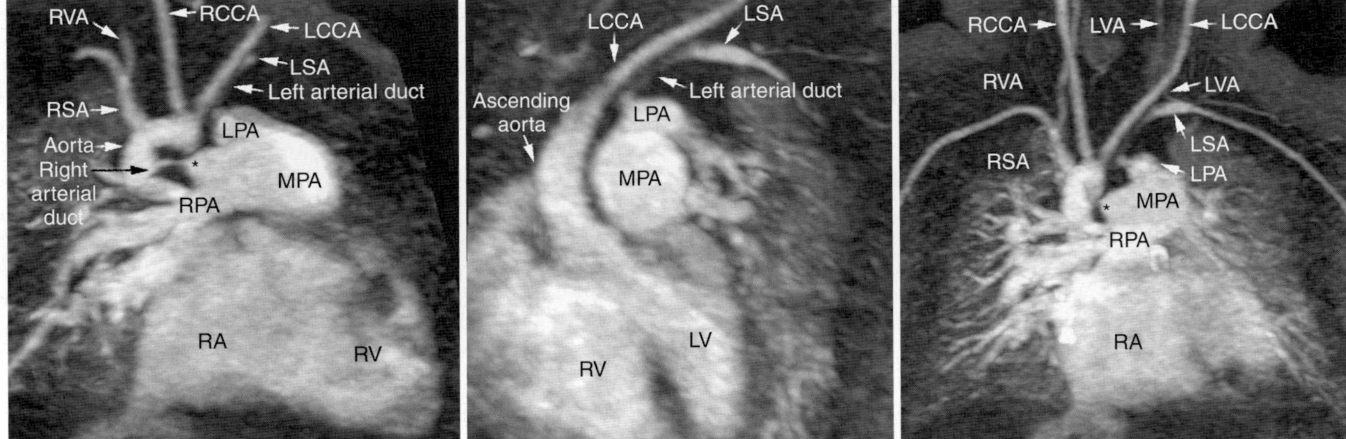

Figure 47-23 These contrast-enhanced magnetic resonance angiograms reformatted in right anterior oblique (*left panel*), left anterior oblique (*middle panel*), and frontal (*right panel*) planes show that there is a right aortic arch that gives rise to the left common carotid, right common carotid, and right subclavian arteries (LCCA, RCCA, RSA) in sequence. The left subclavian artery (LSA) arises from the proximal left pulmonary artery (LPA) through the left-sided arterial duct. The right arterial duct is patent between the right pulmonary artery (RPA) and the descending aorta. Note that the right arterial duct has an ampullary dilatation (*asterisk*) at its pulmonary arterial end. LV, left ventricle; LVA, left vertebral artery; MPA, pulmonary trunk; RA, right atrium; RV, right ventricle; RVA, right vertebral artery. (Reprinted with permission from Sun AM, Alhabshan F, Branson H, Freedom RM, Yoo SJ: MRI diagnosis of isolated origin of the left subclavian artery from the left pulmonary artery. Pediatr Radiol 2005;35:1259–1262.)

on that side through the persistently patent arterial duct (Figs. 47-22 and 47-23).[39–41] It is explained on the basis of abnormal regression at two locations in the hypothetical double arch (Fig. 47-22, left panel), one proximal and the other distal to the origin of the affected subclavian artery. Such isolation occurs more commonly when the aortic arch is right-sided, with the left subclavian artery being the isolated artery in the majority of cases. Flow to the isolated artery varies according to the size of the persistently patent arterial duct, and the patency of the pulmonary outflow tract. When the arterial duct is wide open, and there is no pulmonary obstruction, the left subclavian artery is supplied through the pulmonary arteries. If associated with significant pulmonary obstruction, the flow through the arterial duct may be reversed. Postnatally, when the arterial duct closes, the anomalous artery may lose its primary supply of blood, and can result in vertebral steal on the side of the isolated artery. Brachiocephalic or carotid arteries can also be isolated in comparable fashion.[42]

Double-barreled, or double lumen, aorta is a rare anomaly in which the ascending and descending components of the aorta are connected by two aortic arches on the same side of the trachea (Fig. 47-24).[42–44] It should not be confused with the double aortic arch, in which each arch is to the opposite sides of the trachea. In the past, this anomaly has been interpreted as persistence of the embryological fifth aortic arch.[43] The existence of the fifth aortic arch in human and mammalian embryos, however, remains controversial, never having been encountered during normal development.[45]

Incidence, Genetics and Association with Anomalies

The overall incidence of anomalies involving the aortic arch is difficult to estimate, since an unknown but significant number of individuals having such anomalies do not present with symptoms, and thus remain undiagnosed. The reported incidences of individual anomalies, therefore, vary significantly according to the population studied. A left aortic arch with aberrant origin of the right subclavian artery, which is usually found as an incidental and isolated anomaly, has been reported as the most common condition, being found in 0.5% of a large autopsy series.[2] In patients with other cardiac defects, a right aortic arch with mirror-image branching is the most common malformation.[29]

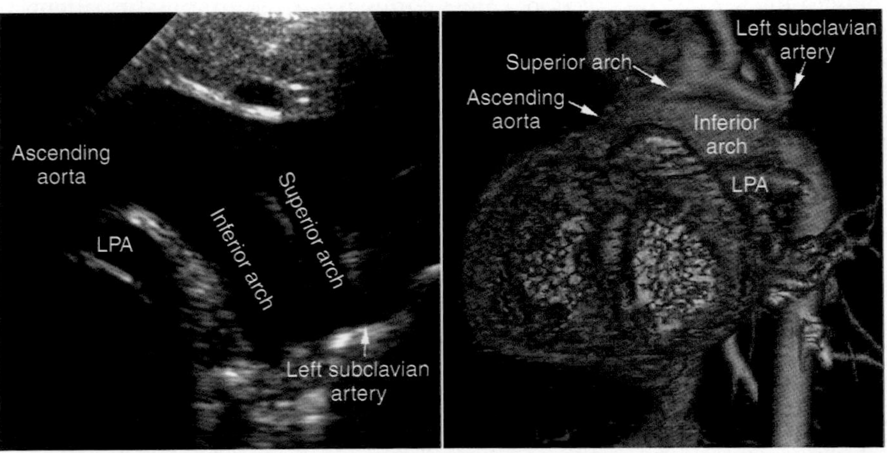

Figure 47-24 The computed tomograms show a double-barreled aortic arch in a patient with tetralogy of Fallot and pulmonary atresia. LPA, left pulmonary artery. (Reprinted with permission from Bernasconi A, Goo HW, Yoo SJ: Double-barrelled aorta with tetralogy of Fallot and pulmonary atresia. Cardiol Young 2006;17:98–101.)

Association with congenitally malformed hearts varies according to the individual lesions. A right aortic arch with mirror-imaged branching is almost always associated with congenital cardiac disease.[29] A right aortic arch is common in tetralogy of Fallot and common arterial trunk, with the incidence ranging from one-sixth to over one-third for both lesions. When tetralogy is associated with pulmonary atresia, the incidence is high at one-third. A mirror-imaged right aortic arch is less frequently seen in transposition, tricuspid atresia, and isolated ventricular septal defect. When not associated with intracardiac anomalies, the mirror-imaged right aortic arch is commonly associated with absence or stenosis of the proximal left pulmonary artery.[29] The rare mirror-imaged right aortic arch with retro-oesophageal left-sided arterial duct is uncommonly associated with other cardiovascular anomalies. Right aortic arch with aberrant left subclavian artery is also less commonly associated with congenital cardiac disease, with the reported incidence ranging from less than one-fifth to over three-fifths.[4,6,7] The most commonly associated malformations are ventricular and atrial septal defects, tetralogy of Fallot, and transposition. Left aortic arch with aberrant right subclavian artery is much less commonly associated with other malformations, and therefore is usually found as an incidental finding. Double aortic arch is associated with other cardiovascular anomalies in up to one-fifth of cases, the most common being atrial and ventricular septal defects, tetralogy of Fallot and patency of the arterial duct.[4–9] Circumflex retro-oesophageal aortic arch is associated with congenitally malformed hearts in up to half of cases.[33] Although uncommon, a right aortic arch with or without an aberrant left subclavian or brachiocephalic artery may be associated with an obstructive lesion of the aortic arch, especially when the arch forms a circumflex retro-oesophageal or high cervical course, or both (see Fig. 47-21).[46–48] Rarely, interruption can be found in a right aortic arch.[47,49]

Non-cardiac anomalies are infrequently associated with anomalies of the aortic arch. The most important non-cardiac anomaly is the oesophageal atresia with or without the VACTERL (vertebral, anal, cardiac, tracheal, oesophageal, renal, and limb anomalies) association.[8,50,51] It has been reported that oesophageal atresia seen in association with such anomalies of the aortic arch tends to have a long gap.[50]

Chromosome 22q11 deletion syndrome is common.[52–54] This deletion is considered to affect migration of cells from the neural crest that contribute to development of the ventricular outflow tracts and pharyngeal arches in the embryo. The precise mechanisms of abnormal development of the aortic arches, however, remain speculative. A fetal series showed an 8% incidence of 22q11 deletion in fetuses with a right aortic arch as an isolated abnormality, and 46% in those with right aortic arch and intracardiac abnormality.[19] Postnatal series showed higher incidences of 22q11 deletion, this being found in up to one-quarter of cases with an isolated anomaly of the aortic arch.[52,53] The higher incidence of 22q11 deletion in postnatal series is explained by selection bias, as these patients are more likely to be referred to a cardiologist.[19] More than half of the patients with an intracardiac anomaly and 22q11 deletion have an anomaly of the aortic arch.[54] In patients with anomalies of the ventricular outflow tracts, anomalies of the subclavian arteries function as an important anatomical marker for chromosome 22q11 deletion, independent of the laterality of the aortic arch.[55] The subclavian arterial anomalies encompass aberrant origin from the descending aorta, isolated origin, distal ductal origin from the pulmonary artery, and cervical origin. Chromosome 22q11 deletion was present in greater than three-quarters of such patients with abnormalities of the ventricular outflow tracts and abnormal subclavian arteries, while it was present in less than three-tenths when there was no subclavian arterial anomaly. The patients with tetralogy of Fallot with chromosome 22q11 deletion show higher incidence of cervical aortic arch.[56] Down syndrome has also been shown to be associated with an increased risk for aberrant right subclavian artery.[5,57,58] In the presence of an anomaly of the aortic arch, therefore, fetal karyotyping is recommended, especially when it is associated with intracardiac anomalies, extracardiac malformations, or an increased nuchal translucency.[19]

Clinical Findings

Patients with a vascular ring or sling may develop symptoms and signs of airway obstruction and/or oesophageal compression.[3–10] Clinical manifestations vary with the severity of encroachment on the trachea, bronchus or oesophagus by the abnormal artery or arteries. The severity of compression of the trachea and oesophagus not only depends on the type of anomaly, but is also affected by the size and shape of the thoracic cage enclosing the vascular structures and airway. For instance, a chest cage with diminished anteroposterior diameter, as in stove chest or straight-back syndrome, is associated with more severe compression than a normally shaped chest cage. In addition, dilation of a vascular component of the anomalous aorta or its neighbouring vessel, and hyperinflation of the lungs, may further compromise the patency of the airway and oesophagus.

Patients with a vascular ring are more frequently symptomatic than those with a vascular sling. Tighter vascular rings usually present early in life with respiratory symptoms, while looser rings or slings may present later with symptoms of oesophageal compression. Patients with a double aortic arch tend to have the earliest onset of symptoms. Common presenting symptoms are respiratory, including stridor, wheezing, and cough. Study of a large cohort showed that symptomatic patients have significantly altered tracheal geometry, with smaller diameters and cross sectional areas compared to asymptomatic patients.[59] The characteristic stridor is inspiratory, but it may be both inspiratory and expiratory. Stridor may not be obvious during sleep or quiet play and is exacerbated by exertion or crying. The severity and pattern of stridor or noisy breathing can change with position. There may be a history of recurrent respiratory infections requiring medical attention, and some patients have been referred for an evaluation of suspected asthma or bronchiolitis. Infants with a tight vascular ring may show life-threatening reflex apnea with feeding. Some infants show opisthotonic posture, with hyperextension of the neck to relieve tracheal compression.[6] Respiratory symptoms seen in infancy or early childhood may disappear with conservative medical treatment as the thoracic cage becomes more spacious as the patient grows.[60]

Symptoms of oesophageal compression, including dysphagia or choking, usually develop later when the patient commences to take solid foods. Dysphagia is often the first symptom in older patients.[16,23] This late onset of dysphagia may be related to the elongation of the aorta, or be secondary to aneurysmal changes of an existing diverticulum of Kommerell or the adjacent descending aorta.[16,24,28] Dysphagia may be associated with frequent aspiration. A vascular ring is occasionally diagnosed at the time of removal of foreign bodies, such as chicken bones and coins. When a diverticulum of Kommerell develops aneurysmal change, it may be complicated by dissection and frank rupture.[16,21,24,28]

The majority of patients with isolated abnormalities grow adequately. Uncommonly there may be failure to thrive and poor physical development due to frequent pulmonary infections, and/or difficulties with feeding. Rarely, the patient may present with the symptoms of compression of a nerve plexus by an abnormally positioned aorta or its branch.[32] Incidental discovery of an anomaly is not uncommon following imaging for other medical problems.

Diagnostic Investigations

The chest radiograph is a simple and logical starting point for the imaging algorithm (Fig. 47-25). It provides information regarding not only the position of the aortic arch, but also the pulmonary complications of the anomaly, if present. The laterality of the aortic arch relative to the trachea is usually readily apparent. The trachea is bent to the other side of the aortic arch. The tracheal air column usually shows a subtle indentation caused by the aortic arch. In most cases, the position of the arch can be traced back from the descending aorta, which can be identified as a vertical linear stripe along the bony spinal column. When the aortic arch and the vertical linear stripe of the proximal descending aorta are seen on the opposite sides, a double aortic arch, or a circumflex retro-oesophageal aortic arch with the descending aorta on the other side, should be suspected. A double aortic arch may cause a concentric narrowing, with bilateral indentation in the lower trachea, but more frequently, the narrowing is asymmetric and the indentation is unilateral. Bilateral indentation by other types of vascular ring is rare. The lateral view may show anterior bowing of the distal trachea when there is a large retro-oesophageal component (Fig. 47-26). A dilated proximal oesophagus containing air may suggest the presence of retro-oesophageal component. The superior mediastinum is wide when there is a cervical aortic arch, and a mediastinal mass can be mistakenly suspected. The superior mediastinum in young children, however, is normally wide because of a large thymus. Atelectasis or pneumonic consolidation involving various lung regions may be present and mask the underlying malformation. In some cases, hyperinflation of the lungs or parts of the lungs may be the predominant radiographic feature.

Although the barium oesophagogram was previously used as a valuable adjunct, its use is almost abandoned now because it does not provide a definitive diagnosis while exposing the patient to radiation.[6]

The definitive diagnosis can be made by using echocardiography, X-ray angiography, computed tomography or magnetic resonance imaging. Echocardiography is always indicated with aortic arch anomalies to exclude any associated intracardiac anomaly. A standardised echocardiographic approach to locate the position of the aortic arch, and its pattern of branching, is always an essential component of the evaluation of suspected congenital cardiac disease.[61] For this purpose, the transducer is positioned transversely in the suprasternal notch and starting with downward angulation, a gentle sweep upward allows identification of the aortic arch position relative to the trachea and the origins and branching pattern of the head and neck branches. In the normal left aortic arch, the first branch heads rightward and bifurcates into the right common carotid and subclavian arteries. Whereas, in the right aortic arch with mirror-image branching, the first branch heads leftward and bifurcates into the left common carotid and subclavian arteries (Fig. 47-27). If the first branch does not bifurcate, then an aberrant subclavian artery should be suspected (Fig. 47-28). Alternatively, a common origin of the right brachiocephalic and left carotid arteries, or a separate origin of the left vertebral artery proximal to the left subclavian artery, can both occur in approximately

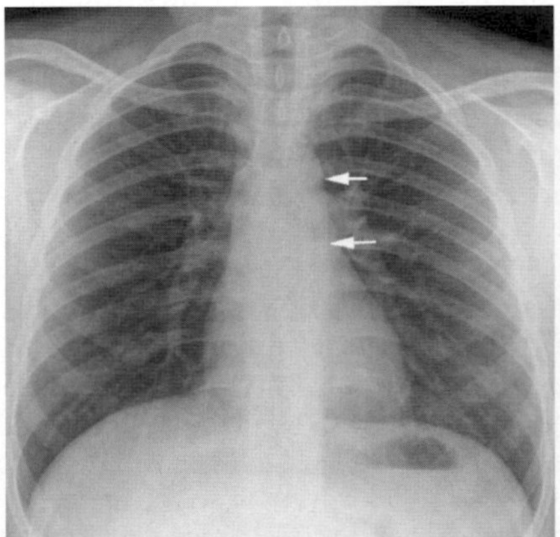
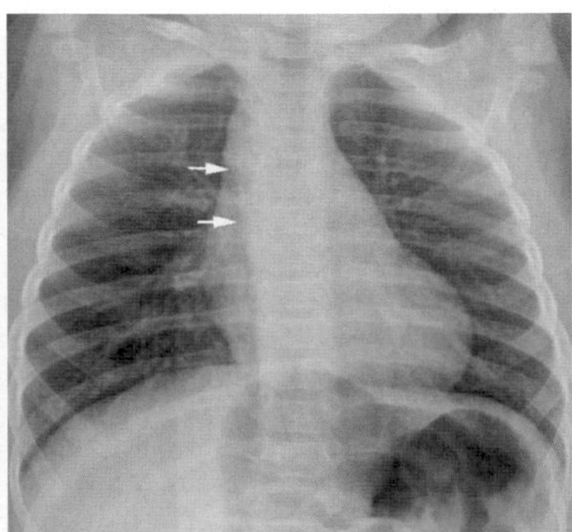
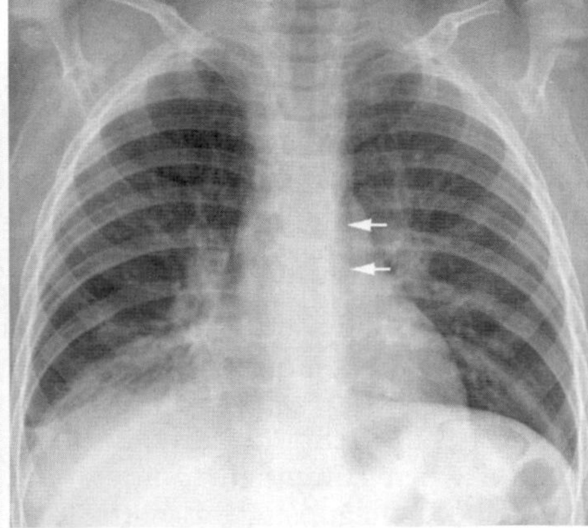

Figure 47-25 The frontal chest radiographs show a normal left aortic arch (*left panel*) and a right aortic arch (*middle panel*). The trachea shows slight indentation on the same side of the aortic arch and is bent slightly to the other side when there is a left or right aortic arch. The aortic arch can be traced downward to the vertical linear stripe of the descending aorta on the same side (*arrows*). In the setting of a double aortic arch (*right panel*), the distal trachea shows narrowing on both sides. In this case, the descending aorta can be traced down the left side (*arrows*) and pneumonic consolidation is seen in the right middle lobe (*right panel*).

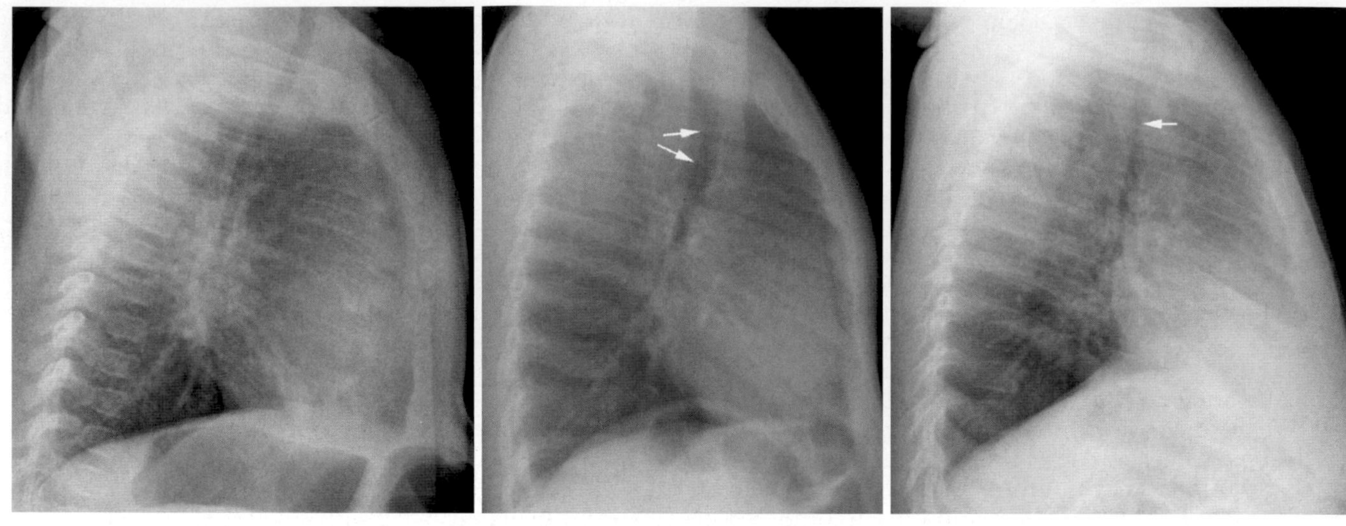

Figure 47-26 These lateral chest radiographs correspond to those shown in Figure 47-25. The left panel shows a normal left aortic arch and a normal trachea, which takes a straight course without narrowing. When the aortic arch is right-sided, and an aberrant left subclavian artery arises from a diverticulum of Kommerell, as in the middle panel, the trachea is bowed forward by the diverticulum (*arrows*). In the setting of a double aortic arch, as shown in the right panel, the distal trachea in this case shows diffuse narrowing (*arrow*), and pneumonic consolidation is seen in the right middle lobe.

one-tenth of otherwise normal left aortic arches. In a double aortic arch, if both are patent, both can be identified in this transverse suprasternal view. Echocardiography has the advantage that it can often be performed with no or minimal sedation at the bedside, and a complete diagnosis can be reached with echocardiography alone when the vascular anatomy is simple, as in classic form of double aortic arch.[8] Often the information provided by echocardiography is incomplete, and the assessment of the anatomy of the airways is not possible with ultrasound.

Although catheterisation with angiography was once the gold standard for the diagnosis, this has almost been completely replaced by computed tomography and magnetic resonance imaging. Both computed tomography and magnetic resonance imaging provide a clear road map allowing the construction of a precise preoperative strategy.[6,62,63]

Computed tomography is perfectly suited for the simultaneous evaluation of the anatomy of the vascular structures and the airways.[62–65] Recent introduction and development of the multi-detector technology in computed tomography has allowed high-resolution acquisition of data from the whole chest within a few seconds. Sedation or general anaesthesia, therefore, is rarely required, even in uncooperative children. Although computed tomography uses a large amount of radiation, the dose can be significantly reduced by carefully adjusting the imaging parameters, scan direction and the volume of coverage.[66] As the vessels in question are rather large structures, artifacts associated with using a low kilo-voltage and low milliampere technique do not significantly reduce the diagnostic accuracy. The volume of tissue covered by computed tomography can be minimised by referring to the already available information. Every effort should be made to reduce the dose of radiation when computed tomography is performed. In performing a diagnostic procedure using radiation, taking beautiful pictures should not be regarded as a virtue. The real virtue is to take images of diagnostic quality, using the lowest possible dose of radiation. The axial images are reviewed by scrolling up and down in the workstation. Three-dimensional reconstruction in various planes is mandatory. Three-dimensional reconstruction is useful, not only for demonstration of the anatomy, but also for more accurate diagnosis. Both maximum-intensity projection and volume-rendering algorithms are useful for the assessment of the vascular structures. Minimum-intensity projection with volume rendering algorithm is used for three-dimensional reconstruction of the airway. The volume rendered images of the vascular structures and airways can be merged to show spatial relationships. Endoluminal volume rendering also allows virtual tracheobronchoscopic demonstration of the airway.[67] The severity of the narrowing seen in the airways at routine computed tomography does not always correlate with symptoms and signs. In addition, a significant discrepancy in severity is often found between bronchoscopic and computed tomographic findings. This is because routine computed tomography has limitations in detecting dynamic airway narrowing. Dynamic narrowing can be assessed by scanning the airway in both inspiratory and expiratory phases when the patient can follow the imaging instructions.[68,69] In infants and uncooperative patients, the suspected pathological region can be repeatedly scanned throughout the respiratory cycle to assess the dynamic nature of the obstruction (Fig. 47-29).[70] It does, however, require significant additional radiation.

Magnetic resonance imaging is also an excellent tool for the assessment of the vascular anatomy.[62,63,71,72] Contrast-enhanced magnetic resonance angiography has been used for the assessment of the vascular structures. Three-dimensional volume data acquisition of the cardiovascular anatomy can be acquired without injection of contrast medium, by using an electrocardiographically gated balanced steady-state free precession sequence and respiratory navigation.[73] Double-inversion recovery sequence is a technique that can be used for the assessment of the airway. Real-time cine magnetic resonance imaging is a future direction for a dynamic airway assessment.[74] Magnetic resonance imaging is the preferred technique in cooperative children because it does not use radiation.

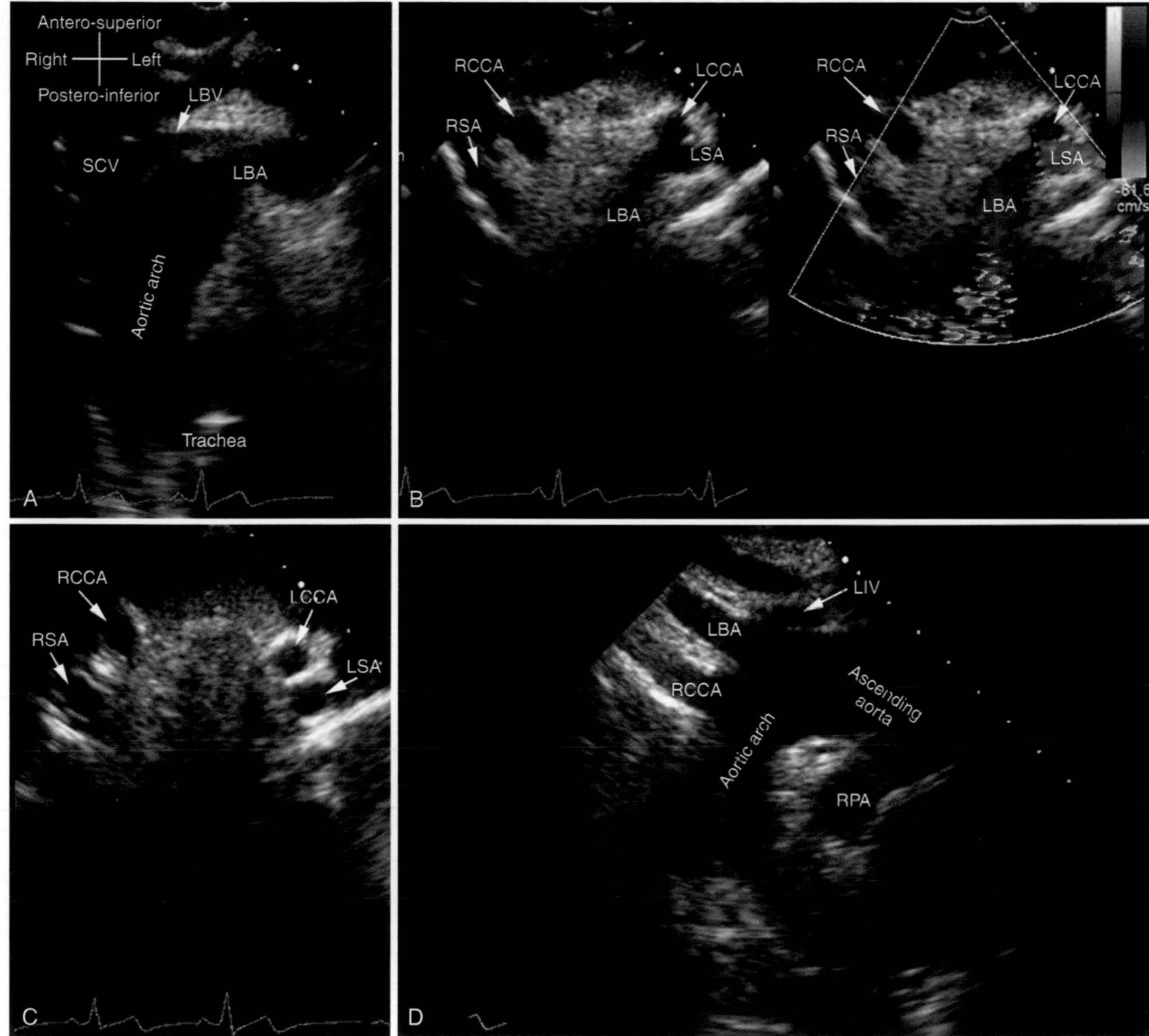

Figure 47-27 The panel of illustrations shows the standardised echocardiographic approach to show the anatomy of the aortic arch in a patient with right aortic arch and mirror-image branching. **A,** The position of the aortic arch relative to the trachea is identified in a downward tilted transverse view from a suprasternal approach. **B,** Sweeping upward with the transducer permits ascertainment of the origins of the brachiocephalic arteries. The first branch in this case is the left brachiocephalic artery (LBA), which bifurcates into the left common carotid and subclavian arteries. **C,** With a further sweep upward, the carotid and subclavian arteries can be imaged in an almost symmetric arrangement in the lower neck. **D,** Then, the transducer is rotated clockwise or counterclockwise to align the ascending and descending aorta with the aortic arch. In this instance, the sonographer has mirror-imaged the transducer clearly to demonstrate that there is a right aortic arch. LBV, left brachiocephalic vein; LCCA, left common carotid artery; LIV, left innominate vein; LSA, left subclavian artery; RCCA, right common carotid artery; RPA, right pulmonary artery; RSA, right subclavian artery; SCV, superior caval vein.

Pre-operative or intra-operative bronchoscopy is still performed in all patients with vascular rings in some institutions.[6,8] Bronchoscopy allows proper positioning of the endotracheal tube, and diagnosis of unrecognised tracheomalacia or bronchomalacia.

It should be noted that none of the currently available imaging modalities is able to visualise of a vascular structure, such as an arterial ligament or an atretic segment of the aortic arch. The presence of such fibrous strands can only be suspected when an arterial branch shows an otherwise unexplainable kinked course or a diverticular outpouching.[15] Presence of a diverticulum of Kommerell indicates that a ligamentous arterial duct extends from the apex of the diverticulum to either the pulmonary artery or an atretic arch on the same side.

Management of Anomalies Causing Tracheal and Oesophageal Compression

The simple existence of a vascular ring is not an indication for surgical intervention. Symptoms of borderline severity may disappear as the child grows. It is generally accepted, however, that surgical intervention should be undertaken whenever the patient is symptomatic, and there is significant compromise to the airways. Unnecessary delay may cause irreversible tracheobronchial damage, leading to

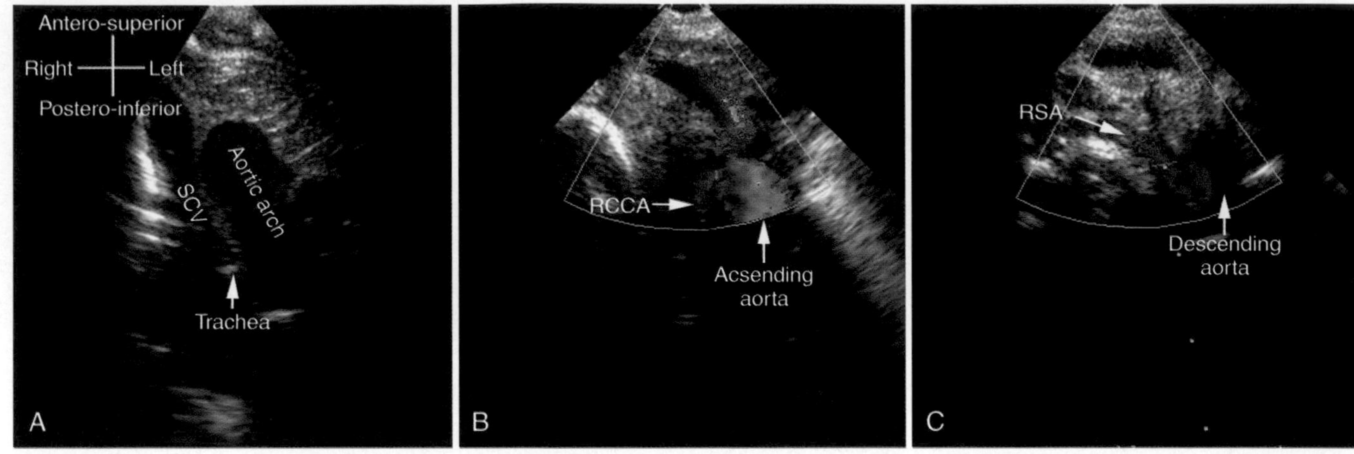

Figure 47-28 This panel of echocardiographic images shows a left aortic arch with an aberrant right subclavian artery. **A,** In the downward transverse view a left aortic arch is displayed with the trachea to the right. **B,** The upward sweep of the transducer reveals the first branch arising from a left aortic arch does not bifurcate, but instead continues forward, upward and rightward, this being characteristic for the right common carotid artery (RCCA). **C,** Inferior angulation of the transducer reveals the aberrant right subclavian artery (RSA) arising more distally from the descending aorta on the left side of the midline. SCV, superior caval vein.

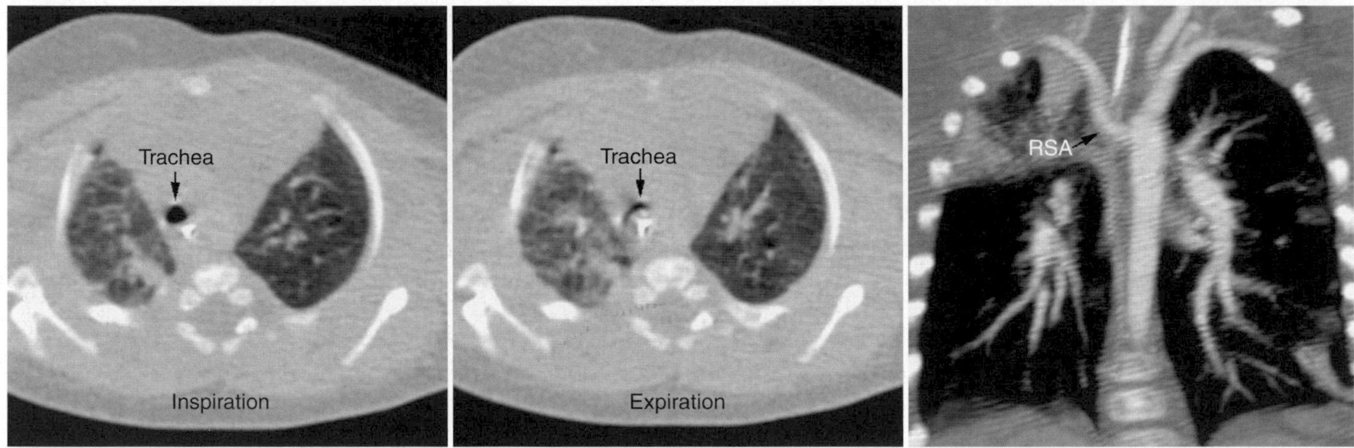

Figure 47-29 The dynamic computed tomographic axial images obtained in inspiration and expiration phases show that the trachea is collapsed during expiration. As shown in the right panel, the patient has an aberrant right subclavian artery (RSA).

chronic compromise of the airways, even after surgical repair of the anomalous arch. In addition, prolonged intubation should be avoided because it may result in erosions into the trachea, aorta, or oesophagus.[10]

When surgical treatment is planned, a judicious decision should be made based on the anatomical information provided by echocardiography, magnetic resonance imaging or computed tomography for the best surgical approach that will allow successful relief of compression of the airway and oesophagus.[6] A left lateral thoracotomy is the most often used surgical approach, but a right thoracotomy or a median sternotomy can be desirable in certain situations. Surgical approaches used for similar conditions vary among surgeons and institutions, often because of the institutional or personal preference and experience.[3–10,16,21–24,27,28,35,36] A muscle sparing thoracotomy is advised as it is associated with less chest discomfort and fast postoperative recovery.[7] Recently, video-assisted thoracoscopic surgery with or without robotic assistance has successfully been performed for division of some vascular rings.[75–77] When there is no associated cardiac defect, the surgery is performed without cardiopulmonary bypass.

A double aortic arch usually requires surgery in early infancy. The smaller of the two arches, or the atretic arch, should be divided. In most cases of double aortic arch, the left arch is the smaller one, or is atretic. The smaller arch is ligated and divided between the subclavian artery and descending aorta through a thoracotomy on that side. The arterial duct is also ligated and divided. Occasionally, aortopexy of either the ascending or descending aorta to the sternum or prevertebral fascia is required for further relief of tracheal or oesophageal compression.

The surgical approach to right aortic arch with aberrant left subclavian artery varies according to the preference of the individual surgeon or the institution. It may be treated by simple division of the ligamentous arterial duct without resection of the diverticulum of Kommerell, but this may be associated with persistent or recurrent symptoms necessitating reoperation. Preferable to this is resection of the diverticulum and reimplantation of the aberrant left subclavian artery to the left common carotid artery, the procedure being performed through a left thoracotomy.[6] Reasons for resection of a diverticulum of Kommerell are to avoid persistent oesophageal compression, and to prevent later development of an aneurysm that may rupture. In symptomatic adults with aberrant left or right subclavian arteries arising directly from the descending aorta without a diverticulum of Kommerell, reimplantation of the aberrant artery to the common carotid artery or ascending aorta on the same side can be performed through a supraclavicular approach.[27] Left aortic arch with aberrant right subclavian artery can be approached through a right thoracotomy. In cases with occlusion or aneurysmal dilation of the aberrant artery, a combined endovascular approach can be considered with endoluminal implantation of a stent.[28]

Circumflex retro-oesophageal aortic arch can be approached through left thoracotomy, but often requires median sternotomy.[34] The retro-oesophageal part of the aortic arch is divided, and the mobilised aortic arch is translocated to the other side of the trachea and anastomosed to the descending aorta.

High cervical arch with tracheal compression requires aortopexy or aortic division, as well as division of the ligamentous arterial duct, resection of a diverticulum of Kommerell, and reimplantation of the aberrant subclavian artery if present.[35–38] The redundant ascending aorta, as well as the aortic arch, should be sutured to the sternum. Relief of obstruction without compression of the airways may require interposition of a prosthetic graft between the ascending and descending aorta.[38]

Operative mortality for relief of vascular rings is now almost zero.[6] Rarely, the surgery is complicated by development of a chylothorax, an aorto-oesophageal fistula, or paralysis of the vocal cords as a result of damage to the recurrent laryngeal nerve. Most patients show immediate symptomatic improvement after surgery. Symptoms related to the airways persist in up to half of patients, and difficulties with feeding in a lesser percentage.[7–9,78] Tracheomalacia is the major determinant for incomplete improvement of the symptoms. Chronic post-operative symptoms are related to age at operation. Symptoms persist most frequently in patients repaired in early infancy, because these patients present early, and therefore tend to have worse pathology. The patients who present later in childhood may also show moderately increased risk of persistent tracheobronchomalacia.

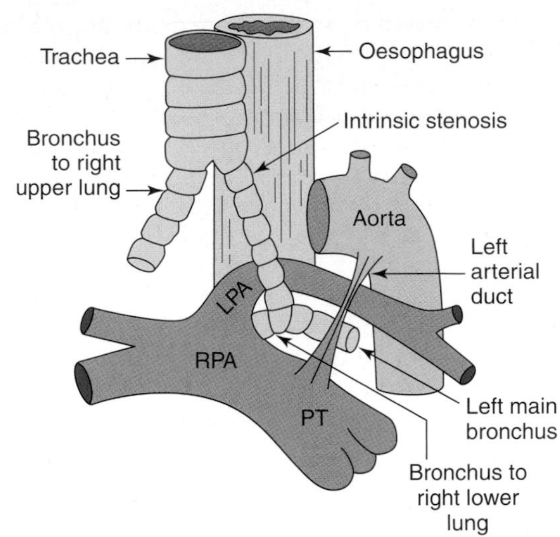

Figure 47-31 The diagram showing a pulmonary arterial sling also illustrates a left-sided arterial ligament connecting the distal left pulmonary artery (LPA) to the descending aorta. PT, pulmonary trunk; RPA, right pulmonary artery.

PULMONARY ARTERIAL SLING

This is a rare congenital anomaly in which the left pulmonary artery does not arise intrapericardially from the pulmonary trunk, but takes its origin extrapericardially from the posterior aspect of the right pulmonary artery, to the right side of the trachea (Figs. 47-30 and 47-31).[79–82] The left pulmonary artery then makes a hairpin turn to the left, and courses toward the hilum of the left lung through the space between the lower trachea and oesophagus. As a consequence, a vascular sling is formed around the right side of the trachea. The arterial duct, or its ligament, connects the pulmonary trunk to the descending aorta on the left side of the trachea. The sling is almost always associated with an abnormality of the airways. The anomalous course of the left pulmonary artery may cause direct mechanical compression of an otherwise normal trachea, resulting in tracheomalacia. An abnormality of the airways, however, occurs far more commonly as an associated lesion. An abnormal branching pattern of the tracheobronchial tree is seen in up to four-fifths of patients with a pulmonary arterial sling.[79–81] Typically the trachea bifurcates into the bronchuses to the right and left lungs at a lower level than normal, with a wide angle between the right and left bronchuses,

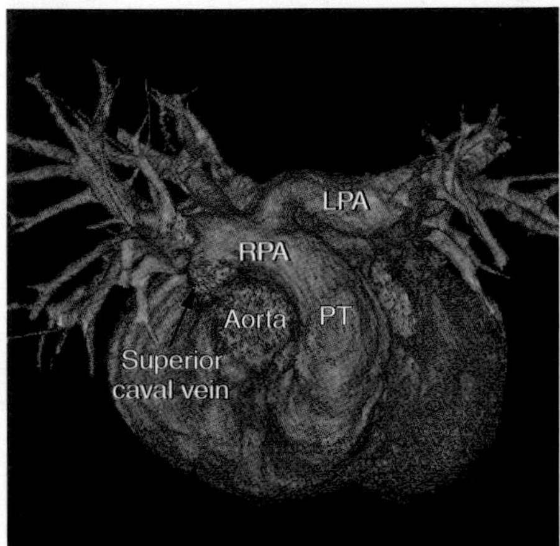

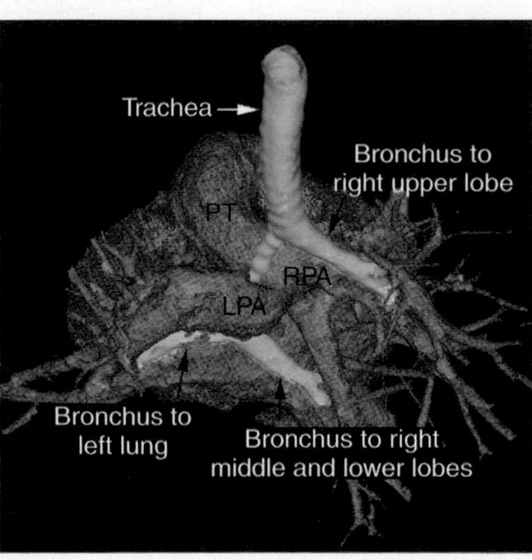

Figure 47-30 The volume rendered computed tomographic angiograms seen from the front and above (*left panel*) and from behind and above (*right panel*) show a pulmonary arterial sling with abnormal tracheobronchial branching and stenosis. The left pulmonary artery (LPA) arises from the proximal right pulmonary artery (RPA), makes a hairpin turn around the airway in the mediastinum and courses to the hilum of the left lung. The airway has two bifurcations in the mediastinum, with a narrow intermediary segment, characteristic of congenital stenosis due to complete cartilaginous rings. PT, pulmonary trunk.

producing an inverted T appearance. In approximately one-third of the cases with a low inverted T bifurcation of the airways, the right upper lobar bronchus arises from the trachea slightly above the level of normal tracheal bifurcation. The left pulmonary artery then forms a sling on the right side of the airway immediately above the lower bifurcation. The low inverted T pattern of bifurcation has previously been described as a bridging bronchus.[80] In this rather confusing concept, it has been considered that this part of the airway between the supposedly normal level of bifurcation and the lower bifurcation into the right and left bronchi is erroneously assumed to be the left main bronchus, and that the bronchus to the entire right lung, or to the right middle and lower lobes, arises abnormally from the left main bronchus. This bronchus, therefore, was thought to create a bridge between the right and left lungs. Almost all cases with the low inverted T bifurcation of the airways, with or without a separate origin of the right upper lobe bronchus, are associated with narrowing of a long segment of the lower airways above the bifurcation. The narrowing is due to complete cartilaginous rings, with absence of the membranous part of the trachea posteriorly. The narrowing may also extend into the main bronchuses. In addition, the right and, less frequently, the left bronchus may show bronchomalacia.[10] One-third of patients with tracheal stenosis due to complete cartilaginous rings have an associated pulmonary arterial sling. The presence of complete rings, however, does not necessarily imply important stenosis, although the trachea is narrower than normal. Imperforate anus is seen in one-sixth of cases with a low inverted T bifurcation, but not in cases with a tracheal bifurcation at normal level.[80]

The left pulmonary artery is often relatively hypoplastic, being considerably smaller than the right pulmonary artery. Stenosis of the right pulmonary artery, with hypoplasia of the right lung, has also been reported.[83] Rarely, the sling is associated with agenesis of the right lung.[84] Also rarely the pulmonary artery to the left upper lobe may arise anomalously from the proximal right pulmonary artery, with normal pulmonary arterial supply to the left lower lobe. In addition, the right upper lobe may have an aberrant supply from the anomalous left pulmonary artery.

The sling is reported to be associated with congenital cardiac disease in from one-third to four-fifths of cases.[81,83,85,86] The most common reported defects are atrial septal defect, patency of the arterial duct, ventricular septal defect, tetralogy of Fallot, coarctation of the aorta, and persistence of the left superior caval vein. The anomaly has also been reported in association with imperforate anus, congenital megacolon, biliary atresia, and genitourinary anomalies. Rarely, an aberrant left pulmonary artery arising distally from the right pulmonary artery does not form a vascular sling but is associated with tracheal stenosis.[87,88] A sling involving the right pulmonary artery has been reported in a case with tetralogy of Fallot and pulmonary atresia when the aortic arch is right-sided.[89] A vascular course similar to the sling has been described involving the arterial duct.[90] In this instance, the duct arose from the right pulmonary artery, and coursed leftward through the space between the distal trachea and oesophagus to connect to the descending aorta on the left side. It is also suggested that an aberrant left subclavian artery can arise from the descending aorta and course through the space between the trachea and oesophagus,[1] but in this instance it is more likely that the artery is a collateral vessel rather than the left subclavian artery itself.[2]

Clinical Manifestations

Pulmonary arterial sling usually presents in the first year of life, although asymptomatic older children and adults have been reported.[81] There is a slight male preponderance.[81] The dominant clinical manifestations are due to obstruction of the airways, and include stridor, wheeze, and cough. Stridor is often expiratory, but can be inspiratory or biphasic. Less commonly, patients present with symptoms from oesophageal compression, such as dysphagia and vomiting. Rarely, the sling is found as an incidental lesion during cardiac or pulmonary investigations for other reasons.

Diagnostic Investigation

The chest radiograph sometimes provides clues to the diagnosis (Fig. 47-32). When present, abnormal branching of the airway can be appreciated in a well-taken frontal image.

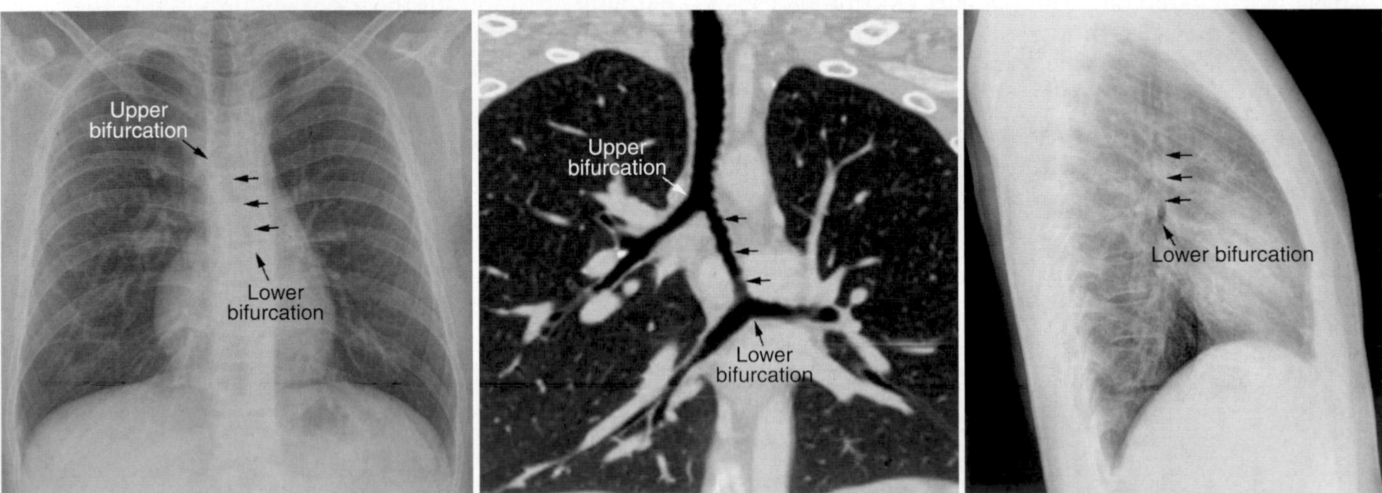

Figure 47-32 The chest radiographs are shown together with computed tomographic correlation of a pulmonary arterial sling. The diagnosis can be entertained when careful observation shows the abnormality seen in the chest radiograph. The *arrows* indicate the narrowed vertical segment of trachea between its upper and lower bifurcations.

The inverted T appearance of the tracheal bifurcation at a level lower than normal is an important sign. Narrowing of long or short tracheal and bronchial segments can also be recognised. The lungs may show various combinations of hyperinflation and/or atelectasis, according to the associated tracheobronchial narrowing and retention of secretions. The pulmonary vascularity may be asymmetric, with the left lung, or less commonly, the right lung, showing less prominent vascularity than its partner. Barium oesophagography is diagnostic.[81] On the lateral view, the left pulmonary artery is seen as a round structure between the air-filled distal trachea and barium-filled oesophagus, causing an anterior indentation in the oesophagus. Barium oesophagography, nonetheless, should be avoided in critically ill neonates, especially if they are ventilator dependent.[82]

Echocardiography reveals continuation of the pulmonary trunk to the right, without origin of the normal left pulmonary artery, a feature which may suggest unilateral absence of the left pulmonary artery, or aberrant origin of the left pulmonary artery from the ascending aorta. The origin of the left pulmonary artery from the right pulmonary artery is appreciated when the pulmonary trunk is followed to the right (Fig. 47-33). Echocardiography is always essential when assessing patients with a sling, since associated congenital cardiac disease is common.

Both computed tomography and magnetic resonance imaging are diagnostic (Fig. 47-34; see also Fig. 47-30).[83,91,92] Contrast-enhanced computed tomography is preferred, not only because of its ability to visualise the pulmonary vessels and airway with great precision, but also because the short time required for scanning obviates the need for general anaesthesia or deep sedation in critically ill patients. Three-dimensional reconstruction of the airways and the contrast-enhanced vascular structures provides complete

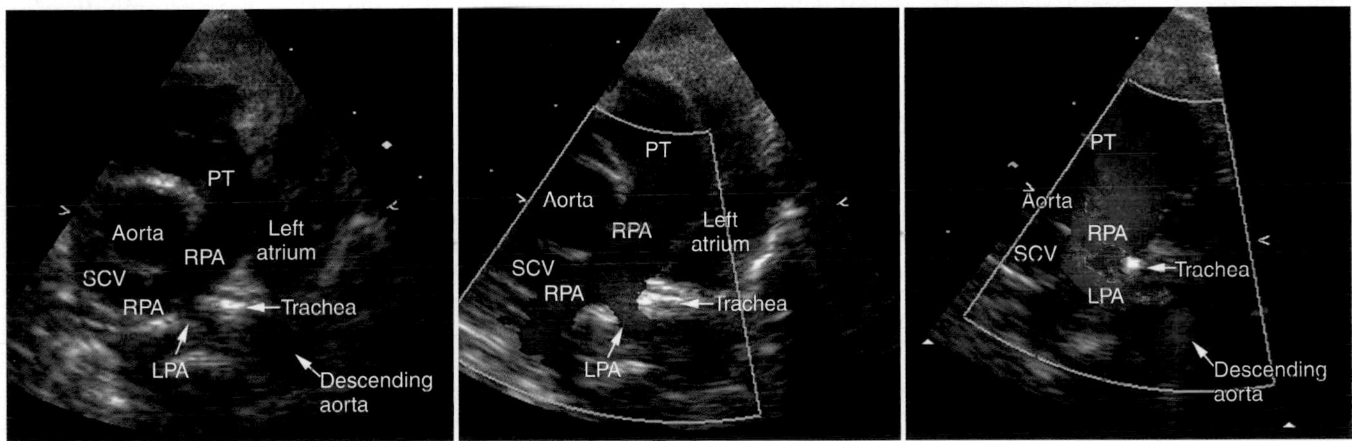

Figure 47-33 The echocardiographic images show a left pulmonary arterial sling. High left parasternal short-axis views of the pulmonary arteries reveal that the pulmonary trunk (PT) continues as the right pulmonary artery (RPA), without giving rise to a normal left pulmonary artery (LPA). The left pulmonary artery arises from the right pulmonary artery behind the ascending aorta. The left pulmonary artery then makes a hairpin turn to course to the left side, encircling the trachea from the right side. This anatomy can be appreciated when the pulmonary trunk is followed as it moves to the right. Note that the proximal part of the LPA is not clearly shown in the cross sectional images because of sonic shadowing from the air-filled trachea. SCV, superior caval vein.

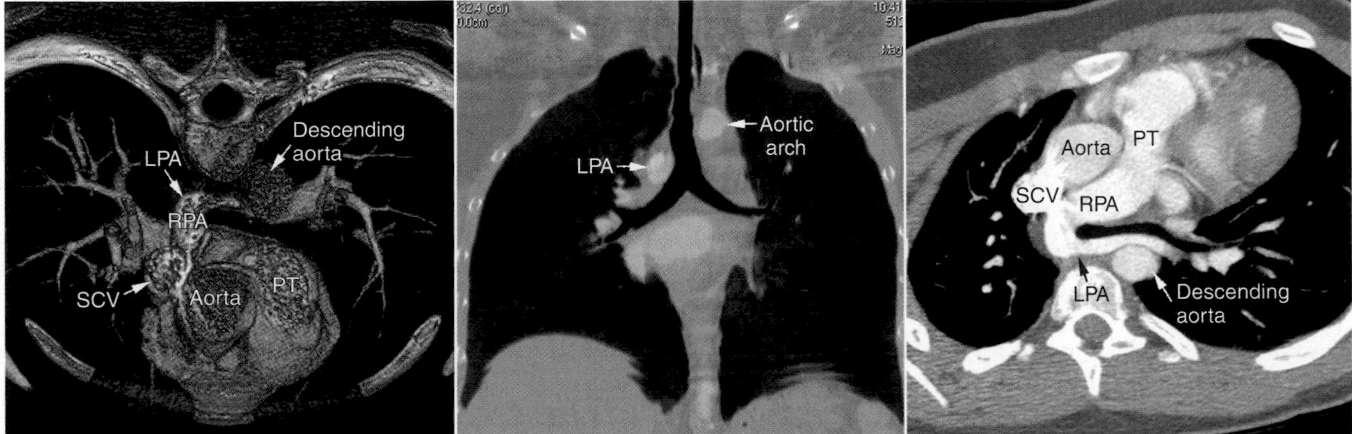

Figure 47-34 These computed tomographic angiograms reformatted in transverse axial and coronal planes show origin of the left pulmonary artery (LPA) from the proximal right pulmonary artery (RPA). The left artery encircles the right side of the distal trachea and courses between the trachea and oesophagus to reach the left hilum. The left pulmonary artery shows mild narrowing in front of the descending aorta. Tracheal branching is at the usual level, but is unusually symmetric. There is no tracheal or bronchial narrowing. PT, pulmonary trunk; SCV, superior caval vein.

information for the subsequent surgical procedure. When the narrowing of the airways is considered dynamic, a few selected slices can be scanned repeatedly for cine-display during respiration.[68,69] Complications such as hyperinflation, collapse, or consolidation of the pulmonary parenchyma due to pneumonia should also be evaluated. Although magnetic resonance imaging can provide comparable information, the time required for scanning is long, and the anatomical detail, especially of the airways and lungs, is not as good as that of computed tomography. Bronchoscopy is recommended when dynamic narrowing due to tracheomalacia or bronchomalacia is suspected. Routine intraoperative bronchoscopy can be useful as the right and left bronchuses distal to the complete cartilaginous rings may also show malacic changes.[10]

Management

Early recognition is important. General supportive respiratory care should be given before proceeding to surgery. Respiratory infection may be difficult to clear completely before surgery because of persistent retention of secretions. Symptomatic patients should undergo surgical intervention without delay.[82,85,86,93–95] The optimal surgical approach is median sternotomy with cardiopulmonary bypass, dividing and mobilising the left pulmonary artery at its origin from the right pulmonary artery, with reimplantation to the pulmonary trunk after complete resection of all ductal tissue. At the same time, associated problems of the airways should be inspected and treated surgically when necessary. Mild tracheal stenosis may not require tracheoplasty. Bronchoscopy after cardiopulmonary bypass can be beneficial because the extent of tracheal stenosis is not always apparent when viewing the trachea externally. Various techniques have been utilised for repairing tracheal stenosis, the length of the stenotic segment dictating the type of reconstruction. Stenosis of a short segment may require simple resection and end-to-end anastomosis. This procedure may obviate the need for division and reanastomosis of the left pulmonary artery, because the undivided left pulmonary artery can be translocated at the time of tracheal resection.[96] This procedure, however, may result in compression of the trachea or left main bronchus. A longer segment of narrowing requires tracheoplasty using a piece of rib cartilage, or more preferably a pericardial patch. In the majority of cases, an excessively long trachea allows resection of a part of the narrowed segment. The resected tracheal piece can also be used to augment the size of the tracheal lumen. This tracheal autograft technique is considered advantageous over other autologous patch materials. Sliding tracheoplasty is also used, transecting the stenotic segment at its midpoint, incising the proximal and distal stenotic segments in vertical direction, anteriorly in one segment and posteriorly in the other. The two spliced extremities are then slid over each other and anastomosed. The optimal surgical technique should be chosen not only according to the extent and nature of the tracheal stenosis, but also according to the institutional expertise. Tracheal repair is not always necessary.[82]

Mortality is variable, with relatively high rates in earlier studies. The postoperative mortality is mainly related to the associated tracheal and bronchial abnormalities, while vascular reconstruction is relatively free of symptomatic complication. Early recognition and surgical intervention may minimise morbidity and mortality. Survivors usually show prompt symptomatic improvement, and are free of significant symptoms at long-term follow-up. Some degree of airway obstruction with granulation tissue often persists, and narrowing of the reimplanted left pulmonary artery is not uncommon.

VASCULAR COMPRESSION OF THE AIRWAY WITHOUT VASCULAR RING OR SLING

As discussed earlier in this chapter, the shape of the thoracic cage is an important factor that contributes to compression of the airway and oesophagus in patients with an anomalous aortic arch or pulmonary arterial sling. In addition, abnormal position or dilation of the otherwise normally formed vessels may cause compression of the airway or oesophagus.

The brachiocephalic arterial compression syndrome refers to a condition in which the brachiocephalic artery arises too far to the left side of the aortic arch, compressing the anterior wall of the trachea as it courses from left to right (Fig. 47-35).[4,97] Such tracheal compression by the brachiocephalic artery is reputed to cause respiratory symptoms, including stridor and bouts of apnoea that may progress to cyanosis, bradycardia, and even death. There has been controversy, nonetheless, regarding its clinical significance. The brachiocephalic artery arises at least partly to the left of the trachea in most normal individuals, and mild indentation of the trachea by the artery is not uncommon.[98] In addition, the majority of individuals with anterior tracheal compression fail to exhibit respiratory symptoms. In congenitally corrected transposition with a left aortic arch, the brachiocephalic artery crosses the midline in front of the trachea because the ascending aorta is typically on the left side. The syndrome is more likely to arise in patients with a crowded superior mediastinum, such as in those patients with cardiomegaly and dilated vessels in the mediastinum or narrow depth of the thoracic cage.[97] Symptomatic compression of the trachea is rare in patients over 2 years of age. In patients with severe symptoms, the artery has been suspended by sutures to the sternal periosteum with or without reimplantation to the more proximal ascending aorta.

An elongated aortic arch may also compress the anterior wall of the trachea significantly, compromising the luminal patency.[99] A classic example is the right aortic arch in congenitally corrected transposition (Fig. 47-36). In this setting, the aorta ascends on the left and takes a long transverse course in front of the trachea to connect to the descending aorta in the right posterior mediastinum. Once the lungs are hyperinflated, they extend to the midline behind the sternum, pushing the mediastinal structures and heart backward, further compromising the tracheal and bronchial patency.

A posteriorly displaced ascending aorta may cause significant compression of the airways (Fig. 47-37).[71,100] The ascending aorta may directly compress the right side of the trachea. In addition, the left main bronchus,

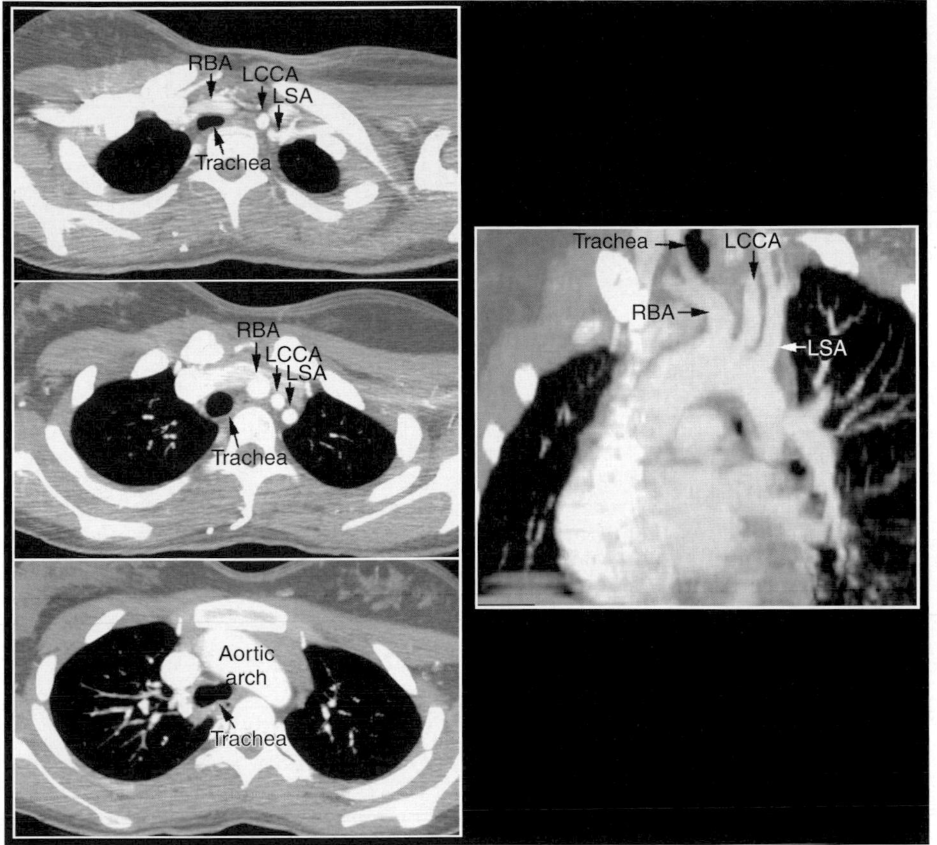

Figure 47-35 The computed tomograms reformatted in transverse axial and coronal planes show the brachiocephalic artery arising from the aorta on the left side of midline and coursing rightward in front of the trachea. The trachea is mildly compressed. Note that the anteroposterior dimension of the thorax is narrow in this case. LCCA, left common carotid artery; LSA, left subclavian artery; RBA, right brachiocephalic artery.

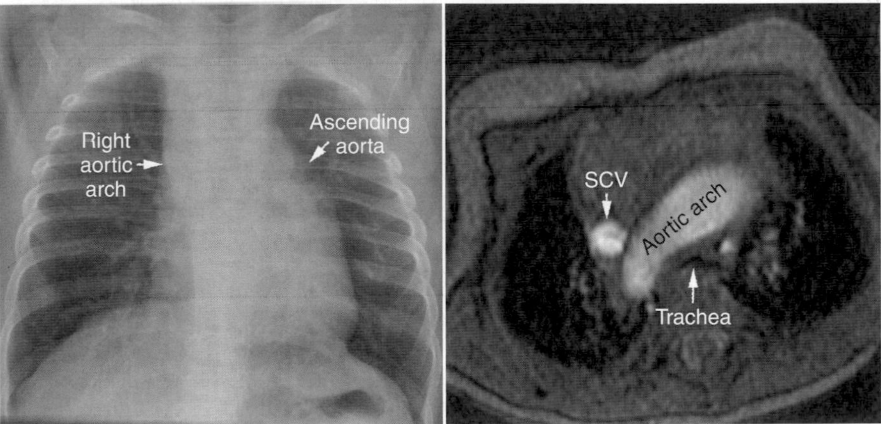

Figure 47-36 In this patient with congenitally corrected transposition and a right aortic arch, an elongated aortic arch compresses the distal trachea. The frontal chest radiograph (*left panel*) shows a right aortic arch. The ascending aorta occupies a far leftward position in the upper mediastinum. Magnetic resonance image in axial transverse plane (*right panel*) shows posterior displacement and narrowing of the distal trachea. Note that the right aortic arch is unusually elongated as it connects the far leftward ascending aorta to the descending aorta on the right side. SCV, superior caval vein.

and less commonly, the right main bronchus, are compressed by the right pulmonary artery which is also displaced backward by the posteriorly displaced ascending aorta.

Absent pulmonary valve syndrome, also associated with bronchial compression, is characterised by severe dilation of the pulmonary arteries in the mediastinum and the hila of the lungs (Fig. 47-38).[101,102] It is most typically associated with tetralogy of Fallot, and in most cases the arterial duct is absent. Most patients present early in life with severe respiratory distress due to the bronchial compression and tracheobronchomalacia. The lungs are typically hyperinflated, with or without scattered areas of segmental or lobar collapse.

As in vascular rings and slings, all these related conditions need a tailored surgical approach and procedure. Contrast-enhanced computed tomography is best suited for investigation of critically ill patients, while magnetic resonance imaging can be used in older and less symptomatic patients.

Figure 47-37 In this patient, posterior displacement of the ascending aorta and the right and left pulmonary arteries compresses the left main bronchus. Transverse axial images of computed tomographic angiography (*left column*) show that the superior mediastinum is crowded with normal vascular structures. The ascending aorta has an unusual posterior location, and the right and left pulmonary arteries are consequently in direct contact with the left main bronchus, compressing it against the spine (*middle and lower panels*). The left main bronchus is squashed in an antero-posterior direction and therefore its vertical dimension is increased (*right column, upper panel*). The diminished antero-posterior diameter of the left main bronchus is well shown in the curved reformatted image seen from below (*right column, lower panel*). LPA, left pulmonary artery; PT, pulmonary trunk; RPA, right pulmonary artery.

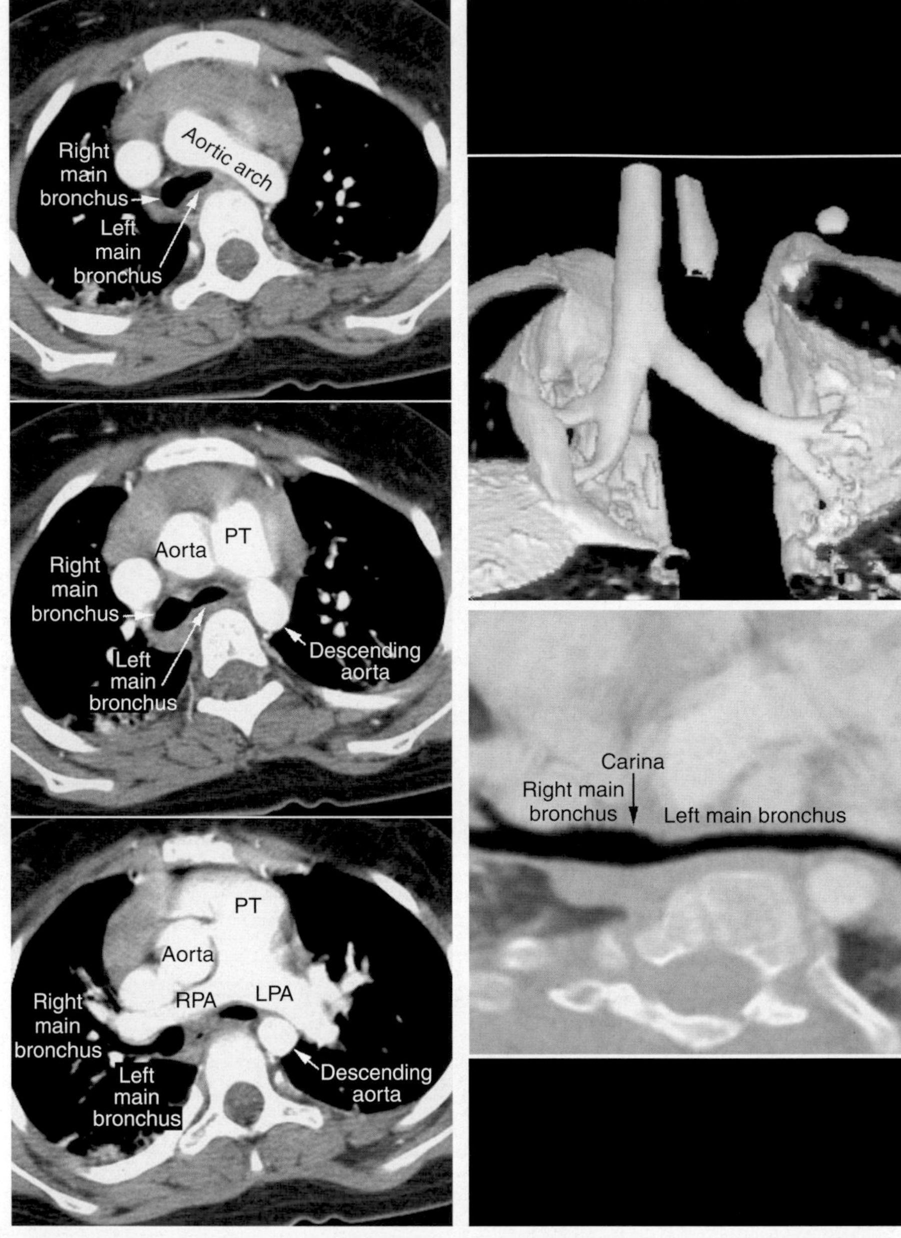

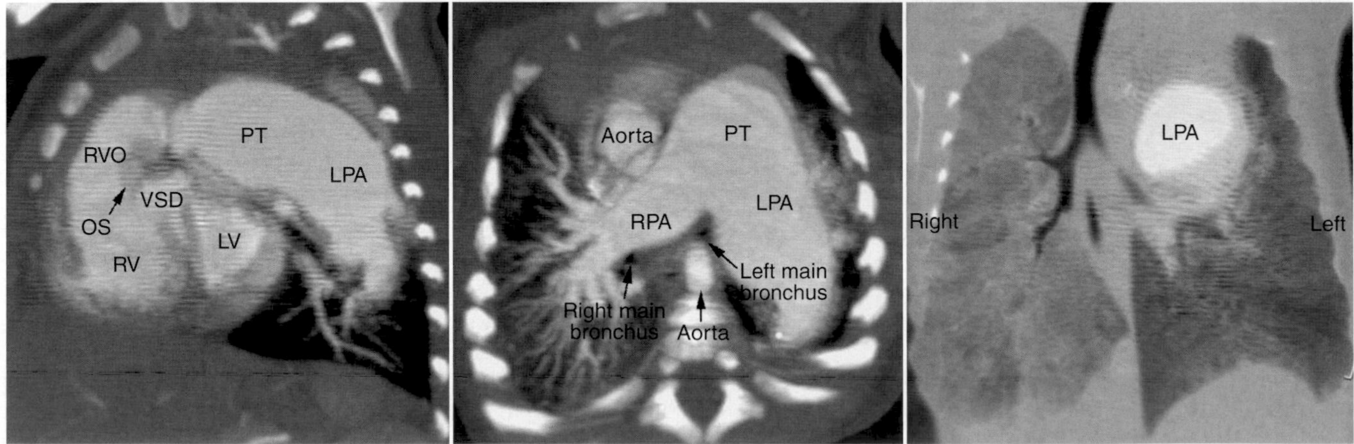

Figure 47-38 These computed tomograms show mild narrowing of the right ventricular outflow (RVO) tract by the anteriorly deviated outlet septum, a ventricular septal defect (VSD; *left panel*), and markedly dilated central pulmonary arteries, consistent with tetralogy of Fallot and absent pulmonary valve syndrome. The left and right bronchi are compressed by the right and left pulmonary arteries (*middle panel*). Reformatted images of the airway in the coronal plane (*right panel*) show severe narrowing of the left main bronchus, with trapping of air in the left lung. LPA, left pulmonary artery; LV, left ventricle; OS, outlet septum; PT, pulmonary trunk; RPA, right pulmonary artery; RV, right ventricle.

ACKNOWLEDGEMENTS

We are very grateful to Dr Eoghan Laffan for valuable comments and corrections on the final manuscript. We thank Ms Jennifer Russell for help with coordination of the references, and Mrs Eul Kyung Kim for making the cartoons which illustrate the hypothetical double arch and its consequence for the fetal and postnatal circulations.

The complete reference list can be found on the companion Expert Consult web site at www.expertconsult.com.

ANNOTATED REFERENCES

- Edwards JE: Anomalies of the derivatives of the aortic arch system. Med Clin N Am 1948;32:925–948.

  In this seminal paper, the pioneer cardiac pathologist, Jesse E. Edwards, introduced a hypothetical model of the double aortic arch that explains the morphogenesis of most anomalies.
- Alsenaidi K, Gurofsky R, Karamlou T, et al: Management and outcomes of double aortic arch in 81 patients. Pediatrics 2006;118:e1336–e1341.

  This original paper reviews the clinical manifestations, associated cardiac and noncardiac anomalies, operative techniques and outcomes in a large cohort of patients with double aortic arch.
- Dodge -Khatami A, Tulevski II, Hitchcock JF, et al: Vascular rings and pulmonary arterial sling: From respiratory collapse to surgical cure, with emphasis on judicious imaging in the hi-tech era. Cardiol Young 2002;12:96–104.

  This review paper presents an excellent overview of the morphology, clinical manifestations, diagnosis and surgical approaches to various vascular rings and the pulmonary arterial sling.
- Yoo SJ, Min JY, Lee YH, et al: Fetal sonographic diagnosis of aortic arch anomalies. Ultraound Obstet Gynecol 2003;22:535–546.
- Patel CR, Lane JR, Spector ML, Smith PC: Fetal echocardiographic diagnosis of vascular rings. J Ultrasound Med 2006;25:251–257.

  These two papers illustrate the fetal echocardiographic findings of various anomalies involving the aortic arches. In the first paper, fetal and postnatal sonographic findings are correlated with morphogenetic mechanisms.
- Momma K, Matsuoka R, Takao A: Aortic arch anomalies associated with chromosome 22q11 deletion (CATCH 22). Pediatr Cardiol 1999;20: 97–102.
- McElhinney DB, Clark BJ 3rd, Weinberg PM, et al: Association of chromosome 22q11 deletion with isolated anomalies of aortic arch laterality and branching. J Am Coll Cardiol 2001;37:2114–2119.

  These two papers show the high incidence of chromosome 22q11 deletion in patients with anomalies of the aortic arch, emphasising the need for screening in patients with or without associated cardiac defects.
- Murdison KA, Andrews BA, Chin AJ: Ultrasonographic display of complex vascular rings. J Am Coll Cardiol 1990;5:1645–1653.

  This original paper illustrates how a suprasternal sweep can assist in echocardiographic evaluation.
- Oddone M, Granata C, Vercellino N, et al: Multi-modality evaluation of the abnormalites of the aortic arches in children: Techniques and imaging spectrum with emphasis on MRI. Pediatr Radiol 2005;35:947–960.
- Hernanz-Shulman M: Vascular rings: A practical approach to imaging diagnosis. Pediatr Radiol 2005;35:961–979.

  These two review papers describe contemporary imaging approaches to anomalies of the aortic arch, with special emphasis on the utility of computed tomography and magnetic resonance imaging.
- Fiore AC, Brown JW, Weber TR, Turrentine MW: Surgical treatment of pulmonary artery sling and tracheal stenosis. Ann Thorac Surg 2005;79:38–46.

  This original paper reviews surgical treatment strategies for pulmonary arterial sling and tracheal stenosis, illustrating the surgical techniques that include patch augmentation of the trachea and slide tracheoplasty. It also emphasises that tracheal repair is not always necessary.
- Backer CL, Mavroudis C, Rigsby CK, Holinger LD: Trends in vascular ring surgery. J Thorac Cardiovasc Surg 2005;129:1339–1347.

  This original paper reviews how diagnostic imaging, operative techniques, and clinical outcomes of vascular rings have evolved in the last 60 years in a large referral center.
- Kim YM, Yoo SJ, Kim TH, et al: Tracheal compression by elongated aortic arch in patients with congenitally corrected transposition of the great arteries. Pediatr Cardiol 2001;22:471–477.
- Kim YM, Yoo SJ, Kim WH, et al: Bronchial compression by posteriorly displaced ascending aorta in patients with congenital heart disease. Ann Thorac Surg 2002;73:881–886.

  These papers assess the mechanism of compression of the airways by an aorta that does not form a vascular ring or sling. The authors emphasise that the trachea can be significantly compressed by the elongated and enlarged aortic arch, when the ascending aorta connects to the descending aorta on the opposite side, and that the main bronchus can be squeezed between the ascending and descending aorta when the ascending aorta has an unusually posterior position.

CHAPTER 48

Abnormal Positions and Relationships of the Heart

ROBERT H. ANDERSON and SHI-JOON YOO

An abnormally positioned heart is not in itself a malformation of major significance. The exceptions are the extreme examples of exteriorisation of the heart, usually described as ectopia cordis, or union of parts of the heart in the setting of conjoined twins. A heart unusually positioned within the chest, an abnormal orientation of the cardiac apex, or the finding of unexpected relationships of structures within the heart, nonetheless, can all lead to considerable diagnostic problems. In the past, such situations created significant confusion. Our philosophy and approach to these situations has been outlined in Chapter 1. Those who have not studied this chapter in detail should, perhaps, return for refreshment concerning our ground rules. In this chapter, we seek to synthesise the value of our concepts in the setting of abnormally positioned hearts, and unexpected intracardiac relationships. We start by discussing the major problems produced by an extrathoracic position of the heart, or ectopia cordis, in its various degrees, following this with a brief account of congenital absence of the pericardium. We then summarise the cardiac problems encountered in the setting of conjoined twins. The location of the heart in an unexpected part of the thoracic cavity, or the orientation of its apex in a disharmonious fashion, the next topics for consideration, are best dealt with simply by description. Having suggested such simple descriptions, we then discuss the problems produced by, and the anomalies associated with, juxtaposition of the atrial appendages, before concluding with a consideration of the arrangements variously described as criss-cross hearts, supero-inferior ventricles, or the topsy-turvy arrangement.

EXTERIORISATION OF THE HEART (ECTOPIA CORDIS)

It is maintained that the famous case of tetralogy of Fallot first reported by Nicolas Steno[1] was the first report of an extrathoracic heart.[2] Rashkind[3] has argued that such malformations were almost certainly recognised long before 1671. In his opinion,[3] they were recorded in the writings of the ancient Babylonians, although there is some dispute concerning the precise translation of the text on the tablet involved. Be that as it may, hearts positioned in part, or completely, out of the thorax fortunately remain very rare. Until recently, with relatively few exceptions, such occurrences proved uniformly fatal. The lesion is usually termed ectopia, but there are deficiencies in such usage.[4] The Greek word *ektopos* simply means away from a place. As such, a heart found in the right chest of an otherwise normal person is ectopic. Despite this semantic failing, which represents yet another example of deficient use of a classical term, and supports the use of the vernacular, ectopia is used universally to account for a heart located in part, or completely, outside the thoracic cavity.

Known cases of an extrathoracic heart have been reviewed extensively and well.[4–6] In terms of categorisation, it was as long ago as 1845 that extrathoracic hearts were grouped according to their location, with description of cervical, thoracic and abdominal subsets.[7] Subsequently, it was suggested that the combined thoracoabdominal position made up a further distinct pattern, with a combined thoracocervical group then added to this list.[4] Cases encountered more recently continue to fall within these groupings.

When the heart is found in the neck, the sternum is usually intact. According to some,[4] this arrangement reflects a retention of the normal initial site of cardiac development. This subset was dismissed by other experts,[2] who argued that it is found only in malformed fetuses. Examples have been recorded, nonetheless, when an infant survived for a few hours with a cervical heart, while one patient with this anomaly was reputed to have survived to adult life.[8] This latter example, however, would probably be better placed in the thoracocervical group. Those dismissing the existence of the cervical subset have suggested the need to distinguish between a cleft to the sternum and an extrathoracic heart.[2] This seems to be unnecessarily divisive, since a heart within the neck is certainly not within the thorax, irrespective of whether or not the sternum is cleft. Irrespective of such niceties, hearts of the cervical type are by far the rarest. There is also a question mark over the group with the heart allegedly contained within the abdomen. Although 38 such hearts were catalogued in one series,[5] re-examination of the original reports suggested that, in all but one, part of the heart was retained within the chest, thus making it better to group them within the combined abdominothoracic subset.[2] The majority of cases, therefore, either protrude from the chest, or else extend through a diaphragmatic defect. All occupy a midline deficiency of the body wall, lying partly in the chest and partly within the abdomen. In the cases exteriorised from the chest, the hearts are usually covered by neither skin nor pericardium (Fig. 48-1). In the past, various means had been employed to provide the lack of moisture ensuing from the absence of a pericardial cavity. Thus, quaint accounts survive from the 18th century, describing exteriorised hearts being covered with a contraption made of pliable osiers and linen, and anointed with wine and melted butter.[9] Hearts were also covered with a pasteboard cone, with oil used for the anointing agent, or else saline sponges.[6] Irrespective of the method employed, most patients survived for only a matter of hours or days.

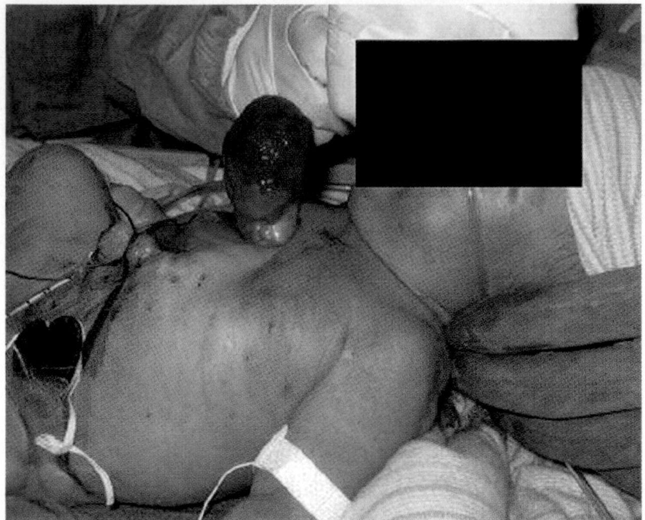

Figure 48-1 A neonate with the heart exteriorised through the thoracic wall. (Courtesy of Dr Marshall Jacobs, Temple University, Philadelphia, Pennsylvania.)

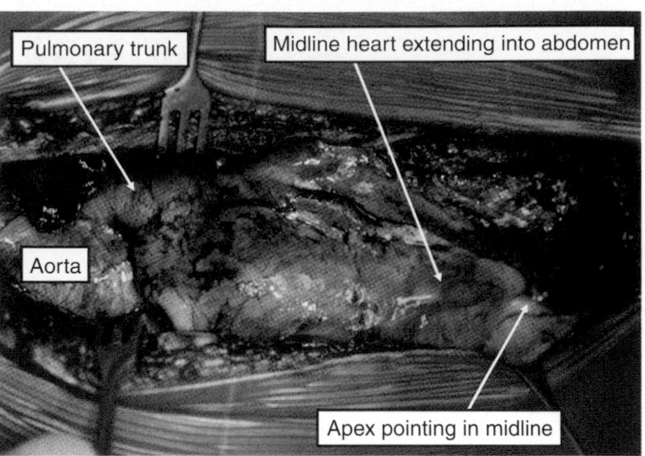

Figure 48-3 Opening the skin in the patient shown in Figure 48-2 revealed a midline heart with it apex also in the midline. There was isomerism of the right atrial appendages and the intracardiac anatomy of tetralogy of Fallot. (Courtesy of Dr Benson R. Wilcox, University of North Carolina, Chapel Hill.)

The difference between exclusively thoracic exteriorisation, and those cases grouped together because the heart is located partly in the thorax and partly in the abdomen (Fig. 48-2), is that in the latter instances the heart is better covered by the body wall, having at least a covering of skin or membrane (Fig. 48-3). It is this group of patients that fall within the syndrome unified by five anomalies, known as the pentalogy of Cantrell. These are a midline deficiency of the abdominal wall, a defect of the lower part of the sternum, a deficiency of the pericardial sac, a deficiency of the diaphragm, and an intracardiac congenital lesion.[10] Not all patients with extrathoracic hearts extending into the abdomen have all of these features. Indeed, the cases can themselves be grouped according to the number of the five features that are present.[11] Lesser forms of the pentalogy include the midline deficiencies shown in Figures 48-2 and 48-3, and protrusions of ventricular diverticula through midline deficiencies of the body wall (Fig. 48-4). Complete exteriorisation of the heart represents the extreme form of the syndrome. Treatment of the patients with the abdominothoracic type of exteriorisation has previously been more successful than for those having exclusively thoracic exteriorisation, although recent experience has shown that the exteriorised thoracic heart can successfully be placed back within the thorax (Fig. 48-5).

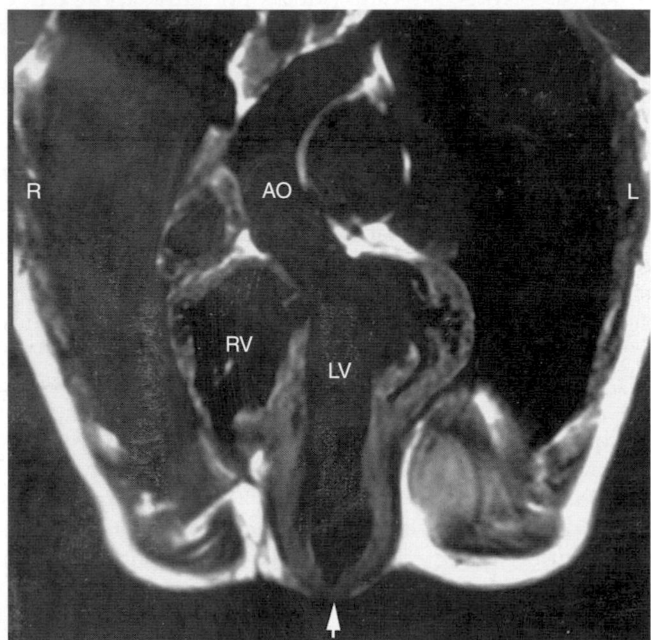

Figure 48-4 This magnetic resonance image shows a left ventricular (LV) diverticulum protruding through a midline deficiency of the body wall (*arrow*). AO, aorta; L, left; R, right; RV, right ventricle. (Courtesy of Dr Walter Duncan, University of British Columbia, Vancouver, British Columbia, Canada.)

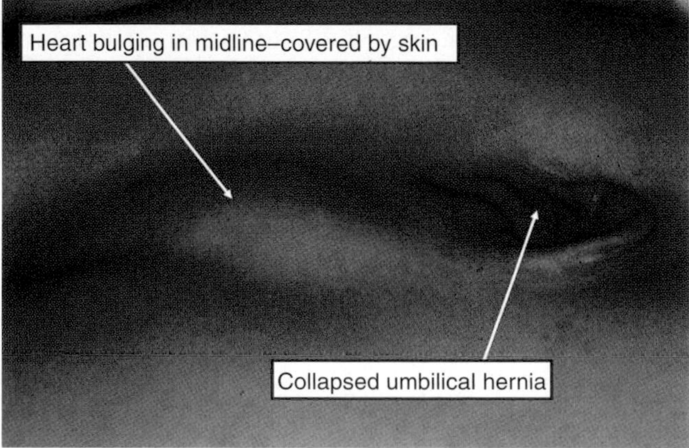

Figure 48-2 This patient has the midline deficiencies of the pentalogy of Cantrell. The heart, occupying both the thorax and the abdomen, is covered by skin and a pericardial cavity. (Courtesy of Dr Benson R. Wilcox, University of North Carolina, Chapel Hill.)

Until recently, very few patients survived reparative surgery, although several persons with abdominal hearts who did not undergo surgery survived into adult life. An example is an old soldier who reputedly fought through several campaigns, and died of suppurative nephritis of the right kidney.[12] The surgical problems encountered in restoring the heart to the body are considerable, including the small size of the deficient thoracic cavity, the excessive length of the venous and arterial connections to the extrathoracic heart, and the

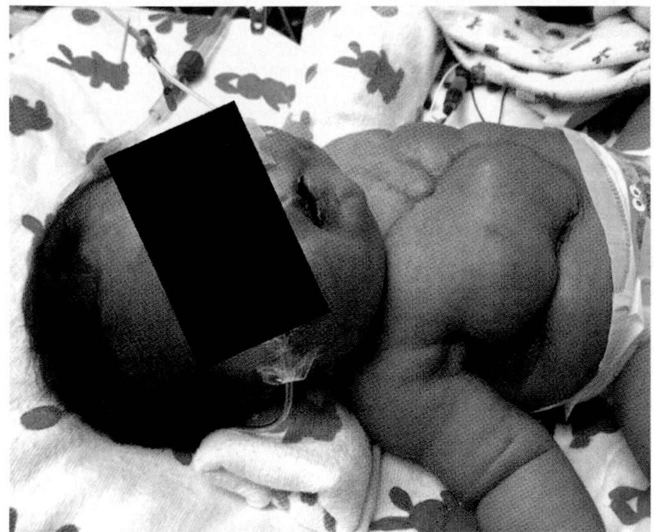

Figure 48-5 The heart in the patient shown in Figure 48-1 was successfully replaced within the thorax. (Courtesy of Dr Marshall Jacobs, Temple University, Philadelphia, Pennsylvania.)

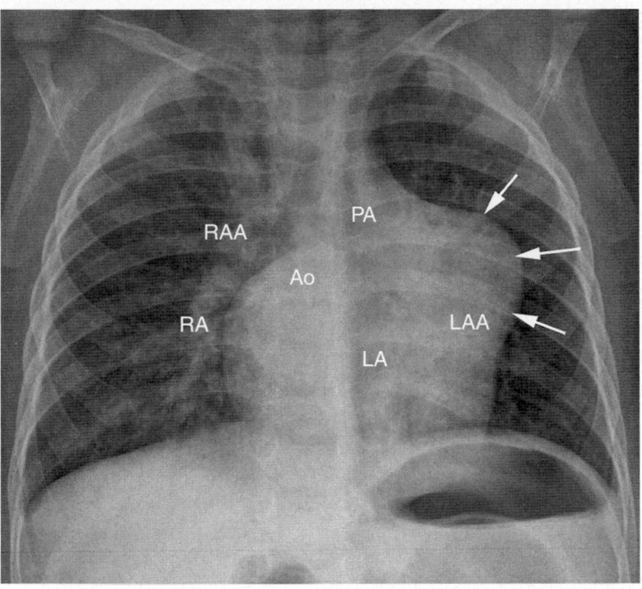

Figure 48-6 The chest radiograph shows an extensive bulge in the left border of the cardiac silhouette (*arrows*). This is very suggestive of herniation of the left atrial appendage through a pericardial deficiency.

frequent co-existence of a large omphalocoele. Recent experience, nonetheless, such as that shown in Figures 48-1 and 48-3, and that of Morales and associates,[13] who reported four successful repairs encountered over a period of 6 years, suggests that the prognosis for those born with exteriorised hearts is now markedly improved, albeit conditioned by the severity of associated intracardiac defects.

CONGENITAL DEFICIENCY OF THE PERICARDIUM

An integral part of the various forms of extrathoracic heart is a gross deficiency of the fibrous pericardial sac. A deficiency of this firm bag can also be found when the heart is in its anticipated intrathoracic position. According to Van Praagh and his colleagues,[2] the anomaly was first observed by Columbus in 1559. Since then, about 150 cases have been described. Hence, the lesion is exceedingly rare. Only three examples were discovered amongst the 1716 hearts in the archive of Boston Children's Hospital.[2] We have knowingly observed only a single case at postmortem, this being a chance finding in a 68-year-old patient.[14] Cases can, therefore, be entirely asymptomatic. Alternatively, such patients may have chest pain that can resemble angina. When associated with other anomalies, such as diaphragmatic hernia or lesions of the heart, it is the associated malformations that dominate the clinical picture. The biggest intrinsic problems occur with relatively localised left-sided deficiencies of the pericardium. Either the ventricles, or the left atrial appendage, can become herniated through a small opening, with strangulation and, in extreme cases, death. Limited deficiency of the fibrous sac on the right side can result in herniation of the lung into the pericardial cavity, with subsequent obstruction of the superior caval vein. The diagnosis is often made, or at least suggested, from the chest radiograph (Fig. 48-6). A large left-sided deficiency permits the entire heart to shift leftwards, with production of three rather than two knuckles on the left heart border as seen on the chest radiograph. When the defect is small, and there is herniation of the left appendage, the heart is normally positioned, but the malpositioned appendage produces an exaggerated bulge in the region of the pulmonary knob. Additional imaging (Fig. 48-7) can confirm herniation of the appendage if it is suspected. Only the small defects require surgical treatment, although large deficiencies may not be entirely benign. This is because the pericardial sac functions as the cardiac seat belt. The heart is more prone to traumatic injury when the pericardium is deficient. Surgical treatment of small defects is done either by enlargement of the defect, then incurring the small risk of losing the seat belt effect, or else by closure using a flap of mediastinal pleura.

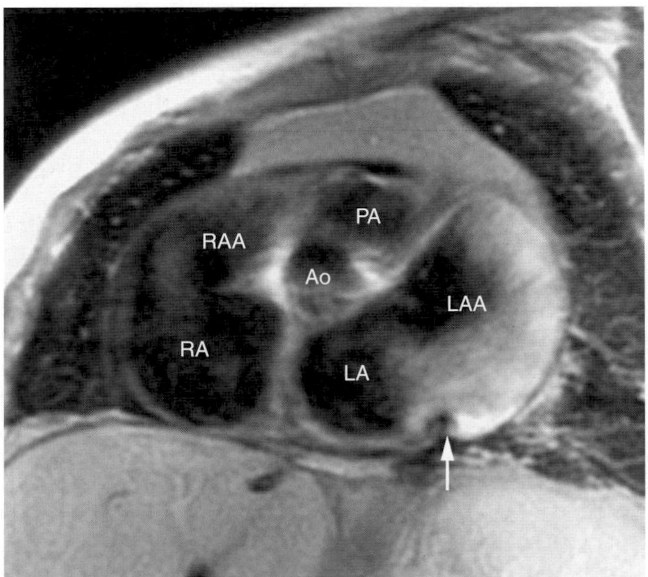

Figure 48-7 Magnetic resonance imaging in the patient shown in Figure 48-6 confirms the herniation of the left atrial appendage (LAA), albeit through a thinned area of pericardium rather than a true pericardial defect (*arrow*). Ao, aorta; LA, left atrium; PA, pulmonary trunk; RA, right atrium; RAA, right atrial appendage.

CONJOINED TWINS

A malformation in the process of monozygotic twinning, which usually produces separate but identical individuals by cleavage of the single fertilised egg, can result in the twins becoming incompletely divided. This produces the rare examples of conjoined twins that, for centuries, have fascinated both medical and lay persons. The incidence is calculated at approximately 1 conjunction in every 50,000 births.[15] The fanciful accounts of monsters and prodigies that appeared in centuries past are not that far removed from reality. The possibilities and sites for conjunction are legion. Accordingly, the categories provided for classification are formidable. The famous Siamese twins, Eng and Chang, who survived into old age, were joined only at the abdomen, sharing no more than a common cord of liver substance. Twins with cardiac involvement are all joined at the chest, although not necessarily with common cardiac chambers. Indeed, those with separate hearts in a common thoracic cavity have the best chance of survival. Even when the hearts themselves are quite separate, there can be extensive intermingling of the circulations between the twins. We have had the opportunity to study three sets of joined twins at autopsy.

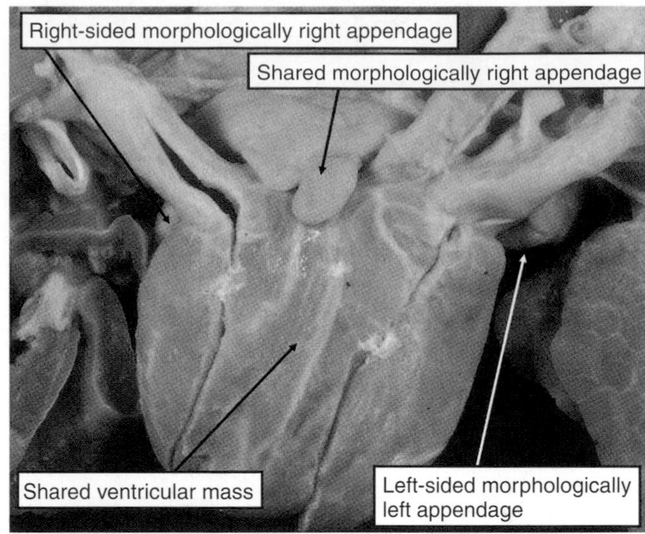

Figure 48-8 The hearts from conjoined twins joined together at atrial and ventricular levels. In the right-sided heart, the right-sided appendage, although not well seen in the photograph, was of right morphology. There is a shared midline appendage, also of right morphology, whilst the left-sided appendage is of left morphology. Thus, the heart of the right-sided twin exhibits right isomerism, whilst the atrial appendages in the heart of the left-sided twin are usually arranged.

In one case, the twins faced each other and were joined at the thorax and abdomen with a common rib cage, with a sternum at each side common to both twins. The right side of one twin faced the left side of the other, and each had its organs arranged in usual fashion. There were separate lungs, but a common liver. Each twin possessed a spleen in its own left side. The hearts were joined at ventricular and atrial level, even though each heart had two atriums and two ventricles. The latter were unconnected, even though set in a common ventricular mass. The interconnections of the great veins, however, were complex in the extreme and would have precluded any attempt at surgical separation.

One of the other sets of twins studied was joined at atrial level in a fascinating fashion. The hearts were joined in the fashion of leaves of a book, rather than faces to face. Within this arrangement, the twins shared a midline morphologically right atrium (Fig. 48-8). Consequently, while the one twin had usual atrial arrangement, the other exhibited isomerism of the right atrial appendages.[16] In keeping with the right isomerism, the right-sided twin also had lungs and bronchuses bilaterally of right morphology, and there was no spleen in its abdominal cavity. Several other examples of conjoined twins have been recorded where the one twin had usual arrangement of its organs and the other had right isomerism. Always it is the right-sided twin that is afflicted by the isomerism. Recent investigations suggest the concept of cross-talk between the conjoined embryos as the basis for failure of lateralisation.[17] The left-sided twin is hypothesised to synthesise an inhibitor of the gene *sonic hedgehog*, activin being proposed as the inhibitor. It is then suggested that diffusion of the inhibitor to the right-sided twin prevents the induction of *nodal*, this latter gene being considered necessary for the formation of morphologically left structures (see also Chapter 22).

Clinical diagnosis of conjunction is not now likely to be a problem. Intra-uterine cross sectional ultrasonography is now likely to reveal the diagnosis in the majority of cases. Although analysis will be difficult, an assessment can be made of the degree of cardiac involvement. If surgical separation is to be attempted, a full investigation will be needed after birth. Angiocardiography and echocardiography should always be performed, along with resonance imaging. Interpretation of the images, considered difficult in the past, should now be very much easier. Even in potentially suitable cases, survivors of attempted separation have thus far been rare. As with exteriorisation of the heart, the situation must be anticipated rapidly to improve, depending of course on the degree of fusion of the cardiac structures, and the severity of the intracardiac lesions in each twin.

ABNORMAL POSITIONING OF THE HEART

The heart is normally located in the mediastinum, with one-third of its bulk to the right, and two-thirds to the left of the midline. With this arrangement, the apex usually points inferiorly and to the left. This combined pattern is traditionally described as levocardia. There are several reasons why the heart can be deviated from this position, or its apex be pointed in an unexpected direction. Although the abnormal position of the heart can be due the cardiac defect, it can also be secondary to a non-cardiac pathology. For example, the heart can be pushed to the right by a space-occupying lesion in the left lung or left pleural cavity, such as hyperinflation of the left lung, or pleural effusion and pneumothorax involving the left pleural cavity. The heart can also be pulled to the right when the right lung is underdeveloped or collapsed. The abnormally rightward position of the heart is typically seen in association with right pulmonary hypoplasia in scimitar syndrome and absence of the right pulmonary artery. The abnormal position is not in itself necessarily an abnormality of the heart. Normal individuals with mirror-imaged arrangement of the organs, for example, normally have a right-sided heart.

When assessing the significance of a right-sided heart, therefore, or a heart with its apex pointing to the right, it is necessary to take account of all these various features. Several questions should be asked. What is the overall arrangement of the organs? Is there an abnormality of the lungs or the thoracic contents? If present, is it of congenital or acquired aetiology? Is the heart itself abnormally structured, or are its chambers grotesquely enlarged? Only when these questions have been posed, and answered, can the significance of an abnormally positioned heart be fully appreciated. Attempts to compress all this information into short phrases or single words have led to complex and confusing usage of the terms dextrocardia, levocardia, dextroversion, evoversion, and dextroposition, particularly when combined with adjectives such as isolated, pivotal, or mixed.[18] For these reasons, it is better not to use these cryptic conventions.

When describing the abnormally positioned heart, it is necessary first to account for its overall location. This can be accomplished by describing it as left-sided, central, or right-sided. Thereafter, it is necessary to account for the orientation of its apex. This also can be left-sided, central, or right-sided. All locations can be categorised solely in terms of the position of the heart, and the orientation of its apex. This information, of course, must be placed in the context of the overall arrangement of the thoracic and abdominal organs, and the presence of acquired or congenital disease of either the heart or the lungs. If, for example, the heart is described as lying mostly in the right chest, and with its apex orientated to the left, there can be little room for misunderstanding this arrangement, irrespective of the precise reason for the abnormal position.

Abnormal positioning of the heart, therefore, should no longer be regarded as a diagnosis in its own right. Finding a right-sided heart, for example, gives no clue as to what is happening inside the organ. The heart itself may be entirely normal. Description of abnormal location is but one part of full sequential segmental analysis (see Chapter 1). Certain well-recognised lesions, or combinations of lesions, nonetheless, are associated with right-sided hearts, or left-sided hearts in those with mirror imagery. The heart is typically right-sided in association with hypoplasia of the right lung in the scimitar syndrome and its variants, known also as the broncho-pulmonary foregut malformation.[19] The heart is also right-sided in well over a third of individuals who have an isomeric arrangement of their organs (see Chapter 22). The single lesion most associated with a right-sided heart, or left-sided heart with mirror-imaged arrangement, is congenitally corrected transposition (see Chapter 39). At best, these are clues to the final diagnosis. The variety of lesions that can exist when the heart is abnormally positioned is protean.

JUXTAPOSITION OF THE ATRIAL APPENDAGES

Although not necessarily representing an abnormal position of the heart itself, but often found when the heart is abnormally located, juxtaposition of the atrial appendages is a potentially confusing feature of a congenitally malformed heart. In the normally constructed heart, the appendages lie one to each side of the arterial pedicle. It is then the morphological nature of each appendage that determines the arrangement of the atrial chambers (see Chapter 1). Juxtaposition of the appendages is seen when both the appendages are to the same side of the arterial pedicle. Such juxtaposition does not interfere with recognition of the structure of each appendage when this feature is assessed on the basis of the extent of the pectinate muscles. Juxtaposition, therefore, can occur in the person with usual atrial arrangement (Fig. 48-9), in the individual with mirror-imaged arrangement, or in the presence of isomeric appendages (Fig. 48-10).

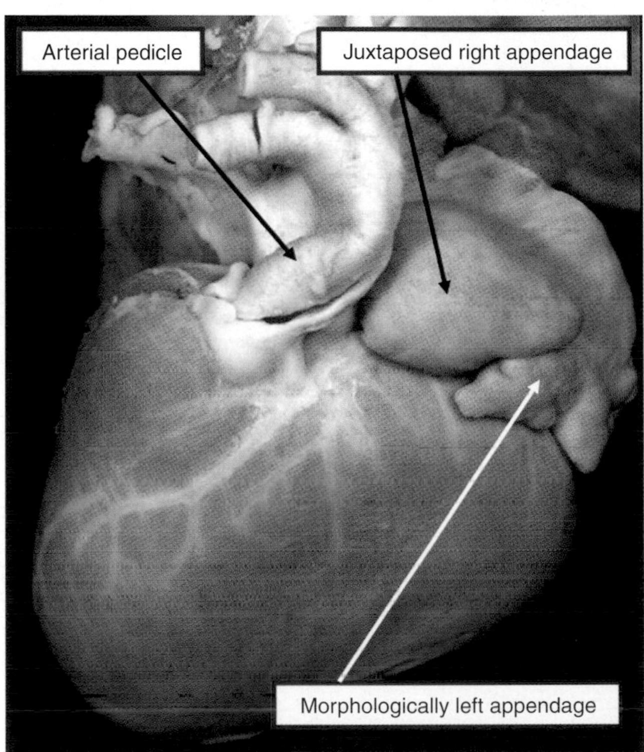

Figure 48-9 In this heart, both the appendages are to the left of the arterial pedicle, albeit that they are still recognised as being morphologically right and morphologically left.

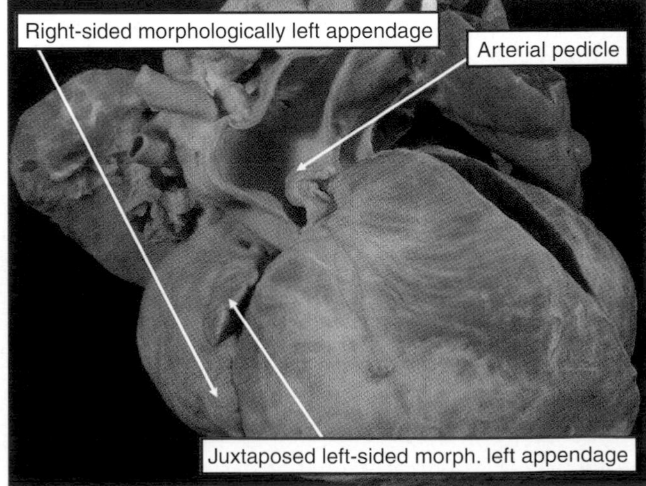

Figure 48-10 In this heart, both the appendages are to the right of the arterial pedicle, and both are recognisably of left morphology. This is right-sided juxtaposition in the setting of left isomerism.

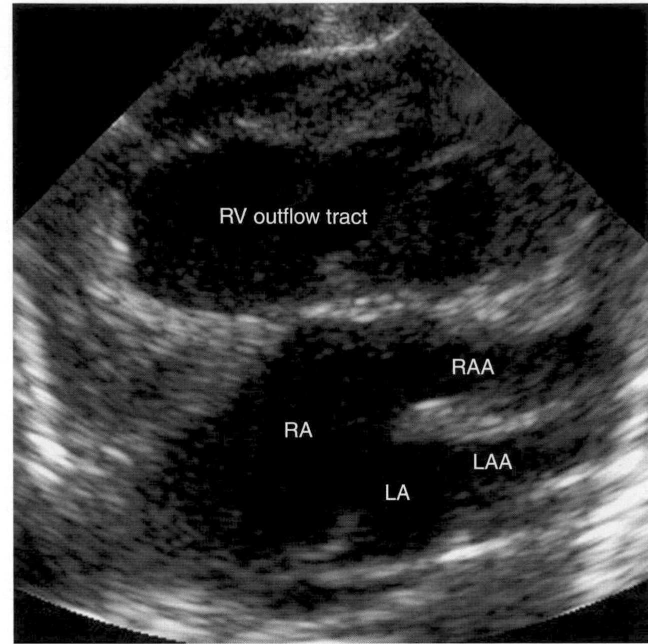

Figure 48-11 This cross sectional echocardiogram, in the short axis of the heart, shows left juxtaposition of the right atrial appendage (RAA) in the setting of double outlet right ventricle (RV). Note that the morphologically right appendage has passed through the transverse sinus to lie alongside the morphologically left appendage (LAA). LA, left atrium; RA, right atrium.

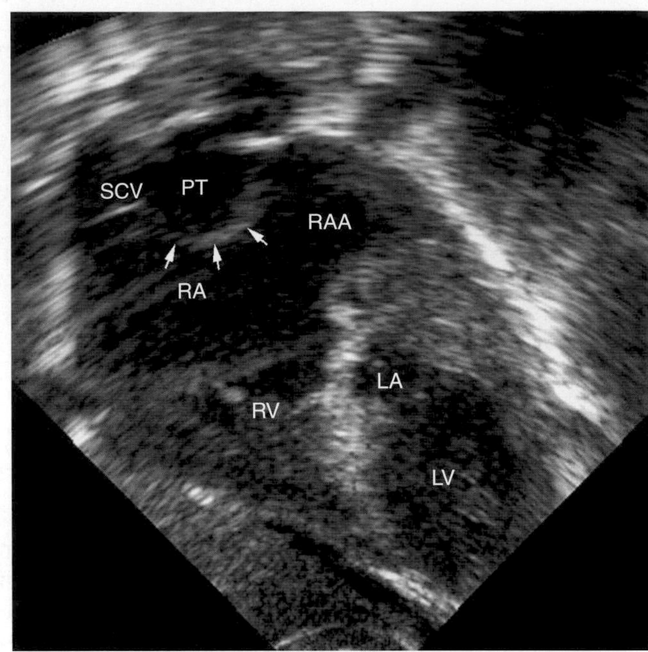

Figure 48-12 The subcostal four-chamber echocardiogram from the patient shown in Figure 48-11 shows that the right atrial appendage (RAA) is displaced to the right. Note that the roof of the right atrium is indented by the arterial trunk (*arrows*), the pulmonary trunk (PT) in this case. LA, left atrium; LV, left ventricle; RA, right atrium; RV, right ventricle; SCV, superior caval vein.

In the presence of usual atrial arrangement, juxtaposition occurs most frequently when the right appendage is deviated leftward through the transverse sinus so that it lies above the left appendage (see Figs. 48-9, 48-11, and 48-12). This is conventionally called left juxtaposition. It tends to be associated with relatively complex anatomical lesions. Noteworthy associated malformations are tricuspid atresia, hypoplasia of the right ventricle, and abnormal ventriculo-arterial connections,[20] such as double outlet right ventricle.

Sometimes the juxtaposition is only partial, with a small pouch of right appendage continuing to protrude forward on the right side of the arterial trunk. The effect of the juxtaposition is to distort the internal morphology of the atrial septum. On opening the relatively small atrial surface, the orifice of the juxtaposed appendage occupies the anticipated site of the oval fossa (Fig. 48-13). The oval fossa is more slit-like, and is deviated postero-inferiorly. The distortion of the right atrium can also produce potential problems in atrial redirection procedures, albeit that nowadays these are usually performed only as part of the double switch procedure, and this is rarely undertaken in patients with juxtaposition. Another consequence of the juxtaposition is to distort the landmarks to the sinus node. The terminal groove is orientated in horizontal rather than vertical fashion, and the sinus node itself is deviated towards the atrioventricular junction. Much more rarely, the appendages can be juxtaposed to the right of the arterial pedicle when there is usual atrial arrangement. It is then the left appendage that occupies the transverse sinus, coming to lie superiorly relative to the right appendage (see Fig. 48-10). In some cases, right juxtaposition is found in hearts when the only associated lesion is an atrial septal defect. In other instances, it may accompany exceedingly complex lesions. In the person with mirror-imaged arrangement, of course, right-sided juxtaposition is the expected variant. It is associated with the same constellation of lesions as is left-sided juxtaposition in the individual with usual atrial arrangement. When there is left juxtaposition, a straight or concave right lower heart border, and a prominent bulging contour of the left mid-heart border, are seen on the chest radiograph because the right atrial appendage is not in its usual place but

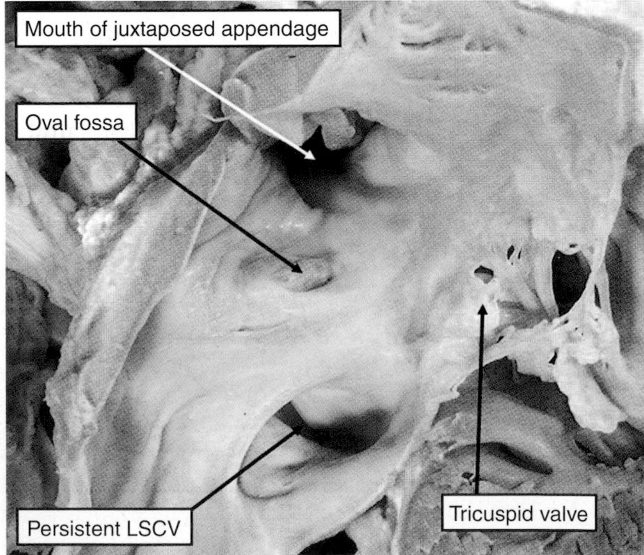

Figure 48-13 The distorted anatomy of the right atrium produced by left juxtaposition of the atrial appendages. The mouth of the appendage is occupying the usual position of the oval fossa. There is a persistent left superior caval vein (LSCV) that drains through the enlarged mouth of the coronary sinus

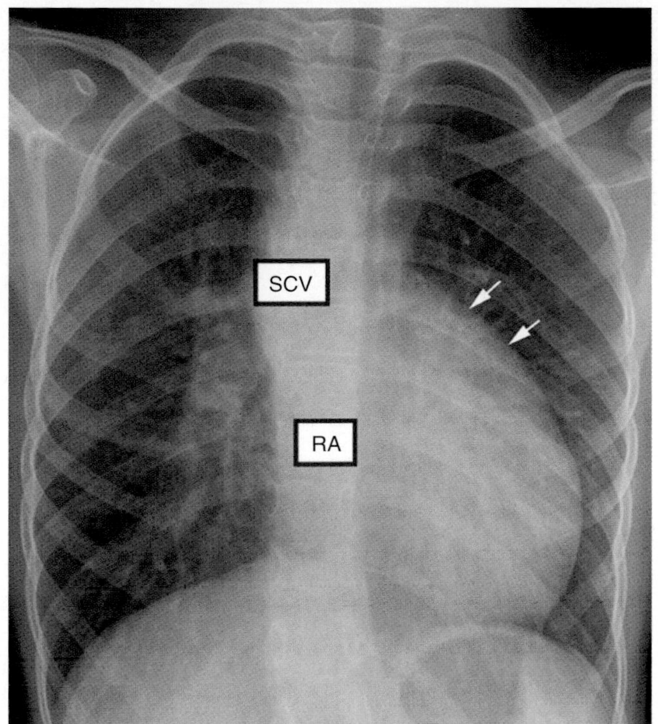

Figure 48-14 The chest radiograph shows the characteristic appearances of left juxtaposition of the atrial appendages. Note the sigmoid configuration of the right border of the cardiac silhouette, and the bulge in the upper part of the left border (*arrows*). RA, right atrium; SCV, superior caval vein.

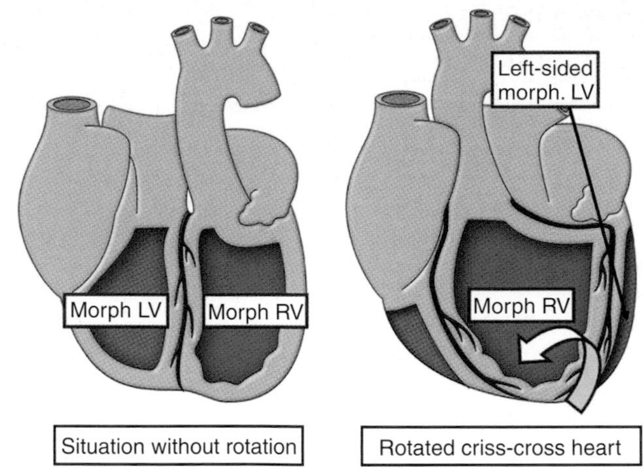

Figure 48-15 The cartoon shows the essence of the criss-cross heart in the setting of usual arrangement and congenitally corrected transposition. Usually the ventricles are positioned side-by-side, with the morphologically left ventricle (LV) to the right. If, however, the ventricular mass becomes twisted (*right cartoon*), then the morphologically right ventricle (RV) assumes an anterior location, the aortic valve is positioned anterior and to the right rather than the left, and part of the morphologically left ventricle can become left-sided. The twisting, in most instances, does not change the segmental connections. Although shown in the setting of congenitally corrected transposition, such twisting can occur in any setting.

displaced to the left (Fig. 48-14; see also Fig. 48-13). The diagnosis is readily made with cross sectional echocardiography (see Figs. 48-10 and 48-11) or magnetic resonance imaging. During cardiac catheterisation, if the diagnosis has not already been made by echocardiography, the first pointer to the diagnosis may be the sampling of systemic venous blood from the left side of the heart in a low pressure zone. If necessary, selective injection of contrast medium into the appendage will establish the diagnosis.

CRISS-CROSS OR TWISTED HEARTS, SUPERO-INFERIOR VENTRICLES, AND RELATED CONDITIONS

The last group of hearts to be considered are those where the relationships of the cardiac chambers, or great arteries, are not as expected for the given segmental connections. The significance of these malformations has diminished markedly since it has been appreciated that segmental connections cannot, and should not, be inferred from abnormal relationships of cardiac structures. The abnormal relationships in themselves, however, can still be a confusing feature. The most commonly encountered is criss-crossing or, more precisely, twisting of the ventricular inlet components, combined with an unexpected relationship of the ventricles.[21,22] There are other arrangements, however, that show an abnormal ventricular relationship without crossing or twisting of the ventricular inlets. There are three mutually exclusive mechanisms that can produce abnormal ventricular relationships for the given segmental connections, namely, twisting, tilting, and rotation. By twisting, we mean a spiral relationship of the atriums and ventricles in which the cardiac chambers and arterial trunks are aligned and arranged as if the heart were twisted clockwise, or anticlockwise, by a hand placed on the cardiac apex with the venous connections of the heart maintained in their normal positions (Fig. 48-15). Tilting, in contrast, produces a supero-inferior relationship of the ventricles, the parallel axes of the ventricular inlet and atrioventricular junctions being preserved as if the apex of the heart were simply lifted by a hand placed on the apex (Fig. 48-16). Rotation describes the much rarer condition, in which the cardiac chambers, arterial trunks and caval veins are all abnormally oriented within the thorax, as if the entire heart were rotated as a block around its long axis.

It is twisting that is the essential feature of the so-called criss-cross heart. The common characteristics of the twisted heart include loss of normal parallel axes of ventricular inlets, with an overt criss-crossed relationship in extreme cases, angulation of the atrial septum, a curved configuration of the ventricular septum, and unusual arterial relationships for the given pathology. The ventricular inlets also adopt a supero-inferior relationship, with the apical components showing the most unusual relationships. In extreme forms, the ventricular apices are displaced to the opposite side, and show a reversed side-by-side relationship. This can occur with any known combination of connections of the cardiac segments. It produces unexpected relationships of the ventricles and great arteries. Twisting is usually in such a direction to place the right ventricular inlet anterior and superior to the left ventricular inlet. In congenitally corrected transposition with usual atrial arrangement, for example, and as shown in Figure 48-15, the morphologically left ventricle is usually a right-sided structure, while the aortic valve most frequently is located anteriorly and to the left. The ventricular mass in the presence of the

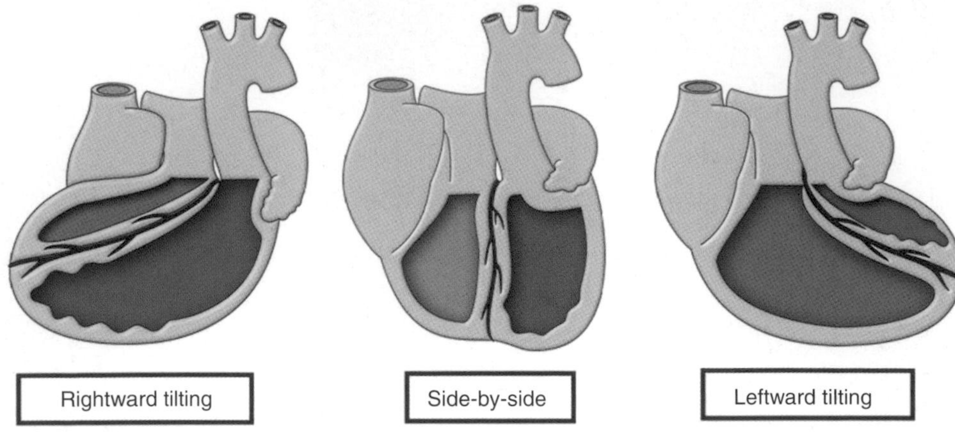

Figure 48-16 The cartoon shows how supero-inferior ventricles are produced, in the setting shown here of congenitally corrected transposition, by tilting of the ventricular mass to either the right or the left. Oftentimes such tilting is combined with a twisting abnormality. The arrangement is also described as upstairs–downstairs heart.

criss-cross malformation is twisted counter-clockwise in such a way that the morphologically right ventricular inlet achieves a rightward and supero-anterior position relative to the left ventricular inlet, while the aortic valve becomes anterior and right-sided. In the presence of usual atrial arrangement, of course, a right-sided and anterior aorta arising from a right-sided morphologically right ventricle is more typically found with the segmental combinations of regular transposition (see Chapter 38). Twisting can also occur with the connections of the segments that normally produce regular transposition. The ventricular mass is twisted clockwise, giving the spurious impression of congenitally corrected transposition. Once the investigator is aware of the possibility, both the abnormal relationships and the true segmental connections are readily demonstrated by current techniques for imaging (Fig. 48-17). The key is first to analyse the connections between the cardiac segments, and only then to take note of the relations of the ventricles and arterial trunks. The secret is not to be surprised when the relationships observed are not as anticipated for the demonstrated segmental connections.

In the typical situation of the criss-cross heart, which can be encountered with any combination of atrioventricular and ventriculo-arterial connections, the ventricular topology is as anticipated for the atrioventricular connections. Thus, in the illustrated situation with concordant atrioventricular connections (see Fig. 48-17), although the morphologically left ventricle is right-sided despite the usual atrial arrangement of the atrial chambers, the morphologically right ventricle will accept only the palmar surface of the right hand of the observer with the thumb, figuratively speaking, in the tricuspid valve. In other words, there is retention of right hand ventricular topology despite the rotation of the ventricular mass along its long axis. Rare cases exist, however, that emphasise the need to distinguish separately on some occasions between the connections of the segments and their topological arrangement.[23,24] These hearts produce a different variant of the criss-cross heart, and one that cannot simply be explained on the basis of rotation of the ventricular mass.

In the examples we have seen, the atrial chambers were arranged in usual fashion. The right atrium connected to the morphologically right ventricle, which as in the heart shown in Figure 48-17, was left-sided relative to the morphologically left ventricle (Fig. 48-18). The left ventricle was connected to the left atrium. Despite

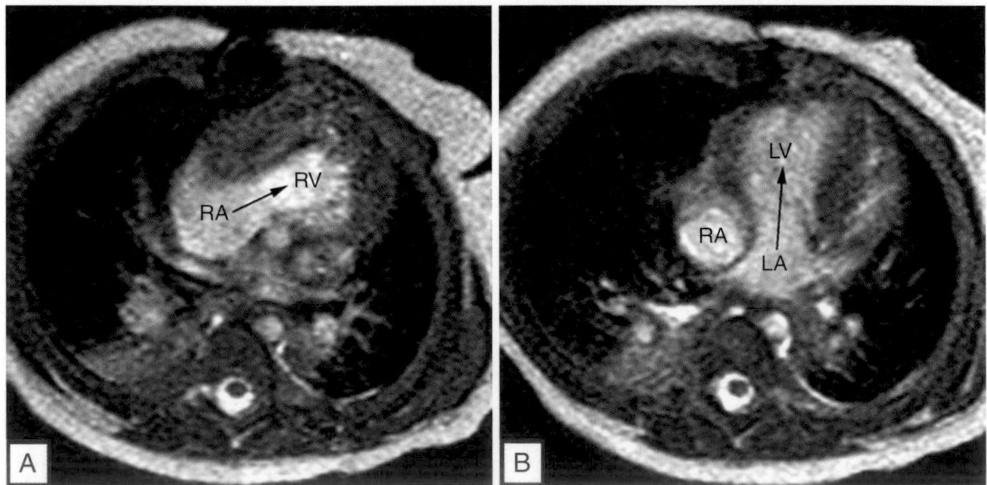

Figure 48-17 These magnetic resonance images in a patient with concordant atrioventricular connections, with the atriums (RA, LA) connected to their appropriate ventricles (RV, LV) show crossing of the atrioventricular inlets (*arrows* in **A** and **B**). This is the essence of the so-called criss-cross heart, the right-sided location of the morphologically left ventricle relative to the right ventricle giving the spurious impression of the discordant atrioventricular connections.

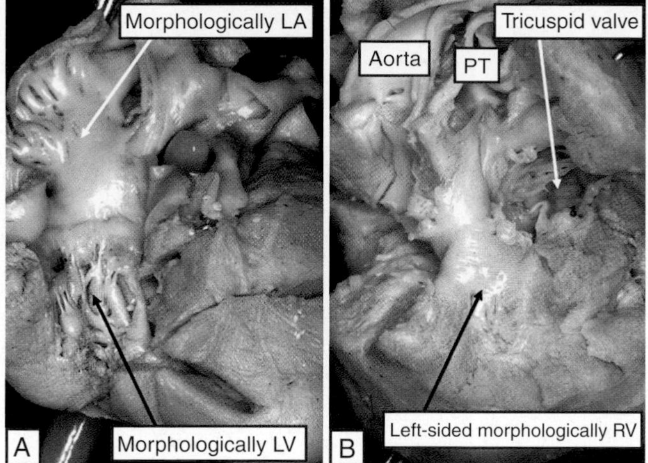

Figure 48-18 The heart illustrated has a very rare form of criss-cross malformation. **A,** The atria are connected to morphologically appropriate ventricles, in other words, the atrioventricular connections are concordant, with the pink probe passing from the usually arranged right atrium to the morphologically right ventricle. **B,** The morphologically right ventricle is left-sided, and gives rise to both arterial trunks in the setting of bilateral infundibula. There is left hand ventricular topology, despite the presence of usual atrial arrangement and concordant atrioventricular connections. Providing that the segmental connections are described separately from the ventricular topology, this arrangement should not cause confusion. LA, left aorta; LV, left ventricle; PT, pulmonary trunk; RV, right ventricle.

the concordant atrioventricular connections, however, there was left hand ventricular topology. In addition, there was double outlet from the morphologically right ventricle and left-sided juxtaposition of the atrial appendages. These rarer, and much more complex, cases emphasise the need, on occasions, to specify the topology of the cardiac segments when they differ from the anticipated arrangement. Provided that all these features are recognised, and accounted for separately, there should be little room for confusion or misunderstanding, irrespective of the specific words used for their description. The term criss-cross itself, however, describes a particular relationship of the ventricular inlets. Indeed, the atrioventricular valvar planes can cross each other even when both valves open to the same ventricle[25] (Fig. 48-19). Simply describing the twisted atrioventricular connections does not account for the morphology of the entire heart. Full sequential segmental description is needed for that purpose.

In comparison with the potential problems encountered with criss-cross hearts, few should be posed by ventricles that are arranged in supero-inferior, or upstairs–downstairs, fashion which simply reflects a tilting of the ventricular mass along its long axis (see Fig. 48-16). Supero-inferior ventricles are usually described in the setting of congenitally corrected transposition, where in most instances the ventricles are arranged in side-by-side fashion. Tilting of the ventricular mass to either side then produces a stacking effect of the ventricles one on top of the other. Like the criss-cross pattern, supero-inferior ventricles are often seen in the presence of straddling and/or overriding atrioventricular valves. As was also the case with the criss-cross arrangement, noting an upstairs–downstairs, or supero-inferior, arrangement does not describe the complete heart, but only a particular ventricular relationship. Sequential segmental description is mandatory for full categorisation of the hearts showing this abnormality.

We now know that a further variation occurs in these unusual ventricular relationships. First described by Freedom and his colleagues in their textbook of angiography, the entirety has now been diagnosed during fetal life, and in a familial setting.[26] Called the topsy-turvy arrangement, the essential feature is rotation of the whole heart around its long axis, with supero-inferior relationships of the atriums and ventricles (Fig. 48-20), but without twisting of the axes of the atrioventricular connections. As the arterial roots, as well as the aortic arch and arterial duct, are displaced downward as a consequence of rotation of the whole heart, the branches of the aortic arch and the superior caval vein are elongated (Fig. 48-21). More importantly, the trachea is elongated and the left bronchus is severely compressed by the low-lying aortic arch and arterial duct (Fig. 48-22).

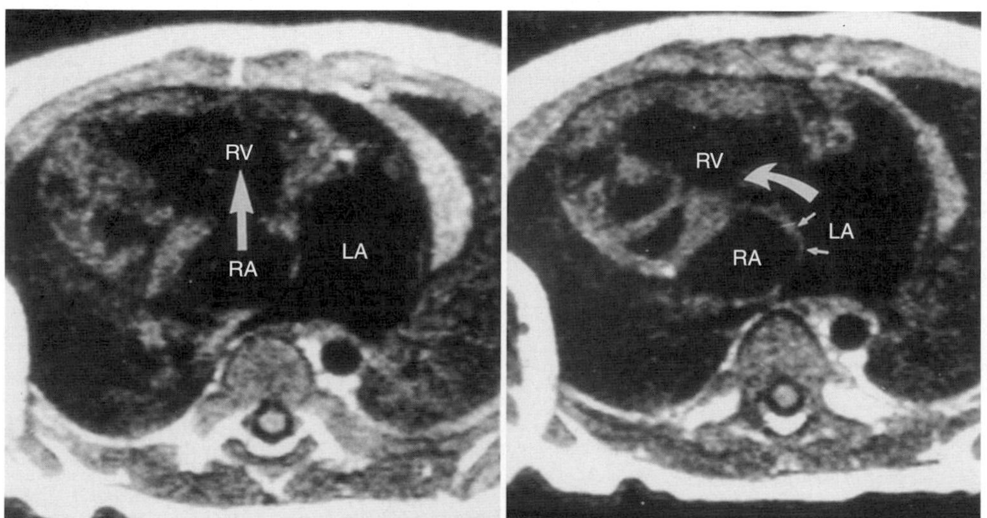

Figure 48-19 These magnetic resonance images from a patient with double inlet right ventricle show how the atrioventricular valves cross each other as they enter the dominant right ventricle (*arrows*), producing twisted double inlet atrioventricular connection. LA, left atrium; RA, right atrium; RV, dominant right ventricle.

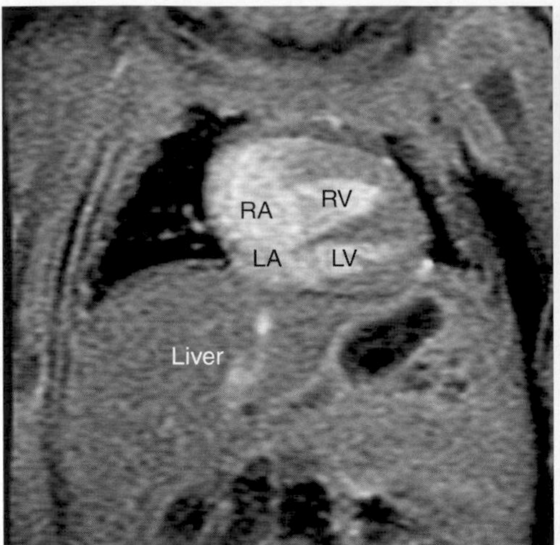

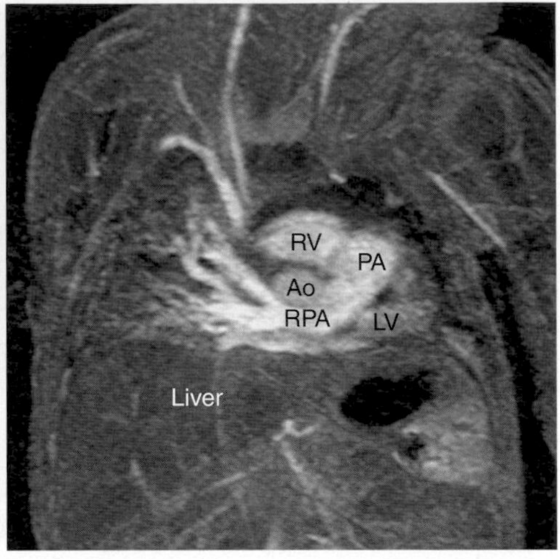

Figure 48-20 These magnetic resonance images show the essence of the topsy-turvy arrangement. The ventricles (RV, LV) are located supero-inferiorly (*left panel*), but without any rotational twisted deformity. The arterial trunks (Ao, PA, RPA), are displaced downwards (*right panel*), with the brachiocephalic arteries and the caval veins elongated as they extend to the mediastinum (see Figure 48-21). LA, left atrium; RA, right atrium.

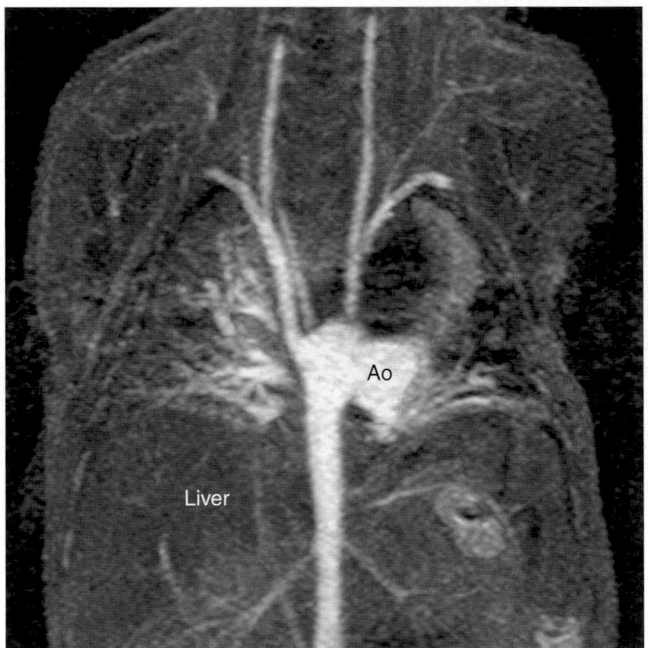

Figure 48-21 This magnetic resonance image shows the elongated brachiocephalic arteries produced in consequence of the topsy-turvy arrangement of the heart. Ao, aorta.

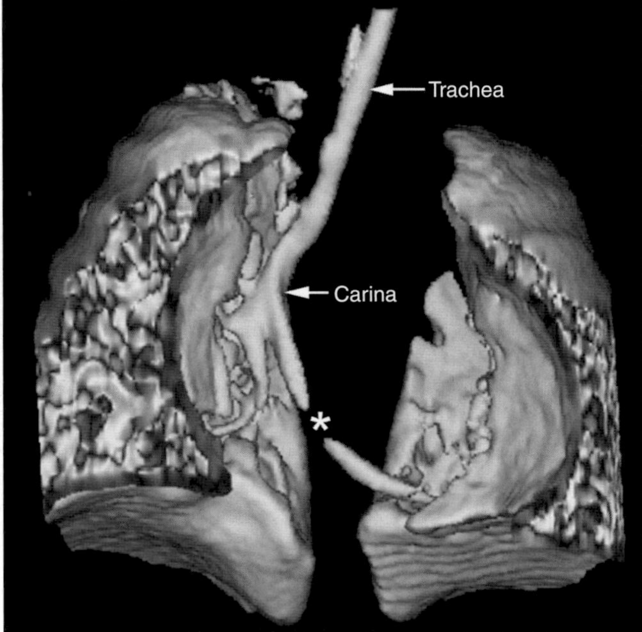

Figure 48-22 The reconstructed computerised tomographic image from the patient shown in Figure 48-20 illustrates the elongation of the trachea and narrowing of the left bronchus (*asterisk*) as a consequence of the low-lying aortic arch and arterial duct produced by the topsy-turvy arrangement.

The complete reference list can be found on the companion Expert Consult web site at www.expertconsult.com.

ANNOTATED REFERENCES

- Kanagasuntheram R, Verzin JA: Ectopia cordis in man. Thorax 1962;17: 159–167.

  An extensive review of the cases described at the time of writing showing the varied patterns for exteriorisation of the heart.

- Cantrell JR, Haller JA, Ravitch MM: A syndrome of congenital defects involving the abdominal wall sternum, diaphragm, pericardium and heart. Surg Gynecol Obstet 1958;107:602–614.

  The initial description of the constellation of lesions now known as the pentalogy of Cantrell, the extreme forms of the syndrome being exteriorisation of the heart, but with lesser forms showing ventricular diverticulums extending through the midline defects of the body wall.

- Toyama WM: Combined congenital defects of the anterior abdominal wall, sternum, diaphragm, pericardium and heart: A case report and review of the syndrome. Pediatrics 1972;50:788–792.

  An erudite review, albeit based on a case report, showing that all five of the features initially described by Cantrell and his colleagues are not present when there are midline deficiencies of the body wall.

- Rossi MB, Burn JL, Ho SY, et al: Conjoined twins and right atrial isomerism. Br Heart J 1987;58:518–524.

  Description of a series of cases of conjoined twins, describing how one of the twins exhibits isomerism of the right atrial appendages.

- Levin M, Roberts DJ, Holmes LB, Tabin C: Laterality defects in conjoined twins. Nature 1996;384:321–324.

  A discussion of the influence of genetic pathways in determining laterality of the bodily organs, and showing how this can produce right isomerism in the setting of conjoined twins.

- Wilkinson JL, Acerete F: Terminological pitfalls in congenital heart disease: Reappraisal of some confusing terms, with an account of a simplified system of basic nomenclature. Br Heart J 1973;35:1166–1177.

  An excellent review of the problems existing with the use of terms such as dextrocardia and levocardia, albeit not going the whole hog and opting for a purely descriptive terminology.

- Freedom RM, Yoo S-J, Woo HW, et al: The bronchopulmonary foregut malformation. Cardiol Young 2006;16:229–251.

  One of the last reviews from the late and much lamented Bob Freedom. Encyclopaedic as usual, it discusses in detail the multiple variants of the Scimitar syndrome.

- Anjos RT, Ho SY, Anderson RH: Surgical implications of juxtaposition of the atrial appendages: A review of forty-nine autopsied hearts. J Thorac Cardiovasc Surg 1990;99:897–904.

An account of the intracardiac malformations, and segmental combinations, encountered when there is juxtaposition of the atrial appendages, with emphasis on the surgical implications of the findings.

- Weinberg PM, Van Praagh R, Wagner HR, Cuaso CC: New form of criss-cross atrioventricular relation: An expanded view of the meaning of d and l-loops. World Congress of Paediatric Cardiology 1980, London (abstract 319).
- Anderson RH, Smith A, Wilkinson JL: Disharmony between atrioventricular connexions and segmental combinations: Unusual variants of 'criss-cross' hearts. J Am Coll Cardiol 1987;10:1274–1277.

  Two accounts, the first, as far as I am aware, appearing only in the form of an abstract, describing the rare hearts in which the segmental combinations are not as expected for the connections between the atrial and ventricular chambers. In these rare situations, clarity is provided by describing separately the connections, the atrial arrangement, and the ventricular topology.

- Jaeggi E, Chitayat D, Golding F, et al: Prenatal diagnosis of topsy-turvy heart. Cardiol Young 2008;18:337–342.

  The first description of the topsy-turvy arrangement, initially described by Freedom and his colleagues, following prenatal diagnosis. The patient described had a sibling with the same malformation. Elongation of the arterial trunks produced marked narrowing of the airways.

- Anderson RH: Criss cross hearts revisited. Pediatr Cardiol 1982;3:305–313.
- Seo J-W, Yoo S-J, Ho SY, et al: Further morphological observations on hearts with twisted atrioventricular connections (criss-cross hearts). Cardiovasc Pathol 1992;1:211–217.

  These two articles review the morphology underscoring the so-called criss-cross arrangement, showing how in most instances the lesions simply reflect twisting of the heart around its long axis.

CHAPTER 49

Cardiomyopathies

JUAN PABLO KASKI and PERRY ELLIOTT

It has become evident that primary myocardial disease represents one of the more neglected aspects of heart disease today. It is often overlooked or misdiagnosed; in addition, it is frequently considered rare, unimportant, or that treatment is of no avail . . . there are misconceptions concerning its rarity or unimportance, as well as treatment.

—W. Proctor Harvey, 1965[1]

The cardiomyopathies are a heterogeneous group of disorders of cardiac muscle (Table 49-1). Previous classifications defined cardiomyopathies as myocardial diseases of unknown cause,[2] but increased understanding of their aetiology and pathogenesis has led to a revised definition of cardiomyopathy as 'a myocardial disorder in which the heart muscle is structurally and functionally abnormal, in the absence of coronary artery disease, hypertension, valvular disease and congenital heart disease sufficient to cause the observed myocardial abnormality'.[3] Cardiomyopathies are classified according to the ventricular morphology and pathophysiology. Four major types are recognised, namely, the dilated, hypertrophic, and restrictive variants and arrhythmogenic right ventricular cardiomyopathy.[4] Diseases that do not fit readily into these groups, such as endocardial fibroelastosis and ventricular non-compaction, are currently considered as unclassified cardiomyopathies. In some circumstances, mixed phenotypes can exist. For example, patients with hypertrophic and dilated cardiomyopathies frequently have restrictive left ventricular physiology; in other cases, hypertrophy and ventricular dilation may co-exist.

HYPERTROPHIC CARDIOMYOPATHY

Definition and Historical Aspects

Hypertrophic cardiomyopathy is defined as left ventricular hypertrophy in the absence of abnormal loading conditions, such as valvar disease, hypertension, or other congenital cardiac malformations, sufficient to explain the degree of hypertrophy.[5] Asymmetrical hypertrophy of the interventricular septum was first described in 1869,[6,7] but hypertrophic cardiomyopathy was only established as a clinical entity in the late 1950s.[8,9] These latter landmark studies were followed by a period of intense clinical investigation, during which the characteristic morphological and haemodynamic features of the disease were defined. Angiographic and M-mode echocardiographic studies focused on dynamic subaortic obstruction, at the time thought to be the defining feature of the condition.[10–13] Use of cross sectional echocardiography demonstrated that any pattern of hypertrophy can occur, and that only a minority have obstruction of the left ventricular outflow tract at rest.[14] The discovery that many patients with hypertrophic cardiomyopathy had familial disease led to a search for the genetic basis of the disease. In 1989, the first mutation in the gene encoding the cardiac β-myosin heavy chain was identified.[15] Since then, more than 400 mutations have been identified in this and other cardiac sarcomeric protein genes.[16]

Epidemiology

Unexplained left ventricular hypertrophy occurs in approximately 1 in every 500 adults.[17–21] The frequency of left ventricular hypertrophy in children is unknown, but population-based studies from Australia[22] and the United States[23] report an incidence between 0.3 and 0.5 cases per 100,000, including cardiomyopathies associated with inborn errors of metabolism, neuromuscular disease, and malformation syndromes. The frequency is greater in males, and highest in the first year of life, with one study showing a second peak in adolescence.[23]

Natural History

Hypertrophic cardiomyopathy can present from infancy to old age.[5,16,24] Many patients follow a stable and benign course, with a low risk of adverse events, but a large number experience progressive symptoms, caused by gradual deterioration in left ventricular systolic and diastolic function and atrial arrhythmias. A proportion of individuals die suddenly, whereas others may die from thromboembolism, progressive cardiac failure, or infective endocarditis.

Sudden Death

Sudden death occurs most commonly in adolescents and young adults.[25] Whilst initial descriptions of the natural history reported annual rates of sudden death from 3% to 6%, recent studies in adults revealed rates of 1% or less per year.[5,26] Similarly, early studies of highly selected populations of children reported rates of sudden death ranging from 2% to 8% per year,[27–29] but recent population-based reports from Australia[30] and the United States[31] report an overall annual rate of sudden death of 1% to 1.5% per year beyond infancy.

Cardiac Failure

Whilst many children and teenagers with hypertrophic cardiomyopathy have few if any symptoms, presentation in infancy can be associated with severe and intractable cardiac failure.[32–35] Some studies have suggested that presentation in infancy itself constitutes an unfavourable prognosis,[33,35] but this finding is not consistent.[34] Progression to an end-stage, or burnt-out, phase is a well-recognised

TABLE 49-1

CLASSIFICATION AND AETIOLOGY OF THE CARDIOMYOPATHIES

Hypertrophic Cardiomyopathy (HCM)	Dilated Cardiomyopathy (DCM)	Arrhythmogenic Right Ventricular Cardiomyopathy (ARVC)	Restrictive Cardiomyopathy (RCM)	Unclassified
		FAMILIAL		
Familial, unknown gene **Sarcomeric protein disease** β-Myosin heavy chain Cardiac myosin binding protein C Cardiac troponin I Troponin-T α-Tropomyosin Essential myosin light chain Regulatory myosin light chain Cardiac actin α-Myosin heavy chain Titin Troponin C Muscle LIM protein **Glycogen storage disease** (e.g., GSD II [Pompe's disease]; GSD III [Forbes' disease], AMP kinase [WPW, HCM, conduction disease]) Danon disease **Lysosomal storage diseases** (e.g., Anderson-Fabry disease, Hurler's syndrome) **Disorders of fatty acid metabolism** **Carnitine deficiency** **Phosphorylase B kinase deficiency** **Mitochondrial cytopathies** (e.g., MELAS, MERFF, LHON) **Syndromic HCM** Noonan's syndrome LEOPARD syndrome Friedreich's ataxia Beckwith-Wiedermann syndrome Swyer's syndrome (pure gonadal dysgenesis) **Other** Phospholamban promoter Familial amyloid	**Familial, unknown gene** **Sarcomeric protein mutations** (see HCM) Zband ZASP Muscle LIM protein TCAP **Cytoskeletal genes** Dystrophin Desmin Metavinculin Sarcoglycan complex CRYAB Epicardin **Nuclear membrane** Lamin A/C Emerin **Mildly dilated CM** **Intercalated disc protein mutations** (see ARVC) **Mitochondrial cytopathy**	**Familial, unknown gene** **Intercalated disc protein mutations** Plakoglobin Desmoplakin Plakophilin 2 Desmoglein 2 Desmocollin 2 **Cardiac ryanodine receptor (RyR2)** **Transforming growth factor-β3** (TGFβ3)	**Familial, unknown gene** **Sarcomeric protein mutations** Troponin I (RCM ± HCM) Essential light chain of myosin **Familial amyloidosis** Transthyretin (RCM + neuropathy) Apolipoprotein (RCM + nephropathy) **Desminopathy** **Pseudoxanthoma elasticum** **Haemochromatosis** **Anderson-Fabry disease** **Glycogen storage disease**	**Left ventricular non-compaction** Barth syndrome Lamin A/C ZASP α-Dystrobrevin
		NON-FAMILIAL		
Obesity **Infant of diabetic mother** **Athletic training** **Amyloid** (AL/prealbumin)	**Myocarditis** (infective/toxic/immune) **Kawasaki disease** **Eosinophilic** (Churg-Strauss syndrome) **Viral persistence** **Drugs** **Pregnancy** **Endocrine** **Nutritional:** thiamine, carnitine, selenium, hypophosphataemia, hypocalcaemia **Alcohol** **Tachycardiomyopathy**	Inflammation?	**Amyloid** (AL/prealbumin) **Scleroderma** **Endomyocardial fibrosis** Hypereosinophilic syndrome Idiopathic Chromosomal cause Drugs: serotonin, methysergide, ergotamine, mercurial agents, busulfan **Carcinoid heart disease** **Metastatic cancers** **Radiation therapy** **Drugs:** Anthracyclines	**Tako-tsubo cardiomyopathy**

Data from Elliott P, Andersson B, Arbustini E, et al: Classification of the cardiomyopathies: A position statement from the European Society of Cardiology Working Group on Myocardial and Pericardial Diseases. Eur Heart J 2008;29:270–276.

complication,[36–49] with a reported prevalence in up to one-sixth of adults.[41,45,47] This end-stage is characterised by progressive left ventricular dilation, mural thinning, and systolic impairment.[50] It is associated with a poor prognosis,[47] with an overall rate of death of up to 11% per year.[41] In children, progression to the burnt-out phase is extremely rare, with only isolated reports.[36,51] Progression to left ventricular systolic dysfunction and dilation may occur in a minority of patients with mitochondrial cardiomyopathies.[52]

Aetiology

Most adolescents and adults with hypertrophic cardiomyopathy have familial disease, caused by autosomal dominantly inherited mutations in sarcomeric protein genes. In less than one-tenth of infants and children, hypertrophic cardiomyopathy can be associated with inborn errors of metabolism, neuromuscular disorders, and malformation syndromes,[31] including Pompe's disease, Friedreich's ataxia, and malformation syndromes such as Noonan's syndrome. Cardiomyopathy associated with metabolic disorders or malformation syndromes is diagnosed earlier in life, usually during infancy or early childhood, whereas neuromuscular diseases tend to be diagnosed in the teenage years. In children with idiopathic hypertrophy, approximately one-third are diagnosed in infancy, one-third during adolescence, and the other third between the ages of 1 year and 11 years.[31]

Sarcomeric Protein Disease

Most individuals with non-syndromic hypertrophic cardiomyopathy have familial disease, inherited in an autosomal dominant manner. Genetic studies have shown that up to three-fifths of adults with the disease have mutations in one of at least 11 genes that encode the proteins of the cardiac sarcomere. These are the MYH7 gene, encoding for β-myosin heavy chain, and carried on chromosome 14; MTBPC3 encoding for myosin-binding protein C and carried on chromosome 11, TNNT2 encoding for cardiac troponin T and carried on chromosome 1; TNNI3 encoding for cardiac troponin I and carried on chromosome 19; TMP1 encoding α-tropomyosin and carried on chromosome 15; ACTC encoding α-cardiac actin and carried on chromosome 15; MYL3 encoding for essential myosin light chain and carried on chromosome 3; MYL2 encoding for regulatory myosin light chain and present on chromosome 12; TNNC1 encoding for cardiac troponin C and carried on chromosome 3; MYH6 encoding for α-myosin heavy chain and carried on chromosome 14[53–56]; and TTN encoding for titin and carried on chromosome 2.[57] There is considerable genetic heterogeneity, with over 400 different mutations identified to date, as well as marked variation in penetrance of the disease, and hence clinical expression.[58] The mechanisms through which mutations in the genes result in the characteristic pathophysiological features are incompletely understood. It has been speculated that the phenotype results from reduced contractile function, but studies of myocytic function in patients who harbour mutations in the genes are inconsistent, with some mutations appearing to depress contractility whereas others enhance sensitivity to calcium and contractility.[59]

The majority of mutations have a dominant negative effect on sarcomeric function; in other words, the mutant protein is incorporated into the sarcomere, but its interaction with the normal wild-type protein disrupts normal sarcomeric assembly and function. Allelic heterogeneity may be explained by the effect of different mutations on the structure and function of the complete peptide. β-Myosin heavy chain, for example, consists of a globular head, an α-helical rod, and a hinge region. The globular head contains binding sites for ATPase and actin, as well as sites for interaction with regulatory and essential light chains in the region of the head-rod. Most mutations in the β-myosin gene are missense DNA nucleotide substitutions that change a single amino acid in the polypeptide sequence. The majority of disease-causing β-myosin heavy chain mutations are found in one of four locations. These are the actin-binding site, the nucleotide-binding pocket, a region in the hinge region adjacent to the binding site for two reactive thiols, and the α-helix close to the essential light chain interaction site. Depending on the position of the mutation, therefore, changes might be expected in ATPase activity, actin-myosin interaction, and protein conformation during contraction.

There is substantial variation in the expression of identical mutations, indicating that other genetic and possibly environmental factors influence expression of the disease. The effect of age is perhaps the best characterised factor, most patients developing electrocardiographic and echocardiographic manifestations of the disease after puberty and before the age of 30. Other modifying factors include gender, polymorphism of the genes regulating the renin-angiotensin-aldosterone system, and the occurrence of homozygosity and compound heterozygotes.

The importance of genetic mutations in children with hypertrophic cardiomyopathy is unknown. The observation that the development of left ventricular hypertrophy in individuals with familial disease often occurs during the period of somatic growth in adolescence[60] has led to the suggestion that sarcomeric protein disease in very young children is rare.[24] There have been no systematic studies, however, evaluating the prevalence of genetic mutations in children with the disease.

Noonan's and LEOPARD Syndromes

Noonan's syndrome is characterised by short stature, dysmorphic facies, skeletal malformations, and a webbed neck.[61–63] Cardiac involvement is present in up to nine-tenths of patients with Noonan's syndrome, most commonly as pulmonary stenosis, frequently secondary to a dysplastic valve, and hypertrophic cardiomyopathy.[64] Some children present with congestive cardiac failure in infancy, which may be associated with biventricular hypertrophy and bilateral obstruction of the ventricular outflow tracts.[64] The histological findings are indistinguishable from idiopathic hypertrophic cardiomyopathy.[65] The syndrome is usually inherited as an autosomal dominant trait with variable penetrance and expression. Recently, mutations in the PTPN11 gene, encoding the protein tyrosine phosphatase SHP-2, a protein with a critical role in RAS-ERK-mediated intracellular signal transduction pathways controlling diverse developmental processes,[66] have been shown to cause the syndrome.[67] To date, at least 39 different mutations have been identified, accounting for approximately half of the cases.[61]

LEOPARD syndrome (an acronym representing lentigines, electrocardiographic abnormalities, ocular hypertelorism, pulmonary stenosis, abnormalities of the genitalia, retardation of growth, and deafness) shares many phenotypic features with Noonan's syndrome. Recent studies have shown that most patients with LEOPARD syndrome also have mutations in the PTPN11 gene.[68] Importantly, only up to one-tenth of individuals with mutations in the PTPN11 gene have hypertrophic cardiomyopathy.[69,70]

Other genes implicated in Noonan's syndrome include SOS1[71], encoding a RAS-specific guanine nucleotide exchange factor, which accounts for up to three-tenths of cases[72,73]; KRAS, which encodes a GTP-binding protein in the RAS-ERK pathway, in less than one-twentieth of cases[74]; and RAF1, a downstream effector of RAS.[75,76]

Danon Disease

This is a lysosomal storage disorder characterised clinically by cardiomyopathy, skeletal myopathy, and developmental delay. It is an X-linked disorder caused by mutations in the gene encoding the lysosome-associated membrane protein-2[77] that result in intracytoplasmic accumulation of autophagic material and glycogen within vacuoles in cardiac and skeletal myocytes.[78] Female carriers usually develop hypertrophic and dilated cardiomyopathy during adulthood, whereas males develop symptoms during childhood and adolescence.[79] The prognosis is generally poor, with most patients dying of cardiac failure. Sudden cardiac death is reported, even in female carriers.[79] Other features, which may aid in differentiating the condition clinically from idiopathic hypertrophic cardiomyopathy, include Wolff-Parkinson-White syndrome, elevated levels of creatine kinase in the serum, and retinitis pigmentosa.[80]

Adenosine Monophosphate–activated Protein Kinase Mutations

Mutations in the gene encoding the γ_2 subunit of the adenosine monophosphate–activated protein kinase[81] can cause a syndrome of hypertrophic cardiomyopathy, abnormalities in conduction, and Wolff-Parkinson-White syndrome. Histologically, there is accumulation of glycogen within cardiac myocytes and conduction tissue. Many affected individuals have a skeletal myopathy, and biopsy of the skeletal muscles shows excess mitochondria and ragged red fibres.[82] Patients develop progressive conduction disease and left ventricular hypertrophy, with complete electrocardiographic expression by the age of 18 years.[82] Atrial arrhythmias are common. Survival in one study was 91% at a mean follow-up of 12 years, with disease-related deaths occurring secondary to thromboembolic stroke related to atrial fibrillation and sudden death.[82] Recent studies suggest that mutations of this gene account for no more than 1% of cases of hypertrophic cardiomyopathy.[82]

Mitochondrial Cardiomyopathies

Primary mitochondrial disorders are caused by sporadic or inherited mutations in nuclear or mitochondrial DNA that may be transmitted as autosomal dominant, autosomal recessive, X-linked, or maternal traits. The most frequent abnormalities occur in genes that encode the respiratory chain protein complexes, leading to impaired utilisation of oxygen and reduced production of energy. The clinical presentation of mitochondrial disease is variable in age at onset, symptoms, and range and severity of involvement of the different organs. Numerous case reports and small series have described cardiovascular abnormalities in patients with primary mitochondrial dysfunction, but data on the prevalence of cardiac disease is sparse, and mostly derived from experience in children. Cardiac involvement is a feature in up to two-fifths of mitochondrial encephalomyopathies,[83] and usually takes the form of a hypertrophic cardiomyopathy,[84] although other cardiomyopathies, including dilated and left ventricular non-compaction, are reported.[83] Children with mitochondrial disease and cardiac involvement present earlier than those with non-cardiac disease[83,84] and have a much worse prognosis, with one study reporting survival of no more than one-fifth at 16 years, compared with 95% for those without cardiac involvement.[83] The cardiac phenotype is usually concentric left ventricular hypertrophy without obstruction of the outflow tract, and rapid progression to left ventricular dilation, systolic impairment, and cardiac failure.[83,84] Sudden arrhythmic death has also been reported.[83,84] Kearns-Sayre syndrome is a mitochondrial disorder comprising the triad of chronic progressive external ophthalmoplegia, retinitis pigmentosa, and atrioventricular block.[85] Cardiac manifestations occur in over half the patients, and include syncope, congestive cardiac failure, and cardiac arrest.[86] The conduction system is frequently affected, with rapid progression to complete heart block associated with death in up to one-fifth.[87]

Friedreich's Ataxia

Friedreich's ataxia is an autosomal recessive condition caused by mutations in the frataxin gene. Cardiac involvement is very common, and is most commonly, but not exclusively, characterised by concentric left ventricular hypertrophy without obstruction to the left ventricular outflow tract.[88] Patients are usually asymptomatic, although progression to left ventricular dilation and cardiac failure is described.[89] Rarely, children with Friedreich's ataxia can present with left ventricular hypertrophy several years before the development of neurological signs.[88] Treatment with the antioxidant idebenone appears to reduce the degree of left ventricular hypertrophy,[90] but further studies are needed to assess the long-term effects.

Anderson-Fabry Disease

Anderson-Fabry disease is an X-linked lysosomal storage disorder caused by mutations in the α-galactosidase A gene. The resultant enzymic deficiency causes progressive accumulation of glycosphingolipid in the skin, nervous system, kidneys, and heart.[91] Cardiac manifestations include progressive left ventricular hypertrophy, valvar disease, and abnormalities of conduction, with supraventricular and ventricular arrhythmias appearing after adolescence in males and females.[91–94] Treatment with recombinant α-galactosidase A improves renal and neurological manifestations, as well as quality of life, but its effect on the cardiac manifestations is still under investigation.[91]

Pompe's Disease

Pompe's disease, or acid maltase deficiency or glycogen storage disease IIa, is an autosomal recessive disorder with infantile, juvenile, and adult variants that differ with respect to age of onset, rate of progression, and extent of involvement of the tissues. The infantile and childhood forms are characterised by deposition of myocardial glycogen, massive cardiac hypertrophy, and cardiac failure. The infantile form presents in the first few months of life with severe skeletal muscular hypotonia, progressive weakness, cardiomegaly, hepatomegaly, and macroglossia, and is usually fatal before 2 years of age owing to cardiorespiratory failure. Obstruction of the left ventricular outflow tract occurs in one-twentieth of patients.[95] The electrocardiogram typically shows broad high-voltage QRS complexes and ventricular pre-excitation. In the variants presenting in juveniles and adults, disease is usually limited to skeletal muscle, with a slowly progressive proximal myopathy and weakness of the respiratory muscles. Replacement with recombinant enzymes appears to cause regression of left ventricular hypertrophy in those with presentation during childhood, and is associated with improved survival.[96]

Infants of Diabetic Mothers

Infants of diabetic mothers can develop transient asymptomatic left ventricular hypertrophy[97] that affects both ventricles, and generally resolves within 3 to 6 months. Rare reports of fatal hypertrophic cardiomyopathy in infants of diabetic mothers are described.[98] The aetiology is unknown, but may relate to increased levels of maternal insulin-like growth factor.[99]

Pathology

Macroscopic Features

In the common form of autosomal dominant hypertrophic cardiomyopathy, myocardial hypertrophy is usually asymmetric, affecting the ventricular septum more than the posterior or lateral walls of the left ventricle.[100,101] Other patterns also occur, including concentric (Fig. 49-1), mid-ventricular, sometimes associated with a left ventricular apical diverticulum,[102] and apical hypertrophy.[103–105] Co-existent right ventricular hypertrophy is present in up to one-fifth of cases.[100] The papillary muscles are often displaced anteriorly, contributing in one-quarter to systolic anterior motion in the resting state of the aortic, and in one-tenth, the mural, leaflets of the mitral valve. There is often an area of endocardial fibrosis on the septum beneath the aortic valve, caused by repeated contact with the aortic leaflet.[100,101] The mitral valve itself is often structurally abnormal, with elongation of the aortic leaflet, an increased number of scallops in the mural leaflet, and occasional direct insertion of the papillary muscle into the ventricular surface of the aortic leaflet.[106] Myocardial bridging of the anterior interventricular coronary artery has been observed in adults and children with hypertrophic cardiomyopathy, and may cause myocardial ischaemia.[107,108]

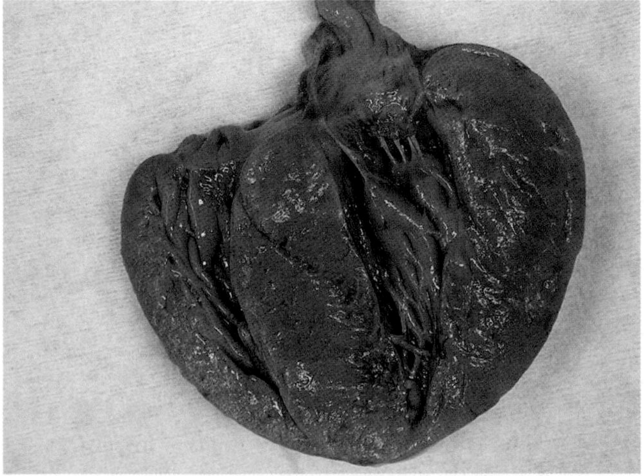

Figure 49-1 The gross pathological specimen shows concentric left ventricular hypertrophy in an 8-week-old infant with mitochondrial disease. (Courtesy of Dr Michael Ashworth, Great Ormond Street Hospital, London, United Kingdom.)

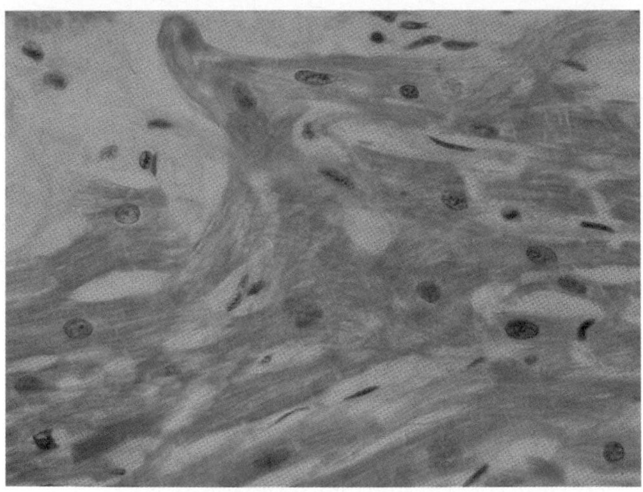

Figure 49-2 Histopathological slide of hypertrophic cardiomyopathy showing myocyte disarray and interstitial fibrosis. (Courtesy of Dr Michael Ashworth, Great Ormond Street Hospital, London, United Kingdom.)

Microscopic Features

The histological hallmarks of the familial variant are the triad of myocytic hypertrophy, myocytic disarray, and interstitial fibrosis (Fig. 49-2).[100,101] Myocytic disarray is characterised by architectural disorganisation of the myocardium, with adjacent myocytes aligned obliquely or perpendicular to each other in association with increased interstitial collagen.[100,101] The myofibrillary architecture within the myocyte itself is also disorganised, with loss of the normal parallel arrangement of the myofibrils. Although disarray occurs in many pathologies, the presence of extensive disarray, more than one-tenth of the ventricular myocardium, is thought to be a highly specific marker for hypertrophic cardiomyopathy.[100,101] Small intramural coronary arteries are often dysplastic and narrowed due to mural thickening by hyperplasia of the smooth muscle cells.[109]

Pathophysiology

Diastolic Function

The major pathophysiological consequence of left ventricular hypertrophy is impairment of left ventricular diastolic properties. Diastolic dysfunction results from abnormalities in both the active component of actin and myosin dissociation in the early filling phase, and the passive properties of the ventricle that affect compliance.[16,110–113] Prolonged or incomplete left ventricular relaxation results in a reduced rate and magnitude of rapid filling. This in turn leads to reduced left ventricular diastolic volume, reduced stroke volume, and altered diastolic relationships of pressure and volume. The net result is elevation of left ventricular end-diastolic pressures and symptoms of reduced exercise tolerance, dyspnoea, and pulmonary oedema.

Systolic Dysfunction

Global measures of left ventricular systolic function are often normal, but progression to left ventricular dilation and systolic impairment is a recognised complication in a subgroup of patients. Predicting which patients are at risk of developing end-stage disease remains a challenge, and the subject of ongoing research. Several studies have identified a number of markers associated with progression to systolic impairment. These include syncope, non-sustained ventricular tachycardia, an abnormal response of the blood pressure to exercise,[47] young age at diagnosis,[37,41] and severe microvascular dysfunction, as assessed by positron emission tomography.[114] A family history of end-stage disease may also be a useful predictor of left ventricular remodelling.[41] Several studies have identified increased left ventricular mural thickness[37,47,48] and cavity dimensions, particularly an increased end-systolic dimension,[41,47] as predictors of progression to left ventricular dilation and systolic impairment, although the predictive value of these and other markers remains to be evaluated in large prospective studies. Although case reports of end-stage disease in children are documented,[36,115] progression to this phase in childhood is extremely rare. Whether onset of hypertrophic cardiomyopathy in infancy or early childhood predisposes individuals to developing end-stage disease is unknown.

Obstruction of the Left Ventricular Outflow Tract

Approximately one-quarter of children and adults with hypertrophic cardiomyopathy have obstructed left ventricular outflow tracts at rest.[16,29,116] The problem is caused by contact between the aortic leaflet, and occasionally the mural leaflet, of the mitral valve and the ventricular septum. The most widely accepted explanation for this phenomenon is that septal hypertrophy and narrowing of the left ventricular outflow tract produce a zone of high velocity anterior to the mitral valve that causes its aortic leaflet to be sucked against the septum by the Venturi effect. This hypothesis does not explain a number of features associated with systolic anterior motion, in particular, the fact that it begins prior to opening of the aortic valve, and that it can occur in patients with little or no septal hypertrophy. Experimental and observational data suggests that anterior displacement of the papillary muscles and submitral apparatus are necessary to create sufficient slack in the leaflets to permit them to move forward in systole. The effect of enhancing contractility in this model is to increase the drag forces on the leaflet, thereby driving rather than sucking it into the septum.

Many patients without obstruction at rest have gradients that can be provoked by physiological and pharmacological interventions that diminish left ventricular end-diastolic volume or increase left ventricular contractility. Labile obstruction refers to the spontaneous appearance and disappearance of obstruction, while latent obstruction describes those gradients that are present only with provocation. The most commonly used techniques used to provoke obstruction are inhalation of amyl nitrate, the Valsalva manoeuvre, and administration of intravenous inotropes. Increasingly, upright exercise is used to provoke gradients in patients with exertional symptoms.[117] Obstruction causes acute reductions in cardiac output, elevated left ventricular filling pressures, and myocardial ischaemia. Corresponding symptoms include chest pain, exertional dyspnoea, presyncope, and syncope.

Arrhythmia

All arrhythmias increase in frequency with advancing age. In adults, atrial fibrillation is the commonest sustained arrhythmia, with an incidence of approximately 2% per year.[118] During follow-up, as many as one-quarter of patients develop paroxysmal or chronic atrial fibrillation, which is associated with increased risk of thromboembolic stroke and death from cardiac failure, but not with sudden death.[5,118] Atrial fibrillation is rare in children and young adults, although paroxysms of haemodynamically compromising atrial fibrillation have been documented in individuals as young as 15 years.[119] Factors that increase the likelihood of atrial fibrillation include older age, worsening functional class, and left atrial enlargement as a result of an obstructed left ventricular outflow tract or severe diastolic left ventricular dysfunction.[118]

The characteristic features of myocytic disarray and interstitial fibrosis seen in hypertrophic cardiomyopathy represent a potent substrate for ventricular arrhythmia. Furthermore, the presence of microvascular and coronary arterial abnormalities identified in some patients, and the haemodynamic alterations caused by the obstructed outflow tract, predispose patients to myocardial ischaemia,[120–122] which is in itself a potential trigger for ventricular arrhythmias. In keeping with this, sudden arrhythmic death is the commonest mode of death, including in children and adolescents.[25] Despite this, ventricular arrhythmia is rarely identified in life in children.[119] Isolated uniform ventricular extrasystoles are documented in up to three-tenths of children and adolescents, multi-form ectopics in one-tenth, and ventricular couplets in another tenth. Frequent ventricular extrasystoles, greater than 100 in 24 hours, however, are exceedingly rare. Furthermore, non-sustained ventricular tachycardia occurs in less than one-tenth of children and adolescents.[119] If present, it is a particularly poor prognostic indicator.[27,29,123] Greater maximal left ventricular mural thickness and left atrial size may be associated with the development of non-sustained ventricular tachycardia.[123]

Patients that have been successfully resuscitated from sustained ventricular arrhythmias such as ventricular tachycardia or ventricular fibrillation are at a high risk of further events.[124] Interrogation of tracings from implantable cardioverter-defibrillators preceding appropriate discharges for sustained ventricular arrhythmias demonstrates that ventricular fibrillation is often preceded by sinus tachycardia, atrial arrhythmia, and ventricular tachycardia.[124,125] The mechanisms by which other tachyarrhythmias trigger ventricular fibrillation have not been fully elucidated, but myocardial ischaemia and abnormal vascular responses may play a role.[124]

Clinical Features

Symptoms

Most individuals with hypertrophic cardiomyopathy have few, if any, symptoms. The initial diagnosis is often made as a result of family screening, following the incidental detection of a heart murmur or an abnormal electrocardiogram. Presentation in infancy can be associated with symptoms of cardiac failure, such as breathlessness, poor feeding, excessive sweating, and failure to thrive.[33–35,126,127] These symptoms usually occur in the presence of apparently normal left ventricular systolic function and are attributable to an obstructed outflow tract or to diastolic dysfunction.

In older children, the most common symptoms are dyspnoea and chest pain. Chest pain is commonly exertional, but may be atypical, and can also occur at rest or following large meals. Typically, there is considerable day-to-day variation in the amount of activity required to produce symptoms.[27,28] Syncope is a relatively common symptom, for which there are multiple mechanisms, including obstruction of the left ventricular outflow tract, abnormal vascular responses, and atrial and ventricular arrhythmias.[16,128,129] Unexplained or exertional syncope is associated with increased risk of sudden death in children and adolescents.

Physical Examination

General physical examination may provide important diagnostic clues in patients with associated syndromes or metabolic disorders. Clinical examination of the cardiovascular system is often normal, but in patients with obstruction of the left ventricular outflow tract, a number of typical features may be identified. The arterial pulse has a rapid upstroke and downstroke, resulting from rapid ejection during the initial phase of systole, followed by a sudden decrease in cardiac output during mid-systole. This is, occasionally, followed by a palpable reflected wave, resulting in a bisferiens pulse. Examination of the jugular venous pulsation may reveal a prominent a wave, caused by reduced right ventricular compliance. Palpation of the precordium may reveal a sustained, or double, apex beat, reflecting a palpable atrial impulse followed by left ventricular contraction. An additional late systolic impulse may rarely result in a triple apical impulse.

On auscultation, patients with the obstructive variant of hypertrophic cardiomyopathy have an ejection systolic murmur that is heard loudest at the left sternal edge, and which radiates to the right upper sternal edge and apex, but usually not to the carotid arteries or axilla. This murmur may be associated with a palpable precordial thrill. As the obstruction in hypertrophic cardiomyopathy is a dynamic phenomenon, the intensity of the murmur is increased by manoeuvres that reduce the preload or afterload, such as standing from a squatting position and the Valsalva manoeuvre. Most patients with obstruction of the left ventricular outflow tract also have mitral regurgitation, resulting from failure of coaptation of the leaflets during systolic anterior motion of the valve. This causes a pansystolic, high-frequency murmur at the apex, radiating to the axilla.

Investigations

The routine investigation comprises a number of noninvasive assessments that aim to establish or confirm the diagnosis, to evaluate the mechanism of symptoms, and to identify predictors of sudden cardiac death and other disease-related complications.

Electrocardiography

The resting 12-lead electrocardiogram is abnormal in up to 95% of individuals. A variety of patterns are recognised (Fig. 49-3). The most common abnormalities include repolarisation abnormalities, pathological Q waves, most frequently in the inferolateral leads, and left atrial enlargement. Common patterns of abnormal repolarisation include inverted T waves and changes in the ST segments in leads I, aVL, V5, and V6, in leads II, III, and aVF, or in leads V1 to V4. Left-axis deviation, with a mean frontal QRS axis between −15 degrees and −90 degrees is common.[10] Intraventricular conduction delay is not uncommon, but bundle branch block, usually involving the left bundle, is infrequent. Voltage criterions for left ventricular hypertrophy alone are not specific for hypertrophic cardiomyopathy, and are often seen in normal, healthy teenagers and young adults. In infants, right ventricular hypertrophy is commonly found. Other recognised patterns include the presence of giant negative T waves in the mid-precordial leads, which are characteristic of hypertrophic cardiomyopathy localised to the distal portion of the left ventricle.[130] It is not uncommon for the corrected QT interval to be slightly prolonged. Some patients have a short PR interval not associated with the Wolff-Parkinson-White syndrome. Atrioventricular conduction delay, including first-degree block, is rare except in particular subtypes, such as in association with PRKAG2 mutations and mitochondrial disease.[131,132]

Echocardiography

The presence on echocardiography of a left ventricular mural thickness greater than two standard deviations above the corrected mean relative to body surface area in any myocardial segment, in the absence of any other cardiac or systemic disease capable of producing a similar degree of hypertrophy, is sufficient for the diagnosis.[5] The focus of early studies using M-mode interrogation was on the detection of asymmetrical septal hypertrophy, using a ratio between the diastolic thickness of the anterior septum and the left ventricular posterior wall of 1.3 to 1 as a diagnostic criterion.[133] Such an increased ratio, however, is commonly found in normal neonates, and in children with congenital cardiac disease.[134] The advent of cross sectional interrogation showed that any pattern of left ventricular hypertrophy is consistent with the diagnosis, including concentric equal hypertrophy across all segments of the left ventricle, eccentric hypertrophy with the lateral and posterior walls more affected than the septum, distal hypertrophy with the distal segments more affected than basal segments, and apical hypertrophy confined to the left ventricular apex (Fig. 49-4).[14,104,135,136]

Dynamic obstruction in the left ventricular outflow tract is associated with mid-systolic closure of the aortic valve, often associated with coarse fluttering of the aortic valve (Fig. 49-5A) on M-mode echocardiography. Obstruction of the left ventricular outflow tract can be detected using colour flow Doppler, and quantified using continuous-wave Doppler (see Fig. 49-5B and C). Due to the dynamic nature of the obstruction of the left ventricular outflow tract, serial measurements of maximal gradients may not provide an accurate reflection of progression or stability. Surrogate measures of severity, such as left atrial dilation, should be documented. In some patients, systolic obliteration of the ventricular cavity may produce a high-velocity gradient in the mid-ventricle. Obstruction of the right ventricular outflow tract may be seen in infants, and in older children and adults with cardiomyopathy associated with Noonan's syndrome and some metabolic disorders.

Most patients with systolic anterior motion of the mitral valve and obstruction of the left ventricular outflow tract have mitral regurgitation with a posteriorly directed jet, which can be detected using colour Doppler imaging. The severity of regurgitation correlates with the degree of obstruction in individual patients, but varies considerably between patients with obstruction of similar severity. The presence of complex mitral regurgitant jets, such as those directed anteriorly or centrally, should trigger a search for other valvar abnormalities, such as prolapse of leaflets.

Left ventricular global systolic function, as assessed from change in ventricular volume during the cardiac cycle, is typically increased. Regional and long-axis function is often

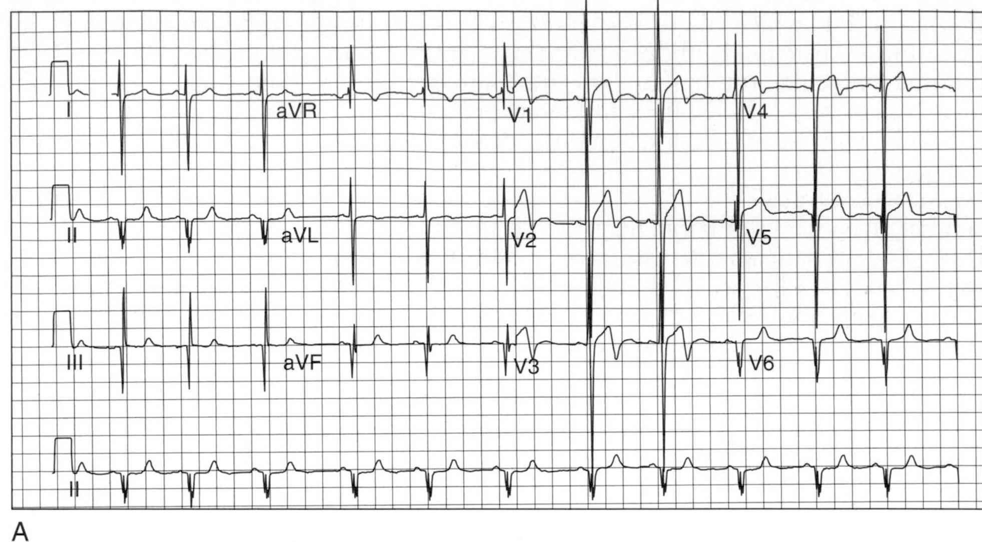

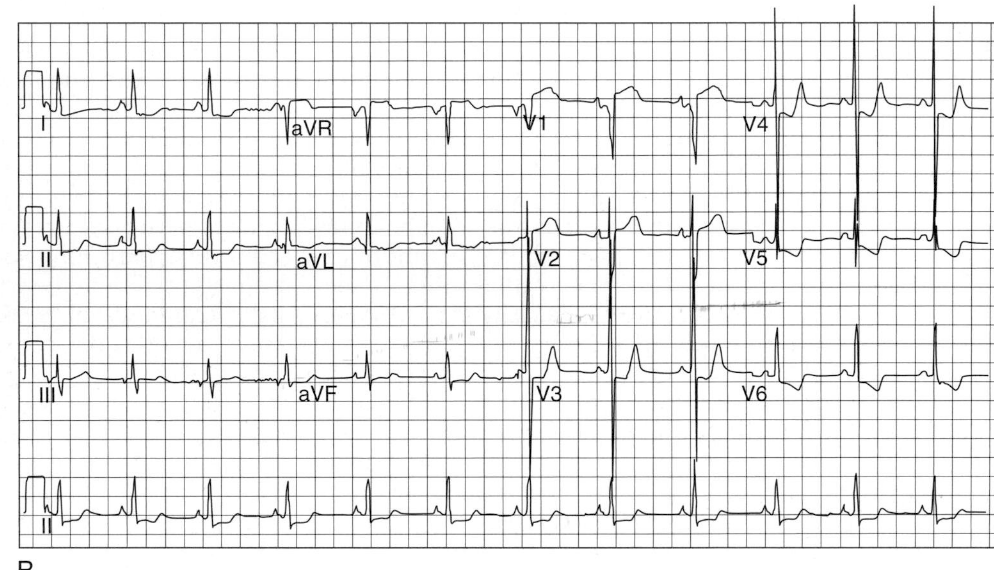

Figure 49-3 Electrocardiographic patterns in hypertrophic cardiomyopathy. **A** shows a 12-lead ECG from a 12-year-old child with asymmetric septal hypertrophy. Note the pathological Q waves in leads II, III, aVF, V5, and V6, and voltage criterions for biventricular hypertrophy. **B** is a 12-lead tracing from an 8-year-old with severe hypertrophic obstructive cardiomyopathy, showing left ventricular hypertrophy and T wave inversion and ST segment abnormalities in leads I, aVL, and V4–V6.

reduced, and responses of cardiac output during exercise may be impaired.[137–139] A small proportion of adults develop progressive thinning of the myocardium, associated with left ventricular systolic impairment and cavity dilation, but progression to this end-stage disease is rare in children.

Diastolic function is commonly assessed using pulsed wave Doppler to interrogate the mitral inflow and pulmonary veins, along with tissue Doppler imaging (Fig. 49-6). Patients may have evidence of impaired relaxation as shown by E/A wave reversal and increased E-wave deceleration time on the Doppler interrogation of the mitral inflow, with a ratio of the systolic to the diastolic waves of greater than 1 on pulmonary vein Doppler, and the duration of the atrial reversal wave seen in the pulmonary veins less than the duration of the mitral inflow A wave (see Fig. 49-6). With worsening diastolic function, a pseudonormal pattern is seen, with normalisation of the mitral inflow E/A ratio and prolongation of the E wave deceleration time, decreased pulmonary venous systolic velocity, increased pulmonary venous diastolic and atrial reversal velocities, pulmonary venous atrial reversal wave duration greater than mitral inflow A wave duration, and decreased velocity of the propagation slope on colour M-mode (see Fig. 49-6). In some patients, a restrictive phenotype is present, characterised by an increased mitral inflow E/A ratio, reduced E wave deceleration time, and increased pulmonary vein A reversal wave velocity.[140] The velocity of the pulmonary venous atrial reversal wave has been shown to correlate with left ventricular filling pressures.[141] Tissue Doppler imaging, and strain and strain rate imaging, can also be used to assess diastolic and systolic function. These techniques have the advantage of being less dependent on loading conditions.[141–145] Characteristically, patients with diastolic left ventricular impairment demonstrate reduced early diastolic velocities in the mitral annulus and septum, and reversal of the ratio of early to late diastolic velocities. In addition, the ratio of mitral inflow E wave to annular early diastolic velocity can be used as a measure of left ventricular end-diastolic pressure, and predicts exercise capacity.[142,143] Tissue Doppler imaging may be useful in detecting mild disease in otherwise phenotypically normal gene carriers.[144,146]

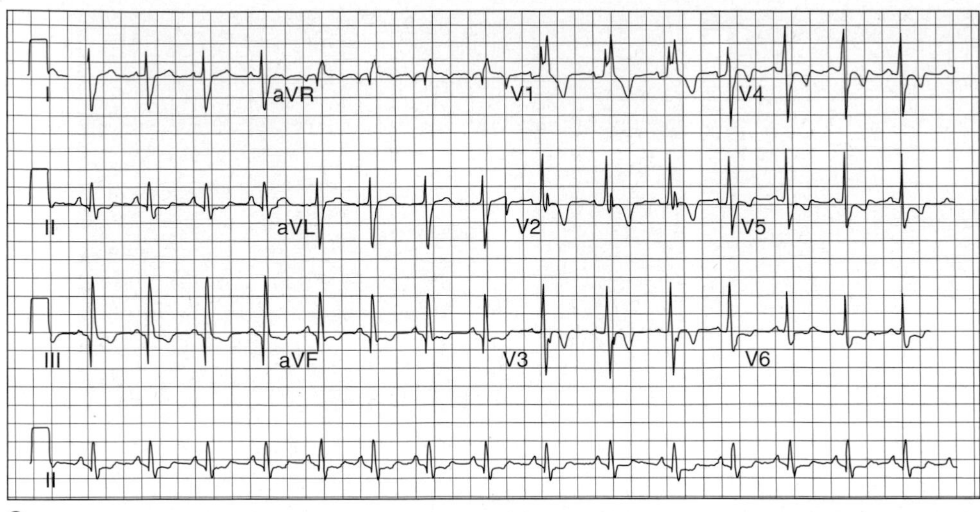

C

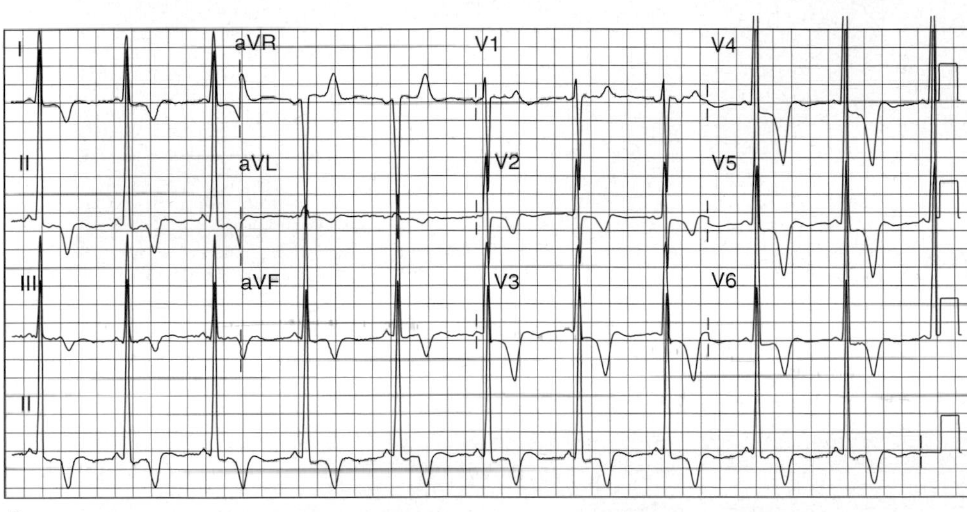

D

Figure 49-3—cont'd C is another 12-lead tracing, but from a 14-year-old with concentric left ventricular hypertrophy. It shows T wave inversion extending from V1 to V5, and deep Q waves in leads III and aVF. **D** is a 12-lead tracing from a young adult with apical hypertrophic cardiomyopathy. It shows widespread T wave inversion, with deep inverted T waves, particularly in the septal leads.

Ambulatory Electrocardiography

The frequency of arrhythmias detected during ambulatory electrocardiographic monitoring is age related.[119,147–149] In adults, 48-hour monitoring reveals supraventricular arrhythmias in up to half the patients, and non-sustained ventricular tachycardia in one-quarter. Most episodes of the latter arrhythmia are relatively slow, asymptomatic, and occur during periods of increased vagal tone. Sustained ventricular tachycardia is uncommon, but may occur in association with apical aneurysms.[150] As discussed above, the frequency of arrhythmia in childhood is much lower, but the presence of ventricular arrhythmia in particular is a marker of poor prognosis.[27,29,119]

Cardiopulmonary Exercise Testing

Individuals usually have a reduced peak consumption of oxygen compared with healthy age-matched controls, even when asymptomatic.[151,152] In children, exercise capacity and peak consumption of oxygen correlate with diastolic impairment.[143,153] Up to one-quarter of adults have an abnormal response of blood pressure to exercise,[154,155] related to abnormal vasodilation of the non-exercising vascular beds, possibly triggered by inappropriate firing of left ventricular baroreceptors[128] and an impaired response of cardiac output.[156] An abnormal response to exercise is associated with an increased risk of sudden death in young adults.[157] In children, the use of cardiopulmonary exercise testing as a tool for stratification of risk has not been evaluated, but there are several problems associated with the technique. Very young children, usually under the age of 7 or 8 years, cannot reliably perform exercise testing, and flat responses are normal in pre-adolescents. The technique, nevertheless, remains a useful tool for the evaluation of severity and response to treatment in older teenagers.

Cardiac Magnetic Resonance Imaging

Like echocardiography, cardiac magnetic resonance imaging can assess the distribution and severity of left ventricular hypertrophy and provide functional measurements of systolic and diastolic function. The technique is particularly useful in the evaluation of patients with hypertrophy of the lateral wall, an area that can be difficult to visualise adequately using cross sectional echocardiography. In addition, magnetic resonance imaging can be used to assess myocardial tissue characteristics during life using gadolinium contrast agents (Fig. 49-7). As many as four-fifths of adults have areas of patchy hyper-enhancement, the extent of which appears to correlate with risk factors

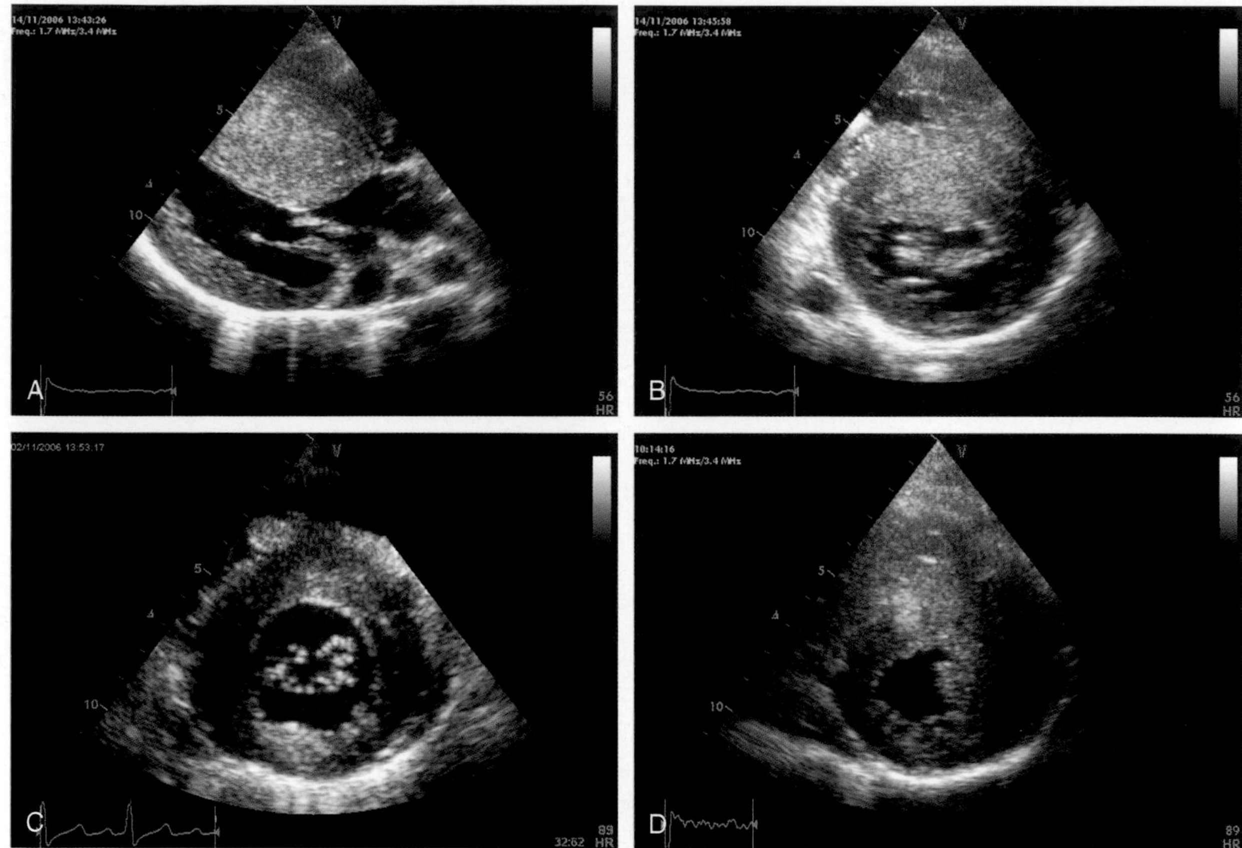

Figure 49-4 Echocardiographic patterns of hypertrophic cardiomyopathy. **A** shows a parasternal long-axis view of a 13-year-old with severe asymmetrical septal hypertrophy. The parasternal short-axis view of the same patient is shown in **B**. **C** shows the parasternal short-axis view from a 12-year-old with concentric left ventricular hypertrophy. **D** is a parasternal short-axis view from a 14-year-old with an eccentric distribution of left ventricular hypertrophy.

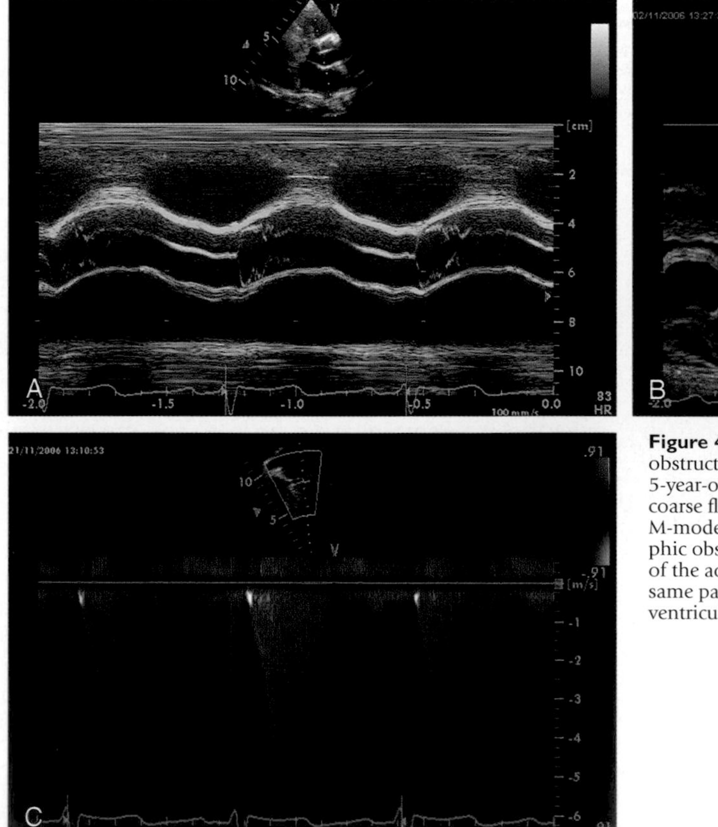

Figure 49-5 Echocardiographic features of left ventricular outflow tract obstruction. **A** shows an M-mode tracing of the aortic valve from a 5-year-old with severe obstructive hypertrophic cardiomyopathy, showing coarse fluttering and mid-systolic closure of the leaflets. **B** is another M-mode recording, but of the mitral valve from a 12-year-old with hypertrophic obstructive cardiomyopathy showing complete systolic anterior motion of the aortic mitral valvar leaflet. **C** is a continuous wave Doppler from the same patient, showing the characteristic waveform of the obstructed left ventricular outflow tract, in this case with a maximal velocity of nearly 5 m/s.

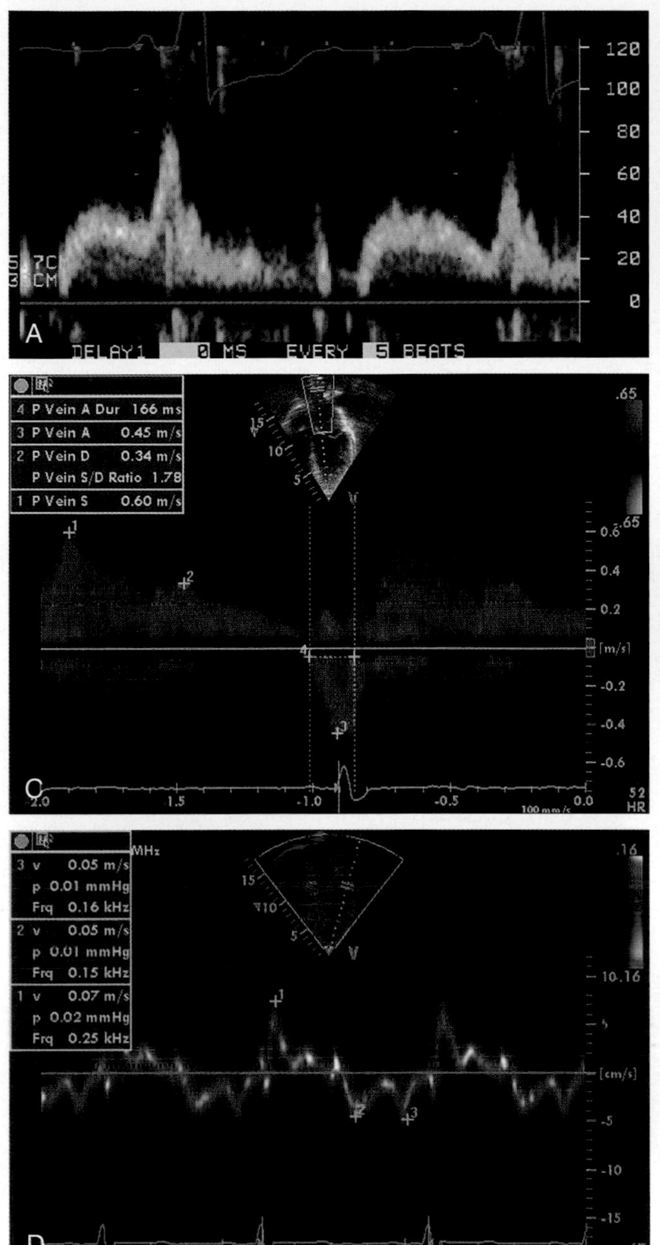

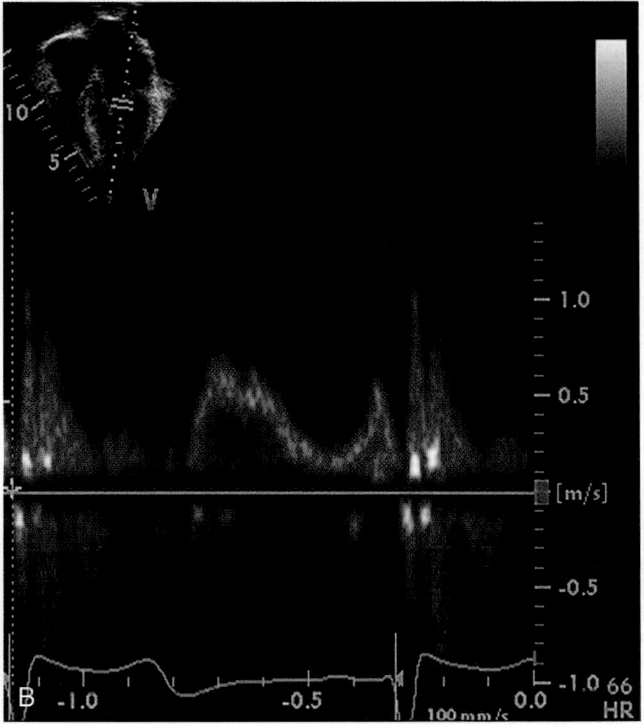

Figure 49-6 The panels show the echocardiographic features of left ventricular diastolic impairment. **A** is a pulsed wave Doppler tracing of the mitral inflow from a 7-year-old with hypertrophic cardiomyopathy. It shows E/A wave reversal and a prolonged E wave deceleration time, characteristic of impaired relaxation of the left ventricle. **B** is another pulsed wave Doppler recording of a 15-year-old, showing pseudo-normalisation of the pattern of mitral inflow, with a normal E/A ratio but prolonged E wave deceleration time. **C** is a pulsed wave Doppler recording in the right upper pulmonary vein in a 14-year-old with severe hypertrophic cardiomyopathy, showing impaired relaxation of the left ventricle, characterised by a reduced diastolic wave and increased atrial reversal wave. **D** is a pulsed wave tissue Doppler recording of the lateral mitral annulus in a 13-year-old with hypertrophic cardiomyopathy showing reduced systolic (Sa), early diastolic (Ea), and late diastolic (Aa) velocities.

for sudden death and with progressive left ventricular remodelling.[158,159]

Other Imaging Modalities

Cardiac catheterisation and angiography are no longer used routinely in the assessment of children, as structural and haemodynamic data is easily obtained using non-invasive techniques. Coronary arteriography may demonstrate myocardial bridging and systolic compression of the epicardial and intramural coronary arteries, but the clinical significance of this observation remains controversial.[108,121,122] Myocardial perfusion scanning using radioisotopes such as thallium-201 has been used to study the pathophysiology of myocardial ischaemia. Although an association between impaired myocardial perfusion and a history of syncope or resuscitated cardiac arrest has been reported in children,[160] larger studies in young adults showed no association between reversible perfusion defects and exertional chest pain or electrocardiographic ST segment changes.[161,162]

Management

Management focuses on three main areas, namely, the counselling of other family members, management of symptoms, and the prevention of disease-related complications.

Family Evaluation

All patients should be counselled on the implications of the diagnosis for their families. Careful analysis of the pedigree can reassure relatives who are not at risk of inheriting the disease.[5] For those who may be at risk, clinical screening with electrocardiograms and echocardiography may be appropriate after counselling. Current guidelines recommend screening with a 12-lead electrocardiogram and echocardiogram at intervals of 12 to 18 months, usually

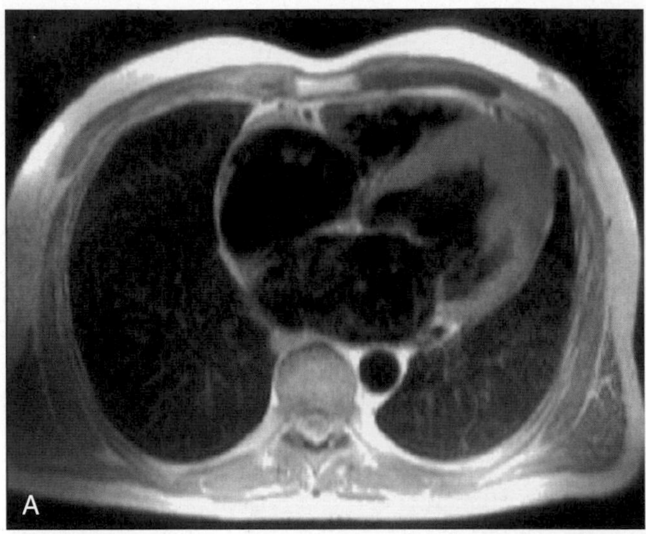

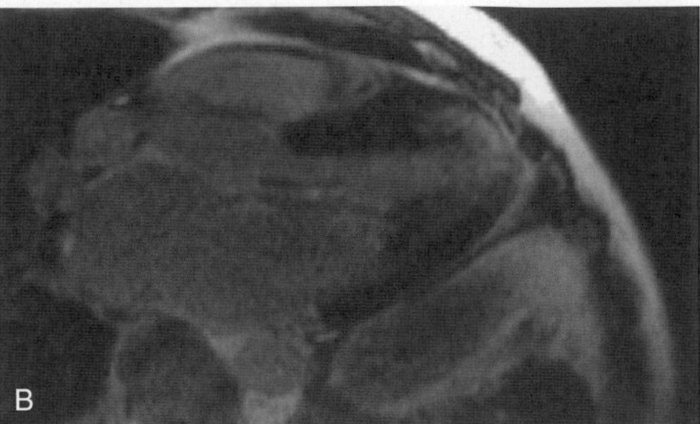

Figure 49-7 Cardiac magnetic resonance imaging in hypertrophic cardiomyopathy. A shows black-blood HASTE imaging of a child with apical hypertrophic cardiomyopathy. **B** shows late gadolinium enhancement of the apical region in the same patient. (Courtesy of Dr Marina Hughes, Great Ormond Street Hospital, London, United Kingdom.)

starting at the age of 12 years, unless there is a malignant family history of premature sudden death, the child is symptomatic or a competitive athlete in intensive training, or there is a clinical suspicion of left ventricular hypertrophy. Screening continues until full growth and maturation are achieved, usually by the age of 18 to 21 years. Following this, if there are no signs of phenotypic expression, screening approximately every 5 years is advised, as the onset of left ventricular hypertrophy may be delayed until well into adulthood in some families.[55,163–168]

It is now possible to offer relatively rapid genetic testing to individuals with unequivocal disease. If a mutation causing disease is identified, relatives can be offered predictive testing. Again, this should be performed only after appropriate genetic counselling and consideration of issues relating to autonomy, confidentiality and psychosocial harm, including loss of self-esteem, stigmatisation or discrimination, and guilt.

Treatment of Symptoms Caused by Obstruction of the Left Ventricular Outflow Tract

By convention, obstruction of the left ventricular outflow tract is defined as a pressure gradient greater than or equal to 30 mm Hg,[12,104] but theoretical models examining the relationship between the gradient and stroke volume predict that only gradients in excess of 50 mm Hg are likely to represent significant obstruction to ventricular ejection.[104] The first-line strategy for control of symptoms in patients with obstructive disease is medical therapy with β-adrenergic receptor blockers, such as propranolol, given at 1 to 2 mg/kg per dose, or more cardioselective drugs such as atenolol, metoprolol, nadolol, and bisoprolol. At standard doses, β-blockers can reduce symptoms of chest pain, dyspnoea, and presyncope on exertion, although they probably do not reduce obstruction under resting conditions. Studies using very large doses of propranolol, up to 23 mg/kg per day, in children and adolescents have reported improved long-term survival,[169] but this is not generally accepted practice, as side effects of β-blockers are common, and even moderate doses can affect growth and school performance in young children, or trigger depression in children and adolescents.[5] If β-blockade is unsuccessful, the addition of the class I antiarrhythmic disopyramide can reduce obstruction and improve symptoms.[170–172] This effect is exerted via its negative inotropic action. Disopyramide is usually well tolerated in children, but initiation at a low dose is recommended, as some patients may experience marked anticholinergic effects. As disopyramide causes accelerated atrioventricular nodal conduction, and may increase the ventricular rate during atrial fibrillation, it is usually administered in combination with a β-blocker. Disopyramide causes prolongation of the QT interval, and so the electrocardiogram must be monitored regularly. Other drugs that prolong the QT interval, such as sotalol or amiodarone, should be avoided.

The calcium antagonist verapamil improves symptoms caused by obstruction, probably by relieving myocardial ischaemia and reducing myocardial contractility.[110,173] Chronic oral therapy has been shown to be effective in children with both obstructive and non-obstructive forms of the disease.[174] Side effects include constipation and hair loss. In patients with severe symptoms caused by large gradients and pulmonary hypertension, verapamil can cause severe haemodynamic deterioration,[175,176] and so should be used with caution.

Several options are available to patients with obstructive hypertrophic cardiomyopathy who do not tolerate drugs, or whose symptoms are refractory to medical therapy. The gold standard[177–181] is septal myotomy or myectomy, in which a trough of muscle is removed from the ventricular septum via an aortic incision. Recently, extended myectomies to the level of the papillary muscle have been performed.[182] In the hands of experienced surgeons, the mortality is less than 1%, and the rate of success is high, with complete and permanent abolition of the gradient, and a marked improvement in symptoms and exercise capacity in over nine-tenths of patients. Non-fatal complications include complete heart block requiring insertion of a permanent pacemaker in less than one-twentieth of patients, and inadvertent creation of small ventricular septal defects. In most cases, a single procedure is required to achieve a permanent reduction in gradient, but repeated operations may be needed in very young children, possibly resulting from a limited initial myectomy due to a small aortic diameter, or from continued remodeling of the left ventricular outflow tract.

Atrioventricular, or dual-chamber, pacing has been shown to reduce gradients in uncontrolled, observational studies including one performed in children,[183–185] and in two randomised controlled clinical trials. The randomised trials showed no objective improvement in exercise capacity and a symptomatic effect no better than placebo,[186,187] except possibly in elderly patients with relatively mild hypertrophy.

An alternative to surgery for adults with obstructive disease is ablation of the ventricular septum by injection of 95% alcohol into a septal perforating coronary artery. This produces an area of localised myocardial necrosis within the basal septum.[188,189] Myocardial damage is kept to a minimum by first visualising the area supplied by the perforator branch using echocardiographic contrast injection.[190] Although short-term results are promising, the long-term effects are unknown, and there is potential for the resulting myocardial scar to act as a substrate for ventricular arrhythmia and sudden death. This, and the fact that the results in children and adolescents are often suboptimal, means that alcohol septal ablation is not recommended for use in this age group.

Management of Symptoms in Non-obstructive Disease

In patients without obstruction of the left ventricular outflow tract, chest pain and dyspnoea are usually caused by diastolic dysfunction and myocardial ischaemia. Treatment in this group of patients is empirical, and often suboptimal. Both β-blockers and calcium antagonists such as verapamil and diltiazem can improve symptoms by improving left ventricular relaxation and filling, reducing left ventricular contractility, and relieving myocardial ischaemia. Other drugs, such as nitrates and inhibitors of angiotensin-converting enzyme, may be beneficial in some patients, but should be used with caution in those in whom obstruction can be provoked, as they can exacerbate the gradient by virtue of their vasodilating effects. Adults who develop end-stage disease should receive conventional treatment for cardiac failure, including inhibition of angiotensin-converting enzymes, and use of angiotensin II receptor antagonists, spironolactone, β-blockers such as carvedilol or metoprolol, digoxin, and if necessary, cardiac transplantation.

Prevention of Sudden Cardiac Death

Although the overall risk of sudden death in children and adults is only approximately 1% per year, a significant minority of individuals have a much greater risk of ventricular arrhythmia and sudden death.[191] The mechanism of sudden death is thought to be ventricular arrhythmia in the majority, and several triggers are recognised, including atrial arrhythmia, myocardial ischaemia, and exercise.[192] The most reliable predictor is a history of previous cardiac arrest.[124,193] In patients without such a history, the most clinically useful markers of risk are a family history of sudden cardiac death,[27,194] unexplained syncope unrelated to neurocardiogenic mechanisms, a flat or hypotensive response of blood pressure to upright exercise,[155,157,195] non-sustained ventricular tachycardia on ambulatory electrocardiographic monitoring or during exercise,[123,147,157] and severe left ventricular hypertrophy on echocardiography, defined as a maximal left ventricular wall thickness of 30 mm or more.[196,197] Importantly, these markers of increased risk can all be identified non-invasively. Studies have shown that patients with none of these features have a low risk of sudden death, less than 1% per year, whereas those with two or more risk factors are at substantially higher risk of dying suddenly, with an estimated annual mortality rate of 3% for those with two risk factors, rising to 6% in those with three or more risk factors.[157] Patients with a single risk factor represent a more difficult group, as the annual death rate in this group is low, but the confidence intervals are wide, suggesting that some individuals with a single risk factor may be twice as likely to die suddenly than patients without risk factors. The evaluation of risk in these patients, therefore, has to be tailored to the individual, taking into account the significance of the risk factor—for example, a particularly malignant family history may be sufficient to trigger primary preventative measures in the absence of a second risk factor—as well as patient specific variables such as age (Fig. 49-8).[157,198] Several studies have shown that obstruction of the left ventricular outflow tract is associated with increased cardiovascular mortality, including sudden death.[199,200] The absolute risk of sudden death associated with obstruction in isolation is low, but it may represent an incremental risk factor in combination with other conventional markers.[199]

Although the algorithm for stratification of risk described above has been applied with some success to children and adolescents,[125] extrapolation of data derived from adults may not always be appropriate for children. Of the conventional markers of an increased risk for sudden death, unexplained syncope, severe left ventricular hypertrophy, and a family history of sudden death have been reported as being particularly relevant to young individuals.[27,157,194,196,197,201] The response of blood pressure to exercise, however, may not be a sensitive marker of the risk in children, and whilst non-sustained ventricular tachycardia is a poor prognostic marker in this population, most children and teenagers who die of hypertrophic cardiomyopathy do not have this arrhythmia.[119]

In patients who are considered to be at high risk, insertion of an implantable cardioverter-defibrillator should be regarded as the treatment of choice.[5] Retrospective registry data demonstrates that implantable cardioverter-defibrillators prevent sudden death in predominantly adult populations, with annual appropriate discharge rates of one-tenth in those undergoing secondary prevention, in other words, those with a history of cardiac arrest or sustained ventricular arrhythmia, and in one-twentieth of groups selected for primary prevention because of risk factors.[202] In children, appropriate discharge rates are higher at 71% per year in those chosen for secondary prevention,[125,203] and 4% per year in those having primary prevention. Despite the life-saving benefits of implantable cardioverter-defibrillators, an increased incidence of complications has been reported in children compared with adults, including a higher rate of inappropriate discharges for supraventricular or sinus tachycardia, an increased risk of infection, complications with leads related to growth,[204–206] and the psychological sequels of appropriate and inappropriate discharges.[207,208] Prior to the advent of implantable cardioverter-defibrillators, amiodarone was used to prevent sudden death in patients considered at

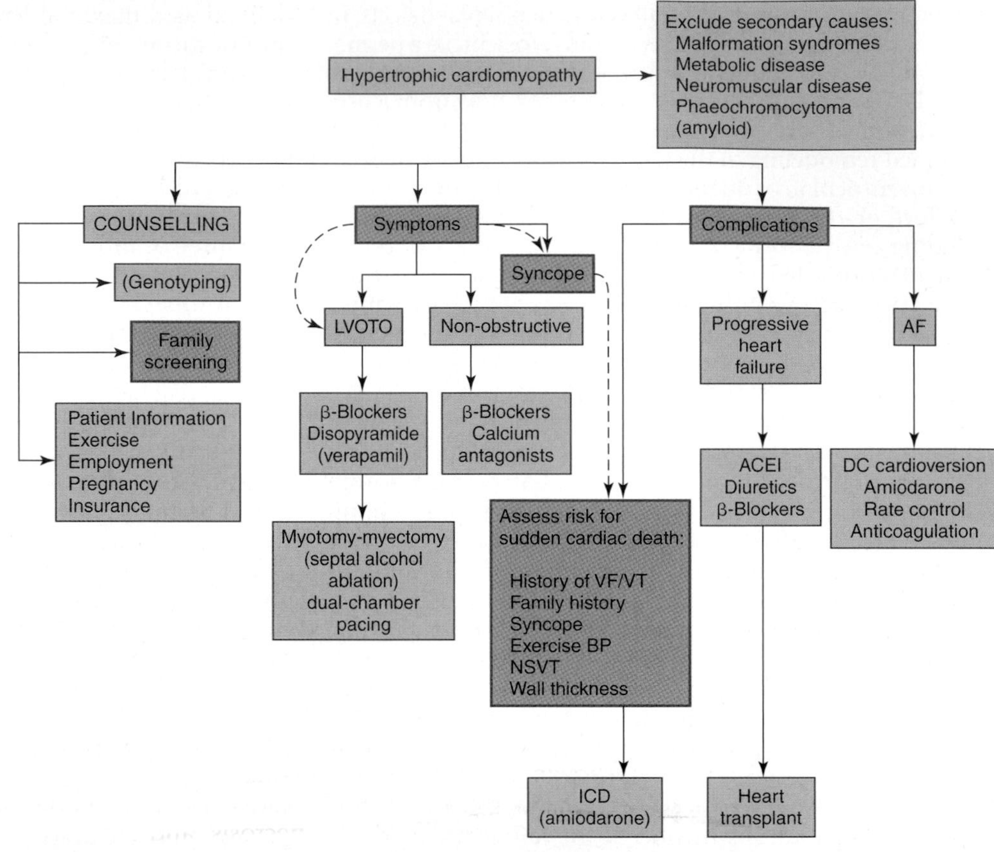

Figure 49-8 The key features in the management of patients with hypertrophic cardiomyopathy. ACEI, angiotensin-converting enzyme inhibitor, AF, atrial fibrillation; BP, blood pressure; ICD, implantable cardioverter-defibrillator; LVOTO, left ventricular outflow tract obstruction; VF/VT, ventricular fibrillation/ventricular tachycardia. (Adapted from Elliott P, McKenna WJ: Hypertrophic cardiomyopathy. Lancet 2004;363: 1881–1891.)

high-risk.[209] The drug, however, does not prevent sudden cardiac death in this group at high-risk.[125] Amiodarone does, nonetheless, remain useful for the treatment of atrial fibrillation.

MYOCARDITIS

Definition and Historical Aspects

The term myocarditis was first used in the early 19th century to describe myocardial diseases not associated with valvar abnormalities, but it now refers to disorders characterised by myocardial inflammation.[210,211] Although a large number of infectious and non-infectious aetiologies of myocarditis have been identified, viruses are thought to be the most important cause in Europe and the United States.[211] Viral myocarditis remains the prototype for the study of the disease,[212] and is the focus of this chapter. Recent advances in molecular biology have revealed new insights into the complex interactions between viral injury and myocardial immune responses, which has led to a better understanding of the pathogenesis of myocarditis, and to the development of novel diagnostic and therapeutic approaches.[213]

Epidemiology

The exact incidence of myocarditis is unknown, since the clinical presentation varies from asymptomatic electrocardiographic abnormalities to haemodynamic collapse and sudden death. Furthermore, the diagnosis can be difficult, as histopathological features[214] have been shown to underestimate its true prevalence.[215] Population estimates of the prevalence range from 1 in 100,000 to 1 in 10,000, with retrospective and prospective postmortem studies reporting myocarditis in up to one-eighth of young victims dying suddenly.[216–220] In children, definite or borderline evidence of myocarditis was found in almost two-fifths of individuals.[221] It has been suggested that infants and young children may be more prone to developing myocarditis, due to a higher rate of enteroviral and adenoviral infections in this age group.[222]

Natural History

The natural history of myocarditis is varied, reflecting its heterogeneous clinical presentation. Most patients probably recover fully, even when they present with a syndrome mimicking acute myocardial infarction.[223,224] Patients presenting with clinical cardiac failure and mild left ventricular systolic impairment typically improve within weeks or months.[212] In patients with more severe left ventricular dysfunction, with an ejection fraction less than 35%, and left ventricular end-diastolic diameters greater than 60 mm, approximately one-quarter progress to transplantation, half develop chronic dilated cardiomyopathy, and the others recover spontaneously.[212,225]

Survival in children ranges from 70% to 100%,[221,226–228] with two-thirds recovering completely.[226] Whilst the prognosis in infants and children with myocarditis is generally good, a high rate of death is reported for neonates with enteroviral myocarditis,[229] suggesting that neonatal myocarditis may represent a higher risk.

Aetiology

Many infectious, inflammatory, and toxic causes of myocarditis have been identified (Table 49-2). Worldwide, the commonest infective myocarditis is Chagas' disease.[230–232] In the Western world, viral myocarditis is the most common cause of inflammatory cardiac disease. Several viruses have been implicated, the most relevant of which are discussed below. Rarer myocarditides in children include giant cell myocarditis, characterised by a giant cell inflammatory infiltrate within the myocardium associated with prominent myocyte necrosis and a high mortality rate, and myocarditis complicating autoimmune disorders such as systemic lupus erythematosus, rheumatoid arthritis, and ulcerative colitis. An important cause in young adults, and increasingly in teenagers, is abuse of cocaine, which can result in acute coronary arterial vasospasm, but may also lead to acute and severe left ventricular systolic dysfunction.[222]

Enterovirus

Historically, the most commonly implicated virus in myocarditis has been the coxsackie B enterovirus.[233] Strains with marked cardiotropic virulence have been identified.[234] A causal association between enteroviruses and myocarditis was initially suggested by studies showing a relationship between rising titres of coxsackievirus B antibodies in the serum and acute symptomatic presentation[235,236] More recently, the enteroviral genome has been detected in myocardial biopsies of patients with myocarditis and dilated cardiomyopathy.[237] The pathogenic mechanism relates cleavage of dystrophin by the coxsackievirus protease, which disrupts the cytoskeletal structural integrity of the cardiac myocyte.[238]

Adenovirus

An early study using viral cultures and serological markers showed the presence of adenovirus in one-sixth of children with acute myocarditis.[239] More recently, adenovirus DNA has been identified using polymerase chain reaction in up to two-fifths of samples from explanted hearts or endomyocardial biopsies in children with acute myocarditis.[240–243] In one study, adenovirus was identified more frequently than enterovirus in both children and adults with myocarditis.[244] Coxsackievirus and adenovirus are known to share a common cellular receptor.[245,246]

Parvovirus

Parvovirus B19 infection is common in humans, usually causing erythema infectiosum. There are several reports of myocarditis associated with parvovirus infection, with one recent study finding viral DNA in one-tenth of endomyocardial biopsy samples taken from adults with histological evidence of myocardial inflammation or left ventricular dysfunction.[247] Childhood parvovirus myocarditis has also been reported with sudden cardiac death.[248–252]

Other Viruses

Many other viruses have been implicated in myocarditis in children, including cytomegalovirus, hepatitis C virus, and herpes simplex virus. In addition, the human immunodeficiency virus has been associated with myocarditis and left ventricular dysfunction.[253–255]

Pathology

Proposed in 1986, the Dallas criterions[214] provide standardised histopathological criterions for classification, defining myocarditis according to the presence of histological evidence of myocytic injury with degeneration or necrosis, and an inflammatory infiltrate not due to ischaemia.[214] Four forms of myocarditis are recognised: active in the presence of both myocytic degeneration or necrosis and definite cellular infiltrate, borderline when there is a definite cellular infiltrate but no evidence of myocardial cellular injury, persistent when active myocarditis is found on a repeat biopsy, and resolving or resolved when there is diminished or absent infiltrates with evidence of connective tissue healing on a repeated biopsy. Despite their widespread use, the criterions have many limitations, including low specificity and sensitivity, with a diagnostic yield as low

TABLE 49-2

COMMON CAUSES OF MYOCARDITIS

Infectious		Immune-mediated		Toxic
Viral	Adenovirus Coxsackievirus Hepatitis C virus Human immunodeficiency virus	Autoantigens	Churg-Strauss syndrome Inflammatory bowel disease Giant cell myocarditis Diabetes mellitus Sarcoidosis Systemic lupus erythematosus Thyrotoxicosis Takayasu's arteritis Wegener's granulomatosis	Anthracyclines Cocaine Interleukin-2 Ethanol Heavy metals
Bacterial	Mycobacteria *Streptococcus* sp. *Mycoplasma pneumoniae* *Treponema pallidum*			
Fungal	*Aspergillus* *Candida* *Coccidioides* *Cryptococcus* *Histoplasma*	Hypersensitivity	Sulphonamides Cephalosporins Diuretics Tricyclic antidepressants Dobutamine	
Protozoal	*Trypanosoma cruzi*			
Parasitic	Schistosomiasis Larva migrans			

Data from Feldman AM, McNamara D: Myocarditis. N Engl J Med 2000;343:1388–1398; and Magnani JW, Dec GW: Myocarditis: Current trends in diagnosis and treatment. Circulation 2006;113:876–990.

as 10% to 20% in some series.[212] Sampling error and variation in interpretation contribute further to the low diagnostic accuracy.[256] Furthermore, some studies have shown a poor association between histological evidence of myocarditis and the presence of autoantibodies in patients with clinically suspected myocarditis.[257] In addition, studies in large cohorts of patients with clinically suspected myocarditis have failed to demonstrate associated positive biopsy findings,[258,259] and a study in children has shown that virus may be present in the myocardium despite a lack of histological evidence of myocarditis.[242] These data suggest that using the Dallas criterions alone to establish a diagnosis of myocarditis may result in significant under-diagnosis of the condition. Newer immunohistochemical and virologic techniques should be used in conjunction with the traditional histological tools to provide a more accurate diagnosis of myocarditis.

Pathophysiology

Studies in animals, mostly mice, have yielded important insights into the pathogenesis of viral myocarditis.[260] Initially, there is direct invasion of the myocardium by cardiotropic viruses, which enter the myocyte via receptor-mediated endocytosis. The viral genome is then translated intracellularly to produce viral protein, or is incorporated into the host cell genome, contributing to myocytic dysfunction by cleaving dystrophin. This is followed by a second phase, in which rapid activation of the host immune system, including recruitment of natural killer cells and macrophages, results in the expression of pro-inflammatory cytokines such as interleukin-1, tumour necrosis factor, and nitric oxide. Activation of CD4+ T lymphocytes, which promotes clonal expansion of B lymphocytes, results in further myocardial damage, local inflammation, and the production of circulating anti-heart antibodies directed against contractile, structural, and mitochondrial proteins.[212,261] This autoimmune response may result in long-term ventricular remodeling through direct effects on myocardial structural components, or through alterations in extracellular matrix turnover, which disrupt the structural integrity of the heart.[262]

Clinical Features

The diagnosis of myocarditis requires a high index of suspicion, particularly in children, as it may mimic other common diagnoses (see Table 49-2). Many individuals with myocarditis may be asymptomatic and manifest only transient electrocardiographic abnormalities. Others may present with symptoms and signs of fulminant cardiogenic shock with acute cardiovascular collapse. In some cases, sudden cardiac death may be the first presentation of myocarditis,[212] and cases of sudden infant death syndrome associated with enterovirus and parvovirus have been reported.[263,264] In other cases, there may be prodromal symptoms of viraemia, including fever, myalgia, coryzal symptoms or gastroenteritis, but the prevalence of these in different series is highly variable, ranging from one-tenth to four-fifths in adults.[211,212,265] A viral prodrome may be more common in children, in whom studies have reported frequencies of up to nine-tenths[226,242] of those with histologically confirmed myocarditis.

Presentation with signs and symptoms of congestive cardiac failure, resulting from an acute impairment of systolic function with our without or left dilation, may differ in adults and children.[266] The prevalence of biopsy-proven myocarditis among adults with acute-onset dilated cardiomyopathy is between one-tenth and one-sixth.[225,267] Prevalence in children ranges from half to four-fifths.[242,244,268]

Investigations

Electrocardiography

Transient electrocardiographic abnormalities occur commonly during community viral endemics, with most patients remaining asymptomatic.[212] In childhood studies, the electrocardiographic changes described include non-specific ST segment and T wave abnormalities, pathological Q waves, T wave inversion, and low QRS voltages.[226,228] Electrocardiographic changes that mimic acute myocardial infarction have also been described.[223,224] Myocarditis also causes atrioventricular block and ventricular arrhythmia, ranging from the presence of frequent ventricular extrasystole to sustained ventricular tachycardia.[212,223,224] These electrocardiographic abnormalities are frequently asymptomatic, but occasionally may be associated with symptoms such as palpitation, presyncope, or syncope. In some cases, the only electrocardiographic manifestation of myocarditis may be a sinus tachycardia.

Chest Radiography

The chest radiograph may show an increased cardiothoracic ratio, increased pulmonary venous markings, and pulmonary oedema in some patients with acute myocarditis. The heart size may be normal in patients with acute, haemodynamically compromising left ventricular dysfunction, and in those with transient electrocardiographic abnormalities.

Echocardiography

Echocardiographic findings are varied and often non-specific, although the echocardiogram is rarely entirely normal in myocarditis, other than in some patients presenting only with ventricular ectopy. Evidence of impaired left ventricular systolic performance, with reduced fractional shortening and ejection fraction, is common.[269] Regional abnormalities of wall motion occur commonly, and functional mitral regurgitation, in the setting of left ventricular dilation, may also be found. Left or right ventricular thrombus may be present. Evidence of left ventricular diastolic impairment may also be detected. Less frequently, right ventricular systolic and diastolic function may also be compromised. Pericardial effusions are common. In the neonatal period and early infancy particularly, echocardiography has an important role in excluding anomalous coronary arterial anatomy, in particular, anomalous origin of the left coronary artery from the pulmonary trunk, as well as left-sided obstructive lesions, which can have a similar clinical presentation to myocarditis.

Cardiac Biomarkers

Routine blood tests such as full blood count and erythrocytic sedimentation rate are not usually helpful in confirming the diagnosis of myocarditis. Markers of myocardial injury may be of use.[270,271] Troponin I has a high specificity for diagnosing myocarditis but a sensitivity of only 34%.[271] Creatine kinase and its cardiac isoform CK-MB are less sensitive and specific than troponin, and are therefore not clinically useful for screening. Increased levels of autoantibodies against myocardial proteins have also been reported, and correlate with progressive worsening of ventricular function.[272,273]

Endomyocardial Biopsy

Cardiac catheterisation with right ventricular endomyocardial biopsy remains the gold standard diagnostic test for myocarditis, albeit the analysis using the Dallas criterions suffers from several important limitations. Immunohistochemical staining of samples can be used to obtain precise characterisation of lymphocyte subtypes.[274] The quantification of major histocompatibility complex and intercellular cell adhesion molecule induction using molecular immunohistochemical techniques has been demonstrated to have a higher sensitivity than the Dallas criterions for diagnosing myocarditis, although this may represent a subgroup of patients with a more chronic form of myocardial injury.[275,276]

Viral Polymerase Chain Reaction

The confirmation of a viral cause for myocarditis has been the subject of much recent interest. The diagnosis of viral myocarditis previously was based on the presence of positive viral cultures or serological confirmation of an antiviral immune response. These methods, however, are time consuming and have a low diagnostic yield. Polymerase chain reaction techniques have been shown successfully and rapidly to detect the presence of viral genome in samples from patients with myocarditis and dilated cardiomyopathy, including children.[242,244,277]

Cardiac Magnetic Resonance Imaging

Cardiac magnetic resonance imaging can demonstrate myocardial inflammation and myocyte injury, including the presence of pericellular and cellular oedema. In addition, the technique can provide useful anatomical and functional information. Although there have been no studies in children with myocarditis, data from adults[278] may be applicable to children.

Management

General Principles

The first-line treatment is supportive. General principles of stabilisation include afterload reduction, anticoagulation, diuresis, and inotropic support. Patients with fulminant acute myocarditis may require intensive intravenous haemodynamic support. Diuretics and vasodilators, such as nitroprusside or glyceryl trinitrate, are the mainstay of afterload reduction. In some cases, mechanical assist devices or extracorporeal membrane oxygenation may be required.[279–282]

Following initial stabilisation, treatment for patients with symptoms and signs of cardiac failure should follow current guidelines set out by the International Society for Heart and Lung Transplantation.[283] This includes the use of inhibitors of angiotensin-converting enzyme and diuretics. The addition of β-blocking agents such as carvedilol should also be considered in patients with compensated cardiac failure. In addition, patients with left ventricular enlargement should receive anticoagulation with aspirin or warfarin. Patients with intractable and deteriorating cardiac failure may require cardiac transplantation.

Immunotherapy

Intravenous immunoglobulin has been considered the standard therapy for children with suspected myocarditis. The reason is that immunoglobulin may help clear the virus directly, or may stimulate the immune response to the viral infection.[284] In support of this, clinically beneficial effects of intravenous immunoglobulin have been reported in both children and adults with acute myocarditis.[285–288] The only double-blind randomised controlled trial, however, failed to show any treatment-related differences in all-cause mortality or any improvement in left ventricular ejection fraction.[289] There are no randomised controlled trials of intravenous immunoglobulin therapy in children with myocarditis. As a result, a recent Cochrane Database review concluded that current evidence does not support the use of intravenous immunoglobulin for the management of presumed viral myocarditis, and that 'intravenous immunoglobulin for presumed viral myocarditis should not be part of routine practice'.[290]

The suggestion that immune responses to viral infection of the myocardium may cause the long-term sequels of viral myocarditis has led to the use of immunosuppression to suppress the acute inflammatory response.[211,212] The contrary argument is that immunosuppression could impair the ability of the host immune system to eradicate virus.[291] Prednisolone increases mortality in mice with acute viral myocarditis.[292] In the Myocarditis Treatment Trial, there was no difference in mortality or improvement in left ventricular function between the control group and those being immunosuppressed,[265] and patients with more robust immune responses had less severe disease and a better outcome. In another study, there was improvement in left ventricular ejection fraction in the immunosuppressed patients, but no difference in mortality, transplantation, or rehospitalisation.[276]

The data in children are scant. Observational case series appear to show a beneficial effect of immunosuppression,[221,228,268,293] but these studies are limited by a lack of randomisation and placebo control.[291]

Novel Therapeutic Strategies

Studies in mice have shown encouraging results with monoclonal antibodies directed against coxsackievirus B[294] and with enterovirus life-cycle inhibitors.[295] In children, preliminary studies using pleconaril, a drug that binds directly to coxsackievirus B and prevents it from infecting target cells, have also shown promise.[296] Ribavirin, started early in the disease process, may also be beneficial in enterovirus myocarditis.[297] More recently, interferon-α[298] and interferon-β[299] have shown encouraging initial results, although their efficacy and long-term side effect profile need to be evaluated in larger randomised controlled trials. Modulation of the renin-angiotensin-aldosterone system using inhibitors of angiotensin-converting enzyme or antagonists of angiotensin receptors has been shown to downregulate autoimmune responses without causing immunosuppression in murine models of myocarditis, suggesting that these agents may be useful in preventing the development of progressive left ventricular remodeling and chronic dilated cardiomyopathy in patients with myocarditis.[300] From a public health perspective, it is possible that vaccines targeting the common viruses associated with myocarditis, such as coxsackievirus B, adenovirus, and parvovirus, might be a more effective strategy.[284]

DILATED CARDIOMYOPATHY

Definition

Dilated cardiomyopathy is a myocardial disorder defined by dilation and impaired systolic function of the left ventricle, or both ventricles, in the absence of coronary arterial disease, valvar abnormalities, or pericardial disease.[4] As will be discussed, a number of different cardiac and systemic diseases are associated with left ventricular dilation and impaired contractility, but in most patients, no identifiable cause is found.[301]

Epidemiology

Dilated cardiomyopathy is the commonest cardiomyopathy in children, accounting for up to three-fifths of cases.[22,23] The annual incidence is between 0.58 and 0.73 cases per 100,000 of the population.[22,23] Overall, males and females are approximately equally affected, but in dilated cardiomyopathy associated with neuromuscular disorders or inborn errors of metabolism, there is a striking male predominance,[302] associated with X-linked inheritance in many cases. The majority of children with dilated cardiomyopathy present before 1 year of age,[302,303] with the exception of the group with an underlying neuromuscular disease, in whom presentation occurs more commonly in adolescence.[302]

Natural History

Early studies of outcome in children reported an actuarial survival from presentation of 79% at 1 year and 61% at 5 years.[304] In a more recent study, freedom from death or transplantation was 69% at 1 year and 54% at 5 years[302] (Fig. 49-9). Actuarial rates of freedom for death or transplantation in a smaller Australian study were 72% at 1 year, and 63% at 5 years.[303] Risk factors for subsequent death or transplantation include older age at diagnosis,[302,303] fractional shortening, congestive cardiac failure at presentation, and familial disease. Patients with idiopathic disease and neuromuscular disorders also do less well.[302]

Aetiology

A number of conditions associated with dilated cardiomyopathy have been described, including neuromuscular disorders, inborn errors of metabolism, and malformation syndromes (see Table 49-1).[302] In the majority of patients, no identifiable cause is found, and the disease is considered idiopathic.[301] Up to one-third of individuals with dilated cardiomyopathy have familial disease, in which at least one other first-degree relative is affected.[305]

Familial Dilated Cardiomyopathy

Familial disease occurs in over a third of adult patients.[305] The reported prevalence of familial dilated cardiomyopathy in children is much lower, from one-twentieth to one-sixth,[302,303] but this is likely to represent an underestimate, resulting from reduced awareness of the inherited nature of the condition among paediatricians, and possibly a higher prevalence of metabolic or syndromic causes in children. A number of genetic mutations can cause dilated cardiomyopathy.[53] In most cases, these are transmitted as an autosomal dominant trait, but other forms of inheritance, including autosomal recessive, X-linked and mitochondrial also occur.

Autosomal Dominant Dilated Cardiomyopathy

Autosomal dominant inheritance accounts for approximately one-quarter of all cases,[306] and was the commonest mode of inheritance in the study from North America,

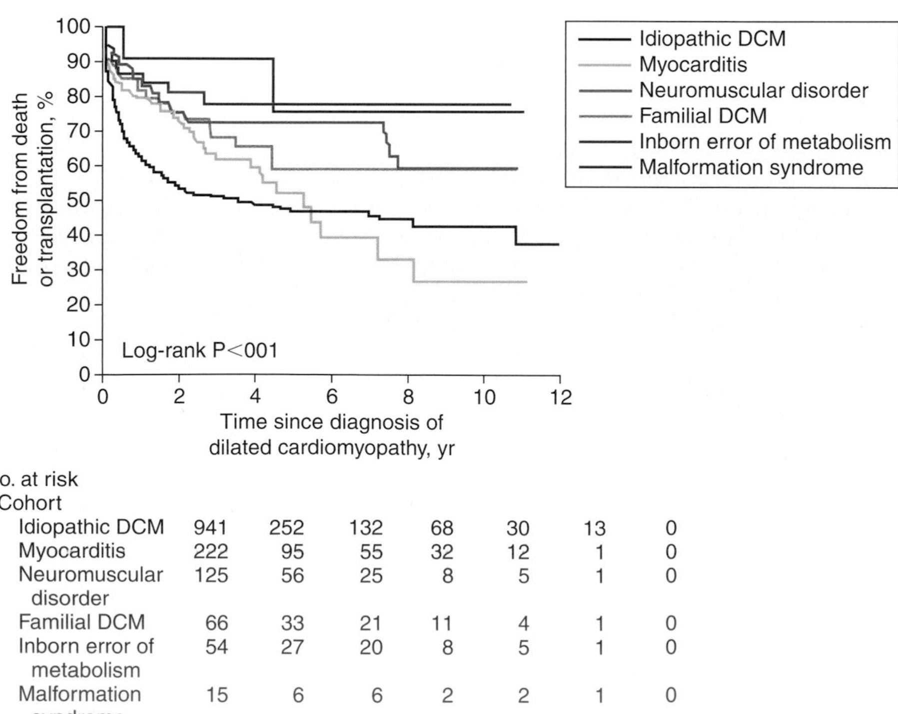

Figure 49-9 Freedom from death or transplantation in children with dilated cardiomyopathy. DCM, dilated cardiomyopathy. (Reproduced with permission from Towbin JA, Lowe AM, Colan SD, et al: Incidence, causes, and outcomes of dilated cardiomyopathy in children. JAMA 2006;296:1867–1876.)

accounting for two-thirds of familial cases.[302] Two major forms of autosomal dominant dilated cardiomyopathy are recognised, namely, isolated (or pure), and dilated cardiomyopathy associated with disease of the cardiac conduction system. In many cases, there may also be a skeletal myopathy.

Genes implicated in the isolated form include cytoskeletal (δ-sarcoglycan,[307] β-sarcoglycan,[308] desmin,[309,310] and sarcomeric protein genes including α-cardiac actin,[311] troponin T,[312] β-myosin heavy chain,[312] troponin C,[313] and α-tropomyosin.[314] Although a number of genes have been mapped when dilated cardiomyopathy is associated with disease of the conduction system,[53,315] only one has been identified to date. Mutations in the lamin A/C gene, which encodes a nuclear envelope intermediate filament protein, usually results in atrial arrhythmia and progressive atrioventricular conduction disease, which precede the development of dilated cardiomyopathy by several years.[316–318] The pathophysiological mechanisms remain poorly understood. Some mutations result in dilated cardiomyopathy and conduction disease alone,[317] whereas others lead to juvenile-onset muscular dystrophies, including Emery-Dreifuss muscular dystrophy[319,320] and familial partial lipodystrophy with insulin-resistant diabetes.[321]

X-linked Dilated Cardiomyopathy

X-linked inheritance accounts for up to one-twentieth of familial cases of dilated cardiomyopathy.[302,322–324] In the study from North America,[302] neuromuscular disorders accounted for one-quarter of cases, and nine-tenths were caused by Duchenne, Becker, and Emery-Dreifuss muscular dystrophies. Patients were significantly older at presentation than children with other causes of dilated cardiomyopathy, and almost all were male, reflecting the X-linked inheritance. Their outcome was poor, with only half surviving or free from transplantation after 5 years.[302] X-linked dilated cardiomyopathy, also caused by mutations in the dystrophin gene, was first described in 1987 in young males with severe disease and rapid progression of congestive cardiac failure to death or transplantation.[325] The condition is characterised by raised isoforms of creatine kinase in the serum, but does not result in clinical signs or symptoms of muscular dystrophy as in Duchenne or Becker muscular dystrophies. Female carriers develop dilated cardiomyopathy in their fifties, and progression of the disease is slower.

Barth syndrome, made up of dilated cardiomyopathy, skeletal myopathy, and neutropaenia, is an X-linked disorder cause by mutations in the G4.5 gene, which encodes the protein tafazzin.[326,327] The condition typically presents in male neonates or young infants, producing congestive cardiac failure, neutropaenia, and 3-methylgutaconic aciduria. Although some children die in infancy, usually due to progressive cardiac failure, sudden death, or sepsis, most survive infancy, but the dilated cardiomyopathy persists. Mutations in the G4.5 gene also cause isolated dilated cardiomyopathy, endocardial fibroelastosis, and left ventricular non-compaction, with or without the other features of Barth syndrome.[328,329]

Other Causes of Dilated Cardiomyopathy in Childhood

Myocarditis is an important cause of dilated cardiomyopathy, accounting for one-sixth to one-third of cases in population-based studies.[302,303] The features of myocarditis were discussed in the preceding section of this chapter. Inborn errors of metabolism account for less than one-twentieth of cases. Of these, mitochondrial disorders are the commonest, accounting for almost half, followed by Barth syndrome, accounting for one-quarter, and primary or systemic deficiency of carnitine, accounting for another tenth.[302] Patients with metabolic disease causing cardiac disease typically present in infancy, and three-quarters are male. Malformation syndromes are rarely associated with dilated cardiomyopathy, accounting for only 1% of cases.[302] Hypocalcaemic rickets, however, can present as an isolated dilated cardiomyopathy in infancy.[330–334]

Pathology

Macroscopically, dilated cardiomyopathy is characterised by the presence of a globular heart, with dilation of the ventricles and diffuse endocardial thickening.[335] Atrial enlargement is also seen, often with thrombus present in the appendages. Overall, myocardial mass is increased, but in the presence of reduced ventricular mural thickness.[335] The histological features are non-specific, but show a combination of myocytic degeneration, interstitial fibrosis, and myocytic nuclear hypertrophy and pleomorphism. Frequently there is an increase in interstitial T lymphocytes, and focal accumulations of macrophages associated with death of individual myocytes. There is often extensive myofibrillary loss, giving the myocytes a vacuolated appearance.[335]

Pathophysiology

The identification of disease-causing mutations in genes encoding various components of the cardiac myocytic cystoskeletal and sarcomeric contractile apparatus shows that the pathogenesis of dilated cardiomyopathy is heterogeneous. Two models have been proposed to explain ventricular remodelling.[53] Those using the concept of a final common pathway argue that the cardiomyopathy reflects a non-specific degenerative state, resulting from a variety of stimuluses, including genetic mutations, viral infections, toxins, and volume overload.[53,306] The mechanisms underlying this final pathway remain speculative, but may include altered myocytic energetics and handling of calcium. Those supporting the alternative hypothesis suggest that a number of distinct, independent pathways can remodel the heart and cause dilated cardiomyopathy, with the different causes of dilated cardiomyopathy sharing common histopathology but having distinct molecular biologic characteristics.[53]

Clinical Features

The symptoms and signs associated with dilated cardiomyopathy are highly variable, and depend on the age of the patient and the degree of left ventricular dysfunction. Whilst the first presentation may be sudden death or a thromboembolic event, most patients present with symptoms of high pulmonary venous pressure and/or low cardiac output which can be acute, sometimes being precipitated by intercurrent illness or arrhythmia,[301] or more chronic, preceding the diagnosis by many months or years. Increasingly, dilated cardiomyopathy is diagnosed incidentally in asymptomatic individuals during family screening.

Symptoms

Infants with dilated cardiomyopathy typically present with poor feeding, tachypnoea, respiratory distress, diaphoresis during feeding, and failure to thrive. Older children and adults initially present with reduced exercise tolerance and dyspnoea on exertion. With worsening left ventricular function, dyspnoea at rest, orthopnoea, paroxysmal nocturnal dyspnoea, peripheral oedema, and ascites develop. In children in particular, symptoms may occur related to mesenteric ischaemia as a result of insufficient cardiac output to perfuse the gastrointestinal tract. This can produce abdominal pain after meals, nausea, vomiting, and anorexia. Symptoms related to arrhythmia, such as palpitation, presyncope, and syncope may occur at any age.

Physical Examination

Features of low cardiac output include persistent sinus tachycardia, weak peripheral pulses, and in advanced disease, hypotension. In older children, the jugular venous pressure may be elevated. Signs of respiratory distress resulting from pulmonary oedema may be present, particularly in infants and younger children, and include intercostal and subcostal recession, nasal flaring, and during acute decompensations, grunting. Palpation of the precordium usually reveals a displaced apical impulse. Hepatomegaly and ascites are common in patients with congestive cardiac failure, including infants. Peripheral oedema may also be seen, affecting the legs and sacrum in older children, and the face and scrotum in infants.

Auscultation of the heart may reveal the presence of a third, and sometimes a fourth, heart sound. In patients with functional mitral regurgitation, there may be a pansystolic murmur at the apex radiating to the axilla, but frequently no murmurs are heard, even in the presence of mitral incompetence, especially if cardiac output is very low. Auscultation of the chest may reveal basal crackles. Indeed, infants may present with wheezing that is difficult to distinguish from asthma or bronchiolitis. Examination of other systems is important, as it may reveal clues to the possible aetiology. In particular, examination of the neuromuscular system may reveal features of mild or subclinical skeletal myopathy. Ophthalmological examination is important if mitochondrial disorders are suspected.

Investigations

Electrocardiography

The electrocardiogram in dilated cardiomyopathy may be normal,[301] but more typically shows sinus tachycardia and non-specific changes in the ST segments and T waves, most commonly in the inferior and lateral leads (Fig. 49-10). In patients with extensive left ventricular fibrosis, abnormal Q waves in the septal leads may be present. Evidence of atrial enlargement and voltage criterions for ventricular hypertrophy, usually involving the left but occasionally both biventricles, are common. All degrees of atrioventricular block may be seen, and raise the possibility of mutations in the *lamin A/C* gene. Supraventricular and ventricular arrhythmias are also common. In children, arrhythmias occur in up to half, and half of these are atrial.[336] Studies in predominantly adult populations have shown a prevalence of non-sustained ventricular tachycardia in just over two-fifths,[337] albeit that ventricular tachycardia is less common in children, occurring in only one-tenth of cases.[336]

Chest Radiography

The chest X-ray is frequently abnormal. An increased cardiothoracic ratio is typical, reflecting left ventricular and left atrial dilation. In addition, patients with pulmonary oedema have signs of increased pulmonary vascular markings. Pleural effusions may also be present.

Echocardiography

In general, the presence of ventricular end-diastolic dimensions greater than two standard deviations above body surface area–corrected means, or greater than 112% of predicted dimension, and fractional shortening of less than 25% are sufficient to make the diagnosis.[4,301,338] These criterions have some limitations, and therefore a number of other useful parameters of left ventricular function are usually measured. These include ejection fraction, myocardial performance index, and assessment of cardiac output, using velocities in the aorta and left ventricular outflow tract as assessed with pulsed and continuous wave Doppler. Cross sectional echocardiography is also used to determine whether intracavitary thrombus is present in the ventricles or atriums (Fig. 49-11). Colour flow Doppler interrogation is used to determine the presence, and quantify the severity, of functional mitral and tricuspid regurgitation.

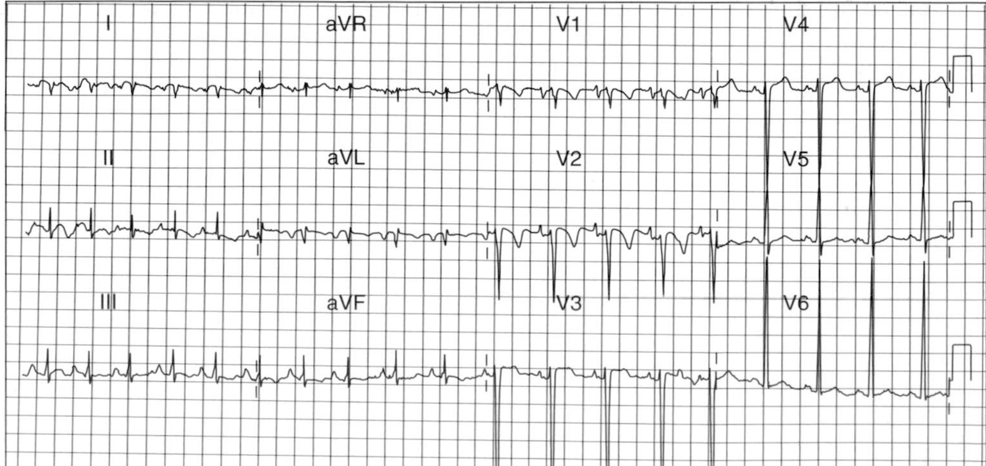

Figure 49-10 The 12-lead electrocardiogram from a 2-year-old with familial idiopathic dilated cardiomyopathy, showing non-specific ST segment and T wave abnormalities.

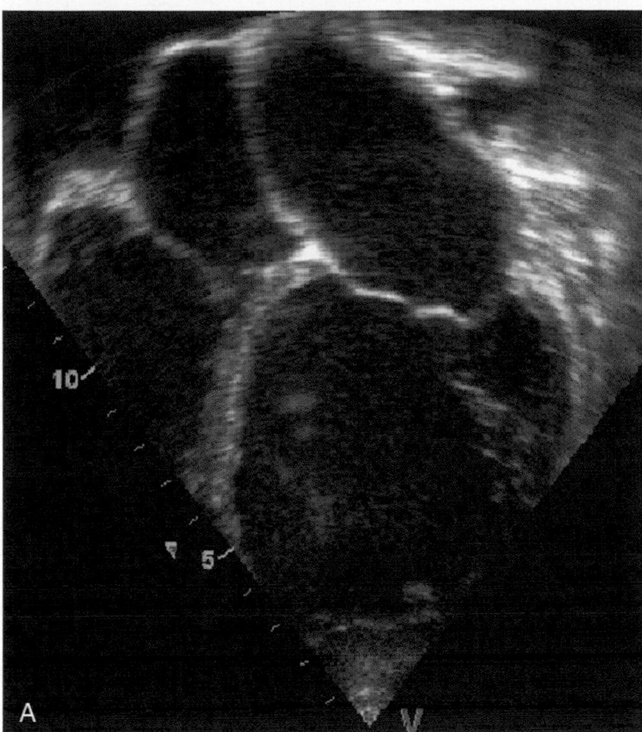

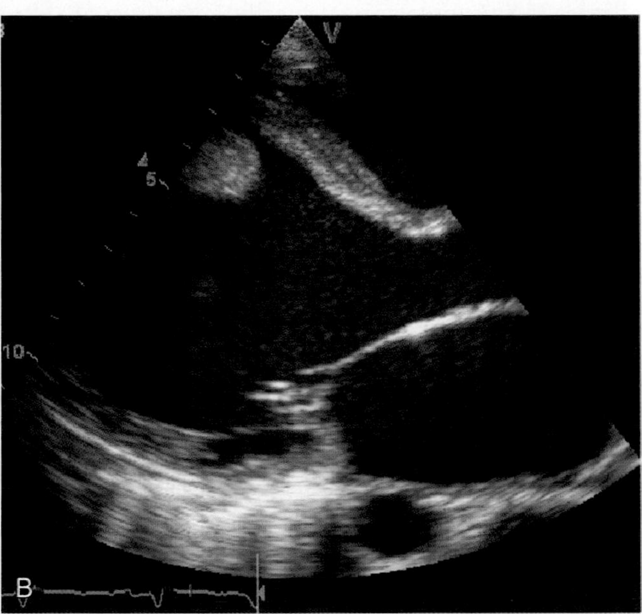

Figure 49-11 Echocardiographic features of dilated cardiomyopathy. **A** shows an apical four-chamber view from a child with dilated cardiomyopathy. Note the dilated left ventricular cavity with thin walls. **B** is a parasternal long-axis view, again showing a dilated, thin-walled left ventricle, but with thrombus in the left ventricular cavity. (Courtesy of Dr Jan Marek, Great Ormond Street Hospital, London, United Kingdom.)

In addition, pulsed and continuous wave Doppler interrogation can be used to estimate pulmonary arterial pressures. Patients frequently have abnormalities of diastolic left ventricular function. These include impaired relaxation or pseudo-normal patterns of mitral inflow and pulmonary venous flow. Occasionally, patients with severe disease have restrictive left ventricular physiology. Tissue Doppler systolic and diastolic annular velocities are significantly lower compared to controls,[339] but further studies are needed to assess whether these parameters have a prognostic role.

Cardiac Biomarkers

Levels of creatine kinase should be measured in the serum of all patients with dilated cardiomyopathy, as this may provide important clues to its aetiology. Other cardiac biomarkers, such as troponin I and troponin T, also may be elevated, suggesting the possibility of inflammatory or ischaemic causes. Levels of B-type natriuretic peptide are elevated in the plasma of children with chronic cardiac failure, and serve to predict rates of survival, hospitalisation, and listing for cardiac transplantation.[340]

Exercise Testing

Symptom limited exercise testing using a treadmill or bicycle, combined with analysis of respiratory gases, is a useful technique to assess functional limitation and progression of disease in those in a stable condition. The children have lower durations of exercise, consume less oxygen, and have lower systolic pressures at peak exercise than their normal peers.[341] The use of the technique as a prognostic tool, however, has not been assessed. Exercise testing remains useful, nonetheless, in the evaluation of children prior to transplantation. The detection of respiratory markers of severe lactic acidaemia during metabolic exercise testing can be caused by mitochondrial or metabolic causes.

Cardiac Catheterisation

Cardiac catheterisation with endomyocardial biopsy may be a useful adjunct in the investigation of some children, but its use is declining with improved non-invasive techniques. Endomyocardial biopsy may be diagnostic for myocarditis, although as already discussed, the diagnostic yield is low. It can also prove valuable in identifying metabolic or mitochondrial disorders. Haemodynamic assessment of left ventricular end-diastolic and pulmonary arterial pressures can be carried out in the catheter laboratory, but this has been superseded by echocardiographic techniques, which are non-invasive and do not require exposure to irradiation or general anaesthesia.

Cardiac Magnetic Resonance Imaging

This is a useful alternative technique for imaging in patients with poor echocardiographic windows. In addition, the detection of fibrosis with gadolinium contrast enhancement may provide an imaging-guided method to improve the diagnostic yield of endomyocardial biopsies.[342]

Management

There are no specific therapies for most patients with dilated cardiomyopathy. The aim of management should be to improve symptoms and prevent progression and complications, such as progressive cardiac failure, sudden death, and thromboembolism. Guidelines for pharmacological therapy of cardiac failure in children are based largely on consensus, coupled with extrapolation of data from studies in adults. Data from children is very limited.[283]

Diuretics

There are no published studies evaluating the effects of diuretics in reducing mortality or improving symptoms in children.[283] Loop and thiazide diuretics, nonetheless, should be used in all patients with fluid retention due to cardiac failure to achieve a euvolaemic state. They should not be used as monotherapy, as they exacerbate neurohormonal activation, which may contribute to progression of the disease.[301] Spironolactone, a specific antagonist of aldosterone, reduces relative mortality by almost one-third in adults with severe cardiac failure and ejection fractions less than 35%.[343] Side effects include hyperkalaemia, although this is infrequent in the presence of normal renal function, and gynaecomastia.

Inhibitors of Angiotensin-converting Enzyme and Blockers of Angiotensin Receptors

Activation of the renin-angiotensin-aldosterone system is central to the pathophysiology of cardiac failure, regardless of the underlying aetiology.[283,301] Multiple large clinical trials have shown that inhibition of angiotensin-converting enzyme improves symptoms, reduces hospitalisations, and reduces cardiovascular mortality in adults with cardiac failure.[344–347] Furthermore, such inhibition or blockade also reduces the rate of progression of disease in asymptomatic patients. A substantial proportion of patients taking inhibitors of angiotensin-converting enzyme in clinical practice are not titrated to the target doses reported in many trials, but evidence suggests that higher doses are associated with a greater reduction in the combined risk of death or transplantation.[348] In most cases, the inhibitors are well tolerated, the most common side effects being a troublesome cough and symptomatic hypotension, which can be prevented with careful up-titration of doses. First-dose hypotension is more problematic when inhibition is obtained using captopril than with the newer agents. A number of small observational studies have reported a beneficial effect in children with cardiac failure.[283,349–352] Only one retrospective report has described the effect of inhibition on mortality in children, showing improved survival during the first year of treatment but not subsequently.[351]

Blockers of the angiotensin receptors have similar haemodynamic effects to inhibitors of angiotensin-converting enzyme, but with fewer side effects. Clinical trials in adults with cardiac failure have shown similar haemodynamic effects, efficacy, and safety,[353,354] and the blockers are currently recommended for adults who do not tolerate inhibition of the angiotensin-converting enzyme. Recent studies have suggested that combined treatment with inhibitors and blockers may be more beneficial in preventing ventricular remodeling than either drug alone, but has no additional impact on survival.[355,356] There is no data relating to efficacy or safety regarding the use of the blockers in children with cardiac failure.

Current recommendations for children with dilated cardiomyopathy are that inhibitors of angiotensin-converting enzyme should be routinely used in all individuals with moderate or severe left ventricular dysfunction regardless of the presence of symptoms. Patients who are intolerant of these agents should be considered for blockade of the angiotensin receptors.[283] The use of inhibitors of angiotensin-converting enzyme is not recommended as initial therapy in patients with decompensated left ventricular dysfunction.[283]

Beta-Blockers

Excess sympathetic activity contributes to cardiac failure, and several multi-centric, placebo-controlled trials using carvedilol,[357,358] metoprolol,[359] and bisoprolol[360] have shown substantial reductions in mortality in adults with symptoms of cardiac failure but in relatively good condition. Beta-blockade is usually well tolerated, but side effects include bradycardia, hypotension, and retention of fluid. The drugs should be started at low doses and carefully uptitrated, and they should not be started in patients with decompensated cardiac failure. A recent trial has suggested that they can be started safely before use of inhibitors of angiotensin-converting enzyme for patients in stable cardiac failure.[361] Their reported use in children with cardiac failure is limited. Small observational studies using carvedilol[362–364] and metoprolol[365] have shown clinically important improvements in left ventricular systolic performance and functional class. In addition, carvedilol appears to delay the time to transplantation or death.[366] The results of the first randomised controlled trial in paediatric cardiomyopathy, from the multi-centre Paediatric Carvedilol Study Group, were recently published.[367] Although there was a trend towards benefit in those receiving carvedilol in terms of all-cause mortality, cardiovascular mortality, and hospitalisation for cardiac failure, this was not statistically significant. It is likely that carvedilol and other β-blockers do improve outcomes for some children with cardiac failure, but larger studies with longer follow-up are needed to confirm this. At present, there are no specific recommendations regarding β-blockade in children with compensated cardiac failure, but their routine use is increasing.

Digitalis

Digoxin improves symptoms in adults with cardiac failure,[368] but no benefit in terms of survival has been demonstrated in studies of large cohorts.[283] High levels of digoxin in the serum may be associated with increased mortality in some patients.[369] The drug is still widely used to treat cardiac failure in infants and children, but there is little data to support its efficacy. Current guidelines recommend the use of low doses to improve symptoms in children with symptomatic cardiac failure, including those with dilated cardiomyopathy, but not for asymptomatic individuals.[283]

Novel Pharmacological Therapies

Nesiritide, a recombinant B-type natriuretic peptide with diuretic, natriuretic, and vasodilator effects, and used in adults with decompensated cardiac failure, has recently been shown to be safe in children, producing improvements in urinary output and functional state.[370,371] Its value over more conventional therapies remains to be determined.

Anticoagulation

The annual risk of thromboembolism in children with dilated cardiomyopathy is unknown, but is likely to be low. The cumulative risk of systemic embolisation in a patient diagnosed at a young age, nonetheless, is substantial.[372] In adults with dilated cardiomyopathy, intramural thrombosis and systemic thromboembolisation are found in up to half, with an incidence between 1.5% and 3.5% per year.[373] Anticoagulation with warfarin is advised in patients in whom an intracardiac thrombus is identified echocardiographically, and in those with a history of thromboembolism. There is no trial data to guide prophylactic anticoagulation in those with dilated cardiomyopathy, but patients with severe ventricular dilation and moderate to severe systolic impairment may benefit from anticoagulation using warfarin.

Treatment of Arrhythmias

Whilst arrhythmias are common in patients with dilated cardiomyopathy, negative chronotropic and proarrhythmic effects limit the use of many commonly used antiarrhythmic agents. Data on the effect of amiodarone on survival in dilated cardiomyopathy is contradictory,[374,375] but the use of implantable cardioverter-defibrillators was associated with a reduction in overall mortality of almost one-quarter.[376] Amiodarone, therefore, appears to be safe in patients with dilated cardiomyopathy, and may be effective at preventing or treating atrial arrhythmias, but does not prevent sudden death. In adults, insertion of an implantable cardioverter-defibrillator is recommended for those having symptomatic ventricular arrhythmias, and in those with ventricular arrhythmias and an ejection fraction less than 35%.[376] This will prevent sudden death, and can serve as a bridge to transplantation. The role of implantable cardioverter-defibrillators as primary prophylaxis in children has not been addressed.

Non-pharmacological Treatment of Advanced Dilated Cardiomyopathy

Cardiac transplantation remains the mainstay of management of children with intractable cardiac failure symptoms and end-stage disease (Fig. 49-12). A number of other approaches aimed at improving symptoms and stabilising the disease or delaying transplantation have now emerged.

Cardiac Resynchronisation Therapy

Many adults with dilated cardiomyopathy have abnormal left ventricular activation that in turn results in prolonged and incoordinate ventricular relaxation. Cardiac resynchronisation therapy using biventricular or multi-site pacing attempts to re-establish synchronous atrioventricular, interventricular, and intraventricular contraction to maximise ventricular efficiency. Studies in adults with severe cardiac failure and left bundle branch block have shown marked improvements in some patients.[377] Similar studies are lacking in children.

Ventricular Assist Devices

In some cases, mechanical assist devices, such as left ventricular assist devices, the Berlin heart, or extracorporeal membrane oxygenation, may be required.[279–281] Studies in children have shown good results with aggressive management of end-stage dilated cardiomyopathy, including bridging to recovery.[282] Ventricular assist devices and transplantation are discussed in detail elsewhere.

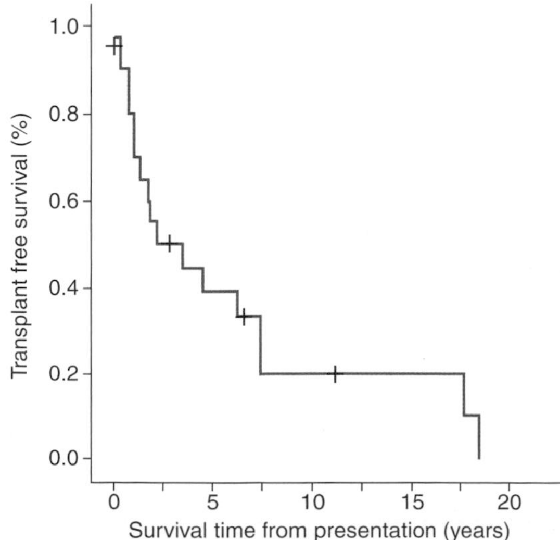

Figure 49-12 Freedom from death or transplantation in 21 patients with idiopathic restrictive cardiomyopathy. (Reproduced with permission from Russo LM, Webber SA: Idiopathic restrictive cardiomyopathy in children. Heart 2005;91: 1199–1202.)

RESTRICTIVE CARDIOMYOPATHY

Definition

Restrictive left ventricular physiology is characterised by a pattern of ventricular filling in which increased stiffness of the myocardium causes ventricular pressure to rise precipitously with only small increases in volume. As restrictive ventricular physiology occurs in a wide range of different pathologies, the definition of restrictive cardiomyopathy has been confusing and variable. For our current purposes, we define restrictive cardiomyopathy on the basis of restrictive ventricular physiology found in the presence of normal or reduced diastolic volumes of one or both ventricles, normal or reduced systolic volumes, and normal ventricular mural thickness.

Epidemiology

The restrictive variant is the rarest of the cardiomyopathies, accounting for less than 3% of cardiomyopathies found in children.[22,23] The total number of children with restrictive cardiomyopathy reported in the literature is less than 150. Their age at presentation ranges from 0 to 19 years, but the majority present between the ages of 2 and 11 years, with a median of 4.7 years. Some reports have suggested a slight female predominance, but this has not been confirmed in other studies.[378]

Natural History

The prognosis when found in children is grave. Without transplantation, approximately half die within 2 years of diagnosis.[379–384] Most children require transplantation within 4 years of diagnosis.[385] Freedom from death or transplantation is 80.5% at 1 year, decreasing dramatically to 39% at 5 years.[383] Pulmonary vascular pressures may rise within a very short period of time following diagnosis,[381,384,385] but this is not easily predicted clinically. All patients with restrictive cardiomyopathy, therefore, should undergo serial assessment of pulmonary vascular resistance, and assessment for potential transplantation should be made early, prior to haemodynamic decompensation.[385] After transplantation, survival is good.[384,385]

Although the majority of deaths in children are caused by rapidly progressive cardiac failure with elevated pulmonary vascular resistance, sudden cardiac death occurs in just over one-quarter, at a rate of 7% per year.[386] Children at risk of sudden death often have no evidence of cardiac failure, but frequently have symptoms and signs of myocardial ischaemia, including chest pain, syncope, and electrocardiographic changes.[386] Individuals with restrictive cardiomyopathy are also at risk of thromboembolic events.[381,385] Risk factors for death from cardiac failure include an increased cardiothoracic ratio on chest radiography,[380] age younger than 5 years at presentation,[380] clinical and radiographic evidence of pulmonary venous congestion,[379] elevated pulmonary vascular resistance index,[381,384,387] and left atrial dilation and elevated ventricular filling pressures.[383]

Aetiology

The disease is caused by many conditions (see Table 49-1), including infiltrative and storage disorders, and endomyocardial disease.[388] In adults, amyloidosis is the commonest cause of restrictive cardiomyopathy in the Western world.[389,390] Cardiac amyloidosis, however, is unheard of in children. In the tropics, endomyocardial fibrosis is the commonest cause in adults, and probably also in children.[388] Outside the tropics, most cases of restrictive cardiomyopathy in children are idiopathic.[388]

Idiopathic Restrictive Cardiomyopathy

The disease is familial in about three-tenths of children.[378] Mutations in the gene encoding desmin, an intermediate filament protein with key structural and functional roles within skeletal and cardiac myocyte myofibrils, are known to cause restrictive cardiomyopathy associated with skeletal myopathy and abnormalities of the cardiac conduction system.[391] The mutations are inherited in an autosomal dominant manner, but sporadic mutations are not infrequent.

Mutations in the gene encoding cardiac troponin I have been identified in over half of adults with the idiopathic variant.[392] Individual examples of these mutations have been reported in children.[392,393]

Endomyocardial Fibrosis and Eosinophilic Cardiomyopathy (Löffler's Endocarditis)

Restrictive ventricular physiology can be caused by endocardial fibrosis, fibroelastosis, and thrombosis. These disorders are subclassified according the presence of eosinophilia as endomyocardial diseases with or without hypereosinophilia. Parasitic infection, drugs such as methysergide, and inflammatory and nutritional factors are implicated in acquired forms of endomyocardial fibrosis. The disease is endemic in tropical and subtropical parts of Africa, India, Asia, and South and Central America, and may account for up to one-quarter of cardiac-related deaths in equatorial Africa.[394] It is rare outside the tropics.[388] Adolescents and young adults are most frequently affected. Onset is usually insidious, with progressive biventricular failure in most cases. The overall prognosis is poor, with almost half dead by 1 year, and almost nine-tenths at 3 years.[395] Typically, fibrous endocardial lesions cause incompetence of the atrioventricular valves, leading to pulmonary congestion and right cardiac failure.

Other Infiltrative and Storage Disorders Associated with Restrictive Cardiomyopathy

Several infiltrative and storage disorders cause restrictive cardiomyopathy (see Table 49-1). These include lysosomal storage disorders such as mucopolysaccharidosis and Anderson-Fabry disease (see Chapter 57), albeit that the latter is more commonly associated with hypertrophic cardiomyopathy.[388]

Cardiac sarcoidosis can produce restrictive cardiomyopathy progressing to systolic impairment, and is also typically associated with conduction disease and a risk of sudden death. The diagnostic tests for sarcoidosis may be normal, and a high index of suspicion is required for diagnosis. Cardiac magnetic resonance imaging and positron emission tomography are the most sensitive imaging techniques, and changes appear to correlate with the activity of the disease. Treatment includes corticosteroids, implantable cardioverter-defibrillators for patients with a history of non-sustained ventricular tachycardia, and cardiac transplantation. Sarcoid granulomatous lesions may recur in the transplanted cardiac allograft.[396] Sarcoidosis is more common in adults than in children, being rare in children below the age of 15 years, and exceedingly rare in those younger than 4 years.[397]

Pathology

The macroscopic features include biatrial dilation in the presence of normal cardiac weight, a small ventricular cavity, and no left ventricular hypertrophy. The morphological spectrum of primary disease includes mild ventricular hypertrophy with increased cardiac weight, sometimes described as hypertrophic restrictive cardiomyopathy, and mild ventricular dilation without hypertrophy.[398] These findings highlight the substantial overlap between restrictive cardiomyopathy and the other cardiomyopathies. In many hearts, there is thrombus in the atrial appendages and patchy endocardial fibrosis.[388] The histological features are classically non-specific, with patchy interstitial fibrosis, which may range in extent from very mild to severe.[388] There may also be fibrosis of the cardiac nodes.[399] Myocytic disarray is not uncommon in patients with pure restrictive cardiomyopathy, even in the absence of macroscopic ventricular hypertrophy.[398] In those with infiltrative and metabolic cardiomyopathies, there will be specific findings appropriate to the disorder.[335]

Pathophysiology

The characteristic feature is the precipitous rise in intraventricular pressures during ventricular filling, caused by a reduction in left ventricular compliance. The result is that ventricular filling is completed in early diastole, and there is little or no filling in late diastole, thereby elevating left ventricular filling pressures and compromising cardiac output. Impaired and delayed active relaxation of the left ventricle may also play a role in the pathophysiology of the idiopathic disease in children.[400]

The finding that mutations in the sarcomeric protein genes cause restrictive cardiomyopathy has provided new insights into the pathophysiology of restrictive left ventricular physiology. Experimental studies have suggested that mutations of troponin I that cause restrictive cardiomyopathy have a greater increase in the sensitivity of calcium ions than those causing hypertrophic cardiomyopathy, resulting in more severe diastolic dysfunction and potentially accounting for the restrictive phenotype in humans.[401,402] In addition, the hearts of troponin I–mutated transgenic mice show increased contractility and impaired relaxation.[403] Similar results have been observed in mice with disease-causing mutations of α-myosin heavy chain.[404] The fact that the same sarcomeric mutation within the same family can result in both restrictive and hypertrophic phenotypes suggests that other genetic and environmental factors are likely to be involved.[140]

Clinical Features

Symptoms

The presentation is usually with symptoms and signs of cardiac failure and arrhythmia. In children, the cardiomyopathy can mimic other, more common, diseases such as asthma or recurrent chest infections, epilepsy, or hepatic conditions. Because of this, referral to the cardiologist is often delayed.[378] Common symptoms include dyspnoea on exertion, recurrent infections of the respiratory tract, and general fatigue and weakness. This may progress rapidly to dyspnoea at rest, orthopnoea, and paroxysmal nocturnal dyspnoea in older children. Symptoms related to increased right-sided pressures may include peripheral oedema and abdominal distention due to ascites. Many patients complain of chest pain and symptoms suggestive of arrhythmia, such as palpitation. Syncope is a presenting symptom in one-tenth of affected children.[386,400] Rarely, sudden death may be the initial manifestation of the disease.

Physical Examination

Clinical examination typically reveals signs of left- and right-sided cardiac failure. Tachypnoea, signs of respiratory distress, and failure to thrive are seen in infants and young children. In older children, the jugular venous pressure is elevated, with a prominent y descent, and fails to fall, or may even rise, during inspiration. The latter is called Kussmaul's sign. Peripheral oedema, ascites, and hepatomegaly are common. The apical impulse is usually normal. Cardiac auscultation reveals a normal first heart sound and normal splitting of the second heart sound. The pulmonary component of the second heart sound may be loud if pulmonary vascular resistance is high. There is usually a third heart sound, and occasionally a fourth heart sound giving rise to a gallop rhythm. The murmurs of atrioventricular valvar regurgitation may be heard.

Investigations

A number of investigations are useful. The purpose is to confirm the diagnosis, to exclude constrictive pericarditis, and to assess suitability for cardiac transplantation.

Electrocardiography

The resting 12-lead electrocardiogram is abnormal in the majority of children with restrictive cardiomyopathy. The most frequent abnormalities include enlargement of the left and right atriums, so-called p-mitrale and p-pulmonale, non-specific changes in the ST segments, and T wave abnormalities. There can be depression of the ST segment and T wave inversion, usually in the inferolateral leads (Fig. 49-13). Voltage criterions for left and right ventricular hypertrophy may also be present. Abnormalities of conduction, including intraventricular conduction delay, and abnormal Q waves may also be seen.

Chest Radiography

The chest radiograph is usually abnormal, showing cardiomegaly caused by atrial enlargement, and pulmonary venous congestion. Interstitial oedema, manifested by the presence of Kerley B lines, may be seen in severe cases.

Echocardiography

Typically, there is marked dilation of both atriums, often dwarfing the size of the ventricles, in the presence of normal or mildly reduced systolic function, and a non-hypertrophied, non-dilated left ventricle (Fig. 49-14A). Severe impairment of left ventricular systolic function, with fractional shortening less than 25%, may develop in up to one-third of children.[380,381,384,400] Many patients with a clinical label of restrictive cardiomyopathy also have mild left ventricular hypertrophy,[380–382,384,400] but in many cases, this may represent part of the spectrum of sarcomeric protein disease.

The flow through the mitral valve as assessed by pulsed-wave Doppler velocities typically shows increased velocities of early diastolic filling, decreased velocities of atrial filling, an increased ratio of early diastolic to atrial filling, a decreased deceleration time, and a decreased isovolumic relaxation time (see Fig. 49-14B). Interrogation of the pulmonary and hepatic veins with pulsed wave Doppler reveals higher diastolic than systolic velocities, increased atrial reversal velocities, and a duration of atrial reversal greater than that of atrial filling (see Fig. 49-14C). Tissue Doppler imaging shows reduced diastolic annular velocities, and an increased ratio of early diastolic tissue Doppler annular velocity to mitral early diastolic filling velocity, reflecting elevated left ventricular end-diastolic pressures. Mitral inflow and pulmonary, hepatic, and tissue Doppler velocities should be evaluated in the context of published normal values for children.

Ambulatory Electrocardiographic Monitoring

Disturbances of atrioventricular conduction, and atrial arrhythmias, are common when restrictive cardiomyopathy is found in childhood, occurring in one-sixth

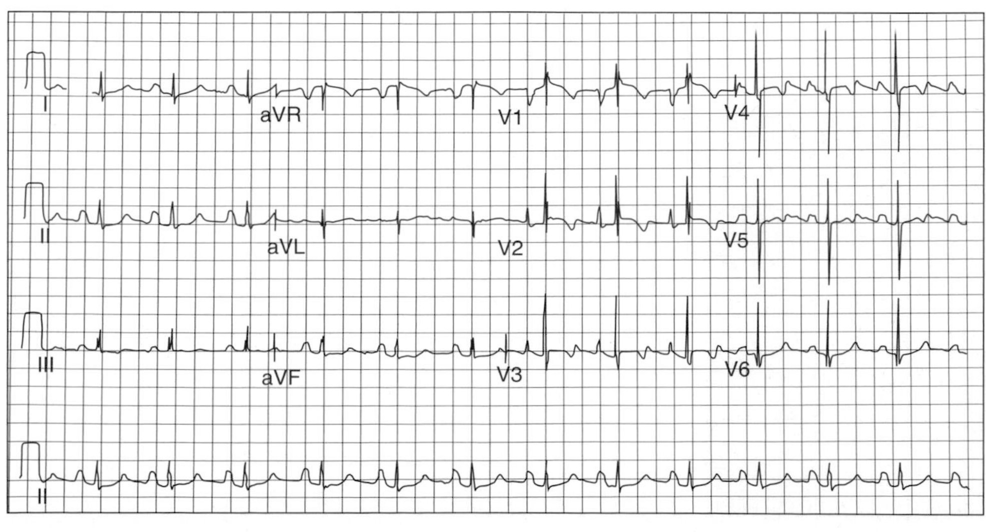

Figure 49-13 This 12-lead electrocardiogram from a 12-year-old with familial restrictive cardiomyopathy shows left and right atrial enlargement and T wave abnormalities extending from leads V1 to V5.

of patients.[378–386] Analysis of the ST segments may reveal evidence of myocardial ischaemia, particularly at higher heart rates, which may precede the development of ventricular arrhythmia.[386]

Cardiopulmonary Exercise Testing

Symptom-limited exercise testing with analysis of respiratory gases provides a useful objective measure of limitation, which can help in management of symptoms and is an important component of assessment prior to transplantation. Peak consumption of oxygen is usually reduced. Exercise testing may also reveal ischaemic electrocardiographic changes at higher heart rates, which may correlate with symptoms such as chest pain.

Cardiac Catheterisation

Cardiac catheterisation is important, particularly prior to consideration for transplantation. The characteristic haemodynamic feature is a deep and rapid early decline in ventricular pressure at the onset of diastole, with a rapid rise to a plateau in early diastole, the so-called dip-and-plateau, or square root, sign.[388] Left ventricular end-diastolic, left atrial, and pulmonary capillary wedge pressures are markedly elevated, and usually 5 mmHg or more greater than right atrial and right ventricular end-diastolic pressures. Volume loading and exercise accentuate the difference between left- and right-sided pressures.

Pulmonary hypertension is frequently present during initial cardiac catheterisation. Elevated indexes of pulmonary vascular resistance are commonly found, and tend to progress during follow-up.[384,385,387] Elevated pulmonary vascular resistance may initially be reversible with nitric oxide or prostacyclin,[385,387] but it is usually not possible to predict the development of fixed pulmonary vascular resistance.[384] Endomyocardial biopsy is usually non-diagnostic, but may be useful in some of the cases due to storage disease or infiltrations.

Management

The prognosis for children with restrictive cardiomyopathy in the absence of transplantation is poor. Medical treatment in severely symptomatic patients is usually supportive until transplantation is performed. Occasionally, patients may remain stable for several months or years before an acute decompensation necessitating transplantation occurs. By that stage, however, pulmonary hypertension may preclude orthotopic transplantation, and heart-lung transplantation or heterotopic cardiac transplantation may be the only options.[405] Medical management should follow guidelines for the management of diastolic cardiac failure set out by the International Society for Heart and Lung Transplantation.[283]

Symptomatic Therapy

Diuretics are useful in patients with symptoms and signs of pulmonary or systemic venous congestion. Over-diuresis, however should be avoided, as it may result in excessive preload reduction and haemodynamic collapse. Careful management of fluids is an important aspect of treatment. In view of atrial enlargement and propensity

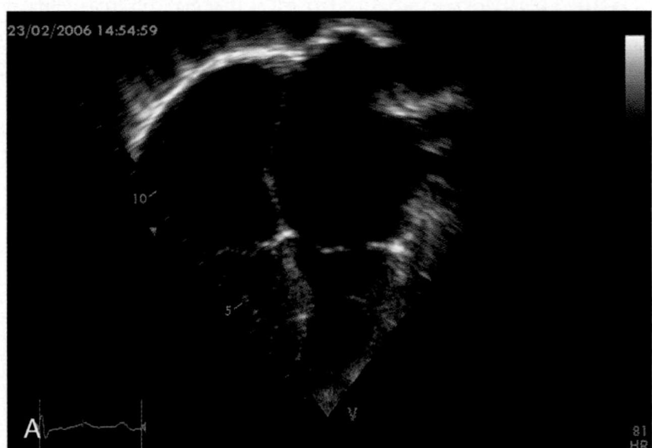

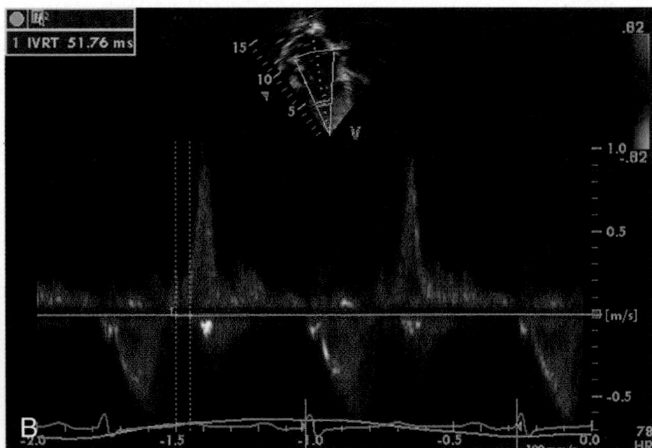

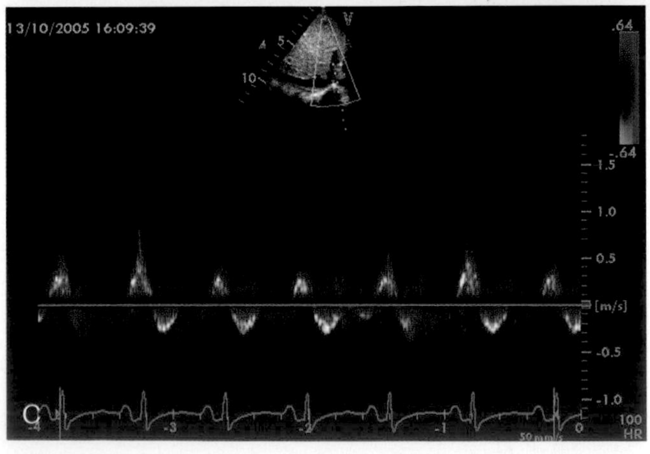

Figure 49-14 Echocardiographic features of restrictive cardiomyopathy. **A** shows an apical four-chamber view from a 6-year-old with restrictive cardiomyopathy. Note the massively dilated left and right atriums without significant left ventricular hypertrophy or dilation. **B** is a continuous wave Doppler recording of mitral inflow and left ventricular outflow from the same patient, showing a short isovolumic relaxation time; the restrictive mitral inflow pattern can also be appreciated, with a peaked E wave, short E wave deceleration time and E/A ratio greater than 2.5. **C** is a pulsed wave Doppler of a hepatic vein in an 8-year-old with restrictive cardiomyopathy, showing an increased atrial reversal wave.

to atrial arrhythmia, prophylactic anticoagulation with warfarin or antiplatelet agents is recommended. Since the atrial contribution to ventricular filling is important, efforts to maintain sinus rhythm with β-blockers and amiodarone may be appropriate. Treatment with afterload-reducing agents, such as inhibitors of angiotensin-converting enzyme, blockers of calcium channels, and nitrates, rarely improves symptoms and can cause deterioration.[349]

Optimisation of Haemodynamics Prior to Transplantation

Transplantation is the only definitive treatment. Whilst fixed and irreversible elevations in pulmonary vascular resistance preclude orthotopic cardiac transplantation,[384] short-term treatment with prostacyclin, for around 2 months, has been shown to reduce transpulmonary gradients sufficiently to allow orthotopic heart transplantation in most children with restrictive cardiomyopathy.[385] While on the waiting list for transplantation, patients should undergo serial Holter monitoring. Cardioverter-defibrillators should be implanted in patients with evidence of ventricular arrhythmia as a bridge to transplantation.

ARRHYTHMOGENIC RIGHT VENTRICULAR CARDIOMYOPATHY

Definition and Historical Aspects

Arrhythmogenic right ventricular cardiomyopathy is a myocardial disease characterised by progressive replacement of right ventricular myocardium by fibrous tissue and fat, initially with regional, and later with global, right and left ventricular involvement. It is associated with ventricular arrhythmias, cardiac failure, and sudden cardiac death. The term arrhythmogenic right ventricular cardiomyopathy now replaces arrhythmogenic right ventricular dysplasia, which was initially used to describe the condition.

Epidemiology

The reported prevalence is approximately 1 in 5000,[406] but emerging data from family studies suggests that this is almost certainly an underestimate caused, in part, by the difficulty in making the diagnosis clinically. In children, arrhythmogenic cardiomyopathies account for less than 3% of all cardiomyopathies.[22,23] The condition has been described, nonetheless, in children as young as 1 year of age,[407] and presentation with sudden death is reported in adolescents as well as in younger children.[408–418] There is a male predominance across all ages.[419]

Natural History

The disease is currently thought to progress through several phases, starting with an early concealed phase, during which patients are asymptomatic, and clinical features are absent. This progresses to an overt electrical disorder, characterised by symptomatic ventricular arrhythmia and morphological abnormalities usually detectable by imaging, followed by a right ventricular phase, characterised by extension of fibro-fatty infiltration throughout the right ventricular myocardium, causing right cardiac failure. The final stage in many patients is a biventricular phase, characterised by left ventricular involvement and biventricular failure, which is often indistinguishable from dilated cardiomyopathy.[420] Studies of families have shown that some patients present for the first time with biventricular dilation, or with predominant, or even exclusive, left ventricular involvement. Sudden cardiac death can occur at any stage, including the concealed phase.[418] Given the progressive nature of the condition, children might be expected to present during the early concealed or arrhythmic phases, rather than with overt cardiomyopathy. Left and right ventricular dilation in children with familial disease, nonetheless, is increasingly recognised.[410,421,422]

Aetiology

Systematic familial studies have shown that this cardiomyopathy is inherited in up to half the cases.[419] The mode of transmission is usually autosomal dominant with variable penetrance, but autosomal recessive forms are also recognised. The first insights into the genetic basis came from the description of an autosomal recessive syndrome characterised by cardiomyopathy, woolly hair, and palmoplantar keratoderma. The afflicted families came from the Greek island of Naxos.[423] The cardiac phenotype demonstrated the typical clinical and histopathological characteristics.[424] Following this initial description, families with a similar phenotype were reported from other Mediterranean areas,[425–428] India,[429] and South America.[430] Subsequent molecular genetic investigations in families with these cardiocutaneous syndromes revealed mutations in the genes encoding plakoglobin and desmoplakin.[425,431,432] These proteins are major components of cell adhesive junctions, with key roles in cell-to-cell communication and transduction of mechanical stress. Mutations in these, and other cell adhesive molecules, including plakophilin-2,[417,433] desmoglein,[434] and desmocollin[413] have been identified in autosomal dominant cases without cutaneous manifestations.[411,435] Rare examples of implicated non-desmosomal genes include the ryanodine receptor-2,[436] more commonly associated with catecholaminergic polymorphic ventricular tachycardia, and transforming growth factor-β.[437] Other aetiopathogenic factors have been suggested to play a role in development. In particular, enteroviral and adenoviral genomes have been identified in a few patients with the condition[438] although other studies have not replicated these findings.[439]

Pathology

In the early stages, abnormal pathological findings are localised to the apical, inflow, and infundibular areas of the right ventricle, initially referred to as the triangle of dysplasia.[440] With progression, the left ventricle may also become involved, with particular involvement of the posterolateral wall and relative sparing of the septum. In some cases, the pathological abnormalities may be confined to the left ventricle.[335,441] Macroscopic examination (Fig. 49-15) may show diffuse or focal thinning of the right ventricular wall, with aneurysms present in up to half the cases.[335,442] Histologically, there is myocardial atrophy and fibro-fatty replacement. Islands or strands of surviving myocytes exhibit a combination of degenerative change with myocytic vacuolation, and are frequently associated with focal infiltrates of mononuclear inflammatory cells.[443–445] In some cases,

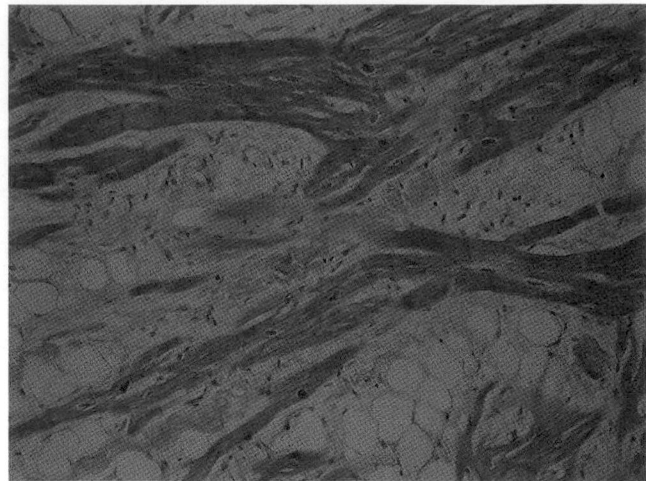

Figure 49-15 Histopathological features of arrhythmogenic right ventricular cardiomyopathy, characterised by fibro-fatty infiltration of the myocardium. (Courtesy of Dr Michael Ashworth, Great Ormond Street Hospital, London, United Kingdom.)

typical histological findings may be present in the absence of any macroscopic features.[446] A second histological pattern, characterised by transmural infiltration of adipose tissue without fibrous replacement or mural thinning, has been suggested to represent an earlier stage of the condition,[443,447] but this is probably a normal finding, particularly in older females.[442]

Clinical Features

The first presentation of the disease is often sudden cardiac death in previously asymptomatic individuals, including young children and teenagers.[408,409,418,448] Occasionally, patients will have experienced syncope in the months preceding their death.[408,449,450] An imbalance of adrenergic activity has been suggested as a possible factor in the genesis of lethal ventricular arrhythmias; thus, exposure to catecholamines, particularly during exercise, may increase the risk of sudden death.[451] Overall, syncope and other symptoms of arrhythmia, including presyncope, palpitation, and chest pain, are common clinical manifestations, but family studies have shown that most affected individuals are asymptomatic, particularly in the early stages.[452] With progression, features of right, and later biventricular, failure may be present, including dyspnoea on exertion.

In children, reports of the condition are biased towards those who have presented with symptoms, and in these patients, arrhythmic symptoms predominate.[410,414,421,450]

Investigations

There is no single diagnostic test, and the diagnosis is based on the presence of major and minor criterions that describe structural, histological, electrocardiographic, arrhythmic, and familial features (Table 49-3).[453] In this scheme, the diagnosis is fulfilled in the presence of two major criterions, or one major plus two minor criterions, or four minor criterions from different categories.[419] Family studies have shown that first-degree relatives of affected individuals may have minor cardiac abnormalities, which, although not fulfilling the above diagnostic criterions, are likely to represent expression in the context of an autosomal dominant disease. Because of this, modified diagnostic criterions have been proposed for diagnosis in family members of affected individuals.[452] Whether these modified criterions are also applicable to pre-adolescent children remains to be evaluated.

Electrocardiography

The most common electrocardiographic abnormality is inversion of the T waves in leads V1 to V3 in the absence of right bundle branch block (Fig. 49-16). This is a normal finding in children, and cannot therefore be used as a diagnostic criterion. Presence of such inversion of T waves beyond lead V3 outside the neonatal period, nonetheless, should raise suspicion of an underlying myocardial pathology. Other electrocardiographic features include abnormalities of depolarisation and conduction such as QRS dispersion, a delay in right intraventricular conduction delay, progressing to right bundle branch block in some patients, and the presence of an epsilon wave. These features are also recognised in children.[450]

Signal-averaged Electrocardiography

The signal-averaged electrocardiogram is used to evaluate the presence of late potentials.[454] Up to four-fifths of patients with arrhythmogenic right ventricular cardiomyopathy have evidence of late potentials on the signal-averaged electrocardiogram,[455,456] and this finding correlates with the risk of ventricular arrhythmia[457] and progression of disease.[458] Normal values for signal-averaged electrocardiography in children have been reported, but to date, there have been no systematic studies evaluating its role in the diagnosis of arrhythmogenic right ventricular cardiomyopathy. Extrapolation from adult data may not be applicable, as late potentials have been shown to be present in less than one-third of individuals with arrhythmogenic right ventricular cardiomyopathy associated with only localised right ventricular abnormalities and normal right ventricular end-diastolic volumes,[458] likely to be the morphology most commonly encountered in children.

Ambulatory Electrocardiographic Monitoring

Perhaps the most useful investigation in children is ambulatory electrocardiographic monitoring. The spectrum of ventricular arrhythmia ranges from frequent ventricular extrasystoles to sustained ventricular tachycardia. The distinctive QRS morphology of ventricular arrhythmia in arrhythmogenic right ventricular cardiomyopathy is a left bundle branch pattern, indicating a right ventricular origin. The morphology of the QRS complex may provide clues as to the site of origin. An inferior axis suggests an origin in the right ventricular outflow tract, whereas a superior axis implies origin in the right ventricular apex or inferior wall. With more advanced disease, several different right ventricular morphologies may be seen, reflecting multiple arrhythmogenic focuses.

Ventricular arrhythmias, ranging from isolated premature ventricular beats to non-sustained or sustained ventricular tachycardia, are common. Suggested arrhythmic mechanisms include re-entry circuits arising from fibro-fatty myocardial replacement, and heterogeneous conduction resulting from destabilisation of cell adhesion complexes and gap junctions.[420] Hot phases are recognised, during which previously stable patients may suffer repeated episodes of ventricular arrhythmia in a short period of

TABLE 49-3

DIAGNOSTIC CRITERIONS FOR ARRHYTHMOGENIC RIGHT VENTRICULAR CARDIOMYOPATHY

	Major	Minor
1. Global and/or regional dysfunction and structural alterations	Severe dilatation and reduction of right ventricular ejection fraction with no (or only mild) left ventricular impairment	Mild global right ventricular dilatation and/or ejection fraction reduction with normal left ventricle
	Localised right ventricular aneurysms (akinetic or dyskinetic areas with diastolic bulging)	Mild segmental dilatation of the right ventricle
	Severe segmental dilatation of the right ventricle	Regional right ventricular hypokinesia
2. Tissue characterisation of walls	Fibro-fatty replacement of myocardium on endomyocardial biopsy	
3. Depolarisation abnormalities	Epsilon waves or localised prolongation (>110 ms) of the QRS complex in right precordial leads (V1–V3)	Late potentials (signal averaged ECG)
4. Repolarisation abnormalities		Inverted T waves in right precordial leads (V2 and V3) (>12 years of age; in absence of right bundle branch block)
5. Arrhythmias		Left bundle branch block type ventricular tachycardia (sustained and nonsustained) on ECG, Holter monitor, or exercise testing
		Frequent ventricular extrasystoles (>1000 in 24 hours)
6. Family history	Familial disease confirmed at postmortem or surgery	Familial history of premature sudden death (<35 years of age) due to suspected right ventricular dysplasia
		Family history, with clinical diagnosis based on present criterions

Adapted from McKenna WJ, Thiene G, Nava A, et al: Diagnosis of arrhythmogenic right ventricular dysplasia/cardiomyopathy. Task Force of the Working Group Myocardial and Pericardial Disease of the European Society of Cardiology and of the Scientific Council on Cardiomyopathies of the International Society and Federation of Cardiology. Br Heart J 1994;71:215–218.

time, and sudden death may occur. In children, isolated ventricular extrasystoles, ventricular couplets and triplets, non-sustained and sustained ventricular tachycardia, and ventricular fibrillation have all been reported.[450]

Exercise Testing

The role of exercise testing in children is primarily to detect ventricular arrhythmias induced by physical activity. Ventricular ectopy and non-sustained ventricular tachycardia of right ventricular origin have been described in young individuals.[450] Cardiopulmonary exercise testing may also be useful as an objective measure of functional capacity in patients with advanced disease.

Echocardiography

A major role of echocardiography in the evaluation of the disease, particularly in children, is the exclusion of congenital cardiac disease in the differential diagnosis, such as partially anomalous venous drainage and Ebstein's malformation.[459–461] The echocardiographic findings include right ventricular dilation and hypokinesia, aneurysms (Fig. 49-17), abnormalities of regional wall motion,

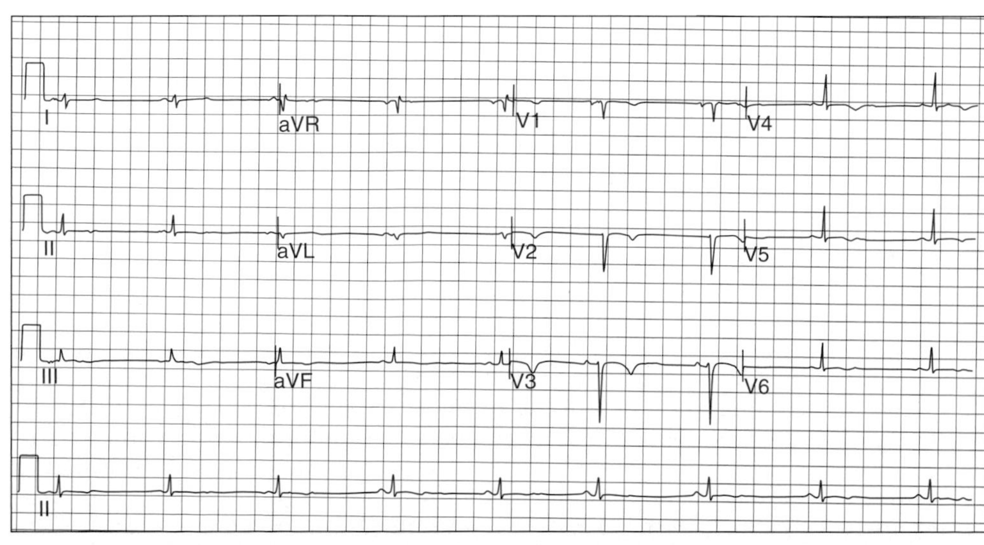

Figure 49-16 The 12-lead electrocardiogram from an undiagnosed 15-year-old who died suddenly, and was found to have arrhythmogenic right ventricular cardiomyopathy on postmortem. There is T wave inversion extending from V1 to V4 with flat T waves elsewhere, reduced right ventricular voltages. and mild QRS dispersion. (Courtesy of Dr Antonis Pantazis, The Heart Hospital, London, United Kingdom.)

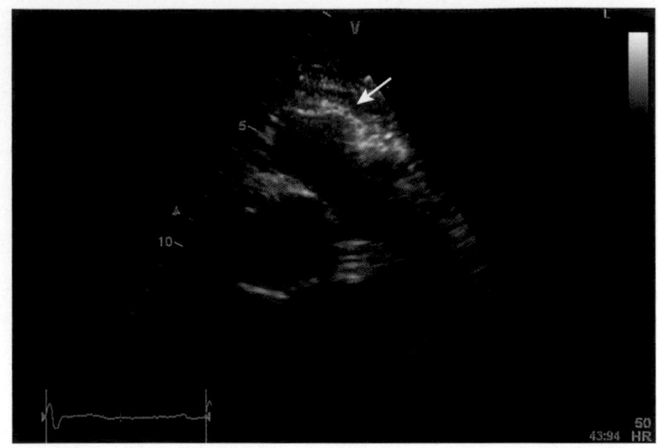

Figure 49-17 This end-systolic parasternal long-axis echocardiographic frame of the right ventricular outflow tract from a young male with arrhythmogenic right ventricular cardiomyopathy shows a small aneurysm of the anterior wall (*arrow*). (Courtesy of Dr Antonis Pantazis, The Heart Hospital, London.)

including dyskinesia of the inferobasal right ventricular segment, increased echogenicity of the moderator band, and right ventricular apical hypertrabeculation.[410,450,461–463] Given the segmental nature of the disease, structure and function should be assessed using multiple views.[464] Left ventricular involvement should also be evaluated. Tricuspid annular early diastolic velocities are reduced.[464]

Cardiac Magnetic Resonance Imaging

Cardiovascular magnetic resonance imaging is an attractive tool, as it is not limited by acoustic windows, and the acquisition of three-dimensional data sets permits accurate determination of right ventricular volumes and function.[465] Late enhancement with gadolinium has been shown to correlate with fibro-fatty changes.[466] There is, nonetheless, an inherent subjectivity in the interpretation of mural thinning, localised abnormalities of wall motion, and intramyocardial fat in the right ventricle.[465,467–469] Reproducibility and accuracy, therefore, are strongly operator dependent.[465]

Endomyocardial Biopsy

Although a histological diagnosis may be definitive, the sensitivity of endomyocardial biopsies is low, since samples are usually taken from the septum, a region that is usually not involved in this disease.[419] Furthermore, there is a high rate of complications, including cardiac perforation and tamponade, resulting from thinning of the right ventricular wall.[453] Endomyocardial biopsies are no longer considered part of the routine diagnostic workup.

Management

Patients with symptomatic, non-life-threatening arrhythmias are usually treated empirically with antiarrhythmic agents, including β-adrenoreceptor blockers and amiodarone.[470] Beta-blockers in particular are effective at treating symptoms related to exercise-induced arrhythmia, and sotalol can suppress ventricular arrhythmia in a high proportion of patients.[470] Patients with severe right ventricular or biventricular involvement should be treated according to current guidelines for cardiac failure, using diuretics, inhibitors of angiotensin-converting enzyme, and anticoagulation. Some patients may become candidates for cardiac transplantation. Patients are discouraged from participating in strenuous physical activities.[418,448,449] Recent studies, however, have shown that most patients who die suddenly do so at rest.[408] Patients considered to be at high risk of sudden cardiac death should be offered an implantable cardioverter-defibrillator. Studies evaluating their role, albeit predominantly in adults, have shown a high rate of appropriate discharges.[471,472] Whilst it is clear that implantation of the cardioverter-defibrillators saves lives in this disease, the problem lies in identifying those individuals at risk who would benefit most from primary prophylaxis. This is particularly important, as implantation of internal defibrillators is not without its side effects, especially in children. A number of markers of increased risk have been proposed, including unexplained syncope, symptomatic ventricular tachycardia, family history of sudden death, young age, left ventricular involvement, and diffuse right ventricular dilation.[473–475] Population-based survival studies are needed to evaluate the significance of these and other factors, such as asymptomatic non-sustained ventricular tachycardia, and to develop an algorithm for stratification of risk for patients with arrhythmogenic right ventricular cardiomyopathy.

UNCLASSIFIED CARDIOMYOPATHIES

The unclassified cardiomyopathies include diseases that do not fit readily into any morphological subgroup. These include left ventricular non-compaction and endocardial fibroelastosis.

Left Ventricular Non-compaction

Left ventricular non-compaction is a disorder of myocardial morphogenesis that results in multiple prominent trabeculations and deep intertrabecular recesses in the left ventricular myocardium.[476–478] The condition, previously termed spongy myocardium or spongiform cardiomyopathy, is thought to result from an arrest in the process of involution of endomyocardial trabeculations, which normally occurs by the end of the 10th week of embryonic development. In infants, as already discussed, left ventricular non-compaction can occur in the X-linked Barth syndrome.[328,479] Mutations in the genes encoding α-dystrobrevin and Cypher/ZASP, two important structural proteins with a role linking the cytoskeleton of the cardiac myocyte to the extracellular matrix, have also been reported in adults with left ventricular non-compaction.[479,480] A family history of non-compaction or dilated cardiomyopathy is present in approximately one-quarter of cases.[481] The abnormality can also occur in congenitally malformed hearts[479,482,483]; indeed, it is probably commoner than thought in these settings. In some cases it is caused by mutations in the NKX2.5 transcription factor.[484,485] It is increasingly becoming recognised as an important cause of cardiomyopathy in children, accounting for nearly one-tenth of cases registered in the Australian study.[22]

Diagnosis can be made using cross sectional echocardiography (Fig. 49-18). Several diagnostic criterions have been proposed. One suggests a ratio of 0.5 or less for the distance from the epicardial surface to the trough of a trabecular recess compared to the distance from the epicardial surface to the peak of the trabeculation measured in end-diastole.[476] Another requires the presence of numerous, excessively prominent trabeculations and deep intertrabecular recesses supplied by blood on colour Doppler, and a bilayered arrangement with a thin compacted layer and a thick non-compacted layer, the ratio of non-compacted to compacted endocardial layers being greater than 2 when measured in end-systole, in the absence of co-existing structural cardiac abnormalities.[486] A third requires the presence of more than three trabeculations protruding from the left ventricular wall distal to the papillary muscles visible in one imaging plane and associated with intertrabecular spaces visualised using colour Doppler.[487] Each proposed criterion has limitations, and the three are probably complementary in making the diagnosis.[481] Although awareness of the condition is increasing, some patients may be misdiagnosed as having distal or apical hypertrophic cardiomyopathy,[488] and an overlap with dilated cardiomyopathy is also recognised.[481] Alternative imaging modalities, particularly cardiac magnetic resonance imaging, may prove useful for distinguishing between left ventricular non-compaction and hypertrophic cardiomyopathy.[488–491] In some children, an undulating phenotype characterised by alternating features of dilated cardiomyopathy and hypertrophic cardiomyopathy has been reported.[483]

The natural history remains to be fully characterised. Initial studies reported a poor prognosis,[492] but subsequent reports in children and adults have suggested a better prognosis.[481,483] Family studies suggest that there may be a prolonged preclinical phase before the onset of symptomatic clinical disease, evidenced by the finding of left ventricular enlargement with preserved systolic function and asymptomatic hypertrabeculation in relatives.[481] In some cases, systolic impairment may have been present early in life, recovering during childhood only to present again in adulthood.[483] The clinical features in adults and children include left ventricular systolic and diastolic dysfunction, thromboembolism, and ventricular arrhythmia.[476,481,483,492–501]

The medical treatment aims to improve symptoms and prevent complications. Aspirin has been recommended in all patients by some groups,[483] with warfarin for patients with documented thromboembolic events. Patients with ventricular dilation and systolic impairment should be managed with vasodilators and β-blockers, according to current guidelines.[283] Patients with evidence of ventricular arrhythmia may benefit from insertion of an implantable cardioverter-defibrillator. In some children refractory to medical therapy, cardiac transplantation may be considered.

Endocardial Fibro-elastosis

Endocardial fibro-elastosis is a rare and poorly understood disease of the endomyocardium. The diagnosis is made histologically, and the pathological hallmarks consist of deposition of collagen and elastin, ventricular hypertrophy, and diffuse endocardial thickening.[502] Sporadic and familial disease has been described.[503] The aetiology is not fully understood. Isolated, or primary, endocardial fibroelastosis often mimics dilated cardiomyopathy.[504] More commonly, it occurs in association with other structural cardiac abnormalities, including left-sided obstructive lesions such as aortic stenosis, and anomalous coronary artery arising from the pulmonary trunk. It is likely that the fibroelastosis represents the end-stage pathological phenotype of a heterogeneous group of conditions, rather than a single disease entity.[505] Possible aetiopathogenic factors include viral infections with agents such as coxsackievirus,[506,507] adenovirus,[508] parvovirus,[509] and mumps virus.[508,510] In addition, it may be associated with metabolic and storage disorders, including primary deficiency of carnitine and respiratory chain abnormalities.[511–515] More recently, it has been recognised in fetal and postnatal life, in association with maternal

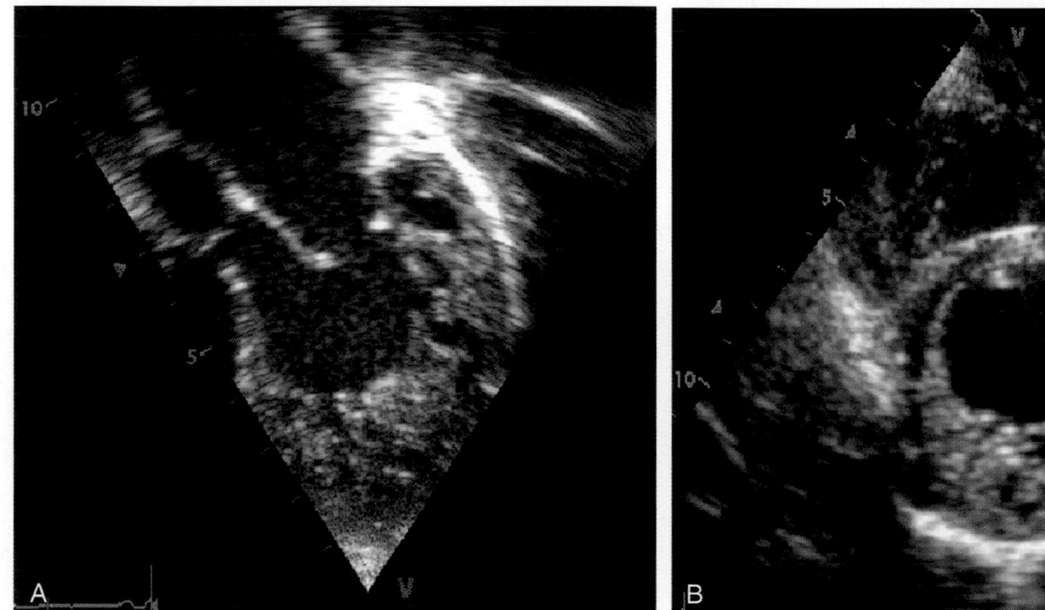

Figure 49-18 Echocardiographic features of left ventricular non-compaction. A is an apical five-chamber frame from a child with left ventricular non-compaction. It shows left ventricular trabeculations and deep recesses extending into the left ventricular mid-cavity. B is a parasternal short-axis view from another child with left ventricular non-compaction, showing a hypertrabeculated area in the distal portion of the left ventricle. (Courtesy of Dr Jan Marek, Great Ormond Street Hospital, London, United Kingdom.)

anti-Ro and anti-La antibodies, in children with and without congenital complete heart block.[516,517]

Endocardial fibroelastosis usually presents in infancy, and the clinical features are typically indistinguishable from those seen in dilated cardiomyopathy.[518] In many cases, patients progress to end-stage cardiac failure and death.[519–521] Survival of three-quarters at 4 years has been reported.[518] The management is symptomatic, and follows that of dilated cardiomyopathy, including diuretics, vasodilators and digoxin.

Tako-tsubo Cardiomyopathy

Stress cardiomyopathy is a recently described cardiomyopathy characterised by transient and rapidly reversible left ventricular apical ballooning and systolic dysfunction in the absence of coronary arterial disease, triggered usually by profound psychological stress.[522–524] It is associated with characteristic elevation of the ST segments on the electrocardiogram that mimics acute myocardial infarction. The condition was first described in Japan as takotsubo cardiomyopathy, after the Japanese name for an octopus trap, *tako-tsubo*, that has a similar configuration to the affected left ventricle. Most affected patients are over 60 years old. Recently, a case of suspected takotsubo cardiomyopathy was reported in a 2-year-old girl, following withdrawal of buprenorphine treatment.[525] The pathogenesis of the condition remains to be elucidated.

The complete reference list can be found on the companion Expert Consult web site at www.expertconsult.com.

ANNOTATED REFERENCES

- Elliott P, Andersson B, Arbustini E, et al: Classification of the cardiomyopathies: A position statement from the European Society of Cardiology Working Group on Myocardial and Pericardial Diseases. Eur Heart J 2008;29:270–276.

  This recent report from the European Society of Cardiology Working Group on Myocardial and Pericardial Diseases provides a comprehensive classification of the cardiomyopathies.
- Nugent AW, Daubeney PE, Chondros P, et al: The epidemiology of childhood cardiomyopathy in Australia. N Engl J Med 2003;348:1639–1646.
- Lipshultz SE, Sleeper LA, Towbin JA, et al: The incidence of pediatric cardiomyopathy in two regions of the United States. N Engl J Med 2003;348:1647–1655.

  These two population-based studies provide novel epidemiological and aetiological data on childhood cardiomyopathies.
- Ahmad F, Seidman JG, Seidman CE: The genetic basis for cardiac remodeling. Annu Rev Genomics Hum Genet 2005;6:185–216.

  This is an excellent and comprehensive review of the genetic basis of cardiomyopathies.
- Elliott PM, Poloniecki J, Dickie S, et al: Sudden death in hypertrophic cardiomyopathy: Identification of high risk patients. J Am Coll Cardiol 2000;36:2212–2218.

  This study reports a non-invasive risk stratification algorithm for identifying patients with hypertrophic cardiomyopathy at risk of sudden death. Although the data is derived from adults, it has been extrapolated to children with some success.
- Maron BJ, Shen WK, Link MS, et al: Efficacy of implantable cardioverter-defibrillators for the prevention of sudden death in patients with hypertrophic cardiomyopathy. N Engl J Med 2000;342:365–373.

  This large study demonstrates that implantation of cardioverter-defibrillators prevents sudden death in a population of patients, mostly adults, with hypertrophic cardiomyopathy.
- Mason JW, O'Connell JB, Herskowitz A, et al: A clinical trial of immunosuppressive therapy for myocarditis. The Myocarditis Treatment Trial Investigators. N Engl J Med 1995;333:269–275.

  This randomised controlled trial of 111 adults with myocarditis showed no improvement in survival in patients given immunosuppressive therapy, suggesting that the routine use of immunosuppressive drugs in patients with myocarditis is not warranted.
- Rosenthal D, Chrisant MR, Edens E, et al: International Society for Heart and Lung Transplantation: Practice guidelines for management of heart failure in children. J Heart Lung Transplant 2004;23:1313–1333.

  These practical guidelines for the management of cardiac failure in children provide an excellent and comprehensive review of the evidence for different drugs available for therapeutic use in children and adults.
- Towbin JA, Lowe AM, Colan SD, et al: Incidence, causes, and outcomes of dilated cardiomyopathy in children. JAMA 2006;296:1867–1876.

  This population-based report provides data on the epidemiology, aetiology, and outcome of children with dilated cardiomyopathy in the current era.
- Shaddy RE, Boucek MM, Hsu DT, et al: Carvedilol for children and adolescents with heart failure: A randomized controlled trial. JAMA 2007;298:1171–1179.

  This is the first randomised controlled trial of medication for the management of cardiac failure in children. Although not statistically significant, the results suggested a trend towards improved survival when patients were treated with carvedilol.

CHAPTER

50

Arterio-venous Fistulas and Related Conditions

SHAKEEL A. QURESHI and JOHN F. REIDY

An arterio-venous fistula is an abnormal connection between an artery and a vein in the absence of any intervening capillary bed. As a result of the low resistance in the veins, a large shunt can occur through such fistulas. The shunting occurs throughout the cardiac cycle, thus producing a continuous flow murmur. Arterio-venous fistulas can involve either the pulmonary or systemic circulations. These are separate entities, and will be considered separately.

EXTRACARDIAC SYSTEMIC ARTERIO-VENOUS MALFORMATIONS

Arterio-venous malformations and fistulas can affect any part of the body. They have a wide range of pathologies, ranging from malformations consisting of abnormal capillaries and dilated venous spaces to direct fistulous communications between major arteries and veins.

Systemic arterio-venous malformations and fistulas can be subdivided into those within and those outside the heart. Extracardiac systemic arterio-venous malformations are of importance to the paediatric cardiologist only when they are haemodynamically significant, and are associated with a large left-to-right shunt. This is a rare situation. Abnormalities with such features are usually congenital in origin. Any large systemic malformation may present with high-output cardiac failure in later life, but rarely in childhood. When a neonate or infant presents with high-output cardiac failure, the most likely extracardiac cause is an aneurysm of the vein of Galen.

Aneurysm of the Vein of Galen

The aneurysmal vein of Galen is an intracerebral arterio-venous malformation. It is the most frequent haemodynamically significant extracardiac arterio-venous shunt encountered in neonates and infants, and affects males three times more frequently than females. It is an uncommon cause of severe cardiac failure in infancy. Affected neonates and infants may present with congestive cardiac failure that suggests a cardiac cause, and this can give rise to diagnostic difficulties. The abnormality consists of multiple feeding arteries, principally the anterior and posterior choroidal arteries and the anterior cerebral artery, which drain directly into an enlarged venous sump. The abnormal vein is considered to be the precursor of the vein of Galen, hence the name of the malformation. The aneurysmal vein drains directly into the straight sinus, and then into the superior sagittal sinus.

Clinical Presentation

The malformations are uncommon. Over a period of almost 20 years, 16 patients with the lesion were encountered at Great Ormond Street Hospital in London,[1] while 29 patients were seen at the Hospital for Sick Children in Toronto over a period of 30 years.[2] Review of the English literature from 1937 to 1981 found only 128 cases. It has been estimated that, in a population of 3 million, it might be expected that one new patient would be seen each year.[3] The cause of these aneurysms is unknown, but they probably result from an early embryonic somatic mutation.

Antenatal scans using ultrasound may occasionally detect the aneurysms in late pregnancy. Colour flow Doppler studies will show the vascular abnormality. Antenatal magnetic resonance imaging will confirm the diagnosis and assess any cerebral damage. Prenatal diagnosis will enable referral to a specialist centre, with all the requisite skills needed to deal with these complex patients.

The majority of cases are diagnosed after birth. Amongst the patients collected from the literature review, about one-third presented in the neonatal period, one-quarter were seen between 3 weeks and 11 months, and the remainder were encountered as older children and adults. Of the neonates, all but two presented with cardiac failure, these patients presenting with subarachnoid haemorrhage and hydrocephalus, respectively. In addition to cardiac failure, which is often refractory to treatment, the neonates showed features of pulmonary hypertension and myocardial ischaemia, as well as cerebral ischaemia resulting from the cerebral steal effect. Compared with the neonates, only two of those presenting as infants had cardiac failure. The majority had hydrocephalus, although one patient presented with a subarachnoid haemorrhage. In the older children and adults, only one had cardiac failure. At these ages, the most common presentation was with subarachnoid haemorrhage, seen in almost half. About one-third developed hydrocephalus, with venous hypertension resulting in epistaxis and distended veins, seen in one-sixth, and generalised neurological deterioration in another sixth thought to be caused by the steal effect of the fistula. In those with the aneurysms, the initial days of life are often unremarkable. If the pulmonary vascular resistance remains high, right-to-left shunting and cyanosis can occur as a result of the grossly increased systemic return. As the run-off from the arterial to venous circulations is of low resistance, there may be bounding pulses, particularly in the carotid arteries, as well as tachycardia. The veins in the neck may be engorged, and a continuous murmur is typically heard over the vault of the skull.

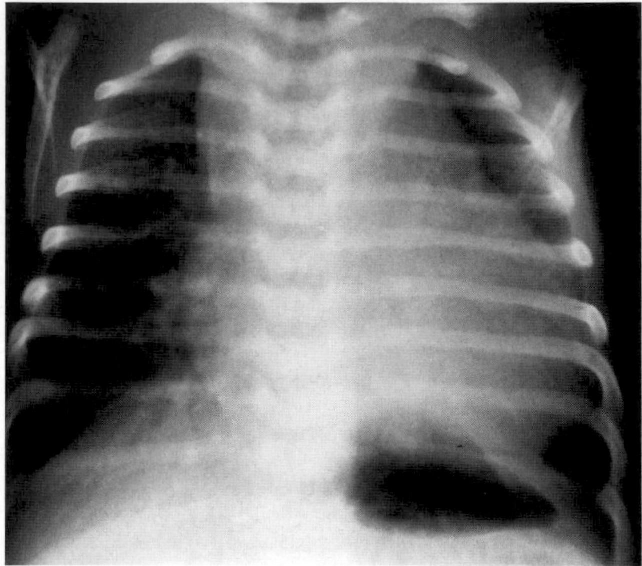

Figure 50-1 This chest radiograph from a neonate shows the non-specific features of marked cardiac enlargement and pulmonary plethora. The absence of any intracardiac abnormality on echocardiography should suggest the diagnosis of an aneurysmal vein of Galen.

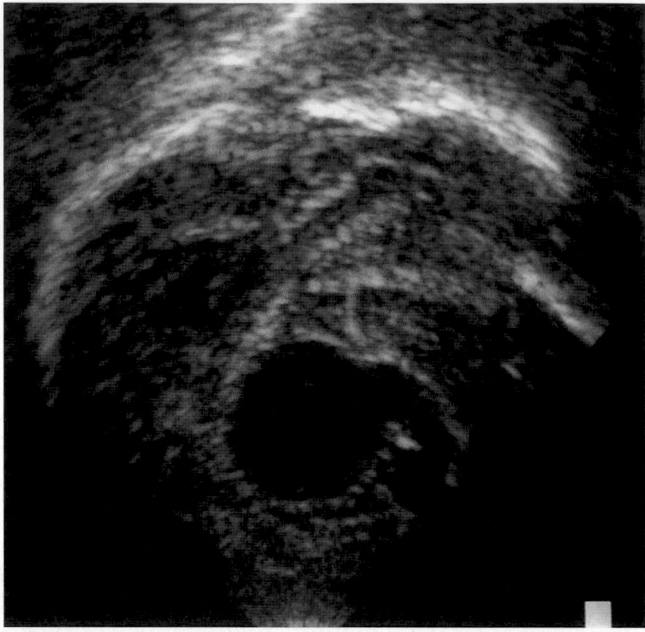

Figure 50-2 Ultrasonic interrogation across the anterior fontanelle shows a large central circular echo-free abnormality typical of an aneurysmal vein of Galen. A large vein is seen draining from the right side. Colour Doppler should demonstrate arterial flow.

Diagnosis

When the fistula is large, the chest radiograph usually shows cardiac enlargement with marked pulmonary plethora (Fig. 50-1). If there is significant right-to-left shunting as a result of an elevated pulmonary vascular resistance, then pulmonary oligaemia may also be present. The electrocardiogram usually shows biventricular hypertrophy. Echocardiography demonstrates enlargement of all four chambers, and excludes a cardiac cause for heart failure. Prior to the availability of ultrasound, the diagnosis was often difficult, and angiography was usually necessary. Angiography should now be performed only with a view to proceeding with embolising the abnormal connection. Ultrasonic scanning of the head across the anterior fontanelle will demonstrate the centrally situated aneurysmal vein. It also often shows the presence of the feeding arteries (Fig. 50-2). Doppler interrogation, and in particular colour Doppler, more readily demonstrates the direction of flow of blood. Where the ultrasound findings are not clear, or when more information is required in older patients, magnetic resonance imaging is indicated. This is now preferred to using computed tomographic (CT) scanning with contrast.

Management

The therapeutic options are embolisation or endovascular treatment. This involves very specialised neuro-interventional techniques, and very few specialised centres achieve the level of expertise and experience required to provide consistent treatment.

The outlook for neonates treated medically is grim.[4] In the series reported from Toronto,[2] all but one of the children treated medically died. Surgery has little or no role nowadays, as the surgical approach also carried a very high mortality, and resulted in significant morbidity. If possible, treatment is initially conservative, as arteriography and embolisation in the neonate is technically very difficult.[5] If the cardiac failure can be managed medically, the therapeutic options are much more encouraging at the age of about 6 months.

Arteriography is performed at the same time as embolisation. Different patterns have been described. In neonates, multiple arteries arise from the internal carotid arterial branches and feed the aneurysm at its antero-superior border (Fig. 50-3). The aneurysm then drains by very large straight and lateral sinuses (Fig. 50-4). Most

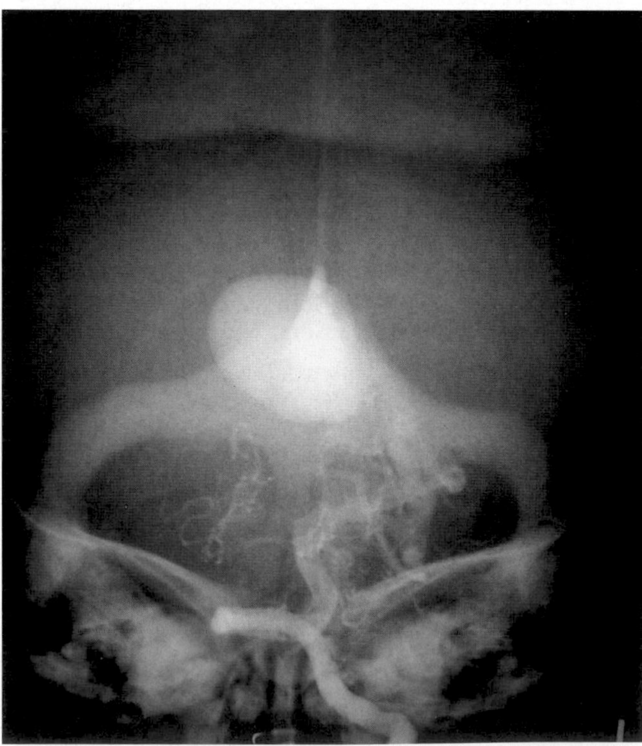

Figure 50-3 Selective carotid arteriography, in the antero-posterior view, shows the aneurysmal vein of Galen filling via multiple small arterial branches. It gained a further supply from the other carotid artery.

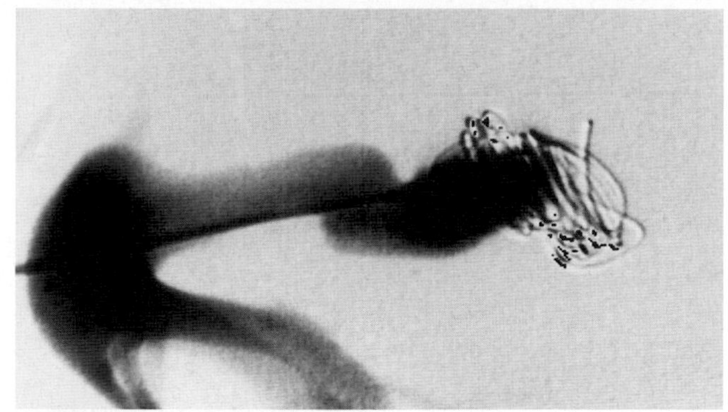

Figure 50-4 The aneurysmal vein of Galen has been catheterised via the transtorcular approach (lateral view). The tip of the catheter is in the aneurysm and multiple large steel coils have been positioned within it. Injection of contrast material demonstrates the large straight sinus draining to the lateral sinuses.

commonly in infants, the feeding artery is situated inferiorly and laterally and consists of a single posterior choroidal artery. In infants and older children, the feeding arteries are usually located anteriorly and superiorly, and consist of one or two posterior choroidal arteries, as well as anterior cerebral arteries. In older children, most commonly the feeding vessels consist of a network of branches arising from the posterior choroidal and thalamic perforating arteries.

The transtorcular venous approach was used at one time directly to access the venous aneurysm,[6–8] but has now largely been superseded by the transarterial route. This involves transfemoral approach and selectively catheterising the small feeding branches to the aneurysm. Embolisation is best performed with liquid embolic agents, such as cyanoacrylate glue. The outlook, if treatment is performed before the onset of cerebral damage, is good.[9] In this the largest series of endovascular treatment, neonates presenting early with severe cardiac failure had the worst prognosis. When there is associated cerebral damage, known as the melting brain syndrome, death or survival with severe cerebral damage is likely. There is often a restriction on the amount of embolisation that can be performed at any one session, particularly in neonates and infants, so multiple embolisations may be necessary. Sometimes these cases may be complicated by stenoses in the jugular bulbs, and stenting has been described in this situation.[10]

CORONARY ARTERIO-VENOUS FISTULAS

These lesions, also known as coronary arterial fistulas or malformations, are connections between one or more of the coronary arteries and a cardiac chamber or great vessel, having bypassed the myocardial capillary bed. They are rare, and usually occur in isolation. The exact incidence is unknown, although they are the most common haemodynamically significant coronary arterial anomaly.[11–13] A majority of the fistulas have a congenital origin, but some may occasionally be detected after cardiac surgery, such as valvar replacement, coronary arterial bypass grafting, and after repeated myocardial biopsies in cardiac transplantation.[14–17] The lesions were discovered in 0.1% of more than 33,000 patients undergoing coronary angiography.[18]

Morphology

It is difficult to provide accurate data on the distribution of the origins and sites of drainage of the fistulas, because reports vary depending on the analysed populations. Patients undergoing interventional or surgical treatment are likely to represent the severe end of the spectrum, whilst information will be unavailable in those with asymptomatic fistulas.

The artery feeding the fistula may be a main coronary artery or one of its branches. The vessel may be dilated and tortuous, and terminates in one of the cardiac chambers or another vessel. The more proximal its origin from the feeding artery, the more dilated the fistula is likely to be. If the fistula drains to the right atrium, and arises proximally from a main artery, it tends to be considerably dilated and less tortuous (Fig. 50-5). When the origin is more distal, and in particular when it arises from the left coronary artery and the drainage is to the right ventricle, the feeding artery may be very tortuous and present a challenge for interventional catheter closure (Fig. 50-6). Multiple arteries can feed into a single coronary arterio-venous fistula, or alternatively the fistula can have multiple sites of drainage.[16,19] The fistulas originate from the right coronary artery in about half the cases, the left anterior interventricular artery being the next most frequently involved, in approximately one-third, and the circumflex artery in about one-fifth.[20] Over nine-tenths of the fistulas, irrespective of their origin, drain to the right side of the heart.[21] In those draining to the right heart, the fistulas open most frequently to the right ventricle, in about two-fifths, followed by the right atrium, coronary sinus, and pulmonary trunk. Multiple fistulas between the three major coronary arteries and the left ventricle have also been reported.[22–24] In adults, fistulas may occasionally be encountered which originate from both the coronary

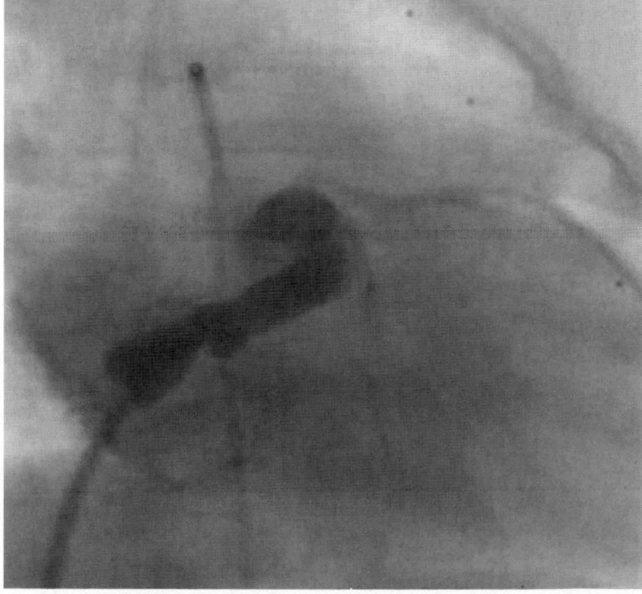

Figure 50-5 Left coronary angiogram in right anterior oblique projection shows a coronary arterio-venous fistula from a dilated branch arising from the circumflex coronary artery draining to the right atrium. The feeding vessel is dilated and less tortuous.

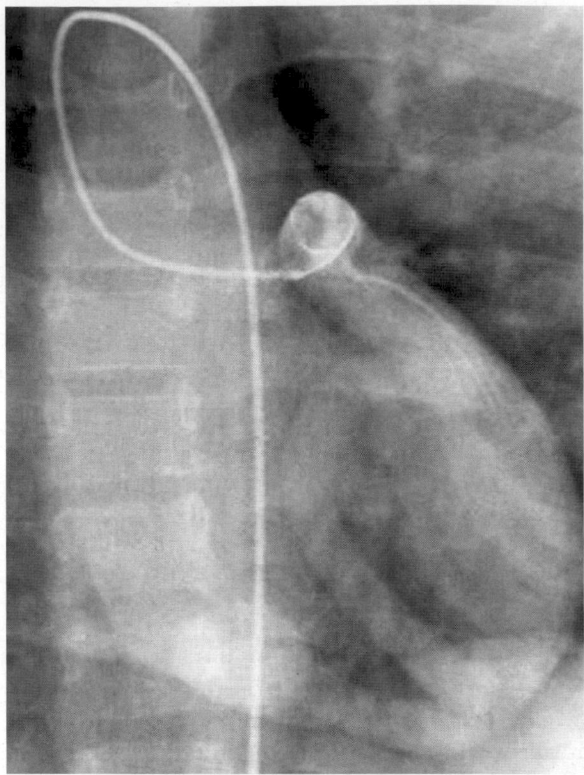

Figure 50-6 Selective left coronary angiogram in antero-posterior projection shows a coronary arterio-venous fistula arising from the left coronary artery. The feeding artery is considerably dilated and tortuous and drains into the right ventricle.

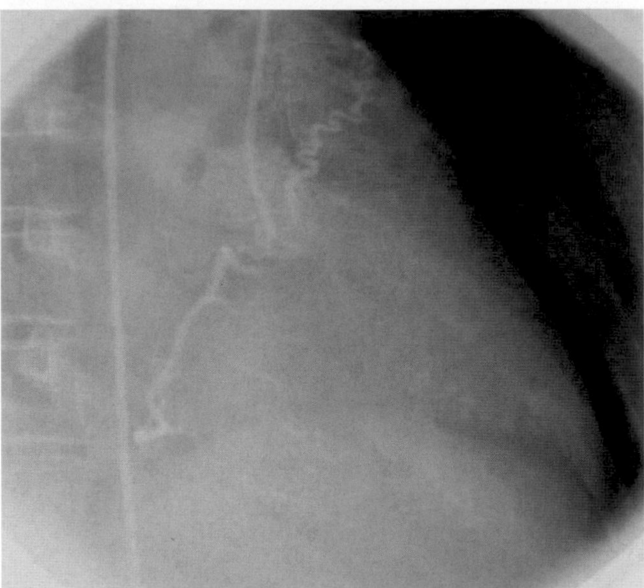

Figure 50-7 Selective right coronary angiogram in the right anterior oblique projection shows a fistula arising from the proximal part of the right coronary artery, which takes a tortuous course and drains into the pulmonary trunk.

arteries and drain into the pulmonary trunk. These fistulas may cause angina even in the absence of coronary arterial disease (Fig. 50-7). They require closure.

Pathophysiology

When the fistula drains to the right side of the heart, the volume load is increased to the right heart, as well as to the pulmonary vascular bed, the left atrium, and the left ventricle. This results in a left-to-right shunt similar to that produced by an atrial or ventricular septal defect, or patency of the arterial duct. When the fistula drains into the left atrium or the left ventricle, there is volume overloading of these chambers but no increase in the pulmonary blood flow. The situation then mimics mitral regurgitation. When the fistula drains into the left ventricle, the haemodynamic effect is similar to that produced by aortic regurgitation. Thus, there may be different echocardiographic appearances, with dilation of different cardiac chambers depending on the sites of the shunts. The size of the shunt is determined by the size of the fistula, and the difference in pressure between the coronary artery and the chamber into which the fistula drains. Occasionally, there may be congestive cardiac failure, while in adults, myocardial ischaemia may rarely occur due to a coronary arterial steal.

Clinical Features

The fistulas are usually asymptomatic in the first two decades, especially when they are haemodynamically small. Indeed a small number may close spontaneously.[25] After the second decade, there is an increase in the frequency of symptoms and complications.[26] Complications include steal from the adjacent myocardium causing myocardial ischaemia, thrombosis and embolism, cardiac failure, atrial fibrillation, rupture, endocarditis or endarteritis, and arrhythmias.[13,20,27–31] Thrombosis within the fistula, although rare, may cause acute myocardial infarction and atrial and ventricular arrhythmias.[32–34] Spontaneous rupture of an aneurysmal fistula has been reported to produce haemopericardium.[35] Recurrent septic pulmonary embolism may occur as a complication of endocarditis of the tricuspid valve if associated with a coronary arterial fistula.[36] Jet lesions may be found on the wall of the coronary sinus opposite the site of entry of the fistula, on the tricuspid valve, or at the orifice of the coronary artery.[36–38]

The fistulas may increase in size over time, although some may be large in the newborn period, and may even be detected prenatally.[39] They may form a short and direct connection with a chamber or a large vessel or form complex long tortuous and aneurysmal cavities. The aneurysmal section of the fistula may dilate progressively, and the feeding artery may become more tortuous.[40] The largest shunts occur when the coronary artery connects to the right rather than the left heart chambers. Even then, the left-to-right shunt is rarely more than 3 to 1.

The presentation varies between finding an asymptomatic continuous murmur, to presentation with congestive cardiac failure or exercise-induced angina.[18] The majority of the patients are asymptomatic, with normal exercise tolerance. Patients with large left-to-right shunts may have symptoms of congestive cardiac failure, especially in infancy, and occasionally in the neonatal period.[41,42] Congestive cardiac failure may also occur in the elderly.[43] Some adult patients may have angina and electrocardiographic evidence of myocardial ischaemia.[16] The mechanism of the angina is presumed to be a steal phenomenon.[28,44,45] Exercise-stress thallium scintigraphy has shown the presence of reversible ischaemia supporting such a phenomenon.[46]

Some patients may be referred because of an asymptomatic murmur, which will be continuous, and heard over the praecordium. Whilst the murmur may sound similar to that of a patent arterial duct, it must be differentiated from the latter. The murmur of a coronary arterial fistula is heard over the mid-chest, rather than below the left clavicle. It may even be audible to the right of the sternal border, and typically peaks in mid-diastole rather than systole, as is the case when the murmur originates from the persistently patent arterial duct. Such findings should alert the physician to the possibility of a coronary arterio-venous fistula. If the fistula connects to the left ventricle, only an early diastolic murmur may be heard. The patient is then referred for echocardiographic assessment.

The differential diagnoses include persistent patency of the arterial duct, ruptured aneurysm of a sinus of Valsalva, ventricular septal defect with aortic regurgitation, venous hums, and other systemic and pulmonary arterio-venous fistulas. Indeed, when it became possible to close patent arterial ducts surgically, the similarities in physical findings led, on occasion, to unintentional surgical exploration of patients with coronary arterial fistulas.

Investigations

The electrocardiogram and chest X-ray are usually unhelpful in the diagnosis and assessment. The electrocardiogram may show the effects of left ventricular volume overload and ischaemic changes. If it is normal, and the patient is old enough to exercise either on the treadmill or a bicycle, changes in the ST segments indicative of ischaemia may become apparent. The chest X-ray is usually normal, but occasionally moderate cardiomegaly may be present when there is a large left-to-right shunt.

When the fistula and the resulting shunt are small, colour Doppler echocardiography may be helpful, demonstrating the chamber or the vessel into which the fistula drains. Conventional pulsed and continuous wave Doppler can then confirm the high velocity of the flow through the fistula. Cross sectional and colour Doppler echocardiography are helpful in demonstrating dilation of the affected coronary artery. As indicated, colour flow mapping may show the site of drainage, but it is difficult to define the detailed anatomy of the fistula with this technique.[47,48] Additional clues may be present when the coronary artery feeding the fistula is enlarged, ectatic or tortuous, or when there is a large shunt. If a dilated coronary artery can be traced from its aortic origin into the fistula, the diagnosis can be confirmed with certainty by conventional Doppler, and in particular by colour flow mapping. Transoesophageal echocardiography has also been used for better definition of the fistulas.[48–51] On colour Doppler interrogation, significant flow may be seen at the origin, or even along the length, of the vessel. It may also be possible to see flow into the chambers of the right heart. Magnetic resonance imaging can confirm, permitting recognition of the proximal coronary arteries, or even the whole length of the fistula.

In patients who are able to exercise, and especially those who complain of angina or dyspnoea, myocardial perfusion or stress thallium scanning may demonstrate reversible ischaemia. It may also determine the size of the territory under threat of ischaemia.[46] In older patients, other areas of acquired coronary arterial disease may be discovered that influence the subsequent management. In these older patients, if a coronary arterial fistula is discovered, even if the coronary arteries are free of atheromatous disease, closure of such a fistula may relieve the symptoms.[52]

The main diagnostic technique remains cardiac catheterisation and angiography, the investigation also helping in planning the appropriate treatment. Initial diagnostic catheterisation is used to assess the haemodynamic significance of the fistula, and to provide details of its anatomy, in particular its size, origin, course, presence of any stenoses, and its site of drainage. Selective angiography of the coronary arteries allows confirmation of the diagnosis, and demonstrates the detailed anatomy of the fistula (Fig. 50-8). Selective injections, however, should be performed only when definitive treatment is planned, such as an interventional procedure or surgery. They should rarely be required nowadays to make the diagnosis. A preliminary aortogram taken in the root helps to determine which coronary artery should be catheterised selectively, but it is usually good practice to perform selective angiography of both the coronary arteries. Visualisation of the fistula may be improved by using the so-called laid-back aortogram.[53] This is obtained by adding caudal angulation at 45 degrees to the frontal view, with slight left or right anterior oblique orientation. A more important reason for detailed selective coronary angiographic assessment is to investigate the possibility of multiple arteries feeding the fistula (Fig. 50-9). Coronary angiography in several planes then assumes great importance. It should be performed as in adults. These views include right anterior oblique, straight antero-posterior, left anterior oblique, left anterior oblique with caudocranial angulation, and left lateral projections.

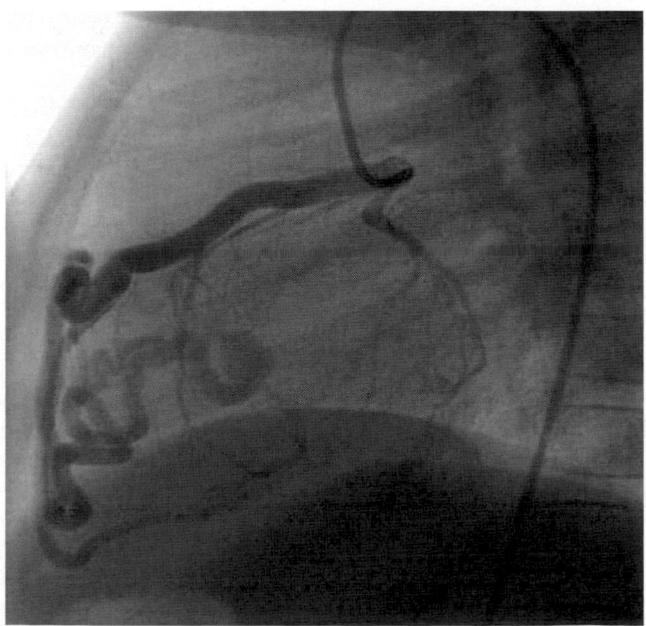

Figure 50-8 Selective angiography of the left coronary artery in the left lateral projection shows a dilated feeding vessel with a tortuous course draining into the right ventricle.

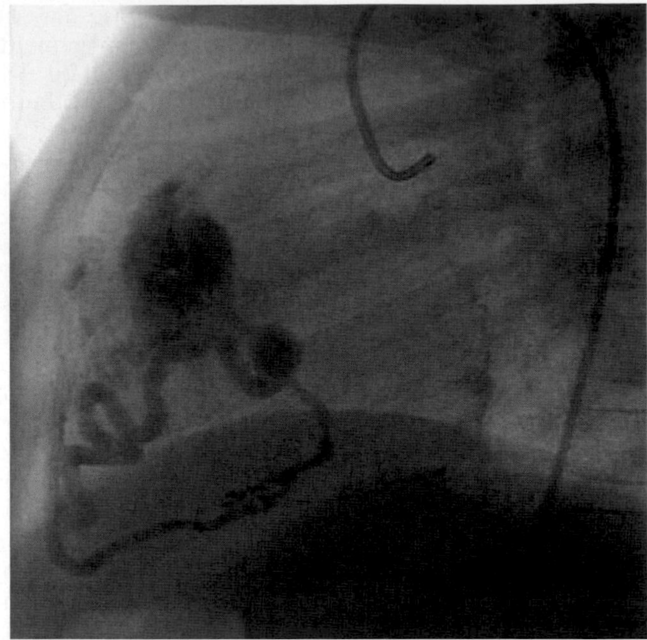

Figure 50-9 Left coronary angiogram with follow-through of the contrast in the left lateral projection in the same patient shown in Figure 50-8. Two vessels drain into the aneurysm, which in turn drains into the right ventricle. In this patient, it is important to close the fistula by deploying coils into the aneurysm.

Management

The options include closure at surgery, or by use of devices inserted through a catheter. The goal of treatment is to occlude the fistula whilst preserving normal coronary arterial flow. The options can be optimised by careful identification of the number of fistulous connections, the nature of the feeding vessel or vessels, the sites of drainage, and quantification of myocardium at risk for injury or loss. The indications for treatment include the presence of a large or increasing left-to-right shunt, left ventricular volume overload, myocardial ischaemia, left ventricular dysfunction, congestive cardiac failure, and prevention of endocarditis or endarteritis.

As techniques for accurately diagnosing coronary arterio-venous fistulas have improved, open heart surgery has become safer, making it even more unlikely that the natural history will ever be clearly defined. In the past, most authors have advocated surgical closure of the fistulas in view of the low operative mortality.[54–57]

Even as long ago as 1979, it had been noted that symptomatic patients over the age of 20 years suffered more problems, as well as more post-operative complications, than did younger patients.[26] This prompted the suggestion that all haemodynamically significant fistulas should be closed, even in the absence of symptoms, to prevent potential complications, such as endarteritis, progressive enlargement of the fistula, secondary atherosclerotic involvement with rupture, and thrombo-embolism. Early surgery also avoids the post-operative problems that can complicate operations performed in later life. The policy of closure, however, has to be balanced against the reports of spontaneous regression or closure, in some younger children with relatively small fistulas draining in particular into the right ventricle.[25, 26, 58–62]

The aim of surgery is to close the fistula while preserving the flow of blood through the normal coronary arterial branches. Different surgical techniques have been used, and all of them appear to be adequate. The fistula is closed at the point of entry into the heart, without interrupting the continuity of the more proximal artery. When the lesion is clearly visible, closure can be achieved, without extracorporeal circulation, by clamping and suturing the fistulous channels on the outside of the heart. This approach does not require opening the fistula, the cardiac chambers, or the coronary arteries, and may be performed with the heart beating. More frequently, however, cardiopulmonary bypass is needed. This may be essential if it becomes necessary to enter a chamber to close the fistula from within, or if insertion of a bypass graft is necessary to maintain viability of the myocardium distal to the ligated artery. A small proportion of patients may develop complications post-operatively. These include ischaemia or infarction downstream from the point of ligation. This may be especially significant when a fistula from the right coronary artery drains to the right atrium or the superior caval vein. Ligation of such a vessel may interrupt the supply to the artery of the sinus node.

Surgical treatment is associated with morbidity, but low mortality rate, which ranges in reported series from zero to 6%.[13,56,57,63–68] Mortality rate, as expected, was higher in the historically older series. Myocardial infarction has been reported in less than one-twentieth of patients,[64] albeit that there is a low, but significant, risk of persistence or recurrence of the fistula.[63–66,69] The true incidence of recurrence, however, is unknown. The reason for the recurrence may be the presence of multiple fistulas, which are difficult to deal with by surgery. Median sternotomy and cardiopulmonary bypass also have their own associated morbidity.[68] Little has been said about the possibility of developing arteriosclerosis in the region of the fistula either subsequent to or prior to surgical treatment.

Until recently, surgery was the only available definitive treatment. In the last two decades, percutaneous transcatheter embolisation has emerged as an effective and safe alternative. When available, it should now be considered the treatment of choice.[16,70–77] The aim of closure by catheterisation is to occlude the artery feeding the fistula as distally, and close to its point of termination, as is possible to avoid occlusion of branches feeding normal myocardium. If the feeding artery is occluded too distally, and if there is no significant stenosis within the artery, then the possibility exists for inadvertent embolisation into the pulmonary circulation. Occlusion should be performed at a precise point, using various materials which include detachable balloons, stainless steel coils, or platinum microcoils.[16,74–79] It is rare nowadays to use detachable balloons, although they proved useful in the past. A large variety of equipment should be available in the catheterisation laboratory to achieve successful closure, because different techniques may be required should the fistula have unusual morphology. It is also necessary to have access to devices of different shapes and sizes, such as the conventional Gianturco coils, controlled-release coils, and a variety of devices normally used to close atrial or ventricular septal defects, persistently patent arterial ducts, or other abnormal vessels.

The choice of the equipment, and the technique to be used, is determined by the morphology of the fistulas.

Other important determinants include the age and size of the patient, the size of the catheter that can be used in the patient, the size of the vessel to be occluded, and the tortuosity of the course required to reach the intended point of occlusion. For example, if the route to the target vessel is tortuous, then superfloppy guide wires combined with Tracker or Micro-ferret infusion catheters are recommended. In the presence of high flow, a stop-flow technique with a balloon is recommended during deployment of a coil or a device. Because of the need for precise occlusion, it is always preferable to use a potentially reversible technique.

For many years, stainless steel coils of 0.038-inch calibre have been widely used for embolisation elsewhere in the vascular system. They can be delivered through standard non-tapered catheters of 5 or 6 French size to occlude coronary arterial fistulas. Positioning such catheters satisfactorily in a distal location in a tortuous fistula, however, may be both difficult and hazardous. In such circumstances,it is safer to insert platinum microcoils, with calibre of 0.018 inch, which are delivered through a co-axial 3 French catheter. Such catheters, used with steerable guidewires, can be manipulated safely through tortuous arteries into very distal locations (Fig. 50-10). Moreover, the high flow that is often encountered in large fistulas makes them difficult to occlude. A mass of platinum coils is frequently necessary. In the last 10 years or so, new interlocking detachable coils have been used, the delivery of which can be controlled.[78,80] Use of such coils makes closure much safer, with the added advantage that they can be retrieved into the catheter if the final position is deemed unsatisfactory. Such coils offer very little resistance to passage through the microcatheters. Even if they embolise inadvertently, they are easy to retrieve with snares. Fistulous arteries permitting very high flow present a particular problem, but temporary occlusion of the proximal portion with a balloon permits safe insertion of an occluding mass of coils (Figs. 50-11 and 50-12).[80,81]

Preliminary arteriography will usually have demonstrated the anatomy of the fistula prior to embolisation. Further detailed, and more selective, coronary angiography is essential to obtain details of the normal coronary arterial branches, which may be small but are at risk during occlusion. The steal from a fistula permitting high flow usually results in poor opacification of the normal branches and possible underestimation of their size. With all the current techniques, occlusion or near occlusion should be

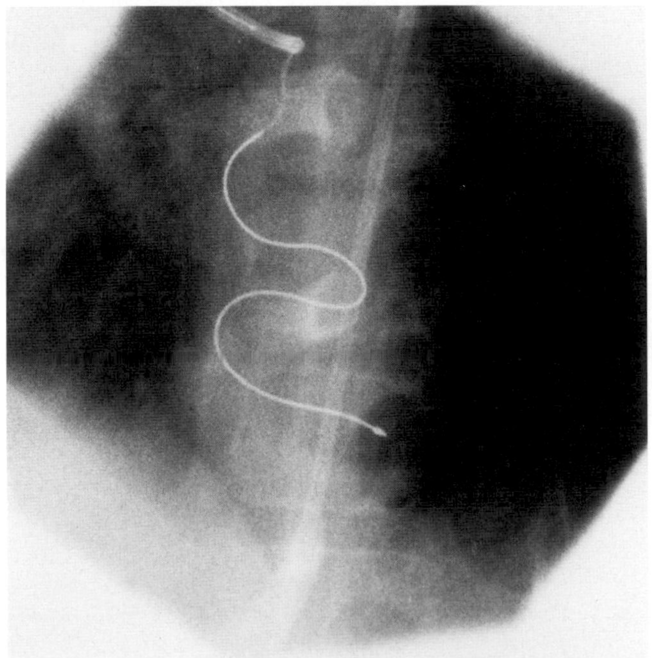

Figure 50-10 A cine frame in the left anterior oblique projection shows a guiding catheter at the origin of the main stem of the left coronary artery. A 3 French Tracker catheter has been passed through the guiding catheter into the tortuous coronary arterio-venous fistula and placed in a distal location. A controlled release coil is seen just protruding through the tip of the Tracker catheter.

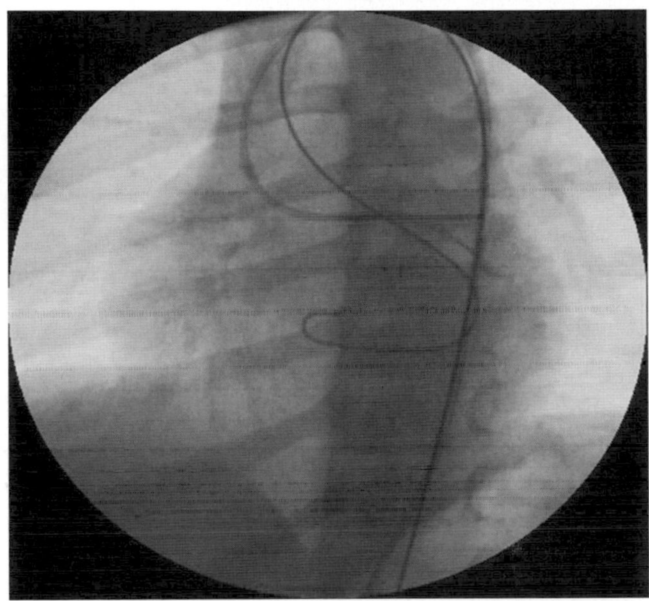

Figure 50-11 A cine frame in the left anterior oblique projection shows a balloon catheter inflated in the proximal part of the left coronary artery in order to allow safe deployment of coils distally in the fistula.

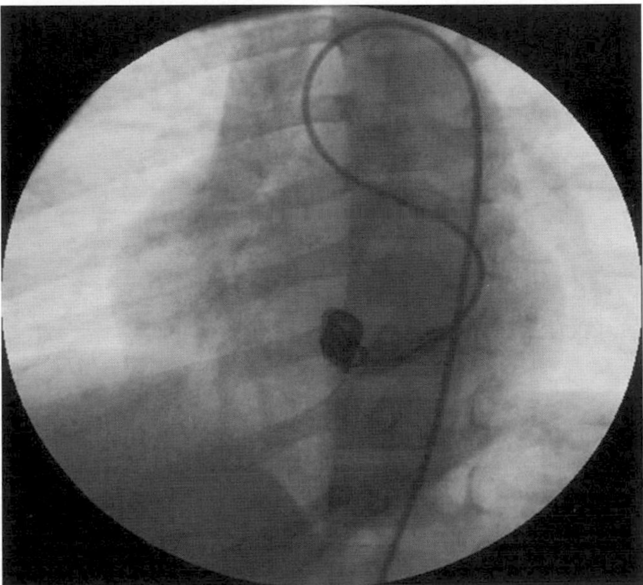

Figure 50-12 A cine frame in the left anterior oblique projection in the same patient shown in Figure 50-11 showing an occluding mass of coils, the balloon having been deflated and removed.

achieved soon after the embolisation. Sometimes, a small second feeding branch to the fistula may only become opacified when the main artery has been occluded (Figs. 50-13 and 50-14). The key to success is to select a technique for embolisation that is suitable for the size and the location of the fistula.

Some fistulas may be more easily closed from the right side of the heart. These fistulas tend to be large, less tortuous, and have a short course to their point of drainage to the right heart (Fig. 50-15). Depending on their size, they may be suitable for occlusion with a vascular plug, a ductal occluder (Fig. 50-16), or an occluder usually used to close atrial or ventricular septal defects.[42,82–86] Fistulas closed in this fashion should be large, and should permit relatively easy and straight access from the right heart. If needed, occlusion can be achieved with the help of an arterio-venous guide wire circuit, using either femoral venous or internal jugular venous access.

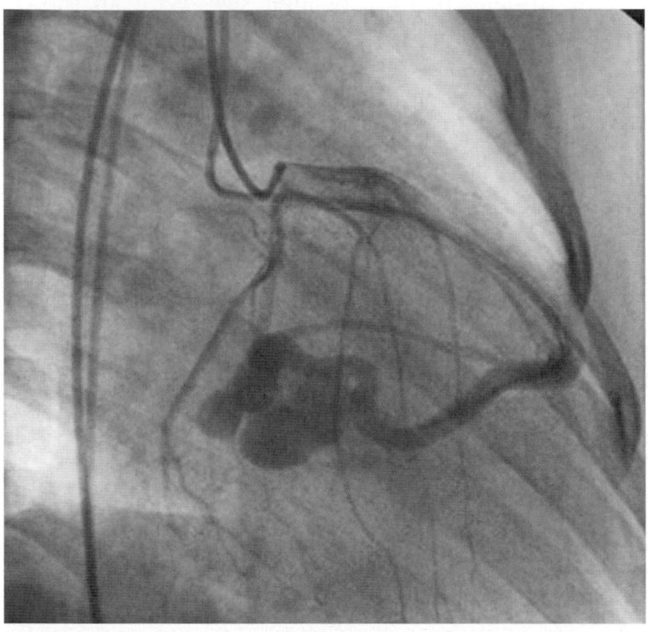

Figure 50-13 A selective left coronary angiogram in the right anterior oblique projection showing a coronary arterio-venous fistula arising from the left anterior descending coronary artery and draining into the right ventricle. There are possibly two feeding vessels supplying the aneurysmal portion, which drains into the right ventricle.

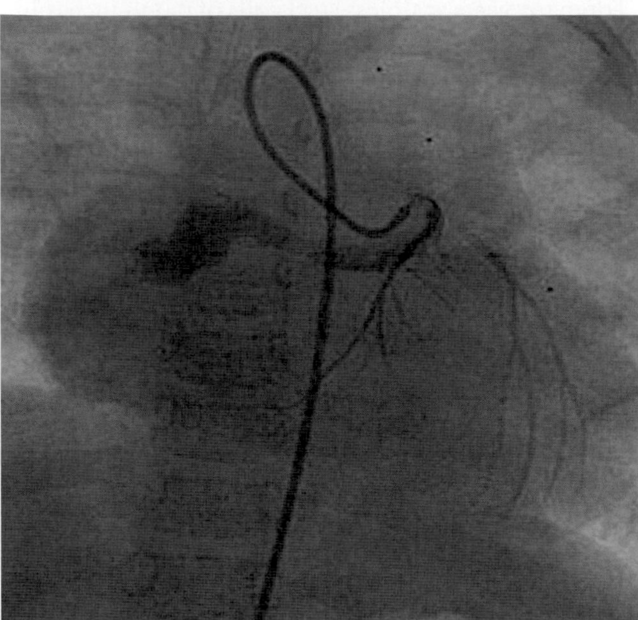

Figure 50-15 A selective left coronary angiogram showing a fistula arising from the left coronary artery. The dilated feeding artery takes a less tortuous course and drains into the right atrium.

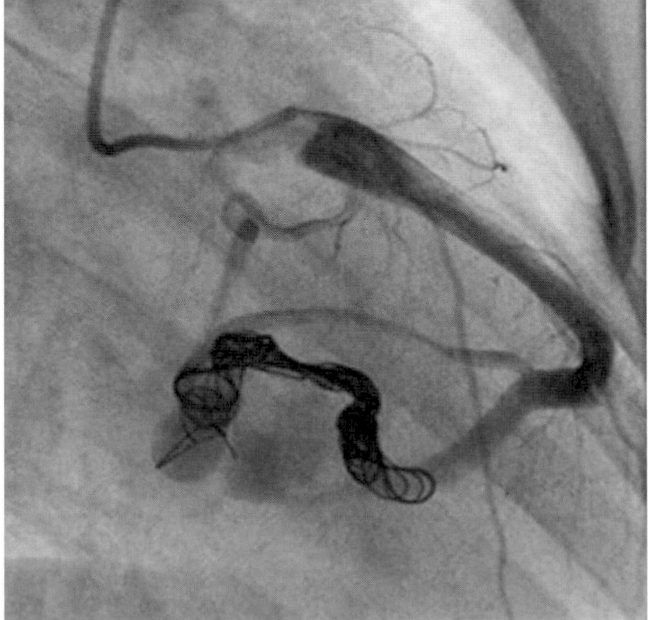

Figure 50-14 A cine frame of the same patient shown in Figure 50-13. After deployment of coils in the aneurysmal part, two further vessels draining into the aneurysm are apparent.

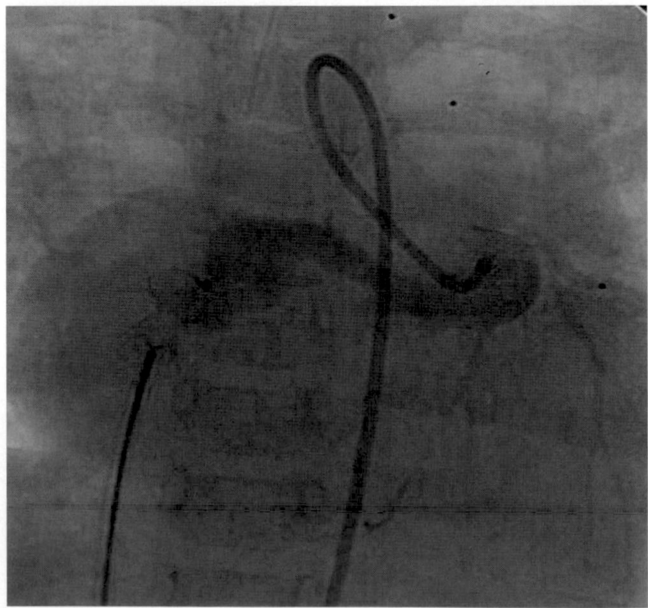

Figure 50-16 A cine frame of the same patient shown in Figure 50-15 demonstrates an Amplatzer duct occluder still attached at the correct location to close the fistula.

After occluding the main fistulous vessel, repeat selective coronary angiography in both the coronary arteries should be performed in order to see if there is a second branch feeding the fistula, which may also need occlusion at the same procedure. When closing fistulas through a catheter, complete occlusion is expected in well over nine-tenths of procedures. The main complications include inadvertent embolisation of coils, transient electrocardiographic T-wave changes, transient bundle branch block, and myocardial infarction. All these complications are rare, apart from inadvertent embolisation, which may result from high flow in the large fistulas, or use of undersized coils.[80] As already discussed, should the coils migrate, they can easily be retrieved with snares.

AORTO–LEFT VENTRICULAR TUNNEL

The aorto–left ventricular tunnel is a rare defect, consisting of an endothelialised communication between the aorta and the left ventricle which bypasses the line of attachment of one of the aortic valvar leaflets. The abnormal channel originates in the ascending aorta, and terminates in the left ventricle (Fig. 50-17).[86] The lesion is found more frequently in males than females, with a ratio of 2:1 to 3:1.[87,88] Although it was originally believed that the lesion was acquired after birth, it is now generally agreed that the entity is congenital,[87,89] having been detected prenatally by echocardiography.[90,91] Detected as early as 19 weeks of gestation, the most important clue to presence of the lesion was colour Doppler evidence of marked aortic regurgitation.

The tunnel usually originates above the right aortic sinus of Valsalva, and can involve the orifice of the right coronary artery. The tunnel courses in the tissue plane between the free-standing muscular right ventricular infundibulum and the aortic sinus, and usually enters the left ventricle through the fibrous triangle between the right and left coronary leaflets of the aortic valve.[92] Occasionally, the tunnel may originate above the origin of the left coronary artery (Fig. 50-18).[93] The tunnel itself may be dilated aneurysmally through part or the entirety of its course. Associated cardiac defects include aortic valves with two leaflets, with aortic stenosis or regurgitation present in the majority of patients. Other defects include patency of the arterial duct, ventricular septal defect, pulmonary stenosis, infundibular right ventricular obstruction, aneurysm of the membranous septum, and critical aortic stenosis.[94,95] Distortion of the aortic valve occurs because of the lack of support of the afflicted leaflet, producing severe regurgitation.

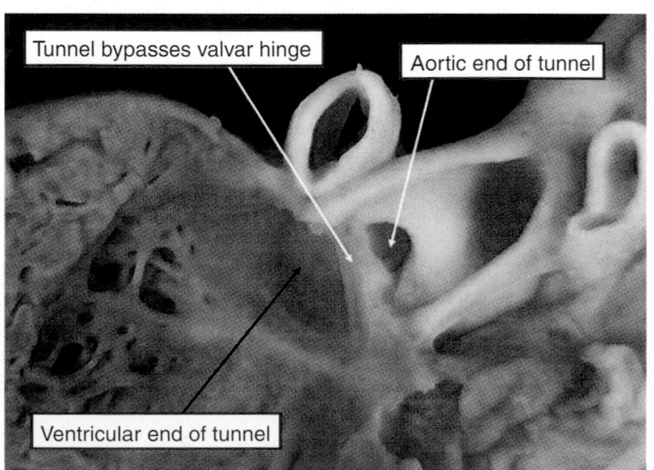

Figure 50-17 As shown in the specimen, the aorto–left ventricular tunnel is a defect bypassing the detached hinge of the aortic valve, which has come apart from the valvar sinus. The tunnel extends through the tissue plane between the aortic sinus and the free-standing muscular subpulmonary infundibulum.

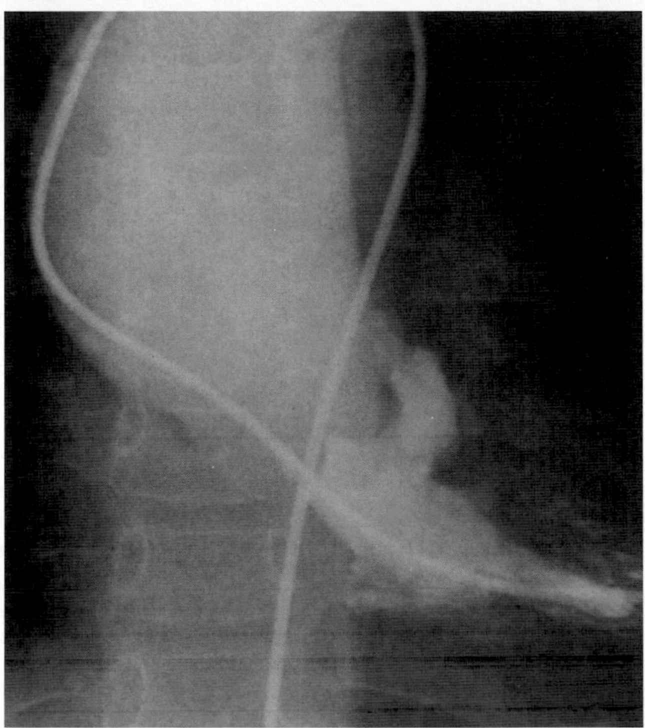

Figure 50-18 This left ventricular angiogram profiled in antero-posterior projection shows an aorto–left ventricular tunnel originating above the left coronary artery. The ascending aorta and the aortic root are very dilated. (Courtesy of Dr Wolfgang Kohler, Erfurt, Germany.)

Clinical Features

The symptoms and signs depend on the size of the tunnel and the severity of aortic regurgitation. Patients with severe regurgitation usually present with symptoms of congestive cardiac failure, with presentation at any point from birth to adult life.[88,96] The signs may include a wide pulse pressure, and loud systolic and diastolic to-and-fro murmurs at the base of the heart, usually with a short interval separating them. The anomaly should be considered in the differential diagnosis of any neonate or infant with systolic and diastolic murmurs along with the signs of aortic regurgitation. The abnormal haemodynamics may produce congestive cardiac failure in the neonate or infant, often with associated left ventricular enlargement and overactivity, with a dilated ascending aorta on a chest radiograph. As emphasised already, the key to diagnosis in fetal life is aortic regurgitation, sometimes with left ventricular dysfunction and hydrops.[90,91]

Investigations

The electrocardiogram shows left ventricular hypertrophy in the majority of patients. Cross sectional and colour Doppler echocardiography usually confirms the diagnosis. In the occasional patient in whom the diagnosis is difficult, magnetic resonance imaging or cardiac catheterisation may be helpful.[97] Angiography in the aortic root usually confirms the diagnosis, although this should be rarely required nowadays. There may be gross dilation and distortion of the aortic sinus, ascending aorta, and the left ventricle. Angiography may also show normal origin of the coronary arteries, thus differentiating the tunnel from a fistula from the coronary artery to the left ventricle. The anterior location of the abnormal tunnel, and the demonstration of a normal aortic sinus of Valsalva, distinguishes the tunnel from ruptured aneurysm of a sinus of Valsalva into the left ventricle.

Management

Surgical closure in early life was first reported over 45 years ago.[87] Presentation with severe regurgitation is at or soon after birth, with early congestive cardiac failure.[88,98] Symptoms of congestive cardiac failure may also appear later, in the second or third decade of life.[87,96] Some patients may die despite medical treatment,[87] but others survive to undergo successful surgical repair. In presence of congestive cardiac failure, surgery is clearly indicated. In asymptomatic neonates, or in those patients in whom cardiac failure is well controlled, surgery can be delayed for a few weeks or months. Early intervention can prevent progressive damage to the aortic valvar leaflets or deformity of the aortic root,[99,100] and early surgery is also required should there be severe aortic stenosis rather than regurgitation.[101]

The technique of repair depends on the type of tunnel. For those with a small aortic opening, closure of the orifice in two layers is advocated.[87] In the setting of larger openings, the aortic end is closed with a patch, while both the aortic and left ventricular ends of the tunnel can be closed.[102] In all the techniques, it is imperative to avoid distortion of the aortic valve and damage to the right coronary artery or the conduction system. The reported operative mortality ranges between zero and 20%.[91,100,102,103] Late complications after repair include aortic regurgitation in up to three-quarters of patients.[100,103] This may necessitate reoperation on the aortic valve. Occasionally, should it be severely stenotic, it may not be possible to preserve the native aortic valve. Replacement with an aortic homograft may then be required to repair both the tunnel and the stenotic valve.[101]

ANEURYSMS OF THE SINUSES OF VALSALVA

Aneurysm of one of the aortic sinuses of Valsalva is a rare defect, which may be congenital or acquired. The incidence varies from 0.14% to 0.35%.[104] Its prevalence appears to be increased in the Asian countries when compared to Western populations.[105] Congenital aneurysms are the result of sinusal mural weakness, which produces downward prolapse of the leaflet. The dilated sinus may bulge into an atrium or ventricle, and may rupture. It is rare in infancy and childhood, being more commonly seen in adults. Aneurysms may be acquired through bacterial endocarditis, albeit that the endocarditis may have occurred on a congenital aneurysm. It can be difficult, therefore, to distinguish between congenital and acquired aneurysms, although frequently the congenital ones are associated with a ventricular septal defect and aortic coarctation. Most aneurysms are single, and most commonly affect the right coronary aortic sinus.

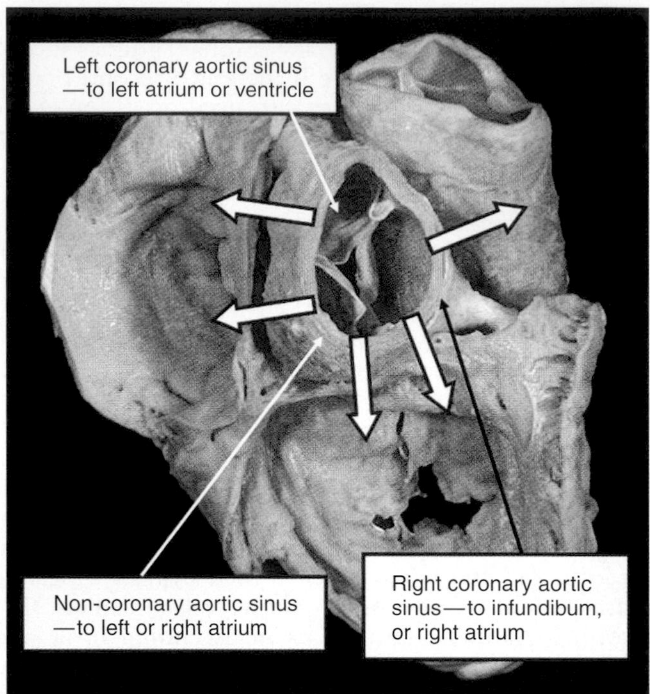

Figure 50-19 The sites of potential rupture of aneurysms of the aortic sinuses of Valsalva, indicated by arrows, have been superimposed on this picture of the short axis of the normal heart viewed from the atrial aspect.

Less commonly, the non-coronary aortic sinus is involved. The left coronary aortic sinus is rarely involved. Aneurysms of the right coronary aortic sinus usually prolapse into the right ventricle or right atrium, and those from the non-coronary sinus into the right atrium. Aneurysms of the left coronary aortic sinus prolapse into the left ventricle. The most common aneurysm, from the right coronary aortic sinus prolapsing into the right ventricle, may be associated with a ventricular septal defect.

As indicated, the aneurysms may rupture, this occurring during childhood or adolescence, and most frequently into the right rather than the left chambers. As expected from their position, aneurysm of the right sinus of Valsalva may rupture into the right ventricle or the right atrium, while those involving the non-coronary sinus tend to rupture into the right or left atrium, and those involving the left coronary aortic sinus rupturing into the left ventricle or the left atrium (Fig. 50-19).[106-108] Rupture can also occur through the septal leaflet of the tricuspid valve, producing an acquired atrioventricular septal defect.[109] There is an increased incidence of rupture when an aneurysm occurs in the presence of a doubly committed subarterial ventricular septal defect. Rupture in these cases may occur into the right ventricular outflow tract.[110] Aneurysms occurring in the setting of Marfan's syndrome are considered as a separate entity. Other associated lesions include an aortic valve with two leaflets, and aortic coarctation. Rupture has also been reported in a patient with Behçet's disease,[111] and as a late complication after repair of dissection of the ascending aorta.[112]

Clinical Features

When the aneurysm has not ruptured, it usually produces no symptoms. It may only be discovered as a chance finding on echocardiography, or angiography, performed during interrogation of another lesion, such as ventricular septal defect. The natural history of unruptured aneurysms is not known. Although rupture has been reported in the neonatal period,[113] it occurs more frequently in the third or fourth decade of life. When the aneurysm ruptures, the majority of the patients become symptomatic. Rupture may produce central precordial chest pain, along with sudden dyspnoea, because of a large left-to-right shunt combined with aortic regurgitation. Very occasionally, rupture may not produce any symptoms. Even rarer still is rupture into the pericardial cavity.[114] Unruptured aneurysms may cause angina, which may be intractable, especially when the aneurysm causes distortion of the origins of the coronary arteries.[115] Myocardial infarction may be the consequence of compression of the coronary arteries, and may occasionally be fatal.[116,117] Other possible complications include transient ischaemic attacks and cerebral embolism.[118–120] Physical examination may reveal a wide pulse pressure and left or right ventricular overactivity. The murmurs vary, with ejection systolic combined with early but long diastolic murmurs, or continuous murmurs heard at the right or left lower sternal borders. Obstruction of the right ventricular outflow tract has occasionally been reported, with or without the presence of a ventricular septal defect.[121,122]

Investigations

The electrocardiogram usually shows left ventricular hypertrophy, occasionally with biventricular hypertrophy. Cross sectional combined with colour Doppler echocardiography is helpful in making the diagnosis,[123] and frequently shows dilation of the aortic root and left ventricular volume overload. A ruptured right coronary aortic sinus may protrude anteriorly, caudally, and leftwards. Severe aortic regurgitation may be present, with turbulent flow into the right ventricle or right atrium seen on colour Doppler.[107] Echocardiography will also show the presence or absence of a ventricular septal defect. Transoesophageal echocardiography shows the anatomy in more detail, and is perhaps superior to the transthoracic approach.[124] Frequently, surgery can be performed without the need for cardiac catheterisation.[119,125] Cardiac catheterisation and angiography merely confirm the echocardiographuc findings, albeit often showing the deformity of the aortic sinus more convincingly. Although filling of the right heart chambers, into which the aneurysm may have ruptured, is frequently seen, occasionally the rapid heart rate and the high cardiac output prevent their opacification. Apart from conventional echocardiography, contrast imaging has also been used for non-invasive diagnosis.[126,127]

Management

The conventional treatment is surgical, although transcatheter approaches have increasingly been used in recent years.[128–130] If the surgical approach is chosen, it is performed on cardiopulmonary bypass. Direct closure can be carried out through an aortotomy, through the right ventricle, or via the right atrium. Sometimes both the aorta and the chamber of entry need to be explored to achieve effective repair.[131,132] Surgical repair may then involve closure of both ends of the aneurysm with patches. If a ventricular septal defect is present, it too should be closed. The aortic valvar leaflets may need resuspension in order to reduce the severity of aortic regurgitation, which may determine the outcome. Even after successful surgical repair, the prognosis is guarded. Recurrence, or an increase, of aortic regurgitation may be seen, and require further surgery. It is debatable whether an aneurysm discovered incidentally in an asymptomatic child should be surgically repaired. Surgical repair can now be achieved without mortality, even though it may be necessary to replace the aortic valve.[133] A more recent surgical experience[134] reported overall survival of 95% at 20 years. In the latter series, reoperation was needed in one-sixth of the patients for replacement of the aortic valve, recurrence of the fistula, or recurrence of a ventricular septal defect.

Transcatheter closure of a ruptured aneurysm of the sinus of Valsalva was first reported in 1994, using a Rashkind umbrella to close the defect.[128] Since then, different devices have been used, and the transcatheter experience has increased.[129, 135] To achieve success, the point of origin of the ruptured sinus needs to be clear of an orifice of a coronary artery by at least half a centimeter. The procedure is usually performed under general anaesthesia, using femoral venous and arterial access, and incorporating selective coronary angiography and an aortogram to delineate the anatomy. Having established an arterio-venous circuit, it is important to size the defect. When the size is uncertain, a balloon can be passed over the guidewire to provide increased accuracy. As discussed, a variety of devices, such as Amplatzer ductal occluder or the device designed for closure of muscular ventricular septal defects, have been used to occlude the ruptured sinus (Figs. 50-20 and 50-21). Having inserted the device, selective coronary angiography is performed to ensure that the aortic end of the device has not encroached on the origin of the coronary arteries.

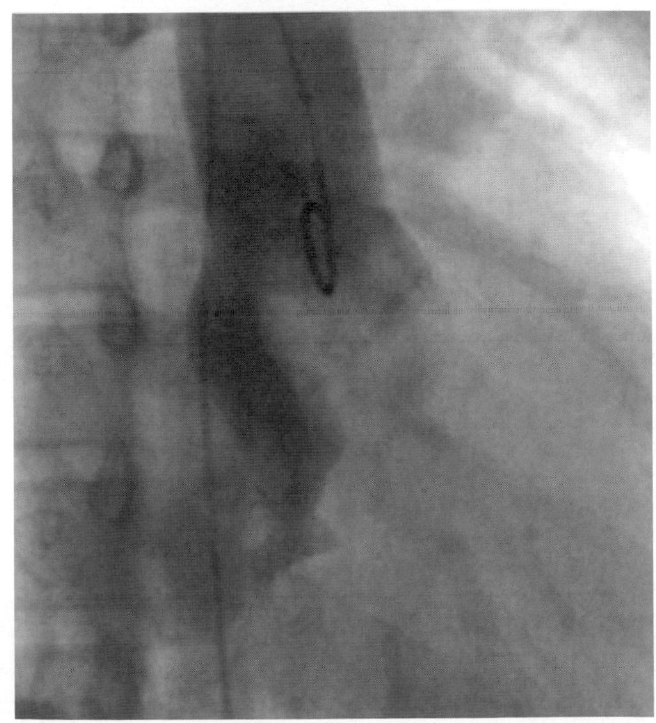

Figure 50-20 An aortogram in the right anterior oblique projection shows a ruptured right sinus of Valsalva draining into the right atrium (Courtesy of Dr Grazyna Brzezinska-Rajszys, Warsaw, Poland.)

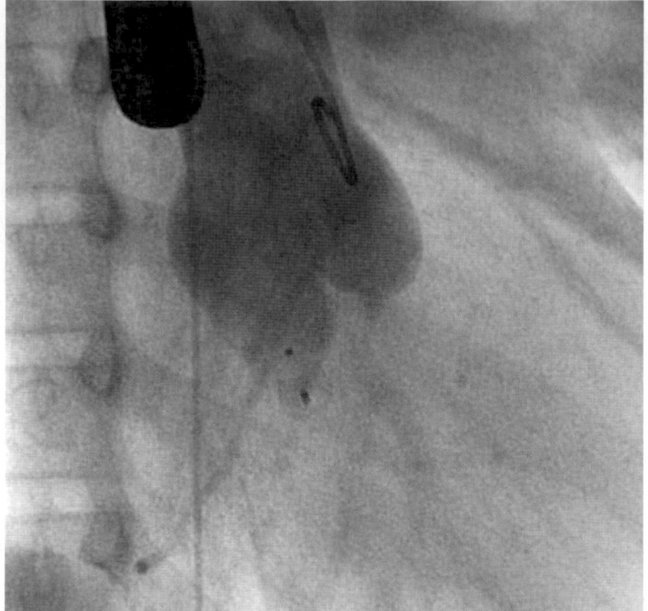

Figure 50-21 A cine frame of an aortogram in the same patient shown in Figure 50-20 showing an Amplatzer duct occluder used to close the ruptured sinus of Valsalva aneurysm. (Courtesy of Dr Grazyna Brzezinska-Rajszys, Warsaw, Poland.)

Insertion of the device should produce complete occlusion of the defect. Haemolysis can occur if there is a significant residual flow, so selection of the most appropriate device is crucial. Reported results have thus far been good.[128–130]

AORTOPULMONARY WINDOW

The aortopulmonary window is an abnormal communication between the intrapericardial components of the ascending aorta and the pulmonary trunk, but in presence of two patent arterial valves. It is a rare defect,[136] and is differentiated from common arterial trunk by the presence of the separate arterial valves arising from discrete subaortic and subpulmonary outflow tracts (Fig. 50-22). The window is usually found between the left lateral wall of the aorta and the right wall of the pulmonary trunk. It can be variable, its dimensions determining the magnitude of the shunt, the pulmonary arterial pressures, and the clinical features.

Morphology

Most frequently the defects are either circular, and positioned midway between the arterial valves and the bifurcation of the pulmonary trunk, helical and in similar position, or large and lacking obvious posterior or distal borders.[137] More rarely, the defect can be tunnel-like.[138] The window is an isolated lesion in about half the patients, but can be found in association with a ventricular septal defect, anomalous origin of the right or left coronary arteries from the pulmonary trunk, aortic coarctation, interruption of the aortic arch (Fig. 50-23), aortic origin of the right pulmonary artery, and in the setting of tetralogy of Fallot or other ventriculo-arterial connections.[139–156] It is unusual, however, to find windows in association with Di George syndrome. An iatrogenic window has now been described following inappropraite balloon dilation of pulmonary arterial stenosis.[157]

Clinical Features

The lesion produces left-to-right shunting comparable to that produced by a large patent arterial duct. The haemodynamic findings are similar to those found in patients with common arterial trunk. Congestive cardiac failure may occur in neonates or infants, with signs suggestive of a persistent patency of the arterial duct, but with a clinical suspicion of common arterial trunk. As the pulmonary vascular resistance falls during the first few weeks of life, the left-to-right shunt through the window increases. Pulmonary hypertension is a frequent complication, depending on the size of the window. The peripheral pulses are bounding, and because of the high pulmonary arterial pressures, there may be a systolic murmur at the base, rather than a continuous murmur.

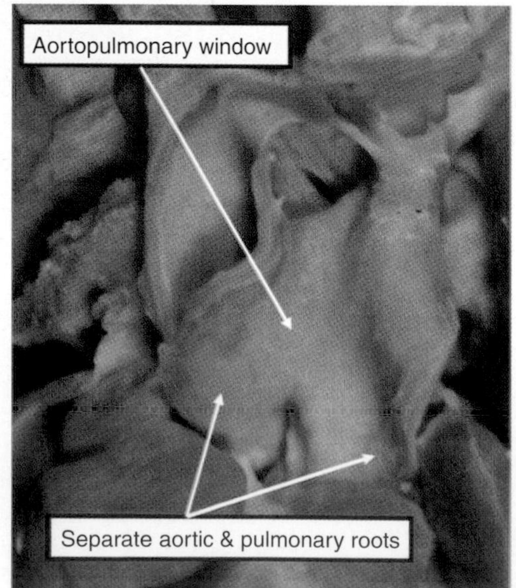

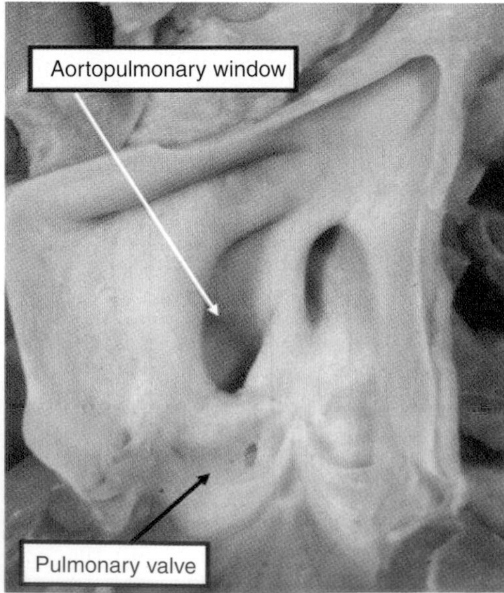

Figure 50-22 These images show a circular aortopulmonary window between the ascending portions of the aorta and the pulmonary trunk. The left panel shows the external features. Note the separate nature of the arterial roots, with a tissue plane between the proximal parts of the aorta and the pulmonary trunk. The right panel shows the view of the window from the pulmonary aspect. Note the separate nature of the pulmonary valve.

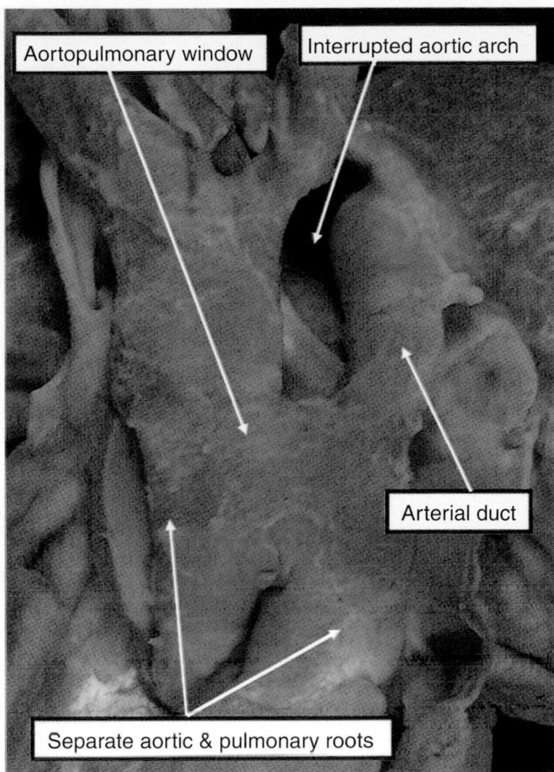

Figure 50-23 The external features of this specimen show an aortopulmonary window in the setting of interruption of the aortic arch at the isthmus. The persistently patent arterial duct is feeding the descending aorta.

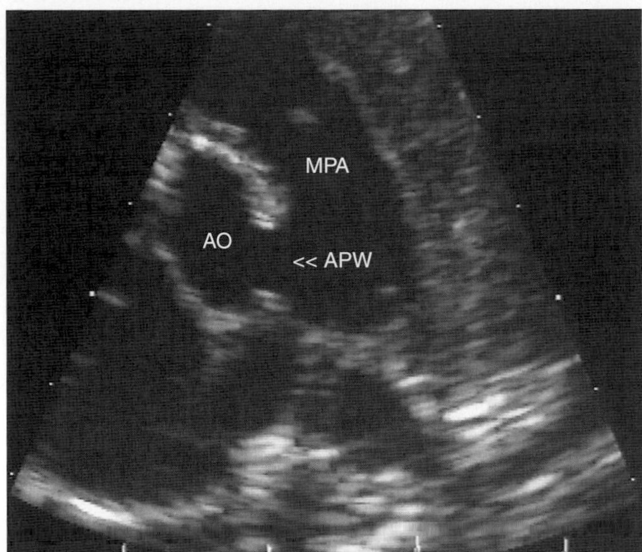

Figure 50-24 The high parasternal short-axis cross sectional echocardiogram shows the morphology of an aortopulmonary window (APW). AO, aorta; MPA, pulmonary trunk.

When the shunt is large, there is often a mid-diastolic murmur as a result of increased flow across the mitral valve. The pulmonary component of the second sound is frequently accentuated. If the window is small, there may be a continuous murmur similar to that generated by an arterial duct. If uncorrected, pulmonary vascular disease may develop within the first few years. Concomitant reversal of the shunt through the window may then cause cyanosis.

Investigations

The electrocardiogram may show left atrial hypertrophy resulting from increased flow. Frequently there is biventricular hypertrophy. The chest radiograph may show generalised cardiomegaly, with plethoric lung fields in those with large windows, but may be normal in those with small windows. The diagnosis is usually easily made with cross sectional echocardiography.[150,158] Parasternal long- and short-axis views usually identify two arterial valves, thus excluding a common arterial trunk. A high left parasternal long-axis view will demonstrate the presence of an arterial duct, as seen in association with interruption of the aortic arch. In between these views, a high parasternal short-axis view will show the window when the transducer is tilted superiorly (Fig. 50-24). Although it is often possible to see the sharp margins of the window on echocardiography, colour Doppler is an essential complementary technique that confirms flow of blood through the window.

Cardiac catheterisation is not usually needed unless there is some doubt about the presence of pulmonary vascular disease, it is performed to delineate other additional defects, or transcatheter closure is to be attempted. If the window is small, the pressures in the right side of the heart may be normal. They may be equal to systemic pressures if the window is large. In these patients, operability may need to be determined by calculation of the pulmonary vascular resistance in air and 100% oxygen. Aortography in the antero-posterior and lateral projections usually demonstrates the window. Other angiograms may be needed to confirm other additional defects, such as anomalous origin of one of the coronary arteries. Magnetic resonance imaging, however, seems a better alternative method for diagnosing additional defects.[155]

Management

Treatment is usually surgical, and there is general agreement that surgery should be performed as early as possible, before the onset of pulmonary vascular disease. The first surgical repair was reported as long ago as 1952.[159] Early experience reported mortality of up to one-fifth,[152] but results have now increased markedly,[156] and deaths after repair are now unexpected. The historical risk factors for death included high pulmonary vascular resistance. Some patients may survive to early adult life without surgery, but will almost certainly have established pulmonary vascular disease. On presentation nowadays, medical treatment is initially needed to control congestive cardiac failure. If cardiac failure cannot be controlled, there is no need to delay surgery. When the window is large, surgery should be carried out at presentation in the first few months, and preferably before 6 months of age.

Repair can usually be performed with cardiopulmonary bypass via a thoracotomy or a sternotomy.[152,156,160,161] Technically, the windows are easy to repair by direct suture when small, or with a patch if large. Direct suture is usually achieved using a transpulmonary approach, while a patch is inserted via either the transpulmonary or a transaortic approach.[152,156] An inverted flap of pulmonary trunk has also been used to repair the window.[162] Repair

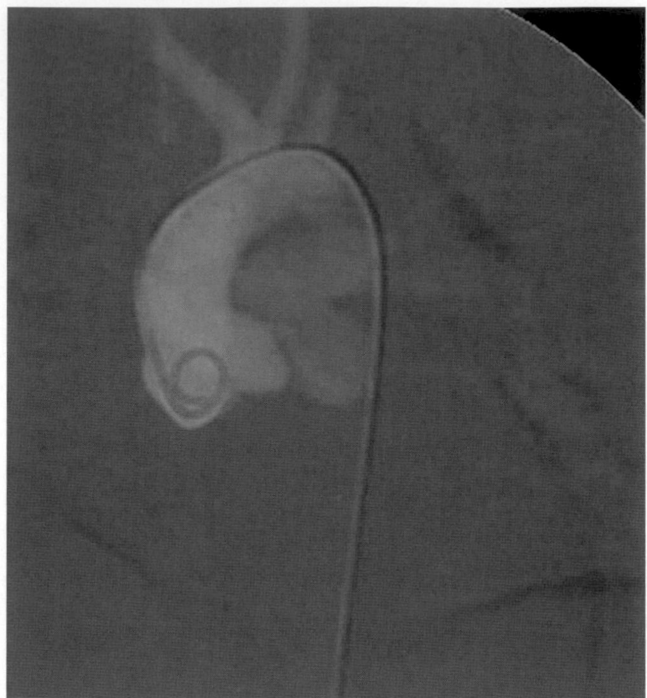

Figure 50-25 A digital subtracted aortogram in the left anterior oblique projection showing opacification of the pulmonary trunk from a small aortopulmonary window. (Courtesy of Dr Mehnaz Atique, Karachi, Pakistan.)

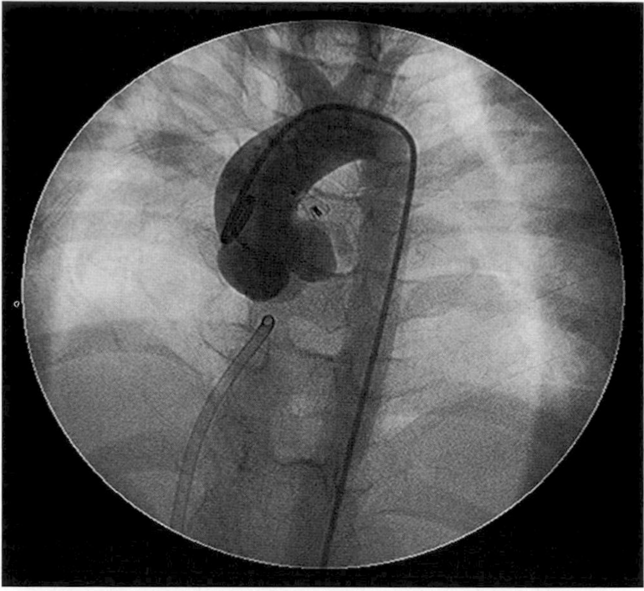

Figure 50-26 A cine frame from an aortogram from the same patient shown in Figure 50-25 showing complete occlusion of the aortopulmonary window with an Amplatzer duct occluder. (Courtesy of Dr Mehnaz Atique, Karachi, Pakistan.)

can also be achieved without cardiopulmonary bypass, the window being ligated with a clip.[161] When associated with other complex defects, then primary repair of the additional defects, along with the closure of the window, is usually undertaken in the neonatal period or in early infancy.[143,144,146,148,149,151,152,154,156,163] It is essential to evaluate the coronary arterial anatomy pre-operatively in order to avoid missing anomalous origin of either coronary artery from the pulmonary trunk. This association may have an important influence on the outcome.[137]

Transcatheter techniques can now be used to close some but not all windows, experience with this method currently being limited. Closure has been performed using a double umbrella, but only for small windows.[164,165] Other devices, such as the Amplatzer variety of devices, have been used, and are a good option for windows of small to medium size (Figs. 50-25 and 50-26).[166,167] Before proceeding with transcatheter closure, it is necessary to make a detailed evaluation of the relationships of the arterial valves, the origins of the coronary arteries, and the positions of the right and left pulmonary arteries. Aortic root angiography is needed to delineate the size of the defect. The defect should be crossed from either the ascending aorta, or from the venous side, but the device is usually delivered from the venous side. After successful closure, anti-platelet agents are given for 6 months.

PULMONARY ARTERIO-VENOUS MALFORMATIONS

Pulmonary arterio-venous malformations are congenital malformations providing an abnormal communication between a pulmonary artery and vein that bypasses the normal pulmonary capillary bed. They may occur as an isolated anomaly or as multiple lesions. Rarely, such abnormalities can be acquired, but are then described not as pulmonary arterio-venous malformations, but as arterio-venous fistulas. Interest in the pulmonary arterio-venous malformations has increased since the mid 1980s with the realisation that they cause more clinical problems, and a greater morbidity, than had been previously recognized. The emergence of transcatheter embolisation as an effective and safe alternative therapy to surgery has also contributed to the increased interest.[168–171]

Incidence

Pulmonary arterio-venous malformations are rare.[172,173] In a survey at the Hospital for Sick Children in Toronto, only 6 cases were found in more than 15,000 cases of congenital cardiac disease.[174] This may well be an underestimate, as small lesions may easily be missed at postmortem, as well as on routine investigations. It is now realised that relatives of patients with known pulmonary arterio-venous malformations, even in the absence of hereditary haemorrhagic telangiectasia, can have incidental and asymptomatic pulmonary arterio-venous malformations.

The malformations may occur as isolated vascular anomalies, or in association with hereditary haemorrhagic telangiectasia, the latter association being more common in some reported series,[171,175] but sporadic cases forming the majority in other series.[172] Now that the relatives of patients with such malformations are being actively screened, it appears that they, too, are commonly afflicted with hereditary haemorrhagic telangiectasia.[171,176] The association with hereditary haemorrhagic telangiectasia is more common in the setting of multiple malformations.[172,177] An incidence of up to one-third has been described in those with hereditary haemorrhagic telangiectasia, and there is also an increased incidence in the apparently unaffected relatives of these patients.

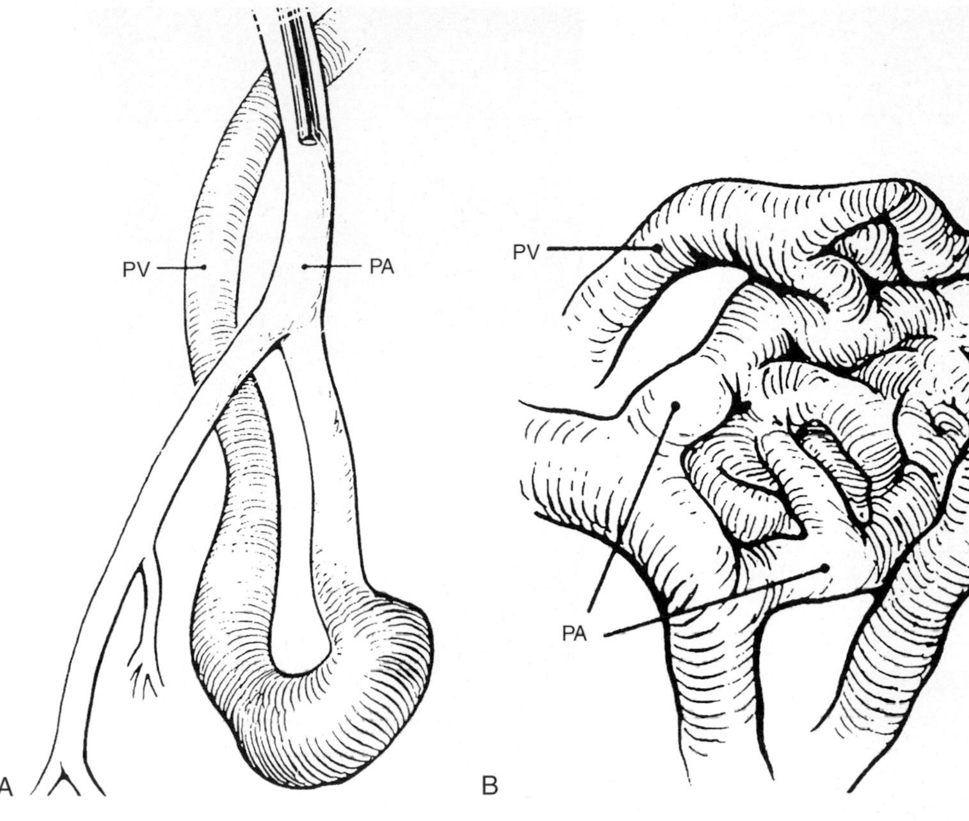

Figure 50-27 Pulmonary arterio-venous malformations can be considered simple (**A**) or complex (**B**). **A,** In the most common form, a large single feeding pulmonary artery (PA) is seen with a single pulmonary vein (PV) draining the non-septated malformation. **B,** In the less common complex type, multiple arteries and veins supply and drain from the septated malformation.

It follows, therefore, that the malformations can be solitary, multiple of varying size, multiple of uniform size, or diffuse.[178] Classification on the basis of structure[179] is simpler, and more appropriate for assessment and evaluation prior to embolisation. Based on angioarchitectural criterions, four-fifths consist of a single pulmonary artery communicating directly with a vein via the malformation, which is usually aneurysmal and non-septated (Fig. 50-27A). This so-called simple type (Figs. 50-28 and 50-29) can usually be cured by embolisation of this single feeding artery. The remaining one-fifth of the lesions are complex (Figs. 50-27B,-50-30 and 50-31), consisting of two or more connecting pulmonary arterial branches feeding aneurysmal and septated malformations, often cirsoid, with two or more draining veins. The malformations more rarely are diffuse, with most of the lungs containing multiple small arterio-venous communications (Figs. 50-32 and 50-33). In the setting of diffuse hepatic disease, such as cirrhosis, right-to-left shunting has sometimes been associated with multiple very small arterio-venous fistulas.[180] It is now well established that similar multiple fistulas can develop after construction of cavopulmonary connections that exclude hepatic flow from the lungs.[181]

Most commonly, the malformations are found in the lower lobes or the right middle lobe, being more common in the right lung.[182,183] They do not generally show much of a tendency to increase in size, albeit that long-term follow-up is not available. Studies using CT scans, however, together with serial measurements of arterial blood gases, have shown that there is little change in the degree of right-to-left shunting, or in the size of the malformations, over a period

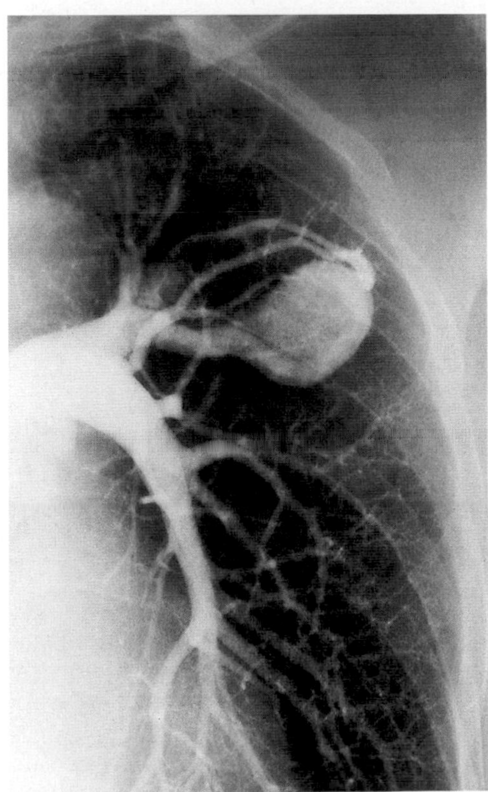

Figure 50-28 A selective injection into the left pulmonary artery shows a pulmonary arterio-venous malformation supplied by a single large feeding artery. The draining vein has not yet opacified (the same patient is shown in Figures 50-29 and 50-35).

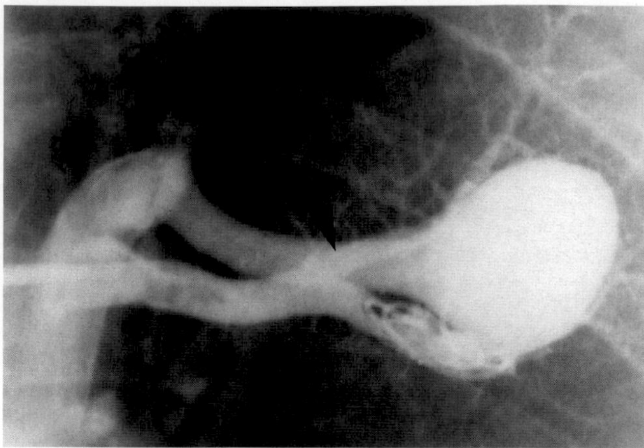

Figure 50-29 The angiographic anatomy of the simple type of pulmonary arterio-venous malformation is best shown on this film with the injection directly into the feeding artery. Despite a collection of coils immediately proximal to the malformation, and further coils within it, the malformation has not been occluded. Note the artery (*black arrow*) supplying normal lung immediately proximal to the coils and the single large vein draining to the left atrium (same patient as in Figures 50-28 and 50-35).

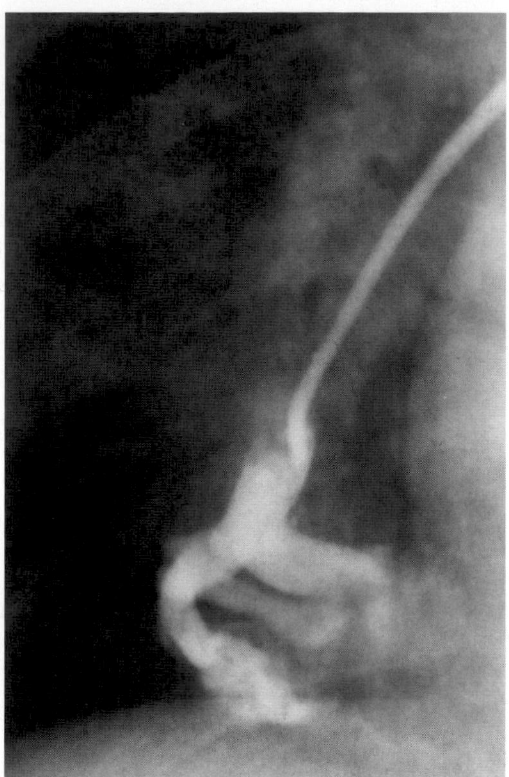

Figure 50-31 A more selective injection into the malformation shown in Figure 50-30 reveals the presence of several feeding arteries.

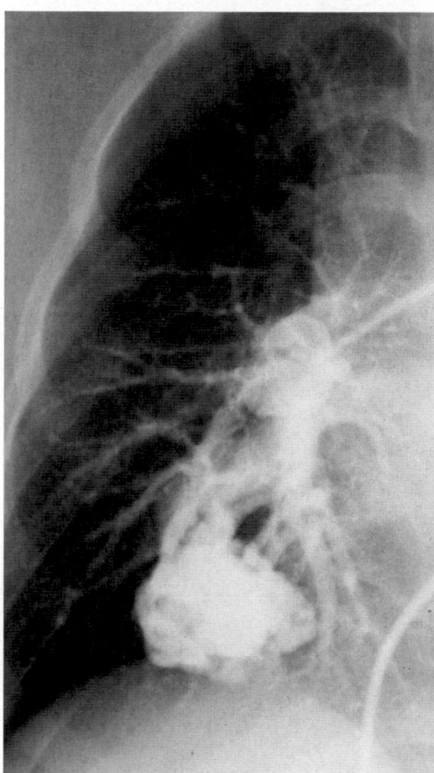

Figure 50-30 Selective injection into the right pulmonary artery shows a complex type of pulmonary arterio-venous malformation with multiple feeding arteries.

of 3 to 4 years.[176,184] Anecdotal experience has shown a gradual increase in size, but at different rates in the two lungs,[185] while several reports have described increases in size during pregnancy, or else the occurrence of significant complications.[186–188] Because of this, it is suggested that young female relatives of affected patients, or members of families with hereditary haemorrhagic telangiectasia, should be screened to exclude asymptomatic malformations, and that this should be carried out before puberty.[188]

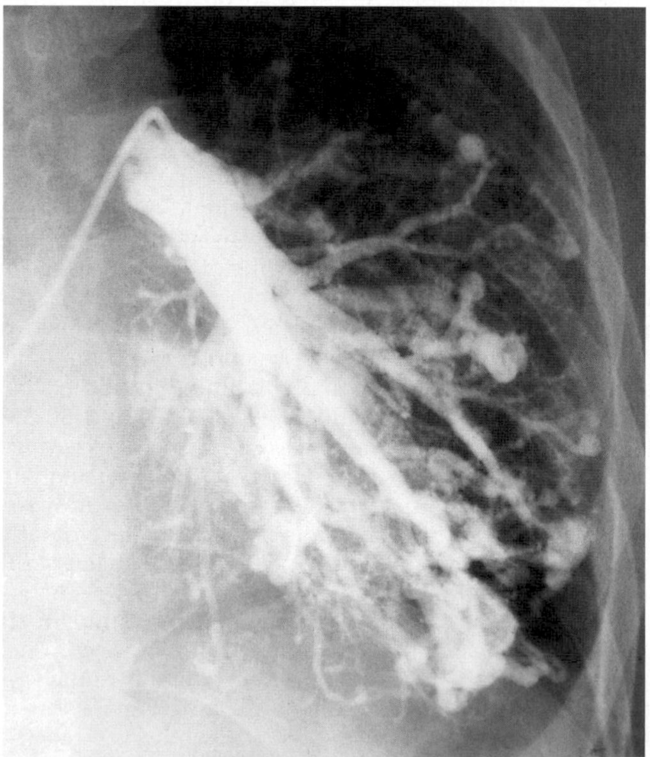

Figure 50-32 A 35-year-old patient with hereditary telangiectasia also had very extensive pulmonary arterio-venous malformations, revealed by an injection into the left descending pulmonary artery.

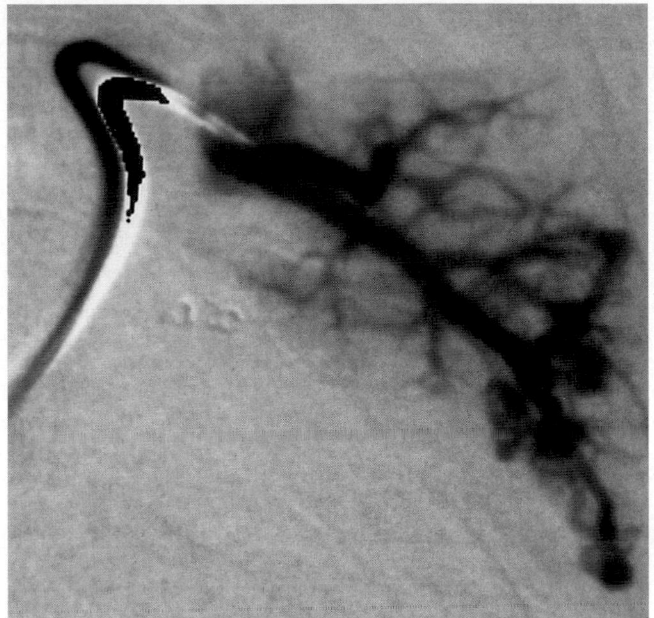

Figure 50-33 A super-selective injection into a branch of the pulmonary artery shows that there are relatively normal appearing arteries arising side by side with abnormal arteries to small pulmonary arterio-venous malformations. This would make selective embolisation very difficult, as normal branches would also be occluded.

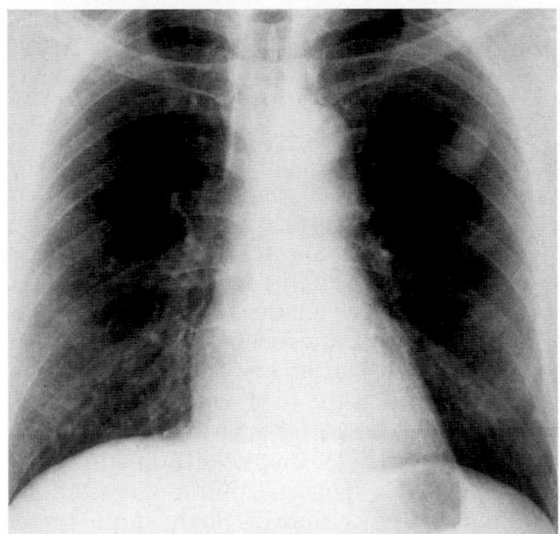

Figure 50-34 Chest radiograph of a 45-year-old man shows a smooth oval density on the left upper zone. It was barely possible to see a tubular structure connecting this with the hilum, suggesting the diagnosis of a pulmonary arterio-venous malformation.

Clinical Presentation

Patients with the malformations present very rarely as neonates and infants, but in this setting cyanosis, respiratory distress, and severe cardiac failure can be found.[189,190] Echocardiography is then needed to rule out congenital cardiac disease. More commonly, presentation is in later childhood, although it is quite common for the malformations to go undetected until mid-adult life. Sometimes the diagnosis is made as an incidental finding on a routine chest X-ray or CT scan (Fig. 50-34). Patients may present with symptoms of dyspnoea and fatigue, which may have been present for some years, even from childhood. Often there is a history of cyanosis on exercise, sometimes with surprisingly good exercise tolerance. A quite common presentation is for a patient to first present with neurological problems.[171,191] This is now recognized to be a major cause of morbidity. It is the single most important reason why such malformations should be actively sought and treated in patients with hereditary haemorrhagic telangiectasia.[176] Some form of cerebrovascular accident, such as a stroke or transient ischaemic attack, may be the initial presenting feature. It has been suggested that up to half of patients are at risk either from some form of paradoxical embolism leading to transient ischaemic attacks or strokes, or from an intracerebral abscess.[176,192] Such an ischaemic episode may be caused by thrombosis associated with polycythaemia or may be caused by a paradoxical embolism related to venous thrombosis and right-to-left shunting. The presence on CT scans of evidence of strokes is not necessarily associated with any symptoms. Haemoptysis rarely occurs from rupture of a malformation, or alternatively may be caused by bleeding from telangiectasia involving the airways.[193] Haemothorax is another rare form of presentation. Bleeding from hereditary haemorrhagic telangiectasia involving the nose and lips may result in an iron deficiency anaemia, and such lesions can affect other parts of the body, including the gut and abdominal organs.

The clinical examination may reveal central cyanosis and clubbing. In the presence of anaemia, the cyanosis may not be obvious. Evidence of hereditary haemorrhagic telangiectasia may be seen involving the nails, skin, and mucous membranes of the mouth, but such changes are rare in children. Examination of the heart and chest will be normal, except that a murmur may be heard associated with a large superficially placed pulmonary arterio-venous malformation. The murmur is usually systolic or continuous.

Screening

Hereditary haemorrhagic telangiectasia is a disorder of vascular development characterised by vascular malformations occurring in the gastrointestinal tract, respiratory system, and the cerebral, hepatic and pulmonary circulations. More than seven-tenths of pulmonary arterio-venous malformations are associated with this condition, and pulmonary arterio-venous malformations occur in one-third of patients with hereditary haemorrhagic telangiectasia. It is important, therefore, that patients with hereditary haemorrhagic telangiectasia are screened for pulmonary arterio-venous malformations.[194] As clinically significant malformations may occur in the absence of dyspnoea, and with normal resting arterial saturations of oxygen, it is important that these patients undergo some form of screening. The accuracy of non-invasive screening tests have been compared against the gold standards of CT angiography or pulmonary angiography.[194] The best test proves to be contrast echocardiography. This reflects the presence of very small microscopic pulmonary arterio-venous malformations that are not detected by CT angiography. A combination of a chest X-ray and contrast echocardiography now permits exclusion of the diagnosis of pulmonary arterio-venous malformations with total confidence.

Should these tests be positive, then CT of the chest should be performed

Investigations

The electrocardiogram is usually normal except in infancy. The echocardiogram, which may also be normal, is important to exclude any intracardiac disease. In many instances, a chest X-ray will either diagnose or strongly suggest the diagnosis. The heart is usually of normal size, and the malformations may be seen in the lungs. Typically they are round, well-defined, homogeneous opacities, often situated peripherally (see Fig. 50-34). Though not always obvious, especially when at the bases of the lungs and behind the heart, abnormal vessels connecting the malformation to the hilum can usually be discerned. Sometimes the chest radiograph is normal when small pulmonary arterio-venous malformations are not visible or, rarely, in the presence of diffuse and very small lesions.[195,196] CT is currently the best modality for demonstrating the malformations.[184,197] If the diagnosis is in doubt, then CT with intravenous contrast will confirm the diagnosis. High-resolution scans through the lungs, and the availability of fast spiral scanners, will now mean that more, and even very small, lesions will be demonstrated.[184] If obvious lesions are seen on the chest radiograph, and the clinical diagnosis is not in doubt, there would seem little point in doing any further tomography, as detailed angiography is necessary to plan for any embolisation of the larger lesions. When a malformation is diagnosed, or strongly suspected, the measurement of arterial blood gases is useful to confirm the presence of hypoxaemia, and to quantify any right-to-left shunting.[168,171,176] The arterial saturations of oxygen should be measured with the patient breathing room air in the erect or sitting position and, after 20 minutes, while breathing 100% oxygen.[198] Orthodeoxia is the term to describe a significant drop in arterial saturations of oxygen in the standing or sitting positions. This is related to the predominantly basal location of pulmonary arterio-venous malformations, and the gravitational shifts of flow that result, as well as the increase in lung volume. Quantitative assessment of the degree of right-to-left shunting can be made from nuclear medicine studies.[199,200] This technique can be used to assess the effectiveness of embolisation, particularly when there are multiple malformations. A further technique to detect right-to-left shunting is to use echocardiography to look for evidence of microcavitation in the left atrium after a peripheral injection of saline.[201]

Pulmonary Angiography

It makes sense to perform angiography and embolisation on the same occasion, especially if there are multiple lesions that may need several attempts at embolisation. Detailed pulmonary angiography is necessary to demonstrate clearly the angioarchitecture of the malformations. Initially, selective right or left pulmonary angiograms are performed (see Figs. 50-28 and 50-30). Selective catheterisation is then needed to demonstrate the feeding artery and its relationship to the adjacent normal pulmonary arterial branches (see Figs. 50-29 and 50-33). Locating the feeding artery may be difficult, especially in the lower zones where many vessels are closely related. Specialised catheter techniques, together with digital angiography, are essential requirements. Injections in varying degrees of obliquity may be needed to show the arterial anatomy.

Treatment

Until 1978, the only treatment available was surgery. The various operations performed included pneumonectomy, transection of the pulmonary trunk, lobectomy, segmentectomy, ligation of feeding vessels, intra-aneurysmal obliteration of the malformations, and wedge resection.[193,202–205] The aim was to be as conservative as possible, for at least two reasons. First, any lung tissue removed is likely to have normal function. Second, the greater the amount of the normal pulmonary circulation that is obliterated, the greater the flow to the rest of the lungs. It is possible that such high flows then cause enlargement of other malformations.[206] Complications of surgery were unusual, even in children.[169,204,205] As the techniques and devices for embolisation have evolved, however, there is now no real role for surgery.

Transcatheter occlusion, or embolisation, of a pulmonary arterio-venous malformation was first described in 1977.[207] Many series have now confirmed the initial encouraging response.[169–171,175,197] There is no place now for diagnostic arteriography alone, as the diagnosis, as well as the number and size of the malformations, will have been usually made on CT scans. Thus, arteriography is performed as a prelude to embolisation. Whenever embolisation is planned, it is essential to obtain informed consent and to detail possible risks. If multiple pulmonary arterio-venous malformation are present, it is advisable to also explain that more than one procedure may be necessary. The aim is to occlude either the feeding artery or the malformation itself (Figs. 50-35 and 50-36). It is vital that techniques are used that prevent any possibility of the material used for embolisation passing through the malformation and ending up in the systemic circulation. Embolisation should not be attempted unless the operator is experienced with embolisation elsewhere in the body. Embolisation of the pulmonary arteries is unique in that, unlike systemic arterial embolisation, where the lungs act as very effective filters for any material that crosses to the venous circulation, the consequences can be catastrophic with a pulmonary arterio-venous malformation. Even with all the necessary precautions, there has to be a very small risk of some systemic embolism, and the patient should be warned of this. If polycythaemia of significant degree is present, then venesection should be performed prior to embolisation. It is also advisable to give a bolus of heparin, approximately 5000 units, at the start of the procedure.

All symptomatic pulmonary arterio-venous malformations, and those associated with hypoxia in the sitting or standing position, should be treated. The risk of paradoxical embolism in small pulmonary arterio-venous malformations in the absence of these problems is very difficult to predict. It has been suggested that, if the feeding artery is greater than 3 mm in diameter on CT, that embolotherapy should be advocated, but this will be influenced by the age of the patient. Embolisation was first described in 1977 using stainless steel coils. In the early experience, detachable balloons and metallic coils were used, but developments with coils and other devices have now rendered balloons obselete.[170]

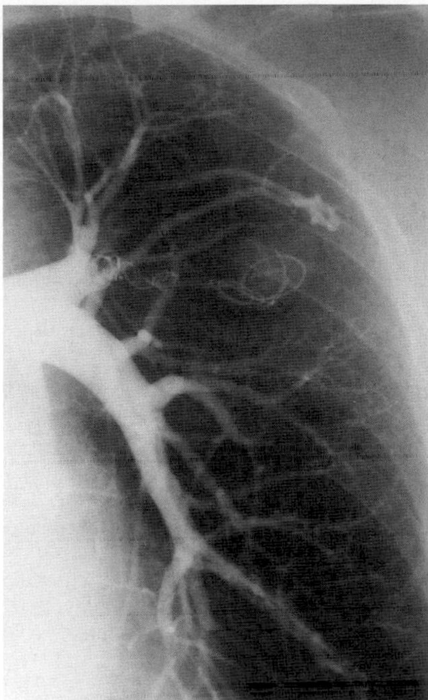

Figure 50-35 A pulmonary arterio-venous malformation is supplied by a single large feeding artery (see earlier catheterisation in the same patient shown in Figure 50-28). At this second embolisation procedure, further coils have been positioned more proximally in the feeding artery. This has occluded the pulmonary arterio-venous malformation, but at the cost of occluding also a small branch supplying normal lung.

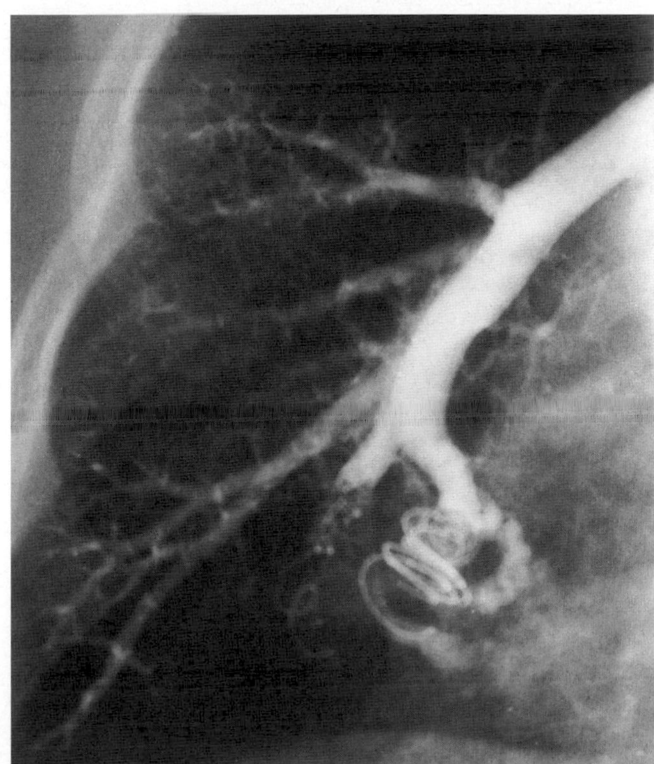

Figure 50-36 Multiple pulmonary arterio-venous malformations in the right lower lobe. These malformations were separately embolised with coils. The film taken after the procedure confirms occlusion of the malformations.

In simple malformation with a single feeding artery, the aim should be to occlude the artery just before it enters the aneurysmal part of the malformation (see Fig. 50-29). More proximal occlusion will be more likely to occlude branches supplying normal lung parenchyma, and result in some pulmonary infarction.[184] It is important to assess the diameter of the artery, as this must not be bigger than the diameter of the coil or occluding device used to occlude it. Too small a coil or device could pass through the malformation and into the single draining vein, which is usually larger than the artery. Whatever technique is used, it is important that the tip of the catheter is precisely placed and that, prior to detaching a balloon or pushing out a coil, this position and its relationship to the feeding artery is confirmed, and also that it is stable. Coils have been most commonly used for occlusion. Until recently, the range of coils was limited, but now platinum microcoils with complex helical shapes and of large diameter are available. There is now a large range of coils available that are detachable or controlled release. This allows the coils to be fully deployed and then retrieved if their position is not optimal. The coil can be repositioned, and only then released or detached when its position is considered satisfactory. Large arteries may need multiple coils to effect occlusion. If occlusion is going to occur, it will usually occur within 15 to 20 minutes of insertion. A large vessel may need several coils of larger diameter to form an anchor point on which several smaller coils can then be trapped to form a nest (see Fig. 50-35). If coils are placed without achieving a critical mass, an artery permitting high flow may not be occluded. A recent development has been to coat coils with a hydrogel polymer. This coating expands five times in about 20 minutes after deployment, thus achieving greater stability, and producing more total mass with fewer coils. Very large diameter coils, up to 2 cm, are now also available. The technique can be varied to place coils directly into the aneurysmal part of the malformation (see Fig. 50-35) rather than in the feeding artery.[208] If the malformation itself is occluded, there is then no risk of revascularisation from opening of unseen small branches. Moreover, no branches to normal lung parenchyma would then be occluded. A theoretical disadvantage of the use of coils is that, when a coil partially occludes the feeding artery, thrombus may form that could embolise into the systemic circulation. There is little evidence to suggest that this occurs. A further significant advance has the development of vascular plugs, such as the Amplatzer Vascular Plug. Such plugs are attached to a nitinol wire. Like the detachable coils, they are retrievable, and are only detached when their position is optimal. A minor disadvantage is that they need to be passed through a slightly larger catheter. A second generation device has now been developed.[209] The feeding artery to a pulmonary arterio-venous malformation will also supply some normal lung parenchyma. Even with very careful and precise embolisation, there is the likelihood of a small amount of normal lung being infarcted (see Figs. 50-33 and 50-35). The more proximal the occlusion, the greater the amount of infarction that will occur.

Pulmonary arterio-venous malformations are not common, and there are few detailed results.[210] In early experiences,[175] failure to restore the arterial oxygen saturations to normal values resulted from persistence of residual malformations too small to be considered for occlusion. Patients with multiple malformations will sometimes have a small lesion that is jointly supplied with a segment of normal lung parenchyma. Occluding the malformation would mean losing that segment of normal lung. In the simple type of malformation, be they single or multiple, embolisation is an effective technique that is safe and usually curative. Embolisation is now the treatment of choice, and surgery should be reserved for those very rare occasions when embolisation is felt to be not technically possible, or when embolisation has failed. Unlike arterio-venous malformations elsewhere in the body, these lesions do not recanalise. In the more complex and diffuse pulmonary arterio-venous malformations, it is much more difficult to eradicate completely all the lesions. By embolising the larger ones, nonetheless, significant clinical improvement can be achieved (see Fig. 50-32). It is always possible to repeat embolisations with no increased risk. Careful monitoring of the effects of embolisation by measuring blood gases and, possibly, by nuclear medicine studies is essential.

The complete reference list can be found on the companion Expert Consult web site at www.expertconsult.com.

ANNOTATED REFERENCES

- Bhattacharya JJ, Thammaroj J: Vein of Galen malformations. J Neurol Neurosurg Psychiatry 2003;74:42–44.

  This article presents an excellent and concise review of this complex malformation.

- Lasjaunias P, Alvarez H, Rodesh G, et al: Aneurysmal malformation of the vein of Galen, follow-up of 120 children healed between 1984 and 1994. Intervent Neuroradiol 1996;2:15–26.

  This is the largest published series that addresses the spectrum of presentations of vein of Galen malformation from the leading neurointerventional group and provides detailed follow-up.

- Jones BV, Ball WS, Tomsick TA, et al : Vein of Galen aneurysmal malformation: Diagnosis and treatment of 13 children with extended clinical follow-up. Am J Neuroradiol 2002;23:1717–1724.

  This study, which has good long-term follow-up data, compares and contrasts the poor results that can be expected in treating this defect in neonates with the much improved results obtained in older children.

- Schleich JM, Rey C, Gewillig M, Bozio A: Spontaneous closure of congenital coronary artery fistulas. Heart 2001;85:E6.

  This paper is an interesting review of cases, in whom spontaneous closure of small coronary arterial fistulas occurred. It emphasises the point that not all fistulas should be closed if they are asymptomatic and small, as they may close spontaneously. Therefore, they should be followed up for a few years to establish that there is no likelihood of closure before attempting catheter closure.

- Liberthson RR, Sagar K, Berkoben JP, et al: Congenital coronary arteriovenous fistula: Report of 13 patients, review of the literature and delineation of management. Circulation 1979;59:849–854.

  The earliest review of the literature. Based on this paper, recommendations were made to close all the fistulas, whether symptomatic or not, as the possibilities of complications increased beyond the second decade.

- Qureshi SA, Reidy JF, Alwi MB, et al: Use of interlocking detachable coils in embolization of coronary arteriovenous fistulas. Am J Cardiol 1996;78:110–113.

  This article makes an important contribution relating to the use of controlled release coils for closing coronary arterial fistulas. This approach is an important advance in the catheter technique.

- Ho SY, Muriago M, Cook AC, et al: Surgical anatomy of aorto-left ventricular tunnel. Ann Thorac Surg 1998;65:509–514.

  This paper shows the various types of aorto–left ventricular tunnels and is of very high educational value for enhancing our understanding of this defect.

- Rao PS, Bromberg BI, Jureidini SB, Fiore AC: Transcatheter sinus of Valsalva aneurysm—innovative use of available technology. Cathet Cardiovasc Intervent 2003;58:130–134.

  This paper highlights the advances in the catheter technology available to close even ruptured sinus of Valsalva aneurysms. This technique opens up an alternative to the traditional surgical approach.

- Backer CL, Mavroudis C: Surgical management of aorto-pulmonary window: A 40 year experience. Eur J Cardiovasc Surg 2002;21:773–779.

  This surgical review of this rare defect highlights surgical techniques used to repair aortopulmonary windows.

- Di Bella I, Gladstone DJ: Surgical management of aortopulmonary window. Ann Thorac Surg 1998;65:768–770.

  This important paper provides details of the surgical treatment of aortopulmonary windows.

- Tkebuchava T, von Segesser LK, Vogt PR, et al: Congenital aortopulmonary window: Diagnosis, surgical technique and long-term results. Eur J Cardiothorac Surg 1997;11:293–297.

  This excellent and detailed paper addresses the various aspects of diagnosis, surgical treatment and the long-term results.

- Naik GD, Chandra SV, Shenoy A, et al: Transcatheter closure of aortopulmonary window using Amplatzer device. Cathet Cardiovasc Intervent 2003;59:402–405.

  This paper describes the use of Amplatzer device in the closure of aortopulmonary window by transcatheter techniques.

- White RI, Mitchell SE, Barth KH: Angioarchitecture of pulmonary arteriovenous malformations: An important consideration before embolotherapy. Am J Roentgenol 1983;140:681–686.

  This landmark original paper gave rise to the commonly used practical classification of pulmonary arterio-venous malformations.

- Cotin V, Plauchu H, Boyle J-Y, et al: Pulmonary arteriovenous malformations in patients with hereditary haemorrhagic telangiectasia. Am J Respir Crit Care Med 2004;169:994–1000.
- Morrell NW: Screening for pulmonary arteriovenous malformations. Am J Respir Crit Care Med 2004;169:978–979.

  The important paper by Cotin et al and an accompanying editorial by Morrell address the issue of screening of patients with hereditary haemorrhagic telangiectasia, which is commonly associated with pulmonary arterio-venous malformations.

- Khurshid I, Downie GH: Pulmonary arteriovenous malformation. Postgrad Med J 2002;78;191–197.

  This paper provides an excellent general review of the subject.

CHAPTER 51

Cardiac Tumours

ELISABETH BÉDARD, ANTON E. BECKER, and MICHAEL A. GATZOULIS

Cardiac tumours in infants and children are rare. Their atypical clinical presentation prevented timely diagnosis in the past, when cardiac tumours were often a postmortem finding. The widespread use of echocardiography, and other non-invasive diagnostic methods, in recent years has resulted in a marked increase in the detection of cardiac tumours during childhood, when the patients are often asymptomatic, and also in fetal life.[1,2] In turn, early recognition of cardiac tumours has resulted in better understanding of their natural history and, combined with advances in surgical techniques, an improved overall outcome.[1,3]

It is difficult to ascertain the true incidence of cardiac tumours because of the tendency to base estimates on postmortem studies, case reports, and experiences of single institutions. The lack of non-invasive diagnostic imaging in earlier reports was another limiting factor. In the general population, and based on the data of 22 large autopsy series, the incidence of cardiac tumours was reported at around 0.02%.[4] The reported incidence in infants and children varied from 0.027% as assessed from autopsy records,[5] to 0.49% in the clinical series analysed in the New England Regional Infant Cardiac Program.[6] Another analysis[2] showed that the incidence of cardiac tumours in children had seemingly increased from 0.06% over the period 1980 to 1984, to 0.32% for the period 1990 to 1995. Review of data from the Armed Forces Institute of Pathology, combined with personal experience from the Cardiovascular Pathology Registry in the Academic Medical Center, Amsterdam, shows that, among a total of 386 primary tumours of the heart collected between 1976 and 1993, only 55 occurred in infants and children below the age of 16 years (Table 51-1).[7] Of these, one-fifth were considered malignant. Table 51-2 shows a detailed breakdown of the types of tumours reported in stillbirths, fetuses, and neonates.[1]

CLINICAL SIGNS AND SYMPTOMS

Although cardiac tumours are usually benign in children, they may induce even life-threatening symptoms. Their clinical manifestations are often non-specific. They may mimic many other diseases of the heart and lungs. Classically, the clinical presentation is divided according to whether it is the consequence of systemic, embolic, or cardiac effects (Table 51-3).

Systemic Manifestations

The systemic manifestations of tumours of the heart are manifold, and include findings such as fever, general malaise, loss of weight, and fatigue. Digital clubbing, Raynaud's phenomenon, myalgia, and arthralgia are usually associated with myxomas. All these features can mimic infective endocarditis, collagen vascular disease, rheumatic heart disease, or malignancy.[8] The constitutional symptoms disappear when the tumour is removed.[8] During the last 15 years, much evidence has accrued to suggest that inflammatory and autoimmune manifestations, seen in the presence of myxomas, may be the result of the production and release of the cytokine interleukin-6 by the tumour.[8–11]

Embolic Manifestations

Embolic signs are not an uncommon manifestation of cardiac tumours, being reported in three-tenths of patients with left atrial myxomas.[12] Embolism is also well described in children,[13] but is infrequent during fetal life or the neonatal period.[1] There can be embolisation of either fragments of the tumour itself (Fig. 51-1), or thrombus aggregated at the surface of the tumour (Fig. 51-2). The distribution of such emboluses depends largely on the localisation of the primary tumour itself, along with the presence or absence of additional cardiac malformations, such as additional shunts or abnormal patterns of flow. Embolisation of tumour fragments occurs only when the tumour itself has an intracavitary extension. Thromboembolic formation, however, can occur also with primary intramural tumours that compromise the endocardium of the cardiac chamber, either by mechanical compression or

TABLE 51-1

DETAILS OF 55 PRIMARY TUMOURS OF THE HEART IN INFANTS AND CHILDREN UNDER 16 YEARS OF AGE AS REGISTERED IN THE FILES OF THE ARMED FORCES INSTITUTE OF PATHOLOGY*

Benign	N = 44	Malignant	N = 11
Rhabdomyoma	20 (19)	Rhabdomyosarcoma	3 (1)
Fibroma	13 (8)	Angiosarcoma	1 (0)
Myxoma	4 (0)	Malignant fibrous histiocytoma	1 (0)
Vascular tumour	2 (1)	Leiomyosarcoma	1 (1)
Tumour of the atrioventricular node	2 (1)	Fibrosarcoma	1 (0)
Purkinje cell tumour	2 (2)	Myxosarcoma	1 (0)
Teratoma	1 (1)	Unclassified	3 (1)

*The numbers of subjects below the age of 1 year are shown in parentheses.

TABLE 51-2

DETAILS OF CARDIAC TUMOURS IDENTIFIED IN FETUSES, STILLBORNS, AND NEONATES*

Type of Tumour	No. (%)	No. Alive	Percent Survival (%)
Rhabdomyoma	120 (53.8)	72	60
Teratoma	40 (17.8)	30	75
Fibroma	28 (12.4)	8	29
Purkinje cell tumour	15 (6.6)	1	7
Vascular tumours	13 (5.8)	11	85
Myxoma	6 (2.7)	1	17
Malignant	2 (0.9)	0	0
Overall number	224 (100)	123	55

*As reviewed by Isaacs H Jr: Fetal and neonatal cardiac tumors. Pediatr Cardiol 2004;25:252–273.

by inducing a functional disturbance. Generally speaking, left-sided tumours embolise to the systemic circulation. Hence, they may affect almost any organ, even the heart itself.[14] Sudden occlusion of a peripheral artery should always alert to the possibility of embolisation from a primary intracardiac tumour, and should alert to the possibility of cerebral embolism.[13] Moreover, multiple systemic embolisation may mimic systemic vasculitis or infective endocarditis, particularly when producing systemic manifestations.

Primary tumours in the right heart chambers may cause pulmonary embolism.[15] This may be indistinguishable from pulmonary embolism secondary to venous thromboembolism. Perfusion defects in the lung due to embolisation from a tumour do not usually resolve within a few weeks, as they do with venous embolisation. Embolisation from a tumour may also be suggested by complete absence of flow to one lung in the presence of a normal perfusion scan on the opposite lung. This is most unusual in patients with recurrent pulmonary venous thromboembolism.

TABLE 51-3

CLINICAL MANIFESTATIONS OF CARDIAC TUMORS

Symptoms/Signs	Remarks
1. Systemic	
Fever	May mimic endocarditis or malignant disease
General malaise	
Weight loss	
Fatigue	
Digital clubbing	May mimic collagen, rheumatic or malignant disease
Raynaud's phenomenon	
Myalgia and arthralgia	
2. Embolic	
Systemic embolism	May affect almost any organ Caused by embolisation of left-sided tumour fragments or thrombi aggregated at its surface
Pulmonary embolism	Caused by embolisation of right-sided tumours
3. Cardiac	
Arrhythmias	Almost any arrhythmias can occur Complete atrioventricular block and sudden death are seen as the extreme
Cardiac failure	May mimic dilated, restrictive, or hypertrophic obstructive cardiomyopathy May present with cardiomegaly, respiratory distress, hydrops, pulmonary oedema, cyanosis
Pericardial effusion and tamponade	Seen mainly in teratoma, malignant tumours, and secondary lesions
Obstruction	May cause outflow tract or atrioventricular valve obstruction and mimic valvar disease May present with new murmur, syncope, sudden death, or acute pulmonary oedema Symptoms and murmur may relate to the patient's position
Tumour plop	Is almost the only specific sign (with the postural variation of a murmur) Results from sudden tension on the stalk of the tumour as it prolapses during diastole into the left ventricular cavity with the possible impact of the mass on the ventricular wall

Cardiac Manifestations

The cardiac events are largely dependent on the location and the extent of the tumour within the heart. Tumours that are localised within the myocardium may occasionally pass unnoticed clinically. They may be discovered as incidental findings at echocardiography or postmortem. Detection of a cardiac mass on routine obstetric sonographic scan is often the initial finding in fetuses.[1]

Arrhythmias

Disturbances of cardiac rhythm can be the first manifestation of a primary cardiac tumour.[16] Should the tumour be located in the region of the atrioventricular node or conduction axis, even small tumours may produce disturbances of atrioventricular conduction. Complete atrioventricular block and sudden death are seen as the extreme clinical manifestation, especially for rhabdomyomas.[1] Moreover, the intramural location of primary tumours may underlie a wide variety of disturbances of rhythm, including atrial fibrillation or flutter, paroxysmal atrial tachycardia, atrioventricular junctional rhythm, Wolff-Parkinson-White syndrome, atrial and ventricular premature beats, ventricular tachycardia, and ventricular fibrillation.[16–19]

Cardiac Failure and Pericardial Effusion

Infiltrative tumours of the myocardium can cause haemodynamic compromise. This tends to occur late in the clinical course when there is substantial involvement of the myocardium or pericardium (Fig. 51-3), producing symptoms of cardiac failure consequent to systolic and or diastolic dysfunction.[1] In some instances, the clinical presentation may mimic that of dilated, restrictive, or hypertrophic obstructive cardiomyopathy.[20,21] Pericardial exudates, eventually with cardiac tamponade, may be the first symptom of the epicardial location of a tumour.[22,23] This is mainly seen with teratomas, malignant tumours, and secondary lesions.

Obstruction

Primary cardiac tumours with intracavitary extension may cause obstruction, or may interfere with valvar closure (Fig. 51-4).[1,3] The signs and symptoms are then highly

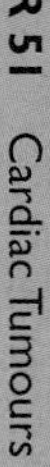

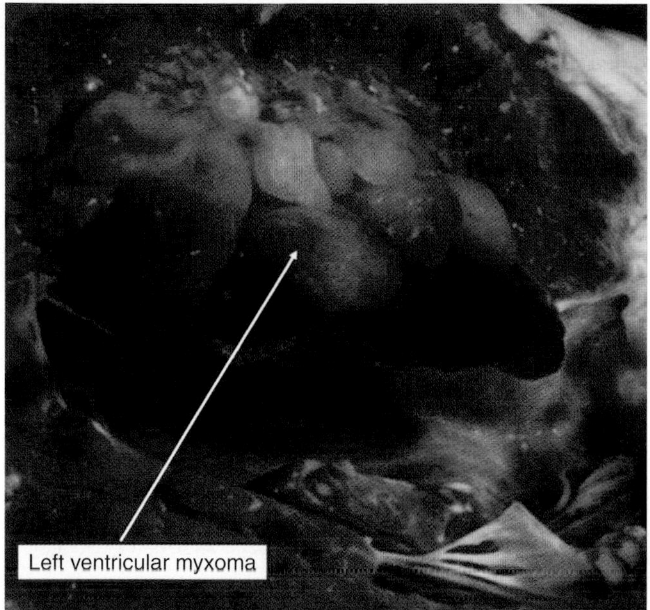

Figure 51-1 The illustration shows a left ventricular myxoma in an adult. It is easy to see how parts of the tumour can fragment and embolise to the systemic circulation.

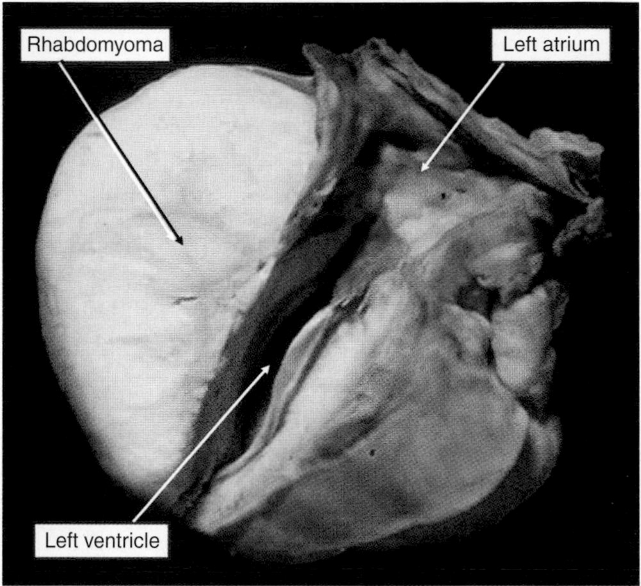

Figure 51-3 The heart is shown from the left side. A huge rhabdomyoma has grown in the antero-superior wall of the left ventricle, compromising the ventricular cavity, and producing cardiac failure.

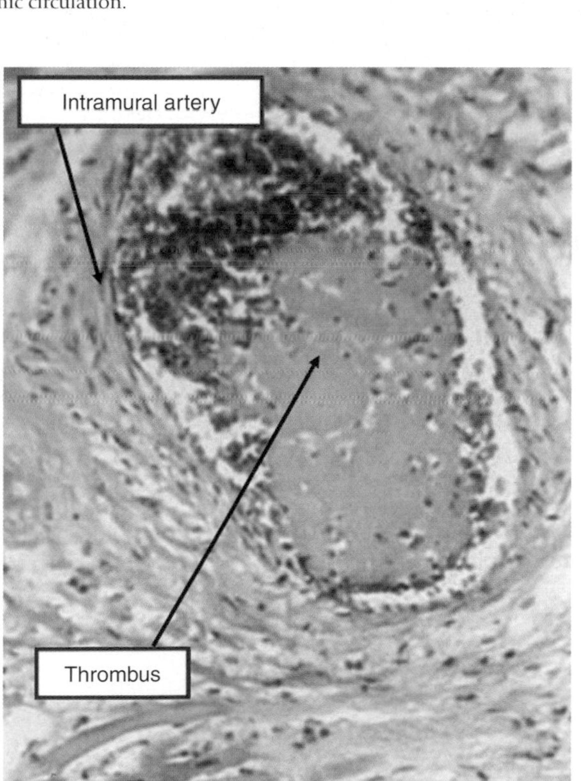

Figure 51-2 The slide shows a section across an intramural coronary artery that is completely occluded by a thrombus detached from the surface of an intracardiac myxoma.

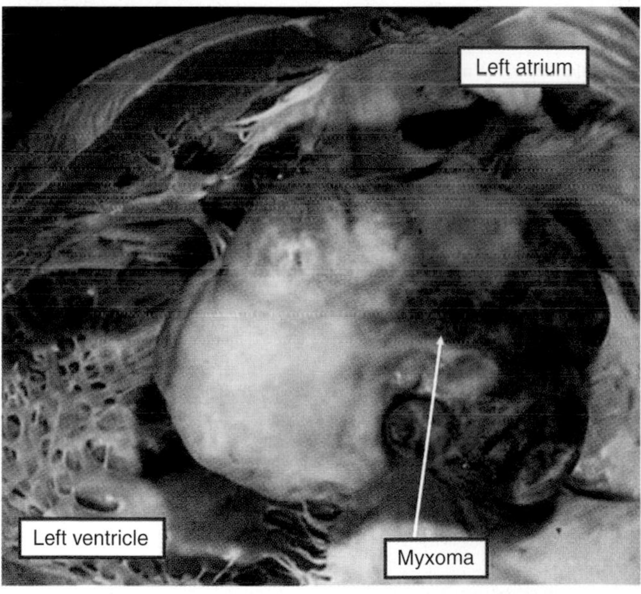

Figure 51-4 The opened left atrioventricular junction in this adult heart is completely blocked by a left atrial myxoma. Note the different colouration of the components of the tumour located in the left atrium and ventricle.

dependent upon the chamber involved, and the size of the tumour. The embolic effects, which are a frequent complication, similarly relate directly to the site of the tumour. Left atrial tumours may produce mitral stenosis (see Fig. 51-4) or insufficiency, and may mimic valvar disease, with new murmurs as a frequent presenting sign in infants and children.[1,24] Intracavitary left ventricular tumours may also cause inflow or outflow obstruction, or atrioventricular valvar insufficiency, along with the anticipated accompanying signs and symptoms. All these obstructive manifestations may have a sudden onset, particularly in the case of a pedunculated highly mobile left atrial tumour, which can cause syncope, sudden unexpected death, or acute pulmonary oedema.[1,3] Such findings are often intermittent, and may relate to the posture of the patient.

Location of Tumour within the Heart

Intracavitary tumours within the right atrium frequently produce symptoms of right-sided cardiac failure.[25] The manifestations may result from either obstruction of the tricuspid orifice or tricuspid valvar insufficiency, the latter secondary to interference with valvar closure. Caval venous obstruction may be seen as a leading feature.[26] Right ventricular intracavitary tumours may similarly produce signs and symptoms of tricuspid valvar obstruction, but can also produce outflow obstruction or atrioventricular valvar insufficiency.[24,27-30] Right-sided failure is often the leading manifestation. As with all cardiac tumours, the physical signs may vary considerably, depending upon their site and size. As stated before, the picture may be further complicated by pulmonary embolism and secondary pulmonary hypertension. Tumours in the right ventricle, therefore, may mimic congenital pulmonary stenosis, restrictive cardiomyopathy, or even cyanotic cardiac disease, especially in the neonate.[1] Atypical chest pain may occur. This is caused by coronary arterial obstruction, either from compression by the tumour itself, or because of coronary arterial embolism (see Fig. 51-2).[14] Hence, intracavitary left ventricular tumours may mimic other conditions, such as aortic and subaortic stenosis, asymmetric septal hypertrophy, and endocardial fibroelastosis.[31-35]

PHYSICAL EXAMINATION

Physical examination is, in general, non-conclusive. Murmurs, when present, are in themselves non-specific, but certain atypical findings may suggest a cardiac tumour rather than primary valvar or myocardial disease. Such findings include postural variation in the intensity of the murmur, and the presence of a so-called tumour plop. The plop has been described particularly in patients with left atrial myxoma, being characteristic of a pedunculated and highly sessile tumour. The plop was heard in one-sixth of the patients in one large series.[12] It most likely results from sudden tension on the stalk of the tumour as it prolapses during diastole into the left ventricular cavity, along with the possible impact of the mass on the ventricular wall.[36]

INVESTIGATIONS

Laboratory Studies

These are non-specific (Table 51-4). Abnormal findings include an elevated erythrocytic sedimentation rate, and increased levels of C-reactive protein in the serum, along with hypergammaglobulinaemia, thrombocytosis or thrombocytopenia, polycythaemia, leucocytosis, and anaemia.

TABLE 51-4

MERITS OF POTENTIAL INVESTIGATIONS IN PATIENTS WITH CARDIAC TUMOURS

Investigation	Remarks
Blood	Non-specific May include elevated erythrocytic sedimentation rate and serum C-reactive protein, hypergammaglobulinaemia, thrombocytosis or thrombocytopenia, polycythaemia, leucocytosis, and anaemia
Electrocardiogram	Non-specific All kinds of rhythm and conduction disturbances or voltage and ST-T wave segmental abnormalities may be seen
Chest radiograph	Non-specific May show abnormal contours of the heart Signs of pulmonary venous obstruction may occur with obstructive left-sided tumours Possible to show calcification of the tumour
Echocardiogram	Main diagnostic modality Allows accurate determination of the size, shape, texture, location, attachment, mobility, and haemodynamic consequences of the tumour
Magnetic resonance imaging	Allows a better soft tissue contrast, and offers a larger field of view, demonstrating the extension to the adjacent structures Requires sedation in children to suppress deep respiration and movements

Electrocardiography

The electrocardiogram is also non-specific. All kinds of disturbances of rhythm and conduction, and abnormalities of voltage and the ST-T segments, may be seen.[1,16] The electrocardiogram may also display the typical pattern of atrial dilation or ventricular hypertrophy.[1,12] Incidental low-voltage complexes may be registered, indicating possible pericardial involvement. Occasionally, it is possible to find the pattern of ventricular pre-excitation.[1] This is particularly the case when the accessory muscular atrioventricular pathways are composed of the intracardiac tumour.[37,38]

Chest Radiography

Cardiac tumours may alter the contours of the heart, but the changes in themselves are most often non-specific. The cardiac contour may be normal, or may display enlargement of either the entire heart or any particular chamber.[39-41] Gross and bizarre distortions of the cardiac contour occasionally occur that are then suggestive of a tumour. The overall picture may be further complicated by the presence of pericardial fluid. Radiographic signs of pulmonary venous obstruction with left atrial enlargement may be observed in patients with obstructive left-sided tumours. Calcification of a primary tumour may occasionally be so intense that it can be noted on the chest radiograph (Fig. 51-5).[39,40]

Echocardiography

Echocardiographic examination is now universally established as the main, and usually the only, diagnostic modality required for children. It allows accurate determination of the size, shape, texture, location, attachment, mobility, and haemodynamic consequences of the tumour. For most patients, it obviates the need for cardiac catheterisation and angiography.[2,3,42,43] Use of the technique, in some hands,[44] has resulted in dramatic increase in the annual incidence of cardiac neoplasms over a period of 5 years, combined with an equally dramatic reduction in unexpected intra-operative findings. Echocardiography is also the method of choice for follow-up, as spontaneous regression of tumours diagnosed during infancy is frequent.[45] The diagnostic sensitivity of transthoracic and transoesophageal approaches has been reported to be 93.3% and 96.8%, respectively.[46] The sensitivity is greatest for endocardial lesions, where the contrast between tumour and an echolucent cavity is most apparent, permitting characterisation of the size and mobility of the masses. In contrast, echocardiographic assessment of the pericardial tumours

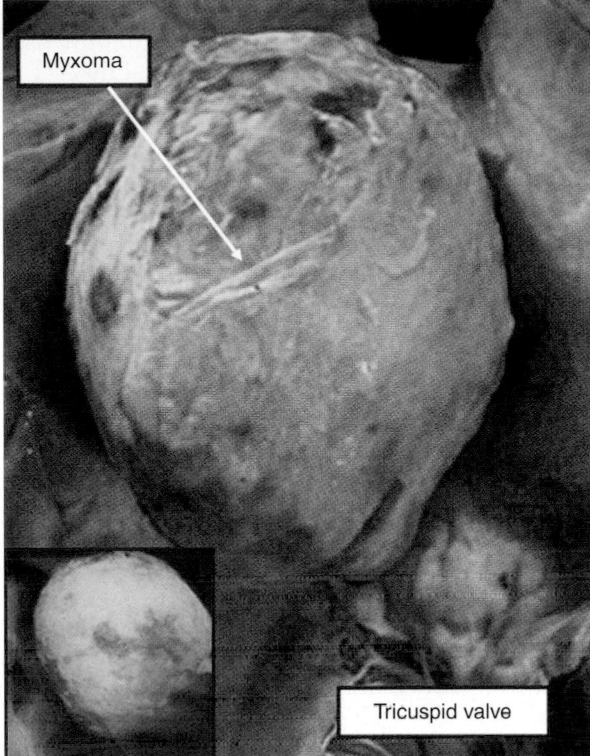

Figure 51-5 This right atrial myxoma from an adult heart is extensively calcified, as shown in the inset, which is a postmortem radiograph. Calcification of this extent can also be seen on chest radiographs during life.

may be limited because of the echo density and their frequent position in the echocardiographic farfield. While involvement of the pericardium, and the extracardiac mediastinum, by the tumour may be revealed by scanning from multiple positions, this being mandatory when assessing any pericardial effusion of unknown aetiology, magnetic resonance imaging is a more capable and reliable technique for this task. Texture may be inferred by the gray-scale appearance, although interpretation remains subjective.[47] Colour processing of the cross sectional gray-scale image has also been applied to distinguish tumour mass from endocardium.[48,49] In recent years, contrast echocardiography has been shown to provide better visualisation of the interface between myocardium and blood.[50] Contrast perfusion imaging of cardiac masses with gray-scale power modulation also facilitates the differential diagnosis.[51] Echocardiography also gives information as to whether the tumour is encapsulated, and whether it is solid or cystic.[52] Cardiac tumours have the tendency to occur at multiple sites. Hence, echocardiographic evaluation should be thorough, encompassing the whole heart and pericardium.[3]

Transoesophageal echocardiography can be a useful adjunct to transthoracic imaging, notably in patients with suboptimal transthoracic windows. It is ideally suited for the examination of suspected tumours involving the atriums, interatrial septum, caval veins, atrioventricular valves, and, to a lesser extent, the great arteries.[53] Another important application is the differentiation of true pathology from normal, or variants of normal, anatomy. For example, a prominent terminal crest may simulate a mass during transthoracic imaging of the morphologically right atrium. Transoesophageal echocardiography can demonstrate this to be a normal structure. In addition, transoesophageal imaging can be used intra-operatively to assist with surgical excision of cardiac tumours, or to guide transvenous biopsy.[3,54] Dynamic three-dimensional echocardiography allows a view of the contents of an intracardiac tumour.[55] It is a valuable way of defining the morphological and spatial characteristics of cardiac and paracardiac tumours, establishing their relationships with adjacent structures, and might be superior to transthoracic echocardiography in the evaluation of the size of intracardiac masses (Fig. 51-6).[42,55–58] When used preoperatively, it may yield important additional information and improve the operative planning.[59] Prenatal echocardiographic screening (Fig. 51-7), performed usually for the assessment of intra-uterine growth, or occasionally as part of investigations for fetal arrhythmias or non-immune hydrops and high-risk pregnancies, has permitted fetal tumours to be diagnosed as early as 19 weeks of gestation,[1,60–62] with two-thirds of the tumours being rhabdomyomas.[1] Prior knowledge of the existence of the tumour in some circumstance has permitted life-saving interventions, such as intra-uterine pericardiocentesis, or even intra-uterine surgery. Prenatal diagnosis

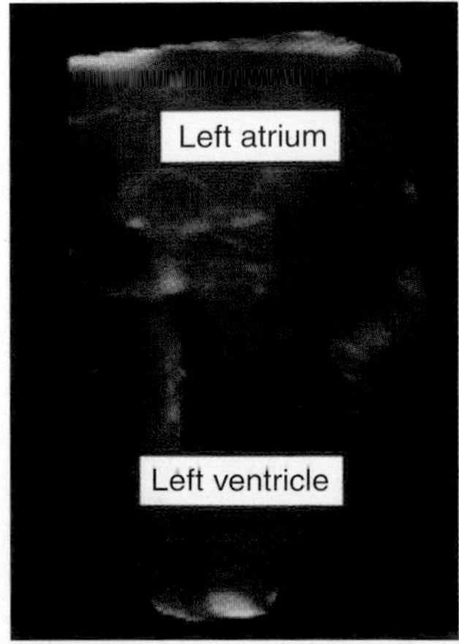

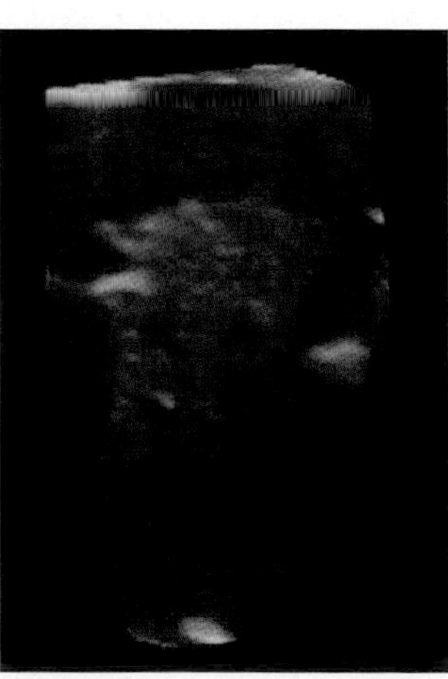

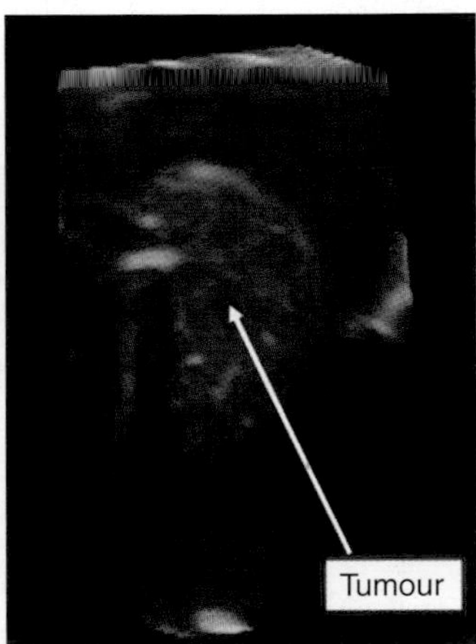

Figure 51-6 Dynamic three-dimensional echocardiography showing a myxoma in a 12-year-old boy, originating in the left atrium and attached to the atrial septum in the region of the oval fossa. The tumour is protruding into the atrioventricular orifice during ventricular diastole. (Courtesy of Dr Jan Marek, Great Ormond Street Hospital, London, United Kingdom.)

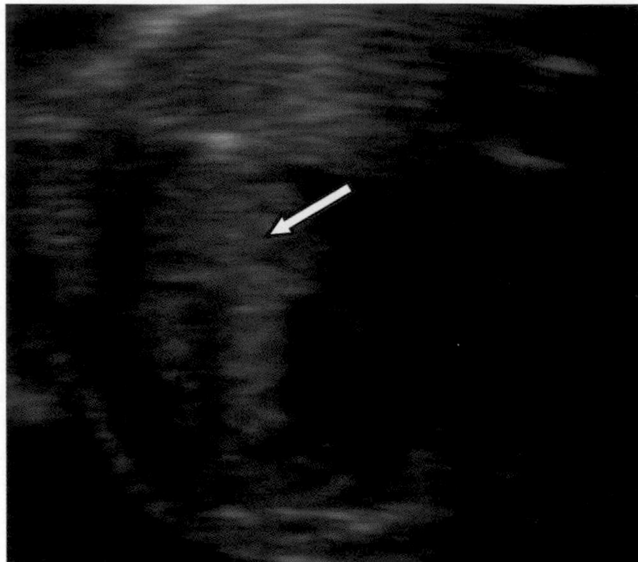

Figure 51-7 This massive right-sided heart tumour (*arrow*) was diagnosed during fetal echocardiography at 21 weeks of gestation. The neoplasm, which is primarily extracardiac, may have an intracardiac extension, and appears to have limited the effective right ventricular cavity, causing some obstruction of the right ventricular outflow tract. A teratoma was suspected, and confirmed at pathology. (Courtesy of Dr Julene Carvalho, Royal Brompton Hospital, London, United Kingdom.)

certainly permits optimisation of postnatal care.[61–64] Spontaneous regression of even symptomatic tumours has also been described when diagnosed during fetal life.[1]

Magnetic Resonance Imaging and Computed Tomography

Since the mid-1980s, magnetic resonance imaging has been increasingly used for the detection and diagnosis of cardiac neoplasms, with various studies comparing its value to transthoracic echocardiography.[40,65–67] Resonance imaging shows better the contrast with soft tissue, and offers a larger field of view, showing the extent of the tumour relative to the adjacent mediastinum, lungs, or vascular structure (Figs. 51-8 and 51-9).[65–70] The inherent natural contrast between the intracardiac and vascular spaces and the surrounding walls of cardiovascular structures enables sharp delineation of the myocardium, with negligible interference by bony or lung tissue.[71] Resonance imaging is unquestionably the superior investigative approach in pericardial lesions, and provides information on the haemodynamic consequences of the tumour. Contrast-enhanced imaging with paramagnetic agents and radio-frequency labelling permits further differentiation of tumour from viable myocardium.[72] With the recent improvement in pulse sequences for cardiac imaging, the motion artefact has been reduced, giving an even better quality to the images.[68] Spin-echo and cine-gradient-echo techniques provide additional valuable information concerning mobility, site of attachment,

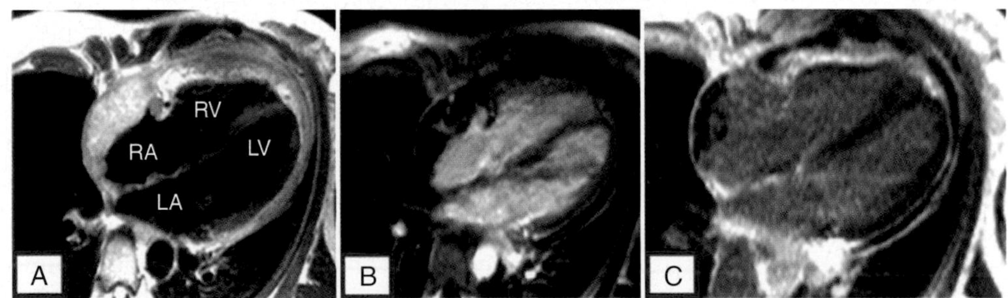

Figure 51-8 Cardiac magnetic resonance imaging showing an angiosarcoma in the free wall of the right atrium in a 45-year-old female. **A**, A spin-echo image in a four-chamber view and the corresponding inversion recovery gradient-echo image acquired 1 min (**B**) and 15 min (**C**) after intravenous injection of gadolinium DTPA. The spin-echo image depicts the anatomical details of the right atrial mass and its relation to surrounding structures. Early and late enhancement (**B** and **C**) indicate increased vascularity, and necrosis and scarring, respectively. LA, left atrium; LV, left ventricle; RA, right atrium; RV, right ventricle. (Courtesy of Dr Raad Mohiaddin, Royal Brompton and Harefield NHS Trust, London, United Kingdom.)

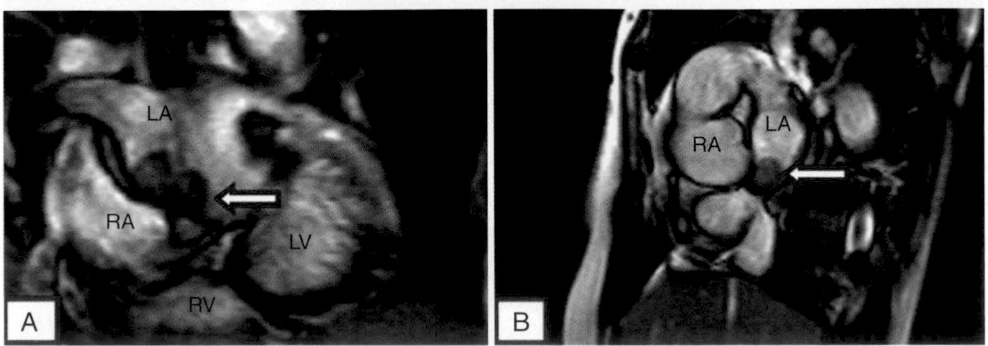

Figure 51-9 Cardiac magnetic resonance imaging of an atrial myxoma. Diastolic frame from dynamic cine studies acquired in the left ventricular horizontal long axis (**A**) and in the short axis of the left atrium (**B**). A solid mass attached to the interatrial septum is clearly seen (*arrow*). LA, left atrium, LV, left ventricle; RA, right atrium; RV, right ventricle. (Courtesy of Dr Raad Mohiaddin, Royal Brompton and Harefield NHS Trust, London, United Kingdom.)

and effects on myocardial and valvar function.[73] The use of resonance imaging in children, nonetheless, is not free of limitations. Heavy sedation is often required to suppress deep respiration and other movements. In those with arrhythmias, interference can still cause significant motion artefact despite electrocardiographic gating, thus compromising the quality of imaging.[68] Furthermore, in contrast to echocardiography, the machine is not portable, and is not suitable for patients requiring intensive care. The technique is also incapable of demonstrating the presence of calcium.[68] Computed tomography, in contrast, is able to detect calcification, of value in the differential diagnosis of cardiac tumours.[67] Computed tomographic scanning is also faster and easier to perform than magnetic resonance imaging.[67] Recently, multi-slice computerised tomography has emerged, permitting detailed delineation of intra- and pericardial masses.[74]

Catheterisation and Angiocardiography

Once accepted as the gold standard for diagnosis, angiocardiography has waned in importance as a result of the availability and reliability of the non-invasive methods of imaging discussed above. One of the last indications remaining is to eliminate the presence of coronary arterial diseases in adults with cardiac tumours.[3,75] Angiocardiography does not demonstrate extension of tumour into the ventricular walls but only the presence of the tumour within the cavities, as demonstrated by filling defects. The possibility of diagnosis by endomyocardial biopsy has been suggested,[76] and may still be used in certain circumstances.[77] This is hardly ever necessary nowadays, as a firm diagnosis can be established using non-invasive imaging. If necessary, diagnosis can be confirmed by peri-operative biopsy should surgical excision of the tumour be justified. Pressure measurements can be obtained with catheterisation, although this has the inherent risk of placing a catheter near or across a friable tumour, a process that may lead to embolisation.[78]

Transthoracic echocardiography, therefore, constitutes the procedure of choice when screening for cardiac tumours. Magnetic resonance and transoesophageal echocardiographic imaging clearly complement one another, and the choice between these techniques depends upon various factors, including the transthoracic echogenicity of the patient, the site of the possible tumour, the availability of these methods, cost, and the physical state and age of the patient.

TYPES OF TUMOUR

Rhabdomyomas

Rhabdomyomas are by far the most frequent tumours found in fetuses, infants and children. They occur almost exclusively in patients under the age of 15 years, and about three-quarters are seen in patients under 1 year of age.[1] They most likely represent hamartomas rather than true neoplasms, being composed of overgrown cardiac muscle.[1,34] They may present as circumscribed non-encapsulated lesions, varying in size from a few millimetres to several centimetres. Occasionally, the lesion may outgrow the size of the heart (see Fig. 51-1). Rhabdomyomas are usually multiple, and have a distinct preference for the ventricular septum and the adjacent ventricular walls (Fig. 51-10).[1,7,34,79] The lesions may be limited to the myocardium, often leading to compression and deformity of the cardiac chambers. Alternatively, they may extend from their intramural location to occupy an intracavitary position (see Fig. 51-10). Nearly half of patients have an intracavitary rhabdomyoma, with marked obstruction to flow of blood in at least one cardiac chamber.[1] Histologically, the lesions are characterised by grotesquely swollen myocytes, which present an almost empty cytoplasm traversed by tiny strands of cross-striated sarcoplasm. The nucleus may thus appear suspended within the cell, giving rise to the so-called spider cell (Fig. 51-11). Spontaneous regression is possible, occurring in most neonates during the first year of life.[1] Echocardiographic follow-up has shown regression within a period as short as 6 weeks.[45,80–83] Tuberous sclerosis is present in over half of those found to have rhabdomyomas. When the tumours are multiple, up to four-fifths have the disease.[1,34]

It is possible to distinguish two main clinical categories. In some patients, the rhabdomyoma is an incidental postmortem finding.[1] In other patients, however, the tumour is the immediate cause of morbidity and/or mortality. In some, it may have led to stillbirth, or death within a few days of birth. In others, the rhabdomyoma may become clinically manifest, usually because of cardiomegaly, intracardiac obstruction, a murmur, congestive cardiac failure, cyanosis, or cardiac arrhythmias, and death may occur suddenly and unexpectedly.[1,7,34,84] Seizures, hydrops, and polyhydramnios have also been described.[34]

The prognosis of children with rhabdomyomas has improved significantly over recent decades due to advances in diagnosis and treatment.[1] Meta-analysis suggests mortality of 25.4%.[34] This, however, is almost certainly an overestimation of the real rate of death, since not all cases are reported. Indeed, survival in some series has been greater than 80%.[1,80,84,85] Once symptoms have appeared suggestive of arrhythmias, obstruction to the outflow tracts, or

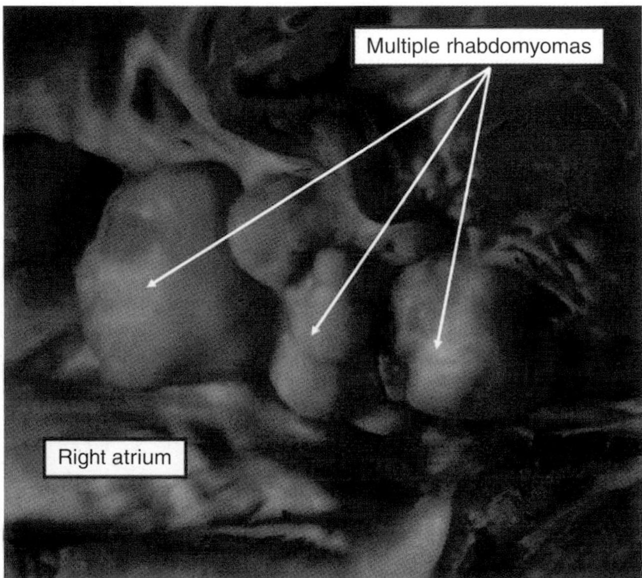

Figure 51-10 These multiple rhabdomyomas, occupying an intracavitary position, are growing from the wall of the right ventricle and the adjacent right atrium.

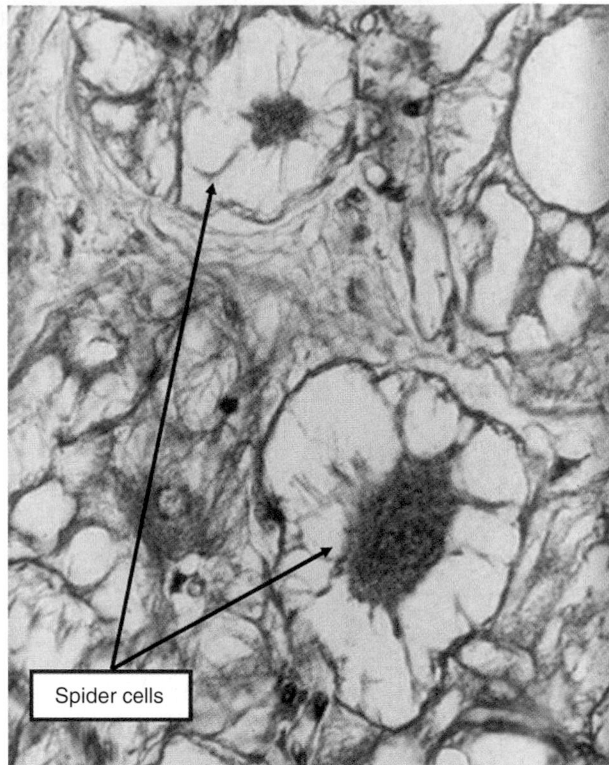

Figure 51-11 This histological section of a rhabdomyoma shows the typical features of the so-called spider cell.

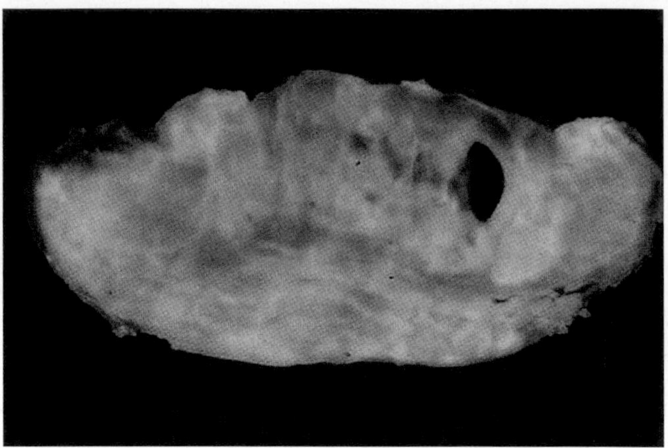

Figure 51-12 The cut edge of this resected fibroma shows the typical fibromatous architecture.

valvar dysfunction, the prognosis becomes worse.[1] It has been suggested, with good reason, that the demonstration of an intracardiac mass in a symptomatic child less than 5 years of age strongly suggests the diagnosis of rhabdomyoma. Since most infants with rhabdomyomas will show a spontaneous regression during the first year of life, surgical intervention should be recommended only in the presence of severe haemodynamic disturbances or persistent arrhythmias.[1] While the cardiac prognosis for fetuses or infants with rhabdomyomas is generally good, concerns are raised because of their common association with tuberous sclerosis. Recent studies suggest that patients with tuberous sclerosis carry a poor neurological prognosis with many of them suffering epilepsy and mental/behavioural disability in childhood and later life.[86,87]

Fibromas

Cardiac fibromas, found in one-quarter of cases, ranked second in frequency amongst tumours identified at postmortem in hearts of children between 1 and 15 years of age (see Table 51-1).[7] The reported prevalence in clinical series has been higher, at one-quarter to one-fifth.[88] These tumours are seen throughout childhood, although they are less common in fetuses and newborns The gross appearance of cardiac fibromas is relatively uniform. They present as solid, firm, whitish lesions, with a distinct fibromatous architecture when seen in cut sections (Fig. 51-12). They may vary in size from 1 to 9 cm.[1] Those producing functional impairment are usually several centimetres in size. Their circumscript appearance suggests an encapsulated nature, but microscopic studies reveal intermingling of the tumour with the adjacent myocardium.[1,7] Moreover, satellite nodules may be present. Calcification within the lesions is not uncommon.[1] Cardiac fibromas, in practical terms, are slow-growing, solitary, but potentially aggressive lesions. Spontaneous regression has not been observed, and surgical excision is often required. Signs and symptoms are largely dependent on the location of the tumour. There is a distinct predilection for the ventricular septum and left ventricular wall. This preference may underlie the presentation of cardiac fibromas with sudden and unexpected death.[89,90] Cardiac arrhythmias and atrioventricular conduction disturbances can occur. The position within the ventricular septum may also lead to compression of the cardiac chambers and, hence, may cause obstruction. Cardiomegaly is often the leading sign when the lesion is localised in the ventricular or atrial free wall. As fibromas and rhabdomyomas may have similar appearances on imaging, complete evaluation for tuberous sclerosis is warranted. In one-twentieth of cases, cardiac fibromas have been associated with the naevoid basal cell carcinoma syndrome, known as Gorlin's syndrome.[1,91] Successful surgical excision of large tumours has been reported in children of all ages, with no recurrence of disease over follow-up of several years, even if the resection was not complete.[7,24,81,88,92,93] Successful transplantation of the heart has also been reported for children with cardiac fibromas.[88,94,95]

Myxomas

Myxomas are the most common type of cardiac tumours in the overall population. They make up approximately one-quarter of all primary tumours of the heart, but their incidence is much lower in infants and children (see Table 51-1).[1,7] They may have a familial trait in perhaps one-twentieth of instances, but most cases are sporadic.[1,8,96] Patients with familial myxomas are younger at the time of diagnosis, and have associated syndromes with mucocutaneous anomalies and endocrinopathy.[7,8,96] Cardiac myxomas are usually attached to the atrial septum in the region of the oval fossa, with three-quarters originating in the left atrium.[8,96] The remaining myxomas arise from the right or left ventricular endocardium with almost equal incidence. Myxomas are multiple in about one-twentieth of cases, most often in those which are familial.

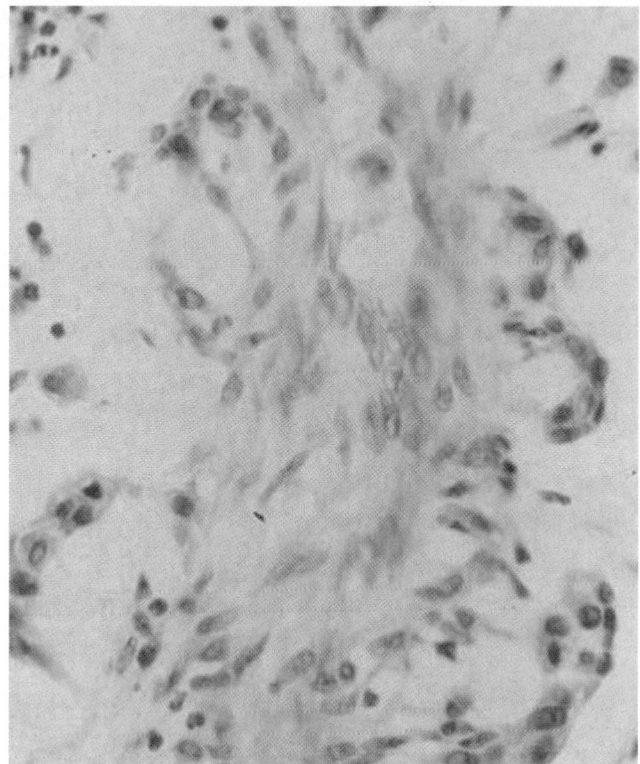

Figure 51-13 The histological section of this myxoma shows the polygonal myxoma cells embedded with a mucoid ground substance rich in glycosaminoglycans.

The tumours typically form a pedunculated mass extending into a cardiac chamber, either with a villous surface (see Fig. 51-1), or with a smooth and lobulated surface (see Fig. 51-5). The friable appearance of the villous surface (see Fig. 51-1) may easily cause detachment and embolisation of either myxomatous fragments or thrombus adherent to the surface.[11] Highly sessile atrial tumours may protrude into the atrioventricular orifice during ventricular diastole, sometimes producing valvar stenosis (see Fig. 51-4). The stalk usually contains vessels of large calibre, which can occasionally be seen on coronary angiograms. Histologically, the tumours are composed of polygonal myxoma cells, embedded within a mucoid ground substance rich in glycosaminoglycans (Fig. 51-13). The cellular make-up within the tumour is quite variable, and they often contain haemorrhagic focuses and cysts.[8] Myxomas are thought to originate from multipotential subendocardial mesenchymal cells.[1,8,96] Their content of abnormal deoxyribonucleic acid suggests a potentially neoplastic nature.[11]

The systemic, embolic, and cardiac manifestations, as previously described, may dominate the clinical profile, although most experience in this respect is based on adults rather than children. In general terms, the signs and symptoms relate directly to their site and size. In overall series, signs and symptoms of mitral valvar disease dominate the clinical presentation. Other features, such as embolic phenomenons, signs and symptoms of tricuspid valvar disease, sudden and unexpected death, pericarditis, myocardial infarction, atrial fibrillation, signs and symptoms of pulmonary valvar disease, and constitutional manifestations such as fever of undetermined origin, may also be the leading manifestation. In a proportion of patients, there are no cardiac symptoms. The tumour may then be detected as an incidental finding. In infancy, cyanosis, cardiomegaly, murmur, and hydramnios have been reported as the presenting feature.[1] Even though myxomas are considered benign, their consequences, such as embolisation or obstruction to flow, can potentially be lethal.[11] Their possible recurrence, local invasion, or extension is also suggestive of a malignant character.[96] The risk of recurrence is less than 1 in 20 for the sporadic myxomas, but 1 in 5 for the familial cases.[8,96] Removal of the tumour is the preferred therapeutic option. The stalk should also be removed completely to reduce the risk of recurrence. Follow-up evaluation for recurrence is warranted.

Teratomas

Most of the studies on primary cardiac tumours place teratomas second or third in frequency, albeit rare in children (see Table 51-1 and Fig. 51-7).[1,7] Most are extracardiac and intrapericardial. They are located at the base of the heart, usually being attached to the root of the arterial pedicle. Intracardiac teratomas do occur, but are exceptionally rare. When found, they can obstruct the ventricular outflow tracts.[28] On gross pathology, teratomas are composed of multilocular cysts separated by solid areas. Microscopically, teratomas contain, by definition, elements derived from all three germ layers of the body.

Infants with intrapericardial teratomas frequently present with tamponade and cardiovascular collapse. The teratomas may grow to bizarre dimensions, leading to impaired cardiac function with or without congestive cardiac failure, or to compression of the airways with respiratory distress. Sudden deaths, severe encroachment by the tumour on the heart and great vessels, and infectious pericarditis have all been reported.[97] The tumours most often present on imaging studies, or because of pericardial effusions when present in fetuses and neonates.[1] Cyanosis, respiratory distress, fetal hydrops, and stillbirth have also been described.[1]

Early and accurate diagnosis is of paramount importance in such critically ill patients, as surgical excision and decompression of the pericardial effusion can be achieved successfully. Furthermore, diagnosis during fetal life allows prompt postnatal, or even prenatal, intervention to the development of cardiopulmonary distress.[61–64,98] In older, asymptomatic children, surgical removal of the tumour is recommended because of the risk of sudden death, and its potential for malignant transformation.

Vascular Tumours

Vascular primary cardiac tumours, such as haemangiomas, represent a heterogeneous group, and can have various pathological characteristics.[99] Vascular tumours arising from the heart are extremely rare, having been documented in less than one-tenth of all primary cardiac tumours seen in children.[99] They occur in the atrial walls, especially of the right atrium (see Fig. 51-8), and may cause haemopericardium and tamponade.[99,100] Intracardiac haemangiomas may also occur.[101] Clinical presentation may be diverse, ranging from no manifestations, or an asymptomatic murmur, to cardiomegaly with pericardial effusions and congestive cardiac failure. When diagnosed after infancy, they rarely present with symptoms.[99]

Gross inspection will usually readily identify the true nature of the lesion. On histology, various vascular lesions can be found, with the most common described as capillary and cavernous types.[1,7] Cardiac vascular tumours are most often diagnosed by echocardiography, but magnetic resonance imaging may provide better tissue characterisation.[101,102] Those presenting in infancy may regress spontaneously, or with anti-angiogenic therapy such as corticosteroids or interferon-alpha.[99] This is not the case in older children. Symptomatic tumours of this type seen in older children should be resected, and do not then seem to recur.[99]

Tumours of the Atrioventricular Node

Cystic tumours of the atrioventricular node, also called mesotheliomas of the atrioventricular node, are exceedingly rare. They are the smallest tumours associated with sudden death, and most of the cases are diagnosed at autopsy.[3] Immunocytochemical studies have demonstrated an epithelial pattern of differentiation, suggesting that the term mesothelioma is incorrect. The cyst wall is covered by a single layer of cuboidal epithelioid cells, and is composed of fibrous connective tissue showing focuses of chronic inflammation. Within the fibrous tissue are smaller cysts lined by similar cuboidal cells, which contain hyaline eosinophilic material.[3,103-105] The majority of patients have partial or complete atrioventricular block, and often die either of complete heart block or of ventricular fibrillation. Cystic tumours of the atrioventricular node have been described as occurring at almost any age, from newborn to 86 years, with a mean age at presentation of 38 years and a ratio of females to males of 3 to 1.[3,103] The tumours, although small, can be detected by echocardiography or magnetic resonance imaging.[103,105] In symptomatic patients with heart block, a pacemaker can be implanted, albeit that pacing has not always prevented death.[103] Indeed, it is not always well tolerated, and ventricular fibrillation may ensue.[105] For these reasons, cystic tumours of the atrioventricular node have recently been surgically excised with success.[103,105]

Purkinje Cell Tumours

These tumours are known under a variety of terms, including oncocytic cardiomyopathy, histiocytoid cardiomyopathy, foamy myocardial transformation, infantile xanthomatous cardiomyopathy, and focal lipid cardiomyopathy.[1,7] They are rare, and to date, less than 100 cases have been described.[1] Most cases were reported in infants under 2 years old, with more than three-quarters found in females.[106] They are associated with tachyarrhythmias, and may give rise to incessant ventricular tachycardia or sudden death. The aetiology remains controversial. It has been proposed that they might arise from a disorder of mitochondrial metabolism. Also, because of the association between histiocytoid cardiomyopathy and an X-linked chromosomal disorder, including microphthalmia with linear skin defect, an abnormality in the p22 region of the X chromosome has been suggested.[106]

Pathological examination of the tumour is characterised by the presence of subendocardial nodules that may be discrete or diffuse throughout the ventricles, with increased weight of the heart.[107] The tumours involve most frequently the conduction system and the left ventricle. Histopathology reveals clusters of vacuolated histiocytoid-like cells with decreased bundles of myofibril.[1,106,107] Ultrastructurally, the cells contain an increased number of mitochondrions.

The most common clinical presentation is with arrhythmia and sudden death.[1,108] Ventricular fibrillation, ventricular tachycardia, Wolff-Parkinson-White syndrome, premature ventricular beats, supraventricular tachycardia, and heart block have all been described.[1,107] Involvement of other organs has been reported. Extracardiac and cardiac malformations, such as ventricular and atrial septal defects, endocardial fibroelastosis, and hypoplastic left heart syndrome, have also been described.[106]

Diagnosis may be difficult, but should be suspected in female infants with tachyarrhythmias, especially if echocardiography reveals nodular deposits on the ventricular endocardium or valves.[1] Accurate examination of the cardiac conduction system is paramount to find the mechanisms responsible for sudden cardiac death in infancy.[1,108] Without treatment, the tumours usually result in death by the age of 2 years.[1,106] When the tumour is resectable, surgical excision has been performed with success.[1,106]

Primary Malignant Tumours

Primary malignant tumours of the heart are extremely rare in infancy and childhood (see Table 51-1). Rhabdomyosarcoma is the leading type.[1] They are characterised clinically by a rapidly downhill course, with death occurring shortly following the onset of symptoms. This is caused by the rapid growth of the tumour, systemic dissemination, and unfavourable response to medical or surgical treatment.[1,24] The tumours have a tendency to invade the myocardium, and to extend within the cardiac chambers. They are difficult to excise completely.[109] Metastasis to the lungs, thymus, and regional lymph nodes can occur.[1] Early, aggressive surgical excision, most often in conjunction with adjunctive chemotherapy and radiation therapy, might result in longer survival in some patients.[1,24,95] This approach, nonetheless, remains palliative because malignant tumours are almost invariably fatal.[1,24] Cardiac transplantation has been performed in a limited number of patients with inconsistent results.[95,110]

Secondary Cardiac Tumours

These are also very rare in children, but are more frequent than the primary type. The clinical picture is nearly always dominated by the underlying disease, albeit that occasionally the cardiac symptoms constitute the basis for the presenting complaints. Cardiac involvement occurs secondary to either direct extension, haematogenous or lymphatic spread, or via extension from the inferior caval vein.[3] Lymphoma is the most common underlying disease in children, followed by Wilms' tumour. Other solid neoplasms, such as malignant hepatic tumour, may also metastasise or grow into the heart.[111,112] The symptoms produced by the metastatic lesions depend on the site and extent of the tumour. Pericardial involvement may give rise to pericardial effusion, which is often blood stained. Cardiac compression may be caused by either an effusion or a solid tumour encasing the heart. Post-operative outcome in patients with secondary cardiac tumours is poor. Surgery should, thus, be reserved for cases with haemodynamic compromise.[111]

SURGICAL THERAPY

The planning of surgical treatment must be based on the accurate assessment of the number, location, size, and extent of the tumour or tumours, on the haemodynamic state of the patient, and on the histological nature of the lesion. Cross sectional echocardiography provides most of this information. Although endomyocardial biopsy has been promoted as a means of histological diagnosis, in most cases the histological nature of the tumour may be predicted accurately from the non-invasive investigations. In infants, multiple nodules nearly always point to a rhabdomyoma, by far the most common tumour of the heart seen in children. The presence of tuberous sclerosis in the infant, or in the family, confirms the diagnosis. A large and well-circumscribed tumour in the septum or ventricular wall is likely to be a fibroma or an intracardiac teratoma.

Because of evolutions in cardiac surgery, complete resection of virtually all primary cardiac tumours is now possible.[24] As a result, the prognosis of children with primary cardiac tumours improved significantly in recent decades. Surgical resection is indicated in all symptomatic patients, in those with significant obstruction of either the ventricular inlet or outlet, or in the setting of life-threatening arrhythmias.[81] Single lesions amenable to surgical resection, especially fibromas, should be considered for removal because of the possibility of arrhythmias, and even sudden cardiac death. If feasible, the aim must be complete resection, but in some series, even incomplete resection of benign tumour has led to good results without recurrence.[24,113] In the setting of myxomas, surgery should be undertaken urgently because of the potential for catastrophic embolisation. Careful examination of the entire heart is necessary to remove concurrent sites of myxomatous tissue. Partial resection for relief of obstruction and amelioration of an increase in chamber size may be indicated when there are significant haemodynamic alterations. Incomplete removal may result later in arrhythmias, and the potential for sudden death will remain. In the presence of multiple lesions, or if there is extensive myocardial involvement, and in the absence of symptoms, surgery is better postponed. Since most rhabdomyomas undergo spontaneous regression, surgical intervention is no longer indicated unless there are significant clinical manifestations.[1,7,24]

OTHER TREATMENTS

When the anatomical location of the tumour precludes curative resection, cardiac transplantation may be considered if there is obstruction to the flow of blood or severe arrhythmias.[95] This option should be considered on a case-by-case basis because of the limited experience to date.[95] Vascular tumours in infants may be treated with anti-angiogenic therapy, such as corticosteroids or interferon-alpha.[99] Very little data is available on chemotherapy or radiation in children with cardiac sarcomas. These therapies, in general, do not appear efficacious.[1,24]

ACKNOWLEDGEMENTS

We thank Drs Julene Carvalho and Raad Mohiaddin, from Royal Brompton Hospital, and Dr Jan Marek, from Great Ormond Street Hospital, for their contribution with illustrations. Dr Bédard has received financial support from the Cardiology Institute of Quebec, Laval University, and the Cardiologists Association of the province of Quebec. Professor Gatzoulis and the Royal Brompton Adult Congenital Heart Center receive support from the British Heart Foundation.

The complete reference list can be found on the companion Expert Consult web site at www.expertconsult.com.

ANNOTATED REFERENCES

- Isaacs H, Jr: Fetal and neonatal cardiac tumors. Pediatr Cardiol 2004;25: 252–273.

  This excellent review discusses the clinical features, findings at imaging, pathology, prognosis, and treatment of fetuses and neonates with cardiac tumours.

- Butany J, Nair V, Naseemuddin A, et al: Cardiac tumours: Diagnosis and management. Lancet Oncol 2005;6:219–228.

  This review addresses the clinical findings, pathology, investigation, and management of patients with benign and malignant cardiac tumours. It provides a good overview of the most common cardiac tumours in the general population, both adult and paediatric.

- Becker AE: Primary heart tumors in the pediatric age group: A review of salient pathologic features relevant for clinicians. Pediatr Cardiol 2000;21:317–323.

  This review summarises the most relevant clinical and pathological information about the commonest primary tumours of the heart found in infants and children.

- Takach TJ, Reul GJ, Ott DA, Cooley DA: Primary cardiac tumors in infants and children: Immediate and long-term operative results. Ann Thorac Surg 1996;62:559–564.

  This important series from a single institution describes 38 surgically excised cardiac tumours in infants and children, and provides immediate and long-term results.

- Verhaaren HA, Vanakker O, De Wolf D, et al: Left ventricular outflow obstruction in rhabdomyoma of infancy: Meta-analysis of the literature. J Pediatr 2003;143:258–263.

  This meta-analysis of 409 published cases of rhabdomyoma reports the symptoms at presentation, the characteristics of the tumour, and mortality.

- Peters PJ, Reinhardt S: The echocardiographic evaluation of intracardiac masses: A review. J Am Soc Echocardiogr 2006;19:230–240.

  This is an excellent review highlighting the role of echocardiography for evaluation of cardiac masses, and focussing on primary and metastatic tumours of the heart.

- Mehmood F, Nanda NC, Vengala S, et al. Live three-dimensional transthoracic echocardiographic assessment of left atrial tumors. Echocardiography 2005;22:137–143.

  This study suggests that live three-dimensional transthoracic echocardiography is better than cross sectional transthoracic echocardiography in assessing the content of an intracardiac tumour.

- Sparrow PJ, Kurian JB, Jones TR, Sivananthan MU: MR imaging of cardiac tumors. Radiographics 2005;25:1255–1276.

  The review discusses the advantages of magnetic resonance imaging for assessment of cardiac tumours, summarising the technique, and describing the expected findings for the most common cardiac tumours.

- Burke AP, Rosado-de-Christenson M, Templeton PA, Virmani R: Cardiac fibroma: Clinicopathologic correlates and surgical treatment. J Thorac Cardiovasc Surg 1994;108:862–870.

  This review of a large series of patients with cardiac fibroma describes the clinical and pathological findings.

- Reynen K: Cardiac myxomas. N Engl J Med 1995;333:1610–1617.

  This review addresses the epidemiology, pathological findings, clinical features, diagnostic tests, and treatment of patients with cardiac myxomas.

CHAPTER 52

Kawasaki Disease

JANE NEWBURGER

Kawasaki disease was first described in 1967, by a Japanese paediatrician, Tomisako Kawasaki.[1] He characterised the illness, then termed mucutaneous lymph node syndrome, as including high fever, non-exudative conjunctivitis, inflammation of the oral mucosa, rash, cervical adenopathy, and findings in the limbs, including swollen hands and feet, red palms and soles, and, later, subungual peeling. At the time, the disease was thought to be self-limited, without long-term consequences. Later, Kawasaki disease was shown to cause coronary arterial aneurysms, which may cause complications of angina, myocardial infarction, and sudden death. Although the disease continues to have the highest relative risk in children of Japanese ancestry, it has been described worldwide in children of all races and ethnicities. In the United States of America, where more than 4000 children with Kawasaki disease are hospitalised annually,[2] Kawasaki disease has surpassed rheumatic fever as a cause of acquired cardiac disease in children. In this chapter, I will summarise current knowledge about the aetiology and pathogenesis, diagnosis, treatment in the acute phase, and natural history of Kawasaki disease.

EPIDEMIOLOGY

The incidence of Kawasaki disease differs according to race and ethnicity. In Japan, Kawasaki disease has an incidence of approximately 138 cases for each 100,000 children under the age of 5 years.[3] In the United States of America, Kawasaki disease has been reported to be most common among Asians and Pacific Islanders, with an incidence of 32.5 cases for each 100,000 children under the age of 5 years, intermediate in non-Hispanic African Americans, where the number is 16.9, and Hispanics, at 11.1 cases, and lowest in Caucasians, with 9.1 cases in each 100,000 children under the age of 5 years.[2] Previous smaller state-based studies suggested similar prevalence according to race.[4,5]

Kawasaki disease is most common in children younger than age 5 years, but one-quarter of cases in the United States of America occur in older children.[2] Young infants have the highest rate of formation of coronary arterial aneurysms, and often present with incomplete features. Children older than age 8 years also have a higher rate of coronary arterial involvement.[6–9] In contrast to young infants, older children generally present with typical findings, but suffer an increased incidence of coronary arterial aneurysms, in part because of delayed diagnosis by physicians, who mistakenly believe that Kawasaki disease only occurs in very young children. Males are affected more than females by a ratio of approximately 1.5 to 1, and the illness is most common during the winter and early spring months.[2,10] Data linking Kawasaki disease to antecedent exposure to carpet cleaning, or to viral infections of the respiratory tract, have been inconsistent.[4,5,11–14] Other studies have suggested that Kawasaki disease is associated with residence near a standing body of water,[15] antecedent eczema,[16] and use of humidifiers.[14]

In Japan, the rate of recurrence of the disease is approximately 3%,[17] and the proportion of cases with a positive family history is approximately 1%.[17,18] Siblings have a relative risk that is 10-fold that of the normal Japanese population, with half developing the disease within 10 days of the first case.[19] The risk of occurrence in twins may be as much as 100-fold higher than in the general population.[19,20] Parents of Japanese children with Kawasaki disease, compared to the general population, have a two-fold higher risk of having had Kawasaki disease themselves in childhood.[19–22] Of note, in the United States, the familial incidence of Kawasaki disease is believed to be far lower than in Japan.

Coronary arterial disease is responsible for almost all deaths in patients with Kawasaki disease.[23] The case fatality rate is 0.08% in Japan.[17] In the United States, reported in-hospital mortality for Kawasaki disease has varied from 0% to 0.17%.[2,24] Although the highest risk of myocardial infarction and death occurs in the first months after illness onset,[25] sudden death from ischaemic heart disease may occur many years later in patients with coronary arterial aneurysms and stenoses.[26]

AETIOLOGY AND PATHOGENESIS

The cause of Kawasaki disease remains unknown, despite decades of investigation and spirited controversy. For many reasons, an infectious cause or trigger seems most likely. The illness is self-limited, and usually non-recurring. Its clinical signs and symptoms overlap with those in known toxin-mediated or viral infections. Its predilection for young children, with rare occurrence in neonates and adults, suggest that immunity is acquired. An infectious agent is further suggested by winter-spring seasonality, outbreaks in the community, and occasional epidemics. Person-to-person transmission does not occur, but infection with a common agent could produce asymptomatic disease in most children, and recognisable signs and symptoms of the disease in a tiny subset of susceptible individuals. It has not been linked to exposure to drugs or to environmental pollutants.

A number of investigations, including reports of selective expansion of Vβ 2 and Vβ 8 T-cell receptor families in the acute stage of the disease, have suggested that the illness may be caused by bacterial superantigens.[27–30]

The prevalence of toxin-producing strains was similar, nonetheless, in patients with the disease and febrile controls in a prospective, multi-centre study.[31] Other investigations have suggested that the immune response in the disease is evoked by a conventional antigen.[32–34] Recently, a cytoplasmic antigen, bound by a synthetic IgA antibody, has been observed in the proximal bronchial epithelium and coronary arteries of the majority of postmortem specimens from children with the disease, but not in postmortem control patients. The nature of the antigen is as yet undetermined.[35] The data suggests that the disease may be caused by a respiratory infectious agent with tropism for vascular tissue.[35] It is also possible that it may be triggered by more than one microbial agent in a susceptible host.

The importance of genetic factors in susceptibility is supported by the influence of race and family history on its incidence (see Epidemiology above). In addition, an increasing literature has explored the association of genetic polymorphisms to susceptibility to the disease, or to development of aneurysms.[22,36–45]

The pathogenesis includes marked immune activation, with release of pro-inflammatory cytokines and growth factors, activation of endothelial cells, and infiltration of coronary arteries and other medium-sized extraparenchymal arteries by CD68+ monocyte/macrophages, CD8+ cytotoxic lymphocytes, and oligoclonal IgA plasma cells.[33,46–55] The integrity of the arterial wall may be disrupted by infiltration of macrophages and release of matrix metalloproteinases.[56]

PATHOLOGY

Mortality peaks between 15 and 45 days after onset of fever, when patients are in a hypercoagulable state and have thrombocytosis and disrupted vascular endothelium.[57] Mortality declines significantly beyond the first year after the onset of the illness. Because of progressive coronary arterial stenosis, however, myocardial infarction may occur many years later. An increasing literature has shown that when diagnosis is not made in childhood, the disease can cause myocardial infarction in young adults.[58]

Because few patients die in the acute phase of the disease in the current era, much of our knowledge about its pathology derives from early studies in Japan.[23,59] In the first 9 days of illness, findings include acute perivasculitis and vasculitis of the microvessels and small arteries, as well as acute perivasculitis and endarteritis of the three major coronary arteries, with influx of neutrophils. Inflammation in the pericardium, myocardium, atrioventricular conduction system, and endocardium are also present. Deaths in this early period are caused by myocarditis and abnormalities of conduction. In the second through fourth weeks of the disease, the coronary arteries are affected by panvasculitis, and aneurysms form, with coronary arterial thrombosis. The cells infiltrating the arterial wall range from neutrophils to large mononuclear cells, and include lymphocytes and plasma cells. At this stage, the internal elastic lamina shows segmental destruction. Pericarditis, myocarditis, inflammation of the atrioventricular conduction system, and endocarditis with valvitis, continue to be present. Mortality in these weeks is most likely to be secondary to ischaemic heart disease, rupture of aneurysms, and myocarditis, including lesions of the conduction system. After 1 month, active inflammation begins to be replaced by progressive neointimal proliferation, neoangiogenesis, and fibrosis with formation of scars. Late deaths are characterised by severe coronary arterial stenosis.

Aneurysms produced by the disease occur in locations that are similar to those of atherosclerotic lesions, that is, in the proximal segments and branches of the coronary arteries, suggesting a role for shear stress in both types of coronary lesions. In addition, growth factors are prominently expressed at the inlets and outlets of the aneurysms, these also being sites of high shear stress.[60] Aneurysms can occur in medium-sized extraparenchymal arteries other than the coronary arteries. In particular, the coeliac, mesenteric, femoral, iliac, renal, axillary, and brachial arteries can be affected.[59] Peripheral arterial aneurysms, however, never occur in the absence of aneurysms involving the coronary arteries.

CLINICAL DIAGNOSIS

General Aspects of Initial Diagnosis

Diagnostic criterions are summarised in Table 52-1.[61] The epidemiologic definition for diagnosis includes fever for 4 days with at least four principal clinical criterions, or fever and fewer than four principal criterions in the presence of coronary arterial abnormalities. By convention, the first day of the disease is considered to be the day on which the fever initially occurs. All clinical features are rarely present at the same time, so the diagnosis requires sequential evaluation of the patient. In the absence of treatment, the mean duration of fever is 11 days, and fever rarely persists beyond 4 weeks. The principal clinical findings are not pathognomonic, so other diseases with similar clinical features should be excluded (Table 52-2).

A diagnosis of incomplete disease may be made in patients who do not fulfill the classic criterions outlined in Table 52-1, whereas the term atypical disease refers to patients who have features not generally seen, for example those presenting with haemophagocytic syndrome, or renal failure. Because coronary arterial disease is now well recognised to occur in children with incomplete or atypical features, and treatment with immunoglobulins must be started early to be effective, a new algorithm for evaluation and treatment of the child with suspected disease was recently developed (Fig. 52-1).[62] The diagnosis may be based upon abnormalities of the coronary arteries by echocardiography when the classic epidemiologic definition is not fulfilled. Because young infants are most likely to have incomplete criterions, and also have the highest risk of aneurysms, echocardiography is recommended for infants less than age 6 months with a fever lasting for 7 or more days without other explanation, in whom there is elevation of either C-reactive protein or the rate of erythrocytic sedimentation.

Laboratory features are reflective of an acute inflammatory response. Virtually all patients at presentation have elevation of the rate of erythrocytic sedimentation or C-reactive protein.[63] The average level of haemoglobin at the time of presentation is two standard deviations below the mean for age, with the anaemia being normocytic and normochromic. The number of white blood cells is generally increased, at a median of 15,000/mm^3, with a leftward shift. The platelet count is usually normal in the

TABLE 52-1

CLINICAL AND LABORATORY FEATURES OF KAWASAKI DISEASE

Epidemiologic Case Definition (Classic Clinical Criterions)
Fever of at least 5 days' duration
Presence of at least four of the following principal features:
Changes in extremities
Polymorphous exanthem
Bilateral conjunctival injection
Changes in the lips and oral cavity
Cervical lymphadenopathy
Exclusion of other diseases with similar findings (see Table 52-2)
Other Clinical and Laboratory Findings
Cardiovascular findings
Congestive heart failure, myocarditis, pericarditis, or valvular regurgitation.
Coronary artery abnormalities
Aneurysms of medium-sized non-coronary arteries
Raynaud's phenomenon
Peripheral gangrene
Musculoskeletal system
Arthritis, arthralgia
Gastrointestinal tract
Diarrhea, vomiting, abdominal pain
Hepatic dysfunction
Hydrops of the gallbladder
Respiratory tract
Pulmonary nodules and interstitial infiltrates
Pleural effusion
Central nervous system
Extreme irritability
Aseptic meningitis
Peripheral facial nerve palsy
Sensorineuronal hearing loss
Genitourinary system
Urethritis/meatitis
Testicular swelling
Other findings
Erythema and induration at Bacille Calmette-Guerin (BCG) inoculation site
Anterior uveitis
Desquamating rash in groin
Laboratory Findings in Acute Kawasaki Disease
Neutrophilia with immature forms
Elevated erythrocyte sedimentation rate
Elevated C-reactive protein
Elevated serum α-l-antitrypsin
Anemia
Hypoalbuminaemia
Thrombocytosis after first week
Sterile pyuria
Elevated serum transaminases
Pleocytosis of CSF
Leukcocytosis in synovial fluid

Reprinted with permission from Newburger JW, Takahashi M, Gerber MA, et al: Diagnosis, treatment, and long-term management of Kawasaki disease: A statement for health professionals from the Committee on Rheumatic Fever, Endocarditis and Kawasaki Disease, Council on Cardiovascular Disease in the Young, American Heart Association. Circulation 2004;110:2747–2771.

first week of the illness, peaking in the third week of the illness to values sometimes higher than 1,000,000/mm^3. After the seventh day of illness, counts are usually at least 450,000/mm^3. Plasma gammaglutamyl transpeptidase, transaminases, and bilirubin, are frequently elevated.[64,65]

TABLE 52-2

DIFFERENTIAL DIAGNOSIS OF KAWASAKI DISEASE

Viral infections including measles and adenovirus
Scarlet fever
Staphylococcal scalded skin syndrome?
Toxic shock syndrome
Bacterial cervical lymphadenitis
Drug hypersensitivity reactions
Stevens-Johnson syndrome
Juvenile rheumatoid arthritis
Rocky Mountain spotted fever
Leptospirosis
Mercury hypersensitivity reaction (acrodynia)

Reprinted with permission from Newburger JW, Takahashi M, Gerber MA, et al: Diagnosis, treatment, and long-term management of Kawasaki disease: A statement for health professionals from the Committee on Rheumatic Fever, Endocarditis and Kawasaki Disease, Council on Cardiovascular Disease in the Young, American Heart Association. Circulation 2004;110:2747–2771.

Synthesis of albumin is decreased in the acute phase, and hypoalbuminaemia is common. Microscopic evaluation of the urine may reveal an elevated count of white blood cells with no identified infectious agent, so-called sterile pyuria. Cerebrospinal fluid contains an increased number of white blood cells, predominantly mononuclear cells, with normal levels of glucose and protein.[66] Serum cardiac troponin[67–69] and brain natriuretic factor[70] may also be elevated in the acute phase of the disease.

Cardiac Findings

The acute phase of the disease may be associated with myocarditis, pericarditis, valvitis, and inflammation in the coronary arterial wall. Cardiac auscultation typically reveals a hyperdynamic praecordium, tachycardia, and a gallop rhythm, even in the absence of fever. Almost all children have an innocent flow murmur related to anaemia and fever. In addition, some children with significant mitral regurgitation have a pansystolic regurgitant murmur at the apex. The disease may occasionally present with low cardiac output syndrome or shock. Electrocardiography may show arrhythmia, prolonged PR interval, or nonspecific ST and T wave changes.

At the time of acute presentation, the maximal z scores for the coronary arteries normalised to body surface area are greater than in the general afebrile population. A maximal z score for the proximal segments of the right or anterior interventricular arteries is at least 2.5 in approximately one-quarter of patients.[71] Coronary arterial dimensions then diminish in the majority of patients treated with immunoglobulins within the first 10 days of illness.

Coronary arterial aneurysms are the most serious long-term complications of the disease. Approximately one in five children who are not treated with high doses of immune globulin given intravenously within the first 10 days of illness develops coronary arterial ectasia or aneurysms. The aneurysms may be detected by echocardiography beginning 7 days after the first appearance of fever, with their diameter usually peaking around 4 weeks after onset of the illness. Independent predictors of development have included age less than 1 year, male gender, delayed treatment with immunoglobulins, persistent or

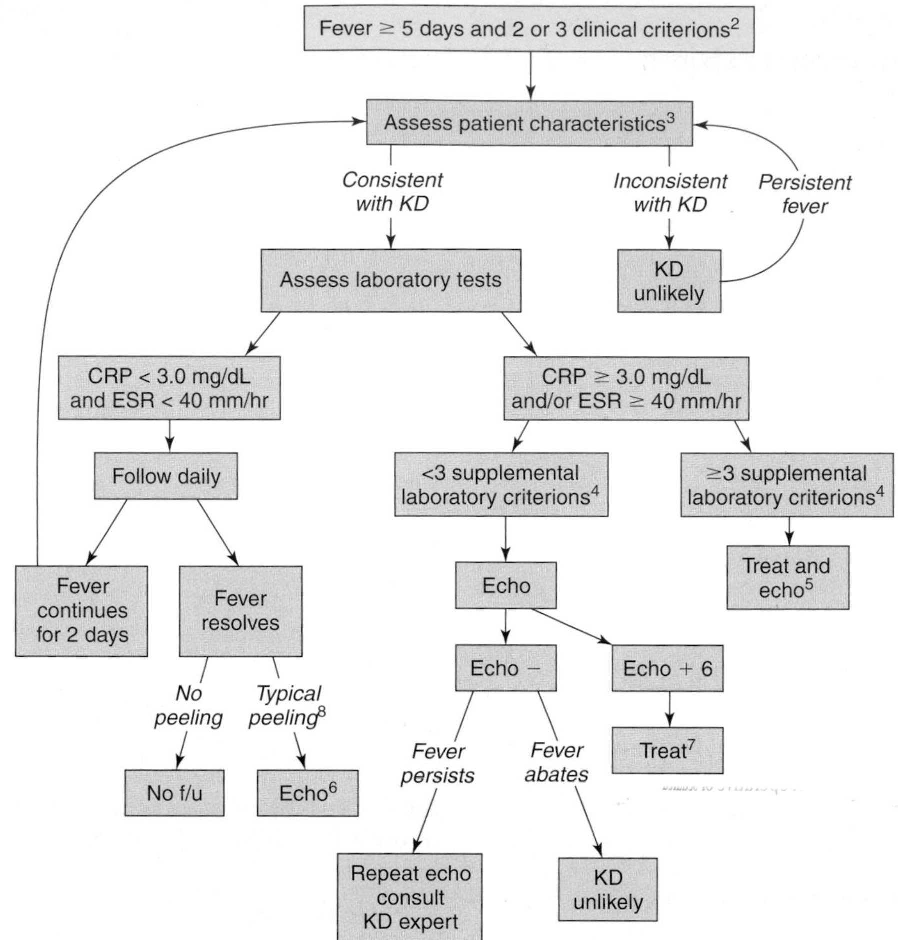

Figure 52-1 Evaluation of suspected incomplete Kawasaki disease (KD). The numbers 2 to 8 in the figure refer to the issues highlighted in the legend. (1) In the absence of gold standard for diagnosis, this algorithm cannot be evidence-based but rather represents the informed opinion of the expert committee. Consultation with an expert should be sought anytime assistance is needed. (2) Infants younger than 6 months old on the seventh day of fever without other explanation should undergo laboratory testing and, if evidence of systemic inflammation is found, an echocardiogram, even if the infants have no clinical criterions for diagnosis. (3) Characteristics suggesting Kawasaki disease are listed in Table 52-1. Characteristics suggesting disease other than Kawasaki disease include exudative conjunctivitis, exudative pharyngitis, discrete intraoral lesions, bullous or vesicular rash, or generalised adenopathy. Consider alternative diagnoses (see Table 52-2). (4) Supplemental laboratory criterions include levels of albumin less than 3.0 g/dL, anaemia for age, elevation of alanine aminotransferase, more than 450,000 platelets per mm^3 after the seventh day, a white blood cell count of greater than 15,000/mm^3, and more than 10 white blood cells per high-power field in the urine. (5) Can treat before performing echocardiogram. (6) Echocardiogram is considered positive for purposes of this algorithm if any of three conditions are met: *z* score for the anterior interventricular or right coronary artery of greater than 2.5, coronary arteries meet Japanese Ministry of Health criterions for aneurysms, or there are more than three other suggestive features, including perivascular brightness, lack of tapering, decreased left ventricular function, mitral regurgitation, pericardial effusion, or *z* scores for the anterior interventricular and right coronary arteries between 2 and 2.5. (7) If the echocardiogram is positive, treatment should be given to children within 10 days of the onset of fever, and those beyond the tenth day with clinical and laboratory signs of ongoing inflammation. (8) Typical peeling begins under nail bed of fingers and then toes. CRP, C-reactive protein; FSR, erythrocyte sedimentation rate; f/u, follow-up. (Reprinted with permission from Newburger JW, Takahashi M, Gerber MA, et al: Diagnosis, treatment, and long-term management of Kawasaki disease: A statement for health professionals from the Committee on Rheumatic Fever, Endocarditis and Kawasaki Disease, Council on Cardiovascular Disease in the Young, American Heart Association. Circulation 2004;110:2747–2771.)

recrudescent fever after immunoglobulins, so-called immunoglobulin resistance, and laboratory measures suggesting worse inflammation.[71–77] Asian/Pacific Islander race and Hispanic ethnicity are also risk factors.[78] Sociodemographic factors appear to play an important role in delayed diagnosis.[79]

Aneurysms are considered to be saccular when their axial and lateral diameters are nearly equal. Fusiform aneurysms occur when there is symmetric dilation, with gradual proximal and distal tapering. Coronary arteries are considered to be ectatic when the dimension is dilated without a segmental aneurysm. Aneurysms are classified as giant when the internal diameter is at least 8 mm.[61,80]

Depression of myocardial function is common in the acute phase of the disease. Endomyocardial biopsies have suggested that myocarditis is a universal feature of Kawasaki disease, and myocardial inflammation is present in from half to three-quarters of patients based upon nuclear imaging. Fortunately, myocardial function usually improves rapidly after administration of intravenous immune globulin, and long-term, clinically significant abnormalities of systolic function are uncommon in the absence of ischaemic heart disease secondary to coronary arterial aneurysms.

In the acute phase, mitral regurgitation may result from valvitis, or from transient dysfunction of the papillary muscles. More than one-quarter of children have mitral regurgitation at the time of presentation.[81] Late mitral regurgitation is usually the result of ischaemic disease. Aortic regurgitation, presumably secondary to valvitis, is infrequently detected by echocardiography in the acute phase.[81] Only rare instances of late mitral regurgitation unrelated to ischaemia or late aortic regurgitation of clinical significance have been reported.[82–84]

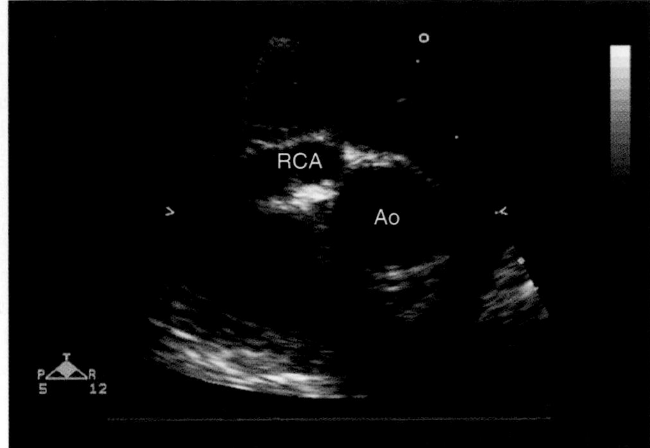

Figure 52-2 The cross sectional echocardiogram shows a giant aneurysm of the right coronary artery (RCA). Ao, aorta.

Echocardiography

Echocardiographic imaging of the coronary arteries is essential in the evaluation of all patients with definite or suspected disease (Fig. 52-2). Its sensitivity and specificity for the detection of dilation of the proximal coronary arterial segments are high when performed with appropriate transducers by experienced sonographers in cooperative or sedated children. Because aneurysms also occur in the absence of the classic criterions, echocardiography has an important role in evaluation of children with protracted fever and some findings consistent with features of Kawasaki disease. Additional echocardiographic features in the acute phase include coronary arterial ectasia, lack of tapering, and perivascular brightness. Left ventricular contractility may also be diminished, and mild valvar regurgitation, particularly mitral regurgitation, is relatively common. [81] Although pericardial effusions may occur, they are infrequently significant in size.[81]

Echocardiography should be performed shortly after diagnosis to provide a baseline examination of coronary dimensions, left ventricular function, valvular regurgitation, and pericardial effusion. In children whose fever resolves after initial treatment with intravenous immune globulin, and who remain afebrile, echocardiography should be repeated at 2 weeks, and again at approximately 6 to 8 weeks after onset of the illness. Children at higher risk, that is those with recrudescent fever, baseline coronary arterial abnormalities, diminished left ventricular function, or pericardial effusion, should undergo more frequent echocardiographic evaluation to guide the need for additional therapies.

Cross sectional echocardiographic imaging should be performed with the transducer of the highest frequency available, and recorded in a dynamic video or digital cine format. The imaging planes and transducer positions required for optimal visualisation of the coronary arterial segments are depicted in Table 52-3. Whenever possible, all major coronary arterial segments should be visualised. The most common site for formation of aneurysms are the proximal segments of the anterior interventricular and right coronary arteries, followed in descending order by the main stem of the left coronary artery, the circumflex artery and the distal part of the right coronary artery, and the junction between the right coronary artery and inferior interventricular artery. Measurements are made from inner edge to inner edge, excluding points of branching.

TABLE 52-3

ECHOCARDIOGRAPHIC VIEWS OF CORONARY ARTERIES IN PATIENTS WITH KAWASAKI DISEASE

- Left main coronary artery: Praecordial short-axis at level of aortic valve; precordial long-axis of left ventricle (superior tangential); subcostal left ventricular long-axis
- Left anterior descending coronary artery: Praecordial short-axis at level of aortic valve; precordial superior tangential long-axis of left ventricle; precordial short-axis of left ventricle
- Left circumflex: Praecordial short-axis at level of aortic valve; apical four-chamber
- Right coronary artery, proximal segment: Praecordial short-axis at level of aortic valve; precordial long-axis (inferior tangential) of left ventricle; subcostal coronal projection of right ventricular outflow tract; subcostal short-axis at level of atrioventricular groove
- Right coronary artery, middle segment: Praecordial long-axis of left ventricle (inferior tangential); apical four-chamber; subcostal left ventricular long-axis; subcostal short-axis at level of atrioventricular groove
- Right coronary artery, distal segment: Apical four-chamber (inferior); subcostal atrial long-axis (inferior)
- Posterior descending coronary artery: Apical four-chamber (inferior); subcostal atrial long-axis (inferior)

Reprinted with permission from Newburger JW, Takahashi M, Gerber MA, et al: Diagnosis, treatment, and long-term management of Kawasaki disease: A statement for health professionals from the Committee on Rheumatic Fever, Endocarditis and Kawasaki Disease, Council on Cardiovascular Disease in the Young, American Heart Association. Circulation 2004;110:2747–2771.

Statistics about the prevalence of aneurysms are based upon criterions set forth by the Japanese Ministry of Health in 1984. These classify coronary arteries as abnormal if the internal luminal diameter is greater than 3 mm in children less than 5 years of age, or 4 mm in children at least 5 years of age, if the internal diameter of a segment measures at least 1.5 times that of an adjacent segment, or if the coronary arterial lumen is clearly irregular.[85]

Because normal dimensions are related to body size, dimensions may also be expressed as units of standard deviation, or *z* scores, adjusted for body surface area (Fig. 52-3).[86] Use of such *z* scores has suggested that the criterions adopted by the Japanese Ministry of Health may result in under-diagnosis and under-estimation of the true prevalence of arterial dilation in the first weeks of the illness. Some limitations should be noted. There is no normative data for febrile patients with other diseases. *Z* scores are available only for the main stem of the left coronary artery and the proximal segments of the anterior interventricular and right coronary arteries. For this reason, the criterion of size 1.5 times that of the surrounding segment is still useful for diagnosis of aneurysms in peripheral sites. Imaging of the coronary arteries may also reveal lack of normal tapering and perivascular echogenicity or brightness, but these qualities are difficult to quantitate and verify.[87]

Stress Testing

Children with aneurysms should undergo periodic stress testing, with assessment of myocardial perfusion or function. Most methods of stress testing used in adult cardiology have been reported in small series of children with Kawasaki disease.[88–98] Because the sensitivity and specificity of tests to provoke myocardial ischaemia have been exhaustively studied in adults with coronary arterial disease, adult guidelines should be followed to choose the best test based upon specific characteristics of the patients.[99] Additional factors in the choice of

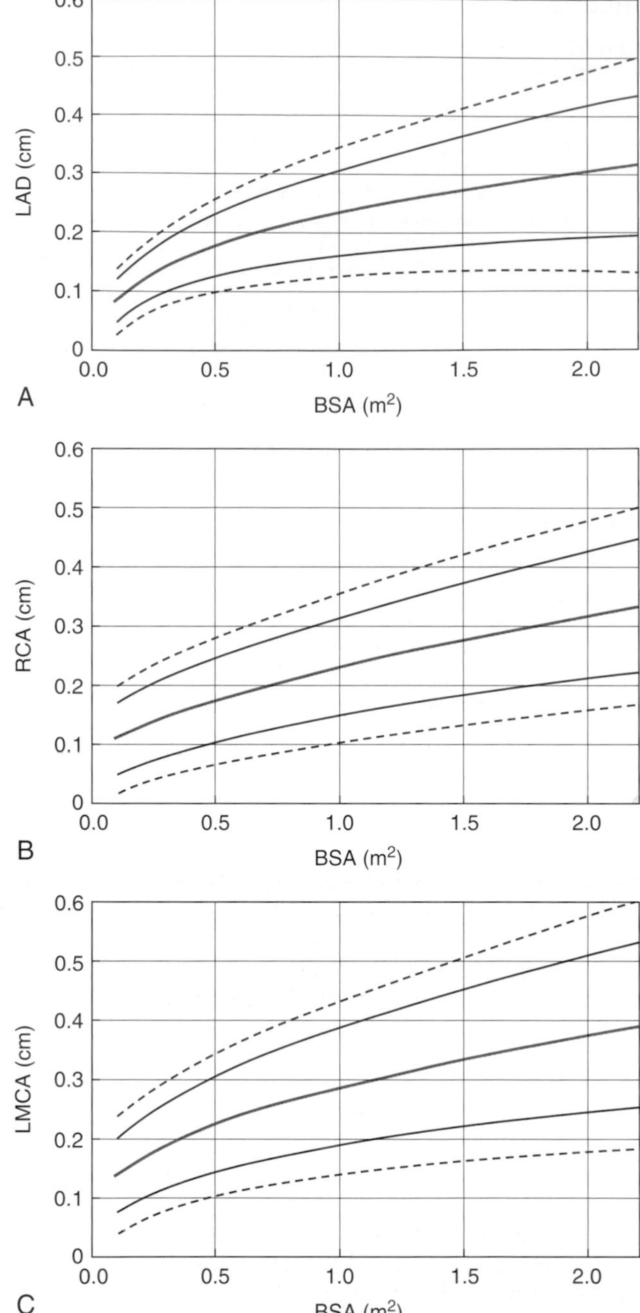

Figure 52-3 Mean and limits for prediction for 2 (*solid purple and blue lines*) and 3 (*dotted purple and blue lines*) standard deviations for the size (*red solid line*) of (**A**) the anterior interventricular artery, (**B**) the proximal right coronary artery (RCA) and (**C**) the main stem of the left coronary artery (LMCA) according to body surface area for children below the age of 18 years. *Z* scores for the main stem should not be based on the dimension at the arterial orifice nor its immediate vicinity. Enlargement of the main stem secondary to Kawasaki disease usually is associated with ectasia of the anterior interventricular or circumflex arteries, or both arteries. (Reprinted with permission from Newburger JW, Takahashi M, Gerber MA, et al: Diagnosis, treatment, and long-term management of Kawasaki disease: A statement for health professionals from the Committee on Rheumatic Fever, Endocarditis and Kawasaki Disease, Council on Cardiovascular Disease in the Young, American Heart Association. Circulation 2004;110:2747–2771.)

modality for testing include institutional expertise with particular techniques, and the age and ability of the child to cooperate with exercise. False positive tests are more likely in patients with a low prior probability of coronary arterial disease. I do not recommend performing stress tests in patients without a history of coronary arterial enlargement.

Other Noninvasive Methods for Imaging the Coronary Arteries

In selected patients, noninvasive imaging methods other than echocardiography may be needed for assessment of the coronary arterial anatomy. In particular, ultrafast computerised tomography, and magnetic resonance imaging and angiography, may provide valuable noninvasive imaging data in patients whose coronary arteries cannot adequately be imaged by echocardiography (Fig. 52-4).[100–104] In addition to imaging, cardiac resonance tests can be performed together with pharmacologic stress, and may allow assessment of myocardial infarction using delayed enhancement (Fig. 52-5).

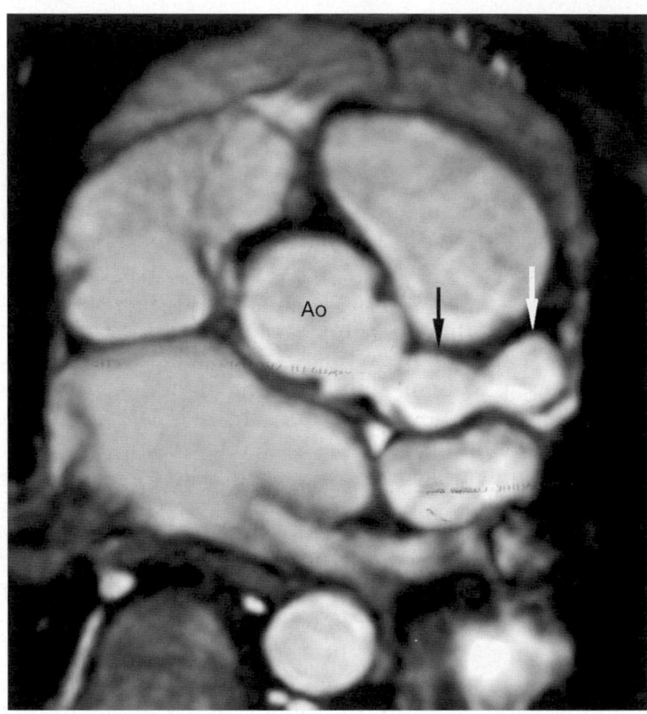

Figure 52-4 The magnetic resonance image shows a giant segmented aneurysm of the anterior interventricular artery, which arises directly from the aortic root. The segments of the aneurysm are depicted by the *arrows* Ao, aorta.

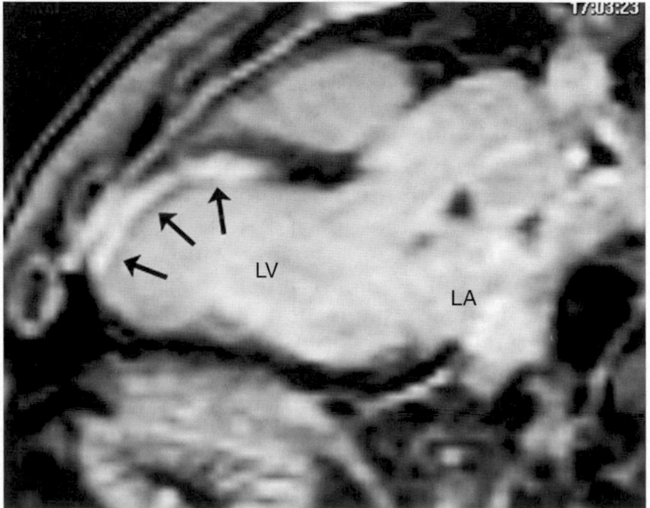

Figure 52-5 Myocardial delayed enhancement imaging shows a large area of nearly transmural hyperenhancement (*arrows*) consistent with an antero-septal myocardial infarction, becoming transmural at the apex. LA, left atrium; LV, left ventricular.

Ultrafast computerised tomography has been shown to have excellent sensitivity for detection of coronary arterial stenoses in patients with the disease.[105] Because the technique is associated with relatively high doses of ionising radiation,[106,107] this test should be reserved for use in circumstances when other non-invasive tests are inadequate for imaging.

Coronary Angiography

Cardiac catheterisation and coronary angiography provide the gold standard for imaging, against which other methods are assessed (Fig. 52-6). Indeed, almost all reports on the natural history of the disease are based upon angiographic studies. In addition to providing better delineation of the distal coronary vasculature than noninvasive tests, angiography is the most reliable method by which to assess coronary arterial stenosis or thrombotic occlusion and the presence of collateral vessels.

Because selective coronary angiography has greater risks than noninvasive imaging, its use should be restricted to selected patients with coronary arterial aneurysms, clinical signs, noninvasive studies indicating myocardial ischaemia, or those in whom noninvasive methods fail to provide adequate images. Angiography is usually performed 6 to 12 months after the onset of the illness in patients with significant aneurysms who have no signs or symptoms of ischaemic heart disease. Angiography can be helpful in guiding anti-thrombotic therapy when proximal aneurysms have regressed, but the distal parts of the coronary arteries cannot be imaged by noninvasive means. Some cardiologists follow patients who have undergone surgical revascularisation or catheter intervention by cardiac catheterisation to evaluate the efficacy of their treatment. To evaluate whether peripheral arterial aneurysms are present,[108] abdominal aortography and subclavian arteriography should be performed in patients undergoing coronary arteriography for the first time.

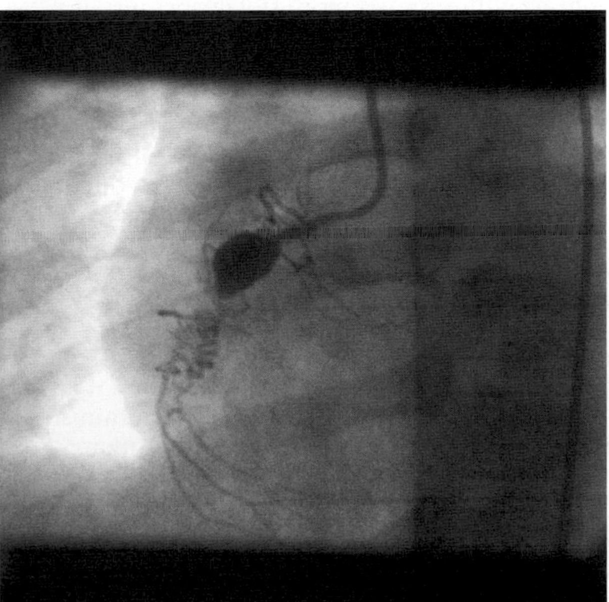

Figure 52-6 The coronary angiogram demonstrates a giant aneurysm of the right coronary artery, with obstruction and bridging collateral arteries in a 4-year-old boy.

NATURAL HISTORY

Patients with Kawasaki disease have had careful follow-up only for the past three decades. It is clear, however, that long-term outcomes are related to the extent of dilation of the coronary arteries in the first month of the illness. Aneurysms reach their peak diameter in the first 4 to 6 weeks after onset of the illness. After this time, a myointimal proliferation results in regression of approximately half to two-thirds of aneurysmal segments.[83,109] The likelihood of regression is primarily determined by the peak luminal diameter, with larger aneurysms being less likely to regress.[110,111] Other factors that predict greater likelihood of regression are younger age, distal location, and fusiform shape.[109] Aneurysms that persist may develop significant stenoses secondary to myointimal proliferation at either end of the aneurysm, calcification, tortuosity, or thrombotic occlusion. Rupture of an aneurysm is rare, and generally occurs early after onset rather than as a late complication.

In patients with persistent aneurysms, the prevalence of coronary arterial stenosis increases over time,[83,108,112] with the highest incidence occurring in patients with giant aneurysms.[112] The principal cause of death is myocardial infarction produced by thrombotic occlusion in a coronary arterial segment with an aneurysm and/or stenosis.[25] The highest risk of myocardial infarction occurs in patients with giant aneurysms, related to sluggish flow in a huge vascular space, often in combination with stenosis at its distal end. Although myocardial infarction occurs most frequently in the first year after onset, patients with aneurysms and/or stenoses have a life-long increased risk for ischaemic events. Indeed, previously undiagnosed Kawasaki disease may become apparent in adulthood at the time of presentation with myocardial infarction.[113,114] Fatalities from myocardial infarction are most likely with obstruction in the main stem of the left coronary artery, or in the proximal segments of both the right and anterior interventricular arteries.[25] Thrombosis of the right, compared to the left, coronary artery is more likely to be silent and to recanalise.

Patients with aneurysms have been found to have stiff and thickened carotid arteries 6 to 20 years after onset, and these changes occur independent of dyslipidaemia.[115] The presence of carotid atherosclerosis suggests that the coronary arteries may be similarly affected. Patients with persistent aneurysms also have been found to have higher levels of high sensitivity C-reactive protein than those without aneurysms or normal children.[116,117] Low-grade ongoing inflammation thus appears to be a late effect in patients with coronary arterial aneurysms.

Regression of the aneurysms restores the internal luminal diameter to normal. The arterial wall, however, shows fibrous intimal thickening on histopathologic examination. Intravascular ultrasound in coronary arteries with regressed aneurysms is characterised by marked symmetric or asymmetric myo-intimal thickening.[118–120] In patients with regressed coronary aneurysms studied by intravascular ultrasound at least 10 years after onset, greater thickening of the intimal and medial layers was significantly associated with larger initial diameter of the coronary arteries.[119]

Regressed aneurysms also have abnormalities of function. Pharmacologic testing with intracoronary arterial administration of isosorbide dinitrate has shown that vascular reactivity is reduced in arterial segments with regressed aneurysms when compared to normal vessels. Vasodilation is progressively impaired as the interval from onset lengthens. In addition, endothelial dysfunction in regressed aneurysms is indicated by constriction of the arteries subsequent to administration of acetylcholine.[120–123] Despite abnormalities of structure and function, children with regressed aneurysms rarely have clinical symptoms or events within the first two decades of follow-up.

Children in whom aneurysms were never detected have normal cardiopulmonary fitness, and careful follow-up in Japan over the past three decades shows that they have no greater likelihood of cardiac or other diseases. Research studies suggest, however, that they should be monitored as an at-risk population. Vascular inflammation is diffuse during the acute disease, and lipid metabolism after the disease is altered for years after resolution of acute symptoms, with a pattern similar to that seen in other vasculitides.[124–126] Increased arterial stiffness in children who never had coronary arterial dilation is suggested by higher mean pulsed wave Doppler velocity in the brachial and radial arteries.[126,127] Coronary physiology may also be disturbed, with lower myocardial flow reserve and higher total coronary arterial resistance found in children with a history of Kawasaki disease in whom coronary dilation was never detected compared to normal controls.[128] Endothelium-dependent brachial arterial reactivity, which often mirrors coronary arterial reactivity, has been reported to be abnormal among children without a history of aneurysms.[129] Reports on endothelial function in the epicardial coronary arteries, as assessed by infusion of acetylcholine, have varied in their findings.[130,131]

TREATMENT

Treatment of the disease in the first weeks after onset is aimed at lowering fever for comfort, reducing inflammation and shear stress in the arterial wall, and preventing thrombosis. To reduce shear stress, children in whom coronary aneurysms are developing should undergo transfusion of red blood cells if they are profoundly anaemic, ideally to achieve a haematocrit of at least 30%, and β-blockers should be administered to reduce myocardial consumption of oxygen. Among patients with aneurysms, prevention and, if needed, treatment of coronary thrombosis are key components of therapy. Patients with coronary arterial stenosis or occlusion and evidence of reversible ischaemia are candidates for interventional catheterisation and surgical procedures. Specific therapies are detailed below.

Anti-inflammatory Therapies in the Acute Phase of Illness

Aspirin

Although aspirin does not affect the prevalence of coronary arterial aneurysms,[132] it has been a cornerstone of therapy because of its anti-pyretic and anti-platelet effects. The agent is given in high doses, 80 mg/kg/day, divided into four daily doses, and this regime is used until the child has been afebrile for at least 48 hours, after which the dose is lowered to 3 to 5 mg/kg/day for its anti-platelet effects. Aspirin in low doses is continued for approximately 6 weeks, and then discontinued in patients without coronary arterial aneurysms. In children with coronary arterial abnormalities, aspirin is continued indefinitely at low doses, and may be used together with other anti-thrombotic therapies, such as clopidogrel or warfarin, in children with coronary arterial lesions placing them at high risk.

Reye syndrome has been reported in children with the disease who are taking aspirin in high doses. Although this syndrome has not been associated with use of aspirin in low doses, annual vaccination against influenza is recommended for all children on chronic treatment with aspirin. When a child medicated on a chronic basis with aspirin develops a flu-like illness, aspirin should be withheld transiently and, if necessary, another anti-platelet medication, such as clopidogrel, should be substituted until resolution of the illness. Because ibuprofen antagonises the inhibitory effect of aspirin on platelets, sustained therapy with ibuprofen should be avoided in children who are taking aspirin in low doses for prophylaxis of coronary arterial thrombosis.[133]

Intravenous Immunoglobulin

Control of inflammation decreases the likelihood of aneurysmal formation, and is the most important aim of therapy in the acute phase of illness. Among the armamentarium of anti-inflammatory agents that have been used, only intravenous immunoglobulin in high doses has been demonstrated to be effective in multiple randomised, multi-centre trials with blinded echo interpretation.[62] When administered in the first 10 days, and ideally within the first 7 days, of illness, intravenous immunoglobulin reduces the prevalence of aneurysms approximately fivefold, to less than 5%. Treatment with intravenous immunoglobulin is also beneficial for children beyond the tenth day of illness in whom fever persists, or who have coronary arterial abnormalities together with persistent clinical and laboratory evidence of inflammation.[134] The standard dosage is 2 g/kg, administered over 8 to 12 hours. In patients who present with diminished left ventricular function, the agent should be administered more slowly, because it provides a considerable volume load. Meta-analyses have demonstrated a dose-response effect,[132] with this data underscoring the current practice of administering a second infusion to the 15% of children who have persistent or recrudescent fever at least 36 hours after completion of the first infusion. For children who defervesce with a second infusion, but in whom fever recurs, a third infusion may be administered. Some children have persistent fever, and develop coronary arterial aneurysms despite treatment, indicating resistance to intravenous gamma globulin. These children should receive alternative anti-inflammatory therapy.

Other Therapies

Corticosteroids are the mainstay of therapy for many childhood vasculitides, and they have been administered to children with Kawasaki disease, both as primary and rescue therapies. Uncontrolled case series, and one open and unblinded multi-centre randomised trial, have suggested that primary treatment may be beneficial.[135–141] In a recent randomised, multi-centre placebo-controlled and blinded trial, primary therapy with pulsed-dose intravenous methylprednisolone did not improve outcomes with regard to coronary arterial lesions in patients who also received standard therapy with immunoglobulins and aspirin.[81]

More often, corticosteroid therapy is administered to the patient resistant to intravenous immune globulin, in whom at least two courses of immunoglobulins are unsuccessful in controlling fever. Once again, retrospective studies and case series suggest that treatment with steroids improves fever and the inflammatory response.[142–146] In a randomised trial in patients with persistent fever after two treatments with immunoglobulins, patients randomised to pulse steroids, compared to those treated with immunoglobulins given at 1 g/kg, had fevers of shorter duration, and reduced length of stay in hospital, but no difference in the incidence of coronary arterial aneurysms.[146] Based upon the currently available literature, treatment with pulse steroids should be reserved for children who have persistent or recrudescent fever despite at least two courses of intravenous gamma globulin given at 2 g/kg.

Abciximab, a murine monoclonal antibody to the platelet glycoprotein IIbIIIa receptor, has been reported in a single-center case series with historical controls to promote regression in the maximal diameter of the aneurysms.[147] This salutary effect is presumed to be secondary to promotion of vascular remodeling through the anti-inflammatory effects of abciximab.

Infliximab, a chimeric monoclonal antibody to TNF-α, is being used increasingly as rescue therapy in those patients who are resistant to immunoglobulins.[148,149] Its efficacy in reducing the prevalence and severity of coronary arterial aneurysms is unknown.

Plasma exchange has been reported to lower the incidence of aneurysms in uncontrolled studies.[150–152] Because this therapy is technically complex to administer, it should be used only when other methods have failed. Rarely, cytotoxic agents have been used to treat refractory patients with acute disease,[145,153] but the risks of such therapies exceed their benefits for the majority of patients.

Prevention of Coronary Arterial Thrombosis

The risk of thrombosis depends upon the size of the coronary arterial aneurysm, as well as the presence of coronary arterial stenosis. Thus, the types of agents used for prophylaxis of thrombosis are tailored to the extent and severity of arterial involvement.[62] Because randomised trials of anti-thrombotic regimes have not been performed, the choice of agents is derived primarily from experience in adults with atherosclerotic disease, including aneurysms, as well as case series and consensus of experts. Patients with small aneurysms are treated with aspirin in doses sufficient to produce an anti-platelet effect (see above). At the other end of the spectrum, giant aneurysms, with a diameter of greater than 8 mm, are characterised by stagnant flow, so anticoagulation with warfarin or low-molecular weight heparin is added to aspirin therapy. For most patients, the international normalised ratio is maintained between 2.0 and 2.5. Patients with giant aneurysms and a history of coronary arterial thrombosis may benefit from treatment similar to that used in patients after replacement of the mitral valve, using, for example, warfarin to maintain the international normalised ratio between 2.5 and 3.5 along with aspirin. The optimal anti-thrombotic regimen for patients with aneurysms intermediate in size between small and giant is controversial. Clopidogrel[154] or anti-coagulation may be added to treatment with aspirin, depending upon the individual situation. For example, treatment of a 3-month-old infant with an aneurysm of 6 mm, with characteristics of flow similar to a giant aneurysm, usually includes anticoagulation together with aspirin. The same-sized aneurysm in an adolescent weighing 80 kg might warrant only anti-platelet therapy. Thus, it is important to consider the *z* scores, although guidelines for their use in choice of an anti-coagulation regimen have not been developed.

Treatment of Coronary Arterial Thrombosis

Thrombolytic therapy in children with coronary arterial thrombosis is primarily guided by studies in adults with acute coronary syndromes. The most common agent used in children is tissue plasminogen activator, at doses of 0.1 to 0.5 mg/kg/hr for 6 hours, administered together with aspirin and heparin or low-molecular-weight heparin.[62] The burden of thrombus in a giant aneurysm is large, and some children have rebound of thrombosis after cessation of thrombolytic therapy. For this reason, treatment may occasionally involve a combination of tissue plasminogen activator and abciximab, given as a bolus of 0.25 mg/kg over 30 minutes, followed by an infusion of 0.125 μg/kg/minute for 12 hours. Mechanical restoration of myocardial perfusion by means of interventional cardiology may be used in patients whose vessels are large enough to accommodate adult-sized catheters.

Interventional Catheterisation Procedures

The indications for interventional catheterisation procedures have not been assessed in randomised trials in children and adults with coronary arterial stenoses secondary to Kawasaki disease. Most of the techniques used in adults with atherosclerotic coronary arterial disease have been applied to the population of children with Kawasaki disease. These include percutaneous transluminal coronary angioplasty, rotational atherectomy, and placement of stents.[155] To provide practical interim suggestions for clinicians until evidence-based guidelines are available, the Research Committee of the Japanese Ministry of Health, Labor and Welfare published recommendations for conditions under which catheter intervention should be considered in such patients.[155] These include presentation with ischaemic symptoms, presence of reversible ischaemia on stress testing, or presence of at least 75% stenosis of the anterior interventricular coronary artery. Contraindications to catheter intervention include severe left ventricular dysfunction, and coronary arteries with multiple, ostial, or long-segment stenoses.

Longer-term results for catheter interventions have now been published with a median follow-up of 3.6 years.[156] For vessels in which angioplasty was used, the early success rate was 86%. For rotational atherectomy, the figure was 96%, and for placement of stents, 90%. At the latest follow-up, stenoses had recurred in 29% of arterial segments in which angioplasty had been performed: in 28% of segments following rotational atherectomy, and in 8% of segments following placement of a stent. Neoaneurysms were noted in 7% of segments treated with angioplasty and rotational ablation, likely related to the high pressure of inflation needed to relieve stenoses in stiff coronary arteries. Procedures are best performed by a multi-disciplinary team that takes advantage of the technical expertise and knowledge of adult cardiologists, working together with paediatric cardiologists, anaesthesiologists, and nurses.

Surgery

As with interventional catheterisation procedures, the indications for bypass grafting in children with Kawasaki disease are based upon experience in adult patients and consensus of experts. Coronary arterial bypass surgery is performed with the goal of improving symptoms of angina, enhancing myocardial perfusion, and lowering the future risk of myocardial infarction or sudden death.[157,158] Children with reversible ischaemia on stress-imaging tests are generally considered for intervention, be it transcatheter or surgical. In addition, high-grade obstructions in at least two major coronary arteries, or in the main stem of the left coronary artery, are indications for surgery because these findings predict a high risk of myocardial infarction. Some experts also consider high-grade stenosis in the anterior interventricular artery to be an indication for intervention. Bypass grafting is contraindicated when there is arterial disease distal to the planned anastomosis, or nonviable myocardium in regions supplied by the affected vessel.[159] Competing flow into arteries supplied by a graft causes a string sign, and may result in occlusion.

Although saphenous venous grafts were used in the earliest surgical series, they are rarely used today because of poor long-term patency in children.[160] Instead, arterial grafts, such as those provided using the internal mammary, radial, and gastroepiploic arteries, have better long-term patency, enlarge in length and diameter as the child grows, and improve myocardial perfusion.[158]

Coronary arterial bypass procedures in children have low morbidity and mortality.[157] In a national survey of such grafting in Japan,[157] long-term rates of patency were shown to be affected by the age of the patient at the time of the graft. Specifically, when performed in children at least 12 years of age, internal mammary arterial grafts had patency rates of 95%, 91%, and 91% at 1, 5, and 15 years after surgery. Lower patency was seen in those who underwent surgery at ages younger than 12 years, at 93%, 73%, and 65%, respectively. Left ventricular ejection fraction of less than 40% was a risk factor for mortality. A recent small series suggests that the use of percutaneous transluminal balloon angioplasty for anastomotic stenosis after bypass grafting improves the long-term patency in small children to rates similar to those in older children.[161]

Cardiac transplantation can be performed in children with Kawasaki disease who have end-stage ischaemic cardiomyopathy in whom severe coronary arterial lesions cannot be treated further with interventional catheterisation or coronary arterial bypass procedures.[162]

RECOMMENDATIONS FOR LONG-TERM FOLLOW-UP

The frequency of follow-up, types of testing, and specific recommendations regarding medications, exercise restrictions, and anticoagulation are summarised in Table 52-4.[163] Certain principles for long-term management are common to patients with all levels of risk. Because the future risk of atherosclerotic coronary disease may be higher in children who have had Kawasaki disease, all children should undergo periodic assessment and counseling about known risk factors.[164] All patients and families should be counseled regarding a heart-healthy diet, the importance of exercise, and the risks of smoking. They should be encouraged to limit adverse effects from passive smoking, so a smoke-free home should be advised. A lipid profile should be obtained approximately 1 year after the onset of the illness. New recommendations from the American Heart Association have established the thresholds at which pharmacologic management of hyperlipidaemia and hypertension should be started, depending upon the severity of coronary arterial disease.[164] Paediatric cardiologists should strive to balance the need for preventive counseling for exercise and a heart healthy diet against the production of cardiac non-disease.

Regular aerobic exercise should be strongly encouraged in all patients to the extent advised in the recommendations of the 36th Bethesda Conference for their level of coronary arterial disease.[165] Those with arteries that were always normal, or only transiently dilated, have no need to restrict their exercise. In patients with coronary arterial disease, participation in competitive sports is guided by the results of non-invasive assessment of left ventricular function and exercise testing with myocardial perfusion imaging. Even patients at the highest categories of risk can participate in some types of competitive sports if they have normal left ventricular function and exercise tolerance, and no evidence of either reversible ischaemia or exercise-induced arrhythmias. Patients taking anti-platelet or anti-coagulant medications should be discouraged from sports involving collisions or high impacts because of the risk of bleeding.

IMPLICATIONS IN ADULT LIFE

Excellent follow-up of patients with Kawasaki disease has occurred only in the last three decades, so data are limited on its implications for life into adulthood. The standardised mortality ratio for males with cardiac complications has been reported to be 2.35, with 95% confidence intervals from 0.96 to 5.19, after long-term follow-up in Japan.[166] The failure of this finding to reach statistical significance may reflect the excellence of therapies for coronary arterial disease, and the rarity of severe coronary arterial aneurysms. Management of anti-coagulation in pregnancy be similar to that in the obstetric patient with a prosthetic valve,[167] and women should have reproductive counseling when they reach childbearing age. The largest series on pregnancy and delivery in women with coronary arterial aneurysms due to Kawasaki disease included 46 deliveries in 30 patients.[168] No patients had coronary arterial complications. To date, patients whose coronary arteries were always normal, or only transiently dilated, have not been found to suffer a higher incidence of cardiac or other diseases in follow-up. Japanese cohorts, nonetheless, will need to be followed into middle age before it is known whether even these patients are at risk for premature atherosclerosis. Continuing surveillance of such patients will be necessary to fully understand the implications of the disease for long-term

TABLE 52-4
RISK STRATIFICATION

Risk Level	Pharmacological Therapy	Physical Activity	Follow-up and Diagnostic Testing	Invasive Testing
I (no coronary artery changes at any stage of illness)	None beyond initial 6–8 weeks	No restrictions beyond initial 6–8 weeks	Cardiovascular risk assessment and counseling at 5-year intervals	None recommended
II (transient coronary artery ectasia that disappears within initial 6–8 weeks)	None beyond initial 6–8 weeks	No restrictions beyond initial 6–8 weeks	Cardiovascular risk assessment and counseling at 3- to 5-year intervals	None recommended
III (small to medium solitary coronary artery aneurysm)	Low-dose aspirin (3–5 mg/kg aspirin per day), at least until aneurysm regression is documented.	For patients in first decade of life, no restriction beyond initial 6–8 weeks. For second decade, physical activity guided by stress testing every other year. Contact or high-impact sports discouraged for patients on anti-platelet agents.	Annual cardiology follow-up with echocardiogram and ECG, combined with cardiovascular risk assessment and counseling. Stress testing with radioisotope perfusion scan or stress echocardiogram every other year.	Angiography, if non-invasive test suggests ischemia
IVa (one or more large or giant coronary artery aneurysms), or IVb (multiple or complex aneurysms, without obstruction)	Long-term anti-platelet therapy and warfarin (target: INR 2.0–2.5) or LMW heparin (target: antifactor Xa level 0.5–1.0 unit/mL) should be combined in giant aneurysms.	Contact or high-impact sports, isometrics, and weight training should be avoided because of the risk of bleeding. Other physical activity recommendations guided by outcome of stress testing or myocardial perfusion scan.	Biannual follow-up with echocardiogram + ECG. Annual pharmacological or exercise stress testing.	Initial angiography at 6–12 months. Repeated angiography if non-invasive test, clinical or laboratory findings suggest ischemia. Elective repeated angiography under some circumstances (see text)
V (coronary artery obstruction)	Long-term low-dose aspirin. Warfarin or LMW heparin if giant aneurysm persists. Use of β-blockers should be considered to reduce myocardial oxygen consumption	Contact or high-impact sports, isometrics, and weight training should be avoided because of the risk of bleeding. Other physical activity recommendations guided by outcome of stress testing or myocardial perfusion scan.	Biannual follow-up with echocardiogram and ECG. Annual pharmacological or exercise stress testing.	Angiography is recommended to address therapeutic options.

Reprinted with permission from Newburger JW, Takahashi M, Gerber MA, et al: Diagnosis, treatment, and long-term management of Kawasaki disease: A statement for health professionals from the Committee on Rheumatic Fever, Endocarditis and Kawasaki Disease, Council on Cardiovascular Disease in the Young, American Heart Association. Circulation 2004;110:2747–2771.

myocardial function, late-onset valvar regurgitation, and the state of the coronary arteries.

The complete reference list can be found on the companion Expert Consult web site at www.expertconsult.com.

ANNOTATED REFERENCES

- Kawasaki T: [Acute febrile mucocutaneous syndrome with lymphoid involvement with specific desquamation of the fingers and toes in children]. Jpn J Allergy 1967;116:78–222.

  The classical first description of the lesion described in this chapter.

- Fujiwara H, Hamashima Y: Pathology of the heart in Kawasaki disease. Pediatrics 1978;61:100–107.

  This manuscript provides the classic description of pathology of the heart in fatal Kawasaki disease in a series of 20 hearts. The authors classify cardiac lesions according to the duration of illness at the time of death. Within the first 9 days of illness, the predominant findings were acute perivasculitis and vasculitis of the microvessels (arterioles, capillaries, and venules) and small arteries, and acute perivasculitis and endarteritis of the three major coronary arteries. Additional findings included pericarditis, myocarditis, inflammation of the atrioventricular conduction system, and endocarditis with valvitis. In the period from 12 to 25 days after illness onset, coronary aneurysms appeared. After 28 days, inflammation in the microvasculature disappeared and coronary arteries began to granulate. In the latest stage, 40 days to 4 years, aneurysms showed scarring with severe stenosis.

- Kato H, Ichinose E, Kawasaki T: Myocardial infarction in Kawasaki disease: Clinical analyses in 195 cases. J Pediatr 1986;108:923–927.

  This manuscript provides the largest series of patients with myocardial infarction resulting from Kawasaki disease. The authors summarise cases in 195 patients with myocardial infarction from 74 hospitals in Japan. Approximately three-quarters of myocardial infarctions occurred within the first year after illness onset. The majority of myocardial infarctions (63%) occurred during sleep or at rest. The most common symptoms included shock, unrest, vomiting, abdominal pain, and chest pain; not surprisingly, older children were much more likely to report chest pain. Almost 40% of patients who suffered myocardial infarctions did not recognise or report symptoms at the time. The mortality rate from the first myocardial infarction was 22%, and 16% of patients had a second myocardial infarction. Fatalities were most likely to occur in those with left main disease or with coronary obstruction in both the proximal right coronary artery and the left anterior descending coronary artery. Survivors were more likely to have single vessel involvement of the right coronary artery.

- Newburger JW, Takahashi M, Gerber MA, et al: Diagnosis, treatment, and long-term management of Kawasaki disease: A statement for health professionals from the Committee on Rheumatic Fever, Endocarditis and Kawasaki Disease, Council on Cardiovascular Disease in the Young, American Heart Association. Circulation 2004;110:2747–2771.

  This scientific statement prepared on behalf of the American Heart Association provides recommendations for the initial evaluation, treatment in the acute phase, and long-term management of patients with Kawasaki disease. It includes a new algorithm to guide clinicians in deciding which children with fever for greater than 5 days, and four or more classic criterions, should undergo echocardiography, receive intravenous gamma globulin, or both, for Kawasaki disease.

- Kato H, Sugimura T, Akagi T, et al: Long-term consequences of Kawasaki disease: A 10- to 21-year follow-up study of 594 patients. Circulation 1996;94:1379–1385.

  This elegant study followed a cohort of 594 consecutive children with acute onset of Kawasaki disease between 1973 and 1983 for 10 to 21 years, with a mean of 13.6 years. All children had coronary angiography after recovery from the acute phase of the disease. Coronary arterial aneurysms initially were present in 146 patients (25%). By approximately 2 years later, 55% of aneurysms had shown regression. Regression was not seen, however, in giant coronary aneurysms. Coronary arterial stenosis increased progressively over time. Among the 448 patients with normal findings at the first angiogram, none developed any cardiac abnormalities over time. Systemic arterial aneurysms occurred in 2% of patients, and valvar heart disease in 1%. During the period of follow-up, 5% of patients developed ischaemic heart disease, and 2% had a myocardial infarction. The mortality rate was 0.8%.

- Tsuda E, Kamiya T, Kimura K, et al: Coronary artery dilatation exceeding 4.0 mm during acute Kawasaki disease predicts a high probability of subsequent late intima-medial thickening. Pediatr Cardiol 2002;23:9–14.

  The authors correlated the maximal coronary arterial diameter in 28 patients during the acute phase of Kawasaki disease with the extent of intima medial thickening by intravascular ultrasound at a mean of 15 years later. The initial coronary arterial diameter was significantly related to late intima medial thickness in the right coronary, the anterior interventricular, and the circumflex arteries. Abnormal intima medial thickness was defined as being equal to or greater than 0.40 mm. Initial coronary arterial dilation exceeding 4.0 mm in any of the main coronary arteries predicted a high likelihood of late abnormalities in intima medial thickness, defined as greater than 0.40 mm, in the corresponding coronary arterial segment at late follow-up.

- Cheung YF, Yung TC, Tam SC, et al: Novel and traditional cardiovascular risk factors in children after Kawasaki disease: Implications for premature atherosclerosis. J Am Coll Cardiol 2004;43:120–124.

  The authors studied a cohort of 102 subjects, 37 having Kawasaki disease with coronary arterial aneurysms, 29 subjects with Kawasaki disease and normal coronary arteries, and 36 healthy age-matched children. The subjects with coronary arterial aneurysms had lower high density lipid cholesterol and levels of apoA-I, and higher levels of apoB and pulse wave velocity than did the control subjects. Those with Kawasaki disease but without aneurysms had higher levels of apoB and pulse wave velocity than did control subjects, but similar levels of high density lipids and apoA-1. These data suggest that children with a history of Kawasaki disease may have an adverse cardiovascular risk profile, as characterised by a proatherogenic alteration of the lipid profile and increased arterial stiffness. Compared to the patients with Kawasaki disease but without aneurysms, those with coronary arterial aneurysms have a worse profile. This study raises concerns that children with a history of Kawasaki disease may be predisposed to premature atherosclerosis later in life.

- Ishii M, Ueno T, Akagi T, et al: Guidelines for catheter intervention in coronary artery lesion in Kawasaki disease. Pediatr Int 2001;43:558–562.

  This manuscript from the Research Committee of the Ministry of Health, Labour, and Welfare in Japan provides guidelines for catheter intervention in those with coronary arterial lesions in Kawasaki disease. The guidelines review the background and natural history of coronary arterial abnormalities; indications and types of interventional cardiology procedures; and recommendations for management after the procedures.

- Tsuda E, Kitamura S: National survey of coronary artery bypass grafting for coronary stenosis caused by Kawasaki disease in Japan. Circulation 2004; 110(11, suppl 1):II61–II66.

  These authors provide information from a national survey of coronary arterial bypass grafting in Japan in calendar year 2002. Among 323 institutions returning the survey instrument, 244 patients who underwent bypass grafting since 1975 were identified. Median age at surgery was 11 years, median interval from onset of Kawasaki disease to surgery was 8 years, and median duration from surgery to follow-up was 5 years. More than one in four patients had had a myocardial infarction prior to surgery. In children whose bypass grafting was performed at an age of at least 12 years, patency rates for internal mammary artery grafting at 1, 5, and 15 years of follow-up were 95%, 91%, and 91%, respectively. The corresponding results for children younger than 12 years at surgery were 93%, 73%, and 65%. Of the children, 6% underwent reoperation. Among 14 late deaths, 9 were sudden. The mortality rate was especially high, at 75%, among children with ejection fraction less than 40%.

- Kavey RE, Allada V, Daniels SR, et al: Cardiovascular risk reduction in high-risk pediatric patients: A scientific statement from the American Heart Association Expert Panel on Population and Prevention Science; the Councils on Cardiovascular Disease in the Young, Epidemiology and Prevention, Nutrition, Physical Activity and Metabolism, High Blood Pressure Research, Cardiovascular Nursing, and the Kidney in Heart Disease; and the Interdisciplinary Working Group on Quality of Care and Outcomes Research: Endorsed by the American Academy of Pediatrics. Circulation 2006;114:2710–2738.

  This scientific statement prepared on behalf of the American Heart Association emphasises that children with certain diagnoses, including Kawasaki disease, are at risk for premature cardiovascular disease, and provides practical recommendations for management of cardiovascular risk. Thresholds for pharmacologic treatment of hyperlipidaemia and hypertension in children with Kawasaki disease are stratified according to whether a child has current coronary arterial aneurysms, regressed aneurysms, or no history of coronary arterial abnormalities.

- Tsuda E, Kawamata K, Neki R, et al: Nationwide survey of pregnancy and delivery in patients with coronary arterial lesions caused by Kawasaki disease in Japan. Cardiol Young 2006;16:173–178.

  The authors provide a survey of pregnancy and delivery in patients with a history of Kawasaki disease in Japan, analysing 46 deliveries in 30 patients from 16 institutions. Coronary arterial bypass grafting had been performed in 4 patients, and 16 patients were receiving low-dose aspirin. No cardiac complications occurred in any patient. The authors recommend that the mode of delivery should be determined primarily by obstetrical considerations, rather than the coronary arterial disease.

SECTION

4

General Disease

CHAPTER 53

Non-rheumatic Inflammatory Diseases of the Heart

EDWARD J. BAKER

In this chapter, I will discuss inflammatory diseases of the heart, excluding rheumatic fever (see Chapter 54), Kawasaki disease (see Chapter 52), and infectious endocarditis (see Chapter 55). Although the heart may be the primary target organ, inflammatory disease of non-rheumatic origin is often more generalised in nature. Usually such diseases affect various structures of the heart in combination. Only rarely will they be limited to the endocardium, the myocardium, or the pericardium. To clarify the discussion, however, I will distinguish between myocarditis and pericarditis.

MYOCARDITIS

Myocarditis is defined as an inflammatory response within the myocardium. Its aetiology and pathogenesis are very variable. In many patients, the precise mechanisms involved still remain unclear. The clinical consequences of myocarditis are largely determined by the degree and extent of myocardial injury. The disease may first present with pump failure, or with abnormalities of rhythm and conduction. In the acute stage, sudden death may occur, often before the diagnosis is made.

The heart is often dilated, with histological studies revealing myocardial necrosis, with accompanying inflammatory reactions (Fig. 53-1). The degree and extent of myocardial necrosis may vary considerably, as may the type of inflammation. Usually, neither one of these histological findings is diagnostic as far as aetiology and pathogenesis are concerned. In more advanced stages of the disease, part of the damaged myocardium may be replaced by scar tissue. Eventually, the histology of the affected heart may be dominated by interstitial fibrosis. In such instances, the condition is often described as chronic myocarditis. Various schemes for the histological grading of myocarditis have been described, most notably the Dallas criterions.[1] Recently, it has been established that the use of these criterions is unreliable when assessing endomyocardial biopsies to diagnose myocarditis.[2] The myocardial changes are not uniform, and the findings depend on the site of sampling. Furthermore, there are significant differences in interpretation of the histology between histopathologists. It is now established that virus may be present in the myocardium without the Dallas criterions for myocarditis being fulfilled.[3] Most importantly, the Dallas classification does not predict prognosis, nor response to immunosuppressive therapy.

Myocarditis may be associated with a variety of aetiological factors including infections, ischaemia, and generalised inflammatory conditions. In children, two main classes of non-rheumatic myocarditis can be recognised: the infectious and generalised autoimmune variants.

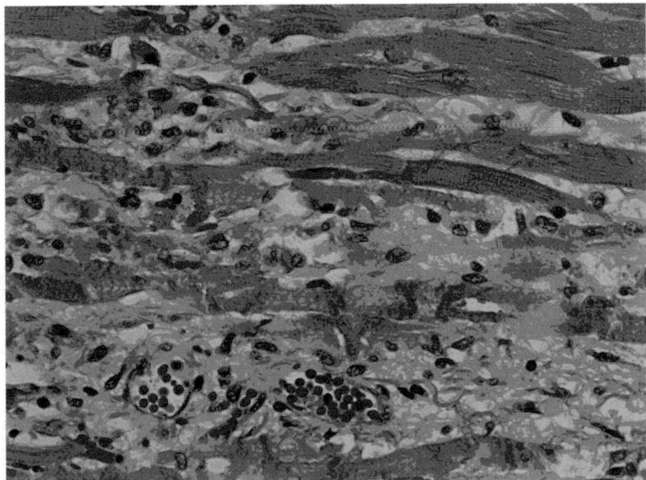

Figure 53-1 The slide shows the typical histologic features of viral myocarditis. There is heavy lymphocytic infiltration with myocardial cell degeneration and necrosis. (Courtesy of Professor Sebastian Lucas, Guy's and St Thomas's Hospital, London, United Kingdom.)

Infectious Myocarditis

Infectious myocarditis can occur as a complication of almost any infectious disease. Viral infections are by far the most important in the industrialised Western world, but in other parts of the world, protozoal infections may rank highest. Many acute bacterial infections can result in myocarditis. It can occur as a complication of tuberculosis, Lyme disease, and haemolytic uraemic syndrome.[1,4–6] Infectious myocarditis is a frequent complication of opportunistic infections in patients with immune deficiencies, either primary or secondary, such as those that occur in patients treated with immunosuppressive drugs. Obviously, therefore, the type and incidence of infectious myocarditis will vary considerably from one part of the world to another. Moreover, its true prevalence in any given population is, as yet, unknown. This is because the disease may take a subclinical course in many patients, and, hence will go undetected. In others, the presence of an infectious myocarditis may be completely masked by the more overt signs and symptoms of other affected organs. Depending on the histological criterions used, evidence of myocarditis has been found in up to one-twentieth of postmortems.[7] It has been demonstrated to be present in approximately one in ten sudden deaths in young adults, and a similar proportion of patients with dilated cardiomyopathy.[8]

Viral Myocarditis

The majority of the cases of myocarditis seen in the West are of viral origin. Almost any viral disease can be complicated by myocarditis. Hence, the clinician should always be alert to this possibility. Viral myocarditis can present with ventricular dysfunction of rapid onset, or with progressive ventricular dysfunction and dilation. Viruses are known to be present in the myocardium of many patients with dilated cardiomyopathy even when the histological criterions for myocarditis are not evident. Enteroviruses, particularly those of Coxsackie group B, have been considered important causes, but molecular studies using the polymerase chain reaction have shown that adenoviruses are more commonly found in the myocardium in patients with clinical myocarditis.[9] Cytomegalovirus, echovirus, hepatitis C, respiratory syncytial virus, and the viruses producing influenza, mumps, and rubella have also been implicated.[10,11] Human immunodeficiency virus also commonly infects the heart.[12] In children, it can cause myocarditis and pericarditis, often presenting with the picture of a dilated cardiomyopathy.[13,14]

The viral infection may be acquired transplacentally or postnatally. The infection may present in neonates and infants, with myocarditis as the leading abnormality. Infections in older children often cause pericarditis as the dominant feature. The mechanisms involved in producing the myocardial injury are complex. Invasion of the myocardial cells by viruses, or elaboration of toxins, may play an important role. Alternatively, cellular immune mechanisms and circulating autoantibodies may be of great importance. A combination, which may vary considerably between individual patients, of viral infection and subsequent abnormal immune response, causing either ineffective viral clearance or autoimmune myocyte damage, seems to underlie the clinical manifestation of the disease. Persistence of the virus, or continuing immune reactions after the viral infection has cleared, may produce chronic myocardial damage and present as chronic dilated cardiomyopathy.

Clinical Features

The clinical onset of myocarditis usually occurs after a latent period following the onset of a systemic viral infection. The signs and symptoms of myocarditis are highly variable, but are principally the result of cardiac failure or disturbances of rhythm. It is understandable, therefore, that there is no single characteristic clinical profile for myocarditis. Indeed, a whole spectrum of abnormalities may exist. At the one end, a child may develop an infectious myocarditis that remains completely unnoticed. At the other end, a child may become acutely ill with signs of both left- and right-sided cardiac failure and low cardiac output, often further complicated by disturbances of rhythm and sudden death.

All signs and symptoms, even the most subtle ones, which indicate failing pump function or abnormalities in rhythm and conduction, should alert the physician to a cardiac complication. This is particularly so when noticed in the setting of a viral disease. In this respect, the important features that may give a clue to the diagnosis are cardiac enlargement, cardiac failure, tachycardia, gallop rhythm, tachypnoea, dyspnoea, fatigue, and the appearance of an apical murmur indicating mitral insufficiency. There may be chest pain from accompanying pericarditis. Non-specific symptoms, such as fever, diarrhoea, problems with feeding, pallor, mild jaundice, and lethargy, often mark the clinical onset of the principal disease. Occasionally, the clinical picture may be dominated by severe respiratory distress secondary to left ventricular failure, so much so that initially a respiratory infection is mistakenly diagnosed. The clinical picture of cardiac failure in a previously well child with often a minor, preceding viral infection is typical.

Laboratory Findings

The sedimentation rate is usually elevated but may be normal. The level of C-reactive protein may also be elevated, and this may be of prognostic significance.[15] The white cell count is variable, as are the levels of the cardiac enzymes, all depending on the severity of the disease and the nature of the infection. Levels of troponin are frequently, but not invariably, elevated.

All available diagnostic procedures should be used, including close collaboration with the bacteriological laboratory, in an attempt to identify an infectious agent. Despite all studies, however, the diagnosis of a viral origin is often based on circumstantial evidence, along with the exclusion of other possible aetiologies, rather than positive identification of an aetiological agent.

Investigations

Radiology

The size of the heart may be normal, particularly in the early period of the disease. More frequently, the heart will be enlarged, with normal lung fields. Occasionally, pulmonary venous congestion will be evident.

Electrocardiography

Electrocardiographic abnormalities are common in myocarditis, but are non-specific (Fig. 53-2). There is often a sinus tachycardia, with lowering of the QRS complexes in the standard leads and/or precordial leads, flattening or inversion of the T waves, and changes in the ST segment. Arrhythmias are often present and may lead to unexpected death. Occasionally, disturbances of conduction are seen, with varying degrees of heart block. Complete atrioventricular block is rare. The QRS complexes may be broadened, with left or right bundle branch block configuration. The electrocardiographic changes may disappear during the course of the disease, or they may show a progressive evolution to overt abnormalities. The abnormalities may persist after the patient has recovered clinically, most likely because of myocardial fibrosis.

Echocardiography

Echocardiography may demonstrate important, albeit non-specific, features. There is usually dilation of the heart chambers, usually predominantly the left ventricle. When the onset is rapid, producing so-called fulminant myocarditis, there may be ventricular dysfunction without dilation. Ventricular dysfunction is usually much more evident in the left ventricle than in the right, and may be either

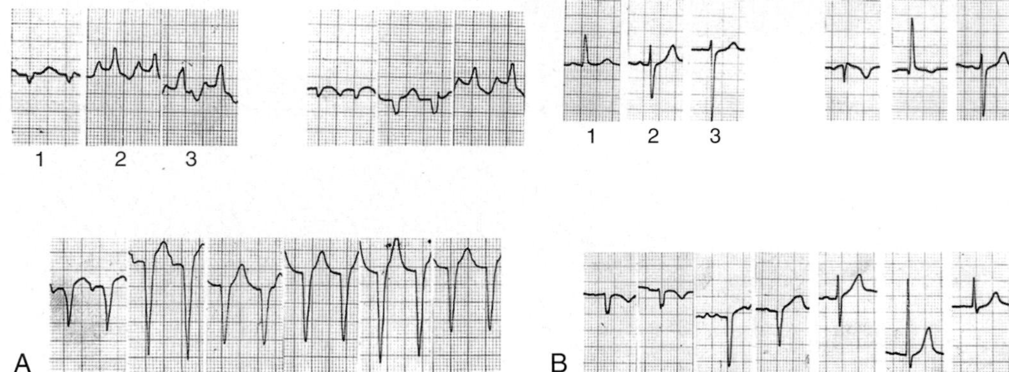

Figure 53-2 The electrocardiogram is from a 9-year-old boy with viral myocarditis. The electrocardiogram on admission (A) showed first-degree atrioventricular block with broad QRS complexes. There is an infarction pattern with QS complexes in all precordial leads. After 30 days, the electrocardiogram had normalised (B), but there was left-axis deviation with slightly broadened QRS complexes, indicative of incomplete left bundle branch block. After 4 years the electrocardiogram had not changed in any important way.

global or segmental. The left atrium may also be enlarged, especially in the presence of mitral insufficiency (Fig. 53-3). The motion of the ventricular septum, and of the ventricular walls, may be reduced and abnormal, while the ejection fraction may be decreased. Echocardiographic tissue characterisation, tissue Doppler imaging, and measurements of myocardial velocity have been shown to differentiate myocarditis from other causes of ventricular dysfunction, albeit that further work will be needed to determine their value in a clinical setting.

The echocardiogram is of great importance in demonstrating or excluding a pericardial effusion and intracardiac thrombosis, and for excluding structural causes of ventricular dysfunction. Identical echocardiographic findings are found in chronic myocarditis and dilated cardiomyopathy.

Other Imaging Techniques

Radionuclide scans have been used for the detection of myocarditis, using either gallium-67 scans or indium-111–labelled monoclonal antimyosin antibody.[16] In practise, the most valuable role of radionuclide imaging is the serial measurement of left ventricular function, where it provides a more reproducible measurement of function than does echocardiography.

Early studies with contrast-enhanced magnetic resonance imaging have shown considerable promise in detecting myocarditis. Focal myocardial enhancement correlates with myocardial injury and histological changes. This has been used to guide biopsy of affected regions, improving the accuracy of histological diagnosis.[17]

Endomyocardial Biopsy

The place of routine endomyocardial biopsy in suspected myocarditis is still unclear. The histological changes of myocarditis are patchy, and so there can never be total confidence that a negative biopsy excludes myocarditis. There is little evidence that biopsy is of value in determining prognosis, or in helping further management.[18] The risk of the biopsy procedure is highest in the acutely unwell young child with severe ventricular dysfunction.[19] After many years of pursuing a policy of routine biopsy in suspected cases, in our own centre we have been unable to demonstrate any benefit, and have abandoned the practise. It is increasingly being used to enable identification of the viral aetiology by analysis of the polymerase chain reaction.[9] Biopsy may be justified in selected cases with unusual or rapidly progressive presentation, or where histology is used to guide therapy.[8]

Treatment

If an infectious agent has been identified as the cause of the myocarditis, and a specific treatment is available, then that should be started. In most cases, the causative agent is not identified. Treatment will then be non-specific, aiming at lowering the cardiac pre- and afterload, and at preventing and controlling complications such as cardiac failure and disturbances of rhythm.

Bedrest is advised for at least 14 days in the acute stage in order to reduce the workload of the heart. A good response is characterised by a sleeping pulse rate of less than 100 beats per minute in children, and of less than 120 beats per minute in infants. Restlessness and hypoxic stress should be avoided. If necessary, oxygen is administered.

Diuretics and inotropic agents may well need to be given intravenously in the initial stages of treatment. In a minority of patients, ventilation and circulatory support may be needed. The place of extracorporeal membrane oxygenation is not well established. As the ventricular function can recover, it should be considered in critically ill patients. Cardiac failure should be treated with diuretics, inhibitors of angiotensin-converting enzyme, and β-blockade.

Patients should be closely monitored for the occurrence of arrhythmias. When present, these disturbances should be treated if they have a deleterious haemodynamic effect. Many antiarrhythmic drugs will further depress myocardial contractility and should be used with care.

Thrombosis can occur in those with very dilated atrial and ventricular chambers. In such patients, transoesophageal echocardiography is needed to exclude intracardiac thrombosis with confidence. Anticoagulation should always be considered in these circumstances. If evidence of intracardiac thrombosis is seen echocardiographically, anti-coagulation should be continued until the left ventricular function has improved.

The value of prescribing drugs that suppress the inflammatory reaction is unclear.[20] Immunosuppression is used more commonly in children than in adults with myocarditis. There is no scientific justification for this diversity of approach. It was advocated in the expectation that

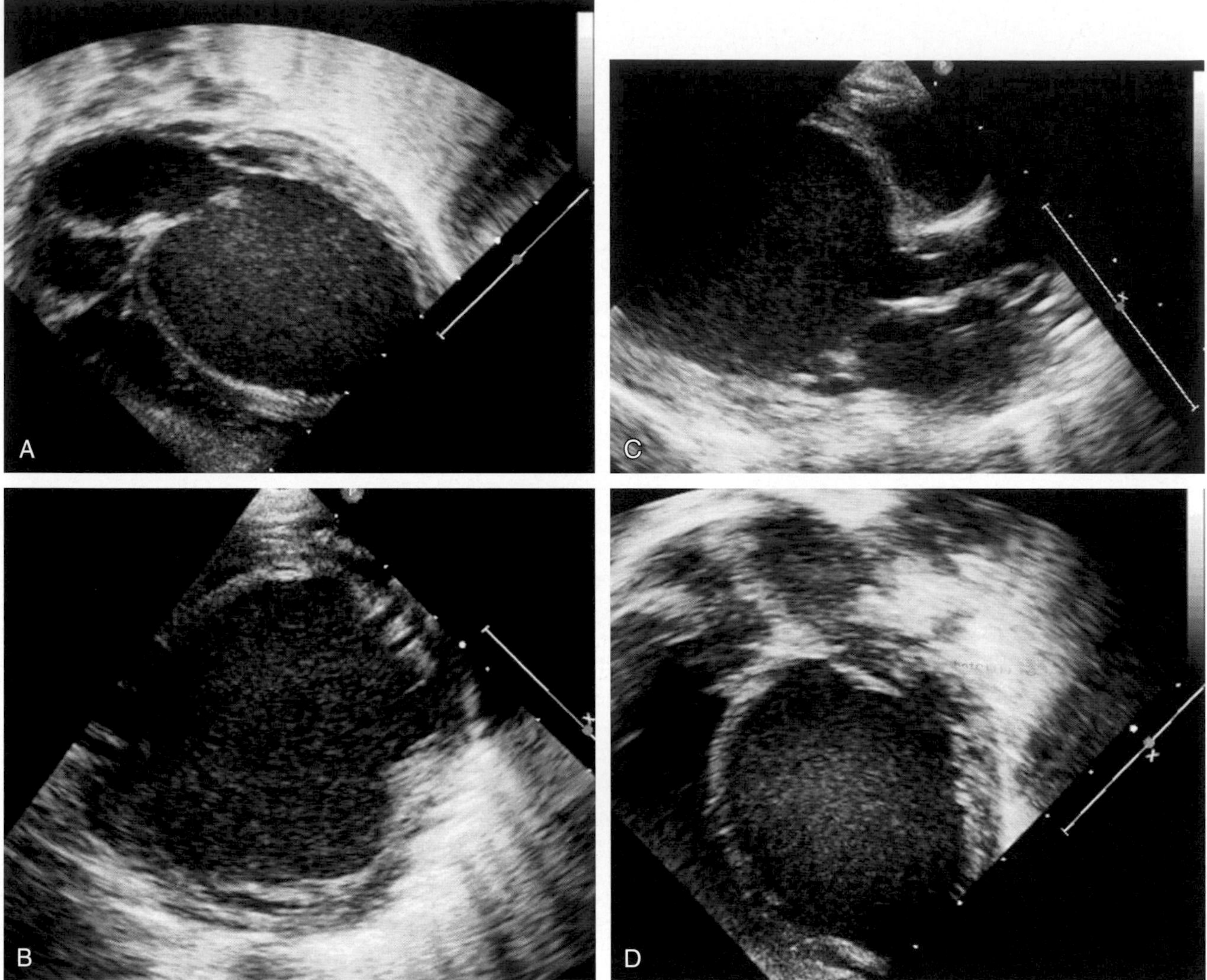

Figure 53-3 These cross sectional echocardiograms are from a child with acute myocarditis, with subcostal (**A**), parasternal short-axis (**B**), parasternal long-axis (**C**), and apical long-axis (**D**) views. The images show dilated cardiomyopathy, each view being dominated by the globular, dilated, left ventricular cavity. Function was very poor, with an estimated left ventricular ejection fraction of 15%. There was moderate mitral incompetence on colour Doppler.

immunosuppressive therapy would resolve the cellular infiltrate in the myocardium and, hence, reduce mortality and morbidity. The use of corticosteroids is advocated for patients with biopsy-proven disease who fail to respond to conventional therapy.[21] Steroids have been reported to help in the treatment of heart block or ventricular tachycardia brought on by myocarditis.[22] Despite this anecdotal evidence, a trial has shown no benefit from the routine use of prednisolone combined with either cyclosporin A or azothioprine.[23] Immunosuppression has been shown to be of value in a rare histological variant of myocarditis—giant cell myocarditis.[24] Immunoglobulin given intravenously in high doses may be beneficial in improving the recovery of ventricular function.[25] It is widely used in children, but clinical trials have not yet shown that it improves the recovery of left ventricular function or the long-term outcome.[26]

Children may die during the acute phase of the illness. In those whose left ventricular function is poor, failing to improve and remaining dependent on diuretics or inotropic agents given in high doses intravenously to control cardiac failure, or in those who develop intractable life-threatening arrhythmias, the option of cardiac transplantation should be considered. Transplantation may also be necessary for those who recover from the acute phase of myocarditis but continue to have poor left ventricular function over the longer term.

Prognosis

Many children make a full recovery from myocarditis. Older children, and those with a lower ejection fraction at presentation, have a worse prognosis.[27] The clinical signs and symptoms usually subside within a few weeks or months. It may take a little longer for the size of the heart and the electrocardiogram parameters to normalise. In some patients, this may take a year or more. Occasionally, the heart may remain enlarged, or episodes of cardiac failure may recur after an initial favourable response. The prognosis in these patients is usually poor. One recent large study showed that two-thirds of children presenting with cardiac myocardial failure were alive without cardiac transplantation at 1 year. Including the patients that had transplantation, more than four-fifths were surviving at 1 year, albeit that most were still on medication 1 year after presentation.[28] A further study showed an overall incidence of dilated cardiomyopathy in children under 18 years of 0.57 cases per 100,000. Of these almost half were diagnosed as myocarditis, three-tenths had died or required transplantation at 1 year, and only just over half were alive at 5 years.[29]

Differential Diagnosis

Myocarditis needs to be distinguished from other anomalies that present with signs and symptoms of acute cardiac failure early in life. A variety of metabolic diseases may present with dilated cardiomyopathy in infancy, and these should be excluded (see Chapters 49 and 57). When the left coronary artery arises anomalously from the pulmonary trunk, the characteristic features are the electrocardiographic signs of an anterolateral myocardial infarction. The diagnosis can be confirmed echocardiographically, or by angiocardiography. Enlargement of the heart and cardiac failure may also be caused by longstanding and severe anaemia of various causes. Dilation of the heart may occur also as a secondary phenomenon in patients with systemic arterio-venous fistulas. Occasionally, a child may present with all the signs and symptoms of dilated cardiomyopathy without a history of an acute disease. Acute cardiac failure accompanied by mitral insufficiency is often the leading symptom. From a clinical viewpoint, there is no difference from chronic myocarditis.

GENERALISED AUTOIMMUNE MYOCARDITIS

Generalised autoimmune myocarditis encompasses a heterogeneous group of diseases. Some cause myocarditis as the dominant feature, while others have an arteritis as the leading pathology. These diseases are also known as collagen, connective tissue, diseases. I discuss here only the cardiac aspects of the two most important diseases relevant to children.

Systemic Lupus Erythematosus

In systemic, or disseminated, lupus erythematosus, the myocardial lesions consist mainly of fibrinoid changes in the connective tissue with a cellular reaction. Similar changes may affect the valves, notably the mitral and aortic valves. The lesions may heal leaving fibrous scars. Libman and Sacks[30] described the distinctive type of valvar and mural endocarditis that occurs in this condition. It is characterised by verrucous lesions along the line of closure of the valves, as well as along the ventricular surface of the leaflets extending onto the mural endocardium. The disease usually has a systematised character and involves many systems, including the heart. Cardiovascular manifestations are infrequent in children.

Cardiac Manifestations

The dominating cardiac feature is pericarditis. A pericardial friction rub is often present, and the chest radiograph will show an enlarged heart. Myocardial involvement may underscore cardiac failure. The latter feature may be complicated further by valvar dysfunction, either as part of the disease or secondary to the ventricular volume overload and accompanying dilation of the chambers. Mitral insufficiency is the most frequent valvar abnormality, although significant aortic insufficiency has been described. The electrocardiogram will usually show non-specific changes of the ST segment. Disturbances of rhythm and conduction are frequent.

Treatment

The treatment of choice is corticosteroids, which also have a favourable effect on the management of cardiac dysfunction. Deleterious effects on the heart have been described, nonetheless, from chronic administration of suppressive doses of prednisone.

Dermatomyositis

Pathology

Dermatomyositis is a multi-systemic disease of uncertain aetiology. It is characterised by diffuse non-suppurative inflammation of striated muscle and skin. Initially, there is oedema of the subendothelial connective tissue, with collection of inflammatory changes round cells in both skin and muscle. Hyalinised material is found in the media of the arterioles, with inflammatory reaction in and around the vessels. In the phase of healing, there may be deposition of calcium salts in skin, subcutaneous tissues, and interfascial planes of muscle. The myocardium may show loss of striations, fragmentation, and vascularisation of myocytes. The interstitial tissues of the heart may also show swelling and oedema.

Cardiac Involvement

Tachycardia is the most common finding. The electrocardiogram may be normal, although occasional abnormal T-waves may be encountered. Complete heart block and arrhythmias have been reported. Murmurs are heard in about one-tenth of cases. Cardiac enlargement and cardiac failure are uncommon. Acute myocarditis, and pericarditis with a pericardial friction rub, have been described.

Treatment and Prognosis

In most instances, long-term treatment with prednisone is beneficial. Other immunosuppressive agents are rarely required. Most children will recover, and medication can be discontinued over 1 or 2 years.

PERICARDITIS

Pericarditis is defined as an inflammatory reaction of the pericardium in response to injury, whether infectious or non-infectious in nature. Its precise incidence is unknown, but there is evidence that, clinically, pericarditis may often pass unnoticed. Indeed, clinical recognition will depend heavily upon the type and severity of the pericardial reaction. When limited, it may easily resolve without attracting notice. It often co-exists with myocarditis. As with myocarditis, the aetiology of pericarditis differs considerably from one part of the world to another. Infectious causes, such as tuberculosis, and pericarditis caused by a generalised autoimmune disease, such as rheumatic fever, are rare in the West. They still form a major threat in other parts of the world.

Pathophysiology

The pericardium is a double-layered sack lined by mesothelial cells and lubricated by a thin film of fluid. This construction enables the heart to move freely without friction.

An accumulation of fluid within the sack, however, may cause cardiac dysfunction, particularly when it occurs over a short period of time. Likewise, a fibrous change within the pericardial layers may have an effect upon cardiac function.

An inflammatory response of pericardium may cause exudation as part of the reaction. This may lead, in turn, to an excessive accumulation of fluid within the pericardial sack. This can cause a rise in intrapericardial pressure. Compression of the heart by the pericardial fluid can cause a decrease of cardiac output, stroke volume, and systolic arterial pressure, resulting in cardiac tamponade. The pericardium is relatively inelastic, and as a result, the pressure-volume relationship of the heart has a progressively rising slope. An initial increase in intrapericardial fluid does not result in a substantial rise in pressure, whereas additional accumulation of fluid will very soon result in a significant elevation of pressure. Likewise, in patients with signs and symptoms of cardiac tamponade owing to excessive intrapericardial fluid, evacuation of a small amount may cause a marked decrease in pressure.

The time during which the fluid accumulates plays a major role. Slow accumulation of fluid will stretch the pericardium gradually. This is much better tolerated than conditions that lead to a rapid increase, and hence equally rapid build-up of pressure. In more severe forms of pericarditis, the increased pressures will lead to impaired venous return during ventricular diastole. This results in a decline in cardiac output. During inspiration, the blood pressure may abnormally fall by more than 10 mm Hg, leading to the so-called paradoxical pulse. In its most severe form, no further filling of the cardiac chambers is possible, and the patient will die with signs of electro-mechanical dissociation. Acute cardiac tamponade is rare in infants and children.

In patients with a haemodynamically significant build-up of pressure within the pericardial sack, several compensatory mechanisms develop in an attempt to maintain an adequate cardiac output. An increase in heart rate, together with peripheral vasoconstriction, increases the afterload of the heart. This results in a higher mean pressure at the expense of a narrow pulse pressure. These compensatory mechanisms are vital. They should not be corrected, as cardiac output may then drop even further. Injudicious use of diuretics in such circumstances can make matters worse rather than better. Constrictive pericarditis was once most commonly seen as a complication of tuberculous pericarditis. Acute viral or idiopathic pericarditis is now a more common antecedent.[31] It is uncommon in childhood.

Clinical Features

In adults with acute fibrinous pericarditis, precordial pain is often the dominant symptom. In childhood, this symptom is less important. When it does occur, the site, radiation, severity, and character of the pain are highly variable. The discomfort may be diminished by sitting up and leaning forward. Other manoeuvres, such as inspiration, deep breathing, and coughing, may increase the sensation of discomfort. At this stage, the pericarditis does not necessarily interfere with the circulation.

At physical examination, the friction rub is the most typical and diagnostic finding, although its absence does not exclude the presence of pericarditis. The rub is maximal along the left sternal border but is often audible over the entire precordium. It is best heard with the patient sitting up or leaning forward. When the pericardial effusion increases, the friction rub may be heard intermittently, or it may disappear totally. The presence of a pericardial rub, however, does not exclude the presence of a large effusion. With marked effusions, the heart sounds are often muffled, and they may become extremely faint. The development of a pericardial effusion does not always produce symptoms. Hence, it may escape clinical notice.

With an increase of fluid, cardiac tamponade will develop. This is characterised by a rise in venous pressure, an enlargement of the liver, and the presence of peripheral oedema. The systolic blood pressure is low, and the pulse pressure is narrow. A paradoxical pulse is often present. The patient usually appears sick, anxious, and distressed, and is cyanosed and dyspnoeic. Moreover, fever, tachycardia and tachypnoea are commonly present. Signs and symptoms of toxicity are often present when the pericarditis is caused by bacterial infection. This condition should be considered an emergency, requiring prompt medical or surgical treatment. A large pericardial effusion can compress the lower part of the lung. This can result in dullness on percussion and bronchial breathing laterally and at the back, a combination known as Ewart's sign.

Investigations

Echocardiography

Cross sectional echocardiography is the most important diagnostic technique. If a pericardial effusion is suspected as a cause of haemodynamic compromise, the examination should be undertaken urgently. In the normal heart, the pericardial sack is hardly identified. The anterior right ventricular wall of the heart is in direct contact with the anterior chest wall, and the inferior and posterior left ventricular walls are in direct contact with the diaphragm, the posterior mediastinal structures, and the pleura. A pericardial effusion will widen the space because of the accumulation of fluid, which does not reflect ultrasound (Fig. 53-4). Echocardiography will show this echo-free space around the heart. Thickening of the pericardium is an uncommon finding. Cross sectional echocardiography permits an approximate estimation of the quantity of the collected fluid.

The majority of patients with small-to-moderate effusions demonstrate essentially normal cardiac motion. Patients with an acute small-volume tamponade produced by a small volume of fluid may demonstrate a limited motion of the cardiac walls. In the presence of large effusions, excessive cardiac displacement may occur. This is observed mainly in benign viral pericarditis and malignancies, but it is rare in children. Cardiac tamponade is a clinical and not an echocardiographic diagnosis.[32] The echocardiographic differentiation of a haemodynamically insignificant effusion from one with tamponade is not easy, but the findings indicating tamponade are diastolic collapse of the right atrial, right ventricular, and left atrial walls.[33] In addition, when there is tamponade, Doppler interrogation of the superior caval vein will show an absence of diastolic flow.[34]

Radiology

The cardiac silhouette may be normal as long as a sizeable effusion is absent. Fluid in the pericardial sack manifests itself radiologically as an enlarged silhouette. In borderline

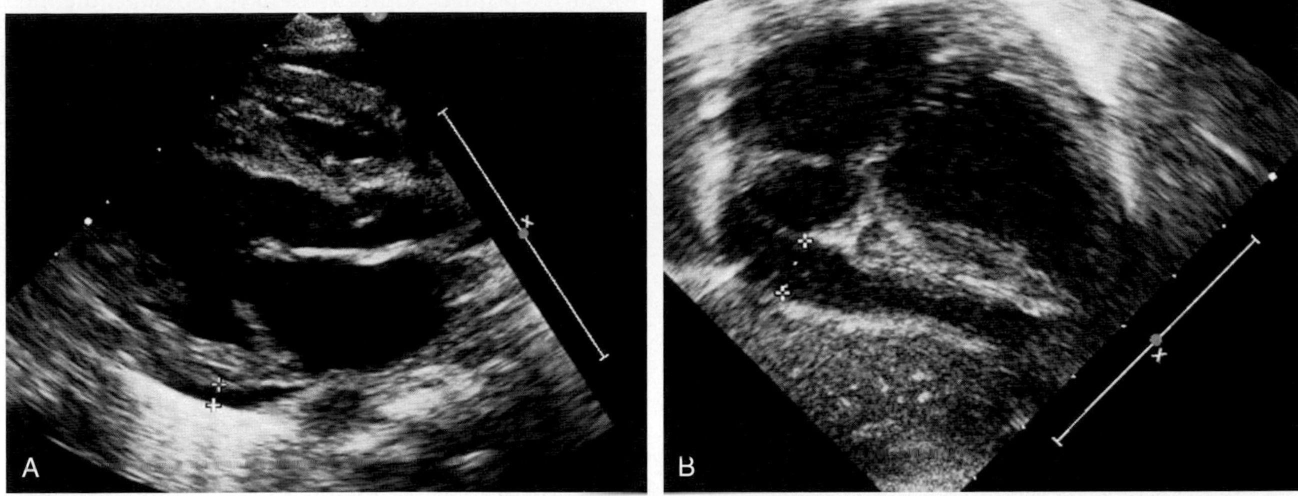

Figure 53-4 The cross sectional echocardiograms show a pericardial effusion. The parasternal long-axis view (**A**) shows a small posterior effusion behind the left ventricular free wall, between the two cross hairs. There is also a collection anterior to the right ventricle. The subcostal view (**B**) shows a large anterior collection of fluid extending from around the right atrium and ventricle to the apex of the heart (between cross hairs). At the level of the right atrium, it measured over 8 mm in width.

cases, comparison with a previous radiograph can be most helpful. As fluid accumulates, the cardiac silhouette increases. This manifests as blunting of the cardiophrenic angles, and disappearance of the sharp angulations between contiguous structures of the heart and great vessels. Changes in the configuration of the cardiac silhouette are occasionally observed when the patient is changed from a recumbent to an upright position. In children, this is not a very reliable finding.

Electrocardiography

Sequential electrocardiographic changes are observed in most patients with pericarditis[35] (Fig. 53-5). They are the result of subepicardial myocardial damage. In the initial stage of the disease, the ST segment is elevated in almost all leads except for leads V_1 and aVR, which often remain unaltered. After a few hours to days, the ST segments may return to the baseline, and the T waves may become flat (Fig. 53-6). In a later stage, the T waves may become inverted. The electrocardiogram may return to normal during convalescence, although the T waves may remain inverted for several months. They may occasionally remain in this form as a permanent change.

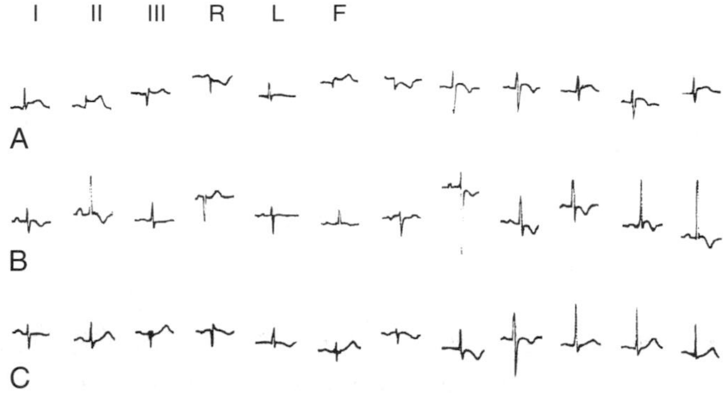

I II III R L F

A

B

C

Figure 53-5 The electrocardiograms are from a 7-year-old boy with pericarditis. On the first day of fever, when he suffered precordial pain, there is ST elevation in nearly all leads (**A**). After 4 weeks (**B**), there are negative T waves, especially in the leads I, II, V_4-V_6. After 1 year (**C**), the electrocardiogram is nearly normal, but there is still a flat T wave in lead I.

In patients with pericardial effusion, the electrocardiogram may have a generalised low voltage. Sinus tachycardia unrelated to fever or other cardiac problems may be present in the initial phase. Supraventricular tachycardias, and ventricular ectopic beats, are a regular phenomenon. None of these changes, however, can be considered specific for pericarditis. Indeed, the electrocardiogram may occasionally remain completely normal.

Pericardiocentesis

Where there is tamponade, or when the pericardial fluid needs to be drained for diagnostic reasons, the choice is between percutaneous aspiration and surgical evacuation. The echocardiographic appearances are of critical importance in determining the correct approach. Where there is tamponade, with a large, tense collection of non-loculated fluid, aspiration is usually the quickest and safest approach.

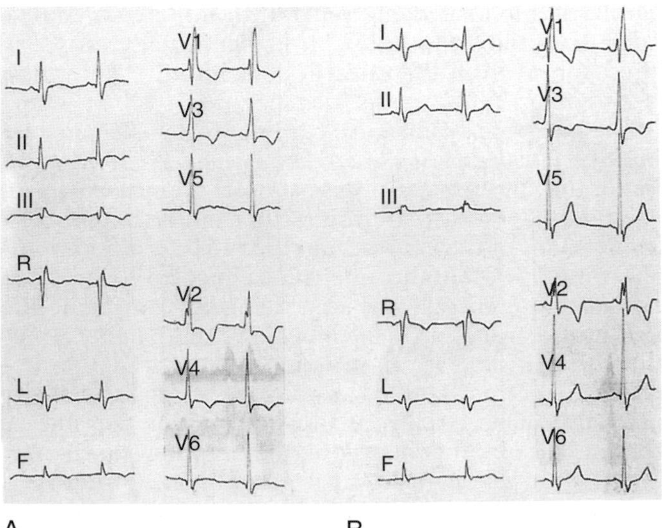

Figure 53-6 The electrocardiogram is taken from a 14-year-old girl with pericarditis. On admission, 1 week after onset of the disease (**A**), the T waves are flat in the leads I, II, V_5, and V_6 and negative in II, III, ACF, and V_4. After 4 weeks (**B**), the electrocardiogram has normalised.

This should always be done with echocardiographic guidance. Screening with X-ray and electrocardiographic guidance are also of value. The safest approach is subxiphoid. Ideally, the patient should be tilted head up, thus encouraging the pericardial fluid to collect anteriorly and inferiorly. Under local anaesthesia, a needle is inserted at about 45 degrees to the abdominal wall. It should be angled cranially, and slightly toward the left. The needle is aspirated as it is advanced. As the pericardium is entered, it is felt to give, and the pericardial fluid will fill the syringe. If the needle is connected to the V lead of an electrocardiogram, the signal will indicate if it has been advanced too far and touched the heart. Radiography can be used, or echocardiographic contrast can be injected, if there is doubt about the position of the tip of the needle.

Once the pericardium is entered, it is best to exchange the needle for a soft pigtail catheter over a wire. The pericardial fluid can then be aspirated. In the setting of recurrent accumulations of fluid, the pigtail catheter can be left in place as a pericardial drain. The fluid should be sent for bacteriologic and cytologic examination. Percutaneous aspiration is a straightforward and safe procedure where there is a large anterior collection of fluid. When the collection is small, or predominantly posterior, aspiration is more difficult and more dangerous. Under these circumstances, or when the fluid is loculated or the accumulation is recurrent, surgical evacuation with the creation of a pericardial window should be considered.

Specific Syndromes

Acute Bacterial Pericarditis

Since the introduction of antibiotics, the incidence of acute bacterial pericarditis has declined drastically. In the West, it has become a rare condition. It remains an important disease, nonetheless, from the point of view of therapy and prognosis. In most instances, bacterial pericarditis is caused by septicaemia, or direct spread from another site of infection, although such a primary site may pass unnoticed. Well-known sources for bacterial pericarditis are pyelonephritis, osteomyelitis, tonsillitis, bacterial pneumonia, and left-sided empyema. Pericarditis may complicate a bacterial endocarditis. It is then usually caused by direct spread from the valvar lesions into the epicardium (see Chapter 55).

The microorganisms most commonly involved are *Haemophilus influenzae, Staphylococcus, Pneumococcus, Meningococcus,* and *Streptococcus* species. Almost any microorganism, however, may cause pericarditis.[36] In children in particular, involvement of the pericardium used to be a most hazardous complication of the tuberculous infection.

Usually the disease has an acute onset with pain, high fever, tachycardia, and tachypnoea. The children often present with signs and symptoms of toxicity. Indeed, the clinical findings of pericardial tamponade and sepsis are highly suggestive of bacterial pericarditis. A friction rub may be present but, on other occasions, the heart may be enlarged with a rapid rate without a friction rub. These findings in the presence of high fever are most suggestive for the presence of bacterial pericarditis. The patient may rapidly deteriorate, and prompt and adequate therapy is required.

Since bacterial pericarditis is often secondary to another infection elsewhere, an intensive search is always necessary for such a primary source. Whenever possible, the medical treatment of bacterial pericarditis should be based on the identification of the primary organism, so that the most effective treatment can be selected. Any previous antibacterial treatment may interfere with this goal. Microbiological and chemical investigations of the pericardial fluid are essential. Cytological studies should be performed to exclude a malignancy.

Blood cultures are important, and from three to five sets should be taken in the first 1 or 2 days after admission. In two-fifths to four-fifths of patients, these cultures will be positive, depending on the organism involved. Specific stains for acid-fast bacteria in the sputum, gastric contents, or urine may disclose tuberculosis as the primary disease. Lumbar puncture may be necessary to prove or eliminate concomitant meningitis.

Appropriate treatment consists of prompt and adequate antibiotic therapy, together with evacuation of the pericardial fluid. The antibiotic therapy should be guided by the sensitivity of the causative organism. If possible, broad-spectrum antibiotics should be avoided. The duration of treatment depends upon the clinical response, but a total period of antibiotic therapy of at least 4 to 6 weeks is usually necessary. The curve of the fever, sedimentation rate, and white blood cell count may be helpful in evaluating the effectiveness of the treatment. A pericardial tap may be sufficient for diagnostic purposes, but a needle or a small-bore pericardiocentesis tube is inadequate for the evacuation of the pericardial fluid. This is because the pus is often loculated or thick. Subxiphoid surgical drainage with a large-bore pericardiostomy tube, or a pericardiectomy, should be performed to obtain the optimal results.

Acute Viral Pericarditis

Viral pericarditis is almost always accompanied by a myocarditis. It is the latter that usually dominates the clinical manifestations. The precise incidence of viral myopericarditis is unknown, but it is probably much higher than can be distilled from the reports in the literature. It is likely that many cases of viral myopericarditis will pass unnoticed. In approximately four-fifths of patients with the typical signs and symptoms of acute pericarditis, the aetiology cannot be established, even after extensive laboratory studies. In many instances, therefore, the viral origin of an acute pericarditis will never be proven. Such cases are better termed acute benign, or idiopathic, pericarditis. Instances of acute pericarditis have been documented with many different viruses.

The typical signs and symptoms of acute viral pericarditis are a low-grade temperature, chest pain, and a friction rub. They often develop after an infection of the upper respiratory tract. The children appear less ill than those seen with bacterial pericarditis. The white blood cell count is usually not elevated, and a relative lymphocytosis may be present. In infants, malaise, problems with feeding, tachycardia, and tachypnoea are often the presenting symptoms.

A pericardial effusion may develop rapidly, but tamponade is rare in the acute phase of viral pericarditis. Every attempt should be made to unravel the aetiology of the pericarditis. Direct proof, however, that the virus is the immediate cause of the pericarditis can only be obtained when the virus is isolated from the pericardium itself. Hence, a diagnostic pericardiocentesis must be considered. Pericardial fluid should be cultured for all types of organism, and extensive biochemical and cytological investigations should be performed.

The therapy of acute pericarditis is symptomatic. It includes bedrest, particularly in those who have myocardial involvement, until the evidence of the infection has disappeared. Precordial pain may be relieved by salicylates, codeine, and other drugs. When there are arrhythmias, antiarrhythmic drugs may be used with care. The use of corticosteroids is best avoided, as it is thought to increase the risk of the development of chronic relapsing pericarditis. Pericardiocentesis is indicated in patients showing signs and symptoms of tamponade.

The prognosis is usually favourable. The disease is often self-limiting, with complete recovery in 3 to 4 weeks. In infants and children with diffuse myocardial involvement, nonetheless, the disease may lead to death. In the fullness of time, a recurrent chronic pericarditis, probably related to a cellular immune mechanism, or a constrictive pericarditis may develop and require surgical intervention.

Post-pericardiotomy Syndrome

Any episode of acute pericarditis may be followed by recurrent pericarditis. This includes the acute pericarditis that accompanies myocardial infarction, when the recurrence is called Dressler's syndrome. Of more relevance in children is the sequence following cardiac surgery involving opening of the pericardium, when it is called the post-pericardiotomy syndrome. The cardiac surgical procedure is followed by an acute illness, with fever, and pericardial and pleural inflammatory reactions. The symptoms develop mostly in the first week after operation, but a febrile period of 2 to 3 weeks is not uncommon. Further relapses are also uncommon, but can appear as long as months or years after the initial event. The pathogenesis of the disease is unclear. Development of anti-heart antibodies in a high percentage of the patients suggests a secondary autoimmune response, possibly in association with a viral infection. There is often an eosinophilia.[37]

The earliest clinical manifestation is a sustained or spiked fever, usually of between 38 and 39 degrees Celsius. Sometimes the children feel ill, with symptoms of general malaise. All the features of pericarditis may be present, including the typical precordial pain. A friction rub is often present. Cardiac tamponade may require pericardiocentesis. Initially, the fluid withdrawn is serosanguineous, but at a later stage only serous fluid is obtained. The fluid is sterile. The chest radiograph and the electrocardiogram show the features of pericarditis. The echocardiogram is indispensable in demonstrating the pericardial fluid, and in differentiating the syndrome from cardiac failure of other causes. Signs and symptoms of pleural involvement are common, especially on the left.

The disease is self-limiting over a period of 2 to 3 weeks. The most important therapeutic measure is bedrest until the fever has disappeared. Salicylates or indomethacin are useful agents in lowering the temperature and diminishing the precordial pain. In the severely ill child, a course of prednisolone, starting at 2 mg/kg per day, and reducing over 2 weeks, is very effective in normalising body temperature and reducing the pain. Colchicine has been used in adults, and has been found to be effective in the treatment of flare-ups and in the prevention of recurrences.[38] There have been reports of its use in children.[39] Diuretics may be useful in reducing the effusion, but should be used with caution. Prompt pericardiocentesis is indicated in patients who develop cardiac tamponade.

The complete reference list can be found on the companion Expert Consult web site at www.expertconsult.com.

ANNOTATED REFERENCES

- Baughman KL: Diagnosis of myocarditis: Death of the Dallas criteria. Circulation 2006;113:593–595.
- Bowles NE, Ni J, Kearney DL, et al: Detection of viruses in myocardial tissues by polymerase chain reaction: Evidence of adenovirus as a common cause of myocarditis in children and adults. J Am Coll Cardiol 2003;42:466–472.

  The approach to the histological diagnosis of myocarditis has changed in recent years with the realisation of the shortcomings of the Dallas criterions. Analysis of myocardial samples using polymerase chain reaction has also changed our views about the common viral aetiologies.
- Magnami JW, Dec W: Myocarditis: Current trends in diagnosis and treatment. Circulation 2006;113:876–890.
- Burch M: Immune suppressive treatment in paediatric myocarditis: Still awaiting the evidence. Heart 2004;90;1103–1104.

  Two reviews about the current approach to treatment of myocarditis. Much of the evidence is based upon studies in the adult population. There is surprisingly little evidence to support much of the treatment commonly used in children.
- Andrews RE, Fenton MJ, Ridout DA, Burch M: New-onset cardiac failure due to heart muscle disease in childhood: A prospective study in the United Kingdom and Ireland. Circulation 2008;117:79–84.
- Towbin JA, April M, Lowe MS, et al: Incidence, causes and outcomes of dilated cardiomyopathy in children. JAMA 2006;296:1867–1876.

  Two recent studies about the incidence and prognosis of dilated cardiomyopathy in children. They are concerned with slightly different populations, but the overall picture is similar. The conventional wisdom that a third of children recover, a third survive with impaired cardiac function, and a third die or need transplantation is in fact not far from the truth. Outcome in both studies is better in younger patients, and in those with better cardiac function at presentation.
- Reddy PS, Curtiss EI, Uretsky BF: Spectrum of hemodynamic changes in cardiac tamponade. Am J Cardiol 1990;66:1487–1491.

  Tamponade is a haemodynamic diagnosis, so understanding the haemodynamic effects of a pericardial effusion is important if the diagnosis is to be made reliably. This is an essential analysis on the progressive haemodynamic changes brought about by a pericardial effusion leading to cardiac tamponade.

Rheumatic Fever

CHAPTER 54A

CLEONICE C. COELHO MOTA, VERA DEMARCHI AIELLO, and ROBERT H. ANDERSON

Rheumatic fever is an acute, diffuse, and non-suppurative inflammatory disease that occurs in susceptible individuals as a late complication after an untreated pharyngotonsillitis, the infection itself sometimes being asymptomatic. It is caused by a group A β-haemolytic *Streptococcus*, specifically, *Streptococcus pyogenes*. The process is triggered by an inadequate immunological response, both humoral and cellular. There are four distinct phases characterizing the disease. The initial streptococcal pharyngotonsillitis is followed by latent period, and then by the acute and chronic phases. The chronic phase is also known as rheumatic heart disease, when the cardiac lesions remain as sequels of the acute phase. The disease has the potential to involve the heart, joints, brain, and subcutaneous and cutaneous tissues. Cardiac injury is the most important manifestation, and it is the injuries to the heart which produce its clinical, social, and economic impact.

Both rheumatic fever and chronic rheumatic heart disease continue to pose serious concerns with regard to health in many parts of the world, and present a significant challenge for those involved in providing health care. In developed countries, although its incidence has been markedly reduced since the 1950s, rheumatic fever remains a risk because of its potential for resurgence.[1] The disease has not yet been completely eradicated. As has been pointed out, prevention will be less than optimal until the pathogenesis of the disease has been totally elucidated.[2,3] In developing countries, this preventable disease remains both socially and clinically devastating, with significant rates of morbidity and mortality. The acute episodes of rheumatic fever are still a cause of death in childhood, and the chronic disease is the most important cause of acquired cardiac disease in children, adolescents, and young adults, besides being considered the most frequent condition necessitating valvar surgery in adults. The repercussions of the disease involve patients of all ages, since the valvar sequels can be carried throughout life. The children and adolescents, who are most frequently admitted to hospital with acute episodes, are the same group of patients who, after the fourth decade of life, form the largest group when analysis is focused on invasive intervention and death. The economic impact must also be considered, not only with regard to the financial cost of clinical and surgical treatments, but also relative to the loss of productivity as the result of disability acquired at an early age.

HISTORICAL BACKGROUND

From the historical perspective, the clinical manifestations of rheumatic fever had been well described prior to the recognition of the complete syndrome. Arthritis had been mentioned since the days of Hippocrates, but only in the 17th century did the French doctor Guillaume de Baillou distinguish acute articular rheumatism from the other forms of rheumatism. In the posthumous edition of the *Liber de Rheumatismo et Pleuritide dorsali*, published in 1642, he was the first author to use the term rheumatism to describe the acute form of arthritis. Thomas Sydenham, in England, in his book *Observationes medicinae*, published in 1676, provided an accurate description of the acute migratory polyarthritis as distinct from gout. He also described, 2 years later, St Vitus's dance, another major manifestation of rheumatic fever, which we now call Sydenham's chorea. Important discoveries in cardiac pathology were made in the 18th century. Warty vegetations, and thickening of the valvar leaflets as an isolated postmortem feature, were recognised in 1709 by Giovanni Maria Lancisi, while Raymond Vieussens, in 1715, contributed a description of mitral stenosis, with calcification of the leaflets. Giovanni Battista Morgagni, in the tome *De Sedibus*, published in 1761, dealt with lesions of all cardiac valves, and described endocardial vegetations. The association of cardiac disease and rheumatism was noted by Morgagni, but deemed coincidental. It was Richard Pulteney, in the same year, who on the basis of his observation of pathology called attention to the association of cardiac involvement and acute articular rheumatism. Matthew Baillie, nonetheless, in his tome entitled *A Series of Engravings Tending to Illustrate the Morbid Anatomy of Some of the Most Important Parts of the Human Body*, gave credit for this recognition of a causal relationship between cardiac disease and rheumatism to David Pitcairn. The first full account of the pathology of rheumatic fever was then provided in 1808 by Dundas, who underscored the relationship of the cardiac features to rheumatism. In 1812, a detailed report was given in *On Rheumatism of the Heart* by William Charles Wells, who in 1813 also described the subcutaneous nodules. This author confirmed that, although Pitcairn had failed to provide a written record, he had already, by 1788, established the association between rheumatism and cardiac lesions. The introduction of the stethoscope by René Laennec, in 1816, facilitated the study of cardiac diseases, but not until 1832 did Jean-Baptiste Bouillaud provide a detailed account of rheumatic cardiac disease, correlating the clinical events with the post-mortem findings. In his treatise *Traité clinique des maladies du coeur* he introduced the term endocarditis and clarified the clinical picture, giving an accurate account of the cardiac involvement and other manifestations in patients with rheumatic fever. The eponym *maladie de Bouillaud* for rheumatic fever recognised his great contribution, distinguished by its exceptional accuracy and clinical significance. In the same year, James Hope, as had already been pointed out by Wells and Dundas, detailed and emphasised the association of acute pericarditis with rheumatic fever. Cheadle, in 1886 described the complete syndrome, emphasising the set of clinical manifestations we currently recognise as major criterians, namely, carditis, arthritis, chorea, subcutaneous nodules, and erythema marginatum. Subsequently, the pathognomonic and distinctive microscopic nodules of rheumatic carditis were described in 1904 by Ludwig Aschoff.[4–8]

The first report of a possible connection between a bacterial infection and rheumatic fever had been suggested by Mantle in 1887, but it was not until 1930 that the causal relationship between infection by the β-haemolytic streptococcus and rheumatic fever was established.[9–11] From then on, data about the disease was gathered in many other fields. Todd, in 1932,[12] introduced a method for measuring one of the antibodies developed by the human body after the contact with the bacteria. Then, 1 year later, Lancefield[13] classified the streptococcus into five distinct groups. Subsequently,[14] continuous administration of sulphanilamide was shown to prevent recurrences, followed in 1950[15] and 1951[16] with demonstration that adequate treatment of the streptococcal pharyngitis with penicillin prevented the disease.

As early as 1944, Thomas Duckett Jones had proposed a set of clinical and laboratorial data to guide and reduce the over-diagnosis of rheumatic fever.[17] The Jones criterians were subsequently modified and updated by the Committee of the American Heart Association.[18–22] They have long been recognised as guidelines for the diagnosis of the first episode of the acute phase. The knowledge of the action of antibiotics in preventing the disease, and the systematisation of the diagnosis by means of the important Jones criterions, heralded a new era of studies.

EPIDEMIOLOGY

Rheumatic fever has a universal distribution, albeit that significant differences in the rates of incidence and prevalence depend on the interaction of characteristics of the aetiologic agent and its human host, besides environmental and socioeconomic conditions. Due to the causal relationship of streptococcal pharyngotonsillitis and rheumatic fever, the epidemiology of the two diseases is closely related. Rheumatic fever is more frequent among children and adolescents between the ages 5 and 15, and has a peak of incidence around the ages of 8 to 9 years. These ages coincide with the peak of streptococcal pharyngotonsillitis in school-aged children, this infection being less common in late adolescence and in adults. Likewise, rheumatic fever is uncommon in children under 4 years of age, and exceedingly rare under the age of 2.[23–25] The increased number of young patients can be attributed to the anticipation of the school years. Data from Brazil revealed that 2.5% of patients had their first episode under the age of 3.[26] In a study from India, Aschoff bodies were found in one-tenth of autopsied cases, the majority from patients between 16 and 40 years of age, indicating a recent attack of carditis.[27] Under special circumstances, such as focal epidemics of streptococcal infections in military populations or closed institutions, the incidence of rheumatic fever can increase in adults.[28,29]

Rheumatic fever occurs in all populations, and shows equal frequency in both genders. The exception is Sydenham's chorea, which is more common in females, and is hardly ever seen in males after puberty.[30] Rheumatic fever has usually been reported as a disease of the temperate climates, but currently it is more prevalent in warm tropical climates, especially in developing countries. Similarly, the influence of seasonal variation in the rates of incidence is now less defined, but in general follows that of streptococcal infections, which are most commonly observed in late winter and early spring.[31,32] The disease is reputed to be more frequent in urban centres than in rural communities, but this is probably due to over-crowding.[33] Although data thus far is inconclusive, it has been suggested that there is an increased susceptibility to rheumatic fever in certain ethnic groups. The aboriginals of Australia's Northern Territory, and the Polynesians, both from rural areas, show a markedly increased incidence of the disease.[31,34] In Hawaii, wide differences in the prevalence of chronic rheumatic heart disease have been documented in the Samoan schoolchildren when compared with the Caucasian Hawaiians[35] Similarly, higher frequencies of rheumatic fever and chronic rheumatic heart disease have been found in the Maori population of New Zealand,[36] and among black schoolchildren in South Africa.[37] Many factors, however, can overlap and interfere in the calculations of the incidence of rheumatic fever and the prevalence of chronic rheumatic heart disease, since different rates can be found under diverse environmental conditions for any given population. In this context, besides the role played by the bacteria and human host, other factors, such as differences in patterns of living condition and streptococcal exposure, in addition to quality of and access to health care, are important and can impact the geographical distribution of the disease, as well as the severity of its sequels.

All over the world, pharyngotonsillitis is one of the most prevalent infections caused by the β-haemolytic streptococcus. It accounts for up to one-third of the throat infections in children, and up to one-tenth in adults [29,38] Although the streptococcal infections are very frequent, only a few individuals develop rheumatic fever. It is calculated that, under endemic conditions, 0.3% of untreated infections, and 3% in epidemics, will lead to a first episode of rheumatic fever.[39] In spite of a marked decrease of rheumatic fever in the developed countries, the incidence of infections of the upper respiratory tract by the group A *Streptococcus* has not been reduced. Even considering that the strains of bacterium producing the infection are often relatively attenuated, more virulent strains can change the characteristics of the infections and their sequels. Emergence of mucoid strains was observed at the close of the 20th century in the United States of America and Western Europe, showing an apparent temporal association with the increase in frequency and severity of the systemic invasive streptococcal infections of the skin and soft tissues such as toxic shock syndrome, sepsis, myositis, and necrotizing fasciitis. The simultaneous resurgence of rheumatic fever in the United States is also highly suggestive of a relation with the appearance of more virulent group A strains.[40–43]

Recurrences of rheumatic fever, as a consequence of inadequate prophylaxis, are more frequent in developing countries, where predisposing factors to streptococcal infections still persist. The risk of subsequent attacks increases with the number of previous attacks, with the continued exposure to streptococcal infections, and falls with age. The recurrence rate is higher during the first 5 years subsequent to the acute episode, particularly in the first 2 years. Likewise, the risk of other attacks is higher in patients receiving oral secondary prophylaxis when compared to parenteral medication. The clinical features of subsequent attacks show a tendency to mimic those seen in the initial attack.[44] Prospective follow-up to identify predictors of significant chronic rheumatic valvar disease[45] shows that almost half recurrences occur in the first 2 years of the disease (Fig. 54A-1).

In spite of a decline in both frequency and severity, rheumatic fever still remains a risk. In 1994, it was estimated by the World Health Organization that a total of 12 million individuals were affected by rheumatic fever and rheumatic heart disease worldwide.[1] In developing countries, the incidence of rheumatic fever is still very high, with a wide variation from 1.0 to 254 for each 100,000 of the population.[1,31,35] More than 336,000 cases of rheumatic fever occur in children and adolescents aged from 5 to 14.[46] Although a downward trend has been noticed worldwide, the rates in some areas are similar to those found in developed countries at the turn of the 20 century.[47,48] Investigations in the aboriginal communities in Northern Australia suggest a lifetime risk for having rheumatic fever to be as high as 5% to 7%.[34]

Rheumatic fever, nonetheless, has now become rare in developed countries, where the incidence is estimated at below 1 for each 100,000 of the population.[49] The reasons for this decline of up to 100 fold over the last 50 to 60 years are not completely understood.[50] Several factors are involved, but none can explain this decline when considered in isolation.[28,43,51,52] It has been attributed to the decreasing rheumatogenic potential of group A streptococcal strains, and to changes in susceptibility of the human host, besides the modifications in the environment. In this context, the increased nutrition and better living conditions, as a consequence of improvements in social and economic standards, have contributed to reduce the spread of the infecting agent. Other determining factors are the better availability of health care, and the advent of antimicrobial agents. The widespread use of antibiotics has accelerated the decrease of the disease, in terms of both morbidity and mortality. A fourfold acceleration of the decline was observed after the introduction of penicillin and other antibiotics.[53] Furthermore, the establishment of stricter clinical criterions enhanced the accuracy of the diagnosis, and consequently reduced over-diagnosis. Technological advances in laboratory diagnosis also improved the differential diagnosis from other cardiac diseases, such as congenital structural diseases, myocarditis, and mitral valvar prolapse, which in a clinical setting had often been misdiagnosed as rheumatic fever.

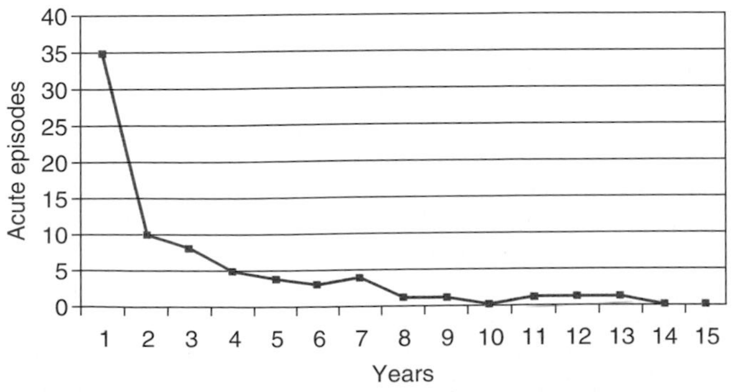

Figure 54A-1 The graph shows the frequency of recurrences in 258 children and adolescents followed up in the Rheumatic Fever Outpatients Clinic, Division of Paediatric Cardiology, Hospital das Clínicas, Federal University of Minas Gerais, Brazil.

Despite the apparent control, the disease had resurged in the United States of America by the mid-1980s. During the last two decades of the 20th century, outbreaks were reported in distinct geographical regions of the country among different age groups, mainly schoolchildren and young adults in military bases.[42,52,54] The outbreaks showed an unexpected pattern, occurring among white, middle-class patients with ready access to health care and antibiotic therapy. Between 1985 and 1988, a national survey was performed in cities of 24 states of the United States, and showed evidence of an increase in the number of cases from 5 to 12 times when compared to the previous decade.[40] Isolated reports of increased frequency of rheumatic fever also came from Europe.[55–57]

No isolated factor can be held responsible for the epidemiological changes in both the disappearance and the reappearance of rheumatic fever, and the underlying reasons have still to be completely explained. It has been questioned whether the outbreaks represented a true risk of return of the disease, or simply were an oscillation in its declining profile of incidence.[51] As was pointed out by Kaplan and Markowitz, the reasons for the virtual disappearance of rheumatic fever have not yet been sufficient to control the disease.[3,52]

AETIOLOGY AND PATHOGENESIS

A broad range of clinical manifestations may occur after a streptococcal infection, varying in severity from mild and superficial dermal infection to necrotizing fasciitis or severe septicaemia. Non-suppurative sequels depend on a delayed immune-mediated host response, and include rheumatic fever, acute glomerulonephritis, and reactive arthritis. As we have already discussed, the association between streptococcal pharyngotonsillitis and the subsequent development of rheumatic fever was recognised in the first half of the twentieth century, but the precise pathogenesis of the disease has still not been completely elucidated. Major advances in the understanding of the pathogenic mechanisms have only recently been achieved from immunological, molecular biologic, and genetic studies. Susceptibility to rheumatic fever depends on the interaction between the streptococcus and host factors, influenced also by environmental conditions. Both humoral and cellular delayed immune responses to the streptococcal throat infection take part in the process. Their extension determines the severity of the disease in one individual. In particular, autoimmunity against the tissues of the host plays a key role in the pathogenesis and progression of the disease. Molecular mimicry between streptococcal antigens and several human tissues, such as cardiac valves and myosin, cartilage, and synovial and cerebral proteins has been proposed and proved to be the basic mechanism triggering autoimmunity. Bacteria are absent from the acute and chronic tissue lesions of rheumatic fever.

STREPTOCOCCUS AND ITS ANTIGENS

Streptococcus pyogenes, or the group A *Streptococcus*, is a Gram-positive extracellular bacterium covered by an outer layer of hyaluronic acid. Its cell wall is composed of repeating units of N-acetyl-D-glucosamine carbohydrates linked to a rhamnose polymer backbone (Fig. 54A-2).

Figure 54A-2 Schematic representation of the cell wall of the group A *Streptococcus*.

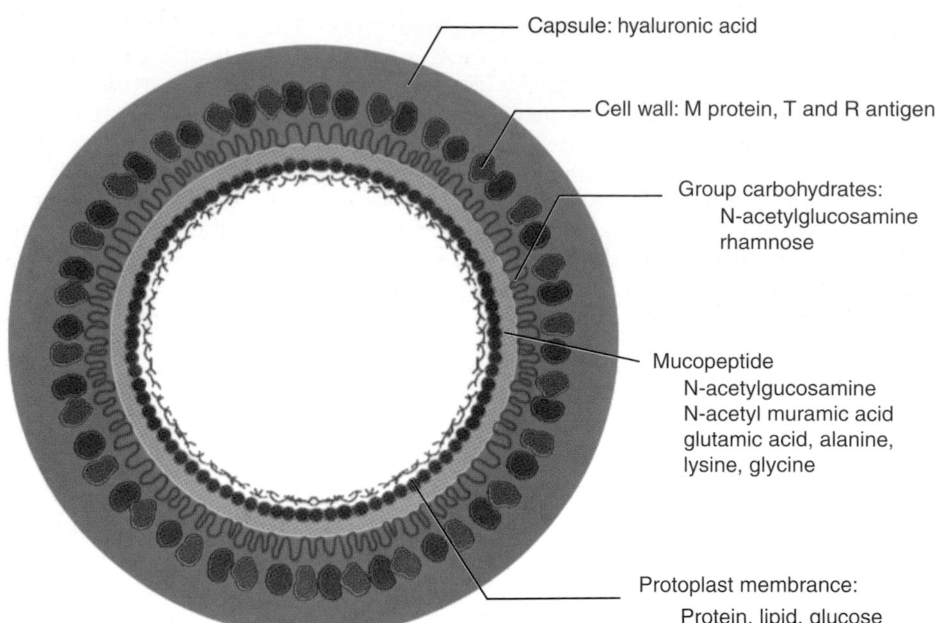

The classification of the microorganism in serogroups is based on studies that distinguished by serology the bacterial mural polysaccharides, giving groups A, B, F, and G. The concept of different bacterial strains causing disease in specific target organs emerged from decades of epidemiological studies, revealing serotypes of group A *Streptococcus* as having a strong tendency to cause pharyngotonsillitis, and others to be associated with impetigo.[41] Although different serogroups may also cause throat infections, there is no evidence linking bacteria from the remaining serological groups with the development of rheumatic fever.[1]

The M, T, and R proteins on the bacterial cell surface, along with lipoteichoic acid, are involved in the adhesion of the bacteria to the host epithelial cells, and in their ability to resist phagocytosis in the human host.[1,58] (see Fig. 54A-2). Thus far, it has proved possible to identify more than 100 M serotypes, based on the antigenic variation of the N-terminal portion.[58] The M protein is particularly important in determining the virulence of the microorganism, since it promotes avid adherence to host tissues. Moreover, it is the M protein that shares structural homology with certain α-helical human molecules such as myosin, tropomyosin, laminin, vimentin, keratin, and laminin, thus forming the basis for the immune-mediated post-infectious sequels. Laminin is an extracellular matrix protein present in the cardiac valves, being secreted by the endothelial cells that line them.

The M protein molecule itself has a variable composition (Fig. 54A-3). As explained, its N-terminal portion contains the A-repeat region that produces antigenic variation.[41] The B-repeat region also varies from serotype to serotype, while the C-repeat regions contain highly conserved epitopes. Classification of the streptococcus into class I or class II depends on whether their M protein reacts with a monoclonal antibody that targets epitopes in the C-repeat region.[1] While class I strains are predominantly negative for the production of serum opacity factor, and are recognised as rheumatogenic, class II strains produce the serum opacity factor, bind fibronectin, and are usually associated with production of glomerulonephritis.[46] Serotypes, such as M types 1, 3, 5, 6, 14, 18, and 24, have also been associated with the development of rheumatic fever. An alternative means of serotyping is to sequence the gene encoding the 5′ terminal end of the M protein. A great range of genetic diversity has been shown in this fashion in isolates recovered from many different geographical locations.[32,59,60] The identification of these so-called *emm* types present in a community at the time of an outbreak of rheumatic fever permitted recognition of the types most commonly associated to the disease, and revealed *emm* types 1, 3, 5, 6, 14, 18, 24, 17, and 29 to be rheumatogenic.[61] This concept of rheumatogenicity, however, has recently been challenged, since some types frequently associated with acute rheumatic fever are infrequently found in several communities with high burdens of the disease, where new, non-M antigen typeable microorganisms have been identified.[46,62] These new types probably result from genetic recombination between different strains of the group A *Streptococcus*. It is not surprising that a clear distinction between the rheumatogenic and non-rheumatogenic strains of the group A *Streptococcus* does not exist in areas of the world with high rates of superficial infections, since multiple genetically distinct strains circulate at the same time. This broad genetic diversity has important implications in the development of a vaccine against streptococcal infections.

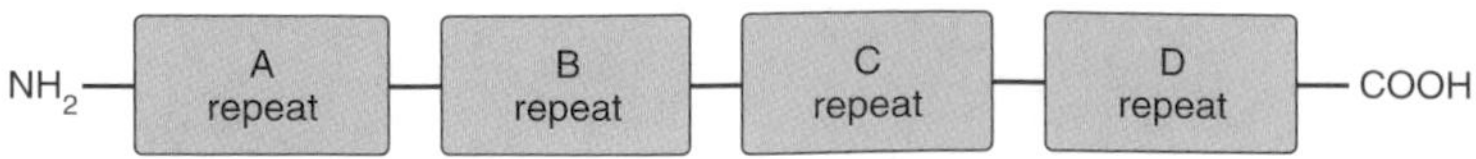

Figure 54A-3 Diagram representing the A, B, C, and D repeat regions of the streptococcal M protein. At the N-terminus, the A repeat region contains the highly variable amino acid sequences that are serotype specific. The C and D regions are highly conserved among the strains of streptococcuses.

THE HUMAN HOST

Alleles of the Human Leucocyte Antigen Associated with Rheumatic Fever

Considering that less than 3% of the patients with acute streptococcal pharyngotonsillitis develop rheumatic fever, it is reasonable to suggest that the genetic predisposition of the individual plays an important role in the pathogenesis of the disease. In the 19th century, it was suggested that both rheumatic fever and rheumatic heart disease were hereditary,[46] possibly transmitted in autosomal recessive fashion. Further studies on the determinants of host susceptibility indicated that the immune response to the streptococcal infection is genetically controlled. More recently, molecular biologic techniques have identified an association between the disease and some alleles of the major histocompatibility complex. These class II human leucocyte antigen molecules are expressed on the surface of antigen-presenting cells, such as macrophages, dendritic cells, and B cells. Together with the bound peptide antigen, they trigger the activation of T lymphocytes. Several such alleles have been associated with rheumatic fever in different countries (Table 54A-1). While DR7 is the allele most frequently associated with rheumatic fever in Brazil, Turkey, and Latvia, the DR4 allele is found in American-Caucasian, Indian, and Saudi-Arabian patients. Recently, in Mexican and Brazilian patients with rheumatic heart disease,[63,64] some alleles of the tumour necrosis factor–α, also located in the region of the major histocompatibility complex, were described with increased frequency. A possible explanation for the frequent association of certain alleles with the development of rheumatic fever and rheumatic heart disease is that these molecules might cause inappropriate activation of the T cells, resulting in autoimmunity.

TABLE 54A-1

CLASS II HLA ALLELES ASSOCIATED WITH THE DEVELOPMENT OF RHEUMATIC FEVER AND RHEUMATIC HEART DISEASE IN DIFFERENT COUNTRIES

HLA Class II Allele	Country
DR1	South Africa Martinique
DR2	USA Mexico
DR3	Turkey India
DR4	USA Saudi Arabia India
DR5	Turkey
DR6	South Africa Egypt
DR7	Brazil Turkey Latvia Egypt
DR9	USA
DQA1*0104	Japan
DQB1*05031	Japan

Modified from Guilherme L, Fae K, Oshiro SE, Kalil J: Molecular pathogenesis of rheumatic fever and rheumatic heart disease. Expert Rev Mol Med 2005;7:1–15.

Interactions Between Host and Pathogens

It is well recognised that the molecular mimicry between some antigens present on the surface of group A *Streptococcus* and specific human tissues triggers the autoimmune response causing acute rheumatic fever. Structural similarities between the streptococcal M protein and myosin are the key for the development of acute carditis. On the other hand, valvar lesions are triggered by immune reactions against human proteins such as laminin, an α-helical coiled-coil molecule present in the valvar subendothelium. Both the humoral and cellular arms of the immune response take part in the host response against these self-proteins sharing some homology with the streptococcus.

Humoral Response

After the adherence of the bacteria to the host cells, the processes of colonisation and invasion supervene, inducing the production of type-specific antibodies by B-derived mononuclear cells, leading to opsonisation and phagocytosis. As pointed out recently,[58] heart-reactive antibodies were first described by Calveti in 1945. The recognition of cross-reactive streptococcal epitopes and human antigens, mainly myosin and laminin, led to a great advance in the studies directed to the knowledge of the mechanism of the disease.

Cross-reaction between antibodies to cardiac valvar tissue and the N-acetylglucosamine of the polysaccharide from group A *Streptococcus* has been clearly demonstrated.[41,65,66] Additionally, some studies have shown that the cross-reacting antibodies bind to the endocardial surface of valves, up-regulating the local expression of adhesion molecules like vascular cell adhesion molecule-1, which facilitates infiltration of inflammatory cells inside the valvar leaflets, which are avascular, leading later to scarring[67] (Fig. 54A-4). The pathogenic mechanism responsible for the Sydenham's chorea present in some patients with acute rheumatic fever is also dependent on the cross-recognition of neuronal tissue proteins by antibodies directed to the N-acetylglucosamine of the streptococcus.[68]

Cellular Response

T lymphocytes of subsets CD4 and CD8 are the main mediators of the myocardial and valvar lesions of rheumatic fever and rheumatic heart disease, participating in a delayed-type hypersensitivity reaction (see Fig. 54A-4). In the acute phase, the pathognomonic histological feature is the Aschoff body, a granulomatous lesion found in both the myocardium and in valvar leaflets, and composed of T lymphocytes, B lymphocytes, macrophages, large mononuclear cells, and polymorphonuclear leucocytes. The nodules develop as a result of cellular infiltration through the endothelium. The presence of activated macrophages inside the bodies is consistent with an immune response of the CD4+ T helper 1 type.[69]

Proinflammatory cytokines, such as tumour necrosis factor–α and interleukin-1, are over-produced by peripheral

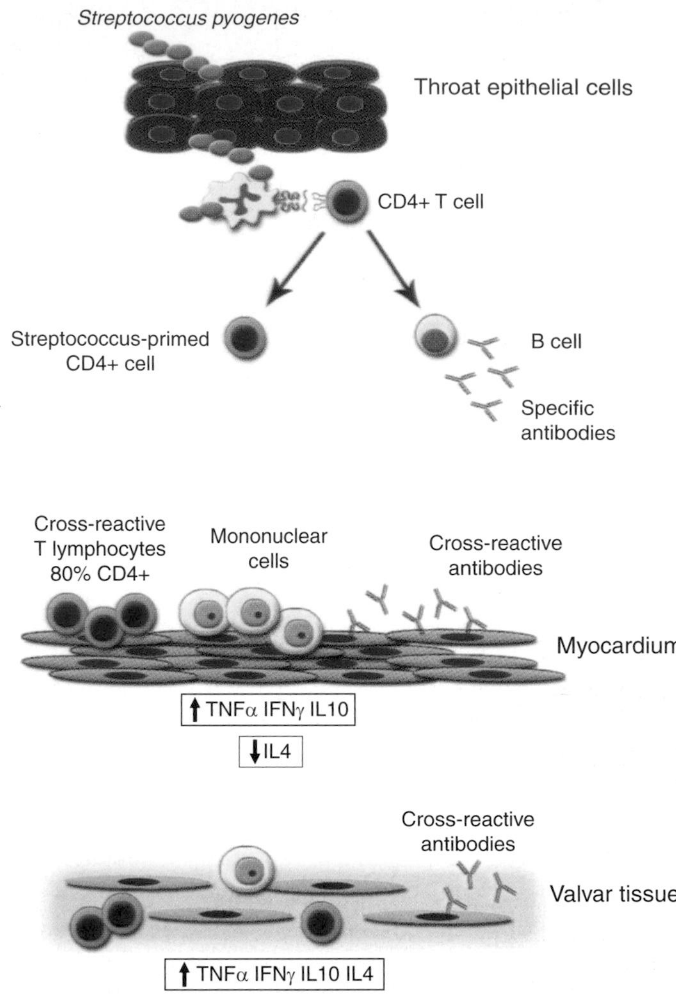

Figure 54A-4 Schematic representation of the cellular and molecular events leading to the development of rheumatic fever and the lesions found in those with rheumatic heart disease. IFN, interferon; IL4, interleukin 4; IL10, interleukin 10, TNF, tumor necrosis factor.

blood mononuclear cells in patients with rheumatic fever. They are also predominantly expressed by mononuclear inflammatory cells inside the chronic valvar lesions, indicating their local role even in the chronic phase of the disease. Cytokines are considered important second signals after infections, triggering effective immune responses in most individuals, but in the context of autoimmune diseases they induce a deleterious response. Differences in the pattern of cytokine production were observed between inflammatory cells derived from valvar and myocardial tissue from patients with rheumatic fever.[70] These findings reinforce the putative role of these regulatory cytokines in the myocardial healing, but not in valves, where the damage is progressive and permanent. The sparing of the right-sided cardiac valves in most cases of rheumatic fever is usually attributed to the lower pressure and shear stress to which they are usually submitted compared to the left-sided valves. Quadrivalvar rheumatic disease has been reported only rarely, and usually then in patients with congenitally malformed hearts.[71] The location of the acute valvar lesions along the lines of closure of the leaflets corroborates the hypothesis that lesions occur at places that are most liable to trauma.

MORPHOLOGY OF THE ACUTE CARDIAC AND EXTRACARDIAC LESIONS

The sequence of immunological events described above culminates in the development of acute rheumatic fever, which presents as exudative and proliferative inflammatory reactions in the connective tissue of the affected organs. These lesions are more distinctive within the heart, but involve also the joints, subcutaneous tissue, brain, and vessels of the lung. Basically, they are characterised by mononuclear inflammatory cells around a focus of fibrinoid necrosis. In the heart, the pericardial, myocardial, endocardial layers are all affected, hence there is a pancarditis. The histological landmark of acute rheumatic fever is the Aschoff body (see Fig. 54-8).

Grossly, the pericarditis is characterised by the deposition of a serofibrinous exudate, giving the so-called bread-and-butter appearance. Acute valvar lesions are found as small vegetations of 1 to 2 millimetres along the lines of closure on the atrial aspect of the atrioventricular valves, and on the ventricular surface of the arterial valves (Fig. 54A-5). These small verrucous lesions may extend to the tendinous cords of the atrioventricular valves, and in rare instances may be associated with cordal rupture, causing severe valvar regurgitation and cardiac failure. Microscopically, the vegetations are composed of fibrin thrombus overlying an area of fibrinoid necrosis of the valvar connective tissue. These areas of necrosis are surrounded by a dense inflammatory infiltrate, containing mononuclear cells and occasional giant cells. Presumably, the fibrin vegetations accumulate on the ulcerated endocardium in areas of extrusion of the damaged collagen (Fig. 54A-6). Although the typical Aschoff bodies, pathognomonic of the disease and most commonly seen in the myocardium, are not usually found in valvar tissues, the acute valvar lesion transforms with time, showing inflammatory cells arranged in palisade around the central necrotic core. These lesions eventually heal, producing local fibrosis. Moreover, the adjacent tissue of the valvar leaflets is oedematous, and shows a diffuse non-specific mononuclear infiltrate. Neovascularisation is not a feature in this phase of the disease, but thin-walled blood vessels can be seen invading at the base of implantation of the leaflet.

In the case of a recurrent attack, the fibrin vegetations still appear on the same structures, but there are already valvar sequels, such as cordal fusion and thickening of the leaflets (Fig. 54A-7). The relative frequency of valvar involvement correlates to the haemodynamic closing pressures, the decreasing order being mitral, aortic, tricuspid, and pulmonary.

Although myocardial involvement in acute rheumatic fever is typically called myocarditis, direct myocytic injury as it is observed in viral myocarditis is not a striking feature. Instead, the finding of multiple Aschoff bodies is the fingerprint of the disease. These granulomatous nodules are usually located in the connective tissue around small vessels (Fig. 54A-8). They show fibrinoid necrosis surrounded by lymphocytes,[58] some plasma cells, and plump macrophages with abundant cytoplasm and a clear nucleus where a central wavy ribbon of condensed chromatin is observed. These are called Anitschkow cells, or caterpillar cells, the latter reflecting their appearance when cut longitudinally.

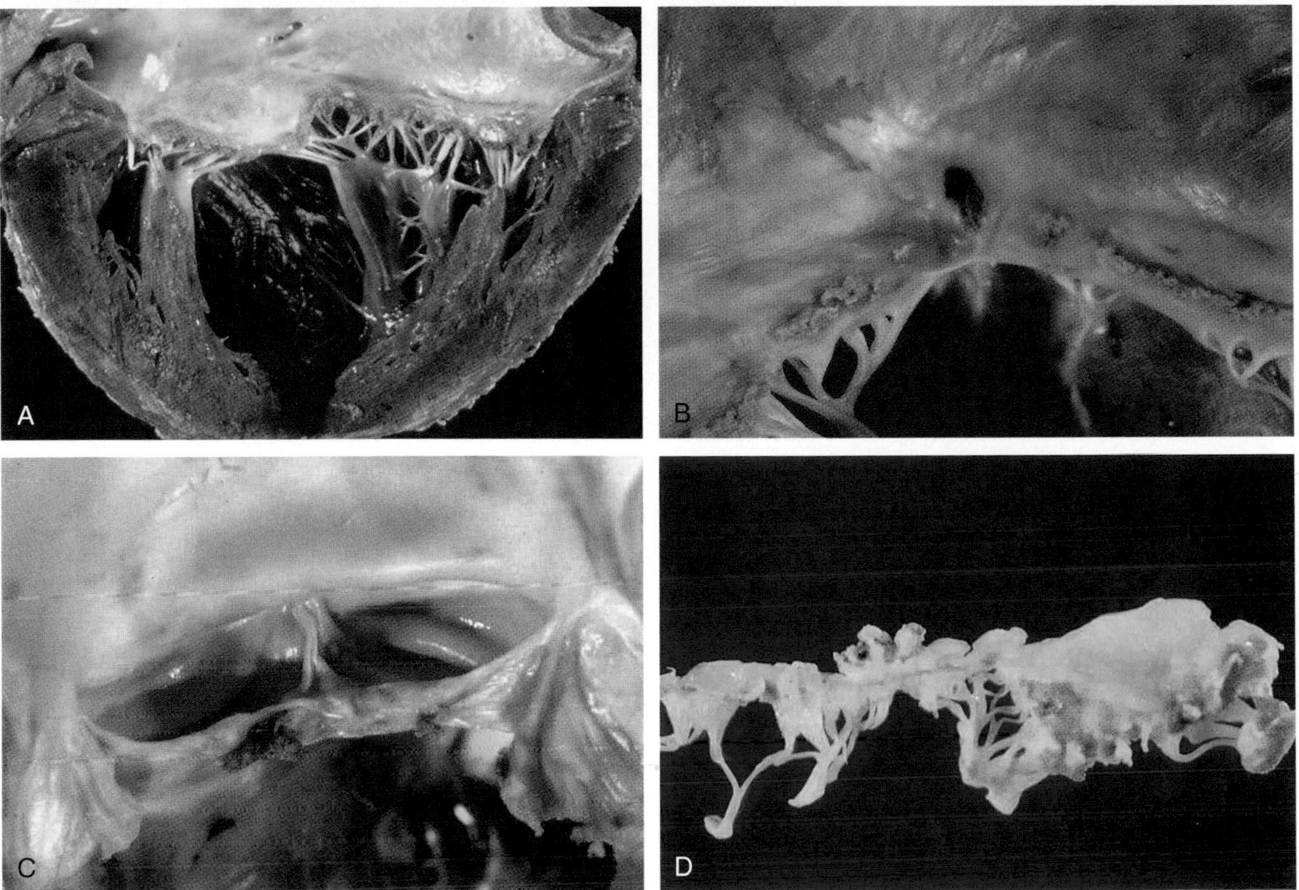

Figure 54A-5 The images show the characteristic lesions in the hearts from children who died in the acute phase of rheumatic fever. Panel **A** shows small vegetations on the line of closure of the mitral valve, with panels **B** and **C** showing similar lesions in the tricuspid and aortic valves, respectively. Note that, in panel **A**, there is moderate dilation of the left atrium and ventricle. The aortic valve shown in panel **C** also shows signs of chronic disease, characterised by partial fusion of the zone of apposition between the non-coronary and right coronary leaflets. Panel **D** shows a surgically excised mitral valve, with massive deposits of fibrin on the line of closure of both leaflets. The tendinous cords are delicate, indicating absence of chronic disease in this valve.

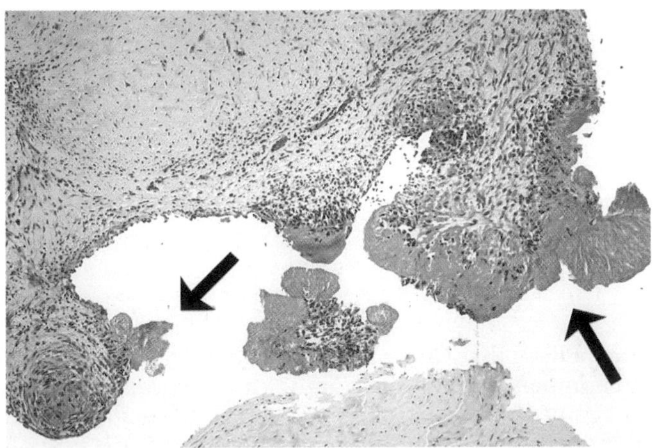

Figure 54A-6 This photomicrograph is taken from a mitral valve excised during the acute phase of rheumatic fever, and showing fibrin vegetations (*arrows*) overlying a densely inflamed valvar stroma. The section is stained with haematoxylin and eosin.

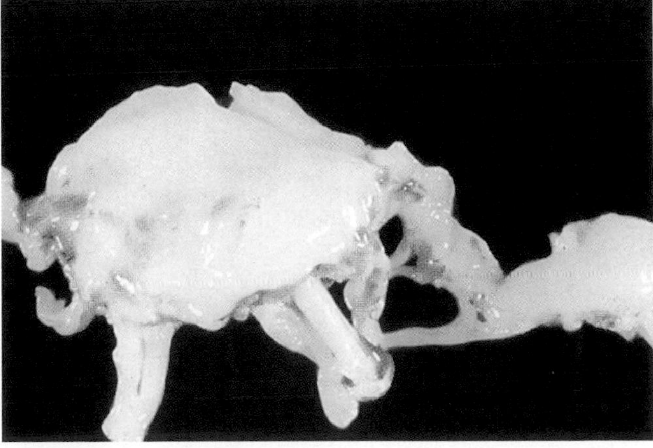

Figure 54A-7 This panel shows a section taken from a surgically excised mitral valve, revealing signs of co-existing chronic disease, with thickened leaflets and fused cords, and superimposed acute rheumatic lesions, with fibrin vegetations on the line of closure.

Multi-nucleated macrophages may also be present, and receive the name of Aschoff giant cells. Aschoff bodies often appear in the myocardium about 4 weeks after the acute onset of rheumatic fever, and may remain in the tissue for as long as 3 to 6 months. Although the earliest lesions show prominent fibrinoid necrosis and inflammation, as described above, the life cycle of the nodule continues with a gradual decrease in the cellular content. The complete healing of those lesions takes the form of a fibrous scar around small myocardial vessels.

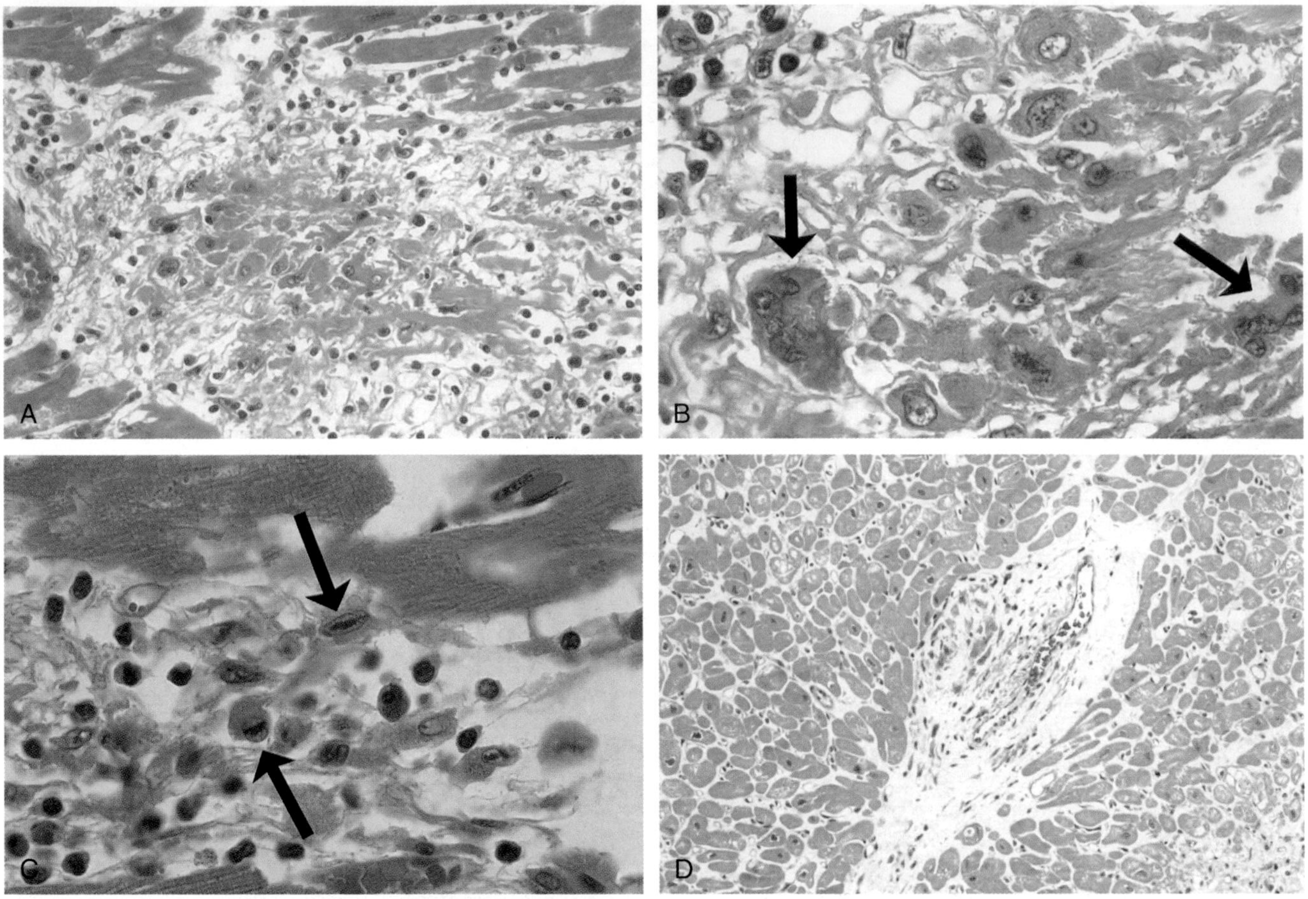

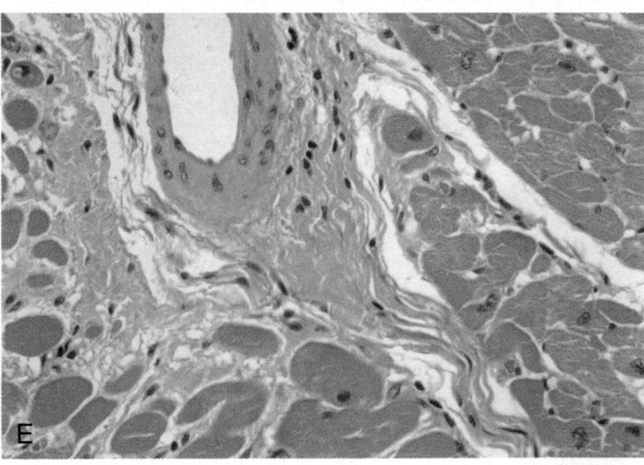

Figure 54A-8 The panels show the histological evolution of the Aschoff body in the myocardium. The exudative phase is shown in panels **A** to **C**. Panel **A** shows the central fibrinoid necrosis surrounded by large mononuclear cells. Panel **B** shows large mononuclear cells, with prominent nucleoluses and also Aschoff's giant cells (*arrows*). Panel **C** illustrates the Anitschkow cells (*arrows*). The proliferative phase is shown in panel **D**, with perivascular accumulation of mononuclear cells and absent fibrinoid necrosis, while panel **E** shows a healed perivascular lesion characterised by fibrosis.

The role of myocarditis in the failure of the heart in acute rheumatic fever has recently been questioned,[72,73] since levels of troponin I are typically within normal limits, which indicates absence of direct damage to cardiomyocytes. Since most patients with heart failure have valvar dysfunction, mainly isolated mitral regurgitation or combined mitral and aortic regurgitation, this in itself could explain the congestive symptoms. Even without direct damage to the contractile cells, nonetheless, the myocardium in the setting of acute rheumatic fever is oedematous and, besides the Aschoff bodies, an interstitial mononuclear inflammatory infiltrate of variable intensity is a common finding. These features could disrupt the myocardial integrity, and possibly interfere with the cardiac function. Dilation of the mitral annulus is also a contentious topic. Some believe that valvar regurgitation precedes dilation of the chambers, while others argue that myocardial impairment comes first, since in the acute phase the leaflets are just mildly deformed by fibrin deposition. Since it is virtually impossible to be certain that a given episode of rheumatic carditis is the first, valvar regurgitation, when present in the context of an acute carditis, could always be the consequence of previous deformity of the leaflets. Another lesion considered characteristic of the acute phase is MacCallum's patch. This is an endocardial lesion on the postero-inferior left atrial wall, frequently containing Aschoff bodies when examined histologically. This thickening, however, is more likely to be a jet lesion from mitral regurgitation than a specific rheumatic lesion. Although the diagnosis of acute rheumatic fever is usually made on clinical grounds, the endomyocardial biopsy is said to have value in diagnosis. Histological diagnosis, however, is based on the presence of Aschoff bodies. These structures were found, in one study, in less than one-third of patients with acute rheumatic fever, and only two-fifths of those with recurrent attacks.[74] This suggests that endomyocardial biopsy is not likely to add important diagnostic information.

DIAGNOSIS

Clinical Manifestations

Since the description provided by Cheadle in 1889, no modification has been incorporated into the clinical profile of rheumatic fever, characterised by its uniformity as a syndrome and by its diversity as a multi-system disease. The clinical presentation, with its variable pattern of symptoms and signs, is determined by the sites of involvement, by the time of appearance along the course of the acute attack, and whether the manifestations occur alone or in combination. Additionally, the clinical picture is also influenced by a wide range in severity of the individual manifestations.

The latent, or asymptomatic, period between the streptococcal infection and the onset of rheumatic fever lasts from 1 to 5 weeks, except for Sydenham's chorea, which may take longer to appear. The acute episodes are time limited, ranging usually from 6 to 12 weeks, but sometimes as long as 6 months in those with severe carditis. All are at risk of recurrence following a subsequent untreated infection with the group A *Streptococcus*. The duration of the acute episode is similar in both the first episode and recurrences.[6]

The diagnosis is made on a clinical basis. The supportive microbiological and serological laboratorial data is then used to characterise the underlying streptococcal infection, besides establishing the presence and resolution of the acute inflammatory process. No single symptom or sign is pathognomonic, nor are there specific laboratory tests. The diagnostic criterions formulated by Jones[17] have been revised over the past years. The reviews have clarified the categorisation of major and minor manifestations, and emphasised the importance of the laboratory evidence of the preceding infection by the group A *Streptococcus*. As a consequence, over-diagnosis has been reduced with provision of more detailed information and improved specificity. In addition, exceptions to the criterions were highlighted with the aim of diminishing the risks of under-diagnosis. The division between major and minor criterions was based on the specificity of the manifestations for the diagnosis, and not on their frequency or prognostic significance.[75] The five most characteristic clinical features constitute the major manifestations, namely, carditis, arthritis, chorea, subcutaneous nodules, and erythema marginatum, independent of their severity. Classically, arthritis and carditis, isolated or in combination, are seen most frequently. Chorea is less common, and the other major manifestations are rare (Fig. 54A-9). The minor manifestations are mostly related to the underlying systemic inflammation. Although non-specific, these clinical and laboratory findings are frequent, and supportive of the diagnosis when accompanying a major manifestation. In the presence of arthritis, however, arthralgia cannot be considered as a minor manifestation. The combination of two major or one major and two minor manifestations, supported by evidence of preceding

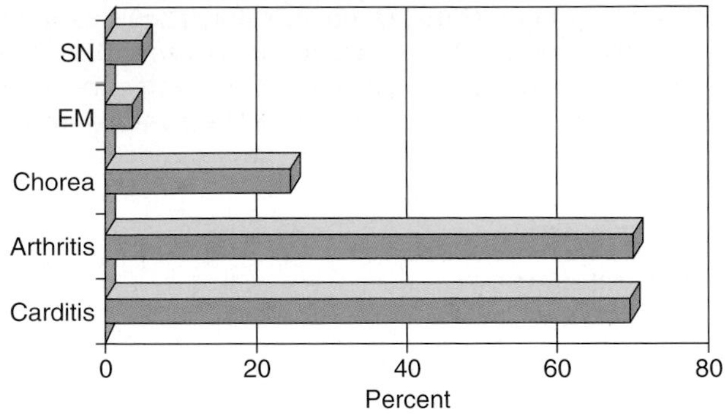

Figure 54A-9 The graph shows the proportional distribution of 1066 children and adolescents with rheumatic fever according to the major manifestations seen in the Rheumatic Fever Outpatients Clinic, Division of Paediatric Cardiology, Hospital das Clínicas, Federal University of Minas Gerais, Brazil. EM, erythema marginatum; SN, subcutaneous nodules.

infection with the group A *Streptococcus*, indicates a high probability for the diagnosis of rheumatic fever[1,21] (Table 54A-2).

The current guidelines are intended for the diagnosis of first attacks. Once other diagnoses are excluded, three situations—Sydenham's chorea, indolent carditis, and recurrent episodes—are exceptions to the strict adherence to the Jones criterions. Since Sydenham's chorea usually occurs as a late manifestation of the disease, the inflammatory process and the immunological response to streptococcal infection could have already subsided when this feature becomes evident, and laboratory evidence is seldom found. Similarly, patients with insidious onset of carditis can delay seeking medical attention. By the time of their clinical evaluation, the acute-phase reactants and levels of antistreptococcal antibodies may be normal. Faced with a reliable history of a previous episode of rheumatic fever, or established chronic rheumatic heart disease, the diagnosis of recurrence constitutes the third exception to

TABLE 54A-2

JONES CRITERIONS, 1992 UPDATE: GUIDELINES FOR THE DIAGNOSIS OF RHEUMATIC FEVER

Major Manifestations	Minor Manifestations
Carditis	Clinical
Polyarthritis	Fever
Chorea	Arthralgia
Subcutaneous nodules	Laboratorial
Erythema marginatum	Prolonged PR interval
	Increased erythrocyte sedimentation rate
	Presence of C-reactive protein

Evidence of a preceding group A beta-haemolytic streptococcal infection: elevated or rising streptococcal antibody titre or positive throat culture or elevated or rapid antigen test for group A streptococci (AHA 992)

Adapted from Guidelines for the diagnosis of rheumatic fever. Jones criteria, 1992 update. Special Writing Group of the Committee on Rheumatic Fever, Endocarditis, and Kawasaki Disease of the Council on Cardiovascular Disease in the Young of the American Heart Association. JAMA 1992;268:2069–2073.

use of the Jones criterions. Diagnosis may then be made in the presence of one major or several minor manifestations, along with supporting evidence of recent infection by the group A *Streptococcus*. In addition to the Jones criterions, other non-specific clinical findings may also be found during the course of the acute episodes.[1,21]

Major Manifestations

Carditis

Carditis is the most serious manifestation, because only in the heart are the lesions potential causes of sequels, such as death during the acute attack or later. The pericardial and myocardial damages carry no long-term morbidity. Carditis in first episodes is more frequent in younger children, and depending on its severity, is characterised by murmurs related to regurgitation of the mitral and aortic valves, enlargement of the heart, pericarditis, and congestive cardiac failure.

Carditis is reported to be seen in up to three-fifths of first attacks, although more recent series have shown higher rates when echocardiography is included in the evaluation.[5,42,45,76] Carditis tends to appear early, and is usually diagnosed within the first 3 weeks of the acute episode. Different patterns of onset can be found. Clinical presentation with fever and arthritis of abrupt onset is observed in older children, with or without indistinct clinical cardiac findings. The involvement of the heart becomes more apparent later over the first 2 weeks of disease. More frequently in young children, the disease begins insidiously, with vague symptoms, slight fever, and a sallow complexion. These children can also present mild arthritic complaints, besides shortness of breath or chest pain. Cardiac findings are present at first examination, are commonly marked, and tend to progress to congestive cardiac failure. Another mode is a late appearance of carditis, concurrent with the manifestations of Sydenham's chorea. This pattern probably represents a progression of a previously unrecognised mild cardiac involvement during the early stages of the acute attack.[6,44] Yet another pattern is that of subclinical, or silent, carditis. Mild cardiac involvement may not be clinically recognised in patients with isolated chorea or arthritis, the valvitis being demonstrated only by Doppler echocardiography.

The cardiac damage in the acute episode is characterised by pancarditis. The determinants of morbidity and mortality, nonetheless, are the degree and extent of endocarditis, represented by the lesions of the cardiac valves. Pericarditis is not common, being found in only one-tenth or less of the patients.[77,78] As with the myocardial participation, this is part of the active pancarditis, and is not found as a sole manifestation. When present, it is invariably associated with valvar dysfunction, so other causes should be investigated if valvar dysfunction is not recognised. Pericardial involvement is diagnosed by the presence of pericardial friction rub, effusion, distant heart sounds and chest discomfort or chest pain. The rub is heard as a scratching or grating sound over the praecordium, especially along the sternal border, and is heard in both phases of the cardiac cycle, having a to-and-fro character. It is less transient in rheumatic fever than in pyogenic infections. In the early stages, the friction rub may obscure the murmur of underlying valvar dysfunction, and the murmur becomes apparent only when the rub subsides.[76] In mild cases, the pericardial injury is sometimes an exclusive echocardiographic finding. Significant effusion is rarely found, and the rheumatic pericarditis does not result in constriction. Despite its low frequency, pericarditis has diagnostic value by providing evidence of an active disease.

Myocarditis has been diagnosed on the basis of signs such as abnormalities of first sound, protodiastolic gallop, cardiomegaly, and congestive cardiac failure. In spite of in the acute process histological and immunological evidences of the myocardial participation, nonetheless, more accurate assessment has provided new insights to the role played by both myocarditis and valvitis in the presentation of symptoms and heart failure.[79] Different from patients with other forms of myocarditis, the ejection fraction and shortening are usually normal in the first episodes. Markers of injury to the myocytes are insignificantly elevated.[72,73,80,81] Patients with congestive cardiac failure unresponsive to clinical treatment throughout the acute phase have shown rapid recovery after valvar surgery.[82] These observations support the notion that the valvar lesions are dominant in the clinical presentation of carditis.[79,83–85]

Endocarditis is the diagnostic hallmark of carditis, being expressed by valvitis. The inflammatory process affects most frequently the mitral and aortic valves. Isolated aortic involvement, however, is rare. Involvement of the right-side valves is unusual. Valvar dysfunctions in the acute phase are represented by regurgitation. Obstructive lesions become established during the chronic phase, the process of cicatrisation taking time to develop. If stenotic lesions are found in the acute phase, this favours the diagnosis of recurrence.

Three murmurs are characteristic of the first acute episode, and they do not represent definitive valvar dysfunction. The apical murmur of mitral regurgitation is pansystolic, beginning with the first sound, and is heard maximally at the apex with the patient in the left lateral decubitus position. It is transmitted to the left axilla, and remains unchanged in both phases of respiration. It has a high-pitched blowing quality, with its loudness roughly proportional to the degree of valvar regurgitation. The Carey Coombs murmur is a low-pitched mid-diastolic murmur, beginning immediately after the third sound, finishing before the first sound, and usually of low intensity. The murmur is best heard at the apex, or just above it, by using the bell portion of the stethoscope applied lightly against the chest wall with the patient again lying in left lateral decubitus. This apical mid-diastolic murmur occurs when there is mitral regurgitation, is transient, and tends to disappear during the recovery from the acute episode. The mechanism is not completely understood. It has been attributed to the inflammatory process and its consequences in the mitral apparatus, besides the high velocity of flow into the dilated left ventricle. The third murmur, the basal diastolic murmur of aortic regurgitation, has a soft, high-pitched, decrescendo quality, and may be found early in the course of the disease. It is difficult to detect, and sometimes has an intermittent character. It is an early diastolic murmur, best heard with the diaphragm of the stethoscope, and is usually loudest at the third space on the left border of the sternum with the patient in the upright position, leaning forward, and after deep expiration. The severity of cardiac findings in the acute episode is variable, going from subclinical lesions to severe presentation with fulminating evolution (Table 54A-3).

TABLE 54A-3

CLASSIFICATION OF RHEUMATIC CARDITIS ACCORDING TO THE MAGNITUDE OF CLINICAL MANIFESTATIONS AND ELECTROCARDIOGRAPHIC, RADIOGRAPHIC, AND DOPPLER ECHOCARDIOGRAPHIC FINDINGS*

Type	Findings
Subclinical carditis	Absence of auscultatory evidence of carditis associated with normal radiographic and electrocardiological examinations, except for the presence of first-degree heart block. Doppler echocardiographical features show mild regurgitation of mitral and/or aortic valves with different characteristics from physiological regurgitation (see Table 54A-4).
Mild carditis	Rapid sleeping pulse, tachycardia out of proportion to fever, possible decrease in the intensity of the first sound, systolic murmur of mild mitral regurgitation, no cardiac enlargement on chest radiography, possible prolongation of the PR interval in the electrocardiographical examination, mild or mild-moderate mitral insufficiency, isolated or associated with mild aortic regurgitation and normal chamber size on echocardiography.
Moderate carditis	Clinical signs are more evident than for mild carditis with persistent tachycardia and a more intense murmur of mitral regurgitation, but without thrill, coming as an isolated lesion or associated with aortic diastolic murmur. The mitral regurgitation can be accompanied by a Carey-Coombs murmur, besides findings of incipient heart failure; a mild or mild-moderate degree of cardiac enlargement in the chest radiography due to left-sided chamber hypertrophy and, if present, the pulmonary congestion is discreet; premature beats, ST segment and T wave changes, low voltage, prolongation of QTc or PR intervals may be observed on the electrocardiogram; mild-moderate mitral regurgitation, isolated or associated with aortic valve incompetence of mild or moderate degree, mild-moderate enlargement of the left-side chambers are seen on echocardiography.
Severe carditis	In addition to the findings of moderate carditis, symptoms and signs of congestive heart failure are found; valvitis is expressed by murmurs related to more severe degrees of mitral and/or aortic regurgitation and can be associated with pericarditis and arrhythmias. There is evident cardiomegaly with prominent vascular markings on chest radiography; a more severe degree of the electrocardiographic changes of left ventricular hypertrophy is sometimes associated with right ventricular hypertrophy. Moderate-severe or severe mitral and/or aortic insufficiency are observed on echocardiography, and the left cardiac chambers show at least moderate enlargement.

*According to the protocol of the Rheumatic Fever Clinic, Department of Paediatrics, Division of Paediatric Cardiology, Hospital das Clínicas/Federal University of Minas Gerais, Brazil.

Subclinical Valvitis

Until the advent of Doppler echocardiography, the diagnosis of rheumatic valvitis had been exclusively based on the presence of auscultatory findings, supported by radiographic and electrocardiographic abnormalities. By the late 1980s, it proved possible positively to identify subclinical valvitis.[86–89] Such silent carditis is found in patients with isolated arthritis and/or pure chorea, without auscultatory findings of valvar dysfunction, but with a pathological pattern of valvar regurgitation revealed by Doppler echocardiographic interrogation (Table 54A-4). Thickening of the valvar leaflets has also been described.[90,91] Subsequently, regurgitant jets have been observed, with a wide range of prevalence.[57,88,92–96] As trivial leaks of pulmonary, tricuspid, and mitral valves are commonly identified by Doppler echocardiographic investigation in normal subjects at all ages, it is essential to use strict criterions to differentiate pathological from physiological regurgitation (see Table 54A-4). Physiological insufficiency can be detected in up to nine-tenths of the normal population, being more frequent in adults than children.[90,97–101] Aortic leaks, however, have rarely been considered physiologic. Mild degrees of mitral and/or aortic regurgitation are most commonly described in rheumatic subclinical valvitis, albeit that mild to moderate degrees have also been identified, mostly involving the aortic valve.[90,102–104] Caution is required when interpreting the evidence of valvar incompetence. Besides the characteristics of the regurgitant jet, it is important to note that the echocardiographic findings do not define the aetiology of the process. They must be considered in the context of the disease, considering associations with other clinical and laboratory manifestations. Although the role of Doppler interrogation has long been recognised, its use without auscultatory support is still controversial.[85,94,105–110] In the last revision of the guidelines for the diagnosis of rheumatic fever by the American Heart Association, in 2002,[22] it was concluded that the existing data was insufficient to include Doppler echocardiographic findings in the absence of clinical manifestations as a criterion for the diagnosis of carditis.

In some patients without auscultatory findings in the early stage of the disease, the murmurs can be identified later.[90,103] Patients, therefore, require serial clinical evaluation, aimed at detecting late clinical evidence of carditis.

TABLE 54A-4

DOPPLER ECHOCARDIOGRAPHIC CRITERIONS FOR THE DIAGNOSIS OF SUBCLINICAL MITRAL AND AORTIC VALVITIS

Type	Criterions
Mitral regurgitation*	Regurgitant jet into the left atrium longer than 1 cm Posterolateral colour jet with a mosaic pattern Identification of colour jet in at least two planes beyond the valvar leaflets Holosystolic regurgitant jet by pulse or continuous Doppler Regurgitant jet with a peak velocity greater than 2.5 mm/sec
Aortic regurgitation*	Identification of colour jet in at least two planes beyond the valvar leaflets Holodiastolic regurgitant jet by pulse or continuous Doppler Regurgitant jet with a peak velocity greater than 2.5 mm/sec

*Thickening of valvar leaflets is an additional finding to support the diagnosis.[90,91]
Data from Veasy LG: Rheumatic fever—T. Duckett Jones and the rest of the story. Cardiol Young 1995;5:293–301; and Ozkutlu S, Ayabakan C, Saraçlar M: Can subclinical valvitis detected by echocardiography be accepted as evidence of carditis in the diagnosis of acute rheumatic fever? Cardiol Young 2001;11:255–260.

As mild valvar dysfunctions are most frequently seen in subclinical valvitis, favourable outcomes are expected for the great majority of patients, with anticipated spontaneous healing of the valvar lesions without sequels.[104,110–113] More recent investigations, nonetheless, have demonstrated that the subclinical valvitis can persist for prolonged periods.[90,102,104,110,114] The valvar lesions can remain subclinical in the chronic phase, characterizing subclinical chronic rheumatic heart disease.[45,105,115] Considering the propensity of recurrences to mimic clinical manifestations of the first episode, the increased risk of more severe involvement of the heart must be borne in mind should there be subsequent attacks.[114]

Recurrent Carditis

Carditis is rarely present for the first time in recurrences. The term mimetic carditis was proposed, considering the heart almost always to be involved in the subsequent attacks in patients exhibiting carditis in the primary episode.[6,52] The diagnosis of recurrent carditis in patients with an established rheumatic valvar disease is often difficult. The clinical presentation includes changes in the character of the murmur, reappearance of a previous murmur, or detection of a new one as the result of the involvement of an additional valve. In addition, detection of a pericardial friction rub or effusion, and a significant increase in the size of the heart, may also be present. Congestive failure is more common in recurrent carditis. Although the heart is invariably involved in recurrences of patients suffering carditis in the first attack, cardiac failure in the chronic phase could also reflect mechanical stress due to valvar dysfunction, being related to the extent of haemodynamic effects. The epidemiological and clinical context, as well as the evidence of a recent streptococcal infection, therefore, must be considered in the diagnosis of recurrent carditis.

Polyarthritis

Polyarthritis is the most frequent major manifestation seen in older children, adolescents, and adults, but constitutes the least specific clinical finding of rheumatic fever. Its frequency increases with age, being seen in up to three-quarters of patients as an isolated presentation, or in association with other manifestations of the disease.[1] The articular involvement usually occurs early in the illness, with duration and severity greater in adults than in children. Polyarthritis is rarely simultaneous with active chorea, the severity of the articular symptoms and signs being inversely proportional to the degree of carditis.[6,44] Polyarthritis is non-suppurative, asymmetrical, migratory, and self-limited, and does not result in permanent deformity. The classical migratory pattern refers to the sequential involvement of joints. While the process is resolving in one joint, another becomes involved, resulting in an overlapping in time with the participation of more than one joint. There is a marked preference to involve the peripheral large joints, and mainly of the legs. Less frequently, the shoulders, hips, spine, and the small joints of the hands and feet are affected. Tenderness and severe pain, out of proportion to the findings of the physical examination, are the most prominent features, and very prompt relief of the symptoms and signs follows the use of anti-inflammatory agents. The pain occurs in both active and passive movements, is usually diffuse, can show radiation to periarticular areas, and is associated with limitation of motion. Other characteristics of inflammation, such as heat, redness, and swelling, although present, are usually less marked. If untreated, the inflammatory findings last from 1 to 5 days in each joint, reach the higher intensity in the first 2 days, with the entire process subsiding over 2 to 4 weeks.[44]

Atypical presentations of arthritis, such as monoarthritis and additive and symmetrical polyarthritis, besides simultaneous participation of several joints, and the longer duration of the inflammatory process, have been described. Involvement of only one joint is often observed if the anti-inflammatory therapy is administered before the migratory characteristic has been established. Jaccoud's arthritis is considered a rare sequel of recurrent attacks of rheumatic fever, and is a possible exception for residual articular deformity. In this situation, periarticular fibrosis of the metacarpophalangeal joint results in marked ulnar deviation and hyperextension of the proximal interphalangeal joints.[116,117] Post-streptococcal reactive arthritis is related as an acute and non-suppurative arthritic condition following a documented group A streptococcal infection. Its characteristics are not typical of rheumatic fever, and do not meet the Jones criterions. There is a latent period, usually shorter than 10 days, and persistence of mono- or polyarthritis for several months with atypical presentation. Clinical findings include an additive and symmetrical rather a migratory pattern and involvement of small and axial joints, besides a poor response to anti-inflammatory therapy.[118,119] An association with mitral valvar dysfunction has been registered in one-twentieth of the patients.[120] Doubts remain whether post-streptococcal reactive arthritis is a different condition from rheumatic fever, or if the two entities represent diverse expressions of the same disease.

Sydenham's Chorea

Sydenham's chorea, chorea minor, or St. Vitus's dance, affects children and adolescents, more frequently females. It is uncommon after puberty, and is rarely seen in postpuberal males.[121] It has been reported in up to one-third of patients, with a peak incidence at around 8 to 9 years of age.[5,122] The latent period after infection is longer than for arthritis and carditis, varying from 1 to 7 months. It may occur as an isolated manifestation, the so-called pure chorea, or less frequently in association with carditis or arthritis.[26] As a late manifestation, the disorder is rarely associated with arthritis, but may co-exist with clinical or subclinical valvitis in up to two-fifths of patients.[1,45,123,124] Chronic rheumatic heart disease has been described in around one-quarter of patients 20 years after the presentation of isolated chorea.[125]

Sydenham's chorea is usually a self-limited disorder, and diagnosis is based exclusively on clinical examination. It is a manifestation of the central nervous system characterised by muscular weakness, hypotonia, and emotional instability, besides involuntary and purposeless but conscious movements of the skeletal muscles. Although the face and the arms and legs are more often involved, any voluntary muscle may be affected. The presentation of facial grimacing is frequent, besides abrupt but not repetitive movements of the limbs, mainly the hands. The uncoordinated movements are mostly evident when the patient is awake, particularly under stress, excitement, or effort. Oculomotor problems have also been reported, which go into remission in most patients after the improvement of the choreiform movements.[126]

The onset is insidious, so that chorea as the first and sole manifestation of rheumatic fever may not be recognised in the early phase, the signs being attributed to behavioural or emotional problems. The child shows attention deficit and inappropriate behaviour, and becomes irritable, restless, and clumsy. Fine muscular incoordination is noted, and voluntary movements, such as unbuttoning clothes or tying shoes laces are difficult to execute. The manifestations become progressively more evident, with disturbances in the speech and handwriting. The signs of muscular weakness and choreiform movements are mostly generalised, sometimes asymmetrical, but one-fifth of patients have hemichorea, with the manifestations limited to one side of the body. So-called chorea paralytica is an expression of generalised and severe presentation, albeit very rare.[122] Certain manoeuvres are helpful to bring out the choreiform movements. When the patient is asked to extend the arms forward, the hands assume the shape of a spoon or dish as a result of wrist flexion and hyperextension of the fingers. The milking sign is demonstrated by alternating increase and decrease in tension when the patient grips the examiner's hand. If the arms are raised above the head, the hands are involuntarily turned outwards. Undulating movements can be observed when the tongue is protruded, resembling a bag of worms. [5,6,44]

Recurrent chorea is not uncommon. More recently, it has been questioned whether all recurrent choreiform episodes are due to rheumatic fever.[127] The severity and the course of the illness up to its resolution are variable. In mild cases, the choreiform movements may subside in few weeks, but most frequently the recovery takes up to 6 months, albeit that in severe cases the manifestation may persist up to more than 2 years.[1] Behavioural abnormalities occur in up to one-third of patients.[128–130] More recently, a broad spectrum of post-streptococcal movement conditions associated with emotional and behaviour disorders have been identified using the acronym PANDAS—paediatric autoimmune neuropsychiatric disorders associated with *Streptococcus*.[131–134]

Subcutaneous Nodules

Other than being useful for diagnosis, subcutaneous nodules have a limited value due to their lower frequency. They are one of the most characteristic major criterions, almost invariably associated with severe carditis.[78,135,136] Seen in only one-tenth of patients, their frequency seems to have been reduced over the last decades.[137] On many occasions, the subcutaneous nodules are not noted by the patients. Sometimes they are found only following careful investigation. They usually appear several weeks after the onset of the acute episode, persist from days to weeks, and rarely last longer than 1 month. They can be seen early in recurrences. The nodules are small, varying in size from millimetres to 2 centimetres, and are firm, painless, and freely movable under the skin. They are encountered in clusters, on the extensor surface of the joints and overlying bone prominences, mainly in the large joints of limbs, knuckles, scalp, and along the spine in the paravertebral areas (Figs. 54A-10 through 54A-12).

Erythema Marginatum

This is an uncommon manifestation, occurring in only one-twentieth of patients. It is a macular rash, sometimes coalescent with a serpiginous or circular form, almost coppery pink at the border, and with a lighter centre. The lesions take the form of enlarging rings, mainly located

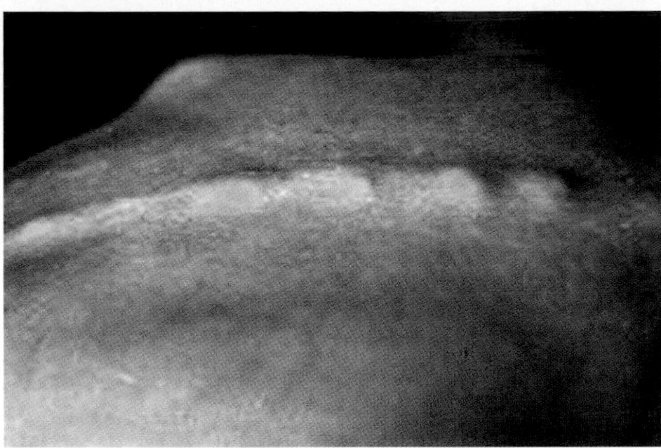

Figure 154A-10 The image shows subcutaneous nodules near bony prominences along the spine, focusing on the thoracic and lumbar vertebras. (Reproduced with permission from Mota CCC, Meira ZMA: Rheumatic fever. Cardiol Young 1999;9:239–248.)

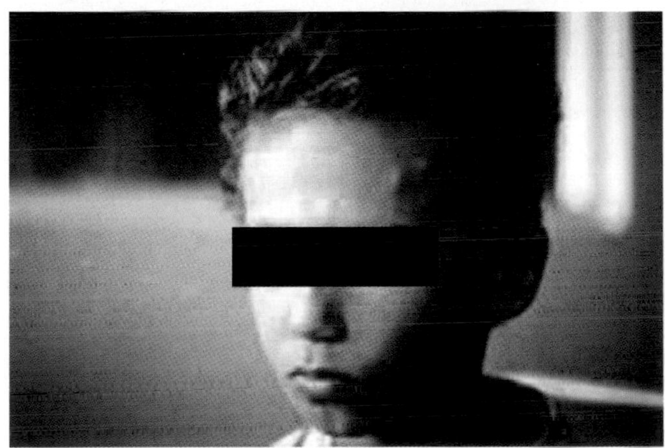

Figure 54A-11 Large subcutaneous nodules as seen on the forehead. (Reproduced with permission from Mota CCC, Meira ZMA, Graciano RN, Silva MC: Diagnostic aspects, carditis and other acute manifestations of streptococcal infection. Cardiol Young 1992;2:222–228.)

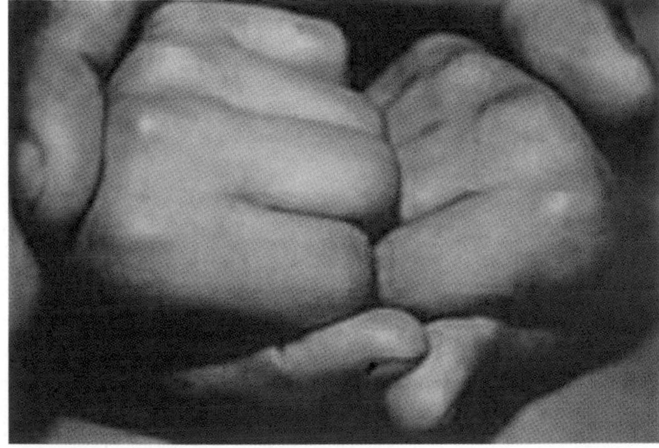

Figure 54A-12 These subcutaneous nodules are found on the extensor surface of tendons near bony prominences in the hands. (Reproduced with permission from From Mota CCC, Meira ZMA, Graciano RN, Silva MC: Diagnostic aspects, carditis and other acute manifestations of streptococcal infection. Cardiol Young 1992;2:222–228.)

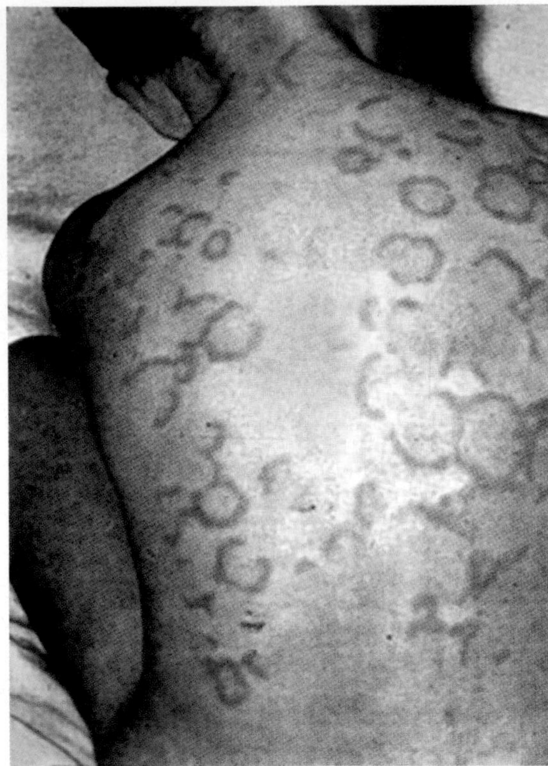

Figure 54A-13 The photograph shows erythema marginatum located on the trunk and proximal limbs. (Reproduced with permission from Mota CCC, Meira ZMA, Graciano RN, Silva MC: Diagnostic aspects, carditis and other acute manifestations of streptococcal infection. Cardiol Young 1992;2:222–228.)

on the trunk and inner surface of the proximal limbs, and are not seen on the face (see Fig. 54A-13). Although the lesion can be seen during the acute phase, it is more often seen in the early stages. Characteristically the manifestation is transient, may last minutes, more usually days, may be intermittent for months, and is not influenced by the use of anti-inflammatory therapy. The lesions are more easily seen in fair-skinned patients, may become more apparent with the application of heat, and are associated most frequently with subcutaneous nodules and carditis.

Minor Manifestations

As isolated features, the minor manifestations are limited by their lack of specificity. When associated with a major manifestation, nonetheless, they can provide support for diagnosis. As already emphasised, arthralgia is considered a minor manifestation only when other signs of inflammation, such as redness, swelling, and heat, are absent. The pain shows the same characteristics as polyarthritis concerning the site and type of joints affected, the migratory pattern and variability in severity. Arthralgia in one or more joints may co-exist with arthritis. In that case, only the major manifestation may be used as a diagnostic criterion. Fever is usually present in the early stage of the disease, commonly of low grade, and can persist for 2 to 3 weeks.[5] There is no characteristic pattern, and it is rare for the temperature to rise higher than 39°C. The laboratory data included among the minor manifestations, as with the clinical findings, are also non-specific.

Other Manifestations

Other symptoms and signs, although less frequent, can be observed, but are not included in the set of minor manifestations of the Jones criterions. Epistaxis is an uncommon presentation, and abdominal pain, mainly around the navel, may precede the major manifestations. Upper abdominal pain, although less common in children than adults, may be a symptom of heart failure. Rheumatic pneumonia is considered a rare event, with high rates of death, and associated with severe carditis.[138–140] Its diagnosis remains controversial considering that similar findings may be present in severe congestive heart failure and that there is an overlapping of clinical and radiographic presentations of the two conditions. Manifestations such as anorexia, listlessness, fatigue, anaemia, weight loss, and pallor are described, but are related to systemic inflammation and to the severity of the clinical presentations, mainly carditis.

Difficulties with the Diagnosis of Rheumatic Fever

The potential for permanent damage to the cardiac valves points to the importance of an accurate and early diagnosis. As no laboratory finding is specific, the history and physical examination remain the basis for the diagnosis. The established guidelines, although very useful, cannot substitute for experience and common sense on behalf of the physician. As a systemic disease of multiple associations, with a wide spectrum of manifestations, diagnostic problems can be present, since several other conditions can fulfil the Jones criterions. On the other hand, not all patients with an acute episode meet these diagnostic requirements. Even in areas where rheumatic fever is still prevalent, its frequency and severity have decreased, resulting in less characteristic presentations. Significant cardiac involvement, particularly if associated with other major manifestations, results in a more characteristic presentation of the disease. On the other hand, characterisation of mild cardiac involvement is difficult. Subclinical or smouldering carditis may not be recognised. As a consequence, the disease is diagnosed in the chronic phase by its valvar sequels. These circumstances have potential implications in prognosis, when the risks of recurrences and worsening of the valvar lesions are considered. Both under- and over-diagnosis of carditis are frequent. Considering the number of adults who present with established rheumatic valvar disease without any preceding history of rheumatic fever, under-diagnosis is particularly common. Over-diagnosis can be equally detrimental when children with innocent murmurs or murmurs caused by congenital cardiac defects associated with sore throats or arthralgia are wrongly labelled as having rheumatic heart disease. Due to the wide group of illnesses with the same presentation, the differential diagnosis of polyarthritis is difficult when the articular involvement is the sole manifestation of the acute phase. The difficulties increase with the presence of monoarthritis as an atypical presentation, or as a consequence of the premature use of anti-inflammatory agents. Usually, the joint involvement is an early and self-limited manifestation along the course of the disease. Mild articular presentation may contribute to misdiagnosis, mainly when the symptoms and signs have already subsided at the clinical examination. Furthermore, the differential diagnosis between polyarthritis and polyarthralgia is difficult if based exclusively on clinical history. In addition, doubts also remain regarding some conditions such as subclinical valvar lesions, post-streptococcal reactive arthritis, and PANDAS. There are many disease processes that may currently fulfill the Jones criterions in their early stage, or mimic the acute rheumatic process very closely. The differential diagnosis includes rheumatoid arthritis, serum sickness, other arthropathies, infective endocarditis, Henoch-Schönlein purpura, acute leucaemia, poliomyelitis and acute appendicitis, viral myocarditis, viral pericarditis, systemic lupus erythematosus, and other collagen disorders that may affect both joints and the heart.

The diagnosis of recurrences can also, on occasion, be challenging. For a presumptive diagnosis, and with the aim of avoiding under-diagnosis, it is important to note the epidemiological context of streptococcal exposure. In patients with cardiac sequels from a previous attack, and when carditis is the sole manifestation of the recurrence, a more precise diagnosis can only be established if pericarditis is found, or if a different valve is damaged. Another consideration is the worsening of previous valvar lesions. In patients with multi-valvar involvement, and with no other associated major manifestations, the question to address is whether the manifestations are due to a recurrence, or whether they represent a higher degree of severity in the evolution of the chronic rheumatic heart disease. The supporting evidence of a recent streptococcal infection is mandatory to confirm the diagnosis of a new attack. Even considering that the acute-phase reactants are not specific for the disease, they are useful to characterise the presence of the inflammatory process. Besides the minor manifestations, other clinical features such as fatigue, anorexia, pallor, and lack of movement contribute to the diagnostic approach when they are not part of the cardiac failure. As the clinical variables are crucial for a better comprehension of the disease, a longer period of close observation sometimes is needed to clarify the diagnosis.

LABORATORY INVESTIGATIONS

Although none of the laboratory tests is specific, they are useful in monitoring the inflammatory process, and contribute to the management of patients, besides providing the evidence of a previous streptococcal infection. There are three categories supporting the clinical diagnosis, namely, tests supporting evidence of a recent group A streptococcal infection, the acute-phase reactants, and a third group of tests, including those examinations evaluating the cardiac involvement.

Supporting Evidence of a Recent Group A Streptococcal Infection

An important requirement for the diagnosis of rheumatic fever is the evidence of the antecedent streptococcal infection, since many other diseases, unrelated to this infection, have a similar clinical profile. Demonstration of infection by the group A *Streptococcus* is necessary because clinical diagnosis of pharyngotonsillitis or scarlet fever due to this cause cannot be made with certainty at the time of the onset of rheumatic fever.[21,29] In the circumstances of Sydenham's chorea and indolent carditis, however, this prerequisite is dispensable.[21] The identification of the bacteria by throat cultures or rapid antigen testing of throat swabs, as well as the documentation of elevated or increasing streptococcal antibody titres, confirms the recent streptococcal infection, but none of these tests is diagnostic of rheumatic fever.

Throat culture remains the most reliable method for identifying the β-haemolytic group A *Streptococcus* in the setting of acute pharyngotonsillitis. The blood agar culture has a sensitivity of 90% to 95% and a specificity of 100%.[29] In contrast with the longer time of 24 to 48 hours needed to obtain a throat culture, a more prompt result is provided by the rapid group A streptococcal antigen detection tests. Most of the available tests, when compared to the blood agar culture, show a specificity greater than 95%, but the sensitivity is variable, from 31% to 95%.[29,141,142] Consequently, when the result is positive, the therapeutic decision can be made with confidence. Nonetheless, considering the wide variation in sensitivity, a blood agar culture is still recommended when the result is negative, particularly in settings where rheumatic fever is highly prevalent.[111,142] In spite of the accuracy, *Streptococcus* is isolated by blood culture at the time of the onset of rheumatic fever in only one-quarter of cases.[21] One reason is the elimination of the bacterium by the defence mechanisms of the body during the latent period, since the streptococcal infectious process usually has already subsided when the diagnosis of rheumatic fever is established. Negative results are also related to the previous use of antibiotics. On the other hand, a positive result cannot distinguish a true streptococcal infection from a streptococcal carrier state.[141]

The determination of the streptococcal antibody titres is the most specific test to confirm a previous infection. Blood titres of antibodies against extracellular products include antistreptolysin O, antideoxyribonuclease B, antihyaluronidase, and antistreptokinase. The range of normal values is variable and related to age, season of the year, and geographical location. Although the bacteria can be found in the upper respiratory tract in both the carrier state and during an acute streptococcal infection, the rising antibody response can be observed only in the case of true infection.[1] The determination of three different antibody tests shows an elevated titre for at least one antibody in up to 95% of patients.[41,77] The antistreptolysin O assay is used most commonly, and provides reliable confirmation of a previous infection in four-fifths or more of patients. Titres tend to be higher in patients with rheumatic fever than in those with uncomplicated streptococcal infections.[5] The titre is considered elevated if it exceeds the upper limit for a given population. This upper limit is defined as the highest value surpassed by only one-fifth of individuals. A single titre of at least 320 Todd units for children, and 240 Todd units for adults, is considered elevated.[21] Although an increased titre is an evidence of a previous streptococcal infection, the demonstration of a rising antibody response from the acute to convalescent phase is a more reliable means to document a recent infection. For the confirmation of rising titres in samples obtained at intervals of 2 to 4 weeks, an increase in titre of two or more dilutions is considered diagnostic.[5] Timing of the determination should also be considered when interpreting the results. The titre usually becomes elevated 2 weeks after the streptococcal infection, peaks at 3 to 4 weeks, and starts to decline after 2 to 3 months.[1,137] As a result, the titres are likely to be normal in the early phase of the disease, as well as in patients with chorea or with indolent carditis, when the titres have usually already returned to normal levels. Borderline or low titres are detected in around one-fifth of patients during the first 2 months after the onset of rheumatic fever, and in about two-fifths of those affected by isolated Sydenham's chorea.[21] Considering the availability, if the titre is not elevated and the diagnosis of rheumatic fever is strongly suggested, another antibody test may be requested to confirm the previous streptococcal infection.[137] The anti-DNAase B titres remain elevated for a longer period of time than do the antistreptolysin O titres, even after uncomplicated streptococcal infection.[141] The streptozyme test is a rapid commercially available slide agglutination test used to detect antibodies to several streptococcal antigens. It has been less well standardised, raising questions about its reliability.[137,141]

Acute-phase Reactants

The acute-phase reactants have been used to identify the presence and degree of the inflammatory process, and to follow the course of the disease activity, as well as its resolution. The most commonly used acute-phase reactants are the erythrocyte sedimentation rate and C-reactive protein. Both these laboratory markers of acute inflammation are sensitive but non-specific, since abnormal results may be produced by many other conditions. Both tests are abnormal in patients with carditis and polyarthritis, whereas they are frequently normal in patients with late presentations of the disease, such as isolated chorea, or only slightly elevated in indolent carditis. In general, the levels normalise after the anti-inflammatory therapy, and the use of corticosteroids results in a quicker return when compared to salicylates.[111] The increase in the erythrocyte sedimentation rate is proportional to the intensity of the inflammatory reaction, but it is unrelated to the site of the clinical manifestation of rheumatic fever.[44,143] The erythrocyte sedimentation rate may be increased in patients with anaemia and suppressed in those with congestive heart failure, neoplasms, and tissue necrosis.

As the C-reactive protein is not usually present in the blood, slightly positive results are significant. It can be an over-sensitive indication of the acute inflammatory process, and is not influenced by anaemia or by heart failure. A C-reactive protein test becomes negative earlier than the decrease of erythrocyte sedimentation rate. Other markers of the inflammatory activity are currently less often used. The serum mucoprotein, and the α_2-globulin fraction in the electrophoretic study, are abnormal along the course of the acute phase, usually show higher levels related to severity of the disease, and are not influenced by medication. The complexity of the quantitative process in the diverse analytic phases is a limitation for the use of the serum mucoprotein. Leucocytosis may occur, but is not sufficiently constant to be of diagnostic value.

Examinations to Evaluate Cardiac Involvement

The third group includes the tests evaluating cardiac involvement. Although the electrocardiogram and chest radiography constitute useful methods, they are characterised by low specificity and sensitivity. Normal results do not exclude the diagnosis of carditis. The chest radiograph is useful in the determination of the presence and degree of the cardiac enlargement in supporting the clinical diagnosis, as is the presence of prominent vascular markings or pulmonary oedema, which characterises the severity of carditis. Variations in cardiac size are also valuable when charting evolution of the disease. Marked cardiomegaly with a rapid increase of the cardiac size, or the configuration of water flask in the erect position, suggest the diagnosis of pericardial effusion even in the absence of a friction rub.[137] In severe cases, this is dubbed rheumatic pneumonia, a rare entity related to multiple radiological patterns, with uni- or bilateral involvement, consolidation, patchy areas of infiltration in the lungs fields, diffuse bilateral and migratory infiltrates, pleural effusion, and confluent nodular lesions.[139]

Electrocardiographic abnormalities are also non-specific, usually temporary, and mainly represented by sinus tachycardia, disturbances in conduction, diffuse ST and T changes, low voltage of the QRS complex and changes in the T wave. There is no correlation with severity, nor do the changes have prognostic significance. Normal tracings do not exclude cardiac involvement, and the diagnosis of carditis should not solely be based on electrocardiographic abnormalities. Arrhythmias are occasionally found, albeit frequently self-limited and benign. In those suffering recurrences, atrial fibrillation can be seen when the left atrium is significantly enlarged.[78] The prolonged PR interval relative to heart rate and age is included as one of the minor manifestations in the Jones criterions. This disturbance may be found with similar frequency in patients with or without carditis, and is also reported in normal children.[5] Advanced conduction delay, including second- and third-degree atrioventricular blocks, is rarely seen. As with the prolonged PR interval, such changes appear as temporary events during the acute episode.[144,145] A prolonged QTc interval has been reported as a more frequent finding in rheumatic fever than first-degree atrioventricular block.[90,146] More recently, the increase in QT dispersion, and its association with cardiac involvement in children with the first episode of rheumatic fever, has been reported. At follow-up, the reduction on the QT dispersion was concomitant with the clinical improvement.[147]

The continuing evolution of technology has allowed the incorporation of non-invasive techniques such as Doppler echocardiography. This now constitutes one of the most important tools for investigating the functional and morphological aspects of patients with rheumatic fever, besides providing support for the management at the first evaluation and follow-up. The technique has added important information regarding the structure of the valvar and subvalvar apparatus, resulting in a better understanding of the mechanisms of valvar dysfunction. Additionally, the technique is useful when evaluating involvement of the pericardium and its repercussions. The evaluation of the degree of severity, and the impact of valvar lesions, by Doppler echocardiography is an integrative process based on multiple parameters, and is dependent of the site and the type of dysfunction.[1,148,149] The accurate assessment of the extension of valvar lesions provides an earlier diagnosis in cases of mild cardiac involvement, identifying subclinical valvar lesions in both the acute and chronic phases (Figs. 54A-14 and 54A-15). A set of Doppler echocardiographic characteristics has been established for the diagnosis of subclinical valvitis, based on patterns of regurgitant jets different from those found in physiological regurgitation (see Table 54A-4). The morphological features of initial involvement include valvar

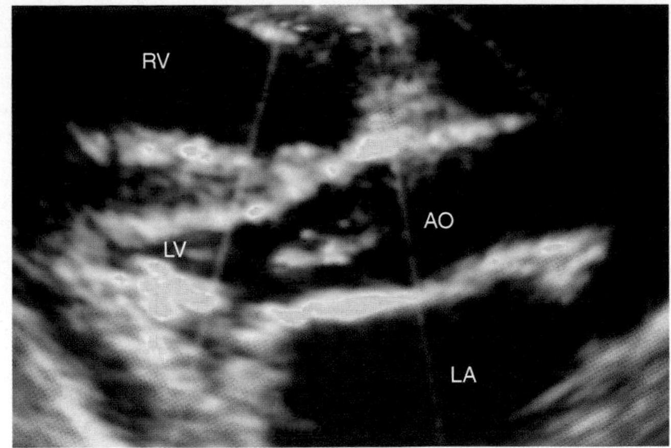

Figure 54A-14 Colour flow mapping in a 9-year-old girl with Sydenham's chorea and subclinical valvitis shows mild aortic regurgitation. AO, aorta; LA, left atrium; LV, left ventricle; RV, right ventricle.

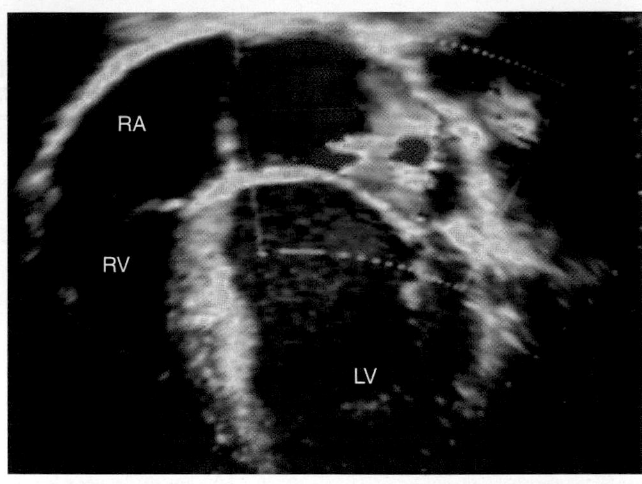

Figure 54A-16 Colour flow mapping in this 14-year-old boy with moderate mitral and aortic regurgitation shows thickening of mitral leaflets, dilation of left-sided chambers, and moderate mitral valvar regurgitation. LV, left ventricle; RA, right atrium; RV, right ventricle.

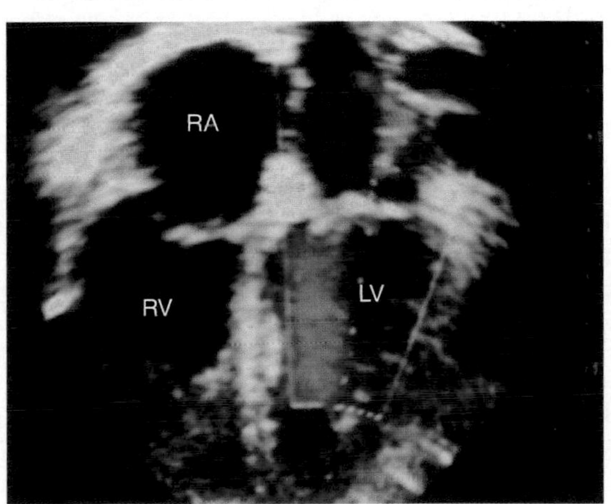

Figure 54A-15 Colour flow mapping in this 7-year-old boy with Sydenham's chorea and subclinical valvitis, with mild thickening of the mitral valvar leaflets, shows mild mitral regurgitation. LV, left ventricle; RA, right atrium; RV, right ventricle.

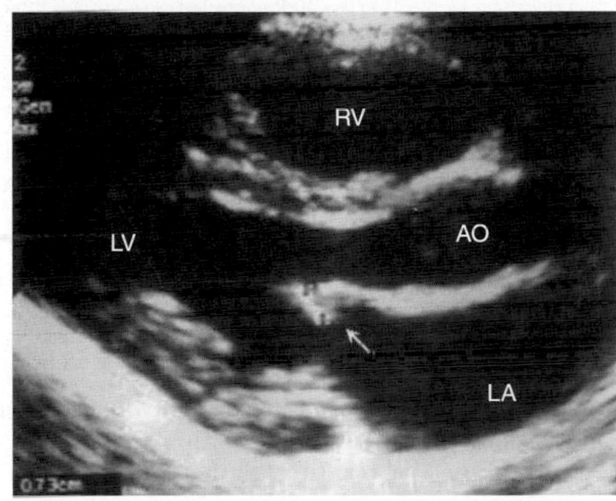

Figure 54A-17 The cross sectional echocardiogram in this 9-year-old girl with mild to moderate mitral regurgitation shows moderate thickening of the aortic leaflet of the mitral valve (*arrow*). AO, aorta; LA, left atrium; LV, left ventricle; RV, right ventricle.

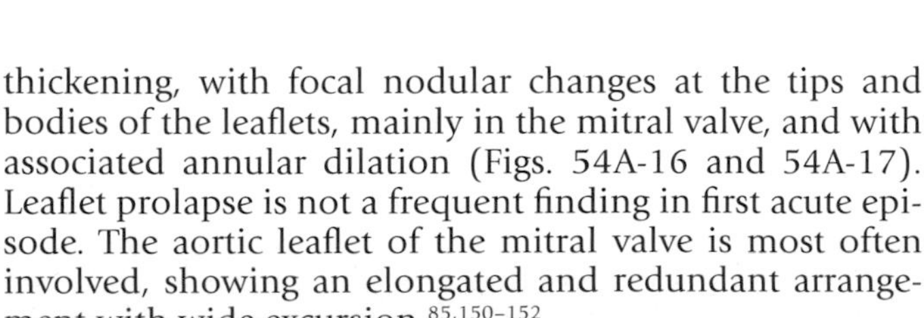

thickening, with focal nodular changes at the tips and bodies of the leaflets, mainly in the mitral valve, and with associated annular dilation (Figs. 54A-16 and 54A-17). Leaflet prolapse is not a frequent finding in first acute episode. The aortic leaflet of the mitral valve is most often involved, showing an elongated and redundant arrangement with wide excursion.[85,150–152]

Rupture of the tendinous cords is a rare event. If seen, it usually involves the aortic leaflet, with resulting severe mitral insufficiency.[151,153,154] In severe cases, monitoring the progress of valvar damage makes it possible to determine the need for intervention during the acute episode, as well as choosing the procedure.[155,156] Doppler echocardiography also contributes to avoidance of over-diagnosis, permitting exclusion of other conditions which, in a clinical setting, could have been misdiagnosed as rheumatic fever.[85,89]

Other modalities for the assessment of cardiac damage include endomyocardial biopsy and radionuclide imaging. As already discussed, the low diagnostic sensitivity of endomyocardial biopsy limits the technique to clinical investigation.[74,111,121] For radionuclide imaging, gallium-67 has shown better diagnostic results when compared to antimyosin scintigraphy, but experience with both methods for imaging myocardial inflammation is limited.[108]

MANAGEMENT

Management of the acute episode includes eradication of tonsillar and pharyngeal group A *Streptococcus*, and treatment of the presenting manifestations. No intervention can be made in the immunological process, however, once it has been triggered. Anti-inflammatory agents can be symptomatically beneficial, but have no curative properties. Considering that the available treatment is supportive, the most effective therapeutic approach is directed towards prophylaxis.[157]

Eradication of the Group A Streptococcal Infection

It is important to eradicate the infecting agent even in the presence of a negative throat culture. Although antimicrobial therapy does not influence the course or severity of the

TABLE 54A-5

PRIMARY PREVENTION OF RHEUMATIC FEVER: TREATMENT FOR GROUP A STREPTOCOCCAL PHARYNGOTONSILLITIS AND ERADICATION OF STREPTOCOCCI[1,141,177]

Agent*	Dose	Route	Duration
Benzathine penicillin	600,000 U for patients <60 lb (27 kg) 1,200,000 U for patients ≥60 lb (27 kg)	Intramuscular	Once
or			
Phenoxymethylpenicillin	250 mg (400,000 U)/dose, for patients <60 lb (27 kg) 500 mg (800,000 U)/dose for patients ≥60 lb (27 kg) Two to three times daily	Oral	10 full days
or			
Amoxicillin	Children: 25–50 mg/kg per day divided into 3 doses Adolescents and adults: total dose of 750–1500 mg/day divided into three doses	Oral	10 full days
For individuals allergic to penicillin:			
Erythromycin estolate	20–40 mg/kg per day divided into 2–4 doses (maximum 1g/day)	Oral	10 full days
or			
Ethylsuccinate	40 mg/kg per day divided into 2–4 doses (maximum 1g/day)	Oral	10 full days

*For other acceptable alternatives, see text. The following agents are not acceptable: sulfonamides, including trimethoprim-sulfamethoxazole, tetracyclines, and chloramphenicol.
Modified from Guidelines for the diagn osis of rheumatic fever. Jones criteria, 1992 update. Special Writing Group of the Committee on Rheumatic Fever, Endocarditis, and Kawasaki Disease of the Council on Cardiovascular Disease in the Young of the American Heart Association. JAMA 1992:268:2069–2073.

disease, it is necessary to avoid the continuous exposure to streptococcal antigens. As soon as the diagnosis is established, patients with any manifestations of the acute rheumatic process, including the late ones such as chorea, should undergo antibiotic therapy to eradicate the streptococcus. The efficacy of eradication is dependent on the choice of the drug, and the length of time in which effective levels are maintained in the blood. In all patients, eradication should be followed by long-term secondary prophylaxis to prevent recurrences. Eradication is similar to treatment recommended for acute streptococcal pharyngotonsillitis (Table 54A-5).

Medical Management of Clinical Manifestations

Apart from a therapeutic course of penicillin needed to eradicate the group A *Streptococcus*, the medical treatment of the clinical manifestations remains supportive, and is based on anti-inflammatory drugs and bedrest. The choice of suppressive medication, duration of bedrest, and subsequent restriction of physical activity is best decided on an individual basis, depending on the severity and clinical response. Corticosteroids and salicylates, the mainstay of therapy, are effective in suppressing the acute signs of inflammation. Corticosteroids have shown a prompter action than salicylates, and can be lifesaving in severe presentations of carditis. There is no evidence that the anti-inflammatory therapy affects the frequency or severity of the valvar lesions, or prevents the cardiac sequels in the chronic phase. When comparing salicylates and corticosteroids, no treatment has been shown definitely to be superior. Meta-analysis showed no statistically significant difference in preventing development of pathological murmurs 1 year after treatment.[158] Likewise, no differences were found concerning the risk of cardiac disease when comparing several corticosteroid agents and intravenous immunoglobulin with aspirin, placebo, or no treatment.[159–161] It is advisable to defer the starting of anti-inflammatory or suppressive treatment until a definitive diagnosis has been established. It is unwise to start a therapeutic trial of either salicylates or steroids prematurely, since this may suppress the inflammatory process sufficiently to make a firm diagnosis almost impossible. It is doubtful if the anti-inflammatory drugs have any effect on either erythema marginatum or subcutaneous nodules.

Bedrest

The recommended duration and strictness of bedrest is variable depending on the manifestations and severity of the clinical presentation. At all stages of treatment, the necessities of patients to participate in recreational activities must be taken into consideration by providing alternatives according to their age and clinical condition. The recommendation of prolonged bedrest is based primarily on reducing cardiac work in those with carditis, and avoiding as much as possible the use of the involved joints in those with arthritis. Strict bedrest should be limited to patients with a more significant involvement of the heart, and to those with arthritis of the legs. Patients with polyarthritis, and without carditis, can be allowed out of bed as soon as the fever and local symptoms have subsided, and laboratory evidence of inflammation has begun to regress, usually after a period of 1 to 2 weeks. If there is no evidence of cardiac involvement in progress, this period is followed by gradual release for activities during the next 2 weeks. In those with carditis, the duration of bedrest depends on the severity of the cardiac lesions and the speed of regression of the acute episode. Patients with carditis, either isolated or associated with polyarthritis, but without cardiomegaly or congestive heart failure, should be made to rest for about a month. The rest need not be strict, and it should be followed by supervised activities for the following weeks. Patients with cardiomegaly, but without definite congestive failure, should be made to rest, with strict enforcement over the first 3 to 4 weeks, before a gradual release. In the presence of carditis and congestive heart failure, patients should be kept on absolute rest until the failure is completely controlled, and they should maintain modified bedrest with slow and gradual restoration of activities, provided there is no rebound.

TABLE 54A-6

TREATMENT OF MAJOR MANIFESTATIONS OF CARDITIS

Clinical Manifestation	Treatment Schedule*
Severe carditis	Prednisone† 2 mg/kg/day once daily
Moderate carditis	Prednisone 1–2 mg/kg/day once daily *or* Aspirin‡ 75–100 mg/day divided into 4 doses
Mild carditis	Aspirin 75–100 mg/day divided into 4 doses
Polyarthritis	Aspirin 75–100 mg/day divided into 4 doses *or* Naproxen 10–20 mg/kg/day
Chorea	Haloperidol§ 2–6 mg/day *or* Valproic acid 20–30 mg/kg/day

*See text for complementary information.
†Maximum dose is 80 mg/day.
‡Serum level should not exceed 30 mg/dL.
§Maximum dose is 6 mg/day.

Carditis

Anti-inflammatory drugs have been extensively employed in the treatment of carditis, showing a prompt effect in terms of cardiac symptoms (Table 54A-6). Salicylates have been used for those with less severe forms of carditis, when there is no necessity for powerful suppression of inflammation.[1,111,137] Corticosteroids have been recommended for patients with at least moderately severe carditis, especially for those with congestive heart failure. Prednisone is usually preferred as it produces less retention of sodium and loss of potassium. The initial dose of prednisone is given for 2 to 3 weeks depending on the severity of the carditis. After this period, a gradual tapering is required. The dose should be slowly withdrawn, decreasing by one-fifth each week, which means a total duration of the treatment of about 8 to 12 weeks, coinciding with the duration of the acute episode. Rebounds are sometimes associated with rapid withdrawal of corticosteroids. Some authors have recommended an overlapping therapy with the aim to prevent rebounds, with the introduction of salicylates as the dose of corticosteroids is reduced.[137,162] The advantage of the use of high doses of methylprednisolone as an alternative treatment remains controversial. It has most frequently been administered as a life-saving therapy for those with severe carditis.[163,164] The use of intravenous gamma-globulin has been reported in patients with carditis, but more investigations are required to evaluate this therapy.[161,165] The lack of clinical improvement due to mechanical factors can be observed in patients with severe valvar lesions, mainly in those with recurrences, and sometimes the treatment is surgical.[26]

Supportive measures include the treatment of congestive heart failure and arrhythmias. Congestive heart failure in rheumatic carditis is often controlled with bedrest and corticosteroids alone. In patients with severe forms of presentation, the use of digoxin, diuretics, and inhibitors of angiotensin-converting enzyme should be considered.[1]

Arthritis

Salicylates are the first-line treatment for patients with established arthritis but without carditis. These agents usually have a dramatic effect on the articular inflammatory process, with a prompt improvement, commonly within 24 to 48 hours. In this context, premature treatment can interfere in the characterisation of the migratory pattern of the arthritis, thus making the diagnosis difficult. The differential diagnosis with other diseases must be considered when the articular symptoms are not responsive to salicylates.[21] An effective and safer dose of aspirin for children usually produces a level of salicylate in the blood of not more than 20 mg, which is well below the toxic range (see Table 54A-6). The full dose is given for the first 2 weeks and subsequently is gradually reduced to up to 60 mg/kg over the next 2 to 3 weeks. A smaller or a larger dose can be used, depending on the clinical response to treatment, and may be maximised for those failing to respond to lower doses. A higher dose, such as 100 mg/kg, is required by few patients. If more massive doses of salicylates are given, toxicity can occur. Rapid breathing is one of the early signs of toxicity. Nausea, vomiting, tinnitus, lassitude and occasionally delirium, convulsion, and coma can occur. Naproxen is an alternative therapy for patients who are allergic to or intolerant of aspirin.[1,166,167]

Sydenham's Chorea

Isolated chorea is treated symptomatically. The patients should be kept in a quiet environment to protect them from external stimulation and stress. Precautions must be taken to prevent accidents and, according to their condition, appropriate sedation can be helpful. Besides barbiturates and chlorpromazine, diazepam has been used in management. Haloperidol and valproic acid are frequently employed, and have been shown to be effective in controlling symptoms,[168,169] albeit requiring longer periods when compared to the time required to control carditis and arthritis[26] after the use of anti-inflammatory drugs (see Table 54A-6).

Anti-inflammatory agents are usually not indicated, because chorea often occurs after the resolution of the systemic inflammatory process. The use of corticosteroids and immunoglobulin in patients with isolated Sydenham's chorea is controversial.[170–174] The need for the eradication of the streptococcus, followed by regular secondary prophylaxis, is as important in chorea as in any other rheumatic manifestation. Due to the more recent observations regarding the neuropsychiatric disorders and persistent disabilities in some patients, a more aggressive treatment has been recommended, along with the need for closer vigilance in the period of follow-up.[128,129,130,175,176]

Rebounds

Clinical or laboratory evidence of rebounds is infrequent. They can be seen after cessation of the anti-inflammatory treatment, and usually occur within 2 to 3 weeks. Some patients show only laboratory abnormalities. Those with clinical rebounds usually show arthralgia, fever, and occasionally arthritis, but severe cardiac manifestations may also occur. Rebounds occur more often after corticosteroid therapy than salicylates. Laboratory rebounds, and most of the clinical rebounds, do not require any treatment. They usually subside spontaneously within a few days. Only the very severe clinical rebounds need a full reinstitution of the earlier treatment.[1,162]

PREVENTION

Prevention of both primary episodes and recurrences is related to the control of the group A streptococcal infections. Primary prevention implicates controlling the initial attack of rheumatic fever by means of the identification and eradication of the group A *Streptococcus* from the tonsillar and pharyngeal tissue during the acute infection, besides promoting means to reduce the exposure of patients to the bacteria. Secondary prevention, by means of the continuous use of antibiotics, is related to the control of recurrences in patients who have already been affected by rheumatic fever, independent from the clinical manifestation or presence of sequels. These patients are particularly susceptible to developing subsequent attacks of the disease when faced with an acute infection by the group A *Streptococcus*, symptomatic or not.

Public education is an important aspect of prevention when the low cost of the prophylactic therapy is compared with the consequences of the disease. In this respect, in Brazil we have followed the concept of vertical programming. Thus, our programme for prophylaxis of rheumatic fever is based on progressive involvement from local through city administrations to the level of a nation-wide programme. In the case of rheumatic fever, the majority of available national resources has been allocated towards diseases specific projects. This is vertical programming, to be contrasted with more broad-based improvements in the health of the population, such as general measures for prevention, and development of primary care services and the health workforce, which represent horizontal programming.

Primary Prevention

Besides preventing rheumatic fever, an accurate diagnosis of a streptococcal pharyngotonsillitis, and the prompt introduction of antibiotic therapy, can shorten the evolution of the infection, with improvement of symptoms. Additionally, adequate management reduces the rate of transmission to close contacts, since after 24 hours of the onset of the treatment, patients are considered noncontagious.[141,177]

Table 54A-7 summarises the clinical features and epidemiological data which may be helpful in identifying the streptococcal pharyngotonsillitis. These characteristics are useful for diagnosis, but none can predict or exclude the streptococcal aetiology with certainty, because the same clinical picture may be produced by other agents which cause exudative pharyngotonsillitis. Hoarseness, conjunctivitis, cough, nasal congestion, and a runny nose are symptoms and signs more usually associated with viral infections.[29,61,177] Considering the difficulties for a precise clinical diagnosis, the laboratory confirmation of group A streptococcal infection should ideally be performed before starting antibiotics. Throat swabs, or the rapid antigen detection test whenever possible, should be obtained with the aim of avoiding excessive use of antibiotics, and consequently the emergence of resistant organisms. The serological examination for streptococcal antibodies to extracellular antigens constitutes a useful method to identify the preceding infection with the group A *Streptococcus* and support the diagnosis of rheumatic fever. The test, however, has limitations in diagnosis, since the results can be interpreted only in retrospect.[1,29,30]

TABLE 54A-7

CLINICAL CHARACTERISTICS OF ACUTE PHARYNGOTONSILLITIS CAUSED BY GROUP A β-HAEMOLYTIC STREPTOCOCCI

Most common in age group of 5–15 years
Sudden onset of acute pharyngeal pain and malaise
Headache
Fever of 102°–104°F (39°–40°C)
Pharyngeal erythema and exudate, soft palatal petechias
Enlarged tender cervical lymph nodes
Scabby erosions on the edges of nostrils
Presence of constitutional signs and symptoms
Acute otitis media
Vomiting
Suppurative sinusitis

Difficulties exist in providing effective primary prevention, since a clinical diagnosis of the streptococcal infection often poses a problem because of the difficulty in ruling out other bacterial and viral causes. Approximately two-fifths of acute throat infections are of bacterial aetiology, and the streptococcus is responsible for about half of these events.[29,178,179] Another difficulty includes the presence of the unrecognised forms of infection, considering that the streptococcal pharyngotonsillitis may not always manifest as a severe infection. A clinically mild sore throat is not uncommon, and sometimes is asymptomatic, but may still lead to rheumatic fever. At least one-third of patients with rheumatic fever have no history of an antecedent streptococcal infection, a limiting condition for primary prophylaxis.[180] In addition, the efficacy of primary prevention is restricted in areas with high rates of exposure. In this context, unfavourable living conditions, such as over-crowding with closer interpersonal contact, constitute a propitious condition for the propagation of the bacteria. Persistence of the streptococcus following the infection as a result of an inappropriate regime for eradication is a cause of failure to prevent rheumatic fever. Streptococcal pharyngotonsillitis, independent of treatment, can present as a self-limited condition. Use of bactericidal drugs, with administration of sufficient doses to ensure therapeutic levels in the serum for 10 days, therefore, is an important requirement to achieve maximal rates of eradication and to prevent rheumatic fever. No single regime achieves the complete eradication in treated patients.[111,141,181] Routine culturing after an adequate treatment with good compliance, nonetheless, is not indicated, except in specific epidemiological situations, such as increased risk of streptococcal infections or presence of streptococcal non-suppurative sequels.[1,29,121,177] Tonsillectomy is not recommended for the primary prevention of rheumatic fever, as no controlled studies have shown its effectiveness in reducing the frequency of the disease.[48]

Recommended regimes for primary prophylaxis are shown in Table 54A-5. Factors to be considered for the selection of therapy include an antimicrobial agent of confirmed clinical and bacteriological efficacy, narrow antimicrobial spectrum, good compliance with therapy, low incidence of side effects, and low cost. The treatment of an acute episode of pharyngotonsillitis before the ninth day of infection is effective in preventing the attack of rheumatic fever.[182] The group A β-haemolytic *Streptococcus* remains remarkably sensitive to penicillin.[52] This antibiotic is considered the drug of choice for treatment, with proven effectiveness in primary prophylaxis. Serious side reactions and major sensitive reactions to penicillin are unusual.[1,30,32,183,184] Drugs other than penicillin offer no advantage for treatment of streptococcal infection, when account is taken of their cost-effectiveness. Intramuscular benzathine penicillin, also known as benzathine penicillin G, is often used, especially for those patients who are unlikely to complete the conventional 10-day course of oral treatment. The oral antibiotic of choice is phenoxymethyl penicillin, or penicillin V. Amoxicillin and ampicillin have been used but have no microbiological advantage over penicillin.[177] The disadvantage, as occurs with phenoxymethyl penicillin, is that oral antibiotics may be taken irregularly or for a shorter period, leading to an inadequate level in the blood, or may be used for insufficient time to achieve maximal rates of eradication of the bacteria. Patients must continue to take the penicillin regularly for the entire period, even though they will probably be completely asymptomatic after the first few days. Another acceptable alternative for a 10-day course of therapy is a first-generation cephalosporin. Besides the disadvantage of the broader spectrum of activity and higher cost, when compared to penicillin, care must be observed, as those who are allergic to penicillin may also be allergic to cephalosporins. Shorter courses of oral penicillin have been reported for the treatment of group A streptococcal pharyngotonsillitis. Although these regimes may be clinically effective in non-epidemic settings, they are not adequate for prevention of rheumatic fever when the treatment of the infection due to rheumatogenic strains is considered.[30] Erythromycin is the first alternative choice for patients allergic to penicillin. It should also be given in divided doses for 10 days, and the dose should not exceed 1 g daily. When a macrolide antibiotic is considered, account should be taken of the rates of resistance in the community. For the rare situation of patients allergic to both penicillin and erythromycin, clindamycin is an option.[29]

Newer macrolides such as azithromycin and clarithromycin are reported as being effective. Azithromycin has a similar antibacterial spectrum to that of erythromycin against the group A *Streptococcus*, has fewer gastrointestinal side effects, and produces high tonsillar tissue concentration. The drawback of these alternatives is cost and their broader spectrum, with the risk of emergence of resistant pathogens.[111] Regarding the shorter courses of azithromycin and some cephalosporins, there is insufficient evidence to recommend these regimes for routine treatment. They should not replace penicillin as the agent of choice.[1,29,32,185] Certain antimicrobials are not recommended for the treatment of streptococcal infections, due to high rates of resistance and consequent failure in eradicating the streptococcus. Tetracycline should not be used because of the high prevalence of resistant strains to this antibiotic. The sulphonamide drugs, although effective as continuous prophylaxis for the prevention of recurrent attacks of rheumatic fever, should not be used for the treatment of streptococcal infection owing to the frequent failure to eradicate the bacteria.[29]

Carriers

Throat carriers can be transient, convalescent, or chronic. Chronic carriers may not show any clinical or serological evidence of infection and, in time, may reveal the organisms in the throat only intermittently. They are known as spotty carriers. The treatment of carriers has questionable value, especially in the absence of clinical or epidemiological evidence of active infection. According to the American Academy of Pediatrics,[177] antimicrobial treatment for throat carriers is an exception, and is indicated only in specific circumstances such as a family history of rheumatic fever, an outbreak of rheumatic fever, or an outbreak of streptococcal pharyngotonsillitis in semiclosed or closed communities.

Secondary Prevention

Secondary prophylaxis should be started soon after the diagnosis of an acute episode of rheumatic fever, or when well-documented rheumatic heart disease is established. The institution of continuous prophylactic regimens to prevent recurrences is mandatory for all patients, independent of the clinical manifestation or presence of sequels, and is based on two premises. First, as it occurs in the primary episodes, there is a causal relationship between the group A streptococcal pharyngotonsillitis and the subsequent attacks. Second, an increased number of recurrences is usually associated with a poor prognosis. Although none of the regimes is able to modify the course or severity of the valvar sequels, prevention of colonisation or streptococcal infections is markedly effective in reducing recurrences and, consequently, the appearance of new valvar lesions or worsening of the preexisting ones. In patients whose diagnosis of rheumatic fever has not completely been elucidated, the need for secondary prophylaxis depends on the judgement of individual risks. Its maintenance should be evaluated during the follow-up.

The regimes for secondary prevention are shown in Table 54A-8. Benzathine penicillin is the first choice, and

TABLE 54A-8

SECONDARY PREVENTION OF RHEUMATIC FEVER: PROPHYLAXIS OF RECURRENT ATTACKS*

Agent	Dose	Route
Benzathine penicillin (benzathine penicillin G)	600,000 units for patients <27 kg (60 lb) 1,200,000 units for patients ≥27 kg (60 lb), single dose, every 3 or 4 weeks†	Instramuscular
or		
Phenoxymethyl penicillin (penicillin V)	250 mg twice daily	Oral
For individuals allergic to penicillin:		
Sulphadiazine (sulfadiazine)	0.5 g for patients <27 kg (60 lb) 1.0 g once daily for patients ≥27kg (60 lb), once daily	Oral
For individuals allergic to penicillin and sulphadiazine:		
Erythromycin	250 mg twice daily	Oral

*See text for complementary information.
†Administration every 3 weeks is recommended in high-risk situations.
Data from World Health Organization: Rheumatic Fever and Rheumatic Heart Disease. Report of a WHO Expert Consultation. Geneva, 29 October-1 November 2001. WHO technical report series No 923. Geneva: WHO, 2004: and Dajani A, Taubert K, Ferrieri P, et al: Treatment of acute Streptococcal pharyngitis and prevention of Rheumatic fever: a statement for health professionals. Committee on Rheumatic Fever, Endocarditis, and Kawasaki Disease of the Council on Cardiovascular Disease in the Young, the American Heart Association. Pediatrics 1995; 96 (4 pt 1): 758-764.

constitutes the most effective strategy to prevent recurrences of acute episodes. Regarding the mode of administration, the monthly use of the repository presentation of penicillin has long been considered an effective form of prophylaxis, and is still currently advocated.[186] Nonetheless, in populations with high prevalence of rheumatic fever, shorter intervals are recommended, supported by observations of higher rates of recurrences related to monthly prophylactic regimens when compared to 3-week intervals.[26,187–189] In addition, pharmacokinetic studies have demonstrated inadequate levels of penicillin in the serum to cover the last week of the month.[190–194] Prevention with regimes at 2-week intervals has shown high levels of penicillin and lower rates of recurrences, but there is the inconvenience of the frequent use of medication, and the adherence to treatment.[26,190,195] The choice of either a 3- or 4-week interval, therefore, must be tailored to the epidemiological context, mainly the frequency of rheumatic fever in the community and individual risks of exposure to the group A *Streptococcus*. In areas where the incidence and prevalence of rheumatic fever are particularly high, the administration of benzathine penicillin every 3 weeks is justified, and is also recommended in special circumstances and for certain individuals deemed to be at high risk.[1,141] For effective prevention, it is necessary to ensure that protective levels will be reached and maintained in the serum during the interval between the doses, besides considering adverse factors such as lack of compliance with continuous medication, bioavailability, and absorption of the drug. In this setting, adequate levels are less predictable when using oral medication. Oral sulphadiazine is recommended for patients allergic to penicillin, and for those allergic to both drugs, erythromycin is the recommended alternative. Sulphadiazine, although effective in preventing colonisation of the upper respiratory tract with streptococcal strains, is not indicated for primary prevention.

Regarding the duration of secondary prophylaxis, lifelong prevention is particularly important in those with established rheumatic heart disease, since patients with cardiac lesions are at higher risk of recurrences. It is known, however, that the risk of subsequent attacks declines with age and the length of time since the last attack. Considering the difficulties of maintaining lifelong treatment, exceptions may be made, especially in older patients. These are determined on an individual basis. In coming to a decision, the physician should carefully take into account a number of factors, such as age, socioeconomic and educational status, the rates of recurrence in the community, the individual risks of acquiring a streptococcal infection, the presence of a recent attack of rheumatic fever, the number of previous attacks, the presence of rheumatic heart disease, and the potential risks of a recurrence in the severity of an established valvar lesion. Adults at an increased risk, such as parents of young children, school teachers, medical and paramedical personnel, and military cadets and servicemen, necessarily need prophylaxis over a longer period of time. In countries with poor socioeconomic development, the environmental factors weigh heavily against effective programmes for secondary prophylaxis. The greatest risk of rheumatic recurrences is in the disadvantaged, which includes children and adolescents, those with established rheumatic heart disease, those who have had multiple attacks in the past, and those suffering crowding at home. Prophylaxis should be continued for prolonged periods in individuals who have had valvar surgery for rheumatic heart disease, even after valvar replacement with prosthetic valves, since they continue to be at risk (Table 54A-9).

TABLE 54A-9

DURATION OF SECONDARY PROPHYLAXIS*

Category of Patient	Duration
Patients without carditis	For 5 years after the last acute episode or until age 21 years, whichever is longer
Patients with carditis but without sequels	For 10 years after the last acute episode or until age 25 years, whichever is longer
Patients with carditis and residual valvar lesion	At least until age 40 years or life-long

*See text for complementary information.

Data from Dajani A, Taubert K, Ferrieri P, et al: Treatment of acute streptococcal pharyngitis and prevention of rheumatic fever: A statement for health professionals. Committee on Rheumatic Fever, Endocarditis, and Kawasaki Disease of the Council on Cardiovascular Disease in the Young, the American Heart Association. Pediatrics 1995;96 (4 Pt 1):758–764; and World Health Organization: Rheumatic Fever and Rheumatic Heart Disease. Report of a WHO Expert Consultation. Geneva, 29 October–1 November 2001. WHO technical report series No. 923. Geneva: WHO, 2004.

One of the main concerns is the adherence of patients to the prophylactic regimens. As a consequence of the use of a medication involving painful administration, or daily oral therapy for long periods of time, sometimes compliance with prophylactic regimens can constitute a challenge, mainly in adolescents. Another reason to discontinue prophylaxis would be incomplete information about the disease and the need of prevention, besides the fear of allergic reactions. Anaphylaxis, however, is a rare event, and the great majority of cases of hypersensitivity are represented by mild reactions, mainly skin rashes. The risk of a serious complication is lower in children than in adults, and long-term prevention does not appear to increase the risk of an allergic reaction.[28,196,197] To improve compliance with the prophylactic regimen, it is important to plan the follow-up with patients and families. Information must be given about the importance of the continuous medication, and why it is necessary to prevent subsequent streptococcal infections.

For the prevention of infective endocarditis, regular evaluation of the oral health is important to avoid the increased risk of bacteraemia associated with dental or gingival diseases. Special attention must be given to patients with valvar lesions and, particularly, in case of prosthetic valves, which are associated with higher predisposition to endocarditis. Additionally, a prosthetic valve is one of the underlying conditions associated with the highest risk of adverse outcome from endocarditis.[198] Patients with previous episodes of endocarditis are at a higher risk of subsequent episodes.[199] Endocarditis prophylaxis should be recommended for patients with rheumatic valvar lesions, depending on the risks of bacteremia, cardiac condition, and the characteristics of the interventional procedure. The updated recommendations for endocarditis prophylaxis have been more restrictive regarding the cardiac conditions warranting prophylaxis.[198,200–202] As the usual dosages used to prevent recurrences of rheumatic fever are lower than those recommended for the prevention of endocarditis, the long-term therapy does not protect from endocarditis.

Additional prevention is necessary. For those on secondary prophylaxis with oral penicillin, it is advisable to administer another class of antibiotic to prevent endocarditis. These patients are likely to harbour viridans streptococci, which are relatively resistant to penicillin and amoxicillin.[198]

Strategies for Immunisation Using Vaccines Against Rheumatic Fever

The efforts to produce a vaccine against infection date from the first decades of the 20th century. The M protein, the principal virulence factor of that bacterium, was initially used as an inducer of protection. The early vaccines, however, despite producing type-specific immune responses, were ineffective in preventing primary or recurrent attacks of rheumatic fever because individuals who have suffered infection with streptococcuses of a given serotype are rarely reinfected with a microorganism of the same M type.[1] The great diversity in M types and *emm* genotypes of *Streptococcus pyogenes* which cause rheumatic fever in different populations, combined with the rapid turnover of its serotypes in endemic regions, make it difficult to obtain an efficacious vaccine.[46]

The key point in production, however, is to avoid the risk of triggering or aggravating rheumatic fever and rheumatic heart disease in the recipients, since antibodies against some M protein sites, the so-called autoimmune epitopes, may cross-react with α-helical human proteins, such as tropomyosin, myosin, and vimentin. One of the recent strategies in the development of vaccines is to use the highly conserved C region of the streptococcal M protein, common to most strains of the bacterium.[203,204] Another attempt to achieve a safe vaccine is the search for protective epitopes of the C-terminal portion of the M protein,[205] aiming at identifying amino-acid residues that could elicit a B-cell response dependent on T-cell signalling, thus providing a protective immune response against *S. pyogenes*.

In a recent communication, use of a recombinant vaccine containing N-terminal M protein fragments from six serotypes of group A *Streptococcus* showed, after a 1-year follow-up period, that the vaccine was well tolerated, did not induce cross-reactivity with human tissues, and increased the antibody levels to M antigens and also the bactericidal serum activity.[206] These preliminary conclusions, however, should not be extrapolated to children, especially those residing in regions of the world with high prevalence of rheumatic fever. Clinical trials directed to this population will be needed. Moreover, there are some other problems in the development of the vaccine that must be over-come, such as the duration of the immunological protection against the bacterial infection, especially in endemic areas from developing countries, routes of administration, and potential side-effects. Still other issues, such as cost and stability of the vaccine under field conditions, must also be addressed, if primary prevention of rheumatic fever is to become effective in a variety of socioeconomic and epidemiological conditions.[1]

ACKNOWLEDGEMENTS

We are indebted to Cleusa C. Lapa Santos, Luiza Guilherme, and Pablo M. Pomerantzeff, for reviewing the text in the light of their specific areas of expertise.

The complete reference list can be found on the companion Expert Consult web site at www.expertconsult.com.

ANNOTATED REFERENCES

- Cunningham MW: Pathogenesis of group A streptococcal infections. Clin Microbiol Rev 2000;13:470–511.

  The author provides an extensive review of the structural and antigenic features of the group A Streptococcus, *discussing the mechanisms of disease, including molecular mimicry with host tissues, which may lead to rheumatic fever and immune-mediated glomerulonephritis. Strategies for production of vaccines are also discussed.*
- Guilherme L, Fae K, Oshiro SE, Kalil J: Molecular pathogenesis of rheumatic fever and rheumatic heart disease. Expert Rev Mol Med 2005;7:1–15.

  This article summarises studies on markers of genetic susceptibility involved in the development of rheumatic fever and rheumatic heart disease, and also focuses on the molecular mimicry mediated by the responses of B and T cells of peripheral blood, and T cells infiltrating heart lesions, against streptococcal antigens and human tissue proteins. The molecular basis of T-cell recognition is assessed through the definition of heart cross-reactive antigens.
- Kotloff KL, Corretti M, Palmer K, et al: Safety and immunogenicity of a recombinant multivalent group A streptococcal vaccine in healthy adults: Phase 1 trial. JAMA 2004;292:709–715.

  This study evaluates the safety and immunogenicity of ascending doses of a recombinant fusion peptide group A streptococcal vaccine containing N-terminal M protein fragments from serotypes 1, 3, 5, 6, 19, and 24 in healthy volunteers. The results provide the first evidence in humans that a hybrid fusion protein is a feasible strategy for evoking type-specific opsonic antibodies against multiple serotypes of group A Streptococcus *without eliciting antibodies that cross-react with host tissues, which represents a critical step in the development of a vaccine.*
- Carapetis JR, Steer AC, Mulholland EK, Weber M: The global burden of group A streptococcal diseases. Lancet Infect Dis 2005;5:685–694.

  The authors evaluate the burden of diseases caused by the group A Streptococcus *on a global scale according to a review of population-based data, highlighting the importance of developing strategies for prevention. It is estimated that more than 336,000 cases of rheumatic fever occur in those aged from 5 to 14 years, and an annual number at more than 471,000 for all ages. About three-fifths of the cases, about 282,000 patients, are expected to develop rheumatic heart disease each year.*
- Guidelines for the diagnosis of rheumatic fever. Jones criteria, 1992 update. Special Writing Group of the Committee on Rheumatic Fever, Endocarditis, and Kawasaki Disease of the Council on Cardiovascular Disease in the Young of the American Heart Association. JAMA 1992:268:2069–2073.

  The diagnostic criterions initially formulated by Jones have been revised over the past years by the American Heart Association. This last review of the guidelines is intended for diagnosis of primary episodes. Nonetheless, when other diseases are excluded, three situations—Sydenham's chorea, indolent carditis, and recurrent episodes—are emphasised as exceptions to the need for strict adherence to the criterions.
- World Health Organization: Rheumatic Fever and Rheumatic Heart Disease: Report of a WHO Expert Consultation, Geneva, 29 October–1 November 2001. WHO technical report series No. 923. Geneva: WHO, 2004.

  This technical report from the World Health Organization comprises a complete and updated review of the epidemiological, pathogenetic, clinical, therapeutic, and prophylactic aspects of rheumatic fever and its cardiac sequels, with an extensive list of references.
- Veasy LG, Tani LY: A new look at acute rheumatic mitral regurgitation. Cardiol Young 2005;15:568–577.

  The authors discuss the role of the pericardium, myocardium, and endocardium in the clinical presentation of rheumatic carditis. In the light of past clinical experience, and the current knowledge of mitral valvar function and structure, the authors analyse the supporting evidence for the newer understanding of the acute mitral regurgitation.
- Stollerman GH: Rheumatic fever. Lancet 1997;349:935–942.

  The unchanged pattern of rheumatic fever regarding the clinical profile, diagnostic criterions, clinical management, and prophylactic approach is reviewed in parallel with the analysis of changes in epidemiological aspects of rheumatic fever, besides the variable pattern of severity of the disease and its sequels among diverse populations. The authors emphasise the importance of an early diagnosis and the prospects for a vaccine.
- Markowitz M: Rheumatic fever—a half-century perspective. Pediatrics 1998;102(Suppl):272–274.

  From a historical perspective, and based on the experience gathered during the past 50 years, the reasons are discussed for the cyclic changes in the incidence of rheumatic fever, as well as the limitations still existing in eradicating the disease.
- Cilliers AM, Manyemba J, Saloojee H: Anti-inflammatory treatment for carditis in acute rheumatic fever. Cochrane Database Syst Rev 2003;(2):CD003176.
- Cilliers AM: Treating acute rheumatic fever. BMJ 2003;327:631–632.

  Randomised trials describing cardiac outcomes in patients treated with several corticosteroid agents, aspirin, intravenous immunoglobulin, and placebo were analysed in a Cochrane review. The results of the comparative analysis did not demonstrate evidences of one therapy to be more effective in reducing the risk of valvar sequels in the long term.

Chronic Rheumatic Heart Disease

CHAPTER 54B

CLEONICE C. COELHO MOTA, VERA DEMARCHI AIELLO, and ROBERT H. ANDERSON

Chronic rheumatic heart disease, representing the permanent lesions of the cardiac valves, is the most serious consequence of rheumatic fever. It accounts for a significant number of repeated hospitalisations and deaths. Recurrences of rheumatic fever play an important role in the worsening of the valvar lesions, but the damage, as a result of the process of cicatrisation, can be progressive even in the absence of subsequent acute episodes. The clinical presentation, the mortality, as well as the frequency and speed of development of an established valvar disease after the acute phase, vary considerably geographically, influenced primarily by the socioeconomic and medical backgrounds of the populations involved. In developed countries, severe rheumatic valvar disease is now uncommon in children and adolescents, and treatment for the advanced form of the disease is usually limited to adults. In contrast, in many developing countries, chronic rheumatic heart disease remains the most important cause of acquired cardiac disease among patients aged between 5 and 30.[1] On a global scale, it has been estimated that around 2 to 4 million patients aged from 5 to 14 are affected with rheumatic heart disease. It is also anticipated that each year an additional 282,000 new patients present with the ravages of chronic disease.[2] The prevalence of chronic disease was mostly based on surveys of schoolchildren, with rates ranging from 0.2 to 77.8 for each 1000 of the population in developing communities.[3–7] The highest rates are registered in the Pacific region and in the Republic of Congo.[8] Among 550 Brazilian students, aged from 10 to 20 years and chosen randomly, the prevalence was calculated at 1.8 cases for each 1000 students.[9] Although progress in diagnosis and management over recent decades has provided a better quality of life, the disease causes significant disabilities and premature deaths in young individuals, with considerable personal and collective costs. The disability-adjusted life years lost to chronic rheumatic heart disease ranged from 27.4 to 173.4 per 100,000 population, giving an estimated 6.6 million life years lost each year throughout the world. The disease is responsible for up to two-thirds of the admissions to hospital due to cardiac problems in some countries. The rates of death because of chronic rheumatic heart disease show a wide variation, from 0.5 to 8.2 for each 100,000 population, according to the area of investigation. For the year 2000, the number of deaths worldwide was estimated at 332,000.[4]

The healing process of rheumatic carditis results in varying degrees of fibrosis and valvar damage. In some instances, fusion and thickening of the pericardium may also occur, but this rarely affects the ultimate cardiac performance. Resolution of the chronic valvar disease has been associated with the degree of the valvar involvement during the acute inflammatory process. Those suffering only mild valvar lesions in the acute phase, with minor degrees of thickening of the valves and tendinous cords, and some fibrosis of the valvar endocardium, are unlikely to suffer abnormal haemodynamic effects in the chronic phase. If recurrences are prevented, mitral insufficiency in patients without cardiomegaly, pericarditis, or cardiac failure is expected to heal without scarring in about four-fifths of cases.[10] On the other hand, more severe valvar damage can occur in the initial acute episode, and the early onset of significant lesions has an important impact on the development and severity of the permanent valvar damage. Considering the clinical and echocardiographic evaluation of cardiac involvement from the acute to the chronic phase, regression of valvar lesions was found mostly in those initially suffering mild carditis, with less regression in those known to have had moderate carditis, and no improvement observed in cases of severe carditis.[11] Poor outcomes for rheumatic heart disease have also shown a causal relation with recurrences.[12–17] Repeated episodes of rheumatic fever usually lead to significant valvar disease in childhood and adolescence, often associated with pulmonary hypertension. The socioeconomic condition is known to be a contributing factor for the high rates of rheumatic fever, recurrences, and rheumatic heart disease.[8,18] In this setting, a low level of maternal schooling also emerged as a variable interacting with recurrences, as well as featuring as an independent risk factor in predicting severe chronic valvar disease in patients without recurrences.[15] It is also likely that episodes of subclinical carditis can result in chronic rheumatic valvar disease. The fact that many adults present with rheumatic heart disease without an earlier history of an acute episode supports this view, although the exact incidence of subclinical attacks is difficult to evaluate. The true incidence of carditis, nonetheless, is probably much higher than previously thought. Failure to recognise the primary episode of rheumatic fever, and inadequate secondary prevention, were identified as the major contributors to the increase in the frequency of recurrences and chronic rheumatic heart disease.[19] More recent studies using echocardiography have consistently documented that subclinical carditis does occur, and have shown a wide variation in prevalence.[20] Similarly, pathological valvar regurgitation detected only by Doppler echocardiography has been reported during the chronic phase in patients not previously suspected to have rheumatic valvar disease after physical examination.[7,15,21,22] Patients with chronic subclinical rheumatic valvar disease, as well as those with subclinical valvitis, are susceptible to infective endocarditis, which, should it occur, significantly alters the cardiac state.

In all age groups, the mitral valve is most commonly affected, followed by a combination of mitral and aortic

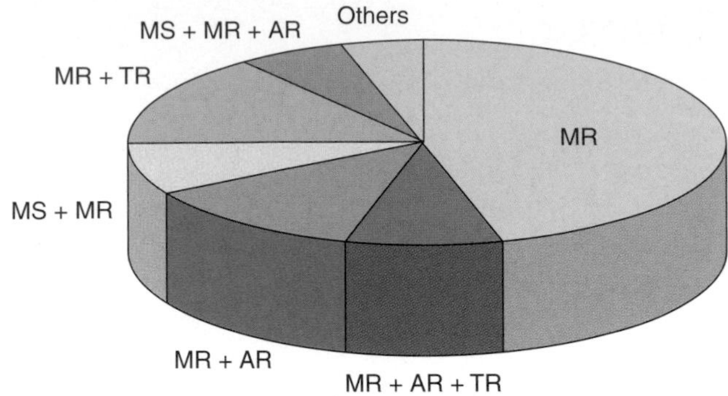

Figure 54B-1 The distribution of children and adolescents with rheumatic heart disease according to the valvar lesions (N = 585) as seen in the Rheumatic Fever Outpatients Clinic, Division of Paediatric Cardiology, Hospital das Clínicas, Federal University of Minas Gerais, Brazil. AR, aortic regurgitation; MR, mitral regurgitation; MS, mitral stenosis; TR, tricuspid regurgitation.

valves, then isolated aortic valvar disease, usually incompetence, and combined mitral, aortic, and tricuspid disease.[23–26] Chronic rheumatic involvement of the pulmonary valve is rare. Analysis of the patients seen in the Rheumatic Fever Outpatients Clinic in Belo Horizonte, Brazil, has revealed isolated mitral regurgitation in almost half of the patients with chronic disease, and the combination of mitral and aortic regurgitation as the second most frequent lesion. Valvar insufficiency was present in almost three-quarters, insufficiency and obstruction in just over one-quarter, and isolated valvar obstruction in only 0.7% (Fig. 54B-1).

Mitral insufficiency is the most frequent valvar lesion involved in paediatric surgical series. In developing countries, mitral stenosis is also a common lesion, and percutaneous balloon valvoplasty, or closed mitral commissurotomy, are procedures frequently carried out in children and adolescents in these regions. Mitral or aortic regurgitation may be sufficiently severe to cause life-threatening haemodynamic effects. These complications may require major cardiac surgery, either electively, or even occasionally as an emergency.[27] The progress in diagnostic methods, catheter interventions, surgical expertise and techniques, and the development of improved valvar prostheses has encouraged the increased use of non-surgical and surgical techniques for the treatment of rheumatic valvar disease in children, adolescents and young adults.

PATHOGENESIS OF CHRONIC LESIONS

Recurrent attacks of acute rheumatic fever lead to rheumatic heart disease, characterised by sequels in the cardiac valves and myocardium. Rheumatic heart disease is estimated to occur in around three-fifths of all patients having acute rheumatic fever. The chronic lesions are the consequence of valvar scarring, and of healing of the pancarditis, including fibrosis of the myocardium and occasionally adhesive pericarditis. In the valves, the organisation of superficial fibrin vegetations from the acute phase results in thickening of the leaflets, fusion of the ends of the zones of apposition, and shortening of tendinous cords. Subsequent damage occurs due to local disturbances of haemodynamics and flow of blood leading to deposition and organisation of thrombus. Once neovascularisation of the valvar leaflets has occurred, inflammatory cells can reach the valvar stroma, not only through the endocardial surface, but also from the endothelium of the newly formed vessels. The predominance of cells producing the regulatory interleukins 4 and 10 in the myocardium, as compared to the valvar tissue, explains at least in part the milder or absent inflammation in the myocardium during the chronic phase of the disease, whereas in valvar tissue inflammation is a permanent finding.[28]

Myocardial remodelling secondary to pressure or volume overload due to valvar dysfunction depends on the severity and duration of the haemodynamic disturbance. If the valvar lesions stand for long periods, as is likely to occur in patients from countries with limited resources for public health, progressive cardiac hypertrophy, chamber dilation, and interstitial myocardial fibrosis may occur, leading to severe cardiac failure that can become irreversible even after later valvar replacement or valvoplasty. In this context, cardiac transplantation is an option to treat these end-stage patients. In a multi-centric study in Brazil, chronic valvar rheumatic heart disease accounted for 3.5% of all cardiac transplants performed over a period of 16 years.[29]

Lesions of the left-sided valves also lead to chronic pulmonary congestion and passive pulmonary hypertension, and consequently to right ventricular hypertrophy and functional tricuspid regurgitation. Atrial fibrillation, a complication present in about half of patients with chronic mitral stenosis as seen in adults, is attributed to the increase of left atrial volume.[30] The disturbed flow of blood in this condition may lead to formation of mural thrombus, and to the risk of systemic thromboembolism. Myocardial dysfunction definitely influences the severity, clinical progress, and prognosis of rheumatic valvar disease.

The potential risk for infective endocarditis in patients with chronic rheumatic disease derives from disruption by the irregular valvar endocardial surface of the normal pattern of laminar flow across the valvar orifice. As stated previously, this progresses to deposition of fibrin. Initially these deposits are sterile and may heal. In the face of significant bacteremia, the microorganisms become enmeshed within the vegetations, leading to infectious endocarditis.

Morphology of Chronic Lesions

The evolution from the initial attack of acute fever to appearance of severe chronic lesions requiring surgical intervention is known to have geographical variation, being shorter in patients from countries with conditions of poor health care because of the greater risk of repeated acute episodes. Although fibrin vegetations and inflammation usually heal, leading to fibrosis of the leaflet, additional damage may be caused by organisation of minute thrombuses deposited on the valvar surface, and also by local haemodynamic disturbances. Moreover, inflammation persists in valvar tissues, perpetuating the process. As discussed already, the mitral valve alone is involved in most children and adults with chronic rheumatic heart disease, but both the mitral and aortic valves are involved in about one-quarter of individuals.[31] Milder lesions can afflict the tricuspid valve, but are rarely seen in the pulmonary valve.

Chronic Rheumatic Mitral Valvar Disease

In the adult patient, isolated mitral stenosis, or stenosis in association with regurgitation, is the most frequent valvar sequel. As with the acute lesions, stenosis is not usually the first presentation of mitral dysfunction, with regurgitation usually seen first. In gross terms, the leaflets are diffusely thickened, and at the early stage of regurgitation, the mural leaflet is retracted, typically showing only one scallop instead of the usual three (Fig. 54B-2). With progression of the disease, the two ends of the zone of apposition between the leaflets fuse together, producing so-called commissural fusion. Varying degrees of shortening and fusion of the cords is also observed, leading, in the most severe cases, to obliteration of the interchordal spaces. In the normal valve, of course, these spaces are wide, and may be considered as part of the valvar orifice (Fig. 54B-3). The morphological feature of obliteration of the intercordal spaces further aggravates the stenosis, and must be given attention during any attempted surgical repair. In severe cases, the valvar apparatus is funnel-like, with the leaflets seemingly inserted directly to the tips of the papillary muscles. Should there be a recurrent acute attack, fibrin vegetations will be found on the already distorted leaflets and cords (see Fig. 54A-7). Deposition of calcium is a late complication of the chronic involvement, usually appearing in adulthood, but it may be present in children with accelerated evolution of the disease. The deposits are seen as large yellow masses on the atrial surface of the leaflets, but especially at the ends of the zone of apposition (Fig. 54B-4). In the setting of severe stenosis, the valvar orifice appears slit-like, and is likened to a fish-mouth or button-hole (Fig. 54B-5). As emphasised, the subvalvar apparatus is also stenotic. The left atrium is usually greatly enlarged, carrying the possibility of formation of thrombus and atrial fibrillation. Thrombuses may be attached to the valve itself (Fig. 54B-6), or be formed inside the tubular left atrial appendage. Rarely, a large free-floating ball thrombus may be found inside the left atrium, with the risk of a fatal systemic embolisation or occlusion of the valvar orifice.

Infective endocarditis is a potential complication of valves afflicted by chronic rheumatic lesions (Fig. 54B-7) because of the disturbed pattern of flow of blood and also the irregular endocardial surface. While large vegetations may be misdiagnosed echocardiographically as thrombuses, small ones may be missed, and the diagnosis confirmed only at histological examination.

The differential diagnosis of rheumatic mitral fibrous scarring includes valvar lesions produced by systemic lupus

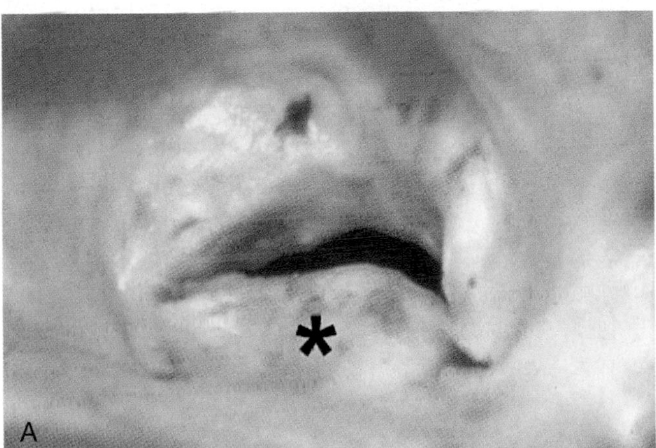

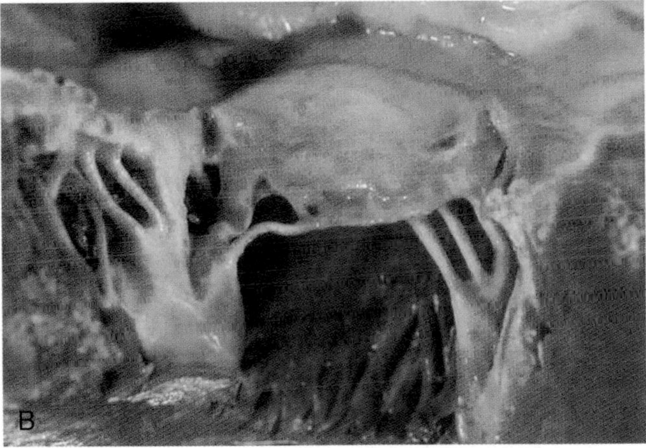

Figure 54B-2 **A,** Left atrium opened to show the thickened mitral valve with a retracted mural leaflet (*asterisk*). **B,** An opened mitral valve with chronic rheumatic lesions characterised by short and thick cords and fusion of the ends of the zone of apposition. (Reproduced with permission from Grinberg M, Sampaio RO [eds]: Doença Valvar. São Paulo, Brazil: Editora Manole, 2006.)

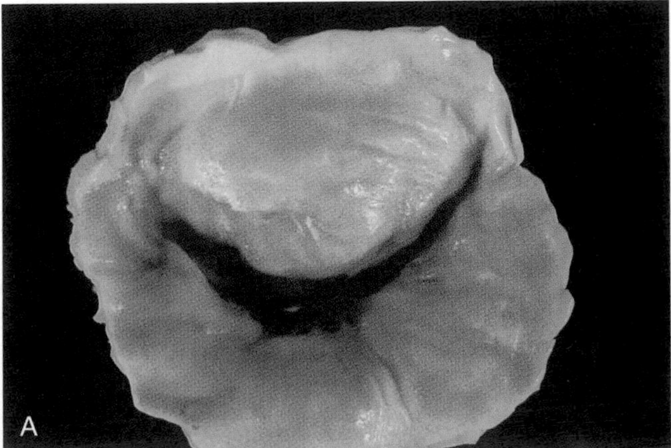

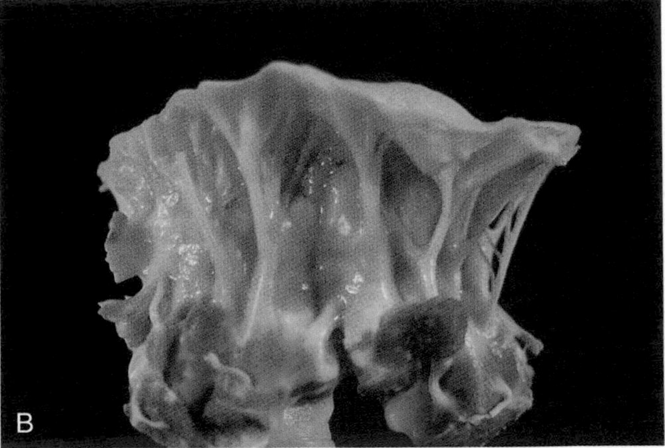

Figure 54B-3 Morphological features of a surgically excised stenotic rheumatic mitral valve. **A,** The atrial aspect, revealing the stenotic orifice and thickened leaflets. **B,** The ventricular aspect, with fused tendinous cords and obliteration of intercordal spaces.

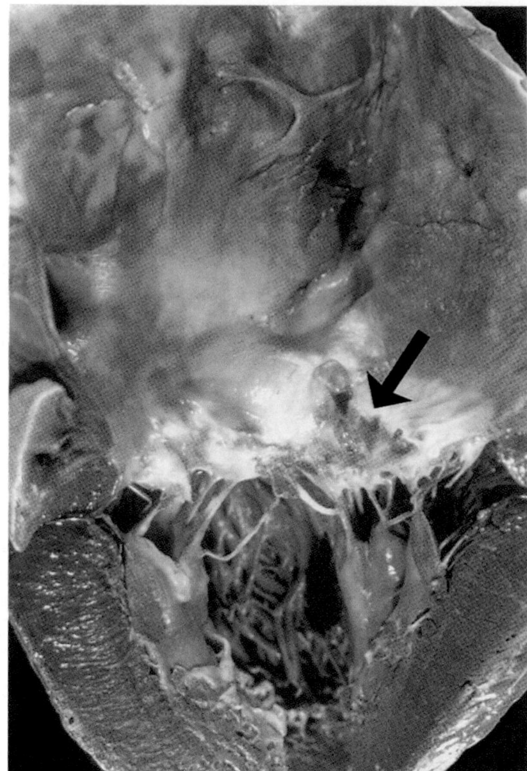

Figure 54B-4 The left-sided cardiac chambers from a patient who died of chronic rheumatic mitral stenosis. There is massive dilation of the left atrium and calcification on the zone of apposition between the leaflets (*arrow*).

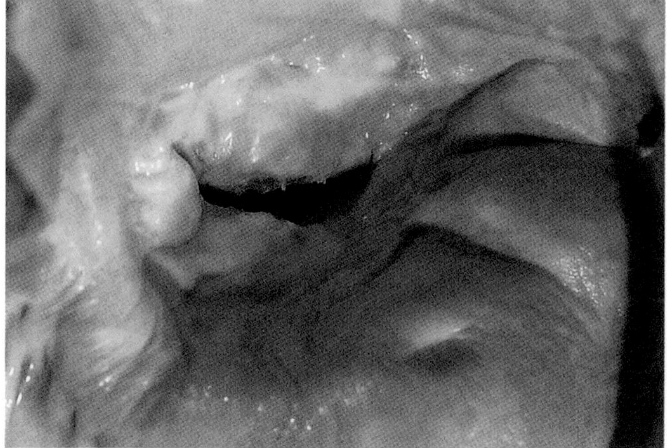

Figure 54B-5 The atrial aspect of a severely stenotic mitral valve, showing a fish-mouth orifice and focal calcification.

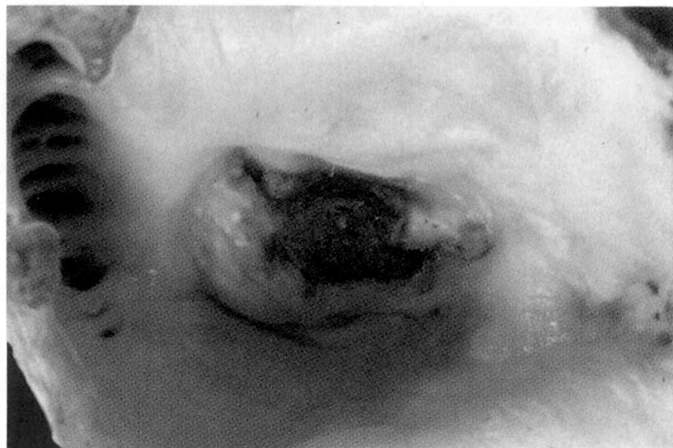

Figure 54B-6 The atrial aspect of a stenotic mitral valve with superimposed thrombosis.

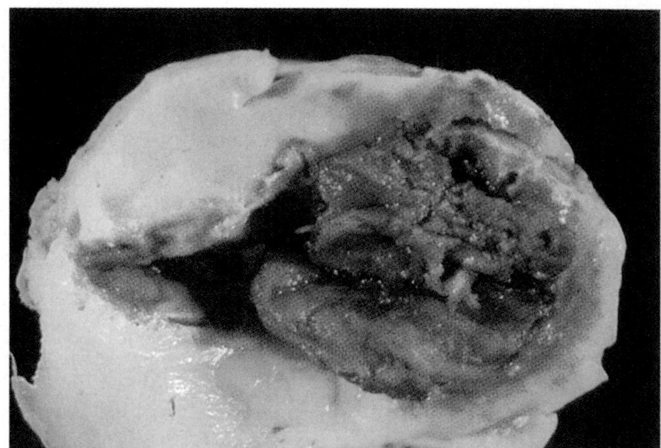

Figure 54B-7 This surgically excised mitral valve shows a chronic rheumatic lesion and a superimposed vegetation of infective endocarditis.

erythematosus, antiphospholipid syndrome, rheumatoid arthritis, post-thoracic irradiation, and carcinoid valvar disease, and those associated with the use of certain appetite suppressants, such as fenfluramine or phentermine. The clinical history and laboratorial findings, nonetheless, usually point to the proper diagnosis.[31]

Chronic Rheumatic Aortic Valvar Disease

As we have discussed, the aortic valve is the second most commonly involved valve, usually in association with involvement of the mitral valve. Isolated aortic lesions are uncommon. In one recent study,[32] solitary involvement of the aortic valve was found in less than 3% of the cases. Rheumatic aortic stenosis is particularly rare in children and adolescents. When seen as an isolated lesion in patients of this age, it is considered to be associated with a congenital lesion.[33]

Macroscopically, the leaflets are diffusely thickened and retracted. Fusion along the zones of apposition between the leaflets begins at their peripheral attachments at the level of the sinotubular junction (Fig. 54B-8). As with the mitral valve, calcification is rare in children, but may involve the free edges of the leaflets, which is different from the finding in degenerative aortic stenosis.

Chronic Rheumatic Tricuspid and Pulmonary Valvar Disease

Functional tricuspid valvar regurgitation is a common finding in patients with significant mitral valvar disease, resulting from right ventricular and annular dilation caused by long-standing pulmonary hypertension. When seen, thickening of the leaflets and shortening of cords are the macroscopical features of the chronic lesion, besides focal fusion of the zones of apposition between the leaflets. Calcific deposits are rare. Chronic organic pulmonary valve involvement is very rare. If found, it almost always involves

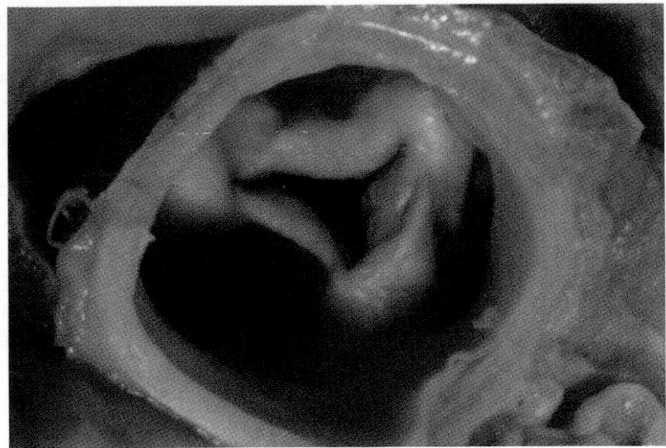

Figure 54B-8 The arterial view of an aortic valve with thickened leaflets and fusion of the ends of the zones of apposition.

rheumatic lesions in the other three valves.[24] Rheumatic fever, nonetheless, can also be found in patients with congenitally malformed hearts, including tetralogy of Fallot, septal defects, and aortic coarctation, with the chronic lesions then being superimposed on the congenital anomalies.[34,35]

HISTOLOGIC FEATURES OF CHRONIC RHEUMATIC VALVAR AND MYOCARDIAL LESIONS

Histologically, valves with chronic rheumatic involvement show dense and diffuse fibrosis, which effaces the typical architecture. It is also possible to recognise newly formed vessels, some with thick walls, along with variable degrees of inflammatory infiltrates made up of lymphocytes and macrophages (Fig. 54B-9). As previously described, the main type of inflammatory cell present is the T lymphocyte of CD4 phenotype,[36] expressing predominantly interferon γ, tumour necrosis factor–α and interleukin 10. Calcium deposits, if seen, are usually surrounded by aggregates of mononuclear cells, including plasma cells. Occasional endocardial ulcerations are covered with thrombus. Aschoff bodies are no longer present at this phase of the disease, unless an acute attack of rheumatic carditis has occurred within the last few weeks. Myocardial fibrous scars result from the organisation of the nodules of the acute phase, and are perivascular in location (see Fig. 54A-8). Additional damage is a consequence of altered haemodynamics, and usually involves variable degrees of myocardial hypertrophy.

Secondary Changes in the Airways and Pulmonary Vasculature

Chronic pulmonary congestion due to left valvar and myocardial dysfunction may be so severe as to result in passive pulmonary hypertension. The alveolar septums become thickened, initially by capillary dilation and later by fibrosis, and alveolar lumens may contain numerous haemosiderin-laden macrophages, the so-called heart failure cells. The interlobular septums show oedema and dilated lymphatic vessels. Venous changes may include intimal and adventitial fibrosis, along with hypertrophy of the medial layer. Long-standing congestion results in extension of the lesions to the arterial territory, with medial hypertrophy, intimal fibrosis, and adventitial enlargement of intra- and pre-acinar arteries.[37]

VALVAR LESIONS

Mitral Regurgitation

Mitral regurgitation, as an isolated lesion or in combination with other valvar defects, is probably, at all ages, the most common valvar dysfunction resulting from the acute rheumatic process. In developing countries, severe forms have necessitated early surgical intervention in young patients.[38,39] In a recent large series of young patients aged under 18 years,[23] isolated mitral regurgitation, as the single most frequent lesion produced by chronic rheumatic heart disease, was found in one-third of the cohort. Analysis of repair of the mitral valve revealed that over one-quarter of operations were performed in patients aged less than 15 years of age.[24] In South Africa, pure mitral regurgitation was the most common lesion in young patients treated by surgery due to rheumatic mitral valve disease, accounting for almost three-fifths of patients aged 20 years or younger, and for almost four-fifths of those who needed surgery in the first 10 years of life.[38] As we have emphasised, it is

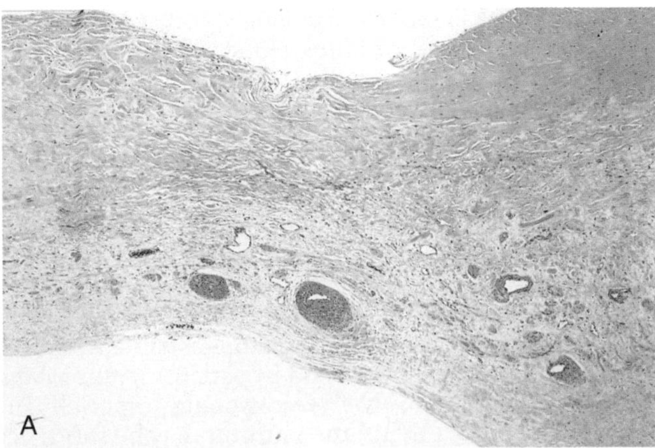

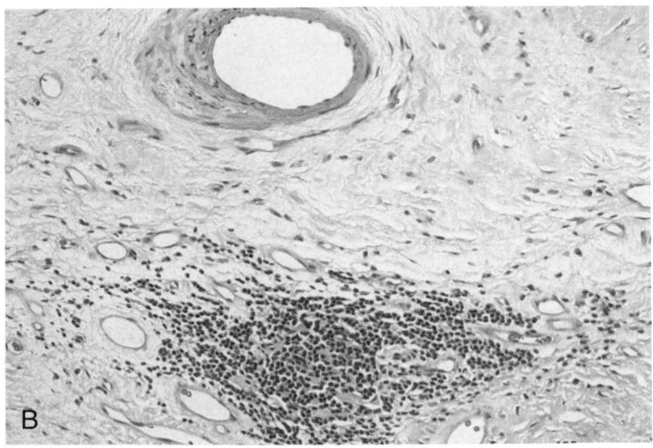

Figure 54B-9 Photomicrographs of cardiac valves with chronic rheumatic involvement. Panel A shows diffuse fibrosis and new vessels, while panel B shows an inflammatory focus made up of mononuclear cells adjacent to a thick-walled vessel. Haematoxylin and eosin stain.

the severity of the acute lesion, and the number of subsequent episodes, that determine the course of the disease. Unlike mitral stenosis, when there is a variable latent period between the establishment of the valvar lesion and the acute episode, mitral regurgitation is frequently present from the onset of the active process. Initial regurgitation has been noted to disappear over periods ranging from 2 months to 9 years, while new lesions such as mitral stenosis, or stenosis combined with regurgitation, appeared over a period of up to 12 years.[26] Patients with mitral regurgitation are far more likely to have suffered a more severe acute episode than those with mitral stenosis.[40] Significant insufficiency may progress rapidly, leading on to congestive heart failure. In contrast, a systolic murmur of mild valvar incompetence may well persist throughout the lifetime of the patient without any symptoms or further complications. In general, mild-to-moderate mitral regurgitation is better tolerated than similar degrees of mitral stenosis. Unlike mitral stenosis, isolated mitral regurgitation affects men more often than women.

Physiology

Mitral valvar regurgitation may be found early in the course of the acute episode, and pathological, haemodynamic, and functional changes are important determinants in the worsening of valvar incompetence. The valvar leaflets become thickened and retracted, with shortening and fusion of the tendinous cords also contributing to restricted valvar closure, which may be aggravated by dilation of the annulus and left atrium. The increased volume overload and output of the left atrium as a result of the regurgitation leads to an increased diastolic volume of the left ventricle, with dilation and hypertrophy of both chambers proportional to the severity of the valvar dysfunction. Hypertrophy of the muscle normalises left ventricular mural stress, and is appropriate for both the degree of volume load and the degree of dilation.[41] In those with moderate valvar incompetence, regurgitant flow from the left ventricle to atrium during systole is approximately half of the total ventricular stroke output. As the left ventricular end-diastolic volume is increased, in spite of the regurgitation into the left atrium, an adequate forward flow is maintained into the aorta during ventricular systole. The size of the left atrium is an important determinant of the rise in pressure in this chamber and in the pulmonary veins. In the setting of chronic disease, as the left atrium has time to dilate, the rise in pressure is relatively low. This factor, coupled with the lower energy cost of ventricular work, probably explains why moderate-to-severe mitral regurgitation is tolerated in many patients for a number of years. In contrast, in acute valvar incompetence with a normally sized left atrium, the left atrial pressure rises suddenly to a marked degree.

Severe mitral regurgitation is much better tolerated than an equal degree of aortic regurgitation. In chronic mitral regurgitation, the increased end-diastolic volume brings in the Frank–Starling mechanism, allowing a larger stroke output and increased left ventricular compliance. The increase in end-diastolic length of the myocytes, without a corresponding elevation in end-diastolic pressure, prevents a marked rise in pulmonary venous pressure.[42] Left ventricular end-diastolic pressure rises relatively minimally because of the compensatory change in left ventricular compliance, and the relations between left ventricular pressure and time remain normal. Ventricular function, therefore, is usually normal in children with mitral regurgitation. The favourable loading conditions often maintain the ejection fraction in the low normal range, and can make the left ventricular dysfunction imperceptible up to the later phases of the disease.[43] At this stage, the mean left atrial and pulmonary venous pressures rise, leading to a decreased pulmonary compliance and, subsequently, to pulmonary vasoconstriction. The mean pulmonary venous pressure is the major determinant of the resulting pulmonary arterial hypertension. Even with moderate-to-severe mitral regurgitation, though pulmonary arterial hypertension does occur, it does not reach the levels found in tight mitral stenosis. The forward stroke volume is maintained until late in the disease, when the regurgitant volume becomes so large that most of the stroke output empties into the left atrium. The forward stroke volume and cardiac output then decrease. A direct relationship exists between the regurgitant volume, the reduction in the forward stroke output, the elevation of the left atrial pressure, and the degree of clinical disability.[44]

Clinical Features

The severity, and to a lesser extent the chronicity, of the regurgitant valve are the main factors in determining the symptoms. Those patients with mild lesions are completely asymptomatic. In patients with even moderate mitral regurgitation, symptoms may be relatively unimpressive. In contrast, in those with severe incompetence, there is effort dyspnoea, easy fatiguability, poor weight gain, palpitations on effort, paroxysmal nocturnal dyspnoea, and finally congestive heart failure. Paroxysmal or chronic atrial fibrillation and infective endocarditis are more common than in mitral stenosis. The susceptibility to thromboembolism, on the other hand, is smaller.[45,46] The jugular venous pressure is normal when there is no congestive heart failure, while normal blood pressure is associated with a slightly widened pulse pressure, giving a brisk pulse. The apical impulse is usually normal in those with mild lesions, with no major precordial pulsations. In significant mitral regurgitation, a hyperdynamic forcible left ventricular heaving apex is palpable, being displaced downwards and laterally. In general, the first heart sound is normal in intensity or somewhat soft. The second heart sound is usually normal, but can be markedly split in those with severe lesions because of the shortening of left ventricular systole. The presence of a loud third heart sound excludes the coexistence of significant mitral stenosis. The most important clinical feature is the characteristic apical systolic murmur. The murmur is pan- or holosystolic, starting with the first sound, which is often muffled. Indeed, it may well extend to the sound of closure of the aortic valve. It is heard best at the apex, radiates to the left axilla and left sternal edge, is unaffected by respiration, and has a blowing quality with no accentuation in mid- or late-systole. There is no definite correlation between the severity of the lesion and the length or intensity of the apical systolic murmur. Some patients with significant mitral regurgitation have a musical seagull murmur. The late systolic murmur of mild mitral regurgitation is often indistinguishable from that of the late systolic murmur found in patients with prolapsing leaflets of the mitral valve.[47] Occasionally, especially in the presence of acute valvitis, the murmur may be short, occurring in early mid- or late-systole. With severe valvar incompetence, a mid-diastolic blowing murmur is audible at the apex, caused by increased diastolic flow through the mitral valve and the turbulence created at the end of the rapid ventricular phase. This murmur, while it may be rumbling, does not extend to late diastole. It is usually shorter than the murmur heard in mitral stenosis. A low-pitched third heart sound, which is often palpable and is caused by the considerable early diastolic filling of the ventricle, is heard in those with significant mitral regurgitation. When there is associated pulmonary hypertension, its signs are present. These include a right ventricular parasternal lift, a loud palpable pulmonary sound, and murmurs of pulmonary and/or tricuspid incompetence. The clinical signs of mitral regurgitation are much less clear-cut than those of mitral stenosis.

The electrocardiogram may be normal when the regurgitation is mild. Even with moderate valvar incompetence, the features may be inconclusive. The P wave is broad, bifid or notched, and usually best seen in lead II or V_1. A more reliable sign of left atrial enlargement is a terminal negative deflection of the P wave in lead V_1 of more than 0.04 seconds in duration and more than 1 mm in depth. Left ventricular hypertrophy occurs when mitral incompetence is more than moderate. There may be changes in the ST and T waves over the lateral chest leads when the valvar lesion is severe. In the presence of associated pulmonary hypertension, right ventricular hypertrophy, and right atrial enlargement are not uncommon (Fig. 54B-10). Although uncommon in children and adolescents, atrial fibrillation occurs in patients with severe disease, and in those with long-standing chronic mitral regurgitation. The chest radiograph may be normal in patients with mild lesions. With well-established mitral regurgitation, the left atrium and the left ventricle are enlarged, their sizes being proportional to the degree of valvar dysfunction. There is

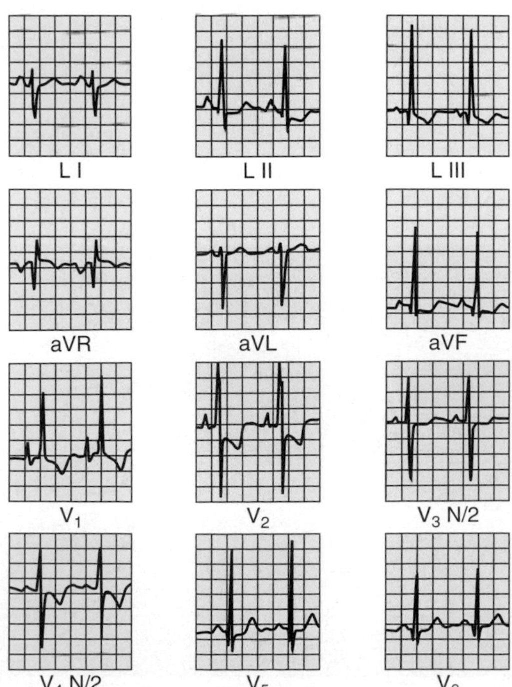

Figure 54B-10 The electrocardiogram from an 8-year-old child with isolated and severe mitral regurgitation complicated by pulmonary hypertension. There is evidence of biventricular hypertrophy and enlargement of both atriums.

pulmonary venous engorgement, especially in the upper lobes (Fig. 54B-11). With the onset of pulmonary hypertension, the pulmonary trunk becomes prominent, and there is dilation of the right ventricle and atrium. Septal lines appear with the onset of cardiac failure.

The Doppler echocardiogram can be very useful, permitting highly sensitive and specific diagnosis of mitral regurgitation. In the M-mode echocardiogram, the EF slope of diastolic closure is not specific, nor does it indicate the severity of the valvar incompetence. There is an increase in the movements of the left ventricular septum and inferior wall because of the large stroke volume. In spite of difficulties in assessing left ventricular function because of the loading conditions in patients with chronic mitral regurgitation, the ejection fraction has been identified as a predictor of survival after surgical correction.[48] Thickening of the leaflets may be seen. Although the rheumatic leaflets may prolapse, the echocardiogram is useful in differentiating rheumatic disease from other causes of valvar prolapse, such as functional mitral regurgitation caused by severe cardiac dilation in primary cardiac muscle disease. The cross sectional echocardiogram in the long-axis view reveals a large, dilated, well-contracting left ventricle, and a dilated pulsatile left atrium. It also provides important information about the morphology of the valvar apparatus. The leaflets of the rheumatic valve are thickened and rigid, and the mural leaflet is frequently noted to be immobile. Cordal rupture, vegetations of infective endocarditis, and either presence or absence of left atrial thrombosis can all be recognised. Besides the morphological data, the severity of valvar incompetence can be assessed by mapping of the regurgitant jet and the width of the vena contracta, in addition to two quantitative methods used for evaluation of the regurgitant volume and calculation of the effective regurgitant orifice area[49–52] (Figs. 54B-12 to 54B-14). In this setting, it is important to avoid over-diagnosis, since trivial incompetence can be seen even in normal subjects. Although rarely needed in children and adolescents, transoesophageal echocardiography is useful in patients in whom evaluation and quantification of the severity of mitral regurgitation has proved difficult when using the transthoracic windows. The valvar apparatus can now be accurately assessed by the three-dimensional technique. Exercise testing may be helpful in evaluating symptoms and establishing changes in exercise tolerance, particularly when it is difficult to obtain a reliable history.[43]

Cardiac catheterisation and angiography are rarely indicated nowadays in patients with isolated mitral regurgitation. If performed, the mean left atrial or pulmonary capillary pressure is usually elevated, but in a small number of cases, aneurysmal dilation of the left atrium can produce a normal left atrial pressure despite significant regurgitation.[53] With significant valvar incompetence, the left atrial pressure is elevated, with a large V wave and a sharp Y descent.[54] A diastolic pressure gradient across the mitral valve can be found even in the absence of significant mitral stenosis. The left ventricular systolic pressures are usually normal, and end-diastolic pressure is normal unless there is left ventricular failure. Calculation of the valvar area by the Gorlin formula is less reliable in the setting of valvar incompetence. The regurgitant volume is measured as the difference between angiographically determined total left ventricular volume and the forward stroke volume using

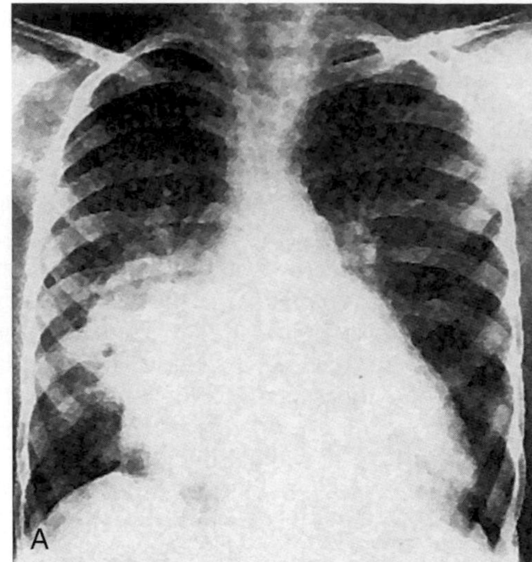

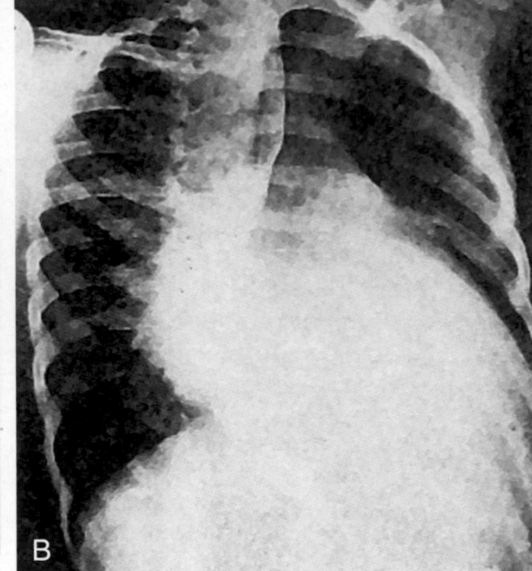

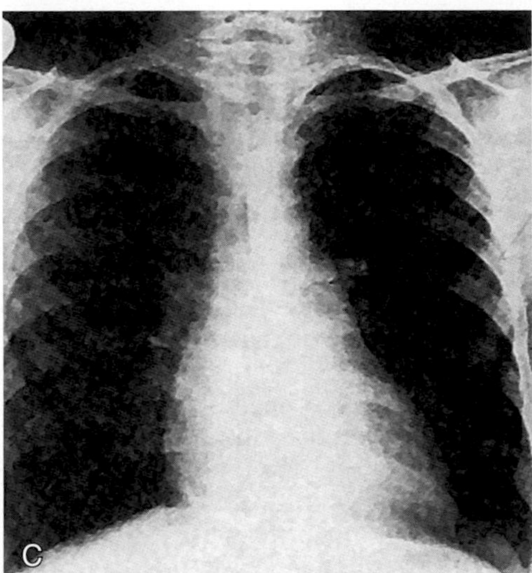

Figure 54B-11 Pre- and post-operative radiographs from an 11-year-old child with severe isolated mitral regurgitation. **A,** The frontal view shows cardiomegaly, marked enlargement of the left atrium with a prominent appendage, and venous congestion of the upper lobes of the lungs. **B,** The barium swallow profiled in right oblique projection confirms the dilatation of the left atrium, with posterior displacement of the oesophagus. **C,** After replacement of the mitral valve, there is regression of all the abnormal features.

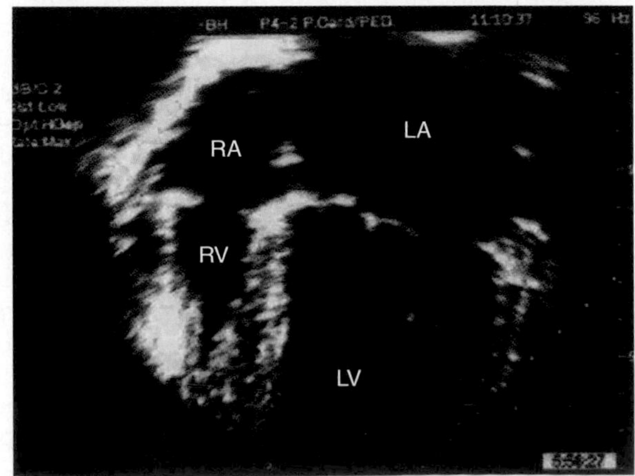

Figure 54B-12 The echocardiogram, in apical four-chamber projection, is from a 16-year-old girl with severe mitral and aortic regurgitation, moderate tricuspid regurgitation, and pulmonary hypertension. The image shows the left-sided chambers greatly enlarged. LA, left atrium; LV, left ventricle; RA, right atrium; RV, right ventricle.

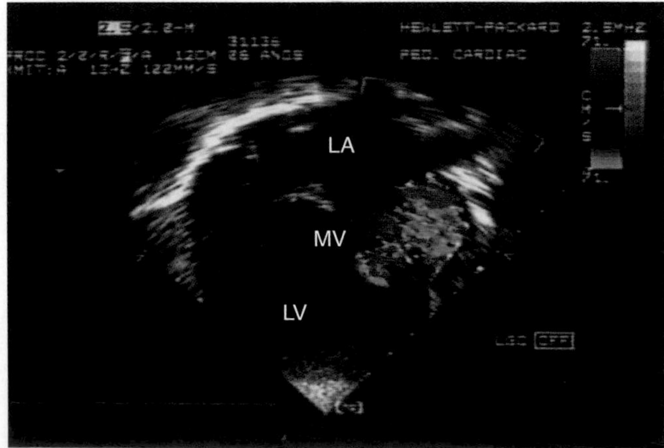

Figure 54B-13 Colour flow mapping in the apical four-chamber view from a 14-year-old boy with moderate to severe mitral regurgitation. LA, left atrium; LV, left ventricle; MV, mitral valve.

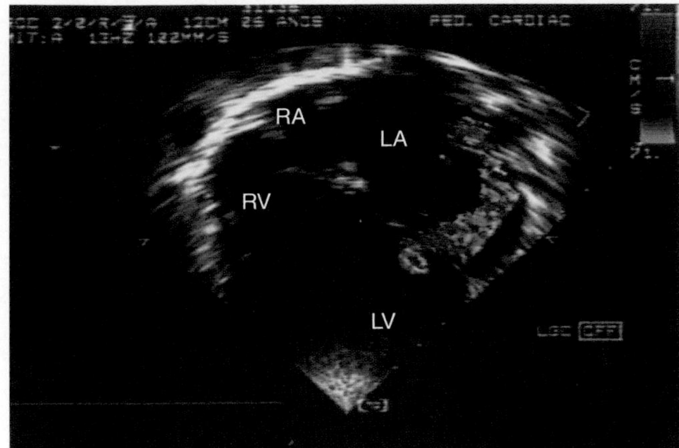

Figure 54B-14 This 6-year-old patient has moderate mitral regurgitation. The Coanda effect is seen in the apical four-chamber view, with the jet stream adhered to the lateral wall of the left atrium. LA, left atrium; LV, left ventricle; RA, right atrium; RV, right ventricle.

the Fick method, the fiberoptic technique, or the indicator dilution technique.[55–57] It can also be achieved by calculating the angiographically measured difference between the right and the left ventricular stroke volumes.[58] Selective left ventricular angiography in the 30-degree right anterior oblique projection profiles the left ventricle, left atrium, and mitral valve (Fig. 54B-15). From a practical point of view, a qualitative estimation of severity from the amount of regurgitation into the left atrium of material injected into the left ventricle has been found useful. The degree of opacification of the left atrium depends on the quantity of blood in this chamber and on its rate of emptying, as well as on the severity of regurgitation. The width of the jet of mitral regurgitation is a good guide to the size of the regurgitant orifice. The left ventricular size, mural thickness and function, besides the degree of movements of the leaflets, can also be assessed. In patients with a decreased left ventricular ejection fraction, there will be an increased end-diastolic volume.

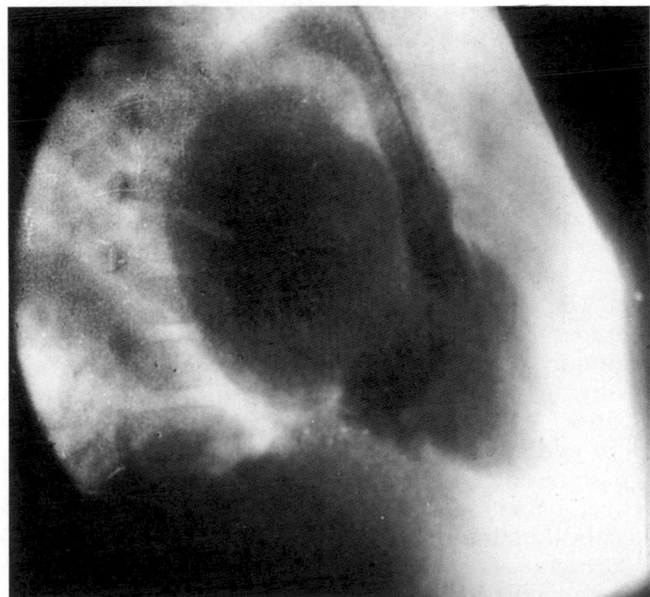

Figure 54B-15 A left ventricular angiogram is profiled in 30-degree right anterior oblique orientation, from the same patient as shown in Figure 54B-11. There is severe regurgitation with a wide jet across the mitral valve, producing dense opacification of the entire left atrium. The aorta appears relatively hypoplastic as a result of the low cardiac output.

Mitral Stenosis

Mitral stenosis is a common chronic rheumatic valvar lesion, becoming established earlier than aortic stenosis. As with the other lesions, there is marked geographic variation. Mitral stenosis, in particular, appears precociously in patients from countries with high rates of the disease, probably due to repeated episodes of acute rheumatic fever associated with poor socioeconomic conditions. This is corroborated by some data from India,[26] showing a change in the pattern of valvar dysfunction according to the phase of the disease. While, in the initial acute attack, mitral regurgitation is frequently the only type of dysfunction present, subsequent episodes are accompanied by different combinations of valvar lesions. In most developing countries, mitral stenosis develops rapidly after the acute event, producing symptomatic young patients, and necessitating early surgical or catheter intervention.[38,59–62] In South Africa, one-fifth of patients with pure mitral stenosis had been treated surgically before the age of 20 years.[38] Similarly, of those treated by balloon valvoplasty in Saudi Arabia, over one-sixth were aged 20 or less.[63] Another series, from the United States,[64] although much smaller, revealed a tendency to milder mitral lesions, and more patients with isolated aortic regurgitation, reflecting the less severe outcome for patients in North America.

Physiology

Mitral stenosis in patients with rheumatic fever is caused by thickening and calcification of the leaflets, along with fusion of the ends of the zone of apposition between the leaflets and obliteration of the intercordal spaces. The resulting narrowing of the valvar orifice produces a barrier in diastolic left ventricular filling from the left atrium, and a gradient is established between the left atrial and left ventricular end-diastolic pressures. The rise in the left atrial pressure is reflected by the elevated pulmonary capillary or pulmonary wedge pressure. With critical mitral stenosis, there is severe left atrial and pulmonary venous hypertension. The pulmonary arterial pressure rises correspondingly to maintain an adequate pulmonary flow. Pulmonary arteriolar constriction, a result of a combination of vasospasm and pulmonary arteriolar disease, results in an elevated pulmonary vascular resistance. In the face of such persistent and significant pulmonary hypertension, there is right ventricular failure. In patients with mild-to-moderate elevation of left atrial pressure, exercise or sudden tachyarrhythmias may diminish the diastolic filling period, resulting in an abrupt elevation of the left atrial pressure. Pulmonary oedema may then occur. Pulmonary hypertension is initially passive. With alteration of pulmonary exchange of gases, and associated hypoxia and arteriolar vasoconstriction, obliterative pulmonary hypertension develops. Since the pulmonary venous pressure in critical mitral stenosis may exceed the oncotic plasma pressure of 30 mm Hg, the increased pulmonary vascular resistance is, to a large extent, a protective mechanism. Thickening of the capillary walls, interstitial tissues, and alveolar membranes produces a barrier at the interface between the capillaries and the alveolar sacs. In isolated mitral stenosis, the relationships between pulmonary pressure and flow are not constant. In some patients, the pulmonary circulation is maintained with only modest elevation of pulmonary arterial pressure, while in others pulmonary vascular disease becomes established, with severe hypertension pushing pulmonary pressures above the systemic level. Most patients with mild-to-moderate mitral stenosis, nonetheless, are able to maintain an adequate cardiac output with moderate exercise. In the presence of critical mitral stenosis, the cardiac output is low at rest. Exercise does not increase the cardiac output, which may even fall in the presence of significant pulmonary hypertension. The increased pulmonary pressure also causes tricuspid regurgitation. In patients who have had repeated episodes of rheumatic carditis, the severity and frequency of congestive heart failure is out of proportion to the severity of the valvar disease alone.

Clinical Features

The symptoms, physical signs, and amount of clinical disability parallel the severity of mitral stenosis. Those with minimal stenosis may be completely asymptomatic. Exercise and atrial fibrillation are among the precipitating causes of the initial presentation of symptoms, even in patients with mild-to-moderate mitral stenosis.[4] Critical or significant mitral stenosis is present when the area of the valvar orifice is reduced to about one-quarter of the expected normal for the age. The common symptoms in critical stenosis are effort dyspnoea, orthopnoea, paroxysmal nocturnal dyspnoea, and episodes of pulmonary oedema. These symptoms may be aggravated by recurrence of carditis, intercurrent infections, and uncontrolled tachycardia or atrial fibrillation. Congestive cardiac failure usually occurs with severe stenosis and more than moderate pulmonary hypertension. The onset of atrial fibrillation usually indicates a relatively advanced stage of disease, and often accounts for worsening in its course. Atrial fibrillation and systemic embolisation, however, are uncommon in children and adolescents.[40,65] The systemic venous pressure is elevated in the presence of cardiac failure and pulmonary hypertension. This elevation is proportional to the severity of stenosis, and it becomes marked with the onset of cardiac failure or atrial fibrillation. The cardiac impulse is usually right ventricular, characteristically described as tapping in nature. When pulmonary hypertension is present, a parasternal lift is found, and pulmonary arterial pulsations, as well as closure of the pulmonary valve, are palpable. There are classic auscultatory findings in mitral stenosis. The first heart sound is accentuated because of an abrupt closure of the leaflets, which are held open until the beginning of ventricular systole. There is a loud, sharp, and high-pitched opening snap caused by a sudden tensing of the leaflets at the limit of their excursion of opening in diastole. A long, rumbling, low-pitched mid-diastolic murmur is heard at the apex, often with presystolic accentuation. In the absence of associated mitral regurgitation, the duration of the diastolic murmur is directly proportional to the severity of the stenosis. The duration of the murmur may be altered by the presence of a fast ventricular rate or congestive heart failure. The murmur is best heard in the lateral position, using the bell of the stethoscope. It is augmented by exercise. Should the patient develop atrial fibrillation, then there is usually loss of the presystolic accentuation. The presence of a pulmonary ejection click and an accentuated pulmonary component of the second sound, along with murmurs of pulmonary and tricuspid regurgitation, indicate severe pulmonary hypertension.

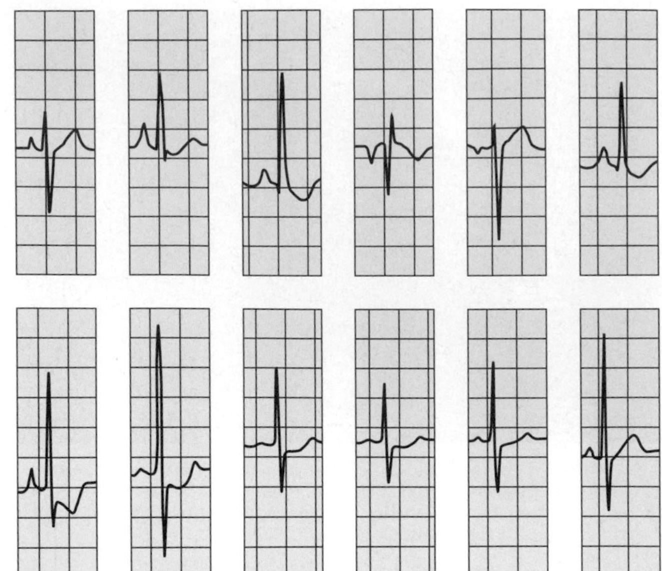

Figure 54B-16 Electrocardiogram from an 11-year-old child with tight mitral stenosis and severe pulmonary hypertension. There is evidence of right-axis deviation, right ventricular hypertrophy, and enlargement of both atrial chambers.

The electrocardiogram shows evidence of left atrial enlargement. Broad, notched P waves are seen in the limb leads, or a biphasic P wave in leads V_1 and V_2, with a marked negative component. Right atrial enlargement, right-axis deviation, and right ventricular hypertrophy of varying degrees reflect the severity of the pulmonary hypertension (Fig. 54B-16). The chest radiograph shows varying degrees of left atrial enlargement, which displaces the oesophagus backwards, with elevation of the left main bronchus and widening of the carina. The enlarged left atrial appendage may be visible on the left cardiac border (Fig. 54B-17). In the presence of pulmonary hypertension, the pulmonary trunk and the right chambers are enlarged. The aorta is usually normal or small. The degree of left atrial enlargement is usually less in isolated mitral stenosis than in mitral incompetence. With mild pulmonary venous hypertension, there is initially distention only of the pulmonary veins from the lower lobes, which may be difficult to identify clearly. Once there is significant pulmonary venous hypertension, there is interstitial oedema in the lower zone, and vasoconstriction in the veins supplying them. The flow of blood is then increased in the veins to the upper lobes, which are dilated, producing differential pulmonary venous circulation. Kerley's A and B lines are seen because of interstitial oedema and small interlobar effusions. Acute pulmonary oedema is recognised by the typical perihilar opacity, with radiations to the periphery. Exercise testing may be helpful in cases with discrepancy between haemodynamic data and symptoms.[43]

Echocardiography has, over the last years, become the most useful tool for both diagnosis and follow-up of patients with mitral stenosis (Figs. 54B-18 and 54B-19). M-mode interrogation still provides information. The valvar leaflets move interiorly during diastole, rather than posteriorly as in the normal situation. The EF slope is decreased, as is the rate of diastolic closure of the aortic leaflet,

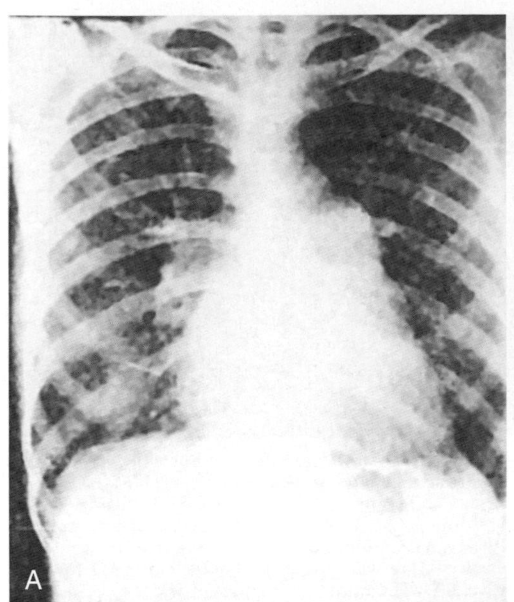

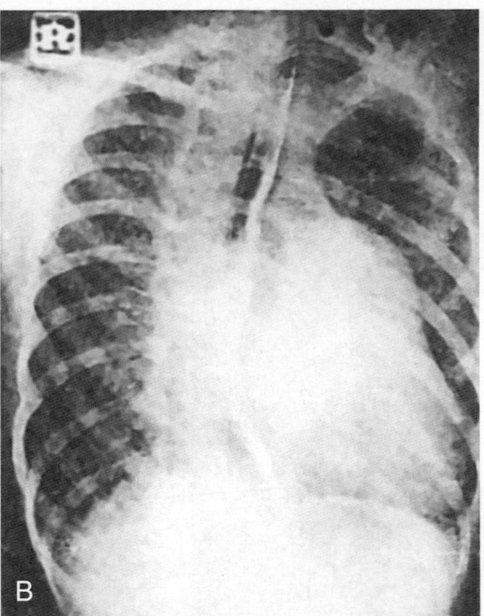

Figure 54B-17 Chest radiograph, shown in postero-anterior and right anterior oblique views, the latter with a barium swallow, from a 12-year-old child with severe mitral stenosis and pulmonary hypertension. The frontal view (**A**) shows cardiomegaly, with an enlarged left atrium, seen as a double density, a dilated pulmonary trunk and venous congestion in the upper lobes of the lungs. The oblique view (**B**) demonstrates the backward displacement of the barium-filled oesophagus caused by left atrial enlargement.

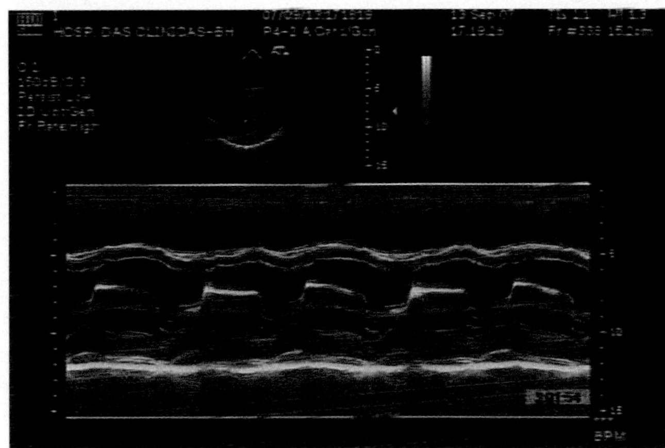

Figure 54B-18 M-mode echocardiogram from a 14-year-old child with severe mitral stenosis shows a decreased EF slope of the aortic leaflet of the mitral valve, and abnormal movement of the mural leaflet. Both leaflets are thickened and move forward parallel to each other during diastole.

generally in relation to the severity of the mitral stenosis. The mural leaflet is frequently tethered to the aortic leaflet, and both can move in parallel fashion during diastole. The amplitude of opening of the aortic leaflet is decreased. The left atrial dimension is increased, but the left ventricular and aortic dimensions are usually normal. There may be evidence of right ventricular dilation, paradoxical septal motion, and deviation of the septum into the left ventricle with the onset of pulmonary hypertension, especially in the presence of tricuspid incompetence. Cross sectional interrogation, combined with Doppler, permit assessment of the severity of the obstruction, the morphology of the valvar apparatus, and the suitability for valvotomy, by providing information concerning the ends of the zone of apposition, and the extent of thickening, tethering, reduced mobility and shrinkage of the leaflets, besides subvalvar fusion. Calcification is uncommon in children and adolescents. An accurate assessment of the anatomy of the valvar orifice, and the thickness of the leaflets, besides planimetry of the orifice area, is obtained using the short-axis view. The relative size and relations of the ventricles and atriums are better seen in the apical four-chamber view. Left ventricular contraction is usually normal, but there may be a reduced rate of filling. Measurements of mean diastolic gradient across the stenotic valve are highly flow and rate dependent, and can be determined from the continuous wave Doppler signal using the modified Bernoulli equation. The Doppler estimation of the valvar area can be obtained from either the diastolic pressure half-time or the continuity methods.[66]

As measurements and other necessary data can now be provided with a high degree of accuracy by echocardiography, cardiac catheterisation and angiography are seldom necessary, and should only be considered if diagnostic questions remain unanswered. If performed, the cardinal abnormality at catheterisation is the diastolic gradient across the mitral valve, measured by simultaneous recording of pressures in the left ventricle and either in the pulmonary capillary wedge or directly in the left atrium. Simultaneous measurements are more useful than measuring pulmonary capillary wedge pressures alone (Fig. 54B-20). The severity of obstruction shown by the degree of the diastolic gradient correlates well with calculated areas of the mitral valve. In sinus rhythm, the late diastolic post-A gradient is the most important measurement. In the presence of atrial fibrillation, however, the A wave disappears. The C wave then becomes prominent, and an X descent is not usually clearly seen. It is useful to calculate the gradient in six or seven consecutive cycles, and to take an average. The level of pulmonary hypertension can be measured from the peak and the mean pulmonary arterial pressure, besides the calculated index of pulmonary vascular resistance. In those who have apparently mild mitral stenosis, as shown by a small gradient, but with significant symptoms, measurement of the gradient is useful subsequent to exercise. If angiography is performed, the mitral valve is best profiled by selective left ventricular angiography in the 30-degree right anterior oblique position. In mitral stenosis with a mobile valve, a clear non-opacified

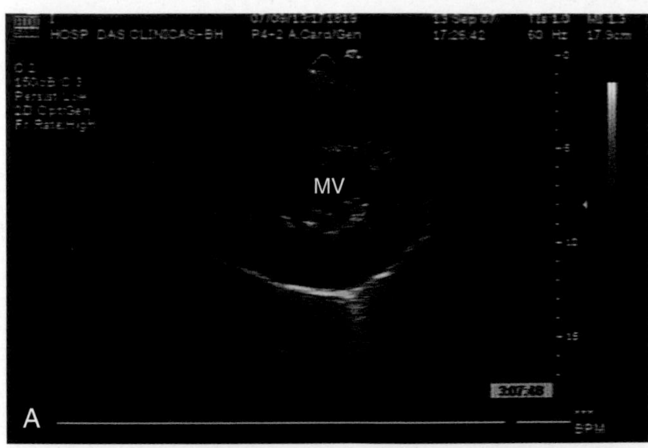

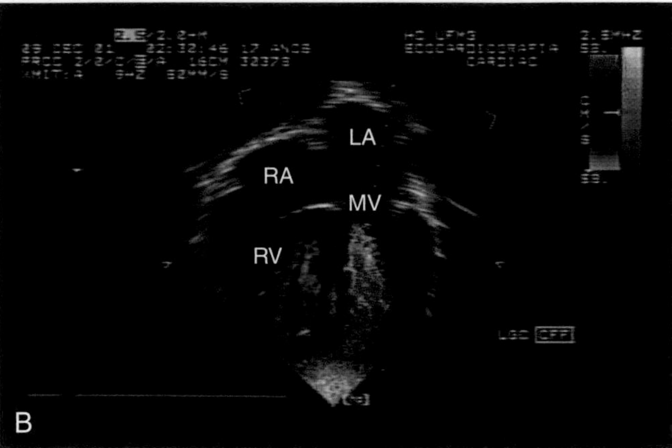

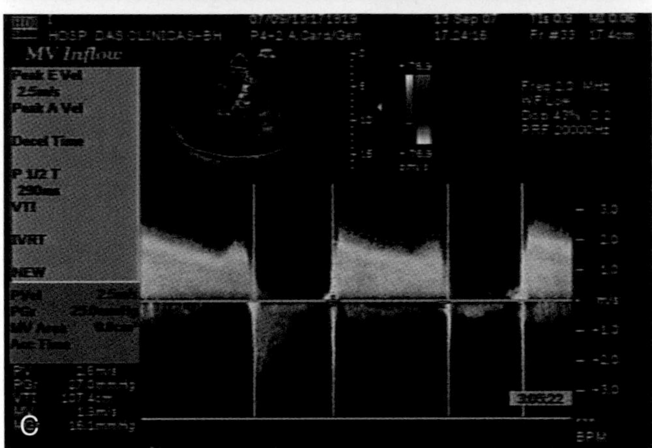

Figure 54B-19 The echograms are from a 17-year-old boy with severe mitral stenosis and moderate regurgitation. The parasternal short-axis view (**A**) shows thickening and tethering of the mitral valve leaflets. Colour flow mapping from the apical four-chamber view (**B**) shows an eccentric high-velocity flow jet. Continuous wave Doppler examination of the stenotic mitral valve (**C**) reveals a valvar area of 0.8 cm^2. LA, left atrium; MV, mitral valve; RA, right atrium; RV, right ventricle.

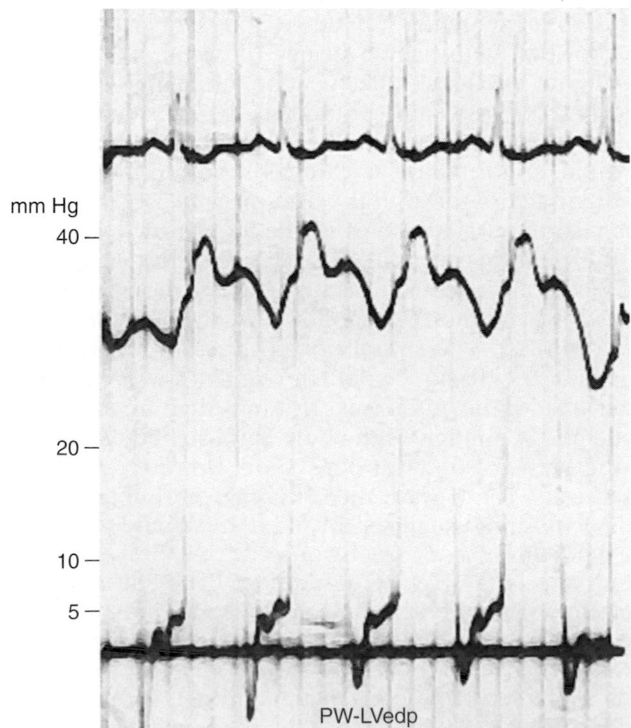

Figure 54B-20 Simultaneously recorded pulmonary capillary wedge and left ventricular pressures reveal a gradient across the mitral valve in a 10-year-old child with severe mitral stenosis. The wedge pressure is markedly elevated, with a high end-diastolic gradient between the pulmonary wedge (PW) and left ventricular end-diastolic pressure (LVedp).

crescent is clearly visualised (Fig. 54B-21). This view is also the best for assessing the degree of mitral regurgitation and the function of the left ventricle. The degree of any associated aortic regurgitation can be assessed by aortic root angiography in the left anterior oblique view.

Aortic Regurgitation

Aortic regurgitation is commonest consequence of rheumatic aortic valvitis, albeit occurring most frequently in combination with mitral valvar disease. Isolated aortic regurgitation was found in only one-twentieth of a large series of patients in India.[67] Likewise, in Brazil it was seen in only 2.7% of patients under 19 years as the unique valvar dysfunction, but in almost half when associated with other valvar lesions.[11] It is commoner in men. Unlike mitral disease, the disappearance of the aortic murmur is relatively uncommon. Aortic regurgitation may range in severity from minimal dysfunction with a faint murmur to severe free aortic regurgitation. The usual natural history is a long asymptomatic period in which mild-to-moderate regurgitation is well tolerated during the compensated phase. In adults, a rate of less than 6% per year is estimated for the progression to symptoms and/or systolic dysfunction. Asymptomatic patients with left ventricular dysfunction develop cardiac symptoms at a rate greater than 25% per year, and the rate of death for symptomatic patients surpasses 20% annually.[43,68] Patients who have recurrent rheumatic episodes may have a more rapid progress. In

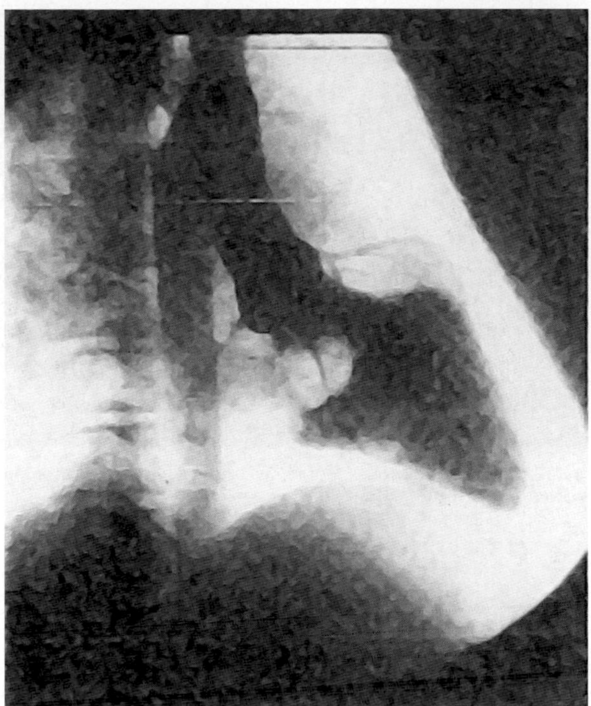

Figure 54B-21 A left ventricular cineangiogram profiled in 30-degree right anterior oblique projection in a patient with tight mitral stenosis. The left ventricular function is normal. A clear crescent is produced by the non-opacified blood from the left atrium crossing a mobile but stenotic valve.

developing countries, as with mitral valvar disease, severe aortic incompetence may become established within 1 to 2 years of the initial episode. Those with associated mitral valvar disease, especially mitral incompetence, have a more rapid downhill course.

Physiology

The volume overload on the left ventricle results in a series of compensatory mechanisms to maintain an adequate forward stroke output, including a large end-diastolic volume, increase in chamber compliance, and both eccentric and concentric hypertrophy of the ventricle.[4,43] The degree of left ventricular dilation is proportional to the severity of the regurgitant volume. There are additional factors such as the size of the regurgitant opening, the phasic nature of the regurgitation, the duration of diastole, the peripheral resistance, the reaction of the left ventricle in diastole, and myocardial perfusion.[69] In chronic aortic regurgitation, since the left ventricle is able to dilate over a period of time, the increase in diastolic compliance permits the left ventricle to accommodate a large regurgitant fraction without a corresponding increase in end-diastolic pressure. The ventricular stress is kept within the normal range through associated ventricular hypertrophy and reduced aortic impedance.[42] Peripheral vasodilation is almost always present with significant aortic lesions. The rapid dissipation of blood into the dilated peripheral vascular bed augments the central aortic regurgitation, resulting in a low diastolic pressure. The lowering of the diastolic pressure has two ill effects. These are reduction of coronary arterial flow and inadequate nutrition of the peripheral tissues. The peak systolic pressure rises as a compensatory mechanism, resulting in a higher mean arterial pressure. The elevated systolic pressure adds a pressure overload to the already existing volume overload of the left ventricle. Both the preload and the afterload are altered, and there are volume and pressure overloads.[46] The wide peripheral arterial pulse pressure in severe incompetence is the result of a combination of the peripheral vasodilation and central aortic regurgitation. The peripheral pulse curve shows a rapid rise to a high peak, with a sharp descending limb and a relatively unimportant dicrotic notch, with a low diastolic pressure and a high systolic peak pressure. The central aortic pressure, however, differs from the peripheral arterial pulse in that there is a sharp early peak followed by a second peak of varying amplitude. With the onset of left ventricular failure, the end-diastolic pressure rises, with an appropriate rise in the left atrial and pulmonary venous pressures, and subsequently of the pulmonary arterial pressures. Severe pulmonary hypertension is not common in chronic aortic incompetence. In contrast, when the aortic regurgitation is acute, there is a sudden rise in the ventricular diastolic pressure, and a sharp rise in pulmonary venous pressure because the left ventricle is relatively unprepared. A sharp and high rise of the end-diastolic pressure may further markedly decrease the flow of blood in the coronary arteries. All these factors added to the systolic dysfunction of the left ventricle result in a low cardiac output with pulmonary oedema and severe congestive heart failure.

Clinical Features

Patients with mild aortic regurgitation are asymptomatic. In some, apart from the murmur, even the peripheral signs may be absent. Those with moderate lesions may remain relatively asymptomatic despite cardiac dilation, as the ventricle is able to increase the cardiac output appropriately on exercise.[70] There may be palpitations on effort or on rest when the aortic regurgitation is severe. Effort dyspnoea occurs early and progresses. With the onset of left ventricular failure, orthopnoea and pulmonary oedema occur. Children and adolescents with severe disease may have nocturnal sweating, tachycardia, and nightmares. Angina is found in those with more severe disease. The blood pressure shows elevated systolic and low diastolic pressures, with a wide pulse pressure. The width of the pulse pressure, and the low diastolic pressure, is roughly proportional to the severity of the lesion. In those with moderate valve dysfunction, however, the width of the pulse pressure does not always correlate with the severity. With severe regurgitation, a water-hammer pulse is present. Other peripheral signs of a wide pulse pressure are increased and marked carotid pulsations; so-called Corrigan's sign; pistol-shot sounds over the femoral pulses; Duroziez's sign of a systolic and diastolic murmur becoming audible when critical pressure is applied to a large artery; visible capillary pulsations in the nail beds; known as Quincke's sign; and the sign of the nodding head. The last, also known as de Musset's sign, is one of the few signs named in honour of a patient. Cardiac enlargement is related to the severity of regurgitation. The apex beat is hyperdynamic and forcible, and there may be expandable pulsations over the entire precordium, with prominence of the left chest. The diagnostic sign of aortic regurgitation is the diastolic high-pitched blowing decrescendo murmur more prominent at the mid left sternal border or the right sternal border. It is best heard with the diaphragm of the stethoscope, with the patient leaning forwards in full expiration. The length and loudness of the murmur are poorly correlated with the severity of the lesion. An aortic systolic ejection flow murmur radiating to the neck, occasionally preceded by an ejection click, is present with severe regurgitation, and the apical mid- and late-diastolic murmur named for Austin Flint often occurs. This is indistinguishable from that of mitral stenosis, but it is usually not accompanied by a thrill. This murmur results from fluttering of the aortic leaflet of the mitral valve, along with antegrade flow of blood through a closing mitral orifice. Premature closure of the mitral valve may occur in severe regurgitation, producing a decreased intensity of the first heart sound. A fourth heart sound is uncommon, and a third sound indicates ventricular failure. With the onset of left ventricular failure, orthopnoea and pulmonary oedema occur. In the presence of severe congestive failure, particularly in acute aortic regurgitation, the peripheral signs are diminished, and murmurs may not be easily audible. Acute aortic regurgitation presents with acute pulmonary oedema and gross congestive heart failure.

The electrocardiogram may be normal, with mild lesions. When there is more severe regurgitation, left ventricular hypertrophy is present, with deep Q waves over the left chest leads. In advanced disease, left atrial P waves and changes in the ST-T segments are present. The chest radiograph shows considerable enlargement of the left ventricle with moderate or severe valvar lesions. The left atrium is usually normal or slightly increased. The ascending aorta and arch are prominent. With advanced disease, enlargement of the left atrium and pulmonary venous congestion are found.

Echocardiography is useful in assessing the dimension, mass, and function of the left ventricle, and quantifies the severity of aortic regurgitation (Figs. 54B-22 and 54B-23). A dilated left ventricular cavity with a normal left atrium, along with increased movement of the ventricular septum and the left ventricular inferior wall, are frequently seen. Wide fluttering of the aortic leaflet of the mitral valve usually occurs in patients who have an Austin Flint murmur. In severe aortic regurgitation, premature closure and delayed opening of the mitral valve are seen. Additionally, semiquantitative assessment and indirect measurements of the severity and width of the aortic regurgitation can be obtained by Doppler interrogation.[66,71]

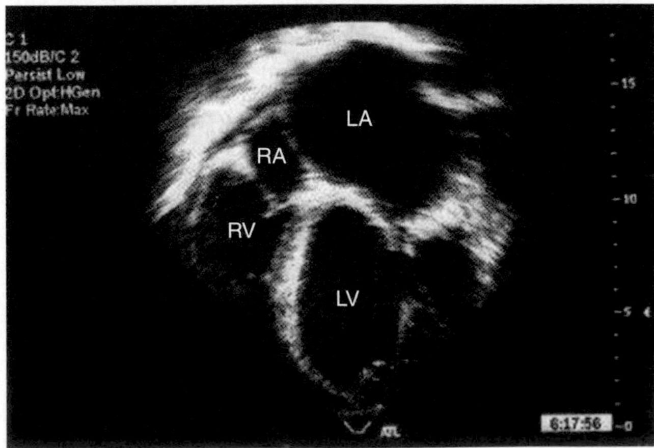

Figure 54B-22 This apical four-chamber view is from a 14-year-old boy with severe mitral and aortic regurgitation. It shows massive dilation of the left chambers and thickening of the mitral valvar leaflets. LA, left atrium; LV, left ventricle; RA, right atrium; RV, right ventricle;.

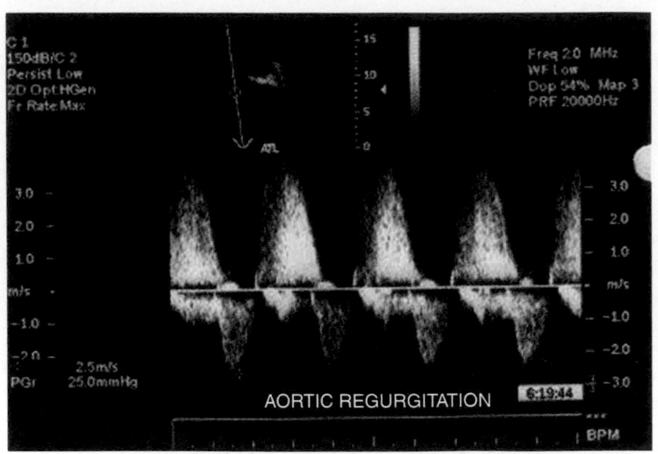

Figure 54B-23 The continuous Doppler recording from a 14-year-old boy shows severe aortic regurgitation.

Cardiac catheterisation and angiography are rarely indicated nowadays in young patients. Should they be performed, the aortic tracings in the face of severe regurgitation reveal a wide pulse pressure and a low diastolic pressure. The left ventricular end-diastolic pressure may be slightly elevated or high, and the pulmonary capillary wedge pressure usually reflects the left ventricular end-diastolic pressure unless there is associated mitral valvar disease. Pulmonary arterial hypertension is uncommon, unless there is chronic long-standing disease, additional mitral valvar disease, or acute aortic incompetence. The cardiac output is relatively normal or slightly decreased. Left ventriculography is useful in assessing the size and the function of the left ventricle, besides the presence or absence of additional mitral incompetence. The left ventricular end-diastolic volume has a close correlation with the regurgitant volume. In the absence of myocardial failure, it is a good index of the severity of the regurgitation.[69] Regurgitation fractions of more than 50%, and an ejection fraction of less than 40%, indicate severe left ventricular dysfunction. Selective aortography in the right and the left anterior oblique projections provides details of the size of the aortic root and the aortic valve, and the degree of regurgitation. In moderate aortic incompetence, the entire left ventricle is opacified for several beats. In those with severe regurgitation, the ventricle is opacified for more than 10 beats.

Aortic Stenosis

Aortic stenosis is a rare rheumatic sequel in childhood. Since this lesion develops slowly and gradually, it often presents at a much later age, usually over decades. Consequently, aortic stenosis occurring as an isolated lesion in children is usually considered to be congenital in origin.[72] In the developing countries, rheumatic aortic stenosis, like rheumatic mitral stenosis, can occur in young patients.[11,73,74]

Physiology

As a consequence of a prolonged latent period for the development of the obstruction, the left ventricle hypertrophies progressively in response to the systolic pressure overload, while a normal systolic mural stress, a normal chamber volume, and an adequate ejection fraction are preserved.[75,76] The increased ratio of volume to mass and mural thickness, besides the reduced compliance, lead to an increasing end-diastolic pressure without dilation, which commonly reflects diastolic rather than systolic dysfunction. The degree of diastolic dysfunction is related to the extent of left ventricle hypertrophy.[77,78] At a more advanced stage, when the hypertrophy and the proportion of the increase of the mural thickness to the pressure are inadequate, the high afterload impairs the systolic function, and consequently the cardiac output. An important contribution to ventricular filling is represented by a forceful atrial contraction. In cases of atrial fibrillation, clinical deterioration can occur with the loss of atrial contraction.

Clinical Features

The mild lesions usually cause no symptoms. In moderate aortic stenosis, there may be effort intolerance of some degree, along with palpitations and angina on extreme effort. With severe stenosis, dyspnoea is present. Palpitations and angina, on effort or at rest, and syncope can occur. Since rheumatic aortic stenosis is most usually seen in association with other lesions, it tends to be the clinical findings of those lesions that dominate the clinical picture. The peripheral pulse volume is low, with an anacrotic and slow-rising pulse. The apical impulse is left ventricular in type, with a sustained thrust and minimal cardiomegaly. Presystolic pulsation from left atrial contraction may be palpable. A systolic thrill of varying intensity and duration is felt in the aortic area, often radiating to the suprasternal notch and into both carotid arteries. The characteristic murmur is rough, coarse, and long, being ejection and systolic in type. It is best heard in the aortic area or in the third left intercostal space. It radiates to the neck. An ejection click may be audible. In case of severe valvar dysfunction it may be inaudible, the long ejection systolic murmur may have a late systolic accentuation, and a loud fourth heart sound may be heard.

The electrocardiogram shows left ventricular hypertrophy of varying degree. With severe disease, there are changes in the ST-T waves. The chest radiography may appear normal in the early stage of the disease. Left ventricular enlargement is apparent with severe disease, and post-stenotic dilation of the aorta can be seen. Pulmonary venous congestion indicates the presence of ventricular failure. Echocardiographic studies show hypertrophy of the left ventricle, with increased thickness of the free wall and septum and good contraction. The ratio of the left ventricular cavity to the ventricular mural thickness can be related to the severity of the aortic stenosis and gradient.[79] Movements of the leaflets are limited, and multiple echoes may be obtained from the thickened leaflets. Unlike congenital aortic stenosis, it is unusual to find an eccentric position of the leaflets. The estimation of the valvar area by the pressure half-time or continuity methods, and Doppler measurement of the gradient, serve to quantify the severity of the obstruction.[66] The systolic gradient may be overestimated in the presence of associated aortic regurgitation. Magnetic resonance imaging may also be useful to assess the severity of the lesion, left ventricular systolic function, mural thickness, volume, and mass.[80] Cardiac catheterisation and angiography are rarely necessary. If performed, the data can document the degree of obstruction by showing the gradient across the valve, permitting calculation of the valvar area, assessment of left ventricular function, and exclusion of other lesions. The left ventricular pressure, besides being elevated, may show an A wave impression on the upstroke. In severe disease, the left ventricular end-diastolic pressures are elevated. Pulmonary hypertension is uncommon, and pulmonary capillary pressures are usually normal or only minimally elevated. Left ventricular angiography shows a relatively normal or small cavity, with vigorous contraction. Selective angiography in the aortic root can demonstrate the presence of three valvar leaflets, and document presence or absence of associated aortic regurgitation.

Tricuspid Valvar Lesions

Primary tricuspid involvement is a rare lesion in rheumatic heart disease. Neither tricuspid incompetence nor stenosis occurs as an isolated dysfunction. Valvar regurgitation is frequently a functional lesion, with right ventricular overload and dilation occurring as a result of severe pulmonary hypertension, though occasionally it can be organic. Functional tricuspid regurgitation generally co-exists with severe left-sided valvar disease and progressing pulmonary hypertension. Such pulmonary hypertension was present in almost half of children and adolescents, and four-fifths of patients older than 18 years in one series,[23] with functional tricuspid regurgitation found in almost two-fifths and four-fifths, respectively. When found, tricuspid stenosis is most frequently associated with mitral stenosis, followed by mitral stenosis and regurgitation, although it does also occur in combination with mitral and aortic valvar disease. Albeit with very few cases present in childhood, one-quarter of patients seen in Saudi Arabia required operations on the tricuspid valve, with half of the valves showing evidence of organic disease.[81]

Physiology

When the tricuspid valve is competent, the annulus usually shortens during systole. In cases of pulmonary arterial hypertension and enlargement of the right ventricular cavity as result of important left-sided disease, the tricuspid annulus dilates and fails to shorten. The leaflets, which remain normal in appearance, fail to coapt.[40,82] With valvar incompetence, there is right atrial volume load, and the increase in the mean right atrial pressure is transmitted to both superior and inferior caval veins. The larger volume in the right atrium increases the size of this chamber. During diastole, the right ventricle is subjected to a higher filling pressure. With consequent dilation to accommodate the extra volume, this intensifies the leak. As with other types of valvar incompetence, the tricuspid regurgitation also shows a tendency to progress, albeit that the ventricular overload on the right side of the heart has a slower deleterious effect than on the left.[40] When present, the tricuspid stenosis adds an additional increment to the right atrial and systemic venous pressures. The large A wave in tricuspid stenosis is caused by increased atrial contraction, and the slow Y descent reflects impairment of the right ventricular filling with inspiration.

Clinical Features

The symptoms of patients with functional tricuspid regurgitation are usually dominated by the associated mitral and/or aortic disease. Occasionally, in some patients, the onset of the valvar incompetence tends to decrease the degree of dyspnoea and orthopnoea. Hepatic enlargement, which is usually present, can produce discomfort or pain in the right upper quadrant of the abdomen. The jugular venous pressure is always elevated, sometimes markedly so, with a dominant V wave and a rapid Y descent. A large C wave may also be seen in the absence of atrial fibrillation. Since the jugular venous pressure represents right atrial pressure, the height of the V wave and the Y descent are good indicators of the severity of the tricuspid regurgitation. The liver is enlarged, tender, and pulsatile in systole. The murmur is pansystolic, blowing in nature, best audible in the fourth left intercostal space, and characteristically increases on inspiration, the so-called Rivero Carvallo sign. With mild lesions, the murmur may be audible only during inspiration. In moderately severe dysfunction, it is present throughout the respiratory cycle, yet increases with inspiration. With severe incompetence, the right ventricle is already maximally overloaded, and inspiration cannot alter the flow of blood across the tricuspid valve. The murmur may then be loud and audible over a large area of the pericardium, including the axilla, and may produce diagnostic difficulties in excluding associated mitral regurgitation. A right ventricular third heart sound may be audible. Mid-diastolic flow murmurs in the tricuspid area are less frequent than in the setting of mitral regurgitation, since the cardiac output is usually low. The combination of low cardiac output and renal congestion can result in a decreased glomerular filtration rate and marked retention of fluid. With severe valvar incompetence, a hypodynamic high-amplitude right ventricular parasternal lift, with retraction along the right sternal border, produces a seesaw rocking motion of the entire precordium.[83] With tricuspid obstruction, a sudden increase in pulmonary flow is less likely, and dyspnoea or orthopnoea may be less prominent. The symptoms are commonly related to those of the associated valvar lesions. With significant tricuspid stenosis, there is a sharp A wave in the jugular venous pressure, and a slow Y descent is found in those patients in sinus rhythm. When atrial fibrillation is present, the prominent A wave, as well as the presystolic murmur, will then disappear. In the presence of severe mitral stenosis and low cardiac output, especially in those patients with atrial fibrillation, the signs of tricuspid stenosis may be masked unless they are looked for carefully. The murmur of tricuspid stenosis usually has a higher pitch than that of mitral stenosis, which it closely resembles. When there is atrial fibrillation, the murmur occurs earlier in diastole. A tricuspid opening snap is often present, but it may be difficult to differentiate it from that of an associated mitral stenosis.

The electrocardiogram in tricuspid regurgitation usually demonstrates right ventricular hypertrophy, right atrial enlargement with a tall spiked P wave in the presence of sinus rhythm, as well as the effects of the left-sided lesions. Although less common in children than in adults, atrial fibrillation may be present. The chest radiograph usually shows considerable generalised cardiomegaly, with right atrial and caval venous engorgement in addition to the signs of underlying mitral and/or aortic valvar disease. Echocardiography shows dilated right ventricular cavities, with paradoxical motion of the ventricular septum and exaggerated movement of the tricuspid valve. Doppler echocardiography permits estimation of the severity of the valvar lesion, right ventricular systolic pressures, and the diastolic gradient, besides aiding the evaluation of the associated lesions (Fig. 54B-24). Cardiac catheterisation,

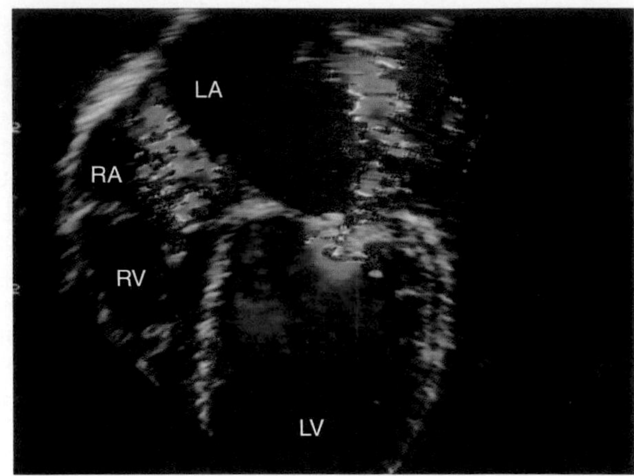

Figure 54B-24 Colour flow mapping from the apical four-chamber view of a 16-year-old boy with mitral valvar dysfunction, aortic regurgitation, and functional tricuspid regurgitation. LA, left atrium; LV, left ventricle; RA, right atrium; RV, right ventricle.

if performed, shows an elevated right atrial mean pressure, with a dominant V wave and a sharp rapid Y descent. The right ventricular end-diastolic pressure is usually elevated. Right ventricular angiography in the 30-degree right anterior oblique projection profiles the tricuspid valve. A dilated right ventricle with regurgitation of the contrast medium into the right atrium is usually found, but the valvar leaflets are not usually easy to visualise.

The electrocardiogram of patients with tricuspid stenosis and sinus rhythm shows severe right atrial enlargement with tall, peaked P waves, in addition to the changes produced by the associated lesions. Similarly, the radiological abnormalities are basically those of the associated lesions but, in addition, show an enlarged right atrium and a distended superior caval vein. The echocardiogram shows a thickened tricuspid valve, with a marked decrease in its rate of diastolic closure. More importantly, it documents the presence or absence of associated mitral stenosis. At cardiac catheterisation, rarely needed nowadays, a diastolic gradient can be demonstrated across the tricuspid valve. The right atrial pressure is increased. Those patients with sinus rhythm show a giant A wave and a slow Y descent. It is preferable to record simultaneous right atrial and right ventricular pressures using a double lumen catheter rather than make a withdrawal from the right ventricle to the right atrium. A selective right atrial angiogram in the 30-degree right anterior oblique projection demonstrates the doming effect of the tricuspid valve into the right ventricle, with the narrow jet of dye passing through the stenosed orifice.

MANAGEMENT

Patients with chronic rheumatic heart disease usually require long-term follow-up. This is based on serial clinical examinations, supplemented by periodic laboratorial evaluations, including electrocardiography, chest radiography, and echocardiography. Medical treatment essentially consists of adequate prevention of recurrences and infective endocarditis, and treatment of congestive cardiac failure and arrhythmias, especially atrial fibrillation. The patients require close observation to detect progression of the disease, besides control of medical therapy, supervision of physical activities, and recognition of complications.

In this setting, complications which should also be considered in the therapeutic approach include embolism, intercurrent infections, and electrolyte imbalance as a consequence of long-term treatment with diuretics.

The ultimate decision of clinical management or invasive therapy is made on an individual basis. The operative risks, and potential post-operative complications, should be balanced against the benefits of an invasive treatment and the risks produced by the valvar lesion in the absence of an invasive approach. The timing and indication for the invasive approach are mostly determined by the severity of the clinical condition, degree of valvar dysfunction, and overall cardiac function. Progression of symptoms, recurrent or persistent congestive cardiac failure, progressive or severe pulmonary hypertension, increasing cardiomegaly on the chest radiograph, progressive evidence of left-sided hypertrophy on the electrocardiogram, atrial fibrillation, and thrombo-embolism are all indicative of severe disease, and make the patient a potential candidate for invasive treatment.[4,43,84] Preservation of ventricular function and adequate pulmonary pressures are the most important factors determining the efficiency of surgical or catheter intervention.

The advances in non-invasive methods, mainly Doppler echocardiography, have had an important role in the selection of patients, along with the choice of the most appropriate invasive intervention. The echocardiographic data has also been used as a prognostic predictor of surgical results, while intra-operative transoesophageal echocardiography has advanced reconstructive surgery, as well as providing a guide during percutaneous balloon valvoplasty.[85–87] The introduction of three-dimensional echocardiography, and pulsed tissue Doppler imaging, have provided new insights into the geometry and spatial relations of the valvar apparatus and myocardial function.

The options now available for invasive treatment include surgery, and percutaneous balloon valvoplasty for stenotic lesions. The percutaneous option became an alternative to surgery in the early 1980s. The excellence of the obtained results led to its increasing use worldwide, with specific indications as discussed below.[88,89] On the other hand, surgical repair retains the advantage of permitting an individual approach to the particular morphological abnormality, and is currently the procedure of choice for valvar insufficiency. Percutaneous valvar implantation is now the new horizon in transcatheter therapeutics, but is rarely used as an alternative to the other approaches, and then only in highly selected cases.[90]

Percutaneous Intervention for the Chronic Valvar Lesions

Approach to Mitral Stenosis

There are currently two techniques, one employing balloons and the other using a metallic device. Valvoplasty with the Inoue balloon is the most popular technique, and has equivalent results to the double balloon technique, which is effective but more demanding.[91] The metallic device has been used for mitral commissurotomy in a large series of patients and has the potential advantage of reutilisation, reducing the cost of the procedure.[92] Percutaneous transvenous mitral valvoplasty proved successful in 94% of patients, with a rate of restenosis of 16% over a mean follow-up of 34.4 months.[93] Restenosis was presumed to be the consequence of turbulent flow, since the patients were receiving appropriate prophylaxis to prevent recurrent attacks of rheumatic fever.

Echocardiography is used to evaluate the valvar anatomy prior to the procedure, aiming to validate the indications for percutaneous treatment, and also to define the prognosis. Scores have been devised to predict the results of percutaneous valvoplasty. Wilkins score is most commonly used, which takes into account the pattern of mobility of the leaflets, the intensity of valvar and subvalvar thickening, and the extent of calcific deposits.[94] Other scores use a more general assessment of the valvar anatomy, taking also in consideration the uneven distribution of the anatomic abnormalities.[95,96] No system, however, has been shown to be superior.[91] Contra-indications to the percutaneous approach include left atrial thrombosis, moderate or severe associated mitral regurgitation, massive calcification of the ends of the zone of apposition between the leaflets, contra-indications for transeptal catheterisation, and the need for surgery on another valve or artery.[91]

Symptomatic patients with moderate to severe mitral stenosis, this representing an area of the valvar orifice of less than 1.5 cm^2, or an indexed area of less than 0.6 cm^2/m^2 of body surface, who are in the second to fourth functional classes of the categorisation established by the New York Heart Association, and with favourable valvar morphology, are all candidates for percutaneous balloon valvoplasty. Children and adolescents with favourable anatomy and mild symptoms can also benefit from the balloon procedure, because it can postpone surgery, avoiding the inherent risks of the surgical procedure, including bypass, as well as avoid scarring of the chest wall and adhesive pericarditis. At the other end of the spectrum of disease, balloon valvotomy has become the procedure of choice for patients with stenotic lesions who are in poor clinical condition and hence present a high surgical risk.[43,52]

The desired end-point of the procedure is to produce a valvar orifice with an area greater than 1 cm^2/m^2 of body surface, opening completely at least one end of the zone of apposition between the leaflets, accompanied by the appearance of, or increment in, mitral regurgitation greater than the first grade in the angiographic classification proposed by Sellers.[97] The results of valvoplasty can be evaluated echocardiographically. Follow-up studies in the immediate, short, and intermediate term show that patients with a score in the Wilkins system equal to or lower than 8 have significantly greater survival and freedom from combined events than patients with scores greater than 8. Some additional features, such as severe mitral regurgitation, high pulmonary arterial pressure after the procedure, and functional classification greater than 4, among others, were identified as predictors of poor outcome.[98] The main complications of the percutaneous approach are haemopericardium, massive mitral regurgitation, and embolism. Severe regurgitation is usually the consequence of tearing the leaflets other than along their zone of apposition, or more rarely rupture of the papillary muscles or tendinous cords. Surgery as an emergency procedure may be required to treat these complications.

Therapeutic Approach to Aortic Stenosis

As we have discussed extensively, significant aortic stenosis is rare in young patients as a sequel of rheumatic carditis. The need for invasive intervention, therefore, usually occurs in adulthood. A few reports have emerged of percutaneous valvotomy for rheumatic aortic stenosis, usually in critically ill patients, or as a bridge to open heart surgery.[99] According to the guidelines for the management of patients with valvar disease provided by the American Heart Association,[43] because of the high rate of complications and restenosis following percutaneous valvoplasty, replacement of the aortic valve is the only effective treatment for degenerative calcific aortic stenosis as seen in the adult. On the other hand, the same publication recommends that younger patients with congenital or rheumatic aortic stenosis could be candidates for the balloon procedure.

Surgery

Surgical intervention adds a considerable burden to the already high cost of management of patients with chronic rheumatic heart disease. The rate of requirement for such surgical intervention in rheumatic valvar dysfunction reflects also the developmental state of the country, with few needs in nations where patients have better access to medical treatment and antibiotic prophylaxis.[64]

Although guidelines for invasive management of patients with valvar disease have been developed and periodically reviewed, they are mostly applicable to adults. In young patients with rheumatic heart disease, several questions remain unsettled. Discussion continues regarding the timing and indications for surgical intervention, since the ideal valvar prostheses are still not currently available. On the other hand, the increased understanding of the mechanics of valvar function, and the advances in surgical techniques, have markedly improved the outcome for children and adolescents. Irreversible myocardial damage, and pulmonary hypertension, need to be prevented because they increase considerably the immediate surgical risk as well as outcomes in the long term.

The potential surgical strategies include open-heart valvar repair or valvar replacement. When the valve is suitable, then repair is the operation of choice. The effort of preserving the native valve is well worthwhile, delaying valvar replacement and its complications in childhood and adolescence. Relative contra-indications to repair or replacement include end-stage lesions with severe ventricular dysfunction, significant fixed pulmonary hypertension, and extensive tissue destruction as a consequence of endocarditis.[4]

Symptomatic children and adolescents with severe mitral regurgitation who are in the third or fourth classes of the categorisation of the New York Heart Association, yet have normal left ventricular function, require surgery. A decline in left ventricular function, even if mild or moderate, has also been taken as an indication for operation in symptomatic or asymptomatic patients with severe rheumatic mitral regurgitation.[40,100,101] Although still controversial, the aim of surgery in asymptomatic patients with severe mitral regurgitation is to prevent deterioration of the contractile state and improve long-term results. According to the American Heart Association and the European Society of Cardiology, surgery should not be undertaken when ejection fraction remains within the lower normal limits,[43,52] and intervention is advised, therefore, when the left ventricular ejection fraction is less than 0.60 and the end-systolic dimension is equal to or greater than 45 mm, adjusted to body surface area. In patients with severe ventricular dysfunction, the possibility of repair should be evaluated before recommending cardiac transplantation. Although there is still divergence of opinion, operation should be contemplated in those patients with severe mitral regurgitation who are in the second class of the categorisation of the New York Heart Association with preserved ventricular function and significant cardiomegaly. In these circumstances, there is a high probability of successful repair at low risk.[40,43,52,102] In children and adolescents who are not candidates for percutaneous valvotomy, the indications for surgical treatment of mitral stenosis include those who are symptomatic, in the third or fourth classes of the New York classification, and have moderate or severe obstruction, defined as an area of the valvar orifice less than 1.5 cm^2, or an indexed area less than 0.6 cm^2/m^2 of body surface, taking into account also the mean mitral valvar gradient and the systolic pulmonary arterial pressure.[4,43,51,52]

In patients with aortic regurgitation, surgery should be considered only in case of severe dysfunction. Hence, intervention is required for symptomatic patients, irrespective of ventricular function. The onset of symptoms such as syncope or near-syncope, dyspnoea, and angina, either on effort or at rest, has important significance in patients with severe valvar regurgitation. When symptoms are mild and their characterisation unclear, clinical judgement is required. Considering the risks of the disease without intervention, and the combined risk of operation and late potential complications of valvar surgery in children and adolescents, but bearing in mind its benefits, a detailed evaluation is necessary to establish the cause and nature of symptoms in the light of haemodynamic and functional parameters. For those who are asymptomatic, with an ejection fraction at rest below the normal lower limit in serial studies, in other words less than 0.50, findings of progressive and severe left ventricular dilation, with an end-systolic dimension greater than 50 mm or 26 mm/m^2 of body surface, should also be considered.[43,52]

Repair of Atrioventricular Valves

Considerable advances have been made in the last decades in the repair as opposed to the replacement of the diseased valves. One of the controversies raised by detailed analysis of the post-surgical evolution is that the late results of repair can be adversely affected by new episodes of rheumatic fever, especially in children and young adults, with ongoing progression of the disease.[39] Thus, the long-term follow-up of repair of the mitral valve in patients with rheumatic disease has not been good when compared to the same procedure used for valvopathies of other aetiologies.[103,104] There remains, nonetheless, a strong incentive towards repair rather than replacement because of the drawbacks of the latter procedure.

Surgery is rarely required during the acute episode of rheumatic fever. If undertaken, it is usually to treat severe mitral insufficiency, typically resulting from the rupture of tendinous cords or prolapse of the aortic leaflet. For chronic lesions, techniques of repair must be tailored to the morphological findings. Débridement of thickened leaflets usually improves their mobility and pliability, while so-called commissurotomy, in reality opening the fused ends of the zone of apposition and sliding plasties of the papillary muscles, increases the area of the valvar orifice. Insufficient valves may require annuloplasty with either prosthetic rings or the De Vega technique, the latter usually applied for regurgitant tricuspid valves. Procedures on the tendinous cords include transposition and shortening. Retracted leaflets can be extended by insertion of patches of autologous or bovine pericardium.[105] Data from a tertiary centre in Brazil demonstrated a significantly greater rate of reoperation at 125 months after repair of the mitral valve in patients aged 16 years and less when compared to those older than 16 years. This probably reflects progression of the rheumatic disease in the younger patients.[39]

Repair of the Aortic Valve

There is limited experience with aortic valvar repair for chronic rheumatic dysfunction. The advantages of repair compared to replacement, nonetheless, include better haemodynamics, the possibility of growth of the aortic root, freedom from anticoagulation, and avoidance in young patients of the complications related to insertion of a prosthetic valve.[60] Compared to repair of the mitral valve, reconstructive techniques are much more demanding for the aortic valve, and are associated with greater rates of failure.[60] Opening of the fused zones of apposition, extension of the leaflets with pericardium, and thinning of the leaflets, are among the techniques that may be applicable in the individual patient. Good results have been reported using fresh autologous pericardium to extend the leaflets.[106] Another series from India, with ages ranging from 6 to 53 years, reported survival free from reoperation of 85.4% at 160 months.[60] Even triple valvar repair is an option to avoid implantation of prostheses.[107]

Valvar Replacement

When repair is not possible because of severely distorted morphology, replacement may be the only available option. Late complications after insertion of prosthetic valves include the need for a new valve as the child overgrows the initial prosthesis, or because of the limited durability of tissue valves, besides the morbidity associated with long-term anticoagulation and the risk of infective endocarditis.[108,109] Mechanical prostheses are generally preferred for children because of their durability compared to the accelerated calcification and dysfunction of bioprostheses[109,110] (Fig. 54B-25). Despite that advantage, mechanical prostheses are known to be thrombogenic, and anticoagulation is thus mandatory. In the setting of poverty, long-term anticoagulation is difficult to manage, and the least thrombogenic prostheses should be implanted.[4] Lower reoperation rates, and fewer complications, have been reported in those who received mechanical prostheses.[111] Insertion of porcine bioprostheses, albeit in adults, achieved an actuarial estimate of freedom from failure equal to 63.7% and 7.7% at 10 and 20 years after surgery, respectively, with a mean duration to failure of over 12 years.[112]

According to the technical report from the World Health Organization, the expected incidence of infective endocarditis on valvar prostheses (Fig. 54B-26) varies from 0.2 to 1.2% per year.[4] Another concern in those with rheumatic heart disease is the best choice whenever there is the need for simultaneous replacement of the mitral and aortic valves. While some groups recommend repair of the mitral valve and replacement of the aortic valve,[113] others prefer double valvar replacement as the standard procedure.[114] The main problem is the need for reoperation on the mitral valve due to the progression of rheumatic lesions in this group of patients. In one series,[115] no potential advantages were identified for preserving rather than replacing the mitral valve when the aortic valve was replaced. According to this group, repair of the mitral valve should be considered only in selected patients in whom the durability of the procedure is expected to be excellent.

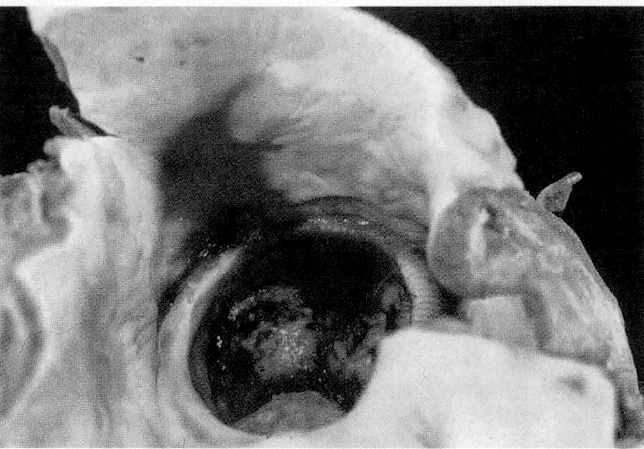

Figure 54B-25 The biological prosthesis inserted in mitral position shows massive calcification (diffuse yellowish colour).

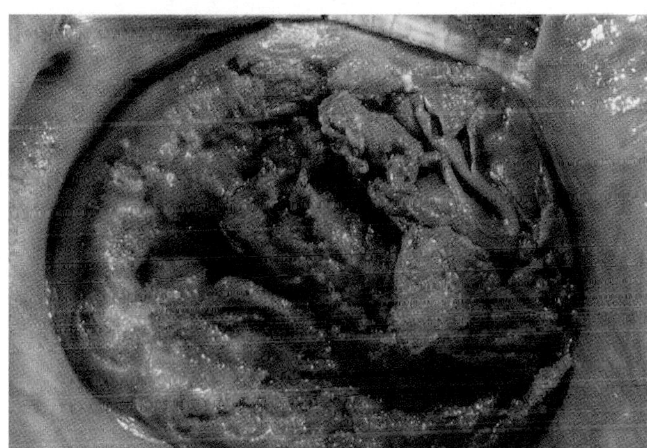

Figure 54B-26 Another biological prosthesis inserted in mitral position shows an extensive vegetation of infective endocarditis.

On the horizon of the interventional approach to valvar disease is percutaneous valvar replacement. Although this procedure is currently limited to a very few centres dealing with highly selected patients, it is a promising alternative to surgery for patients with rheumatic heart disease. The early results with percutaneous replacement of arterial valves have been better than attempts at repairing atrioventricular valves.[116] At the present stage, several questions remain to be answered, mainly regarding the best time for intervention, the technique of implantation, and the best material to be used.[91]

ACKNOWLEDGEMENT

We are indebted to Cleusa C. Lapa Santos, Luiza Guilherme, and Pablo M. Pomerantzeff for reviewing the text in the light of their own specific areas of expertise.

The complete reference list can be found on the companion Expert Consult web site at www.expertconsult.com.

ANNOTATED REFERENCES

- Guilherme L, Cury P, Demarchi LM, et al: Rheumatic heart disease: Proinflammatory cytokines play a role in the progression and maintenance of valvular lesions. Am J Pathol 2000;165:1583–1591.

  This study characterised the cytokine profile of heart-infiltrating T lymphocytes in cases of rheumatic heart disease. The predominant expression of IFN-gamma and TNF-alpha in the heart suggests that Th1-type cytokines could mediate the disease. Unlike in reversible myocardial inflammation, the significantly lower expression of IL-4 in the valvar tissue may contribute to the progression of the disease, leading to permanent valvar damage.

- Kothari SS, Ramakrishnan S, Kumar CK, et al: Intermediate-term results of percutaneous transvenous mitral commissurotomy in children less than 12 years of age. Catheter Cardiovasc Interv 2005;64:487–490.

  The authors review the efficacy of percutaneous transvenous commissurotomy in 100 consecutive children less than 12 years of age, and provide data regarding the follow-up in the intermediate term. The actuarial rate of good functional state, with survival, no repeat interventions, and in the first or second class of the New York categorisation at 100 months was 75.4%. They conclude that the procedure provides excellent intermediate-term palliation even in young children with rheumatic mitral stenosis.

- Steer A, Carapetis J, Molan TM, Shann F: Systematic review of rheumatic heart disease prevalence in children in developing countries: The role of environmental factors. J Paediatr Child Health, 2002;38:229–234.

  Based on surveys with uniform methodology, the authors investigated the prevalence of rheumatic heart disease and the role of the environmental factors in the distribution of the disease in developing countries. The highest prevalence was found in the Pacific region and in the Democratic Republic of Congo. Regarding variations in incidence of rheumatic fever, the differences in streptococcal exposure and treatment seem to be more important than genetic susceptibility in Australian Aborigines.

- American College of Cardiology/American Heart Association Task Force on Practice Guidelines; Society of Cardiovascular Anesthesiologists; Society for Cardiovascular Angiography and Interventions; Society of Thoracic Surgeons; Bonow RO, Carabello BA, Kanu C, et al: ACC/AHA 2006 Guidelines for the management of patients with valvular heart disease: A report of the American College of Cardiology/American Heart Association Task Force on Practice Guidelines (writing committee to revise the 1998 Guidelines for the Management of Patients With Valvular Heart Disease): Developed in collaboration with the Society of Cardiovascular Anesthesiologists: Endorsed by the Society for Cardiovascular Angiography and Interventions and the Society of Thoracic Surgeons. Circulation 2006;114:e84-231. Erratum in Circulation 2007;115:e409.

  This updated report from the American College of Cardiology and the American Heart Association for the long-term management of patients with cardiac valve disease is based on extensive review of the literature. It includes a complete description of each specific valvar lesion. By the definition of practises in several situations, and with the intention of assisting in clinical decision-making, these guidelines discuss the use of diagnostic procedures, prevention, clinical features, and invasive treatments.

- Vahanian A, Baumgartner H, Bax J, et al; Task Force on the Management of Valvular Hearth Disease of the European Society of Cardiology; ESC Committee for Practice Guidelines: Guidelines on the management of valvular heart disease: The Task Force on the Management of Valvular Heart Disease of the European Society of Cardiology. Eur Heart J 28:230–268.

  These guidelines on the management of valvar disease from the European Society of Cardiology aim to present and discuss a set of recommendations to assist the individual patient under specific circumstances. Diagnostic, prophylactic, and therapeutic strategies are discussed, taking into account the risk-benefit of the procedures.

- Chockalingam A, Gnanavelu G, Elangovan S, Chockalingam V: Clinical spectrum of chronic rheumatic heart disease in India. J Heart Valve Dis 2003;12:577–581.

  The clinical spectrum of rheumatic heart disease is described in a large cohort of 10,000 patients, including 2910 children and adolescents. Mitral regurgitation was the most frequent single valvar lesion in the younger group, while mitral stenosis was seen more often in patients aged over 18. Involvement of the four cardiac valves was found in only four cases. The older group of patients showed a higher prevalence of pulmonary hypertension (80.8%) when compared to the younger group (42.4%).

- Meira ZMA, Goulart EM, Colosimo EA, Mota, CCC: Long term follow up of rheumatic fever and predictors of severe rheumatic valvar disease in Brazilian children and adolescents. Heart 2005;91:1019–1022.

  The authors describe the evolution of rheumatic valvar dysfunction since the primary acute episode in a group of 258 children and adolescents, followed up from a period ranging from 2 to 15 years. Chronic valvar disease was seen in 72.1%, of whom 15.9% developed severe valvar dysfunction. Carditis was seen in 40 patients (27.4%), evolving to subclinical chronic valvar disease. Severity of carditis, recurrences, and the maternal educational level were independently associated with severe rheumatic heart disease.

- Essop MR, Nkomo VT: Rheumatic and nonrheumatic valvular heart disease: Epidemiology, management, and prevention in Africa. Circulation 2005;112:3584–3591.

  This extensive review of valvar heart disease in Africa considers the differences in magnitude and pattern when compared with developed countries. The main focuses are the discussion of epidemiological aspects and the huge burden imposed by rheumatic fever and its sequels on limited health care resources. The current concepts on pathogenesis are also discussed, besides considerations regarding controversial issues in the diagnostic and therapeutic approaches.

- Akhtar RP, Abid AR, Zafar H, et al: Prosthetic valve replacement in adolescents with rheumatic heart disease. Asian Cardiovasc Thorac Ann 2007;15:476–481.

  The long-term survival and anticoagulant-related complications following valve replacement are described in patients with rheumatic heart disease and aged less than 18. Thrombosis and stroke were the causes of death in six patients. Survival at 1 and 10 years was 87.5% and 82.9%, respectively. As regards complications, 4.5% of patients had thrombosis, the same percentage as found for haemorrhage.

- Talwar S, Rajesh R, Subramanian A, et al: Mitral valve repair in children with rheumatic heart disease. J Thorac Cardiovasc Surg 2005;129:875–879.

  Based on a cohort of 278 children with rheumatic heart disease, the authors report the experience with repair of the mitral valve. Pre-operative left ventricular dysfunction was associated with greater mortality. The authors report an early mortality of 2.2%, with seven late deaths. Actuarial, reoperation-free, and event-free survivals at 15 years were 95.2, 85.9, and 46.7, respectively.

CHAPTER 55

Infective Endocarditis

ROHAYATI TAIB and DANIEL J. PENNY

Infective endocarditis is a microbial infection of the endocardium. It is a serious and life-threatening disease which is uncommon in childhood. Endocardial infections were formerly known as bacterial endocarditis, but the term infective endocarditis is used in order to encompass both bacterial and fungal causes. The term may also be used to describe infections of the arterial duct, surgically created shunts such as a classical or modified Blalock-Taussig anastomosis, and infection at the site of aortic coarctation, although infective endarteritis would be a more accurate term for this group.

EPIDEMIOLOGY

Prevalence and Incidence

Infective endocarditis is less prevalent in children than in adults, although its incidence in children may be increasing.[1,2] This is in part due to the increased incidence of infective endocarditis in patients with congenitally malformed hearts who are now surviving longer. The epidemiology of infective endocarditis in developed countries has changed. There has been an increase in the survival of children with congenitally malformed hearts, along with a decline in prevalence of rheumatic heart disease, so that in most countries congenital cardiac disease is now the most common substrate for infective endocarditis.

Subsequent to surgical correction of complex congenital cardiovascular malformations, patients have a long-term risk of infective endocarditis, although in up to one-tenth of cases seen in children, no structural cardiac disease or identifiable risk factors exist.[3] The condition in such cases commonly involves infections of the aortic or mitral valves in the setting of bacteraemia due to *Staphylococcus aureus*.[4,5]

The incidence of neonatal endocarditis is also increasing.[6,7] The rate of death in this age group is high, and often the diagnosis is made after death. Early repair of congenital malformations of the heart in neonates and infants has increased the prevalence of perioperative infective endocarditis in this age group.[5] The increased use of indwelling intravenous lines and implantable devices, along with the evolution of more advanced neonatal and paediatric intensive care, has increased the risk of endocarditis related to catheters.[2,7] Indwelling catheters may also predispose to the development of endocarditis in children with cancer.[8]

These changing patterns of infective endocarditis have not occurred in many poor or underdeveloped parts of the world. Rheumatic fever in these countries is still common, and access to congenital cardiac surgery is limited.[9] Rheumatic disease of the mitral and aortic valves, therefore, remains the most common basis for infective endocarditis globally. Abuse of intravenous drugs and degenerative diseases of the heart, which are important causes of endocarditis in adults, are not common predisposing factors in children.

Mortality

Infective endocarditis was universally fatal prior to the introduction of antibiotics. When sulphonamides were introduced, a small proportion of patients were successfully treated. A larger proportion of patients was cured with the introduction of penicillin, when about two-thirds survived the infection, with further increases in survival in more recent decades.[10] This reduction in mortality and morbidity has been due to advances in antimicrobial therapy, early detection of endocarditis, aggressive management of its complications, and improvements in surgical techniques.[10] Despite these improvements, between one-tenth and one-quarter of those suffering endocarditis may still die.[11,12]

PATHOGENESIS

Intact endothelium is resistant to colonisation by microorganisms. Injury or erosion to the endothelial surface, which can occur from haemodynamic or mechanical stress, is a potent inducer of thrombogenesis. The initial deposition of platelets and fibrin over the damaged endothelium is referred to as a nonbacterial thrombotic endocarditis. This is the crucial lesion, which provides a surface for bacteriums to stick to the endothelium, leading to the development of infective endocarditis.[13] When microorganisms enter the bloodstream, colonisation on the altered endothelial surface will ultimately convert the nonbacterial thrombotic endocarditis to infective endocarditis. Trauma to the oral mucosa, particularly the gums, the genitourinary tract, and the gastrointestinal tract are especially associated with increased risk of bacteraemia.

The propensity to adhere to the nonbacterial thrombotic endocarditis depends on the type of microorganism. Gram-positive organisms, such as enterococci or viridans streptococci, have the propensity to adhere to valvar surfaces, whereas gram-negative bacilli, such as *Klebsiella*, do not adhere well.[14] Gram-positive microorganisms, therefore, are the predominant organisms in endocarditis. Other bacterial factors, including dextran produced by the *Streptococcus viridans*, have been identified as promoting adherence to heart valves.[15] Furthermore, the interactions of gram-positive organisms with platelets, and their capacity to resist the antimicrobial properties of platelets, are pivotal to the development and persistence of endocardial infections.[16]

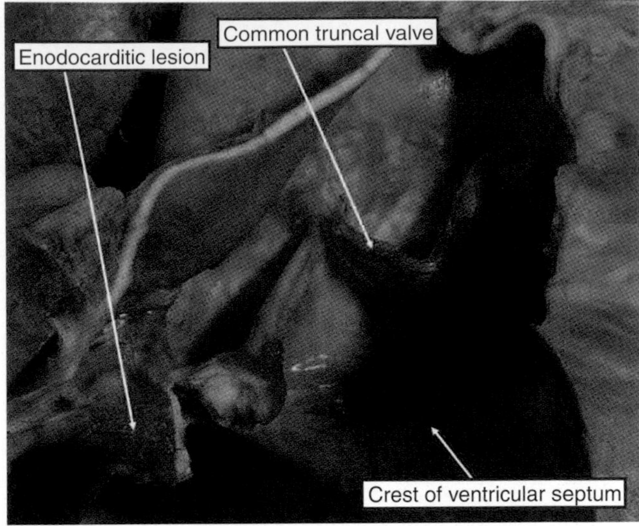

Figure 55-1 There is an endocarditic lesion on the leaflet of the truncal valve in this heart from a patient with common arterial trunk.

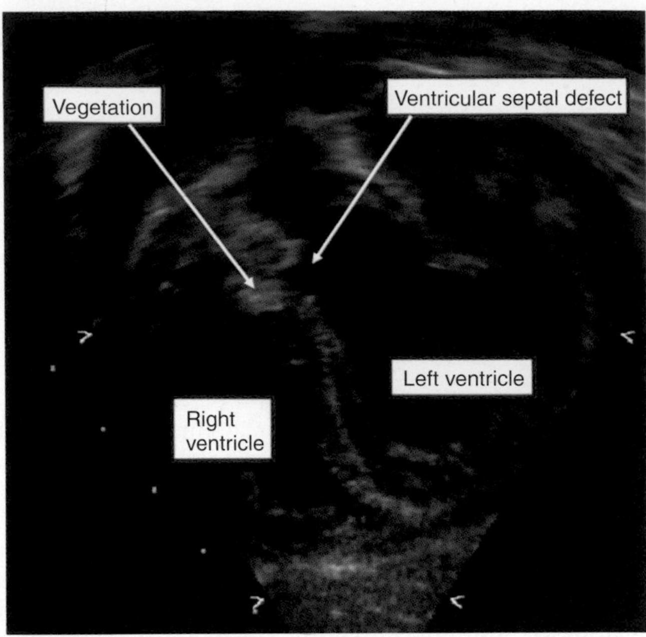

Figure 55-2 This cross sectional echocardiogram was obtained from a patient with endocarditis in the setting of a small ventricular septal defect. The vegetation is on the right ventricular side of the defect, as the jet of high velocity passes from the left to the right ventricle.

The defenses of the host play a major role in the onset of infective endocarditis. In children with cardiac disease, the shear forces associated with a stream of blood with high velocity can damage the endothelium. In damaged valves, the local pattern of flow is altered as a result of changes in the geometry of the valve. Indwelling intravenous catheters positioned in the right side of the heart may traumatise the endocardium, commonly that on the valves, exposing the subendothelial collagen.[17] These factors promote the development of non-bacterial thrombotic endocarditis, allowing adherence of microorganisms during bacteraemia, and the onset of infective endocarditis. Microorganisms, in turn, promote the further deposition of platelets and fibrin, thus enlarging the vegetation (Fig. 55-1). Organisms within the vegetation are protected from the defense mechanisms of the host, which allows them to proliferate rapidly.[18,19]

INFECTIVE ENDOCARDITIS IN THE CONGENITALLY MALFORMED HEART

Congenital cardiac disease is now the major underlying condition predisposing to infective endocarditis during childhood in developed countries. The incidence of infective endocarditis in this group is increasing[5] as more children with congenital cardiac disease survive surgical interventions. Many such patients will have undergone previous cardiac surgery. At highest risk are those who have had repair or palliation of cyanotic disease.[20]

Site of Infection

It has long been known that endocarditis commonly occurs when blood is driven from a source of high pressure, for example, the left ventricle or aorta, through a narrow orifice, for example, aortic coarctation, a small ventricular septal defect or arterial duct, or a regurgitant aortic or mitral valve, at high velocity into a low pressure sink, for example, the atrium, pulmonary trunk, or right ventricle.[21] It has been suggested that the high velocity of the stream of blood immediately beyond the orifice leads to a marked drop in the hydrostatic pressure laterally, so that, consequently, the perfusion of the endothelial intima at this level is reduced. This is then the characteristic site of the infective process. This so-called Venturi effect accounts for the finding that it is the left atrial side of the mitral valve that is affected in mitral incompetence, while in a ventricular septal defect, infection is usually centred on the right ventricular surface of the septum (Fig. 55-2). Small defects are nearly always involved, as large defects dissipate any differences in pressure. Similarly, in an arterial duct, it is commonly the pulmonary arterial end that is infected, while in aortic incompetence, it is the ventricular surface of the leaflet that is involved.

Infective Endocarditis in Unoperated Congenital Heart Disease

The lesions which are most commonly affected by infective endocarditis are small ventricular septal defects, aortic stenosis or incompetence, tetralogy of Fallot, and persistently patent arterial ducts.[22] Conversely, there have been only a few reports of endocarditis possibly related to isolated defects of the atrial septum, although patients with the so-called ostium primum defect, in reality an atrioventricular septal defect with separate valvar orifices for the right and left ventricles, may be affected.[23,24]

In children aged between 5 and 14 years with a ventricular septal defect, the estimated risk is 1 in 500 patient-years, or two infections per 100 patients over a period of 10 years.[25] The risk is increased considerably when there is associated aortic incompetence, or in the setting of defects producing a shunt from the left ventricle to right atrium. When infective endocarditis occurs in those with tetralogy of Fallot and pulmonary atresia, it is usually the aortic valve that is affected. This is also the case in tetralogy with pulmonary stenosis, although the pulmonary valve can also be affected. Prolapse of the mitral valve remains an important underlying cause in children in whom no cardiac anomaly was suspected prior to the development of infective endocarditis. This is also the case in older patients with aortic valves having two leaflets. Infective endocarditis in patients with hypertrophic cardiomyopathy is virtually confined to those with obstruction to the outflow tract, and is more common in those with both obstruction and atrial dilation,[26] although this rarely occurs in childhood.

Infective Endocarditis after Surgery for Congenital Cardiac Disease

When defects such as a ventricular septal defect or the persistently patent arterial duct are completely repaired without residual sequels, the risk of endocarditis is reduced to that for the normal population by 6 months after surgery.[5] For some patients, however, the risks of infective endocarditis may be increased by cardiac surgical procedures, particularly after palliative surgery involving insertion of conduits or creation of shunts to relieve obstruction to the flow of blood to the lungs, and after replacement of the aortic valve with a prosthesis. The risk for infective endocarditis is particularly high in the immediate postoperative period, especially where prosthetic valves or conduits have been used during the repair, or when haemodynamic problems persist.[27]

MICROBIOLOGY

Gram-positive organisms are most commonly responsible for infective endocarditis in children, particularly, streptococcuses, staphylococcuses, and enterococcuses.[28]

Streptococcus

Streptococcus of the Viridans or α-Haemolytic Group

These organisms, which exhibit so-called α-haemolysis on blood agar plates, were responsible for more than nine-tenths of cases before the widespread use of antibiotics.[29]

Oral *Streptococcus* Group

The species that most commonly cause endocarditis are *Streptococcus sanguis, Streptococcus oralis,* also known as *mitis, Streptococcus salivarius, Streptococcus mutans,* and *Gemella morbillorum,* formerly called *Streptococcus morbillorum*. These organisms form part of the normal flora of the mouth and the upper respiratory tract and are almost always susceptible to penicillin G.

Streptococcus milleri Group (*Streptococcus anginosus, Streptococcus intermedius,* and *Streptococcus constellatus*)

Infection with these organisms has the tendency to form abscesses, which disseminate through the bloodstream, for example, visceral abscesses and osteomyelitis.

Abiotrophia defectiva and Infective Endocarditis Produced by *Granulicatella* Species

These agents were formerly known as nutritionally variant streptococci. The strains have nutritional deficiencies that hinder their growth in standard culture media. They often exhibit tolerance to penicillin.

Staphylococcus

Coagulase-positive species, such as *Staphylococcus aureus*, or species which are coagulase negative, such as *Staphylococcus epidermidis* and others, can cause infections in both native and prosthetic valves, indwelling vascular catheters, and prosthetic materials. They are predominantly very resistant to penicillin G and to ampicillin, due to the production of enzymes called β-lactamases

Staphylococcus Aureus

This is one of the most common organisms responsible for infective endocarditis in children. It has virulent properties, and is associated with acute bacterial endocarditis. The organism has the ability to affect normal valves, especially in patients with impaired immunity. Advances in invasive medical treatments, and in particular the increased use of intravascular devices, have resulted in an increased incidence of this form of endocarditis.[30]

Enterococcus

Enterococcus is responsible for endocarditis less frequently in children than in adults, accounting for about one-twentieth of isolates from blood cultures. Faecal organisms are normal commensals in the gut, genitourinary tract, and sometimes the mouth.[31] In older patients, endocarditis may follow procedures within the genitourinary tract, such as urethral catheterisation, abortion, normal delivery, and even insertion of an intra-uterine contraceptive device.

Other Bacterial Organisms

Infection from *Streptococcus pyogenes* was formerly associated with an acute fulminating infection following erysipelas. Infection by this organism is now uncommon, presumably related to the early use of antibiotics in this condition. Similarly, infection with *Streptococcus pneumoniae* was a recognised complication of pneumococcal meningitis or lobar pneumonia, although it is rare following the introduction of antibiotics. Patients with right isomerism and asplenia are still at risk from this infection.

Gram-negative organisms very rarely cause infective endocarditis in children. *Neisseria gonorrhoeae* can cause a fulminating endocarditis, but it is not a major problem in children in the current era. *Pseudomonas aeruginosa* can cause infection in patients on intensive care units, particularly those with indwelling catheters.

Less frequently, endocarditis can be caused by fastidious gram-negative organisms of the so-called HACEK group, specifically, *Haemophilus parainfluenzae, Haemophilus aphrophilus, Haemophilus paraphrophilus, Haemophilus influenzae, Actinobacillus actinomycetemcomitans, Cardiobacterium hominis, Eikenella corrodens, Kingella kingae,* and *Kingella denitrificans.*[32]

Fungal Endocarditis

Fungal endocarditis is rare, but its incidence appears to have increased significantly in recent years due to advances in medical technology. Risk factors include the requirement for prolonged intravenous catheterisation or use of antibiotics, dialysis, hyperalimentation, and immunosuppression, as well as surgical procedures which require implantation of prosthetic devices such as heart valves and pacemakers.[33] The organisms are usually candidal species although aspergillus has been reported. Up to three-quarters of those suffering fungal endocarditis still die. The typical large and friable vegetations contribute to the higher rates of complication. Delay in diagnosis is common and may contribute to the high rates of death.[34]

CLINICAL FEATURES

In paediatric practice, it is still useful clinically to distinguish between acute and subacute presentation. Often no precipitating event or primary focus of infection is found in children. When one is found, dental extractions, orthodontic procedures, or other dental manipulations are the most common.[35] Cardiac catheterisation rarely causes endocarditis, although staphylococcal infection may occur especially at the site of entry of the catheter. The increased use of indwelling intravascular catheters and implantable devices has resulted in many catheter-related infections, bacteraemias, and device-related infections. Endocarditis may follow cardiac surgery, particularly when an artificial material such as external conduit or prosthetic valve is used.

The defense mechanisms of the host, along with the virulence of the infecting organisms, determine the clinical manifestations. Other important factors include the type of valve infected, whether native or prosthetic, whether the infection was acquired in the community or in hospital, and if previous antimicrobial therapy was used. The indiscriminate use of antibiotics in children with congenitally malformed hearts is ill advised unless a genuine cause of illness or pyrexia is found. These factors increase the variability with which infective endocarditis can present. In some patients, infective endocarditis may mimic a wide spectrum of disorders, ranging from other infections to malignancies or diseases of connective tissue. The clinician requires vigilance in keeping infective endocarditis in mind, particularly when a patient with known cardiac disease has an unusual febrile illness, as any delay in diagnosis may lead to a higher rate of complications.

Non-specific Features

Fever

Fever is the most common symptom in patients with endocarditis, particularly in those outside the neonatal period. The fever is initially continuous, but may become recurrent and low grade with asymptomatic intervals, particularly if short courses of antibiotics were given. A low-grade fever is the predominant symptom in the classical presentation of subacute bacterial endocarditis, which is typically caused by the viridans group of streptococcuses. Infection with *Staphylococcus aureus* often causes very high fever. The fever is usually accompanied by a variety of somatic complaints, including fatigue, weakness, arthralgias, myalgias, anorexia, weight loss, rigors, and diaphoresis.

Arthralgias and Arthritis

These features are typical of subacute infective endocarditis, so that it may mimic rheumatologic diseases. Sometimes there is arthritis of a single joint, but more commonly there is generalised arthralgia.[36,37]

Cardiac Features

Congestive Cardiac Failure and Valvitis

Increasing breathlessness and tachycardia may reflect cardiac failure and/or anaemia. Cardiac failure may result from both mechanical and myocardial factors. Valvar involvement may result in destruction of the aortic or mitral valves causing severe regurgitation. Embolism to the coronary circulation may produce myocardial infarction, while occasionally a diffuse myocarditis may also contribute to myocardial dysfunction.

Embolisation

Embolisation of infected or thrombotic material from cardiac vegetations may lead to ischaemia, infarction, or mycotic aneurysms. The site of embolism determines the clinical findings. In patients with endocarditis involving the right side of the heart, embolisation may be misdiagnosed as pneumonia in a patient who presents with chest pain and breathlessness. Typically, the chest radiograph demonstrates multiple, scattered, fluffy infiltrates, which disappear and then reappear on serial films.[38] Vegetations on the mitral valve appear to be particularly associated with a high risk of embolisation. When such embolisation occurs, any organ can be affected. Splenic infarcts present with features typical of an acute abdominal problem.

Neurological Complications

Neurological complications or manifestations are common, being found in more than one-third of patients.[39] These may result from embolisation to the central nervous system, which may result in a stroke or diffuse cerebral vasculitis, which results in a confusional state, headache or psychiatric disturbance. Rarely, mycotic aneurysms within the central nervous system can occur. Their rupture can be catastrophic (Fig. 55-3).

Renal Abnormalities

Renal involvement is most common in patients with staphylococcal infections, resulting in haematuria, glomerulonephritis, or renal infarction, which may occur in up to half of such patients.[40,41]

Physical Findings

Patients appear ill, with a fever. Splenomegaly is present in two-thirds. It is often painless unless the spleen is greatly enlarged. There may be hepatomegaly and other signs of heart failure. Anaemia is common. The auscultatory signs of valvar regurgitation should be carefully sought. The child may have a cardiac anomaly with preexisting murmur. Frequent examinations are necessary if infective endocarditis is suspected, since a change in murmur is one of the classical features of the disease. The classical extracardiac manifestations of infective endocarditis, such as petechial haemorrhages, Roth's spots, Janeway lesions, Osler's nodes, and splenomegaly, are all rare in children.

INFECTIVE ENDOCARDITIS IN THE NEWBORN

Infective endocarditis affecting the newborn commonly occurs in those born prematurely, particularly after a period of prolonged hospitalisation.[42] The incidence appears to be rising, in part due to the increased survival of such premature infants with indwelling catheters,[43] but also due to increased recognition of endocarditis by the application of cross sectional echocardiography. Infections

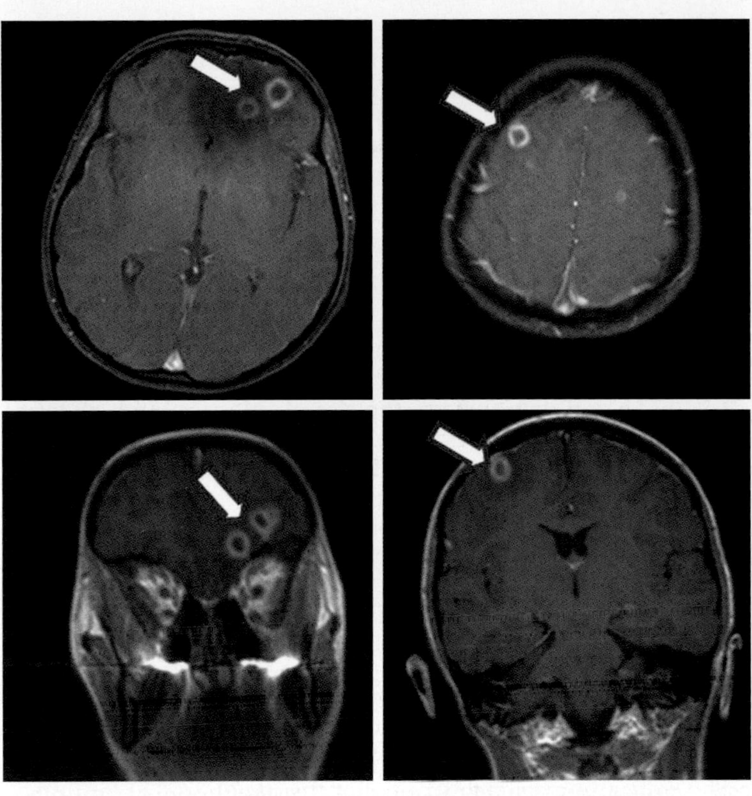

Figure 55-3 Magnetic resonance imaging of the brain in a patient with infective endocarditis involving the aortic valve. The upper panels show transverse images, while the lower panels show frontal images. There are multiple abscesses (*arrows*) involving the inferior part of the left frontal lobe and the superior part of the right parietal lobe.

usually involve the right-sided cardiac structures in babies who have structurally normal hearts. Less than one-third of cases of neonatal endocarditis occurs in the presence of congenital cardiac disease.[44] The most common infecting organisms are *Staphylococcus aureus*, coagulase-negative staphylococcuses, and *Candida* species.

The signs are usually non-specific, particularly in the preterm neonate. Many infants have feeding difficulties, respiratory distress, and tachycardia. Fever is seldom a major feature. Neonates may present with septicaemia, hypotension, congestive cardiac failure, or a changing murmur. Neurological signs and symptoms such as seizures, hemiparesis, and apnoea occur in many infants. Septic embolisms are common, and cause focuses of infection outside the heart, such as osteomyelitis, meningitis, and pneumonia.

LABORATORY DIAGNOSIS

Cultures of Blood

Cultures of blood are of paramount importance in order to isolate the infecting organism. The identity of the organism may suggest the source of bacteraemia, for example, isolation of *Streptococcus viridans* points to an oral source. Based on the organism's sensitivity to antibiotics, initial antibiotic therapy may be corrected, which has been shown to reduce mortality.[45] Blood should be cultured from all patients with fever of unexplained origin and a pathological murmur, a history of cardiac disease, or previous endocarditis. The last indication is because a previous episode of endocarditis is a risk factor for a further episode.[46] Bacteraemia in patients with infective endocarditis is usually continuous. It is not necessary, therefore, to obtain the cultures at any particular phase of the fever cycle. One set of cultures, while better than none, is not sufficient, as it does not demonstrate the continuous nature of the bacteraemia, nor does it maximise the chances of isolating the organism and differentiating between contamination and true bacteraemia.[47] In most units, two or three cultures through separate venipunctures on the first day is considered to be adequate. In the critical situation of acute infective endocarditis, where prompt treatment is crucial, cultures can be obtained within 5 minutes of each other prior to the administration of empiric antibiotic therapy. Pathogens will be grown in cultures in well over seven-tenths of untreated patients, but only from three-fifths of those in whom antibiotics were used before the sample was taken.[48] Further cultures are necessary when results are negative and the clinical suspicion of endocarditis is high, particularly if antibiotics had been given prior to sampling.

False-positive results can be due to contamination by skin flora, or from samples obtained from contaminated intravascular catheters. Such false-positive results can be averted by optimal preparation of the skin before venipuncture. Whenever possible, samples from indwelling catheters should be not be used.[49] Adequate volumes of blood should be obtained. The volume of blood taken should be as large as reasonably possible for the size of the child. Both aerobic and anaerobic cultures should be obtained, though anaerobic cultures are not necessary for all sets.

Other Tests

It is important to determine the sensitivity of the organism to antibiotics and to measure the so-called minimum inhibitory concentration to optimise the choice of antibiotics. Anaemia is common, particularly in those with chronic disease. The number of white cells in the blood is

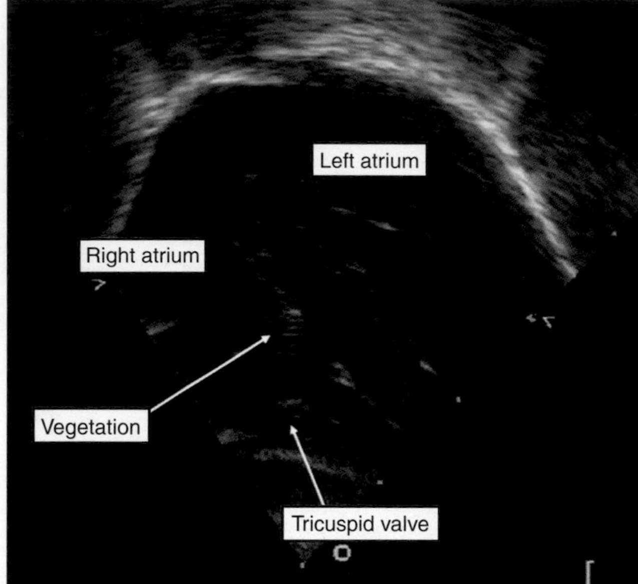

Figure 55-4 Cross sectional echocardiogram from a patient in whom there is a large vegetation within the right atrium, which is prolapsing across the tricuspid valve into the right ventricle.

typically elevated, with a preponderance of polymorphonucleocytes. More than nine-tenths of patients will have at least microscopic haematuria. Haematuria with red blood cell casts, proteinuria, and renal insufficiency may indicate the presence of glomerulonephritis. Elevated levels of acute phase reactants, specifically the rate of erythrocytic sedimentation and levels of C-reactive protein, are common.

In patients who undergo surgery for endocarditis, resected cardiac tissue may be helpful in the identification of so-called fastidious organisms,[50] although it has also been shown that the rate of contamination of such specimens may be high.[51] Amplification of specific bacterial sequences of desoxyribonucleic acid using polymerase chain reaction has also been used for the analysis of blood and tissue samples,[52,53] although this technique is not routine in most laboratories. Cultures of cells may be of use in the identification of intracellular organisms, such as *Bartonella* or *Coxiella*,[54] while serological methods may play a role in the identification of infections with these organisms and others.[54]

IMAGING STUDIES

Echocardiography

Echocardiography is the primary modality for the detection of vegetations and cardiac complications from endocarditis. It can demonstrate the site of infection and extent of damage. Serial assessments can follow the course of infection. Cardiac and valvar function can be monitored and the response to therapy assessed.[55]

Typical echocardiographic findings include the presence of vegetations (Fig. 55-4), abscesses, and new valvar insufficiency. Vegetations are usually seen on the upstream side of the valve, that is, on the atrial side of the atrioventricular valves, on the ventricular side of the arterial valves, and at the points of impingement of high-velocity jets on the valve or cardiac wall. In those with prosthetic valves, vegetations can arise from the prosthetic ring and/or along the edge of the site of a jet with high velocity. The size of the vegetation is likely to predict the likelihood of embolisation, particularly when it is on the mitral valve.[56,57]

Because of superior echocardiographic windows, the sensitivity of transthoracic echocardiography is higher in children than in adults for the detection of vegetations. Transoesophageal echocardiography is more invasive, has a higher cost, and is unnecessary in most cases, especially in younger children. Excellent agreement has been shown between transthoracic and transoesophageal echocardiography, such that, when positive findings at the transoesophageal study are used as the gold standard, the sensitivity of

Figure 55-5 **A,** This cross sectional echocardiogram was taken from a parasternal window in a patient with a para-aortic abscess. **B,** The communication between the cavity of the abscess and the aortic root is demonstrated by colour flow mapping.

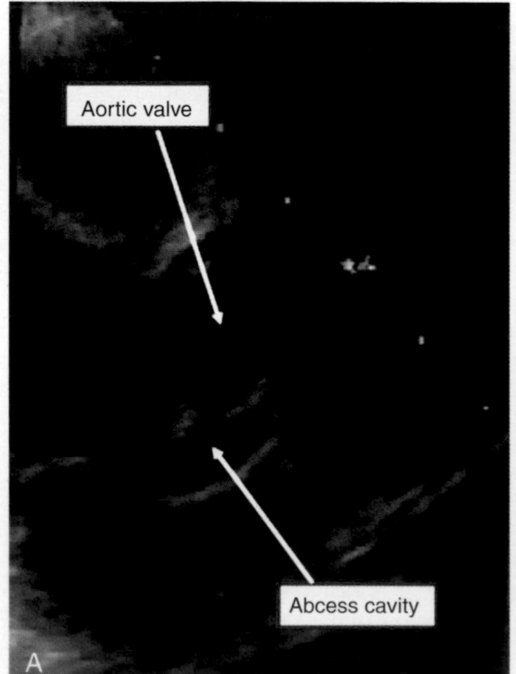

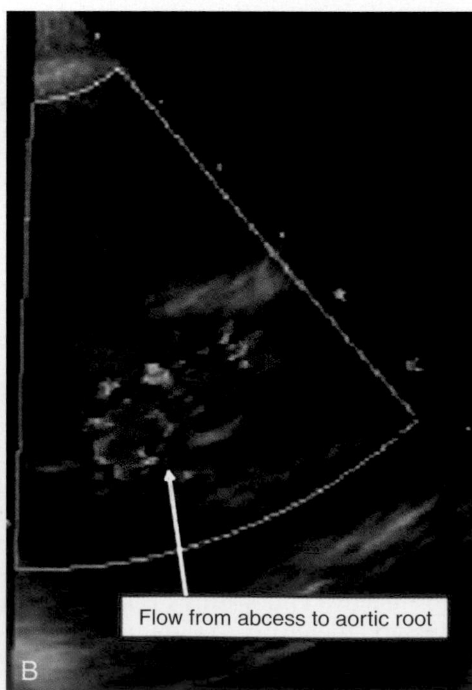

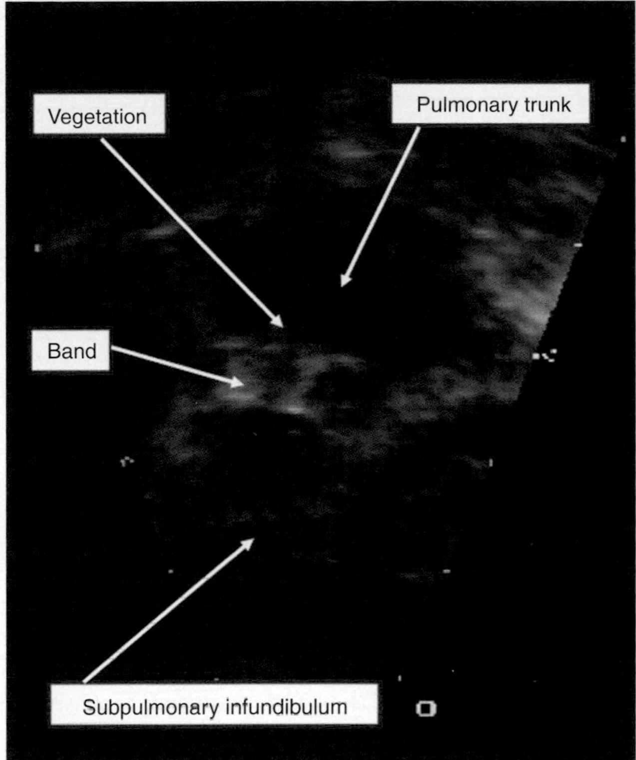

Figure 55-6 Cross sectional echocardiogram demonstrating a vegetation in a patient after surgical palliation involving banding of the pulmonary trunk. The small vegetation, which was difficult to identify, is fixed to the distal side of the band.

transthoracic echocardiography for the detection of vegetations is 93%.[58] A transoesophageal study, therefore, should be reserved for patients in whom transthoracic windows are limited. Transoesophageal echocardiography is particularly useful in the assessment of endocarditis involving the left ventricular outflow tract. In patients with involvement of the aortic valve, a changing dimension of the aortic root on transthoracic examination may indicate the development of an abscess of the aortic root, or involvement of the sinus of Valsalva. A transoesophageal study should be considered in all such patients due to the dangerous consequences of these complications (Fig. 55-5).

Limitations of Echocardiography

The significance of echocardiographic findings should be considered in the setting of the overall clinical picture. Thus, the absence of vegetations on an echocardiogram does not rule out infective endocarditis. Conversely, other types of echogenic masses may resemble a vegetation, for example, a sterile thrombus, sterile prosthetic material, or a normal anatomical variation such as a Eustachian valve.[59] Vegetations are more likely to be identified by transthoracic echocardiography in patients with normal anatomy or isolated valvar pathology than in patients with complex cyanotic disease, as interference of echocardiographic imaging by arterial grafts, conduits, and valves reduces the sensitivity of echocardiography in this group (Fig. 55-6). In such patients transoesophageal studies may be useful (Fig. 55-7).

Magnetic Resonance Imaging and Computerised Tomography

The role of these newer investigative techniques has yet to be established. Anecdotal reports have demonstrated the ability of both modalities to detect complications of infective endocarditis, particularly in the evaluation of intracranial complications, but to the best of our knowledge, there have been no large scale studies. Magnetic resonance imaging may also be of use in the detection of infective endarteritis involving the aortic arch (Fig. 55-8). The length of time currently needed to acquire images, the inability to evaluate motion, and the presence of motion artifact are major limitations of both techniques.[60]

DIAGNOSTIC CRITERIONS

The presentation of infective endocarditis in the majority of patients is non-specific, and does not follow the classical clinical presentation. Much attention was focused, therefore, on the development of a diagnostic criterion for infective endocarditis. The rules known as the Duke criterions[61] are currently the most commonly used, and have been demonstrated to be superior to previous schemes for the diagnosis of infective endocarditis in children.[62]

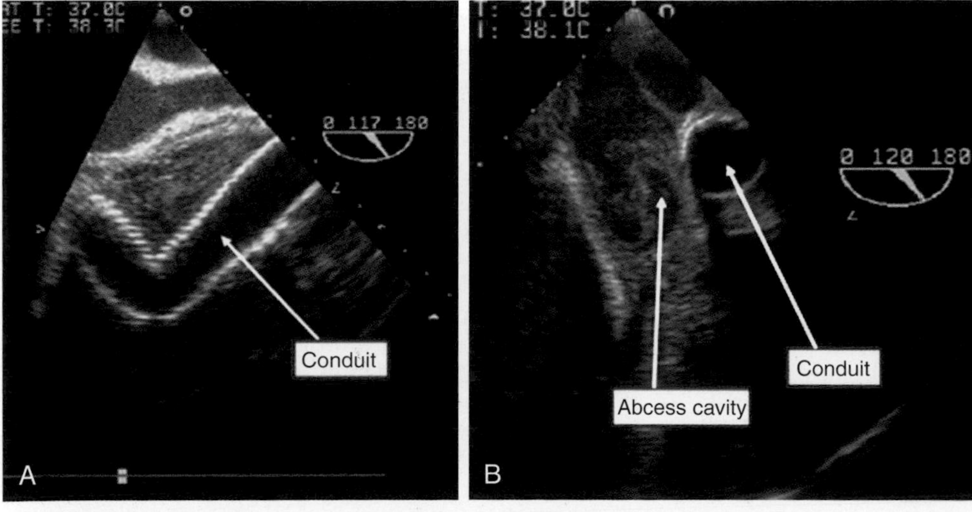

Figure 55-7 A, Transoesophageal echocardiogram in a patient with an extra-anatomic conduit placed between his ascending and descending aorta. B, An abscess cavity can be seen surrounding the conduit.

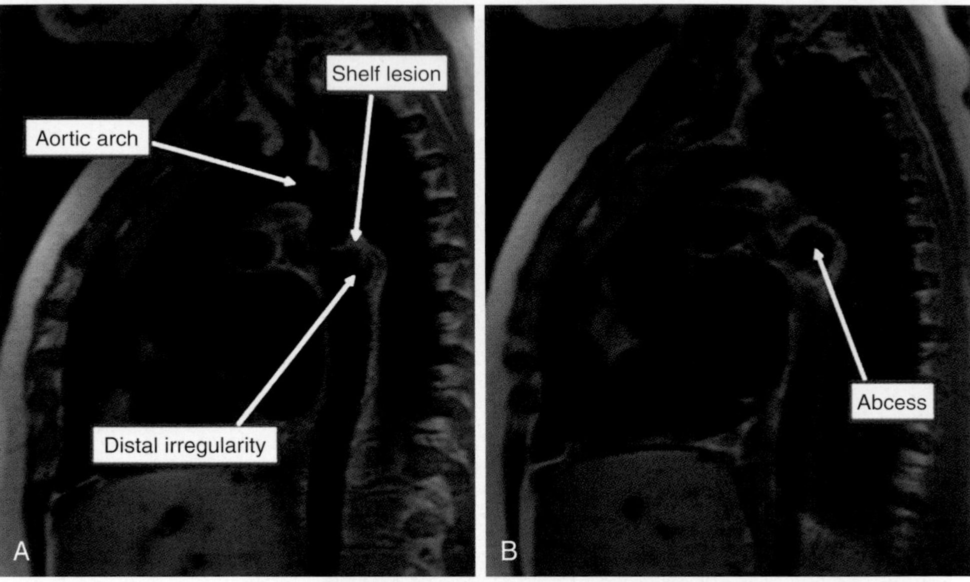

Figure 55-8 Magnetic resonance imaging in a patient who presented with a fever. The femoral pulses were absent, and an echocardiogram demonstrated the present of aortic coarctation. **A,** Magnetic resonance imaging demonstrated the shelf lesion in the aorta, with irregularity and dilation of the aorta distal to it. **B,** Further imaging demonstrated the presence of an abscess.

These criterions use similar principles to the ones employed for the diagnosis of rheumatic fever. They are made up of major and minor criterions (Table 55-1),[63] and incorporate a combination of clinical, microbiological, pathological, and echocardiographic findings. In a modification of the criterions, it has been proposed that the infection caused by *Staphylococcus aureus* should be a major criterion, regardless of whether the infection is nosocomially or community acquired, or whether a primary source of infection is present or absent.[64]

MEDICAL MANAGEMENT OF INFECTIVE ENDOCARDITIS

Therapy consists of prolonged use of the appropriate antibiotics that are adjusted to microbiological findings. In most cases, this is all that is required to cure the infection and prevent life-threatening complications. Surgical intervention may be necessary in selected patients. Optimal management requires early and on-going consultation between multidisciplinary teams consisting of the cardiologist, microbiologist, the specialist in infectious diseases, and the cardiac surgeon.

Principles of Treatment with Antibiotics

Isolation and susceptibility testing of the infecting organism is important in order to guide therapy. Cultures of blood must always be taken before treatment is commenced. In stable patients, treatment may be postponed for up to 48 hours, or even longer, until the results of initial cultures are obtained. This is particularly important if the patient has been treated with antibiotics within the last 8 days.[65] In acutely ill patients, empirical antimicrobial therapy should be commenced after three blood cultures have been obtained. Treatment will later be adjusted according to microbiological test results. Blind therapy should use a combination of antibiotics that are effective against both streptococcuses and staphylococcuses.

Penetration by antibiotics is hampered because the vegetation consists of organisms in very high concentrations embedded within a mixture of fibrin and platelets, often enclosed in a layer of exopolysaccharides. A prolonged course of antibiotics is therefore required for complete eradication, usually between 4 and 8 weeks.

The large inoculum of organisms that exist within the vegetation has relatively low rates of metabolism and division. This results in decreased susceptibility to antibiotics that work against actively growing organisms, such as β-lactam, glycopeptides, and other cell wall–active antimicrobials. There may be variable penetration of antibiotics within the vegetation.

Concentrations of antibiotics within the vegetation must be sufficiently high and sustained in order to be effective. The parenteral route of administration is required for maximal bioavailability. Intravenous administration is preferred over intramuscular injections in infants and children due to their small muscle mass. Therapy should be commenced in hospital to ensure compliance and to monitor the clinical condition. Some patients may have treatment continued out of hospital when they are haemodynamically stable, afebrile with negative cultures, and at low risk of complications.

Whenever possible, bactericidal drugs should be chosen. Bacteriostatic drugs, such as sulphonamides, tetracyclines, and chloramphenicol, may increase the chance of failure of treatment and relapses. Although these agents may suppress fever, the infection is usually not eradicated, and progressive damage to valves may occur.

It is often necessary to monitor the concentrations of antibiotics such as aminoglycosides and vancomycin in the blood in order to achieve therapeutic levels and to prevent potential side effects such as nephrotoxicity and ototoxicity. The efficacy of therapy is indicated by the disappearance of fever, the sterilisation of cultures, and the normalisation of inflammatory markers. Clinical surveillance is necessary to ensure that complications of endocarditis have not occurred. Blood should be cultured during and after treatment. Cessation of bacteraemia generally occurs within several days of appropriate treatment. Bacteraemia produced by *Staphylococcus aureus* may persist for 3 to 5 days subsequent to the start of β-lactam anti-staphylococcal therapy, and from 5 to 10 days when treating with vancomycin. Clinical and

TABLE 55-1

USE OF MODIFIED DUKE CRITERIONS FOR THE DIAGNOSIS OF INFECTIVE ENDOCARDITIS

Major Criterions

I. Positive blood culture for infective endocarditis
- A. Typical microorganism consistent with endocarditis from two separate blood cultures as noted below:
  1. *Viridans* streptococci, *Streptococcus bovis*, or HACEK group,* or
  2. Community-acquired *Staphylococcus aureus* or enterococci, in the absence of a primary focus, or
- B. Microorganisms consistent with endocarditis from persistently positive blood cultures defined as
  1. Two positive cultures of blood samples drawn >12 hours apart, or
  2. All of three or a majority of more than four separate cultures of blood (with first and last sample drawn >1 hour apart)

II. Evidence of endocardial involvement
- A. Positive echocardiogram for endocarditis defined as
  1. Oscillating intracardiac mass on valve or supporting structures, in the path of regurgitant jets, or on implanted material in the absence of an alternative anatomic explanation, or
  2. Abscess, or
  3. New partial dehiscence of prosthetic valve, or
- B. New valvular regurgitation (worsening or changing of pre-existing murmur not sufficient)

Minor Criterions

I. Predisposition: predisposing cardiac condition or intravenous drug use

II. Fever: temperature greater than 38.0°C

III. Vascular phenomena: major arterial embolisation, septic pulmonary infarcts, mycotic aneurysm, intracranial haemorrhage, conjunctival haemorrhages, and Janeway lesions

IV. Immunologic phenomena: glomerulonephritis, Osler's nodes, Roth's spots, rheumatoid factor

V. Microbiological evidence: positive blood culture but does not meet a major criterion as noted above or serological evidence of active infection with organism consistent with endocarditis

VI. Echocardiographic findings: consistent with endocarditis but do not meet a major criterion as noted above

Diagnosis

I. Definite
- A. Pathology or bacteriology of vegetations, major emboli, or intracardiac abscess specimen, or
- B. Two major criterions, or
- C. One major and three minor criterions, or
- D. Five minor criterions

II. Possible
- A. One major and one minor criterion, or
- B. Three minor criterions

III. Rejected
- A. Firm alternative diagnosis, or
- B. Resolution of syndrome after ≤4 days of antimicrobial therapy, or
- C. No pathologic evidence at surgery or autopsy after ≤4 days of antimicrobial therapy, or
- D. Does not meet definite or possible criterions

HACEK indicates *Haemophilus* species, *Actinobacillus* (*Haemophilis*) *actinomycetemcomitans*, *Cardiobacterium hominis*, *Eikenella* species, and *Kingella kingae*.

*Includes nutritionally variant strains (*Abiotrophia* species infective endocarditis). Excludes single positive cultures for coagulase-negative staphylococci and organisms that do not cause endocarditis.

Modified from Haldar SM, O'Gara PT: Infective endocarditis: Diagnosis and management. Nat Clin Pract Cardiovasc Med 2006;3:310–317.

biological surveillance should continue in the subsequent 4 weeks after completion of therapy when the risk of relapse is highest.[66]

Specific Treatment for Infection with Gram-positive organisms

Streptococci

Penicillin G, or ampicillin if penicillin G is unavailable, or ceftriaxone for 4 weeks, results in almost universal recovery. In patients with prosthetic valves, the duration of therapy should be extended to at least 6 weeks. When there is a relative resistance to penicillin, combination with an aminoglycoside is recommended.

Staphylococcus aureus

More than nine-tenths of these organisms are highly resistant to penicillin G and ampicillin as a result of production of β-lactamase. For endocarditis due to methicillin-susceptible *Staphylococcus aureus* involving a native valve or other native cardiac tissue, therapy should include a semisynthetic β-lactamase–resistant penicillin, such as nafcillin or oxacillin, given for a minimum of 6 weeks. There is some evidence that combination with an aminoglycoside might result in earlier sterilisation of the blood and faster resolution of fever, but this does not appear to change the outcome with respect to mortality.[67] Patients with methicillin-resistant strains should be given vancomycin for a minimum of 6 weeks, with or without gentamicin for the first 3 to 5 days of therapy. In patients with endocarditis involving a prosthetic valve, rifampicin should be added for the entire duration of therapy, with the duration of the aminoglycoside treatment being extended to 2 weeks.

Coagulase-negative *Staphylococcus*

Staphylococcal endocarditis on a prosthetic cardiac valve or other cardiac prosthetic material is usually caused by coagulase-negative organisms that are methicillin resistant, especially if the endocarditis develops within 1 year after cardiac surgery. Initial therapy of such patients should include a combination of vancomycin with an aminoglycoside. Therapy should be changed to a β-lactamase–resistant penicillin in proven susceptibility to methicillin.

Enterococci

Such infection is rare in children. These organisms display a relative resistance to penicillin and ampicillin, and a variable resistance to aminoglycosides and vancomycin. In patients with endocarditis on native valves caused by susceptible strains, a combination of penicillin G or ampicillin, together with gentamicin, should be given for 4 to 6 weeks. When prosthetic material is infected, a minimum duration of 6 weeks is recommended.

Fungal Endocarditis

Antimycotic therapy should continue for at least 6 weeks following surgery. Successful medical therapy alone can occur in neonates with mural endocarditis, and occasionally in some older children. The first-line antifungal therapy remains amphotericin B, although it does not penetrate vegetations well. Many patients will require surgery, as medical therapy alone is often unsuccessful.

Anticoagulation and Antiplatelet Treatments

While these treatments have been used to either prevent embolic complications or enhance the effects of antibiotics, there are no systematic studies which support the use of these agents in infective endocarditis. On the contrary, it might be expected that these agents may be detrimental in the acute phase of endocarditis, which is associated with an increased risk of haemorrhage. A number of small studies suggest that the risk of intracerebral haemorrhage following embolisation to the central nervous system may be increased by treatment with anticoagulants.[68,69] It has been recommended that, for patients who require anticoagulants for other reasons (for example, a prosthetic valve) warfarin be replaced with intravenous heparin during the early stages of the disease, until it is clear that all invasive procedures have been completed and that embolisation to the brain has not occurred.[70]

Surgical Management

While it is clear that some patients may benefit from surgical intervention, there is no data which has been prospectively gathered to examine the precise indications for surgical intervention for endocarditis in children. The decision to undertake surgery should be made in consultation with all members of the team caring for the patient. Bacteraemia, or non-completion of antibiotic therapy, should not delay surgery.[71] Several circumstances may require consideration for early surgery.

Severe Uncontrollable Cardiac Failure

Surgical intervention should be considered in patients with infective endocarditis and congestive cardiac failure. This mainly occurs in the setting of left-sided endocarditis, where progressive damage to valves can result in cardiac failure which is not amenable to medical therapy alone. Up to half of these patients may die if they do not undergo surgery.[41] Surgery can substantially reduce this rate of mortality, and is particularly beneficial in those with moderate or severe cardiac failure.

Persistent or Particularly Severe Infection and Fungal Endocarditis

Surgery should be considered if fever and bacteraemia persist for more than 7 to 10 days despite adequate antibiotic therapy. This is a common situation in patients with fungal endocarditis, in whom antifungal therapy and surgery are both commonly required for successful treatment.

Endocarditis on Surgically Created Shunts or Conduits, or Infected Patches and Intracardiac Devices

Endocarditis on prosthetic valves, particularly in the first year after surgery, is commonly due to staphylococcal infection. It may be severe, resulting in dysfunction of the valve, and can be complicated by the formation of an abscess. Infection of shunts or conduits is a potentially life-threatening condition which typically does not respond well to antibiotics alone.[72] Infection on pacing leads is also associated with high mortality and morbidity, commonly necessitating surgical or percutaneous removal of the lead, together with prolonged treatment with antibiotics.

Embolic Indications

The decision for surgery to prevent embolism is more complex, and is made on an individual basis. The greatest risk of embolisation occurs early in the course of the illness, if vegetations are large and mobile, longer than 1 cm, or situated on the aortic leaflet of the mitral valve. Early surgery may be beneficial in such patients, and in those with evidence of recurrent embolism despite appropriate antibiotics.[73]

PREVENTION OF INFECTIVE ENDOCARDITIS

Despite advances in modern antimicrobial and surgical treatments, the morbidity and mortality from endocarditis remain substantial. Prevention, therefore, has become a priority. The organisms that cause endocarditis are part of the normal oral flora, such as *Streptococcus viridans*, as well as the normal gastrointestinal and genitourinary flora. It has long been recognised that certain procedures produce bacteraemia with organisms that can cause endocarditis. Bacteraemia caused by the *viridans* group of streptococcuses is known to follow dental procedures. Bacteraemia also occurs after dental extractions, particularly in patients with periodontal disease and those who undergo multiple extractions.

Bacteraemia and Dental Procedures

Transient bacteraemia produced by streptococcuses of the viridans group may result from any dental procedure that involves manipulation of the gingival or periapical region of the teeth, or perforation of the oral mucosa. The reported frequencies of bacteraemia due to these dental procedures are widely variable, varying from one-tenth to universal bacteraemia. Streptococcal bacteraemia may also occur simply from chewing food, brushing the teeth, or using dental floss, wooden toothpicks, or water irrigation devices.[74]

While the literature emphasises the contribution of dental procedures to the development of endocarditis, this association is difficult to prove conclusively, the evidence being circumstantial. In the majority of patients, dental procedures will not have occurred within 2 weeks before symptoms. Scientific emphasis is now moving towards the cumulative effects of exposures to low inoculations of organisms due to the activities of daily living, rather than to dental treatment itself.[74]

Prophylaxis with Antibiotics

The prophylactic administration of antibiotics to prevent endocarditis in the setting of dental or other procedures has become routine in most developed countries. Guidelines have evolved over the past 50 years, based mainly on expert opinion and case studies. These recommendations have become complicated and varied between different countries, and often contain ambiguities and inconsistencies. Recommendations in the past have recommended the administration of antibiotics at the time of dental treatment for all patients deemed to be at high or moderate risk for infective endocarditis. This is usually a single dose of oral amoxicillin, or clindamycin or azithromycin if allergic, 1 hour prior to the procedure.

The mechanism whereby antibiotics prevent endocarditis is not established, but has been thought to involve effects that occur after circulating organisms have adhered to the endocardium.[75] There is little published data to prove the effectiveness of prophylaxis. Dental prophylaxis and cardiac risk factors have been evaluated in a multicentric case-controlled study, with the conclusion that dental treatment was not a risk factor for infective endocarditis even in patients with valvar cardiac disease, and that few cases could be prevented with prophylaxis even if it were completely effective.[76]

Recommendations

There is now consistent scientific evidence to suggest that the link between dentistry and infective endocarditis is tenuous. Prophylactic antibiotics prior to dental procedures may prevent an exceedingly small number of cases of infective endocarditis even if the prophylaxis was completely successful. New guidelines have now been published to take into account this growing body of evidence.[74,77] Prevention of infective endocarditis is a complex and emotive issue stemming from a prudent attempt to prevent a life-threatening infection. Recent recommendations from the British Society for Antimicrobial Chemotherapy[77] make fewer patients eligible for endocarditis prophylaxis, contrary to long-standing expectations and practices. These new guidelines have been criticised by paediatric cardiologists.[78-80]

Major changes were also included in the recently revised guidelines published by the American Heart Association.[74] The use of antibiotic prophylaxis was limited to patients whom the committee considered to be at highest risk. These include those with prosthetic cardiac valves, those with a previous episode of endocarditis, and those who develop cardiac valvar disease after transplantation. It was recommended that patients with congenital cardiac disease receive prophylaxis only if they had an unrepaired cyanotic defect, including palliative shunts or conduits, were within 6 months of complete repair with prosthetic material or device, or had a residual defect at the site or adjacent to the site of a prosthetic patch or device. For these patients, prophylaxis is recommended for all dental procedures that involve manipulation of gingival tissues or periapical region of teeth, or perforation of oral mucosa. Prophylaxis is also recommended for procedures on respiratory tract or infected skin, dermal structures or musculoskeletal tissue, but not for gastro-urinary or gastrointestinal procedures. It was suggested that the focus should shift towards a greater emphasis on good oral hygiene and access to dental care in patients with underlying cardiac conditions associated with the highest risk of adverse outcome from infective endocarditis, along with those conditions that predispose to the acquisition of infective endocarditis.

Prospective studies will be required to examine the effects of these changes on the incidence of endocarditis, although given the low incidence of the condition, it will be many years before any effects are likely to be demonstrable. Meanwhile, the subject of antibiotic prophylaxis will remain a controversial issue, and guidelines will continue to evolve.

The complete reference list can be found on the companion Expert Consult web site at www.expertconsult.com.

ANNOTATED REFERENCES

- Ferrieri P, Gewitz MH, Gerber MA, et al: Unique features of infective endocarditis in childhood. Pediatrics 2002;109:931–943.

  This excellent review focuses on the features that are particularly relevant to infants and children with endocarditis. It describes its changing epidemiology, laboratory and clinical features, as well as diagnostic and therapeutic considerations.

- Rech A, Loss JF, Machado A, Brunetto AL: Infective endocarditis (IE) in children receiving treatment for cancer. Pediatr Blood Cancer 2004;43: 159–163.

  This useful paper describes the clinical and laboratory features of a large cohort of patients with malignancy who developed endocarditis.

- Ellis ME, Al-Abdely H, Sandridge A, et al: Fungal endocarditis: Evidence in the world literature, 1965–1995. Clin Infect Dis 2001;32:50–62.

  This analysis of a large series of cases describes the characteristic features of fungal endocarditis, including delayed diagnosis and long duration of symptoms before hospitalisation. Mortality was common, with rates of survival being better for patients receiving treatment with combinations of antifungal therapies and surgery.

- Niwa K, Nakazawa M, Tateno S, et al: Infective endocarditis in congenital heart disease: Japanese national collaboration study. Heart 2005;91: 795–800.

  This study provides data on a large cohort of adults and children who developed endocarditis in the setting of congenital heart disease. Mortality was high. The authors recommend that clearer guidelines be developed for the management of endocarditis in this high-risk group.

- Thuny F, Di Salvo G, Belliard O, et al: Risk of embolism and death in infective endocarditis: Prognostic value of echocardiography—a prospective multicenter study. Circulation 2005;112;69–75.

  The difficulties in predicting embolisation of vegetations are widely acknowledged. This multi-centre echocardiographic study identifies bacteriologic and echocardiographic predictors of embolisation in a large cohort of patients.

- Baddour LM, Wilson WR, Bayer AS, et al: Infective endocarditis: Diagnosis, antimicrobial therapy, and management of complications: A statement for healthcare professionals from the Committee on Rheumatic Fever, Endocarditis, and Kawasaki Disease, Council on Cardiovascular Disease in the Young, and the Councils on Clinical Cardiology, Stroke, and Cardiovascular Surgery and Anesthesia, American Heart Association: Endorsed by the Infectious Diseases Society of America. Circulation 2005;111:e394–e434.

This multi-society statement contains guidelines of fundamental importance to the diagnosis and treatment of endocarditis in adults and children.

- Wilson W, Taubert KA, Gewitz M, et al: Prevention of Infective Endocarditis: Guidelines from the American Heart Association: A Guideline from the American Heart Association Rheumatic Fever, Endocarditis, and Kawasaki Disease Committee, Council on Cardiovascular Disease in the Young, and the Council on Clinical Cardiology, Council on Cardiovascular Surgery and Anesthesia, and the Quality of Care and Outcomes Research Interdisciplinary Working Group. Circulation 2007;116:1736–1754.
- Gould FK, Elliott TS, Foweraker J, et al; Working Party of the British Society for Antimicrobial Chemotherapy: Guidelines for the prevention of endocarditis: Report of the Working Party of the British Society for Antimicrobial Chemotherapy. J Antimicrob Chemother 2006;57:1035–1042.

Guidelines for the prevention of infective endocarditis have changed considerably since previous editions of this book. These two articles present these changes. Although the changes have been somewhat controversial, they are now being widely adopted.

CHAPTER 56

Pulmonary Vascular Disease

TILMAN HUMPL and INGRAM SCHULZE-NEICK

Pulmonary hypertension describes a number of different diseases involving the pulmonary vasculature, which have haemodynamic, histological, and therapeutic features in common. The hallmark of these diseases is an abnormally high pulmonary arterial pressure, which—except for large intracardiac shunts permitting transfer of pressure—is due to an increase in the resistance of the pulmonary vasculature, either arterial or venous, to the flow of blood. The histological changes are relatively uniform, and show only vaguely specific dependence on the cause, be it idiopathic, haemodynamic, inflammatory, toxic, or other. The haemodynamic and clinical consequences depend not only on the extent and speed of these changes, but also on the state of the subpulmonary ventricle, which is most usually the morphologically right ventricle.

The different diseases resulting in increased pulmonary vascular resistance show a spectrum of responses to the currently available specific pulmonary antihypertensive substances, with disease-specific profiles of response beginning to emerge. With regard to the individual patient, nonetheless, a correct understanding of the precise pathophysiological situation in which pulmonary vascular resistance is increased and causes pulmonary hypertension is of crucial importance for the correct commencement, and evaluation of efficacy, of treatment.

CLASSIFICATION OF PULMONARY HYPERTENSION

Already in 1891, Ernst von Romberg had described changes in the pulmonary vasculature, which he called sclerosis of the pulmonary arteries.[1] Subsequently, the term primary pulmonary hypertension was coined in 1951.[2] The original classification of chronic cor pulmonale was established by the World Health Organization in 1973,[3] and basically covered three aetiologic groups:

- Diseases primarily affecting the airways of the lung and the alveoluses, such as chronic bronchitis, bronchial asthma, emphysema, pulmonary granulomata, pulmonary resection, congenital cystic disease of the lungs, and high-altitude hypoxia.
- Diseases primarily affecting the movement of the thoracic cage, such as kyphoscoliosis, thoracoplasty, pleural fibrosis, chronic neuromuscular weakness, obesity with alveolar hypoventilation, and idiopathic alveolar hypoventilation.
- Diseases primarily affecting the pulmonary vasculature, such as affections of the arterial wall, thrombotic disorders, embolism, pressure on pulmonary arteries and veins by mediastinal tumours, and so on.

Over the past decades, the classification has been modified, bringing together clinical as well as aetiologic features with the biological expression of the disease. In 1998, during the Second World Symposium on Pulmonary Hypertension, held in Evian, France, the main focus was to establish categories with similar pathophysiological conditions and therapeutic options.[4] From this meeting emerged the following classification:

- Pulmonary arterial hypertension
- Pulmonary venous hypertension
- Pulmonary hypoxaemic hypertension associated with disorders of the respiratory system
- Pulmonary hypertension caused by thrombotic or embolic diseases
- Pulmonary hypertension caused by diseases affecting the pulmonary vasculature itself

The Third World Symposium on Pulmonary Arterial Hypertension, held in Venice, Italy, in 2003, allowed an assessment of the usefulness of the classification produced in Evian and its minor modifications (Table 56-1).[5] The clinically functional classification established by the New York Heart Association for cardiac disease (Table 56-2) is used in an adapted form to assess the clinical severity and progression of the pulmonary vascular disease.[5] Currently, pulmonary arterial hypertension is defined as a mean pulmonary arterial pressure of greater than 25 mm Hg at rest, or greater than 30 mm Hg while exercising, with a normal pulmonary arterial wedge pressure of less than 15 mm Hg, and an increased pulmonary vascular resistance index of greater than 3 Wood units times m^2 body surface area. The Dana Point symposium (2008) introduced the term borderline pulmonary hypertension for those disease states in which mean pulmonary artery pressure exceeds 20 mm Hg (personal communication).

PULMONARY HYPERTENSIVE DISEASES

Idiopathic Pulmonary Arterial Hypertension

Idiopathic pulmonary arterial hypertension is characterised by progressive and sustained elevation of pulmonary arterial pressure in the absence of any distinct cause. The diagnosis is made by exclusion of other aetiologies for pulmonary arterial hypertension. There is also some thought that the disease may be a neoplastic and angioproliferative disorder, rather than a vasomotor model centred on vasoconstriction or impaired vasodilation.[6]

TABLE 56-1

CLASSIFICATION OF PULMONARY HYPERTENSIVE DISEASES AS MADE BY THE WORLD HEALTH ORGANIZATION (VENICE, 2003)

1.	Pulmonary arterial hypertension
1.1.	Idiopathic
1.2.	Familial
1.3.	Associated with
1.3.1.	Collagen vascular disease
1.3.2.	Congenital systemic-to-pulmonary shunts
1.3.3.	Portal hypertension
1.3.4.	Human immunodeficiency viral infection
1.3.5.	Drugs and toxins
1.3.6.	Other (thyroid disorders, glycogen storage disease, Gaucher's disease, hereditary hemorrhagic telangiectasia, hemoglobinopathies, myeloproliferative disorders, splenectomy)
1.4.	Associated with significant venous or capillary involvement
1.4.1.	Pulmonary veno-occlusive disease
1.4.2.	Pulmonary capillary haemangiomatosis
1.5.	Persistent pulmonary hypertension of the newborn
2.	Pulmonary hypertension with left heart disease
2.1.	Left-sided atrial or ventricular heart disease
2.2.	Left-sided valvar heart disease
3.	Pulmonary hypertension associated with lung diseases and/or hypoxemia
3.1.	Chronic obstructive pulmonary disease
3.2.	Interstitial lung disease
3.3.	Sleep-disordered breathing
3.4.	Alveolar hypoventilation disorders
3.5.	Chronic exposure to high altitude
3.6.	Developmental abnormalities
4.	Pulmonary hypertension due to chronic thrombotic and/or embolic disease
4.1.	Thromboembolic obstruction of proximal pulmonary arteries
4.2.	Thromboembolic obstruction of distal pulmonary arteries
4.3.	Non-thrombotic pulmonary embolism (tumor, parasites, foreign material)
5.	Miscellaneous
	Sarcoidosis, histiocytosis X, lymphangiomatosis, compression of pulmonary vessels (adenopathy, tumour, fibrosing mediastinitis)

TABLE 56-2

CLASSIFICATION OF THE CLINICAL FUNCTIONAL STATE IN PATIENTS WITH PULMONARY HYPERTENSION ACCORDING TO THE WORLD HEALTH ORGANIZATION/NYHA

Class I	Patients with pulmonary hypertension, but without resulting limitation of physical activity. Ordinary physical activity does not cause undue dyspnoea or fatigue, chest pain, or near syncope.
Class II	Patients with pulmonary hypertension resulting in slight limitation of physical activity. They are comfortable at rest. Ordinary physical activity causes undue dyspnoea or fatigue, chest pain, or near syncope.
Class III	Patients with pulmonary hypertension resulting in marked limitation of physical activity. They are comfortable at rest. Less than ordinary activity causes undue dyspnoea or fatigue, chest pain, or near syncope.
Class IV	Patients with pulmonary hypertension with inability to carry out any physical activity without symptoms. These patients manifest signs of right heart failure. Dyspnoea and/or fatigue may even be present at rest. Discomfort is increased by any physical activity.

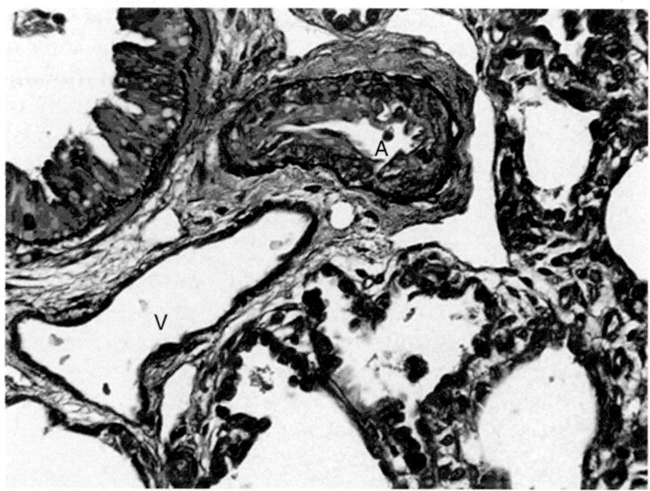

Figure 56-1 Bronchiolovascular unit showing preacinar artery (A) with intimal thickening and adjacent displaced pulmonary vein (V). The alveolar septums are thickened and show centralised capillaries with reduction of alveolar-capillary membranes (original magnification x 100; Movat stain). (Courtesy of Dr. G. Taylor, Hospital for Sick Children, Toronto, Ontario, Canada.)

Pulmonary Veno-occlusive Disease

This is a very rare condition which affects mainly, but not exclusively, children and young adults. Multiple possible factors for its development have been discussed, including infections, genetic aspects, toxic exposure, and autoimmune disorders.[7-13] The clinical presentation is very similar to idiopathic pulmonary arterial hypertension, with shortness of breath, chest pain, syncope, hypoxaemia, and later signs of right-sided cardiac failure. Histological findings (Fig. 56-1) include intimal fibrosis of the pulmonary veins, leading to narrowing and occlusion of affected vessels.[14,15] From the haemodynamic aspect, there is elevated pulmonary arterial pressure, with a normal pulmonary capillary wedge pressure. The chest radiograph (see Fig. 56-3A) typically shows enlargement of the pulmonary trunk, pulmonary oedema with prominent Kerley B lines, and pleural effusions. On computed tomography (see Fig. 56-3B and C), the disease manifests with thickened interlobular septums, enlarged lymph nodes, and ground-glass opacities.[16] Definite diagnosis requires lung biopsy, a high-risk procedure where the benefit for the patient needs to be taken into account. Cardiac catheterisation, with testing for vasodilation, may be indicated, but acute pulmonary oedema has been described.[17] Therapy includes supplemental oxygen and diuresis, as well as anticoagulation.[18] There are also reports on the use of immunosuppressive therapy with corticosteroids[19] and azathioprine,[20] but this approach should be limited to patients with suspected or proven collagen vascular disease. Lung transplantation is most likely the only option for treatment, but the long waiting time for organs may limit the final outcome.

Alveolar Capillary Dysplasia

This is a relatively rare cause of persistent pulmonary hypertension of the newborn, but its incidence is most likely underestimated. A retrospective study on neonates treated with extracorporeal membrane oxygenation in the United Kingdom between 1997 and 2000 identified a total of nine patients with such irreversible lung dysplasia.[21] The aetiology is still uncertain, with familial cases suggesting a possible genetic mutation.[22,23] The histological findings include muscularisation of the pulmonary arterioles, a deficiency in the number of alveolar units and pulmonary capillary vessels with thickening of the interalveolar septums, anomalous pulmonary veins accompanying the pulmonary arteries and bronchuses, and dilated lymphatics.[24–26] The newborn usually presents with severe hypoxaemia, without response to treatment with oxygen or pulmonary vasodilators. Open lung biopsy has been recommended if a neonate with persistent pulmonary hypertension shows no clinical improvement after 72 hours despite maximal medical therapy.[25,26] Cardiac catheterisation may be helpful to complete the diagnostic work-up.[27] Currently the disease is incurable, with a maximum reported survival time of about 3 months, albeit sometimes with a phase of mild improvement with the administration of vasodilating agents.[28,29]

Congenital Diaphragmatic Hernia

This entity is characterised by pulmonary hypoplasia, with structural as well as functional anomalies, leading to a high pulmonary vascular resistance and pulmonary hypertension. A combination of compression of the lungs during fetal life, limited flow of blood to the lungs, and intrinsic pulmonary developmental arrest are essentially responsible for the parenchymal pulmonary hypoplasia.[30–33] In addition, a dysregulation of the expression of the receptors for endothelin-1 has been documented.[34] This leads to failure of postnatal remodelling, resulting in increased right ventricular pressure and perfusion bias to the unaffected side. The clinical management includes surgical repair in the early neonatal phase, followed by care over the long term. With newer options for treatment like high-frequency oscillatory ventilation, intravenous infusion of prostaglandin, inhaled nitric oxide and extracorporeal membrane oxygenation, better neonatal survival is achieved,[35–37] but the number of patients with chronic lung disease, or recurrent or residual pulmonary hypertension, is also increasing. There are no controlled clinical trials on the use of vasodilators in long-term survivors with elevated pulmonary arterial pressures. Maximal exercise capacity was shown to be mildly decreased when a cohort of patients with this problem was compared to normal controls.[38]

Pulmonary Hypertension Associated with Bronchopulmonary Dysplasia or Chronic Lung Disease

Persistently elevated pulmonary arterial pressure related to bronchopulmonary dysplasia is a common finding in ex-preterm infants born with low weight,[39,40] despite preventive therapy,[41] but the pressures tend to fall with increasing age during the first year of life. Improved survival of very immature infants has led to increased numbers of infants with chronic lung disease. Histological findings suggest an arrested alveolar development, or loss of alveoluses, and it was hypothesised that disruption of angiogenesis impairs alveolarisation. In contrast, preservation of vascular growth and endothelial survival may promote growth, and may sustain the architecture of the distal air space.[42] Currently, supplemental oxygen is provided to children with chronic lung disease to prevent hypoxaemia. Other vasodilators, such as oral sildenafil and intravenous or aerosolised prostacyclin, may be considered after careful evaluation and exclusion of fixed pulmonary vascular resistance.

Pulmonary Hypertension Associated with Pulmonary Venous Obstruction

Pulmonary venous obstruction induces both pulmonary arterial and pulmonary venous hypertension. The condition maybe related to anatomical abnormalities of the pulmonary veins, such as partially or totally anomalous pulmonary venous connection or scimitar syndrome, a structural variation such as divided left atrium, or varying occlusion of one or more pulmonary veins, be the occlusion congenital or acquired. In the majority of cases, a surgical or interventional approach is warranted,[43–46] followed by individual assessment for residual pulmonary hypertension and tailored therapy. Whereas the long-term prognosis in the presence of divided left atrium is usually benign, the intrinsic pathology of the pulmonary veins is often progressive.

Pulmonary Hypertension Associated with Congenitally Malformed Hearts: General Considerations

Epidemiology

Pulmonary hypertension in the context of the congenitally malformed heart has a rather small place in the overall classification of pulmonary hypertension (see Table 56-1). Such classification is nowadays seen as insufficient,[47] and is currently under revision. There are a multitude of haemodynamic situations in which pulmonary vascular resistance is increased and plays an important part in the state and prognosis of the patient. Furthermore, almost one in every hundred newborns is born with a congenitally malformed heart, and more than 90% of these now survive well into adulthood, albeit 10% to 18% of these have some form of pulmonary hypertension.[48] These are adults with congenitally malformed hearts and pulmonary hypertension, a combination which is quite complex. The number of these patients is already several-fold higher than the number with idiopathic pulmonary arterial hypertension. The patients with congenitally malformed hearts require their own very specialised cardiopulmonary management.

Pathophysiological Considerations

The pulmonary vasculature is located haemodynamically between the right and left ventricles, with the two ventricles sharing the ventricular septum. This truism results in complex interactions. Damage to the arterial side of the pulmonary endothelium may be the result of shear stress due to pulmonary over-circulation in the setting of congenital interatrial communications, ventricular septal defects, or shunts at arterial level, or to the venous side in the setting of malformations that oppose the blood leaving the lungs, such as stenoses of the pulmonary veins, of the mitral and aortic valve and of the aortic isthmus. This last category includes hypoplasia and systolic and diastolic malfunction of the left heart. The pulmonary vasculature may also be congenitally hypoplastic, as in tetralogy with pulmonary atresia or pulmonary hypoplasia due to diaphragmatic hernia and so on, thus producing an intrinsically increased vascular resistance. In these pathophysiological situations, the pulmonary vascular resistance becomes a major factor influencing morbidity and mortality.[49] To estimate the risk of the development and progression of increased pulmonary vascular resistance in these circumstances, it is necessary to factor in the time, pressure, and volume with which the respective lesion is exerting its damaging stimulus to the pulmonary vasculature. Table 56-3 provides a classification of pulmonary hypertension in the setting of congenital heart disease.

Fontan Physiology

In those with the Fontan circulation, a small change in pulmonary vascular resistance will have an over-proportionate effect. This means that, while being too small to be measured, with the measurement in itself being a challenge, therapeutic reduction may result in palpable clinical benefits. The increase in pulmonary vascular resistance may be due to pulmonary factors or due to ventricular factors, such as disease of the left heart, that may be intricately entangled.

Pulmonary Vascular Resistance in the Child Prior to Operation or Transplantation

This should be low in the child submitted for a timely procedure, but should be measured later, particularly if it cannot be measured accurately in the setting of large shunts, transposition, common arterial trunk, or atrioventricular septal defect. It correlates with the likelihood, as with transplantation, of post-operative pulmonary hypertensive crises or right ventricular failure.

Chronic Postoperative Pulmonary Hypertension

Successful surgery will reconstitute the normal haemodynamic sequence of flow into and out of the two ventricles. In this situation, it is reasonable to transfer most considerations regarding idiopathic pulmonary arterial hypertension. The congenital cardiac malformation itself, nonetheless, coupled with the length of time the pulmonary vasculature was stressed pre-operatively, along with the surgical interventions, increase the vulnerability to abnormal loading conditions and the likelihood of cardiac failure.

Left Heart Disease

This may cause pulmonary venous hypertension, which results in an over-reactive increase of pulmonary vascular resistance. The consequences of the ensuing right ventricular stress, with right ventricular dilation and hypertrophy, result in an important shift of the septum into the left ventricle, which again inhibits left ventricular function. Thus, although the original cause of pulmonary vascular resistance increase is left-sided, an acute test using vasodilators is justified to differentiate the amount of independent overshooting of pulmonary vascular resistance, which may justify pharmacological treatment to increase the overall ventricular performance and cardiac output.

Eisenmenger Physiology

In this setting, changes in pulmonary vascular resistance will not change right ventricular afterload. This is fixed and, by definition, at systemic level due to the large unrestricted shunt. Changes in resistance, nonetheless, will determine the ratio of systemic to pulmonary flows, and thereby the resulting saturation.

Tetralogy with Pulmonary Atresia

If the flow of blood to the lungs is multifocal, through major aortopulmonary collaterals that are mostly mechanically obstructed, as can occur in very cyanosed patients, any amount of successful reduction of pulmonary vascular resistance due to acute vasodilation or chronic

TABLE 56-3

CLASSIFICATION OF PULMONARY HYPERTENSION IN THE SETTING OF CONGENITAL CARDIAC DISEASE

Condition	Fontan Circulation	Pre-operative/ Transplantation	Post-operative	Left Heart Disease	Eisenmenger Physiology	Pulmonary Atresia
Resulting clinical problem of pulmonary vascular resistance elevation	Signs of right heart failure, low cardiac output	Post-operative or post-transplant right heart failure, excluding operation/heart transplantation alone	Increased right ventricular afterload ultimately with circulatory collapse and death	Reduced LV preload, septum pushed to the left ventricle; low cardiac output	Reduced transpulmonary flow of oxygenated blood, increased cyanosis	Less transpulmonary blood flow and pulmonary venous return and systemic oxygenation, increased cyanosis
Treatment aim	Reduced symptoms of right venticular failure	Decreased likelihood of post-operative failure	Decreased RV afterload	Improved LV function and septum position	Increased peripheral saturation	Increased peripheral saturation
Indication	mPAP > 15 mm Hg, low CO	> 3–4 WU × m^2 BSA	RP > 2/3 R_S low RV function	Low cardiac output	PVRI > SVRI saturation <82%–85%	Saturation <82%–85%
End point	mPAP or CO	WU × m^2 BSA	mPAP or PVRI	CO, R/LVEDP	Saturation	Saturation

BSA, body surface area; CO, cardiac output; LV, left ventricular; mPAP, mean pulmonary artery pressure, PVRI, pulmonary vascular resistance index; R/LVEDP, right/left ventricular end-diastolic pressure; RP, pulmonary resistance; R_S, subsystemic resistance; RV, right ventricular; SVRI, systemic vascular resistance index; WU, Wood units.

vascular remodeling will clinically justify pharmacological treatment.

Measurement of Pulmonary Vascular Resistance in Congenital Cardiac Disease

Due to the now established early timing for surgical correction of many congenital cardiac lesions, the likelihood of increased pulmonary vascular resistance in the absence of other risk factors at this early time point is low, and can reasonably be neglected when considering surgery. Late presentation, or presentation without a history of pulmonary over-circulation and cardiac failure despite an unrestrictive shunt, would characterise the typical candidate in whom invasive evaluation of pulmonary vascular resistance is indicated.

The pulmonary vascular resistance is very important, but is not the only criterion on which depend the decisions for the type of cardiac surgery or transplantation, pharmacological treatment, or combinations thereof. The gold standard for obtaining such data remains cardiac catheterisation. This invasive method, however, is increasingly challenged by an increased perception of its risk, especially when compared to the non-invasive measurements and increasingly better and more sophisticated approximations that are provided by magnetic resonance imaging.[50,51] Indeed, the measurement of pulmonary vascular resistance in the setting of congenital cardiac disease presents special challenges regarding the indication for catheterisation, the risk and protocol for anaesthesia, and the techniques of measurement and calculations for pulmonary vascular resistance at baseline and under maximum pharmacological pulmonary vasodilation.

While older patients and children may be catheterised under local anaesthesia, general anaesthesia is usually seen as the safer approach for neonates and infants. Its risk[52] is increasingly perceived as prohibitive, and not justifying the value of the obtained data for clinical decision-making, especially in children in whom the dynamics of the process of disease tend to be more aggressive. As in all patients with increased pulmonary vascular resistance, the risk of general anaesthesia occurs specifically during the phase of induction, and during extubation. The risk is exacerbated by a weak clinical state, especially loss of weight, by specific episodes in the past, and by reduced right ventricular function. A steady state during the procedure, aided by continuous administration of agents to avoid haemodynamic variations, especially towards the end of the examination, is crucial. This should provide stable levels of carbon dioxide, and saturations near those achieved during spontaneous ventilation.

The calculation of pulmonary vascular resistance in the presence of shunts requires meticulous attention to achievement of a steady state, and the site of sampling. Multiple catheters may be used. Correct calculations require the inclusion of the dissolved oxygen into the calculation of the content of a blood sample, and measurement rather than estimation of oxygen consumption, this being especially important for cyanotic patients and candidates for Glenn or Fontan operations.[53,54] The widely used solution of cancelling out the consumption of oxygen from the corresponding equations leads to the fact that flow of blood to the lungs and pulmonary vascular resistance are put in relation to their systemic counterparts, which makes pulmonary vascular resistance a function of systemic vascular resistance. In this way, not only the individual measurements, but also comparisons between multiple catheterisations with the aim of comparing the effects of specific and pulmonary selective treatments, become unreliable.

The difference of mere pulmonary endothelial dysfunction, as opposed to fixed structural decrease and constriction of pulmonary vascular diameter, may be tested with inhalable or intravenous pulmonary vasodilators, providing maximum pulmonary vasodilation. Although, during the last 15 years, a multitude of substances and protocols have been developed for such evaluations and still exist, most institutions use a combination of oxygen and inhaled nitric oxide, nebulised iloprost, or combinations thereof.[55] If normal values are measured during baseline investigations or pulmonary vasodilation, then the surgical and peri-operative risk is assumed to be acceptably low. If, in the presence of increased values for pulmonary vascular resistance, the decrease of either pulmonary vascular resistance, mean pulmonary arterial pressure, or the ratio of pulmonary to systemic vascular resistance ratio exceeds 20%, the patient is considered a responder to pulmonary vasodilation, with the implication that the pulmonary vascular system still possesses endogenous vasodilatory capacity without perivascular fibrosis. This is associated with longer survival, and is an indication for treatment with calcium channel antagonists as an inexpensive therapeutic option.[56,57]

Evaluation of Pulmonary Vascular Resistance Prior to Operative Intervention or Transplantation

In general, pulmonary congestion with cardiac failure in those with shunting defects within the first 3 months of life is taken by most as virtual absence of increased pulmonary vascular resistance. Absence of such an episode, or an age older than 12 months, indicates potentially increased pulmonary vascular resistance needing evaluation. The precise calculation of pulmonary vascular resistance is mandatory for patients considered for operations crucially relying on lowest possible pulmonary vascular resistance, such as creation of a Glenn shunt or conversion to the Fontan circulation.[58] As the results of operation and long-term follow-up depend so much on institutional skill and experience, clear data does not exist as a cutoff for when operation is possible as opposed to being contraindicated. It is customary to assume that values of less than 4 to 6 Wood units times m^2 body surface area, and ratios for pulmonary to systemic resistances from 0.25 to 0.3, indicate operability without the need for further testing using pulmonary vasodilators. Values of up to 7 to 10 Wood units times m^2 body surface area and ratios of resistances in the range of 0.4 to 0.5, are acceptable only if the testing with vasodilators achieves values unequivocally in the lower ranges given above. For those considered for Glenn or Fontan operations, still lower values are required, with less than 3 Wood units times m^2 body surface area and ratios of resistances of 0.2.

Treatment of Pulmonary Hypertension Associated with Congenital Cardiac Disease

Aside from the haemodynamic stressors, other factors such as arterial hypoxaemia in cyanosis, and hypercarbia in hypoventilation, as well as certain syndromes such as Down, Noonan's, and Edwards', are known to enhance or predispose for increased pulmonary vascular resistance. Whatever the precise pathogenetic stimulus, the pulmonary vasculature probably has a limited arsenal of different patterns to react to it. Hence, the result is a uniform change of cellular and histological appearance of the pulmonary vasculature, as delineated by Heath and Edwards[59] or Wagenvoort,[60] beginning with pulmonary endothelial dysfunction, leading to intimal and smooth muscle cell hypertrophy in a complex vascular-adventitial interaction, and eventually ending in complete obstruction of the pulmonary vessel due to the formation of plexiform lesions. The speed of the increase of pulmonary vascular resistance, together with volume loading of the pulmonary circulation, then provides for the macroscopic effects on pulmonary arterial diameter, right ventricular dilation and hypertrophy, and eventually reduction of myocardial contractility. This relative paucity of patterns of reaction is probably the reason that most forms of pulmonary hypertension do react to the current specific options for treatment, which merely replace pulmonary endothelial factors and favour general vasodilation. No drugs yet in routine clinical use provide inhibition or reversal of cell growth. Treatment of the pulmonary vascular resistance is indicated in all those situations where increased flow to the lungs would result in an improvement in delivery of oxygen, or where reduction of the afterload to the right ventricle would increase cardiac output and decrease right-sided cardiac failure. There are also clear contraindications. These include defects permitting large shunts without an increased, and hence protective, pulmonary vascular resistance, and therefore without reduced pulmonary perfusion. In this setting, further pulmonary vasodilation would increase the pulmonary overcirculation and lead to cardiac failure. Pulmonary venous obstructive disease is another contraindication. Because the pulmonary venules in this setting are lined with obstructing non-dilating endothelial cells not reactive to pulmonary vasodilators, pulmonary vasodilation would only inhibit the protective pulmonary arterial capillary vasoconstriction, and thus lead to pulmonary oedema. Hypoplasia or reduced diastolic or systolic function of the left ventricle constitutes a further contraindication, because pulmonary vasodilation would overcome the protective increase in pulmonary vascular resistance and again lead to pulmonary oedema.

Neonatal Pulmonary Hypertension Due to Congenital Cardiac Disease

In some neonates, the high fetal pulmonary vascular resistance does not rapidly fall as is usually the case at birth. This may be due to endothelial and smooth muscle injury as a result of co-existent cardiac anomalies and increased flow of blood to the lungs. The resulting endothelial shear stress may cause alterations of the signaling pathways involving nitric oxide and endothelin, which precede anatomical changes and pulmonary vascular remodeling. In addition, changes in mediators such as transforming growth factor–beta, vascular endothelial growth factor, and vascular potassium channels, as well as upregulation of collagens, have been noted in both animal models and children with congenital cardiac disease with increased flow of blood to the lungs.

Pulmonary hypertension in the presence of large unrestricted shunting in the setting of lesions such as the persistently patent arterial duct, transposition, and common arterial trunk is simply a consequence of communicating tubes, and will be corrected only by surgical treatment. There are a few lesions such as pulmonary hypertension and cyanosis in transposition or Ebstein's malformation, where the use of inhaled nitric oxide may be indicated pre-operatively to enhance the flow to the lungs, enhance oxygenation, and normalise future post-operative right ventricular afterload. Surgical creation of an aortopulmonary shunt may be more effective if the increased pulmonary vascular resistance is due to general pulmonary vascular hypoplasia.[61] In general, the earlier the indicated surgery is performed, the less persistent will be the damage to the pulmonary endothelium and vascular tree. Besides timing, surgical and neonatal intensive care experience will decide on the need for a corrective as opposed to a palliative approach. In doubtful cases, leaving or creating an atrial shunt to bridge the peri-operative period may be useful, the shunt being closed interventionally at a later date.

Acute Post-operative Pulmonary Hypertension

This transient clinical and pathophysiological condition can result from cardiopulmonary bypass surgery. The activation of inflammatory pathways occurs in all organs, with specific problems in each. In the lung, it leads to, and augments, any pre-existing pulmonary endothelial dysfunction. Especially in neonates and infants, but also in larger children, important bronchomechanical interactions exist so that the fluctuations in pulmonary vascular resistance post-operatively have a direct impact on lung compliance and gas exchange. In the high-risk patient, these make the meticulous monitoring of both haemodynamic and pulmonary mechanical parameters mandatory so as to achieve optimal clinical management.

Following cardiopulmonary bypass operations, the pulmonary vascular system experiences for a few days or longer an increase in resistance and sensitivity to vasoconstrictive stimuli. The resistance can be lowered by supplementation of elements from the L-arginine–nitric oxide pathway, and by blockade of the endothelin receptors, suggesting a combined pathophysiology of different pathways as a cause. This pathophysiology persists for several days, making the lung very vulnerable to different stimuli such as handling, suctioning, movement, and hypoventilation. Such stimuli are answered within seconds with an exponential, and very dangerous, life-threatening pulmonary vasospasm. This is the so-called pulmonary hypertensive crisis, which results in a sharp increase in pulmonary vascular resistance and pulmonary arterial pressure, acute right ventricular decompensation with raised central venous pressure, decreased pulmonary blood flow with cyanosis, and left atrial and systemic hypotension (Fig. 56-2A). In infants and young patients, this phase is directly associated with a decrease in lung compliance (see Fig. 56-2B), hypoventilation, hypercarbia, and further pulmonary vascular restriction, producing a vicious circle which can only be interrupted by manual forced and energetic hyperventilation, and which may require other immediate measures aimed at resuscitation. This bronchopulmonary interaction has also been described elsewhere, such as in the variation of both pulmonary compliance and flow of blood to the lungs, and asthma in pulmonary hypertension.

The incidence of life-threatening pulmonary hypertensive crises has markedly decreased, from around 20% of cases in the 1980s to only 1% to 2% 25 years later. This

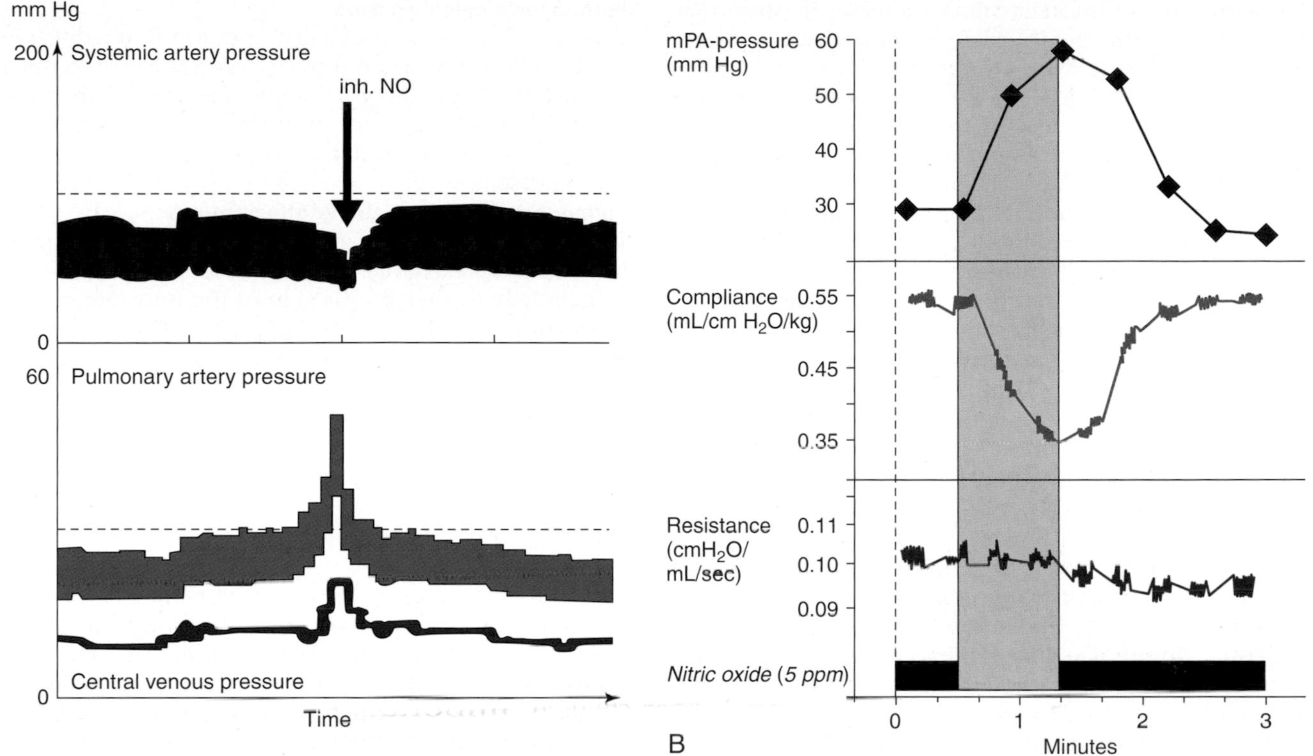

Figure 56-2 A, Original haemodynamic pressure tracing of a pulmonary hypertensive crisis, which resolved with the prompt administration of inhaled nitric oxide (inh. NO). The sharp increase of the pulmonary arterial pressures (lower half of the panel, upper tracing) is accompanied by systemic hypotension (upper half of panel) and an increase of central venous pressure as a sign of acute right heart decompensation (lower half of panel, lower tracing). The situation reverses promptly within less than a minute upon inhalation of 20 ppm nitric oxide. **B**, The bronchopulmonary interaction during such a pulmonary hypertensive crisis. The rise and fall of mean pulmonary arterial pressure (mPA) is accompanied by reverse changes in dynamic lung compliance, in response to the unsuccessful attempt to wean from inhaled nitric oxide (5 ppm) and the decision to recommence the inhalation.

reflects better techniques for surgical repair, cardiopulmonary bypass, post-operative handling, mechanical ventilation, and most importantly, timely operation before the sixth month of life. The pathophysiology nevertheless remains relevant for complex patients, particularly for those with the Fontan circulation. While the basic strategies for avoidance include alkalotic hyperventilation, sedation and paralysis, and sometimes also hypothermia, advanced strategies such as extracorporeal membrane oxygenation are only indicated for bridging a situation that may be expected to recover. Such situations are the post-operative inflammation-related increase of pulmonary vascular resistance, and depressed left or right ventricular function. Other strategies include negative pressure ventilation, ventilation with nitric oxide, and use of specific pulmonary antihypertensive drugs, such as the intravenous or inhaled use of the nucleotide adenosine, the phosphodiesterase 5 inhibitor sildenafil, the calcium channel sensitiser levosimendan, and the endothelin receptor antagonist tezosentan.

Chronic Post-operative Pulmonary Hypertension

The patient in this setting will have a surgically corrected, normal circulation without significant residual shunting defects or obstructions. Pulmonary vascular resistance is increased most likely due to the persisting pre-operative pulmonary vascular damage, as well as the effects of cardiopulmonary bypass surgery. Any left-sided component, such as pulmonary venous stenosis, mitral valvar obstruction or regurgitation, or left ventricular restriction, should clearly be recognised as such, and may warrant cardiac catheterisation to reveal the attributable increase in pulmonary vascular resistance, thus differentiating the increase from the independent overshooting reaction of the arterial pulmonary vascular tree, with the latter potentially accessible to pharmacological treatment.

It is important to make sure that patients and physicians understand that this form of pulmonary hypertension is not idiopathic. It may be stable, regress over time, or progress gradually and then require careful monitoring of cardiac function, which may be more vulnerable because of the surgical repair. The strategies for such treatment are similar to those for idiopathic pulmonary hypertension. This includes the use of anticoagulation, calcium channel blockers, balloon atrioseptostomy, and all specific drugs including phosphodiesterase 5 inhibitors, endothelin receptor antagonists, and intravenous epoprostenol. The reaction to these drugs is probably similar.

Pulmonary Hypertension Due to Left-Sided Cardiac Anomalies

Left-sided obstructions to flow of blood from the lungs includes pulmonary venous stenosis, divided left atrium, mitral valvar stenosis or regurgitation, and left heart systolic or diastolic dysfunction, either without or due to aortic stenosis or coarctation. The increased pressure upstream from the obstruction causes dilation of the involved structures, in other words, the pulmonary veins. Increases in pulmonary venous pressure directly translate into increases of pulmonary arterial pressure, while the transpulmonary gradient, and thus the calculated pulmonary vascular resistance, remains low. Invasive measurement of pulmonary venous pressure or left ventricular end-diastolic pressure, respectively, is necessary, and then calculation of the transpulmonary gradient and pulmonary arterial vascular resistance.

If the lesion is longstanding, the arterial side of the pulmonary vascular tree will react to this increased pressure and develop increased pulmonary vascular resistance via the cellular mechanisms described for idiopathic pulmonary hypertension. This may overshoot and increase out of proportion. The continuing increase of pulmonary vascular resistance will cause an increase of right ventricular diameter, with septal shift into the left ventricle, and reduced cardiac output due to right ventricular failure as described for idiopathic pulmonary arterial hypertension.

Treatment of this form of pulmonary hypertension is only warranted if the primary condition is optimised as far as possible, and invasive demonstration has shown, first, that cardiac output is reduced due to increased pulmonary vascular resistance and, second, that reduction of pulmonary vascular resistance results in improved cardiac output without any increase in pulmonary venous pressure. If the left-sided obstruction is relieved temporarily or chronically by pharmacologic treatment, corrective surgery, or assist devices, the pulmonary vascular resistance may normalise instantly or over a longer time span. In patients with end-stage left-sided cardiac failure, the long-term administration of inotropic agents, or the implantation of ventricular assist devices, to off-load the left ventricle is an accepted and often successful option to permit normalisation of the increased pulmonary vascular resistance and allow for transplantation of the heart in isolation. Unfortunately, the pulmonary hypertension due to pulmonary venous stenosis or mitral valvar disease may persist tenaciously due to the impossibility of completely relieving the lesion surgically or interventionally, this being a far from rare situation.

Fontan Circulation

The serial Fontan circulation amplifies the interdependence of all its circulatory elements. The flow of blood into the thorax and pulmonary vasculature is augmented during inspiration by negative intrathoracic pressure, while the flow of blood out of the thorax is supported by the diastolic function of the systemic ventricle. For both of these mechanisms to function, it is vital to retain as low a pulmonary vascular resistance as possible. Even a mild increase in resistance has an appreciable influence on the Fontan circulation, and leads to its failure. Several factors, with some of them being part of the Fontan state itself, may lead to an increase of pulmonary vascular resistance and reduction on the flow of blood to the lungs.

Anatomical and Mechanical Factors

These include small pulmonary arteries, the presence of stenoses, discontinuous pulmonary arteries, and distal abnormalities of arborisation, all of which increase the pulmonary vascular resistance. The detrimental effect of paralysis of the diaphragm on the dynamics of flow in the Fontan circulation has been clearly demonstrated.

Pathophysiological Factors

Too little flow, or too much flow, can result in either a hypoplastic pulmonary arterial tree or, as a reaction to the additional left-to-right flow, an increased medial thickness of the pulmonary arterioles. Both factors elevate pulmonary vascular resistance, and both have an unknown chronic time course.

Pulmonary Arterio-venous Malformations

These channels occur in around one-sixth of patients, bypassing the exchange of gases by connecting the arterial side directly to the venous side of the pulmonary vasculature. These vessels may be large and allow a right-to-left shunt at low resistance as cyanotic admixture to the systemic blood in patients with increased pulmonary vascular resistance, or in those with previous Glenn operations, where the flow of venous blood from the lower body, including the hepatic contribution, remains connected to the heart, thus bypassing the lung.

Pulsatility of Pulmonary Flow and Pulmonary Endothelial Dysfunction

Pulsatility is greatest in those patients having an atriopulmonary connection. In contrast, the pulsatility is almost lacking in patients with a lateral tunnel or total cavopulmonary connection, causing persistent pulmonary endothelial dysfunction, which can be shown by inhalation of nitric oxide to provoke a fall in pulmonary vascular resistance.[62] Even in those with pulsatile flow, the mean pulmonary arterial pulse pressure is lower than normal.

Reduced Growth of the Pulmonary Arteries

There is insufficient growth of the pulmonary arteries in relation to growth of body surface area over an observation period of 3 to 5 years. This may be due to early reduction of volume from staged cavopulmonary anastomosis to prevent ventricular volume overload and preserve systemic ventricular function. The reduction of pulmonary flow, and early introduction of non-pulsatile flow in the pulmonary circulation, may also affect the growth of the pulmonary arteries.

Micro- and Macro-thrombuses in the Pulmonary Circulation

For several reasons, the Fontan patients are at increased risk for the formation of silent or clinically apparent macro- and micro-thrombus, namely, the low, non-pulsatile systemic venous flow, the thrombogenic material of the conduit itself, and altered hepatic function due to the Fontan state.[63] The threat of pulmonary thromboembolism to a pulmonary circulation with already decreased overall diameter is clear from the experience of increased mortality in such patients with idiopathic pulmonary hypertension, and justifies effective anticoagulation.

Reduced Ventricular Function after the Fontan Operation

The acute reduction in preload resulting from the Fontan operation leads to an increase in the ratio of ventricular mass to volume ratio, with concomitant impaired ventricular relaxation and patterns of filling.[64] Although this hypertrophy has been shown to regress 1 to 3 years after surgery, the abnormal ventricular relaxation and reduced ventricular compliance persist over the long term. A progressive increase in ventricular stiffness, which naturally occurs with age, could also potentially contribute to a steady rise in pulmonary venous pressure, with ensuing increase of pulmonary vascular resistance.

In the attempt to modulate therapeutically pulmonary vascular resistance in patients with the Fontan circulation, both inhaled nitric oxide and the phosphodiesterase inhibitor sildenafil have been used successfully in the acute post-operative setting. Sildenafil was also used for chronic problems like protein-losing enteropathy,[65] improving diastolic mesenteric blood flow, exercise tolerance, pulmonary arterial pressure and pulmonary vascular resistance, and plastic bronchitis, with similar effects as the use of fenestrated stents.[66] Improvement was also reported after treatment with bosentan, an antagonist of endothelin receptors. Although the occurrence of these complications over the long term is correlated in some but not all patients with an increase in pulmonary vascular resistance and central venous and pulmonary arterial pressures, the clinical success of targeted pharmacological modulation of the pulmonary circulation indicates that there may be a role for such treatment on a broader basis, if not even in an anticipatory prophylactic way.

Eisenmenger Syndrome and Its Pathophysiology

Anatomy

The strict definition of Eisenmenger's syndrome as severe systemic cyanosis due to reversal of the shunting at atrial, ventricular or great arterial level theoretically excludes the settings of common atrium and anomalous pulmonary venous drainages, functionally single ventricle, and common arterial trunk, as the cyanosis in these lesions is not a result of shunt reversal, but of obligate intracardiac mixing of desaturated and oxygenised blood. Such considerations are important for proper management. Practically however, the working definition does include the latter diagnoses, and implies inoperability due to suprasystemic pulmonary vascular resistance.[67,68]

The natural history of Eisenmenger's syndrome is quite variable, but eventually leads to severe hypoxaemia, cyanosis, and cardiac failure. In one study, half of a cohort of patients with unrepaired ventricular septal defect was alive 20 years after the diagnosis was made.[69] Other symptoms include progressive shortness of breath, polycythaemia, headache, and haemoptysis. Therapeutic options are limited, and include supplemental oxygen therapy, anticoagulation, vasodilator therapy, and endothelin receptor antagonists.[70–76] There is some controversy about the impact of the drugs. Lung and heart-lung transplantation may be offered with an acceptable risk, and a favourable long-term outcome.[77] Oral contraceptives should be prescribed for females, as pregnancy in such patients has a high incidence of maternal and perinatal death.[78]

While the process is usually interrupted with early surgical correction of the shunting lesion, it may progress in those undergoing late correction. In such cases, a haemodynamic situation similar to idiopathic pulmonary arterial hypertension will result. In cases of significant residual defects, right-to-left shunting can occur, with establishment of the syndrome in a patient who earlier underwent successful surgical correction in the absence of pulmonary vascular disease.

Pathophysiology

The effect of the shunt depends on its exact location and size. This can cause different loading conditions, both to the pulmonary vascular tree and the subpulmonary ventricle, with specific morbidity and mortality.

Atrial Level

The defects with shunting at atrial level deliver large volumes of blood without pressure, causing shear stress to the pulmonary endothelium. In the case of abnormally draining pulmonary veins, the shunt is fixed by the abnormal connection, and only indirectly reflects increasing pulmonary vascular resistance by a reduction of pulmonary flow. In the case of interatrial communications, the left-to-right shunt correlates with the strength of right ventricular systolic opening pull, and right atrial and ventricular diastolic compliance. Due to the continuous venous flow, the shunted volume can be huge, and causes right ventricular dilation. The increase of the pulmonary vascular resistance in the third and fourth decades stretches still further the right ventricular myocytes so that they do not cope well with the increasing afterload, and tend to fail early. The Eisenmenger pathophysiology with cardiac cyanosis is then a result of the atrial right-to-left shunting due to right ventricular failure, and only indirectly due to increased pulmonary vascular resistance.

Ventricular Level

These defects deliver volume and, depending on their restrictive or unrestrictive size, also left ventricular pressure. In systole, and only then, the direction and volume of the shunt is directly ejected into the great arteries, and depends on the ratio of pulmonary to systemic resistance and the ejecting power of the ventricles, ending with closure of the arterial valves. In early and late diastole, there may be different directions and volumes of the shunt depending on ventricular compliance, thus explaining the angiographic and haemodynamic findings of left-to-right shunting during systole and right-to-left shunting in diastole in the presence of a hypertrophied and stiff right ventricle. In an atrioventricular septal defect, the addition of atrial shunting contributes also a volume load, causing ventricular dilation.

In the case of a large defect, the high pressure postnatally maintains a high, near-systemic pulmonary vascular resistance, avoiding severe cyanosis or loud heart sounds, but also avoiding a period of cardiac failure which would stimulate a diagnosis. The cyanosis may not be marked, and may be discovered only later, when pulmonary vascular resistance becomes suprasystemic. Both right and left ventricles deliver blood to both great arteries and thus see the same afterload and work as one unit.[79,80] The peripheral saturation of oxygen is a function of the ratio of pulmonary to systemic flows. Pharmacologically induced pulmonary vasodilation to augment pulmonary venous return may counteract severe cyanosis, but may be hazardous to the oft-compromised myocardial function.

Arterial Level

In the setting of transposition physiology, cyanosis is due to interatrial and intraventricular streaming and morphology, which impairs mixing so that desaturated systemic venous blood enters the subaortic ventricle or the aorta, and pulmonary venous blood returns to the subpulmonary ventricle or the pulmonary artery while pulmonary vascular resistance is low. Saturation can then only be increased anatomically by either separating the atriums in the case of common atrium and anomalously connected pulmonary veins, or in the case of transposition, by creating a left-to-right shunt at atrial level.

All lesions with arterial shunting deliver the shunt flow at systemic pressures to the pulmonary vascular tree continuously during both systole and diastole. They are associated, therefore, with an early and aggressive rise in the pulmonary vascular resistance. Below a certain size, the exact diameter of the defect does matter, and the Eisenmenger syndrome will not be manifest. That threshold appears to be from 2 to 3 cm at atrial level, limiting the ratio of pulmonary to systemic flows to four- to sixfold, and from 1 to 1.5 cm at ventricular level, limiting the ratio to three- or fourfold. The size at arterial level is from 0.5 to 0.7 cm. If the septum is almost entirely missing, as in common atrium, and in those with functionally single ventricles or common arterial trunk, there is complete mixing of the venous and arterialised blood. The resulting saturation is a function of the ratio of pulmonary to systemic flows, and is equal in both great arteries, with univentricular cardiac function. Uncorrected defects of medium size, or residual defects which are neither restrictive nor univentricular, produce a classical Eisenmenger syndrome, where the degree of cyanosis depends on pulmonary vascular resistance.

Differences between Idiopathic and Congenital, Cardiac-Disease–associated Pulmonary Arterial Hypertension

Known Trigger

In contrast to those with idiopathic pulmonary arterial hypertension, the cause for the development of increased pulmonary vascular resistance in patients with congenitally malformed hearts is well known and monitored. In some groups, however, the increase in pulmonary vascular resistance seems to be out of proportion to the stimulus, such as in children with small, persistently patent arterial ducts or insignificant interatrial communications, and in those who have undergone timely correction of transposition.[81–83] It is as yet unclear whether these patients have a latent form of idiopathic pulmonary arterial hypertension, which was triggered by these defects.

Different Dynamics

Those with idiopathic pulmonary arterial hypertension have a broad range of age, with the problem occurring as late as the seventh decade, or as early as the first months of life. The paediatric form shows an aggressive course, which only recently has been modified by available pharmacological treatment.[84–86] In contrast, the development of increased pulmonary vascular resistance in those with congenitally malformed hearts is more predictable, being avoidable by surgical correction at less than 6 months of life, and showing stability over decades in those with the Eisenmenger syndrome.

Right Ventricular Function

When given time, the morphologically right ventricle can adapt to a large extent to increased afterload, and will maintain cardiac output until contractility decreases, at which time the ejection period, stroke volume, and peak systolic pressure correlate with contractility. Morbidity and increased mortality[87–89] are seen when the ventricle is congenitally malformed or surgically altered, with direct effects on the pattern of contraction.

DIAGNOSIS OF PULMONARY HYPERTENSION

Presenting Symptoms

Pulmonary hypertension may be asymptomatic in early stages, but dyspnoea with exertion that progresses over months is the most frequent symptom. Chest pain, syncope, and oedema of the legs may become evident with more severe pulmonary hypertension and impaired right ventricular function. Classifying the limitations in exercise is aided with help of the classification provided by the World Health Organization for clinical severity (see Table 56-2).

Physical Findings

A loud second heart sound is present in most patients with elevated right-sided pressures. Murmurs due to tricuspid regurgitation and pulmonary flow may also be heard. With progression of the disease, jugular venous distension, hepatomegaly, peripheral oedema, and ascites become evident.

Chest Radiography

Typically the central pulmonary arteries are enlarged and the right ventricle is dilated. In addition, there are diminished peripheral pulmonary vascular markings. The presence of underlying conditions, such as interstitial lung disease, may become apparent on the chest film (Fig. 56-3A).

Electrocardiogram

In most patients the electrocardiogram demonstrates right-axis deviation, right atrial enlargement and right ventricular hypertrophy with strain, but the sensitivity and specificity are low. A minority of patients with pulmonary hypertension have a normal electrocardiogram.

Six-minute Walk Test

This test has been used as submaximal exercise test, and as a surrogate marker of physical function. The test is useful for longitudinal follow-up, and to monitor response to treatment.[90] Its disadvantages include its subjective nature, and that cooperation and motivation greatly affect results.[91] Currently, nonetheless, the test is approved by regulatory bodies such as the U. S. Food and Drug Administration as an endpoint for prospective clinical trials in patients with pulmonary hypertension.

Cardiopulmonary Exercise Testing

Over the past years, this form of testing became an additional tool to evaluate patients with pulmonary hypertension.[91] The test includes monitoring of the electrocardiogram and blood pressure, as well as measurement of consumption of oxygen, production of carbon dioxide, and minute ventilation. A change in exercise capacity seems to match other factors of severity, such as survival, haemodynamics, and time to clinical worsening.

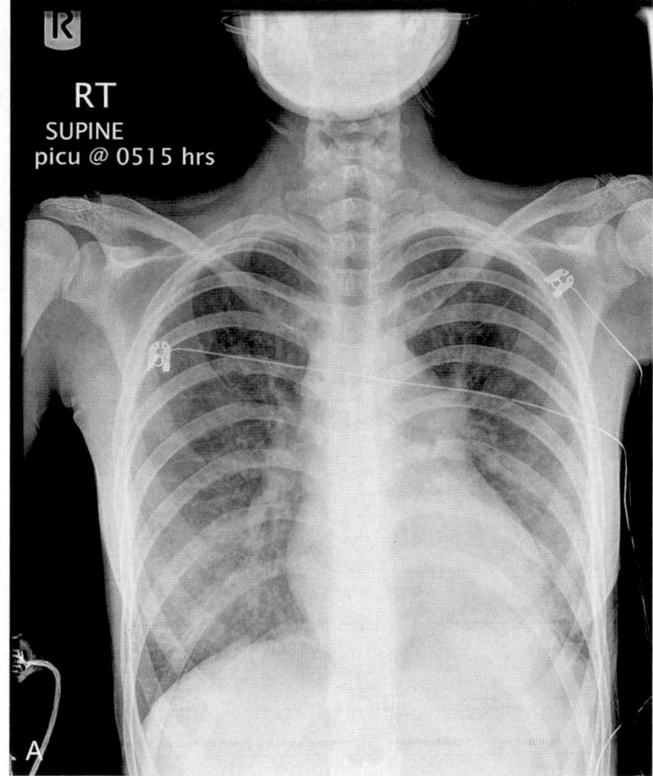

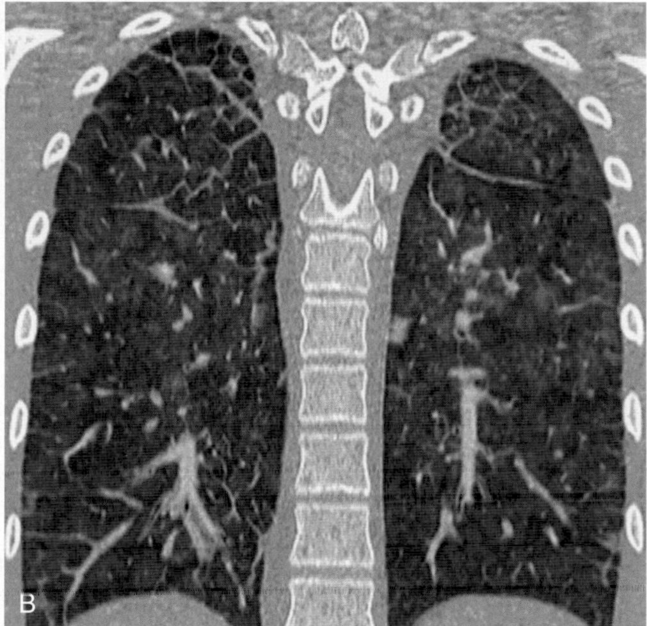

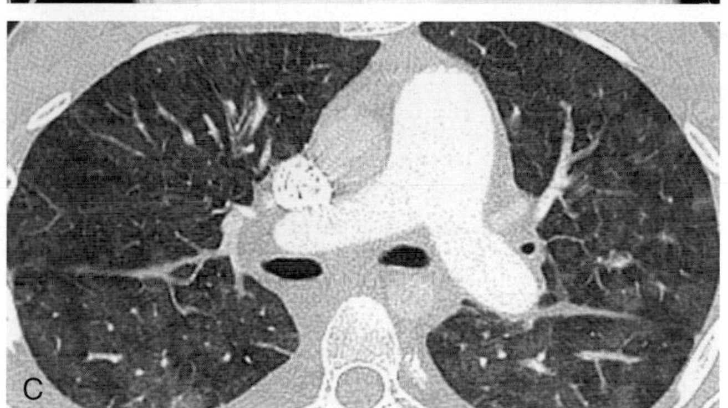

Figure 56-3 A, Chest radiograph from a 16-year-old patient with pulmonary hypertension shows mild cardiomegaly with dilated central pulmonary vessels and increased interstitial markings in both lungs. **B** and **C**, Computed tomogram from the same patient reformatted in axial and coronal plane show ground-glass appearance with a mosaic pattern. The pulmonary arteries in the mediastinum are markedly dilated. Note the diffusely thickened interlobular septums. The thickened septums in the peripheral lungs extend to the pleural surface. The central pulmonary veins were all unobstructed. There is mediastinal oedema. These findings are classic features of pulmonary veno-occlusive disease.

Echocardiography

The hallmark of non-invasive diagnostic imaging for pulmonary hypertension is transthoracic echocardiography. Structural cardiac disease can be diagnosed or excluded, and enlargement of the right atrium, right ventricle and pulmonary arteries may be visualised. In addition, right ventricular function can be assessed. Doppler echocardiography allows estimating the right ventricular systolic pressure by assessing the tricuspid regurgitant jet. Echocardiography fails, however, to detect a measurable tricuspid regurgitant jet in a significant number of patients at high risk, and the absence of the jet does not rule out the presence of severe pulmonary hypertension.[92] Indirect signs of pulmonary hypertension are paradoxical ventricular septal movement, and a decreased or absent collapse of the inferior caval vein. Functional testing involves description of the dimensions and systolic performance of the right ventricle. Size indexed for body surface area should be evaluated in children. Tissue Doppler imaging is able to demonstrate abnormal diastolic and systolic right ventricular function, as well as left ventricular diastolic function. In adults, only right ventricular dysfunctions seem to correlate with pulmonary arterial pressures.[93]

Ventilation-perfusion Lung Scintigraphy

Ventilation-perfusion scintigraphy has high sensitivity and specificity to detect embolic disease, and can reliably differentiate between large-vessel occlusive disease and small-vessel pulmonary vascular disease.[94,95]

Computed Tomography

Findings on computed tomography include cardiomegaly with right-sided cardiac enlargement, enlargement of the central pulmonary arteries, and possible bronchial compression. Major intrapulmonary characteristics are peripheral vasculopathy, with enlarged tortuous vessels and ground-glass centrilobular opacities.[93]

Magnetic Resonance Imaging

Phase-contrast magnetic resonance measurements of flow in the pulmonary trunk seem to correlate with haemodynamic changes, and the average velocity throughout the cardiac circle appears to mirror the pulmonary pressures and resistance.[96] In patients clinically known to have pulmonary hypertension, the cardiac magnetic resonance imaging ratio–derived left ventricular septal-to-free wall curvature was an accurate and reproducible index for estimation of right ventricular systolic pressure if compared to measurement at right heart catheterisation.[97]

Cardiac Catheterisation

Catheterisation of the right heart remains the gold standard for diagnosis of pulmonary hypertension, but the procedure for patients with advanced pulmonary vascular disease carries some risks.[52,98] Right atrial pressure, pulmonary arterial pressures, pulmonary capillary wedge pressure, systemic blood pressure, and mixed venous saturation should be routinely assessed.[99] Cardiac output is determined by thermodilution, or estimated with the modified Fick technique,[100,101] but measurement rather than estimation of oxygen consumption is recommended. Pulmonary vascular resistance, in Woods units times m^2 body surface area, is calculated as mean pulmonary arterial pressure minus pulmonary capillary wedge pressure or left atrial pressure divided by cardiac output. Testing with a short-acting vasodilator allows detection of the remaining potential of reactivity of small pulmonary arteries and arterioles, or demonstrates fixed resistance. Younger children at the time of diagnosis tend to have a more positive response to acute testing, but there is significant variability.[84] Currently, a significant response to acute pulmonary vasodilator testing is defined as a reduction of mean pulmonary arterial pressure of more than 20% without an increase in cardiac output.

Lung Biopsy

Nowadays this procedure is rarely indicated. In some instances, histopathology may establish the diagnosis of vasculitis, pulmonary veno-occlusive disease, or pulmonary capillary hemangiomatosis.[102] The most important limitation of an open lung biopsy is the high risk of mortality during anaesthesia and the surgical procedure.

Genetics

A gene responsible for familial pulmonary hypertension has been found on chromosome 2.[103] The familial form of idiopathic pulmonary hypertension accounts for 5% of all cases. The presentation is usually at younger age. Mutations of the bone morphogenetic receptor 2 gene have been identified in approximately half of patients with the familial form, and in up to 30% of sporadic cases.[104,105] In affected families, half of the siblings or children of patients with the mutation in the familial form have an overall risk of inheriting the gene.[106] In about 30%, however, no mutations can be identified by existing strategies for screening.[13] Carriers with pulmonary arterial hypertension present approximately 10 years earlier than non-carriers, and have more severe haemodynamic compromise at diagnosis.[107] Children with mutations of the bone morphogenetic protein 2 gene are less likely to respond to acute vasodilator testing than mutation-negative patients, and they also seem to have a more severe disease at diagnosis.[108] According to current guidelines, genetic testing and professional counseling should be offered to relatives of those patients with familial disease. Prenatal testing has not been reported.[109] Pulmonary hypertension may also be found in association with hereditary haemorrhagic telangiectasia, which can be caused by mutation in the ALK1 gene.[110]

INTERVENTIONAL AND SURGICAL THERAPIES

Balloon Atrial Septostomy

This procedure is indicated in children with the idiopathic form who are suffering from syncope and/or severe right-sided cardiac failure.[111,112] Careful selection is warranted, as patients with severe right-sided cardiac failure and markedly elevated pulmonary vascular resistance may not tolerate atrial septostomy, the ensuing massive right-to-left shunting potentially resulting in insufficient flow of blood to the lungs and severe hypoxaemia. Puncture of the atrial septum, nonetheless, and subsequent dilations with balloons of increasing diameter, has been shown to relieve symptoms of pulmonary hypertension by increasing systemic flow and reducing right ventricular preload, with improvement of cardiac index and functional class.[113] The incidence of spontaneous decrease in the size of the defect created is relatively high, but insertion of fenestrated devices may help ensure indefinite patency of the atrial communication.

Potts Shunt

In this surgical procedure, which was originally designed to augment blood flow to the pulmonary artery tree, the left pulmonary artery is anastomosed to the descending aorta, permitting the desaturated blood to run from the left pulmonary artery to the lower part of the body.[114] Its purpose is to decrease right ventricular afterload, leading to improvement of right ventricular function, and potential prevention of syncope and sudden death.

Transplantation

It is patients with end-stage pulmonary hypertension, in NYHA classes III and IV who are no longer responding to maximal pharmacological therapy who are generally considered for transplantation. Combined heart-lung transplantation is offered to patients with Eisenmenger's syndrome, albeit that transplantation of both lungs, with repair of the intracardiac defect, may also be considered. Survival at 5 years after transplantation of the heart and lungs has been lower, at around 40%, than that after transplantation only of both lungs, at around 45%.[115] Most centres prefer to transplant both lungs, rather than a single lung, because of the mismatch between ventilation and perfusion that can occur both early from ischaemic reperfusion injury, and later during any rejection of the lung. The timing of transplantation is challenging because of the shortage of organs and the length of the waiting list, but referral to the transplantation team for an initial evaluation is indicated with the initiation of intravenous or subcutaneous prostanoid therapy. Contra-indications include significant extrapulmonary disease, notably renal failure or neurologic conditions, active and uncontrolled extrapulmonary infection, active or recent malignancy, and active infection with the human immunodeficiency virus.

PHARMACOLOGICAL AGENTS

Oxygen

There is currently no consistent data for the effects of long-term treatment with oxygen for patients with pulmonary hypertension. Supplemental oxygen is recommended for patients with chronic hypoxaemia in order to prevent systemic saturations falling below 90%.[116,117] There seems to be a trend towards improved survival for children with Eisenmenger's syndrome receiving long-term treatment with oxygen,[118] whereas in a controlled study, nocturnal administration of oxygen had no effects on haematology, exercise capacity, and quality of life.[75]

Oral Anticoagulation

The benefit of oral anticoagulation has never been documented in a prospective randomised trial.[119] The treatment is based on postmortem observations of embolic thrombosis in small vessels of patients with proven pulmonary hypertension.[109,120] The targeted international normalised ratio in anticoagulated patients varies between centres in North America, aiming at ratios between 1.5 and 2.5, and those working in European centres, who aim at 2.0 to 3.0.[116,117] A lower ratio should be considered for very active children and toddlers because of the higher risk of bleeding complications. There is conflicting data on anticoagulation in Eisenmenger patients, as they are at increased risk of haemoptysis.

Calcium Channel Blockers

These agents inhibit the influx of calcium into vascular smooth muscle cells, and accomplish pulmonary vasodilation. A number of uncontrolled studies have suggested that long-term treatment with such agents given in high doses improves haemodynamics, relieves symptoms, and prolongs survival in children and adults with pulmonary hypertension.[57,84] Only around 40% of children, however, show an acute response during vasodilatory testing in the cardiac catheterisation laboratory, and thus would qualify for chronic therapy.[84] Side effects of treatment include systemic hypotension, tachycardia, shortness of breath, and pulmonary oedema. This therapeutic option is now less used subsequent to the introduction of more targeted drugs.

Prostanoids

Prostacyclin and its analogues play a pivotal role in the treatment of pulmonary arterial hypertension, the approach being supported by the known imbalance of thromboxane A_2 to prostacyclin metabolites in patients with pulmonary hypertension.[121,122] Options for administration include continuous intravenous, continuous subcutaneous, oral, and inhaled applications.

Intravenous Epoprostenol

This agent, when given chronically, improves exercise capacity, haemodynamics, and survival in children with pulmonary arterial hypertension[84,123–125] and is still the most effective substance.[126] This therapeutic pathway usually requires a placement of a permanent central line, and continuous infusion using a small ambulatory pump. The half-time is less than 6 minutes. Major side effects include flushing, hypotension, headache, and jaw and musculoskeletal pain.

Subcutaneous Prostacyclin Analogues

Treprostinil is a stable prostacyclin analogue, with a similar pharmacological spectrum to epoprostenol but with a significantly longer half-time of 3 to 4 hours. It has been shown to be effective in adults,[127] but data in children is still sparse.[128] The drug is usually delivered subcutaneously through the abdominal wall using a portable infusion pump. This limits the use to older children with enough subcutaneous fat, as the development of dermal irritation, or pain at the site of infusion, is frequent. Other side effects are similar to those for epoprostenol.

Oral Prostacyclin Analogues

Beraprost is the first orally active analogue, albeit only approved for treatment of the idiopathic form of the disease in Japan. After oral administration, peak concentrations are reached after 30 minutes. There are two randomised controlled trials using beraprost.[73,129] In the first trial, patients were randomised to receive the maximal tolerated dose of beraprost or placebo for 12 weeks. The agent improved exercise capacity, particularly in patients with idiopathic arterial pulmonary hypertension, while those with associated conditions showed no significant changes. There were, however, no relevant beneficial effects in cardiopulmonary haemodynamics or functional class. The second trial studied the long-term effects of beraprost up to 1 year. During the earlier phases of treatment, the data suggested less progression of the disease, with the effect persisting up to 6 months, but then attenuating with time. After 1 year, there were no longer any differences between the patients receiving beraprost and those having the placebo. Beraprost, therefore, does not play any crucial role in the treatment of pulmonary arterial hypertension related to congenital cardiac lesions and Eisenmenger's syndrome.

Endothelin Receptor Antagonists

The endothelin system has long been implicated in the pathogenesis of pulmonary arterial hypertension.[130–132] It has been shown that antagonism of endothelin receptors improves exercise tolerance, pulmonary haemodynamics, right ventricular hypertrophy, and survival. Other favourable effects are the reduction of pulmonary fibrosis and the remodeling of pulmonary arteries.[133–137] Side effects include flushing, peripheral oedema, both found in less than 10% of patients, and elevations in hepatic function tests, observed in about 3% of children.[138,139] Currently there are three different oral antagonists available for treatment, namely bosentan, which has an almost equal affinity for both endothelin receptors, sitaxsentan, a selective antagonist of endothelin receptor$_A$, and ambrisentan, also a selective antagonist of the A receptor. Several reports have demonstrated the benefits of therapy in children.[138-141] Most of the current knowledge is based on experience with bosentan, with information related to sitaxsentan and ambrisentan mostly gained from experience with adults.[135,142,143]

Phosphodiesterase Inhibitors

This class of drugs inhibits the degradation of cyclic guanosine monophosphate, the second messenger of nitric oxide, by interacting with different subclasses of phosphodiesterases, thus prolonging the effect of endogenous nitric oxide. The currently used sildenafil was developed from its precursor zaprinast, and has a 20-fold higher specificity for phosphodiesterase type 5, which is the subtype acting mainly in the lung. Sildenafil has been studied most often, and may be seen as the prototype of this class of drugs. It has immediate effects when given intravenously, and reaches a maximum after 30 to 45 minutes when given by the usual oral route. It is effective in the short and long term, in infants, adolescents, and adults, immediately post-operatively, and when used chronically. It increases 6-minute walking distance, decreases pulmonary vascular resistance,[144,145] and has remodelling effects on the right ventricle and pulmonary vasculature. Tadalafil is a next-generation phosphodiesterase inhibitor, with even more specificity to phosphodiesterase type 5, and a half-life of 17.5 hours. Udenafil is a newer agent, with a half-life of 34 hours.[146] These substances not only have pulmonary preference as compared with their systemic effect, but also an intrapulmonary selectivity for the ventilated areas. They seem to have some inotropic properties.[147-149]

Combination Therapy

Over the last decade, three classes of substances—prostanoids, endothelin receptor antagonists, and phosphodiesterase 5 inhibitors—have been more closely examined by randomised placebo-controlled trials to prove their beneficial effects.[136,150-156] As these substances act by different modes of action and through different intracellular pathways, it might be expected that combining them would exert synergistic effects, albeit that they can also interfere pharmacologically. For example, when sildenafil and bosentan are combined in individual patients, sildenafil is cleared mostly by hepatic metabolism, predominantly by the P450 enzyme CYP3A4. Bosentan, however, is a known inducer of CYP3A4, as well as a substrate for the enzyme. Thus, steady-state concentrations of sildenafil in the presence of bosentan are 50% lower after 3 to 5 days, probably because of induction.[157] The levels of bosentan, nonetheless, increase in both unaffected people and patients. A recent study assessing the effect of addition of bosentan to existing epoprostenol therapy showed a stronger haemodynamic effect, albeit one which did not translate into clear differences in clinical exercise, functional class, or survival.[153]

Currently, there are two approaches to combination therapy. The first is to start monotherapy with an active substance, and to add a second substance when predefined treatment goals are not met. The alternative concept is immediately to start combination therapy, following the principle to hit hard and early. Despite such advances, pulmonary arterial hypertension remains incurable. Although long-term improvement or stabilisation can be achieved, at least with epoprostenol or bosentan, the idiopathic form remains a progressive disease, and deterioration eventually occurs in a substantial proportion of patients. In two recent studies in adults, survival was 63% after 3 years for the adult form of the disease.[158,159]

All the current questions regarding superiority of combination therapy as opposed to monotherapy, for whom, when, and in what combinations, considering not only pharmacodynamic and kinetic aspects, but also the ratios of cost to benefit, will only be solved in stepwise fashion by major international multi-centric studies in which the most appropriate therapy is used in experienced hands. Indeed, with further progress of development of drugs, a major benefit may be derived not from the effects, but rather out of the meticulous use of the logistics and wider circumstances in which these patients are treated.

OUTLOOK FOR THE FUTURE

While the current therapeutic goal is to use vasodilators and blockers of vasoconstriction in a well thought out way, it is the normal remodelling of the pulmonary vasculature, with the restoration of endothelial function and the growth of new peripheral pulmonary arteries, which should be the ultimate goal of therapy. In the field of paediatric cardiology, combining these drugs with the well-established mechanical method of protecting the pulmonary vascular bed by banding the pulmonary trunk, avoiding extremes of pressure overload to the subpulmonary ventricle, and avoiding systemic desaturation, in patients with congenital shunting lesions and pulmonary vascular resistance too high to operate, may deserve a new and justified interest as a method to allow for recovery of the remodeled pulmonary vascular bed and later surgical correction.

Certainly one important direction for progress is the further development of drug therapy, and while the modes of administration and different formulations have all been exhaustively studied, and while new analogues of existing drugs show some improved effects, other drugs, like vasoactive intestinal peptide, the statins, inhibitors of RhoA and metalloproteinases, openers of the potassium channel, anti-growth factors, as well as stem cell and gene therapy, are all under avid investigation. However, without properly detailed and structured studies, the information in the small groups of patients with pulmonary hypertension will show limited gain and will be repetitive. So, future studies not only need to define valid and practical endpoints but also to look closely into the many possible effects of the studied substances. Finally, the development of dedicated clinical services to optimise the use of drugs and logistics for the care of patients with the different forms of pulmonary hypertension will be as important, if not the predominant aspect, to improve survival and quality of life.

The complete reference list can be found on the companion Expert Consult web site at www.expertconsult.com.

ANNOTATED REFERENCES

- Wood P: The Eisenmenger syndrome or pulmonary hypertension with reversed central shunt. 1. Br Med J 1958;2:701–709, 755–762.
- Heath D, Edwards JE: The pathology of hypertensive pulmonary vascular disease; a description of six grades of structural changes in the pulmonary arteries with special reference to congenital cardiac septal defects. Circulation 1958;18:533–547.
- Haworth SG: Pulmonary vascular disease in different types of congenital heart disease: Implications for interpretation of lung biopsy findings in early childhood. Br Heart J 1984;52:557–571.

These three papers are the pillars on which the current discussions and thoughts on pulmonary hypertension in the setting of congenital heart disease are based. The early date of the papers underlines the fact that the field of pulmonary hypertension was a well-known and integral part of the practice of paediatric cardiology long before it received general and public attention due to the advent of therapeutic pulmonary vasodilators.

- Simonneau G, Galie N, Rubin LJ, et al: Clinical classification of pulmonary hypertension. J Am Coll Cardiol 2004;43(12 Suppl S):5S–12S.
- Galie N, Torbicki A, Barst R, et al: Guidelines on diagnosis and treatment of pulmonary arterial hypertension. The Task Force on Diagnosis and Treatment of Pulmonary Arterial Hypertension of the European Society of Cardiology. Eur Heart J 2004;25:2243–2278.

These papers report on the current classification, diagnosis, and treatment of the different forms of pulmonary hypertension. The authorship illustrates the multicentric and international collaboration in this small but very active subspecialty.

- Rimensberger PC, Spahr-Schopfer I, Berner M, et al: Inhaled nitric oxide versus aerosolized iloprost in secondary pulmonary hypertension in children with congenital heart disease: Vasodilator capacity and cellular mechanisms. Circulation 2001;103:544–548.
- Li J, Bush A, Schulze-Neick I, et al: Measured versus estimated oxygen consumption in ventilated patients with congenital heart disease: The validity of predictive equations. Crit Care Med 2003;31:1235–1240.
- Taylor CJ, Derrick G, McEwan A, et al: Risk of cardiac catheterization under anaesthesia in children with pulmonary hypertension. Br J Anaesth 2007;98:657–661.

These are key papers to the currently recommended approach for cardiac catheterisation in children with pulmonary hypertension. They describe the methodology for measuring maximum pulmonary vasodilatory reserve, and for putting the risk into clinical perspective. The last paper may influence clinical practice in setting the indication for cardiac catheterisation in children.

- Hopkins WE, Ochoa LL, Richardson GW, Trulock EP: Comparison of the hemodynamics and survival of adults with severe primary pulmonary hypertension or Eisenmenger syndrome. J Heart Lung Transplant 1996;15 (1 Pt 1):100–105.
- Khambadkone S, Li J, de Leval MR, et al: Basal pulmonary vascular resistance and nitric oxide responsiveness late after Fontan-type operation. Circulation 2003;107:3204–3208.
- Schulze-Neick I, Beghetti M: Classifying pulmonary hypertension in the setting of the congenitally malformed heart—cleaning up a dog's dinner. Cardiol Young 2008;18:22–25.

These papers discuss different pathophysiological situations involving the congenitally malformed heart and assess the role of pulmonary vascular resistance. While the last paper is a review of the topic, the other two excel in the use of their methodology and the discussion.

CHAPTER 57 Cardiological Aspects of Systemic Disease

ROBERT F. ENGLISH and JOSÉ A. ETTEDGUI

Cardiac involvement in systemic disease can be broadly divided into those conditions in which the heart is involved in the disease process itself, and those in which a structural or functional cardiac abnormality is associated with other anomalies, usually in a recognisable syndrome. Many of the conditions in this latter group have received attention in the sections of this book dealing with aetiology and genetics. These will not be dealt with again, although they may be mentioned, or the discussion amplified, as necessary. A vast number of systemic diseases, nonetheless, can involve the heart during childhood. It is the cardiac aspects of these latter diseases we discuss in this chapter (Table 57-1).

METABOLIC DISORDERS: STORAGE DISEASES

We have chosen to group together here the glycogen storage diseases, the mucopolysaccharidoses, the mucolipidoses, disorders of glycoprotein degradation, acid lipase deficiency, the sphingolipidoses, and the gangliosidoses.

Glycogen Storage Diseases

Glycogen storage diseases can involve the various steps in the storage and degradation of glycogen. There may be an inability to synthesise normal glycogen. Alternatively, there may be an inability to break down glycogen. In the extreme form, abnormal glycogen is synthesised but cannot be broken down. There are eleven described types within this range of disease, and most types involve two or more subtypes. Cardiac involvement has been documented in types I to VIII.

Glycogen Storage Disease Type I (von Gierke's Disease, Glucose-6-Phosphatase Deficiency [Type Ia], Glucose-6-Phosphatase Translocase Deficiency [Type Ib])

Clinical manifestations of type I glycogen storage disease are profound hypoglycaemia, associated with hyperlipidaemia, hyperuricaemia and lactic acidosis. It presents in childhood, primarily involving the liver, kidneys, and mucous layers of the small intestine. Pulmonary hypertension has been described in association with the type Ia variant. Postulated mechanisms include chronic stimulation of the smooth muscle of the pulmonary arterioles by the persistent hepatic metabolism of circulating catecholamines such as serotonin. Levels of serotonin have been shown to be elevated in patients with glycogen storage disease type I. Such elevation of the levels of serotonin in isolation do not appear to confer pulmonary vascular disease on these patients. Rather, it is hypothesised that other mediating factors working in concert with persistently elevated levels of serotonin increase the risk for pulmonary vascular changes.[1–3]

Glycogen Storage Disease Type II (Pompe's Disease, α-1,4-Glucosidase Deficiency)

Pompe's disease is a generalised glycogen storage disease in which glycogen of normal structure is accumulated in the myocardium, skeletal muscle, and liver. The disease is progressive, and is associated with deficiency of lysosomal α-1,4-glucosidase. There are four subtypes based upon age at onset of clinical symptoms. It is the form presenting in infancy that is recognised as classical Pompe's disease, but patients can also present in childhood, adolescence (giving rise to the juvenile form), or adulthood. The age at onset correlates inversely with the measured activity of lysosomal α-1,4-glucosidase in myocytes or fibroblasts. In the infantile form, which is more severe in its cardiac involvement than those forms of later onset, there is generalised accumulation of glycogen in the heart, including the conduction tissues, in skeletal muscle, notably the tongue and diaphragm, and in the liver. Central and peripheral neurons and smooth muscle are also affected. The results are cardiomegaly, hepatomegaly, a thickened diaphragm, and macroglossia. In the heart, the glycogen is deposited mainly in ventricular muscle. There is gross thickening of the ventricular walls, with impairment of both diastolic and systolic performance. The infants typically appear normal at birth, though cases of severe neonatal ventricular hypertrophy have been reported.[4] The median age at onset of clinical symptoms is 1.6 months. Muscular weakness and hypotonia along with loss of motor milestones are noted during the first 6 months of life, and signs of congestive cardiac failure become evident. Although there is excess glycogen in the liver, hepatomegaly is not commonly present until cardiac failure is apparent. The disease is progressive, and most affected babies die before the age of 1 year. The clinical course may be complicated by arrhythmias. Since patients with Pompe's disease appear very sensitive to digoxin, this drug must be used with extreme caution. Irritability and poor feeding often draw attention to the disease. The cardiac physical signs are not characteristic, variable murmurs being heard. Unexplained cardiomegaly and congestive cardiac failure in a generally floppy baby should suggest the diagnosis.[5]

The chest radiograph may be normal at birth, but in all affected infants the heart becomes enlarged within a few weeks. There is no specific cardiac silhouette, but rather a generalised smooth enlargement of the contour. The characteristic electrocardiographic features are a short PR interval, wider than normal QRS complexes, and voltage evidence of left or biventricular hypertrophy, which can be

TABLE 57-1

SYSTEMIC DISEASES WITH CARDIAC INVOLVEMENT

Metabolic Diseases

Storage Diseases

Glycogen storage disease
- Type I: von Gierke's disease
- Type II: Pompe's disease
- Type III: Cori's disease
- Type IV: Andersen's disease
- Type V: McArdle's disease
- Type VI: Hers' disease
- Type VII: Tarui's disease

Mucopolysaccharidoses
- Type I: Hurler's syndrome, Sheie's syndrome, intermediate (Hurler-Scheie) syndrome
- Type II: Hunter's syndrome
- Type III: Sanfilippo's syndrome
- Type IV: Morquio's syndrome
- Type VI: Maroteaux-Lamy syndrome
- Type VII: Sly's syndrome

Mucolipidoses
- Type II: inclusion cell disease
- Type III: pseudo-Hurler polydystrophy

Disorders of glycoprotein degradation
- Mannosidosis
- Fucosidosis
- Sialidosis
- Galactosialidosis
- Aspartylglycosaminuria

Acid lipase deficiency
- Wolman's disease
- Cholesteryl ester storage disease

Sphingolipidoses
- Sphingomyelin lipidosis: Niemann-Pick disease
- Glucosylceramidosis: Gaucher's disease
- α-Galactosidase A deficiency: Fabry's disease

Gangliosidoses
- GM_1 gangliosidosis
- GM_2 gangliosidosis
  - Tay-Sachs disease
  - Sandhoff's disease

Inherited Disorders of Endocrine Function

Diabetes mellitus

Pituitary gigantism and acromegaly

Disorders of thyroid function
- Hypothyroidism
- Hyperthyroidism

Addison's disease

Disorders of Energy Metabolism

Mitochondrial myopathies

Barth syndrome

Propionic acidemia

Methylmalonic aciduria

Disorders of fatty acid metabolism

Disorders of Collagen Synthesis or Extracellular Matrix

Ehlers-Danlos syndrome

Cutis laxa

Osteogenesis imperfecta

Marfan syndrome

Infantile Marfan syndrome

Loeys-Dietz syndrome

Homocystinuria

Neuromuscular Diseases

Muscular dystrophies
- Duchenne's muscular dystrophy
- Childhood limb-girdle muscular dystrophy
- Myotonic muscular dystrophy: Steinert disease
- Autosomal dominant scapuloperoneal myopathy
- Becker's muscular dystrophy
- Facioscapulohumeral muscular dystrophy:
  - Landouzy-Dejerine syndrome
- Emery-Dreifuss muscular dystrophy

Centronuclear myopathy

Nemaline myopathy

Friedreich's ataxia

Arthrogryposis multiplex congenita

Hereditary motor and sensory neuropathy (peroneal muscular atrophy, Charcot-Marie-Tooth disease)

Spinal muscular atrophy type III (juvenile spinal muscular atrophy, Kugelberg-Welander syndrome)

Refsum's disease

Deficiencies

Selenium: Keshan disease

Carnitine

Thiamine: beriberi

Depositions

Haemochromatosis

Autoimmune Diseases

Juvenile idiopathic arthritis

Systemic sclerosis (scleroderma)

Takayasu's arteritis

Polyarteritis nodosa

Systemic lupus erythematosus

Disease Induced by Toxic Mechanisms

Adverse reactions to drugs

Toxic substances

Irradiation

Miscellaneous Systemic Disorders

Hutchinson-Gilford progeria

Arteriohepatic dysplasia: Alagille syndrome

Sickle cell haemoglobinopathy

Anorexia nervosa

severe (Fig. 57-1). In addition, in the majority there are Q waves and inverted T waves in leads I and II and the left chest leads.[6] Electrophysiological studies have shown a short AH interval.[7] Both M-mode and cross sectional echocardiograms demonstrate gross increase in the thickness of the ventricular free walls and the ventricular septum (Fig. 57-2). An impairment of ventricular filling in diastole has been noted,[8] together with reduction of the rate and extent of systolic shortening. Angiocardiography is rarely performed, as it adds little to the diagnosis or management.

The complete clinical picture, together with the characteristic electrocardiographic and echocardiographic findings, will lead immediately to the definitive diagnostic investigation. This is the demonstration of deficiency of lysosomal α-1,4-glucosidase in fibroblasts grown from a skin biopsy. Sometimes the skeletal muscular abnormalities are less evident. The presentation is then as a cardiomyopathy alone. Pompe's disease should be considered in any such case, and skin biopsy performed. Until recently, there was no specific treatment available, and supportive and decongestive measures failed to improve outcomes. Recent studies using recombinant human lysosomal acid α-glucosidase show promise in improving survival.[9] Since the disease appears to be inherited in an autosomal recessive fashion, parents should be advised of the availability of prenatal diagnosis via culture of amniocytes obtained by amniocentesis.

We include Danon disease in this section because it was previously considered to be a variant of Pompe's disease known as glycogen storage disease type IIb with normal acid maltase. The disease is due to a deficiency of lysosome-associated protein 2, and it manifests as a progressive hypertrophic cardiomyopathy with skeletal myopathy. Other similar diseases in this family of autophagic vacuolar myopathies are still being studied. Some demonstrate autosomal recessive inheritance while others are X-linked, and the degree of cardiac and skeletal involvement is variable.[10]

Glycogen Storage Disease Type III (Cori's Disease, Amylo-1, 6-Glucosidase [Debrancher] Deficiency)

In Cori's disease, an autosomal recessive condition, glycogen accumulates in skeletal muscle, in the liver, and in cardiac muscle. The disease is due to a deficiency of amylo-1,6-glucosidase, the enzyme necessary for breaking down branch points in glycogen chains. There are three subtypes dependent upon the primary site of abnormal glycogen storage. Type IIIa involves the liver and muscle, Type IIIb the liver, and Type IIIc the muscle.[4,11] A fourth subtype, IIId, involves normal debrancher enzymic activity but a deficiency of debrancher enzyme transferase activity. Patients with types IIIa and IIIc have a tendency to develop weakness of the skeletal muscles and left ventricular hypertrophy,[12] which is progressive. The clinical course appears to be less severe, with fewer symptoms as compared to hypertrophic obstructive cardiomyopathy.[13,14]

Glycogen Storage Disease Type IV (Andersen's Disease, α-1, 4-Glucan-6-Glucosyltransferase [Brancher] Deficiency)

Andersen's disease is a rare heterogeneous glycogen storage disease characterised by deposition of glycogen of abnormal structure in the liver, leading to cirrhosis. There may also be deposition of polysaccharide in the heart. While liver dysfunction is the most common clinical manifestation, the disease can rarely present with dilated cardiomyopathy, which is typically severe.[15–17]

Glycogen Storage Disease Type V (McArdle's Disease, Muscle Phosphorylase Deficiency)

McArdle's disease results from a deficiency of muscle phosphorylase. It is usually recognised in adolescence or adult life. Its main clinical features are muscular fatiguability, muscular cramps, and myoglobinuria. Rare lethal variants have been reported in infants,[18] but the heart is typically spared. This may be due to activity of a distinct cardiac

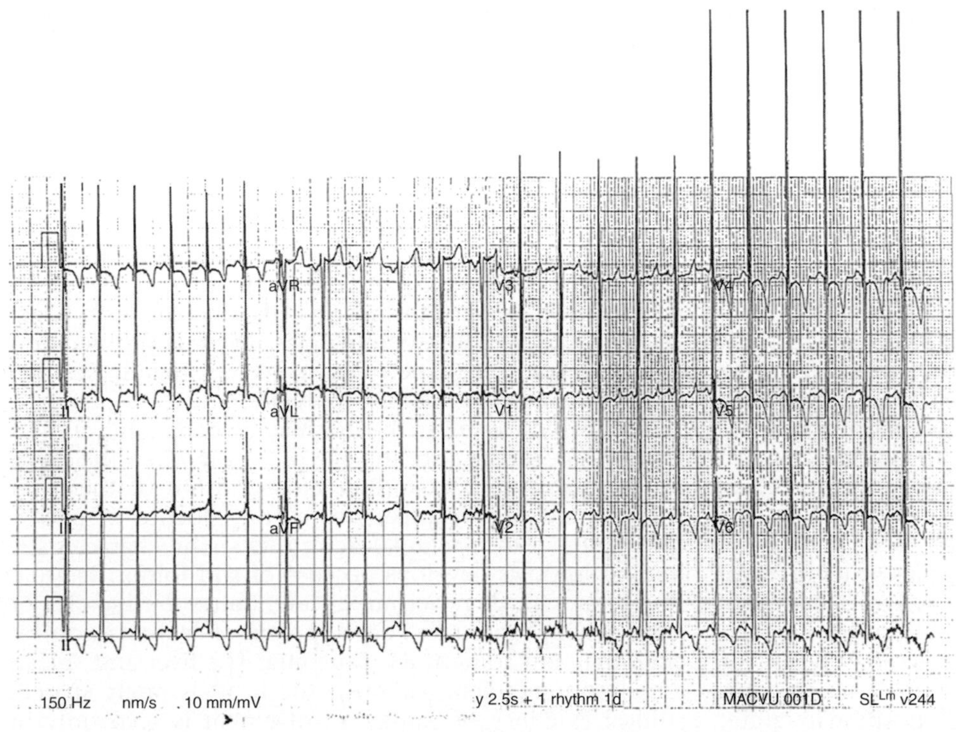

Figure 57-1 The typical electrocardiogram of a patient with Pompe's disease demonstrates striking biventricular hypertrophy.

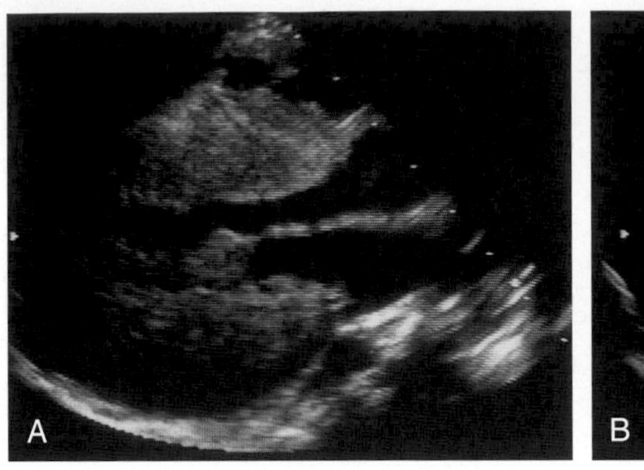

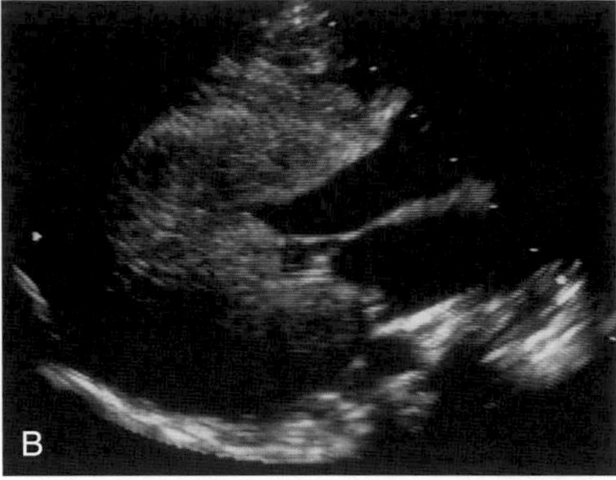

Figure 57-2 Typical echocardiographic findings in glycogen storage disease type II. A shows a diastolic frame in long axis, revealing severe concentric left ventricular hypertrophy, while the systolic frame from the same child (**B**) shows the absence of subaortic obstruction.

phosphorylase isozyme, which retains activity in patients with deficiency of the skeletal isozyme.[19] No clinical cardiac manifestations have been reported, but on occasion the electrocardiogram has features similar to those seen in Pompe's disease.[20]

Glycogen Storage Disease Type VI (Hers' Disease, Phosphorylase B Kinase Deficiency, Liver Phosphorylase Deficiency)

Hers' disease involves both X-linked and autosomal recessive modes of inheritance. It results from deficiency of liver phosphorylase. Both types involve the liver in childhood, whereas involvement of muscles occurs in young adults with the autosomal recessive form of the disease. Rare forms of phosphorylase b kinase deficiency have been described in which deposition of glycogen is limited to the heart.[21]

Glycogen Storage Disease Type VII (Tarui's Disease, Muscle Phosphofructokinase I Deficiency)

Tarui's disease is a rare form of glycogen storage disease that presents in early childhood or adult life with fatiguability, muscular weakness that can be progressive, muscular cramps, and myoglobinuria. Typically, the heart is spared. An infantile form of the disease has also been described in the members of one family. Cardiomyopathy occurred in addition to the progressive muscular weakness, and abnormal deposition of glycogen was noted in the cardiac muscle at autopsy.[22] Progressive cardiomyopathy has also been reported in an adult.[23]

Mucopolysaccharidoses

The mucopolysaccharidoses result from deficiency of lysosomal enzymes involved in the degradation of mucopolysaccharides. The incompletely degraded mucopolysaccharides then accumulate in the tissues. The substances accumulated are dermatan sulphate, heparan sulphate, and keratan sulphate, alone or in combination. In all forms, there is skeletal involvement. In most, there is glaucoma and corneal clouding. Retinal pigmentation frequently occurs. Deafness is a feature of all types. In most, there is hepatosplenomegaly. Involvement of the central nervous system is common, usually with cervical myelopathy as a consequence of pachymeningitis or atlanto-occipital subluxation.

Cardiovascular involvement is a feature of all types. The mucopolysaccharides are deposited in arterial walls, producing lesions similar to atherosclerosis.[24] Deposition in cardiac valves leads to valvar stenosis or regurgitation. The various forms of these diseases are brought about by deficiencies of ten identifiable lysosomal enzymes. Specific deficiencies can be demonstrated in cultured fibroblasts, and prenatal diagnosis from culture of amniocytes is possible. The availability of such diagnosis is important, since there is genetic variability within the different forms of the diseases.

Mucopolysaccharidosis Type I (α-L-Iduronidase Deficiency)

The three major clinical forms of α-L-iduronidase deficiency are Hurler's syndrome, Scheie's syndrome, and a syndrome intermediate between the two, known unsurprisingly as Hurler-Scheie syndrome. These diseases are due to defects in the gene encoding α-L-iduronidase, and multiple defects have been elucidated. These include nonsense, missense, insertional, deletional, and splice-type gene defects. It is thought that the clinical severity of the disease is related to the level of new enzymic activity, which in turn is due to a specific genetic defect.[25,26]

Hurler's Syndrome

The defect in Hurler's syndrome results in a virtual absence of lysosomal α-L-iduronidase. This enzyme is responsible for breakdown of heparan sulfate and dermatan sulfate to heparan and hyaluronic acid, respectively. The enzyme is completely absent in fibroblasts, but some activity is present in the liver. Consequently, traces of the breakdown products of heparan and dermatan may be found in the urine. As a consequence of this enzymic deficiency, both heparan and dermatan sulphates accumulate in the lysosomes of many tissues. When seen in neurons, the lesions bear some resemblance to those found in Tay-Sachs disease. Deposition in the arterial walls is associated with proliferation of smooth muscle cells, and the lesions are described as pseudo-atheromatosis. There is proliferation of both elastic fibres and collagen accompanying the lysosomal accumulation of mucopolysaccharides.

The babies seem to be normal at birth, the clinical features appearing after the age of 1 year when the facial features become coarse. Premature closure of the skull sutures, and hydrocephalus as a consequence of pachymeningitis, lead to cranial deformities. The characteristic lumbar lordosis develops because of stiff joints. Retardation of growth then becomes evident after the age of 2 or 3 years, with subsequent development of deafness, corneal clouding, and sometimes glaucoma. The liver and spleen are always enlarged. Although the heart is rarely spared, clinical evidence of cardiac involvement is seen only in half the patients. Angina is an occasional symptom, but more frequently attention is drawn by the finding of a cardiac murmur or systemic hypertension. The murmurs are variable and usually not loud. Rarely the murmur of aortic or mitral insufficiency may be heard. Cardiac failure has been reported as the presenting feature associated with endocardial fibroelastosis.[27,28]

There are typical skeletal radiological features. The clavicles have wide medial ends. The lower thoracic and upper lumbar vertebras have a flared and hook-shaped appearance. There are also changes in the skull and long bones, the latter being more severely affected in the upper limbs. The heart is usually enlarged, but with no specific silhouette, although left atrial enlargement will occur with severe mitral regurgitation. Similarly, there are no specific electrocardiographic features, although combined ventricular hypertrophy is frequent. A long QT interval has been reported in some patients.[29]

Pathological findings in the heart include deposition of mucopolysaccharide in structures such as the sinus and atrioventricular nodes, as well as in the myocardium and endocardium. The coronary arteries often demonstrate severe luminal narrowing. The mitral valve is most frequently involved, followed by the aortic and tricuspid valves. Pulmonary valvar involvement is only rarely reported. Valvar changes include nodular thickening along the free edges, which may lead to stenosis or regurgitation. Evidence suggests that the accumulation of dermatan sulphate leads to impaired elastogenesis, which may lead to some of the characteristic arterial and valvar deformities.[30]

Thickening of the leaflets of the mitral valve and its annulus is seen echocardiographically. Left ventricular volume load, and diastolic flutter of the mitral valve, are seen when aortic regurgitation is present. Cardiac catheterisation and angiocardiography add little to the diagnostic findings, which include systemic and mild pulmonary hypertension. When present, the haemodynamics and angiography will reflect the severity of valvar insufficiency. The disease progresses inexorably, death occurring by the age of 10 years from cardiac failure, suddenly, or from chest infection. Transplantation of haematopoeitic stem cells has been beneficial in selected patients for many aspects of the disease.[31] The valvar lesions, however, can continue to progress. Enzymic replacement therapy with human recombinant α-L-iduronidase has also been proven beneficial, but, as with transplantation of stem cells, the valvar lesions remain and may progress.[32]

Scheie's Syndrome

Patients with Scheie's syndrome are less severely affected, having normal stature and intellect. They also have a near-normal lifespan. The most striking features are corneal clouding and stiff joints. Typical cardiac manifestations are aortic stenosis and regurgitation, or mitral regurgitation.[33,34] These should be managed in a similar fashion as for otherwise normal subjects. Scheie's syndrome is inherited in autosomal recessive fashion.

Hurler-Scheie Syndrome

Hurler-Scheie syndrome falls in severity between the two extremes of α-L-iduronidase deficiency. The patients are of short stature, with mental retardation and multiple bony defects. There is clouding of the cornea and stiff joints, claw-hand being particularly common. Aortic and mitral valvar involvement are the primary manifestations. Asymmetrical septal hypertrophy has also been reported.[35] The clinical course is intermediate between Hurler's and Scheie's syndromes, with patients living into adolescence or even to the third decade.

Mucopolysaccharidosis Type II (Hunter's Syndrome, Iduronate Sulfatase Deficiency)

Deficiency of iduronate sulfatase results in a block of degradation of dermatan sulphate. The difference in clinical profile between this and Hurler's and Scheie's syndromes, for example, the absence of corneal clouding in Hunter's syndrome, may result from specific variability in the degree of blockage of degradation of the mucopolysaccharide. Furthermore, it may be that the block to degradation caused by the accumulation of iduronate sulfate may be bypassed by hyaluronidase. The severe and mild forms of Hunter's syndrome both have total, or near total, deficiency of iduronate sulfatase. As with mucopolysaccharidosis type I, the clinical phenotype may be representative of the degree of residual enzymic activity specific to certain gene mutations, of which more than 300 have been found for Hunter's syndrome.[36]

The condition can occur with a wide variety in severity. Apart from the extreme rarity of corneal clouding in Hunter's syndrome, and the presence of loss of hearing, the clinical features are those of Hurler's syndrome, although usually less severe. A positive distinguishing physical sign, pointed out by Hunter himself in 1916, is the occurrence of pebble-like ivory-coloured dermal lesions. These are seen over the scapulas and occasionally on the pectoral regions.

Cardiac involvement produces all the manifestations so far mentioned, namely, aortic and mitral regurgitation or stenosis, ischaemic changes, and evidence of myocardial dysfunction. Echocardiography is a useful method for evaluating cardiac involvement. The clinical course is extremely varied. Severely affected individuals die before the age of 15 years. At the opposite end of the spectrum, survival beyond the sixth decade has been reported. Death in younger patients is usually associated with progressive neurological deterioration. The disease is inherited as an X-linked recessive trait, though cases in females have been reported.[37] Since the reproductive fitness of the Hunter gene is low, a large minority of cases must result from new mutations.

A new treatment for Hunter's syndrome has recently emerged with the development of recombinant human iduronate-2-sulfatase. This was well tolerated, and demonstrated improvement in several parameters for outcome, including forced vital capacity, urinary excretion of glycosaminoglycans, the size of the liver and spleen, and 6-minute walk distance.[38,39] The effect of enzymic therapy on the cardiac lesions, however, remains to be determined.

Mucopolysaccharidosis Type III (Sanfilippo's Syndrome)

The degradation of heparan sulphate and N-sulphated or N-acetylated α-linked glucosamine requires four enzymes: heparan N-sulphatase, N-acetyl-α-D-glucosaminidase, acetyl-CoA:α-glucosaminide N-acetyltransferase, and N-acetyl-α-D-glucosamine-6-sulphate sulphatase. Deficiency of one of the four enzymes required for this degradation results in Sanfilippo's syndrome. Consequently, there are four biochemically distinct types of the disease, designated A through D, although they all present the same clinical features.

The onset is usually evident in the first few years of life with behavioural problems. Mental and neurological deterioration are severe and lead to death in the first two decades. Bone, joint, and cardiac involvement are generally less severe than in Hurler's syndrome. Corneal clouding is never seen. There is wide variation in the severity and age at death in all four forms, but type A is likely to be the most severe. Inheritance is in an autosomal recessive fashion. A number of patients with mitral valvar involvement have been reported.[40,41] Cardiac involvement is similar to that of other mucopolysaccharidoses, with thickening of the valvar leaflets. While treatment is primarily supportive, animal studies have been undertaken to assess replacement of the enzymes in a mouse model with mucopolysaccharidosis type III-B.[42]

Mucopolysaccharidosis Type IV (Morquio's Syndrome)

Morquio's syndrome results from defective degradation of keratan sulphate. It occurs in two biochemically distinct forms. The so-called type A is due to a deficiency of N-acetylgalactosamine-6-sulfate sulfatase, while type B results from deficiency of β-galactosidase. The two types have similar clinical features, but type B is less severe, sometimes called the long-legged variant. Despite the generally increased severity of features in type A, more mild forms of type A can occur. Keratan sulphate is excreted in the urine in type A, but this is less evident in type B.

Keratan sulphate is found in cartilage, intervertebral discs, and the cornea. Thus, skeletal involvement with dwarfism, pectus deformities, and bow legs are the most obvious manifestations. Corneal clouding is common. In contrast to the mucopolysaccharidoses described above, the joints in patients with Morquio's syndrome are hyperextensible. Absence or severe hypoplasia of the odontoid process, together with laxity of its associated ligaments, leads to atlanto-occipital subluxation, and consequent cervical myelopathy. The heart is clinically involved only in the severe type. Valves of the heart are primarily involved, with thickening of mitral and aortic leaflets. Concentric left ventricular hypertrophy and, rarely, asymmetrical septal hypertrophy have been described.[40,43] Survival beyond the third or fourth decade is not unusual. The effects of the cervical myelopathy and respiratory problems are the usual cause of death. Experimentation with enzymic replacement therapy in animals has been undertaken and holds some promise.[44]

Mucopolysaccharidosis Type VI (Maroteaux-Lamy Syndrome)

Deficiency of arylsulfatase B results in an inability to hydrolyse the sulfate groups in dermatan sulfate. The clinical picture is similar to that of Hurler's syndrome, but normal intelligence is usually maintained. Although severe in its classical form, milder variations exist. Affected infants can present with an acute cardiopathy.[45] Thickened mitral and aortic valvar leaflets necessitating valvar replacement has been noted in young adults.[46] A left ventricular aneurysm has also been reported.[47] Death usually occurs in the third decade. The condition is inherited in autosomal recessive fashion, though some cases have been presumed to be X-linked.[48] Enzymic replacement therapy with human recombinant arylsulfatase B has been studied, and found to be safe and beneficial in terms of exertional tolerance and urinary excretion of glycosaminoglycan.[49]

Mucopolysaccharidosis Type VII (Sly's Syndrome)

Deficiency of β-glucuronidase results in a clinical syndrome of extremely variable severity. Included in the features are coarse facies, corneal clouding, abdominal and inguinal hernias, puffy hands and feet, hepatosplenomegaly, and a small thoracolumbar hump. Cardiovascular manifestations include hypertension, aortic aneurysm, aortic regurgitation, obstructive arterial disease, and cardiomyopathy.[50,51] Fetal hydrops has also been reported.[52] This extremely rare condition is inherited in autosomal recessive fashion. Duration of survival varies widely, and depends on the severity of the disease. Death as early as 30 months has occurred in one child with severe disease. Animal studies involving enzymic replacement therapy have been performed and are encouraging in terms of improving the cardiovascular changes associated with this disease.[53]

Mucolipidoses

The mucolipidoses present with clinical features similar to the mucopolysaccharidoses, but are biochemically distinct. Leroy and Demars[54] observed inclusions in cultured fibroblasts that occupied the whole cytoplasmic space apart from the Golgi apparatus. It was because of this that the name inclusion cell, or I-cell, disease was coined. The cause of the defect in lysosomal storage is deficiency of several acid hydrolases in the lysosome. But this is not the primary problem, since the plasma abounds in these acid hydrolases, albeit in unstable forms. The problem is failure to locate the hydrolases within the lysosome. Failure of phosphorylation of mannose residues of the hydrolases is the primary defect. Hydrolases without mannose 6-phosphate components are then not recognised by the lysosome, and are not transported across the lysosomal membrane, particularly in connective tissue. In this way, inclusion cell disease and pseudo-Hurler polydystrophy differ from sialidosis, previously called mucolipidosis type I, in which there is a single lysosomal enzyme defect. Mucolipidoses type II, or inclusion cell disease, and type III, or pseudo-Hurler polydystrophy, result from a deficiency of uridine diphosphate-N-acetylglucosamine:lysosomal enzyme N-acetylglucosamine-1-phosphotransferase. The degree to which this enzyme is deficient determines the ultimate phenotype. Diagnosis is suggested by clinical features resembling mucopolysaccharidoses, but without their biochemical abnormalities. Findings of high levels of β-hexosaminidases, iduronate sulphatase, and arylsulphatase A in the serum are diagnostic. The characteristic enzymatic deficiencies in fibroblasts can be identified in cultured cells.

Mucolipidosis Type II (Inclusion Cell Disease, I-Cell Disease)

I-cell disease results from a severe deficiency of the phosphotransferase enzyme due to specific genetic mutations which result in a marked reduction in enzymic activity. Various defects in the gene encoding this enzyme have been discovered in patients with this disorder.[55] The patients with inclusion cell disease present with clinical features very similar to those with Hurler's syndrome. Hepatosplenomegaly is not so obvious, while striking gingival hypertrophy is a feature not encountered in Hurler's syndrome. Furthermore, the disease becomes evident earlier than does Hurler's syndrome. Corneal clouding is the rule. The skeletal and joint abnormalities, together with myocardial infiltration, usually lead to death by the age of 5 years, either from respiratory causes or cardiac failure. Asymmetrical septal hypertrophy has been reported.[56] Treatment of the cardiac manifestations is usually supportive, though surgical management of valvar involvement has been reported.[57] Transplantation of allogeneic stem cells has stemmed the progression of disease in a small number of reported cases.[58]

Mucolipidosis Type III (Pseudo-Hurler Polydystrophy)

Mucolipidosis type III is less severe, and also less common, than type II, and is due to a deficiency of the same phosphotransferase enzyme. In type III, the enzymic activity is less severely reduced, and the manifestations are less severe. There is a fair amount of variability in clinical severity.[59] This is likely due to various genetic defects leading to different levels of enzymic activity. Patients are usually spared the joint manifestations of I-cell disease early in life, and often present with joint stiffness at the age of 4 or 5 years. Growth is moderately retarded, and corneal clouding is present by the age of 7 or 8 years. The patients are disabled by carpal tunnel syndrome and destruction of the hip joints. Cardiac involvement, particularly aortic regurgitation, does occur but is usually not sufficiently severe to cause clinical problems. Patients with pseudo-Hurler polydystrophy survive into the fourth decade.

Disorders of Glycoprotein Degradation

Specific lysosomal enzymic deficiencies result in failure of degradation of glycoproteins, with consequent accumulation of glycoproteins in many tissues, especially the nervous system. They became recognised when patients with appearances similar to those with mucopolysaccharidoses were found to have biochemically distinct diseases.

The five primary disorders of glycoprotein degradation—mannosidosis, fucosidosis, sialidosis, galactosialidosis, and aspartylglycosaminuria—can all be diagnosed by demonstration of the enzyme defect in cultured fibroblasts. Prenatal diagnosis is often possible.

Mannosidosis

Deficiency of α-mannosidase results in the accumulation of oligosaccharides, as their degradation is dependent upon lysosomal activity of this enzyme. Oligosaccharides are excreted in the urine. Several defects in the gene encoding α-mannosidase have been discovered. The specific defect may result in decreased enzymic synthesis, decreased enzymic activity within the lysosomal environment, decreased localisation of the enzyme within the lysosome, or faulty post-translational modification of the enzyme. The patients present with features suggestive of mucopolysaccharidosis but have an increased susceptibility to infections. Progressive mental retardation is typical. Early onset of the disease shown as type I is associated with increased severity. Death occurs between 3 and 10 years of age. Late-onset, or type II, runs a more benign course. Cardiac manifestations are not frequently reported. A short PR interval has been reported in several patients, albeit that its mechanism is unknown.[60] Treatment has been attempted with transplantation of bone marrow, and current strategies under investigation include various forms of enzymic replacement therapy.[61]

Fucosidosis

Deficiency of α-L-fucosidase results in the accumulation of fucosylated oligosaccharides and glycolipids. Two clinical types are recognised. The first type presents in infancy with coarse facies, growth retardation, mental retardation, and neurological deterioration. Convulsions and respiratory infections often occur. The second type has a more benign course and a later onset. Cardiomegaly, probably as a part of a generalised visceromegaly, is the most common cardiac feature. These two types probably represent both ends of a continuum which is dictated by specific enzymic activity as determined by the specific genetic defect. Transplantation of bone marrow has been performed with good results, and further experimentation with enzymic replacement therapy is under way.[62]

Sialidosis

The basic defect in sialidosis is deficiency of α-neuraminidase, with accumulation of sialoglycoconjugates. There are two forms. The first is of late onset. Patients are of normal appearance, but develop the cherry red spot myoclonus syndrome. Decreased visual acuity is associated with a cherry red spot in the macular region. Neurological, and occasionally renal, manifestations dominate the clinical picture. The second type has an early onset, even upon occasion being obvious at birth. The patients have coarse features and enlargement of various organs, including the heart. Echocardiography has shown a thickened left ventricular wall along with thickening of the mitral valve.[63] There is great variability in the spectrum of severity, even in the group with early onset. Survival beyond 20 years is rare, while, occasionally, affected subjects are stillborn. Fetal hydrops has been reported as a presenting feature.[64] Sialidosis is inherited in autosomal recessive fashion. Enzymic replacement therapy and gene transfer are under investigation.[65]

Galactosialidosis

In galactosialidosis, patients have a defect in the production of lysosomal protective protein/cathepsin A, which helps form a stable and activated complex with β-galactosidase and α-neuraminidase.[66] Thus, the symptoms are a combination of those seen in sialidosis and Morquio's syndrome, the severity of which is likely determined by the specific genetic defect and its overall effect on production of functional levels of the protein. An infantile form has been described,[67] though there appears to be clinical variation even in those diagnosed as infants.[68] Complex congenital cardiac malformations have been reported in patients with galactosialidosis.[69] The cardiac manifestations are similar to those seen in Morquio's syndrome and sialidosis, with aortic and mitral valvar thickening which is progressive.[70,71] Recently, the role of these enzymes and protective protein/cathepsin A in elastogenesis has begun to be unraveled, helping further to explain the phenotype associated with these genetic disorders.[72] Early work has begun on therapies involving enzymic replacement or gene transfer.[65,73]

Aspartylglycosaminuria

Aspartylglycosaminuria is a lysosomal storage disease produced by defective or deficient glycosylasparaginase. This enzyme is required for complete breakdown of asparagine-linked glycoproteins within the lysosome.[74] Accumulation of these glycoprotein residues leads to severe and progressive neurologic impairment. It is associated with coarse features, joint laxity, early rapid somatic growth followed by a reduced adolescent growth spurt leading ultimately to short stature, and mental retardation. Animal models demonstrate accumulation of residues within the heart, but clinical cardiac involvement does not appear to predominate. Enzymic replacement is currently being studied in animal models.[75]

Acid Lipase Deficiency (Wolman's Disease and Cholesteryl Ester Storage Disease)

Lysosomal acid lipase is necessary for the cleavage of triglycerides and cholesteryl esters from lipoproteins delivered to the lysosome. Complete or severe deficiency of lysosomal acid lipase results in accumulation of cholesterol in most tissues of the body. The disease occurs in two forms. Wolman's disease is a disease of infancy presenting with vomiting, diarrhoea, hepatosplenomegaly, anaemia and calcification of the adrenal glands. Cardiac manifestations are not usually evident, but microscopic examination of the arteries shows excess fatty deposits. Hepatomegaly is frequently the only sign in the milder form of the disease, known as cholesteryl ester storage disease, though premature atherosclerosis is also seen.[76] The diagnosis of Wolman disease is suggested by the association of hepatosplenomegaly with adrenal calcification. Definitive diagnosis of either disease can be made by assessing acid lipase activity in cultured skin fibroblasts. The disease is inherited in an autosomal recessive fashion. Successful treatment with transplantation of both bone marrow and cord blood has been reported.[77,78]

Sphingolipidoses

Sphingomyelin Lipidosis (Niemann-Pick Disease)

In Niemann-Pick disease, there is accumulation of sphingomyelin in the cells as a result of deficiency of sphingomyelinase. The primary cells affected are those of monocyte-macrophage lineage, as they are frequently employed in the metabolic turnover of these substances. At least four variants exist, but the most frequently encountered is the infantile acute neuronopathic form. Many of these patients are of Ashkenazi Jewish heritage. The disease is characterised by hepatosplenomegaly and the occurrence of foam storage cells in many tissues. The heart is not usually affected, but one infant with acute neuronopathic disease had endocardial fibroelastosis.[79] Since there were no storage cells in the heart, however, this may have been a chance association. Abnormalities in the lipid profile have also been described in children with Niemann-Pick disease types A and B, possibly leading to premature atherosclerosis.[80] Low levels of high density lipid cholesterol were the most consistent finding, while elevated levels of triglyceride and low density lipid cholesterol were seen in approximately two-thirds. These abnormalities were noted at an early age, and may reflect deranged cholesterol metabolism in these cells as a result of sphingomyelin accumulation. Niemann-Pick disease in most of its forms is inherited in an autosomal recessive fashion.

Glucosylceramidosis (Gaucher's Disease)

Gaucher's disease is the most common inherited disorder of glycolipid metabolism. In his original description,[81] Phillippe Gaucher ascribed the changes to a primary epithelioma of the spleen. There is excessive accumulation of glucosylceramide in cells of the reticuloendothelial system in organs throughout the body, resulting from deficiency of the enzyme glucocerebrosidase, which cleaves glucose from glucocerebroside. While over 150 different mutations of the gene encoding glucocerebrosidase have been described, the disease occurs in three varieties based upon the presence or absence of, and rate of progression of, neurologic manifestations. Type I, or the chronic non-neuronopathic form, can be diagnosed at any age. It is the most common form, being characterised by hypersplenism, hepatomegaly with evidence of abnormal hepatic function, and skeletal lesions, including aseptic necrosis of the femoral head. Other long bones and vertebras may also be eroded. In patients with this type of disease, cardiac involvement may be seen with myocardial infiltration or restrictive pericardial disease.[82] The most frequently encountered cardiac problem, however, is cor pulmonale secondary to pulmonary involvement. Mitral and aortic stenosis and insufficiency can also be seen,[83] and severe valvar and aortic arch calcification has been reported.[84] The course is variable. Death may occur in early childhood or, particularly when onset is late, there may be a normal life expectancy. Further variability is apparently the consequence of the non-neuronopathic form at onset changing to one of the other forms with a poorer prognosis.

The acute neuronopathic form, or type II, is usually recognised within the second half of the first year of life. Neurological involvement is evident early, afflicting particularly the cranial nerves and extrapyramidal tracts. The mechanism of death is usually a respiratory infection, since aspiration is common owing to incoordination of the nasopharynx. The subacute neuronopathic form, or type III, falls between the acute and chronic forms. The neurological involvement renders it less benign than the chronic variant, but its course usually stretches over many years.

While describing Gaucher's disease in terms of three distinct phenotypes is convenient, the observed characteristics of this disease are much less well defined. Patients with the same genotype can have widely differing phenotypes, and patients even within a particular type can have markedly differing clinical courses. Thus, while the genetic defects leading to Gaucher's disease are being elucidated, and include over 150 specific mutations already identified, the link between genotype and phenotype is still unclear.

The diagnosis of Gaucher's disease is confirmed by the finding of typical storage cells in the bone marrow, or by liver biopsy. The Gaucher cell is large and lipid laden. The cytoplasm is described as having an appearance of wrinkled tissue paper or crumpled silk. The nucleus is eccentric. These cells have to be differentiated from cells found in multiple myeloma, leucaemia, thalassaemia, and congenital dyserythropoietic anaemia. Demonstration of the enzymic deficiency in cultured skin fibroblasts, or in leucocytes, confirms the diagnosis. Approaches to treatment have included transplantation of organs and enzymic replacement. Improvement in the visceral involvement is common, but neurologic damage is generally not responsive to exogenous enzymic therapy. All three variants are inherited as autosomal recessive traits. Intra-uterine diagnosis is available, and heterozygotes can be identified at least for the acute and chronic types.

α-Galactosidase A Deficiency (Fabry's Disease)

Deficiency of α-galactosidase, a lysosomal enzyme, results in accumulation of phosphosphingolipids in the lysosomes of many tissues and also in the body fluids. The most frequently affected tissue is the vascular endothelium. The disease is of X-linked inheritance, but heterozygous women can show severe manifestations of the disease.[85] The gene locus for the enzyme is on the long arm of the X chromosome.

The disease usually presents in childhood in the male homozygote, often with periodic crises of severe pain of burning character, which usually start in the hands and feet. Crises occur most usually in the afternoon. Development of crises, which become less frequent and severe with time, may be followed by eruption of skin lesions, by angiokeratomas, and by typical opacities of the cornea and the lens. The angiokeratomas are clusters of dark red to purple punctate lesions which are usually flat or slightly raised. They occur most frequently between the umbilicus and the knees. They do not blanch on pressure. Hyperkeratosis and hypohidrosis usually accompany the angiokeratomas. Ocular lesions include typical creamy whorl-like opacities in the cornea. They are frequently found in the female heterozygote as well as the male homozygote. Cardiac disease is manifest with increasing age. Myocardial ischaemia and infarction are common and are secondary to the vascular lesions. Mitral regurgitation and aortic stenosis are the most frequently encountered valvar lesions.[86] Infiltration of the conduction tissues occurs. This results in progressive shortening of the PR interval as in other storage diseases that affect the specialised atrioventricular conduction axis.[87] Myocardial deposition can be detected echocardiographically by demonstration of septal and left ventricular wall thickening.[88] Progressive deposition of glycosphingolipid means that the cardiac problems themselves are also progressive. Since there is concomitant renal involvement, the cardiac effects are exacerbated by, for example, renal hypertension. The clinical course in the male homozygote is one of steady deterioration during early adult life, death being from cardiac or renal disease. The heterozygote female experiences little limitation of style and length of life. The diagnosis can be confirmed, and heterozygotes identified, by demonstrating the enzymic deficiency in leucocytes, and by finding an abnormally high content of accumulated substrates in tears or urinary sediment. Prenatal diagnosis is available. Enzymic replacement was reported in 2002,[89] and positive effects on cardiac involvement are evident.[90]

Gangliosidoses

The gangliosidoses are lysosomal storage diseases characterised by accumulation of gangliosides GM_1 or GM_2, or their related conjugates, owing to deficiency of specific lysosomal hydrolases. The enzyme deficient in GM_1 gangliosidosis is acid β-galactosidase. Deficiency of hexosaminidase A or B, or both, or a deficiency of an enzymic activator, results in GM_2 gangliosidosis.

GM_1 Gangliosidosis

There are many enzymatic and clinical subdivisions of GM_1 gangliosidosis. The gene locus is on the short arm of chromosome 3. Mutation at this locus results in absence of enzymic activity for acid β-galactosidase, leading to accumulation of GM_1 ganglioside in the brain and organs. The wide variation in clinical picture has resulted in a broad classification of infant, juvenile, and adult forms. All forms of GM_1 gangliosidosis are inherited as autosomal recessive traits.

When seen in infancy, the disease is rapidly progressive, characterised by hypotonia, poor feeding, and failure to make motor or intellectual progress. Progressive neurological deterioration results in spastic quadriplegia or decerebrate rigidity. Rarified bones and beaked vertebrae are some of the skeletal lesions encountered. As in Tay-Sachs disease, to be discussed below, a cherry red spot is seen in the macular region of the retina. Death usually occurs by the age of 3 years, frequently from bronchopneumonia. The heart is frequently involved. The spectrum from congestive cardiac failure with systolic dysfunction to isolated valvar thickening has been observed.[91,92] Neonatal ascites has also been reported.[93] Cardiac involvement usually includes cardiomegaly on chest radiography, left ventricular hypertrophy on the echocardiogram, and congestive cardiac failure.[94] Patients with GM_1 gangliosidosis have a defect in the same enzyme which is involved in patients with Morquio's syndrome type B. The clinical heterogeneity among patients with this enzymatic defect is unclear, but probably is related to residual activity of the enzyme, post-processing of the enzyme, and other proteins involved, such as saposin B.[95] A novel therapeutic strategy is under investigation, and involves molecular chaperones, substances which stabilise the configuration of defective enzymes and enable them to remain enzymatically active.[96] Treatment in a mouse model demonstrated improved enzymic activity,[97] and reduced the quantity of substrate in neuronal tissues.[98]

GM_2 Gangliosidoses

The GM_2 gangliosidoses result in variable deficiency of hexosaminidase, the locus for which has been mapped to the q arm of chromosome 5. This enzyme, which is composed of alpha and beta subunits, comes in two forms. Hexosaminidase A, found in the central nervous system, is composed of an alpha and beta subunit, while hexosaminidase B, found in peripheral tissues, is composed of two beta subunits. Thus, the GM_2 gangliosidoses result from a defect in either the alpha subunit, producing Tay-Sachs disease and severe deficiency of hexosaminidase A, or the beta subunit, which produces Sandhoff's disease, with severe deficiency of both types A and B of the enzyme. The juvenile and adult chronic GM_2 gangliosidoses result from less severe deficiencies of hexosaminidase A. Treatment for these disorders is still under investigation and has included gene therapy, substrate reduction, and transplantation of bone marrow.[99–101]

Tay-Sachs Disease

Tay-Sachs disease is the most common of the gangliosidoses. It presents with motor weakness in the first 6 months of life. There is progressive motor and mental deterioration, with convulsions, spasticity, and decerebrate rigidity. Death usually occurs by the age of 3 years, the most frequent cause being bronchopneumonia. The children have doll-like facies. Examination of the retina shows the typical cherry red macula, which later becomes brown. Cardiac accumulation of substrate is usual. Save for a prolonged QT interval and non-specific T wave changes, however, cardiac manifestations are rare. While the hallmark of the disease is accumulation of GM_2 ganglioside in the central nervous system, evidence of involvement of the peripheral and autonomic nervous system has been reported in patients with chronic disease.[102]

Sandhoff's Disease

Sandhoff's disease is similar to Tay-Sachs disease in its presentation and course, but is biochemically distinct. Clinically relevant cardiac involvement is rare, but a cardiomyopathy has been described, along with thickening of the mitral valve and its tension apparatus.[103] Another separate report described a case of congestive cardiac failure due to aortic and mitral valvar thickening with severe mitral regurgitation.[104] The coronary arteries may also be narrowed.[105] As for GM_1 gangliosidoses, inheritance is autosomal recessive.

METABOLIC DISORDERS: INHERITED ENDOCRINE DYSFUNCTION

Diabetes Mellitus

The annual incidence of juvenile diabetes is between 8 and 10 per 100,000 of the population at risk.[106,107] New cases are half as frequent under the age of 10 years as they are between 10 and 20 years of age. Since cardiovascular complications are manifested later in the disease, they are exceedingly rare in childhood.[108] There will be problems presented to the paediatric cardiologist by diabetes because fetal mortality is high in pregnant diabetics. Furthermore, congenital cardiac anomalies occur in approximately one-sixth of offspring of diabetic women, with a wide variety of defects reported. The most frequent cardiac complication is hypertrophic cardiomyopathy,[109] produced by elevated levels of insulin and insulin-like growth factor I.

The most obvious complication, however, is macrosomia. Even in the absence of congenital cardiac disease, infants of diabetic mothers have a host of problems. The syndrome is seen both in mothers with established diabetes and in those who develop the disease during pregnancy. The babies have a characteristic appearance, with high birth weight, plumpness, and puffy plethoric facies. They are jittery owing to hypoglycaemia secondary to hyperinsulinism. The organs, including the heart, are enlarged. The babies are frequently tachypnoeic, but this may not be of cardiac aetiology. Respiratory distress syndrome is quite common. Cardiac murmurs are frequent. Approximately one-third have radiological cardiomegaly. The electrocardiogram is rarely diagnostic.

Echocardiography shows thickening of the right and left ventricular walls together with the septum. Indeed, the ventricular septum is usually thicker than the free walls. Septal thickness, is, in general, most pronounced in those infants in congestive cardiac failure.[110] A spectrum of abnormality exists from that of simple hypertrophy to hypertrophic obstructive cardiomyopathy. Obstruction of the left ventricular outflow tract can occur, as has been demonstrated in the past by cardiac catheterisation. Treatment of the hypertrophic cardiomyopathy is fairly standard in that β-blockade helps in terms of diastolic dysfunction. Diuretics must be used judiciously, as the thickened myocardium requires a higher filling pressure. The clinical and echocardiographic signs of hypertrophic cardiomyopathy usually resolve over the early weeks of life, but myocardial thickening can take up to 6 months to resolve.[111]

More important than diagnosis and treatment is prevention. It is suggested that the most severely affected newborns are those in whom maternal control of diabetes has been poor.[112,113] The importance of late glycaemic control, and the correlation of maternal levels of haemoglobin A_{1C} to severity of disease, has been questioned.[114]

Pituitary Gigantism and Acromegaly

Adenomas of the pituitary that secrete growth hormones cause gigantism in growing children and acromegaly in adults. Acromegalic cardiomyopathy results from elevated levels of growth hormone and the resultant elevated levels of insulin-like growth factor 1. The cardiomyopathy is characterised by biventricular and concentric involvement, which is progressive and may lead to congestive cardiac failure with myocardial fibrosis. The severity of disease relates to the age of the patient. Treatment with somatostatin analogues, which reduce growth levels, is beneficial in terms of clinical symptoms and indexes of myocardial morphology and physiology.[115]

Disorders of Thyroid Function

Hypothyroidism

Congenital Hypothyroidism

Congenital hypothyroidism has many aetiologies. The most common cause is congenital thyroid dysplasia, present in approximately 1 in 6000 live births. There are rarer causes, including endemic deficiency of iodine, diminished responsiveness to thyrotrophin in familial goitre, and administration of antithyroid drugs to pregnant mothers. The cardiac features of cretinism are not dramatic. Normal to slow heart rates, and radiological cardiomegaly, are usually the only manifestations. The enlarged cardiac silhouette is usually caused by pericardial effusion, which is an extremely common feature. Cardiac performance is usually well preserved. Abnormalities of heart rate and the pericardial effusions resolve when substitution treatment of the hypothyroidism is successful. A pericardial effusion can be detected by echocardiography in approximately half of these patients.[116]

Juvenile Hypothyroidism

As with congenital forms, juvenile hypothyroidism has multiple aetiologies. It is generally the result of autoimmune thyroiditis, or Hashimoto's disease. Growth retardation is the most common form of presentation. It can lead to delayed sexual maturation. Cardiac signs and symptoms are few, and cardiac failure is very rare. Bradycardia, low pulse pressure, poor peripheral circulation, and non-specific murmurs may be present. Pericardial effusions, with no evidence of pericarditis, occur in some patients. Tamponade is rarely seen because of the slow rate of fluid accumulation. About one-half of the patients with pericardial effusions have associated pleural effusions. Establishment of a euthyroid state reverses the cardiac manifestations.

Hyperthyroidism

Juvenile Hyperthyroidism

The most common cause of juvenile hyperthyroidism is diffuse toxic goitre, also known as Graves' disease. This is an autoimmune disease in which IgG immunoglobulins, which stimulate excessive production of thyroid hormones, can be demonstrated. It is more common in girls, with a ratio of females to males of approximately 5 to 1. Its greatest incidence is between the ages of 11 and 19 years, and it is rarely seen in children under the age of 3 years. Presenting symptoms include restlessness, poor performance at school, irritability, loss of weight, and occasionally diarrhoea. On examination, patients have warm skin, and a fine tremor is visible in outstretched hands. Enlargement of the thyroid gland is always present, and bruits are audible over the enlarged gland because of its increased vascularity. Exophthalmos is common, but is not marked. Cardiovascular involvement is secondary to an increased adrenergic drive and to direct myocardial stimulation by thyroid hormones. The pulse is fast with a wide pulse pressure. The systolic blood pressure is increased, and the apical impulse is hyperdynamic. On auscultation, the first heart sound is accentuated, and non-specific systolic murmurs may be present. A high incidence of mitral valvar prolapse has been reported in adults with Graves' disease[117,118] but has not been demonstrated in children.[119] This suggests that the appearance of the prolapse is related to the duration of the disease.

The electrocardiogram is atypical. Sinus tachycardia, first-degree atrioventricular block, and non-specific ST segment and T wave changes may be present. Signs of atrial and left ventricular enlargement are more common in children than in adults.[120] Although atrial fibrillation is quite common in adults, it is extremely rare in children. Radiographic cardiomegaly, and a slight increase in pulmonary vascular markings, may be seen, especially in the setting of cardiac failure. The echocardiogram reveals hyperdynamic contractions of the ventricular septum and the left ventricular posterior wall.

Evaluation of cardiac function by radionuclide angiography in the presence of hyperthyroidism has shown a fall in left ventricular ejection fraction with exercise. Upon restoration of a normal thyroid state, the ejection fraction shows its normal exercise-induced increase.[121] In general, the cardiovascular system in childhood tolerates well the effects of hyperthyroidism. In the presence of cardiac failure, however, concomitant cardiovascular lesions must be excluded. Cardiovascular manifestations of hyperthyroidism are reversible with treatment but, if long-standing or poorly treated, the disease may predispose to irreversible cardiac dysfunction.[122]

Addison's Disease

Adrenal insufficiency may occur at any age and demonstrates no predilection for gender. It usually results from autoimmune destruction of the adrenal cortex and is manifested by weakness, hyperpigmentation, nausea, vomiting, loss of weight, and hypotension. When acute in onset, or when seen in patients who are metabolically stressed by a concomitant illness, the disease may present with shock or coma.

Cardiac involvement is due to the chronic hypotension and hypovolemia. Chest radiography may demonstrate diminished cardiac size, presumably due to disuse atrophy.[123] The electrocardiogram may demonstrate diffusely low voltages, sinus bradycardia, and first-degree atrioventricular block. Treatment involves replacement of mineralocorticoid hormones and must be carried out with caution as congestive cardiac failure can ensue. This is presumably due to the acute load of salt and water that is thrust upon the previously unloaded myocardium. This complication is readily treatable and is generally transient.[124]

DISORDERS OF ENERGY METABOLISM

Mitochondrial Myopathies

The mitochondrial myopathies are muscle and systemic disorders characterised by the presence of mitochondria with abnormal structure, number and/or function. They are typically caused by deletions in mitochondrial deoxyribonucleic acid, though some are caused by defects in nuclear deoxyribonucleic acid. These disorders involve complexes of the respiratory chain, and thus affect oxidative phosphorylation.

Chronic progressive ophthalmoplegia, or Kearns-Sayre syndome, is frequently encountered among these diseases. It is associated with pigmentary degeneration of the retina, lack of coordination, facial and limb weaknesses, short stature, and endocrinal anomalies. The disease appears in childhood and has a progressive course. The most frequently reported cardiac anomaly is progressive heart block. Electrocardiograms should be performed frequently for early recognition and appropriate implantation of a pacemaker (see Chapter 19).[125] Cardiomyopathy, prolonged QT interval, torsades de pointes, atrial arrhythmias, and mitral valvar prolapse have also been described.[126–130]

Myoclonic epilepsy with ragged red fibers (MERRF) and mitochondrial encephalopathy, lactic acidosis and stroke-like episodes (MELAS) can present with a dilated cardiomyopathy.[131] Patients with Leigh syndrome, or subacute necrotizing encephalomyelopathy, can develop hypertrophic cardiomyopathy and conduction system defects.[132] Mitochondrial deoxyribonucleic acid is maternally transmitted. Inheritance, therefore, follows non-Mendelian patterns.

Barth Syndrome

Barth syndrome is an X-linked disorder due to a defect in the tafazzin gene, which produces a deficiency of cardiolipin. While the precise pathogenetic mechanism linking this deficiency to the clinical features of Barth syndrome remains to be elucidated, it is known that cardiolipin plays an important role in the processes of mitochondrial energy metabolism.[133] The disease is characterised by a dilated cardiomyopathy, skeletal myopathy, cyclic neutropenia, and retardation of growth. The heart typically displays poor contractility, and is often hypertrabeculated, showing features of ventricular non-compaction. Hypertrophy has also been noted. Cardiac involvement usually becomes manifest in the first decade of life.[134] Sudden death has been reported, and may be due to the increased risk of ventricular arrhythmias, which may require implantation of a defibrillator.[135] Treatment of the cardiomyopathy rests with traditional medical therapy, but cardiac transplantation has been successfully performed.[136] Death typically results from infectious complications or from cardiac disease.

Propionic Acidemia

Propionic acidemia is a rare metabolic disorder due to a deficiency of propionyl-CoA carboxylase, an enzyme involved in the catabolism of valine, leucine, isoleucine, methionine, threonine, cholesterol, and fatty acids. Gene mutations mapped to chromosomes 3 and 13 have been described.[137] Diagnosis is suspected by analysis of urinary organic acids, with elevations of propionate, propionylglycine, and methylcitrate. Confirmation of the diagnosis rests with demonstration of reduced activity of propionyl-CoA carboxylase in skin fibroblasts. There is a wide spectrum in clinical presentation, from severe early onset of the disease in the first days of life to relatively mild forms presenting in adulthood. Patients develop hypoglycinaemia, hyperammonaemia, hypoglycaemia, and deficits in the central nervous system, particularly in times of metabolic stress such as occurs with minor infections. Cardiomyopathy and sudden death are relatively frequent late complications.[138] The latter may be due to an increased prevalence of prolongation of the QT interval in these patients, a phenomenon seen more frequently with age.[139] Because of this, regular electrocardiographic screening is necessary. When involved, the heart is typically dilated with depressed function, though hypertrophy is also seen.[140] Poor ventricular contractility can complicate acute metabolic crises, and patients presenting with encephalopathy should be assessed for left ventricular systolic dysfunction. The precise aetiology of the cardiomyopathy is not known, but disordered carnitine metabolism and toxicity of byproducts in the metabolic pathway of propionyl-CoA carboxylase are leading suspects. Treatment consists of restriction of proteins and supplemental oral carnitine.

Methylmalonic Aciduria

Methylmalonic aciduria is clinically similar to propionic acidaemia and is due to a deficiency of methylmalonyl-CoA mutase. It can also be due to defects in its cofactor, adenosylcobalamin.[141] The enzyme is required for the metabolism of valine, leucine, isoleucine, methionine and threonine and yields succinyl-CoA for the tricarboxylic acid cycle. Deficiency can lead to cardiomyopathy. Some patients, who likely have residual enzymatic activity, or whose disease is the result of defective or deficient cofactor, can respond favorably to supplemental cyanocobalamin. Those with deficiency of the enzyme itself are managed on a low-protein diet with carnitine supplementation. Despite therapy, however, the risk of metabolic crisis during acute illnesses remains high. Recently, hepatocyte-directed gene delivery has been shown to correct the enzymic activity, and may hold promise as a future corrective therapy.[142]

Disorders of Fatty Acid Metabolism

The heart utilises fatty acids for energy production by converting long-chain free fatty acids to long-chain acyl-CoA via acyl-CoA synthetase. These acyl-CoA compounds are then transferred into the mitochondria, where they are degraded to produce acetyl-CoA for use in the tricarboxylic acid cycle.

Carnitine-acylcarnitine translocase mediates entry of fatty acyl-CoA compounds into the mitochondria. Deficiency often results in early death due to severe metabolic collapse with encephalopathy and hypertrophic cardiomyopathy, though patients with milder variants can present later. Treatment with medium chain triglycerides and carnitine supplementation can potentially avert the severe neurologic outcomes usually associated with this disease.[143]

Carnitine palmitoyltransferase II converts acylcarnitine back to acyl-CoA for β-oxidation once it has crossed the inner mitochondrial membrane. Deficiency of this enzyme leads to nonketotic hypoglycaemia with seizures, hepatomegaly, and hypertrophic cardiomyopathy. Milder forms can present later with fasting or during periods of metabolic stress. Treatment consists of a low-fat diet, supplementation with medium-chain triglycerides, carnitine supplementation, and avoidance of fasting.[144]

The acyl-CoA dehydrogenases mediate the reactions yielding acetyl-CoA from acyl-CoA compounds of varying lengths. These enzymes are referred to as short, medium, long, and very long acyl dehydrogenases. Deficiency of any of these can yield a generalised myopathy along with nonketotic hypoglycemia and cardiomyopathy.[91]

DISORDERS OF COLLAGEN SYNTHESIS OR EXTRACELLULAR MATRIX

The group of disorders of collagen synthesis includes several diseases with cardiac involvement. Included in this discussion are Ehlers-Danlos syndrome, cutis laxa, osteogenesis imperfecta, and Marfan syndrome. Alcaptonuria also comes into this general group but, as yet, cardiac disease has not become manifest in childhood. Direct cardiac involvement does not occur in epidermolysis bullosa, but the heart may be affected when the condition is complicated by amyloidosis.

Ehlers-Danlos Syndrome

Phenotypical features unite the biochemically and genetically heterogeneous group of disorders included in Ehlers-Danlos syndrome. The stigmas are hyperextensible skin and joints, easy bruising, and poor healing of wounds. A distinctive facial appearance includes epicanthic folds, a flat bridge of the nose, and prominent downward pointing ears. The skin, apart from the palms and soles, is smooth and rubbery. In later life it may hang in folds from the elbows. Premature death is common in the most severe form, and the babies have poor muscular tone. In addition to the epicanthic folds, ocular signs include easy eversion of the upper eyelid, known as Metenier's sign, blue scleras, and a dislocated lens. A variety of congenital cardiac malformations have been reported,[145–147] being found in approximately one-eighth of patients in one study. Prolapse of the mitral valve had previously been reported to be common in these patients, but a more recent study showed an incidence similar to that of the general population.[148]

More than 10 subtypes of Ehlers-Danlos syndrome have been described, but six major subtypes are recognised and encompass nine-tenths of individuals affected. Patients typically fall into the hypermobility, classical or vascular type. Classic Ehlers-Danlos syndrome, incorporating types I and II, demonstrates the typical cutaneous findings. It most often results from defects in one or more of the collagen or procollagen genes. The hypermobility type is similar, with joint hypermobility the predominant clinical feature. Both of these types, while not characteristically demonstrating vascular changes, have been shown to be associated with dilation of the aortic root and valvar dysfunction.[149] The vascular type, also known as Ehlers-Danlos syndrome type IV, results from mutations in the gene encoding type III procollagen. These patients are at risk for arterial rupture, which typically occurs after the onset of the third decade of life.[150] A more severe recessive form has been reported, and includes both the cutaneous findings of the classic form coupled with cardiac valvar involvement.[151]

Cutis Laxa

Cutis laxa is, again, a genetically heterogeneous group of conditions characterised in the phenotype by the skin being so loose that it appears too large for the body. Unlike the Ehlers-Danlos syndrome, the lax skin is slow to recoil after being stretched. Cutis laxa has some features in common with the Ehlers-Danlos syndrome, such as fragility of the skin, hypermobile joints, and easy bruising. There are characteristic facies, including a long upper lip, a hooked nose, and a short columella. The defect of connective tissue also results in a deep voice owing to lax vocal cords. Hernias and rectal or vaginal prolapse can also be seen. The disease can be inherited in both autosomal dominant and autosomal recessive forms. From the cardiac standpoint, peripheral pulmonary stenosis[152] and aortic dilation have been reported.[153] These findings, coupled with reports of supravalvar aortic stenosis,[154] have helped lead to the discovery that defects in the elastin gene are one cause of this disorder.[155] Defects in other genes, including fibulin-4 and fibulin-5, have also been implicated in some forms.[156,157] Another major complication is cor pulmonale, since emphysema is frequently progressive and severe.[158] Patients with the neonatal variant of cutis laxa can have severe mitral regurgitation with dysplastic valvar leaflets.[159]

Osteogenesis Imperfecta

Bone fragility is the main clinical feature of this condition. Although the fractures are subperiosteal with little displacement, the multiplicity of fractures leads to bowing of the long bones. Additionally, the vertebras are biconcave, with the disc sometimes perforating the vertebral body to give the appearance known as Schmorl's nodes. The skull is frequently made up largely of wormian bones and shows frontal and parietal bossing. The skeletal deformities lead to short stature. The skin is thin but not lax. The sclerae are blue in most types. In the so-called type III variant of the disease, they may become less blue with age. The cardiovascular manifestations include aortic and mitral regurgitation owing to dilation of the valvar hinges or, in the latter, to prolapse from ruptured cords. It has been suggested that aortic root dilation may be present in a certain subset of patients with osteogenesis imperfecta, and that it appears to be nonprogressive.[160] In some patients, aortic or mitral valvar disease is severe and may require replacement surgery. This carries a higher than normal risk due to bleeding complications related to tissue friability. Administration of recombinant factor VIIa may be helpful in controlling bleeding in these patients.[161] Aortic stenosis, defects of the oval fossa, and tetralogy of Fallot have also been reported.[162]

Marfan Syndrome

Marfan syndrome is transmitted as an autosomal dominant disease with variable clinical expression. The prevalence is estimated at 2 to 3 per 10,000. The disease is due to defects in the FBN1 gene on chromosome 15q21, which encodes fibrillin-1, an important component of connective tissues. More than 500 mutations in the gene have been identified, and approximately one-quarter to three-tenths of cases represent new mutations. While the expression of the disease is highly variable, even among family members with the same genetic defect, some correlations between genotype and phenotype have been clarified.[163] More than seven-tenths of those affected are diagnosed before the age of 10 years. Physical features of the syndrome may be present at birth.[164] Affected persons are usually very tall, with an increase in the length of the limbs compared with the trunk. Their arm span exceeds their height (Fig. 57-3A). They have long, thin fingers (Fig. 57-3B), hypermobile joints, kyphoscoliosis, and chest deformities. High arching of the palate, with dental crowding, is commonly seen, as are inguinal hernias. Ocular abnormalities occur in about three-quarters of patients. The most frequent are subluxation of the lenses and myopia. Because of the importance of identifying individuals with this disease, a multidisciplinary group of experts produced diagnostic criterions known as the Ghent nosology.[165] These criterions included skeletal findings as a major criterion, and also introduced molecular diagnostic tools into the clinical diagnosis of this disease (Table 57-2). Patients with a positive family history must meet the major criterions for at least one category, not including the genetic category, plus the criterions for involvement in a second category. Patients with no family history must meet the major criterions for two categories, plus the criterion for involvement in a third category.

Cardiac manifestations in childhood are usually less severe than in adults. Mitral valvar disease in the form of prolapse and incompetence are the most frequent abnormalities. They are present in approximately three-quarters of the patients.[166] Dilation of the aortic root, and fusiform aneurysms of the ascending aorta, are also common, particularly in males. The major consequences of these aortic lesions are valvar regurgitation and aortic dissection. Aortic involvement is progressive, and the risk of aortic dissection increases with increasing diameter due to increases in mural stress. Histopathological examination of the ascending aorta reveals degeneration of the elastic fibres, so-called cystic medial necrosis, which is most severe in patients with aneurysms. The leaflets of the aortic valves contain increased amounts of acid mucopolysaccharide. The mitral valvar annulus is dilated, and may become calcified. Pulmonary arterial dilation and aneurysmal formation have also been reported.[167] The electrocardiogram may show signs of left ventricular and left atrial enlargement when there is significant valvar insufficiency. Disturbances of rhythm, such as first-degree atrioventricular block, atrial ectopic beats, atrial flutter, fibrillation and tachycardia, are common. Ventricular arrhythmias are present in about one-third of the patients during childhood. Progressing with age, they appear to be closely related to mitral valvar prolapse and prolonged ventricular repolarisation.[168] Radiographic examination of the cardiac shadow is difficult in the presence of thoracic skeletal deformities. Cardiac enlargement may be seen in the presence of valvar insufficiency and dilation of the ascending aorta. Echocardiographic evaluation is essential. Mitral valvar prolapse is a very frequent finding. Dilation of the aortic root, sometimes with paradoxical motion of the posterior aortic wall, is common. Mitral and aortic incompetence will lead to left atrial and left ventricular volume overload. Doppler echocardiography should increase the early diagnosis of the valvar abnormalities. Cardiac catheterisation is useful for further assessment of these lesions. Aortic angiography will reveal the dilation of the aortic root. Evaluation with magnetic resonance imaging has demonstrated decreased aortic distensibility and increased stiffness in children with Marfan syndrome.[169]

The pathophysiology of dilation of the aortic root is likely due to a complex interplay between altered vascular mural composition and other destructive processes. The

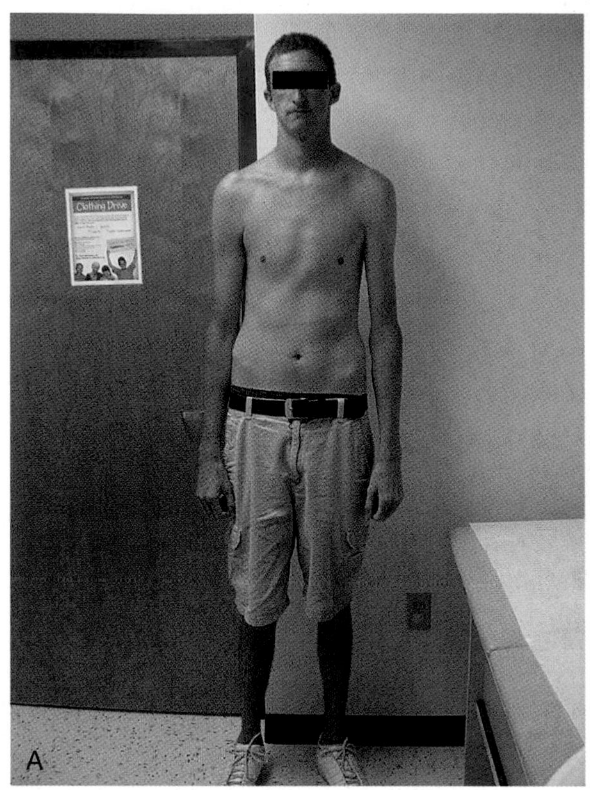

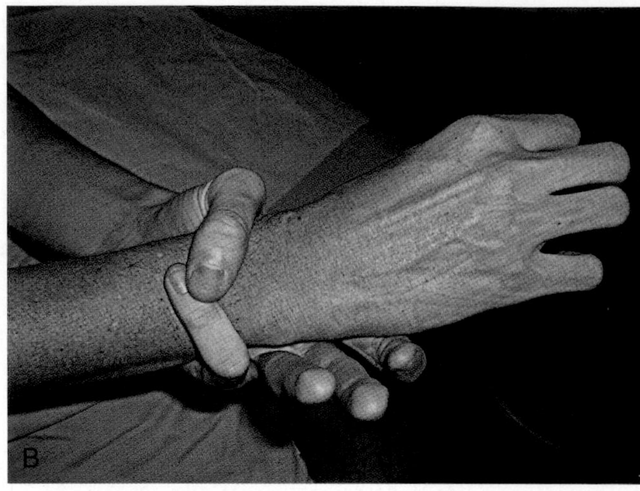

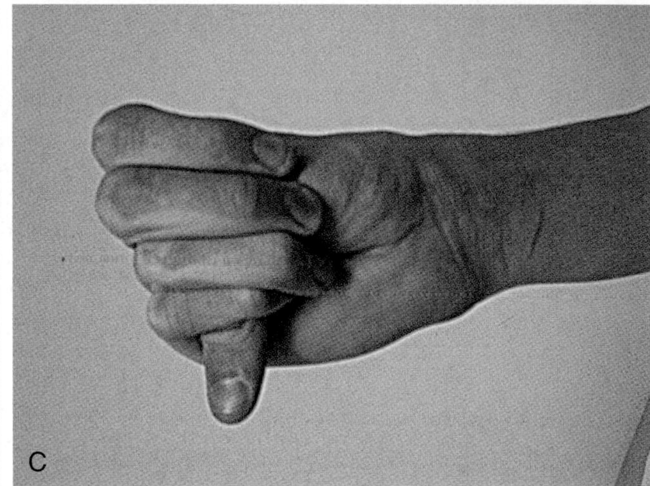

Figure 57-3 Typical body habitus of a patient with Marfan syndrome shows how the arm span exceeds the height by more than 5%,. **B** shows the positive wrist sign, and **C** shows the positive thumb sign.

TABLE 57-2

DIAGNOSTIC CRITERIONS FOR MARFAN SYNDROME

Category	Major Criterions	Minor Criterions
Family history/ genetics	Positive diagnosis in a parent, sibling or child Known FBN1 mutation	None
Cardiac	Aortic root dilation Aortic dissection	Mitral valvar prolapse Calcific mitral valvar annulus (age < 40 years) Pulmonary arterial dilation with no other cause (age < 40 years) Other aortic dilation or dissection (age < 50 years)
Pulmonary	None	Spontaneous pneumothorax Apical blebs
Skin and integument	None	Striae atrophicae Recurrent or incisional hernias
Dura	Lumbosacral dural ectasia	None

defective collagen renders the arterial walls less distensible, but this alone has not proven to lead to arterial dilation. The dilation itself may be related to apoptosis of vascular smooth muscle cells, which has been shown to be related to angiotensin II receptor signaling pathways.[170] Additionally, defective microfibrils result in excessive activity of transforming growth factor–β, which is normally regulated by latent TGF-β binding proteins bound to microfibrils. This excessive TGF-β signaling leads to disordered formation of the matrix, and may be a principal cause of the vascular dilation found in these patients.[171] Patients with Loeys-Dietz syndrome, and other disorders similar to Marfan syndrome, have been found to have defects in the gene encoding the TGF-β receptor.[172] The complex interplay between fibrillin, microfibrils, LTBPs (latent TGF-β binding proteins), TGF-β, and the TGF-β receptor probably accounts for the wide clinical variability in Marfan syndrome and other related disorders.

Life expectancy is very variable. Death usually occurs in the fourth decade, mainly from cardiovascular causes.[173] Cardiac failure, dissection or aneurysms of the aorta, and sudden death are the most frequent causes. Incompetence of both mitral and aortic valves carries a poor prognosis. There is no specific treatment for this condition. Cardiac failure is best treated with diuretics and vasodilators, since the positive inotropic effects of digoxin may further damage the aortic root. Surgical replacement of the diseased valves, and of the ascending aorta, may be necessary. The benefits in children of prophylactic propranolol to delay the dilation of the aorta through its negative inotropic effects has been the subject of some debate. Arguments for[174] and against[175] a beneficial effect have been published. Additionally, with the discovery of a role for angiotensin II and TGF-β in the pathogenesis of aortic aneurysmal formation, investigations into inhibition of angiotensin converting enzyme and blockade of angiotensin receptors have begun.[176,177]

The timing of surgery for repair or replacement of valves, or replacement of the aortic root, must be decided in light of the known risks of surgery, as well of the risks of not performing surgery. Elective replacement of the aortic root can be accomplished with a relatively low risk of mortality.[178] On the other hand, replacing the aortic root emergently due to acute dissection carries a much higher risk of short- and long-term mortality.[179] Early recommendations suggested elective replacement when the root reached an absolute diameter of 60 mm. Many patients suffer dissections at sizes significantly smaller than this, and an annual risk of mortality of nearly 5% has been described for patients with an aortic root greater than 50 mm.[180] Thus, recent recommendations concluded that replacement should occur electively before the root reaches a diameter of 55 mm.[181] Additionally, it is difficult to determine which patients might have an increased risk for dissection at a relatively smaller size of the root. Certainly, for patients with a family history of aortic dissection, or for those in whom pregnancy is likely, intervention is encouraged at a relatively smaller size. Also, women appear to be at risk for dissection at a smaller size.[182] Thus, some are now advocating elective replacement of the aortic root at sizes less than 50 mm.[183] In addition, procedures which allow for replacement while maintaining the native aortic valve have been evaluated and appear to be satisfactory, potentially eliminating the need for chronic anticoagulation.[184,185]

Our group emphasises the importance of early diagnosis and follow-up, with serial measurement of the aortic root, and indexing this to document rates of relative growth, with respect to somatic growth. We institute β-blockade therapy early, and add inhibition of the angiotensin converting enzyme at the first sign of an increased rate of aortic dilation, and in patients with other risk factors such as a family history of aortic dissection. We review each patient carefully when the aortic root measures 45 mm to assess the need for surgical intervention, taking into consideration the specifics of each patient before deciding on the timing of elective repair.

Infantile Marfan Syndrome

An infantile variant of Marfan syndrome is seen on rare occasions. The skeletal and ocular manifestations are similar to the adult forms, but the cardiovascular features are distinct.[186] There is marked myxomatous thickening and redundancy of the leaflets of the mitral and tricuspid valves, with elongation of the tendinous cords leading to severe valvar insufficiency. Morbidity and mortality are primarily related to mitral and tricuspid valvar disease, as opposed to aortic dissection and rupture as seen in the adult form.[187] Additionally, patients with the infantile syndrome frequently exhibit pulmonary emphysematous changes. Because the infantile syndrome carries a poor prognosis, it is important to differentiate it from the classic syndrome, which can occasionally be evident in a neonate. Neonates with the infantile syndrome present in congestive cardiac failure that responds poorly to conventional therapy. Death often occurs within the first 2 years of life, though surgical repair of mitral valvar disease at this age is feasible. A family history of Marfan syndrome is much less common in infants who present with severe cardiovascular symptoms early in life.[188] Most mutations resulting in the infantile syndrome occur between exons 24 and 32 in the fibrillin gene.

Loeys-Dietz Syndrome

Loeys-Dietz syndrome was first described in 2005 in a cohort of 10 families. It is characterised by hypertelorism, bifid uvula and/or cleft palate, and generalised arterial tortuosity with ascending aortic aneurysmal formation and dissection.[189] There is some phenotypical overlap with Marfan syndrome, but the hypertelorism, palatal involvement, and widespread arterial changes help to differentiate this from Marfan syndrome and other similar disorders. Recognition of this disease is critical, as early evaluation for aortic aneurysm formation may lead to operation at a young age. Because of the aggressive nature of root dilation, replacement is recommended at diameters of 40 mm in adults and at even smaller diameters in children.[190]

Homocystinuria

Homocystinuria is an autosomal recessive disorder usually due to deficiency of cystathionine synthase, an enzyme needed for the metabolism of methionine. Affected patients have a bodily habitus similar to those with Marfan syndrome, albeit that their joints usually demonstrate restricted mobility. Cognitive deficits are also common. The primary cardiac complication is that of atherosclerotic disease, which often occurs by adolescence. Endothelial dysfunction contributes to the arterial complications and produces an increased risk for myocardial infarction.[191] Vitamin B_6 helps to reduce levels of homocysteine in approximately half of patients, and this, along with supplementation of vitamin B_{12} and folic acid, forms the mainstay of therapy.

NEUROMUSCULAR DISEASES

Muscular Dystrophies

Duchenne's Muscular Dystrophy

Duchenne's muscular dystrophy is an X-linked recessive disease. Because of this, it almost always afflicts males. Its incidence in male children is calculated at between 13 and 33 cases for each 100,000 live births. Since females with Turner syndrome have only one X chromosome, they too can inherit the disease, and it is seen rarely in this setting. The disease is due to a defect in the gene encoding dystrophin. Dystrophin helps to form a complex which stabilises the sarcolemmal membrane during contraction. While the exact mechanism for muscle degeneration has not been elucidated, abnormal nitric oxide regulation, abnormal sarcolemmal fragility, and increased susceptibility to oxidative stress are felt to play important roles.[192]

The earliest symptoms are clumsiness in walking, a tendency to fall, and an inability to run. Those with the disease also have difficulty in climbing stairs and getting up from the floor. Clinical onset is usually manifested before 4 years of age, and the diagnosis is usually made around 6 years of age. Deterioration is continuous. Most are unable to walk by the age of 10 years. Life expectancy is increasing owing to improved medical therapies, including nocturnal ventilation, early and aggressive management of cardiomyopathy, and perhaps the use of corticosteroids.[193] Muscular weakness and atrophy initially affect the proximal muscle groups of the upper limbs. Involvement of the legs extends from the quadriceps and gluteal muscles to the anterior tibial muscles. Weakness later affects other muscle groups. More power is generally retained in the distal muscles. Slight facial weakness occurs in the late stages. Scapular winging is also a later phenomenon. Muscular hypertrophy of the calves, masticatory muscles, and deltoids is followed by a pseudohypertrophic phase of fatty replacement. Tendon reflexes are lost in the weak muscles. Contractures of the calves and flexor muscles of the hip develop around the age of 8 years. Contractures appear in the hips, knees, elbows, and wrist when the patients are confined to wheelchairs. Severe spinal and thoracic deformities are seen late in the disease. Kyphoscoliosis is common. These result from disuse and abnormal posture. Generalised decalcification of the bones leads to frequent pathological fractures.

Myocardial involvement is common. It is uncertain at what stage it begins, since the physical incapacity limits its manifestation. The heart can be involved from an early age, and in ambulatory patients, subclinical disease may become symptomatic with exercise. In non-ambulatory patients, a resting tachycardia,[194] decreased heart rate variability,[195] echocardiographic evidence of diastolic dysfunction,[196] and myocardial strain changes on magnetic resonance imaging[197] may help to alert the clinician to subclinical myocardial involvement so that medical therapy can be initiated. The roles of cardiac troponins and brain natriuretic peptide are also being evaluated in the assessment of these patients.[198] The cardiac dysfunction is progressive, ultimately resulting in a dilated cardiomyopathy, and the benefits of early medical therapy are controversial. Some advocate early use of afterload reduction therapy,[199,200] but others have shown a benefit only when afterload reduction is combined with β-blockade.[201]

There is a distinctive electrocardiographic pattern in from half to nine-tenths of patients. This includes tall R waves over the right precordial leads with increased R:S amplitude ratios, together with narrow and deep Q waves in the limb and left precordial leads. Female carriers may also have the abnormal electrocardiogram.[202] These findings correspond to pathological observations. There is fatty and fibrous tissue replacement of the myocardium, with selective scarring of the posterolateral wall of the left ventricle and, sometimes, involvement of the posterolateral papillary muscle. Conduction abnormalities are also frequently seen. Among these are prolonged intra-atrial conduction, right bundle branch block, a superior QRS axis, and a short PR interval. Histological studies of the conduction system show multifocal areas of fibrosis, vacuolisation and fatty infiltration.[203] The echocardiogram reveals impairment of both systolic and diastolic function. The thickness of the left ventricular wall is decreased, and this is not related to physical inactivity. The end-diastolic and end-systolic dimensions of the left ventricle increase as systolic function deteriorates.

The diagnosis is made from the clinical characteristics, the high levels of activity of creatine kinase, and biopsy of the skeletal muscles. Creatine kinase activity is from 100 to 300 times the normal when the patients are aged from 1 to 5 years. Other muscle enzymes, like aldolase, glutamic oxalic transaminase, lactic dehydrogenase, and pyruvate kinase are also grossly elevated. The levels of creatine kinase diminish later in the disease, but still remain well above normal limits. Muscle biopsy shows scattered hyaline fibres with active muscular necrosis and regeneration. There is splitting of the muscle fibres, with fatty replacement. The nucleuses are of varied size. The muscle fascicles also become surrounded by perimysial and endomysial connective tissue. Electromyography reveals a decrease in the mean action potential voltage and its duration. An increase in the number of polyphasic potentials is also seen.

Careful general medical management is critical. Since bedrest is harmful, regular physical activity and exercise are to be encouraged. Avoidance of obesity is an important general measure, along with prevention of muscular contractures by passive stretching. Because of the risks of anaesthesia and immobilisation, the benefit from major orthopaedic procedures must be carefully considered. Prevention of scoliosis and thoracic deformities in the wheelchair phase help to avoid respiratory impairment and slow the deterioration of respiratory function. Death is usually from respiratory infections and insufficiency, and cardiac failure or arrhythmias. Detection of carriers is important for appropriate genetic counselling. More than half the carriers can be identified by their elevated levels of creatine kinase, by electromyography and by muscle biopsy. The analysis of the pedigree is particularly useful. Novel treatments for this myopathy are actively being investigated. They include gene therapy,[204] use of inhibitors of proteases,[205] membrane stabilisers,[206] and transplantation of the muscle precursor cells.[207]

Childhood Limb-girdle Muscular Dystrophy

The childhood limb-girdle muscular dystrophies are a heterogeneous group of genetic muscular disorders. At least 17 different types have been described. They can be inherited in either an autosomal dominant or recessive fashion, with 7 genetic defects now identified in the dominant forms, and 11 in the recessive forms. The age at onset is variable, but symptoms generally appear between 5 and 10 years of age. Weakness of the pelvic and shoulder muscles predominates. The disease is slowly progressive, the patients often becoming unable to walk by their twenties. The disease is first suspected when weakness of the limb girdles becomes apparent, although Duchenne's and Becker's muscular dystrophy must be ruled out. An elevated level of creatine kinase will not differentiate between this entity and the dystrophinopathies. This can be done through analysis of the dystrophin gene, and by examination of a muscle biopsy. Various forms of the disease affect the heart. Those with the so-called 1B variant, produced by a mutation in the lamin A/C gene, frequently develop arrhythmias which can be lethal and which may require placement of an implantable defibrillator. Atrioventricular block can also occur, necessitating placement of a pacemaker.[208] This disorder can also result in a dilated cardiomyopathy.

Those with the 2I variant, caused by a defect in the gene encoding the fukutin-related protein, may develop a dilated cardiomyopathy by the third decade. Evidence of arrhythmias is not seen.[209] The precise role of the fukutin-related protein is unknown, but it may play a role in the glycosylation of muscle membrane proteins.

Myotonic Muscular Dystrophy (Steinert Disease)

The involvement of systemic tissues, together with the presence of myotonia and muscular atrophy, separates myotonic muscular dystrophy from the other muscular dystrophies. It has a high incidence, calculated at 13.5 per 100,000 live births. Onset is usually between 20 and 50 years of age, but many cases are clinically apparent during childhood. It is due to an expansion of a CTG trinucleotide repeat on the q arm of chromosome 19.[210] It is transmitted in an autosomal dominant fashion and demonstrates genetic anticipation. Myotonia is the presenting clinical feature in one-third of cases. Others present with weakness of the hands, foot drop, or a tendency to fall. The heart may occasionally become involved prior to diagnosis of the neuromuscular disorder. The facial, masticatory, sternomastoid, forearm, anterior tibial and peroneal muscles are those first affected by weakness. Later it extends to neighbouring muscle groups. The typical facies are characterised by lack of facial expression, and difficulty in closing the eyes and moving the mouth. Ptosis and dysarthria are frequent. Myotonia is often limited to the tongue, forearms and hands, but it may be generalised. The tendon reflexes in the affected muscle groups are reduced.

Cataracts are present in almost all those affected. Impaired pulmonary vital capacity and maximum breathing capacity are common. Abnormal contractions of the oesophagus are thought to be the cause of dysphagia and pulmonary aspiration. Testicular atrophy, diabetes mellitus, increased metabolism of immunoglobulin G with low levels in the serum, progressive dementia, and subnormal intelligence are frequent associations. Cardiac involvement is common and manifests with conduction defects and arrhythmias. First-degree atrioventricular block is commonly seen, and this may progress to complete heart block requiring implantation of a pacemaker.[211] No relationship exists between the degree of involvement of the cardiac and the skeletal muscles. Chest radiography will show the associated deformities of the bony thorax, together with elevated hemidiaphragms. The cardiac silhouette is normal. Death from cardiac involvement is almost always caused by complete atrioventricular block or ventricular tachycardia. It is very rarely caused by myocardial failure.

The most common abnormalities in the electrocardiogram are low amplitudes of the P wave, atrioventricular block of any degree, right and left bundle branch block, abnormal Q waves, and changes in the ST segment and T wave. It is believed that regional myocardial dystrophy is responsible for the abnormal Q waves.[212] Rhythm disturbances include sinus brachycardia, premature atrial beats, atrial fibrillation, atrial flutter, ventricular premature beats and ventricular tachycardia. Four-fifths of the patients have electrophysiological evidence of disease of the atrioventricular conduction axis. A further one-fifth have evidence of intra-atrial conduction disturbances.[213] Disease of the atrioventricular conduction axis progresses with time. A correlative study revealed fibrosis of the right and left bundle branches and fatty infiltration and degeneration around the atrioventricular node, which corresponded accurately with the electrocardiographic and electrophysiological evaluation performed during life.[186]

Mitral valvar prolapse is frequently associated with myotonic muscular dystrophy and is diagnosed echocardiographically. It is present in approximately one-third of patients. There is no relationship, however, between mitral valvar prolapse and the arrhythmias. Systolic and diastolic function are normal. Normal ejection fractions at rest are recorded with radionuclide angiography. Some patients fail to show an increase with exercise. Apical hypokinesia may be present but is of doubtful significance. Careful clinical examination and a high degree of suspicion are required for an early diagnosis. Electromyography and muscle biopsy are useful techniques, as is examination for cataracts using a slit lamp. Cardiological evaluation is required in all patients because of the frequent association of cardiac disease. The disease shows progressive deterioration, with physical incapacity usually occurring 15 to 20 years after the onset of muscular symptoms. Death is usually from respiratory infections, aspiration, cardiac arrhythmias, or anaesthetic complications. There is no specific treatment for the condition. Active exercise and control of weight are important general therapeutic measures. Systemic complications are treated as they arise. Myotonia is relieved by the use of procainamide or phenytoin. Caution must be exerted, however, since procainamide exacerbates pre-existing disturbances of conduction. Electrophysiological studies are warranted in symptomatic patients presenting with syncope or presyncope. A ventricular pacemaker is needed when there are significant abnormalities in the formation or conduction of the cardiac impulse. Myotonic muscular dystrophy appears and progresses during early adult life in the majority of those affected. In a proportion, however, the disease is present at birth. Such congenital cases are often treated as a separate entity. Indeed, as will be seen, they have a totally different presentation and clinical picture. In the fullness of time, they come to resemble the adult form.

The congenital form is characterised by bilateral facial weakness, hypotonia, and mental retardation with delayed motor and speech development. Neonatal respiratory distress is very frequent. Such infants have a high incidence of feeding difficulties owing to muscle weakness. Talipes are a common association. Clinical myotonia is absent but can be demonstrated electromyographically. The adult features of the disease appear during late childhood and adolescence. Cardiac involvement takes the form of a dilated cardiomyopathy. Non-specific electrocardiographic abnormalities appear with progression of the disease. Mortality occurs in the neonatal period as a result of respiratory distress. Beyond this time, there is a tendency to improve, only for the patients to deteriorate as the adult characteristics of the disease appear. The condition is transmitted by the mother. Her clinical involvement has often failed previously to be noted.

Autosomal Dominant Scapuloperoneal Myopathy

Scapuloperoneal myopathy is a very rare form of muscular dystrophy. It is possible to recognise two distinct groups according to the age of onset. They share an autosomal dominant form of inheritance, and involve the same muscle groups. Weakness and atrophy affect the neck, shoulder girdle, and upper arm muscles, together with the tibial and peroneal muscles in the legs. Foot drop and an awkward gait are frequent early symptoms. Deep tendon reflexes are commonly absent. Levels of creatine kinase are slightly elevated in the serum. Electromyography and muscle biopsy show the changes common to muscular dystrophies.

The group of patients with early onset generally present under the age of 10 years. In these, the disease takes a rapid course. Patients develop early contractures and are severely incapacitated by their late teens. They frequently have clinical and electrocardiographic signs of a dilated cardiomyopathy with congestive cardiac failure.[214] Those patients having a late onset present over the age of 40 years, and their clinical course is slow. They seldom develop contractures. Cardiac involvement, usually late, could well be a result of ischaemic heart disease.[215]

Becker's Muscular Dystrophy

Becker's muscular dystrophy is one of the most frequent types of muscular dystrophy. It is inherited in X-linked recessive fashion. The incidence is of the order of 3 to 6 per 100,000 male births. The muscular groups involved are very similar to those in Duchenne's muscular dystrophy. The peroneal and anterior tibial muscles are also affected in the Becker variant. The facial muscles are not involved. Calf hypertrophy and muscle cramps are frequent early symptoms. Club feet are often seen. Contractures appear in the final stages, and scoliosis is rare. Developmental delay is uncommon. The onset of the symptoms is between 5 and 15 years of age, with inability to walk being present by the third decade, and death occurring in the fifth. The individual range, however, is very wide. The diagnosis is primarily clinical. Activity of creatine kinase in the serum is 25 to 200 times the normal. The electromyogram and the muscle biopsy are nonspecific but help to rule out other conditions.

Cardiac abnormalities are infrequent in childhood but are almost always present in some form by the onset of the fourth decade.[216] Electrocardiographic abnormalities are common and include resting tachycardia, interventricular conduction delay, and Q waves in leads II, III, and aVF, suggesting damage to the lateral wall of the left ventricle.[217] Heart rate variability is also decreased and may indicate a risk for sudden death.[218] Dilated cardiomyopathy is seen, and the risk of ventricular dysfunction increases with age, though many patients are asymptomatic from a cardiac standpoint, exhibiting abnormalities only on the electrocardiogram or echocardiogram.[219] Transplantation of the heart for severe left ventricular systolic dysfunction is a well-established palliative option.[220]

Facioscapulohumeral Muscular Dystrophy (Landouzy-Dejerine Syndrome)

Fascioscapulohumeral muscular dystrophy is inherited in an autosomal dominant fashion. It has an incidence of approximately 5 per 100,000 live births. Facial and shoulder weakness generally develop in the second or third decade and progress very slowly. Patients with severe forms of this disease will occasionally present early in life, and progression is then rapid. Characteristically, there are no facial lines and the eyelids are very weak. Winging of the scapulas is seen when the arms are abducted, and there is a marked thoracolumbar lordosis. Affected muscles include the neck flexors, the serrate and pectoral muscles, biceps and triceps in the upper limbs, the hip flexors, and the anterior tibial muscles. In the later stages, the quadriceps and sartorius in the lower limbs are also affected. Retinal vasculopathy is also seen frequently. The levels of creatine kinase in the serum are normal or else only mildly elevated. The precise molecular mechanism for expression has not been elucidated, but patients are known to have a large deletion involving the q arm of chromosome 4. No gene has been identified within this region, and so various hypotheses have been presented to explain the mechanism whereby this deletion induces clinical disease.[221]

Ventricular function is not affected. Supraventricular tachycardia has been reported with a frequency higher than that of the general population.[222] Sinus nodal dysfunction, abnormal atrioventricular nodal or infranodal conduction, and easily inducible atrial fibrillation or flutter have also been reported in around one-quarter of patients studied.[223]

Emery-Dreifuss Muscular Dystrophy

Emery-Dreifuss muscular dystrophy typically presents between 5 and 15 years of age. It can be inherited in an X-linked recessive fashion, or in autosomal dominant or autosomal recessive forms. The biceps and triceps are more severely affected than the deltoid muscle. The peroneals are more involved than the proximal musculature of the legs. Contractures generally develop at the elbows, posterior cervical muscles, and Achilles tendon. Pseudohypertrophy is absent. Levels of creatine kinase are from 3 to 10 times above normal. Progression is very slow, and the physical limitations are minimal. There is normal intellectual function.

The X-linked form is due to a defect in the gene encoding emerin, a nuclear envelope protein which plays a role in the regulation of many cellular and nucleolar processes. Its role in the pathogenesis of muscle damage remains to be elucidated. The autosomal dominant form is due to defects in the lamin A/C gene, similar to variant 1B of limb-girdle muscular dystrophy. Again, the role of lamin A/C mutations in the development of the myopathy is not clear. The recessive form is also due to defects in the gene encoding lamins A and C.[224] How and why defects in the same gene can cause dominant and recessive forms of the disease remains to be discerned.

Cardiac involvement is often manifested by atrial arrhythmias and atrioventricular block. Any degree of atrioventricular block can be present, and a slow junctional escape rhythm is common. Severe sinus bradycardia or sinus arrest is seen and may require implantation of a pacemaker because of the increased risk of sudden death.[225] Atrial paralysis, with the absence of P waves and an inability to electrically pace the atrium, is seen. Ventricular function is often normal, but progressive left ventricular dysfunction occurs due to fibrous infiltration of the myocardium.[226] Cardiac transplantation has been employed for end-stage disease.[227] Those with bradycardia may have hypertrophied and dilated left ventricles, probably as a compensatory physiological response. Electrophysiological studies show prolonged HV intervals and, on some occasions, a complete absence of the His potential. This finding, together with the very slow junctional escape rhythms, suggests that the myopathic process extends into the atrioventricular conduction axis. The high risk of sudden death in this variety of muscular dystrophy makes early recognition important, since insertion of a ventricular pacemaker in patients with bradycardia will improve survival.

Centronuclear Myopathy

This uncommon muscular disorder is characterised by ptosis, strabismus, generalised muscle wasting, and weakness, together with absent or reduced deep tendon reflexes.

Developmental delay and dysarthria are common. A dilated cardiomyopathy has been occasionally observed, and cardiac transplantation has been performed.[228] Patients have a prolonged PR interval and a superior axis on the electrocardiogram. The diagnosis is based on clinical findings, raised levels of creatine kinase in blood, evidence of a myopathy on electromyography, and a typical histological picture. This consists of central location of the nucleus, with variation in the diameter of the muscle fibres and a tendency for predominance of type 1 fibres. Inheritance is variable. The X-linked form is usually the most severe and involves the gene encoding myotubularin. An autosomal recessive form seems to have a milder course, though patients still present in childhood. The autosomal dominant form is milder, with patients reaching adulthood before the onset of symptoms.

Nemaline Myopathy

The nemaline myopathies are so named because muscle specimens demonstrate rods within the myocytes. This group of clinically heterogeneous disorders can result from defects involving actin, troponin, myosin, or tropomyosin. While the skeletal muscles are predominantly involved, cases of hypertrophic and dilated cardiomyopathy are becoming increasingly evident. The main focus is on the α-actin gene, ACTA1, in which numerous defects have been described.[229] Patients can have a very mild course of skeletal muscle weakness or severe neonatal disease leading to respiratory failure. Hypertrophic cardiomyopathy is more commonly seen,[230] but dilated forms of cardiomyopathy have also been reported.[231]

Friedreich's Ataxia

Friedreich's ataxia is a rare spinocerebellar neuromyelopathy occurring in approximately 1 to 2 per 40,000 persons. The disease is inherited in an autosomal recessive fashion, and most cases are due to homozygosity for an expanded GAA triplet on chromosome 9q13.[232] This gene encodes frataxin, a precursor protein which may be involved in the maturation and assembly of iron and sulphur proteins of the mitochondria and cytosol.[233] Children present around the age of 6 years. The most frequent early symptom is an abnormal gait. Neurological signs include the ataxic gait, absent tendon reflexes, incoordination, and a positive Romberg test.[234] Weakness and muscular atrophy of the legs are common, as are dysarthria and loss of vibration and positional sense and extensor plantar responses. Some patients have nystagmus. The presence of brisk tendon reflexes makes the diagnosis of Friedreich's ataxia very unlikely. Skeletal involvement is common, with club feet and scoliosis among the most frequent manifestations. Apart from the clinical aspects of the disease, nerve conduction studies are essential to support the diagnosis. Motor conduction velocity is normal, and sensory conduction is absent or markedly reduced. Since clinical, electrocardiographic, and radiographic examination of the heart are non-specific for the evaluation of cardiac involvement, an echocardiogram is necessary in every patient.

The heart is involved in a very high percentage, and cardiac symptoms are an integral part of the clinical spectrum of the disease. Most usually, the heart exhibits a symmetrical, concentric, and slowly progressive hypertrophic cardiomyopathy. Cardiac involvement may occasionally precede the onset of neurological manifestations.[235] Cardiac symptoms are present in approximately one-third of the patients, and consist mainly of exertional dyspnoea, palpitations, and angina. Clinical findings of cardiac disease are not present in every case. When they are, they include systolic murmurs at the left sternal border and apex, together with third and fourth heart sounds. The pulse may have a rapid upstroke. Evaluation of the severity of disease by physical examination is often difficult because of the presence of scoliosis and the lack of consistent cardiovascular signs. Interestingly, the degree of cardiac involvement appears to correlate with the size of the GAA repeat of the smaller allele, or with the mean size of the repeats in both alleles.[236]

Pathological studies reveal cardiac dilation with ventricular hypertrophy. Histologically, there is a degeneration of myocardial cells with myocardial fibrosis. Intracellular granular deposits of calcium and iron are seen. It is hypothesised that iron-catalysed mitochondrial damage may lead to the pathologic findings in the myocardium.[237] Electrocardiographic changes are present in over two-thirds of patients, and they progress in relation to the duration of the disease. The most frequent changes involve the ST segments and T waves. These are non-specific and are presumably caused by repolarisation disturbances from the underlying myocardial fibrosis. Signs of ventricular hypertrophy are also frequent, and right- or left-axis deviation is common. Arrhythmias are not frequent. When present they include supraventricular and ventricular premature beats, supraventricular tachycardia, atrial flutter and atrial fibrillation.[238]

The presence of scoliosis makes radiographic evaluation of the heart difficult, albeit that its size is usually normal. Most patients have an abnormal echocardiogram. The most common anomalies reflect the presence of symmetrical concentric hypertrophic cardiomyopathy. There is an increase in left ventricular mural and septal thickness. Asymmetrical septal hypertrophy is seen on occasion.[239] Impaired left ventricular function has also been shown echocardiographically and may be the end-stage of the cardiomyopathic process, as reduced fractional shortening of the left ventricle is common. The systolic function of the posterior wall is more severely affected than that of the septum. Abnormal diastolic function may antedate systolic abnormalities. A constant feature is the delay in mitral valvar opening.

The clinical course is marked by steadily progressive deterioration. Cardiac failure, which appears late in the course of the disease, has a poor prognosis and is often a pre-terminal event. Most patients die from cardiac causes. Cardiac failure accounts for half of the deaths. Cardiac arrhythmias and respiratory complications are the other major causes of death. While conventional methods for treating hypertrophic and dilated cardiomyopathy are frequently employed, newer therapeutic options for patients with Friedreich's ataxia have come to light in recent years. Idebenone, a free-radical scavenger, was tested under the hypothesis that iron overload leads to damage of iron-sulfur cluster-containing enzymes, which may lead to the damage seen in the myocardium.[240] Though the treatment remains somewhat controversial and is not universally accepted, several small trials show a consistent benefit in terms of reduction of cardiac mass and improvement in function.[241,242]

Arthrogryposis Multiplex Congenita

Arthrogryposis multiplex congenita presents with joint contractures at birth in at least two different areas of the body. A typical presentation includes equinovarus deformities of the feet, abducted hips, incompletely extended knees and elbows, pronated forearms, and claw hands. The majority of those affected have a neurogenic cause with patchy loss of anterior horn cells, though some cases are caused by primary myopathic disorders. They may result from environmental factors, or may demonstrate a familial propensity. The heart is rarely involved. A report of the myopathic form of arthrogryposis multiplex congenita revealed congenital cardiac disease in one-quarter.[243] These cases resulted from consanguineous matings, and 5 of 6 with congenital cardiac malformations resulted from one pairing.[244] Patency of the arterial duct, congenital aortic stenosis, and mitral stenosis have been reported.[221,245]

Hereditary Motor and Sensory Neuropathy (Peroneal Muscular Atrophy, Charcot-Marie-Tooth Disease)

The hereditary motor and sensory neuropathies are a diverse group of disorders typically inherited in an autosomal or X-linked dominant fashion. Links to defects in connexins and other Schwann cell proteins are well described.[246] They are predominantly a motor neuropathy producing atrophy and weakness of the distal muscles. This determines the typical likeness of the legs to an inverted bottle. Bilateral club foot is a frequent association. The hand and forearm muscles may also be involved. There is a decrease or loss of the deep tendon reflexes. Electromyographic studies show slowing of nerve conduction velocity or signs of denervation. The cardiac involvement has classically been related to supraventricular arrhythmias and conduction system abnormalities. Sick sinus syndrome, right bundle branch block, complete heart block, Wolff-Parkinson-White syndrome, atrial fibrillation, and atrial flutter have been described.[247,248] It has been postulated that there is a primary degeneration of the conduction system rather than changes secondary to a cardiomyopathy.[249] In addition to arrhythmias, left ventricular hypertrabeculation or noncompaction has been reported in a patient with the type 1A variant of Charcot-Marie-Tooth disease, and a duplication defect on chromosome 17 involving the peripheral myelin protein 22.[250] The Roussy-Lévy syndrome is a phenotypic variant of the type 1A, and shares many features with this disease.[251] Dilated cardiomyopathy has been reported.[252]

Spinal Muscular Atrophy Type III (Juvenile Spinal Muscular Atrophy, Kugelberg-Welander Syndrome)

Juvenile spinal muscular atrophy appears in childhood or adolescence. Initially it is manifested by weakness and atrophy of the proximal limb muscles, which is later followed by distal disease. The usual presentation is with difficulty in walking, climbing stairs and lifting the arms. Fasciculation is seen in half those affected. The clinical course is slowly progressive. There is evidence from electromyography and muscle biopsy to indicate disease of the lower motor neurons. Some patients have an associated dilated cardiomyopathy, though this may be secondary to associated respiratory disturbances.[253] Disturbances of rhythm are very frequent and include atrial premature beats, atrial fibrillation, atrial flutter, and advanced degrees of atrioventricular block. Some patients require the implantation of a pacemaker.[254] The electrocardiogram frequently shows a fine tremor on the isoelectric line, which represents fasciculations characteristic of this disease.[255] The syndrome is transmitted in autosomal recessive fashion and is due to defects in the survival motor neuron 1 gene.[256] The infantile form of spinal muscular atrophy, or Werdnig-Hoffman disease, is a lethal variant presenting with severe hypotonia and respiratory failure. Various congenital cardiac malformations have been reported in patients with this disease, but these are likely chance associations.[257,258]

Refsum Disease

Refsum disease is a rare neurological disorder due to the accumulation of phytanic acid in peroxisomes. Phytanic acid is a branched-chain fatty acid which is partially broken down by phytanoyl-CoA 2-hydroxylase. Many cases of the disease are due to defects in the gene encoding this enzyme.[259] This leads to accumulation of phytanic acid in blood and tissues. Symptoms appear in the first and second decade of life, the initial presentation being weakness, unsteady gait and night blindness. These patients have a diagnostic tetrad made up of retinitis pigmentosa, peripheral polyneuropathy with diminished or absent deep tendon reflexes, cerebellar ataxia, and high levels of protein in cerebrospinal fluid without pleocytosis. Other frequent signs are neural deafness, anosmia, nystagmus, and abnormalities of the pupils. The heart is rarely affected. Conduction abnormalities, especially advanced degrees of atrioventricular block requiring pacemaker therapy, are well known. Cardiomyopathy is a rare association.[260] Diets low in phytanic acid produce clinical improvement. Complete recovery is rarely obtained, but treatment will slow the progression of the disease. The addition of plasmapheresis to the diet reduces the levels of phytanic acid more rapidly.[261]

DEFICIENCIES

Selenium

Selenium is a trace element that is an essential component of glutathione peroxidase. The enzyme removes organic hydroperoxides from the cell. Absence of selenium, possibly associated with absence of vitamin E, permits damage to the cell membrane by lipid peroxides. Deficiency of selenium, also known as Keshan disease, affects children living in areas with a poor content of selenium in the soil or those having a poor diet.[262] It gives rise to an endemic cardiomyopathy that affects children between 1 and 9 years of age living in an area extending from the northeast to the southwest of China where the content of selenium in the soil and food is very low. It has also been reported with nutritional changes related to bariatric surgery[263] and with total parenteral nutrition.[264] The incidence has been significantly reduced by supplementing oral sodium selenite in the diet, with no adverse side effects. Once fully developed, the cardiomyopathy is irreversible.[265] Early recognition of the cause of the cardiomyopathy, with timely institution of supplementation with selenium, can bring about resolution.[266] Histopathological features of the heart are areas of myocytic loss with replacement fibrosis in the subepicardial surface of the ventricles.[267]

Carnitine

L-Carnitine, or hydroxy-trimethylammonium butyrate, is an essential cofactor in the transfer of long-chain fatty acids across the inner mitochondrial membrane. Depletion of carnitine blocks the mitochondrial oxidation of fatty acids and leads to cytoplasmic accumulation of lipids. Cardiac and skeletal muscles use fatty acids as their main substrate and, therefore, are very sensitive to carnitine.[268] Primary syndromes due to deficiency of carnitine are divided into myopathic and systemic forms. Patients with muscular deficiency present with progressive weakness and are thought to have abnormal transport of carnitine into skeletal muscle. They have normal levels of carnitine in the plasma, but low concentrations in the muscles. Systemic deficiency presents early in life, with encephalopathy, hypoglycaemia, liver failure, and cardiomyopathy.[269] Muscle weakness and developmental delay are common. Hypotheses for the cause of systemic deficiency include defects in synthesis, renal handling, gastrointestinal absorption and cellular transport, and excessive degradation. At least some cases have been demonstrated to be due to defects in the carnitine transporter gene.[270] Accumulation of triglycerides in muscle often occurs, since fatty acids are not transported effectively into the mitochondrions for oxidation. Patients often have low concentrations of carnitine in the plasma and tissues, though this is not a sensitive marker for the disease.

Cardiomyopathy has frequently been reported in association with either systemic or myopathic deficiency. Many patients are in cardiac failure when they come to medical attention.[271] The electrocardiogram is non-specific, with signs of left ventricular hypertrophy. Very tall and peaked T waves, like those seen in hyperkalaemia, have been described.[272] The echocardiogram reveals left ventricular and left atrial dilation with signs of poor left ventricular function. The last can also be demonstrated by nuclear angiography. Cardiac failure responds poorly to conventional therapy. Endocardial fibroelastosis as a result of systemic deficiency has been described.[273] The diagnosis is dependent on the demonstration of low levels of carnitine in the tissues or blood, though normal levels do not rule out the disorder. Muscle biopsy shows large amounts of lipids in type I muscle fibres and abnormal mitochondrions. The disease is usually fatal without treatment. Oral L-carnitine produces clinical improvement in many patients.[274] Others fail to respond to therapy.[275] Diarrhoea is the main side effect. Diets with only 20% of calories from fat are also useful in long-term treatment. Carnitine deficiency is inherited in autosomal recessive fashion.

Thiamine (Beriberi)

Thiamine, or vitamin B_1, is a water-soluble vitamin that is absorbed from the small intestine. In its active form of thiamine pyrophosphate, it is an essential coenzyme in the metabolism of pyruvate and in the transketolase reaction. Deficiency produces a disease known as beriberi, which has been related to diets consisting of polished rice in oriental societies, and to alcoholism in occidental ones. Classically, the disease has been divided into two major types. In dry beriberi, the patients have peripheral neuropathy with varied disorders of sensation, sometimes amounting to anaesthesia, muscle weakness and atrophy, reduced deep tendon reflexes, fatigue, and difficulty in concentrating. In contrast, in wet beriberi, where the presenting features are a high output cardiac failure with peripheral oedema, the patients have diminished peripheral vascular resistance as a result of muscular arteriolar vasodilation, a wide pulse pressure, and a warm skin. The mechanism leading to a reduction of peripheral vascular resistance is believed to be directly related to the lack of thiamine, since after treatment this parameter returns rapidly to normal.[276] Despite high cardiac output, oliguria is present owing to reduction of renal blood flow and glomerular filtration rate. Increased jugular venous pressure results from peripheral venoconstriction and from an increase in the circulating blood volume.[277] Cutaneous vasoconstriction becomes evident with progression of cardiac failure, and this results in cold hands and peripheral cyanosis. It is not clear whether the cardiac failure results from primary myocardial involvement or whether it is secondary to the vascular changes. In some patients, the additional toxic effects of alcohol make this differentiation very difficult. Histological studies of the heart have shown hydropic degeneration, interstitial and perivascular oedema, and fibrosis and necrosis of myocardial tissue.[278]

An acute variant of the disease with vascular collapse, metabolic acidosis, and variable cardiac output is known as Shoshin beriberi. Patients present in severe biventricular failure. They have renal dysfunction leading to metabolic acidosis. There is a high arterial saturation of oxygen secondary to tachypnoea, which contrasts with peripheral cyanosis caused by cutaneous vasoconstriction.[279] Cardiac catheterisation reveals increased right and left atrial pressures and a low peripheral vascular resistance.[280] Early diagnosis is necessary because patients die rapidly if left untreated. The presentation varies with age. Affected infants are very rarely seen in Western countries. It appears in nursing babies of thiamine-deficient mothers around 1 to 4 months of age. Sometimes the clinical onset is sudden. Acute congestive cardiac failure may then appear in apparently healthy babies following a minor illness. In others, signs and symptoms mimicking meningitis are seen. Administration of thiamine produces a rapid recovery.

Beyond infancy, the dry form is seen in children fed polished rice. Signs and symptoms are of peripheral neuropathy. Cardiovascular involvement and oedema are rare. When presenting in adolescence, alcohol consumption must be considered in addition to poor dietary intake. Patients present with malaise, fatigue, palpitations, dyspnoea, and peripheral oedema. They have an increased jugular venous pressure, a high pulse pressure, a gallop rhythm with non-specific apical systolic murmurs, and a loud pulmonary component to the second sound. There is cardiomegaly on the chest radiograph in half, and the electrocardiogram shows non-specific T wave changes. Haemodynamic studies reveal high cardiac index, stroke index, and circulating blood volume and low peripheral vascular resistance.

Clinical suspicion and a dietary history of poor thiamine intake and/or excessive consumption of alcohol are necessary for diagnosis. Patients with beriberi exhibit low transketolase activity in erythrocytes, which increases after the administration of thiamine pyrophosphate. Patients have low levels of thiamine in blood and urine. An acute response to intravenous thiamine during cardiac catheterisation, with an increase in peripheral vascular resistance and a reduction in cardiac output, has also been used as a diagnostic test.[281]

Beriberi is a treatable cause of cardiac failure. There is a rapid response to administration of thiamine. Parenteral therapy is necessary in extreme cases. Administration can later be continued orally. Bed rest, oxygen, diuretics, and digitalis are useful therapeutic adjuncts. Shoshin beriberi is a medical emergency that is fatal without aggressive medical management. Correction of the acidosis with sodium bicarbonate is essential, together with the measures already described. A balanced diet, with an adequate intake of meat, fresh vegetables and whole grains, will supply the daily requirements of thiamine and prevent beriberi.

DEPOSITIONS

The major disease caused by disordered deposition that arises in childhood is haemochromatosis. The other depositions, such as amyloidosis, do not usually produce difficulties prior to adulthood.

Haemochromatosis

Haemochromatosis results from deposition of iron. It may be primary and hereditary, or secondary. Primary or hereditary haemochromatosis is a rare disease resulting from excessive absorption of iron from the diet. The normal rate of intestinal iron absorption is 1 to 2 mg per day, but this can increase when necessary. In patients with haemochromatosis, intestinal iron absorption can be as high as 8 to 10 mg per day. Also, most iron in the plasma is stored in macrophages, and in patients with haemochromatosis, macrophages more readily release their stores of iron. Intestinal absorption and macrophage release are under control of hepcidin, an antimicrobial peptide which is synthesised by the liver. Hepcidin acts to downregulate absorption and release through its degradation of ferroportin, a membrane protein critical for uptake and release of iron. Synthesis of hepcidin is regulated by multiple proteins in response to the need for and availability of iron. Thus, defects involving the hepcidin gene, the genes encoding its regulator proteins, or the ferroportin gene, can all lead to excessive uptake and release of iron, leading to deposition in the organs. These disorders are inherited in an autosomal recessive fashion. The specific gene affected determines the clinical phenotype.[282]

Secondary haemochromatosis is generally the result of excessive administration of iron through multiple blood transfusions in chronic transfusion-dependent non-haemorrhagic anaemias. The most frequent of these is β-thalassaemia. Each 250 mL of blood delivers approximately 200 mg of iron.[283] Cardiac dysfunction generally occurs after 100 units of blood have been transfused.[284] Though the primary and secondary diseases are quite different, the damaging effects of iron are similar. The excess iron in the tissues weakens the lysosomal membranes and produces damage to the cells.

Damage to organs due to primary haemochromatosis generally appears between 40 and 60 years of age, though those with the more rare juvenile form can exhibit symptoms much earlier. The secondary form may be clinically apparent in the second decade or earlier, depending on the frequency of transfusions. There is widespread deposition of iron in the liver, spleen, pancreas, gonads, skin and heart, which leads to the clinical manifestations. The classic triad consists of hepatic cirrhosis, bronze pigmentation of the skin, and diabetes mellitus. Splenomegaly is present in approximately half the patients with idiopathic haemochromatosis, and in virtually every patient with β-thalassaemia. Cardiac involvement results from excessive deposits of haemosiderin in the heart. This produces a dilated cardiomyopathy with cardiac failure. A restrictive cardiomyopathy has also been described.[285]

The heart is rusty-brown at postmortem, with dilation of all cardiac chambers. Concentration of iron is greater in the subepicardial part of the heart, therefore limiting the use of endomyocardial biopsies.[286] Iron in the form of haemosiderin initially adopts a perinuclear distribution and then extends peripherally as the amount of deposits increases. These are greater in the ventricles than in the atriums and the conduction tissues.[287]

Low-voltage QRS complexes are seen electrocardiographically with non-specific ST segments and T wave changes. A prolonged QT interval may be present. There may be evidence of right or left ventricular hypertrophy. Disturbances of rhythm are common and include atrial and ventricular premature contractions, supraventricular and ventricular tachycardias, and varying degrees of atrioventricular block. Cardiac enlargement and signs of cardiac failure, when present, are seen in the chest radiograph. Echocardiography shows increased left ventricular mural thickness, increased left ventricular and left atrial dimensions, and a reduction in fractional shortening and ejection fraction.[288]

Laboratory studies should include measurements of plasma iron, ferritin, and saturation of transferrin. These typically are elevated. Measurement of the content of iron in samples obtained by needle biopsy of the liver allows accurate estimations of total body iron. Cardiac failure is the cause of death in about one-third of the patients. Early onset of cardiac failure and ventricular arrhythmias presage a poor prognosis. Malignant hepatoma is an important late complication in older patients. Removal of iron by repeated venesection or by chelation with desferroxamine reverses all the cardiac manifestations except the disturbances of conduction.[289] Symptomatic heart block requires insertion of a pacemaker.

AUTOIMMUNE DISEASES

Juvenile Idiopathic Arthritis

Juvenile idiopathic arthritis is the most common form of chronic juvenile arthritis. It is typically characterised by the absence of positive serological tests. The aetiology is unknown, but HLA-B27 histocompatibility antigen is found in approximately one-quarter of patients. The disease is divided into several forms based upon the principal features and onset.

Patients with systemic-onset idiopathic arthritis, or Still's disease, frequently have a quotidian febrile pattern accompanied by an evanescent rash, hepatosplenomegaly, and generalised lymphadenopathy. Arthritis may or may not be present. Pleuritis with interstitial pulmonary disease is frequent. The most common cardiac manifestation is pericarditis.[290]

Polyarticular disease is characterised by symmetrical involvement of the wrist, knee, and ankle joints. The cervical spine is frequently affected. Systemic manifestations are of a milder nature. Rash, splenomegaly, and lymphadenopathy may be present.

The pauci-articular variety affects small children. The joints involved are the knees, ankles, elbows, or wrists. Systemic manifestations are infrequent. Such patients are at risk of blindness from iridocyclitis. This form has the best prognosis. Pericarditis is the most common form of cardiac involvement, though myocarditis can occur as well.[291] Pericarditis is best managed with anti-inflammatories and, when necessary, pericardiocentesis.

Systemic Sclerosis (Scleroderma)

Systemic sclerosis is a disorder of unknown aetiology resulting in tightening and induration of the skin. Visceral manifestations include gastrointestinal disease with dysphagia and reflux related to oesophageal dysmotility; renal disease with azotemia, proteinuria and hypertension; pulmonary disease with interstitial fibrosis and pulmonary vascular changes leading to pulmonary arterial hypertension; and cardiac disease with conduction disturbances, myocardial fibrosis, coronary arterial disease, and autonomic dysfunction.[292,293] Close monitoring for the development of pulmonary hypertension is required, as this remains an important cause of morbidity and mortality, affecting up to one-sixth of patients.[294] Treatment of this complication includes currently available agents aimed at reducing pulmonary vascular resistance, coupled with cyclophosphamide to address the pulmonary interstitial fibrosis.[295]

Takayasu's Arteritis

Takayasu's arteritis, also known as pulseless disease, is a chronic large vessel vasculitis primarily affecting the aorta and the proximal arteries supplying the head and neck, along with the proximal pulmonary arteries. Inflammation of the arterial walls leads to thickening, fibrosis, and ultimately stenosis with formation of thrombus. The disease frequently presents in adolescents or young adults with non-specific symptoms of activation of the inflammatory system. Consequently, the diagnosis may be delayed until more overt evidence of the disease is manifested. This can include reduced pulses, hypertension, vascular bruits and aortic valvar disease.[296] Treatment consists of immunosuppression with corticosteroids. When this is not effective, more aggressive cytotoxic drugs can be used, such as cyclophosphamide, methotrexate, or azathioprine.[297] Angioplasty or implantation of stents is sometimes necessary for severe stenoses unresponsive to medical management.

Polyarteritis Nodosa

Polyarteritis nodosa is a vasculitic syndrome affecting small- to medium-sized arteries, primarily in the kidney, skin, and gastrointestinal tract. The inflammation results in vessel mural necrosis with subsequent fibrosis, thrombosis, and microaneurysm formation. Myocarditis has also been reported.[298] This may be the cause of the left ventricular systolic dysfunction and mitral valvar regurgitation that are frequently seen.[299] Supportive care, coupled with immunomodulatory therapy, are the mainstays of treatment.

Systemic Lupus Erythematosus

Systemic lupus erythematosus is a generalised, progressive, multi-system connective tissue disease of unknown aetiology. During childhood, the mean age of onset is 12 years. Very rarely, is it present before the age of 5 years.[300] The cutaneous, osteoarticular, renal, haematopoietic, central nervous, pulmonary, and gastrointestinal systems are commonly affected. Cardiac involvement is also very frequent and can be present at any time during the course of the disease. The most common manifestations are pericarditis, myocarditis, Libman-Sacks endocarditis leading to valvar stenosis and/or incompetence, disturbances of rhythm, coronary arterial disease, and systemic and pulmonary hypertension. Any of these can lead to congestive cardiac failure, which carries a poor prognosis.[301] Deposition of immune complexes and complement activation have a major pathogenetic role in these lesions. Pericarditis is the most common cardiac manifestation. Up to three-quarters of patients have echocardiographic evidence of pericardial disease. Clinical involvement is seen in one-third, generally as acute pericarditis, which may have a recurrent nature. Serous effusions are common, and complement levels in the fluid are very low. Cases of chronic constrictive pericarditis and tamponade are rare.

Evidence of myocarditis can be seen in about half the patients at postmortem, but clinical involvement is generally silent. Dyspnoea is the most common symptom. The presence of a gallop rhythm, cardiomegaly on the chest radiograph, and ventricular dilation on the echocardiogram complete the clinical picture. The electrocardiogram is non-specific. T wave inversion, ventricular premature beats and first-degree atrioventricular block may all be present. In approximately half the patients, there are non-bacterial verrucous vegetations, so-called Libman-Sacks endocarditis. These are clumps of fibrin with lymphocytes and plasma cell infiltrates which are most frequently seen on the mitral and/or aortic valves. They measure from 0.1 to 4 mm in diameter. Fibrous tissue, which may later become calcified, appears during the process of healing, leading to valvar dysfunction. Mitral and aortic incompetence, and less frequently stenosis, are the most common lesions. Echocardiographic evaluation is a useful non-invasive method for assessment of valvar dysfunction. Doppler examination should increase the sensitivity of early detection of valve disease. The presence of Libman-Sacks vegetations predisposes to bacterial endocarditis. Peripheral embolism is rare. The coronary arteries can be affected by an acute inflammatory arteritic process or, less frequently in childhood, by atherosclerosis. Coronary arteritis can lead to aneurysmal dilation of the arteries, thrombosis, and myocardial infarction. This is an uncommon cause of death. Disturbances of rhythm and conduction are common. Atrial fibrillation or flutter may be seen during acute pericarditis, whereas ventricular ectopic beats and first-degree atrioventricular block are seen in the course of active myocarditis. Complete heart block may result from vasculitis of small vessels, and fibrosis of the conduction system has been described in adults. Systemic hypertension is very frequent. It is generally caused by lupus nephritis or by prolonged steroid therapy.

The revised criterions for the diagnosis of systemic lupus erythematosus require the presence of at least four of the following: malar rash; discoid rash; photosensitivity; oral ulcers; arthritis, pleuritis, or pericarditis; renal disorders such as proteinuria or cellular casts; neurological disorders such as seizures or psychosis; haematological disorders such as haemolytic anaemia, leucopenia, lymphopenia, or thrombocytopenia; immunological disorders such as positive lupus erythematosus cell preparations, antibodies against double-stranded DNA (anti-dsDNA) or Smith protein (anti-Sm), or antinuclear antibodies.[302] A revision to the immunological criterions was made in 1997 to include antiphospholipid and anticardiolipin antibodies.[303]

Long-term prognosis is variable. Boys seem to have a more severe form of the disease than girls. The most common causes of death are renal involvement and sepsis. Death from cardiac lesions is not frequent, but aggressive therapy is warranted when myocarditis is evident, as its course can be fulminant and lethal.[304] Corticosteroids are the basis of treatment. Immunosuppressive therapy with azathioprine or cyclophosphamide can be used as a supplement where there is no response to high doses of steroids or when there is severe renal or central nervous system involvement. Apart from this systemic form of therapy, the management of specific lesions does not differ from the patient without lupus erythematosus.

Neonatal lupus erythematosus is a rare variety of the systemic disease. It is frequently associated with maternal lupus. It is characterised by cutaneous lesions with or without congenital complete heart block and systemic manifestations.[305] Prolongation of the QT interval, sinus bradycardia, lower-grade heart block and dilated cardiomyopathy can also occur. Skin lesions develop within the first 3 months of life and occur mainly in areas exposed to light, thus suggesting photosensitivity. They consist of erythematous macules, papules or plaques that may exhibit the characteristics of discoid lupus, specifically, scaling, atrophy, follicular plugging, and telangiectasia. Later, they have residual hyper- or hypopigmentation and completely resolve within 12 months with minimal atrophy or scarring. Systemic manifestations include hepatosplenomegaly, anaemia, leucopenia and thrombocytopenia. They occur within the first weeks of life and tend to be self-limiting. Specific treatment is rarely necessary. Congenital complete heart block, unlike the cutaneous and systemic manifestations, is irreversible. There is a high correlation with the presence of anti-SS-A/Ro antibodies in maternal serum, these having been demonstrated in over three-quarters of patients.[306] Approximately 5% of babies born to mothers with these antibodies will develop complete heart block.[307] The autoantibodies are frequently found in patients with systemic lupus erythematosus and Sjögren's syndrome, but they are rarely encountered in the general population. Anti-SSA/Ro or anti-SSB/La antibodies are immunoglobulin G forms that reach the fetus by transplacental transfer. They can be detected in babies with congenital complete heart block before 3 months of age, but not after they are 6 months old. The underlying mechanism producing heart block is not clear, but it produces fibrosis of the atrial component of the atrioventricular conduction axis. Pacing may be required in approximately two-thirds.[308] Complete heart block in subsequent pregnancies of mothers with lupus is uncommon, affecting approximately one-sixth. Treatment, both for prevention of heart block and as a treatment for evident evolving heart block, has centered on fluorinated steroids. This remains controversial and has yet to be proven beneficial (see Chapter 16).[309]

HEART DISEASE INDUCED BY TOXIC MECHANISMS

Adverse reactions to drugs and other substances can affect the heart in different ways. These can be classified as hypersensitivity myocarditis, toxic myocarditis, cardiomyopathy, or endocardial fibrosis (Tables 57-3 through 57-5).

The list of drugs in which hypersensitivity myocarditis has been described is very long (see Table 57-3). The true incidence is unknown, since it is rarely recognised clinically and, therefore, tends to be a postmortem finding. Inappropriate sinus tachycardia, mild radiographic cardiomegaly, and ST segment and T wave changes on the electrocardiogram in the presence of other allergic reactions and hypereosinophilia should raise suspicion for clinical diagnosis. Diagnosis is important, since sudden death from heart block or ventricular tachycardia can occur.[310] Hypersensitivity myocarditis is not dose dependent and can occur at any time during administration of drugs. A delayed hypersensitivity reaction is the accepted mechanism. Histopathological examination reveals an interstitial inflammatory infiltrate with eosinophils, atypical lymphocytes, and plasma cells, which mainly affects the ventricles. Myocytic damage is seen, but necrosis is uncommon. Severe cases may exhibit a non-necrotizing vasculitis. These lesions are reversible upon stopping the

TABLE 57-3

DRUGS PRODUCING HYPERSENSITIVITY MYOCARDITIS

Acetazolamide
Amitriptyline
Amphotericin (amphotericin B)
Carbamazepine
Chloramphenicol
Indomethacin (indometacin)
Isoniazid
Methyldopa
Para-aminosalycilic acid
Penicillin
Phenindione
Phenylbutazone
Phenytoin (diphenylhydantoin)
Smallpox vaccine
Spironolactone
Streptomycin
Sulphonamides
Sulphonylureas
Tetracyclines
Thiazide diuretics
Tetanus toxoid

Adapted from Billingham ME: Morphologic changes in drug-induced heart disease. In Bristow MR (ed): Drug-induced Heart Disease. Amsterdam: Elsevier, 1980, pp 127–149; and Taliercio CP, Olney BA, Lie JT: Myocarditis related to drug hypersensitivity. Mayo Clin Proc 1985;60:463–468.

TABLE 57-4

DRUGS AND AGENTS PRODUCING TOXIC MYOCARDITIS

Antimony
Anthracycline antibiotics
Arsenicals
Barbiturates
Caffeine
Catecholamines
Cyclophosphamide
Emetine
5-Fluorouracil
Lithium carbonate
Hydralazine
Paraquat
Phenothiazines
Plasmocid
Quinidine
Rapeseed oil

Adapted from Billingham ME: Morphologic changes in drug-induced heart disease. In Bristow MR (ed): Drug-induced Heart Disease. Amsterdam: Elsevier, 1980, pp 127–149.

TABLE 57-5

DRUGS AND AGENTS PRODUCING ENDOCARDIAL FIBROSIS

Serotonin
Methysergide
Mercury
Busulfan
Irradiation

Adapted from Billingham ME: Morphologic changes in drug-induced heart disease. In Bristow MR (ed): Drug-induced Heart Disease. Amsterdam: Elsevier, 1980, pp 127–149.

drug. Fibrosis, therefore, is not seen. Treatment is centered around discontinuing the offending drug, combined with use of corticosteroids or immunosuppressive therapy.

Many substances have been implicated in the production of toxic myocarditis (see Table 57-4). This is a dose-related condition in which the effects are cumulative. Clinical presentation is that of acute myocarditis. Extensive cellular necrosis occurs over a short period. Histopathological signs include myocardial damage, inflammatory infiltrate, and acute necrotizing vasculitis.[311] Upon recovery, there can be multiple focal scars with residual myocardial dysfunction.

Drug-induced cardiomyopathies are most commonly attributed to alcohol, cobalt, and the anthracycline antibiotics. They produce a dilated cardiomyopathy with poor contractility, leading to congestive cardiac failure. Of these drugs, the anthracycline antibiotics, especially Adriamycin, are important in childhood. Chronic cardiotoxic effects of Adriamycin result in a dose-related cardiomyopathy, which generally appears at a cumulative dose exceeding 450 to 550 mg/m^2. There is great individual variation.[312] Cardiac function should be continually monitored by echocardiography and/or radionuclide angiography. Pathological lesions are focal and disseminated throughout the left ventricular wall and ventricular septum. Myocytes exhibit vacuolar degeneration and/or myofibrillar loss, which may progress to necrosis and interstitial fibrosis. Inflammatory infiltrates are not present. The formation of free radicals and the release of cardio- and vasoactive substances are the most accepted pathogenetic hypotheses. Multiple agents have been proposed to have a protective effect against the cardiotoxic effects of Adriamycin and doxorubicin, but these are still under investigation.[313–315]

Cardiac irradiation during radiotherapy can produce a dose-related heart disease. This appears with doses greater than 4000 to 6000 rad, depending on the amount of cardiac surface exposed. The most common lesion is a delayed pericarditis, which generally appears within the first year of radiation therapy. It adopts the form of an acute pericarditis with fever, pleuritic chest pain, and a pericardial friction rub. Alternatively, it may produce a chronic, generally asymptomatic, pericardial effusion. Treatment is supportive and the disease tends to resolve spontaneously. Some patients develop tamponade requiring pericardiocentesis, and some progress to a chronic constrictive pericarditis necessitating pericardiectomy. Pancarditis is the most severe form of radiation-induced heart disease. There is pericardial and myocardial fibrosis with or without endocardial fibrosis. Patients present in intractable heart failure with the clinical and haemodynamic features of a restrictive cardiomyopathy. Irradiation and Adriamycin have additive cardiotoxic effects that appear at doses of each agent when both forms of therapy are used simultaneously or sequentially. Also, accelerated coronary arterial disease is seen in patients exposed to radiotherapy.[316]

MISCELLANEOUS SYSTEMIC DISORDERS

Hutchinson-Gilford Progeria

Progeria is a disease of premature aging frequently due to a mutation in the lamin A gene. The defective gene product undergoes abnormal post-translational processing and leads to abnormal morphology of the nuclear envelope, with thickening of the nuclear lamina, loss of peripheral heterochromatin, blebbing of the nuclear envelope, and clustering of nuclear pores.[317] How this leads to the clinical phenotype of accelerated aging remains to be elucidated. Affected children are normal during the first months of life, exhibiting evidence of the disease in the second year with failure to thrive, loss of subcutaneous fat, scleroderma, alopecia and development of a typical facies. This consists of a disproportionately large head for the face, a beaked nose, micrognathia, thin lips, and prominent eyes. Skeletal abnormalities include dystrophic clavicles, thoracic deformities, knock-knees, persistent patency of the fontanelle, and osteoarthritis. Intellectual development is normal.[318] The cardiovascular system is affected by premature atherosclerosis of the coronary arteries and the aorta. Most patients have ischaemic heart disease and suffer from myocardial infarctions at a mean age of 13 years. Some present with a dilated cardiomyopathy and cardiac failure with normal coronary arteries. Calcification of the mitral and aortic valves is common.[319] Function of the adrenal, thyroid, parathyroid, and pituitary glands is normal. There is, however, resistance to insulin and abnormal levels of lipids in the serum, with an increase in total lipids, pre-beta, and beta lipoproteins. Dietary treatment with reduction of the lipids to within the normal range does not seem to alter the course of the disease.

Arteriohepatic Dysplasia (Alagille Syndrome)

Arteriohepatic dysplasia is characterised by chronic cholestasis. It usually becomes apparent within the first 3 months of life with prolonged jaundice. Involved infants may present later with a heart murmur.[320] The other features making up this syndrome are a typical facies, vertebral malformations, peripheral pulmonary stenosis, and ocular involvement. Delayed physical, mental, and sexual development have not been consistently reported.[321] The disease is sometimes associated with defects in the *Jagged1* gene, which encodes a ligand for the Notch transmembrane receptor.[322] This signalling mechanism is important for vascular development.[323]

The characteristic facial appearance consists of a prominent forehead, deep-set eyes with mild hypertelorism and a small pointed chin. Ophthalmological examination reveals chorioretinal atrophy and pigment clumping, which may be pathognomonic. Peripheral pulmonary stenosis is the typical cardiovascular anomaly. On physical examination, there is a prominent left parasternal impulse and an ejection systolic murmur at the upper left sternal border radiating to the back, where it may be heard extending into diastole. The electrocardiogram shows right ventricular hypertrophy. Cardiac size may be normal or increased on the chest radiograph, and the lung fields may appear normal or oligaemic. Cardiac catheterisation and angiography confirm the peripheral pulmonary stenosis, which may be single or multiple. The most frequent accompanying cardiovascular lesions are patency of the arterial duct, valvar pulmonary stenosis, and atrial and ventricular septal defects.

Many patients have anomalies of the vertebral arches, usually with a butterfly appearance of the dorsal vertebras. Xanthomas of the palms, extensor surfaces, and skin creases of the hands are seen when hyperlipidaemia is present. Elevated lipids and cholesterol in the serum are controlled by the use of cholestyramine and by the addition of corn oil to the diet. Arteriohepatic dysplasia is confirmed by liver biopsy, which shows the bile ducts to be absent from most portal areas. Periportal fibrosis is absent or mild, and the extrahepatic system is patent. Additional laboratory findings include elevated 5′-nucleotidase, alkaline phosphatase, transaminases, and bilirubin. The peripheral pulmonary stenosis is not progressive, and it does not influence the long-term prognosis of the disease. Half the deaths are from hepatic or cardiac causes.

Sickle Cell Haemoglobinopathy

Sickle cell haemoglobulinopathy is a chronic haemolytic anaemia that predominantly affects those of African descent. The underlying abnormality is the substitution of glutamic acid by valine in the sixth position of the β-chain of haemoglobin. This results in the formation of haemoglobin S. When tension of oxygen is reduced, the haemoglobin S molecules polymerise and produce a crescent, sickle-shaped deformity in the red cells. The pathophysiological consequences of this are vaso-occlusive phenomenons and chronic haemolysis. Organs affected by this process are the kidneys, lungs, liver, spleen, central nervous system, and bones. There are a host of cardiovascular signs and symptoms in patients with sickle cell anaemia, but there is no histopathological evidence of a specific sickle cell cardiomyopathy. Cardiac output is increased, with an increase in stroke volume. The most common symptoms are exertional dyspnoea and palpitations. Physical examination reveals signs of a hyperdynamic circulation.

Peripheral pulses are full, and the apex beat is prominent and displaced laterally. Heart sounds are loud. The second heart sound is widely split and the pulmonary component is often increased. Ejection systolic murmurs are usually present. A third heart sound may be heard, but its presence does not imply cardiac failure. Signs of congestive cardiac failure are rare. Peripheral oedema, pulmonary rales and hepatomegaly may be secondary to venous stasis, pulmonary disease and cholestasis, respectively, and this can confuse the issue.

The electrocardiogram is non-specific. Signs of left ventricular hypertrophy are usually present. First-degree atrioventricular block and ST segment and T wave changes are common. Right ventricular hypertrophy is usually secondary to pulmonary vaso-occlusive disease and is more frequent in older patients. Cardiac enlargement and increased pulmonary vascular markings resembling those seen with a left-to-right shunt are the most frequent radiographic signs. Pulmonary infiltrates produced by infarction and infection may also be present. Echocardiographic examination reveals left atrial and ventricular dilation as a result of the volume overload of chronic anaemia. Left ventricular contraction is very dynamic. Mitral and tricuspid valvar regurgitation are also seen commonly.[324]

Congestive cardiac failure is more common in adults than in children. It appears to be secondary to co-existing renal or cardiovascular disease. Myocardial dysfunction with an abnormal response to exercise has been demonstrated in children, particularly if they suffer from pulmonary hypertension.[325] Approximately one-third suffer from pulmonary hypertension, and this risk probably increases with age.[326] The pulmonary hypertension is multi-factorial, resulting from the effects of chronic vaso-occlusive disease, increased left ventricular filling pressures due to the left-sided chamber enlargement, and probably other as yet undefined effects of vascular dysfunction. The presence of pulmonary hypertension greatly increases long-term risk.[327] Additionally, the risk of sudden death during acute pulmonary vaso-occlusive crises is increased in the presence of pulmonary hypertension, probably secondary to acute increases in the pulmonary vascular resistance related to the crisis.[328] Left ventricular dilation has been shown to normalise following transfusion of packed red cells, further supporting the notion that cardiac abnormalities are related to chronic anaemia, and not specific to sickle cell anaemia.[329] Of course, chronic transfusion can lead to deposition of iron, resulting in ventricular diastolic dysfunction, and it is unclear whether chelation therapy is effective at preventing this complication.[330]

Repair of congenital cardiac malformations is complicated by the presence of sickle cell disease, as cardiopulmonary bypass and hypothermic circulatory arrest can precipitate vaso-occlusive crises. Most recommend a partial or complete exchange transfusion prior to initiation of surgery, with optimisation of blood gases, rates of flow, and volumes. These practices are also often employed even in patients with sickle cell trait. Despite this common practice, there are reports of successful cardiac surgery using cardiopulmonary bypass without the use of exchange transfusion.[331]

Anorexia Nervosa

Anorexia nervosa is a life-threatening disorder in which affected individuals attempt to lose weight through starvation, use of laxatives, and exercise. It affects females more often than males, and typically begins in adolescence. Patients have a distorted body image and fear of weight gain, maintaining a weight less than five-sixths of their ideal weight. While this disorder affects all bodily systems, it carries a high mortality, in part due to its effects on the cardiovascular system. Common findings include sinus bradycardia, reduced volumes, and diminished ventricular mass and cardiac output.[332,333] Despite these changes, left ventricular contractility often remains normal,[334] though cardiomyopathy has been reported.[335] QT prolongation is observed, and may be due to, or exacerbated by, hypokalemia associated with the dietary derangements. This may explain some cases of sudden death.[336] The precise aetiology of reduction in left ventricular mass, volume, and output remains to be elucidated. It may be due to atrophy secondary to malnutrition, or to the effects of chronic loss of preload. Refeeding can normalise many of the cardiac derangements including sinus bradycardia, QT prolongation, and left ventricular changes.[330,337,338] Refeeding by itself can lead to severe cardiopulmonary compromise and must be carried out judiciously.[339]

The complete reference list can be found on the companion Expert Consult web site at www.expertconsult.com.

ANNOTATED REFERENCES

- Shin YS: Glycogen storage disease: Clinical, biochemical and molecular heterogeneity. Semin Pediatr Neurol 2006;13:115–120.

  An excellent description of the glycogen storage diseases, with updates on genetics, biochemistry, and clinical features.
- Scott HS, Bunge S, Gal A, et al: Molecular genetics of mucopolysaccharidosis type I: Diagnostic, clinical, and biological implications. Hum Mutat 1995;6:288–302.

  This paper reviews the genetic mutations leading to MPS I and makes correlations between genotype and phenotype to help explain the clinical heterogeneity of the mucopolysaccharide storage disorders.
- Dangel JH: Cardiovascular changes in children with mucopolysaccharide storage diseases and related disorders: Clinical and echocardiographic findings in 64 patients. Eur J Pediatr 1998;157:534–538.

  The largest descriptive series available for the cardiac findings in patients with mucopolysaccharide storage disorders.
- Michalski JC, Klein A: Glycoprotein lysosomal storage disorders: Alpha and beta mannosidosis, fucosidosis, and alpha-N-acetylgalactosaminidase deficiency. Biochim Biophys Acta 1999;1455:69–84.

  An excellent review of the biochemistry, genetics and clinical features of the glycoproteinoses.
- Eng CM, Germain DP, Banikazemi M, et al: Fabry disease: Guidelines for the evaluation and management of multi-organ system involvement. Genet Med 2006;8:539–548.

  This is a comprehensive review of the issues concerning management of patients with Fabry's disease, and also touches on the genetic and biochemical aspects of the disease.
- Guertl B, Noehammer C, Hoefler G: Metabolic cardiomyopathies. Int J Exp Pathol 2000;81:349–372.

  This is an excellent review of myocardial metabolism, which explores the various metabolic cardiomyopathies in a sequential fashion. It also provides information on other cardiomyopathies due to storage disorders, toxins, and defects of energy metabolism.
- Marin-Garcia J, Goldenthal MJ, Filiano JJ: Cardiomyopathy associated with neurologic disorders and mitochondrial phenotype. J Child Neurol 2002;17:759–765.

  This review of cases provides a good description of the breadth of mitochondrial disorders affecting cardiac function.
- Spencer CT, Bryant RM, Day J, et al: Cardiac and clinical phenotype in Barth syndrome. Pediatrics 2006;118:e337–346.

  A descriptive review of a large series of patients with Barth syndrome, covering genetic, clinical and laboratory findings with a focus on cardiovascular involvement.
- De Paepe A, Devereux RB, Dietz HC, et al: Revised diagnostic criteria for the Marfan syndrome. Am J Med Genet 1996;62:417–426.

  The classic manuscript defining the consensus nosology used to diagnose Marfan syndrome, along with useful indexed tables for measurement of the sinuses of Valsalva.
- Ramirez F, Dietz HC: Marfan syndrome: From molecular pathogenesis to clinical treatment. Curr Opin Genet Dev 2007;17: 252–258.

  This paper is a comprehensive review describing the most recent advances in the understanding of the molecular pathogenesis of the clinical features of Marfan syndrome.
- Wagner KR, Lechtzin N, Judge DP: Current treatment of adult Duchenne muscular dystrophy. Biochim Biophys Acta 2007;1772:229–237.

  This inclusive review covers the important aspects of management for patients with Duchenne's muscular dystrophy, paying particular attention to the cardiopulmonary systems.
- Foster K, Foster H, Dickson JG: Gene therapy progress and prospects: Duchenne muscular dystrophy. Gene Ther 2006;13:1677–1685.

  Here, the latest advances in genetic therapy for patients with Duchenne's muscular dystrophy are described.
- Finsterer J, Stollberger C: The heart in human dystrophinopathies. Cardiology 2003;99:1–19.

  This review covers all aspects of cardiac involvement in the major diseases caused by dystrophin gene mutations. The description of cardiac involvement is accompanied by a thorough assessment of the various modalities available to evaluate and monitor cardiac disease in these patients.
- Pietrangelo A: Hereditary hemochromatosis. Biochim Biophys Acta 2006;1763:700–710.

  This thorough review of haemochromatosis describes the molecular pathogenesis of this disease.
- Casiero D, Frishman WH: Cardiovascular complications of eating disorders. Cardiol Rev 2006;14:227–231.

  An important and useful review of the cardiovascular complications associated with bulimia and anorexia nervosa, including issues related to refeeding syndrome in these patients.

CHAPTER 58

Systemic Hypertension

MANISH D. SINHA and CHRISTOPHER J.D. REID

Systemic hypertension is one of the commonest cardiovascular diseases in adults. Over the past decade, several advances have been made in evaluating the state of blood pressure in children. Paediatric hypertension, nonetheless, remains poorly recognised. Essential hypertension is the most common form of hypertension in adults, but it is becoming increasingly clear that the origin of this condition is in childhood. The prevalence of essential hypertension during childhood is increasing, in keeping with the increasing prevalence of obesity. Secondary hypertension is clinically much more important in children, and is commonly caused by renal disease. Early detection and control not only reduce the general morbidity of hypertension, but also protect the function of the already damaged kidney. Fortunately, recent pharmacological advances enable the blood pressure to be controlled in all patients, with a minimum of undesirable side effects. Consequently, the management of hypertension is particularly rewarding for the practising paediatrician.

EVALUATION OF BLOOD PRESSURE: MEASUREMENT, NORMAL VALUES, AND IMPORTANT INFLUENCES

Measurement of Systemic Blood Pressure

In this section, we discuss issues related to the measurement of blood pressure in the clinic or office, along with 24-hour ambulatory monitoring. Measurement of blood pressure in children is usually first performed at the time of their first presentation to a paediatric department, or as part of their first school physical examination. It is often omitted. Common reasons cited by clinicians include the practical difficulties in making measurements in infants and young children, changing normative limits throughout childhood, and the belief that hypertension is primarily an adult disease. There are several aspects to measurement that need consideration. These include the type of measuring machine, the type of cuff and bladder, the technique of measurement, and variables relating to the patient, the observer, and the environment in which the measurements are made.

Cuff and Bladder

The cuff is the inelastic covering that encases an inflatable rubber bladder. The cuff is usually made of cloth, using semisynthetic or any other material that will reliably and evenly transmit pressure over the artery once the bladder is inflated. A combination that allows removal of the bladder from the cuff so that the cuff can be washed at regular intervals is probably more desirable.[1]

The inflatable bladder, rather than the cuff, needs to be of the correct size. Failure to select the correct size of bladder remains the most common error in the measurement of blood pressure. Miscuffing refers to the inaccuracy introduced as a result of using a bladder that is too small and narrow, or too long relative to the circumference of the upper arm. It is advisable to choose a size of cuff in relation to the circumference of the arm as opposed to its length. Although debated, most researchers in this area agree that the width for children should be about two-fifths of the circumference of the upper arm.[2] This is because measurements made using circumference rather than length as the yardstick correlate best with intra-arterial readings. In both adults and children, use of cuffs which are too small in length, or too narrow in width, will overestimate the pressures measured by errors ranging from 3 over 2 to 12 over 8 mm Hg, with even greater ranges of error in obese individuals.[3] This is sometimes referred to as cuff hypertension. Too large a cuff is increasingly being recognised as a cause of underestimation of pressure in both adults and children.[4–7] Length of the bladder is much more important in children than adults, and also leads to overestimation of the measured pressure.[8]

The suggested solution to the problem of the size of the cuff is to have a range of sizes of bladder available. In the United Kingdom, cuffs and bladders measuring 4 cm in width and 13 cm in length, and then 8 by 18 cm, 12 by 18 cm, 12 by 26 cm, and 12 by 40 cm are available. These usually suffice for arms of all sizes across the paediatric age range, including lean and obese children. Other national societies recommend different sizes.[5] The bladder should be centred over the brachial artery, and should encircle from four-fifths to all of the upper arm.[5,8] In practice, the widest cuff should be used to permit auscultation of the antecubital fossa. The size used should be recorded so that sequential measurements can be compared in the same patient.

Instruments

The mercury sphygmomanometer combined with an inflated cuff and auscultation remains the gold standard for the measurement of blood pressure in children. Widely accepted centiles for normal pressures through childhood have been developed using such a standard mercury sphygmomanometer instrument.[9] Recently, nonetheless, concerns have emerged regarding the safety of mercury for users in the clinical environment, for technicians who have to service the instrument, and for the environment itself.[10,11]

An issue with any method using auscultation is the introduction of the phenomenon of terminal digit preference, and bias of the observer because of knowledge of previous measurements. Any instrument that eliminates or reduces these two is to be welcomed. This initially led to the development of the random-zero sphygmomanometer, which was developed and shown to minimise or eliminate both these items.[12,13] Unfortunately, these devices were shown subsequently significantly to underestimate blood pressure, and were therefore abandoned.[14,15]

Automated oscillometric devices have similarly been developed. These improve on the shortcomings of the auscultatory method by eliminating both terminal digit preference and the bias of the observer. They work by the detection of pressure pulses in the cuff. These are generated as a result of the volume pulses of the artery. When blood starts flowing through the artery at the point of systolic pressure, a pressure pulse is generated. As pressure within the deflating cuff is reduced in a stepwise manner, a series of pressure pulses generate the pulse oscillogram. The pulse amplitudes of this oscillogram provide an envelope curve, with the maximal value on this curve equating to the mean arterial pressure. Systolic and diastolic pressures are calculated from preset algorithms in the instrument microchip, and are a function of the mean. The algorithms are specific to the instrument, and are not declared by the manufacturers.[16,17] Although these automated devices are increasingly being used in primary care and paediatric departments, there are some particular concerns that need to be highlighted. The Dinamap devices are the most commonly studied automated oscillometric devices reported in paediatric series. An earlier version of this device, model 1846 SX, had been shown to have superior correlation with intra-arterial measurements.[18] Other studies, however, reported higher mean systolic measurements using models 1846, 8100, and 845 when compared with the random-zero sphygmomanometer and mercury sphygmomanometer.[19,20] Diastolic measurements had been reported to have better agreement.[19] A more recent report using the Dinamap 8100 monitor highlighted the discrepancy between the two methods, with measurements using the device higher by a mean of 10 mm Hg for systolic and 5 mm Hg for diastolic blood pressure.[21] Although normative limits have been proposed using the Dinamap 8100 instrument, caution needs to be proposed before applying these limits in clinical practice.[22] Another particular practical observation with oscillometric devices is the phenomenon of measurements being higher by about 3 to 5 mm Hg on first measurement, despite control of factors involving the patient, the observer, and the environment.[20,23] The second reading has been reported to be more accurate.

Automatically inflated cuffs have recently been introduced. These measure both systolic and diastolic pressures, recording the results at preset intervals by detecting oscillations in the pressure from the cuff. They are especially useful in the care of the critically ill child, saving nursing time and reducing disturbance to the patient. The calibration needs to be checked frequently if the result is to be regarded as accurate, but they are useful in detecting changes. Indeed, they will alarm automatically if preset parameters are exceeded.

Aneroid sphygmomanometers have also gained in popularity in clinical practice because of their portability and their reliance on techniques similar to the standard mercury sphygmomanometer. Because of this, however, they have no influence on the biases existing with the mercury sphygmomanometer. The devices have proven their accuracy when regular 6-month maintenance is in place to service the instruments.[24]

The majority of devices in clinical use, nonetheless, have not been evaluated independently for accuracy using the two most widely accepted protocols for validation.[25,26] These protocols have been proposed by the British Hypertension Society and the Association for the Advancement of Medical Instrumentation. Several updates of validation have been published, but the best method of finding up-to-date information is on the nonprofit Web site http://www.dableducational.com.[27]

Technique of Measurement

The child should be relaxed and quiet when blood pressure is recorded. Should this not be possible, but readings are made, then the conditions should be recorded. A simple description of the process of measurement to a child at a level appropriate for age will usually lead to a cooperative patient, thus allowing accurate recordings. Measuring pressures in infants who are crying is not useful. The standard position is the sitting position when children are older than 3 years, with the fully exposed arm supported or resting on a table at the level of the heart.[23] An arm higher than the heart will underestimate the pressure, while a lower position will produce overestimations.[28] In younger children and infants, pressure should be routinely measured when the patient is in the supine position. The sphygmomanometer should be placed at the level of the eye of the observer to eliminate error from parallax. The cuff should be inflated about 30 mm Hg above the point at which the radial pulse disappears. In some patients, there will be a silent gap between the systolic and diastolic pressures. Simply inflating the cuff until the sound disappears in such individuals may produce a serious underestimation of systolic pressure. Once inflated, the cuff should be deflated at a rate of 2 to 3 mm Hg per second while auscultating with the stethoscope. The sudden distension of the collapsed artery at the systolic pressure is associated with a clear tapping sound, defined as phase 1 of the Korotkoff sounds. The murmur of turbulent blood flowing through the partially occluded artery is phase 2. Phase 3 is a high-pitched sound produced when the artery, closed during diastole, opens in systole. When the artery no longer closes during diastole, the tapping sounds are low pitched and muffled and quieter. This is phase 4. Phase 5 is when the sounds disappear. This is variable, and may not occur in some children. The fourth phase, however, tends to overestimate the diastolic pressure, while the fifth phase underestimates it. Although the fifth sound is widely accepted as the optimal measurement of diastolic pressure amongst adolescents and adults, there has been considerable debate in the literature concerning its value in children younger than 13 years of age. For these younger children, the fourth sound had generally been preferred, and was recommended by the Task Force Reports on Blood Pressure Control in Children.[29,30] An international committee, nonetheless, recommended the fifth sound,[31,32] and the update of the Task Force Recommendations also advocates using this sound. It is preferred because of its easier identification by observers and the comparability it provides for measuring diastolic pressures across age groups. The two sounds are not equal in most children, and may vary considerably, by up to 10 mm Hg.[33]

The measurement of blood pressure in infants, and in some older children, is sometimes difficult because the sounds are inaudible. The old flush technique is unreliable. It has now been superseded by the use of Doppler ultrasound, using an ultrasonic beam to detect motion of the arterial wall when the cuff is deflated. This technique is remarkably reliable for measurement of the systolic pressure, and corresponds to the intra-arterial pressure better than any other method, including auscultation.[34] It is less reliable in the measurement of diastolic pressure, even when machines specifically designed for diastolic pressure are used.[35] All hospital paediatric departments, especially those specializing in paediatric cardiology, should have an ultrasonic machine for measurement of blood pressure. It is particularly useful in determining pressure in the legs in children with suspected aortic coarctation.[34] Recording of the systolic blood pressure by palpation of the radial artery underestimates the pressure by as much 11 mm Hg.[34] The blood pressure measurement should be recorded immediately, without rounding off the measured value to the nearest preferred whole value.

The number of measurements to be obtained for each visit in order for the observer to be assured that the measured pressure is accurate is also important. In practical terms, an observer should attempt to take at least two or three measurements at each visit. The second measurement is a truer reflection of the pressure, the first being least accurate, especially when measured with an automated oscillometric instrument. Measurements over two, and preferably three, visits should be considered to provide a better reflection of a given blood pressure.[9,20]

Ambulatory Measurement of Blood Pressure

Ambulatory monitoring using a small, portable, programmable monitor, and performed over a continuous 24-hour period, has become a well-accepted method for the diagnosis of hypertension and assessment of treatment in adults. It is now increasingly gaining recognition for its superior role in the diagnosis and evaluation of blood pressure in children. The monitors typically use an oscillometric technique. They can be programmed to record the blood pressure frequently, for example, every 30 minutes during the day and hourly at night. The readings are stored for later downloading, display and analysis by personal computer. The monitor can be worn on the belt or in the pocket, and the recording is made as the children carry on their normal daytime and night-time activities.

There are some inherent disadvantages of recording a single measurement of blood pressure, since pressure itself is a continuous variable. Additionally, there is the phenomenon of white coat hypertension, especially in children. We discuss this in more detail later. Measures made in the clinic also provide no information of pressures when the patient is asleep. Monitoring over a 24-hour period has several advantages over solitary measurements. It is a more accurate representation, being more physiological and detecting the circadian variation in pressure. Multiple measurements are made in the regular environment, including measurements when the patient is both awake and asleep. Measurements are automatically stored, removing observer error and bias. The technique has been shown to have higher reproducibility than measurements made in the clinic in adults.[36–39] This has also been shown in children,[40–44] although reproducing the nocturnal decline in pressure has not been observed as consistently.[37,44] With improving technology, the instruments themselves have become smaller, and this has resulted in their improved tolerability by children, even in infants and toddlers as young as 2 months of age,[45] although there are no normative limits for this population. As normative standards for ambulatory measurements exist only for children older than 5 years of age, we would not recommend such monitoring in younger children.

Increasing age, and higher mean arterial pressures, have previously been described as factors that improve the rate of success of ambulatory measurements made over 24 hours.[46,47] Our own experience is that monitoring is well tolerated, with more successful measurements achieved when patients are asleep than when awake. This is primarily related to the normal unrestricted daytime activity of the child causing errors in measurement due to movement.[48]

Accurate documentation of the waking and sleeping periods is important for correct interpretation of any study made over 24 hours. A number of studies in children have considered measurements only during a fixed waking period, between 08:00 to 20:00, or sleeping, from 24:00 to 06:00, in effect ignoring measurements made over 6 hours during the period of 24 hours. This method has been preferred by some as it improves accuracy in correctly classifying measurements made when the patient is awake and asleep. Our own practice has been to identify correctly the periods when awake or sleeping, using a diary that records such times. Unpublished data from our own series would suggest an error of up to one-tenth in misclassification of measurements made during waking and sleeping. No study has thus far shown the inaccuracy introduced, if any, in ambulatory measurements when ignoring one-quarter of recording time as described above.

Normative data for ambulatory monitoring has now been published.[49] A recent study from the same group using the least mean square method of analysis to account for the non-Gaussian distribution of the original cohort provides 90th and 95th percentiles for daytime and night-time values stratified according to sex and height.[50,51] Our own preference is for the data using the least mean square method. The criterions for defining hypertension in children are different when using data derived from office measurements as opposed to ambulatory monitoring, with higher values for daytime levels using 24-hour monitoring of normotensive children compared to measurements made in the clinic.[52] Findings in children with hypertension, however, are inconsistent.[44,53–56] Ambulatory devices allow assessment of systolic and diastolic pressures, expressed as mean and standard deviation of values during the 24-hour period, including daytime and night-time. The pressure load and dipping state, described below, can also be assessed.

The pressure load as assessed over 24 hours expresses the percentage of measurements above the 95th percentile, but provides no information regarding the amplitude and duration of the pressures above the 95th percentile. In adults, this load has been shown to be more accurate than mean pressures[57,58] in predicting damage to end organs. A recent review[59] suggested a load of less than one-quarter to be normal, and greater than half to be more closely related to damage to the end organs. Attempts have also been made[60] to determine the agreement between mean pressures greater than the 95th percentile and a load of 30% when diagnosing hypertension on the basis of ambulatory monitoring. This data,[60] and that from others,[61–63] suggests that mean pressures above the 95th percentile correlate better with a load in excess of 50%.[61–63]

The physiological nocturnal dip in pressure, and the rise with waking, or the morning surge, has been well described in adults. The absence of any dip in adults is related to cardiovascular and cerebrovascular morbidity and mortality.[64–66] This relationship has not been described in children. A state of non-dipping, however, has been observed in several groups of children with a variety of renal diseases, and after renal transplantation.[67–70] Untreated children with secondary hypertension have been reported to develop nocturnal hypertension and the non-dipping state, as opposed to patients with primary hypertension who maintain their dipping state.[71] The morning surge as described in adults,[72,73] however, is not usually reported in children.

Normal Blood Pressure in Childhood

A large number of studies have been undertaken to establish the range of blood pressure found in normal children,[74–76] with the results for boys summarised in Figure 58-1. As a general rule, a steady increase has been observed with age, with no significant difference between the sexes during childhood. Most studies, unfortunately, differ in some respect, for example, in the sizes of cuff used, with measurements taken with the patient sitting or supine, using different end-points for diastolic pressure, and so on.

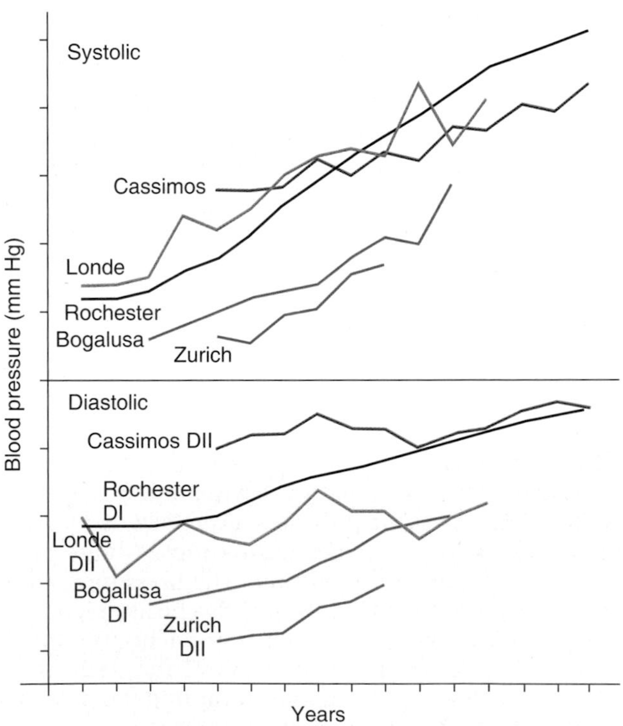

Figure 58-1 The 95th centiles for systolic and diastolic blood pressure in boys taken from various sources. Data from the Rochester (Minnesota) study,[29] including data from the Muscatine study[125]; a Scandinavian study[76]; the Bogalusa study[79]; the Zurich study[75]; and the Londe study[74]. The conditions and measurement parameters varied. Children were seated, except in the study of Londe, where they were supine.[74] The widths of the cuffs used were 9 and 13 cm (Scandinavian),[76] two-thirds of upper arm (Londe),[74] at least two-thirds of upper arm (Rochester),[29] mostly 10 and 12.5 cm (Bogalusa),[79] and the largest possible (Zurich)[75]. Standard mercury sphygmomanometers were used except in the Zurich study, where random zero manometers were used. There is an overlap between use of phase 4, muffling of sounds, and phase 5, cessation of sounds. (Reprinted with permission from Leuman EP: Blood pressure and hypertension in childhood and adolescence. In Frick P, von Harneck GA, Martini GA, et al [eds]: Advances in Internal Medicine and Pediatrics. Berlin: Springer, 1979, pp. 109–183.)

TABLE 58-1

SIZES OF SPHYGMOMANOMETER CUFFS

	Width of Bladder (cm)	Length of Bladder (cm)
Newborns	4	5–10
Infants	6	12
1–5 years	8	15
6–9 years	10	20
10 years and over	13	23
Obese adults	15	30
Adult thigh	18	36

Adapted from Leuman EP: Blood pressure and hypertension in childhood and adolescence. In Frick P, von Harneck GA, Martini GA, et al (eds): Advances in Internal Medicine and Pediatrics. Berlin: Springer, 1979, pp 109–183.

These differences in technique make it difficult to interpret apparent differences between ethnic groups. Adult black individuals have an increased prevalence of hypertension and damage to target organs when compared with whites.[77] Nigerian children were found to have higher pressures than black American children.[78] Higher values for black than white children might be expected in view of the higher prevalence of hypertension in black adults. These were reported by the Bogalusa study,[79] but similar,[30,80–83] lower,[84–86] and no difference in values[87] have also been reported. A significant increase in the proportion of hypertensive 18-year-old black adolescents has also been reported,[88,89] albeit that another study[90] found no difference in the renin-angiotensin-aldosterone system when comparing black and white children and adolescents. It has been suggested[91] that height rather than age is the appropriate standard to which blood pressure should be related. After controlling for height, the effect of age on blood pressure disappears. It is also suggested, therefore, that evaluation of blood pressure in an individual should be based on height and weight rather than age.[80] It is not clear whether sexual maturation has an effect, independent of body mass, on blood pressure.[74]

Obesity poses special problems because of the essential requirement for an adequate cuff in making measurements. Where adequate sizes have been used, obese adolescents have been found to have a higher incidence of hypertension.[86,92–94] Corrections have been made according to the circumference of the arm and the size of the cuff used in the measurement[95] (Table 58-1). Levels of cholesterol and triglyceride in the serum do not correlate well with blood pressure,[79] but levels of glucose in the plasma 1 hour after a glucose load were found to correlate with blood pressure independently of weight.[96] The deleterious influence of salt on blood pressure in children has become clearer, and is discussed briefly later in this chapter. No difference was apparent in blood pressure between bottle- and breast-fed infants.[97]

Normal Values for Blood Pressure Measured in the Clinic

Pressures during childhood vary physiologically with gender, age and height. The practising clinician requires standards with which to compare the blood pressure of individual patients. The most recent Fourth Report from the working group of the National High Blood Pressure Education Program in the United States now provides 50th, 90th, 95th, and 99th centiles for pressures obtained by auscultation in formats specific for gender, age, and height, and is widely accepted as the reference standard for normative values.[9] It provides data over and above that from the previous reports of the Task Force on Blood Pressure Control in Children,[30,32] giving comprehensive values for seven different centiles for height at each age from 1 to 17 years, as shown in Table 58-2 for boys, and Table 58-3 for girls. Despite this addition of new data, there is minimal change in the levels for gender, age, and height for the 90th and 95th percentiles from the last report. Additionally, the new data describes stages of hypertension, defining normotension as below the 90th percentile, pre-hypertension as between the 90th and 95th percentiles, the first stage of hypertension as between the 95th and 99th percentiles plus 5 mm Hg, and the second stage of hypertension as greater than the 99th percentile plus 5 mm Hg, similar to the seventh report of the joint national committee.[98] It provides guidance on the speed at which evaluation, treatment, and referral should be made in a child with elevated blood pressure. The age and gender specific centiles for blood pressure in boys and girls from birth to 12 months of age are shown in Figures 58-2 and 58-3.

Normal Values for Ambulatory Monitoring of Blood Pressure

Data on 24-hour ambulatory monitoring in normal children and adolescents has now been published by several authors.[49,52,83,99–102] These publications contain detailed tables and graphs of mean and standard deviation for systolic and diastolic blood pressure, for day and night, and by sex, height and age. The normative data from a mid-European cohort[49] is most widely accepted. As already discussed, our own preference is to use the data provided by the same group using the least mean square method of analysis.[50,51] There are some common findings in all these series. An important observation is that, in normal children and adolescents, there is a physiological nocturnal dip relative to daytime values as described in adults, with an average fall of one-eighth for systolic, and just over one-fifth for diastolic, pressures.[49,101,102]

As also discussed, the criterions for defining hypertension in children are different when using values obtained in the office as opposed to ambulatory monitoring. Mean values obtained by ambulatory monitoring for both systolic and diastolic pressures are higher during the daytime than those obtained in the clinic for children of the same age and height, probably secondary to the unrestricted physical activity during monitoring over 24 hours. Consequently, normal values based on measurements made in the clinic, such as the Fourth Report described above, should not be used for assessment of readings obtained by ambulatory monitoring. Again, as already emphasised, one study showed higher values in daytime when using 24-hour values for normotensive children,[52] but findings in children with hypertension are inconsistent.[44,53–56] Some[101,102] have also found no differences in pressures between the sexes for ages ranging from 6 to 14 years, while others[83] found higher values for boys at all ages from 10 to 18 years, and still others[49] found higher values for boys when compared to girls at all heights.

Higher values are reported for black teenagers when sleeping compared with white teenagers, though there was no difference during daytime.[83] These observations have been demonstrated both in adults and in younger children, and are shown to persist longitudinally over time.[103–106] It is suggested[107] that this reduced nocturnal fall in black children may represent an increased load, which might contribute to the excess morbidity and mortality from essential hypertension seen in African Americans. Interactions between both genetic and environmental factors are thought to contribute to the ethnic differences in patterns noted with ambulatory monitoring, although much of the variations in levels and patterns remain poorly understood.[108]

White Coat Hypertension and Masked Hypertension

If ambulatory measurements are interpreted in conjunction with those made in the clinic, two further categories are recognised over and above true normotension and true hypertension. White coat hypertension is defined as high measurements made in the clinic but normal values when obtained by self-measurement or using daytime ambulatory monitoring. This phenomenon was first described in children when it was observed that almost half of patients with raised values in the clinic had normal values when assessed using ambulatory monitoring.[109] The observation has since been confirmed in several other studies, albeit with differences in prevalence depending on population studied and the diagnostic criterions.[54,110–112] There is some evidence that such white coat hypertension is potentially a pre-hypertensive state.[113] As opposed to a previous study,[114] those suggesting the pre-hypertensive state reported white coat hypertension in just over half their cohort, with exaggerated values found after exercise, and an increase in the left ventricular mass index in one-tenth of those with white coat hypertension in this predominantly overweight cohort based in a tertiary centre.

Masked hypertension is defined as the finding of normal values in the clinic, but with either systolic or diastolic values obtained during daytime using ambulatory monitoring that are greater than or equal to the 95th centile for sex and height.[49] Such findings[115] were observed in one-tenth of a cohort of normotensive patients aged from 6 to 25 years, with males more commonly affected than females. Similar prevalences were subsequently reported in a series of patients referred because of elevated pressures.[114] Others[112] studied a large cohort of children aged from 6 to 18 years undergoing routine health checks, discovering masked hypertension in almost one-tenth. After follow up of three-quarters of these patients, almost half were shown to be normotensive using ambulatory monitoring, while 13 had persistent masked hypertension, and 3 had sustained hypertension. Those with masked hypertension had higher heart rates over 24 hours and more likelihood of parental hypertension. A small proportion of patients with either white coat or masked hypertension, therefore, may progress to develop sustained hypertension.

When faced with such patients, clinicians should look for co-morbid features, such as diabetes mellitus, obesity, family history of cardiovascular disease, and damage to end

TABLE 58-2

BP LEVELS FOR BOYS BY AGE AND HEIGHT PERCENTILE

Age, yr	BP Percentile	SBP, mm Hg Percentile of Height							DBP, mm Hg Percentile of Height						
		5th	*10th*	*25th*	*50th*	*75th*	*90th*	*95th*	*5th*	*10th*	*25th*	*50th*	*75th*	*90th*	*95th*
1	50th	80	81	83	85	87	88	89	34	35	36	37	38	39	39
	90th	94	95	97	99	100	102	103	49	50	51	52	53	53	54
	95th	98	99	101	103	104	106	106	54	54	55	56	57	58	58
	99th	105	106	108	110	112	113	114	61	62	63	64	65	66	66
2	50th	84	85	87	88	90	92	92	39	40	41	42	43	44	44
	90th	97	99	100	102	104	105	106	54	55	56	57	58	58	59
	95th	101	102	104	106	108	109	110	59	59	60	61	62	63	63
	99th	109	110	111	113	115	117	117	66	67	68	69	70	71	71
3	50th	86	87	89	91	93	94	95	44	44	45	46	47	48	48
	90th	100	101	103	105	107	108	109	59	59	60	61	62	63	63
	95th	104	105	107	109	110	112	113	63	63	64	65	66	67	67
	99th	111	112	114	116	118	119	120	71	71	72	73	74	75	75
4	50th	88	89	91	93	95	96	97	47	48	49	50	51	51	52
	90th	102	103	105	107	109	110	111	62	63	64	65	66	66	67
	95th	106	107	109	111	112	114	115	66	67	68	69	70	71	71
	99th	113	114	116	118	120	121	122	74	75	76	77	78	78	79
5	50th	90	91	93	95	96	98	98	50	51	52	53	54	55	55
	90th	104	105	106	108	110	111	112	65	66	67	68	69	69	70
	95th	108	109	110	112	114	115	116	69	70	71	72	73	74	74
	99th	115	116	118	120	121	123	123	77	78	79	80	81	81	82
6	50th	91	92	94	96	98	99	100	53	53	54	55	56	57	57
	90th	105	106	108	110	111	113	113	68	68	69	70	71	72	72
	95th	109	110	112	114	115	117	117	72	72	73	74	75	76	76
	99th	116	117	119	121	123	124	125	80	80	81	82	83	84	84
7	50th	92	94	95	97	99	100	101	55	55	56	57	58	59	59
	90th	106	107	109	111	113	114	115	70	70	71	72	73	74	74
	95th	110	111	113	115	117	118	119	74	74	75	76	77	78	78
	99th	117	118	120	122	124	125	126	82	82	83	84	85	86	86
8	50th	94	95	97	99	100	102	102	56	57	58	59	60	60	61
	90th	107	109	110	112	114	115	116	71	72	72	73	74	75	76
	95th	111	112	114	116	118	119	120	75	76	77	78	79	79	80
	99th	119	120	122	123	125	127	127	83	84	85	86	87	87	88
9	50th	95	96	98	100	102	103	104	57	58	59	60	61	61	62
	90th	109	110	112	114	115	117	118	72	73	74	75	76	76	77
	95th	113	114	116	118	119	121	121	76	77	78	79	80	81	81
	99th	120	121	123	125	127	128	129	84	85	86	87	88	88	89
10	50th	97	98	100	102	103	105	106	58	59	60	61	61	62	63
	90th	111	112	114	115	117	119	119	73	73	74	75	76	77	78
	95th	115	116	117	119	121	122	123	77	78	79	80	81	81	82
	99th	122	123	125	127	128	130	130	85	86	86	88	88	89	90
11	50th	99	100	102	104	105	107	107	59	59	60	61	62	63	63
	90th	113	114	115	117	119	120	121	74	74	75	76	77	78	78
	95th	117	118	119	121	123	124	125	78	78	79	80	81	82	82
	99th	124	125	127	129	130	132	132	86	86	87	88	89	90	90
12	50th	101	102	104	106	108	109	110	59	60	61	62	63	63	64
	90th	115	116	118	120	121	123	123	74	75	75	76	77	78	79
	95th	119	120	122	123	125	127	127	78	79	80	81	82	82	83
	99th	126	127	129	131	133	134	135	86	87	88	89	90	90	91
13	50th	104	105	106	108	110	111	112	60	60	61	62	63	64	64
	90th	117	118	120	122	124	125	126	75	75	76	77	78	79	79
	95th	121	122	124	126	128	129	130	79	79	80	81	82	83	83
	99th	128	130	131	133	135	136	137	87	87	88	89	90	91	91
14	50th	106	107	109	111	113	114	115	60	61	62	63	64	65	65
	90th	120	121	123	125	126	128	128	75	76	77	78	79	79	80
	95th	124	125	127	128	130	132	132	80	80	81	82	83	84	84
	99th	131	132	134	136	138	139	140	87	88	89	90	91	92	92
15	50th	109	110	112	113	115	117	117	61	62	63	64	65	66	66
	90th	122	124	125	127	129	130	131	76	77	78	79	80	80	81
	95th	126	127	129	131	133	134	135	81	81	82	83	84	85	85
	99th	134	135	136	138	140	142	142	88	89	90	91	92	93	93

(Continued)

TABLE 58-2

BP LEVELS FOR BOYS BY AGE AND HEIGHT PERCENTILE—CONT'D

Age, yr	BP Percentile	SBP, mm Hg							DBP, mm Hg						
		Percentile of Height							Percentile of Height						
		5th	*10th*	*25th*	*50th*	*75th*	*90th*	*95th*	*5th*	*10th*	*25th*	*50th*	*75th*	*90th*	*95th*
16	50th	111	112	114	116	118	119	120	63	63	64	65	66	67	67
	90th	125	126	128	130	131	133	134	78	78	79	80	81	82	82
	95th	129	130	132	134	135	137	137	82	83	83	84	85	86	87
	99th	136	137	139	141	143	144	145	90	90	91	92	93	94	94
17	50th	114	115	116	118	120	121	122	65	66	66	67	68	69	70
	90th	127	128	130	132	134	135	136	80	80	81	82	83	84	84
	95th	131	132	134	136	138	139	140	84	85	86	87	87	88	89
	99th	139	140	141	143	145	146	147	92	93	93	94	95	96	97

Reprinted from the Fourth Report of the National High Blood Pressure Education Program Working Group on High Blood Pressure in Children and Adolescents,[9] with permission.
Copyright © American Academy of Pediatrics.

TABLE 58-3

BP LEVELS FOR GIRLS BY AGE AND HEIGHT PERCENTILE

Age, yr	BP Percentile	SBP, mm Hg							DBP, mm Hg						
		Percentile of Height							Percentile of Height						
		5th	*10th*	*25th*	*50th*	*75th*	*90th*	*95th*	*5th*	*10th*	*25th*	*50th*	*75th*	*90th*	*95th*
1	50th	83	84	85	86	88	89	90	38	39	39	40	41	41	42
	90th	97	97	98	100	101	102	103	52	53	53	54	55	55	56
	95th	100	101	102	104	105	106	107	56	57	57	58	59	59	60
	99th	108	108	109	111	112	113	114	64	64	65	65	66	67	67
2	50th	85	85	87	88	89	91	91	43	44	44	45	46	46	47
	90th	98	99	100	101	103	104	105	57	58	58	59	60	61	61
	95th	102	103	104	105	107	108	109	61	62	62	63	64	65	65
	99th	109	110	111	112	114	115	116	69	69	70	70	71	72	72
3	50th	86	87	88	89	91	92	93	47	48	48	49	50	50	51
	90th	100	100	102	103	104	106	106	61	62	62	63	64	64	65
	95th	104	104	105	107	108	109	110	65	66	66	67	68	68	69
	99th	111	111	113	114	115	116	117	73	73	74	74	75	76	76
4	50th	88	88	90	91	92	94	94	50	50	51	52	52	53	54
	90th	101	102	103	104	106	107	108	64	64	65	66	67	67	68
	95th	105	106	107	108	110	111	112	68	68	69	70	71	71	72
	99th	112	113	114	115	117	118	119	76	76	76	77	78	79	79
5	50th	89	90	91	93	94	95	96	52	53	53	54	55	55	56
	90th	103	103	105	106	107	109	109	66	67	67	68	69	69	70
	95th	107	107	108	110	111	112	113	70	71	71	72	73	73	74
	99th	114	114	116	117	118	120	120	78	78	79	79	80	81	81
6	50th	91	92	93	94	96	97	98	54	54	55	56	56	57	58
	90th	104	105	106	108	109	110	111	68	68	69	70	70	71	72
	95th	108	109	110	111	113	114	115	72	72	73	74	74	75	76
	99th	115	116	117	119	120	121	122	80	80	80	81	82	83	83
7	50th	93	93	95	96	97	99	99	55	56	56	57	58	58	59
	90th	106	107	108	109	111	112	113	69	70	70	71	72	72	73
	95th	110	111	112	113	115	116	116	73	74	74	75	76	76	77
	99th	117	118	119	120	122	123	124	81	81	82	82	83	84	84
8	50th	95	95	96	98	99	100	101	57	57	57	58	59	60	60
	90th	108	109	110	111	113	114	114	71	71	71	72	73	74	74
	95th	112	112	114	115	116	118	118	75	75	75	76	77	78	78
	99th	119	120	121	122	123	125	125	82	82	83	83	84	85	86
9	50th	96	97	98	100	101	102	103	58	58	58	59	60	61	61
	90th	110	110	112	113	114	116	116	72	72	72	73	74	75	75
	95th	114	114	115	117	118	119	120	76	76	76	77	78	79	79
	99th	121	121	123	124	125	127	127	83	83	84	84	85	86	87
10	50th	98	99	100	102	103	104	105	59	59	59	60	61	62	62
	90th	112	112	114	115	116	118	118	73	73	73	74	75	76	76
	95th	116	116	117	119	120	121	122	77	77	77	78	79	80	80
	99th	123	123	125	126	127	129	129	84	84	85	86	86	87	88

(Continued)

TABLE 58-3

BP LEVELS FOR GIRLS BY AGE AND HEIGHT PERCENTILE —CONT'D

Age, yr	BP Percentile	SBP, mm Hg							DBP, mm Hg						
		Percentile of Height							Percentile of Height						
		5th	*10th*	*25th*	*50th*	*75th*	*90th*	*95th*	*5th*	*10th*	*25th*	*50th*	*75th*	*90th*	*95th*
11	50th	00	101	102	103	105	106	107	60	60	60	61	62	63	63
	90th	114	114	116	117	118	119	120	74	74	74	75	76	77	77
	95th	118	118	119	121	122	123	124	78	78	78	79	80	81	81
	99th	125	125	126	128	129	130	131	85	85	86	87	87	88	89
12	50th	102	103	104	105	107	108	109	61	61	61	62	63	64	64
	90th	116	116	117	119	120	121	122	75	75	75	76	77	78	78
	95th	119	120	121	123	124	125	126	79	79	79	80	81	82	82
	99th	127	127	128	130	131	132	133	86	86	87	88	88	89	90
13	50th	104	105	106	107	109	110	110	62	62	62	63	64	65	65
	90th	117	118	119	121	122	123	124	76	76	76	77	78	79	79
	95th	121	122	123	124	126	127	128	80	80	80	81	82	83	83
	99th	128	129	130	132	133	134	135	87	87	88	89	89	90	91
14	50th	106	106	107	109	110	111	112	63	63	63	64	65	66	66
	90th	119	120	121	122	124	125	125	77	77	77	78	79	80	80
	95th	123	123	125	126	127	129	129	81	81	81	82	83	84	84
	99th	130	131	132	133	135	136	136	88	88	89	90	90	91	92
15	50th	107	108	109	110	111	113	113	64	64	64	65	66	67	67
	90th	120	121	122	123	125	126	127	78	78	78	79	80	81	81
	95th	124	125	126	127	129	130	131	82	82	82	83	84	85	85
	99th	131	132	133	134	136	137	138	89	89	90	91	91	92	93
16	50th	108	108	110	111	112	114	114	64	64	65	66	66	67	68
	90th	121	122	123	124	126	127	128	78	78	79	80	81	81	82
	95th	125	126	127	128	130	131	132	82	82	83	84	85	85	86
	99th	132	133	134	135	137	138	139	90	90	90	91	92	93	93
17	50th	108	109	110	111	113	114	115	64	65	65	66	67	67	68
	90th	122	122	123	125	126	127	128	78	79	79	80	81	81	82
	95th	125	126	127	129	130	131	132	82	83	83	84	85	85	86
	99th	133	133	134	136	137	138	139	90	90	91	91	92	93	93

Reprinted from the Fourth Report of the National High Blood Pressure Education Program Working Group on High Blood Pressure in Children and Adolescents,[9] with permission.
Copyright © American Academy of Pediatric.

organs. If none is found, then further follow-up is recommended, making repeated measurements both in the clinic and using ambulatory monitoring, and suggesting changes in lifestyle as for pre-hypertensive patients.[9]

Variability of Blood Pressure

Serial determinations of blood pressure are necessary before concluding that a child is hypertensive, as variability of blood pressure exists even if differences in the devices used for measurement are taken in to account.[88,116,117] There is a general tendency for initially high pressures to regress towards the mean. This tendency is greatest in those with the highest pressures. It is not clear whether the initial recording or the later basal record is the better predictor of hypertensive disease.[118] It is important to recognise that most people have highly labile pressures,[119] with one study reporting that only one-fifth of those identified as having a labile blood pressure when young had definite hypertension in later life.[120]

Most epidemiologic studies in children reporting on the prevalence of hypertension define elevated blood pressure on the basis of at least three measurements done at the time of a single visit, acknowledging the variability of blood pressure. It seems reasonable, at least in children, only to follow up those whose pressures are persistently raised. General advice in relation to weight, smoking, and other risk factors should be given to those adolescents who are persistently borderline.

Tracking

The tendency of the blood pressure of an individual to rise with time along the centile of the initial determination is known as tracking. Such tracking was established by following the blood pressure of two cohorts from South Wales over a period of 8 to 10 years.[121] The rise noted was significantly related to mean pressure at first determination, but only indirectly related to age, conclusions confirmed in a larger study extending over 30 years.[122] The evidence from tracking, therefore, indicates that the blood pressure of an individual is determined from an early age. Any rise that occurs becomes steeper with time and is related to the initial starting pressure. Blood pressure does not rise with age in everyone. Indeed, in some populations it does not rise at all.[123] This emphasises the pathological nature of a raised blood pressure, and of tracking. The importance of tracking in children is firstly, whether it occurs, and if it does, at what age; and secondly, whether tracking enables individuals at risk of

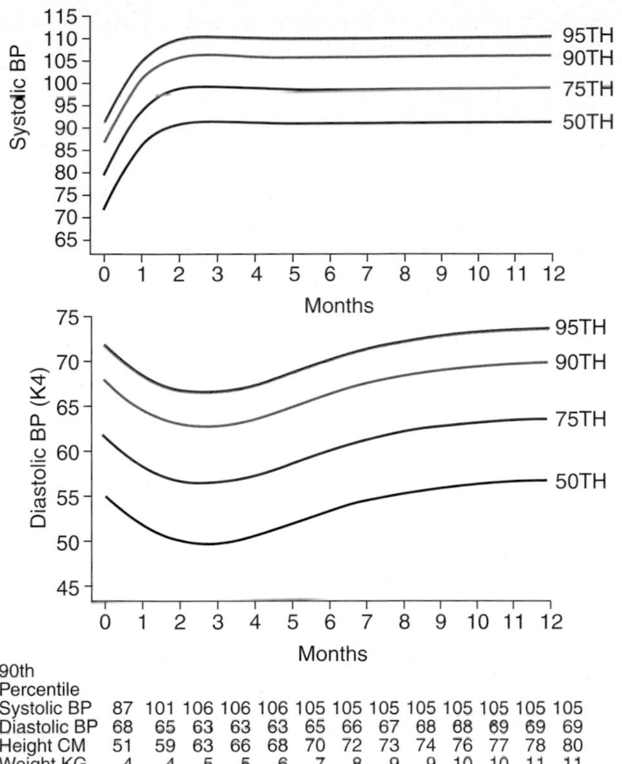

90th Percentile													
Systolic BP	87	101	106	106	106	105	105	105	105	105	105	105	105
Diastolic BP	68	65	63	63	63	65	66	67	68	68	69	69	69
Height CM	51	59	63	66	68	70	72	73	74	76	77	78	80
Weight KG	4	4	5	5	6	7	8	9	9	10	10	11	11

Figure 58-2 Centiles of measurements of blood pressure in boys from birth to the age of 12 months, using phase 4 (K4) for measurement of diastolic pressure. (Reprinted with permission from National Heart, Lung and Blood Institute of the USA: Task Force on Blood Pressure Control in Children [second report]. Pediatrics 1987;79:1–25. ©American Academy of Pediatrics.)

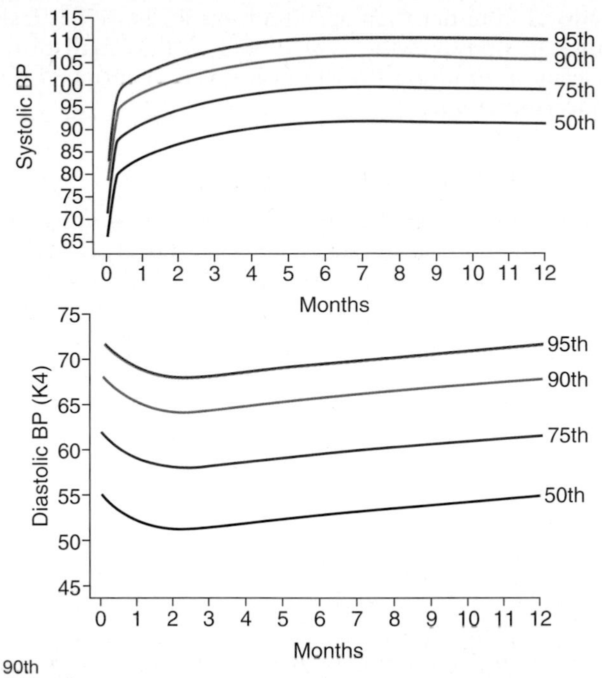

90th Percentile													
Systolic BP	76	98	101	104	105	106	106	106	106	106	106	105	105
Diastolic BP	68	65	64	64	65	65	66	66	66	67	67	67	67
Height (cm)	54	55	56	58	61	63	66	68	70	72	74	75	77
Weight (kg)	4	4	4	5	5	6	7	8	9	9	10	10	11

Figure 58-3 Centiles of measurement of blood pressure in girls from birth to 12 months of age, using phase 4 (K4) for measurement of diastolic pressure. (Reprinted with permission from National Heart, Lung and Blood Institute of the USA: Task Force on Blood Pressure Control in Children [second report]. Pediatrics 1987;79:1–25. ©American Academy of Pediatrics.)

development of hypertensive disease to be identified with reasonable reliability early in life.

A number of studies have demonstrated tracking in childhood.[74,124–129] The phenomenon is not so marked as in adults, but the relation between initial and later pressures increases significantly as the population passes through adolescence. In one study,[128] two-thirds of children with systolic blood pressures more than one standard deviation above the mean at the initial evaluation were above the mean at follow-up. In the Muscatine study, using random zero sphygmomanometer devices,[125] the correlation coefficient for systolic pressures measured 6 years apart was 0.30. In a later report, these investigators reported that pressures in adults correlated with those present during childhood, and change in ponderosity from childhood to adult life. Tracking of blood pressure was more evident for teenagers than for younger children, and for systolic more than for diastolic pressures.[130] The correlation in adults is about 0.7, and this is achieved by about 18 years of age.[128] Others have demonstrated tracking from 5 years of age,[131] or as starting between 1 and 5 years of age.[132] By 4 years, the correlation in repeated measurements was 0.47. A recent retrospective analysis from the Bogalusa Heart Study research group, a community-based investigation of the evolution of cardiovascular disease risk beginning in childhood, has added to the evidence of tracking of blood pressure through childhood to adulthood.[133]

It is becoming increasingly evident, therefore, that increased childhood weight and measurements greater than the 90th centile during early childhood predict with higher accuracy individuals who will be at risk from hypertension, exacerbated by obesity and development of the metabolic syndrome, when they become adults. The realisation that the rise in blood pressure with age is not inevitable, and that individuals at risk might be identified early, so that appropriate avoidance of risk factors might ameliorate their future morbidity, is of considerable potential importance. Further research is required to identify the risk factors to show that their avoidance alters prognosis and to demonstrate the reliability of early identification of a raised blood pressure in predicting future disease.

Familial Clustering

The tendency for parents and children and siblings to have similar blood pressures is well recognised amongst adults. This clustering is also apparent in children, with a correlation between siblings of 0.33 at the age of 2 to 14 years.[134] Significant, though less strong, correlations have been found between mothers and infants as young as 1 week.[135] Studies on adopted children, compared with other members of the family, including non-adopted siblings, have shown no correlation between the blood pressure of adopted children and other members of the family. The blood pressure of the parents and the non-adopted children, in contrast, correlated significantly.[135] This implies that, at least in children, inheritance is more important than environment in determining blood pressure. Environment is not without influence, however, and the duration of adoption rather than age at adoption, as well as resemblance in body weight, was linked to the small positive aggregation of blood pressure observed in adoptees living in the same home.[135,136]

Exercise, Traction, and Hypertension

Isometric rather than dynamic exercise is associated with a greater rise in diastolic pressure.[137] The Task Force Group[29] expressed doubt concerning the advisability of isometric exercise, such as weight lifting, body building, and so on, in hypertensive children. No dangerous rise in either diastolic or systolic pressure was demonstrated, however, during either dynamic or isometric exercise in hypertensive adolescents,[138] with some[139] concluding that maximal exercise testing was safe in hypertensive adolescents. Although the exercise performance of this cohort was normal, systolic and diastolic pressures were higher than in children with labile hypertension. This finding might indicate caution in allowing full participation in physical activity such as competitive sports. With this caveat, exercise is recommended for hypertension because it is associated with a useful reduction in peripheral vascular resistance and blood pressure.[140] Children undergoing orthopaedic immobilisation with plaster casts, and those in traction, have a fourfold greater incidence of hypertension.[141] The rise in blood pressure, averaging 33 mm Hg in one study, was maximal on the fourth day of treatment, but resolved when the treatment was stopped.[142] The cause is not known, but it has been related to increased sympathetic activity from stretching of the sciatic nerve, to retention of salt and water from immobilisation, and to increased production of catecholamines causing increased output of renin from the kidney.[142]

Obesity and Hypertension

The dramatic increase in childhood obesity and overweight state in most developed countries has been an alarming phenomenon over the past two to three decades.[143–146] This phenomenon has been reported worldwide, with recognition that these trends are likely to have major consequence for public health.[147] One major consequence is the development of the metabolic syndrome, this being the association of obesity, hypertension, dyslipidaemia, and diabetes mellitus. Population-based studies have shown that obese and overweight children have much higher rates of hypertension than those who are not overweight.[146,148–151] As we have discussed, levels of blood pressure track from childhood to adulthood. Hypertension, along with other components of the metabolic syndrome, has been shown to lead to the development of early atherosclerosis.[152,153] Lean mass and total body fat mass independently and positively correlate with increased pressures.[154] A positive correlation with blood pressure in this latter cohort was observed across a range of bodily habituses, and not just for overweight or obese children. Others[155] have suggested that loss of weight would help reduce risks of developing hypertension in later life. When evaluating patients with high blood pressure, therefore, note should be taken of the presence of co-morbid features, such as overweight, obesity, and dyslipidaemia. Measures to lose weight should remain an active part of the plan for management of an overweight or obese child with hypertension.

HYPERTENSION

Definition

The precise level defining hypertension during childhood has been debated for some time. Population-based studies have provided some understanding of the physiological changes in blood pressure during childhood. Blood pressure is influenced by gender and age, but the predominant influence of height over age on blood pressure variability, accounting for almost two-fifths of change, has been well demonstrated by the Bogalusa Heart Study.[156] At a given age, taller children have higher pressures. This relationship of increasing blood pressure with body size, therefore, is physiological.

It is possible, nonetheless, to define the statistical likelihood of a pathological event occurring at a given level of blood pressure. If the generally observed rise in blood pressure with advancing age in adult life is itself pathological, then the appropriate cut-off point might be the mean plus 2 standard deviations for a young adult, equating to 140/90 mm Hg. Alternatively, an even lower value of 125/75 mm Hg might be taken, since this represents the mean. Extending this statistical definition in children, the normal can also be defined in relation to the population. Values above the 95th centile are then regarded as being more likely to represent abnormality. This approach necessarily defines 5% of the population as being hypertensive.

The most appropriate definition, therefore, is one that defines values beyond which there is an associated significant risk of developing increased morbidity and mortality in the future. For example, men aged from 40 to 69 years with a blood pressure of 160/100 mm Hg are four times more likely to die than those with a blood pressure of 120/80 mm Hg.[157] A man with a blood pressure of 150/100 mm Hg at the age of 45 years can expect to live 11 years less than a man with a blood pressure of 120/80 mm Hg.[158] No such data exists in children. There is some evidence from the Bogalusa Heart Study that values above the 90th centile will lead to hypertension in adulthood in one-third of patients.[159]

The Fourth Report now provides 50th, 90th, 95th, and 99th centile values obtained by auscultation in gender, age, and height specific format for a large number of children.[9] This guideline has pooled data from several epidemiologic studies, some of whom have measurements made only once. Keeping in mind some of the issues we have already discussed, this is bound to introduce some inaccuracies, with the possibility that some patients may be misclassified.[20] The Fourth Report on measurements of blood pressure, nonetheless, provides the most widely accepted reference standards for normative values.

Which measurement is more important—systolic or diastolic? In children, as in adults, systolic hypertension seems to be more important than diastolic hypertension.[160] Systolic hypertension is more common than diastolic hypertension, and correlates better to left ventricular mass index across a wide range of values.[161–165] Systolic hypertension, when present in combination with normal diastolic blood pressure in a patient, needs to be evaluated and treated.

Another useful definition of hypertension would be values above which treatment was associated with a reduction in morbidity and mortality. Although such values have been established for adults, the lack of damage to end organs, and/or absence of cerebrovascular and cardiovascular endpoints with values during childhood, make it impossible to assign a risk above certain levels. The most common surrogate marker during childhood of hypertensive damage to end organs is the presence of an increased indexed left ventricular mass and/or the presence of left ventricular hypertrophy. Studies of normal and hypertensive children have found that systolic blood pressure and the mass index are positively associated across a wide range of values, with no clear threshold to predict a pathologically increased index.[161–165] It should also be noted that, as blood pressure is a continuous variable within a population, to regard a certain level as pathological is to some extent arbitrary.[166]

Classification

Primary, or essential, hypertension is a term used to describe hypertension for which no obvious cause is apparent. This is the most common type of mild hypertension found in children. Secondary hypertension is hypertension for which an underlying cause can be identified. Such a cause is found in up to nine-tenths of children presenting with severe hypertension, with renal disease being the underlying abnormality in the majority. With the increasing prevalence of childhood obesity, and of the metabolic syndrome as discussed above, changes are occurring in this distribution of primary and secondary hypertension. It is helpful clinically to categorise secondary hypertension as being acute and transient, or chronic and sustained.[167] There is considerable overlap, nonetheless, between children falling into these two groups, and one form may progress to the other.[167]

Patients may show systolic or diastolic hypertension, or both. Isolated systolic hypertension, with a wide pulse pressure, may be a feature of hyperthyroidism, aortic valvar incompetence, patency of the arterial duct, or an arteriovenous shunt. Stress may cause a rise in both systolic and diastolic pressure, or in systolic pressure alone. As we have also discussed, the white coat and masked variants are further diagnostic categories that have been introduced in the field of childhood hypertension.

The severity of the vascular changes observed on retinal examination permits grading of hypertension in childhood. Long-standing hypertension is known to be associated with retinal arteriolar narrowing.[168,169] So-called grade I changes occur with mild venous narrowing at the site of arterial crossing, with slight thickening of the arterial wall. In the changes graded at the second level, there is obvious arteriolar thickening producing the copper wire appearance. Changes of the third grade exist when the arteriolar wall is so thick that no column of blood is visible, this giving the silver wire appearance, with marked venous compression. Grade IV changes are described when the arterioles are thin fibrous cords, with no distal flow. Retinal haemorrhages and exudates are additionally present in changes of the third grade, while papilloedema is a feature of the fourth grade, also considered to be malignant hypertension. Severe retinal changes are less common in children, although papilloedema is observed in hypertensive encephalopathy with headache, drowsiness, and convulsions.[170] Retinal arterioles, as opposed to retinal venules, show better correlation with increasing pressures in both normotensive and hypertensive children. Retinal examination, however, is often difficult in children, who may not be able to tolerate a detailed retinal examination.

Prevalence

The overall prevalence of mild hypertension must be about 5% because this is determined by the definition. The definition, however, requires that the raised blood pressure be persistent. This will tend to lower the prevalence, whereas the inclusion of systolic or diastolic pressure within the definition will tend to raise it.

It is well established that elevated levels can normalise after several measurements are performed over time, with one study,[171] after repeated screening of adolescents, identifying 1.2% of the cohort as having mild systolic, and 2.4% having mild diastolic hypertension. Results from another review[172] showed the range of prevalence dropping from 2% to 13% at initial screening to about 1% showing persistent mild hypertension after repeated measurements. This remains true even now with significant reduction of prevalence of hypertension.[173,174]

Several recent population-based studies from both the developed and the developing world, nonetheless, when using the criterions suggested in the Fourth Report, have found prevalences between 4.5% and 23%.[9,146,148,149,175] Those conducting these studies measured pressures one to three times at one single visit using a mercury sphygmomanometer or an oscillometric device.

The prevalence of severe hypertension is difficult to ascertain. It can only be determined from surveys of populations. Detailed diagnoses are not always provided in such studies. Prevalence for secondary hypertension varied between zero and 0.2% in various surveys.[172] These surveys vary according to their design, and the selection and referral to hospital for investigations. Some studies of normal populations covering thousands of children have revealed no cases of severe secondary hypertension.[172,176] In the Muscatine study,[116] 0.1% had secondary hypertension. Results obtained from other surveys produced figures of 0.07%,[177] 0.11%,[178] and 0.17%.[179]

Causes

Many conditions can be associated with hypertension (Table 58-4), and even this lengthy list is not exhaustive. In Table 58-5, we show the final diagnosis of 100 children referred with severe hypertension to a specialised centre. More recently, an increased incidence of essential hypertension has been associated with overweight and obesity. In practice, if the primary condition is not obvious, coarctation is excluded, and if the hypertension is severe rather than mild or borderline, then renal disease accounts for the vast majority of cases.

In Table 58-5, we show the distribution of ages for the different causes identified. Aortic coarctation, renovascular hypertension, mainly due to thrombosis of the renal artery following umbilical arterial catheterisation, and intracranial haemorrhage are common causes in neonates and infants. In the preschool child, aortic coarctation, renovascular causes, congenital renal abnormalities, tumours, and haemolytic uraemic syndrome predominate. In the older

TABLE 58-4

CAUSES OF HYPERTENSION IN CHILDREN

System	Condition
Renovascular	Renal arterial stenosis Idiopathic Neurofibromatosis type I Williams syndrome Renal arterial thrombosis Renal venous thrombosis Haemolytic uraemic syndrome Fistula External compression
Parenchymal renal disease	Glomerulonephritis Post-infection Henoch-Schoenlein purpura with nephritis IgA nephropathy Systemic lupus erythematosus nephritis Mesangiocapillary glomerulonephritis Focal and segmental glomerulosclerosis Anti-neutrophil cytoplasmic antibody-associated nephritis Anti-glomerular basement membrane nephritis Acute tubular necrosis with secondary salt and water overload Pyelonephritis-related renal scarring, or reflux nephropathy Polycystic kidney disease—autosomal recessive, autosomal dominant Wilms' tumour Obstructive uropathy
Cardiovascular	Aortic coarctation Thoracic Abdominal Fibro-muscular dysplasia Takayasu's arteritis
Endocrine	Catecholamine excess Phaeochromocytoma, neuroblastoma Aldosterone/mineralocorticoid excess Idiopathic mineralocorticoid excess, Conn's syndrome, dexamethasone-suppressive hyperaldosteronism Cortisol/glucocorticoid excess—Cushing's syndrome Steroid therapy, ACTH-producing pituitary tumour, cortisol-producing adrenal tumour Congenital adrenal hyperplasia 17-Hydroxylase deficiency, 11-hydroxylase deficiency Hyperthyroidism Liddle syndrome
Metabolic and drug use	Amphetamine or sympathomimetic overdosage (including nose-drops) Oral contraceptive pill Cyclosporine Monoamine oxidase inhibitors Clonidine withdrawal Acute vitamin D intoxication, hypercalcaemia Chronic vitamin D deficiency Ecstasy (MDMA and derivatives), cocaine Liquorice ingestion
Central nervous system	Convulsions Pain Raised intracranial pressure Guillain-Barré syndrome, dysautonomia
Miscellaneous	Essential

child, chronic nephritis, reflux nephropathy, and end-stage renal disease are more common.

Clinical Features and Complications

The presenting symptoms of hypertension vary according to the severity of the causative disease, the severity of the hypertension, and the age of the child. Raised blood pressure may be an unexpected cause of a common childhood symptom, such as recurrent abdominal pain or headache. It may be an incidental and apparently unconnected finding on physical examination in a child with another complaint. In Table 58-6, we summarise the major clinical symptoms in a cohort of infants and children reviewed from the literature.[172] Inspection of this list emphasises the need to exclude hypertension in any sick child, and should reinforce the importance of routine measurement in the assessment of children.

Severe hypertension may cause congestive cardiac failure with fluid overload, cardiac dilation with impaired ventricular function and mitral incompetence, and pulmonary oedema. This combination is life-threatening and requires intensive care with positive pressure ventilation, diuretic therapy, inotropic support, and sometimes haemofiltration. Paediatric nephrologists, cardiologists, and often paediatric intensivists are usually involved in the investigation and management of severe life-threatening hypertension.

About one-tenth of children with hypertension have neurological symptoms and complications,[180,181] which are frequently the presenting feature. Convulsions were the most frequently encountered complication in one review, occurring in over nine-tenths of the children.[182] Facial palsy and an altered level of consciousness were each encountered in 4%. Visual disturbances may be caused by retinal involvement, vitreous haemorrhage, and infarction of the anterior visual pathways.[183] Cortical blindness is associated with cerebral oedema, which usually resolves, leaving no residual impairment. The posterior leucoencephalopathy syndrome involves oedematous lesions, particularly of the posterior parietal and occipital lobes, and may spread to the basal ganglia, the brainstem, and the cerebellum.[184] It is characterised by headache, nausea and vomiting, seizures, visual disturbances, altered sensory experiences, and occasionally a focal neurological deficit. Whilst there is usually no change seen on computerised tomographic scans, magnetic resonance imaging reveals increased signals predominantly involving the posterior regions of the cerebral hemispheres.

In spite of the relatively good prognosis in survivors, hypertensive encephalopathy is potentially fatal and requires urgent treatment, which we will discuss below. At the other end of the spectrum of severity, mild hypertension, which is usually diagnosed incidentally, may produce no obvious clinical manifestations. Essential hypertension is often mild, and is most commonly seen in the overweight adolescent with a family history of hypertension.

Diagnosis

At diagnosis, it is necessary to establish the severity of the effects of the hypertension, and its cause. A complete family history is important. Essential hypertension is often familial. Some types of renal disease that cause hypertension are inherited, for example, autosomal dominant polycystic

TABLE 58-5

FINAL DIAGNOSIS IN 100 CHILDREN REFERRED FOR HYPERTENSION CONSECUTIVELY OVER A 5-YEAR PERIOD, ACCORDING TO AGE

	AGE (YEARS)			
	0–1	1–5	6–15	All
Chronic glomerulonephritis		2	33	35
Reflux nephropathy			14	14
Obstructive uropathy	1	1	4	6
Haemolytic uraemic syndrome	1	2	3	6
Renovascular	1	3	2	6
Polycystic (infantile and adult)		1	3	4
Dysplastic kidneys		3	3	
Cystinosis		3	3	
Hypoplastic kidneys		1	1	2
Juvenile nephronophthisis			2	2
Wilms' tumour			2	
Papillary necrosis		1		1
Essential hypertension			1	1
Obesity			1	1
Aortic coarctation	8	5	2	15
Total	12	16	72	100

From Gill DG, Mendes de Costa B, Cameron JS, et al: Analysis of 100 children with severe and persistent hypertension. Arch Dis Child 1976;51:951–956.

TABLE 58-6

CLINICAL SYNDROMES OF HYPERTENSION

Syndrome	Percentage (%)
Infants	
Congestive cardiac failure	56
Respiratory distress	36
Failure to thrive, vomiting	29
Irritability	20
Convulsions	11
Children	
Headache	30
Nausea, vomiting	13
Hypertensive encephalopathy	10.6
Polydipsia, polyuria	7.4
Visual problems	5.2
Tiredness, irritability	4.5
Cardiac failure	4.5
Facial palsy	3.4
Epistaxis	3.0
Growth retardation, weight loss	2.7
Cardiac murmur	2.7
Abdominal pain	1.8
Enuresis	1.2

Data from 645 infants and children.
From Leuman EP: Blood pressure and hypertension in childhood and adolescence. In Frick P, von Harneck GA, Martini GA, et al, eds: Advances in Internal Medicine and Pediatrics. Berlin: Springer, 1979, pp. 109–183.

kidney disease, autosomal recessive polycystic kidney disease, and neurofibromatosis type 1. The blood pressure of the parents should be measured. The neonatal history may reveal perinatal asphyxia with low Apgar scores, a risk factor for renal venous thrombosis. Insertion of umbilical arterial and venous catheters in the newborn may lead to reno-vascular thrombosis or embolisation that may be associated with hypertension. A past history of recurrent infections of the urinary tract suggests pyelonephritic scarring as a possible cause. Enquiry should be made for specific symptoms associated with hypertension, such as headaches, epistaxis, or blurred vision. Intermittent episodes of headache, sweating, palpitations and pallor, and rarely flushing may suggest a phaeochromocytoma. A thorough history of potential ingestion of medications should be obtained, and adolescent patients should be asked about use of recreational drugs, such as Ecstasy and cocaine.[185] Maternal use of cocaine may also lead to sustained postnatal hypertension in the newborn.[186]

The physical examination aims to look for signs of the underlying cause of hypertension, and for evidence of damage to end organs. The height and weight should be measured, and the body mass index calculated. Long-standing undiagnosed hypertension may cause poor growth.[187] Initial inspection of the patient may suggest syndromes known to be associated with hypertension, including Cushing's syndrome, Williams syndrome,[188,189] and Turner's syndrome.[190] Peripheral pulses should be assessed, in particular simultaneous palpation of the right brachial and the femoral pulse to exclude brachio-femoral delay as a sign of aortic coarctation. Blood pressure should be measured in the right arm with the patient both lying and standing, and measured in the legs to determine if there is any difference between the upper and lower limbs, a feature again suggestive of coarctation. Close inspection of the skin may reveal the café-au-lait patches and neurofibromas of neurofibromatosis type 1. Palpable kidneys suggest enlarged polycystic kidneys, especially autosomal recessive polycystic kidney disease. Fundoscopy may show changes suggesting long-standing hypertension, such as narrowing or sclerosis of retinal arteries, and changes of arteriovenous crossing. Severe hypertension is associated with retinal haemorrhages and papilloedema.

A strong indication of the cause of the hypertension is often present from the history and examination. As a general rule, essential hypertension is usually mild, while secondary hypertension is severe. Unless the hypertension is mild, the initial investigation and control require admission to hospital. The proportion of children with secondary hypertension caused by aortic coarctation, up to one-third, should be identified clinically. Renal disease, or renal arterial stenosis, is the commonest cause of secondary hypertension in childhood, and this will usually be apparent as the cause after initial routine investigations. The approach to investigation and assessment of neonatal and childhood hypertension have recently been reviewed.[9,191] Routine investigations, and those designed to establish the severity of the hypertension, will include a full blood count, plasma urea, electrolytes, creatinine, and uric acid. A hypokalaemic alkalosis suggests excess activity of aldosterone, either from a mineralocorticoid syndrome or secondary to hyper-reninism. Further blood tests may include measurements of renin, aldosterone, and catecholamines in the plasma. We will discuss such measurements further, but the use of antihypertensive drugs prior to investigation frequently invalidates these assays. The urine should be examined for blood, protein, cells, and casts as markers of renal disease, and should be cultured if urinalysis is abnormal. Unless the cause is obvious, measurements are usually made of vanillylmandelic acid in the urine to exclude either a phaeochromocytoma or hypertension caused by neuroblastoma. A chest radiograph, an electrocardiogram, and an echocardiogram, looking for left ventricular hypertrophy, should be performed,[9,192,193] and ultrasonic investigation made of the kidneys, looking for obvious renal asymmetry, scarring, cysts, or dilation. In addition, a scan using ^{99m}Tc-dimercaptosuccinnic acid is usually performed,[194] this test having a high sensitivity for renal scarring that may not be detected by ultrasonic investigation. As we will discuss, renal arteriography and other specific investigations may be required. As already indicated, the control of the hypertension with drugs may invalidate the determination of renin, aldosterone, and catecholamines in the plasma, as well as the latter agents in the urine,[195,196] so that samples of blood and urine for these investigations, whenever possible, should always be taken prior to initiation of therapy.

Screening

Controversy still exists as to whether normal children should be screened for hypertension. The Fourth Report recommends measurement of blood pressure in all children older than 3 years when seen by a health professional.[9] For children younger than 3 years, measurement of blood pressure has been recommended in specific groups.[9]

Due to some of the inherent problems with measurement of blood pressure discussed previously, the usefulness of routine measurement in children has been questioned.[20,197] As discussed, levels of pressure in children are very variable, and the correlation between initial and follow-up measurements is not sufficiently strong to allow predictions of future values to be made from initial recordings.[198] It has also been suggested that the rate of identification of severe hypertension is too low to justify the expense.[30]

For mild hypertension, the dilemma is considerable, because a large number of such children would be identified by a screening programme. To label an apparently well child as hypertensive could, and probably would, cause great harm. To treat mild hypertension is expensive, and may even be dangerous, but to leave hypertensive children undiagnosed, to become hypertensive adults, may also be undesirable.[199] The issues with severe hypertension are clearer. Early diagnosis allows effective treatment, prevents complications, and improves life expectancy.

In practice, we recommend that children with pressures higher than the 90th centile for age and height should be recalled for further measurement. If found to be normal, no further follow-up is required, though general advice concerning reduction of weight, diet, and so on should be given. The child with severe hypertension should be investigated immediately. As we will discuss, the child with mild hypertension should be followed up. Ambulatory monitoring will help to establish whether such children discovered during visits to the clinic have mild but sustained hypertension at home or at school, or whether they have white coat hypertension.

Hypertension in Infants

The diagnosis of hypertension in infancy requires knowledge of the normal limits for blood pressure. An increasing amount of data is available providing values for premature and term neonates, and in infants in the first year of life.[200–207] A simple guide is that repeated measurements of systolic pressure above 90 mm Hg in neonates at term, and above 80 mm Hg in preterm neonates, are indicative of hypertension.[208] Systemic hypertension in the newborn that is not related to aortic coarctation appears to be increasing. Thromboembolic occlusions of the renal vasculature are commonly related to indwelling umbilical arterial and venous catheters, with four-fifths of cases of renal arterial thrombosis reported in one series associated with indwelling umbilical arterial catheters.[209] Aortic thrombosis has been demonstrated in up to one-third of neonates with indwelling catheters.[210] It is important to check that the tip of the catheter is left below the level of the renal artery, which is between the ninth thoracic and first lumbar vertebras, and immediately to withdraw it below this level if it is found to be incorrectly positioned. The diagnosis of renal vascular involvement may be made by ultrasonic investigation, although computerised tomography or magnetic resonance angiography may give clearer imaging. In some patients, an aortogram and selective renal arteriography may be necessary. Direct dissolution of clot with recombinant human tissue plasminogen activator can also be achieved using the catheter used for the diagnostic study. Infants who suffer an intravascular thrombosis should be screened for inherited thrombophilic disorders.[211]

A relatively common cause of neonatal hypertension is bronchopulmonary dysplasia.[212] Other rarer causes of neonatal hypertension include congenital renal arterial stenosis,[213] renal venous thrombosis, structural renal disorders, raised intracranial pressure from space-occupying lesions, phaeochromocytoma, congenital adrenal hyperplasia, and autosomal recessive polycystic kidney disease. In one study,[214] all infants reviewed with this last diagnosis had established hypertension by 3 months of age. Infants requiring extracorporeal membrane oxygenation are also at risk of hypertension.[215]

Neonates with hypertension are often severely ill, with tachypnoea, cyanosis and congestive cardiac failure. Neurological symptoms are common, with lethargy, apnoea, fits, and focal neurological defects. These symptoms may be related to intracranial bleeding or to hypertensive encephalopathy. One-quarter of affected infants, however, may be asymptomatic.[209] Renal enlargement is uncommon except with renal venous thrombosis. Haematuria and proteinuria occur in about half the infants, but can be present without hypertension. Raised levels of urea or creatinine are common. A consumptive coagulopathy with a microangiopathic haemolytic anaemia may be present, with thrombocytopenia, fragmented red cells and prolonged prothrombin and partial thromboplastin times. Activity of renin is usually raised in the plasma.

Control of the hypertension is vital. Prazosin, in doses up to 500 µg/kg per day, hydralazine up to 10 mg/kg per day, and propranolol up to 2 mg/kg per day are usually successful, though a diuretic may also be required. More potent vasodilator agents, such as minoxidil or captopril, an inhibitor of angiotensin-converting enzyme, may be required. Acute control of severe hypertension can usually be obtained with an intravenous infusion of labetalol, given at 1 to 3 mg/kg per hour, or nitroprusside at 2.5 to 5 µg/kg per minute.

The prognosis for hypertensive neonates and infants is largely determined by the underlying cause. Most studies describe an overall good outcome for neonates. Hypertension is transient in many infants. In one small series,[209] it was possible to discontinue medication in more than three-quarters of hypertensive infants, and at follow-up all but one had normalised their pressures, remaining free from medication. Other investigators[216] followed up a similar series of hypertensive babies discharged from a neonatal intensive care unit. Of the three-quarters requiring drug treatment, all had discontinued medication by the age of 24 months. Similar favourable outcomes were reported for neonates with aortic thrombosis and neonatal renovascular hypertension[217] and for those who developed renal venous thrombosis.[218] Of the latter group, two infants who developed hypertension responded to removal of the abnormal kidney.

Essential, or Primary, Hypertension

The essential form accounts for about nine-tenths of hypertension in adults. It may be defined as a rise in blood pressure of unknown cause that increases risk for cerebral, cardiac, and renal events. In developed countries, the risk of becoming hypertensive during a lifetime, defined for adults as pressures greater than 140/90 mm Hg, exceeds 90%.[219] Essential hypertension is commonly associated with other cardiovascular risk factors such as ageing, being overweight, insulin resistance, diabetes, and hyperlipidaemia. There is a strong genetic component in essential hypertension. Studies in animals have shown an association with excessive ingestion of salt.[220] People with essential hypertension also excrete a salt load more rapidly than do normal subjects, and this abnormality is present in normotensive young relatives.[221] These observations suggest that a renal abnormality may precede the development of essential hypertension in susceptible people. The genetic nature and self-perpetuation of essential hypertension are perhaps the two most recognised characteristics of the condition. As we will discuss, there are well-described monogenic forms of hypertension, but essential hypertension is likely to involve the complex interplay of many genes.[222]

The impact of essential hypertension in adults has led to increasing interest in the early characteristics seen during childhood that are associated with the subsequent development of hypertension. Events during early life[126,130,152] and diet during fetal development, infancy, and childhood probably influence the eventual levels of blood pressure.[133,151,223] Findings relating low weight at birth to an increased risk of death from cardiovascular events in later adult life[224] have led to further studies exploring this relationship.[225] Some[226] have suggested that the link is a deficiency of nephrons at birth in babies born with low weight. Such a deficiency of nephrons may then progress, through hyperfiltration injury in the remaining nephrons, to further glomerulosclerosis and hypertension.[227] Babies born at term with low weight have been shown to have significantly higher blood pressures by the age of 6 years than those born with normal weight.[228] At birth, however, the initial pressures have been found to be significantly lower, and heart rates significantly higher, in those born weighing less than 2500 g.[229] The smaller babies then showed a significantly faster rise in pressure during the first postnatal month, and through the remainder of the first year maintained their pressures at the same levels as the bigger babies, thereby sustaining a higher pressure per kilogram of body weight. Premature birth has also been associated with significantly increased risk of hypertension.[230] A role has been suggested for elevated levels of uric acid, contributing to endothelial dysfunction and leading to microvascular and inflammatory injury to the kidney,[231] this notion being supported by the finding that levels of uric acid correlated with systolic blood pressures.[232]

There is broad recognition that much of the hypertension found in adults relates to dietary intake of salt. The relation between the prevalence of hypertension in a population and the cultural preference for salt in the diet is well established.[233] Processed food accounts for four-fifths of the salt in the average Western diet, and it is argued that the manufacturers of this processed food should reduce this content.[234] A meta-analysis[235] of 10 trials looking at the effect of reducing intake of salt on pressures in infants, children, and adolescents showed that a modest reduction led to an immediate and significant fall in blood pressure.

Investigation and Diagnosis

The majority of children with essential hypertension have only mild elevations of blood pressure, with no clinical signs of hypertension. Only 2 of 74 children reported in one study[236] had left ventricular hypertrophy. Severe hypertension can result from essential hypertension, with almost one-tenth of one cohort[237] having diastolic pressures greater than 122 mm Hg.

Adults with essential hypertension have been classified according to the activity of renin in the plasma,[238] though the significance of this is not established.[239] Low levels of renin are common in blacks with hypertension, and there is some evidence that cardiovascular complications, such as cerebrovascular accidents or myocardial infarcts, are rarer if the activity is low. Activity of renin, however, is usually normal in children with essential hypertension.[74,236,240] Occasional instances of low levels have been reported in children with essential hypertension.[241]

The diagnosis of essential hypertension depends on the exclusion of all known causes of secondary hypertension (see Table 58-4). Cardiovascular causes are usually excluded during the clinical history and examination. Similarly, the problems produced by the central nervous system, and hypertension related to drugs or metabolic causes, do not pose diagnostic difficulties. Renal disease may be apparent from the clinical evaluation, from the examination of urine, or from the measurement of electrolytes in the plasma. A hypokalaemic alkalosis, which suggests either primary or secondary excess of mineralocorticoids, should be excluded in all cases. Activity of renin in the plasma should be carefully determined, and would be expected to be normal in essential hypertension. Ultrasonic and nuclear scans of the kidneys are usually appropriate to exclude major structural abnormalities and to identify parenchymal scarring. If the clinical history and examination, full blood count, plasma electrolytes, examination of urine, urinary excretion of catecholamine metabolites, thyroid function, ultrasonic and nuclear scans, activity of renin in the plasma, and urinary excretion of steroids are all normal, and the hypertension is not severe, then a diagnosis of essential hypertension is usually appropriate. Severe hypertension, particularly with a raised activity of renin in the plasma, will necessitate a careful search for a renal or renovascular cause. This will involve a renal arteriogram, usually with selective sampling from the renal vein to measure levels of renin in the plasma.

Management

There is no question about the desirability of treating children with severe hypertension. We discuss appropriate treatment in our section devoted to this topic. Some common considerations need discussing here, however, as they are of general importance in the management of hypertension in all children, and also because some are of unique significance to children.

The decision to attempt to lower the blood pressure in children must depend, to some extent, on the assessment by the physician of the circumstances of each child. The psychosocial effects on an adolescent of forcing a confrontation with the implications of long-term management for hypertension may exacerbate the problem, as well as causing undesirable alterations in behaviour and growth. Compliance, particularly with medication, may be unsatisfactory.

General dietary and health advice should initially be given. The avoidance of risk factors, such as smoking, should be encouraged. Obesity should be treated with caloric reduction, and regular exercise encouraged. A reduced intake of salt, to 50 mmol per day, with no salt added to cooking or at the table, is important. Some have suggested combining this with a diet high in potassium.[242] A high ratio of polyunsaturated to saturated fats should be encouraged, while foods rich in cholesterol should be avoided, refined carbohydrate reduced, and the content of dietary fibre increased. Such advice may seem a counsel of perfection, but much can usually be achieved by a minimum of intervention, and without generating excessive anxiety or food fads. Compounds known to exacerbate hypertension, such as liquorice, sympathomimetics, and corticosteroids should be avoided. Oral contraceptives must be used with careful monitoring.

Such measures are probably all that is required initially, together with a relaxed but reliable follow-up to check the blood pressure. If the pressure remains obviously unacceptably raised, at more than 99th centile, or continues to be mildly raised over a period of 1 to 2 years, then antihypertensive treatment may be required. We will discuss this in depth below.

Caution regarding treatment of mild hypertension is advisable, not withstanding the reports of successful intervention.[243,244] This is because some studies have failed to demonstrate a significant difference in morbidity from coronary arterial disease between a control group and a group undergoing treatment that involved the reduction in known risk factors and the treatment of hypertension.[245] A reasonable interpretation of available evidence would allow advice concerning smoking, hypercholesterolaemia, obesity, and exercise.[246] The creation of undue anxiety should always be avoided. Treatment with drugs to reduce blood pressure seems reasonable, as indicated above, as long as careful follow-up is guaranteed.

Hypertension induced by oral contraceptives is common, with an incidence of 7.5%. Furthermore, oral contraceptives will exacerbate hypertension in a similar proportion of individuals.[247] The mechanism is thought to involve stimulation of the release of renin and aldosterone, a direct effect of oestrogen on retention of salt and water, and sensitisation of smooth muscle to vasoconstriction produced by angiotensin II. Cardiac output may also increase. Decisions regarding individual patients will need to take account of individual factors, not least the assessment of the risk of pregnancy. It would seem advisable, however, to discontinue oral contraception if hypertension occurs, but not to preclude its use in the presence of preexisting mild hypertension. A formulation containing low levels of oestrogen should be used. A further rise in blood pressure would then be an indication for stopping treatment.

Up to half of the adults receiving antihypertensive therapy become non-compliant. This is probably equally common in children, especially adolescents.[248] The quality of the relationship between doctor and patient, the degree of knowledge of the patient and of participation, and the ease of consultation are important factors. The ease of administration of the medication, including a reduction in the number of drugs and frequency of ingestion, is important. Long-acting formulations requiring once-daily dosage are preferred. Alterations in life style, including diet, must be introduced slowly. Changing habits is often resisted and may also lead to non-compliance in other areas.

Renal Hypertension

Pathophysiology

Renin is a proteolytic enzyme that is produced by the juxtaglomerular cells and stored in the afferent arteriole. After release into the blood, it reacts with angiotensinogen, a substrate in the plasma produced by the liver, to form the decapeptide, angiotensin I. This agent is then further acted upon by converting enzyme in the lung to produce the octapeptide, angiotensin II, which raises blood pressure by direct vasoconstriction and by its indirect effects on the nervous system. It stimulates secretion of aldosterone, promotes retention of sodium by the kidney, and stimulates thirst and the release of catecholamines and vasopressin.[249] Baroreceptors located in the afferent arteriole control the release of renin. This is also affected by other factors, including delivery of sodium in the distal tubule to the macula densa, sympathetic activity, catecholamines, and hypokalaemia. Activity of the renin-angiotensin system is intrinsically related to the balance of sodium and the volume of extracellular fluid.

The importance of renal ischaemia in the generation of hypertension has been appreciated since classic canine experiments.[250] The detailed mechanisms, nonetheless, remain controversial.[249] Unilateral renal arterial constriction in the rat will produce hypertension. If the constriction is removed within a few weeks, the hypertension subsides. If the clip is left for longer, and then removed, the hypertension often persists. Removal of the non-clipped kidney, but not the previously clipped kidney, will often result in a fall in blood pressure. Concentrations of angiotensin II rise in the plasma with the initial unilateral constriction, and this is probably responsible for the initial rise in blood pressure. Thereafter, the concentration slowly decreases, even though the hypertension persists. It is likely that the renin-angiotensin system is still responsible for the hypertension at this stage. This is partly through its vasoconstrictive action, and partly because of retention of salt.[249] Later, after months or years, removal of the abnormal kidney in humans fails to reduce blood pressure. It is likely that renin is not involved in the maintenance of the hypertension. The mechanism by which retention of salt causes hypertension is not certain. It would be expected that a rise in arterial pressure would lead to a pressure natriuresis. If hypertension is maintained without depletion of sodium, therefore, the relation between blood pressure and renal excretion of salt must be reset at a higher level.[251] This is perhaps a result of the effect of angiotensin II in reducing renal perfusion and increasing retention of sodium by the kidney, both directly and by release of aldosterone.[249] The persistence of hypertension after the removal of the initial cause in experimental animals has its clinical counterpart in phaeochromocytoma, Cushing's syndrome, Conn's syndrome and aortic coarctation. In these instances, the blood pressure does not always return to normal after removal of the cause.

The persistent hypertension may be related to damage to the renal vasculature of the non-experimental kidney. This can, in some way which is not yet clear, cause retention of sodium. The mechanism may be similar to that involved in the later stages of essential hypertension, and to the increased peripheral vascular resistance caused by medial and intimal hypertrophy of peripheral arterioles.[252] The complexities of experimental renal hypertension are such that it can cause no surprise that the amelioration of renal ischaemia in the human does not always lead to a reduction in hypertension.[253] Fortunately, in children, perhaps because the period of hypertension is shorter, the results of surgery for renovascular hypertension are more predictable.

Renovascular Hypertension

Renovascular hypertension can be defined as hypertension resulting from obstruction to flow of blood in the renal artery or its branches. The obstruction may be caused by intrinsic disease of the artery, or by compression on the artery from outside. Renovascular lesions account for up to one-tenth of cases of children referred with hypertension,[254–256] and are the third commonest cause of significant hypertension in children after renal scarring and glomerular disease. Fibromuscular dysplasia, or fibromuscular non-atherosclerotic stenosis of the renal vessels, is the main vascular abnormality, and is classified according to the arterial layer in which the lesions predominate.[257,258] Intimal fibroplasia is a rare cause in adults, but occurs primarily in children. Fibromuscular dysplasia, or hyperplasia of the media, is more common, and predominates in adolescents and adults. Overall, the condition is most common in middle-aged females.[172] The lesion in adults is commonly situated in the middle or distal part of the renal artery, whereas stenosis occurs more frequently at the origin of the vessel in children. The aetiology of the condition is unknown, but a cellular reaction to altered dynamics of pressure and flow in the artery has been proposed.[257] Genetic factors may play a role, with the condition being commoner in first-degree relatives of those with involvement of the renal arteries,[259] and in those carrying the ACE-1 allele for the angiotensin-converting-enzyme.[260] It is important to recognise that the condition may be progressive,[261] and may also involve arteries other than the renal vessels.[258,262] A careful search for the involvement of other arteries is mandatory, with particular note taken of absent peripheral pulses or the presence of bruits, especially over the carotids.

A number of cases are associated with neurofibromatosis type 1.[255,263] A careful family history, and clinical examination for other features of the condition, is important. The renal arterial stenosis in neurofibromatosis type 1 is usually caused by intimal proliferation or neurofibromatotic proliferation in the arterial wall.[172] Associated coarctation of the abdominal aorta is common. Occasionally, compression on the artery from outside by a neurofibroma or ganglion neuroma is responsible for hypertension. Other space-occupying lesions that may involve compression of the renal artery include tumours, fibrous bands, haematomas and phaeochromocytomas. Acquired narrowing of the abdominal aorta has been observed following radiotherapy for intra-abdominal malignant disease.[264] Coarctation of the abdominal aorta without neurofibromatosis is often accompanied by renal arterial stenosis.[265] Other vessels originating from the abdominal aorta are usually involved.

Takayasu's arteritis is an important cause of renovascular hypertension in non-white children.[266] The arteritis affects the aorta, the proximal portions of its major branches, and the pulmonary arteries. The onset of the vasculitis is associated with an acute systemic illness, which usually subsides after a few weeks but may recur. The aetiology is unknown, though a link with tuberculosis has been suggested.[267,268] A raised erythrocytic sedimentation rate, and elevated levels of immunoglobulin, indicate active disease. Diagnostic imaging includes Doppler ultrasound and arteriography. More recently, three-dimensional magnetic resonance angiography and positron emission tomography have been shown to reveal early changes in the process of the disease, avoiding the need for intravenous contrast or ionising radiation.[269,270] Therapy of the arteritis is based on the use of corticosteroids,[271] and in some patients the addition of other immunosuppressive drugs such as methotrexate or azathioprine.[272] Following this, management is mainly concerned with control of the hypertension. The prognosis is, to some extent, dependent on the severity of the vasculitis and the resultant damage.

Other miscellaneous causes may be found. Renal arterial stenosis can be present in some cases of infantile hypercalcaemia syndrome.[273] As already discussed, thrombosis or embolism of the renal artery is an important cause of hypertension in infants. Stenosis of arterial branches within the kidney may lead to severe hypertension, and is difficult to diagnose.[274] Diffuse renal arteriolar stenotic lesions can occur in polyarteritis nodosa, haemolytic uraemic syndrome, and following renal irradiation.[275] Renal venous thrombosis in infancy can lead to the development of hypertension.[218,276] Hypertension is common after renal transplantation, but only rarely is caused by renal arterial stenosis. Renal hypertension can occur after traumatic injury to the kidney, causing renal arterial thrombosis or intrarenal vascular damage, or from perinephric inflammation causing constriction on the kidney.[172] Arterio-venous fistulas, either congenital or acquired, following trauma, surgery, or renal biopsy, can all cause hypertension.

A bruit over the renal artery is a useful diagnostic sign, albeit often absent in children with renovascular hypertension. Hypokalaemic alkalosis suggests underlying secondary hyperaldosteronism, which is a consistent feature of renovascular hypertension. Doppler ultrasound has limited sensitivity for detecting renal arterial stenosis.[277,278] Computed duplex sonography is able to measure blood flow velocities as a guide to the presence of stenosis.[279] Overall sensitivity and specificity for Doppler assessment is excellent.[280] Renal scintigraphy may show asymmetry of function and size, with reduced uptake on the side of the stenosed renal artery, but paediatric renovascular disease is often bilateral,[255] and these investigations may not be helpful. Performing the scan before, and then after, a dose of an inhibitor of angiotensin-converting enzyme, such as captopril, may reveal a significant reduction in function of the affected kidney on the second scan. This technique has been found to have sensitivity and specificity of around 90% in adults.[281] A study in children gave comparable findings when compared with renal arteriography.[282]

Direct evidence of renal ischaemia with stimulation of the renin-angiotensin system is derived from the differential determination of renal venous renin. A ratio of 1.5 or more between the affected and the non-affected kidney may predict unilateral renal ischaemia and an anticipated positive response to surgery.[283–285] Using this ratio to predict unilateral disease, however, does not always correlate with the arteriographic findings[255] and in no way removes the need for arteriography. The level of renin in the renal vein of the non-affected kidney is usually suppressed to the level of the systemic concentrations. A ratio of less than 1.5 suggests either bilateral disease, or non-renovascular hypertension, though renovascular hypertension and successful surgery have been reported in some patients.[286] A normal renal arteriogram, with similar activities of renin in both renal veins, will certainly exclude a renal cause for hypertension in most, if not all, cases.

The gold standard investigation for renal arterial stenosis is selective renal arteriography and estimation of renal venous renin. The procedure is usually performed under sedation or general anaesthesia, with access to the renal artery and vein from puncture of the femoral vessels. If the hypertension is mild and easily controlled, and if the other investigations do not suggest renovascular hypertension, it is reasonable not to recommend arteriography, though careful follow-up is essential. The blood pressure should be carefully controlled before attempting arteriography. Adequate hydration should be maintained, and the blood pressure monitored throughout the procedure. Newer techniques include magnetic resonance angiography[287–289] and computed tomographic and spiral angiography.[290] These have the advantage of being less invasive, and can normally be performed without general anaesthesia in children and adolescents.

Interventional treatments of renovascular hypertension include percutaneous transluminal angioplasty (Fig. 58-4)

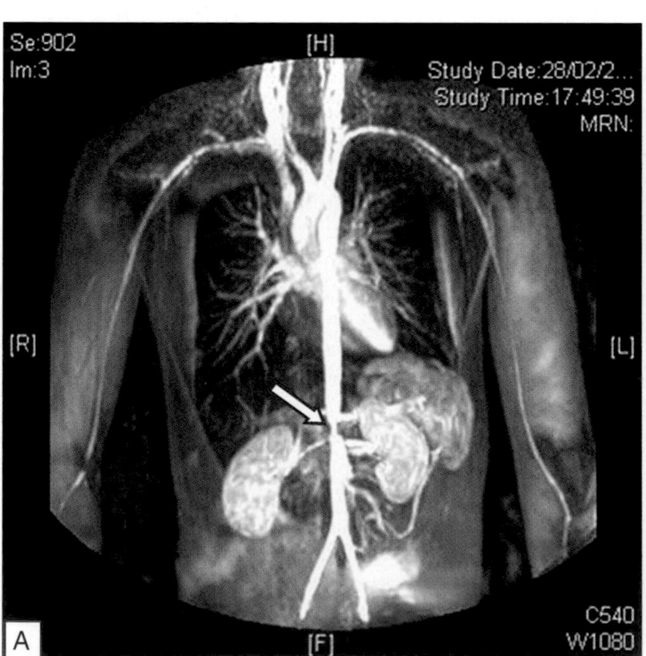

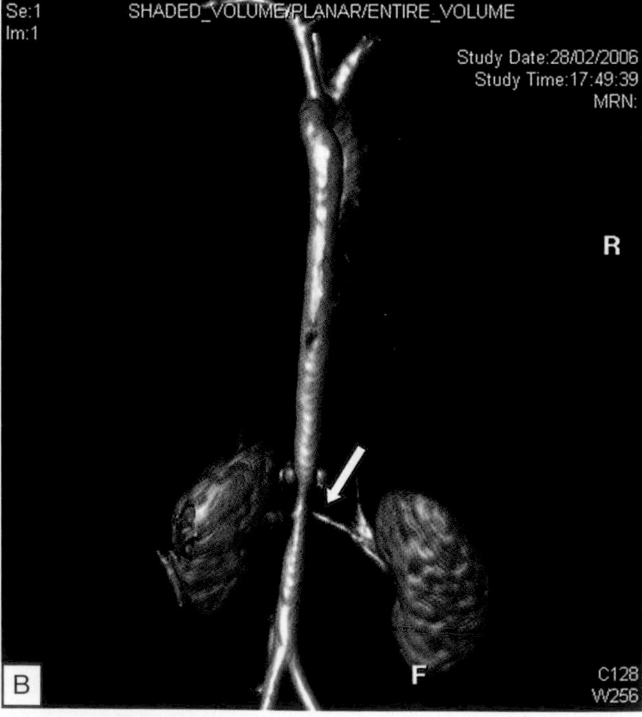

Figure 58-4 This series of images show the steps of treatment for a 9-year-old boy with renovascular hypertension. The areas of interest in each panel are indicated by arrows. A magnetic resonance angiogram (Panel **A**) demonstrates bilateral renal arterial stenosis, combined with the middle aortic syndrome. Panel **B** shows an enhanced image.

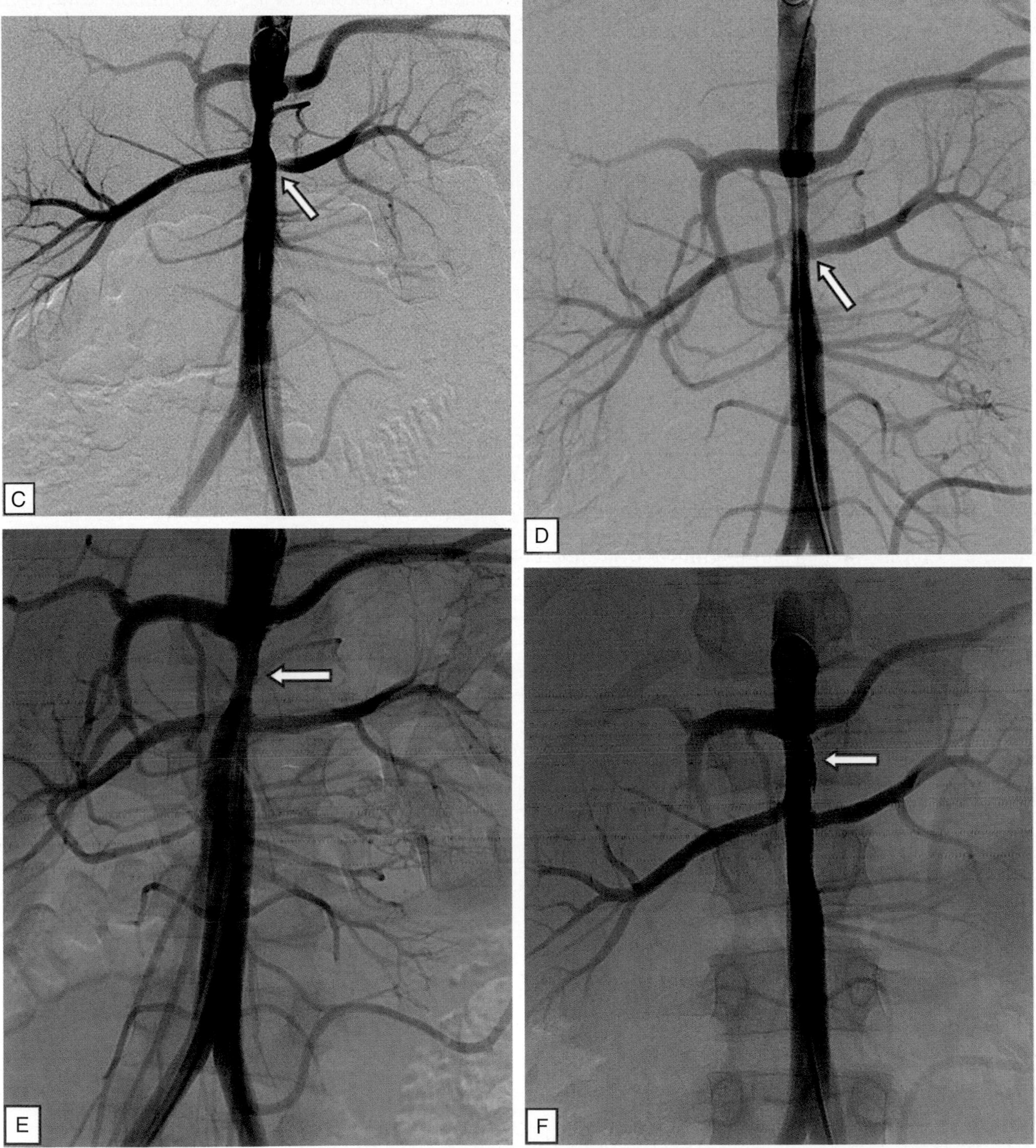

Figure 58-4 Cont'd Panel **C** is a percutaneous renal arteriogram showing severe stenosis of the left proximal renal artery, a normal right renal artery, and stenosis of the middle part of the aorta. Panel **D** shows complete correction of the left renal arterial stenosis subsequent to balloon angioplasty. Panels **E** and **F** show the diameter of the aorta before (**E**) and after (**F**) balloon angioplasty, performed because of persistent hypertension. The patient now has normal blood pressure on a low dose of a single antihypertensive agent 6 months after the aortic balloon angioplasty.

and open surgery. In general, angioplasty is the preferred approach for discrete non-ostial stenoses, whilst open surgery is often needed for ostial, multiple, and extensive stenoses.[291] The rate of cure for surgery in renovascular hypertension in children is high.[172,283,292] It varied between 85% and 100% in various series of properly selected patients, with no operative deaths in one large series.[292] The operative techniques vary according to the nature of the disease. They include renal arterial reconstruction and reimplantation, autotransplantation of the kidney, and venous grafting or prosthetic bypass of the stenosis.[292–295] Decisions regarding treatment where there is abdominal aortic narrowing associated with renal artery stenosis are challenging, because surgical correction of the renal arterial stenosis by vascular shunts from above the coarctation may compromise flow to other organs. Successful outcomes have been reported in the majority of children undergoing surgery for renovascular hypertension associated with abdominal aortic narrowing.[292,294]

Percutaneous transluminal angioplasty is the preferred approach for discrete non-ostial stenoses. The technique is less successful with ostial stenosis, the presence of intrarenal stenoses and abnormalities in other vascular beds, or the long segment renal arterial stenosis often seen in neurofibromatosis type 1. Several published series show an overall favourable outcome, including a number of cases with neurofibromatosis type 1.[253,263,296–301] Restenosis is relatively common, occurring in up to one-quarter of cases[302] and is commoner if a stent has been placed in the vessel. There is relatively little experience of stenting stenosed arteries in children.[301,303] Stenosis may develop in the previously normal renal artery on the unaffected side.[304] The progressive nature of fibromuscular dysplasia in children suggests that every attempt should be made to preserve renal function. Nephrectomy should be performed only if the kidney is small or scarred and has very poor function, accounting for less than one-fifth of total function.

Renal Parenchymal Disease

The renal disease causing hypertension is usually evident from the initial clinical and laboratory evaluation (see Table 58-5). Chronic pyelonephritis with renal scarring is a major cause of childhood hypertension.[180,305,306] Some tertiary centres have reported the development of hypertension in up to one-quarter of patients with severe reflux nephropathy, although other centres have reported a much lower prevalence.[307] A careful search for renal scarring must always be performed using scintigraphic techniques, since renal ultrasound used in isolation may fail to identify renal scarring.[308] If scarring is demonstrated, a contrast micturating cystourethrogram, or indirect radioisotope cystogram, should be considered. Treatment of hypertension is usually medical, as the damage is often bilateral and affects more than one segment of the kidney. Where investigations indicate that the cause of hypertension is a small, scarred and poorly functioning kidney, with a normal unscarred kidney on the other side, then removal of the damaged kidney may cure the hypertension and remove the need for antihypertensive therapy. Occasionally, partial nephrectomy may be indicated for focal scarring where the remainder of the kidney is undamaged; in these cases, sampling of renin in the renal vein is usually required to confirm isolated hyperreninaemia arising from the scarred segment. Obstruction at the pelviureteric junction is occasionally associated with hypertension, which can be cured in some instances by a pyeloplasty.[309–311]

Hypertension is common in acute nephritic syndrome. Indeed, this diagnosis has to be considered in any child with unexplained acute hypertension. Plasma renin is low because of the retention of sodium.[312,313] Hypertension is also common in chronic glomerulonephritis (see Table 58-5), and is almost invariable when renal function declines. Diseases associated with widespread arteriolar damage, such as haemolytic uraemic syndrome, systemic lupus erythematosus, and polyarteritis nodosa, are often accompanied by hypertension. Polycystic kidneys are an important cause of hypertension. The raised pressures are seen early in the autosomal recessive form of the condition encountered in childhood.[314] Hypertension may also develop in childhood in the more common autosomal dominant variant.[315] Hypertension is less common with primary interstitial tubular diseases, such as the Fanconi syndrome or juvenile nephronophthisis, and with the diseases associated with salt wasting, such as renal dysplasia or obstructive uropathy in infancy. When renal insufficiency supervenes, however, even children with these conditions may develop hypertension.

Primary Hyper-reninism

Severe hypertension is uncommon in children with nephroblastoma, also known as Wilms' tumour. It can occur when renal ischaemia is present, or after haemorrhage into the tumour. Occasionally, production of renin by the tumour has been described.[316] Tumours of the juxtaglomerular cells, or haemangiopericytomas, are extremely rare. With these tumours, the activity of renin is elevated in the plasma, and there is often evidence of secondary hyperaldosteronism. The tumours are single, benign and small, measuring from 0.8 to 4 cm.[172] They should be suspected when a raised level of renin is found in the renal vein in association with a normal intravenous urogram. They may be apparent as a translucent area seen during the nephrographic phase of a selective renal arteriogram.[317] Computed tomography may assist in the diagnosis of these lesions.[318] Surgical removal of the tumour is indicated.

Aortic Coarctation

Aortic coarctation is one of the most important causes, after renal disease, of severe hypertension in children.[172,305] The cause of the hypertension in patients with coarctation is complex and not fully explained. The main hypotheses include mechanical obstruction,[319] the neural theory of altered autonomic and baroreceptor function,[320–322] and activation of the renin-angiotensin system.[323,324] Despite apparently successful surgical correction of the aortic narrowing, ongoing or recurrent hypertension is well recognised and common. It may be considered a long-term condition even after surgical correction.[325] In this respect, it is of interest that only 6% of patients with coarctation aged between 1 and 5 years of age had residual hypertension, whereas three-tenths of those undergoing surgery between 6 and 18 years, and almost half of those between 19 and 40 years, had hypertension following surgery.[326] Older age at surgery is also associated with higher risk of subsequent hypertension and cardiovascular morbidity.[327] The pathogenesis of post-operative hypertension is likely to be multifactorial, and involve alterations in the systems described above. The diagnosis and treatment of aortic coarctation is discussed at length in Chapter 46.

Endocrine Disorders

Adrenocortical Hypertension

The adrenal gland synthesises mineralocorticoids, glucocorticoids, and sex hormones from cholesterol. Plasma cortisol feeds back to the pituitary to control the output of adrenocorticotrophic hormone, which stimulates the rate of conversion of cholesterol to pregnenolone. This is an intermediate in the production of all three classes of adrenocortical hormone. Any failure of the control of normal feedback by cortisol will produce an increase in adrenocorticotrophic hormone, giving rise to congenital adrenal hyperplasia. The most useful investigations in the diagnosis of adrenocortical hypertension are a determination of renin in the plasma, which is usually suppressed, along with aldosterone, the exclusion of a hypokalaemic alkalosis, and a careful analysis of the urinary excretion of steroids.

11β-Hydroxylase Deficiency

11-Hydroxylation is the final step in the production of cortisol, also known as compound F, from its immediate precursor corticosterone, or compound S. It is also an essential step in the production of aldosterone from deoxycorticosteroid. Adrenal hyperplasia results from the decreased production of cortisol with an increase in levels of compound S and its urinary metabolites in the plasma. Virilisation is a prominent clinical feature, and hypertension is present in many patients. This is in contrast to the more common variety of congenital adrenal hyperplasia associated with a deficiency in 21-hydroxylase. Hypertension is thought to be caused by an excess of deoxycorticosteroid, which has mineralocorticoid effects. There is evidence of hyperaldosteronism, with a hypokalaemic alkalosis and a low concentration of renin in the plasma.

17α-Hydroxylase Deficiency

17-Hydroxylation is required for the conversion of pregnenolone to 17-hydroxypregnenolone in the production of cortisol and sex hormones. A defect in this process, therefore, results in the diminished secretion of all glucocorticoids and sex hormones, with an increased secretion of mineralocorticoids, leading to hypertension and hypokalaemia. Clinical features include hypogonadism, amenorrhoea, and male pseudohermaphroditism. The production of 17-deoxysteroids, including deoxycorticosteroid and compound B, is increased, but secretion of aldosterone is low, perhaps because of the low levels of renin in the plasma, which is required for the synthesis of aldosterone. It is suppressed by the high concentration of deoxycorticosteroid.[328] The hypertension in both varieties of congenital adrenal hyperplasia resolves with treatment with a glucocorticoid.

Cushing's Syndrome

Cushing's syndrome may be caused by excessive production of adrenocorticotrophic hormone, either pituitary or ectopic, leading to adrenal hyperplasia, by an adrenal tumour such as an adenoma or carcinoma, by primary adrenocortical hyperplasia, or by exogenous administration of glucocorticoids.[329] Hypertension occurs in half of affected children and adolescents.[330] Clinical features include obesity, short stature, hirsutism, and acne. The cause of the hypertension is multi-factorial, and includes the aldosterone-like action of glucocorticoids, activation of the renin-angiotensin system,[331] suppression of various vasodilatory systems including nitric oxide,[332] and enhanced response to pressor effects of vasoactive substances, including catecholamines and angiotensin II.[333] Hypertension may persist after treatment of the underlying cause.

Hyperaldosteronism and Low-renin Hypertension

Concentration of aldosterone in the plasma is high in infancy, decreasing to adult values by 5 years of age.[334,335] Urinary excretion is related to excretion of sodium.[328] The cardinal features of hyperaldosteronism are retention of sodium, hypokalaemia, hypertension, and suppressed activity of renin in the plasma. These changes are seen in a variety of hypertensive syndromes, which share the common feature of low activity of renin in the plasma, but some conditions have high levels of aldosterone and others have low levels (Table 58-7). Several of these syndromes are inherited as single mendelian traits, including dexamethasone-suppressible hypertension and Liddle syndrome, which are autosomally dominant, and apparent mineralocorticoid excess, which is autosomally recessive. The molecular defect has been established for each of these conditions, enabling genetic diagnosis. In addition, the profiles of steroids in the urine for these conditions are characteristic and can aid in diagnosis.[336]

Primary Hyperaldosteronism

Primary hyperaldosteronism is extremely rare in children. It is usually related to nodular hyperplasia rather than to Conn's syndrome, where there is an aldosterone-producing tumour. Hypertension may be severe, and is associated with a low concentration of renin in the plasma and hypokalaemia. Oedema is either absent or minimal. Surgery is recommended for adrenal adenomas. Hypertension frequently recurs after operative treatment for nodular hyperplasia, which may, therefore, respond more satisfactorily to long-term treatment with the antagonist of aldosterone, spironolactone.

Dexamethasone-suppressible Hyperaldosteronism

The hypertension in dexamethasone-suppressible hyperaldosteronism, a dominantly inherited condition that is also known as glucocorticoid-remediable aldosteronism or familial hyperaldosteronism type I, is variable. It is resistant to normal medication, albeit responding to treatment with dexamethasone. Activity of renin is profoundly low in the plasma, and levels of aldosterone are usually, but not always, raised in the serum. The genetic defect is an unequal cross-over event between genes encoding 11β-hydroxylase and aldosterone synthase. This results in a chimeric duplication containing the regulatory elements of 11β-hydroxylase and the coding sequence of aldosterone synthase.[337] Consequently, aldosterone is ectopically synthesised in the adrenal fasciculate zone under the regulation of adrenocorticotrophin hormone, rather than its usual secretagogue, angiotensin II. This chimeric gene product converts cortisol to its 18-oxo and 18-hydroxy metabolites, leading to a pathognomonic profile of urinary steroids, with a raised ratio of 18-oxotetrahydrocortisol to tetrahydroaldosterone.[338] Treatment with dexamethasone leads to suppression of adrenocorticotrophic hormone, and hence suppression of the ectopically produced aldosterone. Direct antagonists of aldosterone, such as spironolactone, have also been used successfully, and may avoid the side effects of dexamethasone.[339]

Liddle's Syndrome

Liddle's syndrome is an autosomal dominant condition with a clinical presentation typical of primary hyperaldosteronism, and yet levels of aldosterone in the serum and urine, as well as activity of renin in the plasma, are suppressed.[340,341] Patients have constitutive activation of the amiloride-sensitive distal renal epithelial sodium channel as a result of mutations in the β- or γ-subunit of the epithelial sodium channel.[342–344] Analysis of urinary steroids reveals negligible aldosterone. Treatment with triamterine or amiloride is successful.

Apparent Mineralocorticoid Excess

A number of children have been observed with hypertension associated with suppressed activity of renin in the plasma, subnormal levels of aldosterone, hypokalaemia with

TABLE 58-7

SYNDROMES OF LOW-RENIN HYPERTENSION

Condition	Inheritance	Aldosterone Level	Potassium Level	Mechanism
11β-Hydroxylase deficiency	Autosomal recessive	Decreased	Low	11β-Hydroxylase deficiency
17α-Hydroxylase deficiency	Autosomal recessive	Decreased	Low	17α-Hydroxylase deficiency
Primary hyperaldosteronism	Sporadic	Increased	Low	Adrenocortical hyperplasia or tumour
Dexamethasone-suppressible hyperaldosteronism	Autosomal dominant	Increased	Low	11β-Hydroxlyase/aldosterone synthase hyperaldosteronism chimeric gene duplication
Liddle syndrome	Autosomal dominant	Decreased	Low	Mutations in β/γ-subunits of epithelial sodium channel conferring increased activity
Apparent mineralocorticoid	Autosomal recessive	Decreased	Low	11β-Hydroxysteroid dehydrogenase excess deficiency with impaired conversion of cortisol to cortisone
Gordon's syndrome	Autosomal dominant	Decreased	High	Increased distal proximal tubular NaCl reabsorption; WNK gene mutations

alkalosis, and a reduced excretion of all known steroids.[328,336] Deficiency of 11β-hydroxysteroid dehydrogenase is the primary defect.[345,346] In this autosomal recessive condition, these mutations cause increased intracellular cortisol that activates the mineralocorticoid receptor.[347] In addition, the cortisol leads to suppression of adrenocorticotrophic hormone, and hence reduced excretion of other corticosteroids. The condition responds to treatment with spironolactone, an antagonist of the mineralocorticoid receptor.

Gordon's Syndrome

Gordon's syndrome is an autosomal dominant condition that is also known as pseudohypoaldosteronism type II. It is characterised by hypertension with low plasma renin activity, hyperkalaemia, metabolic acidosis, and normal glomerular filtration rates.[348] Mutations in the *with-no-lysine kinase 4* gene, or WNK4, are associated with this condition.[349] The gene normally inhibits the thiazide-sensitive sodium-chloride co-transporter in the distal convoluted tubule. Mutated genes fail to inhibit this co-transporter, leading to enhanced reabsorption of sodium chloride and water, with resultant expansion of volume, suppression of renin, and hypertension.[350] The condition responds to restriction of sodium and therapy with thiazide diuretics.

Phaeochromocytoma

Benign phaeochromocytomas, and the malignant phaeochromoblastomas, develop from chromaffin tissue in the adrenal gland or sympathetic ganglions. These tumours produce excessive amounts of catecholamines, and lead to an increase in the excretion of their metabolites in the urine. Abnormal production of catecholamines is also observed with neuroblastomas, and occasionally with ganglion neuromas. Adrenaline and noradrenaline are the principal biologically active catecholamines. Noradrenaline is synthesised from tyrosine via dihydroxyphenylalanine and dopamine. It is then methylated to produce adrenaline, this being the main hormone of the adrenal medulla. Noradrenaline is principally produced by postganglionic sympathetic nerves. Noradrenaline acts mainly on sympathetic α-adrenoceptors, while adrenaline stimulates both α- and β-adrenoceptors. The catecholamines are metabolised to metadrenaline, also called metanephrine, and normetadrenaline, also called normetanephrine, and then oxidised to the principle urinary metabolite 3-methoxy-4-hydroxymandelic acid, also called vanillylmandelic acid. The urine also contains homovanillic acid, produced from dopamine, as well as adrenaline and noradrenaline. Malignant tumours excrete dopamine and homovanillic acid.

Because of the practical difficulties in obtaining accurately timed collections of urine over 24 hours in small children, spot samples may be used, expressing the excretion of vanillylmandelic acid relative to urinary creatinine.[351] Excretion is usually raised in children with phaeochromocytomas, especially if the urine is collected when the patient is hypertensive. Collections over 24 hours may be necessary if the hypertension is episodic. Levels of adrenaline and noradrenaline in the plasma should also be measured. Typically, adrenal tumours produce a rise predominantly in adrenaline, while extra-adrenal tumours lead to raised noradrenaline levels. We show the normal values for excretion of catecholamines in the urine in Table 58-8. Recent publications suggest that measurement of the levels of metanephrine and normetanephrine in the urine and plasma may be the most sensitive and specific assays for the confirmation of phaeochromocytoma.[195,196,352] Whilst catecholamines may be secreted episodically, plasma free metanephrines are produced continuously by the metabolism of catecholamines within phaeochromocytoma tumour cells.[352]

Bananas, and drugs and foods containing vanilla, should be eliminated from the diet before urine is collected. Methyldopa, clofibrate, and inhibitors of monoamine oxidase will reduce excretion of catecholamines. β-Blockers, and blockers of the calcium channels, may increase the levels of catecholamines in the plasma. Labetalol may also interfere with assays. Ideally, the patient should not be receiving these drugs when samples are collected for investigation for phaeochromocytoma. Stress may also lead to increased release of catecholamines, and so collection of blood should be done via a previously inserted cannula, when the child has been resting.

The hypertension is usually ascribed to the increased secretion of noradrenaline. Thus, administration of phentolamine, which blocks α-adrenoceptors, will lower the

TABLE 58-8

URINARY CATECHOLAMINE EXCRETION AND BLOOD CATECHOLAMINES

ADRENALINE, NORADRENALINE, AND DOPAMINE URINARY EXCRETION IN nmol/24 hr

Age (years)	Adrenaline nmol/24 hr	Noradrenaline nmol/24 hr	Dopamine nmol/24 hr
0–1	0–14	0–59	0–555
1–2	0–19	6–100	6–914
2–3	0–33	24–171	261–1697
4–6	1–55	47–266	
7–9	3–76	77–384	
10–14	3–109	89–473	
4–14			424–2612
>15	<100	<470	<2500

ADRENALINE, NORADRENALINE, AND DOPAMINE URINARY EXCRETION IN nmol/mmol OF URINARY CREATININE

Age (years)	Adrenaline nmol/mmol Ur creat	Noradrenaline nmol/mmol Ur creat	Dopamine nmol/mmol Ur creat
0–2	<46	<280	<2216
2–4	<35	<80	<1113
5–9	<22	<59	<774
10–19	<21	<55	<403

VANILLYLMANDELIC ACID (VMA) AND HOMOVANILLIC ACID (HVA) URINARY EXCRETION IN μmol/24 hr, AND μmol/mmol OF URINARY CREATININE

Age (years)	VMA		HVA	
	μmol/24 hr	*μmol/mmol Ur creat*	*μmol/24 hr*	*μmol/mmol Ur creat*
3–5	5–13	2.3–6.2	8–24	3.4–9.6
6–9	10–16	2.3–4.3	12–26	2.7–7.1
10–16	12–26	1.7–50	13–48	2.0–6.4

ADRENALINE AND NORADRENALINE PLASMA LEVELS

Age	Adrenaline pmol/L	Noradrenaline nmol/L
1–7 days	109–710	1.18–2.48
1–16 years	109–628	0.89–2.36

UR creat, urinary excretion of creatinine.
From http://www.calgarylabservices.com/LabTests/AlphabeticalListing/C/Catecholamines-Urine.htm and http://www.calgarylabservices.com/LabTests/AlphabeticalListing/C/Catecholamines-Blood.htm.

blood pressure by more than 20 mm Hg. A starting dose of 0.01 mg/kg body weight is increased to 0.1 mg/kg if no effect is observed. False-positive results are common. The majority of children also have high concentrations of renin in the plasma with secondary aldosteronism. This has been ascribed to depletion of fluid volume, direct stimulation of secretion of renin by adrenaline, compression on the renal artery by the tumour, and associated renal arterial disease in those with neurofibromatosis.[172]

The adrenal medulla is the common site for the tumours, which vary in size from 1 to 10 cm. They are more common on the right, and are bilateral in one-fifth of patients. In one-third, tumours are situated in both the adrenal and extra-adrenal areas, or only in an extra-adrenal site. Boys are affected twice as often as girls, and the incidence is highest between the ages of 11 and 15 years. The most common extra-adrenal site is the aortic bifurcation, or the vicinity of the renal hilum. Bladder tumours are described, which cause paroxysmal hypertension during micturition and, sometimes, haematuria.[353] A dominant mode of inheritance is apparent in some families, and more than half of the patients have multiple tumours. Phaeochromocytoma is frequently associated with other conditions, such as neurofibromatosis and von Hippel–Lindau disease, and with the autosomally dominant multiple endocrine neoplasia syndrome, which includes medullary thyroid carcinoma, islet cell adenoma, and hyperparathyroidism.[354] Hypertension is less common with other neurogenic tumours and only affects about one-tenth of children with neuroblastomas. An increase in urinary dopamine, and its metabolite homovanillic acid, is a characteristic of neuroblastomas.

Clinical features relate to the hypertension, which is sustained in almost nine-tenths of cases, and include headaches, sweating, nausea and vomiting, visual disturbances, abdominal pain, polyuria and polydipsia, convulsions, pallor, and acrocyanosis.

The location of the tumour or tumours can be established with a variety of imaging techniques including ultrasound, scintigraphy, computed tomography, and magnetic resonance imaging.[355] More invasive techniques involve sampling of blood at different levels from the inferior caval vein for determination of levels of catecholamines in the plasma, and arteriography.[356] Invasive investigations should be performed only after full α- and β-adrenoceptor blockade to control the hypertension, and after correction of hypovolaemia. The latter is essential in any case before surgery. Safe anaesthesia and surgery require careful preoperative preparation. Phenoxybenzamine, at 1 mg/kg per day, is used to block α-adrenoceptors, and propranolol, also at 1 mg/kg per day, is used for blockade of β-adrenoceptors. Monitoring of arterial and central venous pressures is required during surgery.[357] Intravenous adrenergic blocking agents such as phentolamine and esmolol should be readily available. Surgical removal of the tumour or tumours results in cure, but the frequency of multiple tumours suggests that long-term follow-up is indicated.

Miscellaneous Endocrine Causes

Primary hyperthyroidism is a rare cause of hypertension in children.[358] Hypertension is also rare in children with primary hyperparathyroidism and is probably related to nephrocalcinosis[359] and to hypercalcaemia which, as we discuss briefly below, raises peripheral vascular resistance.

Neurological Disorders

Severe hypertension can occur in a variety of acute neurological disorders, for example Guillain-Barré syndrome,[360] poliomyelitis, intracranial lesions such as tumours, trauma, asphyxia, and encephalitis.[361] Autonomic dysfunction with overactivity of the sympathetic system is thought to be involved in the pathogenesis in these disorders and in the Riley-Day syndrome of familial dysautonomia,[362] though raised intracranial pressure may be a particular precipitating factor.

Miscellaneous Causes of Hypertension

Drugs

Oral contraceptives have already been discussed. Glucocorticoids and mineralocorticoids are potent causes of hypertension, particularly in children with pre-existing renal disease. Sympathomimetic agents can raise the blood pressure even when used as topical preparations[363] or in nose drops. Mercury poisoning causing acrodynia, or pink disease, is associated with hypertension. Poisoning with heavy metals, such as cadmium and lead, overdosage of reserpine, methyldopa and phenylcyclidine, and cough syrup containing ephedrine have all caused hypertension.[172]

Burns

Systemic hypertension occurs in one-third of children with severe burns.[364] Excessive production of catecholamines, increased renin-angiotensin stimulation, expansion of volume, and hypercalcaemia have been considered in the pathogenesis.[172]

Hypercalcaemia

Hypercalcaemia is associated with hypertension, probably because of a rise in peripheral vascular resistance.[365] The syndrome of infantile hypercalcaemia[273] may be associated with renal arterial stenosis and hypertension.

Other Causes

Hypertension occurs in acute intermittent porphyria.[366] It can be associated with Turner's syndrome, even in the absence of aortic coarctation,[190,367] and with Marfan syndrome.[368] It has been described in pseudoxanthoma elasticum,[369] Stevens-Johnson syndrome,[370] and acrodermatitis enteropathica.[371] It also occurs during sickle cell crisis.[372] Ingestion of liquorice, which contains a substance with a mineralocorticoid effect, may cause hypertension that is similar to the hypertension induced by deoxycorticosteroid.[373]

MEDICAL THERAPY

The importance of non-pharmacological interventions in the management of hypertension has already been discussed, as have the indications for treatment and for surgery. Here we concentrate on pharmacological treatment.

Maintenance Therapy of Chronic Hypertension

Maintenance therapy for chronic hypertension is intended to control the blood pressure at the 90th centile or less for height, age, and sex (Table 58-9). Reference should, therefore, be made to the available tables showing centiles for blood pressure during childhood so that a clear target range for treatment is identified.[9] Compliance is promoted by using the fewest drugs at the lowest dose and frequency. Long-acting formulations requiring once-daily dosing are available for a range of drugs, and liquid or dispersible preparations of most important antihypertensive drugs are also available for use in infants and younger children. If more than one drug is required, the additional drug or drugs should act through a different, and hence complementary, mechanism.

The availability of long-acting inhibitors of angiotensin-converting enzyme, blockers of the calcium channels, and β-blockers provides the majority of hypertensive children with effective and simple treatment that is relatively free of serious side effects. Information on the use of some of the available antihypertensive drugs, however, is limited.

Inhibitors of Angiotensin-converting Enzyme

The inhibitors of angiotensin-converting enzyme are effective antihypertensive agents,[374–376] particularly in renin-mediated hypertension. They also have other benefits in specific situations, such as proteinuric renal impairment and diabetes mellitus.[377,378] The hypotensive effect is not usually seen until some nine-tenths of the enzymic activity has been inhibited. Consequently, there may not be a graded response to the given dose. Captopril is useful initial treatment as the half-life is short, at 2 hours, allowing fairly rapid modification of dose until control is achieved. The recommended dose by body weight for neonates and infants is smaller, as the potency is greater in this group. It is recommended that a small initial test dose be given while the patient is closely observed, as some have shown a profound fall in blood pressure with postural hypotension after a single dose. Enalapril, lisinopril, and ramipril have a long half-life, from 12 to 24 hours, enabling once-daily dosing, which helps compliance in long-term therapy. The reduction in production of aldosterone associated with these drugs may lead to an increase in the levels of potassium, especially with preexisting renal impairment. Rash, neutropenia, loss of taste, and cough are rare side effects. This class of drugs is relatively contraindicated in renal arterial stenosis, as they inhibit the angiotensin II–mediated compensatory efferent arteriolar vasoconstriction, with the risk of a precipitous fall in rates of glomerular filtration.[379] More recently, drugs blocking the receptors to angiotensin II have been

TABLE 58-9

ANTIHYPERTENSIVE DRUGS FOR ORAL USE

Drug	Major Side Effects	Precautions	Dose
Angiotensin II–converting Enzyme Inhibitors			
Captopril	Hypotension, rash, cough, agranulocytosiss	Avoid in renal artery stenosis	Children: 0.1–0.5 mg/kg (maximum 2 mg/kg) three times a day Neonates: 0.01–0.05 mg/kg three times a day
Enalapril	Hypotension, cough	Avoid in renal artery stenosis	0.1 mg/kg (maximum 1.0 mg/kg) once daily (enalapril has been substituted for captopril as 1 mg enalapril per 7.5 mg captopril)
Calcium Channel Blockers			
Nifedipine	Flushing, tachycardia, headache	—	Capsule: 5–10 mg three times a day Modified release tablets: 10–20 mg twice a day Slow release tablets: 30–60 mg once a day
Amlodipine	Flushing, tachycardia, abdominal pain		0.1–0.2 mg/kg once a day; increase to a maximum of 10 mg
Diuretics			
Chlorothiazide	Hypokalaemia, hyperuricaemia	Renal insufficiency	10 mg/kg (maxlmum 40 mg/kg) per day
Furosemide	Hypokalaemia		1–4 mg/kg once or twice a day
Spironolactone	Hyperkalaemia, gynaecomastia	Renal insufficiency	1 mg/kg twice or three times a day
β-Adrenoceptor Blockers			
Propranolol	Reduced cardiac output, bradycardia	Cardiac failure, asthma	0.2–2.0 mg/kg three times a day
Atenolol	As propranolol	As propranolol	1–2 mg/kg (maximum 8 mg/kg) once a day
α-Adrenoceptor Blockers			
Prazosin	Hypotension after first dose, dizziness	First dose reaction	0.01 mg/kg three times a day; increase to a maximum of 0.5 mg/kg three times a day
Mixed α- and β-Adrenoceptor Blockers			
Labetalol	Rash, dry eyes, dizziness	Cardiac failure, asthma	1–2 mg/kg three or four times a day
Vasodilators			
Minoxidil	Fluid retention, tachycardia, hirsutism	—	0.1 mg/kg twice daily; increase by 0.1 mg/kg per dose every 3 days to a maximum of 0.5 mg/kg twice a day
Hydralazine	Flushing, tachycardia, lupus syndrome	—	0.2–1.0 mg/kg

used in children, often in combination with inhibitors of angiotensin-converting enzyme, to produce a combined effect on both hypertension and proteinuria.[380–383]

Blockers of Calcium Channels

These blockers are most effective in low-renin, volume-dependent hypertension. They interfere with the inward displacement of calcium ions through voltage-dependent slow channels in the cell membrane, and reduce blood pressure by causing vasodilation. Nifedipine has been widely used, both in its short-acting form for the rapid lowering of blood pressure in urgent situations, and in its slow-release forms for maintenance treatment of chronic hypertension. These drugs are usually well tolerated. Side effects are mainly related to vasodilatation, and include tachycardia and flushing. Amlodipine is a newer agent that requires only a single daily dose. It has been used successfully for children.[384,385]

Diuretics

These agents are particularly useful in patients with renal disease. They are often required as a second agent to control the retention of fluid associated with long-term use of vasodilators. Thiazide diuretics are effective if the rate of glomerular filtration is over half of normal, but a loop diuretic, such as furosemide, will be needed for more severe degrees of renal impairment. In refractory oedema, especially when associated with congestive cardiac failure, the addition of metolazone to furosemide is usually effective.[386,387] Side effects include hypokalaemia with both groups of diuretics, and ototoxicity when using loop diuretics. The mineralocorticoid antagonist spironolactone is useful in conditions of mineralocorticoid excess. It may also be used in addition to a loop or thiazide diuretic for its potassium sparing effect. Triamterene and amiloride are used specifically for Liddle syndrome.

Blockers of β-Adrenoceptors

The β-blockers have been used as first line therapy for a long time, and are effective in many patients. Cardiac output is reduced, peripheral release of noradrenaline is impaired, release of renin is inhibited, and there is centrally mediated reduction in peripheral sympathetic activity. There is a relatively poor correlation between the antihypertensive effect of the drug and the level of drug in the plasma. Side effects are numerous, and include exacerbation of asthma and cardiac failure, depressed mood, nightmares, and disturbed metabolism of lipids and glucose. Propranolol is useful for initial introduction of β-blockade during in-patient management, where four-times-daily dosing is feasible, and when the shorter half-life makes dose adjustment easier. For long-term treatment, atenolol has a long half-life and need only be given once daily.

Blockers of α-Adrenoceptors

Prazosin is an α-adrenoceptor blocker. It has few serious side effects in children. The antihypertensive effect is through vasodilation. Caution should be observed with the first dose, as it may cause marked postural hypotension. This class of drug is useful in treating catecholamine-induced hypertension. Recently, a long-acting α-adrenoceptor blocker, doxazosin, has been available for once daily dosage. It is not officially licensed for use in children.

Blockers of Both α- and β-Adrenoceptors

Labetalol[388] is a non-selective β-blocker, with less potent α-adrenoceptor blocking properties. Its main use is as an intravenous infusion in the treatment of hypertensive emergencies.[255,389,390]

Vasodilating Agents

The vasodilators are a group of pharmacologically diverse drugs that have vasodilation as their common effect. Some drugs with this effect have already been described above. Hydralazine and minoxidil act directly on the vascular smooth muscle to reduce peripheral vascular resistance. Hydralazine is most often used as an intravenous bolus for rapid control of severe hypertension. Minoxidil is a powerful vasodilator and is usually used as an added agent in resistant hypertension. It causes marked hirsutism. As mentioned above, long-term use of vasodilating drugs is often associated with retention of salt and water, and a diuretic may, therefore, need to be used in addition.

Hypertensive Crisis

The rapid but controlled lowering of blood pressure is essential in children who present with clinically severe hypertension. Clinical features necessitating emergency treatment of hypertension include visual disturbance with retinal haemorrhages and papilloedema; encephalopathy with headache, vomiting, hyper-reflexia, obtunded neurological state, or seizures; and cardiac failure with a dilating heart. Similarly, severely elevated blood pressure that has not yet led to symptomatic damage to target organs should be urgently controlled before an adverse event occurs. It is important initially to assess clinically the extracellular fluid volume. If there is evidence of overload with increased jugular venous pressure or pulmonary oedema, then removal of fluid by a furosemide-induced diuresis or by dialysis is required. The hypertension of acute nephritic syndrome often settles rapidly if an adequate diuresis can be obtained.

Sudden large falls in blood pressure have to be avoided if neurological complications are to be prevented.[255] These complications are more likely if the hypertension has been long standing, though the chronicity of hypertension may not be apparent at initial clinical assessment

TABLE 58-10

DRUGS FOR TREATMENT OF HYPERTENSIVE EMERGENCIES

Drug	Onset of Action	Dose and Route	Mode of Action	Comment
Labetalol	Minutes	1–3 mg/kg per hr as intravenous infusion	Vasodilator	Titrate rate of constant infusion against change in blood pressure
Sodium nitroprusside	Seconds	0.5 μg/kg per min intravenously; increase by 0.2 μg/kg per min to a maximum of 8 μg/kg per min	Vasodilator	1. Titrate rate of constant infusion against change in blood pressure 2. Stop treatment if blood thiocyanate exceeds 100 μg/ml
Hydralazine	Minutes	1. 0.3–0.5 mg/kg as intravenous slow bolus dose; maximum 4-hourly 2. 0.025–0.05 mg/kg per hr intravenously to maximum of 3 mg/kg in 24 hr	Vasodilator	Titrate rate of constant infusion against change in blood pressure
Nifedipine (capsules)	Minutes	0.25–0.5 mg/kg orally	Vasodilator	1. Effect is less controllable than with intravenous infusion 2. Child must bite and swallow capsule, or liquid contents should be removed via a needle and syringe and then swallowed
Minoxidil	Minutes	0.1–0. 2 mg/kg orally	Vasodilator	See (1) for nifedipine
Furosemide	Minutes	2–5 mg/kg intravenously over 20 min	Loop diuretic	For severe intravascular volume expansion states Rapid administration of large doses may be ototoxic

of a child presenting with hypertensive crisis. Some children with malignant hypertension are depleted for salt and fluid and have intense vasoconstriction. They may be especially sensitive to vasodilation and require considerable quantities of saline to maintain and control the blood pressure; therefore, an intravenous line should always be established. Patients should be managed on an intensive care unit or high-dependency unit by staff experienced in treating severe hypertension with intravenous drugs. Clinical improvement is often seen with a relatively small reduction of blood pressure, and the initial aim should not be rapid reduction of blood pressure to normal levels. Rather, as a guide, the eventual target blood pressure should be defined, the total reduction in systolic blood pressure calculated, and then the blood pressure reduced by one-third of this total in the first 6 hours, two-thirds of the total by the next 24 to 36 hours, and the total reduction achieved over a subsequent 48 to 72 hours.

A selection of drugs for use in hypertensive emergencies is shown in Table 58-10. Labetalol is an effective first choice. If it proves insufficient, then sodium nitroprusside may be added. The latter is especially useful because of its very short duration of action. Constant monitoring of the rate of infusion and blood pressure is required during its use. Thiocyanate toxicity can occur with long-term therapy or with renal insufficiency. Although nitroprusside has been used without ill effects for up to 10 days,[391] levels of thiocyanate should be monitored in the blood after 48 hours, and treatment discontinued if the concentration exceeds 100 μg/mL. The solution must be protected from light by shielding the syringe and infusion lines.

Less severe hypertensive crisis is often managed successfully with oral nifedipine in rapid-acting capsule form. Children should be instructed to bite the capsule, as most absorption occurs after swallowing the contained liquid. In young children, a liquid preparation is available, or the contents of a capsule may be aspirated by syringe and fine needle and then administered orally. Intravenous hydralazine may also be used as a rapid acting vasodilator. These agents, however, give less precise control over the rate of fall of blood pressure, and intravenous infusion treatment is preferred where there is symptomatic severe hypertension.

The complete reference list can be found on the companion Expert Consult web site at www.expertconsult.com.

ANNOTATED REFERENCES

- National High Blood Pressure Education Program Working Group on High Blood Pressure in Children and Adolescents: The Fourth Report on the Diagnosis, Evaluation and Treatment of High Blood Pressure in Children and Adolescents. Pediatrics 2004;114:555–576.

  This is a comprehensive review of all aspects of the investigation and management of childhood hypertension, including clinically useful centile charts.
- http://www.dableducational.com.

  This is a non-profit Web site with exhaustive information regarding instruments for measuring blood pressure, of value for patients and professionals.
- Wuhl E, Witte K, Soergel M, et al, for the German Working Group on Pediatric Hypertension: Distribution of 24-h ambulatory blood pressure in children: Normalized reference values and role of body dimensions. J Hypertens 2002;20:1995–2007.

  A widely accepted normative data set for 24-hour ambulatory blood pressure monitoring in children.
- Manger WM: Diagnosis and management of pheochromocytoma—recent advances and current concepts. Kidney Int 2006;70(Suppl 104S):S30–S35.

  This detailed review of the diagnosis and management of phaeochromocytoma includes clinical features, laboratory and imaging methods, treatment, and diagnostic and therapeutic pitfalls.
- Flynn JT: Neonatal hypertension: Diagnosis and management. Pediatr Nephrol 2000;14:332–341.

  A practical review of the diagnosis and management of hypertension in the neonate.
- Staessen JA, Wang J, Bianchi G, Birkenhager WH: Essential hypertension. Lancet 2003;361:1629–1641.

  An in-depth review of essential hypertension, including theories of pathogenesis and an account of the genetics of essential hypertension.
- Srinivasan SR, Myers L, Berenson GS: Changes in metabolic syndrome variables since childhood in prehypertensive and hypertensive subjects: The Bogalusa Heart Study. Hypertension 2006;48:33–39.

  A retrospective study that provides insight in to the natural history of hypertension.
- He FJ, MacGregor GA: Importance of salt in determining blood pressure in children: Meta-analysis of controlled trials. Hypertension 2006;48: 861–869.

  A meta-analysis of 10 trials looking at the effect of reducing the intake of salt on blood pressure in infants, children and adolescents, showing that a modest reduction led to an immediate and significant fall in pressures.
- Barker DJP, Winter PD, Osmond C, et al: Weight in infancy and death from ischaemic heart disease. Lancet 1989;334:577–580.

  Seminal paper that showed the relationship between lower weight at birth and higher mortality from ischaemic heart disease in adult life.
- Mackenzie HS, Brenner BM: Fewer nephrons at birth: A missing link in the etiology of essential hypertension? Am J Kidney Dis 1995;26:91–98.

  This paper details the evidence that reduced nephron numbers at birth is the link between lower birth weight and increased cardiovascular morbidity in later life.
- Deal JE, Snell MF, Barratt TM, Dillon MJ: Renovascular disease in childhood. J Pediatr 1992;121:378–384.

  Detailed review of investigation and management of renovascular hypertension in 54 children treated at a single centre.
- Adelman RD, Coppo R, Dillon MJ: The emergency management of severe hypertension. Pediatr Nephrol 2000;14:422–427.

  Excellent review of the management of paediatric emergency of severe hypertension.
- Silverstein DM, Champoux E, Aviles DH, Vehaskari VM: Treatment of primary and secondary hypertension in children. Pediatr Nephrol 2006;21: 820–827.

  A recent update of the treatment of paediatric hypertension.

CHAPTER 59

Cardiovascular Risk Factors in Infancy and Childhood

MARIETTA CHARAKIDA, JULIAN P. HALCOX, STAVROS P. LOUKOGEORGAKIS, and JOHN E. DEANFIELD

Although the clinical complications of atherosclerosis do not usually occur until adulthood, it is now appreciated that the underlying arterial pathology begins much earlier. Over the last two decades, there have been substantial advances in the understanding of the disturbed vascular biology involved in the initiation and progression of atherosclerosis and its late sequels, with identification of several risk factors on the causal pathway.

In developed countries, better treatment of adults with clinical cardiovascular disease, including reduction of risk factors, has resulted in substantial decrease in morbidity and mortality. This downward trend is slowing, and in developing countries there has been a huge increase in the burden and consequences of atherosclerosis, largely due to a deterioration in the levels of risk factors in the population.[1,2] This has led to increasing interest in the understanding and treatment of the adverse influences promoting atherosclerosis during its long preclinical stage, rather than merely attempting to reverse long-standing atherosclerosis by complex and often expensive interventions which do not fully reverse risk.

The need for identification and treatment of risk factors from childhood is supported by a number of key observations:

- In autopsy studies, atheroma is prevalent in children and young adults who died of non-cardiac causes, from the first decade of life. This has recently been confirmed using intravascular ultrasound, with almost one-fifth of teenagers in the United States being found to have early lesions in their coronary arteries (Fig. 59-1).[3,4]
- The interaction between risk factors and the vessel wall in early life has a strong influence on later cardiovascular outcome. In a recent reanalysis of the Framingham cohort, the risk factor profile at 50 years was associated with a tenfold variation in later event rates.[5]
- Risk factors in early years, such as blood pressure and adiposity, track into adulthood and predict higher rates of events produced by coronary arterial disease.[5]
- Reduction of risk factors in the young, by modification of lifestyle and/or medication, can improve dysfunctional vascular biology, such as endothelial function, and reverse structural changes in the arterial wall, such as the thickness of the carotid intimal and medial layers.[6]
- Early intervention to reduce risk factors is likely to produce greatly leveraged gains in cardiovascular outcome, so that duration of exposure is crucial. In the ARIC study, a genetically determined 28% reduction in lifetime levels of low-density lipoprotein cholesterol levels in subjects with a polymorphism of the PCSK9 gene was associated with a reduction of almost nine-tenths in cardiovascular events.[7]

The study of arterial disease in childhood has been greatly facilitated by the development of non-invasive tests of vascular function and structure using ultrasound, and more recently magnetic resonance. In this chapter, we will review the range of factors which can interact with the arterial wall from early in life, discussing the evidence for a causal role and the opportunity for intervention. This approach to prevention is relevant, not only for the management of children who are at high risk, but also as a population-based strategy to reduce morbidity and mortality from atherosclerosis in later life.

CLASSICAL RISK FACTORS

Classical risk factors identified from adult studies, including hypercholesterolemia, hypertension, cigarette smoking, diabetes, and family history, all have adverse effects on the arterial wall from childhood. Originally it was thought that this occurred only in selected groups with high cardiovascular risk, such as those with familial hypercholesterolaemia, diabetes mellitus types 1 and 2, chronic renal disease, or chronic inflammatory conditions. Large epidemiological studies, however, such as the Bogalusa Heart Study, the Muscatine study, and the Cardiovascular Risk in Young Finns Study in childhood and adolescence, have demonstrated the impact of risk factors even in the general paediatric population. Furthermore, these risk factors tend to tend to track into adulthood.[8–13]

Dyslipidaemia

Cholesterol is absorbed from the intestine, transported to the liver, and taken up by low-density lipoprotein-related proteins.[14] Hepatic cholesterol enters the circulation as very low density lipoprotein, and is metabolised to remnant lipoproteins. Reverse transport of cholesterol from peripheral tissues to the liver is mediated by high-density lipoproteins.[15–17] Cholesterol is recycled to low-density lipoproteins and very low density lipoproteins by cholesteryl-ester transport proteins, or is taken up in the liver by hepatic lipase.[14] Defects in this pathway translate into a range of disordered lipid profiles.

Cholesterol was first postulated to be related to atherosclerosis because it is the major component of advanced atherosclerotic lesions. The causal relationship between

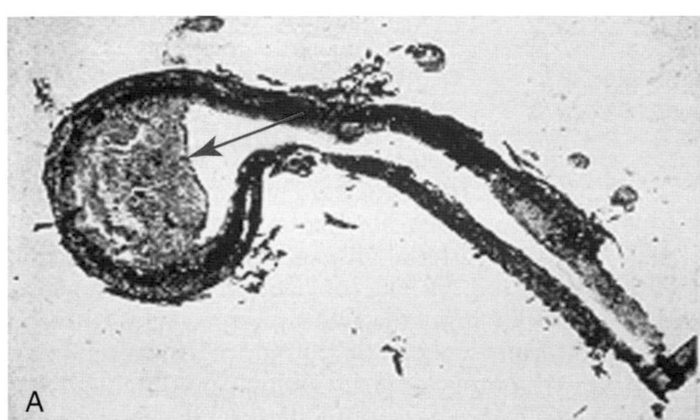

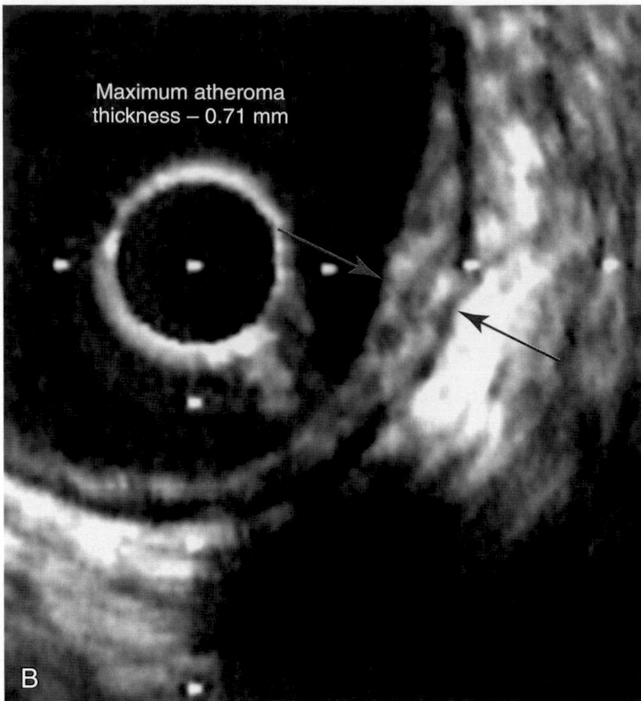

Figure 59-1 The images provide the evidence that atherosclerosis begins in childhood. Coronary atherosclerotic plaques were found in young American soldiers in their teens and early 20s who died in action in the Korean war.[3] The arrow in panel **A** highlights the presence of significant plaque. The intravascular ultrasonic image of the coronary artery of a 17-year-old boy shown in panel **B**, who died of non-cardiac causes, shows the distinct mural thickening of the coronary artery (*arrow*).[4] (**A**, Reproduced with permission from Enos WF, Holms RH, Beyer J: Coronary disease among United States soldiers killed in action in Korea; preliminary report. JAMA 1953;152:1090–1093. Copyright © 1953 Massachusetts Medical Society. All rights reserved. **B**, Reproduced with permission from Tuzcu EM, Kapadia SR, Tutar E, et al: High prevalence of coronary atherosclerosis in asymptomatic teenagers and young adults: Evidence from intravascular ultrasound. Circulation 2001;103:2705–2710.)

cholesterol and the formation of atherosclerotic plaques is now well established, and the impact of cholesterol both in initiation and progression of arterial disease is understood.[18,19] Once lipid subfractions are retained in the intimal layers of the arterial walls, they undergo oxidative modification, and acquire pro-inflammatory actions.[20] Oxidised low-density lipoprotein stimulates the expression of adhesion molecules, such as vascular cell adhesion molecule–1, on endothelial cells, increasing the expression of monocyte chemotactic protein–1 by vascular cells. This promotes infiltration of myocytes into the vascular wall, and proliferation of macrophages. Apart from these initial steps in atherogenesis, oxidised low-density lipoproteins are involved in the progression of atherosclerosis.[20] They promote proliferation of macrophages and smooth muscle cells, as well as the expression and secretion of a variety of growth factors and cytokines from vascular cells. The resulting injury, apoptosis, and necrosis of vascular cells leads to the formation of the lipid core seen in established atherosclerotic lesions.[19]

The association between levels of cholesterol and cardiovascular risk is strong, continuous, and dependent on concentration, even at low levels of cholesterol, from childhood onwards. It is amenable to reversion.[21] Large randomised trials in adults, predominantly using statins, have shown that significant reductions in levels of cholesterol are associated with a tremendous decrease in clinical events.[22–24] A drop of no more than 1% in the level of cholesterol in the serum reduces the risk for coronary arterial disease by 2%.[25]

In children, extreme elevations in the levels of lipids are usually encountered as a result of genetic hyperlipidaemias, whereas modest increases are seen in relation to dietary habits and a sedentary type of life.[26] Reference values for the total concentrations of cholesterol in the serum are available for both sexes from the first few months of life up to 1 year of age, and every 2 years afterwards up to 18 years. At birth, levels of cholesterol are low. They then rise over the first year of life to the level for the rest of childhood before puberty. These normal values in Western societies, even in childhood, are markedly higher than in countries with healthier diets and lifestyles. They may not be therefore healthy and appropriate for prevention of atheroma (Fig. 59-2).[27,28]

Strategies for screening children to establish levels of cholesterol have been reviewed recently in the light of the increasing evidence for the risk in the population, and to identify subjects with familial hypercholesterolaemia. Recent guidelines produced by the National Cholesterol Educational Program, designed to increase sensitivity and specificity of screening programmes, are outlined in Table 59-1.[26] Implementation of national strategies for cascade screening of families, once an index case has been identified, should greatly improve the rate of detection and lead to early and more active treatment from childhood. Family education is important, as eating habits in childhood influence behaviour in later life. The use of drugs, usually statins, in children remains controversial. According to the guidelines, they are not usually advocated until after the first decade of life, and only in children with hyperlipidaemia and two or more other cardiovascular risk factors. Over the past few years, however, a number of randomised controlled trials have demonstrated that treatment with statins is effective and safe in children, albeit with the short-term follow up[29] (see Fig. 59-2). For example, it was shown

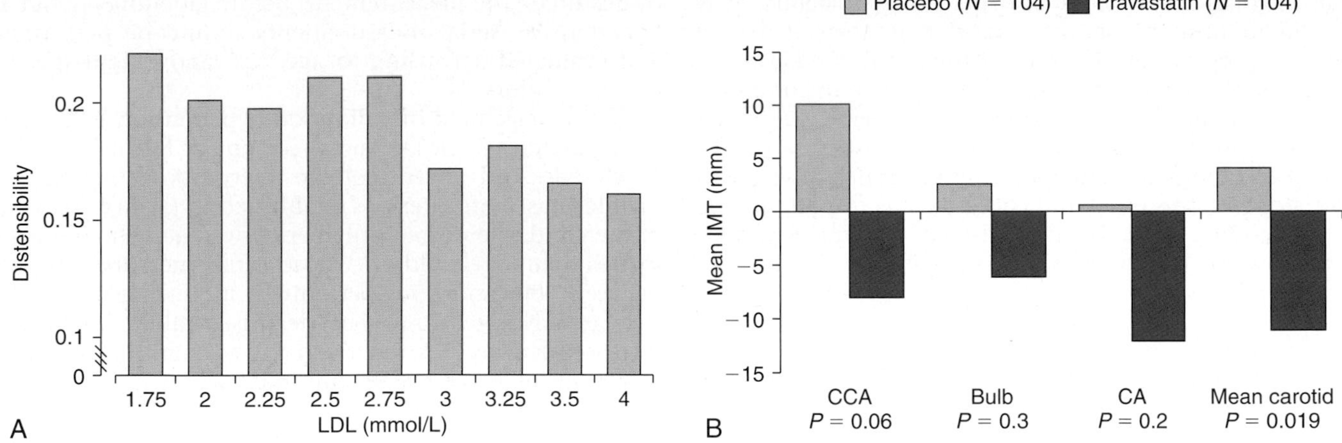

Figure 59-2 Dyslipidaemia in childhood. Panel **A** shows that higher levels of low-density lipoprotein (LDL) cholesterol, even within normal limits, were associated with reduced arterial distensibility in healthy British children aged from 9 to 11 years.[27] Panel **B** shows that treatment over 2 years with pravastatin was associated with a reduction in carotid intimal and medial thickness in children with familial hypercholesterolaemia.[28] CA, carotid artery; CCA, common carotid artery; IMT, intima media thickness. (**A**, Reproduced with permission from Leeson CP, Whincup PH, Cook DG, et al: Cholesterol and arterial distensibility in the first decade of life: A population-based study. Circulation 2000;101:1533–1538.)

TABLE 59-1

RECOMMENDATIONS FOR THERAPEUTIC MANAGEMENT OF HIGH-RISK HYPERLIPIDAEMIA IN CHILDREN AND ADOLESCENTS

Original Recommendations of the National Cholesterol Education Program Expert Panel

1. Consider drug therapy in children ≥10 years of age (usually wait until menarche for females) and after a 6- to 12-month trial of fat- and cholesterol-restricted dietary management
2. Consider drug therapy if
   - Low-density lipoprotein level remains 4.90 mmol/L (190 mg/dL), or
   - Low-density lipoprotein level remains > 4.10 mmol/L (160 mg/dL) and there is a positive family history of premature cardiovascular disease
   - Two other risk factors are present in the child or adolescent after vigorous attempts to control these risk factors
3. Referral to specialized lipid centre may be appropriate
4. Treatment goal
   - Minimal low-density lipoprotein < 3.35 mmol/L (130 mg/dL)
   - Ideal low-density lipoprotein < 2.85 mmol/L (110 mg/dL)

2007 Modifications to National Cholesterol Educational Program recommendations

1. In addition to family history, overweight and obesity should trigger screening with a fasting lipid profile
2. Overweight and obese children with lipid abnormalities should be screened for other aspects of the metabolic syndrome (i.e., insulin resistance and type 2 diabetes, hypertension, and central adiposity)
3. For children meeting criteria for starting lipid-lowering drug therapy, a statin drug is recommended as first-line treatment
4. For children with high-risk lipid abnormalities, the presence of additional risk factors or high-risk conditions may also lower the recommended cutpoint low-density lipoprotein cholesterol level for initiation of drug therapy, lower the desired target low-density lipoprotein cholesterol level, and in selected cases, may prompt consideration for initiation below the age of 10 years

   These risk factors and high-risk conditions may include
   - Male gender
   - Strong family history of premature cardiovascular disease or events
   - Presence of associated low high-density lipoproteins, high triglycerides, small, dense low-density lipoproteins
   - Presence of overweight or obesity and aspects of the metabolic syndrome
   - Presence of other medical conditions associated with an increased atherosclerotic risk such as diabetes, human immunodeficiency virus infection, systemic lupus erythematosus, organ transplantation, survival of childhood cancer
   - Presence of hypertension
   - Current smoking and passive smoke exposure
   - Presence of novel and emerging risk factors and markers, e.g., elevated lipoprotein(a), homocysteine, C-reactive protein
5. Ongoing research of drug therapy of high-risk lipid abnormalities in children is needed, particularly with regard to long-term efficacy and safety, and impact on the atherosclerotic disease process

Adapted from McCrindle BW, Urbina EM, Dennison BA, et al: Drug therapy of high-risk lipid abnormalities in children and adolescents: A scientific statement from the American Heart Association Atherosclerosis, Hypertension, and Obesity in Youth Committee, Council of Cardiovascular Disease in the Young, with the Council on Cardiovascular Nursing. Circulation 2007;115:1948–1967.

that, in children with familial hypercholesterolaemia, early treatment from the age of 8 years was associated with delay in progression of carotid intimal and medial thickness in adolescents and young adults.[30] As far as combined hyperlipidaemias are concerned, no specific guidelines exist for children with persisting hypertriglyceridaemia or low levels of high-density lipoproteins. In such cases, a diet restricted in terms of fat and cholesterol is important, and extra caution is needed in the setting of extreme elevations of triglycerides so as to prevent pancreatitis.[26]

Hypertension

Hypertension is the most common risk factor for clinical cardiovascular disease in both men and women, irrespective of age. Both diastolic and systolic levels of pressure have been associated in a continuous and dose-dependent manner with incidence of stroke, coronary arterial, and peripheral vascular events.[31] The pathophysiology that contributes to cardiovascular risk involves changes in resistance vessels, conduit arteries, and the heart, with alterations in shear stress in the arterial wall, endothelial dysfunction, a procoagulant state, increased oxidative stress, and inflammation.

Recent population studies emphasise the continuous relationship between blood pressure and cardiovascular outcome at levels previously considered safe and effective. This has been termed prehypertension by some, and an excessive response in the levels of blood pressure to exercise has also been shown to predict future cardiovascular events, further broadening the hypertensive phenotype. A wealth of clinical studies have shown that reduction in blood pressure by lifestyle or antihypertensive medication results in substantial fall in cardiovascular complications.

Measurement of blood pressure in childhood is important, as levels from as early as the first year of life track into adulthood. Essential, or idiopathic, hypertension is rare in childhood. It should only be diagnosed when secondary causes have been excluded. In these cases, it is usual to find a strong family history of hypertension. The commonest cause of secondary childhood hypertension is renal disease, but other aetiologies include coarctation of the aorta, endocrine disease, such as pheochromocytoma or hyperthyroidism, and adverse consequences of therapeutic regimes, such as oral contraceptives, sympathomimetics, and so on.[32] Recent reports have shown an association between blood pressure and the index of body mass (see below).[32,33]

According to recommendations made by the National High Blood Pressure Education Program, children older than 3 years should have their blood pressure measured when visiting the doctor. The risk for hypertension, however, cannot be estimated by a single measurement.[34] Blood pressure varies during the day and is influenced by factors of measurement, including the size of cuff, as well as by other less well-controlled factors, such as anxiety and stress. Accurate measurement in childhood requires use of a cuff that is appropriate to the size of the child's right upper arm, with an inflatable bladder having a width that is equal or greater than two-fifths of the circumference of the arm at a point midway between the olecranon and the acromion. The length of the bladder within the cuff should be sufficient to cover at least four-fifths of the circumference of the arm. An oversized cuff can underestimate pressure, whereas an undersized cuff can overestimate the measurement. Before labelling a child as hypertensive, serial measurements should be performed and evaluated according to age, sex, and height-specific percentile plots.[32,34]

The management of childhood hypertension is directed at identifying a cause and any predisposing factors. Changes in lifestyle, and pharmacologic interventions, are recommended based on criterions established according to the age of the child, the degree of hypertension, and the response to treatment. In children whose serial measurements lie between 90th and 95th percentiles, modifications of lifestyle are advocated to achieve decreased caloric intake and increased activity.[34] A reduction in the intake of salt, and increased intake of potassium and calcium, consumption of fresh fruits and vegetables and low-fat dairy products, as well as regular physical exercise and loss of weight, may assist in lowering the blood pressure in children. In adolescents, diets high in polyunsaturated fatty acids are reported to lower both systolic and diastolic measurements. For those found to have measurements lying between the 95th and 99th percentiles plus 5 mm Hg, re-evaluation should occur within 1 or 2 weeks. If this finding is confirmed, pharmacological therapy should be initiated.[34] Antihypertensive medication should also be initiated if there is evidence of damage to end-organs.[34] A number of classes of drugs can be used to lower blood pressure in the young. Blockers of the renin-angiotensin system have been used, particularly in children with co-existing pathology such as diabetes or proteinuria, while β-adrenergic and calcium channel blockers have been successfully administered in children with migraines.[34]

Cigarette Smoking

Cigarette smoking is the most important preventable cause of premature death in Western societies. A strong epidemiological link between cigarette smoking and atherosclerosis has been confirmed in many studies. In young individuals who would otherwise be at very low risk of developing cardiovascular disease,[35] cigarette smoking may cause as many as three-quarters of the events related to atherosclerosis. The longer a person smokes, the higher the risk for coronary arterial disease. In most European countries, 3% of 11-year-olds, 10% of 13-year-olds, and up to one-third of 15-year-olds, are daily smokers, according to the British Medical Association Tobacco Control Resource Centre. There is also evidence that those who begin smoking before the age of 20 years have the highest incidence, and earliest onset, of coronary arterial disease and hypertension.

Tobacco smoke contains hundreds of potential toxic compounds that may accelerate atherogenesis and increase the risk of complications. Endothelial dysfunction occurs early in both active and passive smokers, with a decrease in the bioavailability of nitric oxide.[36] Cigarette smoking also increases pro-inflammatory cytokines and adhesion molecules, and disturbs the coagulation system.[37] Smoking is also associated with other abnormal risk factors, including blood pressure and lipid profile. Cigarette smoking has recently been targeted by many countries, with legislation introduced to ban smoking in public places. Early evidence has shown an impressive rapid reduction in acute coronary arterial events.[38] A major initiative in the young, which includes education in schools on smoking, is a further prerequisite for a successful strategy for reduction of smoking in the population.

Genetics/Family History

The important contribution of genetic make-up in the atherosclerotic process has long been recognised.[39] Identification of single gene disorders, such as familial hypercholesterolaemia, has been important in establishing causal relations between risk factors and disease, and has enormously increased our understanding of atherogenesis.[40] In the absence of overt conventional risk factors, a clear association between family history of premature coronary arterial disease and endothelial dysfunction has been reported, further supporting the importance of the genetic background.[41,42] There has been an explosion of new information from genome-wide association studies, linking a range of genetic polymorphisms to cardiovascular risk in adults.[43,44] This has led to identification of new locuses, which will stimulate research into novel pathways contributing to vascular disease. Large studies of children will be required to determine whether the genetic variations associated with risk in adults operate from an early age to promote atherogenesis or, alternatively, are involved in destabilising established lesions to produce clinical complications.

NOVEL RISK FACTORS

A number of classical risk factors have clearly been linked to the evolution of the preclinical phase of atherosclerosis from childhood. High levels of these individual risk factors, such as cholesterol or hypertension, nonetheless, are uncommon in the absence of specific genetic conditions, such as familial hypercholesterolaemia and other diseases. It is likely, therefore, that a number of previously unrecognised factors, which are more prevalent in the population, may also contribute to initiation and progression of atherosclerosis.

Infection and Inflammation

Atherosclerosis has long been recognised as an inflammatory disorder, and the pathways involved in disturbed vascular biology have been described.[45] Recently, it has become clear that extrinsic inflammatory stimuluses may be involved in vascular inflammation and atherosclerosis. Infection is the commonest inflammatory condition in the young. The first evidence for a causal link with vascular disease came from animal studies in chickens with herpesvirus.[46] Data from human cross sectional epidemiological studies have subsequently implicated a number of viral and bacterial infections. This has led to the concept of the total pathogen burden influencing atherosclerosis, rather than isolated specific agents.[47] Several mechanisms have been proposed. The first is a direct effect of pathogens in the arterial wall, with systemic inflammatory activation leading to secondary arterial mural changes.[48] Most of the clinical studies, including numerous trials using antibiotics, have been performed in adults. They have produced conflicting results and are mostly disappointing.[49] This may be the result of confounding by the burden of other risk factors or, alternatively, because the role of infection may be greatest earlier in the evolution of arterial disease. The latter concept is supported by both animal studies and recent work using surrogate markers of early arterial disease in children and young adults. For example, a reversible effect of even mild infection of the upper respiratory tract on endothelium-dependent flow-mediated dilation has been shown in prepubertal children,[50] and young men who are seropositive for *Chlamydia pneumoniae* have increased thickness of the carotid intimal and medial layers.[51] In addition, other chronic infections, including the human immunodeficiency virus, have been linked with functional and structural arterial abnormalities from childhood and adverse cardiovascular outcome.[52,53] The vascular consequences of childhood infection are likely to depend on a number of factors, including the burden, frequency, and chronicity of infection, the susceptibility of the host, and the presence of other coexisting risk factors for atherosclerosis. Currently, there is no evidence to support a therapeutic strategy against infection for prevention of vascular events in the young, except perhaps in situations of high risk. After transplantation of the heart in children, cytomegalovirus, in particular, has been linked to systemic coronary endothelial dysfunction, and recently to progression of coronary arteriopathy.[54] It may, therefore, become an interesting target for specific treatment in these patients.

Children with chronic inflammatory conditions, such as systemic lupus erythematosus and rheumatoid arthritis, have evidence for abnormalities for arterial structure and function, including reduced flow-mediated dilation and increased thickness of the carotid intimal and medial layers, which are likely to represent accelerated atherosclerosis.[55] Similar abnormalities in the same measures have been associated with increased cardiovascular morbidity and mortality in adults. Childhood vasculitis, including Kawasaki disease, may result in both acute and sustained arterial mural abnormalities, even in the absence of acute coronary arterial complications.[56] Long-term and careful follow-up of these children is important to determine the potential interaction with later acquired risk factors, and the indications for more active preclinical treatment.

Recently, evidence has emerged that chronic periodontal inflammation, which is prevalent in both children and adults, may have adverse effects on the arterial wall. In a randomised controlled trial, reduction in this inflammatory stimulus by periodontal treatment led to recovery of endothelial function, providing evidence for a causal link and a potential new opportunity for population-based reduction of cardiovascular risk.[57]

Early Life Programming

For more than a century, it has been recognised that critical windows in early development may affect permanently later outcome and disease. It was the impact of early nutrition in animal studies that promoted the use of the term programming to describe the potential impact of early influences on later outcome.[58] An association between birth weight and weight at 1 year, and later cardiovascular risk, led to the development of the hypothesis of fetal origins for cardiovascular disease (Fig. 59-3).[59–61] This concept proposed that low birth weight was a surrogate for adverse events that had occurred in intra-uterine life. Blood pressure is the most commonly reported end point in large epidemiological studies examining the developmental origins of cardiovascular disease, since it can be measured easily and non-invasively in different age groups. More than

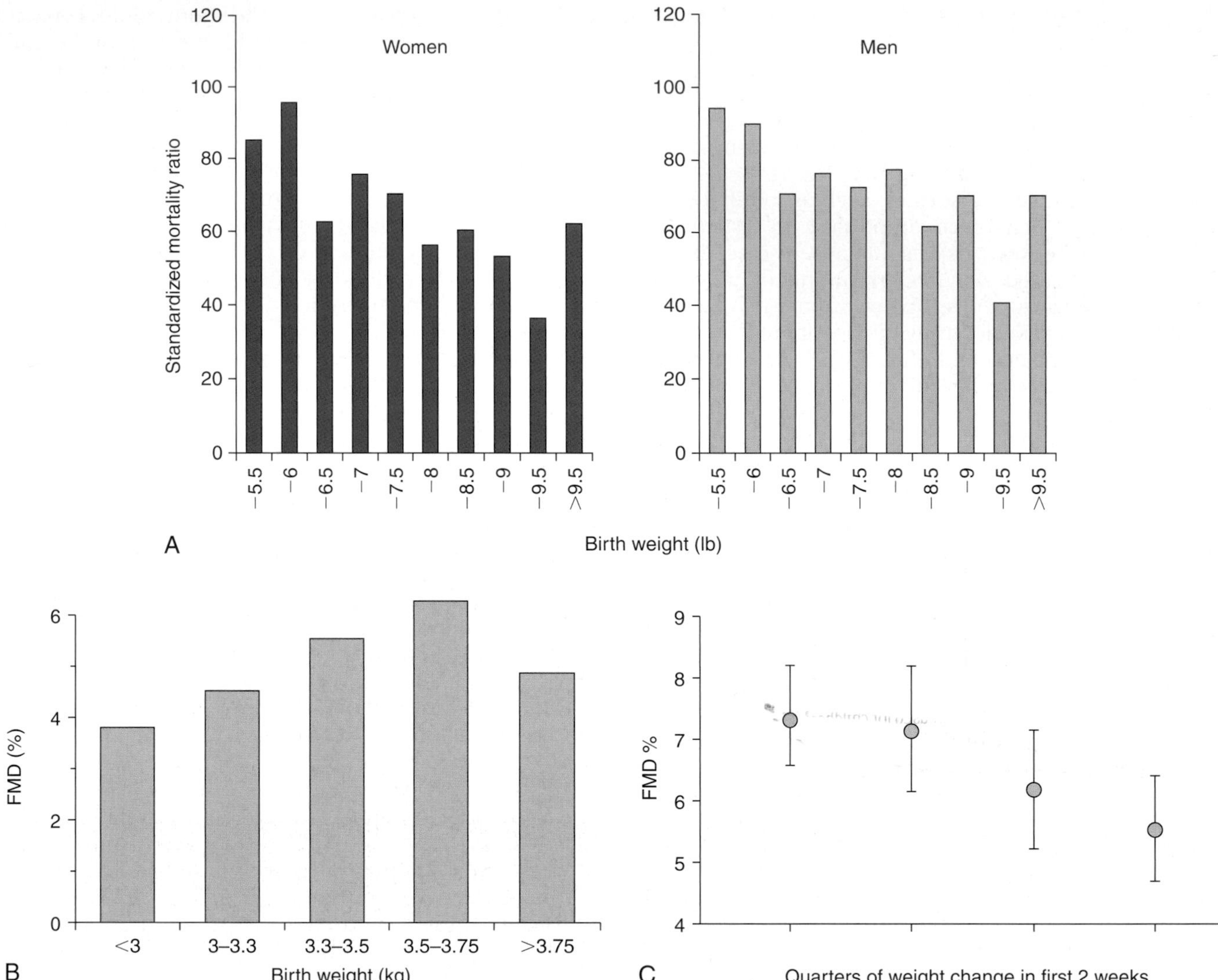

Figure 59-3 Early life programming. Panel **A** shows that low weight at birth was associated with increased cardiovascular mortality in a prospective cohort. There was a continuous relationship between weight at birth and outcome up to the top decile in men and women.[59] Panel **B** shows that weight at birth had a significant graded positive association with flow-mediated dilation (FMD) in a cohort of British children aged from 9 to 11 years when excluding the highest quintile.[60] Panel **C** shows flow-mediated endothelial dependent dilation in adolescence according to quarters of weight change in the initial 2 postnatal weeks. Flow mediated dilation was 4% lower in adolescents who were born prior to term, with the highest compared with the lowest rate of weight gain, in the first 2 weeks after birth. This evidence supports the catch up growth hypothesis.[61] (**B,** Reproduced with permission from Leeson CP, Whincup PH, Cook DG, et al: Flow-mediated dilation in 9- to 11-year-old children: The influence of intrauterine and childhood factors. Circulation 1997;96:2233–2238. **C,** Reproduced with permission from Singhal A, Cole TJ, Fewtrell M, et al: Is slower early growth beneficial for long-term cardiovascular health? Circulation 2004;109:1108-1113.)

50 studies have shown an inverse association between birth weight and blood pressure in adulthood, at the rate of 1 to 2 mm Hg per kilogram.[62] This association is seen in both males and females, and for both systolic and diastolic levels of blood pressure. The causal relationship, however, between adverse fetal environment, intra-uterine retardation of growth, and later cardiovascular disease, has been controversial. As a result of a series of randomised controlled trials, it has been suggested that the postnatal acceleration of growth is the important adverse influence, rather than events occurring antenatally. This has been termed the catch up growth hypothesis.[63,64] The critical postnatal window which affects long-term development may vary from a few weeks to few months (see Fig. 59-3).[59–61] Despite strong evidence for early life programming, both antenatally and postnatally, the mechanisms by which later arterial phenotype and cardiovascular outcome are influenced remain speculative. They may include effects on the growth and development of organs such as the liver or kidney, neurohormonal homeostasis, and levels of cardiovascular risk factors, as well as direct effects on the arterial wall. Evidence for programming has been demonstrated for blood pressure, cholesterol, and insulin resistance, as well as for endothelial function and arterial distensibility.[63,65]

The catch up growth hypothesis has significant implications for science and public health, as postnatal factors, particularly nutrition, are amenable to intervention. The effects of early nutrition may be substantial. For example, the reduction of 3 mm Hg in diastolic blood pressure seen in infants fed a low-nutrient diet is greater than that for all other strategies for reducing blood pressure in the young, including weight loss, restriction of salt, and exercise.[66,67] Feeding strategies for preterm and term infants, including weight gain targets and composition of milk formulas, need to consider not only the short-term effects on health, but also the long-term impact on cardiovascular outcome. Further research should address the relationship between early growth, later growth trajectories, and profiles of cardiovascular risk factors.

Obesity

Over the last two decades, in parallel with advances in reduction of several classical risk factors, there has been an alarming increase in the occurrence of obesity, accompanied by upward shift in the distributions of body fat in the population, especially in the young.[68] This has been a worldwide trend. There is now strong evidence that obesity in adults is associated with coronary arterial disease and cardiovascular events, in association with a high-risk cardiometabolic profile and type 2 diabetes.[69] In the West, the current social distribution of obesity, which is more prevalent in lower socioeconomic groups, suggests that its impact could further exacerbate social inequalities in cardiovascular morbidity and mortality.[70] In developing countries, where obesity is rising in parallel with changes in risk factors associated with urbanisation, the cardiovascular consequences of obesity could be further amplified.[71]

The prevalence of obesity is rising rapidly in children. Specific nomograms which are age and gender specific based on the body mass index are now used for childhood stratification (Table 59-2A).[72] Cut points have been defined. Normal weight is considered to represent those falling between the 5th and 85th percentiles. Those at risk for becoming overweight are those between the 85th and 95th percentiles, while those already overweight are above the 95th percentile. Using this classification, recent data indicates that the prevalence of overweight among children in the United States of America has risen from around one-twentieth in the1980s to almost one-sixth during the last few years.[73]

The epidemic of childhood obesity is likely to have a substantial impact on the future burden of cardiovascular disease within the population for several reasons. Firstly, obesity in childhood tracks to adulthood.[74] Overweight adolescents may be as much as 20 times more likely than their leaner peers to be obese in early adulthood. This has been confirmed in a number of longitudinal studies, including the Muscatine and the Bogalusa heart studies and the Cardiovascular Risk in Young Finns study.[75,76] Of note, the likelihood that an obese child will become an obese adult increases with age and the severity of obesity.[77] Secondly, obesity results in a deranged metabolic profile, which includes dyslipidaemia, hypertension, and insulin resistance (Fig. 59-4).[78,79] The extrapolation of criterions established for adults with the metabolic syndrome to children has been controversial. The International Diabetes Federation has developed a consensus to define metabolic syndrome in children, with thresholds of abnormality being determined according to age. The disturbed metabolic profile seen in obese children is associated with accelerated development of type 2 diabetes.[79] After adjusting for subsequent weight gain, female adolescents aged 18 with an index of body mass of greater than 30 kg/m^2 were 10 times more likely to develop diabetes than those with an index of less than 22 kg/m^2.[79] Thirdly, the cardiovascular effects of obesity are likely to be cumulative, so that both degree and duration of obesity may be important.

TABLE 59-2

A. MANAGEMENT OF WEIGHT AND GOALS OF TREATMENT, BASED ON PERCENTILES FOR THE INDEX OF BODY MASS AND STATE OF HEALTH

Index of Body Mass	Classification	Goal of Treatment
<85th percentile	Normal weight for height	Maintain percentile to prevent obesity
85th–95th percentile	At risk for overweight	Maintain index with aging to reduce to <85th percentile; if index > 25 kg/m^2, maintenance of weight
≥95th percentile	Overweight	Maintenance of weight in younger children, or gradual loss in adolescents, to reduce percentile within the index
≥30 kg/m^2	Adult obesity cut point	Gradual loss of weight by 1–2 kg per month to achieve healthier index
>95th percentile, comorbidity present	Overweight with comorbidity	Gradual loss of weight by 1–2 kg per month to achieve healthier index; assess need for additional treatment of associated conditions

B. GUIDING PRINCIPLES FOR TREATMENT OF OVERWEIGHT CHILDREN

1. Establish individual goals and approaches based on age, degree of overweight, and presence of comorbidities
2. Involve the family or major caregivers in the treatment
3. Provide assessment and monitor frequently
4. Consider behavioural, psychological, and social correlates of weight gain in the plan devised for treatment
5. Provide recommendations for dietary changes and increases in physical activity that can be implemented within the family environment and that foster optimal health, growth, and development

Adapted from Daniels SR, Arnett DK, Eckel RH, et al: Overweight in children and adolescents: Pathophysiology, consequences, prevention and treatment. Circulation 2005;111:1999–2012.

At least four studies have demonstrated that adolescents who are overweight suffer high overall mortality.[80,81] It is likely that the adverse impact of obesity on the population will not be avoided merely by management of its associated risk factors such as hypertension and dyslipidaemia.

A focus on prevention of obesity in childhood rather than in adulthood is more logical, both because it is likely to be more effective and also because it will have a greater benefit for the long-term health of the population. Indeed, children have greater adaptability than adults, and preventing the initial gain in weight is far easier than attempting weight loss once obese. There is little evidence, nevertheless, that current approaches to reduction of weight in the young result in long-term benefits, in terms of either loss of weight or morbidity. Most trials have been short term, and many aspects of adiposity in the young remain unclear. These include the pattern of distribution of fat at different ages and in different ethnic groups, as well as the mechanisms which link adiposity and early vascular mural changes. Understanding these mechanisms is important, as, even if preventative measures to reverse obesity were to be implemented rapidly, at least

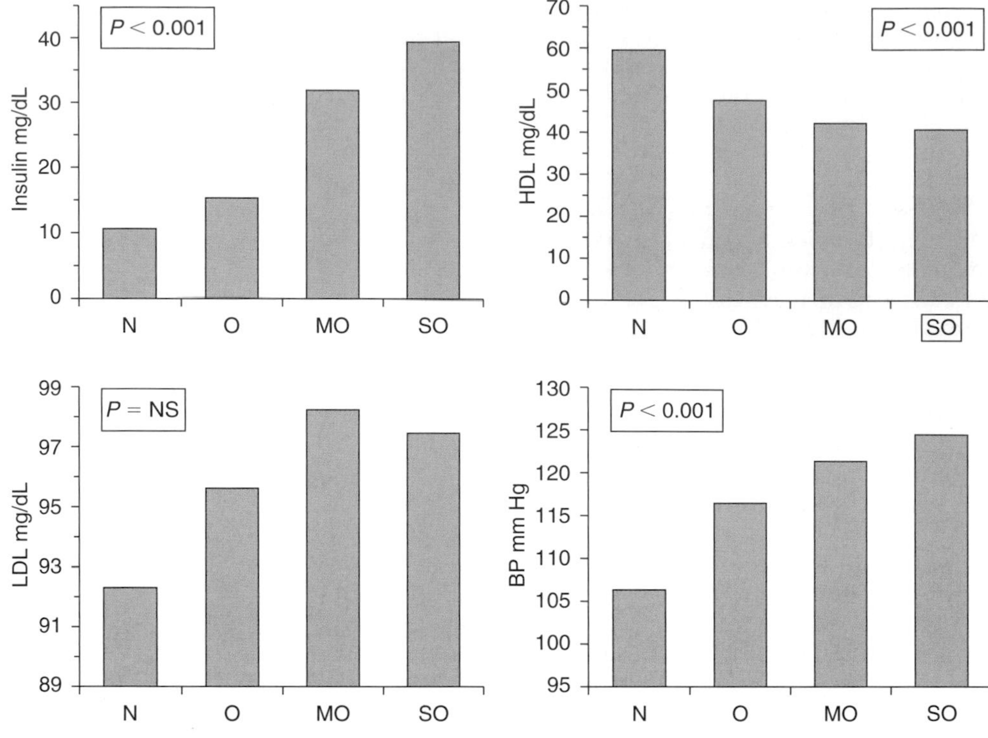

Figure 59-4 Obesity and metabolic syndrome in children and adolescents aged from 4 to 20 years. In children and adolescents in the United States, levels of insulin, blood pressure (BP), and low-density lipoprotein (LDL) cholesterol showed a significant increase with increasing levels of obesity, whereas high-density lipoprotein (HDL) cholesterol showed a graded decrease.[79] MO, moderately obese; N, not obese; O, obese; SO, severely obese. (Reproduced with permission from Weiss R, Dziura J, Burgert TS, et al: Obesity and the metabolic syndrome in children and adolescents. N Engl J Med 2004;350:2362–2374. Copyright © 2004 Massachusetts Medical Society. All rights reserved.)

one generation will end up in adult life with a high prevalence of obesity from childhood. A successful approach to deal with obesity in the young will require concerted political and societal action to alter the obesogenic environment in which children are growing up. There appear to be key windows of opportunity for intervention against obesity, which include pregnancy, the perinatal period to influence programming, infancy, puberty, and adolescence. Current approaches for treatment of obesity in the young include diets, modifications of lifestyle, drugs, and bariatric surgery for the morbidly obese (see Table 59-2B). A better understanding of mechanisms may lead to novel strategies to uncouple obesity and cardiovascular damage.

Diabetes

Although type 1 diabetes was the commonest form of diabetes in childhood, the epidemic of obesity is driving a rapid rise in the early presentation of type 2 diabetes. This is particularly prevalent in Asian, Afro-Caribbean, and Hispanic children, and is a worldwide phenomenon.[82]

The risk for later atherosclerosis and premature cardiovascular death is markedly increased. The pathophysiology of atherosclerosis in diabetes is complex. It involves endothelial activation, inflammation, oxidative stress, and disturbed endogenous vascular repair.[83] In type 2 diabetes, the vascular impact is related to resistance to insulin, and the commonly associated risk profile of hypertension, dyslipidaemia, and disturbed metabolism of fat cells.[84]

The optimal approach to the treatment of children and adolescents with type 1 diabetes, in addition to glycaemic control to retard cardiovascular disease, is uncertain.[55] Trials of statins and the antagonists of the renin-angiotensin system, which have proven benefit in adults, are in progress. In children with type 2 diabetes, modifications in lifestyle to achieve sustained loss of weight are crucial, but difficult to achieve.[55,85] Treatment to restore insulin sensitivity with metformin and thiazolidinediones may be required.[85] Evidence is accumulating for the benefit of reduction of other associated cardiovascular risk factors, including blood pressure and dyslipidaemia, in these high-risk subjects. As a result, more active treatment with statins and antihypertensive agents is likely to be extended to younger subjects, with the aim of lifetime reduction in cardiovascular risk.

SUMMARY

The assessment and management of cardiovascular risk factors from childhood has emerged as a crucial strategy for reduction of the risk from atherosclerosis over the lifetime.[55] Understanding of the evolution of early atherosclerosis, and the impact of interventions at a young age, has been facilitated by the development of non-invasive tests of early changes in arterial function and structure, which are on the causal pathway for later clinical disease. Using this approach, reduction of a range of risk factors in childhood has been shown to be associated with reversibility of early vascular abnormalities. New risk factors are emerging at an early age because of the deterioration in the lifestyle and behaviour of the population. Poor diet and less physical exercise have led to an epidemic of childhood obesity. Paediatricians need to be involved in the characterisation and management of cardiovascular risk factors from childhood, in both high-risk individuals and the general population. The medical profession, in addition, should engage actively with families, teachers, providers of health care, and politicians to promote understanding of the importance of lifetime investment in the reduction of risk factors. Without this, the gains achieved from better management of clinical cardiovascular disease are likely to be overwhelmed by an epidemic driven by deterioration of the profile of risk factors in the next generation of patients.

The complete reference list can be found on the companion Expert Consult web site at www.expertconsult.com.

ANNOTATED REFERENCES

- Tuzcu EM, Kapadia SR, Tutar E, et al: High prevalence of coronary atherosclerosis in asymptomatic teenagers and young adults: Evidence from intravascular ultrasound. Circulation 2001;103:2705–2710.

  This study used intravascular ultrasound to examine the coronary arteries in donor hearts in a transplantation program from subjects dying from non-cardiac causes at different ages. It confirms the literature already extant from autopsy studies, and shows a progressive increase in atheroma from teenage years.

- Cohen JC, Boerwinkle E, Mosley TH, Jr, Hobbs HH: Sequence variations in PCSK9, low LDL, and protection against coronary heart disease. N Engl J Med 2006;354:1264–1272.

  In this large multi-ethnic population, a previously unsuspected genetic variant was associated with a lifetime reduction in low-density lipoprotein cholesterol, and a very large reduction in clinical events. This emphasises the greater potential benefit of early risk factor management for lifetime reduction of risk compared to treatment of patients with clinical disease.

- Oren A, Vos LE, Uiterwaal CS, et al: Cardiovascular risk factors and increased carotid intima-media thickness in healthy young adults: The Atherosclerosis Risk in Young Adults (ARYA) Study. Arch Intern Med 2003;163:1787–1792.

  This large prospective study shows that levels of cardiovascular risk factors in childhood are related to subsequent evidence of structural arterial disease as shown by increased carotid intimal and medial thickness.

- Muntner P, He J, Cutler JA, et al: Trends in blood pressure among children and adolescents. JAMA 2004;291:2107–2113.

  This paper is a systematic meta-analysis of published studies examining the relationship between blood pressure in childhood and in adulthood. It provides strong evidence for the tracking of blood pressure throughout life and highlights the need for early intervention.

- McCarthy MI, Abecasis GR, Cardon LR, et al: Genome-wide association studies for complex traits: Consensus, uncertainty and challenges. Nat Rev Genet 2008;9:356–369.

  Understanding the genetic basis of disease has been revolutionised by the ability to perform genome-wide association studies. This article reviews the opportunities and challenges for this approach.

- Libby P, Ridker PM, Maseri A: Inflammation and atherosclerosis. Circulation 2002;105:1135–1143.

  This article reviews the growing evidence that the vascular biology of atherosclerosis involves inflammatory pathways. This has implications for understanding of the factors involved in progression of atheroma, as well as providing opportunities for new therapeutic approaches.

- Kavey RE, Allada V, Daniels SR, et al: Cardiovascular risk reduction in high-risk pediatric patients: A scientific statement from the American Heart Association Expert Panel on Population and Prevention Science; the Councils on Cardiovascular Disease in the Young, Epidemiology and Prevention, Nutrition, Physical Activity and Metabolism, High Blood Pressure Research, Cardiovascular Nursing, and the Kidney in Heart Disease; and the Interdisciplinary Working Group on Quality of Care and Outcomes Research: Endorsed by the American Academy of Pediatrics. Circulation 2006;114:2710–2738.

  This paper highlights that the atherosclerotic process begins early in life, and addresses the need for reduction of risk factors in childhood. It also provides practical recommendations for management of cardiovascular risk in selected paediatric conditions.

- Singhal A, Lucas A: Early origins of cardiovascular disease: Is there a unifying hypothesis? Lancet 2004;363:1642–1645.

  This review describes the concept of programming, making a strong case for the role of postnatal catch up growth rather than fetal influences, based on a series of randomised clinical trials. The opportunities for intervention are clearly greater after delivery.

- Weiss R, Dziura J, Burgert TS, et al: Obesity and the metabolic syndrome in children and adolescents. N Engl J Med 2004;350:2362–2374.

  This article demonstrates the metabolic consequences of obesity in subjects that are already present in the first two decades of life. The familiar components of metabolic syndrome, including dyslipidaemia, hypertension and insulin resistance, are related to degree of obesity.

- Bibbins-Domingo K, Coxson P, Pletcher MJ, et al: Adolescent overweight and future adult coronary heart disease. N Engl J Med 2007;357:2371–2379.

  This article highlights the potential consequences of childhood obesity on cardiovascular health in adult life. It also suggests that targeting the associated risk factors is unlikely to be sufficient, and that obesity itself should be managed.

Management of Congenital Heart Disease in Pregnancy

CANDICE K. SILVERSIDES, SAMUEL C. SIU, MATHEW SERMER, and JACK M. COLMAN

The successes of paediatric cardiology and cardiac surgery have enabled a new cohort of women, born with congenitally malformed hearts, to reach adulthood. Many of these women differ both anatomically and physiologically from any who have considered pregnancy in the past. Most women in this new cohort can anticipate safe and successful pregnancies. Pregnancy, however, imparts additional haemodynamic loads, changes in mechanisms of clotting, and increased propensity to arrhythmias, all of which increase the risk of adverse maternal cardiac events during pregnancy. In addition, there may be risks for adverse fetal and neonatal events. The recognition and appropriate management of such risks, when present, should optimise outcomes, while the recognition in other cases that a woman with a congenitally malformed heart is not at high risk allows reassurance.

IMPACT OF PREGNANCY ON THE CARDIOVASCULAR SYSTEM

Haemodynamic Changes during Pregnancy

The maternal volume of blood increases by approximately 50%, beginning during the first trimester, and peaking in the third trimester.[1,2] There is also an increase of up to 40% in the mass of erythrocytes.[3] The average heart rate increases by 10 to 20 beats per minute. Beginning early in the first trimester, the systemic vascular resistance and systemic arterial pressure begin to decrease owing to the low-resistance circuit in the uterus and to the effects of endogenous vasodilators. The systemic vascular resistance decreases until mid pregnancy, plateaus, and then rises toward the levels existing prior to pregnancy.[4,5] Systemic arterial pressure also begins to return toward pre-pregnancy levels in the third trimester. The changes in blood volume, vascular resistance, and heart rate all contribute to an increase in cardiac output, which begins early in the first trimester, continues to increase until approximately the end of the second trimester, rising to between one-third and one-half of the levels existing prior to pregnancy,[4,6–11] and then plateaus until term. Cardiac output is affected by position, and is highest when the mother is lying on her left side. The supine gravid uterus can compress the inferior caval vein, which limits venous return, and may lead to a substantial reduction in cardiac output. Women with cardiac disease have been shown to have lower cardiac output during pregnancy when compared to women without such disease.[12] The increased blood volume and systemic vasodilation also affect the flow of blood to other organs, including the skin, uterus, and kidneys. In the kidney, the result is an increase in the effective renal flow of plasma, and a 50% increase in the rate of glomerular filtration.[13]

Labour is associated with a further increase by approximately 10% in basal cardiac output, augmented by an additional surge of up to one-sixth with each uterine contraction.[14] Anxiety, pain, tachycardia, and hypertension or hypotension also contribute to cardiac complications at the time of labour and delivery. Following delivery, there is a further increase in cardiac output due to relief of compression on the inferior caval vein, and auto-transfusion from the now fully contracted uterus. Rapid mobilisation of interstitial fluid in the immediate period following pregnancy may have a significant negative impact on a woman with already compromised cardiac function. Although many of the described changes regress within the first few days after delivery, complete resolution of pregnancy-induced effects on cardiac function may not occur until 6 months after delivery.[15]

Cardiac Symptoms and Signs in Normal Pregnancy

During pregnancy, women often experience fatigue, dyspnea, tachypnoea, palpitations, presyncope, and decreased exercise tolerance. Such symptoms can be identical to those of cardiac decompensation, and clinicians must be careful to differentiate this possibility. Blood pressure decreases during the first part of pregnancy, and then during the last 6 weeks reaches or exceeds pre-pregnancy levels. Blood pressure should be taken when the mother is sitting or lying on her left side to avoid a falsely low reading caused by supine caval venous compression limiting venous return. The diastolic blood pressure falls more than the systolic pressure, resulting in a wide pulse pressure. The heart rate increases. Warm, erythematous hands and feet, nasal congestion, and breast engorgement are due to increased blood flow. Peripheral oedema may be noted. There may be a laterally displaced apical impulse due to modest increase in cardiac size, as well as upward displacement of the heart by the gravid uterus. There is often prominence of the jugular venous pulsation. There may be wide splitting of the first and second heart sounds. The continuous murmur of a venous hum in the right supraclavicular fossa, or a mammary souffle over an engorged breast, can become apparent during pregnancy. A systolic flow murmur is common, secondary to the hyperdynamic circulation, and is best heard at the left lower sternal border.

IMPACT OF PREGNANCY ON COMMON CARDIAC DIAGNOSTIC TESTS

The surface electrocardiogram may show a sinus tachycardia. Because of the change in position of the heart, the electrocardiogram may show a shift in the frontal plane axis, or inversion of the T waves in the inferior leads. The chest radiograph may show a more horizontal cardiac shadow because of elevation of the diaphragm, and an enlarged cardiac silhouette. The pulmonary vascular markings may become more prominent due to increased blood flow, simulating the vascularity produced by a systemic-to-pulmonary shunt. Echocardiographically, the increase in blood volume manifests as mild increases in the dimensions of the atriums and ventricles. The left ventricular mass increases.[7,15,16] The increased cardiac output is associated with increases in velocities of flow across all cardiac valves. Mitral regurgitation may either improve or worsen, according to the relative impact of the fall in systemic vascular resistance versus the change in geometry of the mitral valvar apparatus associated with increasing chamber size. Mild depression of left ventricular contractility has been demonstrated,[11] but left ventricular systolic performance is thought generally to be preserved.[8,10,11]

PRECONCEPTION COUNSELING AND CONTRACEPTION

All women with congenitally malformed hearts should have age-appropriate counseling prior to potential conception, beginning in adolescence.[17] This responsibility often falls to the specialist in congenital cardiac disease caring for the woman at the time, and his or her team, as the patient will often not have access to any others qualified to offer knowledgeable advice. Counseling should address:

- The diagnosis and long-term prognosis for the mother
- The maternal risk of pregnancy
- The risk to the fetus and neonate, including the risk of transmission of congenital cardiac disease to offspring
- Safe and unsafe options for contraception
- The need for high-risk obstetrical and multi-disciplinary care during pregnancy, if appropriate

It is common that information regarding diagnosis, previous procedures, and prognosis are not known to, or are misunderstood by, the patient. Clarification of diagnosis and functional capacity are fundamental to effective preconception counseling. The specialist in congenital cardiac disease is well suited to this task and also to ensuring that this information is provided to, and understood by, other caregivers involved in the management of the pregnancy. Discussion of long-term prognosis of the mother may be straightforward, or very complex and sensitive, depending on the underlying cardiac lesion, the types of surgical interventions, the residual lesions, and co-morbid medical conditions. Because maternal cardiac status can change over time, women with congenitally malformed hearts should be advised to ensure regular follow-up, and in particular to obtain a contemporaneous updated assessment prior to finalizing a decision to pursue pregnancy.[17] We discuss general and lesion-specific maternal and fetal risks associated with pregnancy in the later sections of this chapter.

Family planning needs are often poorly addressed in women with congenitally malformed hearts.[18] The safety and efficacy of various types of contraception need to be considered, but this has not been studied in women with congenitally malformed hearts. Recommendations regarding proper use of contraceptives have been extrapolated from studies in women without cardiac disease, and are based on expert opinion.[19-22] Options include:

- Barrier methods
- Combined oral contraceptives containing oestrogen and progestin
- Oral contraception with progestin alone
- Intra-uterine devices
- Sterilisation
- Emergency contraception

Barrier methods do not pose a health risk to the mother, but are associated with high rates of failure. Up to one-third of women using this technique will have an unintended pregnancy within the first year of use. Barrier methods, therefore, should not be recommended to women in whom there is a significant maternal risk of pregnancy.

Combined oral contraceptives have good efficacy, but the oestrogen component is associated with a risk of both arterial[23,24] and venous[25] thrombosis, which limits their use in women with cyanotic cardiac disease, the Fontan circulation, significant systemic ventricular dysfunction, sustained arrhythmias, mechanical valves, or prior thromboembolic events (Table 60-1). Other forms of combined contraception such as skin patches containing ethinyl estradiol and norelgestromin, and vaginal rings containing ethinyl estradiol and etonogestrel, are also associated with a thrombotic risk. The risk of stroke in association with combined oral contraceptives is further increased if a woman has a history of hypertension, diabetes, obesity, smoking, or migraine headaches.[24] Both oestrogens and progestins can interfere with the metabolism of warfarin, and international normalised ratios need to be monitored more closely in women using these forms of contraception.

Oral contraception using progestin alone is not associated with a risk of arterial or venous thrombosis,[26] but those using these agents suffer higher rates of failure compared to those using combined oestrogens and progestin. Such higher rates of failure are particularly seen with older pills containing only progestin, the so-called mini-pills, which should not be used in women with cardiac disease who face substantial risk of pregnancy.[20] A newer form of pill containing desogestrel is associated with lower rates of failure.[27] Pills containing only progesterone are associated with higher rates of vaginal breakthrough bleeding, and may thus be unacceptable to some patients. Bosentan can reduce the efficacy of pills containing exclusively progestin, so these should not be used alone in patients with pulmonary arterial hypertension undergoing medication with bosentan, in whom the maternal risk associated with pregnancy is substantial. Other forms of contraception using progestin alone include injectable medroxyprogesterone acetate, subcutaneous implants containing etonogestrel, and intra-uterine systems impregnated with levonorgestrel. Depo-Provera, the injectable form of medroxyprogesterone, is given by deep intramuscular injection, and can result in haematomas, a problem for women taking anticoagulants. Implanon, containing etonogestrel, is a subdermal implant that carries less risk of producing haematomas than is seen with intramuscular injection.

Insertion of intra-uterine devices can be associated with bacteraemia. As a result, such devices are contra-indicated in women at high risk for endocarditis, such as those who have suffered previous endocarditis, or those with mechanical heart valves. In approximately one-twentieth

TABLE 60-1

COMBINED HORMONAL CONTRACEPTIVES IN WOMEN WITH CARDIAC DISEASE

Class 1: Always Usable	Class 2: Broadly Usable	Class 3: Caution in Use		Class 4: Do Not Use	
Minor valve lesions: mitral valve prolapse with trivial mitral regurgitation, bicuspid aortic valve with normal function, mild pulmonary stenosis Repaired coarctation with no hypertension or aneurysm Simple congenital lesions successfully repaired in childhood with no sequels	Tissue prosthetic valve lacking any class 3 or 4 features Mild native mitral and aortic valve disease Most arrhythmias other than atrial fibrillation or flutter Hypertrophic cardiomyopathy lacking any class 3 or 4 features Fully recovered past cardiomyopathy including peripartum cardiomyopathy Uncomplicated Marfan syndrome Congenital heart disease lacking any class 3 or 4 features Small left-to-right shunt not reversible with physiological manoeuvres, e.g., small ventricular septal defects	Thrombotic risk, even on warfarin	Mechanical valves: bileaflet valves Previous thromboembolism Atrial arrhythmias, dilated left atrium >4 cm	Thrombotic risk, even on warfarin	Mechanical valves: Starr Edwards valve, Björk Shiley valve, any tricuspid valve Ischemic heart disease Pulmonary hypertension of any cause Dilated cardiomyopathy and left ventricular dysfunction of any cause (left ventricular ejection fraction <30%) Fontan circulation Previous arteritis involving coronary arteries, e.g., Kawasaki disease
		Risk of paradoxical embolism	Potential reversal of left to right shunt: unoperated atrial septal defects	Risk of paradoxical embolism	Cyanotic heart disease, pulmonary arteriovenous malformation

From Thorne S, MacGregor A, Nelson-Piercy C: Risks of contraception and pregnancy in heart disease. Heart 2006;92:1520–1525.

of women, a vasovagal reaction will occur when the cervix is instrumented for placement of a device. This can be particularly hazardous in women with pulmonary hypertension and those with the Fontan circulation.

Sterilisation should be considered for women in whom pregnancy carries a very high risk. This process has a number of limitations, including late rates of failure estimated as high as 1 in 200,[28] though bilateral fimbriectomy is associated with a much lower rate of failure. Further limitations are the associated maternal risks of general anaesthetics or abdominal insufflation with carbon dioxide, poorly tolerated in women with the Fontan circulation, for example, and the psychological impact on the patient. A new alternative utilises hysteroscopic insertion of intratubal stents under oral analgesia.[29] This method may prove useful for women at high risk with other techniques of sterilisation. Vasectomy may not be an ideal solution because a male partner may outlive his spouse and may wish to father children with a new partner.

Emergency contraception, the so-called morning-after pill, available in forms containing oestrogen and progestin, or progestin only, is safe for women with congenitally malformed hearts, and its availability should be made known.[19,30] Termination may be the most appropriate response to pregnancy in infrequent cases, and the possibility should be explored when indicated.

When pregnancy is actively considered, or when the woman presents in a gravid condition, the assessment must incorporate advice about the proper level of obstetric and multi-disciplinary care during pregnancy. Most women with congenitally malformed hearts will benefit from an initial cardiac and high-risk obstetrical consultation. Those with minor lesions and their caregivers can be reassured regarding the low risk of adverse events and the appropriateness of standard obstetrical care. Women at higher risk can be referred appropriately to high-risk obstetrical units, where they will have access to specialists with experience in managing complex cardiac disease through pregnancy.[31]

GLOBAL AND LESION SPECIFIC RISKS AND OUTCOMES

Global Assessment of Maternal and Fetal or Neonatal Risks

Maternal cardiac disease is a risk factor for adverse maternal and fetal events. When evaluating pregnant women with cardiac disease, a global assessment is made of the risk of adverse maternal cardiac events, with fetal and neonatal risks considered separately. This should be supplemented with weighing of lesion-specific risks when these are known.

A Canadian consortium prospectively developed and validated a global risk index for pregnant women with heart disease. A poor functional state defined as New York Heart Association functional class three or four, or cyanosis, systemic ventricular systolic dysfunction, obstruction in the left heart, and history of prior cardiac events such as arrhythmia, stroke, and cardiac failure, were all predictors of adverse maternal cardiac events during pregnancy.[32] A point-score system assigned one point to each of these predictors. Patients with no predictors were at low risk, having a chance of adverse events in only one-twentieth

TABLE 60-2

RISK FACTORS FOR MATERNAL CARDIAC AND NEONATAL ADVERSE EVENTS DURING PREGNANCY IN WOMEN WITH HEART DISEASE

1.1 Adverse Event	1.2 Risk Factor	1.3 Adverse Event	1.4 Risk Factor
Maternal cardiac adverse event*	*General risks* 1. Poor functional class (NYHA class III or IV) or cyanosis 2. Systemic ventricular ejection fraction <40% 3. Left heart obstruction (mitral valve area <2 cm², aortic valve area <1.5 cm², or peak left ventricular outflow tract gradient >30 mm Hg) 4. Cardiac event (arrhythmia, stroke, pulmonary oedema) prior to pregnancy *Lesion specific risks* (see text)	Neonatal adverse event†	1. Poor maternal functional class (NYHA class III or IV) or cyanosis 2. Maternal left heart obstruction (defined above) 3. Maternal age <20 or >35 years 4. Obstetric risk factors‡ 5. Multiple gestation 6. Smoking during pregnancy 7. Anti-coagulant therapy

*Maternal cardiac adverse events include: pulmonary oedema, arrhythmia, stroke and death. The general risk factors can be used to constitute a risk index: the risk of a maternal cardiac adverse event with no risk factors present is <5%, with one risk factor present is 25%, and with more than one risk factor present is 75%. Data from Siu SC, Sermer M, Colman JM, et al: Prospective multicenter study of pregnancy outcomes in women with heart disease. Circulation 2001;104:515–521.
†Neonatal adverse event include premature birth, small-for-gestational age birth weight, respiratory distress syndrome, intraventricular haemorrhage, and fetal or neonatal death. Data from Siu SC, Sermer M, Colman JM, et al: Prospective multicenter study of pregnancy outcomes in women with heart disease. Circulation 2001;104:515–521.
‡History of premature delivery or rupture of membranes, incompetent cervix, or caesarean section; or intra-uterine growth retardation, antepartum bleeding >12 weeks of gestation, febrile illness, or uterine/placental abnormalities during present pregnancy.

of pregnancies, whereas those with one predictor were at intermediate risk, adverse effects being anticipated in one-quarter of pregnancies, and those with more than one predictor were at very high risk, with adverse events anticipated in three-quarters of pregnancies (Table 60-2 and Fig. 60-1). When applying the global score for risk, it should be borne in mind that patients previously known to be at high risk, such as those with Eisenmenger's syndrome, pulmonary hypertension, the Fontan circulation, or Marfan syndrome with a dilated aortic root, were not represented or else under-represented in the populations studied. These previously known markers of high risk, therefore, are not reflected in the global score, and must be separately considered through application of a parallel lesion-specific evaluation of risk. In a recent study, dysfunction of the subpulmonary ventricle and severe pulmonary regurgitation were shown to be additional predictors for adverse maternal cardiac events.[33] Other factors that increase maternal cardiac risk during pregnancy include

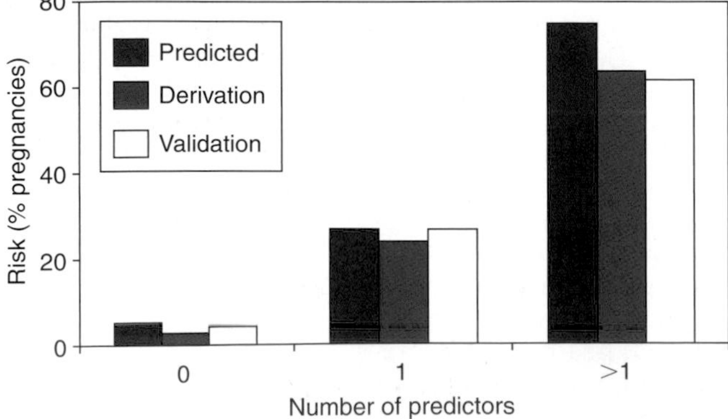

Figure 60-1 Maternal cardiac risk during pregnancy, showing data from the CARPREG Study. (Data from Siu SC, Sermer M, Colman JM, et al: Prospective multicenter study of pregnancy outcomes in women with heart disease. Circulation 2001;104:515–521.)

prosthetic valves, anticoagulant therapy, and co-morbid medical conditions such as diabetes and hypertension.

A British working group has also created a classification of risk for women with cardiac conditions undergoing pregnancy. This categorises the risk during pregnancy using global and lesion-specific elements[19] (Table 60-3). According to these recommendations, pregnancy is contraindicated in women with cardiac lesions associated with extremely high risks of maternal morbidity and mortality. These lesions include systemic ventricular dysfunction producing New York Heart Association functional class, three or four symptoms, an ejection fraction of less than 30%, peripartum cardiomyopathy with any residual left ventricular dysfunction, severe obstruction of the left ventricular outflow tract, Marfan syndrome with an aortic root diameter of greater than 40 mm, and pulmonary arterial hypertension.

General and lesion-specific recommendations for evaluation and management of pregnancy have also been published by the European Society of Cardiology[34] and the Canadian Cardiovascular Society.[35–37] In addition, there are excellent texts available devoted to pregnancy in women with cardiac disease.[38–40]

Although the risks of adverse maternal events during pregnancy and the early peripartal period are reasonably well described, little data is available concerning late maternal outcomes in women with congenitally malformed hearts.[41,42]

Women with cardiac disease also have an increased risk of adverse fetal and neonatal events. In a prospective study,[43] we showed that the risk of neonatal complications, such as premature birth, weight at birth small for gestational age, respiratory distress syndrome, intraventricular haemorrhage, and fetal or neonatal death, is higher in women with cardiac disease, amplified by specific maternal cardiac risk factors, and further amplified by concomitant maternal non-cardiac risk factors for adverse fetal and neonatal outcomes (Fig. 60-2; see also Table 60-2).

TABLE 60-3

PREGNANCY RISK FOR WOMEN WITH CARDIAC DISEASE

Class 1: No Risk	Class 2: Small Increased Risk	Class 2–3: Depending on the Individual	Class 3: Significant Risk	Class 4: Pregnancy Contra-indicated
Uncomplicated, small, or mild pulmonic stenosis, ventricular septal defect or patent ductus arteriosus, mitral valve prolapse with no more than trivial mitral regurgitation	Unoperated atrial septal defect	Mild left ventricular impairment	Mechanical valve	Pulmonary arterial hypertension of any cause
Successfully repaired simple lesions, e.g., atrial septal defect, ventricular septal defect, patent ductus arteriosus, or anomalous pulmonary venous connection	Repaired tetralogy of Fallot	Hypertrophic cardiomyopathy	Systemic right ventricle (e.g., congenitally corrected transposition, complete transposition post-Mustard or post-Senning repair)	Severe systemic ventricular dysfunction associated with New York Heart Association functional class III–IV or left ventricular ejection fraction <30%*
Isolated atrial or ventricular extrasystoles	Most arrhythmias	Native or tissue valvular heart disease not considered class 4	Post-Fontan operation	Previous peripartum cardiomyopathy with any residual impairment of left ventricular function
		Marfan syndrome without dilated aortic root	Cyanotic heart disease	Severe left heart obstruction
		Heart transplant	Other complex congenital lesions	Marfan syndrome with dilated aorta >40 mm

*Risk assessment should be individualized for patients with more complex cardiac anatomy.
Modified from Thorne S, MacGregor A, Nelson-Piercy C: Risks of contraception and pregnancy in heart disease. Heart 2006;92:1520–1525.

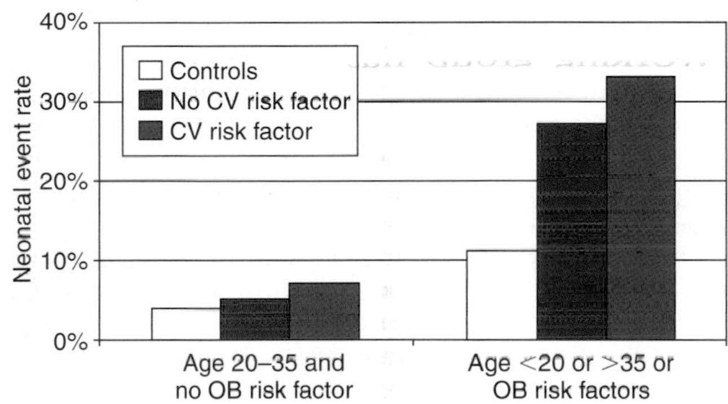

Figure 60-2 Fetal and neonatal risks as amplified by concomitant obstetric risk factors. Obstetric factors include history of premature delivery or rupture of membranes, incompetent cervix, or caesarean section; or intra-uterine growth retardation, antepartum bleeding after 12 weeks of gestation, febrile illness, or uterine/placental abnormalities during the present pregnancy. CV, cardiovascular; OB, obstetric. (Data from Siu SC, Colman JM, Sorensen S, et al: Adverse neonatal and cardiac outcomes are more common in pregnant women with cardiac disease. Circulation 2002;105:2179–2184.)

The risk related to inheritance merits separate discussion. Baseline probability of a congenitally malformed heart in the absence of an affected relative is from 0.4% to 0.6%, but increases about 10-fold when a parent is affected,[44] with some studies suggesting a higher rate of transmission when the mother is the affected parent.[44,45] With certain lesions, the likelihood of transmission is higher. In those with atrioventricular septal defects, the maternal transmission is reported to be 11.6%.[45] In autosomal dominant syndromes such as Noonan's syndrome,[46] Holt-Oram syndrome,[47] Williams syndrome,[48] Marfan syndrome, and the 22q11 deletion syndromes, the risk is 50%, though penetration and phenotypic expression may vary. Because of successful management of patients with congenitally malformed hearts, there is an expanding pool of potential parents who carry higher genetic risk for transmission to offspring. The impact that this will have on rates of congenital cardiac disease in newborns is offset to an unknown extent by advances in diagnosis during early pregnancy through fetal screening that may lead to termination of some affected pregnancies.[49] In our experience, the result of fetal echocardiography in a woman with a known increased risk of carrying a fetus with a congenitally malformed heart is infrequently used to support termination, but rather is applied to facilitate peripartal planning and neonatal management.

We have shown that a careful assessment at least 2 weeks after delivery, supplemented by clinically guided use of echocardiography, can identify additional cases of congenital cardiac disease in offspring of women with congenitally malformed hearts that were not identified by fetal echocardiography.[50]

Lesion-specific Risks, Outcomes, and Strategies for Management

Left-to-right Shunts

Simple left-to-right shunts, including those produced by interatrial communications, ventricular septal defect, and patency of the arterial duct, are generally well tolerated during pregnancy. The increase in volume load is counteracted to some extent by the fall in peripheral vascular resistance, and complications are rare.[51–53] Potential complications include arrhythmias, deterioration in functional class, cardiac failure, and paradoxical embolism. Arrhythmias were reported in only 1 of 123 pregnancies in women with atrial septal defects, and in no pregnancies in women with ventricular septal defects. None of the patients developed cardiac failure during pregnancy.[54]

Atrioventricular septal defects are more complex, and are associated with regurgitation across both the right and left sides of the common atrioventricular junction. Compared to women with simple lesions, those with atrioventricular septal defect are more likely to experience cardiac complications.[53,55] When intracardiac shunts are associated with pulmonary hypertension, the risk again is high, and mainly attributable to the pulmonary hypertension, discussed separately below.

Transposition

Atrial redirection procedures such as the Mustard or Senning operations were the original techniques used to repair patients with transposition, albeit now superseded in most instances by the arterial switch operation (see Chapter 38). Women with arterial switch operations have only recently begun to reach childbearing age, and only limited outcome data is available.[56] Most women with transposition now of childbearing age, therefore, will have had an atrial repair in infancy, and as a consequence will have the morphologically right ventricle and tricuspid valve supporting the systemic circulation. This is associated with variable degrees of systemic ventricular dysfunction and systemic atrioventricular valvar regurgitation. Additional sequels that may impact on pregnancy include atrial arrhythmias, sinus nodal dysfunction, and obstruction or leak across the atrial baffle. Cardiac failure, functional deterioration, and arrhythmias are the main complications reported during pregnancy.[57–64] In addition, obstetric complications, such as premature rupture of membranes, premature labour, premature delivery, and thromboembolic complications, were frequent.[61] Those studying the late effects of pregnancy on the systemic right ventricle found late echocardiographic evidence of systemic ventricular dilation in almost one-third of the women, and deterioration in the function of the systemic ventricle in one-quarter.[63] Premature delivery is reported in one-third of pregnancies, with one-fifth of babies born small for gestational age.[54]

Congenitally Corrected Transposition

Congenitally corrected transposition is also associated with a morphologically right ventricle supporting the systemic circulation. It is also frequent to find regurgitation of the abnormal systemic atrioventricular valve, ventricular septal defect and pulmonary stenosis, and disturbances of atrioventricular conduction (see Chapter 39). Although maternal deaths have not been reported, cardiac failure, arrhythmias, endocarditis, myocardial infarction, and stroke have been described as complications of pregnancy.[65,66]

Those with Functionally Univentricular Hearts and the Fontan Circulation

The Fontan procedure, initially developed as a palliation to improve haemodynamics in patients with tricuspid atresia, has been extended to provide palliation for those with other complex congenital cardiac lesions not amenable to biventricular repair. Despite overall benefit, patients remain with functionally univentricular physiology, and have limited ability to increase cardiac output. Late complications in patients with the Fontan circulation include elevated right atrial and systemic venous pressures, arrhythmias, ventricular dysfunction, protein-losing enteropathy, and thromboembolic events (see Chapter 31). All these problems can be provoked or aggravated by the additional haemodynamic load of pregnancy. Therefore, women with the Fontan circulation need to be educated about the potential maternal risks of pregnancy. If they choose to become pregnant, they must be monitored closely. In one retrospective report on 33 pregnancies including 15 live births, supraventricular tachycardia occurred in one woman.[67] In the same series, two-fifths of women had spontaneous abortions. Others have suggested that maternal cardiac and non-cardiac complications are common,[68,69] with one study reporting miscarriage in half of those becoming pregnant, with amenorrhoea in two-fifths.[69]

Obstruction of the Left Ventricular Outflow Tract

A bifoliate aortic valve (see Chapter 44) is the most common cause of an obstructed left ventricular outflow tract in women of childbearing age. A smaller number of cases are due to subvalvar or supravalvar stenosis, or other abnormalities at the valvar level. Severe obstruction may not be well tolerated during pregnancy because the increased blood volume and stroke volume may provoke left ventricular failure. Furthermore, abrupt changes in preload may be poorly tolerated by the hypertrophied ventricle, so haemorrhage, or the effects of general or regional anaesthetic agents, can lead to profound haemodynamic embarrassment. During pregnancy, women with severe obstruction are at risk for the development of angina, functional deterioration, cardiac failure and arrhythmias, as well as sudden death, though adverse maternal cardiac events are not as common as described in early reports.[70] Our group found adverse maternal cardiac events in around one-twentieth of women during or immediately after pregnancy,[70,71] with similar observations reported by others.[72,73] Our patients frequently required intervention within a few years after pregnancy, up to two-fifths of those with severe stenosis, so this possibility should be addressed during pre-pregnancy counseling.[71] Balloon aortic valvoplasty and aortic valvar surgery have been performed successfully during pregnancy.[74] Because of the risk to the fetus, such interventions should only be performed if there are no other alternatives. Despite relatively reassuring maternal outcomes, fetal, neonatal, and obstetric complications are common in women with aortic stenosis.[71] Aortic insufficiency, on the other hand, is generally well tolerated unless severe and associated with depressed left ventricular function.

Aortic Coarctation

Most women with coarctation of the aorta have had some type of repair (see Chapter 46). Repair may be associated with sequels, in particular development of aneurysms when Dacron has been used for a patch, or pseudoaneurysms.[75] Thus, imaging of the site of repair, optimally by magnetic resonance imaging, is optimal prior to conception.[76] Patients with unrepaired coarctation, or those with repaired coarctation and residual or recurrent obstruction, are subject to upper body hypertension. Antihypertensive treatment directed at the upper body may exacerbate hypotension distal to the coarctation, and thus compromise placental perfusion. This may explain the increased incidence of intra-uterine restriction of growth and prematurity seen in the offspring of such patients.[77] In contemporary studies, maternal mortality in women with repaired coarctation is rare, but women are at increased risk for pregnancy-induced hypertension, pre-eclampsia, and complications related to the associated bifoliate aortic valve.[32,76–78] Dissection of the aorta has been reported.

Marfan Syndrome and Other Aortopathies

Pregnancy-related haemodynamic and hormonal changes impact the structure of the aortic wall, and increase the risk of dilation and dissection. This phenomenon manifests as an increased risk of spontaneous dissection, even in women with no known or diagnosable aortopathy.[79] This is very low in otherwise normal women. Dissection has best been described in those with Marfan syndrome, but women with other aortopathies that have genetic and/or pathologic similarities, such as familial thoracic aortic aneurysm and dissection syndrome, Loeys-Dietz syndrome, the aortopathy associated with the bicuspid aortic valve, Turner's syndrome, and vascular Ehlers-Danlos syndrome, are also at increased risk of aortic complications.[80,81]

In a seminal prospective study of women with Marfan syndrome followed through 45 pregnancies, no significant change was found in the size of the aortic root in those initially having roots of normal size, but one-third of women with dilated roots or those having prior surgery suffered either aortic dissection or progressive aortic dilation.[82] In a recent prospective study, favourable outcomes were reported with no significant changes in aortic root diameter during or following pregnancy when compared to a matched group of childless women. Those with diameters of the root between 40 and 45 mm, however, had a mildly increased rate of growth compared to women with aortic root diameters less than 40 mm.[83] Although there are no trials demonstrating benefit of β-blockade during pregnancy in women with aortopathy, we do recommend such treatment during and after pregnancy in women with Marfan syndrome, coarctation of the aorta, and other aortopathies, in the hope that this may attenuate the risk of aortic dilation or dissection.

Pulmonary Valvar Stenosis

Women with pulmonary valvar stenosis have been reported to tolerate pregnancy well, in spite of the pregnancy-associated increase in preload,[32,72,84] albeit that the risk of hypertensive and neonatal complications may be underappreciated.[85]

Tetralogy of Fallot

Most patients with tetralogy of Fallot will have undergone an intracardiac repair, and many repaired patients will have pulmonary regurgitation and/or right heart dilation and dysfunction in late follow-up. Other potential late complications include surgical scars and patches that can act as a substrate for arrhythmia, residual shunts, and left ventricular dysfunction. One recent study reported adverse cardiac events, including cardiac failure and arrhythmias, in one-eighth of patients.[86] Another study, including 20 pregnancies in women with unrepaired tetralogy of Fallot, reported adverse events such as arrhythmias, cardiac failure, and progressive right ventricular dilation in one-sixth.[87] The presence of severe pulmonic regurgitation and/or a dysfunctional subpulmonary right ventricle is known to be associated with worse maternal outcome during pregnancy.[33] The late effects of pregnancy on the dilated, dysfunctional right ventricle, however, are unknown.

Ebstein's Malformation

Ebstein's malformation can manifest a broad spectrum of severity. Those with severe forms of the disease may present early in life with cyanosis or right-sided cardiac failure, whereas those with mild forms may first be detected incidentally in adulthood (see Chapter 34). The ability of the heart to tolerate the increased demands of pregnancy is dependent on the size and function of the functional right ventricle, the degree of tricuspid regurgitation, and the propensity to arrhythmias. Women with interatrial shunts are at risk for reversal of the flow if they are unable to adapt to the increased preload, and women who enter pregnancy with any degree of right-to-left shunting at the atrial level are likely to demonstrate worsening hypoxaemia and cyanosis as pregnancy proceeds. Despite these potential problems, reported pregnancy outcomes have been favourable.[88,89]

Cyanotic Cardiac Disease

Cyanosis is the visible manifestation of maternal hypoxaemia. In a woman with manifest or potential hypoxemia due to right-to-left shunting, it should be established whether the shunt is due to pulmonary hypertension, in other words, Eisenmenger's syndrome, or another cause, since pulmonary hypertension itself imparts an extremely high risk to pregnancy, as discussed below.

In the absence of pulmonary hypertension, women with cyanotic disease are at risk for adverse maternal cardiac events during pregnancy, in particular cardiac failure, arrhythmias, thrombosis, embolism, and endocarditis, though death is rare.[90–92] The pregnancy-induced fall in systemic vascular resistance will facilitate right-to-left shunting, especially when the shunt is at the level of the ventricles or great arteries. Fetal outcomes are poor. Infants are born small for gestational age.[91] Live births are compromised, and prematurity is common.[90] If maternal saturation of oxygen is less than 0.85, only one-eighth of fetuses progress to be born alive.[90,93]

Pulmonary Hypertension

In spite of advances in treatment, pulmonary hypertension continues to provide a very high risk for pregnancy. When associated with a right-to-left shunt, in other words, Eisenmenger's syndrome, the effects of maternal hypoxaemia and cyanosis play a major additional role.[94] The increased volume load directed through the high-resistance pulmonary circuit will provoke elevations in subpulmonary ventricular pressure, potentially causing subpulmonary ventricular failure, and will augment the right-to-left shunt if present, thereby worsening hypoxaemia. Hypoxaemia acts as a pulmonary vasoconstrictor, thus constituting a vicious cycle. As well, pulmonary thrombosis and pulmonary emboluses are more likely during pregnancy, and may further increase pulmonary vascular resistance. Challenges at delivery, including loss of blood, epidural anesthesia, and vagal responses associated with expulsive efforts of the mother in the second stage of labour, may further facilitate right-to-left shunting, leading to a potential spiral of hypoxaemic pulmonary vasoconstriction, hypotension, and death.

The high mortality of pregnancy in Eisenmenger's syndrome[95] has remained in the range of 30%, even in more recent reports.[96] Outcomes may be better with early diagnosis and comprehensive management.[96,97] In addition, targeted advanced pulmonary vascular therapies applied in specialised centres are likely to provide better outcomes,[94] though reports of such improved outcomes are sparse at the time of writing, and the risk remains high. As a consequence, the widely held consensus is to advise against pregnancy in women with significant pulmonary hypertension of any cause and, in the event of unexpected pregnancy, to offer termination as the safest option.[94,97,98]

Prosthetic Heart Valves

Women with any type of artificial heart valve are at increased risk for complications during pregnancy. Bioprosthetic and mechanical valves each have advantages and disadvantages. Careful consideration of the risks and benefits of each is required prior to selection of the type of prosthetic valve in a woman of childbearing age. During pregnancy, normally functioning bioprosthetic valves are safer than mechanical valves because they are less thrombogenic and do not require ongoing anti-coagulation. Bioprosthetic valves, nonetheless, have limited durability, and women with these valves will generally require repeated surgery in the future.[99,100] Although some studies have suggested that pregnancy accelerates the degeneration of bioprosthetic valves, other studies have not demonstrated this finding.[99,101,102] Less information is available on the safety of homografts during pregnancy, albeit that one study found no valve-related complications occurring during pregnancy.[103]

Mechanical valves have better durability than bioprosthetic ones, but are associated with significantly greater maternal and fetal risks during pregnancy. Because pregnancy is a hypercoagulable state, and because anti-coagulation can be difficult to manage with changing body weight during pregnancy, there is an increased risk of maternal thromboembolic events, occurring on average in one-sixth of pregnancies, of which approximately half is valvar thrombosis.[104–108] Valves in the mitral position give higher thrombotic risks than those in the aortic position, as do early models of mechanical valves, such as those with balls in cages, or the first generation of those with tilting discs. Anti-coagulant therapy is complicated by a risk of bleeding.[109] Specific thrombotic risks are dependent on the type of anti-coagulation used.

Options for anti-coagulants include unfractionated heparin, low-molecular-weight heparin, and oral anti-coagulants such as warfarin and adjunctive aspirin. Heparin does not cross the placenta and therefore is a safer alternative for the fetus. Heparin given subcutaneously, nonetheless, is difficult to manage, and is a less effective anti-coagulant, with higher maternal thrombosis rates than warfarin. Valvar thrombosis, which can be fatal, is less common in pregnancy when oral anti-coagulants are used throughout, when compared to oral anti-coagulants with unfractionated heparin substituted between 6 to 12 weeks of gestation, or heparin is given throughout pregnancy.[109] Heparin may also cause maternal thrombocytopenia and osteoporosis. Warfarin crosses the placenta and is associated with warfarin embryopathy in first trimester use and fetal intracranial bleeding, which is a risk throughout pregnancy.[109] The risk of warfarin embryopathy has been shown to be less if heparin is substituted from 6 until 12 weeks of gestation and also in women whose therapeutic dose of warfarin is less than 5 mg per day.[110,111] Because intracranial bleeding can occur during vaginal delivery in a fetus exposed to maternal warfarin, heparin should be substituted at least 2 weeks prior to delivery, or the fetus must be delivered by caesarean section. Low-molecular-weight heparin is easier to use than unfractionated heparin, and has better bioavailability. It also does not cross the placenta and therefore is safe for the fetus. Initial reports of valvar thrombosis and maternal deaths could have been due to bias in reporting, and to inadequate dosing and monitoring. Recent guidelines suggest that, if low-molecular-weight heparin is used during pregnancy, dosing by weight is not adequate, and careful monitoring of anti-Xa levels is required.[112] Low-dose aspirin is safe and may enhance the effectiveness of heparin in pregnant women with mechanical valves.[112] Both heparin and warfarin are safe in the breastfeeding mother.[112]

There is no consensus on optimal regimes for anti-coagulation in pregnant women with mechanical valves, so the choice should be tailored to the individual after risk and benefits are discussed in detail. No randomised trials are available. Guidelines, predominantly based on expert opinion, have been published by the American Heart Association/American College of Cardiology[112] (Table 60-4), the American College of Chest Physicians[113] (Table 60-5), and the European Society of Cardiology.[34] An alternative approach that incorporates additional risk factors, including the types of valve and their thrombotic potential, was recently recommended.[108]

Arrhythmias

Pregnancy is arrhythmogenic in at least three fundamental ways. As a result of the haemodynamic changes, there is chamber enlargement and stretch. Hormonal changes, in particular increased levels of oestrogen, are proarrhythmic.[114] There are changes in the autonomic milieu in relation to pregnancy.[115] As a consequence, supraventricular and ventricular arrhythmias are more likely to occur during pregnancy in women with preexisting arrhythmias or to appear as new events, and to occur in women with or without structural cardiac disease. If an arrhythmia presents for the first time during pregnancy, the woman should be assessed for structural abnormalities as well, since arrhythmias during pregnancy may be the presenting complaint in a woman with structural cardiac disease, and the impact of a given arrhythmia is more likely to be significant in this setting. It is important to make an accurate diagnosis of the precise mechanism of an arrhythmia, as this is often reassuring, allowing therapy to be withheld, and in any case will guide therapy and avoid application of ineffective and possibly harmful strategies.

Arrhythmias are common in adult patients with congenital cardiac disease, but only a few studies have examined this subject during pregnancy. Studies from our centre have shown that women with a history of arrhythmias, most of whom had structural cardiac disease, were at increased risk for adverse maternal cardiac outcomes during pregnancy.[32,84] In addition, women who had recurrences of arrhythmias during pregnancy were at increased risk for adverse fetal and neonatal events.[116] Nonetheless, because of the potential harmful effects of medications on the fetus, pharmacological therapies should be reserved for patients with significant symptoms, or when sustained episodes result in hypotension. In the case of haemodynamically significant arrhythmias, treatment should not be delayed.

In women of childbearing age, most arrhythmias are supraventricular, and are not life threatening. Recurrence rates of supraventricular tachycardia of up to one-third have been reported during pregnancy.[117,118] In our experience, supraventricular tachycardia recurred in half of women during pregnancy, predominantly those with structural cardiac disease, with half also suffering atrial fibrillation or flutter, this time almost exclusively in those with structural disease.[116] A full discussion of the types of supraventricular tachyarrhythmias and their pharmacological therapies is beyond the scope of this section. Guidelines exist for the treatment of acute exacerbation of atrial arrhythmias in pregnancy.[119,120] Intravenous adenosine, β-blockers, or cardioversion can be used safely, and other therapies considered depending on risk-benefit assessment.

Ventricular arrhythmias during pregnancy in women without heart disease are rare. In those with congenital cardiac disease, in contrast, ventricular arrhythmias may

TABLE 60-4

AMERICAN HEART ASSOCIATION/AMERICAN COLLEGE OF CARDIOLOGY GUIDELINES FOR SELECTION OF ANTI-COAGULANT REGIMES IN PREGNANT PATIENTS WITH MECHANICAL PROSTHETIC VALVES

Class	Recommendations
Class I	1. All pregnant patients with mechanical prosthetic valves must receive continuous therapeutic anti-coagulation with frequent monitoring.
	2. For women requiring long-term warfarin therapy who are attempting pregnancy, pregnancy test should be monitored with discussions about subsequent anti-coagulation therapy, so that anti-coagulation can be continued uninterrupted when pregnancy is achieved.
	3. Pregnant patients with mechanical prosthetic valves who elect to stop warfarin between 6 and 12 weeks of gestation should receive continuous intravenous UFH, dose-adjusted UFH, or dose-adjusted LMWH.
	4. For pregnant patients with mechanical valves, up to 36 weeks of gestation, the therapeutic choice of continuous intravenous or dose-adjusted UFH, dose-adjusted LMWH, or warfarin should be discussed fully. If continuous intravenous UFH is used, the fetal risk is lower, but the maternal risks of prosthetic valve thrombosis, systemic embolization, infection, osteoporosis, and heparin-induced thrombocytopenia are higher.
	5. In pregnant patients with mechanical prosthetic valves who receive dose-adjusted LMWH, the LMWH should be administered twice daily subcutaneously to maintain the anti-Xa level between 0.7 and 1.2 U per ml 4 hours after administration.
	6. In pregnant patients with mechanical prosthetic valves who receive dose-adjusted UFH, the aPTT should be at least twice control.
	7. In pregnant patients with mechanical prosthetic valves who receive warfarin, the INR goal should be 3.0 IU (range, 2.5–3.5)
	8. In pregnant patients with mechanical prosthetic valves, warfarin should be discontinued and continuous intravenous UFH given starting 2–3 weeks before planned delivery.
Class IIa	1. In patients with mechanical prosthetic valves, it is reasonable to avoid warfarin between 6 and 12 weeks of gestation owing to the high risk of fetal defects.
	2. In patients with mechanical prosthetic valves, it is reasonable to resume UFH 4–6 hours after delivery and begin oral warfarin in the absence of bleeding.
	3. In patients with mechanical prosthetic valves, it is reasonable to give low-dose aspirin (75–100 mg per day) in the second and third trimester of pregnancy in addition to anti-coagulation with warfarin or heparin.
Class III	1. LMWH should not be administered to pregnant patients with mechanical prosthetic valves unless anti-Xa levels are monitored 4–6 hours after administration.
	2. Dipyridamole should not be used as an alternative antiplatelet agent in pregnant patients with mechanical prosthetic valves because of its harmful effect on the fetus.

aPTT, activated partial thromboplastin time; INR, international normalized ratio; LMWH, low-molecular-weight heparin; UFH, unfractionated heparin.
From Bonow RO, Carabello BA, Kanu C, et al: ACC/AHA 2006 guidelines for the management of patients with valvular heart disease: A report of the American College of Cardiology/American Heart Association Task Force on Practice Guidelines (writing committee to revise the 1998 Guidelines for the Management of Patients With Valvular Heart Disease): Developed in collaboration with the Society of Cardiovascular Anesthesiologists: Endorsed by the Society for Cardiovascular Angiography and Interventions and the Society of Thoracic Surgeons. Circulation 2006;114:e84–231.

TABLE 60-5

AMERICAN COLLEGE OF CHEST PHYSICIANS GUIDELINES FOR ANTI-COAGULATION REGIMES IN PREGNANT PATIENTS WITH MECHANICAL PROSTHETIC VALVES

1. Aggressive adjusted-dose UFH, given every 12 hours subcutaneously throughout pregnancy; mid-interval aPTT maintained at ≥2 times control levels, or anti-Xa heparin level maintained at 0.35–0.70 IU/mL

or

2. LMWH throughout pregnancy, in doses adjusted according to weight or as necessary to maintain a 4-hour post-injection anti-Xa heparin level of about 1.0 IU/mL

or

3. UFH or LMWH, as above, until the 13th week; change to warfarin until the middle of the third trimester, then restart UFH or LMWH therapy until delivery

aPTT, activated partial thromboplastin time; LMWH, low-molecular-weight heparin; UFH, unfractionated heparin.
From Bates SM, Greer IA, Hirsh J, Ginsberg JS: Use of antithrombotic agents during pregnancy: The Seventh ACCP Conference on Antithrombotic and Thrombolytic Therapy. Chest 2004;126:627S–644S.

develop or recur during pregnancy. We found ventricular tachycardia to recur in one-quarter of women during pregnancy.[116] Medication for preventing such recurrences should be tailored to the type of tachycardia. For instance, women with catecholamine-sensitive ventricular tachycardia, or long QT syndrome, may best be treated with β-blockers. In the case of long QT syndrome, therapy should be continued for several months after delivery, as this is when most of the reported adverse events have occurred, especially in those with the long QT-2 genotype.[121] For acute management, intravenous procainamide, amiodarone, sotalol, or β-blockers can be used.[122] When necessary, cardioversion is considered safe during pregnancy, and cardioverter-defibrillators can also safely be implanted.[123]

PERIPARTAL MANAGEMENT

Detailed discussions about management during and after delivery can be found in other sources.[34–40] For any woman with a congenitally malformed heart at increased risk of adverse maternal cardiac or neonatal complications during pregnancy, there should be timely multi-disciplinary assessment, and a plan should be developed for management which provides recommendations for various contingencies. This plan must be available to the medical team who may be tasked with the care of labour and delivery at unpredictable times, and even in unpredictable places. The plan should therefore be written, widely distributed, with a copy given to the patient to ensure timely access.[31]

General principles of management of labour and delivery for women with congenitally malformed hearts of moderate or great complexity include early effective analgesia by regional techniques, and vaginal delivery in almost every case unless obstetric considerations require caesarean delivery. Induction is considered safe in women with cardiac disease.[124] Assisted vaginal delivery is often indicated in order to limit or avoid maternal expulsive efforts. Caesarean section is rarely indicated for cardiac reasons.

CARDIAC MEDICATIONS AND PROCEDURES DURING PREGNANCY

Drug Use

The use of any drug during pregnancy requires consideration of many factors, including potential fetal toxicity as well as possible pregnancy-related changes in effectiveness of the medication.[125]

Fetal toxicity depends on timing of administration. Prior to implantation, the effect is all-or-none. Teratogenic effects are seen with exposure between 3 and 10 to 12 weeks. Later in pregnancy, effects are mixed and depend on the drug and the magnitude of exposure. General principles with respect to avoiding fetal toxicity include choosing drugs known to be safe when possible, using the least number of drugs for the shortest possible time in the lowest effective dose, and avoiding medications during the first trimester when possible, since the teratogenic effects of most drugs are not well known. The balance of risk to benefit with respect to maternal and fetal health must be calculated. Evaluation subsequent to exposure must consider magnitude of risk. Even if a potentially toxic drug has been used inadvertently, the risk to the fetus may not be high enough to warrant more aggressive steps than earliest possible discontinuation or substitution. Most drugs, except high-molecular-weight molecules such as heparin, are not held back in an important way by the placental barrier, and equilibrate in the fetal circulation over time.

Pregnancy impacts maternal response to a drug through changes in drug absorption, transport, binding, metabolism, and excretion. The impact of these pregnancy-related changes on a specific drug needs independent consideration. For example, drugs predominantly excreted through the kidney will need an increased frequency of administration because of the pregnancy-associated increase in glomerular filtration rate.[13]

Certain common cardiac drugs have known fetal toxicity and should be avoided. Blockers of angiotensin receptors and inhibitors of angiotensin-converting enzyme cause second-trimester fetal nephrotoxicity,[126] and in addition, inhibitors of angiotensin-converting enzyme have been shown to be teratogenic.[127] Warfarin fetal toxicities are to some extent dose related[110] and must be balanced against the maternal need for the drug.

Prophylaxis against Endocarditis

There is a long history of use of prophylactic antibiotics prior to various procedures to prevent endocarditis. The evidence base for such practices has never been robust, and recommendations of guideline committees have changed over time. In consensus documents published between 2004 and 2007, recommendations have become more restrictive. The European Society of Cardiology guidelines from 2004[128] do not recommend prophylaxis for vaginal delivery or hysterectomy, and are silent on the subject of caesarean section. Guidelines from the British Society for Antimicrobial Chemotherapy from 2006[129] propose that prophylactic antibiotics be given for caesarean section or vaginal hysterectomy, but not for vaginal delivery. The guidelines from the American Heart Association/American College of Cardiology appearing in 2007[130] state that prophylaxis solely to prevent endocarditis is not recommended for any type of obstetric delivery.

Diagnostic and Therapeutic Interventions

Diagnostic testing for a woman contemplating pregnancy should optimally be completed before conception. This allows comprehensive assessment without concern about the impact of the testing procedure on the pregnancy, and also allows the application of surgical or therapeutic interventions prior to pregnancy when indicated.[31] This is not always possible. If adequate current information about the cardiac status is not available for a woman who is already pregnant, the investigations should be completed expeditiously. Echocardiography is safe. Exercise stress testing is probably safe,[131] though guidelines on how to interpret and apply results of stress testing done during pregnancy do not exist. Cardiac resonance imaging avoids ionizing radiation, and often produces information of high diagnostic quality, so should be considered, even though fetal risks have not been well characterised. The latter include the effects of heat and noise, and the theoretical effects on fetal development of the fixed and dynamic magnetic fields. Risk may be lessened by avoiding first-trimester studies if possible, by avoiding use of gadolinium contrast, by minimizing time in the coil, and by using lower magnetic energy.[132]

Ionizing radiation, as produced in X-ray and nuclear studies, exposes the fetus to the risk of teratogenesis, and to an increased risk of cancer. The majority of tests that might be contemplated, nonetheless, expose the fetus to radiation doses well below 50 mGy, and no congenital abnormalities have been reported with exposure below this threshold. Shielding should be used, though most fetal irradiation is received through scatter, and thus not prevented by shielding. The incremental lifetime risk for cancer can be calculated, but is exceedingly small. For these reasons, necessary X-ray and nuclear procedures should not be withheld solely because of pregnancy if effective alternative techniques are unavailable.[133,134]

Cardiopulmonary bypass during pregnancy is contemplated only in urgent situations, and the maternal mortality is no higher than for similar emergency procedures in the non-pregnant patient. Fetal mortality is high, in the range of one-third. There is a general belief, although weakly documented, that there has been a trend to reduced fetal mortality in recent years in centres with experience. Outcomes may be improved by applying normothermic techniques involving pulsatile bypass at high rates of flow, and by administering tocolytics preemptively. Interventional or off-pump procedures should be considered instead if feasible. Delivery of the fetus 24 or more hours prior to cardiopulmonary bypass may be preferable in late pregnancy, but prior to 32 weeks of gestation the risk of prematurity may be unacceptable to some patients in spite of the acknowledged risk of cardiopulmonary bypass while the fetus remains in the womb.[134]

The complete reference list can be found on the companion Expert Consult web site at www.expertconsult.com.

ANNOTATED REFERENCES

- Steer PJ, Gatzoulis MA, Baker P: Heart Disease and Pregnancy. London: RCOG Press, 2006.

  This text incorporates the consensus statements developed by an expert panel commissioned by the Royal College of Obstetricians and Gynaecologists of the United Kingdom in 2006, and offers an up-to-date and concentrated review of pregnancy and contraception in women with cardiac disease.

- Oakley C, Warnes C: Heart Disease in Pregnancy, 2nd ed. Malden, MA: BMJ Books/Blackwell Publishing, 2007.

  A multi-authored book, updated as of 2007, which provides an excellent general reference text.

- Siu SC, Colman JM, Sorensen S, et al: Adverse neonatal and cardiac outcomes are more common in pregnant women with cardiac disease. Circulation 2002;105:2179–2184.

  This prospective study showed that maternal cardiac disease increases the risk for adverse fetal and neonatal outcomes and that this risk is amplified by traditional obstetric risk factors. It provides a basis for risk-stratifying women with cardiac disease with respect to adverse fetal and neonatal outcomes.

- Siu SC, Sermer M, Colman JM, et al: Prospective multicenter study of pregnancy outcomes in women with heart disease. Circulation 2001;104: 515–521.

  This multi-centre prospective observational study of 599 pregnancies proposed a risk score derived from maternal characteristics evident prior to pregnancy that predicts the likelihood of adverse maternal cardiac events during pregnancy in women with heart disease. This risk score has been further validated and elaborated in subsequent studies.

- Drenthen W, Pieper PG, Roos-Hesselink JW, et al: Outcome of pregnancy in women with congenital heart disease: A literature review. J Am Coll Cardiol 2007;49:2303–2311.

  A comprehensive review of adverse outcomes of pregnancy reported in the peer-reviewed literature to date. This study examines outcomes of 2491 pregnancies, including miscarriages and elective abortions, in women with congenitally malformed hearts.

- Thorne S, MacGregor A, Nelson-Piercy C: Risks of contraception and pregnancy in heart disease. Heart 2006;92:1520–1525.

  An excellent review of the subject, offering guidelines for appropriate selection of contraception methods in women with various forms of structural cardiac disease.

- Nora JJ: From genetic studies to a multilevel genetic-environmental interaction. J Am Coll Cardiol;23:1468–1471.

  This meta-analysis reports on the rates of transmission of congenital cardiac disease in 13 previously published studies.

CHAPTER 61

Preparing the Young Adult with Complex Congenital Cardiac Disease to Transfer from Paediatric to Adult Care

GARY D. WEBB and JOHN E. DEANFIELD

Most children born with congenitally malformed hearts now survive to adult life, as a result of the spectacular achievements of paediatric cardiology and surgery over the past half-century. This has created a new and growing population of adults who often have complex congenital cardiac malformations which are unfamiliar to conventionally trained adult cardiologists. The need for an integrated strategy of care for such patients with congenitally malformed hearts, who usually require life-long medical care, has been recognised. Several panels of international experts have provided frameworks for provision of services.[1–9] These share a number of common recommendations. First, all recognise the need for management in an adult environment, as the average age of the population of adults with congenital cardiac disease increases. Second, all recommend a hierarchical structure for care, with specialist centres providing a full range of diagnostic facilities and treatments interacting, and often sharing care, with other adult cardiac units. Third, all accept the need for training of a new subspecialty of medical and allied health practitioners with expertise in the management of congenital cardiac disease and the care of adults. Despite the numerous statements expressing consensus, many adolescent patients with congenital cardiac disease still do not have the opportunity to participate in a defined process of transition that aims to optimise clinical education and social outcomes. As a result, few of these patients or their families have learnt what they need to know about their conditions and their responsibilities, and many have been lost to appropriate follow-up.[10] In this chapter, we focus on the steps required for the processes of transition, and then transfer of care, for young adults who have chronic childhood illnesses in general, and complex congenital cardiac diseases (Table 61-1) specifically. We will review important general aspects of transition, as well as the key elements for an orderly programme of transition, which include timing of transfer, location, and staffing. Attention to the provision of care at this important stage of the journey of the patient is essential to maintain the excellent standards of care that are usually provided in the paediatric age group, and to insure that patients become empowered to take over their own issues with health, becoming autonomous and competent young adults.

THE PROCESS OF TRANSITION

Transition is the generic process that applies to all children and adolescents with chronic disease.[11–13] It can be defined as an educational and experiential process that prepares patients to take responsibility for their own health care. The process takes time, and is not necessarily completed on entry to adult care. Its duration varies considerably from patient to patient, and is influenced by a number of factors, including the background, development, and intellect of the patient and the level of support provided by the family. The whole process may take several years, and is only successfully achieved when the patient is fully able to take responsibility for their own health and issues of lifestyle. It is important, therefore, that during the process, young adults with complex congenital cardiac malformations appreciate that, although they have the potential to live healthy and productive lives, most will require life-long cardiac surveillance. They also need to understand the requirement to obtain appropriately skilled care. This remains a challenge in many medical systems. During the

TABLE 61-1

MAJOR TYPES OF COMPLEX CONGENITAL CARDIAC DISEASE

Atrioventricular septal defects
Conduits
Cyanotic congenital cardiac disease
Double outlet ventricle
Ebstein's malformation
Eisenmenger's syndrome
Fontan circulation
Moderate to severe pulmonary regurgitation
Functionally single ventricle
Tetralogy of Fallot
Transposition
Common arterial trunk

process, issues both generic and disease-based need to be addressed. This has an important impact for provision of services, both in terms of location and staffing of the clinic responsible for the transition. Frequently, the coordinated transfer of care from the paediatric to the adult health care environment is the final step in a successful process of transition. This depends importantly on the relationship between the staff of the clinic responsible for transition and the patient, which should have been built up over the years. During and after this time, the nature of the relationship between doctor and patient will change.

Paediatricians tend to consult predominantly with the parents, whereas adult practitioners seek to develop a partnership with the patient. This involves directing information and education towards the patient and, at the same time, encouraging responsibility and self-reliance. It is critical that, during adolescence, in the transition clinic, this connection with the young patient is successfully achieved, so that the patients begin to understand the need for an active role in their own health and cardiac management. If this fails, adolescents and young adults may disappear from medical follow-up and return only when potentially avoidable problems have developed. In a recent review, lapse of medical care, for a median duration of 10 years, occurred during the process of transition in two-thirds of grown-up patients with congenitally malformed hearts. Those who lapsed in this way were three times more likely to require urgent cardiac intervention when next seen. It is the lack of understanding by physicians of the need for continued care into adulthood that may underlie failure of effective communication.[10]

Key Issues for the Process of Transition

When Should Patients Begin the Process of Transition and Transfer?

The timing of entry from a paediatric clinic into a service responsible for transition, and the subsequent transfer to adult clinics, will vary according to the provision of local services and the individual needs of the patient. It is important, however, that transition and transfer occur in a predictable and planned manner.[14] Referral to the clinics responsible for transition should ideally begin by 12 years of age. Attendance at such clinics involves a change in approach from the typical paediatric cardiac clinic. Parents should continue to attend, but there should be greater emphasis on communication with the adolescent, including opportunities for confidential one-on-one discussion with doctors, nurses, and other relevant counsellors. The approach to communication needs to evolve as the teenager grows older, with provision for discussion appropriate to age and maturity. Transfer from the transition clinic to the adult clinic most commonly occurs at the age of 18 years, on completion of schooling. The timing, however, should be flexible so as to meet the needs of the patient. For example, if a patient has developmental delay, or multiple medical problems under active follow-up in the paediatric hospital, transfer may need to occur at an older age.

Patients should understand that transfer to adult care is a natural process and part of growing up. Early discussion, and agreement on an age of transfer, removes the frequent anxiety of families that expert care is being lost, and makes transfer to adult care a development to be viewed optimistically. In some medical systems, provision of adult services for grown-up patients with congenitally malformed hearts is not yet available at a level comparable to that provided during childhood. In these cases, delay of transfer is clearly advisable.

Where Should Care Be Undertaken?

Availability of clinical resources will determine the location of the transition clinic. Ideally, this should be within the paediatric hospital, as this makes the first move from the paediatric clinic less traumatic to the patients and their families. Those staffing the clinic have the opportunity, during several visits over years, to organise the subsequent transfer to adult care, which may need to be to a different hospital.

Facilities for in-patient care should be designed around the needs of young people, and ideally should be separate from paediatric and adult wards, with a different atmosphere and focus. A dedicated adolescent environment for patients with a range of medical conditions can work well for the needs of cardiac patients. This permits provision of facilities, including Internet access, a study area, television, a social area, and kitchen facilities. The adolescent ward should be organised by staff with special awareness and training in the issues of this age group.

Who Should Be Involved in Transitional Care?

The balance of staffing for the transition clinic depends on local resources. It is, however, essential that members of the team providing paediatric care and of the team looking after their future needs as adults with cardiac problems are both involved. This provides an opportunity for discussion between teams of the specific medical needs of the patient, as well as creating a visible connection for the patient and their families. This, in our experience, is a key step to avoiding lapse of care and loss to follow-up when the patient is eventually transferred.

Specialist nurses play a crucial role in successful transition. They should have experience in the needs of adolescents and young adults with congenitally malformed hearts, and should have received training in counselling.[15] There should be facilities for the specialist nurses to consult with the patient separately from the doctor, as this encourages early discussion of sensitive problems and anxieties. The specialist nurses frequently are the main contact with the patient and his or her family, developing a unique relationship with them.

What Is Involved in an Ideal Transitional Programme?

The programme involves both continuation of high-level care for cardiac and non-cardiac problems as well as a specific transitional curriculum designed to prepare the adolescent and young adult for successful transfer. In many centres, a comprehensive transitional curriculum has been developed, which covers education about the cardiac condition, its impact on future life, and strategies to smooth transfer into adulthood.[16]

All children with congenitally malformed hearts should have a plan of care established prior to transfer. Ideally, this is initiated in childhood, and developed during transition. It should be based on a multi-disciplinary process of consultation, and communicated effectively to the adolescent and his or her family. A clear route of transfer to an appropriate level of adult cardiac services is an essential part of this plan. A major potential barrier to successful transition is the belief of patients and families that cardiac surgery or catheter intervention has cured their condition. Patients and families need to have explained to them, in a sensitive manner, that although in many cases life expectancy can be normal or near-normal, the patient's heart is not normal and the patient requires life-long follow-up. It is important that patients understand that, despite treatment, their cardiac condition remains fundamentally different from that of most adult patients, and that relatively few providers have been trained to monitor their care. This should be accompanied by reassurance that their care plan will involve attendance, at least once, at a specialist unit dealing with adults with congenitally malformed hearts. It is equally important at the end of transition to decide which patients do not require long-term cardiac follow-up. Our current policy is to keep patients with conditions deemed to carry low risk on the database, with very infrequent visits. The premised value of this approach is to allow support for issues of life such as employment. Regular cardiac checks of patients with a very low risk of further complications, however, may have adverse consequences. For example, repeated visits may lead to an unnecessarily high level of anxiety about future health. Indeed, there is evidence for this in other medical conditions.

The complexities of the process of transition can seem so daunting that, as a result, little or nothing is done to prepare the young patient. It is clearly important that some steps be taken and that the transition become an integral part of the journey through life of the patient with a congenitally malformed heart, rather than simply being ignored because a comprehensive process seems unachievable. One approach is to adopt a strategy of starting small and aiming to improve. For a disease-based model, some basic information should be put together about the patient and transmitted to him or her clearly and repeatedly. Such a minimalist message might resemble the following:

You have had surgical repair of tetralogy of Fallot. As a result, you have a leaky pulmonary valve. You will need to be followed annually by a cardiologist who knows about congenital cardiac defects. In order to stay healthy, you should see such a person once a year for the rest of your life. If you have any cardiac problems, you should contact this person. You should become knowledgeable about your health history. You should have a copy of your own health information. You should make sure you always have good quality health insurance, and know how to get it. You are at risk for infective endocarditis, and should be sure that your teeth and gums are always healthy to reduce this risk.

The agenda can then be broadened beyond this brief approach by regular consultations with the patient. A more complete curriculum for the transition can be communicated using different strategies, involving the cardiologist and specialist nurses. These strategies can include seminars for patients and families and information provided on paper or online. These methods are invaluable, in particular, when providing access to new information. In many ways, the educational aspects of the transition should continue indefinitely, as patients often feel a greater sense of control over their medical health and management if they are able to seek new knowledge. Close collaboration with support groups for children and adults with congenitally malformed hearts, which have been established in many countries, is invaluable for promoting education.

While the needs of some patients during adolescence are straightforward, others may require cardiac or non-cardiac medical or surgical care. Access to services, including obstetrics and gynaecology, psychiatry, nephrology, respiratory, neurology, and orthopaedics, is important, and this should be provided either within the specialist institution or within a network of linked local centres. A recent model of care developed by the Department of Health in the United Kingdom illustrates a model for primary, secondary, and tertiary provision of care for adults with congenitally malformed hearts (Fig. 61-1).[17]

The clinic providing services during transition should have access to the full range of cardiac diagnostic and treatment modalities, including echocardiography, magnetic resonance imaging, computerised tomography, specialist electrophysiology, interventional catheterisation, and surgery. Easy access to specialists in anticoagulation and, increasingly, provision of anticoagulant management in the home, are also important. As during childhood, optimal management of those with congenitally malformed hearts requires a multi-disciplinary planned approach, involving nurses, technicians, anaesthetists, intensivists, cardiologists, and surgeons. During the years of transition, pathways can be established to ensure standardisation of care and communication. The specialist nurse plays a key role in coordinating this process, including the individual medical and non-medical needs of the patient.

A co-ordinated process of transfer is often the final step in the successful transition to the adult cardiac environment. A carefully prepared summary, or passport, outlining the state of health, is a key element. It should be given to the patient, and should include information on the diagnosis, details of previous treatment, including catheter interventions and surgery, diagnostic tests, as well as current and previous follow-up and medical treatment. It should also include details of contacts for those staffing both the transition clinic and the future clinic for care as an adult with congenital cardiac disease, including a telephone number for the specialist nurse. This is important, as problems often arise between leaving the transition clinic and making the first visit to the adult clinic. The contents of the passport should be discussed with the patient, as it is essential that he or she understand the information and the value of the document. Currently, archiving of and access to important long-term medical records are less than optimal in many health care systems, and similarly communication between centres which may be involved in the care of the adolescent and young adult with congenital heart disease can be poor should the patient move around the country. These situations emphasise the need to empower the patient with understanding of his or her own health care needs as a key part of the process of transition, and to provide effective support when required.

The first visit to the adult cardiac clinic is often very stressful to the patient and his or her family. Patients should know to expect a different experience in the adult cardiac setting, with the focus shifting from the parent to the patient. The style is often perceived as more business-like and less relaxed. Transfer provides an opportunity for the patients to see themselves as young adults. The providers of paediatric services should reassure the patients that the new providers in the adult setting are capable and can be trusted. Support groups can play an important role in alleviating anxiety around this time, as well as providing additional social interaction and help with a range of issues relating to everyday life (see below).

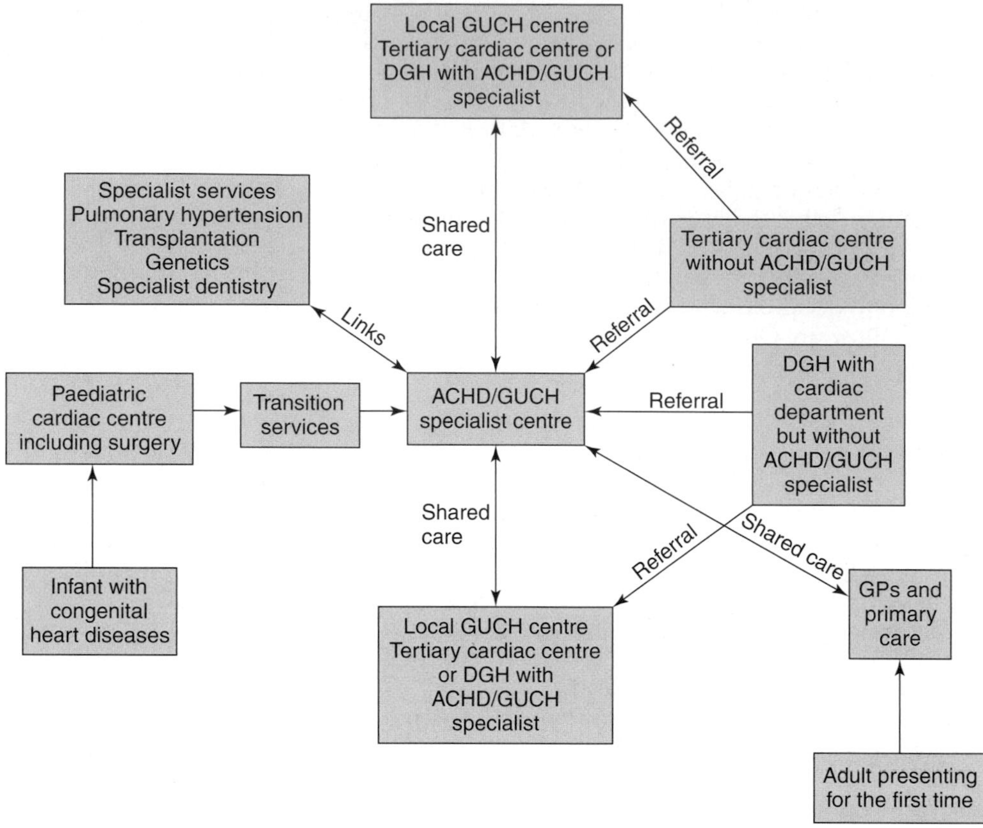

Figure 61-1 A model for transition for adults with congenitally malformed hearts. ACHD, adults with congenital cardiac disease; DGH, district general hospital; GP, general practitioner; GUCH, grown-ups with congenitally malformed hearts. (Adapted from Hudsmith LE, Thorne SA: Transition of care from paediatric to adult services in cardiology. Arch Dis Child 2007;92:927–930.)

Specific Issues during Transition

Adolescence is often the first time that the patient takes responsibility for a wide range of issues relating to medical needs and the continuation of life, and the transition should provide opportunity and sufficient time to address them with nurse specialists, physicians, and other relevant counsellors. Some of the key topics that need to be addressed on a regular basis are listed in Table 61-2.

Cardiac Issues

It is crucial for the patient to understand his or her cardiac defect and its consequences. This is rarely the case when the patient enters the transition clinic. Effective communication requires repetition, especially when patients have learning disabilities, complex cardiac conditions, or low levels of education. Protocols for cardiac care for specific conditions are invaluable to ensure consistency of management, and to explain the reasons for any proposed testing, treatment, and follow-up to the patient. Understanding by the patient of the proposed plan for health care greatly reduces anxieties about unexpected deterioration in his or her condition. Patients should be taught about potential symptoms,and the various options for management which might be required in the future. In addition to the plan for cardiac care, patients need to understand the potential risks involved in non-cardiac medical or surgical treatment. This is particularly important in those with pulmonary hypertension and cyanosis, in whom even innocuous procedures can be life-threatening. Proper planning of procedures, such as anaesthesia for dental care, should involve consultation with the cardiac team responsible for the transition, as the risks are often not appreciated by non-cardiac practitioners.[18]

Contraception

One of the most important issues that is frequently neglected by paediatric cardiologists is contraception and pregnancy. There are now more than 1 million adults living in the United States with malformed hearts, and half are women. Studies show that the cardiologist needs to take the lead in providing information relating to contraception, and the process should begin before the patient reaches adolescence or becomes sexually active. A teenager has a 90% chance of becoming pregnant within a year if sexually active and not using appropriate contraception. The range of options for contraception, with their advantages and disadvantages, should be discussed.[19] This must be conducted in a manner appropriate for the age and maturity of the patient, and needs to take place throughout the transition. It is imperative that there be private opportunities to talk with the doctor or specialist nurse in the absence of parents, and the patient should be reassured that the contents of these discussions will remain confidential.

Pregnancy

Pregnancy is increasingly feasible for many adults with congenitally malformed hearts, and the potential risks to the mother and the unborn child should ideally be discussed before conception. An unwanted pregnancy can be a major medical and psychosocial problem. It should not be the stimulus, as is sometimes the case, for precipitous transfer to adult care. Understanding the impact of pregnancy on the maternal cardiac disease, as well as the risk from her cardiac condition to the fetus, enables the adolescent or young adult to make informed decisions and plan for the future. This will involve consideration of both the

TABLE 61-2

TOPICS FOR THE CURRICULUM FOR THE PROCESS OF TRANSITION

Haemodynamic issues
Outlook
Potential symptoms
Diagnostic tools
Options for management
Issues relating to contraception and pregnancy
Options for contraceptions
Risks of pregnancy
Management of pregnancy
Infective endocarditis
Prevention
Implications, recognition, and response
Issues relating to arrhythmias
Types and implications
Diagnostic tools
Options for management
Noncardiac surgery
Location of surgery
Knowledge and skills of surgical and intensive care teams
Career and vocational planning
Issues relating to lifestyle
Marriage and family planning
Education
Employment
Life and health insurance
Behaviours at high risk
Healthy eating
Physical fitness
Exercise and hobbies
End-of-life decisions
Skills training
Communication
Assertiveness
Self-care

Adapted from Knauth A, Verstappen A, Reiss J, Webb GD: Transition and transfer from pediatric to adult care of the young adult with complex congenital heart disease. Cardiol Clin 2006;24:619–629, vi.

number and timing of pregnancies in the context of the likely future cardiac course. Links between the transition clinic and a clinic specialising in obstetrics should be established. Recent reports have shown not only the potential risks of poorly managed pregnancies but the outstanding results that can be achieved through a multi-disciplinary approach with a team that includes practitioners in congenital cardiac disease, anaesthesia, obstetrics, and fetal medicine.[19,20]

Risk of Recurrence

The risk of recurrence in the offspring of parents with congenitally malformed hearts is one of the most frequently asked questions. Understanding of the genetic basis of complex cardiac malformations is increasing exponentially, and should lead in the near future to a more refined model for prediction of risk. Average values for recurrence in the region of 2% to 4% are often quoted, but the known range is between 2% and 50%.[21] Genetic counselling should be offered to selected patients, particularly when there is a syndrome or a family history. Fetal echocardiography before 18 weeks of gestation plays an important role, often providing reassurance of normal cardiovascular structure and function throughout the remainder of the pregnancy.

Infective Endocarditis

Patients must be educated regarding the importance of dental health, good oral hygiene, and the need for regular dental check-ups. The potential risk of body piercing, acne, tattoos and insertion of intra-uterine contraceptive devices should be explained. Patients should be taught to recognise the symptoms of endocarditis, and how to access care promptly. The recent change in recommendations regarding antibiotic prophylaxis has confused and upset some patients and their families, so clear explanation is important.[22]

Issues Relating to Lifestyle

Adolescence is a time when patients are confronted with many lifestyle issues. For example, they wonder how their cardiac disease will affect their ability to obtain a job, health or life insurance, or a mortgage. Provision of support and counselling on such issues during the transition to adulthood is essential. Many children and young people with congenitally malformed hearts will be able to have any career they may choose. The future of some patients, however, will include physical or other limitations. They may need to be advised to pursue appropriate education and career pathways. For example, a patient with the Fontan circulation should know not to become a bricklayer or a commercial trucker. These patients, and their parents, should have a chance to discuss such issues before the patient reaches high-school age, and before important decisions are made, or actions taken, such as choosing a curriculum or dropping out of school. As the long-term outcome of many complex cardiac conditions becomes clearer, evidence-based recommendations can be made in regard to future careers. These will carry weight with future employers, and represent an opportunity for the clinic staff to act as advocates for their patients, who are often otherwise disadvantaged by the stigma attached to chronic cardiac disease.

Many patients will have difficulty in obtaining both health and life insurance. They may be denied coverage, or offered a heavily loaded premium based on out-of-date information relating to the risk of death. Studies have shown highly variable attitudes to coverage, and patients should be helped to obtain the best deal.[23] Support groups, such as the Grown Up Congenital Heart Disease Association in the United Kingdom (available at: http://www.guch.org.uk), have excellent links with insurance companies. In the United States, the difficulties encountered by young patients with chronic conditions in obtaining health insurance are now recognized. Opportunities vary between states, and it is hoped that legislation to provide a more uniform level of support will be enacted in the next few years.

The importance of a healthy lifestyle, including avoidance of smoking and obesity, should be emphasized. Counseling regarding the use of alcohol or recreational drugs and, in particular, the potential interaction with prescribed drugs such as anticoagulants, requires sensitive private discussion. Maintenance of a healthy lifestyle requires regular physical exercise. During childhood, inappropriate limitations are often imposed. These can have important implications for the confidence of patients, their sense of well-being, and their social interactions.[24] Objective exercise testing should be part of assessment during the process of transition. This should be used to provide recommendations based on the potential beneficial and deleterious effects of exercise on the haemodynamics of the individual patient, as well as on the risk of serious arrhythmia. Standard protocols in adult clinics, often devised for the detection of myocardial ischaemia, are usually inappropriate for adolescents and young adults with congenitally malformed hearts. Advice on travel and driving should also be provided, based on the regularly updated national guidelines.

TRAINING OF PRACTITIONERS TO PROVIDE SERVICES FOR TRANSITION

There is a clear need to develop a new group of specialists to deal with the long-term needs of patients with congenitally malformed hearts. This should include medical practitioners, specialist nurses, and allied health professionals. Recent recommendations emphasise the need for training in adult and paediatric cardiology, as well as familiarity with general medical issues. The provision of services with appropriately trained staff is developing rapidly in some countries but lagging behind in others. Such resources will affect the design and composition of the services. Any necessary compromises, however, should not distract from the need to develop programmes of high quality, which cover seamlessly the entire life course of the patient with a congenitally malformed heart.

SUMMARY

Transition of care from paediatric to adult services is a crucial period for patients with congenital cardiac disease. If managed badly, patients fail to understand their disease, its impact on their life, and the need for long-term follow-up. As a result, they frequently default from care, and their outcome is adversely affected. If managed well, patients can be empowered to graduate from the paediatric environment to take control of their own health. This ensures not only continuity of high-level cardiac treatment, but successful integration into normal adult life. All systems for health care that embark on the treatment of children with congenital cardiac disease must, therefore, undertake to provide an effective service for transition to appropriate adult care.

The complete reference list can be found on the companion Expert Consult web site at www.expertconsult.com.

ANNOTATED REFERENCES

- Celermajer DS, Deanfield JE: Employment and insurance for young adults with congenital heart disease. Br Heart J 1993;69:539–543.

  This study describes the highly variable attitudes of insurance companies and employers towards grown-up patients with congenitally malformed hearts.
- Deanfield J, Thaulow E, Warnes C, et al: Management of grown up congenital heart disease. Eur Heart J 2003;24:1035–1084.

  The most recent European taskforce document on the management of grown-up patients with congenitally malformed hearts, this review includes recommendations on delivery of service as well as brief, lesion-specific lifetime algorithms.
- Knauth A, Verstappen A, Reiss J, Webb GD: Transition and transfer from pediatric to adult care of the young adult with complex congenital heart disease. Cardiol Clin 2006;24:619–629, vi.

  This paper describes the curriculum involved in a successful programme for transition developed at a North American institution.
- Therrien J, Dore A, Gersony W, et al: CCS Consensus Conference 2001 update: Recommendations for the management of adults with congenital heart disease. 1. Can J Cardiol 2001;17:940–959.

  The first comprehensive guideline document for management of adults with congenital heart disease from the Canadian Cardiac Society.
- Thorne S, MacGregor A, Nelson-Piercy C: Risks of contraception and pregnancy in heart disease. Heart 2006;92:1520–1525.

  An excellent review on contraception and pregnancy in the setting of cardiac disease. This is a key issue that needs to be approached throughout the process of transition.
- Viner R: Bridging the gaps: Transition for young people with cancer. Eur J Cancer 2003;39:2684–2687.

  The review provides a good description of protocols for transition and transfer of care, with an emphasis on models of care.

CHAPTER 62

Psychological and Social Aspects of Paediatric Cardiac Disease

KATHLEEN MUSSATTO

What are the outcomes that really matter to patients, families, and societies living with the implications of congenital and acquired paediatric cardiac disease?

Survival and physiological function are certainly paramount. Dramatically improved survival, and reduced morbidity for virtually all lesions, nonetheless, has now shifted focus to the question of quality versus quantity of life. The patients that we follow are not hearts, they are children, incredibly complex and multi-dimensional, and they belong to families of equal complexity. Chronic illness in a child results in psychological stress, not only for the affected child but also for the parents, siblings, caregivers, and social contacts with whom that child interacts. The cumulative effects of the stress of paediatric cardiac disease may impact psychosocial function and quality of life for the child, parents, siblings, and the family as a whole. The process of adjustment to this stress is a complicated, multi-factorial, process that involves an interaction of both risk and resistance factors and, above all, a highly subjective, personal interpretation of the impact of disease on one's life.

In general, children and families are incredibly resilient. They respond to the challenges of chronic disease with a process of adjustment and adaptation that most commonly results in successful normalisation and integration into society. When this process does not occur successfully, a host of problems can result, including psychopathology, reduced quality of life, family disruption, and social discrimination.[1–5] Providers of healthcare to children with paediatric cardiac disease, as well as other social contacts such as teachers, social workers, and play therapists, are in a unique position to assess and intervene with the intention of optimising the adaptation of the child and the family.

Today, the vast majority of congenital cardiac conditions are diagnosed in infancy, and the majority of surgical reconstructive procedures are conducted during the first year of life.[6–9] It is well recognised that only a small minority of congenital cardiac conditions are completely cured despite anatomical repair. In the majority of patients, particularly those with complex lesions, the cardiac malformation results in a chronic condition that requires ongoing medical observation and care. In contrast, acquired paediatric cardiac disease in a previously healthy child can be diagnosed at any age. Although treatment in some situations may afford a complete recovery without cardiac sequels, some conditions, for example cardiomyopathy requiring cardiac transplantation, result in a chronic condition necessitating life-long care. Some postulate that a congenital condition may result in more effective adaptation because the child knows no other existence.[10,11] Other research has not supported this. For example, Varni and Setoguchi[12] found no difference in adjustment for children with congenital versus acquired deficiencies of the limbs. Congenital cardiac disease commonly includes long periods of time during which the child may be relatively asymptomatic. Hence, the child may not be afforded the benefit of adjustment that may occur with a more visible or persistent disorder. The nature of the heart as an organ vital to survival may result in perceptions of stress related to cardiac disease that are out of proportion to the severity of the diagnosis.[13,14] Psychosocial outcomes are inherently subjective in nature. The perspective of the child, the family, and the implications for society must all be considered individually, whilst recognising that significant interactions likely influence the interpretation of the psychosocial impact of cardiac disease in a child.

THE PATIENT

A Developmental Approach to the Psychological Stress of Paediatric Cardiac Disease and Its Treatment

The stress associated with the diagnosis and treatment of congenital or acquired paediatric cardiac disease will vary both with the trajectory of the illness and the natural developmental progression of the child. Chronic illnesses are characterised by relatively stable periods that may be interrupted by acute episodes requiring medical attention or intervention. Thus, there is a risk for both chronic psychological stress and acute crises. The particular stressors and responses of a child receiving care for cardiac disease must be interpreted within the context of the developmental stage. It is well known that children with cardiac disease are at risk for a wide range of cognitive and neurodevelopmental impairments (see Chapter 64). Thus, they may not exhibit age-appropriate responses. Interventions to reduce stress must be targeted to the level of the specific developmental maturity of the child.

It is difficult to assess the psychological stress experienced by sick neonates and young infants. The setting of intensive care required for treatment of these babies is clearly an environment that is alien to the experience of a healthy infant. Hospitalisation and surgery rob an infant of many of the normal stimuli known to foster optimal growth and development, including the physiological protection offered by parents, normal touch and neurological stimulation, and basic satisfaction of needs, for instance feeding and nurturance.[15] In addition, intensive care imposes several noxious stimuli not typically experienced so early in development, including painful interventions, excessive noise and light, sedation, and presence of multiple caregivers. Miranda and colleagues[16–18] have demonstrated that infant rats exposed to repeated painful stimuli demonstrated altered behaviour and visceral hyperalgesia when becoming adults. Of equal concern, however, is evidence that anaesthetic agents commonly used to protect infants from pain during surgery, such as ketamine, isoflurane, and nitrous oxide, may also have a negative impact on neonatal cerebral development.[19–22] It can be concluded that hospitalisation early in life results in an environment that makes the infant vulnerable to disruptions in normal neurobehavioural development, and disturbances of physiological stability. A model for developmental care has been advocated in most neonatal and infant intensive care settings to reduce the inherent risks of hospitalisation. This model promotes minimal handling, reduction of noise and light, support of natural positioning, and individualised care planning with a family centred approach. These interventions have been shown to improve short-term physiological stability. Research on the impact on long-term outcomes, nonetheless, remains inconclusive, and interpretation is problematic due to the presence of multiple confounding variables.[15,23]

In later infancy, babies become increasingly aware of their environment. Hospitalisation at this stage may impart stress due to the anxiety of separation, and the interruption of normal comforting behaviours, such as feeding, cuddling, and non-nutritive sucking. Sedation and physical restraints are often used to prevent an infant from causing harm to themselves during recovery. As the infant is allowed to become fully conscious, immobility and separation from the comforting behaviours of parents may be particularly distressing. An infant may progress through stages in response to separation from their normal environment. Initially there is protest, manifested by excessive irritability and crying. Then there is despair. The crying may stop, but the infant appears despondent and withdrawn, and there may be loss of previously acquired developmental skills. Ultimately, there is detachment. Parental return may be met with apathy, the infant appearing more absorbed with objects and the immediate environment.[24] A shift toward allowing unlimited parental presence in most settings providing healthcare for children has helped to diminish, but cannot eliminate, this stress. Children experiencing prolonged hospitalisations are at increased risk for negative responses. Promoting a home-like environment with family photos and familiar objects may reduce the disruptive effects of hospitalisation.

The toddler and preschool-aged child continue to be extremely sensitive to separation from parents and intrusions by strangers. Painful procedures are met with vehement protests, and the child may be confused by the inability of the parents to rescue them from what seems a treacherous environment.[24] Memories are beginning to be formed, and the young child may associate certain people or places with distress, causing reactions even before anything bad has happened. Refusal to eat or take medications, or excessive combativeness, may reflect the attempt of the young child to regain control of his or her environment. Fear of bodily injury is common in those who have yet to commence schooling. It may be impossible for them to conceptualise that something can allegedly be cured by cutting it open. Illness or hospitalisation may be perceived as punishment for something they have done wrong. At this age, play and exploration are used to help children master their environment and gain autonomy. Opportunities for medical play and socialisation while hospitalised may help to decrease fear and anxiety. Safe places, such as play rooms, must be established in the hospital where the child does not have to fear procedures. Young children often understand far more than they are able to express. The need to prepare them for procedures or experiences should not be underestimated.[24] Specialists in the life of the child, and play therapists, can provide guidance for strategies of preparation that are developmentally appropriate.

The young child beginning school, aged from 6 to 12 years, possesses an immature but developing understanding of his or her body and how it works. The function of the heart as a vital organ is understood by most young children, and the concept of a disease of the heart requiring intervention may be particularly upsetting. Hospitalisation and surgery at this time may invoke fears of bodily injury and death. Children perceive their parents to be their ultimate protectors, and may be frustrated by the inability of their parents to shield them from what they interpret as dangerous invasions of their body. Activities that promote healthy skills for coping, and expression of feelings, will benefit these children. In addition, whenever possible, children at these ages should be allowed to participate in some aspect of decision-making regarding their care, for instance to have a chest tube removed in a procedure room or at their bedside. This may help to provide them with a sense of mastery and control. Many hospitals for children offer classroom experiences, or tutoring at the bedside, to help those hospitalised maintain their academic progress, and to promote normalcy.

In a sample of 182 subjects that had undergone surgery for congenital cardiac disease early in life, and ranging in age from 2 to 18 years at time of survey, parents of children aged 8 to 12 years reported the lowest quality of life on overall, physical, emotional, social, and educational domains.[25] Children aged 8 to 11 with congenital cardiac disease were also found to report lower quality of life and emotional functioning than their counterparts aged 12 to 16.[26] It may not be until the children reach the age of 8 to 10 years that they can conceptualise their own mortality and risk of vulnerability in relation to issues devolving on health.[24] For patients with several forms of congenital cardiac disease, particularly those that require valvar replacement, this age range can be a common time for reintervention. The child may perceive procedures considered to be relatively minor and requiring a short hospital stay as a crisis.[27] Children of these ages are also more sensitive to the levels of anxiety in their parents. The level of distress manifested by their parents, therefore, may influence their own responses.[24]

Adolescents are striving to establish their identity and independence. Restrictions of activity, distorted body image or self-concept, altered peer relationships, the unpredictability of care and treatment for their condition, and uncertainty about prognosis may all serve as threats to these developmental achievements.[28] Denial of the underlying condition and its implications may be a common method of coping, and may manifest itself in poor adherence to recommendations for treatment, or a general lack of knowledge regarding risks and factors promoting health. The natural history of congenital cardiac disease typically consists of periods when the individual is clinically stable, and times that require significant intervention, such as cardiac surgery, to preserve or improve health. The adolescent with stable cardiac disease may view him or herself as well, and may experience the need for treatment as an unwelcome threat to their ability to control their lives and a bitter reminder that their condition is indeed chronic. Dilemmas of normality, social integration, independence, and the development of effective strategies for coping have all been identified as challenges facing adolescents with congenital cardiac disease.[29] Adolescents with a more positive attitude toward their illness have been found to demonstrate lower levels of anxiety and depression.[30] Support from their peers is vital to adolescents. Visitation by friends, and appropriate activities such as access to computers and video games, may lessen the strain of hospitalisation. The Starlight Starbright Children's Foundation is an Internet-based network designed to provide children with chronic illnesses a method to connect with peers facing similar challenges.[31] Issues of privacy and confidentiality are also of great importance. The healthcare team needs to work creatively with parents and children to promote autonomy and participation in planning of treatment through effective programming of adolescent care.

Be they infants, children, or adolescents being treated for paediatric cardiac disease, therefore, all experience stressors related to treatment and hospitalisation. There is great potential to ameliorate this stress with sensitivity to the developmentally appropriate challenges and responses. Developmental aspects of chronic illness and possible supportive interventions are listed in Table 62-1.[32] Explanations of the illness, and necessary care, must be made in a way that the child can easily comprehend. These explanations must be revisited frequently as the child matures.[14] Creation of a nurturing environment specifically designed for children and families, and promoting practices of care centred on the family, should be a goal for all providers of healthcare for children.

Psychological and Behavioural Outcomes for Children with Cardiac Disease

Patterson and Geber[33] stated that 'Children with chronic illnesses or disabilities are normal children in abnormal situations. They have the same developmental needs as all children. But in many different ways, the accomplishment of their developmental tasks is made more difficult by an extra set of demands and hardships associated with the chronic condition'.

The potential for chronic illness in a child to result in abnormal psychological and behavioural outcomes has long been recognised. Emotional disturbances are estimated to be 2 to 2.5 times more common in children with chronic illness than in healthy children.[34] Psychological adjustment of a child to a chronic illness such as cardiac disease is a complex process that is quite difficult to measure and interpret. Multiple factors will influence adjustment, including aspects of the illness and its treatment, characteristics of the child, and factors relating to the parents and family.[3,35,36] A large body of research in children with chronic illnesses in general, and paediatric cardiac disease specifically, has been conducted in an attempt to characterise the long-term psychological and behavioural implications of this experience.[3,35–39]

Coincident with the improved survival of children with congenital cardiac disease in the 1960s and 1970s, it was quickly recognised that these children were at risk for a negative psychological impact.[40–43] Although extensive research has been conducted in this area, findings have been disconcertingly inconsistent, making interpretation quite challenging. The strategy used for sampling, the criterions for inclusion and exclusion, the informant utilised, and the outcomes measured, all bear influence on the generalisability of the findings. A universally agreed upon definition of psychological and behavioural outcomes does not exist. Hence, several different criterions have been used to characterise children with cardiac disease and other chronic illnesses as having normal or abnormal outcomes.[35,36,39] Very few studies have systematically assessed all of these components simultaneously. Assessment of long-term outcomes is needed. There is little agreement in the paediatric literature, however, as to when long-term starts or finishes. Outcomes have been measured in children as young as toddlers to those of adults living with congenital cardiac conditions. The impact of confounding variables on psychological and behavioural outcomes is likely to increase with age. Continual shifts in care-giving practices, and changes in biomedical technology, also impact the interpretability of the findings. The children of today benefit from an armamentarium of strategies designed to impart neuropsychological protection during care for cardiac disease. Findings based on investigation of older survivors may not be representative of outcomes for a newborn today. There is also a much broader awareness and attention to these issues in children with chronic illness in general. This will hopefully result in early recognition and intervention for problems whose course can potentially be reversed.

The most widely used measure of psychological and behavioural outcomes has been the Child Behaviour Checklist.[44] An estimate of overall emotional and behavioural problems is calculated from a report on items relating to both competence and problems. The score can be further categorised to reflect the degree of internalising problems, for example, anxiety, depression, and social withdrawal, as opposed to externalising problems such as hyperactivity, inattention, and aggression. There are four versions of the instrument available to allow for responses from the parent, via the Child Behaviour Checklist, from the patient, using the Youth or Young-Adult Self-Report, or from the teacher, using the Teacher's Report Form. The measure has been widely used in samples of both healthy and chronically ill children, and has excellent psychometric properties. Caution has been advised, however, in using the Checklist in children with a chronic illness.[45] Skills for social function may be underestimated because of the reliance on social activities as a measure of competence. Symptoms of a somatic nature may be overly emphasised

TABLE 62-1

DEVELOPMENTAL ASPECTS OF CHRONIC ILLNESS OR DISABILITY IN CHILDREN

Developmental Tasks	Potential Effects of Chronic Illness or Disability	Supportive Interventions
Infancy		
Develop a sense of trust	Multiple caregivers and frequent separations, especially if hospitalised	Encourage consistent caregivers in hospital or other care settings
Attach to parent	Deprived of consistent nurturing	Encourage parents to visit frequently or room-in during hospitalisation, and to participate in care
Learn through sensorimotor experiences	Delayed because of separation, parental grief for loss of dream child, parental inability to accept the condition, especially a visible defect	Emphasise healthy, perfect qualities of infant
Begin to develop a sense of separateness from parent	Increased exposure to more painful experiences than pleasurable ones	Help parents learn special care needs of infant to enable them to feel competent
	Limited contact with environment from restricted movement or confinement	Expose infant to pleasurable experiences through all senses (touch, hearing, sight, taste, movement)
	Increased dependency on parent for care	Encourage age-appropriate developmental skills (e.g. holding bottle, finger feeding, crawling)
	Over-involvement of parent in care	Encourage all family members to participate in care to prevent over-involvement of one member
		Encourage periodic respite from demands of care responsibilities
Toddlerhood		
Develop autonomy	Increased dependency on parent	Encourage independence in as many areas as possible (e.g. toileting, dressing, feeding)
Master locomotor and language skills	Limited opportunity to test own abilities and limits	Provide gross motor skill activity and modification of toys or equipment, such as modified swing or rocking horse
Learn through sensorimotor experience, beginning preoperational thought	Increased exposure to painful experiences	Give choices to allow simple feeling of control (e.g. choice of what book to look at or what kind of sandwich to eat)
		Institute age-appropriate discipline and limit-setting
		Recognise that negative and ritualistic behaviors are normal
		Provide pleasurable sensory experiences (e.g. water play, sandbox, finger paint)
Preschool		
Develop initiative and purpose	Limited opportunities for success in accomplishing simple tasks or mastering self-care skills	Encourage mastery of self-help skills
Master self-care skills	Limited opportunities for socialisation with peers; may appear like a baby to age-mates	Provide devices that make tasks easier (e.g., self-dressing)
Begin to develop peer relationships	Protection within tolerant and secure family may cause child to fear criticism and withdraw	Encourage socialisation, such as inviting friends to play, day care experiences, trips to park
Develop sense of body image and sexual identification	Awareness of body may center on pain, anxiety, and failure	Provide age-appropriate play, especially associative play opportunities
Learn through pre-operational thought (magical thinking)	Sex role identification focused primarily on mothering skills	Emphasise child's abilities; dress appropriately to enhance desirable appearance
	Guilt (thinking he or she caused the illness or disability, or is being punished for wrong-doing)	Encourage relationships with same-sex and opposite-sex peers and adults
		Help child deal with criticisms; realise that too much protection prevents child from learning realities of world
		Clarify that cause of child's illness or disability is not his or her fault or a punishment

School Age		
Develop a sense of accomplishment Form peer relationships Learn through concrete operations	Limited opportunities to achieve and compete (e.g., many school absences or inability to join regular athletic activities) Limited opportunities for socialisation Incomplete comprehension of the imposed physical limitations or treatment of the disorder	Encourage school attendance; schedule medical visits at times other than school; encourage child to make up missed work Educate teachers and classmates about child's condition, abilities and special needs Encourage sports activities (e.g., Special Olympics) Encourage socialisation (e.g., Girl Scouts, Campfire, Boy Scouts, 4-H Clubs, having a best friend or a club) Provide child with knowledge about his or her condition Encourage creative activities (e.g., VSA arts)
Adolescence		
Develop personal and sexual identity Achieve independence from family Form heterosexual relationships Learn through abstract thinking	Increased sense of feeling different from peers and less able to compete with peers in appearance, abilities, special skills Increased dependency on family; limited job or career opportunities Limited opportunities for heterosexual friendships; fewer opportunities to discuss sexual concerns with peers Increased concern with issues such as why he or she got the disorder, whether he or she can marry and have a family Decreased opportunity for earlier stages of cognition may impede achieving level of abstract thinking	Realise that many of the difficulties the teenager is experiencing are part of the normal adolescence (rebelliousness, risk taking, lack of cooperation, hostility toward authority) Provide instruction on interpersonal and coping skills Encourage socialisation with peers, including peers with special needs and those without special needs Provide instruction on decision-making, assertiveness, and other skills necessary to manage personal plans Encourage increased responsibility for care and management of the disease or condition, such as assuming responsibility for making and keeping appointments (ideally alone), sharing assessment and planning stages of healthcare delivery, and contacting resources Encourage activities appropriate for age, such as attending mixed-gender parties, sports activities, driving a car Be alert to cues that signal readiness for information regarding implications of condition on sexuality and reproduction Emphasise good appearance and wearing stylish clothes, use of makeup Understand that adolescent has same sexual needs and concerns as any other teenager Discuss planning for the future and how condition can affect choices

From Whaley and Wong's Nursing Care of Infants and Children, Sixth Edition (pp. 1006–1007), by D. Wong, M. Hockenberry-Eaton, D. Wilson, M. Winkelstein, and E. Ahmann, 1999, St. Louis, MO: Mosby. Reprinted with permission.

in children that have symptoms related to their condition. The instrument may lack the sensitivity to detect mild problems with adjustment.[45] Methodological issues, therefore, must be considered when interpreting findings using these instruments. Other indicators of psychopathology used in research in paediatric cardiac disease have included diagnostic criterions for psychiatric disorders, and measures of anxiety, depression, self-concept, and general psychosocial functioning.

Sample characteristics, variables assessed, and measures utilised have varied widely in studies of children with cardiac disease. Consequently, findings have been highly variable. Despite this, several important themes have emerged that warrant attention. Some well-designed studies with fairly large samples have revealed virtually no or very small differences in psychosocial function in subjects treated for paediatric cardiac disease compared to normative values or healthy controls.[46–48] Multiple studies, in contrast, have identified a higher than expected incidence of behavioural problems in children with cardiac disease.[49–59] Internalising problems, in particular, social withdrawal, anxiety, and somatic complaints, and externalising problems, most commonly, attention deficits and hyperactivity, have both been reported. The impact of severity has been inconsistent, with some studies reporting more problems in children with more severe cardiac disease,[47,52,55,58–61] and others demonstrating little to no effect of severity.[39,46,48–50,62] In general, it has been found that factors relating to the specific disease have lower correlations with adjustment than do the characteristics of the child or the parent and family themselves.[35] Some authors have speculated that factors related to the underlying diagnosis contribute to a cumulative risk that moderates the relationship between the stress experienced by a child and their ultimate level of adjustment.[35,36,47,63]

General deficits in psychosocial functioning in children with cardiac disease have been identified. Psychiatric disorders such as anxiety and depression were present in just over one-quarter of a sample awaiting transplantation or cardiac surgery. The prevalence of disorders decreased in those undergoing conventional cardiac surgery postoperatively, but persisted in those undergoing transplantation.[64,65] A higher rate of psychiatric problems was found in children with severe cardiac disease compared to those with repaired atrial septal defects, the effects on psychological functioning considered moderated by both physical capacity and family difficulties.[60] Similarly, children at approximately 6 years of age were found to have more problems than healthy controls, albeit that the differences disappeared when taking account of the effects of intelligence and neurological impairment.[66] Concomitant conditions, including behaviour, learning, anxiety, attention problems, and depression were also shown to contribute to a score for psychosocial function that was significantly lower than population norms, with lower familial socioeconomic state also having a negative impact on psychosocial outcomes.[67]

Temperament or general life view may impact on psychosocial adjustment. Anxiety, and medical fears, in the child have been found to be closely related to maternal anxiety and behavioural problems.[61,68] High trait anxiety has been shown to contribute to biases in the perception of stress-induced cardiac symptoms in those treated for congenital cardiac conditions.[69] Altered self-concept has also been reported in children with cardiac disease.[70–73] Children with congenital cardiac disease rated themselves as weaker, more frightened, and more ill than a comparison of healthy controls. These differences disappeared, however, when assessed 1 year after surgery.[73] Physical self-concept was lower in children with cardiac disease than healthy controls, albeit that family, school, appearance, emotional and general self-concept did not differ from controls.[72] A lower self-concept was found in male adolescents with cardiac disease that was speculated to be directly related to diminished physical capacity. On a more positive note, adolescents with cardiac disease were found to have less anxiety, and a higher sense of self-control, than healthy controls, reflecting the development of positive skills for coping with the challenges of their condition.[70]

Meta-analytic techniques[39] have revealed that only older patients, with a mean age of greater than 10 years, demonstrate more total, internalising, and to a lesser extent, externalising behavioural problems, with severity of the disease not related to the behavioural problems. The problems demonstrated are more likely related to a cumulative experience of life, with both risk and protective factors related only in part to the cardiac disease. Longitudinal studies in children with cardiac disease are needed to illuminate further the contributions of important variables, such as self-perception, social experiences, parenting style, and collective life stress on psychological and behavioural outcomes.

Quality of Life

Quality of life has been frequently cited as an important measure of outcome for children living with paediatric cardiac disease.[74–77] Despite this, it remains poorly conceptualised in the literature. Lack of a uniform definition for quality of life, and inconsistent strategies of measurement, have resulted in problematic methodological issues for many studies purporting to address this concept. Moons and colleagues[78] reviewed 70 studies relating to paediatric cardiac disease published between January 1980 and October 2003 which discussed quality of life as an outcome. They evaluated the studies using 10 previously published criterions to evaluate validity and methodological rigour in the assessment of quality of life.[79] Overall, the findings revealed a collection of work that was inconclusive, difficult to interpret, and not generalisable to the population of patients with paediatric cardiac disease. Of the articles, one-quarter presented conclusions about quality of life, but did not explicitly measure it. More than two-fifths discussed quality of life in their abstract or discussion sections, but did not account for its measurement in the methods or results sections. Only one study provided a conceptual definition of quality of life that served as a basis for the investigation. On the whole, just over half of the manuscripts reviewed did not meet any of the 10 criterions evaluated, and only 2 had a summary score of 50 or higher out of a possible 100.

An evaluation of the variables or measurements used to assess quality of life for a patient with paediatric cardiac disease is a critical starting point when attempting to interpret the extant literature. Traditionally, researchers have focused on objective measures as indicators of quality of life. These have included functional state, general health, severity of disease, exercise tolerance, categorisation with the system devised by the New York Heart Association,[80] socioeconomic level, state of employment, educational level, size of support network, marital state, and number of offspring, among others. Clinical variables, such as the need for reoperation, number of hospitalisations, life expectancy, and need for chronic medication, have also been used as proxy indicators of quality of life.[81–88] Although each of these variables may have an influence on quality of life, alone they are not an adequate substitution for a more comprehensive measurement. None of the variables used as proxies for quality of life has been shown to have a reproducible predictive relationship. Physical functional state has been the most significant predictor of quality of life, whereas severity of illness has been repeatedly shown to have only a minor association with self or parent-reported outcomes.[25,89,90]

It is currently thought that quality of life is primarily determined by subjective mechanisms and interpretations, such as attitudes, perceptions, aspirations, and the personal degree of importance assigned to various domains of life.[91,92] In general, it is agreed that quality of life is multidimensional in nature and represents a global assessment of several core domains including physical, emotional, social, spiritual, and achievement, the latter measured both educationally or occupationally.[92–95] Using these criterions, quality of life has been defined as 'the subjective and personally derived assessment of overall well-being that results from evaluation of satisfaction across an aggregate of personally or clinically important domains'.[92] Hence, the personal and subjective analysis of the individual regarding his or her situation is the primary force guiding the perception of quality of life, not the objectively measured criterion. For this reason, some have argued that quality of life cannot be quantitatively measured and that assessment must also capture a qualitative evaluation of the importance of functional outcomes to the individual.[67,87,96] In children, however, it is difficult to obtain a subjective assessment of the importance of various domains from the children themselves. They may be too young or too ill to respond directly. They may lack the conceptual maturity to comprehend the value of varying levels of function. Their present-focused attention may limit their ability to conceive of the long-term implications of different functional states.[95] For this reason, parents are the most commonly employed proxy reporters for the quality of life of their children. Teachers and other providers of healthcare have also been used. Use of alternative respondents, although necessary at times, has significant drawbacks. Objective observers such as parents tend to report more visible aspects of behaviour and functioning. Child self-reports may identify more internal experiences and symptoms. In addition, self-assessment of functioning may be different from that perceived by the parent or other observer.[95] Despite these limitations, several well-validated instruments exist to measure functional state in the various domains known to be directly related to quality of life. Both generic and disease-specific measures exist that allow conclusions to be drawn regarding quality of life in physical and psychosocial realms.[97,98]

Since the call of Moons and colleagues[78] for increased methodological rigour in the assessment of quality of life in subjects with paediatric cardiac disease, several studies have emerged that have systematically pursued a greater understanding of this important outcome. In a sample of 321 attendees of a paediatric cardiac clinic representing a mix of diagnostic backgrounds, parents completed the Child Health Questionnaire[99] and reported overall physical and psychosocial quality of life to be similar to a normative sample. Better outcomes for the children with cardiac disease were reported for the subscales self-esteem, family cohesion, and bodily pain/discomfort, but worse outcomes were demonstrated with respect to physical functioning, general health perceptions, family activities, and parental impact—emotional. The greatest impact on physical quality of life was noted in those with the greatest functional limitations, namely children with cardiomyopathy and those requiring major interventions.[100] Parent-report of quality of life for children with paediatric cardiac disease was found to be significantly lower than a healthy normative sample for overall, physical, emotional, social, and school function in two studies with large samples using the generic module of Pediatric Quality of Life Inventory.[25,94] Child self-reports were similar to those of parents. Children, nonetheless, rated their physical function better than did their parents.[94] The instrument was able to distinguish between levels of severity in those subjects who had undergone multiple cardiac operations, with those having functionally univentricular or complex biventricular anatomy reporting lower quality of life than those who had undergone a single reparative surgery, namely the arterial switch procedure.[25] Parents identified anxiety relative to treatment and cognitive problems as the most concerning disease-specific areas of function.[94] In children with functionally univentricular anatomy, quality of life has been reported to be lower than healthy controls, particularly in the areas of social and emotional function, behaviour, and cognition.[67,101,102] In contrast, assessments of patients after repair of transposed arterial trunks have demonstrated quality of life to be essentially equivalent to the general population.[81,103]

Quality of life, therefore, is an important assessment of outcome for children with paediatric cardiac disease, but it presents many challenges for measurement. If perceptions of quality of life are to be used to guide counselling for families, it is crucial for research to utilise sound methods to assess this outcome. Strategies to incorporate the level of importance assigned by the child and family to various areas of function must continue to be developed. Providers of healthcare must suspend their assumptions regarding the impact of state of health on overall quality of life, and seek the subjective interpretation of the individual. It must be recognised that overall adjustment and well-being are determined by complex relationships between multiple factors relating to the child, the family, and the illness that may impart either risk or resistance.[1,35,36,104] Ideally, assessment of quality of life in children with paediatric cardiac disease will become a routine part of clinical follow-up, and ultimately will serve as a guide for clinical decision-making.

THE FAMILY

Adjustment and Adaptation

Paediatric cardiac disease results in distress not only for the affected child, but also for the entire family network of which that child is a part. Individual family members, including mothers, fathers, and siblings, as well as the family unit as a whole, are required to adapt to the complex challenges of chronic illness, and each will likely follow their own trajectory of adjustment.[105] Similar to the responses of individual children, the response of the family to the diagnosis and management of chronic illness in a child is a complex and multi-faceted process.[1,2,5,104,106,107] Overwhelmingly, families demonstrate incredible resilience, and ultimately most will successfully adapt to the challenges of the condition.[5,107] When this does not occur, poor adaptation may be manifested by excessive stress, psychological illness, negative impact on quality of life for the child or family members, and negative impact on the overall adjustment of the affected child.[1,3,35,36,108,109]

Specific phases of a chronic condition such as paediatric cardiac disease will present unique challenges to families. The time of diagnosis, exacerbation of symptoms, need for intervention, or even routine clinical follow-up may each present as critical times requiring response from the family.[107,110] Additionally, the routine progression through normal developmental stages for the affected child may cause the family to view the illness within a new context. Specifically, entering school, adolescence, and successful transition to adulthood may be times when the family must reassess their appraisal of the impact of the cardiac disease on the ability of the child to function.[111,112] Family units and individual members typically move in and out of stages of adjustment that range from helpless floundering to developing expertise, and ultimately to successful normalisation and incorporation of illness-management strategies into their everyday lives.[106] Several child, family, and illness-related characteristics will influence the perception by the family of stress, abilities to cope, and their eventual adaptation. A model proposed to account for these factors is presented in Figure 62-1.[5,113–115]

The appraisal of the stress of chronic illness in a child, or its perceived threat to integrity and ability to function, is a significant factor in determining response.[2,5,106–108,116] Illness-related variables to consider include age of onset, severity and prognosis of the disease, predictability of symptoms, the type and degree of limitations, and the effectiveness and consequences of treatment.[2,5,106,107] The uncertainty regarding long-term outcomes for several forms of paediatric cardiac disease may pose additional stress for families.[74,117] Age, gender, developmental stage, and ability of the child to comprehend the condition and treatment will also influence the interpretation of these illness-related factors.[1,2,35] Prior experience with stress may have a positive or negative influence on adaptation. Previous success with managing stress in particular, previous health-related challenges, may provide a family with a sense of mastery and practiced skills for coping with new situations. It is recognised that families typically experience a pile-up of various types of stress related to both normal and unexpected transitions. For the family dealing with an excessive burden of stress, the addition of a child with a complex cardiac disease could overwhelm their resources to cope.[2,107] Individual levels of anxiety at baseline, and in response to stressful situations, are likely to influence how the impact of cardiac disease is perceived.[118] The developmental stage of the family accounts for the evolution of families over time as they are exposed to a variety of life events. Child-rearing families are challenged with developing a family identity that is both flexible and stable.[119,120] Flexibility is needed to incorporate changes and face stress, allowing the family to evolve to a new level of functioning. Stability defines the ability of the family to maintain its identity, and re-establish equilibrium, despite the need for ongoing adaptation. Maturity in families promotes higher levels of organisation, and thereby improves flexibility and stability.[119] First-time parents facing the diagnosis of paediatric cardiac disease may lack the skills necessary to differentiate between normal behaviour or symptoms of their infant and those that are a result of the underlying condition.[121–123] They may also lack an established style of parenting that promotes optimal development of the child.[58]

The ability to cope with the stress perceived to be associated with the diagnosis of cardiac disease in a child will be influenced by characteristics inherent to the family, and aspects of the socio-cultural network in which that family exists. Demographic variables, such as socioeconomic state, structure and size of the family, and culture will exert an

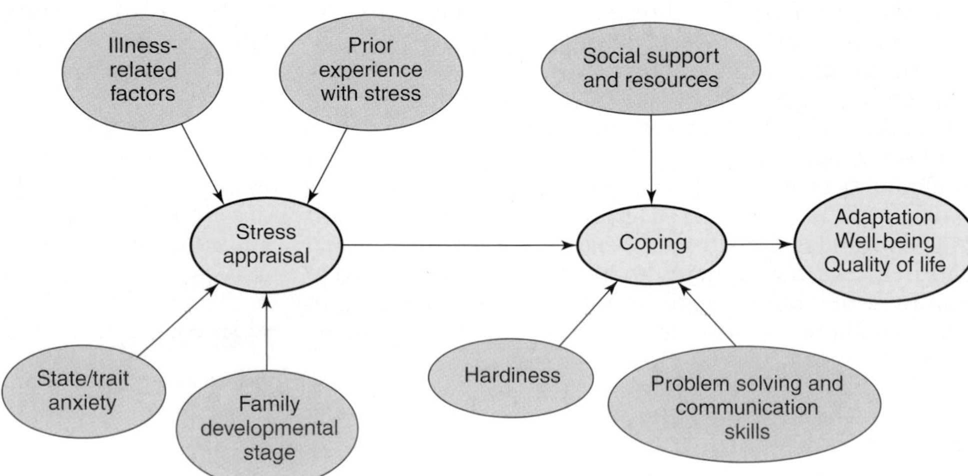

Figure 62-1 Adaptation by the family to cardiac disease in a child. (Adapted from McCubbin, Thompson, and McCubbin, 1996; Leske, 2000; Leske, 2003{{1335 McCubbin, Hamilton I. 1996;701 Leske, J.S. 2000; 700 Leske, J.S. 2003; }} Cardiol Young 2006;16(suppl 3):110–116, with permission.)

influence on adaptation in addition to social and community support networks on which the family can rely. Characteristics unique to the individual family, such as their established patterns of functioning, their skills for solving problems and communication, and their innate degree of hardiness or resiliency, will also guide their process of adaptation.[1,2,5,35,107] Both what the family has, their strengths and resources, and what the family does, their behaviours for coping, will influence their potential for successful adaptation. The degree of social support perceived by the family is an important illustration. It is not merely the presence of a strong social network that is beneficial, but the perception that this network effectively meets specific needs, which may be for emotional, self-esteem, or practical family support.[4,5] Maternal perceptions of the implications of cardiac disease in a child, whether warranted or not, have proven to be more significant predictors of child and family adjustment than the medical severity of the condition.[108,116,124,125] Helping families to achieve realistic perspectives through education and guidance regarding expectations for their children with cardiac disease may have important implications for improving adjustment in children and families.

Effects on Parenting

From the moment of diagnosis, parents of children with cardiac disease are thrust into a world that requires them to adjust expectations dramatically, gather information, and make decisions in an area in which the great majority of them are exceedingly unfamiliar. Parents experience a vast array of emotions during their early adjustment to the diagnosis of cardiac disease in a child. These may include denial or disbelief, intense helplessness over their inability to prevent the condition and protect the child from harm, guilt over their role in causing or failing to recognise the disease, dismay and dread at witnessing pain and suffering, fear that the child will die, and anxiety about the uncertainty of what the child and family will endure in the future.[126,127] Persistent symptoms of post-traumatic stress disorder have been identified in parents of children diagnosed with life-threatening conditions.[128–130] Higher trait anxiety, smaller social networks, and greater perceived intensity of treatment and threat to the life of the child were identified as risk factors for post-traumatic stress disorder in parents of children with childhood cancer.[130] While this phenomenon has not been extensively explored in parents of children with cardiac disease, it is clear that their experiences would put them at risk for extreme distress. Recently, moderate to severe symptoms of post-traumatic stress disorder were found in nearly two-fifths of parents sampled at a median time of 2½ years after cardiac transplantation.[131]

Providers of healthcare must be extremely sensitive to the needs of parents during this critical time. The antenatal diagnosis of cardiac disease results in a uniquely sensitive and challenging situation. Individual parents will have different approaches to decision-making that are influenced by their prior experiences, internal characteristics, and general beliefs about parenting.[132,133] When forced to make decisions, even for an unborn child, parents are assuming a parenting role, and desire to make the best decision for their baby and family.[110] Some families may prefer a more paternalistic approach from those providing healthcare, with clear guidance toward the best option. Other parents may have predetermined opinions about what would or would not be acceptable to them, and may be offended by options that do not fit with their lifestyle, or those perceived to be presented in a biased fashion. Rempel and colleagues[110] provided eloquent insight into the process of decision-making for parents receiving an antenatal diagnosis of cardiac disease. They cautioned that providers of information 'must gain an understanding of each family's beliefs and values and provide information and counselling that is responsive to parents' different decision-making approaches'. This advice also applies to families facing a postnatal diagnosis. Of note, both parents receiving an antenatal diagnosis of congenital cardiac disease, and those receiving a postnatal diagnosis, were shown to demonstrate similar elevated psychological distress at the time of diagnosis.[134] At 6 months after birth, the levels of distress in those receiving postnatal diagnosis had returned to normative values, while those receiving the news prior to birth continued to demonstrate elevated distress.

In an effort to cope with the diagnosis of cardiac disease in a newborn, parents may respond by distancing themselves from the infant, or demonstrating altered attachment to the baby as a way of protecting themselves from the pain and loss that they fear.[132] This has important implications for bonding and later parent-infant interactions. Infants with congenital cardiac disease and their mothers were shown to demonstrate less positive affect and engagement during interaction than a non-cardiac group when assessed both prior to and 6 months after corrective surgery.[122] The temperament of infants with cardiac disease has been described by mothers as more withdrawn, more intense, and as having lower thresholds to stimulation than healthy infants.[123] These characteristics may impact parental involvement with the child, and could have a negative influence on development.

Exploration of styles of parenting for parents of children with moderate-to-severe cardiac disease has identified lower expectations[58,112] and lower levels of discipline[58] than in parents of healthy children. Mothers reported high levels of vigilance with their children and a desire to normalise the child and their family life as much as possible. Interestingly, aside from these acknowledgements of the impact of the cardiac disease, in this study, mothers of children with cardiac disease and mothers of healthy children were otherwise notably similar on both self-reported measures of parenting and child behaviour and videotaped interactions.[112]

The vulnerable child syndrome originally described by Green and Solnit[135] is defined as a reaction characterised by disturbance in psychosocial development often occurring in children whose parents expect them to die prematurely. It has been described in several populations of children with chronic illnesses, and may contribute to long-term behavioural and social problems.[113] Over-protection and reduced expectations of a child with a complex condition may be a very normal response. When overdone, this could have a negative influence on physical, emotional, and social development, and eventually the quality of life. Counselling and reinforcement for parents to treat their child with cardiac disease as a normal child may help to reduce this impact. Although most parents adjust effectively to the challenges of having a child with a complex condition such as cardiac disease, the adjustment may come at a significant emotional and psychological cost that may manifest itself in other aspects such as marital satisfaction, depression, or personal fulfillment. Opportunities to provide support, anticipatory guidance, and ongoing education, regarding both the cardiac condition and strategies for parenting, should be incorporated into the routine follow-up of children with cardiac disease.

Psychological Responses of Parents and Families of Children with Cardiac Disease

The responses of parents and families to the challenges imposed by cardiac disease in a child are influenced by multiple variables, as previously described, and are inherently difficult to predict or generalise. The last decade has witnessed a flourish of research designed to shed light on these responses. Lawoko and Soares [136–138] studied reports from a large sample of Swedish parents of children with congenital cardiac disease, parents of children with other diseases, and parents of healthy children. Higher levels of distress, hopelessness, and reduced quality of life were identified in the parents of the children with cardiac disease, being more prevalent in mothers than fathers. Socioeconomic factors, such as the financial burden imposed by the disease and changes in career trajectories due to the illness, have demonstrated an influence on perceptions of quality of life by both the child and the parents.[137,139,140] Parental perceptions of their individual quality of life may have an effect on how they perceive quality of life for their child.[141] In one-fifth of families surveyed, Wray and Maynard[13] identified significant negative influences related to the presence of paediatric cardiac disease on several aspects of family functioning, particularly recreational and social activities, and negative effects on siblings of the affected child. Of note, however, over two-fifths of the sample reported that their family had been drawn closer together by their experience. The presence of additional health problems, not uncommon in children with cardiac disease, added a significant negative contribution to overall family morbidity. Little information is available on marital satisfaction and stability in families living with paediatric cardiac disease. The presence of chronic illness in a child has been related to greater marital role strain, but does not necessarily result in marital dissatisfaction or depression.[142,143]

As one might expect, several groups have documented higher than expected levels of stress for parents of children with cardiac disease. Goldberg and colleagues[144] found that parents of young infants with cardiac disease reported the highest scores for stress on the child domain of the Parenting Stress Index[145] in the areas of child acceptance, mood, distractibility/hyperactivity, and reinforcement of parent compared to parents of healthy children or children with cystic fibrosis. Similarly, parents of older children with cardiac disease demonstrated higher than expected levels of stress in the child domain.[146] This domain assesses qualities of the child that may make them difficult to parent such as extreme temperament[123] and may impact parent-infant interactions and attachment.[122] Level of stress in the child domain has been found to be correlated significantly with the presence of child behavioural problems in school-aged children with surgically treated complex congenital cardiac disease.[109,113,147] Excessive stress in a parent may influence the development of such problems. Strategies to alleviate stress, or to help parents develop skills for management of stress, may benefit the individual parent, the affected child, and the family as a whole.

The severity of the underlying cardiac disease has not been found to be a reliable predictor of parenting stress,[146,148,149] with daily stress and more emotional methods of coping being significantly predictive of maternal adjustment to children with cardiac disease.[148] Differences in reports of mothers versus fathers regarding demands of care-giving for infants with cardiac disease have also been studied.[122] Although similar levels of demands were reported by both parents, mothers and fathers identified different aspects of care as the most time-consuming or stressful. Mothers spent the majority of their time addressing the physical needs of their infants, especially feeding. Fathers reported the most time spent attending to the infants' emotional and developmental needs. Interestingly, families with other children experienced higher levels of stress and transitions than did first-time parents. Fathers have been traditionally underrepresented in family outcomes research. In two qualitative studies exploring the experience of fathers of children with cardiac disease, several conflicting themes were identified including joy versus sadness, feeling powerful versus helpless, and maintaining versus losing control.[150,151] Interventions to provide psychological support for the unique needs of fathers are ripe for further investigation.

Effects on Siblings

Brothers and sisters of a child with paediatric cardiac disease experience a wide range of emotions in response to the illness. How they interpret the impact of cardiac disease will be influenced by a number of variables, including their age and level of development, the nature of the illness, the degree of change in routines and interactions with the parents that the illness imposes, the relationship with their ill sibling, and the resources available to the family both in terms of socioeconomic state and social support.[24] Unrecognised stress in siblings may manifest itself as behavioural problems, changes in school performance, alterations in eating or sleeping habits, or heightened anxiety at separation.[152]

Young children may be most vulnerable to stress due to their inability to conceptualise causation. They may fear that they will also become ill, or worry that through some action or thought they have caused the illness in their sibling. Younger children are also more distressed by separation from parents and alterations in routines. Older children may experience greater anxiety over the health and prognosis of their ill sibling. Anger and resentment over attention paid to the ill child, and the change in responsibilities for the older child, might also occur.[152] Typically, paediatric cardiac disease is not highly visible. Healthy siblings, therefore, may have difficulty understanding how the ill child is different, or why they require special care or attention. As an example, the family of a young boy that had undergone cardiac transplantation as an infant had always explained his condition by saying that he had received 'the heart of an angel'. His mother reported that his younger sibling protested loudly in anger one day, 'I want an angel heart too!' Healthy siblings of children with cardiac disease are more likely to exhibit behavioural problems when the illness has a high impact on family life, and the intensity of treatment or visibility of the condition is low.[52] Behavioural problems have been identified more frequently in siblings of transplanted patients than in those of children with congenital conditions.[13] Greater visibility of a chronic condition and regular treatment routines may facilitate better sibling acceptance and adaptation.

Hospitalisation and need for surgery result in physical separation from both the ill sibling and the parents. The well children left behind may feel abandoned and helpless. Structuring responsibilities so that there is minimal disruption to the routine of the healthy child is beneficial. The level of maternal education has been demonstrated to lessen anxiety amongst siblings, likely due to a greater sense of responsibility to provide support and information, as well as access to more resources.[152] To facilitate positive adjustment, it is important for parents to provide siblings with accurate and developmentally appropriate explanations of the cardiac condition and its treatment.[52] When a newborn requires immediate hospitalisation, the siblings at home may have difficulty believing the baby is real. The healthy children should be provided with opportunities to visit, see pictures of the baby, and to send them special things such as drawings or toys, in order to build a sense of connection to the new family member. The healthcare team, in particular child life specialists, should provide guidance to the family to facilitate visits by the siblings, age-appropriate preparation, and to provide siblings an opportunity to express their feelings and concerns.[24]

Meeting the Needs of Families

Awareness of the potential psychological and social burdens for families living with the diagnosis of cardiac disease in a child is critical for the entire team of those providing healthcare. We will fall far short of our potential to support our patients and their families if we focus only on the physical needs of the affected child. Parents and other family members should be made to feel welcome to express their greatest fears, concerns, and questions.[14,153] Frequent communication from consistent caregivers is needed to allow families to gain a detailed understanding of the condition of their child and its implications.[14,154–156] Information delivered at times of high stress is not fully absorbed or retained, yet parents may be unwilling to volunteer that they do not understand aspects of the condition. Asking parents to describe what they know or believe about the condition may provide insight into areas where they need further education or clarification. This education needs to be revisited frequently as the child progresses through normal developmental stages, and when the cardiac condition or plan for management acutely changes.

When a child has an uncertain prognosis, or remains critically ill for an extended period of time, parents look to providers of healthcare for accurate information and reason to maintain hope.[14] At these times, professionals must cope with their own frustrations at their inability to predict every outcome, and attempt to provide families with the most realistic information possible. Frequently, a plethora of caregivers becomes involved in the care of children with complex malformations. Parents may ask the same questions of multiple providers, and begin to compare and contrast answers. Inconsistencies in information will decrease trust and increase anxiety. Remember that parents are also at risk for stress related to events they witness in the critical care environment, and sharing of experiences with acquaintances made in the waiting room. Conferences for interdisciplinary care that include parents are needed to facilitate planning that accounts for the information needed by the family.

Psychosocial support for families may come from many sources. Support groups coordinated by the hospital or other families may provide valuable opportunities to share experiences and feelings. Today it is common for people to seek information on-line from formal support networks, and from individuals that share information regarding their personal experiences. Parents should be cautioned to evaluate critically the quality of information received from non-medical sources, and reminded that no two children undergo the exact same experience. Parents should be provided with directions to reliable sources of electronic information, such as hospital websites, the American Heart Association,[157] the Congenital Heart Information Network,[158] the European Congenital Heart Disease Organisation,[159] or the Children's Heart Federation,[160] among others. Often the experience of meeting another parent and child that have been through a similar course of events can be incredibly helpful. A cohort of parents and children that are willing to speak with newly diagnosed families can be coordinated by liaison nurses, social workers, psychologists, or child life specialists. DeMaso and colleagues[153] used an electronic journal to link families and children to personal narratives that were similar to their own experience. Results included decreased social isolation, increased understanding of feelings related to the illness, and more positive reactions in mothers.

Efforts should be made to support the confidence of the parents in their ability to master the needs for care of their child, and to recognise signs and symptoms that may require attention. Systematic discharge planning that includes living in hospital, and caring for the child while he or she is still hospitalised, provides an opportunity for parents to practice their skills and receive important feedback.[155] Home visits by trained nurses and follow-up phone calls can also provide valuable reassurance. Ideally, parents should be provided with clearly defined parameters that should prompt contact with the system providing healthcare, and a reliable method to reach someone who will understand the cardiac condition, for instance a cardiac nurse hot-line.[161] Ongoing information was the most common area of need identified by families.[154] Parents desired written information and diagrams about diagnosis and previous operations, information for both themselves and their child on the practical implications of the diagnosis such as activity restrictions, side-effects of medications, details to share with schools, and updated information on prognosis and the development of new approaches to treatment.

When a Child Is Dying

Despite our best efforts, there are times in the management of paediatric cardiac disease when no cure or palliation is possible, and it becomes inevitable that the child will die. These situations pose a profound challenge for health professionals. Communication with children and their families at these times is critical yet delicate. Many health professionals may not be well trained in how to approach these situations.[133,162] Consultation with experts in mental health, palliative care, and bereavement to support the child, parents, and siblings can provide invaluable assistance. If the affected child is at an age where they are aware of their condition, they should be provided with opportunities to express concerns about their future without fear that they will upset their family members or members of the team providing care. Children may have fear of impending pain or abandonment that can be alleviated with assurances from trusted adults.[14,163] Parents, although inherently hopeful, may find some comfort in hearing that death may be unavoidable. This acknowledgement may help them to address their fears and begin the process of grieving. Total denial of impending death will only make its acceptance more difficult, and may leave parents with feelings of guilt or blame.[14] Because parents are the ultimate makers of decisions regarding the care of their child, they may experience regret over a choice to pursue surgery or a specific treatment. An opportunity to review with staff the situation and care after a child has died may help parents gain comfort in knowing that they made the best decisions possible, and that their child has not been forgotten by those who provided care.

Attention must also be directed to the emotional needs of siblings at this difficult time. Opportunities for siblings to express their feelings by asking questions, drawing pictures, telling stories, and spending time with the ill child should be provided. Parents should be given information on the typical responses of children to the loss of a sibling which commonly include attention-seeking behaviour, irritability, sleeping difficulties, guilt at surviving, health complaints, and confusion over their new role in the changed family.[163] Whenever possible, families should be supported in their desire to fulfil culturally or spiritually important traditions when a child is dying. Choices of how the family wants to say goodbye, and support for the departure of the family from the hospital, should be provided. Leaving their child in the arms of a favourite or trusted staff member may help a family conclude this final visit.[163] Provision of bereavement support should be made available by those providing care for as long as the family finds it beneficial.

SOCIAL ISSUES

Every child and family affected by paediatric cardiac disease exists within a network of social structures that include financial, legal, political, educational, cultural, religious, and healthcare systems. The impact of chronic illness in a child must be considered within the context of each of these systems.

The financial implications of paediatric cardiac disease are associated with the expense of delivering care, the impact of lost wages and contribution to society from a parent that leaves the work force to care for an ill child, and the long-term abilities of the affected children to gain employment and support themselves. Although children with special needs comprise less than one-fifth of the overall population of children in the United States of America, they account for more than four-fifths of the costs of providing healthcare.[164] Whether this burden is absorbed by private health insurance, national health plans, or individual families, it is a formidable expense that, in some form or another, is transferred to society. Many private insurance plans have a cap of $1 million or less for lifetime coverage of an individual. Although this may sound generous to most parents, it is not uncommon for children that require multiple hospitalisations and surgeries to reach this limit before they reach school age. This may result in a job-lock phenomenon, where parents are unable to leave their current job for fear of losing insurance coverage.[165] Social work services should be made available to parents of children with complex cardiac disease to ensure that they are aware of the support programmes available to them. Adolescents with cardiac disease require career counselling regarding appropriate educational and vocational goals, and adults should be informed of the legal protections in place to reduce discrimination based on disability.[166–168] They may also need guidance regarding their needs and eligibility for insurance once they are no longer covered by the policies of their parents. Further legal protections, such as the Americans with Disabilities Act,[169] are in place to ensure civil rights for persons with disabilities regarding their access to education, employment, and other public benefits.

Systems providing public education are mandated to provide full access to all educational opportunities for children with special needs, albeit that these services are often limited by the economical constraints of the system. Whilst the majority of children with cardiac disease will achieve educational accomplishments similar to their peers of the same age, it is clear that some will demonstrate learning challenges that may require special education services (see Chapter 64). Individual tutoring, and strategies for specialised teaching, may be cost-prohibitive in some school systems. Children with relatively minor learning problems may be grouped with more severely retarded children in order to conserve scant resources. School teachers may also lack the training necessary to deal with issues associated with chronically ill children in the school system.[170] It is important that parents are equipped with the information necessary to communicate with educators of their child to assure that children with cardiac disease are encouraged to reach their full potential.

Providers of care to children and families living with cardiac disease must be sensitive to diversity in several aspects of family life, including differences in ethnicity, race, cultural beliefs and mores, socioeconomic state, spirituality, and religious affiliations and traditions. Sensitivity requires more than just the recognition of individual differences, and must also include an attempt to understand the implications of these differences for the care of the child. Certain treatments, such as blood transfusion for a Jehovah's witness, may put the individual at risk of being ostracised from his or her community. Other recommendations including dietary changes, or accepting support from non–family members, may be so incongruent with the culture that they become nearly impossible to implement. Health beliefs, behaviours, and expectations or acceptance of various outcomes will also vary by cultural background. Improved relationships will result from recognition of culturally driven assumptions, and sensitive consideration to appropriate strategies for treatment.[171–173]

Providers of healthcare for children face personal and ethical challenges associated with the care of patients with paediatric cardiac disease. The ethical principals of justice and beneficence relate to equitable treatment and allocation of resources for individuals, as well as the mandate for providers of healthcare to promote good at both the individual and societal level.[167] Whilst infants are rarely restricted from needed care, access to resources may diminish as children mature.[167] Disparities in access to paediatric specialists have been associated with both economic state and race.[174–176] Balancing the greatest good for society with that of the individual is a delicate task. Preserving the life of a child with a complex condition will undoubtedly impart future costs in terms of morbidity, and the potential for transmission of the condition to future generations. It is not possible, however, to value the benefits of the contribution of any individual to society.

The burden to staff looking after children in terms of emotional stress may be exceptional. Paediatric nurses and physicians are at risk for compassion fatigue and burn-out due to their repeated exposure to difficult procedures and treatments performed on children, and the emotional burden of caring for families.[177] More than half of surveyed paediatric critical care physicians reported to be at risk or burned out with perceptions about the value of their work, and feelings of success and satisfaction, being highly associated with those considering themselves burned out.[178]

Suffering by, or demise of, a child can be one of the most emotionally devastating events of which anyone can be a part. Staff form attachments to both patients and families, and need to recognise their own feelings and grief when they are unable to save the child. Given the medical technology available to sustain life today, many deaths in the paediatric intensive care unit will be related to decisions to limit or withdraw life-sustaining treatment. These decisions typically follow a prolonged course in the intensive care environment, and the relationships developed between patients, family members, and staff must be acknowledged. Nurses are commonly at the bedside of critically ill children on a continual basis. Family members often share concerns or fears with nurses that they are not able or willing to express to physicians. Disagreement and poor communication among staff may occur when there is conflicting information about what families have been told or their understanding of treatment decisions.[14,179] It is helpful to encourage discussion of psychosocial and ethical issues when planning daily care in those with complex malformations among the entire medical and non-medical team. Documentation about what families have been told, and the concerns they have expressed, can help to reduce missteps in communication. Formal meetings with the family must be conducted to achieve a consensus on the plan of care when benefit from further therapy appears futile.[179] The goal of a humane and dignified death that corresponds as much as possible to the wishes and beliefs of the family should be paramount for all caregivers that face this regrettable situation.

SUMMARY

The outcomes that really matter to patients, families, and societies living with the implications of congenital and acquired paediatric cardiac disease extend far beyond mere survival. Psychosocial outcomes for patients include the perception of stress related to treatment, psychological and behavioural development, quality of life, and the societal consequences of life with a chronic illness. Families face unique challenges as they are called upon to adapt to life with a child with paediatric cardiac disease. There may be effects on parenting and psychological well-being, as well as important implications for siblings and other family members. Social systems also need to adapt to and accommodate the needs of children with special needs and the growing population of adults that survive paediatric cardiac disease.

Psychosocial outcomes are highly subjective in nature and are determined by complex interactions between factors concerning risk and resistance inherent to the child, the family, the illness, and the social systems in which they exist. Individual perceptions and values must be recognised as an important determinant of successful adaptation. Professionals caring for these patients and families must support communication, and explore the psychosocial needs and concerns. The entire team providing care must also acknowledge its own feelings in order to meet the needs of the patients and families served. Building on the strengths of an individual child and family, and supporting efforts in coping, will enhance adaptation and well-being. The human spirit is incredibly resilient, even in times of great adversity. May the strength of the children and families we care for be an inspiration to all of us.

"Our greatest glory is not in never falling, but in rising every time we fall."

—Confucius

The complete reference list can be found on the companion Expert Consult web site at www.expertconsult.com.

ANNOTATED REFERENCES

- Spijkerboer AW, Utens EM, De Koning WB, et al: Health-related quality of life in children and adolescents after invasive treatment for congenital heart disease. Qual Life Res 2006;15:663–673.

  The authors have extensive history in the evaluation of psychological and social outcomes for children with cardiac disease. In this manuscript, the health-related quality of life was examined for 113 children aged 8 to 15 years that had undergone surgical intervention for repair of a congenital cardiac defect. Quality of life was reported as worse than a healthy reference group. Children aged 8 to 11 years scored lower than adolescents aged 12 to 15 years. There were no differences based on gender or diagnostic group.

- Karsdorp PA, Everaerd W, Kindt M, Mulder BJ: Psychological and cognitive functioning in children and adolescents with congenital heart disease: A meta-analysis. J Pediatr Psychol 2007;32:527–541.

  In a meta-analytic review of the literature from 1980 to May, 2005, addressing psychological and cognitive functioning of children and adolescents with cardiac disease, the authors found that only older children demonstrated an increased risk for behavioural problems. They concluded that the presence of cardiac disease alone does not necessarily impart problems with psychological function. They recommend longitudinal study of children with cardiac disease to improve understanding of the complex factors that influence long-term adjustment of children.

- McCrindle BW, Williams RV, Mitchell PD, et al: Relationship of patient and medical characteristics to health status in children and adolescents after the Fontan procedure. Circulation 2006;113:1123–1129.

  The investigators of the Pediatric Heart Network conducted a cross sectional study of 537 patients that had undergone Fontan palliation for complex paediatric cardiac disease to examine the relationships of patient and medical characteristics to perceived state of health. Problems with attention, learning, development, behaviour, anxiety and depression were identified. Both physical and psychosocial function scores were lower than the instrument norms. Lower socioeconomic state added an independent negative impact on outcome.

- Moons P, VanDeyk K, Budts W, DeGeest S: Caliber of quality-of-life assessments in congenital heart disease: A plea for more conceptual and methodological rigor. Arch Pediatr Adolesc Med 2004;158:1062–1069.

  Moons and colleagues reviewed 70 studies relating to paediatric cardiac disease published between January, 1980, and October, 2003, which discussed quality of life as an outcome. They evaluated the studies using 10 previously published criterions to evaluate validity and methodological rigour in the assessment of quality of life. Few studies met the specified criterions, resulting in a collection of work that was inconclusive, difficult to interpret, and not generalisable to the population of patients with paediatric cardiac disease. A call for greater methodological rigor in the assessment of this important outcome was issued.

- DeMaso DR, Campis LK, Wypij D, et al: The impact of maternal perceptions and medical severity on the adjustment of children with congenital heart disease. J Pediatr Psychol 1991;16:137–149.

  The authors, psychologists, and paediatric cardiologists at Children's Hospital, Boston, examined the hypothesis that maternal perceptions would be more significant predictors of emotional adjustment for children with cardiac disease than the clinical severity of their illness. In the 99 mothers sampled, maternal perceptions were the most potent predictor of emotional adjustment in the children accounting for 33 percent of the variability in adjustment whereas severity of illness accounted for only 3 percent. The mother-child relationship and accurate perceptions of the impact of the condition appear to be critical factors in adjustment.

- Visconti KJ, Saudino KJ, Rappaport LA, et al: Influence of parental stress and social support on the behavioral adjustment of children with transposition of the great arteries. J Dev Behav Pediatr 2002;23:314–321.

  The authors, part of the Boston Circulatory Arrest Study group, examined the relationships between parental stress, social support, and behaviour problems at 4 years of age in children that had undergone surgical repair of transposed arterial trunks. Outcomes were favourable with parents reporting less stress, more social support, and fewer behaviour problems than normative samples. Families with less social support reported higher levels of stress related to parenting. Higher levels of stress reported by parents correlated with a greater number of behaviour problems in the children. This manuscript illustrates the multiple factors that contribute to adjustment of children and families.

- Lawoko S, Soares JJ: Quality of life among parents of children with congenital heart disease, parents of children with other diseases and parents of healthy children. Qual Life Res 2003;12:655–666.

  In a large sample of parents in Sweden, the authors compared quality of life for parents of children with cardiac disease, parents of children with other diseases, and parents of healthy children. Parents of children with cardiac disease reported significantly lower quality of life than parents of healthy children. Mothers reported worse outcomes than fathers. Distress, hopelessness, and financial stress were more important than the presence or severity of the condition of the child in predicting outcomes.

- Goldbeck L, Melches J: The impact of the severity of disease and social disadvantage on quality of life in families with congenital cardiac disease. Cardiol Young 2006;16:67–75.

  Psychologists in Ulm, Germany, investigated the combined impact of social disadvantage and severity of the cardiac condition of the child on quality of life for 132 children and their caregivers. A significant interaction effect between the two predictors was identified, such that mild disease with social risk had virtually the same impact as severe disease with no social risk. Both medical and social risks for a poor response to the stress of cardiac disease in a child must be considered.

- Wray J, Maynard L: The needs of families of children with heart disease. J Dev Behav Pediatr 2006;27:11–17.

  Psychologists from the United Kingdom conducted a mailed survey to examine the perceived needs of children with cardiac disease and their families. The greatest need identified by two-fifths of the sample was for information about the child's condition. Nearly three-fifths of the sample had one or more unmet need and this increased with the age of the child. Provision of ongoing support and education for children with cardiac disease and their families is emphasised.

- Kamphuis M, Vogels T, Ottenkamp J, et al: Employment in adults with congenital heart disease. Arch Pediatr Adolesc Med 2002;156:1143–1148.

  This group provding paediatric cardiac care in the Netherlands examined job participation and career-related problems in adults with complex and mild congenital cardiac disease. They found a higher rate of unemployment, and problems with career, due to health in those with complex malformations. This highlights just one aspect of the social consequences of congenital cardiac disease. The need for counselling related to education and career planning is emphasised.

CHAPTER 63

Ethics and Consent

MARTIN J. ELLIOTT and TONI ELLIS

In his introduction to the equivalent of this chapter in the second edition of this book, G. R. Dunstan[1] pointed out the increasing role and understanding of ethical principles in paediatric cardiology. At that time, it might have been tempting to think that the specialty had encountered all the ethical issues it could reasonably expect to face. Not so. The last few years have seen new ethical issues emerge, and new thinking is needed. These issues include improved prenatal diagnosis, more genetic and epidemiological information, the increased use of mechanical circulatory support and a reduction of available organs for transplantation, and, with the evolution of the Internet, the rise of the expert patient or family. Interactions between physician, parents and child are complex and challenging. They have been described poetically[2] as 'a dance with three partners', in which the physician must learn both to lead and to follow. Ethical treatment in the context of a child within a family must take into account all relevant aspects. The physician must be aware not only of the consequences of the diagnosis but also of the quality of life after treatment, as well as its quantity. The physician must help the family understand the consequences of decisions both to treat and not to treat. As the Royal College of Paediatricians and Child Health pointed out in 1997,[3] generally the physician will ask, 'How shall we help this baby to live?' Sometimes he or she must ask, 'Ought we to help this baby to live, given the means we have and the predictable outcome?'

In many countries and cultures, legal frameworks have evolved to attempt to deal with these developments and changing relationships, and these are usually expressed as changes to the rules for obtaining consent. Yet there is variation in practice, and as ethical behaviour remains, at least in part, culture-dependent, the reader is reminded that the general points made in this chapter are delivered from the perspective of United Kingdom residents with a largely European bias. We have attempted to highlight different practice where possible.

International and intercultural differences in economic and political factors also influence clinical practice, and these may have significant ethical implications over which the physician may have little control. For example, if a country has major problems with water supply, or an excessive incidence of malaria or acquired immunodeficiency syndrome, it may be considered unethical to offer treatment to children with hypoplastic left heart syndrome. Not to do so in, for example, the United States might induce the opposite interpretation. This ethical relativity must always be understood and allowed for.

Despite the evolving success of our relatively young specialty, one of the most distressing aspects of our work is the persistent uncertainty of long-term outcome. Uncertainty is very difficult to cope with, and if combined, as it often is, with a series of interventions involving considerable risk, it is not surprising that families find uncertainty stressful. The physician has to exercise informed judgement in the face of this uncertainty, in partnership with the family.[4] In every aspect of the above discussion, a key element is the relationship developed between physician and family, a relationship which must be built on trust. It is all about communication.

COMMUNICATION WITH PATIENTS AND FAMILIES

Paediatric cardiology presents specific difficulties in communication with families. Not only are congenital heart disease and its treatment difficult to understand, but the language we professionals use is beset by shorthand and abbreviations, for example, hypoplast, VSD, DORV, SVR, and so on. Even if we use these only between ourselves at the bedside, they can have the apparent effect of excluding the family, and thus lay us open to accusations of elitism or paternalism. Those of us dealing with children need to understand these problems, but as has been pointed out in an excellent recent review,[5] few of us have had any explicit training in such three-way communications. This chapter is not the place to teach the basics, and we recommend this piece of work[5] as a good foundation. Much of it is common sense. For example, making sure the environment is child- and family-friendly, peaceful and calm. Always make a point of introducing yourself. Always be well prepared, making sure you have read the notes. Ask questions, listen, share information, explain carefully with visual aids or models as needed, and always ensure that the family understands by asking them to report back to you what you have said. Good understanding is expressed by maintaining eye contact, the asking of questions, and a positive body language, such as is achieved by leaning forward. Poor understanding can be inferred from opposite behaviours. Our own anecdotal observations demonstrate the fact that even these basic techniques are patchily applied. In our own unit, we have found role-play and video analysis helpful in reversing the practice of bad communication. A key question you might ask yourself is, 'Would this standard of care, or communication, be acceptable to me or my family?' If the answer is 'no', then you should take responsibility and change your behaviour. Other good summaries of these basic aspects of effective communication are presented elsewhere,[6,7] and in the Framework of Competencies for Basic Specialist Training in Paediatrics, published in October 2004 (Available at: http://www.rcpch.ac.uk/doc.aspx?id_Resource=2429).

CONSENT

The principle of informed consent, aimed at the lawfulness of health assistance, reflects the concept of autonomy and decisional auto-determination of the person requiring and requesting medical or surgical interventions.[8] Evidence exists that forms of consent probably existed in classical cultures, and are certainly implied in that fundamental element of the Hippocratic oath: 'First, do no harm'. Informed consent requires the giving of information, the certainty of the understanding of that information, time for reflection, and the actual giving of consent for the therapeutic intervention. Whilst there is variation in the mode of application of these components in different countries, particularly in the need for the signing of consent forms, which are compulsory in the United Kingdom and the United States, but not currently needed in Sweden or Belgium, the basic principles are consistent.

The concept of consent has changed over time.[9] Until the 1970s, consent was a rather paternalistic process. The doctor knew best, and was not afraid to say so, and society accepted this role. Society trusted doctors, who were perceived as figures of professional authority to whom respect was owed for their knowledge and wisdom. As decisions became more complex, and doctors less well trusted, this paternalistic model began to fade, and was replaced by one reflecting the autonomy of the patient in decision-making. This model presumes that the physician can translate his or her knowledge and experience in a manner that allows patients and families to grasp the implications and nuances of a particular decision. Sadly, this presumption has proved impossible to achieve, since as has been pointed out,[9] you would need to be able 'to infuse the patient with the contents of a textbook and the accumulated experience of the physician' for this really to be possible. Thus, a new model has emerged, that of shared decision-making. This model assumes that the physician and family will, and can, evaluate the available options in a systematic way, arriving at a clear and logical decision aware of the burdens as well as the benefits of treatment. The model still assumes a high degree of information availability, but more accurately reflects the realities of current practice.

There are three situations in paediatric cardiology that need to be considered in understanding the potential of the last model in our practice. These are prenatal counselling, a previously undiagnosed postnatal surgical or medical emergency, and an elective procedure to someone after regular clinical review.

Prenatal Counselling

In this situation, the family, previously happily looking forward to a new child, are suddenly thrust into a situation in which anxiety, sadness, guilt, and numbness dominate their emotions. In the midst of this psychological turmoil, they are expected to grasp the complexities of the congenitally malformed heart, acquire some understanding of the treatments and their consequences, and begin to understand concepts of risk and uncertainty, which are difficult enough under the happiest of circumstances. It is not surprising that families are vulnerable to the imposition of the preferences of the medical team involved. The impact of cultural influences on the given advice, or the response to it, has been described in the context of hypoplastic left heart, comparing religious and pro-life America with more secular and pro-choice Europe.[10] Such a societal bias to a pro-life stance means that abortion or termination of pregnancy is likely to be chosen much less frequently. This is just an example of the need to provide information in as many ways as possible to aid understanding. In fetal practice, nurse specialists, professional counsellors, and specific physicians combine to aid the family in making their decision. Most families will also search the Internet, consult friends or other family members, and require time to decide with regard to termination or continuance of pregnancy. The mother, particularly, will experience all sorts of emotions at this time. Because she lacks the medical knowledge of the physician, her assessment of risk must be even less certain than the professional view.

The duty of the doctor is not done when a factual explanation has been provided, and a request made for the mother's consent or decision. Should things not turn out well, her burden of regret or loss will be heavier than that of the professional. It is not to her good if she adds to it a burden of guilt. Guilt may be lessened or avoided if she can feel that her decision had the warrant of the approval or support of her doctor. Certainty cannot be required. Indeed, it is unattainable. But if a doctor feels sufficiently encouraged by the data to suggest the procedure in the first place, there seems to be no reason why, without over-reaching, that encouragement cannot be shared with a responsible parent. The same consideration is apt, although it is not the only one, in discussing the option of terminating a pregnancy after the detection of grave fetal abnormality. It has even stronger force when a medical decision is taken, as licitly it may be in ethics and in law, to desist from further efforts to keep alive a severely ill baby. Doctors have to learn to live with such decisions. Parents should not be obliged to. Most teams have no problems understanding parents who opt for termination if they so wish, but in societies which have adopted a primarily pro-life stance, this may become a significant source of tension. Such tension is more evident in the postnatal emergency example.

Postnatal Medical or Surgical Emergency

In this setting, and in the absence of prenatal diagnosis, the parents are confronted with new and shocking information, and little time to decide. The cardiologist or surgeon is aware that a procedure can be performed, palliative or otherwise, which will undoubtedly permit life, but which may often form just one step in a longer-term strategy of uncertain outcome but with certain shortening of life. The doctors will know little of the family circumstances, and less of their personalities and beliefs. Information may be given, but may well be less understood than when more time is available. The family will have little time to consult elsewhere, or to conduct their own Internet research. This is a situation closer to the old paternalistic model, and places specific demands upon those obtaining consent. Attempts to transfer an understanding of risk, uncertainty, and predicted outcomes should be made, and great care must be exercised in trying not to impose treatment for which there may be little or guarded enthusiasm. Unit policy may be invoked as a rationale for treatment, but in the absence of family context, this could be interpreted as persuasion rather than consent. Again, the quality of the consent process is dependent upon a team of people, usually doctors and nurses, being willing and able to take the time to help the parents understand the problem, along with the consequences of any decision. Sympathy, care, and understanding are key elements in the process. We find it wise to think of creating a relationship which allows for questioning and mutual respect.

There is no substitute for the truth, and certainly no place for lies, yet we know that huge bias exists in the information provided to parents by physicians.[11] Physicians promote treatments that they believe work, that are done well in their own institution, and yet whose results may bear little relationship to their estimates of outcomes. Thus, both doctors and patients may base decisions on estimates of outcome and risk that may have little accurate foundation in fact. We could argue that it is like the partially sighted leading the blind. Over the coming years, we need to place the outcomes of our work into the public arena in much more interpretable and accessible forms to improve the quality of this process of consent.

Elective Treatment after Regular Review

In this situation, consent is more clearly and appropriately a chronic process, in which the family and child are gradually educated over time by their cardiologist and his or her team in the vagaries of the condition and its treatment. Such understanding evolves with exposure to echocardiography, sharing images and explanations, review of pre-prepared patient information, and, in the current era, parent- or child-driven Internet research. As an example, in our clinic only recently, a child was busy searching the Internet on his iPhone as the interview with his parents proceeded. The subsequent questions from the child were profound, searching, and relevant.

After such longer-term, chronic evolution of understanding of what is going to happen, and with the resultant greater opportunity to build a relationship, the subsequent consent to a procedure might be considered to be a formality. Sadly, this has not been our experience. Often, cardiologists have indeed taught the family the general issues associated with treatment, and the benefits and significant risks of the procedure to come may well have been covered. But the surgeon obtaining consent at a pre-admission clinic, or the day before surgery, may well be faced with a situation in which, for the first time, the family is asked to confront such specific risks as cerebral damage associated with open-heart surgery, the risk of delayed closure of the chest, mediastinitis, long stay in the intensive care unit, and so on. The obtaining of consent turns into a litany of risk, rather than a confirmation of an understood balance of risk and benefit. This becomes even more of an issue if consent is also being sought for any or several research projects, since research governance mandates specific and detailed consent for all studies. At this time, it can be very difficult for a family to see the wood from the trees. They are anxious, having thought that the procedure had been decided, and have come to terms with it. Then, suddenly, the benefits of the procedure may be lost in the welter of risk which they are forced, by the legislation of consent, to hear. It seems that the process of consent may sometimes become a burden all of its own, and great care should be exercised to avoid that. Whenever possible, time should be allowed between the consent and the procedure, allowing a period for reflection, further questioning, and confirmation of understanding. Once again, the pressures on hospitals to be efficient may make such demands difficult to meet, but in our view such difficulties should be overcome by the process of change, rather than by bad practice in obtaining consent.

EXPLAINING AND UNDERSTANDING RISK

Understanding risk is one of the most difficult things to do. This is reflected by the recent decision of the University of Cambridge to establish a Professorial Chair in The Human Understanding of Risk. Predicting risk is notoriously difficult. Thus, if poor prediction is combined with poor understanding, it is not surprising that there can be important misunderstandings in communication. In obtaining consent, or in defining the optimal treatment, it is also important to rank risk and to balance it against benefit. This tends to be done intuitively by physicians, but for the frightened family, these issues of balance need to be laid out with care and patience, using as many techniques as necessary to ensure understanding.

Who Should Get Consent and How?

In the United Kingdom, the General Medical Council has issued an outstanding document entitled 'Consent; patients and doctors making decisions together', which provides guidance to cover these issues. Its title reflects that change towards consensus, rather than patronage or autonomy. The following list, paraphrased from that document, describes what the General Medical Council concluded the doctor must explain to the patient and family:

You, the doctor, must give patients the information they want or need about:

- The diagnosis and prognosis
- Any uncertainties about the diagnosis or prognosis, including options for further investigations
- Options for treating or managing the condition, including the option not to treat
- The purpose of any proposed investigation or treatment and what it will involve
- The potential benefits, risks, and burdens, and the likelihood of success, for each option; this should include information, if available, about
  - Whether the benefits or risks are affected by which organisation or doctor is chosen to provide care
  - Whether a proposed investigation or treatment is part of a research programme or is an innovative treatment designed specifically for their benefit
  - The people who will be mainly responsible for and involved in their care, what their roles are, and to what extent students may be involved
  - Their right to refuse to take part in teaching or research
  - Their right to seek a second opinion

- Any bills they will have to pay
- Any conflicts of interest that you, or your organisation, may have
- Any treatments that you believe have greater potential benefit for the patient than those you or your organisation can offer

Clearly this is an extensive list. It takes time and commitment to take consent on these terms, and the consenter must clearly be well informed, able to explain but also to listen. It is impossible to obtain informed consent if one is oneself uninformed! The General Medical Council also provides important guidance on the issue of delegation of the responsibility for consenting. The General Medical Council states:

> If you are the doctor undertaking an investigation or providing treatment, it is your responsibility to discuss it with the patient. If this is not practical, you can delegate the responsibility to someone else, provided you make sure that the person you delegate to
> - is suitably trained and qualified
> - has sufficient knowledge of the proposed investigation or treatment, and understands the risks involved
> - understands, and agrees to act in accordance with, the guidance [in this booklet]
>
> If you delegate, you are still responsible for making sure that the patient has been given enough time and information to make an informed decision, and has given their consent, before you start any investigation or treatment.

The doctor has to explain all this information in a way that is understandable, and allow the family and the patient to question, and develop understanding of, the issues. These rules apply equally to children and adults who may well be able to grasp the issues, and who should be involved in any decision-making. Specific allowance must be made to help them understand, either by additional teaching materials, or with the help of colleagues, such as nurses or play specialists, even if the ultimate legal responsibility rests with the parent or guardian.

Knowing whether a child is able to give consent on his or her own behalf is a skill and also depends on the legal rulings in the country concerned. In the United Kingdom, a child may be judged able to give consent if he or she is so-called Gillick competent. This follows from a case in the 1980s, in which Mrs Gillick challenged the lawfulness of guidance provided by the Department of Health that doctors could provide contraceptive advice and treatment to girls under the age of 16 without parental consent or knowledge in some circumstances, after her daughter had been given contraceptives by the family doctor without her knowledge. The House of Lords decided against the mother, on the grounds that it was lawful if, amongst other issues, 'the child had sufficient maturity and intelligence to understand the nature and implications of the proposed treatment'. This advice was initially limited to the issue of contraception, but a later judgement widened it to include other aspects of sexual health, and the term Gillick competent was born. It has provided a good rule of thumb in clinical practice for many of us to help ensure true partnership in decision-making with children of any age, clearly able to understand the issues. The message is simple. Respect the child and family, and treat them as you would wish to be treated, namely with respect and care.

Current Ethical Dilemmas

The management of patients with congenitally malformed hearts has produced some important ethical issues over the years. In finishing, we discuss a representative selection of some of the current problems.

Hypoplastic Left Heart Syndrome

Despite improving results at all stages of the treatment of this condition, there remain sufficient doubts over the long-term results, quality of life, and limited options for end-stage treatment that many doctors feel that the decisions regarding termination of pregnancy after prenatal diagnosis, and the provision of so-called comfort care rather than therapy postnatally, remain extremely difficult. These concerns relate to the perceptions of the quality of life, strains on the family, and beliefs that the non-cardiac associations of the treatment and condition will also make the burden of disease too great. In some countries, notably France, these views are widely held, and contrast strongly with attitudes in the United States.[10] As with many ethical debates, there is no correct answer, and hopefully detailed studies of quality of life and the burden of disease will effectively influence debate in the future. Nonetheless, we have heard arguments forwarded at professional meetings in the United States that the hospital concerned ought to put the child into the care of the courts if the parents refuse treatment, in order that the child can benefit from the Norwood strategy. The ethics of refusing treatment, or forcing it upon an unwilling family in this setting, have not yet been tested. The issue has been reviewed in excellent fashion.[12] Clearly, the decision not to allow the child to undergo surgery, when everything and everyone around seems devoted to providing that care, is difficult, a kind of environmental coercion. These issues have been movingly described by a parent who opted for no treatment for a child with hypoplastic left heart syndrome.[13] Although times have moved on since then, and attitudes to treatment have altered, the emotions presented in this article make important reading.

Prenatal Diagnosis, and Difficult Decisions in Neonatal and Infant Critical Care

The attitude of doctors towards termination of pregnancy at various fetal ages and for various conditions is, perhaps surprisingly, highly variable and as a result very contentious. What data or values are they using to support their advice? This issue has recently been debated, with the conclusion reached that this area needs greater research both legally and medically.[14] Importantly, it was also stated that doctors must guard against forcing their own values onto the wider society. Most Western societies abort more normal fetuses than they do abnormal ones, and yet prenatal diagnosis can provide considerable reassurance for those seeking to have a normal baby. Excellent prenatal scans can raise difficult dilemmas for the parents, particularly as they may have to choose from options including initial treatments which carry high risks, or significant uncertainty over the long term. The ethics around this have been widely reviewed, recently by the Nuffield Council on Bioethics,[15] which concluded, 'We consider that a pregnant woman who has chosen to continue her pregnancy has strong ethical obligations to protect the health of the future child. We are not persuaded, however, that the law should require pregnant women to submit to medical or surgical interventions to benefit a fetus against their will'. It seems to us that this statement represents an accurate summary of ethical attitudes in most of the world.

BRIDGING TO TRANSPLANTATION

Ethical issues sometimes emerge so quickly, as a result of rapid medical progress, that we are unprepared to deal with them, and discover too late that we should have undertaken ethical review in parallel with the medical development. Such a situation is emerging with the use of ventricular assist devices as a bridge to transplantation in children. The mismatch between supply of, and demand for, donor hearts to manage end-stage cardiac failure from whatever cause in children prompted the development of devices to support the circulation until an organ became available, or recovery occurred.

The success of the Berlin Heart Device throughout the world has surprised us all, and now it has become the support of choice in many centres. Yet, simultaneously, the number of donors has fallen, and thus an increasing number of children exists, waiting on such support and hoping for the appearance of a heart. All the patients in whom a Berlin Heart has been inserted in the United Kingdom are on an urgent list. Cynics may say that the only way to obtain a transplant is to be supported on a Berlin Heart. Where does this lead? What should we tell families? Who should be given a Berlin Heart—all or few? Are all those on such support equal, or should scoring be introduced to rank urgency, such as on the basis of the duration of support? How do we deal with the massive costs, and thus the opportunity cost to other groups of patients? Who should decide about rationing? There are of course no simple answers, but we do have a responsibility to address the issue, and to find frameworks for dealing with it which are rational and fair. So far we have failed, driven perhaps by the need to make progress, or to do better than our peers. The balance between progress, resources, ambition and expectations, real or unreal, is hard to find, but is a responsibility of medicine. This dilemma is often characterised by the question 'Just because we can, should we?'

There will, of course, be many other examples which any reader might wish to propose. It is not the purpose of this chapter to provide guidance for all situations. Rather, we wanted to emphasise the need for ethical review and self-criticism. We should make ourselves open to comment and criticism, and learn to use the expertise and advice of those in society who are trained to consider without bias the wider issues. We wish again to emphasise the importance of putting the patient and family at the centre of thinking, sublimating personal ambition or greed to that greater good.

Intuition: Personal and Corporate

Decision is a day-to-day, hour-to-hour reality in practice. Decisions are taken at every step throughout the course of treatment, to the time of discharge or allocation to long-term or short-term nursing care. These decisions are often taken rapidly, and in the heat of battle. The doctor is trained to gather relevant information, to interpret it, and to frame his or her duty accordingly. As time has passed, we have become able to access ever more information, and outcomes are much better understood. We have a responsibility to be aware of these results, and to make them available to whomsoever needs them, including families. The Internet has greatly contributed to this freedom.

Reflection, and an elementary self-awareness, teach that the strictly scientific element in reaching decisions is sometimes limited. Such scientific data, such as readings from scans, dials, graphs, biochemical values and the like, rarely dictate decision. Indeed, they may paralyse decision, for they may pull in different directions. Only a personal decision can resolve the conflict. Scientific logic might argue that, given one gap in a particular pattern of knowledge, experiment or research in one direction might fill it. If the research would require the violation of some vulnerable interest, however, it cannot be undertaken. And, of course, in an individual patient, there would not be time. Scientific logic cannot have the last word.

Decisions, therefore, though grounded as they are in medical science, contain an important intuitive element. The acquisition and sharpening of a disciplined intuition are part of a thorough medical and social training. Medical intuition is essential to the humane practice of medicine. When autonomous, however, it can be a menace.

There is, therefore, another ethical demand. It is for what might be called a corporate intuition, a community of minds working together by which personal intuitions and subjective judgements may be checked, validated, or countermanded. Paediatric cardiology requires work in a multi-disciplinary team, within which consultation and discussion precede decision-making. The development of a corporate conscience, a facility in moral reasoning together, is a necessary condition if decisions are to be made that, on the one hand, take the empirical data into account, and, on the other, amount to the best apparent choice possible from the available options, none of which may be ideal. Such common possession of wisdom is not acquired without discipline. The present organization of specialist hospital medicine should, in theory, favour it. The balance between experienced, senior team members, and new, often transient, staff provides a good basis for new ideas to be tested against experience and policy. Between them there is an interchange not only in terms of science and technical education, but also in values, generating the necessary tensions that constrain and encourage the transmission of ethics from generation to generation.

Medical ethics is first a corporate possession, that of a profession. It is embodied personally as each member makes it his or her own. Codes like the Helsinki Declaration governing medical research are markers of minimum demand and social expectation. The living practice of the ethics, and its necessary development, is ideally an activity of the functional team. The individual works best as a moral agent in small, tangible societies. The Latin root of that word is societas, for which the old English translation is fellowship, as old, incidentally, as the translation of mores, or morals, as manners. Models of collegiate fellowship exist within the common experience, in which knowledge is valued, pursued, ordered, and transmitted. Standards, intellectual and professional, are set, acquired and maintained. Members are disciplined. Persons are fulfilled. Ethics is an activity proper to humans as rational and social beings. It is vital for staff involved in the care of patients with congenitally malformed hearts.

The complete reference list can be found on the companion Expert Consult web site at www.expertconsult.com.

ANNOTATED REFERENCES

- Pantell CL, Lewis CC: Talking with children: How to improve the process and outcome of medical care. Medical Encounter 1993;10: 3–7.

  This paper outlines with great clarity the issues which one needs to take into account when talking to children and their families. Like many good reviews on this subject, it emphasises the need to listen and to respect.

- Royal College of Paediatricians and Child Health: Withholding or Withdrawing Life Saving Treatment in Children: A Framework for Practice. London, 1997.

  Reports from working parties can be dry and of little help. This one is different. The group has addressed many of the practical and ethical problems we face as front-line cardiologists and surgeons, and their advice is of great importance. As presented, they reflect the law of the United Kingdom, and provide indications of what must be considered when terminal care is required.

- Maguire P, Pitceathly C: Key communication skills and how to acquire them. BMJ 2002;325:697–700.

  This paper presents an excellent summary and checklist for all of us needing to communicate with patients and relatives. It is straightforward and well written.

- Mallardi V: The origin of informed consent. Acta Otorhinolaryngol Ital 2005;25:312–327.

  An interesting diversion into the history of consent, providing a context for current ethical thinking. There is little new in history, but plenty of advice!

- Mercurio MR, Peterec SM, Weeks B: Hypoplastic left heart syndrome, extreme prematurity, comfort care only, and the principle of justice. Pediatrics 2008;122:186–189.

  This important paper covers all aspects of decision-making when comfort care is being considered. The principles of justice, applied to all participants, are clearly explained, and the subsequent balance which emerges is of great common sense.

- Vuillemot L: The fate of baby Amy. New York Times 1988; 25 Sept.

  Although rather dated in context, this article by a parent encompasses pretty well all that a parent might feel, and leaves the reader with a profound sense of respect, which can be carried into daily interactions with families.

CHAPTER 64

The Central Nervous System in Children and Young Adults with Congenital Cardiac Disease

AMANDA J. SHILLINGFORD and GIL WERNOVSKY

Prior to the early 1980s, it was uncommon for children with complex congenitally malformed hearts to survive into later childhood. The nearly simultaneous advances in congenital cardiac surgery, echocardiography, and intensive care were coupled with the availability of prostaglandins and the developing discipline of interventional cardiology. Together, these factors resulted in a dramatic fall in surgical mortality, with complex repairs taking place at increasingly younger ages. At many large centers, palliative surgery followed by later repair was replaced by primary repair in infancy, while staged reconstructive surgery for various forms of functionally univentricular heart, including those with hypoplastic left heart syndrome, was improving with steadily falling rates of surgical mortality.[1-4] As a result, the early part of the 21st century has seen an increasing number of children entering primary and secondary schooling. Research into their academic and behavioural outcomes has revealed some sobering realisations about the outcomes in these survivors of paediatric cardiac surgery.

For the purposes of this chapter, complex congenital cardiac disease will refer to morphological abnormalities significant enough to require surgical or catheter intervention as neonates or young infants. As a group, patients with such malformations have a significantly higher incidence of academic difficulties, behavioural abnormalities, fine and gross motor delays, problems with visual motor integration and executive planning, speech delays, inattention, and hyperactivity.[5-17] Abnormalities of the central nervous system in infants with congenital cardiac disease is characterised by abnormalities of tone, difficulties with feeding, delays in major motor milestones, and speech deficits.[5,8,18,19] In children with congenital cardiac disease, the need for special services in school is significantly increased compared to the general population.[6,11,13,20] As children progress through school, low scores in terms of academic achievement, learning disabilities, behavioural problems, difficulties with social cognition and attention deficit/hyperactivity disorder may result in academic failure, development of poor skills in both the classroom and socially, low self-esteem, behavioural disinhibition, and ultimate delinqunecy.[21-23] Recent reports have also shown that quality of life is affected in children with complex malformations.[24]

Dependent upon a number of factors, including the underlying congenital lesion and the associated surgical management, genetic contributions, additional perinatal events such as profound hypoxia-ischaemia from a delayed diagnosis,[25] or post-operative events such as low cardiac output syndrome,[26] the incidence of abnormalities may range from infrequent to ubiquitous. For example, in studies of children with transposition, a small fraction may have severe developmental impairment, perhaps one-half are normal in all respects, and nearly one-half will have a combination of speech, motor, behaviour or learning issues.[6,27] Compared to children with transposition, the proportion of children with other forms of complex disease, such as obstructed totally anomalous pulmonary venous connection, hypoplastic left heart syndrome, or interruption of the aortic arch who are developmentally normal is significantly decreased, with perhaps only one-third of those tested having no dysfunction in any domain.[11,12] While most of these abnormalities are relatively mild, and may only be determined by formal testing, they result in a so-called high-prevalence, low-severity developmental signature. A schematic representation is shown in Figure 64-1.

Importantly, the combined outcomes of developmental delay, academic difficulties, and behavioural abnormalities represent the single most common morbidity affecting the quality of life in surviving patients with congenital cardiac disease when they reach school age. This complication is more common than late mortality, severe exercise impairment, unplanned reoperations, bacterial endocarditis, or significant arrhythmias. The later implications of these findings through adulthood are uncertain, and must continue to be a robust area of research. Our current understanding of the aetiology of these findings is discussed below.

SCOPE OF THE PROBLEM IN ADULTS WITH CONGENITAL CARDIAC DISEASE

Surprisingly, although the current number of adults with congenital cardiac disease is at least as many as the number of children with congenital cardiac disease, there is a paucity of studies investigating outcomes relating to the central nervous system, particularly with regard to behaviour and cognition. In contrast, there is an increasing number of investigations evaluating employment, physical activity, insurability, and quality of life in these adults, which complement nicely the recent data on younger children. The results of these studies in adults are mixed. Some suggest over-achievement in life-related activities, employment, and quality of life, while others describe deficits in social functioning, lifetime earnings, and health-related quality of life.[28-32] These mixed results are most likely due to the heterogeneous nature of congenital cardiac malformations, as well as the multiple non-cardiac reasons for suboptimal outcomes. As patients are further removed from surgery, it

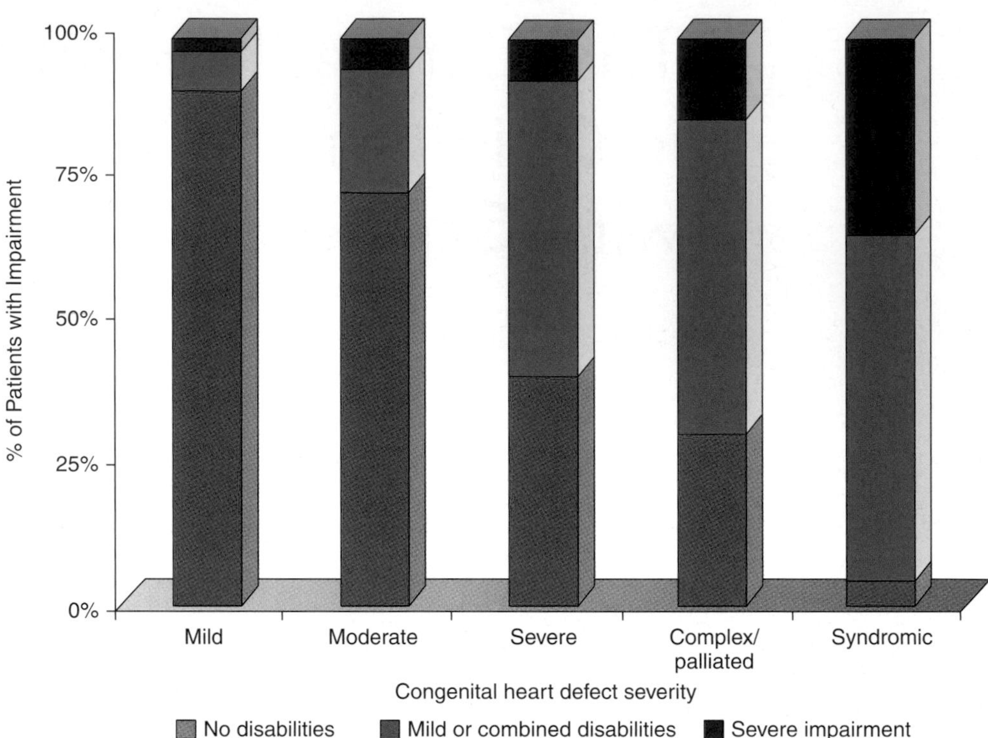

Figure 64-1 Schematic representation of developmental abnormalities in children with congenital cardiac disease. Children with milder forms of congenital cardiac disease, for example, ventricular septal defect without an associated genetic syndrome, as a group, have a low incidence of developmental abnormalities, and more than mild abnormalities are rare. Increasingly complex forms of congenital cardiac disease, for example transposition or totally anomalous pulmonary venous return, are associated with increasing numbers of children with developmental deficits, and only the minority of children with extremely complex heart disease, for example, functionally univentricular heart, are completely normal in all respects. Those having congenital cardiac disease associated with chromosomal abnormalities, for example Down and DiGeorge syndromes, or multiple congenital anomalies, are nearly always associated with developmental abnormalities, in many cases, severe. (From Wernovsky G: Current insights regarding neurological and developmental abnormalities in children and young adults with complex congenital cardiac disease. Cardiol Young 2006;16[Suppl 1]:92–104.)

is likely that the social and environmental milieu are more responsible for shaping long-term outcomes, compared to the underlying structure of the brain, or the effects of hypoxaemia, low cardiac output, and cardiac surgery.

At this point, it must be emphasised that it is ill-advised to suggest that the current findings in adults are applicable to current children, or will be predictive of later dysfunction in the next generation of patients with congenital cardiac disease. The diagnostic capabilities, surgical techniques, and importantly, interventional philosophy were quite different when current adults with congenital cardiac disease were children. For example, a child born in the 1960s or 1970s with tetralogy of Fallot would most likely have been managed with one or more systemic-to-pulmonary arterial shunts prior to a complete repair in later childhood. The outcomes 30 years on in these patients are likely to be different than those for a child born in the current era who undergoes a single-stage correction in early infancy.

We believe, nonetheless, that the recent reports of adverse outcomes in children currently of school age, such as behavioural and academic difficulties, deficits in motor function, social cognition and social interactions, set the stage for functional difficulties seen later in adult life. One model that has been proposed for analysis of outcomes in patients with cancer is that the ultimate outcome of interest results from a combination of environmental influences in the susceptible host. In patients with congenital cardiac disease, environmental influences include, but are not limited to, the effects of cardiac surgery in general and cardiopulmonary bypass in particular, hypoxaemia, low cardiac output, hospital complications, social class, psychosocial interactions, and the implications of chronic disease on the family unit. Host, or patient-related, factors similarly include, but are not limited to, birth weight, the physiology caused by the underlying cardiac malformation, genetic abnormalities including recognised syndromes and allele polymorphisms, and additional congenital anomalies, especially in the brain, which affect long-term outcomes.

CONGENITAL CEREBRAL DISEASE

Given that the central nervous and cardiovascular systems form nearly simultaneously in early gestation, it is not surprising that there is an increased incidence of structural abnormalities of the brain in children with co-existing structural abnormalities of the heart. Many children with multiple congenital anomalies or chromosomal abnormalities, many of whom have co-existing congenital cardiac disease, will have developmental delay and behavioural issues as a significant component of late morbidity. In addition to genetic factors which may affect both systems from a macroscopic perspective, congenital cardiac disease may alter cerebral blood flow, delivery of oxygen, or both, and result in secondary effects of the vulnerable fetal central nervous system.

The brain of the full-term neonate with congenital cardiac disease structurally resembles that of a preterm neonate,[32] and interestingly, survivors of complex cardiac surgery, when they reach school age, have developmental findings which are very similar to survivors of premature birth, suggesting a similar pathological response to injury. Serial studies of the fetal brain, using ultrasound and magnetic resonance imaging, are currently underway, and are increasing our understanding of the interactions between the abnormal fetal cardiovascular system and cerebral development.

Microcephaly

The circumference of the head at birth is a surrogate for growth of the brain, and in neonates without congenital cardiac disease, microcephaly is independently associated with later developmental delays and academic difficulties.

Multiple studies have shown the incidence of microcephaly at birth is increased in children with congenital cardiac disease, approaching one-fourth of children in some reports,[33-36] and persists into later infancy.[37,38] In a group of 318 neonates with various forms of congenital cardiac disease evaluated at our institution between 1992 and 1997, the incidence of congenital microcephaly, defined as a circumference of the head at or below the second percentile, was nearly 1 in 10.[34] More complex lesions have a higher incidence. In a series of consecutive neonatal autopsies at The Children's Hospital of Philadelphia, approximately one-third of infants with hypoplastic left heart syndrome were noted to have congenital anomalies of the central nervous system and/or were microcephalic.[39] While the causes are speculative, and most certainly multifactorial, a recent report in children with hypoplastic left heart syndrome, where the median circumference of the head at birth is only at the 18th percentile of that reported for normal neonates, revealed that patients with microcephaly had significantly smaller ascending aortas than those without, suggesting that reduced flow to the brain from the left ventricle secondary to anatomical hypoplasia of the ascending aorta may result in diminished brain growth.[33]

The Open Operculum

The opercular region is that covering the so-called insulae Relie, and is made up of frontal, temporal, and parietal cortical convolutions. In magnetic resonance and computed tomographic imaging studies of neonates with complex congenital cardiac disease, underdevelopment of the operculum may be seen in nearly one-quarter of the patients, and is a marker for functional immaturity of the brain.[35,40] This may be a unilateral or bilateral finding, and has been termed underoperculinisation, or an open operculum (Fig. 64-2). The operculum is thought to be related to oral motor coordination, taste, and speech, particularly to expressive language. In adults who develop a stroke in this area of the brain, the so-called Foix-Chavany-Marie syndrome, deficits include impairment of voluntary movements such as chewing and deglutition, dysarthria, and problems with taste.[41] In macaque monkeys, receptive fields on the tongue, lips and palate have been mapped to the operculum.[42] Given the high prevalence of problems with feeding,[36] delay with expressive language, and oral-motor apraxia in children with complex cardiac malformations,[5,12,27] as well as the increasing recognition of a high prevalence of an open operculum, we speculate that some patients with these developmental disabilities may have a structural underdevelopment of the operculum. We are currently pursuing this hypothesis.

Periventricular Leucomalacia

Injury to the white matter, a common finding in premature infants, has been increasingly recognised in full-term neonates with congenitally malformed hears.[40] It has also been suggested that decreased flow to the brain pre-operatively was significantly associated with lesions in the white matter, affecting slightly over one-quarter of neonates before surgery.[35] Periventricular leukomalacia was also found in slightly over half of a cohort of patients who underwent surgery for congenital cardiac disease as neonates, but was rarely detected in those who underwent surgery between 1 and 6 months of age.[43]

All of these studies were carried out using populations of children who underwent cardiac surgery with deep hypothermic circulatory arrest. Because of concerns that the use of this technique during cardiac surgery is directly related to cerebral injury, many centres have adopted regional perfusion of the brain using low flow as an alternate strategy which decreases the period of cerebral ischaemia during cardiac surgery. Studies using magnetic resonance imaging of patients corrected with this technique[44] showed evidence of ischaemic lesions in one-quarter of the cohort prior to cardiac surgery, and in almost three-quarters after surgery. The majority of the ischaemic injury seen after surgery was in the form of periventricular leucomalacia, a proportion that is similar to those patients undergoing deep hypothermic circulatory arrest.[45] In another study,[46] injury to the white matter and/or stroke were identified in 22 infants pre-operatively, while another one-third of the survivors developed new evidence of brain injury on post-operative imaging. More sophisticated magnetic resonance imaging[32] has shown not only a high incidence of injury to the white

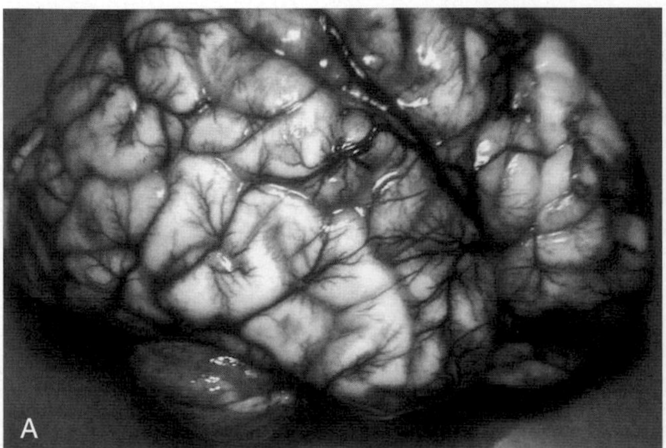

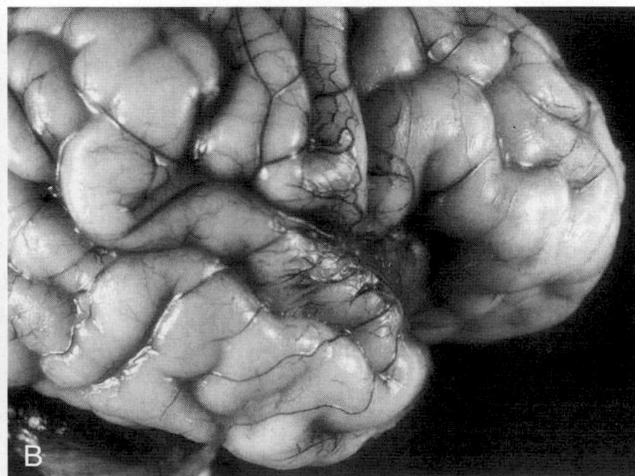

Figure 64-2 The normal external appearance of the brain (A) is compared with underdevelopment of the operculum (B). (From Wernovsky G: Current insights regarding neurological and developmental abnormalities in children and young adults with complex congenital cardiac disease. Cardiol Young 2006;16[Suppl 1]:92–104.)

matter, but also evidence of immature brain metabolism and microstructure, which are strikingly similar to findings seen in the premature population.

Periventricular leucomalacia is believed to arise from several factors, including the high susceptibility of the immature oligodendrocyte to hypoxic ischaemic injury, as well as the watershed distribution of flow of blood to this area between the small arteries that penetrate from the cortex and those that arise centrally and run radially outward. This watershed area is particularly prone to ischaemia during decreases in cerebral perfusion pressure. In premature infants, severe degrees of periventricular leucomalacia have been associated with cerebral palsy, while mild degrees of injury have been associated with developmental delay,[47] motor difficulties, and behavioural disorders,[48] a developmental signature remarkably similar to school-age children with congenital cardiac disease.

Additional Anatomical Findings at Birth

Congenital anatomical anomalies of the central nervous system are known to be coincident with malformations of the heart.[39,49–51] Cerebral abnormalities have been noted in one-quarter of a cohort of infants, with nearly half, such as holoprosencephaly and agenesis of the corpus callosum, present prior to any surgery.[52]

Fetal Cerebrovascular Physiology and Delivery of Oxygen

Ultrasound studies in the fetus have revealed that cerebral vascular resistance is altered in the presence of congenital cardiac disease. Fetuses with left-sided disease, for example, hypoplastic left heart syndrome, were shown to have decreased cerebral vascular resistance compared to normal.[53,54] In patients with aortic atresia, the fetal cardiac output from the arterial duct must deliver flow cephalad to the brain as well as caudad to the low resistance placenta. It is speculated that cerebral vascular resistance must therefore be lower than normal to allow adequate blood flow to the developing brain. Fetuses with right-sided obstructive lesions, for example, tetralogy of Fallot, were also shown to have increased fetal cerebral vascular resistance.[53] In these children, it is speculated that the obstruction to flow into the pulmonary arteries changes the usual delivery from the patent arterial duct caudad to the placenta. In these cases, the left ventricle must contribute to placental blood flow antegrade from the ascending aorta, with a resultant increase in cerebral vascular resistance. The impact of these alterations in fetal cerebral vascular resistance is unclear, but almost certainly plays a role in subsequent neurological development.

In the normal fetus, the intracirculatory patterns created by the normal fetal connections result in preferential streaming of the most highly oxygenated fetal blood to the developing brain, and most desaturated blood to the placenta. When significant structural disease exists within the heart, these beneficial patterns are likely to be altered. Although not yet confirmed by fetal magnetic resonance spectroscopy, fetuses with transposition are likely to have the blood with the lowest saturation of oxygen returning to the ascending aorta and brain, while blood with the highest saturation will return to the abdominal organs and placenta. Speculation on the consequences of the transposed fetal circulation as an explanation for the high incidence of macrosomia in these infants dates back 40 years,[55] and has also been offered as an explanation for the increased incidence of relative microcephaly seen in transposition.[56] Complete mixing, as seen in those with functionally univentricular hearts, will produce intermediate values of fetal cerebral saturations of oxygen, but lower than those seen in the normal fetus (Fig. 64-3).

PERI-OPERATIVE CONTRIBUTORS

Pre-operative Factors

Neonates with complex congenital cardiac disease frequently require hospitalisation immediately after birth, many to receive intravenous infusions of prostaglandin, some requiring intubation, mechanical ventilation, or invasive interventions such as balloon atrial septostomy. All of these interventions carry risks to the central nervous system, especially the potential for paradoxical embolus to the brain of air or particulate matter in children with intracardiac right-to-left shunts. These patients also have saturations of oxygen that are below normal, potentially compromising cerebral delivery of oxygen. In addition to diminished content of oxygen, neonates with critical congenital cardiac disease also have diminished flow of blood to the brain.[35] Such a finding of reduced flow to the brain, and abnormal vascular reactivity, has recently been confirmed in a neonatal piglet model of functionally univentricular physiology.[57]

Intra-operative Factors

The conduct of cardiopulmonary bypass, and other support techniques used during open heart surgery, has received considerable attention, and has been the subject of active research. As opposed to all of the risk factors for abnormal neurological development discussed thus far, variation in intra-operative support, such as the conduct of cardiopulmonary bypass, is one of the few modifiable risk factors which may be altered to improve long-term neurological outcomes. Potential modifiable technical features of cardiopulmonary bypass are shown in Table 64-1, and we pay particular attention to three of these.

pH Management

In one very important trial at Children's Hospital, Boston, developmental and neurological outcomes were evaluated in infants undergoing repair of a variety of cardiac defects at less than nine months of age who were randomised to either alpha-stat or pH-stat management during deep hypothermic cardiopulmonary bypass. Eligibility was limited to children undergoing various forms of biventricular repair in the first 9 months of life. Although there were some benefits reported with the use of pH-stat management for outcomes in the immediate peri-operative period,[58] the use of either strategy was not consistently related to either improved or impaired neurodevelopmental outcomes at one to four years of age.[59] On the Bayley Scales of Infant Development, there was no effect of treatment on the Psychomotor Development Index. The Mental Developmental Index, in contrast, varied significantly depending on the underlying anatomical diagnosis. For patients with transposition and tetralogy of Fallot, use of pH-stat resulted in a slightly higher mental developmental index, although the

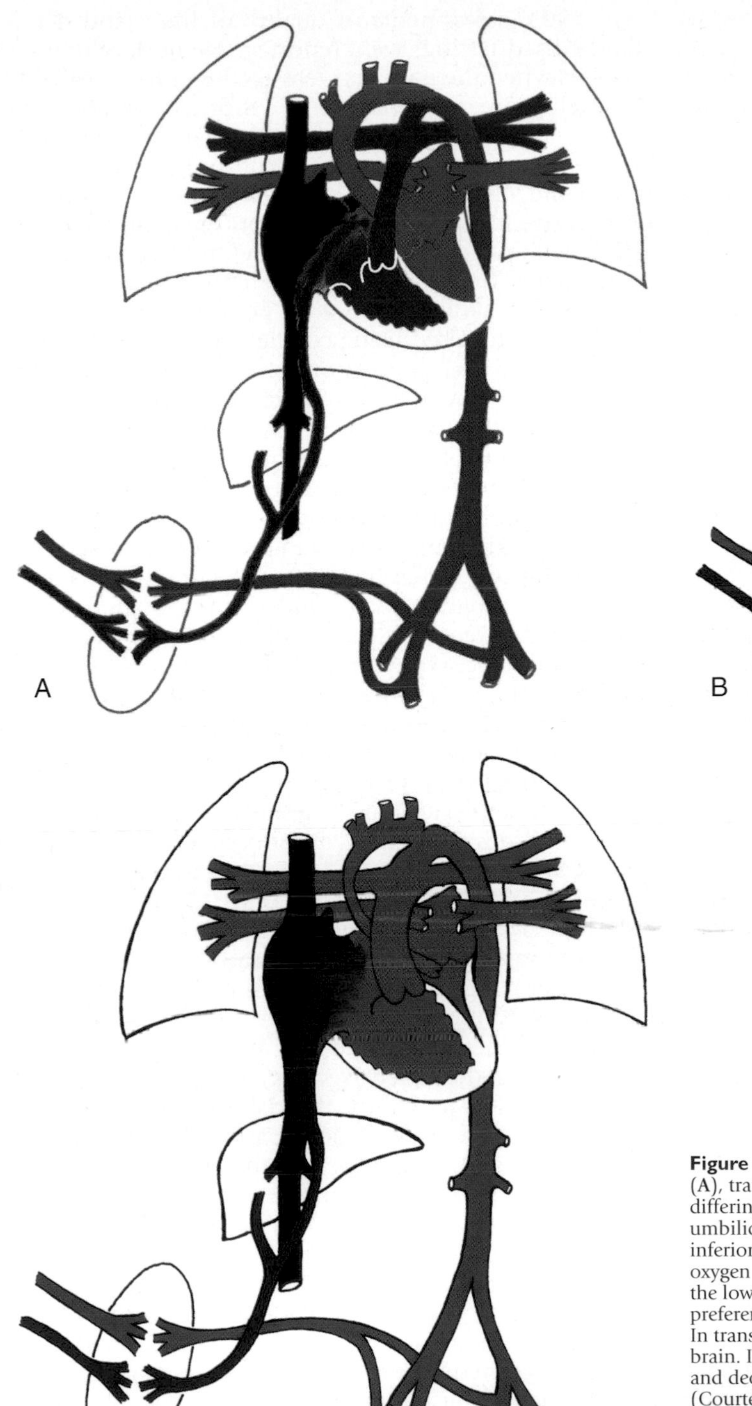

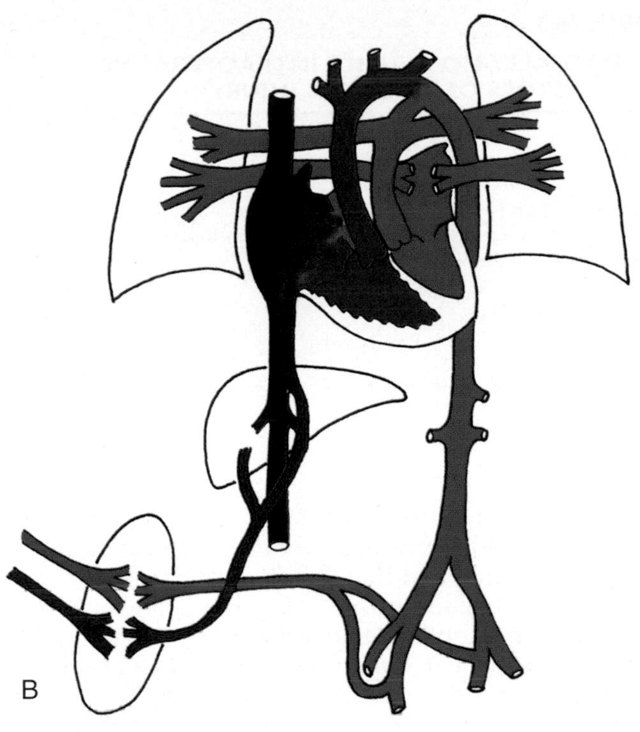

Figure 64-3 The fetal circulation is compared between the normal heart (**A**), transposition (**B**), and hypoplastic left heart (**C**). Colours represent differing levels of oxygenation, with the highest oxygen content, from the umbilical vein, in *red*, and the lowest oxygen content, from the superior and inferior caval veins, in *blue*. In the normal heart, the blood with the highest oxygen content is preferentially directed to the fetal brain, while blood with the lowest oxygen content is directed to the placenta. The benefits of this preferential streaming are altered in the face of many congenital heart lesions. In transposition, blood with the lowest content is redirected back to the fetal brain. In hypoplastic left heart syndrome, complete mixing of oxygenated and deoxygenated blood takes place in the fetal atrium. See text for details. (Courtesy of PA-C Eliot May. Reproduced and modified with permission from Johnson BA, Ades A: Delivery room and early postnatal management of neonates who have prenatally diagnosed congenital heart disease. Clin Perinatol 2005;32:921–946, ix.)

difference was not statistically significant. In patients with a ventricular septal defect, the effect was opposite, with use of alpha-stat management resulting in significantly improved scores. There was a significant effect of cardiac diagnosis on outcomes. Both scores of the Bayley examinations were significantly higher in those with transposition compared to the other cardiac defects. Despite the equivocal data in this early report, with no longer-term follow-up yet available, many centers are currently utilising pH-stat management exclusively in all operations on neonates and infants.[60–62] Further research in this area, based upon additional potential modifiers, for example, cardiac diagnosis, age, pre-operative hypoxaemia, or presence of major systemic-to-pulmonary collateral arteries, should continue.

Deep Hypothermic Circulatory Arrest

Much has been written on the potentially deleterious effects of prolonged circulatory arrest with profound hypothermia in cardiac surgery for neonates and infants. It is generally agreed that very prolonged periods of uninterrupted circulatory arrest may have adverse neurological outcomes.

TABLE 64-1

POTENTIALLY MODIFIABLE INTRAOPERATIVE RISK FACTORS OF CEREBRAL INJURY

Air or particulate embolus
Rate and depth of core cooling (if utilized)
Deep hypothermic circulatory arrest (if utilized)
pH management during cardiopulmonary bypass
Hematocrit management during cardiopulmonary bypass
Reperfusion injury and inflammation
Rate of core rewarming/hyperthermia
Postoperative delivery of oxygen
Hypoglycaemia
Hyperoxia/hypoxaemia

Close inspection of the data shows that the effects of short durations of circulatory arrest are inconsistently related to adverse outcomes, and that the effect of circulatory arrest is not a linear phenomenon.[63,64] The effects are most likely modified by other pre-operative and post-operative factors related to the patient. Some reports, most in an earlier era of cardiac surgery demonstrate a detrimental effect of circulatory arrest on a variety of outcomes relating to the central nervous system,[7,9,65–68] while some demonstrate either an inconsistent effect or no effect.[12,37,69,70] Some have taken the stance that, since the majority of studies suggest a negative effect of circulatory arrest, it should be avoided at all costs. Innovative and challenging strategies have been designed to provide continuous cerebral perfusion during reconstruction of the aortic arch or intracardiac repair. The avoidance of circulatory arrest, however, by necessity requires an increased duration of cardiopulmonary bypass.[71] This has consistently been shown to have an adverse effect on outcomes in both the short and longer term.[72,73] A randomised trial comparing circulatory arrest to continuous cerebral perfusion has recently been completed at the University of Michigan.[74] This demonstrated no improvement in developmental scores at one year of age. Similar findings were reported in a contemporaneous but non-randomised study at Children's Hospital of Boston.[75]

It seems imprudent to change practice based upon studies with only short-term developmental assessment. Developmental studies in infants have very limited predictive validity for long-term outcomes, either for patients with[6,76] or without[77] congenital cardiac disease. Perhaps the best conducted study in this regard, which emphasises this point, is the Boston Circulatory Arrest Study.[5,6,63,76,78–81] In this study, a cohort of children with transposition undergoing an arterial switch were randomly assigned to intra-operative support predominantly by deep hypothermic circulatory arrest or predominantly by cardiopulmonary bypass at low flow. Earlier reports suggested that the group as a whole was performing below expectations in many aspects of evaluation, with worse outcomes for the those undergoing circulatory arrest in the areas of post-operative seizures,[80] motor skills at 1 year of age,[79] as well as behaviour, speech, and language at the age of 4 years.[5] Mean intelligence quotient at the age of 4 was lower than expected at 93, with no difference according to assignment. Many centers began avoiding even short periods of circulatory arrest based upon these and other reports.

In 2003, assessments of quality of life,[82] and detailed standardised testing[6] were reported. Neurodevelopmental analyses when the patients were aged 8 years revealed that the intelligence quotients for the cohort as a whole are now closer to normal, at 98 versus the population mean of 100. The patients did demonstrate significant deficits in visual-spatial and visual-memory skills, as well as in components of executive functioning such as working memory, hypothesis generation, sustained attention, and higher-order language skills. In other words, the children had difficulty coordinating skills in order to perform complex operations. Those repaired using circulatory arrest scored worse on motor and speech functioning, while those undergoing bypass at low flow demonstrated worse scores for impulsivity and behaviour. When compared to a normative sample, parents of the entire cohort reported significantly higher frequencies of attention problems, developmental delay, and problems with learning and speech. More than one-third of the population required remedial services at school, and one in ten had repeated a grade. Thus, in this population of patients who underwent the arterial switch operation between 1988 and 1992, there appears to be a correlation between congenital cardiac disease and its surgical repair, with difficulties occurring later with speech and language, behavioural difficulties, and execution planning in childhood.[6,16,63,82] Whether current modifications of techniques will improve the outcomes in the long term remains the subject of ongoing study.

This well-designed trial, with superb follow-up, enrolled neonates who were planned to undergo an arterial switch operation between 1988 and 1992. Hence, the results reflect the peri-operative and surgical care delivered in that era, and thus may not be generalisable to the current era, or to other congenital cardiac lesions. For example, some features of routine post-operative care, including extension of the anaesthetic period for at least 48 hours,[83] active rewarming in the intensive care unit after surgery, and hyperventilation to reduce the risk of pulmonary hypertension, may each independently and adversely affect neurodevelopmental outcomes. In addition, those patients randomised to predominantly continuous bypass did undergo a brief period of circulatory arrest. Thus, the study does not compare use of circulatory arrest to no circulatory arrest. The results, nonetheless, serve to show the multiple factors which influence developmental outcome at school age, and show that factors related to poorer outcome, such as deep hypothermic circulatory arrest, which seem apparent and significant on early testing, may be attenuated or even abolished during longer-term follow-up, as other factors assume a more important role.

Haematocrit During Bypass

During cardiopulmonary bypass, haemodilution has been widely applied based upon the notion that increased viscosity would be detrimental during periods of profound or even moderate hypothermia. Work in animals suggesting that higher levels for the haematocrit confirmed better cerebral protection[84] was recently investigated in two randomised clinical trials.[85] The results of these trials indicated that levels for the haematocrit up to 24% were associated with increasing scores in the psychomotor development index, although the improvement was not linear at levels greater than 24%. In addition, lower levels were associated with higher fluid balance and higher levels of lactate in the serum.[61,85,86]

Post-operative Factors

It has long been recognised that systemic flow is reduced in the first 24 to 48 hours following cardiac surgery, typically reaching a nadir in the first post-operative night.[73,87,88] At this time, the central nervous system may be especially vulnerable to secondary insults of decreased delivery of oxygen, particularly after circulatory arrest. To minimise the potential effects of low cardiac output following intra-operative ischaemia and reperfusion, the routine use of extracorporeal membrane oxygenation has been proposed for neonates at particularly high risk, such as those with hypoplastic left heart syndrome.[89] Post-operative mechanical support, however, has the potential to produce multiple deleterious effects, and the relative risks and benefits of this approach, as well as short- and long-term outcomes, are currently under investigation by those who performed the initial study.[89] Currently, close attention to cardiac output, and delivery and consumption of oxygen, seems warranted from the stance of the central nervous system, albeit that techniques for quantitative assessment of these parameters at the bedside is limited, particularly if there are residual intracardiac shunts.

Following cardiopulmonary bypass, with or without circulatory arrest, autoregulation of cerebral flow may be impaired, making the neonate and infant particularly vulnerable to periods of low cardiac output and/or hypoxaemia.[90] Although many studies in laboratory animals demonstrated various factors that adversely affect cerebral flow following cardiopulmonary bypass, it has previously been difficult to reproduce these studies in post-operative neonates and infants. Recently, transcranial Doppler and cerebral near-infrared spectroscopy techniques have been used to study cerebral flow in the cardiac intensive care unit following biventricular repair.[91] Approximately one in six of the patients studied demonstrated abnormalities of cerebrovascular pressure autoregulation, with risk factors including hypercapnia and higher mean arterial pressure during the time of the measurements. To date, the potentially deleterious effects of significant hypocapnia, which decreases total flow to the brain, and hypotension, the latter for ethical reasons, have not been studied in post-operative neonates. Further research is needed to determine the combined effects of cardiac output, mechanical ventilation, and cerebral flow, especially in the immediate post-operative period.

There have been recent reports following cardiac surgery in adults, as well in critically ill children with non-cardiac disease, suggesting that hyperglycemia is associated with adverse outcomes. These reports had stimulated some centers to develop protocols to control glycaemia, including continuous infusions of insulin, following congenital cardiac surgery in neonates and infants. However, recent reports have shown that hyperglycaemia is not a risk factor for adverse neurological or non-neurological outcomes in children after cardiac surgery.[92,93] In fact, hypoglycaemia may be more detrimental to the neonatal myocardium and brain. Thus, the treatment may be worse than the disease. This emphasises the point that extrapolation of research and management from patients without congenital cardiac disease to the neonatal and infant population following cardiac surgery should be undertaken with great care, skepticism, and after well-designed specific research.

Seizures have been reported to occur in the immediate post-operative period in up to one-fifth of neonates, depending upon the method used for detection. Clinical seizures are significantly less prevalent than those detected on continuous electroencephalographic monitoring.[78,94] The aetiology is most likely multi-factorial, but likely to be more prevalent in younger patients, those with prolonged periods of circulatory arrest, or those with co-existing abnormalities of the central nervous system. Peri-operative seizures are a marker for early injury, and have previously been reported to be associated with worse scores on developmental testing in children with transposition studied in the Boston Circulatory Arrest Trial,[5,79] although more recent data may show less of an impact than previously identified.[95]

In addition to the identified factors above, the immediate post-operative period typically requires invasive monitoring, mechanical ventilation and significant medical support, especially in the neonate and young infant.[4] While these therapies have resulted in significant improvements in mortality,[96] they increase the risk factors which may adversely affect the central nervous system, including paradoxical embolus of air or particulate matter from peripheral or central intravenous access, fever, hypoglycaemia and swings in cerebral flow brought on by acute changes in mechanical ventilation. As was previously reported in a group of children who underwent the Fontan procedure,[9] longer stay in hospital and in the intensive care unit in the neonatal period was associated with worse developmental outcomes at the age of 8 years.[81] These effects were significant, even when controlling for other factors known to adversely affect long-term outcome, such as seizures, intra-operative support duration, reoperations and other post-operative events. Children with transposition whose length of stay was in the fourth quartile had mean intelligence quotients 7.6 points lower than those in the first quartile. Further investigation into the multiple potential mechanisms of injury to the central nervous system in the intensive care environment must continue.

There has been increasing interest in monitoring of the central nervous system in the intensive care unit, with interventions aimed at improving short-term cardiac outcomes, as well as longer-term neurodevelopmental outcomes.[96,97] In particular, the increasing use of cerebral near infrared spectroscopy holds great promise in this regard.[98,99] The benefits and risks of near-infrared spectroscopy, as well as the longer-term predictive validity of lower scores has not yet been studied in detail. Nonetheless, this technology is currently in use in a large number of centres caring for neonates and infants with critical congenital cardiac disease.[100]

Continuous recording of the electroencephalogram, either with multiple channels or in an integrated fashion, also holds promise for peri-operative monitoring of the central nervous system. Abnormalities of the background electroencephalogram have been shown to be significantly related to other morbidities in the cardiac intensive care unit, such as the duration of mechanical ventilation, a longer length of stay in the hospital, and the need for supplemental tube feedings at hospital discharge.[101] These surrogate markers of injury are likely to be predictive of later neurological and developmental abnormalities.

Following discharge from hospital, some neonates remain at risk for ongoing injury to the central nervous system. Chronic hypoxaemia, as a result of ongoing palliation and/or residual intracardiac right-to-left shunting, may result in neurodevelopmental impairment. In children with transposition, older age at repair, as a surrogate for duration of hypoxaemia, has been associated with worse outcomes during follow-up.[102] Studies, many from a much earlier era of cardiac surgery when delayed repair was common, consistently show lower scores in children with cyanotic as opposed to acyanotic lesions.[103–113] Simple comparisons of defects with and without associated hypoxaemia, however, are confounded by the multiple factors present in children with cyanotic disease, including earlier age at repair and exposure to bypass, more complex surgical procedures, abnormal fetal patterns of flow, and many of the factors mentioned in this review. In children with structurally normal hearts and hypoxaemia from other causes, such as chronic lung disease, sleep disordered breathing, or high altitude, chronic or intermittent hypoxaemia has been associated with adverse effects on development, behaviour, and academic achievement.[114] The presence of hypoxaemia undoubtedly plays some role in patients with congenital cardiac disease, but is most likely modified by other factors, as it is difficult to measure the effect of hypoxaemia in isolation. The most recent studies comparing neurodevelopmental outcomes following repair of tetralogy of Fallot with those following isolated ventricular septal defect, support the potential impact of chronic hypoxaemia in these children.[27,115–117]

GENETIC AND ENVIRONMENTAL FACTORS

Socioeconomic state is perhaps the strongest predictor of eventual neurodevelopmental outcome, and is a reflection of both the environment and the genetic factors for development inherited from the parents. Multiple studies have shown the relationship between socioeconomic state and/or parental intelligence and outcome in children with congenital cardiac disease.[6,7,9,117,118] In adolescents and young adults who have undergone the Fontan procedure, socioeconomic state accounted for one-sixth of the variability in scores for intelligence quotient, whereas the percent variability explained by circulatory arrest and all other surgical variables accounted for only just over one-twentieth.[119] Curiously, this effect was not seen in a small cohort of teenagers with hypoplastic left heart syndrome.[69]

Children with identified genetic syndromes with known chromosomal abnormalities, such as Down, Williams, and DiGeorge syndromes and trisomy 13 and 18, as well as multiple associations of congenital anomalies, such as the CHARGE and VACTERL associations, frequently have co-existing congenital cardiac disease. In total perhaps one-third of all children with complex congenital cardiac disease have additional abnormalities besides their cardiac disease. Subchromosomal genetic abnormalities are being discovered with increasing frequency in this population, and most studies report worse outcome in children with associated congenital anomalies compared to children with the same lesion without additional anomalies.

Trisomy 21 is universally associated with mental retardation and other neurological impairments,[120,121] and is associated with a variety of cardiac defects, some associated with hypoxaemia, and many which require cardiopulmonary bypass for repair. Microdeletion of the 22nd chromosome has been shown to result in the phenotype of DiGeorge or velo-cardio-facial syndrome, with many of these children having abnormalities of the ventricular outflow tracts, such as tetralogy of Fallot, interruption of the aortic arch, and common arterial trunk, isolated ventricular septal defects, or abnormalities of branching of the aortic arch.[122] While some of the developmental delay and behavioural problems seen in these patients may be related to the underlying congenital cardiac disease and/or its treatment, as discussed above, and some of the speech delay may be related to the associated palatal abnormalities, recent reports suggest that there is an increased incidence of abnormalities in the white matter,[123] as well as a predisposition to psychiatric abnormalities.[124,125] Studies are currently underway to determine the relationship of these findings to the haploinsufficiency of genes on chromosome 22q11.[126]

Apolipoprotein E is also known to be important in the regulation of cholesterol metabolism, and is thought to effect neurological recovery following a variety of injuries to the central nervous system. Genetic polymorphisms of apolipoprotein E are related to abnormal neurological development, with a significantly smaller head circumference found in children aged 1 year who underwent open heart surgery as neonates or young infants.[127] The effect of the genotype was independent of ethnicity, socioeconomic state, cardiac defect, and the use of deep hypothermic circulatory arrest.

CURRENT OUTCOMES IN CHILDREN AND YOUNG ADULTS FOLLOWING REPAIR OF TETRALOGY OF FALLOT

Despite a nearly 60-year history of surgical intervention for tetralogy of Fallot, there are surprisingly few studies documenting neurodevelopmental outcome in this population. In addition, follow-up studies in such patients are confounded by the era in which surgery was conducted. For the contemporary population of adults, surgical management often entailed initial placement of a shunt as a source of supplemental pulmonary flow, followed by a more complete repair in later childhood. These patients, therefore, remained hypoxaemic for a longer duration of time. In the current era, most centers elect to perform a complete repair in infancy.

In spite of these limitations, patterns of deficiencies are emerging. Reports of patients in their third and fourth decades reveal that the mean scores for intelligence quotient are generally in the low normal range. This population, however, is facing challenges with respect to academic achievement and employment.[128,129] Comprehensive neurodevelopmental testing in such patients revealed significant deficits in executive function, including problem solving and planning strategies. In addition, a relatively small number of subjects pursued higher education and most did not have employment commensurate with the level of education. Interestingly, there was a correlation between the occurrence of pre-operative cyanotic spells and low self esteem and problems with executive functioning in adults.[128] Follow-up testing of early school age children who underwent surgical repair in the 1990s similarly indicates that while scores for intelligence are lower compared to the general population, the mean for the group is still within the normal range. Problems with executive function, attention, memory, language, visual-spatial skills, and sensory motor skills, nonetheless, are prevalent.[115,117,130]

Another important consideration when describing the neurodevelopmental and behavioural patterns in patients with tetralogy of Fallot is that approximately one-quarter have an extracardiac abnormality, including a genetic syndrome or a chromosome abnormality, which is independently associated with neurological impairment.[131] In particular, microdeletion of chromosome 22q11.2 is present in one-eighth of all patients with tetralogy of Fallot, and up to half of those patients who also have a right aortic arch.[122] Microdeletion of chromosome 22q11, in the absence of congenital cardiac disease, is associated with lower intelligence, learning disabilities, attention deficit hyperactivity disorder, and schizophrenia.[132] Accordingly, the association of genetic alterations in patients with tetralogy of Fallot adversely affects neurological outcomes.[70,133]

CURRENT OUTCOMES IN CHILDREN WITH TRANSPOSITION

In addition to the well documented longitudinal findings in the Boston Circulatory Arrest cohort, a number of additional studies have demonstrated similar findings. These include cognitive outcomes in the normal range in the majority of survivors, with a relatively high prevalence of mild learning disabilities, speech and language delays, behavioural problems, and inattention/hyperactivity.[118,134–138] The majority of a cohort undergoing an arterial switch as neonates between 1986 and 1992 described a good quality of life, and had not required a cardiac reintervention.[134,135] Similar to the findings from the Boston Circulatory Arrest Study, patients had normal scores on formal cognitive testing, but had significant deficiencies in the areas of language and speech, gross and fine motor coordination, as well as behavioural problems. A correlation was also found between peri-operative events, such as significant hypoxaemia or acidosis, prolonged cardiopulmonary bypass, or low cardiac output, and adverse neurodevelopmental and behavioural testing.[118,135]

CURRENT OUTCOMES IN CHILDREN FOLLOWING THE FONTAN PROCEDURE

Children with a functionally univentricular heart manifest many, if not all, of the risk factors for adverse long-term neurological and developmental outcomes. Most have abnormal fetal cerebral physiology, as well as ductal-dependant circulation at birth, require intensive care, early cardiac surgery with cardiopulmonary bypass with or without circulatory arrest, have prolonged and multiple hospitalisations, and a prolonged period of hypoxaemia. Thromboembolic complications and stroke may occur at any stage of surgical reconstruction and during follow-up.[139,140] Studies investigating the risk factors for adverse long-term outcomes in these patients are hampered by the interrelationship of most of the risk factors, and the frequent changes in surgical management. Studies of teenage children and young adults with the Fontan circulation have shown a higher than expected incidence of neurological problems. It is impossible to know if these outcomes represent sequels of management in the late 1980s and early 1990s, are inherent to the central nervous system of children with a functionally univentricular heart, or are a combination of these features. More recent studies have suggested better results,[141] but the predictive validity of preschool testing for the long-term is limited.[77]

As reported in children with transposition, deficits in visual-motor integration were common in those with the Fontan circuit,[67] and as a group, patients with the Fontan circulation and hypoplastic left heart syndrome had low-normal intelligence and difficulties with adaptive behaviour.[142] The largest series of children and young adults with a Fontan circulation to be studied to date underwent formal testing at Children's Hospital in Boston.[9] The results in these patients reflect the management of the 1970s and 1980s, with an average age at conversion to the Fontan circuit of 7.3 years. Intermediate superior cavopulmonary connections were performed in only a minority of the patients, as were fenestrations of the baffle. Over the duration of the study, a number of different surgical modifications were undertaken, hospital mortality was high, and prolonged pleural effusions were common in the survivors.[143] Thus, the generalisability of these outcomes to current patients may be questioned, the more so since only five patients had been included with hypoplastic left heart syndrome. Given these limitations, the majority of these patients had intelligence quotients and scores for achievement in the normal range, although the group performed lower than expected compared to their peers in the normal population. Risk factors for adverse outcomes in cognitive function included lower socioeconomic state, anatomical diagnosis, and the prior use of circulatory arrest. The risk factors for worse performance on testing for achievement included lower socioeconomic state, diagnosis, and circulatory arrest, as well as a number of post-operative factors such as the need for an early reoperation, longer length of stay, and higher right atrial pressures on the first post-operative day. Duration of hypoxaemia, that is the age at conversion to the Fontan circuit, in contrast, was not associated with adverse outcomes. The cohort has now been expanded to include patients from a more recent era, specifically with more patients who had undergone an interim superior cavopulmonary connection, as well as more patients with hypoplastic left heart syndrome.[7] These patients were considerably younger at the time of the Fontan procedure, and had scores slightly lower than the previously reported cohort. Longer total duration of circulatory arrest was significantly associated with lower scores. If one patient with a cumulative duration of 158 minutes was excluded from the analysis, however, the relationship was no longer significant. Interestingly, socioeconomic state was not associated with scores for intelligence. The conclusion reached was that the current approach to children with functionally univentricular hearts, with increasingly complex patients and a planned three-stage approach in most patients, has not significantly adversely affected outcomes compared to the historical cohort.

A contemporary cross sectional study has also been performed of patients who underwent a Fontan operation at The Children's Hospital of Philadelphia between 1992 and 1999.[144] Median age at follow-up was 8 years, and over half of the cohort included patients with hypoplastic left heart syndrome. A majority of children had required additional hospitalisations, and yet 9 out of 10 parents still rated the health of their child as excellent or good. Although standard testing for achievement was not performed in this cohort, two-thirds of parents rated school performance of the children as average or above average. Furthermore, there were no significant peri-operative predictors of poor school performance, including the diagnosis of hypoplastic left heart syndrome.

The increasing number of survivors among children with hypoplastic left heart syndrome undergoing staged reconstruction is one of the significant advances in paediatric cardiology and cardiac surgery in the past two decades. The oldest survivors from The Children's Hospital of Philadelphia have now been studied.[69] Mean scores on standardised testing were significantly lower than that in normative populations, two-thirds were thought to have attention deficit-hyperactivity, and one in five had clinically important scores for anxiety and depression. On multivariate analysis, it was the pre-operative state of the patient that most strongly predicted outcome, and intra-operative variables, such as duration of cardiopulmonary bypass or circulatory arrest, were not found to be associated with poorer scores. The authors argued that, with recent prenatal, intra-operative and post-operative advances, current results were likely to be better. This has now been confirmed by a recent study showing the average intelligence quotient to be 94 in the setting of hypoplastic left heart syndrome.[141]

It is of interest to examine the developmental abnormalities seen in groups of children with hypoplastic left heart syndrome, and compare them to the findings following infants undergoing transplantation for the same disease.[145,146] The patterns of dysfunction are remarkably similar, despite the markedly different therapeutic strategies. This suggests that factors other than the surgical approach and intra-operative support, such as congenital cerebral disease and abnormal fetal physiology, may play a more significant role in long-term outcome.

FUTURE DIRECTIONS

While advances in the medical and surgical fields have allowed the ability to mend children born with congenital cardiac disease, the increasing number of survivors has created a growing cohort of children with potential academic difficulties. The causes are clearly multi-factorial, additive, and incompletely understood. Much has been learned about cardiopulmonary bypass and the relatively short period of time these children spend in surgery. Much more work needs to be done to understand the modifiable risk factors in the peri-operative period, the influences of the timing of surgery, and whether or not improved monitoring of the central nervous system in the intensive care unit setting will improve neurological and developmental outcomes.

CONCLUSIONS

In Figure 64-4, we show some of the current understanding regarding the multiple factors which may adversely affect the central nervous system in children with complex congenital cardiac disease. There is a growing body of literature showing suboptimal outcomes in school age children, particularly with respect to attention, behaviour, higher order executive function, handwriting and school performance. Many of the

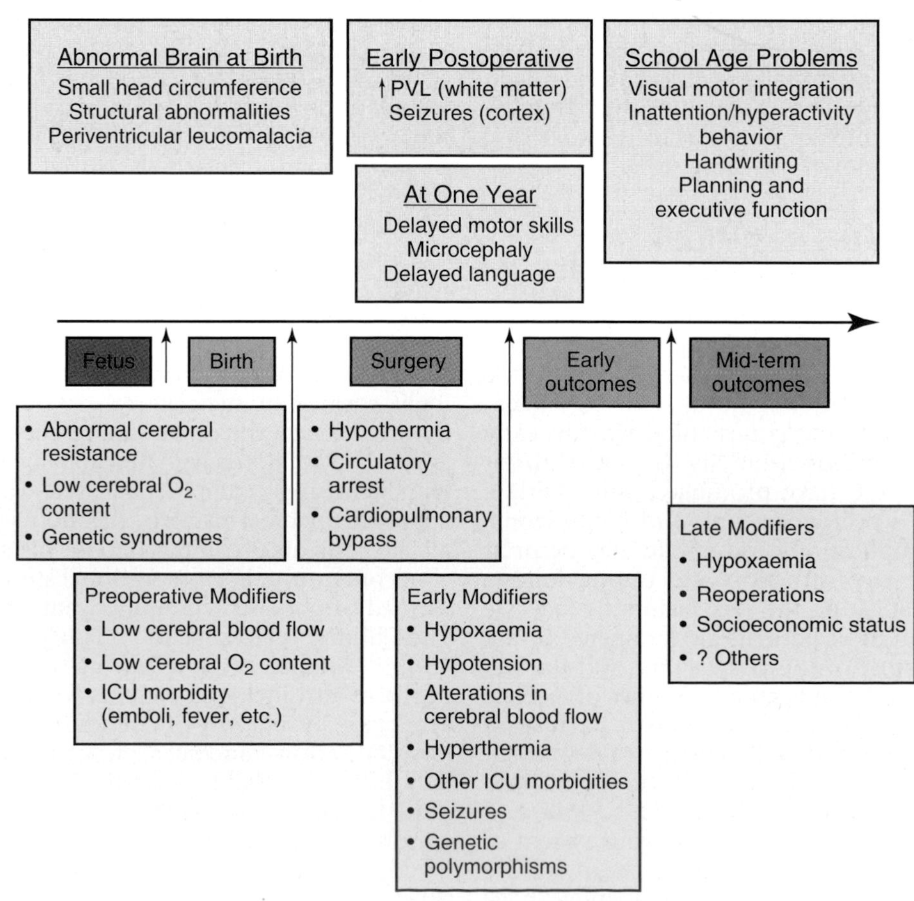

Figure 64-4 Currently identified factors that, in total, adversely affect long-term neurological and developmental outcomes in children with complex congenital cardiac disease. ICU, intensive care unit; PVI, periventricular leucomalacia. (From Wernovsky G: Current insights regarding neurological and developmental abnormalities in children and young adults with complex congenital cardiac disease. Cardiol Young 2006;16[Suppl 1]:92–104.)

risk factors for adverse outcomes are interrelated, such as abnormalities of the fetal circulation, the need for prolonged intensive care, complex operations with cardiopulmonary bypass with or without deep hypothermia and circulatory arrest, prolonged hypoxaemia and multiple reoperations. Thus, it is difficult to conclude which, if any, are most explanatory. Many of the reports on the effects of cerebral consequences of cardiopulmonary bypass in particular are conflicting, and there is a need for ongoing laboratory experiments and controlled clinical trials before sweeping changes to intra-operative management are undertaken, with particular attention to long-term outcomes in school age children. Neurodevelopmental abnormalities are widely prevalent, and are major contributors to adverse health-related outcomes concerning quality of life. Further research must continue, in the laboratory, inpatient, and outpatient settings.

The complete reference list can be found on the companion Expert Consult web site at www.expertconsult.com.

ANNOTATED REFERENCES

- Bellinger DC, Bernstein JH, Kirkwood MW, et al: Visual-spatial skills in children after open-heart surgery. J Dev Behav Pediatr 2003;24:169–179.

  This study is part of the series of reports from the Boston Circulatory Arrest Study group, in which a total of 171 children born with transposition were randomised to undergo the arterial switch operation with either low-flow cardiopulmonary bypass or a predominant deep hypothermic circulatory arrest strategy between 1988 and 1992. The cohort has been followed prospectively, and various aspects of the 8 year follow-up data are published. In this report, Bellinger and colleagues have explored the clinical significance of visual-spatial deficits, which were not only found in this population of patients with transposition from the Boston Circulatory Arrest Study, but are patterns reported for other forms of congenital cardiac disease as well. The authors used the Rey-Osterrieth Complex Figure, which is a standardised design-copy task developed to elicit more complex processes required for visual-perception and visual-motor skills. Additional testing was performed in order to delineate the neuropsychological origins of poor performance on the copy task. The results revealed that over one half of the children in the cohort scored at the lowest level, which is twice as many as expected in a normal population of 8-years-olds. Impaired visual-perception skills, rather than motor or cognitive skills, were implicated as the primary contributor to the poor performance on the Rey-Osterrieth Complex Figure test. Of note, neither peri-operative events nor intra-operative strategy were significantly associated with poor performance. Visual-spatial deficits and specifically visual-perception deficits are associated with difficulties in specific academic areas, such as mathematics. This study provides unique insight into the practical implications for children and their families, and the findings from the adolescent follow-up of this cohort should present even more information about how visual-spatial deficits identified in the early school years affect later academic achievement and social integration.

- Limperopoulos C, Majnemer A, Shevell MI, et al: Predictors of developmental disabilities after open heart surgery in young children with congenital heart defects. J Pediatr 2002;141:51–58.

  This study is part of a series of published reports from Montreal Children's Hospital describing ongoing follow-up of a cohort of children who underwent cardiac surgery requiring cardiopulmonary bypass, with or without deep hypothermic circulatory arrest, before the age of 2 years. Neurodevelopmental evaluations were performed prior to surgery, and follow-up occurred at 12 to 18 months after surgery. Of note, patients with hypoplastic left heart syndrome were excluded. The authors found that fine and gross motor deficits were present in two-fifths of the tested cohort, and significant deficits in language, eye-hand coordination, practical reasoning, locomotor, and personal social difficulties were also present. Microcephaly was present in three-tenths of the group, and global developmental delays were identified in nearly one quarter. The pre-operative neurological status was found to be predictive of delay at the follow-up, and specifically the presence of pre-operative microcephaly was a strong predictor of adverse outcomes. A longer duration of deep hypothermic circulatory arrest time was associated with worse outcomes. In addition, prolonged length of stay and need for intensive care was associated with worse outcomes. The findings from this study add to the growing body of data outlining the potential deficits facing survivors of early cardiac surgery, while also highlighting the importance of identifying patients in the peri-operative period who are at higher risk of later neurodevelopmental impairment, which will ultimately prove valuable for educating and counseling families.

- Creighton DE, Robertson CM, Sauve RS, et al: Neurocognitive, functional, and health outcomes at 5 years of age for children after complex cardiac surgery at 6 weeks of age or younger. Pediatrics 2007;120:e478–e486.

  Creighton and colleagues from Alberta Children's Hospital report the 5-year follow-up of 85 infants who underwent cardiac surgery prior to 6 weeks of age between 1996 and 1999. Of the initial infants enrolled, 61 were available for assessment, and represented five surgical groups: arterial switch operation, arterial switch operation with ventricular septal defect closure, Norwood procedure, simple total anomalous pulmonary venous repair, and a miscellaneous group. The Norwood patients scored lower than both the arterial switch operation groups and the total anomalous pulmonary venous return repair group for full scale intelligence quotient and verbal intelligence quotient. The duration of deep hypothermic circulatory arrest and cardiopulmonary bypass did not correlate with cognitive outcomes. The authors previously published the results of developmental assessments at 2 years of age from this cohort, and were able to demonstrate that subjects receiving normal assessments at 2 years of age continued to do well at 5 years of age. In addition, fewer subjects had impaired cognitive scores at 5 years than at 2 years. An important strength of this study is that multiple forms of cardiac defects are represented, and therefore allows for comparison of differences between cardiac defects in the setting of relatively standardised peri-operative management.

- Uzark K, Jones K, Slusher J, et al: Quality of life in children with heart disease as perceived by children and parents. Pediatrics 2008;121:e1060–e1067.

  Uzark and colleagues from Cincinnati administered the Pediatric Quality of Life Inventory Generic Core Scales and Cardiac Module to 475 families and 347 school age children with varying levels of cardiac disease. Overall, children self-reported significantly lower scores for psychosocial and physical functioning compared to normal healthy populations. While subscale scores for emotional and social functioning were also lower than normal children, the most dramatic differences were for school function. Children with more severe cardiac disease reported lower scores for physical functioning, but there were only small differences in psychosocial scores among disease severity. In contrast, parental reports of quality of life varied based on the age group of the child. Total quality of life scores in the toddler and child age group were not significantly different compared to the normal children, while reports from parents of teenagers did reveal a significant difference. Moreover, lower scores from parents correlated with more significant cardiac disease. This extensive evaluation in a large sample provides a contemporary review of how cardiac disease affects children as they progress through school and provides compelling evidence for ongoing assessments not only of physical health, but also school performance and social functioning. In addition, the discrepancy between parental and child reports suggests that children with cardiac disease may have more impairment than parents realise.

- Moons P, Van Deyk K, De Bleser L, et al: Quality of life and health status in adults with congenital heart disease: A direct comparison with healthy counterparts. Eur J Cardiovasc Prev Rehabil 2006;13:407–413.

  Moons and associates from Leuven, Belgium, have published several reports challenging the notion that adults with congenital cardiac disease universally have a poor quality of life. The authors propose that traditional measures of quality of life have concentrated too heavily on functional outcomes such as employment or education level, rather than focusing on the individual's perception of life satisfaction. In this study, 404 adult patients with varying forms of congenital heart disease and 404 healthy matched controls were recruited to participate in a questionnaire study to assess both quality of life and perceived health status (three different standardised scales were used and are described in detail in the manuscript). Overall, the patients reported high scores for subjective health status. Patients reported that the most important determinant of quality of life was 'feeling that one's body is less capable than one would wish'. When compared to the healthy controls, the patients actually reported a better quality of life, while there was no significant difference for self-perceived health status between the groups. The authors note that the adults with congenital heart disease may have different values or coping skills with respect to quality of life perceptions compared to the general population and thus measures of quality of life should not be limited to functional outcomes only. As the number of adult patients with congenital heart disease increases, outcome evaluations will become increasingly important. Moons and colleagues have shown that the quality of life for this population is not significantly different from the general population if the assessment is based on the individual's perceptions.

- Miller SP, McQuillen PS, Hamrick S, et al: Abnormal brain development in newborns with congenital cardiac disease. N Engl J Med 2007;357:1928–1938.

  The authors from University of California, San Francisco utilised advanced techniques, such as magnetic resonance spectroscopy and diffusion tensor imaging, to analyse the brains of 41 newborns with either transposition or functionally single ventricle prior to cardiac surgery. One-third of the cohort had evidence of pre-operative neurological injury in the form of white matter injury, stroke, or haemorrhage, while new post-operative injuries were identified in an additional three-tenths of the cohort. Abnormalities were identified using both techniques indicative of immature brain metabolism and microstructural development. The findings suggest that full-term infants with complex congenital cardiac disease have impaired cerebral development with patterns that are similar to preterm infants at birth. Since the neurodevelopmental outcomes in congenital cardiac disease are strikingly similar to those described in premature infant follow-up studies, the finding of brain immaturity is congruent. Moreover, the studies were performed in pre-operative infants, and thus the brain abnormalities are presumably related to impaired fetal central nervous system development. Understanding patterns of cerebral blood flow and delivery of oxygen to the fetal brain will be an important area of research in light of the findings from this study.

- Rosenthal GL: Patterns of prenatal growth among infants with cardiovascular malformations: Possible fetal hemodynamic effects. Am J Epidemiol 1996;143:505–513.

Geoffrey Rosenthal examined newborn infants with four types of congenital cardiac disease who had been enrolled in the Baltimore–Washington Infant Study, which was a population based case-control study designed to explore environmental and genetic risk factors for congenital cardiac disease. Eligible subjects included full-term infants without associated extracardiac abnormalities and comprised 69 patients with transposition, 66 patients with tetralogy of Fallot, 51 patients with hypoplastic left heart syndrome, 65 patients with coarctation of the aorta, and 276 controls. Anthropometric measurements, as well as the ponderal index, a measure of relative thinness, were abstracted from patient records. Potential confounders such as maternal weight gain, smoking, pre-pregnancy weight gain and diabetes mellitus, as well as infant sex, race, and gestational age were also included in the statistical model. Compared to controls, infants with transposition had a smaller head circumference, shorter birth length, and greater birth weight given birth length, as well as a smaller head volume relative to birth weight. Thus these infants tended to have smaller head circumference, but greater birth weight. Infants with tetralogy of Fallot had lower birth weight, shorter birth length, and smaller head circumference compared to controls. Infants with hypoplastic left heart syndrome similarly had smaller head circumference, lower birth weight, and shorter birth length, with a more striking difference in the head volume relative to birth weight. Thus infants with hypoplastic left heart syndrome were small in all dimensions, but the head size was relatively smaller compared to the other dimensions. Infants with coarctation were found to have larger head volume relative to birth weight, but overall lower birth weight and shorter birth length. This study is an eloquent demonstration of variances of patterns of fetal growth among four different forms of congenital cardiac disease that presumably maintain unique alterations of fetal circulatory patterns which affect cerebral blood flow. More information is needed regarding fetal brain development in congenital cardiac disease in order to correlate the observations from this study with later neurological impairment.

- Hoffman GM, Mussatto KA, Brosig CL, et al: Systemic venous oxygen saturation after the Norwood procedure and childhood neurodevelopmental outcome. J Thorac Cardiovasc Surg 2005;130:1094–1100.

Hoffman and associates from Children's Hospital, Wisconsin investigated the neurodevelopmental status of 13 patients with hypoplastic left heart syndrome at a mean age of 4.5 years after a Fontan completion. The specific aim of this study was to assess the influence of systemic venous saturation of oxygen in the post-operative period as a measure of systemic delivery of oxygen. In other words, is there a correlation between post-operative hypoxaemia and later neurodevelopmental outcome. Mean scores for all developmental measures (McCarthy Scale of Children's Abilities–Motor and General Cognitive, Beery Test of Visual-Motor Integration, and Achenbach's Child Behaviour Checklist) in this cohort were within the normal range, but overall lower than expected in the normal population. Statistically significant differences were observed for the McCarthy scale of Children's Abilities–Motor and the Composite score. Of the peri-operative variables assessed, only systemic venous saturation of oxygen correlated with abnormal outcomes significantly. Moreover, a longer duration with a low systemic venous saturation of oxygen was associated with a greater relative risk of abnormal outcome. Although a significant limitation of this study is the small sample size, the data suggests a valid link between the post-operative state and later neurodevelopmental outcomes, as well as suggests the benefits of non-traditional monitoring in the post-operative period.

- Hovels-Gurich HH, Konrad K, Skorzenski D, et al: Long-term neurodevelopmental outcome and exercise capacity after corrective surgery for tetralogy of Fallot or ventricular septal defect in infancy. Ann Thorac Surg 2006;81:958–966.

Hovels-Gurich and colleagues from Aachen University of Technology have published a series of follow-up studies in children who underwent cardiac surgery in infancy in order to investigate the longer-term effects of pre-operative hypoxaemia compared to infants without pre-operative hypoxaemia, but with pre-operative symptoms of cardiac failure due to pulmonary over-circulation. No subject had an identifiable chromosome abnormality or genetic syndrome. One-third of the total cohort had evidence of central nervous system abnormalities, but there was not a statistically significant difference between those with tetralogy of Fallot or ventricular septal defect. The total group also had significantly worse scores compared to age-matched published controls. Gross motor dysfunction was higher for those with tetralogy of Fallot compared to ventricular septal defect, but there were no differences between the groups for the other domains. Exercise capacity was not significantly different compared to the normal population. Although the cohort is relatively small in this study, the conformity of the peri-operative management between the two groups provides a basis for assessing the impact that prolonged hypoxaemia may have on outcomes. Additional published reports from this group have investigated behaviour, quality of life, and speech and language outcomes. There continues to be a trend toward those with tetralogy of Fallot scoring worse than those having a ventricular septal defect, although the effects on behavioural outcomes appear to be more related to attention problems.

- Gaynor JW, Gerdes M, Zackai EH, et al: Apolipoprotein E genotype and neurodevelopmental sequelae of infant cardiac surgery. J Thorac Cardiovasc Surg 2003;126:1736–1745.

Gaynor and associates enrolled 368 infants, who underwent cardiac surgery before 6 months of age at The Children's Hospital of Philadelphia between 1998 and 2001. Pre-operative data was obtained on all subjects, and 1-year neurodevelopmental evaluations were performed in 244 of the survivors. The primary aim was to evaluate whether genetic polymorphisms are associated with longer-term outcomes. Apolipoprotein E is a regulator of cholesterol metabolism and specifically involved in lipid transport in the central nervous system. In adults, specific isoforms of apolipoprotein E have been associated with Alzheimer's disease, as well as recovery after neurological injury. The results of this study revealed a significant association between the presence of the APOE ε2 allele and a lower Psychomotor Development Index from the Bayley Scales of Infant Development. The implications of this association suggest that infants at risk for more significant neurological injury may be identified pre-operatively or even antenatally based on genetic testing, and these findings may impact counseling as well as management techniques in the future. However, more definitive evaluations in older children will provide valuable information. The 4-year follow-up of this cohort is underway.

CHAPTER 65

Communication with the Referring Teams Providing Health Care

PAUL STEPHENS, Jr., TYRA BRYANT-STEPHENS, and GIL WERNOVSKY

Communication between the cardiologist and providers of primary care is an essential component of the medical care of the patient, and is of increasing importance in the current era, which is marked by increased complexity of medical testing and polypharmacy. Breakdowns in this vital area of communication can result in delayed or missed diagnoses, repeated or unnecessary testing, and increased risk of litigation.[1] The challenges that face patients with congenitally malformed hearts go beyond their particular pathophysiology. All patients with important cardiovascular defects require healthcare delivered by multiple teams. The providers of primary care, general practitioners, and general paediatricians, are usually the first line of defense against morbidity and mortality for these patients, and usually are based close to the area of residence of the patient. The cardiac specialist may be located a great distance from the patient, and therefore must maintain constant and consistent interaction with the team providing primary services in order to optimise the delivery of healthcare. Difficulties in communication between generalists and specialists have been extensively documented. Many physicians learn how to perform effective consultations through trial and error, resulting in considerable variability in consultation skills[2] and frustrated referring physicians. Paediatricians have generally been slow in developing an infrastructure for effective consultation, and most of the landmark literature in this area comes from experience with adult patients. Explicit instructions have been developed for internists in how to perform effective consultations.[2] In this chapter, we review some of the challenges encountered when multiple teams care for a mutual patient. Some common problems are highlighted by making reference to hypothetical cases. We also offer some thoughts on potential solutions.

CASE I

Dr. John has referred a patient to you. On completing your evaluation, you feel sure that the patient has a small haemodynamically insignificant ventricular septal defect that does not require surgical intervention. At the consultation with the parents, you assured them that their child was well, required no intervention or restrictions of exercise, and recommended reassessment in from 2 to 3 years. Now the child wants to participate in competitive athletics, and the parents are concerned about the cardiac defect, and if the child should be allowed to compete at a level of high intensity.

Whose Patient Is This?

The overall health of the child is, first and foremost, the responsibility of the team providing primary healthcare, and consultants must recognise their subsidiary role.[2] This is always the case, irrespective of whether the cardiac disease is trivial or complex. Prolonged stays in hospital, particularly soon after birth in the neonatal intensive care and step-down units, often result in the accumulations of multiple problems. The complexity of those problems facing the parents makes the assimilation of medical information a difficult task for hospital-based specialists, let alone the provider of primary care, who must eventually assume this responsibility after the patient is discharged from the hospital. In the present era of improved surgical outcomes, and higher rates of survival, a common scene experienced by the generalist is the follow-up visit subsequent to the hospitalisation of the infant with complex congenital cardiac disease. After appropriate visits with the supervising cardiologist, these infants require visits with their providers of primary care for mandatory immunisations, anticipatory guidance for young and new parents, as well as surveillance of other organ systems that are critical for normal growth and development. Complex medical problems can be intimidating for any caregiver, but the team providing primary healthcare typically possesses a very balanced fund of medical knowledge and expertise in a number of areas, enabling those persons to be the most qualified medically to supervise the child subsequent to discharge. The potential disconnection between those providing primary care and the patient subsequent to prolonged hospitalisations, nonetheless, may lead to a lack of confidence on the part of the primary caregiver. In consequence of this disconnection, the needs of the patient, with the exception of immunisations, may be left in part to the specialist, who cares for the most complex, or most potentially life-threatening, of the medical problems. This relinquishment of the overall care of the patient to the specialist should be avoided. The specialist team can play a major role in ensuring that the generalist remains the confident primary provider of healthcare. Timely, and collegial, communications from the specialist in paediatric cardiology, including details of the precise diagnosis and plans for treatment, may help the team providing primary healthcare to feel empowered to provide ongoing care for the patient.[3]

In the hypothetical situation outlined above, the provider of primary care, with guidance from the paediatric cardiologist, should make the decision regarding participation in sports. The cardiologist, for example, may not be aware of other conditions, such as absence of, or damage to, one of paired organs that may preclude participation in certain competitive sports. Because of this, the specialist may give inappropriate approval for the patient to participate in activities that could be detrimental to health in the event of injury. The team providing primary services is most important in this framework of a tiered approach to comprehensive provision of health care. Dysfunction may ensue if roles and responsibilities are not appropriately assumed.

Parental Concerns: Who Should I Call to Discuss a Medical Problem?

Although the paediatric cardiac specialist knows that the overall surveillance of the health of the child is primarily the responsibility of the team providing primary care,[4] parental confusion, and at times unrealistic expectations, are occasionally encountered by the cardiac specialist. The dilemma of which specialist to call for symptoms and signs of illness may be a problem even for physicians. Parents, who for the most part have no formal medical training, also share in this dilemma. Telephone calls, and increasingly, email correspondence to cardiac specialists that should be directed toward the primary team, and communications in the opposite direction, are not uncommon events, particularly when made by parents who have children with newly diagnosed cardiac disease. A substantial number of parents of children with serious cardiac disease may believe that the provider of primary care is unable to meet many of the needs of their child.[5] It is important for the cardiac specialist to have patience with the parents, grandparents, and guardians of children with cardiac disease when family concerns result in what can seem to be endless or inappropriate telephone calls, and frequent visits.

Many times, it is the level of parental anxiety, rather than the complexity of the cardiac disease, which is the determining factor for frequent contact with the specialist. The number of telephone calls and visits expressing anxiety correlate inversely with the length of experience that the parents have in managing their child with cardiac disease. The number of telephone calls, however, does not appear to vary directly with the complexity of the cardiac conditions. In our experience, even simple congenital cardiac malformations not requiring surgical treatment have produced high levels of anxiety in family members, who have needed constant reassurance regarding the well-being of the child. More parental experience with children with congenital cardiac disease appears to translate into a lower level of anxiety, and fewer telephone calls to the cardiac specialist. The majority of parents of teenagers with congenital cardiac malformations preferred using their provider of primary care rather than their paediatric cardiologist as a point of first contact for all concerns relating to general health, as well as for many potential concerns relating to the heart.[6]

Parental anxieties seem to escalate whenever a sudden unexpected, or unsolved, death occurs in the community or nationally, and gains significant attention in the media. The cardiac specialist should not be surprised when urgent referrals are needed to rule out cardiac disease, particularly after the unexpected death of a local or well-known athlete prior to the start of the school season when pre-participatory evaluations for sport are in full swing in the offices of providers of primary care. A plethora of referrals to the cardiac specialist typically follows for a short period of time whenever such an event occurs. The ebb and flow of such referrals are, and will likely always be, a part of the practice of the primary team, as well as the cardiac specialist. These physicians can take advantage of available ancillary tests in the face of such an epidemic of the need for cardiac consultation. Many families are very uncomfortable waiting for the elective appointment to rule out cardiac disease, and can be reassured if preliminary tests are normal. The cardiac specialist can advise the primary team so as to alleviate some of these concerns by taking advantage, in this particular situation, of the availability of an electrocardiogram. A normal electrocardiogram makes unlikely the diagnoses of hypertrophic cardiomyopathy, this being the leading cause of sudden death in competitive athletes in the United States of America. Electrocardiographic testing can be used in many cases transiently to alleviate some parental concerns until the time that the child can be seen by the cardiologist.

CASE 2

A child aged 2 years, having chronic lung disease and stridor, is referred for exclusion of cardiac disease. The parents relate that the paediatric pulmonologist, who had seen the child approximately one week previously, was concerned about a possible vascular ring, and had referred the child for a cardiac consultation. The physician providing primary care had not yet received written correspondence from the paediatric pulmonologist, and did not understand the need for the referral.

Modes of Communication

The nature of the correspondence from the cardiologist should reflect the tiered system of provision of care. Irrespective of who has referred the patient to the cardiac specialist, the primary team should be the primary addressee for all correspondence. The type of correspondence can be variable. Some consultants choose to send a preliminary short communication, delineating the diagnostic impression and suggested therapeutic plan, while others choose to communicate to the referring physician via an electronic medical record. Irrespective of the mode of communication, the paediatric cardiologist is encouraged to have the communication transcribed as soon as possible after the encounter with the patient. Although the busy cardiologist may find time short, and possibly delay the communication to a more convenient time, such an approach results in more time being spent in trying to recall the details of the encounter. Prompt communication is also frequently helpful to the provider and family in the event that cardiac disease is excluded and the patient needs referrals to additional specialists, or requires completion of forms allowing participation in competitive sports. Many studies have documented inadequate feedback from the consulting physicians in rural settings, and also in university medical centres.[7–9] A study of the communication between oncologists and general practitioners found problems with the timeliness of communication and suggested interventions included greater use of telephone or fax, improved secretarial support, the use of email, nurse-led communications, universal patient records, and revisiting the option of patient-held medical records.[10] In one study, referring physicians who enclosed an addressed envelope with the request for consultation increased the percentage of consultant feedback from two-fifths to three-fifths.[9] In the past, electronic mail had not been widely accepted by specialists or generalists as a preferred method of communication,[11] albeit that this pattern may change in the future. Even with the use of electronic correspondence, one study cited the lack of timely information as a major reason for dissatisfaction among providers of primary care.[12] If promptly performed soon after the visit, electronic transfer of information has the potential to induce major cultural changes in the delivery of healthcare.[13] Although quite difficult to perform for most busy specialists, most referring physicians prefer direct verbal communication, a type of communication for which there is likely no substitute, especially if the consultant thinks that the recommendations are crucial or controversial.[2,14] Goldman and colleagues,[2] in their landmark article, stated succinctly 'talk is cheap, and effective'. Despite the previously well-documented observation that direct communication by phone is a highly valued activity by generalists, the minority of specialists shared this opinion.[11] In one study, the satisfaction ratings for the referring physicians was found to be highest for referrals involving specialist feedback by both telephone and letter.[15] Consulting physicians are more likely to respond to the referring physician by phone, or in person, if they were directly contacted by the referring physician.[7] Studies have also shown that attention to these factors influences the choice made by the primary team concerning specialist referral. A comprehensive detailed prompt communication, clearly delineating the plans for treatment, the natural course of disease, and issues related to management, is associated with a greater level of satisfaction for the primary team.[16]

The cardiac consultant must also develop a style of communication that suits himself or herself, and that is appropriate for the recipient. A brief informal survey of a clinical practice at the Children's Hospital of Philadelphia revealed that most clinicians prefer communications that are both informative of the particulars of their patient, and also instructional in a general sense. In this survey, the majority of the respondents of this hospital-based centre for primary care reported reading the letter from the consultant in its entirety, both for information about the patient as well as for didactic purposes The latter point may come as a surprise to many cardiac specialists, who have been under the impression that only the initial impression, and the component relating to therapeutic plans at the conclusion of the letter, are read by the primary team. Although the didactic, instructional, letter requires more time from the cardiac specialist, at least one such letter, among the many which will accrue for a patient with complex cardiac disease, will likely aid and equip the referring provider, which may lead to more confidence in the care of these patients. This concept of teaching with tact, an instructional letter that is not overly simplistic, was one of the original ten commandments for effective consultation.[2,14] Furthermore, referring letters which have elements of anticipatory guidance, for example listing of the typical symptoms to be expected for pulmonary over-circulation in patients with an unrestrictive ventricular septal defect, may help the primary provider be on guard for these symptoms, and help to guarantee that certain patients are not lost to follow-up. Generalists and specialists agree that consultation letters should include information about how to manage acute problems in patients with chronic disease.[11] Citations of literature in the communication have not generally been felt to be helpful.[14]

Additional correspondence detailing results of tests not immediately available on the initial day of consultation day, such as the outcome of 24-hour ambulatory electrocardiographic monitoring, have also been a challenge for the busy cardiac specialist. Every effort should be made, nonetheless, to assure the written completion of the medical record. Well-formulated diagnostic summaries, and plans for treatment, in the medical record also help to eliminate potentially extra work in the form of telephone calls and repeated referrals. There is also less anxiety on the part of both the referring provider and the parents if sufficient information from the consultant is provided in a timely fashion.

Long lists of problems, particularly complex medical problems involving multiple subspecialties, as well as fear of making major, and even minor, errors, may elicit anxiety on the part of providers of primary care. Good communication can minimise this anxiety. The cardiac specialist can play a major role in alleviating the stress associated with managing patients with complex medical problems by frequently updating the primary team during prolonged hospitalisations, and also by prompt communication of the results of outpatient visits. Likewise, the cardiac specialist may feel intimidated when patients are noted to have non-cardiac illnesses that can cause significant morbidity, and or mortality. Asthma, influenza, developmental delay, and complications from neoplastic disorders, are not uncommon medical problems which are encountered in patients with cardiac disease. Although once skilled in the care of these problems, most cardiologists, particular ones furthest away from medical training, may not possess the appropriate skills to manage such medical problems, and may inadvertently place the patient at risk. Parents frequently feel that the cardiologist, particularly those providers who have cared for their child since the diagnosis of the illness, appear to have medical knowledge that extends beyond the discipline of cardiology. The reasons for this sentiment are not entirely understood, but perhaps relate to the recognition by the parents that their cardiac consultant knows their child exquisitely well, which is quite true. This knowledge of the medical history of the child, however, does not always translate into proficiency in managing non-cardiac medical conditions. The cardiac specialist, therefore, should not feel incompetent or inferior when faced with a non-cardiac condition that is perplexing, or even simple, but nonetheless beyond his or her expertise. The specialist should always suggest to the parents to seek the advice of their primary team, rather than potentially to mismanage non-cardiac maladies.

Involvement of the primary team in the entire process of managing complex patients not only should be exercised when non-cardiac problems surface, but should also be a process that occurs early in the care of the patient. A discussion to involve the primary team at an early stage in the process of care is not the usual mode of operation in large tertiary centres. Furthermore, there can even be arrogance on the part of the subspecialist. Such arrogance may manifest as disparaging remarks made behind doors, or lack of appropriate and timely communications. This type of behavior is probably not rare among today's medical professionals, and runs counter to the first code of ethics of the American Medical Association, which stated in 1847:

> *A physician who is called upon to consult, should observe the most honorable and scrupulous regard for the character and standing of the practitioner in attendance: the practice of the latter, if necessary, should be justified as far as it can be, consistently with a conscientious regard for truth, and no hint or insinuation should be thrown out, which could impair the confidence reposed in him, or affect his reputation.*

Unless there is incompetence that can affect the health of the patient, consulting physicians should avoid denigrating colleagues.[4]

As already discussed, the tension that can occur when providers of primary care are invited into the planning of care at a relatively late stage may result in such a degree of discomfort and difficulty that a critical error can occur in management. Late involvement of the primary team may lead to more work for the cardiologist, and at times less expertise in the care of the patient, thus placing the patient at risk for missed diagnoses or inappropriate treatment. The cardiac specialist should recognise this bias and, although more time costly in the short term, interact with the primary team on a professional level at all times. Ultimately, time, and respect, will be gained with such an approach.

Similar lessons are important for the team providing primary care. Some high-volume general practices may refer patients to the specialist, rather than discuss the case personally, via either phone calls or emails, so as to assess if the referral is necessary. Such an approach may lead to a pattern of over-referral, frequently of relatively non-complex medical problems. Potentially long waiting times for the appointment with the specialist may increase the anxiety of both physician and parents, which may have been minimised with a personal communication with, and reassurance from, the cardiac specialist. The cardiac specialist should encourage an open communication with those providing primary care, either by telephone or email, which may potentially reduce unnecessary referrals. A plan for open communication may also facilitate the delivery of results in a timely fashion for patients who require only an electrocardiogram, and who do not require a formal complete cardiac assessment, such as children who are medicated with drugs having cardiac side-effects requiring serial electrocardiographic monitoring. Some patients enter the office of the cardiac specialist with a collection of reports from recent tests aimed at diagnosing the problem at hand. The cardiac specialist is occasionally faced with weeding through the results of tests that may have not been necessary. Rather than perseverating over the necessity of the tests, and even perhaps the referral itself, an available cardiac specialist can play a role earlier in the process of referral.

Increasingly, written correspondence from the specialist to those providing primary care is also sent to the families of the patient. Possession of the relevant letters by the parents, or even the patient him or herself, may improve the overall care, and involve the patient and their families in their own healthcare. Written correspondence serves to reinforce what was discussed in the office visit, and may not have been remembered or was misinterpreted.[17] In a recent study, patients appreciated receiving a copy of the letter sent to the team providing primary care.[18] Although patients do not always understand fully the content of the letter,[19,20] a certain level of understanding is nevertheless achieved, and comprehension is improved when a second, less complex, letter is sent directly to the patient from the specialist. This letter also opens up dialogue between the parent and physician by triggering questions about things that might not have been understood. Many times, it is hard for parents to comprehend all of the information and instructions that are given to them at the first visit with the specialist. By receiving a copy of the letter, they are able to review the diagnosis and instructions, as well as ask questions for clarification. This interpretation is confirmed by studies concluding that most parents of children were satisfied when they received a copy of the letter that was sent to their general practitioner,[21] although it did not necessarily improve compliance with future visits.[22] Fewer errors in information have occurred when the letter was dictated in the presence of the patient.[19] The letter allows families to carry a copy of the cardiac details when travelling, so that all of the details of complex disease do not need to be remembered. Despite evidence that satisfaction amongst patients is improved when they receive a copy of the correspondence from the specialist to the generalist, physicians remain largely resistant to performing it.

CASE 3

A generalist desires an appointment for an infant of 6 months, who was noted to have a murmur during a regular check up. The parents have become more anxious after learning that the earliest available appointment with the cardiac specialist requires a waiting time of 2 months. The parents request that the paediatrician intervene.

How Long Is Too Long?

Generally speaking, most referrals to the cardiac specialist do not represent emergencies, while few are urgent. Truly emergent referrals are quite rare. One of the more common dilemmas for the team providing primary care involves determining the appropriate waiting time for referrals to subspecialists. The team may not feel qualified to ascertain if a few months of waiting time is too long. The cardiac specialist can play a key role in helping to solve this problem. Cardiac specialists, and providers of primary care, agree that a child who is failing to thrive, and has evidence of pulmonary over-circulation, requires an urgent referral, whereas an undiagnosed cyanotic patient, or one who is desaturated, needs to be seen immediately. Asymptomatic patients who have femoral pulses that are difficult to palpate, or absent, usually require urgent consultation. Patients with tachyarrhythmias or significant bradyarrhythmias usually require direct treatment in the emergency room, while those with arrhythmias and haemodynamic instability require immediate treatment in the office.

In our experience, infants who are not cyanosed, are gaining weight appropriately, and have strong femoral arterial pulses by palpation, rarely have immediately life-threatening congenital cardiac disease. In the hypothetical case highlighted above, the cardiac specialist can reassure the family and those providing primary care, that, in the absence of the above findings, the probability for significant cardiac disease is low. The patient can be given a routine appointment, and the family can be given the option of an earlier appointment in the event that another family cancels their appointment. The level of anxiety suffered by the parents, nonetheless, despite the reassurance of those providing primary care, needs to be factored in to the timing of the appointment.

There are a few helpful adjustments or modifications in the arena of rapid accessibility that the cardiac specialist may offer to the providers of primary healthcare. The availability of satellite clinics may give the generalist more options in securing an appointment for their patients, especially when these visits can be arranged during non-traditional hours, such as appointments in the evening, or at week-ends. The outpatient physicians at the centres organised by Children's Hospital of Philadelphia saw 22,839 patients during the past academic year. Of these, one-third of the encounters occurred in satellite clinics closer to the homes of the patients. A significant increase in the outpatient visits during the past few years was a direct result of encounters at satellite clinics. Increased availability of appointments has resulted in improved satisfaction for both the patients and the referring physicians.[23]

THE CARDIOLOGIST AS A RESOURCE OF THE COMMUNITY, AND AN ADVOCATE FOR THE PATIENT

Barriers to communication can be chipped away when the cardiac specialist serves more than just a consulting role in the direct care of patients, but also as a resource for the community. Making the generalist, parents, and community-at-large aware of available professional resources specifically designed for the patient with cardiac disease has proven to be helpful at the Children's Hospital of Philadelphia, which regularly sponsors seminars providing information about the cardiac problems for parents, and conferences providing continuing medical education for professionals. Sponsoring the patients with complex malformations for the Make-a-Wish Foundation, a benevolent organisation that attempts to deliver the once in a lifetime experience for terminally ill children, is a worthwhile activity. The cardiac specialist can also make parents aware of other resources, including summer camps for patients with cardiac disease, internet chat sites, or web logs for parents and patients with congenitally malformed hearts, along with other resources which have helped the child to reintegrate back into his or her community after cardiac interventions. Our group has brought attention to the neurological and psychological issues faced by patients with cardiac disease. Studies on hyperactivity attention deficit disorder in patients with palliated or repaired defects have revolutionised the need for early intervention, prompting teachers, parents, and communities to recognise the potential need for remedial services for this vulnerable population.[24] A programme has been established for surveillance in the home that reduced interstage mortality and improved the survival of patients with functionally single ventricles.[25,26] Efforts have been made to place automated external defibrillators in schools in an attempt to reduce the risk of sudden catastrophic events in high school athletes.[27] Programmes such as these, which go into the community for the provisions of service, have redefined the notion of how large hospitals providing tertiary care can provide for their patients. These ventures, and others, have helped to forge alliances among providers of primary care, cardiac specialists, and community-based workers.

CONCLUSIONS

Optimal care involves a collaborative approach between the team providing primary care and the specialist. Open lines of communication are the cornerstone of this approach, and should optimally involve various combinations of direct, written, faxed and electronic forms. All parties benefit when the provision of healthcare is shared amongst the providers. The teams providing primary care usually gain a higher level of professional satisfaction and confidence when intricately involved in the making of decisions involving their medically complex patients. Most importantly, the patients derive the most benefit when communication is timely, complete, and neither overly simplistic nor pedantic. When lines for communication are firmly in place, it is possible to maximise satisfaction for both the provider, the patients, and the families.

The complete reference list can be found on the companion Expert Consult web site at www.expertconsult.com.

ANNOTATED REFERENCES

- Epstein RM: Communication between primary care physicians and consultants. Arch Fam Med 1995;403–409.

  A frequently cited article that explores some of the core issues pertinent in problems of communication among physicians, including the different subcultures that have evolved among physicians providing primary care and specialists. Case scenes highlighting the communication barriers are given.

- Goldman L, Lee T, Rudd P: Ten commandments for effective consultations. Arch Intern Med 1983;143:1753–1755.

  Excellent and frequently cited opinion article from a major teaching hospital in Boston, Massachusetts, that serves as a guide, not meant to be all-inclusive, of some of the essential features of an effective consultation. The consultant is encouraged to determine the question, establish urgency, gather the data ('look for yourself'), be as brief as possible, be specific, provide contingency plans, not covet the patient ('honour thy turf'), teach with tact without condescension, contact directly with the referring physician and provide appropriate follow-up.

- Pearson SD: Principles of generalist-specialist relationships. J Gen Intern Med 1999;14(suppl 1):S13–S20.

  An opinion article promoting the general principles which should guide the interaction between the specialist and generalist. Duties of the referring and consulting physicians, joint duties and responsibilities of healthcare plans in supporting this relationship are discussed.

- McPhee SJ, Lo B, Saika GY, Meltzer R: How good is communication between primary care physicians and subspecialty consultants? Arch Intern Med 1984;144:1265–1268.

  Prospective study of 464 consecutive patient referrals from 27 practitioners of a general internal medicine group at a university medical centre in San Francisco, California. Despite referring physicians provision of background information in 98% of the cases, communication of the findings by the consultants occurred in only 55% of the consultations.

- Cummins RO, Smith RW, Inui TS: Communication failure in primary care. JAMA 1980;243:1650–1652.

  Survey of 233 referrals to specialists from a two-physician practice within 80 km of two university medical centres. The overall rate of receiving follow-up information was 62%. Private specialists provided more follow up information (78%) than either university affiliated emergency rooms (48%) or university affiliated specialty clinics (59%).

- Curry RW, Crandall LA, Coggins WJ: The referral process: A study of one method for improving communication between rural practitioners and consultants. J Fam Pract 1980;10:287–291.

Randomised prospective study of 235 patient referrals from three rural primary care clinics to a university medical centre in Gainesville, Florida. Receipt of specialist feedback occurred at a higher percentage (60%) when a mailer was included in the consultation request than with patient referrals in which a request for feedback and a return mailer was not included (39%). Private specialists were also more likely to provide feedback.

- Farquhar MC, Barclay SI, Earl H, et al: Barriers to effective communication across the primary/secondary interface: Examples for the ovarian cancer patient journey. Eur J Cancer Care (Engl) 2005;14:359–366.

This study explored the views of general practitioners regarding the process of communication from specialists in patients with ovarian cancer. Nine general practitioners experienced in the care of patients with ovarian cancer from predominantly semi-rural regions in the United Kingdom participated in a structured interview process within 6 months of the death of their patient. The main challenge of communication reported by the practitioners was the tardiness of the written or oral communication which led to handcuffing of the general practitioners in their ability to provide appropriate care. General practitioners reported inadequacies in their knowledge of test results and felt out of touch with the state of the patient. Subsequent to the insufficient communication, the practitioners reported feeling inadequate in their ability to provide moral support, crisis management, patient advocacy, and end of life care. Suggested communication improvements are reported in the text. General practitioners as a group welcomed calls from doctors or nurses.

- Stille CJ, Primack W, Savageau JA: Generalist-subspecialist communication for children with chronic conditions. Pediatrics 2003;112:1314–1320.

A survey of 403 paediatricians, specialists and generalists, in New England identifying target areas to improve communications between the two groups when sharing care of chronically ill patients. Differences in perception about the adequacy, timing and type of the communication were found. Suggestions for targeted interventions are given.

- Gandhi TK, Sittig DF, Franklin M, et al: Communication breakdown in the outpatient referral process. J Gen Intern Med 2000;15:626–631.

A survey of providers of primary care and specialists at a major teaching hospital in Boston, Massachusetts. Of the providers of primary care, 63% were dissatisfied with their current referral process, citing the major problems of communication being the lack of timeliness of information and inadequate referral letter content. Two weeks after the referral visit, two-fifths of the providers of primary care had received no information from the specialists and 4 weeks after the referral visit, one-quarter still had yet to receive written correspondence.

- Salerno SM, Hurst FP, Halvorson S, Mercado DL: Principles of effective consultation. Arch Intern Med 2007;167:271–275.

An anonymous survey of 323 providers of adult medicine in the United States of America exploring the ideal relationships between referring and consulting physicians. Specialty-dependent differences in referring and consulting practices were noted. A modified ten commandments for effective consultation is proposed.

- Forrest CB, Glade GB, Baker AE, et al: Coordination of specialty referrals and physician satisfaction with referral care. Arch Pediatr Adolesc Med 2000;154:499–506.

A survey of 122 pediatricians located in 85 practices throughout 34 states in the United States of America conducted by the Pediatric Research in Office Settings, a research based network established by the American Academy of Pediatrics. This survey examined the bidirectional transfer of information between referring and specialist physicians. Referring physicians were most satisfied when specialists communicated results by both telephone and letter, however this occurred in only 7% of the 964 referrals. Only 51% of the referrals were completed (defined as when the referring physician received written feedback from the specialist) within 3 months after the specialist visit.

- Kinchen K, Cooper L, Levine D, et al: Referral of patients to specialists: Factors affecting choice of specialists by primary care physicians. Ann Fam Med 2004; 2:245–252.

This was a national cross sectional study of primary care physicians in the United States via questionnaire. Respondents identified factors of major importance when choosing a specialist, with a response rate of 59%. The medical skill of the specialist was identified as the most important variable when choosing a specialist. Timeliness of the appointment, prior experience with the specialist and the quality of the specialist communication to the primary care physician were also deemed to be of major importance.

- Cowper DM, Lenton SW: Letter writing to parents following paediatric outpatient consultation: A survey of parent and GP views. Child Care Health Dev 1996;22:303–310.

A survey of parents and general practitioners of paediatric outpatient clinic patients at a major teaching hospital in Bath, United Kingdom. All 103 parents were in favor of receiving a letter from their child's specialist and most general practitioners considered that the letters would improve parental satisfaction and compliance.

- Saunders NC, Georgalas C, Blaney SP, et al: Does receiving a copy of correspondence improve patients' satisfaction with their outpatient consultation? J Laryngol Otol 2003;117:126–129.

A cohort of 200 patients in the United Kingdom were randomly assigned to receive a copy of the letter that was sent from the specialist providing treatment of diseases of the ear, nose, and throat to their general practitioner and were asked to complete a satisfaction survey. Compared to those that did not receive a copy of the letter, recipients had a higher satisfaction score. The only other factors predictive of a higher level of satisfaction were spending more time with the doctor or having a detailed explanation of the problem.

- Roberts, NJ, Partridge, MR: How useful are post consultation letters to patients? BMC Med 2006;4:2.

This study was performed in the United Kingdom involving 62 patients and the aim was to assess the utility of letters sent from the specialist to both the general practitioner and patient. Separate letters which summarised the encounter between the specialist and the patient were sent to both the general practitioner and the patient. The recipients were asked to evaluate these letters in terms of readability and accuracy of content. The majority of the patients expressed satisfaction about receiving a letter at their reading level, while the minority of patients preferred receiving copies of both letters. Few general practitioners desired receiving both letters, reporting that there was an increased workload, having to read both. Patients and general practitioners were also asked to circle items that were not comprehensible or inaccurate. Very few letters had inaccuracies, and as expected, most patients circled more items that were not comprehensible on the general practitioner's letters compared to the letters sent specifically to them. The article concluded that patient satisfaction improved when they received letters from the specialist despite the lack of full comprehension of the letter.

- O'Reilly M, Cahill M, Perry I: Writing to patients: A randomized controlled trial. Clin Med 2006;6:178–182.

This is a randomised controlled study of 150 patients in a general hematology clinic in Limerick, Ireland, to determine whether a brief letter of thanks for attending the clinic visit versus a detailed letter from the consultant recounting the visit would enhance recall of the visit. The majority of the patients were more satisfied with the detailed letter from the consultant, but there was no substantial difference in recall of information among the two groups.

- Waterson T, San Lazaro C. Sending parents outpatient letters about their children: Parents' and general practitioners' view. Qual Health Care 1994;3:142–146.

The study assessed the impact of letters from the general paediatric specialist to the families of the referred paediatric patient and also to the general practitioner. The majority of the families reported that the letter from the specialist improved their understanding of the medical problem and they were happy to have received a letter. The majority of the general practitioners favored the idea, however many of the general practitioners expressed reservations about direct communication between the specialist and the parents of the patient.

CHAPTER 66

Growth and Nutrition

LISA M. KOHR and NANCY J. BRAUDIS

Nutrition is fundamental for ensuring adequate energy for basal metabolism, growth, and physical activity. Infants and children possess high metabolic rates and limited reserves of endogenous substrates at baseline, and are at risk for developing deficiencies of energy during episodes of acute or chronic illness.[1] Infants and children with congenitally malformed hearts are at significant risk for developing such energetic imbalance due to increased expenditure of energy, and poor or inadequate nutrition.[2] Energetic imbalance leads to the development of malnutrition, which can adversely affect somatic growth, along with cognitive and motor development.[3] Failure of growth alters the metabolic response to injury and, for children with congenitally malformed hearts, increases the risk of post-operative morbidity and mortality, contributing to longer lengths of hospitalisation and times needed for recovery.[1]

MALNUTRITION

Malnutrition is defined as a state of poor nutrition and failure of growth (Table 66-1). Failure of growth exists when weight, or weight for height, is less than 2 standard deviations below the mean for sex and age, weight is less than the third centile, or weight for age has a *z* value of less than −2.0.[4] Criterions for the diagnosis of malnutrition also apply to children whose curve for gain in weight crosses more than 2 centiles from baseline on the growth charts created by the National Center for Health Statistics after having previously achieved a stable pattern. The baseline centile is the maximum weight achieved between 4 and 8 weeks of age, as studies have shown that the gain in weight during this time period correlates with the weight at the age of 12 months.[4]

Malnutrition is a well-known consequence of congenital cardiac disease. It is estimated that four-fifths of hospitalised infants with congenitally malformed hearts suffer from acute or chronic malnutrition.[5] Prior to the 1980s, when such children underwent surgical correction at an older age, those with acyanotic and cyanotic lesions exhibited failure of growth at birth that persisted well into childhood.[6] In the current era of neonatal surgery, there has been a shift in the severity of pre-operatively delayed growth from the infants with cyanotic lesions to those having congestive cardiac failure. This is due primarily to the earlier age at surgical intervention.[7] The cause of malnutrition in these children is multi-factorial, albeit that the magnitude of the disturbed growth appears to be related to the anatomical lesion.[1]

Significance of Malnutrition in Those with Congenitally Malformed Hearts

Malnutrition, specifically failure of growth, has been reported in more than half the children with congenitally malformed hearts.[2] The amount and type of retardation in somatic growth varies depending on the haemodynamic impact of the defect. In one study,[8] factors impacting on the extent of malnutrition included gender, the type of cardiac disease, weight at birth, thickness of the subscapular and triceps muscles, and cephalic circumference. The index of weight for length was found rapidly to decrease in those with cyanotic lesions, albeit that no differences in anthropometric measurements were noted between those having cyanotic and acyanotic lesions. Boys showed greater deterioration in weight for age, suggesting more acute malnutrition, while girls had lower linear growth for age, indicative of more chronic malnutrition. In another study,[9] somatic growth was shown to be most affected in patients with large ventricular septal defects and tetralogy of Fallot, improving after operative repair, but failing to normalise. Catch-up growth for length was strongly correlated with severity of pre-operative growth failure, but not with age at operation.[9] In yet another study,[10] weight was found to be below the third centile in half of those studied, height in one-third, and skin fold thicknesses in from one-eighth to one-fifth, thus endorsing the findings of Chen and colleagues.[2]

MECHANISMS OF FAILURE TO GROW

Congenital Cardiac Disease

As discussed already, at birth, infants with both cyanotic and acyanotic cardiac lesions are more likely to have low weight.[2,8] The Baltimore-Washington Infant Study[11] found that infants with tetralogy of Fallot, atrioventricular septal defects, ventricular septal defects, and hypoplastic left heart syndrome had the lowest weights at birth, even when corrected for gestational age, findings endorsed in another study, this one showing also that those with transposition had normal weights at birth.[12]

Failure to grow after birth is dependent on the haemodynamic effects of the cardiac lesion. The growth curve of neonates with mild malformations may be minimally affected, while those with severe cyanotic disease are at

TABLE 66-1

WATERLOW CLASSIFICATION OF MALNUTRITION

Range	Acute Malnutrition (Wasting) (% Median of Weight for Height)	Chronic Malnutrition (Stunting) (% Median of Height for Age)
Normal	>90	>95
Mild	80–90	90–95
Moderate	70–80	85–90
Severe	<70	<85

Adapted from Waterlow JC: Classification and definition of protein-calorie malnutrition. Br J Med 1972;3:566–569.

highest risk for malnutrition.[13] Pulmonary hypertension appears to be an important risk factor for failing growth in those with both acyanotic and cyanotic lesions, such children tending to suffer severe growth failure.[14]

Congestive cardiac failure causes a hypermetabolic state and subsequent growth failure.[1] Cardiac lesions commonly resulting in congestive cardiac failure include hypoplastic left heart syndrome, patency of the arterial duct, totally anomalous pulmonary venous connection, critical valvar aortic stenosis, coarctation of the aorta, and ventricular septal defects.[15,16] With large and unrestrictive left-to-right shunts, excessive flow of blood to the lungs causes increased pulmonary and left heart pressures, along with elevated left ventricular end-diastolic pressures, resulting in a high-output state and failure to grow.[14]

Children with cyanotic defects frequently have decreased weight and height compared to healthy infants.[15] Cyanotic lesions such as transposition and tetralogy of Fallot with and without pulmonary atresia usually have right-to-left shunting resulting in hypoxaemia. The duration of hypoxaemia in years is directly related to the retardation of growth.[2] Children who are both hypoxaemic and have congestive cardiac failure are more severely affected.[2]

Children with multiple anomalies, in addition to congenital cardiac disease, are at the highest risk for acute and chronic malnutrition.[2] Genetic syndromes frequently associated with congenital cardiac disease, including trisomies 21, 13, and 18, Turner's syndrome, Williams syndrome, Noonan's syndrome, and DiGeorge syndrome, may also impact the rate of growth due to alterations in caloric intake, gastrointestinal absorption, metabolism, and expenditure of energy.[1,2]

Inadequate Caloric Intake

Inadequate caloric intake is believed to be the main cause of infants with congenital cardiac disease failing to grow. The feeding patterns of such children have been compared to matched subgroups of normal infants.[1,17] For infants with congenitally malformed hearts, feeding is equivalent to an exercise test, demanding increased amounts of energy. Intolerance of feeding can be attributed to an inability to expend sufficient energy on feeding, as exhibited by tachycardia, tachypnoea, shortness of breath, and vomiting. Other contributing factors include early satiety, decreased gastric capacity caused by hepatosplenomegaly, delayed gastric emptying time secondary to low cardiac output and an uncoordinated suck, and abnormal patterns of swallowing and breathing due to tachypnoea. Additionally, fluid restrictions and diuretic therapy as part of the medical management may limit caloric intake.

Hypermetabolism

Energetic imbalance is a major contributing factor to failure of growth and malnutrition in children with congenitally malformed hearts.[18] The energy available for metabolism is the sum of total energy expenditure and energy stored. Basal metabolic rate represents the major component of total energy expenditure and metabolisable energy. In general, children have a higher metabolic rate, placing them at high risk for energetic deficiencies during episodes of acute illness.[1] The basal metabolic rate of infants is almost twice that of an adult per kilogram of body weight.

Children with congestive cardiac failure have been reported to have up to five times higher basal metabolic rates than children without cardiac disease.[18] The elevated basal metabolic rate may be due to the increased workload of the cardiac and respiratory systems. Resting expenditure of energy represents consumption of oxygen per kilogram of body weight, and has been shown to be increased in malnourished infants with congestive cardiac failure.[1] This increase has been attributed to a dilated or hypertrophied cardiac muscle, which can use up to one-third of the total oxygen consumed by the body, compared to one-tenth used by the healthy child.[10] Other conditions which have been attributed to an elevation in the total body metabolic rate in children with congestive cardiac failure include increased activity of the sympathetic nervous system, haematopoietic tissue, and respiratory muscles.[1]

Frequent respiratory infections and fever will also contribute to a state of hypermetabolism and failure of growth. In infants, total expenditure of energy is increased due to an increase in physical activity from 5% of total metabolisable energy intake at 6 weeks of age to 34% at 12 months of age.[19] A marked rise in total energy expenditure relative to resting energy expenditure occurs in 3- to 5-month-olds with left-to-right shunting lesions due to increased cardiac workload, increased work of breathing, diminished myocardial efficiency, and increased stimulation of the sympathetic nervous system.[1]

Malabsorption

Malabsorption is another condition which contributes to the malnutrition seen in children with congenitally malformed hearts. This can result from gastrointestinal tissue hypoxia, and causes feeding intolerance, limits caloric intake, and decreases absorption of nutrients.[13] The presence of hepatosplenomegaly may cause decreased gastric capacity and altered oral intake of nutrients. Those with cardiac lesions resulting in right-sided cardiac failure and increased systemic venous pressure due to right-to-left shunting may develop oedema of the intestinal wall and mucosal surfaces. These changes in the intestinal wall will lead to impaired nutrient extraction and malabsorption, affecting the timing, volume, and caloric density of feedings.[13]

Growth Factor Hormone

Endocrine factors have been investigated as a possible cause for the growth delay in children with congenital heart disease.[20] Others found a positive correlation between low saturations of oxygen and levels of IGF-1 in the serum, indicating that hypoxaemia may be an independent factor contributing to growth failure.[21–23]

ASSESSMENT OF GROWTH DELAY

Physical Growth

Physical growth is a direct reflection of nutritional well-being and is the single most important parameter used in assessing nutritional growth. Periodic assessments should be made to determine whether weight, height, length, and head circumference are within normal limits for age and gender. Anthropometric measurements can assess the longitudinal speed of growth. Length is the most useful indicator, and is most reliable after 2 years of age due to the difficulty in obtaining accurate measurements in infants.[4] Weight for height, the ratio of true weight to the ideal weight for height, is used to differentiate stunted growth from wasting independent of age. Stunting caused by chronic malnutrition, chronic illness, and genetic or endocrine abnormalities results in a child who is small for age but proportional for weight to height.[4] Body mass index is the best indicator of excess weight and obesity in children and adolescents. Children with an index between the 85th and 95th centiles are considered at risk for being overweight, whilst those with an index greater than or equal to the 95th centile are considered obese.[24] Head circumference is a useful tool until the child reaches 3 years of age. It is particularly important for children who have undergone a bidirectional Glenn procedure, and may provide information regarding the patency of the shunt. Measurements of the skinfolds at the triceps and the suprailiac crest are useful for estimating total body fat. Their application is limited in infants and young children, however, due to their lack of validity.[4] Other tools exist, but are rarely used routinely in children, again due to lack of validity, coupled with lack of accessibility, invasiveness, or cost.

Anthropometry

For children who are hospitalised, anthropometry may occur on a daily or biweekly basis to track tolerance of oral feedings, or effectiveness of breast-feedings, high-calorie diet, or anti-congestive therapy. Standard guidelines point to a target gain of weight of 10 to 35 grams per day for infants, depending on their age in months[25] (Table 66-2). Infants who are undernourished have weights that plot at 2 standard deviations below the mean for gender and age on the growth charts compiled by the National Center for Health Statistics.[4] The rate of gain in weight of children with congenitally malformed hearts is typically affected more than the height. If the nutritional deficit is severe and long term, weight and height are equally affected.[8] Currently, there are no standard measurements which have been established for the population with congenitally malformed hearts. Interpreting data collected for this population, and evaluating any delayed growth on the basis of standards derived from healthy children, therefore, may exaggerate the degree of malnutrition.

Prealbumin

Prealbumin, also known as thyroxine-binding prealbumin, or transthyretin, is a sensitive marker for assessing the severity of illness in children who have critical or chronic disease, and correlates with outcomes and recovery.[26] Specifically, levels of prealbumin have been shown to be a sensitive indicator of protein-calorie nutrition. The marker is more sensitive than either albumin or transferrin in measuring intake of protein and calories.[26] Being a negative acute phase reactant, its levels will decrease in presence of inflammation. It also decreases in the presence of hepatic dysfunction, since it reflects the ability of the liver to synthesise protein. Due to the accessibility of the test, and the rapid turnover in results, measuring levels of prealbumin allows for a more accurate and timely assessment of change in diet.[26] Serial levels obtained once or twice a week can assist in identifying nutritional adequacy.[27] The test should be used when there is suspicion of subclinical or marginal levels of protein-calorie nutrition, to assess the nutritional response to diet, including parenteral nutrition, and as a biochemical marker of nutritional adequacy in premature infants.

TABLE 66-2

EXPECTED GAINS IN WEIGHT FOR INFANTS AND OLDER CHILDREN

Age	Weight (g/day)	Length (cm/mo), Crown to Heel
Newborns (gestational age)		
31 wk	24	3.2–4.4
34 wk	35	
>36 wk	30	
Infants		
0–3 mo	25–35	2.6–3.5
4–6 mo	15–21	1.6–2.5
7–12 mo	10–13	1.2–1.7
Children		
1–3 yr	4–10	0.7–1.1
4–6 yr	5–8	0.5–0.8
7–10 yr	5–12	0.4–0.6

NUTRITIONAL MANAGEMENT

Requirements of Nutrients in Infancy

There are six classes of nutrients that influence the patterns of growth in infants and children: carbohydrates, fats, proteins, vitamins, minerals, and water, which in combination provide optimal nutrition and allow somatic growth (Table 66-3). Nutritional options in infancy include breast-feeding along with a host of commercial formulas prepared specifically for premature and term infants, as well as for specific medical conditions. For healthy infants up to 6 months of age, the recommended dietary allowance in terms of calories is from 108 to 117 kilocalories per kilogram of body weight (kcal/kg) per day.[25] The need for protein during early infancy is high, due to rapid muscular and skeletal growth, and approximately 2.2 grams per kilogram of body weight[4] (see Table 66-3). Neonates with haemodynamically significant congenital cardiac malformations require substantially more nutritional support to sustain and catch up growth than do their healthy counterparts.[1] Those with mild to moderate disease may require from 130 to 150 kcal/kg per day, while those having moderate to severe lesions may require as much as 175 to 180 kcal/kg

TABLE 66-3

RECOMMENDED MACRO AND MICRO NUTRIENTS FOR GROWTH

Component	Function	Recommended Daily Intake	Special Considerations for CHD
Calories	Provides energy for all metabolic processes and to support growth.	Calorie levels based on EER and activity levels from the Institute of Medicine, Dietary Reference Intakes (DRI) Macronutrient Report, 2000. *Premature infant* 110–130 kcal/kg *RDA* 0–6 mo, 108 kcal/kg 7–12 mo, 98 kcal/kg 1–3 yr, 102 kcal/kg 4–6 yr, 90 kcal/kg Females 11–14 yr, 47 kcal/kg; 15–18 yr, 40 kcal/kg Males 11–14 yr, 55 kcal/kg; 15–18 yr, 45 kcal/kg	Children with CHD may require up to 50% more calories due to increased metabolic needs. Catch-up growth in children with growth failure is determined by ideal body weight for height and using indirect calorimetry or calorie levels based on EER. Caloric requirement for infants with poor growth: kcal/kg = RDA for age (kcal/kg) × ideal weight for height divided by actual weight Supplementation may be required with calorie-dense formula, supplemental NGT/GT feedings, or high-calorie diet.
Protein	Major structural component of all cells, acts as transport carrier.	Protein requirements are based on metabolic needs. Preterm infant 1.1–1.5 g/kg *RDA* 0–6 mo, 1.52 g/kg 7–12 mo, 1.2 g/kg 1–3 yr, 1.05 g/kg 4–6 yr, 0.95 g/kg Females 11–13 yr, 0.95 g/kg; 14–18 yr, 0.85 g/kg Males 11–13 yr, 0.95 g/kg; 14–18 yr, 0.85 g/kg	Children with CHD may require twice the recommended amount of protein due to malnutrition and severe protein losses. When protein modular is used for caloric supplementation, monitor for increased solute load.
Carbohydrate	Calorie source to maintain body weight. Primary source of energy for the brain.	RDA 55%–60% of total calories Children and adults, 130 g/day Added sugars should not exceed 25% of total calories consumed.	Carbohydrate modular use for caloric supplementation may cause increased fecal output due to high osmolarity.
Fat	Increases absorption of fat soluble vitamins. Source of n-3 and n-6 polyunsaturated fatty acids (essential component of cell membrane, involved in cell signaling).	*AMDR* *Children* 1–3 yr, 30–40 g 4–8 yr, 25–35 g Males and females >9 yr, 25–35 g	Fat modular use may cause delayed gastric emptying and decreased appetite. Use with caution in patients with history of gastroesophageal reflux or aspiration.
Fluids/Water	Essential for maintaining vascular volume.	Fluid (volume/24 hr) *Premature infant* 80 mL/kg/day on day 1 of life Increase by 10–20 mL/kg/day as infant matures. Weight ≤10 kg = 100 mL/kg Weight ≤20 kg = 1000 mL + 50 mL/kg for each kg above 10 kg Weight >20 kg = 1500 mL + 20 mL/kg for each kg above 20 kg	Preterm infants have increased fluid requirements (up to 130–150 mL/kg/day depending on birth weight. Neonates and children with unrepaired CHD may require fluid restrictions. Following complete repair, fluid may be liberalized as tolerated.
Vitamins			
Vitamin A	Antioxidant, important in protecting mitochondria and cells from reactive oxygen intermediates. Essential for normal vision, gene expression, embryonic development, growth and immune function.	0–6 mo, 400 μg 7–12 mo, 500 μg 1–3 yr, 300 μg 4–8 yr, 400 μg Females 9–13 yr, 900 μg; 14–18 yr, 600 μg Males 9–13 yr, 600 μg; 14–18 yr, 900 μg	Children with heart failure may require higher amounts of certain micronutrients to optimize cardiac function. Serum levels of micronutrients may not reflect adequacy of nutrients at the tissue level.
B_1, thiamine	Coenzyme for carbohydrate metabolism and maintenance of myelin for nerve and muscle function.	0–6 mo, 0.2 mg 7–12 mo, 0.3 mg 1–3 yr, 0.5 mg 4–8 yr, 0.6 mg 9–13 yr, 0.9 mg Females 14–18 yr, 1.0 mg Males 14–18 yr, 1.2 mg	Endogenous antioxidants include enzymatic antioxidants (zinc in superoxide dismutase or selenium in glutathione peroxidase), free radical scavengers (vitamins A, C, and E) and metal chelators.
B_3, niacin	Functions in intracellular respiration, fatty acid synthesis, and glucose oxidation. Decreases cholesterol and lipoprotein levels.	0–6 mo, 2 mg 7–12 mo, 4 mg 1–3 yr, 6 mg 4–8 yr, 8 mg 9–13 yr, 12 mg Females 14–18 yr, 14 mg Males 14–18 yr, 16 mg	During stress, free radical production exceeds normal clearance. Antioxidants limit deleterious effect of free radicals.

TABLE 66-3—CONT'D

RECOMMENDED MACRO AND MICRO NUTRIENTS FOR GROWTH—CONT'D

Component	Function	Recommended Daily Intake	Special Considerations for CHD
B_6	Reduces homocysteine levels and improves endothelial function	0–6 mo, 0.1 mg 7–12 mo, 0.3 mg 1–3 yr, 0.5 mg 4–8 yr, 0.6 mg 9–13 yr, 1 mg Females 14–18 yr, 1.2 mg Males 14–18 yr, 1.3 mg	
B_{12}	Improves endothelial function by reducing homocysteine levels.	0–6 mo, 0.4 μg 7–12 mo, 0.5 μg 1–3 yr, 0.9 μg 4–8 yr, 1.2 μg 9–13 yr, 1.8 μg 14–18 yr, 2.4 μg	
Vitamin C	Antioxidant. Helps maintain tissue levels of vitamins A and E.	0–6 mo, 40 mg 7–12 mo, 50 mg 1–3 yr, 15 mg 4–8 yr, 25 mg 9–13 yr, 45 mg Females 14–18 yr, 65 mg Males 14–18 yr, 75 mg	
Vitamin D	Essential for calcium absorption from the intestine.	0 mo–18 yr, 5 μg	
Vitamin E	Antioxidant working to prevent propagation of lipid peroxidation.	0–6 mo, 4 mg 7–12 mo, 5 mg 1–3 yr, 6 mg 4–8 yr, 7 mg 9–13 yr, 11 mg 14–18 yr, 15 mg	
Vitamin K	Promotes liver synthesis of clotting factors (II, VII, IX, X).	0–6 mo, 2 μg 7–12 mo, 2.5 μg 1–3 yr, 30 μg 4–8 yr, 55 μg 9–13 yr, 60 μg 14–18 yr, 75 μg	
Folate	Necessary for DNA synthesis and replication.	0–6 mo, 65 μg 7–12 mo, 80 μg 1–3 yr, 150 μg 4–8 yr, 200 μg 9–13 yr, 300 μg 14–18 yr, 400 μg	Inadequate concentrations may decrease circulating levels of homocysteine.
Minerals			
Calcium	Essential for bone metabolism and muscle contraction.	*Preterm infant:* 0–6 mo, 210 mg 7–12 mo, 270 mg 1–3 yr, 500 mg 4–8 yr, 800 mg 9–18 yr, 1300 mg	
Chromium	Potentiates the action of insulin. Plays role in protein and lipid metabolism. Required for growth.	0–6 mo, 0.2 g 7–12 mo, 5.5 μg 1–3 yr, 11 μg 4–8 yr, 15 μg Females 9–13 yr, 21 μg; 14–18 yr, 24 μg Males 9–13 yr, 25 μg; 14–18 yr, 35 μg	Decrease intake in presence of renal dysfunction.
Copper	Functions in iron metabolism.	0–6 mo, 200 μg 7–12 mo, 220 μg 1–3 yr, 340 μg 4–8 yr, 440 μg 9–13 yr, 700 μg 14–18 yr, 890 μg	

(Continued)

TABLE 66-3—CONT'D

RECOMMENDED MACRO AND MICRO NUTRIENTS FOR GROWTH—CONT'D

Component	Function	Recommended Daily Intake	Special Considerations for CHD
Iron	Necessary for ATP to be synthesized.	0–6 mo, 0.27 mg 7–12 mo, 11 mg 1–3 yr, 7 mg 4–8 yr, 10 mg 9–13 yr, 8 mg Females 14–18 yr, 15 mg Males 14–18 yr, 11 mg	
Magnesium	Active component of antioxidant enzymes.	0–6 mo, 30 mg 7–12 mo, 75 mg 1–3 yr, 80 mg 4–8 yr, 130 mg 9–13 yr, 240 mg Females 14–18 yr, 360 mg Males 14–18 yr, 410 mg	
Manganese	Cofactor in many enzyme functions. Stimulates synthesis of cholesterol and fatty acids in liver. Influences mucopolysaccharide synthesis.	0–6 mo, 0.003 mg 7–12 mo, 0.6 mg 1–3 yr, 1.2 mg 4–8 yr, 1.5 mg Females 9–18 yr, 1.6 mg Males 9–13 yr, 1.9 mg; 14–18 yr, 2.2 mg	
Phosphorus	Antioxidant that works in concert with vitamin E to protect cells from peroxidase damage. Required in all cellular reproduction and protein synthesis.	0–6 mo, 100 mg 7–12 mo, 275 mg 1–3 yr, 460 mg 4–8 yr, 500 mg 9–18 yr, 1250 mg	Vital to the structure of bones and teeth. Primary constituents of cellular membranes. Required for the production of ATP, the major physiologic molecule used in the storage and transport of energy. Key buffering system used to ensure acid-base balance.
Selenium	Antioxidant component of glutathione peroxidase that protects cell components from oxidative damage.	0–6 mo, 15 μg 7 mo–3 yr, 20 μg 4–8 yr, 30 μg 9–13 yr, 40 μg 14–18 yr, 55 μg	
Zinc	Needed for DNA and RNA synthesis and other enzyme functions. Necessary for optimal wound healing.	0–6 mo, 2 mg 7 mo–3 yr, 3 mg 4–8 yr, 5 mg 9–13 yr, 8 mg Females 14–18 yr, 9 mg Males 14–18 yr, 11 mg	
Other			
Carnitine	Essential for transport of long-chain fatty acids from cytoplasm to β-oxidation sites within the mitochondrial matrix.	No established RDA	
Taurine	Nonessential amino acid that participates in controlling cellular calcium levels.	No established RDA	
Fiber	Assists in maintaining normal glucose levels and bowel regularity.	1–3 yr, 19 g 4–8 yr, 25 g Males 9–13 yr, 31 g; 14–18 yr, 38 g Females 9–18 yr, 26 g	

AMDR, acceptable macronutrient distribution range; CHD, congenital cardiac disease; EER, estimated energy requirement; GT, gastrostomy tube; NGT, nasogastric tube; RDA, recommended dietary allowance.
Adapted from Miller TL, Neri D, Extein J, et al: Nutrition in pediatric cardiomyopathy. Prog Pediatr 2007;24;59–71.

per day.[2] Diets that contain a deficient amount of carbohydrates, fats, and protein will result in poor weight gain, while linear growth is retarded when the dietary intake of protein is deficient.[4]

Fluid requirements for the normal neonate are 120 mL/kg per day for those weighing less than 3 kilograms, and 100 mL/kg per day for heavier neonates.[28] Once intravenous access is secured, intravenous fluids are started at 80 mL/kg per day, and generally advanced to a goal of 100 mL/kg per day over the course of 72 hours for all neonates except those with functionally univentricular circulations, or those with excessive insensible losses, fluids in these latter cases generally being started at 100 mL/kg per hour.[29] Neonates with congestive heart failure have losses of fluids up to one-sixth greater than those of a normal neonate due to their increased work of breathing, vomiting, and diuretics.[29] Achieving an optimal fluid balance in children with congenitally malformed hearts, therefore, is challenging, in part because of their insensible losses, but also because of the potential for protein imbalance and the role it plays in the retention of fluid.

Management of In-patients

It is axiomatic that timely nutritional support is needed for patients with congenitally malformed hearts so as to maintain an adequate nutritional state, and to minimise the physiologic consequences of undernutrition. Goals for neonates considered to be at risk, therefore, are to provide adequate nutrition to promote growth, and to correct nutrient deficiency. Goals for children include providing adequate nutrition to meet current metabolic demands, as well as for catch-up growth.[30] The challenge is to calculate energy requirements to maintain metabolism, this requiring 40 to 70 kcal/kg per day, as well as synthesis of tissues and storage of energy for growth, requiring an additional 50 to 70 kcal/kg per day, and to cope with routine losses of approximately 20 kcal/kg per day as well as any further expenditures related to illness.[28] A compromised nutritional state may delay surgical intervention and increase the risk of post-operative complications. In the neonate, poor nutrition negatively impacts cerebral development, cognitive function, and attainment of motor skills.[29]

Types of Nutrition

Parenteral Nutrition

Parenteral nutrition and intralipids should be started when the initiation of enteral feedings is not an option for ensuring metabolic needs.[28] Due to the high incidence of respiratory problems, limited gastric capacity, and intestinal hypomotility of premature infants, enteral feeds should be initiated and advanced in slow fashion.[29] Parenteral nutrition supplements the calories provided by limited enteral feedings to ensure the nutritional needs. The nutritional content of the parenteral supply is limited by the type of vascular access available. The content of dextrose in peripheral parenteral nutrition should not exceed 12.5%, and amino acids should not exceed 2%, because of the potential of producing venous irritation. Lipid tolerance of 20% solutions is superior to that of 10% solutions due to their lower content of phospholipid emulsifiers.[28] For term infants born with low weight, parenteral nutrition should be instituted within the initial 3 days of life if enteral feeds are contra-indicated due to concerns of necrotizing enterocolitis or extracardiac anomalies such as tracheoesophageal fistula, duodenal atresia, and gastroschisis.[29] In such infants born with low weight, it has been shown that the average retention of nitrogen improved even when the intake of energy was less than 30 kcal/kg per day when protein, 1.15 g/kg per day, was initiated on the first day of life.[28]

The rate of glomerular filtration, and the distal and proximal tubular function, are decreased in infants of less than 34 weeks of gestation. Premature infants have a decreased ability to concentrate urine compared to those born at term.[4] This produces a risk for hyperkalaemia during the first few days of life. Electrolytes, therefore, are generally not added to intravenous fluids for the first 24 hours of life.[4] Neonates born at term may require supplementation of calcium over the first 24 to 48 hours after birth due to the sudden cessation of placental delivery of calcium, the decreased release of parathyroid hormone, and elevated levels of calcitonin.[30] Infants who are premature, infants who required phototherapy or were exposed to anticonvulsants during fetal life, and infants of diabetic mothers or mothers with a history of hyperparathyroidism are all at risk for prolonged periods of hypocalcaemia. Preventative therapy consists of doses of 25 to 75 mg/kg per day of intravenous elemental calcium added to intravenous fluid or parenteral nutrition.[30]

For children and adolescents, parenteral nutrition and intralipids should be initiated when a delay of up to 1 week is anticipated before enteral feedings can be started.[4] Parenteral nutrition should be implemented in children who exhibit signs of malnutrition pre-operatively to avoid deficiencies of fatty acids and to promote optimal nutrition.[30] If a delay of longer than 1 week is anticipated before the initiation of enteral feedings, consideration should be given to placing a central venous line so as to optimise the caloric density of the parenteral solution.[4]

Prolonged administration of parenteral nutrition is associated with cholestasis, hepatocellular necrosis, and in advanced cases, hepatic disease or cirrhosis.[4] After 2 to 3 weeks of parenteral nutrition, infants are at risk for developing cholestasis as evidenced by hyperbilirubinaemia and elevated transaminaemia.[28] Older children and adolescents develop steatosis and steatohepatitis.[30] The severest hepatic pathological changes are found in patients with the poorest enteral intake. Enteral feedings, therefore, should be commenced as soon as possible, even if only as trophic feeds, to minimise the risk of hepatic dysfunction.[4]

Infant Nutrition

Breast Milk

The Department of Health and Human Services of the United States and the American Academy of Pediatrics recommend exclusive breast-feeding during the first year of life.[31,32] Human milk provides optimal fat, protein, and carbohydrates for the infant born at term. Breast milk possesses anti-infective properties, reducing the incidence of acute illness, pathogenic bacterial faecal flora, necrotizing enterocolitis, otitis media, and infections of the lower respiratory and urinary tracts.[32] It has been suggested that immune-mediated diseases, such as diabetes mellitus, Crohn's disease, eczema, asthma, and allergic gastroenteritis, are lower among breast-fed infants.[32] The bond between mother and infant is enhanced, and cognitive scores consistently improve in direct relation to the duration of breast-feeding.[33] When the mother is unable to produce sufficient supply, or when breast-feeding is contra-indicated due to maternal health reasons, banked donor breast milk is available. Possible reasons for using donor breast milk may include prematurity, allergies, inborn errors of metabolism, and renal disease. Despite the well-known benefits of breast-feeding, infants with congenitally malformed hearts are often unable to meet their caloric needs by this method. Despite this caveat, parents should be educated about the benefits of breast milk, provided either by bottle or a supplemental device.

Paralysis of the Vocal Cords

Paralysis of the vocal cords has been reported in 2% of children under the age of 1 year undergoing cardiac surgery.[60] Such paralysis is a significant post-operative complication because it can compromise the ability of the infant to effectively swallow and increase the risk of aspiration.[61] Dysfunction may be related to operative injury to the recurrent laryngeal nerve, or direct trauma from prolonged intubation.[60] The most common presenting symptom of unilateral paralysis is a weak cry following extubation. Diagnosis is made by bedside fiberoptic laryngoscopy.[60] In one series involving patients less than 12 months old, all infants had paralysis on the left side, consistent with the anatomical position of the laryngeal nerve.[62] Strategies for management include study of swallowing to evaluate for aspiration, thickened oral feedings, and in severe cases the implementation of nasogastric or gastrostomy feedings.[61]

Gastroesophageal Reflux

Gastroesophageal reflux is commonly seen in children with congenitally malformed hearts, especially during the immediate post-operative period.[4] It is characteristically seen in neonates with haemodynamically significant lesions in the setting of delayed gastric emptying. The impact of any non-cardiac factors must be identified early in life in order to institute appropriate interventions and optimise the nutritional state.[63] Children with congenitally malformed hearts are known to have a high rate of gastroesophageal reflux, primary aspiration, and growth failure.[64] Clinical signs include recurrent vomiting, poor weight gain, dysphasia, abdominal pain and persistent respiratory symptoms.[63] Diagnosis is made based on history and physical examination, study of the upper gastrointestinal tract, and monitoring of oesophageal pH, or by endoscopy and, occasionally, biopsy.[63]

Options for treatment include prone positioning after the age of 12 months, supplementation with tube feeding, pharmacological therapies, and surgical interventions.[63] The use of thickened feedings, either commercially prepared or by adding cereal, remains controversial. Fewer episodes of emesis have been reported with the use of such thickened feeds, albeit that data suggests that thickened feeds may contribute to longer episodes of reflux.[65–67] The so-called reflux index was significantly reduced when infants were placed in the prone rather than the supine position.[68]

Pharmacological agents used for treatment are suppressants of acid and prokinetic agents.[63] The most common surgical intervention for severe and persistent symptoms is the Nissen fundoplication.[63] Surgical repair has been shown to be safe and effective, resulting in greater weight gain and improved oral intake.[64] Occasionally, these interventions do not alleviate the condition. In such circumstances, the patient may require supplemental feedings through a nasogastric, gastrostomy, or jejunostomy tube to achieve adequate caloric intake and growth.

When to Feed: Myths and Realities

Umbilical Arterial Catheters

The practice of using umbilical arterial catheters is widespread, although the evidence to support the safety of concurrently introducing enteral nutrition remains controversial. A survey of neonatal intensive care directors showed that one-sixth of neonates with such catheters in place received enteral feedings most of the time, one-third for some of the time, and half never.[68] No difference has been shown in flow through the superior mesenteric artery in neonates with or without such catheters,[69] and others have found no increased incidence of problems with feeding.[70] Despite the preliminary evidence supporting the use of enteral nutrition in premature infants with these catheters, nonetheless, the practice remains unclear.

Prostaglandin E_1

In one study, evidence of increased difficulties in feeding was observed in neonates receiving prostaglandin E_1 as a continuous intravenous infusion for longer than 2 weeks.[71] Persistent gastric distention has been documented with short-term treatment at high doses, albeit that the problem resolved once the infusions were discontinued.[72] Prolonged duration and dosing, nonetheless, is associated with an increased risk of developing obstruction of the gastric outlet.[71–74] Neonates receiving prostaglandin E_1 therefore, should be closely monitored for signs of intolerance in feeding.

Neuromuscular Blockade

Although gastric emptying is often delayed in critically ill patients, the capacity of the gut to absorb is not reduced by the effects of neuromuscular blockade.[75] Such treatment is held by some to produce only a slight increase in abdominal distention in post-operative patients,[76] albeit that others observed abdominal distention or excessive gastric residuals in one-third of patients, with most feedings having to be discontinued.[77] The decision to provide enteral nutrition to patients receiving neuromuscular blockade, therefore, remains uncertain, as does the debate over the usefulness of gastric residuals as an indicator of feeding intolerance.

Post-operative Nutritional Challenges

Necrotizing Enterocolitis

Infants with congenitally malformed hearts are at much greater risk for developing necrotizing enterocolitis.[78,79] The overall incidence is reported at around 3%, but was doubled in infants with functional single ventricles.[80,81] The aetiology is thought to reflect hypoxia and hypoperfusion of the gut.[82] Cardiopulmonary bypass alters the intestinal barrier and increases permeability.[83] Reduced splanchnic flow may also contribute to its development in the post-operative period.[83] Infants who developed the complication had at least one other associated risk factor, including prematurity, prostaglandins infused at high doses, multiple episodes of poor systemic perfusion, and shock.[80] Medical management involves antibiotic therapy and parenteral nutrition. Surgical intervention is indicated when there is necrosis of the bowel or perforation.[84,85]

Chylothorax

The incidence of chylothorax following surgery for congenital cardiac lesions ranges from 0.85% to 3.8%,[86–90] and is usually the consequence of direct injury to the thoracic duct, this being the leading cause,[86] or an alteration in lymphatic flow.[87,88] The proximity of the thoracic duct to important anatomical structures such as the aorta renders the duct vulnerable to injury during surgical procedures. Higher rates of chylous effusions occur in patients requiring the more complex surgical repairs. Strategies for

TABLE 66-5

LOW LONG-CHAIN TRIGLYCERIDE FORMULAS

Formula	Supplier	Percentage of Calories from Fat	MCT:LCT Ratio	Indications for Use
Monogen 20 kcal/oz	Nutricia	25	90:10	Infant formula. Optimal essential fats (omega-6:omega-3 = 4.6:1).
Portagen 20 kcal/oz	Mead Johnson	40	86:14	Infant formula. Taste may hinder achievement of goal volume.
Lipisorb 40.5 kcal/oz	Mead Johnson	35	85:14	Must be reconstituted to use as infant formula. Vanilla flavored.
Pregestimil 20 kcal/oz	Mead Johnson	50	55:45	Infant formula. Hypoallergenic with low renal solute load. Lactose and sucrose free.
Vivonex Pediatric 24 kcal/oz	Nestle	25	68:32	For infants and toddlers requiring hydrolyzed protein source. Lactose free.
Tolerex 30 kcal/oz	Nestle	1	0:10	For children aged 1–10 yr requiring hydrolyzed protein source. Lactose free.
Peptamen Junior 30 kcal/oz	Nestle	33	60:40	For children aged 1–10 yr. Contains 100% hydrolyzed whey peptides. Lactose free.
Vital HN 30 kcal/oz	Ross	9.4	45:55	For older children. Partially hydrolyzed protein source. Low residue and gluten free.

kcal, kilocalorie; LCT, long chain triglyceride; MCT, medium chain triglyceride; oz, ounce.

management include a low-fat diet, medium-chain triglycerides to reduce lymphatic flow, total parenteral nutrition, octreotide therapy, and surgical intervention[89] (Table 66-5). Most cases resolve with conservative nutritional management. Advanced therapies and surgical interventions are implemented for prolonged chylous drainage.[87,88]

Special Populations

Infants Born with Low Weight

Almost one-tenth of infants are born weighing less than 2500 grams, and then pose a nutritional challenge for caregivers when also having a congenitally malformed heart.[29] A strong association is reported between cardiac disease and a low weight at birth, infants who are small for gestational age, and prematurity.[11,12] Nutritional management of this group at high risk must take into account the haemodynamic impact of the congenital cardiac lesion, the degree of prematurity and its associated sequels, intra-uterine retardation of growth, and the presence of anomalies or syndromes.[28] Premature infants are at highest risk for developing necrotizing enterocolitis,[91] with hyperosmolarity of feeds, bowel ischaemia, infection, and immature intestinal host defenses all identified as potentially causative.[29] Studies in infants who are small for gestational age[70,92] have documented the presence of abnormal flow in the mesenteric or umbilical arteries prior to surgical intervention, providing one explanation for the increased rate of bowel ischaemia in this population when compared to infants born at term.

Patients Requiring Mechanical Support

Parenteral nutrition has historically been the choice of support for critically ill patients on extracorporeal membrane oxygenation.[93] Clinicians often withhold enteral nutrition out of concern for decreased gut perfusion, hypoxia, and the vasoconstrictive effects of cardiovascular medications,[94] albeit that levels of intestinal hormones were shown to be comparable in neonates supported or not supported with extracorporeal oxygenation.[95] Several studies of critically ill children and adults supported either with venoarterial or venovenous oxygenation have shown that enteral nutrition is generally well tolerated, producing no serious adverse events.[95–98]

Patients supported by a ventricular assist device, however, suffer from a variety of conditions associated with cardiac failure, which place them at risk for malnutrition.[99,100] Conditions include poor pre-operative nutritional state, anorexia, nausea, and early satiety from the weight of the intra-abdominally implanted device as well as delayed gastric emptying.[101] The determination of nutritional requirements must take into account their pre-operative nutritional state as well as their current health. The Society of Critical Care Medicine supports use of evidence-based protocols for feeding.[101] Such a standardised regime has been developed for adults who require support with a ventricular assist device.[102] In conjunction with the interdisciplinary team that includes a registered dietician, nutritional management for each patient is determined by the score they receive based on severity of illness and a subjective global assessment of the degree of malnutrition. Once a score is assigned, requirements are calculated for calories and proteins, and enteral feedings are started at low levels and advanced while maintaining metabolic stability. Due to the generally poor nutritional state of such patients, enteral nutrition should be started as soon as possible. If enteral feedings are not tolerated, parenteral nutrition should be initiated.[102]

Nutritional Challenges for the Out-patient

Challenges for these patients vary depending on their baseline, their current metabolic needs taking into account the presence of a residual cardiac defect or progression of disease, and the need for catch-up growth.

In this work, Anne Ades and colleagues reviewed the impact of low birth weight on outcomes following surgical correction of congenital cardiac disease. Causes of postnatal failure to gain weight are discussed, along with strategies for management.

- Einarson KD, Arthur HM: Predictors of oral feeding difficulty in cardiac surgical infants. Pediatr Nurs 2003;29:315–319.

  The time to discharge from hospital for infants after open heart surgery is contingent on the ability to consume and tolerate enteral nutrition. This study identifies factors influencing oral feedings in infants less than 1 month of age following congenital cardiac surgery. The authors determined that difficulties in feeding occurred most often in infants with injured vocal cords, prolonged intubation, and low weight at the time of surgical intervention.

- Kogon BE, Ramaswamy V, Todd K, et al: Feeding difficulty in newborns following congenital heart surgery. Congenit Heart Dis 2007;2:332–337.

  In this study, the investigators showed that difficulties in feeding were common after congenital cardiac surgery, especially in patients with complex disease and those requiring prolonged intubation. A significant number of patients required a prolonged time to reach the goals of feeding, prolonged time to transition to oral feeds, and procedures to facilitate feeding.

- Meert KL, Daphtary KM, Metheny NA: Gastric vs small-bowel feeding in critically ill children receiving mechanical ventilation: A randomized controlled trial. Chest 2004;126:872–878.

  This randomised clinical trial evaluated the effect of positioning a feeding tube in the stomach as opposed to the small bowel on the delivery of nutrition and associated complications in critically ill children. The authors found a significant increase in the amount of nutrition delivered in those having the tube placed in the small bowel, but found no difference in the tolerance of feedings or aspiration.

- McElhinney DB, Hedrick HL, Bush DM, et al: Necrotizing enterocolitis in neonates with congenital heart disease: Risk factors and outcomes. Pediatrics 2000;106:1080–1087.

  This study demonstrated that risk factors for developing necrotizing enterocolitis include prematurity, hypoplastic left heart syndrome, common arterial trunk, and periods of low cardiac output. Necrotizing enterocolitis led to longer stays in hospital, but was not associated with higher mortality.

- Chan EH, Russell JL, Williams WG, et al: Postoperative chylothorax after cardiothoracic surgery in children. Ann Thorac Surg 2005;80:1864–1870.

  In this study the authors identified the incidence of chylothorax in children following congenital cardiac surgery, and discuss risk factors and strategies for management, including a care map. The documented increased incidence may be related to differences in the characteristics of the patients and more complex surgical procedures.

- Vogt K, Manlhiot C, Van Arsdell G, et al: Somatic growth in children with single ventricle physiology. J Am Coll Cardiol 2007;50:1876–1883.

  In this study, the investigators showed that infants with functionally univentricular physiology have impaired gain in weight, but that catch-up growth occurred after the bidirectional Glenn procedure. The group at highest risk included those with systemic venous collateral channels.

- Ono M, Dietmar B, Goerler H, et al: Somatic development long after the Fontan operation: Factors influencing catch-up growth. J Thorac Cardiovasc Surg 2007;134:1199–1206.

  In this study, the investigators showed that somatic growth declined before conversion to the Fontan circulation, but catch-up growth occurred during long-term follow-up. Early unloading appeared to be related to improved somatic growth. A prior atrioseptectomy, construction of a central shunt, and reconstruction of the pulmonary arteries were all associated with impaired growth.

- Rychik J: Protein-losing enteropathy after Fontan operation. Congenit Heart Dis 2007;2:288–300.

  In this work, Jack Rychik proposed a causative theory that includes a combination of mechanisms leading to the development of protein losing enteropathy following conversion to the Fontan circulation. These conditions include altered haemodynamics, mesenteric vascular resistance, and enterocyte basal membrane glycosaminoglycan, as well as systemic inflammation. Manifestations of the disease and clinical management are discussed.

- Pinto NM, Marino BS, Wernovsky G, et al: Obesity is a common comorbidity in children with congenital and acquired heart disease. Pediatrics 2007;120: e1157–e1164.

  In this study, Nelangi Pinto and colleagues showed that obesity is common in children with congenitally malformed hearts. The long-term impact of obesity on various types of congenital cardiac disease is discussed, as well as the implications for out-patient follow-up and treatment.

CHAPTER 67

Formulary

EDWARD J. BAKER

Clinical trials of medicines for children have been limited, and often therapeutic decisions are made on the basis of evidence of efficacy and safety in adult patients. Caution in the use of new, unlicensed medicines, without evidence in children is therefore inevitable. This means that the choice of medicines is much more limited than in adult practice. Here, I present a summary of medicines commonly used for cardiovascular disorders in children (Table 67-1). This list does not attempt to be comprehensive, as practice will vary internationally, and some drugs in common use in one part of the world are hardly used elsewhere. The paucity of evidence makes this unavoidable. This summary, therefore, is not a replacement for local guidelines. To avoid confusion, I have used the recommended international non-proprietary names for the medicines covered. Where there is a common alternative name, I have included it, but I have not tried to include local or proprietary names, as these vary internationally.

I have included the important cardiac indications for the medicines covered, and their major contra-indications and side effects. I have not been able to cover all possibilities, and readers are advised to consult detailed prescribing information and the information sheets for these medicines before prescribing them. As a guide, I have included the typical regime for dosing children between birth and 10 years, but prescribers should consult their local guidelines for more details, particularly for preterm neonates and older children, for whom the dosage may vary. The formulary does not include medicines that have a much wider application than cardiac conditions, such as antibiotics and anti-coagulants, but focuses purely on the cardiovascular use of the drugs described.

TABLE 67-1

SUMMARY OF MEDICINES COMMONLY USED FOR CARDIOVASCULAR DISORDERS IN CHILDREN

Drug	Indications	Contra-indications	Major Side Effects	Typical Dose and Frequency	Comments
Adenosine	Diagnosis of arrhythmias and termination of supraventricular arrhythmias	Heart block, asthma	Chest pain, dyspnoea, bronchospasm, severe bradycardia	Fast intravenous bolus of 100 μg/kg to maximum of 300 μg/kg for the neonate, or 500 μg/kg for the older child	Electrocardiographic monitoring and recording during the administration of the bolus is essential. The bolus can be repeated after 2 minutes with the dose increased progressively until electrocardiographic changes occur.
Alprostadil (prostaglandin E_1)	Maintenance of the patency of the ductus arteriosus in the neonate		Apnoea, tachycardia, hypotension, fever, cortical proliferation of long bones, necrotising enterocolitis	Intravenous infusion of initially 10 ng/kg per minute, can be increased to 50 ng/kg per minute according to response	Monitor heart rate, respiration, and temperature. Ventilation may be required for apnoea.
Amiloride	Potassium sparing diuretic	Hyperkalaemia, renal failure	Hyponatraemia, hyperkalaemia, hypotension	Orally 200 μg/kg twice per day Maximum of 20 mg per day	Weak diuretic used in combination with thiazide or loop diuretics
Amiodarone	Supraventricular and ventricular arrhythmias	Bradycardia, heart block, hypotension	Bradycardia, thyroid disorders, hepatotoxicity, corneal microdeposits, photosensitivity, gray skin discolouration, neuropathy, anaemia	Orally initially 5 mg/kg two to three times per day, reduce to maintenance dose after 7 days Maintenance 5 mg/kg once per day or based on measurement of plasma levels Intravenous infusion initially 25 μg/kg per hour for 4 hours then 5 to 15 μg/kg per minute. Maximum of 1.2 g per day	Long-term administration should be avoided because of the incidence of side effects. Careful monitoring of hepatic, thyroid and visual function is required. Photosensitivity and skin discolouration can be severe, and sun block is required. Monitor the heart rate during intravenous infusions, and adjust the dose as necessary. Therapeutic plasma level of amiodarone and its active metabolite is 0.6 to 2.5 mg/L.
Aspirin	Low-dose antiplatelet prophylaxis against thrombosis High dose anti-inflammatory agent for Kawasaki disease	Viral infections, with the risk of Reye's syndrome, peptic ulceration bleeding disorders	Reye's syndrome, bleeding especially gastrointestinal, bronchospasm	Low-dose antiplatelet: orally 5 mg/kg (maximum of 75 mg) once per day High-dose antiplatelet: orally 20 to 25 mg/kg 4 times per day for approximately 14 days, then reduce to low dose	High-dose aspirin is also used in acute rheumatic fever (see Chapter 54A) and post-pericardectomy syndrome (see Chapter 53).
Atenolol	Hypertension, supraventricular and ventricular tachycardias	Asthma, heart block, hypotension, depressed myocardial function	Bradycardia, heart failure, bronchospasm, heart block, peripheral vasoconstriction, fatigue	Orally 1 to 2 mg/kg once per day Maximum of 100 mg per day	Use smaller doses in renal and hepatic impairment.
Captopril	Cardiac failure, hypertension	Renal impairment, renovascular disease, coarctation, left ventricular outflow or inflow obstruction	Hypotension particularly with initial doses, renal impairment, tachycardia, photosensitivity, persistent dry cough	Orally initially 100 μg/kg three times per day, increasing to 1 mg/kg three times per day	ACE inhibitor, in heart failure usually combined with a loop diuretic Do not give with potassium sparing diuretics. Initiate carefully under close supervision, usually in an in-patient to ensure close monitoring of blood pressure and renal function.
Carvedilol	Cardiac failure	Asthma, heart block, hypotension, depressed myocardial function	Bradycardia, cardiac failure, bronchospasm, heart block, peripheral vasoconstriction, fatigue	Orally initially 50 μg/kg (maximum of 3.125 mg) twice per day. Increase at 2-week intervals eventually up to 350 μg/kg (maximum of 25 mg) twice per day	Used as a third-line treatment for chronic cardiac failure as an adjunct to diuretics and inhibitors of angiotensin-converting enzyme As yet, there is no evidence of long-term benefit in children.
Clopidogrel	Antiplatelet prophylaxis against thrombosis as an alternative to low-dose aspirin		Haemorrhage, neutropenia	Orally 1 mg/kg once per day (maximum of 75 mg)	Used as a second-line treatment after aspirin

Digoxin	Supraventricular arrhythmias, cardiac failure	Heart block, renal failure, Wolff-Parkinson-White syndrome, ventricular tachycardia	Anorexia, abdominal pain, heart block, arrhythmias	Orally, neonates to 5 years: 10 μg/kg/day Children 5 to 10 years: 6 μg/kg/day Maximum 250 μg/day	In urgent circumstances, loading doses (digitalisation) may be needed over first 24 hours. Dose should be reduced in preterm neonates and renal failure. Is of limited value in cardiac failure, and rarely used as first choice Intravenous administration is rarely justified. Therapeutic plasma digoxin concentration 0.8 to 2.0 μg/L
Dinoprostone (prostaglandin E_2)	Maintaining the patency of the ductus arteriosus in the neonate		Apnoea, tachycardia, hypotension, fever, cortical proliferation of long bones, necrotising enterocolitis	Intravenous infusion of initially 5 ng/kg/min, can be increased to 20 ng/kg/min according to response	Monitor heart rate, respiration, and temperature. Ventilation may be required for apnoea.
Dipyridamole	Antiplatelet prophylaxis against thrombosis as an alternative to low-dose aspirin	Heart failure, aortic stenosis	Hypotension, tachycardia, bronchospasm	Orally 2.5 mg/kg twice per day Over age 12 years: 100 to 200 mg three times per day	Dipyridamole has also been used to treat pulmonary hypertension. Antiplatelet action may be synergistic with aspirin.
Dobutamine	Inotropic support in low cardiac output	Left ventricular outflow obstruction	Tachycardia, hypotension	Intravenous infusion 2 to 20 μg/kg/min	
Dopamine	Hypotension and low cardiac output	Tachycardia, arrhythmia	Hypertension, tachycardia, arrhythmias	Intravenous infusion 2 to 20 μg/kg/min	There is little evidence that low doses have beneficial vasodilatory effects in clinical practice.
Enalapril	Heart failure, hypertension	Renal impairment, renovascular disease, coarctation, left ventricular outflow or inflow obstruction	Hypotension particularly with initial doses, renal impairment, tachycardia, Raynaud's syndrome, Stevens-Johnson syndrome, alopecia, muscle cramps, persistent dry cough	Orally initially 0.1 mg/kg/day, increasing according to response up to a maximum of 1.0 mg/kg/day	ACE inhibitor, in heart failure usually combined with a loop diuretic. Do not give with potassium sparing diuretics. Initiate carefully under close supervision, usually as an in-patient to ensure close monitoring of blood pressure and renal function.
Epinephrine (adrenaline)	Acute hypotension	Hypertension	Tachycardia, hypertension, arrhythmias	Intravenous infusion of 100 ng/kg/min, up to 1.5 μg/kg/min	
Esmolol	Emergency management of arrhythmias and hypertension, cyanotic spells in tetralogy of Fallot	Asthma, heart block, hypotension, depressed myocardial function	Bradycardia, heart failure, bronchospasm, heart block	Intravenously initial dose of 500 μg/kg administered over 1 to 2 minutes Can be followed by an infusion of 25 to 50 μg/kg/min Can be increased to a maximum of 200 μg/kg/min in resistant cases	Relatively cardioselective β-blocker Reduce dose if hypotension or bradycardia occurs. Higher dose of infusion may be required to terminate severe cyanotic spells in tetralogy of Fallot.
Flecainide	Ventricular tachycardia, arrhythmias in Wolff-Parkinson-White syndrome, atrioventricular re-entry tachycardias	Heart failure, heart block, hypokalaemia	Precipitation of life-threatening arrhythmias particularly in structural heart disease Depression of myocardial function especially when used with β-blockers or calcium-channel blockers	Orally 2 mg/kg two to three times per day Adjust dose according to plasma levels Intravenously 2 mg/kg per dose Infusion of 100 to 250 μg/kg/hr until arrhythmia controlled (maximum total dose of 600 mg in first day)	Monitor electrocardiogram during slow intravenous administration. If intravenous infusion lasts more than 24 hours, monitor plasma levels (therapeutic range 200 to 800 μg/L).

(Continued)

TABLE 67-1

SUMMARY OF MEDICINES COMMONLY USED FOR CARDIOVASCULAR DISORDERS IN CHILDREN—CONT'D

Drug	Indications	Contra-indications	Major Side Effects	Typical Dose and Frequency	Comments
Furosemide (frusemide)	Cardiac failure, pulmonary oedema, hypertension	Hypokalaemia, hypotension	Hyponatraemia, hypokalaemia, hypomagnesaemia, nephrocalcinosis, hypotension, deafness (with rapid intravenous infusion)	Orally 0.5 to 2 mg/kg two to three times per day (maximum of 12 mg/kg/day or 80 mg/day in total, whichever is lower) Intravenously 0.5 to 1 mg/kg up to four times per day, or continuous infusion of 0.1 to 2 mg/kg/hr	In oliguria, much higher doses may be needed, titrated against the urine output.
Ibuprofen	Closure of the patent arterial duct in preterm neonates	Hepatic impairment, pulmonary hypertension, bleeding disorders, necrotising enterocolitis, infection	Bleeding especially intracranial bleeding, renal impairment, necrotising enterocolitis	Slow intravenous infusion of 10 mg/kg Second and third doses at 24 and 48 hours of 5 mg/kg	Reduce dose with renal impairment, and monitor hepatic function.
Indomethacin	Closure of the patent arterial duct in preterm neonates	Renal impairment, infection, bleeding, especially intracranial bleeding, necrotising enterocolitis	Haemorrhage, including intracranial bleeding, oliguria or anuria, fluid retention	Intravenous infusion over 30 minutes Neonate under 48 hours: 200 μg, followed by two doses of 100 μg separated by 12 to 24 hours Neonate 2 to 7 days: 200 μg, followed by two doses of 200 μg separated by 12 to 24 hours Neonate over 7 days: 200 μg, followed by two doses of 250 μg separated by 12 to 24 hours	Monitor urinary output, and delay second and third doses until it recovers. Indomethacin is also used as an anti-inflammatory agent in post-pericardiectomy syndrome.
Isoprenaline	Bradycardia, complete heart block	Hypotension	Hypotension, tachycardia, arrhythmias	0.02 μg/kg/min increasing to a maximum of 0.5 μg/min (neonate maximum of 0.2 μg/kg/min)	
Lidocaine (lignocaine)	Ventricular fibrillation, ventricular tachycardia	Heart block, myocardial dysfunction, hepatic failure, renal failure	Central nervous system depression, respiratory depression, hypotension bradycardia	Intravenous bolus of 500 μg to 1 mg/kg over 1 minute Repeat at 5-minute intervals up to a maximum of 3 mg/kg, followed by an intravenous infusion of 1 to 3 mg/kg/hr	Monitor electrocardiogram during administration. Reduce dose in presence of hepatic or renal impairment.
Lisinopril	Heart failure, hypertension	Renal impairment, renovascular disease, coarctation, left ventricular outflow or inflow obstruction	Hypotension particularly with initial doses, renal impairment, tachycardia, alopecia, persistent dry cough	Orally initially 0.1 mg/kg/day, increasing according to response to 0.5 to 1.0 mg/kg/day. Maximum 40 mg/day	ACE inhibitor, in heart failure usually combined with a loop diuretic. Do not give with potassium sparing diuretics. Initiate carefully under close supervision, usually as an in-patient to ensure close monitoring of blood pressure and renal function.
Losartan	Heart failure, hypertension	Renal impairment, renovascular disease, coarctation, left ventricular outflow or inflow obstruction	First-dose hypotension, hyperkalaemia	Orally 0.5 mg/kg once per day, increasing to a maximum of 2 mg/kg once per day	Angiotensin II receptor antagonist with similar effects to inhibitors of angiotensin-converting enzyme, but it does not cause the characteristic dry cough of the inhibitors of the enzyme and is a useful alternative. Use a lower dose in renal or hepatic impairment. Introduce with caution because of the risk of hypotension

Milrinone	Heart failure, low cardiac output, shock	Renal failure, hypotension	Arrhythmias, hypotension	Intravenous infusion of 30 to 45 μg/kg/hr	Phosphodiesterase inhibitor with positive inotropic and vasodilator effects Loading dose of 50 to 75 μg/kg for first hour, omit if hypotension occurs Reduce dose in renal failure. Short-term use only
Norepinephrine (noradrenaline)	Hypotension secondary to severe vasodilation	Hypertension	Hypertension, severe vasoconstriction and peripheral ischaemia, arrhythmias	20 to 100 ng/kg/min up to maximum of 1 μg/kg/min	
Propranolol	Hypertension, supraventricular and ventricular tachycardias, cyanotic spells in tetralogy of Fallot	Asthma, heart block, hypotension, depressed myocardial function	Bradycardia, heart failure, bronchospasm, heart block, peripheral vasoconstriction, fatigue	Tetralogy of Fallot: intravenously 15 to 20 μg/kg, increasing to 100 to 200 μg/kg given slowly under electrocardiographic control Arrhythmias: orally 250 to 500 μg/kg three times per day Can increase up to 1 mg/kg three times per day Intravenously 10 to 50 μg/kg slowly under electrocardiographic control	Do not give with verapamil. Use smaller doses in renal and hepatic impairment.
Sildenafil	Pulmonary hypertension	Hypotension	Dyspepsia, headache, visual disturbances, priapism	Orally 0.5 mg/kg every 4 to 6 hours, increasing according to response to a maximum of 2 mg/kg every 4 hours	Reduce dose in hepatic or renal impairment. Used to treat pulmonary hypertension following cardiac surgery and to wean from inhaled nitric oxide
Sotalol	Atrial flutter, supraventricular and ventricular tachycardias	Asthma, heart block, hypotension, depressed myocardial function, hypokalaemia, hypomagnesaemia, prolonged QT interval	Bradycardia, heart failure, bronchospasm, heart block, arrhythmias, prolongation of QT interval, torsades de pointes	Orally 1 mg/kg twice daily, increasing as needed every 3 to 4 days to maximum of 4 mg/kg twice per day (maximum of 80 mg twice per day)	Monitor the QT interval. Do not administer with other drugs that prolong the QT interval. Therapeutic range is 0.04 to 2.0 mg/L
Spironolactone	Potassium sparing diuretic (aldosterone antagonist)	Hyperkalaemia, hyponatraemia	Hyperkalaemia, hyponatraemia, hepatotoxicity, gynaecomastia, osteomalacia	Orally 0.5 to 1 mg/kg up to three times per day	Typically used with loop diuretics Should not be given simultaneously with inhibitors of angiotensin-converting enzyme

Index

Page numbers followed by b indicate boxes; f, figures; t, tables.

J

K

L